KU-005-675

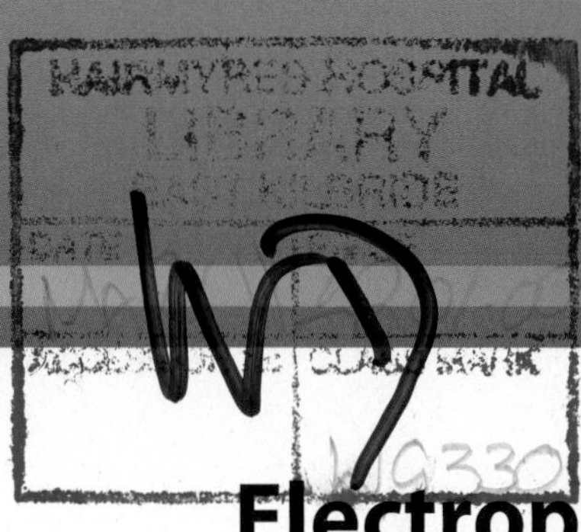

Cardiac Electrophysiology

From Cell to Bedside

Fifth Edition

Cardiac Electrophysiology
From Cell to Bedside

DOUGLAS P. ZIPES, MD
Distinguished Professor
Emeritus Professor of Medicine, Pharmacology, and Toxicology
Emeritus Director, Division of Cardiology and the Krannert Institute of Cardiology
Indiana University School of Medicine
Indianapolis, Indiana
Editor-in-Chief, Heart*Rhythm*

JOSÉ JALIFE, MD
Cyrus and Jane Farrehi Professor of Cardiovascular Research
Professor of Internal Medicine
Professor of Molecular and Integrative Physiology
University of Michigan Medical School
Co-Director, University of Michigan Center for Arrhythmia Research
Ann Arbor, Michigan

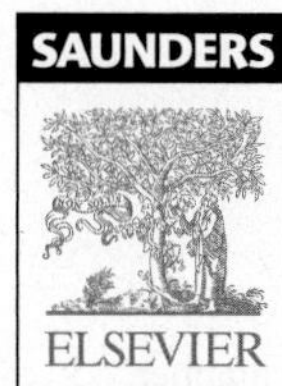

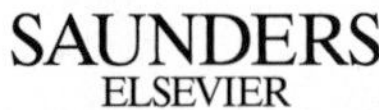

1600 John F. Kennedy Blvd.
Ste 1800
Philadelphia, PA 19103-2899

CARDIAC ELECTROPHYSIOLOGY:
FROM CELL TO BEDSIDE

ISBN: 978-1-4160-5973-8

Notice

Knowledge and best practice in this field are constantly changing. As new research and experience broaden our knowledge, changes in practice, treatment, and drug therapy may become necessary or appropriate. Readers are advised to check the most current information provided (i) on procedures featured or (ii) by the manufacturer of each product to be administered, to verify the recommended dose or formula, the method and duration of administration, and contraindications. It is the responsibility of the practitioner, relying on his or her experience and knowledge of the patient, to make diagnoses, to determine dosages and the best treatment for each individual patient, and to take all appropriate safety precautions. To the fullest extent of the law, neither the Publisher nor the Editors assume any liability for any injury and/or damage to persons or property arising out of or related to any use of the material contained in this book.

The Publisher

Library of Congress Cataloging-in-Publication Data

Cardiac electrophysiology : from cell to bedside / [edited by] Dougles P. Zipes, Jose Jalife. – 5th ed.
p. ; cm.
Includes bibliographical references and index.
ISBN 978-1-4160-5973-8
1. Arrhythmia. 2. Heart conduction system. 3. Electrophysiology. I. Zipes, Douglas P. II. Jalife, Jose.
[DNLM: 1. Arrhythmias, Cardiac. 2. Cardiac electrophysiology. 3. Heart—physiology.
WG 330 C26925 2009]
RC685.A65C286 2009
616.1′28—dc22 2008037595

Acquisitions Editor: Natasha Andjelkovic
Developmental Editor: Janice Gaillard
Publishing Services Manager: Frank Polizzano
Project Manager: Jeff Gunning
Design Direction: Lou Forgione

Printed in Canada

Last digit is the print number: 9 8 7 6 5 4 3 2 1

Contributors

Michael J. Ackerman, MD, PhD
Professor of Pediatrics, Medicine, and Molecular Pharmacology, Mayo Clinic School of Medicine; Director, Long QT Syndrome Clinic; Director, Windland Smith Rice Sudden Death Genomics Laboratory; Consultant in Pediatrics and Medicine, Mayo Clinic, Rochester, Minnesota
Single Nucleotide Polymorphisms and Cardiac Arrhythmias; Progressive Cardiac Conduction Disease

Mark E. Alexander, MD
Assistant Professor of Pediatrics, Harvard Medical School; Associate in Cardiology, Children's Hospital Boston, Boston, Massachusetts
Arrhythmias in Pediatrics

Mark E. Anderson, MD, PhD
Professor of Medicine and Physiology and Potter-Lambert Chair in Cardiology, University of Iowa Carver College of Medicine; Director, Division of Cardiovascular Medicine; Associate Director, UI Cardiovascular Research Center, University of Iowa Hospitals and Clinics, Iowa City, Iowa
Intracellular Signaling and Regulation of Cardiac Ion Channels; Ventricular Tachycardia in Patients with Heart Failure

Charles Antzelevitch, PhD
Professor of Pharmacology, State University of New York Upstate Medical University College of Medicine, Syracuse; Executive Director and Director of Research, Masonic Medical Research Laboratory, Utica, New York
Drug-Induced Channelopathies

Justus M. B. Anumonwo, PhD
Assistant Professor of Internal Medicine (Cardiovascular), University of Michigan Medical School; University of Michigan Center for Arrhythmia Research, Ann Arbor, Michigan
Biophysical Properties of Inwardly Rectifying Potassium Channels

Michael Artman, MD
Professor and Chair, Department of Pediatrics, University of Iowa Carver College of Medicine; Physician-in-Chief, University Iowa Children's Hospital, Iowa City, Iowa
Developmental Regulation of Cardiac Ion Channels

Felipe Atienza, MD, PhD
Assistant Professor, School of Medicine, Universidad Complutense de Madrid; Cardiac Electrophysiologist, Cardiology Department, Hospital General Universitario Gregorio Marañón, Madrid, Spain
Atrial Flutter

Peter H. Backx, DVM, PhD
Professor, Richard Lewar Centre of Excellence, and Department of Physiology, University of Toronto; Staff Scientist, Toronto General Hospital Research Institute, Toronto, Ontario, Canada
Voltage-Regulated Potassium Channels

Jeffrey R. Balser, MD, PhD
Associate Vice Chancellor for Health Affairs; Dean, School of Medicine; and James Tayloe Gwathmey Clinician Scientist Professor, Vanderbilt University Medical Center, Nashville, Tennessee
Biophysics of Normal and Abnormal Cardiac Sodium Channel Function

David G. Benditt, MD
Professor of Medicine, University of Minnesota Medical School, Minneapolis, Minnesota
Head-up Tilt Table Testing

Edward J. Berbari, PhD
Professor of Biomedical Engineering, Indiana University–Purdue University Indianapolis, Indianapolis, Indiana
High-Resolution Electrocardiography

Omer Berenfeld, PhD
Assistant Professor of Internal Medicine and Biomedical Engineering, University of Michigan Medical School; University of Michigan Center for Arrhythmia Research, Ann Arbor, Michigan
Dominant Frequency and the Mechanisms of Maintenance of Atrial Fibrillation

Donald M. Bers, PhD
Silva Chair for Cardiovascular Research and Distinguished Professor and Chair, Department of Pharmacology, University of California, Davis, School of Medicine, Davis, California
Cardiac Calcium Channels

Raffaella Bloise, MD, PhD
Department of Molecular Cardiology, IRCCS Fondazione Salvatore Maugeri, Pavia, Italy
Timothy Syndrome

Martin Borggrefe, MD
Director, First Department of Medicine–Cardiology, University Hospital Mannheim, Mannheim, Germany
Idiopathic Ventricular Fibrillation

Tim Boussy, PhD
Electrophysiology Fellow, University of Barcelona, Spain
The Brugada Syndrome

Mark R. Boyett, BSc, PhD
Professor of Cardiac Electrophysiology, University of Manchester, Manchester, United Kingdom
The Sinoatrial Node: Its Complex Structure and Unique Ion Channel Gene Program

Noel G. Boyle, MD, PhD
Professor of Medicine, David Geffen School of Medicine at UCLA; Director, Cardiac Electrophysiology Labs, UCLA Cardiac Arrhythmia Center; Ronald Reagan UCLA Medical Center, Los Angeles, California
Lesion-Forming Technologies for Catheter Ablation

Günter Breithardt, MD
Professor of Medicine (Cardiology), Medical Faculty, University of Münster; Head, Department of Cardiology and Angiology, Hospital of the University of Münster, Münster, Germany
Drug-Induced Ventricular Tachycardia

Peter R. Brink, PhD
Professor and Chairman, Department of Physiology and Biophysics, Stony Brook University School of Medicine, Stony Brook, New York
Biologic Pacing

Josep Brugada, MD
Chairman, Cardiovascular Center, and CFO, Ramon Brugada Senior Foundation; Professor, Fundacio Clinic; Medical Director, Hospital Clinic, Barcelona, Spain
The Brugada Syndrome

Pedro Brugada, MD
CEO, Ramon Brugada Senior Foundation; Professor of Cardiology and Physiology, Heart Rhythm Management Center, Free University of Brussels, Brussels, Belgium
The Brugada Syndrome

Ramon Brugada, MD
CSO, Ramon Brugada Senior Foundation; Dean, Medical Faculty and Director, Genetics Center, University of Girona Faculty of Medicine; Cardiologist, Hospital Trueta, Girona, Spain
The Brugada Syndrome

Brett Burstein, PhD
McGill University Faculty of Medicine; Montreal Heart Institute, Montreal, Quebec, Canada
Molecular Remodeling and Chronic Atrial Fibrillation

Hugh Calkins, MD
Nicholas J. Fortuin Professor of Cardiology and Professor of Medicine, Johns Hopkins University School of Medicine; Director of Electrophysiology, Johns Hopkins Hospital, Baltimore, Maryland
Syncope

David Callans, MD
Professor of Medicine, University of Pennsylvania School of Medicine; Associate Director of Electrophysiology, University of Pennsylvania Health System, Philadelphia, Pennsylvania
Ventricular Tachycardia in Patients with Coronary Artery Disease

A. John Camm, MD, FRCP
British Heart Foundation Professor of Clinical Cardiology, St. George's University of London; Honorary Consultant Cardiologist, St. George's Healthcare Trust, London, United Kingdom
Introduction: Progress in Antiarrhythmic Therapies

Sean M. Caples, DO
Assistant Professor of Medicine, Mayo Clinic College of Medicine; Consultant, Division of Pulmonary and Critical Care Medicine, Mayo Clinic, Rochester, Minnesota
Sleep-Disordered Breathing and Arrhythmias

Sheila J. Carroll, MD
Assistant Professor of Pediatrics (Pediatric Cardiology), Weill Cornell Medical College; Assistant Attending Pediatrician (Pediatric Cardiology), NewYork-Presbyterian Hospital, New York, New York
KCNQ1/KCNE1 Macromolecular Signaling Complex: Channel Microdomains and Human Disease

Agustin Castellanos, MD, FACC, FAHA
Professor of Medicine, Division of Cardiology, University of Miami Leonard F. Miller School of Medicine, Miami, Florida
Sudden Cardiac Death; Parasystole

William A. Catterall, PhD
Professor and Chair, Department of Pharmacology, University of Washington School of Medicine, Seattle, Washington
Voltage-Gated Sodium Channels and Electrical Excitability of the Heart

David Cesario, MD, PhD
Assistant Professor of Medicine, David Geffen School of Medicine at UCLA; Ronald Reagan UCLA Medical Center, Los Angeles, California
Lesion-Forming Technologies for Catheter Ablation

Philippe Charron, MD, PhD
Associate Professor/Master Lecturer, CHU La Salpétrière, Paris, France
Arrhythmogenic Right Ventricular Cardiomyopathies

Lan S. Chen, MD
Professor of Clinical Neurology, Department of Neurology, Indiana University School of Medicine; Pediatric Neurologist, Riley Hospital for Children, Indianapolis, Indiana
Nerve Sprouting and Cardiac Arrhythmias

Lei Chen, MD, PhD
Associate Research Scientist, Department of Pharmacology, Columbia University College of Physicians and Surgeons, New York, New York
KCNQ1/KCNE1 Macromolecular Signaling Complex: Channel Microdomains and Human Disease

Peng-Sheng Chen, MD
Professor of Medicine and Medtronic Zipes Chair of Cardiology; Chief, Krannert Institute of Cardiology and Division of Cardiology, Department of Medicine, Indiana University School of Medicine, Indianapolis, Indiana
Nerve Sprouting and Cardiac Arrhythmias

Xiongwen Chen, PhD
Assistant Professor, Temple University School of Medicine, Philadelphia, Pennsylvania
Pharmacology of L-type and T-type Calcium Channels in the Heart

Nipavan Chiamvimonvat, MD
Professor of Medicine and Roger Tatarian Endowed Professor of Cardiovascular Medicine, University of California, Davis, School of Medicine, Davis; Staff Cardiologist, Department of Veterans Affairs, Northern California Health Care System, Mather, California
Adrenergic Signaling and Cardiac Ion Channels

Aman Chugh, MD
Assistant Professor of Medicine, University of Michigan Medical School; Co-Director, Electrophysiology Fellowship Program, University of Michigan Cardiovascular Center, Ann Arbor, Michigan
Antrioventricular Reentry and Variants

Jacques Clémenty, MD
Professor of Cardiology, University Victor Segalen Bordeaux II; Hôpital Cardiologique du Haut-Lévêque, Bordeaux, France
Role of Cardiac and Thoracic Veins in Arrhythmogenesis

William A. Coetzee, DSc
Professor, Departments of Pediatrics, Physiology and Neuroscience, and Pharmacology, New York University School of Medicine, New York, New York
Developmental Regulation of Cardiac Ion Channels

Ira S. Cohen, MD, PhD
Leading Professor of Physiology and Biophysics, Stony Brook University School of Medicine; Director, Institute of Molecular Cardiology, Stony Brook, New York
Biologic Pacing

Lia Crotti, MD, PhD
Assistant Professor of Cardiology, University of Pavia Medical School; Cardiologist, Policlinico San Matteo, Pavia, Italy
Long QT and Short QT Syndromes

Phillip Cuculich, MD
Clinical Fellow, Department of Internal Medicine, Cardiovascular Division, Washington University in St. Louis School of Medicine, St. Louis, Missouri
Noninvasive Electrocardiographic Imaging (ECGI): Clinical Applications

Dawood Darbar, MBChB, MD
Associate Professor of Medicine, Vanderbilt University School of Medicine; Director, Vanderbilt Arrhythmia Service, Vanderbilt University Medical Center, Nashville, Tennessee
Standard Antiarrhythmic Drugs

Mithilesh K. Das, MD
Associate Professor of Clinical Medicine, Indiana University School of Medicine; Director, Cardiac Electrophysiology, Roudebush VA Medical Center, Indianapolis, Indiana
Differential Diagnosis for Wide QRS Complex Tachycardia; Assessment of the Patient with a Cardiac Arrhythmia

Mario Delmar, MD, PhD
Frank N. Wilson Professor of Cardiovascular Medicine and Professor of Internal Medicine and of Molecular and Integrative Physiology, University of Michigan Medical School; Co-Director, University of Michigan Center of Arrhythmia Research, Ann Arbor, Michigan
Molecular Organization and Regulation of the Cardiac Gap Junction Channel Connexin 43; Connexins as Potential Targets for Cardiovascular Pharmacology

Dobromir Dobrev, MD
Professor of Medicine and Lecturer, Department of Pharmacology and Toxicology, Carl Gustav Carus Medical Faculty, Dresden University of Technology, Dresden, Germany
Molecular Remodeling and Chronic Atrial Fibrillation

Halina Dobrzynski, PhD
Lecturer in Cardiac Electrophysiology, University of Manchester, Manchester, United Kingdom
The Sinoatrial Node: Its Complex Structure and Unique Ion Channel Gene Program; Mechanisms of Atrioventricular Nodal Excitability and Propagation

Derek J. Dosdall, PhD
Instructor, Department of Medicine, Division of Cardiovascular Disease, University of Alabama at Birmingham School of Medicine, Birmingham, Alabama
Mechanisms of Defibrillation

Lars Eckardt, MD, PhD
Peter Osypka Professor of Experimental and Clinical Electrophysiology; Professor of Cardiology, Medical Faculty, University of Münster/Medizinische Clinic C, Münster, Germany
Drug-Induced Ventricular Tachycardia

Igor R. Efimov, PhD
Lucy and Stanley Lopata Distinguished Professor of Biomedical Engineering, Cell Biology and Physiology, and Radiology, Washington University in St. Louis School of Engineering, St. Louis, Missouri
Mechanisms of Atrioventricular Nodal Excitability and Propagation

Kenneth A. Ellenbogen, MD
Kontos Professor of Cardiology, Virginia Commonwealth University School of Medicine; Director, Electrophysiology and Pacing, Medical College of Virginia, Richmond, Virginia
Atrial Tachycardia

N. A. Mark Estes III, MD
Professor of Medicine, Tufts University School of Medicine; Director, Cardiac Arrhythmia Service, Division of Cardiology; Tufts Medical Center, Boston, Massachusetts
Sudden Cardiac Death in Athletes, Including Commotio Cordis

Susan P. Etheridge, MD
Professor of Pediatrics–Cardiology, University of Utah School of Medicine, Salt Lake City, Utah
Andersen-Tawil Syndrome

Thomas H. Everett IV, PhD
Adjunct Assistant Professor of Cardiac Electrophysiology, Division of Cardiology, Department of Medicine, University of California, San Francisco, School of Medicine, San Francisco, California
Structural Atrial Remodeling Alters the Substrate and Spatiotemporal Organization of Atrial Fibrillation

Vladimir G. Fast, PhD
Associate Professor, Department of Biomedical Engineering, University of Alabama at Birmingham School of Medicine, Birmingham, Alabama
Mechanisms of Defibrillation

Glenn I. Fishman, MD
William Goldring Professor of Medicine, Professor of Pharmacology, and Professor of Neuroscience and Physiology, New York University School of Medicine; Director, Leon H. Charney Division of Cardiology, NYU Langone Medical Center, New York, New York
Gap Junction Distribution and Regulation in the Heart

Guy Fontaine, MD, PhD, HDR
Formerly at CHU La Salpétrière, Paris, France
Arrhythmogenic Right Ventricular Cardiomyopathies

Michael R. Franz, MD, PhD
Professor of Pharmacology, Georgetown University School of Medicine; Director, Electrophysiology and Cardiac Research, Washington DC VA Medical Center, Washington, DC
Monophasic Action Potential Recording

Paul Friedman, MD
Professor of Medicine, Mayo Clinic College of Medicine; Consultant, Division of Cardiovascular Diseases, Mayo Clinic, Rochester, Minnesota
Implantable Cardioverter-Defibrillator: Clinical Aspects

Joseph M. Galvin, MBBCh, LRCP&SI, FESC, FACC, FRCPI
Lecturer in Medicine, Royal College of Surgeons in Ireland; Consultant Cardiologist and Electrophysiologist, Connolly and Mater Hospitals, Dublin, Ireland
Ventricular Tachycardia in Patients with Dilated Cardiomyopathy

Apoor S. Gami, MD, MSc
Cardiac Electrophysiologist, Midwest Heart Specialists, Elmhurst, Illinois
Sleep-Disordered Breathing and Arrhythmias

Alfred L. George, Jr., MD
Grant W. Liddle Professor of Medicine and Pharmacology and Chief, Division of Genetic Medicine, Vanderbilt University of School of Medicine, Nashville, Tennessee
Inheritable Sodium Channel Diseases

Subham Ghosh, MS
Research Scientist, Cardiac Bioelectricity and Arrhythmia Center, Washington University in St. Louis School of Engineering, St. Louis, Missouri
Noninvasive Electrocardiographic Imaging: Methodology and Excitation of the Normal Human Heart

Michael R. Gold, MD, PhD
Michael E. Assey Professor of Medicine, School of Medicine; Chief of Cardiology; Associate Dean, Interdisciplinary Clinical Programs, Medical University of South Carolina, Charleston, South Carolina
Newer Applications of Pacemakers

Jeffrey J. Goldberger, MD
Professor of Medicine, Department of Medicine, Division of Cardiology, Northwestern University Feinberg School of Medicine; Director, Cardiac Electrophysiology Section, Northwestern Memorial Hospital, Chicago, Illinois
Impact of Nontraditional Antiarrhythmic Drugs on Sudden Cardiac Death

Richard A. Gray, PhD
Associate Professor, Department of Biomedical Engineering, University of Alabama at Birmingham School of Medicine, Birmingham, Alabama
Rotors and Spiral Waves in the Heart

William J. Groh, MD, MPH
Associate Professor of Medicine, Indiana University School of Medicine, Indianapolis, Indiana
Arrhythmias in Patients with Neurologic Disorders

Michel Haïssaguerre, MD
Professor of Cardiology, University Victor Segalen Bordeaux II; Hôpital Cardiologique due Haut-Lévêque, Bordeaux, France
Role of Cardiac and Thoracic Veins in Arrhythmogenesis; Atrial Substrate Ablation in Atrial Fibrillation

David L. Hayes, MD
Professor of Medicine, Mayo Clinic College of Medicine; Chair, Cardiovascular Diseases, Mayo Clinic, Rochester, Minnesota
Implantable Pacemakers

Stefan Herrmann, PhD
Research Fellow, Institut für Experimentelle und Klinische Pharmakologie und Toxikologie, Friedrich-Alexander-Universitat Erlangen-Nürnberg, Erlangen, Germany
Hyperpolarization-Activated, Cyclic Nucleotide–Gated (HCN) Channels: From Genes to Function

Gerhard Hindricks, MD, PhD
Adjunct Professor of Internal Medicine, Medical Faculty, University of Leipzig; Director of Electrophysiology, Heart Center Leipzig, Leipzig, Germany
Catheter Ablation of Ventricular Arrhythmias in Patients without Structural Heart Disease

Siew Yen Ho, PhD, FRCPath
Professor of Cardiac Morphology, National Heart and Lung Institute, Imperial College London; Honorary Consultant, Royal Brompton and Harefield Hospitals, London, United Kingdom
Morphologic Correlates of Atrial Arrhythmias

Méléze Hocini, MD
University Victor Segalen Bordeaux II; Hôpital Cardiologique du Haut-Lévêque, Bordeaux, France
Role of Cardiac and Thoracic Veins in Arrhythmogenesis

Denice M. Hodgson-Zingman, MD
Assistant Professor of Medicine, University of Iowa Carver College of Medicine; Clinical Cardiac Electrophysiologist, University of Iowa Hospitals and Clinics, Iowa City, Iowa
Ventricular Tachycardia in Patients with Heart Failure

Stefan H. Hohnloser, MD
Professor of Medicine–Cardiology, Medical Faculty, J. W. Goethe University; Director, Section of Clinical Electrophysiology, J. W. Goethe University Hospital, Frankfurt, Germany
T Wave Alternans

Steven R. Houser, PhD
Professor and Chair, Department of Physiology, Temple University School of Medicine, Philadelphia, Pennsylvania
Pharmacology of L-type and T-type Calcium Channels in the Heart

Larry V. Hryshko, PhD
Professor of Medicine, University of Manitoba Faculty of Medicine; Principal Investigator, Institute of Cardiovascular Sciences, St. Boniface Hospital Research Centre, Winnipeg, Manitoba, Canada
Membrane Pumps and Exchangers

William J. Hucker, PhD
Department of Biomedical Engineering, School of Engineering, Washington University in St. Louis, St. Louis, Missouri
Mechanisms of Atrioventricular Nodal Excitability and Propagation

Gary D. Hutchins, PhD
John W. Beeler Professor of Radiology, Indiana University School of Medicine, Indianapolis, Indiana
Neurocardiac Imaging

Raymond E. Ideker, MD, PhD
Jean V. Marks Professor of Medicine, Professor of Biomedical Engineering, and Professor of Physiology, Department of Medicine, Division of Cardiovascular Disease, University of Alabama at Birmingham School of Medicine, Birmingham, Alabama
Mechanisms of Defibrillation

Warren M. Jackman, MD
George Lynn Cross Research Professor Emeritus, University of Oklahoma School of Medicine, Oklahoma City, Oklahoma
Electrophysiologic Characteristics of Atrioventricular Nodal Reentrant Tachycardia: Implications of Reentrant Circuits

Pierre Jaïs, MD
Professor of Cardiology, University Victor Segalen Bordeaux II; Hôpital Cardiologique du Haut-Lévêque, Bordeaux, France
Role of Cardiac and Thoracic Veins in Arrhythmogenesis

José Jalife, MD
Cyrus and Jane Farrehi Professor of Cardiovascular Research, Professor of Internal Medicine, and Professor of Molecular and Integrative Physiology, University of Michigan Medical School; Co-Director, University of Michigan Center for Arrhythmia Research, Ann Arbor, Michigan
Fibrosis and Fibroblast Infiltration: An Active Structural Substrate for Altered Propagation and Spontaneous Tachyarrhythmias; Dynamics and Molecular Mechanisms of Ventricular Tachycardia and Fibrillation in Normal Hearts

Craig T. January, MD, PhD
Professor of Medicine and Physiology, University of Wisconsin School of Medicine and Public Health; Attending, University of Wisconsin Hospital and Clinics, Madison, Wisconsin
Pharmacology of the Cardiac Sodium Channel

Alan H. Kadish, MD
Chester and Deborah Cooley Professor of Medicine, Northwestern University Feinberg School of Medicine; Director, Clinical Trials Unit, Northwestern Memorial Hospital, Chicago, Illinois
Impact of Nontraditional Antiarrhythmic Drugs on Sudden Cardiac Death

Jérôme Kalifa, MD, PhD
Assistant Professor, Department of Internal Medicine, University of Michigan Medical School/University of Michigan Center for Arrhythmia Research, Ann Arbor, Michigan
Electrophysiologic Basis of Electrogram Fragmentation in Atrial Fibrillation

Jonathan M. Kalman, MBBS, PhD
Professor of Medicine, University of Melbourne Faculty of Medicine; Director, Cardiac Electrophysiology, Royal Melbourne Hospital, Melbourne, Victoria, Australia
Catheter Ablation of Supraventricular Arrhythmias

Mohamed H. Kanj, MD
Staff, Cleveland Clinic, Cleveland, Ohio
Implantable Cardioverter-Defibrillator: Technical Aspects

Robert S. Kass, PhD
Hosack Professor of Pharmacology, Alumni Professor of Pharmacology, and Chair, Department of Pharmacology, Columbia University College of Physicians and Surgeons, New York, New York
KCNQ1/KCNE1 Macromolecular Signaling Complex: Channel Microdomains and Human Disease

Paulus Kirchhoff, MD
Associate Professor of Medicine, Medical Faculty; University of Münster; Attending Physician and Head, Cardiac Catheterization Laboratory, Department of Cardiology and Angiology, University Hospital Münster, Münster, Germany
New Antiarrhythmic Drugs and New Concepts for Old Drugs

André G. Kléber, MD
Professor of Physiology, Medical Faculty, University of Bern, Bern, Switzerland
Intercellular Communication and Impulse Propagation

George J. Klein, MD
Professor of Medicine, Division of Cardiology, University of Western Ontario Faculty of Medicine; Cardiologist, London Health Sciences Center, London, Ontario, Canada
The Use of Implantable Loop Recorders

Sébastien Knecht, MD
Service de Rhythmologie, Hôpital Cardiologique du Haut-Lévêque, Bordeaux, France
Atrial Substrate Ablation in Atrial Fibrillation

Michael Koa-Wing, BSc, MRCP
Clinical Research Fellow, Imperial College Healthcare NHS Trust, St. Mary's Hospital, London, United Kingdom
Mapping and Imaging

Peter Kohl, MD, PhD
Tutor in Biomedical Sciences, Department of Physiology, Anatomy and Genetics, Balliol College, University of Oxford, Oxford, United Kingdom; Adjunct Associate Professor, University of Maryland School of Medicine/Biotechnology Institute, Baltimore, Maryland
Cardiac Stretch–Activated Channels and Mechano-Electric Transduction

Hans Kottkamp, MD, PhD
Adjunct Professor of Internal Medicine, Medical Faculty, University of Leipzig, Leipzig, Germany; Director of Electrophysiology, Clinic Hirslanden/Heart Center, Zurich, Switzerland
Catheter Ablation of Ventricular Arrhythmias in Patients without Structural Heart Disease

Andrew D. Krahn, MD
Professor of Medicine, Division of Cardiology, University of Western Ontario Faculty of Medicine; Cardiologist, London Health Sciences Center, London, Ontario, Canada
The Use of Implantable Loop Recorders

John D. Kugler, MD
D. B. and Paula Vanner Professor of Pediatrics and Professor of Internal Medicine, University of Nebraska College of Medicine; Clinical Professor of Pediatrics, Creighton University School of Medicine; University of Nebraska and Creighton University Chief of Joint Division of Pediatric Cardiology; Director of Cardiology, Children's Hospital, Omaha, Nebraska
Catheter Ablation in Pediatric and Congenital Heart Disease Patients

Junko Kurokawa, PhD
Associate Professor, Department of Bio-informational Pharmacology, Medical Research Institute, Tokyo Medical and Dental University, Tokyo, Japan
KCNQ1/KCNE1 Macromolecular Signaling Complex: Channel Microdomains and Human Disease

Edward G. Lakatta, MD
Chief, Laboratory of Cardiovascular Science, Intramural Research Program–NIH, National Institute on Aging, Baltimore, Maryland
A New Functional Paradigm for the Heart's Pacemaker: Mutual Entrainment of Intracellular Calcium Clocks and Surface Membrane Ion Channel Clocks

Paul D. Lampe, PhD
Research Professor, Global Health Department, University of Washington School of Medicine; Member and Associate Program Head, Molecular Diagnostics Program, Public Health Sciences and Human Biology, Fred Hutchinson Cancer Research Center, Seattle, Washington
Gap Junction Distribution and Regulation in the Heart

Kenneth R. Laurita, PhD
Associate Professor of Medicine and Biomedical Engineering, Case Western Reserve University School of Medicine; Metrohealth Medical Center, Cleveland, Ohio
Cardiac Alternans as a Pathophysiologic Mechanism of Arrhythmias

Bruce R. Lerman, MD
H. Altschul Master Professor of Medicine, Weill Cornell College of Medicine; Chief, Division of Cardiology, NewYork–Presbyterian Hospital; Director, Cardiac Electrophysiology Laboratory, Cornell University Medical Center, New York, New York
Ventricular Tachycardia in Patients with Structurally Normal Hearts

Rebecca Lewandowski, PhD
Department of Pharmacology, State University of New York Upstate Medical University MD/PhD Program, Syracuse, New York
Connexins as Potential Targets for Cardiovascular Pharmacology

Ronald A. Li, PhD
Associate Professor, Department of Cell Biology and Human Anatomy, University of California, Davis, School of Medicine, Davis; Associate Investigator, Institute of Pediatric Regenerative Medicine, Shriners Hospital, Sacramento, California
Adrenergic Signaling and Cardiac Ion Channels

Kang Teng Lim, MD
Service de Rhythmologie, Hôpital Cardiologique du Haut-Lévêque, Bordeaux, France
Atrial Substrate Ablation in Atrial Fibrillation

Mark S. Link, MD
Professor of Medicine, Tufts University School of Medicine; Co-Director, Cardiac Electrophysiology Laboratory; Director, Center for the Evaluation of Athletes, Division of Cardiology, Tufts Medical Center, Boston, Massachusetts
Sudden Cardiac Death in Athletes, Including Commotio Cordis

Nian Liu, MD, PhD
Researcher in Cardiovascular Genetics, Leon H. Charney Division of Cardiology, NYU Langone Medical Center/Smilow Research Center, New York, New York
Inheritable Disease of Intracellular Calcium Regulation

Deborah J. Lockwood, BM, BCh, MA
Assistant Professor of Medicine, University of Oklahoma College of Medicine, Oklahoma City, Oklahoma
Electrophysiologic Characteristics of Atrioventricular Nodal Reentrant Tachycardia: Implications for Reentrant Circuits

Fei Lü, MD, PhD
Associate Professor of Medicine, University of Minnesota Medical School, Minneapolis, Minnesota
Head-up Tilt Table Testing

Andreas Ludwig, MD
Professor, Institut für Experimentelle und Klinische Pharmakologie und Toxikologie, Friedrich-Alexander-Universitat Erlangen-Nürnberg, Erlangen, Germany
Hyperpolarization-Activated, Cyclic Nucleotide–Gated (HCN) Channels: From Genes to Function

Sebastian K. G. Maier, MD
Medizinsche Klinik und Poliklinik I, Universität Würzburg, Würzburg, Germany
Voltage-Gated Sodium Channels and Electrical Excitability of the Heart

Jonathan C. Makielski, MD
Professor of Medicine and Physiology, University of Wisconsin School of Medicine and Public Health; Cardiovascular Medicine, University of Wisconsin Hospital and Clinics, Madison, Wisconsin
Pharmacology of the Cardiac Sodium Channel; Sudden Infant Death Syndrome

Marek Malik, PhD, MD, DSc, DSc(Med), FACC, FESC, FHRS
Professor of Cardiac Electrophysiology and Head, Noninvasive Electrocardiology, Cardiac and Vascular Sciences, St. George's University of London; Chairman, St. Paul's Cardiac Electrophysiology, London, United Kingdom
Electrocardiographic and Autonomic Testing of Cardiac Risk

Victor Maltsev, PhD
Staff Scientist, Laboratory of Cardiovascular Science, Intramural Research Program–NIH, National Institute of Aging, Baltimore, Maryland
A New Functional Paradigm for the Heart's Pacemaker: Mutual Entrainment of Intracellular Calcium Clocks and Surface Membrane Ion Channel Clocks

Francis E. Marchlinski, MD
Professor of Medicine, University of Pennsylvania School of Medicine; Director of Electrophysiology Laboratory, Hospital of the University of Pennsylvania; Director of Electrophysiology, University of Pennsylvania Health System, Philadelphia, Pennsylvania
Gender Differences in Arrhythmias

Vias Markides, MD, FRCP
Honorary Senior Lecturer, National Heart and Lung Institute; Consultant Cardiologist and Clinical Lead in Cardiac Electrophysiology, Royal Brompton and Harefield Hospitals, London, United Kingdom
Mapping and Imaging

Barry J. Maron, MD
Adjunct Professor of Medicine, Tufts University School of Medicine, Boston, Massachusetts; Director, Hypertrophic Cardiomyopathy Center, Minneapolis Heart Institute Foundation, Minneapolis, Minnesota
Ventricular Arrhythmias in Hypertrophic Cardiomyopathy

James B. Martins, MD
Professor of Medicine, University of Iowa Carver College of Medicine; Attending, Iowa City VA Medical Center, Iowa City, Iowa
Neural Mechanisms Initiating and Maintaining Arrhythmias: Summarizing Data from Animal Models and Human Diseases

Argelia Medeiros-Domingo, MD, PhD
Postdoctoral Fellow, Windland Smith Rice Sudden Death Genomics Laboratory, Mayo Clinic, Rochester, Minnesota
Progressive Cardiac Conduction Disease

John M. Miller, MD
Professor of Medicine, Indiana University School of Medicine; Director, Clinical Cardiac Electrophysiology, Clarian Health Partners, Indianapolis, Indiana
Differential Diagnosis for Wide QRS Complex Tachycardia

Michael A. Miller, PhD
Assistant Research Professor, Imaging Sciences, Department of Radiology, Indiana University School of Medicine, Indianapolis, Indiana
Neurocardiac Imaging

Michele Miragoli, PhD
Research Assistant, Medical Faculty, University of Bern, Bern, Switzerland
Cardiac Myofibroblasts and Arrhythmogenesis

Peter J. Mohler, PhD
Associate Professor, Departments of Medicine and Molecular Physiology and Biophysics, University of Iowa Carver College of Medicine, Iowa City, Iowa
Intracellular Signaling and Regulation of Cardiac Ion Channels

Fred Morady, MD
Professor of Internal Medicine, University of Michigan Medical School, Ann Arbor, Michigan
Atrioventricular Reentry and Variants

Hiroshi Morita, MD, PhD
Assistant Professor, Department of Cardiovascular Medicine, Okayama University Graduate School of Medicine, Dentistry and Pharmaceutical Sciences, Okayama City, Okayama, Japan
Insight into Mechanisms of Ventricular Tachycardia from Isolated Wedge Preparations

Viviana Muñoz, PhD
Postdoctoral Fellow, Department of Internal Medicine–Cardiology, University of Michigan Center for Arrhythmia Research, Ann Arbor, Michigan
Fibrosis and Fibroblast Infiltration: An Active Structural Substrate for Altered Propagation and Spontaneous Tachyarrhythmias; Dynamics and Molecular Mechanisms of Ventricular Tachycardia and Fibrillation in Normal Hearts

Robert J. Myerburg, MD, FACC, FAHA
Professor of Medicine and Physiology, Division of Cardiology, and American Heart Association Chair in Cardiovascular Research, University of Miami Leonard F. Miller School of Medicine, Miami, Florida
Sudden Cardiac Death; Parasystole

Hiroshi Nakagawa, MD, PhD
Professor of Medicine, University of Oklahoma College of Medicine; Co-Director, Heart Rhythm Institute, Oklahoma City, Oklahoma
Electrophysiologic Characteristics of Atrioventricular Nodal Reentrant Tachycardia: Implications of Reentrant Circuits

Carlo Napolitano, MD, PhD
Department of Molecular Cardiology, IRCCS Fondazione Salvatore Maugeri, Pavia, Italy
Inheritable Disease of Intracellular Calcium Regulation; Catecholaminergic Polymorphic Ventricular Tachycardia; Timothy Syndrome

Stanley Nattel, MD, FACC, FRCPC, FRSC
Professor of Medicine and Paul-David Chair in Cardiovascular Electrophysiology, University of Montreal Faculty of Medicine; Cardiologist and Director, Electrophysiology Research Program, Montreal Heart Institute, Montreal, Quebec, Canada
Molecular Remodeling and Chronic Atrial Fibrillation

Jeanne M. Nerbonne, PhD
Alumni Endowed Professor of Molecular Biology and Pharmacology, Department of Developmental Biology, Washington University in St. Louis School of Medicine, St. Louis, Missouri
Heterogeneous Expression of Repolarizing Potassium Currents in the Mammalian Myocardium

Ernst Niggli, MD
Professor of Physiology, Medical Faculty, University of Bern, Bern, Switzerland
Sacroplasmic Reticulum Ion Channels

Sami F. Noujaim, PhD
Research Fellow, Department of Internal Medicine–Cardiology, University of Michigan Center for Arrhythmia Research, Ann Arbor, Michigan
Dynamics and Molecular Mechanisms of Ventricular Tachycardia and Fibrillation in Normal Hearts

Jeffrey E. Oligin, MD
Professor of Medicine, University of California, San Francisco, School of Medicine; Chief, Cardiac Electrophysiology, Division of Cardiology, Department of Medicine, UCSF Medical Center, San Francisco, California
Structural Atrial Remodeling Alters the Substrate and Spatiotemporal Organization of Atrial Fibrillation

Hakan Oral, MD
Frederick G. L. Huetwell Professor of Cardiovascular Medicine, University of Michigan Medical School; Director, Cardiac Electrophysiology Service, University of Michigan Health System, Ann Arbor, Michigan
Atrial Fibrillation: Mechanisms, Features, and Management

Gavin Y. Oudit, MD, PhD, FRCPC
Assistant Professor of Medicine, University of Alberta Faculty of Medicine; Staff Cardiologist and Clinical Investigator, Mazankowski Alberta Heart Institute, Edmonton, Alberta, Canada
Voltage-Regulated Potassium Channels

Alexander V. Panfilov, PhD
University Hoofddocent, Department of Theoretical Biology, Utrecht University, Utrecht, The Netherlands
Theory of Reentry

Carlo Pappone, MD, PhD, FACC
Director, Department of Arrhythmology, San Raffaele University Hospital, Milan, Italy
Pulmonary Vein Isolation for Atrial Fibriallation

Nicholas S. Peters, MD, FRCP
Professor of Cardiology, Imperial College London; National Heart and Lung Institute; Head, Cardiac Electrophysiology, and Consultant Cardiologist, Imperial College Healthcare NHS Trust, St. Mary's Hospital, London, United Kingdom
Mapping and Imaging

Robert W. Peters, MD
Professor of Medicine, University of Maryland School of Medicine; Chief of Cardiology, Baltimore Department of Veterans Affairs Medical Center, Baltimore, Maryland
Newer Applications of Pacemakers

Jørgen Søberg Petersen, MD, PhD
Senior Vice President, Research, and Global Head, Autoimmune and Inflammatory Diseases, Merck Serono International S.A., Geneva, Switzerland
Connexins as Potential Targets for Cardiovascular Pharmacology

Eckard Picht, MD
Postdoctoral Fellow, University of California, Davis, School of Medicine, Davis, California
Cardiac Calcium Channels

Gernot Plank, PhD
Institute of Biophysics, Medical University of Graz, Graz, Austria
Modeling Cardiac Defibrillation

Silvia G. Priori, MD, PhD
Associate Professor of Cardiology, University of Pavia Medical School, Pavia, Italy; Professor of Medicine, New York University School of Medicine; Director, Cardiovascular Genetics Program, Leon H. Charney Division of Cardiology, NYU Langone Medical Center, New York, New York; Director, Molecular Cardiology and Electrophysiology Laboratories, IRCCS Fondazione Salvatore Maugeri, Pavia, Italy
Inheritable Disease of Intracellular Calcium Regulation; Catecholaminergic Polymorphic Ventricular Tachycardia; Timothy Syndrome

Zhilin Qu, PhD
Associate Professor of Medicine, David Geffen School of Medicine at UCLA, Los Angeles, California
Nonlinear Dynamics of Excitation and Propagation in Cardiac Muscle

Charulatha Ramanathan, PhD
Vice President, CardioInsight Technologies, Cleveland, Ohio
Noninvasive Electrocardiographic Imaging: Methodology and Excitation of the Normal Human Heart

Richard B. Robinson, PhD
Professor of Pharmacology, Columbia University College of Physicians and Surgeons, New York New York
Biologic Pacing

Dan M. Roden, MD
Professor of Medicine and Pharmacology, Vanderbilt University School of Medicine; Director, Oates Institute for Experimental Therapeutics; Assistant Vice-Chancellor for Personalized Medicine, Vanderbilt University Medical Center, Nashville, Tennessee
Pharmacogenomics of Cardiac Arrhythmias and Effect on Drug Therapy

Stephan Rohr, MD
Professor of Physiology, Medical Faculty, University of Bern, Bern, Switzerland
Cardiac Myofibroblasts and Arrhythmogenesis

Michael R. Rosen, MD
Professor of Pediatrics and Gustavus A. Pfeiffer Professor of Pharmacology, Department of Pharmacology; Director, Center for Molecular Therapeutics, Columbia University College of Physicians and Surgeons, New York, New York
Biologic Pacing

David S. Rosenbaum, MD
Professor of Medicine, Biomedical Engineering, Physiology, and Biophysics, Case Western Reserve University School of Medicine; Director and Chief, Heart and Vascular Center, Metro Health Medical Center, Cleveland, Ohio
Cardiac Alternans as a Pathophysiologic Mechanism of Arrhythmias

Yanfei Ruan, MD, PhD
Researcher in Cardiovascular Genetics, Leon H. Charney Division of Cardiology, NYU Langone Medical Center/ Smilow Research Center, New York, New York
Catecholaminergic Polymorphic Ventricular Tachycardia

Yoram Rudy, PhD
Fred Saigh Distinguished Professor of Engineering, Department of Biomedical Engineering, Washington University in St. Louis School of Engineering; Director, Cardiac Bioelectricity and Arrhythmia Center, St. Louis, Missouri
Ionic Mechanisms of Ventricular Action Potential Excitation; Noninvasive Electrocardiographic Imaging: Methodology and Excitation of the Normal Human Heart; Noninvasive Electrocardiographic Imaging (ECGI): Clinical Applications

Jeremy N. Ruskin, MD
Associate Professor of Medicine, Harvard Medical School; Director, Cardiac Arrhythmia Service, Massachusetts General Hospital, Boston, Massachusetts
Ventricular Tachycardia in Patients with Dilated Cardiomyopathy

Andrea M. Russo, MD
Clinical Associate Professor of Medicine, University of Pennsylvania School of Medicine; Director, Electrophysiology Laboratory, Penn-Presbyterian Medical Center, University of Pennsylvania Health System, Philadelphia, Pennsylvania
Gender Differences in Arrhythmias

Scott Sakaguchi, MD
Associate Professor of Medicine, University of Minnesota Medical School, Minneapolis, Minnesota
Head-up Tilt Table Testing

Prashanthan Sanders, MBBS
University Victor Segalen Bordeaux II; Hôpital Cardiologique du Haut-Lévêque, Bordeaux, France
Role of Cardiac and Thoracic Veins in Arrhythmogenesis

Michael C. Sanguinetti, PhD
Professor of Physiology, University of Utah School of Medicine; Associate Director, Nora Eccles Harrison Cardiovascular Research and Training Institute, Salt Lake City, Utah
Gating of Cardiac Delayed Rectifier Potassium Channels

Vincenzo Santinelli, MD
Professor of Cardiology, San Raffaele University; Scientific Director, Department of Arrhythmology, San Raffaele University Hospital, Milan, Italy
Pulmonary Vein Isolation for Atrial Fibrillation

Rainer Schimpf, MD
First Department of Medicine–Cardiology, University Hospital Mannheim, Mannheim, Germany
Idiopathic Ventricular Fibrillation

Peter J. Schwartz, MD
Professor and Chairman, Department of Cardiology, and Director, School for the Board in Cardiology, School of Medicine, University of Pavia; Chief Coronary Care Unit, Fondazione IRCCS Policlinico S. Matteo, Pavia, Italy
Long QT and Short QT Syndromes

Kalyanam Shivkumar, MD, PhD
Professor of Medicine and Radiology, David Geffen School of Medicine at UCLA; Director, UCLA Cardiac Arrhythmia Center and EP Program, Ronald Reagan UCLA Medical Center, Los Angeles, California
Lesion-Forming Technologies for Catheter Ablation

Jonathan Silva, PhD
Research Scientist, Department of Biomedical Engineering, Washington University in St. Louis School of Engineering, St. Louis, Missouri
Ionic Mechanisms of Ventricular Action Potential Excitation

Allan C. Skanes, MD
Associate Professor, Department of Medicine, Division of Cardiology, University of Western Ontario Faculty of Medicine; Cardiologist, London Health Services Centre, London, Ontario, Canada
The Use of Implantable Loop Recorders

Richard L. Snowdon, MD
Consultant Electrophysiologist/Cardiologist, Liverpool Heart and Chest Hospital NHS Trust, Liverpool, United Kingdom
Catheter Ablation of Supraventricular Arrhythmias

Virend K. Somer, MD, PhD
Professor of Medicine, Mayo Clinic School of Medicine, Rochester, Minnesota
Sleep-Disordered Breathing and Arrhythmias

Paul Sorge, PhD
Associate Professor of Biochemistry and Molecular Biology, University of Nebraska College of Medicine, Omaha, Nebraska
Molecular Organization and Regulation of the Cardiac Gap Junction Channel Connexin 43

Igor Splawski, PhD
Assistant Professor, Harvard Medical School; Scientific Associate, Children's Hospital Boston, Boston, Massachusetts
Timothy Syndrome

Bruce S. Stambler, MD
Cardiologist, University Hospitals of Cleveland, Cleveland, Ohio
Atrial Tachycardia

William G. Stevenson, MD
Professor of Medicine, Harvard Medical School; Physician, Cardiovascular Division, Brigham and Women's Hospital, Boston, Massachusetts
Catheter Ablation for Ventricular Tachycardia in Patients with Structural Heart Disease

Juliane Stieber, MD
Assistant Professor, Institut für Experimentelle und Klinische Pharmakologie und Toxikologie, Friedrich-Alexander-Universitat Erlangen-Nürnberg, Erlangen, Germany
Hyperpolarization-Activated, Cyclic Nucleotide–Gated (HCN) Channels: From Genes to Function

Richard Sutton, DScMed
Professor, Imperial College London; Cardiovascular Medicine, St. Mary's Hospital, London, United Kingdom
Head-up Tilt Table Testing

Michael O. Sweeney, MD
Associate Professor of Medicine, Harvard Medical School; Cardiac Arrhythmia Service, Brigham and Women's Hospital; Boston, Massachusetts
Cardiac Resynchronization Therapy

Charles Swerdlow, MD
Clinical Professor of Medicine, David Geffen School of Medicine at UCLA; Electrophysiocardiologist, Cedars-Sinai Medical Center, Los Angeles, California
Implantable Cardioverter-Defibrillator: Clinical Aspects

Hanno L. Tan, MD
Department of Cardiology and Heart Failure Research Center, Academic Medical Center, University of Amsterdam, Amsterdam, The Netherlands
Inheritable Potassium Channel Diseases

Usha Tedrow, MD
Instructor of Medicine, Harvard Medical School; Associate Director, Clinical Cardiac Electrophysiology Program, Brigham and Women's Hospital, Boston, Massachusetts
Catheter Ablation for Ventricular Tachycardia in Patients with Structural Heart Disease

James O. Tellez, BSc, PhD
Postdoctoral Fellow in Cardiac Electrophysiology, University of Manchester, Manchester, United Kingdom
The Sinoatrial Node: Its Complex Structure and Unique Ion Channel Gene Program

David J. Tester, BS
Senior Research Technologist and Supervisor, Windlow Smith Rice Sudden Death Genomics Laboratory, Mayo Clinic, Rochester, Minnesota
Single Nucleotide Polymorphisms and Cardiac Arrhythmias

Natalia A. Trayanova, PhD
Institute for Computational Medicine, Johns Hopkins University, Baltimore, Maryland
Modeling Cardiac Defibrillation

John K. Triedman, MD
Associate Professor of Pediatrics, Harvard Medical School; Senior Associate, Department of Cardiology, Children's Hospital Boston, Boston, Massachusetts
Atrial Arrhythmias in Congenital Heart Disease

Martin Tristani-Firouzi, MD
Associate Professor of Pediatrics, University of Utah School of Medicine; Investigator, Nova Eccles Harrison Cardiovascular Research and Training Institute, Salt Lake City, Utah
Gating of Cardiac Delayed Rectifier Potassium Channels; Andersen-Tawil Syndrome

Miguel Valderrábano, MD
Associate Professor of Medicine, Weill Cornell Medical College, New York, New York; Director, Division of Cardiac Electrophysiology, Department of Cardiology, The Methodist Hospital, Houston, Texas
Exercise-Induced Arrhythmias

George F. Van Hare, MD
Louis Larrick Ward Professor of Pediatrics, Washington University in St. Louis School of Medicine; Director, Pediatric Cardiology, St. Louis Children's Hospital, St. Louis, Missouri
Ventricular Tachycardia in Patients after Surgery for Congenital Heart Disease

Prakash C. Vishwanathan, PhD
Grant Writer, College of Sciences, Old Dominion University, Norfolk, Virginia
Biophysics of Normal an Abnormal Cardiac Sodium Channel Function

Albert L. Waldo, MD
Walter H. Pritchard Professor of Cardiology, Professor of Medicine, and Professor of Biomedical Engineering, Case Western Reserve University School of Medicine; Associate Chief of Cardiology for Academic Affairs; Immediate Past Director, Clinical Cardiac Electrophysiology Program, University Hospitals Case Medical Center, Cleveland, Ohio
Atrial Flutter

Paul J. Wang, MD
Professor of Medicine, Stanford University School of Medicine; Director, Cardiac Arrhythmia Service, Stanford University Medical Center, Stanford, California
Implantable Pacemakers

Yong Wang, MS
Research Scientist, Department of Biomedical Engineering, Washington University in St. Louis School of Engineering, St. Louis, Missouri
Noninvasive Electrocardiographic Imaging (ECGI): Clinical Applications

Mark D. Warren, PhD
Postdoctoral Research Associate, Nora Eccles Harrison Cardiovascular Research and Training Institute, University of Utah, Salt Lake City, Utah
Mechanisms of Ischemic Ventricular Fibrillation

Robert Weingart, PhD
Professor of Physiology, Medical Faculty, University of Bern, Bern, Switzerland
Biophysical Properties of Gap Junctions

James N. Weiss, MD
Professor of Medicine and Physiology, David Geffen School of Medicine at UCLA; Chief, Division of Cardiology, UCLA Medical Center Cardiovascular Research Laboratories, Los Angeles, California
Nonlinear Dynamics of Excitation and Propagation in Cardiac Muscle

Arthur A. M. Wilde, MD, PhD
Department of Cardiology and Heart Failure Research Center, Academic Medical Center, University of Amsterdam, Amsterdam, The Netherlands
Inheritable Potassium Channel Diseases

Bruce L. Wilkoff, MD
Professor of Medicine, Cleveland Clinic Lerner College of Medicine of Case Western Reserve University; Co-Director, Section of Cardiac Electrophysiology and Pacing, and Director, Cardiac Pacing and Tachyarrhythmia Devices, Cleveland Clinic, Cleveland, Ohio
Implantable Cardioverter-Defibrillator: Technical Aspects

Lance D. Winson, MD
Associate Professor of Emergency Medicine, Case Western Reserve University School of Medicine; Attending Physician, Metro Health Medical Center, Cleveland, Ohio
Cardiac Alternans as a Pathophysiologic Mechanism of Arrhythmias

Christian Wolpert, MD
First Department of Medicine–Cardiology, University Hospital Mannheim, Mannheim, Germany
Idiopathic Ventricular Fibrillation

Mark A. Wood, MD
Professor of Medicine, Virginia Commonwealth University School of Medicine, Richmond, Virginia
Atrial Tachycardia

Matthew Wright, MBBS, PhD
Service de Rhythmologie, Hôpital Cardiologique du Haut-Lévêque, Bordeaux, France
Atrial Substrate Ablation in Atrial Fibrillation

Jiashin Wu, PhD
Assistant Professor of Molecular Pharmacology and Physiology, University of South Florida College of Medicine, Tampa, Florida
Insight into Mechanisms of Ventricular Tachycardia from Isolated Wedge Preparations

Alexey V. Zaitsev, PhD
Research Associate Professor of Bioengineering, College of Engineering/Nora Eccles Harrison Cardiovascular Research and Training Institute, University of Utah, Salt Lake City, Utah
Mechanisms of Ischemic Ventricular Fibrillation

Douglas P. Zipes, MD
Distinguished Professor and Emeritus Professor of Medicine, Pharmacology, and Toxicology; Emeritus Director, Division of Cardiology and the Krannert Institute of Cardiology, Indiana University School of Medicine, Indianapolis, Indiana; Editor-in-Chief, Heart*Rhythm*
Neurocardiac Imaging; Insight into Mechanisms of Ventricular Tachycardia from Isolated Wedge Preparations; Assessment of the Patient with a Cardiac Arrhythmia

Sharon Zlochiver, PhD
Senior Lecturer, Department of Biomedical Engineering, Tel-Aviv University, Tel-Aviv, Israel
Fibrosis and Fibroblast Infiltration: An Active Structural Substrate for Altered Propagation and Spontaneous Tachyarrhythmias

Preface

In the five years since the fourth edition of this book was published, advances in cardiac electrophysiology have been impressive. A broadening understanding of the fundamental electrophysiologic mechanisms underlying normal and abnormal cardiac excitation and impulse propagation is emerging, thanks in part to leapfrog improvements in technology, from the use of voltage clamping and the Ling Gerard microelectrode, through patch clamping and molecular biology, to optical mapping, computer modeling, and molecular genetics. A wide variety of basic mechanisms of normal and abnormal cardiac excitation, impulse propagation, and arrhythmias have been well described as a result of such improvements. In addition, basic cardiac electrophysiology has contributed to identification of disease loci for currently known mutations in proteins that form sarcolemmal and sub-sarcolemmal ion channels, discoveries that have greatly improved current understanding of the substrate for cardiac arrhythmias in both inherited and acquired diseases. The first part of *Cardiac Electrophysiology: From Cell to Bedside* addresses all of these issues and offers a conglomerate of comprehensive reviews on modern concepts in basic cardiac electrophysiology. This in-depth background is provided to help the reader integrate knowledge from the molecular to the organ level and to support translation of that knowledge into clinical practice.

The second half of the book focuses on clinical progress, which has been equally remarkable, with continued elucidation of pathophysiologic mechanisms responsible for many arrhythmias, including the different types of atrial fibrillation and many ventricular tachyarrhythmias, as well as new approaches to their management. Development of drugs, devices, and ablation techniques continues to advance at a startling pace. Perhaps no area has progressed as much as research into the genetic underpinning of many arrhythmias, not just those clearly related to ion channel abnormalities such as long and short QT syndromes, catecholaminergic ventricular tachycardia, right ventricular and hypertrophic cardiomyopathies, and Brugada syndrome, but the more common arrhythmias such as atrial fibrillation, ventricular tachycardia, and those related to sudden cardiac death. The growth of new imaging modalities has been breathtaking and has kept pace with the need for better pictures of cardiac anatomy, particularly of the left atrium and pulmonary veins. Advances in recording electrical signals from the heart can be marked by three phases: development of the electrocardiograph, catheter-based intracardiac recordings, and now ECG imaging. The last phase has opened a new era into noninvasive assessment of cardiac activation.

The format of the book continues to evolve as well. The use of color throughout maximizes accessibility of information presented in the figures and diagrams, as well as providing a more attractive appearance overall. In addition, the electronic format facilitates availability for ready reference. As before, the authors of the chapters are the leaders in their areas, and we are pleased that they consider writing for *Cardiac Electrophysiology: From Cell to Bedside* a happy task. We thank them for their contributions, which continue to make this book an important reference text for basic and clinical scientists, clinicians, and general cardiologists. We strive to craft it as the all-inclusive knowledge source, literally "from cell to bedside," for those interested in heart rhythms. We think it is one of the few books accomplishing that goal with such an authoritative list of experts.

Finally, we thank our wives, Joan Zipes and Paloma Jalife, whose constant support allows us to undertake such endeavors as this, and the people at Elsevier, particularly Natasha Andjelkovic, Janice Gaillard, and Jeff Gunning, for all their help.

In the final analysis, the reader determines the success or failure of a book, and we are pleased that so many of you liked the previous editions and have made this publication an important part of your educational resources. We hope that this edition meets your expectations equally well.

Douglas P. Zipes
José Jalife

Contents

Introduction: Progress in Antiarrhythmic Therapies

A. JOHN CAMM

CHAPTER OUTLINE

Background

Cardiac arrhythmias can be diagnosed and treated far better today than 50 years ago. For example, it is now the 50th anniversary of the implantation of the first cardiac pacemaker, an impressive life-saving invention. Other impressive examples of therapies introduced during the past several decades that save lives or dramatically reduce suffering are antiarrhythmic drugs such as amiodarone, the implantable cardioverter-defibrillator (ICD), and the many techniques of ablation.

Both basic and clinical research in the field of cardiac arrhythmology have been particularly prolific, especially over the past 3 decades (Fig. I-1). Highly successful, albeit imperfect and expensive, therapies have emerged. The success of these treatments, which are largely empirical and nonspecific in nature, has led to the notion that the medical problems associated with cardiac arrhythmias have been solved—but such is not the case, especially because the implementation of these therapies has been patchy at best.

The arrhythmology community has failed to stimulate the development of more specifically targeted and potentially much better therapies. What is worse, the empirical yet seemingly effective therapies that have emerged have been grudgingly and often inadequately investigated, and the results and implications have been poorly promulgated. Although professional guidelines have embraced the modest evidence base and eagerly put forward positive recommendations, little attempt has been made to use these guidelines to their full extent by ensuring their widespread implementation and by auditing the value they bring to the health care system.

Successful Therapeutics

Pacemaker

Swedish engineers designed the first miniature pacemaker, which was implanted in 1958. The first device lasted only a few hours, but the patient survived. In fact, he lived for almost half a decade supported by increasingly sophisticated, smaller, yet longer-lived pacemakers. Millions of these gadgets have now been implanted, and very many lives are saved at relatively little cost. No drug can match this empirical performance for the treatment of any bradycardia, whereas the pacemaker can prevent every bradycardia, irrespective of its etiology or mechanism. This is confidently stated, although no controlled clinical trials whatsoever have been conducted that bear on the efficacy of pacemaker therapy.

Nevertheless, the success of the pacemaker rendered efforts to develop any pharmaceutical solution seemingly unnecessary and commercially futile. Yet the pacemaker has problems and is far from the ideal solution. It is a manmade machine and can fail; it requires continual surveillance and eventual replacement; and it is inserted into the body, from which it may be rejected or where it may become infected. Long-term ectopic electrical stimulation of the ventricle may result in cardiac failure, requiring the institution of more complex stimulation modalities such as biventricular stimulation.

A better solution may now emerge—the biologic pacemaker ("biopacemaker").[1] Stem cells may be modified in a variety of ways to mature into sinus node, atrioventricular node, or conduction system tissue, which may then be seeded to appropriate locations and become integrated and connected within the defective natural tissue. Eventually, when problems related to safety and reliability have been solved, "natural" impulse generation and conduction may be restored. Such specific, targeted treatment is not available today but may emerge as mainline therapy that will replace electronic devices in the not-too-distant future. Alternatively, because the genetic basis for some conduction disorders is known, gene modification also offers the opportunity for therapy that specifically corrects the underlying genetic disorder responsible for the disease.

Implantable Cardioverter-Defibrillator

The miniaturization of the cardioverter-defibrillator in 1981 led to implantation of the device in humans. The first demonstrations of ICDs in animals and later in humans led to the eponym "Lazarus device," because of its seemingly miraculous efficacy in restoring life. Such devices initially were large, poorly programmable, difficult to implant, and relatively short-lived. Most of these early problems were quickly solved, and early trials proved convincingly that the ICD saved lives.[2-5] For the first time, this very effective therapy was able to demonstrate the comparative inefficacy of so-called antiarrhythmic drugs that seemed to do little to prevent loss of life.[6] The ICD is now popular for treatment for most patients at risk for sudden tachyarrhythmic death, irrespective of the mechanism underlying the arrhythmia. Nonetheless, use of these devices is not a perfect solution. In many instances, the patient must literally die or come very close to death to benefit from its ability to restore life; moreover, inappropriate and often painful discharges still occur; and the device may fail, or may excite biologic reactions. Worst of all, it is expensive, and inequality of access to this treatment is obvious despite a welter of guidelines attesting to the value of this therapy.

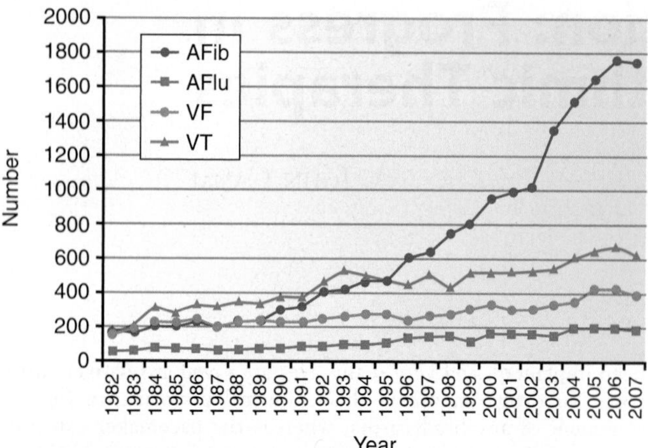

Figure I-1 PubMed citations for the search terms *atrial fibrillation* (AFib), *atrial flutter* (AFlu), *ventricular tachycardia* (VT), and *ventricular fibrillation* (VF) from 1982 to 2007. The data were accessed on May 1, 2008. Publications, particularly relating to atrial fibrillation, have been prolific.

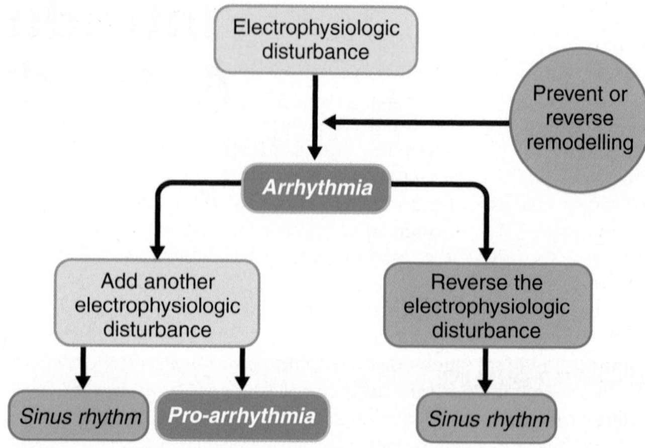

Figure I-2 Graphical illustration of current and future strategic approaches to the prescription of antiarrhythmic therapy. At present, most antiarrhythmic therapy is chosen empirically (with respect to efficacy), whereas the ideal approach toward which current investigations should move is targeting of therapy to prevent, reverse, or correct specific electrophysiologic abnormalities. See text for details.

The outstanding efficacy of ICD treatment has stifled research into alternative therapies for life-threatening ventricular arrhythmias. Practically no drug discovery or development activity has been related to the treatment of ventricular tachyarrhythmias in the pharmaceutical industry. Antiarrhythmic drugs are positioned as complementary to background ICD therapy, in the sense that such treatment may reduce the occurrence of rapid ventricular arrhythmias and lessen the discharge rate of the device, calm ventricular storms, prevent the delivery of inappropriate therapies, or reduce the defibrillation threshold. A similar subsidiary role has been assigned to ventricular ablation therapy, although some evidence suggests that such treatment may in some instances be sufficiently curative to render additional ICD therapy unnecessary. Of importance, it is now becoming apparent that targeted drug therapy may be able to play a definitive role in the reduction of sudden cardiac death in important although small subgroups of patients at risk from well-described and understood mechanisms of ventricular arrhythmogenesis.

Antiarrhythmic Drugs

During the past 50 years or so, cardiologists and arrhythmologists have explored the use of dozens of antiarrhythmic drugs. According to the Vaughan Williams classification,[7] most of these were sodium channel (class 1) or potassium channel (class 3) blockers. If a drug from one category was unsuccessful, the physician often would try an alternative from the other group. No specific patient characteristic provided any clue to the likely efficacy of antiarrhythmic drugs, and the choice of therapy was made most often on the basis of possible adverse effects. Although it often was theorized that therapy was designed to block conduction or to increase refractoriness, by mechanisms of action readily demonstrable in experimental animal models, the clinician, with few exceptions such as atrioventricular reentry in the Wolff-Parkinson-White syndrome, had no idea how or why therapy was either effective or ineffective in a particular patient. It was clear only that the antiarrhythmic drug further disturbed the abnormality that generated the trigger or substrate for the arrhythmia (Fig. I-2). Physicians hoped that the result would be antiarrhythmic but began to realize that all too often, the additional drug-induced disturbance to the electrophysiologic milieu would have, worst of all, a proarrhythmic consequence.

This sense of the "blunderbuss" approach to the drug treatment of arrhythmias became increasingly clear when multi-channel blockers, which often also had other major cardiovascular effects, became available. Amiodarone is the best example, blocking as it does the sodium channel and several potassium channels in addition to being a calcium antagonist, a nonspecific antiadrenergic agent, and a coronary artery vasodilator. Although clinical trial data on this drug were relatively scarce, it rapidly became popular because physicians perceived it to be effective. The drug was administered for the treatment of almost any arrhythmia, and because it appeared to be safe to give to patients with ischemia, hypertrophy, or cardiac dilatation, amiodarone became a drug of choice in every therapeutic cascade, relegated to a subsidiary position only because of its extracardiac side effects. Not surprisingly, many recent attempts have been made to improve amiodarone—for example, by increasing its solubility or reducing its elimination half-life and metabolic interactions. Another avenue of research has been the development of a similar multichannel molecule that retains or improves the efficacy of the drug while reducing its extracardiac complications, its long half-life, and its numerous interactions. The attempt has been to produce a "drug for all seasons," which may, of course, be clinically valuable but is intellectually unsatisfactory because of its empirical application.

Instead, a new approach to drug development may be evolving. Because electrophysiologic disturbance of the atria is the pathomechanism responsible for atrial fibrillation, it would seem logical to use an antiarrhythmic agent that targets the atrium in attempting to treat the condition. This approach would avoid negative inotropic and proarrhythmic side effects on the ventricle. Thus, drugs intended to block the ultra-rapid component of the outward potassium rectifier current, which is present only in the atrium, are being developed. Unfortunately, some of these drugs have proved to be insufficiently specific for this channel.

On the other hand, newer molecules, at present on the drawing board, in preclinical development, or in normal volunteer studies, seem more promising. Because atrial fibrillation seems to be supported largely by left atrial substrate, researchers are now exploring the possibility that drugs may potentially be developed that specifically affect left atrial tissue. More realistically, drug design is focusing on specificity to remodel atrial tissue that supports atrial fibrillation. For example, I_{KACh} is constitutively active in atrial fibrillation and provides a tempting target for the possible suppression of atrial fibrillation.[8] Other drugs are being developed with the aim of suppression of pulmonary vein triggers, or with the intention of inhibiting substrate development in order to halt or even reverse progressive deterioration from first-onset atrial fibrillation, through recurrent forms of the arrhythmia, eventually to permanent atrial fibrillation.

Drug development for the management of ventricular tachycardia has been far more restrained. Multichannel blockers have not been much investigated, and obviously those drugs designed to target atrial mechanisms have not been pursed for ventricular arrhythmias. Gap junction modulators and stretch receptor antagonists have been proposed but little investigated. Some interesting and highly targeted treatments, however, have been evaluated for the treatment of ventricular arrhythmia associated with subtypes of the long QT syndrome. For example, potassium channel openers such as nicorandil have been advocated for LQT1; spironolactone and supplementary potassium have value in LQT2; and mexiletine, flecainide, and most recently ranolazine have been used in patients with LQT3.[9-11] The delayed inward sodium current, I_{NaL}, is upregulated in LQT3, and ranolazine specifically inhibits this current at therapeutic concentrations. This example nicely illustrates the principle of targeting the specific abnormality, rather than swamping the electrophysiologic milieu and hoping for the best.

Ablation Therapy

Surgeons introduced antiarrhythmic ablation therapy in the 1970s. For patients with symptomatic or dangerous Wolff-Parkinson-White syndrome, accessory atrioventricular connections could be identified by means of epicardial mapping techniques, and the pathway could then be physically interrupted by cutting or freezing. The abnormal tissue linking the atrium directly to the ventricle was thereby removed from the conduction circuit, leaving the patient with a normal heart. This approach resulted in a clinical cure, and the patient could then expect to lead and live a normal life. It was not long before cardiologists developed catheter-based techniques, initially using barotrauma energy from intracardiac discharges, so-called *fulguration*, and then radiofrequency energy, which could be more carefully controlled, for *ablation*.

It was soon realized that ablation therapy could be applied to more arrhythmia substrates than Wolff-Parkinson-White syndrome alone. Junctional tachycardias supported by probably redundant duality of atrioventricular node conduction could be as easily treated with a procedure that again left the patient with essentially a normal heart and life expectancy. Other arrhythmias, whether automatic or reentrant in nature, that emanated from a focal source could be eradicated relatively easily, especially when sophisticated mapping systems began to evolve. Other macro reentrant arrhythmias, such as atrial flutter or ventricular tachycardias, that use critical conduction pathways also became targets of ablation therapy, because the tachycardia could be effectively treated even if the underlying pathology for the most part remained.

Destruction of the atrioventricular node–His bundle conduction pathway is a less satisfactory application of ablation therapy. Normal tissue is destroyed, and the patient becomes dependent on pacemaker therapy to support the ventricular rate. Of greater importance, the arrhythmia and its associated pathology remain in place, and the arrhythmia may itself worsen—for example, paroxysmal atrial fibrillation often converts to persistent or permanent forms of the arrhythmia, with consequent atrial dilatation and a potential for worsening thromboembolic risk. The expression of the arrhythmia is affected only at the level of the ventricle. Nevertheless, the treatment is effective, and the patient's quality of life usually is much improved. Physicians, however, are not comfortable with this procedure, particularly because of its irreversible nature. Attempts to modify rather than destroy the atrioventricular node—intuitively a much more satisfactory approach—have not been successful.

Atrial fibrillation is an arrhythmia with a potentially large substrate, and initially it was difficult to imagine how this could easily be treated by ablation. Surgeons led the way and, following the suggestions of basic scientists and using projections from computer models, demonstrated that reducing the contiguous atrial mass, using operations such as the maze procedure, led to abolition of atrial fibrillation in a high proportion of cases. Electrophysiologists attempted to emulate this effect in the catheter laboratory, but it proved very difficult to accomplish. It was then realized that most episodes of atrial fibrillation are triggered by rapidly firing ectopic foci, usually located within the pulmonary veins. Attempts were made to locate and destroy these foci, and although this approach was successful in some hands, post-procedural pulmonary vein stenosis was common. This technique was largely abandoned, and instead conduction from the pulmonary vein was blocked by encircling the pulmonary veins with lines of ablation. Additional lines to break up the substrate often are thought to be necessary if the fibrillation is longstanding or if underlying atrial or ventricular disease is present.

Other investigators have taken different approaches to the ablation treatment of atrial fibrillation by identifying and extirpating areas with low voltage or complex fractionated electrograms. Another technique is to locate and destroy the autonomic ganglia that overlie atrial myocardium, on the basis that autonomic modulation is critical to the triggering and sustenance of atrial fibrillation. Still other investigators have emphasized that it may be critical to destroy or isolate the electrophysiologic abnormalities of other venoatrial structures and junctions, and interrupt major inter- and intra-atrial conduction pathways. In many centers, all of these techniques (the ablation blunderbuss) are applied to difficult cases. Similar, virtually empirical techniques may be applied to ventricular arrhythmias that emerge from diffuse substrates, especially in dilated or arrhythmogenic cardiomyopathies. The techniques may certainly be effective, but they are not carefully targeted and from a theoretical perspective are inherently unsatisfactory. Better solutions are required.

Despite the increasingly empirical nature of some of these ablation procedures, they do appear to be outstandingly effective. For example, recent trials comparing ablation treatment with conventional antiarrhythmic drug therapy for suppression of the recurrence of atrial fibrillation[12-14] have uniformly demonstrated that pulmonary vein isolation was much the better treatment (Table I-1).

Proving Therapeutic Efficacy

Atrial Fibrillation

Atrial fibrillation may be highly symptomatic, particularly when the rhythm is rapid and irregular, underlying heart disease is present, or the patient is female, hypertensive, or young. In others, particularly the older patient with persistent or permanent atrial fibrillation and a slower and a more regular ventricular rate, the arrhythmia may be relatively asymptomatic, although the patient's quality of life may still be degraded.

Until recently, electrocardiographic documentation of a recurrence of the arrhythmia was thought to be the appropriate method by which to assess the value of an antiarrhythmic agent or an ablation procedure for the treatment of atrial fibrillation. The time to a symptomatic recurrence of atrial fibrillation (or atrial tachycardia or flutter) has been the outcome parameter of choice. This has been relatively easily accomplished by providing patients with transtelephonic event monitors. Because

Table I-1 Randomized Clinical Trials of Ablation Therapies versus Antiarrhythmic Drug Therapies for Atrial Fibrillation

Study	No. of Patients	Mean Age, Years	Type of AF	Previous Use of AAD	Ablation Technique	Follow-up	Crossed over to Ablation	AF Free at 1 Year	
								Ablation	AAD
Krittayaphong et al, 2003	30	52	Paroxysmal or persistent	Yes	PVI±LACA	1 year	Not stated	79%	40%
Wazni et al, 2005 (RAAFT)	70	53±8 (ablation) 54±8 (AAD)	Mainly paroxysmal	No	PVI	1 year	49%*	87%	37%
Stabile et al, 2005 (CACAF)	137	62±9 (ablation) 62±10 (AAD)	Paroxysmal or persistent	Yes, ≥2 AAD failure	LACA	1 year	57%	56%	9%
Pappone et al, 2006 (APAF)	198	55±10 (ablation) 57±10 (AAD)	Paroxysmal	Yes, ≥2 AAD failure (mean 2±1)	CPVA	1 year	42%	86%	22%
Jaïs et al, 2006 (A4 study)	112	51±11	Paroxysmal	Yes, ≥1 AAD failure	PVI±LACA/CTI	1 year	63%	89%	23%
Forleo et al, 2008	70†	63±9 (ablation) 65±6 (AAD)	Paroxysmal or persistent	Yes, ≥1 AAD failure	PVI	1 year	Not stated	80%	43%

*After 1 year; †with diabetes mellitus type 2.

AAD, antiarrhythmic drugs; AF, atrial fibrillation; APAF, Ablation for Paroxysmal Atrial Fibrillation study; A4, Atrial fibrillation Ablation versus AntiArrhythmic drugs; CACAF, Catheter Ablation for the Cure of Atrial Fibrillation study; CPVA, circumferential pulmonary vein ablation; CTI, cavotricuspid isthmus; LACA, left atrial catheter ablation; PVI, pulmonary vein isolation; RAAFT, Radiofrequency Ablation Atrial Fibrillation Trial.

such recurrences are not randomly distributed, however, it has been proposed that the time to the first, second, and subsequent recurrences should be evaluated in order to provide a more comprehensive assessment of antiarrhythmic efficacy. This assessment approach has proved to be much more difficult to accomplish because patients often are not willing to remain on the same, possibly placebo treatment, and to suffer multiple symptomatic recurrences.

Antiarrhythmic drugs (or other strategies such as pulmonary vein ablation) may slow and regularize the ventricular response rate, thereby rendering the arrhythmia asymptomatic rather than suppressing the atrial fibrillation itself. To ensure that the agent under testing is "antiarrhythmic" rather than merely "rate-slowing," it has become necessary to capture asymptomatic episodes. This is impossible without long-term continuous monitoring, but investigators have been satisfied with several weeks of continuous monitoring or with random sampling over longer periods using intermittent event monitoring.

When an implanted device (pacemaker, ICD, or implantable loop recorder) has been fitted, it is possible to detect and to store records of events (derived measures, such as the duration of fast and irregular rhythms [atrial fibrillation equivalent], or atrial, ventricular, or subcutaneous electrograms themselves) that are time- and date-stamped. The sensitivity and specificity of the identification of such events are not yet perfect and for trial purposes usually will require adjudication by a core laboratory or event committee.

The consequences of arrhythmia recurrence on functional outcomes such as exercise tolerance (e.g., a 6-minute walk test), cognitive function, symptomatic status (e.g., specific activity scale, European Heart Rhythm Association [EHRA] classification), and quality of life (general instruments, e.g., SF-36 and Euro-Qol, or specific atrial fibrillation questionnaires) must be assessed. Although it has been possible to show that patients in fibrillation at the time have degraded scores, it has proved difficult to show that a reduction in the likelihood of recurrence improves functional capacity of any sort, including "quality of life."

The treatment of atrial fibrillation recurrences may require hospitalization for cardioversion or rate control. Possible complications of atrial fibrillation include thromboembolic events (cerebrovascular accidents, transient ischemic attacks, formation of systemic or pulmonary emboli), congestive heart failure (tachycardiomyopathy or aggravation of other forms of heart failure), and ventricular arrhythmias, all of which may lead to either death or requirement for hospitalization. It is therefore suggested that ablation and antiarrhythmic drug trials for atrial fibrillation (such as trials of antithrombotic drugs in patients with atrial fibrillation) should use these as their primary outcome events.[15]

Trials of this nature have now been conducted to inform the rate-versus-rhythm debate (the Atrial Fibrillation Follow-up Investigation of Rhythm Management [AFFIRM][16] and the Atrial Fibrillation and Congestive Heart Failure [AF-CHF] trial). Of surprise to many, rate control proved not to be inferior to rhythm control, at least in the population of relatively elderly patients enrolled in these trials. Recently, results from the first antiarrhythmic drug trial to use these hard endpoints were reported. When tested against placebo control in the ATHENA (A placebo-controlled, double-blind, parallel arm

Trial to assess the efficacy of dronedarone 400 mg bid for the prevention of cardiovascular Hospitalization or death from any cause in patiENts with Atrial fibrillation/atrial flutter) trial, dronedarone proved to be remarkably effective in reducing the composite endpoint of cardiovascular-related hospitalization and all-cause mortality.[17] Adequate trials of atrial fibrillation ablation, controlled against either antiarrhythmic drug therapy or rate control therapy, are awaited. Such trials are in the design or pilot phase, but for the time being, the clinician must rely on data from essentially inadequate trials that use subjective or surrogate endpoints, short follow-up periods, and small numbers of subjects.

Ventricular Tachyarrhythmias

Originally, antiarrhythmic drug trials were conducted in small cohorts of cardiac arrest survivors or patients with life-threatening ventricular tachycardias. Typically, two antiarrhythmic drugs were pitched against each other, because it was unethical to leave patients wholly unprotected against their arrhythmia. The endpoint in these trials was a recurrence of the arrhythmia or sudden cardiac death. In general, amiodarone proved to be the most effective therapeutic agent in this setting.

Many other large trials with mortality endpoints and placebo controls were conducted in populations at risk of ventricular arrhythmia (primary prevention trials). These populations were usually defined as being at high risk because they consisted of post–myocardial infarction patients with depressed left ventricular function or high ambient ventricular ectopy. In this setting, only sotalol[18] proved to be effective, whereas others such as azimilide,[19] dofetilide,[20] and probably amiodarone[21] proved to be ineffective, although amiodarone did seem to reduce sudden cardiac death, especially when combined with a beta-blocker. Of importance, flecainide, encainide,[22] and *d*-sotalol[23] were associated with adverse outcomes, probably because of proarrhythmic effects.

Dofetilide[24] and dronedarone were evaluated in high-risk heart failure populations. The effect of dofetilide was neutral, but dronedarone seemed to be associated with excess mortality in this setting, subsequently explained by inappropriate termination of angiotensin-converting enzyme (ACE) inhibitor or adrenergic receptor blocker (ARB) therapy in response to a small increase in serum creatinine levels, which should have been anticipated. When amiodarone therapy was systematically evaluated in a placebo- and ICD-controlled secondary prevention trial in patients with heart failure, amiodarone proved to be no more effective than placebo and considerably less effective than ICD treatment.[6]

The ICD seemed to be self-evidently effective to many physicians, who were therefore reluctant to subject their patients to a trial of the ICD against the prevailing antiarrhythmic drug therapy. On the other hand, some physicians and scientists successfully argued that such trials were essential to proper validation of treatment efficacy of the device. Three secondary prevention trials of the ICD versus therapy with antiarrhythmic drugs, predominantly amiodarone and sotalol, were conducted. The AVID (Antiarrhythmics Versus Implantable Defibrillators) trial was demonstrated unequivocal mortality reduction associated with ICD therapy and was supported in meta-analysis by the other two trials, which had similar efficacy point estimates.[2-5]

Three major primary prevention trials and a number of smaller trials[6,25-32] were undertaken against the background of optimal medical therapy, and in one case (see earlier) with randomized amiodarone or placebo controls (Fig. I-3). Two of the trials, the Multicenter Automatic Defibrillator Implantation Trial (MADIT II) and the Sudden Cardiac Death in Heart Failure Trial (SCD-HeFT), were positive, and the third trial,

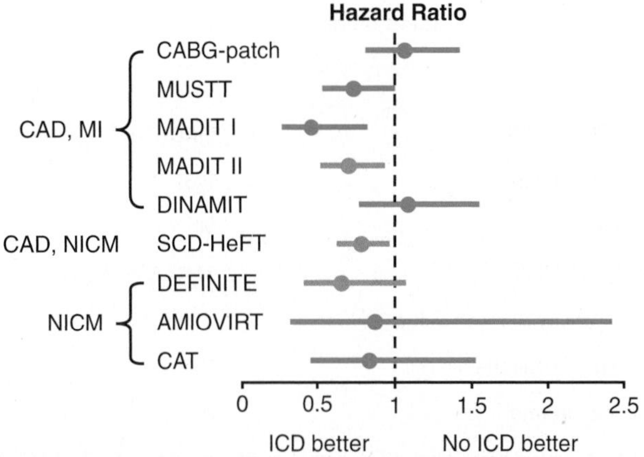

Figure I-3 Hazard ratios and confidence intervals for primary prevention implantable cardioverter-defibrillator (ICD) trials. The CABG-Patch trial and DINAMIT were conducted in very specific populations (post–coronary artery bypass grafting, for coronary artery disease [CAD], and immediately post–myocardial infarction [MI], respectively), and the MUSTT design did not incorporate true randomization between ICD and an alternative treatment. AMIOVIRT, CAT, and MADIT I were small trials. MADIT II, SCD-HeFT, and DEFINITE were large trials in important clinical populations (remote post–myocardial infarction and/or heart failure). AMIOVIRT, Amiodarone versus Implantable Cardioverter-Defibrillator: Randomized Trial; CABG Patch, Coronary Artery Bypass Graft Patch trial; CAT, CArdiomyopathy Trial; DEFINITE, DEFibrillators In Non-Ischemic cardiomyopathy Treatment Evaluation; DINAMIT, Defibrillator IN Acute Myocardial Infarction Trial; MADIT, Multicenter Automatic Defibrillator Implantation Trial; MUSTT, Multicenter Unsustained Tachycardia Trial; NICM, nonischemic cardiomyopathy; SCD-HeFT, Sudden Cardiac Death in Heart Failure Trial.

the DEFibrillators In Non-Ischemic cardiomyopathy Treatment Evaluation (DEFINITE), showed a positive trend in favor of device therapy, thereby establishing the effectiveness of the ICD. A surprising finding was that only a relatively small number of patients were required for investigators and clinicians to reach a high level of confidence in this form of therapy (Table I-2).

It is now established that trials of antiarrhythmic drug therapy for patients with life-threatening ventricular arrhythmias should be undertaken in patients who are protected by previous ICD implantation. Sotalol, amiodarone, and azimilide have been tried against placebo in ICD recipients.[33-35] All three drugs, as well as amiodarone plus a beta-blocker, in particular, have proved to be effective in reducing the number of device interventions, implying some antiarrhythmic activity. Such trials, however, cannot provide sufficient evidence of antiarrhythmic efficacy outside the setting of ICD treatment. If an antiarrhythmic agent virtually eliminated ICD interventions, a trial of ICD versus such therapy would then be justified. Unfortunately, no candidate therapy is available at present, and it is such a demanding level of expectation that development of such a drug may not be achieved for many years.

Implementing Successful Therapy

The usual sequence of medical student education, postgraduate specialist training, and additional continuing medical education must be supplemented by careful analysis of the evidence base for medical diagnosis and therapeutic management. The synthesis of tools designed to simplify and improve education is necessary. The development of management guidelines is a critical step in this process. Professional societies, health care providers, and health care payers all are legitimate stakeholders in guideline production and their utilization. Other stakeholders include patients, who may be able to contribute important insight into

Table I-2 Baseline Features of Major Primary Prevention ICD Trials: MADIT II, DEFINITE, and SCD-HeFT

	Study		
Study Feature	**MADIT II**	**DEFINITE**	**SCD-HeFT**
No. of patients	1232	458	2521
Disease	MI	DCM	CHF
NYHA I/II/III/IV	37/34.5/24/4.5	21.6/57.4/21.0/...	.../70/30/...
LVEF (%), with mean value	≤30 (23)	≤35 (21)	≤35 (25)
Ischemic/nonischemic (%)	100/...	.../100	52/48
Follow-up (mo)	20	29	45.5

CHF, congestive heart failure; DCM, dilated cardiomyopathy; DEFINITE; DEFibrillators In Non-Ischemic cardiomyopathy Treatment Evaluation; ICD, implantable cardioverter-defibrillator; LVEF, left ventricular ejection fraction; MADIT, Multicenter Automatic Defibrillator Implantation Trial; MI, myocardial infarction; NYHA, New York Heart Association (class); SCD-HeFT, Sudden Cardiac Death in Heart Failure Trial.

the recommendations considered by guideline writers, and the medical industry, which may be able to provide further information and evidence on which to base recommendations. All stakeholders should be provided with an opportunity to contribute. Most international guidelines written by professional societies on matters related to arrhythmias have been heavily dominated by medical input; it is not surprising, therefore, that acceptance of the guidelines by other stakeholders often has been little more than notional.

Guideline writers generally base their recommendations on evidence relating to the efficacy and safety of diagnostic or therapeutic procedures.[36-39] Issues such as cost and ease of implementation of guideline recommendations are not considered when the guidelines are written but are left to others to consider at a later stage. Occasionally the entire process is combined, but this inevitably gives rise to awkward compromise. The alternative, however, is a multiplicity of divergent guidelines dealing with the same issues. Such has often been the case with guidelines relating to the expensive management of cardiac arrhythmias when governments and health care payers have produced their own more affordable guidelines, which usually require that therapies cost less than $50,000 per quality-adjusted life-year saved. Unfortunately many otherwise highly effective antiarrhythmic strategies are more expensive, especially over the short term.

In most parts of the world, little infrastructure is in place to introduce and implement guidelines. Educators may expose and popularize the guidelines, but care pathways, funding issues, and other resources needed for guidelines implementation may not be available. These limitations have certainly been evident in efforts at widespread introduction of ICD therapy, cardiac resynchronization therapy with defibrillation (CRT-D), and atrial fibrillation–ventricular tachycardia ablation in many parts of the world.

Guideline implementation should stimulate active audit against guideline recommendations. Physicians are strongly recommended to participate in this process in order to reveal inadequacies of education, referrals, funding, equipment, follow-up, databases, and so on. Provided with such information, physicians and their professional society representatives are better armed to argue for improved resources. Those providing care for patients with cardiac arrhythmias must be actively involved in this process to improve the outlook for their patients.

Conclusions

Although major advances in clinical arrhythmology have been achieved, available therapies have remained or have become empirical, blunderbuss, and nonspecific. Such therapies may harm as well as help. Only when the mechanism of the arrhythmia is directly addressed will therapy cure patients without the risk of killing them.

Clinical trials in the arena of arrhythmology have too often used surrogate endpoints, often of a subjective nature. Trials generally have been too small and poorly controlled. Regulators and clinical scientists are now agreed that large, well-controlled trials with objective and clinically relevant endpoints are needed to validate therapeutic mandates.

The management of arrhythmias often has relied on clinical experience, and only recently have guidelines been drawn up to assist the physician to provide optimal care for patients with cardiac arrhythmias. The value of accurate data-based information on the clinical practice of arrhythmology is now well recognized, and such information is beginning to accrue. Nevertheless, systematic and widespread audit of these achievements remains to be conducted.

The increasing quality of the evidence base, derived from well-designed clinical trials and directed toward specific correction of electrophysiologic abnormalities that are responsible for arrhythmias, will inevitably lead to much-improved therapies that can be expected to achieve a reduction in mortality and morbidity rates and in the monetary investment necessary to maintain arrhythmia-free survival.

References

1. Plotnikov AN, Sosunov EA, Qu J, et al: Biological pacemaker implanted in canine left bundle branch provides ventricular escape rhythms that have physiologically acceptable rates. Circulation 109:506-512, 2004.
2. A comparison of antiarrhythmic-drug therapy with implantable defibrillators in patients resuscitated from near-fatal ventricular arrhythmias. The Antiarrhythmics Versus Implantable Defibrillators (AVID) Investigators. N Engl J Med 337: 1576-1583, 1997.
3. Connolly SJ, Gent M, Roberts RS, et al: Canadian Implantable Defibrillator Study (CIDS): A randomized trial of the

implantable cardioverter defibrillator against amiodarone. Circulation 101:1297-1302, 2000.

4. Kuck KH, Cappato R, Siebels J, Rüppel R: Randomized comparison of antiarrhythmic drug therapy with implantable defibrillators in patients resuscitated from cardiac arrest: The Cardiac Arrest Study Hamburg (CASH). Circulation 102:748-754, 2000.
5. Connolly SJ, Hallstrom AP, Cappato R, et al: Meta-analysis of the implantable cardioverter defibrillator secondary prevention trials. AVID, CASH and CIDS studies. Antiarrhythmics vs Implantable Defibrillator study. Cardiac Arrest Study Hamburg. Canadian Implantable Defibrillator Study. Eur Heart J 21:2071-2078, 2000.
6. Bardy GH, Lee KL, Mark DB, et al, Sudden Cardiac Death in Heart Failure Trial (SCD-HeFT) Investigators: Amiodarone or an implantable cardioverter-defibrillator for congestive heart failure. N Engl J Med 352:225-237, 2005.
7. Vaughan Williams EM: Classifying antiarrhythmic actions: By facts or speculation. J Clin Pharmacol 32:964-977, 1992.
8. Etheridge SP, Compton SJ, Tristani-Firouzi M, Mason JW: A new oral therapy for long QT syndrome: Long-term oral potassium improves repolarization in patients with *HERG* mutations. J Am Coll Cardiol 42:1777-1782, 2003.
9. Shimizu W, Aiba T, Antzelevitch C: Specific therapy based on the genotype and cellular mechanism in inherited cardiac arrhythmias. Long QT syndrome and Brugada syndrome. Curr Pharm Des 11:1561-1572, 2005.
10. Moss AJ, Windle JR, Hall WJ, et al: Safety and efficacy of flecainide in subjects with long QT-3 syndrome (deltaKPQ mutation): A randomized, double-blind, placebo-controlled clinical trial. Ann Noninvasive Electrocardiol 10(4 Suppl): 59-66, 2005.
11. Schwartz PJ, Priori SG, Locati EH, et al: Long QT syndrome patients with mutations of the *SCN5A* and *HERG* genes have differential responses to Na+ channel blockade and to increases in heart rate. Implications for gene-specific therapy. Circulation 92:3381-3386, 1995.
12. Wazni OM, Marrouche NF, Martin DO, et al: Radiofrequency ablation vs antiarrhythmic drugs as first-line treatment of symptomatic atrial fibrillation: A randomized trial. JAMA 293:2634-2640, 2005.
13. Pappone C, Augello G, Sala S, et al: A randomized trial of circumferential pulmonary vein ablation versus antiarrhythmic drug therapy in paroxysmal atrial fibrillation: The APAF Study. J Am Coll Cardiol 48:2340-2347, 2006.
14. Stabile G, Bertaglia E, Senatore G, et al: Catheter ablation treatment in patients with drug-refractory atrial fibrillation: A prospective, multi-centre, randomized, controlled study (Catheter Ablation for the Cure of Atrial Fibrillation Study). Eur Heart J 27:216-221, 2006.
15. Singh BN, Connolly SJ, Crijns HJ, et al, EURIDIS and ADONIS Investigators: Dronedarone for maintenance of sinus rhythm in atrial fibrillation or flutter. N Engl J Med 357:987-999, 2007.
16. Wyse DG, Waldo AL, DiMarco JP, et al, Atrial Fibrillation Follow-up Investigation of Rhythm Management (AFFIRM) Investigators: A comparison of rate control and rhythm control in patients with atrial fibrillation. N Engl J Med 347:1825-1833, 2002.
17. Honhnloser SH: Effects of dronedarone on cardiovascular outcomes in high-risk patients with atrial fibrillation or atrial flutter—results of the ATHENA trial. Session SP07. Presented at Heart Rhythm Society 29th Annual Scientific Sessions, San Francisco, May 14-17, 2008.
18. Julian DG, Jackson FS, Szekely P, Prescott RJ: A controlled trial of sotalol for 1 year after myocardial infarction. Circulation 67:I61-I62, 1983.
19. Camm AJ, Pratt CM, Schwartz PJ, et al, AzimiLide post Infarct surVival Evaluation (ALIVE) Investigators: Mortality in patients after a recent myocardial infarction: A randomized, placebo-controlled trial of azimilide using heart rate variability for risk stratification. Circulation 109:990-996, 2004.
20. Køber L, Bloch Thomsen PE, Møller M, et al, Danish Investigations of Arrhythmia and Mortality on Dofetilide (DIAMOND) Study Group: Effect of dofetilide in patients with recent myocardial infarction and left-ventricular dysfunction: A randomised trial. Lancet 356:2052-2058, 2000.
21. Julian DG, Camm AJ, Frangin G, et al: Randomised trial of effect of amiodarone on mortality in patients with left-ventricular dysfunction after recent myocardial infarction: EMIAT. European Myocardial Infarct Amiodarone Trial Investigators. Lancet 349:667-674, 1997. Erratum in Lancet 349:1180, 1997.
22. Echt DS, Liebson PR, Mitchell LB, et al: Mortality and morbidity in patients receiving encainide, flecainide, or placebo. The Cardiac Arrhythmia Suppression Trial. N Engl J Med 324:781-788, 1991.
23. Waldo AL, Camm AJ, deRuyter H, et al: Effect of *d*-sotalol on mortality in patients with left ventricular dysfunction after recent and remote myocardial infarction. The SWORD Investigators. Survival with Oral *d*-Sotalol Lancet 348:7-12, 1996. Erratum in Lancet 348:416, 1996.
24. Møller M, Torp-Pedersen CT, Køber L: Dofetilide in patients with congestive heart failure and left ventricular dysfunction: Safety aspects and effect on atrial fibrillation. The Danish Investigators of Arrhythmia and Mortality on Dofetilide (DIAMOND) Study Group. Congest Heart Fail 7:146-150, 2001.
25. Kadish A, Dyer A, Daubert JP, et al, Defibrillators in Non-Ischemic Cardiomyopathy Treatment Evaluation (DEFINITE) Investigators: Prophylactic defibrillator implantation in patients with nonischemic dilated cardiomyopathy. N Engl J Med 350:2151-2158, 2004.
26. Moss AJ, Zareba W, Hall WJ, et al, Multicenter Automatic Defibrillator Implantation Trial II Investigators: Prophylactic implantation of a defibrillator in patients with myocardial infarction and reduced ejection fraction. N Engl J Med 346:877-883, 2002.
27. Buxton AE, Lee KL, Fisher JD, et al: A randomized study of the prevention of sudden death in patients with coronary artery disease. Multicenter Unsustained Tachycardia Trial Investigators. N Engl J Med 341:1882-1890, 1999. Erratum in N Engl J Med 342:1300, 2000.
28. Moss AJ, Hall WJ, Cannom DS, et al: Improved survival with an implanted defibrillator in patients with coronary disease at high risk for ventricular arrhythmia. Multicenter Automatic Defibrillator Implantation Trial Investigators. N Engl J Med 335:1933-1940, 1996.
29. Hohnloser SH, Kuck KH, Dorian P, et al, DINAMIT Investigators: Prophylactic use of an implantable cardioverter-defibrillator after acute myocardial infarction. N Engl J Med 351:2481-2488, 2004.
30. Bigger JT Jr: Prophylactic use of implanted cardiac defibrillators in patients at high risk for ventricular arrhythmias after coronary-artery bypass graft surgery. Coronary Artery Bypass Graft (CABG) Patch Trial Investigators. N Engl J Med 337:1569-1575, 1997. PMID: 9371853.
31. Strickberger SA, Hummel JD, Bartlett TG, et al, AMIOVIRT Investigators: Amiodarone versus implantable cardioverter-defibrillator: Randomized trial in patients with nonischemic dilated cardiomyopathy and asymptomatic nonsustained ventricular tachycardia—AMIOVIRT. J Am Coll Cardiol 41:1707-1712, 2003.
32. Bänsch D, Antz M, Boczor S, et al: Primary prevention of sudden cardiac death in idiopathic dilated cardiomyopathy: The Cardiomyopathy Trial (CAT). Circulation 105:1453-1458, 2002.
33. Pacifico A, Hohnloser SH, Williams JH, et al: Prevention of implantable-defibrillator shocks by treatment with sotalol. d,l-Sotalol Implantable Cardioverter-Defibrillator Study Group. N Engl J Med 340:1855-1862, 1999.
34. Dorian P, Borggrefe M, Al-Khalidi HR, et al, SHock Inhibition Evaluation with AzimiLiDe (SHIELD) Investigators: Placebo-controlled, randomized clinical trial of azimilide for prevention of ventricular tachyarrhythmias in patients with an implantable cardioverter defibrillator. Circulation 110:3646-3654, 2004.
35. Connolly SJ, Dorian P, Roberts RS, et al, Optimal Pharmacological Therapy in Cardioverter Defibrillator Patients (OPTIC) Investigators: Comparison of beta-blockers, amiodarone plus beta-blockers, or sotalol for prevention of shocks from implantable cardioverter defibrillators: The OPTIC Study: A randomized trial. JAMA 295:165-171, 2006.
36. Fuster V, Rydén LE, Cannom DS, et alfor the American College of Cardiology, American Heart Association Task Force, European Society of Cardiology Committee for Practice Guidelines, European Heart Rhythm Association, Heart Rhythm Society: ACC/AHA/ESC 2006 guidelines for the management of patients with atrial

fibrillation: Full text: A report of the American College of Cardiology/American Heart Association Task Force on Practice Guidelines and the European Society of Cardiology Committee for Practice Guidelines (Writing Committee to Revise the 2001 Guidelines for the Management of Patients with Atrial Fibrillation) developed in collaboration with the European Heart Rhythm Association and the Heart Rhythm Society. Europace 8:651-745, 2006.

37. Blomström-Lundqvist C, Scheinman MM, Aliot EM, et al, for the American College of Cardiology, American Heart Association Task Force on Practice Guidelines, European Society of Cardiology Committee for Practice Guidelines, Writing Committee to Develop Guidelines for the Management of Patients With Supraventricular Arrhythmias: ACC/AHA/ESC guidelines for the management of patients with supraventricular arrhythmias—executive summary: A report of the American College of Cardiology/American Heart Association Task Force on Practice Guidelines and the European Society of Cardiology Committee for Practice Guidelines (Writing Committee to Develop Guidelines for the Management of Patients with Supraventricular Arrhythmias). Circulation 108:1871-1909, 2003.

38. Brignole M, Alboni P, Benditt DG, et al, for the Task Force on Syncope, European Society of Cardiology: Guidelines on management (diagnosis and treatment) of syncope—update 2004. Europace 6:467-537, 2004.

39. Zipes DP, Camm AJ, Borggrefe M, et al, for the American College of Cardiology, American Heart Association Task Force, European Society of Cardiology Committee for Practice Guidelines, European Heart Rhythm Association, Heart Rhythm Society: ACC/AHA/ESC 2006 guidelines for management of patients with ventricular arrhythmias and the prevention of sudden cardiac death: A report of the American College of Cardiology/American Heart Association Task Force and the European Society of Cardiology Committee for Practice Guidelines (Writing Committee to Develop Guidelines for Management of Patients with Ventricular Arrhythmias and the Prevention of Sudden Cardiac Death) developed in collaboration with the European Heart Rhythm Association and the Heart Rhythm Society. Europace 8: 746-837, 2006.

40. Krittayaphong R, Raungrattanaamporn O, Bhuripanyo K, et al: A randomized clinical trial of the efficacy of radiofrequency catheter ablation and amiodarone in the treatment of symptomatic atrial fibrillation. J Med Assoc Thai 86 Suppl 1:S8-S16, 2003.

41. Jaïs P, Cauchemez B, Macle L, et al: Catheter ablation versus antiarrhythmic drugs for atrial fibrillation: the A4 study. Circulation 118:2498-2505, 2008.

42. Forleo GB, Mantica M, De Luca L, et al: Catheter ablation of atrial fibrillation in patients with diabetes mellitus type 2: results from a randomized study comparing pulmonary vein isolation versus antiarrhythmic drug therapy. J Cardiovasc Electrophysiol 20:22-28, 2009.

Structural and Molecular Bases of Ion Channel Function

PART I

Voltage-Gated Sodium Channels and Electrical Excitability of the Heart

1

William A. Catterall and Sebastian K. G. Maier

CHAPTER OUTLINE

Voltage-gated sodium channels initiate action potentials in cardiac myocytes and other excitable cells, and they are responsible for propagation of action potentials through the atria, conduction system, and ventricles of the heart. They are complexes of a large pore-forming α subunit and smaller β subunits. The importance of their functional role is illustrated by mutations in them that cause long QT syndrome type 3 and Brugada syndrome.

Much is now known about the mechanisms of activation, inactivation, and ion conduction by the sodium channel protein, as summarized in this chapter. Multiple genes, several of which are expressed in the mammalian heart, encode sodium channel subunits, and the distinct sodium channel subtypes have subtle differences in functional properties and differential distribution in subcellular compartments of cardiac myocytes. These differences in function and localization may contribute to specialized functional roles of sodium channels in cardiac physiology and pharmacology.

Subunit Structure of Sodium Channels

Sodium channel proteins purified from excitable cells are complexes composed of an approximately 260-kD α subunit in association with one or two auxiliary β subunits approximately 33 to 39 kD in size.[1] Purified sodium channel complexes of α and β subunits are sufficient for voltage-dependent gating and ion conduction in artificial lipid membranes,[1,2] and expression of the α subunit alone is sufficient for physiologic function in recipient nonexcitable cells,[3] indicating that this subunit has all of the necessary structural elements for voltage-dependent gating and ion conduction. The primary sequence predicts that the sodium channel α subunit folds into four internally repeated domains (I to IV), each of which contains six α-helical transmembrane segments, S1 to S6[3-6] (Fig. 1-1). In each domain, segments S1 through S4 serve as the voltage-sensing module, and the S5 and S6 segments and the reentrant P loop between them serve as the pore-forming module. One large extracellular loop connects either the S5 or S6 transmembrane segment to the P loop in each domain; the other extracellular loops are small. Large intracellular loops link the four homologous domains, and the large amino-terminal (N-terminal) and carboxyl-terminal (C-terminal) domains also contribute substantially to the mass of the internal face of sodium channels. This view of sodium channel architecture, originally derived from hydrophobicity analysis of the amino acid sequence,[4] has been largely confirmed by biochemical, electrophysiologic, and structural experiments.[6]

The auxiliary β subunits were identified in the initial purification studies of sodium channels.[1] These subunits have a single transmembrane segment, a large N-terminal extracellular domain that is homologous in structure to a variable chain (V-type) immunoglobulin-like fold, and a short C-terminal intracellular segment (see Fig. 1-1).[7-10] The β subunits interact with α subunits through their extracellular immunoglobulin-like domains, modulate α subunit function, and enhance their cell surface expression.[11] Like other proteins with an extracellular immunoglobulin-like fold, they also serve as cell adhesion molecules by interacting with extracellular matrix proteins, cell adhesion molecules, and cytoskeletal linker proteins.[12-17] These interactions are thought to localize and stabilize sodium channels in specific subcellular compartments and to bring crucial signaling molecules to the sodium channel to regulate it. Deletion of the genes encoding β subunits causes alterations in sodium channel function; reduced action potential conduction and abnormal development of myelin folds in axons; hyperexcitability and epilepsy in the brain; and arrhythmias in the heart.[18-20]

Three-Dimensional Structure of Sodium Channels

The three-dimensional structure of the sodium channel is not yet completely known, but some limited structural information has emerged. Structural determination at 1.9-nm resolution by cryoelectron microscopy and image reconstruction techniques shows sodium channels as having a bell shape from a side

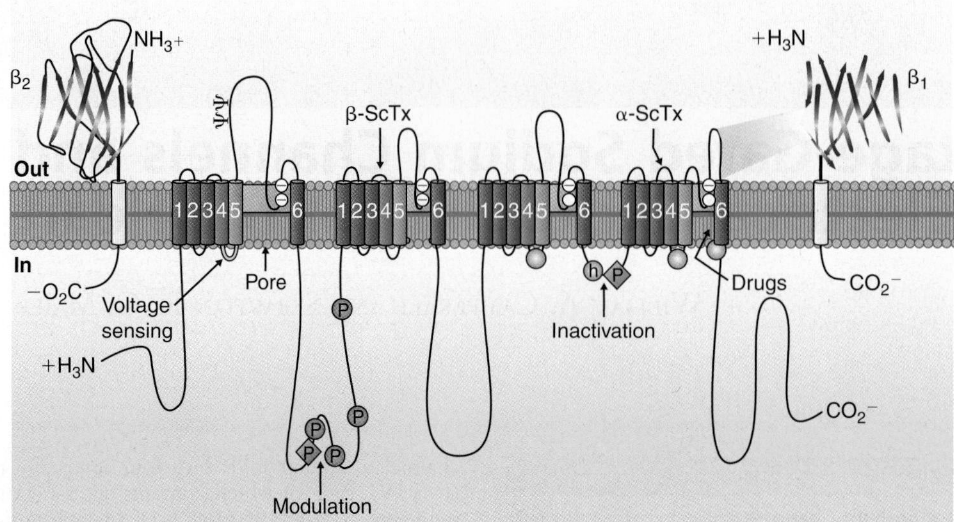

Figure 1-1 Transmembrane organization of sodium channel subunits. The primary structures of the subunits of the voltage-gated ion channels are illustrated as transmembrane folding diagrams. *Cylinders* represent probable α-helical segments: S1-S3, *blue*; S4, *green*; S5, *orange*; S6, *purple*; outer pore loop, *shaded orange area.* **Bold** lines represent the polypeptide chains of each subunit, with length approximately proportional to the number of amino acid residues in the brain sodium channel subtypes. The extracellular domains of the β_1 and β_2 subunits are shown as immunoglobulin-like folds; Ψ, sites of probable *N*-linked glycosylation; P, sites of demonstrated protein phosphorylation by protein kinase A *(red circles)* and protein kinase C *(red diamonds)*; *white circles*, the outer (EEDD) and inner (DEKA) rings of amino residues that form the ion selectivity filter and the tetrodotoxin binding site; ++, S4 voltage sensors; "h" in *blue circle*, inactivation particle in the inactivation gate loop; *empty blue circles*, sites implicated in forming the inactivation gate receptor. The structure of the extracellular domain of the β subunits is illustrated as an immunoglobulin-like fold based on amino acid sequence homology to the myelin P0 protein.[8,24] Sites of binding of α and β scorpion toxins (α-ScTx, β-ScTx) and a site of interaction between α and β_1 subunits also are shown.

view, a four-fold symmetry of transmembrane masses as viewed from above the membrane, and large intracellular and extracellular masses through which several inlets and outlets allow aqueous access[21] (Fig. 1-2A). Unexpectedly, this image of sodium channels reveals a central pore that does not directly connect the intracellular and extracellular spaces, instead splitting into four branches near the membrane surface. Moreover, it suggests the presence of four peripherally located narrow transmembrane pores, which may function as gating pores for voltage-sensor movement as described below.

The global fold of the sodium channel is predicted to be similar to that of voltage-gated potassium channels (see Fig. 1-2B). The structure of the open state of this channel has been determined by x-ray crystallography,[22] and the structure of the closed state has been predicted using the Rosetta method of structural modeling.[23] This structural view shows the S5 and S6 region of channel arrayed in four-fold symmetry around the aqueous ion conduction pathway (red, orange, and yellow in Fig. 1-2B). The selectivity filter of the pore at its narrow extracellular end is formed by the P loops (tan), whereas the wider vestibule in the center of the pore is formed mostly by the S6 segments (red). A single voltage-sensor module is illustrated for simplicity (blue and green in Fig. 1-2B). In the resting (closed) state of the channel, the S4 segment is in an inward position. Activation of the voltage sensor by depolarization causes outward and rotational movement of the S4 segment and complementary movement of the S1, S2, and S3 segments around it (see movies 1 and 2 at www.pnas.org/cgi/content/full/0602350103/DC1). These coupled molecular movements translocate the gating charges in the S4 segment from exposure to the intracellular milieu to exposure to the extracellular milieu, as required for voltage-dependent gating.[23]

Comparison of the primary structures of the auxiliary β subunits with those of other proteins revealed a close structural relationship to the family of proteins that contain immunoglobulin-like folds.[8] The extracellular domains of these type I single-membrane-spanning proteins are predicted to fold in a manner similar to that for myelin protein P0, whose immunoglobin-like fold is known to be formed by a sandwich of two β sheets held together by hydrophobic interactions (see Fig. 1-1).[24] P0 is a cell adhesion molecule involved in tight wrapping of myelin sheets, and many related cell adhesion molecules with extracellular immunoglobulin-like folds and a single-membrane-spanning segment are involved in cell-cell interactions among neurons and glial cells.[24] As expected from their structure, $Na_V\beta$ subunits also interact with extracellular matrix molecules and other cell adhesion molecules.[12-16,25]

Sodium Channel Function

Classical work by Hodgkin and Huxley[26] defined the three key functions of sodium channels: (1) voltage-dependent activation, (2) fast inactivation, and (3) selective ion conductance. Building on this foundation, detailed biophysical studies revealed the ion selectivity of the channel pore, detected the movement of the voltage sensors as gating current, and developed mechanistic models for these essential channel functions.[27,28] As described next, more recent structure-function studies using molecular, biochemical, structural, and electrophysiologic techniques have

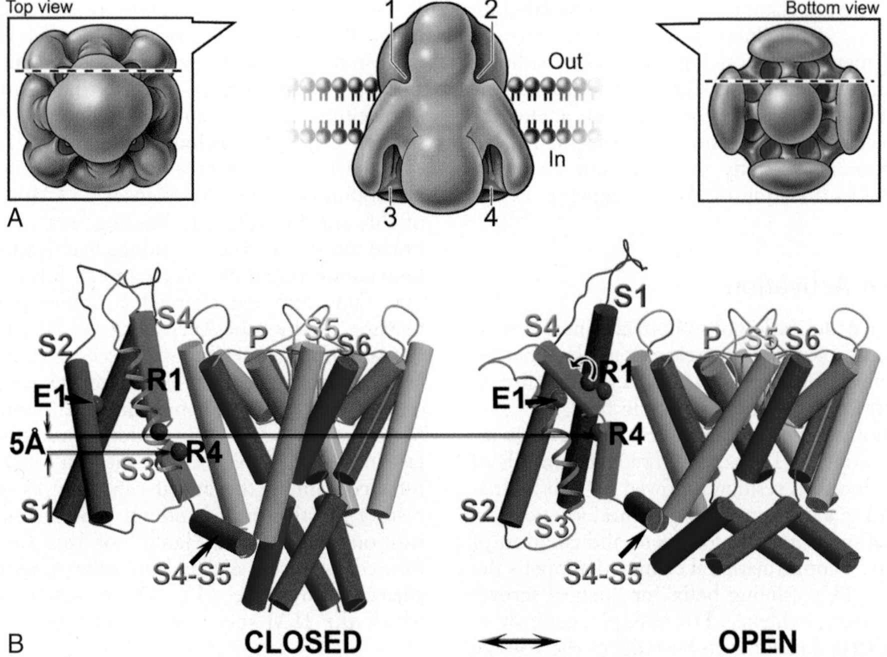

Figure 1-2 Three-dimensional structure of sodium channels. **A,** The three-dimensional structure of the Na_V channel α subunit at 200-nm resolution, drawn from electron micrograph reconstructions. **B,** Models of the closed and open states of voltage-gated potassium (K_V1 2) channels, depicted in cylinder representation. Only a single voltage-sensing module is shown attached to the tetramer of the pore-forming module for clarity. Transmembrane segments S1 through S6 and the P loop are colored by rainbow scheme from *blue* to *red*, as in Figure 1-1. The S4-S5 linker is *purple*. Approximate positions of the α carbon atoms of the first and fourth gating charge–carrying arginines in the S4 (labeled R1 and R4, in *blue*) and glutamate 226 in the S2 (labeled E1, in *red*) are depicted in sphere representation. All intracellular and extracellular loops, except for the S4-S5 linker, are represented by *curved lines* for simplicity. Vertical translation of the R4 between the closed and open states along the membrane normal vector and relative to the plane of the membrane is indicated by *arrows*. The S3 segment is represented by a *ribbon* pattern to show clearly the positions of the gating charge–carrying arginines in the adjacent S4 segment. (**A,** Adapted from Sato C, Ueno Y, Asai K, et al: The voltage-sensitive sodium channel is a bell-shaped molecule with several cavities. Nature 409:1047-1051, 2001.)

provided clear understanding of the molecular basis for these sodium channel functions.

Outer Pore and Selectivity Filter

Voltage clamp studies showed that sodium channels are highly selective for sodium versus potassium and other monovalent cations.[28,29] Analysis of ion selectivity and block by tetrodotoxin and saxitoxin led to development of a model of tetrodotoxin and saxitoxin as plugs of the selectivity filter in the outer pore of sodium channels.[28] Mutational analysis identified a key glutamate residue in the membrane-reentrant loop in domain I as a crucial residue for tetrodotoxin and saxitoxin binding.[30] Further studies revealed a pair of important amino acid residues, mostly negatively charged, in analogous positions in all four domains (small white circles in Fig. 1-1).[31] Mutation of a set of four residues in analogous positions in each domain—aspartate in domain I, glutamate in domain II, lysine in domain III, and alanine in domain IV (i.e., DEKA)—to glutamates confers calcium selectivity,[32] indicating that the side chains of these amino acid residues determine the specificity for sodium ions as they are conducted through the ion selectivity filter of the pore. These results showed that the narrow selectivity filter in the outer pore is formed by the reentrant P loops between transmembrane segments S5 and S6 of each domain (see Fig. 1-1). These amino acid residues form outer and inner rings that serve as the receptor site for tetrodotoxin and saxitoxin as well as the selectivity filter in the outer pore of sodium channels.[33,34] Mutations in this postulated ring of amino acid residues have strong effects on selectivity for organic and inorganic monovalent cations, in agreement with the idea that they form the selectivity filter, and structure-function studies suggest specific structural interactions and functional roles for the P loops from the four domains.[35-38]

These conclusions about the structure of the outer pore of sodium channels also derive strong support from work on potassium channels. A corresponding pore loop was identified in potassium channels and shown to control ion conductance and selectivity,[39] and the three-dimensional structure of a bacterial potassium channel reveals a narrow ion selectivity filter formed by the pore loop from its four identical subunits.[22,40] In the potassium channel, the backbone carbonyl groups of the peptide bonds of three consecutive amino acid residues form the narrow part of the selectivity filter. It will be of great interest to learn how the structure of the outer pore of potassium channels is modified to yield the different ion selectivity of sodium and calcium channels.

The Inner Pore and Local Anesthetic-Antiarrhythmic Drug Receptor Site

Voltage clamp studies led to the conclusion that local anesthetics enter from the intracellular side and bind in the inner pore of sodium channels,[28] and similar work revealed analogous intracellular block of calcium and potassium channels. As with the outer pore, the first indication that the S6 segments form the inner pore of the voltage-gated ion channels came from locating a pore blocker receptor site—in this case, the phenylalkylamine receptor site of L-type calcium channels.[42] Photoaffinity labeling with these high-affinity, intracellular pore blockers showed that only the IVS6 segment of the calcium channel α_1 subunit was labeled. Subsequently, mutagenesis studies of sodium channels revealed the local anesthetic receptor site in an analogous position in the sodium channel.[43] Mutations in S6 segments also affect ion permeation and selectivity of potassium channels, further supporting the identification of the S6 segments as the inner pore lining.[44]

Voltage-Dependent Activation

The voltage dependence of activation of sodium channels derives from outward movement of approximately 12 gating charges occurring as a consequence of depolarization of the membrane and consequent reduction of membrane electric field.[27,45] The S4 segments of each homologous domain serve as the primary voltage sensors for activation.[4,5] They contain repeated motifs of a positively charged amino acid residue followed by two hydrophobic residues, creating a transmembrane spiral of positive charges. On depolarization, outward movement and rotation of S4 are thought to initiate a conformational change that opens the sodium channel pore.[4,5] This "sliding helix" or "helical screw" model is supported by strong evidence. For example, neutralization of the positively charged residues in S4 reduces the voltage dependence of gating.[46] The outward and rotational gating movement of S4 segment has been detected directly by reaction of substituted cysteine residues in S4 segments with extracellular sulfhydryl reagents after channel activation and by analysis of the movement of fluorescent probes incorporated into these substituted cysteine residues.[47,48] A structural model of the voltage-sensing and pore-forming modules of sodium channels in the resting and activated states is illustrated in Figure 1-2, and videos of the gating movements of the voltage sensor and pore modules during activation and opening of the sodium channel are available online[23] (see movies 1 and 2 at www.pnas.org/cgi/content/full/0602350103/DC1).[49] As in the sliding helix model, the S4 segment (green in Fig. 1-2B) moves outward and rotates as the channel moves from the closed to the open state. This movement translocates the S4 gating charges (blue circles in Fig. 1-2B) outward such that they move from exposure to the intracellular side of the membrane in the closed state to the extracellular side of the membrane in the open state. As the S4 segments move outward, the S1, S2, and S3 segments rotate in the converse direction to aid in changing the exposure of the gating charges from the intracellular to the extracellular side of the membrane.

Pore Opening

During activation of the voltage sensors of sodium channels, the S4 and S5 intracellular linkers in each domain (purple in Fig. 1-2B) exert a force on the adjacent S6 segments, and the pore opens by bending the S6 segment (red in Fig. 1-2B). In bacterial voltage-gated potassium channels and sodium channels, bending of the S6 segment occurs at a critical hinge glycine residue approximately one-third down the S6 segment[50-52]; this bending motion allows the opening of the inner mouth of the pore (see movies 1 and 2 at www.pnas.org/cgi/content/full/0602350103/DC1) and rapid ion movement across the membrane.

Fast Inactivation

Fast inactivation of the sodium channel is a critical process that occurs within milliseconds of channel opening. The generally accepted model of this process involves a conserved inactivation gate formed by the intracellular loop connecting domains III and IV (see Fig. 1-1), which serves as a hinged lid that binds to the intracellular end of the pore and blocks it (Fig. 1-3). Intracellular perfusion of proteases prevents fast inactivation.[27] Site-directed antipeptide antibodies against the short, highly conserved intracellular loop connecting domains III and IV of the sodium channel α subunit (see Fig. 1-1), but not antibodies directed to other intracellular domains, were found to prevent fast sodium channel inactivation.[53,54] Moreover, the accessibility of this site for antibody binding was reduced when the membrane was depolarized to induce inactivation, suggesting that the loop connecting domains III and IV forms an inactivation "gate" that folds into the channel structure during inactivation.[53,54] Cutting the loop between domains III and IV by expression of the sodium channel in two pieces greatly slows inactivation.[46] Mutagenesis studies of this region revealed a hydrophobic triad of isoleucine, phenylalanine, and methionine—denoted I, F, and M in Figure 1-3A in single-letter notation—that is critical for fast inactivation (blue circle with "h" in Fig. 1-1B),[55] and peptides containing this motif can serve as pore blockers and can restore inactivation to sodium channels having a mutated inactivation gate.[56] The "latch" of this fast inactivation gate is formed by three key hydrophobic residues (i.e., IFM) and an adjacent threonine (T). These results support a model in which the IFM motif serves as a tethered pore blocker that

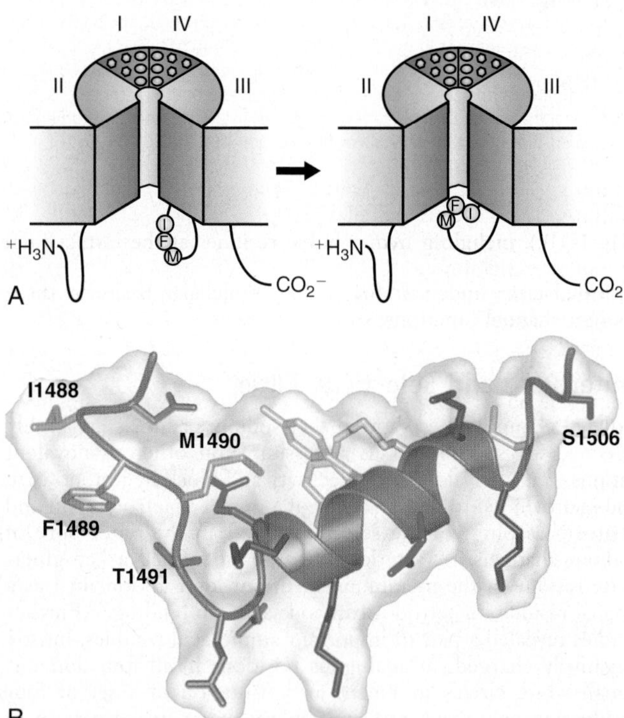

Figure 1-3 The molecular mechanism of fast sodium channel inactivation. **A,** The hinged-lid mechanism. The intracellular loop connecting domains III and IV of the sodium channel is depicted as forming a hinged lid with the critical phenylalanine (Phe1489, designated F1489 in the figure) within the IFM motif shown occluding the mouth of the pore during the inactivation process. The *circles* represent the transmembrane helices. **B,** Three-dimensional structure of the central segment of the inactivation gate as determined by multidimensional nuclear magnetic resonance (NMR) studies. Isoleucine (I1488), phenylalanine (F1489), and methionine (M1490) (i.e., IFM) are illustrated in *yellow*. Threonine (T1491), which is important for inactivation, and serine (S1506), which is a site of phosphorylation and modulation by protein kinase C, also are indicated. (**A** and **B,** Adapted from Catterall WA: From ionic currents to molecular mechanisms: The structure and function of voltage-gated sodium channels. Neuron 26:13-25, 2000.)

binds to a receptor in the intracellular mouth of the pore. Inactivation is impaired in proportion to the hydrophilicity of amino acid substitutions for the key phenylalanine residue (Phe1489) (denoted F1489 in Fig. 1-3B), suggesting that it forms a hydrophobic interaction with an inactivation gate receptor during inactivation.[57] Voltage-dependent movement of the inactivation gate has been detected by measuring the accessibility of a cysteine residue substituted for F1489.[58] This substituted cysteine residue becomes inaccessible to reaction with sulfhydryl reagents as the inactivation gate closes. Glycine and proline residues that flank the IFM motif may serve as molecular hinges to allow closure of the inactivation gate like a hinged lid (see Fig. 1-3A).[59]

The three-dimensional structure of the central portion of the inactivation gate has been determined by expression as a separate peptide and analysis by multidimensional nuclear magnetic resonance (NMR) methods.[60] These experiments reveal a rigid α helix flanked on its N-terminal side by two turns, the second of which contains the IFM motif (see Fig. 1-3B). The fold of the inactivation gate peptide projects F1489 into the solvent away from the core of the peptide, an unusual position for a hydrophobic residue in a short peptide. In this position, F1489 is poised to serve as a tethered ligand that occludes the pore. The nearby threonine (T1491), which is an important residue for inactivation,[57] also is in position to interact with the inactivation gate receptor in the pore. By contrast, the methionine of the IFM motif (M1490) is buried in the core of the peptide, interacting with two tyrosine residues in the α helix. This hydrophobic interaction stabilizes the fold of the peptide and forces F1489 into its exposed position. The structure of the inactivation gate peptide in solution suggests that the rigid α helix serves as a scaffold to present the IFM motif and T1491 to a receptor in the mouth of the pore as the gate closes.

Scanning mutagenesis experiments have revealed multiple amino acid residues that may form the inactivation gate receptor within and near the intracellular mouth of the pore (blue circles in Fig. 1-1B,), including hydrophobic residues at the intracellular end of transmembrane segment IVS6[61] and amino acid residues in intracellular loops IIIS4-S5[62] and IVS4-S5.[63-66] Mutations of residues in each of these positions impair inactivation by destabilizing the inactivated state, as expected for disruption of the inactivation gate receptor. In addition, mutations in intracellular loop IVS4-S5 impair closed channel blocking by IFM-containing peptides, consistent with function as the inactivation gate receptor,[64] and paired insertions of charged residues in the IIIS4-S5 loop and in the IFM motif indicate that these peptide segments interact during inactivation.[62] Evidently, multiple peptide segments form a complex inactivation gate receptor into which the inactivation gate closes to occlude the inner pore.

Coupling of Activation to Inactivation

Sodium channel inactivation derives most or all of its voltage dependence from coupling to the activation process driven by transmembrane movements of the S4 voltage sensors.[27] Increasingly strong evidence implicates the S4 segment in domain IV in this process. Mutations of charged amino acid residues at the extracellular end of the IVS4 segment have strong and selective effects on inactivation.[67] Both α-scorpion toxins and sea anemone toxins uncouple activation from inactivation by binding to a receptor site at the extracellular end of the IVS4 segment and preventing its normal gating movement,[68,69] evidently trapping it in a position that is permissive for activation but not for fast inactivation. The gating movements of the IIIS4 and IVS4 segments, detected by covalently incorporated fluorescent probes, are immobilized in the outward position by fast inactivation, arguing that their movement is coupled to the inactivation process.[70] Together, these results provide strong evidence that outward movement of the S4 segment in domain IV is the signal to initiate fast inactivation of the sodium channel by closure of the intracellular inactivation gate. The molecular mechanism for coupling of this movement of IVS4 to inactivation gate closure is an interesting subject for further investigation.

Sodium Channel Genes

Sodium channels are the founding members of an ion channel superfamily that includes voltage-gated calcium channels; TRP (transient receptor potential) channels; voltage-gated, inward rectifying, and two-pore-domain potassium channels; and cyclic nucleotide–regulated (CNG and HCN) channels.[71] In evolution, the four-domain sodium channel was last among the voltage-gated ion channels to appear, and it is found only in multicellular organisms. Sodium channels are thought to have evolved by two rounds of gene duplication from ancestral single-domain bacterial sodium channels. Voltage-gated sodium channel genes are present in a variety of metazoan species, including fly, leech, squid, and jellyfish. The biophysical properties, pharmacology, gene organization, and even intron splice sites of these invertebrate sodium channels are largely similar to those of the mammalian sodium channels.

Ten related sodium channel genes are found in vertebrates[71,72] (Fig. 1-4). More than 20 exons comprise each of the sodium channel α subunit genes in mammals. Genes encoding sodium channels $Na_V1.1$, $Na_V1.2$, $Na_V1.3$, and $Na_V1.7$ are located on chromosome 2 in humans, and these channels share similarities in sequence, biophysical characteristics, block by nanomolar concentrations of tetrodotoxin, and broad expression in neurons. A second cluster of genes encoding $Na_V1.5$, $Na_V1.8$, and $Na_V1.9$ channels is localized to 3p21-24. Although they are more than 75% identical in sequence to the group of channels encoded by genes residing on chromosome 2, these sodium channels all contain amino acid substitutions that confer varying degrees of resistance to the pore blocker tetrodotoxin. In $Na_V1.5$, the principal cardiac isoform,[73] a single-amino-acid change, from phenylalanine to cysteine, in the pore region of domain I is responsible for 200-fold reduction in tetrodotoxin sensitivity from that in channels encoded by genes on chromosome 2.[74] At the identical position in $Na_V1.8$ and $Na_V1.9$, the amino acid residue is serine, and this change results in even greater resistance to tetrodotoxin.[75] These two channels are expressed primarily in peripheral sensory neurons. In comparison with the sodium channels encoded by genes on chromosomes 2 and 3, $Na_V1.4$—which is expressed in skeletal muscle—and $Na_V1.6$—which is highly abundant in the central nervous system—have greater than 85% sequence identity and similar functional properties, including tetrodotoxin sensitivity in the nanomolar concentration range. A tenth sodium channel, Na_x, whose gene is located near those of the sodium channels of chromosome 2, is evolutionarily more distant.[72] Key differences in functionally important regions of voltage sensor and inactivation gate and lack of functional expression of voltage-gated sodium currents in heterologous cells suggest that Na_x may not function as a voltage-dependent sodium channel. Consistent with this conclusion, targeted deletion of the Na_x gene in mice causes functional deficits in regulation of plasma salt levels.[76]

The $Na_V\beta$ subunits are encoded by four distinct genes in mammals.[7-10] The gene encoding β_1 maps to chromosomal band 19q13; β_2 and β_4 genes are located on 11q22-23; and the β_3 gene is located nearby on 11q24. The β_1 and β_3 subunits associate noncovalently with the α subunits, whereas β_2 and β_4 are covalently linked by a disulfide bond These distinct modes of

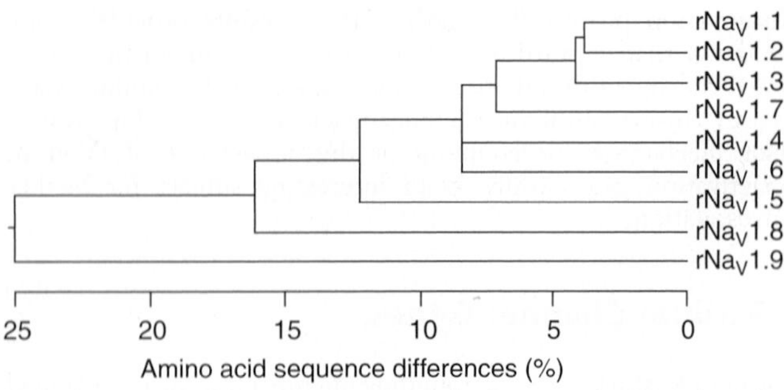

Figure 1-4 Amino acid sequence similarity of voltage-gated sodium channel α subunits. Comparison of amino acid identity for rat sodium channels $Na_V1.1$ to $Na_V1.9$ was performed with Megalign in the program DNAStar (using the Clustal method) for the four domains and the cytoplasmic linker connecting domains III and IV.

association and the corresponding similarities in amino acid sequence suggest that the similar pairs of β subunits (β_1 and β_3 versus β_2 and β_4) may be able to substitute for each other in interaction with sodium channel α subunits.

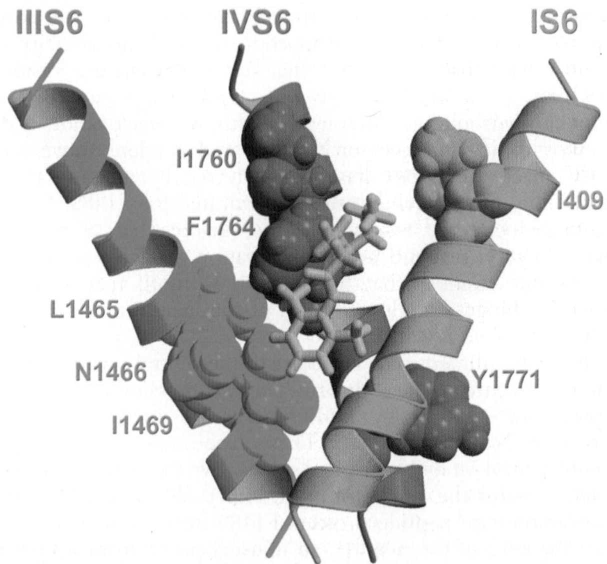

Figure 1-5 Model of etidocaine binding to the local anesthetic receptor site: Three-dimensional model of proposed orientation of amino acid residues within the sodium channel pore for etidocaine. Only transmembrane segments IS6 (*red*), IIIS6 (*green*), and IVS6 (*blue*) are shown. Residues important for etidocaine binding are shown in space-filling representation.

Molecular Pharmacology of Sodium Channels

Sodium channels are the molecular targets for drugs used in control of cardiac arrhythmias as well as in local anesthesia, prevention of acute pain, and treatment of epilepsy and bipolar disorder. Sodium channel-blocking drugs are also in development for treatment of chronic pain. Sodium channel-blocking drugs bind to a specific receptor within the pore of sodium channels, formed by the S6 segments in domains I, III, and IV[43,77-80] (Fig. 1-5). Their binding blocks ion movement through the pore and stabilizes the inactivated state of sodium channels. Antiarrhythmic drugs and antiepileptic drugs share similar, overlapping receptor sites. Complete block of sodium channels would be lethal; however, these drugs selectively block sodium channels in depolarized or rapidly firing cells, such as axons carrying high-intensity pain information and rapidly firing nerve and cardiac muscle cells that drive epileptic seizures or cardiac arrhythmias.[81-83] This selective block arises because the drugs can reach their binding site in the pore of the sodium channel more rapidly when the pore is repetitively opened, and they bind with high affinity to inactivated sodium channels that are generated in rapidly firing or depolarized cells. This use-dependent action of the sodium channel-blocking drugs is essential for their therapeutic efficacy.

High-affinity binding of local anesthetics to the inactivated state of sodium channels requires two critical amino acid residues, Phe1764 and Tyr1771, $Na_V1.2$ channels, which are located on the same side of the IVS6 transmembrane segment two α-helical turns apart (in Fig. 1-5, F1764 and Y1771 in blue, etidocaine in yellow).[43,78-80] It is likely that the tertiary amino group of local anesthetics interacts with Phe1764, which is located more deeply in the pore, and that the aromatic moiety of the local anesthetics interacts with Tyr1771, which is located nearer to the intracellular end of the pore (blue residues in Fig. 1-5). Subsequent work has shown that sodium channel-blocking drugs of diverse structure that are used as antiarrhythmic agents and as anticonvulsants also interact with the same site as for local anesthetics but engage in additional interactions with other nearby amino acid residues as well.[84-88]

In addition to these important pharmaceutical agents, sodium channels are the molecular targets for a large number of neurotoxins that paralyze prey by preventing neuromuscular function.[89,90] These toxins act at five or more distinct receptor sites, either blocking the pore of the channel or altering the kinetics or voltage dependence of gating. The pore blockers tetrodotoxin and saxitoxin bind to neurotoxin receptor site 1, which is formed by the P loops in the four domains as described above.

Expression, Localization, and Function of Sodium Channel Subtypes

The 10 sodium channel subtypes are differentially expressed in tissues and differentially localized within individual cells.[71,72] Two sodium channel subtypes are predominant in muscle tissues: $Na_V1.4$ in skeletal muscle and $Na_V1.5$ in the heart. $Na_V1.5$ is transiently expressed in developing skeletal muscle but is replaced by $Na_V1.4$ in the adult. In contrast with these muscle sodium channel genes, most sodium channel subtypes are expressed primarily in neurons. $Na_V1.3$ is highly expressed in fetal nervous tissues, whereas $Na_V1.1$, $Na_V1.2$ and $Na_V1.6$ are abundant in juvenile and adult central nervous systems. Generally, $Na_V1.1$ and $Na_V1.3$ are localized primarily in neuronal cell bodies, where they may control the neuronal excitability through integration of synaptic impulses to set the threshold for action potential generation and propagation to the dendritic and axonal compartments. $Na_V1.2$ is localized primarily in unmyelinated axons. During development, $Na_V1.6$ replaces $Na_V1.2$ in maturing nodes of Ranvier in myelinated axons. $Na_V1.1$, $Na_V1.2$, and $Na_V1.6$ also are expressed at low level in the peripheral nervous system. However, three isoforms that have been cloned from sympathetic and dorsal root ganglion neurons, $Na_V1.7$, $Na_V1.8$, and $Na_V1.9$, are more abundant and are the principal sodium channels in the peripheral nervous system. The $Na_V1.7$ channel is localized in axons, where it functions in initiating and conducting the action potential. More restricted expression patterns are observed for $Na_V1.8$ and $Na_V1.9$; these channels are highly expressed in small sensory neurons of dorsal root ganglia and trigeminal ganglia, where they have a key role in nociception.

Although $Na_V1.5$ channels are expressed primarily in the heart and often are termed the "cardiac" sodium channels,[73] several of the "brain" sodium channel subtypes also are expressed at lower levels in the heart, where they are differentially localized in subcellular compartments in a cell-specific and species-specific manner. In human atrial myocytes, $Na_V1.5$ channels are localized in a striated pattern on the cell surface at the Z lines in each sarcomere (Fig. 1-6). By contrast, $Na_V1.2$ channels are localized primarily at the intercalated disks, but at lower concentration, and $Na_V1.1$ channels are localized at low density in a scattered punctate pattern over the cell surface (see Fig. 1-6). Because all of the "brain" and "skeletal muscle" sodium channel subtypes are inhibited by nanomolar concentrations of tetrodotoxin, whereas $Na_V1.5$ channels require micromolar concentrations of tetrodotoxin for inhibition, the contribution of the tetrodotoxin-sensitive sodium channels to cardiac contractility can be tested in careful dose-response experiments. Such experiments indicate that 12% to 27% of sodium current is conducted by the tetrodotoxin-sensitive sodium channels, and that block of these channels reduces the amplitude and velocity of contraction of atrial muscle strips by approximately 15%.[91] The differential localization of these subtypes suggests specific functions for the $Na_V1.2$ channels in initiation of the action potential at intercalated disks and the $Na_V1.5$ channels in depolarizing the atrial membrane near the voltage-gated calcium channels at the Z lines in order to efficiently initiate excitation-contraction coupling.

In human ventricular myocytes, a similar pattern of localization of sodium channels is observed, with $Na_V1.2$ channels localized primarily at the intercalated disks and the predominant $Na_V1.5$ channels localized in a striated pattern at the Z lines (see Fig. 1-6). In contrast with atrial myocytes, which have no transverse tubules (T tubules), the $Na_V1.5$ channels are localized at the cell surface and extend into the T tubules in ventricular myocytes. It is likely that these two channel types have similar functions as in atrial myocytes, $Na_V1.2$ initiating the action potential at the intercalated disk and $Na_V1.5$ conducting the action potential along the myocyte surface and into the T tubule to reach the calcium channels and activate excitation-contraction coupling.

The distribution of sodium channels in mouse ventricular myocytes is quite different from that in human cardiac myocytes.[92-94] In the mouse heart, $Na_V1.5$ channels are localized in high density in the intercalated disks, whereas $Na_V1.1$ channels are localized in lower density at the Z lines.[92] The high concentration of sodium channels at the ends of mouse ventricular myocytes suggests that they conduct action potentials in a saltatory manner, as in a myelinated nerve; that is, the large sodium current entering at the intercalated disk instantaneously depolarizes the entire myocyte and directly activates the high density of sodium channels at the intercalated disks at the other end of the cell, rather than being conducted progressively across the cell. The instantaneous depolarization of the entire cell surface would then initiate action potentials in the T tubules conducted by the tetrodotoxin-sensitive sodium channels there. This altered mode of initiation and conduction of the cardiac action potential may be a specialization that supports the rapid beating rate of the mouse heart (600 beats per minute) without loss of synchrony and force of contraction.

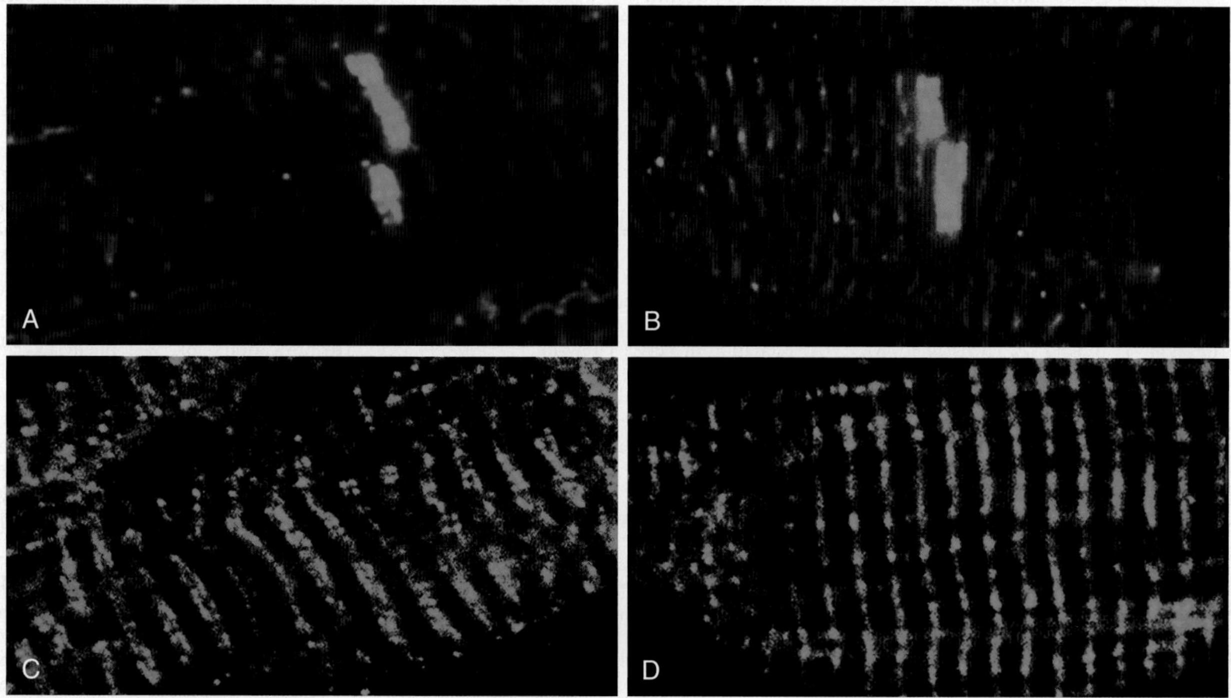

Figure 1-6 Localization of sodium channels in cardiac myocytes. **A,** Human atrial tissue labeled with anti-$Na_V1.2$, illustrating staining of $Na_V1.2$ in the intercalated disk region. **B,** Human ventricular tissue labeled with anti-$Na_V1.2$, illustrating labeling of the channel at the end of each myocyte in the intercalated disk region, with lower levels of staining at the Z lines. **C,** Human atrial tissue labeled with anti-$Na_V1.5$, illustrating staining of $Na_V1.5$ in a striated pattern near the Z lines. **D,** Human ventricular tissue double-labeled with anti-$Na_V1.5$, illustrating staining of $Na_V1.5$ in a striated pattern near the Z lines.

References

1. Catterall WA: The molecular basis of neuronal excitability. Science 223:653-661, 1984.
2. Hartshorne RP, Keller BU, Talvenheimo JA, et al: Functional reconstitution of the purified brain sodium channel in planar lipid bilayers. Proc Natl Acad Sci USA 82:240-244, 1985.
3. Numa S, Noda M: Molecular structure of sodium channels. Ann N Y Acad Sci 479:338-355, 1986.
4. Guy HR, Seetharamulu P: Molecular model of the action potential sodium channel. Proc Natl Acad Sci USA 508: 508-512, 1986.
5. Catterall WA: Molecular properties of voltage-sensitive sodium channels. Annu Rev Biochem 55:953-985, 1986.
6. Catterall WA: From ionic currents to molecular mechanisms: The structure and function of voltage-gated sodium channels. Neuron 26:13-25, 2000.
7. Isom LL, DeJongh KS, Patton DE, et al: Primary structure and functional expression of the β1 subunit of the rat brain sodium channel. Science 256:839-842, 1992.
8. Isom LL, Ragsdale DS, De Jongh KS, et al: Structure and function of the β2 subunit of brain sodium channels, a transmembrane glycoprotein with a CAM-motif. Cell 83:433-442, 1995.
9. Morgan K, Stevens EB, Shah B, et al: Beta 3: An additional auxiliary subunit of the voltage-sensitive sodium channel that modulates channel gating with distinct kinetics. Proc Natl Acad Sci USA 97:2308-2313, 2000.
10. Yu FH, Westenbroek RE, Silos-Santiago I, et al: Sodium channel β4, a new disulfide-linked auxiliary subunit with similarity to β2. J Neurosci 23:7577-7585, 2004.
11. McCormick KA, Srinivasan J, White K, et al: The extracellular domain of the β1 subunit is both necessary and sufficient for modulation of the activity of voltage-gated sodium channels. J Biol Chem 274:32638-32646, 1999.
12. Ratcliffe CF, Qu Y, McCormick KA, et al: A sodium channel signaling complex: Modulation by associated receptor protein tyrosine phosphatase β. Nat Neurosci 3:437-444, 2000.
13. Srinivasan J, Laeng P, Schachner M, Catterall WA: Interaction of voltage-gated sodium channels with the extracellular matrix molecules tenascin-C and tenascin-R. Proc Natl Acad Sci USA 95:15753-15757, 1998.
14. Ratcliffe CF, Westenbroek RE, Curtis R, Catterall WA: Sodium channel β1 and β3 subunits associate with neurofascin through their extracellular immunoglobulin-like domain. J Cell Biol 154:427-434, 2001.
15. Kazarinova-Noyes K, Malhotra JD, McEwen DP, et al: Contactin associates with sodium channels and increases their functional expression. J Neurosci 21:7517-7525, 2001.
16. Malhotra JD, Koopmann MC, Kazen-Gillespie KA, et al: Structural requirements for interaction of sodium channel beta 1 subunits with ankyrin. J Biol Chem 277:26681-26688, 2002.
17. Xiao Z-C, Ragsdale DS, Malhotra JD, et al: Tenascin-R is a functional modulator of sodium channel β subunits. J Biol Chem 274:26511-26517, 1999.
18. Chen C, Bharucha V, Chen Y, et al: Reduced sodium channel density, altered voltage dependence of inactivation, and increased susceptibility to seizures in mice lacking sodium channel β2-subunits. Proc Natl Acad Sci USA 99:17072-17077, 2002.
19. Chen C, Westenbroek E, Xu X, et al: Mice lacking sodium channel β1 subunits display defects in neuronal excitability, sodium channel expression, and nodal architecture. J Neurosci 24:4030-4042, 2004.
20. Lopez-Santiago LF, Meadows L, Ernst SJ, et al: Sodium channel Scn1b null mice exhibit prolonged QT and RR intervals. J Mol Cell Cardiol 43:636-647, 2007.
21. Sato C, Ueno Y, Asai K , et al: The voltage-sensitive sodium channel is a bell-shaped molecule with several cavities. Nature 409:1047-1051, 2001.
22. Long SB, Campbell EB, Mackinnon R: Crystal structure of a mammalian voltage-dependent Shaker family potassium channel. Science 309:897-903, 2005.
23. Yarov-Yarovoy V, Baker D, Catterall WA: Voltage sensor conformations in the open and closed states in ROSETTA structural models of K^+ channels. Proc Natl Acad Sci USA 103:7292-7297, 2006.
24. Shapiro L, Doyle JP, Hensley P, et al: Crystal structure of the extracellular domain from P_0, the major structural protein of peripheral nerve myelin. Neuron 17:435-449, 1996.
25. Isom LL: Sodium channel beta subunits: Anything but auxiliary. Neuroscientist 7:42-54, 2001.
26. Hodgkin AL, Huxley AF: A quantitative description of membrane current and its application to conduction and excitation in nerve. J Physiol 117:500-544, 1952.
27. Armstrong CM: Sodium channels and gating currents. Physiol Rev 61:644-682, 1981.
28. Hille B: Ionic Channels of Excitable Membranes, 3rd ed. Sunderland, MA, Sinauer, 2001.
29. Hille B: The permeability of the sodium channel to metal cations in myelinated nerve. J Gen Physiol 59:637-658, 1972.
30. Noda M, Suzuki H, Numa S, Stühmer W: A single point mutation confers tetrodotoxin and saxitoxin insensitivity on the sodium channel II. FEBS Lett 259:213-216, 1989.
31. Terlau H, Heinemann SH, Stühmer W, et al: Mapping the site of block by tetrodotoxin and saxitoxin of sodium channel II. FEBS Lett 293:93-96, 1991.
32. Heinemann SH, Terlau H, Stühmer W, et al: Calcium channel characteristics conferred on the sodium channel by single mutations. Nature 356:441-443, 1992.
33. Lipkind GM, Fozzard HA: A structural model of the tetrodotoxin and saxitoxin binding site of the Na^+ channel. Biophys J 66:1-13, 1994.
34. Penzotti JL, Fozzard HA, Lipkind GM, Dudley SC Jr: Differences in saxitoxin and tetrodotoxin binding revealed by mutagenesis of the Na^+ channel outer vestibule. Biophys J 75:2647-2657, 1998.
35. Chiamvimonvat N, Pérez-García MT, Ranjan R, et al: Depth asymmetries of the pore-lining segments of the Na^+ channel revealed by cysteine mutagenesis. Neuron 16:1037-1047, 1996.
36. Pérez-García MT, Chiamvimonvat N, Marban E, Tomaselli GF: Structure of the sodium channel pore revealed by serial cysteine mutagenesis. Proc Natl Acad Sci USA 93:300-304, 1996.
37. Schlief T, Schönherr R, Imoto K, Heinemann SH: Pore properties of rat brain II sodium channels mutated in the selectivity filter domain. Eur Biophys J 25:75-91, 1996.
38. Sun YM, Favre I, Schild L, Moczydlowski E: On the structural basis for size-selective permeation of organic cations through the voltage-gated sodium channel—effect of alanine mutations at the DEKA locus on selectivity, inhibition by Ca^{2+} and H^+, and molecular sieving. J Gen Physiol 110:693-715, 1997.
39. Miller C: Annus mirabilis for potassium channels. Science 252:1092-1096, 1991.
40. Doyle DA, Cabral JM, Pfuetzner RA, et al: The structure of the potassium channel: Molecular basis of K^+ conduction and selectivity. Science 280:69-77, 1998.
41. Zhou Y, Morais-Cabral JH, Kaufman A, MacKinnon R: Chemistry of ion coordination and hydration revealed by a K^+ channel-Fab complex at 20 Å resolution. Nature 414:43-48, 2001.
42. Striessnig J, Glossmann H, Catterall WA: Identification of a phenylalkylamine binding region within the α_1 subunit of skeletal muscle Ca^{2+} channels. Proc Natl Acad Sci USA 87:9108-9112, 1990.
43. Ragsdale DS, McPhee JC, Scheuer T, Catterall WA: Molecular determinants of state-dependent block of Na^+ channels by local anesthetics. Science 265:1724-1728, 1994.
44. Lopez GA, Jan YN, Jan LY: Evidence that the S6 segment of the Shaker voltage-gated K^+ channel comprises part of the pore. Nature 367:179-182, 1994.
45. Hirschberg B, Rovner A, Lieberman M, Patlak J: Transfer of twelve charges is needed to open skeletal muscle Na^+ channels. J Gen Physiol 106:1053-1068, 1995.

46. Stuhmer W, Conti F, Suzuki H, et al: Structural parts involved in activation and inactivation of the sodium channel. Nature 339:597-603, 1989.
47. Yang N, Horn R: Evidence for voltage-dependent S4 movement in sodium channel. Neuron 15:213-218, 1995.
48. Yang NB, George AL Jr, Horn R: Molecular basis of charge movement in voltage-gated sodium channels. Neuron 16:113-122, 1996.
49. Tombola F, Pathak MM, Isacoff EY: How does voltage open an ion channel? Annu Rev Cell Dev Biol 22:23-52, 2006.
50. Jiang Y, Lee A, Chen J, et al: Crystal structure and mechanism of a calcium-gated potassium channel. Nature 417:515-522, 2002.
51. Jiang Y, Lee A, Chen J, et al: The open pore conformation of potassium channels. Nature 417:523-526, 2002.
52. Zhao Y, Yarov-Yarovoy V, Scheuer T, Catterall WA: A gating hinge in sodium channels: A molecular switch for electrical signaling. Neuron 41:859-865, 2004.
53. Vassilev PM, Scheuer T, Catterall WA: Identification of an intracellular peptide segment involved in sodium channel inactivation. Science 241:1658-1661, 1988.
54. Vassilev P, Scheuer T, Catterall WA: Inhibition of inactivation of single sodium channels by a site-directed antibody. Proc Natl Acad Sci USA 86:8147-8151, 1989.
55. West JW, Patton DE, Scheuer T, et al: A cluster of hydrophobic amino acid residues required for fast Na^+ channel inactivation. Proc Natl Acad Sci USA 89:10910-10914, 1992.
56. Eaholtz G, Scheuer T, Catterall WA: Restoration of inactivation and block of open sodium channels by an inactivation gate peptide. Neuron 12:1041-1048, 1994.
57. Kellenberger S, West JW, Scheuer T, Catterall WA: Molecular analysis of the putative inactivation particle in the inactivation gate of brain type IIA Na^+ channels. J Gen Physiol 109:589-605, 1997b.
58. Kellenberger S, Scheuer T, Catterall WA: Movement of the Na^+ channel inactivation gate during inactivation. J Biol Chem 271:30971-30979, 1996.
59. Kellenberger S, West JW, Catterall WA, Scheuer T: Molecular analysis of potential hinge residues in the inactivation gate of brain type IIA Na^+ channels. J Gen Physiol 19:607-617, 1997a.
60. Rohl CA, Boeckman FA, Baker C, et al: Solution structure of the sodium channel inactivation gate. Biochemistry 38:855-861, 1999.
61. McPhee JC, Ragsdale DS, Scheuer T, Catterall WA: A critical role for transmembrane segment IVS6 of the sodium channel α subunit in fast inactivation. J Biol Chem 270:12025-12034, 1995.
62. Smith MR, Goldin AL: Interaction between the sodium channel inactivation linker and domain III S4-S5. Biophys J 73:1885-1895, 1997.
63. Lerche H, Peter W, Fleischhauer R, et al: Role in fast inactivation of the IV/S4-S5 loop of the human muscle Na^+ channel probed by cysteine mutagenesis. J Physiol (Lond) 505:345-352, 1997.
64. McPhee JC, Ragsdale D, Scheuer T, Catterall WA: A critical role for the S4-S5 intracellular loop in domain IV of the sodium channel α subunit in fast inactivation. J Biol Chem 273:1121-1129, 1998.
65. Tang LH, Chehab N, Wieland SJ, Kallen RG: Glutamine substitution at alanine1649 in the S4-S5 cytoplasmic loop of domain 4 removes the voltage sensitivity of fast inactivation in the human heart sodium channel. J Gen Physiol 111:639-652, 1998.
66. Filatov GN, Nguyen TP, Kraner SD, Barchi L: Inactivation and secondary structure in the D4/S4-5 region of the SkM1 sodium channel. J Gen Physiol 111:703-715, 1998.
67. Chen LQ, Santarelli V, Horn R, Kallen RG: A unique role for the S4 segment of domain 4 in the inactivation of sodium channels. J Gen Physiol 108:549-556, 1996.
68. Rogers JC, Qu Y, Tanada TN, et al: Molecular determinants of high affinity binding of α-scorpion toxin and sea anemone toxin in the S3-S4 extracellular loop in domain IV of the Na^+ channel α subunit. J Biol Chem 271:15950-15962, 1996.
69. Sheets MF, Kyle JW, Kallen RG, Hanck DA: The Na channel voltage sensor associated with inactivation is localized to the external charged residues of domain IV, S4. Biophys J 77:747-757, 1999.
70. Cha A, Ruben PCG Jr, George AL, et al: Voltage sensors in domains III and IV, but not I and II, are immobilized by Na^+ channel fast inactivation. Neuron 22:73-87, 1999.
71. Yu FH, Catterall WA: The VGL-chanome: A protein superfamily specialized for electrical signaling and ionic homeostasis. Science STKE 2004(253):re15, 2004.
72. Goldin AL, Barchi RL, Caldwell JH, et al: Nomenclature of voltage-gated sodium channels. Neuron 28:365-368, 2000.
73. Rogart RB, Cribbs LL, Muglia LK, et al: Molecular cloning of a putative tetrodotoxin-resistant rat heart Na^+ channel isoform. Proc Natl Acad Sci USA 86:8170-8174, 1989.
74. Satin J, Kyle JW, Chen M, et al: A mutant of TTX-resistant cardiac sodium channels with TTX-sensitive properties. Science 256:1202-1205, 1992.
75. Sivilotti L, Okuse K, Akopian AN, et al: A single serine residue confers tetrodotoxin insensitivity on the rat sensory-neuron-specific sodium channel SNS. FEBS Lett 409:49-52, 1997.
76. Hiyama TY, Watanabe E, Okado H, Noda M: The subfornical organ is the primary locus of sodium-level sensing by Na_x sodium channels for the control of salt-intake behavior. J Neurosci 24:9276-9281, 2004.
77. Ahern CA, Eastwood AL, Dougherty DA, et al: Electrostatic contributions of aromatic residues in the local anesthetic receptor of voltage-gated sodium channels. Circ Res 102:86-94, 2008.
78. Li G, Yarov-Yarovoy V, Qu Y, et al: Differential interactions of lamotrigine and related drugs with transmembrane segment IVS6 of voltage-gated sodium channels. Neuropharmacology 44:413-422, 2003.
79. Yarov-Yarovoy V, Brown J, Sharp EM, et al: Molecular determinants of voltage-dependent gating and binding of pore-blocking drugs in transmembrane segment IIIS6 of the Na channel α subunit. J Biol Chem 276:20-27, 2001.
80. Yarov-Yarovoy V, McPhee JC, Idsvoog D, et al: Role of amino acid residues in transmembrane segments IS6 and IIS6 of the Na^+ channel α subunit in voltage-dependent gating and drug block. J Biol Chem 277:35393-35401, 2002.
81. Hille B: Local anesthetics: Hydrophilic and hydrophobic pathways for the drug-receptor reaction. J Gen Physiol 69:497-515, 1977.
82. Hondeghem LM, Katzung BG: Antiarrhythmic agents: The modulated receptor mechanism of action of sodium and calcium channel-blocking drugs. Annu Rev Pharmacol Toxicol 24:387-423, 1984.
83. Catterall WA: Common modes of drug action on Na^+ channels: Local anesthetics, antiarrhythmics and anticonvulsants. Trends Pharmacol Science 8:57-65, 1987.
84. Ragsdale DS, McPhee JC, Scheuer T, Catterall WA: Common molecular determinants of local anesthetic, antiarrhythmic, and anticonvulsant block of voltage-gated Na^+ channels. Proc Natl Acad Sci USA 93:9270-9275, 1996.
85. Wright SN, Wang SY, Wang GK: Lysine point mutations in Na^+ channel D4-S6 reduce inactivated channel block by local anesthetics. Mol Pharmacol 54:733-739, 1998.
86. Nau C, Wang SY, Wang GK: Point mutations at L1280 in Nav1.4 channel D3-S6 modulate binding affinity and stereoselectivity of bupivacaine enantiomers. Mol Pharmacol 63:1398-1406, 2003.
87. Weiser T, Qu Y, Catterall WA, Scheuer T: Differential interaction of R-mexiletine with the local anesthetic receptor site on brain and heart sodium channel alpha-subunits. Mol Pharmacol 56:1238-1244, 1999.
88. Lipkind GM, Fozzard HA: Molecular modeling of local anesthetic drug binding by voltage-gated sodium channels. Mol Pharmacol 68:1611-1622, 2005.
89. Cestèle S, Catterall WA: Molecular mechanisms of neurotoxin action on voltage gated sodium channels. Biochimie 82:883-892, 2000.
90. Catterall WA, Cestèle S, Yarov-Yarovoy V, et al: Voltage-gated ion channels and gating modifier toxins. Toxicon 49:124-141, 2007.
91. Westenbroek RE, Kaufmann S, Lange V, et al.: Localization and function of sodium channel subtypes in human heart. Circulation 116:11-12, 2007.
92. Maier S, Westenbroek RE, Schenkman KA, et al: An unexpected role for brain type sodium channels in coupling of cell surface depolarization to contraction in the heart. Proc Natl Acad Sci USA 99:4073-4078, 2002.
93. Maier SKG, Westenbroek RE, Yamanushi TT, et al: An unexpected requirement for brain-type sodium channels for control of heart rate in the mouse sinoatrial node. Proc Natl Acad Sci USA 100:3507-3512, 2003.
94. Maier SKG, Westenbroek RE, McCormick KA, et al: Distinct subcellular localization of different sodium channel α and β subunits in single ventricular myocytes from mouse heart. Circulation 109:1421-1427, 2004.

Cardiac Calcium Channels 2

DONALD M. BERS AND ECKARD PICHT

CHAPTER OUTLINE

Calcium channels are essential contributors to cardiac electrophysiologic properties and also constitute the critical initiator of cardiac excitation-contraction coupling, by triggering sarcoplasmic reticulum (SR) release of Ca^{2+} ions. The SR Ca^{2+} release channels that are activated by transsarcolemmal Ca^{2+} influx are described in Chapter 6. Additional detail on cardiac calcium channels and excitation-contraction coupling can be found in other sources.[1-4]

Calcium Channel Types

At least 10 calcium channel genes are recognized, designated by several different nomenclatures (Fig. 2-1). Some of these channels are expressed primarily in neurons; two main types of calcium channels are expressed in cardiac myocytes, L- and T-type (both of which also conduct barium).[1,5] The L-type calcium channels are characterized by a large single-channel conductance (approximately 25 picosiemens [pS] in 110 mM barium), long-lasting openings (with Ba^{2+} as the charge carrier), sensitivity to 1,4-dihydropyridines (DHPs) (see Chapter 16), and activation at larger depolarizations (i.e., at more positive membrane potential, E_m). T-type calcium channels are characterized by a smaller single-channel conductance (approximately 8 pS in 110 mM barium), more transient openings, insensitivity to DHPs, and activation at more negative E_m. Further distinctions among L- and T-type calcium channels in heart are recognized: L-type calcium current (I_{Ca}) is due mainly to α_{1C} (and, to a lesser extent, α_{1D}), and T-type I_{Ca} is due to α_{1G} and α_{1H}. The $Ca_V1.2$ nomenclature is more formally accepted now (versus α_{1C}), but L- and T-type are still widely used for the groups $Ca_V1.x$ and $Ca_V3.x$, respectively.

Functional $I_{Ca,L}$ is present in all cardiac myocytes, whereas cardiac $I_{Ca,T}$ is more prominent in atrial cells and cardiac Purkinje cells.[6,7] The two current types can be separated by using voltage protocols with different holding potentials (Fig. 2-2A). A negative holding potential (e.g., −70 mV) allows the activation of both $I_{Ca,L}$ and $I_{Ca,T}$. The apparent hump at negative E_m reflects $I_{Ca,T}$ (see Fig. 2-2B). A more positive holding potential (e.g., −40 mV) inactivates $I_{Ca,T}$ and allows the selective measurement of $I_{Ca,L}$. The difference between these two measurements is then used to determine $I_{Ca,T}$ (see Fig. 2-2C). Purkinje cells have abundant $I_{Ca,T}$[8]; pacemaker and some atrial myocytes also have significant amounts.[5,9] The amount of $I_{Ca,T}$ in mature ventricular myocytes, however, is either modest in guinea pig[10] or undetectable in bullfrog, calf, cat, rabbit, rat, mouse, and ferret[5,11-14] as well as in human atrial myocytes.[15] Neonatal rat and mouse ventricular myocytes exhibit $I_{Ca,T}$,[11,16-18] and significant $I_{Ca,T}$ may reappear in ventricular myocytes during the development of ventricular hypertrophy in cat[12] and rat.[19] Additionally, small ventricular myocytes expressing $I_{Ca,T}$ may represent new myocytes (due to proliferative regeneration) on their way to maturity.[20] Only T- and L-type I_{Ca} currents are apparent in cardiac myocytes, whereas intracardiac neurons may express N-, P/Q- or R-type currents.[21]

The relative prominence of $I_{Ca,T}$ in pacemaker and conducting cells, and its activation at E_m in the diastolic pacemaker range has led to suggestions of and evidence for a role of $I_{Ca,T}$ in atrial pacemaking.[9,22,23] Because $I_{Ca,T}$ is relatively small and inactivates very rapidly, the total amount of Ca^{2+} flux by way of $I_{Ca,T}$ is small compared with that by way of $I_{Ca,L}$ and negligible in most ventricular myocytes (from the standpoint of overall Ca^{2+} fluxes). This may reflect different functional roles, wherein $I_{Ca,L}$ is more involved in triggering SR Ca^{2+} release and refilling SR Ca^{2+} stores, rather than pacemaking or myocyte development.

When calcium is the charge carrier of $I_{Ca,L}$, inactivation is rapid (see Fig. 2-5 and "I_{Ca} Inactivation" later on), and the $I_{Ca,L}$ kinetics can be confused with $I_{Ca,T}$. Therefore, $I_{Ca,L}$ versus $I_{Ca,T}$ can be best distinguished when barium is the charge carrier, because $I_{Ca,L}$ inactivation is then especially slow (e.g., see Fig. 2-5). When T-type current is prominent, it also can be resolved by the difference in holding E_m dependence (see Fig. 2-2).

Cardiac cell types in which $I_{Ca,T}$ is prominent also have less extensive transverse tubules (T tubules). It is not known explicitly whether T-type calcium channels are excluded from T tubules, but L-type calcium channels in cardiac and skeletal muscle are concentrated there.

Thus far, human calcium channelopathies have been associated with five α_1 calcium channel subunit genes and with two of the auxiliary subunit genes.[24,25] Two missense mutations in the sixth transmembrane segment of domain I were recently identified in $Ca_V1.2$ (G402S and G406R), leading to reduced channel inactivation. Clinically, these mutations are associated with Timothy syndrome, a severe multisystem disorder. Patients carrying such mutations demonstrate QT prolongation (LQT8) and cardiac arrhythmias. Because of the widespread expression of $Ca_V1.2$ throughout the body, patients also are affected with numerous functional and developmental abnormalities including those affecting the heart, central nervous system, skin, and teeth.[24,26,27]

Unless otherwise specified, subsequent discussion of calcium channels and I_{Ca} refers to L-type calcium channels or $I_{Ca,L}$ for cardiac myocytes.

	Type	Channel Name	Pore Subunit	Gene Name	Chromosomal Locus	Tissue
HVA	L	$Ca_V1.1$	α_{1S}	*CACNA1S*	1q31-32	Skeletal muscle
		$Ca_V1.2$	α_{1C}	*CACNA1C*	12p13	**Heart**, brain, lung, smooth muscle, glands
		$Ca_V1.3$	α_{1D}	*CACNA1D*	3p14.3	Neurons, **heart** (atrium, SA and AV nodes)
		$Ca_V1.4$	α_{1F}	*CACNA1F*	Xp11.23	Retina, spinal cord, lymphoid tissue
	P/Q	$Ca_V2.1$	α_{1A}	*CACNA1A*	19p13.1	Neurons
	N	$Ca_V2.2$	α_{1B}	*CACNA1B*	9q34	Neurons
	R	$Ca_V2.3$	α_{1E}	*CACNA1E*	1q25-31	Neurons, **heart**, testes, pituitary
LVA	T	$Ca_V3.1$	α_{1G}	*CACNA1G*	17q22	Neurons
		$Ca_V3.2$	α_{1H}	*CACNA1H*	16p13.3	**Heart** (Purkinje fibers), kidney, liver
		$Ca_V3.3$	α_{1I}	*CACNA1I*	22q13	Neurons

Figure 2-1 Dendrogram of calcium channel types. The two main evolutionary branches are high voltage– and low voltage–activated (HVA and LVA). The HVA channels are divided into L-type and non–L-type (including P/Q, N, and R types); the LVA channels all are referred to as T-type calcium channels. Several different nomenclatures are indicated, along with the human chromosome location. AV, atrioventricular; SA, sinoatrial.

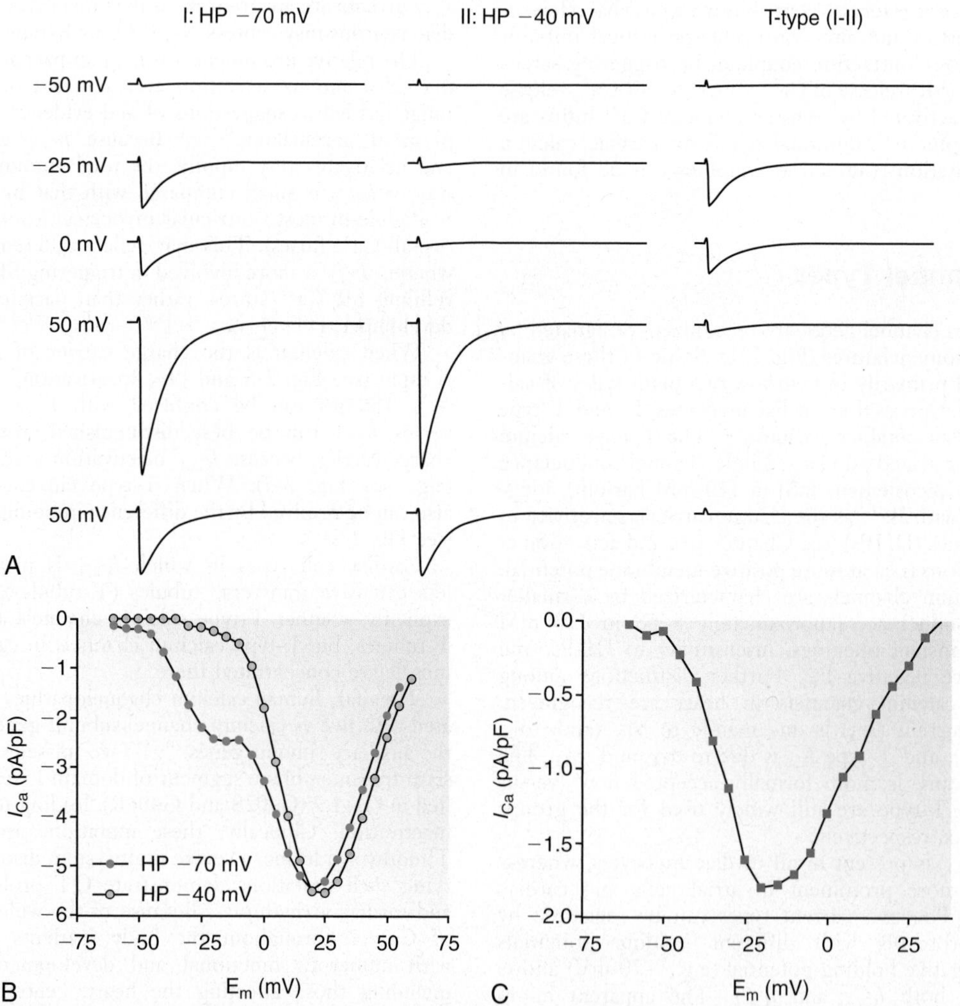

Figure 2-2 L- and T-type calcium channel currents in heart. **A,** $I_{Ca,L}$ and $I_{Ca,T}$ can be separated by different holding potentials. Voltage steps from a holding potential of −70 mV activate both $I_{Ca,L}$ and $I_{Ca,T}$. The apparent hump in the current-voltage relation at −30 mV obtained by this voltage protocol is due to $I_{Ca,T}$. A holding potential of −40 mV inactivates $I_{Ca,T}$, allowing the isolated measurement of $I_{Ca,L}$. The difference of the currents represents $I_{Ca,T}$. **B,** Calcium current-voltage relationships measured in dog Purkinje fibers using square pulses from a holding potential of −70 mV and −40 mV. **C,** $I_{Ca,T}$ calculated from the difference of the two curves shown in **B**. (Data in **B** and **C** from Rosati B, Dun W, Hirose M, et al: Molecular basis of the T- and L-type Ca^{2+} currents in canine Purkinje fibres. J Physiol 579:465-471, 2007.)

Molecular Characterization of Calcium Channels

Five protein subunits—α_1, α_2, β, γ, and δ—make up the skeletal muscle calcium channel, and all have been sequenced.[28-32] The α_1 subunit of skeletal muscle (α_{1S}) is distinct from the cardiac channel clone (α_{1C}).[33] The α_1 subunit contains the conduction pore and binding sites for dihydropyridines (DHPs), phenylalkylamines (PAAs), and benzothiazepines (BTZs), as well as main regulatory sites. Its structure is similar to that of E_m-dependent sodium channel and potassium channels (Fig. 2-3). That is, α_{1C} has four homologous domains, I to IV, each of which has six transmembrane spans—S1 to S6, with charged S4 serving as the main voltage sensor, and pore loops (P loops) between S5 and S6.

The long carboxyl tail (C terminus) contains an EF-hand and an IQ motif, as well as binding sites for calmodulin, calmodulin kinase II (CaMKII), sorcin, and protein phosphatase 2A. The A-kinase anchoring protein AKAP15 interacts with the C terminus of $Ca_V1.2$ by way of a leucine zipper-like motif and targets protein kinase A (PKA) near the serine PKA phosphorylation site (Ser1928).[34] The distal C terminus undergoes proteolytic cleavage and forms a non–covalently bound complex with the truncated C terminus of the α_{1C} subunit between the proximal and distal C-terminal domains (PCRD and DCRD in Fig. 2-3).[35] The formation of this autoinhibitory complex reduces the coupling efficiency of voltage sensing to channel opening and shifts the voltage dependence of activation to more positive membrane potentials.[35] In addition to regulating the calcium channel itself, the C-terminal fragment may further regulate other cellular functions. Recently, it was shown in neurons that this fragment translocates to the nucleus and regulates the expression of genes involved in signaling and excitability.[36]

The numerous splice variants identified for the human *CACNA1C* gene may lead to altered biophysical, biochemical, or pharmacologic properties.[37,38] The α_{1D} subunit also is expressed in the heart,[39,40] but the functional consequence of α_{1D} versus α_{1C} (or splice variants) is not entirely clear. The α_{1D} protein is expressed at relatively high levels in pacemaker-type cells,[23,41] and I_{Ca} from this channel activates at E_m between that for $I_{Ca,T}$ and the $I_{Ca,L}$ derived from α_{1C}.[41,42] Pacemaker depolarization in sinoatrial node cells may include $I_{Ca,T}$ activation relatively early during diastolic depolarization, with subsequent sequential recruitment of $I_{Ca,L}$ from α_{1D} and then $I_{Ca,L}$ from α_{1C}, to contribute to depolarization.[23,43,44]

The α_2 subunit and the δ subunit are produced by the same $\alpha_2\delta$ gene.[45] The $\alpha_2\delta$ protein gets cleaved (but retains α_2-δ interaction by means of disulfide links), and the δ portion anchors the complex in the membrane (see Fig. 2-3). Different $\alpha_2\delta$ variants also are recognized (α_{2A} predominates in skeletal muscle, α_{2B} in brain, and α_{2C} and α_{2D} in heart). Coexpression of $\alpha_2\delta$ with α_{1C}

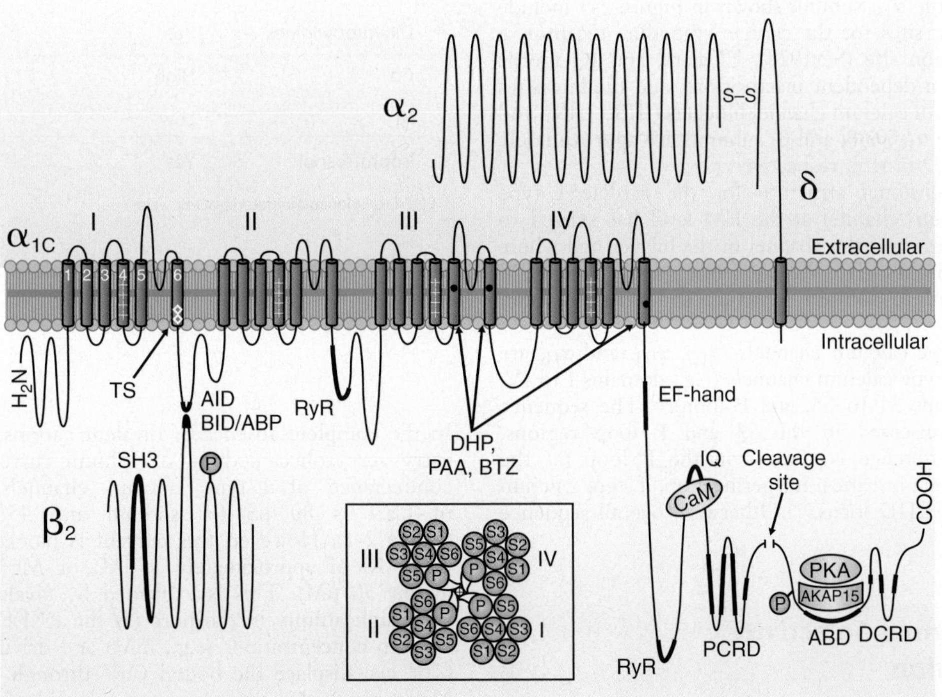

Figure 2-3 Subunit structure of cardiac L-type calcium channel. The α_1 subunit has four domains, I to IV, each with six transmembrane spans (S1 to S6) and a pore loop. Positively charged gating regions in S4 of each domain are indicated by +. Calcium channel antagonists—dihydropyridines, phenylalkylamines, and benzothiazepines (DHPs, PAAs, and BTZs)—bind to IIIS5, IIIS6, and IVS6 regions. Possible interaction sites between the α_1 subunit and the ryanodine receptor (RyR) are indicated, as well as a protein kinase A (PKA) phosphorylation site (serine S1928), an EF-hand region, and an IQ motif at which calmodulin (CaM) can bind. The distal carboxyl (C) terminus (COOH) is cleaved from the α_1 subunit and forms a complex with the proximal C terminus. The proximal and distal C-terminal regulatory domains (PCRD and DCRD) that mediate this interaction also are indicated. PKA binds distal to the PKA phosphorylation site by means of A-kinase anchoring protein-15 (AKAP15) to an AKAP-binding domain (ABD). TS indicates the approximate localization of mutations associated with Timothy syndrome. The β_2 subunit is cytosolic, can be phosphorylated (P), and interacts with α_1 at the α and β interaction domains (AID, BID/ABP). *Inset,* A top view of the calcium channel showing a likely organization of transmembrane regions around the pore. SH3, Src homology domain 3. (Some data in this figure from Durell SR, Hao Y, Guy HR: Structural models of the transmembrane region of voltage-gated and other K^+ channels in open, closed, and inactivated conformations. J Struct Biol 121:263-284, 1998.)

increases DHPR-binding sites, gating currents, and I_{Ca}.[46-48] Thus, $\alpha_2\delta$ may help in the formation of functional sarcolemmal channels, but it also may alter calcium channel gating.[49] The γ subunit is a prominent part of the skeletal muscle calcium channel,[30,31] but clear evidence for a functionally important cardiac γ subunit is lacking.

Multiple β subunit genes (encoding subunits β_1 to β_4) also are known, but the main cardiac isoform is β_2, and alternative splice variants have been identified.[50] Coexpression of β_2 with α_{1C} causes a 10-fold increase in current, accelerates activation and inactivation kinetics, shifts steady-state inactivation, and greatly increases the number of high-affinity DHP-binding sites.[51-53] The β subunit is a completely cytosolic protein without any membrane-anchoring region. Its interaction with the α_1 subunit occurs by means of the β-interaction domain (BID), which binds tightly to the α-interaction domain (AID) in the I-II linker of the α_{1C} subunit.[54,55] Recently however, the structure of the molecular interaction of the β_2 conserved core in complex with the AID was resolved.[56] This work showed that the BID is unavailable for protein-protein interaction because it is buried in the β_2 core. Rather, the AID engages with the β_2 subunit through a conserved hydrophobic cleft named the *α-binding pocket* (ABP).

The β subunit serves as a molecular chaperone by antagonizing an endoplasmic reticulum retention signal in the I-II linker of the α_1 subunit, helping nascent α_{1C} molecules to fold properly and reach the sarcolemma.[57] The β_{2A} subunit is phosphorylated by PKA at S459, S478, and S479. Furthermore, a CaMKII phosphorylation site was described at T498 and has been implicated in mediating calcium-dependent I_{Ca} facilitation.[58]

Other sites on the α_{1C} subunit shown in Figure 2-3 include possible interacting sites for the cardiac ryanodine receptor, a PKA phosphorylation site (Ser1928), EF-hand and IQ motifs (involved in calcium-dependent inactivation), and binding sites for the main classes of calcium channel blockers (IIIS$_5$, IIIS$_6$, and IVS$_6$). In heart, the α_{1C}, $\alpha_2\delta$, and β_2 subunits are approximately 200, 175, and 60 kD in size, respectively.

The three-dimensional structure for the cardiac L-type voltage-gated calcium channel at the EM level has started to identify the orientation of the channel in the bilayer and where the auxiliary subunits associate.[59] More work is needed to obtain the structural detail to connect structure and function more comprehensively.

The three T-type calcium channels, α_{1G}, α_{1H}, and α_{1I}, are structurally like L-type calcium channels (e.g., domains I to IV, transmembrane spans S1 to S6, and P loop).[60] The sequence is most highly conserved in the S4 and P loop regions, although a key difference is present in the P loop (at the "EEEE" locus, which is critical for permeation, T-type calcium channels have an EEDD locus.[61]) Otherwise, overall sequence identity is low.

Table 2-1 Properties of Cardiac L- and T-type Calcium Channels

Property	L-type	T-type
Activation range		
5 mM Ca^{2+}	Positive to −30 mV	Positive to −60 mV
110 mM Ba^{2+}	Positive to −10 mV	Positive to −50 mV
Inactivation		
Range	Positive to −40 mV	−90 to −60 mV
Calcium-dependent	Yes	No
Voltage-dependent	Slow	Fast
Tail deactivation	Fast	Slow
Conductance		
110 mM Ba^{2+}	25 pS	8 pS
110 mM Ca^{2+}	8 pS	8 pS
150 mM Na^+, EDTA	80 pS	50 pS
Mean open time	Typically <1 ms	Short, 1-2 ms
Kinetics (Ba^{2+})	Multiple bursts per pulse	1 burst per pulse (inactivation)
Pharmacologic sensitivity		
Dihydropyridines	Yes	No
Cd	High	Low
Ni	Low	High
Isoproterenol	Yes	No

EDTA, ethylenediaminetetra-acetic acid.

Calcium Channel Selectivity and Permeation

The narrowest point in the calcium channel pore is approximately 0.6 nm in diameter (as established by the finding that tetramethylammonium can permeate).[62] Nevertheless, calcium channels show greater than 1000-fold selectivity over small monovalent cations such as Li^+, Na^+, Ba^{2+}, K^+, and Cs^+, so size is not the critical factor in selectivity. A key factor in calcium channel selectivity appears to be a ring of glutamates in the pore (the EEEE locus at the selectivity filter), with each of the four P loops contributing one glutamate.[63,64] In the complete absence of divalent cations, calcium channels carry very robust sodium or lithium current (single-channel conductance of L-type calcium channels in the absence of Ca^{2+} is 80 pS for sodium and 45 pS for lithium) (Table 2-1). However, this current is blocked by extracellular Ca^{2+} (K_i of approximately 1 μM) or Mg^{2+} (K_i of approximately 50 μM). This is explained by divalent cation binding with high affinity in the pore (at the EEEE locus). At higher calcium concentrations (e.g., mM) and driving force, a second Ca^{2+} can displace the bound Ca^{2+} through the pore (whereas Na^+ cannot); this accounts for perceptible I_{Ca}. Barium current through L-type calcium channels is greater than calcium current (single-channel conductance 25 pS versus 8 pS), but barium current is more susceptible to block by cobalt. This finding is consistent with barium binding within the channel (with weaker affinity than that observed for calcium), such that Co^{2+} competes with Ba^{2+} more effectively. This feature also explains the higher barium versus calcium current: Because Ba^{2+} doesn't "stick" in the channel as well, it can go through more quickly.

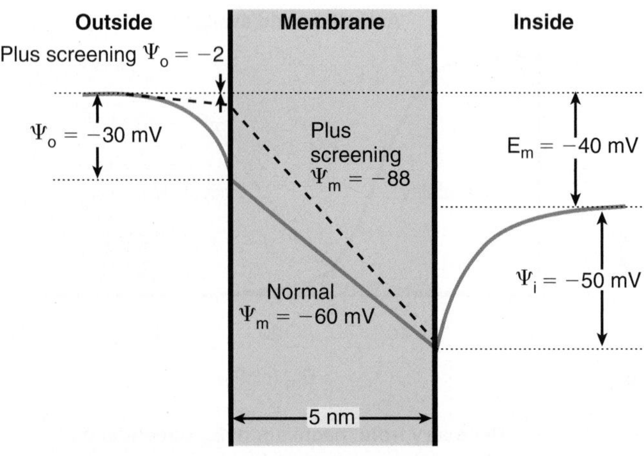

Figure 2-4 Surface potential and channel gating. At higher extracellular divalent ion concentration, external surface charge is screened thereby decreasing ψ_o and making transbilayer potential (ψ_m) more negative for the same membrane potential, E_m. Thus, greater E_m depolarization is required to reach the same ψ_m. (From Bers DM: Excitation-Contraction Coupling and Cardiac Contractile Force, 2nd ed. Dordrecht, Kluwer, 2001.)

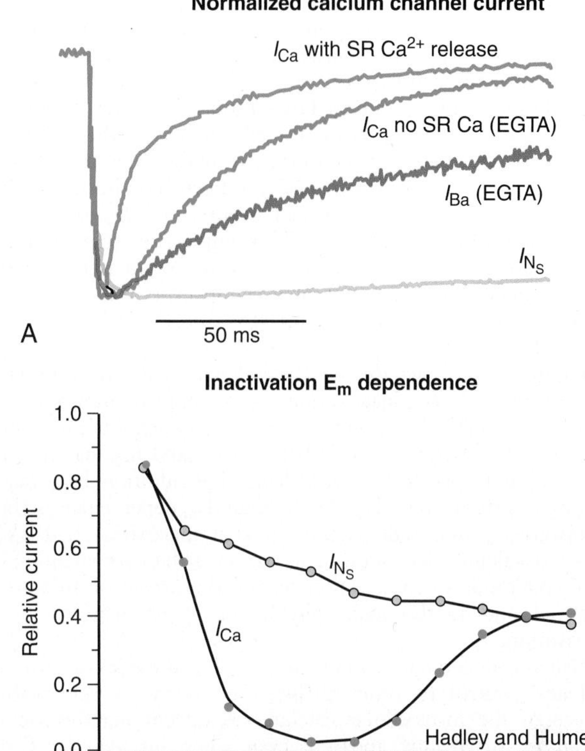

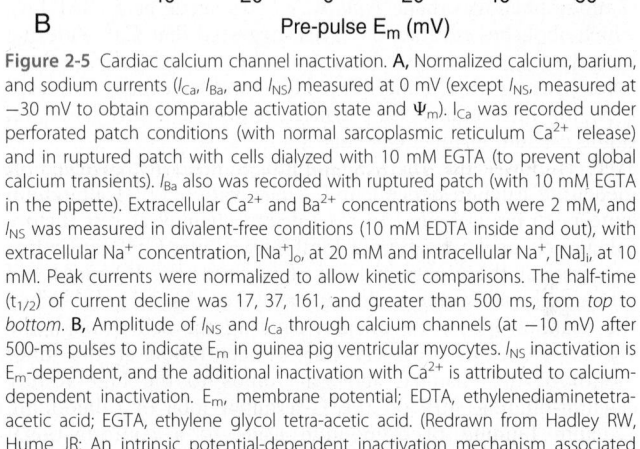

Figure 2-5 Cardiac calcium channel inactivation. **A,** Normalized calcium, barium, and sodium currents (I_{Ca}, I_{Ba}, and I_{NS}) measured at 0 mV (except I_{NS}, measured at −30 mV to obtain comparable activation state and Ψ_m). I_{Ca} was recorded under perforated patch conditions (with normal sarcoplasmic reticulum Ca^{2+} release) and in ruptured patch with cells dialyzed with 10 mM EGTA (to prevent global calcium transients). I_{Ba} also was recorded with ruptured patch (with 10 mM EGTA in the pipette). Extracellular Ca^{2+} and Ba^{2+} concentrations both were 2 mM, and I_{NS} was measured in divalent-free conditions (10 mM EDTA inside and out), with extracellular Na^+ concentration, $[Na^+]_o$, at 20 mM and intracellular Na^+, $[Na]_i$, at 10 mM. Peak currents were normalized to allow kinetic comparisons. The half-time ($t_{1/2}$) of current decline was 17, 37, 161, and greater than 500 ms, from *top* to *bottom*. **B,** Amplitude of I_{NS} and I_{Ca} through calcium channels (at −10 mV) after 500-ms pulses to indicate E_m in guinea pig ventricular myocytes. I_{NS} inactivation is E_m-dependent, and the additional inactivation with Ca^{2+} is attributed to calcium-dependent inactivation. E_m, membrane potential; EDTA, ethylenediaminetetra-acetic acid; EGTA, ethylene glycol tetra-acetic acid. (Redrawn from Hadley RW, Hume JR: An intrinsic potential-dependent inactivation mechanism associated with calcium channels in guinea-pig myocytes. J Physiol 389:205-222, 1987; and Bers DM: Excitation-Contraction Coupling and Cardiac Contractile Force, 2nd ed. Dordrecht, Kluwer, 2001.)

Calcium Channel Gating

Surface Potential and Activation

Cardiac I_{Ca} is rapidly activated by depolarization, reaching a peak in approximately 2 to 7 ms, depending on the temperature and E_m. Calcium channel activation depends on E_m, but as for all voltage-dependent channels, is also sensitive to changes in surface potential. Surface potential arises from fixed negative charges on the membrane surface (e.g., due to charged membrane phospholipids). Figure 2-4 shows how changing extracellular and intracellular surface potential (ψ_o and ψ_i) affects the electric field within the membrane (ψ_m), which is what the channel voltage sensors sense. This diagram depicts the situation near threshold of I_{Ca} activation (E_m = −40 mV) at physiologic Ca^{2+} concentration and ionic strength. The surface potentials correspond to surface charge densities of 0.3 to $1/nm^2$. This range corresponds to the surface densities of acidic phospholipids and sugars and agrees with experimental estimates. The more negative ψ_i reflects preferential distribution of negatively charged phospholipids on the inner sarcolemmal leaflet in cardiac muscle and lower intracellular divalent cation concentration. Divalent cations are particularly effective in screening surface charge because they are concentrated by the negative ψ_m and can bind to negatively charged sites, thereby neutralizing them.

At E_m = −40 mV in Figure 2-4, the transbilayer potential (ψ_m) is −60 mV. If extracellular calcium concentration is increased such that ψ_o is nearly abolished, then ψ_m is considerably more polarized (−88 mV) for the same E_m = −40 mV. Thus, the channel protein senses a more negative voltage, and a greater depolarization will be required for the channel to reach the threshold for activation. This effect applies to all E_m-dependent channels and applies equally to the E_m dependence of inactivation. It explains the increased excitability of cells in low calcium concentrations. Conversely, high extracellular Ca^{2+} concentration stabilizes E_m-dependent channels and reduces excitability (a rightward shift of the curves in Fig. 2-6A).

I_{Ca} Inactivation

Inactivation of calcium channels is time-, E_m-, and intracellular Ca^{2+} concentration–dependent.[65-67] Figure 2-5A shows that inactivation of nonselective monovalent current through calcium channels (I_{NS} measured without divalent cations) is very slow (half-time, $t_{1/2}$, longer than 500 ms), reflecting purely E_m-dependent inactivation. The barium current (I_{Ba}) in Figure 2-5A inactivates more rapidly ($t_{1/2}$ = 161 ms) than I_{NS}; this may reflect a modest ability of barium to mimic calcium-dependent inactivation. When Ca^{2+} is the charge carrier, with 10 mM ethylene glycol tetra-acetic acid (EGTA) in the pipette to abolish calcium transients (and SR Ca^{2+} release), inactivation is faster still ($t_{1/2}$ = 37 ms). This probably reflects calcium-dependent inactivation due to entry of Ca^{2+} through the channel itself. EGTA is a slow Ca^{2+} buffer and therefore cannot prevent a rise in local intracellular Ca^{2+} concentration near the calcium channel mouth. During normal excitation-contraction coupling, calcium also is released from the SR, which further elevates local intracellular Ca^{2+} concentration near the calcium channel. The top I_{Ca} trace in Figure 2-5A reflects conditions under which a normal calcium transient occurs, and I_{Ca} inactivates much faster still ($t_{1/2}$ = 17 ms). This emphasizes that SR Ca^{2+} release also plays a major role in I_{Ca} inactivation in a physiologic setting. Indeed, in action potential clamp experiments, normal SR Ca^{2+} release reduces the integrated Ca^{2+} influx by way of $I_{Ca,L}$ by 50%.[68]

Figure 2-5B shows the E_m dependence of inactivation as a function of E_m.[66] I_{NS} inactivation was incomplete after 500 ms, even at +60 mV. At strong positive E_m (when little calcium enters), little difference is seen between I_{Ca} and I_{NS} inactivation (i.e., it is more purely E_m dependent). The additional I_{Ca} inactivation at intermediate E_m has the same E_m dependence as that for inward I_{Ca} amplitude (e.g., maximal at approximately 0 mV). This fast calcium-dependent inactivation is the overwhelmingly dominant mode of inactivation on the time scale of an action potential and is the main physiologic mechanism of $I_{Ca,L}$ inactivation.

Calcium-dependent inactivation of I_{Ca} provides a sort of feedback control to limit further Ca^{2+} entry. A remarkable feature of the intracellular calcium–dependent inactivation is that it is still readily apparent even when intracellular Ca^{2+} concentration is fairly heavily buffered by EGTA or 1,2-bis (2-aminophenoxy)ethane *N,N,N′,N′*-tetra-acetic acid (BAPTA), which abolishes contraction. This suggested that Ca^{2+} entering by way of I_{Ca} must cause inactivation by acting locally, perhaps before mixing with "bulk" Ca^{2+}. Höfer and colleagues estimated a K_i for intracellular Ca^{2+} concentration of 4 μM based on single calcium channel currents.[69]

It is now clear that calmodulin is centrally involved in mediating calcium-dependent I_{Ca} inactivation.[70,71] Calmodulin appears to be prebound to the calcium channel at rest (before calcium channel activation or local intracellular Ca^{2+} concentration rise) at the C-terminal tail of α_{1C} near the IQ motif and serves as the constituent calcium sensor (see Fig. 2-7).[72,73] When the channel opens, the calcium entering the cell through the channel increases the local Ca^{2+} concentration at the inner mouth of the channel, and Ca^{2+} binds to the high-affinity calcium-binding sites on the C-terminal lobe of calmodulin. Calcium binding of calmodulin leads to a conformational change that relieves the EF-hand–mediated inhibition of the I-II linker, which has been proposed to be the pore occluder.[74]

If voltage clamp pulses (or action potentials) are very long, I_{Ca} can be largely inactivated during the cytosolic calcium transient but then can partly recover as intracellular Ca^{2+} concentration declines.[75] This sort of reactivation of L-type calcium channels during long action potentials may contribute to arrhythmogenic early afterdepolarizations (EADs).[76-78]

Steady-state activation and availability (or inactivation) curves for I_{Ca} in rabbit ventricular myocytes are shown in Figure 2-6A. The calcium channel activation variable (d_∞) starts increasing at approximately −40 mV and is maximal by 0 mV. The inactivation variable (f_∞) begins decreasing at −45 mV and is nearly 0 at −15 mV. The slight overlap of these two curves indicates a "window current." That is, at approximately −28 mV, the conductance is approximately 1% of maximum ($d_\infty \times f_\infty$), such that a steady-state I_{Ca} that is approximately 1% of maximal would flow at this E_m. During action potential repolarization, as E_m enters this shaded region in Figure 2-6A, it is possible (especially with long action potential durations) for some I_{Ca} currents

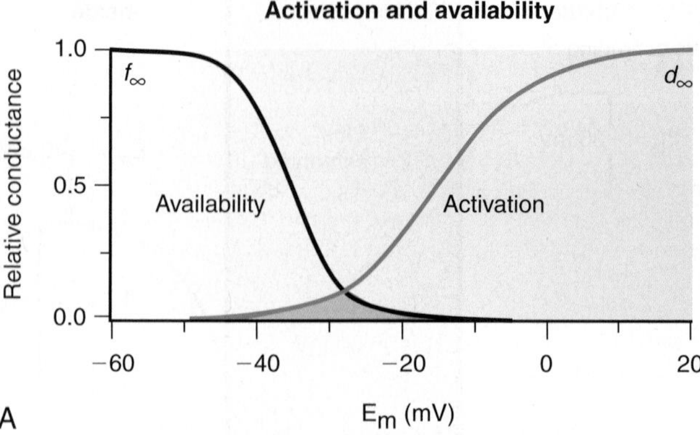

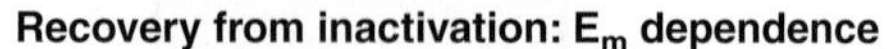

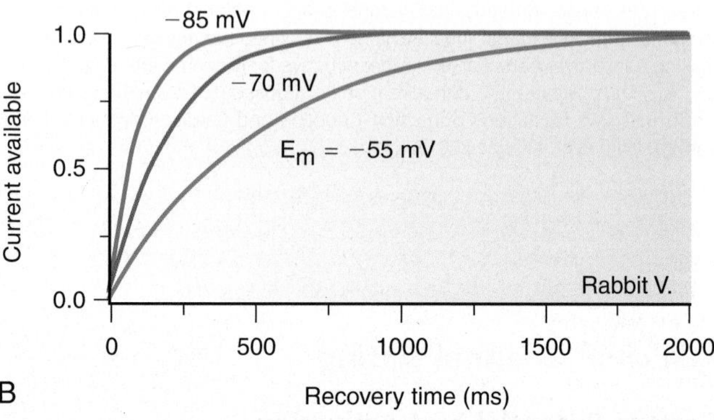

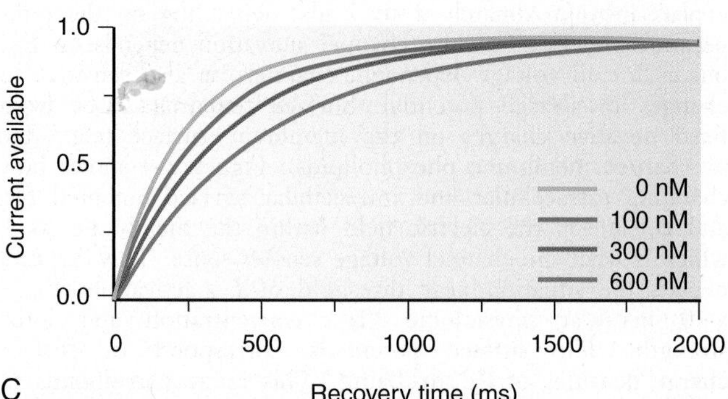

Figure 2-6 Cardiac calcium channel activation, availability, and recovery from inactivation. **A,** I_{Ca} availability is measured by depolarizing from −90 mV to the indicated E_m for 2 seconds and then testing the remaining available I_{Ca} at E_m = 0 mV (extracellular Ca^{2+} concentration = 2 mM). The result is referred to as a steady-state inactivation or availability curve. Activation is measured by dividing the peak current by the apparent driving force ($E_m - E_{rev}$) according to Ohm's law ($G = I/\Delta V$). **B,** Time and E_m dependence of recovery from inactivation of rabbit ventricular I_{Ca}. After a 2-second pulse to +10 mV to induce inactivation, E_m is held at the values indicated for different times before testing I_{Ca} available with a pulse to 0 mV. **C,** $[Ca^{2+}]_i$ dependence of recovery from inactivation of rabbit ventricular I_{Ca}. Recovery from inactivation was measured at 0, 100, 300, and 600 nM intracellular calcium, and holding potential was −70 mV. $[Ca^{2+}]_i$, intracellular calcium concentration. (Data for **A** from Yuan W, Ginsburg KS, Bers DM: Comparison of sarcolemmal calcium channel current in rabbit and rat ventricular myocytes. J Physiol 493:733-746, 1996; data for **B** and for **C** at 2 mM $[Ca^{2+}]_o$ and 23° C from Altamirano J, Bers DM: Effect of intracellular Ca^{2+} and action potential duration on L-type Ca^{2+} channel inactivation and recovery from inactivation in rabbit cardiac myocytes. Am J Physiol Heart Circ Physiol 293:H563-H573, 2007.)

to recover from inactivation and cause net depolarization. This is a leading mechanistic hypothesis for the basis of EADs.

After a calcium channel inactivates, recovery from inactivation also is intracellular calcium– and E_m-dependent.[65] Figure 2-6B shows that recovery is much slower at $E_m = -55$ mV than at −85 mV. This means that calcium channel recovery becomes very fast only as action potential repolarization is nearly complete. At −55 mV it can be appreciated that frequency-dependent accumulation of inactivated channels may occur (e.g., at 1 Hz). This can reduce I_{Ca} in a protocol-dependent way experimentally and in a frequency-dependent way physiologically. At a given E_m, elevated concentration of intracellular Ca^{2+} also slows recovery from inactivation (see Fig. 2-6C). Thus, the combination of slowed (or incomplete) decline in intracellular Ca^{2+}concentration and reduced diastolic interval (due to action potential prolongation and high heart rate), as often occurs in heart failure, would tend to limit I_{Ca} availability. This may contribute to reduced contractility and to the negative force-frequency relationship typically observed in heart failure.[65,79]

Calcium-Dependent I_{Ca} Facilitation or I_{Ca} Staircase

With increased pacing frequency from a holding potential of approximately −40 mV, a progressive decline in I_{Ca} amplitude typically is observed.[80,81] This negative I_{Ca} "staircase" probably reflects incomplete calcium channel recovery from inactivation between pulses (at −40 mV). By contrast, at physiologic holding E_m (−80 mV), a pulse-dependent progressive increase in I_{Ca} amplitude and a prominent slowing of inactivation that accumulates over 5 to 10 pulses at 1 Hz are characteristic.[65,80,82,83] This positive I_{Ca} staircase is calcium-dependent (does not occur with barium current), occurs even without SR Ca^{2+} release, and is mediated by CaMKII-dependent phosphorylation.[13,84-86] This facilitatory effect of Ca^{2+} entry on subsequent I_{Ca} is distinct from but coexists with the intercellular calcium–dependent inactivation described earlier. The physiologic role of this calcium-dependent facilitation is not entirely clear, but it may partly offset direct calcium-dependent inactivation and create calcium channel memory on a time scale of a few seconds. The exact molecular mechanism underlying I_{Ca} facilitation is not fully resolved, but the calmodulin-activating CaMKII in this process is likely to be distinct from the calmodulin involved in calcium-dependent inactivation (Fig. 2-7). Activated CaMKII can associate with multiple CaMKII interaction sites on the C-terminal tail of the α_{1C} subunit adjacent to the calmodulin-binding IQ motif.[87,88] CaMKII phosphorylation sites mediating I_{Ca} facilitation have been described on the N and C termini of the α_{1C} subunit[87] as well as on the accessory β_2 subunit.[58]

Voltage-dependent facilitation of I_{Ca} also has been described for cardiac I_{Ca}.[89-91] This facilitation occurs with pulses to very positive potentials (e.g., greater than +100 mV) and also dissipates extremely rapidly on repolarization to physiologic E_m in ventricular myocytes. Thus, it is less clear that voltage-mediated I_{Ca} facilitation is physiologically important in normal cardiac myocytes.

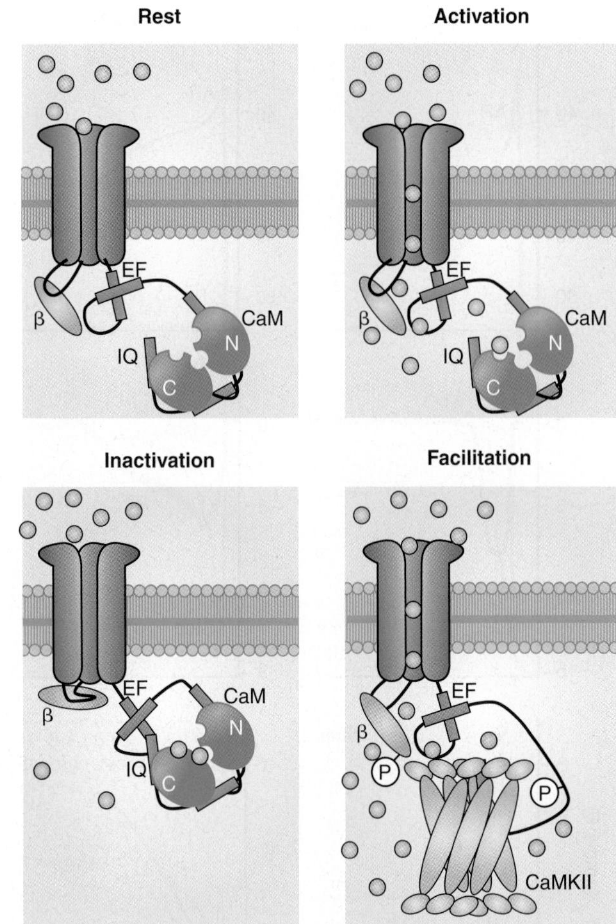

Figure 2-7 Inactivation and facilitation of the cardiac L-type calcium channel (LTCC). At rest, the calcium channel is closed, and calmodulin (CaM) is prebound to the C-terminal end of the α_1 subunit serving as the constituent calcium sensor. On depolarization, Ca^{2+} influx occurs, and calcium binds to the high-affinity calcium-binding sites at the C terminus of calmodulin. A conformational change then relieves the EF-hand–mediated inhibition of the I-II linker, allowing interaction of the I-II linker with the pore and inducing inactivation. Calcium/calmodulin also can activate CaMKII, leading to phosphorylation of the LTCC, thereby slowing inactivation and causing I_{Ca} facilitation. Different CaMKII phosphorylation sites (indicated by encircled P) inducing facilitation have been proposed, including at the α_1 C and N termini, as well as at the β subunit.

Amount of Ca^{2+} Entry through Calcium Channels

Usually, single calcium channel current is recorded at unphysiologically high concentrations of Ca^{2+} or Ba^{2+}. Under more physiologic conditions, single-channel I_{Ca} probably is approximately 0.2 pA in cardiac myocytes. That means that for a typical whole-cell peak I_{Ca} value of 1 nA in physiologic solution, approximately 5000 calcium channels need to be open simultaneously. Approximately 15 calcium channels are present per μm^2 of cell membrane,[92] although these are mainly concentrated in T tubule and at junctional complexes between the sarcolemma and SR (where they play a central role in excitation-contraction coupling). This means that there are approximately 300,000 L-type calcium channels per ventricular myocyte, and that only approximately 3% are open during the peak of measured I_{Ca}.

The quantity and time course of Ca^{2+} entry through I_{Ca} are functionally important with respect to the action potential, excitation-contraction coupling, and calcium requirements for myofilament activation. During a square voltage clamp pulse to 0 mV, the I_{Ca} waveform can be integrated to infer a Ca^{2+} influx of approximately 10 μmol/L of cytosol (this is equivalent to peak I_{Ca} = 1 nA of triangular shape, 120 ms in duration, in a

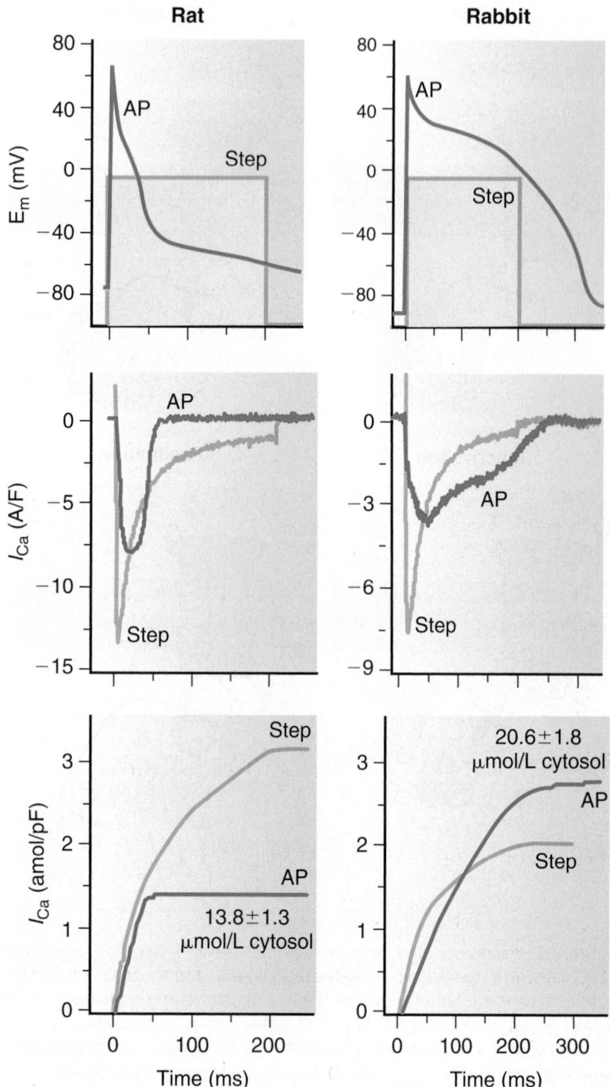

Figure 2-8 I_{Ca} during square pulses and action potentials (APs). Rat and rabbit ventricular myocytes (at 25°C) were voltage clamped with either a square voltage step or an AP waveform. All other currents were blocked (e.g., by replacement of potassium with cesium and of sodium with tetraethylammonium [TEA], inside and outside of the cell), and cells were dialyzed with 10 mM ethylene glycol tetra-acetic acid (EGTA) to prevent calcium transients. Running integrals of calcium influx during AP clamp are shown, along with mean values. (Data from Yuan W, Ginsburg KS, Bers DM: Comparison of sarcolemmal calcium channel current in rabbit and rat ventricular myocytes. J Physiol 493:733-746, 1996.)

myocyte with 30 pL of cytosol). Ca^{2+} influx during the action potential, however, may differ significantly from the usual square pulse. Figure 2-8 compares square pulses and action potential waveforms used as command potentials in voltage clamp.[14,68,93,94] Peak I_{Ca} during the action potential clamp is lower and occurs later than with the square pulse. This is because at the action potential peak (+50 mV), calcium channels activate rapidly, but the driving force for calcium initially is low because E_m is close to the reversal potential for I_{Ca} (approximately +60 mV). As E_m falls, the driving force for I_{Ca} apparently increases faster than the channels inactivate, producing a larger current at later times during the action potential. In rabbit ventricle, I_{Ca} also is more sustained during the action potential than a square pulse. The bottom panels in Figure 2-8 show running integrals of calcium influx. In rat ventricular myocytes, the amount of calcium influx for the same 200-ms square pulse is higher than in rabbit.[14] This is due to species differences in I_{Ca} activation and inactivation. However, the rat ventricular action potential is very brief, and with species-appropriate action potential waveforms, the calcium influx is much higher in rabbit than in rat ventricular myocytes (21 versus 14 μmol/L cytosol).

The I_{Ca} results in Figure 2-8 overestimate physiologic Ca^{2+} influx because I_{Ca} was measured in cells dialyzed with EGTA (which reduces calcium-dependent inactivation of I_{Ca}). Integrated I_{Ca} also was measured during action potential clamp in rabbit ventricular myocyte at 25°C and 35°C, when normal SR Ca^{2+} release occurred, but all other currents, including $I_{Na/Ca}$ and $I_{Cl(Ca)}$, were blocked.[68] For steady-state action potential clamps (and contractions), I_{Ca} peaks earlier and higher at 35°C than at 25°C, but the values for integrated Ca^{2+} influx at the two temperatures are almost the same. Also measured in this experiment was how I_{Ca} changes during action potentials as the SR is refilled (after prior depletion) and contractions recover to steady state. As the contractions and SR Ca^{2+} release got larger, I_{Ca} inactivated more rapidly and completely during the action potential (reducing I_{Ca} especially late in the action potential). At both 25°C and 35°C, integrated I_{Ca} decreased from 12 to 6 μmol/L of cytosol as the SR goes from empty to steady-state loading. This finding indicates that I_{Ca} inactivation due to SR Ca^{2+} release decreases net Ca^{2+} influx by approximately 50% at both temperatures.

The kinetics of the SR Ca^{2+} release–induced I_{Ca} inactivation also provided information about the timing of SR Ca^{2+} release.[68,94] The investigators inferred that the local SR Ca^{2+} release flux sensed by the L-type calcium channel reaches a peak in 5 ms at 25°C (or 2.5 ms at 35°C). This is much faster than the rate of rise of the global cellular calcium transient but is not surprising because SR Ca^{2+} release by way of ryanodine receptors would be expected to occur very near the L-type Ca channel. It also emphasizes that Ca^{2+}-sensitive ionic currents can be excellent sensors of local Ca^{2+} concentration in the cell.

In conclusion, L-type I_{Ca} is the main route of Ca^{2+} entry into the cell (versus leak, Na^+-Ca^+ exchange, or $I_{Ca,T}$). I_{Ca} plays a central role in cardiac electrophysiology, affecting action potential configuration and arrhythmogenesis (by EADs). I_{Ca} also is central to excitation-contraction coupling and overall cellular Ca^{2+} regulation and contraction. The kinetics and amplitude of the I_{Ca} during the action potential are critical factors both in controlling Ca^{2+} released by the SR and in contributing directly to the replenishment of SR Ca^{2+} stores.

References

1. Bers DM: Calcium cycling and signaling in cardiac myocytes. Annu Rev Physiol 70:23-49, 2008.
2. Bodi I, Mikala G, Koch SE, et al: The L-type calcium channel in the heart: The beat goes on. J Clin Invest 115:3306-3317, 2005.
3. Catterall WA: Structure and regulation of voltage-gated Ca^{2+} channels. Annu Rev Cell Dev Biol 16:521-555, 2000.
4. Catterall WA, Perez-Reyes E, Snutch TP, Striessnig J: International Union of Pharmacology. XLVIII. Nomenclature and structure-function relationships of voltage-gated calcium channels. Pharmacol Rev 57:411-425, 2005.
5. Bean BP: Classes of calcium channels in vertebrate cells. Annu Rev Physiol 51:367-384, 1989.
6. Bean BP: Two kinds of calcium channels in canine atrial cells. Differences in kinetics,

selectivity, and pharmacology. J Gen Physiol 86:1-30, 1985.

7. Hirano Y, Fozzard HA, January CT: Characteristics of L- and T-type Ca^{2+} currents in canine cardiac Purkinje cells. Am J Physiol 256:H1478-H1492, 1989.
8. Rosati B, Dun W, Hirose M, et al: Molecular basis of the T- and L-type Ca^{2+} currents in canine Purkinje fibres. J Physiol 579:465-471, 2007.
9. Hagiwara N, Irisawa H, Kameyama M: Contribution of two types of calcium currents to the pacemaker potentials of rabbit sino-atrial node cells. J Physiol 395:233-253, 1988.
10. Mitra R, Morad M: Two types of calcium channels in guinea pig ventricular myocytes. Proc Natl Acad Sci U S A 83:5340-5344, 1986.
11. Niwa N, Yasui K, Opthof T, et al: $Ca_V3.2$ subunit underlies the functional T-type Ca^{2+} channel in murine hearts during the embryonic period. Am J Physiol Heart Circ Physiol 286:H2257-H2263, 2004.
12. Nuss HB, Houser SR: T-type Ca^{2+} current is expressed in hypertrophied adult feline left ventricular myocytes. Circ Res 73:777-782, 1993.
13. Yuan W, Bers DM: Ca-dependent facilitation of cardiac Ca current is due to Ca-calmodulin–dependent protein kinase. Am J Physiol 267:H982-H993, 1994.
14. Yuan W, Ginsburg KS, Bers DM: Comparison of sarcolemmal calcium channel current in rabbit and rat ventricular myocytes. J Physiol 493:733-746, 1996.
15. Skasa M, Jüngling E, Picht E, et al: L-type calcium currents in atrial myocytes from patients with persistent and non-persistent atrial fibrillation. Basic Res Cardiol 96:151-159, 2001.
16. Cribbs LL, Martin BL, Schroder EA, et al: Identification of the t-type calcium channel ($Ca_V3.1d$) in developing mouse heart. Circ Res 88:403-407, 2001.
17. Gaughan JP, Hefner CA, Houser SR: Electrophysiological properties of neonatal rat ventricular myocytes with α_1-adrenergic-induced hypertrophy. Am J Physiol 275:H577-H590, 1998.
18. Wetzel GT, Chen F, Klitzner TS: Ca^{2+} channel kinetics in acutely isolated fetal, neonatal, and adult rabbit cardiac myocytes. Circ Res 72:1065-1074, 1993.
19. Martinez ML, Heredia MP, Delgado C: Expression of T-type Ca^{2+} channels in ventricular cells from hypertrophied rat hearts. J Mol Cell Cardiol 31:1617-1625, 1999.
20. Chen X, Wilson RM, Kubo H, et al: Adolescent feline heart contains a population of small, proliferative ventricular myocytes with immature physiological properties. Circ Res 100:536-544, 2007.
21. Jeong SW, Wurster RD: Calcium channel currents in acutely dissociated intracardiac neurons from adult rats. J Neurophysiol 77:1769-1778, 1997.
22. Lipsius SL, Huser J, Blatter LA: Intracellular Ca^{2+} release sparks atrial pacemaker activity. News Physiol Sci 16:101-106, 2001.
23. Mangoni ME, Couette B, Marger L, et al: Voltage-dependent calcium channels and cardiac pacemaker activity: From ionic currents to genes. Prog Biophys Mol Biol 90:38-63, 2006.
24. Adams PJ, Snutch TP: Calcium channelopathies: Voltage-gated calcium channels. In Carafoli E, Brini M (eds): Calcium Signalling and Disease. New York, Springer, 2007, pp 215-251.
25. Bidaud I, Mezghrani A, Swayne LA, et al: Voltage-gated calcium channels in genetic diseases. Biochim Biophys Acta 1763:1169-1174, 2006.
26. Splawski I, Timothy KW, Decher N, et al: Severe arrhythmia disorder caused by cardiac L-type calcium channel mutations. Proc Natl Acad Sci U S A 102:8089-8096, 2005.
27. Splawski I, Timothy KW, Sharpe LM, et al: $Ca_V1.2$ calcium channel dysfunction causes a multisystem disorder including arrhythmia and autism. Cell 119:19-31, 2004.
28. Bosse E, Regulla S, Biel M, et al: The cDNA and deduced amino acid sequence of the γ subunit of the L-type calcium channel from rabbit skeletal muscle. FEBS Lett 267:153-156, 1990.
29. Ellis SB, Williams ME, Ways NR, et al: Sequence and expression of mRNAs encoding the α_1 and α_2 subunits of a DHP-sensitive calcium channel. Science 241:1661-1664, 1988.
30. Jay SD, Ellis SB, McCue AF, et al: Primary structure of the γ subunit of the DHP-sensitive calcium channel from skeletal muscle. Science 248:490-492, 1990.
31. Ruth P, Rohrkasten A, Biel M, et al: Primary structure of the β subunit of the DHP-sensitive calcium channel from skeletal muscle. Science 245:1115-1118, 1989.
32. Tanabe T, Takeshima H, Mikami A, et al: Primary structure of the receptor for calcium channel blockers from skeletal muscle. Nature 328:313-318, 1987.
33. Mikami A, Imoto K, Tanabe T, et al: Primary structure and functional expression of the cardiac dihydropyridine-sensitive calcium channel. Nature 340:230-233, 1989.
34. Hulme JT, Lin TW, Westenbroek RE, et al: β-Adrenergic regulation requires direct anchoring of PKA to cardiac $Ca_V1.2$ channels via a leucine zipper interaction with A kinase–anchoring protein 15. Proc Natl Acad Sci U S A 100:13093-13098, 2003.
35. Hulme JT, Yarov-Yarovoy V, Lin TW, et al: Autoinhibitory control of the $Ca_V1.2$ channel by its proteolytically processed distal C-terminal domain. J Physiol 576:87-102, 2006.
36. Gomez-Ospina N, Tsuruta F, Barreto-Chang O, et al: The C terminus of the L-type voltage-gated calcium channel $Ca_V1.2$ encodes a transcription factor. Cell 127:591-606, 2006.
37. Abernethy DR, Soldatov NM: Structure-functional diversity of human L-type Ca^{2+} channel: perspectives for new pharmacological targets. J Pharmacol Exp Ther 300:724-728, 2002.
38. Tang ZZ, Liang MC, Lu S, et al: Transcript scanning reveals novel and extensive splice variations in human l-type voltage-gated calcium channel, $Ca_V1.2$ α_1 subunit. J Biol Chem 279:44335-44343, 2004.
39. Takimoto K, Li D, Nerbonne JM, Levitan ES: Distribution, splicing and glucocorticoid-induced expression of cardiac α_{1C} and α_{1D} voltage-gated Ca^{2+} channel mRNAs. J Mol Cell Cardiol 29:3035-3042, 1997.
40. Wyatt CN, Campbell V, Brodbeck J, et al: Voltage-dependent binding and calcium channel current inhibition by an anti-α_{1D} subunit antibody in rat dorsal root ganglion neurones and guinea-pig myocytes. J Physiol 502:307-319, 1997.
41. Zhang Z, Xu Y, Song H, et al: Functional roles of $Ca_V1.3$ (α_{1D}) calcium channel in sinoatrial nodes: Insight gained using gene-targeted null mutant mice. Circ Res 90:981-987, 2002.
42. Xu W, Lipscombe D: Neuronal $Ca_V1.3\alpha_1$ L-type channels activate at relatively hyperpolarized membrane potentials and are incompletely inhibited by dihydropyridines. J Neurosci 21:5944-5951, 2001.
43. Huser J, Blatter LA, Lipsius SL: Intracellular Ca^{2+} release contributes to automaticity in cat atrial pacemaker cells. J Physiol 524:415-422, 2000.
44. Lipsius SL, Bers DM: Cardiac pacemaking: I_f vs. Ca^{2+}, is it really that simple? J Mol Cell Cardiol 35:891-893, 2003.
45. Jay SD, Sharp AH, Kahl SD, et al: Structural characterization of the dihydropyridine-sensitive calcium channel α_2-subunit and the associated δ peptides. J Biol Chem 266:3287-3293, 1991.
46. Bangalore R, Mehrke G, Gingrich K, et al: Influence of L-type Ca channel a_2/δ-subunit on ionic and gating current in transiently transfected HEK 293 cells. Am J Physiol 270:H1521-H1528, 1996.
47. Singer D, Biel M, Lotan I, et al: The roles of the subunits in the function of the calcium channel. Science 253:1553-1557, 1991.
48. Wei X, Pan S, Lang W, et al: Molecular determinants of cardiac Ca^{2+} channel pharmacology. Subunit requirement for the high affinity and allosteric regulation of dihydropyridine binding. J Biol Chem 270:27106-27111, 1995.
49. Felix R: Voltage-dependent Ca^{2+} channel $a_2\delta$ auxiliary subunit: Structure, function and regulation. Receptors Channels 6:351-362, 1999.
50. Arikkath J, Campbell KP: Auxiliary subunits: Essential components of the voltage-gated calcium channel complex. Curr Opin Neurobiol 13:298-307, 2003.
51. Mitterdorfer J, Froschmayr M, Grabner M, et al: Calcium channels: The β-subunit increases the affinity of dihydropyridine and Ca^{2+} binding sites of the α_1-subunit. FEBS Lett 352:141-145, 1994.
52. Neely A, Wei X, Olcese R, et al: Potentiation by the β subunit of the ratio of the ionic current to the charge movement in the cardiac calcium channel. Science 262:575-578, 1993.
53. Perez-Reyes E, Castellano A, Kim HS, et al: Cloning and expression of a cardiac/brain β subunit of the L-type calcium channel. J Biol Chem 267:1792-1797, 1992.

54. De Waard M, Pragnell M, Campbell KP: Ca^{2+} channel regulation by a conserved β subunit domain. Neuron 13:495-503, 1994.
55. Pragnell M, De WM, Mori Y, et al: Calcium channel β-subunit binds to a conserved motif in the I-II cytoplasmic linker of the α_1-subunit. Nature 368:67-70, 1994.
56. Van Petegem F, Clark KA, Chatelain FC, Minor DL Jr: Structure of a complex between a voltage-gated calcium channel β-subunit and an α-subunit domain. Nature 429:671-675, 2004.
57. Bichet D, Cornet V, Geib S, et al: The I-II loop of the Ca^{2+} channel α_1 subunit contains an endoplasmic reticulum retention signal antagonized by the β subunit. Neuron 25:177-190, 2000.
58. Grueter CE, Abiria SA, Dzhura I, et al: L-type Ca^{2+} channel facilitation mediated by phosphorylation of the β subunit by CaMKII. Mol Cell 23:641-650, 2006.
59. Wang MC, Collins RF, Ford RC, et al: The three-dimensional structure of the cardiac L-type voltage-gated calcium channel: Comparison with the skeletal muscle form reveals a common architectural motif. J Biol Chem 279:7159-7168, 2004.
60. Perez-Reyes E: Molecular characterization of T-type calcium channels. Cell Calcium 40:89-96, 2006.
61. Talavera K, Nilius B: Biophysics and structure-function relationship of T-type Ca^{2+} channels. Cell Calcium 40:97-114, 2006.
62. McCleskey EW, Almers W: The Ca channel in skeletal muscle is a large pore. Proc Natl Acad Sci U S A 82:7149-7153, 1985.
63. Chen XH, Tsien RW: Aspartate substitutions establish the concerted action of P-region glutamates in repeats I and III in forming the protonation site of L-type Ca^{2+} channels. J Biol Chem 272:30002-30008, 1997.
64. Sather WA, McCleskey EW: Permeation and selectivity in calcium channels. Annu Rev Physiol 65:133-159, 2003.
65. Altamirano J, Bers DM: Effect of intracellular Ca^{2+} and action potential duration on L-type Ca^{2+} channel inactivation and recovery from inactivation in rabbit cardiac myocytes. Am J Physiol Heart Circ Physiol 293:H563-H573, 2007.
66. Hadley RW, Hume JR: An intrinsic potential-dependent inactivation mechanism associated with calcium channels in guinea-pig myocytes. J Physiol 389:205-222, 1987.
67. Kass RS, Sanguinetti MC: Inactivation of calcium channel current in the calf cardiac Purkinje fiber. Evidence for voltage- and calcium-mediated mechanisms. J Gen Physiol 84:705-726, 1984.
68. Puglisi JL, Yuan W, Bassani JW, Bers DM: Ca^{2+} influx through Ca^{2+} channels in rabbit ventricular myocytes during action potential clamp: Influence of temperature. Circ Res 85:e7-e16, 1999.
69. Hofer GF, Hohenthanner K, Baumgartner W, et al: Intracellular Ca^{2+} inactivates L-type Ca^{2+} channels with a Hill coefficient of approximately 1 and an inhibition constant of approximately 4 microM by reducing channel's open probability. Biophys J 73:1857-1865, 1997.
70. Peterson BZ, DeMaria CD, Adelman JP, Yue DT: Calmodulin is the Ca^{2+} sensor for Ca^{2+} -dependent inactivation of L-type calcium channels. Neuron 22:549-558, 1999.
71. Zuhlke RD, Pitt GS, Deisseroth K, et al: Calmodulin supports both inactivation and facilitation of L-type calcium channels. Nature 399:159-162, 1999.
72. Erickson MG, Alseikhan BA, Peterson BZ, Yue DT: Preassociation of calmodulin with voltage-gated Ca^{2+} channels revealed by FRET in single living cells. Neuron 31:973-985, 2001.
73. Pitt GS, Zuhlke RD, Hudmon A, et al: Molecular basis of calmodulin tethering and Ca^{2+}-dependent inactivation of L-type Ca^{2+} channels. J Biol Chem 276:30794-30802, 2001.
74. Kim J, Ghosh S, Nunziato DA, Pitt GS: Identification of the components controlling inactivation of voltage-gated Ca^{2+} channels. Neuron 41:745-754, 2004.
75. Sipido KR, Callewaert G, Carmeliet E: Inhibition and rapid recovery of Ca^{2+} current during Ca^{2+} release from sarcoplasmic reticulum in guinea pig ventricular myocytes. Circ Res 76:102-109, 1995.
76. January CT, Riddle JM: Early afterdepolarizations: Mechanism of induction and block. A role for L-type Ca^{2+} current. Circ Res 64:977-990, 1989.
77. Tanskanen AJ, Greenstein JL, O'Rourke B, Winslow RL: The role of stochastic and modal gating of cardiac L-type Ca^{2+} channels on early after-depolarizations. Biophys J 88:85-95, 2005.
78. Ter Keurs HE, Boyden PA: Calcium and arrhythmogenesis. Physiol Rev 87:457-506, 2007.
79. Hasenfuss G, Pieske B: Calcium cycling in congestive heart failure. J Mol Cell Cardiol 34:951-969, 2002.
80. Hryshko LV, Bers DM: Ca current facilitation during postrest recovery depends on Ca entry. Am J Physiol 259:H951-H961, 1990.
81. Tseng GN: Calcium current restitution in mammalian ventricular myocytes is modulated by intracellular calcium. Circ Res 63:468-482, 1988.
82. Picht E, DeSantiago J, Huke S, et al: CaMKII inhibition targeted to the sarcoplasmic reticulum inhibits frequency-dependent acceleration of relaxation and Ca^{2+} current facilitation. J Mol Cell Cardiol 42:196-205, 2007.
83. Zygmunt AC, Maylie J: Stimulation-dependent facilitation of the high threshold calcium current in guinea-pig ventricular myocytes. J Physiol 428:653-671, 1990.
84. Anderson ME, Braun AP, Schulman H, Premack BA: Multifunctional Ca^{2+}/calmodulin-dependent protein kinase mediates Ca^{2+}-induced enhancement of the L-type Ca^{2+} current in rabbit ventricular myocytes. Circ Res 75:854-861, 1994.
85. Dzhura I, Wu Y, Colbran RJ, et al: Calmodulin kinase determines calcium-dependent facilitation of L-type calcium channels. Nat Cell Biol 2:173-177, 2000.
86. Xiao RP, Cheng H, Lederer WJ, et al: Dual regulation of Ca^{2+}/calmodulin-dependent kinase II activity by membrane voltage and by calcium influx. Proc Natl Acad Sci U S A 91:9659-9663, 1994.
87. Hudmon A, Schulman H, Kim J, et al: CaMKII tethers to L-type Ca^{2+} channels, establishing a local and dedicated integrator of Ca^{2+} signals for facilitation. J Cell Biol 171:537-547, 2005.
88. Pitt GS: Calmodulin and CaMKII as molecular switches for cardiac ion channels. Cardiovasc Res 73:641-647, 2007.
89. Kamp TJ, Hu H, Marban E: Voltage-dependent facilitation of cardiac L-type Ca channels expressed in HEK-293 cells requires β-subunit. Am J Physiol Heart Circ Physiol 278:H126-H136, 2000.
90. Lee TS, Karl R, Moosmang S, et al: Calmodulin kinase II is involved in voltage-dependent facilitation of the L-type $Ca_V1.2$ calcium channel: Identification of the phosphorylation sites. J Biol Chem 281:25560-25567, 2006.
91. Sculptoreanu A, Rotman E, Takahashi M, et al: Voltage-dependent potentiation of the activity of cardiac L-type calcium channel α_1 subunits due to phosphorylation by cAMP-dependent protein kinase. Proc Natl Acad Sci U S A 90:10135-10139, 1993.
92. Lew WY, Hryshko LV, Bers DM: Dihydropyridine receptors are primarily functional L-type calcium channels in rabbit ventricular myocytes. Circ Res 69:1139-1145, 1991.
93. Grantham CJ, Cannell MB: Ca^{2+} influx during the cardiac action potential in guinea pig ventricular myocytes. Circ Res 79:194-200, 1996.
94. Linz KW, Meyer R: Control of L-type calcium current during the action potential of guinea-pig ventricular myocytes. J Physiol 513:425-442, 1998.
95. Durell SR, Hao Y, Guy HR: Structural models of the transmembrane region of voltage-gated and other K^+ channels in open, closed, and inactivated conformations. J Struct Biol 121:263-284, 1998.
96. Bers DM: Excitation-Contraction Coupling and Cardiac Contractile Force, 2nd ed. Dordrecht, Kluwer, 2001.

Voltage-Regulated Potassium Channels 3

Gavin Y. Oudit and Peter H. Backx

CHAPTER OUTLINE

The cardiac action potential profile is governed by the complex interaction between depolarizing inward currents and repolarizing outward currents. Repolarizing currents originate primarily from potassium channels, although currents generated by the Na^+-Ca^{2+} exchanger and the Na^+,K^+-ATPase also make small contributions (Fig. 3-1). Cardiac potassium channels are divided into three main categories: voltage-gated (K_V) currents, inward rectifiers, and background potassium currents. Specific subunits of these currents, discussed later on, are listed in Table 3-1 (see also Fig. 3-1). Quantitative and qualitative variations in the expression and biophysical properties of voltage-regulated potassium channels appear to be largely responsible for action potential differences, observed during development, between regions of the heart and between normal and diseased myocardium.

Cardiac voltage-regulated potassium channels are dynamic macromolecular structures consisting of four α subunits (pore-forming) assembled with a variety of accessory subunits, the cytoskeleton, and various signaling complexes (Fig. 3-2; Table 3-2). Functional changes in these channels lead to the modulation of the electrical and contractile properties of the heart and are the molecular targets of various pharmacologic agents, such as class III antiarrhythmic drugs. Mutations in these channels are associated with a number of cardiovascular disorders, including the long QT syndromes.

Dr. Backx's research for this chapter was supported by operating grants from the Canadian Institutes for Health Research; funds for equipment from the Tiffin Trust and the Heart & Stroke/Richard Lewar Centre (HSRLC) are gratefully acknowledged. Dr. Oudit's work also was supported by the Canadian Institutes for Health Research and by the Heart & Stroke Foundation of Canada.

Biophysical Properties of Voltage-Gated Potassium Channels

Voltage-gated potassium (K_V) channels consist of a tetrameric assembly of α subunits. Each α subunit contains six membrane-spanning segments, S1 to S6, with both amino (N) and carboxyl (C) termini located on the intracellular side of the membrane. Segments S1 to S4 confer voltage-sensing properties to these channels, whereas S5 and S6 are critical for forming the channel pore (Fig. 3-3; see also Fig. 3-2). K_V channels typically fluctuate stochastically between open conducting (activated) conformational state(s) and nonconducting conformational state(s), with the kinetics of the transitions depending critically on membrane voltage and channel structure (see Fig. 3-4F). Nonconducting states can be classified as either closed (deactivated) or inactivated states. Typically, during the course of an action potential, closed K_V channels activate or open in response to membrane depolarization and subsequently enter the inactivated state in a time-dependent manner. Reentry into the closed state requires membrane repolarization. The voltage- and time-dependent transition between these different conformational functional states is referred to as *gating*. The molecular mechanisms and regulation of channel gating vary widely among the different K_V channels.

Mechanism of Activation Gating

The central feature of K_V channel activation (opening) (as with voltage-dependent sodium and calcium channels) is a temporal coupling of a voltage sensor to the movement of an "activation gate." The voltage sensor resides in the highly conserved fourth transmembrane segment (S4)[1] of the α subunits which have positively charged arginine or lysine residues at every third or fourth position (see Fig. 3-3A). Previous models predict that the S4 segment is embedded in a protein-lined canal formed by the other transmembrane helices, thereby sequestering the gating charges away from the low-dielectric membrane environment.[2-4] More recent studies have established that these voltage sensors appear as "paddle structures" formed by an antiparallel arrangement of the S3 and S4 segments, with several of the gating charges directly exposed to lipid environment, apparently at the charged interface between the membrane and the aqueous phase.[5-9] This arrangement of voltage sensors explains the important effects of membrane lipid composition on voltage-dependent channel function.[10] Channel activation following depolarization involves relatively large displacements of S4 leading to channel opening by means of direct coupling between the S4-S5 linker region and the C-terminal end of S6,[1] which along with S5 lines the intracellular vestibule of the channel pore, resulting in a very short selectivity filter (see Fig. 3-3B).[1,11] The C-terminal segment of S6 contains a highly conserved proline sequence (PxP or PxG), which is critically involved in coupling movement of the voltage sensor to channel opening.[1] Once channel opening has occurred, K^+ ions are able to rapidly traverse the membrane, whereas large organic

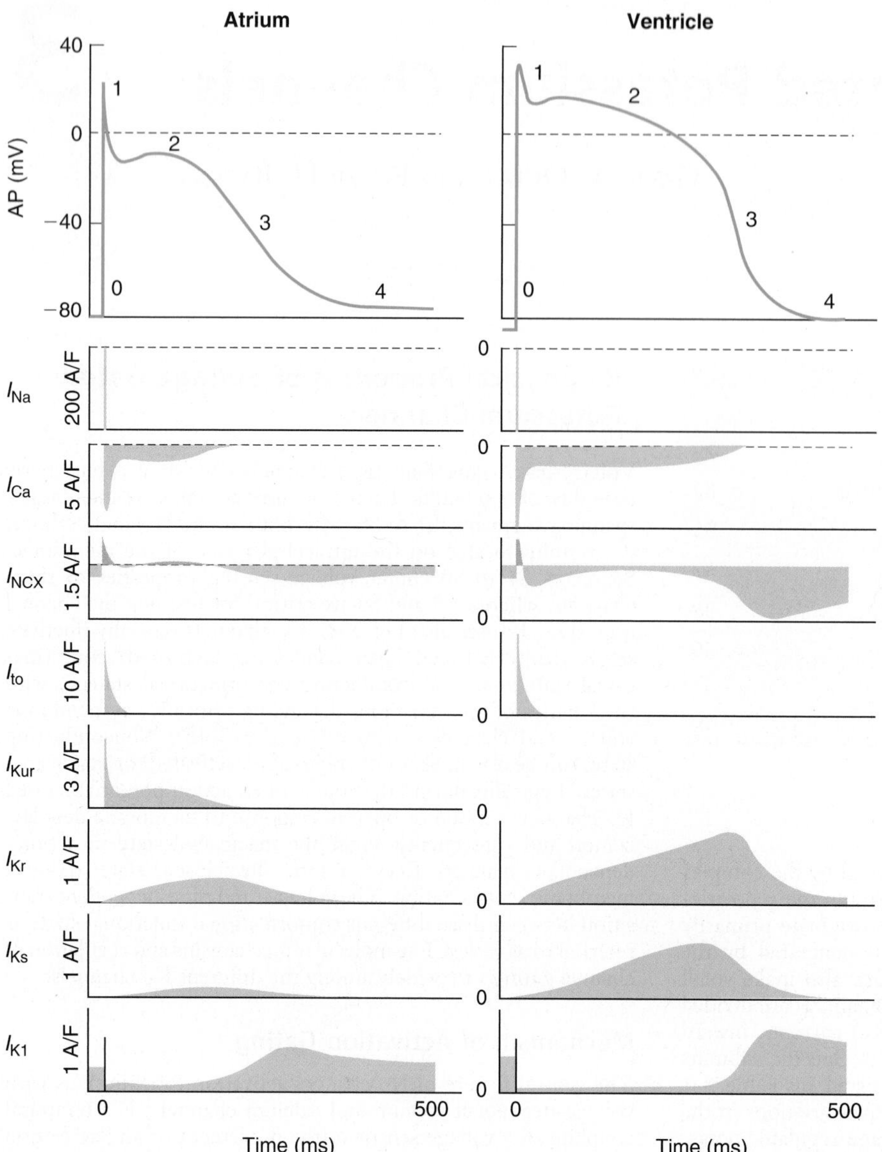

Figure 3-1 Representative cardiac action potential (AP) waveforms, from atrial *(left)* and ventricular *(right)* myocytes. **Top panel,** The five phases of the AP are labeled: 0, upstroke of the AP, representing depolarization of the membrane; 1, initial repolarization; 2, plateau phase; 3, late repolarization phase; and 4, the resting (diastolic) phase. **Lower panels,** The rate of change of the AP is directly proportional to the sum of the underlying transmembrane ion currents. Inward currents (currents below the line) depolarize the membrane; outward currents (currents above the line) contribute to repolarization. Compared with an atrial AP, the ventricular AP typically has a longer duration, higher plateau potential (phase 2), and a more negative resting membrane potential (phase 4). The presence of an ultrarapid delayed rectifier potassium current (I_{Kur}) in atrial myocytes contributes to the lower plateau phase in the atrial AP. Greater inward rectifier potassium current (I_{K1}) in ventricular cells provides a faster phase 3 repolarization and a more negative resting membrane potential (phase 4). A/F, ampere/farad; I_{Na}, Na^+ current; I_{Ca}, Ca^{2+} current; I_{NCX}, NCX current; I_{to}, transient outward K^+ current; I_{Kur}, ultrarapid delayed rectifier K^+ current; I_{Kr}, rapid delayed rectifier K^+ current; I_{Ks}, slow delayed rectifier K^+ current; I_{Ki}, inward rectifier K^+ current; NCX, Na^+-Ca^{2+} exchanger.

cations, drugs, and inactivation particles are permitted to enter, and bind to the intracellular face of, the pore.

Selectivity Filter and Permeation Pore

Potassium channels catalyze selective transport of K^+ ions across lipid bilayers at near diffusion-limited rates while remaining largely impermeable to other biologic cations. The pore of K_V channels is formed by the S5 and S6 transmembrane domains along with their linker region (P loop), which are contributed symmetrically from each subunit, as observed in the KcsA potassium channel (see Fig. 3-3A).[12] The overall length of the pore is approximately 4.5 nm. The pore itself consists of four parts (from inside to outside): a cytoplasmic tunnel that splays open during activation, a large water-filled central cavity (1 nm in diameter), a narrow selectivity filter, and a wide, shallow extracellular vestibule (see Fig. 3-3B). The narrow selectivity filter is largely formed by the carbonyl backbone of residues, with their oxygen atoms pointing inward toward the ion conduction pathway (from inside to outside): threonine-X-glycine-tyrosine-glycine (TXGYG) (i.e., the "signature sequence"), where X represents a variable residue and the GYG sequence is an absolute requirement for K^+ selectivity (see Fig. 3-3B).[12] These carbonyl oxygens in the signature sequence from the four α subunits are symmetrically positioned and rigidly and spatially arranged to allow optimal interaction with K^+ ions, although other channel domains can modulate the structural rigidity of this region, thereby altering channel selectivity.

Inactivation Gating

Inactivation is a feature of many voltage-gated potassium channels and refers to the process whereby channel opening after depolarization leads to a conformational transition to a stable nonconducting state that is distinct from the closed state. Inactivated channels generally are incapable of reopening again unless the membrane potential is repolarized, allowing channels to "recover" back to the closed state (see Fig. 3-4F). Three types of distinct conformation-related changes have been identified with inactivation gating of K_V channels: N-type, C-type, and U-type inactivation.

3

Table 3-1 α (Pore-Forming) Subunits of Cardiac Potassium Channels

Current	Description	Gene(s)	AP Phase	Activation Mechanism	Clone	Molecular Structure/ Assembly
$I_{to,f}$	Transient outward current, fast	*KCND2* *KCND3*	Phase 1	Voltage (depolarization)	K_V4.2/4.3	Single-pore; 6 TM domains; tetramer
$I_{to,c}$	Transient outward current, slow	*KCNA4* *KCNA7* *KCNC4*	Phase 1	Voltage (depolarization)	K_V1.4/1.7/3.4	Single-pore; 6 TM domains; tetramer
I_{Kur}	Ultrarapid delayed rectifier	*KCNA5* *KCNC1*	Phase 2	Voltage (depolarization)	K_V1.5/3.1	Single-pore; 6 TM domains; tetramer
I_{Kr}	Rapid delayed rectifier	*KCNH2*	Phase 3	Voltage (depolarization)	HERG	Single-pore; 6 TM domains; tetramer
I_{Ks}	Slow delayed rectifier	*KCNQ1*	Phase 3	Voltage (depolarization)	K_VLQT1	Single-pore; 6 TM domains; tetramer
I_{K1}	Inward rectifier, strong	*KCNJ2* *KCNJ12*	Phases 3 and 4	Voltage (depolarization)	Kir2.1/2.2	Single-pore; 2 TM domains; tetramer
I_{KATP}	ADP-activated potassium channel*	*KCNJ11*	Phases 1 and 2	Increased ADP/ATP ratio (ATP depletion)	Kir6.2 (+ SUR2A)	Single-pore; 2 TM domains; tetramer
I_{KACh}	M2 receptor—gated potassium channel* †	*KCNJ3* *KCNJ5*	Phase 4	Acetylcholine (vagal tone)	Kir3.1/3.4	Single-pore; 2 TM domains; tetramer
I_{Kp}	Background potassium channels	*KCNK1/6* *KCNK3* *KCNK4*	All phases	Metabolic parameters Membrane stretch	TWIK-1/2* TASK-1 TRAAK	Single-pore; 4 TM domains; dimer
I_h	Pacemaker channel‡	*HCN2* *HCN4*	Phase 4	Voltage (hyperpolarization)	HCN2/4	Single-pore; 6 TM domains; tetramer

ADP, adenine diphosphate; AP, action potential; ATP, adenine triphosphate; SUR2A, sulfonylurea receptor isoform 2A (forms octameric complex with Kir6.2 subunits); TM, transmembrane.

*Weak inward rectifiers.

†Muscarinic receptor (type 2) in atrial and nodal cells.

‡Nonselective (permeates both Na^+ and K^+ ions), with HCN2 and four isoforms being present in myocytes and nodal cells.

N-Type Inactivation: Ball and Chain Gating

N-type inactivation was first described in Shaker K_V channels and was found to satisfy many of the tenets of the "ball-and-chain" mechanism including its rapid kinetics. In this type of inactivation, the N-terminal domain (inactivation "ball" tethered to a "chain") binds to its receptor on the inner vestibule of the channel, thereby physically blocking the pore,[13] as originally described in squid axon sodium currents.[14] Inactivation domains are contributed by either the pore-forming α subunit or certain auxiliary β subunits.[1,13] Because of the steric hindrance posed by the β subunit–T1 domain ($T1_4\beta_4$) on the intracellular side of the pore (see Fig. 3-3C), inactivation peptides appear to gain access to the channel pore through lateral openings between the cytoplasmic domains of the four α subunits.[15] Despite evidence for occlusion of the inner vestibule, it is clear that the process of N-terminal interaction with the channel allosterically catalyzes additional molecular changes identified as C-type inactivation.

C-Type Inactivation: Molecular Transitions in the Selectivity Region

A second mechanism for channel inactivation involves conformational changes in the outer mouth of the pore called C-type inactivation.[1,13] C-type inactivation can be strongly accelerated by N-type inactivation but persists in K_V1.x channels when the inactivation "ball" is deleted. Distinct from N-type inactivation, C-type inactivation is sensitive to extracellular K^+ concentration and mutations at the extracellular entryway to the pore and also may underlie a physiologic response to accumulation of extracellular K^+.[1,13] This inactivation process (normally slower than N-type inactivation) functions by regulating repetitive electrical activity, while its sensitivity to K^+ concentration confers a physiologic sensitivity to accumulation of extracellular K^+.

U-Type Inactivation

In addition to N- and C-type inactivation, K_V1.x channels also show a U-shaped voltage dependence of inactivation with prolonged stimulation rates.[16,17] Specifically, long depolarizations above 0 mV favor entry into the U-type inactivated conformation, which recovers rapidly back to the closed state. Moreover, the fraction of channels in a U-type inactivated state is increased by extracellular tetraethylammonium (TEA) and high extracellular K^+ concentration.[16,17] Although the fundamental conformational changes underlying U-type inactivation remain unclear, the cytosolic T1 domain of K_V channels appears to be intimately involved. Mechanisms underlying U-type inactivation play an important physiologic role in ion channel function.[16,17]

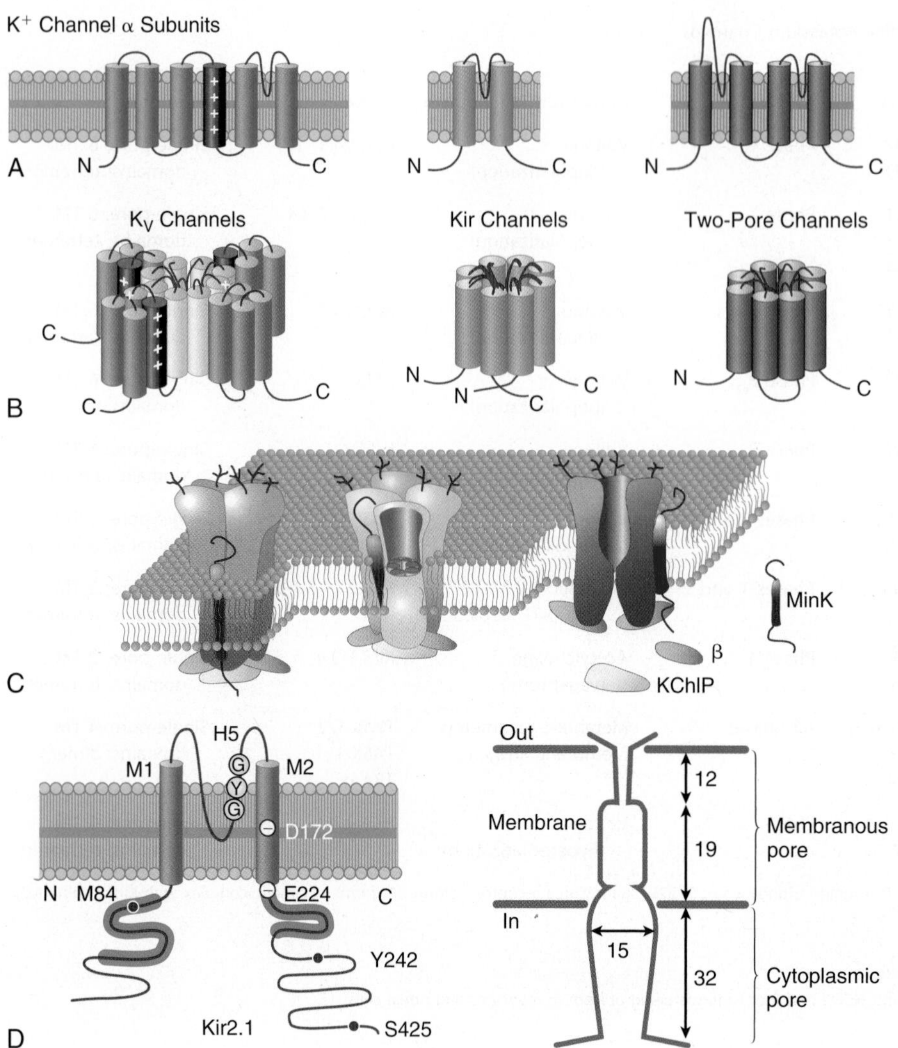

Figure 3-2 Molecular composition of cardiac potassium channels. **A** and **B,** Amino termini (N) and carboxyl termini (C) are indicated. **A,** K_V, Kir, and two-pore α subunits are integral membrane proteins with six, two, and four membrane-spanning domains, respectively. **B,** These α subunits assemble as tetramers or dimers to form K^+-selective pores. **C,** Accessory subunits such as the intracellular K_V β subunit and KChIP2 and the transmembrane MinK also contribute to the formation of functional cardiac potassium channels. **D,** Schematic of Kir2.1 topology (M1 and M2 membrane-spanning segments and the connecting H5 pore-forming loop), with key amino acid residues shown. D172 (aspartate) and E224 (glutamate) residues are critical for the strong inward rectification of the Kir2.x channels, and the *green* regions are involved in the formation of the cytoplasmic pore *(left)* and geometry of the ion conduction pathway in Kir2.x channels. M84 (methionine), Y242 (tyrosine), and S425 (serine) are also important for channel activity. Selectivity filter, 1.2 nm; inner pore, 1.9 nm; cytoplasmic pore, 3.2 nm (maximum diameter of the cytoplasmic pore is 1.5 nm) *(right)*. (**D,** Modified from Nishida M, MacKinnon R: Structural basis of inward rectification. Cytoplasmic pore of the G protein–gated inward rectifier GIRK1 at 1.8 Å resolution. Cell 111:957-965, 2002.)

Subunits of Voltage-Gated Potassium Channels

α Pore-Forming Subunits

Voltage-regulated potassium channel α subunits are transmembrane pore-forming proteins that assemble as tetramers with accessory subunits to form functional potassium channels. After the identification of four *Drosophila* subfamilies of K_V channels (Shaker, Shab, Shaw, Shal), homologous families of α subunits were uncovered in mammals: K_V1.x (*KCNA*), K_V2.x (*KCNB*), K_V3.x (*KCNC*), and K_V4.x (*KCND*); members of the K_V5, K_V6, K_V8, and K_V9 subfamilies do not express currents by themselves and are thought to regulate the activity of the other K_V subfamilies.[18,19] The pore-forming α subunit (K_V α) contains six transmembrane domains (S1-S6) flanked by cytoplasmic amino and carboxyl termini (see Figs. 3-2 and 3-3A). Most evidence suggests that only K_Vα belonging to the same subfamily (K_V1.x, K_V2.x, K_V3.x, and K_V4.x) can coassemble as heteromultimers to form a functional channel which depends critically on a highly conserved 120-amino-acid N-terminal region called T1 or Nab domain.[18,19] Assembly of four K_V α subunits from the K_V1.x and K_V4.x subfamilies forms the slow ($I_{to,s}$) and fast ($I_{to,f}$) components of the transient outward K^+ current, respectively (see Figs. 3-2 and 3-3A and Table 3-1).[18,19] K_V1.5 α subunits, which encode the ultrarapid delayed rectifier current (I_{Kur}), coassemble to form a tetramer with similar topology and organization to those of the I_{to}-encoding K_V1.4 and K_V4.x subunits (see Figs. 3-2 and 3-3A and Table 3-1).[20,21] The distribution of I_{to}-encoding K_V channels in the sarcolemmae is heterogeneous and tissue-specific. In atrial myocytes, K_V4.2 is located in the peripheral sarcolemmae and intercalated disks, whereas in ventricular myocytes, K_V4.2 is found predominantly in the transverse-axial tubular system.[22] Membrane-targeting signals that are responsible for differential targeting and glycosylation of the K_V α subunits and their interaction with K_V β subunits reside in the C terminus of K_V channels.[18]

The other major class of KV α subunits belongs to the HERG (encoded by the human *ether-a-go-go*–related gene) (*KCNH2*) and KvLQT1 (*KCNQ1*) subfamilies.[23-25] Like the K_V1.x to K_V4.x subfamilies, these channel proteins also are integral membrane proteins with six transmembrane domains, intracellular N and C termini, and a positively charged voltage sensor

3

Table 3-2 Auxiliary (Accessory) Subunits of Voltage-Gated Potassium Channels

Subunit	Gene	Molecular Structure	CBD	Current	Surface Expression	Activation/ Inactivation
KChAP	*KCHAP*	Intracellular (85 kD)	No	I_{to} (K_V4.3)* ↑	↑	↔ROA, ↔ROI, ↔RFI
KChIP2†‡	*KCNIP2*	Intracellular (220-270 aa)	Yes	I_{to} (K_V4.3) ↑	↑	↓ROI,§ ↑RFI, DVA
Frequenin		Intracellular (22 kD)	Yes	I_{to} (K_V4.2)§ ↑	↑	↓ROI,§ ↑RFI
Neuronal Ca^{2+} sensor-1		Intracellular (25 kD)	Yes	I_{to} (K_V4.3) ↑	↑	↓ROI, ↔RFI, DVA
β subunit 1 (K_Vβ1.2)‡	*KCNAB1*	Intracellular	No	I_{to} (K_V1.4) ↓ I_{Kur} ↓¶	NR NR	↑ROI, ↓RFI NR
β subunit 1 (K_Vβ1.3)‡	*KCNAB1*	Intracellular (419 aa)	No	I_{Kur} ↔	NR	↑ROI, HVA
β subunit 3 (K_Vβ3)	*KCNAB2*	Intracellular (408 aa)	No	I_{to} (K_V1.4) I_{to} (K_V4.3) ↑ I_{Kur} ↔	NR ↑ NR	↑ROI ↑ROI, ↓RFI ↑ROI, HVA
MiRP1**	*KCNE2*	Single TM domain (EC N-terminal) (123 aa)	No	I_{Kr} ↓ I_{Ks} ↓ I_{to} (K_V4.3) ↑	 NR NR	DVA ↓ROA ↓ROI
MinK	*KCNE1*	Single TM domain (EC N-terminal) (129-130 aa)	No	I_{Kr} ↑ I_{Ks} ↑	↔ ↔	HVA ↓ROA

aa, amino acids; CBD, calcium-binding domain; DVA, depolarizing shift in voltage activation; EC, extracellular; HVA, hyperpolarizing shift in voltage activation; NR, not reported; RFI, recovery from inactivation; ROA, rate of activation; ROI, rate of inactivation; TM, transmembrane.
*Effect inhibited by K_Vβ1.2.
†Spliced variants.
‡Single-nucleotide polymorphisms exist in humans.
§Dependent on Ca^{2+}.
¶Anatagonized by KChAP expression.
**Expressed predominantly in Purkinje system.
↑, increase; ↔, no change; ↓, decrease.

S4 region (see Figs. 3-2 and 3-3A). However, they have a different domain structure from that of the K_V1.x to K_V4.x subfamilies, characterized by the absence of a T1 domain and the presence of a sensor domain in the C terminus (see Fig. 3-3D).[1,24,25] The α subunits coassemble as homotetramers (with their accessory subunits) to form functional channels: HERG (I_{Kr}), the rapid component of the delayed rectifier current, and KvLQT1 (I_{Ks}), the slow component of the delayed rectifier current.[24,25] HERG also has a large N-terminal domain that has a structural similarity to PAS (Per-Arnt-Sim) domain, which is involved in signal transduction (see Fig. 3-3D).[23,24] By contrast, the intracellular N-terminal segment of K_VLQT1 is short and lacks a PAS domain.[1,23] The HERG C-terminal region also contains a cyclic nucleotide–binding domain. Two N-terminal splice variants and one C-terminal splice variant of HERG are present in the human heart and can regulate the gating kinetics of HERG without forming functional channels.[24,26] The N-terminal truncated isoform of K_VLQT1 (isoform 2) is expressed in the human heart and functions as a dominant-negative regulator of I_{Ks}.[25] The role of these spliced variants in regulating the delayed rectifiers in vivo is currently unclear.[24,26]

In contrast with I_{to}-encoding K_V α subunits, which are preferentially localized in the region of the intercalated disks, HERG appears to be distributed uniformly in the sarcolemmal and T tubule membranes.[26] This suggests that distinct mechanisms regulate membrane targeting of different potassium channels in the mammalian myocardium.

Auxiliary (Accessory) Subunits

The level of expression as well as the biophysical properties of K_V1.x to K_V4.x subfamilies is modulated by accessory cytoplasmic proteins, such as β subunits, KChAP, KChIPs, and other Ca^{2+}-sensing proteins (see Table 3-2). The three highly homologous β subunit families, K_Vβ1, K_Vβ2, and K_Vβ3, have multiple alternatively spliced variants.[27,28] Each β subunit contains a conserved core region with a variable N-terminal peptide and functions as a complete oxidoreductase enzyme, with its active site positioned to potentially interact with the potassium channel voltage sensor.[15,28] The β subunits also can assemble with a fourfold symmetrical structure and are able to coassemble with the T1 domain of the N termini of K_V α subunit ($T1_4β_4$) (see Fig. 3-3C).[15] KVβ1.2, KVβ1.3, and KVβ3 are expressed in the human heart, with twofold higher expression of K_V3 in the ventricle than in the atrium but with no chamber-specific difference in expression seen for K_V1.2.[27,29] K_V channels also can be regulated by K_V channel–associated protein (KChAP), a member of the transcription

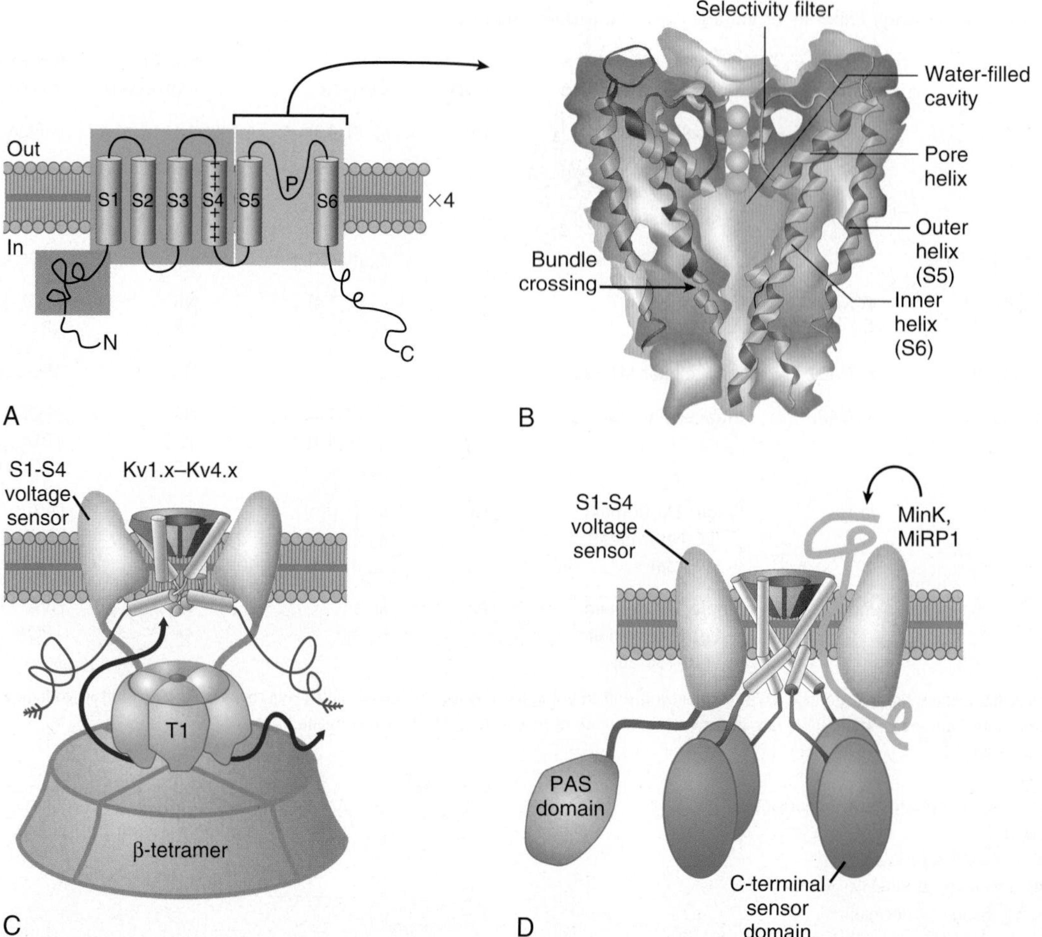

Figure 3-3 Molecular architecture of the voltage-gated potassium channel. **A,** Each α subunit has six transmembrane segments, S1 to S6, with the narrowest part of the pore, the selectivity filter, formed by a loop between S5 and S6, and the voltage sensor includes the S4 region with its multiple positive charges. **B,** The bacterial KcsA potassium channel with its outer helix homologous to S5 and the inner helix to S6 is the prototype for the pore-forming domain of the voltage-gated potassium channels. The interior of the protein is dark gray, with secondary structure shown as ribbons for three of the four subunits, and the water-exposed surface of the protein is light gray. The narrow selectivity filter is seen at the *top*, with the extended selectivity filter loop supported by the pore helices. The four *spheres* mark the four potassium-binding sites. The four *inner helices* cross to constrict the channel at the *bottom* (bundle crossing). Between the selectivity filter and bundle crossing is the water-filled cavity. **C,** The K_V1.x–K_V4.x subfamily has at its N terminus a tetramerization domain (T1, *blue/green*) that determines the specificity of subunit tetrameric assembly and also serves as a platform for protein interactions and intracellular signaling. The C terminus (*green*) has a PDZ-binding motif that determines the physical localization of the channel and its association into large signaling complexes. **D,** The voltage-gated K_VLQT1 and HERG channels also have a tetrameric organization but with a different domain structure, characterized by the absence of a T1 domain and the presence of a sensor domain in the C terminus.

factor–binding protein family, by increasing the functional cell surface expression of specific K_V channels without affecting other channel properties (see Table 3-2).[18] KChAP is a potassium channel modulatory protein that exhibits "chaperone-like" behavior toward a subset of potassium channels. KChAP, a soluble protein, binds transiently to the cytoplasmic N termini of its target channels, thereby increasing channel expression in a transcription-independent manner.[18,29]

K_V channel–interacting proteins (KChIPs) are calcium-binding proteins that interact with the cytoplasmic N termini of K_V4 α subunits and reconstitute several features of native cardiac currents generated by these channels by modulating their density and inactivation kinetics.[18,30] KChIP2 is the main isoform expressed in the heart, which co-localizes and co-immunoprecipitates with the native K_V channel (see Table 3-2).[30] In cardiac myocytes, KChIP2 has two spliced variants and is expressed predominantly in the T tubules and nuclei.[31] Coexpression of K_V4.2 and KChIP2 was observed to increase the density of K_V4.2 currents, indicating that KChIP2 may promote or stabilize expression of K_V4.2 at the cell surface, in addition to modulating the biophysical properties so that it closely correspond to $I_{to,f}$ in cardiac myocytes (see Table 3-2).[30,32] Two other KChIP-related calcium-binding proteins, frequenin and neuronal calcium sensor-1, also are expressed in heart, and both increase I_{to} density and alter the inactivation characteristics (see Table 3-2).[18,33,34]

Similarly, the HERG and KvLQT1 subfamilies are regulated by accessory subunits that belong to the KCNE family and include MinK (minimal K^+ channel), MinK-related peptide 1 (MiRP1), MiRP2, and MiRP3, encoded by the *KCNE* genes (*KCNE1* through *KCNE4*, respectively), with MinK, MiRP1, and *KCNE3* being expressed in the heart (see Table 3-2).[23-25,35] These proteins are not cytoplasmic but represent single-domain transmembrane proteins with extracellular N termini, which are intimately associated with the α subunit and may displace the voltage sensor domain or interact with it directly.[1,24,25]

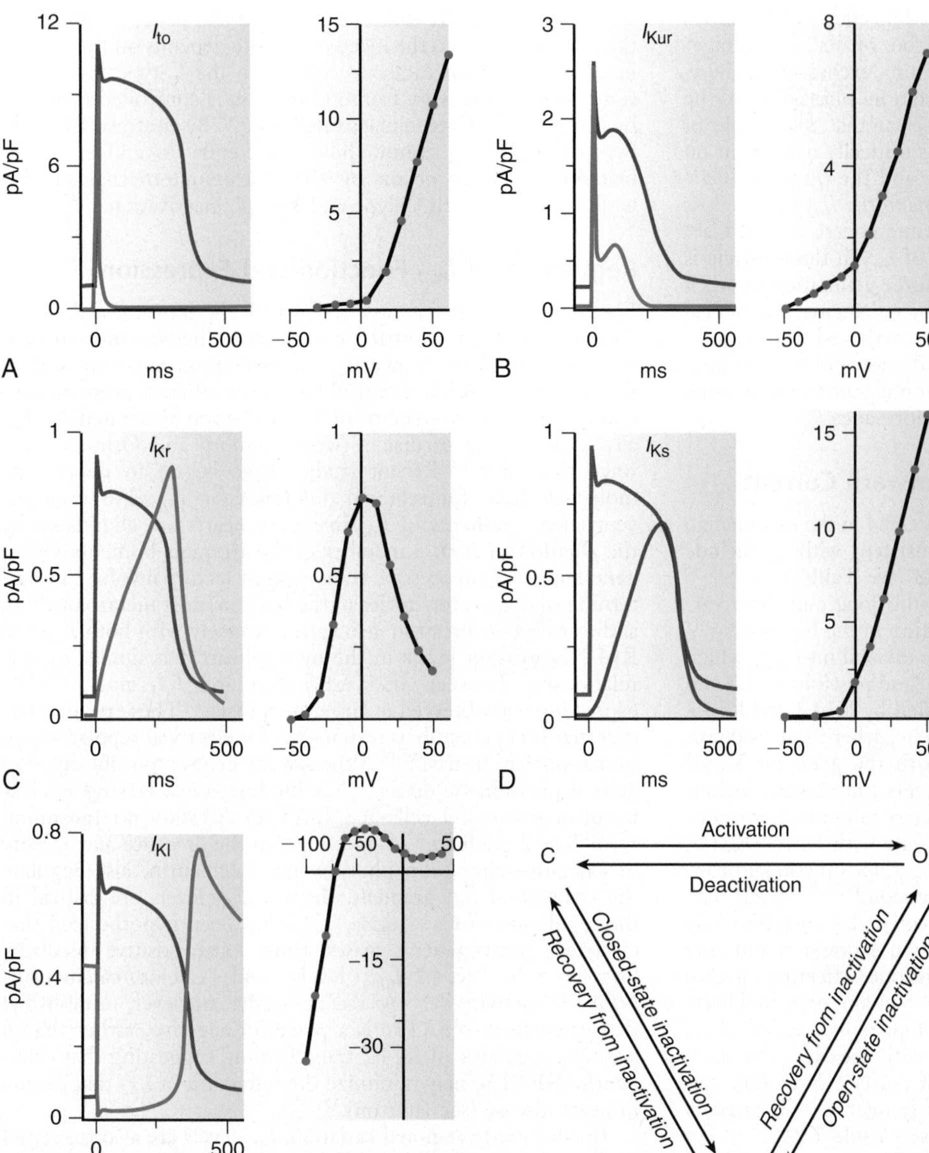

Figure 3-4 Current-voltage relationships in voltage-regulated potassium channels. **A–E,** The time courses of major potassium currents during an action potential (AP) *(superimposed purple line)*, as well as steady-state current-voltage relationships. **A,** Ventricular transient outward potassium current (I_{to}); **B,** atrial ultra-rapid delayed rectifier potassium current (I_{Kur}); **C,** ventricular rapid delayed rectifier potassium current (I_{Kr}); **D,** ventricular slow delayed rectifier potassium current (I_{Ks}); and **E,** ventricular inward rectifier potassium current (I_{K1}). These currents can be described by transitions of the protein between different conformational states. **F** depicts ion channel activity: Activation of the channel from a nonconducting closed state (C) to an open (O) conformation allows ion permeation. Both open and closed channels may enter a nonconducting inactive conformation (I). Transition of a channel from an open to a closed conformation is referred to as channel deactivation. pA/pF, picoampere/picofarad.

Initial functional expression experiments suggested that MiRP1 could associate with HERG and modulate the channel function. More recently, it has been shown that MiRP1 also can associate with K_VLQT1.[25] Similarly, MinK can associate with both HERG and K_VLQT1 subunits and modulate their function.[24,25,36] Accordingly, the KCNE subunits may engage in promiscuous interactions with α subunits from different gene families.

Transient Outward Currents

Physiologic Role of Transient Outward Current

The transient outward current, I_{to}, in cardiomyocytes consists of two components: a calcium-activated chloride current (I_{to2}) and a classical calcium-independent potassium current (I_{to1}) (referred to hereafter as I_{to}). The calcium-independent I_{to} is of two types: a "rapid" or "fast" I_{to}, called $I_{to,f}$, and a slower form, $I_{to,s}$. $I_{to,f}$ and $I_{to,s}$ activate rapidly, with an activation time constant, τ_a, of approximately 2 to 10 ms, but have differing time constants for inactivation kinetics (25 to 80 ms for $I_{to,f}$ and 80 to 200 ms for $I_{to,s}$) and for recovery from steady-state inactivation (25 to 80 ms for $I_{to,f}$ and 1 to 2 seconds for $I_{to,s}$).[18,37] $I_{to,s}$ is smaller than $I_{to,f}$ in most species, including humans. $I_{to,f}$ is the primary determinant of the time course of early repolarization (phase 1) of atrial and ventricular action potentials (Fig. 3-4; see also Fig. 3-1), and $I_{to,f}$ varies greatly between regions of the heart. For example, $I_{to,f}$ expression is favored in epicardial regions, the right ventricle and the base of the heart,[18,37] compared with the septum, left ventricular endocardium, and apex of the heart.[38] Regional variations in $I_{to,f}$ underlie the heterogeneity of action potential profiles, which are responsible for orderly ventricular repolarization. Variation in $I_{to,f}$ also is responsible for much of the regional modulation of contractility,[18] which has been linked to ability of early repolarization to strongly modulate L-type calcium current magnitude, thereby regulating excitation-contraction coupling and myocardial contractility.[39] The effects of $I_{to,f}$ levels on contractility also may potentially be related to voltage-dependent modulation of sodium-calcium exchanger activity, particularly during the early repolarization phase, when the exchanger reverses direction.[18,39] It is clear that the profile of the early repolarization period, which is critically dependent on $I_{to,f}$ levels, controls both the amplitude and the timing of Ca^{2+} release from the SR.[39] Indeed, reductions in the $I_{to,f}$ and the loss of the notch lead to a slowing of the time course for SR Ca^{2+} release. Consequently, the distribution of $I_{to,f}$ in the ventricle is predicted to synchronize the timing of force generation between different regions of the ventricle, thereby enhancing mechanical efficiency. Of note in this regard, the generalized downregulation of $I_{to,f}$, as occurs in advanced heart disease and heart failure, is predicted to slow the time course of force generation, thereby contributing to reduced myocardial performance.

Molecular Basis of Transient Outward Current

The pore-forming channel proteins expressed in the mammalian heart having biophysical properties consistent with I_{to} include $K_V1.4$, $K_V1.7$, $K_V3.4$, $K_V4.2$, and $K_V4.3$ (see Table 3-1),[18,19,40] with $K_V4.3$ being alternatively spliced into long and short variants differing by a 19-amino-acid insertion in the C terminus.[41] As already mentioned, cardiac I_{to} can be divided into $I_{to,s}$, which is encoded primarily by the $K_V1.4$ gene (and possibly $K_V1.7$ and $K_V3.4$ genes),[18] and $I_{to,f}$, which is encoded by $K_V4.2$ and $K_V4.3$ genes. $I_{to,f}$ is encoded by the $K_V4.3$ gene, whereas in rodents, both $K_V4.2$ and $K_V4.3$ are present, with the gene for $K_V4.2$ being dominant.[18,19] $I_{to,f}$ and $I_{to,s}$ channels can contain various accessory subunits that associate with K_V α subunits. For example, K_V β subunits can specifically associate with $K_V1.4$, $K_V1.5$, and $K_V4.3$ α subunits, thereby modifying their functional properties, stability, and cell surface expression.[18,27,42] $K_V\beta3$ can increase the rate of inactivation of human $K_V1.4$ currents.[27] By contrast, $K_V\beta1$ and $K_V\beta3$ increase protein expression and current density of $K_V4.3$ channel without affecting gating (see Table 3-2).[18,42] $K_V\beta1$ and $K_V\beta3$ contain protein kinase A (PKA) and protein kinase C (PKC) phosphorylation sites, which may modulate their interaction with the K_V subunits.[18] MiRP-1, the endogenous β subunit of I_{Kr} (see later on), can promiscuously increase the density of human $K_V4.3$ currents with a modest slowing of inactivation (see Table 3-2).[42]

KChAP also enhances the functional expression, without altering gating or voltage dependence, of a subset of K_V channels including $K_V4.3$, without increasing $K_V1.5$, Kir2.2, HERG, or K_VLQT1 currents.[43] Complexes of KChAP and $K_V4.3$ have been co-immunoprecipitated from heart samples, implying that KChAP is an important regulatory subunit for the native cardiac I_{to}.[43] $K_V\beta1.2$ inhibits the increase in $K_V4.3$ current produced by KChAP, suggesting that different accessory subunits may interact in their regulation of I_{to} (see Table 3-2).[29] Coassembly of $K_V4.3$ with KChIP2 may underlie the regional transmural heterogeneity in $I_{to,f}$ expression in canine and human heart,[44] although no gradient of KChIP2 expression at the protein level has been observed.[31] Loss of KChIP2 expression leads to downregulation and loss of transmural gradient of I_{to}, action potential prolongation, and increased susceptibility to ventricular arrhythmias.[32] Although I_{to} traditionally has been considered to be a calcium-independent current, association with KChIP2 and other related calcium-binding proteins (frequenin and neuronal calcium sensor-1) suggests that native I_{to} is regulated by intracellular Ca^{2+} dynamics (see Table 3-2).[18,31,34]

The prominent inactivation properties of I_{to} currents originate primarily from the biophysical properties of the pore-forming α subunits. Specifically, $K_V1.4$, $K_V1.7$, and $K_V3.4$ channels undergo both N- and C-type inactivation, which are kinetically linked.[13] For example, in $K_V1.4$ channels, the rate of entry into the inactivated state depends on the N-type inactivation, which catalyzes entry into the C-type inactivated state, whereas recovery from inactivation is controlled primarily by exit from the C-type inactivated state.[13] By contrast, all members of the K_V4.x family show rapid entry to and exit from inactivation, which occurs by way of a unique mechanism that is distinct from both C-type and N-type inactivation.[13,45]

Regulation of $I_{to,f}$ Function and Expression

Electrical heterogeneity associated with the transmural $I_{to,f}$ gradient is expected to contribute to the coordination and synchronization of repolarization and force generation across the wall of the ventricle,[39] which is critical for energy efficient pressure generation. The heterogeneity of repolarization generated by $I_{to,f}$ also explains the cardiac T wave memory and Osborne or J wave formation.[18] Recent studies have begun to dissect the molecular basis for regional differences in $I_{to,f}$. For example, ventricular gradients of $I_{to,f}$ in mouse hearts are eliminated by the ablation of *Irx5*, a member of the Iroquois homeobox (Irx) gene family of suppressive transcription factors involved in patterning of diverse territories of the body in most metazoans.[46] In addition, Irx5 expression also varies inversely with both $I_{to,f}$ and Kv4.2 expression levels in the mouse heart[46]; a similar inverse relationship between Irx5 expression and $I_{to,f}$ and KChIP2 expression was observed in larger mammals.[47] These results suggest that Irx5 generally is responsible for electrical repolarization in mammalian hearts.[46,47] Although *Irx* genes typically suppress gene expression by direct DNA binding, mice lacking nuclear factor of activated T cells-3c (NFAT3c) also show no transmural I_{to} or $K_V4.2$ gradient,[48] suggesting that the presence and activity of calcium–calmodulin phosphatase, calcineurin, also regulate the transmural $I_{to,f}$ gradient. Because $I_{to,f}$ levels are critical in the regulation of Ca^{2+} levels,[49,50] it has been hypothesized that electrical heterogeneity arises from local positive feedback between the $K_V4.2$-$I_{to,f}$ levels and calcium-calcineurin-NFAT3c activity.[48,51] A recent study, however, established that calcineurin-NFAT3c is a powerful negative, rather than a positive, regulator of $K_V4.2$ transcription, suggesting that calcineurin-NFAT3c may minimize the reduction in $I_{to,f}$ that occurs in heart disease (see later on).[52]

In addition to regional variation, $I_{to,f}$ levels are also regulated in the development of heart disease as well as by various neurohumoral and hormonal factors. For example, chronic exposure of ventricular myocytes to α-adrenergic agonists (such as phenylephrine) reduces $I_{to,f}$ in association with decreased $K_V4.2$, $K_V4.3$, and KChIP2 expression.[18,53] Of interest, α-adrenergic agonists mediate increased $I_{to,s}$ and $K_V1.4$ expression.[18,53] The mechanism for reduced $I_{to,f}$ is unlikely to be related to the simultaneous activation of calcineurin-NFAT, because this transcriptional pathway upregulates $K_V4.2$ expression while having no effect on $K_V4.3$ or KChIP2 expression levels. $I_{to,f}$ reductions after the acute application of α-adrenergic agonists occur in several species by way of both PKC-dependent and PKC-independent pathways,[18,54] with reductions in human cardiomyocytes requiring PKC-dependent phosphorylation of the long isoform of $K_V4.3$.[41]

Angiotensin II (AT-II) stimulation of AT-II type 1 (AT-1) receptors not only reduces $I_{to,f}$ but also modulates its kinetics. For example, incubation of canine epicardial ventricular myocytes with AT-II transforms epicardial fast $I_{to,f}$, assumed to be $K_V4.3$-based, into a current with much slower kinetics without changing either $K_V1.4$ or $K_V4.3$ messenger RNA (mRNA) levels.[55] Conversely, treatment of the endocardial myocytes with the AT-1 blocker, losartan, converts slow endocardial I_{to} currents (presumably $I_{to,f}$) into the faster $I_{to,f}$ of the epicardium.[55] These observations suggest that biophysical properties of $I_{to,f}$ can dynamically change without alterations in expression of the underlying genes. These biophysical changes of $I_{to,f}$ induced by AT-II may involve redox changes or sulfhydryl modification of $I_{to,f}$ channels, possibly as a result of NADPH oxidase activation.[56]

Thyroid hormone also profoundly affects $I_{to,f}$. Hypothyroidism prolongs action potential duration in conjunction with a marked reduction in $I_{to,f}$ density along with decreased $K_V4.2$ expression, whereas hyperthyroidism has the reverse effect.[54,57-60] The perinatal surge in the thyroid hormone T_3 (triiodothyronine) leads to major changes in $K_V4.2$ and $K_V4.3$ expression that are largely responsible for postnatal action potential changes and electrical remodeling.[18,57] In contrast to thyroid hormone, aldosterone, which is a member of the steroid hormone superfamily, induces downregulation of $I_{to,f}$ in ventricular myocytes.[61]

One central feature of heart disease is the electrical remodeling that involves downregulation of $I_{to,f}$ in conjunction with reductions in $K_V4.2$, $K_V4.3$, and KChIP2,[18,39,62] which in turn have been linked to the hypertrophy associated with heart disease, possibly through the activation of the calcineurin–nuclear factor of activated T cells (NFAT) pathway.[49,62,63] Consistent with this idea, enhancing $K_V4.2$ or $K_V4.3$ expression in cardiomyocytes or whole hearts prevents hypertrophy.[50,64] These observations further suggest that $I_{to,f}$ and calcineurin-NFAT activation participate in a positive feedback mechanism for simultaneously driving electrical and mechanical remodeling in heart disease.[48] Of note, however, calcineurin-NFAT positively regulates $K_V4.2$ transcription, thereby minimizing the reductions in $I_{to,f}$ and $K_V4.2$ expression observed in cardiac hypertrophy and heart disease.[52] Nevertheless, inhibition of calcineurin signaling after myocardial infarction can prevent hypertrophy and $I_{to,f}$ downregulation,[62] suggesting that calcineurin effects may depend on the disease process. It also is conceivable that other Ca^{2+}-dependent processes may play a role in $I_{to,f}$ regulation, because inhibition of the multifunctional calcium-calmodulin–dependent protein kinase II (CaMKII) increases myocardial $K_V4.2$-4.3 expression and $I_{to,f}$ density.[65,66] A potential "master switch" in the regulation of gene expression in heart disease is thyroid hormone: The changes in the expression of many genes, particularly $K_V4.2$ and $K_V4.3$, occurring in heart disease closely mimic the alterations observed in hypothyroidism.[60] Consistent with this observation, heart-specific elevations in thyroid hormone in the heart were found to reverse both the functional and genetic changes observed in hypertrophic mouse hearts, suggesting that altered thyroid hormone signaling may be responsible for many of the genetic, mechanical, and electrical changes that occur in heart disease.[60]

Delayed Rectifiers

Physiologic Role of Delayed Rectifier Current

The cardiac delayed rectifier potassium current (I_K) initially was identified on the basis of its relatively slow (delayed) onset compared with other cardiac potassium currents. I_K consists of three component currents, I_{Kur}, I_{Kr}, and I_{Ks}, each with distinct voltage and time-dependent properties (see Figs. 3-1 and 3-4B to D). I_K is a primary determinant of the late phase 2 and phase 3 repolarization in cardiomyocytes,[24,25] with slow deactivation of I_{Ks}, and particularly I_{Kr}, also contributing briefly to enhanced conductance and the membrane refractoriness in early phase 4. Regional variations and species differences in action potential configuration have been associated with differential expression patterns of I_{Kur}, I_{Kr}, and I_{Ks} channels.[20] For example, the short action potentials typically seen in atrial myocytes are associated with relatively high levels of the rapidly activating and very slow inactivating I_{Kur} (see Figs. 3-1 and 3-4A).[17,20] Moreover, although atrial I_K contains both I_{Kr} and I_{Ks} components, I_{Kr} is reported to be larger in left than in right atrial myocytes, resulting in relatively shorter action potentials in the left atrium.[20] In the ventricle, I_{Kr} appears to be more abundant in the epicardial and apical myocytes, where action potentials are relatively shorter,[67] whereas the longer action potentials in midmyocardial cells are associated with decreased I_{Ks}.[20] I_{Kr} activates rapidly and displays marked inward rectification compared with I_{Ks}. These properties of I_{Kr} result from very rapid inactivation, which proceeds at a rate faster than channel activation at positive membrane potentials.[24] Consequently, I_{Kr} has a relatively low conductance during the action potential plateau (phase 2) but increases during phase 3 repolarization (see Figs. 3-1 and 3-4C). By contrast, I_{Ks} increases gradually during the plateau phase of the action potential because of its slow activation kinetics, but remains activated during phase 3 repolarization as a result of slow deactivation (see Figs. 3-1 and 3-4D).[25] The slow deactivation of I_{Kr} and I_{Ks} may be an important contributor to the shortening of atrial and ventricular action potentials at rapid heart rates.[24,68] These channels remain in the activated state during the shortened diastolic interval, thereby contributing to a faster rate of repolarization.[24,68] The important role of delayed rectifiers in cardiac repolarization is illustrated by the congenital and acquired long and short QT syndromes resulting from loss-of-function and gain-of-function mutations, respectively, in these channels (see later on).

Molecular Basis for Delayed Rectifier Currents

I_{Kur} has been definitively identified in human and canine atrial myocytes, where it is encoded by $K_V1.5$ and $K_V3.1$ channel genes, respectively.[20,21] In other species such as the mouse, delayed rectifier-like currents are found in both atrial and ventricular myocytes and include $I_{K,slow1}$, encoded by the $K_V1.5$ gene, and $I_{K,slow2}$, encoded by the $K_V2.1$ gene.[19] In the heart, $K_V\beta1.2$ co-immunoprecipitates with $K_V1.5$ subunits, whereas KChAP attenuates the depression of $K_V1.5$ currents produced by $K_V\beta1.2$.[29] The N-terminal peptide in $K_V\beta1.3$ and $K_V\beta3$ subunits confers a rapid inactivation to $K_V1.5$ subunits by means of a proposed N-type inactivation.[27] In addition, both $K_V\beta1.3$ and $K_V\beta3$ subunits cause a hyperpolarizing shift in the voltage activation curve of human $K_V1.5$ current, suggesting that these channels can open at more negative membrane potentials.[27] The association of $K_V1.5$ subunits with accessory K_V β subunits also confers a significant degree of sensitivity of I_{Kur} to the intracellular redox state.[28] $K_V1.5$ undergoes C-type inactivation, which is typical of the $K_V1.x$ subfamily.[13] The rapid U-type inactivation also has been demonstrated in members of the $K_V1.x$ subfamily including $K_V1.5$, which has been postulated to involve interaction of the N-terminal T1 domain with the channel pore.[17]

In cardiac myocytes, HERG (KCNH2) coassembles with MinK-related peptide 1 (MiRP1) (i.e., KCNE2), thereby giving HERG channels their gating, reduced unitary conductance, regulation, and distinctive biphasic inhibition by the methanesulfonilide class III antiarrhythmic drug E4031 observed for native cardiac I_{Kr} (see Tables 3-1 and 3-2).[24,69] Inherited loss-of-function mutations in HERG (LQT2) or MiRP1 (LQT6) causing defects in I_{Kr} are associated with congenital long QT syndromes,[23-25,69] whereas gain-of-function mutations in HERG (*KCNH2*) are associated with short QT syndrome 1 (SQTS1).[70] A high propensity for drug-induced block and acquired long QT syndrome is associated with HERG channels, which may be related to the unique pore structure and function of HERG.[23,24] Unlike the rapid inactivation of $K_V1.x$ subfamily, HERG channel inactivation is unaffected by truncation of its N-terminal region but seems to involve conformational changes in the outer pore region similar to those of C-type inactivation. HERG inactivation, however, shows several properties, biophysically distinct from those of "classic" C-type inactivation, that may be related to the unique amino acid residues in the pore region, including the absence of a tyrosine residue in the signature sequence.[13,24] In addition, the PAS domain of HERG may be important in mediating the slow rate of channel deactivation.[23]

Cardiac I_{Ks} is generated by coassembly of K_VLTQ1 (*KCNQ1*) with minimal potassium channel protein or MinK (*KCNE1*) (see Tables 3-1 and 3-2).[25,35] Coexpression of MinK reverses the regulation by pH while altering the pharmacologic sensitivity to blockers and temperature sensitivity of K_VLQT1 channels.[25] K_VLQT1 also can coassemble with MiRP1 and KCNE3, both of which are expressed in human atrium and ventricle,[35] and HERG can coassemble with MinK.[24] Inherited loss-of-function mutations in K_VLQT1 (LQT1) or MinK (LQT5) causing defects in I_{Ks} are associated with congenital long QT syndromes,[23,25] whereas gain-of-function mutations in K_VLQT1 (*KCNQ1*) are associated with short QT syndrome 2 (SQTS2).[70] MinK localizes to the T tubules surrounding the Z line in ventricular myocytes, where it is linked to the myofibrillar components by an adaptor protein; this array may form a mechanoelectrical feedback system by means of stretch-dependent regulation of I_{Ks}.[71] Gating of the K_VLQT1 channels is characterized by rather slow activation kinetics and a delayed, incomplete, and intrinsically voltage-independent inactivation, which are modulated by the association of K_VLQT1 with MinK: Activation becomes extremely slow, inactivation appears to be abolished, and the single-channel conductance is increased (see Table 3-2).[25]

Regulation of Delayed Rectifier Currents

Both β- and α-adrenergic stimulation increase I_{Kur} by PKA and PKC effects, respectively,[72] whereas activation of Src family of protein tyrosine kinases reduces I_{Kur} by the phosphorylation of Src homology 3 (SH3) domains in the N terminus of $K_V1.5$ channels.[73] The steroid hormone superfamily, including glucocorticoids, thyroid hormone and androgens, can alter the transcription of $K_V1.5$ subunit. Hyperthyroidism can lead to transcriptional upregulation while hypothyroidism leads to decreased expression of $K_V1.5$ channel genes, although it remains to be shown whether these changes occur in atrial myocytes.[59,74] The effects of male sex hormones lead to a reduction in the density of I_{Kur} and $K_V1.5$ expression, which may play an important role in gender-specific differences in atrial repolarization.[75] HERG channels are regulated by PKA at phosphorylation sites located in the N and C termini, as well as by cyclic adenosine monophosphate (cAMP) at a cyclic nucleotide–binding domain (CNBD) in the C terminus.[24] PKA activation reduces HERG current, whereas a direct binding of cAMP to the HERG channel increases current. The summation of these effects results in a net decrease in the current.[76] These opposing effects of PKA and cAMP also are observed as voltage shifts in the activation curves. When HERG is coexpressed with MiRP1 or minK, however, cAMP produces a net increase in the current, consistent with the observation that loss-of-function mutations in the CNBD of HERG channels are associated with LQT2 syndrome.[24,76,77]

By contrast, α-adrenergic stimulation reduces HERG currents, which is prevented by excess phosphatidylinositol 4,5-biphosphate (PIP_2). This finding suggests that the mechanism is due to G protein–coupled receptor stimulation of PLC, resulting in the consumption of endogenous PIP_2. PIP_2-dependent effects are due primarily to altered channel gating, with no significant change in single channel conductance.[78] The physiologic relevance of PIP_2-HERG interactions is supported by the observations that endothelin-1 decreases I_{Kr} (and prolongs action potentials) in human ventricular myocytes, possibly by the local depletion of PIP_2.[78,79] β-Adrenergic stimulation also increases I_{Ks} by means of PKA-dependent phosphorylation of K_VLQT1 channels which involves a macromolecular complex that includes PKA, protein phosphatase 1, and the targeting protein yotiao.[80] β-Adrenergic upregulation of I_{Kr} and I_{Ks} provides a possible mechanistic link between increased adrenergic drive and shortening of the cardiac action potential duration. I_{Ks} also can be modulated by PKC activation.[25] Altered thyroid hormone status results in changes in I_{Ks}-encoding subunits, with hypothyroidism resulting in increased expression and hyperthyroidism resulting in decreased expression of K_VLQT1 and MinK.[59]

Voltage-Regulated Inward Rectifier

Physiologic Role and Mechanism of Inward Rectification

Owing to the inability of voltage-regulated inward rectifier (I_{K1}) channels to support outward potassium currents at positive potentials, which is called inward rectification (see Fig. 3-4E), I_{K1} plays a major role in the late phase of repolarization (phase 3) of the cardiac action potential and in setting the resting membrane potential (phase 4) (see Fig. 3-1).[81] Clear chamber-specific differences in I_{K1} are recognized, with a higher density of I_{K1} occurring in ventricular myocytes but very little I_{K1} current in atrial myocytes (see Fig. 3-1), which may be related to differential expression of Kir2.x subunits.[20,82] The strong rectification properties of I_{K1} currents are necessary to prevent these channels from counteracting the membrane depolarization that typically occurs in the myocardium after Na^+ influx through voltage-gated sodium channels. I_{K1} rectification has been linked to blockade of the channel pore by the intracellular cation Mg^{2+} and linear polyamines (putrescine, spermidine, and spermine).[81] These blocking particles enter the pore from the cytoplasm, and their ability to block the Kir2.x channels is relieved by membrane repolarization, allowing outward potassium currents during phase 3 of the action potential (see Figs. 3-1 and 3-4E).[81] Accordingly, Kir2.x channels are voltage-regulated despite not having the classic voltage-sensing mechanism—namely, the S1 to S4 segments—of the K_V channels.

Molecular Basis of Inward Rectifier

The inward rectifier potassium channel family comprises at least seven subfamilies, Kir1 to Kir7 (i.e., KCNJ-1 to KCNJ-16).[19,81] The pore-forming α subunits of channels in this family are distinct from the K_V channels and possess two transmembrane segments, M1 and M2, connected by a pore-forming P loop (H5), along with cytoplasmic N and C termini (see Fig. 3-2D).[81] The inward rectifier channel membrane structure is analogous to the S5, S6, and P loop regions of K_V channels. The Kir channels having the most pronounced (strong) inward rectification belong to the Kir2.x subfamily, which underlie cardiac I_{K1} (Kir2.1 to Kir2.4) (KCNJ-2, KCNJ-12, KCNJ-4, and KCNJ-14, respectively).[19,82,83] In the heart, Kir2.1 (with variants Kir2.1a and Kir2.1b), Kir2.2, and Kir2.3 channels appear to coassemble as heterotetramers, which may account for the wide range of conductances observed for I_{K1} channels in the heart.[83-85] In contrast with K_V channels, the proximal C terminus and the transmembrane segment M2 appear to determine homo- and heteromultimerization.[86] An intrasubunit disulfide bond between the extremities of the P loop (Cys122 and Cys154 in Kir2.1) is required for Kir2.x channel function presumably by contributing to proper protein folding.[87] Stability of tertiary structure of the selectivity filter in Kir2.x channels also depends on an electrostatic interaction between two conserved residues in the P loop region.[88] Intracellular polyamine and Mg^{2+}-induced rectification depends strongly on the presence of negatively charged residues situated in the M2 domain and the proximal C terminus[81] (see Fig. 3-2D) and also is modulated by intracellular Ca^{2+} and by the cytoskeleton.[89] These channels contain a conduction pore that is nearly 6 nm long (as a result of an extended cytoplasmic pore), which governs inward rectification by allowing access of the polyamines and Mg^{2+} to the membranous pore region (see Fig. 3-2D).[90] In addition to Kir2.x channels, three other notable inward rectifier (weak) potassium channels are present in the myocardium: the TWIK-1 background potassium channels (*KCNK1*), which help to set the resting membrane potential (discussed later on); I_{KACh} channels (*KCNJ3, KCNJ5*), which regulate heart rate and conduction through the atrioventricular node in response to acetylcholine (ACh); and I_{KATP} channels (*KCNJ11*), which respond to changes in metabolic state (see Table 3-1).

Regulation of Inward Rectification

Native I_{K1} in human ventricular myocytes is reduced by β-adrenergic receptor stimulation and by the intracellular application of catalytic subunit of PKA.[91] The catalytic subunit of PKA can completely inhibit Kir2.1 currents by means of the phosphorylation of a serine residue in the C terminus.[92] Stimulation of α-adrenergic receptors in human atrial myocytes also reduces I_{K1} current,[93] which may depend on a PKC-dependent phosphorylation of the Se64 (N-terminus) and Thre353 residue (C terminus) of Kir2.1b channel[85] or the Thre53 residue (N-terminus) in Kir2.3 channels.[94] In addition to adrenergic control of I_{K1}, activation of the AT-1 receptors by angiotensin II also appears to downregulate cardiac I_{K1}.[95] Depletion of PIP_2 has been reported to cause "rundown" (disappearance) of I_{K1} activity, and direct application of PIP_2-containing liposomes to membrane patches reactivates rundown channels.[96] Activation of cardiac phospholipase C and phosphoinositide 3-kinase enzyme systems can lead to depletion of PIP_2 from the plasma membrane, which may limit Kir2.x channel activity.[96,97] This regulation appears to depend on positively charged basic residues residing in both the C and the N termini of the Kir2.x channels, which are postulated to interact with the anionic phospholipid head groups of PIP_2 at the cytoplasmic face of the membrane, thereby maintaining channel activity.[96,97] Indeed, interference between PIP_2 and cardiac Kir2.1 appears to underlie the loss-of-function phenotype for several mutations associated with Andersen's syndrome (*LQT7*),[97,98] whereas gain-of-function mutations in Kir2.1 (*KCNJ2*) result in short QT syndrome 3 (SQTS3).[70] PIP_2 interaction with the individual Kir2.x subunits also may be important for the subunit assembly.[86,98]

Background Potassium Currents

In addition to I_{K1}, other background K^+-selective currents also contribute to action potential repolarization and establishing the diastolic (resting) membrane potential. In this family of channels, the basic structure is a tandem repeat of *two* α subunits (a dimer), each with four transmembrane domains, and a pore region, with at least three members identified in the human heart: TWIK-1/2 (*KCNK1/6*), TASK-1 (*KCNK3*), and TRAAK (*KCNK4*) (see Table 3-1 and Fig. 3-2A and B).[82,99,100] These channels produce currents that are quasi-instantaneous and noninactivating. A distinguishing feature of TWIK-1 (*KCNK1*) is its weak inward rectification, which results in significant outward currents between −60 and 0 mV.[82,99] These channels are activated by PKC and inhibited by intracellular acidification.[99] By contrast, TASK-1 (*KCNK3*) and TRAAK (*KCNK4*) currents show little rectification, making them more active through the depolarization period of the action potential. TASK-1 currents are extremely sensitive to variations in external pH in a narrow physiologic range, whereas TRAAK form mechanosensitive channels that are modulated by arachidonic acid and polyunsaturated fatty acids.[99] The properties of these channels suggest that in cardiac myocytes, they may be involved in responding to cellular metabolism and mechanical activity.[82,99]

Voltage-Regulated Potassium Channels in Cardiac Disease

Due to their widespread role in regulating myocardial excitability, voltage-regulated potassium channels are key players in the genesis of atrial and ventricular arrhythmias, as well as possibly impaired myocardial contractility seen in end-stage heart disease.[18,39,101,102] Although alteration in potassium channel function can occur by gain- or loss-of-function mechanisms, a majority of changes in voltage-regulated potassium channels involve reduction in potassium currents. Reduced function can be the result of decreased expression of pore-forming α subunit or accessory subunits (or both), altered regulatory pathways, or changes in cellular metabolism.[18,32,56,101,103] Congenital long QT syndromes can result from decreased I_{Kr} (*LQT2* and *LQT6*), I_{Ks} (*LQT1*and *LQT5*)[23,69] and I_{K1} (*LQT7*).[97,98] In acquired heart disease, downregulation in expression of $K_V4.2/4.3$,[18,103] HERG,[24] KChIP2,[32] and MinK[24] have been described in association with reduced I_{to}[18,103] and I_{Kr}.[24,104] The only gain-of-function potassium channelopathy involves increased I_{Ks}, leading to action potential shortening and reentry in association with familial atrial fibrillation.[35]

Downregulation of voltage-regulated potassium channels can lead to action potential prolongation, which can promote *triggered arrhythmias* by the generation of early and delayed afterdepolarizations (EADs and DADs, respectively).[23,102] In addition, regional changes in dispersion of refractoriness can lead to unidirectional block of a wave of electrical excitation, thereby creating a substrate for arrhythmia—the pathomechanism for *reentrant arrhythmias*.[23,32] In large species, such as humans and dogs, rapid early repolarization may be necessary physiologically for adequate recruitment and synchronization of Ca^{2+} release events that contribute to the whole-cell calcium transient.[39] On the other hand, slowing the rate of phase 1 repolarization (due to decreased I_{to}) can reduce trigger $I_{Ca,L}$ (by the voltage-gated calcium channels), which increases the dispersion of SR Ca^{2+} release, thereby exacerbating impaired Ca^{2+} cycling in heart disease.[39] Accordingly, the impact of voltage-regulated potassium channels on cardiac function should not be considered in isolation but must be integrated in the context of the other ion channel-exchangers in both physiologic and pathophysiologic conditions.

References

1. Yellen G: The voltage-gated potassium channels and their relatives. Nature 419: 35-42, 2002.
2. Bezanilla F: Voltage sensor movements. J Gen Physiol 120:465-473, 2002.
3. Horn R: Coupled movements in voltage-gated ion channels. J Gen Physiol 120: 449-553, 2002.
4. Gandhi CS, Isacoff EY: Molecular models of voltage sensing. J Gen Physiol 120:455-463, 2002.
5. Jiang Y, Lee A, Chen J, et al: X-ray structure of a voltage-dependent K^+ channel. Nature 423:33-41, 2003.
6. Jiang Y, Ruta V, Chen J, et al: The principle of gating charge movement in a voltage-dependent K^+ channel. Nature 423:42-48, 2003.
7. Lee SY, Lee A, Chen J, MacKinnon R: Structure of the K_VAP voltage-dependent K^+ channel and its dependence on the lipid membrane. Proc Natl Acad Sci U S A 102:15441-15446, 2005.
8. Long SB, Campbell EB, Mackinnon R: Voltage sensor of Kv1.2: Structural basis of electromechanical coupling. Science 309:903-908, 2005a.
9. Long SB, Campbell EB, Mackinnon R: Crystal structure of a mammalian voltage-dependent Shaker family K^+ channel. Science 309:897-903, 2005b.
10. Schmidt D, Jiang QX, MacKinnon R: Phospholipids and the origin of cationic gating charges in voltage sensors. Nature 444:775-779, 2006.
11. Jiang Y, Lee A, Chen J, et al: The open pore conformation of potassium channels. Nature 417:523-526, 2002.
12. Doyle DA, Morais Cabral J, Pfuetzner RA, et al: The structure of the potassium channel: Molecular basis of K^+ conduction and selectivity. Science 280:69-77, 1998.
13. Rasmusson RL, Morales MJ, Wang S, et al: Inactivation of voltage-gated cardiac K^+ channels. Circ Res 82:739-750, 1998.
14. Bezanilla F, Armstrong CM: Inactivation of the sodium channel. I. Sodium current experiments. J Gen Physiol 70:549-566, 1977.
15. Gulbis JM, Zhou M, Mann S, MacKinnon R: Structure of the cytoplasmic beta subunit-T1 assembly of voltage-dependent K^+ channels. Science 289:123-127, 2000.
16. Klemic KG, Kirsch GE, Jones SW: U-type inactivation of K_V3.1 and Shaker potassium channels. Biophys J 81:814-826, 2001.
17. Kurata HT, Soon GS, Eldstrom JR, et al: Amino-terminal determinants of U-type inactivation of voltage-gated K^+ channels. J Biol Chem 277:29045-29053, 2002.
18. Oudit GY, Kassiri Z, Sah R, et al: The molecular physiology of the cardiac transient outward potassium current (I(to)) in normal and diseased myocardium. J Mol Cell Cardiol 33:851-872, 2001.
19. Nerbonne JM, Nichols CG, Schwarz TL, Escande D: Genetic manipulation of cardiac K(+) channel function in mice: What have we learned, and where do we go from here? Circ Res 89:944-956, 2001.
20. Schram G, Pourrier M, Melnyk P, Nattel S: Differential distribution of cardiac ion channel expression as a basis for regional specialization in electrical function. Circ Res 90:939-950, 2002.
21. Nitabach MN, Llamas DA, Araneda RC, et al: A mechanism for combinatorial regulation of electrical activity: Potassium channel subunits capable of functioning as Src homology 3-dependent adaptors. Proc Natl Acad Sci U S A 98:705-710, 2001.
22. Takeuchi S, Takagishi Y, Yasui K, et al: Voltage-gated K(+) channel, Kv4.2, localizes predominantly to the transverse-axial tubular system of the rat myocyte. J Mol Cell Cardiol 32:1361-1369, 2000.
23. Keating MT, Sanguinetti MC: Molecular and cellular mechanisms of cardiac arrhythmias. Cell 104:569-580, 2001.
24. Tseng GN: I(Kr): The hERG channel. J Mol Cell Cardiol 33:835-849, 2001.
25. Kurokawa J, Abriel H, Kass RS: Molecular basis of the delayed rectifier current I(ks)in heart. J Mol Cell Cardiol 33:873-882, 2001.
26. Pond AL, Nerbonne JM: ERG proteins and functional cardiac I(Kr) channels in rat, mouse, and human heart. Trends Cardiovasc Med 11:286-294, 2001.
27. Deal KK, England SK, Tamkun MM: Molecular physiology of cardiac potassium channels. Physiol Rev 76:49-67, 1996.
28. Pongs O, Leicher T, Berger M, et al: Functional and molecular aspects of voltage-gated K^+ channel beta subunits. Ann N Y Acad Sci 868:344-355, 1999.
29. Kuryshev YA, Wible BA, Gudz TI, et al: KChAP/$K_V$beta1.2 interactions and their effects on cardiac Kv channel expression. Am J Physiol Cell Physiol 281: C290-C299, 2001.
30. An WF, Bowlby MR, Betty M, et al: Modulation of A-type potassium channels by a family of calcium sensors. Nature 403:553-556, 2000.
31. Deschenes I, DiSilvestre D, Juang GJ, et al: Regulation of K_V4.3 current by KChIP2 splice variants: A component of native cardiac I(to)? Circulation 106:423-429, 2002.
32. Kuo HC, Cheng CF, Clark RB, et al: A defect in the Kv channel–interacting protein 2 (KChIP2) gene leads to a complete loss of I(to) and confers susceptibility to ventricular tachycardia. Cell 2001; 107:801-813, 2001.
33. Guo W, Malin SA, Johns DC, et al: Modulation of Kv4-encoded K(+) currents in the mammalian myocardium by neuronal calcium sensor-1. J Biol Chem 277: 26436-26443, 2002.
34. Nakamura TY, Pountney DJ, Ozaita A, et al: A role for frequenin, a Ca^{2+}-binding protein, as a regulator of K_V4 K^+-currents. Proc Natl Acad Sci U S A 98:12808-12813, 2001.
35. Chen YH, Xu SJ, Bendahhou S, et al: KCNQ1 gain-of-function mutation in familial atrial fibrillation. Science 299: 251-254, 2003.
36. Tinel N, Diochot S, Borsotto M, et al: KCNE2 confers background current characteristics to the cardiac KCNQ1 potassium channel. EMBO J 19:6326-6330, 2000.
37. Nabauer M, Beuckelmann DJ, Uberfuhr P, Steinbeck G: Regional differences in current density and rate-dependent properties of the transient outward current in subepicardial and subendocardial myocytes of human left ventricle. Circulation 93: 168-177, 1996.
38. Di Diego JM, Sun ZQ, Antzelevitch C: I(to) and action potential notch are smaller in left vs. right canine ventricular epicardium. Am J Physiol 271:H548-H561, 1996.
39. Sah R, Ramirez RJ, Oudit GY, et al: Regulation of cardiac excitation-contraction coupling by action potential repolarization: Role of the transient outward potassium current (I(to)). J Physiol 546: 5-18, 2002.
40. Han W, Bao W, Wang Z, Nattel S: Comparison of ion-channel subunit expression in canine cardiac Purkinje fibers and ventricular muscle. Circ Res 91:790-797, 2002.
41. Po SS, Wu RC, Juang GJ, et al: Mechanism of alpha-adrenergic regulation of expressed hK_V4.3 currents. Am J Physiol Heart Circ Physiol 281:H2518-H2527, 2001.
42. Deschenes I, Tomaselli GF: Modulation of Kv4.3 current by accessory subunits. FEBS Lett 528:183-188, 2002.
43. Kuryshev YA, Gudz TI, Brown AM, Wible BA: K_{ChAP} as a chaperone for specific K(+) channels. Am J Physiol Cell Physiol 278:C931-C941, 2000.
44. Rosati B, Pan Z, Lypen S, et al: Regulation of KChIP2 potassium channel beta subunit gene expression underlies the gradient of transient outward current in canine and human ventricle. J Physiol. 2001;533:119-125.
45. Bahring R, Boland LM, Varghese A, et al: Kinetic analysis of open- and closed-state inactivation transitions in human K_V4.2 A-type potassium channels. J Physiol 535:65-81, 2001.
46. Costantini DL, Arruda EP, Agarwal P, et al: The homeodomain transcription factor Irx5 establishes the mouse cardiac ventricular repolarization gradient. Cell 123:347-358, 2005.
47. Rosati B, Grau F, McKinnon D: Regional variation in mRNA transcript abundance within the ventricular wall. J Mol Cell Cardiol 40:295-302, 2006.
48. Rossow CF, Dilly KW, Santana LF: Differential calcineurin/NFATc3 activity contributes to the Ito transmural gradient in the mouse heart. Circ Res 98:1306-1313, 2006.
49. Kassiri Z, Zobel C, Nguyen TT, et al: Reduction of I(to) causes hypertrophy in neonatal rat ventricular myocytes. Circ Res 90:578-585, 2002.
50. Zobel C, Kassiri Z, Nguyen TT, et al: Prevention of hypertrophy by overexpression of K_V4.2 in cultured neonatal cardiomyocytes. Circulation 106:2385-2391, 2002.
51. Perrier E, Perrier R, Richard S, Benitah JP: Ca^{2+} controls functional expression of the cardiac K^+ transient outward current via the calcineurin pathway. J Biol Chem 279:40634-40639, 2004.
52. Gong N, Bodi I, Zobel C, et al: Calcineurin increases cardiac transient outward K^+

currents via transcriptional up-regulation of $K_V4.2$ channel subunits. J Biol Chem 281:38498-38506, 2006.
53. Zhang TT, Takimoto K, Stewart AF, et al: Independent regulation of cardiac $K_V4.3$ potassium channel expression by angiotensin II and phenylephrine. Circ Res 88: 476-482, 2001.
54. Shimoni Y: Hormonal control of cardiac ion channels and transporters. Prog Biophys Mol Biol 1999;72:67-108, 1999.
55. Yu H, Gao J, Wang H, et al: Effects of the renin-angiotensin system on the current *I*(to) in epicardial and endocardial ventricular myocytes from the canine heart. Circ Res 86:1062-1068, 2000.
56. Oudit GY, Trivieri MG, Backx PH: Sulfhydryl modulation of K(+) currents: A possible cross-link between oxidative stress and altered cardiovascular function. J Mol Cell Cardiol 35:1-4, 2003.
57. Wickenden AD, Kaprielian R, Parker TG, et al: Effects of development and thyroid hormone on K^+ currents and K^+ channel gene expression in rat ventricle. J Physiol (Lond) 504:271-286, 1997.
58. Wickenden AD, Kaprielian R, You X-M, Backx PH: The thyroid hormone analog DITPA restores Ito in rats after myocardial infarction. Am J Physiol Heart Circ Physiol 278:H1105-H1116, 2000.
59. Le Bouter S, Demolombe S, Chambellan A, et al: Microarray analysis reveals complex remodeling of cardiac ion channel expression with altered thyroid status: Relation to cellular and integrated electrophysiology. Circ Res 92:234-242, 2003.
60. Trivieri MG, Oudit GY, Sah R, et al: Cardiac-specific elevations in thyroid hormone enhance contractility and prevent pressure overload–induced cardiac dysfunction. Proc Natl Acad Sci U S A 103:6043-6048, 2006.
61. Benitah JP, Perrier E, Gomez AM, Vassort G: Effects of aldosterone on transient outward K^+ current density in rat ventricular myocytes. J Physiol 537:151-160, 2001.
62. Rossow CF, Minami E, Chase EG, et al: NFATc3-induced reductions in voltage-gated K^+ currents after myocardial infarction. Circ Res 94:1340-1350, 2004.
63. Wickenden AD, Kaprielian R, Kassiri Z, et al: The role of action potential prolongation and altered intracellular calcium handling in the pathogenesis of heart failure. Cardiovasc Res 37:312-323, 1998.
64. Lebeche D, Kaprielian R, del Monte F, et al: In vivo cardiac gene transfer of $K_V4.3$ abrogates the hypertrophic response in rats after aortic stenosis. Circulation 110:3435-3443, 2004.
65. Colinas O, Gallego M, Setien R, et al: Differential modulation of $K_V4.2$ and $K_V4.3$ channels by calmodulin-dependent protein kinase II in rat cardiac myocytes. Am J Physiol Heart Circ Physiol 291:H1978-H1987, 2006.
66. Li J, Marionneau C, Zhang R, et al: Calmodulin kinase II inhibition shortens action potential duration by upregulation of K^+ currents. Circ Res 99:1092-1099, 2006.
67. van Ginneken AC, Veldkamp MW: Implications of inhomogeneous distribution of IKS and IKr channels in ventricle with respect to effects of class III agents and beta-agonists. Cardiovasc Res 43:20-22, 1999.
68. Gintant GA: Two components of delayed rectifier current in canine atrium and ventricle. Does I_{Ks} play a role in the reverse rate dependence of class III agents? Circ Res 78:26-37, 1996.
69. Abbott GW, Sesti F, Splawski I, et al: MiRP1 forms IKr potassium channels with HERG and is associated with cardiac arrhythmia. Cell 97:175-187, 1999.
70. Schimpf R, Wolpert C, Gaita F, et al: Short QT syndrome. Cardiovasc Res 67:357-366, 2005.
71. Furukawa T, Ono Y, Tsuchiya H, et al: Specific interaction of the potassium channel beta-subunit MinK with the sarcomeric protein T-cap suggests a T-tubule–myofibril linking system. J Mol Biol 313:775-784, 2001.
72. Yue L, Feng J, Wang Z, Nattel S: Adrenergic control of the ultrarapid delayed rectifier current in canine atrial myocytes. J Physiol 516:385-398, 1999.
73. Nitabach MN, Llamas DA, Thompson IJ, et al: Phosphorylation-dependent and phosphorylation-independent modes of modulation of Shaker family voltage-gated potassium channels by SRC family protein tyrosine kinases. J Neurosci 22:7913-7922, 2002.
74. Takimoto K, Levitan ES: Glucocorticoid induction of $K_V1.5$ K^+ channel gene expression in ventricle of rat heart. Circ Res 75:1006-1013, 1994.
75. Brouillette J, Trepanier-Boulay V, Fiset C: Effect of androgen deficiency on mouse ventricular repolarization. J Physiol 546:403-413, 2003.
76. Cui J, Melman Y, Palma E, et al: Cyclic AMP regulates the HERG K(+) channel by dual pathways. Curr Biol 10:671-674, 2000.
77. Satler CA, Walsh EP, Vesely MR, et al: Novel missense mutation in the cyclic nucleotide–binding domain of HERG causes long QT syndrome. Am J Med Genet 65:27-35, 1996.
78. Bian J, Cui J, McDonald TV: HERG K(+) channel activity is regulated by changes in phosphatidyl inositol 4,5-bisphosphate. Circ Res 89:1168-1176, 2001.
79. Magyar J, Iost N, Kortvely A, et al: Effects of endothelin-1 on calcium and potassium currents in undiseased human ventricular myocytes. Pflügers Arch 441:144-149, 2000.
80. Marx SO, Kurokawa J, Reiken S, et al: Requirement of a macromolecular signaling complex for beta adrenergic receptor modulation of the KCNQ1-KCNE1 potassium channel. Science 295:496-499, 2002.
81. Lopatin AN, Nichols CG: Inward rectifiers in the heart: An update on *I*(K1). J Mol Cell Cardiol 33:625-638, 2001.
82. Wang Z, Yue L, White M, et al: Differential distribution of inward rectifier potassium channel transcripts in human atrium versus ventricle. Circulation 98:2422-2428, 1998.
83. Zobel C, Cho HC, Nguyen TT, et al: Molecular dissection of the inward rectifier potassium current (I_{K1}) in rabbit cardiomyocytes: Evidence for heteromeric co-assembly of Kir2.1 and Kir2.2. J Physiol 550:365-372, 2003.
84. Preisig-Muller R, Schlichthorl G, Goerge T, et al: Heteromerization of Kir2.x potassium channels contributes to the phenotype of Andersen's syndrome. Proc Natl Acad Sci U S A 99:7774-7779, 2002.
85. Karle CA, Zitron E, Zhang W, et al: Human cardiac inwardly-rectifying K^+ channel Kir(2.1b) is inhibited by direct protein kinase C–dependent regulation in human isolated cardiomyocytes and in an expression system. Circulation 106: 1493-1499, 2002.
86. Tinker A, Jan YN, Jan LY: Regions responsible for the assembly of inwardly rectifying potassium channels. Cell 87:857-868, 1996.
87. Cho HC, Tsushima RG, Nguyen TT, et al: Two critical cysteine residues implicated in disulfide bond formation and proper folding of Kir2.1. Biochemistry 39:4649-4657, 2000.
88. Yang J, Yu M, Jan YN, Jan LY: Stabilization of ion selectivity filter by pore loop ion pairs in an inwardly rectifying potassium channel. Proc Natl Acad Sci U S A 94:1568-1572, 1997.
89. Mazzanti M, Assandri R, Ferroni A, DiFrancesco D: Cytoskeletal control of rectification and expression of four substates in cardiac inward rectifier K^+ channels. FASEB J 10:357-361, 1996.
90. Nishida M, MacKinnon R: Structural basis of inward rectification. Cytoplasmic pore of the G protein–gated inward rectifier GIRK1 at 1.8 Å resolution. Cell 111:957-965, 2002.
91. Koumi S, Backer CL, Arentzen CE, Sato R: β-Adrenergic modulation of the inwardly rectifying potassium channel in isolated human ventricular myocytes. Alteration in channel response to beta-adrenergic stimulation in failing human hearts. J Clin Invest 96:2870-2881, 1995.
92. Wischmeyer E, Karschin A: Receptor stimulation causes slow inhibition of IRK1 inwardly rectifying K^+ channels by direct protein kinase A–mediated phosphorylation. Proc Natl Acad Sci U S A 93:5819-5823, 1996.
93. Sato R, Koumi S: Modulation of the inwardly rectifying K^+ channel in isolated human atrial myocytes by alpha 1-adrenergic stimulation. J Membr Biol 148:185-191, 1995.
94. Zhu G, Qu Z, Cui N, Jiang C: Suppression of Kir2.3 activity by protein kinase C phosphorylation of the channel protein at threonine 53. J Biol Chem 274:11643-11746, 1999.
95. Rials SJ, Xu X, Wu Y, et al: Restoration of normal ventricular electrophysiology in renovascular hypertensive rabbits after treatment with losartan. J Cardiovasc Pharmacol 37:317-323, 2001.
96. Rohacs T, Chen J, Prestwich GD, Logothetis DE: Distinct specificities of inwardly rectifying K(+) channels for phosphoinositides. J Biol Chem 274: 36065-36072, 1999.
97. Lopes CM, Zhang H, Rohacs T, et al: Alterations in conserved Kir channel–PIP_2 interactions underlie channelopathies. Neuron 34:933-944, 2002.

98. Ai T, Fujiwara Y, Tsuji K, et al: Novel KCNJ2 mutation in familial periodic paralysis with ventricular dysrhythmia. Circulation 105:2592-2594, 2002.
99. Lesage F, Lazdunski M: Molecular and functional properties of two-pore-domain potassium channels. Am J Physiol Renal Physiol 279:F793-F801, 2000.
100. Ozaita A, Vega-Saenz de, Miera E: Cloning of two transcripts, HKT4.1a and HKT4.1b, from the human two-pore K^+ channel gene *KCNK4*. Chromosomal localization, tissue distribution and functional expression. Brain Res Mol Brain Res 102:18-27, 2002.
101. Nabauer M, Kaab S: Potassium channel down-regulation in heart failure. Cardiovasc Res 37:324-334, 1998.
102. Pogwizd SM, Bers DM: Na/Ca exchange in heart failure: Contractile dysfunction and arrhythmogenesis. Ann N Y Acad Sci 976:454-465, 2002.
103. Kaab S, Dixon J, Duc J, et al: Molecular basis of transient outward potassium current downregulation in human heart failure: A decrease in $K_V4.3$ mRNA correlates with a reduction in current density. Circulation 98:1383-1393, 1998.
104. Tsuji Y, Opthof T, Kamiya K, et al: Pacing-induced heart failure causes a reduction of delayed rectifier potassium currents along with decreases in calcium and transient outward currents in rabbit ventricle. Cardiovasc Res 48:300-309, 2000.

Intracellular Signaling and Regulation of Cardiac Ion Channels

4

Peter J. Mohler and Mark E. Anderson

CHAPTER OUTLINE

Signaling Overview

Ion channels, ionic exchangers, and ion-motive ATPases all exist in cells as macromolecular complexes. These electrical current–generating protein complexes can be studied precisely and in real time using high-resolution voltage clamp methods.[1] The advent of patch clamp and molecular cloning allowed measurements of ionic currents in heterologous cells. The extent of biophysical information generated by these approaches was unprecedented and allowed for detailed structure-function analysis of the molecular physiology underlying the cardiac action potential and cardiac arrhythmias. On the other hand, assays of electrical proteins in heterologous cells were performed without knowledge of the membership or stoichiometry of the entire signaling complex. Historically, the initial focus of ion channel studies was on the pore-forming α subunit; widespread appreciation that α subunits are coordinately regulated by auxiliary β subunits, protein kinases and phosphatases, and redox signaling, scaffolding, and anchoring proteins emerged more recently.

Cardiac electrophysiology has entered an era of increasing nuance and greater complexity, with the important task of quantitatively explicating the biology of macromolecular electrical protein complexes. This chapter examines some of the highlights in this rapidly advancing field and presents examples that illustrate the (sometimes surprising) importance of the contribution of auxiliary proteins in regulating cardiac electrophysiology.

Signaling Regulation for Disease

The first long QT syndromes were identified as genetic mutations that altered the ion channel activity (gating) properties of potassium channel α subunits (reviewed in Chapter 49).[2] Other long QT syndromes due to mutations in auxiliary potassium channel subunits were identified later.[3] Recognition that genetic arrhythmias are linked to defects in non–pore-forming ion channel subunits is now widespread. Several such examples, including ankyrin syndrome, caveolin-3, and yotiao, are examined in detail later in the chapter. Dynamic, reversible regulation of electrical protein complexes is accomplished by phosphorylation, and oxidation. Normal physiologic regulation of electrical protein complexes occurs in part because kinases and phosphatases, and oxidases and reductases participate in these macromolecular complexes. Dysregulation of kinase-[4] and of redox-mediated signaling[5] to ion channel complexes has now been implicated in establishing proarrhythmic substrates in acquired heart disease. The role of one such proarrhythmic kinase, the multifunctional calmodulin–dependent protein kinase II (CaMKII), is explored later in the chapter.

Local Myocyte Signaling Regulates Global Cardiac Function

Compartmentalization of local signaling pathways in the vertebrate cardiomyocyte is critical for global cardiac function. This concept is well exemplified by the regulation of local calcium concentrations during cardiomyocyte systole and diastole.[6] After initiation of cardiomyocyte depolarization, calcium enters the cardiomyocyte cytosol through L-type calcium channels ($Ca_V1.2$) localized in clusters along the transverse (T) tubule membrane (Fig. 4-1). This increase in cytosolic calcium is detected by tightly juxtaposed (approximately 15 nm) sarcoplasmic reticulum (SR) ryanodine receptor calcium release channels (see Fig. 4-1). On stimulation, ryanodine receptors release calcium down an approximately 10,000-fold concentration gradient into the myocyte cytosol to bind and activate the thin-filament protein troponin and initiate cardiomyocyte contraction. Myocyte relaxation is initiated by multiple molecular pathways that remove calcium from the cytosol. The primary molecular mechanism for cytosolic calcium extrusion is the sarcoplasmic-endoplasmic reticulum (SR-ER) Ca^{2+}-ATPase (SERCA2), which pumps calcium against its concentration gradient into the ER-SR.[6] Calcium extrusion also is mediated by the sarcolemmal Na^+-Ca^{2+} exchanger, and to a lesser extent by the plasma membrane Ca^{2+}-ATPase (PMCA2).[7] The electrochemical gradient required for this excitation-contraction coupling is maintained in an ATP-dependent process by the sarcolemmal Na^+,K^+-ATPase.

Cardiomyocyte Local Membrane Organization: Form Fits Function

The structural and molecular properties of cardiomyocyte membrane domains represent a central feature for regulation of local ion channel signaling pathways. Of interest, each specific vertebrate cell type (ventricular myocyte, atrial myocyte, sinoatrial node myocyte) has evolved unique structural elements

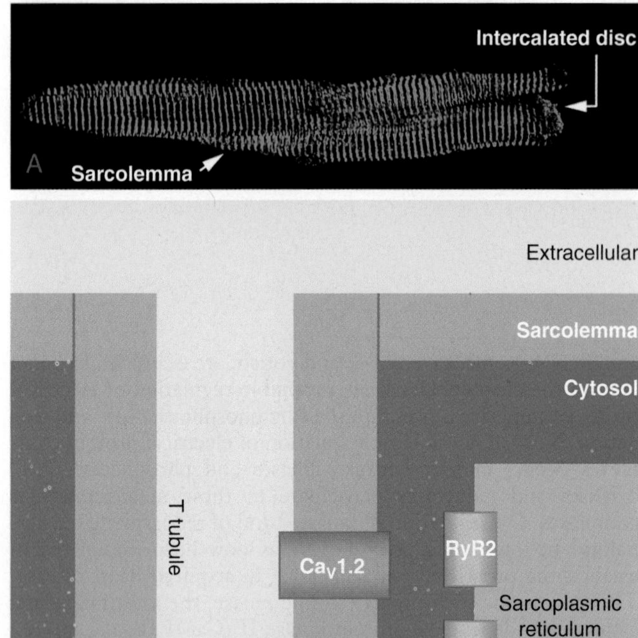

Figure 4-1 Ventricular cardiomyocyte membrane organization. **A,** The adult ventricular cardiomyocyte (stained with α-actinin) displays a complex membrane structure. The sarcolemmal membrane contains invaginations, the transverse (T) tubules, that regulate excitation-contraction coupling. **B,** Ryanodine receptors, localized on the interior sarcoplasmic reticulum membrane, are tightly coupled with L-type calcium channels ($Ca_V1.2$) on the T tubule membrane. Recent findings suggest that the cardiomyocyte nuclear envelope is coupled with the sarcoplasmic reticulum. (From Wu X, Zhang T, Bossuyt J, et al: Local $InsP_3$-dependent perinuclear Ca^{2+} signaling in cardiac myocyte excitation-transcription coupling. J Clin Invest 116:675-682, 2006.)

and molecular machinery to regulate intracellular signaling to control unique functions.[8] Although the unique features of each cell type place limits on the generic discussion of electrical protein complexes, some general points and representative cell-specific elements that illustrate key concepts are discussed next.

The vertebrate ventricular cardiomyocyte is composed of an external membrane, or *sarcolemmal membrane*. The sarcolemmal membrane is further divided into the external membrane (sarcolemma) and regularly organized membrane invaginations—the T tubules (see Fig. 4-1)—that play an essential role in cardiomyocyte *excitation-contraction* coupling. Additionally, ventricular cardiomyocytes display a highly organized *intercalated disc* at the terminal boundary of adjacent cells that regulates both electrical and mechanical signaling (see Fig. 4-1).

The complexity of the ventricular cardiomyocyte external membrane is matched by the organization of the intracellular membrane. Specifically, the ventricular cardiomyocyte SR-ER is a web-like organelle critical for regulating intracellular calcium (see Fig. 4-1).[9] This internal membrane is tightly juxtaposed with the external T tubule network to regulate intracellular calcium and excitation-contraction coupling (see later). Moreover, recent findings demonstrate that this internal membrane network is likely tightly coupled to the ventricular cardiomyocyte nuclear envelope to modulate myocyte transcriptional programs (termed *excitation-transcription* coupling).[10]

Cardiomyocyte ultrastructure has been extensively covered in multiple reviews.[11] Moreover, the basic principles of excitation contraction are well defined in various texts and reviews.[6,7] Therefore, this section focuses on recent discoveries in cardiomyocyte signaling including the role of ankyrin polypeptides in the biogenesis and maintenance of ion channel signaling domains in cardiomyocytes, the role of caveolae-enriched membrane compartments for compartmentalization of ion channel and associated signaling molecules, and yotiao-dependent regulation of potassium channel activity.

Cardiac Ankyrins Organize Ion Channel Signaling Complexes

Ankyrins are a family of adapter proteins required for the targeting of ion channels and transporters in a number of cell types, including erythrocytes, Purkinje neurons, renal epithelial cells, cardiomyocytes, and pancreatic beta cells.[12-15] Ankyrin-associated membrane proteins include voltage-gated sodium channels $Na_V1.1$, $Na_V1.2$, $Na_V1.5$, and $Na_V1.6$; voltage-gated potassium channels KCNQ2 and KCNQ3; inositol 1,4,5-trisphosphate ($InsP_3$) receptor; Na^+-Ca^{2+} exchanger; anion exchanger, and Na^+,K^+-ATPase.[16,17] Moreover, ankyrins associate with cell adhesion molecules including neurofascin.[15] In addition to binding membrane proteins, ankyrins associate with the beta-spectrin family of actin-binding proteins[15] and cytoskeletal proteins obscurin and titin.[18,19] Finally, ankyrins have been linked with the targeting of signaling proteins including Fas, clathrin, protein phosphatase 2, and the cellular co-chaperone Hdj-1.[15,20-22]

Ankyrin-B Coordinates Local Organization of Na^+-Ca^{2+} Exchanger, Na^+,K^+-ATPase, and $InsP_3$ Receptor

In heart, ankyrin-B is required for the local organization of ion channel-transporter signaling complexes at the T tubule–SR membrane (Fig. 4-2). Specifically, cardiac ankyrin-B directly associates with, and targets Na^+-Ca^{2+} exchanger and Na^+,K^+-ATPase to the T tubule membrane, and $InsP_3$ receptor to the sarcoplasmic membrane domain (see Fig. 4-2).[23,24] Mice lacking ankyrin-B die as neonates, and cardiomyocytes derived from these neonatal mice before death display abnormal expression and localization of Na^+,K^+-ATPase, Na^+-Ca^{2+} exchanger, and $InsP_3$ receptor.[24,25] Additionally, ankyrin-B–null cardiomyocytes display aberrant calcium dynamics and abnormal spontaneous contraction rates.[25] Cardiomyocytes derived from adult ankyrin-$B^{+/-}$ mice (heterozygotes with approximately 50% reduction in ankyrin-B protein) display reduced targeting of Na^+,K^+-ATPase, Na^+-Ca^{2+} exchanger, and $InsP_3$ receptor.[24] Moreover, ankyrin-$B^{+/-}$ adult mouse cardiomyocytes display elevated SR calcium levels and increased SR calcium transients, likely resulting from abnormal targeting of Na^+,K^+-ATPase and Na^+-Ca^{2+} exchanger.[24] Finally, although displaying normal baseline action potentials, ankyrin-$B^{+/-}$ cardiomyocytes display afterdepolarizations after treatment with isoproterenol.[24] Conscious ankyrin-$B^{+/-}$ mice display bradycardia with minor elevations in QT_c at rest, but no spontaneous arrhythmias.[24] In contrast, ankyrin-$B^{+/-}$ mice treated with catecholamines display polymorphic arrhythmia, syncope, and sudden death.[24]

Human *ANK2* gene variants are associated with a potentially fatal polymorphic ventricular arrhythmia termed *ankyrin-B syndrome*.[24,26,27] Cardiac clinical manifestations in variant carriers include sinus bradycardia, heart rate variability, atrial fibrillation, polymorphic ventricular arrhythmia, and sudden cardiac death.[24,26,27] Clinical phenotypes vary, however, depending on the specific *ANK2* gene variant, and variability of phenotype occurs across patient populations.[28] Sinus node dysfunction and risk of catecholaminergic ventricular arrhythmia are consistent clinical features. To date, nine human *ANK2* variants have

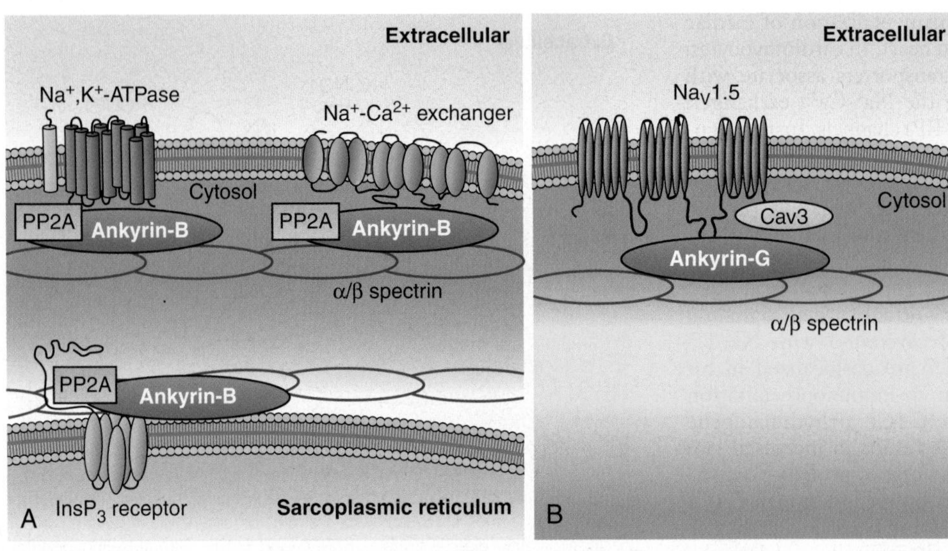

Figure 4-2 Ankyrin-based macromolecular signaling complex. **A,** Ankyrin-B is required for the targeting of Na^+-Ca^{2+} exchanger and Na^+,K^+-ATPase to transverse tubule membrane domains. Additionally, ankyrin-B is required for targeting $InsP_3$ receptors to the myocyte sarcoplasmic reticulum. Recent findings support a role of ankyrin-B for the targeting of protein phosphatase 2A (PP2A) in myocytes.[20] Ankyrin-B dysfunction results in abnormal cytosolic calcium and human arrhythmia. **B,** $Na_V1.5$ localization at the intercalated disc membrane requires direct interaction with ankyrin-G. Recent data demonstrate that caveolin-3 (Cav3) also is associated with $Na_V1.5$.

4

been identified.[24,26,27] Three represent severe ankyrin-B loss-of-function mutations when introduced into cardiomyocytes.[26]

In addition to a central role of cardiac ankyrin-B for organizing key ion channels and transporters in heart, recent evidence suggests that it may serve a key role in organizing ion channel-transporter macromolecular signaling complexes. Bhasin and colleagues recently identified B56 alpha, the regulatory subunit for protein phosphatase 2A (PP2A) as a binding partner for ankyrin-B in cardiomyocytes (see Fig. 4-2).[20] PP2A is not properly localized in primary cardiomyocytes lacking ankyrin-B.[20] Although the role of protein phosphorylation for ankyrin-B–associated protein Na^+-Ca^{2+} exchanger is controversial, ankyrin-B partners Na^+,K^+-ATPase and $InsP_3$ receptor are known phosphoproteins.[29,30] Additionally, ankyrin-B itself is likely a target for post-translational protein phosphorylation regulation. An important future goal for the field is to determine the targets of ankyrin-B–targeted PP2A in heart.

Ankyrin-G is Required for Coordinating $Na_V1.5$ Signaling at the Cardiomyocyte Intercalated Disc

Compartmentalization of $Na_V1.5$ at the intercalated disc membrane of cardiomyocytes requires ankyrin-G (see Fig. 4-2). Evidence for a potential role for ankyrin-G in cardiac Na_V channel organization at the intercalated disc includes direct association of ankyrin-G membrane-binding domain with brain Na_V channel isoforms ($Na_V1.2$, $Na_V1.6$)[31,32] and clustering of ankyrin-G with brain Na_V channel isoforms at nodes of Ranvier, axon initial segments, and neuromuscular junction.[32-35] Independent work by Dargent and Lambert laboratories identified the ankyrin-binding motif in the $Na_V1.2$ α subunit.[36,37] This nine amino acid motif is conserved across most voltage-gated sodium channel α isoforms including $Na_V1.1$, $Na_V1.2$, $Na_V1.4$, $Na_V1.5$, and $Na_V1.6$.[38]

Based on the conservation of the ankyrin-G–binding motif in cardiac $Na_V1.5$, Bennett and colleagues characterized the expression pattern of ankyrin-G in vertebrate heart.[38] Consistent with findings from brain, ankyrin-G is coexpressed with $Na_V1.5$ at the cardiomyocyte intercalated disc membrane.[38] Moreover, ankyrin-G copurifies with $Na_V1.5$ from detergent-soluble lysates of heart and directly binds $Na_V1.5$ in in vitro binding assays.[38] Removal of the 9-amino-acid ankyrin-binding motif from $Na_V1.5$ inhibits ankyrin-G–binding activity for the channel.[38]

In 2002, Priori and colleagues identified a mis-sense variant in *SCN5A* in a female proband with the Brugada syndrome.[39] This single variant resulted in substitution of a highly conserved glutamic acid to lysine in the $Na_V1.5$ ankyrin-binding motif.[38] Subsequent biochemical experiments demonstrated that this mutant $Na_V1.5$ variant lacked ankyrin-binding activity in vitro and was not efficiently targeted to the intercalated disc membrane surface of adult rat cardiomyocytes.[38] Therefore, similar to ankyrin-B, ankyrin-G is required for the biogenesis of ion channel signaling domains in excitable cardiomyocytes. In keeping with the multivalent role of ankyrin-B in heart for coordinating ion channel, transporter, cytoskeletal, and signaling molecules, ankyrin-G probably is responsible for the targeting of additional proteins to the $Na_V1.5$ protein intercalated disc complex.

Caveolae Compartmentalize Local Signaling Complexes

Caveolae are small (less than 100 nm in diameter) omega-shaped lipid and cholesterol membrane domains. In a host of tissues, caveolar function has been linked with cell signaling and endocytosis.[40] Recent findings in cardiac tissue illustrate a potentially important role for caveolae in the compartmentalization of ion channels, signaling proteins, and effector proteins. The primary coat protein of caveolae is the polypeptide caveolin. In humans, three genes encode caveolin-1, caveolin-2, and caveolin-3. Caveolin-3 is the principal caveolin polypeptide expressed in diaphragm, cardiac muscle, smooth muscle, and skeletal muscle.[41]

Caveolin-3 is required for normal muscle physiology. Mice homozygous for a caveolin-3–null mutation display mild to moderate cardiomyopathy[42] as well as disorganized T tubules.[43,44] Additionally, these mice display mild skeletal muscle myopathy.[43,45] In humans, the *CAV3* gene (encoding caveolin-3) variants are associated with rippling muscle disease, hyperCKemia (i.e., unexplained, persistently high levels of creatine kinase),[42] distal myopathy, and limb-girdle muscular dystrophy. Recently, Vatta and colleagues identified human long QT probands with four unique *CAV3* gene variants.[46] *CAV3* proband phenotypes included prolonged QT_c, sinus bradycardia, and nonexertional syncope. More recently, both Arnestad and Cronk and their coworkers identified an association between *CAV3* gene variants and the sudden infant death syndrome.[47,48]

Caveolae are critical for the compartmentalization of cardiac ion channels and signaling molecules in heart. In cardiomyocytes, a number of key ion channels and transporters associate with caveolae-enriched domains, including the Na^+-Ca^{2+} exchanger, $Na_V1.5$, transient receptor potential (TRP) channels, $InsP_3$ receptors, plasma membrane Ca^{2+}-ATPase, $K_V1.5$, HCN4, and $Ca_V1.2$.[49-57] Moreover, caveolae compartmentalize ion channels-transporters with key signaling molecules, including protein kinase C (PKC), adenylyl cyclase, endothelial nitric oxide synthase (eNOS), PP2A, protein kinase A (PKA), β_2-adrenergic receptors, and the G-protein αs subunit (Gαs).[58-64]

The importance of caveolin-3 for normal cardiac signaling is illustrated by recent association of caveolin-3 with $Na_V1.5$ (see Fig. 4-2). Caveolin-3 and $Na_V1.5$ are co-localized in rat and human heart[46,57] and associate in co-immunoprecipitation experiments.[46] Expression of human *CAV3* arrhythmia gene variants with $Na_V1.5$ in HEK293 cells results in increased late (sustained) sodium current. These phenotypes probably constitute the molecular basis of arrhythmia observed in human *CAV3* variant carriers. The role of caveolin-3 for $Na_V1.5$ signaling is currently unknown. Caveolin-3 may allosterically regulate the activity of $Na_V1.5$, and human variants may affect this activity. Alternatively, caveolin-3 may recruit additional ion channels or signaling proteins to a caveolar $Na_V1.5$ macromolecular complex. Although future experiments will be required to resolve these specific issues, these findings clearly illustrate the importance of compartmentalized signaling complexes for normal cardiac function.

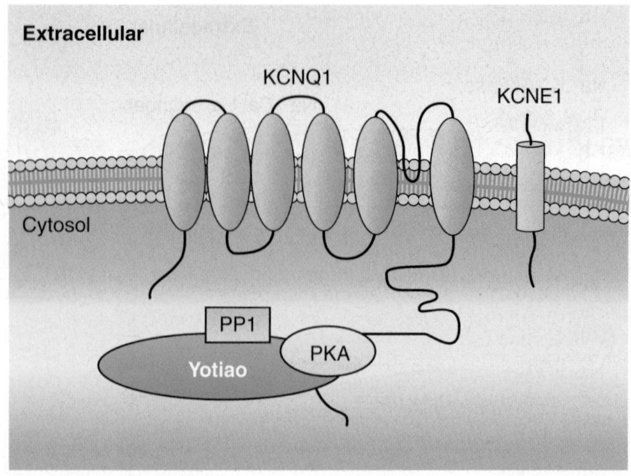

Figure 4-3 Cardiac yotiao protein complex regulates I_{Ks} signaling. The adaptor protein yotiao serves as a signaling scaffold for adrenergic regulation of I_{Ks}. Specifically, yotiao directly couples KCNQ1 and KCNE1 with signaling proteins, including protein kinase A (PKA) and protein phosphatase 1 (PP1). Human KCNQ1 variants that affect interaction with yotiao display abnormal adrenergic regulation.

Local Regulation of I_{Ks} is Required for Cardiac Function

Regulation of local ion channel signaling complexes is required for normal cardiac repolarization. *KCNQ1* and *KCNE1* encode the α and β subunits of the slowly activating and deactivating I_{Ks} current in heart.[65-67] Human loss-of-function variants in *KCNQ1* are linked with human long QT syndrome type 1 arrhythmia, whereas gain-of-function mutations are associated with atrial fibrillation[68] and short QT syndrome.[69] Loss-of-function variants in *KCNE1* are associated with long QT syndrome type 5. Although both syndromes may be clinically managed, both *LQT1* and *LQT5* variant carriers are at risk for polymorphic ventricular arrhythmia and sudden cardiac death in response to catecholamines.[70] Of interest, in both cardiomyocytes and heterologous cells, I_{Ks} is highly sensitive to PKA. Specifically, β-adrenergic stimulation augments I_{Ks}, thereby promoting action potential repolarization.

Yotiao is a large, multivalent adapter protein required for organizing ion channel signaling complexes in neuron[71,72] (Fig. 4-3). Specifically, work from multiple groups of investigators implicates yotiao activity critical for the recruitment of the regulatory subunit of PKA (an A kinase–anchoring protein [AKAP]) to neuronal channel complexes. More recent data demonstrate that yotiao-dependent protein compartmentalization also is required for I_{Ks} channel signaling in heart.[73] Kass and colleagues demonstrated that in addition to recruiting PKA activity to regulate I_{Ks} (as an AKAP), yotiao directly associates with and targets protein phosphatase 1 (PP1) to the KCNQ1–KCNE1 protein complex, consistent with previous findings in neurons.[72] In an elegant set of experiments, Kurokawa and colleagues demonstrated that yotiao activity was required for both scaffolding activity of the channel complex with signaling molecules and regulation of channel gating.[74,75]

Several years ago, a mis-sense variant was identified in a large cohort of Finnish patients with long QT syndrome type 1.[76] *KCNQ1* (G589D) variant carriers displayed significant arrhythmia events associated with catecholaminergic stimulation. Subsequent electrophysiological analysis of the channel variant in heterologous cells revealed that the channel variant displayed increased threshold of activation and a significant reduction in channel membrane expression.[76] A striking finding is that the *KCNQ1* channel G589D variant lacks yotiao-binding activity and therefore disrupts local ion channel signaling mechanisms.[73] Specifically, the *KCNQ1* G589D variant renders the I_{Ks} channel complex less sensitive to β-adrenergic regulation.[73] Mathematical modeling demonstrated that the mutant channel behaved appropriately at rest (i.e., no resting QT instability was noted). In the context of sympathetic stimulation, however, the mutant channel could produce electrical instability, prolongation of QT_c, and extrasystoles.[77] These findings with I_{Ks} channel signaling complexes clearly demonstrate the importance of local ion channel signaling domains for normal cardiomyocyte electrical stability.

Calmodulin-Dependent Protein Kinase II Targets $Ca_V1.2$ by Way of an Adapter Sequence Embedded in β Subunits

CaMKII regulates key Ca^{2+}-homeostatic proteins and a wide variety of ion channel proteins. The contributions of CaMKII to cardiac arrhythmias and heart failure are addressed in detail in Chapter 65. In brief, CaMKII activity and expression are increased in human heart failure, and in many animal models of heart failure.[78] CaMKII exerts a variety of proarrhythmic influences, but one key effect is that CaMKII causes $Ca_V1.2$ to enter a highly active gating mode that induces early afterdepolarizations and contributes to cellular Ca^{2+} overload.[79] This section focuses specifically on a recently recognized novel mechanism for CaMKII association to $Ca_V1.2$ β subunits that illustrates the potential complexity and rich possibilities for signaling within macromolecular protein complexes.

Despite the large number of CaMKII target proteins in heart, CaMKII is not homogeneously distributed in cardiac myocytes. CaMKII is enriched along the Z lines, consistent with association to T tubule proteins,[80] where it is anticipated to regulate excitation-contraction coupling[81] and L-type calcium channels (predominantly $Ca_V1.2$ in ventricular myocytes).[82]

CaMKII actions on $Ca_V1.2$ require cytoskeletal proteins[83] and are highly dependent upon the ultrastructural organization of SR Ca^{2+} release in ventricular myocytes.[84] Most protein kinases participate in macromolecular ion channel complexes by way of adapter proteins (e.g., yotiao or caveolin-3, as discussed previously). CaMKII adapter proteins ("CaMKaps") have not been reported, however. CaMKII is inactive under basal conditions because the kinase domain is bound to a "pseudosubstrate" amino acid sequence in the regulatory domain.[85]

We used this sequence as a template to search for candidate proteins with the capacity for direct CaMKII binding, without the requirement for an intervening adapter protein. Two important "hits" were the two main $Ca_V1.2$ β subunit isoforms (types 1 and 2). A predicted CaMKII phosphorylation target (T498) also was present in this predicted binding domain for all $Ca_V1.2$ β subunit isoforms (β1 to β4). Our studies showed that CaMKII binds directly to a highly restricted target sequence and that phosphorylation of T498 is necessary for CaMKII facilitation of $Ca_V1.2$ current in adult ventricular myocytes (Fig. 4-4).[86] These data reveal a previously unrecognized, parsimonious association mechanism whereby a kinase recognizes a macromolecular complex by way of an embedded target sequence.

Of interest, the biophysical effect of CaMKII on $Ca_V1.2$ is mimicked by overexpression of a calmodulin-binding sequence on the $Ca_V1.2$ intracellular carboxyl (C) terminus.[84] $Ca_V1.2$ "autoactivation" by these embedded agonists requires binding to an unstructured amino (N)-terminal segment of the β subunit.[87] This binding and activation are prevented by calmodulin, showing that calmodulin (also part of the $Ca_V1.2$ macromolecular complex) (see Fig. 4-4)[88] plays a dual role to activate CaMKII, while also negatively regulating $Ca_V1.2$ channel stimulating α-β subunit interactions. More information is necessary before a global understanding of the regulation of the $Ca_V1.2$ macromolecular complex by CaMKII and calmodulin is achieved. The dynamic nature of these interactions means that a variety of approaches will be required, in addition to static structural information, to accomplish this quest. Improved understanding of macromolecular interactions of electrically active proteins in heart is a necessary step for developing the next generation of antiarrhythmic medications.

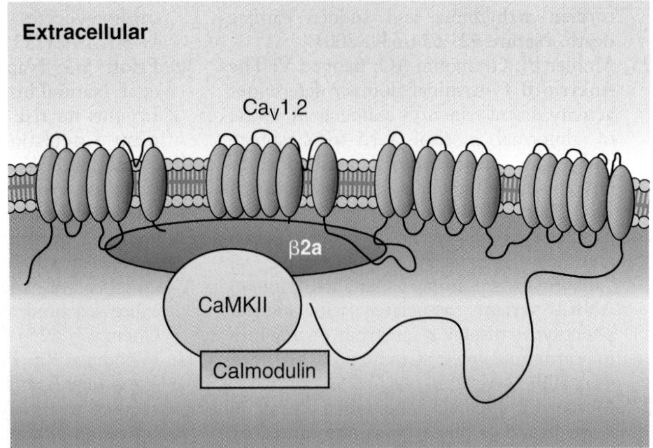

Figure 4-4 Calcium-calmodulin kinase II (CaMKII) targets $Ca_V1.2$ by means of an adaptor sequence in β-subunits. $Ca_V1.2$ β2a targets the multifunctional CaMKII to the L-type calcium channel macromolecular complex to modulate cardiomyocyte $Ca_V1.2$ activity.

References

1. Hamill OP, Marty A, Neher E, et al: Improved patch-clamp techniques for high-resolution current recording from cells and cell-free membrane patches. Pflügers Arch 391:85-100, 1981.
2. Sanguinetti MC, Jiang C, Curran ME, Keating MT: A mechanistic link between an inherited and an acquired cardiac arrhythmia: HERG encodes the I_{Kr} potassium channel. Cell 81:299-307, 1995.
3. Splawski I, Tristani-Firouzi M, Lehmann MH, et al: Mutations in the hMinK gene cause long QT syndrome and suppress I_{Ks} function. Nat Genet 17:338-340, 1997.
4. Anderson ME, Higgins LS, Schulman H: Disease mechanisms and emerging therapies: Protein kinases and their inhibitors in myocardial disease. Nat Clin Pract 3:437-445, 2006.
5. Heinemann SH, Hoshi T: Multifunctional potassium channels: Electrical switches and redox enzymes, all in one. Sci STKE 2006 (350):pe33, 2006.
6. Bers DM: Excitation-Contraction Coupling and Cardiac Contractile Force, 2nd ed. Dordrecht, Kluwer, 2001.
7. Bers DM: Cardiac excitation-contraction coupling. Nature 415:198-205, 2002.
8. Song LS, Guatimosim S, Gomez-Viquez L, et al: Calcium biology of the transverse tubules in heart. Ann N Y Acad Sci 1047:99-111, 2005.
9. Sun XH, Protasi F, Takahashi M, et al: Molecular architecture of membranes involved in excitation-contraction coupling of cardiac muscle. J Cell Biol 129:659-671, 1995.
10. Wu X, Zhang T, Bossuyt J, et al: Local InsP3-dependent perinuclear Ca^{2+} signaling in cardiac myocyte excitation-transcription coupling. J Clin Invest 116:675-682, 2006.
11. Frank JS, Garfinkel A: Immunological and structural configuration of membrane and cytoskeletal proteins involved in excitation-contraction coupling of cardiac muscle. In Langer GA, (ed): The Myocardium, 2nd ed. San Diego, Academic Press, 1997, pp 1-32.
12. Mohler PJ, Healy JA, Xue H, et al: Ankyrin-B syndrome: Enhanced cardiac function balanced by risk of cardiac death and premature senescence. PLoS ONE 2:e1051, 2007.
13. Kizhatil K, Davis JQ, Davis L, et al: Ankyrin-G is a molecular partner of E-cadherin in epithelial cells and early embryos. J Biol Chem 282:26552-26561, 2007.
14. Kizhatil K, Yoon W, Mohler PJ, et al: Ankyrin-G and beta2-spectrin collaborate in biogenesis of lateral membrane of human bronchial epithelial cells. J Biol Chem 282: 2029-2037, 2007.
15. Bennett V, Baines AJ: Spectrin and ankyrin-based pathways: Metazoan inventions for integrating cells into tissues. Physiol Rev 81:1353-1392, 2001.
16. Mohler PJ, Wehrens XH: Mechanisms of human arrhythmia syndromes: abnormal cardiac macromolecular interactions. Physiology 22:342-350, 2007.
17. Cunha SR, Mohler PJ: Cardiac ankyrins: Essential components for development and maintenance of excitable membrane domains in heart. Cardiovasc Res 71:22-29, 2006.
18. Kontrogianni-Konstantopoulos A, Jones EM, Van Rossum DB, Bloch RJ: Obscurin is a ligand for small ankyrin 1 in skeletal muscle. Mol Biol Cell 14:1138-1148, 2003.
19. Bagnato P, Barone V, Giacomello E, et al: Binding of an ankyrin-1 isoform to obscurin suggests a molecular link between the sarcoplasmic reticulum and myofibrils in striated muscles. J Cell Biol 160:245-253, 2003.
20. Bhasin N, Cunha SR, Mudannayake M, et al: Molecular basis for PP2A regulatory subunit B56α targeting in cardiomyocytes. Am J Physiol Heart Circ Physiol 293:H109-H119, 2007.
21. Mohler PJ, Hoffman JA, Davis JQ, et al: Isoform specificity among ankyrins: An amphipathic alpha-helix in the divergent regulatory domain of ankyrin-B interacts with the molecular co-chaperone Hdj1/Hsp40. J Biol Chem 279:25798-25804, 2004.
22. Del Rio M, Imam A, DeLeon M, et al: The death domain of kidney ankyrin interacts with Fas and promotes Fas-mediated cell death in renal epithelia. J Am Soc Nephrol 15:41-51, 2004.
23. Mohler PJ, Davis JQ, Bennett V: Ankyrin-B coordinates the Na/K ATPase, Na/Ca exchanger, and InsP(3) receptor in a cardiac T-tubule/SR microdomain. PLoS Biol 3:e423, 2005.
24. Mohler PJ, Schott JJ, Gramolini AO, et al: Ankyrin-B mutation causes type 4 long-QT

cardiac arrhythmia and sudden cardiac death. Nature 421:634-639, 2003.

25. Mohler PJ, Gramolini AO, Bennett V: The Ankyrin-B C-terminal domain determines activity of ankyrin-B/G chimeras in rescue of abnormal inositol 1,4,5-trisphosphate and ryanodine receptor distribution in ankyrin-B(–/–) neonatal cardiomyocytes. J Biol Chem 277:10599-10607, 2002.
26. Mohler PJ, Le Scouarnec S, Denjoy I, et al: Defining the cellular phenotype of "ankyrin-B syndrome" variants: Human ANK2 variants associated with clinical phenotypes display a spectrum of activities in cardiomyocytes. Circulation 115:432-441, 2007.
27. Mohler PJ, Splawski I, Napolitano C, et al: A cardiac arrhythmia syndrome caused by loss of ankyrin-B function. Proc Natl Acad Sci U S A 101:9137-9142, 2004.
28. Mohler PJ: Ankyrins and human disease: What the electrophysiologist should know. J Cardiovasc Electrophysiol 17:1153-1159, 2006.
29. DeSouza N, Reiken S, Ondrias K, et al: Protein kinase A and two phosphatases are components of the inositol 1,4,5-trisphosphate receptor macromolecular signaling complex. J Biol Chem 277: 39397-39400, 2002.
30. Lecuona E, Dada LA, Sun H, et al: Na,K-ATPase alpha1-subunit dephosphorylation by protein phosphatase 2A is necessary for its recruitment to the plasma membrane. FASEB J 20:2618-2620, 2006.
31. Davis JQ, Lambert S, Bennett V: Molecular composition of the node of Ranvier: Identification of ankyrin-binding cell adhesion molecules neurofascin (mucin+/third FNIII domain–) and NrCAM at nodal axon segments. J Cell Biol 135:1355-1367, 1996.
32. Kordeli E, Lambert S, Bennett V: AnkyrinG. A new ankyrin gene with neural-specific isoforms localized at the axonal initial segment and node of Ranvier. J Biol Chem 270:2352-2359, 1995.
33. Flucher BE, Daniels MP: Distribution of Na^+ channels and ankyrin in neuromuscular junctions is complementary to that of acetylcholine receptors and the 43 kD protein. Neuron 3:163-175, 1989.
34. Kordeli E, Ludosky MA, Deprette C, et al: AnkyrinG is associated with the postsynaptic membrane and the sarcoplasmic reticulum in the skeletal muscle fiber. J Cell Sci 111:2197-2207, 1998.
35. Wood SJ, Slater CR: β-Spectrin is colocalized with both voltage-gated sodium channels and ankyrinG at the adult rat neuromuscular junction. J Cell Biol 140: 675-684, 1998.
36. Garrido JJ, Giraud P, Carlier E, et al: A targeting motif involved in sodium channel clustering at the axonal initial segment. Science 300:2091-2094, 2003.
37. Lemaillet G, Walker B, Lambert S: Identification of a conserved ankyrin-binding motif in the family of sodium channel alpha subunits. J Biol Chem 278: 27333-27339, 2003.
38. Mohler PJ, Rivolta I, Napolitano C, et al: $Na_V1.5$ E1053K mutation causing Brugada syndrome blocks binding to ankyrin-G and expression of $Na_V1.5$ on the surface of cardiomyocytes. Proc Natl Acad Sci U S A 101:17533-17538, 2004.
39. Priori SG, Napolitano C, Gasparini M, et al: Natural history of Brugada syndrome: Insights for risk stratification and management. Circulation 105:1342-1347, 2002.
40. Razani B, Woodman SE, Lisanti MP: Caveolae: From cell biology to animal physiology. Pharmacol Rev 54:431-467, 2002.
41. Tang Z, Scherer PE, Okamoto T, et al: Molecular cloning of caveolin-3, a novel member of the caveolin gene family expressed predominantly in muscle. J Biol Chem 271:2255-2261, 1996.
42. Woodman SE, Park DS, Cohen AW, et al: Caveolin-3 knock-out mice develop a progressive cardiomyopathy and show hyperactivation of the p42/44 MAPK cascade. J Biol Chem 277:38988-38997, 2002.
43. Galbiati F, Engelman JA, Volonte D, et al: Caveolin-3 null mice show a loss of caveolae, changes in the microdomain distribution of the dystrophin-glycoprotein complex, and T-tubule abnormalities. J Biol Chem 276:21425-21433, 2001.
44. Volonte D, Peoples AJ, Galbiati F: Modulation of myoblast fusion by caveolin-3 in dystrophic skeletal muscle cells: Implications for Duchenne muscular dystrophy and limb-girdle muscular dystrophy-1C. Mol Biol Cell 14:4075-4088, 2003.
45. Hagiwara Y, Sasaoka T, Araishi K, et al: Caveolin-3 deficiency causes muscle degeneration in mice. Hum Mol Genet 9:3047-3054, 2000.
46. Vatta M, Ackerman MJ, Ye B, et al: Mutant caveolin-3 induces persistent late sodium current and is associated with long-QT syndrome. Circulation 114:2104-2112, 2006.
47. Arnestad M, Crotti L, Rognum TO, et al: Prevalence of long-QT syndrome gene variants in sudden infant death syndrome. Circulation 115:361-367, 2007.
48. Cronk LB, Ye B, Kaku T, et al: Novel mechanism for sudden infant death syndrome: Persistent late sodium current secondary to mutations in caveolin-3. Heart Rhythm 4:161-166, 2007.
49. Barbuti A, Gravante B, Riolfo M, et al: Localization of pacemaker channels in lipid rafts regulates channel kinetics. Circ Res 94:1325-1331, 2004.
50. Bossuyt J, Taylor BE, James-Kracke M, Hale CC: The cardiac sodium-calcium exchanger associates with caveolin-3. Ann N Y Acad Sci 976:197-204, 2002.
51. Bossuyt J, Taylor BE, James-Kracke M, Hale CC: Evidence for cardiac sodium-calcium exchanger association with caveolin-3. FEBS Lett 511:113-117, 2002.
52. Fujimoto T: Calcium pump of the plasma membrane is localized in caveolae. J Cell Biol 120:1147-1157, 1993.
53. Fujimoto T, Nakade S, Miyawaki A, et al: Localization of inositol 1,4,5-trisphosphate receptor–like protein in plasmalemmal caveolae. J Cell Biol 119:1507-1513, 1992.
54. Lockwich TP, Liu X, Singh BB, et al: Assembly of Trp1 in a signaling complex associated with caveolin-scaffolding lipid raft domains. J Biol Chem 275:11934-11942, 2000.
55. Martens JR, Sakamoto N, Sullivan SA, et al: Isoform-specific localization of voltage-gated K^+ channels to distinct lipid raft populations. Targeting of $K_V1.5$ to caveolae. J Biol Chem 276:8409-8414, 2001.
56. Teubl M, Groschner K, Kohlwein SD, et al: Na(+)/Ca(2+) exchange facilitates Ca(2+)-dependent activation of endothelial nitric-oxide synthase. J Biol Chem 274: 29529-29535, 1999.
57. Yarbrough TL, Lu T, Lee HC, Shibata EF: Localization of cardiac sodium channels in caveolin-rich membrane domains: Regulation of sodium current amplitude. Circ Res 90:443-449, 2002.
58. Balijepalli RC, Foell JD, Hall DD, et al: Localization of cardiac L-type Ca(2+) channels to a caveolar macromolecular signaling complex is required for beta(2)-adrenergic regulation. Proc Natl Acad Sci U S A 103:7500-7505, 2006.
59. Barouch LA, Harrison RW, Skaf MW, et al: Nitric oxide regulates the heart by spatial confinement of nitric oxide synthase isoforms. Nature 416:337-339, 2002.
60. Crossthwaite AJ, Seebacher T, Masada N, et al: The cytosolic domains of Ca^{2+}-sensitive adenylyl cyclases dictate their targeting to plasma membrane lipid rafts. J Biol Chem 280:6380-6391, 2005.
61. Ostrom RS, Violin JD, Coleman S, Insel PA: Selective enhancement of beta-adrenergic receptor signaling by overexpression of adenylyl cyclase type 6: Colocalization of receptor and adenylyl cyclase in caveolae of cardiac myocytes. Mol Pharmacol 57:1075-1079, 2000.
62. Rybin VO, Xu X, Lisanti MP, Steinberg SF: Differential targeting of beta-adrenergic receptor subtypes and adenylyl cyclase to cardiomyocyte caveolae. A mechanism to functionally regulate the cAMP signaling pathway. J Biol Chem 275:41447-41457, 2000.
63. Rybin VO, Xu X, Steinberg SF: Activated protein kinase C isoforms target to cardiomyocyte caveolae: Stimulation of local protein phosphorylation. Circ Res 84:980-988, 1999.
64. Xiang Y, Rybin VO, Steinberg SF, Kobilka B: Caveolar localization dictates physiologic signaling of beta 2-adrenoceptors in neonatal cardiac myocytes. J Biol Chem 277:34280-34286, 2002.
65. Jespersen T, Grunnet M, Olesen SP: The KCNQ1 potassium channel: From gene to physiological function. Physiology 20:408-416, 2005.
66. Barhanin J, Lesage F, Guillemare E, et al: K(V)LQT1 and IsK (minK) proteins associate to form the I(Ks) cardiac potassium current. Nature 384:78-80, 1996.
67. Sanguinetti MC, Curran ME, Zou A, et al: Coassembly of K(V)LQT1 and minK (IsK) proteins to form cardiac I(Ks) potassium channel. Nature 384:80-83, 1996.
68. Chen YH, Xu SJ, Bendahhou S, et al: KCNQ1 gain-of-function mutation in familial atrial fibrillation. Science 299:251-254, 2003.
69. Hong K, Piper DR, Diaz-Valdecantos A, et al: De novo KCNQ1 mutation responsible for atrial fibrillation and short QT syndrome in utero. Cardiovasc Res 68: 433-440, 2005.
70. Schwartz PJ, Priori SG, Spazzolini C, et al: Genotype-phenotype correlation in the

long-QT syndrome: Gene-specific triggers for life-threatening arrhythmias. Circulation 103:89-95, 2001.

71. Feliciello A, Cardone L, Garbi C, et al: Yotiao protein, a ligand for the NMDA receptor, binds and targets cAMP-dependent protein kinase II(1). FEBS Lett 464:174-178, 1999.
72. Westphal RS, Tavalin SJ, Lin JW, et al: Regulation of NMDA receptors by an associated phosphatase-kinase signaling complex. Science 285:93-96, 1999.
73. Marx SO, Kurokawa J, Reiken S, et al: Requirement of a macromolecular signaling complex for beta adrenergic receptor modulation of the KCNQ1-KCNE1 potassium channel. Science 295:496-499, 2002.
74. Kurokawa J, Chen L, Kass RS: Requirement of subunit expression for cAMP-mediated regulation of a heart potassium channel. Proc Natl Acad Sci U S A 100: 2122-2127, 2003.
75. Kurokawa J, Motoike HK, Rao J, Kass RS: Regulatory actions of the A-kinase anchoring protein Yotiao on a heart potassium channel downstream of PKA phosphorylation. Proc Natl Acad Sci U S A 101:16374-16378, 2004.
76. Piippo K, Swan H, Pasternack M, et al: A founder mutation of the potassium channel KCNQ1 in long QT syndrome: Implications for estimation of disease prevalence and molecular diagnostics. J Am Coll Cardiol 37:562-568, 2001.
77. Saucerman JJ, Healy SN, Belik ME, et al: Proarrhythmic consequences of a KCNQ1 AKAP-binding domain mutation: Computational models of whole cells and heterogeneous tissue. Circ Res 95:1216-1224, 2004.
78. Zhang T, Brown JH: Role of Ca^{2+}/calmodulin-dependent protein kinase II in cardiac hypertrophy and heart failure. Cardiovasc Res 63:476-486, 2004.
79. Anderson ME: Multiple downstream proarrhythmic targets for calmodulin kinase II: Moving beyond an ion channel–centric focus. Cardiovasc Res 73:657-666, 2007.
80. Wu Y, MacMillan LB, McNeill RB, et al: CaM kinase augments cardiac L-type Ca^{2+} current: A cellular mechanism for long Q-T arrhythmias. Am J Physiol 276: H2168-H2178, 1999.
81. Wu Y, Colbran RJ, Anderson ME: Calmodulin kinase is a molecular switch for cardiac excitation-contraction coupling. Proc Natl Acad Sci U S A 98:2877-2881, 2001.
82. Dzhura I, Wu Y, Colbran RJ, et al: Calmodulin kinase determines calcium-dependent facilitation of L-type calcium channels. Nat Cell Biol 2:173-177, 2000.
83. Dzhura I, Wu Y, Colbran RJ, et al: Cytoskeletal disrupting agents prevent calmodulin kinase, IQ domain and voltage-dependent facilitation of L-type Ca^{2+} channels. J Physiol 545:399-406, 2002.
84. Wu Y, Dzhura I, Colbran RJ, Anderson ME: Calmodulin kinase and a calmodulin-binding 'IQ' domain facilitate L-type Ca^{2+} current in rabbit ventricular myocytes by a common mechanism. J Physiol 535:679-687, 2001.
85. Yang E, Schulman H: Structural examination of autoregulation of multifunctional calcium/calmodulin-dependent protein kinase II. J Biol Chem 274:26199-26208, 1999.
86. Grueter CE, Abiria SA, Dzhura I, et al: L-type Ca(2+) channel facilitation mediated by phosphorylation of the beta subunit by CaMKII. Mol Cell 23:641-650, 2006.
87. Zhang R, Dzhura I, Grueter CE, et al: A dynamic alpha-beta inter-subunit agonist signaling complex is a novel feedback mechanism for regulating L-type Ca^{2+} channel opening. FASEB J 19:1573-1575, 2005.
88. Hudmon A, Schulman H, Kim J, et al: CaMKII tethers to L-type Ca^{2+} channels, establishing a local and dedicated integrator of Ca2+ signals for facilitation. J Cell Biol 171:537-547, 2005.

Membrane Pumps and Exchangers 5

LARRY V. HRYSHKO

CHAPTER OUTLINE

Overview of Membrane Pumps and Exchangers

The electrical activity of cardiac muscle reflects the carefully orchestrated gating of distinct ion channels that activate and control cardiac contractions. Moreover, the nuances of channel gating allow for wide variability in cardiac output and heart rates while still providing intrinsic protective mechanisms to prevent the occurrence of electrical malfunction. Coincident changes in many channels are essential to maintain the temporal relationships between diastole and systole so that adequate ventricular filling can occur over a broad range of heart rates. However, for ion channels to repetitiously perform their tasks, ion gradients must exist to enable this electrical signaling. Furthermore, for healthy cellular function, the ionic environment within cells must be carefully maintained to optimize the numerous secondary processes that are occurring and are coupled to these ion gradients. In large part, membrane pumps and exchangers are responsible for this maintenance of ion gradients and the intracellular ionic environment.

In comparison with many ion channels, far less information is available concerning the molecular operation of membrane pumps and exchangers. Usually, the basis for this disparity stems from the inability to assess the elementary activity of single transport molecules or the dearth of pharmacologic tools to modify their behavior. Thus, the usual circuit whereby drugs facilitate the understanding of structure-function relationships and these relationships facilitate drug development is much less developed for membrane pumps and exchangers. Molecular insight into how various exchangers and pumps accomplish their functions is increasing but still lags behind the comparatively straightforward understanding of ion channel permeation. Nevetheless, numerous studies have demonstrated the therapeutic potential of modifying specific transport molecules to counter various kinds of cardiovascular pathology.

A comprehensive review of all membrane pumps and exchangers of relevance to cardiac physiology and pathophysiology is beyond the scope of this chapter. Accordingly, only two membrane pumps and two ion exchangers that are representative of these transport families are considered. As examples of membrane ion pumps, the sarcolemmal Na^+,K^+-ATPase and Ca^{2+}-ATPase are discussed. For membrane ion exchangers, the sarcolemmal Na^+-Ca^{2+} exchanger and Na^+-H^+ exchanger are described. In common to all, these pumps or exchangers can influence intracellular calcium homeostasis either directly by transporting Ca^{2+} or indirectly through their influence on intracellular Na^+ levels. These proteins have received considerable attention by the research community, and many are subjects of clinical interest. It is noteworthy that the operation of these selected membrane pumps and exchangers is inextricably linked in a manner that is of considerable importance toward explication of cardiac physiology and pathophysiology. By necessity, cited references often are current and comprehensive review articles, rather than original works.

Historically, the pharmacologic manipulation of specific membrane pumps and exchangers includes agents, such as digitalis, that have been used for centuries. At the experimental level, many novel pharmacologic agents show promise or opportunity for the treatment of various cardiac ailments by their modulation of these transporters. By comparison with ion channels, fewer pharmacologic tools are available, hindering elucidation of specific transport and regulatory mechanisms. Theoretically, however, the manipulation of distinct ion pumps and exchangers offers a range of therapeutic possibilities equal to or greater than that realized through the modification of ion channels.

Na^+,K^+-ATPase

Physiology and Regulation

The Mg^{2+}-activated Na^+,K^+-ATPase constitutes the sodium pump of cardiac sarcolemma, an enzyme responsible for the maintenance of Na^+ and K^+ concentration gradients in these cells. This function is of paramount importance to normal cellular operation, because the existence of these ion gradients underlies electrical excitability, cell volume and pH regulation, and the provision of energy for numerous secondary active transport processes. Under physiologic conditions, the operation of this transporter is electrogenic, producing an outwardly directed current as 3 Na^+ are removed from the cell in exchange for the influx of 2 K^+. Thus, the normal mode of operation of the sodium pump helps to maintain the resting potential of cardiac cells, and its short-term inhibition leads to a slight depolarization of several millivolts.[1] Although ion fluxes through potassium channels (and, to a lesser extent, sodium channels) exert far greater influences on cardiac resting potential, it is noteworthy that their operation is entirely dependent on the ion gradients established by the sodium pump. Inhibition of the sodium pump typically prolongs the cardiac action potential, owing to a direct reduction in hyperpolarizing currents.[1] These effects are complicated by the additional electrophysiologic influences of changing intracellular Ca^{2+} levels, which can directly produce action potential shortening. The sodium pump is of particular importance in cardiac muscle performance because its operation is a critical determinant of intracellular Na^+ levels and, consequently, cardiac inotropic status. Subtle changes in intracellular Na^+ levels exert considerable effects on cardiac contractility, because these levels directly influence the activity of the cardiac Na^+-Ca^{2+} exchanger.[2]

Regulation of sodium pump activity is very complex and is only beginning to become understood. In large part, this complexity originates from the presence of several distinct sodium pump isoforms, found throughout the heart, with unique functional attributes and expression levels, differential regulation, developmental and disease-related changes, and distinct cellular and subcellular localization patterns.[3-7] Moreover, sodium pump activity not only influences global cytoplasmic Na^+ levels but also appears to critically influence Na^+ levels within restricted subsarcolemmal "fuzzy" spaces,[8] which can significantly alter the activity of co-localized Na^+-sensitive transporters such as the Na^+-Ca^{2+} exchanger.[4,9-13]

The role of FXYD proteins as modulators of the Na^+,K^+-ATPase is becoming increasingly well established,[14,15] and these proteins are now known to mediate the effects of α- and β-adrenergic stimulation. Phospholemman, or FXYD1, is a member of this larger FXYD family and is the end-effector of protein kinase A (PKA)- and protein kinase C (PKC)-mediated sodium pump regulation in cardiac muscle.[14,16-21] PKA phosphorylates serine 68 of phospholemman, which ultimately leads to an activation of the sodium pump by increasing the affinity for Na^+, whereas PKC phosphorylates serine 63 and serine 68, leading to an increase in pump maximal velocity (V_{max}) with unchanged Na^+ affinity. Overall, a comprehensive understanding of how the sodium pump is regulated in discrete locations within the heart, and how this ultimately influences contractility and conduction, is only beginning to emerge.

Transport Mechanism

The Post-Albers model of ion transport by the Na^+,K^+-ATPase is widely accepted and has received substantial verification through distinct experimental techniques. Details of this transport cycle and their underlying experimental basis have been reviewed extensively[1,22,23] and are only briefly reiterated here. Intracellular Na^+ binds to the E_1 conformation of the enzyme, which has intracellularly oriented ion-binding sites and bound Mg^{2+}–adenosine triphosphate (ATP). Sodium binding results in ATP hydrolysis, phosphorylation of the enzyme, and occlusion of bound Na^+ such that these ions are no longer accessible to either aqueous compartment. From this configuration, the enzyme shifts to the E_2 conformation, wherein ion-binding sites are oriented to the extracellular compartment and Na^+ unbinding can occur. This latter conformation of the enzyme is believed to constitute a narrow, high-field access channel, and the unbinding and release of Na^+ from this channel constitute the electrogenic step of the reaction cycle.[24,25] The phosphorylated enzyme (E_2P) is now available to bind extracellular K^+ which ultimately leads to occlusion of these ions, dephosphorylation of the enzyme, and reorientation of the binding sites to the intracellular surface. Intracellular ATP then catalyzes the release of K^+ ions, and the enzyme becomes available for a subsequent transport cycle. Under physiologic conditions, the sodium pump is thought to transport ions exclusively in this Na^+ efflux–K^+ influx direction, although the reverse reaction can be readily induced experimentally.[26] Notably, several characteristics of the sodium pump are altered depending on the conformation (i.e., E_1 or E_2) being evaluated. Such characteristics include the affinities for both Na^+ and K^+, sensitivity to ATP and adenine diphosphate (ADP), and proteolytic cleavage patterns.[22,27]

Palytoxin has been an increasingly important tool used to investigate the electrophysiologic properties of the sodium pump. This marine toxin converts the sodium pump into a channel-like protein, permitting the electrophysiologic analysis of "pump channel" elementary currents[28] by uncoupling the intracellular and extracellular gates that normally restrict ion accessibility to a single membrane surface at any given time. This agent has been very useful in studying the specific ionic residues involved in ion translocation through the pump and in determining specific aspects of the selectivity filter and pore structure, vestibule structure, and the nature of partial reactions.[28-31] The numerous advances in characterization of both structural and functional features of the sodium pump have led to a continuous refinement of the Post-Albers cycle to explain pump function and to elucidate how the Na^+,K^+-ATPase accomplishes its critical task at the molecular level.[26,27,30,32-39]

Biochemistry and Molecular Biology

The Na^+,K^+-ATPase is a member of the P-type ATPase superfamily, characterized by their transient ATP-mediated phosphorylation during a transport cycle. In the case of the sodium pump, this occurs on aspartate D376 in a region of the protein that is highly conserved within the P-type ATPase family. The sodium pump is a heterodimeric protein composed of an α subunit and a β subunit. A third, γ subunit also has been identified, although its expression either does not occur (e.g., in humans) or is minimal (e.g., in rat and *Xenopus*) in cardiac tissue and it is unlikely to represent an essential component of the Na^+,K^+-ATPase enzyme complex.[40] Of interest, however, related members of the FXYD family of proteins, such as phospholemman, may subserve the role of the γ subunit in cardiac muscle.[41,42]

All three subunits show distinct isoforms. For the α and β subunits, up to four distinct isoforms have been identified.[22] Any pairing of α and β subunits results in a functional sodium pump, although both subunits must be present for functional activity. In cardiac muscle, there are considerable species-dependent differences in isoform expression patterns. In human atrial and ventricular tissue, for example, the α_1, α_2, and α_3 isoforms all are expressed (in association with the β_1 subunit), and chamber-specific variations in expression levels are observed.[43] Furthermore, in cardiac tissue, the expression pattern of distinct isoforms can be regionally specific, even at the level of individual cardiac cells.[44] Although several studies have been able to identify functional differences for distinct isoform combinations, the consequences of such specialization and localization are poorly understood.

The various α subunits are roughly 1000 amino acids in length, with a molecular mass of approximately 110 kD, and conduct ion transport and ATPase activity. They also are the receptors for digitalis-like compounds. Hydropathy analyses and chemical labeling studies indicate that the α subunit possesses 10 transmembrane-spanning segments, with both the amino terminus (N terminus) and the carboxyl terminus (C terminus) facing intracellularly. Numerous important functional domains and residues have been identified by protein biochemistry and structure-function studies. In brief, ATP binding and hydrolysis are mediated by the large cytoplasmic domain between transmembrane segments 4 and 5, and the highly conserved aspartate residue that is the specific phosphorylation target has been identified. Cation binding occurs within the transmembrane segments, with major contributions mediated by carboxyl-containing residues in transmembrane segments 5 and 6. A tremendous advance in the study of P-type ATPases has been the determination of a high-resolution crystal structure of the sarcoplasmic reticulum–endoplasmic reticulum Ca^{2+}-ATPase

(SERCA) pump, a related P-type ATPase family member.[45] Several general principles of operation of SERCA may extend directly to the Na^+,K^+-ATPase, including the large conformational changes that couple ion occlusion and ATP hydrolysis.[22,46] This has been largely confirmed with the recent report of a crystal structure of the renal Na^+,K^+-ATPase at 3.5 Å resolution.[47] Notably, the binding of rubidium ions (as K^+ analogues) within this structure occupies the same cavity and uses homologous amino acid residues used by the SERCA pump for Ca^{2+} binding. This study also identified the physical relationships among the α, β, and γ subunits and postulated a novel regulatory mechanism whereby the C terminus of the α subunit resides within a pocket formed by the transmembrane segments and possibly controls Na^+ affinity.[47]

In cardiac muscle, the β_1 subunit is the predominant isoform found in association with the various α subunits. It is a type II membrane protein, having a single transmembrane segment, an intracellular N terminus, with the major portion of its mass located extracellularly. The functional role of the β subunit is largely unknown. It is clearly required for the functional activity of the α subunits and also plays a role in trafficking and correct membrane insertion of these subunits. Efforts to define a functional role beyond that of protein processing have yielded some clues. For example, mutagenesis of the β subunit or alteration of its disulfide bridges (three such bridges are present in its extracellular domain) can alter functional properties of the sodium pump. Furthermore, protease cleavage sites for the β subunit are altered in response to unique enzyme conformations adopted by the α subunit, indicative of conformational coupling between these proteins.[22] From the recently determined crystal structure, the β subunit has been shown to interact with transmembrane helices 7 and 10 of the α subunit.[47]

Pharmacology

The cardiac Na^+,K^+-ATPase has been targeted for pharmacologic intervention for more than 2 centuries, long before any recognition of its existence. Specifically, digitalis and various cardiac glycosides (e.g., digoxin, ouabain) have historically been used for the treatment of congestive heart failure. At present, cardiac glycosides continue to serve a prominent role in treating cardiac insufficiency and also are widely used to control ventricular response rates for specific supraventricular arrhythmias (e.g., atrial fibrillation). The primary effects of digoxin with respect to rate control are mediated through parasympathetic effects on the atrioventricular node. Despite the long history of use for heart failure, there seems to be a continual reevaluation of the clinical benefits associated with cardiac glycoside use as well as continued interest in the scientific basis for its therapeutic effects.[4,6,48-50] Most recently, pharmacologic modulation of the sodium pump also has garnered interest as a potential treatment for hypertension, various cancers, and certain neurologic disorders.[51-57]

The identification of the sodium pump as the target protein inhibited by cardiac glycosides was achieved approximately 40 years ago. Mechanistically, these compounds exert their inotropic effects indirectly through the consequences of altering the Na^+ electrochemical gradient. This, in turn, alters the ability of the sarcolemmal Na^+-Ca^{2+} exchanger to remove cytoplasmic Ca^{2+}. Specifically, the diminution of the Na^+ electrochemical gradient reduces the extent of forward-mode Na^+-Ca^{2+} exchange (i.e., Ca^{2+} efflux) and augments the prevalence of reverse-mode Na^+-Ca^{2+} exchange (i.e., Ca^{2+} influx). During cardiac relaxation, myoplasmic Ca^{2+} removal is accomplished through two competing transport mechanisms—namely, reuptake into the sarcoplasmic reticulum and removal from the cell by Na^+-Ca^{2+} exchange. Because cardiac glycosides reduce the net effectiveness of Na^+-Ca^{2+} exchange in removing Ca^{2+}, Ca^{2+} reuptake by the sarcoplasmic reticulum increases. This minor change in the competitive balance between Ca^{2+} removal mechanisms is greatly amplified by the increase in diastolic Ca^{2+} levels also associated with cardiac glycoside treatment. During systole, a greater amount of Ca^{2+} is released from the sarcoplasmic reticulum, adding to the elevated background level of diastolic Ca^{2+}. Cardiac contractility is exceptionally sensitive to intracellular Na^+ concentrations, and considerable increases in force are accomplished with very minor changes in intracellular Na^+ levels of a few millimolar.[2] Moreover, toxicity from these compounds incurred by way of intracellular Ca^{2+} overload simply reflects the overzealous accomplishment of the intended inotropic effect.

Alternative mechanisms have been proposed for the inotropic effects of cardiac glycosides including direct alterations of sarcoplasmic reticulum Ca^{2+} release channels[58] and the induction of a significant calcium conductance through sodium channels.[59] These possibilities remain highly controversial, because other experimental results argue strongly against their importance or even existence.[52] For example, it has been shown that cardiac glycosides are without effect in cells devoid of Na^+,[2] indicating that a sodium-dependent phenomenon is responsible. However, this result may be species-specific, because glycoside inotropy has been observed in feline myocytes under Na^+-free conditions.[60] In cardiac myotubes from mice with cardiospecific knockout of Na^+-Ca^{2+} exchange, cardiac glycosides are without effect, indicating that Na^+-Ca^{2+} exchange is essential for their action.[61] Even though this result argues strongly in favor of the accepted notion for glycoside action, its applicability to other species is unknown. Overall, the accepted dogma for glycoside action seems widely applicable with respect to its inotropic effects, although the latest discoveries regarding the role of the sodium pump in cell signaling, growth modulation, and apoptosis have yet to be incorporated into current understanding of the overall clinical spectrum of effects.

Despite a considerable history of cardiac glycoside use to increase cardiac contractility, it is still unlikely that this approach has been optimized. In a major clinical trial evaluating digoxin in the treatment of heart failure, mortality rates were not decreased, although reductions in hospitalization and in the progression of heart failure were evident.[62] Additional analysis from the Digitalis Investigation Group (DIG) trial[62] suggested a significant gender-based difference in response to digoxin treatment, with females showing a 4.2% increase in mortality rate over that observed with placebo.[63] Finally, additional post hoc analyses of the DIG trial support the notion that serum digoxin concentrations between 0.5 and 0.9 ng/mL do indeed reduce both mortality and hospitalization due to heart failure. The utility of digoxin therapy remains hindered by its narrow therapeutic index, however, and the continued obscurity regarding its optimal clinical use may simply reflect the tottering about an optimal serum concentration.

From a scientific perspective, it is clear that a great deal remains to be learned regarding cardiac glycosides. Furthermore, evidence supporting the existence of endogenous ouabain-like compounds continues to amass,[53,54,64] which may greatly complicate the clinical picture. The notion that low levels of endogenous or exogenous cardiac glycosides may stimulate rather than inhibit the sodium pump has reemerged.[65] Prominent gender-based differences with respect to cardiac injury susceptibility continue to be reported.[63] Moreover, the "usual suspects" such as sodium pumps, Na^+-Ca^{2+} exchangers, and intracellular Na^+ levels all show considerable changes during the progression of heart failure.[6,13,66-68] In view of just these few examples, rather erratic responsiveness to cardiac glycosides may be anticipated. Because cardiac glycosides are likely to remain an important component of the treatment for heart failure, it seems imperative to refine current understanding of their actions and optimal utilization.

Sarcolemmal Ca^{2+}-ATPase

Physiology

Plasmalemmal calcium pumps serve prominent roles in Ca^{2+} extrusion in most, if not all, eukaryotic cells. The sarcolemmal Ca^{2+}-ATPase is a member of the P-type ATPase superfamily, and in cardiac muscle, this enzyme removes intracellular Ca^{2+} in parallel with the Na^+-Ca^{2+} exchange system. Ca^{2+} efflux is absolutely essential for myocardial cell survival, so it is somewhat surprising that many studies have failed to identify a prominent role for the sarcolemmal Ca^{2+}-ATPase in beat-to-beat Ca^{2+} efflux from heart. That is, the Ca^{2+}-ATPase does not appear to contribute substantially to diastolic Ca^{2+} removal in cardiac tissue in a majority of species, because this role is played primarily by the cardiac Na^+-Ca^{2+} exchanger.

The current understanding of the role played by the sarcolemmal Ca^{2+}-ATPase in myocardial relaxation has been obtained primarily by two general approaches. The pharmacologic approach is somewhat limited by the dearth of available agents, and the use of existing agents has not been widespread. Most commonly, eosin and carboxyeosin have been used as inhibitors to establish this role.[69,70] These pharmacologic studies identified a significant role for the sarcolemmal Ca^{2+}-ATPase, which was found to account for 24% to 45% of Ca^{2+} removal.[71] By contrast, in studies in which the contribution of the sarcolemmal Ca^{2+}-ATPase to cardiac relaxation has been deduced after inhibition of other identified Ca^{2+} removal mechanisms, its role seems almost negligible.[72] In transgenic rats in which the sarcolemmal calcium pump was overexpressed twofold, no effects were observed on either systolic or diastolic cardiac performance. Finally, knockout of *PMCA1* is embryonic lethal, precluding a detailed analysis of the cardiovascular effects of the expressed protein.[73,74] On balance, the larger part of the evidence does not support a major role for this transport system in mediating cardiac relaxation. It is noteworthy that the equivalent overexpression of the Na^+-Ca^{2+} exchanger also is benign with respect to physiologic cardiac function, yet its importance in cardiac relaxation has been unequivocally accepted.[75] A surprising finding is that conditional knockout of the cardiac Na^+-Ca^{2+} exchanger (NCX1) leads to viable animals with reasonably normal cardiac function.[76] Thus, under specific conditions, the sarcolemmal Ca^{2+}-ATPase may have the ability to enact cardiac relaxation, despite a marked compensatory reduction in Ca^{2+} entry in the NCX1–conditional KO mice.[77-79]

Alternative physiologic roles for the sarcolemmal Ca^{2+}-ATPase have recently been proposed. For example, in neonatal myocytes from transgenic mice overexpressing this pump, the rates of protein synthesis were markedly increased, implying a role in myocardial cell growth.[72] This result has been extended to show a role of the calcium pump in regulating endothelin-1–mediated growth responses. The calcium pump also may constitute the voltage-independent B-type calcium channel that has been demonstrated to modulate apoptosis in cardiac cells.[80-82] Newer studies suggest a prominent role for plasma membrane Ca^{2+}-ATPase 4 (PMCA-4) in neuronal nitric oxide synthase (nNOS)-mediated signaling in heart.[83] Overall, however, the importance of this transporter in cardiac physiology remains relatively obscure, in large part owing to the multiplicity of splice variants and their unique regulatory properties and cellular localizations.[84,85] Of interest, in NCX1-knockout mice, embryonic lethality occurs at roughly 9 to 10 days post coitum, indicating that the PMCA cannot rescue calcium homeostasis within the heart unless NCX1 knockout occurs conditionally.[76] Before embryonic lethality, however, these cardiac cells do indeed undergo rhythmic contractions.[86] Thus, the sarcolemmal calcium pump shows considerable variability in its capacity as a Ca^{2+} transport mechanism in the heart.

Biochemistry and Molecular Biology

Although the sarcolemmal and sarcoplasmic reticulum Ca^{2+}-ATPases both are members of the P-type ATPase family, these proteins are structurally quite distinct. That is, they bear the same degree of similarity to other P-type ATPases (e.g., Na^+,K^+-ATPase, H^+,K^+-ATPase) as they do to each other. Functionally, they are related by the formation of an aspartyl phosphate intermediate during the transport cycle.[87] Four nonallelic genes of the sarcolemmal Ca^{2+}-ATPase have been identified in humans, and in conjunction with extensive alternative splicing, the proteins encoded by these genes constitute a very large family of distinct calcium pumps. The physiologic basis for this tremendous diversity is unknown, although numerous functional or regulatory differences have been observed for distinct variants.[88,89] The structural diversity also is thought to underlie the differential membrane localization of unique PMCAs[85] and their interactions with several other signaling molecules.[90]

Topological models of the sarcolemmal calcium pump predict 10 transmembrane segments with intracellularly oriented N and C termini. Three major intracellular domains constitute the major portion of the protein mass. The first of these (located between transmembrane segments 2 and 3) appears to participate as a "transduction domain" involved in long-range conformational changes associated with transport and in regulation by acidic phospholipids. The second and largest intracellular domain is found between transmembrane segments 4 and 5. It is the major catalytic domain in which ATP binding and formation of the acyl phosphate intermediate occur. The final intracellular domain is the C terminus of the protein and is a major site for regulation, including that mediated by Ca^{2+}-calmodulin.[89,91,92] This latter domain serves an autoinhibitory role through its interactions with the catalytic core of the pump.[85]

Na^+-H^+ Exchange

Physiology

The regulation of intracellular pH is of critical importance to tissues, particularly those with prodigious energy utilization. Such tissue is exemplified by cardiac muscle, in which metabolic acids are continuously generated during repetitious contractile activity. To deal with the requirement of maintaining pH, several independent mechanisms exist in cardiac sarcolemmal membranes, including the Na^+-H^+ exchanger, the Na^+-HCO_3^- cotransporter, the Cl^--OH^- exchanger, and the Cl^--HCO_3^- exchanger. Of these systems, the Na^+-H^+ exchanger and the Na^+-HCO_3^- cotransporter are responsible for alleviating intracellular acidosis, whereas the latter two transporters are involved with offsetting increases in intracellular alkalinity.[13,93] This section discusses the Na^+-H^+ exchanger, because it remains an attractive and aggressively pursued target for pharmacologic intervention. Numerous recent studies have identified intriguing new roles for the Na^+-H^+ exchanger protein 1 (NHE1) beyond that of pH regulation.[94-99]

The Na^+-H^+ exchanger is an electroneutral ion counter-transporter that stoichiometrically exchanges one intracellular proton for one extracellular Na^+.[13,100] Of the nine identified isoforms of the Na^+-H^+ exchanger (NHE1 to NHE9), cardiac muscle primarily expresses the NHE1 isoform in the sarcolemma.[100,101] This isoform is exquisitely sensitive to activation by increases in the intracellular proton concentration, and its activation is mediated by conformational changes associated with proton binding to a pH sensor region. This transport system has a very large capacity for proton efflux–Na^+ influx, far in excess of the pumping capacity of the sodium pump.[13,93] Moreover, an amazingly complex variety of regulatory mechanisms influence the pH sensitivity of NHE1, primarily through phosphorylation reactions targeting the large intracellular C-terminal domain of the protein.[102,103] The resultant allosteric modifications of NHE1 can dramatically alter a variety of physiologic responses, because this isoform is ubiquitously expressed in mammalian cells.[100,101,104]

Overall, the NHE1 counter-transporter accounts for the greater part of proton efflux from cardiac cells under physiologic conditions.[13,93] Of note, clinical interest in this transporter was originally focused on its operation under pathophysiologic conditions, because NHE1 has been shown to play a major role in mediating cardiac ischemia-reperfusion injury. Specifically, in response to ischemia, a rapid intracellular and extracellular acidification occurs in association with the conversion to anaerobic metabolism. The intracellular acidification alone accounts for a substantial proportion of the contractile dysfunction associated with ischemia, because the myofilament Ca^{2+} sensitivity and force-generating capabilities are markedly impaired. Although reperfusion of ischemic tissue is essential for salvaging myocardium, this maneuver paradoxically induces a brief period of more rapid cellular injury. With reperfusion, the extracellular pH is rapidly restored, creating favorable conditions for NHE1 to restore intracellular pH. Consequently, a large and rapid influx of Na^+ occurs that markedly impairs the efficiency of the cardiac Na^+-Ca^{2+} exchanger as a Ca^{2+} removal mechanism. This transient diminution of the Na^+ electrochemical gradient reduces the ability of the Na^+-Ca^{2+} exchanger to operate in the forward (Ca^{2+} efflux) mode, and the reverse mode of operation of Na^+-Ca^{2+} exchange also becomes promoted. Depending on severity, this can rapidly lead to cellular Ca^{2+} overload, associated with dangerous arrhythmias and cell death. Accordingly, the inhibition of NHE1 represented a very attractive means of limiting the cell damage associated with reperfusion of ischemic cardiac tissue and numerous experimental studies validated the utility of this approach. Unfortunately, the clinical application of NHE1 inhibitors has been far less successful than would have been predicted from these enticing experimental findings.[95,105-107]

Biochemistry and Molecular Biology

The cardiac Na^+-H^+ exchanger is a member of the NHE superfamily that currently is recognized to have nine distinct isoforms (NHE1 to NHE9), some of which are found intracellularly.[93,100,102,108] NHE1 represents the major isoform found in cardiac sarcolemma and appears ubiquitously as the "housekeeping" NHE in other cell types. This 110-kD glycoprotein is composed of approximately 815 amino acids and is modeled to possess 12 transmembrane-spanning regions, with both N- and C-terminal domains located intracellularly.[102,109] These transmembrane regions and their corresponding connecting loops constitute the major portion of the protein (roughly 500 amino acids) and are thought to mediate ion transport and proton sensing for activation. The remainder of the protein (approximately 315 amino acids) appears in a large hydrophilic C-terminal domain. Structure-function studies of NHE1 have demonstrated that the C-terminal domain possesses a number of subdomains responsible for the allosteric modification of NHE1 function through various signaling cascades. A crystal structure has been reported for the Na^+-H^+ antiporter from *Escherichia coli*,[110] although it has very low sequence identity to mammalian NHE1.[111] From structural studies and mutagenesis experiments, information is increasing with respect to identifying the sites of inhibitor action, ion-binding sites, and sites of interaction with other regulatory molecules.[96,100,111-116]

The regulation of NHE1 by a variety of signaling networks has been studied and reviewed extensively and therefore is not reiterated here.[94,98,102,103,117] Several recent findings, however, appear to be of particular relevance to cardiac pathophysiology. For example, NHE1 is thought to serve a prominent role in cardiac hypertrophy, fibrosis, and remodeling in heart failure.[103,118] Moreover, increasing evidence suggests that NHE1 is involved in regulating cell proliferation and hypertrophy.[102] Of interest, sarcolemmal polyphosphoinositides (i.e., 4,5-phosphatidylinositol biphosphate [PIP_2]) also appear to regulate NHE1 activity,[109] a response similar to that observed for the cardiac Na^+-Ca^{2+} exchanger[119] and one that may profoundly influence both of their behaviors during ATP depletion. Finally, the importance of NHE1 as a multifunctional protein with numerous nontransport roles is increasingly recognized. These roles include functions in scaffolding or anchoring for ensemble of signaling molecules to coordinate their activities.[96,114,116]

Pharmacology

A vast body of experimental evidence has been accumulated demonstrating a contributory role for NHE1 in reperfusion-induced injury of cardiac muscle. With the advent of specific inhibitors targeting this molecule, these studies have almost unanimously demonstrated cardioprotective effects against ischemic injury using a variety of indices. These indices include improvements in the recovery of contractility, reduction in infarct size and the extent of hypercontracture, and reduced ionic disturbances and arrhythmias. Based on this compelling and tantalizing evidence, the evaluation of Na^+-H^+ exchange inhibitors in cardioprotection for ischemia-reperfusion injury resulted in four clinical trials.[103,120] Overall, although a modest degree of cardioprotection was observed in several of these studies, particularly in high-risk patients undergoing coronary artery bypass surgery, the final outcome from these trials was not favorable owing to unanticipated increases in the number of postsurgical cerebrovascular events.[95,120-122] Continued interest in the therapeutic potential of NHE inhibitors stems from the recognition of their potential involvement in cardiac hypertrophy and heart failure.[94,95,99]

Two general classes of NHE1 inhibitors are recognized: *amiloride*, as well as various congeners such as ethylisopropylamiloride and 5-*N*-(methylpropyl)amiloride, and *benzoylguanidines* and various congeners such as HOE694 and HOE642.[117] These inhibitors show considerable specificity for NHE1 compared with other NHE family members. Novel derivatives of both classes of NHE1 inhibitors are being introduced very rapidly, and experimental evidence continues to support powerful cardioprotective, antihypertrophic, and antiproliferative effects for these agents.[95,97,98,107,116]

Na^+-Ca^{2+} Exchange

Physiologic Role of Na^+-Ca^{2+} Exchange

Cardiac Na^+-Ca^{2+} exchange is thought to be the primary mechanism for transsarcolemmal Ca^{2+} removal, an absolute requirement for cardiac muscle relaxation. Quantitatively, this exchange has been shown to remove the same amount of Ca^{2+}

that enters cardiac cells with each heartbeat.[123] Because Ca^{2+} entry levels are dynamically regulated to control cardiac inotropy, the Na^+-Ca^{2+} exchanger must be able to vary the amount of Ca^{2+} efflux to coincide with these changes. This capability is essential to avoid intracellular Ca^{2+} overload or Ca^{2+} depletion. Among different species and during developmental changes, considerable differences are observed in the proportion of activating Ca^{2+} derived from L-type Ca^{2+} channels versus that from the sarcoplasmic reticulum. Irrespective of this variability, however, the requirement for Ca^{2+} influx equaling Ca^{2+} efflux over any extended period remains essential for viable cardiac function.

As a reversible ion counter-transporter, Na^+-Ca^{2+} exchange also can serve as a Ca^{2+} entry mechanism. That is, depending on the existing electrochemical gradients, the exchanger is capable of bringing Ca^{2+} into cells to support or augment cardiac contractions. This reverse mode of Na^+-Ca^{2+} exchange has been postulated to contribute to cardiac excitation-contraction coupling by directly contributing to calcium-induced Ca^{2+} release from the sarcoplasmic reticulum.[124] Although the physiologic relevance of this mechanism has been debated actively over the past several years, a consensus seems to be emerging. That is, reverse Na^+-Ca^{2+} exchange is not a primary, or even prominent, contributor to calcium-induced Ca^{2+} release during activation. However, its operation exerts a considerable influence on cardiac inotropy by directly influencing sarcoplasmic reticulum Ca^{2+} levels and by controlling intracellular Ca^{2+} levels, particularly near the subsarcolemmal sites where L-type calcium channels and sarcoplasmic reticulum release channels are in close proximity. Both of these roles for the exchanger directly influence the gain or efficiency of cardiac excitation-contraction coupling, in addition to a small but direct contribution to calcium-induced Ca^{2+} release.[2,72,75,125-127]

During cardiac relaxation, the sarcoplasmic reticulum and Na^+-Ca^{2+} exchange systems compete for cytoplasmic Ca^{2+}. It has been demonstrated experimentally that both of these systems have the independent capability of mediating complete cardiac relaxation.[128] The sarcoplasmic reticulum can accomplish this at near-physiologic rates, whereas the rate is somewhat reduced when the Na^+-Ca^{2+} exchanger works independently. This finding has several important physiologic implications. Of most importance, both systems have considerable reserve capacity to achieve diastolic Ca^{2+} levels. Second, no obvious redundancies have been noted in Ca^{2+} removal capabilities from other transport systems, because blockade of both Na^+-Ca^{2+} exchange and sarcoplasmic reticular Ca^{2+} uptake severely impairs cardiac relaxation. Although the mitochondria and sarcolemmal Ca^{2+}-ATPase can contribute to lowering intracellular Ca^{2+} levels, they do not appear to do so at physiologically meaningful rates. Of note, independent sarcoplasmic reticulum function can relax cardiac muscle quickly—but this could not occur for sequential beats, because intracellular Ca^{2+} overload would rapidly develop. By contrast, the Na^+-Ca^{2+} exchanger can accomplish this repetitively, because its forward operation removes Ca^{2+} from cardiac cells. These relationships and limitations between sarcoplasmic reticulum Ca^{2+} uptake and Na^+-Ca^{2+} exchange–mediated Ca^{2+} efflux are likely to contribute to the overt alterations in cardiac performance and Ca^{2+} handling that occur during heart failure.

Transport Mechanism

The Na^+-Ca^{2+} exchanger is an electrogenic ion counter-transporter with a generally accepted stoichiometry of 3 Na^+:1 Ca^{2+}. As a consequence of this coupling ratio, the operation of the exchanger both influences and is influenced by the transmembrane potential. The contribution of Na^+-Ca^{2+} exchange to the characteristics of the cardiac action potential has been somewhat difficult to ascertain owing to the lack of suitable inhibitors. In its forward mode of operation, Na^+-Ca^{2+} exchange generates inward currents that would prolong the action potential. Conversely, reverse Na^+-Ca^{2+} exchange would produce hyperpolarizing currents, thereby shortening the action potential. Beyond this simple description, the direction and activity of Na^+-Ca^{2+} exchange during an action potential can be presumed to be markedly influenced by several factors. These include dynamic changes in Ca^{2+} and Na^+ at the subsarcolemmal space, the concomitant changes in voltage, and any or all kinetic variations imparted by intrinsic regulatory mechanisms. Although these factors pose formidable barriers to analysis, significant progress is occurring with respect to understanding dynamic Na^+-Ca^{2+} exchange operation.[2,72]

The generally accepted stoichiometry of the Na^+-Ca^{2+} exchanger has been questioned recently by studies demonstrating a 4:1 or variable stoichiometry.[129,130] If additional studies were to support these findings, the consequences with regard to current understanding of physiologic Na^+-Ca^{2+} exchange function would be considerable. Specifically, a profound impact could be expected on accepted hypotheses regarding the quantitative coupling between Ca^{2+} influx and efflux, the exchanger transport rates, its contribution to the action potential characteristics, the likelihood of reverse exchange contributing to Ca^{2+} entry, and the necessity for regulating this more potent Ca^{2+} efflux mechanism. At present, most current studies addressing this issue provide compelling support for the original 3:1 stoichiometry, although uncertainty still remains.[131-135] An intriguing recent set of observations suggests that the stoichiometry may be variable, allowing for a background inward Na^+ conductance to occur through the exchanger.[13,132,136]

The most widely accepted transport mechanism for Na^+-Ca^{2+} exchange is a consecutive model whereby a single ion-binding site is alternatively exposed to the intracellular and extracellular membrane surfaces. On binding of either Na^+ or Ca^{2+}, the exchanger and bound ion(s) gain the ability to translocate to the opposite membrane surface, where the bound ion can be released; then the ion binding site becomes available for subsequent translocation events. Within the constraints of this model, both Na^+ and Ca^{2+} have the ability to compete for the single binding site. The conformation of the exchanger and its affinities for the transported ions differ according to which membrane surface these ion-binding sites reside upon. Several experimental studies are consistent with the consecutive transport model. Moreover, these data generally are inconsistent with a simultaneous transport whereby both Na^+ and Ca^{2+} must be bound for translocation to occur. For example, several groups have identified ionic currents associated with partial reactions of the exchanger transport cycle with electrogenicity being reported for both limbs of the transport cycle.[137-142] Also, the apparent ion affinity is influenced by the concentration of the counter-ion, an essential feature of a consecutive transport model.[137]

Several groups of investigators have attempted to determine the turnover rates for Na^+-Ca^{2+} exchange, and a fairly broad range of values have been reported.[75] In many cases, these turnover rates have been derived from studies examining exchanger partial reactions; consequently, these do not provide information on turnover rates for the entire reaction cycle or those under physiologic conditions.[137,140,143] At present, a reliable means of unambiguously counting Na^+-Ca^{2+} exchangers is lacking. An accurate assessment of physiologic turnover rates for the exchanger would be exceptionally useful in elucidating the minimal required exchanger densities required to accomplish diastolic Ca^{2+} efflux. Moreover, they would lend great insight into the transport capacity of the Na^+-Ca^{2+} system and the necessity, if any, for regulating its function by active regulatory mechanisms. Meanwhile, current understanding of how Na^+-Ca^{2+} exchanger efflux is coupled to varying Ca^{2+} influx remains very limited.

Molecular Properties of the Cardiac Na^+-Ca^{2+} Exchanger

The cardiac Na^+-Ca^{2+} exchanger is a member of a much larger superfamily of cation-Ca^{2+} exchangers.[144,145] The prototypical cardiac exchanger, now referred to as NCX1.1, was first cloned in 1990 from a canine cardiac complementary DNA (cDNA) library.[146] Within the NCX branch of this superfamily, three unique genes, located on different chromosomes, that encode Na^+-Ca^{2+} exchangers—NCX1, NCX2, and NCX3—have been identified in mammals. Both NCX1 and NCX3 are subject to alternative splicing, and several individual exchangers are expressed in a tissue-specific manner.[147-150] For NCX1, splicing occurs by the requisite expression of one of two mutually exclusive exons, A and B, followed by different combinations of four cassette exons, C to F. NCX1.1 is the only exchanger expressed in cardiac muscle and contains exons A and C to F.

The mature NCX1.1 protein consists of 938 amino acids and is approximately 110 kD in size. Current topological models suggest that the Na^+-Ca^{2+} exchanger has nine transmembrane segments and a large cytoplasmic loop between transmembrane segments 5 and 6 that constitutes slightly more than half of the protein mass.[147,151,152] The site of alternative splicing occurs toward the C terminus of the large cytoplasmic loop beginning at amino acid residue 570. Several important functional domains have been identified, and the exchanger is crudely divided into the ion-translocating transmembrane domains and the regulatory cytoplasmic domain.[153,154] Within the transmembrane domains, two reentrant loops exist on opposite membrane surfaces that may serve an important role in ion translocation.[154-156] Several functionally important domains have been identified within the large cytoplasmic loop, including the high-affinity regulatory calcium-binding sites, the site involved with intracellular Na^+–dependent inactivation (XIP region), and the alternative splicing region.[147,154]

Both solution and crystal structures of the regulatory calcium-binding sites in NCX1 have recently been reported using NMR spectroscopy and x-ray crystallography, respectively.[157-159] Of interest, both approaches have revealed the presence of two calcium-binding domains (CBDs), each capable of binding multiple Ca^{2+} ions. Although small discrepancies initially were noted regarding the number of bound Ca^{2+} ions obtained from these two different approaches, both studies localized the coordination sites to the same general area and confirmed the importance of several Ca^{2+}-coordinating residues previously identified by mutagenesis. At present, it is agreed that CBD1 is capable of binding four Ca^{2+} ions, whereas two Ca^{2+} ions are bound at CBD2.[157-160] The functional significance of the two distinct CBDs remains poorly understood at this time, although mutagenesis at both sites dramatically alters calcium-dependent regulation.[158] Considerable unfolding of the CBD1 domain was reported in the absence of Ca^{2+}, whereas CBD2 remained relatively intact.[157,158,160] Of note, the alternative slicing region of NCX1 comprises a portion of the second CBD, and alternative splicing is known to alter ionic regulation of several NCX1 members.[157,158,161] The XIP region of the exchanger has been extensively characterized by mutagenesis of the native region, as well as mutagenesis of the exogenous peptide.[162-164] Mutations within this region can prominently influence the kinetics of Na^+-dependent inactivation, as discussed next. Several studies also have determined the specific details of helix packing for several transmembrane segments of NCX1.[154,165,166]

Regulation of Na^+-Ca^{2+} Exchange

Despite a central role for Na^+-Ca^{2+} exchange in cardiac excitation-contraction coupling, very little is known concerning the physiologic regulation of this transport system. A major question to be answered is how the Na^+-Ca^{2+} exchange system can adjust Ca^{2+} efflux levels to match changes in Ca^{2+} entry. To date, two forms of ionic regulation have been identified, and these autoregulatory mechanisms are mediated by the transport ions themselves. These intrinsic mechanisms are currently attractive candidates for providing the coupling of Ca^{2+} influx and efflux, as their operation can dramatically alter the population of functional exchangers. Na^+_i-dependent or I_1 regulation of Na^+-Ca^{2+} exchange describes the ability of cytoplasmic Na^+_i to promote an inactive state of the exchanger, although this response occurs only at high concentrations of cytoplasmic Na^+.[167] Ca^{2+}-dependent or I_2 regulation describes the stimulatory effects of cytoplasmic Ca^{2+} on both inward and outward exchange currents, an effect noted within the ranges of Ca^{2+} normally observed in myocytes.[75,147,168] This latter effect is evident in both whole-cell recordings and isolated membrane patches and may constitute the means by which the Na^+-Ca^{2+} exchanger can respond to changes in Ca^{2+} entry levels.[169] Ionic regulation of NCX1 is complex, and prominent interactions are observed with both mechanisms.[13,170-172]

Na^+-Ca^{2+} exchange activity is regulated by several additional factors including pH, β-adrenergic stimulation (but see reports by Ginsburg and Bers[173] and Lin and colleagues[174]), ATP levels, PKA, PKC, calcineurin, phospholemman, acyl-coenzyme As (acyl-CoAs), and membrane phospholipids (most notably PIP_2).[168,175-182] In most cases, how these regulatory responses are mediated or how they affect the physiologic operation of the heart remains unclear. For example, although both PKA- and PKC-mediated modulation of Na^+-Ca^{2+} exchange activity have been reported, it is uncertain whether this effect involves phosphorylation of the exchanger per se or other unidentified targets, and the physiologic relevance, if any, is unknown. PIP_2-mediated regulation of the exchanger involves an alleviation of Na^+-dependent or I_1-dependent inactivation of the exchanger. Because the role of I_1 inactivation in normal cardiac physiology remains unknown, however, the relevance of this type of regulation remains obscure. Regulation of the Na^+-Ca^{2+} exchanger by ATP also appears to involve this latter PIP_2-mediated mechanism. Overall, current understanding of Na^+-Ca^{2+} exchange regulation in physiology and pathophysiology is minimal.

Role of Na^+-Ca^{2+} Exchange in Cardiac Pathophysiology

Ample experimental evidence implicates the Na^+-Ca^{2+} exchanger in contributing to specific types of cardiac injury. The role played by Na^+-Ca^{2+} exchange in ischemia-reperfusion injury is best understood among these distinct types of injury. During ischemia, the switch to anaerobic metabolism with concomitant reduction or elimination of metabolite washout leads to an acidification of cardiac cells. During this period, intracellular Na^+ rises, although the extent to which this occurs presumably is model- and time-dependent. On reperfusion, the extracellular pH is rapidly restored, leading to a considerable pH gradient. The sarcolemmal Na^+-H^+ exchanger restores intracellular pH after ischemia, leading to a further increase in intracellular Na^+ levels. The consequent reduction in the transmembrane Na^+_i electrochemical gradient reduces the driving force for

Ca^{2+} efflux by forward exchange and facilitates the ability of reverse exchange to mediate Ca^{2+} influx. Depending on severity, the net reduction in Ca^{2+} efflux capacity can rapidly produce calcium overload or cell death. In view of this scenario, inhibition of the reverse mode of Na^+-Ca^{2+} exchange is an extremely attractive target for pharmacologic intervention as an adjunct to reperfusion therapy.[105,183-185]

In most models of heart failure, Na^+-Ca^{2+} exchange levels have been demonstrated to increase, with a reciprocal reduction in the levels of the sarcoplasmic reticulum Ca^{2+}-ATPase. This relationship also has been frequently observed in human heart failure.[186,187] A developing notion is that reverse Na^+-Ca^{2+} exchange serves a prominent role in supporting contractions in the failing heart to compensate for the decline in Ca^{2+} derived intracellularly. Although this increase in Na^+-Ca^{2+} exchange may support contractions, it also can predispose the heart to dangerous arrhythmias, because forward-mode Na^+-Ca^{2+} exchange constitutes a major, if not exclusive, component of transient inward currents.[188] In light of this risk, an appropriate strategy for pharmacologic intervention is not obvious. Within the context of cardiac glycoside therapy, improvements in contractility by means of indirect Na^+-Ca^{2+} exchange inhibition would be difficult to separate from the promotion of arrhythmias.[189]

Pharmacologic Manipulation of Na^+-Ca^{2+} Exchange

Historically, the ability to directly manipulate the function of Na^+-Ca^{2+} exchange proteins has been very elusive. A majority of compounds previously used for this purpose were completely lacking in specificity for the exchanger compared with other ion transport systems. Experimentally, the most common means of inhibiting exchange function was either to eliminate extracellular Na^+ and Ca^{2+} or to apply high concentrations of Ni^{2+} or La^{3+}. In 1996, however, two groups of investigators reported on a novel isothiourea compound, now known as KB-R7943.[190,191] This compound has been studied extensively since its introduction in an effort to glean mechanistic insight and to evaluate its therapeutic potential. Relatively little consensus has evolved with respect to its site of action, transport mode selectivity, mechanism of action, and isoform selectivity. In stark contrast, the cardioprotective effects of KB-R7943 have been established almost unanimously in a wide variety of cardiac injury models.[75]

Recently, a more potent Na^+-Ca^{2+} exchange inhibitor called SEA0400 has been described. This compound inhibits Na^+-Ca^{2+} exchange activity in the low nanomolar range in both cardiac and neuronal cell preparations.[151,192] The actions of this compound on a number of different ion channels and transporters have been examined, and considerable specificity for the Na^+-Ca^{2+} exchanger was observed. Notably, however, this compound also influenced Ca^{2+} transients and excitability in cardiac myotubes from NCX1.1-knockout mice, indicating a broader spectrum of effects than pure exchange inhibition.[193] Nevertheless, in a recent comparison of the cardioprotective effects of SEA0400 and KB-R7943, clear benefits were observed with SEA0400. Specifically, SEA0400 was found to exert a decrease infarct size by up to 75% in a coronary artery ligation protocol. This effect was concentration-dependent (median effective concentration [EC_{50}] = 5.7 nM) and occurred whether the compound was applied before or after regional ischemia. Considerably less efficacy was observed with KB-R7943, and functional recovery was impaired at higher concentrations.[194]

SEA0400 shows an apparent selectivity for reverse-mode Na^+-Ca^{2+} exchange current, a process mediated by its interaction with the sodium-dependent inactivation mechanism. That is, under ionic conditions that favor reverse exchange (i.e., elevated intracellular Na^+ levels such as those occurring during ischemia-reperfusion injury), SEA0400 prominently inhibits the exchanger. By contrast, under physiologic conditions in which intracellular Na^+ concentration is low, the potency of SEA0400 is greatly reduced. Thus, SEA0400 acts as a "conditional" NCX inhibitor, and this characteristic seems highly desirable with respect to the treatment of ischemia-reperfusion injury. Of note, however, NCX1 inhibition is not truly mode-selective, and the drug-inhibited exchangers will be unavailable in either transport mode.[195-197]

Manipulation of Na^+-Ca^{2+} exchange activity appears to be a promising approach toward minimizing reperfusion injury. Although the pharmacologic tools to accomplish this goal currently are limited, the initial results show effects similar to those observed with Na^+-H^+ exchange blockers. It is interesting to compare and contrast these different strategies with respect to ischemia-reperfusion injury. In both cases, the intent is to prevent reverse Na^+-Ca^{2+} exchange from producing intracellular Ca^{2+} overload with consequent cellular necrosis. In the case of utilizing Na^+-H^+ exchange blockers, this is accomplished by preventing or reducing the accumulation of intracellular Na^+, although an obvious consequence is a prolongation of an acidotic state. By contrast, with inhibition of the reverse mode of Na^+-Ca^{2+} exchange inhibition, the recovery from acidosis would proceed normally, although intracellular Na^+ levels would be anticipated to rise substantially, until corrected by the Na^+,K^+-ATPase. If the reverse mode of Na^+-Ca^{2+} exchange could be selectively inhibited, the acute influx of Ca^{2+} entry might be prevented, although the efficacy of forward mode Na^+-Ca^{2+} exchange might temporarily be compromised. Anticipated consequences range from a desirable positive inotropy to overt Ca^{2+} overload. Obviously, such speculations grossly oversimplify a complex and diverse set of sequelae during reperfusion injury. Nevertheless, early experimental results have established, in principle, that selective modification of Na^+-Ca^{2+} exchange activity is a promising cardioprotective strategy. Although cautious optimism seems warranted, the pharmacologic tools to address this approach remain scarce, and closing major gaps in the current understanding would require such tools. Moreover, lessons learned from clinical trials with Na^+-H^+ exchange blockers clearly demonstrate the difficulty in moving from bench to bedside.

Outlook and Future Directions

Other than prevention, the plethora of cardiac ailments facing today's aging population is most economically treated by pharmacologic approaches. In this regard, the manipulation of ion transporters appears promising, particularly with respect to reducing the damage associated with myocardial infarction, hypertrophy, and heart failure. Abnormalities in intracellular Na^+ and Ca^{2+} homeostasis are consistently observed in all of these diseases. To counter these changes, a greater understanding of the alterations in various ion pumps and exchangers is required, as well as a coincident increase in chemical modifiers of their function. Recent progress in the manipulation of Na^+-H^+ exchange and Na^+-Ca^{2+} exchange and the promising experimental results lend credence to the idea that these targets merit further investigation.

5

References

1. Glitsch HG: Electrophysiology of the sodium-potassium-ATPase in cardiac cells. Physiol Rev 81:1791-1826, 2001.
2. Bers DM: Excitation-Contraction Coupling and Cardiac Contractile Force. London, Kluwer, 2001.
3. Despa S, Bers DM: Functional analysis of Na^+/K^+-ATPase isoform distribution in rat ventricular myocytes. Am J Physiol Cell Physiol 293:C321-C327, 2007.
4. Dostanic I, Schultz JE, Lorenz JN, et al: The α1 isoform of Na,K-ATPase regulates cardiac contractility and functionally interacts and co-localizes with the Na/Ca-exchanger in heart. J Biol Chem 279:54053-54061, 2004.
5. Berry RG, Despa S, Fuller W, et al: Differential distribution and regulation of mouse cardiac Na^+/K^+-ATPase α1 and α2 subunits in T-tubule and surface sarcolemmal membranes. Cardiovasc Res 73:92-100, 2007.
6. Muller-Ehmsen J, McDonough AA, Farley RA, et al: Sodium pump isoform expression in heart failure: Implication for treatment. Basic Res Cardiol 97(:Suppl 1):I25-I30, 2002.
7. Srivastava S, Cala SE, Coetzee WA, et al: Phospholemman expression is high in the newborn rabbit heart and declines with postnatal maturation. Biochem Biophys Res Commun 355:338-341, 2007.
8. Barry WH: Na "Fuzzy space": Does it exist, and is it important in ischemic injury? J Cardiovasc Electrophysiol 17(Suppl 1): S43-S46, 2006.
9. Swift F, Tovsrud N, Enger UH, et al: The Na^+/K^+-ATPase a2-isoform regulates cardiac contractility in rat cardiomyocytes. Cardiovasc Res 75:109-117, 2007.
10. Despa S, Kockskamper J, Blatter LA, et al: Na/K pump-induced $[Na]_i$ gradients in rat ventricular myocytes measured with two-photon microscopy. Biophys J 87:1360-1368, 2004.
11. Despa S, Brette F, Orchard CH, et al: Na/Ca exchange and Na/K-ATPase function are equally concentrated in transverse tubules of rat ventricular myocytes. Biophys J 85:3388-3396, 2003.
12. Matchkov VV, Gustafsson H, Rahman A, et al: Interaction between Na^+/K^+-pump and Na^+/Ca^{2+}-exchanger modulates intercellular communication. Circ Res 100: 1026-1035, 2007.
13. Hilgemann DW, Yaradanakul A, Wang Y, et al: Molecular control of cardiac sodium homeostasis in health and disease. J Cardiovasc Electrophysiol 17(Suppl 1): S47-S56, 2006.
14. Geering K: FXYD proteins: New regulators of Na-K-ATPase. Am J Physiol Renal Physiol 290:F241-F250, 2006.
15. Li C, Grosdidier A, Crambert G, et al: Structural and functional interaction sites between Na,K-ATPase and FXYD proteins. J Biol Chem 279:38895-38902, 2004.
16. Fuller W, Shattock MJ: Phospholemman and the cardiac sodium pump: protein kinase C, take a bow. Circ Res 99: 1290-1292, 2006.
17. Pavlovic D, Fuller W, Shattock MJ: The intracellular region of FXYD1 is sufficient to regulate cardiac Na/K ATPase. FASEB J 21:1539-1546, 2007.
18. Jia LG, Donnet C, Bogaev RC, et al: Hypertrophy, increased ejection fraction, and reduced Na-K-ATPase activity in phospholemman-deficient mice. Am J Physiol Heart Circ Physiol 288: H1982-H1988, 2005.
19. Han F, Bossuyt J, Despa S, et al: Phospholemman phosphorylation mediates the protein kinase C–dependent effects on Na^+/K^+ pump function in cardiac myocytes. Circ Res 99:1376-1383, 2006.
20. Bossuyt J, Despa S, Martin JL, et al: Phospholemman phosphorylation alters its fluorescence resonance energy transfer with the Na/K-ATPase pump. J Biol Chem 281:32765-32773, 2006.
21. Bibert S, Roy S, Schaer D, et al: Phosphorylation of phospholemman (FXYD1) by protein kinase A and C modulates distinct Na,K-ATPase isozymes. J Biol Chem 283:476-486, 2008.
22. Kaplan JH: Biochemistry of Na,K-ATPase. Annu Rev Biochem 71:511-535, 2002.
23. Scheiner-Bobis G: The sodium pump. Its molecular properties and mechanics of ion transport. Eur J Biochem 269:2424-2433, 2002.
24. Holmgren M, Wagg J, Bezanilla F, et al: Three distinct and sequential steps in the release of sodium ions by the Na^+/K^+-ATPase. Nature 403:898-901, 2000.
25. Hilgemann DW: Channel-like function of the Na,K pump probed at microsecond resolution in giant membrane patches. Science 263:1429-1432, 1994.
26. De WP, Gadsby DC, Rakowski RF: Voltage dependence of the apparent affinity for external Na^+ of the backward-running sodium pump. J Gen Physiol 117:315-328, 2001.
27. Horisberger JD: Recent insights into the structure and mechanism of the sodium pump. Physiology (Bethesda) 19:377-387, 2004.
28. Rakowski RF, Artigas P, Palma F, et al: Sodium flux ratio in Na/K pump-channels opened by palytoxin. J Gen Physiol 130: 41-54, 2007.
29. Reyes N, Gadsby DC: Ion permeation through the Na^+,K^+-ATPase. Nature 443:470-474, 2006.
30. Harmel N, Apell HJ: Palytoxin-induced effects on partial reactions of the Na,K-ATPase. J Gen Physiol 128:103-118, 2006.
31. Guennoun-Lehmann S, Fonseca JE, Horisberger JD, et al: Palytoxin acts on Na^+,K^+-ATPase but not nongastric H^+,K^+-ATPase. J Membr Biol 216: 107-116, 2007.
32. Apell HJ: How do P-type ATPases transport ions? Bioelectrochemistry 63:149-156, 2004.
33. Clarke RJ, Kane DJ: Two gears of pumping by the sodium pump. Biophys J 93: 4187-4196, 2007.
34. Li C, Capendeguy O, Geering K, et al: A third Na^+-binding site in the sodium pump. Proc Natl Acad Sci U S A 102: 12706-12711, 2005.
35. Li C, Geering K, Horisberger JD: The third sodium binding site of Na,K-ATPase is functionally linked to acidic pH-activated inward current. J Membr Biol 213:1-9, 2006.
36. Ingwall JS, Balschi JA: Energetics of the Na^+ pump in the heart. J Cardiovasc Electrophysiol 17 Suppl 1:S127-S133, 2006.
37. Fonseca J, Kaya S, Rakowski R: Modeling of binding sites and electrostatics in the ion-motive sodium pump. Sixth Conference on Nanotechnology. 2006 IEEE-NANO 2006 1:154-157, 2006.
38. Martin DW: Structure-function relationships in the Na^+,K^+-pump. Semin Nephrol 25:282-291, 2005.
39. Rakowski RF, Sagar S: Found: Na^+ and K^+ binding sites of the sodium pump. News Physiol Sci 18:164-168, 2003.
40. Therien AG, Blostein R: Mechanisms of sodium pump regulation. Am J Physiol Cell Physiol 279:C541-C566, 2000.
41. Crambert G, Fuzesi M, Garty H, et al: Phospholemman (FXYD1) associates with Na,K-ATPase and regulates its transport properties. Proc Natl Acad Sci U S A 99:11476-11481, 2002.
42. Therien AG, Pu HX, Karlish SJ, et al: Molecular and functional studies of the gamma subunit of the sodium pump. J Bioenerg Biomembr 33:407-414, 2001.
43. Wang J, Schwinger RH, Frank K, et al: Regional expression of sodium pump subunits isoforms and Na^+-Ca^{++} exchanger in the human heart. J Clin Invest 98: 1650-1658, 1996.
44. McDonough AA, Zhang Y, Shin V, et al: Subcellular distribution of sodium pump isoform subunits in mammalian cardiac myocytes. Am J Physiol 270:1221-1227, 1996.
45. Toyoshima C, Nakasako M, Nomura H, et al: Crystal structure of the calcium pump of sarcoplasmic reticulum at 2.6 Å resolution. Nature 405:647-655, 2000.
46. Kaplan JH, Hu YK, Gatto C: Conformational coupling: the moving parts of an ion pump. J Bioenerg Biomembr 33:379-385, 2001.
47. Morth JP, Pedersen BP, Toustrup-Jensen MS, et al: Crystal structure of the sodium-potassium pump. Nature 450:1043-1049, 2007.
48. Gheorghiade M, Adams KF Jr, Colucci WS: Digoxin in the management of cardiovascular disorders. Circulation 109: 2959-2964, 2004.
49. Hamad E, Mather PJ, Srinivasan S, et al: Pharmacologic therapy of chronic heart failure. Am J Cardiovasc Drugs 7:235-248, 2007.
50. Dostanic I, Paul RJ, Lorenz JN, et al: The α_2-isoform of Na-K-ATPase mediates ouabain-induced hypertension in mice and increased vascular contractility in vitro. Am J Physiol Heart Circ Physiol 288: H477-H485, 2005.
51. Aperia A: New roles for an old enzyme: Na,K-ATPase emerges as an interesting drug target. J Intern Med 261:44-52, 2007.

52. Altamirano J, Li Y, DeSantiago J, et al: The inotropic effect of cardioactive glycosides in ventricular myocytes requires Na^+-Ca^{2+} exchanger function. J Physiol 575:845-854, 2006.
53. Schoner W, Scheiner-Bobis G: Endogenous and exogenous cardiac glycosides and their mechanisms of action. Am J Cardiovasc Drugs 7:173-189, 2007.
54. Schoner W, Scheiner-Bobis G: Endogenous and exogenous cardiac glycosides: Their roles in hypertension, salt metabolism, and cell growth. Am J Physiol Cell Physiol 293:C509-C536, 2007.
55. Wattenberg EV: Palytoxin: Exploiting a novel skin tumor promoter to explore signal transduction and carcinogenesis. Am J Physiol Cell Physiol 292:24-32, 2007.
56. Kaplan JH: The sodium pump and hypertension: A physiological role for the cardiac glycoside binding site of the Na,K-ATPase. Proc Natl Acad Sci U S A 102: 15723-15724, 2005.
57. Mijatovic T, Roland I, Van QE, et al: The α1 subunit of the sodium pump could represent a novel target to combat non–small cell lung cancers. J Pathol 212:170-179, 2007.
58. Jorgensen PL: Aspects of gene structure and functional regulation of the isozymes of Na,K-ATPase. Cell Mol Biol (Noisy-le-grand) 47:231-238, 2001.
59. Santana LF, Gomez AM, Lederer WJ: $Ca2^+$ flux through promiscuous cardiac Na^+ channels: Slip-mode conductance. Science 279:1027-1033, 1998.
60. Nishio M, Ruch SW, Wasserstrom JA: Positive inotropic effects of ouabain in isolated cat ventricular myocytes in sodium-free conditions. Am J Physiol Heart Circ Physiol 283:H2045-H2053, 2002.
61. Reuter H, Henderson SA, Han T, et al: The Na^+-Ca^{2+} exchanger is essential for the action of cardiac glycosides. Circ Res 90:305-308, 2002.
62. The effect of digoxin on mortality and morbidity in patients with heart failure. The Digitalis Investigation Group. N Engl J Med 336:525-533, 1997.
63. Rathore SS, Wang Y, Krumholz HM: Sex-based differences in the effect of digoxin for the treatment of heart failure. N Engl J Med 347:1403-1411, 2002.
64. Schoner W: Endogenous cardiac glycosides, a new class of steroid hormones. Eur J Biochem 269:2440-2448, 2002.
65. Gao J, Wymore RS, Wang Y, et al: Isoform-specific stimulation of cardiac Na/K pumps by nanomolar concentrations of glycosides. J Gen Physiol 119:297-312, 2002.
66. Muller-Ehmsen J, Wang J, Schwinger RH, et al: Region specific regulation of sodium pump isoform and Na,Ca-exchanger expression in the failing human heart—right atrium vs left ventricle. Cell Mol Biol (Noisy-le-Grand) 47:373-381, 2001.
67. Despa S, Islam MA, Weber CR, et al: Intracellular Na^+ concentration is elevated in heart failure but Na/K pump function is unchanged. Circulation 105:2543-2548, 2002.
68. Wang J, Velotta JB, McDonough AA, et al: All human Na^+-K^+-ATPase α-subunit isoforms have a similar affinity for cardiac glycosides. Am J Physiol Cell Physiol 281:C1336-C1343, 2001.
69. Gatto C, Hale CC, Xu W, et al: Eosin, a potent inhibitor of the plasma membrane Ca pump, does not inhibit the cardiac Na-Ca exchanger. Biochemistry 34: 965-972, 1995.
70. Choi HS, Eisner DA: The role of sarcolemmal Ca^{2+}-ATPase in the regulation of resting calcium concentration in rat ventricular myocytes. J Physiol (Lond) 515:109-118, 1999.
71. Choi HS, Eisner DA: The effects of inhibition of the sarcolemmal Ca-ATPase on systolic calcium fluxes and intracellular calcium concentration in rat ventricular myocytes. Pflügers Arch 437:966-971, 1999.
72. Bers DM: Cardiac excitation-contraction coupling. Nature 415:198-205, 2002.
73. Tempel BL, Shilling DJ: The plasma membrane calcium ATPase and disease. Subcell Biochem 45:365-383, 2007.
74. Prasad V, Okunade GW, Miller ML, et al: Phenotypes of SERCA and PMCA knockout mice. Biochem Biophys Res Commun 322:1192-1203, 2004.
75. Hryshko LV: The cardiac Na^+-Ca^{2+} exchanger. In Page E, Fozzard HA, Solaro RJ (eds): Handbook of Physiology. Section 2: The Cardiovascular System. Vol 1: The Heart. Oxford, Oxford University Press, 2002, pp 388-419.
76. Henderson SA, Goldhaber JI, So JM, et al: Functional adult myocardium in the absence of Na^+-Ca^{2+} exchange. Cardiac-specific knockout of NCX1. Circ Res 95:604-611, 2004.
77. Pott C, Philipson KD, Goldhaber JI: Excitation-contraction coupling in Na^+-Ca^{2+} exchanger knockout mice: Reduced transsarcolemmal Ca^{2+} flux. Circ Res 97:1288-1295, 2005.
78. Pott C, Ren X, Tran DX, et al: Mechanism of shortened action potential duration in Na^+-Ca^{2+} exchanger knockout mice. Am J Physiol Cell Physiol 292:C968-C973, 2007.
79. Pott C, Yip M, Goldhaber JI, et al: Regulation of cardiac L-type Ca^{2+} current in Na^+-Ca^{2+} exchanger knockout mice: functional coupling of the Ca^{2+} channel and the Na^+-Ca^{2+} exchanger. Biophys J 92:1431-1437, 2007.
80. Henaff M, Antoine S, Mercadier JJ, et al: The voltage-independent B-type Ca^{2+} channel modulates apoptosis of cardiac myocytes. FASEB J 16:99-101, 2002.
81. Antoine S, Pinet C, Coulombe A: Are B-type Ca^{2+} channels of cardiac myocytes akin to the passive ion channel in the plasma membrane Ca^{2+} pump? J Membr Biol 179:37-50, 2001.
82. Pinet C, Antoine S, Filoteo AG, et al: Reincorporated plasma membrane Ca^{2+}-ATPase can mediate B-type Ca^{2+} channels observed in native membrane of human red blood cells. J Membr Biol 187:185-201, 2002.
83. Oceandy D, Stanley PJ, Cartwright EJ, et al: The regulatory function of plasma-membrane Ca^{2+}-ATPase (PMCA) in the heart. Biochem Soc Trans 35:927-930, 2007.
84. Strehler EE, Caride AJ, Filoteo AG, et al: Plasma membrane Ca^{2+} ATPases as dynamic regulators of cellular calcium handling. Ann N Y Acad Sci 1099:226-236, 2007.
85. Strehler EE, Filoteo AG, Penniston JT, et al: Plasma-membrane Ca^{2+} pumps: Structural diversity as the basis for functional versatility. Biochem Soc Trans 35:919-922, 2007.
86. Philipson KD: Na^+-Ca^{2+} exchange: Three new tools. Circ Res 90:118-119, 2002.
87. Carafoli E, Brini M: Calcium pumps: Structural basis for and mechanism of calcium transmembrane transport. Curr Opin Chem Biol 4:152-161, 2000.
88. Caride AJ, Filoteo AG, Penheiter AR, et al: Delayed activation of the plasma membrane calcium pump by a sudden increase in Ca^{2+}: Fast pumps reside in fast cells. Cell Calcium 30:49-57, 2001.
89. Strehler EE, Zacharias DA: Role of alternative splicing in generating isoform diversity among plasma membrane calcium pumps. Physiol Rev 81:21-50, 2001.
90. Williams JC, Armesilla AL, Mohamed TM, et al: The sarcolemmal calcium pump, α-1 syntrophin, and neuronal nitric-oxide synthase are parts of a macromolecular protein complex. J Biol Chem 281:23341-23348, 2006.
91. Monteith GR, Roufogalis BD: The plasma membrane calcium pump—a physiological perspective on its regulation. Cell Calcium 18:459-470, 1995.
92. Penniston JT, Enyedi A: Modulation of the plasma membrane Ca^{2+} pump. J Membr Biol 165:101-109, 1998.
93. Vaughan-Jones RD, Villafuerte FC, Swietach P, et al: pH-regulated Na^+ influx into the mammalian ventricular myocyte: The relative role of Na^+-H^+ exchange and Na^+-HCO co-transport. J Cardiovasc Electrophysiol 17(:Suppl 1):S134-S140, 2006.
94. Leineweber K, Heusch G, Schulz R: Regulation and role of the presynaptic and myocardial Na^+/H^+ exchanger NHE1: Effects on the sympathetic nervous system in heart failure. Cardiovasc Drug Rev 25:123-131, 2007.
95. Karmazyn M, Sawyer M, Fliegel L: The Na^+/H^+ exchanger: A target for cardiac therapeutic intervention. Curr Drug Targets Cardiovasc Haematol Disord 5:323-335, 2005.
96. Meima ME, Mackley JR, Barber DL: Beyond ion translocation: Structural functions of the sodium-hydrogen exchanger isoform-1. Curr Opin Nephrol Hypertens 16:365-372, 2007.
97. Cardone RA, Casavola V, Reshkin SJ: The role of disturbed pH dynamics and the Na^+/H^+ exchanger in metastasis. Nat Rev Cancer 5:786-795, 2005.
98. Jung YS, Kim HY, Kim J, et al: Physical interactions and functional coupling between Daxx and sodium hydrogen exchanger 1 in ischemic cell death. J Biol Chem 283:1018-1025, 2008.
99. Javadov S, Choi A, Rajapurohitam V, et al: NHE-1 inhibition-induced cardioprotection against ischaemia/reperfusion is associated with attenuation of the mitochondrial permeability transition. Cardiovasc Res 77:416-424, 2008.

100. Slepkov ER, Rainey JK, Sykes BD, et al: Structural and functional analysis of the Na^+/H^+ exchanger. Biochem J 401: 623-633, 2007.
101. Orlowski J, Grinstein S: Diversity of the mammalian sodium/proton exchanger SLC9 gene family. Pflügers Arch 447:549-565, 2004.
102. Putney LK, Denker SP, Barber DL: The changing face of the Na^+/H^+ exchanger, NHE1: Structure, regulation, and cellular actions. Annu Rev Pharmacol Toxicol 42:527-552, 2002.
103. Karmazyn M, Gan XT, Humphreys RA, et al: The myocardial Na^+-H^+ exchange. Structure, regulation, and its role in heart disease. Circ Res 85:777-786, 1999.
104. Alexander RT, Grinstein S: Na^+/H^+ exchangers and the regulation of volume. Acta Physiol (Oxf) 187:159-167, 2006.
105. Doggrell SA, Hancox JC: Is timing everything? Therapeutic potential of modulators of cardiac Na^+ transporters. Expert Opin Invest Drugs 12:1123-1142, 2003.
106. Allen DG, Xiao XH: Role of the cardiac Na^+/H^+ exchanger during ischemia and reperfusion. Cardiovasc Res 57:934-941, 2003.
107. Masereel B, Pochet L, Laeckmann D: An overview of inhibitors of Na^+/H^+ exchanger. Eur J Med Chem 38:547-554, 2003.
108. Numata M, Orlowski J: Molecular cloning and characterization of a novel $(Na^+,K^+)/H^+$ exchanger localized to the trans-Golgi network. J Biol Chem 276:17387-17394, 2001.
109. Aharonovitz O, Zaun HC, Balla T, et al: Intracellular pH regulation by Na^+/H^+ exchange requires phosphatidylinositol 4,5-bisphosphate. J Cell Biol 150: 213-224, 2000.
110. Hunte C, Screpanti E, Venturi M, et al: Structure of a Na^+/H^+ antiporter and insights into mechanism of action and regulation by pH. Nature 435:1197-1202, 2005.
111. Landau M, Herz K, Padan E, et al: Model structure of the Na^+/H^+ exchanger 1 (NHE1): Functional and clinical implications. J Biol Chem 282:37854-37863, 2007.
112. Ammar YB, Takeda S, Hisamitsu T, et al: Crystal structure of CHP2 complexed with NHE1-cytosolic region and an implication for pH regulation. EMBO J 25:2315-2325, 2006.
113. Mishima M, Wakabayashi S, Kojima C: Solution structure of the cytoplasmic region of Na^+/H^+ exchanger 1 complexed with essential cofactor calcineurin B homologous protein 1. J Biol Chem 282:2741-2751, 2007.
114. Baumgartner M, Patel H, Barber DL: Na^+/H^+ exchanger NHE1 as plasma membrane scaffold in the assembly of signaling complexes. Am J Physiol Cell Physiol 287:844-850, 2004.
115. Slepkov E, Fliegel L: Structure and function of the NHE1 isoform of the Na^+/H^+ exchanger. Biochem Cell Biol 80:499-508, 2002.
116. Fliegel L, Karmazyn M: The cardiac Na-H exchanger: A key downstream mediator for the cellular hypertrophic effects of paracrine, autocrine and hormonal factors. Biochem Cell Biol 82:626-635, 2004.
117. Orlowski J: Na^+/H^+ exchangers. Molecular diversity and relevance to heart. Ann N Y Acad Sci 874:346-353, 1999.
118. Engelhardt S, Hein L, Keller U, et al: Inhibition of Na^+/H^+-exchange prevents hypertrophy, fibrosis and heart failure in β_1-adrenergic receptor transgenic mice. Naunyn-Schmiedebergs Arch Pharmacol 365:343, 2002.
119. Hilgemann DW, Ball R: Regulation of cardiac Na^+,Ca^{2+} exchange and K_{ATP} potassium channels by PIP_2. Science 273:956-959, 1996.
120. Avkiran M, Marber MS: Na^+/H^+ exchange inhibitors for cardioprotective therapy: progress, problems and prospects. J Am Coll Cardiol 39:747-753, 2002.
121. Zeymer U, Suryapranata H, Monassier JP, et al: The Na^+/H^+ exchange inhibitor eniporide as an adjunct to early reperfusion therapy for acute myocardial infarction. Results of the Evaluation of the Safety and Cardioprotective Effects of Eniporide in Acute Myocardial Infarction (ESCAMI) trial. J Am Coll Cardiol 38:1644-1650, 2001.
122. Theroux P, Chaitman BR, Danchin N, et al: Inhibition of the sodium-hydrogen exchanger with cariporide to prevent myocardial infarction in high-risk ischemic situations. Main results of the GUARDIAN trial. Circulation 102: 3032-3038, 2000.
123. Bridge JH, Smolley JR, Spitzer KW: The relationship between charge movements associated with I_{Ca} and $I_{Na\text{-}Ca}$ in cardiac myocytes. Science 248:376-378, 1990.
124. Leblanc N, Hume JR: Sodium current-induced release of calcium from cardiac sarcoplasmic reticulum. Science 248: 372-376, 1990.
125. Goldhaber JI: Sodium-calcium exchange: The phantom menace. Circ Res 85: 982-984, 1999.
126. Blaustein MP, Lederer WJ: Sodium/calcium exchange: Its physiological implications. Physiol Rev 79:763-854, 1999.
127. Sobie EA, Cannell MB, Bridge JH: Allosteric activation of Na^+-Ca^{2+} exchange by L-type Ca^{2+} current augments the trigger flux for SR Ca^{2+} release in ventricular myocytes. Biophys J 94:L54-L56, 2008.
128. Bers DM, Bassani JW, Bassani RA: Competition and redistribution among calcium transport systems in rabbit cardiac myocytes. Cardiovasc Res 27: 1772-1777, 1993.
129. Fujioka Y, Komeda M, Matsuoka S: Stoichiometry of Na^+-Ca^{2+} exchange in inside-out patches excised from guinea-pig ventricular myocytes. J Physiol (Lond) 523:339-351, 2000.
130. Dong H, Dunn J, Lytton J: Stoichiometry of the cardiac Na^+/Ca^{2+} exchanger NCX1.1 measured in transfected HEK cells. Biophys J 82:1943-1952, 2002.
131. Hinata M, Yamamura H, Li L, et al: Stoichiometry of Na^+-Ca^{2+} exchange is. 3:1 in guinea-pig ventricular myocytes. J Physiol 545:453-461, 2002.
132. Hilgemann DW: New insights into the molecular and cellular workings of the cardiac Na^+/Ca^{2+} exchanger. Am J Physiol Cell Physiol 287:C1167-C1172, 2004.
133. Hinata M, Kimura J: Forefront of Na^+/Ca^{2+} exchanger studies: Stoichiometry of cardiac Na^+/Ca^{2+} exchanger; 3:1 or. 4:1? J Pharmacol Sci 96:15-18, 2004.
134. Kang TM, Steciuk M, Hilgemann DW: Sodium-calcium exchange stoichiometry: Is the noose tightening? Ann N Y Acad Sci 976:142-151, 2002.
135. Bers DM, Ginsburg KS: Na:Ca stoichiometry and cytosolic Ca-dependent activation of NCX in intact cardiomyocytes. Ann N Y Acad Sci 1099:326-338, 2007.
136. Kang TM, Hilgemann DW: Multiple transport modes of the cardiac Na^+/Ca^{2+} exchanger. Nature 427:544-548, 2004.
137. Hilgemann DW, Nicoll DA, Philipson KD: Charge movement during Na^+ translocation by native and cloned cardiac Na^+/Ca^{2+} exchanger. Nature 352:715-718, 1991.
138. Niggli E, Lederer WJ: Molecular operations of the sodium-calcium exchanger revealed by conformation currents. Nature 349:621-624, 1991.
139. Kappl M, Hartung K: Rapid charge translocation by the cardiac Na^+-Ca^{2+} exchanger after a Ca^{2+} concentration jump. Biophys J 71:2473-2485, 1996.
140. Haase A, Wood PG, Pintschovius V, et al: Time resolved kinetics of the guinea pig Na-Ca exchanger (NCX1) expressed in Xenopus oocytes: Voltage and Ca^{2+} dependence of pre-steady-state current investigated by photolytic Ca^{2+} concentration jumps. Pflügers Arch 454:1031-1042, 2007.
141. Kappl M, Hartung K: Kinetics of Na-Ca exchange current after a Ca^{2+} concentration jump. Ann N Y Acad Sci 779: 290-292, 1996.
142. Kappl M, Nagel G, Hartung K: Voltage and Ca^{2+} dependence of pre-steady-state currents of the Na-Ca exchanger generated by Ca^{2+} concentration jumps. Biophys J 81:2628-2638, 2001.
143. Hilgemann DW: Unitary cardiac Na^+,Ca^{2+} exchange current magnitudes determined from channel-like noise and charge movements of ion transport. Biophys J 71:759-768, 1996.
144. Cai X, Lytton J: The Cation/Ca^{2+} exchanger superfamily: Phylogenetic analysis and structural implications. Mol Biol Evol 21:1692-1703, 2004.
145. Marshall CR, Fox JA, Butland SL, et al: Phylogeny of Na^+/Ca^{2+} exchanger (NCX) genes from genomic data identifies new gene duplications and a new family member in fish species. Physiol Genomics 21:161-173, 2005.
146. Nicoll DA, Longoni S, Philipson KD: Molecular cloning and functional expression of the cardiac sarcolemmal Na^+-Ca^{2+} exchanger. Science 250:562-565, 1990.
147. Philipson KD, Nicoll DA: Sodium-calcium exchange: A molecular perspective. Annu Rev Physiol 62:111-133, 2000.
148. Kofuji P, Lederer WJ, Schulze DH: Mutually exclusive and cassette exons

underlie alternatively spliced isoforms of the Na/Ca exchanger. J Biol Chem 269:5145-5149, 1994.
149. Lytton J: Na^+/Ca^{2+} exchangers: Three mammalian gene families control Ca^{2+} transport. Biochem J 406:365-382, 2007.
150. Lee SL, Yu AS, Lytton J: Tissue-specific expression of Na^+-Ca^{2+} exchanger isoforms. J Biol Chem 269:14849-14852, 1994.
151. Tanaka H, Nishimaru K, Aikawa T, et al: Effect of SEA0400, a novel inhibitor of sodium-calcium exchanger, on myocardial ionic currents. Br J Pharmacol 135: 1096-1100, 2002.
152. Iwamoto T, Uehara A, Imanaga I, et al: The Na^+/Ca^{2+} exchanger NCX1 has oppositely oriented reentrant loop domains that contain conserved aspartic acids whose mutation alters its apparent Ca^{2+} affinity. J Biol Chem 275: 38571-38580, 2000.
153. Matsuoka S, Nicoll DA, Reilly RF, et al: Initial localization of regulatory regions of the cardiac sarcolemmal Na^+-Ca^{2+} exchanger. Proc Natl Acad Sci U S A 90:3870-3874, 1993.
154. Nicoll DA, Ren X, Ottolia M, et al: What we know about the structure of NCX1 and how it relates to its function. Ann N Y Acad Sci 1099:1-6, 2007.
155. Nicoll DA, Ottolia M, Lu L, et al: A new topological model of the cardiac sarcolemmal Na^+-Ca^{2+} exchanger. J Biol Chem 274:910-917, 1999.
156. Shigekawa M, Iwamoto T, Uehara A, et al: Probing ion binding sites in the Na^+/Ca^{2+} exchanger. Ann N Y Acad Sci 976:19-30, 2002.
157. Hilge M, Aelen J, Vuister GW: Ca^{2+} regulation in the $Na+/Ca^{2+}$ exchanger involves two markedly different Ca^{2+} sensors. Mol Cell 22:15-25, 2006.
158. Besserer GM, Ottolia M, Nicoll DA, et al: The second Ca^{2+}-binding domain of the Na^+-Ca^{2+} exchanger is essential for regulation: Crystal structures and mutational analysis. Proc Natl Acad Sci U S A 104:18467-18472, 2007.
159. Nicoll DA, Sawaya MR, Kwon S, et al: The crystal structure of the primary Ca^{2+} sensor of the Na^+/Ca^{2+} exchanger reveals a novel Ca^{2+} binding motif. J Biol Chem 281:21577-21581, 2006.
160. Hilge M, Aelen J, Perrakis A, et al: Structural basis for Ca^{2+} regulation in the Na^+/Ca^{2+} exchanger. Ann N Y Acad Sci 1099:7-15, 2007.
161. Dyck C, Omelchenko A, Elias CL, et al: Ionic regulatory properties of brain and kidney splice variants of the NCX1 Na^+-Ca^{2+} exchanger. J Gen Physiol 114:701-711, 1999.
162. Dyck C, Maxwell K, Buchko J, et al: Structure-function analysis of CALX1.1, a Na^+-Ca^{2+} exchanger from Drosophila. Mutagenesis of ionic regulatory sites. J Biol Chem 273:12981-12987, 1998.
163. He Z, Petesch N, Voges K, et al: Identification of important amino acid residues of the Na^+-Ca^{2+} exchanger inhibitory peptide, XIP. J Membr Biol 156: 149-156, 1997.
164. Matsuoka S, Nicoll DA, He Z, et al: Regulation of cardiac Na^+-Ca^{2+} exchanger by the endogenous XIP region. J Gen Physiol 109:273-286, 1997.
165. Ren X, Nicoll DA, Philipson KD: Transmembrane segments I, II, and VI of the canine cardiac Na^+/Ca^{2+} exchanger are in proximity. Ann N Y Acad Sci 1099:40-42, 2007.
166. Ren X, Nicoll DA, Philipson KD: Helix packing of the cardiac Na^+-Ca^{2+} exchanger: Proximity of transmembrane segments 1, 2, and 6. J Biol Chem 281:22808-22814, 2006.
167. Hilgemann DW, Matsuoka S, Nagel GA, et al: Steady-state and dynamic properties of cardiac sodium-calcium exchange. Sodium-dependent inactivation. J Gen Physiol 100:905-932, 1992.
168. Hilgemann DW, Collins A, Matsuoka S: Steady-state and dynamic properties of cardiac sodium-calcium exchange. Secondary modulation by cytoplasmic calcium and ATP. J Gen Physiol 100: 933-961, 1992.
169. Matsuoka S, Hilgemann DW: Inactivation of outward Na^+-Ca^{2+} exchange current in guinea- pig ventricular myocytes. J Physiol (Lond) 476:443-458, 1994.
170. Urbanczyk J, Chernysh O, Condrescu M, et al: Sodium-calcium exchange does not require allosteric calcium activation at high cytosolic sodium concentrations. J Physiol 575:693-705, 2006.
171. Kim BJ, Jun JY, So I, et al: Involvement of mitochondrial Na^+-Ca^{2+} exchange in intestinal pacemaking activity. World J Gastroenterol 12:796-799, 2006.
172. Matsuoka S, Nicoll DA, Hryshko LV, et al: Regulation of the cardiac Na^+-Ca^{2+} exchanger by Ca^{2+}. Mutational analysis of the Ca^{2+}-binding domain. J Gen Physiol 105:403-420, 1995.
173. Ginsburg K, Bers DM: Isoproterenol does not enhance Na/Ca exchange current in intact rabbit ventricular myocytes. Biophys J 86:26a-27a, 2004.
174. Lin X, Jo H, Sakakibara Y, et al: β-Adrenergic stimulation does not activate Na^+-Ca^{2+} exchange current in guinea-pig, mouse and rat ventricular myocytes. Am J Physiol Cell Physiol 290:C601-C608, 2006.
175. Riedel MJ, Baczko I, Searle GJ, et al: Metabolic regulation of sodium-calcium exchange by intracellular acyl CoAs. EMBO J 25:4605-4614, 2006.
176. Doering AE, Lederer WJ: The action of Na^+ as a cofactor in the inhibition by cytoplasmic protons of the cardiac Na^+-Ca^{2+} exchanger in the guinea-pig. J Physiol (Lond) 480:9-20, 1994.
177. Zhang XQ, Ahlers BA, Tucker AL, et al: Phospholemman inhibition of the cardiac Na^+/Ca^{2+} exchanger. Role of phosphorylation. J Biol Chem 281:7784-7792, 2006.
178. Pulina MV, Rizzuto R, Brini M, et al: Inhibitory interaction of the plasma membrane Na^+/Ca^{2+} exchangers with the 14-3-3 proteins. J Biol Chem 281: 19645-19654, 2006.
179. Shigekawa M, Katanosaka Y, Wakabayashi S: Regulation of the cardiac Na^+/Ca^{2+} exchanger by calcineurin and protein kinase C. Ann N Y Acad Sci 1099:53-63, 2007.
180. Shen C, Lin MJ, Yaradanakul A, et al: Dual control of cardiac Na^+-Ca^{2+} exchange by PIP_2: Analysis of the surface membrane fraction by extracellular cysteine PEGylation. J Physiol 582:1011-1026, 2007.
181. Yaradanakul A, Feng S, Shen C, et al: Dual control of cardiac Na^+-Ca^{2+} exchange by PIP_2: Electrophysiological analysis of direct and indirect mechanisms. J Physiol 582:991-1010, 2007.
182. Ruknudin AM, Wei SK, Haigney MC, et al: Phosphorylation and other conundrums of Na/Ca exchanger, NCX1. Ann N Y Acad Sci 1099:103-118, 2007.
183. Iwamoto T: Sodium-calcium exchange inhibitors: Therapeutic potential in cardiovascular diseases. Future Cardiol 1:519-529, 2005.
184. Iwamoto T, Watanabe Y, Kita S, et al: Na^+/Ca^{2+} exchange inhibitors: A new class of calcium regulators. Cardiovasc Hematol Disord Drug Targets 7: 188-198, 2007.
185. Lee C, Dhalla NS, Hryshko LV: Therapeutic potential of novel Na^+-Ca^{2+} exchange inhibitors in attenuating ischemia-reperfusion injury. Can J Cardiol 21:509-516, 2005.
186. Hasenfuss G, Schillinger W, Lehnart SE, et al: Relationship between Na^+-Ca^{2+}-exchanger protein levels and diastolic function of failing human myocardium. Circulation 99:641-648, 1999.
187. Dipla K, Mattiello JA, Margulies KB, et al: The sarcoplasmic reticulum and the Na^+/Ca^{2+} exchanger both contribute to the Ca^{2+} transient of failing human ventricular myocytes. Circ Res 84:435-444, 1999.
188. Pogwizd SM, Schlotthauer K, Li L, et al: Arrhythmogenesis and contractile dysfunction in heart failure: Roles of sodium-calcium exchange, inward rectifier potassium current, and residual b-adrenergic responsiveness. Circ Res 88:1159-1167, 2001.
189. Venetucci LA, Trafford AW, O'Neill SC, et al: Na/Ca exchange: Regulator of intracellular calcium and source of arrhythmias in the heart. Ann N Y Acad Sci 1099: 315-325, 2007.
190. Iwamoto T, Watano T, Shigekawa M: A novel isothiourea derivative selectively inhibits the reverse mode of Na^+/Ca^{2+} exchange in cells expressing NCX1. J Biol Chem 271:22391-22397, 1996.
191. Watano T, Kimura J, Morita T, et al: A novel antagonist, No. 7943, of the Na^+/Ca^{2+} exchange current in guinea-pig cardiac ventricular cells. Br J Pharmacol 119:555-563, 1996.
192. Matsuda T, Arakawa N, Takuma K, et al: SEA0400, a novel and selective inhibitor of the Na^+-Ca^{2+} exchanger, attenuates reperfusion injury in the in vitro and in vivo cerebral ischemic models. J Pharmacol Exp Ther 298:249-256, 2001.
193. Reuter H, Henderson SA, Han T, et al: Knockout mice for pharmacological screening: testing the specificity of

Na^+-Ca^{2+} exchange inhibitors. Circ Res 91:90-92, 2002.
194. Magee WP, Deshmukh G, DeNinno MP, et al: Differing cardioprotective efficacy of the Na^+-Ca^{2+} exchanger inhibitors, SEA0400 and KB-R7943. Am J Physiol Heart Circ Physiol 284:H903-H910, 2003.
195. Bouchard R, Omelchenko A, Le HD, et al: Effects of SEA0400 on mutant NCX1.1 Na^+-Ca^{2+} exchangers with altered ionic regulation. Mol Pharmacol 65:802-810, 2004.
196. Noble D, Blaustein MP: Directionality in drug action on sodium-calcium exchange. Ann N Y Acad Sci 1099:540-543, 2007.
197. Lee C, Visen N, Dhalla NS, et al: Inhibitory profile of SEA0400 [2-[4-[(2,5-difluorophenyl)methoxy]phenoxy]-5-ethoxyaniline] assessed on the cardiac Na^+-Ca^{2+} exchanger, NCX1.1. J Pharmacol Exp Ther 311:748-757, 2004.

5

Sarcoplasmic Reticulum Ion Channels 6

Ernst Niggli

CHAPTER OUTLINE

The Sarcoplasmic Reticulum

Structure and Overall Function of the Cardiac Sarcoplasmic Reticulum

The sarcoplasmic reticulum (SR) is a cellular organelle present in cardiac myocytes of almost all species. Its most important function is to amplify the transient Ca^{2+} signals that initiate muscle contraction. The primary Ca^{2+} signal is generated by Ca^{2+} influx through voltage-dependent L-type calcium channels during the action potential. This Ca^{2+} signal is subsequently amplified by Ca^{2+} release from the SR in a process termed *excitation-contraction coupling*.[1] The mechanism driving the amplification is calcium-induced Ca^{2+} release (CICR).[2,3] The SR lumen contains a millimolar concentration of Ca^{2+}, with a large fraction bound to the low-affinity calcium-binding protein calsequestrin.[4] Depending on the species, the SR occupies up to approximately 8% of the cardiomyocyte volume.[1]

On the ultrastructural level, the SR is organized in several distinct compartments exhibiting regularly repeating arrangements along the cell axis and sarcomeres. The excitation-contraction coupling and Ca^{2+} release events occur preferentially in the regions in which the SR is in close contact with the sarcolemma, in dyads and in peripheral couplings. Dyads are present in myocytes containing transverse (T) tubules, such as ventricular myocytes. In the dyadic region, the SR is separated from the sarcolemma by a very narrow cleft (approximately 15 nm). Peripheral couplings are more often observed in myocytes containing no or only few T tubules, such as atrial myocytes. Between the T tubules of adjacent sarcomeres the SR forms a reticular structure. Whereas the junctional domains of the SR are thought to contain a very large fraction of all SR Ca^{2+} release channels (also known as ryanodine receptors [RyRs]), the longitudinal SR network contains a high density of Ca^{2+}-ATPases (also called sarcoplasmic-endoplasmic reticulum calcium pumps [SERCAs]). Together with the nuclear envelope, the entire SR seems to form a well-connected, continuous network throughout each myocyte.[5]

*Work on which this chapter is based was supported by the Swiss National Science Foundation and the Swiss Foundation for Research on Muscle Diseases.

Methods and Preparations to Measure Sarcoplasmic Reticulum Ion Channel Function

Sarcoplasmic Reticulum Vesicles and Artificial Lipid Bilayers

Because the SR is an intracellular organelle, functional and biophysical studies of its ion channels are not straightforward but rather challenging. Unlike channels located in the sarcolemma, intracellular channels are not directly accessible to electrophysiologic methods, such as the patch clamp technique (patch clamp recording from the nuclear envelope[6] and from skeletal muscle SR "sarcoballs"[7] has been described). Sucrose density gradient centrifugation of homogenized cardiac muscle allows the separation of light and heavy SR vesicles. The latter contain RyRs at a high density, in addition to SR calcium pumps and other SR ion channels. They have been used in numerous biochemical and tracer flux assays to study various features and pharmacologic properties of SR Ca^{2+} release and of other ion conductances in the SR membrane.[4,8]

The incorporation of channels into artificial lipid membranes (e.g., by fusion of SR vesicles into the bilayer) has turned out to be the most powerful electrophysiologic technique to record ion channel activity from intracellular organelles, such as the SR. This technique has allowed the characterization of many biophysical features of the RyRs on the molecular level and in great detail.[9-11] As with any other technique, however, some specific limitations need to be recognized. Often, these experiments had to be carried out under conditions that were quite far from physiologic (e.g., absence of Mg^{2+} and adenine triphosphate (ATP)—but see the report by Mejia-Alvarez and colleagues[12]). Furthermore, a single RyR may behave differently than it does when acting as a member of a channel cluster exhibiting cooperativity.[13] Moreover, some modulatory proteins may have been lost during purification and isolation of the channel proteins.[14] Nevertheless, this method is still the most powerful and direct approach to study single RyR channel biophysics. Also, other channels of the SR, such as potassium and chloride channels, have been extensively examined with this technique.[15-17] These monovalent anion and cation channels have been implicated in the movement of countercharge during SR Ca^{2+} release, to maintain electroneutrality (see later on).

Ca^{2+} Imaging

Imaging of cellular Ca^{2+} signaling events has allowed the monitoring of function of RyRs in a more native environment. Elementary events of Ca^{2+} signaling, such as Ca^{2+} sparks, are thought to closely reflect the behavior of a small group of RyRs[18,19]; from the analysis of such elementary Ca^{2+} signals, a great deal has been learned about SR Ca^{2+} release in cardiac muscle, but also in other tissues (reviewed by Niggli and Shirokova[20]). One initial expectation, the temporal and spatial quantitative reconstruction of the underlying Ca^{2+} release flux based on the imaging data, has been a dauntingly difficult task because of many unknowns, such as subcellular Ca^{2+} buffering capacities, and also because of signal-to-noise issues of the confocal image data.[21,22] An alternative approach originally developed to estimate SR Ca^{2+} release fluxes in skeletal muscle fibers[23] has recently been adapted to examine subcellular Ca^{2+} release events, such as so-called sparks. Fluorescence signals that quantitatively reflect the SR Ca^{2+} release flux can itself be observed using a fluorescent Ca^{2+} indicator with fast kinetics of calcium binding, in combination with an excess of a nonfluorescent slow Ca^{2+} buffer, such as ethylene glycol tetra-acetic acid (EGTA). Such signals have been termed "Ca^{2+} spikes."[24,25]

Electron Microprobe Analysis

Changes of Ca^{2+} and other ions within the SR also have been analyzed using an ultrarapid freezing technique. This has been combined with electron microprobe analysis of the cytosolic and intra-SR ionic composition in electron micrographs obtained from tissue frozen at different time points.[26] Such experiments have contributed valuable information about ion fluxes, particularly regarding the extent of SR Ca^{2+} depletion and the amount of countercharge movements into the SR during Ca^{2+} release (see later on).

Ca^{2+} Imaging inside the Sarcoplasmic Reticulum

More recently, several techniques have been developed to measure the Ca^{2+} concentration inside the SR. Loading the SR with the low-affinity Ca^{2+} indicator fluo-5-N by exposure to the acetoxymethyl (AM) ester form of the dye has enabled measurements of the Ca^{2+} concentration inside the cardiac muscle SR[27] and even resolution of the local depletion resulting from a Ca^{2+} spark, called a "Ca^{2+} blink".[28] This technique also can provide information about the function of the Ca^{2+} store and will be a valuable tool in future studies of Ca^{2+} signaling alterations during cardiac diseases, such as congestive heart failure (for example, see reports by Kubalova and Guo and their coworkers[29,30]). The precise procedures and conditions needed to successfully load the SR with the Ca^{2+} indicator are very delicate, however, and seem to depend critically on temperature, dye concentration, loading time, species, and other unknown factors.

The Sarcoplasmic Reticulum Calcium Release Channel (Ryanodine Receptor-2)

Structure and Components of the Ryanodine Receptor-2 Macromolecular Complex

The cardiac RyR is a huge protein comprising 4996 amino acids, with a molecular mass of 565 kD for each of the four RyR monomers, totaling 2.2 MD for the entire tetramer. The tetramer forms a macromolecular complex with several associated proteins that frequently have a regulatory function. As of today, known associated proteins include protein kinase A (PKA), muscle A kinase–anchoring protein (mAKAP), protein phosphatases PP1 and PP2A, phosphodiesterase, calmodulin, calcium-calmodulin–dependent protein kinase II (CamK-II), calstabin2 (i.e., FKPB12.6), junctin, and triadin (recently reviewed by Bers[31]). Three mammalian isoforms are known: RyR1, RyR2, and RyR3. RyR1 is found mainly in skeletal muscle; RyR2 is the dominant isoform in cardiac muscle and also is found in smooth muscle; and RyR3 is expressed to a variable extent in brain and skeletal, cardiac, and smooth muscle but also in other tissues.[32] The complementary DNA (cDNA) of the cardiac RyR2 has been cloned and sequenced,[33] and various studies on the secondary and three-dimensional structure suggest the presence of 4 to 12 segments spanning the SR membrane and a huge cytosolic domain located in the dyadic cleft[34,35] (Fig. 6-1). This domain is thought to

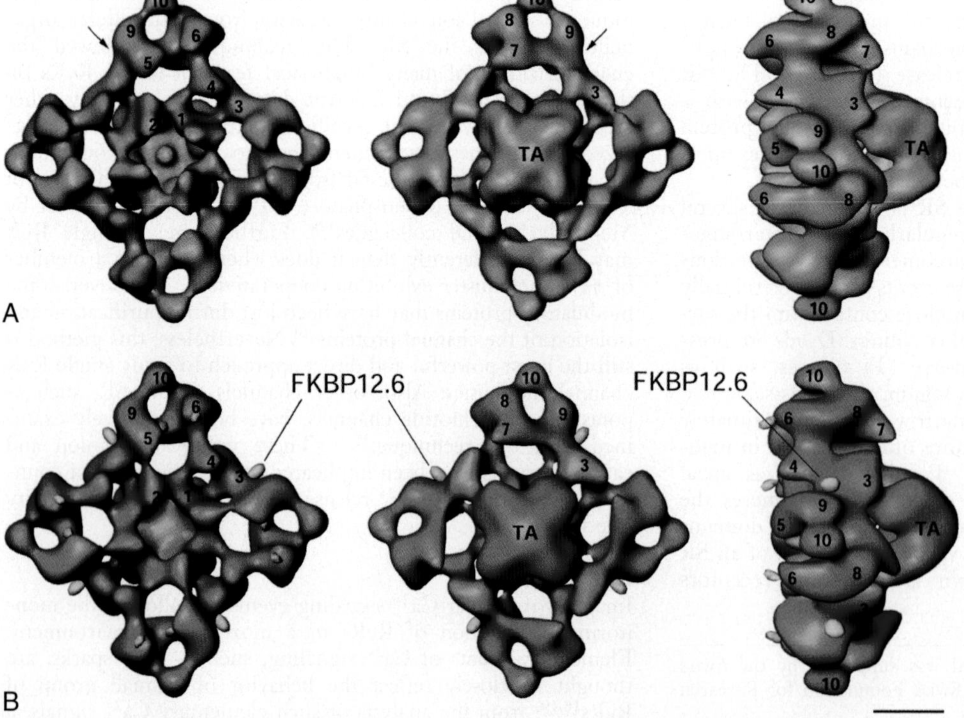

Figure 6-1 Three dimensional surface representations of RyR2 **(A)** without and **(B)** with calstabin2 (a.k.a. FKBP12.6) bound. *Left:* cytoplasmic view; *middle:* SR junctional face; *right:* side view. TA: transmembrane assembly. Numbers: established nomenclature of domains. Scale bar: 10 nm. (From Sharma MR, Jeyakumar LH, Fleischer S, Wagenknecht T: Three-dimensional visualization of FKBP12.6 binding to an open conformation of cardiac ryanodine receptor. Biophys J 90:164-172, 2006.)

correspond to the dense particles identified in electron micrographs (sometimes called *feet* because of their resemblance to the "feet" of a caterpillar as seen on cross section of a skeletal muscle T tubule).[36] Cryoelectron microscopy, combined with volume-rendering reconstruction techniques, has provided a three-dimensional view of the RyR2 protein, showing a large and square-shaped "foot" domain (29 × 29 × 12 nm) spanning the dyadic cleft and a smaller domain crossing the SR membrane (see Fig. 6-1).[37,38]

Activation and Gating of Ryanodine Receptor-2

In lipid bilayer experiments, cardiac RyRs are half-maximally activated at Ca^{2+} concentrations of approximately 1 to 10 μM, with a large variability depending on experimental conditions such as solution composition, luminal Ca^{2+} concentration, channel isolation, and reconstitution procedures.[9,11,14] Often in such studies, a monovalent current (e.g., K^+, Cs^+) through the RyR is recorded because of the large monovalent conductance of the RyR (approximately 750 picosiemens (pS) for high K^+ concentrations). The calcium current through a single RyR under near-physiologic conditions, however, was estimated to be very small, less than 0.6 pA (Fig. 6-2).[12,39] Furthermore, most bilayer studies were carried out at steady or only slowly changing Ca^{2+} concentrations. Of interest, when rapid Ca^{2+} concentration jumps were applied to RyRs incorporated in lipid bilayers with photolytic methods, it seemed that the instantaneous Ca^{2+} sensitivity of the RyRs was several-fold higher, and the open probability of the channel subsequently slowly decayed to a lower steady-state level by a mechanism termed *adaptation*[10,40] (but see the work of Lamb and Schiefer and their coworkers[41,42]).

In cardiac myocytes, RyRs are assembled in a paracrystalline lattice in each dyad, containing from 80 to 260 channels, depending on the species.[36,43] Each array of RyRs is faced by several DHPRs located in the T tubule plasmalemma. Calcium entering by way of one or more DHPRs is thought to activate opening of RyRs by the CICR mechanism to form a Ca^{2+} spark (Fig. 6-3).[3] Current data indicate that two Ca^{2+} ions are required to open an RyR.[44] Once activated, Ca^{2+} sparks are all-or-none events that are generated by a few RyR channels opening within the cluster.[45] Near-simultaneous activation of several RyRs is ensured by CICR spreading within the channel array or by coupled gating, mediated by allosteric interactions, presumably involving the small accessory protein calstabin2 (FKBP12.6).[13] Whether and why only a few channels out of this cluster become activated during each Ca^{2+} spark is at present a mystery and not understood. After approximately 10 ms, Ca^{2+} release from the SR terminates, and the Ca^{2+} spark signal starts to decay, mostly owing to diffusion of Ca^{2+} away from its source. Possible mechanisms governing termination of CICR and Ca^{2+} sparks are discussed later in the chapter.

Since the discovery of the Ca^{2+} sparks, several methods have been developed to characterize the signal transduction between the L-type Ca^{2+} current and the CICR and to examine its possible impairments during various cardiac diseases. Because excitation-contraction coupling by CICR is in essence a Ca^{2+} signal amplification system, these methods commonly are referred to as *excitation-contraction coupling gain measurements*. Although initially the "macroscopic" (or whole-cell) gain has been defined as the ratio of SR Ca^{2+} release to Ca^{2+} influx by way of the L-type calcium current, the notion of Ca^{2+} sparks and the underlying local control theory have led to a conceptually new understanding of excitation-contraction coupling gain in terms of "Ca^{2+} spark trigger probability" per single L-type calcium channel (i.e., the dihydropyridine receptor [DHPR]) opening.[46] This "microscopic" parameter is expected to depend much less on SR Ca^{2+} content than on the macroscopic gain, and should provide more direct information about the molecular events governing signal transduction across the dyadic cleft and its possible impairments in disease. It appears that in experiments in which only a very small number of DHPRs are allowed to open

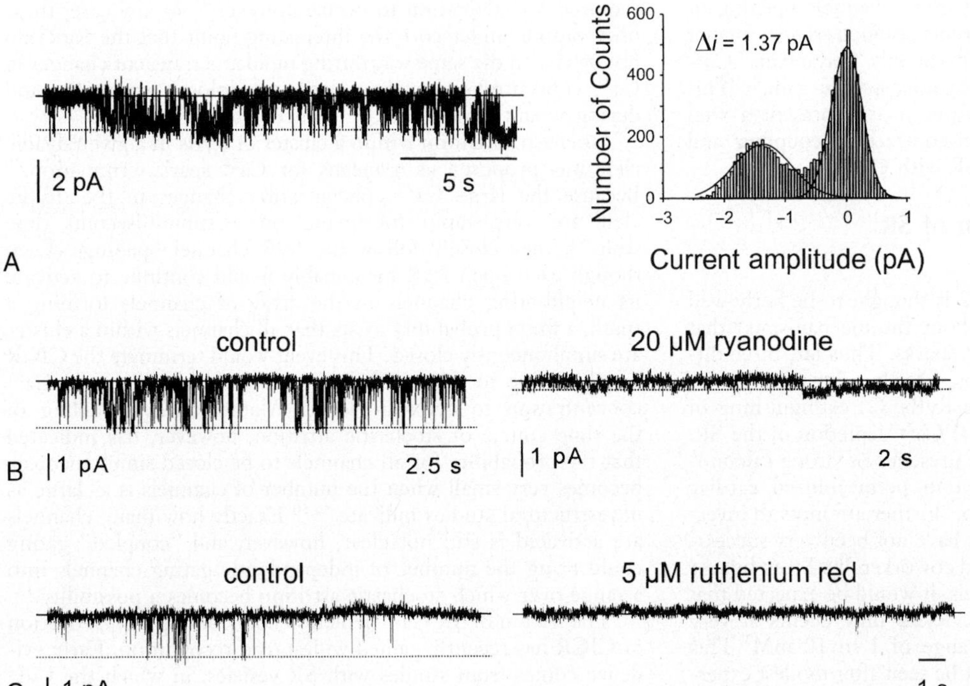

Figure 6-2 Unitary Ca^{2+} current via RyR2 with 2 mM Ca^{2+} as the current carrier. **A**, Representative current trace and amplitude histogram (*right*). **B** and **C**, Identification of the channel by ryanodine and ruthenium red, respectively. (From Mejia-Alvarez R, Kettlun C, Rios E, et al: Unitary Ca^{2+} current through cardiac ryanodine receptor channels under quasi-physiological ionic conditions. J Gen Physiol 113:177-186, 1999.)

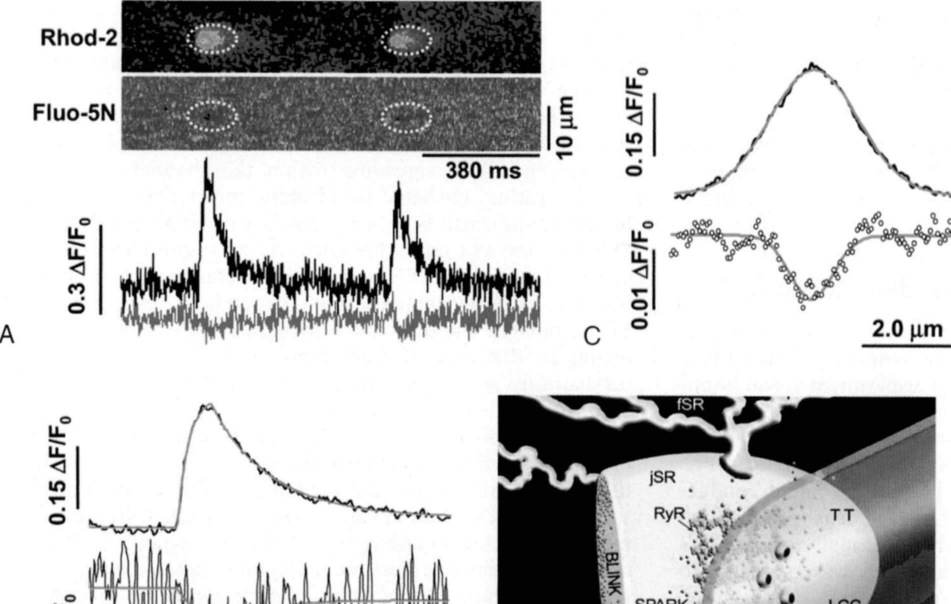

Figure 6-3 Complementary Ca^{2+} spark and Ca^{2+} blink signal pairs. **A,** Simultaneous recordings of Ca^{2+} sparks and Ca^{2+} blinks with rhod-2 and fluo-5-N. **B,** Average time-course of spark and blink. **C,** Average spatial profile of spark and blink. **D,** Overview of the structures involved (T-tubule [TT], L-type Ca^{2+} channel [LCC] and SR). (From Brochet DX, Yang D, Di Maio A, et al: Ca^{2+} blinks: Rapid nanoscopic store calcium signaling. Proc Natl Acad Sci U S A 102:3099-3104, 2005. Copyright 2005, National Academy of Sciences, U S A.)

(e.g., on average, less than one channel per dyad, in the presence of a calcium channel antagonist), the Ca^{2+} spark trigger probability depends largely on the amplitude of the calcium current through each single DHPR and on the RyR sensitivity.[46] Of note, however, when several DHPRs belonging to a given dyad open (as is the case under physiologic conditions), the Ca^{2+} spark trigger probability may already be very high (i.e., approaching 1). Under these conditions, larger L-type calcium currents (either as a result of more channels opening or owing to larger single-channel currents) cannot trigger further SR Ca^{2+} release and therefore contribute only "redundant" Ca^{2+} influx, which, by definition, reduces microscopic gain.[25] This "redundant" calcium current, however, may represent a vital safety feature of cardiac excitation-contraction coupling and may be important for loading the SR with Ca^{2+}.

Inactivation and Termination of SR Calcium Release

Although the activation of the RyR2 is thought to be fairly well understood, much less is known about the mechanism(s) that terminate SR Ca^{2+} release and Ca^{2+} sparks. Thus far, three different mechanisms have been proposed to shut down CICR: (1) calcium-induced inactivation of the RyRs, (2) extinguishing of CICR by stochastic attrition, and (3) Ca^{2+} depletion of the SR. Although initial data suggesting the presence of strong calcium-induced inactivation were obtained in permeabilized cardiac muscle preparations a long time ago,[3] further attempts to investigate this mechanism in intact cells have not been very successful[47] (but see the report by Sham and coworkers[48]). From bilayer experiments of reconstituted channels, it would be expected that calcium-induced inactivation of the RyR2 only occurs at very high Ca^{2+} concentrations, in the range of 1 to 10 mM. This may explain why inactivation cannot be seen after modest experimental elevations of the cytosolic Ca^{2+} level. Very high Ca^{2+} concentrations, however, are in fact expected to occur within the limited space of the dyadic cleft during influx and release of Ca^{2+}.[49] A process similar to inactivation is adaptation of the RyRs, a time-dependent reduction of the single-channel-open probability after activation. Adaptation has been observed after flash photolytic liberation of Ca^{2+} from caged compounds[40] and may be related to previous observations of calcium-induced inactivation. Extremely high Ca^{2+} concentration jumps seem to be required for adaptation to occur, however.[41] In any case, these observations underscore the interesting point that the RyRs do not behave in the same way during rapid and transient changes in Ca^{2+} concentration, such as with physiologic activation, and during steady changes in Ca^{2+} concentration.

Stochastic attrition within a cluster of RyRs in a given dyadic cleft was proposed as a means for Ca^{2+} spark termination.[50] Because the large Ca^{2+} concentration changes in the dyadic cleft are very rapid (occurring on a submillisecond time scale[49]), they closely follow the RyR channel openings. Even though each open RyR presumably would continue to activate its neighboring channels in the array of channels forming a spark, a finite probability exists that all channels within a cluster are simultaneously closed. This event would terminate the CICR locally owing to the rapid drop of the very high dyadic Ca^{2+} concentration to cytosolic levels. Mathematical modeling of the time course of stochastic attrition, however, has indicated that the probability for all channels to be closed simultaneously becomes very small when the number of channels is as large as ultrastructural studies indicate.[36,50] Exactly how many channels are activated is still not clear, however, and "coupled" gating could bring the number of independently gating channels into a range over which stochastic attrition becomes a possibility.[13]

The notion of SR Ca^{2+} depletion contributing to inactivation of CICR has recently gained widespread recognition. Early evidence comes from studies with SR vesicles, in which the Ca^{2+} release was seen to exhibit kinetic variation as a function of vesicular calsequestrin content.[4] On the basis of this observation, it has been proposed that calcium-induced conformational changes of calsequestrin initiate a backwards signal affecting the RyRs. On the cellular level, an early observation consistent with this idea was that global Ca^{2+} transients required much longer to recover from refractoriness than local signals, such as Ca^{2+} sparks,[51,52] presumably because the SR has to reload its Ca^{2+} by means of SERCA after a global release, whereas a single dyad can refill Ca^{2+} much faster by intra-SR Ca^{2+} diffusion. Indeed, modifying the SERCA pharmacologically or by ablating the SERCA-inhibitory protein phospholamban provided supporting evidence for this notion.[53]

More recently, further support for the importance of such a retrograde signaling pathway has been obtained by transiently overexpressing calsequestrin (or inhibiting its expression) in cultured cardiomyocytes. Large amounts of calsequestrin delayed Ca^{2+} spark termination, whereas low calsequestrin levels led to premature Ca^{2+} spark termination, again consistent with the idea of RyR deactivation as a consequence of SR Ca^{2+} depletion.[54] In lipid bilayer studies, the luminal Ca^{2+} sensitivity found in native RyRs could be "rescued" for purified RyRs when calsequestrin, together with junctin and triadin, was added to the side corresponding to the SR lumen.[14] Thus, the pathway signaling SR depletion seems to involve calsequestrin as the "sensor" and junctin as well as triadin as intermediate and allosterically coupled proteins enabling this "retrograde" signal. At present, it is thought that CICR terminates before the SR is completely empty and that approximately 50% of the total Ca^{2+} remain inside the store.[27,55] The extent of Ca^{2+} remaining in the SR and of the corresponding fractional Ca^{2+} release, however, probably depends on several factors and may be altered in a variety of cardiac conditions and diseases.[29,30,56] With the recent availability of intra-SR Ca^{2+} measurements, these features will certainly be investigated in detail in the near future.

Regulation of the Channel

Phosphorylation

Many cellular proteins are regulated by means of phosphorylation by various protein kinases. On the RyR2, several potential phosphorylation sites for PKA and CaMK-II have been identified.[57-60] Regulation of the cardiac SR Ca^{2+} release mechanism in health and disease through phosphorylation of key proteins is at present the focus of intensive investigation in several laboratories. It is particularly important, because maladaptive changes in the RyR Ca^{2+} sensitivity may be an important element in the pathophysiology of a number of diseases, such as hypertrophy and congestive heart failure—conditions that are expected to reach almost endemic proportions in today's aging population. Although several older studies reported modifications of RyR gating after phosphorylation,[9,10] more specific hypotheses regarding the consequences of such changes have been advanced more recently.[57] In one proposed scenario, PKA-dependent phosphorylation of the RyR at Ser2808 (or Ser2809, depending on the species) during β-adrenergic stimulation was proposed to lead to dissociation of the calstabin2 proteins from the RyRs, making their closed state less stable and the channels more Ca^{2+}-sensitive. Although it may seem beneficial to increase the RyR open probability and efficiency of Ca^{2+} signaling in cases of emergencies ("fight-or-flight" reaction), a prolonged or excessive stimulation may finally lead to "hyperphosphorylation" of the RyR, partly also owing to reduced availability of phosphodiesterase and phosphatase,[61] making the release channels overly Ca^{2+}-sensitive. Hyperphosphorylated channels could spontaneously open and represent a pathway for Ca^{2+} to leak out from the SR (partly visible as Ca^{2+} sparks). In the long run, such an extra leak would result in SR Ca^{2+} depletion, followed by a reduction of the calcium transient amplitudes, a change that would clearly be maladaptive. With hyperphosphorylation of the RyRs, however, comes the elevated risk to trigger arrhythmias, particularly in combination with other conditions that lead to enhanced Ca^{2+} sensitivity of the RyRs, such as RyR mutations (see later on). Even though a substantial body of evidence supports this scenario, also backed by observations made in transgenic animals with deleted or constitutively phosphorylated Ser2808 sites,[58] certain aspects of its entire framework are still highly controversial. Several research laboratories have not been able to reproduce specific aspects of the experimental findings or have made diverging observations. This includes reports of PKA-dependent phosphorylation at sites different from Ser2008,[59] phosphorylation by kinases other than PKA (e.g., CamK-II, protein kinase G) or the absence of subsequent functional consequences, such as calstabin2 dissociation, change of RyR-open probability, or Ca^{2+} spark frequency.[62-64] Other studies found similar functional adjustments of excitation-contraction coupling but associated them with CamK-II–dependent phosphorylation of the RyRs.[60] At present, it is not clear why these discrepancies exist among different studies. Most likely, valuable and important information may be obtained about the system by sorting out the details underlying these discrepancies. As is so often the case, the divergent findings may be related to the specifics of the methods used or the reagents and tools used but may also arise from the underestimated complexity of the involved regulatory mechanisms. The functional studies may have similar difficulties and depend on particular experimental conditions and methods but also on the animal species and the particular disease model used. Because some of the expected modifications of Ca^{2+} signaling occurring after β-adrenergic stimulation or during the development of cardiac pathology may have a biphasic or multiphasic time course, the precise timing of the experiments is most likely of particular importance as well. Related to that, the behavior of the RyRs under steady-state conditions is known to be different than during more physiologic experimental protocols mimicking the cyclic activity of the beating heart. For example, the initial and steady-state RyR open probability changed in opposite ways after PKA-dependent phosphorylation, with a higher open probability (P_o) immediately after activation, but a lower P_o in the steady state.[10] Furthermore, basic features of the measured functional parameter may be able to mask the consequences of RyR phosphorylation. We found that global (whole-cell) calcium transients are, to a large extent, governed by the SR Ca^{2+} content, whereas changes of RyR gating could be more readily detected in local Ca^{2+} signals, such as Ca^{2+} sparks and two-photon photolytically induced Ca^{2+} release signals.[65] This study found enhanced SR Ca^{2+} release after β-adrenergic stimulation, despite the fact that total SR Ca^{2+} load and global Ca^{2+} release were reduced under these conditions, probably as a result of enhanced SR Ca^{2+} leak. These findings imply a change of RyR gating due to PKA-dependent phosphorylation of the channel itself, or of a closely associated protein.[66]

SR Ca^{2+} Content

The fraction of the SR Ca^{2+} content that usually is released with each heartbeat seems to strongly depend on the SR Ca^{2+} load.[67] It also is known that whenever the SR Ca^{2+} load becomes very high, spontaneous Ca^{2+} release events, such as frequent Ca^{2+} sparks and Ca^{2+} waves, occur that are thought to play an important proarrhythmogenic role under pathologic conditions (see below). As already mentioned, the open probability of the RyRs also was found to depend on the luminal Ca^{2+} concentration in bilayer studies, particularly in the presence of calsequestrin, junctin, and triadin.[14] Thus, the mechanism increasing the sensitivity of the RyRs at abnormally high SR Ca^{2+} loads may be intimately related (or even identical) to the one governing Ca^{2+} release termination due to store emptying and RyR deactivation, as discussed earlier. Thus, elevated SR Ca^{2+} load may "sensitize" the RyRs above normal, such that they become activated even by the resting cytosolic Ca^{2+} concentration. We found indirect evidence for the importance of such an intra-SR sensitization mechanism in experiments in which the SERCA of Ca^{2+}-overloaded cardiomyocytes was rapidly blocked by photorelease of an inhibitor from a caged precursor.[68] Blocking the SERCA immediately slowed down the speed of Ca^{2+} waves, suggesting that SR Ca^{2+} uptake has a facilitating effect on Ca^{2+} wave propagation, possibly by way of RyR sensitization on SR Ca^{2+} loading. Similarly, slowing down the SERCA pharmacologically delayed recovery of CICR from refractoriness, whereas in transgenic animals lacking phospholamban, the associated unrestrained SERCA activity greatly accelerated recovery.[53]

Several small proteins have been identified in preparations of SR membrane and are associated with the RyRs. Some have identified modulatory roles, whereas the precise function of others is more elusive. Some features of the small proteins triadin, junctin, calstabin2, and other proteins of the macromolecular RyR complex are discussed earlier, in the paragraphs dealing with phosphorylation of the RyR and with CICR termination. Other proteins localizing into the dyadic regions include sorcin, a 21.6-kD calcium-binding protein that binds to the RyR with high affinity and completely inhibits channel activity.[69] The high concentration of Ca^{2+} prevailing in the dyadic cleft promotes translocation of sorcin from a soluble to a membranous compartment, and this protein may therefore play a role in calcium-induced inactivation of the RyRs. Calmodulin and S100A1, two other calcium-binding proteins, also were found to inhibit RyR activity and may therefore play a role in calcium-mediated CICR termination.[11,70] In addition, some loops of the sarcolemmal DHPRs and the protein Homer may interact with the RyR2, and several reports have suggested a communication between DHPRs and RyRs by means other than through Ca^{2+} influx.[71-73] Similarly, imperatoxin A and parts of the DHPR α_1 subunit II-III loop, which appear to have structural similarities, affect RyR2 gating.[74,75]

Modulation of Ryanodine Receptor Activity

Experimentally and pharmacologically, the RyRs are modulated by a large range of extra- and intracellular constituents, and detailed recent excellent reviews cover most aspects of this function.[76,77] The boundary between RyR modulation and regulation is not always very well defined. Several of the known modulatory constituents, however, do not normally change in a regulated way or to a large extent inside a healthy cardiomyocyte (e.g., Mg^{2+}, pH, ATP, redox potential) but may do so under pathologic conditions, such as prolonged ischemia. Lipid bilayer and [^{3}H]-ryanodine binding studies indicate that free Mg^{2+} and protons tend to inhibit the cardiac RyR, whereas ATP promotes its activity. This ATP effect occurs by way of an adenine-binding site on the RyRs and is not due to phosphorylation of the protein, because it also is seen with other adenosine nucleotides, including nonhydrolyzable ATP analogues.[78] The fall in pH and ATP, together with the concomitant rise in free Mg^{2+}, would be expected to seriously limit CICR during periods of ischemia. This effect may actually be beneficial and protective, because it would reduce the energy consumption of the affected cells. Analogous studies with these modulators are thus far rather limited on the level of intact cells and Ca^{2+} sparks. In one study with permeabilized cardiac myocytes, ATP removal appeared to decrease the frequency of Ca^{2+} sparks independently of changes in the SR Ca^{2+} load, which would be consistent with the known ATP effects mediated by the adenine nucleotide–binding site on the RyRs.[79]

The RyRs contain a large number of free sulfhydryl groups that normally are in a reduced state because of the low redox potential of the cardiac cytosol. Therefore, the RyRs are potentially easy targets for oxidation by reactive oxygen species (ROS) or for *S*-nitrosylation.[80,81] ROS typically are generated during various forms of cellular stress, most notably during ischemia and reperfusion, but also during congestive heart failure.[82,83] Redox modifications of the cardiac RyRs are known to increase its Ca^{2+} sensitivity dramatically,[8,84] possibly by interfering with interdomain interactions, such as molecular zipping and unzipping within the RyR protein, that are important for gating of the channel. In this model, zipped domains are thought to stabilize the closed state of the channel. Related to this hypothesis, it has recently been noted that this type of defective gating is prominently present during congestive heart failure and can be normalized with antioxidant therapy.[85]

Furthermore, the second messengers originally studied in sea urchin eggs, cyclic ADP (cADP) ribose, and nicotinic acid adenine dinucleotide phosphate (NAADP) have been suggested to play a role as activating modulators for RyR2 and Ca^{2+} sparks.[86,87]

Pathology of the Ryanodine Receptor

SR Ca^{2+} Overload

It has been known for a long time that SR Ca^{2+} overload can generate arrhythmias, which manifest themselves as early afterdepolarizations on the cellular level.[88] In voltage clamp experiments, spontaneous Ca^{2+} release from the overloaded SR and Ca^{2+} waves were then found to elicit calcium-activated currents (so-called transient inward currents, I_{ti}).[89,90] A variety of channels and transporters located on the sarcolemma seem to underlie these currents, depending on the species, but also on the type of cells (i.e., Purkinje versus working cardiomyocytes). Identified possible charge carriers include calcium-activated chloride channels,[91] unspecific cation channels,[92,93] and, most notably, the electrogenic Na^+-Ca^{2+} exchanger (I_{NCX}).[94-96] Although the precise mechanism eliciting "spontaneous" SR Ca^{2+} release and Ca^{2+} waves is not yet known, some evidence suggests that it may be related to the regulation of the Ca^{2+} sensitivity of the RyR by intra-SR Ca^{2+}, the same mechanism that normally contributes to CICR termination by RyR deactivation (see earlier). Thus, SR Ca^{2+} overload may shift the termination mechanism in the opposite direction, making the RyRs excessively sensitive for Ca^{2+} such that the resting cytosolic Ca^{2+} concentration (or only a slightly elevated concentration) is sufficient to open the Ca^{2+} release channels.[68] As with SR Ca^{2+} overloading, other pathologic stimuli also may induce an abnormal propensity to arrhythmias through RyR sensitization and SR Ca^{2+} release, such as RyR hyperphosphorylation, redox modifications of the release channels, or mutations of the RyR2 (Fig. 6-4). These mechanisms are discussed elsewhere in this chapter.

Ryanodine Receptor Mutations

Mutations of the skeletal muscle RyR1 have been known to be linked to malignant hyperthermia for quite some time. Only recently, however, were corresponding mutations discovered in analogous regions of the RyR2 protein.[97-99] These mutations give rise to abnormal Ca^{2+} sensitivity of the RyRs, particularly when the SR becomes overloaded; this results in a high prevalence of arrhythmias during β-adrenergic stimulation.[100] These arrhythmias usually are manifested as exercise-induced catecholaminergic polymorphic ventricular tachycardias (CPVTs), which may cause sudden cardiac death. For patients so affected, but probably for those with many other conditions characterized

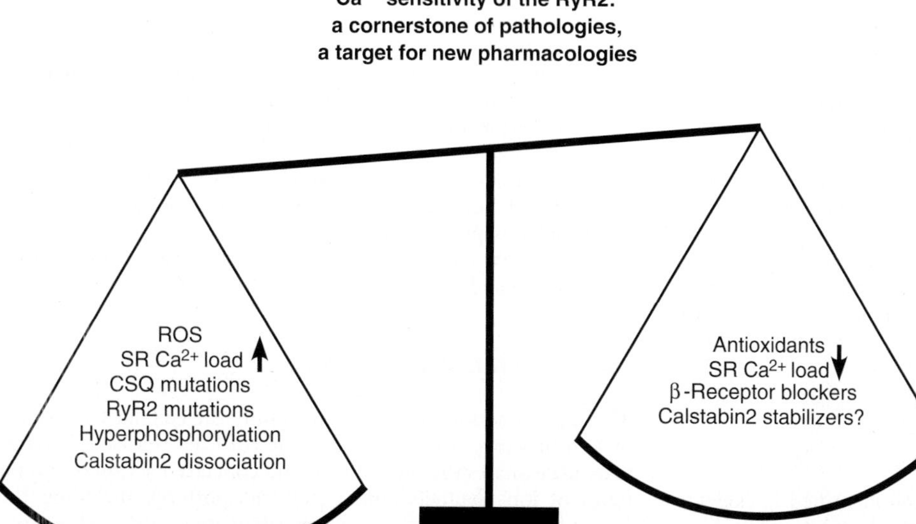

Figure 6-4 Summary of the balance between RyR2 destabilizing pathologies and RyR2 stabilizing options. Many pathologies converge into a common final end point, a sensitization of the RyRs for cytosolic Ca^{2+} leading to hyperexcitability, SR Ca^{2+} leak, and arrhythmogenesis.

by abnormally high Ca^{2+} sensitivity of the RyRs, drugs that can stabilize the channels may potentially be very beneficial, opening a new avenue for treatment (as discussed in the next section), in addition to the β-blockers, which can attenuate the adrenergic input.

Pharmacology and Toxicology of the Ryanodine Receptor

The cardiac RyRs are direct targets for a variety of pharmacologic compounds and toxins (reviewed in detail by Sutko and associates[101]). All of these drugs are used as experimental pharmacologic tools; thus far, no compounds in clinical use are known to directly target the RyR2. Most notably, the plant alkaloid ryanodine has helped with the functional characterization but also the isolation and sequencing of the channel. Each RyR has both a very-high-affinity (dissociation constant [K_D] of approximately 1 to 10 nM) and a low-affinity (K_D of approximately 1 to 10 μM) binding site for ryanodine.[101] Binding of ryanodine to the RyR is use-dependent, suggesting that the sites are accessible only when the channels are open. At the high-affinity site, ryanodine induces long-lasting channel openings at a subconductance state, whereas high concentrations block the channel. For experimental purposes, the ryanodine effect is essentially irreversible.

Caffeine, in high concentrations (5 to 20 mM), leads to immediate opening of all RyRs by making them very sensitive to Ca^{2+} and often is used experimentally to estimate SR Ca^{2+} content. At micromolar concentrations, caffeine increases the Ca^{2+} sensitivity of the RyRs; this property can be used experimentally to mimic some features of the modified Ca^{2+} signaling during heart failure.[102] Tetracaine inhibits the RyRs, but its block can be overcome by elevated SR luminal Ca^{2+} concentrations. It has been used experimentally to reduce and quantify the spontaneous SR Ca^{2+} leak (by way of RyRs).[103] Ruthenium red, another inhibitor of the RyR2, was found to prolong the time the channel spends in the closed state. At micromolar concentrations, it reduces the Ca^{2+} spark frequency.[104]

Several toxins, such as the scorpion toxins imperatoxin A and imperatoxin I, seem to affect the gating of RyR2.[75] Some anticancer drugs (e.g., doxorubicin) with cardiac side effects are suspected to cause redox modification of the RyRs and other proteins, which seriously limits their therapeutic use.[105] The immunosuppressants FK506 and rapamycin are known to have cardiotoxic effects that are thought to arise partly from their ability to interfere with the stability of calstabin2 binding to the RyRs.[13]

On the positive side, it has recently been reported that the benzothiazepine derivative JTV-519 (K201) can stabilize calstabin2 on the RyR2 protein and slow down or prevent its dissociation.[106] Because a multitude of pathologic conditions appear to affect the RyR2 by converging to a common end point, the alteration of its gating behavior with a destabilization of its closed state, this or similarly acting compounds may represent a new class of therapeutic tools targeting the RyR for treating a variety of pathologic conditions that lead to arrhythmogenic RyR hypersensitivity,[107] including mutations of the RyR2, hyperphosphorylation of the RyR2 during congestive heart failure, SR Ca^{2+} overload, redox modifications of the RyRs, and others.

Monovalent Cation Channels

In SR vesicles, a substantial monovalent ion conductance has been determined by various techniques, and extensive redistributions of K^+ (but not Na^+ and Cl^-) during SR Ca^{2+} release were noted with electron microprobe analysis.[26] It has been evident for a long time that Ca^{2+} release from the SR cannot possibly be entirely electrogenic, because the electrical potential of the SR membrane would rapidly reach the equilibrium for Ca^{2+}, which would preclude further SR Ca^{2+} release.[108] Thus, the need for countercharge movement mediated by ions other than Ca^{2+} is obvious, to maintain electroneutrality or at least limit the changes of the SR membrane potential. Although several types of K^+ and Cl^- channels have been discovered in SR vesicles and examined in lipid bilayer reconstitution experiments, their structure and identity remain elusive (see the section on the recently identified trimeric intracellular cation channel [TRIC] later in the chapter).

The SR membrane contains a large-conductance potassium channel that is blocked by Cs^+ and by decamethonium, gallamine, and neomycin, but also by millimolar concentrations of Ca^{2+}.[16,109-112] Depending on the SR Ca^{2+} content, relief from Ca^{2+} block may be a physiologically relevant mechanism facilitating countercharge movement by way of these channels. Some studies described block of the SR potassium channel by 4-aminopyridine (4-AP),[113] whereas others reported the absence of 4-AP sensitivity in an SR potassium channel isolated from atrial cardiac tissue.[114] At present, it is not clear whether these are in fact two different types of channels.

Chloride Channels

Two types of chloride channels have been identified in skeletal muscle SR with lipid bilayer experiments, based on their biophysical properties: a large-conductance (250 pS) channel and a small-conductance (70 pS) channel.[15] In another study, a cardiac chloride channel also has been reported to conduct larger anions, such as phosphate and even ATP.[115] As mentioned earlier, the Cl^- concentration inside the SR does not change appreciably during Ca^{2+} release, at least in skeletal muscle.[26] Therefore, the physiologic role of these channels is not well defined at present.

The Trimeric Intracellular Cation Channel

Several small proteins located inside the SR or closely associated with the RyR macromolecular complex were discovered, purified, and characterized with biochemical techniques in the past. In many instances, the function of these proteins initially was unknown. The role of one of these proteins, previously termed mitsugumin 33, has recently been resolved. This 33-kD protein has three proposed transmembrane segments and forms a trimeric intracellular cation channel (TRIC) that is located in the SR and endoplasmic reticulum membranes.[17] The two subtypes TRIC-A and TRIC-B are expressed mainly in excitable tissues, including the SR of cardiac and skeletal muscle, and in the brain (TRIC-A) or the endoplasmic reticulum of many different tissues (TRIC-B). In bilayer experiments, TRIC-A was found to be only moderately selective for K^+ over Na^+ (permeability ratio, 1.5) with a K^+ conductance of approximately 110 pS in 200 mM K^+. TRIC-A is neither blocked by nor permeable to Ca^{2+} and Mg^{2+} and is not inhibited by decamethonium. Thus, in terms of permeability and pharmacology, the TRICs are clearly distinct from the well-known potassium channel of the SR. Initial functional studies also were carried out in transgenic animals lacking either TRIC-A or TRIC-B, or both channels. TRIC-A–knockout mice were viable and fertile, whereas TRIC-B knockout was associated with neonatal lethality. Embryos of the double-knockout mice died at embryonic day 10. Their cardiomyocytes showed swollen SR structures and abnormally small Ca^{2+}-oscillation amplitudes. In addition, recordings of Ca^{2+} signals suggested impaired CICR in skeletal muscle fibers of TRIC-A–knockout mice, in which the Ca^{2+} spark amplitude was reduced but the duration of Ca^{2+} release (i.e., the spark rise time) was prolonged. Taken together, these findings seem to indicate that countercharge movement by way of TRIC plays a permissive and very important role for SR Ca^{2+} release.

Conclusion and Outlook

The main function of the SR, to amplify the cellular Ca^{2+} signal by continuously going through cycles of Ca^{2+} release and reuptake, necessitates the finely tuned and concerted action of several types of ion channels (and other transporters), including the RyRs, but also channels for monovalent ions. Although a large body of knowledge about many aspects of the basic function of the RyRs has been accumulated, the role of the other channels is still rather mysterious. This extensive knowledge of many basic functions of the RyR channels also contrasts sharply with the still limited knowledge regarding their regulation, adaptation, and maladaptation in cardiac disease. Furthermore, it would appear that several SR ion channels offer themselves as potentially important therapeutic targets but may also mediate cardiotoxicity of several drugs. Unfortunately, at present, pharmacologic options targeting SR channels directly are almost nonexistent.

More specifically, what are the important and burning questions regarding SR channel function that need to be answered in the future? First of all, both the activation and the inactivation of the RyRs in situ are still not completely understood. It would be important to know why only few RyRs from within an apparently cooperatively well-coupled cluster of channels open. Because some arrhythmias are thought to be triggered by undue spontaneous SR Ca^{2+} release, it is essential to establish which mechanisms govern CICR termination and what the kinetics are for both shutdown of Ca^{2+} release and recovery from refractoriness. Also needed is a clearer picture of the vast array of molecular interactions and regulatory changes within the RyR macromolecular complex to elucidate the almost certainly critical alterations of excitation-contraction coupling and Ca^{2+} signaling in cardiac disease. Regarding the function and regulation of the other SR membrane channels and the question of membrane potential changes across the SR membrane, current knowledge is very limited, but these channels may be important regulators of CICR as well. Overall, much progress has been made during the last few decades, but many burning questions regarding the basic function, regulation, and pharmacology of SR ion channels remain unanswered.

References

1. Bers DM: Cardiac excitation-contraction coupling. Nature 415:198-205, 2002.
2. Endo M, Tanaka M, Ogawa Y: Calcium induced release of calcium from the sarcoplasmic reticulum of skinned skeletal muscle fibres. Nature 228:34-36, 1970.
3. Fabiato A: Time and calcium dependence of activation and inactivation of calcium-induced release of calcium from the sarcoplasmic reticulum of a skinned canine cardiac Purkinje cell. J Gen Physiol 85:247-289, 1985.
4. Ikemoto N, Ronjat M, Meszaros LG, Koshita M: Postulated role of calsequestrin in the regulation of calcium release from sarcoplasmic reticulum. Biochemistry 28:6764-6771, 1989.
5. Wu X, Bers DM: Sarcoplasmic reticulum and nuclear envelope are one highly interconnected Ca^{2+} store throughout cardiac myocyte. Circ Res 99:283-291, 2006.
6. Mazzanti M, DeFelice LJ, Cohn J, Malter H: Ion channels in the nuclear envelope. Nature 343:764-767, 1990.
7. Stein P, Palade P: Sarcoballs: Direct access to sarcoplasmic reticulum Ca^{2+}-channels in skinned frog muscle fibers. Biophys J 54:357-363, 1988.
8. Sanchez G, Hidalgo C, Donoso P: Kinetic studies of calcium-induced calcium release in cardiac sarcoplasmic reticulum vesicles. Biophys J 84:2319-2330, 2003.
9. Hain J, Onoue H, Mayrleitner M, et al: Phosphorylation modulates the function of the calcium release channel of sarcoplasmic

reticulum from cardiac muscle. J Biol Chem 270:2074-2081, 1995.
10. Valdivia HH, Kaplan JH, Ellis-Davies GC, Lederer WJ: Rapid adaptation of cardiac ryanodine receptors: Modulation by Mg^{2+} and phosphorylation. Science 267: 1997-2000, 1995.
11. Xu L, Meissner G: Mechanism of calmodulin inhibition of cardiac sarcoplasmic reticulum Ca^{2+} release channel (ryanodine receptor). Biophys J 86:797-804, 2004.
12. Mejia-Alvarez R, Kettlun C, Rios E, et al: Unitary Ca^{2+} current through cardiac ryanodine receptor channels under quasi-physiological ionic conditions. J Gen Physiol 113:177-186, 1999.
13. Marx SO, Gaburjakova J, Gaburjakova M, et al: Coupled gating between cardiac calcium release channels (ryanodine receptors). Circ Res 88:1151-1158, 2001.
14. Gyorke I, Hester N, Jones LR, Gyorke S: The role of calsequestrin, triadin, and junctin in conferring cardiac ryanodine receptor responsiveness to luminal calcium. Biophys J 86:2121-2128, 2004.
15. Kourie JI, Laver DR, Junankar PR, et al: Characteristics of two types of chloride channel in sarcoplasmic reticulum vesicles from rabbit skeletal muscle. Biophys J 70:202-221, 1996.
16. Coronado R, Miller C: Decamethonium and hexamethonium block K+ channels of sarcoplasmic reticulum. Nature 288:495-497, 1980.
17. Yazawa M, Ferrante C, Feng J, et al: TRIC channels are essential for Ca^{2+} handling in intracellular stores. Nature 448:78-82, 2007.
18. Cheng H, Lederer WJ, Cannell MB: Calcium sparks—elementary events underlying excitation-contraction coupling in heart-muscle. Science 262:740-744, 1993.
19. Niggli E: Localized intracellular calcium signaling in muscle: Calcium sparks and calcium quarks. Annu Rev Physiol 61:311-335, 1999.
20. Niggli E, Shirokova N: A guide to sparkology: The taxonomy of elementary cellular Ca^{2+} signaling events. Cell Calcium 42:379-387, 2007.
21. Blatter LA, Huser J, Rios E: Sarcoplasmic reticulum Ca^{2+} release flux underlying Ca^{2+} sparks in cardiac muscle. Proc Natl Acad Sci U S A 94:4176-4181, 1997.
22. Soeller C, Cannell MB: Estimation of the sarcoplasmic reticulum Ca^{2+} release flux underlying Ca^{2+} sparks. Biophys J 82:2396-2414, 2002.
23. Struk A, Szucs G, Kemmer H, Melzer W: Fura-2 calcium signals in skeletal muscle fibres loaded with high concentrations of EGTA. Cell Calcium 23:23-32, 1998.
24. Song LS, Sham JS, Stern MD, et al: Direct measurement of SR release flux by tracking 'Ca^{2+} spikes' in rat cardiac myocytes. J Physiol 512:677-691, 1998.
25. Altamirano J, Bers DM: Voltage dependence of cardiac excitation-contraction coupling: Unitary Ca^{2+} current amplitude and open channel probability. Circ Res 101:590-597, 2007.
26. Somlyo AV, Gonzalez-Serratos HG, Shuman H, et al: Calcium release and ionic changes in the sarcoplasmic reticulum of tetanized muscle: An electron-probe study. J Cell Biol 90:577-594, 1981.
27. Shannon TR, Guo T, Bers DM: Ca^{2+} scraps: Local depletions of free $[Ca^{2+}]$ in cardiac sarcoplasmic reticulum during contractions leave substantial Ca^{2+} reserve. Circ Res 93:40-45, 2003.
28. Brochet DX, Yang D, Di Maio A, et al: Ca^{2+} blinks: Rapid nanoscopic store calcium signaling. Proc Natl Acad Sci U S A 102:3099-3104, 2005.
29. Kubalova Z, Terentyev D, Viatchenko-Karpinski S, et al: Abnormal intrastore calcium signaling in chronic heart failure. Proc Natl Acad Sci U S A 102: 14104-14109, 2005.
30. Guo T, Ai X, Shannon TR, et al: Intra-sarcoplasmic reticulum free $[Ca^{2+}]$ and buffering in arrhythmogenic failing rabbit heart. Circ Res 101:802-810, 2007.
31. Bers DM: Macromolecular complexes regulating cardiac ryanodine receptor function. J Mol Cell Cardiol 37:417-429, 2004.
32. Ledbetter MW, Preiner JK, Louis CF, Mickelson JR: Tissue distribution of ryanodine receptor isoforms and alleles determined by reverse transcription polymerase chain reaction. J Biol Chem 269: 31544-31551, 1994.
33. Otsu K, Willard HF, Khanna VK, et al: Molecular cloning of cDNA encoding the Ca^{2+} release channel (ryanodine receptor) of rabbit cardiac muscle sarcoplasmic reticulum. J Biol Chem 265:13472-13483, 1990.
34. Tunwell RE, Wickenden C, Bertrand BM, et al: The human cardiac muscle ryanodine receptor-calcium release channel: Identification, primary structure and topological analysis. Biochem J 318:477-487, 1996.
35. Dulhunty AF, Pouliquin P: What we don't know about the structure of ryanodine receptor calcium release channels. Clin Exp Pharmacol Physiol 30:713-723, 2003.
36. Franzini-Armstrong C, Protasi F, Ramesh V: Shape, size, and distribution of Ca^{2+} release units and couplons in skeletal and cardiac muscles. Biophys J 77:1528-1539, 1999.
37. Serysheva II, Hamilton SL, Chiu W, Ludtke SJ: Structure of Ca^{2+} release channel at 14 Å resolution. J Mol Biol 345: 427-431, 2005.
38. Sharma MR, Jeyakumar LH, Fleischer S, Wagenknecht T: Three-dimensional visualization of FKBP12.6 binding to an open conformation of cardiac ryanodine receptor. Biophys J 90:164-172, 2006.
39. Tinker A, Lindsay AR, Williams AJ: Cation conduction in the calcium release channel of the cardiac sarcoplasmic reticulum under physiological and pathophysiological conditions. Cardiovasc Res 27:1820-1825, 1993.
40. Gyorke S, Fill M: Ryanodine receptor adaptation: Control mechanism of Ca^{2+}-induced Ca^{2+} release in heart. Science 260:807-809, 1993.
41. Lamb GD, Laver DR, Stephenson DG: Questions about adaptation in ryanodine receptors. J Gen Physiol 116:883-890, 2000.
42. Schiefer A, Meissner G, Isenberg G: Ca^{2+} activation and Ca^{2+} inactivation of canine reconstituted cardiac sarcoplasmic reticulum Ca^{2+}-release channels. J Physiol 489:337-348, 1995.
43. Soeller C, Crossman D, Gilbert R, Cannell MB: Analysis of ryanodine receptor clusters in rat and human cardiac myocytes. Proc Natl Acad Sci U S A 104:14958-14963, 2007.
44. Santana LF, Cheng H, Gomez AM, et al: Relation between the sarcolemmal Ca^{2+} current and Ca^{2+} sparks and local control theories for cardiac excitation-contraction coupling. Circ Res 78:166-171, 1996.
45. Wang SQ, Song LS, Lakatta EG, Cheng H: Ca^{2+} signalling between single L-type Ca^{2+} channels and ryanodine receptors in heart cells. Nature 410:592-596, 2001.
46. Gomez AM, Valdivia HH, Cheng H, et al: Defective excitation-contraction coupling in experimental cardiac hypertrophy and heart failure. Science 276:800-806, 1997.
47. Nabauer M, Ellis-Davies GC, Kaplan JH, Morad M: Modulation of Ca^{2+} channel selectivity and cardiac contraction by photorelease of Ca^{2+}. Am J Physiol 256:H916-H920, 1989.
48. Sham JS, Song LS, Chen Y, et al: Termination of Ca^{2+} release by a local inactivation of ryanodine receptors in cardiac myocytes. Proc Natl Acad Sci U S A 95:15096-15101, 1998.
49. Cannell MB, Soeller C: Numerical analysis of ryanodine receptor activation by L-type channel activity in the cardiac muscle dyad. Biophys J 73:112-122, 1997.
50. Stern MD: Theory of excitation-contraction coupling in cardiac muscle. Biophys J 63:497-517, 1992.
51. DelPrincipe F, Egger M, Niggli E: Calcium signalling in cardiac muscle: Refractoriness revealed by coherent activation. Nat Cell Biol 1:323-329, 1999.
52. Sobie EA, Song LS, Lederer WJ: Local recovery of Ca^{2+} release in rat ventricular myocytes. J Physiol 565:441-447, 2005.
53. Szentesi P, Pignier C, Egger M, et al: Sarcoplasmic reticulum Ca^{2+} refilling controls recovery from Ca^{2+}-induced Ca^{2+} release refractoriness in heart muscle. Circ Res 95:807-813, 2004.
54. Terentyev D, Viatchenko-Karpinski S, Gyorke I, et al: Calsequestrin determines the functional size and stability of cardiac intracellular calcium stores: Mechanism for hereditary arrhythmia. Proc Natl Acad Sci U S A 100:11759-11764, 2003.
55. Varro A, Negretti N, Hester SB, Eisner DA: An estimate of the calcium content of the sarcoplasmic reticulum in rat ventricular myocytes. Pflügers Arch 423:158-160, 1993.
56. MacQuaide N, Dempster J, Smith GL: Measurement and modeling of Ca^{2+} waves in isolated rabbit ventricular cardiomyocytes. Biophys J 93:2581-2595, 2007.
57. Marx SO, Reiken S, Hisamatsu Y, et al: PKA phosphorylation dissociates FKBP12.6 from the calcium release channel (ryanodine receptor): Defective regulation in failing hearts. Cell 101:365-376, 2000.
58. Wehrens XH, Lehnart SE, Reiken S, et al: Ryanodine receptor/calcium release channel PKA phosphorylation: A critical

mediator of heart failure progression. Proc Natl Acad Sci U S A 103:511-518, 2006.
59. Xiao B, Zhong G, Obayashi M, et al: Ser-2030, but not Ser-2808, is the major phosphorylation site in cardiac ryanodine receptors responding to protein kinase A activation upon β-adrenergic stimulation in normal and failing hearts. Biochem J 396:7-16, 2006.
60. Ai X, Curran JW, Shannon TR, et al: Ca^{2+}/calmodulin-dependent protein kinase modulates cardiac ryanodine receptor phosphorylation and sarcoplasmic reticulum Ca^{2+} leak in heart failure. Circ Res 97:1314-1322, 2005.
61. Wehrens XH, Lehnart SE, Huang F, et al: FKBP12.6 deficiency and defective calcium release channel (ryanodine receptor) function linked to exercise-induced sudden cardiac death. Cell 113:829-840, 2003.
62. Stange M, Xu L, Balshaw D, et al: Characterization of recombinant skeletal muscle (Ser-2843) and cardiac muscle (Ser-2809) ryanodine receptor phosphorylation mutants. J Biol Chem 278: 51693-51702, 2003.
63. Li Y, Kranias EG, Mignery GA, Bers DM: Protein kinase A phosphorylation of the ryanodine receptor does not affect calcium sparks in mouse ventricular myocytes. Circ Res 90:309-316, 2002.
64. Benkusky NA, Weber CS, Scherman JA, et al: Intact β-adrenergic response and unmodified progression toward heart failure in mice with genetic ablation of a major protein kinase A phosphorylation site in the cardiac ryanodine receptor. Circ Res 819-829, 2007.
65. Lindegger N, Niggli E: Paradoxical SR Ca^{2+} release in guinea-pig cardiac myocytes after β-adrenergic stimulation revealed by two-photon photolysis of caged Ca^{2+}. J Physiol 565:801-813, 2005.
66. Ogrodnik J, Niggli E: Enhanced SR Ca^{2+} release after β-adrenergic stimulation in guinea-pig ventricular myocytes attributed to PKA-mediated phosphorylation. Biophys J 90:71a, 2006.
67. Shannon TR, Ginsburg KS, Bers DM: Potentiation of fractional sarcoplasmic reticulum calcium release by total and free intra-sarcoplasmic reticulum calcium concentration. Biophys J 78:334-343, 2000.
68. Keller M, Kao JP, Egger M, Niggli E: Calcium waves driven by sensitization wave-fronts. Cardiovasc Res 74:39-45, 2007.
69. Farrell EF, Antaramian A, Benkusky N, et al: Regulation of cardiac excitation-contraction coupling by sorcin, a novel modulator of ryanodine receptors. Biol Res 37:609-612, 2004.
70. Volkers M, Loughrey CM, MacQuaide N, et al: S100a1 decreases calcium spark frequency and alters their spatial characteristics in permeabilized adult ventricular cardiomyocytes. Cell Calcium 41:135-143, 2007.
71. Katoh H, Schlotthauer K, Bers DM: Transmission of information from cardiac dihydropyridine receptor to ryanodine receptor: Evidence from BayK 8644 effects on resting Ca^{2+} sparks. Circ Res 87: 106-111, 2000.
72. Copello JA, Zima AV, Diaz-Sylvester PL, et al: Ca^{2+} entry–independent effects of L-type Ca^{2+} channel modulators on Ca^{2+} sparks in ventricular myocytes. Am J Physiol Cell Physiol 292:C2129-C2140, 2007.
73. Huang G, Kim JY, Dehoff M, et al: Ca^{2+} signaling in microdomains: Homer1 mediates the interaction between RyR2 and cav1.2 to regulate excitation-contraction coupling. J Biol Chem 282:14283-14290, 2007.
74. Dulhunty AF, Curtis SM, Watson S, et al: Multiple actions of imperatoxin A on ryanodine receptors: Interactions with the II-III loop A fragment. J Biol Chem 279:11853-11862, 2004.
75. Tripathy A, Resch W, Xu L, et al: Imperatoxin A induces subconductance states in Ca^{2+} release channels (ryanodine receptors) of cardiac and skeletal muscle. J Gen Physiol 111:679-690, 1998.
76. Meissner G: Ryanodine receptor/Ca^{2+} release channels and their regulation by endogenous effectors. Annu Rev Physiol 56:485-508, 1994.
77. Meissner G: Molecular regulation of cardiac ryanodine receptor ion channel. Cell Calcium 35:621-628, 2004.
78. Xu L, Mann G, Meissner G: Regulation of cardiac Ca^{2+} release channel (ryanodine receptor) by Ca^{2+}, H+, Mg^{2+}, and adenine nucleotides under normal and simulated ischemic conditions. Circ Res 79:1100-1109, 1996.
79. Yang Z, Steele DS: Effects of cytosolic ATP on Ca^{2+} sparks and SR Ca^{2+} content in permeabilized cardiac myocytes. Circ Res 89:526-533, 2001.
80. Xu L, Eu JP, Meissner G, Stamler JS: Activation of the cardiac calcium release channel (ryanodine receptor) by poly-S-nitrosylation. Science 279:234-237, 1998.
81. Lim G, Venetucci L, Eisner DA, Casadei B: Does nitric oxide modulate cardiac ryanodine receptor function? Implications for excitation-contraction coupling. Cardiovasc Res E-pub, 2007.
82. Hare JM, Stamler JS: NO/redox disequilibrium in the failing heart and cardiovascular system. J Clin Invest 115:509-517, 2005.
83. Oda T, Yano M, Yamamoto T, et al: Defective regulation of interdomain interactions within the ryanodine receptor plays a key role in the pathogenesis of heart failure. Circulation 111:3400-3410, 2005.
84. Zima AV, Blatter LA: Redox regulation of cardiac calcium channels and transporters. Cardiovasc Res 71:310-321, 2006.
85. Yano M, Okuda S, Oda T, et al: Correction of defective interdomain interaction within ryanodine receptor by antioxidant is a new therapeutic strategy against heart failure. Circulation 112:3633-3643, 2005.
86. Macgregor A, Yamasaki M, Rakovic S, et al: NAADP controls cross-talk between distinct Ca^{2+} stores in the heart. J Biol Chem 282:15302-15311, 2007.
87. Cui Y, Galione A, Terrar DA: Effects of photoreleased cadp-ribose on calcium transients and calcium sparks in myocytes isolated from guinea-pig and rat ventricle. Biochem J 342:269-273, 1999.
88. Ferrier GR, Moe GK: Effect of calcium on acetylstrophanthidin-induced transient depolarizations in canine Purkinje tissue. Circ Res 33:508-515, 1973.
89. Kass RS, Lederer WJ, Tsien RW, Weingart R: Role of calcium ions in transient inward currents and aftercontractions induced by strophanthidin in cardiac Purkinje fibres. J Physiol 281:187-208, 1978.
90. Berlin JR, Cannell MB, Lederer WJ: Cellular origins of the transient inward current in cardiac myocytes. Role of fluctuations and waves of elevated intracellular calcium. Circ Res 65:115-126, 1989.
91. Sipido KR, Callewaert G, Carmeliet E: $[Ca^{2+}]_i$ transients and $[Ca^{2+}]_i$-dependent chloride current in single Purkinje cells from rabbit heart. J Physiol 468:641-667, 1993.
92. Ehara T, Noma A, Ono K: Calcium-activated non-selective cation channel in ventricular cells isolated from adult guinea-pig hearts. J Physiol 403:117-133, 1988.
93. Niggli E: Strontium-induced creep currents associated with tonic contractions in cardiac myocytes isolated from guinea-pigs. J Physiol 414:549-568, 1989.
94. Kimura J, Noma A, Irisawa H: Na-Ca exchange current in mammalian heart cells. Nature 319:596-597, 1986.
95. Lipp P, Pott L: Transient inward current in guinea-pig atrial myocytes reflects a change of sodium-calcium exchange current. J Physiol 397:601-630, 1988.
96. Niggli E, Lederer WJ: Activation of Na-Ca exchange current by photolysis of caged calcium. Biophys J 65:882-891, 1993.
97. Laitinen PJ, Brown KM, Piippo K, et al: Mutations of the cardiac ryanodine receptor (RyR2) gene in familial polymorphic ventricular tachycardia. Circulation 103:485-490, 2001.
98. Priori SG, Napolitano C, Tiso N, et al: Mutations in the cardiac ryanodine receptor gene (hRyR2) underlie catecholaminergic polymorphic ventricular tachycardia. Circulation 103:196-200, 2001.
99. George CH, Jundi H, Walters N, et al: Arrhythmogenic mutation-linked defects in ryanodine receptor autoregulation reveal a novel mechanism of Ca^{2+} release channel dysfunction. Circ Res 98:88-97, 2006.
100. Jiang D, Xiao B, Yang D, et al: RyR2 mutations linked to ventricular tachycardia and sudden death reduce the threshold for store-overload–induced Ca^{2+} release (SOICR). Proc Natl Acad Sci U S A 101:13062-13067, 2004.
101. Sutko JL, Airey JA, Welch W, Ruest L: The pharmacology of ryanodine and related compounds. Pharmacol Rev 49:53-98, 1997.
102. Eisner DA, Choi HS, Diaz ME, et al: Integrative analysis of calcium cycling in cardiac muscle. Circ Res 87:1087-1094, 2000.
103. Overend CL, O'Neill SC, Eisner DA: The effect of tetracaine on stimulated contractions, sarcoplasmic reticulum Ca^{2+} content and membrane current in isolated rat ventricular myocytes. J Physiol 507:759-769, 1998.

104. Lukyanenko V, Gyorke I, Subramanian S, et al: Inhibition of Ca^{2+} sparks by ruthenium red in permeabilized rat ventricular myocytes. Biophys J 79:1273-1284, 2000.
105. Zuppinger C, Timolati F, Suter TM: Pathophysiology and diagnosis of cancer drug induced cardiomyopathy. Cardiovasc Toxicol 7:61-66, 2007.
106. Lehnart SE, Terrenoire C, Reiken S, et al: Stabilization of cardiac ryanodine receptor prevents intracellular calcium leak and arrhythmias. Proc Natl Acad Sci U S A 103:7906-7910, 2006.
107. Wehrens XH, Marks AR: Novel therapeutic approaches for heart failure by normalizing calcium cycling. Nat Rev Drug Discov 3:565-573, 2004.
108. Oetliker H: An appraisal of the evidence for a sarcoplasmic reticulum membrane potential and its relation to calcium release in skeletal muscle. J Muscle Res Cell Motil 3:247-272, 1982.
109. Coronado R, Rosenberg RL, Miller C: Ionic selectivity, saturation, and block in a K^+-selective channel from sarcoplasmic reticulum. J Gen Physiol 76:425-446, 1980.
110. Cukierman S, Yellen G, Miller C: The K^+ channel of sarcoplasmic reticulum. A new look at Cs+ block. Biophys J 48:477-484, 1985.
111. Hill JA Jr, Coronado R, Strauss HC: Potassium channel of cardiac sarcoplasmic reticulum is a multi-ion channel. Biophys J 55:35-45, 1989.
112. Oosawa Y, Sokabe M: Voltage-dependent aminoglycoside blockade of the sarcoplasmic reticulum K^+ channel. Am J Physiol 250:C361-C364, 1986.
113. Liu QY, Rasmusson RL, Liu QX, Strauss HC: Voltage-dependent, open channel blockade of the cardiac sarcoplasmic reticulum potassium channel by 4-aminopyridine. Can J Cardiol 14:275-280, 1998.
114. Picard L, Cote K, Teijeira J, et al: Sarcoplasmic reticulum K^+ channels from human and sheep atrial cells display a specific electro-pharmacological profile. J Mol Cell Cardiol 34:1163-1172, 2002.
115. Kawano S, Kuruma A, Hirayama Y, Hiraoka M: Anion permeability and conduction of adenine nucleotides through a chloride channel in cardiac sarcoplasmic reticulum. J Biol Chem 274:2085-2092, 1999.

Hyperpolarization-Activated, Cyclic Nucleotide–Gated (HCN) Channels: From Genes to Function

7

JULIANE STIEBER, STEFAN HERRMANN, AND ANDREAS LUDWIG

CHAPTER OUTLINE

Sinoatrial cells of the heart display a unique action potential characterized by a slow depolarizing phase that renders these cells spontaneously active. The depolarizing phase is mediated by an interaction between different ion channels and transporters, such as *h*yperpolarization-activated, *c*yclic *n*ucleotide–gated (HCN) channels, T- and L-type calcium channels, ryanodine receptors, and Na^+/Ca^{2+} exchangers. This chapter gives an overview of HCN channels. The four members of this family of proteins generate a current termed I_f in the heart and I_h in the brain. After the identification of HCN channels, knowledge about the molecular diversity, structure, and physiologic role of these proteins has grown tremendously. In addition, recent efforts to create a "biopacemaker" are based mainly on transduction of cardiac tissue with HCN channel genes.

Molecular Identification of HCN Channels

The electrophysiologic properties of I_f have been well characterized (e.g., in reviews by DiFrancesco[1] and Pape[2]). A distinguishing feature of the I_f channel is that it is activated not on depolarization of the membrane (as are most voltage-gated ion channels) but on membrane hyperpolarization. The channel is permeable for K^+ and Na^+ ions, with a three-fold higher selectivity for K^+ than for Na^+. At the maximum diastolic potential of sinoatrial node cells (approximately −60 to −75 mV), I_f channels carry an inward current that depolarizes the membrane potential toward the activation range of T-type and then L-type calcium channels (Fig. 7-1). The voltage dependence of I_f activation is regulated by cyclic adenosine monophosphate (cAMP). Direct binding of cAMP to the channel shifts the activation curve to more depolarized voltages, so the channel opens more completely. In addition, the activation kinetics of the channel are strongly accelerated. The increase in heart rate in response to β-adrenergic agonists (which increase the intracellular cAMP level) has been attributed to this direct effect of cAMP on the I_f channel (see Fig. 7-1).[3] Similarly, lowering the cAMP level by muscarinic agonists inhibits opening of the channel and is thought to result in a reduced heart rate.[4]

The molecular basis of I_f was identified by cloning the HCN channel gene family.[5-9] Four different genes termed *HCN1* to *HCN4* have been identified in mammals, and closely related genes have been found in a wide variety of species.[10] The HCN family of channel proteins belongs to the superfamily of voltage-gated cation channels and is distantly related to the cyclic nucleotide–gated and the eag potassium channel family. The channels are composed of six transmembrane segments (S1 to S6), including a positively charged S4 segment constituting the voltage sensor[11] (Fig. 7-2). Between the fifth and sixth membrane-spanning segments lies the ion-conducting pore region. The proteins contain a cyclic nucleotide–binding domain (CNBD) in the carboxyl (C)-terminal region, the structure of which was recently determined.[12] Hence, HCN channels contain structural features of both voltage- and cyclic nucleotide–gated ion channels, in accordance with their modulation by both membrane potential and cyclic nucleotides.

Structure-Function Relations of HCN Channels

Each HCN isoform generates a hyperpolarization-activated current in heterologous expression systems with the typical features of native I_f (HCN1,[7] HCN2,[5,6] HCN3,[13,14] HCN4[6,8,9]). However, the currents differ in their activation kinetics, voltage dependence of activation, and extent of cAMP modulation.

Activation Kinetics

Individual HCN isoforms can be differentiated according to their speed of activation. HCN1 is the most rapidly activating channel (activation time constant, τ between 30 and 300 ms at potentials ranging from −70 to −140 mV), HCN2 and HCN3 have intermediate activation kinetics (τ = 200 to 500 ms), HCN4 is the most slowly gating channel (τ = 300 ms to several seconds). Single amino acids located in transmembrane segments S1 and S2 and the loop between S1 and S2 were identified as major determinants of the difference in activation kinetics between HCN2 and HCN4.[15] The speed of channel opening is strongly dependent on the membrane potential—being faster at more hyperpolarized potentials. Another factor influencing the kinetics of HCN channel activation is temperature, with a temperature coefficient (Q_{10}) of approximately 4.5.[16]

Voltage Dependence of Activation

All four channels are activated on membrane hyperpolarization below −40 mV. The data on the exact potential of half-maximal channel activation ($V_{1/2}$) vary even for the same channel. For example, $V_{1/2}$ values from −75 mV to −110 mV for HCN4

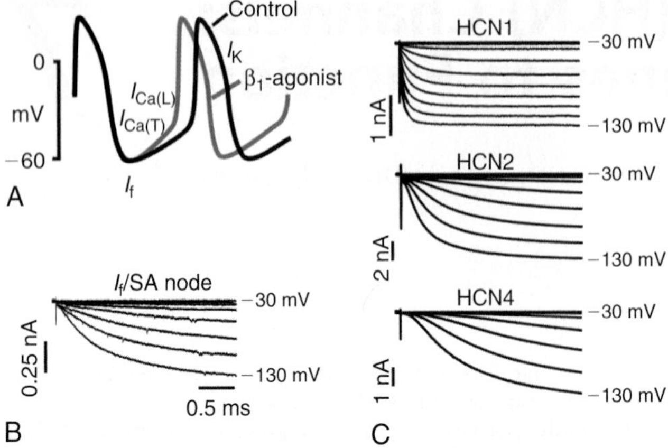

Figure 7-1 **A,** Action potential of a sinoatrial node cell under control conditions *(black)* and in the presence of a β_1-adrenoceptor agonist *(dark red)*. The four types of currents that may contribute to pacemaker activity of the sinoatrial node are indicated: I_f, hyperpolarization-activated cation current; $I_{Ca(T)}$, T-type Ca^{2+} current; $I_{Ca(L)}$, L-type Ca^{2+} current; I_K, delayed-rectifier K^+ current. **B** and **C,** Representative recordings of I_f are from a murine sinoatrial (SA) node cell (**B**) and of murine HCN1, human HCN2, and human HCN4 expressed in HEK293 cells (**C**). Shown are whole-cell voltage recordings measured under identical conditions at room temperature. From a holding potential of −40 mV, voltage steps ranging from −30 to −130 mV were applied.

have been reported, depending on, among other parameters, the pulse protocol used to (pre)activate the channel and on the ionic composition of the solutions.[5,8,9,13,17] Generally, HCN1 and HCN3 show a $V_{1/2}$ value 10 to 20 mV more positive than that for HCN2 and HCN4 when analyzed in heterologous expression systems.[18]

It is assumed that hyperpolarization-activated gating of HCN channels is initiated by a movement of the strongly positively charged S4 segment.[11] This "charge sensor" detects the change in membrane potential and should move inward on hyperpolarization and outward on depolarization (i.e., the direction of the

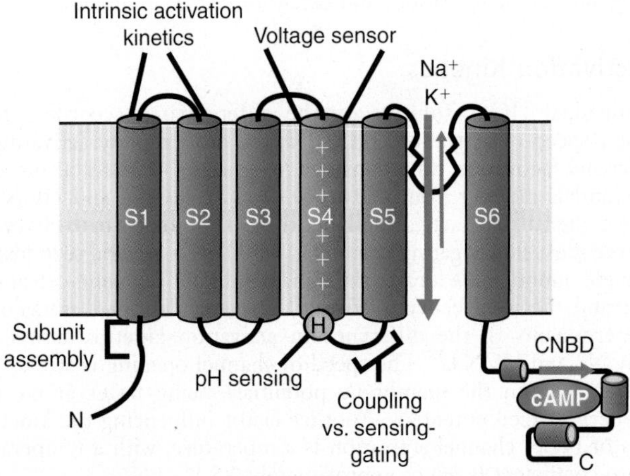

Figure 7-2 Primary structure of an HCN channel. *Cylinders* depict the six transmembrane segments S1 to S6. The positively charged S4 segment represents the voltage sensor *(red)*. The pH sensor of the channel is a histidine residue (the circled "H") located at the boundary between the S4 segment and the S4-S5 linker. The cytoplasmic S4-S5 linker, which is important for coupling between the S4 movement and opening and closing of the activation gate, also is labeled. C, carboxyl terminus; cAMP, cyclic adenine monophosphate; CNBD, cyclic nucleotide–binding domain; N, amino terminus.

S4 movement in HCN channels would be the same as in depolarization-activated channels). In HCN channels, however, the inward movement of S4 is thought to open the activation gate, whereas in depolarization-activated channels, it closes the gate. Direct experimental evidence supporting this model comes from a study examining the voltage-dependent accessibility of cysteine residues introduced in the S4 segment of spHCN.[11] It was shown that the S4 segment makes indeed an inward (or outward) movement in response to hyperpolarization (or depolarization). This finding indicates that the coupling mechanism between voltage sensor and activation gate in HCN channels must be different from that in depolarization-activated channels.

Alanine-scanning mutagenesis of the intracellular S4-S5 linker indicated that this region is important for coupling between S4 movement and opening and closing of the activation gate.[19] The activation gate itself may be localized at the intracellular side of the channel pore.[20,21]

Ion Selectivity

HCN channels contain a pore region carrying the glycine-tyrosine-glycine (GYG) amino acid motif, which provides the selectivity filter in potassium channels. In contrast with these channels, HCN channels have a low selectivity for K^+,[5,7] meaning that HCN channels carry a depolarizing Na^+ current under physiologic conditions. It is unknown why HCN channels display a low selectivity for K^+ despite the presence of the GYG motif in the pore. Homology modeling indicates that the reduced selectivity for K^+ ions may be caused by an increased flexibility of the inner pore of the channels.[22]

Modulation by Cyclic Nucleotides

The channels possess a CNBD in their carboxyl terminus (C terminus) mediating the modulatory effect of cAMP. The cAMP shifts the voltage dependence of activation to more positive voltages and enhances the speed of channel activation. The four channels vary in the extent of their response to cAMP, however. HCN2 and HCN4 are strongly modulated (shift of $V_{1/2}$ by approximately +10 to +15 mV). By contrast, the activation curve of HCN1 is only minimally shifted,[23-25] and HCN3 is not positively modulated by cyclic nucleotides.[13,14]

Deletion of the CNBD has been shown to shift the voltage dependence to more positive voltages, an effect similar to that of cAMP on wild-type channels.[25,26] This observation indicates that the CNBD in the cAMP unbound state inhibits activation of the channel core by shifting gating to more hyperpolarized potentials. Binding of cAMP to the CNBD relieves this inhibition. The difference in the cAMP response between HCN1/3 and HCN2/4 can be explained by the difference in the extent of inhibition. HCN1 is weakly inhibited by the CNBD (minimal positive shift on deletion of the CNBD), whereas HCN2 is strongly inhibited (large positive shift on CNBD deletion). Therefore, HCN2 channels reveal a large response to cAMP, whereas HCN1 channels are only weakly affected by the presence of cAMP. In addition to cAMP, cyclic guanosine monophosphate (cGMP) also stimulates HCN channels.[5] The sensitivity for cGMP of HCN2 (K_a = 6 μM), however, is approximately 10-fold lower than that for cAMP (K_a = 0.5 μM).

Other Cellular Factors Modulating HCN Channels

HCN channels are modulated by various other endogenous factors and mechanisms, such as intracellular pH,[27] tyrosine phosphorylation,[28] and membrane phospholipids.[29,30] Acidic pH values shift the channel activation curve to more hyperpolarized potentials, thereby inhibiting channel activity. A conserved histidine residue localized at the boundary between S4 and the S4-S5 linker (His321 of HCN2) is the major determinant of pH sensitivity.[31] The modulation by intracellular protons may be important during cardiac ischemia, when cytosolic pH values drop to 6.0 or lower. Inhibition of HCN channel activity in the conduction system may potentially then disturb rhythm generation and provoke arrhythmias. Both tyrosine phosphorylation by Src kinases and PIP_2 have an activity-enhancing effect on HCN currents, not only on heterologously expressed channels but also on native channels in embryonic cardiomyocytes or adult sinoatrial cells.[28-30]

The foregoing mechanisms are not HCN channel–specific but rather are universal regulatory mechanisms. Their relevance for the modulation of cardiac pacemaker function in vivo has yet to be determined.

Channel Complex Formation

By analogy to CNG and potassium channels, it is most likely that HCN subunits assemble to form tetramers.[32] A dominant-negative pore mutant of HCN suppressed coexpressed wild-type HCN1 in a dose-dependent manner consistent with tetramer formation.[33] In addition, the crystallized CNBD regions from HCN2 assembled as tetramers with a four-fold axis of rotational symmetry.[12] Interaction between a conserved domain in the amino-terminal region of HCN channels also has been suggested to be important for subunit coassembly.[34,35]

Because several HCN isoforms are coexpressed in a single cell type (e.g., HCN1, 2+4 in sinoatrial node cells),[36] the question arises whether HCN subunits can coassemble to form heteromers. Expression of a tandem construct of HCN1+HCN2[24] and coexpression of single HCN1 and HCN2 subunits in *Xenopus* oocytes[37] yielded currents with characteristics intermediate between those of HCN1 and HCN2 homomers. In addition, a dominant-negative pore mutant of HCN[33] suppressed coexpressed HCN2, indicating that HCN subunits are able to form heteromeric complexes. The formation of heteromers of various dimeric combinations of HCN isoforms also has been demonstrated in a mammalian heterologous expression system.[38] In addition, immunoprecipitation experiments indicated that at least HCN1 and HCN2 can form heteromeres also in vivo.[38] A native cell that expresses several HCN genes, however, also may produce homomeric channels. Of note, several cell types, such as cerebellar basket cells and retinal photoreceptors, express only a single HCN isoform. This finding supports the hypothesis that native HCN channels also can exist as homomers.

A potential auxiliary subunit of HCN channels may be the MinK-related peptide 1 (MiRP1) (i.e., KCNE2). Coexpression of MiRP1 with HCN1 or HCN2 was found to increase current density and to accelerate activation kinetics in heterologous expression systems and transfected cardiomyocytes.[39,40]

HCN Channel Expression in Heart

Expression of HCN1, HCN2, and HCN4 has been found in the adult heart. The expression pattern of HCN channel subunits differs in various cardiac regions and also displays some species-dependent variations. In the sinoatrial node, HCN4 is by far the most highly expressed isoform in all species studied up to now. It represents greater than 80% of the total HCN message.[18,41] In addition to HCN4, HCN2 and low levels of HCN1 also are expressed in the murine sinoatrial node.[18,36,41] In the rabbit sinoatrial node, expression of HCN1 is significantly higher than in mouse.[23] HCN4 transcript and protein also were detected in canine cardiac Purkinje fibers.[42] HCN4 messenger RNA (mRNA) was significantly more highly expressed compared with HCN2 in these cells; expression of HCN1 was not detected. HCN channel transcripts also have been found in atrial and ventricular myocytes. HCN2 is the predominant isoform in these nonpacing cells. Besides HCN2, low expression of HCN4 has been detected in murine, canine, and human working myocardium.[6,18,42]

Cardiac HCN Channels and Native I_f

The comparison of HCN channel properties reported in the literature with those of native I_f has to take into account that the current is dependent on various experimental parameters. This is illustrated by the wide range of $V_{1/2}$ values (e.g., −65 to −92 mV) and activation time constants reported for sinoatrial I_f.[43] A direct comparison of HCN channels in HEK293 cells with sinoatrial I_f channels under identical conditions is shown in Figure 7-1. Obviously, sinoatrial I_f mainly resembles the HCN4 current. The slightly faster activation kinetics of the native current are in accordance with the hypothesis that sinoatrial I_f is generated by the combined activity of HCN4 (predominating, slow activating) and HCN2 (minor contribution, fast-activating). In some species, such as rabbit, HCN1 also may contribute.[23] Additional studies using, for example, gene deletion experiments (see later on) are necessary to define unequivocally the molecular basis of cardiac I_f.

I_f in ventricular cells has a much lower current density and more negative $V_{1/2}$ (−95 to −135 mV) than have been measured for sinoatrial I_f. It has been reported that ventricular cells from patients with ischemic cardiomyopathy have a two-fold higher I_f density and an activation curve shifted to positive potentials compared with those from control subjects.[44,45] This finding raises the possibility that I_f in ischemic hearts may represent an arrhythmogenic mechanism by generating a pathologic depolarizing current.[46]

The different $V_{1/2}$ values of ventricular and sinoatrial I_f can not be sufficiently explained by the differential expression of HCN2 and HCN4 in these regions since the voltage dependence of both channels is quite similar.[13] Other cellular factors such as PIP_2 and auxiliary subunits may influence the voltage dependence of HCN isoforms. This feature has been illustrated in a study of overexpression of HCN2 in newborn and adult ventricular myocytes.[47] It is known that I_f in newborn cardiomyocytes activates at less negative voltages than in adult cells. Remarkably, overexpressed HCN2 exhibited a similar difference in activation (+20 mV) between adult and neonate cells, which did not result from differing cAMP levels. Thus, the developmental state of the myocyte determines the voltage dependence of the HCN2 isoform.

I_f Blockers as Bradycardic Drugs

HCN currents are thought to underlie, together with other ion channels, the spontaneous slow diastolic depolarization rate (DDR) of the sinus node. Thus, substances that block this current can delay the DDR, thereby prolonging diastole. Recently, an HCN blocker, ivabradine (Procoralan), was approved as the first bradycardic drug using this mechanism, which influences only chronotropy but not inotropy. Ivabradine, like the related experimental drugs cilobradine and zatebradine, blocks HCN currents in dose- and use-dependent fashion[48,49] (Fig. 7-3). Even though different modes of channel block onset have been described,[50] this drug does not discriminate among the four HCN subtypes—all HCN isoforms are equally efficiently blocked once steady state has been reached.[49] Nevertheless, the main action of administered ivabradine seems to be the block of sinoatrial I_f. As indicated by the relative lack of side effects, neuronal HCN channels are not efficiently reached, with the exception of retinal HCN1, so that visual signs and symptoms may result. Remarkably, these I_f blockers are not able to completely arrest the heart but merely lower the heart rate to a basal level and leave the heart rate–accelerating response to β-adrenergic stimulation intact.[49] Higher doses, however, induce a cardiac arrhythmia in mice characterized by repetitive sinus pauses, similar to the phenotype of HCN4-deficient mice as described next.

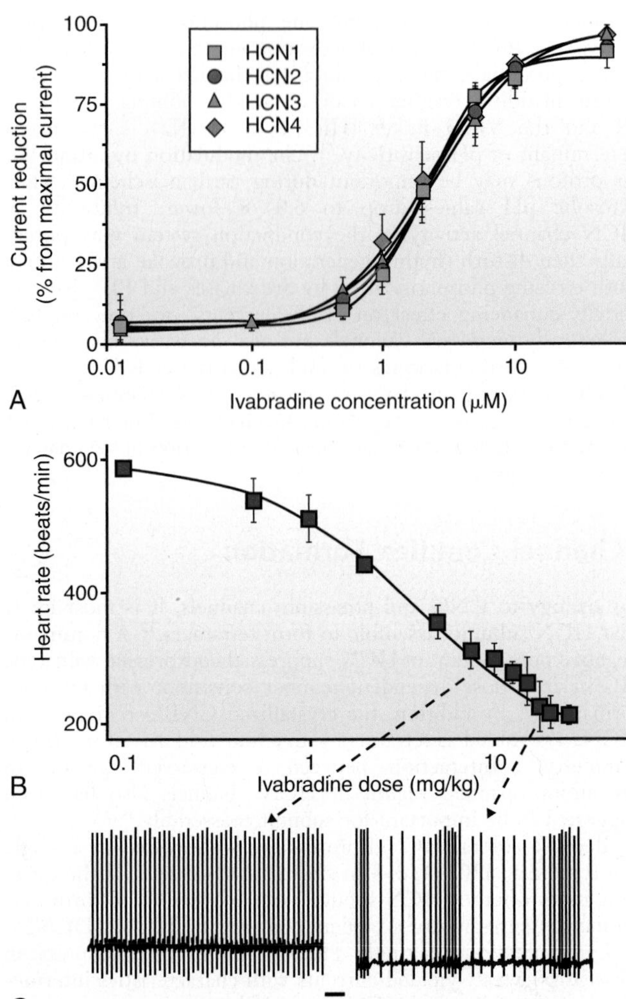

Figure 7-3 **A**, Steady-state inhibition of the human HCN1, HCN2, HCN3, and HCN4 channels expressed in HEK293 cells by ivabradine. Values at *symbols* are for mean reduction ± SD of currents at the indicated drug concentration determined after steady-state inhibition was reached (50 to 500 activating steps to −100 mV). *N* = 17 to 56 cells for each HCN subtype. Superimposed dose-response curves represent logistic fits of means. **B**, Dose-dependent heart rate reduction after intraperitoneal injection of ivabradine, assessed by telemetric ECG recordings in mice. *Symbols* represent mean ± SD, and the superimposed dose-response curve represents the logistic fit of the means. The heart rate is regular and rhythmic up to a dose of approximately 12.5 mg/kg. **C**, Representative electrocardiographic tracings recorded 30 minutes after intraperitoneal injection of the indicated ivabradine dose. *Left tracing*, 7.5 mg/kg ivabradine induces bradycardia but no arrhythmia. *Right tracing*, 25 mg/kg induces bradycardia and arrhythmia. Scale bar: 1 s. (Figures 7-3A and B modified from Stieber J, Wieland K, Stoeckl G, et al: Bradycardic and proarrhythmic properties of sinus node inhibitors. Mol Pharmacol 69:1328-1337, 2006. © American Society for Pharmacology and Experimental Therapeutics.)

Deletion of HCN Channels in Mice

To analyze the role of cardiac HCN channels in vivo, we generated and analyzed HCN2- and HCN4-knockout mice using a Cre/loxP-based approach. Because the global and heart-specific knockout of HCN4 is associated with embryonic lethality,[51] we deleted HCN4 in the adult mouse using a tamoxifen-inducible Cre line that showed high recombination efficiency in the sinoatrial node area.

HCN2

The electrocardiogram (ECG) of resting (but not active) HCN2-deficient mice displayed sinus arrhythmia with varying RR intervals and unaltered ECG complexes.[52] This kind of dysrhythmia also is seen in ECGs of wild-type mice but occurred much more often in HCN2-knockout animals. Heart rates at rest and during spontaneous activity were not different between wild-type and knockout. Furthermore, β-adrenergic agonists and atropine increased heart rate in $HCN2^{-/-}$ mice to the same extent as in wild-type mice. A prime role ascribed to I_f has been the modulation of heart rate in response to sympathetic stimulation. The results suggest that HCN2 is not necessary for mediating the chronotropic effect of β-adrenergic agonists. The reason could be that I_f in isolated sinoatrial node cells from HCN2-knockout mice was reduced by only approximately 30% compared with wild-type. This finding suggested that (1) HCN2 generates part of sinoatrial I_f but that (2) the main component of sinoatrial I_f is produced by another HCN channel, presumably HCN4.

Nevertheless, the maximum diastolic potential of HCN2-knockout cells was approximately 5 mV more hyperpolarized than that for wild-type cells. Hence, the primary role of HCN2 in sinoatrial cells may be to control resting membrane properties. The following mechanism may underlie the arrhythmia of HCN2-deficient mice: The loss of HCN2 hyperpolarizes the membrane and may destabilize the regular generation of action potentials. Excess hyperpolarizations (e.g., by increased potassium channel activity or influences from connected atrial cells) may not be limited fast enough, potentially resulting in the delayed generation of the next action potential.

HCN4

Conditional deletion of HCN4 in the adult mouse heart[36] resulted in a more pronounced phenotype than that associated with deletion of HCN2 but was still surprisingly mild in view of the importance of HCN4 during embryonic pacemaker cell development and the postulated role of I_f as a key determinant of heart rate modulation.[51] Both basic and β-adrenergic agonist–stimulated heart rates of HCN4-deficient mice did not differ from those in wild-type mice (Fig. 7-4A). During basic heart rates, however, repetitive sinus pauses occurred in the HCN4-knockout cells, both in vivo and in isolated hearts. They were characterized by normal ECG complexes with irregular prolongations of the diastolic phase (T to P duration). Those pauses appeared to increase in number proportionately

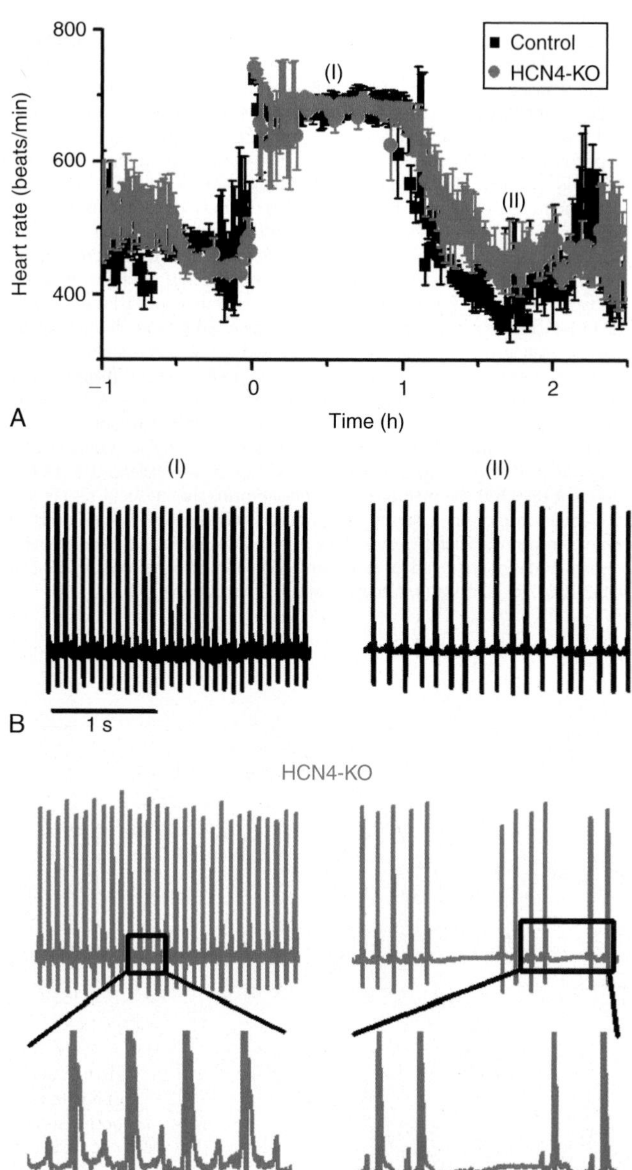

Figure 7-4 Cardiac phenotype of HCN4-deficient mice. **A,** Injection of 0.5 mg/kg isoproterenol at t = 0 increased the heart rate in both wild-type (control) and HCN4-deficient (HCN4-KO) mice. **B,** Representative electrocardiographic tracings of wild-type *(black)* and HCN4-deficient *(dark red)* mice during β-adrenergic-stimulated (I) and basal (II) heart rate. **C,** Sinus pauses appear primarily during basal heart rates. Scale bar: 1 s. (Modified from Herrmann S, Stieber J, Stoeckl G, et al: HCN4 provides a 'depolarization reserve' and is not required for heart rate acceleration in mice. EMBO J 26:4423-4432, 2007. © European Molecular Biology Organization.)

with decreasing heart rates but completely disappeared during stimulated heart rates (see Fig. 7-4B and C). Moreover, bradycardic agents such as carbachol or adenosine not only slowed down the heart rate more markedly than in wild-type cells but also resulted in an increased number and duration of sinus pauses. Analysis of isolated sinoatrial node cells revealed a strong reduction in I_f by approximately 75% relative to control cells (Fig. 7-5A). Both the analysis of electrophysiologic parameters and expression studies on mRNA and protein level confirmed that the residual current in HCN4-knockout mice was not carried by HCN4 but possibly was carried by HCN2 or HCN1, or both. As in HCN2-deficient sinoatrial node cells, the membrane potential of isolated HCN4-deficient sinoatrial node cells was approximately 8 mV more negative than in control cells. As a functional consequence, HCN4-deficient pacemaker cells did not discharge action potentials as readily as did wild-type sinoatrial node cells. Under basal conditions, approximately 90% of the analyzed HCN4-knockout sinoatrial node cells showed only a stable resting potential of approximately −65 mV. Of interest, these cells depolarized and started to generate normal sinoatrial action potentials when isoproterenol (see Fig. 7-5B) or a short depolarizing current pulse (not shown) was applied, suggesting a correctly functioning sinoatrial node cell once spontaneous activity was triggered. Is the small residual I_f, however, the mediator for this triggering and for the acceleration of the heart rate in the HCN4-knockout mouse? This does not seem very likely, because even though the current-voltage (*I-V*) curve of the residual HCN4-knockout I_f responded to isoproterenol-cAMP application by a rightward shift, the small current amplitude could not be significantly increased (see Fig. 7-5C).

According to these results, we propose a refined model for the function of the HCN4 channel in sinoatrial node cells (see Fig. 7-5D): To ensure stable pacemaking over time, depolarizing currents are in a dynamic balance with repolarizing currents. In most situations, and particularly during sympathetic stimulation, HCN4 is not required to promote stable pacemaking. Increased repolarizing currents, resulting, for example, from muscarinic or adenosine receptor stimulation, normally are counterregulated by an increased I_f, which provides the additional depolarisation required in this situation. HCN4-deficient cells cannot provide this current, resulting in a prolonged diastolic depolarization phase, a delay in the appearance of the next sinoatrial action potential, and the appearance of sinus pauses.

Physiologic Role of HCN Channels in Humans

Experimental results from knockout mice may or may not have limited significance for human physiology. Therefore, the functional role of HCN channels in the human heart is still under investigation. To date, four studies reported mutations of HCN4 in humans.[53-56] The clinical features of these patients range from asymptomatic bradycardia[55,56] to severe syncope.[53,54] In a single patient with bradycardia and atrial fibrillation, a truncated channel lacking the CNBD was identified.[53] In another patient with bradycardia, QT prolongation, and episodes of torsade de pointes, a mis-sense mutation in the C-linker connecting S6 and the CNBD was detected.[54] In addition, two reports described inherited familial bradycardia associated with a point mutation in the CNBD[55] and a pore mutation[56] of HCN4. The CNBD point mutation shifted channel activation to more hyperpolarized potentials. It was suggested that this changed activation behavior decreases the inward diastolic current in sinoatrial node cells, thereby slowing the heart rate.[55] Of note, affected family members with the HCN4 pore mutation showed no evidence of chronotropic incompetence.[56]

Taken together, these reports indicate that in the human heart, HCN4 is important in determining basal heart rate. This seems at odd with the results with deletion of HCN4 in mice, in which no bradycardia was detected[36]; several factors may account for this difference. The human patients have all heterozygous mutations, whereas in the mouse model, a

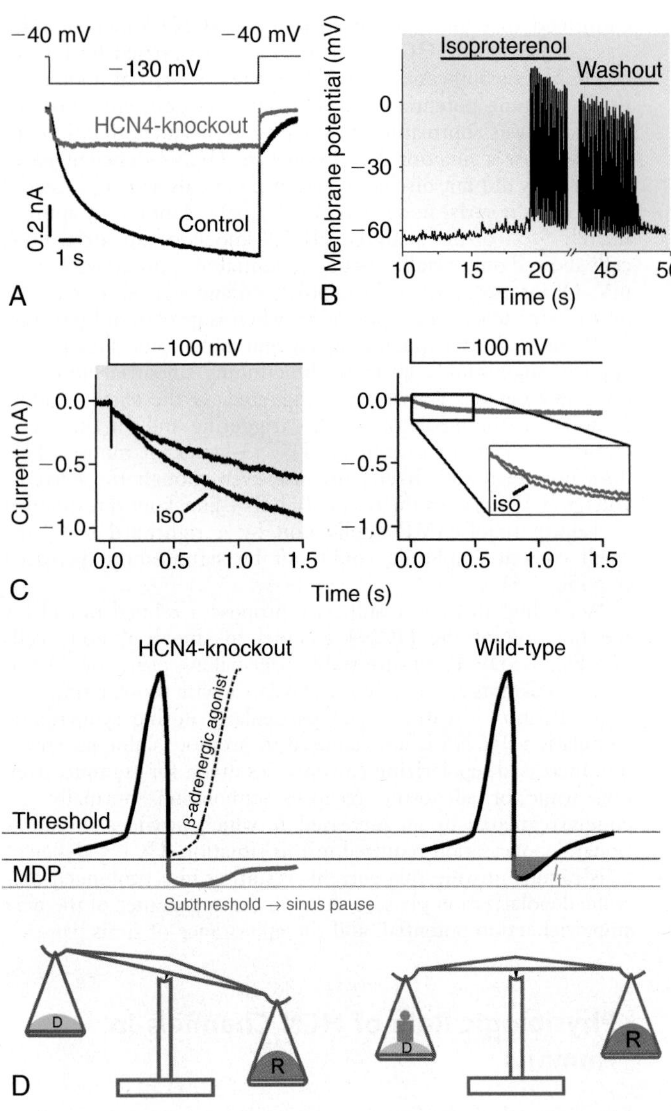

Figure 7-5 **A,** I_f in sinoatrial node cells. Representative current tracings from sinoatrial node cells for wild-type (black) and HCN4-deficient mice *(dark red)*. Whole-cell voltage clamp currents were measured by "stepping" from a holding potential of −40 mV to −130 mV. **B,** Representative membrane potential–action potential (AP) recorded from an HCN4-deficient sinoatrial node cell. The cell showed a stable resting membrane potential of approximately −65 mV; superfusion with bath solution containing 1 μM isoproterenol initiated regular AP firing. Washout of isoproterenol led to hyperpolarization of the cell membrane and cease of AP discharge. **C,** Examples of I_f tracings elicited at −100 mV from control *(left)* and knockout *(right)* sinoatrial node cells before and after application of 1 μM isoproterenol (iso). An enlargement of the I_f current in the HCN4-knockout cells is shown in the inset *(right)*. Residual I_f in HCN4-deficient sinoatrial cells is not significantly increased by isoproterenol. **D,** Proposed role of HCN4 channels in sinoatrial node cells. *Lower part*, Scale illustrating the overall relationship between depolarizing and repolarizing currents. *Upper part*, Schemes of spontaneous APs under basal *(solid line)* and β-adrenergic–stimulated *(broken line)* conditions. Shown are sinoatrial node APs after an increase in repolarizing (R) currents (e.g., muscarinic stimulation, *dark red weight*). In wild-type cells *(right)*, HCN4 is activated and provides a depolarizing (D) current (*dark green weight*), keeping the system well balanced. In HCN4-deficient cells *(left)*, the membrane potential remains subthreshold, resulting in the appearance of sinus pauses. MDP, maximum diastolic potential. (Modified from Herrmann S, Stieber J, Stoeckl G, et al: HCN4 provides a 'depolarization reserve' and is not required for heart rate acceleration in mice. EMBO J 26:4423-4432, 2007. © European Molecular Biology Organization.)

complete deletion of the channel was analyzed. The phenotype resulting from the presence of a normal and a differently modulated channel versus complete lack of the protein has to be analyzed in more detail—for example, in animal models carrying the foregoing mutations. In addition, the roughly 10-fold difference in heart rate between mice and humans also may contribute. This possibility is supported by the finding that HCN4-knockout mice displayed the most pronounced sinoatrial dysfunction at low heart rates, whereas no arrhythmia was detected at high heart rates.

References

1. DiFrancesco D: Pacemaker mechanisms in cardiac tissue. Annu Rev Physiol 55: 455-472, 1993.
2. Pape HC: Queer current and pacemaker: The hyperpolarization-activated cation current in neurons. Annu Rev Physiol 58:299-327, 1996.
3. DiFrancesco D, Tortora P: Direct activation of cardiac pacemaker channels by intracellular cyclic AMP. Nature 351:145-147, 1991.
4. DiFrancesco D, Ducouret P, Robinson RB: Muscarinic modulation of cardiac rate at low acetylcholine concentrations. Science 243:669-671, 1989.
5. Ludwig A, Zong X, Jeglitsch M, et al: A family of hyperpolarization-activated mammalian cation channels. Nature 393: 587-591, 1998.
6. Ludwig A, Zong X, Stieber J, et al: Two pacemaker channels from human heart with profoundly different activation kinetics. EMBO J 18:2323-2339, 1999.
7. Santoro B, Liu DT, Yao H, et al: Identification of a gene encoding a hyperpolarization-activated pacemaker channel of brain. Cell 93:717-729, 1998.
8. Ishii TM, Takano M, Xie LH, et al: Molecular characterization of the hyperpolarization-activated cation channel in rabbit heart sinoatrial node. J Biol Chem 274:12835-12839, 1999.
9. Seifert R, Scholten A, Gauss R, et al: Molecular characterization of a slowly gating human hyperpolarization-activated channel predominantly expressed in thalamus, heart, and testis. Proc Natl Acad Sci U S A 96:9391-9396, 1999.
10. Jackson HA, Marshall CR, Accili EA: Evolution and structural diversification of hyperpolarization-activated cyclic nucleotide–gated channel genes. Physiol Genomics 29:231-245, 2007.
11. Mannikko R, Elinder F, Larsson HP: Voltage-sensing mechanism is conserved

among ion channels gated by opposite voltages. Nature 419:837-841, 2002.
12. Zagotta WN, Olivier NB, Black KD, et al: Structural basis for modulation and agonist specificity of HCN pacemaker channels. Nature 425:200-205, 2003.
13. Stieber J, Stockl G, Herrmann S, et al: Functional expression of the human HCN3 channel. J Biol Chem 280:34635-34643, 2005.
14. Mistrik P, Mader R, Michalakis S, et al: The murine HCN3 gene encodes a hyperpolarization-activated cation channel with slow kinetics and unique response to cyclic nucleotides. J Biol Chem 280:27056-27061, 2005.
15. Stieber J, Thomer A, Much B, et al: Molecular basis for the different activation kinetics of the pacemaker channels HCN2 and HCN4. J Biol Chem 278:33672-33680, 2003.
16. Magee JC: Dendritic hyperpolarization-activated currents modify the integrative properties of hippocampal CA1 pyramidal neurons. J Neurosci 18:7613-7624, 1998.
17. Santoro B, Chen S, Luthi A, et al: Molecular and functional heterogeneity of hyperpolarization-activated pacemaker channels in the mouse CNS. J Neurosci 20:5264-5275, 2000.
18. Moosmang S, Stieber J, Zong X, et al: Cellular expression and functional characterization of four hyperpolarization-activated pacemaker channels in cardiac and neuronal tissues. Eur J Biochem 268: 1646-1652, 2001.
19. Chen J, Mitcheson JS, Tristani-Firouzi M, et al: The S4-S5 linker couples voltage sensing and activation of pacemaker channels. Proc Natl Acad Sci U S A 98:11277-11282, 2001.
20. Rothberg BS, Shin KS, Phale PS, Yellen G: Voltage-controlled gating at the intracellular entrance to a hyperpolarization-activated cation channel. J Gen Physiol 119:83-91, 2002.
21. Rothberg BS, Shin KS, Yellen G: Movements near the gate of a hyperpolarization-activated cation channel. J Gen Physiol 122:501-510, 2003.
22. Giorgetti A, Carloni P, Mistrik P, Torre V: A homology model of the pore region of HCN channels. Biophys J 89:932-944, 2005.
23. Moroni A, Gorza L, Beltrame M, et al: Hyperpolarization-activated cyclic nucleotide–gated channel 1 is a molecular determinant of the cardiac pacemaker current I(f). J Biol Chem 276:29233-29241, 2001.
24. Ulens C, Tytgat J: Functional heteromerization of HCN1 and HCN2 pacemaker channels. J Biol Chem 276:6069-6072, 2001.
25. Wainger BJ, DeGennaro M, Santoro B, et al: Molecular mechanism of cAMP modulation of HCN pacemaker channels. Nature 411:805-810, 2001.
26. Wang J, Chen S, Siegelbaum SA: Regulation of hyperpolarization-activated HCN channel gating and cAMP modulation due to interactions of COOH terminus and core transmembrane regions. J Gen Physiol 118:237-250, 2001.
27. Munsch T, Pape HC: Modulation of the hyperpolarization-activated cation current of rat thalamic relay neurones by intracellular pH. J Physiol 519:493-504, 1999.
28. Zong X, Eckert C, Yuan H, et al: A novel mechanism of modulation of hyperpolarization-activated cyclic nucleotide–gated channels by Src kinase. J Biol Chem 280:34224-34232, 2005.
29. Zolles G, Klocker N, Wenzel D, et al: Pacemaking by HCN channels requires interaction with phosphoinositides. Neuron 52:1027-1036, 2006.
30. Pian P, Bucchi A, Robinson RB, Siegelbaum SA: Regulation of gating and rundown of HCN hyperpolarization-activated channels by exogenous and endogenous PIP2. J Gen Physiol 128:593-604, 2006.
31. Zong X, Stieber J, Ludwig A, et al: A single histidine residue determines the pH sensitivity of the pacemaker channel HCN2. J Biol Chem 276:6313-6319, 2001.
32. Biel M, Schneider A, Wahl C: Cardiac HCN channels: Structure, function, and modulation. Trends Cardiovasc Med 12:206-212, 2002.
33. Xue T, Marban E, Li RA: Dominant-negative suppression of HCN1- and HCN2-encoded pacemaker currents by an engineered HCN1 construct: Insights into structure-function relationships and multimerization. Circ Res 90:1267-1273, 2002.
34. Proenza C, Tran N, Angoli D, et al: Different roles for the cyclic nucleotide binding domain and amino terminus in assembly and expression of hyperpolarization-activated, cyclic nucleotide–gated channels. J Biol Chem 277:29634-29642, 2002.
35. Tran N, Proenza C, Macri V, et al: A conserved domain in the NH2 terminus important for assembly and functional expression of pacemaker channels. J Biol Chem 277:43588-43592, 2002.
36. Herrmann S, Stieber J, Stockl G, et al: HCN4 provides a 'depolarization reserve' and is not required for heart rate acceleration in mice. EMBO J 26:4423-4432, 2007.
37. Chen S, Wang J, Siegelbaum SA: Properties of hyperpolarization-activated pacemaker current defined by coassembly of HCN1 and HCN2 subunits and basal modulation by cyclic nucleotide. J Gen Physiol 117:491-504, 2001.
38. Much B, Wahl-Schott C, Zong X, et al: Role of subunit heteromerization and N-linked glycosylation in the formation of functional hyperpolarization-activated cyclic nucleotide–gated channels. J Biol Chem 278:43781-43786, 2003.
39. Yu H, Wu J, Potapova I, et al: MinK-related peptide. 1: A beta subunit for the HCN ion channel subunit family enhances expression and speeds activation. Circ Res 88:E84-E87, 2001.
40. Qu J, Kryukova Y, Potapova IA, et al: MiRP1 modulates HCN2 channel expression and gating in cardiac myocytes. J Biol Chem 279:43497-43502, 2004.
41. Shi W, Wymore R, Yu H, et al: Distribution and prevalence of hyperpolarization-activated cation channel (HCN) mRNA expression in cardiac tissues. Circ Res 85:E1-E6, 1999.
42. Han W, Bao W, Wang Z, Nattel S: Comparison of ion-channel subunit expression in canine cardiac Purkinje fibers and ventricular muscle. Circ Res 91:790-797, 2002.
43. Ludwig A, Zong X, Hofmann F, Biel M: Structure and function of cardiac pacemaker channels. Cell Physiol Biochem 9:179-186, 1999.
44. Cerbai E, Sartiani L, DePaoli P, et al: The properties of the pacemaker current I(f) in human ventricular myocytes are modulated by cardiac disease. J Mol Cell Cardiol 33:441-448, 2001.
45. Hoppe UC, Jansen E, Sudkamp M, Beuckelmann DJ: Hyperpolarization-activated inward current in ventricular myocytes from normal and failing human hearts. Circulation 97:55-65, 1998.
46. Cerbai E, Mugelli A: I(f) in non-pacemaker cells: Role and pharmacological implications. Pharmacol Res 53:416-423, 2006.
47. Qu J, Barbuti A, Protas L, et al: HCN2 overexpression in newborn and adult ventricular myocytes: Distinct effects on gating and excitability. Circ Res 89:E8-E14, 2001.
48. Bucchi A, Baruscotti M, DiFrancesco D: Current-dependent block of rabbit sino-atrial node I(f) channels by ivabradine. J Gen Physiol 120:1-13, 2002.
49. Stieber J, Wieland K, Stockl G, et al: Bradycardic and proarrhythmic properties of sinus node inhibitors. Mol Pharmacol 69:1328-1337, 2006.
50. Bucchi A, Tognati A, Milanesi R, et al: Properties of ivabradine-induced block of HCN1 and HCN4 channels. J Physiol 572:335-346, 2006.
51. Stieber J, Herrmann S, Feil S, et al: The hyperpolarization-activated channel HCN4 is required for the generation of pacemaker action potentials in the embryonic heart. Proc Natl Acad Sci U S A 100:15235-15240, 2003.
52. Ludwig A, Budde T, Stieber J, et al: Absence epilepsy and sinus dysrhythmia in mice lacking the pacemaker channel HCN2. EMBO J 22:216-224, 2003.
53. Schulze-Bahr E, Neu A, Friederich P, et al: Pacemaker channel dysfunction in a patient with sinus node disease. J Clin Invest 111:1537-1545, 2003.
54. Ueda K, Nakamura K, Hayashi T, et al: Functional characterization of a trafficking-defective HCN4 mutation, D553N, associated with cardiac arrhythmia. J Biol Chem 279:27194-27198, 2004.
55. Milanesi R, Baruscotti M, Gnecchi-Ruscone T, DiFrancesco D: Familial sinus bradycardia associated with a mutation in the cardiac pacemaker channel. N Engl J Med 354:151-157, 2006.
56. Nof E, Luria D, Brass D, et al: Point mutation in the HCN4 cardiac ion channel pore affecting synthesis, trafficking, and functional expression is associated with familial asymptomatic sinus bradycardia. Circulation 116:463-470, 2007.

Molecular Organization and Regulation of the Cardiac Gap Junction Channel Connexin 43

8

Mario Delmar and Paul Sorgen

CHAPTER OUTLINE

Gap junction channels provide a pathway for direct cell-to-cell communication between adjacent cells. These channels are involved in a number of biologic functions, such as electrical conduction, embryogenesis, and cell growth. The last 50 years have seen significant advances in elucidation of some basic properties of gap junctions such as molecular composition, three-dimensional structure, regulation, single-channel permeability, conductance, and selectivity. At the macroscopic level, several investigators have studied the role of gap junctions in electrical synchrony and arrhythmias. More recently, studies have been aimed at characterizing the interrelation of gap junctions with other molecular partners. The emerging picture is that of a sophisticated network wherein the structure that maintains electrical coupling crosstalks with other molecules involved in electrical excitability, as well as those molecules that maintain mechanical coupling, working together to achieve functional synchrony.

This chapter reviews the structural aspects of cardiac gap junctions, first within the functional-morphological complex where they are hosted—the intercalated disk—and then as elements that are key to the normal function and regulation of the heart.

The Cardiac Intercalated Disk: Structure and Function

The first description of the intercalated disk was in 1866, by Ebhert, who considered this structure to be a homogeneous "cementing material" at cell boundaries between cardiocytes. This view was challenged by the concept that the cardiac muscle was a continuous syncytium with no cell boundaries. It was not until the electron microscopic observations of Sjöstrand and Anderson in 1954 and 1958 that the theory of the anatomic syncytium was replaced by the demonstration that heart muscle cells are individually separated from one another and that the intercalated disk represents a "special differentiation of the sarcoplasm in connection with transversally oriented cell boundaries."[1] The work of these investigators led to the description of the intercalated disk as containing three separate structures, now called desmosomes, adherens junctions, and gap junctions. Reviews of the historical aspects of this work are available in the literature.[1,2] This section presents a brief overview of the general properties of each of these structures.

Gap Junctions

In 1958, Sjöstrand and colleagues described an area of specialization in the cardiac intercalated disk composed of "three dark lines with two intervening less dense lines." This structure, which was similar to the one previously identified in the giant axon of the crayfish, was named the "longitudinal connexion" by these investigators. Years later, Revel coined the term "gap junctions," a designation emphasizing the two key features: a gap between the cells and yet a junction between them (reviewed by Delmar and coworkers[2]).

Gap junctions are involved in a number of biologic functions. Most relevant in the context of this discussion is the fact that gap junctions form intercellular channels that provide a low-resistance pathway for direct cell-to-cell passage of electrical current between cardiac myocytes. Each gap junction channel is composed of two hexameric structures called connexons that dock across the extracellular space and form a permeable pore isolated from the extracellular space. Each connexon results from oligomerization of an integral membrane protein, *connexin*. The most abundant connexin isotype in the heart, brain, and other tissues is the 43-kD protein connexin 43 (Cx43). Excellent reviews on various aspects of gap junctions are available in the literature.[3,4]

The importance of Cx43 in the propagation of the cardiac action potential is well established. If Cx43 channels are not present, normal propagation is disrupted and lethal arrhythmias can ensue.[5,6] The recent observation that gap junctions are significantly diminished in the hearts of patients with Naxos disease and Carvajal syndrome,[7,8] as well as in boxer dogs afflicted with arrhythmogenic right ventricular cardiomyopathy (ARVC),[9] supports the notion that the absence (or reduction) of gap junction plaques may be a key substrate responsible for the high incidence of sudden cardiac death in at least some clinical cases in which the integrity of the intercalated disk is compromised.[8-10]

Adherens Junctions

Adherens junctions are specialized structures essential for the mechanical coupling between neighboring cells. The three morphologically different forms of adherens junctions are *puncta adherentia*, *zonula adherens*, and *fascia adherens*, the last-named corresponding to the morphology commonly found in the cardiac intercalated disk.[11] Cell-cell mechanical anchoring occurs at two crucial points: the extracellular space, within which cadherins tightly bind to each other, and the intracellular space, within which the cytoplasmic end of cadherin is indirectly attached to the actin cytoskeleton. The association between cadherin and the cytoskeleton involves at least two molecular "hinges": Cadherin binds to β-catenin and plakoglobin, and both molecules in turn bind to α-catenin (among others), the latter being in direct contact with actin. This is only a simplified description, however, because other interactions are likely to occur.[12] This string of intermolecular interactions provides mechanical continuity between cells, allowing for the mechanical work of individual myocytes to be integrated into the pumping function of the whole heart.

Desmosomes

The desmosome (*macula adherens*) appears as two parallel tripartite plaques containing an intercellular gap of approximately 30 nm bisected by a distinct line, parallel to the apposed cell membranes.[13] Desmosomes contribute to the mechanical continuity between cardiac cells. Whereas adherens junctions link the actin cytoskeleton of adjacent cells, desmosomes provide continuity to the intermediate filament network (mainly desmin, in the case of heart).[13,14] In the extracellular space, desmosomal cadherins (desmocolins and desmogleins) bind tightly to each other. In the intracellular space, the intermediate filaments bind to desmoplakin. The interaction between desmoplakin and the desmosomal cadherin can be in some cases direct but mostly occurs through their association with plakophilin and plakoglobin.[13,14] The topological organization of desmosomal molecules was studied by North and associates[15] using quantitative immunogold electron microscopy. These investigators localized the amino (N) terminus of desmoplakin within the outer dense plaque and the carboxyl (C) terminus at the site of attachment with the intermediate filament. Plakoglobin was localized together with the C termini of the desmosomal cadherins, and plakophilin-1 was found deep within the outer plaque, near the plasma membrane. Consistent with this map, biochemical evidence has demonstrated that desmoplakin binds to plakophilin through their N-terminal domains,[13,16] whereas desmoplakin binds to the intermediate filament by way of its C-terminal domain.[13]

In their 2001 "News and Views" article, Sarah Hatsell and Pamela Cowin described the desmosome complex as "... a system as staid and solid as the queen's corsets."[14] With that analogy, it is easy to imagine the loss of containment that would follow in its absence. Mice deficient in either plakoglobin, desmoplakin, or plakophilin-2 (PKP2) die during embryonic development as a result of severe myocardial rupture.[17-19] More relevant from the point of view of clinical cardiology, cardiomyopathy in humans has been linked to mutations in desmosomal proteins.[20] In a number of cases, loss of mechanical integrity is associated with severe arrhythmias. This observation led to the hypothesis that normal electrical coupling of cardiac myocytes depends on normal mechanical coupling.[8] Recent studies strongly support this notion.[21,22] The next section reviews some of the recent observations documenting the morphologic and functional integration that occurs between the individual structures of the intercalated disk.

The Intercalated Disk as a Functional Unit

The original description of the intercalated disk identified three structures. Research over the last 50 years supports the notion that rather than being separate entities, these may be three elements of a single functional unit.[23] The dependence of desmosome formation on adherens junctions is well documented.[24] Studies on epithelial cells have shown that cadherin-dependent contact (a "cadherin kiss")[25] is a necessary initial step in cell adhesion. These "puncta" serve as nucleation sites at which other adherens junction plaque components aggregate as a prelude for desmosomal formation.[25] Results from experiments in N-cadherin–deficient mice also show that in the absence of adherens junctions, no desmosomal formation occurs.[26] Additional evidence suggests the reverse process: Under certain experimental conditions, desmosomal disruption can interfere with adherens junction formation. Indeed, Vasioukhin and colleagues have shown that in keratinocytes, cell adhesion formation is interrupted in the absence of desmoplakin.[27] Moreover, cell adhesion can be reestablished by expression of the N-terminal domain of desmoplakin.[27] The question arises of whether desmosomal disruption may prevent gap junction formation, either directly or by interfering with cell adhesion. Recent studies provide the first piece of evidence demonstrating that two main components of these structures, Cx43 and PKP2, associate within the same molecular complex and that absence of one (PKP2) leads to significant remodeling of the other.[22]

Strong evidence shows, on the other hand, that cell-cell adhesion represents an important component of gap junction formation in both cardiac[7] and noncardiac systems.[28,29] In 1990, Musil and associates showed that communication-deficient cells can convert to a communication-competent phenotype by transfection with a complementary DNA (cDNA) encoding E-cadherin.[28] Meyer and associates used Cx43-expressing Novikoff hepatoma cells to show that cell-cell dye transfer could be prevented by Fab fragments of antibodies against N-cadherin.[29] The laboratory of Cecilia Lo also showed that coupling was significantly reduced in cells from the cardiac neural crest of mouse embryos deficient in N-cadherin.[30] More recently, Kosteskii and Li and their coworkers demonstrated that conditional knockout of N-cadherin leads to significant loss of cardiac gap junctions and the consequent development of severe ventricular arrhythmias.[26,31]

Although data have accumulated on the dependence of gap junctions on cell-cell adhesion, evidence regarding whether the integrity of the desmosome itself is relevant to cardiac gap junction structure and function in the heart is less clear. In their 1997 study of the developmental changes in intercalated disk proteins, Angst and colleagues showed that significantly higher levels of N-cadherin and desmoplakin at the cell termini preceded the co-localization of Cx43.[32] In 1999, Kostin and coworkers reported results of a study in which they followed the time course of reassembly of intercellular junctions after dissociation of adult rat cardiac myocytes.[33] These investigators observed a "temporal intermingling" of the reassembling of adherens junctions and desmosomes, with the subsequent development of gap junctions. They concluded that the formation of mechanical junctions was a prerequisite for gap junction formation. They were not able to establish the relative importance of desmosomes versus adherens junctions, however.

More specific to desmosomal integrity is the study by Grossman and colleagues, who characterized the structure of the intercalated disk in embryonic mouse hearts lacking PKP2.[17] Their results showed that in the absence of PKP2, fascia adherens–like and desmosome-like structures were difficult to distinguish. These investigators postulated an overall reduction "in the architectural stability of the intercalated disc." They did not characterize either the gap junction structure or the abundance and distribution of Cx43. Yet, given the overall importance of cell adhesion on gap junction formation, it is reasonable to speculate that the absence of PKP2 may have affected the integrity of the gap junction plaques. Recent results strongly support the latter hypothesis.[22]

Of interest, although gap junction formation and function seem to be dependent on the presence of mechanical coupling, the integrity of adherens junctions or desmosomes is not affected by the absence of Cx43. A case in point is the study by Gutstein and coworkers[34] showing that the expression and localization of several intercalated disk proteins in the mouse heart were not altered by the absence of Cx43 expression. This finding suggests

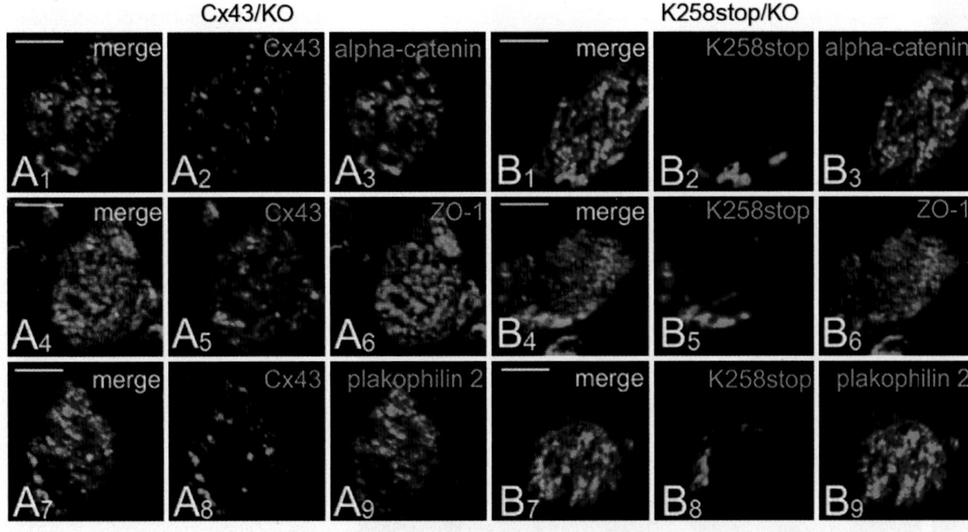

Figure 8-1 En face confocal microscopic images of cardiac intercalated disk obtained from mice expressing either connexin 43 (Cx43) or a Cx43 mutant lacking the carboxyl-terminal (regulatory) domain. Note the intermingling of proteins in the case of the mice expressing the full-length protein *(left)* and the segregation of Cx43 from other components of the disk in those cases in which the C-terminal domain (CT) has been truncated from Cx43 *(right)*. KO, knockout. Images in panels A and B obtained from murine hearts expressing either wild-type Cx43 (A panels, Cx43/KO) or the truncated form (B panels, K258stop/KO) (From Maass K, Shibayama J, Chase S, et al: Truncation of connexin43 changes number, size and localization of cardiac gap junction plaques. Circ Res 101:1283-1291, 2007.)

that the systems are not completely interdependent. Although functional gap junctions require mechanical integrity, the intercellular communication provided by gap junctions is not a requirement for the formation of mechanical coupling.

Although gap junctions are not a necessary requirement for mechanical coupling, disruption of connexin integrity does affect the intermolecular interactions that take place within the intercalated disk. Indeed, the studies by Maass and coworkers[35] show that loss of the C-terminal domain of Cx43 (which acts as the regulatory domain of the protein) causes a change in the morphologic features of the cardiac gap junctions. In this instance, the number of gap junction plaques within the intercalated disk is reduced, although the size of each plaque is increased. Moreover, other intercalated disk proteins are segregated from their characteristic position. Figure 8-1 shows confocal immunofluorescence microscopy images from this study. The pictures on the left correspond to the localization of Cx43 (green) and other intercalated disk proteins (red) in a heart obtained from mice expressing Cx43. The images on the right are of structures in the heart of a mouse in which the Cx43 gene was replaced with a construct coding for a Cx43 protein lacking the C-terminal domain. (For reasons of viability, heterozygous mice—null in one allele—were used as control animals.) The control images show the characteristic alternating pattern of staining. Loss of the C-terminal domain, on the other hand, caused significant segregation of the structures, where mechanical junction proteins clustered together and apart from the zone occupied by Cx43 (see the report by Maass and coworkers[35] for further details). The functional consequences of this segregation remain to be determined. The data do show that intermolecular interactions within the intercalated disk, involving Cx43, determine the ultimate morphology of the overall structure.

The original description of the intercalated disk was based on its morphologic features at the electron microscopic level. Yet as an organelle, the intercalated disk seems to include other molecular complexes that also are fundamental to the success of intercellular synchrony. A case in point is that of the sodium channel complex. Recent observations suggest that some $Na_V1.x$ channel proteins, as well as some of their β subunits, reside at the sites of end-to-end cell apposition and physically interact with Cx43.[36] This observation further strengthens the view of the intercalated disk not as a collection of molecules that localize to the same place in the cell while ignoring each other, but rather more like a highly specialized subcellular organelle, in which different components interact with each other to achieve a synchronized function. Just as the mitochondria, or the endoplasmic reticulum, or the Golgi apparatus, are molecular collections embedded in membranous structures that work together to achieve a certain function, so the intercalated disk acts as the specialized structure that accomplishes a fundamental function for the survival of the heart: electromechanical communication between neighboring cells.

More than 50 years since the original studies of Weidmann showed electrotonic propagation in the heart, a high-resolution structural and molecular picture of intercellular communication has begun to emerge. The following section focuses on the high-resolution molecular structure of the connexin molecules.

Molecular Structure of Connexin 43

The advent of molecular cloning led to the identification of the genes that code for gap junction proteins and allowed for a correlation between the primary sequence of gap junctions and their function and molecular identity. Yet a number of functional domains conserve similar high-order structures, although the level of amino acid identity is very limited. A step forward in elucidating the intimate mechanisms of molecular function requires identification of the secondary and tertiary structures of the domains involved. Recently, a significant effort has been placed in identifying the high-order structures of connexin domains. In this section, general aspects of the functional relevance of Cx43 are presented first, followed by a summary of recent and current efforts aimed at further elucidation of its structure and function.

Hydropathy and topological studies originally predicted that a connexin subunit traverses the membrane four times (transmembrane domains M1 to M4), with both the C terminus and the N terminus projecting into the cytoplasmic space. Two extracellular loops, E_1 and E_2, provide continuity between domains M1 and M2 and between M3 and M4, respectively whereas the region between M2 and M3 (the "cytoplasmic loop" [CL]) also is located in the intracellular space.

Separate investigations have aimed at characterizing the high-order structure of the gap junction channel. Early studies showed that a connexin hemichannel has a six-fold symmetry, with a pore in the center.[37,38] The initial observations were

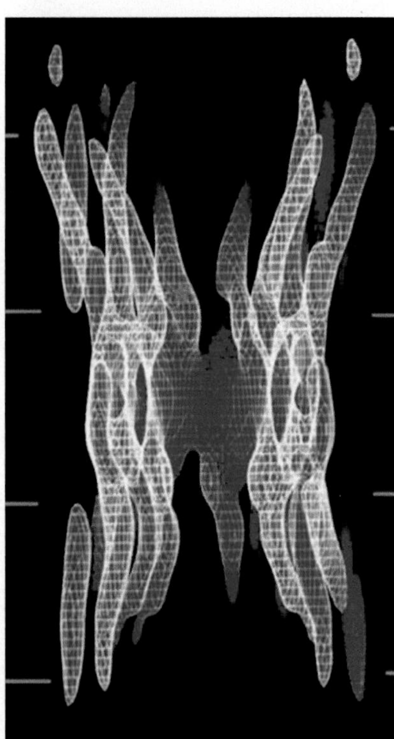

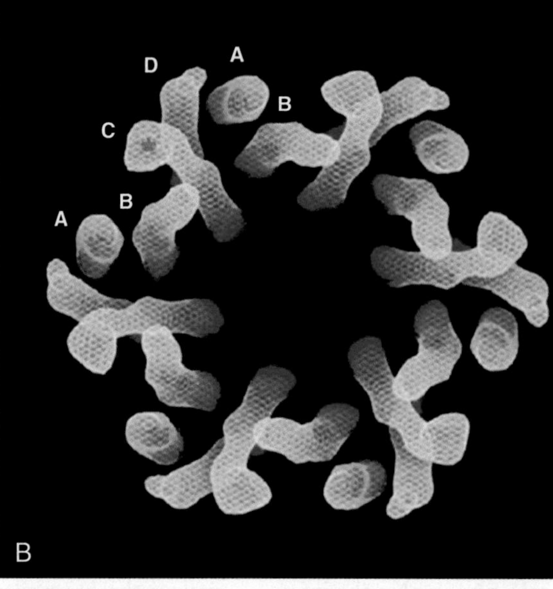

Figure 8-2 Ultrastructure of the connexin 43 (Cx43) channel determined by electron crystallography. The resolution was 75 nm in the membrane plane and 210 nm in the vertical direction. **A,** Side view of the entire channel. The *red lines* represent the lipid bilayers. The *red asterisk* indicates the point at which the pore diameter is estimated to be the smallest. **B,** View from the cytoplasmic side. The channel is formed by six repeats of four identifiable densities (A to D), each density corresponding to one transmembrane domain. (From Unger VM, Kumar NM, Gilula NB, Yeager M: Three-dimensional structure of a recombinant gap junction membrane channel. Science 283:1176-1180, 1999, with permission.)

confirmed and expanded in several subsequent studies.[39-41] A major step forward came from the work of Unger and colleagues.[42] These investigators used electron crystallography to solve the three-dimensional structure of gap junction channels formed by Cx43 subunits that lacked the C-terminal domain. The assembled gap junction channels were observed at a resolution of 7.5 Å in the membrane plane and 21 Å in the vertical direction. The study clearly showed the electron densities corresponding to 24 transmembrane domains in α-helical order. As shown in Figure 8-2, these 24 transmembrane α helices are organized as six repeats of four transmembrane domains (labeled A to D), consistent with the notion that a connexon is formed by the oligomerization of six connexins, each with four transmembrane domains. The images from Unger and colleagues' study further revealed that the pore narrows from 40 Å to 15 Å at the boundary with the extracellular gap. This narrowing (initially proposed by the low-angle x-ray diffraction analysis of Makowski and colleagues[43] and also suggested by the data of Unwin and Zampighi[44]) is due to the tilting of the channel-lining transmembrane domain (labeled C in the right panel of Fig. 8-2). Whether the pore structure revealed by the images of Unger's group[42] corresponds to that of an open or a closed channel remains to be determined. The accompanying data published by these investigators[42] further showed that the C helix extends beyond the putative boundary of the bilayer and into the cytoplasm. If this C domain corresponds to the third transmembrane domain (see later on), a possible conclusion is that the second half of the cytoplasmic loop also is an α helix, which conforms part of the vestibule of the pore. The latter concept would be consistent with observations of this domain using nuclear magnetic resonance techniques[45] and with the functional mapping of this area.[46]

The landmark paper of Unger and colleagues[42] provided a fundamental framework for understanding the gap junction pore from a structural point of view. Of note, however, the investigators needed to truncate the C terminus of Cx43 in order to achieve an adequate view of the pore-forming region. Hence, with the exception of a small fragment of the cytoplasmic loop, intracellular regions were not characterized within this structure. Additional work has shown that the C-terminal domain is mostly a random coil, although two well-defined areas of α-helicity have been described.[47] Moreover, changes in the pH of the solvent causes dimerization of the C-terminal domain,[48] which may be a relevant step in the regulation of Cx43 by intracellular factors such as low pH.[49]

Correlating the Primary Sequence with the High-Order Structure of the Channel Pore

The correlation between the structure of the pore as solved by electron cryo-crystallography and the domains of connexin as identified topologically has been difficult. Which transmembrane domain in the primary sequence (M1 to M4) corresponds to which transmembrane domain in the structure (A to D)? (See Fig. 8-2.) The answer to this question remains elusive, despite extensive research in this area. A recent excellent critical review of this subject is highly recommended for the interested reader.[50] In this publication, Yeager and Harris cite the different studies implicating regions in N-terminal, M1, E_1, and M3 as pore-lining domains. These investigators also address possible methodologic and functional aspects that may possibly underlie the lack of convergence of all available data.

In a recent study, Fleishman and associates[51] used data from an improved cryoelectron microscopy map (resolution of 5.7 Å

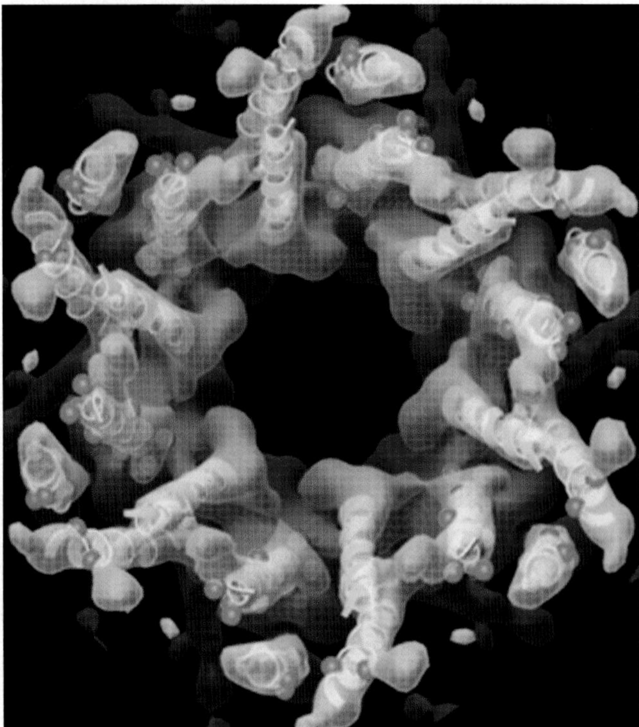

Figure 8-3 Molecular model of a connexon (a hemichannel). The constraints obtained from the three-dimensional cryoelectron micrograph map of Unger and coworkers[42] are shown in *blue*. α-Helical domains (*yellow*) are fitted within the electron density map with the following assignments: M1 = B, M2 = A, M3 = C, and M4 = D, where M1 to M4 are the primary sequence transmembrane domains of a connexon and the letters A to D correspond to the electron density assignments described by Unger and colleagues[42] (see assignments A-D in Figure 8-2). *Red spheres* identify the predicted location of amino acids that, when mutated, result in diseases such as Charcot-Marie-Tooth disease. (From Yeager M, Harris AL: Gap junction channel structure in the early 21st century: Facts and fantasies. Curr Opin Cell Biol 19:1-6, 2007; adapted from Fleishman SJ, Unger VM, Yeager M, Ben-Tal N: A C-alpha model for the transmembrane alpha-helices of gap junction intercellular channels. Mol Cell 15:879-888, 2004.)

in the plane of the membrane and 19.8 Å in the vertical direction) to model the different α-helical domains within a connexon. These workers took into consideration the relative spatial locations of conserved and variable residues within the connexin family, as well as some of the functional data available, to predict the correspondence between primary sequence and three-dimensional electron density maps. The results, presented in Figure 8-3, are consistent with the notion that the C helix (as assigned by Unger's group)[42] is indeed the third transmembrane domain, and helices A, B, and D would correspond to M2, M1, and M4, respectively. Further data will be necessary to confirm these assignments. An important point is that the structural data represent a snapshot of what is, on the other hand, a dynamic, functional channel that is subject to regulation by a variety of factors in the cellular space. The next section describes structural data relevant to the regulation of gap junction channels. Although some of the cited studies have been conducted in connexin 26 (Cx26), which is not found in the heart, significant conservation in the structure and function of connexins has been observed, so conclusions obtained from one connexin may be cautiously applied to others.

Connexin Structure during Gap Junction Regulation

Obtaining suitable three-dimensional crystals for oligomerized connexins remains a major hurdle to achieving a high-resolution structure of gap junctions. Electron crystallography, cryoelectron microscopy, and atomic force microscopy (AFM) offer alternative approaches (albeit of lower resolution) to the determination of membrane protein structures without the need for the generation of three-dimensional crystals. Over the past few years, the laboratories of Sosinsky and Lal and their associates have taken advantage of these methods to provide novel insight into how chemical mediators of gap junction regulation (e.g., Ca^{2+} and pH) affect the structure of Cx43 and Cx26 channels and hemichannels. Some of these results are outlined next.

In a recent study, the Sosinsky laboratory used AFM to image the conformational changes of the cytoplasmic and extracellular surfaces of native Cx26 gap junction plaques in response to changes in calcium concentration.[52] Calcium has long been postulated to play a crucial role in the gating of gap junction intercellular communication by decreasing or suppressing electrical coupling. In the absence of calcium, the cytoplasmic domains formed a hexameric pore (with inner diameter of 2.8 nm) protruding 1.7 nm from the membrane bilayer, which exhibited a high degree of structural flexibility. Similar to the cytoplasmic domains, the extracellular connexon surface formed a hexameric pore, exhibiting an inner diameter of 1.5 nm, that protruded 1.6 nm from the lipid bilayer (Fig. 8-4A). When the extracellular hemichannel surface was imaged in the presence of calcium (0.5 mM), the entrance narrowed significantly as evident in the reduced pore size (from 1.5 to 0.6 nm) (see Fig. 8-4B). The conformational change was fully reversible and specific among other divalent cations tested (e.g., magnesium). The conformational change did not alter the height, nor did it cause a rotation of the extracellular domains. Calcium also had a profound but different effect on the cytoplasmic surface, inducing the formation of microdomains and an increase in the plaque height. The cytoplasmic surface was too flexible, however, to be imaged at sufficiently high resolution to assign structural changes. These observations, together with the differences in intracellular and extracellular hemichannel sensitivity to calcium concentrations (intracellular, μM range; extracellular, mM range), support the idea that the gating mechanism for channel closure at the extracellular surface differs from the one that operates at the cytoplasmic surface.

AFM also has been used to examine the three-dimensional molecular surface topology of nontruncated Cx43 hemichannels reconstituted in lipid membranes.[53] In this study, the investigators concluded that the extracellular surface reaches a height of 1.3 nm from the membrane plane, whereas the intracellular surface rises to a height of 4.7 nm. Using this model, they explored the conformational modifications that result from changes in the concentration of calcium at the mouth of the channel. In calcium-free buffer, AFM images of the extracellular face showed a well-defined doughnut-like structure consisting of six subunits and a central pore-like depression. The pore diameter was 2.5 nm, with a depth of 0.8 nm. This pore size was not changed in the presence of magnesium or nickel; however, 73% and 26% of the channels showed a pore diameter reduction (to 1.8 nm) at calcium concentrations of 1.4 and 1 mM, respectively. The results suggested that the channel pore can occupy two states, one open (pore diameter of 2.5 nm) and one closed (pore diameter of 1.8 nm), and that the preferred state is a function of the concentration of calcium. It is worth noting that the open and closed channel diameters (2.5 and 1.8 nm) were similar to those predicted from the electron

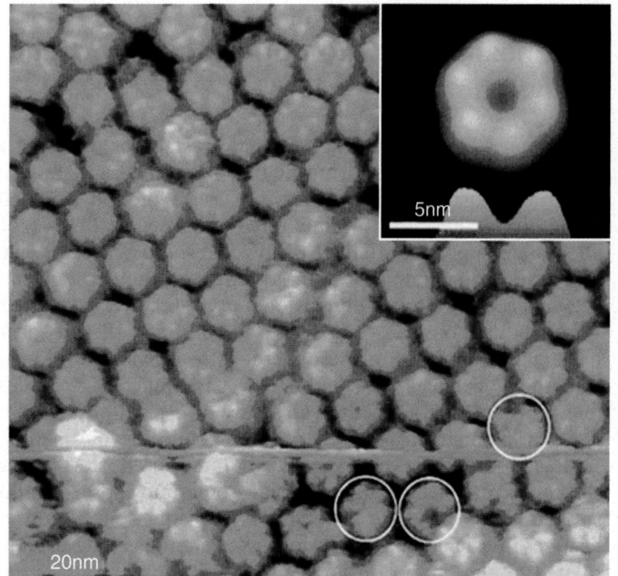

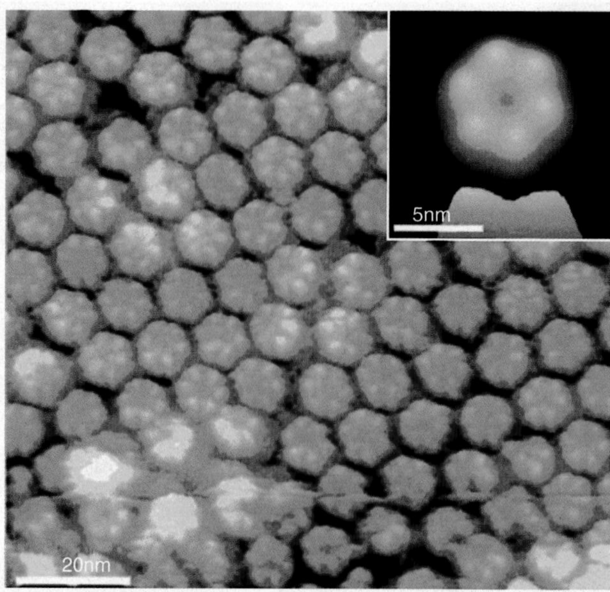

Figure 8-4 Conformational changes in connexin 26 (Cx26) hemichannels observed in low- and high-calcium buffers by atomic force microscopy (AFM). **A,** AFM topograph showing the extracellular connexon surface imaged in a calcium-free buffer solution. Individual connexons exhibit defects in the number of subunits, as indicated by the *circles*. **B,** Same connexon surface imaged in **A,** but in the presence of 0.5 mM calcium. *Inset,* The channel diameter has changed significantly, as seen in the correlation-averaged *top view* and the profile at the *bottom*. All images were displayed as relief tilted by 5 degrees. (Adapted by permissions from Macmillan Publishers Ltd: Muller DJ, Hand GM, Engel A, Sosinsky GE: Conformational changes in surface structures of isolated connexin 26 gap junctions. EMBO J 21:3598-3607, 2002.)

microscopy study by Unger's group[42] but quite different from the open and closed diameters for isolated Cx26 gap junction channels (1.5 nm to 0.6 nm).[52] Also, Muller and associates[52] showed that Cx26 hemichannels closed at a lower calcium concentration than that observed for Cx43 hemichannels (0.5 and 1.8 mM, respectively), suggesting that this difference in calcium sensitivity may be related to the functional differences between the two hemichannels.

A different mechanism underlying Cx26 channel closure was observed in response to alterations in pH.[54] High-resolution imaging by AFM of Cx26 hemichannels revealed that the pore was closed in response to acidification, but only in the presence of an aminosulfonate buffer (e.g., HEPES). The overall diameter of the hexameric hemichannel did not change, yet the depth of the channel decreased concomitant with an increase in the width of the connexon lobes under the more acidic conditions. For example, at pH 7.6, the channel entrance diameter was 1.7 nm, whereas at pH 6.0, the diameter was 0.6 nm, with approximately 6.5 degrees of rotation in the hemichannel lobes. These results support the model of a physical gate close to the extracellular surface, because not only does the pore diameter decrease on acidification, but also its depth is shallower.

More recently, the Sosinsky laboratory has reported the electron crystallographic structure of a human Cx26 mutant (M34A).[55] This point mutation has been linked to cases of prelingual nonsyndromic hereditary deafness. Of interest, although the Cx26 mutant was purified as a hemichannel, during the crystallization process, full Cx26 gap junction channels were formed, suggesting that hydrophobic interactions in the extracellular domains drive hemichannels to redock into full-length gap junctions. The three-dimensional structure of this channel was determined at a resolution of 100 nm in the *x-y* plane, which allowed fitting of the density to the four transmembrane helices (Fig. 8-5A). The results showed strong similarity between the structure of the Cx26M34A mutant and that of the Cx43 truncation mutant previously studied by Unger and colleagues.[42] The three-dimensional structure of Cx26M34A also displayed a prominent density in the pore of each hemichannel, suggesting that a plug physically blocks the channel within the membrane (see Fig. 8-5B). This result is consistent with the notion of regulation of connexin channels by intramolecular interactions that involve cytoplasmic domains (a "particle-receptor" or "ball-and-chain-like" model; see the report by Delmar and coworkers[56]). In the case of the Cx26 channel, the most likely candidate was thought to be the N-terminal domain, whereas functional studies suggest that in Cx43, the C-terminal domain acts as the regulatory unit.[56]

In this regard, the recent work of Lal and colleagues is of interest.[57] These investigators used AFM-based single-molecule spectroscopy with antibody-modified AFM tips to examine the flexibility of the Cx43 C-terminal domain. They surmised that if the C-terminal domain acts as a gating particle, it should be a flexible domain that can move to open or close the channel. To explore this possibility, they used Cx43 antibodies targeted to the C-terminal domain (anti-$CT_{252\text{-}270}$ or anti-$CT_{360\text{-}382}$ [CT = C-terminal]). The antibodies were connected to the AFM tip with a flexible polyethylene glycol (PEG) spacer and were presented to Cx43 hemichannels reconstituted in a lipid bilayer. A large extension (approximately 105 nm) was detected when Cx43 interacted with anti-$CT_{360\text{-}382}$. The anti-$CT_{252\text{-}270}$–Cx43 interaction caused a shorter extension (approximately 57 nm)—an expected result, given that the site of interaction was located in the middle portion of the flexible Cx43 C-terminal domain. Moreover, an increase in the calcium concentration in the medium (to 1.8 mM) significantly decreased the occurrence of the C-terminal–antibody interactions, which may have resulted from conformational changes in the Cx43 C-terminal domain, leading to steric hindrance effects that prevented binding. This finding is consistent with studies from the laboratory of

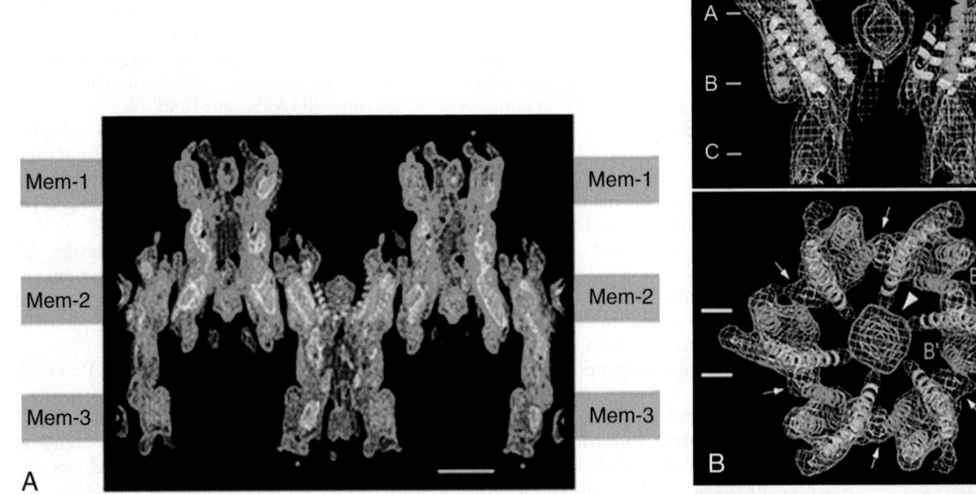

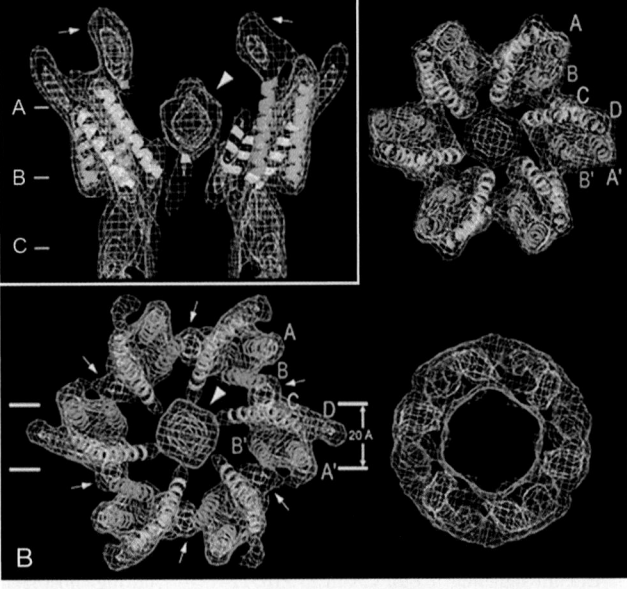

Figure 8-5 Structural details of the Cx26 gap junction. **A**, View of the Cx26 density map perpendicular to the membrane plane. The three membranes, indicated by the gray bars, surround two extracellular gap regions. **B**, (inset) 20 Å-thick section perpendicular to the membrane plane through the density map of a hemichannel from Mem-2 in panel A. The arrowhead and white arrows represent the plug and the inner cytoplasmic protrusions from helices B and C, respectively. A-C, Slabs through the density map corresponding to the lines shown in inset. The four helices are labeled A-D. (Adapted from Oshima A, Tani K, Hiroaki Y, et al: Three-dimensional structure of a human connexin26 gap junction channel reveals a plug in the vestibule. Proc Natl Acad Sci U S A 104:10034-10039, 2007. Copyright 2007, National Academy of Sciences, U S A.)

Sorgen and coworkers showing that residues 376 to 379 (i.e., within the region covered by the $CT_{360-382}$ antibody) are involved in the interaction with the Cx43 cytoplasmic loop domain under low-pH conditions.[49] Taken together, the stretch length, the presence of antibody–C-terminal domain interactions at 0 mM calcium, and the lack of such interaction at 1.8 mM calcium support the model of the Cx43 C-terminal domain acting as a gating particle to regulate the channels.

Conclusions and Future Directions

This chapter summarizes some of the key findings in the search for an understanding of the structure and function of the cardiac gap junction channel.[1] Of course, any attempt to review the literature carries the risk of omission. To cite all of the authors who have contributed to this field would be impossible. Accordingly, only some names were selected for inclusion here, although certainly the work of many others is of equal importance. For this necessary "minimization" of the relevant literature, we apologize in advance.

It has been more than 50 years since the demonstration of electrotonic propagation in the heart by Silvio Weidmann, and the first microscopic observations of gap junctions by Sjöstrand, with Andersson in 1954 and with others in 1958. Today, the ultrastructural resolution reaches the level of the molecule, so current understanding of function expands to the whole organ lacking the gene. Much has been learned, and much more remains to be answered. As technology and science progress, a higher resolution of structural details, along with an integration of the information obtained through different methods, is likely. Furthermore, the field of gap junctions may be approaching a stage at which targeted, structure-based drug design may be possible. This may allow for a significant step forward in elucidation of the specific functional consequences of gap junction channel gating both in health and in disease.

References

1. Sjostrand, Anderson-Cedergen: Intercalated discs of heart muscle. In Bourne GH (ed): The Structure and Function of Muscle. New York, Academic Press, 1960.
2. Delmar M, Duffy HS, Soren PL, et al: Molecular organization and regulation of the cardaic gap junction channel connexin43. In Zipes DP, Jalife J (eds): Cardiac Electrophysiology: From Cell to Bedside, 4th ed. Philadelphia, Saunders, 2004, pp 66-76.
3. Harris AL: Emerging issues of connexin channels: Biophysics fills the gap. Q Rev Biophys 34:325-472, 2001.
4. Harris AL, Locke D: Gap Junctions. Secaucus, NJ, Humana Press, in press.
5. Danik SB, Liu F, Zhang J, et al: Modulation of cardiac gap junction expression and arrhythmic susceptibility. Circ Res 95:1035-1041, 2004.
6. Yao JA, Gutstein DE, Liu F, et al: Cell coupling between ventricular myocyte pairs from connexin43-deficient murine hearts. Circ Res 93:736-743, 2003.
7. Kaplan SR, Gard JJ, Protonotarios N, et al: Remodeling of myocyte gap junctions in arrhythmogenic right ventricular cardiomyopathy due to a deletion in plakoglobin (Naxos disease). Heart Rhythm 1:3-11, 2004.
8. Kaplan SR, Gard JJ, Carvajal-Huerta L, et al: Structural and molecular pathology of the heart in carvajal syndrome. Cardiovasc Pathol 13:26-32, 2004.
9. Basso C, Fox PR, Meurs KM, et al: Arrhythmogenic right ventricular cardiomyopathy causing sudden cardiac death in boxer dogs: A new animal model of human disease. Circulation 109:1180-1185, 2004.
10. Saffitz JE: Dependence of electrical coupling on mechanical coupling in cardiac myocytes. In Thiene G, Pessina AC (eds): Advances in Cardiovascular Medicine.

Padua, Italy, Universita degli Studi di Padova, 2003, pp 15-28.
11. Gottardi CJ, Niessen CM, Gumbiner BM: The adherens junction. In Beckerle MC (ed): Cell Adhesion, 1st ed. Oxford, Oxford University Press, 2001, pp 259-287.
12. Gates J, Peifer M: Can 1000 reviews be wrong? Actin, alpha-catenin, and adherens junctions. Cell 123:769-772, 2005.
13. Bannon LJ, Goldfinger LE, Jones JCR, Green KJ: Desmosomes and hemidesmosomes. In Beckerle MC (ed): Cell Adhesion, 1st ed. Oxford, Oxford University Press, 2001, pp 324-368.
14. Hatsell S, Cowin P: Deconstructing desmoplakin. Nat Cell Biol 3:E270-E272, 2001.
15. North AJ, Bardsley WG, Hyam J, et al: Molecular map of the desmosomal plaque. J Cell Sci 112:4325-4336, 1999.
16. Chen X, Bonne S, Hatzfeld M, et al: Protein binding and functional characterization of plakophilin 2. Evidence for its diverse roles in desmosomes and beta-catenin signaling. J Biol Chem 277:10512-10522, 2002.
17. Grossmann KS, Grund C, Huelsken J, et al: Requirement of plakophilin 2 for heart morphogenesis and cardiac junction formation. J Cell Biol 167:149-160, 2004.
18. Gallicano GI, Kouklis P, Bauer C, et al: Desmoplakin is required early in development for assembly of desmosomes and cytoskeletal linkage. J Cell Biol 143: 2009-2022, 1998.
19. Ruiz P, Brinkmann V, Ledermann B, et al: Targeted mutation of plakoglobin in mice reveals essential functions of desmosomes in the embryonic heart. J Cell Biol 135:215-225, 1996.
20. Sen-Chowdhry S, Syrris P, McKenna WJ: Genetics of right ventricular cardiomyopathy. J Cardiovasc Electrophysiol 16: 927-935, 2005.
21. Oxford EM, Everitt M, Coombs W, et al: Molecular composition of the intercalated disc in a spontaneous canine animal model of arrhythmogenic right ventricular dysplasia/cardiomyopathy. Heart Rhythm 4:1196-1205, 2007.
22. Oxford EM, Musa H, Maass K, et al: Connexin43 remodeling caused by inhibition of Plakophilin-2 expression in cardiac cells. Circ Res 101:703-711, 2007.
23. Delmar M: The intercalated disk as a single functional unit. Heart Rhythm 1:12-13, 2004.
24. Gumbiner B, Stevenson B, Grimaldi A: The role of the cell adhesion molecule uvomorulin in the formation and maintenance of the epithelial junctional complex. J Cell Biol 107:1575-1587, 1988.
25. Vasioukhin V, Bauer C, Yin M, Fuchs E: Directed actin polymerization is the driving force for epithelial cell-cell adhesion. Cell 100:209-219, 2000.
26. Kostetskii I, Li J, Xiong Y, et al: Induced deletion of the N-cadherin gene in the heart leads to dissolution of the intercalated disc structure. Circ Res 96:346-354, 2005.
27. Vasioukhin V, Bowers E, Bauer C, et al: Desmoplakin is essential in epidermal sheet formation. Nat Cell Biol 3: 1076-1085, 2001.
28. Musil LS, Cunningham BA, Edelman GM, Goodenough DA: Differential phosphorylation of the gap junction protein connexin43 in junctional communication-competent and -deficient cell lines. J Cell Biol 111:2077-2088, 1990.
29. Meyer RA, Laird DW, Revel JP, Johnson RG: Inhibition of gap junction and adherens junction assembly by connexin and A-CAM antibodies. J Cell Biol 119: 179-189, 1992.
30. Xu X, Li WE, Huang GY, et al: Modulation of mouse neural crest cell motility by N-cadherin and connexin 43 gap junctions. J Cell Biol 154:217-230, 2001.
31. Li J, Patel VV, Kostetskii I, et al: Cardiac-specific loss of N-cadherin leads to alteration in connexins with conduction slowing and arrhythmogenesis. Circ Res 97:474-481, 2005.
32. Angst BD, Khan LU, Severs NJ, et al: Dissociated spatial patterning of gap junctions and cell adhesion junctions during postnatal differentiation of ventricular myocardium. Circ Res 80:88-94, 1997.
33. Kostin S, Hein S, Bauer EP, Schaper J: Spatiotemporal development and distribution of intercellular junctions in adult rat cardiomyocytes in culture. Circ Res 85:154-167, 1999.
34. Gutstein DE, Liu FY, Meyers MB, et al: The organization of adherens junctions and desmosomes at the cardiac intercalated disc is independent of gap junctions. J Cell Sci 116:875-885, 2003.
35. Maass K, Shibayama J, Chase S, et al: Truncation of connexin43 changes number, size and localization of cardiac gap junction plaques. Circ Res 101:1283-1291, 2007.
36. Malhotra JD, Thyagarajan V, Chen C, Isom LL: Tyrosine-phosphorylated and nonphosphorylated sodium channel beta1 subunits are differentially localized in cardiac myocytes. J Biol Chem 279: 40748-40754, 2004.
37. Makowski L: Structural domains in gap junctions: Implications for the control of intercellular communication. In Bennett MVL, Spray DC (eds): Gap Junctions. Cold Spring Harbor, NY, Cold Spring Harbor Laboratory Press, 1985, pp 5-12.
38. Zampighi GA, Simon SA: The structure of gap junctions as revealed by electron microscopy. In Bennett MVL, Spray DC (eds): Gap Junctions. Cold Spring Harbor, NY, Cold Spring Harbor Laboratory Press, 1985, pp 13-22.
39. Tibbitts TT, Caspar DL, Phillips WC, Goodenough DA: Diffraction diagnosis of protein folding in gap junction connexons. Biophys J 57:1025-1036, 1990.
40. Hoh JH, Lal R, John SA, et al: Atomic force microscopy and dissection of gap junctions. Science 253:1405-1408, 1991.
41. Hoh JH, Sosinsky GE, Revel JP, Hansma PK: Structure of the extracellular surface of the gap junction by atomic force microscopy. Biophys J 65:149-163, 1993.
42. Unger VM, Kumar NM, Gilula NB, Yeager M: Three-dimensional structure of a recombinant gap junction membrane channel. Science 283:1176-1180, 1999.
43. Makowski L, Caspar DLD, Phillips WC, Goodenough DA: Gap junction structures. II. Analysis of the X-ray diffraction data. J Cell Biol 74:629-645, 1977.
44. Unwin PN, Zampighi G: Structure of the junction between communicating cells. Nature 283:545-549, 1980.
45. Duffy HS, Sorgen P, Girvin M, et al: pH-dependent intramolecular binding and structure involving Cx43 cytoplasmic domains. J Biol Chem 277:36706-36714, 2002.
46. Shibayama J, Gutierrez C, Gonzalez D, et al: Effect of charge substitutions at residue his142 on voltage gating of connexin43 channels. Biophys J 91:4054-4063, 2006.
47. Sorgen PL, Duffy HS, Sahoo P, et al: Structural changes in the carboxyl terminus of the gap junction protein connexin43 indicates signaling between binding domains for c-Src and zonula occludens-1. J Biol Chem 279:54695-54701, 2004.
48. Sorgen PL, Duffy HS, Spray DC, Delmar M: pH-dependent dimerization of the carboxyl terminal domain of Cx43. Biophys J 87:574-581, 2004.
49. Hirst B, Sahoo P, Kieken F, et al: Characterization of the pH-dependent interaction between the gap junction protein connexin43 carboxyl terminal and cytoplasmic loop domains. J Biol Chem 282:5801-5813, 2007.
50. Yeager M, Harris AL: Gap junction channel structure in the early 21st century: Facts and fantasies. Curr Opin Cell Biol 19:1-6, 2007.
51. Fleishman SJ, Unger VM, Yeager M, Ben-Tal N: A C-alpha model for the transmembrane alpha-helices of gap junction intercellular channels. Mol Cell 15: 879-888, 2004.
52. Muller DJ, Hand GM, Engel A, Sosinsky GE: Conformational changes in surface structures of isolated connexin 26 gap junctions. EMBO J 21:3598-3607, 2002.
53. Thimm J, Mechler A, Lin H, et al: Calcium-dependent open/closed conformations and interfacial energy maps of reconstituted hemichannels. J Biol Chem 280:10646-10654, 2005.
54. Yu J, Bippes CA, Hand GM, et al: Aminosulfonate modulated pH-induced conformational changes in connexin26 hemichannels. J Biol Chem 282: 8895-8904, 2007.
55. Oshima A, Tani K, Hiroaki Y, et al: Three-dimensional structure of a human connexin26 gap junction channel reveals a plug in the vestibule. Proc Natl Acad Sci U S A 104:10034-10039, 2007.
56. Delmar M, Coombs W, Sorgen P, et al: Structural bases for the regulation of connexin43 channels. Cardiovasc Res 62: 268-275, 2004.
57. Liu F, Arce FT, Ramachandran S, Lal R: Nanomechanics of hemichannel conformations: connexin flexibility underlying channel opening and closing. J Biol Chem 281:23207-23217, 2006.

Biophysics of Cardiac Ion Channel Function

PART II

Biophysics of Normal and Abnormal Cardiac Sodium Channel Function

9

PRAKASH C. VISWANATHAN AND JEFFREY R. BALSER

CHAPTER OUTLINE

Voltage-gated sodium channels are transmembrane proteins responsible for the rapid upstroke of the cardiac action potential and therefore underlie impulse conduction through much of the myocardium. Thus, sodium channels are key molecular substrates in both inherited and acquired disorders of cardiac excitability. Ongoing efforts to reconcile emerging sodium channel structural data with assays revealing insights into biophysical function are forming a framework for the development of more precise interventions to modify cardiac excitability and to treat disorders of cardiac rhythm.

The availability of detailed crystal structures for pore-forming regions of potassium channels is increasing,[1] and structural data are now becoming available for small segments of the sodium channel.[2,3] While these static structures emerge, dynamic analyses are providing detailed functional models that explain how these large, pore-forming proteins drastically change their structural conformation on a submillisecond time scale in response to the membrane electrical field—a process termed *gating*. As genomic strategies increasingly link disorders in electrical excitability to cardiac sodium channel mutations, functional studies of the "diseased" channels reveal unique pathologic gating defects. Of note, both the salutary and the toxic effects of antiarrhythmic drugs hinge critically on the dynamic features of sodium channel gating, so progress in drug design will require integration of both static and dynamic sodium channel structure.

This chapter presents an emerging view of normal and abnormal cardiac sodium channel gating function. The chapter content draws on the detailed discussion of sodium channel structure and permeation in Chapter 1 and develops more fully the structure-function relationships relating to dynamic channel function, to prepare for later discussion of the mechanisms of arrhythmogenesis due to inherited sodium channel mutations (Chapter 50), as well as the molecular pharmacology of sodium channel–blocking agents (Chapter 16). The discussion and citations are selective; the reader is referred to more thorough treatments of related topics, including sodium channel regulation by second messengers and enzymes, details of cation permeation, and modulation by auxiliary subunits.[4-7]

Salary support was provided by the National Institutes of Health (Grant R01 GM56307) and The James Tayloe Gwathmey Physician-Scientist Chair.

FAST GATING PROCESSES: A SYMPHONY OF STRUCTURE AND FUNCTION

Our understanding of how sodium channel structure relates to gating function has escalated with cloning and expression of the channel protein. The tetrodotoxin-"insensitive" human cardiac sodium channel ($Na_V1.5$), encoded by the gene *SCN5A*, is composed of a principal (α) subunit that includes four homologous domains numbered I through IV (Fig. 9-1A), each with six transmembrane α-helical segments, S1 to S6, of which S4 bears several positive charges comprising either arginine or lysine residues. The four domains, attached to one another by cytoplasmic linker sequences, wrap around a central pore such that the pore (P) loops (SS1 and SS2) between S5 and S6 of each domain form part of the pore lining. Over the past 2 decades, site-directed mutagenesis has been used, along with patch clamp electrophysiologic measurements and amino acid fluorescence labeling methods, to define the location and motion of specific

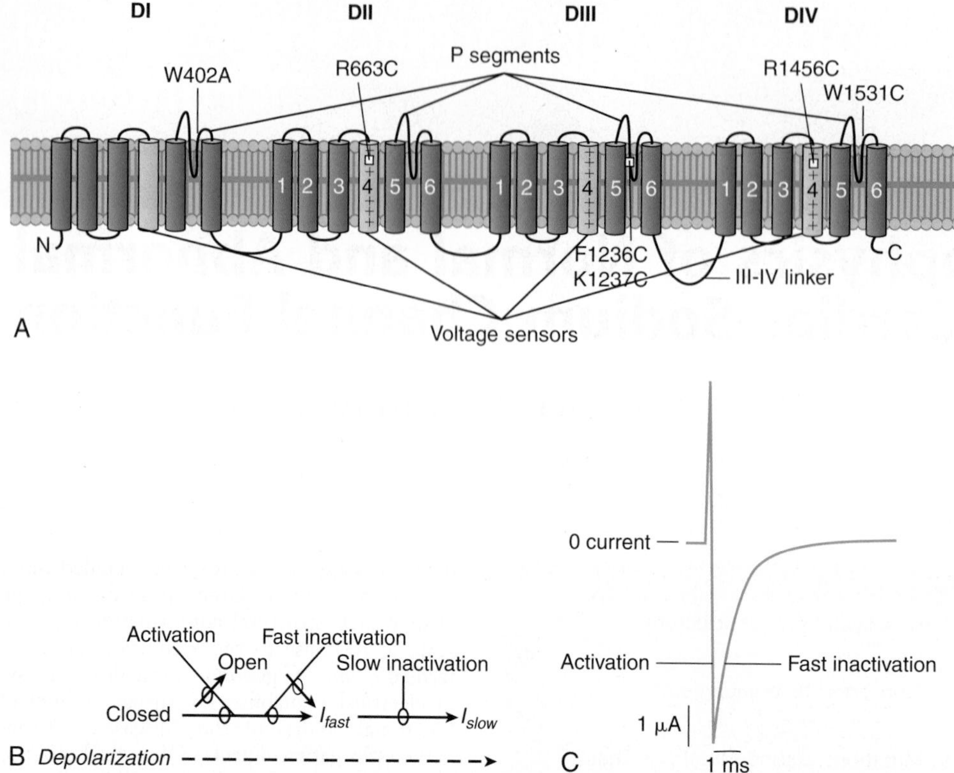

Figure 9-1 Sodium channels. **A,** Topology of the voltage-gated sodium channel. The S4 segments in each of the four homologous domains (DI to DIV) contain positively charged lysine and arginine residues that detect changes in the transmembrane field. The S5-S6 linker sequences are P segments that line the outer pore. The III-IV linker plays a major role in fast inactivation. Individual amino acid residues discussed in the chapter are numbered according to the original rat skeletal muscle clone.[8] C = carboxyl terminus; N = amino terminus. **B,** Simplified scheme of the sodium channel gating conformational changes in response to membrane depolarization. Activation and fast inactivation occur nearly simultaneously, such that channels sometimes reach the fast inactivated state (I_{fast}) without opening (closed-state inactivation). Sustained depolarization induces channels to occupy stable, slow inactivated states (I_{slow}). **C,** Whole-cell current recorded from a cultured (HEK293) cell expressing recombinant human cardiac sodium channels. The current was elicited by a sudden depolarization, analogous to the stimulus of a cardiac action potential. Note that the current rapidly increases (coincident with activation gating) and then decays as channels undergo fast inactivation.

amino acid residues during voltage-dependent gating function.[5,8]

The fundamental properties of sodium channels that enable them to carry out their physiologic roles are illustrated in Figure 9-1B, which shows the principal gated states occupied by sodium channels as the cell membrane is depolarized. On depolarization, channels undergo a process termed *activation*, involving the concerted, outward movement of all four charged S4 segments (see Fig. 9-1A), leading to opening of the channel pore.[9] At nearly the same time, depolarization initiates fast inactivation (see Fig. 9-1B), a distinct form of channel closure that also depends on outward movement of the S4 sensors, but primarily those in domains III and IV (D3S4 and D4S4, respectively; this notation is used throughout the chapter).[8,10] In addition to outward motion of the S4 segments, a critical structure in fast inactivation is the III-IV linker (see Fig. 9-1A), which may function as a "lid" that occludes the inner pore.[11] A triplet of hydrophobic residues (IFM) near the center of the III-IV linker (see Fig. 9-1A) may comprise a "latch" that holds the lid in a closed position over the inner pore.[3] The docking site for the lid consists of multiple regions, including the cytoplasmic linkers connecting segments 4 and 5 (S4-S5) in domains III and IV and the cytoplasmic end of the S6 segment in domain IV.[12,13]

Fast inactivation is, on average, slightly delayed relative to activation. This delay has two consequences. First, it allows time for a transient inward sodium current to pass before the channel closes (see Fig. 9-1C). Second, although a majority of sodium channels open before inactivating, a smaller but significant percentage actually inactivate without ever opening (see Fig. 9-1B). This latter process, denoted *closed-state inactivation*, has been identified as a fundamental gating process that critically distinguishes cardiac sodium channels from other sodium channel isoforms. Both neuronal and skeletal muscle sodium channels exhibit far less closed-state inactivation at potentials close to the normal cardiac resting potential. Moreover, closed-state inactivation is modified by inherited mutations associated with congenital arrhythmia syndromes and modifies the action of antiarrhythmic compounds when channels are modified by mutations (discussed later).[14,15]

What is the relationship between outward motion of the charged S4 segments and pore closure during fast inactivation? Studies of gating current, produced by the movement of charged arginine residues through the membrane electric field, are providing new insights into the relationship between S4 motion and the inactivation lid. Gating currents are slowed or "immobilized" by fast inactivation, suggesting the possibility that binding of the III-IV linker may lock the S4 sensors in an outward position. Recent studies, hoever, indicate that the D4S4 gating charge is immobilized by inactivation, independent of whether the III-IV linker lid is bound,[16] suggesting that other domains may function during fast inactivation to immobilize the gating charge.

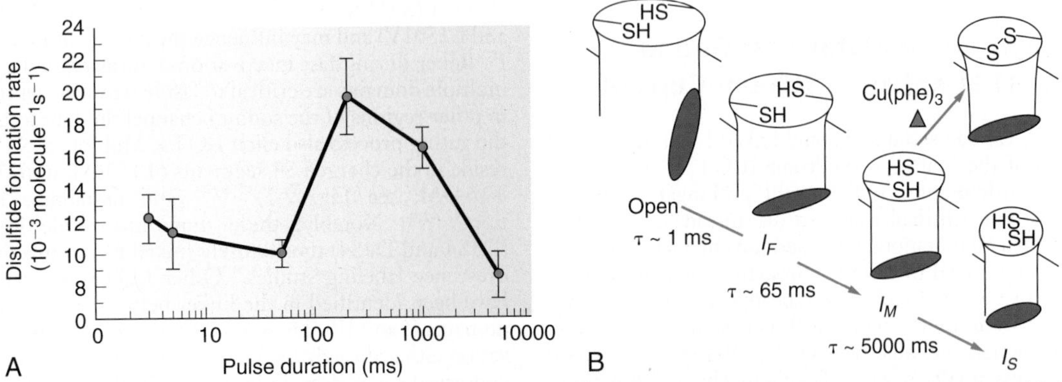

Figure 9-2 Disulfide bond formation in the outer pore catalyzed by 100 μM copper phenanthroline (Cu(phe)$_3$). **A,** Sodium current was generated in *Xenopus* oocytes expressing K1237C-W1531C channels at a pulse rate of 0.05 Hz. The rate at which sodium current decreased reflected the rate of interdomain disulfide bond formation *(ordinate)*. Changing the pulse duration *(abscissa)* from 3 ms to 5000 ms altered the rate of bond formation: Disulfide bond formation was greatest at intermediate pulse widths. **B,** The diagram illustrates sequential occupancy of three inactivated states (fast, intermediate, and slow—I_F, I_M, and I_S) as the length of the depolarization is extended. Time constants for entry into the three inactivated states were derived from experimental protocols[23] and from the literature.[30] The scheme suggests that when the intermediate I_M state is occupied, the 1237 and 1531 cysteines are spatially optimized for disulfide bond formation. (Modified from Benitah JP, Chen Z, Balser J, et al: Molecular dynamics of the sodium channel pore vary with gating: Interactions between P segment motions and inactivation. J Neurosci 19:1577-1585, 1999.)

Several mutations that cause long QT syndrome by destabilizing fast inactivation have been localized to the carboxyl (C) terminus.[17,18] Using mathematical modeling and circular dichroism measurements, Cormier and coworkers identified six α-helical segments in the proximal half of the C terminus.[2] Deletion of the sixth helical segment destabilized fast inactivation implicating the proximal C terminus as an essential cofactor in the fast inactivation mechanism.[2] Furthermore, multiple sequence alignments, homology modeling, and biophysical data have revealed the presence of EF-hand motifs in the proximal part of the C terminus.[19] EF-hands are helix-loop-helix motifs that typically bind to calcium in the loops between the helices and provide a means for calcium-dependent regulation of the protein containing the EF-hand. Binding of Ca^{2+} to this EF-hand motif was found to affect channel function by inducing a depolarizing shift in the voltage dependence of channel availability. These studies provide not only strong support for the role of calcium in modulating sodium channel inactivation but also evidence that serves as a basis for understanding why genetic mutations in this region lead to dramatic changes in channel function, probably by influencing calcium dependence.

Slow Inactivation: A Concerted Rearrangement in the Pore

Whereas fast inactivated sodium channels recover rapidly (within 10 ms) during the hyperpolarized interval between stimuli, on prolonged depolarization, sodium channels progressively enter slow inactivated states; collectively, these states are referred to as I_S (see Fig. 9-1B). These more stable, nonconducting states have diverse lifetimes ranging from hundreds of milliseconds to many seconds.[20,21] An intermediate kinetic component of slow inactivation (I_M) develops in cardiac sodium channels with a time course relevant to the duration of the cardiac action potential (hundreds of milliseconds).[17,22] Although fast inactivation seems primarily to involve cytoplasmic structures, both site-directed mutations and chimeric analyses suggest a key role for the *P segments* in slow inactivation.[23-26] These linker sequences between the S5 and S6 segments in each domain bend back into the membrane and line the outer pore (see Fig. 9-1A).

In potassium channels, slow C-type inactivation involves a dynamic rearrangement of the P segments[27] that critically alters the characteristics of the permeation pathway.[28] Studies of outer pore residues in the sodium channel during slow inactivation also reveal a dynamic picture,[29,30] suggesting an analogy between C-type inactivation in potassium channels and slow inactivation in sodium channels.[24] A channel engineered to include P segment cysteine substitutions across the pore in domains III and IV (Fig. 9-2; see also Fig. 9-1A, K1237C-W1531C) forms an internal disulfide bond that occludes the pore when it is exposed to oxidizing catalysts.[29] Disulfide bond formation was dependent on channel depolarization, and the reaction was most rapid with depolarizations of intermediate length (200 ms) (see Fig. 9-2A), suggesting that the two P segment cysteinyls are approximated more closely in the I_M inactivated state than in either the fast inactivated (I_F) or slower inactivated (I_S) state (see Fig. 9-2B).[24] The emerging view of the sodium channel pore incorporates a high degree of conformational flexibility during both gating and permeation and may even suggest analogies between sodium channels and enzymes.[31]

Just as the S4 segments "transduce" the membrane potential to the fast inactivation gating structures, the D4S4 sensor seems to have an analogous role in slow inactivation. Here again, structure-function motifs in the potassium channel parallel those in the sodium channel. Recent studies using patch clamp recording and voltage clamp fluorometry reveal that the potassium channel outer pore interacts directly with the S4 voltage sensor during slow (C-type) inactivation.[32] In sodium channels, slow inactivation gating is amplified by sulfhydryl modification of a cysteine engineered at the third outermost arginine residue in D4S4 (R1456C; see Fig. 9-1A).[33] This effect was antagonized by alanine substitution in the domain I P segment (W402A) (see Fig. 9-1A),[33] a substitution known to inhibit the I_M component of slow inactivation.[34] Hence, a consistent theme that encompasses both fast and slow gating is the linkage between the initial voltage-sensing motion of the S4 segments, leading to the ensemble motion of several gating structures that operate over a range of time scales to enable, and then disable, Na^+ permeation through the pore.

Long QT Syndrome Mutations: Gating Mutations That Enhance Sodium Current

Mutations in the cardiac sodium channel linked to an autosomal dominant form of the long QT syndrome (LQT3)[35] (Fig. 9-3) produce electrocardiographic QT interval prolongation and a peculiar polymorphic ventricular tachycardia (torsade de pointes). To date, more than 50 mutations in the sodium channel gene have been identified and linked to LQT3. These mutations invariably disrupt fast inactivation[36-38] and allow repeated reopening during sustained depolarization, evoking a small, persistent sodium current during the action potential plateau (Fig. 9-4A). This excess inward current, essentially a gain of sodium channel function, delays cellular repolarization and predisposes patients to polymorphic ventricular tachycardia. Surprisingly, the size of this sustained current is miniscule (approximately 0.5% to 2%) compared with the peak sodium current that develops immediately on depolarization.[18,37,38] Nonetheless, linkage among this sustained current, action potential prolongation, and proarrhythmic activity has been validated in quantitative modeling[39] illustrating the highly nonlinear relationship between sodium channel function and cardiac excitability. Although a majority of the mutations destabilize fast inactivation, others lead to gain of function by modifying gating processes such as voltage-dependence of activation or inactivation or recovery from inactivation. The net effect of these gating changes, however, is always a gain of sodium channel function.

Consistent with the role of the III-IV linker in fast inactivation, the first reported LQT3 mutation was a deletion of three residues in this region (1505 to 1507 ΔKPQ; see Fig. 9-3).[36] At least seven other mutations reside near the cytoplasmic face of the channel (S941N, A997S, D1114N, N1325S, A1330P, DK1500, and L1501V) and may influence the motion or binding of the III-IV linker during fast inactivation. Consistent with the view that multiple domains are critical to fast inactivation gating, mutations in other regions of the sodium channel thought to be essential to the gating process also elicit LQT3. Multiple SCN5A mutations reside in the charged S4 segments (T1304M, R1623Q, R1644H, T1645M; see Fig. 9-3)[37,40,41] and destabilize fast inactivation.[37,42,43] Notably, these mutations reside in the sensors (D3S4 and D4S4) most closely linked to fast inactivation in fluorescence labeling studies.[8] Other LQT3-associated mutations have been identified in the linker between domains I and II and domains II and III. These mutations probably modify fast inactivation either directly or through allosteric mechanisms. A highly conserved acidic domain in the proximal C terminus also harbors a number of LQT3 mutations (see Fig. 9-3), consistent with the emerging role of this region in the fast inactivation gating described earlier. The structural mechanism whereby the C terminus influences fast inactivation remains uncertain; studies of multiple simultaneous charge neutralizations in the C terminus do not elicit a more severe or additive effect,[18] suggesting that this acidic region may not participate in fast inactivation as a large, charged particle. Support for this concept has come from recent studies that demonstrate an interaction between the proximal C terminus and the domain III-IV linker.[44] Mutations in the C terminus that disrupt this interaction enhance channel reopening, leading to gain of function and long QT syndrome. Additionally, molecular modeling has identified two EF-hand motifs in the proximal C terminus that binds to calcium (see Fig. 9-6).[19] Mutations within this motif reduce Ca^{2+} affinity and alter inactivation properties, revealing a molecular basis for the long QT mutations that occur in this key region of the sodium channel.

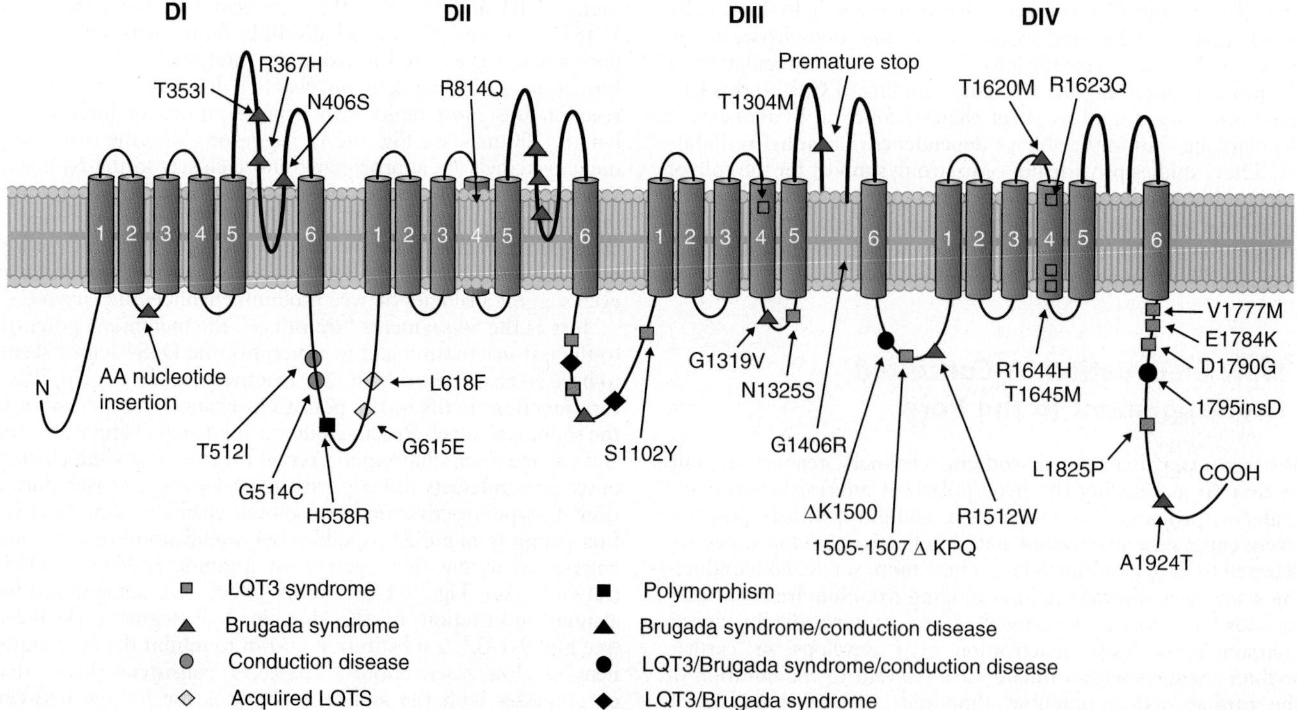

Figure 9-3 Inherited mutations in the cardiac sodium channel. The topology of the sodium channel is shown in the same style as Figure 9-1 and indicates mutations, discussed in the text (numbering follows the human cardiac sodium channel, $Na_V1.5$), linked to the long QT syndrome and Brugada syndrome. The mutations shown represent only a small subset of the SCN5A mutations linked to these inherited syndromes. Mutations tend to cluster in and around the S4 segments, the cytoplasmic linkers, the C terminus, and the P loops, consistent with the important roles of these loci in channel gating.

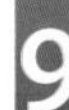

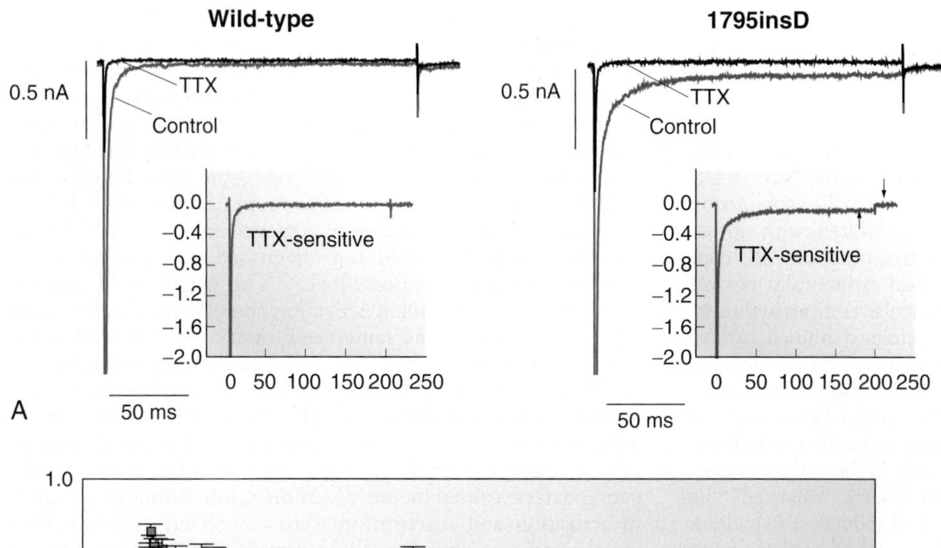

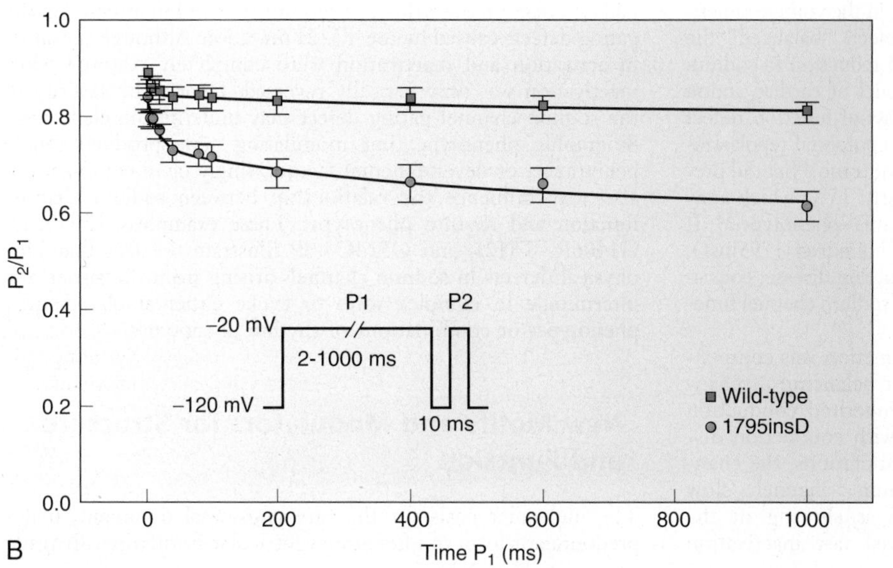

Figure 9-4 A mutation in the C terminus alters two gating processes and provokes LQT3 and Brugada syndrome.[17] **A,** Similar to other LQT3 mutations, the 1795insD mutation induces a sustained component of inward current. *Insets* show the tetrodotoxin (TTX)-sensitive current (30 μM), obtained by subtraction, with a significantly larger TTX-sensitive persistent current *(left, arrows)* for the mutant. **B,** An enhanced slow kinetic component of inactivation also was seen in 1795insD. Development of slow inactivation was evaluated using the voltage clamp protocol (see inset), whereby channels were depolarized for variable time intervals (P_1) and then allowed to recover for 10 ms from fast inactivation but not from slow inactivation. The remaining sodium current stimulated by the P_2 pulse reflects the extent of intermediate (I_M) slow inactivation induced in the P1 pulse. The mutation increased the magnitude of the slow inactivation component. (Modified from Veldkamp MW, Viswanathan PC, Bezzina C, et al: Two distinct congenital arrhythmias evoked by a multidysfunctional Na^+ channel. Circ Res 86:E91-E97, 2000.)

Brugada Syndrome: Gating Mutations That Reduce Sodium Current

The origin of a distinct class of idiopathic ventricular arrhythmias, collectively known as *Brugada syndrome*,[45] can be traced to recently identified SCN5A mutations. Unlike patients with the LQT3, patients with this condition manifest distinctive electrocardiographic features that include right bundle branch block and elevation of the ST segment in leads V1 to V3 and experience idiopathic ventricular tachycardia and fibrillation. The full scope of cellular and ion channel biophysical mechanisms that underlie Brugada syndrome are discussed in detail in Chapters 50 and 68; however, a consistent theme that has emerged is that Brugada syndrome mutations, in contrast with LQT3 mutations, elicit a loss of sodium channel function.

Further insight into the linkage between loss and gain of function and these diverse arrhythmia syndromes has resulted from analysis of a large kindred in which affected persons manifest heart rate–dependent features of both LQT3 and Brugada syndrome: The QT interval is prolonged at slow heart rates, and distinctive ST segment elevations occur with exercise.[17,46] Consistent with the notion that LQT3 is elicited by a gain of function and Brugada syndrome by loss of function, the C-terminal mutation, 1795insD, has opposite effects on the two distinct kinetic components of sodium channel inactivation (fast and slow).[17] Like many other LQT3 mutations, 1795insD disrupts fast inactivation, causing sustained sodium current throughout the action potential plateau (see Fig. 9-4A), which prolongs cardiac repolarization at slow heart rates. At the same time, 1795insD augments the intermediate kinetic component of slow inactivation (see Fig. 9-4B; denoted I_M in Fig. 9-2). This gating effect slows the recovery of sodium channels between stimuli, causing loss of function mainly at rapid heart rates (consistent with the 1795insD clinical phenotype)[17] attributable to the relatively brief diastolic interval during tachycardia. Studies of the Brugada syndrome–associated mutations, G1406R, G1319V, T1620M, and D1714G, also reveal, in addition to other loss-of-function features, enhancement of the I_M component of slow inactivation.[47-50] It is noteworthy that studies of sodium channel gating function in myocytes isolated from the epicardial border zone of the 5-day infarcted canine heart reveal a delay in recovery from inactivation that resembles enhanced slow (I_M) inactivation and is consistent with the postrepolarization refractoriness seen in that model.[51] Taken together, these results suggest that enhanced sodium channel slow inactivation is a proarrhythmic biophysical mechanism that deserves detailed evaluation in more common, acquired forms of sudden cardiac death, such as cardiac ischemia.

Cardiac Conduction Disease: A Biophysical Compromise?

Not all SCN5A mutations that evoke loss of function elicit Brugada syndrome. A Dutch family carrying a mutation in the $Na_V1.5$ I-II linker (G514C) (see Fig. 9-3) exhibited isolated cardiac conduction disease requiring pacemaker therapy in two children, with slowed conduction throughout the myocardium (atria, ventricles, and conduction system).[52] All family members had structurally normal hearts and exhibited no tendency for ventricular tachyarrhythmias. Patch clamp studies of heterologously expressed human cardiac sodium channels ($Na_V1.5$) mutated to include G514C revealed changes in the voltage dependence of sodium channel activation (stronger depolarizations required to open channels) that mirrored the loss-of-function defects associated with other Brugada mutations.[53] However, a parallel depolarizing shift in the voltage dependence of inactivation (a gain-of-function defect) "balanced" the primary activation defect, causing the overall reduction in sodium current to be small. In a computational model of cardiac action potential conduction (Fig. 9-5), this mild loss-of-function defect was not sufficient to induce the marked action potential repolarization abnormalities associated with Brugada syndrome[53] but did predict myocardial conduction slowing of nearly 15% which may potentially contribute to the bradyarrhythmia phenotype.[52] It should be noted that in the Brugada-LQT3 kindred 1795insD, affected carriers also exhibit features of conduction disease, consistent with a causal relationship between loss of sodium channel function and conduction disease.

Although the G514C-imposed loss of function was compensated for by opposing gating defects, other balancing mechanisms may be operative in this and other inherited conduction disease syndromes. In two other families with conduction disease, associated with G298S and D1595N mutations, the channel mutants exhibited increased sodium channel slow inactivation (a loss of function), as well as slowing of the sodium current decay rate due to delayed fast inactivation (hence, a balancing gain of function).[54] On the other hand, SCN5A mutations identified in two other families with isolated conduction disease would, on the basis of large deleted segments, produce entirely nonfunctional sodium channels.[55] Similarly, members of another large kindred heterozygous for a mutation in the domain III P segment (G1406R) (see Fig. 9-3) that entirely eliminates the expressed I_{Na} included four patients with Brugada syndrome, as well as seven patients who exhibited only conduction disturbance.[50] A novel mutation, T512I, was identified in a 2-year-old boy diagnosed with second-degree atrioventricular conduction block.[56] The mutation, in addition to hyperpolarizing shifts in activation and inactivation, enhanced slow inactivation to the same extent as in the 1795insD mutation. Yet the patient in this case did not exhibit features typical of the Brugada syndrome. Further analysis revealed the existence of a common polymorphism, H558R, also in the sodium channel gene and present in 25% of the population. The polymorphism had no effect on the wild-type sodium current but attenuated the gating defects caused by the T512I mutation. Although the shifts in activation and inactivation were completely restored, slow inactivation was only partially reversed. Hence, the severity of the sodium channel gating defect may underlie the electrocardiographic phenotype, but modulating gene products, allele penetrance, or developmental factors, singly or in combination, also may influence the relationship between sodium channel function and rhythm phenotype. These examples—1795insD, G1406R, T512I, and G514C—all illustrate the fact that biophysical defects in sodium channels arising from mutations can intermingle in complex ways to evoke either single, distinct phenotypes or combinations of rhythm phenotypes.

New Motifs and Modulators for Structure and Function

The molecular basis for the rare autosomal dominant, male-predominant form of idiopathic ventricular fibrillation, Brugada

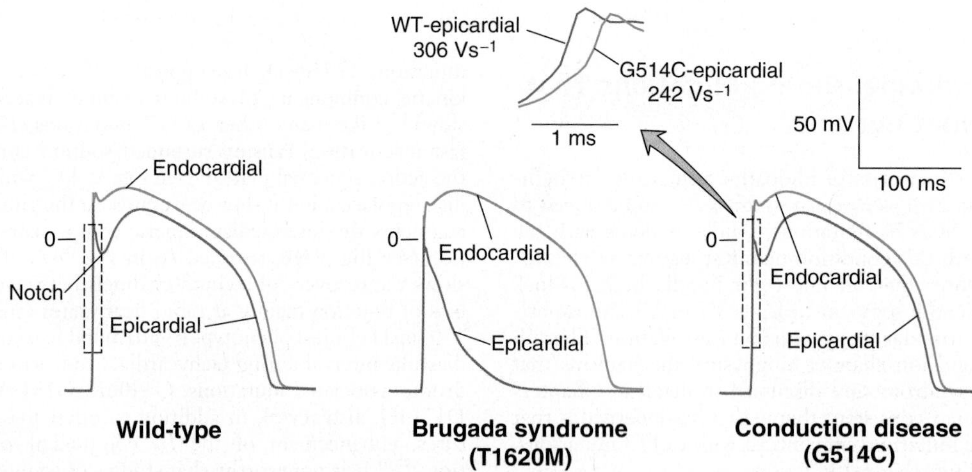

Figure 9-5 Action potentials in a model cardiac cell simulating Brugada syndrome and conduction disease. Endocardial and epicardial action potentials are shown. **Left graph,** Wild-type action potentials, for which the epicardial "notch" resulting from a larger transient potassium current (I_{to}) is indicated. **Middle panel,** T1620M, in which activation gating is compromised but fast inactivation is hastened, causing a marked reduction in sodium current. This results in early repolarization in the epicardium but not the endocardium, with a resultant transmural voltage gradient and Brugada syndrome.[49] **Right panel,** G514C, in which activation is compromised (as with T1620M) but fast inactivation is decreased. The latter effect tends to increase the sodium current and offset the activation defect. The net reduction in sodium current is therefore smaller than that for T1620M, such that the epicardial action potential plateau is maintained, although the action potential upstroke *(dashed boxes)* is delayed. Action potential upstroke (the *dashed boxes* on wild-type and G514C action potentials) is shown on an expanded time base to illustrate that the mutation slows the rate of the action potential upstroke (dV/dt_{max}) and thereby slows myocardial conduction. (From Tan HL, Bink-Boelkens MTE, Bezzina CR, et al: A sodium channel mutation causes isolated cardiac conduction disease. Nature 409:1043-1047, 2001.)

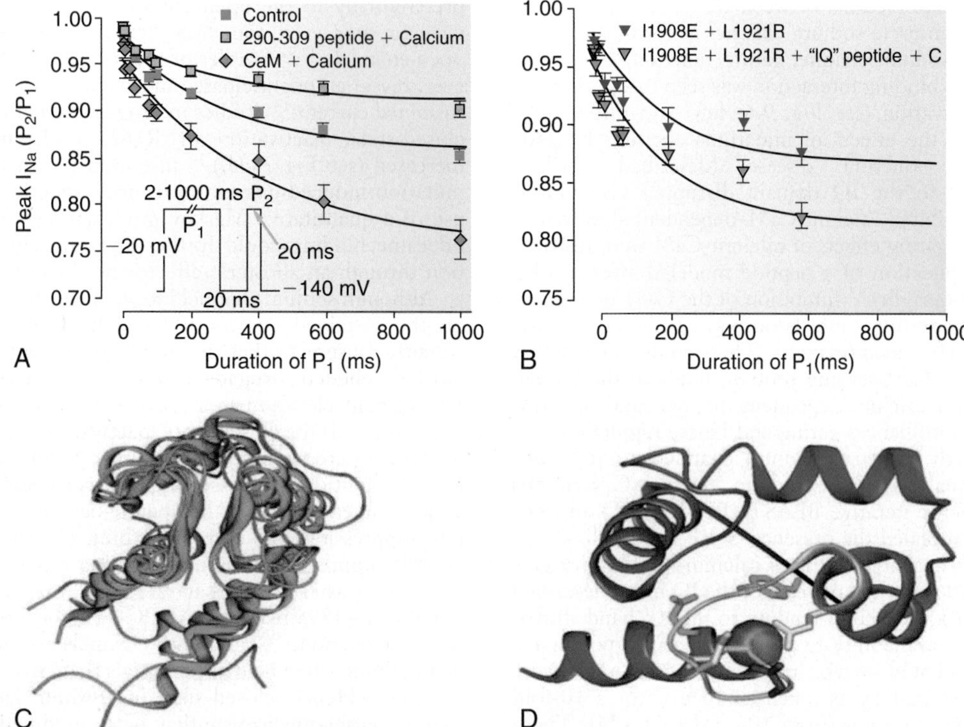

Figure 9-6 Calcium and calmodulin (CaM) kinase modulate cardiac sodium channel. **A,** Slow inactivation was measured in a manner identical to that for Figure 9-4B (see voltage clamp protocol, *inset*) in wild-type cardiac sodium channels expressed in cultured (HEK293) cells. In the presence of intracellular calcium, a CaM kinase peptide inhibitor (290-309 peptide), also exposed intracellularly, inhibited slow inactivation. By contrast, CaM in the presence of calcium increased slow inactivation in a manner similar to that seen with Brugada syndrome mutations. **B,** A mutant $Na_V1.5$ sodium channel with two key residues in the putative carboxyl (C)-terminal "IQ" domain were modified (I1908E + L1921R). This double mutation rendered the channel resistant to CaM-induced slow inactivation *(not shown)*; however, the slow inactivation gating effect of CaM was restored by including a wild-type "IQ" peptide in the intracellular solution *(open inverted triangles)*. **C,** Energy-minimized three-dimensional model of the sodium channel C terminus *(green ribbon)* superimposed on the backbone structure of the calcium-binding proteins *(red)*. **D,** Predicted model for the $Na_V1.5$ proximal C terminus highlighting the features of the EF-hand loop region. The *red* residue represents the long QT syndrome mutation, D1790G. Positions at which mutations elicit arrhythmia phenotypes are shown in *green*. A *translucent cyan sphere* represents the Ca^{2+} ion location in the EF-hand.

syndrome, is still poorly understood. Although more than 80 mutations of the cardiac sodium channel gene (*SCN5A*) at chromosomal locus 3p21 have been identified and linked to Brugada syndrome, these mutations cause only approximately 20% of the Brugada syndrome cases. Using positional cloning, Weiss and coworkers identified a new locus on 3p24 in a large family with Brugada syndrome.[57] Direct sequencing identified a mutation (A280V) in the glycerol-3-phosphate dehydrogenase 1–like (GPD1-L) gene.[58] Compared to wild-type GPD1-L, expression of A280V GPD1-L in HEK cells expressing SCN5A reduced inward sodium currents by approximately 50%. By contrast, A280V GPD1-L had no effect on the current through the skeletal muscle sodium channel or the rapid delayed rectifier potassium channel, HERG. Further analysis revealed that this reduction in sodium current was a result of reduced sodium channel trafficking. The exact mechanism by which GPD1-L reduces the expression of the cardiac sodium current is still unclear, but this instance is the first in which a non–ion channel–related gene has been linked to the Brugada syndrome. Screening for disease-causing mutations has therefore become quite a useful tool for identifying potential interacting and modulating proteins.

Most voltage-gated ion channels consist of a macromolecular complex of proteins, each of which plays a role in modulating the current through the pore-forming subunit. The β subunit of the cardiac sodium channel plays a crucial role in the regulation of sodium current.[59] The β_1 subunit, which is expressed in the heart, increases the functional expression of the sodium current, accelerates channel inactivation, and alters the voltage dependence of activation and inactivation. The extracellular domain of the β_1 subunit is thought to play a role in this modulation. By contrast, the intracellular domain of β_2 subunit has been shown to modulate the gating of cardiac sodium channels, suggesting multiple levels of sodium channel regulation. Subsequently, a number of proteins have been found to interact and regulate the cardiac sodium channel. These include ankyrin proteins, fibroblast growth factor homologous factor 1B, Nedd4-like ubiquitin-protein ligase, syntrophin proteins, and 14-3-3, a member of highly conserved cytosolic acidic proteins expressed in a wide range of organisms and tissues including the heart.[60-62]

Calcium ions (Ca^{2+}) have a fundamental role in cardiac myocyte excitation-contraction coupling, yet mechanisms whereby intracellular Ca^{2+} may directly modulate sodium channel gating function have only recently emerged. Through binding of calcium in a cooperative manner (by way of four E-F hand motifs), calmodulin (CaM) undergoes conformational rearrangements that allow interactions with substrates participating in a wide range of adaptive responses. Calcium-dependent CaM binding to the C terminus of sarcolemmal calcium channels, at a C-terminal locus called an "IQ" domain, allows calcium-dependent inactivation of the channel, providing important feedback control over intracellular Ca^{2+}.[63,64] Voltage-gated sodium channels also contain a putative C-terminal IQ CaM-binding domain.[65]

Specific binding interactions between the C terminus of the cardiac and skeletal muscle sodium channel isoforms and CaM critically influence sodium channel gating function.[66,67] In the cardiac channel, this binding interaction was seen to significantly enhance slow inactivation (see Fig. 9-6, left) and did so in a manner resembling the effects of mutations eliciting Brugada syndrome and conduction disease (described earlier). Mutations targeted to the IQ domain disrupted CaM binding[66,67] and also inhibited calcium-CaM–dependent slow inactivation, whereas the gating effects of calcium-CaM were restored by intracellular application of a peptide modeled after the IQ domain (see Fig. 9-6, right).[67] Inhibition of the CaM-dependent protein kinase had additional effects on $Na_V1.5$ channel gating, independent of CaM overexpression.[66] These studies clarify that CaM, an ubiquitous Ca^{2+}-sensing protein, binds to the human sodium channel in a calcium-dependent manner, and that this binding interaction influences gating and kinase regulation.

Ca^{2+} also directly binds to sodium channels to influence channel gating. Analysis of the sodium channel C terminus using position specific iterative BLAST (PSI-BLAST) and homology modeling revealed the presence of EF-hand helix-loop-helix motifs, which is characteristic of calcium-binding proteins including CaM, 120 residues upstream of the IQ motif described earlier (see Fig. 9-6).[19] Calcium binding to the EF hand shifted the sodium channel availability to more depolarized potentials. The membrane potential at which 50% of the channels were available to open shifted by as much as 10 mV for a 10-fold change in Ca^{2+} concentration (from 100 nM to 1 μM). These effects also were found to be independent of CaM. The LQT3 mutation D1790G, which is located in the EF-hand motif, was found to reduce Ca^{2+} affinity by reducing the calcium-dependent shift in channel availability. An EF-hand knockout (mutant sodium channel lacking the EF-hand calcium-binding residues) completely abolished calcium dependence. Further analysis is required to establish the relative importance of the calcium-mediated effects on sodium channel gating. It is known that oxidative stress during ischemia or infarction reduces sodium channel availability. At the same time, ischemia also inacreases intracellular calcium. Therefore, the depolarizing shift in channel availability with increasing Ca^{2+} level could be a protective mechanism to maintain normal excitation during ischemic conditions. This hypothesis remains to be tested, however.

Inherited Cardiac Arrhythmias Inform Antiarrhythmic Pharmacologic Mechanisms

Whereas the inherited SCN5A mutations provide valuable insights into sodium channel function, these mutant channels also are now proving to be useful as probes to investigate the molecular pharmacology of antiarrhythmic drugs. A full discussion of sodium channel pharmacology is provided in Chapter 16; this section provides examples that illustrate how abnormal sodium channel gating function, manifest in inherited arrhythmia syndromes, may fundamentally affect the consequences of drug therapy.

Sodium channel blockers have been useful in managing patients with LQT3 disorders.[68,69] The binding site for therapeutically active sodium channel blockers, such as lidocaine, has been localized to amino acid residues residing in the cytoplasmic portion of the S6 segment (Fig. 9-7C, left), mainly in domain IV.[70] At the same time, the pathologic sustained currents through LQT3 channels (see Fig. 9-4A) are potently inhibited by lidocaine and its analogues,[37,71] even though these LQT3 mutations (see Fig. 9-3) are distant from the S6 binding locus. Studies of drug action in LQT3 posited that lidocaine may bind preferentially to the open conformation of the LQT3 mutant pore or may even somehow "repair" the fast inactivation of open channels.[42,72] Studies of the R1623Q LQT3 mutant, however, reveal an unanticipated mechanism for lidocaine action on sustained current.[14] Studies in drug-free conditions revealed that closed-state inactivation of R1623Q channels was actually increased (see Fig. 9-1B),[14] in contrast with the more obvious mutation-induced disruption in open-state inactivation.[42] With use of a quantitative Markov model, it was demonstrated that lidocaine binding could further augment closed-state inactivation through an allosteric effector mechanism.[14]

Although sodium channel blockers may have beneficial effects on the sustained current induced by LQT3 mutants, it was recently observed that flecainide, a potent sodium channel blocker, elicited Brugada syndrome–like electrocardiographic ST segment elevation in a number of patients carrying LQT3 mutations.[73] If the closed-state inactivation gating characteristics of R1623Q are recapitulated in other sodium channels carrying LQT3 mutations, the associated pharmacologic sensitivity may at once engender both a therapeutic benefit (from sustained current suppression) and a proarrhythmic risk (due to peak sodium current suppression). In corroborating this result at an in vitro level, it was shown that at least two LQT3 syndrome mutations—1795insD and ΔKPQ—exhibit pronounced closed-state inactivation,[15,74] and both channels exhibit enhanced block by flecainide when held at potentials that favor closed-state inactivation.[15] Hence, closed-state inactivation gating is a sodium channel gating mechanism that, when modified, may profoundly influence the clinical response to drug therapy.

Slow Inactivation and the P Segments: A Mechanism for Local Anesthetic Use Dependence?

Local anesthetics inhibit the current through voltage-dependent sodium channels and are widely used to provide regional anesthesia and to treat disorders of cellular excitability. Although these drugs are clinically important, the detailed mechanisms by which they exert their inhibitory effects on sodium channels are still poorly understood. It has long been observed that sodium current gradually decreases during repetitive trains of action potentials—an effect termed *use dependence*—and that this effect is greatly augmented by sodium channel–blocking drugs. Studies that exploit cysteine labeling of fast inactivating gating structures (i.e., the III-IV linker) have clarified that, contrary to earlier proposals, use dependence does not result from trapping of sodium channels in the fast-inactivated state.[75] Recently, by recording the sodium channel gating currents, it was determined that movement of S4 voltage sensors primarily in domains III and IV is associated with high-affinity lidocaine block.[76] Binding of lidocaine stabilized the S4 segments in an outward, depolarized position. These results suggested that the position of the D3S4 and D4S4 segments promoted the formation of a high-affinity lidocaine-binding site. This effect also was observed in channels lacking fast inactivation, lending support to the studies showing that use dependence does not result from trapping of sodium channels in the fast inactivated states.

At the same time, studies of sodium channel use dependence during a number of interventions (mutations and cation substitutions) that modify slow inactivation[34,77] suggest that slow recovery of channels between depolarizing stimuli may involve an interaction between sodium channel blockers and slow inactivated conformational states. As a more direct test, investigators[78] used an engineered cysteine (F1236C) (see Fig. 9-1A) as a sentinel for slow inactivated motion of P segments and

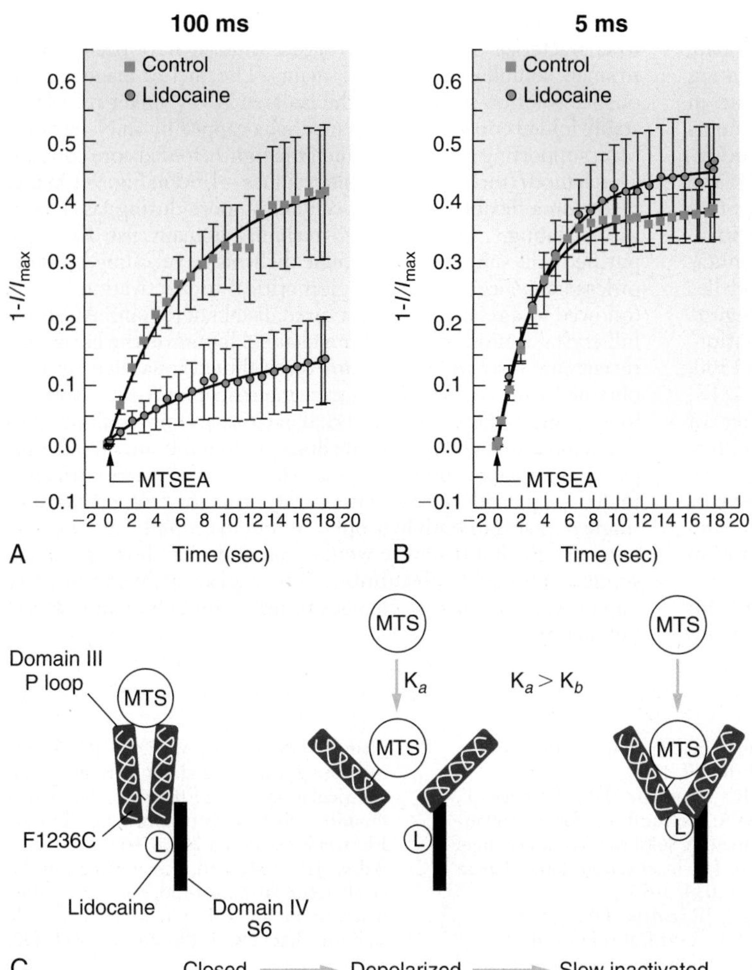

Figure 9-7 Methanethiosulfonate-ethylammonium (MTSEA) modification of F1236C channels is modulated by slow inactivation and use-dependent lidocaine block. **A,** HEK293 cells expressing F1236C channels are exposed to trains of either brief (5-ms) or intermediate-length (100-ms) depolarizations. Peak sodium current (relative to pre-MTSEA) is plotted relative to cumulative depolarization time. In lidocaine-free conditions, MTSEA modification was more rapid when the pulse duration was brief, suggesting that slow inactivation renders the 1236 cysteine less accessible (compare *rising phase* and *solid symbols* in **A** and **B**). In addition, lidocaine (100 μM) markedly reduced the depolarization-dependent MTSEA modification rate when the pulse duration was 100 ms but not 5 ms *(open symbols)*. **C,** A conceptual model of P segment motion and MTS accessibility during slow inactivation and lidocaine (L) block. According to this model, an engineered P loop cysteinyl near the selectivity filter is exposed when channels open but becomes less exposed during slow inactivation, suggesting that this portion of the selectivity filter rearranges during slow inactivation. Lidocaine, when bound to its putative S6 domain receptor on the cytoplasmic side of the selectivity filter, may at the same time stabilize the P segment rearrangement that occurs during slow inactivation, thereby promoting use dependence. (Modified from Ong BH, Tomaselli GF, Balser JR: A structural rearrangement in the sodium channel pore linked to slow inactivation and use dependence. J Gen Physiol 116:653-661, 2000.)

demonstrated state-dependent accessibility of this residue to covalent modification by methanethiosulfonate-ethylammonium (MTSEA). Trains of brief, 5-ms depolarizations sufficient to open and induce fast inactivation of channels (but not to induce slow inactivation) produced more rapid MTSEA modification (see Fig. 9-7B) than did longer (100-ms) pulse widths (see Fig. 9-7A), suggesting that slow inactivation inhibits depolarization-induced MTSEA accessibility of the cysteine side chain (see Fig. 9-7C). Of importance, lidocaine further inhibited the depolarization-dependent sulfhydryl modification induced by these sustained (100-ms) depolarizations, but not by brief (5-ms) depolarizations (see Fig. 9-7A and B). Electrostatic interactions between the adjacent P segment residue (K1237) and the lidocaine amino (N) terminus suggest that S6 residues forming a putative lidocaine receptor lie in proximity to the P segments.[79] Hence, it was postulated that the structural rearrangements associated with slow inactivation move the sodium channel P segments into positions that stabilize the interaction between lidocaine and the pore (see Fig. 9-7C). This was further corroborated by more recent studies that used kinetic differences in the rate of recovery from slow inactivation between two local anesthetic (LA) compounds (lidocaine and bupivacaine) in use-dependent block.[80] The experiments were designed to test whether the kinetic differences correlated with cysteine side chain accessibility in the P loop during gating. Using lidocaine and bupivacaine in a high-speed solution exchange system, it was shown that under identical pulse-train conditions, sulfhydryl protection is conditionally dependent on the degree of use-dependent block. The data suggested that pore conformational changes that alter MTSEA accessibility track the differences in rate of recovery from use-dependent block and implicate slow inactivation in the compound-specific differences in use-dependent drug block. It was proposed that LA compounds may produce their kinetically distinct voltage-dependent behavior by modulating slow inactivation gating to varying degrees. The association of Brugada syndrome with enhanced slow inactivation in specific families (e.g., T1620M and 1795insD)[17,48] raises the possibility that this gating defect exacerbates the Brugada phenotype during exposure to sodium channel blockers, such as flecainide.[15]

The Future: A Dynamic Cardiac Sodium Channel Structure

Inspection of Figure 9-3 suggests an intriguing nonrandom clustering of Brugada syndrome and LQT3 loci. For example, T1620M, associated with Brugada syndrome, resides on the external linker between S3 and S4 in domain IV, only three residues C-terminal to the outermost S4 arginine, R1623Q, associated with LQT3. The observed gating effects of R1623Q on fast inactivation[42,43] and T1620M on both fast and slow inactivation[42,43,48,53] are consistent with the structure-function data (discussed earlier) supporting the role of D4S4 in both gating processes.[10,33,81] Brugada syndrome mutations also occur in domains I and II but preferentially in the S5 and S6 segments (P loops), where they probably reduce sodium current by modifying the pore structure. Analogous clustering of LQT3 and Brugada syndrome mutations appears in the III-IV linker (see Fig. 9-3). Although III-IV linker mutations typically disrupt inactivation (LQT3), a recently identified Brugada syndrome mutation, R1512W, slowed recovery from inactivation[82,83] and lies only five residues away from the ΔKPQ LQT3 deletion, suggesting a more complex role of this linker in channel inactivation. Consistent with this hypothesis, another mutation, ΔK1500, was identified proximal to the ΔKPQ mutation causing LQT3, Brugada syndrome, and conduction disease.[84] A number of LQT3 and Brugada mutations also lie side by side in the C terminus and influence both fast and slow inactivation (see Fig. 9-3). In fact, mutation of a C-terminal tyrosine (Y1795) to cysteine or histidine evokes LQT-3 or Brugada syndrome, respectively and in vitro evokes gain- or loss-of-function effects on inactivation gating that are consistent with these in vivo phenotypes.[85]

The surprisingly diverse effects of these vicinal mutations and multifunctional loci emphasize the importance of future studies aimed at defining three-dimensional protein structure. Efforts to characterize the channel structure thus far have been limited to small, soluble cytoplasmic domains. The nuclear magnetic resonance solution structure of the isolated III-IV linker revealed a stably folded core comprising an α helix capped by an N-terminal turn, supporting a model in which the tightly folded core contains a latch motif (three hydrophobic residues—IFM in Fig. 9-1A) that pivots on a flexible hinge to occlude the pore during fast inactivation gating.[3] The soluble C-terminal domain also has been purified and subjected to circular dichroism, revealing a highly ordered α-helical proximal region critical to inactivation gating, followed by a relatively unstructured distal tail region.[2] Although full crystallization of the sodium channel looms on the horizon, a recent low-resolution (190-nm) three-dimensional density map obtained with use of cryoelectron microscopy reveals a surprisingly complex network of internal cavities and pores along both the cytoplasmic and the extracellular membrane surfaces.[86] This complex structure foreshadows a structure comprising intricately folded loops and helices, with rapid alternation of exposure of single domains to both hydrophobic and hydrophilic microenvironments. Such a structure would readily explain how seemingly subtle amino acid substitutions, albeit adjacent in the primary sequence, evoke diverse changes in protein function and cardiac excitability.

References

1. Doyle DA, Cabral JM, Pfuetzner RA, et al: The structure of the potassium channel: Molecular basis of K^+ conduction and selectivity. Science 280:69-77, 1998.
2. Cormier JW, Rivolta I, Tateyama M, et al: Secondary structure of the human cardiac Na^+ channel C terminus: Evidence for a role of helical structures in modulation of channel inactivation. J Biol Chem 277:9233-9241, 2002.
3. Rohl CA, Boeckman FA, Baker C, et al: Solution structure of the sodium channel inactivation gate. Biochemistry 38:855-861, 1999.
4. Balser JR: Structure and function of the cardiac sodium channels. Cardiovasc Res 42:327-338, 1999.
5. Catterall WA: From ionic currents to molecular mechanisms: The structure and function of voltage-gated sodium channels. Neuron 26:13-25, 2000.
6. Fozzard HA, Hanck DA: Structure and function of voltage-dependent sodium channels: comparison of brain II and cardiac isoforms. Physiol Rev 76:887-926, 1996.
7. Marban E, Yamagishi T, Tomaselli GF: Structure and function of voltage-gated sodium channels. J Physiol (Lond) 508:647-657, 1998.
8. Cha A, Ruben PC, George AL Jr, et al: Voltage sensors in domains III and IV, but not I and II, are immobilized by Na^+ channel fast inactivation [see comments]. Neuron 22:73-87, 1999.
9. Kontis KJ, Rounaghi A, Goldin AL: Sodium channel activation gating is affected by substitutions of voltage sensor positive charges in all four domains. J Gen Physiol 110:391-401, 1997.
10. Yang N, Horn R: Evidence for voltage-dependent S4 movement in sodium channels. Neuron 15:213-218, 1995.
11. Kellenberger S, Scheuer T, Catterall WA: Movement of the Na^+ channel inactivation gate during inactivation. J Biol Chem 271:30971-30979, 1996.
12. McPhee JC, Ragsdale DS, Scheuer T, Catterall WA: A critical role for transmembrane segment IVS6 of the sodium channel α subunit in fast inactivation. J Biol Chem 270:12025-12034, 1995.
13. McPhee JC, Ragsdale DS, Scheuer T, Catterall WA: A critical role for the S4-S5 intracellular loop in domain IV of the sodium channel alpha-subunit in fast inactivation. J Biol Chem 273:1121-1129, 1998.
14. Kambouris NG, Nuss HB, Johns DC, et al: A revised view of cardiac sodium channel blockade in the long-QT syndrome. J Clin Invest 105:1133-1140, 2000.
15. Viswanathan PC, Bezzina CR, George AL Jr, et al: Gating-dependent mechanisms for flecainide action in SCN5A-linked arrhythmia syndromes. Circulation 15:542-544, 2001.
16. Sheets MF, Kyle JW, Hanck DA: The role of the putative inactivation lid in sodium channel gating current immobilization. J Gen Physiol 115:609-620, 2000.
17. Veldkamp MW, Viswanathan PC, Bezzina C, et al: Two distinct congenital arrhythmias evoked by a multidysfunctional Na(+) channel. Circ Res 86:E91-E97, 2000.
18. Wei J, Wang DW, Alings M, et al: Congenital long-QT syndrome caused by a novel mutation in a conserved acidic domain of the cardiac Na^+ channel. Circulation 99:3165-3171, 1999.
19. Wingo TL, Shah VN, Anderson ME, et al: An EF-hand in the sodium channel couples intracellular calcium to cardiac excitability. Nat Struct Mol Biol 11:219-225, 2004.
20. Cannon SC: Slow inactivation of sodium channels: more than just a laboratory curiosity. Biophys J 71:5-7, 1996.
21. Cummins TR, Sigworth FJ: Impaired slow inactivation in mutant sodium channels. Biophys JJ 71:227-236, 1996.
22. Shander GS, Fan Z, Makielski JC: Slowly recovering cardiac sodium current in rat ventricular myocytes: Effects of conditioning duration and recovery potential. J Cardiovasc Electrophysiol 6:786-795, 1995.
23. Balser JR, Nuss HB, Chiamvimonvat N, et al: External pore residue mediates slow inactivation in m1 rat skeletal muscle sodium channels. J Physiol 494:431-442, 1996.
24. Benitah JP, Chen Z, Balser J, et al: Molecular dynamics of the sodium channel pore vary with gating: Interactions between P-segment motions and inactivation. J Neurosci 19:1577-1585, 1999.
25. Todt H, Dudley SC Jr, Kyle JW, et al: Ultra-slow inactivation in mu1 Na^+ channels is produced by a structural rearrangement of the outer vestibule. Biophys J 76:1335-1345, 1999.
26. Vilin YY, Makita N, George AL Jr, Ruben PC: Structural determinants of slow inactivation in human cardiac and skeletal muscle sodium channels. Biophys J 77:1384-1393, 1999.
27. Liu Y, Jurman ME, Yellen G: Dynamic rearrangement of the outer mouth of a K^+ channel during gating. Neuron 16:859-867, 1996.
28. Kiss L, LoTurco J, Korn SJ: Contribution of the selectivity filter to inactivation in potassium channels. Biophys J 76:253-263, 1999.
29. Benitah JP, Ranjan R, Yamagishi T, et al: Molecular motions within the pore of voltage-dependent sodium channels. Biophys J 73:603-613, 1997.
30. Tsushima RG, Li RA, Backx PH: P-loop flexibility in Na^+ channel pores revealed by single- and double-cysteine replacements. J Gen Physiol 110:59-72, 1997.
31. Marban E, Tomaselli GF: Ion channels as enzymes: Analogy or homology? Trends Neurosci 20:144-147, 1997.

32. Loots E, Isacoff EY: Molecular coupling of S4 to a K(+) channel's slow inactivation gate. J Gen Physiol 116:623-636, 2000.
33. Mitrovic N, George AL Jr, Horn R: Role of domain 4 in sodium channel slow inactivation. J Gen Physiol 115:707-718, 2000.
34. Kambouris N, Hastings L, Stepanovic S, et al: Mechanistic link between local anesthetic action and inactivation gating probed by outer pore mutations in the rat M1 sodium channel. J Physiol 512:693-705, 1998.
35. Wang Q, Shen J, Splawski I, et al: SCN5A mutations associated with an inherited cardiac arrhythmia, long QT syndrome. Cell 80:805-811, 1995.
36. Bennett PB, Yazawa K, Naomasa M, George AL: Molecular mechanism for an inherited cardiac arrhythmia. Nature 376:683-685, 1995.
37. Dumaine R, Wang Q, Keating MT, et al: Multiple mechanisms of Na^+ channel–linked long-QT syndrome. Circ Res 78:916-924, 1996.
38. Wang DW, Yazawa K, George AL, Bennett PB: Characterization of human cardiac Na^+ channel mutations in the congenital long QT syndrome. Proc Natl Acad Sci U S A 93:13200-13205, 1996.
39. Clancy CE, Rudy Y: Linking a genetic defect to its cellular phenotype in a cardiac arrhythmia. Nature 400:566-569, 1999.
40. Matsuoka R, Yamagishi H, Furutani M, et al: A de novo missense mutation of the SCN5A gene in long QT syndrome. Circulation 96:1-56, 1997.
41. Wattanasirichaigoon D, Vesely MR, Duggal P, et al: Sodium channel abnormalities are infrequent in patients with long QT syndrome: Identification of two novel SCN5A mutations. Am J Med Genet 86:470-476, 1999.
42. Kambouris NG, Nuss HB, Johns DC, et al: Phenotypic characterization of a novel long QT syndrome mutation in the cardiac sodium channel. Circulation 97:640-644, 1998.
43. Makita N, Shirai N, Nagashima M, et al: A de novo missense mutation of human cardiac Na^+ channel exhibiting novel molecular mechanisms of long QT syndrome. FEBS Lett 423:5-9, 1998.
44. Motoike HK, Liu H, Glaaser IW, et al: The Na^+ channel inactivation gate is a molecular complex: A novel role of the COOH-terminal domain. J Gen Physiol 123:155-165, 2004.
45. Brugada P, Brugada J: Right bundle branch block, persistent ST segment elevation and sudden cardiac death: A distinct clinical and electrocardiographic syndrome. A multicenter report. J Am Coll Cardiol 20: 1391-1396, 1992.
46. Bezzina C, Veldkamp MW, van Den Berg MP, et al: A single Na(+) channel mutation causing both long-QT and Brugada syndromes. Circ Res 85:1206-1213, 1999.
47. Casini S, Tan HL, Bhuiyan ZA, et al: Characterization of a novel SCN5A mutation associated with Brugada syndrome reveals involvement of DIIIS4-S5 linker in slow inactivation. Cardiovasc Res 76: 418-429, 2007.
48. Wang DW, Makita N, Kitabatake A, et al: Enhanced sodium channel intermediate inactivation in Brugada syndrome. Circ Res 87:e37-e43, 2000.
49. Amin AS, Verkerk AO, Bhuiyan ZA, et al: Novel Brugada syndrome–causing mutation in ion-conducting pore of cardiac Na^+ channel does not affect ion selectivity properties. Acta Physiol Scand 185: 291-301, 2005.
50. Kyndt F, Probst V, Potet F, et al: Novel SCN5A mutation leading either to isolated cardiac conduction defect or Brugada syndrome in a large French family. Circulation 104:3081-3086, 2001.
51. Pu J, Balser JR, Boyden PA: Lidocaine action on Na^+ currents in ventricular myocytes from the epicardial border zone of the infarcted heart. Circ Res 83:431-440, 1998.
52. Tan HL, Bink-Boelkens MTE, Bezzina CR, et al: A sodium channel mutation causes isolated cardiac conduction disease. Nature 409:1043-1047, 2001.
53. Dumaine R, Towgin JA, Burgada P, et al: Ionic mechanisms responsible for the electrocardiographic phenotype of the Brugada syndrome are temperature dependent. Circ Res 85:803-809, 1999.
54. Wang DW, Viswanathan PC, Balser JR, et al: Clinical, genetic, and biophysical characterization of SCN5A mutations associated with atrioventricular conduction block. Circulation 105:341-346, 2002.
55. Schott JJ, Alshinawi C, Kyndt F, et al: Cardiac conduction defects associate with mutations in SCN5A. Nat Genet 23: 20-21, 1999.
56. Viswanathan PC, Benson DW, Balser JR: A common SCN5A polymorphism modulates the biophysical effects of an SCN5A mutation. J Clin Invest 111:341-346, 2003.
57. Weiss R, Barmada MM, Nguyen T, et al: Clinical and molecular heterogeneity in the Brugada syndrome: A novel gene locus on chromosome 3. Circulation 105:707-713, 2002.
58. London B, Michalec M, Mehdi H, et al: Mutation in glycerol-3-phosphate dehydrogenase 1 like gene (GPD1-L) decreases cardiac Na^+ current and causes inherited arrhythmias. Circulation 116:2260-2268, 2007.
59. Hanlon MR, Wallace BA: Structure and function of voltage-dependent ion channel regulatory beta subunits. Biochemistry 41:2886-2894, 2002.
60. Allouis M, Le Bouffant F, Wilders R, et al: 14-3-3 is a regulator of the cardiac voltage-gated sodium channel $Na_V1.5$. Circ Res 98:1538-1546, 2006.
61. van Bemmelen MX, Rougier JS, Gavillet B, et al: Cardiac voltage-gated sodium channel $Na_V1.5$ is regulated by Nedd4-2 mediated ubiquitination. Circ Res 95:284-291, 2004.
62. Abriel H, Kass RS: Regulation of the voltage-gated cardiac sodium channel $Na_V1.5$ by interacting proteins. Trends Cardiovasc Med 15:35-40, 2005.
63. Lee A, Wong ST, Gallagher D, et al: Ca^{2+}/calmodulin binds to and modulates P/Q-type calcium channels. Nature 399:155-159, 1999.
64. Zuhlke RD, Reuter H: Ca^{2+}-sensitive inactivation of L-type Ca^{2+} channels depends on multiple cytoplasmic amino acid sequences of the alpha1C subunit. Proc Natl Acad Sci U S A 95:3287-3294, 1998.
65. Mori M, Konno T, Ozawa T, et al: Novel interaction of the voltage-dependent sodium channel (VDSC) with calmodulin: Does VDSC acquire calmodulin-mediated Ca^{2+}-sensitivity? Biochemistry 39:1316-1323, 2000.
66. Deschenes I, Neyroud N, DiSilvestre D, et al: Isoform-specific modulation of voltage-gated Na(+) channels by calmodulin. Circ Res 90:E49-E57, 2002.
67. Tan HL, Kupershmidt S, Zhang R, et al: A calcium sensor in the sodium channel modulates cardiac excitability. Nature 415: 442-447, 2002.
68. Benhorin J, Taub R, Goldmit M, et al: Effects of flecainide in patients with new SCN5A mutation: Mutation-specific therapy for long-QT syndrome? Circulation 101:1698-1706, 2000.
69. Shimizu W, Antzelevitch C: Sodium channel block with mexilitine is effective in reducing dispersion of repolarization and preventing torsade de pointes in LQT2 and LQT3 models of the long-QT syndrome. Circulation 96:2038-2047, 1997.
70. Ragsdale DS, McPhee JC, Scheuer T, Catterall WA: Molecular determinants of state-dependent block of Na^+ channels by local anesthetics. Science 265:1724-1728, 1994.
71. An RH, Bangalore R, Rosero SZ, Kass RS: Lidocaine block of LQT-3 mutant human Na channels. Circ Res 79:103-108, 1996.
72. Wang DW, Yazawa K, Makita N, et al: Pharmacological targeting of long QT mutant sodium channels. J Clin Invest 99:1714-1720, 1997.
73. Priori SG, Napolitano C, Schwartz PJ, et al: The elusive link between LQT3 and Brugada syndrome: The role of flecainide challenge. Circulation 102:945-947, 2000.
74. Chen T, Sheets MF: Enhancement of closed-state inactivation in long QT syndrome sodium channel mutations delta KPQ. Am J Physiol Heart Circ Physiol 283:H966-H975, 2002.
75. Vedantham V, Cannon SC: The position of the fast-inactivation gate during lidocaine block of voltage-gated Na^+ channels. J Gen Physiol 113:7-16, 1999.
76. Sheets MF, Hanck DA: Outward stabilization of the S4 segments in domains III and IV enhances lidocaine block of sodium channels. J Physiol 582:317-334, 2007.
77. Chen Z, Ong B-H, Kambouris NG, et al: Lidocaine induces a slow inactivated state in rat skeletal muscle sodium channels. J Pharmacol 524:37-49, 2000.
78. Ong BH, Tomaselli GF, Balser JR: A structural rearrangement in the sodium channel pore linked to slow inactivation and use dependence. J Gen Physiol 116:653-661, 2000.
79. Sunami A, Dudley SC Jr, Fozzard HA: Sodium channel selectivity filter regulates antiarrhythmic drug binding. Proc Natl Acad Sci U S A 94:14126-14131, 1997.
80. Fukuda K, Nakajima T, Viswanathan PC, Balser JR: Compound-specific Na^+ channel pore conformational changes induced by local anaesthetics. J Physiol 564:21-31, 2005.

9

81. Chahine M, George AL, Zhou M, et al: Sodium channel mutations in paramyotonia congenita uncouple inactivation from activation. Neuron 12:281-294, 1994.
82. Deschenes I, Baroudi G, Berthet M, et al: Electrophysiological characterization of SCN5A mutations causing long QT (E1784K) and Brugada (R1512W and R1432G) syndromes. Cardiovasc Res 46:55-65, 2000.
83. Rook MB, Alshinawi CB, Groenewegen WA, et al: Human SCN5A gene mutations alter cardiac sodium channel kinetics and are associated with the Brugada syndrome. Cardiovasc Res 44:507-517, 1999.
84. Grant AO, Carboni MP, Neplioueva V, et al: Long QT syndrome, Brugada syndrome, and conduction system disease are linked to a single sodium channel mutation. J Clin Invest 110:1201-1209, 2002.
85. Rivolta I, Abriel H, Tateyama M, et al: Inherited Brugada and long QT-3 syndrome mutations of a single residue of the cardiac sodium channel confer distinct channel and clinical phenotypes. J Biol Chem 276:30623-30630, 2001.
86. Sato C, Ueno Y, Asai K, et al: The voltage-sensitive sodium channel is a bell-shaped molecule with several cavities. Nature 409:1047-1051, 2001.

Gating of Cardiac Delayed Rectifier Potassium Channels 10

MICHAEL C. SANGUINETTI AND MARTIN TRISTANI-FIROUZI

CHAPTER OUTLINE

Overview of Potassium Channel Activity

The combined activities of several different potassium channels are required for repolarization of cardiomyocyte action potentials. Repolarization occurs in three overlapping phases. Phase 1 repolarization is very rapid and initiated by activation of a transient outward potassium current (I_{to}). The duration of phase 2, also called the plateau phase, varies considerably with heart rate and size. Small rodents have very rapid heart rates, necessitating an extremely brief plateau phase. At the slower heart rates typical of large mammals, including canines and humans, action potentials have a much longer plateau phase that can last for hundreds of milliseconds. In large mammals, I_{to} has relatively small amplitude and rapidly inactivates during the plateau phase. In all species, the inward rectifier potassium current (I_{K1}) is blocked by internal Mg^{2+} and polyamines[1] and therefore contributes only negligible outward current during phases 1 and 2 of the action potential. Termination of the plateau phase requires activation of other voltage-gated potassium (Kv) channels, specifically one or more types of delayed rectifier potassium currents (I_K). Three types of I_K are now commonly recognized based on their variable rates of activation: I_{Kur} (ultra-rapid), I_{Kr} (rapid), and I_{Ks} (slow). The end of the plateau phase merges with the onset of the faster phase 3 repolarization as I_{K1} recovers from block by internal Mg^{2+} and polyamines and joins I_K to terminate the action potential. An ionic current model for human ventricular myocytes provides a representative example of the relative densities of repolarizing potassium currents (Fig. 10-1). However, the relative contribution of the different delayed rectifier potassium currents to cardiomyocyte repolarization differs between species and regions of the heart and varies with heart rate. For example, in rabbit ventricular muscle, I_{Kr} density is greatest in the apex, whereas I_{Ks} predominates in the base.[2]

I_{Kur}, also referred to as the steady-state (I_{ss}), sustained (I_{sus}), or persistent plateau (I_{Kp}) current,[3-5] is characterized by fast activation (activation time constant, τ_{act} approximately 10 ms at 0 mV) and sensitivity to block by 4-aminopyridine (4-AP).[4] I_{Kur} is half-activated at −4 mV and has a single-channel conductance of 17 picosiemens (pS). The specific properties of I_{Kur} vary between species, suggesting diversity in the molecular basis of the channel underlying the macroscopic current. In humans, I_{Kur} is the predominant delayed rectifier current responsible for repolarization of the atrium,[4] but this current is absent or very small in the ventricle.[6] In other mammals, I_{Kur} also can be an important repolarizing current in the ventricle.[7,8]

Cardiac I_K originally was defined as two overlapping outward currents described as "i_{x1}" and "i_{x2}" in Purkinje fibers[9] and chick atrial myocytes.[10] I_{Kr} was later defined in guinea pig heart as a component of I_K blocked by methanesulfonanilides[11] and at the single-channel level in rabbit atrial node cells.[12] I_{Kr} is half-activated at −30 mV and has a single-channel conductance of 2 pS. Voltage-dependent inactivation reduces outward I_{Kr} during the plateau phase of the action potential, but channels rapidly recover from inactivation and current magnitude rebounds during phase 3 repolarization (see Fig. 10-1). Slow deactivation of I_{Kr} after repolarization of atrial nodal myocytes also contributes to the slow diastolic depolarization of these pacemaker cells.[12]

I_{Ks} can easily be distinguished from I_{Kr} by its distinct biophysical properties and lack of sensitivity to methanesulfonanilides.[11,13-15] I_{Ks} activates very slowly at transmembrane potentials positive to −30 mV and reaches its half-maximal activation at approximately +20 mV; thus, it contributes most to repolarization late in the plateau phase of a cardiac action potential (see Fig. 10-1). I_{Ks} is half-activated at +20 mV, has a single-channel conductance of 4.5 pS, and is specifically blocked by chromanol 293B[16] and the benzodiazepine L-735821.[17]

A detailed description of the biophysical and pharmacologic properties of cardiac delayed rectifier potassium channels is available elsewhere,[18] and an abbreviated summary is presented in Table 10-1. The remainder of this chapter describes the molecular basis of cardiac delayed rectifier potassium channels and reviews studies using cloned channels to determine the mechanisms and structural basis of their voltage-dependent gating.

Molecular Basis of Single Channels

Ultrarapid Delayed Rectifier Channel

Identification of the molecular basis of I_{Kur} has been complicated by substantial overlap in the biophysical properties of several other potassium channels as well as additional heterogeneous properties imparted by modulatory K_V β subunits. In humans, *KCNA5* encodes a 613-amino-acid α subunit that coassembles as a tetramer to form the $K_V1.5$ channel, which has biophysical and pharmacologic properties similar to those of native I_{Kur} in human atria. Whole-cell and single-channel currents for $K_V1.5$ are shown in Figure 10-2A. Experiments utilizing antisense oligodeoxynucleotides targeted against $K_V1.5$ provide additional evidence that $K_V1.5$ α subunits contribute to I_{Kur}. Functional knockdown of $K_V1.5$ with antisense oligodeoxynucleotides selectively attenuated I_{Kur} in cultured human, rat and mouse atrial myocytes by 50% to 70%.[19-21] The inability to completely abolish I_{Kur} using this approach suggests the possibility of molecular

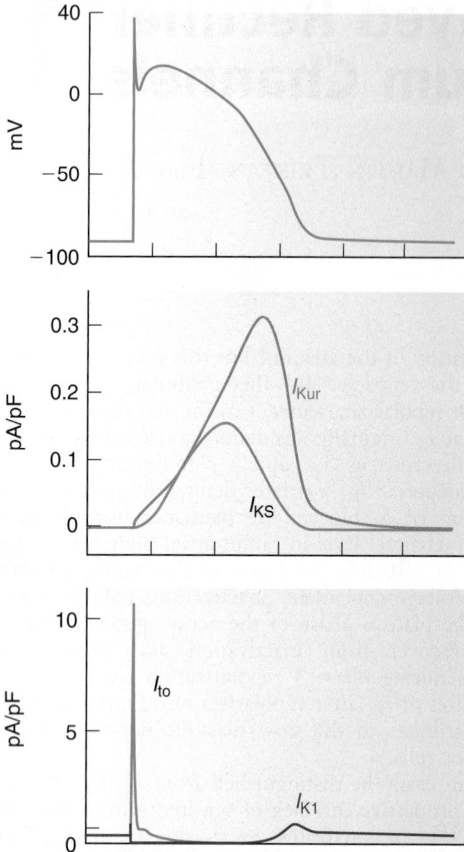

Figure 10-1 Multiple potassium currents mediate repolarization of human ventricular action potentials. *Upper panel* shows action potential curve. Potassium currents are plotted in the two *lower panels*. Atrial myocytes also have an ultrarapid delayed rectifier current (I_{Kur}). Simulations are based on a model for a human ventricular myocyte. (Figure adapted from Sanguinetti MC, Tristani-Firouzi M: hERG potassium channels and cardiac arrhythmia. Nature 440:463-469, 2006; human ventricular myocyte model described in Priebe L, Beuckelmann DJ: Simulation study of cellular electric properties in heart failure. Circ Res 82:1206-1223, 1998.)

heterogeneity in the genesis of I_{Kur}. In mouse atrial myocytes, anti-K_V2.1 oligodeoxynucleotides also inhibit a rapidly activating, sustained component of I_K,[20] and two-pore domain potassium (K_{2P}) channels also may contribute to this current.[22] Gene-targeting approaches, however, further support the notion that K_V1.5 is the major molecular correlate of I_{Kur}. A functional knockout of K_V1.5 resulted in elimination of the rapidly activating, 4-AP–sensitive component of I_K in mouse ventricle.[23] The ability of K_V1.5 α subunits to coassemble with K_V β subunits allows for additional modulation and may potentially account for some of the species heterogeneity in the properties of I_{Kur}. Coassembly of K_V1.5 with K_Vβ1.3 accessory subunits induces a 13-mV hyperpolarizing shift in activation, slows deactivation three-fold, and significantly accelerates channel inactivation.[24] K_Vβ1.3 also reduces the binding affinity for several channel blockers[25] by competition at a binding site located in the central cavity.[26] Thus, the regulatory K_V β subunits allow for cell- or species-specific modulation of K_V1.5 and may account for some of the discrepant properties reported for I_{Kur}. In addition, heteromultimeric assembly of K_V1.5 with other K_V1 α subunits (e.g., K_V1.2) also may account for the diversity in I_{Kur} properties.

Rapid Delayed Rectifier Channel

The human ether-à-go-go–related gene (*HERG*) was first cloned from human hippocampus based on sequence homology with *Drosophila* eag (ether-à-go-go) potassium channels.[27] *KCNH2* encodes an 1158-amino-acid α subunit that coassembles as a tetramer to form the HERG (K_V11.1) channel. When heterologously expressed in oocytes, HERG induces a current with properties similar to those of cardiac I_{Kr}, including rectification of the current-voltage (i.e., *I-V*) relationship, single-channel conductance, and voltage dependence of gating.[28,29] Whole-cell and single-channel currents for HERG are shown in Figure 10-2B. HERG channels are specifically blocked by dofetilide, E-4031, MK-499, and several peptide toxins (see Table 10-1). In heterologous expression systems, HERG can coassemble with the β subunit MiRP1 (MinK-related protein 1), encoded by *KCNE2*.[30] Compared with HERG alone, HERG-MiRP1, exhibits a decreased single-channel conductance and a slower rate of deactivation.[30]

Investigators disagree over the importance of MiRP1 as a modulatory subunit for HERG. Weerapura and colleagues[31] reported that the biophysical and pharmacologic properties of HERG channels were similar to those of guinea pig I_{Kr}, and the discrepancies that remained were not significantly altered by coexpression with MiRP1. MiRP1 also can interact with greater affinity to other cardiac ion channel subunits, including the transient outward potassium channel K_V4.2[32] and the hyperpolarization-activated cation pacemaker channel HCN2.[33] MiRP1 is expressed at high levels in sinoatrial node but is poorly expressed in ventricle.[33] In canines, MiRP1 mRNA and protein are far more abundant in Purkinje fibers than in ventricular tissue.[34] Thus, the physiologic role of MiRP1 as a modulator of HERG channels may differ between species and tissue type. Two isoforms of HERG are expressed in the heart. HERG1a is a full-length isoform, whereas HERG1b[35,36] has a much shorter N terminus (36 amino acids for the 1b form, compared with 376 amino acids for 1a). HERG1b does not express well on its own but coassembles with HERG1a subunits to form a channel with faster kinetics of deactivation.

Slow Delayed Rectifier Channel

When MinK, a putative ion channel subunit cloned from rat kidney, was expressed in oocytes, it induced a slow potassium current with properties similar to those of I_{Ks}. Human MinK has only 129 amino acids and a single transmembrane domain, however, so it seemed unlikely that coassembly of these subunits alone could form functional channels. Moreover, MinK does not induce currents when transfected into mammalian cells. The hypothesized protein partner of MinK[37] was discovered during a positional cloning search for a gene associated with long QT syndrome by Keating and colleagues.[38] This gene, *KCNQ1*, encodes a 676-amino-acid α subunit (KCNQ1, K_VLQT1, or K_V7.1). Coexpression of KCNQ1 α subunits with MinK β subunits induced I_{Ks} in mammalian cells and increased the magnitude of I_{Ks} in oocytes by greater than six-fold that for MinK alone.[39-41] KCNQ1 subunits can coassemble to form functional tetrameric channels in the absence of minK; however, coassembly with MinK increases single-channel conductance, slows the rate of activation, and removes inactivation. Whole-cell and single-channel currents for KCNQ1-MinK are shown in Figure 10-2C. KCNQ1-MinK heteromultimeric channels also are more sensitive than KCNQ1 to block by certain drugs such as chromanol 293B.[42] Heteromultimerization also alters the sensitivity of channels to an activator. The benzodiazepine R-L3 increases the magnitude and slows

Table 10-1 Summary of Biophysical and Pharmacologic Properties of Human Cardiac Delayed Rectifier Potassium Currents

	Potassium Current		
Property	I_{Kur}	I_{Kr}	I_{Ks}
Protein(s)	$K_V1.5$	ERG (+ MiRP1?)	KCNQ1 + MinK
Alternate protein name(s)		$K_V11.1$	$K_V7.1$ + IsK
Human gene(s)	*KCNA5*	*KCNH2* + *KCNE2*	*KCNQ* + *KCNE1*
Blockers (IC_{50})	4-Aminopyridine (0.27 mM) Diphenyl phosphine oxide (0.6 μM)[a] S0100176 (0.7 μM)[b] AVE0118 (5.6 μM)[c]	Dofetilide (15-35 nM) E4031 (8 nM) Astemizole (1 nM) Ergtoxin (12 nM)[d] BeKM-1 (3 nM)[e] APETx1 (34 nM)[f]	Chromanol 293B (1 μM) L-735821 (80 nM) HMR-1556 (34 nM)[g]
$V_{1/2}$ for activation	−4 mV	−30 mV	+20 mV
Rate of activation (τ_{act}); 0 mV	10 ms	200 ms	800 ms
$V_{1/2}$ for inactivation	−25 mV*	−80 mV*	NA
Rate of inactivation (τ_{inact}); 0 mV	250, 3000 ms*	10 ms*	NA
Single-channel conductance†	17 pS*	2 pS*	4.5 pS*

*Values were obtained using human cardiac myocytes or the corresponding heterologously expressed human cloned channels.

†Determined using physiologic K^+ concentration.

[a]Data from Lagrutta A, Wang J, Fermini B, Salata JJ: Novel, potent inhibitors of human $K_v1.5$ K^+ channels and ultrarapidly activating delayed rectifier potassium current. J Pharmacol Exp Ther 317:1054-1063, 2006.

[b]Data from Decher N, Pirard B, Bundis F, et al: Molecular basis for $K_v1.5$ channel block: Conservation of drug binding sites among voltage-gated K^+ channels. J Biol Chem 279:394-400, 2004.

[c]Data from Decher N, Kumar P, Gonzalez T, et al: Binding site of a novel $K_v1.5$ blocker: A "foot in the door" against atrial fibrillation. Mol Pharmacol 70:1204-1211, 2006.

[d]Data from Pardo-Lopez L, Zhang M, Liu J, et al: Mapping the binding site of a human ether-à-go-go-related gene–specific peptide toxin (ErgTx) to the channel's outer vestibule. J Biol Chem 277:16403-16411, 2002.

[e]Data from Korolkova YV, Kozlov SA, Lipkin AV, et al: An ERG channel inhibitor from the scorpion *Buthus eupeus*. J Biol Chem 276:9868-9876, 2001.

[f]Data from Diochot S, Loret E, Bruhn T, et al: APETx1, a new toxin from the sea anemone *Anthopleura elegantissima*, blocks voltage-gated human ether-à-go-go–related gene potassium channels. Mol Pharmacol 64:59-69, 2003.

[g]Data from Gogelein H, Bruggemann A, Gerlach U, et al: Inhibition of I_{Ks} channels by HMR 1556. Naunyn Schmiedebergs Arch Pharmacol 362:480-488, 2000.

IC_{50}, half maximal (50%) inhibitory concentration; NA, not applicable; $V_{(1/2)}$, half maximal voltage.

the gating of KCNQ1 channels but not KCNQ1-MinK channels.[43]

The sites of subunit interaction and number of MinK subunits that coassemble with KCNQ1 subunits to form a functional channel are not known with certainty. Several studies suggest that two MinK subunits are present in each channel based on interaction of wild-type and mutant subunits,[37,44] whereas characterization of KCNQ1-MinK fusion proteins suggests that the stoichiometry of the heteromultimeric channels may not be a fixed number.[45] Cys-scanning mutagenesis of minK and altered block of KCNQ1-MinK channels by thiol-reactive Cd^{2+} suggest that MinK resides near the pore region of KCNQ1[46] and interacts with the S6 domain.[47] Mutagenesis studies indicate a clear and important role for Thr58 of MinK in altering KCNQ1 channel gating.[48] Despite extensive and laborious work,[49-51] however, the structural details of KCNQ1-MinK interactions remain uncertain.

Structural Features of Voltage-Gated Potassium Channels

Current understanding of the biophysical and structural basis of ion channel gating was advanced tremendously by elucidation of the high-resolution crystal structures of the bacterial potassium channels KcsA,[52,53] MthK,[54,55] and K_VAP[56] and more recently from the voltage-gated mammalian channel $K_V1.2$.[57,58] Like all K_V channels, $K_V1.5$, HERG, and KCNQ1 α subunits coassemble to form homotetramers. Each subunit has six transmembrane α helices and forms two functionally distinct modules, one that senses transmembrane potential (S1 to S4 domains) and one that forms the K^+-selective pore (S5 and S6 domains). The transmembrane electrical field provides the force that activates, deactivates, and, in some cases, inactivates K_V channels. The S4 domain, with a basic

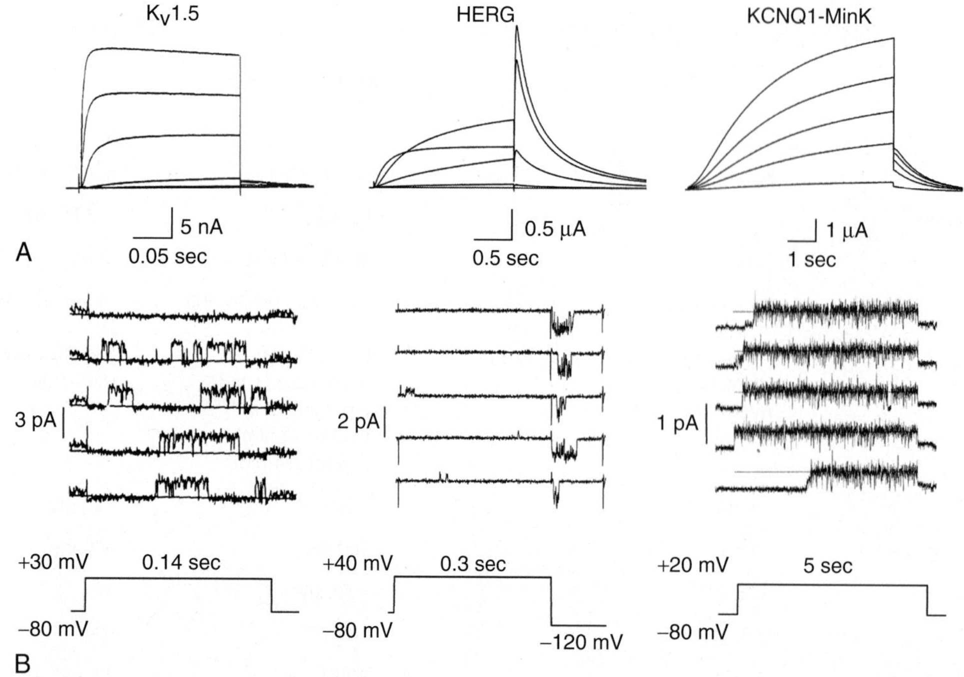

Figure 10-2 Representative examples of whole-cell (**A**) and single-channel currents (**B**) for cardiac delayed rectifier potassium channels. K_V1.5 channels were expressed in HEK293 cells, and whole-cell currents were recorded with the patch clamp technique.[109] HERG and KCNQ1-MinK channels were expressed in *Xenopus* oocytes, and whole-cell currents were recorded with the two-microelectrode voltage clamp technique. Single K_V1.5[110] and HERG[111] channels were recorded in a cell-attached patch, and single KCNQ1–rat MinK[98] channels were recorded in an inside-out patch. Voltage pulses used to elicit currents are depicted in the *bottom panel* in **B**. (Data for patch clamp technique from Zhang S, Kehl SJ, Fedida D: Modulation of K_v1.5 potassium channel gating by extracellular zinc. Biophys J 81:125-136, 2001. Data for recorded single K_V1.5[110] channels from Fedida D, Wible B, Wang Z, et al: Identity of a novel delayed rectifier current from human heart with a cloned K^+ channel current. Circ Res 73:210-216, 1993. Data for recorded single HERG[111] channels from Kiehn J, Lacerda AE, Brown AM: Pathways of HERG inactivation. Am J Physiol 277:H199-H210, 1999. Data for single KCNQ1–rat MinK channels from the article by Yang and Sigworth.[98])

amino acid located at every third position in the α helix, functions as the primary voltage sensor. A change in membrane potential induces movement of the S4 domains that drive channel opening and closing. Whether the S4 movement is a small rotation or translation[59-61] or a large "paddle-like" motion[62,63] remains a subject of debate.

The pore module (S5 and S6 domains) includes an activation gate that, when in an open position, permits ion conduction and a selectivity filter that dictates K^+-specific permeation. The selectivity filter contains a so-called signature sequence, Thr-Val-Gly-Tyr-Gly. The backbone carbonyl oxygens from these residues form multiple coordination sites for dehydrated K^+ ions as they pass in single file through the filter.[52] Although the Thr and Tyr residues are substituted with Ser and Phe in HERG, the channel remains highly K^+-selective. The narrow selectivity filter is located near the extracellular side of the membrane and leads to a wider, water-filled central cavity that is lined by the S6 α helices. The closed state of the activation gate is generated by criss-crossing of the C-terminal ends of the S6 helices, thereby creating a narrow aperture that prevents ion diffusion from the cytosol to the central cavity. Based on electroparamagnetic resonance (EPR) studies of KcsA channel opening[64] and the crystal structures of channels in the open (K_VAP, K_V1.2, MthK)[54,56,58] or closed (KcsA)[52] state, channel opening probably involves outward splaying of the S6 helices, thereby widening the aperture to allow ions to flow into or out of the central cavity. The hinge point from which the S6 helices splay outward usually is a conserved Gly residue located just beneath the selectivity filter.[52] KCNQ1 channels have an Ala in the homologous position, however, and mutation of the conserved Gly in HERG to Ala does not markedly alter channel opening. Apparently, a Gly is not an absolute requirement for operation of the activation gate. The S6 domain of many K_V channels, including K_V1.5, contains a Pro-Val-Pro motif near the location of the putative activation gate. The Pro-Val-Pro motif is postulated to disrupt the α-helical structure of the S6 domain and is a critical component of the activation gate in these K_V channels.[65,66] In KCNQ1, the homologous sequence (Pro-Ala-Gly) may have a similar function. HERG channels do not have this motif. Thus, the S6 α helices likely form the activation gate and participate in channel opening; however, no universal structural feature defining the activation gate has been identified.

Although considerable progress has been made in defining the structure of K_V channels, the mechanism of coupling voltage sensor movement to channel opening (electromechanical coupling) remains less well understood. The cytoplasmic loop between the voltage sensing and pore domains (S4-S5 linker) is an amphipathic α helix that is located near the C-terminal portion of the S6 α helix.[58] MacKinnon and colleagues[57] proposed that the S4-S5 linker functions as a lever driven by voltage-induced changes in S4 that pushes against the S5 and S6 helices to close the channel. Studies in a variety of voltage-gated ion channels,[67-69] including HERG,[70-72] support an important role for the S4-S5 linker in channel gating. Crosslinking of cysteine residues introduced into the S4-S5 linker and the C-terminal portion of the S6 domain of HERG suggests that the S4-S5 linker is the structural link that couples voltage sensing to channel opening.[70]

Gating Mechanisms

$K_V1.5$

Single-channel and whole-cell ionic currents are used to define the kinetics of channel opening and closing. Gating currents are generated by intramembrane charge (voltage sensor) displacement and provide insight into conformational changes in channels that precede their opening. These small, transient currents can be measured only after ionic currents are eliminated, either by ion substitution or pharmacologic block or by studying mutant channels that are incapable of conducting ionic currents.

The salient features of $K_V1.5$ gating currents are illustrated in Figure 10-3A, and a more detailed analysis is provided by Wang and Fedida and colleagues.[73-75] Step depolarization to a potential of −20 mV, at which less than 50% of the channels are open, elicits small outward gating currents (Ig_{ON}) that rise and decay rapidly, whereas membrane repolarization elicits inward gating currents (Ig_{OFF}) that also rise and decay rapidly. Depolarization to more positive potentials at which all channels are open (e.g., +80 mV) elicits large Ig_{ON} as channels rapidly undergo transit through multiple closed states into the open state. After a strong depolarization, however, Ig_{OFF} shows a slowing rising phase, followed by a slow decay. Thus, charge movement between closed states is relatively fast, but once channels undergo transit into their open state, the return of gating charge (Ig_{OFF}) is slowed. Longer depolarizations result in a reduction in the amount of return gating charge with hyperpolarization, a process called charge immobilization, as channels very slowly convert to a "C-type" inactivated state.[74] However, the duration of the cardiac action potential is sufficiently short that C-type inactivation of $K_V1.5$ channels is negligible.

HERG

The slow activation and rapid inactivation of HERG ionic current imply that the underlying movement of the voltage sensor is different from that of other K_V channels. Gating currents can be observed as very small outward currents that occur before the relatively slow onset of ionic currents (see Fig. 10-3B). Voltage clamp fluorimetry[76] and direct measurement of gating currents[77] of HERG reveal two distinct components of charge displacement with a slow component approximately 100 times slower than $K_V1.5$ gating current (compare parts A and C in Fig. 10-3). The slow gating component carries approximately 90% of the gating charge and is responsible for the slow rate of HERG activation and implies that a large energy barrier exists in the intermediate transitions that precede channel opening. The source of the fast gating component is not clear but probably represents rapid transitions between channel states during the early steps of the activation pathway. Most of the gating charge displacement is due to rearrangements in the highly charged S4 domain. As illustrated in Figure 10-3D, the voltage dependence of charge movement (i.e., the charge-voltage relationship, Q-V) occurs at more negative potentials than the voltage dependence of ionic currents (the conductance-voltage relationship, G-V). The most critical S4 residue for HERG gating appears to be R531, because neutralization of this residue markedly increases the energy required for channel opening.[78-80]

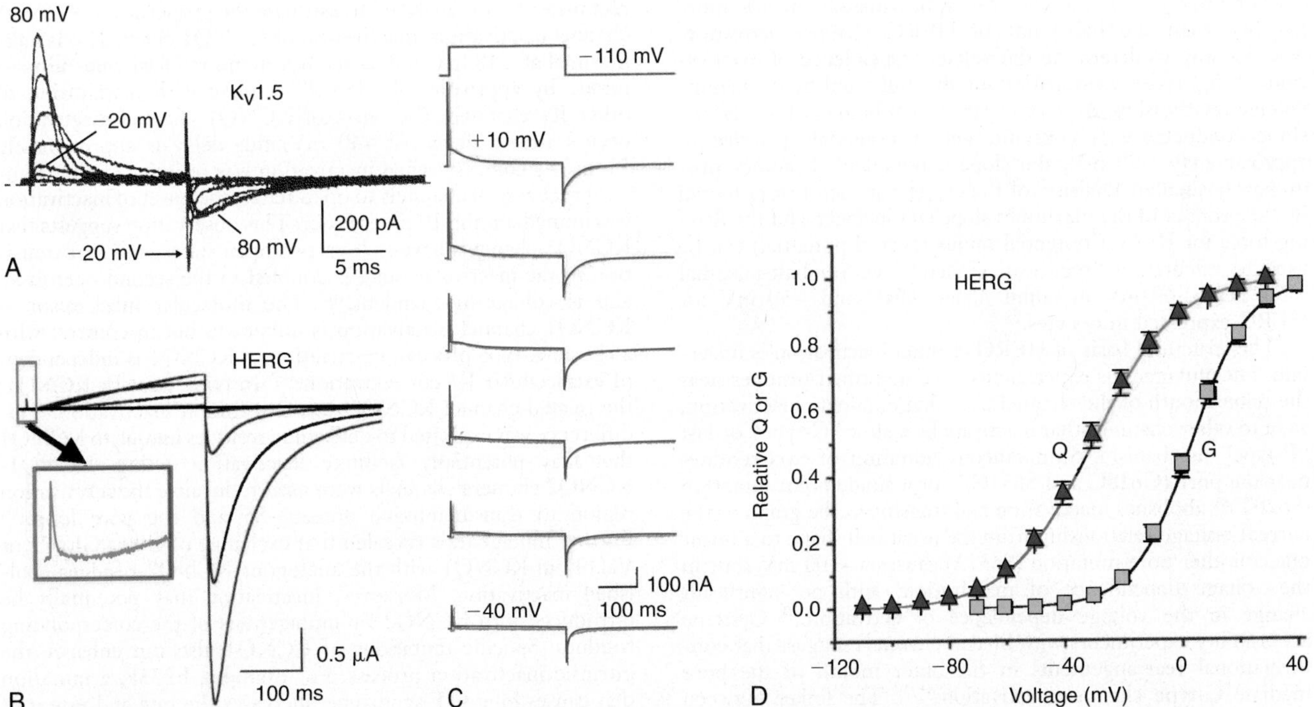

Figure 10-3 Gating currents for $K_V1.5$ and HERG channels. **A,** "On" gating currents (Ig_{ON}) for $K_V1.5$ channels activated by membrane depolarization to potentials ranging from −60 mV to +80 mV; "off" gating currents (Ig_{OFF}) were activated when the cell was repolarized to −100 mV. Channels were expressed in HEK cells.[109] **B,** Outward HERG ionic currents were elicited by depolarizing pulses from −50 to +30 mV (20-mV increments), and inward tail currents were measured after repolarization to −110 mV. *Boxed area* represents gating currents that develop much faster than ionic currents. Channels were expressed in *Xenopus* oocytes.[77] **C,** HERG gating currents. **D,** Comparison of voltage dependence of charge (Q) and conductance (G) for HERG channels.

Movement of the S4 during depolarization is facilitated by negative countercharges in adjacent domains of the voltage-sensing module. Negatively charged aspartate residues in domains S1 to S3 stabilize the closed, intermediate, and open states of HERG and other K_V channels.[81-83] Aspartate residues near the extracellular ends of the S2 and S3 domains form a coordination site for divalent cations, such as Mg^{2+} and Ca^{2+}, that modulate channel opening.[81,84,85]

A slow rate of activation usually is associated with a slow rate of deactivation. Of note, however, deletion of the first 354 amino acids in the N terminus of HERG accelerates the rate of channel deactivation but does not cause a corresponding change in activation. The crystal structure of the HERG N terminus revealed a basic helix-loop-helix structure typical of other Per-Arnt-Sim (PAS) domains that are critical for protein-protein interactions.[86] How the PAS domain of HERG influences deactivation remains unclear; however, it may interact with an accessory protein or another region of HERG to slow channel closure.

HERG exhibits inward rectification, a property critical for limiting outward K^+ conductance during the plateau phase of the cardiac action potential. In typical inward rectifier potassium (Kir) channels, rectification derives from block by intracellular polyamines and Mg^{2+}. However, rectification of HERG channels results from a combination of slow activation and very rapid (τ, less than 20 ms) inactivation. HERG inactivation can be quantified using a triple-pulse voltage clamp protocol. Channels are first activated or inactivated by a prepulse to a positive potential (e.g., +40 mV); then a short second pulse (e.g., 10 ms) is applied to a variable potential, thereby allowing channels to partially recover from inactivation but not to deactivate appreciably. Finally, a third pulse is applied to a positive potential to measure the relative proportion of channels that were in the open state at the end of the second pulse.[87,88] The half-point for inactivation of HERG estimated with this protocol is between −80 and −90 mV, approximately 70 mV more negative than the half-point of HERG channel activation. Another way to determine the voltage dependence of inactivation of I_{Kr} is by examination of the fully activated current-voltage relationship. At very negative membrane potentials, the slope conductance is constant, but at potentials positive to approximately −90 mV, the slope conductance becomes progressively smaller. Division of the current at each test potential by the product of the maximum slope conductance and the driving force for K^+ (test potential minus reversal potential) can be used to calculate a "rectification factor" with a half-maximal value near −60 mV in rabbit nodal cells[12] and −50 mV for HERG expressed in oocytes.[28]

The structural basis of HERG channel inactivation is uncertain, but mutagenesis experiments have identified residues near the outer mouth of the channel pore that eliminate inactivation, as in to other channels that inactivate by a slow "C-type" or fast "P-type" mechanism. Simultaneous mutation of two residues near the pore (G628C and S631C)[87] or a single point mutation (S620T)[89] abolishes inactivation and transforms the graph of the current-voltage relationship from the usual bell shape to a linear one. Another pore mutation (S631A) causes a +100 mV shift in the voltage dependence of inactivation, with no significant change in the voltage dependence of activation.[90] Cysteine accessibility experiments with Shaker channels suggest that conformational rearrangements in the outer mouth of the pore mediate C-type channel inactivation.[65,91] The linker between S5 and the pore helix (S5-P linker) in HERG is approximately 30 amino acids longer than in most K_V channels and is proposed to form an α-helical structure that lies adjacent to the outer vestibule of the channel. The S5-P linker may play a role in the steps leading to channel inactivation[92-95] that involves an alteration, perhaps partial constriction, of the selectivity filter. HERG channels are permeable to Na^+ when in the inactivated state, consistent with a narrowed selectivity filter.[96] In addition, HERG channel gating is unusually sensitive to extracellular Na^+ concentration. External Na^+ blocks outward current, and competition with external K^+ for a binding site near the external pore[97] explains the finding that elevation of extracellular K^+ concentration paradoxically enhances outward flux of K^+ despite the decrease in driving force.[28]

KCNQ1-MinK

MinK (KCNE1) alters several biophysical properties of KCNQ1 channels. MinK increases single-channel conductance, slows the rate of current activation, and suppresses channel inactivation. Single KCNQ1 channels open and close extremely rapidly (i.e., flicker), preventing accurate measurement of their amplitude or open and closed dwell times. Yang and Sigworth[98] and Sesti and Goldstein[99] reported that the single-channel conductance of KCNQ1-MinK channels was four to six times larger than that of homomultimeric KCNQ1 channels. For example, the single-channel conductance was estimated to be 0.7 pS for KCNQ1 alone and 4.5 pS for KCNQ1-MinK channels.[98] Slow activation of I_{Ks} appears to result from an unusually slow movement of the S4 voltage sensor, as though minK stabilizes the closed state of the KCNQ1 channel. The rate of state-dependent modification of Cys residues introduced into the S4 domain of KCNQ1 by methanethiosulfonates was found to be 13 times faster for KCNQ1 homotetramers than for KCNQ1-MinK heteromultimeric channels.[100]

KCNQ1 channel inactivation is not obvious from inspection of currents activated by membrane depolarization but is revealed by tail current analysis. Membrane repolarization causes a transient increase in KCNQ1 channel conductance that precedes deactivation, resulting in a "hook" in the tail current. This indirect measure was analyzed to estimate the properties of KCNQ1 channel inactivation. Inactivation of KCNQ1 channels was half-maximal at −18 mV and, at its maximum, reduced current magnitude by approximately 35%.[101] Unlike with inactivation of other Kv channels, the onset of KCNQ1 channel inactivation occurs after a delay. At +40 mV, this delay is approximately 75 ms. By contrast, when inactivation was re-induced after transient recovery of channels to open states, the onset of inactivation was immediate and 10 times faster. This observation suggests that KCNQ1 channels have at least two open states, and that transition to the inactivated state is coupled to the second open state and is voltage-independent.[102] The molecular mechanism of KCNQ1 channel inactivation is unknown, but in contrast with a classic C-type process, inactivation of KCNQ1 is independent of extracellular K^+ concentration.[102] In contrast with KCNQ1, the related channel KCNQ2 does not exhibit inactivation. This difference was exploited to determine residues unique to KCNQ1 that may potentially facilitate inactivation gating. KCNQ1-KCNQ2 chimera channels were used to localize the inactivation region to transmembrane domain S5 and the pore loop.[103] Further mutagenesis revealed that exchange of either Gly272 or Val307 in KCNQ1 with the analogous KCNQ2 residues abolished inactivation. Moreover, inactivation may potentially be introduced into KCNQ2 by mutagenesis of the corresponding residues. Specific mutations of KCNQ1 also can enhance the intrinsic inactivation process. For example, L273F, a mutation that causes long QT syndrome, increases the rate and extent of KCNQ1 inactivation, thereby explaining its ability to decrease I_{Ks} in the heart.[103] Further work is needed to determine if inactivation of KCNQ1 channels involves a narrowing of the selectivity filter as postulated for other channels that undergo C-type inactivation, such as $K_V1.5$ and perhaps HERG.

The mechanism by which MinK (KCNE1) suppresses inactivation of KCNQ1 channels is unknown. KCNQ1-MinK channels do not appear to inactivate, as indicated by a lack of a hook in the tail current. As noted by Pusch and colleagues,[101] however, it is possible that I_{Ks} inactivates on a much slower time scale than that noted for KCNQ1 current. The other known KCNE subunits (KCNE2 to KCNE 5) also are expressed in the heart and modify KCNQ1 channel gating.[104] KCNE4 and KCNE5 stabilize the closed state of the channel, whereas KCNE3 makes the channel remain open. Investigators disagree regarding the relative abundance of the different subunits in the human ventricle, with KCNE1 > KCNE4 > KCNE5 ≅ KCNE3 >> KCNE2 reported in one study[105] and KCNQ1 >> KCNE4 > *or* = KCNE1 > KCNE3 > KCNE2 > KCNE5 in another.[106] Regardless, the physiologic relevance of KCNQ1 channel regulation by KCNE subunits other than KCNE1 (MinK) in the heart merits further investigation.

References

1. Nichols CG, Lopatin AN: Inward rectifier potassium channels. Annu Rev Physiol 59:171-191, 1997.
2. Cheng J, Kamiya K, Liu W, et al: Heterogeneous distribution of the two components of delayed rectifier K^+ current: A potential mechanism of the proarrhythmic effects of methanesulfonanilide class III agents. Cardiovasc Res 43:135-147, 1999.
3. Boyle WA, Nerbonne JM: A novel type of depolarization-activated K^+ current in isolated adult rat atrial myocytes. Am J Physiol 260:H1236-H1247, 1991.
4. Wang Z, Fermini B, Nattel S: Sustained depolarization-induced outward current in human atrial myocytes: Evidence for a novel delayed rectifier K^+ current similar to $K_V1.5$ cloned channel currents. Circ Res 73:1061-1076, 1993.
5. Yue DT, Marban E: A novel cardiac potassium channel that is active and conductive at depolarized potentials. Pflügers Arch 413:127-133, 1988.
6. Li G-R, Feng J, Yue L, et al: Evidence for two components of delayed rectifier K^+ current in human ventricular myocytes. Circ Res 78:689-696, 1996.
7. Yue L, Feng J, Li G, Nattel S: Characterization of an ultrarapid delayed rectifier potassium channel involved in canine atrial repolarization. J Physiol (Lond) 496:647-662, 1996.
8. Backx PH, Marban E: Background potassium current active during the plateau of the action potential in guinea pig ventricular myocytes. Circ Res 72:890-900, 1993.
9. Noble D, Tsien RW: Outward membrane currents activated in the plateau range of potentials in cardiac Purkinje fibres. J Physiol 200:205-231, 1969.
10. Clay JR, Hill CE, Roitman D, Shrier A: Repolarization current in embryonic chick atrial heart cells. J Physiol 403:525-537, 1988.
11. Sanguinetti MC, Jurkiewicz NK: Two components of cardiac delayed rectifier K^+ current: Differential sensitivity to block by class III antiarrhythmic agents. J Gen Physiol 96:195-215, 1990.
12. Shibasaki T: Conductance and kinetics of delayed rectifier potassium channels in nodal cells of the rabbit heart. J Physiol 387:227-250, 1987.
13. Clay JR, Ogbaghebriel A, Paquette T, et al: A quantitative description of the E-4031–sensitive repolarization current in rabbit ventricular myocytes. Biophys J 69:1830-1837, 1995.
14. Liu D-W, Antzelevitch C: Characteristics of the delayed rectifier current (I_{Kr} and I_{Ks}) in canine ventricular epicardial, midmyocardial, and endocardial myocytes: A weaker I_{Ks} contributes to the longer action potential of the M cell. Circ Res 76:351-365, 1995.
15. Gintant GA: Two components of delayed rectifier current in canine atrium and ventricle (does I_{Ks} play a role in the reverse rate dependence of class III agents?). Circ Res 78:26-37, 1996.
16. Busch AE, Suessbrich H, Waldegger S, et al: Inhibition of I_{Ks} in guinea pig cardiac myocytes and guinea pig I_{sK} channels by the chromanol 293B. Eur J Physiol 432:1094-1096, 1996.
17. Salata JJ, Jurkiewicz NK, Sanguinetti MC, et al: The novel class III antiarrhythmic agent, L-735,821 is a potent and selective blocker of I_{Ks} in guinea pig ventricular myocytes. Circulation 1996;94:1529, 1996.
18. Nerbonne JM, Kass RS: Molecular physiology of cardiac repolarization. Physiol Rev 85:1205-1253, 2005.
19. Bou-Abboud E, Nerbonne JM: Molecular correlates of the calcium-independent, depolarization-activated K^+ currents in rat atrial myocytes. J Physiol 517:407-420, 1999.
20. Bou-Abboud E, Li H, Nerbonne JM: Molecular diversity of the repolarizing voltage-gated K^+ currents in mouse atrial cells. J Physiol 529:345-358, 2000.
21. Feng J, Wible B, Li G, et al: Antisense oligodeoxynucleotides directed against $K_v1.5$ mRNA specifically inhibit ultrarapid delayed rectifier K^+ current in cultured adult human atrial myocytes. Circ Res 80:572-579, 1997.
22. Goldstein SA, Bockenhauer D, O'Kelly I, Zilberberg N: Potassium leak channels and the KCNK family of two-P-domain subunits. Nat Rev Neurosci 2:175-184, 2001.
23. London B, Guo W, Pan X, et al: Targeted replacement of $K_V1.5$ in the mouse leads to loss of the 4-aminopyridine–sensitive component of $I_{K,slow}$ and resistance to drug-induced Qt prolongation. Circ Res 88:940-946, 2001.
24. England SK, Uebele VN, Kodali J, et al: A novel K^+ channel β-subunit ($hK_V\beta1.3$) is produced via alternative mRNA splicing. J Biol Chem 270:28531-28534, 1995.
25. Gonzalez T, Navarro-Polanco R, Arias C, et al: Assembly with the $K_v\beta1.3$ subunit modulates drug block of $hK_V1.5$ channels. Mol Pharmacol 62:1456-1463, 2002.
26. Decher N, Kumar P, Gonzalez T, et al: Structural basis for competition between drug binding and $K_V\beta1.3$ accessory subunit–induced N-type inactivation of $K_V1.5$ channels. Mol Pharmacol 68:995-1005, 2005.
27. Warmke J, Drysdale R, Ganetzky B: A distinct potassium channel polypeptide encoded by the *Drosophila* eag locus. Science 252:1560-1564, 1991.
28. Sanguinetti MC, Jiang C, Curran ME, Keating MT: A mechanistic link between an inherited and an acquired cardiac arrhythmia: HERG encodes the I_{Kr} potassium channel. Cell 81:299-307, 1995.
29. Trudeau M, Warmke JW, Ganetzky B, Robertson GA: HERG, a human inward rectifier in the voltage-gated potassium channel family. Science 269:92-95, 1995.
30. Abbott GW, Sesti F, Splawski I, et al: MiRP1 forms I_{Kr} potassium channels with HERG and is associated with cardiac arrhythmia. Cell 97:175-187, 1999.
31. Weerapura M, Nattel S, Chartier D, et al: A comparison of currents carried by HERG, with and without coexpression of MiRP1, and the native rapid delayed rectifier current. Is MiRP1 the missing link? J Physiol 540:15-27, 2002.
32. Zhang M, Jiang M, Tseng GN: minK-related peptide 1 associates with $K_V4.2$ and modulates its gating function: Potential role as beta subunit of cardiac transient outward channel? Circ Res 88:1012-1019, 2001.
33. Yu H, Wu J, Potapova I, et al: MinK-related peptide 1: A beta subunit for the HCN ion channel subunit family enhances expression and speeds activation. Circ Res 88:E84-E87, 2001.
34. Pourrier M, Zicha S, Ehrlich J, et al: Canine ventricular KCNE2 expression resides predominantly in Purkinje fibers. Circ Res 93:189-191, 2003.
35. London B, Trudeau MC, Newton KP, et al: Two isoforms of the mouse ether–à-go-go–related gene coassemble to form channels with properties similar to the rapidly activating component of the cardiac delayed rectifier K^+ current. Circ Res 81:870-878, 1997.
36. Lees-Miller JP, Kondo C, Wang L, Duff HJ: Electrophysiological characterization of an alternatively processed ERG K^+ channel in mouse and human hearts. Circ Res 81:719-726, 1997.
37. Wang K-W, Goldstein SAN: Subunit composition of minK potassium channels. Neuron 14:1303-1309, 1995.
38. Wang Q, Curran ME, Splawski I, et al: Positional cloning of a novel potassium channel gene: KVLQT1 mutations cause cardiac arrhythmias. Nat Genet 12:17-23, 1996.
39. Barhanin J, Lesage F, Guillemare E, et al: KvLQT1 and IsK (minK) proteins

associate to form the I_{Ks} cardiac potassium channel. Nature 384:78-80, 1996.
40. Sanguinetti MC, Curran ME, Zou A, et al: Coassembly of KvLQT1 and minK (IsK) proteins to form cardiac I_{Ks} potassium channel. Nature 384:80-83, 1996.
41. Yang WP, Levesque PC, Little WA, et al: KvLQT1, a voltage-gated potassium channel responsible for human cardiac arrhythmias. Proc Natl Acad Sci U S A 94:4017-4021, 1997.
42. Lerche C, Seebohm G, Wagner CI, et al: Molecular impact of MinK on the enantiospecific block of I(Ks) by chromanols. Br J Pharmacol 131:1503-1506, 2000.
43. Salata JJ, Jurkiewicz NK, Wang J, et al: A novel benzodiazepine that activates cardiac slow delayed rectifier K^+ channels. Mol Pharmacol 53:220-230, 1998.
44. Chen H, Kim LA, Rajan S, et al: Charybdotoxin binding in the I(Ks) pore demonstrates two MinK subunits in each channel complex. Neuron 40:15-23, 2003.
45. Wang W, Xia J, Kass RS: MinK-KvLQT1 fusion proteins, evidence for multiple stoichiometries of the assembled IsK channel. J Biol Chem 273:34069-34074, 1998.
46. Tai KK, Goldstein SAN: The conduction pore of a cardiac potassium channel. Nature 391:605-608, 1998.
47. Tapper AR, George AL Jr: Location and orientation of minK within the I_{Ks} potassium channel complex. J Biol Chem 276:38249-38254, 2001.
48. Melman YF, Krumerman A, McDonald TV: A single transmembrane site in the KCNE-encoded proteins controls the specificity of K_VLQT1 channel gating. J Biol Chem 277:25187-25194, 2002.
49. Chen H, Goldstein SA: Serial perturbation of MinK in I_{Ks} implies an alpha-helical transmembrane span traversing the channel corpus. Biophys J 93:2332-2340, 2007.
50. Gage SD, Kobertz WR. KCNE3 truncation mutants reveal a bipartite modulation of KCNQ1 K^+ channels. J Gen Physiol 124:759-771, 2004.
51. Rocheleau JM, Gage SD, Kobertz WR: Secondary structure of a KCNE cytoplasmic domain. J Gen Physiol 128:721-729, 2006.
52. Doyle DA, Morais Cabral J, Pfuetzner RA, et al: The structure of the potassium channel: Molecular basis of K^+ conduction and selectivity. Science 280:69-77, 1998.
53. Zhou Y, Morais-Cabral JH, Kaufman A, MacKinnon R: Chemistry of ion coordination and hydration revealed by a K^+ channel–Fab complex at 2.0 Å resolution. Nature 414:43-48, 2001.
54. Jiang Y, Lee A, Cadene M, et al: The open pore conformation of potassium channels. Nature 417:523-526, 2002.
55. Jiang Y, Lee A, Chen J, et al: Crystal structure and mechanism of a calcium-gated potassium channel. Nature 417:515-522, 2002.
56. Jiang Y, Lee A, Chen J, et al: X-ray structure of a voltage-dependent K^+ channel. Nature 423:33-41, 2003.
57. Long SB, Campbell EB, Mackinnon R: Voltage sensor of K_V1.2: Structural basis of electromechanical coupling. Science 309:903-908, 2005a.
58. Long SB, Campbell EB, Mackinnon R: Crystal structure of a mammalian voltage-dependent Shaker family K^+ channel. Science 309:897-903, 2005b.
59. Posson DJ, Ge P, Miller C, et al: Small vertical movement of a K^+ channel voltage sensor measured with luminescence energy transfer. Nature 436:848-851, 2005.
60. Ahern CA, Horn R: Specificity of charge-carrying residues in the voltage sensor of potassium channels. J Gen Physiol 123:205-216, 2004a.
61. Ahern CA, Horn R: Stirring up controversy with a voltage sensor paddle. Trends Neurosci 27:303-307, 2004b.
62. Jiang Y, Ruta V, Chen J, et al: The principle of gating charge movement in a voltage-dependent K^+ channel. Nature 423:42-48, 2003.
63. Ruta V, Chen J, Mackinnon R: Calibrated measurement of gating-charge arginine displacement in the K_vAP voltage-dependent K^+ channel. Cell 123:463-475, 2005.
64. Perozo E, Cortes DM, Cuello LG: Structural rearrangements underlying K^+-channel activation gating. Science 285:73-78, 1999.
65. Yellen G: The moving parts of voltage-gated ion channels. Q Rev Biophys 31:239-295, 1998.
66. del Camino D, Holmgren M, Liu Y, Yellen G: Blocker protection in the pore of a voltage-gated K^+ channel and its structural implications. Nature 403:321-325, 2000.
67. Chen J, Mitcheson J, Tristani-Firouzi M, et al: The S4-S5 linker couples voltage sensing and activation of pacemaker channels. Proc Natl Acad Sci U S A 98:11277-11282, 2001.
68. Decher N, Chen J, Sanguinetti MC: Voltage-dependent gating of HCN pacemaker channels: Molecular coupling between the S4-S5 and C-linkers. J Biol Chem. 279:13859-13865
69. McCormack K, Tanouye MA, Iverson LE, et al: A role for hydrophobic residues in the voltage-dependent gating of Shaker K^+ channels. Proc Natl Acad Sci U S A 88:2931-2935, 1991.
70. Ferrer T, Rupp J, Piper DR, Tristani-Firouzi M: The S4-S5 linker directly couples voltage sensor movement to the activation gate in the human ether-à-go-go–related gene (hERG) K^+ channel. J Biol Chem 281:12858-12864, 2006.
71. Tristani-Firouzi M, Chen J, Sanguinetti MC: Interactions between S4-S5 linker and S6 transmembrane domain modulate gating of HERG K^+ channels. J Biol Chem 277:18994-19000, 2002.
72. Sanguinetti MC, Xu QP: Mutations of the S4-S5 linker alter activation properties of HERG potassium channels expressed in *Xenopus* oocytes. J Physiol 514:667-675, 1999.
73. Wang Z, Fedida D: Uncoupling of gating charge movement and closure of the ion pore during recovery from inactivation in the K_V1.5 channel. J Gen Physiol 120:249-260, 2002.
74. Wang Z, Fedida D: Gating charge immobilization caused by the transition between inactivated states in the K_V1.5 channel. Biophys J 81:2614-2627, 2001.
75. Fedida D, Bouchard R, Chen FS: Slow gating charge immobilization in the human potassium channel K_V1.5 and its prevention by 4-aminopyridine. J Physiol 494:377-387, 1996.
76. Smith PL, Yellen G: Fast and slow voltage sensor movements in HERG potassium channels. J Gen Physiol 119:275-293, 2002.
77. Piper DR, Varghese A, Sanguinetti MC, Tristani-Firouzi M: Gating currents associated with intramembrane charge displacement in HERG potassium channels. Proc Natl Acad Sci U S A 100:10534-10539, 2003.
78. Zhang M, Liu J, Tseng GN: Gating charges in the activation and inactivation processes of the HERG channel. J Gen Physiol 124:703-718, 2004.
79. Subbiah RN, Kondo M, Campbell TJ, Vandenberg JI: Tryptophan scanning mutagenesis of the HERG K^+ channel: The S4 domain is loosely packed and likely to be lipid exposed. J Physiol 569:367-379, 2005.
80. Piper DR, Hinz WA, Tallurri CK, et al: Regional specificity of human ether-à-go-go–related gene channel activation and inactivation gating. J Biol Chem 280:7206-7217, 2005.
81. Silverman WR, Roux B, Papazian DM: Structural basis of two-stage voltage-dependent activation in K^+ channels. Proc Natl Acad Sci U S A 100:2935-2940, 2003.
82. Tiwari-Woodruff SK, Schulteis CT, Mock AF, Papazian DM: Electrostatic interactions between transmembrane segments mediate folding of Shaker K^+ channel subunits. Biophys J 72:1489-1500, 1997.
83. Seoh S-A, Sigg D, Papazian DM, Bezanilla F: Voltage-sensing residues in the S2 and S4 segments of the Shaker K^+ channel. Neuron 16:1159-1167, 1996.
84. Tang CY, Bezanilla F, Papazian DM: Extracellular Mg^{2+} modulates slow gating transitions and the opening of *Drosophila* ether-à-go-go potassium channels. J Gen Physiol 115:319-338, 2000.
85. Silverman WR, Tang CY, Mock AF, et al: Mg^{2+} modulates voltage-dependent activation in ether-à-go-go potassium channels by binding between transmembrane segments S2 and S3. J Gen Physiol 116: 663-678, 2000.
86. Morais Cabral JH, Lee A, Cohen SL, et al: Crystal structure and functional analysis of the HERG potassium channel N terminus: A eukaryotic PAS domain. Cell 95:649-655, 1998.
87. Smith PL, Baukrowitz T, Yellen G: The inward rectification mechanism of the HERG cardiac potassium channel. Nature 379:833-836, 1996.
88. Spector PS, Curran ME, Zou A, et al: Fast inactivation causes rectification of the I_{Kr} channel. J Gen Physiol 107:611-619, 1996.
89. Ficker E, Jarolimek W, Kiehn J, et al: Molecular determinants of dofetilide block of HERG K^+ channels. Circ Res 82:386-395, 1998.
90. Zou A, Xu QP, Sanguinetti MC: A mutation in the pore region of HERG K^+ channels reduces rectification by shifting the voltage dependence of inactivation. J Physiol 509:129-138, 1998.

91. Liu Y, Jurman ME, Yellen G: Dynamic rearrangement of the outer mouth of a K^+ channel during gating. Neuron 16:859-867, 1996.
92. Clarke CE, Hill AP, Zhao J, et al: Effect of S5P alpha-helix charge mutants on inactivation of hERG K^+ channels. J Physiol 573:291-304, 2006.
93. Jiang M, Zhang M, Maslennikov IV, et al: Dynamic conformational changes of extracellular S5-P linkers in the hERG channel. J Physiol 569:75-89, 2005.
94. Liu J, Zhang M, Jiang M, Tseng GN: Structural and functional role of the extracellular S5-P linker in the HERG potassium channel. J Gen Physiol 120:723-737, 2002.
95. Torres AM, Bansal PS, Sunde M, et al: Structure of the HERG K^+ channel S5P extracellular linker: Role of an amphipathic alpha-helix in C-type inactivation. J Biol Chem 278:42136-42148, 2003.
96. Gang H, Zhang S: Na^+ permeation and block of hERG potassium channels. J Gen Physiol 128:55-71, 2006.
97. Numaguchi H, Johnson JP Jr, Petersen CI, Balser JR: A sensitive mechanism for cation modulation of potassium current. Nat Neurosci 3:429-430, 2000.
98. Yang Y, Sigworth FJ: 19 Single-channel properties of I_{Ks} potassium channels. J Gen Physiol 112:665-678, 1998.
99. Sesti F, Goldstein SA: Single-channel characteristics of wild-type I_{Ks} channels and channels formed with two minK mutants that cause long QT syndrome. J Gen Physiol 112:651-663, 1998.
100. Nakajo K, Kubo Y: KCNE1 and KCNE3 stabilize and/or slow voltage sensing S4 segment of KCNQ1 channel. J Gen Physiol 130:269-281, 2007.
101. Tristani-Firouzi M, Sanguinetti MC: Voltage-dependent inactivation of the K^+ channel KvLQT1 is eliminated by association with minK subunits. J Physiol 510:37-45, 1998.
102. Pusch M, Magrassi R, Wollnik B, Conti F: Activation and inactivation of homomeric KvLQT1 potassium channels. Biophys J 75:785-792, 1998.
103. Seebohm G, Scherer CR, Busch AE, Lerche C: Identification of specific pore residues mediating KCNQ1 inactivation. A novel mechanism for long QT syndrome. J Biol Chem. 276:13600-13605, 2001.
104. Jespersen T, Grunnet M, Olesen SP: The KCNQ1 potassium channel: From gene to physiological function. Physiology (Bethesda) 20:408-416, 2005.
105. Lundquist AL, Manderfield LJ, Vanoye CG, et al: Expression of multiple *KCNE* genes in human heart may enable variable modulation of I_{Ks}. J Mol Cell Cardiol 38:277-287, 2005.
106. Bendahhou S, Marionneau C, Haurogne K, et al: In vitro molecular interactions and distribution of KCNE family with KCNQ1 in the human heart. Cardiovasc Res 67:529-538, 2005.

Cardiac Stretch–Activated Channels and Mechano-Electric Transduction

11

Peter Kohl

CHAPTER OUTLINE

Background

The heart is an exquisitely mechanosensitive organ, as anyone who has ever come in contact with cardiac tissue will appreciate. Langendorff-perfused heart preparations, for example (unfortunately a vanishing commodity of modern biomedical training), can be stopped or restarted literally at the flick of a finger. This is not a phenomenon restricted to small animals or the isolated heart. Reinstatement of normal sinus node rhythm in patients who are being weaned from cardiac bypass is regularly prompted by finger-tapping of the exposed ventricular wall. As with electrical stimulation that may be used to pace, "cardiovert," or fibrillate a heart, mechanical stimuli also can contribute to the initiation and maintenance of arrhythmias. Mechanically induced arrhythmias are of variable severity and duration, including premature ventricular beats (PVBs), tachycardia, and fibrillation. Manifestations of this behavior are exploited, inadvertently at times, for example in judging the final approach of cardiac catheters to the heart by monitoring the occurrence of PVBs.

In conceptual terms, cardiac mechano-electric transduction can be taken to complement the process of excitation-contraction coupling, thereby integrating cardiac mechano-electric behavior (Fig. 11-1). Manifestations of cardiac mechanosensitivity are present at all levels of structural and functional integration, from in situ findings in patients and whole-animal experiments, to ex situ tissue and organ studies, in vitro cells or culture systems, and subcellular domains such as membrane patches. Indeed, patch clamp identification of cardiac stretch–activated ion channels (SACs), by Sachs and coworkers,[1] was pivotal not only for development of insight into mechanisms underlying cardiac mechano-electric transduction but also for advancement of a topic that had long been viewed as "artifact" or a matter of clinical curiosity, rather than a relevant component of cardiac electro-mechanic integration.

The UK Medical and Biotechnology & Biosciences Research Councils provide continued support for work on which this chapter is based. The author is a Senior Fellow of the British Heart Foundation.

As it turns out, effects of SACs on cardiomyocyte electrophysiology are theoretically sufficient to quantitatively explain a majority of known acute manifestations of cardiac mechano-electric transduction, both proarrhythmic and antiarrhythmic. Such plausibility does not confirm, of course, that SACs are the only, or even the major, contributor to mechanosensitive responses in cardiac electrophysiology. On the contrary, a multitude of mechanisms are involved in functional and structural adaptation of myocardium to its mechanical environment. These non–SAC-mediated cardiac mechanosensitive responses recently have been addressed in several excellent reviews.[2-6]

This chapter focuses on acute electrophysiologic responses of the heart to mechanical stimulation, and on the roles that SACs play as mediators of cardiac mechano-electric transduction.

Functional Relevance of Cardiac Mechano-Electric Transduction

Effects of cardiac mechanical stimulation on heart rate and rhythm have been reported in the medical literature for well over a century. To name but a few core contributions (a more complete review is available[7]), pioneering work by Felice Meola and by Ferdinand Riedinger identified, in the late 19th century, *commotio cordis* (or *commotio thoracica*) as an independent pathologic entity wherein cardiac rhythm disturbances of variable severity were caused by nonpenetrating mechanical stimulation of the chest in the absence of structural damage to the heart. In the early 20th century, Eduard Schott and Luigi Condorelli reported independently that precordial fist thumps could be used to pace otherwise asystolic ventricles, such as in Adams-Stokes syndrome sufferers, and Francis Bainbridge famously identified the positive chronotropic response of the heart to increased venous return. This response was subsequently confirmed in isolated cardiac tissue by John Blinks and by Klaus Deck, who showed that this mechanosensitive behavior was encoded, in part at least, at the level of cardiac tissue.

Thus, from the very beginning of published reports on the subject, mechanical stimulation of the heart has been found to have the potential for both causing and terminating heart rhythm disturbances, as well as for modulating normal pacemaking rate.

Mechanical Induction of Nonphysiologic Rhythms

Diastolic stretch of cardiac tissue generally causes membrane depolarization (if the stretch is strong enough to induce any change), whether in working myocardium[8] (where such depolarization may trigger PVB) or in conduction[9] and pacemaker tissue[10] (where, in many, but not all species, an increase in pacemaking rate is observed).[11] The rate of rise in intensity of transient mechanical stimuli enhances electrophysiologic efficacy.

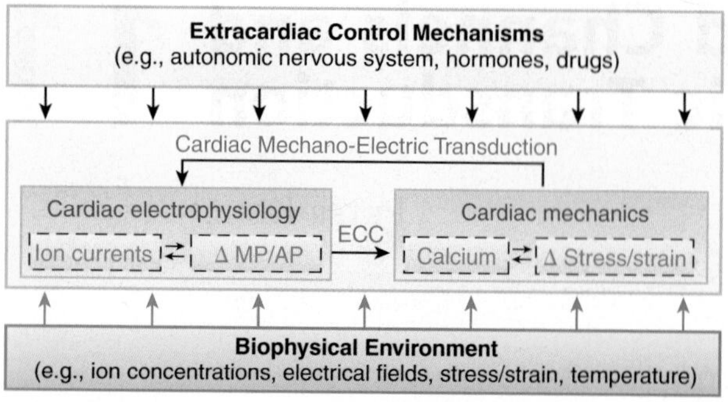

Figure 11-1 Schematic view of cardiac electro-mechanic integration. Within the heart itself *(center box)*, electrical behavior steers mechanical activity by means of excitation-contraction coupling (ECC), but it is in turn affected by mechano-electric transduction. The process involves a multitude of interdependent feed-forward and feedback pathways that affect ion transport, membrane potential (MP), and action potential (AP) configuration (Δ MP/AP), calcium handling, and stress-strain dynamics (*not shown* in detail, for simplicity). Intracardiac electro-mechanic interactions are modulated by the biophysical environment of the heart *(bottom box)*, and they form a target of extracardiac control *(top box)*.

This effect involves mechanisms beyond those known from electrical stimulation and includes the viscoelastic coupling between macroscopic mechanical commands and electrophysiologically relevant microscopic effects on mechano-electric transducers.[6] The fact that mechanical stimuli of sufficient amplitude can be used to pace otherwise asystolic hearts has been elegantly illustrated by Franz and colleagues using Langendorff-perfused rabbit heart preparations in which the ventricles, rendered asystolic by ablation of the atrioventricular node, were stimulated by periodic inflation of an intraventricular balloon (Fig. 11-2).

Similar behavior is understood to underlie so-called fist pacing in asystolic patients. Energy levels required for mechanical PVB induction by precordial impact have been established by defibrillation pioneer Zoll and colleagues in human volunteers as 0.04-1.5 J.[12] For comparison, the lower end of this energy range is roughly equivalent to dropping a 50-g laser pointer from a height of just over 8 cm (3 inches).

The same study found that in anesthetized dogs, impacts with energies 10 times the PVB induction threshold do not induce repetitive responses, tachycardia, or fibrillation, even if applied

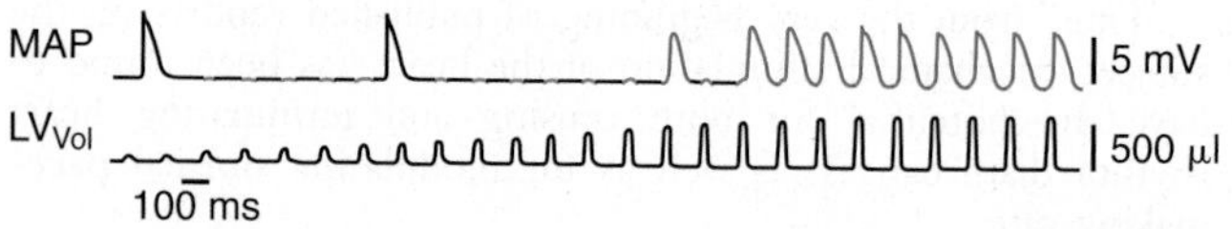

Figure 11-2 Mechanical pacing of the asystolic heart (rabbit isolated Langendorff-perfused preparation). Pulsatile left ventricular (LV) distention (*bottom trace*, showing increasing LV balloon inflation volumes) causes diastolic membrane depolarization (*top trace, blue highlights*). The amplitude of diastolic depolarization increases with that of the mechanical stimulus and, on reaching threshold levels, gives rise to generation of action potentials with each volume stimulus (*top trace, red*). *Note*: The first two action potentials are spontaneous escape beats, unrelated to the mechanical stimulus. LV_{Vol}, LV volume increase; MAP, monophasic action potential. (Modified from Franz MR, Cima R, Wang D, et al: Electrophysiological effects of myocardial stretch and mechanical determinants of stretch-activated arrhythmias. Circulation 86:968-978, 1992.)

in the relative refractory period.[12] Overall, this finding is in keeping with the notion that arrhythmogenesis requires the combination of *trigger* and *sustaining mechanisms*, so that consequences of isolated ectopic beats, whether mechanically induced or not, usually are benign.

Although the foregoing examples illustrate effects of the external mechanical environment on cardiac mechano-electric transduction (see Fig. 11-1, bottom box), mechanical induction of PVBs also may occur as a result of the heart's own contractile activity (see Fig. 11-1, middle box). This is illustrated in Figure 11-3A, which shows monophasic action potential (MAP) recordings from a patient undergoing pulmonary balloon valvuloplasty, a procedure whereby the stenosed right ventricular outflow valve is widened by insertion and inflation of a balloon. During balloon inflation, right ventricular contractions are isovolumic (no ejection) and give rise to significantly increased right ventricular peak pressures. This generally is associated with action potential shortening and occurrence of early afterdepolarization (EAD)-like events. If suprathreshold, these can give rise to PVBs.[13] As before, against an otherwise inconspicuous myocardial background, repetitive activity is not normally induced.

In contrast, in the presence of preexisting pathology, PVBs may give rise to sustained arrhythmias. Figure 11-3B shows an example of a whole-animal model of pathologically prolonged QT intervals (long QT syndrome—here, LQT1). QT interval prolongation is induced acutely by pharmacologic block (HMR1556) of the slowly activating component of the delayed rectifier potassium current (I_{Ks}). On this background, additional β-adrenergic stimulation (see Fig. 11-1, top box), here by bolus injection of isoproterenol, gives rise to ventricular aftercontractions of increasing amplitude (up to 25 mm Hg). Originating from near-endocardial locations, their onset may precede (by tens of milliseconds) epicardial afterdepolarizations or alterations in descending T-wave morphology (when visible). With increasing amplitude, afterdepolarizations eventually reach threshold for PVB generation, followed by induction of torsades de pointes arrhythmic activity.[14]

Under certain conditions, acute mechanical stimulation alone is sufficient to give rise to both trigger *and* sustaining mechanisms for maintained arrhythmias, even in otherwise healthy myocardium—for example, in *commotio cordis*.[15] A number of risk factors for the mechanical induction of such rhythm disturbances have been identified, based on experimental observations from the pioneering work of Schlomka[16] to modern-day studies by Link and colleagues.[17] Key risk factors are (1) type of impact (impulse-like stimulation whose arrhythmogenic risk is inversely related to projectile compliance and contact area), (2) impact location (chest areas that offer efficient energy transmission from body surface to myocardium), (3) impact energy (large subcontusional forces, reaching more than 100 J in competitive sports), and (4) impact timing (before peak of the electrocardiographic T-wave). The first three factors may be regarded as permissive: Only if they are present does timing become decisive,[18] which may explain why the vast majority of chest impacts result in relatively benign heart rhythm changes, if any. In addition, the time window for induction of ventricular fibrillation, the most severe outcome of commotio cordis, is very narrow indeed (a duration of about 15 ms has been observed in an anesthetized pig model).[19]

Quantitative model considerations suggest that arrhythmogenesis is favored, during this narrow time window, by a critical overlap of the mechanically stimulated tissue region with the trailing end of the excitation wave.[20,21] Sustained arrhythmogenesis occurs when, in addition to mechanical induction of PVBs in myocardium that has regained excitability (trigger), the intersection of mechanically affected myocardium and the trailing

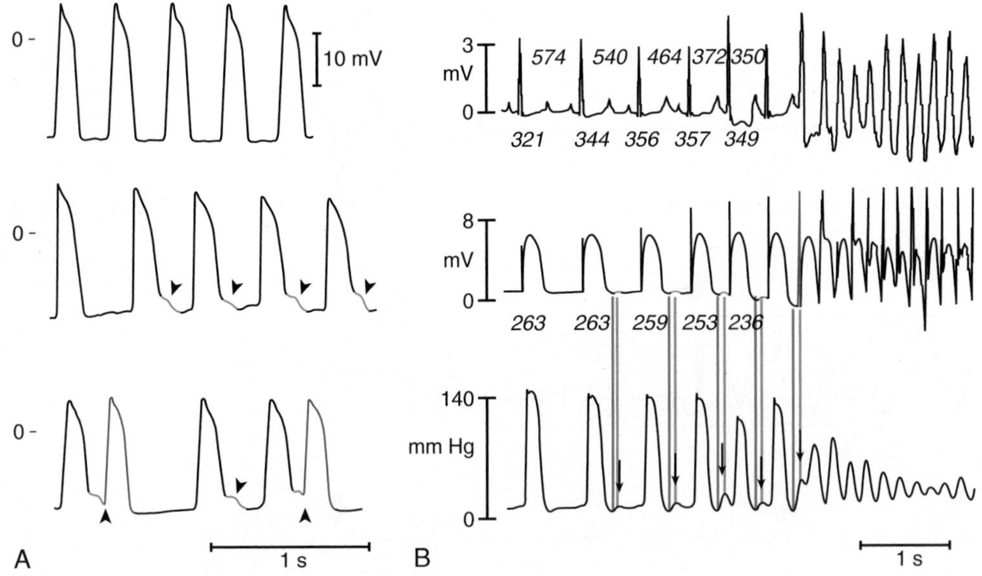

Figure 11-3 Cardiac contraction–induced tissue depolarization *(blue)* and induction of premature ventricular beats (PVBs) *(red)*. **A,** Early afterdepolarization-like events *(slanted arrow heads)* and induction of PVBs *(upward arrow heads)* during right ventricular (RV) outflow tract occlusion in a patient. Monophasic action potential (MAP) recordings from RV epicardium before (*top trace*) and during (*middle* and *bottom traces*) inflation of a balloon in the RV outflow tract. **B,** Incremental left ventricular (LV) aftercontractions precede induction of torsades de pointes (TdP) during β-adrenergic stimulation in an anesthetized dog model of long QT syndrome (LQT1). The onset of LV aftercontractions (*bottom trace, arrows*) precedes the occurrence of epicardial afterdepolarizations (*middle trace, blue*); once above threshold, these afterdepolarizations trigger a PVB (*middle trace, red*) inducing TdP (*top trace*). *From top to bottom*: Electrocardiogram (numbers indicate RR interval, above, and QT duration, below [in ms]); MAPs recorded from LV epicardium (numbers show MAP duration at 90% repolarization [in ms]); LV pressure. The *green* and *orange marker lines* indicate onset and peak LV aftercontractions, respectively. (**A** modified from Levine JH, Guarnieri T, Kadish AH, et al: Changes in myocardial repolarization in patients undergoing balloon valvuloplasty for congenital pulmonary stenosis: Evidence for contraction-excitation feedback in humans. Circulation 77:70-77, 1988. **B** modified from Gallacher DJ, Van de Water A, van der Linde H, et al: In vivo mechanisms precipitating torsades de pointes in a canine model of drug-induced long-QT1 syndrome. Cardiovasc Res 76:247-256, 2007.)

repolarization wave gives rise to a functional block zone around which reentry can develop (sustaining mechanism).

In contrast with these acute stretch effects, contributions of mechano-electric transduction to arrhythmogenesis in *chronic* cardiac overload are more difficult to uncover. Usually, pathologic conditions that involve cardiac pressure or volume overload tend to develop relatively slowly, and they are associated with pronounced structural and functional remodeling of the myocardium. The causes of both overload and tissue remodeling may be proarrhythmogenic in their own right. Nonetheless, mechanical factors have been implicated in the domestication of atrial fibrillation,[22] and in ventricular arrhythmogenesis in pressure- or volume-overloaded hearts.[23,24]

A conceptually interesting approach to probing the relevance of mechanical factors for arrhythmogenesis in the chronically overloaded heart is the temporary removal of tissue distention—for example, by the Valsalva maneuver (an attempt to forcefully exhale against the closed glottis). Intrathoracic pressure increases during the strain phase of the maneuver, reducing venous return and favoring arterial drainage from the chest, which leads to a measurable reduction in cardiac dimensions. On this background, ventricular tachycardia can be converted to sinus rhythm. By way of example, in the study illustrated in Figure 11-4, 7 of 15 patients showed sustained and 2 patients showed transient cardioversion.[23] Relief of ventricular wall stress, rather than autonomic nervous system–mediated responses, appears to be a causal contributor to this antiarrhythmic effect, because successful cardioversion also can be observed in the presence of pharmacologic[23] or surgical denervation of the heart (as in transplant recipients).[25]

Thus, acute diastolic stretch can trigger ectopic excitation, and systolic or sustained stretch may contribute to arrhythmia sustenance by causing heterogeneity in excitability, refractoriness, and electrical load. These observed effects have implications for preventive measures (chest protector design), as well as for interventions such as hemodynamic unloading, active and passive cardiac assist, biventricular pacing, or defibrillation, when defibrillation threshold increases with ventricular preload.[26,27] Of note, the recommendation in the 2005 International Liaison Committee on Resuscitation (ILCOR)

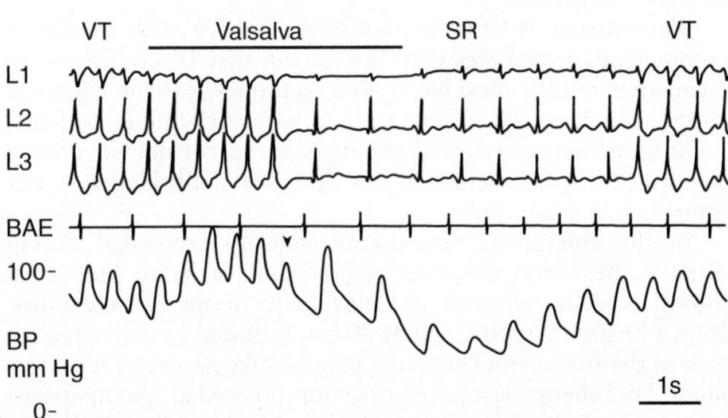

Figure 11-4 Temporary conversion of ventricular tachycardia (VT) to sinus rhythm (SR) by intrathoracic pressure–induced reduction in cardiac dimensions. The Valsalva maneuver is performed for the period indicated by the *horizontal line (at top)*, causing reduction in cardiac dimensions (confirmed independently), on the background of which VT is converted to SR (*arrowhead* indicating last ectopic beat). After termination of the maneuver, ventricles become re-distended, and VT resumes. BAE, bipolar atrial electrogram; BP, arterial blood pressure; L1 to L3, ECG leads 1 to 3. (From Waxman MB, Wald RW, Finley JP, et al: Valsalva termination of ventricular tachycardia. Circulation 62:843-851, 1980.)

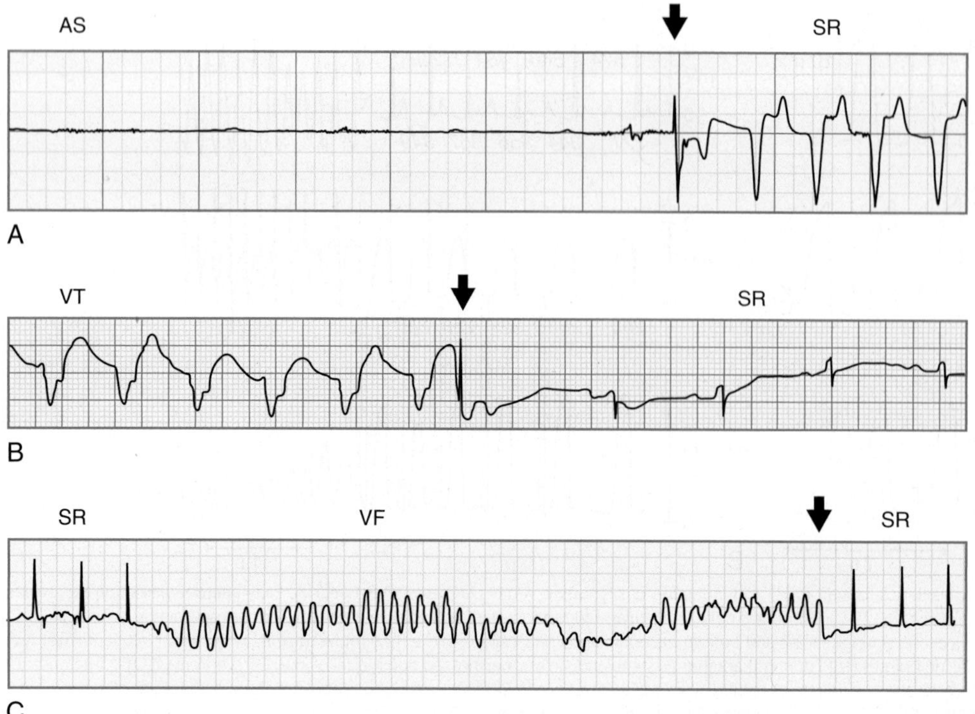

Figure 11-5 ECG recordings of precordial thump–induced cardioversion in patients. **A,** Conversion of ventricular asystole (AS) to sinus rhythm (SR) by precordial thump. **B,** Precordial thump–version of ventricular tachycardia (VT). **C,** Precordial thump–induced termination of early ventricular fibrillation (VF). *Arrows* indicate timing of precordial thump. (**A,** From Pellis T, Kette F, Lovisa D, et al: Utility of precordial thump for treatment of out of hospital cardiac arrest: A prospective study. Resuscitation 80:17-23, 2009. **B,** from Pennington JE, Taylor J, Lown B: Chest thump for reverting ventricular tachycardia. N Engl J Med 283:1192-1195, 1970; **C,** from Barrett JS: Chest thumps and the heart beat. N Engl J Med 284:393, 1971.)

guidelines, to apply cardiac compression before attempted defibrillation in adults with prolonged out-of-hospital cardiac arrest (for longer than 4 to 5 minutes), also may be beneficial in this context.

Mechanical Termination of Nonphysiologic Rhythms

Acute mechanical stimulation, usually by precordial thump, can be used as a means of advanced cardiopulmonary resuscitation to terminate arrhythmias, including ventricular asystole, ventricular tachycardia, and ventricular fibrillation (Fig. 11-5A,[28] B,[29] and C,[30] respectively).

The current ILCOR consensus on science with treatment recommendations states that "fist pacing may be considered in haemodynamically unstable bradyarrhythmias, until an electrical pacemaker is available," whereas in tachyarrhythmic patients, "one immediate precordial thump may be considered after a monitored cardiac arrest, if an electrical defibrillator is not immediately available."

In the emergency resuscitation setting, precordial thump often is the fastest resuscitative procedure at hand. Precordial thump is delivered with the ulnar side of the clenched fist, from a height of approximately 20 cm, followed by active retraction of the fist to emphasize the impulse-like nature of the stimulus. The energy levels required for precordial thump–based termination of ventricular tachycardia and ventricular fibrillation are one to two orders of magnitude higher than those involved in fist pacing of the asystolic ventricle (4 to 10 J versus approximately 0.04 to 1.5 J in the adult),[31,32] and these more powerful thumps are applied preferentially to the lower sternum, rather than the left sternal edge (which tends to be targeted by fist pacing and precordial percussion).[33]

The mechanism of action of precordial thumps differs from chest compression in that precordial thumps are aimed, in the asystolic heart, at triggering cardiac excitation to cause active contraction, rather than at expelling ventricular content via externally applied deformation of the heart. The hemodynamic efficacy of mechanically triggered cardiac contractions is not different from that of electrically stimulated beats,[34] and both are approximately twice as productive (in terms of volume output) as optimally performed chest compressions.[35] Precordial thump for termination of tachyarrhythmias is believed also to act primarily by depolarizing excitable tissue, in this case, however, with the effect of removing excitable gap(s).[29] Of interest, a common manifestation of precordial thump effects in electrocardiogram (ECG) recordings is a stimulus-related "artifact" that tends to point in the same direction as that of the major component of the normal QRS complex. This suggests that mechanically induced excitation may proceed along a general pathway in bulk myocardium that has an overall trajectory similar to that of normal electrical excitation. It is possible, therefore, that earliest excitation is triggered either in cells of the secondary or tertiary pacemaker and conduction tissue axes of the heart (such as Purkinje fibers, that have long been known to be mechanosensitive)[9] or in subendocardial locations (which, according to many reports, appear to show more pronounced responses to mechanical stimulation than subepicardial sites).[14]

Efficacy of precordial thumps in the real-life clinical setting is difficult to calibrate and compare because patient backgrounds vary over a large range of parameters, and mechanical impact properties are not normally monitored. The current ILCOR guidelines highlight the lack of controlled prospective studies in this area. Available data from systematic observations on tens[36] to 100 patients,[37] and retrospective data collections from even larger populations,[38] suggest that fist pacing of the bradycardic heart has higher success rates (up to 90%)[37] than precordial thump–version of tachyarrhythmias (between 60% and 1%).[36,39] At the same time, negative side effects (such as increases in ventricular tachycardia frequency) are relatively rare, and these do not usually include induction of ventricular fibrillation, unless there is pronounced preexisting metabolic impairment of cardiac tissue (such as in digitalis intoxication[31] or after asphyxia[40]). The mechanisms and determinants of the different effects of precordial mechanical stimulation on heart rhythm are the subjects of ongoing experimental research and computer modeling, but available data remain compatible with the notion of a mandatory involvement of SACs.[41]

Mechanical Modulation of Cardiac Pacemaking

A positive chronotropic response of the heart to stretch has been observed in many mammals with "low" resting heart rates, such as the guinea pig, rabbit, cat, dog, and human, but not in the fast-beating mouse heart, in which stretch actually reduces beating rate, although apparently involving the same underlying substrate—namely, SACs.[11]

From a systemic standpoint, early induction of the next beat in response to increased venous return is advantageous (unless volume throughput is inflow-limited, such as in species with already very high heart rates). In species with an "upright" body posture, however, a chief (and evidently overriding) requirement for survival is the control of cardiac output *pressure*, to ensure brain blood supply. Therefore, heart rate responses to hemodynamic stimuli that affect both venous return and arterial pressure (such as most changes in body posture—for example, in tilt-table experiments) will be determined primarily by arterial pressure control patterns. This obscured the identification of a positive chronotropic response to stretch in humans until Donald and Shepherd dissociated the increase in venous return from arterial pressure changes by passively elevating the legs of healthy volunteers in supine position, confirming the positive chronotropic response in humans.[42]

Cardiac mechano-electric transduction also is believed to underlie the component of respiratory sinus arrhythmia (RSA) that is independent of the autonomic nervous system. Here, dynamic changes in thoracoabdominal pressure gradients favor venous blood return to the heart during inspiration, causing a relative increase in right atrial filling and an associated rise in heart rate. Although this mechanical component contributes little to RSA at rest (when modulation of vagal innervation is the dominant driver), it becomes a major cause of RSA during peak exercise in healthy subjects (when vagal tone is reduced while respiratory effort and associated pressure gradient changes are enhanced),[43] as well as in transplant recipients.[44]

If mechanical modulation of heart rate were the only manifestation of "physiologic relevance," it might be tempting to ask why cardiac mechano-electric transduction has been preserved during evolution, against its clear proarrhythmic potential, which presumably would exert a negative selection bias. This question is somewhat misleading, of course, because the evolutionary cost of removing any trait is unknown (in particular, if it does not per se conflict with reproductive potential). It is possible, however, that the electrophysiologic manifestations of cardiac mechano-electric transduction are side effects, rather than main targets, of underlying mechanisms (akin to the arrhythmogenic potential, conferred on the Na^+-Ca^{2+} exchanger in calcium-overloaded cells as a consequence of its electrogenicity, whereas its physiologic function is to maintain ion concentration gradients). Thus, it is conceivable that mechano-electric transduction is a "side effect" of mechano-mechanic transduction, perhaps required for the adjustment of individual cells' calcium concentration to external mechanical demand, as discussed later (see "Conclusions and Outlook" section).

Overall, the range of cardiac electrophysiologic responses to mechanical stimuli is not different, in principle, from that caused by electrical energy delivery. Both can be used to pace, "cardiovert," or arrest the heart. Concepts such as the vulnerable window for the induction of particularly severe rhythm disturbances apply to both electrical and mechanical stimulation. Even the effective energy ranges required for pacing, cardioversion, and defibrillation are not entirely dissimilar (external electrical defibrillation, for example, usually is achieved by extracorporeal application of 150 to 250 J; only 4% of the induced currents actually traverse the heart,[45] yielding a cardiac energy delivery level of 6 to 10 J, as applied for precordial thump–version). These similarities are, perhaps, less surprising if one recalls that mechanical energy is converted into a transmembrane current by ion fluxes through SACs, occurring at the very target of the intervention—the cardiac cell.

Cardiac Stretch-Activated Ion Channels

Mechanosensitive ion channels can be found in most prokaryotic and eukaryotic cell types. They can be either activated, or inactivated, by mechanical stimuli such as stretch or cell swelling. Swelling-activated channels in particular are believed to be a phylogenetically ancient theme, required to allow single-celled organisms to adapt to potentially drastic changes in osmotic pressure in their external environment.

Types of Mechanosensitive Ion Channels

The mammalian heart contains ion channels that are activated by stretch in the absence of cell volume changes (SACs), and cell volume-activated channels (VACs). SACs respond to mechanical stimuli within milliseconds, whereas VACs tend to show a significant lag time (minutes) between the onset of cell volume changes and ion channel activation. SACs have therefore been implicated as a substrate underlying electrophysiologic responses to dynamic changes in the cardiac mechanical environment (the focus of this chapter), whereas VACs are understood to contribute in chronic settings such as (post)ischemic swelling or hypertrophy (in which VACs are constitutionally active).[46] Differences in activation time courses may indeed have prevented the observation of further similarities between the two channel populations, and this is a subject of current investigation.[47]

Cardiac SACs were discovered in the 1980s, initially in cultured avian skeletal muscle by Guharay and Sachs[1] and then in mammalian myocardium by Craelius and colleagues.[48] SACs either show little selectivity for (predominantly monovalent) cations (SAC_{NS}, for nonselective) or preferentially conduct potassium ions (SAC_K). These selectivity profiles determine their transmembrane current reversal potentials, which are halfway between action potential plateau and resting potentials for SAC_{NS} (usually between 0 and −30 mV) or close to the potassium equilibrium potential for SAC_K (approximately −95 mV).

Like other "descriptive" ion channel classifications, these categories are not absolute, and overlap with other types of ion channels is inevitable, as several mechanosensitive ion channels also are voltage- or ligand-sensitive (and vice versa). Thus, the hyperpolarization-activated cyclic nucleotide–sensitive channel (HCN) is mechanically modulated,[49] as is the adenosine triphosphate (ATP)-inactivated potassium channel (K_{ATP}), whose open probability is increased by stretch in atrial[50] and ventricular myocytes.[41] Mechanosensitivity may explain why these two ion channel populations appear to be less active when studied in vitro, compared with their expected behavior in situ. The contribution of the so-called *funny current*, i_f (HCN equivalent of cardiac pacemaker cells), to pacemaking, for example, could be underestimated under conditions of reduced external load (as is normally the case for isolated cell and tissue preparations).

Likewise, activation of K_{ATP} channels may occur only after reaching unusually low ATP levels in mechanically unloaded cardiac cells in vitro. This arrangement would be in keeping with the in situ observation that prevention of systolic stretch (paradoxical segment lengthening) of ischemic tissue, achieved using a tripod-like mechanical clamp, reduces or delays extracellular potassium accumulation in the anesthetized pig.[24] For practicality, SACs are therefore regarded as those channels whose open probability is affected *primarily* by the mechanical environment, and for whom mechanical stimulation normally is *sufficient* to promote opening.

SACs respond to a range of external stimuli, including local membrane deformation, changes in cell curvature, lateral compression, and axial stretch. Whether transfer of mechanical energy to the ion channel protein occurs mainly via the cytoskeleton or the lipid bilayer is a matter of debate (in all likelihood, both are involved, to individually varying degrees). Some SACs (such as a transient receptor potential channel [TRPC1]) can be activated mechanically in pure lipid bilayers.[51] Other SACs are sensitive to cytoskeletal integrity, which may either promote or prevent channel openings.[52]

The molecular level mechanisms of cardiac SAC activation are not well established. Open- and closed-state data from large-conductance prokaryotic mechanosensitive channels (MscL) have identified one mode of action: An iris-like increase in pore dimensions occurs during channel opening, involving an increase in the outer circumference of the protein in the plane of the sarcolemma, combined with a reduction in transsarcolemmal dimensions.[53] These changes would be favored by increased lipid bilayer tension and by membrane thinning, both of which could underlie the mechanosensitive gating of the channel. In this context, any channel whose projection in the plane of the cell membrane increases during opening *should* be sensitive to lipid bilayer tension. The question "Why do SAC channels exist?" could be replaced, therefore, by "How is it possible that certain channels show little mechanical modulation?" Recent reports indicate that the range of mechanosensitive channels may indeed be significantly larger than has been customarily assumed.[54]

No sequence or structure homologies of MscL have been identified in mammalian myocardium. Recent evidence, however, suggests that TRPC channels (such as TRPC1[51] or TRPC6[55]) may underlie cardiac SAC_{NS}, and cardiac SAC_K subtypes appear to include two-pore-domain channels (such as TREK-1)[56], inwardly rectifying channels (such as Kir),[57] and ligand-activated ones (e.g., K_{ATP}).[50]

A more detailed functional description of individual SACs has thus far been complicated by the fact that some channel populations (in particular, SAC_{NS}) appear to be located in membrane areas that are not easily accessible to patch clamp investigations in adult mammalian ventricular cells. These areas may include T tubules[58] and caveolae.[59] Single-channel data have therefore been obtained mainly in neonatal or atrial cells (which show few T tubules).

Pharmacologic Probes

In the absence of direct access to several of the relevant ion channel populations by the patch clamp technique, SAC contributions to cardiac electrophysiology have been studied by pharmacologic block, largely using the ionic form of gadolinium (Gd^{3+}) (typically 10 to 100 μM), aminoglycosidic antibiotics (e.g., streptomycin, in a dose of 30 to 50 μM), or a tarantula venom peptide, *Grammostola spatulata* mechanotoxin (GsMTx-4) (effective at concentrations ranging from 100 nM for the native peptide to 1 to 5 μM for the commercially available synthetic form). All of these substances have drawbacks. Gadolinium suffers from a lack in specificity (overlapping concentration range for block of L-type calcium, sodium, and rapid delayed rectifier potassium channels, as well as of the Na^+-Ca^{2+} exchanger), and precipitation in bicarbonate- or phosphate-buffered solutions (although it is possible that both Gd^{3+} and gadolinium salts may affect SACs). Aminoglycosidic antibiotics are not strictly selective (e.g., L-type calcium channel block with a half-maximal inhibitory concentration, IC_{50}, of 1 to 2 mM), nor are they necessarily reliable tools for acute SAC block in situ (if they were, they would be unlikely to be prescribed as antibiotics). Finally, GsMTx-4—although highly selective and effective in both D and L configurations—suffers from limited availability and high cost.

In view of the foregoing limitations, streptomycin has emerged as a popular pharmacologic probe to study SACs in vitro, where it efficiently and reasonably specifically (at micromolar concentrations) blocks whole-cell currents activated by axial stretch (Fig. 11-6). In this context, caution is advised when using cultured cells to study mechanosensitive behavior, because many culture media contain streptomycin.

The mechanisms of action of SAC blockers have not been fully resolved, but appear to include screening of negative charges (all known blockers are cations with net charges ranging from 2+ for streptomycin to 5+ for GsMTx-4), interactions with the lipid bilayer, and open channel block (a recent in-depth review by White[60] details the potential of SACs as targets for pharmacologic interventions).

Manifestations of Cardiac SAC Activation

Cellular-Level Responses

Whole-cell SAC currents have been recorded from most cardiomyocyte types, including sinoatrial node pacemaker cells, Purkinje fibers, and atrial and ventricular myocytes. Their effects on cellular electrophysiology depend on the effective stretch *target* (SAC_{NS}, SAC_K) and stretch *timing* relative to the cardiac cycle, as well as on rate of rise, amplitude, and profile of the *stimulus* (Fig. 11-7).

As a rule, diastolic stretch—if of sufficient amplitude to cause any changes in membrane potential at all—gives rise to depolarization. This can best be explained by activation of SAC_{NS}, whose pharmacologic blockade prevents these membrane potential changes.

Effects of stretch during the course of the action potential are less clear-cut, because shortening, crossover of repolarization, and action potential lengthening all have been reported. Some of this discrepancy may be explained by differences in recording techniques, because sharp electrodes and perforated or ruptured patch may give rise to opposite action potential duration changes, hinging on differential effects of these techniques on the interaction between SAC and calcium handling.[61] Crossover of action potential repolarization and EAD-like behavior are seen in particular when more severe stretch is applied and maintained throughout the course of the action potential (Fig 11-8). In this context, the repolarization level at which action potential duration is measured may also give rise to (apparently) conflicting data, because early action potential shortening can coincide with late action potential prolongation.

Although stretch of normal myocardium appears to preferentially target SAC_{NS} (whose block often fully eradicates acute whole-cell current responses in isolated cells) (see Fig. 11-6), different effects may be observed under conditions of metabolic impairment. Thus, K_{ATP} channels that normally are quiescent in atrial and ventricular cardiomyocytes respond to pipette suction[50] and axial stretch[41] when preactivated by a reduction in

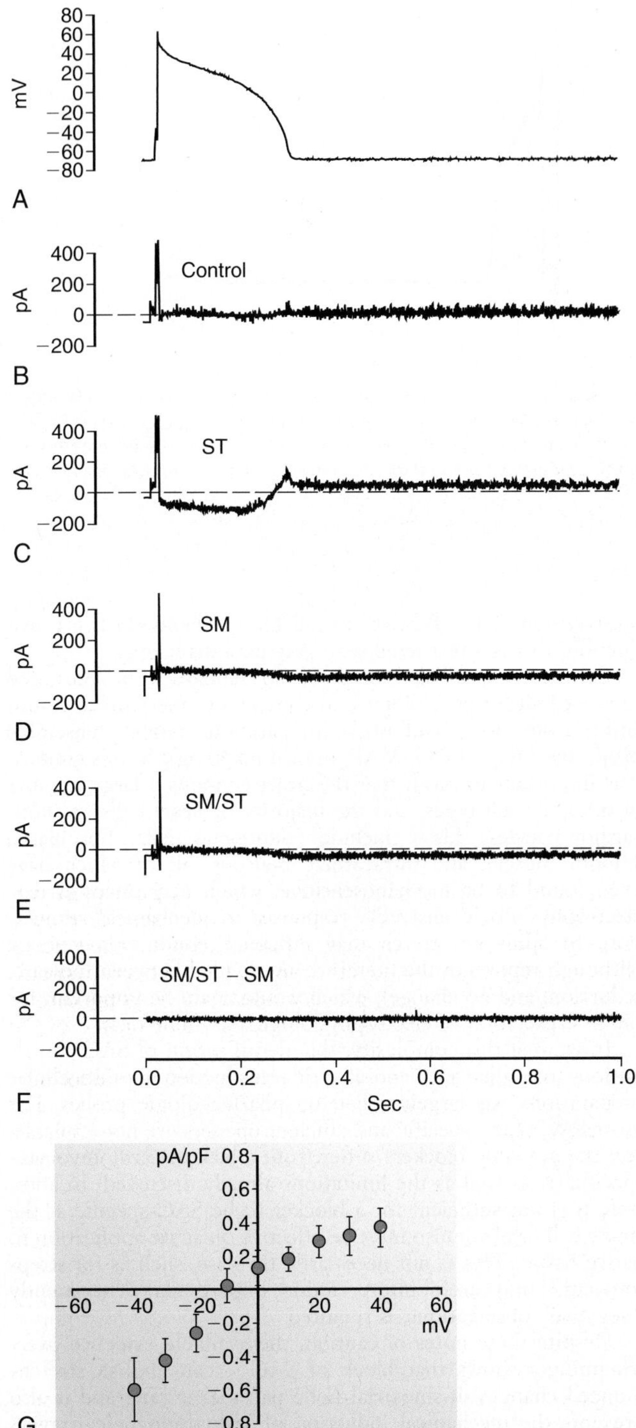

Figure 11-6 Action potential (AP) clamp recording of whole-cell current, induced by axial stretch of guinea pig ventricular myocyte, in the absence and presence of 40 μM of streptomycin. **A,** AP recorded in control conditions and reapplied to the same cell as a voltage clamp command (AP clamp). Compensation currents (**B** to **E**) illustrate the cell's response to interventions (*compensation* current polarity is opposite that of native *transmembrane* currents): **B,** absence of any intervention (Control); **C,** after application of 5% stretch (ST); **D,** after return to control length and application of streptomycin (SM); **E,** during 5% stretch in the presence of streptomycin (SM/ST); **F,** difference current (SM/ST − SM), illustrating that any streptomycin-resistant stretch-induced current is near 0 pA; **G,** current-voltage relation of the stretch-induced whole-cell current during AP repolarization from +40 to −40 mV; this current appears commensurate with SAC_{NS}, and it is completely abolished by 40 μM streptomycin *(not shown)*. (From Lei M, Cooper PJ, Kohl P: Unpublished data.)

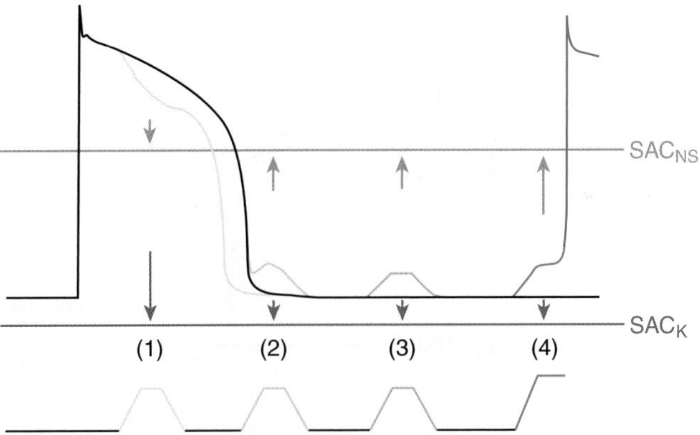

Figure 11-7 Schematic representation of transient stretch effects on whole-cell membrane potential (MP, black curve) with contributions by cation nonselective and potassium-selective stretch-activated channels (SAC_{NS} and SAC_K, respectively). SAC_{NS} *(orange)* have a reversal potential about halfway between plateau and resting MP. Depending on the timing of mechanical stimuli *(bottom curve)*, their activation may shorten action potential (AP) duration (1), cause early (2) or delayed (3) afterdepolarization-like behavior, or—if strong enough— trigger excitation (4) *(red)*. The reversal potential of SAC_K *(violet)* is negative to the resting MP. Their activation, during *any* part of the cardiac cycle, would tend to re- or hyperpolarize cardiac cells, in particular during the AP plateau (when their electrotonic driving force is largest; compare lengths of *arrows* indicating SAC effects on MP). Given that diastolic stretch, if it causes any change in MP at all, tends to depolarize resting membranes, the response of cardiomyocytes to stretch appears to be dominated by SAC_{NS} under normal circumstances.

ATP concentration. Such coactivation of a potassium-selective channel by ATP reduction and stretch could give rise to a less positive reversal potential of the net current induced by stretch in the ATP-starved heart. This may potentially explain the reduced efficacy of precordial thump (less efficient eradication of excitable gaps by reduced net inward current) in myocardium with severe metabolic impairment.[41]

Stretch effects vary not only with disease but also with age, cell type and location, and animal species. Subendocardial ventricular cardiomyocytes, for example, appear to be more likely than subepicardial cells to respond to mechanical stimulation by EAD-like behavior, both in single cells (see Fig. 11-8) and in whole animals.[14] Differences in mechanosensitivity may be caused by (1) variable expression, or responsiveness, of mechanotransducers; (2) different mechanical properties of components involved in transmission of mechanical stimuli to the transducers; or (3) distinct electrophysiologic background properties of affected cells and tissues. This last factor appears to underlie species differences in sinoatrial node pacemaker responses to mechanical stimulation.

The response of sinoatrial node pacemaker cells to stretch seems to chiefly involve SAC_{NS} activation, as shown in rabbit sinoatrial node isolated cells during axial stretch.[62] The principal effects of stretch on sinoatrial node action potential configuration are qualitatively equivalent to those observed in ventricular cells. They include an acceleration both of spontaneous diastolic depolarization and of early action potential repolarization rates (both with the ability to increase pacemaker rate), combined with a slowing of late action potential repolarization from approximately −15 mV (i.e., past the SAC_{NS} reversal potential) to maximum diastolic potentials (which would prolong the pacemaker cycle and reduce beating rate, if it dominated the response). In other words, spontaneous sinoatrial node pacemaker potential changes that move *toward* the reversal potential of SAC_{NS} (−11 mV in rabbit sinoatrial node cells)[62] are accelerated by

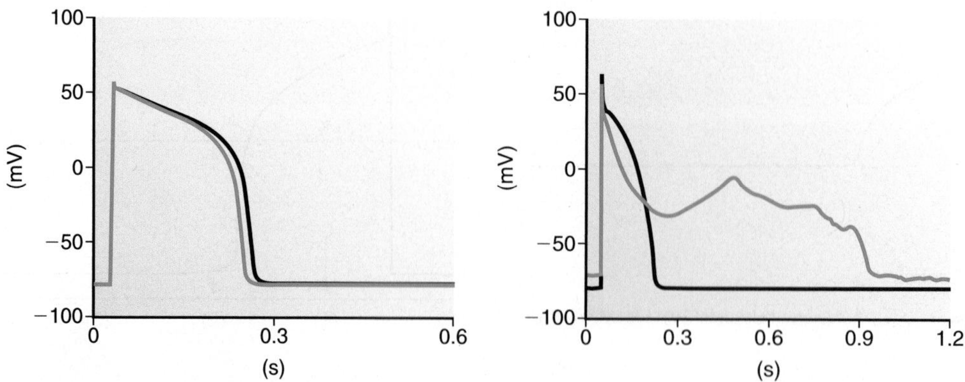

Figure 11-8 Effects of sustained moderate (4% to 5%) and severe (10% to 12%) stretch on guinea pig isolated ventricular myocyte action potential (AP) configuration. Perforated patch clamp recordings show AP shortening in the absence of diastolic membrane potential changes during moderate stretch, applied to a ventricular subepicardial myocyte using a pair of carbon fibers *(left)*; severe axial distention causes diastolic membrane depolarization, early AP shortening, and subsequent crossover of AP repolarization, yielding early afterdepolarization-like behavior in a subendocardial myocyte *(right)*. *Black*, control AP; *blue*, AP during stretch. Note different time scales on left and right. (From Cooper PJ, Cheng L-X, Kohl P: Unpublished data.)

stretch, whereas those that move away from the reversal potential are slowed.

If the sinoatrial node pacemaker potential waveforms of slow- and fast-beating mammals are compared (e.g., guinea pig or rabbit versus mouse), it is apparent that murine sinoatrial node pacemaker potentials have a very different inherent morphology: Both action potential upstroke and initial repolarization are very fast, followed by an extended late repolarization phase. The percentage of the pacemaker cycle during which the membrane potential moves *away* from the reversal potential of SAC_{NS} dominates murine sinoatrial node pacemaking (71%, compared with only 46% in the rabbit).[11] This property may underlie the negative chronotropic response to stretch, observed in murine sinoatrial node (even when beating rates are reduced experimentally, to be comparable to species that show a positive chronotropic response). Of importance, both the negative and the positive chronotropic responses to stretch can be abolished by application of GsMTx-4.[11] Thus, identical mechanisms may give rise to opposite responses, depending on the electrophysiologic background of affected cells and tissue—an observation that reemphasizes the need for caution in extrapolating observations between species, such as from mouse to human.

Tissue- and Organ-Level Effects

Cardiac arrhythmias are inherently multicellular phenomena, and it is therefore necessary to investigate mechanisms, modulators, and outcomes of cardiac mechano-electric transduction at tissue and organ levels. However, relating insight to lower levels of integration can be difficult in multicellular biologic systems.

On the "input" side, quantification of mechanical interventions is even more difficult in tissue than it is in cells (where sarcomere length can be used as an index of applied whole-cell strain) or membrane patches (where membrane deformation may be monitored). In most tissue preparations (except trabeculae or very thin papillary muscles), effective mechanical deformation usually cannot be monitored or graded at (sub)cellular levels. In the absence of cell deformation data, characterization of externally applied mechanical stimuli is helpful. Owing to the complex visco-elastic tissue properties which confer a strong time-varying component to the translation of external interventions into effective stimuli for mechano-electric transduction, this is a restricted surrogate parameter only.

On the "output" side, many of the standard techniques used to record electrophysiologic consequences of mechanical stimulation from tissue and organ preparations report "ensemble properties" (e.g., ECG, MAP, optical mapping). In this context, it is important to recall that the heart contains a large number of different cell types, and the majority of heart cells are non-cardiomyocytes. These include endothelial cells, fibroblasts, smooth muscle, and intracardiac neurons, all of which have been found to be mechanosensitive, which may affect cardiac electrophysiologic ensemble responses to mechanical stimulation. In addition, stretch may influence conduction velocity (although reports in the literature are divided between increase, reduction, and no change), which would again be important for the interpretation of electrophysiologic ensemble data.

In view of this complexity, the identification of SAC contributions to cardiac mechano-electric transduction in multicellular preparations has largely relied on pharmacologic probes. For most SAC types, specific and efficient openers are not available, and the available blockers suffer from a lack in cardiomyocyte-specificity, as well as the limitations already discussed. In addition, it is not sufficient for a blocker to be SAC-specific at the single cell level—it also must be effective on acute application to native tissue. This is not necessarily the case, such as for streptomycin,[11] and careful interpretation, in particular of apparently "negative" observations, is required.

Despite these notes of caution, the available evidence overwhelmingly shows that block of SAC_{NS} can abolish stretch-induced changes in sinoatrial node pacemaker rate, and it also prevents the mechanical induction of arrhythmogenic triggers (such as single PVBs)[63] or the mechanical promotion of sustained arrhythmias (such as in preload-dependent amplification of burst-pacing–induced AF).[64] Block of SAC_K can prevent mechanically induced development of ventricular fibrillation,[65] probably by removal of an arrhythmia-sustaining effect, or by modification of the vulnerable window for induction of vetricular fibrillation.[18]

Integration of cardiac mechano-electric transduction across levels of structural and functional complexity benefits from quantitative computational models that address behavior from SAC effects on cardiomyocyte activity[66] to regional stress-strain distribution in whole heart.[67] These models have been used to assess the biophysical plausibility of cause-and-effect predictions, and have aided hypothesis formation and experimental design for subsequent validation.[41] This combination of "wet" and "dry" research also has helped to identify engineering needs for improved experimental models to study cardiac mechano-electric transduction. The range of novel or improved tools, developed over the past two or three years, includes single-cell force-length clamps for cardiomyocyte work-loop investigations, structured tissue cultures grown on elastic membranes for control of the mechanical environment, mechanically coupled heterogeneous cardiac muscle strips, and isolated heart models of commotio cordis. These developments hold significant promise for new insight into cardiac mechano-electric transduction in the next few years.

Conclusions and Outlook

The currently available data suggest that mechanical stimulation, acting via sarcolemmal SACs, gives rise to changes in cardiomyocyte membrane or action potential configuration, which appear to be sufficient to quantitatively explain a majority of acute expressions of cardiac mechano-electric transduction (Fig. 11-9). Sufficiency should not, however, be confused with necessity, validity, or exclusivity. Thus, in addition to sarcolemmal SACs that allow ion flux between cell interior and extracellular space, channels in subcellular compartments may be mechanosensitive (such as in the sarcoplasmic reticulum,[68] or mitochondria[69]), as may channels that link neighboring cells (thus far shown for noncardiac connexin isoforms).[70]

Furthermore, there are complex interactions of SAC effects with other mediators of mechano-electric integration,

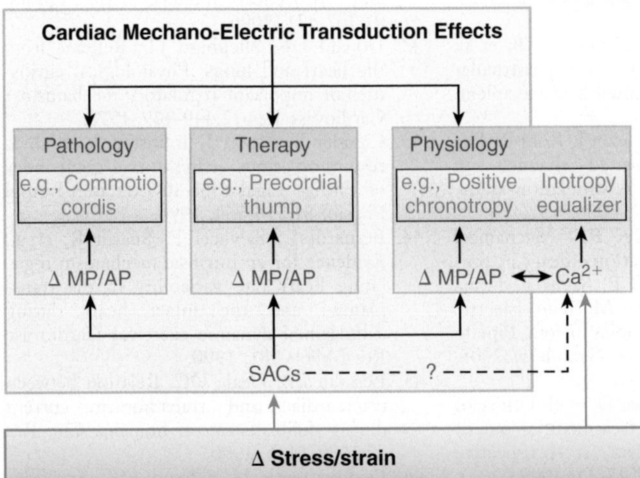

Figure 11-9 Schematic representation of functional relevance *(blue)* and key mechanisms *(red)* of acute cardiac mechano-electric transduction. Effects of mechano-electric transduction are particularly striking in the context of induction and termination of dysrhythmia (*left* and *middle*, respectively) and can be explained by the effects of stretch-activated ion channels (SACs) on cardiomyocyte electrophysiology. Less well documented is the physiologic relevance of cardiac SACs *(right)*, which—in addition to preload-dependent modulation of pacemaking rate—could include an additional role in the matching of individual cell contractility to external demand by modulating cellular calcium content (far right, see text). AP, action potential; MP, membrane potential. SACs, stretch-activated ion channels.

in particular calcium.[71] SACs may affect cellular calcium load either directly, or through changes in membrane or action potential configuration, with "knock-on" effects on voltage-sensitive calcium fluxes. This could, in fact, hold the key to a better understanding of the physiologic relevance of cardiac SACs. If, for example, an individual myocyte in situ was less contractile than its neighbors, then it would be stretched (or prevented from shortening) during systole. If this allowed the affected cell to either gain (possibly by way of calcium influx through SACs), or preserve, intracellular calcium (e.g., by way of sodium influx through SACs, reducing the driving force for calcium extrusion by the Na^+-Ca^{2+} exchanger), then this cell would be able to adapt its contractility to external demand, probably within a small number of beats. Such matching of local contractility to varying external loads has been shown experimentally in mechanically linked isolated cardiac muscle strips,[72] and it could act as an equalizer of the inotropic state of individual cardiomyocytes (see Fig. 11-9). This mechanism may underlie the efficient matching of microscopic function to regionally and temporally varying myocardial stress-strain gradients, which clearly is required to support externally homogeneous pump function in an inherently heterogeneous organ such as the heart. Interactions of sarcolemmal SACs with other mediators of mechano-electric function remain a key target for research into cardiac electro-mechanic integration.

In spite of recent progress in the description of SACs and their effects on cardiac mechano-electric transduction, the list of open questions is long. To name but a few:

- Current mechanical stimulation techniques generally are limited in their ability to control levels of stress or strain applied to individual cells or channels.
- The question whether stress or strain is the key modulator of SAC opening remains unanswered.
- Although the molecular-genetic identity of mammalian cardiac SACs is beginning to emerge, proteomic insight into channel structure and function is still scarce.
- The roles of regional differences in mechano-electric transduction, tissue heterogeneity, nonmyocyte cellular contributions, and so on, all are ill explored.
- Changes during development, aging, and disease are only beginning to be addressed.
- Pharmacologic tools for modulating SAC activity are neither organ-specific nor able to target individual cell types or disease states, and they suffer from a range of limitations that restrict their use in systemic investigations.
- Techniques to report electrophysiologic effects of in situ SAC activation should provide cell type–specific signals with high spatiotemporal resolution, perhaps through development of genetically encoded fluorescent markers.

All of these factors already constitute targets of ongoing research and development. These investigations are motivated not merely by the desire to better comprehend a constituent part of cardiac mechano-electric integration, but by their wider relevance for prevention and treatment of arrhythmias. A better grasp of cardiac mechano-electric transduction may open interesting opportunities for novel device developments, and it could hold significant promise for pharmacologic interventions, in particular if these could target areas of abnormal tissue motility, such as ischemic foci, aneurysms, or scars.

Acknowledgment

I thank Patricia J. Cooper and Alan Garny for their helpful comments during the preparation of this chapter.

References

1. Guharay F, Sachs F: Stretch-activated single ion channel currents in tissue-cultured embryonic chick skeletal muscle. J Physiol 352:685-701, 1984.
2. Linke WA: Sense and stretchability: The role of titin and titin-associated proteins in myocardial stress-sensing and mechanical dysfunction. Cardiovasc Res 77:637-648, 2008.
3. Spinale FG: Myocardial matrix remodeling and the matrix metalloproteinases: Influence on cardiac form and function. Physiol Rev 87:1285-1342, 2007.
4. Seddon M, Shah AM, Casadei B: Cardiomyocytes as effectors of nitric oxide signalling. Cardiovasc Res 75:315-326, 2007.
5. ter Keurs HE, Boyden PA: Calcium and arrhythmogenesis. Physiol Rev 87:457-506, 2007.
6. Suzuki T, Yamazaki T: Stretch effects on second messengers and early gene expression. In Kohl P, Sachs F, Franz MR (eds): Cardiac Mechano-Electric Feedback and Arrhythmias: From Pipette to Patient, Philadelphia: Saunders, 2005, pp 63-69.
7. Kohl P, Hunter P, Noble D: Stretch-induced changes in heart rate and rhythm: Clinical observations, experiments and mathematical models. Prog Biophys Mol Biol 71:91-138, 1999.
8. Franz MR, Cima R, Wang D, et al: Electrophysiological effects of myocardial stretch and mechanical determinants of stretch-activated arrhythmias. Circulation 86:968-978, 1992.
9. Kaufmann R, Theophile U: Automatiefördernde Dehnungseffekte an Purkinje-Fäden, Papillarmuskeln und Vorhoftrabekeln von Rhesus-Affen. Pflügers Archiv 297:174-189, 1967.
10. Deck KA: Dehnungseffekte am spontanschlagenden, isolierten Sinusknoten. Pflügers Archiv 280:120-130, 1964.
11. Cooper PJ, Kohl P: Species- and preparation-dependence of stretch effects on sino-atrial node pacemaking. Ann N Y Acad Sci 1047:324-335, 2005.
12. Zoll PM, Belgard AH, Weintraub MJ, Frank HA: External mechanical cardiac stimulation. N Engl J Med 294: 1274-1275, 1976.
13. Levine JH, Guarnieri T, Kadish AH, et al: Changes in myocardial repolarization in patients undergoing balloon valvuloplasty for congenital pulmonary stenosis: Evidence for contraction-excitation feedback in humans. Circulation 77:70-77, 1988.
14. Gallacher DJ, Van de Water A, van der Linde H, et al: In vivo mechanisms precipitating torsades de pointes in a canine model of drug-induced long-QT1 syndrome. Cardiovasc Res 76:247-256, 2007.
15. Maron BJ, Gohman TE, Kyle SB, et al: Clinical profile and spectrum of commotio cordis. JAMA 287:1142-1146, 2002.
16. Schlomka G: Commotio cordis und ihre Folgen. Die Einwirkung stumpfer Brustwandtraumen auf das Herz. Ergeb Inn Med Kinderheilkd 47:1-91, 1934.
17. Link MS, Estes III NAM, Maron BJ: Sudden death caused by chest wall trauma (commotio cordis). In Kohl P, Sachs F, Franz MR (eds): Cardiac Mechano-Electric Feedback and Arrhythmias: From Pipette to Patient. Philadelphia, Saunders, 2005, pp 270-276.
18. Kohl P, Nesbitt AD, Cooper PJ, Lei M: Sudden cardiac death by commotio cordis: Role of mechano-electric feedback. Cardiovasc Res 50:280-289, 2001.
19. Link MS, Wang PJ, Pandian NG, et al: An experimental model of sudden cardiac death due to low-energy chest-wall impact (commotio cordis). N Engl J Med 338:1805-1811, 1998.
20. Garny A, Kohl P: Mechanical induction of arrhythmias during ventricular repolarization: modelling cellular mechanisms and their interaction in 2D. Ann N Y Acad Sci 1015:133-143, 2004.
21. Li W, Kohl P, Trayanova N: Induction of ventricular arrhythmias following a mechanical impact: a simulation study in 3D. J Mol Histol 35:679-686, 2004.
22. Allessie MA, Ausma J, Schotten U: Electrical, contractile and structural remodeling during atrial fibrillation. Cardiovasc Res 54:230-246, 2002.
23. Moreno J, Zaitsev AV, Warren M, et al: Effect of remodelling, stretch and ischaemia on ventricular fibrillation frequency and dynamics in a heart failure model. Cardiovasc Res 65:158, 2005.
24. Lab MJ: Regional stretch effects in pathological myocardium. In Kohl P, Sachs F, Franz MR (eds): Cardiac Mechano-Electric Feedback and Arrhythmias: From Pipette to Patient. Philadelphia, Saunders, 2005, pp 108-118.
25. Ambrosi P, Habib G, Kreitmann B, et al: Valsalva manoeuvre for supraventricular tachycardia in transplanted heart recipient. Lancet 346:713, 1995.
26. Trayanova N, Li W, Eason J, Kohl P: The effect of stretch-activated channels on defibrillation efficacy: A simulation study. Heart Rhythm 1:67-77, 2004.
27. Doppalapudi H, Ideker RE: Mechanical modulation of defibrillation efficacy by preload changes. In Kohl P, Sachs F, Franz MR (eds): Cardiac Mechano-Electric Feedback and Arrhythmias: From Pipette to Patient. Philadelphia, Saunders, 2005, pp 321-331.
28. Pellis T, Kette F, Lovisa D, et al: Utility of precordial thump for treatment of out of hospital cardiac arrest: A prospective study. Resuscitation 80:17-23, 2009.
29. Pennington JE, Taylor J, Lown B: Chest thump for reverting ventricular tachycardia. N Engl J Med 283:1192-1195, 1970.
30. Barrett JS: Chest thumps and the heart beat. N Engl J Med 284:393, 1971.
31. Sclarovsky S, Kracoff OH, Agmon J: Acceleration of ventricular tachycardia induced by a chest thump. Chest 80: 596-599, 1981.
32. Kohl P, King AM, Boulin C: Antiarrhythmic effects of acute mechanical stimulation. In Kohl P, Sachs F, Franz MR (eds): Cardiac Mechano-Electric Feedback and Arrhythmias: From Pipette to Patient. Philadelphia, Saunders, 2005, pp 304-314.
33. Eich C, Bleckmann A, Schwarz SKW: Percussion pacing—an almost forgotten procedure for haemodynamically unstable bradycardias? A report of three case studies and review of the literature. Br J Anaesth 98:429-433, 2007.
34. Chan L, Reid C, Taylor B: Effect of three emergency pacing modalities on cardiac output in cardiac arrest due to ventricular asystole. Resuscitation 52:117-119, 2002.
35. Iseri LT, Allen BJ, Baron K, Brodsky MA: Fist pacing, a forgotten procedure in bradysystolic cardiac arrest. Am Heart J 113:1545-1550, 1987.
36. Befeler B: Mechanical stimulation of the heart: Its therapeutic value in tachyarrhythmias. Chest 73:832-838, 1978.
37. Klumbies A, Paliege R, Volkmann H: Mechanische Notfallstimulation bei Asystolie und extremer Bradykardie. Z Gesamte Inn Med 43:348-352, 1988.
38. Kohl P: A hard beat to make the heart beat. Resuscitation Council (UK) Newsletter 10:2-4, 2005.
39. Amir O, Schliamser JE, Nemer S, Arie M: Ineffectiveness of precordial thump for cardioversion of malignant ventricular tachyarrhythmias. PACE 30:153-156, 2007.
40. Yakaitis RW, Redding JS: Precordial thumping during cardiac resusitation. Crit Care Med 1:22-26, 1973.
41. Kohl P, Bollensdorff C, Garny A: Effects of mechano-sensitive ion channels on ventricular electrophysiology: Experimental and theoretical models. Expl Physiol 91:307-321, 2006.
42. Donald DE, Shepherd JT: Reflexes from the heart and lungs: Physiological curiosities or important regulatory mechanisms? Cardiovasc Res 12:449-469, 1978.
43. Casadei B, Moon J, Johnston J, et al: Is respiratory sinus arrhythmia a good index of cardiac vagal tone in exercise? J Appl Physiol 81:556-564, 1996.
44. Bernardi L, Salvucci F, Suardi R, et al: Evidence for an intrinsic mechanism regulating heart rate variability in the transplanted and the intact heart during submaximal dynamic exercise? Cardiovasc Res 24:969-981, 1990.
45. Lerman BB, Deale OC: Relation between transcardiac and transthoracic current during defibrillation in humans. Circ Res 67:1420-1426, 1990.
46. Baumgarten CM, Clemo HF: Swelling-activated chloride channels in cardiac physiology and pathophysiology. Prog Biophys Mol Biol 82:25-42, 2003.
47. Seol CA, Kim WT, Ha JM, et al: Stretch-activated currents in cardiomyocytes isolated from rabbit pulmonary veins. Prog Biophys Mol Biol 97:217-231, 2008.
48. Craelius W, Chen V, El-Sherif N: Stretch activated ion channels in ventricular myocytes. BioSci Rep 8:407-414, 1988.
49. Lin W, Laitko U, Juranka PF, Morris CE: Dual stretch responses of mHCN2

pacemaker channels: Accelerated activation, accelerated deactivation. Biophys J 92:1559-1572, 2007.
50. van Wagoner DR, Lamorgese M: Ischemia potentiates the mechanosensitive modulation of atrial ATP-sensitive potassium channels. Ann N Y Acad Sci 723:392-395, 1994.
51. Maroto R, Raso A, Wood TG, et al: TRPC1 forms the stretch-activated cation channel in vertebrate cells. Nat Cell Biol 7:179-185, 2005.
52. Janmey PA: The cytoskeleton and cell signalling: Component localization and mechanical coupling. Physiol Rev 78:763-781, 1998.
53. Perozo E, Kloda A, Cortes DM, Martinac B: Physical principles underlying the transduction of bilayer deformation forces during mechanosensitive channel gating. Nat Struct Biol 9:696-703, 2002.
54. Morris CE, Juranka PF: Na_V channel mechanosensitivity: Activation and inactivation accelerate reversibly with stretch. Biophys J 93:822-833, 2007.
55. Dyachenko V, Christ A, Gubanov R, Isenberg G: Bending of Z-lines by mechanical stimuli: An input signal for integrin dependent modulation of ion channels? Prog Biophys Mol Biol 97:196-216, 2008.
56. Terrenoire C, Lauritzen I, Lesage F, et al: TREK-1–like potassium channel in atrial cells inhibited by β-adrenergic stimulation and activated by volatile anesthetics. Circ Res 89:336-342, 2001.
57. Tamargo J, Caballero R, Gomez R, et al: Pharmacology of cardiac potassium channels. Cardiovasc Res 62:9-33, 2004.
58. Zeng T, Bett GCL, Sachs F: Stretch-activated whole cell currents in adult rat cardiac myocytes. Am J Physiol 278:H548-H557, 2000.
59. Kohl P, Cooper PJ, Holloway H: Effects of acute ventricular volume manipulation on in situ cardiomyocyte cell membrane configuration. Prog Biophys Mol Biol 82:221-227, 2003.
60. White E: Mechanosensitive channels: Therapeutic targets in the myocardium? Curr Pharm Des 12:3645-3663, 2006.
61. Calaghan SC, Belus A, White E: Do stretch-induced changes in intracellular calcium modify the electrical activity of cardiac muscle? Prog Biophys Mol Biol 82:81-95, 2003.
62. Cooper PJ, Lei M, Cheng L-X, Kohl P: Axial stretch increases spontaneous pacemaker activity in rabbit isolated sinoatrial node cells. J Appl Physiol 89:2099-2104, 2000.
63. Hansen DE, Borganelli M, Stacy GPJ, Taylor LK: Dose-dependent inhibition of stretch-induced arrhythmias by gadolinium in isolated canine ventricles. Evidence for a unique mode of antiarrhythmic action. Circ Res 69:820-831, 1991.
64. Bode F, Sachs F, Franz MR: Tarantula peptide inhibits atrial fibrillation. Nature 409:35-36, 2001.
65. Link MS, Wang PJ, VanderBrink BA, et al: Selective activation of the K^+_{ATP} channel is a mechanism by which sudden death is produced by low-energy chest-wall impact (commotio cordis). Circulation 100: 413-418, 1999.
66. Healy SN, McCulloch AD: An ionic model of stretch-activated and stretch-modulated currents in rabbit ventricular myocytes. Eropace 7:S128-S134, 2005.
67. Remme EW, Nash MP, Hunter PJ: Distributions of myocyte stretch, stress, and work in models of normal and infarcted ventricles. In Kohl P, Sachs F, Franz MR (eds): Cardiac Mechano-Electric Feedback and Arrhythmias: From Pipette to Patient. Philadelphia, Saunders, 2005, pp 381-390.
68. Iribe G, Ward CW, Camelliti P, et al: Axial stretch of rat single ventricular cardiomyocytes causes an acute and transient increase in $Ca2^+$ spark rate. Circ Res 104:787-795, 2009.
69. Belmonte S, Morad M: 'Pressure-flow'–triggered intracellular Ca^{2+} transients in rat cardiac myocytes: Possible mechanisms and role of mitochondria. J Physiol 586:1379-1397, 2008.
70. Bao L, Sachs F, Dahl G: Connexins are mechanosensitive. Am J Physiol Cell Physiol 278:C1389-C1395, 2004.
71. ter Keurs HE, Wakayama Y, Sugai Y, et al: Role of sarcomere mechanics and Ca^{2+} overload in Ca^{2+} waves and arrhythmias in rat cardiac muscle. Ann N Y Acad Sci 1080:248-267, 2006.
72. Solovyova O, Katsnelson L, Konovalov P, et al: Activation sequence as a key factor in spatio-temporal optimization of myocardial function. Phil Trans R Soc (Ser A) 364:1367-1383, 2006.

The Sinoatrial Node: Its Complex Structure and Unique Ion Channel Gene Program

12

Mark R. Boyett, James O. Tellez, and Halina Dobrzynski

CHAPTER OUTLINE

The sinoatrial node, in order to fulfill its function as the pacemaker of the heart, has both a complex structure and a unique ion channel gene program, and these are the focus of this chapter. Clues concerning both have recently emerged from study of the embryonic development of the heart.

Development, Structure, and Function of the Sinoatrial Node

In medical textbooks, the sinoatrial node is always shown as a small tissue at the junction of the superior vena cava with the right atrium (for example, see the illustration from the famous medical illustrator, Frank H. Netter), but this is inconsistent with electrophysiologic findings: Both in patients and in normal human volunteers, the leading pacemaker site (identified by mapping extracellular potentials across the atria in patients during open heart surgery, or by mapping body surface potentials in normal human volunteers) can be at any site along the crista terminalis (a thick atrial muscle bundle) between the superior and inferior vena cava.[1] Similarly, in experimental animals, the leading pacemaker site can be at any site between the superior and the inferior vena cava, as shown in Figure 12-1A.[2] This variability suggests that the sinoatrial node is a much more extensive structure than was originally thought. Consistent with this idea, in order to ablate the sinoatrial node in the dog, an extensive lesion along the length of the crista terminalis from the superior to the inferior vena cava has to be made.[1]

From serial sections (some stained with Masson's trichrome to show histologic features and others immunolabeled for marker proteins), we have constructed a detailed computer model of the anatomy of the sinoatrial node of the rabbit.[3] The model, shown in Figure 12-1B, demonstrates that, in the rabbit at least, the sinoatrial node is an extensive structure, encompassing tissue from the superior to the inferior vena cava, as consistent with relevant electrophysiologic findings. The extensive nature of the sinoatrial node is a vestige of the embryologic development of the cardiac conduction system: In the embryo, the heart begins as a simple linear tube made of *primary myocardium*. The cardiac chambers (atria and ventricles), made of *working myocardium*, develop by budding off from the tube of primary myocardium.[4] Two transcription factors, Tbx2 and Tbx3, are expressed in the primary myocardium, but not in the working myocardium of the developing chambers (Tbx2 is expressed transiently during embryonic development and Tbx3 perhaps throughout life).[4] Tbx2 and Tbx3 are transcriptional repressors—their absence in the developing chambers allows the expression of a working myocardium-specific program of gene expression (involving perhaps more than 1500 genes[5]—see later on), resulting in low automaticity, high conduction velocity, high sarcoplasmic reticulum (SR) activity, and high contractility.[4] By contrast, the presence of Tbx2 and Tbx3 in the primary myocardium allows the primary myocardium to retain its characteristics: high automaticity, low conduction velocity, low SR activity, and low contractility.[4]

The Tbx3-expressing primary myocardium forms much of the cardiac conduction system. The Tbx3-expressing primary myocardium in a 12.5-day mouse embryo is shown in Figure 12-1C in red; it extends from the superior vena cava to the ventricles.[6] From the superior vena cava, the Tbx3-expressing primary myocardium extends down the dorsal wall of the right atrium—it is this tissue that forms the sinoatrial node in the adult (see Figure 12-1B). At the atrioventricular junction, there is a large mass of Tbx3-expressing primary myocardium: in the adult, this forms the atrioventricular node as well as the tricuspid, mitral and aortic ring bundles. Finally, the Tbx3-expressing primary myocardium in the ventricles forms the proximal bundle branches. Both the sinoatrial node alone[1] and the cardiac conduction system as a whole behave as a hierarchy of pacemakers, and the more superior the leading pacemaker site, the faster the heart rate. It is possible that this gradient in pacemaking is the result of a gradient in Tbx transcription factors.[5]

Ionic Currents and Ion Channels in the Sinoatrial Node

Many differences exist in electrical activity in the center of the sinoatrial node and the surrounding atrial muscle (Fig. 12-2). During diastole, in atrial muscle, a stable resting potential of approximately −80 mV has been measured (Fig. 12-2). By contrast, in the sinoatrial node, during diastole, the membrane is more depolarized (the maximum diastolic potential, the peak negative potential after the action potential, typically is approximately −60 mV); furthermore, during diastole, a slow depolarization occurs (see Fig. 12-2). This *diastolic depolarization* (or pacemaker potential) is ultimately responsible for pacemaking: When the membrane potential reaches the threshold potential

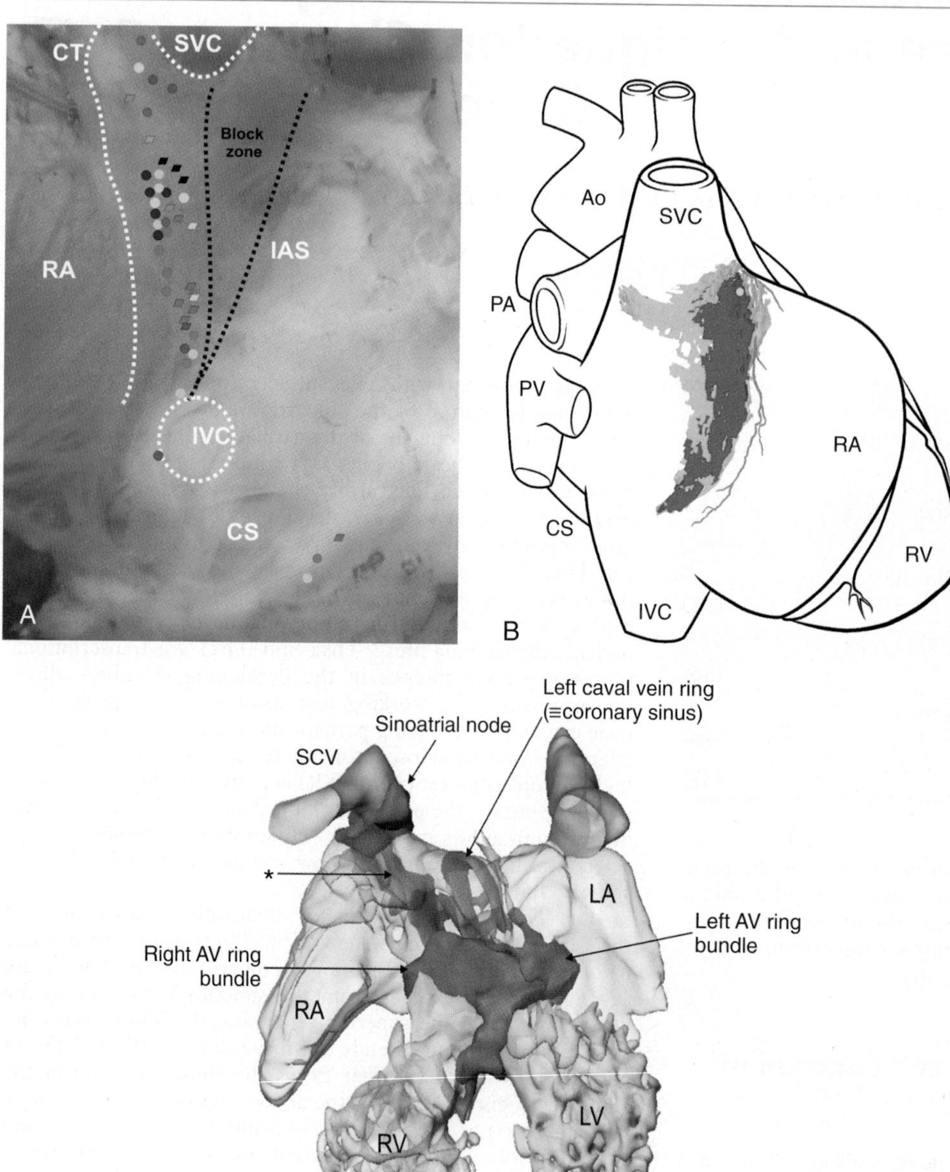

Figure 12-1 The sinoatrial node is an extensive structure. **A,** Position of the leading pacemaker site in the sinoatrial node of the rabbit. The *colored symbols* show the position of the leading pacemaker site in different preparations, and they are superimposed on a photograph of one of the right atrial preparations used. **B,** Model of the sinoatrial node of the rabbit superimposed on a dorsal view of the heart. *Red,* central sinoatrial node tissue; *blue,* peripheral sinoatrial node tissue. **C,** Ventral view of a three-dimensional reconstruction of Tbx3-positive tissue *(red)* in relation to the lumen of the right and left atria *(blue)* and the right *(green)* and left *(yellow)* ventricles of an E12.5 mouse heart. Ao, aorta; AV, atrioventricular; CS, coronary sinus; CT, crista terminalis; IAS, interatrial septum; IVC, inferior vena cava; LA, left atrium; LV, left ventricle; PA, pulmonary artery; PV, pulmonary vein; RA, right atrial free wall or right atrium; RV, right ventricle; SVC/SCV, superior vena cava/superior caval vein. (**A,** From Fedorov VV, Hucker WJ, Dobrzynski H, et al: Postganglionic nerve stimulation induces temporal inhibition of excitability in the rabbit sinoatrial node. Am J Physiol 291:H612-H623, 2006; **B,** from Dobrzynski H, Li J, Tellez J, et al: Computer three-dimensional reconstruction of the sinoatrial node. Circulation 111:846-854, 2005; **C,** from Hoogaars WM, Tessari A, Moorman AF, et al: The transcriptional repressor Tbx3 delineates the developing central conduction system of the heart. Cardiovasc Res 62:489-499, 2004.)

during the diastolic depolarization, another spontaneous action potential is initiated (see Fig. 12-2). Other differences in electrical activity have been recognized (see Fig. 12-2). For example, the upstroke of the action potential in the atrial muscle is rapid—the maximum upstroke velocity (dV/dt_{max}) is greater than 100 V/s. In the sinoatrial node, the upstroke of the action potential is slow (see Fig. 12-2)—for example, in the human, dV/dt_{max} is approximately 5 V/s.[7] Recent studies of messenger RNA (mRNA) levels for ion channels and associated subunits in the sinoatrial node using quantitative polymerase chain reaction (PCR) assay have greatly improved current understanding of the electrophysiologic character of this region; the studies by Tellez and colleagues[8,9] on the rabbit and rat and by Marionneau and coworkers[10] on the mouse are discussed later on. Figure 12-2 summarizes ion channel expression in the sinoatrial node and atrial muscle.

Sodium and Calcium Channels

The inward sodium current (I_{Na}) is responsible for the rapid upstroke of the action potential in the atrial muscle. The upstroke of the action potential in the centre of the sinoatrial node is slow, as a result of the absence of I_{Na} (Fig. 12-3B).[11,12] In the rabbit, the selective blocker of I_{Na}, tetrodotoxin (TTX), has no detectable effect on the electrical activity of tissue from the center of the sinoatrial node (see Fig. 12-3B).[13] In all species studied (rabbit, rat, and mouse—see earlier), at the mRNA level, the cardiac isoform of the sodium channel, $Na_V1.5$, is the most abundantly expressed sodium channel isoform in the atrial muscle, and the amount of $Na_V1.5$ mRNA is lower in the sinoatrial node than in the atrial muscle. Figure 12-3D shows the distribution of $Na_V1.5$ mRNA in the rabbit sinoatrial node as determined by in situ hybridization—it is present in the atrial muscle but is not detected in the center of the sinoatrial node.

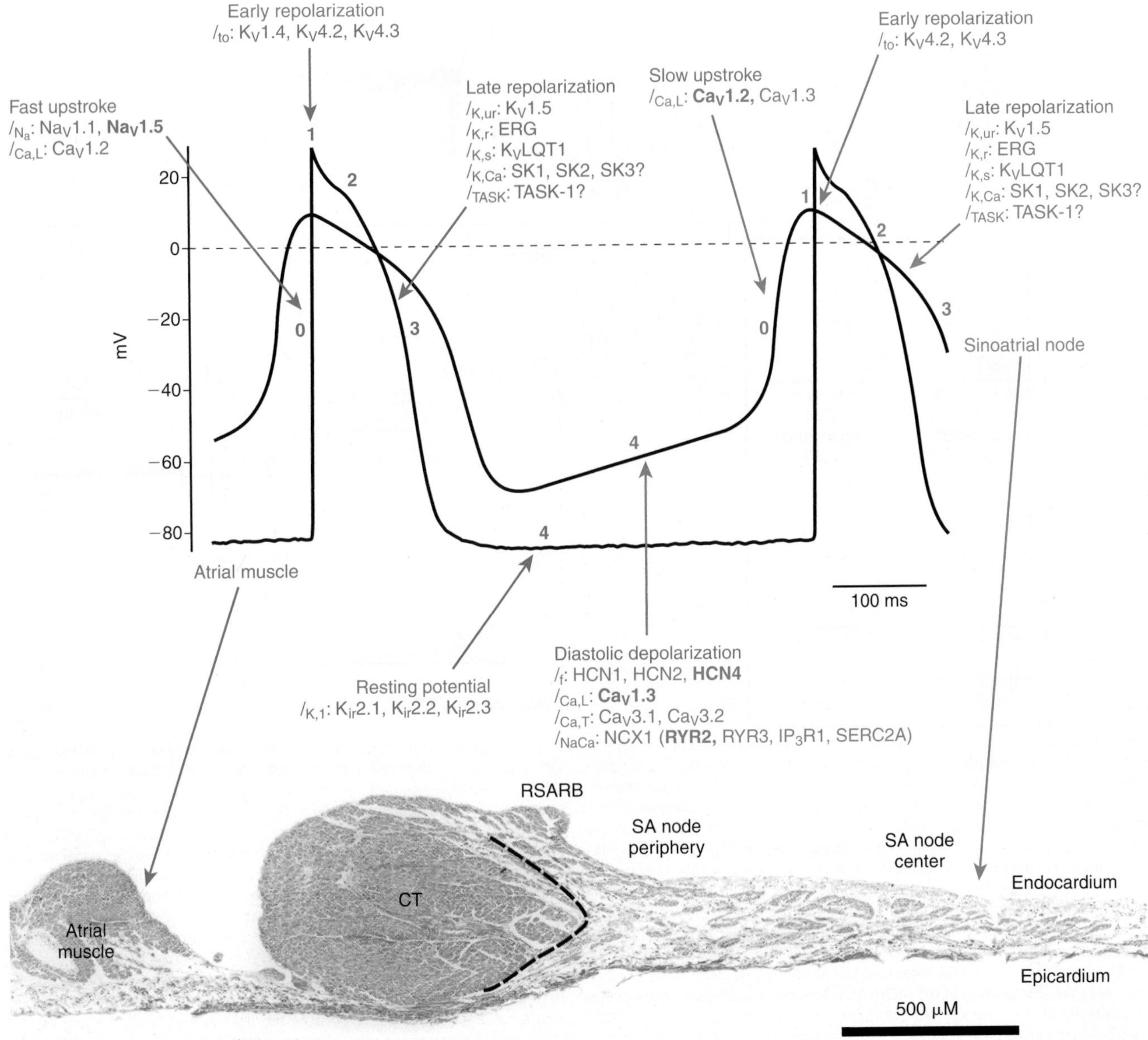

Figure 12-2 Summary of ionic currents and ion channels involved in the different phases of the sinoatrial node action potential. **Top,** Superimposed action potentials recorded from the center of the rabbit sinoatrial node and from the surrounding atrial muscle. *Green* annotations relate to the atrial action potential, and the *blue* annotations relate to the sinoatrial node action potential. The phases of the action potentials are *numbered*. Ionic currents and ion channels involved in the different phases are shown. More important ion channels are shown in **bold**. We have attempted to generalize, and the ionic currents and ion channels do not relate to a particular species (of note, however, important species differences exist). **Bottom,** Masson's trichrome–stained section through the rabbit sinoatrial node cut perpendicular to the crista terminalis (CT) approximately at the level of the leading pacemaker site. RSARB, right branch of the sinoatrial ring bundle.

$Na_V1.5$ protein also has been shown to be absent from the center of the (mouse) sinoatrial node.[12] The reduced level or absence of $Na_V1.5$ mRNA and protein in the center of the sinoatrial node is consistent with the absence of I_{Na} in this region. Despite the reduced level or absence of $Na_V1.5$ in the center of the sinoatrial node, the heterozygous $Na_V1.5$-knockout mouse has sinoatrial node dysfunction, manifested as bradycardia and increased sinoatrial node conduction time (Table 12-1). Furthermore, various families with familial (i.e., hereditary) sick sinus syndrome have been identified; in some instances, the sick sinus syndrome is linked to loss-of-function mutations in the gene (*SCN5A*) responsible for $Na_V1.5$ (see Table 12-1). A possible explanation for this unexpected sinoatrial node dysfunction is presented later in the chapter.

At the mRNA level, other isoforms of the sodium channel ($Na_V1.1$, $Na_V1.2$, $Na_V1.3$, $Na_V1.4$, and $Na_V1.6$) also have been detected in the sinoatrial node. In all species, however, they are weakly expressed in comparison with $Na_V1.5$. Nevertheless, in the rat and mouse sinoatrial node at least, $Na_V1.1$ protein is detectable throughout the sinoatrial node (and in the atrial muscle), and in the mouse, block of TTX-sensitive sodium channels (such as $Na_V1.1$—but not $Na_V1.5$) results in a slowing of pacemaking.[12] $Na_V\beta_1$ (at the mRNA level) has been shown to be the most abundantly expressed sodium channel accessory

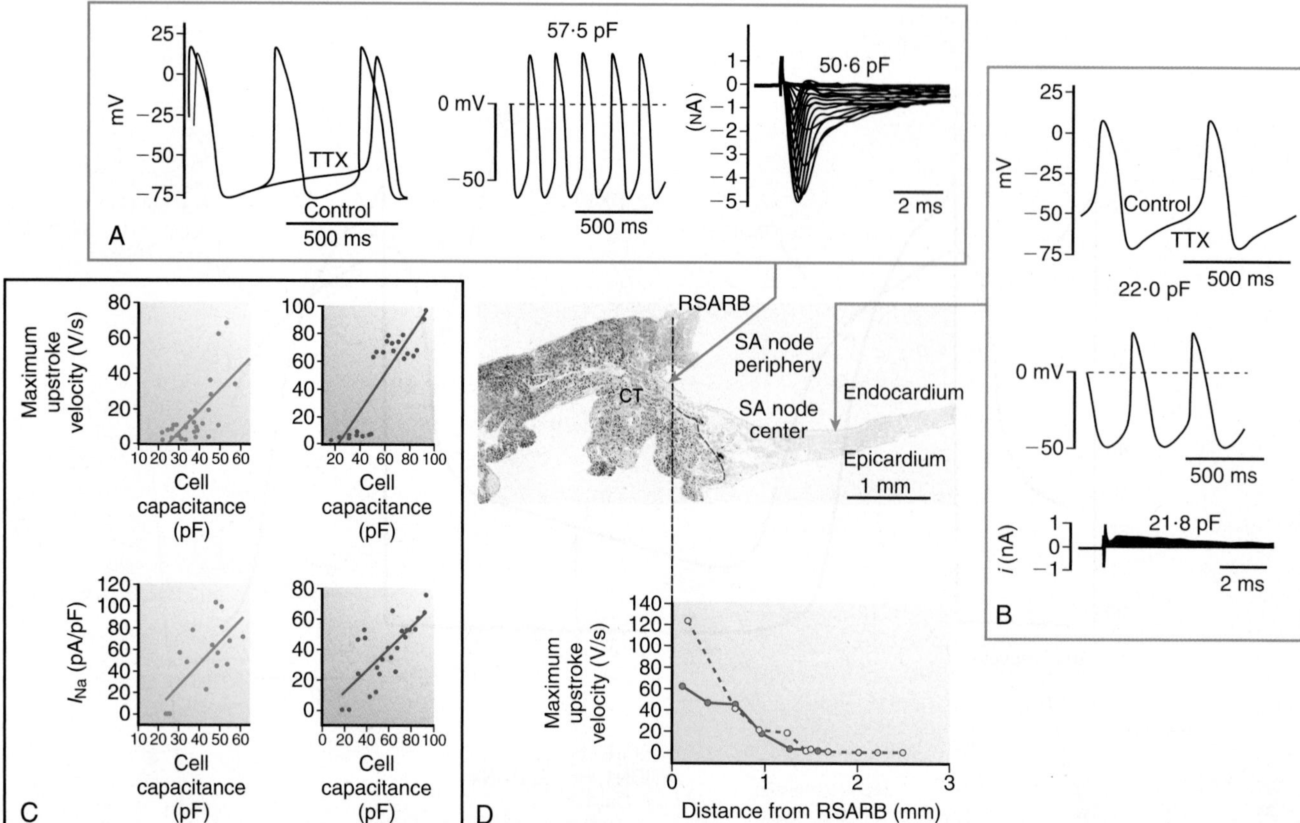

Figure 12-3 The action potential upstroke, I_{Na} and $Na_V1.5$ in the rabbit sinoatrial node. **A**, Role of I_{Na} in the periphery of the sinoatrial (SA) node. *Left*, Block of I_{Na} by tetrodotoxin (TTX) slows pacemaking in the periphery of the SA node; action potentials (recorded from a small ball of tissue isolated from the periphery of the SA node) under control conditions and in the presence of 20 μM TTX are superimposed. *Middle*, Action potentials recorded from a large SA node cell (cell capacitance, 57.5 pF) likely to be from the periphery of the SA node. *Right*, I_{Na} recorded from a large SA node cell (cell capacitance, 50.6 pF) likely to be from the periphery of the SA node. I_{Na} was recorded during pulses to −55 to +30 mV in 5-mV increments (holding potential, −60 mV). **B**, Role of I_{Na} in the center of the SA node. *Top*, Block of I_{Na} by TTX does *not* slow pacemaking in the center of the SA node; action potentials (recorded from a small ball of tissue isolated from the center of the SA node) under control conditions and in the presence of 20 μM TTX are superimposed. *Middle*, Action potentials recorded from a small SA node cell (cell capacitance, 22 pF) likely to be from the center of the SA node. *Bottom*, Currents recorded from a small SA node cell (cell capacitance, 21.8 pF) likely to be from the center of the SA node; I_{Na} is not present (voltage clamp protocol same as for **A**, *Right*). **C**, Cell size dependence of dV/dt_{max} of the action potential and the density of I_{Na} in rabbit SA node cells *(blue graphs)* and rabbit atrioventricular node cells *(red graphs)*. dV/dt_{max} in the *top graphs* and I_{Na} density at −5 (SA node cells) or −30 (atrioventricular node cells) mV in the *bottom graphs* are plotted against the cell capacitance (each point is from a different cell). **D**, Distribution of $Na_V1.5$ messenger RNA (mRNA) and dV/dt_{max} in the rabbit SA node. *Top*, Distribution of $Na_V1.5$ mRNA (as determined by in situ hybridization) in a section cut perpendicular to the crista terminalis (CT) approximately at the level of the leading pacemaker site. The labeling of the mRNA is in the form of black spots (corresponding to the rough endoplasmic reticulum)—labeling is seen in the atrial muscle and in the periphery of the SA node, but not in the center of the node. *Bottom*, dV/dt_{max} plotted as a function of distance from the right branch of the SA ring bundle (RSARB)—the graph is aligned with the tissue section. *Open circles*, values from the intact sinoatrial node; *closed circles*, values from small balls of tissue isolated from the different regions. (**A** and **B**, From Kodama I, Nikmaram MR, Boyett MR, et al: Regional differences in the role of the Ca^{2+} and Na^+ currents in pacemaker activity in the sinoatrial node. Am J Physiol 272:H2793-H2806, 1997; and Honjo H, Boyett MR, Kodama I, Toyama J: Correlation between electrical activity and the size of rabbit sinoatrial node cells. J Physiol 496:795-808, 1996. **C**, From Honjo H, Boyett MR, Kodama I, Toyama J: Correlation between electrical activity and the size of rabbit sinoatrial node cells. J Physiol 496:795-808, 1996; and Ren FX, Niu XL, Ou Y, et al: Morphological and electrophysiological properties of single myocardial cells from Koch triangle of rabbit heart. Chin Med J (Engl) 119:2075-2084, 2006. **D**, From Tellez JO, Dobrzynski H, Greener ID, et al: Differential expression of ion channel transcripts in atrial muscle and sinoatrial node in rabbit. Circ Res 99:1384-1393, 2006; and Kodama I, Boyett MR: Regional differences in the electrical activity of the rabbit sinus node. Pflügers Arch 404:214-226, 1985.)

subunit in the sinoatrial node of rat and mouse. However, $Na_V\beta_2$ has been shown to be functionally important in the mouse sinoatrial node—knockout results in "sick sinus–like syndrome," with a variable cycle length (see Table 12-1).

Two different inward calcium currents have been recorded in sinoatrial node cells. One current remains active for approximately 300 ms after activation; this is the long-lasting (L) type calcium current ($I_{Ca,L}$). The second current remains active for only approximately 30 ms after activation and is therefore known as the transient (T)-type calcium current ($I_{Ca,T}$). In the rabbit, block of $I_{Ca,L}$ with nifedipine results in the complete cessation of spontaneous activity in tissue from the center of the rabbit sinoatrial node.[13] This is because $I_{Ca,L}$ is the main contributor to the upstroke of the action potential in the center of the rabbit sinoatrial node as a result of the lack of I_{Na}. As well as the action potential upstroke, $I_{Ca,L}$ also is in part responsible for the plateau (phase 2) of the action potential, as it is elsewhere in the heart. At the mRNA level, the cardiac isoform of the L-type calcium channel, $Ca_V1.2$, is the most abundantly expressed L-type calcium channel isoform in the sinoatrial node of rat and mouse. In all species, however, the amount of $Ca_V1.2$ mRNA is lower in the sinoatrial node than in the atrial muscle. In addition, $Ca_V1.2$ protein has been reported to be undetectable within a region of the guinea pig sinoatrial node.[14] The mRNA for another L-type

Table 12-1 Ion Channels Associated with Bradycardia in Mice and Humans*

Channel Protein	Mouse	Human
$Na_V1.5$	•	•
$Na_V\beta_2$	•	
$Ca_V1.3$	•	
$Ca_V3.1$	•	
HCN2	•	
HCN4	•	•
ERG	•	
Ankyrin-B	•	•
RYR2		•
Connexin40	•	

Data from Dobrzynski H, Boyett MR, Anderson RH: New insights into pacemaker activity: Promoting understanding of sick sinus syndrome. Circulation 115:1921-1932, 2007; Lees-Miller JP, Guo J, Somers JR, et al: Selective knockout of mouse ERG1 B potassium channel eliminates I_{Kr} in adult ventricular myocytes and elicits episodes of abrupt sinus bradycardia. Mol Cell Biol 23:1856-1862, 2003; Postma AV, Denjoy I, Kamblock J, et al: Catecholaminergic polymorphic ventricular tachycardia: RYR2 mutations, bradycardia, and follow up of the patients. J Med Genet 42:863-870, 2005; and Zhang Z, Xu Y, Song H, et al: Functional roles of $Ca_V1.3$ α_{1D} calcium channel in sinoatrial nodes: Insight gained using gene-targeted null mutant mice. Circ Res 90:981-987, 2002.

*In humans, families have been identified with a history of sick sinus syndrome resulting from a mutation in an ion channel. In mice, bradycardia results from knockout of the gene encoding the ion channel protein.

ERG, ether-à-go-go–related gene; HCN, hyperpolarization-activated, cyclic nucleotide–gated; RYR2, ryanodine receptor-2.

calcium channel isoform, $Ca_V1.3$, is more abundant in the sinoatrial node than in the atrial muscle in all species. The importance of $Ca_V1.3$ has been shown by the $Ca_V1.3$-knockout mouse—the mouse has sinoatrial node dysfunction (bradycardia and spontaneous arrhythmias) (see Table 12-1).

$I_{Ca,T}$ has been recorded in sinoatrial node cells from several species.[15] Block of $I_{Ca,T}$ by Ni^{2+} slows the spontaneous activity of rabbit sinoatrial node cells.[15] This effect is due to the slowing of the last two thirds of the diastolic depolarization.[15] A role for $I_{Ca,T}$ in diastolic depolarization is consistent with its activation threshold of approximately −60 mV, which is within the diastolic range (see Fig. 12-2). The density of $I_{Ca,T}$ tends to be greater in smaller animals.[15] The ion channels responsible for $I_{Ca,T}$ are $Ca_V3.1$ and $Ca_V3.2$. $Ca_V3.1$ mRNA is equally abundant in the sinoatrial node and in atrial muscle in the rat. In the mouse, however, $Ca_v3.1$ mRNA is more abundant in the sinoatrial node than in the atrial muscle. In the rat and mouse, $Ca_V3.1$ mRNA is present at levels equal to those of $Ca_V1.2$ mRNA. The importance of $Ca_V3.1$ to sinoatrial node function in the mouse has been shown using the $Ca_V3.1$-knockout mouse, which has bradycardia (see Table 12-1). In the rabbit, $Ca_V3.1$ mRNA is undetectable in the sinoatrial node—this suggests that $Ca_V3.2$ is the dominant isoform, but mRNA data for $Ca_V3.2$ in the rabbit sinoatrial node are not available. In the mouse, the abundance of $Ca_V3.2$ mRNA is comparable to that of $Ca_V3.1$ mRNA.

The calcium channel complex includes several accessory subunits. In the mouse, $Ca_V\alpha_2\delta_2$ mRNA is more abundant in the sinoatrial node than in the atrial muscle, but this pattern is not seen in the other species. Messenger RNA for three Ca_V β subunits—$Ca_V\beta_1$ to $Ca_V\beta_3$—has been detected in the sinoatrial node, and $Ca_V\beta_2$ mRNA is the most abundant in the rat and mouse. The abundance of $Ca_V\gamma_4$ mRNA is lower in the sinoatrial node than in the atrial muscle in rat and mouse.

HCN Channels

One of the ionic currents underlying the diastolic depolarization in the sinoatrial node is the so-called *funny current* (I_f) (Fig. 12-4B). I_f has unusual properties that have earned the current its "funny" name and fit those required to generate the diastolic depolarization: It is activated in the diastolic range of potentials (negative to approximately −40 mV), it is inward in direction, and it is carried by both Na^+ and K^+ ions. I_f can be enhanced by adrenergic agonists; these agents increase intracellular cyclic AMP (cAMP), which can interact directly with the ion channel responsible for I_f.[16] Block of I_f by Cs^+ or ivabradine, for example, slows the spontaneous activity of sinoatrial node cells[16]—for example, in the human, the cycle length of sinoatrial node cells is increased by 26% with exposure to 2 mM Cs^+ (see Fig. 12-4A).[7] The hyperpolarization-activated, cyclic nucleotide–gated (HCN) family of ion channels is responsible for I_f. The four members of this family are HCN1 to HCN4. In all species, including the human,[17] at the mRNA level, HCN4 is the most abundantly expressed isoform in the sinoatrial node, and it is more abundant in the sinoatrial node than in the atrial muscle (e.g., see Fig. 12-4C). HCN4 protein is distributed in the same manner in the mouse and human (see Fig. 12-4D and E).[18] The importance of HCN4 has been demonstrated using the HCN4-knockout mouse: In the embryo, I_f is reduced by 85% in the sinoatrial node and the heart rate is reduced by 37%, and death occurs between embryonic days 9.5 and 11.5 (see Table 12-1). Three reports of familial sick sinus syndrome have been linked to mutations in HCN4 (see Table 12-1).

In all species, including the human,[17] HCN1 mRNA, like HCN4 mRNA, is more abundant in the sinoatrial node than in the atrial muscle (see Fig. 12-4C). In the rat, mouse, and human,[17] HCN2 mRNA also is present in the sinoatrial node, but at a lower level than that observed for HCN1 and HCN4 mRNAs. Nevertheless, the HCN2-knockout mouse displays sinus dysrhythmia (see Table 12-1). In the mouse and human[17] sinoatrial node, HCN3 mRNA is present at very low levels.

Transient Outward Potassium Channels

The transient outward potassium current (I_{to}) activates and inactivates rapidly on depolarization and is responsible for the early phase of repolarization (phase 1) during the course of the action potential and can control action potential duration. In the rabbit, I_{to} has been shown to be present in sinoatrial node cells, although at a lower density than in atrial cells.[8] In the rabbit sinoatrial node, block of I_{to} by 4-aminopyridine slows the initial rapid phase of repolarization and abolishes the notch (if present), prolongs action potential duration, and decreases the maximum diastolic potential.[19] The ion channels $K_V1.4$, $K_V4.2$, and $K_V4.3$ are responsible for I_{to}; the relative abundance of the three isoforms is species-dependent. In rabbit atrial muscle, at the mRNA level, $K_V1.4$ is the most abundant isoform, but it is less abundant in the sinoatrial node. Conversely, in the rabbit, $K_V4.2$ mRNA is more abundant in the sinoatrial node than in the atrial muscle.

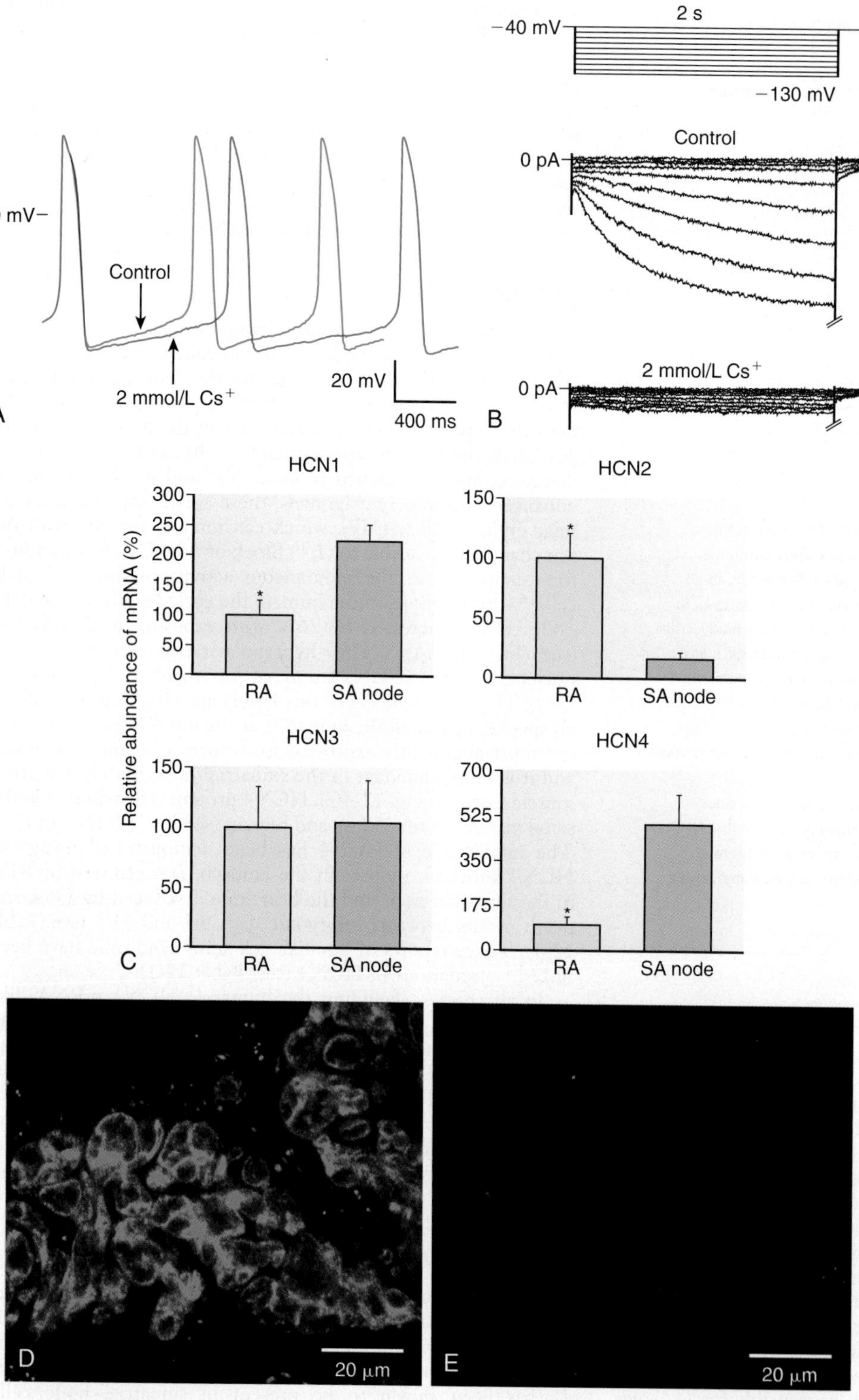

Figure 12-4 Funny channels and funny current in the human sinoatrial node: Superimposed action potentials (**A**) and recordings of I_f (during the voltage clamp pulses shown) (**B**) from a human sinoatrial node cell under control conditions and after block of I_f by 2 mM Cs^+. **C,** Relative abundance of messenger RNA for HCN1 to HCN4 (measured using quantitative polymerase chain reaction assay) in the atrial muscle and sinoatrial node of the human. Messenger RNA abundance is expressed as a percentage of that in the atrial muscle. **D** and **E,** Immunofluorescence labeling of HCN4 in the sinoatrial node (**D**) and atrial muscle (**E**) of the human. RA, right atrium; SA, sinoatrial. (**A** and **B,** From Verkerk AO, Wilders R, van Borren MM, et al: Pacemaker current (I_f) in the human sinoatrial node. Eur Heart J 28:2472-2478, 2007; **D** and **E,** from Chandler NJ, Molenaar P, Boyett MR, Dobrzynski H: Mapping of the human sinus node. Europace 9(Suppl 5):v10, 2007.)

Therefore, an isoform switch occurs from $K_V1.4$ to $K_V4.2$ from atrial muscle to sinoatrial node; this is consistent with relevant electrophysiologic findings: Whereas I_{to} recovers slowly from inactivation in the atrial muscle (time constants, 1.5 and 6.7 s), consistent with the properties of $K_V1.4$, it recovers rapidly in the sinoatrial node (time constant, 45 ms), consistent with the properties of $K_V4.2$.[8] In mouse atrial muscle, at the mRNA level, $K_V4.2$ is the most abundant isoform, and $K_V4.2$ mRNA is less abundant in the sinoatrial node than in the atrial muscle. The accessory subunits, KChAP and KChIP2, associate with K_V4 subunits[20] and mRNA for both KChAP and KChIP2 have been detected in the sinoatrial node.

Delayed Rectifier Potassium Channels

Three types of outward delayed rectifier potassium current are known to exist: ultra-rapid ($I_{K,ur}$), rapid ($I_{K,r}$), and slow ($I_{K,s}$). The currents are activated ultra-rapidly, rapidly, and slowly, respectively, on depolarization. Activation of the delayed rectifier potassium currents during the action potential helps bring about repolarization (and thereby helps determine action potential duration) and, in the absence of $I_{K,1}$ (see later on), sets the maximum diastolic potential. During diastole, the time-dependent deactivation (or decay) of $I_{K,r}$, and perhaps $I_{K,ur}$ and $I_{K,s}$, plays a permissive role in the diastolic depolarization—that is, it allows inward current to depolarize the membrane ("K^+ decay hypothesis"). The relative importance of $I_{K,r}$ and $I_{K,s}$ is species-dependent: $I_{K,r}$ is more important in the rabbit (however, although the role of $I_{K,s}$ is small under control conditions, it is significant during β-adrenergic stimulation), whereas $I_{K,s}$ is more important in the guinea pig.[21] Partial block of $I_{K,r}$ with the class III antiarrhythmic agent E-4031 in the rabbit sinoatrial node results in an increase in action potential duration, a more positive maximum diastolic potential, and a slowing of pacemaking.[19] $K_V1.5$ is the ion channel responsible for $I_{K,ur}$; $K_V11.1$, more commonly known as the ether-à-go-go–related gene (ERG) protein, is responsible for $I_{K,r}$; and $K_V7.1$, more commonly known as K_VLQT1, is responsible for $I_{K,s}$. Relative abundances in the sinoatrial node, at the mRNA level, are as follows: in the rabbit, ERG > K_VLQT1 ≈ $K_V1.5$; in the rat, ERG ≈ K_VLQT1 ≈ $K_V1.5$; and in the mouse, ERG ≈ K_vLQT1 > $K_V1.5$. $K_V1.5$ protein has been shown to be present in the guinea pig and ferret sinoatrial node.[8] The ERG-knockout mouse can experience spontaneous episodes of sinus bradycardia (see Table 12-1).

Inward Rectifier Potassium Channels

In the working myocardium, the background inward rectifier potassium current ($I_{K,1}$) is responsible for the stable resting potential, and its property of inward rectification facilitates the long plateau of the action potential. The maximum diastolic potential of sinoatrial node tissue is more positive than the resting potential of the working myocardium, and in the rabbit, this is the result of the absence of $I_{K,1}$ in the sinoatrial node.[1] Curiously, however, $I_{K,1}$ has been measured in rat and mouse sinoatrial node cells.[21] The absence of $I_{K,1}$ plays a permissive role in the diastolic depolarization—knockout of $I_{K,1}$ in the ventricles has been proposed as a strategy to create a biopacemaker (an engineered biologic pacemaker) in the ventricles.[22] The Kir2 ion channel family is responsible for $I_{K,1}$ and has four members: Kir2.1 to Kir2.4. In all species, at the mRNA level, Kir2.1, Kir2.2, and Kir2.3 are expressed in the atrial muscle, and in general (but not in all cases), the amount of Kir2 mRNA is lower in the sinoatrial node than in the atrial muscle. This finding is consistent with data for green fluorescent protein–tagged Kir2.1, which was abundantly expressed in the atrial muscle of the mouse but not in the sinoatrial node.[23] Similarly, in the human, native Kir2.1 protein is expressed in the atrial muscle but not in the sinoatrial node.[1] It is not clear if Kir2.4 is expressed in cardiac tissue.

Acetylcholine (ACh) released from parasympathetic vagal nerves causes a decrease in the heart rate. ACh achieves this by binding to M_2 muscarinic receptors. This activates G protein, which in turn activates the ACh-activated potassium current, I_{KACh}. Activation of I_{KACh} leads to a shortening of the action potential and an increase in the maximum diastolic potential, as well as a slowing of pacemaking. The channel responsible for I_{KACh} is a heteromultimer of Kir3.1 and Kir3.4 subunits. Kir3.1 mRNA is abundantly expressed in the sinoatrial node of all species, and Kir3.4 mRNA has been detected in the mouse sinoatrial node. Kir3.1 and Kir3.4 proteins have been detected in the rat sinoatrial node.[21] Studies in the Kir3.4-knockout mouse have demonstrated that I_{KACh} is responsible for approximately half of the negative chronotropic effect of vagal stimulation on heart rate.[24]

Cardiac tissue also is known to express an inward rectifier potassium channel that is inhibited by physiologic levels of cytosolic adenosine triphosphate (ATP). Under conditions of metabolic stress, such as hypoxia or ischemia, ATP levels fall, leading to the opening of this channel and the generation of the ATP-sensitive potassium current, I_{KATP}. I_{KATP} has been recorded from rabbit sinoatrial node cells, and activation of the current leads to a slowing or cessation of pacemaker activity.[21] Kir6.1 or Kir6.2 is responsible for the I_{KATP} channel. Messenger RNA for both isoforms is present in the sinoatrial node of the rabbit and mouse, but Kir6.2 mRNA is more abundant than Kir6.1 mRNA. The I_{KATP} channel complexes with the sulfonylurea receptor 2 (SUR2) subunit in cardiac tissue. At the mRNA level, in the rabbit and mouse, Kir6.2 is less abundant in the sinoatrial node than in the atrial muscle. In the rabbit at least, SUR2a mRNA also is less abundant in the sinoatrial node than in the atrial muscle.

More Potassium Channels

Additional potassium channels also have been identified in the sinoatrial node. The function of twin-pore-domain potassium channels in the sinoatrial node is unclear, but some evidence suggests that TASK-1 can regulate action potential duration in rat ventricular myocytes by contributing to repolarization.[25] TWIK-1 mRNA has been detected in the rabbit sinoatrial node, although it is weakly expressed compared with ERG mRNA. Messenger RNA for TWIK-1, TWIK-2, TASK-1, and TREK-1 has been detected in the rat sinoatrial node, and the mRNA abundance for these ion channels is similar to that of ERG. TASK-2 mRNA has been detected in the mouse sinoatrial node, although it is less abundant than other ion channels such as ERG.

Ca^{2+}-sensitive potassium current ($I_{K,Ca}$) has been shown to contribute to repolarization during the action potential in cardiac myocytes.[26] It has yet to be shown, however, if $I_{K,Ca}$ is present in the sinoatrial node. The SK family of channels is responsible for $I_{K,Ca}$ and has three members, SK1 to SK3. Messenger RNA for all three isoforms has been detected in rat and mouse sinoatrial node, but the SK mRNA is less abundant than ERG mRNA.

Calcium-Handling Proteins

The link between electrical excitation and contraction of a cell is provided by Ca^{2+}. The arrival of the action potential causes the cytoplasmic Ca^{2+} concentration to increase from approximately 10^{-7} to 10^{-6} M. This is brought about by entry of extracellular Ca^{2+} into the cell through activated calcium channels in the cell membrane. The Ca^{2+} influx triggers release of stored Ca^{2+} from the SR by way of a calcium channel known as the ryanodine receptor (RYR). The resultant increase in cytosolic Ca^{2+} results in activation of the contractile machinery and contraction. Once the membrane begins to repolarize, extracellular Ca^{2+} entry into the cytosol occurs at a reduced rate, and Ca^{2+} is removed from the cytosol back into the SR by means of the sarcoendoplasmic reticulum Ca^{2+}-ATPase (SERCA). Thus, cytosolic Ca^{2+} level drops and the contractile machinery relaxes. In the sinoatrial node, Ca^{2+} release from the SR also has been implicated in pacemaking.[27] It has been suggested that some SR Ca^{2+} release occurs during the diastolic depolarization. This occurs either in response to $I_{Ca,T}$ or spontaneously (as a result of the high cAMP level in the sinoatrial node).[1] The diastolic Ca^{2+} release activates the Na^+-Ca^{2+} exchanger. Because the Na^+-Ca^{2+} exchanger is electrogenic, an inward Na^+-Ca^{2+} exchanger current (I_{NaCa}) results, which contributes to the diastolic depolarization. It has been postulated that the positive chronotropic effect of β-adrenergic stimulation occurs by means of this mechanism: β-adrenergic stimulation increases $I_{Ca,L}$ and the Ca^{2+} content of the SR, leading to greater diastolic SR Ca^{2+} release and consequently more inward I_{NaCa}.[27] However, the extent to which intracellular Ca^{2+} release and the resultant I_{NaCa} contribute to diastolic depolarization in the sinoatrial node is still the subject of controversy.

Ryanodine has been used to "block" SR Ca^{2+} release—in all studies on rabbit and guinea pig sinoatrial node, this agent slows pacemaking.[1] In rabbit sinoatrial node cells, Lyashkov and colleagues,[28] for example, reported that 30 μM ryanodine causes pacemaking to stop; Honjo and coworkers,[29] however, reported that it slows pacemaking by only approximately 22%. This discrepancy may be the result of a difference in the duration of exposure to ryanodine: Lyashkov and colleagues[28] applied it for longer than 15 minutes, whereas Honjo and coworkers[29] applied it for 5 to 10 minutes only—it is possible that "rundown" may contribute to the slowing of pacemaking during a long exposure to ryanodine.

Three RYR isoforms, RYR1 to RYR3, have been identified. RYR2 mRNA is abundantly expressed in the atrial muscle and it is less abundant in the sinoatrial node. Conversely, RYR3 mRNA is more abundant in the sinoatrial node than in the atrial muscle in the rabbit and mouse[30] (although, in the rabbit sinoatrial node at least, the abundance of RYR3 mRNA is still lower than that of RYR2 mRNA). RYR2 protein has been detected in the sinoatrial node of the rabbit and guinea pig.[31]

Intracellular Ca^{2+} release can also occur by way of inositol 1,4,5-trisphosphate receptors (IP_3Rs). Three isoforms are known to exist: IP_3R1 to IP_3R3. The mRNA for all three isoforms has been detected in the rat sinoatrial node. IP_3R1 is more abundant in the rat sinoatrial node than in the atrial muscle. Three isoforms of the Na^+-Ca^{2+} exchanger (NCX) have been identified: NCX1 to NCX3. NCX1 mRNA is present in the sinoatrial at the same abundance as in the atrial muscle, and NCX1 protein also has been detected in the rabbit sinoatrial node.[31] Information on the expression of the other isoforms is lacking. SERC2A mRNA is abundantly expressed in the sinoatrial node; in the rabbit and mouse sinoatrial node, SERC2A mRNA is equally abundant in the sinoatrial node and in the atrial muscle, but in the rat, the amount of the mRNA is lower in the sinoatrial node than in the atrial muscle. SERC2A protein has been detected in the rabbit sinoatrial node.[31]

Depletion of intracellular Ca^{2+} stores can increase influx of extracellular Ca^{2+} by way of store-operated calcium channels (SOCCs). This process has been implicated in sinoatrial node function in the mouse, and SOCCs can potentially contribute to pacemaking.[32] The TRPC family of ion channels has been proposed to be responsible for SOCCs. This family is made up of seven members, TRPC1 to TRPC7. Messenger RNA for TRPC1, TRPC3, and TRPC6 has been detected in the rat sinoatrial node (TRPC1 mRNA is the most abundant), and mRNA for all TRPC isoforms (with the exception of TRPC5) has been detected in the mouse sinoatrial node.[32] Protein for TRPC1, TRPC3, TRPC4, and TRPC6 also has been detected in mouse sinoatrial node cells.[32] Orai1 (also known as CRACM1) also has been proposed to be responsible for SOCCs[33]; STIM1 is thought to be important for Orai1 function,[33] and STIM1 mRNA is present in the rat sinoatrial node.

Connexins

Electrical coupling between cardiac myocytes allows the propagation of the action potential through the heart and is provided by gap junctions. The gap junction is made up of two hemichannels (connexons) in the cell membranes of the two neighboring cells. Each connexon is composed of six connexin subunits. Electrical coupling is strong in the atrial muscle (to allow rapid propagation of the atrial action potential), and mathematical modeling demonstrates that electrical coupling should be poorer within the sinoatrial node: If electrical coupling were strong in the sinoatrial node, the electrotonic interaction with the more hyperpolarized atrial muscle would suppress the pacemaking of the sinoatrial node.[34] Good evidence indicates that electrical coupling in the sinoatrial node is indeed weak.[19] The gap junctions in the sinoatrial node of several species are less numerous and smaller in size than those in the surrounding atrial tissue.[34] The major cardiac connexin isoform is the medium-conductance Cx43, and Cx43 mRNA is abundant in the atrial muscle in all species. As expected, the abundance of Cx43 mRNA is lower in the sinoatrial node than in the atrial muscle in all species—for example, see Figure 12-5C, which shows the distribution of Cx43 mRNA in the rabbit sinoatrial node as determined by in situ hybridization. This is consistent with protein data: Cx43 protein is absent from rabbit, rat, mouse, human, and guinea pig sinoatrial nodes (see Fig. 12-5A and B).[34,35] Again as expected, the abundance of mRNA for large-conductance Cx40 is lower in the sinoatrial node than in the atrial muscle in all species (with the exception of the rat, in which no difference has been observed between the two tissues—however, Cx40 mRNA is of low abundance). Nevertheless, an increase in the sinoatrial node recovery time and evidence of a bradycardia have been observed in the Cx40-knockout mouse (see Table 12-1). Cx30.2 and Cx45 are low-conductance connexins, and as expected, both are present at the mRNA level in the sinoatrial node of the rat and mouse. In the rat, the abundance of Cx30.2 mRNA is greater in the sinoatrial node than in the atrial muscle. Cx30.2 protein has been detected in the mouse sinoatrial node,[34] and Cx45 protein has been detected in rabbit and human sinoatrial node.[34,35]

Plasticity of Ion Channel Expression in the Sinoatrial Node

Ion channel expression in the sinoatrial node is not static—it varies depending on circumstances, as it does elsewhere in the heart. Changes in ion channel expression have been observed in a wide range of circumstances.

Postnatal Development During postnatal development, both the normal heart rate and the intrinsic heart rate (heart rate in the absence of autonomic tone) decline. For example, in humans, the normal heart rate at birth is approximately 140 beats per minute, whereas in the young adult it is approximately 70 beats per minute. In the rabbit sinoatrial node, postnatal development culminates in a 36% decrease in the density of I_f and a 32% decrease in the density of $I_{Ca,L}$.[36] Perhaps consistent with this, a 69% decrease in the expression of HCN4 and a 58% decrease in the expression of $Ca_V1.3$ have been observed in the rabbit sinoatrial node during postnatal development.[37] In the center of the sinoatrial node of the adult rabbit, as is well known, no I_{Na} is detected, and pacemaker activity is insensitive to block of I_{Na} by TTX (see earlier). In neonatal rabbit sinoatrial node cells, however, I_{Na} has been recorded, and the pacemaker activity is sensitive to TTX; the I_{Na} disappears by the 40th postnatal

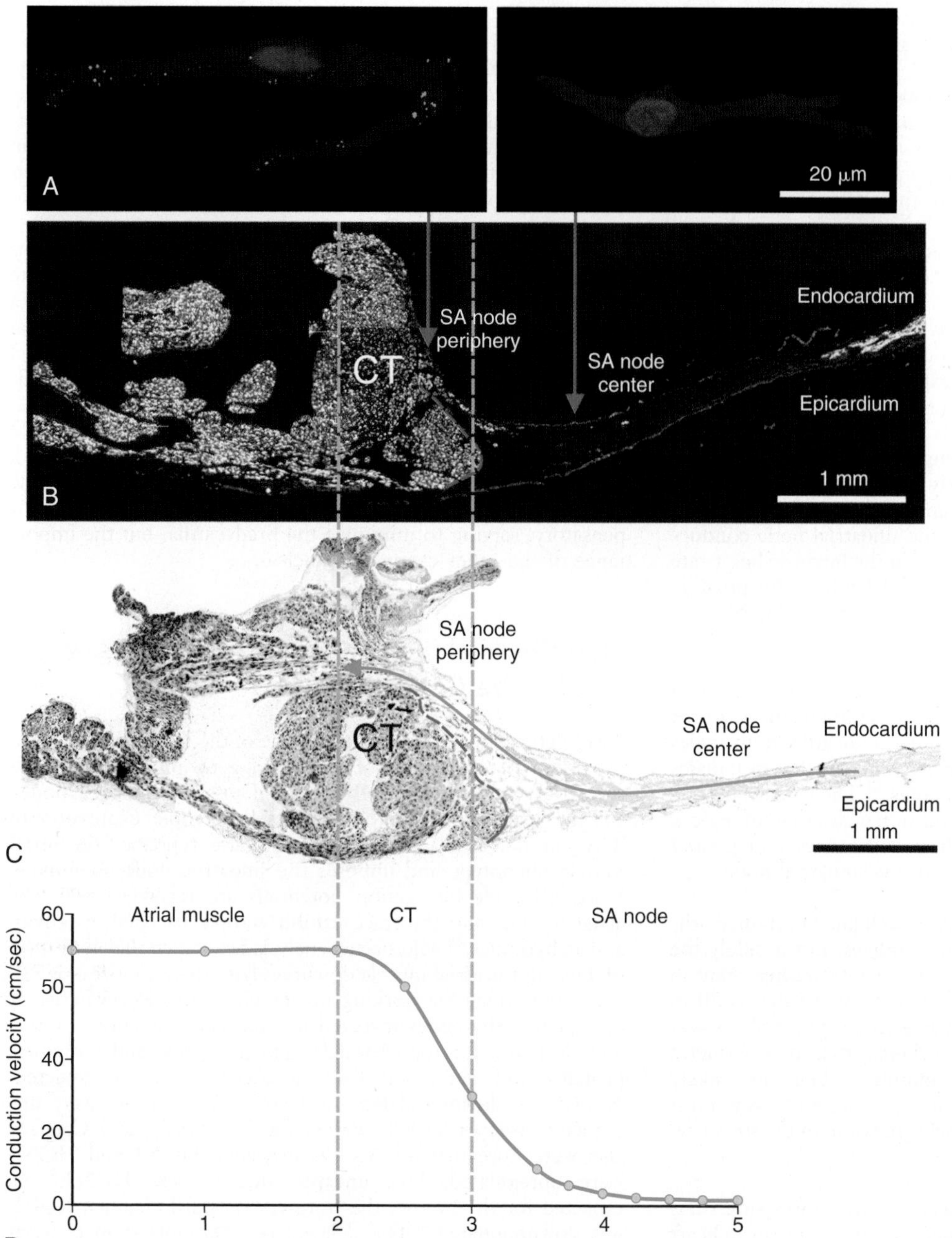

Figure 12-5 Electrical coupling in the rabbit sinoatrial (SA) node. **A,** Immunofluorescence labeling of connexin43 (Cx43) *(green spots)* in large and small SA node cells, probably from the periphery and center of the SA node, respectively. Cx43 is expressed in the large cell but not in the small cell. The nuclei are stained *red.* **B** and **C,** Distribution of Cx43 protein (**B**) and messenger RNA (mRNA) (**C**) in sections cut perpendicular to the crista terminalis (CT) approximately at the level of the leading pacemaker site in the SA node. Protein was labeled using immunohistochemistry staining, and mRNA was labeled using in situ hybridization. The *red dashed lines* in **B** and **C** show the connective tissue isolating the peripheral SA node tissue (on the endocardial surface of the CT) from the atrial muscle making up the bulk of the CT. **D,** Conduction velocity plotted as a function of distance along the conduction pathway (*blue line* in **C**) from the center of the SA node (leading pacemaker site), through the periphery of the SA node to the atrial muscle—the graph is aligned with the tissue section. (**A,** From Honjo H, Boyett MR, Coppen SR, et al: Heterogeneous expression of connexins in rabbit sinoatrial node cells: Correlation between connexin isotype and cell size. Cardiovasc Res 53:89-96, 2002; **B,** from Musa H, Lei M, Honjo H, et al: Heterogeneous expression of Ca^{2+} handling proteins in sinoatrial node. J Histochem Cytochem 50:311-324, 2002; **C,** from Tellez JO, Dobrzynski H, Greener ID, et al: Differential expression of ion channel transcripts in atrial muscle and sinoatrial node in rabbit. Circ Res 99:1384-1393, 2006; **D,** from Sano T, Yamagishi S: Spread of excitation from the sinus node. Circ Res 16:423-430, 1965.)

day.[36] The I_{Na} shows unusually high sensitivity to TTX and is attributed to $Na_V1.1$.[36] A 61% decline in NCX1 mRNA in the rabbit sinoatrial node during postnatal development also has been reported.[37] The declines in I_{Na}, $I_{Ca,L}$, I_f, $Ca_V1.3$, HCN4, and NCX1 all could potentially be responsible for the decline in heart rate during postnatal development.

Aging During aging (from the young adult to senescence), a decline occurs in the function of the sinoatrial node. Although the normal heart rate is constant during aging, in the human and other mammals, there continues to be a decline in the intrinsic heart rate, as well as an increase in the sinoatrial node conduction time and also, in the rabbit and cat at least, an increase in action potential duration.[19] The incidence of sick sinus syndrome increases in an exponential-like manner with age, and a majority of cases of sick sinus syndrome occur in the elderly. Previously, the age-dependent decline in sinoatrial node function has been attributed to fibrosis and a loss of sinoatrial node cells, but this has been disputed, with evidence of changes in the expression of ion channels reported in several studies.[9,14,38] In the sinoatrial node of the rabbit and cat, an enlargement of the sinoatrial node area with a slow action potential (dV/dt_{max} less than 5 V/s) has been observed.[19] This finding suggests an enlargement of the sinoatrial node area lacking $Na_V1.5$, and such an enlargement has been described in the rat.[39] In the rat, an age-dependent enlargement of the sinoatrial node area lacking Cx43 and expressing HCN4 also has been described.[39] In the guinea pig, an age-dependent enlargement of the sinoatrial node area lacking Cx43 and $Ca_V1.2$ has been reported.[38] In the guinea pig, the enlargement is much greater than can be explained by any increase in heart size,[38] whereas in the rat, although the enlargement is in proportion to an increase in heart size, it possibly involves hyperplasia (increase in the number of sinoatrial node cells).[39] In the rat, quantitative PCR assay has revealed age-dependent changes in 15 ion channel subunits in the sinoatrial node—for example, decreases in HCN1, $K_V1.5$, and Cx30.2 mRNAs.[9] It is possible that the changes in ion channel expression in the sinoatrial node may be involved in the age-dependent decline in sinoatrial node function: The age-dependent increase of the sinoatrial node conduction time has been linked to the expansion of sinoatrial node tissue lacking Cx43[38]—in the old (as compared to the young) guinea pig, the action potential has been shown to propagate a greater distance from the leading pacemaker site through Cx43-negative (and therefore slowly conducting) tissue to the atrial muscle.[38] The expansion of sinoatrial node tissue lacking $Na_V1.5$ also is expected to increase the sinoatrial node conduction time. The age-dependent decrease in the intrinsic heart rate could be the result of the decrease in HCN1 mRNA (or possibly the expansion of sinoatrial node tissue lacking Cx43, $Na_V1.5$, and $Ca_V1.2$).

Gender The normal heart rate as well as the intrinsic heart rate in men is less than that in women. For example, in a study of subjects 21 to 30 years of age, the intrinsic heart rate in males was approximately 93 beats per minute, whereas that in females was approximately 101 beats per minutes.[40] The sinoatrial node recovery time also is different (greater in females than in males). The most likely explanation of these differences is a gender difference in ion channel expression in the sinoatrial node.

Training-Induced Bradycardia As is well known, trained athletes have a lower heart rate than nonathletes; this is solely the result of a decrease in the intrinsic heart rate, rather than an increase in parasympathetic tone.[41] In a study of subjects 20 to 26 years of age, the intrinsic heart rate in rowing athletes was approximately 80 beats per minute, whereas that in nonathletes was approximately 100 beats per minute.[41] The most likely explanation of the difference in the intrinsic heart rate is a training-induced difference in ion channel expression in the sinoatrial node.

Heart Failure In the human, heart failure causes sick sinus syndrome: During heart failure, a decrease in the intrinsic heart rate, an increase in the corrected sinus node recovery time, a caudal shift of the leading pacemaker site, and abnormal propagation of the action potential from the sinoatrial node have been documented.[42] Sudden cardiac death is a significant problem in patients with congestive heart failure, and bradyarrhythmias account for approximately 42% of in-hospital sudden deaths in this group.[42] In animal models, a decrease in the intrinsic heart rate also has been observed during heart failure.[43] Block of I_f by zatebradine causes a smaller decrease in the heart rate in the rabbit in heart failure,[1] and a decrease in sinus node pacemaking in the rabbit in heart failure has been attributed to a decrease in I_f.[43] In the dog, a decrease in HCN2 and HCN4 mRNA and protein by up to approximately 80% is observed in the sinoatrial node in heart failure.[44]

Atrial Fibrillation In patients, sick sinus syndrome frequently is associated with atrial fibrillation, forming the basis of the "tachycardia-bradycardia syndrome."[45] For example, prolonged sinus pauses can occur on termination of atrial fibrillation.[45] The sick sinus syndrome may be caused by the atrial fibrillation: In the dog, pacing-induced atrial fibrillation for 2 to 6 weeks results in sinoatrial node dysfunction—namely, a decrease in the intrinsic and maximal heart rates and a prolongation of the sinoatrial node recovery time.[46] Atrial fibrillation is well known to result in a remodeling of ion channels in the atria, so it also may result in a remodeling of ion channels in the sinoatrial node.

Bradycardia Leoni and colleagues[47] showed that in conscious mice, a moderate but chronic reduction in heart rate of 16% (caused by ivabradine, a blocker of I_f) resulted in a complex remodeling of ion channel transcripts in the sinoatrial node (but not in the ventricles). Nine ion channel subunits, including $Na_V\beta_1$ (−25%), $Ca_V3.1$ (−29%), $K_V\beta_2$ (−41%), $K_V\beta_3$ (−30%), and Kir6.1 (−28%), were downregulated, whereas eight were upregulated, including HCN2 (+24%), HCN4 (+52%), $K_V1.1$ (+30%), Kir2.1 (+29%), Kir3.1 (+41%), RYR2 (+15%), and Cx43 (+26%). It is possible that the upregulation of HCN2, HCN4, and RYR2 was compensatory, serving to minimize the bradycardia, but the importance of the other changes is unclear.

Ion Channels in the Sinoatrial Node Are under the Control of Tbx3

Tbx3 deficiency in the sinoatrial node of the mouse results in an expansion of expression of the atrial gene program into the sinoatrial node region, and in partial loss of sinoatrial node–specific gene expression.[48] Conversely, ectopic expression of Tbx3 in the atrial muscle of the mouse represses the atrial muscle phenotype and imposes the sinoatrial node phenotype: Sinoatrial node–like action potentials are recorded from the atrial muscle, and the mice exhibit ectopic pacemaker activity and arrhythmias.[48] Microarray analysis has shown that activation of Tbx3 in the atrial muscle downregulates the expression of 737 genes important for working myocardium function, whereas it upregulates 809 genes involved in pacemaker function.[5] These include genes for ion channels, gap junctions, and structural proteins and genes involved in metabolism. As expected, $Na_V1.5$ was downregulated and $Ca_V3.1$ and $Ca_V\alpha_2\delta_2$ were upregulated (see earlier); however, $Ca_V3.2$, $Ca_V\beta_2$, and $Ca_V\alpha_2\delta_1$ also were upregulated.[5] Also as expected, HCN1 and HCN4 were upregulated, but, unexpectedly, so was HCN2.[5] As expected for the mouse, the transient outward channel, $K_V4.2$, was downregulated.[5] The delayed rectifier potassium channel ERG was upregulated[5] (ERG is more abundant in the sinoatrial node than in the atrial muscle in the rabbit,[8] but not in the mouse[10]). Perhaps as expected, the inward rectifier potassium channel subunits, Kir2.1, Kir2.2, Kir3.1, Kir6.1, Kir6.2, and SUR2a, all were downregulated; Kir3.4 was upregulated.[5] The twin-pore-domain potassium channel, TASK-1, was downregulated.[5] Also perhaps as expected, RYR2 and SERCA2a were downregulated.[5] As expected, the gap junction subunits, Cx40 and Cx43, were downregulated, whereas Cx30.2 was upregulated; Cx45 also was upregulated.[5]

Interfacing the Sinoatrial Node with the Atrial Muscle

Theoretically, it is difficult for the sinoatrial node to exhibit pacemaking and drive the surrounding large mass of more hyperpolarized atrial muscle,[34] so in order for the sinoatrial node to function, specializations are necessary. The following discussion relates to the rabbit, for which we have information.

Figure 12-1B shows that the sinoatrial node consists of an inner central region (in red) and an outer peripheral region (in blue). The central region consists of a homogeneous population of smaller sinoatrial node cells[3] with an average length of approximately 63 μm and an average capacitance (calculated) of 40 pF.[49] The cells are "empty," and the percentage volume of myofilament is only approximately 20%[50]; the SR also is relatively poorly developed, and RYR2 is present at the cell perimeter only.[31] As described earlier, because $Na_V1.5$ and Cx43 are not expressed in the central region, the cells are weakly coupled and have a slow Ca^{2+}-dependent action potential. The importance of the weak electrical coupling has already been explained. The absence of $Na_V1.5$ may be a vestige of embryonic development, or it may be functionally important: Purkinje fibers, which express $Na_V1.5$, show prominent overdrive suppression that is ultimately the result of $Na_V1.5$,[51] whereas the sinoatrial node, which does not express $Na_V1.5$, does not (it would be potentially fatal if the sinoatrial node could be overdriven by an ectopic focus).

In contrast with the central region, the peripheral region contains larger sinoatrial node cells—the cells have an average length of approximately 101 μm and an average capacitance (calculated) of 64 pF.[49] The cells are not "empty," and the percentage volume of myofilaments is approximately 40%[50]; the SR is well developed, and RYR2 is present in the cell interior as well as at the cell perimeter (same as in atrial myocytes).[31] The peripheral region also is heterogeneous, and sinoatrial node cells are interdigitated with atrial myocytes.[3,34] It has been argued that the interdigitations help the sinoatrial node to show pacemaking and drive the atrial muscle.[34] In addition, in the peripheral region (which includes the right branch of the sinoatrial ring bundle [RSARB]), both $Na_V1.5$ and Cx43 are expressed (e.g., see Figs. 12-3D and 12-5B and C)[34]; furthermore, large sinoatrial node cells (likely to be from the periphery) have a substantial I_{Na}[11] and express Cx43 (see Figs. 12-3A and 12-5A).[35] In terms of cell size (and percentage volume of myofilaments and SR development) as well as I_{Na} and Cx43, peripheral cells are therefore transitional. As a result of the expression of $Na_V1.5$ and Cx43 in the peripheral region, both dV/dt_{max} and the conduction velocity (which is dependent on electrical coupling) are greater[19,52]—Figure 12-3D shows that whereas dV/dt_{max} is less than 10 V/s in the center, it is greater than 60 V/s in the periphery, and Figure 12-5D shows that whereas the conduction velocity is less than 10 cm/s in the center, it is greater than 30 cm/s in the periphery. Furthermore, Figure 12-3A shows that pacemaker activity in peripheral tissue is slowed after block of I_{Na} by TTX. The expression of $Na_V1.5$ and Cx43 in the peripheral region may help the sinoatrial node to drive the atrial muscle: To accomplish this, the sinoatrial node must generate and deliver depolarizing current to the atrial muscle—$Na_V1.5$ may generate it and Cx43 may deliver it. Loss of $Na_V1.5$ results in a bradycardia (see Table 12-1)—perhaps this is a reflection of the importance of $Na_V1.5$ in the peripheral region of the sinoatrial node.

As is evident from Figure 12-3C (blue graphs), in cells isolated from the whole of the sinoatrial node (center and periphery), significant correlations exist between dV/dt_{max} and the density of I_{Na} and cell capacitance. Almost identical relationships have been observed in rabbit atrioventricular node cells (see Fig. 12-3C, red graphs).[53] A significant correlation between the density of I_{Na} and cell capacitance also has been observed in mouse sinoatrial node cells.[12] It is known that Tbx3 directly controls the *SCN5A* gene responsible for I_{Na} (see earlier)—perhaps it also controls cell size, and perhaps Tbx3 expression varies from the center to the periphery.

Conclusions

The sinoatrial node is perhaps a much more extensive structure (probably including tissue from the superior to the inferior vena cava) than is depicted in today's textbooks, and this notion is consistent with the electrophysiologic findings and the embryologic development of the sinoatrial node. The function of the sinoatrial node is an electrical one and, therefore, dependent on ion channels; over the past few years, understanding of ion channel expression in the sinoatrial node has increased dramatically. The differences in electrical activity between the working myocardium and the sinoatrial node are now known to be the result of many differences in ion channel expression. The significance of some of the differences (e.g., HCN4) has been elucidated, but understanding is still lacking for many other such differences. It appears that many of the differences in ion channel expression are rather surprisingly the result of a single transcription factor, Tbx3. Clearly, ion channel expression in the sinoatrial node is not static—it is plastic and varies in many different circumstances, including sick sinus syndrome. A focus of current research is to develop a biopacemaker and convert working myocardium into a pacemaker tissue. This is being attempted by the manipulation of a *single* gene.[22] It is now known, however, that more than 1500 differences in gene expression between the working myocardium and the sinoatrial node are likely[5]; therefore, the manipulation of a single gene in the working myocardium is unlikely to convert it into a fast and robust pacemaker tissue. Perhaps the expression of Tbx3 offers an alternative strategy.[48]

Acknowledgments

We thank Natalie J. Chandler, Eman S. H. Abd Allah, and Joseph F. Yanni for their contributions to this chapter.

References

1. Dobrzynski H, Boyett MR, Anderson RH: New insights into pacemaker activity: Promoting understanding of sick sinus syndrome. Circulation 115:1921-1932, 2007.
2. Fedorov VV, Hucker WJ, Dobrzynski H, et al: Postganglionic nerve stimulation induces temporal inhibition of excitability in the rabbit sinoatrial node. Am J Physiol 291:H612-H623, 2006.
3. Dobrzynski H, Li J, Tellez J, et al: Computer three-dimensional reconstruction of the sinoatrial node. Circulation 111:846-854, 2005.
4. Hoogaars WM, Christoffels VM, Moorman AFM: Morphogenesis of the vertebrate heart. Adv Dev Biol 18:31-68, 2007.
5. Hoogaars WMH: The role of Tbx3 in the formation of the cardiac conduction system. PhD thesis, University of Amsterdam, 2007.
6. Hoogaars WM, Tessari A, Moorman AF, et al: The transcriptional repressor Tbx3 delineates the developing central conduction system of the heart. Cardiovasc Res 62:489-499, 2004.
7. Verkerk AO, Wilders R, van Borren MM, et al: Pacemaker current (I_f) in the human sinoatrial node. Eur Heart J 28:2472-2478, 2007.
8. Tellez JO, Dobrzynski H, Greener ID, et al: Differential expression of ion channel transcripts in atrial muscle and sinoatrial node in rabbit. Circ Res 99:1384-1393, 2006.
9. Tellez JO, Dobrzynski H, Yanni J, et al: Effects of aging on gene expression in the rat sinoatrial node. J Mol Cell Cardiol 40:982, 2006.

10. Marionneau C, Couette B, Liu J, et al: Specific pattern of ionic channel gene expression associated with pacemaker activity in the mouse heart. J Physiol 562:223-234, 2005.
11. Honjo H, Boyett MR, Kodama I, Toyama J: Correlation between electrical activity and the size of rabbit sinoatrial node cells. J Physiol 496:795-808, 1996.
12. Lei M, Jones SA, Liu J, et al: Requirement of neuronal- and cardiac-type sodium channels for murine sinoatrial node pacemaking. J Physiol 559:835-848, 2004.
13. Kodama I, Nikmaram MR, Boyett MR, et al: Regional differences in the role of the Ca^{2+} and Na^{+} currents in pacemaker activity in the sinoatrial node. Am J Physiol 272:H2793-H2806, 1997.
14. Jones SA, Boyett MR, Lancaster MK: Declining into failure: The age-dependent loss of the L-type calcium channel within the sinoatrial node. Circulation 115:1183-1190, 2007.
15. Ono K, Iijima T: Pathophysiological significance of T-type Ca^{2+} channels: Properties and functional roles of T-type Ca^{2+} channels in cardiac pacemaking. J Pharmacol Sci 99:197-204, 2005.
16. Barbuti A, Baruscotti M, DiFrancesco D: The pacemaker current: From basics to the clinics. J Cardiovasc Electrophysiol 18:342-347, 2007.
17. Chandler NJ, Molenaar P, Boyett MR, Dobrzynski H: Mapping of the human sinus node. Europace 9(Suppl 5):v10, 2007.
18. Liu J, Dobrzynski H, Yanni J, et al: Organisation of the mouse sinoatrial node: Structure and expression of HCN channels. Cardiovasc Res 73:729-738, 2007.
19. Boyett MR, Honjo H, Kodama I: The sinoatrial node, a heterogeneous pacemaker structure. Cardiovasc Res 47:658-687, 2000.
20. Pourrier M, Schram G, Nattel S: Properties, expression and potential roles of cardiac K^{+} channel accessory subunits: MinK, MiRPs, KChIP, and KChAP. J Membr Biol 194:141-152, 2003.
21. Satoh H: Sino-atrial nodal cells of mammalian hearts: Ionic currents and gene expression of pacemaker ionic channels. J Smooth Muscle Res 39:175-193, 2003.
22. Rosen MR, Brink PR, Cohen IS, Robinson RB: Genes, stem cells and biological pacemakers. Cardiovasc Res 64:12-23, 2004.
23. Dobrzynski H, Billeter R, Greener ID, et al: Expression of Kir2.1 and Kir6.2 transgenes under the control of the α-MHC promoter in the sinoatrial and atrioventricular nodes in transgenic mice. J Mol Cell Cardiol 41:855-867, 2006.
24. Wickman K, Nemec J, Gendler SJ, Clapham DE: Abnormal heart rate regulation in GIRK4 knockout mice. Neuron 20:103-114, 1998.
25. Putzke C, Wemhoner K, Sachse FB, et al: The acid-sensitive potassium channel TASK-1 in rat cardiac muscle. Cardiovasc Res 75:59-68, 2007.
26. Xu Y, Tuteja D, Zhang Z, et al: Molecular identification and functional roles of a Ca^{2+}-activated K^{+} channel in human and mouse hearts. J Biol Chem 278:49085-49094, 2003.
27. Vinogradova TM, Maltsev VA, Bogdanov KY, et al: Rhythmic Ca^{2+} oscillations drive sinoatrial nodal cell pacemaker function to make the heart tick. Ann N Y Acad Sci 1047:138-156, 2005.
28. Lyashkov AE, Juhaszova M, Dobrzynski H, et al: Calcium cycling protein density and functional importance to automaticity of isolated sinoatrial nodal cells are independent of cell size. Circ Res 100:1723-1731, 2007.
29. Honjo H, Inada S, Lancaster MK, et al: Sarcoplasmic reticulum Ca^{2+} release is not a dominating factor in sinoatrial node pacemaker activity. Circ Res 92:e41-e44, 2003.
30. Masumiya H, Yamamoto H, Hemberger M, et al: The mouse sino-atrial node expresses both the type 2 and type 3 Ca^{2+} release channels/ryanodine receptors. FEBS Lett 553:141-144, 2003.
31. Musa H, Lei M, Honjo H, et al: Heterogeneous expression of Ca^{2+} handling proteins in sinoatrial node. J Histochem Cytochem 50:311-324, 2002.
32. Ju Y-K, Chu Y, Chaulet H, et al: Store-operated Ca^{2+} influx and expression of TRPC genes in mouse sinoatrial node. Circ Res 100:1605-1614, 2007.
33. Smyth JT, Dehaven WI, Jones BF, et al: Emerging perspectives in store-operated Ca^{2+} entry: Roles of Orai, Stim and TRP. Biochim Biophys Acta 1763:1147-1160, 2006.
34. Boyett MR, Inada S, Yoo S, et al: Connexins in the sinoatrial and atrioventricular nodes. Adv Cardiol 42:175-197, 2006.
35. Honjo H, Boyett MR, Coppen SR, et al: Heterogeneous expression of connexins in rabbit sinoatrial node cells: Correlation between connexin isotype and cell size. Cardiovasc Res 53:89-96, 2002.
36. Baruscotti M, Robinson RB: Electrophysiology and pacemaker function of the developing sinoatrial node. Am J Physiol 293:H2613-H2623, 2007.
37. Abd Allah ESH, Tellez JO, Dobrzynski H, Boyett MR: Post-natal developmental changes in the sinoatrial node. Biophys J 94:2236, 2008.
38. Jones SA, Lancaster MK, Boyett MR: Ageing-related changes of connexins and conduction within the sinoatrial node. J Physiol 560:429-437, 2004.
39. Yanni JF, Tellez JO, Dobrzynski H, Boyett MR: Age-dependent changes in HCN4 and $Na_V1.5$ in the sinoatrial node. J Mol Cell Cardiol 42:S15, 2007.
40. Burke JH, Goldberger JJ, Ehlert FA, et al: Gender differences in heart rate before and after autonomic blockade: Evidence against an intrinsic gender effect. Am J Med 100:537-543, 1996.
41. Katona PG, McLean M, Dighton DH, Guz A: Sympathetic and parasympathetic cardiac control in athletes and nonathletes at rest. J Appl Physiol 52:1652-1657, 1982.
42. Sanders P, Kistler PM, Morton JB, et al: Remodeling of sinus node function in patients with congestive heart failure: Reduction in sinus node reserve. Circulation 110:897-903, 2004.
43. Verkerk AO, Wilders R, Coronel R, et al: Ionic remodeling of sinoatrial node cells by heart failure. Circulation 108:760-766, 2003.
44. Zicha S, Fernandez-Velasco M, Lonardo G, et al: Sinus node dysfunction and hyperpolarization-activated (HCN) channel subunit remodeling in a canine heart failure model. Cardiovasc Res 66:472-481, 2005.
45. Hocini M, Sanders P, Deisenhofer I, et al: Reverse remodeling of sinus node function after catheter ablation of atrial fibrillation in patients with prolonged sinus pauses. Circulation 108:1172-1175, 2003.
46. Elvan A, Wylie K, Zipes DP: Pacing-induced chronic atrial fibrillation impairs sinus node function in dogs. Electrophysiological remodeling. Circulation 94:2953-2960, 1996.
47. Leoni AL, Marionneau C, Demolombe S, et al: Chronic heart rate reduction remodels ion channel transcripts in the mouse sinoatrial node but not in the ventricle. Physiol Genom 24:4-12, 2005.
48. Hoogaars WM, Engel A, Brons JF, et al: Tbx3 controls the sinoatrial node gene program and imposes pacemaker function on the atria. Genes Dev 21:1098-1112, 2007.
49. Lancaster MK, Jones SA, Trafford AW, Boyett MR: Cellular statistics of heterogeneity within the rabbit right atrium and sinoatrial node. J Physiol 551:PC2, 2003.
50. Masson-Pévet MA, Bleeker WK, Besselsen E, et al: Pacemaker cell types in the rabbit sinus node: A correlative ultrastructural and electrophysiological study. J Mol Cell Cardiol 16:53-63, 1984.
51. Boyett MR, Fedida D: Changes in the electrical activity of dog cardiac Purkinje fibres at high heart rates. J Physiol 350:361-391, 1984.
52. Sano T, Yamagishi S: Spread of excitation from the sinus node. Circ Res 16:423-430, 1965.
53. Ren FX, Niu XL, Ou Y, et al: Morphological and electrophysiological properties of single myocardial cells from Koch triangle of rabbit heart. Chin Med J (Engl) 119:2075-2084, 2006.
54. Kodama I, Boyett MR: Regional differences in the electrical activity of the rabbit sinus node. Pflügers Arch 404:214-226, 1985.
55. Lees-Miller JP, Guo J, Somers JR, et al: Selective knockout of mouse ERG1 B potassium channel eliminates I_{Kr} in adult ventricular myocytes and elicits episodes of abrupt sinus bradycardia. Mol Cell Biol 23:1856-1862, 2003.
56. Postma AV, Denjoy I, Kamblock J, et al: Catecholaminergic polymorphic ventricular tachycardia: RYR2 mutations, bradycardia, and follow up of the patients. J Med Genet 42:863-870, 2005.
57. Zhang Z, Xu Y, Song H, et al: Functional roles of $Ca_V1.3$ α_{1D} calcium channel in sinoatrial nodes: Insight gained using gene-targeted null mutant mice. Circ Res 90:981-987, 2002.

Biophysical Properties of Inwardly Rectifying Potassium Channels 13

JUSTUS M. B. ANUMONWO

CHAPTER OUTLINE

Background

In the heart, inwardly rectifying potassium (Kir) channels play a critical role in stabilizing the resting membrane potential, determining excitation threshold, and modulating the repolarization process of the cardiac cell action potential.[1,2] Inward rectification in potassium channels is a phenomenon in which the conductance of the Kir channel increases with membrane hyperpolarization but decreases with depolarization to potentials above the potassium equilibrium potential (E_K). Thus, by preferentially passing current in one direction, Kir channels behave as "bio-diodes" in the cell membrane. It is generally believed that the molecular basis of rectification is the depolarization-induced movement of intracellular cations, such as magnesium or polyamines (spermine and spermidine, or putrescine and cadaverine) into the cytoplasmic mouth of the channel, resulting in a physical occlusion of the ion permeation pathway.[1,3] This diode-like characteristic of channel "gating" forms a defining biophysical fingerprint of the Kir channel. The property enables the Kir conductance to stabilize the membrane potential of the cell at rest, as well as to protect the cell from an excessive loss of K^+ ions during the plateau phase of the cardiac action potential. Nevertheless, the relatively small outward current through the channel is critical for its electrophysiologic function.

Studies in past decades have described three important Kir currents in the heart: the classical inward rectifier (I_{K1}), the acetylcholine-activated potassium current (I_{KACh}), and the adenosine triphosphate (ATP)-sensitive potassium current (I_{KATP}). For these channels, the primary (α) subunits have been identified and are encoded by the *KCNJ* family of genes. A variety of disorders, the so-called ion channel diseases, have been associated with mutations in the *KCNJ* genes.[4] This chapter begins with a brief discussion of the general characteristics of the Kir currents that are native to myocardial cells. This is followed by a description of the biophysical properties of the underlying channels in heterologous expression systems. Details on other aspects of this subject are available in excellent reviews.[3,5-7]

Cardiac Inward Rectifier Potassium Currents

Classical Inward Rectifier Potassium Current: I_{K1}

The resting potassium conductance in the cardiac cell is primarily determined by a voltage-independent, inwardly rectifying potassium current, I_{K1}. This extensively studied, classical inward rectifier channel current is thought to be poorly expressed or absent in nodal (sinus node and atrioventricular node) cells but robustly expressed in atrial and ventricular cells. Furthermore, although evidence indicates that ventricular cells have the higher expression levels of the current, this observation may be species-dependent.[8] The general properties of I_{K1} have been reviewed extensively.[1] Rectification of I_{K1} depends on the block of the underlying channel pore by intracellular cations, specifically Mg^{2+} and polyamines. The I_{K1} channel also is blocked by Cs^+ and Ba^{2+}, acting from the extracellular mouth of the channel pore.

The unitary conductance values reported for the channel surprisingly varies according to the group of investigators. In an extensive characterization of I_{K1} in guinea pig ventricular myocytes,[9] a conductance value of 27 pS was reported. Also, it was reported that the channel underlying I_{K1} has a unitary conductance of 40 pS and a long mean open time of 100 ms.[10] Yet, in another study on guinea pig ventricular cell I_{K1},[11] a unitary conductance value of 33 to 34 pS was reported. The reason for the differences in unitary conductance values is not currently clear; however, tissue- and species-specific differences in expression patterns in the underlying molecular mechanisms may exist. This issue is addressed further in a later section.

Acetylcholine-Activated Potassium Current: I_{KACh}

As the name implies, I_{KACh} is activated by acetylcholine (ACh), which is released from the vagus nerve. The effect of ACh is mediated through the stimulation of M2 muscarinic receptors in heart cells. Although usually referred to as acetylcholine-gated potassium channel, the channels can be stimulated by other agents such as α_2-adrenergic agonists, somatostatin, and adenosine. I_{KACh} unitary conductance is similar to that recorded for I_{K1} and is approximately 30 to 40 pS.[12,13] The inwardly rectifying channels underlying I_{KACh} are expressed predominantly in sinus nodal, atrial, and Purkinje cells, and when activated in the pacemaker cells of the sinus node, I_{KACh} permits K^+ efflux, resulting in membrane hyperpolarization and in the slowing of heart rate. This activation process of the channel is membrane-delimited and rapid and is thought to be important in the beat-to-beat control of the heart rate. Some evidence indicates that ventricular cells in a number of species, including humans, also express I_{KACh}; however, in ventricular cells, the underlying channels are much less sensitive to ACh compared with those in sinus nodal, atrial, and Purkinje cells.[14,15]

Adenosine Triphosphate–Sensitive Potassium Current: I_{KATP}

The I_{KATP} channels have a primary role of coupling cell excitability to the metabolic state of the cell. The channels are rapidly and reversibly blocked by the binding of adenosine nucleotides present in the cytoplasm, and the potency of inhibition by the nucleotides increases from adenosine monophosphate (AMP) to adenosine diphosphate (ADP) and is maximal for ATP. The underlying channels interact with a variety of intracellular factors to "gate" the ion channel. By acting at different binding sites, it has been shown that a nonhydrolytic association of the channel with ATP blocks the channel, whereas the channels are activated by magnesium-bound nucleotides. It is noteworthy that in the myocardial cell, intracellular ATP concentration is in the millimolar range, whereas the half-maximal inhibitory concentration (IC_{50}) for ATP-dependent inhibition is in the micromolar range. Thus, under physiologic conditions, the channels are essentially closed. During metabolic stress in the heart, such as that occurring in hypoxia and ischemia, intracellular I_{KATP} is reduced, thereby favoring the activation of the channels. The resultant efflux of potassium ions leads to a shortening of the action potential duration (APD). The APD shortening will reduce contraction, a desirable effect for a myocardium with compromised function. The unitary conductance of an I_{KATP} channel with symmetrical (150 mM) K^+ ions in cardiac myocytes is 70 to 90 pS,[16] with a mean open time of approximately 1 ms.[17]

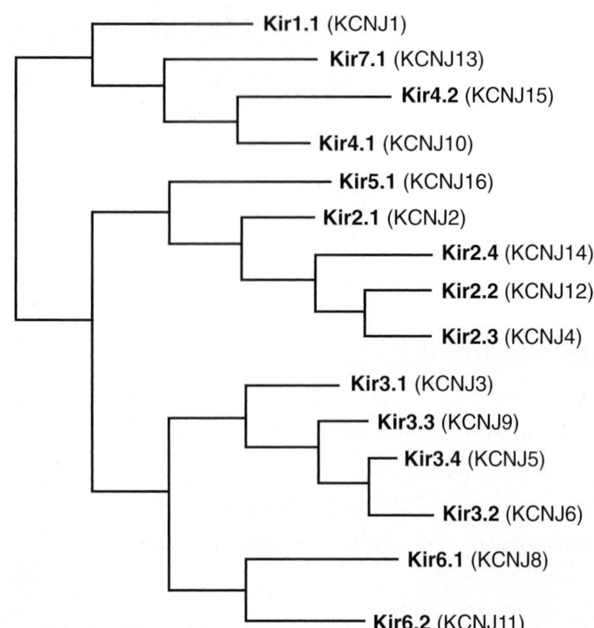

Figure 13-1 A dendrogram showing the relatedness of human inwardly rectifying potassium channel. (Modified from Kubo Y, Adelman JP, Clapham DE, et al: International Union of Pharmacology. LIV. Nomenclature and molecular relationships of inwardly rectifying potassium channels. Pharmacol Rev 57:509-526, 2005.)

Subunit Structure and Molecular Properties of Inward Rectifier Potassium Channels

The molecular correlates of Kir currents in the myocardium are the Kir family of proteins. The Kir family of ion channels comprises a large group of potassium channels that are structurally and functionally different from the voltage-gated (Kv) potassium channels.[18-20] After the cloning of the *Drosophila* Shaker locus, homology screening with the Kv subunits did not result in any Kir channels. A breakthrough came in 1993, when three different laboratories used expression cloning to obtain and characterize, for the first time, the molecular properties of Kir channels.[21-23] At least seven subfamily members of the Kir channels are now recognized (Fig. 13-1; Table 13-1). In general, Kir channels share approximately 40% amino acid identity, whereas similarity is greater (approximately 60%) within each subfamily. Kir4 and Kir5 form inwardly rectifying currents in the brain. The other members of the Kir family, Kir1, Kir2, Kir3, and Kir6, are expressed in the heart. Relatively little is known about the role of Kir1 in the heart; more information is available on Kir2, Kir3, and Kir6 channels.

It is noteworthy, however, that Lesage and colleagues[24-26] cloned the first of another group of inwardly rectifying potassium channels, which consist of two Kir channels in tandem. The channels (dubbed "TWIK" for *t*andem of P domains in *w*eakly *i*nward rectifier potassium (*K*⁺) channels) are weak inward rectifiers and dimerize to form ion channels. The channels are expressed in both atrial and ventricular tissue, with a greater expression in the latter. TWIK channels have a weak sensitivity to Ba^{2+}, and rectification is Mg^{2+}-dependent. Several other TWIK-related channels have been described that belong to the *KCNK* family of genes.[24] The channels are regulated by a variety of agents such as polyunsaturated fatty acid and stretch (TRAAK), and by acid (TASK). Increasing evidence indicates that the channels may contribute significantly to the background current in the heart. (Owing to space limitations, TWIK and the related channels are not discussed further in this chapter.) The cardiac Kir channels expressed in the heart, in particular, the Kir2 subfamily, constitute the main focus of later sections of this chapter.

Kir2 Subfamily Underlies the Classical Inward Rectifier

The Kir2 subfamily members have approximately 60% sequence homology within the subfamily members (Kir2.1 to Kir2.4, or Kir2.x); however, one important difference lies in the length of the cytoplasmic tail. Important tissue- and species-specific differences in expression of the Kir2 isoforms have been recognized.[27-30] Even in view of the relatively high degree of sequence homology among the subfamily members, important differences exist in the biophysical and regulatory properties of Kir2 channels expressed in myocardial cells, which are summarized in Table 13-2.

Kir2.1 Channels

The expression-cloning technique was used in the mouse macrophage cell line to isolate a cDNA encoding a 428–amino acid protein.[21] The protein underlies an inward rectifier channel, dubbed IRK1 (Kir2.1), and was shown to have two transmembrane segments per subunit and a 40% sequence similarity to the ATP-regulated potassium channel.[22] The channels conducted inward potassium current below the K^+ equilibrium potential but passed little outward current positive of the equilibrium potential, were selective for K^+ ions, and had a unitary conductance of 23 pS in cell-attached oocyte membrane patches. (The mechanisms underlying Kir2 channel rectification have been, for the most part, studied using heterologously expressed Kir2.1 channels and are dealt with more extensively in a subsequent section.) A voltage- and time-dependent channel block by extracellular Na^+, Cs^+, and Ba^{2+}, properties of which suggest

Table 13-1 Diversity of α Subunit Proteins in Inward Rectifier Potassium Channels

Chromosome Family	Cardiac Subfamily	Protein	Gene	Human	Mouse	Current
Kir	Kir1	Kir1.1	*KCNJ1*	11q25		?
	Kir2	Kir2.1	*KCNJ2*	17q23	11	I_{K1}
		Kir2.2	*KCNJ12*	17p11.2	11	I_{K1}
		Kir2.3	*KCNJ4*	22U		?
		Kir2.4	*KCNJ14*	19q13.4		?
	Kir3	Kir3.1	*KCNJ3*		2	I_{KACh}
		Kir3.2	*KCNJ6*	21q22		
			KCNJ7		16	
		Kir3.3	*KCNJ9*	1q21	1	
		Kir3.4	*KCNJ5*	11q25	9	I_{KACh}
	Kir4	Kir4.1	*KCNJ10*	1q21	1	
		Kir4.2	*KCNJ15*	21q22	16	
	Kir5	Kir5.1	*KCNJ16*	17q25		
	Kir6	Kir6.1	*KCNJ8*	12p11.1	6	
		Kir6.2	*KCNJ11*	11p15		I_{KATP}

From Nerbonne JM, Nichols CG, Schwarz TL, Escande D: Genetic manipulation of cardiac K^+ channel function in mice: What have we learned, and where do we go from here? Circ Res 89:944-956, 2001.

open channel block, also was reported.[21] The extracellular Cs^+ block was steep, indicating multiple binding sites for the cation in the channel pore.

In another study,[31] the time-dependent outward currents through Kir2.1 channels in the murine fibroblast (L) cells were extensively characterized. Specifically, the study examined outward currents in the presence of Mg^{2+}, putrescine, and endogenous spermine. Repolarizing the cell membrane from depolarized potentials resulted in a time-dependent change in outward current: A transient increase and then a decrease in the outward currents were observed. The initial increase was attributed to a transient relief of channel block by the divalent cations (Mg^{2+} and putrescine), whereas the reblock was attributable to block by spermine. It was concluded that this effect of Mg^{2+} at the plateau range of potentials should be important for repolarization of the cardiac action potential.

Table 13-2 Biophysical and Regulatory Properties of Individual Kir2.x Channel Isoforms

Property	Kir2.1	Kir2.2	Kir2.3
Unitary conductance (pS)	25	35	10
Barium block: IC_{50} (mM)	3.2	0.5	10.3
Arachidonic acid effect: EC_{50} (μM)	Insensitive	Insensitive	447
Proton block (pK_a)	4.95	—	6.8

EC_{50}, median effective concentration; IC_{50}, median inhibitory concentration (half-maximal block).

More recently, the unitary conductance and pharmacologic block of guinea pig Kir2.1 channels heterologously expressed in HEK293 were studied in mammalian cells and in oocytes.[28] The investigators reported a unitary conductance of 30.6 pS in symmetrical K^+ (140 mM). The barium concentration required for IC_{50} at −100 mV was 3.24 mM. Overall, these data show that within the Kir2 subfamily expressed in myocardial cells, Kir2.1 channels have intermediate conductance properties and pharmacologic sensitivity to Ba^{2+}. Notably, an important, frequent observation from several of these studies is the different unitary conductance values reported for Kir2.1 channels. Furthermore, the values are not identical to the unitary conductance values for I_{K1} recorded in native cardiac myocytes. One possibility is the interaction of the Kir2 channel proteins with other proteins in the expression systems, resulting in the modulation of unitary conductance values.[28,32]

Kir2.2 Channels

Compared with Kir2.1 channels, relatively less information is available for the Kir2.2 isoforms. Molecular cloning and functional expression of Kir2.2 channels were performed in the mouse[33] and in the rat brain.[34] The latter study showed that the amino acid sequence of the channel, which was named RB-IRK2, has 70% identity to the mouse Kir2.1 channel. Murine Kir2.2 clone was reported to encode a 427–amino acid protein, and when expressed in oocytes, the channels had a unitary conductance of 34.2 pS in equimolar (140 mM) K^+ solutions.[33] During their recording conditions, Kir2.1 channels had a relatively smaller unitary conductance of 22.2 pS. It also was reported that, in contrast with the Kir2.1 channels, a significant amount of inactivation of the Kir2.2 channels was observed in the presence of hyperpolarizing pulses. The study by Koyama and colleagues[34] also showed that Kir2.2 channels were sensitive to extracellular Cs^+ and Ba^{2+}, and that the channels were blocked in a time- and voltage-dependent manner.

The biophysical properties of Kir2.2 channels cloned from the guinea pig heart were recently described.[28] Unitary conductance values averaged 40 pS, and the channels showed a high sensitivity to extracellular Ba^{2+}. It also was reported that IC_{50} for extracellular Ba^{2+} block (0.51 mM) was the lowest among the Kir2 isoforms. The study also suggested that although the guinea pig cardiac muscle expressed Kir2.1, Kir2.2, and Kir2.3 channels, Kir2.2 was the major contributor to the inward rectifier current (however, see later discussion).

Kir2.3 Channels

Properties of an inward rectifier channel HIRK1 (Kir2.3) cloned from human hippocampus were studied by following heterologous expression.[35] The clone was reported to have 60% sequence similarity to the previously cloned Kir2.1 and to encode a 445–amino acid protein. Expression studies in oocytes showed a unitary conductance that averaged 10 pS, measured from on-cell membrane patches either directly or by noise analysis. The channels also were blocked by intracellular, but not extracellular, tetraethylammonium (TEA) ions. From the mouse brain complementary DNA (cDNA) library, a study by Morishige and coworkers[36] characterized the MB-IRK3 clone for the Kir2.3 channel, which also was reported to encode a 445–amino acid protein. This study also described a unitary conductance of 10 pS, with 140 mM extracellular K^+, and a clear concentration- and voltage-dependent block of the channels by extracellular Ba^{2+} and Cs^+. In the same year, properties of a strongly rectifying Kir channel isolated from the human hippocampus were described after expression in oocytes.[37] The channel had a sequence homology of 67% when compared with Kir2.1. The investigators also reported that the Kir2.3 currents were blocked by extracellular Ba^{2+} and Cs^+. Analysis of Cs^+ block showed that the theoretical fractional electrical distance (*d*) was 1.4 for the Cs^+ binding site within the electrical field across the membrane. Kir2.3 channels had a unitary conductance of 13 pS, and channel gating kinetics were slow, with long open times at negative potentials.[37] Both channel conductance and channel rectification depended on extracellular K^+. It is noteworthy that an important property of Kir2.3 channels is their proton sensitivity. Unlike Kir2.1 and Kir2.2, the Kir2.3 subunit is sensitive to pH.[27,30] Therefore, sequence homology notwithstanding, significant differences exist in the properties of individual Kir2 isoforms. It is almost certain that these differences in the isoforms have important implications in the properties of I_{K1} in the native environment.[27,30] Such implications currently are being examined in our laboratory.

Physiological Function of the Classical Inward Rectifier Requires a Heteromeric Assembly of Kir2 Channels

It generally is assumed that Kir2 subfamily members primarily underlie I_{K1}, given that in heterologous expression systems the channel proteins have time- and voltage-dependent rectification properties that are very similar to the properties recorded for native I_{K1} in the heart.[1,3] Of the four Kir2 subfamilies described, only Kir2.1, Kir2.2, and Kir2.3 are expressed in myocardial cells.[28] Immunocytochemical analysis with polyclonal antibodies showed that Kir2.4 expression was demonstrable only in cardiac neuronal cells.[28] The role of Kir2.1 and Kir2.2 in I_{K1} was given further support by the gene knockout approach.[38] Ventricular myocytes from Kir2.1$^{-/-}$ mice lacked detectable I_{K1} in whole-cell recordings. Furthermore, a 50% reduction in I_{K1} was observed in Kir2.2$^{-/-}$ mice, suggesting the possibility that Kir2.2 also can contribute to I_{K1}. The role of Kir2.3 in I_{K1} is not clear[7]; however, the report by Dhamoon and colleagues[27] is of interest in this regard.

The manner in which Kir2.x proteins assemble to form the channels that underlie I_{K1} is still not clear. Kir2 members are thought to exist as homotetramers,[39] or heterotetramers[40,41] in vivo. Evidence for heteromerization in Kir2 channels was provided after coexpression of pairs of Kir2 channels (Kir2.x and Kir2.y) as individual channels or as concatamers.[42] The roles of the individual isoforms were identified on the basis of their pharmacologic block by Ba^{2+}. Of interest, the investigators found that after coexpression of Kir2.1 and Kir2.2 in oocytes, the IC_{50} for Ba^{2+} block of the channels differed significantly from the value expected when the channels are independently expressed as homomeric channels. In addition, the two-yeast hybrid system was used to show that the N and C termini of different Kir2 channel isoforms do indeed interact.

A consistent finding is that the unitary conductance of I_{K1} from different laboratories vary markedly, ranging from 10 to 40 pS.[9-11,27] Is it possible that the differences in unitary conductance values for I_{K1} can be attributed to the different Kir2.x channels expressed in these cells/tissues? Also intriguing is the observation that the reported unitary conductances do not match the values reported for heterologously expressed Kir2.x proteins. One possible explanation for apparent differences in reported unitary conductances is the presence of other interacting proteins in the various cell environments.

A recent study by Munoz and associates[43] has provided further support for heteromerization as well as for its functional significance in the physiologic function of I_{K1}. Voltage clamp experiments were performed to test the pH sensitivity of whole-cell and unitary currents in HEK293 cells stably expressing guinea pig Kir2.1 or Kir2.3 isoforms. Additional experiments were carried out on sheep cardiac ventricular myocytes, which predominantly express the two isoforms. The investigators reported that whole-cell Kir2.1/Kir2.3 currents rectified in a manner reminiscent of Kir2.1 but were significantly inhibited by extracellular acidification in the physiologic range (p*Ka* =7.4). At extracellular pH (pH_o) = 6.0, unitary conductances of heteromeric channels were reduced. The ovine cardiac ventricular cell I_{K1} also was pH_o- and CO_2-sensitive, consistent with the expression of Kir2.3 in the species. It was therefore concluded that Kir2.1 and Kir2.3 isoforms form heteromeric channels in HEK293 and in the sheep ventricular myocardium. It also was concluded that the presence of Kir2.3 subunit(s) in heteromeric channels confers pH sensitivity to the channels.

Kir3 Subfamily Underlies I_{KACh}

The Kir3 isoforms are thought to mediate I_{KACh}.[7] The channels are directly coupled to the M2 receptors by a membrane-delimited (and hence fast) pathway, and the coupling mechanism involves a pertussis toxin–sensitive guanosine triphosphate (GTP)-binding protein (i.e., G protein). Activation of I_{KACh} channel occurs when the $\beta\gamma$ subunits of the G protein bind to the Kir3.x channels.[44]

Support for the role of the Kir3.x channels in I_{KACh} also has been obtained from mice with targeted deletion of the Kir3.4 gene. Electrophysiologic experiments in the animals show that they lack any measurable I_{KACh}.[45] How do the Kir3 channel isoforms come together in the I_{KACh} channel complex? Some evidence indicates that the I_{KACh} channels in the heart formed by Kir3.1 and Kir3.4 proteins are heteromeric channel complexes with a stoichiometric ratio of 1:1. Kir3.1 and Kir3.4 channels also are known, respectively, as GIRK1 and GIRK4. (GIRK stands for *G protein–coupled, inwardly rectifying potassium channel.*) However, the Kir3.x nomenclature is used in this chapter. Other evidence indicates that of the two Kir3 isoforms, Kir3.4 is important for channel processing and for localization on the cell surface. Furthermore, the binding site for the G protein βγ subunits is located on Kir3.4.

I_{KATP} Channel: A Complex of Kir6 Subfamily and the Sulfonylurea Receptor

Some evidence indicates that the molecular correlate of I_{KATP} is a composite of two Kir6 subfamily members, KCNJ8 (Kir6.1) and KCNJ11 (Kir6.2), and the ATP-binding cassette proteins that encode the sulfonylurea receptor (SUR).[46,47] The significance of the Kir6.2 protein in the complex is reasonably well established: I_{KATP} channel activity is absent in Kir6.2$^{-/-}$ mice.[48,49] Kir6.1 also is expressed in the heart, and the experiments show that I_{KATP} is reduced in ventricular cells in the presence of antisense against SUR1. The heteromultimeric channel complex consists of two Kir6.2 proteins and two SURs, with each Kir member associated with each SUR member. The channel is sensitive to several agents: ATP inhibits the channel, whereas phosphatidylinositol 4,5-bisphosphate (PIP_2) activates it by the direct interactions with the Kir6.2 subunits. It has been suggested[47,50] that PIP_2 and ATP bind to the cytoplasmic domains of each Kir6.2 to stabilize channel in the open and closed states, respectively. They also have suggested a total of four binding sites created at the interfaces of the Kir6.2 subunits. The manner by which binding of PIP_2 and ATP leads to channel gating remains to be resolved.

Architecture of Kir Channel Proteins Revealed by X-ray Crystallography

X-ray crystallographic studies have provided new insight into the molecular structures of Kir channel proteins.[20,51-54] These studies have confirmed results from earlier investigations showing that Kir family members are structurally and functionally different from the voltage-gated potassium channels. Members of the Kir family are composed of four subunits, and each subunit has two transmembrane domains (M1 and M2), cytoplasmic N and C termini, and a pore-forming structure between M1 and M2.[55] The pore structure contains a pore helix (P) and the characteristic GYG (or GFG) stretch that determines K^+ selectivity in all potassium channels.[19,20] In Figure 13-2, the side view of a bacterial Kir channel (KirBac1.1[53]) is schematized, showing the transmembrane domains of two subunits (blue and green) and the C-terminal regions of neighboring subunits (red and yellow). The transmembrane domains from each subunit are arranged as an antiparallel coiled-coil and make contact with each other. This structure shows that a very significant portion (approximately 70%) of the channel residues forms a cytoplasmic pore important for intracellular channel regulation and rectification.

How does this structure relate to the structure of other Kir channel proteins? Other Kir channels within the family may have slight variations of this general architecture.[54] For example, in the KirBac channel, in addition to the M1 and M2 helices, a "slide helix" is located in the cytoplasmic face of the cell, which may not be present in all other Kir channels. Also, evidence from mutagenesis and functional analysis indicates that the pore of the Kir2.1 channel may be different from that of another bacterial channel, the KcsA, the crystal structure of which has recently been deduced.[20,51,52] The protein structure formed by the N and C termini of Kir3.1 (GIRK1) was investigated at a resolution of 0.18 nm.[52] It was reported that the channel has a cytoplasmic pore lined with acid and hydrophobic residues that could play a role in rectification. Furthermore, it was shown that the cytoplasmic pore extended the overall length of the channel approximately two-fold, to approximately 6 nm.

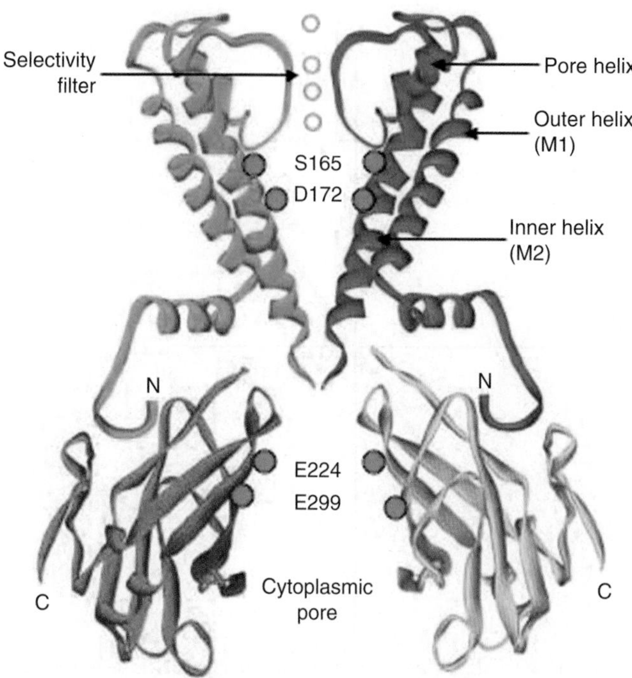

Figure 13-2 Architecture of a typical Kir channel. This is a general structure *(side view)* adapted from the KirBac1 channel. The transmembrane domains of two subunits are shown in *green* and *blue*. The C-terminal domains of the other two subunits are shown in *red* and *yellow*. Residues important for rectification are shown as *red circles*. C, carboxyl terminus; N, amino terminus. (Modified from Bichet D, Haass FA, Jan LY: Merging functional studies with structures of inward-rectifier K(+) channels. Nat Rev Neurosci 4:957-967, 2003.)

Mechanisms of Rectification in Inward Rectifier Potassium Channels

Inward rectification was first proposed to result from a voltage-dependent block of channel pore by a cytoplasmic particle, and subsequent studies have indeed demonstrated that rectification results from a voltage-dependent block by intracellular Na^+, Mg^{2+}, and polyamines.[1] The sensitivity of this block is different among the different Kir subfamilies,[56] and although every Kir channel shows the property of inward rectification, Kir channels can be grouped as "strongly" rectifying (Kir2 and Kir3) or "weakly" rectifying (Kir1 and Kir6) channels.[1,5,6] Weak inward rectifiers turn on or "activate" instantaneously with membrane hyperpolarization; by contrast, the strong rectifiers activate in a time-dependent manner. The "activation" kinetics of strong inward rectifiers during membrane hyperpolarization is reflective of the time-dependent unblocking characteristics of the channel.

In later studies, extensive characterization of the mechanism of inward rectification of the classical inward rectifier current and the role of intracellular cations was carried out in a variety of cardiac cells.[57-59] Results from these studies provided additional support for the role of intracellular Mg^{2+} on inward rectification.

Magnesium- and Polyamine-Induced Rectification

With the availability of Kir channel clones, the role of intracellular Mg^{2+} in inward rectification was further tested and

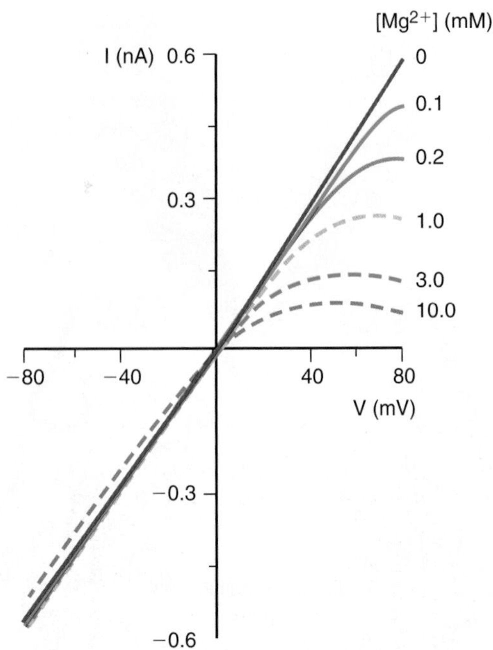

Figure 13-3 Effects of intracellular magnesium on inward rectification. Intracellular magnesium caused a dose-dependent inhibition of outward (but not inward) current through Kir1.1 channels. Currents were recorded with equimolar potassium (100 mM) on both sides of the membrane. (Modified from Lu Z, MacKinnon R: Electrostatic tuning of Mg^{2+} affinity in an inward-rectifier K^+ channel. Nature 371:243-246, 1994; and Ashcroft F: Inwardly rectifying K^+ channels. In Ion Channels and Disease. San Diego, Academic Press, 2000, pp 135-159.)

confirmed on channels expressed in oocytes or in mammalian cells.[60] For example, investigators examined the effect of Mg^{2+} on inward rectification in Kir1.1 channels heterologously expressed in oocytes (Fig. 13-3). Currents were recorded in cell membrane patches, with equimolar (100 mM) K^+ on both sides of the membrane. Mg^{2+} caused a concentration-dependent block of outward currents through the channels. Figure 13-3 shows that increasing concentrations of Mg^{2+} cause a decrease in outward but not inward component of the channel.

Thus, the role of intracellular Mg^{2+} channel block of inward rectification is reasonably well established. However, it has been consistently observed that inward rectification is evident in some Kir channels even in the absence of intracellular Mg^{2+}. Moreover, results from other studies point to an additional "intrinsic" mechanism of rectification that was voltage- (but not intracellular Mg^{2+}-) dependent.[59] It was subsequently reported that the "intrinsic" rectification of strong inward rectifiers was caused by intracellular organic cations known as polyamines.[61] The investigators suggested that the so-called intrinsic rectification was caused by a voltage-dependent channel block by the organic cations. Channel block was much steeper with spermine and spermidine, respectively, with four and three positive charges, compared with putrescine or Mg^{2+}, each with two positive charges.

Rectification Properties are Related to Electrostatic Interactions in the Cytoplasmic Pore of a Kir Channel

What structural components of the channel are involved in the polyamine (or Mg^{2+})-induced inward rectification? Also, what is the physical location of the polyamine-binding site(s) and what is responsible for the steep voltage dependence of the polyamine-induced rectification? One study[60] showed that mutations at one position in the second transmembrane segment of the Kir channel altered Mg^{2+} sensitivity. The mutation also converted the weakly rectifying (Kir1.1) channel into a strong rectifier. In Kir2 subfamily members, some evidence suggests that strong inward rectification by intracellular polyamines and Mg^{2+} depends on three negatively charged residues located in the second transmembrane domain D172 (the rectification controller) and in the carboxyl-terminal tail (E224 and E299) (see Fig. 13-2).[62-64] Polyamines enter the Kir channel pore to physically occlude it. Among the polyamines, spermine is the most voltage-dependent blocker and also has the highest potency for blocking the channel.

Recent studies involving a combination of mutagenesis and X-ray crystallography have provided better insight into electrostatic interactions in the ion permeation pathway, especially within the cytoplasmic pore, revealing the role of other cytoplasmic residues.[52,53,65] In a comparative analysis of the cytoplasmic structures of Kir2.1 and Kir3, a flexible cytoplasmic pore-facing loop (Fig. 13-4) was described (G loop) that forms a girdle around the central axis of the Kir channel pore.[52,53,65] It was reported that this girdle constricts the ion permeation pathway

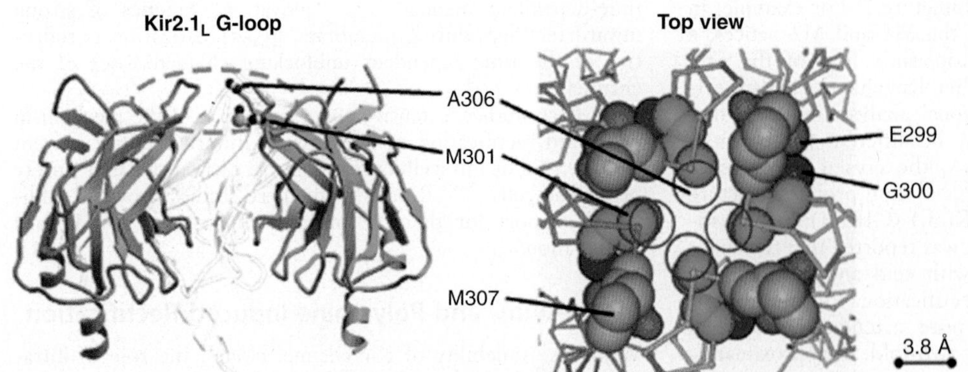

Figure 13-4 A flexible "girdle," or G loop, in the cytoplasmic pore of a Kir2.1 channel. A306 of the G loop is situated at the narrowest part of the pore. Other labeled residues are part of the G loop. (Modified from Pegan S, Arrabit C, Zhou W, et al: Cytoplasmic domain structures of Kir2.1 and Kir3.1 show sites for modulating gating and rectification. Nat Neurosci 8:279-287, 2005.)

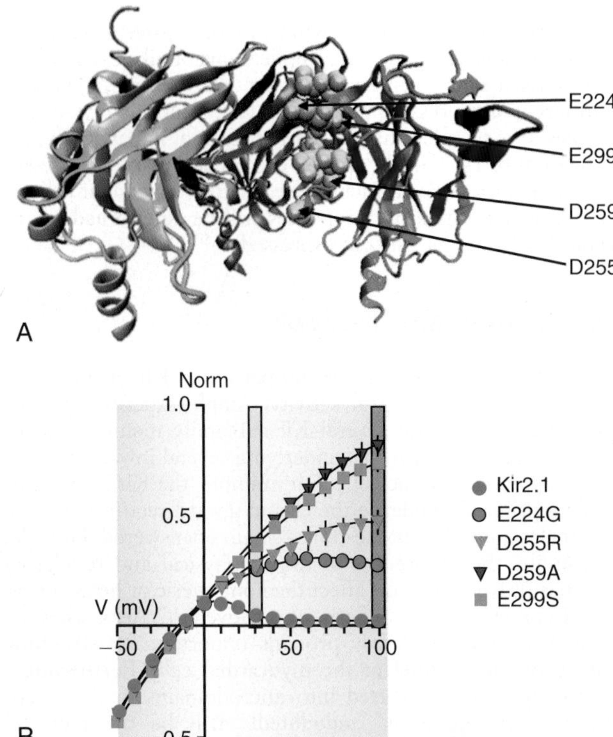

Figure 13-5 A cluster of negatively charged residues involved in rectification of a Kir2.1 channel. A di-aspartate cluster (D255 and D259) profoundly modulates rectification. In the *top panel*, amino acids lining the permeation pathway are highlighted onto a Kir2.1 channel (only three subunits are illustrated). *Bottom panel* shows normalized whole-cell currents of Kir2.1 wild type and mutants (E22G, D255R, D259A, E299S). Rectification at +30 mV (gray) and +100 mV (*dark gray*) are shown as bars. (Modified from Pegan S, Arrabit C, Zhou W, et al: Cytoplasmic domain structures of Kir2.1 and Kir3.1 show sites for modulating gating and rectification. Nat Neurosci 8:279-287, 2005.)

in a manner similar to the acetylcholine channel. Whereas the G loop in the Kir3.1 has an opening of 90 nm, the G loop in Kir2.1 is only 57 nm. In the study, mutations in the G-loop were shown to disrupt inward rectification. In the same study, a set of di-aspartate residues were shown to significantly affect rectification of the Kir2.1 channel (Fig. 13-5). Thus, in addition to the previously described glutamate 224 and glutamate 299 residues, a set of aspartate 255 and aspartate 259 located farther away from the pore than the glutamates of the channels are involved in channel rectification.

The precise mechanism involved in this rectification is not known but may be attributable to providing addition negative charges in the cytoplasmic pore, thereby attracting mono-, di- and polyvalent cations. Several models have subsequently been proposed to explain polyamine-binding sites and voltage dependence of channel block. Thus, polyamines may bind at a deep site (between the rectification controller and the selectivity filter), or they may bind at a shallow site in the cytoplasmic pore of the channel. In either case, displacement of potassium ions would be responsible for the voltage dependence of block. A relatively recent study[66] aimed at determining the polyamine binding site in a Kir channel investigated the effects of polyamine blockade on the rate of (2-aminoethyl) methanethiosulfonate (MTSEA) modification of cysteine residues engineered into the pore of a mutant Kir6.2 channel (N160D). The results showed that spermine binds at a deep site beyond the rectification controller residue, a site that is very close to the extracellular mouth of the pore.

Rectification Properties of Kir2.x Subfamily

Consistent with their significant sequence homology, all Kir2 channels have the three residues important for rectification. Heterologous expression studies also have demonstrated that Kir2.x channel unitary conductances inwardly rectify in a strong manner at potentials positive to E_K.[21,33,35] Recent laboratory experiments, however, unexpectedly showed that whole-cell current rectification properties are different in the three isoforms.[27] Voltage clamp ramps from −100 to +10 mV were used, and barium-sensitive outward current profiles were compared in the Kir2 isoforms. Figure 13-6A shows representative

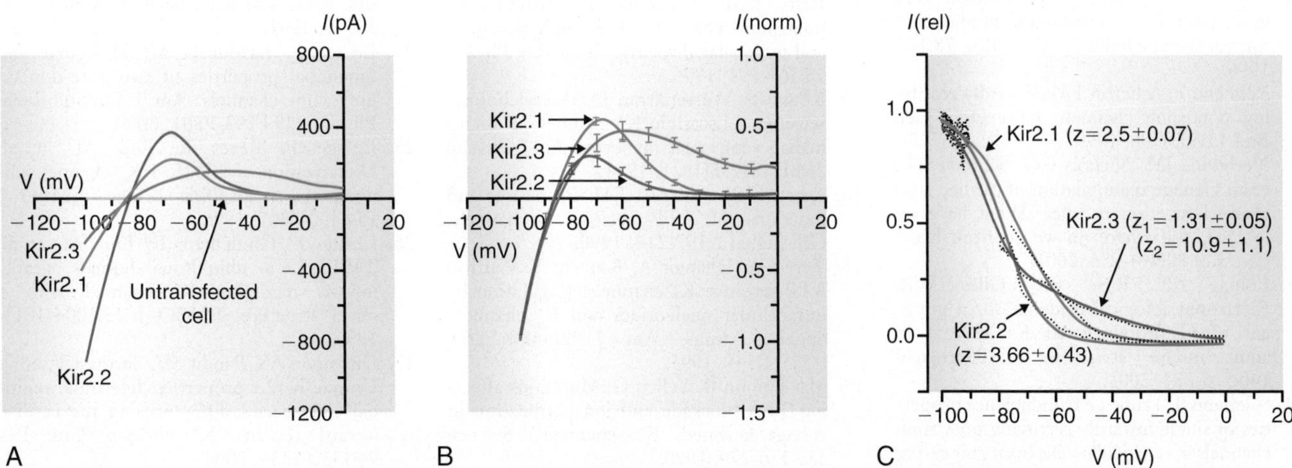

Figure 13-6 Current-voltage (*I-V*) relations of Kir2.x channels expressed in HEK293 cells. **A,** Comparison of ramp-generated, barium-sensitive currents in cells expressing Kir2.x channels. Current in an untransfected cell is superimposed. **B,** Average data for cells expressing Kir2.1 (*n* = 6), Kir2.2 (*n* = 6), and Kir2.3 (*n* = 4) channels. Data were normalized to current at −100 mV. **C,** Average relative (rel) current as a function of voltage. Data were fitted with a single (Kir2.1 and Kir2.2) or a double (Kir2.3) Boltzmann function. (**A-C,** Modified from Dhamoon AS, Pandit SV, Sarmast F, et al: Unique Kir2.x properties determine regional and species differences in the cardiac inward rectifier K^+ current. Circ Res 94:1332-1339, 2004.)

current-voltage (I-V) relationships of the Kir2 isoforms, as well as current-voltage relations in an untransfected cell. Figure 13-6B illustrates the rectification profiles of Kir2.x currents normalized to their respective currents at −100 mV. Outward current peaked at similar voltages for Kir2.1 (−68 mV) and Kir2.2 (−74 mV). However, outward current in Kir2.3 channels peaked at a more positive potential (−55 mV) than the other two isoforms. The degree of rectification of the Kir2.x channels was quantified by fitting with the Boltzmann equation (see Fig. 13-6C). The investigators reported that whereas a single Boltzmann function was sufficient to fit Kir2.1 and Kir2.2 currents (z = 2.5 and 3.7, respectively), Kir2.3 currents could be fitted only by a double Boltzmann function (z_1 = 1.3; z_2 = 10.9). Their results also showed that Kir2.2 channels had stronger voltage dependence of rectification than that observed for Kir2.1 channels. These observations have been confirmed by work from other laboratories.[67,68]

A detailed characterization of steady-state and kinetic properties of block of Kir2.1, Kir2.2, and Kir2.3 channels by spermine was undertaken in recent studies.[67,68] The investigators reported that although rectification in Kir2 channels followed a general mechanism, significant and physiologically relevant quantitative differences existed among the different Kir2 isoforms, attributable to differences in isoform sensitivity to polyamines. In one of these studies,[68] spermine block of Kir2.1 and Kir2.2 channels was examined. These investigators were interested in determining the importance of the low-affinity block in mediating outward Kir2 currents. Results from that study showed important differences in rectification properties of Kir2 channels examined. The results also were consistent with the idea that the Kir2 channel exists in two states having different susceptibilities to internal cationic blockers. The implications of all of these findings discussed earlier can be significant. For example, in view of the differential expression patterns of Kir2 isoforms in a variety of tissues, it is possible that I_{K1} properties and, in particular, the rectification of I_{K1} will depend on the predominantly expressed Kir2 channel isoform. In such a case, the I_{K1}-dependent cellular excitability and regulatory properties will be determined by the specific Kir2 channel isoform expressed.[27,30]

Conclusions and Outlook

The biophysical and regulatory properties of Kir channels are crucial for cardiac electrical activity. Ample experimental evidence clearly implicates several Kir subfamily members as the major molecular mechanisms underlying several inward rectifier currents in native cardiac cells. For example, the Kir2 subfamily members primarily underlie the classic inward rectifier current. Nevertheless, significant questions remain unanswered. How do, for example, the differences in the biophysical and regulatory properties of Kir2 isoforms affect the homomeric or heteromeric channel complexes that underlie the native I_{K1}? Also, what are the ancillary and regulatory proteins important for structural integrity of the channel in the myocardial cell? Furthermore, how are the channels sorted into microdomains in the sarcolemma? These questions undoubtedly will be the focus of much investigation in the near future.

References

1. Lopatin AN, Nichols CG: Inward rectifiers in the heart: An update on I(K1). J Mol Cell Cardiol 33:625-638, 2001.
2. Lu Z: Mechanism of rectification in inward-rectifier K+ channels. Annu Rev Physiol 66:103-129, 2004.
3. Stanfield PR, Nakajima S, Nakajima Y: Constitutively active and G-protein coupled inward rectifier K+ channels: Kir2.0 and Kir3.0. Rev Physiol Biochem Pharmacol 145:47-179, 2002.
4. Ashcroft FM: Ion Channels and Disease. San Diego, Academic Press, 2000.
5. Nichols CG, Makhina EN, Pearson WL, et al: Inward rectification and implications for cardiac excitability. Circ Res 78:1-7, 1996.
6. Reimann F, Ashcroft FM: Inwardly rectifying potassium channels. Curr Opin Cell Biol 11:503-508, 1999.
7. Nerbonne JM, Nichols CG, Schwarz TL, et al: Genetic manipulation of cardiac K(+) channel function in mice: What have we learned, and where do we go from here? Circ Res 89:944-956, 2001.
8. Lomax AE, Rose RA, Giles WR: Electrophysiological evidence for a gradient of G protein–gated K+ current in adult mouse atria. Br J Pharmacol 140:576-584, 2003.
9. Sakmann B, Trube G: Conductance properties of single inwardly rectifying potassium channels in ventricular cells from guinea-pig heart. J Physiol 347:641-657, 1984.
10. Kurachi Y: Voltage-dependent activation of the inward-rectifier potassium channel in the ventricular cell membrane of guinea-pig heart. J Physiol 366:365-385, 1985.
11. Shioya T, Matsuda H, Noma A: Fast and slow blockades of the inward-rectifier K+ channel by external divalent cations in guinea-pig cardiac myocytes. Pflügers Arch 422:427-435, 1993.
12. Shimoni Y, Clark RB, Giles WR: Role of an inwardly rectifying potassium current in rabbit ventricular action potential. J Physiol 448:709-727, 1992.
13. Kurachi Y, Nakajima T, Sugimoto T: Acetylcholine activation of K+ channels in cell-free membrane of atrial cells. Am J Physiol 251:H681-H684, 1986.
14. Barry DM, Nerbonne JM: Myocardial potassium channels: Electrophysiological and molecular diversity. Annu Rev Physiol 58:363-394, 1996.
15. Koumi S, Wasserstrom JA: Acetylcholine-sensitive muscarinic K+ channels in mammalian ventricular myocytes. Am J Physiol 266:H1812-H1821, 1994.
16. Ashcroft SJ, Ashcroft FM: Properties and functions of ATP-sensitive K-channels. Cell Signal 2:197-214, 1990.
17. Terzic A, Jahangir A, Kurachi Y: Cardiac ATP-sensitive K+ channels: Regulation by intracellular nucleotides and K+ channel–opening drugs. Am J Physiol 269:C525-C545, 1995.
18. MacKinnon R, Yellen G: Mutations affecting TEA blockade and ion permeation in voltage-activated K+ channels. Science 250:276-279, 1990.
19. Yool AJ, Schwarz TL: Alteration of ionic selectivity of a K+ channel by mutation of the H5 region. Nature 349:700-704, 1991.
20. Doyle DA, Morais Cabral J, Pfuetzner RA, et al: The structure of the potassium channel: Molecular basis of K+ conduction and selectivity. Science 280:69-77, 1998.
21. Kubo Y, Baldwin TJ, Jan YN, et al: Primary structure and functional expression of a mouse inward rectifier potassium channel. Nature 362:127-133, 1993.
22. Ho K, Nichols CG, Lederer WJ, et al: Cloning and expression of an inwardly rectifying ATP-regulated potassium channel. Nature 362:31-38, 1993.
23. Dascal N, Schreibmayer W, Lim NF, et al: Atrial G protein-activated K+ channel: Expression cloning and molecular properties. Proc Natl Acad Sci U S A 90:10235-10239, 1993.
24. Lesage F, Lazdunski M: Molecular and functional properties of two-pore-domain potassium channels. Am J Physiol Renal Physiol 279:F793-F801, 2000.
25. Lesage F, Reyes R, Fink M, et al: Dimerization of TWIK-1 K+ channel subunits via a disulfide bridge. EMBO J 15:6400-6407, 1996.
26. Lesage F, Guillemare E, Fink M, et al: TWIK-1, a ubiquitous human weakly inward rectifying K+ channel with a novel structure. EMBO J 15:1004-1011, 1996.
27. Dhamoon AS, Pandit SV, Sarmast F, et al: Unique Kir2.x properties determine regional and species differences in the cardiac inward rectifier K+ current. Circ Res 94:1332-1339, 2004.
28. Liu GX, Derst C, Schlichthorl G, et al: Comparison of cloned Kir2 channels with native inward rectifier K+ channels from guinea-pig cardiomyocytes. J Physiol 532:115-126, 2001.

29. Wang Z, Yue L, White M, et al: Differential distribution of inward rectifier potassium channel transcripts in human atrium versus ventricle. Circulation 98:2422-2428, 1998.
30. Melnyk P, Zhang L, Shrier A, et al: Differential distribution of Kir2.1 and Kir2.3 subunits in canine atrium and ventricle. Am J Physiol Heart Circ Physiol 283:H1123-H1133, 2002.
31. Ishihara K: Time-dependent outward currents through the inward rectifier potassium channel I_{RK1}. The role of weak blocking molecules. J Gen Physiol 109:229-243, 1997.
32. Nehring RB, Wischmeyer E, Doring F, et al: Neuronal inwardly rectifying K^+ channels differentially couple to PDZ proteins of the PSD-95/SAP90 family. J Neurosci 20:156-162, 2000.
33. Takahashi N, Morishige K, Jahangir A, et al: Molecular cloning and functional expression of cDNA encoding a second class of inward rectifier potassium channels in the mouse brain. J Biol Chem 269:23274-23279, 1994.
34. Koyama H, Morishige K, Takahashi N, et al: Molecular cloning, functional expression and localization of a novel inward rectifier potassium channel in the rat brain. FEBS Lett 341:303-307, 1994.
35. Makhina EN, Kelly AJ, Lopatin AN, et al: Cloning and expression of a novel human brain inward rectifier potassium channel. J Biol Chem 269:20468-20474, 1994.
36. Morishige K, Takahashi N, Jahangir A, et al: Molecular cloning and functional expression of a novel brain-specific inward rectifier potassium channel. FEBS Lett 346:251-256, 1994.
37. Perier F, Radeke CM, Vandenberg CA: Primary structure and characterization of a small-conductance inwardly rectifying potassium channel from human hippocampus. Proc Natl Acad Sci U S A 91:6240-6244, 1994.
38. Zaritsky JJ, Redell JB, Tempel BL, et al: The consequences of disrupting cardiac inwardly rectifying K(+) current (I(K1)) as revealed by the targeted deletion of the murine Kir2.1 and Kir2.2 genes. J Physiol 533:697-710, 2001.
39. Tinker A, Jan YN, Jan LY: Regions responsible for the assembly of inwardly rectifying potassium channels. Cell 87:857-868, 1996.
40. Cohen NA, Sha Q, Makhina EN, et al: Inhibition of an inward rectifier potassium channel (Kir2.3) by G-protein beta gamma subunits. J Biol Chem 271:32301-32305, 1996.
41. Fink M, Duprat F, Heurteaux C, et al: Dominant negative chimeras provide evidence for homo and heteromultimeric assembly of inward rectifier K^+ channel proteins via their N-terminal end. FEBS Lett 378:64-68, 1996.
42. Preisig-Muller R, Schlichthorl G, Goerge T, et al: Heteromerization of Kir2.x potassium channels contributes to the phenotype of Andersen's syndrome. Proc Natl Acad Sci U S A 99:7774-7779, 2002.
43. Munoz V, Vaidyanathan R, Tolkacheva EG, et al: Kir2.3 isoform confers pH sensitivity to heteromeric Kir2.1/Kir2.3 channels in HEK293 cells. Heart Rhythm 4:487-496, 2007.
44. Logothetis DE, Kurachi Y, Galper J, et al: Nature 325:321-326, 1987.
45. Wickman K, Nemec J, Gendler SJ, et al: Abnormal heart rate regulation in GIRK4 knockout mice. Neuron 20:103-114, 1998.
46. Inagaki N, Gonoi T, Clement JPt, et al: Reconstitution of IKATP: An inward rectifier subunit plus the sulfonylurea receptor. Science 270:1166-1170, 1995.
47. Nichols CG: KATP channels as molecular sensors of cellular metabolism. Nature 440:470-476, 2006.
48. Miki T, Nagashima K, Tashiro F, et al: Defective insulin secretion and enhanced insulin action in KATP channel–deficient mice. Proc Natl Acad Sci U S A 95:10402-10406, 1998.
49. Suzuki M, Li RA, Miki T, et al: Functional roles of cardiac and vascular ATP-sensitive potassium channels clarified by Kir6.2-knockout mice. Circ Res 88:570-577, 2001.
50. Enkvetchakul D, Nichols CG: Gating mechanism of KATP channels: Function fits form. J Gen Physiol 122:471-480, 2003.
51. Zhou Y, Morais-Cabral JH, Kaufman A, et al: Chemistry of ion coordination and hydration revealed by a K^+ channel–Fab complex at 2.0 Å resolution. Nature 414:43-48, 2001.
52. Nishida M, MacKinnon R: Structural basis of inward rectification: Cytoplasmic pore of the G protein-gated inward rectifier GIRK1 at 1.8 Å resolution. Cell 111:957-965, 2002.
53. Kuo A, Gulbis JM, Antcliff JF, et al: Crystal structure of the potassium channel KirBac1.1 in the closed state. Science 300:1922-1926, 2003.
54. Bichet D, Haass FA, Jan LY: Merging functional studies with structures of inward-rectifier K(+) channels. Nat Rev Neurosci 4:957-967, 2003.
55. Yang J, Jan YN, Jan LY: Determination of the subunit stoichiometry of an inwardly rectifying potassium channel. Neuron 15:1441-1447, 1995.
56. Fakler B, Brandle U, Bond C, et al: A structural determinant of differential sensitivity of cloned inward rectifier K^+ channels to intracellular spermine. FEBS Lett 356:199-203, 1994.
57. Matsuda H, Saigusa A, Irisawa H: Ohmic conductance through the inwardly rectifying K channel and blocking by internal Mg^{2+}. Nature 325:156-159, 1987.
58. Vandenberg CA: Inward rectification of a potassium channel in cardiac ventricular cells depends on internal magnesium ions. Proc Natl Acad Sci U S A 84:2560-2564, 1987.
59. Oliva C, Cohen IS, Pennefather P: The mechanism of rectification of i_{K1} in canine Purkinje myocytes. J Gen Physiol 96:299-318, 1990.
60. Lu Z, MacKinnon R: Electrostatic tuning of Mg2+ affinity in an inward-rectifier K^+ channel. Nature 371:243-246, 1994.
61. Lopatin AN, Makhina EN, Nichols CG: Potassium channel block by cytoplasmic polyamines as the mechanism of intrinsic rectification. Nature 372:366-369, 1994.
62. Stanfield PR, Davies NW, Shelton PA, et al: A single aspartate residue is involved in both intrinsic gating and blockage by Mg_{2+} of the inward rectifier, I_{RK1}. J Physiol 478:1-6, 1994.
63. Yang J, Jan YN, Jan LY: Control of rectification and permeation by residues in two distinct domains in an inward rectifier K^+ channel. Neuron 14:1047-1054, 1995.
64. Kubo Y, Murata Y: Control of rectification and permeation by two distinct sites after the second transmembrane region in Kir2.1 K^+ channel. J Physiol 531:645-660, 2001.
65. Pegan S, Arrabit C, Zhou W, et al: Cytoplasmic domain structures of Kir2.1 and Kir3.1 show sites for modulating gating and rectification. Nat Neurosci 8:279-287, 2005.
66. Kurata HT, Marton LJ, Nichols CG: The polyamine binding site in inward rectifier K^+ channels. J Gen Physiol 127:467-480, 2006.
67. Panama BK, Lopatin AN: Differential polyamine sensitivity in inwardly rectifying Kir2 potassium channels. J Physiol 571:287-302, 2006.
68. Ishihara K, Yan DH: Low-affinity spermine block mediating outward currents through Kir2.1 and Kir2.2 inward rectifier potassium channels. J Physiol 583:891-908, 2007.

Biophysical Properties of Gap Junctions 14

Robert Weingart

CHAPTER OUTLINE

Background

Cardiac impulse propagation is determined by source and sink factors. The former involve the excitatory inward currents carried by Na^+ or Ca^{2+} (or both), the latter the passive electrical properties of cells and the tissue architecture (see Chapter 25) (reviewed by Kléber and Rudy[1]). A modification of each of these elements alters the conduction velocity, θ, in the heart. The passive electrical properties include the intracellular longitudinal resistance, $r_i = r_j + r_c$, where r_j is gap junction resistance and r_c is cytoplasmic resistance. Gap junctions form intercellular connections and thus are prominent elements of the passive electrical properties. This chapter summarizes the current knowledge on the biophysical properties of gap junctions and gap junction channels.

Gap junctions are assemblies of intercellular channels. Each gap junction channel consists of two connexons or *hemichannels*; each hemichannel is made of six proteins called *connexins*. Cardiac myocytes express four different connexin isoforms. The cardiac connexins Cx40, Cx43, and Cx45 have long been known.[2] An additional isoform, Cx31.9 (homologue to mouse Cx30.2), has been discovered only recently.[3,4] Connexins are differentially expressed in cardiac tissue (see Chapter 29). Most cardiomyocytes express more than one kind of connexin. This opens the possibility to form a spectrum of structurally different gap junction channels with putatively different properties. The term *homomeric* describes a hemichannel composed of a single connexin type; *heteromeric* means a hemichannel made of more than one connexin type. The channel as a whole may be *homotypic* (matching hemichannels) or *heterotypic* (nonmatching hemichannels).

Cell pairs are most useful to study the electrical properties of gap junctions and gap junction channels. Figure 14-1 illustrates the concept of the whole-cell dual-voltage clamp technique[5] (for additional considerations, see the 1981 article by Spray and colleagues[6]). Each cell of a pair is attached to a patch pipette. After formation of a gigaohm-seal (GΩ), the membrane patch under the pipettes is ruptured, thereby establishing functional contact with the cytosol. The pipettes are connected to separate amplifiers, allowing the membrane potential of each cell to be controlled (V_1, V_2) and current flow through each pipette to be measured (I_1, I_2). Initially, the membrane potential of both cells is clamped to the same voltage, $V_1 = V_2$. A junctional voltage (V_j) is then established by depolarizing or hyperpolarizing cell 1 while the membrane potential of cell 2 is maintained. Under this condition, V_j corresponds to the difference voltage between the cells: $V_j = V_2 - V_1$. The current recorded from cell 1 is the sum of two components, the gap junction current, I_j, and the membrane current, $I_{m,1}$; the current gained from cell 2 corresponds to $-V_j$. The conductance of the gap junction or gap junction channel is determined as $g_j = I_j/V_j$ or $\gamma_j = I_j/V_j$, respectively.

This method is applicable to dispersed cardiomyocytes from adult or neonatal hearts, communication-deficient cells transfected to express desired connexins, or connexin RNA–injected oocytes.[7] In the first two cases, attention has to be paid to series resistance problems arising from high pipette resistances versus low values of r_j and r_m.[8]

This work was supported by the Swiss National Science Foundation (grant 3100A0-108175).

Homomeric-Homotypic Channels

Gap junction channels have a voltage-dependent gating mechanism. At rest, when V_j = 0 mV, the channels usually are open. During the course of a propagated action potential, when $V_j \neq 0$ mV, they tend to close in a voltage- and time-dependent manner. The conductance, the sensitivity to voltage, and the kinetics vary among channels made of different connexins.

Multichannel Properties

Figure 14-2 illustrates the behavior of gap junctions made of Cx43, the most abundant connexin in the heart. The data presented were obtained using pairs of transfected HeLa cells.[9] The upper panel in the figure shows gap junction currents, I_j, recorded when one cell of a pair was depolarized or hyperpolarized (downward or upward signals), to establish a negative or positive V_j, respectively. The traces show that I_j grows larger and inactivates faster with increasing V_j, giving rise to an instantaneous component, $I_{j,inst}$, and a steady-state component, $I_{j,ss}$, respectively.

The lower panel shows the results of the analysis. For each I_j trace, the amplitude of $I_{j,inst}$ and $I_{j,ss}$ was determined to calculate the conductances $g_{j,inst} = I_{j,inst}/V_j$ and $g_{j,ss} = I_{j,ss}/V_j$, respectively. The normalized values of $g_{j,inst}$ (*blue circles*) and $g_{j,ss}$ (*green circles*) were then plotted as a function of V_j. The functions $g_{j,inst} = f(V_j)$ and $g_{j,ss} = f(V_j)$ both were symmetrical with respect to the polarity of V_j. The smooth curve corresponds to the best fit of data to a function predicting that the hemichannels obey an exponential conductance-voltage relationship (see equation [29] in the 1998 article by Vogel and Weingart,[10] or equation [1] in their 2002 report[11]). The bell-shaped curve represents the best fit of data to

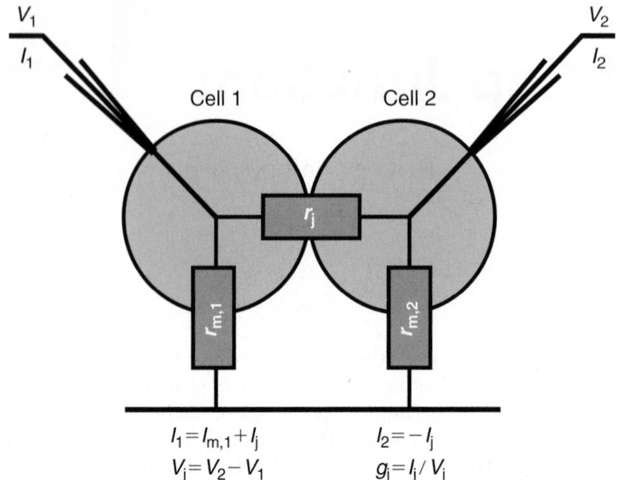

Figure 14-1 Dual-voltage clamp method. Cell pair preparation with attached patch pipettes and superimposed equivalent circuit underlying the analysis of the resistive elements involved. $r_{m,1}$, $r_{m,2}$, membrane resistance of cells 1 and 2; r_j, gap junction resistance; V_1, V_2, membrane of cells 1 and 2; I_1, I_2, currents measured with pipettes 1 and 2; V_j, transjunctional voltage; I_j, gap junction current; g_j, gap junction conductance. For further explanation, see text.

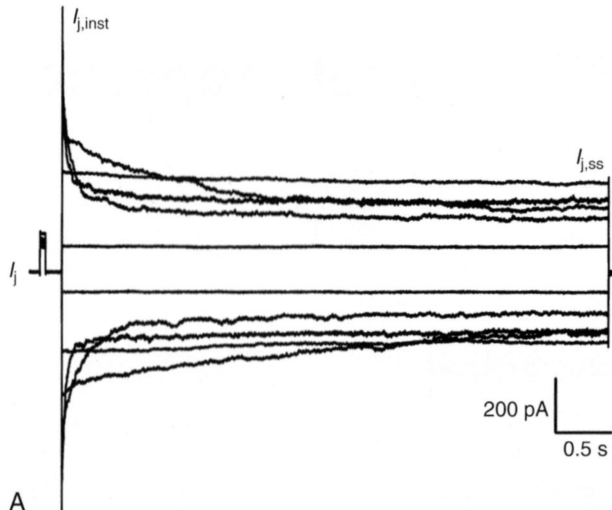

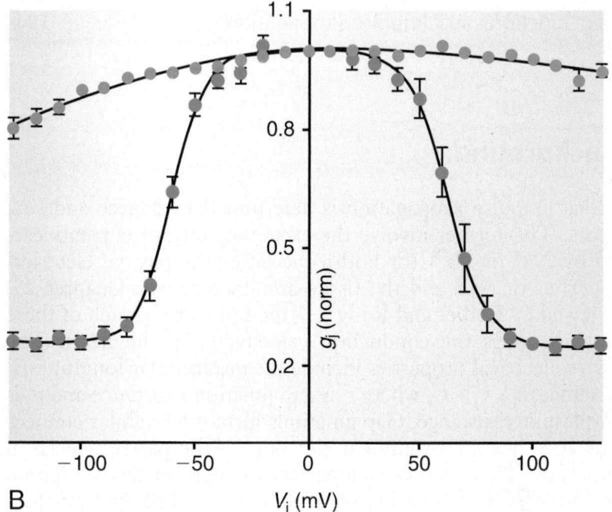

Figure 14-2 Multichannel currents of Cx43-Cx43 channels. A, Family of gap junction current signals I_j recorded at V_j = ±10, ±40, ±70, ±100, and ±130 mV. $I_{j,inst}$: instantaneous current; $I_{j,ss}$: steady-state current. B, Normalized instantaneous conductance $g_{j,inst}$ (*blue circles*) and steady-state conductance $g_{j,ss}$ (*green circles*) as functions of V_j. (From Desplantez T, Halliday D, Dupont E, Weingart R: Cardiac connexins Cx43 and Cx45: Formation of diverse gap junction channels with diverse electrical properties. Pflügers Arch 448:363-375, 2004, with permission.)

the Boltzmann equation separately applied to both V_j polarities. This is based on the view that each gap junction channel contains two symmetrical gates in series.[12]

Table 14-1 presents typical Boltzmann parameters for cardiac connexins, with data derived from various studies.[3-5,9,13-23,25-28,39] These parameters are useful to describe the process of V_j-sensitive gating.[6] $V_{j,0}$ is the voltage at which $g_{j,ss}$ is half-maximally inactivated, z is the number of positive charges moving through the electrical field applied, and $g_{j,min}$ is the minimal $g_{j,ss}$ at large V_j. The smaller $V_{j,0}$, the more pronounced is the V_j sensitivity of $g_{j,ss}$; the larger z, the steeper is the maximal slope of the V_j-dependent decay of $g_{j,ss}$. Data comparison reveals that the V_j sensitivity of $g_{j,ss}$ follows the sequence Cx45 > Cx40 > Cx43 > Cx30.2. Hence, during propagated action potentials, the V_j-dependent decay of $g_{j,ss}$ exerts an impairment of θ that is most prominent for Cx45 and virtually absent for Cx30.2.

The gap junction currents also can be used to study the kinetics of V_j-dependent gating. I_j undergoes a time-dependent inactivation during V_j pulses and a time-dependent recovery from inactivation thereafter. With regard to inactivation, I_j remains constant at small V_j and inactivates slowly at intermediate V_j (see Fig. 14-2, upper panel). The decay follows an exponential time course, giving rise to a time constant, τ_i. At large V_j, I_j inactivates rapidly. The decay follows the sum of two exponentials, leading to two time constants, τ_{i1} and τ_{i2}. The available data suggest that τ_{i1} follows the sequence Cx40 < Cx43 < Cx45 << Cx30.2. Thus, during propagated action potentials, the kinetics of I_j inactivation exerts an impairment of θ, which is most prominent for Cx40 and virtually absent for Cx30.2.

Data on recovery of I_j from inactivation for cardiac connexins are rudimentary. A more complete study of Cx46 gap junction channels is available.[29] The investigators reported that I_j recovers exponentially with time, giving rise to a time constant, τ_r, and demonstrated that large inactivation of I_j is accompanied by slow recovery, and vice versa. By analogy, cardiac gap junction channels are expected to follow the same pattern. Nevertheless, it would be desirable to have quantitative data on kinetics of I_j recovery for cardiac gap junction channels. This is crucial because during tachycardia, incomplete recovery of I_j may lead to a sustained decrease in g_j and hence maintained impairment of θ.

Single-Channel Properties

Cell pairs expressing cardiac connexins also have been used to explore the properties of single gap junction channels. Reliable data were obtained first from induced cell pairs[5,23] and later also from preformed cell pairs weakly coupled or normally coupled and exposed to submaximal doses of uncoupling agents, such as *n*-heptanol (reviewed by Harris[7]).

Figure 14-3 shows unitary currents gained from induced pairs of HeLa cells expressing Cx40.[5] Two cells in close proximity were sealed onto separate patch pipettes. The cells were then maneuvered against each other to form a cell pair. The formation of a GJ began within tens of minutes. Figure 14-3A shows

Table 14-1 Multichannel and Single-Channel Data for Various Types of Gap Junctions and Gap Junction Channels

Channel Type	$V_{j,o}$ (mV)	z	$g_{j,min}$	$\gamma_{j,main}$ (pS)	$\gamma_{j,residual}$ (pS)
Cx30.2-Cx30.2	>±100	n.d.	n.d.	10	n.d.
Cx40-Cx40	±48	±3.84	±0.30	165	33
Cx43-Cx43	±59	±2.93	±0.33	90	28
Cx45-Cx45	±24	±2.47	±0.10	35	12
Cx40-Cx43	−82/n.d.	−1.9/n.d.	−0.31/n.d.	60/100	14/20
Cx40-Cx45	n.d./50	n.d./3.3	n.d./0.06	30/40	n.d.
Cx43-Cx45	−12/134	−2.1/0.6	0.05/n.d.	40	11

Values represent averages derived from representative studies (multichannel/single-channel).
Data for Cx30.2-Cx30.2, respectively Cx31.9-Cx31.9, from references 3, 4/3, 4; for Cx40-Cx40, from references 5, 13, 14, 15, Desplantez et al., in preparation/5, 14, 18, 25; for Cx43-Cx43, from references 9, 16-20, 23, 26, 27; for Cx45-Cx45, from references 9, 19-22, 28, Desplantez et al., in preparation; for Cx40-Cx43, 15, 19, Desplantez et al; in preparation/15, 19, 38, Desplantez et al., in preparation; for Cx40-Cx45, from references 9, 19, 20/V. Valiunas, personal communication, 2000; and for Cx43-Cx45, from references 9, 19, 20/20, Desplantez et al., in preparation. n.d., not determined.
Experimental conditions: room temperature; *pipette solution*: potassium aspartate, if available. For further explanation, see text.

two examples of current records documenting the first channel insertion. The slow transition (tens of ms) reflects the first opening of a newly formed channel. Subsequent closings and openings were fast (ms) and correspond to V_j-dependent channel operation. During this activity, I_j fluctuated between two discrete levels corresponding to the channel main state and residual state, the latter attributable to incomplete channel closure. Figure 14-3B illustrates single-channel records elicited by a V_j pulse of −50 mV, obtained early during the process of gap junction formation when one (upper I_1 trace) and two channels (lower I_1 trace) were present. In the former case, two discrete current levels were present, reflecting $I_{j,main}$ and $I_{j,residual}$, indicating one channel. In the latter case, three discrete current levels were apparent, reflecting $2 \times I_{j,main}$, $I_{j,main} + I_{j,residual}$, and $2 \times I_{j,residual}$, indicating two channels. Figure 14-3C summarizes the results from many I_j records. The amplitudes of the current steps were determined to calculate channel conductances. The values of $\gamma_{j,main}$ and $\gamma_{j,residual}$ were then collected and sampled in 4-picosiemens (pS) bins. The resulting conductance histogram yielded two separate peaks corresponding to $\gamma_{j,residual}$ (left-hand distribution) and $\gamma_{j,main}$ data (right-hand distribution). Measurements at different V_j showed that $\gamma_{j,main}$ is slightly V_j sensitive,[31,32] in agreement with the slight curvature of $g_{j,inst} = f(V_j)$ in Figure 14-2.

On occasion, subconductance states can be observed between $\gamma_{j,main}$ and $\gamma_{j,residual}$.[5,29] A systematic study on Cx30 gap junction channels reported five substate conductances unevenly spaced between $\gamma_{j,main}$ and $\gamma_{j,residual}$, suggesting that each of the six

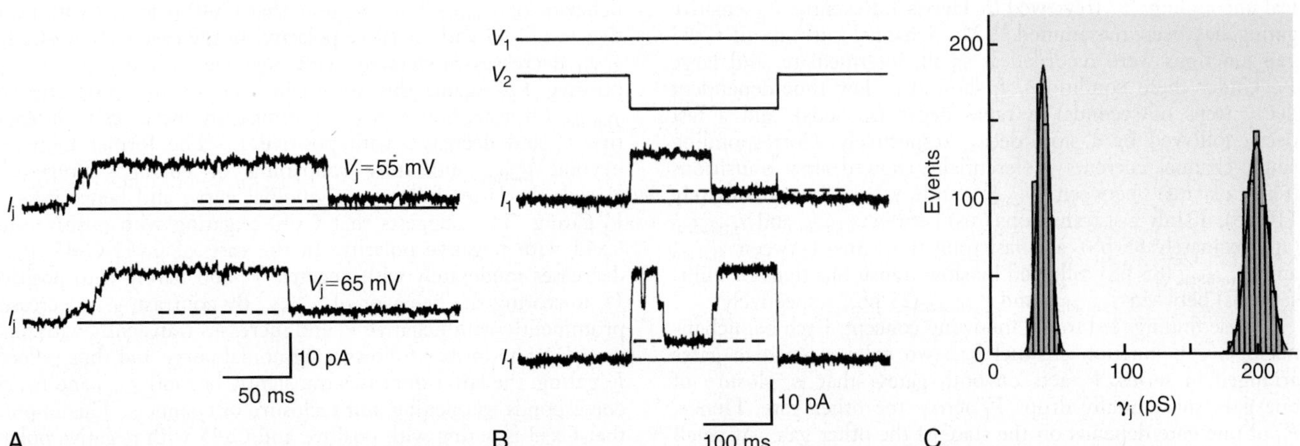

Figure 14-3 Single-channel currents of Cx40-Cx40 channels. **A,** De novo formation of a GJC. **B,** Single-channel currents elicited by a transjunctional voltage, V_j, of −50 mV (V_1 = −50 mV, V_2 = −100 mV). Single-channel currents, I_j, in the presence of one *(upper trace)* and two *(lower trace)* functional channels undergoing fast transitions between the residual state (- - - -) and main state. **C,** Frequency histogram of channel conductance, γ_j. Left-hand distribution: $\gamma_{j,residual}$; mean value = 36.5 pS; right-hand distribution: $\gamma_{j,main}$; mean value = 198.2 pS. Bin width = 4 pS. (**A-C,** From Bukauskas FF, Elfgang, Willecke K, Weingart R: Biophysical properties of gap junction channels formed by mouse connexin40 in induced pairs of transfected human HeLa cells. Biophys J 68:2289-2298, 1995, with permission.)

connexins of a hemichannel acts as a subgate.[24] Current transitions involving substates also were fast (milliseconds). Of interest, substate events always started from and ended at $\gamma_{j,main}$.

Table 14-1 also presents typical values of unitary conductance for homomeric-homotypic gap junction channels. The values of $\gamma_{j,main}$ and $\gamma_{j,residual}$ vary widely. Both follow the sequence Cx40 > Cx43 > Cx45 > Cx30.2. Of interest, $\gamma_{j,main}$ of the least-conducting channel (Cx30.2) is smaller than $\gamma_{j,residual}$ of the best conducting channel (Cx40). The residual state explains the incomplete decay of $g_{j,ss}$ at large V_j (see Fig. 14-2). Channel gating provides a selectivity filter for solute permeation.

Standard Gating Concept

The studies described led to a generalized concept of V_j gating.[10,11] The gating mechanism consists of six subgates. Their operation gives rise to fast current transitions involving $\gamma_{j,main}$, $\gamma_{j,substate}$, and $\gamma_{j,residual}$. Transitions always initiate from and terminate at $\gamma_{j,main}$. Substates are short-lasting and infrequent. Hence, $g_{j,ss}$ is determined mainly by $\gamma_{j,main}$ and $\gamma_{j,residual}$. The probability that channels are in the open state, P_o, is governed by V_j. At small V_j, it is close to 1—nearly all channels are in the main state. At large V_j, it approaches 0—that is, all channels are in the residual state. The latter state explains why $g_{j,ss}$ at large V_j does not decline to zero. At steady state, $g_{j,ss}$ approximates $\gamma_{j,residual}/\gamma_{j,main}$. For reasons of symmetry, only one or the other hemichannel of a gap junction channel is gating at a given V_j polarity. Thus, at $\gamma_{j,residual}$, one hemichannel is residing in a low-conductance configuration and the other one in a high-conductance configuration. Alternatively, at $\gamma_{j,main}$, both hemichannels are residing in the high-conductance configuration.

Expanded Concept

Over the last several years, evidence has emerged requiring a modification of the standard gating model.[28,32] Although the recent findings are crucial for a complete biophysical description of gap junction channels, their impact on cardiac gap junctions may be marginal. The new observations are summarized briefly next.

On rare occasions, slow transitions (tens of milliseconds) between $\gamma_{j,main}$ and a closed state, $\gamma_{j,closed}$, were noticed, preferentially at large V_js.[5,33] The V_j-sensitive slow transitions resembled the opening transitions seen during de novo formation of gap junction channels[5,23] (see earlier) and during chemical uncoupling[23,34] (reviewed by Harris[7]). Recently, V_j-sensitive gating has been reexamined.[35] Multichannel currents of Cx43 gap junctions were recorded at small, intermediate, and large V_j. Under these conditions, I_j showed a slow time-dependent decay (tens of seconds), a rapid decay (seconds), and a fast decay followed by a slow decay, respectively. Corresponding single-channel currents preferentially showed slow transitions (tens of ms) between $\gamma_{j,main}$ and $\gamma_{j,closed}$ (approximately 110 pS), mainly fast transitions (ms) between $\gamma_{j,main}$ and $\gamma_{j,residual}$ (approximately 85 pS), and fast transitions (ms) between $\gamma_{j,main}$ and $\gamma_{j,residual}$ (85 pS) followed by slow transitions (tens of milliseconds) between $\gamma_{j,residual}$ and $\gamma_{j,closed}$ (25 pS), respectively.

These findings led to the following concept. Each hemichannel of a gap junction channel has two voltage-sensitive gates arranged in series. V_j acts on both gates—that is, closure of one gate substantially drops V_j across the other gate. Hence, P_o of one gate depends on the state of the other gate. At small voltage, V_j gating is mediated mainly through a slow V_j gate; at intermediate voltage, through the fast V_j gate; and at large voltage, first through the fast V_j gate and then through a slow V_j gate. Owing to weak sensitivity to voltage and slow kinetics, the slow V_j gate plays a small effect on g_j, preferentially at low and large voltage. As a result of strong sensitivity to voltage and fast kinetics, the fast V_j gate plays a large effect on g_j, preferentially at intermediate and large voltage. Thus, during the course of a cardiac action potential, the fast V_j gate is essential while the slow V_j gate is negligible.

Mixed Channels

Most cardiomyocytes coexpress more than one connexin type (see Chapter 29). The presence of multiple connexins within the same channel opens the possibility of a wide range of mixed channels. Although homomeric-heterotypic gap junction channels have been studied extensively, little is known about heteromeric-homotypic and heteromeric-heterotypic channels.

Homomeric-Heterotypic Channels

It has been shown that Cx40, Cx43, and Cx45 hemichannels establish functional homomeric-heterotypic gap junction channels with each other[9,15,19,20] (see also the 2007 article by Rackauskas and colleagues[36] for Cx40-Cx43 channels). Recently, it was reported that Cx30.2 also forms channels with Cx40, Cx43, and Cx45.[4,37]

Figure 14-4A to C illustrates the behavior of the homomeric-heterotypic gap junction channels Cx40-Cx43, Cx40-Cx45, and Cx43-Cx45, respectively. The upper panels show I_j records induced by different V_j pulses. For each cell pair, the size and time course of I_j were sensitive to the size and polarity of V_j. In the case of Cx40-Cx43, I_j was larger and showed a more prominent inactivation when cell Cx43 was negative inside (upward signals). In the case of Cx40-Cx45, I_j was smaller and inactivated when cell Cx40 was positive inside (upward signals) and activated when it was negative inside (downward signals). In the case of Cx43-Cx45, I_j was smaller and inactivated when cell Cx45 was negative inside (downward signals).

The lower panels show the analysis of the I_j records plotting the normalized $g_{j,inst}$ (*blue circles*) and $g_{j,ss}$ (*green circles*) as a function of V_j. For each type of cell pair, both relationships were asymmetrical. In the case of Cx40-Cx43, $g_{j,inst}$ increased transiently with negative V_j and decreased gradually with positive V_j, reflecting the V_j sensitivity of $\gamma_{j,main}$. By contrast, $g_{j,ss}$ decreased prominently with negative V_j and moderately with positive V_j. The former followed a sigmoidal curve and hence represents V_j gating; the latter followed $g_{j,inst} = f(V_j)$ and hence resembles the behavior of $\gamma_{j,main}$. This suggests that Cx40 is gating with positive and Cx43 with negative polarity. In the case of Cx40-Cx45, $g_{j,inst}$ decreases moderately with negative V_j and slightly with positive V_j. Again, this is attributable to the properties of $\gamma_{j,main}$. Of note, however, $g_{j,ss}$ prominently increases with negative V_j and decreases with positive V_j. The former increases beyond $g_{j,inst}$, indicating reopening of channels previously closed; the latter follows a sigmoidal curve and hence reflects V_j gating. This suggests that Cx40 is gating with positive and Cx45 with negative polarity. In the case of Cx43-Cx45, $g_{j,inst}$ decreases moderately with negative V_j and barely with positive V_j, mirroring the behavior of $\gamma_{j,main}$. By contrast, $g_{j,ss}$ decreases prominently with negative V_j and increases transiently with positive V_j. The former follows a sigmoidal curve and thus reflects V_j gating; the latter increases transiently beyond $g_{j,inst}$ and hence corresponds to opening and reclosure of channels. This implies that Cx43 is gating with positive and Cx45 with negative polarity. To rescue this interpretation, it has to be assumed that hemichannel docking affects the gating polarity of Cx43[9] (of note, however, see also the 2007 article by Rackauskas and colleagues[36] for gating polarity of Cx40). The smooth curves represent the best fit of data to the Boltzmann equation. Values for the

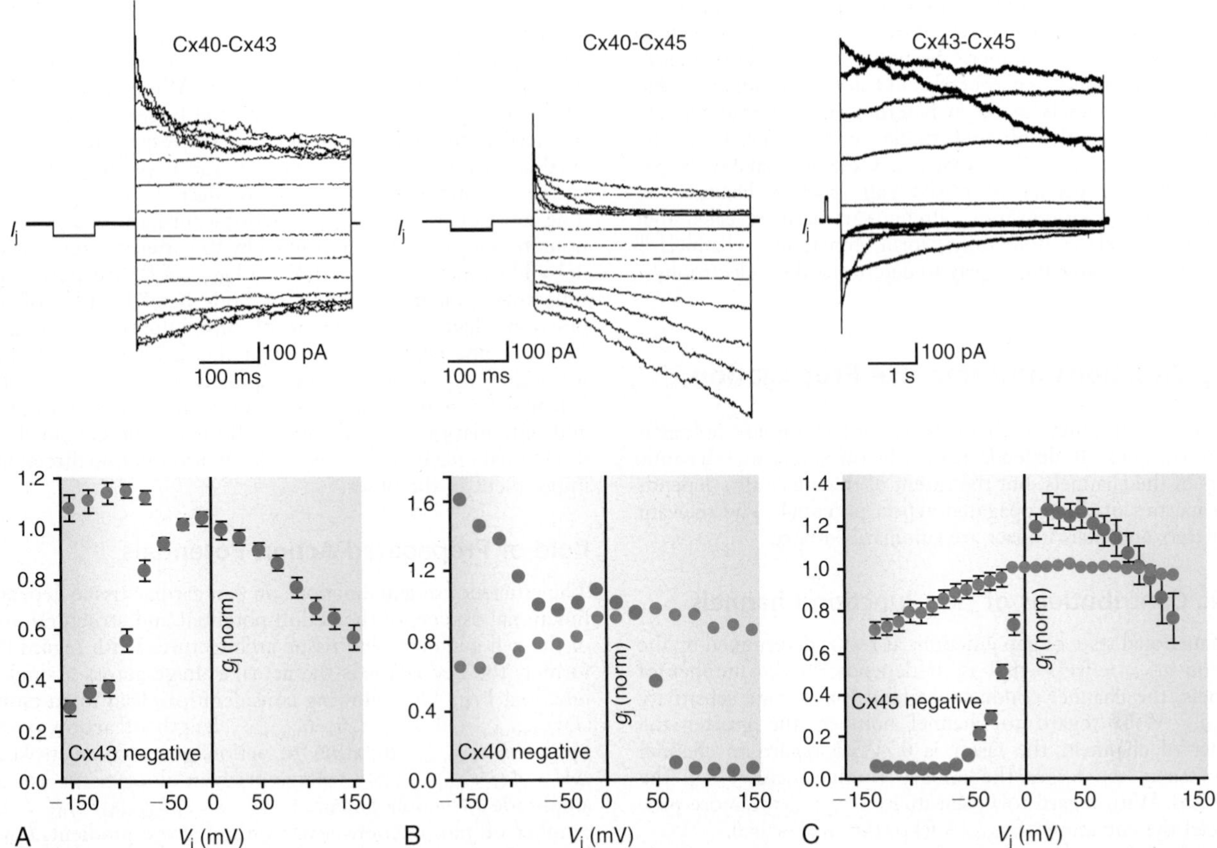

Figure 14-4 Multichannel currents of homomeric-heterotypic channels involving Cx40, Cx43, and Cx45. Dependence of gap junction conductance, g_j, on junctional voltage, V_j, for Cx40-Cx43 (**A**), Cx40-Cx45 (**B**), and Cx43-Cx45 (**C**) channels. *Upper panels*: Family of gap junction currents, I_j, elicited by a standard pulse protocol. *Lower panels*: Plots of normalized instantaneous (*blue circles*) and steady-state (*green circles*) conductance. (**A** and **B**, From Valiunas V, Weingart R, Brink PR: Formation of heterotypic gap junction channels by connexins 40 and 43. Circ Res 86:e42-e49, 2000; **C**, from Desplantez T, Halliday D, Dupont E, Weingart R: Cardiac connexins Cx43 and Cx45: Formation of diverse gap junction channels with diverse electrical properties. Pflügers Arch 448:363-375, 2004., with permission.)

Boltzmann parameters are given in Table 14-1. By and large, they are between those of the respective homomeric-homotypic gap junction channels.

The complexity of I_j records hampers a quantitative kinetic analysis. In the case of Cx40-Cx43, however, I_j records and $g_{j,ss} = f(V_j)$ indicate that channel gating occurs almost exclusively at negative V_j, giving rise to a rapid I_j inactivation. This suggests *superimposed* gating: Both gates of a channel respond quasi-simultaneously. In the case of Cx40-Cx45, I_j records and $g_{j,ss} = f(V_j)$ indicate that channel gating occurs at negative *and* positive V_j, reflecting rapid inactivation and slow recovery from inactivation, respectively. This suggests *sequential* gating: One gate of a channel is responding after the other. In the case of Cx43-Cx45, I_j records and $g_{j,ss} = f(V_j)$ indicate that channel gating occurs mainly at negative but also at positive V_j, leading to rapid inactivation and slow recovery from inactivation, respectively. This suggests *partial overlap* of superimposed and sequential gating.

Data on single channels are scarce (see Table 14-1). Cx40-Cx43 has been most extensively studied.[15,19,25,36] Unitary currents are larger when cell Cx43 is negative inside and smaller when it is positive—that is, $\gamma_{j,main}$ is 100/60 pS at $V_j = \pm 70$ mV. In the latter case, residuals are virtually absent. The channels exhibit a strong dependence on V_j polarity but a weak dependence on V_j amplitude. These properties are consistent with the behavior of Cx40-Cx43 at the multichannel level. In the case of Cx40-Cx45, the only measurement available is a $\gamma_{j,main}$ of 30 to 40 pS (V. Valiunas, personal communication, 2000). In the case of Cx43-Cx45, the situation is similar. These channels have a $\gamma_{j,main}$ of 40 pS and a $\gamma_{j,residual}$ of 11 pS (Desplantez et al., in preparation).

In conclusion, $g_{j,inst} = f(V_j)$ and $g_{j,ss} = f(V_j)$ are asymmetrical for Cx40-Cx43, Cx40-Cx45, and Cx43-Cx45. This means that during propagated action potentials, gap junction channels can affect θ. Depending on the extent and direction of the asymmetry of $g_{j,inst} = f(V_j)$ and $g_{j,ss} = f(V_j)$, θ is weakly or moderately facilitated or impaired. Specifically, impulse propagation Cx45 → Cx40 is facilitated (sinoatrial node → atrial muscle) and Cx40 → Cx45 is impaired (atrial muscle → atrioventricular node); Cx45 → Cx43 is facilitated (sinoatrial node → atrial muscle) and Cx43 → Cx45 is impaired (atrial muscle → atrioventricular node); and Cx40 → Cx43 is facilitated (Purkinje fiber → ventricular muscle).

Heteromeric-Homotypic and Heteromeric-Heterotypic Channels

Although biochemical studies suggest that heteromeric-homotypic and heteromeric-heterotypic channels exist,[38,39] thus far only indirect functional evidence has been obtained. Hints at their existence emerged from experiments on transfected cells coexpressing two types of connexins: Cx40/Cx43[15,38] or Cx43/Cx45.[9,20,39] Pairing of Cx40/Cx43 cells with themselves or with Cx40 or Cx43 cells and pairing of Cx43/Cx45 cells with themselves or with Cx43 or Cx45 yielded a broad spectrum of functional behavior. Some relationships, $g_{j,inst} = f(V_j)$ and $g_{j,ss} = f(V_j)$, and unitary conductances observed could be ascribed to combinations of homomeric-homotypic and homomeric-heterotypic channels, but others could not. This suggests that gap junction channels made of heteromeric hemichannels are operational. Recently initiated studies with connexin-tandem constructs made of Cx40, Cx43, and Cx45 will enable assessment of the properties of mixed gap junction channels of known connexin composition. Preliminary tests revealed that all hemichannel combinations form functional channels.[40] Experiments are now under way to determine their electrophysiologic properties.

Gap Junctions and Impulse Propagation

The role of gap junction channels on cardiac impulse propagation is complex. It depends primarily on static and dynamic factors of the channels, but the extent of the effect also depends on properties of the propagated action potential. The relevant parameters and their impact are summarized next.

Static Contributions of Gap Junction Channels

The functional state of gap junctions at rest is determined by the function $g_{j,inst} = f(V_j)$—that is, it depends on the number of channels, the channel conductance, and the voltage sensitivity of $g_{j,inst}$. With regard to channel number, the greater the number of channels, the faster is θ. With regard to channel conductance, the larger the unitary conductance, $\gamma_{j,main}$, the faster is θ. With regard to V_j sensitivity of $g_{j,inst}$, the more pronounced the curvature of $g_{j,inst} = f(V_j)$, the smaller is θ.

Dynamic Contributions of Gap Junction Channels

V_j gating of gap junction channels introduces a variable source of gap junction modulation. Hence, the functional state of gap junctions during propagated action potentials is determined not only by static parameters but also by dynamic parameters arising from the transition between the functions $g_{j,inst} = f(V_j)$ and $g_{j,ss} = f(V_j)$—that is, it depends on the voltage sensitivity of $g_{j,ss}$ and the kinetics of its inactivation. With respect to V_j sensitivity of $g_{j,ss}$, the smaller $V_{j,0}$ and the larger z, the more pronounced is the impairment on θ. With respect to kinetics, the smaller τ_i, the more pronounced is the impairment on θ. The situation is more complex for homomeric-heterotypic channels. The functional state of gap junctions during propagated action potentials is now also determined by the orientation of the channels. The functions $g_{j,inst} = f(V_j)$ and $g_{j,ss} = f(V_j)$ are asymmetrical, reflecting concurrent gating of both hemichannels of a gap junction channel as a result of superimposed V_j sensitivity. Hence, some channels may be in the residual state at $V_j = 0$ mV—that is, channel reopening occurs at one V_j polarity. Likewise, V_j gating may occur preferentially at one V_j polarity and only marginally at the other. Both situations contribute to directional effects on θ—that is, facilitation in one direction and impairment in the other.

Role of Propagated Action Potentials

The efficiency of gap junctions on θ in cardiac tissue depends on functional aspects of the action potential and structural aspects of the cell geometry and tissue architecture. With regard to the former, the key factor is the actual voltage across a single gap junction, V_{GJ}. The following considerations lead to an estimate: (1) $l_{upstroke} = \theta \times t_{upstroke}$ ($l_{upstroke}$, length of action potential upstroke; $t_{upstroke}$, duration of action potential upstroke); (2) $\Delta V = A_{AP}/l_{upstroke}$ (ΔV, voltage gradient along tissue axis; A_{AP}, amplitude of action potential); (3) $n = [(l_{upstroke}/l_{cell}) - 1]$ (n, number of gap junctions sensing the voltage gradient; l_{cell}, cell length); and (4) $V_{GJ} = \Delta V/n$. Under physiologic conditions, calculated values of V_{GJ} range from approximately 1.5 mV (for sinoatrial and atrioventricular nodes) to approximately 20 mV (for auricular and ventricular muscle).[41] At pathophysiologic conditions leading to slow impulse propagation, the effect will be substantially larger.

References

1. Kléber AG, Rudy Y: Basic mechanisms of cardiac impulse propagation and associated arrhythmias. Physiol Rev 84:431-488, 2004.
2. Severs NJ, Coppen SR, Dupont E, et al: Gap junction alterations in human cardiac disease. Cardiovasc Res 62:368-377, 2004.
3. White TW, Srinivas M, Ripps H, et al: Virtual cloning, functional expression, and gating analysis of human connexin31.9. Am J Physiol Cell Physiol 283:C960-C970, 2002.
4. Kreuzberg MM, Söhl G, Kim J-S, et al: Functional properties of mouse connexin30.2 expressed in the conduction system of the heart. Circ Res 96:1169-1177, 2005.
5. Bukauskas FF, Elfgang, Willecke K, Weingart R: Biophysical properties of gap junction channels formed by mouse connexin40 in induced pairs of transfected human HeLa cells. Biophys J 68:2289-2298, 1995.
6. Spray DC, Harris AL, Bennett MVL: Equilibrium properties of a voltage-dependent junctional conductance. J Gen Physiol 77:77-93, 1981.
7. Harris AL: Emerging issues of connexin channels: Biophysics fills the gap. Quart Rev Biophys 34:325-472, 2001.
8. Van Rijen HVM, Wilders R, Van Ginneken ACG, Jongsma HJ: Quantitative analysis of dual whole-cell voltage-clamp determination of gap junction conductance. Pflügers Arch 436:141-151, 1998.
9. Desplantez T, Halliday D, Dupont E, Weingart R: Cardiac connexins Cx43 and Cx45: Formation of diverse gap junction channels with diverse electrical properties. Pflügers Arch 448:363-375, 2004.
10. Vogel R, Weingart R: Mathematical model of vertebrate gap junctions derived from electrical measurements on homotypic and heterotypic channels. J Physiol 510: 177-189, 1998.
11. Vogel R, Weingart R: The electrophysiology of gap junctions and gap junction channels and their mathematical modeling. Biol Cell 94:501-510, 2002.
12. Harris AL, Spray DC, Bennett MVL: Kinetic properties of a voltage-dependent junctional conductance. J Gen Physiol 77:95-117, 1981.
13. Beblo DA, Wang HZ, Beyer EC, et al: Unique conductance, gating, and selective permeability properties of gap junction channels formed by connexin40. Circ Res 77:813-822, 1995.
14. Anumonwo JMB, Taffet SM, Gu H, et al: The carboxyl terminal domain regulates the unitary conductance and voltage dependence of connexin40 gap junction channels. Circ Res 88:666-673, 2001.
15. Cottrell GT, Wu Y, Burt JM: Cx40 and Cx43 expression ratio influences heteromeric/heterotypic gap junction channel properties. Am J Physiol Cell Physiol 282:C1469-C1482, 2002.
16. Wang HZ, Li J, Lemanski LF, Veenstra RD: Gating of mammalian cardiac gap junction channels by transjunctional voltage. Biophys J 63:139-151, 1992.
17. Banach K, Weingart R: Connexin43 gap junctions exhibit asymmetrical gating properties. Pflügers Arch 431:775-785, 1996.
18. He DS, Jiang JX, Taffet SM, Burt JM: Formation of heteromeric gap junction channels by connexins 40 and 43 in vascular smooth muscle cells. Proc Natl Acad Sci U S A. 96:6495-6500, 1999.
19. Valiunas V, Weingart R, Brink PR: Formation of heterotypic gap junction channels by connexins 40 and 43. Circ Res 86:e42-e49, 2000.
20. Elenes S, Martinez AD, Delmar M, et al: Heterotypic docking of Cx43 and Cx45

connexons blocks fast voltage gating of Cx43. Biophys J 81:1406-1418, 2001.
21. Moreno AP, Laing JG, Beyer EC, Spray DC: Properties of gap junction channels formed of connexin 45 endogenously expressed in human hepatoma (SKHep1) cells. Am J Physiol Cell Physiol 268:C356-C365, 1995.
22. Barrio LC, Capel J, Jarillo JA, et al: Species-specific voltage-gating properties of connexin-45 junctions expressed in Xenopus oocytes. Biophys J 73:757-769, 1997.
23. Valiunas V, Bukauskas FF, Weingart R: Conductance and selective permeability of connexin43 gap junction channels examined in neonatal rat heart cells. Circ Res 80:708-719, 1997.
24. Vogel R, Valiunas V, Weingart R: Subconductance states of Cx30 gap junction channels: Data from transfected HeLa cells versus data from a mathematical model. Biophys J 91:2337-2348, 2006.
25. Cottrell GT, Burt JM: Heterotypic gap junction channel formation between heteromeric and homotypic Cx40 and Cx43 connexons. Am J Physiol Cell Physiol 281:C1559-C1567, 2001.
26. Moreno AP, Sáez JC, Fishman GI, Spray DC: Human connexin43 gap junction channels. Regulation of unitary conductances by phosphorylation. Circ Res 74:1050-1075, 1994.
27. Moreno AP, Chanson M, Anumonwo J, et al: Role of carboxyl tail of connexin43 in transjunctional fast voltage gating. Circ Res 90:450-457, 2002.
28. Bukauskas FF, Bukauskiene A, Verselis VK, Bennett MVL: Coupling asymmetry of heterotypic connexin 45/connexin 43-EGFP gap junctions: Properties of fast and slow gating mechanisms. Proc Natl Acad Sci U S A 99:7113-7118, 2002.
29. Sakai R, Elfgang C, Vogel R, et al: The electrical behaviour of rat connexin46 gap junction channels expressed in transfected Hela cells. Pflügers Arch 446:714-727, 2003.
30. Valiunas V, Manthey D, Vogel R, et al: Biophysical properties of mouse connexin30 gap junction channels studied in transfected human HeLa cells. J Physiol 519:631-644, 1999.
31. Valiunas V: Biophysical properties of connexin-45 gap junction hemichannels studied in vertebrate cells. J Gen Physiol 119:119-147, 2002.
32. Bukauskas FF, Verselis VK: Gap junction channel gating. Biochim Biophys Acta 1662:42-60, 2004.
33. Banach K, Weingart R: Connexin43 gap junction channels exhibit fast and slow current transitions. Pflügers Arch 439: 248-250, 2000.
34. Weingart R, Bukauskas FF: Long-chain n-alkanols and arachidonic acid interfere with the V_m-gating mechanism of gap junction channels. Pflügers Arch 510:177-189, 1997.
35. Bukauskas FF, Bukauskiene A, Bennett MVL, Verselis VK: Gating properties of gap junction channels assembled from connexin43 and connexin43 fused with green fluorescent protein. Biophys J 81:137-152, 2001.
36. Rackauskas M, Kreuzberg MM, Pranevicius M, et al: Gating properties of heterotypic gap junction channels formed of connexins 40, 43 and 45. Biophys J 92:1952-1965, 2007.
37. Rackauskas M, Verselis VK, Bukauskas FF: The permeability of homotypic and heterotypic gap junction channels formed of cardiac connexins, mCx30.2, Cx40, Cx43 and Cx45. Am J Physiol Heart Circ Physiol 293:H1729-H1736, 2007.
38. Valiunas V, Gemel J, Brink PR, Beyer EC: Gap junction channels formed by coexpressed connexin40 and connexin43. Am J Physiol Heart and Circ 281:H1675-H1689, 2001.
39. Martinez AD, Hayrapetyan V, Moreno AP, Beyer EC: Connexin43 and connexin45 form heteromeric gap junction channels in which individual components determine permeability and regulation. Circ Res 90:1100-1107, 2002.
40. Desplantez T, Dupont E, Thomas N, et al: Tandem constructs of Cx40, Cx43 and Cx45 to probe properties of heteromeric channels of known composition. Paper presented at the 2005 International Gap Junction Conference, Whistler, BC, Canada, Aug 13-18, 2005.
41. Desplantez T, Dupont E, Severs NJ, Weingart R: Gap junction channels and cardiac impulse propagation. J Membr Biol 218:13-28, 2007.

Intermolecular Interactions and Pharmacology of Cardiac Ion Channels

PART III

Developmental Regulation of Cardiac Ion Channels

15

MICHAEL ARTMAN AND WILLIAM A. COETZEE

CHAPTER OUTLINE

Perinatal development brings about many important biologic changes, including alterations in cardiovascular structure and function. In addition to the increasingly well-characterized morphologic changes in molecular embryology,[1] the immature heart also has tremendous plasticity and capacity for remodeling in the mechanisms and regulation of excitability, contraction, relaxation, and conduction. This chapter summarizes the experimental studies describing these differences. The reader is referred to various reviews[2-6] on this subject to supplement the chapter content. The term *developmental* often is used loosely in the literature, which leads to discrepancies in data reporting and interpretation. In the following discussion, the focus is on the perinatal period of cardiac development.

Changes in Cellular Morphology and Ultrastructure

In addition to the functional alterations, changes also occur at the cellular and ultrastructural levels. Neonatal cardiac cells are smaller in size and diameter than adult myocytes and contain fewer contractile myofilaments.[7,8] Although these differences can partly explain the diminished contractile performance of the immature myocardium, many other functional changes have to be taken into consideration (as described later on). Another significant difference is that the transverse tubule (T tubule) network, which is responsible for propagating electrical impulses deep into the myocyte, is poorly developed in the immature cardiac myocyte. From this perspective, the immature ventricular myocyte resembles myocytes from adult atria or cells from the conduction system (or cells from the nonmammalian heart), in which a T tubule system also is largely lacking. The mitochondrial content of the immature myocyte also is less,[7] which is interesting in view of the enhanced mitochondrial Ca^{2+} uptake in immature heart.[9] The lower mitochondrial volume also is consistent with the finding that during gestation, glycolysis and lactate oxidation constitute the major sources of adenosine triphosphate (ATP) for the fetal heart and with the rapid shift that occurs around birth from carbohydrate to fatty acid utilization. Other subcellular differences include a less well-developed sarcoplasmic reticular network and a larger surface area–to–volume ratio.[8]

The Action Potential, "Resting" Membrane Potential, and Intracellular Ion Activities

Results from a mosaic of experimental studies, each designed to investigate an individual ionic current system or specific ion channel, have provided clear evidence that the immature heart differs significantly from the adult heart in the ionic nature of pacemaker activity and in mechanisms of Ca^{2+} influx as a trigger for contractility.

The "Resting" Membrane Potential

Virtually all cells, even nonexcitable cells, have negative resting membrane potentials, crucial for regulating complex physiologic processes such as secretion, impulse propagation, and contraction. In most cells, this negative potential is caused predominantly by a large K^+ permeability of the membrane relative to other ions, which in cardiac myocytes (as is the case for many other cell types) is caused by inward rectifying "background" potassium channels (denoted I_{K1}). Cardiac myocytes isolated from fetuses and neonates have a less negative maximum diastolic (or "resting") potential than that for myocytes from the adult.[10] It is before birth, however, that the largest changes in membrane potential and K^+ conductance seem to occur. For example, the largest change in membrane potential occurs between fetal days 12 and 18 in fetal rat ventricle (−55 mV to −80 mV).[11] This increasing resting potential during fetal cardiac development must have important functional electrophysiologic consequences in the developing embryonic, fetal, and neonatal heart, such as during the generation of spontaneous beating of the heart in the presence of an underdeveloped conduction system.

Action Potential Duration

In addition to the more depolarized resting membrane potential, the immature heart often displays a longer action potential duration (APD) than that characteristic of adult myocardium. Age-dependent increases in the APD have been noted in heart muscle cells from cat,[12] mouse,[13] rat,[14] rabbit,[15] and human.[16]

Membrane Currents Responsible for the Cardiac Action Potential

Many different ionic currents are responsible for orchestrating the heart beat. Among others, these include the inward rectifying potassium current that is responsible for setting a negative membrane potential, the sodium current that is responsible for the initial upstroke of the cardiac action potential, the rapidly inactivating transient outward potassium current (I_{to}) that causes an early repolarization of the action potential, the L-type calcium current responsible for Ca^{2+} influx during the action potential, the T-type calcium current that may be involved in pacemaker activity, and the bidirectional Na^+-Ca^{2+} exchanger.

A very large diversity of the molecular components of ion channels has been recognized—many of these give rise to ion channels with similar (yet subtly different) features. Furthermore, association of ion channel subunits with accessory subunits often leads to altered expression levels, function, regulation, and pharmacologic properties of these channels. Despite the relatively large body of data describing changes in the activity of specific ion channels during development (see later), much less is known regarding the expression of molecular components of these ion channel subunits, which is even more diverse than the limited number of functional ion channel systems described in the heart.[17] An understanding of the nature of the ion channel transcriptome in the heart, and of how it changes during development, is essential for a realistic approach to important clinical issues related to neonatal cardiology, such as congenital abnormalities, cardiomyopathies, heart failure, arrhythmias, and cardiac drug therapy.

Potassium Channels

Inwardly Rectifying Potassium Channels

Inwardly rectifying potassium channels are critically important for heart function by setting the maximum diastolic potential, which in turn helps to determine the upstroke velocity of the action potential and hence the conduction velocity. Furthermore, they carry a small but significant outward current during late stages of the action potential, thereby contributing significantly to final repolarization. Under experimental conditions, comparatively less outward potassium current is passed than current in the inward direction, a property termed *inward rectification*. Several types of inwardly rectifying potassium currents have been identified in cardiac tissue.

The Cardiac Inward Rectifier: I_{K1}

The maximum diastolic potential becomes progressively more negative before birth (see earlier) and the difference between membrane resting potential and the calculated K^+ equilibrium potential decreases with embryonic development. This is due partly to an increase in the membrane K^+ permeability (e.g., the permeability ratio of Na^+ to K^+ more than doubles from day 4 to day 18 in the embryonic chick heart).[18] Voltage clamp studies have shown that the whole-cell I_{K1} density, which is the primary current responsible for the negative resting potential of adult myocytes, is low in the fetus, and that it increases during pre- and postnatal development.[5,19]

Members of the Kir2 subfamily (particularly Kir2.1, Kir2.3, and Kir2.4) generally are thought to be molecular candidates of I_{K1} channels, owing to their strong rectification properties and pronounced Ba^{2+} block when expressed in heterologous expression systems.[17] Using RNAse protection assays and competitive reverse transcriptase–polymerase chain reaction (RT-PCR) methods, we reported strong upregulation of Kir2.1 messenger RNA (mRNA) levels with perinatal development in the mouse heart.[20] In a more recent ion channel mRNA profiling study, one of us [WAC] also found upregulation of Kir2.1 mRNA levels. Curiously, however, Kir2.1 expression levels *decreased* after birth before increasing again in the adult. Because the membrane potential and I_{K1} density do not follow this pattern (see earlier), other subunits may contribute to the I_{K1} during early development. This contention is supported by the observation that mouse cardiac myocytes from Kir2.1$^{-/-}$ mice have a fairly negative maximum diastolic membrane potential.[21] It is possible that this redundancy may be fulfilled by other Kir members (such as the Kir4 subfamily) or two-pore potassium channels, which demonstrate interesting developmental changes. Future experiments should be directed at determining the rôles of these subunits in generating membrane potential during early development.

G Protein–Activated Potassium Channels

Binding of acetylcholine (ACh) to M2 muscarinic receptors opens G protein–activated I_{KACh} channels, which are responsible for the negative chronotropic and inotropic cardiac effects on vagal stimulation. On agonist binding, βγ subunits dissociate, which directly activates the channel.[22] Functional data suggest that this signaling axis is not well represented in the developing heart. For example, ACh has little effect on the resting membrane potential and APD of immature chick embryonic ventricle.[10] In isolated membrane patches of neonatal rat ventricular myocytes, ACh readily activates I_{KACh} channels.[19] In ventricular myocytes, the current density (number of channels per unitary area of membrane) of whole-cell currents induced by ACh was reported not to be different in 1- to 5-day neonatal hearts and in adult rat hearts.[19] By contrast, marked upregulation of I_{KACh} occurs in developing atrial myocytes, which persists after birth.[23] These data would therefore suggest that incomplete vagal innervation may only be partly responsible for the underdeveloped response to this neurotransmitter, and that channel expression levels also should be considered.

In the heart, I_{KACh} channels are thought to consist of heteromeric Kir3.1 and Kir3.4 subunits,[17] although expression of homomeric Kir3 channels may occur. An interesting report demonstrated that the molecular composition of the G protein–activated I_{KACh} channel may be dynamically regulated during development.[24] It was reported that fetal I_{KACh} channels may be formed by Kir3.1 subunits and that upregulation of Kir3.4 subunits (which also was observed by one of us [WAC][25]) may account for the adult phenotype of the channel. The potential functional consequences of this finding are interesting to consider. Channels composed of Kir3.1 are strong rectifiers and as a consequence do not produce much outward repolarizing current on depolarizations (during the action potential plateau). Therefore, even when activated by ACh, these channels will not contribute as much as the Kir3.4-containing I_{KACh} channels (which rectify weakly) to action potential shorting. This is a fine example of how these molecular studies may provide interesting insights into the previously observed insensitivity of developing cardiac myocytes to exogenously applied ACh.

K_{ATP} Channels

The ATP-sensitive potassium (K_{ATP}) channels in cardiac tissue open mainly under pathophysiologic or stress conditions and protect against ischemia-induced damage. Their opening is promoted by (among other factors) an increase in the cytosolic adenosine diphosphate (ADP)-ATP ratio,[26] as occurs during ischemia or hypoxia. A role for K_{ATP} channels in exercise-induced stress also has been identified.[27] Activation of these channels contributes significantly to action potential shortening during hypoxia. A strong age-dependence in the sensitivity of the action potential to hypoxia has been recognized. For example, whereas hypoxia shortened the action potential duration in 15-day chick hearts, no effect of hypoxia was observed on the APD in 3-day-old hearts.[28] In the 3-day-old hearts, APD shortening could be elicited only by the combination of hypoxia and glucose deprivation.[28] These effects may partly be explained by the dependency of the developing heart on anaerobic glycolysis, instead of oxidative phosphorylation, as well as the known tolerance of the developing heart to ischemia and hypoxia.[29] The well-described changes in the levels of K_{ATP} channel expression (and perhaps even their molecular composition), however, also must be taken into consideration. For example, in a study on developing rat heart, we reported that K_{ATP} channel activity can be recorded only after fetal day 12 (no detectable K_{ATP} channel was observed at earlier ages), after which the K_{ATP} current density dramatically increases with age throughout fetal development and after birth. No further increases are observed after day 20 after birth.[19] A similar developmental increase in K_{ATP} channel current density was reported to occur in the chick[30] and rabbit.[31] Of interest, in the latter study, the unitary conductance of K_{ATP} channels was reported also to be smaller in fetal hearts. In the mouse fetus, K_{ATP} channel were recorded as early as day 11, and the K_{ATP} channel current density was reported to be remarkably high (compared with other channels) and to exhibit strong upregulation with developmental age.[32]

Subunits of the K_{ATP} channel include the pore-forming Kir6.1 or Kir6.2 subunits that heteromultimerize with regulatory sulfonylurea receptor-1 (SUR1) and -2 (SUR2) subunits.[17] Expression of each of these subunits in the heart has been documented, with clear upregulation of these subunits during development.[25,33] It remains to be seen to what extent the developmental expression of these subunits correlates with the developmental changes in the biophysical properties of K_{ATP} channels,[31] or with other possible differences. The homeobox transcription factor Tinman plays an important role in the initiation of heart development. Of interest, the SUR homologue (dSUR) in the fruitfly *Drosophila* is a target of Tinman.[34] Defining the transcription factors and regulatory elements that determine ion channel expression during development is obviously important in order to elucidate the nature of the developmental genetic program, but no similar studies have been performed in mammals to date.

Repolarizing (Voltage-Activated) Potassium Currents

Transient Outward Potassium Current, I_{to}

The cardiac action potential repolarizes in part owing to the voltage-dependent activation of outward potassium currents. Developmentally, a progressive increase occurs in the amplitudes of these repolarizing potassium currents, and a strong correlation exists between the developmental upregulation of repolarizing potassium currents and action potential shortening.[14] Under voltage-clamp conditions, these repolarizing currents either are transient (i.e., they exhibit rapid spontaneous inactivation during a sustained depolarization) or are of the type referred to as delayed rectifiers (i.e., with little or no inactivation). Two distinct transient outward potassium currents, $I_{to,f}$ and $I_{to,s}$ (fast and slow, respectively), are known.

High concentrations of 4-aminopyridine (4-AP) (approximately 2 mM), which blocks $I_{to,f}$ and I_{Kur}, have a more pronounced effect on the APD in rat cardiac myocytes at 10 days than at 1 day, suggesting a progressive contribution of these currents to the repolarization process during development.[14] The effect of 4-AP on the action potential also has been reported to be less pronounced in developing mouse cardiac myocytes.[35] In keeping with this finding, strong upregulation of I_{to} density occurs during perinatal development, which continues after birth (with a four-fold change in the first 10 days after birth), and the increase continues until the adult stage.[14,35] It should be noted that the I_{to} is less prominent in the ventricles of larger animals, and the high I_{to} density in rodent hearts may be an evolutionary adaptation to their high heart rates and the requirement for a short action potential. In mouse ventricular cells, the rate of I_{to} inactivation was reported to be significantly slower with increasing developmental age.[35] Additionally, developmental changes occur in the time course of recovery from inactivation and the voltage dependence of the steady-state inactivation characteristics.[14,35] These changes in I_{to} density, kinetics, and other biophysical properties may largely account for their role in action potential shortening during perinatal development.

In general, gene expression of repolarizing potassium channels is significantly greater in the mature heart than in the immature heart.[36] Molecularly, $I_{to,f}$ channels are thought to be composed of members of the Kv4 subfamily (mainly Kv4.2 and Kv4.3) of potassium channel subunits.[17] The accessory subunit KChIP2 is thought to be mandatory for surface expression and function of the channel, but subunits such as MIRP1 also may regulate the I_{to} channel.[37] In rat ventricle, $I_{to,f}$ is not present in early embryonic (E12) hearts, and appearance after birth (day 10) is, of interest, not correlated with an increase in Kv4.2 and Kv4.3 mRNA but rather is associated with a huge upregulation of KChIP2 mRNA levels.[38] Furthermore, because exogenously expressed KChIP2 subunits were shown in the latter study to similarly increase $I_{to,f}$ amplitudes in embryonic myocytes, the possibility is raised that KChIP2 expression regulates the appearance of $I_{to,f}$ channels during development.

Studies regarding the developmental changes of $I_{to,f}$ in human heart are conflicting. In an early study, a lack of $I_{to,f}$ was reported in atrial myocytes isolated from children between 2 months and 5 years of age,[39] which is consistent with the reported developmental increase in $I_{to,f}$ density from neonatal (1 day to 10 months) to adult.[40] Other studies, however, reported no developmental changes in human atrial $I_{to,f}$ between ages 4 days to 14 years[41] or even the possibility that the atrial $I_{to,f}$ may be larger in the neonate (3 to 10 months of age) than in the adult.[42] It remains to be seen to what extent the various clinical conditions or medications contributed to these reported inconsistencies.

Delayed Rectifier Potassium Currents

I_{to} is not strongly expressed in the ventricles of larger animals, such as rabbits. Because APD shortening also occurs after birth in these larger animals (see earlier), other changes in potassium currents may contribute. For example, the developmental increase of I_{K1} (see earlier) partially accounts for the APD prolongation with development.[14] Several distinct delayed rectifier potassium currents in mammalian ventricle are recognized to contribute to repolarization. In an early study, these delayed rectifiers (collectively termed I_K) were described to increase in amplitude with age. When corrected for the progressively increasing cell size with development, however, the I_K density increased only up to 15 days postnatally, after which the current density declined.[43] At least three separate noninactivating delayed rectifier potassium currents—I_{Kr}, I_{Ks}, and I_{Kur}—are now known to exist, with distinct pharmacologic profiles.

The sensitivity of the cardiac action potential to dofetilide, which selectively blocks I_{Kr}, was examined in developing mouse heart.[44] The drug caused significant action potential prolongation in fetal and neonatal cardiac myocytes but had little effect on adult action potentials. In parallel, [^{3}H]dofetilide binding was high in immature heart isolates but was not detected in adult mouse heart. Finally, patch clamp recordings directly demonstrated I_{Kr} to be downregulated in mouse cardiac myocytes after birth. In a separate study, it was found that electrocardiogram (ECG) changes (ST segment elevation and prolongation of QT and QTc intervals) that occur at approximately 1 day after birth were abolished by dofetilide,[45] which again is strongly supportive of an important functional role for I_{Kr} at this early developmental period. This is a clinically relevant finding in view of the embryotoxic effects of class III antiarrhythmic drugs that block I_{Kr}.

Other delayed rectifier potassium currents contribute to repolarization, including I_{Ks} and I_{Kur}. In mouse ventricle, indapamide (which blocks I_{Ks}) had no effect on action potentials at any age (fetal to adult), suggesting that this repolarizing current is functionally insignificant in the mouse ventricle at all developmental stages.[44] By contrast, I_{Kur} (which is blocked by low concentrations of 4-AP) is robustly expressed in immature (3 postnatal days) cardiac myocytes, after which the current density decreases until it cannot be detected in adult mouse ventricle.[46] Of interest, these delayed rectifier currents are not downregulated in the mouse atrium (by contrast, developmental upregulation is reported[47]), which raises the possibility that chamber-specific regulation of channel expression occurs during development.

Molecularly, the delayed rectifier potassium channels are not extensively characterized but may be due to channels assembled by Kv1.5, Kv1.2, Kv2.1, erg, or KvLQT subunits.[17,48,49] In the rat ventricle, Kv1.2, Kv1.5, and Kv2.1 mRNA abundances all are increased postnatally,[43] which is not consistent with the declining densities of delayed rectifier potassium channels (see earlier). In situ hybridization experiments demonstrated the presence of erg mRNA (and also the accessory subunit MiRP1) in embryonic rat heart,[50] but a longitudinal study was not performed to assess how the expression of these subunits may contribute to developmental changes in delayed rectifiers. In a recent study, relatively high mRNA expression levels of Kv1.1, Kv2.1, and Kv1.5 were found in the adult mouse heart.[25] The high Kv1.1 mRNA expression level may point to additional complexity of molecular components of the mouse repolarizing potassium currents. Some of the two-pore potassium channels, such as TASK,[17] also may potentially contribute to a "plateau" repolarizing potassium current. TASK-1 is expressed in early embryonic heart tube, but its expression has been reported to be restricted to the conducting system as the heart matures.[51] Additional studies are needed to characterize the mRNA and protein expression levels of these subunits (as well as accessory subunits such as the potassium channel regulatory protein MinK and MiRPs).

Voltage-Activated Calcium Channels

Voltage-activated calcium channels open in response to membrane depolarization (during an action potential) and contribute to pacemaker activity and the relatively long-lasting ventricular cardiac action potential. In adult myocytes, the resulting Ca^{2+} influx serves as a trigger for graded calcium release from the sarcoplasmic reticulum, thereby regulating contractile strength. Strong evidence, however, suggests that the immature rabbit heart may be less reliant on calcium channel influx as a trigger for sarcoplasmic reticulum calcium release, and that instead, contraction is much more dependent upon transsarcolemmal influx of calcium (by way of Na^+-Ca^{2+} exchange and calcium channels) for direct activation of the contractile elements. Thus, the role and contribution of voltage-activated calcium channels to the action potential and to excitation-contraction coupling change significantly during cardiac maturation.

L-type Calcium Channels

An alphabetical nomenclature has evolved for distinct functional classes of calcium currents recorded in different cell types.[52] L-type calcium currents require a strong depolarization for activation, are long-lasting, and are blocked by specific antagonists, such as dihydropyridines. Developmental changes in the L-type calcium currents ($I_{Ca,L}$) are fairly well documented, but data are not always internally consistent. During the embryonic period, a fairly large increase in the $I_{Ca,L}$ in mouse heart has been observed (a doubling occurs from E11 to E18).[32] After birth, however, changes appear to be modest. In the rat, early reports suggested that the $I_{Ca,L}$ amplitude is larger in isolated myocytes from neonatal (2 to 7 days) rat heart than in those from young adult heart (6 to 8 weeks).[53] Subsequent studies, however, reported that the $I_{Ca,L}$ density increased by approximately 25% from the neonatal (3 to 5 days) to adult rat (see Figure 3 in the paper by Katsube and colleagues[54]) or that the peak $I_{Ca,L}$ density was constant over this age range.[55] In rabbit, some controversy also exists. Although some reports suggested a fairly substantial increase of $I_{Ca,L}$ amplitude density from birth to adult,[56,57] others noted a modest increase of only approximately 30% to 70% over the same developmental period.[58-60] In human atrial myocytes, the $I_{Ca,L}$ density is largely unaltered between ages 3 days to 79 years, suggesting that the channels are already functionally mature at the time of birth.[61]

Even though controversy exists regarding $I_{Ca,L}$ peak density during development, most studies agree that the voltage dependence is largely unchanged. In the rabbit, shifts in the voltage dependence of the steady-state kinetic variables also have been reported,[58] such that the "window" $I_{Ca,L}$ is smaller in the neonate than in the adult. The time constant of inactivation is smaller in atrial cells from pediatric human patients[61] but is not different in rat[62] or rabbit.[59] Of interest, however, the immature $I_{Ca,L}$ generally lacks a response to interventions that act on the sarcoplasmic reticulum. In the adult, a feedback of Ca^{2+} released from the sarcoplasmic reticulum alters the kinetics of $I_{Ca,L}$, such that the released Ca^{2+} contributes to the calcium-dependent inactivation mechanism. Inhibiting sarcoplasmic reticulum function with ryanodine and caffeine, for example, expectedly abolishes contractions in the adult, but it also causes an increase the calcium current amplitude, changes in the inactivation time constant, and a positive shift in the voltage dependence of the steady-state inactivation parameter. In neonatal rat ventricular myocytes, ryanodine or caffeine had no effect on contractions or any of the afore-mentioned parameters.[53] In rabbit ventricular myocytes, the transition to the mature phenotype of coupling between $I_{Ca,L}$ and sarcoplasmic reticulum Ca^{2+} occurs only at 2 to 3 weeks after birth.[59] Thus, even though the immature calcium channel may have pharmacologic and biophysical properties similar to those in the adult, major differences exist in the manner in which the channels couple to the rest of the calcium-homeostatic machinery such as the sarcoplasmic reticulum. These differences may reside in the late developmental onset of T tubule formation, which necessitates a different calcium-homeostatic mechanism in the immature heart (see later on).

Molecularly, cardiac L-type calcium channels are thought to be composed of the pore-forming $Ca_V1.2$ (α_{1C}) subunit and several regulatory components, including β_2, $\alpha_2\delta$, and γ subunits.[63]

Disruption of the Cacna1c ($Ca_V1.2$) gene results in embryonic lethality, with death occurring at 14 days after conception,[64] underscoring the importance of this channel after this developmental age. Consistent with these data, Harrell and colleagues found highest expression levels of $Ca_V1.2$ in mouse heart.[25] An interesting possible isoform switch of $Ca_V1.2$ may occur during embryonic development.[65] Isoform switching from $Ca_V1.3$ to $Ca_V1.2$ during embryonic development also has been reported.[66] Of interest, at E12.5, a functional $I_{Ca,L}$ (that is stimulated by Bay K 8644 and inhibited with low sensitivity by nisoldipine) can be recorded from cardiac myocytes isolated from hearts of $Ca_V1.2$-null mice.[64] This current also is present in $Ca_V1.3$-null mice,[64] and its molecular nature remains to be established; other subunits present in the embryonic heart (such as $Ca_V1.1$[67]) need to be considered. Other Ca_V subunits also may be important for heart function, as suggested by the finding that arrhythmias occur in prenatal hearts after ablation of the $Ca_V2.3$ (α_{1E}) subunit.[68] The low expression level of $Ca_V2.3$ reported by Harrell and colleagues, however,[25] is suggestive of restricted or regional expression patterns (such as the conduction system), or of expression occurring predominantly at earlier developmental time points (e.g., 10 to 12 days after conception, when arrhythmias were observed in the latter study).

T-type Calcium Channels

The rapidly activating calcium current—the T-type calcium current ($I_{Ca,T}$)—is activated at more negative voltages than those observed for $I_{Ca,L}$ and is less sensitive to block by dihydropyridines. Clear evidence exists for the presence of an important role for $I_{Ca,T}$ in the immature heart.[69] First, $I_{Ca,T}$ is more frequently observed in embryonic or neonatal atrial and ventricular myocytes, and it is rarely observed in adult cardiac myocytes.[70,71] Important developmental changes in current density also are seen. For example, in rat atrial myocytes, $I_{Ca,T}$ peak current density was roughly similar to that of $I_{Ca,L}$ at 8 days after birth, after which a steady decline in current density occurred up to adulthood, whereas $I_{Ca,L}$ density was marginally upregulated during the same time period.[72] Clear evidence also points to regional variations in expression patterns during ontogeny. In the latter study, for example, $I_{Ca,L}$ was small relative to $I_{Ca,L}$ in the rat neonatal ventricle (at 8 days of age) and was virtually undetectable in the adult ventricle.[72] Most of the changes appear to occur after birth: A robust $I_{Ca,T}$ can be recorded before birth in rat ventricular myocytes, followed by a progressive and rapid decline after birth until it is virtually undetectable in the 21-day-old neonate.[71] These data suggest that $I_{Ca,T}$ may be associated with development and postnatal growth of cardiac myocytes. Other evidence indicates that in chick heart, $I_{Ca,T}$ can directly contribute to excitation-contraction coupling and Ca^{2+} signaling.[73] The function of $I_{Ca,T}$, however, is best described in the conduction system, where it may contribute to impulse initiation of propagation.[74,75] It is perhaps therefore not surprising that in the rabbit atrioventricular node, the amplitude of $I_{Ca,T}$ remains unchanged during ontogeny, whereas developmental changes in $I_{Ca,L}$ occur.[76]

Channels responsible for the cardiac T-type calcium current are thought to be composed of $Ca_V3.1$ ($\alpha 1_G$) or $Ca_V3.2$ ($\alpha 1_H$) subunits, or both.[77] In a profiling study of cardiac expression of ion channels during mouse perinatal development, Harrell and colleagues saw expression of both of these in mouse heart. Expression was higher in the immature than in the adult heart, suggesting an important role for these channels in electrophysiology of the immature heart.[25] Other studies also reported expression of these subunits in developing heart[69,76] and declining expression after birth.[71] In humans, $Ca_V3.2$ mRNA is expressed in fetal heart, and expression also declines during pregnancy and after birth.[78]

Sodium Channels

Sodium channels contribute significantly to the initiation, rapid repolarization, and rapid propagation of the cardiac action potential. A "window" sodium current also contributes to the APD. As with many other ion channels, sodium channels are subject to developmental changes. This was suggested by early studies in which the maximum upstroke velocity of the action potential (V_{max}) was found to be smaller in isolated Purkinje strands of neonatal (9 days of age) dog hearts than in those of adult animal hearts.[79] In the latter study, the membrane potential also was more depolarized, which may have partially inactivated the sodium current to decrease V_{max}. However, injection of hyperpolarizing currents to normalize the membrane potential relative to that of the adult did not restore V_{max}, suggesting a de facto developmental change in sodium channel density or kinetics. A similar finding has been reported for atrial and ventricular myocytes isolated from developing guinea pigs, with the difference that the I_{Na} changes were reported to occur during the embryonic period rather than during the neonatal period.[80] This finding is not surprising in view of the relative maturity of the guinea pig at birth (67-day gestational period). Under voltage clamp conditions, developmental changes in I_{Na} have been demonstrated directly in chick embryo.[11] The sodium current density and maximal conductance are increased with age, suggesting an increase in channel number. Of interest, the voltages at which inactivation occurs is more positive in the embryo than in the adult, which allows the sodium current to directly contribute to automatic activity in the chick embryo.[11]

The relative contribution of I_{Na} to electrical activity in the immature heart was assessed using tetrodotoxin (TTX), a specific blocker of I_{Na}. Of interest, TTX had remarkable effects. As expected, the V_{max} is substantially reduced,[81] suggesting a direct role for I_{Na} in conduction velocity. However, TTX also caused changes in the APD,[81] which is consistent with the slower inactivation caused by reopenings of sodium channels during depolarization.[82] Furthermore, TTX caused a slowing of the rate of spontaneous depolarization and firing rate of immature (but not adult) rabbit sinoatrial nodal cells,[83] consistent with a major role for I_{Na} in pacemaker activity.

The sensitivity of I_{Na} to TTX is much higher in the immature heart than in the adult heart.[81] This current also is significantly more sensitive to block by class I antiarrhythmic drugs (lidocaine and phenytoin).[81,84,85] The differential pharmacologic sensitivity of the immature I_{Na} is suggestive of a different molecular composition. Of the 10 sodium channel pore-forming (α) subunits, cardiac (with low TTX sensitivity) sodium channels are thought to be composed mainly of $Na_V1.5$ subunits.[86] Recent data also suggest a role for "neuronal" (with higher TTX sensitivity) sodium channel subunits in the heart.[87] In an investigation of the expression of different types of sodium channel subunits during development, robust expression of several of these neuronal sodium channel subunits, including $Na_V1.3$, $Na_V1.4$, $Na_V1.2$, and $Na_V1.6$, was observed in immature mouse heart.[88] The $Na_V1.1$ subunit also was found to be expressed at high levels in the immature rabbit sinoatrial node.[89] These findings may partly explain the altered pharmacologic profile of the immature I_{Na}.

In a recent ion channel profiling of the immature heart, Harrell and colleagues found expression of $Na_V1.5$, $Na_V1.4$, and $Na_V1.8$ in the adult mouse heart.[25] They also found high expression levels of $Na_V2.3$, which has a weak sequence similarity to the Na_V1 subfamily and has previously been detected in mouse heart.[90] These data demonstrated fairly large changes in sodium channel gene expression, with $Na_V1.5$, $Na_V1.4$, and $Na_V2.3$ being expressed at higher levels in adult heart than in immature heart. Although expressed at lower levels, $Na_V1.8$

mRNA was present at higher levels in the immature heart than in the adult heart.

Sodium channels are heterotrimers and also contain two auxiliary β subunits in addition to the pore-forming α subunits. These β subunits have multiple functions and affect channel expression level and kinetics but also have other diverse roles such as cytoskeletal interactions, regulation of cell migration, and others.[91] A previous study has demonstrated that the β1 subunit is upregulated during perinatal development,[92] which could partly account for developmental changes in I_{Na} amplitude and kinetics.

Chloride Channels

Cardiac tissue expresses a range of anion channels, including cyclic adenosine monophosphate (cAMP)-activated chloride channels, protein kinase C (PKC)-activated chloride channels, volume-regulated anion channels (VRACs), Ca^{2+}-activated chloride channels, chloride channels activated by purinergic receptors, and voltage-activated chloride channels (ClCs).[93] Fairly strong evidence indicates that chloride channels are developmentally regulated. For example, when recordings of the I_{NaCa} were made under Cl^--containing and nominally Cl^--free conditions, the contribution of a substantial Ca^{2+}-activated chloride current was identified in neonatal (1 to 9 days of age) rabbit ventricular myocytes.[94] Developmental regulation of cAMP-activated chloride channels (at least in some species) also is possible, because no evidence of this current has been found in adult canine,[95] rat,[96,97] or mouse hearts,[98] despite reports in neonatal rat[99] and mouse[100] myocytes. The strongest evidence comes from single-channel studies performed on isolated rat cardiac myocytes, in which a large (400-pS) chloride channel could consistently be recorded in myocytes from neonatal (less than 12 days) hearts but was not observed in older rats.[101]

Several genes code for chloride channel subunits.[93] Evidence is available for strong upregulation of CFTR expression during development.[102] The ion channel profiling study by Harrell and colleagues[25] found expression of a range of chloride channel genes in the mouse heart, including the CLC family. In general, the CLC family members all were upregulated with perinatal development (with the exception of CLC-5, which was expressed at slightly higher levels in immature heart). This was in contrast with the Clca family, which generally was expressed at higher levels in immature myocardium than in adult heart. It is of interest that members of the Clca family express Ca^{2+}-activated chloride channels in heterologous expression systems. These data, together with functional measurements,[94] suggest the possibility that a link exists between calcium homeostasis, chloride channels activity and maintenance of the immature action potential duration, which could present a novel therapeutic target for regulating immature excitability. Despite these changes in chloride channel gene expression, however, the functional role of chloride channels in the immature heart remains to be elucidated.

Other Channels

Pacemaker Channels

Several ion channels, including sodium channels, calcium channels, and pacemaker channels, contribute to impulse initiation in the heart. Important changes occur during development regarding the relative contribution of these channels to pacemaker activity in the sinoatrial node (as reviewed recently by Baruscotti and Robinson[89]). Pacemaker channels, which contribute to the pacemaker current (I_f), are predominantly functionally active in the pacemaker and conducting tissue of the heart. These cation channels activate with membrane hyperpolarization, thus leading to a progressive spontaneous depolarization that characterizes phase 4 of the cardiac action potential. These channels are also strongly activated by cAMP, which is one of the major mechanisms responsible for an increased slope of phase 4 depolarization and accelerated pacemaker activity in response to adrenergic responses. The density of I_f is greater in SA nodal myocytes isolated from rabbit neonatal (9- to 10-day) hearts than in myocytes from adult hearts,[103] suggesting an important role for these channels in the immature conduction system and the slowing of the heart rate during development. These data are consistent with the observation that Cs^+ (a I_f blocker) has a more pronounced effect on pacemaker activity in the immature heart.[104] The pacemaker current also is present in mouse embryonic ventricular myocytes (as early as E9.5), and its expression is markedly decreased during fetal development, which is associated with a loss of spontaneous ventricular pacemaker activity.[105]

Hyperpolarization-activated, cyclic nucleotide–gated (HCN) subunits are thought to be components of pacemaker channels.[106] HCN1, HCN2, and HCN4 all are expressed in the heart, with HCN4 being the major component in the pacemaker region (where they may heteromultimerize with HCN1 subunits). Although pacemaker channels are present in the ventricle, they are not normally thought to operate as pacemaker channels in this tissue. The HCN2 transcript expression is comparable in conducting and ventricular tissue.[107] Harrell and colleagues found predominant expression of HCN2 in adult mouse heart, which is most likely to reflect the larger mass of ventricular tissue relative to conduction or pacemaker tissue.[25] The upregulation of HCN transcripts during development[25] suggests less emphasis on these channels for the generation of pacemaker activity in the immature myocardium (as supported by the work of Schanne and associates[108]). The HCN4 subunit is thought to be the major subunit of sinoatrial node pacemaker channels[89] and is even used as a marker for sinoatrial nodal development,[109] but the presence of HCN2 also has been described.[104] Both HCN2 and HCN4 expression levels are downregulated during development,[104] consistent with a major role of pacemaker channels during early development. Indeed, cardiac-specific knockout of HCN4 leads to embryonic death at days 9.5 to 11.5 as a result of severe bradycardia,[110] underscoring the importance of pacemaker channel function in embryonic development.

Intracellular Calcium Homeostasis

The contractile performance of immature heart differs significantly from the adult. This may be due in part to contractile properties of the myocardium itself. For example, the maximal active tension developed by papillary muscles isolated from neonatal kittens (less than 24 hours old) is significantly less that in the adult cat.[111] In the same species, however, significant age-dependent differences exist in which the papillary muscle responds to changes in the rate of stimulation, suggesting an increasing role of internal Ca^{2+} stores with age.[8] These observations are paralleled by increased development of the sarcoplasmic reticulum and age-dependent formation of T tubules[8] (see earlier). An increase in maximal developed force also was noted in rabbit heart (fetal to adult), which was correlated with an increasing sarcoplasmic reticulum function.[9]

Consistent with increasing sarcoplasmic reticulum dependence of contractility with age, blocking sarcoplasmic reticular function with ryanodine had little effect on contractions in perfused rabbit hearts before the age of 28 days after birth.[112] During voltage clamp conditions, age-dependent differences are seen in the kinetics of contractile force development in rabbit heart, such that the early peak contraction (which is largely due to sarcoplasmic reticulum Ca^{2+} release) is less well developed in immature papillary muscle.[5] These and other data led to the conclusion that tension development in the immature myocardium is supported largely by the influx of Ca^{2+} across the sarcolemma. As the myocardium matures, intracellular Ca^{2+} uptake and re-release by the sarcoplasmic reticulum play an increasingly important role in tension development.

The Sarcoplasmic Reticulum and the Sarcoplasmic Reticulum Ca^{2+} Release Channel

Histologically, very clear evidence shows that the sarcoplasmic reticulum is poorly developed and sparse in the immature heart (see earlier) and that subunits of the sarcoplasmic reticulum Ca^{2+} release channel (RyR2) are upregulated after birth,[113,114] consistent with a lesser functional role of the sarcoplasmic reticulum in the immature heart. Pharmacologic data also support this notion. For example, ryanodine and thapsigargin (which block sarcoplasmic reticulum Ca^{2+} release and uptake, respectively) exert much less depression of contractions or calcium transient amplitude in immature hearts (or cardiac myocytes isolated from immature hearts) than in the adult in a variety of species.[5,6]

Despite the fact that the sarcoplasmic reticulum does not fully participate in excitation-contraction coupling in the immature heart, however, evidence suggests that it is primed with releasable Ca^{2+}. For example, rapid application of caffeine (which at high concentrations opens sarcoplasmic reticulum calcium channels and is used as a tool to assess the releasable sarcoplasmic reticulum Ca^{2+} pool) causes a robust increase in cytosolic Ca^{2+} in neonatal (1 to 2 days of age) rabbit ventricular myocytes.[115] A similar observation has been made for fetal rat ventricular myocytes.[116] Some evidence also suggests that the immature sarcoplasmic reticulum contains a greater amount of stored Ca^{2+} compared with the adult sarcoplasmic reticulum.[117] Functionally, active sarcoplasmic reticulum Ca^{2+} release channels also can be detected by the localized transient increase in intracellular Ca^{2+} (an event termed *calcium sparks*[118]). In the adult heart, these calcium sparks can be detected as isolated events even during diastole. As would be expected for an immature sarcoplasmic reticulum, spontaneous calcium sparks are rarely observed in the immature rabbit or rat ventricular cells, and when detected, they occur solely at the cell periphery.[115,116] The sarcoplasmic reticulum calcium channels therefore appear to be fully functional in the immature heart. Indeed, when single sarcoplasmic reticulum calcium channels were incorporated into planar lipid membranes, no differences were observed in biophysical or pharmacologic properties of the channels in 1-day-old rat heart versus the adult heart.[119]

Collectively, these data suggest that functional coupling between the sarcoplasmic reticulum calcium release channels and L-type calcium channels is diminished in the immature heart as a consequence of spatial segregation of these two populations of calcium channels. The transition to a mature excitation-contraction coupling phenotype in ventricular myocardium (primary dependency on triggered sarcoplasmic reticulum calcium release) depends on development of the T tubule system to bring the sarcolemmal L-type calcium channels into close proximity with the intracellular Ca^{2+} release channels in the junctional sarcoplasmic reticulum.

The Na^+-Ca^{2+} Exchanger

Early reports have suggested that myocardial mechanical function of neonatal rabbit heart was more sensitive that adult hearts to manipulations of extracellular Na^+ and that this is due to a larger role of the Na^+-Ca^{2+} exchanger to contractions in the immature heart.[120] The Na^+-Ca^{2+} exchange activity, measured as a sodium-dependent Ca^{2+} uptake in crude membranes from chick heart, also has been demonstrated to increase linearly from embryonic day 4 to day 10 of the newborn stage.[121] Similarly, using sarcolemmal membranes from late fetal, neonatal and adult rabbit hearts an increase in sodium-dependent Ca^{2+} uptake also was demonstrated in the rabbit.[122] These functional changes are matched by developmental increases in the Na^+-Ca^{2+} exchanger mRNA and protein levels.[6]

The Na^+-Ca^{2+} exchanger is electrogenic because 3 Na^+ ions are exchanged for every Ca^{2+} ion transported, and it therefore carries electronic charge that can be measured under patch clamp conditions.[123] In directly measuring the Na^+-Ca^{2+} exchanger current (I_{NaCa}), it was found that the Na^+-Ca^{2+} exchange density was high in neonatal (1 to 2 days after birth) rabbit ventricular myocytes and declined significantly within the first 3 weeks after birth.[94,124]

In the rabbit, a functional role of Ca^{2+} entry across the sarcolemma as a source of Ca^{2+} for directly activating the contractile elements (as opposed to triggering Ca^{2+} release from the sarcoplasmic reticulum, as is well documented in the adult) is demonstrated by several findings:

1. After a period of Ca^{2+} removal, contractions are restored more readily in neonatal myocytes than in adult cells.[125]
2. The immature contractile response and intracellular calcium transient are relatively resistant to interventions that affect the sarcoplasmic reticulum (exposure to ryanodine and thapsigargin—see earlier).
3. Under voltage clamp conditions, tension of neonatal papillary muscle increases linearly as the membrane potential is made more depolarized,[5,6] whereas this relationship is bell-shaped in the adult. In subsequent studies, a direct correlation between the magnitude of the calcium current and the amplitude of the intracellular calcium transient was demonstrated, which resulted in a bell-shaped function of the calcium transient as a function of voltage. In 3-day old rabbit ventricular myocytes, however, the amplitude of the calcium transient was progressively increased with increasing depolarization, despite the fact that the calcium current amplitude decreased.[59]
4. During maintained depolarization, tension is augmented with time in the developing myocardium,[126] which is not consistent with a sarcoplasmic reticulum Ca^{2+} release process.
5. The neonatal calcium transient is not affected by $I_{Ca,L}$ blockade (e.g., with nifedipine) but is strongly inhibited by I_{NaCa} blockade (e.g., with Ni^{2+}).[5,6]
6. Ca^{2+} entry by way of I_{NaCa} (when all other Ca^{2+} entry pathways are blocked) can directly support normal contractions in immature myocytes.[5,6]

Collectively, these data provide compelling evidence for lack of functional coupling between Ca^{2+} influx through L-type calcium channels and sarcoplasmic reticulum Ca^{2+} release in the neonate, and for the direct participation of Ca^{2+} influx through "reverse" I_{NaCa} to effect contraction in the immature rabbit heart.

The Na^+-Ca^{2+} exchanger also may have additional functions during development. For example, although knockout of *NCX1* (the gene coding for the Na^+-Ca^{2+} exchanger protein) is embryonically lethal (at approximately 9.5 days), transgenic re-expression of NCX1 in cardiac myocytes (driven by the α-HMC promoter) does not rescue this phenotype.[127] It should be noted that important species differences (or differences at earlier developmental time points), in terms of the relative importance of different calcium-homeostatic pathways during development, are possible. For example, although calcium transients in mouse embryonic (E9.5) myocytes are expectedly unaffected by ryanodine and thapsigargin (see the foregoing for comparison), they are unaffected by I_{NaCa} blockade (with KB-R 7943) and abolished by $I_{Ca,L}$ (with nisoldipine), which suggests that in the early embyonic mouse heart, activator Ca^{2+} for contraction depends almost exclusively on L-type calcium channels.[114] In addition to an important role for I_{NaCa} in developing rat myocardium, Ca^{2+} influx through both L- and T-type calcium channels also is significant.[128]

Calcium Pumps

Relaxation in adult ventricular myocardium is caused predominantly by the taking back up of Ca^{2+} ions into the sarcoplasmic reticulum (after its release) by an ATP-dependent calcium pump, *sarcoplasmic-endoplasmic reticulum Ca^{2+}-ATPase (SERCA)*.[129] In keeping with the lesser role of sarcoplasmic reticulum generally ascribed to Ca^{2+} cycling in the immature heart (see earlier), a lesser role of sarcoplasmic reticulum Ca^{2+} uptake also is expected. Consistent with this finding, we found the relaxation rate to be significantly slower in newborn (1- to 12-day) rabbit ventricular myocytes than in the mature heart.[130] In the same study, we also investigated the contribution of different Ca^{2+}-extruding pathways by applying a pulse of caffeine, which empties the sarcoplasmic reticulum Ca^{2+} stores, and then assessing the rates of relaxation. In the presence of caffeine, the relaxation rate was markedly prolonged in the adult heart, but not in the immature heart, consistent with a smaller contribution of sarcoplasmic reticulum Ca^{2+} reuptake as the predominant mechanism of cytosolic Ca^{2+} removal from neonatal cardiac myocytes. When, in addition, the Na^+-Ca^{2+} exchanger also was blocked, the relaxation rate was slowed in the neonatal heart, suggesting an important role for Ca^{2+} removal by this pathway during early development. Of interest, however, relaxation still occurred in the immature heart (albeit at a slow rate, but faster than in the adult) when both of these pathways were blocked, which suggests that other pathways exist in the immature heart for removal of Ca^{2+} from the cytosol (either into other cytosolic compartments or by other sarcolemmal pathways). A reduced role of sarcoplasmic reticulum Ca^{2+} uptake in immature heart also was determined by Ca^{2+} flux assays.[131]

Consistent with a reduced role of sarcoplasmic reticulum Ca^{2+} uptake in the immature heart, the sarcoplasmic reticulum calcium pump mRNA and protein levels are reduced in immature heart compared with the adult heart.[114,132] The sarcoplasmic reticulum calcium pump is composed of subunits that are formed by at least three genes (*SERCA1* to *SERCA3*), with several different splice variants. During early development, interesting isoform switching of these subunits takes place. For example, using situ hybridization techniques, it was shown that SERCA3 mRNA is highly expressed in the heart tube and also is present in the yolk sac, but that cardiac expression disappears by embryonic days 14 to 16.[133] By contrast, SERCA2a mRNA is coexpressed with SERCA3 in the heart tube but also remains expressed in the cardiomyocytes throughout life. The functional significance of this finding remains to be identified.

Ion Channel Expression in the Early Fetus

Barring a few exceptions, most of the published studies on ion channels during cardiac development that are reviewed here relate to the perinatal period (late fetus and immediately after birth). To directly address ion channel expression during fetal development, we turned to publicly available microarray databases. We analyzed the benchmark cardiac development microarray data, available as part of the National Institutes of Health (NIH)-sponsored CardioGenomics project.* These data were obtained using RNA isolated from the hearts of fetal C57B/6 mice at different developmental stages, including the heart tube at days E10.5 and E11.5 and ventricles at 12.5, 13.5, 14.5, 16.5, and 18.5 days after fertilization (three microarrays per time point). We normalized the data using the robust multichip analysis (RMA) algorithm (ArrayAssist). A list of 313 ion channel genes was used to compile a subset of data, which then were normalized to the expression values of several reference ("housekeeping") genes, including the β-actin gene, *DHFR*, *G6PD*, the histone H_3 gene, *HMBS*, the HGPRTase gene, and the cyclophilin B gene. Hierarchical clustering was performed after log2 transformation (no other data adjustment or normalization was performed) and visualized using TreeView (software by Dr. Michael B. Eisen, University of California at Berkeley). Of the 313 genes, genes that code for the following subunits did not appear to be present in the dataset: Na-K ATPase α4, $Ca_V3.3$, *CLC4*, *CNGA3*, *CNGB1*, *KChIP3*, *HCN4*, *IP3R4*, Kv1.8, Kv6.2, Kv6.3, Kv12.3, Kv11.2, Kir7.1, *K2P10*.1, *K2P15*.1, *K2P17*.1, *K2P18*.1, *K2P9*.1, slo-beta-3, ENac-δ, Slc26a9, NBCe2, *NHE10*, *NHE2*, *NHE7*, *TRPV1*, *TRPV3*, and *TRPV5*. The fetal developmental expression profiles of the remaining genes are shown in Figure 15-1.

The vast majority of the ion channel and exchanger genes are expressed in the immature heart, and expression generally is upregulated during fetal development. Genes with a marked upregulation during development code for calcium channel subunits ($Ca_V3.1$), K_{ATP} channel subunits (Kir6.1, Kir6.2, and SUR2), inward rectifier potassium channel subunits (Kir2.1 and Kir2.2), voltage-gated potassium channel subunits (Kv1.4 and Kv9.1), and a potassium channel regulatory protein (MinK), and a connexin (Cx46). Of interest, another group of genes has high expression levels early, and expression declines with embryonic development. Subunits encoded by this group of genes include ClC-2 (a chloride channel), Nav1.3 and $Nav\beta_3$ (components of sodium channels), Cav3.1 and $Ca_V1.3$ (calcium channels), sloβ1 and Kv7.1 (components of potassium channels), Cx37 (a connexin), RyR3 and calsequestrin 1 (components of sarcoplasmic reticulum calcium regulation), PMCA1 (a sarcolemmal calcium pump), AE1 (i.e., SLC4A1—an anion exchanger), and CAII (i.e., SLC4A7—a sodium-bicarbonate cotransporter). In some instances, a good correlation is found between published data and these findings obtained with the microarray analysis, and in others, novel changes are predicted that may have functional consequences during embryonic development. These data remain to be independently verified experimentally but may point the way for future directions.

Perspectives and Future Directions

It is apparent that expression and functional activity of a number of cardiac ion channels change significantly during perinatal maturation and that these changes have profound effects on cardiac electrophysiology and mechanical function. What is less apparent, however, are the factors that underlie some of these developmental changes. The developmental pattern and program of normal gene expression are undoubtedly influenced by environmental influences (hormonal fluxes, nutritional support to the developing embryo, maternal illnesses or infections, and so on). Evidence has emerged recently to support the concept of epigenetic modification of genes during fetal development that may have life-long consequences for increasing an individual patient's risk for coronary artery disease, hypertension, and diabetes. It seems likely that changes in ion channel expression or activity may be involved in some of these adult-onset diseases that

*http://cardiogenomics.med.harvard.edu/groups/proj1/pages/embryo_home.html.

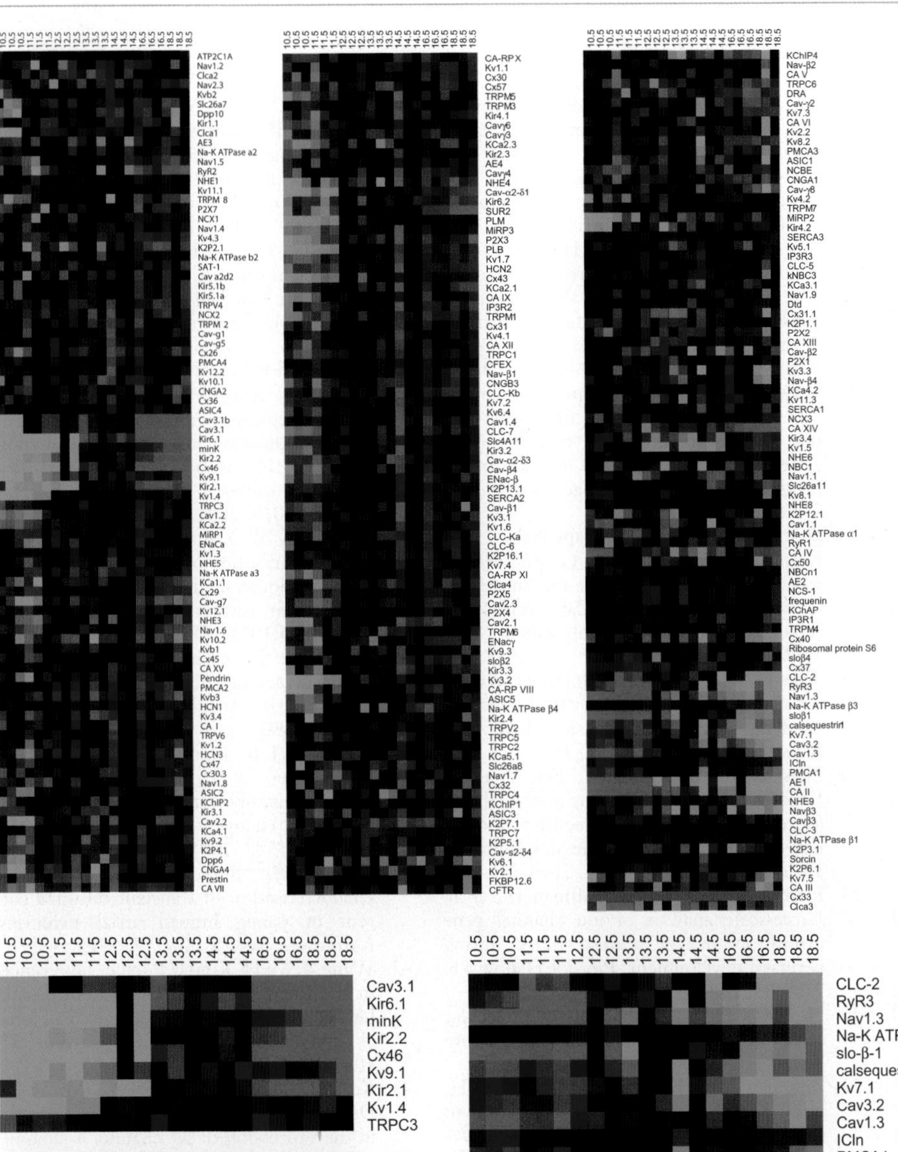

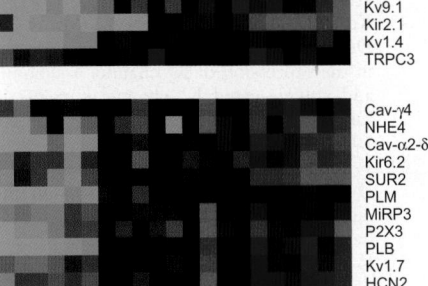

Figure 15-1 A heat map depicting the expression levels of 266 genes coding for subunits of ion channels, exchangers, and pumps during embryonic development. Gene expression levels were normalized to those of selected reference genes. See text for details.

have their roots in fetal development. This is an area that is ripe for future study.

An understanding of the normal developmental regulation of cardiac ion channels is important for understanding normal maturation of cardiac rhythm and excitation-contraction coupling and, hence, contractile function in the developing heart. Implications may be broader for the mature heart as well. After myocardial injury and in the setting of heart failure, changes in excitation-contraction coupling ion channel expression mimic a reversion to an immature pattern of expression and function. Furthermore, attempts at myocardial regeneration involving stem cell therapy are likely to involve a maturational process and developmental program for these cells as they progress from pluripotent cells to mature cardiac myocytes. Unraveling the normal developmental processes probably will be important for optimizing therapeutic strategies for myocardial cellular regeneration or replacement. Transcript expression in the embryonic murine heart provide a foundation for future studies to define these developmental processes and the factors that influence normal and abnormal expression and regulation of cardiac ion channels. In addition to the traditional promoter-based developmental regulation of expression, changes in protein trafficking, post-transcriptional regulation, and signaling pathways are likely to occur during normal and abnormal development and will be critical to define before developmental ion channel biology in the heart can be fully elucidated.

References

1. Olson EN: Gene regulatory networks in the evolution and development of the heart. Science 313:1922-1927, 2006.
2. Tibbits GF, Xu L, Sedarat F: Ontogeny of excitation-contraction coupling in the mammalian heart. Comp Biochem Physiol A Mol Integr Physiol 132:691-698, 2002.
3. Tohse N, Seki S, Kobayashi T, et al: Development of excitation-contraction coupling in cardiomyocytes. Jpn J Physiol 54:1-6, 2004.
4. Vornanen M, Shiels HA, Farrell AP: Plasticity of excitation-contraction coupling in fish cardiac myocytes. Comp Biochem Physiol A Mol Integr Physiol 132:827-846, 2002.
5. Wetzel GT, Klitzner TS: Developmental cardiac electrophysiology recent advances in cellular physiology. Cardiovasc Res 31:E52-E60, 1996.
6. Artman M, Haddock PS, Coetzee WA: Calcium regulation in the developing heart. In Clark EB, Nakazawa M, Takao A (eds): Etiology and Morphogenesis of Congenital Heart Disease. Armonk, NY, Futura Publishing, 2000, pp 289-291.
7. Cullen M, Sheridan D, Tynan M: Post-natal ultrastructural development of the cat myocardium. J Physiol 265:16P-17P, 1977.
8. Maylie JG: Excitation-contraction coupling in neonatal and adult myocardium of cat. Am J Physiol 242:H834-H843, 1982.
9. Nakanishi T, Jarmakani JM: Developmental changes in myocardial mechanical function and subcellular organelles. Am J Physiol 246:H615-H625, 1984.
10. Sperelakis N, Shigenobu K: Changes in membrane potential of chick embryonic hearts during development. J Gen Physiol 60:430-453, 1972.
11. Kojima M, Ishima T, Taniguchi N, et al: Developmental changes in beta-adrenoceptors, muscarinic cholinoceptors and Ca^{2+} channels in rat ventricular muscles. Br J Pharmacol 99:334-339, 1990.
12. Sheridan DJ: Postnatal developmental changes in the electrophysiological properties of cat right ventricular papillary muscles. Cardiovasc Res 14:700-709, 1980.
13. Trepanier-Boulay V, Lupien MA, St-Michel C, Fiset C: Postnatal development of atrial repolarization in the mouse. Cardiovasc Res 64:84-93, 2004.
14. Kilborn MJ, Fedida D: A study of the developmental changes in outward currents of rat ventricular myocytes. J Physiol Lond 430:37-60, 1990.
15. Haddock PS, Artman M, Coetzee WA: Influence of postnatal changes in action potential duration on Na-Ca exchange in rabbit ventricular myocytes. Pflügers Arch–Eur J Physiol 435:789-795, 1998.
16. Escande D, Loisance D, Planche C, Coraboeuf E: Age-related changes of action potential plateau shape in isolated human atrial fibers. Am J Physiol 249:H843-H850, 1985.
17. Coetzee WA, Amarillo Y, Chiu J, et al: Molecular diversity of K^+ channels. Ann N Y Acad. Sci 868:233-285, 1999.
18. Sperelakis N, Pappano AJ: 1983. Physiology and pharmacology of developing heart cells. Pharmacol Ther 22:1-39, 1983.
19. Xie LH, Takano M, Noma A: Development of inwardly rectifying K^+ channel family in rat ventricular myocytes. Am J Physiol 272:H1741-H1750, 1997.
20. Nakamura TY, Lee K, Artman M, et al: The Role of Kir2.1 in the genesis of native cardiac inward rectifier K^+ currents during pre- and postnatal development. Ann N Y Acad Sci 868:434-437, 1999.
21. Zaritsky JJ, Redell JB, Tempel BL, Schwarz TL: The consequences of disrupting cardiac inwardly rectifying K^+ current (I(K1)) as revealed by the targeted deletion of the murine Kir2.1 and Kir2.2 genes. J Physiol 533:697-710, 2001.
22. Stehno-Bittel L, Krapivinsky G, Krapivinsky L, et al: The G protein beta gamma subunit transduces the muscarinic receptor signal for Ca^{2+} release in Xenopus oocytes. J Biol Chem 270: 30068-30074, 1995.
23. Takano M, Noma A: Development of muscarinic potassium current in fetal and neonatal rat heart. Am J Physiol Heart Circ Physiol 272:H1188-H1195, 1997.
24. Fleischmann BK, Duan Y, Fan Y, et al: Differential subunit composition of the G protein–activated inward-rectifier potassium channel during cardiac development. J Clin Invest 114:994-1001, 2004.
25. Harrell MD, Harbi S, Hoffman JF, et al: Large-scale analysis of ion channel gene expression in the mouse heart during perinatal development. Physiol Genom 28: 273-283, 2007.
26. Nichols CG: K_{ATP} channels as molecular sensors of cellular metabolism. Nature 440:470-476, 2006.
27. Zingman LV, Hodgson DM, Bast PH, et al: Kir6.2 is required for adaptation to stress. Proc Natl Acad Sci U S A 99:13278-13283, 2002.
28. Kasuya Y, Matsuki N, Shigenobu K: Changes in sensitivity to anoxia of the cardiac action potential plateau during chick embryonic development. Dev Biol 58: 124-133, 1977.
29. Tripp ME: Developmental cardiac metabolism in health and disease. Pediatr Cardiol 10:150-158, 1989.
30. Haddad GE, Petrich ER, Zumino AP, Schanne OF: Background K^+ currents and response to metabolic inhibition during early development in rat cardiocytes. Mol Cell Biochem 177:159-168, 1997.
31. Chen FH, Wetzel GT, Friedman WF, Klitzner TS: ATP-sensitive potassium channels in neonatal and adult rabbit ventricular myocytes. Pediatr Res 32:230-235, 1992.
32. Davies MP, An RH, Doevendans P, et al: Developmental changes in ionic channel activity in the embryonic murine heart. Circ Res 78:15-25, 1996.
33. Morrissey A, Parachuru L, Leung M, et al: Expression of K(ATP) channel subunits during perinatal maturation in the mouse heart. Pediatr Res 58:185-192, 2005.
34. Akasaka T, Klinedinst S, Ocorr K, et al: The ATP-sensitive potassium (KATP) channel-encoded dSUR gene is required for Drosophila heart function and is regulated by Tinman. Proc Natl Acad Sci U S A 103:11999-12004, 2006.
35. Wang L, Duff HJ: Developmental changes in transient outward current in mouse ventricle. Circ Res 81:120-127, 1997.
36. Roberds SL, Tamkun MM: Developmental expression of cloned cardiac potassium channels. FEBS Lett 284:152-154, 1991.
37. Zhang M, Jiang M, Tseng GN: MinK-related peptide 1 associates with $K_V4.2$ and modulates its gating function: Potential role as beta subunit of cardiac transient outward channel? Circ Res 88:1012-1019, 2001.
38. Kobayashi T, Yamada Y, Nagashima M, et al: Contribution of KChIP2 to the developmental increase in transient outward current of rat cardiomyocytes. J Mol Cell Cardiol 35:1073-1082, 2003.
39. Mansourati J, Le Grand B: Transient outward current in young and adult diseased human atria. Am J Physiol 265:H1466-H1470, 1993.
40. Crumb WJ Jr, Pigott JD, Clarkson CW: Comparison of I_{to} in young and adult human atrial myocytes: Evidence for developmental changes. Am J Physiol 268: H1335-H1342, 1995.
41. Gross GJ, Burke RP, Castle NA: Characterisation of transient outward current in young human atrial myocytes. Cardiovasc Res 29:112-117, 1995.
42. Wang Y, Xu H, Kumar R, et al: Differences in transient outward current properties between neonatal and adult human atrial myocytes. J Mol Cell Cardiol 35: 1083-1092, 2003.
43. Xu HD, Dixon JE, Barry DM, et al: Developmental analysis reveals mismatches in the expression of K^+ channel α subunits and voltage-gated K^+ channel currents in rat ventricular myocytes. J Gen Physiol 108:405-419, 1996.
44. Wang L, Feng ZP, Kondo CS, Sheldon RS, Duff HJ: Developmental changes in the delayed rectifier K^+ channels in mouse heart. Circ Res 79:79-85, 1996.
45. Wang L, Swirp S, Duff H: Age-dependent response of the electrocardiogram to K^+ channel blockers in mice. Am J Physiol Cell Physiol 278:C73-C80, 2000.
46. Guo WN, Kamiya K, Liu MR, Toyama J: Developmental changes of the ultrarapid delayed rectifier K^+ current in rat ventricular myocytes. Pflügers Arch. 433:442-445, 1997.
47. Grandy SA, Trepanier-Boulay V, Fiset C: Postnatal development has a marked effect on ventricular repolarization in mice. Am J Physiol Heart Circ Physiol 293:H2168-H2177, 2007.
48. London B, Guo W, Pan X, et al: Targeted replacement of $K_V1.5$ in the mouse leads to loss of the 4-aminopyridine-sensitive component of I(K,slow) and resistance to drug-induced qt prolongation. Circ Res 88:940-946, 2001.

49. Kodirov SA, Brunner M, Nerbonne JM, et al: Attenuation of I(K, slow1) and I(K, slow2) in Kv1/Kv2DN mice prolongs APD and QT intervals but does not suppress spontaneous or inducible arrhythmias. Am J Physiol Heart Circ Physiol 286:H368-H374, 2004.
50. Chun KR, Koenen M, Katus HA, Zehelein J: Expression of the IKr components KCNH2 (rERG) and KCNE2 (rMiRP1) during late rat heart development. Exp Mol Med 36:367-371, 2004.
51. Graham V, Zhang H, Willis S, Creazzo TL: Expression of a two-pore domain K^+ channel (TASK-1) in developing avian and mouse ventricular conduction systems. Dev Dyn 235:143-151, 2006.
52. Catterall WA, Perez-Reyes E, Snutch TP, Striessnig J: International Union of Pharmacology. XLVIII. Nomenclature and structure-function relationships of voltage-gated calcium channels. Pharmacol Rev 57:411-425, 2005.
53. Cohen NM, Lederer WJ: Changes in the calcium current of rat heart ventricular myocytes during development. J Physiol Lond 406:115-146, 1988.
54. Katsube Y, Yokoshiki H, Nguyen L, Sperelakis N: Differences in isoproterenol stimulation of Ca^{2+} current of rat ventricular myocytes in neonatal compared to adult. Eur J Pharmacol 317:391-400, 1996.
55. Vornanen M: Contribution of sarcolemmal calcium current to total cellular calcium in postnatally developing rat heart. Cardiovasc Res 32:400-410, 1996.
56. Osaka T, Joyner RW: Developmental changes in calcium currents of rabbit ventricular cells. Circ Res 68:788-796, 1991.
57. Wetzel GT, Chen FH, Klitzner TS: L-type and T-type calcium channels in acutely isolated neonatal and adult cardiac myocytes. Pediatr Res 30:89-94, 1991.
58. Wetzel GT, Chen FH, Klitzner TS: Ca^{2+} channel kinetics in acutely isolated fetal, neonatal, and adult rabbit cardiac myocytes. Circ Res 72:1065-1074, 1993.
59. Huang J, Xu L., Thomas M, et al: L-type Ca^{2+} channel function and expression in neonatal rabbit ventricular myocytes. Am J Physiol Heart Circ Physiol 290: H2267-H2276, 2006.
60. Collis LP, Srivastava S, Coetzee WA, Artman M: β2 Adrenergic receptor agonists stimulate L-type calcium current independent of PKA in newborn rabbit ventricular myocytes. Am J Physiol Heart Circ Physiol 293:H2826-H2835, 2007.
61. Roca TP, Pigott JD, Clarkson CW, Crumb WJ: L-type calcium current in pediatric and adult human atrial myocytes: Evidence for developmental changes in channel inactivation. Pediatr Res 40: 462-468, 1996.
62. Cohen NM, Lederer WJ: Calcium current in isolated neonatal rat ventricular myocytes. J Physiol Lond 391:169-191, 1987.
63. Arikkath J, Campbell KP: Auxiliary subunits: Essential components of the voltage-gated calcium channel complex. Curr Opin Neurobiol 13:298-307, 2003.
64. Seisenberger C, Specht V, Welling A, et al: Functional embryonic cardiomyocytes after disruption of the L-type alpha1C ($Ca_V1.2$) calcium channel gene in the mouse. J Biol Chem 275:39193-39199, 2000.
65. Haase H, Pfitzmaier B, McEnery MW, Morano I: Expression of Ca^{2+} channel subunits during cardiac ontogeny in mice and rats: Identification of fetal alpha(1C) and beta subunit isoforms. J Cell Biochem 76:695-703, 2000.
66. Takemura H, Yasui K, Opthof T, et al: Subtype switching of L-type Ca^{2+} channel from $Ca_V1.3$ to $Ca_V1.2$ in embryonic murine ventricle. Circ J 69:1405-1411, 2005.
67. Klugbauer N, Welling A, Specht V, et al: L-type Ca^{2+} channels of the embryonic mouse heart. Eur J Pharmacol 447: 279-284, 2002.
68. Lu ZJ, Pereverzev A, Liu HL, et al: Arrhythmia in isolated prenatal hearts after ablation of the $Ca_V2.3$ (alpha1E) subunit of voltage-gated Ca^{2+} channels. Cell Physiol Biochem 14:11-22, 2004.
69. Cribbs LL, Martin BL, Schroder EA, et al: Identification of the T-type calcium channel (Ca(v)3.1d) in developing mouse heart. Circ Res 88:403-407, 2001.
70. Vassort G, Talavera K, Alvarez JL: Role of T-type Ca^{2+} channels in the heart. Cell Calcium 40:205-220, 2006.
71. Ferron L, Capuano V, Deroubaix E, et al: Functional and molecular characterization of a T-type Ca^{2+} channel during fetal and postnatal rat heart development. J Mol Cell Cardiol 34:533-546, 2002.
72. Leuranguer V, Monteil A, Bourinet E, et al: T-type calcium currents in rat cardiomyocytes during postnatal development: Contribution to hormone secretion. Am J Physiol Heart Circ Physiol 279: H2540-H2548, 2000.
73. Kitchens SA, Burch J, Creazzo TL: T-type Ca^{2+} current contribution to Ca^{2+}-induced Ca^{2+} release in developing myocardium. J Mol Cell Cardiol 35:515-523, 2003.
74. Hagiwara N, Irisawa H, Kameyama M: Contribution of two types of calcium currents to the pacemaker potentials of rabbit sino-atrial node cells. J Physiol Lond 395:233-253, 1988.
75. Zhou Z, Lipsius SL: T-type calcium current in latent pacemaker cells isolated from cat right atrium. J Mol Cell Cardiol 26:1211-1219, 1994.
76. Protas L, DiFrancesco D, Robinson RB: L-type but not T-type calcium current changes during postnatal development in rabbit sinoatrial node. Am J Physiol Heart Circ Physiol 281:H1252-H1259, 2001.
77. Yunker AM, McEnery MW: Low-voltage-activated ("T-type") calcium channels in review. J Bioenerg Biomembr 35:533-575, 2003.
78. Qu Y, Boutjdir M: Gene expression of SERCA2a and L- and T-type Ca channels during human heart development. Pediatr Res 50:569-574, 2001.
79. Rosen MR, Reder RF, Hordof AJ, et al: Age-related changes in Purkinje fiber action potentials of adult dogs. Circ Res 43:931-938, 1978.
80. Agata N, Tanaka H, Shigenobu K: Developmantal changes in action potential properties of the guinea-pig myocardium. Acta Physiol Scand 149:331-337, 1993.
81. Reder RF, Miura DS, Danilo P, Rosen MR: The electrophysiological properties of normal neonatal and adult canine cardiac Purkinje fibers. Circ Res 48:658-668, 1981.
82. Zhang JF, Robinson RB, Siegelbaum SA: Sympathetic neurons mediate developmental change in cardiac sodium channel gating through long-term neurotransmitter action. Neuron 9:97-103, 1992.
83. Baruscotti M, DiFrancesco D, Robinson RB: A TTX-sensitive inward sodium current contributes to spontaneous activity in newborn rabbit sino-atrial node cells. J Physiol 492:21-30, 1996.
84. Xu YQ, Pickoff AS, Clarkson CW: Evidence for developmental changes in sodium channel inactivation gating and sodium channel block by phenytoin in rat cardiac myocytes. Circ Res 69:644-656, 1991.
85. Xu YQ, Pickoff AS, Clarkson CW: Developmental changes in the effects of lidocaine on sodium channels in rat cardiac myocytes. J Pharmacol Exp Ther 262:670-676, 1992.
86. Catterall WA, Goldin AL, Waxman SG: International Union of Pharmacology. XXXIX. Compendium of voltage-gated ion channels: Sodium channels. Pharmacol Rev 55:575-578, 2003.
87. Maier SK, Westenbroek RE, Schenkman KA, et al: An unexpected role for brain-type sodium channels in coupling of cell surface depolarization to contraction in the heart. Proc Natl Acad Sci U S A 99:4073-4078, 2002.
88. Haufe V, Camacho JA, Dumaine R, et al: Expression pattern of neuronal and skeletal muscle voltage-gated Na^+ channels in the developing mouse heart. J Physiol 564:683-696, 2005.
89. Baruscotti M, Robinson RB: Electrophysiology and pacemaker function of the developing sinoatrial node. Am J Physiol Heart Circ Physiol 293:H2613-H2623, 2007.
90. Knittle TJ, Doyle KL, Tamkun MM: Immunolocalization of the $mNa_V2.3$ Na^+ channel in mouse heart: Upregulation in myometrium during pregnancy. Am J Physiol 270:C688-C696, 1996.
91. Isom LL: Sodium channel beta subunits: Anything but auxiliary. Neuroscientist 7:42-54, 2001.
92. Dominguez JN, Navarro F, Franco D, et al: Temporal and spatial expression pattern of beta1 sodium channel subunit during heart development. Cardiovasc Res 65:842-850, 2005.
93. Hume JR, Duan D, Collier ML, et al: Anion transport in heart. Physiol Rev 80:31-81, 2000.
94. Haddock PS, Coetzee WA, Artman M: Na^+/Ca^{2+} exchange current and contractions measured under Cl^--free conditions in developing rabbit hearts. Am J Physiol 273:H837-H846, 1997.
95. Sorota S, Siegal MS, Hoffman BF: The isoproterenol-induced chloride current and cardiac resting potential. J Mol Cell Cardiol 23:1191-1198, 1991.
96. Dukes ID, Cleemann L, Morad M: Tedisamil blocks the transient and

delayed rectifier K^+ currents in mammalian cardiac and glial cells. J Pharmacol Exp Ther 254:560-569, 1990.
97. Kaneda M, Fukui K, Doi K: Activation of chloride current by P2-purinoceptors in rat ventricular myocytes. Br J Pharmacol 111:1355-1360, 1994.
98. Levesque PC, Hume JR: ATP_o but not $cAMP_i$ activates a chloride conductance in mouse ventricular myocytes. Cardiovasc Res 29:336-343, 1995.
99. Walsh KB: Activation of a heart chloride current during stimulation of protein kinase C. Mol Pharmacol 40:342-346, 1991.
100. Prat AG, Cunningham CC, Jackson GR Jr, et al: Actin filament organization is required for proper cAMP-dependent activation of CFTR. Am J Physiol 277:C1160-C1169, 1999.
101. Coulombe A, Coraboeuf E: Large-conductance chloride channels of newborn rat cardiac myocytes are activated by hypotonic media. Pflügers Arch–Eur J Physiol 422:143-150, 1992.
102. Wong KR, Trezise AE, Vandenberg JI: Developmental regulation of the gradient of CFTR expression in the rabbit heart. Mech Dev 94:195-197, 2000.
103. Accili EA, Robinson RB, DiFrancesco D: Properties and modulation of I_f in newborn versus adult cardiac SA node. Am J Physiol 272:H1549-H1552, 1997.
104. Huang X, Yang P, Du Y, et al: Age-related down-regulation of HCN channels in rat sinoatrial node. Basic Res Cardiol 102:429-435, 2007.
105. Yasui K, Liu W, Opthof T, et al: I(f) current and spontaneous activity in mouse embryonic ventricular myocytes. Circ Res 88:536-542, 2001.
106. Baruscotti M, Bucchi A, DiFrancesco D: Physiology and pharmacology of the cardiac pacemaker ("funny") current. Pharmacol Ther 107:59-79, 2005.
107. Han W, Bao W, Wang Z, Nattel S: Comparison of ion-channel subunit expression in canine cardiac Purkinje fibers and ventricular muscle. Circ Res 91:790-797, 2002.
108. Schanne OF, Boutin L, Derosiers J: Effects of K-channel blockers, calcium, and verapamil suggest different pacemaker mechanisms in cultured neonatal rat and embryonic chick ventricle cells. Can J Physiol Pharmacol 67:795-800, 1989.
109. Mommersteeg MT, Hoogaars WM, Prall OW, et al: Molecular pathway for the localized formation of the sinoatrial node. Circ Res 100:354-362, 2007.
110. Stieber J, Herrmann S, Feil S, et al: The hyperpolarization-activated channel HCN4 is required for the generation of pacemaker action potentials in the embryonic heart. Proc Natl Acad Sci U S A 100:15235-15240, 2003.
111. Davies P, Dewar J, Tynan M, Ward R: Post-natal developmental changes in the length-tension relationship of cat papillary muscles. J Physiol 253:95-102, 1975.
112. Nakanishi T, Seguchi M, Takao A: Development of the myocardial contractile system. Experientia 44:936-944, 1988.
113. Brillantes AM, Bezprozvannaya S, Marks AR: Developmental and tissue-specific regulation of rabbit skeletal and cardiac muscle calcium channels involved in excitation-contraction coupling. Circ Res 75:503-510, 1994.
114. Liu W, Yasui K, Opthof T, et al: Developmental changes of Ca^{2+} handling in mouse ventricular cells from early embryo to adulthood. Life Sci 71:1279-1292, 2002.
115. Haddock PS, Coetzee WA, Cho E, et al: Sub-cellular $[Ca^{2+}]_i$ gradients during excitation-contraction coupling in newborn rabbit ventricular myocytes. Circ Res 85:415-427, 1999.
116. Seki S, Nagashima M, Yamada Y, et al: Fetal and postnatal development of Ca^{2+} transients and Ca^{2+} sparks in rat cardiomyocytes. Cardiovasc Res 58:535-548, 2003.
117. Huang J, Hove-Madsen L, Tibbits GF: Na^+/Ca^{2+} exchange activity in neonatal rabbit ventricular myocytes. Am J Physiol Cell Physiol 288:C195-C203, 2005.
118. Cheng H, Lederer WJ, Cannell MB: Calcium sparks: Elementary events underlying excitation-contraction coupling in heart muscle. Science 262:740-744, 1993.
119. Perez CG, Copello JA, Li Y, et al: Ryanodine receptor function in newborn rat heart. Am J Physiol Heart Circ Physiol 288:H2527-H2540, 2005.
120. Nakanishi T, Jarmakani JM: Effect of extracellular sodium on mechanical function in the newborn rabbit. Dev Pharmacol Ther 2:188-200, 1981.
121. Vetter R, Will H: Sarcolemmal Na-Ca exchange and sarcoplasmic reticulum calcium uptake in developing chick heart. J Mol Cell Cardiol 18:1267-1275, 1986.
122. Artman M: Sarcolemmal Na^+-Ca^{2+} exchange activity and exchanger immunoreactivity in developing rabbit hearts. Am J Physiol 263:H1506-H1513, 1992.
123. Kimura J, Noma A, Irisawa H: Na-Ca exchange current in mammalian heart cells. Nature 319:596-597, 1986.
124. Artman M, Ichikawa H, Avkiran M, Coetzee WA: Na^+-Ca^{2+} exchange current density in cardiac myocytes isolated from rabbits and guinea pigs during postnatal development. Am J Physiol 268: H1714-H1722, 1995.
125. Chin TK, Friedman WF, Klitzner TS: Developmental changes in cardiac myocyte calcium regulation. Circ Res 67:574-579, 1990.
126. Klitzner TS, Chen F, Raven RR, et al: Calcium current and tension generation in immature mammalian myocardium: Effects of diltiazem. J Mol Cell Cardiol 23:807-815, 1991.
127. Conway SJ, Kruzynska-Frejtag A, Wang J, et al: Role of sodium-calcium exchanger (NCX1) in embryonic heart development: A transgenic rescue? Ann N Y Acad Sci 976:268-281, 2002.
128. Escobar AL, Ribeiro-Costa R, Villalba-Galea C, et al: Developmental changes of intracellular Ca^{2+} transients in beating rat hearts. Am J Physiol Heart Circ Physiol 286:H971-H978, 2004.
129. Periasamy M, Kalyanasundaram A: SERCA pump isoforms: Their role in calcium transport and disease. Muscle Nerve 35:430-442, 2007.
130. Balaguru D, Haddock PS, Puglisi JL, et al: Role of the sarcoplasmic reticulum in contraction and relaxation of immature rabbit ventricular myocytes. J Mol Cell Cardiol 29:2747-2757, 1997.
131. Prakash P, Meera P, Tripathi O: Developmental changes in Ca^{2+} uptake, Na^+,Ca^{2+} exchange and Ca^{2+} ATPase in freshly isolated embryonic, newborn and adult chicken heart. Reprod Fertil Dev 8:71-78, 1996.
132. Vetter R, Studer R, Reinecke H, et al: Reciprocal changes in the postnatal expression of the sarcolemmal Na^+-Ca^{2+}exchanger and SERCA2 in rat heart. J Mol Cell Cardiol 27:1689-1701, 1995.
133. Anger M, Samuel JL, Marotte F, et al: In situ mRNA distribution of sarco(endo)-plasmic reticulum Ca^{2+} ATPase isoforms during ontogeny in the rat. J Mol Cell Cardiol 26:539-550, 1994.

Pharmacology of the Cardiac Sodium Channel 16

CRAIG T. JANUARY AND JONATHAN C. MAKIELSKI

CHAPTER OUTLINE

Sodium Channels

The cardiac sodium channel is composed of the α (pore-forming) subunit protein, $Na_V1.5$ (a product of the gene *SCN5A*[1] at chromosome locus 3p21), and associated β (accessory) subunit proteins. This sodium channel is found predominantly in heart but also occurs in parts of the brain and the gastrointestinal tract. *SCN5A* belongs to a family of genes encoding structurally similar voltage-dependent sodium channels that are found predominantly in other tissues, including skeletal muscle ($Na_V1.4$), brain ($Na_V1.1$, Na_V 1.2, and Na_V 1.6), and peripheral nerve ($Na_V1.7$, Na_V 1.8, and Na_V 1.9).[2] The α subunit protein controls properties including channel selectivity for Na^+ ions and voltage-dependent activation and inactivation, and it has the major drug- and toxin-binding sites. The channel also has β subunit proteins encoded by separate genes that may influence its kinetics and pharmacology. Furthermore, as shown in Figure 16-1, the sodium channel resides in the cell membrane in complex macromolecular structures composed of multiple additional putative interacting and regulatory proteins.[3] Thus, regulation of the sodium channel depends not only on its α and β subunits but also on multiple cytoskeletal, membrane, and extracellular matrix signaling pathways that are incompletely understood but offer additional targets for pharmacologic manipulation. Complex membrane macromolecular microdomains have been proposed for several other ion channels as well.[3-5]

Ionic current through the sodium channel (I_{Na}) determines excitability and conduction in atrium, His-Purkinje system, and ventricle, and Na^+ entry through sodium channels also modulates intracellular Na^+ and through Na^+-Ca^{2+} exchange, intracellular Ca^{2+} and cell contraction. Sodium channels are voltage-activated—the channel protein responds within a millisecond to the initiation of cell membrane depolarization by opening, leading to cell excitation and cell-to-cell conduction. The sodium current then normally decreases to less than 1% of its peak value over the next several milliseconds because of voltage-dependent inactivation. The small amount of I_{Na} remaining, along with slowly inactivating L-type calcium current, helps maintain the cardiac action potential plateau. With repolarization of the action potential, the sodium channel normally recovers rapidly from inactivation (within 10 ms) and is ready to open again. Sodium channel–blocking drugs tend to decrease excitability and conduction by inhibiting peak I_{Na} and also may shorten action potential duration by blocking late I_{Na}. Drugs or toxins that increase late I_{Na} would tend to prolong the action potential and refractoriness.

Inhibition of Sodium Channels

Vaughn Williams class 1 antiarrhythmic drugs act by decreasing I_{Na}. This inhibition, or block, is divided into two types: tonic block and use-dependent block. *Tonic block* is induced by drug exposure before application of a single depolarization. *Use-dependent block* is the block produced by repetitive or more frequent depolarizations, and it is use-dependent block of I_{Na} that is central to antiarrhythmic drug action. These types of block are illustrated in Figure 16-2, in which sodium current was recorded from a voltage-clamped heart cell. After a control I_{Na} trace was recorded, lidocaine was applied while the cell was maintained at rest; this was followed by a train of depolarizing steps to repetitively activate I_{Na}. The decrease in I_{Na} noted in response to the first depolarization is tonic block. With repetitive depolarizations, additional block develops, as is illustrated by a trace from the 50th depolarization in the pulse train. The additional block is use-dependent block (also called *frequency-dependent block*, *voltage-dependent block*, or *state-dependent block*, among other terms).[6] Use-dependent block is thought to be crucial to antiarrhythmic drug action because the effect will be more prominent at rapid heart rates during tachycardia.

Use-dependent block occurs because block develops during depolarization (electrical systole) and dissipates after repolarization (electrical diastole). Figure 16-3 shows three cardiac action potentials at a slower rate (see Fig. 16-3A) and a faster rate (see Fig. 16-3B). Block develops exponentially during depolarization (see Fig. 16-3C) and recovers exponentially during repolarization. If block has not recovered completely before the next depolarization occurs, then the new block develops from a higher level than in the previous cycle, and block accumulates (solid line in Fig. 16-3C). For the faster rate depicted in Figure 16-3B, the block for the second and third action potentials develops from higher levels (dashed line in Fig. 16-3B) because of less time for recovery from drug block. The amount of block that develops depends on several factors, including the frequency of depolarization and the duration of each action potential; of importance, it also depends on the recovery characteristics of the drug used to induce block. A drug with rapid recovery will give less block with the next depolarization than one with slower recovery. Furthermore, for

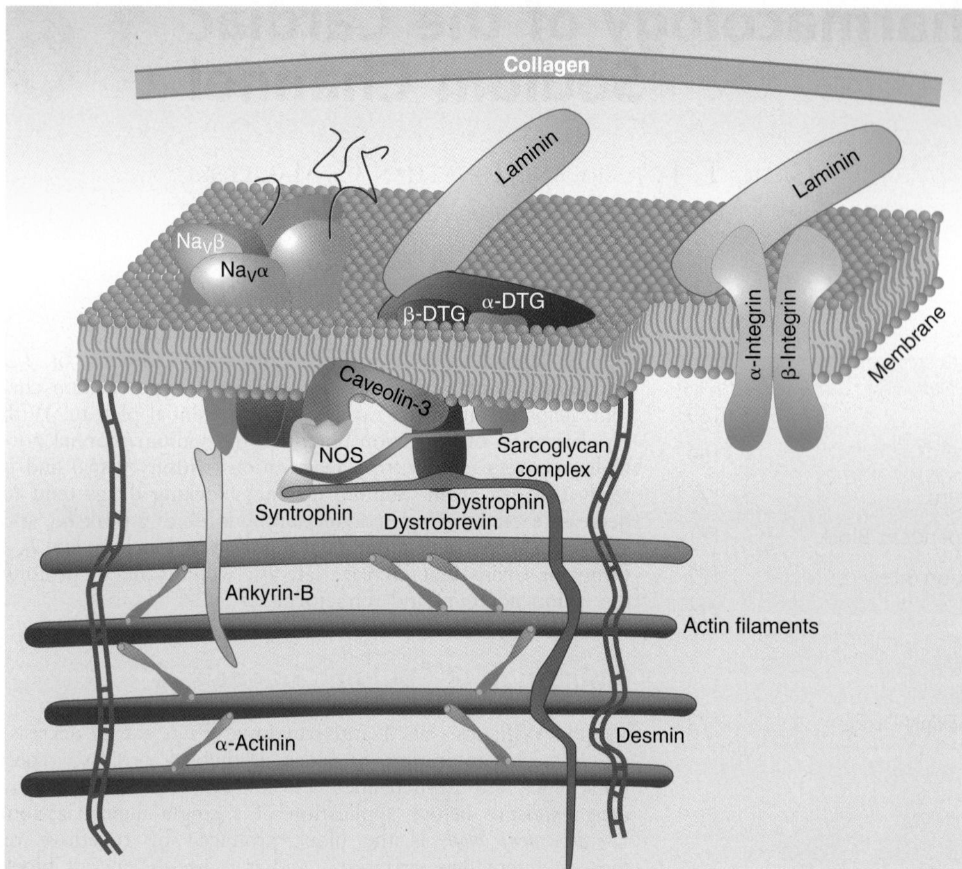

Figure 16-1 The sodium channel macromolecular complex. The sodium channel α and β subunits in the cell membrane undergo regulation by a complex array of interacting proteins and signaling pathways. (Modified from Adamson PB, Barr RC, Callans DJ, et al: The perplexing complexity of cardiac arrhythmias: Beyond electrical remodeling. Heart Rhythm 2:650-659, 2005.)

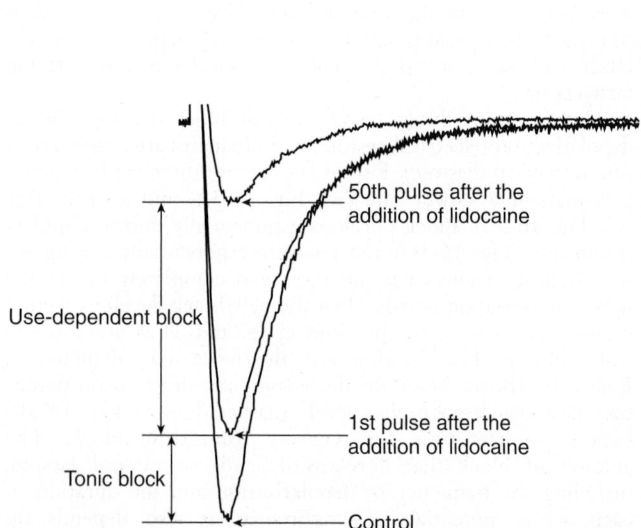

Figure 16-2 Picture of sodium current with block by lidocaine. Recordings show control I_{Na} and then I_{Na} after drug was added for the 1st and 50th depolarizations of a pulse train. Holding potential, −140 mV; depolarizing step to 20 mV.

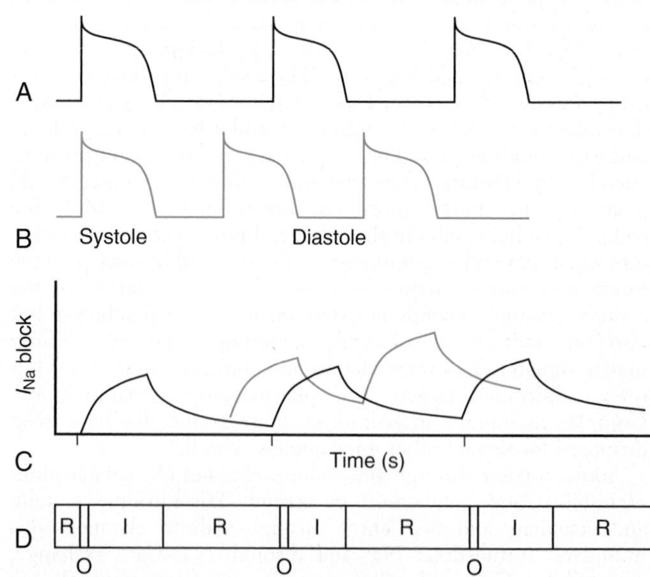

Figure 16-3 Use-dependent block of I_{Na}. **A** and **B** diagram ventricular action potentials applied at two rates. **C** shows the effect of rate on the use dependence of block. Block develops during depolarization (systole) and is relieved during repolarization (diastole). The faster rate is associated with greater accumulation of block. **D** shows a model of channel state transitions that correspond to those depicted in **A**. *Channel states*: R, resting; O, open; I, inactivated.

antiarrhythmic drugs, it is important to recognize that the recovery rate is dependent on parameters such as membrane voltage and generally is slowed by clinically important events such as membrane depolarization, ischemia, and acidosis.[7] Thus, antiarrhythmic drugs may have greater channel-blocking effects in disease states. This idea of phasic ion channel blockade incorporates very few assumptions about the underlying molecular mechanism, and in fact the molecular mechanisms behind use-dependent block are still a matter of debate, because interpretation of experimental data is necessarily model-dependent, and often the same set of data can be interpreted differently in the context of different models.

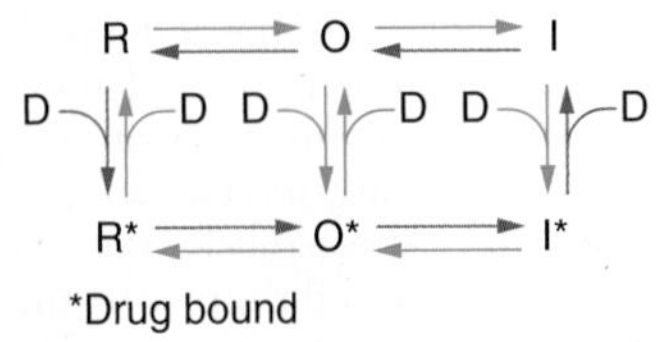

R ⇌ O ⇌ I

D D D D D D

R* ⇌ O* ⇌ I*

*Drug bound

Figure 16-4 Modulated-receptor model. This model postulated that the affinity of the drug (D) for the channel varied according to the kinetic state of the channel: R (resting), O (open), or I (inactivated). Kinetic transitions between drug-unbound and drug-bound states can be modeled by a series of rate constants.

Classification of Antiarrhythmic Drugs

Vaughn Williams proposed a classification scheme for antiarrhythmic drugs based on their effects on cardiac action potentials that has been modified and challenged through the past few decades but remains useful and is widely cited. Class I drugs (Table 16-1) originally were described as those that tended to decrease the upstroke velocity of the cardiac action potential and slow conduction velocity, and it was recognized that the mechanism was sodium current inhibition. Harrison[8] subdivided the classification for class I drugs into IA, IB, and IC on the basis of their effect on the electrocardiogram (ECG), conduction slowing, and action potential duration, as noted in Table 16-1. Campbell[9] demonstrated experimentally, using action potential upstroke velocity, that the kinetics of the onset of use-dependent block determined the classification and could account for the effects on the QRS duration. The clinical importance of this subclassification was emphasized in the wake of the Cardiac Arrhythmia Suppression Trial,[10] wherein class IC drugs, those with the slowest kinetics for onset of block, were found to increase mortality rate among patients with minor ventricular ectopy following myocardial infarction. In the Vaughan Williams classification, drugs that prolong action potential duration and prolong the QT interval are in class III, and these drugs generally block potassium channels. Drugs in class IA such as quinidine also have been shown to block potassium channels, and this is the most likely mechanism for action potential and QT interval prolongation. Of note, most drugs in the Vaughn Williams classification scheme are now known to block multiple ion channels, with varying affinities and kinetics.

Molecular Mechanisms for Use-Dependent Block

The *modulated-receptor model* for use-dependent block was derived independently by Hille for nerve tissue[11] and by Hondeghem and Katzung[12] for heart tissue (Fig. 16-4). This model postulated that the affinity of the drug for the channel varied according to the kinetic state of the channel. During each cardiac cycle, sodium channels go through multiple distinct "states" (see Fig. 16-3D). At resting potentials, the channel is in a closed or resting state (R). With the initiation of depolarization, the channel transiently changes to the open state (O), in which it conducts Na^+ ions to generate I_{Na}. With continued depolarization, the channel changes to an inactivated state (I) in which it does not conduct Na^+ ions, and with membrane repolarization, the channel quickly recovers to R. These states are thought to correspond to specific molecular configurations of the channel protein. If the affinity of a drug to bind to the O or I conformation of the channel is greater than for R, then drug binding will be favored during systole and unbinding will be favored during diastole. In the context of the modulated-receptor model, it is of interest to determine whether or not the drug interacts preferentially with the O or I conformation (or both). Some drugs show increased binding as a depolarizing step is prolonged; this effect is taken to suggest preferential binding to the I conformation because this state is maintained during depolarization. Other drugs do not depend on the duration of the depolarization; this lack of correlation is interpreted as interaction of the drug with the O conformation channel, because the dwell time in the transient open state does not depend on the duration of the depolarization. Other interpretations are

Table 16-1 Harrison/Campbell Class I Modifications of the Vaughn Williams Scheme

Class	Examples	ECG Effect	Harrison	Campbell	Primary State Dependence
1A	Quinidine Procainamide Disopyramide	Prolong QT interval	Slow conduction, Prolong APD	Intermediate use-dependent kinetics	Open state
1B	Lidocaine Mexiletine Tocainide	Little effect	Little effect on conduction or APD in physiologic conditions	Rapid use-dependent kinetics	Inactivated state
1C	Flecainide Propafenone	Prolong QRS duration	Markedly slow conduction	Slow use-dependent kinetics	Open state

APD, action potential duration; ECG, electrocardiogram.

possible however. The kinetics of the sodium channel are not as simple as in a three-state model. The channel actually passes through several "pre-O" transient states on the way to opening, and the drug could preferentially interact with the channel in one or another of these states. Alternatively, the drug could interact very quickly and come to equilibrium with the channel within even a very short depolarization and thus exhibits no interactions with longer depolarizations. The sodium channel gating scheme also contains potentially numerous "slow" or "intermediate" inactivated states. The classification into fast or slow inactivated states may be useful for clinical action, because in general, open channel–blocking drugs tend to be positively charged and have slower recovery kinetics than inactivated state blockers (see Table 16-1). Interaction with the R conformation channel would produce tonic block, which is not considered here because tonic block is not a feature of antiarrhythmic drugs at therapeutic doses.

An alternative model for antiarrhythmic drug effect, the *guarded-receptor model*,[13] was proposed as a potential simplifying explanation for use-dependent block. It postulated a fixed affinity of drug for the channel, as is typical of many ligand-mediated receptors, but with access to the channel receptor varied by drug trapping and guarding functions to produce apparent state-dependent differences in drug affinity. This model could reproduce many of the use-dependent properties of drug block of I_{Na}. In the end, however, the guarded-receptor model alone probably cannot account for all of the experimental data, such as altered gating of drug-bound channels,[14] a key implication of the modulated-receptor model.

Another, often unstated assumption of these drug block models is that a drug-bound channel is "plugged" and cannot conduct. It also is possible that drug binding simply favors maintenance of a nonconducting channel conformation. Indeed, Khodorov and coworkers originally proposed drug block of sodium channels as "stabilization of the inactivated state,"[15] and later investigators have proposed variations on this concept to account for drug effects.[16] Another possibility is that the drug decreases single-channel conductance, but in those few instances in which this appeared to occur, more detailed studies showed that this effect was due to "flicker block," a rapid opening and closing of the channel that when filtered only appeared to decrease conductance.

These differences may be of kinetic and biophysical interest, but as a matter of practicality, the effects of the drugs in patients may be dominated by regional, tissue, and cellular differences such as the effect of the longer action potentials in heart, different resting potentials, and frequency of the rhythm, rather than an intrinsic difference in channel affinity. A simple example is lidocaine, whose effect increases with longer depolarizations because of prominent inactivated state binding. Thus, lidocaine affects ventricular tissue more than atrial tissue owing to the longer action potential duration in the ventricle than in atrium, and it would affect nerve and muscle tissue even less owing to the very short action potentials in those tissues. Recently, heterogeneity in cardiac sodium channel structure, including very common genetic polymorphisms and ubiquitous splice variants, has been reported.[17] The possible differential pharmacology of these channels has not yet been described.

Molecular Biology of Drug Interaction Sites

Earlier studies had suggested a drug interaction site on the intracellular side of the pore of the sodium channel because membrane nonpermeable drugs acted only from the inside and not the outside, and external Na^+ could compete with the drug block presumably by accessing the site through the pore.[18] The cloning and sequencing of $Na_V1.5$ and other sodium channels allowed testing of this idea by the expression of channels with mutations designed to alter putative interaction sites.

Site-directed mutagenesis first suggested that domain IVS6[19] was important for local anesthetic block, and later evidence also showed a role for S6 in the other domains.[20,21] The same sites on S6 were shown to be important for many Vaughan Williams class I drugs, and more recently for the antianginal drug ranolazine.[22] The linker between domains III and IV was shown to be involved with inactivation and to affect drug interaction,[23] and further studies showed that part of the III-IV inactivation linker may be directly involved with the interaction site,[24] rather than acting by altering inactivation. The pore region of domain I[25] and domain III[26] also has been implicated in antiarrhythmic drug binding. The connector between S4 and S5 in domain III also is involved in inactivation,[27] and recent evidence suggests that the S4-S5 connector in all domains of the cardiac sodium channel play a role in lidocaine interaction with the channel.[28]

The voltage dependence of inactivation affects drug block; a negative shift in inactivation will increase apparent block, and a positive shift will decrease it. Accordingly, mutations that shift inactivation may potentially be misinterpreted as a direct effect at the binding site. Separating these two can be very difficult, but when inactivation is unshifted, or when the shift in inactivation is in the opposite direction for the effect on block, then the mutation can be interpreted as being at the interaction site. The β1 subunit affected lidocaine block of the channel[29] independently of effects on gating. Effects of the β2, β3, and β4 subunits on drug binding are unknown.

Finally, recent elegant molecular models of drug interaction with the sodium channel have been developed. For example, molecular models of lidocaine binding suggest that it docks within the channel with its positive charge below the selectivity filter to partially occlude the channel pore but also to generate an electrostatic barrier to Na^+ permeation.[29a,29b] Thus, these models suggest that the mechanism of sodium channel block by lidocaine involves drug binding within the open/inactivated channel to narrow of the pore lumen (steric block) and to create an electrostatic barrier to Na^+ movement through the pore.

Block of Late Sodium Channels

A small (less than 1% of peak) I_{Na} persists during a long depolarization, and this may be a target for selective blockade. The late opening of single sodium channels under these conditions was shown many years ago, and block of late I_{Na} by tetrodotoxin (TTX) was shown to shorten action potential duration.[30] Increase in late I_{Na} by various toxins (ATX-II, APA, and others) can cause prolongation of cardiac action potentials, thereby generating experimental models of acquired and congenital long QT syndrome (LQT3) (see Chapters 19 and 49). More recently it has been appreciated that entry of Na^+ through late I_{Na} may affect sodium-calcium homeostasis to play a role in contractility and ischemia.[31] Selective block of late I_{Na} over peak I_{Na} has been shown for drugs such as mexiletine[32] and flecainide,[33] which were about three times more potent for block of late I_{Na} over peak I_{Na} when studied in heterologously expressed LQT3 mutations. Ranolazine, in similar experiments, exerted approximately 10-fold preferential block of late I_{Na} over peak I_{Na} for two LQT3 mutations.[22] When studied in native myocytes from failing dog hearts, the relative selectivity for late I_{Na} over peak I_{Na} was approximately 3-fold for lidocaine, approximately 13-fold for amiodarone, and approximately 38-fold for ranolazine.[34]

Drug Effects on Channel Trafficking: Novel Antiarrhythmic Drug Effects

Drug- and temperature-dependent modification (improvement, correction, or "rescue") of post-translational ion channel protein trafficking within mammalian cells has been described for the cystic fibrosis chloride channel[35] and the HERG (human ether-à-go-go) potassium channel. For the sodium channel, mexiletine increases messenger RNA (mRNA) for the channel[36] in rat cardiac muscle. Mexiletine also is capable of rescuing expression of a human trafficking–deficient sodium channel mutation, M1766L.[37] This may be a more general effect, because for the Brugada mutation, G1743R, the expression also is rescued by drugs.[38] Although in their infancy, drug-induced transcriptional modification and post-translational rescue of ion channel protein biogenesis and trafficking have the potential for development as new antiarrhythmic therapeutic agents for use in human heart disease.

Specificity of Sodium Channel–Blocking Drugs

Virtually all clinically relevant sodium channel–blocking drugs lack perfect specificity for sodium channels. Sodium channel–blocking drugs or those in Vaughn Williams class I (see Table 16-1) usually are thought to have sodium channel block as their primary mode of action at therapeutic doses in vivo, but many of these drugs also block other channels and receptors. Potassium channel block by the class IA drugs is widely recognized and can be a source of significant toxicity. Many sodium channel blockers suppress calcium (mainly L-type) channels. Drugs such as propafenone act as β-adrenergic receptor–blocking agents. Amiodarone usually is considered to exert mainly a class III effect, but it has prominent effects on the sodium channel, and it also blocks calcium channels, potassium channels, and β-adrenergic receptors and has effects in several noncardiac tissues and organs. Hence, pharmacologic effects of sodium channel–active antiarrhythmic drugs are complex, and effects on other channels or receptors must be considered in assessing their clinical actions.

References

1. Goldin AL: Evolution of voltage-gated Na(+) channels. J Exp Biol 205:575-584, 2002.
2. Maier SK, Westenbroek RE, Schenkman KA, et al: An unexpected role for brain-type sodium channels in coupling of cell surface depolarization to contraction in the heart. Proc Natl Acad Sci U S A 99:4073-4078, 2002.
3. Adamson PB, Barr RC, Callans DJ, et al: The perplexing complexity of cardiac arrhythmias: Beyond electrical remodeling. Heart Rhythm 2:650-659, 2005.
4. Balijepalli RC, Foell JD, Hall DD, et al: Localization of cardiac L-type Ca(2+) channels to a caveolar macromolecular signaling complex is required for beta(2)-adrenergic regulation. Proc Natl Acad Sci U S A 103:7500-7505, 2006.
5. Balijepalli RC, Delisle BP, Balijepalli SY, et al: Kv11.1 (ERG1) K^+ channels localize in cholesterol- and sphingolipid-enriched membranes and are modulated by membrane cholesterol. Channels 1:263-272, 2007.
6. Courtney KR: Mechanism of frequency-dependent inhibition of sodium currents in frog myelinated nerve by the lidocaine derivative GEA. J Pharmacol Exp Ther 195:225-236, 1975.
7. Campbell TJ, Wyse KR, Hemsworth PD: Effects of hyperkalemia, acidosis, and hypoxia on the depression of maximum rate of depolarization by class I antiarrhythmic drugs in guinea pig myocardium: Differential actions of class Ib and Ic agents. J Cardiovasc Pharmacol 18:51-59, 1991.
8. Harrison DC: Symposium on the perspectives on treatment of ventricular arrhythmias: Introduction. Am J Cardiol 52:1C-2C, 1983.
9. Campbell TJ: Subclassification of class I antiarrhythmic drugs: Enhanced relevance after CAST. Cardiovasc Drugs Ther 6:519-528, 1992.
10. The Cardiac Arrhythmia Suppression Trial (CAST) investigators: Preliminary report: Effect of encainide and flecainide on mortality in a randomized trial of arrhythmia suppression after myocardial infarction. N Engl J Med 321:406-412, 1989.
11. Hille B: Local anesthetics: Hydrophilic and hydrophobic pathways for the drug-receptor reaction. J Gen Physiol 69: 497-515, 1977.
12. Hondeghem LM, Katzung BG: Time- and voltage-dependent interactions of antiarrhythmic drugs with cardiac sodium channels. Biochim Biophys Acta 472:373-398, 1977.
13. Starmer CF, Grant AO, Strauss HC: Mechanisms of use-dependent block of sodium channels in excitable membranes by local anesthetics. Biophys J 46:15-27, 1984.
14. Hanck DA, Makielski JC, Sheets MF: Lidocaine alters activation gating of cardiac Na channels. Pflügers Arch 439:814-821, 2000.
15. Khodorov BI, Shishkova E, Peganov E, Revenko S: Inhibition of sodium currents in frog Ranvier node treated with local anesthetics. Role of slow sodium inactivation. Biochim Biophys Acta 433:409-435, 1976.
16. Balser JR, Nuss HB, Orias DW, et al: Local anesthetics as effectors of allosteric gating. Lidocaine effects on inactivation-deficient rat skeletal muscle Na channels. J Clin Invest 98:2874-2886, 1996.
17. Makielski JC, Ye B, Valdivia CR, et al: A ubiquitous splice variant and a common polymorphism affect heterologous expression of recombinant human SCN5A heart sodium channels. Circ Res 93:821-828, 2003.
18. Strichartz GR: The inhibition of sodium currents in myelinated nerve by quaternary derivatives of lidocaine. J Gen Physiol 62:37-57, 1973.
19. Ragsdale DS, Mcphee JC, Scheuer T, Catterall WA: Molecular determinants of state-dependent block of Na^+ channels by local anesthetics. Science 265:1724-1728, 1994.
20. Yarov-Yarovoy V, Brown J, Sharp EM, et al: Molecular determinants of voltage-dependent gating and binding of pore-blocking drugs in transmembrane segment IIIS6 of the Na(+) channel alpha subunit. J Biol Chem 276:20-27, 2001.
21. Yarov-Yarovoy V, Mcphee JC, Idsvoog D, et al: Role of amino acid residues in transmembrane segments IS6 and IIS6 of the Na^+ channel alpha subunit in voltage-dependent gating and drug block. J Biol Chem 277:35393-35401, 2002.
22. Fredj S, Sampson KJ, Liu H, Kass RS: Molecular basis of ranolazine block of LQT-3 mutant sodium channels: Evidence for site of action. Br J Pharmacol 148:16-24, 2006.
23. Bennett PB, Valenzuela C, Chen LQ, Kallen RG: On the molecular nature of the lidocaine receptor of cardiac Na^+ channels. Modification of block by alterations in the alpha-subunit III-IV interdomain. Circ Res 77:592, 1995.
24. Fan Z, George ALJ, Kyle JW, Makielski JC: Two human paramyotonia congenita mutations have opposite effects on lidocaine block of Na^+ channels expressed in a mammalian cell line. J Physiol (Lond) 496:275-286, 1996.
25. Sunami A, Glaaser IW, Fozzard HA: A critical residue for isoform difference in tetrodotoxin affinity is a molecular determinant of the external access path for local

anesthetics in the cardiac sodium channel. Proc Natl Acad Sci U S A 97:2326-2331, 2000.

26. Sunami A, Dudley SC Jr, Fozzard HA: Sodium channel selectivity filter regulates antiarrhythmic drug binding. Proc Natl Acad Sci U S A 94:14126-14131, 1997.
27. Smith MR, Goldin AL: Interaction between the sodium channel inactivation linker and domain III S4-S5. Biophys J 73:1885-1895, 1997.
28. Ye B: Structure-function of the cardiac sodium channel (*SCN5A*/Nav 1.5)—the common background sequence and the effects of naturally ocurring and designed mutations. PhD thesis, University of Wisconsin–Madison, 2002.
29. Makielski JC, Limberis JT, Chang SY, et al: Coexpression of β1 with cardiac sodium channel α subunits in oocytes decreases lidocaine block. Mol Pharmacol 49:30-39, 1996.

29a. McNulty MM, Edgerton GB, Shah RD, et al: Charge at the lidocaine binding site residue Phe-1759 affects permeation in human cardiac voltage-gated sodium channels. J Physiol 581:741-755, 2007.

29b. Lipkind GM, Fozzard HA: Molecular modeling of local anesthetic drug binding by voltage-gated sodium channels. Mol Pharmacol 68:1611-1622, 2005.

30. Dudel J, Peper K, Rudel R, Trautwein W: Effect of tetrodotoxin on membrane currents in mammalian cardiac fibres. Nature 213:296-297, 1967.
31. Saint DA: The cardiac persistent sodium current: An appealing therapeutic target?. Br.J.Pharmacol 153:1133-1142, 2008.
32. Dumaine R, Wang Q, Keating MT, et al: Multiple mechanisms of Na^+ channel–linked long-QT syndrome. Circ Res 78:916-924, 1996.
33. Nagatomo T, January CT, Makielski JC: Preferential block of late sodium current in the LQT3 ΔKPQ mutant by the class I(C) antiarrhythmic flecainide. Mol Pharmacol 57:101-107, 2000.
34. Undrovinas AI, Belardinelli L, Undrovinas NA, Sabbah HN: Ranolazine improves abnormal repolarization and contraction in left ventricular myocytes of dogs with heart failure by inhibiting late sodium current. J Cardiovasc Electrophysiol 17(Suppl 1):S169-S177, 2006.
35. Denning GM, Anderson MP, Amara JF, et al: Processing of mutant cystic fibrosis transmembrane conductance regulator is temperature-sensitive. Nature 358:761-764, 1992.
36. Delisle BP, Anson BD, Rajamani S, January CT: Biology of cardiac arrhythmias: Ion channel protein trafficking. Circ Res 94:1418-1428, 2004.
37. Valdivia CR, Ackerman MJ, Tester DA, et al: A novel *SCN5A* arrhythmia mutation, M1766L, with expression defect rescued by mexiletine. Cardiovasc Res 54:624-629, 2002.
38. Valdivia CR, Tester DA, Makielski JC, Ackerman MJ: Clinical, molecular, and functional characterization of a *SCN5A* Brugada syndrome mutation with expression defect rescued by mexiletine [abstract]. Circulation 106:II-283, 2002.

Pharmacology of L-type and T-type Calcium Channels in the Heart 17

XIONGWEN CHEN AND STEVEN R. HOUSER

Overview of L-type and T-type Calcium Channels

Calcium influx during the early phases of the cardiac action potential is essential, because it triggers the release of Ca^{2+} from the sarcoplasmic reticulum, thereby elevating cytoplasmic Ca^{2+} to initiate contraction. Two types of voltage-dependent calcium channels, L-type and T-type calcium channels (L and T for "long-opening" and "tiny-conductance," respectively), have been found in the heart. The L-type calcium channel (LTCC), also referred to as Ca_V1,[1] is the predominant calcium channel in adult ventricle and is the principal focus of this chapter. Much less is known about the functional significance of the T-type calcium channel (TTCC).

LTCCs are present in every cardiac myocyte, and Ca^{2+} influx through these channels has many important functions. In sinoatrial node cells, the current through the LTCC, $I_{Ca,L}$, contributes to their pacemaker activity and is primarily responsible for the upstroke of the action potential. $I_{Ca,L}$ also is responsible for the upstroke of the action potential in cells in the atrioventricular node and is the principal determinant of conduction velocity through this region of the heart. In atrial, ventricular, and His-Purkinje myocytes, the sodium current is responsible for the rapid upstroke of the action potential, and the slower activation of $I_{Ca,L}$ makes a significant contribution to the shape of the action potential plateau phase, which prevents reentry arrhythmias.

The LTCC is centrally involved in many signaling pathways. The best-understood Ca^{2+} influx–mediated signaling function is excitation-contraction coupling. Ca^{2+} influx through the LTCC is necessary for inducing and grading Ca^{2+} release from the sarcoplasmic reticulum and is the major source of Ca^{2+} to load the sarcoplasmic reticulum.[2] It is now believed that in the normal heart, sufficient LTCC activation occurs with each heart beat to induce Ca^{2+} release from all regions of sarcoplasmic reticulum.[3] This triggering effect is a major function of the LTCC. The magnitude of the $I_{Ca,L}$ also is a major determinant of the strength of the heart beat (contractility). Usually the increase in the $I_{Ca,L}$ results from increased sympathetic nerve stimulation, which, by a β-adrenergic signaling cascade, leads to an increase in LTCC opening probability. This additional Ca^{2+} influx results in an increase in sarcoplasmic reticulum Ca^{2+} loading and release, to produce increased cardiac contractile function.

Recently, we have shown that persistent increases in Ca^{2+} influx through the LTCC can induce ventricular myocyte hypertrophy,[4] and that if the Ca^{2+} influx is excessive, it can produce myocyte death through both apoptosis[5] and necrosis.[4] Because of the central role of the LTCC in the initiation of the heart beat, conduction of the action potential through the atrioventricular node, duration of the plateau phase of the action potential, regulation of cardiac contractility, and induction of myocyte death pathways, drugs that modify the behavior of these channels have significant impact on the electrical, contractile, and survival functions of heart.

TTCCs (collectively named Ca_V3 according to the nomenclature of calcium channels[1]) are activated and inactivated at membrane potentials about 30 mV more negative than for the LTCCs. Compared with LTCCs, TTCCs have lower unit conductance, faster inactivation, and slower deactivation kinetics. TTCCs are encoded by three genes, $\alpha 1_G$ ($Ca_V3.1$), $\alpha 1_H$ ($Ca_V3.2$), and $\alpha 1_I$ ($Ca_V3.3$), with alternative splicing.[1,6] Whether or not TTCCs have auxiliary subunits is not clear because the pore-forming α subunit is adequate to constitute the channel activity in heterologous expression systems,[6] although γ5 subunit has been shown to be able to regulate $\alpha 1_G$.[7] The channel proteins encoded by these genes have slightly different biophysical and pharmacologic properties.[8] For example, $Ca_V3.2$ is more sensitive to Ni^{2+}, with a half-maximal inhibitory concentration (IC_{50}) of approximately 10 μM, whereas $Ca_V3.1$ and $Ca_V3.3$ have an IC_{50} of greater than 100 μM.[6]

Much less is known about the functional roles of TTCC in cardiac myocytes, especially in ventricular myocytes (see Chapter 2). These channels are much less abundant than LTCCs, and they are not expressed in all cardiac myocytes in the adult heart. An interesting feature of these channels is that their expression is developmentally regulated.[9] TTCCs are abundant in the fetal and neonatal heart, but the channels disappear fairly rapidly—in ventricular myocytes, after birth.[10] Most studies have shown that in the adult heart, current through the TTCC ($I_{Ca,T}$) is not present in ventricular myocytes. TTCCs are found in the adult heart in myocytes of the sinoatrial node, atrioventricular node, Purkinje fibers, and atria. In these cells, $I_{Ca,T}$ is involved in spontaneous rhythm generation and in conduction.[10] Mice in which the $\alpha 1_G$ TTCC has been knocked out exhibit sinus bradycardia, consistent with the pacemaking role of the TTCC.

We also have shown that $I_{Ca,T}$ is reexpressed in the adult heart with hypertrophy in response to persistent pressure overload.[11] These results suggest that TTCCs may be involved in hypertrophic growth signaling. The functional role of $I_{Ca,T}$ in hypertrophied ventricular myocytes is still not well understood. It is now clear, however, that $I_{Ca,T}$ is not an efficient inducer for Ca^{2+} release from the sarcoplasmic reticulum,[12] consistent with

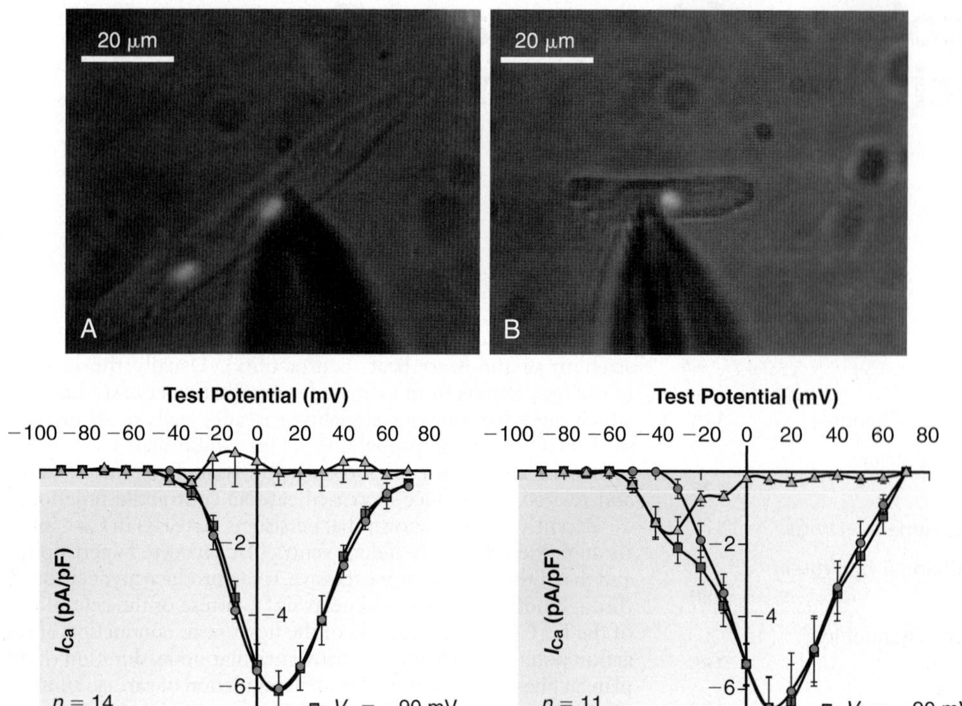

Figure 17-1 T-type calcium current is expressed in small mononucleated myocytes (approximately 12% of all ventricular myocytes) but not in large binucleated (approximately 87% of all ventricular myocytes) adolescent feline ventricular myocytes. **A** and **B**, Representative small mononucleated (**A**) and large binucleated feline ventricular myocytes (**B**), used for electrophysiologic measurements, are shown. The nucleus in live ventricular myocytes is stained with a DNA dye, Hoechst 33258. **C** and **D**, Average data from calcium current recordings at the holding potentials of −90 mV (*purple square*) and −50 mV (*red circle*), respectively, and the differences ($I_{Ca,T}$, *blue triangle*) in these cells.

the idea that it may be involved in Ca^{2+} signaling in ways that are fundamentally different from those for $I_{Ca,L}$.

Recent studies have shown that the TTCC is uniquely expressed in subpopulations of small mononucleated ventricular myocytes in the adolescent heart[13] (Fig. 17-1). These studies suggest that TTCCs are involved in the proliferation of newly forming cardiac myocytes, through a yet-to-be-determined signaling pathway.[13] Supporting this idea is the observation that the TTCC also is expressed in the newly formed cardiac myocytes differentiated from c-Kit–positive cardiac stem cells.[13] These recent findings indicate that in the adult heart, the TTCC may play an important role in the hypertrophy of mature cardiac myocytes and also may be involved in the generation of new cardiac myocytes that are derived from a resident cardiac stem cell. If this is so, drugs that influence Ca^{2+} influx through the TTCC could be of benefit in patients with pathologic cardiac hypertrophy and cardiac rhythm disturbances and for promoting cardiac regeneration.

Structure and Function of the L-type Calcium Channel

Structure and function of the L-type calcium channel are described in detail in Chapter 2 and are reviewed here only to provide appropriate context for understanding the effects of drugs and signaling pathways that alter the properties of LTCC, as discussed next.

Structure

The cardiac LTCC (also named $Ca_V1.2$[1]) is composed of four subunits: α1 β, γ, and α2/δ. The α1 subunit is the pore-forming subunit, with a molecular mass of approximately 230 kD. It was first cloned in 1989.[14] The molecular structure and the functional roles of different portions of the α subunit have been well studied.[15] The α1 subunit of the LTCC has the prototypical structure of other voltage-sensitive ion channels, such as sodium channels. It is a large membrane protein with four domains (I to IV) of similar structure, each having six transmembrane segments, S1 to S6. The α1 subunit is arranged within the membrane to form a Ca^{2+}-selective pore, with the S5 and S6 segments of each domain lining the channel pore. The S4 segments of each domain contain charged amino acids that are thought to impart the voltage-sensing function of the channel. Both the amino (N) and carboxyl (C) termini of the molecule are intracellular and are importantly involved in the regulation of channel function.

The α1 subunit is capable of mediating $I_{Ca,L}$ without the involvement of other subunits. However, strong evidence exists for auxiliary LTCC subunits that serve to modulate the expression and the gating of the α subunit. The β subunit is a small (51- to 71-kD) protein without transmembrane-spanning domains. This cytosolic protein influences the behavior of the LTCC and also appears to serve as a molecular chaperone to traffic the α subunit to the appropriate location on the surface membrane.[16] Four β genes with many different splicing variants when expressed have been found in cardiac myocytes.[16] Eight γ subunit genes have been cloned as well. This subunit has been believed to be associated with the $\alpha 1_C$. The functional role of this subunit is not entirely clear, however.[7] It may modulate the $\alpha 1_C$ subunit to a small extent and have some nonchannel functions.[17] The α_2 and δ subunits are from one gene product that undergoes post-translational cleavage. They are linked to each other with disulfide bonds. The δ subunit has a transmembrane segment that anchors the extracellular α2 subunit to the membrane. The α2 subunit interacts with α1 and influences its biophysical properties (activation time of $I_{Ca,L}$).[18] Four genes encoding α2/δ subunit have been cloned.

Functions

Ca^{2+} influx through the LTCC involves voltage- and Ca^{2+}-dependent transitions in channel conformation that cause the pore-forming α1 subunit to transiently allow permeation of Ca^{2+} into the myocyte. At the normal resting potential of cardiac myocytes (approximately −80 mV), the LTCC is primarily in a closed (C) but available (to open with depolarization) state. Depolarization of the surface membrane (and of the transverse tubules [T tubules]) causes an LTCC conformational change that leads to opening (O) of the α1 subunit pore, and Ca^{2+} moves into the cell down its electrochemical gradient. As with many other voltage-sensitive ion channels, depolarization also leads to channel inactivation, so that the channel open time is short-lived. Inactivation of the LTCC is more complex than that of many other voltage-regulated ion channels, however, because it has a very strong Ca^{2+}-dependent component.[19] This Ca^{2+}-dependent component causes larger calcium currents to inactivate at a faster rate than tha observed for smaller ones, providing a potent negative feedback effect on Ca^{2+} influx, which prevents sarcoplasmic reticulum Ca^{2+} overload. With each action potential, Ca^{2+} permeates the LTCC, and the Ca^{2+} influx, together with the induced Ca^{2+} release from the sarcoplasmic reticulum, regulates LTCC inactivation.

Drugs and signaling cascades that influence $I_{Ca,L}$ do so by altering these LTCC state transitions. The size of the whole-cell $I_{Ca,L}$ during any set of conditions is determined by the number (N) of available channels, the average probability (P_0) at any time (t) that LTCCs will open, and the magnitude of the current through a single channel (i).

$$I_{Ca,L} = N(t) \times i \times P_0(t)$$

Modulation of the L-type Calcium Channel by Drugs

The LTCC plays critical roles in the regulation of cardiac contractility and in the constriction of vascular smooth muscle. The molecular identity of the LTCC in these two tissues is the same, but the resting potential in cardiac myocytes is more negative than in smooth muscle. The relatively depolarized state of the vascular smooth muscle cells enhances the inactivated state of LTCC, so many LTCC-blocking drugs affect smooth muscle without altering cardiac myocytes.

Drugs modifying the LTCC have been developed to treat cardiovascular diseases, such as hypertension, angina, and arrhythmia.[20] These drugs function primarily by blocking Ca^{2+} influx into smooth muscle cells in the vasculature, with minimal effects on the heart. New drugs with higher specificity are still under development for disease treatments. This section summarizes the LTCC drugs already developed and provides some information on those ones still under development.

Classes of L-type Calcium Channel Agonists and Antagonists

At present, three major classes of structurally unrelated chemical compounds are in clinical use to alter the behavior of LTCC—namely, dihydropyridines (DHPs), phenylalkylamines (PAAs or ΦAAs), and benzothiazepines (BZTs) (Fig. 17-2). Common DHP derivatives include amlodipine, azidopine, Bay K 8644, CGP 28392, FRC-8653, H-160-51, iodipine, nifedipine, nimodipne, nisoldipine, nitredipine, PN 200-110, S-202-791, and YC-170. Most DHPs are LTCC antagonists that block L-type calcium current. The exceptions are (−)Bay K 8644, CGP 28392, FRC-8653, H-160-51, (+)S-202-791, and YC-170, which can increase the L-type calcium current and have thus been termed LTCC agonists. All PAAs and BZTs are LTCC antagonists. PAAs include verapamil, D600, D888, and D890. BZTs have fewer derivatives, the most common of which is diltiazem. These LTCC agonists and antagonists have specific binding sites on LTCC that have been defined using either membrane impermeant techniques (using permanently charged forms of drugs or photoaffinity labeling) or molecular biology techniques to generate deletion mutants or chimeric channels.[21] These studies have lead to the development of current structural and functional models of the LTCC.[21]

Drug-Binding Sites

The mechanism of the actions of these three classes of LTCC agonists and antagonists can be well explained with classical ligand receptor models. This theory predicts that charged or uncharged drugs gain access to their specific binding sites either from the aqueous phase (intra- and extracellular, or intrapore) or by dissolving in the membrane lipid phase, respectively. The binding of these drugs to the α1 subunit of the LTCC has now been well established, and it is this binding that influences the permeation of Ca^{2+} into cardiac myocytes during the course of the action potential.

Charged or uncharged forms of LTCC antagonists were first used to gain insight into the location of drug binding. These studies showed that extracellular application of charged forms of DHPs or PAAs was ineffective[21] and that the effectiveness was increased when the fraction of uncharged forms was augmented.[22] Intracellular application of the charged form of DHPs also was ineffective, suggesting that *uncharged forms of DHPs* are favored and a location for binding that involves the membrane lipid environment. Intracellular application of charged PAAs[21,23] effectively blocks $I_{Ca,L}$, indicating that PAAs have to enter the cytoplasm in their charged form to access their binding sites and that *charged forms of PAAs* are favored for binding. Diltiazem is able to block $I_{Ca,L}$ from both outside and inside of the cell, but the charged form (quaternary form) has a much lower LTCC affinity,[21,23] which indicates that the *uncharged form of diltiazem* is favored for binding.

Recombinant techniques, together with photoaffinity labeling and antibody mapping, have identified much more specific regions for binding of each of the three classes of calcium channel antagonists (or agonists)[21] (Fig. 17-3). DHPs, PAAs, and BZTs each appear to have separate binding sites, and the binding of one class of compound influences the others. Photoaffinity labeling has shown that the binding sites for DHPs, PAAs, and BZTs all are on α1 subunit. IIIS6 and IVS6 are the regions to which BZTs and DHPs appear to bind.[21] Experiments using chimeric channels from skeletal and cardiac forms of the LTCC revealed that IIIS5[24] also is required for DHP binding to the cardiac LTCC. Both IIIS6 and IVS6 are required for PAA binding.[25] The common feature of all of these experiments is that they suggest that these drugs impart their effects by binding to regions of the LTCC that are thought to be in or near the pore-forming portion of the channel (S5 and S6 segments).

Mutation analysis has further pinpointed the amino acid residues necessary for drug binding.[21,23] Residues that appear to be critical for DHP binding are Thr1039 and Gln1043 in IIIS5; Tyr1152, Ile1156, and Met1161 in IIIS6; and Asn1472 in IVS6. Recently it was shown that Ser1115 in the IIIS5-S6

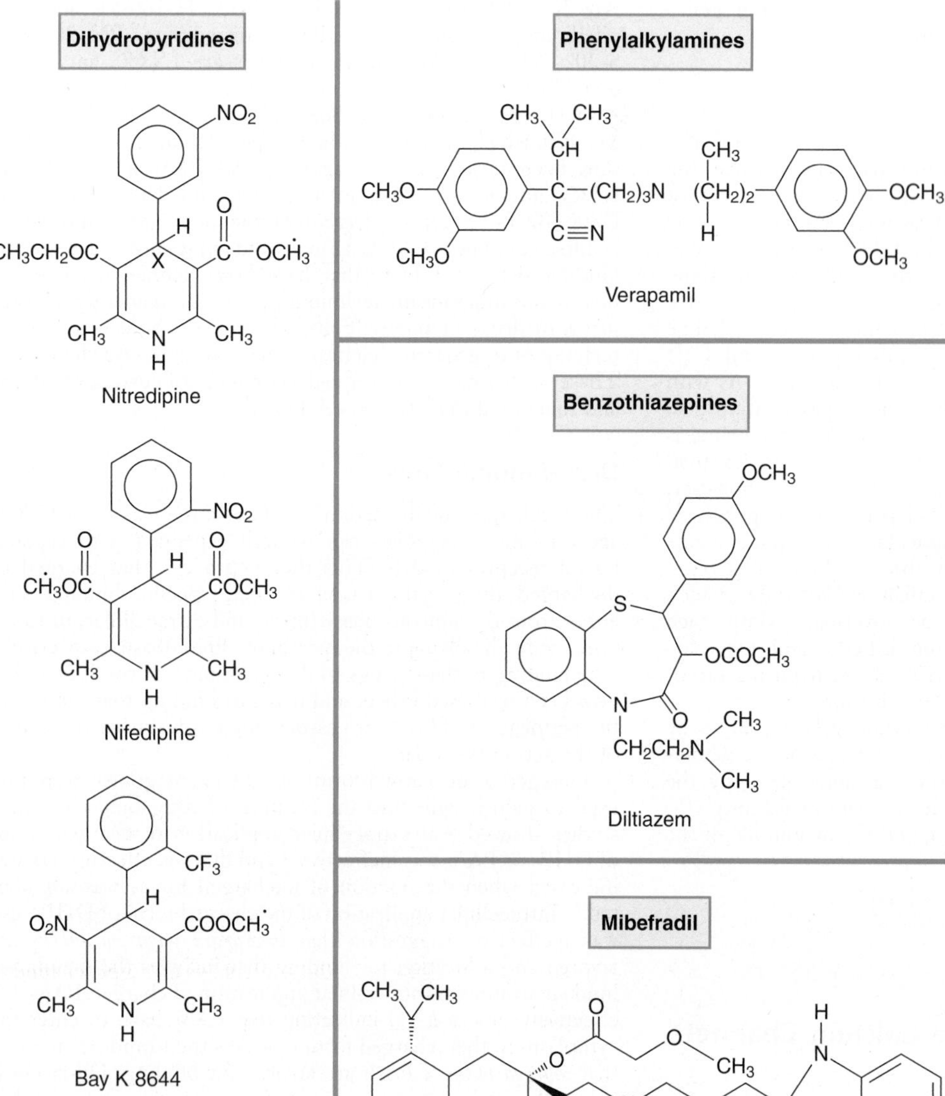

Figure 17-2 Chemical structures of representative agonists and antagonists of L- and T-type calcium channels (LTCC and TTCC). Mibefradil is an antagonist of the TTCC; the others are antagonists of the LTCC, except Bay K 8644, which is an LTCC agonist.

linker of α1 subunit also plays a critical role in DHP binding and in the action of DHP agonists.[26] The amino acid residues for PAA binding include Tyr1463, Ala1467, Ile1470, and Met1464 in IVS6 and Tyr1152, Ile1153, Phe1164, and Val1165 in IIIS6. For BZT binding, Tyr1463, Ala1467, and Ile1470 in IVS6 are necessary. A very recent study showed that IVS5 contributes to the blockade of $I_{Ca,L}$ by diltiazem.[27] These studies all suggest that the binding of these three classes of LTCC agonists and antagonists involves S6 segments that presumably participate in the formation of the channel pore. Furthermore, the common involvement of IVS6 may explain the interaction of binding of different classes of agonists and antagonists.

DHP and PAA binding is influenced by the extracellular concentration of Ca^{2+} and other cations. High concentrations of Ca^{2+} inhibit drug binding, indicating one or more calcium-binding sites should be included in an "allosterical model" of drug binding. Further studies in this regard led to a newer biochemical model that assumes two calcium-binding sites in the LTCC selectivity filter domain, one with high affinity and the other with relatively low affinity for Ca^{2+}. The model predicts that when only the high-affinity binding site is occupied, the LTCC is in a nonconductive state (inactivated state), and DHP antagonist binding is favored. In the presence of high concentrations of extracellular Ca^{2+}, the low-affinity binding site also would be occupied and permeation through LTCC is enabled. This model predicts that LTCC agonists influence the second Ca^{2+} binding to produce a highly conductive state and that antagonists stabilize calcium binding to the high-affinity binding site.[21,23]

Mechanisms of Actions of L-type Calcium Channel Agonists and Antagonists

LTCC antagonists are able to partially or completely block the whole-cell calcium current ($I_{Ca,L}$) without decreasing the amplitude of the current through a single LTCC ($i_{Ca,L}$). Experiments using single-channel recording techniques showed that both LTCC agonists and antagonists did not change the amplitude of the single-channel LTCC current ($i_{Ca,L}$). These studies show that Ca^{2+} antagonists and agonists do not change the

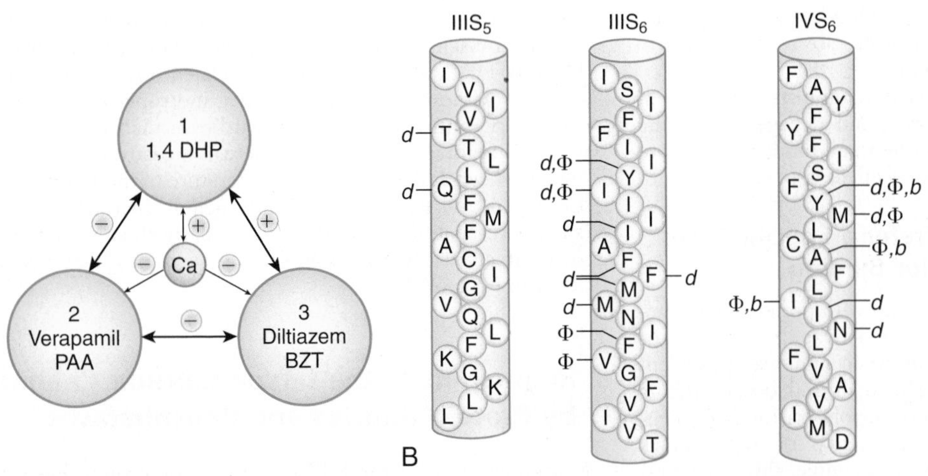

Figure 17-3 Antagonist binding to the L-type calcium channel (LTCC). **A**, Interactions of antagonist binding by a dihydropyridine (DHP), a phenylalkylamine (PAA), and a benzathiazepine (BZT) to the LTCC. For example, DHP binding to the LTCC enhances BZT and Ca^{2+} binding. **B**, Antagonist binding sites on IIIS5, IIIS6, and IVS6, transmembrane segments that are critical for DHP (*d*), PAA (Φ), and BZT (*b*). (**A** and **B**, From Bers DM: Excitation-Contraction Coupling and Cardiac Contractile Force, 2nd ed. Dordrecht, Kluwer Academic, 2001.)

conductance of individual charge-carrying channels but rather alter their ability to open and close. Partial block of $I_{Ca,L}$ by LTCC antagonists has little or no effect on the time course of activation,[28] but DHP antagonists accelerate $I_{Ca,L}$ inactivation by decreasing channel openings during prolonged depolarizations. PAAs and diltiazem (DLT) do not change the rate of decay of $I_{Ca,L}$, but some studies reported enhanced inactivation when Ba^{2+} was used as the charge carrier or in the presence of high concentration of antagonists.

All three classes of antagonists cause a negative shift of voltage dependence of inactivation, suggesting that they stabilize the channel in its inactivated state. This effect decreases the availability[29] and probability of opening (P_o) at the single channel level, and reduces the charge movement associated with channel activation (gating charge). At the single-channel level, DHP antagonists have little effect on open and closed times[30] but PAAs (e.g., D-600)[29] significantly shorten open time and prolong closed time. Less is known about the effects of BZTs on single LTCC but it has been suggested that diltiazem decreases P_o, with no significant effect on $i_{Ca,L}$ amplitude.[31] An important feature of all calcium channel antagonists is that binding (and associated effects) are significantly affected by membrane potential, with hyperpolarization (e.g., +100 mV) reducing antagonist binding. The dependency of LTCC antagonist binding and blocking on the membrane potential is the rationale for using LTCC antagonists to lower blood pressure in hypertension. At therapeutic concentrations, these LTCC antagonists relax vascular smooth muscle without reducing the contractility of the heart because, as stated earlier, vascular smooth muscle cells have relatively more depolarized resting membrane potentials (approximately −60 mV).

An interesting feature of the DHP drugs that have been developed to modify the behavior of LTCC is that molecules with similar structures can be either agonists (LTCC activators) or antagonists. The most intensively studied LTCC agonist is Bay K 8644, which has (−) and (+) stereoisomers. The agonist effect is due to the (−) form of Bay K 8644, which increases maximal $I_{Ca,L}$ two- to four-fold.[32] This effect is caused by prolonging the channel open time (which has been termed "mode 2" gating), thereby increasing P_0.[33] Bay K 8644 also accelerates $I_{Ca,L}$ activation and slows its deactivation (i.e., it brings out a prominent tail current).[33] Because Bay K 8644 prolongs LTCC open time at the single-channel level, the decay of whole-cell $I_{Ca,L}$ should be slower. However, increasing $I_{Ca,L}$ accelerates the rate of decay, as a consequence of calcium-dependent inactivation. As a result, the $I_{Ca,L}$ inactivation is accelerated after Bay K 8644 application. Bay K 8644 also shifts the voltage dependence of $I_{Ca,L}$ activation and inactivation ($d_\infty$and f_∞ to more hyperpolarized potentials.[32] Of importance, although Bay K 8644 increases $I_{Ca,L}$, it has no effect on LTCC charge movement, implying no increase in the total number of LTCCs.[34] The DHP LTCC agonist (+)-202-791 has similar effects on $I_{Ca,L}$ and on $i_{Ca,L}$.[32] Recently a new DHP agonist, Bay Y 5959, has been studied, and its effect on LTCC gating is different from that of Bay K 8644, in that it increases both the mean open time and the mean closed time, resulting in a reduced rate of calcium current activation, an increased peak current, and a slowing of LTCC deactivation with repolarization.[35]

Studies of LTCC agonists and antagonists on single channels have led to a theory of gating "modes" (Fig. 17-4) that is still somewhat controversial.[21] According to this theory, LTCC "gates" in three distinct patterns or "modes." In mode 0, the LTCC is primarily in an inactivated (unavailable) state, with long periods without channel activation. Mode 1 is the normal mode of LTCC gating. It is characterized by periods of short openings in rapid bursts following a depolarizing step. Mode 2 gating is characterized by long openings.[33] Experiments in which repetitive voltage steps were applied to membrane patches containing single LTCCs show that the rates of switching between different modes are much slower than the rates of transition between different states (C1, C2, O, and I states) within a gating mode. Under normal conditions mode 1 gating is most common, with occasional periods of mode 0. Mode 2 gating is relatively rare under native conditions but can be induced by DHP LTCC agonists such as BAY K 8644, by protein kinase A (PKA)-dependent phosphorylation, and by high-voltage prepulse depolarization.

Dual Effects of Drugs on the L-type Calcium Channel

The fact that drugs that modulate the behavior of LTCC can act as either an agonist or an antagonist was first described for (−)Bay K 8644.[36] This molecule has antagonist effects on $I_{Ca,L}$ when (1) its concentration is high, (2) it is applied to the membrane when it is held at positive potentials, and (3) the frequency of test pulses is high.[36] Other studies have shown that the stereoisomers (−)Bay K 8644 and (+)S-202-791 are more selective agonists and exert antagonist effects only when cells are held at positive membrane potentials.[37] These results suggest[36] that drug-bound channels have a slower rate of repriming to an available state, after repolarization.

LTCC antagonists also can behave as agonists, especially at low concentration, at slow pacing rate, and at negative holding potentials. Usually this effect is transient and moderate (30% to 40%) and appears before the blocking effect is observed.[29]

Agonists and Antagonists Prefer a Specific State of L-type Calcium Channel for Binding

All LTCC agonists and antagonists bind with preference to specific channel states (open, closed, or inactivated). For antagonists, this preference leads to both tonic and use-dependent $I_{Ca,L}$ block.[32] *Tonic block* is relatively small and occurs after a long rest or during very slow rates of depolarization from negative membrane potentials. The efficiency of tonic block depends on membrane potential. As an example, the concentration of DHPs that can fully block $I_{Ca,L}$ at relatively positive holding potentials (e.g., −50 mV) blocks only 10% to 20% of $I_{Ca,L}$ at the normal resting potential of −80 mV.[38] When the resting potential was −80 mV, the K_d for nitrendipine binding to LTCC was 730 nM, whereas a K_d of 0.36 nM was observed at the holding potential (V_h) of −10 mV.[39] These and other studies provide strong support for the idea that DHPs bind with the highest affinity to the *inactivated* state of the LTCC, which is promoted by a depolarized membrane potential.

The accumulation of inhibition with repetitive depolarization is called *use-dependent block*. Increases in pulse duration, frequency, and positive holding or conditioning potentials all enhance the blocking effects of DHP, PAA, and BZT blockers, documenting that drugs of all classes bind with preference to the LTCC in open or inactivated states. PAAs (such as verapamil) appear to have the highest preference for the *open* state of the LTCC (i.e., they require voltage pulses to induce open state and subsequent block) because they show much more use dependence than do DHPs.[40]

Clinical Uses of L-type Calcium Channel Agonists and Antagonists

LTCC agonists are positive inotropic drugs (they increase Ca^{2+} influx and sarcoplasmic reticulum Ca^{2+} loading). These drugs are not useful clinically for the treatment of heart failure. Although Bay K 8644 causes increases in cardiac function via its positive inotropy, it increases patient mortality by inducing other adverse effects. The adverse effects of Bay K 8644 include increases in peripheral vascular resistance accompanied by hypertension; prolongation of action potentials, which is proarrhythmic; and activation of neuronal LTCC, which induces seizures.[15] These effects all were predictable, in view of the functional significance and ubiquitous distribution of the LTCC. Although some relatively new DHP agonists such as Bay Y 5959 are available,[15] it seems unlikely that these drugs will ever have widespread clinical usefulness because of their lack of tissue specificity. Novel LTCC agonist drugs for the treatment of poor cardiac function would need to specifically target the heart, probably the ventricle. This possibility seems unlikely because the molecular nature of the LTCC is identical in different tissues.

By contrast, LTCC antagonists have long been used for treating hypertension, effort-related angina, and atrial arrhythmias.[41] In all of these clinical uses, the beneficial effects appear to be derived from the fact that LTCC antagonists have a higher affinity for open or inactivated states of the LTCC, and these states vary with resting potential, which varies significantly in different tissues. The antihypertensive and antianginal effects take advantage of the fact that the resting membrane potential of smooth muscle is more depolarized than cardiac myocytes. Thus, LTCC block and the associated vasodilation can be achieved without significant negative inotropy. However, some cautionary notes about excess cardiovascular mortality, high myocardial infarction rate, and increased gastrointestinal bleeding have been added to the safety literature of these drugs.[20] The use-dependent nature of certain calcium channel antagonists (such as verapamil) makes them particularly effective in the treatment of atrial tachyarrhythmia. These topics are covered in detail in Chapter 98.

Regulation of the L-type Calcium Channel by Protein Kinases and Phosphatases

Phosphorylation of the LTCC complex by protein kinases and dephosphorylation by protein phosphatases are physiologically and pathologically relevant processes in cardiac myocytes. The primary physiologic regulation of LTCC is by means of β-adrenergic signaling pathways mediated by the sympathetic nervous system, which activate PKA. Phosphorylation of the LTCC complex by means of these pathways causes an increase in Ca^{2+} influx, sarcoplasmic reticulum Ca^{2+} loading, and sarcoplasmic reticulum Ca^{2+} release and underlies the associated increase in cardiac contractility.

Abnormalities of this signaling cascade are well described in the context of cardiac diseases that lead to congestive heart failure. Many clinically useful drugs, particularly β-adrenergic antagonists, are likely to impart a portion of their beneficial effects by influencing the phosphorylation state of the LTCC complex. The regulation of the LTCC complex by way of well-described signaling cascades is briefly reviewed next, with the understanding that drugs that activate or block these pathways will impart at least a portion of their cardiac effects through their influence on the cardiac LTCC. It should be noted in this regard that calmodulin-dependent kinase II (CaMKII) is an important regulator of the LTCC. These effects are reviewed in Chapter 2 and are not discussed further here.

Effects of β-Adrenergic (cAMP/PKA) Signaling Pathways on the L-type Calcium Channel

Activation of the sympathetic nervous system is a major mechanism for controlling the rate and contractility of the normal heart. Catecholamines released from sympathetic nerves bind to β-adrenergic receptors on the cell surface, leading to phosphorylation of LTCC complex through activation of PKA (Fig. 17-5). Tsien and workers initially[42] proposed that the stimulatory effect of cAMP in heart cells was caused by PKA-mediated phosphorylation of LTCC. These ideas were subsequently confirmed in many other laboratories. PKA-dependent phosphorylation of LTCC causes several-fold increases in $I_{Ca,L}$ and also shifts the voltage dependence of both activation and inactivation to more negative membrane potentials (see Fig. 17-5, "NF"). Because PKA-dependent phosphorylation prolongs single-channel open time, the whole-cell $I_{Ca,L}$ should decay more slowly. As discussed earlier, however, this effect is offset by enhanced Ca^{2+}-dependent inactivation, owing to the increase in $I_{Ca,L}$. Single-channel experiments have shown that PKA-dependent LTCC phosphorylation increases channel availability and open probability and induces mode 2 gating without a change in single-channel conductance.[32] These effects can be blocked by PKA inhibitors such as H-89 and Rp-cAMP, as well as by polypeptides such as PKA-I.

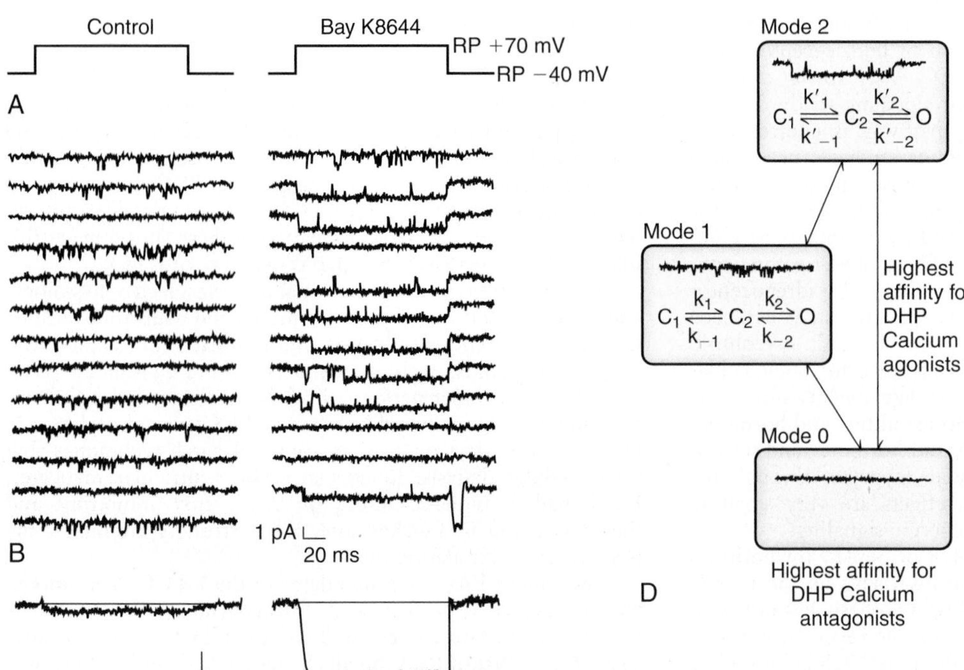

Figure 17-4 The effect of Bay K 8644, an L-type calcium channel (LTCC) agonist, on channel gating. **A,** Voltage clamp protocol for single-channel recording referenced to the resting potential of −60 mV. **B,** Single-channel recordings in the absence *(left)* and presence *(right)* of 5 μM Bay K 8644. Notice the very long openings induced by Bay K 8644. **C,** Average current from all sweeps. **D,** Modal theory of LTCC gating. The rate of transitions between modes is much slower than the rates of switching between states. C_1 and C_2 are two closed states, and O is the open state. DHP, dihydropyridine. (**A** to **D,** From Bers DM: Excitation-Contraction Coupling and Cardiac Contractile Force, 2nd ed. Dordrecht, Kluwer Academic, 2001.)

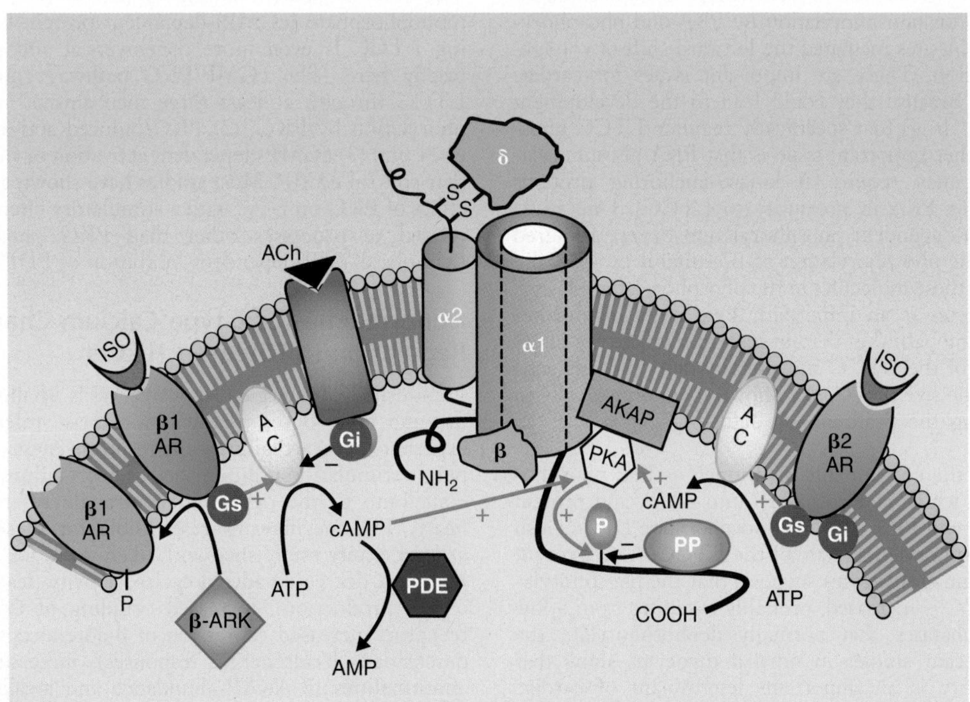

Figure 17-5 Scheme of the cyclic adenosine monophosphate (cAMP)/protein kinase A (PKA) pathway for LTCC regulation with β-adrenergic system as an example. When an agonist (e.g., isoproterenol [ISO]) binds to β-adrenergic receptors, β_1- and β_2-adrenergic receptors (β1 AR and β2 AR), the associated stimulatory G proteins (Gs) is activated, and inhibitory Gβγ subunits are dissociated from Gαs. Activated Gαs then diffuses to activate adenyl cyclase (AC) that is attached to cell membrane. Active AC catalyzes the production of cAMP; therefore, local cAMP concentration increases dramatically. Elevated cAMP concentration activates PKA anchored close to LTCC by A kinase–anchoring proteins (AKAPs), and subsequently PKA phosphorylates LTCC. This cartoon shows PKA-dependent phosphorylation of α1 subunit at the C-terminus. (PKA sites present on the β subunit are omitted for simplicity.) Phosphorylated LTCC is dephosphorylated by protein phosphatase 2A (PP2A) and protein phosphatase 1 (PP1). The cAMP is cleaved by phosphodiesterases (PDE). Activation of M2 cholinergic receptor may inhibit AC activity by means of Gi proteins. ACh, acetylcholine; β-ARK, β-adrenergic receptor kinase; COOH, carboxyl terminus; NH_2, amino terminus; PP, protein phosphatase.

Two major subtypes of β-adrenoceptors, β_1 and β_2, are present in cardiac myocytes and activation of both receptors have been reported to phosphorylate LTCC. Very strong evidence supports a major role for β_1 receptor signaling to the LTCC. The functional relevance of the β_2 pathway is controversial, however, and needs further study. Some studies[43] have found that zinterol, a β_2-adrenoceptor agonist, increases $I_{Ca,L}$. Nagykaldi and associates[44] recently showed, however, that the effects of zinterol on $I_{Ca,L}$ were blocked by β_1-antagonist CGP 20712A but not by β_2-antagonists. These investigators concluded that zinterol exerted its effect by way of β_1-adrenoceptor owing to its relatively low specificity. Of interest, it has been shown that β_2-adrenergic receptor, the LTCC, caveolin-3, Gαs, adenyl cyclase, PKA, and PP2A form a macromolecular complex in caveolae, indicating locally regulated β_2-adrenergic effects on the LTCC.[45] Other neurotransmitters and hormones such as histamine, glucagons, parathyroid hormone, and serotonin also can modulate $I_{Ca,L}$ in cardiac myocytes through the cAMP/PKA signal pathway. These effects are very small in comparison with those due to β-adrenergic signaling.

Ser1928 on $\alpha 1_C$ subunit and Ser478 or Ser479 (or both) on the β2 subunit are thought to be the PKA sites on the LTCC mediating the increase in $I_{Ca,L}$.[46] This hypothesis has not been well established with direct measurements, however. In addition, the role of the C terminus of $\alpha 1_C$, where Ser1928 is located, is controversial, because this portion of the protein can be cleaved by proteases or truncated by alternative splicing. This cleaved cytoplasmic C terminus of LTCC appears to remain tethered to the membrane-embedded α1 subunit[47] through protein-protein interactions. The relative roles of α1 and β2 phosphorylation to regulation of LTCC remain largely undetermined. Naguro and associates[48] found that Ser1901 in the so-called rat brain type II $\alpha 1_C$ (corresponding to Ser1928 in cardiac $\alpha 1_C$) is responsible for the increase in P_0 on phosphorylation by PKA and phosphorylation of other PKA sites mediated the leftward shift of voltage-dependent activation. These are important issues for cardiac calcium channels because they could lead to the development of cardiac-specific drugs that specifically regulate LTCC phosphorylation. Another important issue is that PKA phosphorylation of LTCCs may require A kinase–anchoring proteins (AKAPs) to anchor PKA in proximity to LTCCs. One study showed that PKA-dependent phosphorylation of $\alpha 1_C$ required AKAP, whereas the phosphorylation of β2 subunit by PKA did not.[47] The role of these molecules in the phosphorylation defects in diseased myocytes is an important topic requiring further study. The signaling pathways that interact to regulate the phosphorylation state of the LTCC and thereby determine its activation state and the size of $I_{Ca,L}$ are shown diagrammatically in Figure 17-5, using the β-adrenergic signaling pathway as an example.

In addition to the components mentioned earlier, phosphodiesterase (PDE), which cleaves cAMP into AMP, and protein phosphatases PP1 and PP2, which dephosphorylate LTCC, also influence the phosphorylation state of the LTCC. A very recent study in failing human myocytes suggests that the phosphorylation state of LTCC is increased, probably resulting from a low activity of phosphatases that normally dephosphorylate the LTCC. Other recent studies in normal myocytes show that phosphatase activity is an important determinant of cardiac LTCC properties.[49]

Regulation of the L-type Calcium Channel by Protein Kinase C in Cardiac Myocytes

Unlike the effect of PKA, the effect of protein kinase C (PKC) on $I_{Ca,L}$ is controversial. Some studies revealed stimulatory effects of PKC, whereas others show inhibitory effects or biphasic responses.[46] In vitro, both the α1 and β2 subunits of LTCC are good substrates for PKC-mediated phosphorylation, with a stoichiometry of 2 to 3 moles of phosphate per mole of α1 subunit and 1 to 2 moles of phosphate per mole of β2 subunit.[46] The PKC sites are possibly located at N terminus (Thγ-27 and Thγ-31), and phosphorylation of these sites by PKC has been shown to cause $I_{Ca,L}$ inhibition.[50] Other studies suggest that PKC sites at regions other than N terminus inhibit LTCC activity in the dephosphorylated state,[51] and that phosphorylation of these sites relieves this inhibition and increases the open probability of LTCC.

PKC has been proposed to mediate the electrophysiologic and contractile effects of many hormones and neurotransmitters, including α-adrenergic agonists, intracellular ATP, angiotensin II, glucocorticoids, arginine vasopressin, and endothelin (ET). Angiotensin II under perforated patch conditions (no cell dialysis) enhances $I_{Ca,L}$, possibly through PKC phosphorylation,[52] but has little effect on $I_{Ca,L}$ in ruptured patch techniques that cause cellular dialysis. In normal rabbit ventricular myocytes, ET-1 had a biphasic effect on $I_{Ca,L}$, first inhibiting and then increasing it. Furthermore, ET-1 strongly attenuates the β-adrenergic stimulation on $I_{Ca,L}$.[53]

The role of PKC as a modulator of the LTCC is an important unresolved issue that needs further study. What is clear is that the quantitative effect of PKC on LTCC is significantly smaller than that of PKA. Small changes in Ca^{2+} influx, however, can have significant effects on the heart, and modulating these phosphorylation sites represents a novel approach to drug targeting.

Regulation of L-type Calcium Channel by Protein Kinase G in Cardiac Myocytes

The role of protein kinase G (PKG) (i.e., cyclic guanosine monophosphate [cGMP]-dependent protein kinase) in regulating LTCC is even more controversial and is discussed only briefly here. The cGMP/PKG pathway could influence the LTCC through at least three mechanisms[46]: (1) direct phosphorylation by PKG, (2) PKG-induced activation of phosphatases, and (3) cGMP-dependent activation or inhibition of PDEs that control cAMP. Most studies have shown a direct inhibitory effect of PKG on $I_{Ca,L}$, with a stimulatory effect of cGMP being related to processes other than PKG phosphorylation—for example, cGMP-dependent inhibition of PDEIII.

Abnormalities of L-type Calcium Channel Regulation in Diseased Hearts

Diminished adrenergic responsiveness is a hallmark of heart failure and contributes to the low exercise tolerance of patients experiencing heart failure. The responsiveness of $I_{Ca,L}$ to β-adrenergic stimulation is diminished in heart failure[54] (Fig. 17-6) and contribute to the depressed contractile reserve of the failing heart. The mechanisms responsible for these blunted effects are not firmly established with likely roles for reduced receptor numbers, decreased adenyl cyclase activity (leading to decreased cAMP production), increased coupling of G_i to β-adrenergic receptor, increased expression of β-adrenoceptor kinase (which desensitizes β-adrenergic responses), increased PDE activity, abnormalities in AKAP abundance and localization, increased activity of signaling pathways (such as the cGMP/PKG pathway) that antagonize the cAMP/PKA pathway,[55] and abnormalities of LTCC phosphorylation state caused by reduced phosphatase activity.[56] These processes all are worthy of future investigation. Of interest, currently effective heart failure therapies such as use of β-adrenergic receptor blockers may impart part of their clinical benefit by altering the phosphorylation state of PKA target protein such as the LTCC.[54]

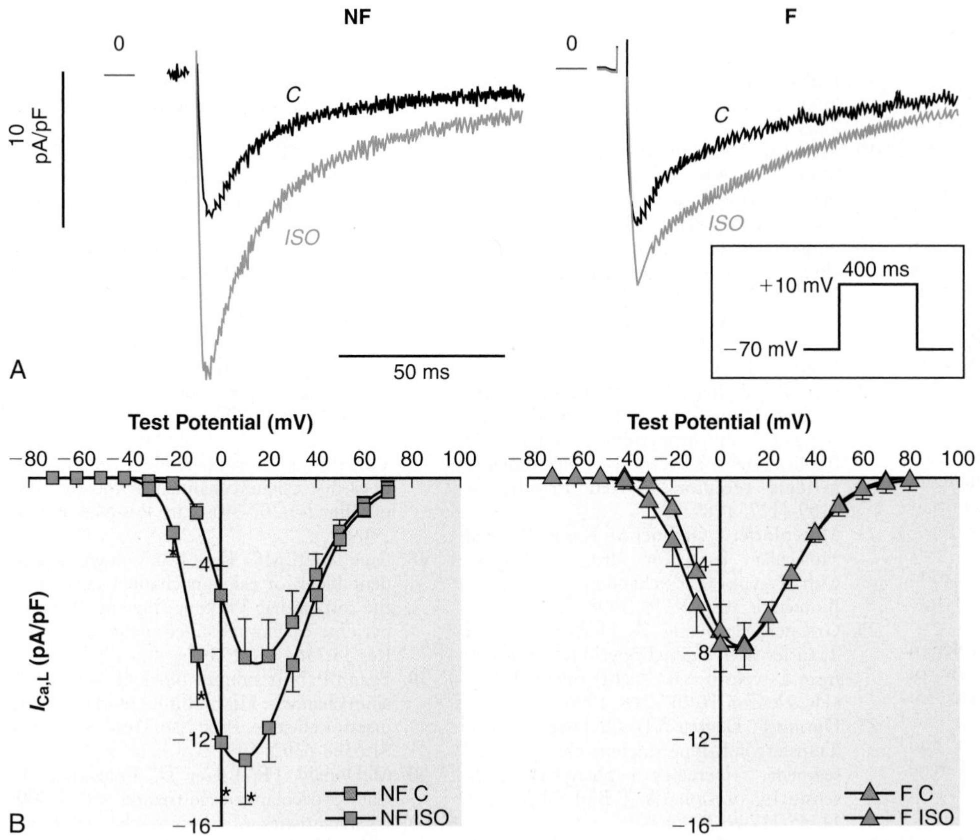

Figure 17-6 The effect of 1 μM isoproterenol (ISO) on $I_{Ca,L}$ in nonfailing (NF) (n = 12, N = 6) and failing (F) (n = 9, N = 4) human ventricular myocytes. **A,** Example current traces before and after bath application of 1 μM ISO. ISO increased $I_{Ca,L}$ significantly in the NF myocytes but had little effect in the F myocytes. The effect of ISO on peak calcium current was significantly less in F cells (124% ±12%) myocytes than in NF (190% ± 15%) myocytes. **B,** The effect of ISO on $I_{Ca,L}$-voltage relationship in NF and F myocytes. ISO significantly increased maximal $I_{Ca,L}$ in NF myocytes but had minimal effect in F myocytes ($I_{Ca,L,ISO}/I_{Ca,L,ctr}$ in NF versus F, compared with 1.57 versus 1.08). n, the number of myocytes studied; N, the number of hearts studied; *, $P < 0.05$ using post hoc T-test after two-way repeated ANOVA showed a significant difference. (**A** and **B,** From Chen X, Piacentino V 3rd, Furukawa S, et al: L-type Ca^{2+} channel density and regulation are altered in failing human ventricular myocytes and recover after support with mechanical assist devices. Circ Res 91:517-524, 2002.)

Pharmacology of the T-type Calcium Channel in the Heart

The TTCC is not widely expressed in all types of cardiac myocytes in the adult heart. Three genes, $\alpha 1_G$, $\alpha 1_H$, and $\alpha 1_I$, have been found to encode TTCCs, and they exhibit subtle differences in biophysical and pharmacologic properties. The regulation of these TTCCs by hormones and neurotransmitter are modest. In general, it is believed that the current through TTCCs ($I_{Ca,T}$) is insensitive to adrenergic (or PKA) stimulation in cardiac tissue.[57] $I_{Ca,T}$ through Cav3.2 is regulated by signaling pathways. ET-1 is able to increase $I_{Ca,T}$ in rat ventricular myocytes, whereas atrial natriuretic factor inhibits $I_{Ca,T}$ in frog atrial cells.[57] Both of these signaling pathways are likely to be upregulated in cardiac disease states, when TTCCs are re-expressed in ventricular myocytes.

TTCCs have been implicated in the development of heart disease and in the secretion of neurohormones, such as aldosterone, renin, atrial naturetic factor, and insulin, all of which regulate heart function.[58] Therefore, TTCC antagonists could be therapeutically valuable. TTCC pharmacology is not well developed, however, with no highly specific T-type calcium channel antagonists yet devised. Mibefradil (also named Ro 40-5967) is the most specific antagonist available, but it still has potent effects on the LTCC. Structurally, mibefradil is a derivative of tetralol and is unrelated to the three categories of classic LTCC antagonists (see Fig. 17-1). It suppresses TTCC and shifts the steady-state inactivation to more negative voltages.[59] Mibefradil induces peripheral vasodilation and heart rate reduction but no decrease in cardiac contractility in patients with heart failure. In addition, mibefradil inhibits neurohormonal releases of aldosterone from adrenal medulla and cortex and of norepinephrine from the sympathetic nerves.[60] Clinical trials have shown that mibefradil is an effective antianginal, antihypertensive, and anti-ischemic agent. Trials in patients with congestive heart failure, however, have been disappointing.[61] Unexpected metabolic drug interaction with the cytochrome P-450 3A4 complicates the putative beneficial effects of mibefradil and has resulted in its withdrawal from the market. A recent study indicates that a mibefradil metabolite inhibits the LTCC, and a nonhydrolyzable analogue is able to selectively inhibit the TTCC.[62] Whether or not this will lead to a clinically effective TTCC therapeutic agent is unclear.

Dihydropyridines generally are specific for the LTCC, without inhibition of the TTCC, but recently efonidipine, a dihydropyridine derivative, has been found to inhibit both LTCC and TTCC.[58] New specific TTCC antagonists without such drug interaction might be clinically useful and would help in basic research because they would allow the functional role of this channel to be more clearly defined.

Summary

LTCC antagonists are widely used drugs in the treatment of cardiovascular disorders. Their pharmacology and mechanisms of action on the heart and vasculature are well studied and well established. TTCC pharmacology is almost nonexistent. In view of the role of TTCC in cardiac hypertrophy and their potential role in cardiac and smooth muscle regeneration, drugs that specifically modulate these ion channels would certainly serve as valuable research tools and could provide novel therapies for certain forms of cardiovascular disease.

References

1. Ertel EA, Campbell KP, Harpold MM, et al: Nomenclature of voltage-gated calcium channels. Neuron 25:533-535, 2000.
2. Bers DM: Excitation-Contraction Coupling and Cardiac Contractile Force, 2nd ed. Dordrecht, Kluwer Academic, 2001.
3. Inoue M, Bridge JH: Ca^{2+} sparks in rabbit ventricular myocytes evoked by action potentials: Involvement of clusters of L-type Ca^{2+} channels. Circ Res 92:532-538, 2003.
4. Nakayama H, Chen X, Baines CP, et al: Ca^{2+}- and mitochondrial-dependent cardiomyocyte necrosis as a primary mediator of heart failure. J Clin Invest 117:2431-2444, 2007.
5. Chen X, Zhang X, Kubo H, et al: Ca^{2+} influx-induced sarcoplasmic reticulum Ca^{2+} overload causes mitochondrial-dependent apoptosis in ventricular myocytes. Circ Res 97:1009-1017, 2005.
6. Perez-Reyes E: Molecular characterization of T-type calcium channels. Cell Calcium 40:89-96, 2006.
7. Black JL 3rd: The voltage-gated calcium channel gamma subunits: A review of the literature. J Bioenerg Biomembr 35: 649-660, 2003.
8. Talavera K, Nilius B: Biophysics and structure-function relationship of T-type Ca^{2+} channels. Cell Calcium 40:97-114, 2006.
9. Qu Y, Boutjdir M: Gene expression of SERCA2a and L- and T-type Ca channels during human heart development. Pediatr Res 50:569-574, 2001.
10. Vassort G, Talavera K, Alvarez JL: Role of T-type Ca^{2+} channels in the heart. Cell Calcium 40:205-220, 2006.
11. Nuss HB, Houser SR: T-type Ca^{2+} current is expressed in hypertrophied adult feline left ventricular myocytes. Circ Res 73:777-782, 1993.
12. Sipido KR, Carmeliet E, Van de Werf F: T-type Ca^{2+} current as a trigger for Ca^{2+} release from the sarcoplasmic reticulum in guinea-pig ventricular myocytes. J Physiol 508:439-451, 1998.
13. Chen X, Wilson RM, Kubo H, et al: Adolescent feline heart contains a population of small, proliferative ventricular myocytes with immature physiological properties. Circ Res 100:536-544, 2007.
14. Mikami A, Imoto K, Tanabe T, et al: Primary structure and functional expression of the cardiac dihydropyridine-sensitive calcium channel. Nature 340:230-233, 1989.
15. Striessnig J: Pharmacology, structure and function of cardiac L-type Ca(2+) channels. Cell Physiol Biochem 9:242-269, 1999.
16. Hidalgo P, Neely A: Multiplicity of protein interactions and functions of the voltage-gated calcium channel beta-subunit. Cell Calcium 42:389-396, 2007.
17. Qiao X, Meng H: Nonchannel functions of the calcium channel gamma subunit: Insight from research on the Stargazer mutant. J Bioenerg Biomembr 35:661-670, 2003.
18. Klugbauer N, Marais E, Hofmann F: Calcium channel alpha$_2$delta subunits: Differential expression, function, and drug binding. J Bioenerg Biomembr 35:639-647, 2003.
19. Anderson ME: Ca^{2+}-dependent regulation of cardiac L-type Ca^{2+} channels: Is a unifying mechanism at hand?. J Mol Cell Cardiol 33:639-650, 2001.
20. Triggle DJ: Calcium channel antagonists: clinical uses—past, present and future. Biochem Pharmacol 74:1-9, 2007.
21. Catterall WA, Striessnig J: Receptor sites for Ca^{2+} channel antagonists. Trends Pharmacol Sci 13:256-262, 1992.
22. Kass RS, Arena JP: Influence of pH_o on calcium channel block by amlodipine, a charged dihydropyridine compound. Implications for location of the dihydropyridine receptor. J Gen Physiol 93: 1109-1127, 1989.
23. Mitterdorfer J, Grabner M, Kraus RL, et al: Molecular basis of drug interaction with L-type Ca^{2+} channels. J Bioenerg Biomembr 30:319-334, 1998.
24. Grabner M, Wang Z, Hering S, et al: Transfer of 1,4-dihydropyridine sensitivity from L-type to class A (BI) calcium channels. Neuron 16:207-218, 1996.
25. Doring F, Degtiar VE, Grabner M, et al: Transfer of L-type calcium channel IVS6 segment increases phenylalkylamine sensitivity of alpha1A. J Biol Chem 271: 11745-11749, 1996.
26. Yamaguchi S, Okamura Y, Nagao T, Adachi-Akahane S: Serine residue in the IIIS5-S6 linker of the L-type Ca^{2+} channel alpha 1C subunit is the critical determinant of the action of dihydropyridine Ca^{2+} channel agonists. J Biol Chem 275: 41504-41511, 2000.
27. Bodi I, Koch SE, Yamaguchi H, et al: The role of region IVS5 of the human cardiac calcium channel in establishing inactivated channel conformation: Use-dependent block by benzothiazepines. J Biol Chem 277:20651-20659, 2002.
28. Lee KS, Tsien RW: Mechanism of calcium channel blockade by verapamil, D600, diltiazem and nitrendipine in single dialysed heart cells. Nature 302:790-794, 1983.
29. McDonald T, Pelzer D, Trautwein W: Dual action (stimulation, inhibition) of D600 on contractility and calcium channels in guinea-pig and cat heart cells. J Physiol 414:569-586, 1989.
30. Brown AM, Kunze DL, Yatani A: Dual effects of dihydropyridines on whole cell and unitary calcium currents in single ventricular cells of guinea-pig. J Physiol 379:495-514, 1986.
31. Zahradnikova A, Zahradnik I: Interaction of diltiazem with single L-type calcium channels in guinea-pig ventricular myocytes. Gen Physiol Biophys 11:535-543, 1992.
32. McDonald TF, Pelzer S, Trautwein W, Pelzer DJ: Regulation and modulation of calcium channels in cardiac, skeletal, and smooth muscle cells. Physiol Rev 74: 365-507, 1994.
33. Hess P, Lansman JB, Tsien RW: Different modes of Ca channel gating behaviour favoured by dihydropyridine Ca agonists and antagonists. Nature 311:538-544, 1984.
34. Josephson IR, Sperelakis N: Fast activation of cardiac Ca^{++} channel gating charge by the dihydropyridine agonist, BAY K 8644. Biophys J 58:1307-1311, 1990.
35. Bechem M, Goldmann S, Gross R, et al: A new type of Ca-channel modulation by a novel class of 1,4-dihydropyridines. Life Sci 60:107-118, 1997.
36. Hadley RW, Hume JR: Calcium channel antagonist properties of Bay K 8644 in single guinea pig ventricular cells. Circ Res 62:97-104, 1988.
37. Kamp TJ, Sanguinetti MC, Miller RJ: Voltage- and use-dependent modulation of cardiac calcium channels by the dihydropyridine (+)-202-791. Circ Res 64:338-351, 1989.
38. Sanguinetti MC, Kass RS: Voltage-dependent block of calcium channel current in the calf cardiac Purkinje fiber by dihydropyridine calcium channel antagonists. Circ Res 55:336-348, 1984.
39. Bean BP: Nitrendipine block of cardiac calcium channels: High-affinity binding to the inactivated state. Proc Natl Acad Sci U S A 81:6388-6392, 1984.
40. McDonald TF, Pelzer D, Trautwein W: Cat ventricular muscle treated with D600: Characteristics of calcium channel block and unblock. J Physiol 352:217-241, 1984.
41. Clusin WT, Anderson ME: Calcium channel blockers: Current controversies and basic mechanisms of action. Adv Pharmacol 46:253-296, 1999.
42. Tsien RW: Adrenaline-like effects of intracellular iontophoresis of cyclic AMP in cardiac Purkinje fibres. Nat New Biol 245:120-122, 1973.
43. Chen-Izu Y, Xiao RP, Izu LT, et al: G(i)-dependent localization of beta(2)-adrenergic receptor signaling to L-type Ca(2+) channels. Biophys J 79:2547-2556, 2000.
44. Nagykaldi Z, Kem D, Lazzara R, Szabo B: Canine ventricular myocyte beta$_2$-adrenoceptors are not functionally coupled to L-type calcium current. J Cardiovasc Electrophysiol 10:1240-1251, 1999.
45. Balijepalli RC, Foell JD, Hall DD, et al: Localization of cardiac L-type Ca(2+) channels to a caveolar macromolecular signaling complex is required for beta(2)-adrenergic regulation. Proc Natl Acad Sci U S A 103:7500-7505, 2006.
46. Keef KD, Hume JR, Zhong J: Regulation of cardiac and smooth muscle Ca(2+) channels (Ca(V)1.2a,b) by protein kinases. Am J Physiol Cell Physiol 281:C1743-C1756, 2001.
47. Gao T, Yatani A, Dell'Acqua ML, et al: cAMP-dependent regulation of cardiac L-type Ca^{2+} channels requires membrane targeting of PKA and phosphorylation of channel subunits. Neuron 19:185-196, 1997.
48. Naguro I, Nagao T, Adachi-Akahane S: Ser(1901) of alpha(1C) subunit is required for the PKA-mediated enhancement of

L-type Ca(2+) channel currents but not for the negative shift of activation. FEBS Lett 489:87-91, 2001.

49. duBell WH, Lederer WJ, Rogers TB: Dynamic modulation of excitation-contraction coupling by protein phosphatases in rat ventricular myocytes. J Physiol 493:793-800, 1996.

50. McHugh D, Sharp EM, Scheuer T, Catterall WA: Inhibition of cardiac L-type calcium channels by protein kinase C phosphorylation of two sites in the N-terminal domain. Proc Natl Acad Sci U S A 97:12334-12338, 2000.

51. Shistik E, Keren-Raifman T, Idelson GH, et al: The N terminus of the cardiac L-type Ca(2+) channel alpha(1C) subunit. The initial segment is ubiquitous and crucial for protein kinase C modulation, but is not directly phosphorylated. J Biol Chem 274:31145-31149, 1999.

52. Kurata S, Ishikawa K, Iijima T: Enhancement by arginine vasopressin of the L-type Ca^{2+} current in guinea pig ventricular myocytes. Pharmacology 59:21-33, 1999.

53. Watanabe T, Kobayashi K, Suzuki T, et al: A preliminary report on continuous recording of salivary pH using telemetry in an edentulous patient. Int J Prosthodont 12:313-317, 1999.

54. Chen X, Piacentino V3rd, Furukawa S, et al: L-type Ca^{2+} channel density and regulation are altered in failing human ventricular myocytes and recover after support with mechanical assist devices. Circ Res 91:517-524, 2002.

55. Port JD, Bristow MR: Altered beta-adrenergic receptor gene regulation and signaling in chronic heart failure. J Mol Cell Cardiol 33:887-905, 2001.

56. Schroder F, Handrock R, Beuckelmann DJ, et al: Increased availability and open probability of single L-type calcium channels from failing compared with nonfailing human ventricle. Circulation 98:969-976, 1998.

57. Chemin J, Traboulsie A, Lory P: Molecular pathways underlying the modulation of T-type calcium channels by neurotransmitters and hormones. Cell Calcium 40:121-134, 2006.

58. Tanaka H, Shigenobu K: Pathophysiological significance of T-type Ca^{2+} channels: T-type Ca^{2+} channels and drug development. J Pharmacol Sci 99:214-220, 2005.

59. Pinto JM, Sosunov EA, Gainullin RZ, et al: Effects of mibefradil, a T-type calcium current antagonist, on electrophysiology of Purkinje fibers that survived in the infarcted canine heart. J Cardiovasc Electrophysiol 10:1224-1235, 1999.

60. Clozel JP, Ertel EA, Ertel SI: Voltage-gated T-type Ca^{2+} channels and heart failure. Proc Assoc Am Physicians 111: 429-437, 1999.

61. Levine TB, Bernink PJ, Caspi A, et al: Effect of mibefradil, a T-type calcium channel blocker, on morbidity and mortality in moderate to severe congestive heart failure: The MACH-1 study. Mortality Assessment in Congestive Heart Failure Trial. Circulation 101:758-764, 2000.

62. Huang L, Keyser BM, Tagmose TM, et al: NNC 55-0396 [(1S,2S)-2-(2-(N-[(3-benzimidazol-2-yl)propyl]-N-methylamino) ethyl)-6-fluoro-1,2,3,4-tetrahydro-1-isopropyl-2-naphtyl cyclopropanecarboxylate dihydrochloride]: A new selective inhibitor of T-type calcium channels. J Pharmacol Exp Ther 309:193-199, 2004.

17

KCNQ1/KCNE1 Macromolecular Signaling Complex: Channel Microdomains and Human Disease 18

LEI CHEN, SHEILA J. CARROLL, JUNKO KUROKAWA, AND ROBERT S. KASS

CHAPTER OUTLINE

Background

Autonomic nervous system control of heart rate and cardiac contractility, through sympathetic and parasympathetic activity, is a fundamental property of the cardiovascular system. Exercise or emotional stress stimulates the sympathetic nervous system (SNS), resulting in a rapid and dramatic increase in heart rate, which, in order to ensure adequate diastolic filling time, is accompanied by a concomitant reduction of the ventricular action potential duration and the corresponding QT interval on the electrocardiogram (ECG). Defective regulation of cardiac electrical activity in the face of SNS activity can lead to arrhythmias.[1]

SNS control of cardiac electrical activity is mediated by the activation of β-adrenergic receptors, which regulate the function of select ion channel proteins by means of phosphorylation by cyclic adenosine monophosphate (cAMP)-dependent protein kinase A (PKA). PKA phosphorylation modulates the activity of L-type calcium channels, allowing calcium entry to be augmented on a beat-to-beat basis. This enhanced Ca^{2+} entry contributes to action potential prolongation as well as an increase in intracellular Ca^{2+} available for subsequent uptake by the cardiac sarcoplasmic reticulum. PKA phosphorylation also activates the major intracellular calcium release channel on the sarcoplasmic reticulum, the type 2 ryanodine receptor (RyR2),[2] which is responsible for releasing calcium to trigger muscle contraction.

Sympathetic stimulation also leads to cAMP-dependent increase of a slowly activating potassium channel current, I_{Ks} (Fig. 18-1). This modulation increases repolarization current, which is essential to counter the stimulatory effects of PKA on L-type calcium channels.[3] Regulation of ventricular action potential duration and QT interval in response to SNS stimulation results from a balance of inward and outward membrane currents. The duration of the action potential indirectly controls cell calcium, and this balance of modulated currents can be thought of as a necessary mechanism to regulate calcium homeostasis in the face of sympathetic activity.

Inherited mutations in ion channel proteins have been associated with disorders that are exacerbated by SNS activity. For example, the genes that encode the subunit components of the I_{Ks} channel—the pore-forming α subunit, KCNQ1, and the auxiliary β subunit,[4,5] KCNE1—have been linked to congenital long QT syndrome. This syndrome, a rare disease in which the QT interval of the ECG is prolonged as a result of dysfunctional ventricular repolarization, can precipitate polymorphic ventricular tachycardia and is associated with syncope, seizures, and sudden death.[6] Mutations in *KCNQ1*, which codes for the α subunit of the I_{Ks} channel (i.e., KCNQ1), cause long QT syndrome type 1 (LQT1), and mutations in *KCNE1*, the gene encoding the auxiliary β subunit (i.e., KCNE1), cause LQT5.[7] In affected patients, triggers of arrhythmias are gene-specific, and persons with mutations in either *KCNQ1* or *KCNE1* are at greatest risk of experiencing a fatal cardiac arrhythmia in the face of elevated SNS activity.[8] Unraveling the molecular links between the SNS and regulation of the KCNQ1/KCNE1 channel has direct implications for the mechanistic basis of triggers of arrhythmias in LQTS.

β-Adrenergic Receptor Signaling: Coordination of Localized Regulation of Channel Proteins by A Kinase–Anchoring Proteins

The complex regulation of key ion channel proteins by β-adrenergic receptor stimulation is mediated by compartmentalization of cAMP-dependent PKA and protein phosphatases[9,10] which is achieved through association with targeting proteins, the A kinase–anchoring proteins (AKAPs).[11] AKAPs are a group of structurally diverse proteins with the common function of binding to PKA, protein phosphatase 1 (PP1), and protein kinase C (PKC).[12-14] The binding of these anchoring proteins to protein partners determines their localization and substrate specificity. This enables regulatory enzymes to be present at high concentrations at the site of their substrates within the cell.[15] Discrete local signaling complexes are formed that are required for the proper processing of signaling events. Disruption of the local complexes can imbalance the response, leaving some, but not all, pathways intact. Uncoupling of local complexes by disruption of targeting protein–mediated protein-protein interactions is an example of such a mechanism.

Leucine-Isoleucine Zippers Coordinate Protein-Protein Interactions

Marks and colleagues[2,16] were the first to show that the cardiac calcium release channel–ryanodine receptor (RyR2) is regulated by way of a macromolecular signaling complex in which kinases and phosphatases are targeted to the channel through leucine-

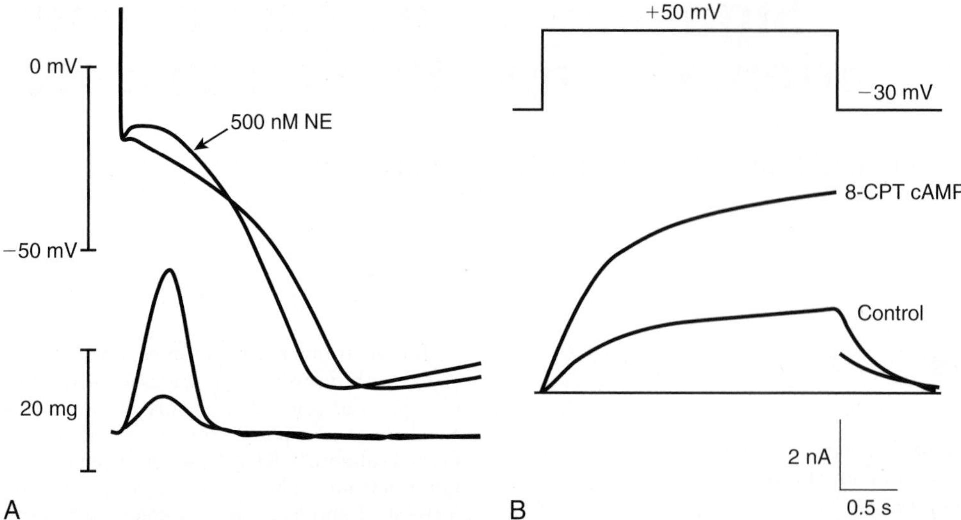

Figure 18-1 Sympathetic nervous system regulation of I_{Ks} currents. **A,** Norepinephrine (NE) increases plateau height and shortens action potential duration and increases the force of contraction in isolated calf Purkinje fibers. **B,** The membrane permeant cyclic adenosine monophosphate (cAMP) analogue 8-CPT–cAMP increases slow outward currents in isolated guinea pig myocytes. Currents shown are in response to a voltage pulse to +50 mV from a holding potential of −30 mV. Recordings were carried out in the same cell in the absence (control) and presence of 8 CPT–cAMP. (**A,** From Kass RS, Wiegers SE: The ionic basis of concentration-related effects of noradrenaline on the action potential of calf cardiac Purkinje fibres. J Physiol 322:541-558, 1982; **B,** from Walsh KB, Kass RS: Regulation of a heart potassium channel by protein kinase A and C. Science 242:67-69, 1988.)

isoleucine zipper–mediated protein-protein interactions, and to suggest that this may be a common motif for coordination of ion channel signaling complexes.[17] Other investigators subsequently showed that this is in fact the case for at least two other ion channels that are regulated by PKA: L-type calcium channels[18] and KCNQ1/KCNE1 potassium channels.[19]

The leucine-isoleucine zipper domain is an α-helical structure that forms coiled coils and originally was identified as highly conserved motifs mediating the binding of transcription factors to DNA.[20] Coiled coils are composed of heptad repeats $(abcdefg)_n$ in which hydrophobic residues occur at positions *a* and *d* and form the hydrophobic face of the helix, whereas *b*, *c*, *e*, *f*, and *g* are hydrophilic residues and form the solvent exposed part of the coiled coil.[21] Leucine zippers classically contain a leucine in position *d* because of a flexible side chain, although the canonical leucine residue can be replaced by an isoleucine or valine (as is the case in mixed-lineage kinase-3).[22] Electrostatic interactions between side chains in the *e* and *g* sites from neighboring helices are believed to help specify binding partners,[23] and charged residues at these positions may be destabilizing when not involved in ion pairs.[24] In addition, residues occupying the *e* and *g* positions exhibit a restricted range of substitutions based on the volume occluded by adjacent structures.[25] In vitro site-directed mutagenesis studies successfully revealed the sequence specificity of interacting helices in proteins such as GCN4 DNA-binding domain,[26] phospholamban,[25] myosin-binding subunit/cGMP-dependent protein kinase Iα (cGKIα),[27] ryanodine receptor types 1 and 2,[17] and the KCNQ1/KCNE1 channel.[19] Substitution of an alanine for one or more of the *d* position leucines or isoleucines in the motif diminished the ability of the leucine zipper to mediate protein-protein interaction without disrupting the native α-helical structure.[26,28]

I_{Ks} Channels Form a Macromolecular Complex with A Kinase–Anchoring Protein Yotiao

I_{Ks} channel forms a macromolecular signaling complex that is coordinated by the binding of the AKAP yotiao[29] by way of a leucine zipper motif in the KCNQ1 carboxyl-terminal (C-terminal) domain (Figs. 18-2A and 18-3A).[19] PKA and PP1, which bind to yotiao, are thus recruited directly to the channel microdomain and regulate it principally by phosphorylation of a single amino-terminal (N-terminal) KCNQ1 residue, Ser27.[19] Reconstitution of PKA- and PP1-mediated regulation of the KCNQ1/KCNE1 current in Chinese hamster ovary (CHO) cells requires coexpression of KCNQ1/KCNE1 channel and yotiao (see Fig. 18-2B) and is ablated by mutation of the KCNQ1 leucine zipper, which prevents yotiao binding to the channel, resulting in ablation of PKA phosphorylation of serine.[27]

The physiologic consequences of PKA phosphorylation of the KCNQ1/KCNE1 channel complex include a profound increase in the activity of these channels, a hyperpolarizing shift in the voltage dependence of channel activation, and a slowing of the return of activated (open) to resting (closed) channels during diastole. This combination of effects ensures that during voltage depolarization, KCNQ1/KCNE1 channel activity is increased in the presence of SNS stimulation over such activity in its absence. Consequently, the substantial repolarization reserve is activated in the face of SNS-mediated activity, and this reserve potassium channel current can offset SNS-mediated increases in calcium channel currents, which, by themselves, would prolong action potential duration.[3]

Pathologic Consequences of Disruption of the I_{Ks}/Yotiao Complex

It is now evident that disruption of the I_{Ks}/yotiao complex may have severe pathologic consequences. Naturally occurring mutations in KCNQ1, KCNE1, and yotiao have been identified to compromise the physical or functional integrity of the macromolecular complex and are associated with long QT syndrome.

Disruption of I_{Ks}/Yotiao Complex by KCNQ1 Mutations in Patients with Long QT Syndrome

Just as artificial mutations such as substitution of alanine residues for the leucines in the second and third *d* positions within

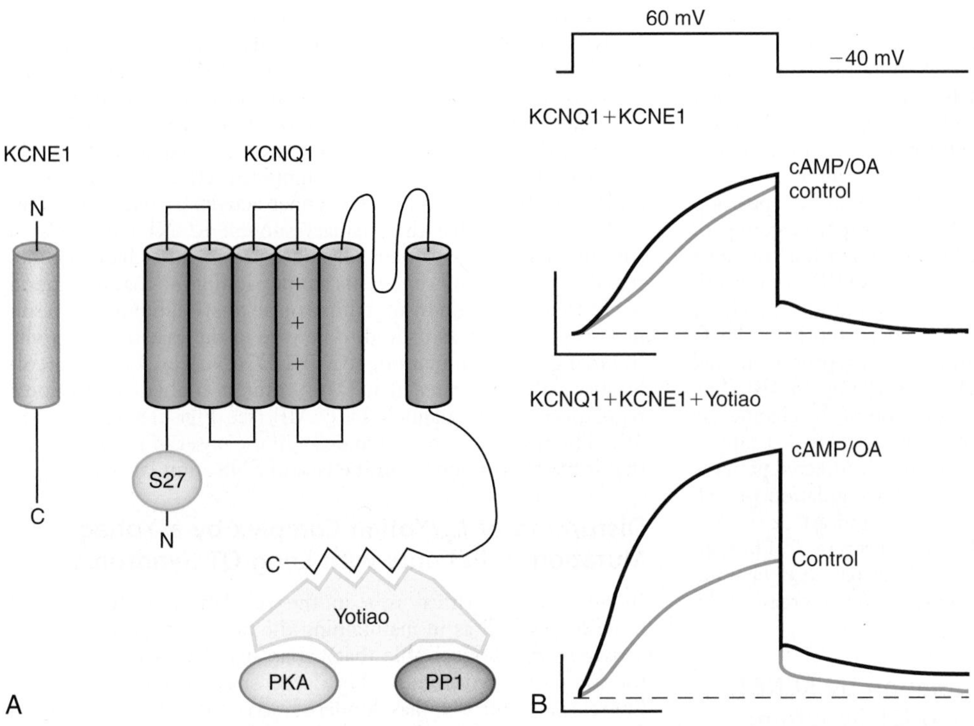

Figure 18-2 **A,** The KCNE1/KCNQ1/yotiao macromolecular complex. **B,** Membrane currents recorded in the absence (control) and presence of intracellular cyclic adenosine monophosphate (cAMP)/okadaic acid (OA) in cells transfected with KCNE1/KCNQ1 *(upper)* and KCNE1/KCNQ1/yotiao *(lower)*. Transfection of cells with yotiao was necessary for regulation of the expressed currents.

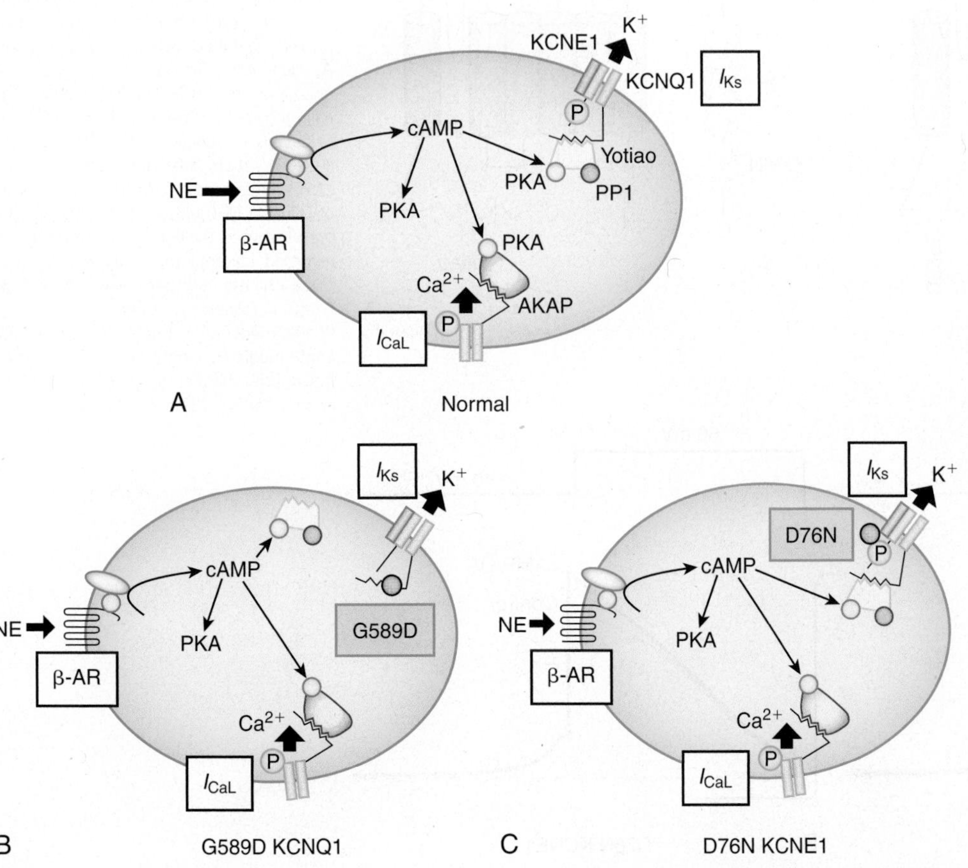

Figure 18-3 Schematic diagrams of cardiac myocytes indicating signaling microdomains for L-type calcium channels ($I_{Ca,L}$) and KCNE1/KCNQ1/yotiao complexes (I_{Ks}). **A,** In wild-type cells, stimulation of β-adrenergic receptors (β-AR) elevates intracellular cyclic adenosine monophosphate (cAMP), which in turn leads to protein kinase A (PKA)-dependent phosphorylation of both calcium and potasium channels. **B,** Uncoupling yotiao through the LQT1 G589D mutation precludes I_{Ks}, but not $I_{Ca,L}$, channels from β-adrenergic receptor–mediated phosphorylation. **C,** The LQT5 D76N mutation does not uncouple I_{Ks} channels from PKA-mediated phosphorylation but ablates the functional response to β-adrenergic stimulation. L-type calcium channels are not affected by this mutation. NE, norepinephrine.

the human KCNQ1 (hKCNQ1) leucine zipper motif abrogate its interaction with yotiao, without disturbing the α-helical structure of the motif, so too inherited mutations can disrupt leucine zippers and uncouple signaling molecules from their substrates. As noted earlier, residues occupying the *e* and *g* positions in the leucine zipper motif exhibit a limited range of substitutions based on the volume occluded by adjacent structures.[26] Thus, the naturally occurring G589D mutation at an *e* position in the leucine zipper motif of hKCNQ1 disrupts targeting of yotiao to hKCNQ1. The inherited G589D mutation has been linked to long QT syndrome variant 1 (LQT1) in Finnish families.[30] Moreover, the KCNQ1 G589D mutation, by virtue of the fact that it disrupts the leucine zipper motif in the C terminus of KCNQ1, nullifies β-adrenergic receptor–mediated regulation of the channel (Fig. 18-4A; see also Fig. 18-3B). The G589D mutation causes a defect in regulation of the channel by preventing assembly of the macromolecular complex that targets PKA and PP1 to the C terminus of the channel. Affected patients with this mutation suffer from dysfunctional regulation of QT duration during mental and physical stress[31] and are at risk for arrhythmia and sudden cardiac death during exercise.[30] Thus, an inherited mutation of a single residue on the KCNQ1 channel disrupts the I_{Ks}/yotiao signaling complex, thereby increasing the risk of arrhythmia in patients with this mutation.

Disruption of I_{Ks} Channel Regulation by KCNE1 Mutations in Patients with Long QT Syndrome

Kurokawa and colleagues demonstrated that cAMP-mediated functional regulation of KCNQ1/KCNE1 channels requires the expression of KCNQ1 with its auxiliary subunit KCNE1.[32] Dialysis of patch-clamped CHO cells expressing hKCNQ1, hKCNE1, and yotiao with exposure to cAMP and phosphatase inhibitor okadaic acid (OA) results in almost a twofold increase in channel activity as well as a negative shift in the voltage dependence of the channels.[19] In cells expressing yotiao and hKCNQ1 without hKCNE1, however, no significant effect of intracellular cAMP and OA on KCNQ1 channel activity is observed. This finding suggests that the auxiliary subunit KCNE1 may play a role in transducing protein phosphorylation into channel functional regulation and represents a new paradigm—that disruption of channel regulation by mutations on auxiliary subunit may result in diseases. This was proved to be true in the case of a naturally occurring LQT5 mutation, KCNE1 D76N. Kurokawa and colleagues[32] demonstrated that D76N mutation ablated functional regulation of the channels by cAMP (see Figs. 18-3C and 18-4B). The result is an expected delay in the onset of repolarization that is more pronounced in the face of SNS stimulation.

Disruption of I_{Ks}/Yotiao Complex by a Yotiao Mutation in Patients with Long QT Syndrome

In view of its critical role in the regulation of I_{Ks} channel function, as well as in maintaining the normal cardiac electrical activities, it is conceivable that yotiao may be a candidate gene for long QT syndromes. The large size, however, of yotiao (more than 200 kD) has hindered screening affected patients for novel mutations. In a recent study, Chen and associates characterized the molecular mechanism of KCN1-yotiao interaction. The interaction between the two molecules is a

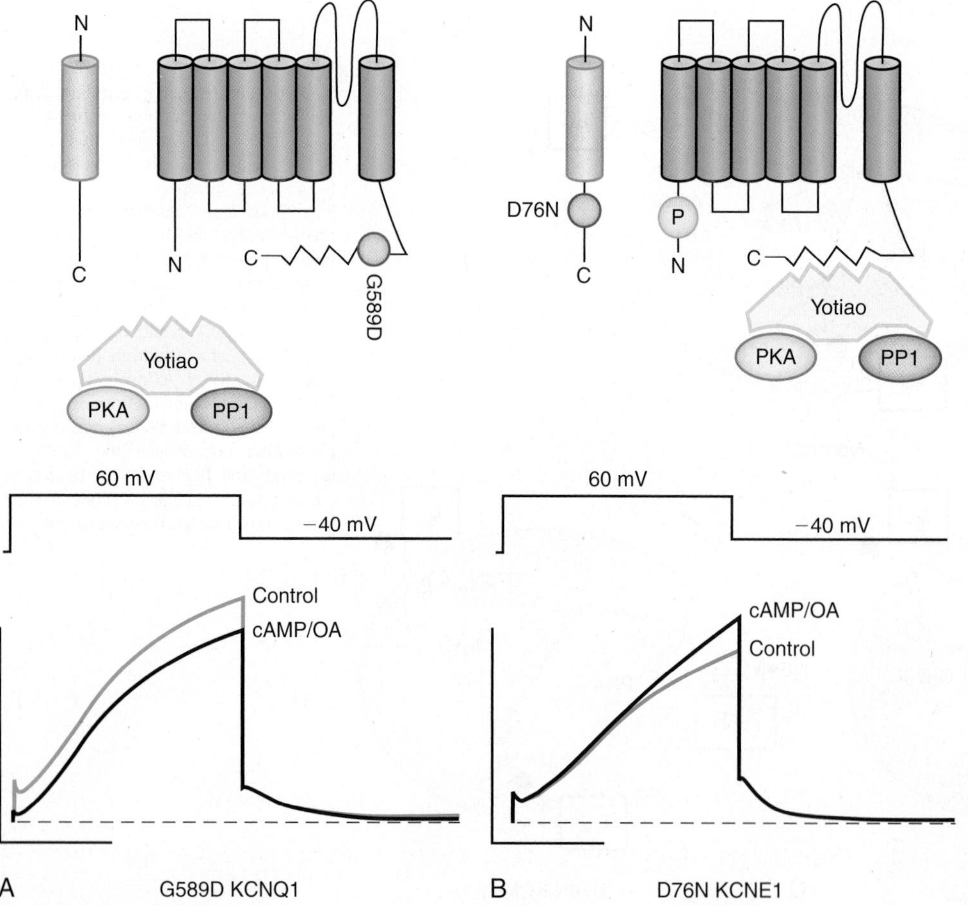

Figure 18-4 Direct experimental evidence for uncoupling of I_{Ks} (KCNE1/KCNQ1) channels from cyclic adenosine monophosphate (cAMP)-dependent modulation. **A,** *Upper panel*: The G589D LQT-3 mutation uncouples the KCNE1/KCNQ1/yotiao signaling complex. *Lower panel*: Currents in CHO cells transfected with KCNE1 G589D (KCNQ1)/yotiao are not responsive to cAMP/okadaic acid (OA). **B,** Coexpression of D76N KCNE1 with KCNQ1/yotiao *(upper panel)* ablates the functional response of recorded currents to cAMP/okadaic acid. CHO, Chinese hamster ovary. (**A** and **B,** From Kurokawa J, Chen L, Kass RS: Requirement of subunit expression for cAMP-mediated regulation of a heart potassium channel [abstract]. Proc Natl Acad Sci U S A 100:2122-2127, 2003.)

three-way binding that involves both yotiao N and C termini as well as the leucine zipper on KCNQ1 C terminus. Of particular interest, the yotiao C-terminal binding site (residue 1574-1643) contains a leucine zipper motif that potentially matches the reciprocal counterpart in KCNQ1. The identification of yotiao binding motifs enabled the quick screening in specific exons of Yotiao gene that encode for these important binding modules. In 50 patients with a strong clinical diagnosis of long QT syndrome (QTc of 480 ms or greater, or Schwartz[16] score of 3.0 or higher) but negative for mutations in all relevant genes including *KCNQ1* and *KCNE1*, a mis-sense mutation (S1570L) was identified in one patient but was absent in 1320 ethnic-matched reference alleles. The patient had experienced episodes of syncope and exhibited a prolonged QTc of 485 ms, and had a positive family history. Similar to the case of G589D mutation in KCNQ1, yotiao S1570L mutation is located close to its C-terminal binding site and has a negative impact on the formation of the I_{Ks}/yotiao complex. The mutation also reduced PKA-induced phosphorylation of KCNQ1 and rendered the I_{Ks} channels insensitive to PKA regulation. Moreover, computational modeling study revealed that yotiao S1570L mutation significantly prolonged the cardiac action potential duration, especially under the impact of SNS innervations (Fig. 18-5). These findings not only established yotiao as a novel causal gene in long QT syndrome but also reinforced the idea the AKAPs play critical roles in many physiologic processes. Yotiao S1570L mutation is the first disease mutation found in AKAPs.

Uncoupling of I_{Ks} Channels from Sympathetic Nervous System–Mediated Regulation: Novel Mechanisms of Arrhythmia

PKA-dependent regulation of at least three key ion channels in the heart (RyR2, L-type channels, and KCNQ1/KCNE1 channels) requires assembly of leucine zipper–mediated macromolecular signaling complexes. Disruption of a subset of these complexes can lead to an imbalanced response to SNS stimulation. The KCNQ1 mutation, G589D, is the first-described example of disease-associated disruption of a macromolecular signaling complex. Yotiao S1570L, on the other hand, disrupts the same complex by changing the structure of the adapter protein. KCNE1 D76N represents a novel mechanism of disrupting regulation of an ion channel by mutation on an auxiliary subunit.

How might the disruption of I_{Ks} (KCNQ1/KCNE1 channels) regulation contribute to the arrhythmia risk? Phosphorylation of wild-type KCNQ1/KCNE1 channel, mediated by the SNS, causes at least two important functional changes in channel activity: an increase in current density during and after activating depolarizing pulses and, of importance, a slowing of the deactivation of channels after the termination of activating pulses.[33] Because KCNQ1/KCNE1 channels activate with a slow time course during depolarization (in vivo, the depolarizing event is the ventricular action potential), during each action potential the accumulation of open KCNQ1/KCNE1 channels will ultimately be one of the key determinants of ventricular action potential and hence QT interval duration. SNS-mediated increase in channel activity provides more channel activity per action potential and hence tips the balance of currents in favor of repolarization earlier than in the absence of SNS stimulation, leading to action potential duration shortening. Additionally, because β-adrenergic stimulation slows the deactivation of this channel activity between beats, the accumulation of open KCNQ1/KCNE1 channels will be faster on a beat-by-beat basis with SNS stimulation.[34] Thus, β-adrenergic receptor–mediated stimulation of the activity of KCNQ1/KCNE1 channels provides a reserve of outward current that acts to speed the repolarization process in the face of increased activity of L-type calcium channels.[3]

Regulation of the cardiac ventricular action potential duration by the SNS is due in part to β-adrenergic receptor–mediated stimulation of the activity of KCNQ1/KCNE1 channels, which provides a reserve of outward current that hastens the repolarization process.[3] This stimulation, a consequence of PKA phosphorylation of a single residue (Ser27) of the KCNQ1 subunit, is coordinated by a C-terminal domain macromolecular signaling complex.[19] The importance of the KCNQ1/KCNE1 channel and its regulation is apparent, because mutations in either KCNQ1 (LQT1) or KCNE1 (LQT5), which reduce the activity of KCNQ1/KCNE1 channels in general or specifically disrupt the signaling complex, put patients with long QT syndrome at the greatest risk for triggered arrhythmias and sudden death in the setting of increased sympathetic activity.

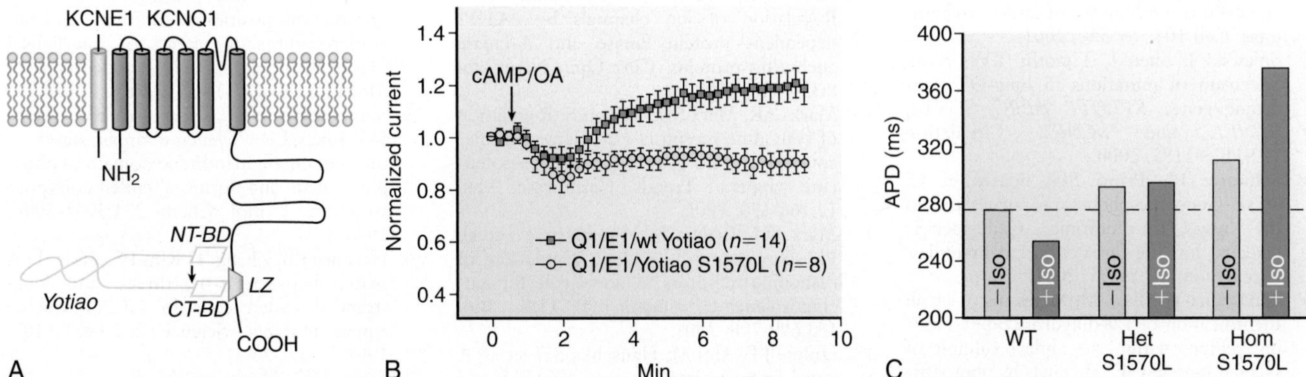

Figure 18-5 Disruption of I_{Ks} signaling complex by a mutation in A kinase–anchoring protein (AKAP) yotiao causes long QT (LQT) syndrome. **A,** The interaction between KCNQ1 and yotiao is mediated by a leucine zipper (LZ) motif on KCNQ1 C terminus and two binding sites on yotiao N and C termini (NT-BD and CT-BD). An LQT mutation S1570L is located near yotiao CT-BD and is indicated by a *black arrow*. **B,** S1570L mutation on yotiao disrupts functional regulation of I_{Ks} channels by protein kinase A (PKA). cAMP, cyclic adenosine monophosphate; OA, okadaic acid. **C,** Computational simulation shows abnormal cardiac action potential duration (APD) prolongation in S1570L alleles under isoproterenol (iso) stimulation.

The G589D mutation, which falls within the KCNQ1 C-terminal leucine zipper, uncouples the KCNQ1/KCNE1 channel from SNS-mediated regulation without affecting RyR2 or the L-type calcium channel; both retain the ability to be regulated by SNS activity. Thus, the activity of both the L-type calcium and RyR2 channels is enhanced, but without normal SNS-stimulated increase in reserve repolarizing potassium channel current. The D76N mutation in KCNE1 severely disrupts the important, physiologically relevant functional consequences of KCNQ1 phosphorylation. It ablates functional regulation of the KCNQ/KCNE1 channels by cAMP and reduces the basal current density. This mutation would be expected to reduce repolarizing current, prolong cellular action potentials, and contribute to prolonged QT intervals in affected patients even in the absence of SNS stimulation. Patients affected with this mutation would be expected to have inadequate reserve potassium channel activity to offset SNS stimulation of L-type calcium channels, resulting in inability to adequately control action potential duration in the face of elevated sympathetic tone. The D76N mutation, although not uncoupling the channel from SNS-mediated phosphorylation, effectively uncouples the functional response of the channel to SNS activity. In effect, the end result is very similar to that of the G589D mutation of KCNQ1: imbalance in ionic currents in the face of SNS stimulation.

This imbalance in calcium regulatory mechanisms predisposes cells to two types of calcium-mediated rhythm disturbances, early afterdepolarizations (EADs)[35,36] and delayed afterdepolarizations (DADs),[37-39] both of which can lead to triggered arrhythmias in affected cells. Two novel mechanisms by which point mutations in the KCNQ1/KCNE1 macromolecular signaling complex can lead to disease have been recognized: Leucine zipper mutations in KCNQ1 *physically* disrupt and mutations in KCNE1 *functionally* disrupt the response of the I_{Ks} channels to SNS stimulation. Thus, an inherited mutation of a single residue in the KCNQ1 leucine zipper or in the KCNQ1 auxiliary subunit KCNE1 can disrupt local communication between the brain and the heart, leading to unstable electrical activity driven by calcium-mediated proarrhythmic events.

Local signaling domains, coordinated by the assembly of leucine zipper–mediated macromolecular signaling complexes, thus become important to an understanding of both the genesis of cardiac arrhythmias and of novel targets to permit their treatment and prevention at the molecular level.

References

1. Wit AL, Hoffman BF, Rosen MR: Electrophysiology and pharmacology of cardiac arrhythmias. IX. Cardiac electrophysiologic effects of beta adrenergic receptor stimulation and blockade. Part C. Am Heart J 90:795-803, 1975.
2. Marx SO, Reiken S, Hisamatsu Y, et al: PKA phosphorylation dissociates FKBP12.6 from the calcium release channel (ryanodine receptor): Defective regulation in failing hearts. Cell 101:365-376, 2000.
3. Kass RS, Wiegers SE: The ionic basis of concentration-related effects of noradrenaline on the action potential of calf cardiac Purkinje fibres. J Physiol 322:541-558, 1982.
4. Sanguinetti MC, Curran ME, Zou A, et al: Coassembly of K_VLQT1 and minK(I_{sK}) proteins to form cardiac I_{Ks} potassium channel. Nature 384:80-83, 1996.
5. Barhanin J, Lesage F, Guillemare E, et al: K(v)LQT1 and I_{sK} (minK) proteins associate to form the I-Ks cardiac potassium current. Nature 384:78-80, 1996.
6. Keating MT, Sanguinetti MC: Molecular and cellular mechanisms of cardiac arrhythmias. Cell 104:569-580, 2001.
7. Splawski I, Shen J, Timothy KW, et al: Spectrum of mutations in long-QT syndrome genes: *KVLQT1, HERG, SCN5A, KCNE1,* and *KCNE2.* Circulation 102:1178-1185, 2000.
8. Schwartz PJ, Priori SG, Spazzolini C, et al: Genotype-phenotype correlation in the long-QT syndrome: Gene-specific triggers for life-threatening arrhythmias. Circulation 103:89-95, 2001.
9. Nakayama H, Taki M, Striessnig J, et al: Identification of 1,4-dihydropyridine binding regions within the alpha1 subunit of skeletal muscle Ca^{2+} channels by photoaffinity labeling with diazepine. Proc Natl Acad Sci U S A 88:9203-9207, 1991.
10. Fleckenstein A: Specific pharmacology of calcium in myocardium, cardiac pacemakers, and vascular smooth muscle. Annu Rev Pharmacol Toxicol 17:149-166, 1977.
11. Bayer R, Hennekes R, Kaufmann R, Mannhold R: Ionotropic and electrophysiological actions of verapamil and D600 on mammalian myocardium: I. Pattern of inotropic effects of the racemic compounds. Naunyn Schmiedebergs Arch Pharmacol 290:49-68, 1975.
12. Potet F, Scott JD, Mohammad-Panah R, et al: AKAP proteins anchor cAMP-dependent protein kinase to KvLQT1/IsK channel complex. Am J Physiol Heart Circ Physiol 280:H2038-H2045, 2001.
13. Edwards AS, Scott JD: A-kinase anchoring proteins: Protein kinase A and beyond. Curr Opin Cell Biol 12:217-221, 2000.
14. Scott JD, Dell'Acqua ML, Fraser ID, et al: Coordination of cAMP signaling events through PKA anchoring. Adv Pharmacol 47:175-207, 2000.
15. Gray PC, Scott JD, Catterall WA: Regulation of ion channels by cAMP-dependent protein kinase and A-kinase anchoring proteins. Curr Opin Neurobiol 8:330-334, 1998.
16. Marks AR, Marx SO, Reiken S: Regulation of ryanodine receptors via macromolecular complexes: a novel role for leucine/isoleucine zippers. Trends Cardiovasc Med 12:166-170, 2002.
17. Marx SO, Reiken S, Hisamatsu Y, et al: Phosphorylation-dependent regulation of ryanodine receptors. A novel role for leucine/isoleucine zippers. J Cell Biol 153:699-708, 2001.
18. Hulme JT, Ahn M, Hauschka SD, et al: A novel leucine zipper targets AKAP15 and cyclic AMP–dependent protein kinase to the C terminus of the skeletal muscle Ca^{2+} channel and modulates its function. J Biol Chem 277:4079-4087, 2002.
19. Marx SO, Kurokawa J, Reiken S, et al: Requirement of a macromolecular signaling complex for beta adrenergic receptor modulation of the KCNQ1-KCNE1 potassium channel. Science 295:496-499, 2002.
20. Landschulz WH, Johnson PF, McKnight SL: The leucine zipper: A hypothetical structure common to a new class of DNA binding proteins. Science 240:1759-1764, 1988.
21. Lupas A: Coiled coils: New structures and new functions. Trends Biochem Sci 21:375-382, 1996.
22. Leung IW, Lassam N: Dimerization via tandem leucine zippers is essential for the activation of the mitogen-activated protein kinase kinase kinase, MLK-3. J Biol Chem 273:32408-32415, 1998.
23. Walshaw J, Woolfson DN: Open-and-shut cases in coiled-coil assembly: Alpha-sheets and alpha-cylinders. Protein Sci 10:668-673, 2001.
24. Kohn WD, Kay CM, Hodges RS: Orientation, positional, additivity, and oligomerization-state effects of interhelical ion pairs in alpha-helical coiled-coils. J Mol Biol 283:993-1012, 1998.
25. Simmerman HK, Kobayashi YM, Autry JM, Jones LR: A leucine zipper stabilizes the pentameric membrane domain of phospholamban and forms a coiled-coil pore structure. J Biol Chem 271:5941-5946, 1996.
26. Harbury PB, Zhang T, Kim PS, Alber T: A switch between two-, three-, and four-stranded coiled coils in GCN4 leucine zipper mutants. Science 262:1401-1407, 1993.
27. Surks HK, Mochizuki N, Kasai Y, et al: Regulation of myosin phosphatase by a specific interaction with cGMP-dependent

protein kinase Ialpha. Science 286:1583-1587, 1999.
28. Moitra J, Szilak L, Krylov D, Vinson C: Leucine is the most stabilizing aliphatic amino acid in the d position of a dimeric leucine zipper coiled coil. Biochemistry 36:12567-12573, 1997.
29. Lin JW, Wyszynski M, Madhavan R, et al: Yotiao, a novel protein of neuromuscular junction and brain that interacts with specific splice variants of NMDA receptor subunit NR1. J Neurosci 18:2017-2027, 1998.
30. Piippo K, Swan H, Pasternack M, et al: A founder mutation of the potassium channel KCNQ1 in long QT syndrome: Implications for estimation of disease prevalence and molecular diagnostics. J Am Coll Cardiol 37:562-568, 2001.
31. Paavonen KJ, Swan H, Piippo K, et al: Response of the QT interval to mental and physical stress in types LQT1 and LQT2 of the long QT syndrome. Heart 86:39-44, 2001.
32. Kurokawa J, Chen L, Kass RS: Requirement of subunit expression for cAMP-mediated regulation of a heart potassium channel [abstract]. Proc Natl Acad Sci U S A 100:2122-2127, 2003.
33. Walsh KB, Kass RS: Regulation of a heart potassium channel by protein kinase A and C. Science 242:67-69, 1988.
34. Viswanathan PC, Shaw RM, Rudy Y: Effects of I_{Kr} and I_{Ks} heterogeneity on action potential duration and its rate dependence: A simulation study. Circulation 99:2466-2474, 1999.
35. January CT, Moscucci A: Cellular mechanisms of early afterdepolarizations. Ann N Y Acad Sci 644:23-32, 1992.
36. January CT, Riddle JM: Early afterdepolarizations: Mechanism of induction and block. A role for L-type calcium current. Circ Res 64:977-990, 1989.
37. January CT, Fozzard HA: Delayed afterdepolarizations in heart muscle: Mechanisms and relevance. Pharmacol Rev 40:219-227, 1988.
38. Wit AL, Rosen MR: Pathophysiologic mechanisms of cardiac arrhythmias. Am Heart J 106:798-811, 1983.
39. Kass RS, Lederer JW, Tsien RW, Weingart R: Role of calcium ions in transient inward currents and aftercontactions induced by strophanthidin in cardiac Purkinje fibres. J Physiol (Lond) 281:187-208, 1978.

Drug-Induced Channelopathies 19

Charles Antzelevitch

CHAPTER OUTLINE

Introduction

Drug-induced modulation of ion channel activity can compromise conduction, amplify dispersion of repolarization, and induce triggered activity, thereby contributing to the development of both passive and active cardiac arrhythmias. Inhibition of inward currents with sodium and calcium channel blockers generally slows conduction, reduces excitability, and leads to the development of bradyarrhythmias secondary to sinoatrial and atrioventricular block. Inward current inhibition also can lead to active arrhythmias by creating the substrate for reentry in the form of unidirectional block and slow conduction, or by causing loss of the action potential dome and marked abbreviation of the action potential in epicardium. In the latter case, sodium and calcium channel block can give rise to transmural as well as epicardial dispersion of repolarization, leading to the development of phase 2 reentry-mediated extrasystoles, ST segment elevation, and polymorphic ventricular tachycardia, all electrophysiologic features of the Brugada syndrome.[1] Inhibition of outward repolarizing current generally gives rise to an increase in action potential duration (APD) as well as early afterdepolarization (EAD)-induced triggered activity. Because APD prolongation usually is inhomogeneous, drugs that inhibit outward repolarizing currents commonly amplify transmural dispersion of repolarization (TDR), thus providing the substrate for the development of torsade de pointes arrhythmias, characteristic of the long QT syndrome.[2] Drug-induced augmentation of late inward current can do likewise, contributing to the development of EADs, TDR, and torsade de pointes.[3] The focus in this chapter is on the acquired long QT syndrome, the most frequently encountered form of drug-induced channelopathy.

Drug-Induced Long QT Syndrome

The QT interval is a body surface measure of the time required for the ventricles of the heart to repolarize. Prolongation of the QT interval occurs when the action potential of a significant proportion of cells in the ventricular myocardium is prolonged, as a result of a reduction in one or more repolarizing currents or an augmentation of inward currents, or both. The effect of a drug on APD is determined by the balance between its action to alter inward and outward currents. A prolonged APD can be caused by drug effects on a single or many ion channels, pumps, or exchangers. Inhibition of the rapidly activating delayed rectifier potassium channels (I_{Kr}) is the most common cause of drug-induced QT prolongation.[4] As discussed later, many drugs block multiple cardiac ion channels, thus causing a more complex alteration of action potential morphology.

I_{Kr} block and QT prolongation have attracted considerable attention in recent years due to their association with life-threatening cardiac arrhythmias, such as torsade de pointes.[5] Antiarrhythmic drugs with class III action, which prolong cardiac repolarization by blocking potassium channels, were among the first to be linked to this arrhythmogenic syndrome. The incidence of torsade de pointes in patients who receive quinidine is estimated to range between 2.0% and 8.8%. Therapy with DL-sotalol has been associated with an incidence ranging from 1.8% to 4.8%. A similar incidence has been described for newer class III agents, such as dofetilide and ibutilide.[6]

An ever-increasing number and spectrum of noncardiovascular agents, most acting by inhibition of I_{Kr}, also have been shown to aggravate or precipitate torsade de pointes.[5] More than 50 commercially available or investigational noncardiovascular and 20 cardiovascular non-antiarrhythmic drugs have been implicated. This problem appears to arise more frequently with newer drugs, and a number of agents have been withdrawn from the market in recent years (e.g. prenylamine, terodiline, and in some countries sertindole, grepafloxacin, terfenadine, astemizole and cisapride).

Table 19-1 presents a list of drugs known to prolong the QT interval and to induce torsade de pointes. Most of these agents block I_{Kr}, many also block slowly activating delayed rectifier current (I_{Ks}), and some augment late I_{Na}, so that in many ways their action is similar to the pathophysiologic changes encountered in the three principal congenital forms of long QT syndrome. The acquired form of the disease is far more prevalent than the congenital form and in some cases may have a genetic predisposition.

Although antidepressants are widely recognized in their ability to precipitate an acquired form of the Brugada syndrome,[7-15] they are only weakly associated with an ability to prolong the QT interval and to induce torsade de pointes. Among antidepressants agents, aminotryptyline, imipramine, and maprotiline are the agents most commonly associated with torsade de pointes; the greatest prolongation of QT interval is observed with maprotiline.[16] Antidepressant-induced torsade de pointes typically is observed in the presence of drug combinations. Antipsychotic drugs generally have a higher torsadogenic potential than antidepressants. Ray and colleagues[17] (2001) conducted a retrospective cohort study of half a million Medicaid patients between 1988 and 1993, before the introduction of atypical antipsychotics, and observed that the risk for sudden death increased 2.39 times in persons receiving

Table 19-1 Drugs Associated with Increased Risk of Long QT Syndrome and Torsade de Pointes

Generic Name	Clinical Use
Amiodarone	Antiarrhythmic
Arsenic trioxide	Anticancer/leukemia
Bepridil	Antianginal
Chloroquine	Antimalarial
Chlorpromazine	Antipsychotic/antiemetic/schizophrenia/nausea
Cisapride	GI stimulant
Clarithromycin	Antibiotic
Disopyramide	Antiarrhythmic
Dofetilide	Antiarrhythmic
Domperidone	Antinausea
Droperidol	Sedative; antinausea
Erythromycin	Antibiotic; GI stimulant
Halofantrine	Antimalarial
Haloperidol	Antipsychotic/schizophrenia, agitation
Ibutilide	Antiarrhythmic
Levomethadyl	Opiate agonist/pain control
Mesoridazine	Antipsychotic/schizophrenia
Methadone	Opiate agonist/pain control
Pentamidine	Anti-infective/*Pneumocystis* pneumonia
Pimozide	Antipsychotic/Tourette's syndrome tics
Procainamide	Antiarrhythmic
Quinidine	Antiarrhythmic
Sotalol	Antiarrhythmic
Sparfloxacin	Antibiotic
Thioridazine	Antipsychotic/schizophrenia

Modified from www.QTdrugs.org, a link to "QT Drug Lists" on the website of the Arizona Center for Education and Research on Therapeutics (funded by the U.S. Agency for Healthcare Research and Quality).
GI, gastrointestinal (tract).

antipsychotic drugs over that observed in those who did not receive these agents. Although the study did not demonstrate causality, it suggested that the potential adverse cardiac effects of antipsychotics should be considered in clinical practice, particularly for patients with cardiovascular disease. Hennessy and associates,[18] in a study of 90,000 patients, observed that patients who received pharmacologic treatment for schizophrenia had a higher incidence of cardiac arrest and ventricular arrhythmias than in non-schizophrenia patients. The drugs used were clozapine, haloperidol, risperidone, and thioridazine. Liperoti and coworkers,[19] in a study of nursing homes residents in six states, observed that the use of conventional antipsychotics led to a two-fold increase in risk of hospitalization for ventricular arrhythmias and cardiac arrest, especially in patients with preexisting cardiac disease.

Mechanism of Drug-Induced QT Interval Prolongation and Torsade de Pointes

Drug-induced torsade de pointes arises as a consequence of the development of a substrate in the form of augmented spatial dispersion of repolarization and a trigger in the form of early or delayed afterdepolarization-induced triggered activity.[2,20,21] Augmentation of spatial dispersion of repolarization may be in the form of exaggerated transmural, transseptal, or apicobasal dispersion of repolarization.[22-25] The past couple of decades have witnessed significant advances in appreciation of the cellular diversity of the ventricular myocardium. A number of studies have highlighted regional differences in electrical properties of ventricular cells, as well as differences in the response of the different cell types to pharmacologic agents and pathophysiologic states (as summarized in published reviews[22,26]). Among the heterogeneities uncovered are electrical and pharmacologic distinctions between endocardium and epicardium of the canine, feline, rabbit, rat, mouse, and human heart, as well as differences in the electrophysiologic characteristics and pharmacologic responsiveness of M cells located in the deep structures of the ventricles of the heart.

M cells are distinguished by the ability of their action potential to prolong more than those of epicardial and endocardial cells in response to a slowing of rate or in response to drugs with QT-prolonging actions (or both).[27] The ionic basis for these features include the presence of a smaller slowly activating delayed rectifier current (I_{Ks}), a larger late sodium current (late I_{Na}), and a larger electrogenic sodium-calcium exchange current ($I_{Na\text{-}Ca}$). Cells with M cell characteristics have been reported in canine, guinea pig, rabbit, pig, and human ventricles.[28]

Differences in the time course of repolarization of the three ventricular myocardial cell types generate voltage gradients that are responsible for the inscription of the T wave in the ECG. Preferential prolongation of the M cell APD is thought to provide the principal substrate for arrhythmogenesis under long QT conditions. Studies using the arterially perfused wedge preparation have developed experimental models of acquired long QT syndrome (Fig. 19-1). The wedge model is capable of developing and sustaining a variety of arrhythmias, including torsade de pointes.

I_{Ks} block alone produces a homogeneous prolongation of repolarization across the ventricular wall, but does not induce arrhythmias (see Fig. 19-1A). The addition of a β-adrenergic agonist such as isoproterenol leads to abbreviation of epicardial and endocardial APD with little or no change in the APD of the M cell, resulting in a marked augmentation of TDR and the development of spontaneous and stimulation-induced torsade de pointes.[29] These cellular changes generally give rise to a broad-based T wave and a long QT interval characteristic of the type 1 long QT syndrome variant, LQT1. The development of torsade de pointes in this model is exquisitely sensitive to β-adrenergic stimulation, consistent with the high sensitivity of patients with congenital long QT syndrome, LQT1 in particular, to sympathetic stimulation.[30]

I_{Krs} block with D-sotalol also causes a greater prolongation of the M cell action potential and a slowing of phase 3 of the action potential of all three cell types, resulting in low-amplitude T waves, prolonged QT interval, large transmural dispersion of repolarization, and the development of spontaneous as well as stimulation-induced torsade de pointes (see Fig. 19-1B).

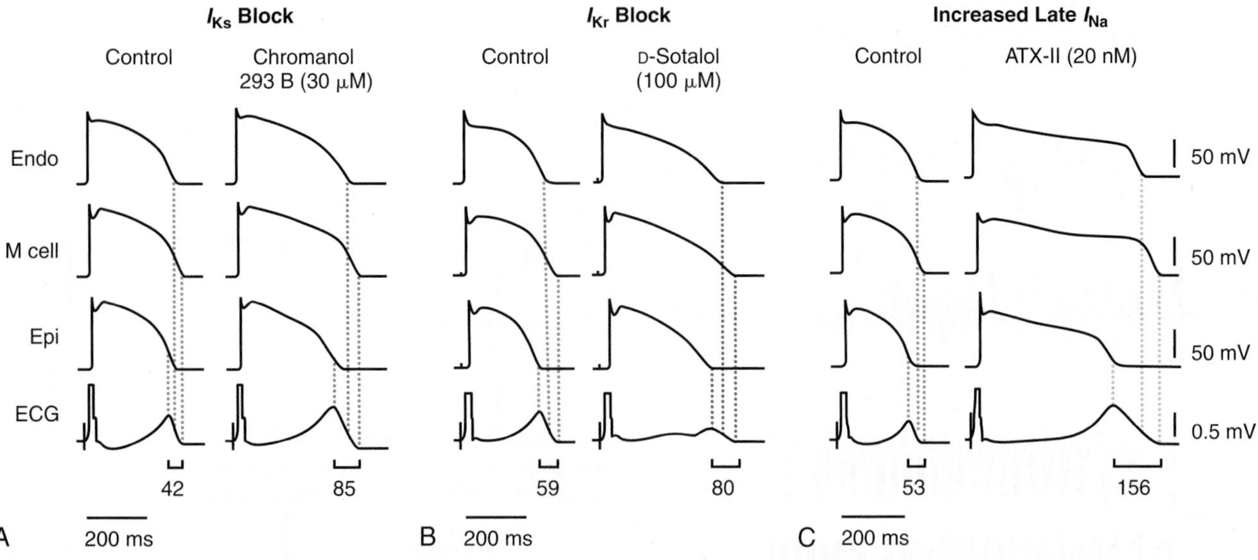

Figure 19-1 Transmembrane action potentials and transmural electrocardiogram (ECG) traces in control and after I_{Ks} block (**A**), I_{Kr} block (**B**), and increase in late I_{Na} (**C**), in arterially perfused canine left ventricular wedge preparations. **A** to **C** depict action potentials simultaneously recorded from endocardial (Endo), M cell, and epicardial (Epi) sites, together with a transmural ECG trace. Basic cycle length (BCL) = 2000 ms. In all cases, the peak of the T wave in the ECG is coincident with the repolarization of the epicardial action potential, whereas the end of the T wave is coincident with the repolarization of the M cell action potential. Repolarization of the endocardial cell is intermediate between that of the M cell and epicardial cell. Transmural dispersion of repolarization across the ventricular wall, defined as the difference in the repolarization time between M and epicardial cells, is denoted below the ECG traces. (Modified from Shimizu W, Antzelevitch C: Cellular basis for the ECG features of the LQT1 form of the long QT syndrome: Effects of β-adrenergic agonists and antagonists and sodium channel blockers on transmural dispersion of repolarization and torsade de pointes. Circulation 98:2314-2322, 1998; and Shimizu W, Antzelevitch C: Sodium channel block with mexiletine is effective in reducing dispersion of repolarization and preventing torsade de pointes in LQT2 and LQT3 models of the long-QT syndrome. Circulation 96:2038-2047, 1997.)

The addition of hypokalemia further accentuates the reduction in the amplitude of the T wave, giving rise to a deeply notched or bifurcated appearance, similar to that commonly seen in patients with the LQT2 variant of the syndrome.[31,32]

Augmentation of late I_{Na} with the sea anemone toxin (ATX-II)[32] markedly prolongs the QT interval, delays the onset of the T wave, in some cases also widening it, and causes a sharp rise in TDR as a result of a greater prolongation of the APD of the M cell (see Fig. 19-1C). A relatively large effect of ATX-II to prolong the APD of epicardium and endocardium leads to a relatively long delay in the onset of the T wave, consistent with the late-appearing T wave pattern and prolonged isoelectric ST segment commonly observed in patients with the LQT3 form of the long QT syndrome.

The tachyarrhythmia most commonly encountered in congenital and acquired long QT syndrome is torsade de pointes, an atypical polymorphic ventricular tachycardia. Torsade de pointes most commonly develops in patients receiving an I_{Kr} blocker, especially in the presence of hypokalemia and slow heart rates or long pauses, conditions similar to those under which I_{Kr} blockers induce EADs and triggered activity in isolated Purkinje fibers and M cells. An EAD-induced extrasystole is believed to be responsible for the premature beat that initiates torsade de pointes, but the maintenance of the arrhythmia generally is thought to be due to circus movement reentry.[22] In the wedge model, torsade de pointes occurs spontaneously or can be electrically induced. Figure 19-2 illustrates an example of drug-induced torsade de pointes in a wedge preparation perfused with Tyrode's solution warmed to a physiologic temperature. When the perfusate is cooled, all focal extrasystolic activity is suppressed and spontaneous torsade de pointes is no longer observed, but the arrhythmia can be readily induced with a single premature beat applied to the epicardium, the site of briefest refractoriness. The action potential recordings demonstrate the persistence of a substrate for reentry in the form of a TDR. Taken together these observations are provide strong evidence for reentry as the basis for torsade de pointes.

Although polymorphic ventricular tachycardia can arise as a consequence of both focal and reentrant mechanisms, in both the presence and the absence of a prolonged QT interval, the available data point to the following hypothesis as the basis for most cases of long QT syndrome–related torsade de pointes (Fig. 19-3). The hypothesis presumes the presence of electrical heterogeneity in the form of transmural dispersion of repolarization under baseline conditions. This intrinsic heterogeneity is amplified by agents that reduce net repolarizing current by means of a reduction in I_{Kr} or I_{Ks} or augmentation of late I_{Ca} or late I_{Na}. Conditions leading to a reduction in I_{Kr} or augmentation of late I_{Na} produce a preferential prolongation of the M cell action potential. As a consequence, the QT interval prolongs and is accompanied by a dramatic increase in transmural dispersion of repolarization, which creates a vulnerable window for the development of reentry. The reduction in net repolarizing current also predisposes to the development of EAD-induced triggered activity in M and Purkinje cells, which provide the extrasystole that triggers torsade de pointes when it falls within the vulnerable period. β-Adrenergic agonists further amplify transmural heterogeneity (transiently) in the case of I_{Kr} block but reduce it in the case of I_{Na} promoters.[33] By contrast, conditions leading to a reduction in I_{Kr} cause a homogeneous prolongation of APD throughout the ventricular wall, leading to a prolongation of the QT interval but with no increase in transmural dispersion of repolarization. Torsade de pointes does not occur spontaneously, nor can it be induced by programmed stimulation under these conditions until a β-adrenergic agonist is introduced. Isoproterenol dramatically increases transmural dispersion of

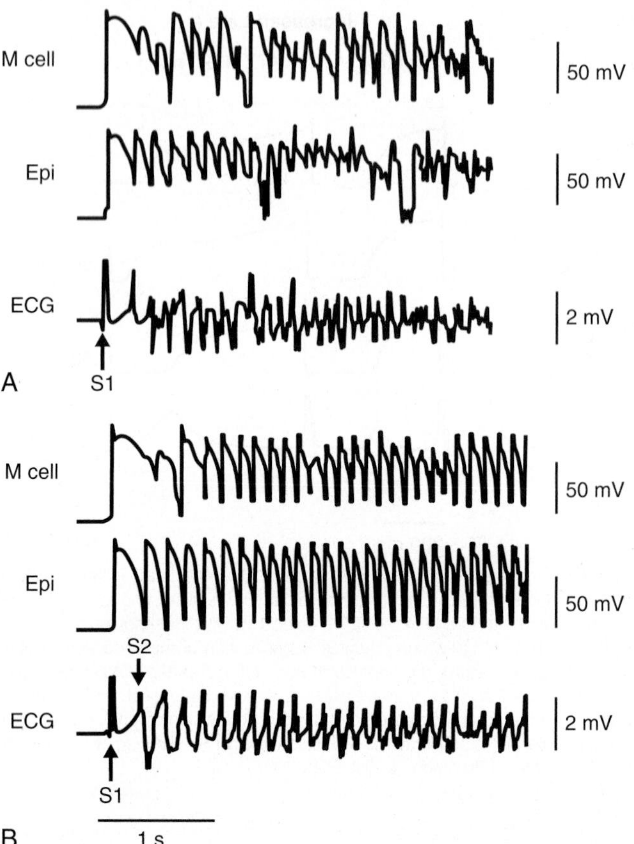

Figure 19-2 Spontaneous and stimulation-induced polymorphic ventricular tachycardia with features of torsade de pointes occurring in a canine arterially perfused left ventricular wedge preparation. **A,** Spontaneous torsade de pointes in a preparation pretreated with chromanol (30 μmol/L) plus isoproterenol (100 nmol/L). A spontaneous premature beat with a coupling interval of 285 ms, probably originating from subendocardial Purkinje system, initiates an episode of torsade de pointes. **B,** The perfusate temperature was cooler (36° C) and extrasystolic activity was absent, presumably owing to absence of early afterdepolarization–induced triggered activity. The presence of a reentrant substrate in the form of a transmural dispersion of repolarization is evidenced by the capability to induce torsade de pointes with a single extrasystole applied to epicardium (site of briefest refractoriness). S1-S1 interval = 2000 ms. (Modified from Antzelevitch C, Shimizu W: Cellular mechanisms underlying the long QT syndrome. Curr Opin Cardiol 17:43-51, 2002.)

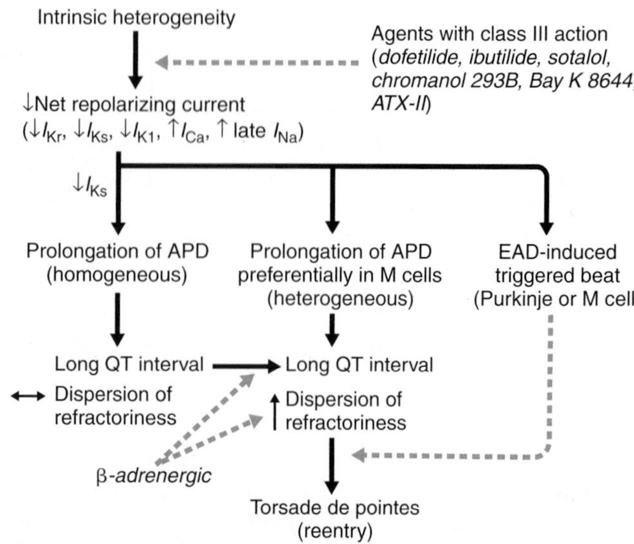

Figure 19-3 Proposed cellular mechanism for the development of torsade de pointes in the acquired long QT syndrome. APD, action potential duration; EAD, early afterdepolarization.

repolarization and refractoriness under these conditions by abbreviating the APD of epicardium and endocardium, thereby creating a vulnerable window that an EAD-induced triggered response can invade to generate torsade de pointes. The β-adrenergic stimulation also facilitates the development of a triggered response that initiates torsade de pointes.

Drugs Affecting Multiple Ion Channels

Drugs affecting two or more ion channels, such as quinidine, pentobarbital, amiodarone, ranolazine, and azimilide, produce a more complex response. In the case of quinidine, relatively low therapeutic levels of the drug (3 to 5 μM) produce a marked prolongation of the M cell APD but not of epicardium and endocardium, consistent with a predominant effect of the drug to block I_{Kr} at this concentration. At higher concentrations, quinidine produces a further prolongation of the epicardial and endocardial action potential, consistent with an effect of the drug to block I_{Ks}, but an *abbreviation* of the APD of the M cell, owing to its action to suppress late I_{Na}.[34] Thus, at low concentrations, quinidine prolongs QT and TDR, whereas at higher concentrations the prolongation of QT is not accompanied by an increase in TDR. This may be the reason why quinidine produced torsade de pointes at low therapeutic concentrations but not at high therapeutic or toxic concentrations.[6]

An example of an agent that prolongs the QT interval but reduces transmural dispersion of repolarization is sodium pentobarbital[35] (Fig. 19-4). As with high concentrations of quinidine, pentobarbital does this by inhibiting I_{Kr}, I_{Ks}, and I_{Na} most prominently.[35] This multichannel inhibition leads to a greater prolongation of APD in epicardial and endocardial cells than in M cells, causing a significant reduction in the transmural dispersion of repolarization. The effect of the drug on late I_{Na} (and I_{Ca}) also suppresses D-sotalol–induced EAD activity in M cells. Thus, despite its actions to prolong QT, pentobarbital does not induce torsade de pointes.[35] By virtue of its actions to reduce transmural dispersion and inhibit EAD-induced triggered activity, the anesthetic is effective in suppressing D-sotalol–induced torsade de pointes.[36]

Amiodarone is another agent that acts to prolong the QT interval, but which induces torsade de pointes only rarely. Amiodarone is a potent antiarrhythmic drug used in the management of both atrial and ventricular arrhythmias. In addition to itsβ-blocking properties, amiodarone is known to block the sodium, potassium, and calcium channels in the heart. Its antiarrhythmic efficacy and low incidence of proarrhythmia relative to other agents with class III actions are attributed to its complex pharmacology. When administered chronically (30 to 40 mg/kg per day orally for 30 to 45 days), amiodarone produces a greater prolongation of APD in epicardium and endocardium of the dog heart, but less of an increase, or even a decrease at slow rates, in the M region, thereby reducing TDR.[37] Chronic amiodarone therapy also suppresses the ability of the I_{Kr} blocker, D-sotalol,

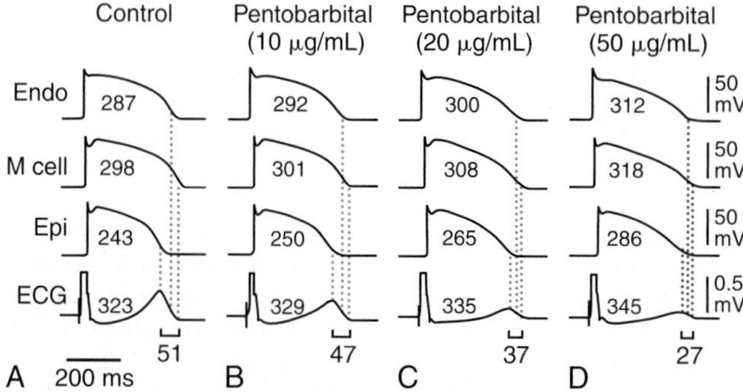

Figure 19-4 Dose-dependent effect of sodium pentobarbital (at concentrations of 10, 20, and 50 μg/mL) on transmembrane and elecrocardiogram (ECG) activity in an arterially perfused canine left ventricular wedge preparation. All ECG traces show action potentials simultaneously recorded from endocardial (Endo), M cell, and epicardial (Epi) sites, together with a transmural ECG. BCL = 2000 ms. Pentobarbital prolongs the QT interval and increases action potential duration (APD) of the endocardial and epicardial cells more than that of the M cell, thus reducing transmural dispersion of repolarization and flattening the T wave in a dose-dependent manner. *Numbers* associated with each action potential indicate the APD_{90} value. *Numbers* associated with the ECG denote the QT interval, and those beneath the ECG represent the transmural dispersion of repolarization. APD_{90}, action potential duration at 90% repolarization. (From Shimizu W, McMahon B, Antzelevitch C: Sodium pentobarbital reduces transmural dispersion of repolarization and prevents torsade de pointes in models of acquired and congenital long QT syndrome. J Cardiovasc Electrophysiol 10:156-164, 1999.)

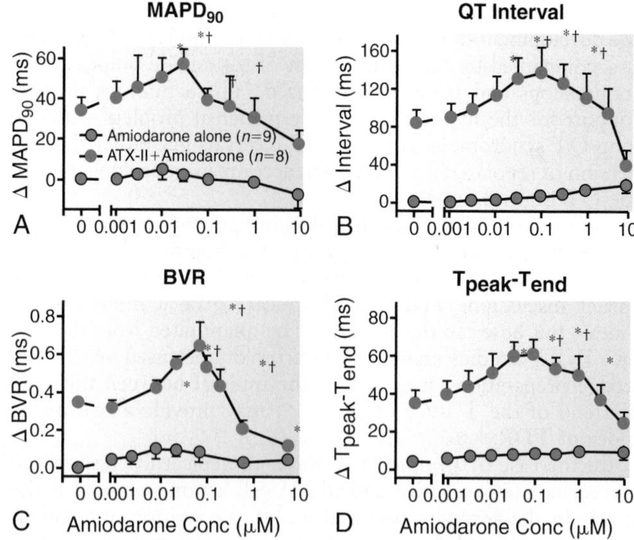

Figure 19-5 Amiodarone-induced prolongation of the QT interval and torsade de pointes. Concentration-response relationships for amiodarone on monophasic action potential duration at 90% repolarization ($MAPD_{90}$) (**A**), QT interval (**B**), beat-to-beat variability (BVR) (**C**), and $T_{peak} - T_{end}$ on the electrocardiogram (**D**) in female rabbit isolated hearts in the absence and presence of 3 nmol/L sea anemone toxin ATX-II (n = 6 in each group). Values were calculated as changes from control in individual hearts and are represented as mean ± SEM. *Asterisks* indicate the significance (P <.05) of the difference from either control (amiodarone alone) or ATX-II (ATX-II + amiodarone). † indicates the occurrence of torsade de pointes. (Modified from Wu L, Rajamani S, Shryock JC, et al: Augmentation of late sodium current unmasks the proarrhythmic effects of amiodarone. Cardiovasc Res 77:481-488, 2008.)

to induce a marked dispersion of repolarization or early afterdepolarization activity. Thus, chronic amiodarone treatment differentially alters the cellular electrophysiology of ventricular myocardium so as to produce an important decrease in TDR, especially under conditions in which dispersion is exaggerated. Amiodarone is the only class III antiarrhythmic agent that has thus far failed to produce torsade de pointes in the canine model of chronic atrioventricular block (CAVB).[38]

Wu and coworkers recently developed a female isolated rabbit heart model in which the proarrhythmic potential of amiodarone and other QT-prolonging drugs with a low proarrhythmic risk could be identified. They used low concentrations (1 to 3 nmol/L) of the sea anemone toxin (ATX-II), which increases late I_{Na} and thus mimics the gain of function of sodium channels caused by various *SCN5A* polymorphisms and mutations.[39] As illustrated in Figure 19-5, in the presence of low levels of ATX-II, amiodarone exhibits a biphasic concentration-dependent effect to induce and then suppress arrhythmic activity, secondary to inhibition of I_{Kr} and then I_{Na} currents. This is the first preclinical model to demonstrate the potential for amiodarone to induce torsade de pointes.[39] The ability of low concentrations of ATX-II to unmask the arrhythmogenic potential of amiodarone is consistent with the finding of an increased incidence of torsade de pointes among patients receiving amiodarone who have an *SCN5A* polymorphism (S1102Y) that causes a "gain of function" of late I_{Na}.[40]

Ranolazine, an experimental antianginal agent, has been shown to possess ionic and cellular actions similar to those of amiodarone.[41,42] Like amiodarone, ranolazine produces block of late I_{Na} (half-maximal inhibitory concentration [IC_{50}] = 5.9 μM), I_{Kr} (IC_{50} = 11.4 μM), and I_{Ca} (IC_{50} = 296 μM). Despite potent block of I_{Kr}, the drug produces little QT prolongation, owing to its equally potent effect to block inward currents, particularly late I_{Na}. Its effect to prolong the QT interval notwithstanding, ranolazine reduces transmural dispersion of repolarization and is capable of suppressing D-sotalol–induced EAD activity in experimental models of torsade de pointes.[42-45] Moreover, ranolazine does not induce spontaneous torsade de pointes in experimental models, nor does it permit induction of the arrhythmia by programmed electrical stimulation. These results highlight the fact that I_{Kr} block, even if potent, does not in and of itself predict the arrhythmogenic potential of pharmacologic agents.

This conclusion is further supported by a study evaluating the I_{Kr}-blocking potency of a series of antiarrhythmics associated with a range of clinical risks of torsade de pointes in mouse AT-1 and Ltk cells transfected with HERG (human ether-à-go-go–related gene) (i.e., the cardiac potassium channel protein encoded by KCNH2).[46] The results indicate that not all drugs that cause torsade de pointes are potent I_{Kr} blockers, and that I_{Kr} block is not necessarily associated with this dysrhythmia, suggesting that other properties of the drugs contribute to their propensity to cause torsade de pointes.

Antiarrhythmic drugs that prolong QT without inducing torsade de pointes have in common the ability to inhibit I_{Ks}, I_{Kr}, and I_{Na} (and/or I_{Ca}) and thus to prolong repolarization without increasing TDR. Indeed, in some cases, transmural dispersion may be reduced.

Another pharmacologic agent capable of prolonging the QT interval without increasing TDR is the I_{Ks} blocker chromanol 293B. Chromanol 293B produces a homogeneous prolongation of APD across the ventricular wall.[29] Despite a prominent prolongation of QT, chromanol 293B never produces torsade de pointes in experimental models, either spontaneously or in response to programmed stimulation. The addition of a β-adrenergic agent leads to a marked abbreviation of APD of epicardium and endocardium, but not of the M cell, resulting in the development of a marked dispersion of repolarization, which is accompanied by the development of torsade de pointes, both spontaneous and stimulation-induced. These findings provide support for the hypothesis that the principal problem with the long QT syndrome is not long QT intervals but rather the dispersion of repolarization that often accompanies prolongation of the QT interval.

If QT prolongation and I_{Kr}-blocking potency are not reliable indices for predicting the proclivity of a drug to induce torsade de pointes, are better surrogates available? As suggested by the earlier discussion, TDR would appear to be a more reliable index—but how can this parameter be quantitated from the surface ECG? Studies conducted in arterially perfused ventricular wedge preparations suggest that the interval between the peak and end of the T wave (T_{peak}-T_{end}) may provide a reasonable index of TDR.

In the case of an upright T wave, the epicardial response is the earliest to repolarize and the M cell action potential is the latest. In the coronary-perfused wedge preparation, repolarization of the epicardial action potential coincides with the peak of the T wave and repolarization of the M cells is coincident with the end of the T wave, so that the interval from the peak to the end of the T wave provides a measure of TDR. These studies suggested that the T_{peak}-T_{end} interval in precordial ECG leads could provide an index of spatial dispersion of repolarization, transmural dispersion in particular. Recent studies have provided guidelines for the estimation of TDR in the case of more complex T waves, including negative, biphasic, and triphasic T waves. In such cases, the interval from the nadir of the first component of the T wave to the end of the T wave was shown to provide an electrocardiographic approximation of TDR.[22]

Although relatively straight forward in the coronary-perfused wedge preparation, extrapolation of these relationships to the surface ECG recorded in vivo must be approached with great caution. The T_{peak}-T_{end} interval is unlikely to provide an absolute measure of transmural dispersion in vivo, as elegantly demonstrated by Xia and coworkers.[47] However, changes in this parameter are thought to be capable of reflecting changes in spatial dispersion of repolarization, particularly TDR, and thus may be prognostic of arrhythmic risk under a variety of conditions.[22] Direct evidence in support of T_{peak}-T_{end} as an index to predict torsade de pointes in patients with long QT syndrome was provided by Yamaguchi and coworkers.[48] These investigators concluded that T_{peak}-T_{end} is more valuable than QTc and QT dispersion as a predictor of torsade de pointes in patients with the acquired syndrome.

Shimizu and coworkers demonstrated that T_{peak}-T_{end}, but not QTc, predicts sudden cardiac death in patients with hypertrophic cardiomyopathy.[49] In a case-control study comparing 30 cases of acquired bradyarrhythmias complicated by torsade de pointes and 113 cases with uncomplicated bradyarrhythmias, Topilski and colleagues found that QT, QTc, and T_{peak}-T_{end} intervals were strong predictors of torsade de pointes, with the best single discriminator being a prolonged T_{peak}-T_{end}.[50] Watanabe and associates demonstrated that prolonged T_{peak}-T_{end} is associated with inducibility, as well as with spontaneous development of ventricular tachycardia in high-risk patients with organic heart disease.[51]

Although an association between increased T_{peak}-T_{end} and arrhythmic risk is emerging, direct validation of T_{peak}-T_{end} measured at the body surface as an index of TDR is still lacking. Because the precordial leads view the electrical field across the ventricular wall, T_{peak}-T_{end} would be expected to be most representative of TDR in these leads. The precordial leads are unipolar leads placed on the chest that are referenced to the Wilson central terminal. The direction of these leads is radially toward the "center" of the heart, the center of the Einthoven triangle. Unlike the precordial leads, the bipolar limb leads, including leads I, II, and III, do not look across the ventricular wall. Although T_{peak}-T_{end} intervals measured in these limb leads may provide an index of TDR, they are more likely to reflect global dispersion, including apicobasal and interventricular dispersion of repolarization.[47,52]

A prominent augmentation of TDR is likely to be arrhythmogenic, because the dispersion of repolarization and refractoriness occurs over a very short distance (the width of the ventricular wall), creating a steep repolarization gradient.[53,54] It is the steepness of the repolarization gradient, rather than the total magnitude of dispersion, that determines arrhythmogenic potential. Apicobasal or interventricular dispersion of repolarization is less informative because it may or may not be associated with a steep repolarization gradient and thus may or may not be associated with arrhythmic risk. Steep apicobasal repolarization gradients are more likely to arise in smaller hearts, such as rabbit or guinea pig, and less likely to arise in larger hearts, such as dog and human.

Another important factor to consider is that TDR can be highly variable in different regions of the ventricular myocardium, particularly under pathophysiologic conditions. Consequently, it is important to measure T_{peak}-T_{end} independently in each of the precordial leads, and it is not advisable to average T_{peak}-T_{end} among several leads.[47] Because long QT syndrome is principally a left ventricular or septal disorder, TDR is likely to be greatest in the mid- to left ventricular wall. Yamaguchi and colleagues, in their study of acquired long QT syndrome, targeted lead V_5.[48] By contrast, because Brugada syndrome is a right ventricular disorder, TDR is greatest in the right ventricular free wall and therefore is best reflected in the right precordial leads. For this reason, Castro and coworkers targeted lead V_2 in their study.[55]

The extent to which TDR exists in the normal heart *in vivo* has been a matter of considerable debate.[26,56,57] The controversy derives in large part from the fact that quantitation of TDR in animals *in vivo* is hampered by (1) the inability to record local repolarization accurately and (2) the unavoidable use of anesthesia that reduces TDR. These same constraints apply to the measurement of TDR in the human heart. Indirect evidence for the presence of a prominent TDR in the human heart in the absence of general anesthesia was provided in a recent study.[58] Theoretical studies have been helpful in understanding the role of electrical coupling in the expression of TDR under *in vivo* conditions.[59]

The available data support the hypothesis that augmentation of TDR, rather than QT prolongation, is responsible for the principal substrate that underlies the development of torsade de pointes.[2,20-23,60] Figure 19-6 presents a qualitative comparison of the effects of different classes of drugs on QT interval and TDR. In the case of pure I_{Kr} blockers such as dofetilide, sotalol, and ibutilide, QT prolongation is proportional to drug concentration, and dose-dependent prolongation of the QT interval is paralleled by an increase in TDR; when TDR achieves the threshold for reentry, torsade de pointes develops. In the case of multichannel blockers, including quinidine, cisapride, and amiodarone, in the setting of augmented late I_{Na}, QT prolongation generally is a biphasic function of drug concentration. When the IC_{50} for outward current block (e.g., I_{Kr} block) is smaller than the IC_{50} for inward current block (e.g., late I_{Na} block), QT and TDR increase at low concentrations of the drug and decrease at higher concentrations of drug. Torsade de pointes develops only during a "window" of drug concentrations at which TDR exceeds the threshold for reentry. Finally, when the IC_{50} for late I_{Na} block is smaller than the IC_{50} for I_{Kr} block, as in the case of pentobarbital, ranolazine, and

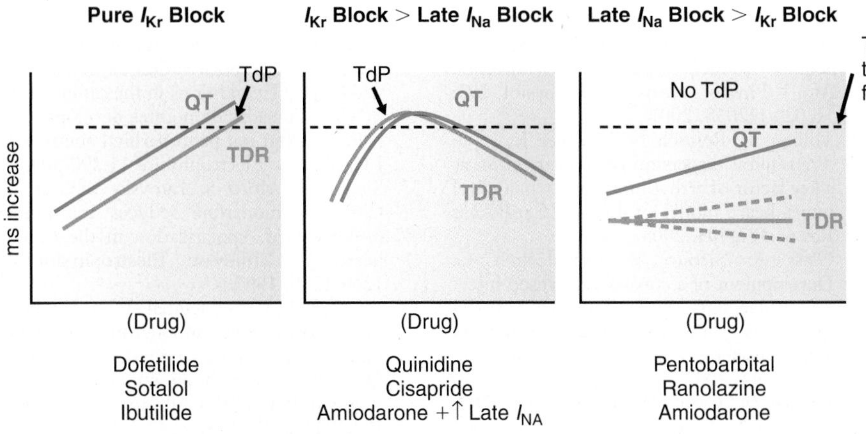

Figure 19-6 Correlation of QT interval and transmural dispersion of repolarization (TDR) in response to different classes of QT-prolonging agents. TdP, torsade de pointes.

amiodarone, dose-dependent QT prolongation is tempered, and augmentation of TDR no longer parallels the prolongation of QT interval; consequently, torsade de pointes does not develop. TDR does not increase under these conditions because of failure of the M cell action potential to prolong preferentially, owing to inhibition of late I_{Na}, which is most intense in this cell type.

Influence of Genetics on Drug-Induced QT Interval Prolongation

The degree to which a genetic predisposition contributes to the clinical manifestation of a drug-induced long QT interval and torsade de pointes is not well defined. Available data suggest that up to 10% to 15% of persons in whom torsade de pointes develops after exposure to QT-prolonging drugs possess mutations associated with the long QT syndrome and may be considered to have a subclinical form of the congenital syndrome.[61]

Abbott and coworkers were among the first to show that a polymorphism (i.e., a genetic variation that is present in greater than 1% of the population) in an ion channel gene is associated with a predisposition to drug-induced torsade de pointes.[62] These investigators identified a polymorphism (T8A) of the *KCNE2* gene coding for MiRP1, a β subunit of the I_{Kr} channel that is present in 1.6% of the population and is associated with torsade de pointes related to quinidine and sulfamethoxazole-trimethoprim administration. This finding suggests that common genetic variations may increase the risk for developmental of drug-related arrhythmias. Yang and associates[63] showed that DNA variants in the coding regions of congenital long QT disease genes predisposing to acquired long QT syndrome can be identified in approximately 10% to 15% of affected persons, predominantly in genes encoding ancillary subunits, providing further support for the hypothesis that subclinical mutations and polymorphisms may predispose to drug-induced torsade de pointes. As discussed earlier, Splawski and colleagues[40] further advanced this concept by identifying a heterozygous polymorphism involving substitution of serine with tyrosine in codon 1103 (S1103Y) in the sodium channel gene *SCN5A* (S1102Y in the shorter splice variant of *SCN5A*) among Africans and African Americans that increases the risk for acquired torsade de pointes. The polymorphism was present in 57% of 23 patients with proarrhythmic episodes but in only 13% of control subjects. These findings suggest that carriers of such polymorphisms can be identified and excluded from treatment with drugs that are associated with a risk of proarrhythmia. It is conceivable that such testing could be applied widely, because accurate results could be made available rapidly at relatively low cost.

Another common polymorphism that has been associated with acquired forms of long QT syndrome and torsade de pointes is K897T in KCNH2.[64] Most functional expression studies have reported that K897T reduces I_{Kr},[65-67] although one study has reported an increase in HERG current.[68]

Genetic defects also can contribute to drug-induced channelopathies by influencing the metabolism of drugs. In the case of relatively pure I_{Kr} blockers, a clear relationship has been recognized between plasma levels of drug and the incidence of torsade de pointes. Genetic variants of the genes coding for enzymes responsible for drug metabolism could alter pharmacokinetics so as to cause wide fluctuations in plasma levels, thus exerting a significant proarrhythmic influence.[69] For example, in the case of cytochrome CYP2D6, which is involved in the metabolism of some QT-prolonging drugs (terodiline, thioridazine), multiple polymorphisms have been reported that reduce or eliminate its function; 5% to 10% of whites and African Americans lack a functional CYP2D6. Numerous proteins, including drug transport molecules and other drug-metabolizing enzymes, are involved in drug absorption, distribution, and elimination, and genetic variants of each of these have the potential to modulate drug concentrations and effects. Multiple substrates and inhibitors of the cytochrome P-450 enzymes have been identified (a comprehensive database can be found at http://medicine.iupui.edu/flockhart).

References

1. Antzelevitch C: Brugada syndrome. PACE 29:1130-1159, 2006.
2. Antzelevitch C: Heterogeneity and cardiac arrhythmias: An overview. Heart Rhythm 4:964-972, 2007.
3. Novosel D, Hof A, Zierhut W, Hof RP: Proarrhythmic effects of DPI 201-106 elicited with programmed electrical stimulation—a comparison with sotalol. J Cardiovasc Pharmaco l21:967-972, 1993.
4. Bednar MM, Harrigan EP, Anziano RJ, et al: The QT interval. Prog Cardiovasc Dis 43:1-45, 2001.
5. Haverkamp W, Breithardt G, Camm AJ, et al: The potential for QT prolongation

and proarrhythmia by non-antiarrhythmic drugs: Clinical and regulatory implications. Report on a Policy Conference of the European Society of Cardiology. Cardiovasc Res 47:219-233, 2000.
6. Antzelevitch C: Drug-induced channelopathies. In Zipes DP, Jalife J (eds): Cardiac Electrophysiology: From Cell to Bedside, 4th ed. Philadelphia, Saunders, 2004, pp 151-157.
7. Goldgran-Toledano D, Sideris G, Kevorkian JP: Overdose of cyclic antidepressants and the Brugada syndrome. N Engl J Med 346:1591-1592, 2002.
8. Rouleau F, Asfar P, Boulet S, et al: Transient ST segment elevation in right precordial leads induced by psychotropic drugs: Relationship to the Brugada syndrome. J Cardiovasc Electrophysiol 12:61-65, 2001.
9. Babaliaros VC, Hurst JW: Tricyclic antidepressants and the Brugada syndrome: An example of Brugada waves appearing after the administration of desipramine. Clin Cardiol 25:395-398, 2002.
10. Akhtar M, Goldschlager NF: Brugada electrocardiographic pattern due to tricyclic antidepressant overdose. J Electrocardiol 39:336-339, 2006.
11. Chow BJ, Gollob M, Birnie D: Brugada syndrome precipitated by a tricyclic antidepressant. Heart 91:651, 2005.
12. Bolognesi R, Tsialtas D, Vasini P, et al: Abnormal ventricular repolarization mimicking myocardial infarction after heterocyclic antidepressant overdose. Am J Cardiol 79:242-245, 1997.
13. Tada H, Sticherling C, Oral H, Morady F: Brugada syndrome mimicked by tricyclic antidepressant overdose. J Cardiovasc Electrophysiol 12:275, 2001.
14. Bigwood B, Galler D, Amir N, Smith W: Brugada syndrome following tricyclic antidepressant overdose. Anaesth Intensive Care 33:266-270, 2005.
15. Darbar D, Yang T, Churchwell K, et al: Unmasking of Brugada syndrome by lithium. Circulation 112:1527-1531, 2005.
16. Vieweg WV, Wood MA: Tricyclic antidepressants, QT interval prolongation, and torsade de pointes. Psychosomatics 45:371-377, 2004.
17. Ray WA, Meredith S, Thapa PB, et al: Antipsychotics and the risk of sudden cardiac death. Arch Gen Psychiatry 58:1161-1167, 2001.
18. Hennessy S, Bilker WB, Knauss JS, et al: Cardiac arrest and ventricular arrhythmia in patients taking antipsychotic drugs: Cohort study using administrative data. BMJ 325:1070, 2002.
19. Liperoti R, Gambassi G, Lapane KL, et al: Conventional and atypical antipsychotics and the risk of hospitalization for ventricular arrhythmias or cardiac arrest. Arch Intern Med 165:696-701, 2005.
20. Antzelevitch C: Ionic, molecular, and cellular bases of QT-interval prolongation and torsade de pointes. Europace 9:iv4-iv15, 2007.
21. Belardinelli L, Antzelevitch C, Vos MA: Assessing predictors of drug-induced torsade de pointes. Trends Pharmacol Sci 24:619-625, 2003.
22. Antzelevitch C: The role of spatial dispersion of repolarization in inherited and acquired sudden cardiac death syndromes. Am J Physiol Heart Circ Physiol 293: H2024-H2038, 2007.
23. Milberg P, Reinsch N, Wasmer K, et al: Transmural dispersion of repolarization as a key factor of arrhythmogenicity in a novel intact heart model of LQT3. Cardiovasc Res 65:397-404, 2005.
24. Glass A, Sicouri S, Antzelevitch C: Development of a coronary-perfused interventricular septal preparation as a model for studying the role of the septum in arrhythmogenesis. J Electrocardiol 40: S142-S144, 2007.
25. Restivo M, Caref EB, Kozhevnikov DO, El-Sherif N: Spatial dispersion of repolarization is a key factor in the arrhythmogenicity of long QT syndrome. J Cardiovasc Electrophysiol 15:323-331, 2004.
26. Antzelevitch C, Shimizu W, Yan GX, et al: The M cell: Its contribution to the ECG and to normal and abnormal electrical function of the heart. J Cardiovasc Electrophysiol 10:1124-1152, 1999.
27. Sicouri S, Antzelevitch C: A subpopulation of cells with unique electrophysiological properties in the deep subepicardium of the canine ventricle. The M cell. Circ Res 68:1729-1741, 1991.
28. Antzelevitch C, Shimizu W: Cellular mechanisms underlying the long QT syndrome. Curr Opin Cardiol 17:43-51, 2002.
29. Shimizu W, Antzelevitch C: Cellular basis for the ECG features of the LQT1 form of the long QT syndrome: Effects of β-adrenergic agonists and antagonists and sodium channel blockers on transmural dispersion of repolarization and torsade de pointes. Circulation 98:2314-2322, 1998.
30. Schwartz PJ, Priori SG, Spazzolini C, et al: Genotype-phenotype correlation in the long-QT syndrome: Gene-specific triggers for life-threatening arrhythmias. Circulation 103:89-95, 2001.
31. Yan GX, Antzelevitch C: Cellular basis for the normal T wave and the electrocardiographic manifestations of the long QT syndrome. Circulation 98:1928-1936, 1998.
32. Shimizu W, Antzelevitch C: Sodium channel block with mexiletine is effective in reducing dispersion of repolarization and preventing torsade de pointes in LQT2 and LQT3 models of the long-QT syndrome. Circulation 96:2038-2047, 1997.
33. Shimizu W, Antzelevitch C: Differential effects of beta-adrenergic agonists and antagonists in LQT1, LQT2 and LQT3 models of the long QT syndrome. J Am Coll Cardiol 35:778-786, 2000.
34. Balser JR, Bennett PB, Hondeghem LM, Roden DM: Suppression of time-dependent outward current in guinea-pig ventricular myocytes. Actions of quinidine and amiodarone. Circ Res 69:519-529, 1991.
35. Shimizu W, McMahon B, Antzelevitch C: Sodium pentobarbital reduces transmural dispersion of repolarization and prevents torsade de pointes in models of acquired and congenital long QT syndrome. J Cardiovasc Electrophysiol 10:156-164, 1999.
36. Weissenburger J, Nesterenko VV, Antzelevitch C: Transmural heterogeneity of ventricular repolarization under baseline and long QT conditions in the canine heart in vivo: Torsades de pointes develops with halothane but not pentobarbital anesthesia. J Cardiovasc Electrophysiol 11:290-304.
37. Sicouri S, Moro S, Litovsky SH, et al: Chronic amiodarone reduces transmural dispersion of repolarization in the canine heart. J Cardiovasc Electrophysiol 8: 1269-1279, 1997.
38. van Opstal JM, Schoenmakers M, Verduyn SC, et al: Chronic amiodarone evokes no torsade de pointes arrhythmias despite QT lengthening in an animal model of acquired long-QT syndrome. Circulation 104:2722-2727, 2001.
39. Wu L, Rajamani S, Shryock JC, et al: Augmentation of late sodium current unmasks the proarrhythmic effects of amiodarone. Cardiovasc Res 77:481-488, 2008.
40. Splawski I, Timothy KW, Tateyama M, et al: Variant of SCN5A sodium channel implicated in risk of cardiac arrhythmia. Science 297:1333-1336, 2002.
41. Antzelevitch C, Belardinelli L, Zygmunt AC, et al: Electrophysiologic effects of ranolazine: A novel anti-anginal agent with antiarrhythmic properties. Circulation 110:904-910, 2004.
42. Antzelevitch C, Belardinelli L, Wu L, et al: Electrophysiologic properties and antiarrhythmic actions of a novel anti-anginal agent. J Cardiovasc Pharmacol Ther 9(Suppl 1):S65-S83, 2004.
43. Belardinelli L, Shryock JC, Fraser H: Inhibition of the late sodium current as a potential cardioprotective principle: Effects of the late sodium current inhibitor ranolazine. Heart 92 Suppl 4:iv6-iv14, 2006.
44. Song Y, Shryock JC, Wu L, Belardinelli L: Antagonism by ranolazine of the pro-arrhyhtmic effects of increasing late I_{Na} in guinea pig ventricular myocytes. J Cardiovasc Pharmacol 44:192-199, 2004.
45. Wu L, Shryock JC, Song Y, et al: Antiarrhythmic effects of ranolazine in a guinea pig in vitro model of long-QT syndrome. J Pharmacol Exp Ther 310: 599-605, 2004.
46. Yang T, Snyders D, Roden DM: Drug block of I(kr): Model systems and relevance to human arrhythmias. J Cardiovasc Pharmacol 38:737-744, 2001.
47. Xia Y, Liang Y, Kongstad O, et al: In vivo validation of the coincidence of the peak and end of the T wave with full repolarization of the epicardium and endocardium in swine. Heart Rhythm 2:162-169, 2005.
48. Yamaguchi M, Shimizu M, Ino H, et al: T wave peak-to-end interval and QT dispersion in acquired long QT syndrome: A new index for arrhythmogenicity. Clin Sci (Lond) 105:671-676, 2003.
49. Shimizu M, Ino H, Okeie K, et al: T-peak to T-end interval may be a better predictor of high-risk patients with hypertrophic cardiomyopathy associated with a cardiac troponin I mutation than QT dispersion. Clin Cardiol 25:335-339, 2002.
50. Topilski I, Rogowski O, Rosso R, et al: The morphology of the QT interval predicts

torsade de pointes during acquired bradyarrhythmias. J Am Coll Cardiol 9:320-328, 2007.

51. Watanabe N, Kobayashi Y, Tanno K, et al: Transmural dispersion of repolarization and ventricular tachyarrhythmias. J Electrocardiol 37:191-200, 2004.
52. Opthof T, Coronel R, Wilms-Schopman FJ, et al: Dispersion of repolarization in canine ventricle and the electrocardiographic T wave: T(p-e) interval does not reflect transmural dispersion. Heart Rhythm 4:341-348, 2007.
53. Akar FG, Yan GX, Antzelevitch C, Rosenbaum DS: Unique topographical distribution of M cells underlies reentrant mechanism of torsade de pointes in the long-QT syndrome. Circulation 105:1247-1253, 2002.
54. Aiba T, Shimizu W, Hidaka I, et al: Cellular basis for trigger and maintenance of ventricular fibrillation in the Brugada syndrome model: High-resolution optical mapping study. J Am Coll Cardiol 47:2074-2085, 2006.
55. Castro HJ, Antzelevitch C, Tornes BF, et al: Tpeak-Tend and Tpeak-end dispersion as risk factors for ventricular tachycardia/ventricular fibrillation in patients with the Brugada syndrome. J Am Coll Cardiol 47:1828-1834, 2006.
56. Anyukhovsky EP, Sosunov EA, Gainullin RZ, Rosen MR: The controversial M cell. J Cardiovasc Electrophysiol 10:244-260, 1999.
57. Coronel R, de Bakker JM, Wilms-Schopman FJ, et al: Monophasic action potentials and activation recovery intervals as measures of ventricular action potential duration: Experimental evidence to resolve some controversies. Heart Rhythm 3: 1043-1050, 2006.
58. Fish JM, Brugada J, Antzelevitch C: Potential proarrhythmic effects of biventricular pacing. J Am Coll Cardiol 46:2340-2347, 2005.
59. Viswanathan PC, Shaw RM, Rudy Y: Effects of I_{Kr} and I_{Ks} heterogeneity on action potential duration and its rate-dependence: A simulation study. Circulation 99:2466-2474, 1999.
60. Fenichel RR, Malik M, Antzelevitch C, et al: Drug-induced torsade de pointes and implications for drug development. J Cardiovasc Electrophysiol 15:475-495, 2004.
61. Roden DM: Long QT syndrome: Reduced repolarization reserve and the genetic link. J Intern Med 259:59-69, 2006.
62. Abbott GW, Sesti F, Splawski I, et al: MiRP1 forms I_{Kr} potassium channels with HERG and is associated with cardiac arrhythmia. Cell 97:175-187, 1999.
63. Yang P, Kanki H, Drolet B, et al: Allelic variants in long-QT disease genes in patients with drug-associated torsades de pointes. Circulation 105:1943-1948, 2002.
64. Pollevick GD, Oliva A, Viskin S, et al: Genetic predisposition to post-myocardial infarction long QT intervals and torsade de pointes [abstract]. Heart Rhythm 4:S121, 2007.
65. Crotti L, Lundquist AL, Insolia R, et al: KCNH2-K897T is a genetic modifier of latent congenital long-QT syndrome. Circulation 112:1251-1258, 2005.
66. Anson BD, Ackerman MJ, Tester DJ, et al: Molecular and functional characterization of common polymorphisms in HERG (KCNH2) potassium channels. Am J Physiol Heart Circ Physiol 286:H2434-H2441, 2004.
67. Paavonen KJ, Chapman H, Laitinen PJ, et al: Functional characterization of the common amino acid 897 polymorphism of the cardiac potassium channel KCNH2 (HERG). Cardiovasc Res 59:603-611, 2003.
68. Bezzina CR, Verkerk AO, Busjahn A, et al: A common polymorphism in KCNH2 (HERG) hastens cardiac repolarization. Cardiovasc Res 59:27-36, 2003.
69. Roden DM: Pharmacogenetics and drug-induced arrhythmias. Cardiovasc Res 50:224-231, 2001.

Connexins as Potential Targets for Cardiovascular Pharmacology 20

Rebecca Lewandowski, Jørgen Søberg Petersen, and Mario Delmar

CHAPTER OUTLINE

Background

Intercellular current flows between cardiac cells—thus enabling an effective heart beat—by way of gap junction channels. Functionally, cardiac cells form a syncytium that allows for the propagation of both electrical and metabolic signals throughout the tissue. From that perspective, coupling is a desired physiologic state, and closure of gap junctions constitutes an "abnormal" condition that ought to be prevented or reversed. Using this train of thought, various investigators have proposed that closure of gap junctions during pathologic conditions such as ischemia could lead to malignant ventricular arrhythmias.[1-5] Yet loss of coupling under ischemic conditions also could be seen as cardioprotective, because it could preserve the integrity of tissue adjoining an area of damage ("healing over").[6] If gap junctions were to remain open at the ischemic border zone, apoptosis-triggering signals could move through gap junctions, thereby extending the area of damage beyond that lacking oxygen supply. Studies on brain ischemia have shown that this "bystander effect" may be responsible, at least in part, for the area of penumbra surrounding ischemic tissue.[7] (Of interest, penumbra is not observed in cardiac ischemia, whereas healing over is well demonstrated.[8-10]) Opposite to this view is the argument that although cell death signals can move through gap junctions, so do molecular signals that can preserve cell integrity, thereby helping cell survival within the area at risk. Part of today's lack of a clear understanding of the beneficial or deleterious effect of gap junction regulation on pathophysiology is consequent to the lack of experimental tools that can selectively modulate gap junction channels. Much has been learned, for example, from the use of tetrodotoxin to validate the relevance of sodium channels in health and disease.[11-15] Yet, although the list of pharmacologic tools to modulate sodium, potassium, or calcium channels (among others) is extensive, the pharmacology of gap junctions is a nascent field.

This chapter reviews previous studies demonstrating chemically induced modification of gap junctions and discusses the potential use of gap junctions as targets for cardiovascular pharmacology. Although most agents described thus far induce gap junction closure in a rather nonselective manner, peptide-based and oligonucleotide-based strategies have yielded new, promising approaches for the design of gap junction modifiers that can either reduce[16,17] or enhance intercellular communication. Specifics are outlined in the following discussion.

Chemical Agents That Induce Gap Junction Closure

Long-Chain Alcohols, Fatty Acids, and General Anesthetics

At micromolar concentrations, heptanol, octanol, myristoleic acid, decanoic acid, and palmitoleic acid all are capable of uncoupling cardiac gap junction channels,[18-20] concurrent with a decrease in open channel probability.[21] Similarly, halothane and isoflurane are two general anesthetics that reversibly close gap junction at concentrations used in clinical practice.[22] A 90% reduction in initial gap junction conductance was seen within 15 seconds after incubation of neonatal rat cardiomyocytes with 2 mM halothane.[22] Additionally, He and Burt showed that halothane reduced the mean open time and increased the mean closed time, whereas single-channel conductance remained unaffected.[23] It has been proposed that the mechanism of action of these agents is rather nonspecific, perhaps by disrupting the fluidity of the plasma membrane or affecting the hydrophobic lipid-protein interface.[22,24] Studies in other ion channels, however, suggest that general anesthetics interact directly with the channel protein, probably within selected binding pockets in pore-forming domains.[25] Although structure-function studies of gap junction closure by these agents are lacking, a direct interaction with the channel protein is a likely mechanism.[26] Because of the rapid effects and complete reversibility of these agents, they commonly are used as "uncouplers." Of note, they also affect various other ion channels, making them highly nonselective.[24,27-29]

Glycyrrhizic Acid Metabolites

Davidson and colleagues used a metabolic cooperativity assay in human fibroblasts to determine that the glycyrrhizic acid metabolites 18α-glycyrrhetinic acid, 18β-glycyrrhetinic acid (αGA and βGA), and carbenoxolone reversibly inhibited coupling at concentrations as low as 2 μM.[30] These compounds require a longer exposure time than that for alkanols and general anesthetics. Their mechanism of action remains unclear, although it has been proposed that they may affect the phosphorylation state of the protein or may modify the ability of connexin subunits to aggregate within the cellular environment.[30] A recent study by Sagar and associates further investigated the effects of carbenoxolone on junctional dye transfer in bovine aortic endothelial cells (BAECs), which express connexin43 (Cx43).[31] These workers found that staurosporine inhibited the carbenoxolone-induced increase in Cx43 content. This result suggested a role for kinases in the mechanism of carbenoxolone. As with other compounds, the effect of these metabolites is not selective for gap junctions.[31]

Receptor Ligands

Gap junction coupling also is regulated by a number of endogenous mediators, including acetylcholine (ACh), norepinephrine, angiotensin (AT), and the angiogenic vascular endothelial growth factor (VEGF), as well as many others. The ACh analogue carbachol (100 μM) causes a reduction in electrical coupling in neonatal heart, similar to that observed after application of 8-Br–cyclic guanosine monophosphate (cGMP), which supports the possibility that the mechanism of action may be mediated by protein kinase G (PKG).[32] Gap junctional coupling has also been shown to decrease in adult rat ventricular cardiomyocytes on α-adrenergic stimulation with phenylephrine in a protein kinase C (PKC)-dependent manner.[33] Similarly, angiotensin has been shown to acutely decrease gap junction coupling in cardiac cells, most likely by way of AT-1 receptors coupled to $G_{q/11}$ proteins and PKC.[34] Additional studies have shown that VEGF acts through the tyrosine kinase–coupled VEGF receptors (type 2) to reversibly inhibit gap junction dye transfer in endothelial cells within 15 to 30 minutes (50 ng/mL VEGF). An accompanying change in the phosphorylation of Cx43 was also observed.[35] Also acutely acting, a thromboxane A_2 mimetic reduced dye transfer between human endothelial cells and showed internalization of Cx43 concurrent with capillary formation.[36] Finally, insulin, and insulin-like growth factor, can cause decreases in Cx43 gap junction coupling.[37] As with other phosphorylation-mediated mechanisms, this process is dependent on the integrity of the carboxyl-terminal (C-terminal) domain and follows a "ball-and-chain"–like mechanism.[38,39]

Antimalarials

The effects of the antimalarials on gap junction coupling, particularly quinine and quinine-derivatives such as mefloquine, are interesting because they seem to be connexin subtype–specific. A study by Srinivas and coworkers showed that quinine dramatically blocks channels formed by Cx36 and Cx50 and moderately blocks Cx45 channels (shown by a 50% decrease in gap junction conductance), whereas the other connexin subtypes were insensitive to quinine exposure.[40] This study represented the first demonstration of connexin-specific gap junction block by a pharmacologic agent.

Fenamates

Fenamates are nonsteroidal agents generally known for their anti-inflammatory effects at nanomolar concentrations, but at higher concentrations (10 to 100 μM) they also have been shown to block membrane ion channels.[41] Recently, they also were found to have uncoupling effects in monolayer cultured cells expressing gap junction channels. Hark and associates showed that flufenamic acid (FFA), niflumic acid (NFA), and meclofenamic acid (MFA) caused uncoupling in Cx43-expressing normal rat kidney cells (NRKs). The block was rapid but not entirely reversible. The order of potency was MFA > NFA > FFA for block of electrical and dye coupling.[42] Unlike in the case with antimalarials, little selectivity with regard to connexin subtype was observed. Also, the mechanism of action remains largely unknown, because the uncoupling did not seem to be attributable to membrane potential, PKC, cyclo-oxygenase activation, or intracellular Ca^{2+} levels. The sites of blockade were compared for antimalarials and fenamates. The fenamates appeared to involve actual gating, whereas quinine and its derivatives appeared to work through open-channel block.[43]

Cannabinoids

A reduction in electrical coupling and dye transfer also was shown in cultured endothelial cells within 15 minutes of treatment with the cannabinoid receptor agonist δ^9-tetrahydrocannabinol (10 to 30 μM) or a synthetic version HU210 (10 μM). This effect was attributed to Cx43 phosphorylation in an ERK1/ERK2 (extracellular-regulated kinases 1 and 2)-dependent manner.[44] Further studies would be necessary to assess whether such effects are relevant to biologic conditions.

Cardiac Glycosides

It has been suggested that cardiac glycosides strophanthidin, ouabain, and digitoxin decrease intercellular coupling,[45] perhaps by a mechanism that involves an increase in intracellular Ca^{2+} concentration.[46] Studies in this area of research have not been pursued further in recent years, although it would be interesting to assess the sensitivity of specific connexins to determine whether a connexin-specific effect (perhaps for those connexins expressed in the atrioventricular node) could be observed.

Molecular Approaches to Reduction of Cell-Cell Coupling

Although the foregoing agents reduce coupling in a rather nonselective manner, some investigators have specifically targeted Cx43 RNA by antisense-directed strategies. These experiments have not been conducted in models directly relevant to cardiac electrophysiology; nevertheless, they are presented here because they represent a growing body of evidence showing that downregulation of Cx43 channels may be of therapeutic potential. Small oligonucleotides (typically comprising 20 bases or fewer) have been shown to effectively decrease the amount of gap junction channel protein expressed. Recently, Qiu and colleagues correlated the level of local Cx43 expression with the time course of skin wound healing in mouse.[16] These investigators showed that a single topical application of Cx43 antisense gel brought about a transient downregulation of Cx43 protein levels, ultimately resulting in a dramatic increase in the rate of skin wound closure. The results showed a damped inflammatory response and a simultaneously enhanced rate of re-epithelization. Figure 20-1 shows the macroscopic appearance of the healing process in pairs of antisense-treated and untreated incisional and excisional wounds (see Fig. 20-1A to J). As can be seen in the Cx43 antisense-treated samples, knockdown resulted in attenuated macroscopic inflammation, as evidenced by reduced swelling and redness. A significant reduction in wound gape was seen within hours of injury, and almost complete wound closure occurred by 1 and 2 days. Microscopically, a significant reduction in neutrophil numbers was seen in the tissue around the wound. The added therapeutic benefits included a significant reduction in the extent of granulation tissue deposition and the subsequent formation of a smaller, less distorted scar. The findings of Law and colleagues are consistent with these observations.[17] Whether reduction in Cx43 levels could change the time course and formation of scar in other tissues (such as

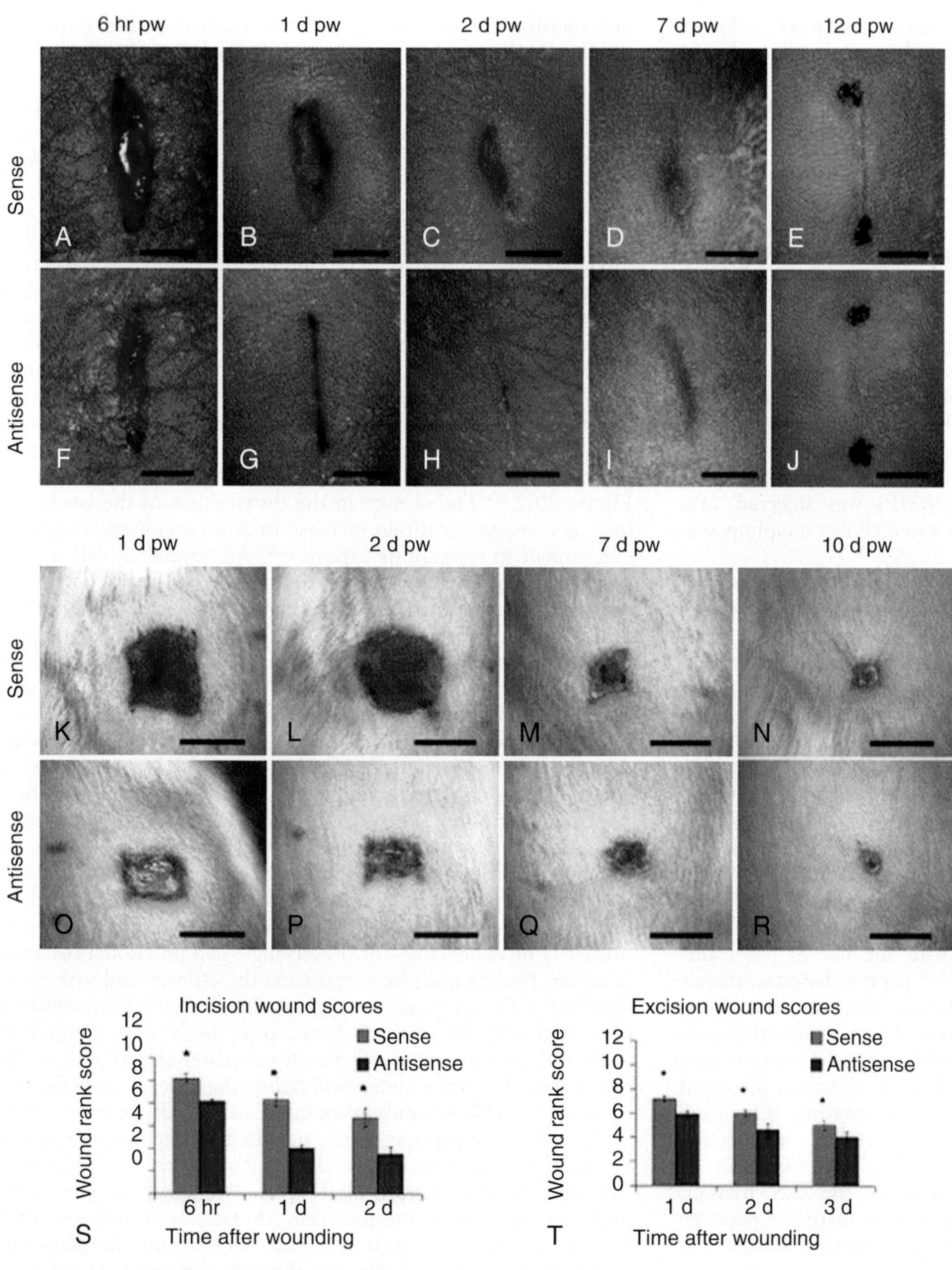

Figure 20-1 The healing process in treated and untreated wounds (incisional and excisional). **A** to **E,** Macroscopic images of full-thickness, incisional lesions on the backs of neonatal mice from control pairs. **F** to **J,** Images of wounds treated with antisense. The images were compared at different time points after wounding (pw = post wounding): 6 hours (**A** and **F**), 1 day (**B** and **G**), 2 days (**C** and **H**), 7 days (**D** and **I**), and 10 days (**E** and **J**). **K** to **N,** Macroscopic images of excisional lesions on the backs of adult mice from control pairs. **O** to **R,** Images of antisense-treated counterparts of **K** to **N.** Incision wound scores were quantified by histograms for the mean wound rank score for both Cx43 antisense-treated wounds and control wounds in the neonatal incisional model (**S**) and the adult excisional model (**T**). Significant differences were seen between Cx43 antisense-treated wounds and control wounds (n = 8) when these were analyzed with the Wilcoxon signed rank test. The *asterisks* indicate P values, as follows: P =.028, 6 hours; P =.001, 1 day; and P =.012, 2 days. *Scale bars* in **A** to **J** represent 1 mm, and those in **K** to **R** represent 0.5 mm. (Adapted from Figure 2 of Qiu C, Coutinho P, Frank S, et al: Targeting connexin43 expression accelerates the rate of wound repair. Curr Biol 13:1697-1703, 2003.)

heart) remains to be determined. It is worth noting that decreased Cx43 expression (in this case by gene haplodeficiency) also decreased the progression of atherosclerotic plaque formation in a murine model of the disease.[47]

Peptide-Based Strategies for Reduction of Gap Junction–Mediated Intercellular Communication

In 1994, studies showed that extracellular application of peptides corresponding to relevant extracellular domains of connexins decreased the extent of cell-cell coupling.[48,49] Specifically, synthetic peptides representing the extracellular loop sequences of Cx32 inhibited cell-cell channel formation.[48] More recently, a review by Evans and associates[50] highlighted the advances (and limitations) of connexin-mimetic peptides, including their effectiveness as tools in blocking not only Cx37, Cx40, and Cx43 channels but also connexin hemichannels. Various groups of investigators have shown these peptides to effectively inhibit gap junctional transfer of fluorescent dyes, electrical coupling, and synchronized Ca^{2+} oscillations in smooth muscle cells.[50] The two most widely used peptides are Gap26 and Gap27, which correspond respectively to sequences on the first and second extracellular loops of Cx43. These two peptides also have been shown to inhibit the intercellular propagation of Ca^{2+} waves in monolayer cell cultures.[50] Yet recent studies suggest that these peptides may not be as specific as originally thought. Indeed, in examining the effects of connexin- and pannexin-mimetic peptides, Wang and colleagues[51] recently showed an attenuation of channel currents that was not consistent with sequence-specific actions of the peptides. These workers found that connexin-mimetic peptides inhibited pannexin channel currents but did not inhibit the connexin currents of the channels from which the sequence was derived. Similarly, pannexin-mimetic peptides did inhibit pannexin channel currents but also extended promiscuously to Cx46 channels.[51]

Agents That Increase Gap Junction Coupling

Although several agents have been found to decrease coupling (albeit with limited specificity), less is known about chemical modification intended to increase electrical communication in the heart. The studies by De Mello and by Burt and Spray showed that activation of phosphorylation pathways (specifically, PKA) enhanced intercellular coupling.[52-54] Similarly, when cyclic adenosine monophosphate (cAMP) was injected into canine Purkinje fibers, gap junction intercellular coupling was increased.[52]

In a separate study, Darrow and coworkers demonstrated that a 24-hour treatment with dibutyryl cAMP leads to enhanced expression of Cx45 and Cx43 in cardiac myocytes.[55] Other mediators shown to affect connexin expression include endothelin (ET),[58] AT,[56] tumor necrosis factor-α (TNF-α),[57] basic fibroblast growth factor (bFGF),[58] and VEGF.[59] Ultimately, these mediators (and potential pharmacologic targets) can alter normal connexin expression by changing the typical connexin ratios (e.g., Cx43/Cx40), the overall total connexin expression, or the connexin distribution at the regional and subcellular levels. All of these agents have non-connnexin molecules as targets, however, and act on complex intracellular signaling pathways that affect a number of cellular processes.

Specificity of targeting remains an important challenge in connexin pharmacology today. As with the use of connexin-mimetic molecules (see also earlier),[48,49] peptide-based strategies have been developed to identify molecules that can enhance intercellular communication in the heart. The use of peptides as pharmaceutical agents has become widely accepted over the past decade, and exenatide (Byetta), teriparatide (Fortéo), lisinopril (Prinivil, Zestril), octreotide acetate (Sandostatin), zafirlukast (Accolate), eptifibatide (Integrilin), hirudin, enfuvirtide (Fuzeon), and goserelin acetate (Zoladex) are examples of successful peptide-based pharmaceuticals in the U.S. market. A review of recent progress and the current status of peptidic sequences that enhance or preserve gap junction function is presented next.

Peptide-Based Strategies to Increase or Preserve Gap Junctional Communication

Antiarrhythmic Peptides

In the early 1980s, Aonuma and colleagues characterized the ability of a series of natural peptides derived from bovine atria to synchronize the beating of cultured chick cardiomyocytes.[60,61] Because these compounds were shown to have an effect on the synchronization of pacemaker activity of cardiac cells, they were dubbed "antiarrhythmic peptides" (AAPs). A series of follow-up studies led to the characterization of AAP10 and its D-amino acid analogue ZP123, later named *rotigaptide*, as potential antiarrhythmic agents.[62] The experiments of Eloff and associates suggested that ZP123 (rotigaptide) may act by preserving intercellular communication under conditions of metabolic stress.[63] Separate experiments indicated that this peptide does not modify the morphology of the cardiac action potential; moreover, the peptide was shown not to interact with a panel of integral membrane proteins.[64,65]

In a recent review, Haugan and Petersen examined the experimental and clinical data obtained using rotigaptide in four different animal models of atrial fibrillation (AF).[66] Treatment with rotigaptide was shown to increase atrial conduction velocity—with no proarrhythmogenic effect—in animal models of AF and congestive heart failure–related AF. More specifically, in dog models of both atrial ischemia-induced AF and chronic atrial dilatation, rotigaptide treatment was associated with a significant antiarrhythmic effect. Additionally, it was shown that rotigaptide prevented conduction slowing and reverted established conduction slowing in the isolated rat atrium in a concentration-dependent manner. The effects of rotigaptide also were examined in rabbit atria with chronic atrial dilatation using high-resolution optical mapping on isolated Langendorff-perfused rabbit hearts. An example of the results is shown in Figure 20-2.[67] The change in the distribution of the isochrone lines is consistent with an increase in atrial conduction velocity consequent to rotigaptide exposure.[68] Additional animal studies showed that pretreatment with rotigaptide prevented both ventricular and atrial arrhythmias during conditions of acute cardiac ischemia. As Figure 20-3 shows, VT was prevented by rotigaptide treatment during reperfusion in dogs.[69] Open-chest dogs were subjected to 1 hour of ligation of the left circumflex coronary artery, followed by 4 hours of reperfusion. Ten minutes before reperfusion, rotigaptide or saline were given, and premature ventricular complexes (PVCs) and VT episodes were counted for 2-minute periods every 5 minutes during the first hour of reperfusion. The occurrence of PVCs and VT was suppressed by the two highest doses of rotigaptide, with a maximal reduction in the highest group by approximately 95%.[69]

The experience with rotigaptide was recently summarized by Kjolbye and coworkers.[70] Rotigaptide is the first drug that acts primarily by enhancing—or preserving—gap junctional communication. Phase I trials have evaluated the efficacy and toxicity of the drug, with highly encouraging results. Recent reports, thus far presented only in abstract form, describe a new compound (GAP134) as a potential gap junction opener that can be orally administered. Future studies will define the efficacy and selectivity of this compound and its potential use as a therapeutic agent.

Although rotigaptide seems to enhance gap junction communication, its cellular or molecular target is unknown. Attempts to demonstrate binding of rotigaptide to the Cx43 molecule have been unsuccessful. In fact, it is believed that rotigaptide does not exert its effect directly on the connexin molecule but does so indirectly through activation of yet unidentified kinases. It is known that rotigaptide modifies the phosphorylation state of Cx43.[71] The latter carries a high risk of connexin-unrelated effects on cell function, because kinases are likely to interact with a variety of substrates, not only Cx43. The cumulated evidence for rotigaptide-induced effects on Cx43-mediated junctional conductance is substantial.[63-68,70,71] Dye transfer studies suggest that rotigaptide stimulates Cx43-mediated intercellular communication but that it is devoid of activity on Cx26 and Cx32—connexins with a short C-terminal tail lacking several of the regulatory domains of Cx43 and Cx40.[72] Overall, the studies with rotigaptide strongly support the notion that enhancement of gap junction communication, particularly under conditions of metabolic stress, may have an important antiarrhythmic effect. Yet the lack of knowledge of the cellular target of rotigaptide and its possible effects on cellular pathways other than PKC activation amply justifies the development of a new generation of drugs with a defined structure-activity relation that can serve as tools to elucidate the role of gap junction regulation in the electrophysiology of

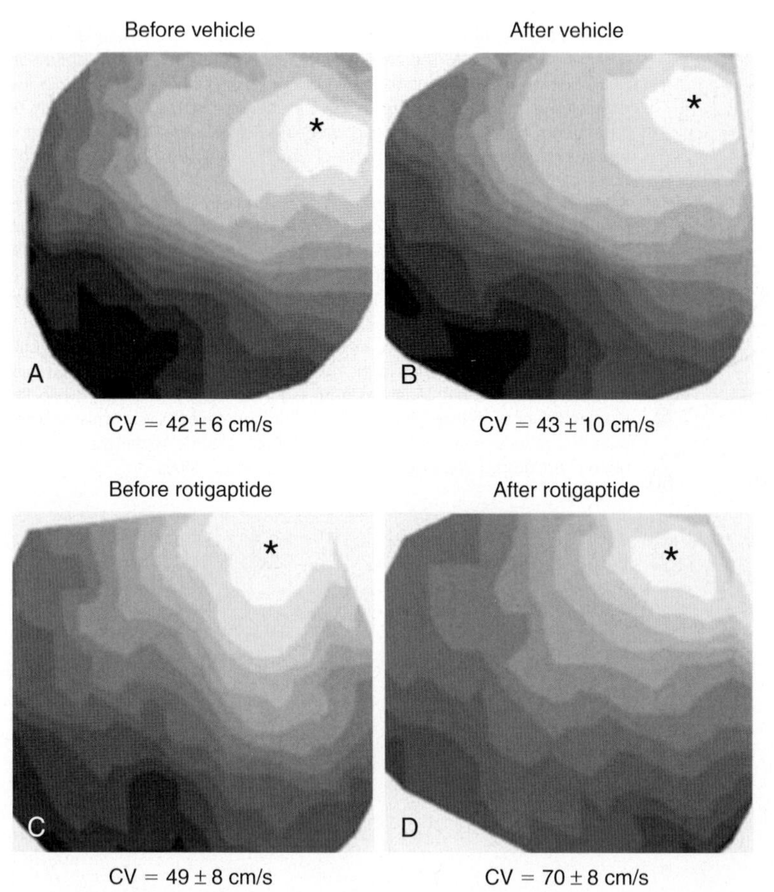

Figure 20-2 Atrial conduction is increased after treatment with rotigaptide in chronic volume-overloaded rabbit hearts. **A** to **D**, Isochronal maps from the right atrial free wall during steady-state pacing at a cycle length of 100 ms before and after treatment with a control vehicle (**A** and **B**) or rotigaptide (**C** and **D**). The *asterisk* indicates the position of the pacing electrode. Large areas of marked conduction slowing (illustrated by relative crowding of isochrones) are shown in both atria before treatment (**A** and **C**). After treatment with the vehicle control, the activation pattern was unchanged (**C**). **D**, however, shows a marked increase in conduction velocity (CV) in the rotigaptide treatment group, as evidenced by broader isochrones. The mean CV was calculated from local CV vectors at 20 sites in the center of the mapping field and is depicted by the numerical data at the *bottom* of each isochrone map. The *isochronal lines* each represent 2 ms. (Adapted from Figure 1 from Haugan K, Miyamoto T, Takeishi Y, et al: Rotigaptide (ZP123) improves atrial conduction slowing in chronic volume overload-induced dilated atria. Basic Clin Pharmacol Toxicol 99:71-79, 2006.)

the heart, both in normal and in diseased states. To this effect, we have applied the knowledge accumulated on the structural bases for Cx43 regulation to identify peptidic molecules that can affect channel function. The following paragraphs summarize our current thinking and the results obtained thus far on the development of new peptides of potential value as future pharmacologic agents.

The Carboxyl-Terminal Domain of Connexin43 as a Target for Drug Design

Previous studies from our laboratory have shown that the C-terminal region of Cx43 (Cx43CT) acts as the major regulatory domain of the cardiac gap junction channel (reviewed by Delmar and coworkers[39]). Our experiments further support the hypothesis that chemical regulation of Cx43 follows a "particle-receptor" model, similar to the ball-and-chain model for voltage gating of sodium and potassium channels.[73,74] We propose that the C-terminal domain acts as a gating particle (Fig. 20-4). Under normal conditions, the particle resides away from the pore, and the channel is open, as seen in Figure 20-4A. Yet, as illustrated in Figure 20-4B, changes in the intracellular environment (such as activation of specific kinases[75,76] or changes in intracellular pH[39,77,78]) causes the intramolecular binding of the C-terminal domain with a separate region of the protein, affiliated with the pore. This "receptor" domain is located in the second half of the cytoplasmic loop.[77,79,80] On the basis of this model, we proposed that interfering with the particle-receptor interaction could be an effective strategy for the prevention of gap junction closure. We therefore aimed to develop a molecule that, by binding to the C-terminal domain, prevents channel closure.

The search for a new Cx43CT binder of potential pharmacologic use was based on a high-throughput assay called "phage display." This method has previously been used in drug discovery with great success. Compounds such as adalimumab (Humira) were first identified by phage display. By applying this method, an estimated 2.5 billion peptidic sequences were tested for their ability to bind to Cx43CT. After a process of additional testing and selection (described in Shibayama and colleagues[26]), we focused our attention on a 34-amino-acid peptide, dubbed "RXP-E." Our studies showed that this compound prevented the closure of gap junctions induced by alkanols as well as by intracellular acidification.[26] We further documented that in the presence of the peptide, the open time of Cx43 channels was drastically prolonged.[26] Experiments in progress suggest that this molecule can be introduced into cultured cells by using translocating sequences,[81,82] and that the size of the active molecule can be significantly reduced. Accordingly, future generations of compounds, based on the RXP-E sequence, will allow us to study the role of gap junction closure on the initiation and maintenance of arrhythmic events.

A peptide-based strategy, grounded on a structure-activity relation, also was used by Hunter and coworkers to characterize the interaction of Cx43CT with the scaffolding protein zonula occludens-1 (ZO-1).[83] The interaction between these two proteins occurs specifically between the second PDZ domain of ZO-1 and the last nine amino acids of Cx43 (the "PDZ-binding domain"),[83] as supported by the work of Sorgen and associates.[80]

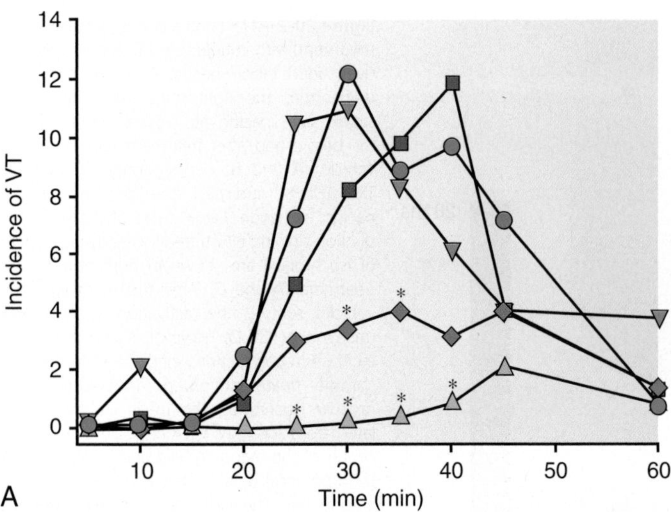

Figure 20-3 Ventricular tachycardia (VT) is prevented by rotigaptide during reperfusion in dogs. A, The concentration-dependent effect of rotigaptide on the incidence of VT in the first 60 minutes of reperfusion. Incidence values are expressed as the mean. The trends in VT incidence over the first 60 minutes of reperfusion in control and rotigaptide-treated dogs were compared using a repeated-measures one-way analysis of variance (ANOVA). The control conditions *(green circles)* achieved the highest incidence of VT; the highest concentration of rotigaptide *(yellow upward-pointing triangles)* prevented VT. B, The quantitative total VT episodes. Total VT values are expressed as means ± SEM (*n* = 5 to 8 animals). Again, the control group saw the highest occurrence of PVCs and VT, which were suppressed by the two highest doses of rotigaptide. The total numbers of VT episodes in control and rotigaptide-treated dogs were compared using a one-way ANOVA, followed by Dunnet's post hoc test. *, statistically significant difference in VT compared with control ($P < .05$); †, statistically significant difference in the overall trend of VT during the first 60 min. of reperfusion ($P < .05$). (Adapted from Figure 3 from Hennan JK, Swillo RE, Morgan GA, et al: Rotigaptide (ZP123) prevents spontaneous ventricular arrhythmias and reduces infarct size during myocardial ischemia/reperfusion injury in open-chest dogs. J Pharmacol Exp Ther 317:236-243, 2006.)

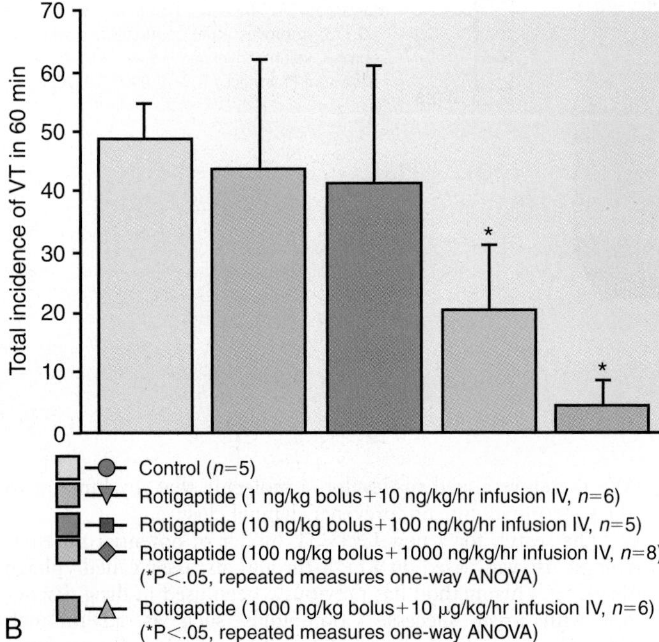

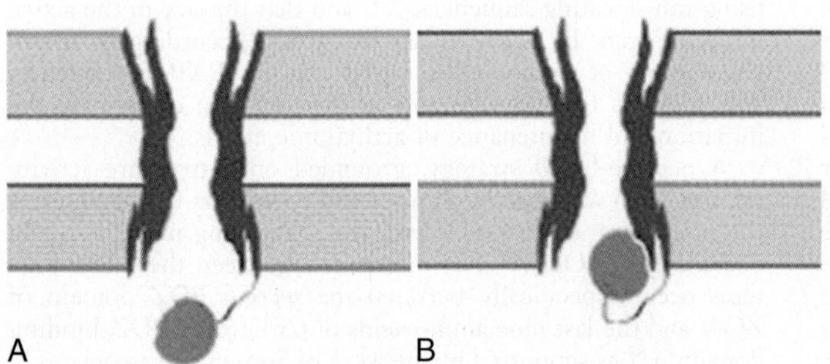

Figure 20-4 The concept of a ball-and-chain model is schematically depicted for the chemical regulation of connexins. This diagram demonstrates the flexible intracellular domain (the carboxyl-terminal domain) that acts as a gating particle. In A, the gate is away from the pore under normal conditions. As shown in B, however, certain stimuli (including conditions such as low pH or phosphorylation) can cause the gate to swing toward the mouth of the channel and bind to a "receptor" affiliated with the pore, thereby closing (or modifying) the channel. (Adapted from Figure 1 from Delmar M, Coombs W, Sorgen P, et al: Structural bases for the chemical regulation of connexin43 channels. Cardiovasc Res 62:268-275, 2004.)

Accordingly, introduction of a peptide corresponding to the PDZ-binding sequence of Cx43 into cells prevented the Cx43-ZO1 interaction. With this model, Hunter and coworkers demonstrated that prevention of the interaction of Cx43 with ZO-1 leads to a reduction of peripherally associated ZO-1, accompanied by a significant increase in plaque size. Further analysis indicated that this increased plaque size was not due to increased protein expression or decreased turnover, but rather to unregulated accumulation of gap junctional channels from nonjunctional pools. Using this model, it may be possible to increase intercellular communication between cells. Further experiments will be necessary to assess the latter hypothesis.

Summary and Conclusions

Despite substantial progress in elucidation of gap junction regulation in the past decade, few novel pharmacologic agents have been identified that are specific to connexin molecules. As a major player in intercellular communication, gap junctions represent an ideal target for pharmacologic modification. Because of their rapid gating properties and short half-life, pharmacologic approaches can be directed at both acute and long-term levels. The dichotomous nature of intercellular signaling suggests that at times, channel closure may be beneficial to prevent the spread of inappropriate signals, whereas in other situations, maximal cellular coupling may be required to maintain cardiac electrical synchrony.

It is unclear whether holding gap junctions open under pathologic conditions such as ischemia would be ultimately beneficial or deleterious, although initial data seem to indicate that preservation of gap junction communication in the heart may have an antiarrhythmic effect.[66,70] One of the reasons why such a gap in knowledge exists, however, is the limited availability of pharmacologic agents that can, with at least some partial selectivity, interfere with gap junction regulation. Rotigaptide represented a major breakthrough, setting the stage for new generations of structure-based molecules that could affect gap junction function.[26,83] Future research will show whether any of these molecules—or their derivatives—will become effective therapy for actual use in the practice of medicine.

References

1. Gutstein DE, Morley GE, Tamaddon H, et al: Conduction slowing and sudden arrhythmic death in mice with cardiac-restricted inactivation of connexin43. Circ Res 88:333-339, 2001.
2. Gutstein DE, Morley GE, Vaidya D, et al: Heterogeneous expression of gap junction channels in the heart leads to conduction defects and ventricular dysfunction. Circulation 104:1194-1199, 2001.
3. Danik SB, Liu F, Zhang J, et al: Modulation of cardiac gap junction expression and arrhythmic susceptibility. Circ Res 95:1035-1041, 2004.
4. Eckardt D, Theis M, Degen J, et al: Functional role of connexin43 gap junction channels in adult mouse heart assessed by inducible gene deletion. J Mol Cell Cardiol 36:101-110, 2004.
5. van Rijen HV, Eckardt D, Degen J, et al: Slow conduction and enhanced anisotropy increase the propensity for ventricular tachyarrhythmias in adult mice with induced deletion of connexin43. Circulation 109:1048-1055, 2004.
6. Rohr S, Kucera JP, Fast VG, Kleber AG: Paradoxical improvement of impulse conduction in cardiac tissue by partial cellular uncoupling. Science 275:841-844, 1997.
7. Nakase T, Fushiki S, Naus CC: Astrocytic gap junctions composed of connexin 43 reduce apoptotic neuronal damage in cerebral ischemia. Stroke 34:1987-1993, 2003.
8. Cascio WE, Yang H, Muller-Borer BJ, Johnson TA: Ischemia-induced arrhythmia: The role of connexins, gap junctions, and attendant changes in impulse propagation. J Electrocardiol 38:55-59, 2005.
9. Dekker LR, Coronel R, VanBavel E, et al: Intracellular Ca^{2+} and delay of ischemia-induced electrical uncoupling in preconditioned rabbit ventricular myocardium. Cardiovasc Res 44:101-112, 1999.
10. Kleber AG, Riegger CB, Janse MJ: Electrical uncoupling and increase of extracellular resistance after induction of ischemia in isolated, arterially perfused rabbit papillary muscle. Circ Res 61:271-279, 1987.
11. Delmar M, Michaels DC, Jalife J: Slow recovery of excitability and the Wenckebach phenomenon in the single guinea pig ventricular myocyte. Circ Res 65:761-774, 1989.
12. Delmar M, Ibarra J, Davidenko J, et al: Dynamics of the background outward current of single guinea pig ventricular myocytes. Ionic mechanisms of hysteresis in cardiac cells. Circ Res 69:1316-1326, 1991.
13. Akopian AN, Sivilotti L, Wood JN: A tetrodotoxin-resistant voltage-gated sodium channel expressed by sensory neurons. Nature 379:257-262, 1996.
14. Cummins TR, Dib-Hajj SD, Black JA, et al: A novel persistent tetrodotoxin-resistant sodium current in SNS-null and wild-type small primary sensory neurons. J Neurosci 19:R43, 1999.
15. Duff HJ, Sheldon RS, Cannon NJ: Tetrodotoxin: Sodium channel specific anti-arrhythmic activity. Cardiovasc Res 22:800-807, 1988.
16. Qiu C, Coutinho P, Frank S, et al: Targeting connexin43 expression accelerates the rate of wound repair. Curr Biol 13:1697-1703, 2003.
17. Law LY, Zhang WV, Stott NS, et al: In vitro optimization of antisense oligodeoxynucleotide design: An example using the connexin gene family. J Biomol Tech 17:270-282, 2006.
18. Burt JM, Massey KD, Minnich BN: Uncoupling of cardiac cells by fatty acids: Structure-activity relationships. Am J Physiol 260:439-448, 1991.
19. Delmar M, Michaels DC, Johnson T, Jalife J: Effects of increasing intercellular resistance on transverse and longitudinal propagation in sheep epicardial muscle. Circ Res 60:780-785, 1987.
20. Dhein S, Krusemann K, Schaefer T: Effects of the gap junction uncoupler palmitoleic acid on the activation and repolarization wavefronts in isolated rabbit hearts. Br J Pharmacol 128:1375-1384, 1999.
21. Takens-Kwak BR, Jongsma HJ, Rook MB, Van Ginneken AC: Mechanism of heptanol-induced uncoupling of cardiac gap junctions: A perforated patch-clamp study. Am J Physiol 262:1531-1538, 1992.
22. Burt JM, Spray DC: Volatile anesthetics block intercellular communication between neonatal rat myocardial cells. Circ Res 65:829-837, 1989.
23. He DS, Burt JM: Mechanism and selectivity of the effects of halothane on gap junction channel function. Circ Res 86: E104-E109, 2000.
24. Firestone LL, Miller JC, Miller KW: Tables of physical and pharmacological properties of anesthetics. In: Roth SH, Miller KW (eds): Molecular and Cellular Mechanisms of Anesthetics. New York, Plenum Publishing, 1984, pp 455-470.
25. Mascia MP, Trudell JR, Harris RA: Specific binding sites for alcohols and anesthetics on ligand-gated ion channels. Proc Natl Acad Sci U S A 97:9305-9310, 2000.
26. Shibayama J, Lewandowski R, Kieken F, et al: Identification of a novel peptide that interferes with the chemical regulation of connexin43. Circ Res 98:1365-1372, 2006.
27. Burt JM, Spray DC: Volatile anesthetics block intercellular communication between neonatal rat myocardial cells. Circ Res 65:829-837, 1989.
28. Rusy BF, Komai H: Anesthetic depression of myocardial contractility: A review of possible mechanisms. Anesthesiology 76:745-766, 1987.
29. Nelson WL, Makielski JC: Block of sodium current by heptanol in voltage-clamped canine cardiac Purkinje cells. Circ Res 68:977-983, 1991.
30. Davidson JS, Baumgarten IM, Harley EH: Reversible inhibition of intercellular junctional communication by glycyrrhetinic

acid. Biochem Biophys Res Commun 134:29-36, 1986.
31. Sagar GD, Larson DM: Carbenoxolone inhibits junctional transfer and upregulates connexin43 expression by a protein kinase A–dependent pathway. J Cell Biochem 98:1543-1551, 2006.
32. Takens-Kwak BR, Jongsma HJ: Cardiac gap junctions: Three distinct single channel conductances and their modulation by phosphorylating treatments. Pflügers Arch 422:198-200, 1992.
33. De Mello WC: Influence of alpha-adrenergic-receptor activation on junctional conductance in heart cells: Interaction with beta-adrenergic adrenergic agonists. J Cardiovasc Pharmacol 29:273-277, 1997.
34. De Mello WC: Is an intracellular renin-angiotensin system involved in control of cell communication in heart? J Cardiovasc Pharmacol 23:640-646, 1994.
35. Suarez S, Ballmer-Hofer K: VEGF transiently disrupts gap junctional communication in endothelial cells. J Cell Sci 114:1229-1235, 2001.
36. Ashton AW, Yokota R, John G, et al: Inhibition of endothelial cell migration, intercellular communication, and vascular tube formation by thromboxane A(2). J Biol Chem 274:35562-35570, 1999.
37. Homma N, Alvarado JL, Coombs W, et al: A particle-receptor model for the insulin-induced closure of connexin43 channels. Circ Res 83:27-32, 1998.
38. Morley GE, Taffet SM, Delmar M: Intramolecular interactions mediate pH regulation of connexin43 channels. Biophys J 70:1294-1302, 1996.
39. Delmar M, Coombs W, Sorgen P, et al: Structural bases for the chemical regulation of connexin43 channels. Cardiovasc Res 62:268-275, 2004.
40. Srinivas M, Hopperstad MG, Spray DC: Quinine blocks specific gap junction channel subtypes. Proc Natl Acad Sci U S A 98:10942-10947, 2001.
41. Schultz BD, Singh AK, Devor DC, Bridges RJ: Pharmacology of CFTR chloride channel activity. Physiol Rev 79:S109-S144, 1999.
42. Harks EG, de Roos AD, Peters PH, et al: Fenamates: A novel class of reversible gap junction blockers. J Pharmacol Exp Ther 298:1033-1041, 2001.
43. Srinivas M, Spray DC: Closure of gap junction channels by arylaminobenzoates. Mol Pharmacol 63:1389-1397, 2003.
44. Brandes RP, Popp R, Ott G, et al: The extracellular regulated kinases (ERK) 1/2 mediate cannabinoid-induced inhibition of gap junctional communication in endothelial cells. Br J Pharmacol 136:709-716, 2002.
45. De Mello WC: Influence of the sodium pump on intercellular communication in heart fibres: Effect of intracellular injection of sodium ion on electrical coupling. J Physiol (Lond) 263:171-197, 1976.
46. Weingart R, Maurer P: Cell-to-cell coupling studied in isolated ventricular cell pairs. Experientia 43:1091-1094, 1987.
47. Kwak BR, Veillard N, Pelli G, et al: Reduced connexin43 expression inhibits atherosclerotic lesion formation in low-density lipoprotein receptor-deficient mice. Circulation 107:1033-1039, 2003.
48. Dahl G, Nonner W, Werner R: Attempts to define functional domains of gap junction proteins with synthetic peptides. Biophys J 67:1816-1822, 1994.
49. Monaghan P, Perusinghe N, Carlile G, Evans WH: Rapid modulation of gap junction expression in mouse mammary gland during pregnancy, lactation, and involution. J Histochem Cytochem 42:931-938, 1994.
50. Evans WH, De Vuyst E, Leybaert L: The gap junction cellular internet: Connexin hemichannels enter the signalling limelight. Biochem J 397:1-14, 2006.
51. Wang J, Ma M, Locovei S, et al: Modulation of membrane channel currents by gap junction protein mimetic peptides: Size matters. Am J Physiol Cell Physiol 293:1112-1119, 2007.
52. De Mello WC: Effect of intracellular injection of calcium and strontium on cell communication in heart. J Physiol (Lond) 250:231-245, 1975.
53. De Mello WC: Cyclic AMP and junctional communication viewed through a multibiophysical approach. In Peracchia C, (ed): Biophysics of Gap Junction Channels. Boca Raton, FL, CRC Press, 1991, pp 229-239.
54. Burt JM, Spray DC: Inotropic agents modulate gap junctional conductance between cardiac myocytes. Am J Physiol 254:H1206-H1210, 1988.
55. Darrow BJ, Fast VG, Kleber AG, et al: Functional and structural assessment of intercellular communication. Increased conduction velocity and enhanced connexin expression in dibutyryl cAMP–reated cultured cardiac myocytes. Circ Res 79: 174-183, 1996.
56. Polontchouk L, Ebelt B, Jackels M, Dhein S: Chronic effects of endothelin 1 and angiotensin II on gap junctions and intercellular communication in cardiac cells. FASEB J 16:87-89, 2002.
57. Lerner DL, Chapman Q, Green KG, Saffitz JE: Reversible down-regulation of connexin43 expression in acute cardiac allograft rejection. J Heart Lung Transplant 20:93-97, 2001.
58. Doble BW, Kardami E: Basic fibroblast growth factor stimulates connexin-43 expression and intercellular communication of cardiac fibroblasts. Mol Cell Biochem 143:81-87, 1995.
59. Pimentel RC, Yamada KA, Kleber AG, Saffitz JE: Autocrine regulation of myocyte Cx43 expression by VEGF. Circ Res 90:671-677, 2002.
60. Aonuma S, Kohama Y, Akai K, et al: Studies on heart. XIX. Isolation of an atrial peptide that improves the rhythmicity of cultured myocardial cell clusters. Chem Pharm Bull (Tokyo) 28:3332-3339, 1980.
61. Aonuma S, Kohama Y, Makino T, Fujisawa Y: Studies of heart. XXI. Amino acid sequence of antiarrhythmic peptide (AAP) isolated from atria. J Pharmacobiodyn 5:40-48, 1982.
62. Herve JC, Dhein S: Pharmacology of cardiovascular gap junctions. Adv Cardiol 42:107-131, 2006.
63. Eloff BC, Gilat E, Wan X, Rosenbaum DS: Pharmacological modulation of cardiac gap junctions to enhance cardiac conduction: Evidence supporting a novel target for antiarrhythmic therapy. Circulation 108:3157-3163, 2003.
64. Kjolbye AL, Knudsen CB, Jepsen T, et al: Pharmacological characterization of the new stable antiarrhythmic peptide analog Ac-D-Tyr-D-Pro-D-Hyp-Gly-D-Ala-Gly-NH2 (ZP123): in vivo and in vitro studies. J Pharmacol Exp Ther 306:1191-1199, 2003.
65. Xing D, Kjolbye AL, Nielsen MS, et al: ZP123 increases gap junctional conductance and prevents reentrant ventricular tachycardia during myocardial ischemia in open chest dogs. J Cardiovasc Electrophysiol 14:510-520, 2003.
66. Haugan K, Petersen JS: Gap junction modifying antiarrhythmic peptides: Therapeutic potential in atrial fibrillation. Drugs Fut 32:245-260, 2007.
67. Haugan K, Miyamoto T, Takeishi Y, et al: Rotigaptide (ZP123) improves atrial conduction slowing in chronic volume overload-induced dilated atria. Basic Clin Pharmacol Toxicol 99:71-79, 2006.
68. Haugan K, Kjolbye AL, Hennan JK, Petersen JS: Rotigaptide (ZP123) reverts established atrial conduction velocity slowing. Cell Commun Adhes 12:271-278, 2005.
69. Hennan JK, Swillo RE, Morgan GA, et al: Rotigaptide (ZP123) prevents spontaneous ventricular arrhythmias and reduces infarct size during myocardial ischemia/reperfusion injury in open-chest dogs. J Pharmacol Exp Ther 317:236-243, 2006.
70. Kjolbye AL, Haugan K, Hennan JK, Petersen JS: Pharmacological modulation of gap junction function with the novel compound rotigaptide: A promising new principle for prevention of arrhythmias. Basic Clin Pharmacol Toxicol 101:215-230, 2007.
71. Xing D, Kjolbye AL, Petersen JS, Martins JB: Pharmacological stimulation of cardiac gap junction coupling does not affect ischemia-induced focal ventricular tachycardia or triggered activity in dogs. Am J Physiol Heart Circ Physiol 288:H511-H516, 2005.
72. Clarke TC, Thomas D, Petersen JS, et al: The antiarrhythmic peptide rotigaptide (ZP123) increases gap junction intercellular communication in cardiac myocytes and HeLa cells expressing connexin 43. Br J Pharmacol 147:486-495, 2006.
73. Armstrong CM, Bezanilla F: Inactivation of the sodium channel. II. Gating current experiments. J Gen Physiol 70:567-590, 1977.
74. Zagotta WN, Hoshi T, Aldrich RW: Restoration of inactivation in mutants of Shaker potassium channels by a peptide derived from ShB. Science 250:568-571, 1990.
75. Lampe PD, TenBroek EM, Burt JM, et al: Phosphorylation of connexin43 on serine368 by protein kinase C regulates gap junctional communication. J Cell Biol 149:1503-1512, 2000.
76. Lau AF: c-Src: Bridging the gap between phosphorylation- and acidification-induced

gap junction channel closure. Sci STKE 2005:e33, 2005.

77. Duffy HS, Sorgen PL, Girvin ME, et al: pH-dependent intramolecular binding and structure involving Cx43 cytoplasmic domains. J Biol Chem 277:36706-36714, 2002.
78. Ek-Vitorin JF, Calero G, Morley GE, et al: PH regulation of connexin43: Molecular analysis of the gating particle. Biophys J 71:1273-1284, 1996.
79. Sorgen PL, Duffy HS, Cahill SM, et al: Sequence-specific resonance assignment of the carboxyl terminal domain of connexin43. J Biomol NMR 23:245-246, 2002.
80. Sorgen PL, Duffy HS, Sahoo P, et al: Structural changes in the carboxyl terminus of the gap junction protein connexin43 indicates signaling between binding domains for c-Src and zonula occludens-1. J Biol Chem 279:54695-54701, 2004.
81. Wadia JS, Stan RV, Dowdy SF: Transducible TAT-HA fusogenic peptide enhances escape of TAT-fusion proteins after lipid raft macropinocytosis. Nat Med 10:310-315, 2004.
82. Kim D, Jeon C, Kim JH, et al: Cytoplasmic transduction peptide (CTP): New approach for the delivery of biomolecules into cytoplasm in vitro and in vivo. Exp Cell Res 312:1277-1288, 2006.
83. Hunter AW, Barker RJ, Zhu C, Gourdie RG: Zonula occludens-1 alters connexin43 gap junction size and organization by influencing channel accretion. Mol Biol Cell 16:5686-5698, 2005.

Cell Biology of Cardiac Impulse Initiation and Propagation

PART IV

Fibrosis and Fibroblast Infiltration: An Active Structural Substrate for Altered Propagation and Spontaneous Tachyarrhythmias

21

Viviana Muñoz, Sharon Zlochiver, and José Jalife

CHAPTER OUTLINE

Cardiac injuries such as myocardial infarction (MI) and cardiomyopathies can lead to structural remodeling, with fibroblast activation, differentiation into myofibroblasts, and proliferation leading to increased production and accumulation of extracellular matrix (ECM), that is, fibrosis.[1] Although compact fibrosis can arise in an infarct scar, it usually exhibits a mixture of collagen, myofibroblasts, and myocardial fibers. Such a structure increases the complexity of electrical conduction within a labyrinth of surviving myocardial bundles.[2] In addition to MI, fibrosis develops in other pathologies: Dilated cardiomyopathy is often associated with mild focal interstitial fibrosis. Hypertrophic cardiomyopathy and arrhythmogenic right ventricular cardiomyopathy (ARVC) are genetic disorders characterized by widespread fibrosis and myocardial fibrofatty replacement, respectively.

It is highly probable that under physiologic conditions, at least one fibroblast is in contact with every myocyte.[3] Because myocytes do not proliferate, during fibrosis the ratio of fibroblasts and myofibroblasts to myocytes increases even further. In addition to the well-recognized arrhythmogenic effect of loss of myocyte connectivity due to the excessive ECM, the possible electrical coupling between myocytes and fibroblasts, or more specifically the myofibroblast phenotype, plays a role in the mechanisms of arrhythmias. From this perspective, cardiac fibroblasts and myofibroblasts are potential targets for regulation. In chapter 26, Rohr and Miragoli review recent in-vitro studies aimed at characterizing the way electrical coupling between fibroblasts and cardiomyocytes affects electrical impulse initiation and conduction. Here we take advantage of that knowledge to analyze the arrhythmogenic consequences of fibroblast-cardiomyocyte coupling, or lack thereof, and review experimental and numerical results regarding the role of fibrosis in the mechanisms of spontaneous initiation and maintenance of atrial and ventricular tachyarrhythmias.

This research is supported by National Heart, Lung, and Blood Institute grants P01-HL039707, P01-HL87226 and R01-HL070074.

Cardiac Fibrosis and Fibroblasts as Electrical Insulators

During fibrosis, the increased collagen acts as an electrically insulating barrier, impeding electrical propagation and electrotonic continuity within the myocardium. This has been suggested as a substrate for reentrant arrhythmias, due to both the formation of passive obstacles for conduction and the increase in cardiac electrical heterogeneity.[4]

Ventricular Fibrosis

De Bakker and colleagues showed in Langendorff-perfused human hearts with healed infarcts that the surviving fibers within the infarct form an anatomic substrate for initiation and maintenance of reentry.[5] In such hearts, arrhythmogenesis is the result of very long conduction delays over short distances due to zigzag conduction in small muscle bundles separated by fibrotic deposits.[6] In a simulation study, Turner and coworkers linked the distribution and structure of fibrosis barriers to action potential abnormalities and dispersion of action potential duration, which can lead to ventricular fibrillation (VF). Longitudinal and transverse fibrosis depositions at various densities were simulated and found to block the activation wave fronts, diverting propagation into a wiggly pathway. This in turn was manifested as fractionated electrograms with multiple delayed deflections, known in the clinical setting as a harbinger of VF.[7]

Additional support for the role of fibrosis as a structural substrate for ventricular arrhythmias arises from the anatomic remodeling of a healed MI.[8] At the margin of the infarction, fibrosis interspersed with ventricular muscle provides the anchors for reentrant circuits that give rise to ventricular tachycardia (VT) and, subsequently, VF.[9] Modern therapeutic approaches have successfully reduced the size of infarct areas, concomitantly reducing the incidence of VT to 1% of revascularized patients. Despite such reduction, the number of patients at risk for ventricular arrhythmias has remained fairly stable due to an aging population with greater number of MI survivors at risk.[10]

Atrial Fibrosis

The remodeling of the cardiac tissue due to heart failure is characterized by substantial collagen accumulation and fibrosis in the atria. In one study, the spatial distribution of fibrosis was found to govern fibrillation wave dynamics in the posterior left atrium during heart failure in sheep.[11] A combined simulation and experimental study further established the role of fibrosis and fibroblast distribution on arrhythmia maintenance and propagation dynamics. The study suggested that the amount, spatial distribution, and type of fibrosis—that is, diffuse (homogeneously distributed small fibrotic deposits) or patchy (large fibrous obstacles)—affected the patterns and types of arrhythmia.

Whether the mechanism of atrial fibrillation (AF) was reentrant or focal, the large size of the fibrous patches in heart failure provided the major factor responsible for different dynamics of AF waves in heart-failure hearts. In those hearts, activation breakthroughs were closer to the pulmonary vein ostia than in control hearts, and the architecture of fibrosis in the posterior left atrium consisted primarily of patches, with the larger fibrotic obstacles found preferentially in the vicinity of the pulmonary vein ostia (Fig. 21-1). Both large posterior left atrium fibrous patches and the pulmonary vein ostia acted to anchor reentrant circuits and impair wave propagation to generate delays, wave breaks, and signal fractionation.

Computer simulations reconstituted these findings and showed that the patches need not be confluent to be the central pivoting attachment of reentry, because simple heterogeneous distribution of diffuse fibrosis could also attach a reentry circuit at a specific posterior left atrium location. Simulations also showed that the patches of fibrosis dramatically increased the variability and complexity of the activation patterns, being responsible for propagation delays and unidirectional blocks, in accordance with the experimental observations.

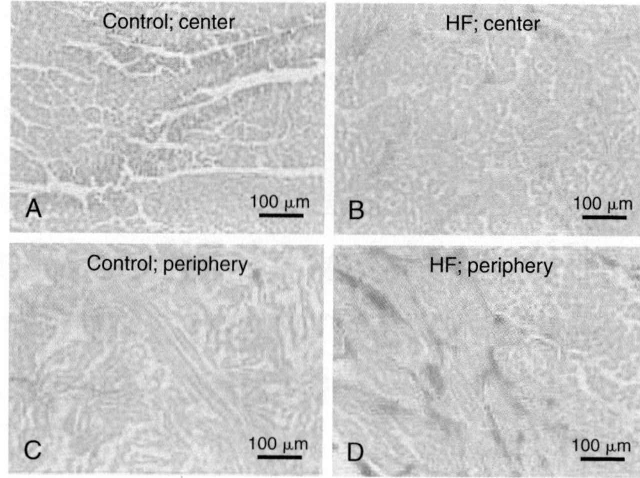

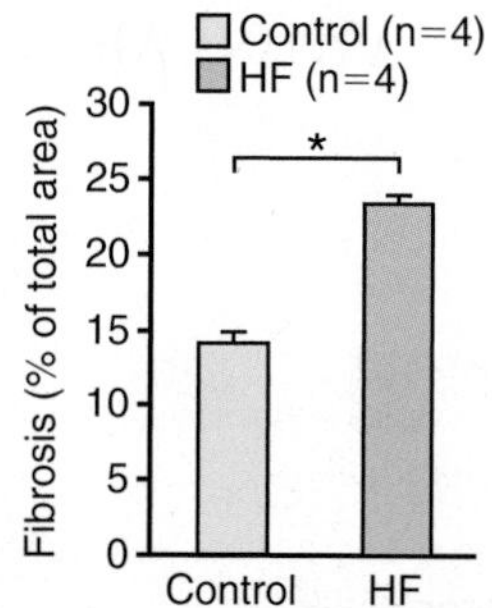

Figure 21-1 Micrographs showing distribution of fibrosis in the center (**A** and **B**) and periphery (**C** and **D**) of the posterior left atrium of a sheep heart (picrosirius red staining). **A** and **C**, control. **B** and **D**, heart failure. **E**, Morphometric quantification of fibrous tissue content in control and heart failure (HF) specimens. $^*P < 0.001$. (From Tanaka K, Zlochiver S, Vikstrom KL, et al: Spatial distribution of fibrosis governs fibrillation wave dynamics in the posterior left atrium during heart failure. Circ Res 101:839-847, 2007.)

Cardiac Fibroblasts

In addition to the role of the increased extracellular volume on the electrical propagation in the heart, which was the focus of the above-mentioned studies, it is important to assess how fibroblasts themselves affect normal cardiac function. Although cardiac myocytes make up the bulk of myocardial volume, the cardiac fibroblasts are the most numerous cell type in the mammalian heart.[12] They form a highly organized network within the myocardium to provide mechanical and structural support. Fibroblasts produce interstitial collagen (I and III), and therefore traditionally their role has been relegated to the synthesis and remodeling of the ECM.[13] The fibroblast-to-myocyte cell number ratio makes it reasonable to assume that in the working heart, each myocyte is adjacent to at least one fibroblast, a condition that becomes even more prominent in heart failure.[4]

Electrophysiologically, the fibroblasts are passive cells with smaller capacitance than myocytes, exhibiting a relatively low resting membrane potential of about −15 mV and high membrane resistance of more than 4 GΩ due primarily to the conductance of several potassium ion channels.[11,14-17] When these cells are electrotonically uncoupled from their neighboring myocytes, as is the probable condition in most regions of the normal heart, their effect on electrical impulse propagation is similar to that of fibrosis and extracellular collagen accumulation—that is, acting as insulating barriers.

Evidence for in-vivo coupling between myocytes and fibroblasts has been suggested in the rabbit sinoatrial node, a region particularly rich in connective tissue.[18] Yet, during cardiac remodeling, relatively quiescent fibroblasts can differentiate into myofibroblasts, which have been demonstrated to express several smooth-muscle markers and connexins (gap junction proteins) in vitro, opening the possibility for electrical connectivity of myocytes to myofibroblasts during heart disease and making these cells active participants in electrical conduction via formation of gap junctions with myocytes.

Cardiac Activity Modulation by Heterocellular Electrotonic Coupling

Already in the early 1970s Goshima and colleagues showed coupling between myocytes and other cell types.[19,20] In 1992, Rook and coworkers[21] measured the gap junction conductivity between myofibroblasts and between myofibroblast-myocyte (heterologous) pairs of neonatal rats. They found a conductance of 21 pS between two fibroblasts and 32 pS in the heterologous pair, each of which could not be explained solely by connexin43 (the major connexin in myocytes). The authors then suggested the existence of an unknown connexin. Later works have

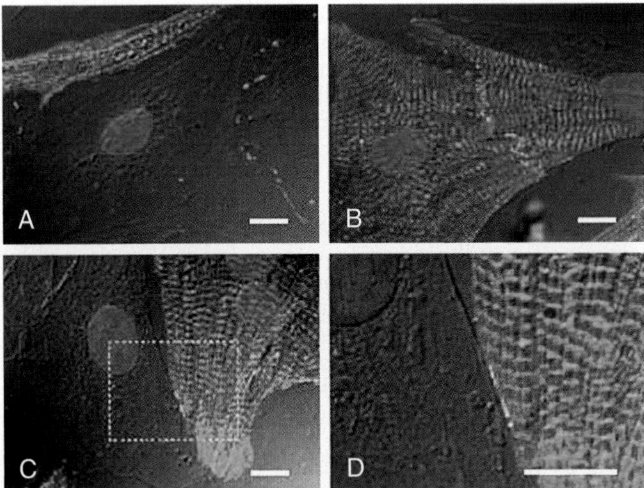

Figure 21-2 Immunofluorescence samples showing connexin43-positive staining *(green)* between two myofibroblasts **(A)**, between two myocytes **(B)**, and between a myocyte and a myofibroblast (**C** and **D**). **D** is a higher magnification of the *boxed area* in **C**. Myocyte-specific sarcomeric ?-actinin in *red* and nuclei in *blue*. Scale bars, 10 μm. (From Zlochiver S, Munoz V, Vikstrom K, et al: Electrotonic myofibroblast-to-myocyte coupling increases propensity to reentrant arrhythmias in 2-dimensional cardiac monolayers. Biophys J 95:4469-4480, 2008.)

identified connexin40 and connexin45 coupling myofibroblasts,[22,23] which by formation of heteromerized gap junctions with connexin43 might explain the heterologous gap junction conduction. The existence of gap junction proteins between myofibroblast homologous pairs and myofibroblast-myocyte heterologous pairs in vitro has been also confirmed independently in immunohistochemical studies.[22,24,25] As an example, Figure 21-2 shows that connexin43 (Cx43 - green) was present at junctions between neighboring myofibroblasts (panel A), between myocytes (Fig. 21-2B), and between myocytes and - myofibroblasts (Fig. 21-2C; higher magnification in Fig. 21-2D).

Several in-silico and in-vitro models have specifically quantified the effects of heterocellular coupling between myofibroblasts and myocytes on the electrical activity and passive properties of myocardial tissue. MacCannell and colleagues showed in a mathematical model that myofibroblasts cause a shortening of the adjacent myocytes' action potential duration (APD), reducing the plateau height of the action potential.[15] The resting potential of the myofibroblasts was significantly hyperpolarized to become close to that of the coupled ventricular myocyte. This is consistent with the findings of Rook and coworkers showing that within a coculture, the resting potential of myofibroblasts hyperpolarized approximately to that of connected myocytes.

A different result was presented in the study of Miragoli and colleagues,[22] in which the impulse conduction velocity and maximal upstroke gradient were assessed in cultured strands of myocytes coated with myofibroblasts from neonatal rat hearts. Increasing the density of myofibroblasts increased conduction velocity and upstroke gradient up to a certain threshold, followed by a decline of these two properties. The group found that this nonlinear effect is due to the gradual depolarization of the myocyte resting membrane potential from –78 mV to –50 mV as the density of myofibroblasts increases. This study has demonstrated the role of myofibroblasts as current sinks to electrical propagation.

A previous study from the same group[24] showed a different possible effect of myofibroblast deposits within the myocardium: as long-range conductors. The investigators cocultured neonatal rat ventricular myocytes and fibroblasts in a pattern of myocyte strands interrupted with fibroblasts over various distances. They concluded that successful, albeit delayed, conduction along such a disturbed myocyte strand is possible if the myofibroblast patch is shorter than 300 μm.

Electrical Propagation Patterns and Coupling

In a study conducted in our laboratory,[25] myofibroblast infiltration significantly modified the spatiotemporal characteristics of reentry in cultured monolayers of cardiac origin. We have reproduced in Figure 21-3A representative examples recorded in monolayers with varying myofibroblast-to-myocyte ratios. They show that both frequency of reentry and complexity of wave propagation depended on the relative area occupied by myofibroblasts. In the phase maps on the top row, in which each color represents a phase of the action potential, the convergence of all colors at any given location is a phase singularity.[26] Clearly, the number of phase singularities and wavelets multiplied as the myofibroblast-to-myocyte ratio increased from 0.1 to 0.5 and 0.7. In the middle row, time-space plots[27] were constructed for activity recorded along the horizontal white lines in the phase maps. They demonstrate that increasing the myofibroblast-to-myocyte ratio increased complexity but decreased reentry frequency. The latter is reflected by the gradual increase in the time intervals between any two consecutive activations in the respective time-space plot. Yet, despite wave fragmentation, the signals were highly periodic for all cases (see panel A, bottom row).

The relationship between rotation frequency and myofibroblast-to-myocyte ratio was found to be linear (see Fig. 21-3B and C). However, the effect of electrical coupling was nonlinear and in fact nonmonotonic in numerical simulations. Regression analysis revealed that the most dramatic decreases in frequency were observed at intermediate coupling levels (see Fig. 21-2C).

Numerical simulations also established a similar dependency of phase singularity myofibroblast-to-myocyte ratios. Simulations also showed that higher values of heterocellular coupling supported conduction at higher levels of myofibroblast infiltration (see Fig. 21-2C).

Heterocellular Coupling and Conduction Velocity

Conduction velocity is an important dynamic property with respect to propagation and wave-break formation. We investigated the effect of heterocellular coupling on conduction velocity during steady-state pacing in cocultures. In Figure 21-4, measured conduction velocities are shown for three myofibroblast coupling levels (silenced Cx43, control, and overexpressed Cx43) and pacing frequencies of 3 Hz and 4 Hz. Each symbol corresponds to one experiment, and the solid lines connect the mean conduction velocities in each coupling condition and pacing frequency. A clear biphasic dependency of conduction velocity on myofibroblast Cx43 expression level, and thus on heterocellular coupling level, was observed. An increase in coupling from silenced to control myofibroblasts resulted in significantly reduced conduction velocities, whereas a further increase in coupling level from control to overexpressed myofibroblasts resulted in increased conduction velocities.

The relationship between conduction velocity and myofibroblast coupling was determined in parallel simulations using similar pacing rates and myofibroblast-to-myocyte ratio (see Fig. 21-4B). Gradually increasing myofibroblast coupling revealed a biphasic dependence of conduction velocity on coupling. These numerical results suggest that for a given myofibroblast-to-myocyte area ratio, a similar value of conduction velocity can be observed for two different levels of heterocellular coupling.

These data lead to the following interpretation regarding the biphasic dependence of conduction velocity on myofibroblast-to-

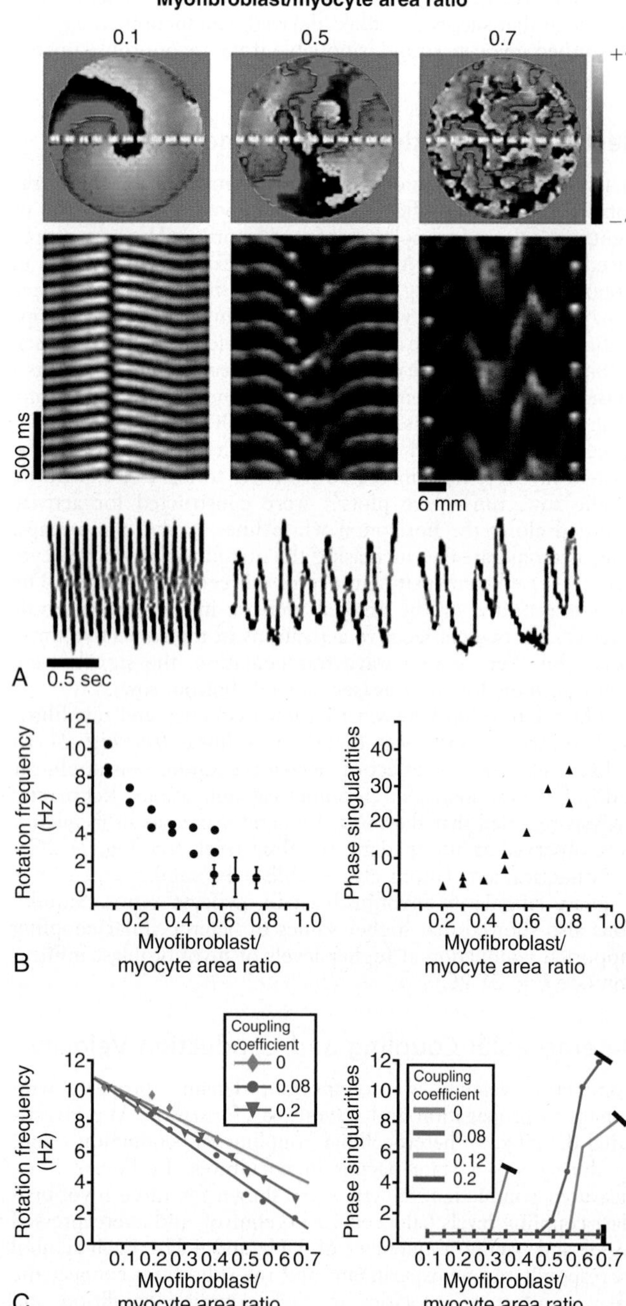

Figure 21-3 **A,** Phase maps (top), time-space plots (middle) and single-pixel recordings (bottom) show increasing numbers of singularity points with increasing numbers of myofibroblasts; myofibroblast-to-myocyte area ratios: 0.1, 0.5, and 0.7. **B,** Rotation frequency (*left*, n = 19) and number of phase singularities (*right*, n = 14) as functions of myofibroblast-to-myocyte area ratio in experiments. **C,** Rotation frequency *(left)* and number of phase singularities *(right)* as functions of myofibroblast-to-myocyte area ratio and heterocellular coupling in numerical simulations. (Modified from Zlochiver S, Munoz V, Vikstrom K, et al: Electrotonic myofibroblast-to-myocyte coupling increases propensity to reentrant arrhythmias in 2-dimensional cardiac monolayers. Biophys J 95:4469-4480, 2008.)

myocyte coupling (see Fig. 21-4B): At very low levels of coupling, the wave front entering the myofibroblasts is insufficient to transmit enough depolarizing current downstream to the neighboring myocytes. Thus, at these levels the myofibroblasts behave as current sinks that hamper successful propagation. In a one-dimensional cable, this condition resulted in propagation block.[25] However, in two dimensions, the wavefront finds alternative pathways and circumnavigates the myofibroblast. Therefore, conduction is maintained via these alternative pathways at the expense of overall conduction velocity and is characterized by heterogeneous wave propagation. As coupling increases toward the threshold level, myofibroblasts drain more and more charge from their neighboring myocytes, resulting in further conduction velocity decrease, which explains the left half of the curve in Figure 21-4B. Above threshold, however, the excitation wave provides enough charge through the myofibroblasts to excite downstream myocytes. At this point the myofibroblasts switch from being charge sinks to become short-range charge transmitters that facilitate downstream excitation with increasing levels of coupling. Hence, wavefronts become smoother, and velocity increases, explaining the right half of the curve in Figure 21-4B.

Initiation of Arrhythmias

Electrotonically coupled myofibroblasts might have an intriguing role in initiating arrhythmias. Similar to the effect of injury current in the border zone of acute infarct, depolarization-induced automaticity is a plausible mechanism for initiation of triggered activity in remodeling cardiac tissue due to the higher resting membrane potential of myofibroblasts compared to myocytes. In an in-vitro study where cultured patterned strands of neonatal ventricular myocytes were coated with myofibroblasts, spontaneous activity at low frequencies of about 1 Hz was induced in a myofibroblast density–dependent manner.[28] Increasing the density of myofibroblasts resulted in a biphasic effect on the percentage of active preparations: An initial increase up to a density level of 50% was followed by a decrease. The effect on the frequency of focal discharges was linear, whereby increasing myofibroblast density resulted in lower frequency of spontaneous activity.

The mechanisms of arrhythmia initiation in the setting of fibrotic deposits and electrotonic coupling between myofibroblasts and myocytes were investigated in our laboratory in an in-silico model of a human papillary muscle from an infarcted heart. A transverse section of the papillary muscle,[6] halfway between the base and the tip, was digitized into a realistic two-dimensional model (Fig. 21-5) incorporating substantial deposits of clustered myofibroblasts.

Electrical activity was computed by considering both ventricular myocytes and myofibroblast kinetics. During dynamic pacing, reentry was initiated only in the settings of heterocellular coupling—see Figure 21-6. Figure 21-6A shows two isochronal maps for a simulation in which myofibroblast to myocyte coupling was set. The two maps correspond to just before and immediately after unidirectional block occurred, which resulted in reentry at 6.8 seconds after the onset of pacing. Before reentry initiated, electrical propagation dispersed from the stimulated tissue along two pathways—upper and lower—due to the large fibrotic obstacle to the right of the pulse location. At 6.8 seconds, the impulse blocked in one direction and failed to propagate along the lower branch. Anatomic and functional factors combined to result in a source-to-sink mismatch that led to the unidirectional block.

Anatomically, the morphology of the active cardiac tissue at the block location was funnel-like, with the lower propagation branch starting as a narrow stripe that abruptly expanded. The stripe was bordered on the upper side by a highly resistive

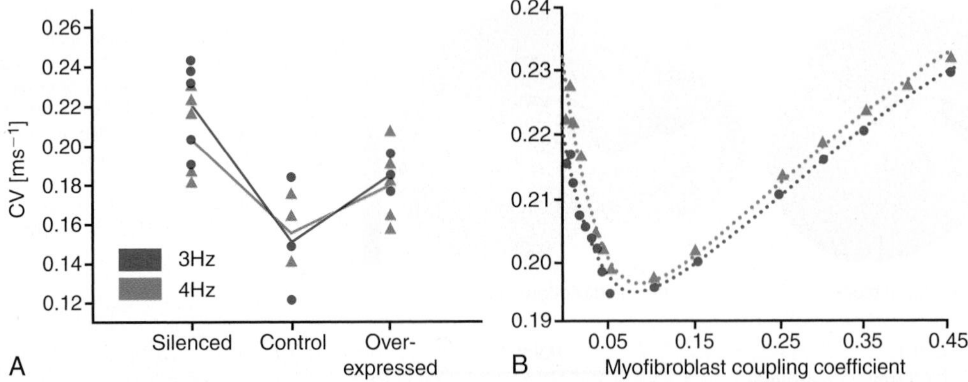

Figure 21-4 Effects of heterocellular electrical coupling during pacing in two-dimensional monolayers and simulations. **A,** Experimental conduction velocity (CV) vs. myofibroblast coupling coefficient for pacing at 3 Hz *(red)* and 4 Hz *(blue)*. Three levels of myofibroblast coupling were achieved using connexin43 (Cx43) siRNA-treated myofibroblasts (silenced), nontreated myofibroblasts (control), and Cx43 overexpressed myofibroblasts (overexpressed). **B,** Numerical results for CV vs. myofibroblast coupling coefficient for pacing at 3 Hz *(red)* and 4 Hz *(blue)*. All simulations and experiments were performed for a myofibroblast-to-myocyte area ratio of 0.25. (From Zlochiver S, Munoz V, Vikstrom K, et al: Electrotonic myofibroblast-to-myocyte coupling increases propensity to reentrant arrhythmias in 2-dimensional cardiac monolayers. Biophys J 95:4469-4480, 2008.)

fibrotic patch and on the bottom side by insulating external boundary. Functionally, during repetitive stimulation there was a gradual reduction of the maximum diastolic potential proximate to the site of block. The two tracings in Figure 21-6B correspond to point 1 (near the site of unidirectional block) and point 2 (approximately at the same distance from the stimulation source, but on the upper propagation branch). The gradual reduction in diastolic potential was accompanied by a decrease in action potential amplitude due to reduced availability of sodium channels, which reduced the source charge (this is not shown in the figure). Without heterocellular coupling, the reduced excitability was absent, as was suggested by repeating the simulation with the same ionic conditions except for assuming complete isolation between the two cell types (see Fig. 21-6C). No block was seen at any time anywhere in the heterogeneous sheet under these conditions. Similar to the depolarization-induced automaticity mechanism mentioned earlier, electrical coupling between myofibroblasts and myocytes depolarized the resting membrane potential of the myocytes adjacent to fibrotic patches by passive electrotonic diffusion, because myofibroblasts have an appreciably less negative resting membrane potential than myocytes (~−15 mV vs. ~−80 mV).

Other than promoting unidirectional block, the fibrotic deposits also produced large conduction delays that eventually enabled reentrant propagation. At the location marked by the green arrow in Figure 21-6A, a delay of about 40 ms was formed by a passive fibrotic patch connecting two myocardial segments, thus serving as a long-range conductor. The delay prevented interactions between wave fronts and wave tails and thus enabled sustained reentry within a relatively short path.

Overall, these simulations demonstrate and confirm the roles of electrically coupled myofibroblasts as current sinks, long-range conductors, and delay sources, as well as in the anchoring of reentrant waves; all such effects potentially contribute to initiation and maintenance of arrhythmias.

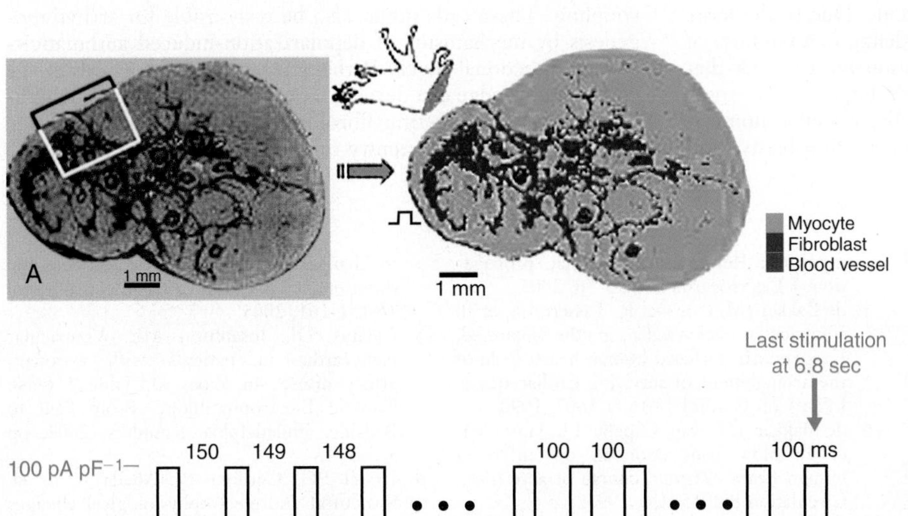

Figure 21-5 **A.** Digitization of a papillary muscle section of an infarcted human heart *(left)* into a two-dimensional computer model *(right)*. Stimulation location is marked by ⎍. **B.** Pacing protocol. (**A** *left* from de Bakker JM, Coronel R, Tasseron S, et al: Ventricular tachycardia in the infarcted, Langendorff-perfused human heart: Role of the arrangement of surviving cardiac fibers. J Am Coll Cardiol 15:1594-1607, 1990.)

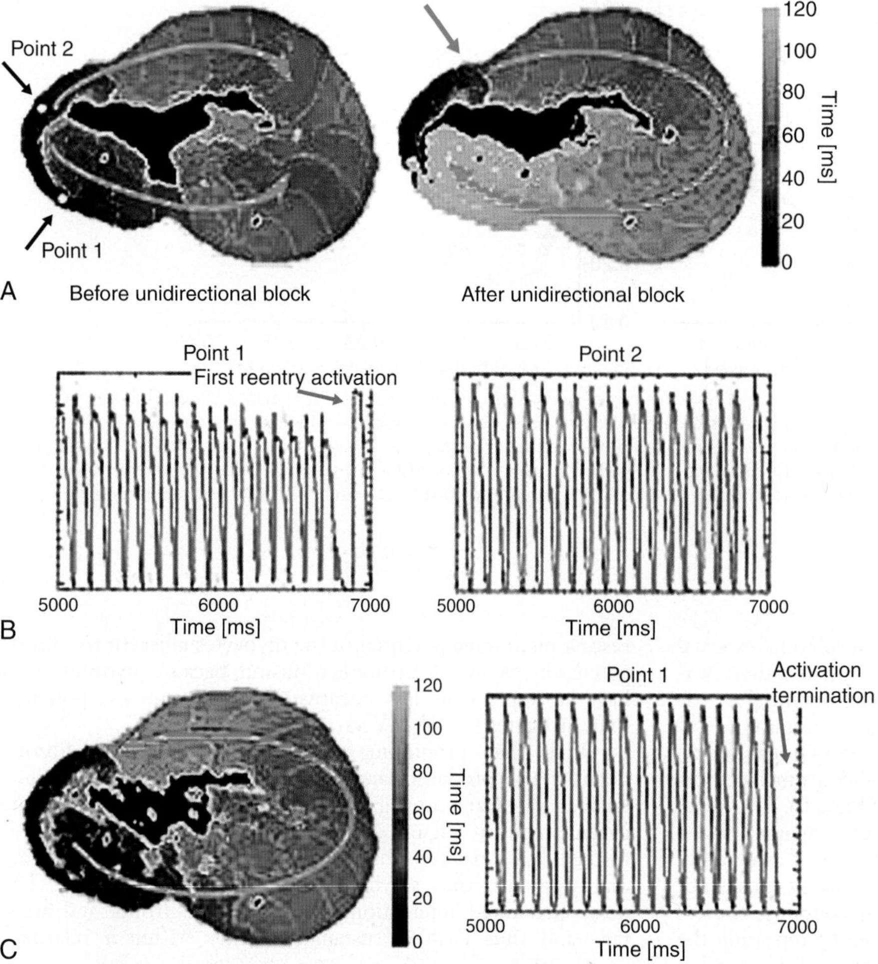

Figure 21-6 **A**, Isochronal maps of activation times before *(left)* and after *(right)* the formation of unidirectional block. Contours are separated by 5 ms. The *green arrow* marks a propagation delay caused by a fibrotic patch. **B**, Two-second transmembrane voltage traces (during pacing and following pacing termination) at points 1 and 2 indicated in A. **C**, Isochronal map and transmembrane voltage tracing, similar to those in A and B, for the case of no myofibroblast-to-myocyte electrical coupling.

Summary

It is clear that fibrosis with fibroblast proliferation and differentiation into myofibroblasts is arrhythmogenic. Due to the large propensity of this type of structural remodeling in a plethora of cardiac diseases as well as aging, it is reasonable to think that fibroblasts may be important therapeutic targets. The work detailed in this chapter shows experimentally, as well as numerically, that the interactions among myocytes, fibroblasts, and myofibroblasts affect electrical wave propagation in a highly complex, nonlinear manner, increasing or decreasing conduction velocity, depending on the degree of heterocellular electrical coupling. These cells might also be responsible for arrhythmogenesis by mechanisms of depolarization-induced automaticity and unidirectional block. Perhaps researchers taking advantage of such knowledge can develop a new generation of antiarrhythmic approaches targeting fibroblasts and their myofibroblastic phenotype to prevent reentry initiation.

References

1. Diez J, Lopez B, Gonzalez A, et al: Clinical aspects of hypertensive myocardial fibrosis. Curr Opin Cardiol 16:328-335, 2001.
2. Kawara T, Derksen R, de Groot JR, et al: Activation delay after premature stimulation in chronically diseased human myocardium relates to the architecture of interstitial fibrosis. Circulation 104: 3069-3075, 2001.
3. Camelliti P, Borg TK, Kohl P: Structural and functional characterisation of cardiac fibroblasts. Cardiovasc Res 65:40-51, 2005.
4. Kohl P, Camelliti P, Burton FL, et al: Electrical coupling of fibroblasts and myocytes: Relevance for cardiac propagation. J Electrocardiol 38:45-50, 2005.
5. de Bakker JM, Coronel R, Tasseron S, et al: Ventricular tachycardia in the infarcted, Langendorff-perfused human heart: Role of the arrangement of surviving cardiac fibers. J Am Coll Cardiol 15:1594-1607, 1990.
6. de Bakker JM, van Capelle FJ, Janse MJ, et al: Slow conduction in the infarcted human heart. 'Zigzag' course of activation. Circulation 88:915-926, 1993.
7. Turner I, Huang H, Saumarez RC: Numerical simulation of paced electrogram fractionation: Relating clinical observations to changes in fibrosis and action potential duration. J Cardiovasc Electrophysiol 16:151-161, 2005.
8. Callans DJ, Josephson ME: Ventricular tachycardia in patients with coronary artery disese. In Zipes D, Jalife J (eds): Cardiac Electrophysiology: From Cell to Bedside. Philadelphia: Saunders, 2004, pp 569-574.
9. Ursell PC, Gardner PI, Albala A, et al: Structural and electrophysiological changes in the epicardial border zone of canine myocardial infarcts during infarct healing. Circ Res 56:436-451, 1985.

10. Zheng ZJ, Croft JB, Giles WH, et al: Sudden cardiac death in the United States, 1989 to 1998. Circulation 104: 2158-2163, 2001.
11. Tanaka K, Zlochiver S, Vikstrom KL, et al: Spatial distribution of fibrosis governs fibrillation wave dynamics in the posterior left atrium during heart failure. Circ Res 101:839-847, 2007.
12. Baudino TA, Carver W, Giles W, et al: Cardiac fibroblasts: friend or foe? Am J Physiol Heart Circ Physiol 291: H1015-H1026, 2006.
13. Brown RD, Ambler SK, Mitchell MD, et al: The cardiac fibroblast: Therapeutic target in myocardial remodeling and failure. Annu Rev Pharmacol Toxicol 45:657-687, 2005.
14. Shibukawa Y, Chilton EL, Maccannell KA, et al: K^+ currents activated by depolarization in cardiac fibroblasts. Biophys J 88:3924-3935, 2005.
15. MacCannell KA, Bazzazi H, Chilton L, et al: A mathematical model of electrotonic interactions between ventricular myocytes and fibroblasts. Biophys J 92:4121-4132, 2007.
16. Kamkin A, Kiseleva I, Wagner KD, et al: Mechanically induced potentials in fibroblasts from human right atrium. Exp Physiol 84:347-356, 1999.
17. Chilton L, Ohya S, Freed D, et al: K^+ currents regulate the resting membrane potential, proliferation, and contractile responses in ventricular fibroblasts and myofibroblasts. Am J Physiol Heart Circ Physiol 288:H2931-H2939, 2005.
18. De Maziere AM, van Ginneken AC, Wilders R, et al: Spatial and functional relationship between myocytes and fibroblasts in the rabbit sinoatrial node. J Mol Cell Cardiol 24:567-578, 1992.
19. Goshima K: Synchronized beating of and electrotonic transmission between myocardial cells mediated by heterotypic strain cells in monolayer culture. Exp Cell Res 58:420-426, 1969.
20. Goshima K: Formation of nexuses and electrotonic transmission between myocardial and FL cells in monolayer culture. Exp Cell Res 63:124-130, 1970.
21. Rook MB, van Ginneken AC, de Jonge B, et al: Differences in gap junction channels between cardiac myocytes, fibroblasts, and heterologous pairs. Am J Physiol 263:C959-C977, 1992.
22. Miragoli M, Gaudesius G, Rohr S: Electrotonic modulation of cardiac impulse conduction by myofibroblasts. Circ Res 98:801-810, 2006.
23. Camelliti P, Green CR, LeGrice I, et al: Fibroblast network in rabbit sinoatrial node: Structural and functional identification of homogeneous and heterogeneous cell coupling. Circ Res 94:828-835, 2004.
24. Gaudesius G, Miragoli M, Thomas SP, et al: Coupling of cardiac electrical activity over extended distances by fibroblasts of cardiac origin. Circ Res 93:421-428, 2003.
25. Zlochiver S, Munoz V, Vikstrom K, et al: Electrotonic myofibroblast-to-myocyte coupling increases propensity to reentrant arrhythmias in 2-dimensional cardiac monolayers. Biophys J 95:4469-4480, 2008.
26. Gray RA, Pertsov AM, Jalife J: Spatial and temporal organization during cardiac fibrillation. Nature 392:75-78, 1998.
27. Pertsov AM, Davidenko JM, Salomonsz R, et al: Spiral waves of excitation underlie reentrant activity in isolated cardiac muscle. Circ Res 72:631-650, 1993.
28. Miragoli M, Salvarani N, Rohr S: Myofibroblasts induce ectopic activity in cardiac tissue. Circ Res 101:755-758, 2007.

Biologic Pacing 22

MICHAEL R. ROSEN, PETER R. BRINK, IRA S. COHEN, AND RICHARD B. ROBINSON

CHAPTER OUTLINE

The Natural Pacemaker

The natural pacemaker of the heart, the sinoatrial node (the true biologic pacemaker) is a complex structure whose anatomy is geared to facilitating the transmission of impulses to the rest of the heart while protecting it from excitation by ectopic impulses arising elsewhere. Its unique complement of ion channels regularly and rhythmically initiates impulses throughout the life cycle, and its autonomic neural supply ensures a ready adjustment to physiologic demands for altering heart rate. Yet, like any biologic system, the sinoatrial node is affected by aging and pathology in ways that can lead to dysfunction. For much of human history this dysfunction, expressed as sinoatrial arrest or block or atrioventricular (AV) block, was accompanied by syncope and—over a relatively short time—death.[1,2] The major therapy of these conditions in the mid 20th century was ephedrine and then sublingual isoproterenol, administered every 2 hours. Not only was death a constant threat, but quality of life was marginal.

In the 1960s, electronic pacing became available not as the cumbersome and painful therapy it had been previously (see later), but as a device that could be implanted transvenously and with little risk.[3,4] Early units were relatively massive—rather like hockey pucks in appearance—but they were lifesaving. Technology improved and the size of units diminished over the second half of the 20th century; improvement and innovation continue in the current era.

However, electronic pacing is not perfect: although it restores to individuals their lives, their families, and their society, it is not the seamlessly functioning structure exemplified by the sinoatrial node. This has led investigators to explore gene and cell therapies that replace or mimic the sinoatrial node as possible alternatives to the electronic pacemaker. The intent, in brief, is to fully replace the sinoatrial node's function, albeit not its structure.

One might almost say that cardiac pacemaking is attempting to come full circle—from biologic to electronic and back to biologic—but success is not yet within our grasp. To provide a perspective and a view of future directions we first discuss the mechanisms underlying the function of the sinoatrial node, consider pathologies affecting pacemaker function, and consider the rationale for developing biologic pacemakers. We then proceed to strategies for building biologic pacemakers, including the successes and failures to date. We finish with a discussion of challenges for the future.

The Normal Pacemaker of the Heart

The mammalian sinoatrial node was identified structurally in 1907 by Keith and Flack[5] and its function as the primary source of the cardiac impulse was demonstrated electrophysiologically by Lewis and colleagues in 1910.[6] In describing the structure and function of the sinoatrial node, these investigators recognized they were dealing with a heterogeneous structure that appeared to provide the dominant site of origin of the normal heartbeat. Yet the mechanisms determining the function of the sinoatrial node remained a mystery for some time. One school of thought held that the node—and indeed all the cardiac specialized conducting system—consisted of specialized neural fibers, with a neural impulse being responsible for initiating the heartbeat.[7] Sinus rhythm persisted after cardiac denervation,[8] which argued against thoughts of central neural origin, although the possibility of local neuronal activity being the cause of the heartbeat was a continuing belief.[7]

The modern era of molecular biophysics has determined the reasons for the origin of cardiac impulses, although the origin of the sinoatrial node cells themselves remains a subject of active investigation.[e.g.9] As shown in Figure 22-1A, multiple currents contribute to the sinoatrial node action potential.[10-13] The resting membrane potentials of normal sinoatrial node cells are more depolarized than those of most other cardiac myocytes, no doubt as the result of a small inward rectifier current, I_{K1}. The action potential initiated at these voltages has calcium rather than sodium as its inward charge carrier. This generates a slowly propagating impulse the like of which is seen as well only in the AV node, AV valves, and coronary sinus of the normal heart.

As sinoatrial node cells repolarize to their maximum diastolic potentials, their hyperpolarization permits the opening of hyperpolarization-activated cyclic nucleotide–gated (HCN) channels through which an inward sodium current, referred to as I_f, flows and begins to depolarize the membrane (see Fig. 22-1).[10-12] Also contributing to diastolic depolarization are the Na^+-Ca^{2+} exchanger and inward currents carried via T- and L-type calcium channels.[12-14] All this occurs against the backdrop of outward (repolarizing) potassium current, such that any increase in inward current or decrease in outward current increases the slope of phase 4 depolarization and the pacemaker rate.

Among the major modulators of phase 4 depolarization are the sympathetic and parasympathetic nervous systems.

These studies were supported by USPHS-NHLBI grant HL-28958 and the Boston Scientific Corporation.

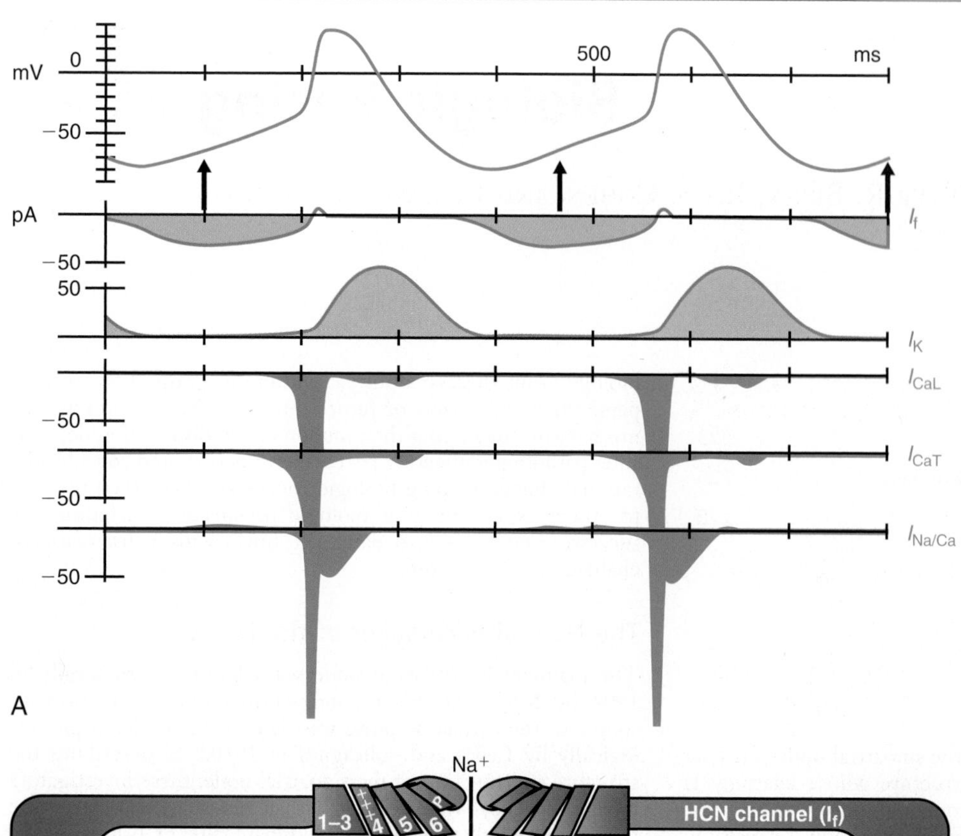

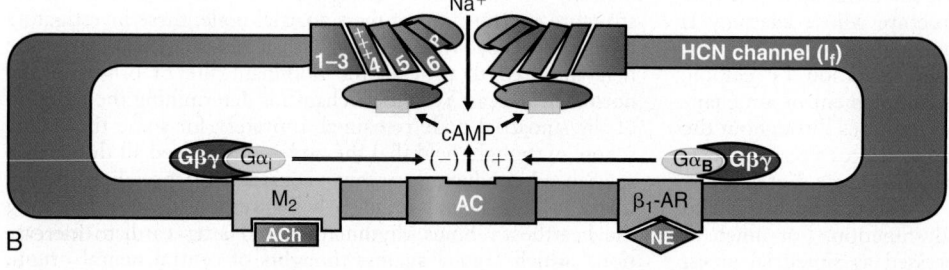

Figure 22-1 **A,** The sinoatrial node action potential and the currents contributing to impulse generation. **B,** The HCN channel. See text for discussion. AC, alternating current; ACh, acetylcholine; β_1-AR, β_1-adrenergic receptor; cAMP, cyclic adenosine monophosphate; $G\alpha_i$, inhibitory Gα protein subunit; Gβγ, G protein βγ subunit; HCN, hyperpolarization-activated cyclic nucleotide–gated [channel]; I_f, fast current; I_{CaL}, L-type calcium current; I_{CaT}, T-type calcium current; I_K, potassium current; $I_{Na/Ca}$, sodium-calcium current; M_2, muscarinic receptor; NE, norepinephrine. (Reproduced and modified with permission from DiFrancesco D, Camm AJ: Heart rate lowering by specific and selective I_f current inhibition with ivabradine: A new therapeutic perspective in cardiovascular disease. Drugs 64:1757-1765, 2004; and Biel M, Schneider A, Wahl C: Cardiac HCN channels: Structure, function, and modulation. Trends Cardiovasc Med 12:202-216, 2002.)

Their respective neurohumors, norepinephrine and acetylcholine, act via β-adrenergic or muscarinic receptor–G protein-linked pathways to increase (β-adrenergic) or decrease (muscarinic) cyclic adenosine monophosphate (cAMP) synthesis (see Fig. 22-1B). The binding of cAMP to a site near the carboxy terminus of the HCN channel shifts channel activation positively, which results in an increase in phase 4 depolarization.[12]

Whereas all the currents described contribute to the slope of phase 4 depolarization and to pacemaker rate, the initiator of the process appears to be I_f.[10-11] That all pacemaker activity is not attributable to I_f has been demonstrated in experiments using I_f-blocking drugs. In experimental models and in the clinic, the result is significant slowing of sinus rate but not termination of the rhythm.[15,16] Indeed, the inability to suppress sinus node function using any one blocker highlights the redundancy within the system such that it continues to function even under challenge.

The HCN channels that initiate pacemaker function have six transmembrane-spanning domains, are ubiquitous in heart, and are found elsewhere in the body as well (see Fig. 22-1B). There are four channel isoforms, HCN1-4, with HCN4 and HCN1 in sinoatrial node, HCN2 in much of the conducting system and myocardium, and HCN3 largely in neural tissues.[12] Each has differing activation and deactivation kinetics and differing cAMP sensitivity. The critical aspects of these channels with regard to pacemaker activity are their activation on hyperpolarization and their modulation by autonomic neurohumors.

To summarize, the primary biologic pacemaker is both structurally and functionally complex. In settings of disordered sinoatrial node impulse initiation or propagation that interfere with normal cardiac function, one has the choice of attempting to remake or repair the sinoatrial node—a difficult and as yet impossible task—or to reproduce aspects of its function. The overall goals are to restore the quality of life and to prolong life itself.

Pathologies Affecting Normal Pacemaker Function and a Brief History of Therapies

In 1827 and 1846, respectively, Adams[1] and Stokes[2] noted the clinical characteristics of an event that had likely afflicted humanity for centuries: They described patients who became pale, whose pulse became slow or was absent, and who then collapsed. We now recognize the pathology here was high-degree heart block. In the 20th century, the availability of synthetic catecholamines and later of β-agonists afforded one form of treatment: sublingual isoproterenol every 2 hours.[17] Although this therapy increased the rate of idioventricular pacemakers to a more physiologic range in many patients, it also could and did cause ventricular tachycardia. Moreover, this stopgap therapy could not ensure any long-term survival: Most patients in complete heart block who could not generate stable idioventricular rhythms of 50 beats per minute or more in the absence of medication died within months of diagnosis.

The answer to the dilemma faced by these patients and their physicians was the electronic pacemaker. Discovery of this device is traced to the 1889 report of McWilliam of a means for delivering shocks at about 60 to 70 times per minute to a patient in whom the heartbeat had failed.[18] In 1928, Lidwell and Booth used an electrical power source attached to a needle plunged into the heart to revive "a stillborn infant."[19] The term *cardiac pacemaker* is attributed to Hyman, who used a hand-cranked device to generate electrical shocks in 1932.[20] The modern era in pacing commenced in the early 1950s when Hopps[21] in Canada and then Zoll[22] in the United States reported devices that delivered transcutaneous shocks. Pacing via shocks delivered through an intramyocardial needle in the setting of postsurgical complete heart block was reported by Weirich and colleagues in 1957,[23] the same year in which Bakken fabricated the first portable external pacemaker.[24]

The first pacemakers implanted in the human heart required thoracotomies for intramyocardial electrode placement.[4] The first report of temporary transvenous approaches was in 1959[3]; the early 1960s then saw the rapid adoption of transvenous pacing with implanted units. Early units had no sensing function, paced at a fixed rate, and, although internally implanted, were cumbersome and required frequent power pack changes because they used mercury batteries. Their failure to sense often led to competition between implanted and idioventricular pacemakers and, in far too many instances, arrhythmogenesis. But in the 1960s and 1970s, batteries, electrodes, and software were rapidly improved so that pacemakers could be placed in a demand mode, sensing spontaneously occurring beats in the heart and resetting appropriately.[4,24,25]

Advances continued through the 20th century and into the 21st, bringing AV sequential pacing that synchronized the sequence of atrial and ventricular activation in patients having normal sinus node function and AV block; the exploration of the epicardial veins of the heart as sites for biventricular pacing to improve cardiac output; and the evolution of cardioverter defibrillators that could sense, shock, and then pace if needed, for patients who had potentially lethal tachyarrhythmias.

Innovation continues through the present. For example, units are being tested that vary heart rate according to the body's physiologic needs,[26] and leadless electrodes are being developed that hold the promise of stimulating the heart without incorporating a catheter. So the history of electronic pacing has been meteoric and its future is bright.

Rationale for Developing Biologic Pacemakers

Given this description of electronic pacemakers, why even bother with biologic pacing—or indeed with any other approach? Simply because the electronic pacemaker, although a wonderful treatment, remains a panacea and not a cure. Box 22-1 summarizes why biologic pacemakers are being investigated to normalize cardiac rhythm in a way that more nearly approximates the physiologic state than do electronic pacemakers. If biologic pacing succeeds, then the two technologies would likely be used in tandem for some time to maximize patient safety. However, the eventual goal would be to see the phasing out of electronic pacing. Biologic pacemaking represents a truly disruptive technology.

Box 22-1 Limitations of Cardiac Pacemakers

- Not responsive to the autonomic nervous system (i.e., to the demands of exercise and emotion)
- Require monitoring and maintenance, including battery or electrode replacement
- Not optimal for pediatric patients
- Problems with infection, interference from other devices
- Often cannot implant a pacemaker at sites that optimize contraction in individual patients
- Palliate the problem but do not cure it

Strategies for Building Biologic Pacemakers

In the late 1980s, biologic pacing was a pipe dream occasionally discussed around coffee tables among investigators working on mechanisms of impulse initiation. The discussions were likely stimulated by Dario DiFrancesco's discovery of the pacemaker current, I_f,[10,11] and usually began with statements like, "Wouldn't it be wonderful if we could put pacemaker currents into diseased sinus nodes or ventricles and create a site of normal impulse initiation." Surely this was the stuff of science fiction, but as we've learned time and again, science fiction often explores desirable outcomes before the needed technology has been developed, the works of Jules Verne being a prime example.

By the late 1990s, advances in genetic manipulation and stem cell science brought the concept of biologic pacing to the realm of the possible, as we and others ventured to state in lectures and in print rather than simply at the coffee table. The template for exploration of biologic pacing is suggested in Figure 22-1. In brief, β-adrenergic stimulation can modulate I_f to increase pacemaker rate, and muscarinic stimulation slows rate. Indeed the first published science on biologic pacing used as a strategy the overexpression of β_2-adrenergic receptors in murine and then porcine hearts.[27,28] When a naked plasmid incorporating the β_2-receptor was injected into pig atria the basal rate and the response to catecholaminergic stimulation were increased. Clearly, overexpressing β-adrenergic receptors could augment sinus node function and increase the rate of normal rhythms. The investigators recognized several major concerns: In a diseased heart in which the sinus node is not functioning well or in which there is AV block, there is the very real possibility that β-receptor overexpression can be arrhythmogenic; upregulating β-receptors implies there are pacemaker cells already in the heart that will respond normally to increased catecholaminergic effect, which might or might not be the case; and success in transfecting using naked plasmids is often marginal in the heart in situ.

Hence, although these early studies provided proof of concept for biologic pacing, the strategy was not one that could be advanced. All subsequent strategies have depended on the manipulation of ion channels delivered via viral vectors or stem cell platforms or on the properties of channels resident in stem cells or other cell types to perform biologic pacing.

Viral Vector–Based Delivery of Constructs

Referring to Figure 22-1A, the initial ion channel–based approach reported transfection of guinea pig ventricles with an adenoviral vector incorporating a dominant negative construct to reduce the repolarizing current, I_{K1}.[29] As shown on electrocardiograms in the intact heart and with microelectrode and ion current recordings, an ectopic ventricular rhythm was expressed that was associated with phase 4 depolarization and reduced I_{K1} in myocytes. However, there were shortcomings, in the main associated with the effect of reducing repolarizing current to increase the duration of the action potential. A subsequent publication by the same group showed that the repolarization characteristics of Anderson's syndrome were also produced by this approach to biologic pacing,[30] so that its continued development was undesirable.

Concurrently with these reports, our own group had been working with means to modify and magnify the pacemaker current, I_f, originally reported by DiFrancesco.[10,11] We first demonstrated in neonatal rat myocytes in cell culture that using an adenoviral vector to overexpress the HCN2 channel isoform resulted in a robust and rapid pacemaker that far exceeded in rate and stability the rhythm normally seen in nontransfected cultures.[31,32] For this reason we adopted the strategy of using HCN genes as the basis for building biologic pacemakers and centered the approach on HCN2.[33] An additional attraction of working with HCN channels in this fashion was that the inward current flows only during diastole; hence, although we were increasing an inward current, this would not result in prolongation of the action potential. This avoided the problem that had afflicted the downregulation of I_{K1}.

Our initial in vivo study involved injecting adenoviral HCN2 and green fluorescent protein (GFP) constructs into canine left atria and several days later using vagal stimulation to shut down the sinus node.[33] The result was escape beats originating from the implant site. Cells disaggregated from this site showed I_f (actually I_{HCN2}) about 100 times greater in magnitude than that in native atrial myocytes. Additional vagal stimulation terminated firing of this pacemaker locus, suggesting the likelihood of vagal control.

In a follow-up study we used a custom-designed electrode catheter to locate the left bundle branch system in dogs and to inject the same adenoviral-HCN2 complex into the bundle branch.[34] When the vagal nerves were stimulated to terminate sinus rhythm and induce AV block, a rhythm emerged from the injection site. Follow-up studies demonstrated spontaneous and rapid impulse initiation at these bundle branch sites. In a later study we found that in dogs in radiofrequency ablation–induced complete heart block, the biologic pacemaker inserted into the left bundle branch system could drive the heart regularly and stably.[35] These rhythms were mapped to their bundle branch origins (Fig. 22-2).

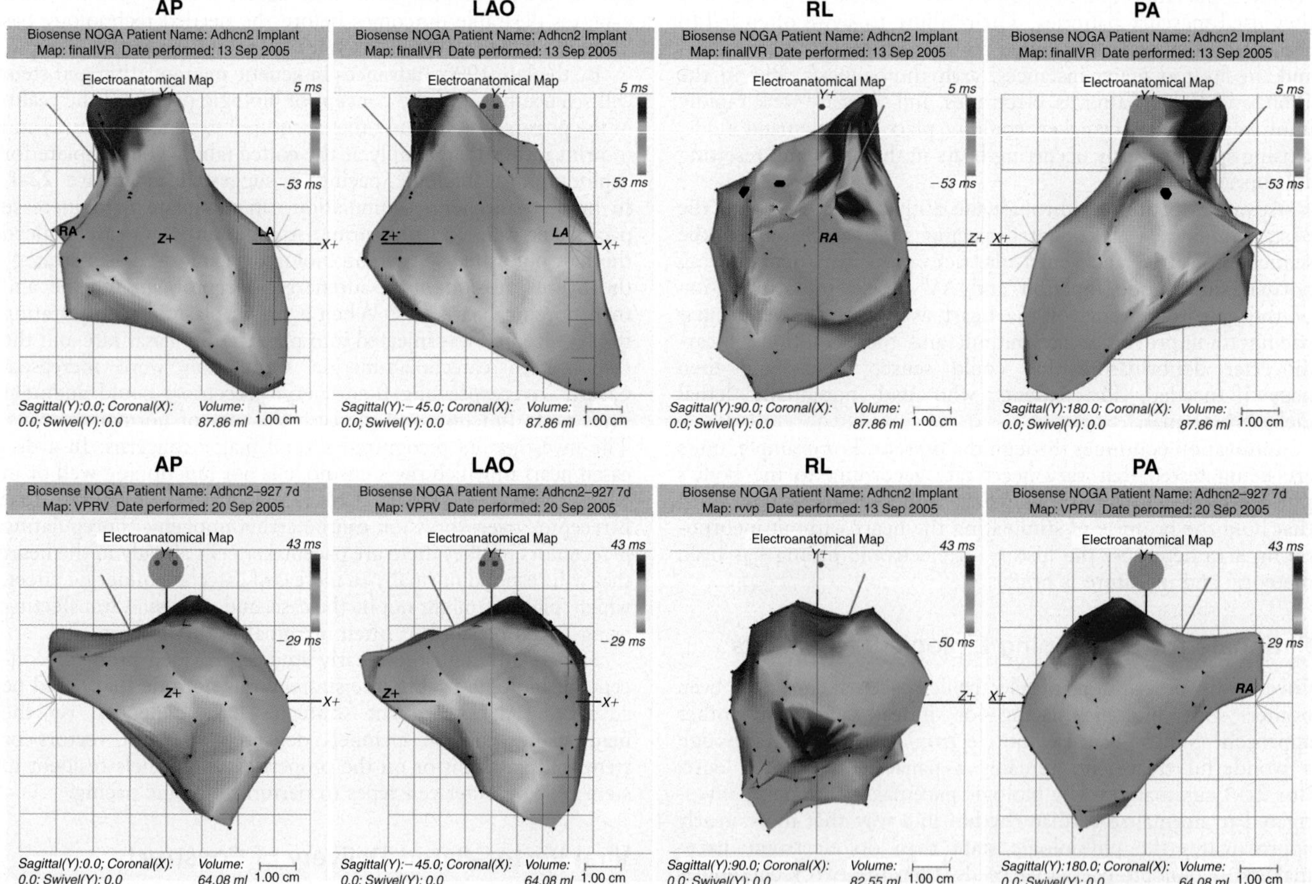

Figure 22-2 Noncontact mapping of left ventricle with the CARTO system in a dog with complete heart block, an electronic right ventricular apical endocardial pacemaker, and an HCN2 adenoviral construct administered into the proximal left bundle branch. Panels demonstrate four projections, showing early *(red)* through late *(blue)* activation. *Upper panels* show an impulse-activating left ventricular endocardium at several sites simultaneously, reflecting arrival of an impulse initiated in the left bundle branch system. *Lower panels* show early activation of left ventricular septum via the electronic pacemaker. AP, anteroposterior; IV, intraventricular; LAO, left anterior oblique; PA, posteroanterior; RL, right lateral.

During the 2-week life span of the adenovirus, about 70% of beats originated from the injection site. Their basal rates averaged 50 to 60 beats per minute.[35] The remaining 30% of beats were provided by the demand electronic pacemaker, which was set at an escape rate of 45 beats per minute. A control group of saline-injected animals with electronic pacemakers also set at 45 beats per minute had 90% of beats electrically stimulated, with the remainder arising from various idioventricular sites. The biologic pacemaker manifested a brisk response to catecholamine injection, seen as an approximate 50% rate increase. Taking this together with our earlier report,[33] we concluded that both vagal and sympathetic (or at least β-adrenergic) control of biologic pacing was possible.

More recent studies have attempted to replicate or improve on the function of HCN2 using designer-based potassium-channel genes[36] or else mutant or chimeric HCN channels.[35,37,38] None of these has shown clear superiority to HCN2 and one chimera—HCN212—resulted in ventricular tachycardias often exceeding rates of 200 beats per minute.[38] The latter were readily suppressed by the I_f blocking drug ivabradine. Although not resulting in an improved biologic pacemaker, the experiments on HCN212 provided two useful lessons: The first was that continued attempts to identify a pacemaker gene that might have basal rates of 60 to 80 beats per minute and good autonomic responsiveness should be possible; the second was that should biologic pacemaker toxicity ever be seen as a tachycardia, this would respond to I_f blockade.

Experiments using viral vectors and various HCN constructs, including HCN4 and HCN1, are continuing, and it is likely that one will provide an effective and autonomically responsive pacemaker. Although many of the experiments reported have used adenoviral vectors, there is increasing use of adeno-associated virus and lentivirus. The advantage of the former is that it provides relatively long-lasting expression of constructs; however, to what extent this expression is episomal rather than genomic is as yet unsolved. The most certain means for obtaining genomic incorporation of constructs is with lentivirus. Although members of this family are used clinically for a variety of experimental gene therapies, there is still concern about its long-term safety.

Cell Therapies

Two differing philosophies have provided the framework for using cell therapies in biologic pacing. The first uses cells that appear to have a normal complement of ion-channel genes to develop a biologic pacemaker. The most far-advanced therapy reported uses human embryonic stem cells that have been forced along a cardiogenic lineage.[39] Within this lineage, a subset of cells manifests typical pacemaker characteristics, including action potentials showing prominent phase 4 depolarization.[39] The underlying populations of ion channels include a very weak I_{K1} and a robust I_f, which together would tend to generate depolarization during phase 4.[40] Unlike sinoatrial node, however, the major contributor of inward current is reportedly sodium, rather than L-type calcium current.[40]

Clusters of these cells in culture have been shown to originate and propagate spontaneous rhythms, and when implanted into the ventricles of pigs in complete heart block they have initiated stable spontaneous rhythms that persist for up to 3 months.[39] The major issues regarding this approach have been and remain the need to use immunosuppression as well as questions regarding the eventual fate of the cells (will they persist as pacemaker cells or will they mature into nonbeating ventricular myocytes or into other inimical cell types?).

Other attempts to work with cells containing full ion channel complements have included the grafting of fetal[41] or neonatal[42] pacemaker cells. These research directions have not yet been published in sufficient detail to permit an objective evaluation of the possibilities they offer.

The second philosophy for cell therapy uses a cell type that does not have the proper ion channel population to generate pacemaker function but that has other characteristics that make it a candidate for exploitation as a platform therapy. By this we mean that it can be loaded with a gene or genes of interest that result in its delivering a pacemaker signal to adjacent cells. Some work has been reported using fibroblasts as platforms and fusing them with ventricular myocytes,[43] but the more completely reported approach to date has been our own, using adult human mesenchymal stem cells (hMSCs).[44-46]

Gene chip analysis of hMSCs has shown them not to have any appreciable signal for the pacemaker genes, HCN1-4, but they do have a robust signal for the cardiac connexins, Cx40 and Cx43.[45] In deciding to work with hMSCs as biologic pacemakers, we hypothesized that if we could load them with a pacemaker gene, they might couple adequately to myocytes such that the depolarizing signal generated by I_f would be transmitted to adjacent myocytes, causing them to depolarize (Fig. 22-3).[47,48] Using both dye transfer and current injection experiments in cell pairs, we showed that hMSCs could indeed communicate with myocytes.[45] This prompted us to load them with HCN2 via electroporation (avoiding any viral vector) (Fig. 22-4A-C) and to implant them in canine left ventricle.[44,46]

In an initial study we used vagal stimulation to suppress sinoatrial node impulse initiation and AV conduction. Here, an escape rhythm that pace mapped to the injection site was generated by the hMSC-based pacemakers (see Fig. 22-4D). We also demonstrated the presence of connexins at interstices between hMSCs and muscle cells (see Fig. 22-4E). In a subsequent study of dogs in complete heart block we found that hMSCs generate pacemaker function for at least 6 weeks when a critical mass of 700,000 or more cells, approximately 50% of which were loaded with HCN2, were implanted at a single site in the left ventricle.[46] Longer-term follow-up has not yet been performed.

Critical questions regarding these and any stem cells are not only the possibility of evolution into other, inimical or ineffective cell types but also the possibility of rejection or apoptosis.[47,48] In a 6-week trial of human MSCs xenotransplanted into canine hearts, we have seen no rejection (Fig 22-5).[46] This is consistent with the hypothesis that hMSCs are immunoprotected, most likely by one of several humoral factors released by them.[49-53] However, we have seen robust rejection of some lots of hMSCs by canine hearts,[41] which is not unexpected with xenotransplantation. As a result, longer-term study in dogs is now ongoing using canine MSCs loaded with human HCN2. As for the eventual human application of hMSCs, studies of their allogeneic administration to human subjects for myocardial repair have not reported any rejection response, but there has been a high degree of cell loss.[49,50] Clearly, issues remain regarding how to best bring this therapy to human subjects.

Optimizing Biologic Pacemaker Function

Research on biologic pacemakers has shown that the human embryonic stem cell and hMSC approaches, as well as viral vector administration, all support cardiac rhythm and physiologic demands effectively over limited periods of time.[35,39,46] We have investigated a mutant HCN2 (E324A), which we tested in the hope that it would further optimize pacemaker properties.[35] This showed some enhanced catecholamine responsiveness, but overall it had only modest advantage over the wild-type channel.

We also tested a chimeric channel, HCN212, which incorporated the transmembrane portion including the pore of

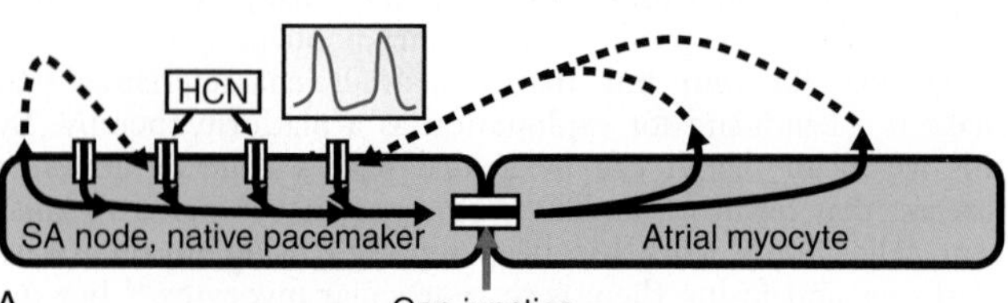

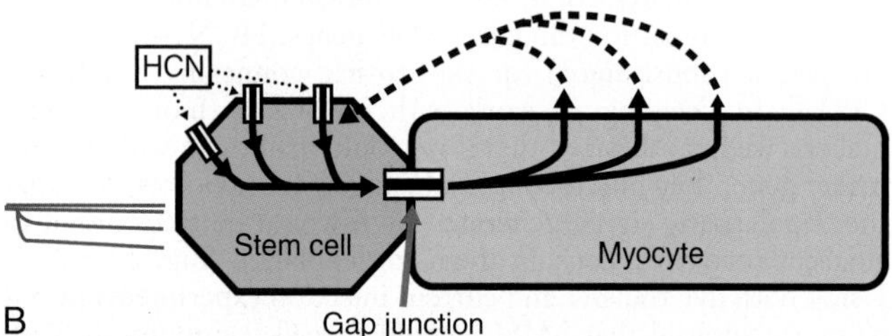

Figure 22-3 Initiation of spontaneous rhythms by wild-type pacemaker cells and by genetically engineered stem cell pacemakers. **A**, In a native pacemaker cell (or in a myocyte engineered to incorporate pacemaker current via gene transfer), action potentials *(inset)* are initiated via inward current flowing through transmembrane HCN channels. These open when the membrane repolarizes to its maximum diastolic potential and close when the membrane has depolarized during the action potential. Current flowing via gap junctions to adjacent myocytes results in their excitation and the propagation of impulses through the conducting system. **B**, A stem cell has been engineered to incorporate HCN channels in its membrane. These channels can only open, and current can only flow through them *(inset)* when the membrane is hyperpolarized; such hyperpolarization can only be delivered if an adjacent myocyte is tightly coupled to the stem cell via gap junctions. In the presence of such coupling and the opening of the HCN channels to induce local current flow, the adjacent myocyte is excited and initiates an action potential that then propagates through the conducting system. The depolarization of the action potential results in the closing of the HCN channels until the next repolarization restores a high negative membrane potential. In summary, wild-type and genetically engineered pacemaker cells incorporate in each cell all the machinery needed to initiate and propagate action potentials. In contrast, in the stem cell–myocyte pairing, two cells together work as a single functional unit whose operation critically depends on the gap junctions that form between the two disparate cell types. HCN, hyperpolarization-activated cyclic nucleotide–gated [channel]. (Reproduced with permission from Rosen MR, Brink PR, Cohen IS, et al: Genes, stem cells and biological pacemakers. Cardiovasc Res 64:12-23, 2004.)

HCN1 (which has more positive activation than HCN2) and the amino- and carboxy-termini (the latter incorporating the cAMP binding site) of HCN2.[38] The hypothesis was that this channel would generate faster basal pacemaker rates than HCN2, which typically are around 45 to 60 bpm, while exhibiting greater autonomic responsiveness than HCN1 alone. In fact, this approach resulted in an overshoot, such that ventricular tachycardias having rates in excess of 200 bpm occurred. Although the result here was unfortunate with regard to our search for a more ideal construct, it did permit us to test whether I_f blockade might suppress any arrhythmias generated by the biologic pacemaker. We found that the I_f blocker ivabradine was effective here.[38]

Another mutant gene has been developed by Marban and colleagues. They used a potassium channel engineered to carry inward sodium current having many of the properties of I_f.[36] The shortcoming was the absence of a cAMP binding site, without which there is no autonomic modulation. Although these and other constructs so far developed have not offered advantage over the wild type, it is likely that continued efforts at discovery will develop robust alternatives.

Another aspect of optimization involves the relationship between biologic and electronic pacing. When and if biologic pacing is ready for clinical trial, it cannot simply be administered to human subjects who need support for their ventricular rate. Rather, it will have to be used together with electronic pacemakers, because these are the current state of the art. For this reason we have tested integration of biologic and electronic pacemakers in tandem operation.[35] We found that tandem biologic-electronic pacemaker therapy manifests a seamless interface between biologic and electronic components, maintaining heart rate >45 bpm; conservation of total electronic beats delivered (which should prolong battery life); the possibility of using the memory function of the electronic pacemaker to track the function of the biologic component; and a more physiologic and catecholamine-responsive heart rate than is provided by electronic pacemakers alone.

The need to reclaim normal cardiac activation in the setting of normal sinus rhythm and complete heart block has also led investigators to engineer bypass tracts so that sinus impulses can gain access to the ventricles. This design would facilitate AV conduction and would potentially rival the function of AV sequential electronic pacing. However, this work is still in its infancy relative to biologic pacemaking. In one innovative approach, rat skeletal myoblasts were placed in an artificial matrix and inserted into the AV groove of rats whose adjacent atrium and ventricle had been denuded of epicardium. AV conduction and survival of transplanted cells was then documented.[54] Replication of results and information regarding long-term success of this approach are awaited.

Challenges

Some of the challenges are unique to biologic pacing: others hold for a variety of other approaches to gene and cell therapy. A major challenge is to identify the optimal construct. Overall, HCN2, itself, manifests properties that likely are adequate for first-generation biologic pacing. However, it might be preferable to have a construct that maintains basal rates in the 60- to 70-bpm range and reaches peaks of 120 to 140 bpm on catecholamine stimulation. It is for this reason that the groups working in this area continue attempts at optimizing mutant and chimeric constructs.

Although we have demonstrated that vagal and β-adrenergic responsiveness are characteristics of HCN2-based biologic pacemakers, further understanding of autonomic control is required. Preliminary data using HCN2 in both viral and hMSC constructs have demonstrated that vagal control depends on the site at which the pacemaker is implanted.[55] That is, in vagally innervated regions, Poincaré plots of heart rate variability are consistent with vagal-sympathetic input. In contrast, on the lateral free wall of the left ventricle, where there is little to no vagal innervation, there is no evidence of vagal input, and only sympathetic responsiveness is seen.

Preclinical and clinical testing of biologic pacing also are major challenges. At the preclinical level, the questions that arise relate largely to duration of action and the presence or absence of toxicity. The availability of electronic pacing is a major help here, as it removes any sense of urgency from the field. The only factor of importance is to get the process right—if biologic pacing works, then it should supplant the electronic, and if ultimately it doesn't, then the electronic will suffice.

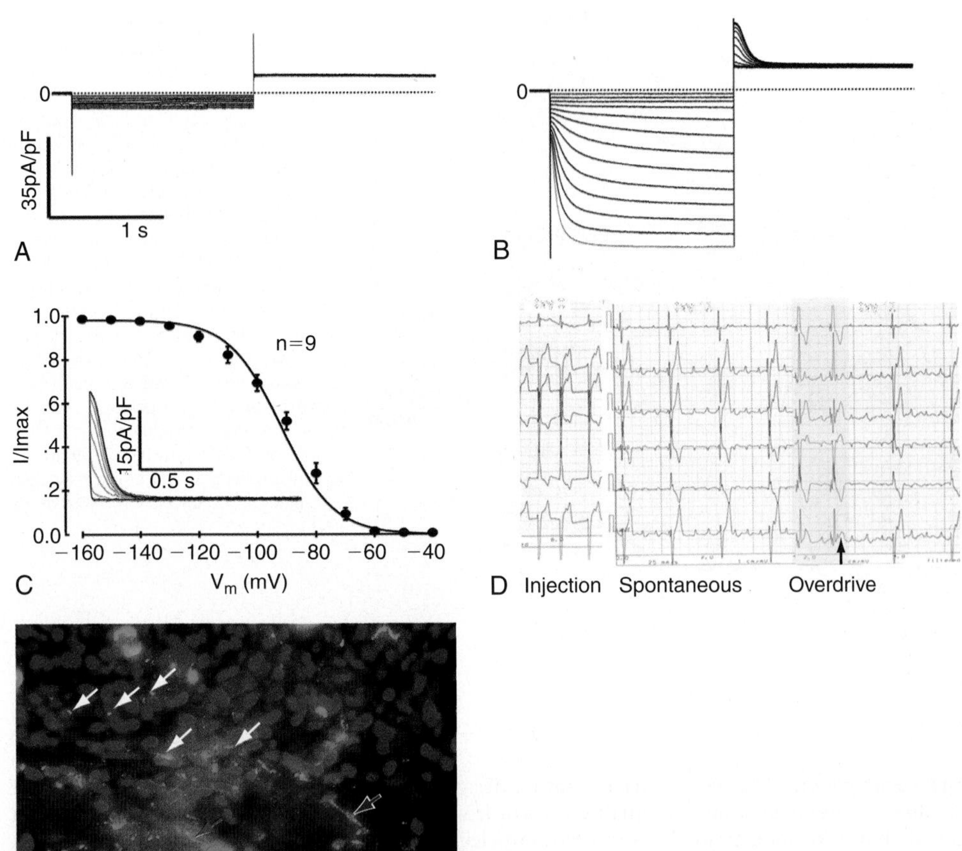

Figure 22-4 Example of loading hMSC with a gene of interest, studying it biophysically, and determining its effect on the heart. **A,** Pacemaker current, I_f, is not seen in a nonelectroporated hMSC. **B,** Functional expression of I_f in hMSC transfected with the *mHCN2* gene. **C,** Fit by the Boltzmann equation to the normalized tail currents of I_f gives a midpoint of −91.8 ± 0.9 mV and a slope of 8.8 ± 0.5 mV (n = 9). I_f is fully activated around −140 mV and has an activation threshold of −60 mV. *Inset* shows representative tail currents used for activation curves. Voltage protocol: Hold at −30 mV, hyperpolarize × 1.5 s to −40 to −160 mV in 10-mV increments followed by 1.5 s voltage step to +20 mV. **D,** Pacemaker function in canine heart in situ. *Top to bottom,* ECG leads I, II, III, aVR, aVL, and aVF. *1,* Pacing from hMSC injection site showing ECG configuration; *2,* spontaneous rhythm pace maps to site of injection, suggesting it is initiated at the injection site; *3,* last two beats of overdrive pacing *(blue highlight)* at 80 bpm followed by escape rhythm. Escape time = 1.3 sec. **E,** Immunostaining for connexin43 in a region of interface between an injection site and myocardium. DAPI staining reveals nuclei. *Purple arrows* are intercalated discs; *white arrows* show connexin43 staining between hMSCs; *red arrows* show connexin43 staining between hMSCs and myocytes. ECG, electrocardiogram; hMSC, human mesenchymal stem cell. (Modified with permission from Potapova I, Plotnikov A, Lu Z, et al: Human mesenchymal stem cell as a gene delivery system to create cardiac pacemakers. Circ Res **94**:841-959, 2004.)

What do we and others need to show if biologic pacing is to move into clinical testing? We need 1-year trials of either viral or stem-cell constructs showing that there is no toxicity and reliable effect. The hallmark for comparison is the electronic pacemaker. At the preclinical level, such comparisons are needed for 6 to 12 months in a large-animal model. These should show that regardless of whether a viral vector or a cell platform delivery system or a pacemaker cell is used, it provides function that supports life with an adequate basal rate and adequate responses to autonomic input. This activity must emanate uniquely from the site implanted with no evidence of wandering of constructs or cells to other sites in the heart that might compete or to other sites in the body.

Satisfying these demands is no mean feat: it requires that we follow the beat-by-beat function of the heart for 6- to 12-month periods while concurrently ensuring that viral vectors are not causing untoward effects on the heart or other tissues and that cells—whether hMSCs or ESC-derived or other—are not being destroyed, migrating elsewhere, or transforming into forms that are malignant or if not malignant, then nonfunctional.

A variety of methods are available for tracking cells (Table 22-1). Ideally, tracking should use markers that stay with the cell forever, that cannot pass from cell to cell, and whose signal can be read from the body surface via imaging techniques. To date, no method has been adequate. Methods most often used for in vivo studies have been variations on magnetic resonance imaging (MRI) to track iron or ferritin particles loaded into stem cells. The shortcoming is that if a cell dies, these particles can be taken up by or reside in other cells or can reside outside the cells. On being read via MRI, these particles may be correctly identified as a persistent signal and as a result give rise to a false-positive conclusion of continued presence of the stem cells.

We have worked recently with quantum dots as a tracking method (Fig. 22-6).[56] These nanoparticles have the advantages of passive loading into cells, inability to pass through gap junctions, uptake and removal by the reticuloendothelial system if host cells die, and a strong emission signal that can be readily detected. Although these are readily identified in tissue sections, tracing the fate of cells loaded with quantum dots using standard imaging techniques in vivo remains a major challenge.

Another issue important to large animal research and to future applicability to human subjects is delivery of constructs. Although catheters are available for delivering viral vectors in specific settings, the ideal flexible catheter with electrode recording capability at its tip and a large enough bore to not inflict damage on stem cells has not been reported.

Viral vectors remain a problem because adenoviral vectors express only episomally and are of use largely for proof of concept or transient gene delivery. Adeno-associated virus provides

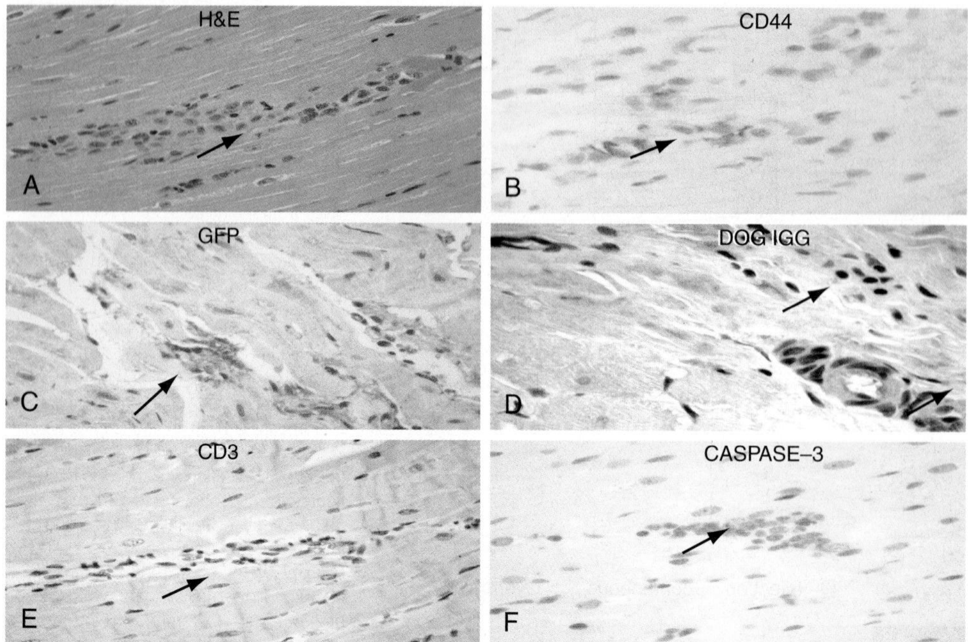

Figure 22-5 hMSCs 6 weeks after LV anterior wall intramyocardial injection. Hematoxylin and eosin (H&E) identifies basophilic cells *(upper left)* that are CD44 positive *(upper right)* and GFP positive (peroxidase stain, *middle left*). hMSCs do not display labeling or binding of dog-IGG to their surface *(middle right)*, evidence against humoral rejection. CD3-positive T lymphocytes are rarely noted in association with clusters of hMSCs *(lower left)*, evidence against cellular rejection. Staining is negative for activated CASPASE–3 *(lower right)*, evidence against apoptosis. hMSC, human mesochymal stem cell. (Original magnification: ×400). (Reproduced with permission from Plotnikov AP, Shlapakova I, Szabolcs MJ, et al: Xenografted adult human mesenchymal stem cells provide a platform for sustained biological pacemaker function in canine heart. Circulation 116:706-713, 2007.)

more long-term expression, but episomal versus genomic expression remain issues. Lentivirus, which does result in genomic incorporation, appears to be the vector of choice for long-term maintenance of an effect, although safety issues remain a concern.

Cell systems must be optimized and their persistence documented. Autologous cells elicit no immune response when readministered to the donor. However, they would make biologic pacing into a designer therapy whose expense and insurance of quality control from patient to patient would be nightmarish in comparison to electronic pacing. It has been shown that hMSCs can be administered allogeneically to human subjects with no adverse reactions, although long-term persistence is still an issue.[49] These might ultimately offer a readily standardized cell type, but more research is needed to test this. Human ESCs have required the use of immunosuppression in experiments to date.[39] Whether this will be the case in human experimentation remains to be seen, but a lifetime of electronic pacing appears far preferable to a lifetime of immunosuppression.

Table 22-1 Methods of Cell Tracking

Agent	Limitations
Reporter Proteins	
LacZ, b-gal	Require secondary detection
GFP	Unstable, may be weaker than autofluorescence
Ex vivo Staining	
FISH	Expensive, false positives
Surface markers	Lost or unexpressed over time; require secondary detection
Inorganic	
Radiometals	Toxicity, uniformity of loading
Fluorescent microspheres	Significant aggregation, unstable signal
Nanoparticles (i.e., quantum dots)	New technology, many unknowns

FISH, fluorescent in situ hybridization; GFP, green fluorescent protein.

The choice of promoter and regulation of nucleic acids are additional issues. To date many of us have worked with a cytomegalovirus (CMV) promoter. However, there can be temporal changes in the expression of promoters,[57] and CMV might not be the best long-term choice. Moreover, because of safety concerns, the idea of a cardiac-specific (and maybe even cardiac region–specific) promoter would be of importance. This would seem especially relevant with regard to viral delivery.

Duration of effect and robustness of expression will be influenced by processes regulating protein expression. MicroRNA might reduce expression; alterations in protein degradation alter expression of proteins and can affect RNA and DNA expression, DNA regulatory sequences, and the modulation of expression. All of these will continue to be explored over the coming years.

One issue on which some progress has been made is the design of preclinical and clinical trials of biologic pacemakers. One could not envisage a standard phase 1 trial in which healthy volunteers are sought. Rather, a reasonable trial design in human subjects would enroll patients in chronic atrial fibrillation and complete heart block in whom demand ventricular pacing is needed. The canine equivalent of this trial would have animals in ablation-induced complete heart block. Either setting would incorporate implantation of a right ventricular apical endocardial demand pacemaker, as well as implantation of the biologic pacemaker. The biologic pacemaker would be implanted at a site that prior electrophysiologic testing identified as the site that

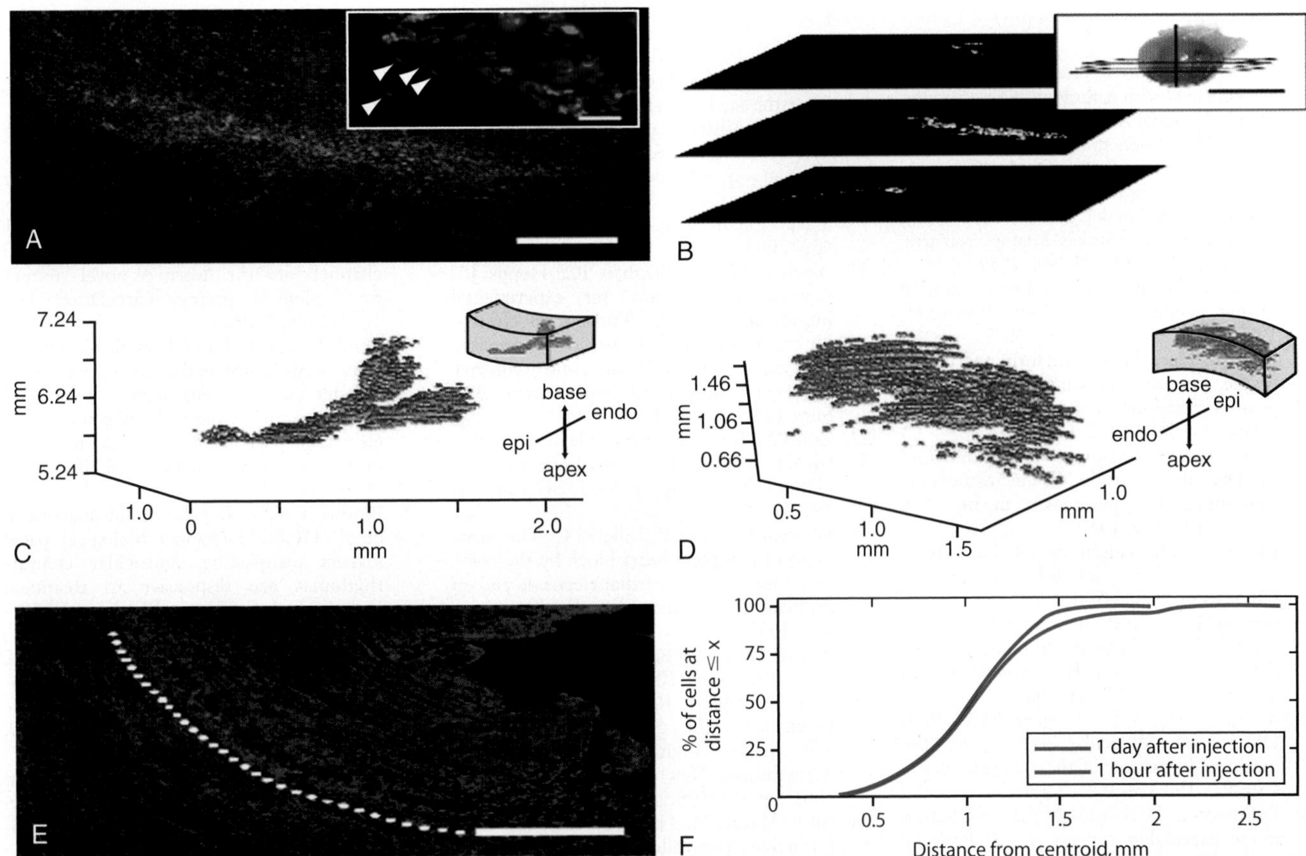

Figure 22-6 Quantum dots (QD) are used to identify single hMSCs after injection into the rat heart and further used to reconstruct the three-dimensional (3D) distribution of all delivered cells. Rat hearts were injected with QD-hMSCs. Fixed frozen sections were cut transversely (plane shown in **B**, *inset*) at 10 μm and mounted onto glass slides. Sections were imaged for QD fluorescence emission (655 nm) with phase overlay to visualize tissue borders. QD-hMSCs can be visualized at **(A)** low power, and **(A**, *inset***)** high power (Hoechst 33342 dye used to stain nuclei blue). **A** *(inset)*, Endogenous nuclei can be seen adjacent to the delivered cells in the midmyocardium *(arrows)*. Serial low power images were registered with respect to one another. **B**, Binary masks were generated where white pixels depict the QD-positive zones in the images. The vertical line *(inset)* represents the *z* axis, which has a zero value at the apex of the heart. The binary masks for all of the QD-positive sections of the heart were compiled and used to generate the 3D reconstruction of delivered cells in the tissue. QD-hMSCs remaining in the tissue adhesive on the epicardial surface (and not within the cardiac syncytium) were excluded from the reconstruction. **C**, QD-hMSC reconstruction in an animal that was euthanized 1 hour after injection. **D**, Reconstruction from an animal euthanized 1 day after injection, with orientation noted in inset. Our reconstructions in **C** and **D** do not account for all of the approximately 100,000 hMSCs delivered through the needle. Some of these cells undoubtedly leaked out of the needle track, and others might not have survived the injection protocol. The views of reconstructions **C** and **D** are oriented for optimal static visualization; they have different scales and are situated at different positions along the *z*-axis depending on the distance of the injection site from the apex of the heart. **E**, One day after injection of QD-hMSCs into the heart, the pattern of QD-hMSCs is well organized and appears to mimic the endogenous myocardial orientation (*dotted white line* highlights myofibril alignment). Complete representations of the spatial localization of QD-hMSCs in the heart permits further quantitative analyses. **F**, One parameter that can be computed is the distance of individual cells from the centroid of the total cell mass. The plots show the percentage of cells at a distance ≤X for both the 1-hour and 1-day rats. At both time points, most of the cells are within 1.5 mm of the centroid. Scale bars: **A** *(inset)*, 1 cm; **B** *(inset)*, 20 μm; **E**, 500 μm. hMSC, human mesenchymal stem cell. (Reproduced with permission from Rosen AB, Kelly DJ, Schuldt AJ, et al: Finding fluorescent needles in the cardiac haystack: Tracking human mesenchymal stem cells labeled with quantum dots for quantitative in vivo 3-D fluorescence analysis. Stem Cells 25:2128-2138, 2007.)

optimizes cardiac output in that individual subject. The electronic pacemaker provides a safety net if there is temporary or permanent failure in the biologic one. In addition, the electronic pacemaker can be used to track and record the function of the biologic pacemaker. The biologic unit, in turn, would likely conserve battery power in the electronic unit; our work to date has shown that tandem biologic-electronic operation sees the electronic unit firing only 30% of the time, which would indeed prolong the life of the battery.[35] In addition, the biologic component would be the heart's primary pacemaker, would provide autonomic responsiveness, and would provide cardiac activation and output characteristics superior to that provided by the electronic unit. Proof-of-concept experiments of this tandem pacing approach have been promising and have shown no competition between biologic and electronic units.[35]

Conclusions

The hyperbolic world we inhabit expects this morning's ideas to be this afternoon's cures. It would be irresponsible to try to make biologic pacing fit this mold. Because electronic pacing provides the luxury of a competent backstop, biologic pacing should be optimized and adequately tested before human experimentation begins. Indeed, our own prejudice is that this should be true of all therapies in a profession whose dictum is purportedly primum non nocere. The advantage of this more cautious approach is that the difficult questions that must be asked and the difficult experiments that must be done will not merely aid in advancing our knowledge in this circumscribed field but likely will find beneficial application in a variety of areas of gene and cell therapy.

References

1. Adams R: Cases of diseases of the heart, accompanied with pathological observations. Dublin Hospital Reports 4:353-453, 1827.
2. Stokes W: Observations on some cases of permanently slow pulse. Dublin Quarterly Journal of Medical Science 2:73-85, 1846.
3. Furman S, Schwedel JB: An intracardiac pacemaker for Stokes-Adams seizures. N Engl J Med 261:943-948, 1959.
4. Jeffrey K: The invention and reinvention of cardiac pacing. Cardiol Clin 10:561-571, 1992.
5. Keith A, Flack MW: The form and nature of the muscular connections between the primary divisions of the vertebrate heart. J Anat Physiol 41:172-189, 1907.
6. Lewis T, Oppenheimer BS, Oppenheimer A: The site of origin of the mammalian heart-beat; The pacemaker in the dog. Heart 2:147-169, 1910.
7. Fye WB: The origin of the heart beat: A tale of frogs, jellyfish, and turtles. Circulation 76:493-500, 1987.
8. Geison G: The Royal Institution Lectures of 1869. In Michael Foster and the Cambridge School of Physiology. Princeton, Princeton University Press, 1978, p 200.
9. Mommersteeg MT, Hoogaars WM, Prall OW, et al: Molecular pathway for the localized formation of the sinoatrial node. Circ Res 100:354-362, 2007.
10. DiFrancesco D: A study of the ionic nature if the pacemaker current in calf Purkinje fibres. J Physiol 314:377-393, 1981.
11. DiFrancesco D: Block and activation of the pacemaker channel in calf Purkinje fibres: Effects of potassium, caesium and rubidium. J Physiol 222:329-347, 1982.
12. Biel M, Schneider A, Wahl C: Cardiac HCN channels: Structure, function, and modulation. Trends Cardiovasc Med 12:202-216, 2002.
13. Boyett MR, Dobrzynski H, Lancaster MK, et al: Sophisticated architecture is required for the sinoatrial node to perform its normal pacemaker function. J Cardiovasc Electrophysiol 14:104-106, 2003.
14. Bogdanov KY, Maltsev VA, Vinogradova TM, et al: Membrane potential fluctuations resulting from submembrane Ca^{2+} releases in rabbit sinoatrial nodal cells impart an exponential phase to the late diastolic depolarization that controls their chronotropic state. Circ Res 99:979-987, 2006.
15. Thollon C, Bedut S, Villeneuve N, et al: Use-dependent inhibition of hHCN4 by ivabradine and relationship with reduction in pacemaker activity. Br J Pharmacol 150:37-46, 2007.
16. Borer JS, Fox K, Jaillon P, et al for the Ivabradine Investigators Group: Antianginal and antiischemic effects of ivabradine, an I_f inhibitor, in stable angina. A randomized, double-blind, multicentered, placebo-controlled trial. Circulation 107:817-823, 2003.
17. Scherf D, Schott A: Extrasystoles and Allied Arrhythmias, 3rd ed. Chicago, Year Book Medical Publishers, 1973.
18. McWilliam JA: Electrical stimulation of the heart in man. Brit Med J 1:348-350, 1889.
19. Lidwell MC: Cardiac Disease in Relation to Anaesthesia. In Transactions of the Third Session. Australasian Medical Congress, Sydney, Australia, Sept. 2-7 1929, p 160.
20. Furman S, Szarka G, Layvand D: Reconstruction of Hyman's second pacemaker. Pacing Clin Electrophysiol 28:446-453, 2005.
21. Bigelow WG, Callaghan JC, Hopps JA: General hypothermia for experimental intracardiac surgery: The use of electrophrenic respirations, an artificial pacemaker for cardiac standstill, and radio-frequency rewarming in general hypothermia. Ann Surg 132:531-537, 1950.
22. Zoll PM: Resuscitation of the heart in ventricular standstill by external electric stimulation. New Engl J Med 247:768-771, 1952.
23. Weirich W, Gott V, Lillehei C: The treatment of complete heart block by the combined use of a myocardial electrode and an artificial pacemaker. Surg Forum 8:360-363, 1957.
24. Nelson G: A brief history of cardiac pacing. Tex Heart Inst J 20:12-18, 1993.
25. Zivin A, Mehra R, Bardy GH: Cardiac pacemakers. In Spooner PM, Rosen MR (eds): Foundations of Cardiac Arrhythmias. New York, Marcel Dekker, 2001, pp 571-598.
26. Alt E, Matula M, Theres H, et al: The basis for activity controlled rate variable cardiac pacemakers: An analysis of mechanical forces on the human body induced by exercise and environment. Pac Clin Electrophysiol 12:1667-1680, 1989.
27. Edelberg JM, Aird WC, Rosenberg RD: Enhancement of murine cardiac chronotropy by the molecular transfer of the human β_2-adrenergic receptor cDNA. J Clin Invest 101:337-343, 1998.
28. Edelberg JM, Huang DT, Josephson ME, et al: Molecular enhancement of porcine cardiac chronotropy. Heart 86:559-562, 2001.
29. Miake J, Marbán E, Nuss HB: Gene therapy: Biological pacemaker created by gene transfer. Nature 419:132-133, 2002.
30. Miake J, Marbán E, Nuss HB: Functional role of inward rectifier current in heart probed by Kir2.1 overexpression and dominant-negative-suppression. J Clin Invest 111:1529-1536, 2003.
31. Yu H, Wu J, Potapova I, et al: MinK-related peptide. 1: A β subunit for the HCN ion channel subunit family enhances expression and speeds activation. Circ Res 88:E84-E87, 2001.
32. Qu J, Barbuti A, Protas L, et al: HNC2 overexpression in newborn and adult ventricular myocytes: Distinct effects on gating and excitability. Circ Res 89:E8-E14, 2001.
33. Qu J, Plotnikov AN, Danilo P Jr, et al: Expression and function of a biological pacemaker in canine heart. Circulation 107:1106-1109, 2003.
34. Plotnikov AN, Sosunov EA, Qu J, et al: A biological pacemaker implanted in the canine left bundle branch provides ventricular escape rhythms having physiologically acceptable rates. Circulation 109:506-512, 2004.
35. Bucchi A, Plotnikov AN, Shlapakova I, et al: Wild-type and mutant HCN channels in a tandem biological-electronic cardiac pacemaker. Circulation 114:992-999, 2006.
36. Kashiwakura Y, Cho HC, Barth AS, et al: Gene transfer of a synthetic pacemaker channel into the heart: A novel strategy for biological pacing. Circulation 114: 1682-1686, 2006.
37. Tse HF, Xue T, Lau CP, et al: Bioartificial sinus node constructed via in vivo gene transfer of an engineered pacemaker HCN channel reduces the dependence on electronic pacemaker in a sick-sinus syndrome model. Circulation 114:1000-1011, 2006.
38. Plotnikov AN, Bucchi A, Shlapakova I, et al: HCN212-channel biological pacemakers manifesting ventricular tachyarrhythmias are responsive to treatment with I_f blockade. Heart Rhythm 5(2):282-288, 2008.
39. Kehat I, Khimovich L, Caspi O, et al: Electromechanical integration of cardiomyocytes derived from human embryonic stem cells. Nat Biotechnol 22:1282-1289, 2004.
40. Satin J, Kehat I, Caspi O, et al: Mechanism of spontaneous excitability in human embryonic stem cell derived cardiomyocytes. J Physiol 559:479-496, 2004.
41. Lin G, Cai J, Jiang H, et al: Biological pacemaker created by fetal cardiomyocyte transplantation. J Biomed Sci 12:513-519, 2005.
42. Cai J, Lin G, Jiang H, et al: Transplanted neonatal cardiomyocytes as a potential biological pacemaker in pigs with complete atrioventricular block. Transplantation 81:1022-1026, 2006.
43. Cho HC, Kashiwakura Y, Marbán E: Creation of a biological pacemaker by cell fusion. Circ Res 100:1112-1115, 2007.
44. Potapova I, Plotnikov A, Lu Z, et al: Human mesenchymal stem cell as a gene delivery system to create cardiac pacemakers. Circ Res 94:952-959, 2004.
45. Valiunas V, Doronin S, Valiuniene L, et al: Human mesenchymal stem cells make cardiac connexins and form functional gap junctions. J Physiol 555:617-626, 2004.
46. Plotnikov AP, Shlapakova I, Szabolcs MJ, et al: Xenografted adult human mesenchymal stem cells provide a platform for sustained biological pacemaker function in canine heart. Circulation 116:706-713, 2007.
47. Rosen MR, Brink PR, Cohen IS, et al: Genes, stem cells and biological pacemakers. Cardiovasc Res 64:12-23, 2004.
48. Rosen M: Biological pacemaking: In our lifetime? Heart Rhythm 2:418-428, 2005.
49. Zimmett JM, Hare JM: Emerging role for bone marrow derived mesenchymal stem cells in myocardial regenerative therapy. Basic Res Cardiol 100:471-481, 2005.
50. Rosen MR: Are stem cells drugs? The regulation of stem cell research and development. Circulation 114:1992-2000, 2006.

51. Groh ME, Maitra B, Szekely E, et al: Human mesenchymal stem cells require monocyte-mediated activation to suppress alloreactive T cells. Exp Hematol 33: 928-934, 2005.
52. Di Nicola M, Carlo-Stella C, Magni M, et al: Human bone marrow stromal cells suppress T-lymphocyte proliferation induced by cellular or nonspecific mitogenic stimuli. Blood 99:3838-3843, 2002.
53. Tse WT, Pendleton JD, Beyer WM, et al: Suppression of allogeneic T-cell proliferation by human marrow stromal cells: Implications in transplantation. Transplantation 75:389-397, 2003.
54. Choi YH, Stamm C, Hammer PE, et al: Cardiac conduction through engineered tissue. Am J Pathol 169:72-85, 2006.
55. Shlapakova IN, Verrier RL, Danilo P Jr, et al: Autonomic control of HCN2-based biological pacemakers. Heart Rhythm 4:S55, 2007.
56. Rosen AB, Kelly DJ, Schuldt AJ, et al: Finding fluorescent needles in the cardiac haystack: Tracking human mesenchymal stem cells labeled with quantum dots for quantitative in vivo 3-D fluorescence analysis. Stem Cells 25:2128-2138, 2007.
57. Reinhard E, Nedivi E, Wegner J, et al: Neural selective activation and temporal regulation of a mammalian GAP-43 promoter in zebrafish. Development 120:1767-1775, 1994.

A New Functional Paradigm for the Heart's Pacemaker: Mutual Entrainment of Intracellular Calcium Clocks and Surface Membrane Ion Channel Clocks 23

EDWARD G. LAKATTA AND VICTOR MALTSEV

CHAPTER OUTLINE

Different types of cells within the heart—pacemaker cells within the sinoatrial (SA) node and ventricular myocytes—determine how fast and strong, respectively, the heart beats. The heart's pacemaker cells normally generate spontaneous rhythmic changes of their membrane potential, thereby producing roughly periodic spontaneous action potentials, or normal automaticity. Pacemaker cells within the heart having clocks with the briefest rhythmic periods capture or trigger other excitable cells. SA node pacemaker cells are the dominant cardiac pacemaker cells, because they exhibit shorter periods between spontaneous action potentials than do atrioventricular (AV) node cells or His-Purkinje cells. Thus, SA node pacemaker cells initiate the cardiac impulses by generating spontaneous action potentials that are conducted to the ventricle and entrain the duty cycle of ventricular cells.

The heart pacemaker generates billions of uninterrupted beats at greatly varying rates during the human life span and therefore must be a robust system. It has become apparent from the application of systems approaches to biologic functions[1] that pacemaker function robustness results from the timely integration of signaling events at several levels of the pacemaker, including subcellular, cellular (surface membrane), and tissue architecture. Robustness of SA node pacemaker cells (fail-safe properties conserved during evolution of the animal kingdom) and flexibility of these cells (the ability to react to demands for faster or slower firing rate) require multiple interactions among intrinsic cell mechanisms. This interactive network of mechanisms intrinsic to SA node pacemaker cells must also interpret and react to signals arising extrinsic to the cell, such as stretch, electrotonic impulses, or neurotransmitter or hormonal stimulation of surface membrane receptors. The predominant view of initiation of the heart beat, for the past several decades,[2] however, has been that it resides solely in the realm of surface membrane ion channels of SA node pacemaker cells (Fig. 23-1A).

However, evidence that an intracellular clock may be implicated in the initiation of the cardiac impulse stems from discoveries at the turn of the 20th century.[3] Multiple subsequent clues indicated that this intracellular clock was a Ca^{2+} oscillator[4,5] and that it produced an (oscillatory) inward current[6] that could result in spontaneous Ca^{2+} release–ignited excitation of the cell membrane to initiate action potentials.[7] However, the brute force experimental Ca^{2+} overload that was often employed in earlier studies of pacemaker tissue relegated the relevance of such intracellular Ca^{2+} release to abnormal automaticity.[8]

Recent experimental evidence, derived from the simultaneous confocal imaging of submembrane Ca^{2+} and the membrane potential of SA node pacemaker cells and supported by numerical modeling, indicates that the sarcoplasmic reticulum (SR), the major Ca^{2+} store in SA node pacemaker cells, can operate as yet another *physiologic* clock within cardiac pacemaker cells: It generates spontaneous, rhythmic, local Ca^{2+} releases (see Fig. 23-1B and C) in the absence of Ca^{2+} overload. These tightly regulated but rhythmic local Ca^{2+} releases begin to occur beneath the surface membrane during the later part of diastolic depolarization, and they activate electrogenic operation of the Na^+-Ca^{2+} exchanger; the Na^+-Ca^{2+} exchanger inward current imparts an exponential increase to the late diastolic depolarization, leading to activation of L-type calcium channel current (I_{CaL}).

The I_{CaL} generates the next action potential upstroke and membrane excitation; via its Ca^{2+} influx, it also triggers Ca^{2+}-induced Ca^{2+} release, which synchronizes the intracellular Ca^{2+} oscillators of the local SR fragments in a relatively Ca^{2+}-depleted state, thus ensuring the uniform functional integrity of the SR, which permits the generation of powerful spontaneous subsarcolemmal Ca^{2+} signals at a crucial time later in diastole. Our review summarizes evidence for a novel mechanism of cardiac pacemaker function and regulation based on the idea that the cardiac pacemaker clock is a robust complex system of coupled oscillators—Ca^{2+} and membrane clocks—controlled by the kinetics of multiple regulatory feedback and feed-forward interactions of the system components via their complex dependencies on Ca^{2+}, cyclic adenosine monophosphate (cAMP), phosphorylation, and the membrane potential.

This research was supported by the Intramural Research Program of the National Institutes of Health, National Institute on Aging.

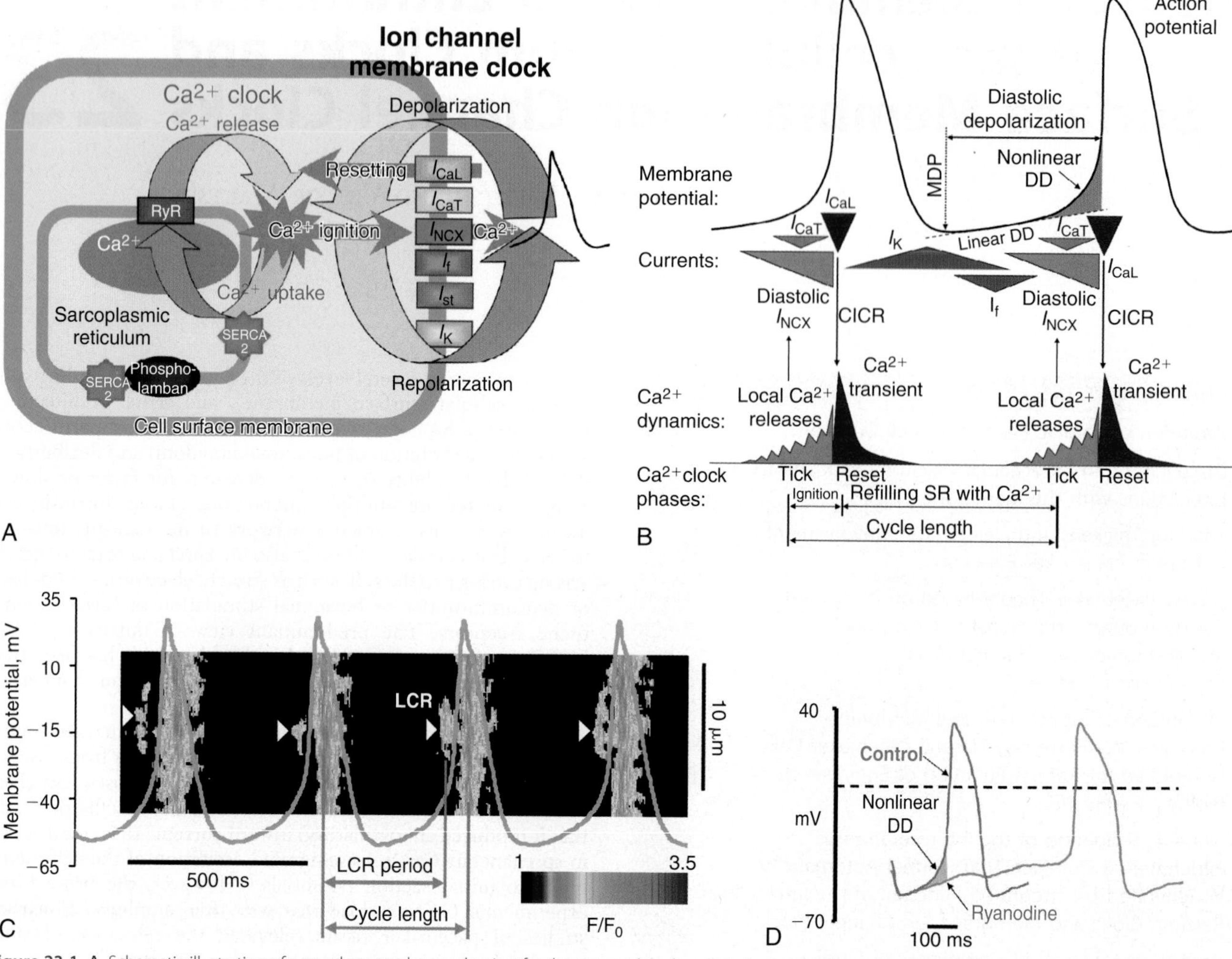

Figure 23-1 **A,** Schematic illustration of a novel pacemaker mechanism for the sinoatrial node cell. A classic membrane ion channel clock operates not in isolation but in tight cooperation with yet another clock (calcium clock) located under the cell membrane. The dynamically coupled clocks produce robust heartbeats, because the calcium clock ignites membrane excitations but the membrane clock resets the calcium clock each pacemaker cycle via Ca^{2+}-induced Ca^{2+} release. (Modified from Maltsev VA, Lakatta EG: Normal heart rhythm is initiated and regulated by an intracellular calcium clock within pacemaker cells. Heart Lung Circ 16:335-348, 2007.) **B,** Schematic illustration of the key phases of the interactions between the membrane clock (membrane potential and ion currents) and the calcium clock (Ca^{2+} dynamics and calcium clock phases) comprising the pacemaker mechanism. (Modified from Maltsev VA, Lakatta EG: Cardiac pacemaker cell failure with preserved I_f, I_{CaL}, and I_{Kr}: A lesson about pacemaker function learned from ischemia-induced bradycardia. J Mol Cell Cardiol 42:289-294, 2007.) **C,** Linescan confocal Ca^{2+} image with superimposed spontaneous action potentials measured in rabbit SA node pacemaker cells. *White arrowheads* show local Ca^{2+} releases. Time increases from left to right and vertical displacement correspond to position along the scan line. (Modified from Bogdanov KY, Maltsev VA, Vinogradova TM, et al: Membrane potential fluctuations resulting from submembrane Ca^{2+} releases in rabbit sinoatrial nodal cells impart an exponential phase to the late diastolic depolarization that controls their chronotropic state. Circ Res 99:979-987, 2006.) **D,** Ryanodine abolishes the calcium clock–mediated action potential ignition by inhibition of the nonlinear diastolic depolarization *(gray area* shown by *arrows).* (Modified from Lakatta EG, Vinogradova T, Lyashkov A, et al: The integration of spontaneous intracellular Ca^{2+} cycling and surface membrane ion channel activation entrains normal automaticity in cells of the heart's pacemaker. Ann N Y Acad Sci 1080:178-206, 2006.) CICR, Ca^{2+}-induced Ca^{2+} release; DD, diastolic depolarization; F/F_0, ratio of measured fluorescence to basal fluorescence; I_{CaL}, L-type calcium current; I_{CaT}, T-type calcium current; I_f, hyperpolarization-activated funny current; I_K, potassium current; I_{NCX}, Na^+-Ca^{2+} exchanger current; I_{st}, sustained current; LCR, local subsarcolemmal Ca^{2+} release; MDP, maximum diastolic potential; RyR, ryanodine receptor; SA, sinoatrial; SR, sarcoplasmic reticulum.

Evolution of Cardiac Pacemaker Cell Dogma

Myogenic Origin of Cardiac Impulse Initiation

The current dogma of the initiation and regulation of rhythmic heartbeats has evolved for almost 200 years from the intertwining of theory and experimentation.[9] In the early 1880s, Gaskell, applying heat to the tortoise heart, demonstrated that heart automaticity was myogenic rather than neurogenic. Specifically, he noted that the automaticity could occur in all different regions of the heart including the ventricle, indicating that—in contrast to skeletal muscle, which strictly followed the paradigm of nerve-mediated excitation inducing contraction—cardiac tissues possess their own internal excitatory oscillator. The area of the turtle heart with the greatest automaticity was the sinus venosus, which emanated impulses that entrained the entire heart.

Initial Idea of an Intracellular Origin for the Pacemaker Action Potential

The unique feature of the action potentials of pacemaker cells is that they arise spontaneously due to events that precede the rapid action-potential upstroke. A slow potential change preceding the discharge of cardiac impulses was first observed by Arvanitaki working on the snail heart in 1937. Later, in 1943, Bozler, employing monophasic potential recordings, observed a similar phenomenon in sinus venosus of turtle.[10] He called the slow depolarizing potential change a "prepotential" and suggested that it was "the basis underlying automaticity" including "normal rhythmicity." In rhythmically active strips of cardiac muscle (from turtles, rabbits, cats, and dogs) and sinus venosus (from turtle, high K^+) he noted oscillatory monophasic subthreshold potentials of relatively (compared to nerve) low frequency of approximately 1 Hz, which were enhanced by increasing extracellular calcium ($[Ca^{2+}]_o$) or by adding adrenaline. Discharging impulses on the top of oscillatory potentials were accompanied by synchronized variations in isometric force (tonus).[11] Bozler postulated that

> *the tonus changes and the local potentials are probably manifestations of a more fundamental process, a fluctuation in resting metabolism. . . . Their chief interest lies in their relation to the automaticity and rhythmicity of the muscle. It may be assumed that an increase in metabolism causes a rise in tonus and a decreased surface polarization. The decrease in polarization in turn may be considered as the last link in the chain of processes leading to the discharge of an impulse.*

Quantitative Theory of Membrane Excitation

In 1952, Hodgkin and Huxley applied the voltage-clamp approach to giant squid nerve cells and established current-voltage relationships for Na^+ and K^+ currents. Based on these data they formulated a new quantitative theory of membrane excitation. According to the Hodgkin-Huxley formalism, surface membrane ion channels are opened (or activated) by a change in membrane voltage and undergo a time-dependent transition into an inactivated state. Noble adapted the Hodgkin-Huxley formulation for the heart, using Purkinje fibers as a pacemaker model.[12] The kinetics of activation and inactivation of the channels are the timing mechanisms of the currents, which compose the membrane clock in cardiac pacemaker cells (see Fig. 23-1A and B).

Membrane Clock of Sinoatrial Nodal Cells, the Heart's Primary Pacemaker Cells

The membrane-delimited pacemaker mechanism derived from the Hodgkin-Huxley theory became the subject of extensive experimental search driven by the successful application of the voltage clamp technique to SA node cells and later to single SA node pacemaker cells. These voltage clamp studies have successfully identified numerous ion current components in SA node pacemaker cells.[2,8] Voltage-gated Na^+ current (I_{Na}), however, is absent in cells of the primary pacemaker region of the SA node, and the action potential upstroke is mainly formed by activation of L-type Ca^{2+} current (I_{CaL}) in these cells. The depolarization activates outward K^+ currents, which eventually prevail over inward currents and repolarize the membrane toward its lowest level within the cycle, the *maximum diastolic potential*. The maximum diastolic potential of about −65 mV is higher than the resting potential of about −90 mV in ventricular myocytes, or the maximum diastolic potential in Purkinje fibers, within ranges from −70 to −85 mV, because SA node pacemaker cells express either no inward rectifier K^+ current (I_{K1}) or, in some species, a very small I_{K1}.

Studies of the initiating event of normal automaticity of the heart's pacemaker cells had originally intensely focused upon ion currents that determine the maximum diastolic potential and early diastolic depolarization events that are caused by the prior action potential and essentially reflect a membrane *recovery* process. The early diastolic depolarization of SA node pacemaker cells is mainly attributable to the g_K decay mechanism.[12] Following achievement of the maximum diastolic potential, the conductance for delayed rectifier K^+ current (I_K) decreases as the potassium channels inactivate after their activation during action potential. This shifts the balance in favor of inward currents driven by a background (i.e., voltage-dependent and time-independent) membrane permeability—for example, to sodium ions[12]—resulting in a depolarization immediately after the maximum diastolic potential. This response is essentially an afterpotential (or afterhyperpolarization), which is also observed in other cardiac cell types.[3]

The repolarization during the later part of the action potential also activates another early-mid diastolic depolarization mechanism, the hyperpolarization-activated *funny current* (I_f).[13,14] In the past, this current was referred to as the *pacemaker current*, but it is not the dominant pacemaker mechanism in SA node pacemaker cells:[8,15] experimental blockade of I_f results only in a minor increase of the cycle length (5%-20%) in SA node pacemaker cells.[2] Due to its low activation voltage (<−65 mV) and slow activation kinetics, I_f contributes to a slower diastolic depolarization in a more negative (compared to SA node pacemaker cells) voltage range in subsidiary pacemaker cells and Purkinje cells.

Events following the recovery process of the prior action potential that occur during the late part of the diastolic depolarization and ignite the subsequent action potential were not initially recognized. A contribution of I_{CaL} (referred to as I_s at the time) to diastolic depolarization was suggested in 1980 by Yanagihara and colleagues.[16] I_{CaL} activation indeed occurs before the membrane excitation, as the threshold of I_{CaL} lies within the mid-late diastolic depolarization range, at around −50 mV.[14,17,18] This relatively low activation threshold of I_{CaL} in rabbit SA node pacemaker cells might be explained, at least in part, by two factors: L-type calcium channels appear to be phosphorylated in the basal state by highly active protein kinase A (PKA),[19,20] and a low activation threshold L-type calcium channel isoform, Cav1.3, can operate, as shown in mouse SA node pacemaker cells.[21] It has also been suggested that because T-type Ca^{2+} current (I_{CaT}) has a low activation threshold (~−60 mV), its activation during the mid-late diastolic depolarization might trigger a depolarization leading to activation of the conventional I_{CaL}.[22] Finally, a nonselective sustained current (I_{st})[23] was identified as yet another potential late diastolic depolarization mechanism. However, the identity of I_{st} remains unclear because it exhibits many properties of I_{CaL} and Na^+-Ca^{2+} exchanger current (see later), and neither its molecular origin nor specific blockers have been discovered.

Although the voltage- and time- dependent interplay of the ion channel currents could explain the spontaneous diastolic depolarization in pacemaker cells such as SA node pacemaker cells,[2] the interplay of these channels turns out to be extremely complex. Many previously identified currents are, in fact, ensembles of subcomponents; others are species dependent or are expressed only in some SA node pacemaker cells. For example, Cl^- current was observed only in one third[24] and I_{CaT} in one fifth of the rabbit SA node pacemaker cells (in 5 from 25 cells tested[17]). I_K was resolved into rapid and slow components, I_{Kr} and I_{Ks}, respectively. Bullfrog sinus venosus cells lack I_f. An I_{K1} of small amplitude is present in mouse, rat, and monkey; I_{Ks} is present in porcine SA node pacemaker cells, but I_{Kr} operates in rat and rabbit (under basal conditions).

I_{CaT} likely contributes to pacemaker function in relatively small animals having high basal beating rate (e.g., mouse or rat), but its contribution decreases as the size of the animal increases. For example, I_{CaT} is absent in human and porcine SA node pacemaker cells and it makes only a minor contribution to rabbit SA node pacemaker cell function, because similar to blockade of I_f, blockade of I_{CaT} results in a minor cycle length increase of 14% to 16%. Currently there is no consensus as to which of the SA node pacemaker cell ion channels makes the major contribution to pacemaker activity. Various viewpoints on the membrane clock (see Fig. 23-1A) essentially include combinations of previously suggested diastolic depolarization mechanisms: the original g_K decay mechanism of 1962,[12] I_{CaL} activation,[16] I_f activation,[13,14] I_{CaT} activation,[22] or I_{st} activation.[23] Numerous numerical models, based upon gating schema of ensembles of SA node pacemaker cell membrane ion currents, have been devised, and any of these models, featuring different contributions of the ion currents to the diastolic depolarization, can indeed generate spontaneous action potentials.[2]

Because the idea of a uniquely important pacemaker mechanism was not confirmed in the extensive experimental studies of ion channels across numerous species, could it be that there is no uniquely important pacemaker ion channel? Or is it possible that regardless of combination or contributions of the different ion channel types, not all of the crucial mechanisms that are implicated in spontaneous excitation of pacemaker cells are embodied in the ensemble properties of cell surface ion channels? Could it be that the formal cause of spontaneous rhythmic action potentials in SA node pacemaker cells (the initiating step of their normal automaticity) is an intracellular process, possibly similar to the one that Bozler had suggested earlier in 1943?[11]

Discovery of an Intracellular Calcium Clock and Its Interactions with the Membrane Clock

The discovery and initial characterization of an intracellular clock within cardiac cells required that it must essentially be disengaged from entrainment by the membrane clock. As early as in 1897, irregularity of heart contractions was induced experimentally by digitalis in dogs; extrasystoles induced by digitalis, barium, or veratrine were extensively studied during the first four decades of the twentieth century.[3] Early pharmacologic experimental approaches to studying heart rhythm mechanisms in human patients, whole animal models, and isolated cardiac muscle (studies of 1939-1943 by Segers and Bozler) produced cell Ca^{2+} overload. Abnormal, rather than normal, automaticity was being explored in these earlier studies.

In the late 1970s to early 1980s, as the importance of intracellular Ca^{2+} transients (as the trigger for cell contractions) in primarily contractile cardiac cells came into focus, the idea that an intracellular oscillator could drive membrane excitations in Purkinje fibers was temporarily revived.[5] Pharmacologic microelectrode studies of action potentials in the early 1970s[3] rediscovered the triggered activity described approximately 30 years earlier in the monophasic recordings.[10,11] These studies to probe a role for Ca^{2+} in pacemaker cell automaticity continued to employ brute force experimental Ca^{2+} overload in their approach to create easily measurable Ca^{2+} oscillations. It was shown that the action potentials of Purkinje fibers exposed to ouabain or to acetylstrophanthidin develop delayed afterdepolarizations and aftercontractions in the context of increased Ca_o or decreased K_o and was depressed by Mg^{2+} and that the amplitude of these was enhanced by driving the fiber at a faster rate.

Voltage clamp studies that employed Ca^{2+} overload to disconnect the surface membrane processes from intracellular ones demonstrated that an intracellular oscillatory process produces spontaneous membrane current oscillations. It was proposed[5,6] that the intracellular oscillatory mechanism involves cycles of Ca^{2+} movement between SR and myoplasm, as previously suggested for skinned cardiac preparations by Fabiato and Fabiato.[25] Furthermore, the observation that oscillatory currents were inhibited by Ca^{2+}-current blockers gave rise to a new and important idea that Ca^{2+} oscillations might represent the result of "a two-way interaction between surface membrane potential and intracellular Ca^{2+} stores."[6] Such spontaneous Ca^{2+} signals, including Ca^{2+} oscillations, were then indeed measured directly by aequorin in Purkinje fibers.[26]

An important issue that needed to be addressed was how Ca^{2+} oscillatory signals are transformed into respective electrical signals of cell membrane? It turned out that major ion (K^+ and Ca^{2+}) currents in cardiac cells, including SA node pacemaker cells, were modulated by Ca^{2+} and cyclic nucleotides. Based on this knowledge, researchers speculated that intracellular Ca^{2+} oscillations could be linked to membrane potential via a Ca^{2+}-dependent K^+ conductance,[4] a nonselective Na^+ and K^+ cation channel,[6] or Na^+-Ca^{2+} exchanger current (I_{NCX}).[8] Interestingly, early studies following the discovery of Na^+-Ca^{2+} exchanger in cardiac muscle by Reuter in 1968, suggested that the Na^+-Ca^{2+} exchanger function was electrically neutral (two sodium ions for each calcium ion). An electrogenic ion exchange stoichiometry of 3:1 instead of 2:1, as well as its contribution into the slow inward current (I_s) was realized later, around 1981,[8] and was first introduced into the DiFrancesco-Noble model of Purkinje fiber.

But because oscillatory current became manifest only in the Ca^{2+} overload state, similar to that described by Lewis, Rothberger, Scherf, Segers, and Bozler in their studies in the 1920s to 1940s,[3] such current fluctuations were primarily interpreted as a disturbance of normal cardiac function.[6] Upon testing an integration of a simple Ca^{2+} oscillator scheme into a pacemaker model, Noble concluded that "clarification of these abnormal rhythm mechanisms required additional experiments."[8] Other pacemaker cognoscenti of the day, although basically in agreement with this view, were somewhat more liberal in their vision. Cranefield[3] reasoned that "the true automaticity of the SA node or of Purkinje fibers might have a close connection with triggered activity." Irisawa speculated that subthreshold oscillations contribute to a "safety margin to prevent the SA node cell from becoming quiescent."[4]

However, because spontaneous, localized, oscillatory Ca^{2+} signals of the Ca^{2+} clock within SA node pacemaker cells could not be measured under normal conditions at that time, the concept that an internal Ca^{2+} oscillator provides the initiating signals for normal automaticity was again abandoned.

The Plot Thickens: Intracellular Ca^{2+} Involvement in Normal Pacemaker Function

In the late 1980s, experimental investigation of the role of Ca^{2+} in pacemaker function began to shift from experimental Ca^{2+} overload paradigms to more physiologic conditions. Afterdepolarizations and aftercontractions were recorded in Purkinje fibers under normal Ca^{2+} loading conditions,[27] and these fibers demonstrated localized, spontaneous myofilament motion caused by spontaneous local Ca^{2+} oscillations.[28] Subsequently, it was discovered that ryanodine (by disabling ryanodine receptor function and depleting SR Ca^{2+} content) has a profound negative chronotropic effect on automaticity of subsidiary atrial pacemakers.[29] Analyses of the ryanodine effect on action potential shape led to the suggestion that Ca^{2+} released from the SR contributes to diastolic depolarization, primarily during its *later* half (see Fig. 23-1B to D) and plays a prominent role in bringing the late diastolic depolarization to the action potential activation threshold. Further voltage clamp experiments in perforated patch configuration in isolated cat atrial latent pacemaker cells demonstrated the occurrence of an inward current during the late diastolic depolarization, which was sensitive to ryanodine.[30] It was suggested that this current component contributes to the diastolic depolarization in these cells and is linked to SR Ca^{2+} release and presumably due to I_{NCX}.

When it became possible to routinely measure intracellular Ca^{2+} in spontaneously firing SA node pacemaker cells, it was observed that a cytosolic Ca^{2+} transient is evoked by each spontaneous action potential and that Ca^{2+} influx via L-type calcium channels affects Ca^{2+} loading of the SR; chelation of intracellular Ca^{2+} in rabbit SA node pacemaker cells by BAPTA (1,2-bis [2-aminophenoxy]ethane-*N,N,N,N*-tetraacetic acid)[18,31] (but not EGTA [ethylene glycol bis(P-aminoethyl ether)-*N, N'*-tetraacetic acid])[18] applied intracellularly, markedly slowed or abolished spontaneous beating by SA node pacemaker cells. A strong negative chronotropic effect of EGTA, however, has been reported in guinea pig (SA node pacemaker cells[32] and AV node cells).[33] Intracellular Ca^{2+} buffering blocks spontaneous action potential generation, which is strong evidence that normal automaticity of these cells is tightly linked to intracellular Ca^{2+} dynamics.

Additional studies made a compelling argument that rhythmic Ca^{2+} cycling within mammalian SA node pacemaker cells is crucial for their normal automaticity. Ca^{2+}-cycling proteins, sarcoplasmic/endoplasmic reticulum calcium adenosine triphosphatase (SERCA), ryanodine receptor, and Na^{+}-Ca^{2+} exchanger, previously identified in atrial or ventricular cells, were also identified in SA node pacemaker cells.[34,35] The potential importance of SR Ca^{2+} release for function of SA node pacemaker cells was demonstrated directly by ryanodine effects on Ca^{2+} cycling in these cells.[36] The importance of ryanodine receptor–mediated Ca^{2+} release and I_{NCX} for normal spontaneous beating was also demonstrated in amphibian toad pacemaker cells.[37] Changes in the cytosolic Ca^{2+} transient in response to β-adrenergic receptor stimulation were correlated with changes in the beating rate.[34,37] Thus, it was becoming recognized that intracellular Ca^{2+} cycling within pacemaker cells is somehow involved in *normal* pacemaker function of SA node pacemaker cells.

A New Pacemaker Theory Based on Integrated Function of an Intracellular Calcium Clock and Membrane Ion Channel Clock: Experimental Evidence

Calcium Clocks in Sinoatrial Node Pacemaker Cells Ignite Rhythmic Action Potentials via Activation of Na^{+}-Ca^{2+} Exchanger Current

Fluorescence imaging of intracellular Ca^{2+} in rabbit SA node pacemaker cells over the last decade has documented the occurrence of not only action potential–induced global cytosolic Ca^{2+} transients[31] but also the occurrence of localized Ca^{2+} releases beneath the cell surface membrane during *late* diastolic depolarization of spontaneously firing SA node pacemaker cells in the absence of Ca^{2+} overload (see Fig. 23-1C). Such local Ca^{2+} releases occur in pacemaker cells in the form of multiple locally propagating wavelets beneath the cell membrane,[38,39] larger than the spontaneous Ca^{2+} sparks in ventricular cells, but markedly less than well-organized Ca^{2+} waves that can propagate the length of ventricular cells.[7] Occurrence of local Ca^{2+} release in spontaneously firing rabbit SA node pacemaker cells during the late diastolic depolarization does not require triggering by the depolarization,[40] because local Ca^{2+} releases are observed in the absence of membrane potential changes, namely in voltage-clamped SA node pacemaker cells in physiologic solutions, and in skinned SA node pacemaker cells, bathed in 100 nM [Ca^{2+}].[20,40]

Local Ca^{2+} releases occurring during the late diastolic depolarization begin to boil and then explode at this phase of pacemaker cycle,[39,41,42] and they are accompanied by inward currents that produce miniature membrane voltage fluctuations. These rhythmic oscillatory currents are activated by rhythmic local Ca^{2+} releases, because during voltage clamp both local Ca^{2+} releases and the currents exhibit fluctuations of the same frequency,[20,40] and both are abolished by ryanodine.[43] Because the scale of Na^{+}-Ca^{2+} exchanger current activated by the calcium clock during the diastolic depolarization in SA node pacemaker cells is only about 10 pA,[40] it might have easily been distorted or missed in earlier whole-cell patch clamp experiments. However, a 10-pA current has crucial importance during diastolic depolarization, because membrane electrical resistance during this phase of the cycle is very high: A tiny current change of approximately 3 pA is enough to drive the critical diastolic depolarization change in rabbit SA node pacemaker cells.[14]

Although the effect of individual stochastic local Ca^{2+} releases on the diastolic depolarization is relatively small (~0.2 mV), a synchronized or cooperative action of the local Ca^{2+} release ensemble imparts the exponentially rising phase to the diastolic depolarization,[39,41,42] thereby initiating the subsequent action potential (see Fig. 23-1B). A failure to generate diastolic I_{NCX} signals leads to failure to generate an exponentially rising late diastolic depolarization phase, resulting in pacemaker failure, even when Ca^{2+} influx via I_{CaL} is normal (e.g., when ryanodine receptors are disabled by ryanodine [see Fig. 23-1D] or during short-term Na^{+}-Ca^{2+} exchanger blockade[39]) or enhanced (e.g., in ischemic-like conditions[44]).

Morphologic Evidence for Tight Functional Integration of Components of Calcium and Membrane Clocks

The morphologic background for this functional crosstalk between the calcium clock and the Na^{+}-Ca^{2+} exchanger has been demonstrated in rabbit SA node pacemaker cells (Fig. 23-2).[45] The average relative whole-cell immunolabeling density of ryanodine receptors and SERCA2 is similar in SA node pacemaker cells, in atrial and ventricle myocytes, and among SA node pacemaker cells of all sizes. Labeling of Na^{+}-Ca^{2+} exchanger 1 (NCX1) is also similar among rabbit SA node pacemaker cells of all sizes and exceeds that in atrial and ventricular myocytes. Relative submembrane colocalization of NCX1 and cardiac ryanodine receptor in all SA node pacemaker cells exceeds that in the other cell types.[45] Furthermore, the connexin43 negative primary pacemaker area of the intact rabbit SA node exhibits robust immunolabeling for cardiac ryanodine receptor, NCX1, and SERCA2.[45] Thus, there is a dense association of SERCA2, ryanodine receptors, and NCX1 in small SA node pacemaker cells, thought to reside within the SA node center, the site of SA node impulse initiation.

Factors That Govern the Calcium Clock's Ticking Speed and Payload: Calcium and Protein Kinase A–Dependent Protein Phosphorylation

The delay between the onset of the prior action potential–triggered global Ca^{2+} transient and the subsequent occurrence

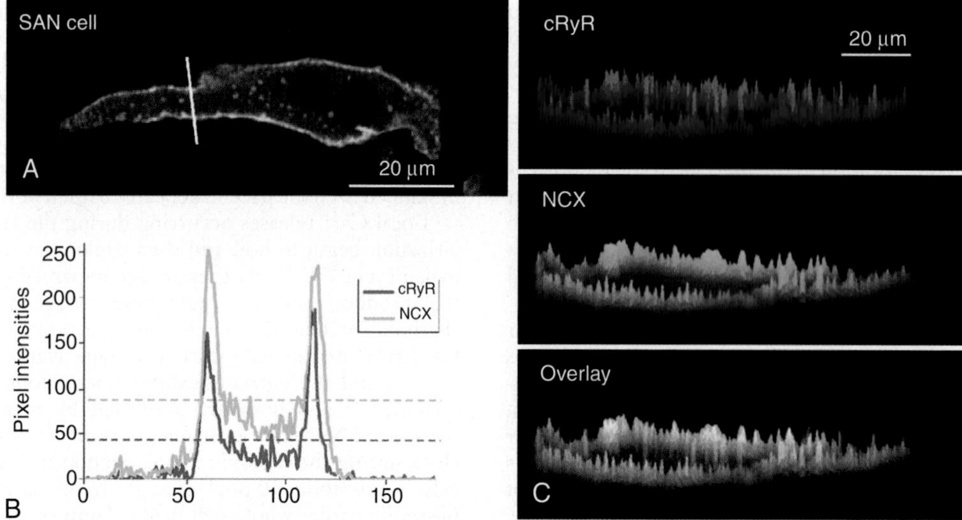

Figure 23-2 Morphologic integration of Ca^{2+} cycling proteins with cell surface membrane proteins. **A,** Confocal whole-cell image of cells doubly immunolabeled for Na^{+}-Ca^{2+} exchanger and ryanodine receptor. **B,** Graphed pixel-by-pixel fluorescence intensities of labeling along an arbitrary line, positioned as indicated by the *thick white line* in A. The *horizontal dashed lines* indicate the average pixel intensity. **C,** Topographical profiles of the pixel intensity levels of each antibody labeling and overlay of the small sinoatrial node pacemaker cells. The maximum height represents the brightest possible pixel in the source image (using an 8-bit image intensity scale). Less-bright pixels are accordingly scaled to a smaller height. cRyR, cardiac ryanodine receptor; NCX, Na^{+}-Ca^{2+} exchanger; SAN, sinoatrial node. (From Lyashkov AE, Juhaszova M, Dobrzynski H, et al: Calcium cycling protein density and functional importance to automaticity of isolated sinoatrial nodal cells are independent of cell size. Circ Res 100:1723-1731, 2007.)

of local Ca^{2+} releases during the late diastolic depolarization—shortly before the subsequent action potential—is the local Ca^{2+} release period (see Fig. 23-1C) and reflects the speed at which the rhythmic calcium clock within cardiac cells is ticking. The likelihood for spontaneous SR Ca^{2+} release to occur increases as a function of the SR Ca^{2+} load, determined, in a physiologic context, by the Ca^{2+} available for pumping and the phosphorylation status of the SR Ca^{2+} cycling proteins.[7] Thus, the convergence of multiple factors governs the local Ca^{2+} release period, including the rate at which Ca^{2+} is pumped into the SR, the threshold SR Ca^{2+} load required to initiate spontaneous Ca^{2+} release, and the availability of SR calcium-release channels, namely, ryanodine receptors. The rate of Ca^{2+} refilling of the SR, which increases the SR free [Ca^{2+}], determines the time to achieve a threshold Ca^{2+} level for the spontaneous Ca^{2+} release to occur (Fig. 23-3A).

Basal diastolic cytosolic Ca^{2+} levels in rabbit SA node pacemaker cells are low (~150 nM), and they do not differ from those of rabbit ventricular cells. However, the basal state SR calcium clock within SA node pacemaker cells restitutes and generates local Ca^{2+} releases with a period less than 0.5 seconds, which is substantially less than in ventricular myocytes under basal conditions (~10 sec). One discovery provides the clue as to why the SR calcium clock ticks so rapidly in SA node pacemaker cells and why local Ca^{2+} releases are larger than Ca^{2+} sparks of ventricular myocytes: Basal state levels of cAMP and cAMP-dependent phosphorylation within SA node pacemaker cells are high, even in the absence of β-adrenergic receptor stimulation.[20]

High basal cAMP levels within SA node pacemaker cells are high due to high constitutive adenylyl cyclase activity (see Fig. 23-3C).[20] Ca^{2+}-activated adenylyl cyclase isoforms, highly expressed in the brain, are expressed in rabbit[46] and guinea pig[47] SA node pacemaker cells. Interestingly, basal phosphodiesterase activity also appears to be markedly elevated in SA node pacemaker cells,[48] serving as a brake to keep basal cAMP levels in check. High levels of constitutive A cyclase and phosphodiesterase (PDE) activity enable the SA node pacemaker cells to rapidly respond to demands for a change in the cAMP level and cycle length.

Basal-state PKA-dependent protein phosphorylation is obligatory for basal occurrence of local Ca^{2+} releases, and gradations in basal PKA-dependent phosphorylation result in gradations in the local Ca^{2+} release period and signal mass.[20] Stimulation of β-adrenergic receptors extends the range of PKA dependence of local Ca^{2+} release periods. The PKA dependence of the local Ca^{2+} release period and signal mass is attributable to at least three (and probably several more) potential mechanisms: augmentation of Ca^{2+} influx via phosphorylation of L-type calcium channels, augmentation of Ca^{2+} pumping into the SR via phospholamban phosphorylation, and increased availability of ryanodine receptors via their phosphorylation. In spontaneously beating SA node pacemaker cells, inhibition or activation of PKA results in gradations in phospholamban phosphorylation, paralleled by gradations in local Ca^{2+} release period[20]; but graded phosphorylation of L-type channels and ryanodine receptors also likely occurs in such experiments. The dependence of L-type calcium channel period on PKA inhibition or the addition of cAMP to skinned SA node pacemaker cells or during voltage clamp[20] demonstrates the role of PKA-dependent mechanisms distinct from those of L-type calcium channels. However, there have been no experiments to date that separate the roles of Ca^{2+} pumping from ryanodine receptor availability in the generation of spontaneous local Ca^{2+} releases.

PKA-dependent phosphorylation of SR cycling proteins and L-type calcium channels leads to synchronization of ryanodine receptor firing. Phosphorylated ryanodine receptors exhibit not only increased open probability[49] but also more synchronized activation than in the nonphosphorylated state.[50] Concomitant phosphorylation of phospholamban permits more rapid achievement of the SR Ca^{2+} load presented to ryanodine receptors. Phosphorylated L-type calcium channels provide more Ca^{2+} influx and thereby permit more Ca^{2+} to be pumped (at a faster

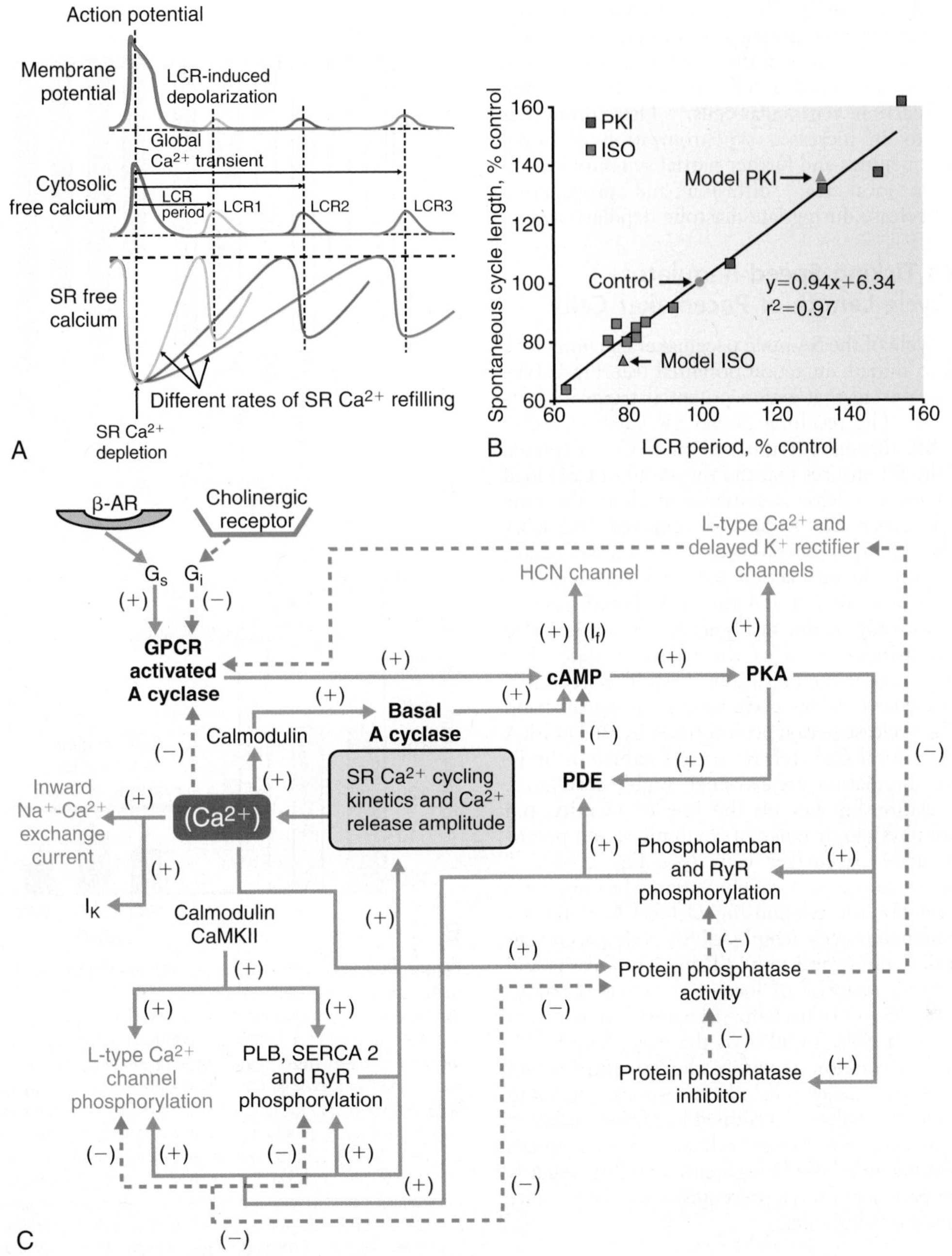

Figure 23-3 Control of SA node pacemaker cells function. **A,** Schematic illustration of the idea that the rate of SR Ca^{2+} refilling controls the local Ca^{2+} release period and the timing of the local Ca^{2+} release–induced depolarization. **B,** The relative effects of protein kinase A inhibitor (PKI) and isoproterenol (ISO) to alter cycle length over a wide range are linked to their effects on the local Ca^{2+} release period within the same cells. Squares and solid line depict the experimentally obtained data; triangles depict data simulated by a numerical SA node pacemaker cell model using experimentally measured changes in local Ca^{2+} release characteristics and phase. (Modified from Vinogradova TM, Lyashkov AE, Zhu W, et al: High basal protein kinase A–dependent phosphorylation drives rhythmic internal Ca^{2+} store oscillations and spontaneous beating of cardiac pacemaker cells. Circ Res 98:505-514, 2006.) **C,** Schematic illustration of the interplay of basal Ca^{2+}-activated adenylyl cyclase (A Cyclase [AC]), cyclic adenosine monophosphate (cAMP), and phosphodiesterase (PDE) cast in the context of sarcoplasmic reticulum Ca^{2+} cycling, L-type calcium channels and Na^+-Ca^{2+} exchanger activation and other membrane ion channels that generate spontaneous SA node pacemaker cells action potential (see text for details). The Ca^{2+}-cAMP interaction results in a feed-forward fail-safe system: cAMP and cAMP-PKA (protein kinase A)-dependent phosphorylation of Ca^{2+} cycling proteins (phospholamban, ryanodine receptors, L-type calcium channels, and crosstalk of these) generates local, spontaneous submembrane Ca^{2+} releases and increases global cytoplasmic Ca^{2+} transients triggered by action potentials. Increased Ca^{2+} activates ACs that further increase cAMP. The dual basal Ca^{2+} and cAMP-PKA feed-forward regulation is kept in check by a high basal PDE activity, which prevents cAMP-PKA signaling to become excessive (i.e., acts as a negative-feedback mechanism to prevent an excessive basal beating rate and to ensure reserve cAMP-PKA modulation of spontaneous beating via activation of β-adrenergic receptors (β-AR). Phosphatase activity likely constitutes an additional intrinsic brake on PKA signaling in SA node pacemaker cells, but this has not yet been measured. Note that since the cAMP increase induced by β-AR stimulation is not reduced by Ca^{2+} chelation, the ACs that couple to β-ARs (and associated PDEs) are depicted in the schema in a separate location from the basal Ca^{2+}-activated ACs. The properties of membrane ion channels, in addition to the Na^+-Ca^{2+} exchanger, are modulated by local [Ca^{2+}] and cAMP or cAMP-mediated, PKA-dependent phosphorylation. ISO, isoproterenol; LCR, local subsarcolemmal Ca^{2+} release; PKI, protein kinase inhibitor; PLB, phospholamban; SA, sinoatrial; SERCA, sarcoplasmic/endoplasmic reticulum calcium adenosine triphosphatase; SR, sarcoplasmic reticulum; RyR, ryanodine receptor.

rate and subsequently released!). The result of enhanced functional status of SR Ca^{2+} cycling proteins of SA node pacemaker cells and L-type calcium channels in the basal state is that local Ca^{2+} releases in SA node pacemaker cells are more frequent and broader than Ca^{2+} sparks in ventricular cells.[39] These properties can be attributed to an increased synchronization of initial ryanodine receptor openings and further partial synchronization of the releases via local Ca^{2+} diffusion and propagating Ca^{2+}-induced Ca^{2+} release during late diastolic depolarization.

Calcium Clock's Ticking Speed Regulates Spontaneous Cycle Length of Pacemaker Cells

Each spontaneous cycle of the SA node pacemaker calcium clock can be envisioned to initiate an action potential (see Fig. 23-1). Ca^{2+} influx via I_{CaL} during that action potential triggers Ca^{2+}-induced Ca^{2+} release. The resulting global SR Ca^{2+} depletion synchronizes the SR throughout the cell in a Ca^{2+}-depleted state. Refilling of the SR ensures that the threshold of Ca^{2+} load required for spontaneous release is achieved at about the time when ryanodine receptor inactivation is removed following prior activation; then the spontaneous local Ca^{2+} releases occur, activating I_{NCX} to ignite the next action potential, and so on.

The local Ca^{2+} release period and the cycle length remain strongly coupled, not only in the steady-state beating but also during stringent transitions, such as the transient state after removal of voltage clamp at the maximum diastolic potential.[40] Further, the relative change in the cycle length among cells and the relative local Ca^{2+} release period prolongation by PKI (a PKA inhibitor), or relative local Ca^{2+} release period reduction by β-adrenergic receptor stimulation, are extremely highly correlated, (r^2 = 0.97); this relationship lies on the line of identity and embraces the entire physiologic range of rhythmic action potential firing of SA node pacemaker cells (see Fig. 23-3B).[20] Regardless of the conditions and widely varying beating rates from about 1.2 to 4 Hz, the relationship of local Ca^{2+}-release periods to the spontaneous cycle lengths of SA node pacemaker cells is nearly identical and is near unity (Table 1 in Lakatta and coworkers[51]): The vast majority of local Ca^{2+} releases always appear synchronously 65 to 110 ms before the next action potential upstroke, that is, at 80% to 90% of the cycle length.[40,41] Interestingly, this time window is within the 1:1 entrainment zone in the SA node pacemaker cells' phase response curves to external rhythmic electric pulses determined in earlier studies.[52] The persistent occurrence of local Ca^{2+} release and I_{NCX} signals within this time window of relatively high entrainability, regardless of the absolute cycle length, is a prerequisite for their ability to regulate spontaneous firing rate.

Interfering with the Calcium Clock or Critical Components of the Membrane Clock Prevents Normal Automaticity and Rate Regulation

Fig. 23-4A summarizes experimental data clearly showing critical importance of both Ca^{2+} and membrane clocks for normal automaticity of SA node pacemaker cells. Interfering with the calcium clock by buffering intracellular Ca^{2+}, disabling ryanodine receptors, blocking I_{NCX}, or slowing the SR calcium clock ticking speed by inhibiting SR Ca^{2+} pump,[32] adenylyl cyclase, or basal PKA activity has marked effects to slow or to halt rhythmic action potentials. Increasing PKA signaling via stimulation of β-adrenergic receptors, exposure to a membrane- permeable analogue of cAMP, or inhibition of phosphodiesterase activity accelerates the action potential firing rate (see Fig. 23-4B). These maneuvers that increase PKA signaling require an intact calcium clock to effect an increase in the spontaneous action potential firing rate (see Fig. 23-4B).

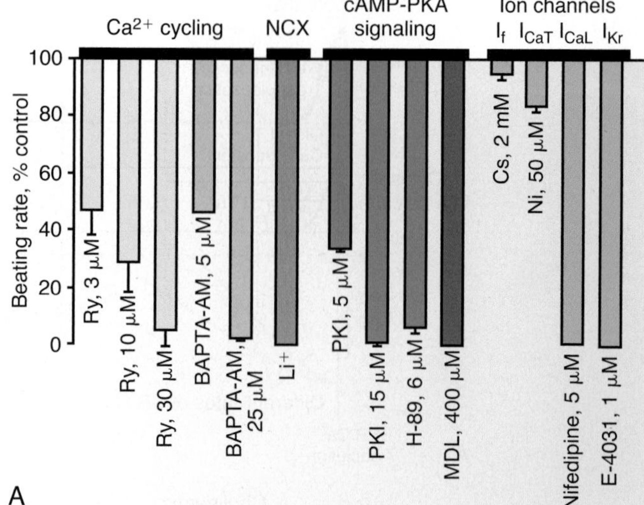

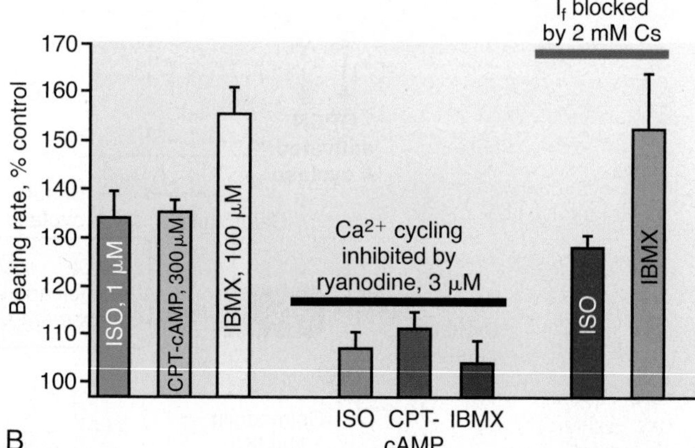

Figure 23-4 Spontaneous beating and rate regulation of rabbit SA node pacemaker cells critically depends upon Ca^{2+}-related mechanisms, protein phosphorylation, and major components of the membrane clock. Each bar shows a change in the beating rate (percentage of control) induced by different drugs that affect different components of the SA node pacemaker system. **A,** Ryanodine receptors (ryanodine, Ry), cytosolic Ca^{2+} (BAPTA), Na^+-Ca^{2+} exchanger (Li^+ substitution for Na^+), protein phosphorylation (PKI, H-89, MDL), or ion channels: I_f (Cs^+), I_{CaT} (Ni^{2+}), I_{CaL} (nifedipine), I_{Kr} (E-4031). IBMX is a phosphodiesterase inhibitor, PKI and H-89 are PKA inhibitors, and MDL is an adenylyl cyclase inhibitor. (Modified from Lakatta EG, Vinogradova T, Lyashkov A, et al: The integration of spontaneous intracellular Ca^{2+} cycling and surface membrane ion channel activation entrains normal automaticity in cells of the heart's pacemaker. Ann N Y Acad Sci 1080:178-206, 2006.) **B,** Chronotropic effects of isoproterenol (ISO), a membrane-permeable cAMP (CPT-cAMP), and IBMX require intact Ca^{2+} cycling (ryanodine, 3 μM), but not I_f (2 mM Cs^+). (Data from Vinogradova TM, Lyashkov AE, Zhu W, et al: High basal protein kinase A–dependent phosphorylation drives rhythmic internal Ca^{2+} store oscillations and spontaneous beating of cardiac pacemaker cells. Circ Res 98:505-514, 2006; Vinogradova TM, Sirenko S, Lyashkov AE, et al: Constitutive phosphodiesterase activity restricts spontaneous beating rate of cardiac pacemaker cells by suppressing local Ca^{2+} releases. Circ Res 102:761-769, 2008.) BAPTA, 1,2-bis[2-aminophenoxy]ethane-*N,N,N,N*-tetraacetic acid; cAMP, cyclic adenosine monophosphate; CPT, chlorophenylthio; IBMX, isobutylmethylxanthine; I_f, hyperpolarization-activated funny current; I_{CaL}, L-type calcium current; I_{CaT}, T-type calcium current; I_{Kr}, rapid potassium current; ISO, isoproterenol; MDL, adenylate cyclase inhibitor; NCX, Na^+-Ca^{2+} exchanger; PKA, protein kinase A; PKI, protein kinase A inhibitor; SA, sinoatrial.

Because I_{CaL} and I_K are the major contributors to the action potential, their blockade, as expected, abrogates spontaneous action potential firing. Inhibition of I_f or I_{CaT}, in contrast, has only minor effects to slow the action potential firing rate, suggesting that these are not critical components of either the membrane clock or of the entire pacemaker mechanism of coupled oscillators (Ca^{2+} and membrane clocks). Whereas in humans a mutation of *HCN4* close to the cAMP-binding site substantially reduces I_f (by shifting its voltage-dependence of activation), it does not preclude a specific phenotype beyond a modest reduction of basal heart rate.[53] Maneuvers that enhance cAMP and PKA signaling do not require I_f, because they remain effective to accelerate action potential firing rate in the presence of I_f blockade (see Fig. 23-4B).[15,45,54] The dependence of the β-adrenergic receptor chronotropic effect on Ca^{2+} cycling pertains not only to isolated SA node pacemaker cells but also to intact cells in dogs.[20] More recent studies in genetically manipulated mice[55,56] have also been interpreted to indicate that I_f is not required for robust chronotropic response to perturbations that increase cAMP. However, depolarization reserve conferred by I_f[55] might explain the requirement of I_f for normal embryonic development of the SA node.[57] An abnormal SA node development may be related to the reduced beating rate associated with I_f knockout at the onset of embryogenesis.[58]

Integration of Intracellular and Membrane Processes Manifested by Natural Pacemaker Cells Is Required for Robust Function of Engineered Biologic Pacemakers

There has been explosive interest in embryonic spontaneously active cardiac myocytes (and stem cell–derived cardiomyocytes) with respect to engineering cardiac tissue, particularly regarding the idea of creating a *simple* biologic pacemaker for clinical use: a cellular oscillator with manipulated or adjusted membrane clock components such as I_{K1} and I_f.[59]

However, experimental studies clearly show that function of these cells, including automaticity, greatly depends on cell Ca^{2+} cycling. Ca^{2+} cycling proteins (RyR2 and SERCA2a) are expressed very early in cardiomyocyte development, and SR Ca^{2+} cycling is crucially important in the developmental regulation of Ca^{2+} transients and contraction in developing cardiomyocytes.[60] I_{CaL} is present in the stem cell–derived cardiomyocytes when they first beat, and its density dramatically (~3 times) increases during further differentiation.[61] Ryanodine receptors and L-type calcium channels establish tight functional coupling in stem cell–derived cardiomyocytes, which is characterized by gradual I_{CaL}-triggered Ca^{2+}-induced Ca^{2+} release.[62] Ca^{2+}-induced Ca^{2+} release serves to couple excitation to contraction in adult cardiac cells, but a novel function of Ca^{2+}-induced Ca^{2+} release in developing cardiomyocytes (as in adult SA node pacemaker cells) is to support cell automaticity by synchronization of local SR Ca^{2+} oscillators, resulting in powerful and rhythmic ignition of action potentials via Na^+-Ca^{2+} exchanger current.[63]

Knocking out *RyR2* in mice results in death of the embryos,[64] the cause of which was interpreted to be perturbed Ca^{2+} homeostasis. A specific explanation of this lethality is gleaned from studies of cardiomyocytes derived from mouse embryonic stem cells. *RyR2* knockout causes a failure of spontaneous Ca^{2+} release in embryonic cardiac cells and suppresses spontaneous cell beating,[65] and it also leads to a marked depression of the obligatory developmental increase in heart rate and cardiac output that support continued cardiac embryonic differentiation.[65] As in adult SA node pacemaker cells, a crucial regulatory role of *RyR2*-mediated Ca^{2+} releases in pacemaker function is demonstrated in *RyR2* knockout cells, because β-adrenergic receptor stimulation is ineffective in these cells.[60] In addition to the ryanodine receptor, another type of Ca^{2+} release channel activated by inositol 1,4,5-trisphosphate (IP3) has been also found to be critically important for spontaneous initiation of Ca^{2+} release in the embryonic and stem cell–derived cardiomyocytes.[66-68] One study[67] suggested that IP3 initiates the release, and ryanodine receptors amplify the IP3 signaling.

A relatively higher functional density of I_{NCX} has been reported in early embryonic cardiomyocytes.[69] The vital importance of Na^+-Ca^{2+} exchanger function in embryonic cardiomyocytes is supported by the observation that Na^+-Ca^{2+} exchanger knockout mice produce embryos that die in utero without evidence of the heart ever beating.[70]

These data indicate that the mechanism of automaticity of embryonic cardiac cells is not as simple as previously interpreted: Automaticity is not solely generated by a membrane clock via a reciprocal activation of a few voltage-gated membrane ion currents.[61] Rather automaticity is a complex integration of ryanodine receptor- and IP3-based Ca^{2+} oscillators with the membrane clock via I_{NCX} (similar to adult pacemakers).[66-68] Thus, it is our opinion that serious consideration of Ca^{2+}-cycling is critical for future bioengineering of viable, stable and robust, and responsive cellular pacemakers for clinical applications.

Numeric Validation of the Interpretation of Experimental Evidence That Normal Automaticity Is Generated by Integrated Function of the Intracellular Calcium Clock and Membrane Ion Channel Clock

Numeric Modeling of the Membrane Clock: Limitations and Previous Attempts of Integration with Intracellular Processes

One review[2] lists no fewer than 12 different, but essentially surface membrane–delimited SA node pacemaker cell models that have been published since 1980. Despite an apparent triumph of the application of the Hodgkin-Huxley formalism to describe the shape of action potential and diastolic depolarization of SA node pacemaker cells, these different numerical models react differently to the perturbations (e.g., ion channel blockade), and a unique, definitive formulation has not been found.

Both fundamental and technical limitations of the membrane-delimited approach were recognized long ago.[8] When formulations for ion transporters and intracellular Ca^{2+} release from SR were ultimately included into SA node pacemaker cell models, these models better approximated cell ion homeostasis. However, because of the absence of Ca^{2+} measurement in SA node pacemaker cells at the time, Ca^{2+} release formulations in these models were adopted from models of atrial or ventricular myocytes. Although formulations of such models closely predict a Ca^{2+} transient initiated by the action potential,[31] this Ca^{2+} transient has almost no contribution to the diastolic depolarization. This led Zhang and colleagues[71] to conclude that "inclusion of intracellular Na^+ and Ca^{2+} handling in the models is not essential," and they excluded Ca^{2+}-release formulations from their model, in which ion concentrations were ascribed constant values as they had been in the earliest pacemaker models of the 1960s.[12]

When it became evident that local Ca^{2+} gradients,[38,39] rather than the bulk cytosolic Ca^{2+} transient, are important for the pacemaker cell membrane function, a more recent Kurata and colleagues model[72] described [Ca^{2+}] changes specifically in the submembrane space. But simulations of Ca^{2+} dynamics by this model showed that while bulk cytosol Ca^{2+} transient decay continues for some time during the early diastolic depolarization, the Ca^{2+} transient in the submembrane space ends sharply at the maximum diastolic potential (see Fig. 5 in Kurata et al[72]). Because it is the submembrane Ca^{2+} that interacts with surface membrane proteins (including the Na^{+}-Ca^{2+} exchanger) to affect diastolic depolarization, this model predicts no contribution of the action potential–induced Ca^{2+} transient to any part of the diastolic depolarization that follows the maximum diastolic potential. This also indicates that measurements of submembrane Ca^{2+} dynamics are critical for instructive modeling of pacemaker activity.

Confocal Ca^{2+} imaging has documented the occurrence of abundant submembrane local Ca^{2+} releases during the late diastolic depolarization.[38,39] Simulated action potentials can be easily entrained to fire with the frequency of the diastolic local Ca^{2+} releases, when the experimental local Ca^{2+}-release waveforms[73] or their sinusoidal approximations[20,41] are included in the models. Furthermore, when local Ca^{2+}-release characteristics change, as PKA signaling is graded, the model closely predicts the beating rate change observed experimentally (see Fig. 23-3B).[20] Still, these initial models were somewhat naive because they lacked terms to account for calcium clocks that generate spontaneous, timely local Ca^{2+} releases.

Novel Theoretical Modeling of the Calcium Clock and Its Interactions with the Membrane Clock

A unique, novel numerical model of rabbit primary SA node pacemaker cells[74] simulates the SR function to pump Ca^{2+} and to effect rhythmic spontaneous Ca^{2+} releases via ryanodine receptors. The model predicts that in the absence of membrane clock function, SR can operate as a self-sustained Ca^{2+} oscillator ("free running" SR clock). The rate and amplitude of the oscillations are controlled by the SR Ca^{2+} pumping rate, the amount of free Ca^{2+} in the system, and the kinetics and the amount of ryanodine receptors. The Ca^{2+} oscillator is extremely flexible: It operates over a wide range of frequencies (1.25-8.9 Hz) that extends over the entire range of heart rates.

When the surface membrane in the model is operative, it intimately interacts with the Ca^{2+} lock. The spontaneous diastolic Ca^{2+} releases of the calcium clock remain periodic and bring the membrane to its excitation threshold to generate rhythmic action potentials via activation of I_{NCX}. The coupling of these two heterogeneous systems—the Ca^{2+} and surface membrane clocks—is the essence of the pacemaker mechanism in this new model. Although the calcium clock pumps and spontaneously releases Ca,$^{2+}$ providing rhythmic ignition signals for the membrane clock, the membrane clock modulates the rate, rhythm, and amplitude of Ca^{2+} releases via its multiple interactions with the calcium clock: the tight L-type calcium channel–ryanodine receptor crosstalk in submembrane space via Ca^{2+}-induced Ca^{2+} release; refueling or rewinding the calcium clock of the model, which is achieved during the action potential, as Ca^{2+} influx of I_{CaL} is pumped into SR (SR refueling); Na^{+}-Ca^{2+} exchanger–assisted Ca^{2+} removal from the submembrane space after global Ca^{2+} transient prepares the subspace for the next spontaneous release cycle.

The spontaneous cycle length of the coupled Ca^{2+} and membrane clocks in the model simulation comprises the sum of the action potential duration, the time needed to refill the SR with Ca,$^{2+}$ and the time needed for the action potential ignition. Concomitant changes in the cycle length of SA node pacemaker cells and in the period and signal mass of local Ca^{2+} releases that have been observed experimentally in response to graded PKA activity[20] are closely predicted by the model. The model also predicts that the speed of the SA node pacemaker calcium clock can be graded by the degree of phosphorylation of Ca^{2+} cycling proteins, including phospholamban modulation of the SR Ca^{2+} pumping rate, to produce gradations in the action potential firing rate to match the chronotropic demand for a given condition. This new rate-regulation mechanism is fundamentally different from that of classical models, which attribute the rate change mainly to voltage-dependent shift in I_f activation that leads to the early diastolic depolarization slope change (e.g., see Fig. 9A in Demir et al[75]). In contrast to the classic models, this new model predicts the major rate regulation via late diastolic depolarization acceleration, as shown experimentally.[42]

An Additional Level of Complexity of Cardiac Pacemaker Function Arises within the Sinoatrial Nodal Tissue

Although our focus has mainly been on mechanisms of spontaneous activity of individual pacemaker cells, it would be an oversimplification to limit consideration of cardiac pacemaker function only to the intrinsic properties of these cells. The SA node tissue is a highly heterogeneous structure characterized by complex cell-to-cell interactions and extremely robust impulse generation. It has been well established that in the intact SA node the initiation of electrical activity of each beat originates from the central area, which contains mostly small SA node pacemaker cells,[76,77] and that in the intact SA node the shape of the membrane potential impulses varies between the center and the periphery of the SA node.[78,79] These observations have spawned two hypotheses regarding the structure and function relationships of individual cells within intact SA node tissue: a gradual transition of cell structure and function from the center of the SA node to its periphery (gradient model)[79] or a diffuse population of atrial cells that interacts with SA node pacemaker cells within the SA node tissue (mosaic model).[80,81] Another view embraces both hypotheses: Within the SA node center there is a gradient of pacemaker properties, whereas in the periphery the mosaic model is more plausible.[77]

An interesting proposal regarding the SA node impulse is that it is initiated by a democratic type of synchronous firing of cells within the SA node, with each pacemaker cell contributing to an aggregate signal, and involving mutual entrainment among cells.[82] Mutual phase resetting of neighboring pacemaker cells can still be the underlying mechanism of pacemaker synchronization in either the gradient or mosaic model, because the *late diastolic depolarization acceleration* is the earliest observed event within SA node pacemaker cells in the SA node region where electrical activity first occurs.[79]

A perspective gleaned from measurements in a large number of SA node pacemaker cells in isolation is that substantial random variation occurs about the average of Ca^{2+} cycling protein densities and action potential characteristics (e.g., the standard deviation for the rate of the action potential is about 25% of its average) of smaller and larger cells.[45] Although it is not possible to know whether some local neighborhoods within the SA node have distributions of SA node pacemaker cells that are skewed from the average, it is possible that small SA node pacemaker cells with the shortest cycle lengths are clustered together within the center of the node. If this were the case, SA node pacemaker cells within such a cluster would become mutually entrained by the electrotonic signal derived from the operation of their calcium clocks to generate local releases of Ca^{2+} during the late diastolic depolarization. The resultant synchronization of this cell depolarization resulting from the mutual entrainment then becomes sufficient for that cluster to generate an action potential that is conducted through the node.

Studies have demonstrated the occurrence of robust action potential–induced Ca^{2+} transients and spontaneous late diastolic depolarization local Ca^{2+} releases in small cells thought to reside within the central SA node region. The crucial effects of Ca^{2+} chelation, Na^+-Ca^{2+} exchanger blockade, or ryanodine on the function of SA node pacemaker cells have been also demonstrated in these SA node pacemaker cells.[45] Thus, it is reasonable to infer that the diastolic Ca^{2+} signals that have the proven ability to generate late diastolic depolarization acceleration in individual SA node pacemaker cells are critically important not only for automaticity of isolated SA node pacemaker cells (see earlier) but also for cell interactions that occur to form the leading pacemaker region within the SA node.

The function of SA node pacemaker cells within the intact SA node is determined by intrinsic cell properties, but these intrinsic properties are modulated by factors of the local environment in which SA node pacemaker cells reside. Extrinsic modulators include mechanical and electrotonic forces and the autonomic milieu, which are heterogeneous throughout the SA node. For example, differences in the action potential shape of SA node pacemaker cells within the SA node tissue could be a result of the mutual entrainment between the depolarizing charge, transferred by ion channels of single SA node cells, and structural properties of the surrounding inexcitable tissue that imposes the electrical load on a depolarizing cell. It is possible that small cells with less capacitance, and correspondingly with smaller charges, could be more affected by the surrounding electrical load than big cells.

SA node tissue contains numerous fibroblasts and extensive connective tissue that can occupy as much as 25% to 90% of the SA node.[76] In cardiomyocytes, an increase in the fibroblast density decreases the rate of action potential upstroke and depolarizes resting potential.[83] If this were also true for SA node pacemaker cells, then small SA node pacemaker cells within the SA node center might have a less-negative maximum diastolic potential and a less-steep action potential upstroke, because the SA node primary pacemaker area has the highest connective tissue density.[76] In addition to bands of fibrous tissue, variable densities and types of gap junction proteins within the node also contribute to local variations in intracellular resistances and the formation of local neighborhoods where clusters of SA node pacemaker cells reside.[84] After SA node pacemaker cells are activated, heterogeneous mechanical stress occurs within the node because the myofilament density within SA node pacemaker cells decreases from the peripheral to the central area.[85] The autonomic milieu is heterogeneous throughout the node, with the central area having the greatest density of nerve endings and autonomic receptors on SA node pacemaker cells.

In the final analysis, a requirement for the supremacy of the central SA node area in initiating the SA node impulse is that the mutually entrained rate of its cells,[86] determined by the net balance of intrinsic mechanisms and their modulation by extrinsic factors, exceeds that of other neighborhoods to which the impulse spreads. A phase shift in mutually entrained action potential, generated within an SA node neighborhood, must account for the often-observed shift in the leading pacemaker site after interventions that act differentially among neighborhoods within the SA node to alter intrinsic properties of SA node pacemaker cells such as vagal or sympathetic stimulation.[79]

Summary

Cardiac pacemaker cells possess two oscillators that differ in nature: *chemical* calcium clocks of the SR and *electrical* clocks of the surface membrane ion channels. Flexible, yet robust, cardiac pacemaker cell function emerges from tightly coupled operation of these two oscillators: They each entrain, optimize, and support short-term and long-term operation of the other to generate rhythmic spontaneous Ca^{2+} releases and action potentials over the entire range of physiologic heart rates. These coupled oscillators that differ in nature thus represent heterogeneous redundancy within SA node pacemaker cells, which confers extremely high robustness to their pacemaker function. Yet another level of complexity ensuring even higher level of robustness and flexibility of the heart's pacemaker is the heterogeneous interactive network of cells within the SA node.

The hypothesis of interacting clocks presented here for pacemaker cells can be extended to ventricular cells in which mutual entrainment of membrane and calcium clocks drive rhythmic contractions. Thus, a general theory of heart function emerges from the concept of coupled Ca^{2+} and membrane potential oscillators.[9,87] The heart rate and the strength of each heart beat are regulated by coupled oscillators composed of the same components. In SA node pacemaker cells, sequential operation of calcium clock components excites the membrane clock via these molecules (SERCA → ryanodine receptor → Na^+-Ca^{2+} exchanger → L-type calcium channel) to initiate the cardiac impulse. In ventricular cells, the membrane clock activates the calcium clock via these molecules (L-type calcium channel → ryanodine receptor → SERCA and Na^+-Ca^{2+} exchanger) to produce a global cytosolic Ca^{2+} transient that drives contraction. This general theory of heart function provides a new conceptual framework to resolve the plethora of unsolved mysteries of normal and pathologic heart function.

References

1. Carlson JM, Doyle J: Complexity and robustness. Proc Natl Acad Sci U S A 99(Suppl 1):2538-2545, 2002.
2. Wilders R: Computer modelling of the sinoatrial node. Med Biol Eng Comput 45: 189-207, 2007.
3. Cranefield PF: Action potentials, afterpotentials, and arrhythmias. Circ Res 41:415-423, 1977.
4. Irisawa H: Comparative physiology of the cardiac pacemaker mechanism. Physiol Rev 58:461-498, 1978.
5. Tsien RW, Kass RS, Weingart R: Cellular and subcellular mechanisms of cardiac pacemaker oscillations. J Exp Biol 81:205-215, 1979.
6. Kass RS, Tsien RW: Fluctuations in membrane current driven by intracellular calcium in cardiac Purkinje fibers. Biophys J 38: 259-269, 1982.
7. Lakatta EG: Functional implications of spontaneous sarcoplasmic reticulum Ca^{2+} release in the heart. Cardiovasc Res 26: 193-214, 1992.
8. Noble D: The surprising heart: A review of recent progress in cardiac electrophysiology. J Physiol 353:1-50, 1984.
9. Maltsev VA, Vinogradova TM, Lakatta EG: The emergence of a general theory of the initiation and strength of the heartbeat. J Pharmacol Sci 100:338-369, 2006.
10. Bozler E: The initiation of impulses in cardiac muscle. Am J Physiol 138:273-282, 1943.
11. Bozler E: Tonus changes in cardiac muscle and their significance for the initiation of impulses. Am J Physiol 139:477-480, 1943.
12. Noble D: A modification of the Hodgkin-Huxley equations applicable to Purkinje fibre action and pace-maker potentials. J Physiol 160:317-352, 1962.
13. Maylie J, Morad M, Weiss J: A study of pace-maker potential in rabbit sino-atrial node: Measurement of potassium activity under voltage-clamp conditions. J Physiol 311:161-178, 1981.

14. DiFrancesco D: The contribution of the "pacemaker" current (I_f) to generation of spontaneous activity in rabbit sino-atrial node myocytes. J Physiol 434:23-40, 1991.
15. Noma A, Morad M, Irisawa H: Does the "pacemaker current" generate the diastolic depolarization in the rabbit SA node cells? Pflugers Arch 397:190-194, 1983.
16. Yanagihara K, Noma A, Irisawa H: Reconstruction of sino-atrial node pacemaker potential based on the voltage clamp experiments. Jpn J Physiol 30:841-857, 1980.
17. Mangoni ME, Fontanaud P, Noble PJ, et al: Facilitation of the L-type calcium current in rabbit sino-atrial cells: Effect on cardiac automaticity. Cardiovasc Res 48:375-392, 2000.
18. Vinogradova TM, Zhou YY, Bogdanov KY, et al: Sinoatrial node pacemaker activity requires Ca^{2+}/calmodulin-dependent protein kinase II activation. Circ Res 87:760-767, 2000.
19. Petit-Jacques J, Bois P, Bescond J, Lenfant J: Mechanism of muscarinic control of the high-threshold calcium current in rabbit sino-atrial node myocytes. Pflugers Arch 423:21-27, 1993.
20. Vinogradova TM, Lyashkov AE, Zhu W, et al: High basal protein kinase A–dependent phosphorylation drives rhythmic internal Ca^{2+} store oscillations and spontaneous beating of cardiac pacemaker cells. Circ Res 98:505-514, 2006.
21. Mangoni ME, Couette B, Bourinet E, et al: Functional role of L-type Cav1.3 Ca^{2+} channels in cardiac pacemaker activity. Proc Natl Acad Sci U S A 100:5543-5548, 2003.
22. Nilius B: Possible functional significance of a novel type of cardiac Ca^{+} channel. Biomed Biochim Acta 45:K37-K45, 1986.
23. Guo J, Ono K, Noma A: A sustained inward current activated at the diastolic potential range in rabbit sino-atrial node cells. J Physiol 483(Pt 1):1-13, 1995.
24. Verkerk AO, Wilders R, Zegers JG, et al: Ca^{2+}-activated Cl^{-} current in rabbit sino-atrial node cells. J Physiol 540:105-117, 2002.
25. Fabiato A, Fabiato F: Calcium-induced release of calcium from the sarcoplasmic reticulum of skinned cells from adult human, dog, cat, rabbit, rat, and frog hearts and from fetal and new-born rat ventricles. Ann N Y Acad Sci 307:491-522, 1978.
26. Wier WG, Kort AA, Stern MD, et al: Cellular calcium fluctuations in mammalian heart: Direct evidence from noise analysis of aequorin signals in Purkinje fibers. Proc Natl Acad Sci U S A 80:7367-7371, 1983.
27. Lipsius SL, Gibbons WR: Membrane currents, contractions, and aftercontractions in cardiac Purkinje fibers. Am J Physiol 243:H77-H86, 1982.
28. Lakatta EG, Lappe DL: Diastolic scattered light fluctuation, resting force and twitch force in mammalian cardiac muscle. J Physiol 315:369-3941, 1981.
29. Rubenstein DS, Lipsius SL: Mechanisms of automaticity in subsidiary pacemakers from cat right atrium. Circ Res 64:648-657, 1989.
30. Zhou Z, Lipsius SL: Na^{+}-Ca^{2+} exchange current in latent pacemaker cells isolated from cat right atrium. J Physiol 466:263-285, 1993.
31. Li J, Qu J, Nathan RD: Ionic basis of ryanodine's negative chronotropic effect on pacemaker cells isolated from the sinoatrial node. Am J Physiol 273:H2481-H2489, 1997.
32. Sanders L, Rakovic S, Lowe M, et al: Fundamental importance of Na^{+}-Ca^{2+} exchange for the pacemaking mechanism in guinea-pig sino-atrial node. J Physiol 571:639-649, 2006.
33. Hancox JC, Levi AJ, Brooksby P: Intracellular calcium transients recorded with Fura-2 in spontaneously active myocytes isolated from the atrioventricular node of the rabbit heart. Proc Biol Sci 255:99-105, 1994.
34. Rigg L, Heath BM, Cui Y, Terrar DA: Localisation and functional significance of ryanodine receptors during β-adrenoceptor stimulation in the guinea-pig sino-atrial node. Cardiovasc Res 48:254-264, 2000.
35. Musa H, Lei M, Honjo H, et al: Heterogeneous expression of Ca^{2+} handling proteins in rabbit sinoatrial node. J Histochem Cytochem 50:311-324, 2002.
36. Rigg L, Terrar DA: Possible role of calcium release from the sarcoplasmic reticulum in pacemaking in guinea-pig sino-atrial node. Exp Physiol 81:877-880, 1996.
37. Ju YK, Allen DG: How does β-adrenergic stimulation increase the heart rate? The role of intracellular Ca^{2+} release in amphibian pacemaker cells. J Physiol 516 (Pt 3):793-804, 1999.
38. Huser J, Blatter LA, Lipsius SL: Intracellular Ca^{2+} release contributes to automaticity in cat atrial pacemaker cells. J Physiol 524 Pt 2:415-422, 2000.
39. Bogdanov KY, Vinogradova TM, Lakatta EG: Sinoatrial nodal cell ryanodine receptor and Na^{+}-Ca^{2+} exchanger: Molecular partners in pacemaker regulation. Circ Res 88:1254-1258, 2001.
40. Vinogradova TM, Zhou YY, Maltsev V, et al: Rhythmic ryanodine receptor Ca^{2+} releases during diastolic depolarization of sinoatrial pacemaker cells do not require membrane depolarization. Circ Res 94:802-809, 2004.
41. Maltsev VA, Vinogradova TM, Bogdanov KY, et al: Diastolic calcium release controls the beating rate of rabbit sinoatrial node cells: Numerical modeling of the coupling process. Biophys J 86:2596-2605, 2004.
42. Bogdanov KY, Maltsev VA, Vinogradova TM, et al: Membrane potential fluctuations resulting from submembrane Ca^{2+} releases in rabbit sinoatrial nodal cells impart an exponential phase to the late diastolic depolarization that controls their chronotropic state. Circ Res 99:979-987, 2006.
43. Lakatta EG, Vinogradova T, Lyashkov A, et al: The integration of spontaneous intracellular Ca^{2+} cycling and surface membrane ion channel activation entrains normal automaticity in cells of the heart's pacemaker. Ann N Y Acad Sci 1080:178-206, 2006.
44. Maltsev VA, Lakatta EG: Cardiac pacemaker cell failure with preserved I_f, I_{CaL}, and I_{Kr}: A lesson about pacemaker function learned from ischemia-induced bradycardia. J Mol Cell Cardiol 42:289-294, 2007.
45. Lyashkov AE, Juhaszova M, Dobrzynski H, et al: Calcium cycling protein density and functional importance to automaticity of isolated sinoatrial nodal cells are independent of cell size. Circ Res 100:1723-1731, 2007.
46. Vinogradova TM, Ruknudin AM, Zhu W, et al: High basal cAMP content markedly elevates PKA-dependent protein phosphorylation and sustains spontaneous beating in rabbit sinoatrial nodal pacemaker cells (SANC) [abstract]. Biophys J 90:155a, 2006.
47. Mattick P, Parrington J, Odia E, et al: Ca^{2+}-stimulated adenylyl cyclase isoform AC1 is preferentially expressed in guinea-pig sino-atrial node cells and modulates the I_f pacemaker current. J Physiol 582: 1195-1203, 2007.
48. Vinogradova TM, Sirenko S, Lyashkov AE, et al: Constitutive phosphodiesterase activity restricts spontaneous beating rate of cardiac pacemaker cells by suppressing local Ca^{2+} releases. Circ Res 102:761-769, 2008.
49. Takasago T, Imagawa T, Shigekawa M: Phosphorylation of the cardiac ryanodine receptor by cAMP-dependent protein kinase. J Biochem (Tokyo) 106:872-877, 1989.
50. Song LS, Wang SQ, Xiao RP, et al: β-Adrenergic stimulation synchronizes intracellular Ca^{2+} release during excitation-contraction coupling in cardiac myocytes. Circ Res 88:794-801, 2001.
51. Lakatta EG, Vinogradova TM, Maltsev VA: The missing link in the mystery of normal automaticity of cardiac pacemaker cells. Ann N Y Acad Sci 1123:41-57, 2008.
52. Anumonwo JM, Delmar M, Vinet A, et al: Phase resetting and entrainment of pacemaker activity in single sinus nodal cells. Circ Res 68:1138-1153, 1991.
53. Milanesi R, Baruscotti M, Gnecchi-Ruscone T, DiFrancesco D: Familial sinus bradycardia associated with a mutation in the cardiac pacemaker channel. N Engl J Med 354:151-157, 2006.
54. Vinogradova TM, Bogdanov KY, Lakatta EG: β-Adrenergic stimulation modulates ryanodine receptor Ca^{2+} release during diastolic depolarization to accelerate pacemaker activity in rabbit sinoatrial nodal cells. Circ Res 90:73-79, 2002.
55. Herrmann S, Stieber J, Stockl G, et al: HCN4 provides a "depolarization reserve" and is not required for heart rate acceleration in mice. Embo J 26:4423-4432, 2007.
56. Rose RA, Kabir MG, Backx PH: Altered heart rate and sinoatrial node function in mice lacking the cAMP regulator phosphoinositide 3-kinase-γ. Circ Res 101(12):1274-1282, 2007.
57. Mommersteeg MT, Hoogaars WM, Prall OW, et al: Molecular pathway for the localized formation of the sinoatrial node. Circ Res 100:354-362, 2007.
58. Stieber J, Herrmann S, Feil S, et al: The hyperpolarization-activated channel HCN4 is required for the generation of pacemaker action potentials in the embryonic heart. Proc Natl Acad Sci U S A 100:15235-15240, 2003.

59. Miake J, Marban E, Nuss HB: Biological pacemaker created by gene transfer. Nature 419:132-133, 2002.
60. Fu JD, Li J, Tweedie D, et al: Crucial role of the sarcoplasmic reticulum in the developmental regulation of Ca^{2+} transients and contraction in cardiomyocytes derived from embryonic stem cells. FASEB J 20:181-183, 2006.
61. Maltsev VA, Wobus AM, Rohwedel J, et al: Cardiomyocytes differentiated in vitro from embryonic stem cells developmentally express cardiac-specific genes and ionic currents. Circ Res 75:233-244, 1994.
62. Maltsev VA, Sirenko SG, Maltseva LA, Crider DG, Boheler KR, Stern MD, Lakatta EG: Cardiomyocytes differentiated in vitro from mouse embryonic stem cells develop the adult type Ca^{2+}-induced Ca^{2+} release [abstract]. Biophys J 90:2695, 2006.
63. Maltsev VA, Zahanich I, Maltseva LA, et al: L-type Ca^{2+} current synchronizes local intracellular Ca^{2+} oscillators which trigger rhythmic action potentials in developing cardiomyocytes. American Heart Association Meeting. Circulation 116: part II, 186, 2007.
64. Takeshima H, Komazaki S, Hirose K, et al: Embryonic lethality and abnormal cardiac myocytes in mice lacking ryanodine receptor type 2. EMBO J 17:3309-3316, 1998.
65. Yang HT, Tweedie D, Wang S, et al: The ryanodine receptor modulates the spontaneous beating rate of cardiomyocytes during development. Proc Natl Acad Sci U S A 99:9225-9230, 2002.
66. Mery A, Aimond F, Menard C, et al: Initiation of embryonic cardiac pacemaker activity by inositol 1,4,5-trisphosphate–dependent calcium signaling. Mol Biol Cell 16:2414-2423, 2005.
67. Kapur N, Banach K: Inositol-1,4,5-trisphosphate–mediated spontaneous activity in mouse embryonic stem cell–derived cardiomyocytes. J Physiol 581:1113-1127, 2007.
68. Sasse P, Zhang J, Cleemann L, et al: Intracellular Ca^{2+} oscillations, a potential pacemaking mechanism in early embryonic heart cells. J Gen Physiol 130:133-144, 2007.
69. Reppel M, Sasse P, Malan D, et al: Functional expression of the Na^+/Ca^{2+} exchanger in the embryonic mouse heart. J Mol Cell Cardiol 42:121-132, 2007.
70. Koushik SV, Wang J, Rogers R, et al: Targeted inactivation of the sodium-calcium exchanger (NCX1) results in the lack of a heartbeat and abnormal myofibrillar organization. FASEB J 15:1209-1211, 2001.
71. Zhang H, Holden AV, Kodama I, et al: Mathematical models of action potentials in the periphery and center of the rabbit sinoatrial node. Am J Physiol 279: H397-H421, 2000.
72. Kurata Y, Hisatome I, Imanishi S, Shibamoto T: Dynamical description of sinoatrial node pacemaking: Improved mathematical model for primary pacemaker cell. Am J Physiol 283:H2074-H2101, 2002.
73. Lakatta EG, Maltsev VA, Bogdanov KY, et al: Cyclic variation of intracellular calcium: A critical factor for cardiac pacemaker cell dominance. Circ Res 92: e45-e50, 2003.
74. Maltsev VA, Lakatta EG: Synergism of coupled subsarcolemmal Ca^{2+} clocks and sarcolemmal voltage clocks confers robust and flexible pacemaker function in a novel pacemaker cell model. Am J Physiol Heart Circ Physiol 2009, Epub ahead of print.
75. Demir SS, Clark JW, Giles WR: Parasympathetic modulation of sinoatrial node pacemaker activity in rabbit heart: A unifying model. Am J Physiol 276: H2221-H2244, 1999.
76. Opthof T, de Jonge B, Jongsma HJ, Bouman LN: Functional morphology of the mammalian sinuatrial node. Eur Heart J 8:1249-1259, 1987.
77. Dobrzynski H, Li J, Tellez J, et al: Computer three-dimensional reconstruction of the sinoatrial node. Circulation 111:846-854, 2005.
78. Boyett MR, Honjo H, Kodama I: The sinoatrial node, a heterogeneous pacemaker structure. Cardiovasc Res 47:658-687, 2000.
79. Bleeker WK, Mackaay AJ, Masson-Pevet M, et al: Functional and morphological organization of the rabbit sinus node. Circ Res 46:11-22, 1980.
80. Verheijck EE, Wessels A, van Ginneken AC, et al: Distribution of atrial and nodal cells within the rabbit sinoatrial node: Models of sinoatrial transition. Circulation 97:1623-1631, 1998.
81. Boyett MR, Honjo H, Yamamoto M, et al: Downward gradient in action potential duration along conduction path in and around the sinoatrial node. Am J Physiol 276:H686-H698, 1999.
82. Jalife J: Mutual entrainment and electrical coupling as mechanisms for synchronous firing of rabbit sino-atrial pace-maker cells. J Physiol 356:221-243, 1984.
83. Miragoli M, Gaudesius G, Rohr S: Electrotonic modulation of cardiac impulse conduction by myofibroblasts. Circ Res 98:801-810, 2006.
84. James TN: The sinus node. Am J Cardiol 40:965-986, 1977.
85. Masson-Pevet MA, Bleeker WK, Besselsen E, et al: Pacemaker cell types in the rabbit sinus node: A correlative ultrastructural and electrophysiological study. J Mol Cell Cardiol 16:53-63, 1984.
86. Michaels DC, Matyas EP, Jalife J: Mechanisms of sinoatrial pacemaker synchronization: A new hypothesis. Circ Res 61:704-714, 1987.
87. Lakatta EG: Beyond Bowditch: The convergence of cardiac chronotropy and inotropy. Cell Calcium 35:629-642, 2004.

Mechanisms of Atrioventricular Nodal Excitability and Propagation 24

William J. Hucker, Halina Dobrzynski, and Igor R. Efimov

CHAPTER OUTLINE

Zipes refers to the atrioventricular node as both the "soul of the heart" and, paraphrasing Churchill, as a "riddle wrapped in a mystery inside an enigma," which succinctly sums up the central importance of the atrioventricular (AV) junction in cardiac electrophysiology, as well as the incredibly complex heterogeneity that defines its structure and function.[1] Despite a century of investigation since its discovery, many aspects of AV nodal physiology have indeed remained mysterious. Nonetheless, advances in imaging modalities and molecular biology are beginning to decipher the true nature of AV conduction. Specifically, fluorescent imaging of voltage-sensitive dyes, intact structural imaging with new imaging modalities such as optical coherence tomography, molecular imaging with immunohistochemistry, and high-throughput molecular biology techniques have contributed significantly to the field of AV nodal electrophysiology. The combination of these techniques has begun to build a global framework characterizing the structure and function of the AV node, which might finally unravel the mysteries of AV nodal electrophysiology.

Structure and Function of the Atrioventricular Junction

A century of research has occurred since Tawara's discovery of the AV node,[2] and many of Tawara's exquisite initial descriptions have been expanded upon and refined. Morphologically, tissue surrounding the node Tawara described is composed of cell layers with various morphologies as well as fibrous and fatty tissue. The endocardium consists of a layer of normal working myocardium. However below this superficial layer, the normal myocardial cells merge into an envelope of transitional cells surrounding the AV node. The node itself can be divided into different structures based on cell morphology and the morphology of the overall structure. Using the central fibrous body as the demarcation between the His bundle and the AV node as Tawara suggested, the AV nodal portion can be further divided into the lower nodal bundle and the compact AV node.[3]

In the lower nodal bundle, cells are longer and arranged more parallel to each other than in the compact node. In the compact node, cells are small and spindle shaped and have no clear cellular orientation. Extending proximally from the lower nodal bundle toward the coronary sinus is the inferior nodal extension. In rabbits, this is the only inferior nodal extension, but in humans, it is one of two[4] and is referred to as the *rightward inferior nodal extension*. The second inferior nodal extension of humans extends from the compact node toward the coronary sinus and is usually shorter than the rightward extension.[4] The complexity of the AV junction is further enhanced by an extensive heterogeneous nervous network of both parasympathetic and sympathetic neurons surrounding the myocytes of the nodal structures.[5]

Functionally, a different nomenclature has developed based on the marked heterogeneity in the action potential waveform at the AV node.[6,7] Three main types of AV node cell have been described based on action potential morphology: atrionodal, nodal, and nodo-His cells (Fig. 24-1A).[6,7] Nodal cells have a low resting potential, a small amplitude action potential with a slow upstroke, and pacemaker activity. Atrionodal cells are transitional cells in that they have electrophysiologic characteristics midway between those of atrial muscle and nodal cells: The resting potential is higher and the action potential upstroke is larger and faster than in nodal cells. nodo-His cells are also transitional cells in that they have electrophysiologic characteristics midway between those of nodal cells and the cells of the bundle of His. Again, the resting potential of nodo-His cells is higher and the action potential upstroke is larger and faster than in nodal cells.

Relating the functional characterization of cells in the AV junction with specific structures defined morphologically is challenging, and was succinctly stated by Meijler and Janse, who said "we are faced with a paradoxical situation that the most *typical* nodal action potential has not yet been linked to the most *typical* nodal cell."[3] Nevertheless, attempts have been made to correlate the action potential morphology to the morphologic characteristics of a particular cell through the combination of microelectrodes and histology,[8] and it appears that the nodo-His cell matches the lower nodal bundle, nodal cells are predominantly in the compact node, and atrionodal cells are the transitional cells.[8] However, the heterogeneity in the action potential waveform at the AV node is likely to be the result of heterogeneity in ion-channel densities and kinetics. Therefore one method to relate functional properties, such as action-potential morphology, to specific cells within the AV junction is to characterize the expression of ion channels throughout the AV junction.

These studies were supported by the National Institutes of Health, Whitaker Foundation, American Heart Association, Stanley and Lucy Lopata Endowment, British Heart Foundation, and Medtronic Inc.

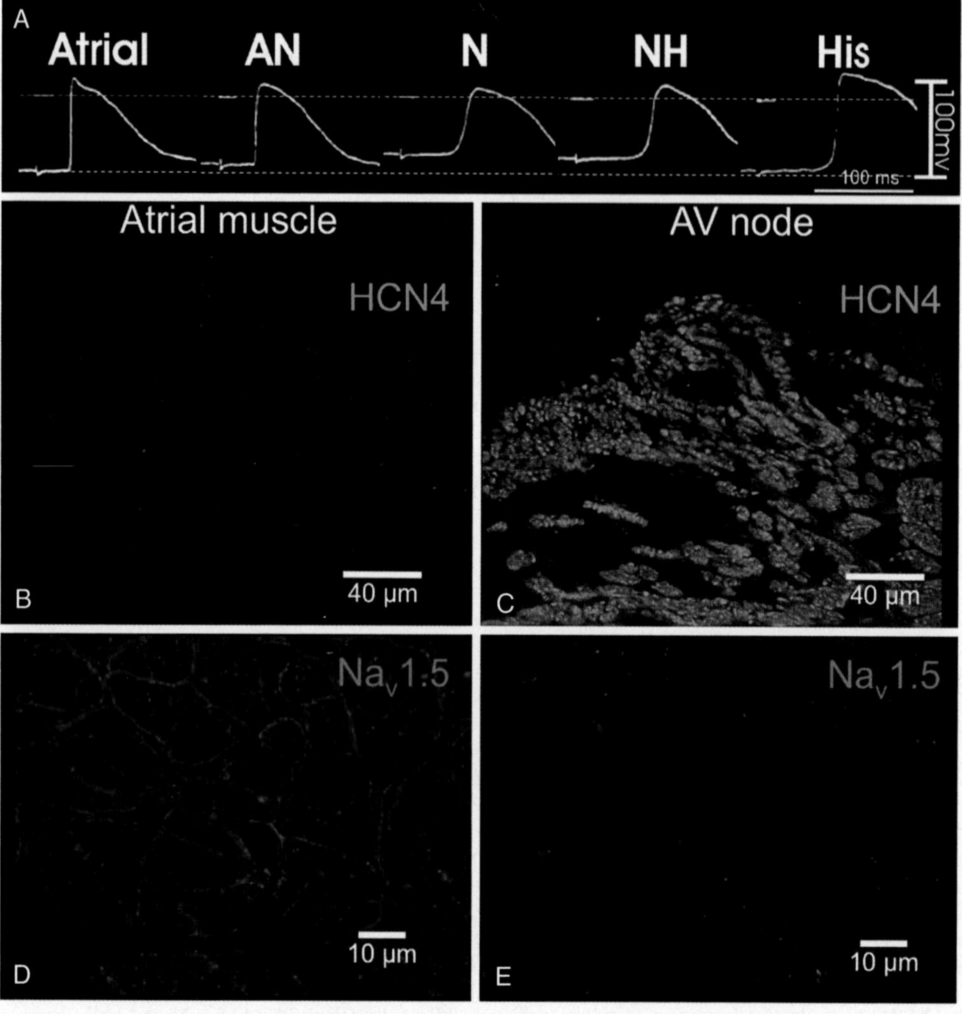

Figure 24-1 Action potentials and immunofluorescence labeling of ion channel proteins in the atrial muscle *(left)* and atrioventricular (AV) node *(right)* in the human. **A,** Action potential recordings from atrial, atrionodal (AN), nodal (N), nodo-His (NH), and His cells at the rabbit AV junction. (From de Carvalho AP, de Almeida DF: Spread of activity through the atrioventricular node. Circ Res 8:801-809, 1960.) **B** and **C,** Hyperpolarization-activated cyclic nucleotide–gated cation channel 4 (HCN4) *(green signal).* HCN4 is expressed at the AV node (primarily within the cell membrane), but it is less expressed in the atrial muscle. **D** and **E,** Voltage-gated sodium channel 1.5 ($Na_V1.5$) *(red signal).* $Na_V1.5$ is expressed in the atrial muscle (primarily within the cell membrane), but it is less expressed at the AV node.

Molecular Heterogeneity in the Atrioventricular Junction

Pacemaker Current and Hyperpolarization-Activated Cyclic Nucleotide–Gated Cation Channels

The AV node is known to be a subsidiary pacemaker. I_f is carried by hyperpolarization-activated cyclic nucleotide–gated cation (HCN) channels and is partly responsible for the diastolic depolarization (pacemaker potential) in pacemaker cells. Pacemaking in the AV node of the rabbit and mouse shows sensitivity to block of I_f by Cs^+ ions.[9,10] I_f has been recorded from cells isolated from the AV node of the rabbit and guinea pig.[11-13] In a study by Hancox and Levi,[11] 10% to 20% of cells isolated from the rabbit AV node possessed I_f. Munk and colleagues[12] discriminated between ovoid and rod-shaped cells isolated from the rabbit AV node; the majority of ovoid cells, presumed to be nodal cells, possessed I_f, whereas the majority of rod-shaped cells, presumed to be atrionodal or nodo-His cells, did not.[12] In the rabbit, both HCN4 messenger RNA (mRNA)[14] and protein[9] are highly expressed in the AV node, with the highest expression in the inferior nodal extension. Expression of HCN4 mRNA and protein at the AV node has also been seen in the human and rat.[15,16] Immunolabeling experiments revealed labeling of HCN4 protein in the human AV node but not in the atrial muscle, as shown in Figure 24-1B-C. In the rabbit, HCN1 mRNA is also highly expressed at the AV node.[14] It is possible, therefore, that the I_f channel may be a heteromultimer of HCN1 and HCN4.

Sodium Current and Voltage-Gated Sodium Channels

I_{Na} is responsible for the fast upstroke of the action potential in the working myocardium. In the rabbit, Munk and coworkers[12] reported I_{Na} to be present in all rod-shaped cells, presumed to be atrionodal or nodo-His cells, but absent from the majority of ovoid cells, presumed to be nodal cells. In cells isolated from the rabbit AV node, Ren and colleagues[17] showed a significant correlation between I_{Na} density and cell size; small cells (with the properties of nodal cells) lacked I_{Na}, and larger cells (with the properties of atrionodal or nodo-His cells) possessed substantial I_{Na}. The sodium channel isoform responsible for I_{Na} in the working myocardium is the cardiac isoform, $Na_V1.5$.

In the human, rabbit, and rat, immunohistochemistry shows $Na_V1.5$ protein to be undetectable or poorly expressed in the compact node (see Fig. 24-1D and E).[15,16] In the AV junction in the rabbit, $Na_V1.5$ mRNA is least abundant in the inferior nodal extension.[14] These data suggest that $Na_V1.5$, and therefore I_{Na}, is absent in the nodal cell, whereas $Na_V1.5$ and I_{Na} may be present in atrionodal and nodo-His cells (but perhaps at a reduced level compared to atrial muscle); this explains the low upstroke velocity of the nodal cell and the higher upstroke velocity of atrionodal and nodo-His cells (see Fig. 24-1A). The heterozygous $Na_V1.5$ knockout mouse shows AV conduction disturbances.[18] Furthermore, in the human, mutations in $Na_V1.5$ are associated with varying degrees of AV block.[19] These disturbances in AV conduction are presumably the result of reduced excitability caused by the loss of functional $Na_V1.5$ in the atrionodal and nodo-His regions.

As well as the cardiac sodium channel isoform, $Na_V1.5$, neuronal sodium channel isoforms have been shown to be expressed in the heart.[20] $Na_V1.1$ mRNA is more highly expressed in the rabbit AV node (as compared to the working myocardium).[14] Mouse AV node also shows higher expression of $Na_V1.1$ and $Na_V1.7$ mRNA.[21] However, in the rat, $Na_V1.1$ protein is expressed in the atrial muscle and inferior nodal extension but not in the compact node.[15] In the rat, $Na_V1.3$ protein is highly expressed in the AV node, but it is expressed by neuronal tissue rather than cardiac myocytes.[15]

Calcium Currents and Calcium Channels

The L-type calcium current, $I_{Ca,L}$, is responsible for the upstroke of the action potential of the nodal cell.[22] The major cardiac L-type calcium channel isoform is $Ca_V1.2$, which is abundant in the working myocardium. However, in the AV node of the rabbit and mouse, there is reduced expression of $Ca_V1.2$ mRNA in the nodal tissue (as compared to the working myocardium).[14,21] Nonetheless, human subjects with Timothy syndrome, which is the result of a mutation in $Ca_V1.2$, display 2:1 AV block.[23] There is evidence of an isoform switch from $Ca_V1.2$ to $Ca_V1.3$, an alternative L-type calcium channel isoform, at the AV node: $Ca_V1.3$ mRNA shows relatively high expression in the AV node of the human, rabbit, and mouse as compared to the working myocardium.[14,16,21,24] $Ca_V1.3$ has a more negative activation threshold than $Ca_V1.2$,[25] and this may be advantageous to a tissue lacking $Na_V1.5$. The importance of $Ca_V1.3$ in AV node conduction has been shown by the $Ca_V1.3$ knockout mouse, in which a prolonged PR interval is seen.[24] In addition, newborn infants with autoimmune antibodies against $Ca_V1.3$ show varying degrees of AV block.[26]

Another calcium current, the T-type calcium current, $I_{Ca,T}$, also plays an important role in the AV node. $I_{Ca,T}$ has been measured in rabbit AV node cells and is proposed to be responsible for certain types of AV block due to concealed conduction.[27] Substantial $I_{Ca,T}$ (comparable in amplitude to $I_{Ca,L}$) has also been recorded in mouse AV node cells. In the mouse, $Ca_V3.1$ appears to be the channel mediating $I_{Ca,T}$ in the AV node, because the $Ca_V3.1$ knockout mouse lacks $I_{Ca,T}$ in nodal cells and shows profound AV node conduction disturbances. High levels of $Ca_V3.1$ mRNA are detected in the mouse AV node.[21]

Transient Outward Potassium Current and Potassium Channels

The transient outward potassium current, I_{to}, is a major cardiac repolarizing current. Mitcheson and Hancox[28] observed I_{to} in AV node cells from the rabbit and Munk and coworkers[12] also reported that rabbit nodal cells contain the I_{to} current in the majority of rod-shaped cells, presumed to be atrionodal or nodo-His cells, but found it to be absent from the majority of ovoid cells, presumed to be nodal cells. Furthermore, even in rod-shaped cells, the density of I_{to} was low as compared to that in atrial cells.[12]

In the rabbit atrium, $K_V1.4$ is the principal I_{to} channel, and $K_V1.4$ mRNA expression is reduced in the AV node of the rabbit as compared to the atrial muscle.[14] $K_V4.2$ and $K_V4.3$ are alternative I_{to} channels; in the rabbit, $K_V4.2$ and $K_V4.3$ mRNAs in the AV node are the same as in the atrial muscle. However in the rabbit, an auxiliary subunit required for K_V4 channel surface expression, K_V channel-interacting protein 2 (KChIP2), is present in the atrial muscle but is absent from the AV node.[14] These results are consistent with the low density or absence of I_{to} at the AV node of the rabbit. I_{to} is also reported to be absent in guinea pig AV node cells.[13] The potassium channel isoform responsible for I_{to} is species dependent, and therefore the pattern of expression of $K_V1.4$, $K_V4.2$, and $K_V4.3$ channels in other species may be different from that in the rabbit.

Delayed Rectifier Potassium Current and $K_V1.5$, ERG, and K_VLQT1 channels

The delayed rectifier potassium currents, $I_{K,ur}$, $I_{K,r}$, and $I_{K,s}$, are also major repolarizing currents in the heart. In addition, in the absence of $I_{K,1}$ (see later), they are important in determining the maximum diastolic potential. In AV node cells from the guinea pig, both $I_{K,r}$ and $I_{K,s}$ have been recorded,[13] whereas in AV node cells from the rabbit, only $I_{K,r}$ has been recorded. $K_V1.5$, ERG, and K_VLQT1 are responsible for $I_{K,ur}$, $I_{K,r}$ and $I_{K,s}$, respectively. In the human, rabbit, and mouse, the expression of $K_V1.5$, ERG, and K_VLQT1 mRNA is equal between the atrial muscle and AV node.[21] However, the relative abundance of the three mRNAs is species dependent: In the rabbit, ERG $\approx$ $K_V1.5$ > K_VLQT1; in the mouse, ERG $\approx$ K_VLQT1 > $K_V1.5$.[14,16,21]

Inward Rectifier Potassium Currents and Potassium Channels

The background inward rectifier current, $I_{K,1}$, is responsible for the resting potential of approximately -80 mV in the working myocardium. In AV node cells from the rabbit, $I_{K,1}$ is absent,[12,29] which facilitates pacemaking. Consistent with this, there is evidence that $K_{ir}2.1$ is not expressed in the AV node of the mouse.[30] The lack of $I_{K,1}$ and $K_{ir}2.1$ in the AV node explains why the nodal cell is more depolarized than atrial muscle (see Fig. 24-1A). Curiously, $I_{K,1}$ is present in guinea pig AV node cells.[13] $K_{ir}6.2$ and SUR2A are the two subunits composing the channel responsible for the ATP-sensitive potassium current, $I_{K,ATP}$. Interestingly, there is reduced expression of $K_{ir}6.2$ and SUR2A mRNAs in the rabbit AV node (as compared to the working myocardium).[14]

Summary

The heterogeneous expression of specific ion channels throughout the AV junction can explain the unique features of the various action potential morphologies recorded in this region. For instance, the lack of I_{Na} and the presence of $I_{Ca,L}$ in the AV node is consistent with the slow upstroke of the nodal cell. The low resting membrane potential of the nodal cell can be explained by the presence of HCN4 and the lack of I_{K1}. Similarly, the action potential morphologies of atrionodal and nodo-His cells are consistent with the presence of I_{Na} and I_{to} in the rod-shaped cells observed by Munk and colleagues.[12] A summary of the ion channel expression and ion currents of the AV node, as well as the working myocardium of the atrium and ventricle, is shown in Figure 24-2. To truly decipher ion channels and ion currents in particular morphologic cell types throughout the AV

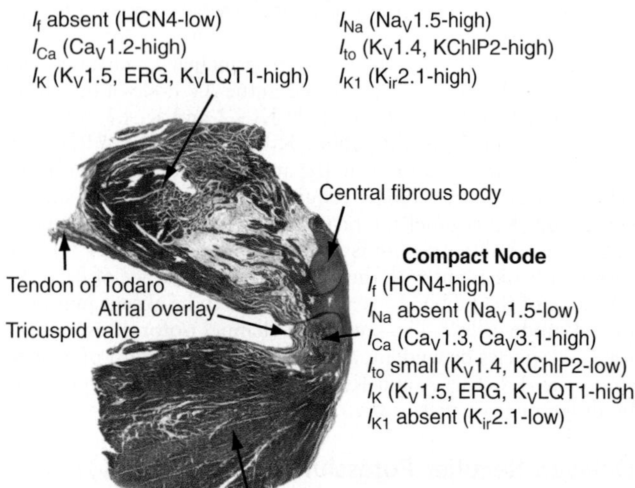

Figure 24-2 Summary of ionic currents and ion channels in the atrioventricular (AV) node. A section through the compact node of the human heart stained with Masson's trichrome is shown. Ionic currents and ion channels in the atrial muscle compact node are listed. The ionic currents and ion channels listed are for the mammalian AV node and not specifically for the human; there are important species differences; see text for details. Ca$_V$, voltage-gated calcium channel; ERG, ether-a-go-go -related gene; HCN, hyperpolarization-activated cyclic nucleotide–gated cation channel; I_{Ca}, calcium current; I_f, hyperpolarization-activated funny current; I_K, potassium current; I_{Na}, sodium current; I_{to}, transient outward current; K$_{ir}$, inward-rectifier potassium channel; K$_V$, voltage-gated potassium channel; KChIP, K$_V$ channel–interacting protein; LQT, long QT [syndrome]; Na$_V$, voltage-gated sodium channel.

junction, such as lower nodal bundle cells, transitional cells, or compact nodal cells, mRNA or protein measurements will have to be made from cells in situ using laser-dissection techniques that allow the precise localization of the cell types that are studied.

Cell-to-Cell Coupling in the Atrioventricular Junction

Four cardiac connexins have been identified, and each has been shown to be present in the AV junction in various species.[31] In human, rabbit, and rat, Cx40 mRNA or protein is abundantly expressed in the AV node.[16] In the human, Cx40 mRNA is more abundantly expressed in the AV node than in the working myocardium.[16] The abundance of Cx40 in the AV node suggests that it plays an important role in AV node conduction. Consistent with this, the Cx40 knockout mouse shows AV block.[32] Cx45 mRNA and protein are also expressed in the AV node of the rabbit, mouse, and rat.[14] Cx30.2 protein is abundantly expressed in the mouse AV node, and the Cx30.2 knockout mouse shows profound AV conduction disturbances.[33] However, mRNA for Cx31.9 (the human equivalent of Cx30.2) is expressed at a low level (e.g., as compared to Cx40, Cx43, and Cx45 mRNAs) in the AV node of the human[16]; this suggests that Cx31.9 plays a negligible role in the human.

In the human, immunohistochemical investigations of the AV junction have shown that Cx43 is expressed heterogeneously.[34] As shown in Figure 24-3, the leftward nodal extension and the compact nodal region both express very little Cx43, whereas the rightward extension, lower nodal bundle, and His bundle all express Cx43 similarly to each other and significantly higher than the compact node and leftward extension. Likewise in the rabbit, it has been shown that Cx43 is present in the inferior nodal extension (which is the correlate of the rightward extension in the human) and lower nodal bundle, but it is absent from the compact node.[35] The transitional cells that surround the nodal structures in the human all express high levels of Cx43. Inferior transitional cells were often in close proximity to the rightward extension, which may be the interface between the rightward extension and the atrial myocardium.

Figure 24-3G displays a three-dimensional reconstruction of the human AV junction that was constructed from histology slides that were adjacent to those stained for Cx43. Various structures within the AV junction are depicted with their relative Cx43 expression. The rightward extension and lower nodal bundle are shown as a continuous structure, as are the leftward extension and compact node, based on the similarities of Cx43 expression in these structures.

Functional Heterogeneity of the Atrioventricular Junction

The molecular heterogeneity of cells within the AV junction gives rise to a diverse range of macroscopic functions during AV conduction, such as very slow propagation, low-pass filtering properties, and discrete rate-dependent pathways. These pathways form the substrate for AV node reentrant tachycardia (AVNRT), which is the most common cause of paroxysmal supraventricular tachycardia and the impetus for much of the clinical attention given to the AV junction. However, despite clinical and scientific interest in this arrhythmia and AV conduction in general, mechanisms of AV conduction are still not fully understood.

Fortunately, current technology has created a host of new techniques to bridge the gap between AV node structure and function. For instance, optical mapping techniques now allow hundreds or thousands of simultaneous recordings at a time. The disadvantage of optical imaging as compared to microelectrodes is that an optical action potential is a summed average of the electrical activity from many cells with different morphologic and molecular characteristics. To distinguish the contributions of different cells and tissue layers to optical recordings, optical mapping can be coupled with high-resolution structural imaging to capture the intact tissue architecture that generates optical signals. One imaging modality with the cellular resolution and the depth penetration to image tissue layers contributing to optical action potentials is optical coherence tomography (OCT).[36] Current state-of-the-art OCT systems have spatial resolution down to 1 to 2 μm,[37] but depth penetration is limited to approximately 2 mm in cardiac tissue.[38] Other techniques, such as photoacoustic microscropy or ultrasound-modulated optical tomography, may be able overcome this limitation while preserving adequate spatial resolution.[39] Finally, combining functional imaging and structural imaging with molecular imaging such as immunohistochemistry and mRNA analysis from functionally characterized regions will truly integrate macroscopic function with molecular distributions.

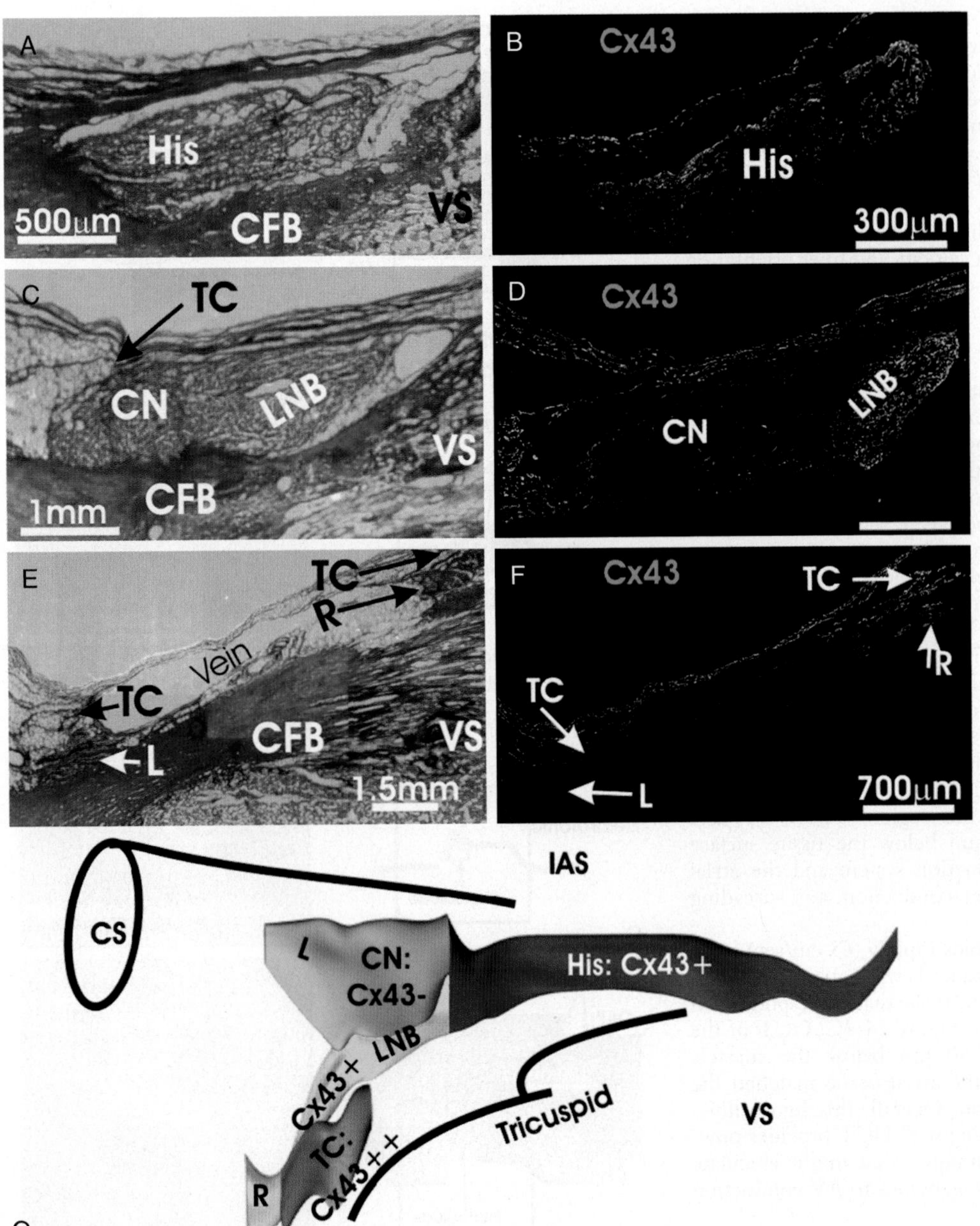

Figure 24-3 Connexin43 (Cx43) in the human atrioventricular junction. **A** and **B**, The His bundle **(A)**, completely surrounded by the fibrous tissue of the central fibrous body (CFB), expresses Cx43 heterogeneously throughout **(B)**. **C**, The AV node can be divided into the compact node *(CN)* and the lower nodal bundle *(LNB)* based on cell morphology and tissue architecture. Transitional cells *(TC)* can be seen connecting superficial atrial layers to the CN. **D**, Cx43 is highly expressed in the LNB, and it is only present in small amounts in the CN. Cx43 is present in both the TC and the endocardial atrial layer. **E** and **F**, The leftward and rightward inferior nodal extensions (*L* and *R*, respectively) are separated by several millimeters of connective and adipose tissue, and each extension has nearby transitional cells *(TC)*. Cx43 is present in the rightward extension and transitional cells but is almost absent from the leftward extension. **G**, A three-dimensional reconstruction of the AV conduction system was created from histology of this preparation. The His bundle is shown in *green*. The compact AV node *(CN)* and the leftward extension are depicted as one structure in *cyan* based on the low presence of Cx43 in these structures. The lower nodal bundle *(LNB)* and the rightward extension are shown in *yellow* as one structure based on their similar Cx43 levels. Transitional cells *(TC)* that were closely related to the rightward extension are shown in *orange;* this may be the interface between the atrial myocardium and the rightward extension. (Modified from Hucker WJ, McCain M, Laughner JI, et al: Connexin43 expression delineates two discrete pathways in the human atrioventricular junction. Anat Rec [Hoboken] 291[2]:204-215, 2008.)

Mechanisms of Atrioventricular Conduction

The slow AV nodal conduction was explained by a decremental conduction hypothesis of Hoffman and Cranefield.[40] Such decremental conduction may be due to reduced intercellular coupling between nodal myocytes, as compared to atrial or ventricular tissue, or the absence of I_{Na} within the node. A different hypothesis was put forward by Rosenblueth, who postulated that a step delay in conduction at a particular location in the node could explain the appearance of Wenkebach cycles at fast atrial rates and could explain the slow conduction of the node under normal conditions.[41] A seminal microelectrode study by Billette[6] provided experimental evidence for this theory, showing that the majority of the AV delay was at the interface of atrionodal cells with nodal cells. A theoretical study demonstrated that a reduction in intercellular conductance (such as that seen in the AV node) could produce a step delay in conduction, reduce conduction velocity, and paradoxically increase the safety factor of conduction.[42] Although the step delay hypothesized by Rosenblueth cannot explain all rate-dependent AV nodal properties, experimental and theoretical studies have provided evidence in a variety of species that the step delay is an important component of AV nodal conduction.[43]

The Cx43 staining shown in Figure 24-3 illustrates that there is an abrupt transition of Cx43 expression from the transitional cells that surround the AV node to the adjacent compact nodal tissue, which has very little Cx43. Such an abrupt change in intercellular coupling could be partially responsible for a step delay in conduction.[42] Also, recent OCT data have suggested that structural features of the AV junction might also play a role in a step delay.[38]

Figure 24-4 illustrates an example where retrograde conduction through the AV junction was optically mapped, and the preparation was subsequently imaged with OCT. In Figure 24-4A, an activation map of retrograde AV conduction was constructed from the three-dimensional (3D) optical signals recorded from the AV junction. Figure 24-4B displays the volume of OCT data that was recorded from this preparation. As can be seen in Figure 24-4C to E, components of the activation map can be correlated with different layers of tissue in the OCT volume based on conduction velocity and fiber orientation vectors. In Figure 24-4C, conduction spreads from the His bundle on the right toward the AV node and inferior nodal extension on the left at 20 cm/sec, as indicated with conduction velocity vectors.

An example optical action potential (OAP) is also shown in Figure 24-4C. This OAP exhibits two distinct upstrokes: The initial upstroke is followed by a small plateau and then a larger upstroke. The portion of the activation map shown in Figure 24-4C was constructed from any OAP containing the initial upstroke. In the deep tissue layers seen in OCT (700-1100 μm below the surface), the fibers of the conduction system were oriented approximately parallel to the conduction velocity vectors, as shown in Figure 24-4C. Even at a depth of 800 μm below the surface, the OCT signal from the conduction system was easily detectable, whereas the signal from the surrounding myocardium was significantly lower.

In Figure 24-4D, conduction propagated very slowly (~2 cm/sec), and OAPs show no distinct upstroke during this period. Instead, there is a small initial depolarization in the OAP illustrated in Figure 24-5D, which is consistent with electrotonic activation of the myocardium in this region. The OCT data from this region show that 400 μm below the tissue surface is the interface between the conduction system and the atrial myocardium, where it appears that conduction was spreading transverse to fiber orientation.

In Figure 24-4E, activation spreads rapidly (65 cm/sec) in all directions. The activation map in panel E was constructed from OAPs that only contained a single upstroke that corresponded in time to the second upstroke seen in Figure 24-4C. OCT of the superficial layer of atrial tissue, 50 μm below the surface, revealed that fiber orientation in the atrial tissue matched the initial direction of rapid conduction. Overall, this figure illustrates that combining optical mapping with OCT provides powerful bimodal optical imaging techniques that might elucidate the contribution of structural heterogeneities to AV conduction in 3D mapping.

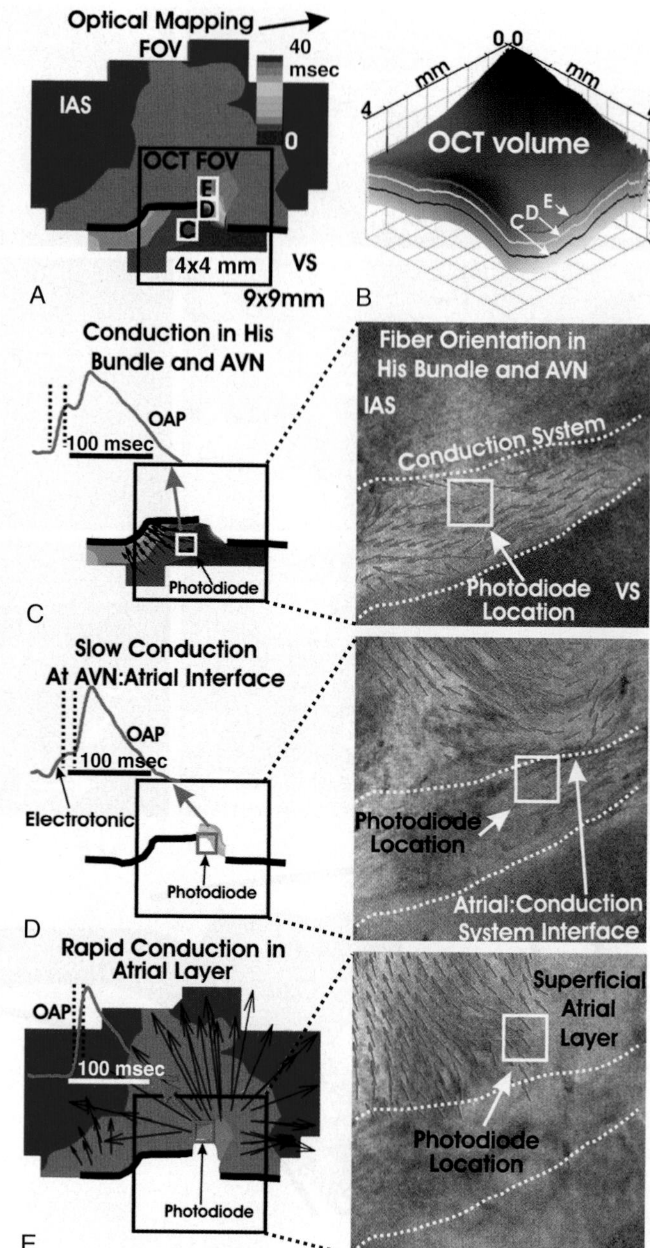

Figure 24-4 Optical mapping of retrograde atrioventricular (AV) conduction coupled with optical coherence tomography (OCT). **A,** Activation map recorded in the rabbit AV junction during retrograde AV conduction. *Blue map* shows conduction over the His-AVN-INE (His bundle, AV node, and inferior nodal extension) axis; the *red map* shows conduction after the retrograde fast pathway breakthrough, which activated atrial tissue. **B,** Volume of optical coherence tomography data showing the three layers of tissue illustrated in **C, D,** and **E. C,** Map of conduction and OCT images from the deep structure of the His-AVN-INE. Left panel shows representative dual-component optical signal and pattern of activation. Right panel shows vectors of fiber orientation reconstructed from OCT data. Note that conduction propagates along the fibers. **D,** Map of conduction and fiber orientation in the intermediate layer containing the fast pathway. Note that very slow conduction occurs transverse to fiber orientation. **E,** Conduction over the atrial layer of tissue. Note very rapid conduction along the fiber orientation. FOV, field of view; IAS, interatrial septum; OAP, optical action potential; VS, vagal stimulation. (Reproduced with permission from Hucker WJ, Ripplinger C, Fleming C, et al: Multimodal biophotonic imaging to correlate structure and function in cardiac tissue. J Biomed Opt 13:054012, 2008.)

Dual Pathways

The first clear and elegant description of AV nodal reentry belongs to Mines, who described longitudinal dissociation preceding the onset of reentry and leading to its initiation.[44] More than half a century later, reentry was induced by premature stimulation and documented by Moe and colleagues in dogs,[45] Coumel and coworkers in humans,[46] and Janse and colleagues in rabbit preparations.[47] Unlike the painstaking work of several-site microelectrode recordings that were originally used to investigate the substrate of dual pathways,[6,47] optical techniques can generate hundreds of recordings, providing a thorough documentation of AV nodal reentry. Using optical methods in the rabbit, it has been demonstrated that there is not a single distinct structural substrate of the fast pathway; rather, the atrial layer and the transitional cells surrounding the AV node are involved in fast pathway conduction.[48]

The substrate for the slow pathway in the rabbit appears to be inferior nodal extension.[48] In the human however, the true anatomic substrates of the functional circuits involved in AVNRT

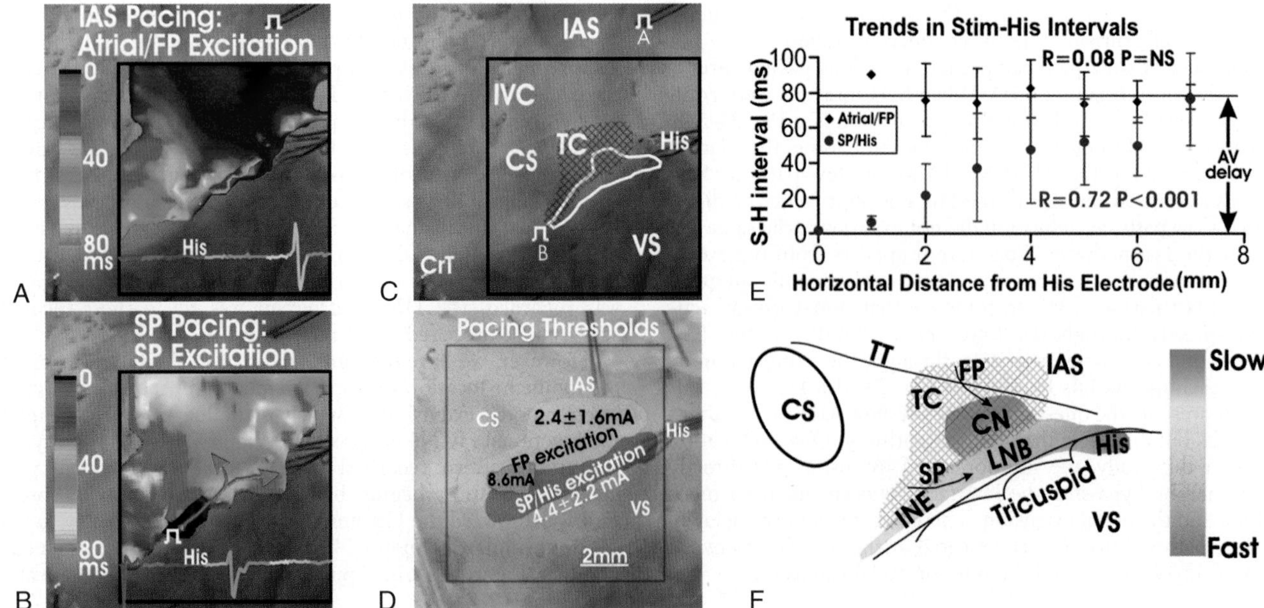

Figure 24-5 Atrioventricular (AV) conduction with and without the AV delay. **A,** Pacing the interatrial septum produced a wave of excitation across the triangle of Koch and fast pathway (FP) activation of the AV node. After a delay, His excitation is seen in *orange*. The His electrogram at the bottom of the panel indicates that the delay between the pacing stimulus and His excitation (the S-H interval) was 70 ms. **B,** Pacing stimuli applied near the tricuspid valve within the triangle of Koch produced linear slow pathway (SP) conduction that spread retrogradely across the triangle of Koch and proceeded directly toward the His bundle with S-H interval = 43 ms. The His electrogram had a different morphology than with fast-pathway activation. **C,** Schematic outline of the AV conduction system in the preparation shown in **A** and **B** consisting of the His bundle, compact AV node, and inferior nodal extension with the approximate location of transitional cells *(TC)* depicted as the *crosshatched area.* A and B, location of pacing electrode in panel A and B. CS, coronary sinus; IAS, interatrial septum; IVC, inferior vena cava; VS, ventricular septum. **D,** Fast pathway *(FP)* or slow pathway *(SP)* activation was produced in separate areas of the triangle of Koch and had different pacing thresholds. FP activation had a predominantly lower pacing threshold; however one area below the coronary sinus *(CS)* had high pacing thresholds. Pacing stimuli applied close to the His bundle directly excited the His bundle with pacing thresholds statistically the same as SP pacing. **E,** S-H intervals were measured for each pacing location throughout the triangle of Koch. Pacing that produced FP activation of the AVN had a constant S-H interval, due to the AV delay, which was not correlated with the distance from the His bundle (or His electrode). SP pacing, however, produced S-H intervals that were highly correlated with the distance from the His bundle and decreased linearly as the His electrode was approached. No nonlinear AV delay was observed with slow pathway pacing. **F,** We hypothesize that SP excitation passes through the inferior nodal extension *(INE)* and lower nodal bundle *(LNB)* directly to the His bundle, whereas FP activation travels through transitional cells *(TC)* and the compact node *(CN)*, where the AVN delay occurs. TT, tendon of Todaro. (Modified with permission from Hucker WJ, Sharma V, Nikolski VP, Efimov IR: Atrioventricular conduction with and without AV nodal delay: Two pathways to the bundle of His in the rabbit heart. Am J Physiol Heart Circ Physiol 293:H1122-H1130, 2007.)

are still debated.[49] As shown in Figure 24-3, Cx43 delimiting two structures in the human AV junction might imply that these structures have different conduction properties that contribute to AVNRT. However, more-detailed mapping of other connexin isoforms, as well as ion channel expression in these structures, will be necessary to fully understand conduction in these tissues.

His Bundle Excitation in the Context of Dual Pathways

Due to the limitations of right ventricular pacing,[50] new pacing strategies such as cardiac resynchronization therapy with biventricular pacing and direct His bundle pacing have been explored to pace the ventricles synchronously. Both methods produce a significantly narrower QRS complex, but lead placement with both techniques can be challenging. Also, a deeper understanding of the influence of AV nodal dual pathway conduction on His excitation is desirable to design new pacing strategies centered around His excitation.

Previous studies have illustrated that the activating pathway of the AV node determines the magnitude of the His electrogram.[51] This indicates that the influence of the activating pathway does not end at the AV node itself, but instead determines either the manner of His depolarization or which domain of the His is activated. Previous studies have shown that the activation patterns of the slow pathway and the fast pathway in the rabbit can be recognized optically in the context of premature (S2) stimuli.[48] However, these activating pathways can also be visualized by pacing them directly within the triangle of Koch.[52] For typical fast pathway activation (see Fig. 24-5A), a rapid wave of depolarization spreads across the superficial atrial myocardium, followed by a period where usually no conduction is detectible due to low-amplitude optical signals during AV conduction, and finally His activation occurs (shown in orange). The corresponding His electrogram is shown, indicating His activation approximately 70 ms after stimulation.

Typically, slow pathway conduction is only seen in the context of premature stimuli: S1-S2 pacing protocols.[48] However, *directly pacing* the slow pathway is also possible, and the typical activation pattern is shown in Figure 24-5B. Slow pathway activation spreads from the pacing electrode linearly toward the His bundle and bifurcates, with activation continuing toward the His bundle as well as spreading retrogradely across the interatrial septum. The His electrogram occurred 43 ms after stimulation with a characteristic change in electrogram morphology from fast pathway to slow pathway activation.[51] Paradoxically, the interval between the pacing stimulus and His activation (S-H interval) was *shorter* with slow pathway activation than with fast pathway activation. A schematic of the conduction system in this rabbit AV junctional preparation is shown in Figure 24-5C for clarity.

The crosshatched area denotes the approximate location of transitional cells surrounding the conduction system.

The zone of slow pathway pacing, as well as pacing thresholds, is shown in Figure 24-5D. When S-H intervals were compared between fast and slow pathway activation (see Fig. 24-5E), fast-pathway S-H intervals remained constant across the triangle of Koch, reflecting the AV delay. However slow pathway S-H intervals decreased linearly as the His was approached, indicating that slow pathway activation did not experience the same AV delay as the fast pathway. Therefore it appears from these data that the slow pathway is connected to the His bundle uniquely from the fast pathway. We hypothesize that slow-pathway activation spreads through the lower nodal bundle to the His, whereas the fast pathway passes through the compact node before reaching the His bundle (see Fig. 24-5F). However, this scenario presents the question of how the slow pathway conducts to the His bundle faster than the fast pathway. One explanation is that in this study, the inferior nodal extension was directly paced, thereby bypassing the interface between the atrial myocardium and the nodal extension. Therefore, most of the delay in the slow pathway may be accumulated at the interface between the atrial myocardium and the inferior nodal extension.

Pacemaking Activity in the Atrioventricular Junction

When Tawara published his discovery of the AV node in 1902, his mentor Ludwig Aschoff postulated that the AV node may be the pacemaker of the heart.[2] Indeed since that time, many studies have confirmed that the AV junction can act as a pacemaker.[9] In fact, Meijler and colleagues have hypothesized that the primary role of the AV junction is not conduction, but rather it is to act as an oscillator, or pacemaker, which is electrotonically modulated by the atrial myocardium.[53] Historically it was presumed that the AV junctional pacemaker was predominately located in the nodo-His or His region because when a junctional rhythm was recorded, the His electrogram was the earliest recorded activity that preceded atrial activation.

However, we have demonstrated that in the rabbit heart, the predominant location of the AV junctional pacemaker is in the inferior nodal extension,[5,9] which is the location of the highest AV junctional HCN4 expression.[14] Figure 24-6A shows a typical activation pattern recorded from the rabbit junctional pacemaker: Activation begins below the coronary sinus, spreads rightward toward the His bundle with no apparent delay in conduction, similar to Figure 24-5B, and produces the His electrogram in Figure 24-6B. Approximately 55 ms after activation

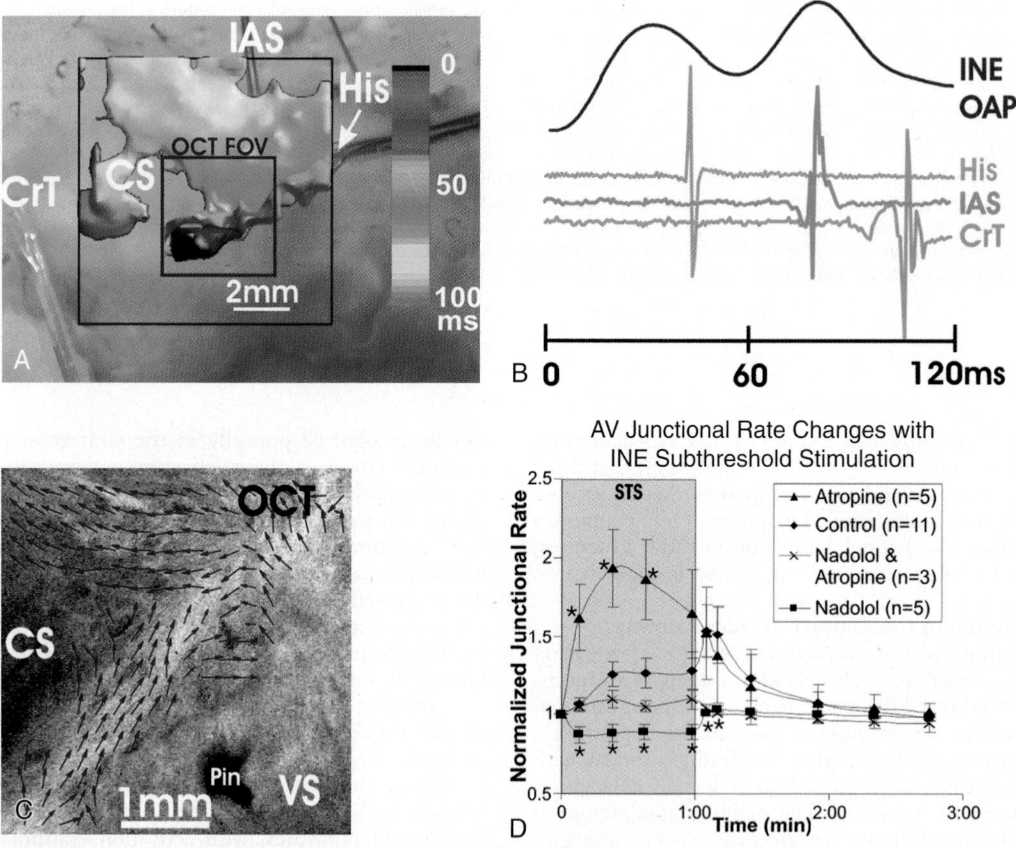

Figure 24-6 Pacemaking activity in the atrioventricular (AV) junction. **A,** The AV junctional pacemaker most often originates beneath the coronary sinus. Activation spreads linearly toward the His bundle (similar to Fig. 24-5B) and activates the His bundle, and it spreads retrogradely across the triangle of Koch and the interatrial septum *(IAS)*. **B,** The optical action potential (OAP) recorded from the leading pacemaker location, as well as the His, IAS, and lower crista terminalis (CrT) electrograms are shown. CS, coronary sinus; FOV, field of view; INE, inferior nodal extension. **C,** Optical coherence tomography (OCT) of this preparation 150 μm below the surface revealed the interface of the conduction system and the superficial atrial tissue, with fiber orientation that matched the activation pattern shown in **A**. VS, ventricular septum. **D,** Subthreshold stimulation (STS) was used to autonomically modulate the AV junctional pacemaker in the inferior nodal extension (INE). The effects of STS could be pharmacologically separated: Atropine blocked parasympathetic stimulation, and STS with atropine doubled the rate of the AV junction pacemaker. Nadolol blocked sympathetic stimulation and when coupled with STS reduced the junctional rate by 13%. (Modified with permission from Hucker WJ, Nikolski VP, Efimov IR: Autonomic control and innervation of the atrioventricular junctional pacemaker. Heart Rhythm 4:1326-1335, 2007.)

begins, retrograde activation spreads across the interatrial septum and wraps around the CS to activate the lower crista terminalis. OCT imaging of this preparation (see Fig. 24-3C) revealed the junction of the superficial atrium with the conduction system 100 to 200 μm below the tissue surface. The fiber orientation at this depth (see Fig. 24-6C) matchs the pattern of excitation seen in Figure 24-6A. The conduction system of this preparation could be seen in OCT images for another 800 μm below the surface.

The AV nodal pacemaker is controlled by the autonomic nervous system. Applying high-frequency subthreshold stimulation is a commonly used technique to stimulate intracardiac postganglionic neurons, and this technique was used to investigate the response of the AV junctional pacemaker to autonomic stimulation.[5] In control conditions, subthreshold stimulation (STS) induces changes in the junctional rate that depend on the interplay between the sympathetic and parasympathetic branches of the autonomic nervous system. As shown in Figure 24-6D, STS applied with no drugs present (control) increased the junctional rate during STS, and after STS the junctional rate transiently increased further before decreasing to prestimulation rates. STS with atropine (blocking parasympathetic innervation) doubled the junctional rate during STS, and STS with nadolol (blocking the sympathetic innervation) caused a decrease in rate. Using STS, the rabbit junctional rhythm was accelerated to 412 ±29 ms, which is similar to sinus rates in rabbits.[5] However unlike the SA node under autonomic modulation,[54] the junctional pacemaker did not shift in the majority of cases with STS. The stability and sympathetic tone of the junctional pacemaker may have clinical implications for patients undergoing AV nodal ablations: Preserving the junctional pacemaker during ablation leaves a backup pacemaking mechanism in the event of a device failure, and an alternative pacing strategy could exploit the sympathetic tone of the junctional pacemaker to accelerate it to sinus rates, which would excite the ventricles physiologically through the ventricular conduction system.[55,56]

Our investigations in rabbit hearts indicate that the role of the AV junctional pacemaker may be underappreciated. It has classically been assumed that the junctional pacemaker only operated when SA nodal activity ceased; however, in our experience, a rabbit right atrial preparation containing both the SA and AV nodes exhibits a leading pacemaker in the inferior nodal extension in approximately 30% of experiments. Likewise, vagal stimulation of the SA node in this preparation can induce the dominant pacemaker to shift to the inferior nodal extension in the majority of cases.

The molecular basis of pacemaking activity has also been investigated in the AV junction. As indicated earlier, HCN4, which carries the I_f current, is widely expressed throughout the AV junction, with its highest levels in the inferior nodal extension.[14] Also it has been suggested that sarcoplasmic reticulum calcium release (via the ryanodine receptor, RYR2), plays a role in pacemaking at the sinoatrial node by activating the inward Na^+-Ca^{2+} exchange current. It might also play a substantial role at the AV node: In the isolated AV node of the mouse, 2 μM ryanodine (a functional blocker of sarcoplasmic reticulum calcium release) increases the cycle length (time between spontaneous beats) by approximately 240%.[10] In the rabbit AV node, mRNAs for the calcium-handling proteins—RYR2, RYR3, and SERCA2a—are all reduced (as compared to the working myocardium).[14] On the other hand, expression of NCX1 mRNA in the rabbit AV node is similar to that in the working myocardium.[14] However, additional studies are needed to deduce the role of calcium-handling proteins in AV junctional pacemaking activity.

Conclusions

Multiple imaging modalities and new molecular biology techniques have certainly begun to bridge the gap between AV node structure and function. The successful imaging of AV node conduction during AV nodal reentry, dual pathway conduction, and junctional rhythm has enhanced our understanding of electrophysiology in the AV junction. Applying fluorescent mapping to the human AV junction might soon provide answers to questions that surround pathways of AVNRT. Likewise, the application of OCT to the AV junction where pathways of conduction have been visualized can provide direct evidence of the tissue involved in conduction and allow truly three-dimensional real-time imaging of electrical activity in the AV junction, as well as in other structures of the heart. Similarly, rapid developments in molecular biology techniques have generated a wealth of information regarding the ionic basis of AV conduction in normal and pathologic states. The increased level of understanding of the profound complexity in the three-dimensional structure of the AV junction will provide the basis for a comprehensive mathematical model, allowing for quantitative investigation of AV nodal pathophysiology that might lead to the development of novel treatment strategies.

References

1. Mazgalev TN, Tchou P: Atrial-AV Nodal Electrophysiology: A View from the Millenium. Armonk, NY: Futura Publishing, 2000.
2. Tawara S: Das Reizleitungssystem des Saugetierherzens: Eine Anatomische-Histologische Studie über das Atrioventrikularbundel und die Purkinjeschen Faden. Jena: Gustav Fischer Verlag, 1906.
3. Meijler FL, Janse MJ: Morphology and electrophysiology of the mammalian atrioventricular node. Physiol Rev 68:608-647, 1988.
4. Inoue S, Becker AE: Posterior extensions of the human compact atrioventricular node: A neglected anatomic feature of potential clinical significance. Circulation 97: 188-193, 1998.
5. Hucker WJ, Nikolski VP, Efimov IR: Autonomic control and innervation of the atrioventricular junctional pacemaker. Heart Rhythm 4:1326-1335, 2007.
6. Billette J: Atrioventricular nodal activation during periodic premature stimulation of the atrium. Am J Physiol 252:H163-H177, 1987.
7. de Carvalho AP, de Almeida DF: Spread of activity through the atrioventricular node. Circ Res 8:801-809, 1960.
8. Anderson RH, Durrer D, Janse MJ, et al: A combined morphological and electrophysiological study of the atrioventricular node of the rabbit heart. Circ Res 35:909-922, 1974.
9. Dobrzynski H, Nikolski VP, Sambelashvili AT, et al: Site of origin and molecular substrate of atrioventricular junctional rhythm in the rabbit heart. Circ Res 93:1102-1110, 2003.
10. Nikmaram MR, Liu J, Abdelrahman M, et al: Characterization of the effects of ryanodine, TTX, E-4031 and 4-AP on the sinoatrial and atrioventricular nodes. Prog Biophys Mol Biol 96(1-3):452-464, 2008.
11. Hancox J, Levi A: The hyperpolarization-activated current, I_f, is not required for pacemaking in single cells from the rabbit atrioventricular node. Pflügers Arch 427:121-128, 1994.
12. Munk AA, Adjemian RA, Zhao J, et al: Electrophysiological properties of morphologically distinct cells isolated from the rabbit atrioventricular node. J Physiol 493:801-818, 1996.
13. Yuill KH, Hancox JC: Characteristics of single cells isolated from the atrioventricular node of the adult guinea-pig heart. Pflugers Arch 445:311-320, 2002.
14. Greener ID, Tellez JO, Dobrzynski H, et al: Distribution of ion channel transcripts in the rabbit atrioventricular node as

studied using in situ hybridisation and quantitative PCR. J Mol Cell Cardiol 40:982-983, 2006.

15. Yoo S, Dobrzynski H, Fedorov VV, et al: Localisation of Na^+ channel isoforms at the atrioventricular junction and atrioventricular node. Circulation 114:1360-1371, 2006.
16. Greener ID, Chandler NJ, Tellez JO, et al: Expression profile of ion channels and gap junctional proteins in the human atrioventricualr node. Heart Rhythm 4(suppl S):S141-S168, 2007.
17. Ren FX, Niu XL, Ou Y, et al: Morphological and electrophysiological properties of single myocardial cells from Koch triangle of rabbit heart. Chin Med J (Engl) 119:2075-2084, 2006.
18. Papadatos GA, Wallerstein PM, Head CE, et al: Slowed conduction and ventricular tachycardia after targeted disruption of the cardiac sodium channel gene *Scn5a*. Proc Natl Acad Sci U S A 99:6210-6215, 2002.
19. Wang DW, Viswanathan PC, Balser JR, et al: Clinical, genetic, and biophysical characterization of *SCN5A* mutations associated with atrioventricular conduction block. Circulation 105:341-346, 2002.
20. Maier SKG, Westenbroek RE, Yamanushi TT, et al: An unexpected requirement for brain-type sodium channels for control of heart rate in the mouse sinoatrial node. Proc Natl Acad Sci U S A 100:3507-3512, 2003.
21. Marionneau C, Couette B, Liu J, et al: Specific pattern of ionic channel gene expression associated with pacemaker activity in the mouse heart. J Physiol 562: 223-234, 2005.
22. Zipes DP, Mendez C: Action of manganese ions and tetrodotoxin on atrioventricular nodal transmembrane potentials in isolated rabbit hearts. Circ Res 32:447-454, 1973.
23. Splawski I, Timothy KW, Decher N, et al: Severe arrhythmia disorder caused by cardiac L-type calcium channel mutations. Proc Natl Acad Sci U S A 102:8089-8096, 2005.
24. Mangoni ME, Couette B, Bourinet E, et al: Functional role of L-type Cav1.3 Ca^{2+} channels in cardiac pacemaker activity. Proc Natl Acad Sci U S A 100:5543-5548, 2003.
25. Xu W, Lipscombe D: Neuronal $Ca_V1.3\alpha1$ L-type channels activate at relatively hyperpolarized membrane potentials and are incompletely inhibited by dihydropyridines. J Neurosci 21:5944-5951, 2001.
26. Qu Y, Baroudi G, Yue Y, Boutjdir M: Novel molecular mechanism involving $\alpha1D$ ($Ca_V1.3$) L-type calcium channel in autoimmune-associated sinus bradycardia. Circulation 111:3034-3041, 2005.
27. Liu Y, Zeng W, Delmar M, Jalife J: Ionic mechanisms of electronic inhibition and concealed conduction in rabbit atrioventricular nodal myocytes. Circulation 88:1634-1646, 1993.
28. Mitcheson JS, Hancox JC: Characteristics of a transient outward current (sensitive to 4-aminopyridine) in Ca^{2+}-tolerant myocytes isolated from the rabbit atrioventricular node. Pflugers Arch 438:68-78, 1999.
29. Hancox JC, Yuill KH, Mitcheson JS, Convery MK: Progress and gaps in understanding the electrophysiological properties of morphologically normal cells from the cardiac atrioventricular node. Int J Bifurcation Chaos 13:3675-3691, 2003.
30. Dobrzynski H, Billeter R, Greener ID, et al: Expression of Kir2.1 and Kir6.2 transgenes under the control of the α-MHC promoter in the sinoatrial and atrioventricular nodes in transgenic mice. J Mol Cell Cardiol 41:855-867, 2006.
31. Boyett MR, Inada S, Yoo S, et al: Connexins in the sinoatrial and atrioventricular nodes. Adv Cardiol 42:175-197, 2006.
32. Simon AM, Goodenough DA, Paul DL: Mice lacking connexin40 have cardiac conduction abnormalities characteristic of atrioventricular block and bundle branch block. Curr Biol 8:295-298, 1998.
33. Kreuzberg MM, Schrickel JW, Ghanem A, et al: Connexin30.2 containing gap junction channels decelerate impulse propagation through the atrioventricular node. Proc Natl Acad Sci U S A 103:5959-5964, 2006.
34. Hucker WJ, McCain M, Laughner JI, Iaizzo P, Efimov I: Connexin43 expression delineates two discrete pathways in the human atrioventricular junction. Anat Rec (Hoboken) 291(2):204-215, 2008.
35. Ko YS, Yeh HI, Ko YL, et al: Three-dimensional reconstruction of the rabbit atrioventricular conduction axis by combining histological, desmin, and connexin mapping data. Circulation 109:1172-1179, 2004.
36. Huang D, Swanson EA, Lin CP, et al: Optical coherence tomography. Science 254:1178-1181, 1991.
37. Fujimoto JG: Optical coherence tomography for ultrahigh resolution in vivo imaging. Nat Biotechnol 21:1361-1367, 2003.
38. Hucker WJ, Ripplinger C, Fleming C, et al: Multimodal biophotonic imaging to correlate structure and function in cardiac tissue. J Biomed Opt 13:054012, 2008.
39. Zhang HF, Maslov K, Stoica G, Wang LV: Functional photoacoustic microscopy for high-resolution and noninvasive in vivo imaging. Nat Biotech 24:848-851, 2006.
40. Hoffman B, Cranefield P: Electrophysiology of the Heart. New York: McGraw-Hill, 1960.
41. Rosenblueth A: Mechanism of the Wenckebach-Luciani cycles. Am J Physiol 194:491-494, 1958.
42. Shaw RM, Rudy Y: Ionic mechanisms of propagation in cardiac tissue. Roles of the sodium and L-type calcium currents during reduced excitability and decreased gap junction coupling. Circ Res 81:727-741, 1997.
43. Choi BR, Salama G: Optical mapping of atrioventricular node reveals a conduction barrier between atrial and nodal cells. Am J Physiol 274:H829-H845, 1998.
44. Mines GR: On dynamic equilibrium in the heart. J Physiol 46:349-383, 1913.
45. Moe GK, Preston JB, Burlington H: Physiologic evidence for a dual A-V transmission system. Circ Res 4:357-375, 1956.
46. Coumel P, Carbol C, Fabiato A, et al: Tachycardie permanente par rythme reciproque. Archives des Maladies du Coeur et des Vaisseaux 60:1830-1864, 1967.
47. Janse MJ, Capelle FV, Freud GE, Durrer D: Circus movement within the AV node as a basis for supraventricular tachycardia as shown by multiple microelectrode recording in the isolated rabbit heart. Circ Res 28:403-414, 1971.
48. Nikolski VP, Jones SA, Lancaster MK, et al: Cx43 and dual-pathway electrophysiology of the atrioventricular node and atrioventricular nodal reentry. Circ Res 92:469-475, 2003.
49. Katritsis DG, Becker A: The atrioventricular nodal reentrant tachycardia circuit: A proposal. Heart Rhythm 4:1354-1360, 2007.
50. Manolis AS: The deleterious consequences of right ventricular apical pacing: Time to seek alternate site pacing. Pacing Clin Electrophysiol 29:298-315, 2006.
51. Zhang Y, Bharati S, Mowrey KA, et al: His electrogram alternans reveal dual-wavefront inputs into and longitudinal dissociation within the bundle of His. Circulation 104:832-838, 2001.
52. Hucker WJ, Sharma V, Nikolski VP, Efimov IR: Atrioventricular conduction with and without AV nodal delay: two pathways to the bundle of His in the rabbit heart. Am J Physiol Heart Circ Physiol 293:H1122-H1130, 2007.
53. Meijler FL, Fisch C: Does the atrioventricular node conduct? Br Heart J 61:309-315, 1989.
54. Fedorov VV, Hucker WJ, Dobrzynski H, et al: Postganglionic nerve stimulation induces temporal inhibition of excitability in rabbit sinoatrial node. Am J Physiol Heart Circ Physiol 291:H612-H623, 2006.
55. Strohmer B, Hwang C, Peter CT, Chen PS: Selective atrionodal input ablation for induction of proximal complete heart block with stable junctional escape rhythm in patients with uncontrolled atrial fibrillation. J Interv Card Electrophysiol 8:49-57, 2003.
56. Swenne CA, Schalij MJ: Pacemaking in the AV node. Heart Rhythm 4:1336-1337, 2007.

Intercellular Communication and Impulse Propagation 25

André G. Kléber

CHAPTER OUTLINE

Rapid propagation of the electrical impulse through the atrial myocardium, the atrioventricular-conduction system, and the ventricular myocardium coordinates excitation and contraction of the ventricles. Knowledge about the process of electrical propagation is necessary to understand normal cardiac function and arrhythmogenesis. Disturbances of impulse propagation, especially propagation slowing and propagation block, lead to circulating excitation with reentry, a self-perpetuating mechanism involved in the initiation and maintenance of the majority of cardiac arrhythmias. The major determinants of electrical impulse propagation are the electrical properties of the individual cardiac myocytes that generate transmembrane electrical charge movement, the gap junctions that provide the functional electrical contacts between the myocytes, and the two-dimensional and three-dimensional anisotropic structure of the network of excitable cells.[1,2]

This chapter focuses specifically on the involvement of connexins in the mechanism of normal and slowed electrical propagation. It assumes knowledge about the structural, molecular, biophysical, and pharmacologic properties of gap junction channels and the variability of connexin distribution in various regions of the heart. All these topics are specifically addressed in other chapters of this book. Although it is useful to discuss the role of gap junctions in propagation in a separate chapter, it is important to recognize that there is a complex interaction among all the determinants of impulse propagation. As a consequence, the effect of a change in electrical cell-to-cell coupling by gap junction channels on propagation strongly depends on the state of the other determinants.[2]

The Role of Cell-to-Cell Coupling in Uniform Propagation

The Single-Cell Chain

The chain of single cells is a simple model that can help us understand the principle of cardiac impulse propagation, and especially the involvement of gap junctions in propagation. Studies in a single chain of cardiomyocytes have been performed either using computer models or synthetic cardiac cell strands.[3]

Figure 25-1 shows the results of experiments using multisite high-resolution optical mapping of transmembrane potential to measure microscopic propagation.[3] The figure illustrates the measurement of action potentials within the cytoplasm of a single myocyte and across the border to the adjacent cell. Panel C depicts the histograms of the corresponding cytoplasmic and intercellular conduction times. From the comparison of the two measurements, average conduction times of 38 μsec along a distance of 30 μm in the cytoplasm and of 80 μsec across an end-to-end cell border were calculated. These results indicate that the time taken for normal propagation across a cell-to-cell connection is of the same order of magnitude as the time taken to activate a cell along its main axis, and they confirm previous computer simulations carried out in a simulated cell chain using the Luo-Rudy models as a basis to the ventricular action potential.[4]

Taking into account that cytoplasmic conduction takes place along an intracellular path of about 100 μm and cell-to-cell conduction across a gap junction of only 8 nm in width, these and other theoretical and experimental studies demonstrated that the process of electrical propagation at the cellular level is discontinuous even in the normal state, with a slow velocity across the gap junction. Interestingly, these significant delays recorded at end-to-end gap junctions in single cell chains are masked to a major extent in cell strands that are several cells in width. Thus, lateral apposition of cell strands in synthetic cellular networks and introduction of lateral coupling reduced the average conduction time across an end-to-end cell junction from 50% total conduction time in single cell strands to 20% in strands of five cells in width.[3] This reduction in the degree of propagation discontinuity is due to compensatory flow of small currents through lateral gap junctions (lateral averaging), which smoothes the effect of the electrical discontinuities caused by the end-to-end connections.

The Anisotropic Cellular Network

Electrical anisotropy, the dependence of electrical propagation velocity θ and other electrical parameters on the direction of impulse spread, is a consequence of the cardiospecific architecture of the cellular network. It is important for understanding normal electrical cardiac function and has been implicated in the mechanisms responsible for initiation and maintenance of re-entry.[1,2] On a macroscopic scale (velocities measured over a distance of several cell lengths[1]), the mean anisotropic velocity ratio, defined as the ratio of longitudinal velocity to transverse velocity, V_L:V_T, ranges from 8.9 (atrial crista terminalis) and 2.7 (ventricular myocardium) to 2.0 (anisotropic cell cultures). At the cellular level, electrical anisotropy is affected by the shape and the size of the anisotropic cells and by the amount and the distribution pattern of gap junctions.

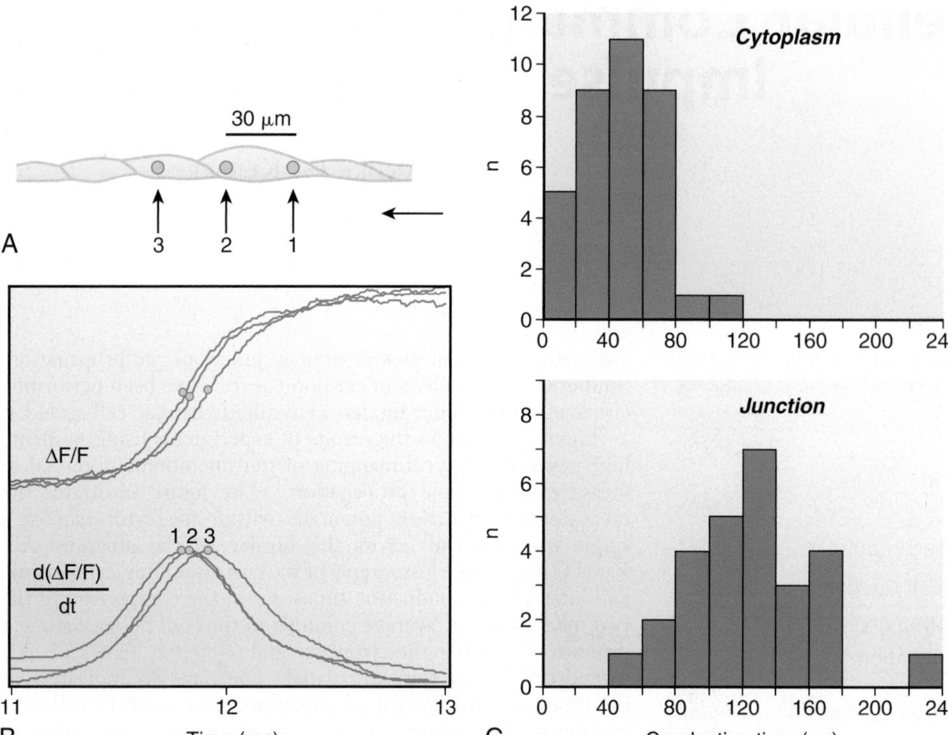

Figure 25-1 Electrical propagation in a cell strand. **A,** Microscopic appearance (reproduction) of a cultured synthetic chain of neonatal cardiac myocytes. Numbered dots superimposed on the cell chain depict positions of light-sensitive diodes 1 to 3 (diameter of a single circular diode = 6.5 μm) separated by a distance of 30 μm. **B,** Optical recording of action potential upstrokes from diodes 1 to 3, measured as fluorescence change ΔF/F of a voltage-sensitive dye *(upper traces)* and the first time derivatives [d(ΔF/F)/dt, lower traces]. Numbers 1, 2, and 3 denote maximal values of (ΔF/F)/dt taken as times of local activation. **C,** Histograms of cytoplasmic (time between diodes 1 and 2, upper graph) and junctional (time between diodes 2 and 3, lower graph) conduction times. The difference between the mean conduction times amounts to approximately 80 μsec and reflects the mean conduction time across the end-to-end cell junctions. (Modified from Fast VG, Kléber AG: Microscopic conduction in cultured strands of neonatal rat heart cells measured with voltage-sensitive dyes. Circ Res 73(5):914-925, 1993.)

Figure 25-2, taken from an elegant theoretical study by Spach and colleagues,[5] illustrates the separate effects of the size, the anisotropic shape of the cardiac cells, and the distribution pattern of gap junctions on propagation. In adult ventricular and atrial myocardium, gap junctions are preferentially located at cell ends and are scarcer along the lateral cell boundaries in most cardiac regions.[6] In contrast, gap junctions in neonatal myocardium show a dot-like appearance with a regular spacing around the cell perimeter.[7] A distribution pattern similar to the neonatal pattern is also found in the remodeled tissue surrounding myocardial infarction.[8] Spach's group first simulated propagation in networks of adult canine ventricular cells (see Fig. 25-2, column a) and neonatal rat ventricular cells (see Fig. 25-2, column d) based on experimental data. Subsequently they created two *virtual* cellular networks, a *first* exhibiting the large cell size of the adult dog ventricle and the gap junction distribution of neonatal rat hearts (see Fig. 25-2, column b) and a *second* showing the small cell size of the rat neonatal ventricular myocytes and the gap junction distribution pattern of the adult dog (see Fig. 25-2, column c).

Although the four patterns showed a similar electrical behavior during longitudinal propagation, the behavior during transverse propagation was distinctly different among the four groups. Importantly, *cell size was the major determinant* of both the activation delay between individual cells along the axis of propagation and dV_m/dt_{max}, and the distribution pattern of gap junctions had a significant but only small effect. The important effect of cell size on propagation velocity is further underlined by the experimental observation that average conduction velocity in neonatal *isotropic* cell cultures (being composed of nonaligned and nonelongated cells) is slower than longitudinal velocity in anisotropic cultures (composed of anisotropically aligned and elongated cells).[9]

The Role of Cell-to-Cell Uncoupling in Slow Conduction

The Safety Factor for Propagation

The classic principle of conduction of the electrical impulse is based on sequential excitation of cardiac cells by local circuit currents, which are driven by the voltage gradient between excited and resting cells and scaled by the cell-to-cell resistance. This principle has been used to define the safety factor of conduction (SF), a parameter providing important information about the dependence of propagation velocity on the state of the ion channels, cell-to-cell coupling, and cell geometry. The formal definition of SF is given by the equation:[4]

$$SF = \frac{\int_A I_c dt \bullet + \bullet \int_A I_{out} dt}{\int_A I_{in} \bullet dt} \qquad A|Q_m > 0 \qquad (1)$$

In principle, this equation corresponds to a ratio of time integrals of electrical currents, that is, to electrical charges, flowing during the period A, when the cell contributes to the propagation process (Q_m>0). The denominator in this equation corresponds to the electrical charge that a cell receives from the upstream tissue. This charge serves to depolarize the cell to the threshold of excitation. The numerator equals the charge that the excited cell generates by activation of ion channels. It splits into two components, the charge that the cell generates for

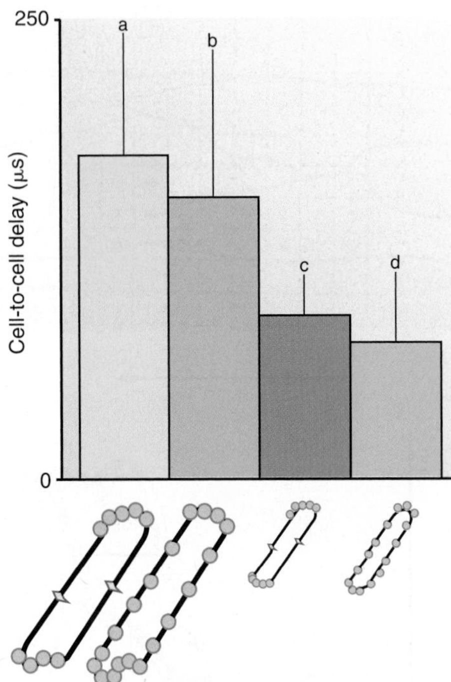

Figure 25-2 Effect of cell size and distribution pattern of gap junctions on cell-to-cell propagation delay. Column *a* represents values simulated from a model of the normal adult dog heart cell, with gap junctions located predominantly at the longitudinal ends. Column *d* represents values of the normal neonatal rat heart cell with regularly spaced gap junctions around the cell perimeter. Column *b* corresponds to a virtual cell with the cell size of a dog myocyte and the gap junction pattern of a neonatal rat heart cell; column *c* corresponds to a virtual cell with the cell size of a neonatal rat myocyte and the gap junction pattern of an adult dog myocyte. Note that cell size has a significantly larger effect than gap junction pattern on both parameters. (Modified from Spach MS, Heidlage JF, Dolber PC, Barr RC: Electrophysiological effects of remodeling cardiac gap junctions and cell size: experimental and model studies of normal cardiac growth. Circ Res 86[3]:302-311, 2000.)

its own depolarization ($Q_c = \int I_c dt$) and for the depolarization of downstream cells ($Q_{out} = \int I_{out} dt$). The repartition of these two components depends on downstream electrotonic load. Propagation is successful (SF >1) if the charge produced by excitation of a cell (numerator) exceeds the charge required to cause excitation (denominator).

This concept of propagation safety is very useful for the definition and explanation of the role of cell-to-cell coupling in propagation. For normal conduction velocities, SF is approximately 1.5, which means that the total electrical charge produced by depolarizing ion channels of a cell exceeds the excitatory charge flowing into the cell from upstream by 50%.[4]

Conduction Slowing Due to Cell-to-Cell Uncoupling

Acute cell-to-cell uncoupling follows closure of gap junctions consequent to ischemia, hypoxia, intracellular acidification,[1,2] and application of uncoupling drugs, such as alcohols and fatty acids. Most of these experimental interventions, with the exception of the external-loop-specific oligopeptides,[10] produce a run down of the gap junctional conductance, g_0, which renders the quantitative correlation of a given level of reduced gap junction conductance to the corresponding propagation velocity difficult. Therefore, quantitative information about the relationship between the level of coupling and propagation velocity stems from theoretical simulations and from experiments involving genetic ablation of connexins.[7,11-13]

The relation between cell-to-cell coupling and propagation velocity θ, obtained in a computational model, is depicted in Figure 25-3A. The decrease of θ reveals two major facts. First, θ is relatively insensitive to changes in coupling resistance (square root relationship[1,2]). This theoretical result has been supported by several experimental studies. Thus, conditional knockout of Cx43, in which a small residual expression of Cx43 (~10%-15%) was observed, was associated with only moderate conduction slowing,[14] and heterozygote germline ablation of Cx43 to about 50% of normal Cx43 protein level produced a significant reduction of g_0, but no or only a small decrease in velocity.[12]

The second observation relates to the fact that very small velocities can be achieved by an extreme reduction of cell-to-cell coupling to levels of 100-fold or more. The persistence of propagation at such a level of uncoupling is explained by the increase in the safety factor, as shown in Figure 25-3A. This figure also illustrates the usefulness of the safety-factor algorithm, as formulated by equation 1, to explain changes in propagation. Decreases in gap junction conductance (g_0) will reduce local circuit current and the denominator term in equation 1. At the same time, uncoupling of cells *prevents a downstream dissipation* of local axial current (reduction of the second term in the numerator of eq. 1) and counteracts this decrease.

As a third factor, the decrease of local current flowing into the downstream membrane sites delays the subthreshold capacitive loading of the membranes and produces an almost simultaneous excitation of the cells. This marked intercellular delay underlies propagation slowing. Also, the marked contrast between the intercellular delay and the almost instantaneous cellular excitation produces the typical patterned of discontinuous saltatory conduction that follows the discontinuity in axial electrical resistance (low cytoplasmic vs. very high gap junction resistance), as depicted in Figure 25-3B.

The saltatory excitation pattern typical for uncoupled tissue is shown in Figure 25-4A. It provides an example of high resolution optical mapping of action potential upstrokes in a synthetic strand of murine ventricular myocytes with genetic ablation of Cx43. In such strands, residual coupling of less than 5% of normal is due to the presence of Cx45.[7] Action potentials recorded from cell 1 (blue) and cell 2 (red) show almost simultaneously (space-clamped) excited cells. A long delay at the cell border (~1 ms) can be observed, very similarly to the saltatory type of propagation suggested from theoretical work. The persistence of slow propagation and the absence of propagation block with more than 95% decreased cell-to-cell coupling is a consistent finding in strands synthesized from ventricular myocytes with genetic ablation of Cx43.[7]

Importantly, the behavior of the safety factor and the decrease in propagation velocity during cell-to-cell uncoupling are markedly different from the changes observed with inhibition of depolarizing membrane current. Thus, the inhibition of Na^+ inward current causes a rapid decrease in safety factor and conduction block at velocities that are an order of magnitude higher than those observed with marked uncoupling of gap junctions.[1,15] As a further consequence of cell-to-cell uncoupling, charge flowing through L-type Ca^{2+} channels is increasingly involved in propagation and, inversely, the involvement of Na^+ decreases. It is well known that conduction is driven by the inward sodium current, I_{Na}, in the normal electrical state of the atrial and the ventricular myocardium. If large delays across cell borders appear, the depolarization of a given cluster of cells (driven cells) occurs at a time when the membrane potential of the previous cluster (driver cells) is already depolarized to

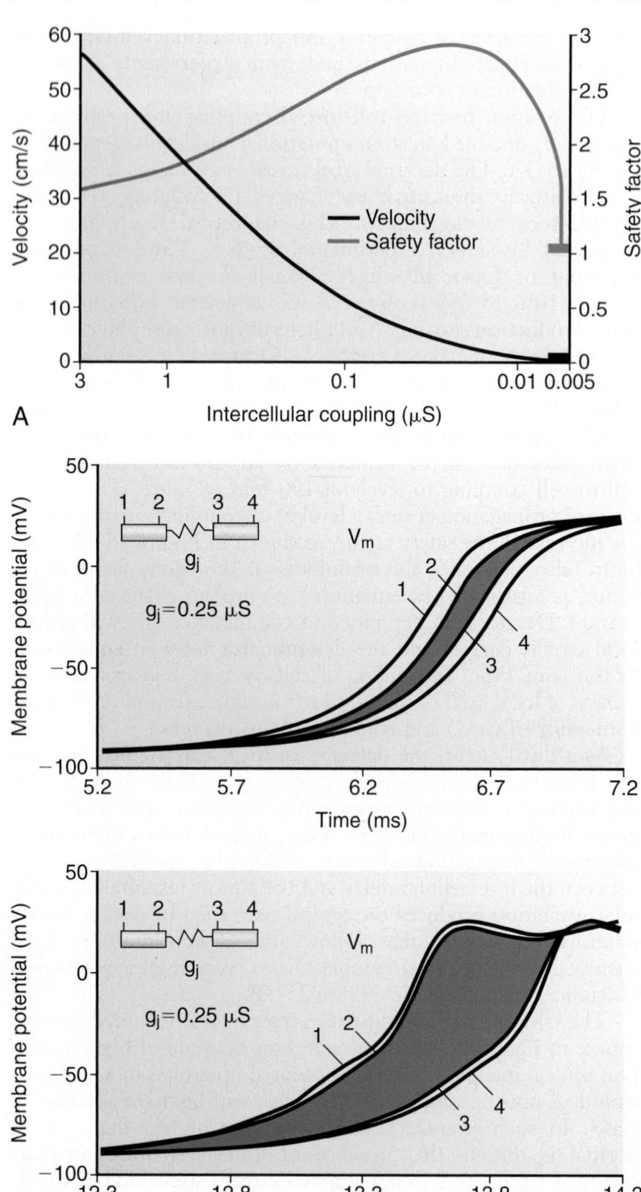

Figure 25-3 A, Simulated dependence of electrical propagation velocity *(solid line)* and safety factor *(dotted line)* on intercellular coupling. The safety factor of propagation increases with decreasing cell-to-cell coupling. A rapid decrease of the safety factor is only observed at approximately a 100-fold uncoupling. Note the logarithmic scale on the abscissa. **B,** Change of cellular excitation pattern with cell-to-cell uncoupling. *Top,* Two action potential upstrokes simulated in a upstream cell (*1* and *2*) and two action potential upstrokes simulated in the adjacent down stream cell (*3* and *4*) in a normal state of electrical coupling (gap junction conductance = 2.5 µS). *Bottom,* Two action potential upstrokes simulated in a upstream cell (*1* and *2*) and two action potential upstrokes simulated in the adjacent downstream cell (*3* and *4*) with a 10-fold decrease in cell-to-cell coupling (gap junction conductance = 0.25 µS). Note that the conduction delay has decreased within the cells and increased between the cells following cell-to-cell uncoupling. (Reproduced from Shaw RM, Rudy Y: Ionic mechanisms of propagation in cardiac tissue. Roles of the sodium and L-type calcium currents during reduced excitability and decreased gap junction coupling. Circ Res 81(5):727-741, 1997.)

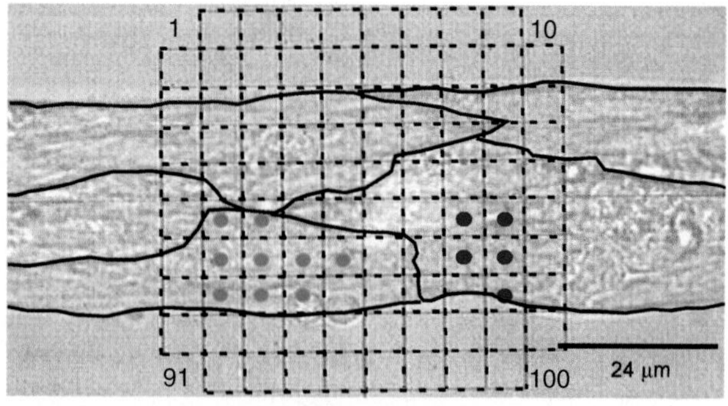

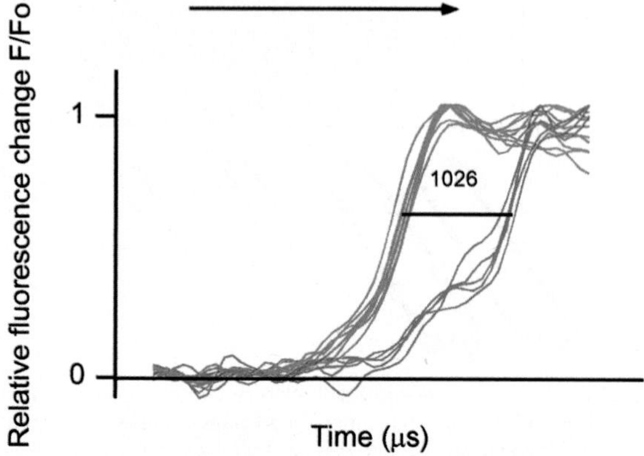

Figure 25-4 Effect of germline connexin43 (Cx43) ablation on propagation in a synthetic strand of murine neonatal ventricular myocytes. *Top,* Image of a synthetic murine strand showing outlined cell borders and position of light-sensitive diodes in an upstream *(red)* and downstream *(blue)* cell. *Bottom,* Action potential upstrokes showing a typical excitation pattern with almost simultaneous excitation of the two cells and a long (1026 ms) excitation delay at the cell border. The degree of uncoupling caused by genetic Cx43 ablation was >95%, the decrease in macroscopic velocity was approximately 25-fold. (Reproduced from Beauchamp P, Choby C, Desplantez T, et al: Electrical propagation in synthetic ventricular myocyte strands from germline connexin43 knockout mice. Circ Res 95[2]:170-178, 2004.)

its plateau level. As a consequence, the L-type Ca^{2+} current, I_{CaL}, carries the main charge responsible for the depolarization of the downstream cluster to the main extent. This switch from Na^{+}-dependent to Ca^{2+}-dependent conduction was shown in theoretical studies by Joyner and colleagues[16] and Shaw and Rudy[4] and has been experimentally demonstrated for the analogous situation in macroscopic discontinuities. The local delay required for I_{CaL} to become the dominant charge carrier amounts to approximately 2 ms.[17]

Field Effect Propagation of the Cardiac Impulse

In the 1950s and 1960s, when the functional role of intercalated disks as electrical low-resistance cell-to-cell junctions was experimentally defined,[18] the hypothesis of transmission of the electrical impulse by an "electrical field mechanism" (i.e., cell-to-cell transmission in the absence of electrical coupling by open connexin channels) was put forward by Sperelakis[19] as an alternative mechanism to explain gap junction channel-dependent propagation. The principle of this mechanism is based on the assumption of a very high electrical

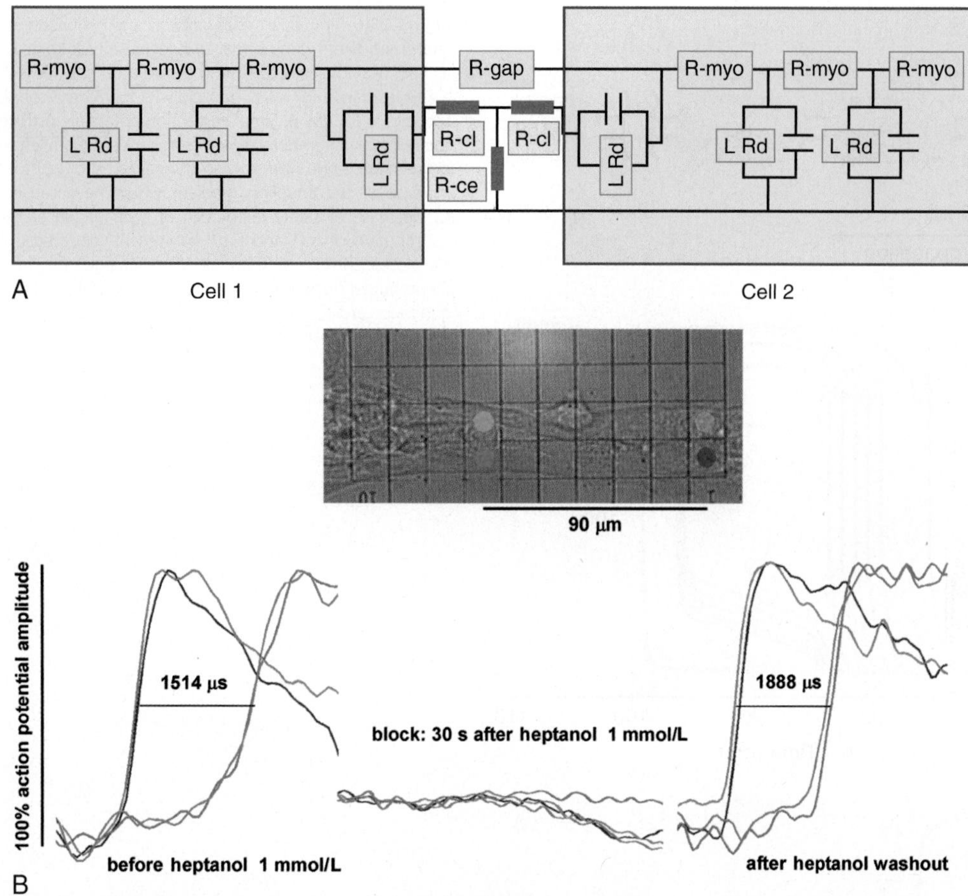

Figure 25-5 Is field effect transmission of the electrical impulse possible in cardiac tissue? **A,** Electrical equivalent circuit taken to simulate field effect transmission. The circuit represents two cells, each consisting of myoplasmic resistances *(R-myo)* and circuit elements simulating the behavior of the surface cell membrane (*L Rd* elements in parallel with membrane capacitance). The cell-to-cell interface is simulated, in addition to the usual gap junction resistance, *R-gap*, by L Rd elements that are linked to a resistance of the intercellular cleft *(R-cl)*. In turn, R-cl is connected to the extracellular space by a resistance *R-ce*. (Modified from Kucera JP, Rohr S, Rudy Y: Localization of sodium channels in intercalated disks modulates cardiac conduction. Circ Res 91[12]:1176-1182, 2002.) **B,** Total uncoupling of gap junction resistance produces conduction block in cultured synthetic strands of murine neonatal ventricular myocytes. *Top*, Measurement of action potential upstrokes in an upstream cell *(red, blue)* and a downstream cell *(green, light blue)*. *Bottom*, Action potential upstrokes before application *(left part)*, during application (after 30 sec, *middle part*), and after washout *(right part)* of heptanol (1 mmol) in a strand composed of connexin re (Cx43)- ablated myocytes. Genetic ablation produces a large intercellular conduction delay *(left and right parts)* that is due to the presence of Cx45 (not shown). Application of the uncoupling agent heptanol produces immediate propagation block, indicating absence of field effect transmission in this condition. (Reproduced from Beauchamp P, Choby C, Desplantez T, et al: Electrical propagation in synthetic ventricular myocyte strands from germline connexin43 knockout mice. Circ Res 95[2]:170-178, 2004.)

resistance in the intercellular clefts and between the intercellular cleft and the remainder of the extracellular space (see Fig. 25-5A). In such a case, the voltage divider formed by these resistances can increase the voltage of the downstream cells to threshold of excitation and thus produce propagation without current flow through gap junction channels.

A theoretical study suggested that the conditions at which field effect transmission in heart can occur are restricted with respect to localized distribution of Na^+ channels and assumptions about the resistive properties of the intercalated disk.[20] In this theoretical study, the Na^+ channels driving electrical field transmission had to be almost exclusively clustered at the intercalated disk. However, the presence of Na^+ channels has been described also in T-tubules.[21,22] Furthermore, electrical field transmission occurred within a limited range of cleft resistances if the extracellular resistance was neglected. In the myocardium in vivo, the high resistance of the extracellular space remote from the cell-to-cell junctions[23] is predicted to counteract the effect of the high resistance in the intercalated disk. In synthetic strands of ventricular myocytes with genetic ablation of Cx43, application of a gap junction blocker produced immediate conduction block and excluded the existence of field affect transmission in this experimental model (see Figure 25-5B).

Uniform versus Nonuniform Cell-to-Cell Coupling

Electrical propagation in the heart may be nonuniform in several respects. First, normal cardiac structures contain discontinuities in tissue geometry. Such sites produce source-to-sink mismatch, a mismatch between the amount of upstream tissue that has to produce the excitatory current and the amount of downstream tissue. Second, the mismatch can involve a boundary between zones of different degrees in cell-to-cell coupling. Both types of

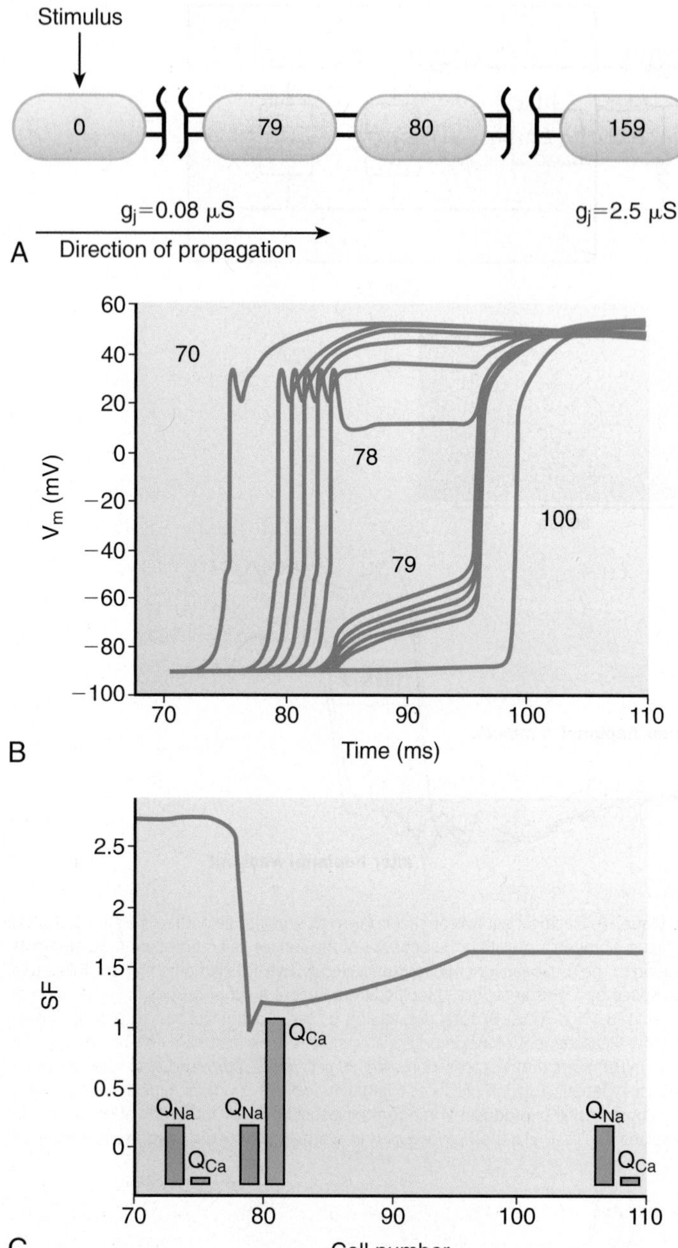

Figure 25-6 Simulation of asymmetrical propagation at a boundary between strand segments with normal and decreased cell-to-cell coupling. **A,** Sketch of a chain of single cells consisting of two segments. Cells 0 to 78 are coupled by a low resistance (g_j = 0.08 μS); cells 79 to 159 are coupled by a normal resistance (g_j = 2.5 μS). **B,** Simulated action potential upstrokes in cells denoted by the respective numbers, showing propagation from left to right. Note the large delay at transition from low to normal levels of cell-to-cell coupling (a slight increase of the coupling gradient would have caused propagation block). **C,** Decrease of safety factor (SF) of propagation at the transition site, and contribution of Na^+ and Ca^{2+} movement *(black bars)* to propagation. Note the localized contribution of Ca^{2+} charge, Q_{Ca}, at the transition site. (Reproduced from Wang Y, Rudy Y: Action potential propagation in inhomogeneous cardiac tissue: Safety factor considerations and ionic mechanism. Am J Physiol Heart Circ Physiol 278[4]:H1019-H1029, 2000.)

discontinuities are known to occur in the normal heart[2] and may be amplified in cardiac disease.

Theoretical work suggests that the biophysical laws that govern propagation at a site of mismatch in tissue geometry or cell-to-cell coupling are very similar for both of these types, and numerous theoretical and experimental studies have been published on geometrical mismatch.[2] The effect of mismatch due to heterogeneity in cell-to-cell coupling is illustrated in Figure 25-6.[24] In this situation, propagation is depicted at the boundary between two segments of a simulated cardiac strand with low (left segment) and normal (right segment) cell-to-cell coupling. The marked conduction delay observed at the boundary (followed by propagation block if the gradient in coupling is made slightly larger) is due to the relatively low local current density produced by the upstream elements with lower cell-to-cell coupling. In other words, the gradient in cell-to-cell coupling causes a mismatch between electrotonic current produced upstream (source) and the downstream load (sinks).

Comparing the mechanism of development of unidirectional block, as illustrated in Figure 25-6, with the situation of ubiquitous uncoupling (Fig. 25-4), reveals an important difference. Ubiquitous cell-to-cell uncoupling is resistant against the development of propagation block due to the continuous recurrence of high-resistance cell-to-cell junctions, while interfaces between regions of cells with different degrees of coupling produce unidirectional block. Transition from bidirectional propagation to unidirectional block, as shown in Figure 25-6, occurs at a boundary showing an approximately 10-fold change in coupling, while at least 100-fold increase of gap junction conductance is required for production of very slow conduction and block in ubiquitous

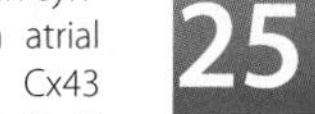

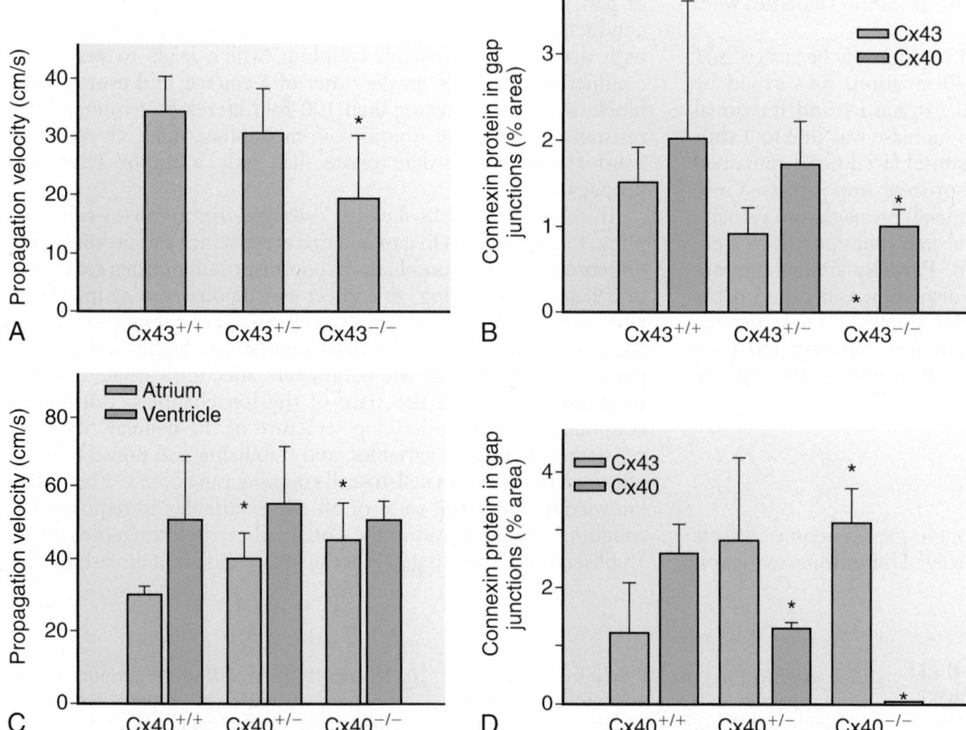

Figure 25-7 Complex effects of coexpressed connexin (Cx) 43 and Cx40 in synthetic atrial strands. **A**, Change in atrial propagation velocity with genetic Cx43 ablation. **B**, Changes in Cx43 and Cx40 signal in gap junctions with genetic Cx43 ablation. **C**, Change in atrial and ventricular propagation velocity with genetic Cx40 ablation. **D**, Changes in Cx43 and Cx40 signal in gap junctions with genetic Cx40 ablation. (Reproduced from reference Beauchamp P, Yamada KA, Baertschi AJ, et al: Relative contributions of connexins 40 and 43 to atrial impulse propagation in synthetic strands of neonatal and fetal murine cardiomyocytes. Circ Res 99[11]: 1216-1224, 2006.)

uncoupling. A similarly high sensitivity of unidirectional block to uncoupling has been observed at geometrical tissue discontinuities.[25]

Evidence that heterogeneity of cell-to-cell uncoupling is associated with propagation disturbances was provided by studies using various types of conditional cardiospecific genetic ablation of Cx43.[26-28] Danik and colleagues produced mice that are born with a normal phenotype, start to develop lethal arrhythmias by approximately 5 to 7 weeks of age, and die within of approximately 7 months. Within the same time frame, these mice develop nonuniform ablation of Cx43 in the ventricles, suggesting an important role for heterogeneity in connexin expression in arrhythmogenesis.

The Role of Coexpression of Connexins43, 45, and 40 in Ventricular and Atrial Propagation

Cardiac murine myocardium expresses four types of connexins: Cx43, Cx45, Cx40, and Cx30.12. Ventricular working myocardium expresses Cx43 and Cx45, whereas Cx43, Cx40, and Cx45 are detectable in atrial myocardium. Gradients in expression of connexins have been described between right and left atrial tissue and within ventricular myocardium.[29] Cx43 and Cx40 are connexins with a relatively large single channel conductance, and Cx45 has a small single channel conductance.[30]

The fact that connexin molecules with different biophysical properties are coexpressed in the same cell junction raises questions about whether heteromeric and heterotypic gap junction channels are formed in the heart, and about the general functional significance of such channels. Although such channels have been produced in artificial cell lines, the role of such channels in cardiac tissue has not been fully elucidated. In ventricular myocardium, the dominating role of Cx43 is generally acknowledged, whereas the role of Cx45 is still largely unclear. Ablation of Cx43 of approximately 90% in conditional knockout mice leads to marked conduction slowing, and full germline ablation of Cx43 leads to very slow propagation caused by small residual levels of Cx45 (see Fig. 25-4). Upregulation of Cx45 might play an important role in heart failure.[31] Also, Cx45 might modulate intercellular exchange of small regulatory molecules or mediate signals to cell junctions.

In atrial myocardium, the role of coexistence of Cx43 and Cx40 seems more complex and more controversial. Atrial tissue shows a large spectrum of propagation velocities, ranging from at least 1 m/sec in the crista terminalis and the Bachmann's bundle to approximately 0.2 m/sec in the trabeculated appendages,[1] and the possibility that the relative expression levels of these connexins plays a role in modulating atrial velocity has to be taken into consideration. Measurements of propagation velocity in whole atria of Cx40 knockout mice have produced controversial results. In the first reports, a decrease of propagation velocity was demonstrated. Subsequently, it was shown that ablation of Cx40 did not significantly change the duration of atrial excitation and produced local conduction slowing only at circumscribed sites in the right atrium.[13]

One reason for these discrepancies may be that Cx40 ablation is accompanied by malformations that might affect macroscopic measurements of propagation.[32] Work carried out in human atria suggests that atrial propagation velocity is determined by a balance between Cx40 and Cx43 coexpression.[33] A high level of Cx40 relative to Cx43 was associated with a decrease in atrial propagation velocity, whereas the opposite, an increased expression of Cx43 relative to Cx40, was associated with an increase in propagation velocity. These findings are supported by recent experiments carried out in synthetic strands of neonatal cardiac myocytes. Thus, germline ablation of Cx40 produced an upregulation of propagation velocity, as shown in Figure 25-7C, to a level where atrial and ventricular propagation velocities were not significantly different.

Part of this seemingly paradoxical finding was because Cx43 in gap junctions increased with Cx40 ablation. As verified by immunohistochemistry, TritonX-100 extraction, and fractional Western blotting, at least part of this increase was due to a shift of Cx43 to the cell junctions, whereas total atrial Cx43 remained unchanged. With Cx43 ablation, a process opposite to Cx40 ablation took place, inamely both atrial propagation velocity and the amount of Cx40 in the atrial gap junctions decreased, as illustrated in Figures 25-7A and B. Partially similar interactions between Cx40 and Cx43 were also shown in experiments using Cx43- and Cx40-transfected HeLa cells.[34] These experiments illustrate the complexities of connexin biology and their impact on cardiac electrical cell-to-cell coupling and on the regional variability in propagation.

Summary

Electrical cell-to-cell coupling through gap junctions affects impulse propagation in a complex way. Ubiquitous reduction of gap junctional conductance in uniform structures decreases conduction velocity. The safety factor for propagation increases with decreased cell-to-cell coupling, which leads to very slow conduction velocities on the order of 1 cm/sec, and propagation block occurs at a greater than 100-fold increase of intercellular resistance. Moderate ubiquitous uncoupling, such as reported from remodeled cardiac tissue, has only a minor effect on propagation.

In cellular networks showing *heterogeneities* in cell-to-cell coupling, local gradients in gap junctional resistance can produce unidirectional conduction block. In contrast to ubiquitous reduction in cell-to-cell coupling, this effect can be observed at interfaces with more moderate gradients in cell-to-cell coupling (~10-fold), suggesting that such local heterogeneities are highly arrhythmogenic. Importantly, all the parameters affecting cardiac impulse propagation, such as the state of the ion channels, cell-to-cell coupling, and the underlying structure of the cellular network, represent interacting variables, and stabilizing and nonstabilizing effects of reduction in cell-to-cell coupling can coexist. Therefore, knowledge about the state of all these variables is required for weighing and interpreting the potentially arrhythmogenic role of an observed change in gap junction expression in a diseased state.

References

1. Kléber AG, Janse MJ, Fast VG: Normal and abnormal conduction in the heart. In Page E, Fozzard HA, Solaro J (eds): Handbook of Physiology: The Cardiovascular System: The Heart. New York, Oxford University Press, 2002, pp 455-530.
2. Kléber AG, Rudy Y: Basic mechanisms of cardiac impulse propagation and associated arrhythmias. Physiol Rev 84(2):431-488, 2004.
3. Fast VG, Kléber AG: Microscopic conduction in cultured strands of neonatal rat heart cells measured with voltage-sensitive dyes. Circ Res 73(5):914-925, 1993.
4. Shaw RM, Rudy Y: Ionic mechanisms of propagation in cardiac tissue. Roles of the sodium and L-type calcium currents during reduced excitability and decreased gap junction coupling. Circ Res 81(5):727-741, 1997.
5. Spach MS, Heidlage JF, Dolber PC, Barr RC: Electrophysiological effects of remodeling cardiac gap junctions and cell size: experimental and model studies of normal cardiac growth. Circ Res 86(3):302-311, 2000.
6. Hoyt RH, Cohen ML, Saffitz JE: Distribution and three-dimensional structure of intercellular junctions in canine myocardium. Circ Res 64:563-574, 1989.
7. Beauchamp P, Choby C, Desplantez T, et al: Electrical propagation in synthetic ventricular myocyte strands from germline connexin43 knockout mice. Circ Res 95(2):170-178, 2004.
8. Peters NS, Coromilas J, Severs NJ, Wit AL: Disturbed connexin43 gap junction distribution correlates with the location of reentrant circuits in the epicardial border zone of healing canine infarcts that cause ventricular tachycardia. Circulation 95(4):988-996, 1997.
9. Fast VG, Kléber AG: Anisotropic conduction in monolayers of neonatal rat heart cells cultured on collagen substrate. Circ Res 75(3):591-595, 1994.
10. Kwak BR, Jongsma HJ: Selective inhibition of gap junction channel activity by synthetic peptides. J Physiol 516(Pt 3):679-685, 1999.
11. Thomas SP, Bircher-Lehmann L, Thomas SA, et al: Synthetic strands of neonatal mouse cardiac myocytes: structural and electrophysiological properties. Circ Res 87(6):467-473, 2000.
12. Thomas SP, Kucera JP, Bircher-Lehmann L, et al: Impulse propagation in synthetic strands of neonatal cardiac myocytes with genetically reduced levels of connexin43. Circ Res 92(11):1209-1216, 2003.
13. Beauchamp P, Yamada KA, Baertschi AJ, et al: Relative contributions of connexins 40 and 43 to atrial impulse propagation in synthetic strands of neonatal and fetal murine cardiomyocytes. Circ Res 99(11):1216-1224, 2006.
14. Gutstein DE, Morley GE, Tamaddon H, et al: Conduction slowing and sudden arrhythmic death in mice with cardiac-restricted inactivation of connexin43. Circ Res 88(3):333-339, 2001.
15. Rohr S, Kucera JP, Kléber AG: Slow conduction in cardiac tissue: I. Effects of a reduction of excitability vs. a reduction in cell-to-cell coupling on microconduction. Circ Res 83:781-794, 1998.
16. Joyner RW, Kumar R, Wilders R, et al: Modulating L-type calcium current affects discontinuous cardiac action potential conduction. Biophys J 71(1):237-245, 1996.
17. Rohr S, Kucera J: Involvement of the calcium inward current in cardiac impulse propagation: induction of unidirectional conduction block by nifedipine and reversal by Bay K 8644. Biophys J 72(2 Pt 1): 754-766, 1997.
18. Weidmann S: The diffusion of radiopotassium across intercalated disks of mammalian cardiac muscle. J Physiol (London) 187:323-342, 1966.
19. Sperelakis N, Hoshiko T: Electrical impedance of cardiac muscle. Circ Res 9: 1280-1283, 1961.
20. Kucera JP, Rohr S, Rudy Y: Localization of sodium channels in intercalated disks modulates cardiac conduction. Circ Res 91(12):1176-1182, 2002.
21. Brette F, Orchard CH: No apparent requirement for neuronal sodium channels in excitation-contraction coupling in rat ventricular myocytes. Circ Res 98(5): 667-674, 2006.
22. Maier SK, Westenbroek RE, Schenkman KA, et al: An unexpected role for brain-type sodium channels in coupling of cell surface depolarization to contraction in the heart. Proc Natl Acad Sci U S A 99(6):4073-4078, 2002.
23. Kléber AG, Riegger CB: Electrical constants of arterially perfused rabbit papillary muscle. J Physiol (London) 385:307-324, 1987.
24. Wang Y, Rudy Y: Action potential propagation in inhomogeneous cardiac tissue: Safety factor considerations and ionic mechanism. Am J Physiol Heart Circ Physiol 278(4):H1019-H1029, 2000.
25. Fast VG, Kléber AG: Block of impulse propagation at an abrupt tissue expansion: Evaluation of the critical strand diameter in 2- and 3-dimensional computer models. Cardiovasc Res 30:449-459, 1995.
26. Gutstein DE, Morley GE, Vaidya D, et al: Heterogeneous expression of gap junction channels in the heart leads to conduction defects and ventricular dysfunction. Circulation 104(10):1194-1199, 2001.
27. Danik SB, Liu F, Zhang J, et al: Modulation of cardiac gap junction expression and arrhythmic susceptibility. Circ Res 95(10):1035-1041, 2004.
28. Gutstein DE, Danik SB, Lewitton S, et al: Focal gap junction uncoupling and spontaneous ventricular ectopy. Am J Physiol Heart Circ Physiol 289(3):H1091-H1098, 2005.
29. Vozzi C, Dupont E, Coppen SR, et al: Chamber-related differences in connexin expression in the human heart. J Mol Cell Cardiol 31(5):991-1003, 1999.

30. Harris AL: Emerging issues of connexin channels: Biophysics fills the gap. Q Rev Biophys 34(3):325-472, 2001.
31. Yamada KA, Rogers JG, Sundset R, et al: Up-regulation of connexin45 in heart failure. J Cardiovasc Electrophysiol 14(11):1205-1212, 2003.
32. Gu H, Smith FC, Taffet SM, Delmar M: High incidence of cardiac malformations in connexin40-deficient mice. Circ Res 93(3):201-206, 2003.
33. Kanagaratnam P, Rothery S, Patel P, et al: Relative expression of immunolocalized connexins 40 and 43 correlates with human atrial conduction properties. J Am Coll Cardiol 39(1):116-123, 2002.
34. Valiunas V, Gemel J, Brink PR, Beyer EC: Gap junction channels formed by coexpressed connexin40 and connexin43. Am J Physiol Heart Circ Physiol 281(4): H1675-H1689, 2001.

Cardiac Myofibroblasts and Arrhythmogenesis 26

Stephan Rohr and Michele Miragoli

CHAPTER OUTLINE

A variety of pathologic conditions including pressure overload, volume overload, and infarction induce structural remodeling of the heart, which can lead to heart failure and cardiac arrhythmias.[1,2] Clinically, structural remodeling is characterized by changes in the shape, size, and function of the heart. These changes are based on diverse and complex cellular reactions to injury and involve cardiomyocytes and noncardiac cells. Histopathologically, remodeling typically involves cardiomyocyte hypertrophy, activation and proliferation of fibroblasts, increased extracellular matrix deposition, and cell death.[3] Functionally, structural remodeling induces mechanical dysfunction and is accompanied by an increased likelihood of occurrence of life-threatening cardiac arrhythmias.[1]

Arrhythmogenic mechanisms in structurally remodeled hearts can be divided into mechanisms related to altered electrophysiologic properties of the cardiomyocytes (electrical remodeling) and mechanisms related to remodeling of the extracellular matrix (fibrotic remodeling). Electrical remodeling affects a large number of ion channels, exchangers, and calcium-handling proteins and ultimately predisposes the heart to arrhythmias by inducing activity triggered by calcium overload or by causing dispersion of repolarization and thereby enabling reentrant electrical activity.[1,4] Connexin redistribution as observed in remodeled tissue following infarction affects impulse propagation and predisposes the heart to arrhythmias.[5] Fibrotic remodeling, in turn, favors the initiation and perpetuation of arrhythmias by the presence of collagenous septa that separate bundles of cardiomyocytes over substantial distances, thus inducing structural discontinuities at the cellular level.[6,7]

Based on the tenet that fibrotic laminae act as electrical insulators that induce interstitial resistive discontinuities, the spread of electrical activity under these conditions is impeded and results in nonuniform conduction[7,8] or zigzag activation of the myocardium.[9] Both of these conditions induce slow conduction and conduction blocks, which are key ingredients of arrhythmogenesis. All of these important and well-established arrhythmogenic mechanisms in structurally remodeled myocardia are *cardiomyocyte centered* in the sense that they concern either adverse changes in active membrane properties of the cardiomyocytes (electrical remodeling) or changes in their passive electrical properties (altered three-dimensional [3D] organization of cardiomyocytes; extent and topography of gap junctional coupling). But what about fibroblasts?

The Swiss National Science Foundation (grant #320000-118247) and the Swiss University Conference (Heart Remodeling in Health and Disease project) support this research.

Fibroblasts and Myofibroblasts in the Working Myocardium

The normal myocardium is composed of fibroblasts, cardiomyocytes, vascular smooth muscle cells, endothelial cells, and nerve cells. This somewhat unorthodox sequence of cell types reflects, in descending order, their relative numbers in the myocardium. As an example, it has been shown using fluorescence-activated cell sorting that adult rat ventricular tissue is mainly composed of fibroblasts (64%) and cardiomyocytes (30%), with the remaining 6% consisting of other cell types.[10] Similar relative abundances have been reported for normal human hearts, where fibroblasts were shown to outnumber cardiomyocytes by a factor of about two to three while occupying about 20% of the volume of the working myocardium.[11,12]

Functionally, interstitial fibroblasts are of central importance for the structural integrity of the myocardium because they are responsible for the production and maintenance of the extracellular matrix. This matrix consists of a complex 3D network of fibrillar collagen and elastin, which serves as a scaffold for cardiomyocytes and integrates contractile forces to result in an efficient pump function of the entire organ. The fibrillar network is subjected to a continuous and substantial turnover that can amount up to approximately 5% per day.[13] Under physiologic conditions, tight control of formation and degradation of fibrillar collagen by fibroblasts is therefore of utmost importance in order to maintain the structural and functional integrity of the myocardium over time. In addition to this central role in cardiac structure, fibroblasts are thought to be involved in the function of the sinoatrial node where there is evidence that they establish heterocellular gap-junctional coupling with cardiomyocytes in situ.[14] Being an ongoing research field on its own, the effects of fibroblasts on sinoatrial nodal function are not further discussed in this chapter.

In contrast to fibroblasts, myofibroblasts are not normally present in healthy hearts, with the exception of valve leaflets.[15] Myofibroblasts were first described by Gabbiani and coworkers as fibroblastic cells located within granulation tissue of skin wounds, where they initiate contraction of the granulation tissue and disappear thereafter by programmed cell death.[16,17] Myofibroblasts express several smooth muscle cell markers,

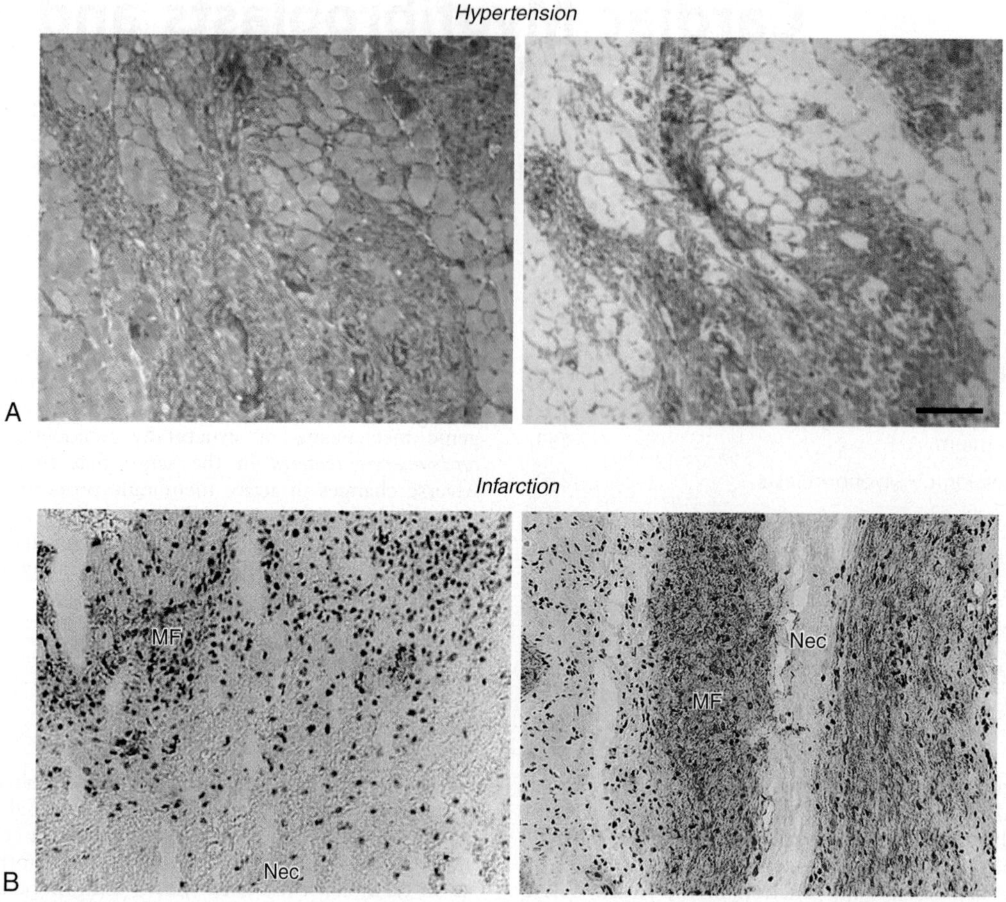

Figure 26-1 Presence of myofibroblasts in fibrotic and infarcted hearts. **A,** Adjacent sections of fibrotic myocardium of rats with renin-dependent hypertension are stained with Masson's trichrome (*left;* collagen = blue) and with antibodies against α–smooth muscle actin to identify myofibroblasts (*right*). Bar = 50 μm. (Modified from Clement S, Chaponnier C, Gabbiani G: A subpopulation of cardiomyocytes expressing α-skeletal actin is identified by a specific polyclonal antibody. Circ Res 85:51e-58e, 1999, with permission.) **B,** Sections of infarcted rat myocardium labeled for α–smooth muscle actin. Myofibroblasts (MF) appear at the border of necrotic tissue (Nec) after 3 days (*left*) and substantially proliferate thereafter (*right;* 2 weeks) (×400). (Modified from Sun Y, Weber KT: Angiotensin converting enzyme and myofibroblasts during tissue repair in the rat heart. J Mol Cell Cardiol 28:851-858, 1996, with permission.)

among which α–smooth muscle actin (α-SMA) is considered to be the most reliable immunocytochemical marker.[18,19] The incorporation of α-SMA into newly formed stress fibers permits myofibroblasts to develop tensile forces that ultimately lead to the development of fibrocontractive diseases such as renal, hepatic, and cardiac fibrosis as well as asthma-related airway remodeling.[20] Apart from synthesizing extracellular matrix components and exerting mechanical forces, myofibroblasts also exhibit a broad range of paracrine activities. In a review by Powell and colleagues, intestinal myofibroblasts were reported to produce cytokines (four types), growth factors (12 types), chemokines (seven types) and mediators of inflammation (eight types). The secretion of these 31 substances is paralleled by an equally impressive repertoire of at least 25 different receptors for partly the same as well as other humoral factors.[21]

Whereas myofibroblasts are not normally present in the working myocardium, this situation changes drastically in the context of pathologic heart conditions like pressure overload and infarction. In both instances, myofibroblasts appear in large numbers in the myocardium, where they are thought to contribute importantly to the establishment of fibrosis.[22,23] In animal models of pressure overload, it was shown that early inflammatory changes are followed by myofibroblast proliferation (within days) and the subsequent development of perivascular and interstitial fibrosis (Figure 26-1A).[24-27] Similarly, at sites of myocardial infarctions, myofibroblasts appear in large numbers a few days after the ischemic event (Figure 26-1B) and locally persist for many years due to incomplete apoptosis.[28-32] In infarcts, myofibroblasts are crucially involved in the initial scar formation and the continuous rebuilding of the scar thereafter.[33] Although the exact origin of myofibroblasts is still not entirely clear (circulating or resident adventitial or interstitial fibroblasts undergoing a phenotype switch to myofibroblasts, circulating bone marrow–derived progenitor cells),[33-35] there is ample evidence that their appearance is triggered by local inflammatory reactions, mechanical stress, and humoral factors.[34-38] Among the humoral factors, induction of myofibroblasts is triggered in particular by transforming growth factor (TGF)-β_1, but other humoral factors such as basic fibroblast growth factor (bFGF/FGF-2), angiotensin II, catecholamines, and insulin-like growth factor-1 (IGF-1) are involved in the determination of phenotype and function of cardiac fibroblasts as well.[38]

Connexin Expression by Myofibroblasts

Expression of connexins is a well-established feature of myofibroblasts[39] that has been found in a variety of tissues such as suburothelial tissue,[40] intestine,[41] breast cancer stroma,[42] and healing skin wounds.[43] In these tissues, myofibroblasts form a 3D network of cells communicating with each other via gap junctions.

In the intact heart, investigations of connexin expression by connective tissue cells within the working myocardium are scarce and mostly concern the question whether fibroblasts in healthy tissue establish homocellular gap junctional coupling among themselves, or heterocellular gap junctional coupling with cardiomyocytes, or both. In this regard, recent immunocytochemical studies produced controversial results. One study showed homo-and heterocellular connexin expression by fibroblasts in neonatal rat ventricles (Cx43 and Cx45),[44] but another investigation performed with sheep ventricular tissue found no immunocytochemical evidence for Cx43 expression by fibroblasts in the myocardium.[45] Interestingly, however, the latter study reported that fibroblasts residing in infarct scars show abundant expression of Cx43 and Cx45.[45] By combining this finding with the results of other immunohistochemical studies showing that fibroblasts in infarct scars are in fact myofibroblasts,[29,31] the interesting perspective emerges that the connexin-expressing fibroblasts observed in infarct scars in the former study were in fact connexin-expressing *myo*fibroblasts. This interpretation would be in line with observations in other tissues mentioned earlier, where it was found that myofibroblasts form homocellular gap junctions.

But what about heterocellular coupling of myofibroblasts to cardiomyocytes? Whereas comprehensive studies dedicated specifically to this question are not yet available, an immunohistologic study of infarcts in rat ventricles has shown that cardiomyocytes bordering the infarcted area formed tentacle-like extensions that seemed to end blind but that displayed extensive Cx43 labeling.[46] Whether these Cx43-decorated tentacles belong to regions where cardiomyocytes establish gap junctional coupling with noncardiomyocytes in the infarct zone, correspond to newly formed hemichannels, or are remnants of earlier intercalated disks was not further investigated in that study. Nevertheless, it is tempting to speculate that these sites might correspond to gap-junctional contact sites between border-zone cardiomyocytes and myofibroblasts within the infarct.

In contrast to the still-open question of gap junctional myofibroblast-to-cardiomyocyte coupling in diseased cardiac tissue in vivo, cardiac myofibroblasts in vitro readily establish gap junctional contacts both among themselves and with neighboring cardiomyocytes. In cell culture, fibroblasts isolated from healthy neonatal rat ventricles undergo a rapid phenotype switch to α-SMA–expressing myofibroblasts as illustrated in Figure 26-2. In addition to α-SMA, these cells also express vimentin but generally not desmin (VA-type myofibroblasts). The phenotype switch from fibroblasts to myofibroblasts was shown to be elicited by, for example, mechanical stress imposed on the fibroblasts by rigid culture substrates,[47] and it is triggered by humoral factors like TGF-β_1.[48] As shown in Figure 26-3, cultured myofibroblasts of cardiac origin express both Cx43 and Cx45,[49] which is identical to the profile of connexins expressed by connective tissue cells within infarcts in sheep ventricle.[45]

The connexins are targeted to both homocellular contact sites and to regions of heterocellular contact between myofibroblasts and cardiomyocytes. Typically, the connexin staining has a fine-punctate appearance. This suggests that myofibroblasts form relatively small gap junctions comprising only a few channels. If, also in vivo, myofibroblasts form small gap junctions or if gap junctional channels exist in dispersed form, this might contribute to the explanation why there are as yet no electron-microscopic evidence of homo- or heterocellular coupling of myofibroblasts in intact cardiac tissue, because such a distribution possibly escapes electron-microscopic detection.[50]

Given that myofibroblasts are capable of establishing gap junctional coupling both among themselves and with cardiomyocytes in vitro, the question arises whether and to what extent such coupling might influence cardiac electrophysiology. Unfortunately, investigations of this question in vivo are hampered by severe methodologic difficulties. Apart from problems in visualizing myofibroblasts in intact tissue with the purpose, for example, to perform patch clamp recordings, the electrophysiologic signature of myofibroblasts in vivo would be different from cardiomyocytes only if they were not coupled by gap junctions. Upon coupling, electrotonic current flow would force their membrane potential to closely follow the dynamic fluctuations in membrane potentials of the neighboring cardiomyocytes, therefore rendering a differentiation between myofibroblast signal and cardiomyocyte signal difficult.[51]

The complex and variable cellular microarchitecture of structurally remodeled myocardium in vivo precludes a systematic investigation of structure-function relationships between cardiomyocytes and myofibroblasts with currently available experimental approaches. Because of these difficulties, systematic studies aimed at characterizing the influence of myofibroblasts on cardiomyocyte electrophysiology have so far been limited to in vitro experimental systems. These systems have the distinct advantage that the two cell types can be clearly identified and that spatial interactions between cardiomyocytes and myofibroblasts can be reproducibly controlled using patterned growth techniques as outlined in more detail later.[52]

Myofibroblasts Reestablish Conduction in Severed Cardiac Tissue

Previous studies in patients with donor hearts have shown that electrical activity between recipient and donor tissue can undergo synchronization even though they are separated by scar tissue.[53] This raised the question whether connective tissue cells of the scar might possibly serve as conductors for excitatory current flow between donor and recipient cardiac tissue.

We investigated this hypothesis in vitro by establishing a tissue model of the scar region of transplanted heart as illustrated in Figure 26-4A. The model consisted of strands of cultured ventricular cardiomyocytes that were interrupted over defined distances by inserts consisting of myofibroblasts.[54] The preparations were stained with voltage sensitive dyes, and, following extracellular stimulation, impulse propagation across the myofibroblast insert was monitored with an array of photodetectors at high spatiotemporal resolution. A typical example of such an experiment is shown in Figure 26-4B. Action potential upstrokes along the preparation were monophasic in the regions of cardiomyocytes. Along the 130-μm-long insert consisting of myofibroblasts, upstrokes were biphasic, with the first rapid component being due to electrotonic current flow from the proximal cardiomyocyte segment and the second rapid component being evoked by electrotonic current flow from the distal cardiomyocyte segment that was activated with a delay. Delays, which amounted to approximately 30 ms in this particular example, were positively correlated to insert lengths up to 300 μm (Figure 26-4C). At lengths greater than 300 μm, myofibroblasts failed to sustain conduction. Similar to myofibroblasts, electrical synchronization between cardiomyocyte strands was also supported by Cx43-transfected HeLa cells but not by communication-deficient HeLa wild-type cells. This indicates that not the cell type per se but its ability to establish heterocellular gap-junctional coupling was essential for the nonexcitable myofibroblasts to support impulse transmission.

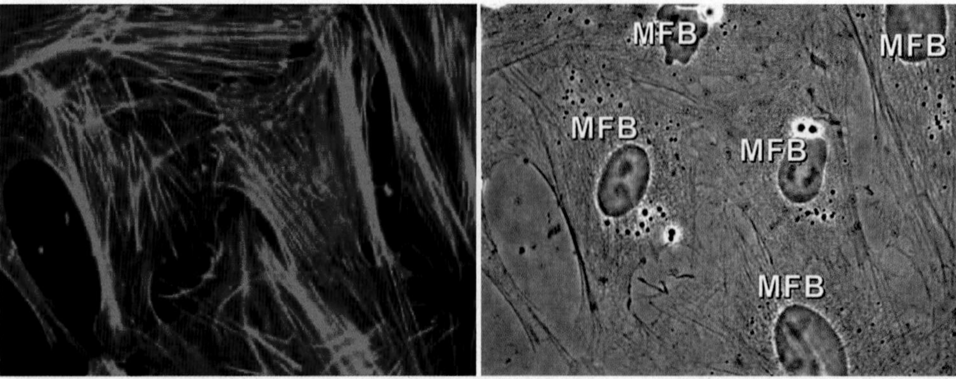

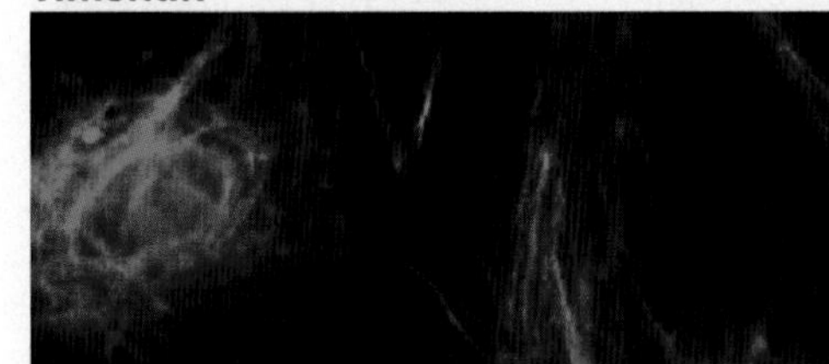

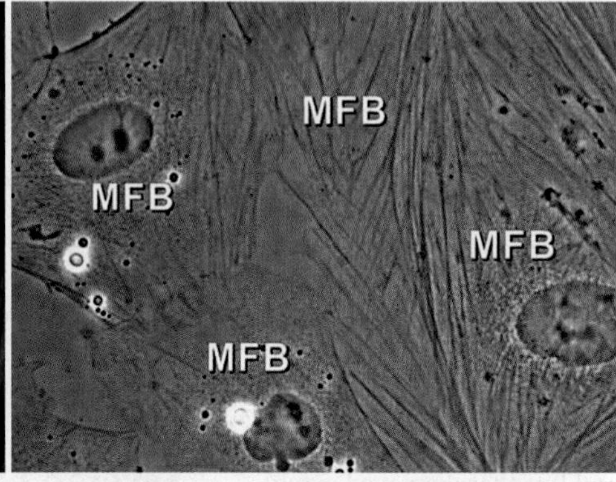

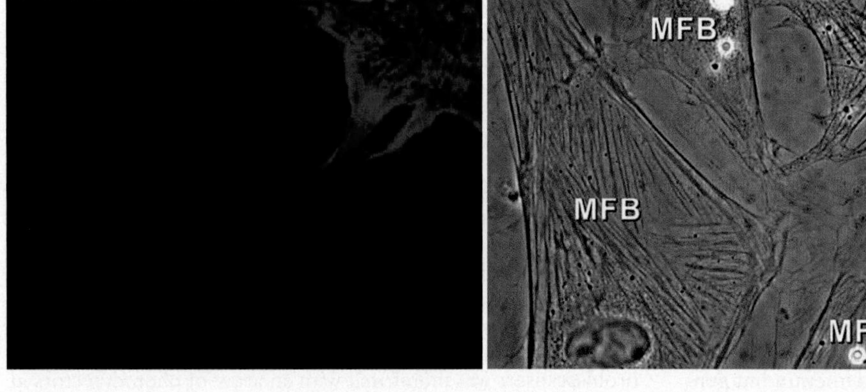

Figure 26-2 Fibroblasts of cardiac origin in cell culture. The expression of α-smooth muscle actin and vimentin as well as the absence of desmin expression identifies the cultured cardiac fibroblasts as myofibroblasts (MFB). The desmin-positive cell in the *upper right corner of the bottom left panel* corresponds to a cardiomyocyte (CM) *(bottom right panel)*.

Taken together, these findings suggest that myofibroblasts in intact diseased hearts might influence the spatial patterns of electrical activation not only by producing electrical barriers consisting of collagenous septa but also by forming cellular pathways for excitatory current flow. In this respect, myofibroblasts might have an antiarrhythmic effect by supporting propagation in tissue areas that otherwise would cause conduction blocks. On the other hand, because conduction across myofibroblasts is substantially delayed, they might in fact have a proarrhythmic effect by inducing slow and discontinuous conduction. Accordingly, if myofibroblasts in intact diseased hearts exert effects on conduction similar to those observed in vitro, then whether their net effect is proarrhythmic or antiarrhythmic ultimately depends on the specific cellular microarchitecture.

Myofibroblasts Slow Impulse Conduction

Given that myofibroblasts are capable of establishing heterocellular gap-junctional communication with cardiomyocytes, and given that the two cell types exhibit highly different electrical phenotypes,[55] it is likely that ensuing electrotonic interactions influence impulse propagation. This question was investigated by uniformly coating dense monolayer strands of cultured ventricular cardiomyocytes with cardiac fibroblasts.[49] An example of such a preparation is shown in Figure 26-5A. Even though cultured on a soft substrate consisting of cardiomyocytes, fibroblasts underwent a phenotype switch to myofibroblasts similar to cells cultured on rigid substrates, as evidenced by the robust

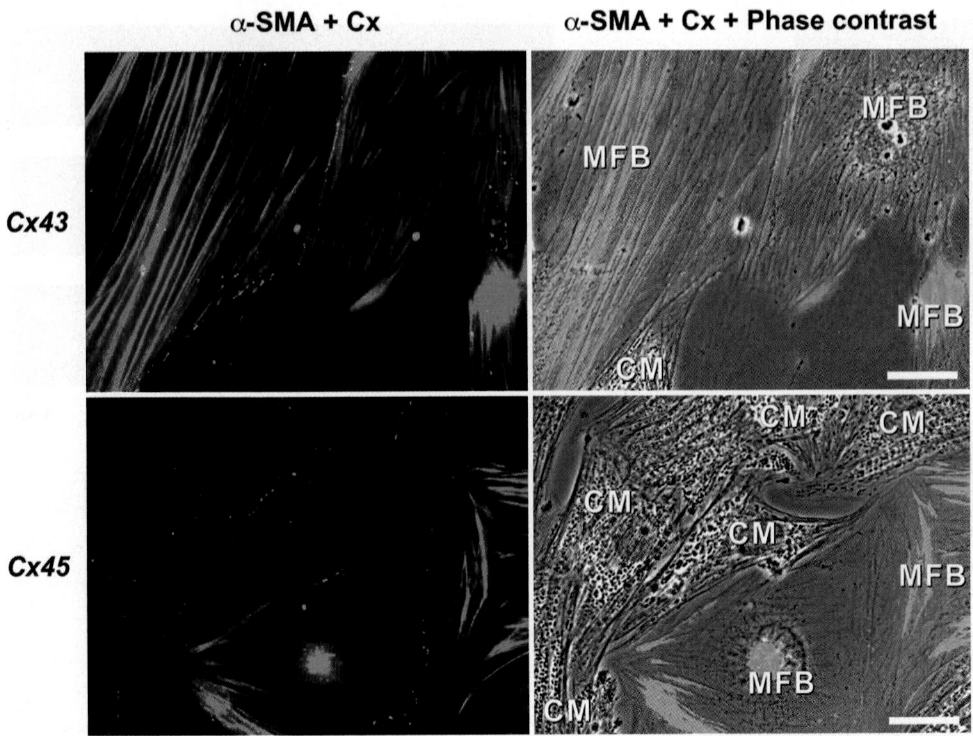

Figure 26-3 Connexin (Cx) expression by cardiac myofibroblasts in culture. Cocultures of cardiomyocytes and fibroblasts were stained for α–smooth muscle actin (α-SMA; *red*), connexin 43 *(green; upper row)*, and connexin 45 *(green; lower row)*. Fibroblasts stain intensely for α-SMA, which identifies them as myofibroblasts (MFB). Myofibroblasts express Cx43 and Cx45 at contact sites both among themselves and with cardiomyocytes (CM). Bar = 5 μm. (Modified from Miragoli M, Gaudesius G, Rohr S: Electrotonic modulation of cardiac impulse conduction by myofibroblasts. Circ Res 98:801-810, 2006 with permission.)

and stress fiber–like expression of α-SMA. Conduction velocity and maximal upstroke velocities in these preparations showed a biphasic dependence on myofibroblast density (Figure 26-5B), and maximal conduction velocities (~45 cm/sec) were reached at myofibroblast densities between 5% and 10%.

This biphasic behavior is reminiscent of the phenomenon of supernormal conduction as observed during gradual depolarization of cardiac tissue with potassium.[56,57] It suggests that myofibroblasts induce a density-dependent gradual depolarization of cardiomyocytes toward levels of membrane potentials, giving rise to slow conduction based on L-type calcium inward currents. In accordance with this hypothesis, measurements of membrane potentials using intracellular impalements at normal extracellular potassium concentrations showed that an increase in myofibroblast densities from about 5% to about 55% was accompanied by a parallel decrease of maximal diastolic membrane potentials of cardiomyocytes from about −80 mV to about −55 mV (Figure 26-5C).

These findings suggest that regions of intimate contact between myofibroblasts and cardiomyocytes as found, for example, in the infarct border zone or in fibrotic myocardia (cf. Figure 26-1) might contribute, in addition to electrical remodeling and redistribution of gap junctions as described by others before,[58,59] to local arrhythmogenic slowing of conduction by inducing partial depolarization of adjacent cardiomyocytes. Interestingly, such a depolarization has in fact been observed in multicellular preparations isolated from the epicardial border zone of 5-day-old infarcts[60] but not in dispersed single cardiomyocytes from the same zone.[61] Whereas it was suggested that this difference might be due to ion accumulation in the multicellular preparations,[58] the findings described here offer an alternate explanation, namely, that reduced resting potentials in the multicellular preparations of the epicardial border zone might have been due to the depolarizing influence of myofibroblasts, which, obviously, was lost upon isolation of single cardiomyocytes.

Myofibroblasts Elicit Ectopic Activity

Focal ectopic activity in cardiac tissue is a key factor in the initiation and perpetuation of tachyarrhythmias. In fact, the majority of ventricular tachycardias in nonischemic heart failure and a fraction of tachycardias in ischemic heart failure are thought to be based on ectopic pacemakers firing at a rate faster than the sinus node.[62] Moreover, premature ectopic beats can trigger the establishment of reentrant electrical activity underlying atrial and ventricular tachyarrhythmias.[63,64] Origins and the mechanisms of ectopic activity vary in different parts of the heart.

In atrial fibrillation (AF), it has been shown that ectopic activity arising at the muscular sleeves that extend into the atrial veins plays an important role.[63,65] Accordingly, ablation of these sleeves has become a widely accepted procedure to prevent recurrence of AF, even though the exact nature of the cell types and the cellular electrophysiologic mechanisms underlying ectopic activity are still a matter of debate.[66,67]

In the ventricles, ectopic activations have been shown to originate in the endocardium or epicardium in nonischemic heart failure[68,69] and at the border zone of acute infarcts.[70] Whereas ectopic activity in nonischemic heart failure is related to early or delayed afterdepolarizations secondary to intracellular calcium handling dysfunction,[62,71] ectopic activity arising at the border zone of acute infarcts is thought to depend on injury currents.[72-74] These currents, which flow from depolarized ischemic tissue to adjacent normal tissue, cause the normal tissue to undergo partial depolarization. Depending on the magnitude of this depolarization, excitability of the normal tissue adjacent to the ischemic region is increased (subthreshold) or, if suprathreshold, an ectopic beat is elicited.

Because myofibroblasts induce partial depolarization of cardiomyocytes by electrotonic interaction similar to injury currents present in ischemic tissue, it is conceivable that they might evoke ectopic activity based on the same basic mechanism.

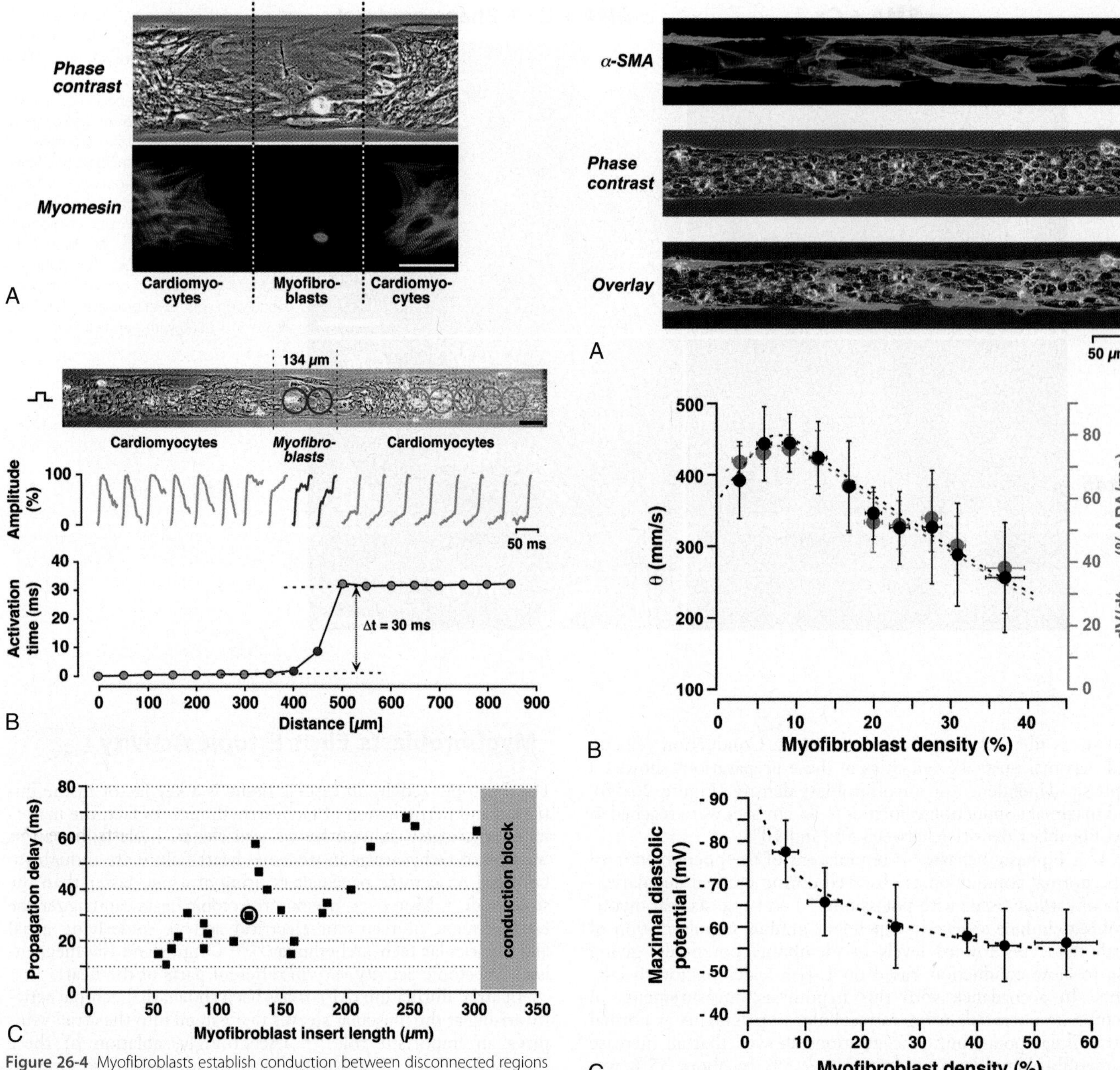

Figure 26-4 Myofibroblasts establish conduction between disconnected regions of cardiomyocytes. **A,** Phase contrast image of a strand of cardiomyocytes being interrupted by a patch of myofibroblasts. The myomesin staining *below* illustrates the spatial extent of separation between the two cardiomyocyte strands. Bar = 50 μm. **B,** Optical recording of impulse propagation along a strand of cardiomyocytes, which is interrupted by an insert of myofibroblasts. *Upper row,* Phase-contrast picture of the preparation. rings indicate the position of individual photodetectors (*orange:* sites on cardiomyocytes; *blue:* sites on myofibroblasts). *Middle row,* Optically recorded action potential upstrokes along the preparation following stimulation at the left. *Lower row,* Plot of local activation times along the preparation as a function of distance. At the site of the myofibroblast insert, conduction is delayed by about 30 ms. **C,** Propagation delays across myofibroblast inserts as a function of insert length. Conduction block occurs at insert lengths >300 μm. (Modified from Gaudesius G, Miragoli M, Thomas SP, Rohr S: Coupling of cardiac electrical activity over extended distances by fibroblasts of cardiac origin. Circ Res 93:421-428, 2003 with permission.)

Figure 26-5 Myofibroblasts induce slow conduction. **A,** Images depicting the morphology of an experimental preparation consisting of a strand of cardiomyocytes coated with a layer of myofibroblasts that stain positive for α-smooth muscle actin (α-SMA; *green*). **B,** Optically measured impulse conduction velocity (α; *black*) and maximal upstroke velocity (dV/dt$_{max}$; *red*) as a function of myofibroblast density. **C,** Maximal diastolic potentials measured with intracellular electrodes as a function of myofibroblast density. (Modified from Miragoli M, Gaudesius G, Rohr S: Electrotonic modulation of cardiac impulse conduction by myofibroblasts. Circ Res 98:801-810, 2006 with permission.)

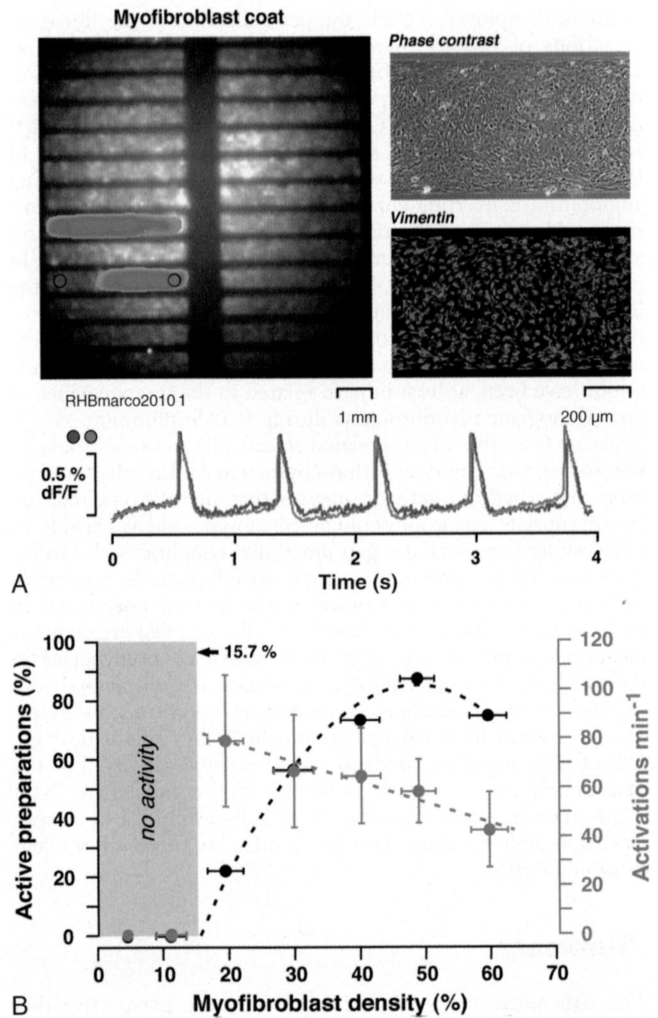

Figure 26-6 Myofibroblasts induce ectopic activity in cardiac tissue. A, Overview of an experimental preparation consisting of individual strands of cardiomyocytes (4.5 × 0.6 mm each) that were coated with myofibroblasts of cardiac origin. Propagating spontaneous activation is shown in *green*. The phase-contrast picture on the *right* demonstrates the dense cellular microarchitecture of the strands, and the vimentin staining illustrates the distribution of myofibroblasts. The optical action potential recordings shown *below* were obtained from the strand marked with a *red and a blue disk*. This particular strand exhibited spontaneous activity at 1.2 Hz, which was propagating from right to left. B, Percentage of active preparations (*black*, binomial fit) and frequency of spontaneous activations (*red*, linear fit) as a function of myofibroblast density. (Modified from Miragoli M, Salvarani N, Rohr S: Myofibroblasts induce ectopic activity in cardiac tissue. Circ Res 101:755-758, 2007, with permission.)

This hypothesis was investigated in strands of cultured neonatal rat ventricular cardiomyocytes as shown in Figure 26-6A.[75] Whereas control preparations with minimal contamination by endogenous myofibroblasts were invariably quiescent, coating of cardiomyocyte strands with increasing numbers of myofibroblasts caused a density-dependent increase in the percentage of spontaneous active preparations. As shown in Figure 26-6B, spontaneous ectopic activity was induced at myofibroblast densities greater than 15% and involved more than 80% of the preparations at densities around 50%. Over the same range of myofibroblast densities, frequencies of spontaneous activations decreased from about 80 to about 50 beats per minute.

Mechanistically, induction of ectopic activity was likely related to the graded depolarization of cardiomyocytes by myofibroblasts because pharmacologic opening of adenosine triphosphate (ATP)-dependent potassium channels caused cessation of spontaneous activity and because spontaneous activity could be induced in current clamped single cardiomyocytes at clamp potentials (~−67 mV), highly similar to those expected for strands coated with 15% myofibroblasts (~−66 mV). Induction of spontaneous activity was not specific for myofibroblasts because communication-competent HeLa cells, which likewise have a reduced intrinsic membrane potential, were similarly able to elicit ectopic activity when cultured on top of strands of cardiomyocytes.[75]

These findings expand the concept of arrhythmogenic injury currents flowing within *homocellular* networks of cardiomyocytes with spatially heterogeneous electrophysiologic properties to *heterocellular* networks in which injury currents arise as a consequence of the electrophysiologic differences between different cell types.[76] For dense monolayer cultures of cardiomyocytes, it is in fact this type of interaction between myofibroblasts and cardiomyocytes that is responsible for the hallmark of this experimental system: the presence of spontaneous activity. If myofibroblast densities are low, cultures are completely quiescent, which is in fact the expected result if ventricular cardiomyocytes retain their quiescent in vivo phenotype also in cell culture. This finding has implications for interpreting experimentally induced beat-rate changes in spontaneously active cardiomyocyte monolayers because such changes are not necessarily cardiomyocyte-related but might occur secondary to changes in the electrophysiologic phenotype of myofibroblasts.

Implications, Open Questions, and Perspectives

From this research, it emerges that myofibroblasts have the potential to exert substantial proarrhythmic activity based on mechanisms that are summarized schematically in Figure 26-7. Once myofibroblasts are recruited to the myocardium in sufficient numbers due to inflammatory processes, mechanical stress, and humoral factors, they are likely to contribute to arrhythmogenesis by collagen secretion that leads to cardiac fibrosis[22,23] and, hence, to arrhythmogenic slow conduction and conduction blocks. Myofibroblasts can also contribute to arrhythmogenesis by inducing electrical remodeling of cardiomyocytes based on

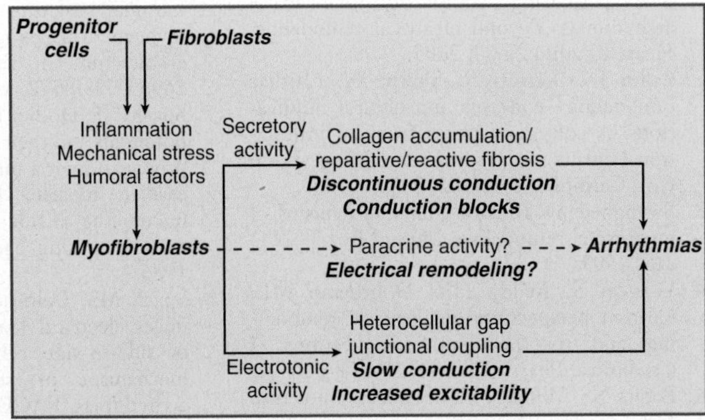

Figure 26-7 Scenario of the involvement of myofibroblasts in cardiac arrhythmogenesis.

paracrine activity. In this context, it has been shown that myofibroblast-related humoral factors such as tumor necrosis factor (TNF)-α, nerve growth factor (NGF), IGF-1, angiotensin-II, bFGF, and TGF-β_1 afflict various potassium and calcium ion channels of cardiomyocytes.[77-82] To what extent, however, electrical remodeling induced by these humoral factors is involved in arrhythmogenesis in vivo is still not entirely clear. As shown in this chapter, myofibroblasts might additionally be involved in arrhythmogenesis by directly affecting cardiomyocyte electrophysiology by electrotonic interaction following establishment of heterocellular gap-junctional coupling. This interaction results in slow conduction and in ectopic activity. Accordingly, myofibroblasts might not only set the stage for focal tachyarrhythmias but also might initiate reentrant activation whose perpetuation would subsequently be supported by the simultaneous presence of myofibroblast-induced uniform or discontinuous slow conduction.

Whether and to what extent such arrhythmogenic consequences of electrotonic interactions between myofibroblasts and cardiomyocytes as observed in vitro can ultimately be translated to intact diseased myocardium in vivo crucially depends on finding answers to the following questions. Of primary importance is the need to find unambiguous evidence for the presence of heterocellular gap junctional coupling between myofibroblasts and cardiomyocytes in structurally remodeled myocardia. Secondly, it will be important to find experimental approaches permitting the determination of the degree of heterocellular gap junctional coupling in intact tissues in order to get an estimate of the extent of electrotonic crosstalk between cardiomyocytes and myofibroblasts. Thirdly, it will be necessary to compare the in vitro cell model to intact tissue in respect to the spatial organization and the relative numbers and cell sizes of myofibroblasts and cardiomyocytes. This comparison will permit researchers to make predictions as to the likelihood that effects observed at specific myofibroblast densities in vitro also occur in intact tissue. Finally, it will be important to assess whether the depolarizing capacity of myofibroblasts as observed in vitro is preserved in intact hearts. Circumstantial evidence in favor of such a depolarization is provided by previous findings of a reduction in resting potentials of cardiomyocytes in infarct border zones,[60] but further investigations into this question are clearly needed.

If the concept of myofibroblast induced arrhythmogenesis applies to intact cardiac tissue as well, myofibroblasts might emerge as a new target for specific antiarrhythmic therapies. Present therapeutic efforts concerning cardiac fibroblasts are aimed at reducing fibrosis and counteracting heart failure.[83] Strategies employed include the neutralization of the fibrogenic actions of various autocrine and paracrine factors such as angiotensin II, aldosterone, endothelin, TGF-β_1, TNF-α, bFGF, platelet-derived growth factor (PDGF), connective-tissue growth factor (CTGF), interleukins, and osteopontin.[38] Interestingly, it has been found that decreasing the activity of the renin-angiotensin-aldosterone system (RAAS) by inhibiting angiotensin-converting enzyme (ACE) or by blocking angiotensin or aldosterone receptors ameliorates fibrosis[84] and reduces atrial fibrillation in a dog model of congestive heart failure.[85] In parallel, a different set of studies showed that antagonizing the RAAS reduces the transition from fibroblasts to myofibroblasts.[86,87] In the context of this chapter, it is tempting to speculate that the reduction of atrial fibrillation in the former study might have been, at least in part, related to the disappearance of arrhythmogenic myofibroblasts during RAAS inhibition.

Apart from these issues related specifically to myofibroblasts, the finding that communication-competent HeLa cells similarly exert proarrhythmic activity suggests that any cell type that has an appropriate electrophysiologic phenotype and is capable of establishing heterocellular gap-junctional coupling with cardiomyocytes has the potential to elicit arrhythmias. In particular, such arrhythmogenic mechanisms might become operational in the context of cell therapies based on cell types that are communication competent but differ from native cardiomyocytes in their cellular electrophysiologic properties. If transplanted cells exhibit a reduced membrane potential, as was shown, for example, for human mesenchymal stem cells,[88] they might bear the risk of inducing slow conduction and ectopic activity. For the case of cell therapies with communication-competent cells, it seems therefore desirable that these cells exhibit, also at rest, electrophysiologic characteristics similar to those of resident cardiomyocytes.

Summary

The data presented in this chapter open the perspective that myofibroblasts appearing during structural remodeling of the heart might be involved in arrhythmogenesis in a way that goes beyond the mere secretion of collagen and thus the establishment of a nonuniform substrate for impulse propagation. If future experiments show that myofibroblast-dependent arrhythmogenesis is likely to occur also in intact hearts, this cell type might emerge as a specific *noncardiomyocyte* target for treating arrhythmias in structurally remodeled myocardium.

References

1. Adamson PB, Barr RC, Callans DJ, et al: The perplexing complexity of cardiac arrhythmias: Beyond electrical remodeling. Heart Rhythm 2:650, 2005.
2. Cohn JN, Ferrari R, Sharpe N: Cardiac remodeling—concepts and clinical implications: A consensus paper from an international forum on cardiac remodeling. J Am Coll Cardiol 35:569-582, 2000.
3. Swynghedauw B: Molecular mechanisms of myocardial remodeling. Physiol Rev 79:215-262, 1999.
4. Wasson S, Reddy HK, Dohrmann ML: Current perspectives of electrical remodeling and its therapeutic implications. J Cardiovasc Pharm Ther 9:129-144, 2004.
5. Peters NS, Wit AL: Myocardial architecture and ventricular arrhythmogenesis. Circ 97:1746-1754, 1998.
6. LeGrice IJ, Smaill LL, Chai LZ, et al: Laminar structure of the heart: Ventricular myocyte arrangement and connective tissue architecture in the dog. Am J Physiol 269:H571-H582, 1995.
7. Spach MS, Dolber PC: Relating extracellular potentials and their derivatives to anisotropic propagation at a microscopic level in human cardiac muscle. Evidence for electrical uncoupling of side-to-side fiber connections with increasing age. Circ Res 58:356-371, 1986.
8. Spach MS, Boineau JP: Microfibrosis produces electrical load variations due to loss of side-to-side cell connections: A major mechanism of structural heart disease arrhythmias. PACE 20:397-413, 1997.
9. De Bakker JMT, Van Capelle FJL, Janse MJ, et al: Slow conduction in the infarcted human heart—zigzag course of activation. Circulation 88:915-926, 1993.
10. Banerjee I, Fuseler JW, Price RL, et al: Determination of cell types and numbers during cardiac development in the neonatal and adult rat and mouse. Am J Physiol Heart Circ Physiol 293:H1883-H1891, 2007.
11. Adler CP, Ringlage WP, Böhm N: DNS-Gehalt und Zellzahl in Herz und Leber von Kindern. Pathol Res Pract 172:25-41, 1981.
12. Maisch B: Extracellular matrix and cardiac interstitium: Restriction is not a restricted phenomenon. Herz 20:75-80, 1995.
13. McAnulty RJ, Laurent GJ: Collagen synthesis and degradation in vivo. Evidence for rapid rates of collagen turnover with extensive degradation of newly synthesized

collagen in tissues of the adult rat. Coll Relat Res 7:93-104, 1987.
14. Camelliti P, Green CR, LeGrice I, Kohl P: Fibroblast network in rabbit sinoatrial node: Structural and functional identification of homogeneous and heterogeneous cell coupling. Circ Res 94:828-835, 2004.
15. Aikawa E, Whittaker P, Farber M, et al: Human semilunar cardiac valve remodeling by activated cells from fetus to adult: Implications for postnatal adaptation, pathology, and tissue engineering. Circulation 113:1344-1352, 2006.
16. Gabbiani G: The myofibroblast in wound healing and fibrocontractive diseases. J Pathol 200:500-503, 2003.
17. Gabbiani G, Ryan GB, Majno G: Presence of modified fibroblasts in granulation tissue and their possible role in wound contraction. Experientia 27:549-550, 1971.
18. Darby I, Skalli O, Gabbiani G: α-Smooth muscle actin is transiently expressed by myofibroblasts during experimental wound healing. Lab Invest 63:21-29, 1990.
19. Tomasek JJ, Gabbiani G, Hinz B, et al: Myofibroblasts and mechanoregulation of connective tissue remodelling. Nat Rev Mol Cell Biol 3:349-363, 2002.
20. Desmouliere A, Darby IA, Gabbiani G: Normal and pathologic soft tissue remodeling: Role of the myofibroblast, with special emphasis on liver and kidney fibrosis. Lab Invest 83:1689-1707, 2003.
21. Powell DW, Mifflin RC, Valentich JD, et al: Myofibroblasts. I. Paracrine cells important in health and disease. Am J Physiol 277:C1-C19, 1999.
22. Weber KT: Extracellular matrix remodeling in heart failure: A role for de novo angiotensin II generation. Circulation 96:4065-4082, 1997.
23. Weber KT: Fibrosis in hypertensive heart disease: Focus on cardiac fibroblasts. J Hypertens 22:47-50, 2004.
24. Clement S, Chaponnier C, Gabbiani G: A subpopulation of cardiomyocytes expressing α-skeletal actin is identified by a specific polyclonal antibody. Circ Res 85:51e-58e, 1999.
25. Leslie KO, Taatjes DJ, Schwarz J, et al: Cardiac myofibroblasts express alpha smooth muscle actin during right ventricular pressure overload in the rabbit. Am J Pathol 139:207-216, 1991.
26. Kuwahara F, Kai H, Tokuda K, et al: Transforming growth factor function blocking prevents myocardial fibrosis and diastolic dysfunction in pressure-overloaded rats. Circulation 106:130-135, 2003.
27. Tokuda K, Kai H, Kuwahara F, et al: Pressure-independent effects of angiotensin II on hypertensive myocardial fibrosis. Hypertension 43:499-503, 2004.
28. Peterson DJ, Ju H, Panagia M, et al: Expression of Gi-2α and Gsα in myofibroblasts localized to the infarct scar in heart failure due to myocardial infarction. Cardiovasc Res 41:575-585, 1999.
29. Sun Y, Weber KT: Angiotensin converting enzyme and myofibroblasts during tissue repair in the rat heart. J Mol Cell Cardiol 28:851-858, 1996.
30. Sun Y, Weber KT: Infarct scar: A dynamic tissue. Cardiovasc Res 46:250-256, 2000.
31. Willems IE, Havenith MG, De Mey JG, Daemen MJ: The α–smooth muscle actin–positive cells in healing human myocardial scars. Am J Pathol 145:868-875, 1994.
32. Takemura G, Ohno M, Hayakawa Y, et al: Role of apoptosis in the disappearance of infiltrated and proliferated interstitial cells after myocardial infarction. Circ Res 82:1130-1138, 1998.
33. Sun Y, Kiani MF, Postlethwaite AE, Weber KT: Infarct scar as living tissue. Basic Res Cardiol 97:343-347, 2003.
34. Desmouliere A, Chapponier C, Gabbiani G: Tissue repair, contraction, and the myofibroblast. Wound Rep Reg 13:7-12, 2005.
35. Hinz B, Phan SH, Thannickal VJ, et al: The myofibroblast: One function, multiple origins. Am J Pathol 170:1807-1816, 2007.
36. Weber KT: From inflammation to fibrosis: A stiff stretch of highway. Hypertension 43:716-719, 2004.
37. Kuwahara F, Kai H, Tokuda K, et al: Hypertensive myocardial fibrosis and diastolic dysfunction. Hypertension 43:739-745, 2004.
38. Manabe I, Shindo T, Nagai R: Gene expression in fibroblasts and fibrosis. Circ Res 91:1103-1113, 2002.
39. Eyden B: The myofibroblast: An assessment of controversial issues and a definition useful in diagnosis and research. Ultrastruct Pathol 25:39-50, 2001.
40. Sui GP, Rothery S, Dupont E, et al: Gap junctions and connexin expression in human suburothelial interstitial cells. BJU Int 90:118-129, 2003.
41. Powell DW, Mifflin RC, Valentich JD, et al: Myofibroblasts. II. Intestinal subepithelial myofibroblasts. Am J Physiol 277:C183-C201, 1999.
42. Jamieson S, Going JJ, D'Arcy R, George WD: Expression of gap junction proteins connexin 26 and connexin 43 in normal human breast and in breast tumours. J Pathol 184:37-43, 1998.
43. Gabbiani G, Chaponnier C, Huttner I: Cytoplasmic filaments and gap junctions in epithelial cells and myofibroblasts during wound healing. J Cell Biol 76:561-568, 1978.
44. Goldsmith ED, Hoffman A, Morales MO, et al: Organization of fibroblasts in the heart. Dev Dyn 230:787-794, 2004.
45. Camelliti P, Devlin GP, Matthews KG, et al: Spatially and temporally distinct expression of fibroblast connexins after sheep ventricular infarction. Cardiovas Res 62:415, 2004.
46. Matsushita T, Takamatsu T: Ischaemia-induced temporal expression of connexin43 in rat heart. Virchows Archiv V431:453, 1997.
47. Wang J, Chen H, Seth A, McCulloch CA: Mechanical force regulation of myofibroblast differentiation in cardiac fibroblasts. Am J Physiol Heart Circ Physiol 285:H1871-H1881, 2003.
48. Ronnov-Jessen L, Petersen OW: Induction of α–smooth muscle actin by transforming growth factor-beta 1 in quiescent human breast gland fibroblasts. Implications for myofibroblast generation in breast neoplasia. Lab Invest 68:696-707, 1993.
49. Miragoli M, Gaudesius G, Rohr S: Electrotonic modulation of cardiac impulse conduction by myofibroblasts. Circ Res 98:801-810, 2006.
50. Beny JL, Connat JL: An electron-microscopic study of smooth muscle cell dye coupling in the pig coronary arteries. Role of gap junctions. Circ Res 70:49-55, 1992.
51. Rohr S, Salzberg BM: Multiple site optical recording of transmembrane voltage (MSORTV) in patterned growth heart cell cultures: Assessing electrical behavior, with microsecond resolution, on a cellular and subcellular scale. Biophys. J 67:1301-1315, 1994.
52. Rohr S, Flückiger-Labrada R, Kucera JP: Photolithographically defined deposition of attachment factors as a versatile method for patterning the growth of different cell types in culture. Eur J Physiol 446:125-132, 2003.
53. Lefroy DC, Fang JC, Stevenson LW, et al: Recipient-to-donor atrioatrial conduction after orthotopic heart transplantation: Surface electrocardiographic features and estimated prevalence. Am J Cardiol 82:444-450, 1998.
54. Gaudesius G, Miragoli M, Thomas SP, Rohr S: Coupling of cardiac electrical activity over extended distances by fibroblasts of cardiac origin. Circ Res 93:421-428, 2003.
55. Hyde A, Blondel B, Matter A, et al: Homo- and heterocellular junctions in cell cultures: An electrophysiological and morphological study. Prog Brain Res 31:283-311, 1969.
56. Kagiyama Y, Hill JL, Gettes LS: Interaction of acidosis and increased extracellular potassium on action potential characteristics and conduction in guinea pig ventricular muscle. Circ Res 51:614-623, 1982.
57. Shaw R, Rudy Y: Electrophysiologic effects of acute myocardial ischemia. A mechanistic investigation of action potential conduction and conduction failure. Circ Res 80:124-138, 1997.
58. Pinto JMB, Boyden PA: Electrical remodeling in ischemia and infarction. Cardiovas Res 42:284-297, 1999.
59. Peters NS, Coromilas J, Severs NJ, Wit AL: Disturbed connexin43 gap junction distribution correlates with the location of reentrant circuits in the epicardial border zone of healing canine infarcts that cause ventricular tachycardia. Circulation 95:988-996, 1997.
60. Ursell PC, Gardner PI, Albala A, et al: Structural and electrophysiological changes in the epicardial border zone of canine myocardial infarcts during infarct healing. Circ Res 56:436-451, 1985.
61. Lue WM, Boyden PA: Abnormal electrical properties of myocytes from chronically infarcted canine heart. Alterations in V_{max} and the transient outward current. Circulation 85:1175-1188, 1998.
62. Rubart M, Zipes DP: Mechanisms of sudden cardiac death. J Clin Invest 115:2305-2315, 2005.
63. Tsai C-F, Tai C-T, Hsieh M-H, et al: Initiation of atrial fibrillation by ectopic beats originating from the superior vena cava: Electrophysiological characteristics and results of radiofrequency ablation. Circulation 102:67-74, 2000.

64. Gorenek B, Kudaiberdieva G, Birdane A, et al: Initiation of monomorphic ventricular tachycardia: Electrophysiological, clinical features, and drug therapy in patients with implantable defibrillators. J Electrocardiol 36:213-218, 2003.
65. Haïssaguerre M, Jaïs P, Shah DC, et al: Spontaneous initiation of atrial fibrillation by ectopic beats originating in the pulmonary veins. New Engl J Med 339:659-666, 1998.
66. Coutu P, Chartier D, Nattel S: Comparison of Ca^{2+}-handling properties of canine pulmonary vein and left atrial cardiomyocytes. Am J Physiol 291:H2290-H2300, 2006.
67. Nattel S: Basic electrophysiology of the pulmonary veins and their role in atrial fibrillation: Precipitators, perpetuators, and perplexers. J Cardiovasc Electrophysiol 14:1372-1375, 2003.
68. Pogwizd SM: Nonreentrant mechanisms underlying spontaneous ventricular arrhythmias in a model of nonischemic heart failure in rabbits. Circulation 92:1034-1048, 1995.
69. Pogwizd SM, McKenzie JP, Cain ME: Mechanisms underlying spontaneous and induced ventricular arrhythmias in patients with idiopathic dilated cardiomyopathy. Circulation 98:2404-2414, 1998.
70. Coronel R, Wilms-Schopman FJG, deGroot JR: Origin of ischemia-induced phase 1b ventricular arrhythmias in pig hearts. J Am Coll Cardiol 39:166-176, 2003.
71. Yano M, Ikeda Y, Matsuzaki M: Altered intracellular Ca^{2+} handling in heart failure. J Clin Invest 115:556-564, 2005.
72. Coronel R, Wilms-Schopman FJ, Opthof T, et al: Injury current and gradients of diastolic stimulation threshold, TQ potential, and extracellular potassium concentration during acute regional ischemia in the isolated perfused pig heart. Circ Res 68:1241-1249, 1991.
73. Janse MJ, van Capelle FJ, Morsink H, et al: Flow of "injury" current and patterns of excitation during early ventricular arrhythmias in acute regional myocardial ischemia in isolated porcine and canine hearts. Evidence for two different arrhythmogenic mechanisms. Circ Res 47:151-165, 1980.
74. Katzung BG, Hondeghem LM, Grant AO: Cardiac ventricular automaticity induced by current of injury. Pflügers Arch 360:193-197, 1975.
75. Miragoli M, Salvarani N, Rohr S: Myofibroblasts induce ectopic activity in cardiac tissue. Circ Res 101:755-758, 2007.
76. Carmeliet E: Cardiac ionic currents and acute ischemia: From channels to arrhythmias. Physiol Rev 79:917-1017, 1999.
77. Hatada K, Washizuka T, Horie M, et al: Tumor necrosis factor-α inhibits the cardiac delayed rectifier K current via the asphingomyelin pathway. Biochem Biophys Res Com 344:189, 2006.
78. Heath BM, Xia J, Dong E, et al: Overexpression of nerve growth factor in the heart alters ion channel activity and beta-adrenergic signalling in an adult transgenic mouse. J Physiol (Lond) 512:779-791, 1998.
79. Sun H, Kerfant B-G, Zhao D, et al: Insulin-like growth factor-1 and PTEN deletion enhance cardiac L-type Ca^{2+} currents via increased PI3Ka/PKB signaling. Circ Res 98:1390-1397, 2006.
80. Ferron L, Capuano V, Ruchon Y, et al: Angiotensin II signaling pathways mediate expression of cardiac T-type calcium channels. Circ Res 93:1241-1248, 2003.
81. Guo W, Kamiya K, Toyama J: bFGF promotes functional expressions of transient outward currents in cultured neonatal rat ventricular cells. Pflügers Arch V430:1015-1017, 1995.
82. Avila G, Medina IM, Jimenez E, et al: Transforming growth factor-β_1 decreases cardiac muscle L-type Ca^{2+} current and charge movement by acting on the $Ca_V1.2$ mRNA. Am J Physiol 292:H622-H631, 2007.
83. Brown RD, Ambler SK, Mitchell MD, Long CS: The cardiac fibroblast: Therapeutic target in myocardial remodeling and failure. Ann Rev Pharm Toxicol 45:657-687, 2005.
84. Sun Y, Weber KT: RAS and connective tissue in the heart. Int J Biochem Cell Biol 35:919, 2003.
85. Li D, Shinagawa K, Pang L, et al: Effects of angiotensin-converting enzyme inhibition on the development of the atrial fibrillation substrate in dogs with ventricular tachypacing-induced congestive heart failure. Circulation 104:2608-2614, 2001.
86. Kurikawa N, Suga M, Kuroda S, et al: An angiotensin II type 1 receptor antagonist, olmesartan medoxomil, improves experimental liver fibrosis by suppression of proliferation and collagen synthesis in activated hepatic stellate cells. Br J Pharmacol 139:1085-1094, 2003.
87. Yamada T, Kuno A, Masuda K, et al: Candesartan, an angiotensin II receptor antagonist, suppresses pancreatic inflammation and fibrosis in rats. J Pharmacol Exp Ther 307:17-23, 2003.
88. Heubach JF, Graf EM, Leutheuser J, et al: Electrophysiological properties of human mesenchymal stem cells. J Physiol 554:659-672, 2004.

Cardiac Alternans as a Pathophysiologic Mechanism of Arrhythmias 27

KENNETH R. LAURITA, LANCE D. WILSON, AND DAVID S. ROSENBAUM

CHAPTER OUTLINE

T wave alternans, a repetitive beat-to-beat change of electrocardiographic (ECG) T wave morphology, has been recognized as a precursor of ventricular arrhythmias and sudden death for more than 100 years. In 1872 Traube reported pulsus alternans, now known to be the mechanical correlate of T wave alternans, and an ominous sign in patients with heart failure.[1] T wave alternans was described shortly after the ECG was introduced into clinical medicine,[2] and is associated with susceptibility to sudden cardiac death in humans.[3,4]

The recognition that cardiac alternans (including mechanical and T wave alternans) as a marker for poor prognosis in disease was initially based only on anecdotal clinical observations.[3-6] The original experiments of Hellerstein provided the first evidence that cardiac alternans is a reproducible and quantifiable phenomenon when induced by myocardial ischemia. These experiments suggested that, in fact, cardiac alternans may be a common precursor to electrical instability in the heart.[7] In the 1980s, Cohen and coworkers[8-10] established a close quantitative relationship between T wave alternans and vulnerability to ventricular fibrillation (VF) during myocardial ischemia in the dog. These findings were confirmed by Nearing and colleagues,[11] who measured T wave alternans with intracavitary electrodes. T wave alternans was, therefore, established as a quantitative marker of electrical instability in the heart.

Clinical Significance of T Wave Alternans

The demonstration that visually undetectable, microvolt-level T wave alternans is common in patients at risk for sudden cardiac death[12] provided the impetus for implementing T wave alternans testing in clinical practice and motivated intense interest in determining mechanisms that underlie T wave alternans. It is now recognized that subtle microvolt-level T wave alternans can be reliably detected and quantified on the surface ECG in approximately 50% of patients who have impaired systolic function and who are at heightened risk for ventricular fibrillation.[13] T wave alternans independently predicts susceptibility to sudden cardiac death (SCD) in these patients.[13,14] T wave alternans is absent in approximately 30% of patients with indications for prophylactic implantable cardioverter defibrillator (ICD) therapy (based on left ventricle ejection fraction <0.35), and such patients are at remarkably low risk (2%-5%) of events.[13] These findings have been verified in several independent clinical trials,[12,13,15-19] suggesting that cardiac alternans plays a role in triggering cardiac electrical instability and might have a role in risk stratification of patients for SCD. The clinical findings suggest that cardiac alternans reflects a pathophysiologic mechanism responsible for triggering cardiac arrhythmias in a variety of disease processes, which is the focus of this chapter.

Alternans in Heart Disease

In normal hearts it has been demonstrated experimentally that T wave alternans detected on the surface ECG is a physiologic rate-dependent property of the heart that arises from the level of the single cell.[20] T wave alternans develops when heart rate is elevated past a threshold level.[21] In fact, in clinical T wave alternans testing, the presence of significant T wave alternans is defined by the threshold heart rate at which it is induced; in humans, T wave alternans occurring at heart rates less than 110 beats per minute defines an abnormal test.

Both myocyte calcium handling and sarcolemmel ionic currents governing repolarization demonstrate rate dependence and have been implicated in the mechanism of cardiac alternans. Importantly, a variety of cardiac diseases where cardiac alternans has been observed are also associated with impaired function of one or more aspects of these cellular processes (Table 27-1). These include congestive heart failure,[22] and cardiomyopathies,[23-25] long QT syndrome,[26,27-30] and Brugada syndrome.[31,32] T wave alternans has been observed in acute ischemic cardiac syndromes, including acute myocardial infarction[33,34] and coronary vasospasm.[35,36] Numerous other arrhythmogenic conditions are associated with T wave alternans including electrolyte imbalances,[37,38] alcoholism,[37,39] drug intoxication[40-43] and hypothermia.[10] In such patients, the appearance T wave alternans often precedes the onset of ventricular arrhythmias, suggesting a causal relationship.

Microvolt and visible T wave alternans have been associated with ventricular arrhythmias in diverse experimental and clinical settings[44,45,46] and are common in patients at risk for sudden cardiac death.[12] This raises the speculation that T wave alternans may be a universal precursor to cardiac arrhythmias in multiple pathologic states associated with electrical instability in the heart (see Table 27-1).[47] It is quite unlikely that there is *one* mechanism of cardiac alternans, because there are data that potentially explain specific cellular or subcellular abnormalities that underlie cardiac alternans in a variety of clinical conditions (see Table 27-1). Most experimental studies that have elucidated mechanisms of cardiac alternans have focused on normal myocardium but, nonetheless, have provided important insights into novel pathophysiologic mechanisms of alternans-mediated arrhythmias in heart disease.

Table 27-1 Alternans in Heart Disease

Disease State	Alternans Associated with Susceptibility to Arrhythmias	Proposed Mechanisms of Alternans	Heart Rates Required to Induce Alternans	Evidence with Selected References
Normal	Yes	Calcium cycling	Very fast	Clinical observation, experimental studies, simulation studies[20,21,52,72,79,105]
Heart failure	Yes	Calcium cycling, impaired repolarization, conduction slowing,structural barriers	Moderately increased	Clinical trials, minimal experimental studies[13,14,119]
Hypertrophic Cardiomyopathy	Yes	Unknown	Moderately increased	Clinical studies[23,24]
Long QT syndrome; Brugada syndrome	Yes	Impaired repolarization, autonomic influences	Slow	Case reports, modeling studies, minimal experimental studies[27,59,62,101]
Acute myocardial ischemia	Yes	Repolarization, refractoriness; calcium cycling, conduction slowing	Normal	Experimental studies, clinical observations[7,11,35,36,60,115,140,144]
Electrolyte imbalance, drug intoxication, hypothermia	Yes	Largely unknown, conduction slowing, impaired repolarization	Fast or slow, unknown	Case reports limited to experimental studies[10,37-43]

Mechanisms of Cardiac Alternans

Cardiac alternans involves interdependent processes linking cellular sarcoplasmic reticulum (SR) calcium-cycling machinery (causing pulsus or mechanical alternans) to sarcolemmal ionic fluxes (causing T-wave alternans). These processes are diagramed in Figure 27-1. There is considerable evidence suggesting that beat-to-beat fluctuations in T-wave morphology, which characterizes T wave alternans, arise from action potential alternans at the cellular level, which, in turn, coincides with alternations in ionic flux through the cell membrane and sarcomere (Fig 27-1).[20,48,49] The involvement of such interdependent and complex processes present challenges in identifying specific cellular, subcellular, and molecular mechanisms underlying alternans.

There are two prevailing hypotheses for the generation of alternans on the cellular level. One mechanism for repolarization alternans is beat-to-beat oscillations of current flux through sarcolemmal ion channels responsible for repolarization (e.g., represented by I_K in Fig. 27-1), which can be directly related to the kinetics of individual or combined repolarization currents. For example, incomplete recovery from time-dependent inactivation of an ion channel can lead to beat-to-beat alternation in ion flux through that channel. This will, in turn, cause alternating calcium flux through the SR. Alternatively, alternans can arise primarily from beat-to-beat oscillations in the amount of calcium released from the SR through the ryanodine receptor (RyR).

As can be imagined, what makes the investigation of cardiac alternans particularly challenging is that regulation of repolarization currents and SR calcium are closely intertwined. This complex relationship is determined by numerous sarcolemmal ion channels and sarcomere regulatory proteins. All sarcolemmal currents that are sensitive to intracellular calcium can play a role, but the primary currents (see Fig. 27-1) are the Na^+-Ca^{2+} exchanger (I_{NCX}) and L-type calcium current (I_{CaL}). For example, a large calcium release inactivates more I_{CaL} and shortens the duration of the action potential (APD). In addition, a large calcium release activates more I_{NCX} operating in the forward mode (removing calcium) and lengthens APD. By convention, such coupling from calcium to voltage (see Fig. 27-1) is negative when APD shortens in response to a large calcium release, and positive when APD lengthens in response to a large calcium release.[50]

Mechanisms of alternans becomes further complicated because coupling between calcium and voltage is bidirectional. That is, APD can also influence SR calcium release (Vm-to-Ca coupling). For example, given a constant heart rate, a prolongation of repolarization shortens the following diastolic interval and shortens the recovery time for I_{CaL}. As a result, I_{CaL} is less and calcium release from the SR is less as well. Despite the complex bidirectional nature of calcium and voltage coupling, it is possible (as outlined later) to describe separately the cellular mechanisms of alternans based on repolarization kinetics and intracellular calcium cycling.

Cellular Mechanisms of Alternans

The Action Potential Duration Restitution Hypothesis

When heart rate exceeds the ability of a repolarization channel to fully recover from time-dependent inactivation, the ion channel is partially open upon initiation of the next beat. As a result, APD of this beat is shorter and the recovery (diastolic) interval greater. For the next beat, the channel is more recovered and thus is less open upon initiation (less net repolarization current), resulting in longer APD and shorter diastolic interval, perpetuating action potential alternans.

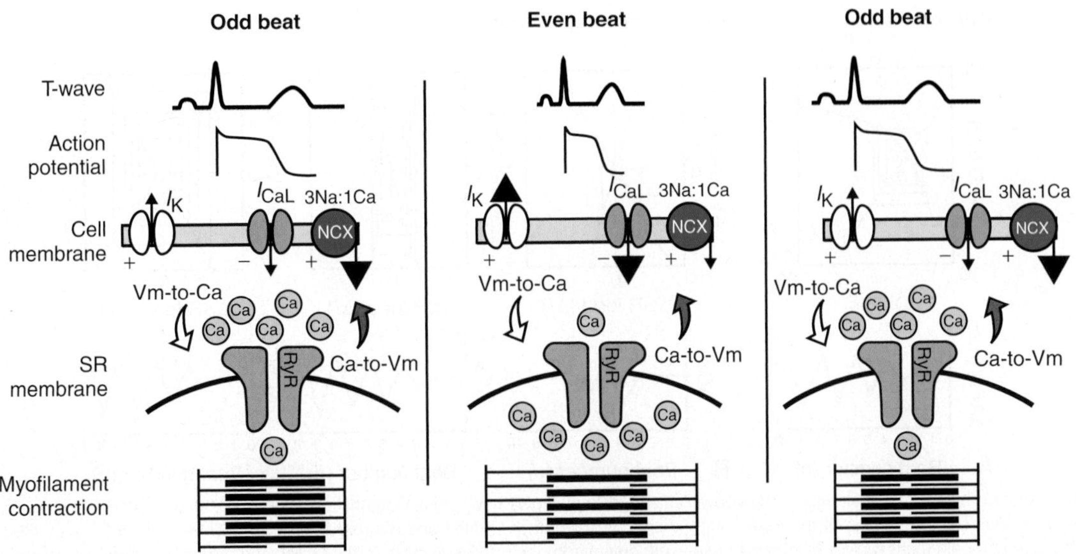

Figure 27-1 Schematic diagram depicting cellular processes underlying cardiac alternans. The clinical manifestation of cardiac alternans can be electrical in the form of T-wave alternans *(top);* beat-to-beat oscillation in T-wave shape, or mechanical as pulsus alternans *(bottom);* or beat-to-beat oscillation in pulse pressure or generated force. The general mechanisms of T-wave and pulses alternans are described as the figure progresses from top and bottom (respectively) to the center, where mechanisms intertwine. T-wave alternans corresponds with beat-to-beat fluctuations in action potential duration. Similarly, mechanical alternans coincides with beat-to-beat fluctuation in sarcoplasmic reticulum (SR) calcium flux. In this schema, alternans can occur via one of two processes. It can be driven primarily by beat-to-beat fluctuations in membrane currents (e.g., I_K in figure), which, through a process of voltage-to-calcium coupling (Vm-to-Ca), secondarily causes alternans in SR calcium flux. Conversely, alternans can arise primarily from beat-to-beat fluctuations in SR calcium release from the ryanodine release channel (RyR), which, through a process of Ca-to-Vm coupling, secondarily causes alternans of one or more calcium-sensitive ion channels, typically L-type calcium channel (I_{CaL}) and the Na^+-Ca^{2+} exchanger. In response to the large SR calcium release *(odd beats)*, the Na^+-Ca^{2+} exchanger causes action potential prolongation (positive Ca-to-Vm coupling), whereas action potentials would have shortened on odd beats if I_{CaL} were the predominant electrogenic mechanism (negative Ca-to-Vm coupling). See text for details.

The way alternans occurs as a function of APD and diastolic interval (DI) can be depicted in an APD restitution curve (Fig. 27-2A).[51,52] Typically APD shortens exponentially with decreasing DI. Using this relationship, APD of the preceding DI can be predicted as long as heart rate is constant (see Fig. 27-2A, red line). Alternans can be predicted as well. As shown in Figure 27-2A, given an initial condition (asterisk), the arrows track the evolution of APD on a beat-by-beat basis until steady state alternans is achieved (outermost points). Importantly, based on APD restitution, alternans can only occur when the restitution slope exceeds unity. This theoretical relationship has led to several important paradigms. For example, it may be possible to suppress alternans by reducing the slope of the restitution curve.[53] The restitution hypotheses is also consistent with the well-described heart-rate dependence of alternans. For example, as heart rate increases, the CL line moves toward the origin where the slope of restitution is greatest, making alternans more likely to occur.

Several theoretical[54,55] and experimental[56-58] studies support a relationship between alternans and APD restitution. Studies by Dilly and colleagues[59] and Saitoh and colleagues[60] were among the earliest to correlate repolarization alternans with APD restitution. Interestingly, these same studies suggest intracellular calcium regulation as an important factor as well. More recently, Hua and coworkers[61] demonstrated how overexpression of I_{Kr}, an important determinant of APD restitution, can suppress alternans. Finally, in a clinical study, Koller and colleagues[62] demonstrated steeper dynamic restitution in patients with structural heart disease, which was also associated with action potential alternans and ventricular tachycardia.

Although there is considerable support for the APD restitution hypothesis from computer simulations, experimental evidence has been somewhat conflicting. In particular, ventricular myocytes that are most susceptible to alternans do not necessarily exhibit a steep restitution slope.[63] Also, many conditions that *reduce* APD restitution slope (e.g., ischemia) are potent stimuli for alternans.[64,65] There are other important limitations to the APD restitution hypothesis for alternans. Although there are several ways to measure restitution, including standard,[66] dynamic restitution,[67] and restitution portrait,[68] the most appropriate method has not been established. Also, it can be difficult to define a unique APD restitution property of individual myocytes, because under certain conditions (e.g., during alternans) a single myocyte can take on two restitution properties.[69] It is also uncertain that the restitution hypothesis is applicable to T wave alternans in humans. Narayan and coworkers[70] observed that in patients with LV dysfunction, standard action potential duration restitution (measured using intracardiac MAPs), did not exhibit a restitution slope greater than 1 when T wave alternans was manifest in patients. Finally, due to the numerous nonspecific ionic mechanisms that influence APD restitution, its utility for identifying specific ionic or molecular mechanisms is limited,[71-73] can yield conflicting results,[74] and might not be the best approach.[75]

The Calcium-Cycling (Calcium Restitution) Hypothesis

The calcium-cycling hypothesis states that cellular alternans occurs when heart rate exceeds the capacity of the myocyte's intracellular machinery to cycle calcium on an every-beat basis. Consequently, SR and cytoplasmic calcium flux alternate from beat to beat. *Calcium cycling* refers to calcium release from the SR, which initiates systolic contraction, and the subsequent reuptake of calcium back into the SR for diastolic relaxation (for detailed review, see Laurita and Rosenbaum[76]). The magnitude and rate of SR calcium release and reuptake determine the rate at which calcium can be cycled to maintain intracellular

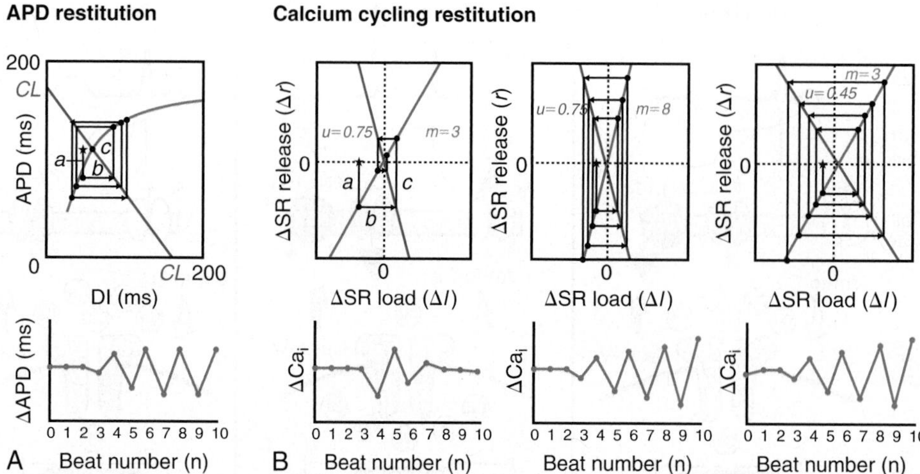

Figure 27-2 A, Restitution hypothesis of alternans. The cobweb diagram *(top)* shows how action potential duration (APD) alternans arises from an exponential APD restitution curve *(blue line)*. The *red line* shows the relationship among cycle length (CL), APD, and diastolic interval (DI), where APD = CL − DI. Given a set of initial conditions for APD and DI *(*)*, alternans evolves as intersecting lines are drawn from the restitution curve to the CL line and back to the restitution curve (lines *a, b,* and *c*). The *bottom graph* shows the development and persistence of APD alternans with beat number as derived from the cobweb diagram. For the restitution hypothesis, the slope of the steep portion of the restitution curve determines the stability of alternans. See text for details. **B,** The calcium cycling (calcium restitution) hypothesis of alternans. The *blue line* shows the relationship between SR calcium release and load, and the *red line* depicts the efficiency of calcium uptake. As with APD restitution **(A)**, a cobweb diagram can be drawn from initial conditions *(*)*, with line segments intersecting the calcium release *(blue)* and reuptake *(red)* lines (lines *a, b,* and *c*). In the first plot at the *bottom left*, the slopes for SR calcium uptake (*u*) and release (*m*) are such that only transient alternans of calcium release occurs. However, an increase in SR calcium restitution slope (*blue line*, middle) or an impairment of SR calcium reuptake (*red line*, right) can lead to persistent alternans. See text for details. (From Weiss JN, Karma A, Shiferaw Y, et al: From pulsus to pulseless: The saga of cardiac alternans. Circ Res 98:1244-1253, 2006.)

calcium homeostasis. For example, if an action potential is initiated before calcium returns to diastolic levels (i.e., before all calcium released can be reclaimed), then the amount of calcium available in the SR is reduced. As a result, calcium release on the subsequent beat is reduced. Given a smaller release but the same time to reclaim calcium, more calcium will end up in the SR and result in a larger release. That is, the amount of released calcium can only be fully reclaimed on an alternating-beat basis, giving rise to self-perpetuating calcium alternans.

The calcium-cycling hypothesis for cardiac alternans can be explained by impaired SR calcium release or reuptake. For example, as with APD restitution, the dynamic properties of SR calcium regulation can predict alternans of calcium release, as described by Weiss and coworkers.[52] Shown in Figure 27-2B are calcium cycling restitution curves, where SR calcium release is plotted as a function of SR load (blue line). To predict SR calcium release alternans, two relationships must be considered. First, the efficiency of calcium uptake is shown in figure 27-2 (panel B) as a red line, whose slope (u) is directly related to the rate of SR reuptake. Second, the gain of SR calcium release for a given SR load must be taken into account as well (slope of blue line, m), which can be considered to be a form of calcium restitution.

As with APD restitution, a cobweb diagram can be drawn to demonstrate the occurrence of calcium release alternans. In the first plot (Fig. 27-2B, left) the slopes for SR calcium uptake (u = 0.75) and release (m = 3) are such that a small perturbation of rate from initial conditions (asterisks) produces transient alternans that dampens within a few beats because the calcium restitution slope is not sufficiently steep. However, as shown in Figure 27-2B (middle panel), with an increase in SR calcium restitution slope (m = 5, blue line), a perturbation in heart rate (asterisks) leads to persistent alternans. Similarly, impairment of SR calcium reuptake (Figure 27-2B, right panel) can lead to persistent alternans even when SR calcium-release dynamics are unchanged. This paradigm has been supported by theoretical studies[52,77] and suggests that excitation-contraction coupling proteins responsible for SR release and reuptake are centrally involved in mechanisms of cardiac alternans.

Subcellular and Molecular Mechanisms of Calcium Transient Alternans

Calcium Uptake into the Sarcoplasmic Reticulum

To maintain homeostasis, the amount of calcium released through the RyR to initiate contraction must be matched by an equivalent about of calcium reclaimed during diastole via either sarcolemmal membrane (Na^+-Ca^{2+} exchanger) or SR calcium reuptake (SERCA2a) processes. If SR calcium uptake is impaired, then cytosolic calcium cannot be fully reclaimed on each beat, and alternans dynamics ensues. Considerable experimental data support this mechanism.

Shown in Figure 27-3 is an example of calcium alternans that depends on the rate of calcium uptake by the SR. Shown are calcium transients measured near the epicardium and endocardium in the canine left ventricular wedge preparation during an abrupt decrease in pacing cycle length. At baseline, the decay phase of calcium transients recorded just before the step change demonstrates a reduced rate of calcium decline to diastolic levels (larger Tau) in endocardium myocytes compared to the epicardium myocytes. As stimulus rate was increased (see Fig. 27-3, arrow), calcium transient alternans was substantially greater near the endocardium compared to the epicardium, suggesting that myocytes with reduced capacity for SR calcium reuptake are most susceptible to alternans. Such findings have been reaffirmed by several other studies.[78-80]

Transmural heterogeneities of alternans that we and others have reported can provide potential clues to molecular mechanisms of alternans. To determine the molecular mechanisms of calcium alternans, we compared protein expression in tissue samples taken from alternans-prone and alternans-resistant myocytes.[79,81] In several mammalian species, myocytes that were

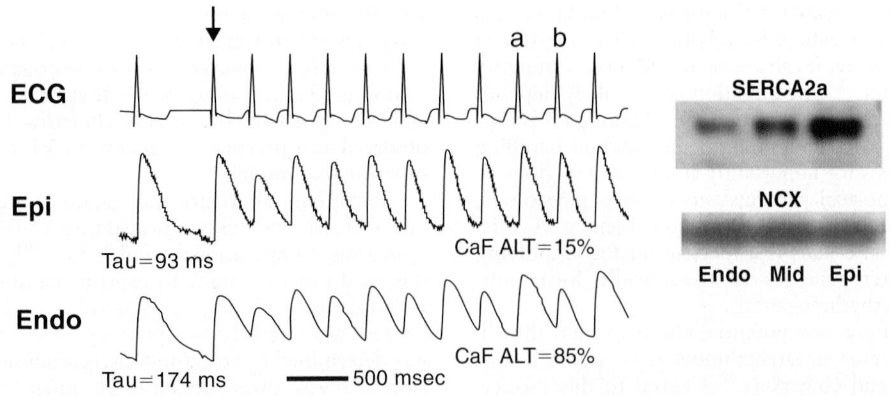

Figure 27-3 Electrocardiogram (ECG) and calcium transients recorded near the epicardium (Epi) and endocardium (Endo) during an abrupt increase in pacing cycle length from 600 to 300 ms *(arrow)*. At Endo, where the decay of the calcium transient (Tau) was slower (174 ms) compared to Epi (93 ms), the magnitude of calcium transient alternans (CaF Endo; compare amplitude of beat a to beat b) was greater. Representative Western blot *(right)* indicating the expression of SERCA2a (110 kDa) and a proteolytic fragment of Na^+-Ca^{2+} exchanger (70 kDa) across the transmural wall, each loaded with equal amounts of protein. Subendocardial layers (Endo) and midmyocardial layers (Mid) showed less expression of SERCA2a compared to subepicardial layers (Epi). In contrast, no significant difference in transmural Na^+-Ca^{2+} exchanger expression was observed.

most susceptible to alternans also exhibited reduced SERCA2a expression (example shown in Fig. 27-3, right).[63,79,81] These data are consistent with previous studies that have shown significantly less SERCA2a mRNA in canine subendocardium compared to the subepicardium[82] and a trend toward less SERCA2a expression near the endocardium in normal human hearts.[83] We have also found that enhancement of SERCA2a using targeted gene transfer markedly attenuates susceptibility to alternans and cardiac arrhythmias,[84] establishing a causal mechanistic relationship between specific molecules responsible for SR calcium reuptake, alternans, and arrhythmogenesis.

Calcium Release from the Sarcoplasmic Reticulum

It is well established that SR calcium content is a major determinant of SR calcium release. Diaz and colleagues[85] used a voltage clamp protocol that was designed to intentionally weaken the calcium-induced calcium-release (CICR) response by using a lower-than-normal activation voltage for I_{CaL}. This caused most RyR channels to open by a calcium wave (i.e., calcium released from neighboring RyR clusters) rather than by CICR, resulting in spatially desynchronized calcium release. Given that calcium waves only occur when SR calcium content is above a threshold value, when release does occur the SR will become depleted below this threshold such that on the subsequent voltage clamp pulse, no release will occur. The absence of a release will maintain enough calcium in the SR such that on the next voltage clamp, a release will occur, perpetuating alternans of calcium release. Importantly, under these conditions, calcium transient alternans occurs at stimulation rates much slower than what is required during normal CICR, presumably because of the very steep relationship between SR calcium content and SR calcium release.

In a theoretical study, Shiferaw and coworkers[86] used similar local dynamics of calcium release and also found that alternans is dependent on a steep, nonlinear, relationship between SR calcium release and content. These findings suggest that the SR calcium store is an important mechanism of alternans.[87] This conclusion, however, is controversial because others have shown that alternans in SR calcium release does not depend solely on SR calcium load. Picht and colleagues[88] used direct measurements of intra-SR free calcium to show that calcium release alternans does not require SR calcium content alternans but, rather, might depend more on RyR recovery.[89] In either case, taken together, these findings suggest that molecules involved in SR calcium reuptake and release are centrally involved in the mechanism of cellular alternans.

Alternans Caused by Direct Mechanoelectrical Feedback

In addition to the role intracellular calcium plays, the direct effect mechanical contraction has on APD (mechanoelectrical feedback) might also play a role in repolarization alternans. In a novel study, Murphy and colleagues[90,91] observed electrical alternans during simulated pulse alternans obtained by mechanically clamping the aorta on every other beat. In this case, alternans of SR calcium release was probably not occurring. If so, some other form of direct mechanoelectrical feedback is the underlying mechanism of electrical alternans. For example, mechanosensitive ion channels, such as stretch-activated channels, can significantly change membrane potential on a beat-to-beat basis and may be playing a role.[92] It is also possible that by alternating contraction or relaxation, the binding affinity of troponin C and, thus, free calcium alternates as well.[93] This could directly affect several calcium-sensitive ion channels and, thus, alternans of APD. Finally, some clinical data suggest that T-wave alternans can be enhanced by mechanoelectrical feedback during acute volume overload in structurally normal hearts.[94] Despite these possibilities, the exact mechanisms by which mechanical alternans can directly affect electrical alternans are not well understood and need to be further investigated. However, it is unlikely that direct mechanoelectrical feedback is a singular mechanism of alternans, because alternans clearly occurs even when contraction is completely inhibited.[63,74]

Mechanisms Linking Alternans to Arrhythmogenesis

Tissue heterogeneities, whether attributable to structural discontinuities, ischemia, or heterogeneous expression of sarcolemmal ionic currents form a critical component of the electrophysiologic substrate for reentrant excitation in the heart. A premature or ectopic beat in the presence of sufficient heterogeneity of repolarization can cause a propagating impulse to block at areas of increased refractoriness (unidirectional block); it can also propagate into less-refractory areas, and after a sufficient time delay, it can re-excite the more refractory zone and initiate reentry.[95] The initiation of VF likely depends on enhanced dispersion of repolarization.[95-97] Although it is now abundantly clear that electrophysiologic and calcium-handling properties of myocytes vary importantly in different regions of myocardium, under normal circumstances these physiologic heterogeneities are not sufficient to promote reentry. As discussed below, cardiac alternans is a mechanism for amplifying electrophysiologic heterogeneities to dynamically form substrates for reentrant arrhythmogenesis.

A mechanism linking action potential alternans (and thus T wave alternans) to reentrant arrhythmogenesis and VF was described by Pastore and coworkers.[20] Central to this mechanism is the development of spatially discordant alternans, where action potential alternans occurs in opposite phase between regions of neighboring cells (Fig. 27-4A).[20] When action potential alternans is first initiated above a particular threshold heart rate, it occurs with identical phase (APD either prolongs or shortens simultaneously in all cells) in a region of ventricular myocardium. This is termed *spatially concordant action potential alternans* (see Fig. 27-4A). Concordant action potential alternans itself is not arrhythmogenic because repolarization remains spatially synchronized and, consequently, spatial dispersion of repolarization does not differ substantially from baseline (see Fig. 27-4B). However, in response to further acceleration of heart rate or a premature impulse, spatially concordant alternans is transformed to spatially discordant alternans, where myocytes in neighboring regions of myocardium exhibit action potentials that alternate with opposite phase (see Fig. 27-4A). Discordant alternans has a significant impact on the spatial organization of repolarization across the ventricle (see Fig. 27-4B).

Discordant alternans creates steep gradients of repolarization[20] that are sufficient to cause conduction block, promoting reentrant excitation. Therefore, discordant alternans serves as a mechanism for dynamically amplifying electrophysiologic heterogeneities in the heart to produce conditions for reentrant excitation.[20,98,99] This is illustrated in Figure 27-5, where the development of discordant alternans is associated with marked amplification of the repolarization gradient (shaded red) between myocytes at two ventricular locations. Under these conditions, a premature beat (asterisks) fails to propagate against the repolarization gradient, leading to the first beat of reentrant excitation and VF. Spatially discordant alternans has been consistently observed as a precursor to reentrant VF and VT in a variety of experimental models.

Discordant alternans was demonstrated experimentally in intact heart and tissue preparations[20,58,98,100] as well as in numerous computational models.[71,77,101] This same paradigm was used experimentally to explain the initiation of a variety of arrhythmias, including polymorphic and monomorphic VT, because although the morphology of the resultant arrhythmias was determined by structural discontinuities in tissue, discordant alternans was always required to initiate reentry.[98] In patients with impaired left ventricular function, discordant action potential alternans has been suggested by intracardiac activation-recovery interval recordings[102] and potentially underlies phase reversal induced by a premature stimulus observed in clinical T wave alternans, which itself predicts increased susceptibility to arrhythmias and mortality.[103]

Mechanisms of Discordant Alternans between Cells

Because spatially discordant alternans is the key step linking cardiac alternans to arrhythmogenesis, it is important to understand its underlying mechanisms. Spatially discordant alternans typically arises after spatially concordant alternans is already established. Therefore, for discordant alternans to develop, the phase of action-potential alternans must change in one region of myocardium but not in others. There are three mechanism by which neighboring cells, under apparently identical conditions, would respond differently with respect to their alternans phase leading to spatially discordant alternans: conduction velocity restitution,[71,104] intracellular uncoupling,[98] and spatial heterogeneities of calcium cycling and the sarcolemmal ionic currents that govern repolarization. These mechanisms are not mutually

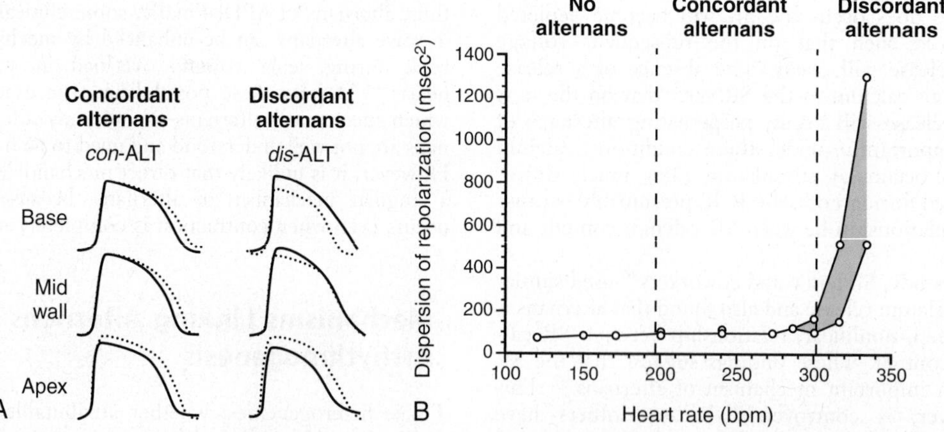

Figure 27-4 Development of discordant alternans promotes dispersion of repolarization. **A,** Optical action potentials from epicardial cells from the base, apex, and mid wall of guinea pig heart during two consecutive beats *(solid* and *stippled lines)* of action potential alternans. Above a critical heart rate, concordant alternans (*left*, all action potential in phase) is transformed to discordant alternans, where action potentials are in opposite phase between base and apex. **B,** Development of discordant alternans markedly amplifies spatial gradients of repolarization. con-ALT, concordant alternans; dis-ALT, discordant alternans. (Adapted from Pastore JM, Girouard SD, Laurita KR, et al: Mechanism linking T-wave alternans to the genesis of cardiac fibrillation. Circulation 99:1385-1394, 1999.)

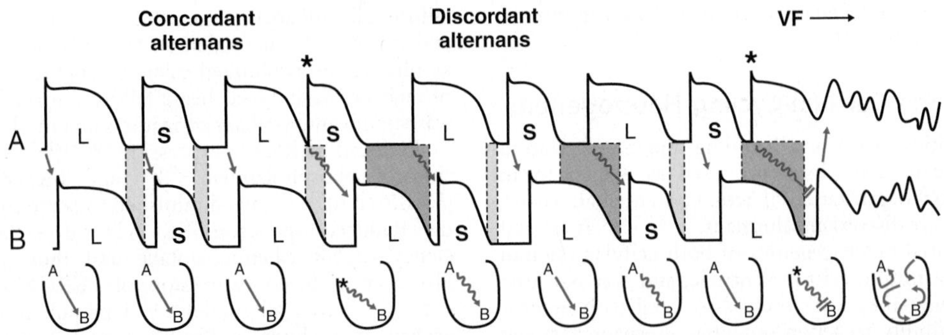

Figure 27-5 Mechanism of discordant alternans in arrhythmogenesis. Action potential propagation between two ventricular sites (*A* to *B*) are shown. *L* indicates long action potential duration, and *S* indicates a short action potential. Dispersion of repolarization between sites is indicated by *shaded bars*. Transition from concordant to discordant alternans and the development of ventricular fibrillation (VF) is shown. Premature beats are represented by the *asterisks*. See text for details. (Adapted from Oshodi GO, Wilson LD, Costantini O, Rosenbaum DS: Microvolt T wave alternans: Mechanisms and implications for prediction of sudden cardiac death. In Gussak I, Antzelevitch C, Wilde AAM, et al (eds): Electrical Diseases of the Heart: Genetics, Mechanisms, Treatment, Prevention. New York, NY: Springer-Verlag, 2007, pp 394-408.)

exclusive; they can coexist and be complementary. Importantly, different mechanisms could be operative or more important under different conditions or disease states.

Restitution of Conduction Velocity

Theoretical computer modeling studies have suggested a mechanism for discordant alternans based on restitution of conduction velocity.[104] These simulations predict that conduction velocity restitution alone, even in the absence of spatially heterogeneous properties of action potentials across the heart can explain spatially discordant alternans.[71,101,104-106] *Conduction velocity restitution* refers to the slowing of conduction velocity occurring in response to progressively premature stimuli. According to the conduction velocity restitution hypothesis for cardiac alternans, a premature beat or sudden acceleration of rate causes conduction slowing, such that cardiomyocytes distant but not proximal to the pacing site experience preferentially delayed activation and, in turn, preferentially longer diastolic intervals.

This mechanism is illustrated in Figure 27-5, where discordant alternans arises from concordant alternans in response to a premature stimulus. During the prematurely stimulated beat, despite the shorter stimulus interval, cells distant from the pacing site (site B) undergo action potential prolongation (according to APD restitution) because they are preceded by longer diastolic intervals (according to conduction velocity restitution). Consequently, the short-long-short sequence of APD is transformed to a short-long-long sequence at site B while retaining the short-long-short sequence at site A. Selective resetting of APD alternans phase at sites downstream but not upstream to the site of the premature beat results in spatially discordant alternans. Spatially discordant alternans, therefore, is characterized by two myocardial zones undergoing APD alternans with opposite phase, separated by a zone exhibiting no alternans, referred to as the *node*.[20,77,104] The conduction velocity restitution hypothesis can explain why cells that change phase are located distal to the ectopic beat, how the location of the node depends on premature stimulus interval or pacing rate, and how multiple nodes can develop in the same heart.[71]

The conduction velocity restitution hypothesis has several limitations. Although, according to conduction velocity restitution, heterogeneous electrophysiologic properties are not required for inducing discordant alternans, normal and, particularly, diseased myocardium clearly possesses considerable heterogeneities. There is evidence that conduction velocity restitution still plays a role under these circumstances.[104] Another issue is that conduction velocity restitution may be minimal relative to APD restitution, because premature stimulus-induced conduction slowing leads to block or fails to capture myocardium before substantial conduction velocity slowing occurs.[20,107]

Intracellular Uncoupling

Another mechanism promoting discordant alternans is attributable to intercellular uncoupling.[71,98] Cardiac myocytes are electrically coupled via gap junctions that allow the flow of electrotonic current between cells. In general, electrotonic coupling acts to homogenize repolarization between cells. In contrast, cell-to-cell uncoupling unmasks intrinsic differences in cellular electrophysiologic properties between neighboring myocytes.[108] Cell-to-cell uncoupling has an important effect on spatial synchronization of repolarization.[19,110] Any tendency for neighboring myocytes to alternate with opposite phase because of intrinsic differences in calcium cycling properties or APD restitution, for example, is opposed by electrotonic coupling between these cells. In a guinea pig model of alternans, the introduction of a structural barrier to electrotonically uncouple neighboring cells greatly facilitated the development of discordant alternans,[98] suggesting that structural barriers such as those imposed by myocardial infarction can impose regional intercellular uncoupling to promote spatially discordant alternans.[98] For example, the maintenance of marked APD gradients between epicardial and midmyocardial layers has been attributed to reduced expression of cardiac gap junctions in this region.[109,110] Conversely, disease or drug-induced uncoupling (as is observed in heart failure and ischemia, for example) between cells can promote discordant alternans.

In addition to regional uncoupling by structural barriers, microscopic uncoupling on a cellular scale can also promote spatially discordant alternans. For example, discordant alternans associated with ischemia-induced intercellular uncoupling was attributable to reduced gap-junction conductance from intracellular acidification during ischemia.[111] Discordant alternans was suppressed by pharmacologically increasing gap-junction conductance with a compound that inhibited ischemia-induced phosphorylation of gap junctions, thereby maintaining intercellular coupling.[111] This is in accordance with previous findings showing an increased level of alternans during ischemia,[59,112] and it supports the hypothesis that the transition from concordant to discordant alternans is affected by the degree of gap junction intercellular conductance as suggested by experimental[98] and modeling studies.[104]

Regional Ionic and Calcium-Cycling Heterogeneity

Spatial heterogeneities of calcium handling and repolarization properties of myocytes have been proposed as a mechanism underlying the spatial organization of action potential alternans, potentially leading to discordant alternans.[52,63,77,113] It is well established that spatial heterogeneities of both cellular calcium handling and repolarization exist in ventricle, and that—at least for calcium handling—they are closely associated with heterogeneities in susceptibility to action potential alternans between myocytes.[81] Just as intrinsic heterogeneities of cellular calcium cycling or repolarization properties in myocytes can potentially explain spatial differences in susceptibility to action potential alternans, these same heterogeneities might also explain the spatial organization of discordant alternans,[20] although experimental evidence for this hypothesis remains limited.[49] However, patterns of discordant alternans are not random, but rather orient themselves along gradients of APD and restitution[20] and patterns of discordant alternans can be independent of pacing site in intact hearts. These two observations support a mechanism for discordant alternans related to intrinsic differences in myocyte properties across the heart.

Computer modeling studies have suggested a novel mechanism in which spatial heterogeneity in the phase of Ca-to-Vm coupling during alternans could result in discordant alternans.[52,77] As discussed earlier, cellular calcium and action potential alternans can be positively or negatively coupled (depending on the relative balance between calcium-sensitive sarcolemmal ionic currents). Spatially discordant alternans could result when calcium alternans is homogeneous in tissue but Ca-to-Vm coupling is positive (i.e., large calcium transient associated with a long action potential) in some cells and negative (i.e., a large calcium transient associated with a short action potential) in others. This mechanism has yet to be demonstrated experimentally, although negative Ca-to-Vm coupling has been demonstrated in ischemia.[114] Interestingly, discordant subcellular alternans, in which calcium alternans is out of phase within regions of a single myocyte, has been observed.[115] How this relates to the organization of calcium alternans on the level of the intact heart or on patterns of action potential alternans remains unclear.[52,77]

Clearly, the aforementioned mechanisms of discordant alternans are not mutually exclusive and are likely interrelated in the whole heart. It is possible that heterogeneity of APD restitution between myocytes plays a critical role in discordant alternans, but under circumstances where conduction velocity is pathologically slowed (by myocardial disease, ischemia, or drugs), conduction velocity restitution might play a more prominent or even a primary role. Similarly, intercellular uncoupling by structural barriers or gap-junction remodeling might not only promote spatially discordant alternans from a primary effect on reducing synchronization of repolarization (i.e., reduced electrotonic modulation between myocytes) but also can secondarily slow conduction, thereby favoring the development of discordant alternans that is dependent on restitution of conduction velocity.

Mechanisms of Alternans in Cardiac Disease

Heart Failure

Because heart failure produces fundamental alterations in cellular calcium-handling properties, it is no surprise that heart failure can enhance susceptibility to cardiac alternans. We[116] and others[117,118] have demonstrated reduced calcium transient amplitude and prolonged calcium reuptake in the canine model of tachycardia-induced heart failure. Susceptibility to alternans was significantly enhanced in the same model.[119,120]

Reduced SERCA2a expression,[80,121-123] as well as the expression of phospholamban[124-126] and FK506 binding protein (FKBP 12.6)[127,128] are diminished in some models of heart failure. Reduced expression SERCA2a is expected to lower the efficiency of SR calcium uptake and thus promote alternans. However, reduced expression of SERCA2a is not a finding common across all models.[129] Upregulation of the Na^+-Ca^{2+} exchanger is almost uniformly reported in human and animal models of heart failure.[121,130] In heart failure, increased Na^+-Ca^{2+} exchanger may be a compensatory response to decreased SERCA2a expression or a leaky RyR (i.e., increased open probability during diastole) in order to extrude calcium and improve diastolic function.[22]

The effect of increased Na^+-Ca^{2+} exchanger on alternans may be primarily through Ca-to-Vm coupling. That is, positive coupling of Ca-to-Vm is expected to be greater in heart failure compared to normal and thus could amplify repolarization alternans. In addition, the expression of the Na^+-K^+ pump[131] and its modulation by phospholemma[132] might influence intracellular Na^+ levels. Changes in intracellular Na^+ alters the driving force for forward mode Na^+-Ca^{2+} exchanger[133,134] and could influence the balance (net polarity) of Ca-to-Vm coupling.[135]

Enhanced susceptibility to alternans in heart failure has also been associated with a reduction of FKBP12.6. Lehnart and colleagues[136] have shown that FKBP12.6–deficient mice, which can develop heart failure, are less prone to electrical alternans when pretreated with JTV519, a compound that increases the binding affinity of FKBP12.6 for RyR. However, the role FKBP12.6 plays in heart failure and arrhythmogenesis is controversial.[137] It is possible that other changes associated with heart failure can affect calcium-transient alternans, such as detubulation[138] and disruption of the regular organization of transverse tubules.[139]

Myocardial Ischemia

Myocardial ischemia creates an important substrate for alternans.[66,140,141] Qian and colleagues[140,142] have shown that the development of significant alternans can develop during the acute phases of ischemia. Interestingly, they found that during acute ischemia, spatially discordant alternans occurred at a much slower heart rate than under normal conditions and that repolarization alternans occurred in the absence of conduction alternans.[142] These effects may be attributable to metabolic inhibition of RyR leading to calcium cycling alternans.[114,143] These studies highlight RyR channel dysfunction as a possible mechanism of calcium-transient alternans irrespective of SR calcium load. Interestingly, it is unlikely that the mechanisms of alternans associated with ischemia involves abnormal repolarization given that ischemia shortens APD and flattens the APD restitution curve.[64] Ischemia can also induce alternating conduction block into ischemic beds due to post-repolarization refractoriness.[144] However, in contrast to other settings where cardiac alternans occurs, a causal relationship between ischemia-induced alternans and arrhythmogenesis has yet to be established.

Long-QT Syndrome

Patients with prolonged repolarization (long-QT syndrome) are susceptible to T-wave alternans.[26-30,145] It is not obvious how calcium handling could be a primary mechanism of alternans in

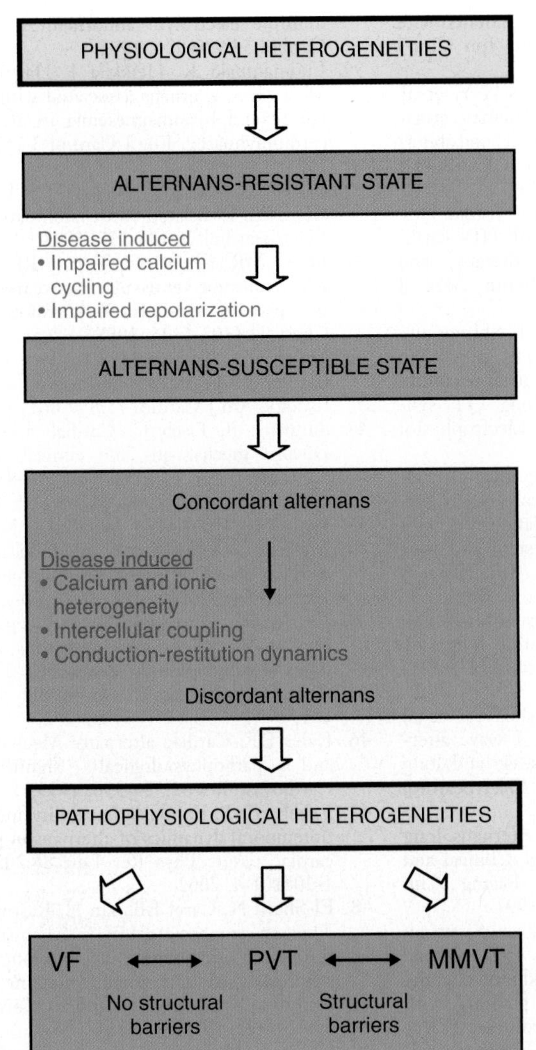

Figure 27-6 Paradigm for cardiac alternans in the mechanism of arrhythmogenesis. MMVI, monomorphic ventricular tachycardia; PVT, polymorphic ventricular tachycardia; VF, ventricular fibrillation.

patients with long QT syndrome; nevertheless, despite a lesion in repolarization, intracellular calcium alternans might also be an important mechanism.[100] Long-QT syndrome is somewhat unusual in that T-wave alternans and arrhythmias are provoked at slow rather than increased heart rates (see Table 27-1). The autonomic nervous system seems to play an important modulatory role in cardiac alternans in long-QT syndrome.[27]

Drug Toxicity

Cardiac alternans has been observed secondary to toxicity or even therapeutic exposure to multiple classes of drugs. Therefore, alternans may be involved in the mechanism of drug-induced proarrhythmia. Cardiotoxic drugs might have multiple effects that would predispose to cardiac alternans, including effects on conduction slowing (class Ia antiarrhythmics), impairing repolarization (type Ic antiarrhythmic drugs, I_{Kr}-blocking drugs), or alterations in electrolytes or autonomic regulation (expected to have downstream effects on calcium cycling). For example, flecainide-induced conduction slowing can evoke local activation sequence alternans[146] or ST segment alternans[147] that precedes VF. Drugs that affect repolarization have also been observed to promote cardiac alternans in the presence of abnormal electrolytes or cardiomyopathies, all of which represent multiple impairments of repolarization reserve.[42]

Drug-induced promotion or suppression of cardiac alternans might be a potential method of differentiating proarrhythmic from nonproarrhythmic I_{Kr}-blocking drugs during drug development.[148] Experimentally, proarrhythmic I_{Kr}-blocking drugs promoted cardiac alternans, while I_{Kr}-blocking drugs associated with low clinical risk of proarrhythmia either did not promote or suppressed cardiac alternans. This suggests that cardiac alternans may be a mechanism for sudden cardiac death secondary to drugs that impair repolarization reserve. T-wave alternans related to drug toxicity might have multifactorial mechanisms, depending on the specificity of the drug for altering conduction, repolarization, contractile function, or other effects.

Conclusions

Cardiac alternans is a precursor to arrhythmias in remarkably diverse clinical and experimental conditions. A proposed paradigm for the cascade of events linking cellular alternans to arrhythmogenesis is shown in Figure 27-6. The normal ventricle is composed of myocytes with physiologic heterogeneous ionic and calcium-cycling properties that ordinarily produce spatial gradients of repolarization that are insufficient to cause conduction block and reentrant arrhythmias. Therefore, under normal circumstances, cardiac myocytes are in a state of relative alternans resistance. However, heart diseases such as heart failure can enhance susceptibility to cardiac alternans by impairing cellular calcium cycling or ion channel function. Susceptibility to alternans is manifested clinically and experimentally by a reduction in the heart rate threshold required to induce it. When spatially discordant alternans is triggered from concordant alternans, electrophysiologic heterogeneities are dynamically amplified to form pathophysiologic heterogeneities of repolarization of sufficient magnitude to promote conditions for conduction block and reentrant excitation. A broad range of arrhythmias can ensue, including VF or monomorphic VT, depending on whether structural discontinuities (barriers or scars) are present in the tissue and can serve as an anchor for stabilizing reentrant rotors.

References

1. Traube L: Ein Fall von Pulsus Bigeminus nebst Bemerkungen über die Leberschwellungen bei Klappenfehlern und über acute Leberatrophie. Berlin Klin Wochenschr 9:185-188, 1872.
2. Herring H: Experimentelle Studien an Saugetieren über das Electrocardiogramm. Z Exp Med 7:363, 1909.
3. Lewis T: Notes upon alternation of the heart. Q J Med 4:141-144, 1910.
4. Windle JD: The incidence and prognostic value of the pulsus alternans in myocardial and arterial disease. Q J Med 6:453-462, 1913.
5. Kalter HH, Schwartz ML: Electrical alternans. N Y State J Med 98:1164-1166, 1948.
6. Hamburger WW, Katz LN, Saphir L: Electrical alternans, clinical study with report of two necropsies. JAMA 106:902-905, 1936.
7. Hellerstein HK, Leibow IM: Electrical alternation in experimental coronary artery occlusion. Am J Physiol 160:366-374, 1950.

8. Adam D, Smith J, Akselrod S, et al: Fluctuations in T-wave morphology and susceptibility to ventricular fibrillation. J Electrocardiol 17:209-218, 1984.
9. Ritzenberg AL, Adam DR, Cohen RJ: Period multupling—evidence for nonlinear behaviour of the canine heart. Nature 307:159-161, 1984.
10. Smith JM, Clancy EA, Valeri R, et al: Electrical alternans and cardiac electrical instability. Circulation 77:110-121, 1988.
11. Nearing B, Huang AH, Verrier RL: Dynamic tracking of cardiac vulnerability by complex demodulation of the T-wave. Science 252:437-440, 1991.
12. Rosenbaum DS, Jackson LE, Smith JM, et al: Electrical alternans and vulnerability to ventricular arrhythmias. N Engl J Med 330:235-241, 1994.
13. Bloomfield DM, Steinman RC, Namerow PB, et al: Microvolt T-wave alternans distinguishes between patients likely and patients not likely to benefit from implanted cardiac defibrillator therapy: A solution to the Multicenter Automatic Defibrillator Implantation Trial (MADIT) II conundrum. Circulation 110:1885-1889, 2004.
14. Klingenheben T, Zabel M, D'Agostino RB, et al: Predictive value of T-wave alternans for arrhythmic events in patients with congestive heart failure. Lancet 356:651-652, 2000.
15. Verrier RL, Nearing BD, La Rovere MT, et al: ATRAMI Investigators. Ambulatory electrocardiogram-based tracking of T wave alternans in postmyocardial infarction patients to assess risk of cardiac arrest or arrhythmic death. J Cardiovasc Electrophysiol 14:705-711, 2003.
16. Hohnloser SH, Klingenheben T, Bloomfield D, et al: Usefulness of microvolt T-wave alternans for prediction of ventricular tachyarrhythmic events in patients with dilated cardiomyopathy: Results from a prospective observational study. J Am Coll Cardiol 41:2220-2224, 2003.
17. Bloomfield DM, Hohnloser SH, Cohen RJ: Interpretation and classification of microvolt T wave alternans tests. J Cardiovasc Electrophysiol 13:502-512, 2002.
18. Hohnloser SH, Klingenheben T, Zabel M, et al: T wave alternans during exercise and atrial pacing in humans. J Cardiovasc Electrophysiol 8:987-993, 1997.
19. Ikeda T, Saito H, Tanno K, et al: T-wave alternans as a predictor for sudden cardiac death after myocardial infarction. Am J Cardiol 89:79-82, 2002.
20. Pastore JM, Girouard SD, Laurita KR, et al: Mechanism linking T-wave alternans to the genesis of cardiac fibrillation. Circulation 99:1385-1394, 1999.
21. Rubenstein DS, Lipsius SL: Premature beats elicit a phase reversal of mechanoelectrical alternans in cat ventricular myocytes: A possible mechanism for reentrant arrhythmias. Circulation 91:201-214, 1995.
22. Hobai IA, O'Rourke B: Enhanced Ca^{2+}-activated Na^{+}-Ca^{2+} exchange activity in canine pacing-induced heart failure. Circ Res 87:690-698, 2000.
23. Momiyama Y, Hartikainen J, Nagayoshi H, et al: Exercise-induced T-wave alternans as a marker of high risk in patients with hypertrophic cardiomyopathy. Jpn Circ J 61:650-656, 1997.
24. Kon-No Y, Watanabe J, Koseki Y, et al: Microvolt T wave alternans in human cardiac hypertrophy: Electrical instability and abnormal myocardial arrangement. J Cardiovasc Electrophysiol 12:759-763, 2001.
25. Kent S, Ferguson M, Trotta R, Jordan L: T wave alternans associated with HIV cardiomyopathy, erythromycin therapy, and electrolyte disturbances. South Med J 91:755-758, 1998.
26. Shimizu W, Ohe T, Kurita T, Shimomura K: Differential response of QTU interval to exercise, isoproterenol, and atrial pacing in patients with congenital long QT syndrome. Pacing Clin Electrophysiol 14:1966-1970, 1991.
27. Schwartz PJ, Malliani A: Electrical alternation of the T-wave: Clinical and experimental evidence of its relationship with the sympathetic nervous system and with the long Q-T syndrome. Am Heart J 89:45-50, 1975.
28. Zareba W, Moss AJ, Le Cessie S, Hall WJ: T wave alternans in idiopathic long QT syndrome. J Am Coll Cardiol 23:1541-1546, 1994.
29. Burattini L, Zareba W, Rashba EJ, et al: ECG features of microvolt T-wave alternans in coronary artery disease and long QT syndrome patients. J Electrocardiol 31(Suppl):114-120, 1998.
30. Habbab MA, el-Sherif N: T alternans, long QT, and torsades de pointes: Clinical and experimental observations. Pacing Clin Electrophysiol 15:916-931, 1992.
31. Tada T, Kusano KF, Nagase S, et al: Clinical significance of macroscopic T-wave alternans after sodium channel blocker administration in patients with Brugada syndrome. J Cardiovasc Electrophysiol J Cardiovasc Electrophysiol 19(1):56-61, 2008.
32. Morita H, Nagase S, Kusano K, Ohe T: Spontaneous T wave alternans and premature ventricular contractions during febrile illness in a patient with Brugada syndrome. J Cardiovasc Electrophysiol 13:816-818, 2002.
33. Puletti M, Curione M, Righetti G, Jacobellis G: Alternans of the ST-segment and T-wave in acute myocardial infarction. JElectrocardiology 13:297-300, 1980.
34. Salerno JA, Previtali M, Panciroli C, et al: Ventricular arrhythmias during acute myocardial ischemia in man. The role and significance of R-ST-T alternans and the prevention of ischemic sudden death by medical treatment. Euro Heart J 7:63-75, 1986.
35. Cheng TC: Electrical alternans: An association with coronary artery spasm. Arch Intern Med 143:1052-1053, 1983.
36. Kleinfeld MJ, Rozanski JJ: Alternans of the ST-segment in Prenzmetal's angina. Circulation 55:574-577, 1977.
37. Reddy CVR, Kiok JP, Khan RG, El-Sherif N: Repolarization alternans associated with alcoholism and hypomagnesemia. Am J Cardiol 53:390-391, 1984.
38. Shimoni Z, Flateau E, Schiller D, et al: Electrical alternans of giant U waves with multiple electrolyte abnormalities. Am J Cardiol 54:920-921, 1984.
39. Luomanmaki K, Heikkila J, Hartikainen M: T-wave alternans associated with heart failure and hypomagnesemia in alcoholic cardiomyopathy. Eur J Cardiol 3:167-170, 1975.
40. Bardaji A, Vidal F, Richart C: T wave alternans associated with amiodarone. J Electrocardiol 26:155-157, 1993.
41. Bibler MR, Chou TC, Toltzis RJ, Wade PA: Recurrent ventricular tachycardia due to pentamidine-induced cardiotoxicity. Chest 94:1303-1306, 1988.
42. Orban Z, MacDonald LL, Peters MA, Guslits B: Erythromycin-induced cardiac toxicity. Am J Cardiol 75:859-861, 1995.
43. Surawicz B, Fisch C: Cardiac alternans: Diverse mechanisms and clinical manifestations. J Am Coll Cardiol 20:483-499, 1992.
44. Rashba EJ, Cooklin M, MacMurdy K, et al: Effects of selective autonomic blockade on T-wave alternans in humans. Circulation 105:837-842, 2002.
45. Verrier RL, Nearing BD: Electrophysiologic basis for T wave alternans as an index of vulnerability to ventricular fibrillation. J Cardiovasc Electrophysiol 5:445-461, 1994.
46. Euler DE: Cardiac alternans: Mechanisms and pathophysiological significance. Cardiovasc Res 42:583-590, 1999.
47. Echebarria B, Karma A: Instability and spatiotemporal dynamics of alternans in paced cardiac tissue. Phys Rev Lett 88:208101-1-208101-4, 2002.
48. El-Sherif N, Caref EB, Yin H, Restivo M: The electrophysiological mechanism of ventricular arrhythmias in the long QT syndrome—tridimensional mapping of activation and recovery patterns. Circ Res 79:474-492, 1996.
49. Chinushi M, Kozhevnikov D, Caref EB, et al: Mechanism of discordant T wave alternans in the in vivo heart. J Cardiovasc Electrophysiol 14:632-638, 2003.
50. Shiferaw Y, Sato D, Karma A: Coupled dynamics of voltage and calcium in paced cardiac cells. Phys Rev E Stat Nonlin Soft Matter Phys 71:021903, 2005.
51. Nolasco JB, Dahlen RW: A graphic method for the study of alternation in cardiac action potentials. J Appl Physiol 25:191-196, 1968.
52. Weiss JN, Karma A, Shiferaw Y, et al: From pulsus to pulseless: The saga of cardiac alternans. Circ Res 98:1244-1253, 2006.
53. Mahajan A, Sato D, Shiferaw Y, et al: Modifying L-type calcium current kinetics: Consequences for cardiac excitation and arrhythmia dynamics. Biophys J 94(2): 411-423, 2008.
54. Karma A: Electrical alternans and spiral wave breakup in cardiac tissue. Chaos 4:461-472, 1994.
55. ten Tusscher KH, Panfilov AV: Alternans and spiral breakup in a human ventricular tissue model. Am J Physiol Heart Circ Physiol 291:H1088-H1100, 2006.
56. Koller M, Riccio M, Gilmour R: Dynamic restitution of action potential duration during electrical alternans and ven-

tricular fibrillation. Am J Physiol 275 (5 Pt 2):H1635-H1642, 1998.

57. Tolkacheva EG, Anumonwo JM, Jalife J: Action potential duration restitution portraits of mammalian ventricular myocytes: Role of calcium current. Biophys J 91:2735-2745, 2006.
58. Chinushi M, Restivo M, Caref EB, El-Sherif N: Electrophysiological basis of arrhythmogenicity of QT/T alternans in the long-QT syndrome—tridimensional analysis of the kinetics of cardiac repolarization. Circ Res 83:614-628, 1998.
59. Dilly SG, Lab MJ: Electrophysiological alternans and restitution during acute regional ischaemia in myocardium of anaesthetized pig. J Physiol 402:315-333, 1988.
60. Saitoh H, Bailey J, Surawicz B: Action potential duration alternans in dog Purkinje and ventricular muscle fibers. Circulation 80:1421-1431, 1989.
61. Hua F, Johns DC, Gilmour RF Jr: Suppression of electrical alternans by overexpression of HERG in canine ventricular myocytes. Am J Physiol Heart Circ Physiol 286:H2342-H2351, 2004.
62. Koller ML, Maier SK, Gelzer AR, et al: Altered dynamics of action potential restitution and alternans in humans with structural heart disease. Circulation 112:1542-1548, 2005.
63. Pruvot EJ, Katra RP, Rosenbaum DS, Laurita KR: Role of calcium cycling versus restitution in the mechanism of repolarization alternans. Circ Res 94:1083-1090, 2004.
64. Kurz RW, Ren XL, Franz MR: Dispersion and delay of electrical restitution in the globally ischaemic heart. Eur Heart J 15:547-554, 1994.
65. Mohabir R, Lee HC, Kurz RW, Clusin WT: Effects of ischemia and hypercarbic acidosis on myocyte calcium transients, contraction, and pHi in perfused rabbit hearts. Circ Res 69:1525-1537, 1991.
66. Bass BG: Restitution of the action potential in cat papillary muscle. Am J Physiol 228:1717-1724, 1975.
67. Koller ML, Riccio ML, Gilmour RF Jr: Dynamic restitution of action potential duration during electrical alternans and ventricular fibrillation. Am J Physiol 275:H1635-H1642, 1998.
68. Kalb SS, Dobrovolny HM, Tolkacheva EG, et al: The restitution portrait: A new method for investigating rate-dependent restitution. J Cardiovasc Electrophysiol 15:698-709, 2004.
69. Pastore JM, Laurita KR, Rosenbaum DS: Importance of spatiotemporal heterogeneity of cellular restitution in mechanism of arrhythmogenic discordant alternans. Heart Rhythm 3:711-719, 2006.
70. Narayan SM, Franz MR, Lalani G, et al: T-wave alternans, restitution of human action potential duration, and outcome. J Am Coll Cardiol 50:2385-2392, 2007.
71. Watanabe MA, Fenton FH, Evans SJ, et al: Mechanisms for discordant alternans. J Cardiovasc Electrophysiol 12:196-206, 2001.
72. Garfinkel A, Kim YH, Voroshilovsky O, et al: Preventing ventricular fibrillation by flattening cardiac restitution. Proc Natl Acad Sci U S A 97:6061-6066, 2000.
73. Riccio ML, Koller ML, Gilmour RF Jr: Electrical restitution and spatiotemporal organization during ventricular fibrillation. Circ Res 84:955-963, 1999.
74. Banville I, Gray RA: Effect of action potential duration and conduction velocity restitution and their spatial dispersion on alternans and the stability of arrhythmias. J Cardiovasc Electrophysiol 13:1141-1149, 2002.
75. Laurita KR: Role of action potential duration restitution in arrhythmogenesis. J Cardiovasc Electrophysiol 15:464-465, 2004.
76. Laurita KR, Rosenbaum DS: Mechanisms and potential therapeutic targets for ventricular arrhythmias associated with impaired cardiac calcium cycling. J Mol Cell Cardiol 44:31-43, 2008.
77. Sato D, Shiferaw Y, Garfinkel A, et al: Spatially discordant alternans in cardiac tissue: Role of calcium cycling. Circ Res 99:520-527, 2006.
78. Cordeiro JM, Malone JE, Di Diego JM, et al: Cellular and subcellular alternans in the canine left ventricle. Am J Physiol Heart Circ Physiol 293(6):H3506-H3516, 2007.
79. Wan X, Laurita KR, Pruvot E, Rosenbaum DS: Molecular correlates of repolarization alternans in cardiac myocytes. J Mol Cell Cardiol 39:419-428, 2005.
80. Kihara Y, Morgan JP: Abnormal Ca_i^{2+} handling is the primary cause of mechanical alternans: Study in ferret ventricular muscles. Am J Physiol 261:H1746-H1755, 1991.
81. Laurita KR, Katra R, Wible B, et al: Transmural heterogeneity of calcium handling in canine. Circ Res 92:668-675, 2003.
82. Igarashi-Saito K, Tsutsui H, Takahashi M, et al: Endocardial versus epicardial differences of sarcoplasmic reticulum Ca^{2+}-ATPase gene expression in the canine failing myocardium. Basic Res Cardiol 94:267-273, 1999.
83. Prestle J, Dieterich S, Preuss M, et al: Heterogeneous transmural gene expression of calcium-handling proteins and natriuretic peptides in the failing human heart. Cardiovasc Res 43:323-331, 1999.
84. Cutler MJ, Wan X, Hajjar RJ, Rosenbaum DS: Targeted SERCA2a gene overexpression identifies mechanism and potential therapy for arrhythmogenic cardiac alternans. Circulation 116:(II):217, 2007.
85. Diaz ME, O'Neill SC, Eisner DA: Sarcoplasmic reticulum calcium content fluctuation is the key to cardiac alternans. Circ Res 94:650-656, 2004.
86. Shiferaw Y, Watanabe MA, Garfinkel A, et al: Model of intracellular calcium cycling in ventricular myocytes. Biophys J 85:3666-3686, 2003.
87. Sipido KR: Understanding cardiac alternans: The answer lies in the Ca^{2+} store. Circ Res 94:570-572, 2004.
88. Picht E, DeSantiago J, Blatter LA, Bers DM: Cardiac alternans do not rely on diastolic sarcoplasmic reticulum calcium content fluctuations. Circ Res 99:740-748, 2006.
89. Dumitrescu C, Narayan P, Efimov IR, et al: Mechanical alternans and restitution in failing SHHF rat left ventricles. Am J Physiol Heart Circ Physiol 282:H1320-H1326, 2002.
90. Murphy CF, Lab MJ, Horner SM, et al: Regional electromechanical alternans in anesthetized pig hearts: Modulation by mechanoelectric feedback. Am J Physiol 267:H1726-H1735, 1994.
91. Murphy CF, Horner SM, Dick DJ, et al: Electrical alternans and the onset of rate-induced pulsus alternans during acute regional ischaemia in the anaesthetised pig heart. Cardiovasc Res 32:138-147, 1996.
92. Kohl P, Sachs F: Mechanoelectric feedback in cardiac cells. Philosoph Trans Royal Soc Lond Series A Mathemat Phys Eng Sci 359:1173-1185, 2001.
93. Housmans PR, Lee NK, Blinks JR: Active shortening retards the decline of the intracellular calcium transient in mammalian heart muscle. Science 221:159-161, 1983.
94. Narayan SM, Drinan DD, Lackey RP, Edman CF: Acute volume overload elevates T-wave alternans magnitude. J Appl Physiol 102:1462-1468, 2007.
95. Han J, Moe G: Nonuniform recovery of excitability in ventricular muscle. Circ Res 14:44-60, 1964.
96. Kuo C, Atarashi H, Reddy P, Surawicz B: Dispersion of ventricular repolarization and arrhythmia: Study of two consecutive premature complexes. Circulation 72:370-376, 1985.
97. Kuo C, Munakata K, Reddy CP, Surawicz B: Characteristics and possible mechanisms of ventricular arrhythmia dependent on the dispersion of action potential durations. Circulation 67:1356-1357, 1983.
98. Pastore JM, Rosenbaum DS: Role of structural barriers in the mechanism of alternans-induced reentry. Circ Res 87:1157-1163, 2000.
99. Walker ML, Rosenbaum DS: Repolarization alternans: Implications for the mechanism and prevention of sudden cardiac death. Cardiovasc Res 57:599-614, 2003.
100. Shimizu W, Antzelevitch C: Cellular and ionic basis for T-wave alternans under long-QT conditions. Circulation 99:1499-1507, 1999.
101. Cao JM, Qu ZL, Kim YH, et al: Spatiotemporal heterogeneity in the induction of ventricular fibrillation by rapid pacing importance of cardiac restitution properties. Circ Res 84:1318-1331, 1999.
102. Selvaraj RJ, Picton P, Nanthakumar K, et al: Endocardial and epicardial repolarization alternans in human cardiomyopathy: Evidence for spatiotemporal heterogeneity and correlation with body surface T-wave alternans. J Am Coll Cardiol 49:338-346, 2007.
103. Narayan SM, Smith JM, Schechtman KB, et al: T-wave alternans phase following ventricular extrasystoles predicts arrhythmia-free survival. Heart Rhythm 2:234-241, 2005.
104. Qu Z, Garfinkel A, Chen P, Weiss J: Mechanisms of discordant alternans and

induction of reentry in simulated cardiac tissue. Circulation 102:1664-1670, 2000.
105. Podrid PJ, Fuchs T, Candinas R: Role of the sympathetic nervous system in the genesis of ventricular arrhythmia. Circulation 82:I-103-I-113, 1990.
106. Bellavere F, Ferri M, Guarini L, et al: Prolonged QT period in diabetic autonomic neuropathy: A possible role in sudden cardiac death? Br Heart J 59:379-383, 1988.
107. Laurita KR, Girouard SD, Rudy Y, Rosenbaum DS: Role of passive electrical properties during action potential restitution in the intact heart. Am J Physiol 273:H1205-H1214, 1997.
108. Lesh MD, Pring M, Spear JF: Cellular uncoupling can unmask dispersion of action potential duration in ventricular myocardium. A computer modeling study. Circ Res 65:1426-1440, 1989.
109. Poelzing S, Akar FG, Baron E, Rosenbaum DS: Heterogeneous connexin43 expression produces electrophysiological heterogeneities across ventricular wall. Am J Physiol Heart Circ Physiol 286:H2001-H2009, 2004.
110. Poelzing S, Rosenbaum DS: Altered connexin43 expression produces arrhythmia substrate in heart failure. Am J Physiol Heart Circ Physiol 287:H1762-H1770, 2004.
111. Kjolbye AL, Dikshteyn M, Eloff BC, Deschenes I, Rosenbaum DS: Maintenance of intercellular coupling by the antiarrhythmic peptide rotigaptide suppresses arrhythmogenic discordant alternans. Am J Physiol Heart Circ Physiol 294(1):H41-H49, 2008.
112. Kurz RW, Mohabir R, Ren X-L, Franz MR: Ischaemia induced alternans of action potential duration in the intact heart: Dependence on coronary flow, preload, and cycle length. Eur Heart J 14:1410-1420, 1993.
113. Pastore JM., Rosenbaum DS: Spatial and temporal heterogeneities of cellular restitution are responsible for arrhythmogenic discordant alternans. Circulation 100:I-51, 1999.
114. Hüser J, Wang YG, Sheehan KA, et al: Functional coupling between glycolysis and excitation-contraction coupling underlies alternans in cat heart cells. JPhysiol (Lond) 524:795-806, 2000.
115. Aistrup GL, Kelly JE, Kapur S, et al: Pacing-induced heterogeneities in intracellular Ca^{2+} signaling, cardiac alternans, and ventricular arrhythmias in intact rat heart. Circ Res 99:e65-e73, 2006.
116. Hoeker GS, Katra RP, Laurita KR: Imaging cellular calcium dysfunction in the heart using multi-modal optical mapping. Conf Proc IEEE Eng Med Biol Soc 1:571-575, 2006.
117. Jiang MT, Lokuta AJ, Farrell EF, et al: Abnormal Ca^{2+} release, but normal ryanodine receptors, in canine and human heart failure. Circ Res 91:1015-1022, 2002.
118. O'Rourke B, Kass DA, Tomaselli GF, et al: Mechanisms of altered excitation-contraction coupling in canine tachycardia-induced heart failure. I—Experimental studies. Circ Res 84:562-570, 1999.
119. Wilson LD, Wan X, Rosenbaum DS: Cellular alternans: A mechanism linking calcium cycling proteins to cardiac arrhythmogenesis. Ann N Y Acad Sci 1080:216-234, 2006.
120. Wilson LD, Jeyaraj D, Xiaoping X, et al: Heart failure enhances susceptibility to arrhythmogenic cardiac alternans. Heart Rhythm, in press.
121. Tomaselli GF, Marbán E: Electrophysiological remodeling in hypertrophy and heart failure. Cardiovasc Res 42:270-283, 1999.
122. Davies CH, Davia K, Bennett JG, et al: Reduced contraction and altered frequency response of isolated ventricular myocytes from patients with heart failure. Circulation 92:2540-2549, 1995.
123. De La Bastie D, Levitsky D, Rappaport L, et al: Function of the sarcoplasmic reticulum and expression of its Ca^{2+}-ATPase gene in pressure overload-induced cardiac hypertrophy in the rat. Circ Res 66:554-564, 1990.
124. Studer R, Reinecke H, Bilger J, et al: Gene expression of the cardiac Na^+-Ca^{2+} exchanger in end-stage human heart failure. Circ Res 75(3):443-453, 1994.
125. Flesch M, Schwinger RHG, Schiffer F, et al: Evidence for functional relevance of an enhanced expression of the Na^+-Ca^{2+} exchanger in failing human myocardium. Circulation 94:992-1002, 1996.
126. Schwinger RHG, Böhm M, Schmidt U, et al: Unchanged protein levels of SERCA II and phospholamban but reduced Ca^{2+} uptake and Ca^{2+}-ATPase activity of cardiac sarcoplasmic reticulum from dilated cardiomyopathy patients compared with patients with nonfailing hearts. Circulation 92:3220-3228, 1995.
127. Yano M, Ono K, Ohkusa T, et al: Altered stoichiometry of FKBP12.6 versus ryanodine receptor as a cause of abnormal Ca^{2+} leak through ryanodine receptor in heart failure. Circulation 102:2131-2136, 2000.
128. Marx SO, Reiken S, Hisamatsu Y, et al: PKA phosphorylation dissociates FKBP12.6 from the calcium release channel (ryanodine receptor): Defective regulation in failing hearts. Cell 101:365-376, 2000.
129. Belevych A, Kubalova Z, Terentyev D, et al: Enhanced ryanodine receptor-mediated calcium leak determines reduced sarcoplasmic reticulum calcium content in chronic canine heart failure. Biophys J 93(11):4083-4092, 2007.
130. Hasenfuss G: Alterations of calcium-regulatory proteins in heart failure. Cardiovasc Res 37:279-289, 1998.
131. Bossuyt J, Ai X, Moorman JR, et al: Expression and phosphorylation of the Na-pump regulatory subunit phospholemman in heart failure. Circ Res 97:558-565, 2005.
132. Despa S, Bossuyt J, Han F, Ginsburg KS, et al: Phospholemman-phosphorylation mediates the beta-adrenergic effects on Na/K pump function in cardiac myocytes. Circ Res 97:252-259, 2005.
133. Despa S, Islam MA, Weber CR, et al: Intracellular Na^+ concentration is elevated in heart failure but Na/K pump function is unchanged. Circulation 105:2543-2548, 2002.
134. Valdivia CR, Chu WW, Pu J, et al: Increased late sodium current in myocytes from a canine heart failure model and from failing human heart. J Mol Cell Cardiol 38:475-483, 2005.
135. Baartscheer A, Schumacher CA, Belterman CN, et al: $[Na^+]_i$ and the driving force of the Na^+/Ca^{2+}-exchanger in heart failure. Cardiovasc Res 15:986-995, 2003.
136. Lehnart SE, Terrenoire C, Reiken S, et al: Stabilization of cardiac ryanodine receptor prevents intracellular calcium leak and arrhythmias. Proc Natl Acad Sci U S A 103:7906-7910, 2006.
137. Xiao B, Sutherland C, Walsh MP, Chen SR: Protein kinase A phosphorylation at serine-2808 of the cardiac Ca^{2+}-release channel (ryanodine receptor) does not dissociate 12.6-kDa FK506-binding protein (FKBP12.6). Circ Res 94:487-495, 2004.
138. Louch WE, Bito V, Heinzel FR, et al: Reduced synchrony of Ca^{2+} release with loss of T-tubules—a comparison to Ca^{2+} release in human failing cardiomyocytes. Cardiovasc Res 62:63-73, 2004.
139. Song LS, Sobie EA, McCulle S, et al: Orphaned ryanodine receptors in the failing heart. Proc Natl Acad Sci U S A 103:4305-4310, 2006.
140. Qian YW, Clusin WT, Lin SF, et al: Spatial heterogeneity of calcium transient alternans during the early phase of myocardial ischemia in the blood-perfused rabbit heart. Circulation 104:2082-2087, 2001.
141. Kurz RW, Mohabir R, Ren XL, Franz MR: Ischaemia induced alternans of action potential duration in the intact-heart: Dependence on coronary flow, preload and cycle length. Eur Heart J 14:1410-1420, 1993.
142. Qian YW, Sung RJ, Lin SF, et al: Spatial heterogeneity of action potential alternans during global ischemia in the rabbit heart. Am J Physiol Heart Circ Physiol 285:H2722-H2733, 2003.
143. Kockskamper J, Blatter LA: Subcellular Ca^{2+} alternans represents a novel mechanism for the generation of arrhythmogenic Ca^{2+} waves in cat atrial myocytes. J Physiol 545:65-79, 2002.
144. Janse MJ, Van Capelle F, Morsink H, et al: Flow of "injury" current and patterns of excitation during early ventricular arrhythmias in acute regional myocardial ischemia in isolated porcine and canine heart. Circ Res 47:151-165, 1980.
145. Platt SB, Vijgen JM, Albrecht P, et al: Occult T wave alternans in long QT syndrome. J Cardiovasc Electrophysiol 7:144-148, 1996.
146. Watanabe T, Yamaki M, Kubota I, et al: Relation between activation sequence fluctuation and arrhythmogenicity in

sodium-channel blockade. Am J Physiol Heart Circ Physiol 277:H971-H977, 1999.

147. Tachibana H, Yamaki M, Kubota I, et al: Intracoronary flecainide induces ST alternans and reentrant arrhythmia on intact canine heart: A role of 4-aminopyridine-sensitive current. Circulation 99:1637-1643, 1999.

148. Fossa AA, Wisialowski T, Wolfgang E, et al: Differential effect of HERG blocking agents on cardiac electrical alternans in the guinea pig. Eur J Pharmacol 486:209-221, 2004.

149. Oshodi GO, Wilson LD, Costantini O, Rosenbaum DS: Microvolt T wave alternans: Mechanisms and implications for prediction of sudden cardiac death. In Gussak I, Antzelevitch C, Wilde AAM, et al (eds): Electrical Diseases of the Heart: Genetics, Mechanisms, Treatment, Prevention. New York, NY: Springer-Verlag, 2007, pp 394-408.

Heterogeneous Expression of Repolarizing Potassium Currents in the Mammalian Myocardium 28

JEANNE M. NERBONNE

CHAPTER OUTLINE

In the mammalian myocardium, there are marked regional differences in action potential waveforms, durations, and frequency dependences. These differences influence excitation-contraction coupling and affect the normal propagation of excitation through the myocardium and the dispersion of repolarization in the ventricles. Electrophysiologic studies on isolated mammalian cardiac myocytes have identified multiple types of voltage-gated K^+ (Kv) channel currents with distinct time- and voltage-dependent properties. A number of nonvoltage-gated, inwardly rectifying K^+ (Kir) channels have also been identified.

The various Kv channels appear to be differentially expressed in different cardiac cell types, contributing to cellular and regional differences in action potential waveforms and refractoriness. In the diseased myocardium, K^+ current remodeling can be pronounced, influencing propagation and rhythmicity, effects that can lead to increased dispersion of repolarization and create substrates for reentrant arrhythmias. The molecular cloning of a large number of Kv and Kir channel pore-forming (α) and accessory (β) subunits, as well as the more recently identified two-pore domain K^+ (K2P) channel subunits, has provided molecular insights into the composition of the functionally distinct types of K^+ channels in cardiac myocytes and facilitated efforts focused on exploring the molecular mechanisms controlling the properties and the functional cell surface expression of these channels in the normal and in the diseased myocardium.

Action-potential waveforms vary markedly in different regions of the mammalian heart (Fig. 28-1). In atrial and ventricular myocardium, for example, the action-potential upstroke, attributed to inward currents through voltage-gated Na^+ channels, is rapid (see Fig. 28-1). In nodal tissues, in contrast, which lack functional voltage-gated Na^+ channels, the upstroke of the action potential is substantially slower (see Fig. 28-1) and is dominated by Ca^{2+} influx through voltage-gated Ca^{2+} channels. There are also marked regional differences in action potential heights and durations, as well as in the time course(s) of action potential repolarization (see Fig. 28-1). These differences, which affect the normal spread of excitation in the myocardium and influence the dispersion of repolarization in the ventricles, primarily reflect regional differences in the functional expression or the properties (or both) of the outward K^+ currents, as well as the inward (voltage-gated Na^+ and Ca^{2+}) currents.[1]

Cellular electrophysiologic studies have detailed the properties of the major inward (Na^+ and Ca^{2+}) and outward (K^+) currents (see Fig. 28-1) that shape the waveforms of myocardial action potentials. In contrast to cardiac Na^+ and Ca^{2+} currents, there are multiple types of myocardial K^+ currents, and, of the various K^+ currents, the Kv currents are the most numerous and diverse (Table 28-1). Indeed, multiple types of Kv channels, as well as nonvoltage-gated Kir channels, have been distinguished physiologically and pharmacologically in cells from different species and from different regions of the heart (see Table 28-1) in the same species. The differential expression of Kv and Kir channels contributes to regional variations in myocardial action potential waveforms (see Fig. 28-1) and refractoriness.[1-3] In addition, changes in the densities, distributions, and properties of Kv and Kir channels are evident in a variety of myocardial diseases, and these changes affect repolarization, influence propagation, and decrease rhythmicity, effects that can produce substrates for the generation of life-threatening arrhythmias.[1] There is, therefore, considerable interest in defining the molecular mechanisms controlling the biophysical properties and the functional cell surface expression of these channels.

A large number of Kv (Table 28-2) and Kir (Table 28-4) pore-forming α subunits and accessory β subunits (Table 28-3) have been identified,[4,5] and considerable progress has been made in defining the relationships between these subunits and the functional myocardial Kv and Kir channels.[3,6,7] Importantly, the studies completed to date have revealed that the molecular correlates of the various types of Kv and Kir channels distinguished electrophysiologically (see Table 28-1) are, indeed, distinct.[3,7] In the long term, defining the molecular compositions of myocardial Kv and Kir channels will also facilitate future studies focused on determining the molecular mechanisms controlling the marked regional differences in the functional expression of these channels in the normal myocardium, as well as the derangements in the expression or the functioning of these channels that occur with myocardial disease. In this chapter, the electrophysiologic and molecular diversity of repolarizing myocardial Kv and Kir channels is reviewed, with emphasis on the K^+ channels that are differentially distributed, and the molecular mechanisms controlling regional heterogeneities in K^+ channel expression are explored.

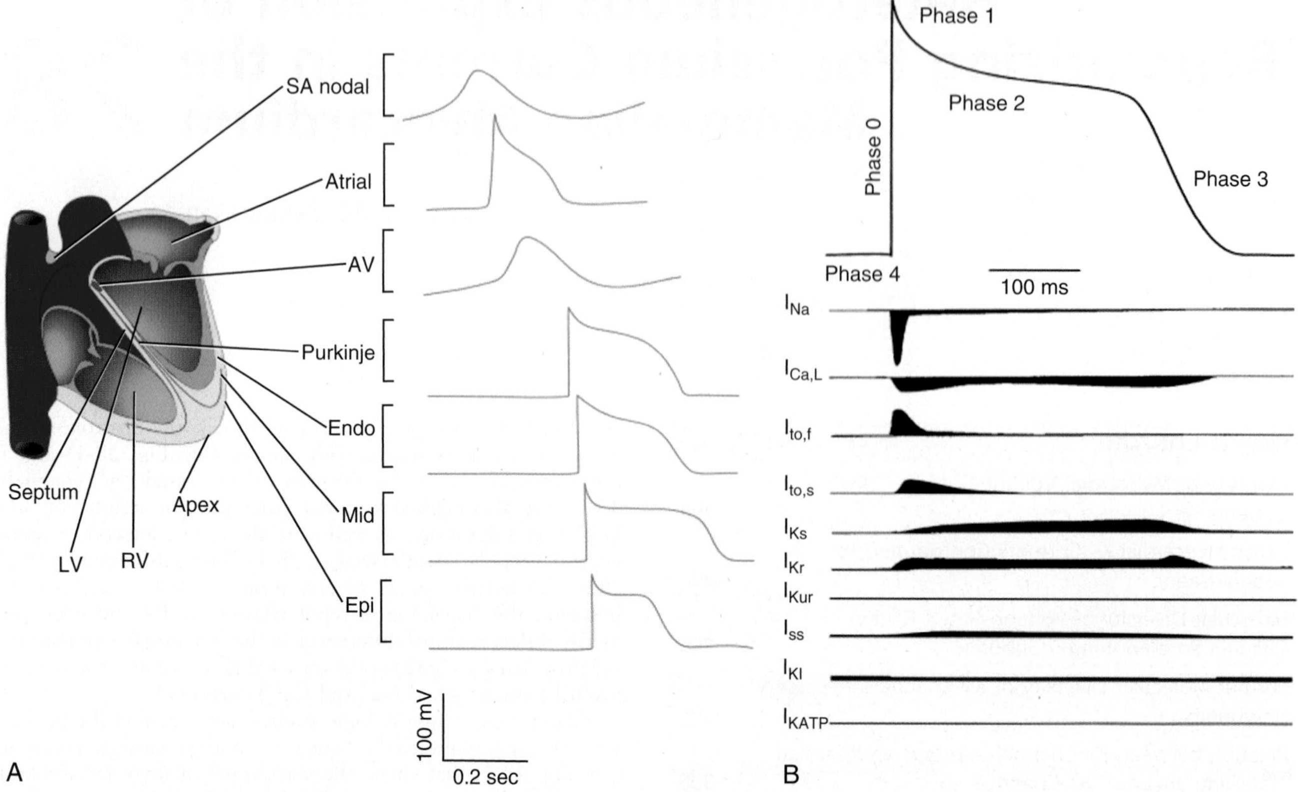

Figure 28-1 **A,** Action-potential waveforms, displaced in time to reflect the temporal sequence of propagation, vary in different regions of the heart. **B,** Schematic of a typical action potential in a human ventricular myocyte and the underlying ionic currents. As discussed in the text, the contribution of each of the various K^+ currents to shaping action potential waveforms and controlling repolarization varies in different cell types and different regions of the myocardium. AV, atrioventricular; endo, endocardial; epi, epicardial; LV, left ventricle; mid, midmyocardial; SA, sinoatrial.

Table 28-1 Cationic Currents Underlying Myocardial Action Potential Generation

Current	Activation	Inactivation	Recovery	Pharmacology*	Expression	Heterogeneity
Inward						
I_{Na}	Fast	Fast	Fast	TTX	Atria, Ventricles, Purkinje	Yes
I_{CaL}	Fast	Ca^{2+}-dependent	Fast	DHP Cd^{2+}	Atria, Ventricles, Nodes, Purkinje	No
I_{CaT}	Fast	Fast	Fast		Atria, Nodes	No
I_f	Fast	Slow	Fast	Cs^+	Nodes	No
Outward						
$I_{to,f}$	Fast	Fast	Fast	μM 4-AP, HaTX, HpTX	Atria, Ventricles, Purkinje	Yes
$I_{to,s}$	Fast	Slow	Slow	μM 4-AP	Ventricles	Yes
I_{Kr}	Moderate	Fast	Slow	E-4031, dofetilide	Ventricles	Yes
I_{Ks}	Very slow	No		NE-10064, E-10133	Ventricles	Yes
I_{Kur}	Fast	No	No	μM 4-AP	Atria	No
I_{Kp}	Fast	No		Ba^{2+}	Ventricles	??
I_K	Slow	Slow	Slow	μM TEA	Ventricles	??
$I_{K,slow1}$	Fast	Slow	Slow	μM 4-AP	Atria, Ventricles	No
$I_{K,slow2}$	Fast	Very slow	Slow	μM TEA	Atria, Ventricles	No
I_{ss}	Slow	No		μM TEA	Atria, Ventricles	No
I_{KI}				Ba^{2+}	Atria, Ventricles	Yes
I_{KATP}				SUR	Atria, Ventricles	Yes

*4-AP, 4-aminopyridine; DHP, dihydropyridines; HaTX, hanatoxin; HpTX, heteropodatoxin; SUR, sulfonylureas; TEA, tetraethylammonium; TTX, tetrodotoxin.

Table 28-2 Voltage-Gated Potassium (Kv) Channel Pore-Forming α Subunits

Protein	Gene	Cardiac Current
Kv1 Subfamily		
Kv1.1	*KCNA1*	
Kv1.2	*KCNA2*	I_{Ks} (rat) ($I_{K,DTX}$)
Kv1.3	*KCNA3*	
Kv1.4	*KCNA4*	$I_{to,s}$
Kv1.5	*KCNA5*	I_{Kur} (human/rat) $I_{K,slow1}$ (mouse)
Kv1.6	*KCNA6*	
Kv1.7	*KCNA7*	??
Kv1.10	*KCNA10*	
Kv2 Subfamily		
Kv2.1	*KCNB1*	I_{Ks} (mouse)
Kv2.2	*KCNB2*	??
Kv3		
Kv3.1	*KCNC1*	??
Kv3.2	*KCNC2*	
Kv3.3	*KCNC3*	
Kv3.4	*KCNC4*	
Kv4 Subfamily		
Kv4.1	*KCND1*	??
Kv4.2	*KCND2*	$I_{to,f}$ (mouse/rat)
Kv4.3	*KCND3*	$I_{to,f}$ (human)
Kv5 Subfamily		
Kv5.1	*KCNF1*	??
Kv6 Subfamily		
Kv6.1	*KCNG1*	
Kv6.2	*KCNG2*	
Kv7 Subfamily		
KCNQ1 (KvLQT1)	*KCNQ1*	I_{Ks}
KCNQ2	*KCNQ2*	
KCNQ3	*KCNQ3*	
KCNQ4	*KCNQ4*	
KCNQ5	*KCNQ5*	
Kv8 Subfamily		
Kv8.1	*KCNV1*	
Kv8.2	*KCNV2*	
Kv9 Subfamily		
Kv9.1	*KCNS1*	
Kv9.2	*KCNS2*	
Kv9.3	*KCNS3*	
Kv11 (erg) Subfamily		
Kv11.1	*KCNH1*	
Kv11.2	*KCNH2*	I_{Kr}
Kv11.3	*KCNH3*	
Kv11.4	*KCNH4*	
Kv11.5	*KCNH5*	

Note: Bold type indicates proteins expressed in mammalian heart.

Table 28-3 Voltage-Gated Potassium (K_V) Channel Accessory β Subunits

Subunit / Protein	Gene	Cardiac Current
Kvβ Family		
Kvβ1	*KCNAB1*	$I_{to,f}$?, $I_{K,slow2}$?
Kvβ2	*KCNAB2*	??
Kvβ3	*KCNAB3*	
KCNE Family		
minK	*KCNE1*	I_{Ks}
MiRP1	*KCNE2*	I_{Ks}??, $I_{to,f}$??
MiRP2	*KCNE3*	I_{Kr}?, $I_{to,f}$?, I_f?
MiRP3	*KCNE4*	??
MiRP4	*KCNE5*	??
KChAP Family		
KChAP	PIAS3	$I_{to,f}$?, I_K?, $I_{K,slow1}$?, $I_{K,slow2}$?
KChIP Family		
KChIP1	*KCNIP1*	
KChIP2	*KCNIP2*	$I_{to,f}$
KChIP3	*KCNIP3*	
KChIP4	*KCNIP4*	
NCS Family		
NCS-1	*FREQ*	$I_{to,f}$, others??
DPP Family		
DPP6	DPP6	$I_{to,f}$, others?
DPP10	DPP10	$I_{to,f}$, others?

Note: Bold type indicates proteins expressed in mammalian heart.

DPP, dipeptidyl aminopeptidase-like protein; KChAP, voltage-gated K^+ channel accessory protein; KChIP, voltage-gated K^+ channel interacting protein; NCS, neuronal Ca^{2+}-sensing (protein).

Table 28-4 Inward Rectifier K^+ (Kir) and Two-Pore K^+ (K2P) Channel α Subunits

Protein	Gene	Cardiac Current	Protein	Gene	Cardiac Current
Kir Family			*TWIK Subfamily*		
Kir1 Subfamily			**TWIK-1**	*KCNK1*	??
Kir1.1	*KCNJ1*	??	TWIK-2	*KCNK6*	
Kir2 Subfamily			**TWIK-3**	*KCNK7*	
Kir2.1	*KCNJ2*	I_{K1}	TWIK-4	*KCNK8*	
Kir2.2	*KCNJ12*	I_{K1}	*TREK Subfamily*		
Kir2.3	*KCNJ4*	??	**TREK-1**	*KCNK2*	??
Kir2.4	*KCNJ14*		**TREK-2**	*KCNK3*	??
Kir3 Subfamily			*TASK Subfamily*		
Kir3.1	*KCNJ3*	??	**TASK-1**	*KCNK10*	I_{Kp}
Kir3.2	*KCNJ6*		TASK-2	*KCNK5*	
Kir3.3	*KCNJ7*		TASK-3	*KCNK9*	
Kir3.4	*KCNJ9*		TASK-4	*KCNK14*	
Kir4 Subfamily			TASK-5	*KCNK15*	
Kir4.1	*KCNJ5*		*TRAAK Subfamily*		
Kir4.2	*KCNJ10*		TRAAK-1	*KCNK4*	
Kir5 Subfamily			*THIK Subfamily*		
Kir5.1	*KCNJ15, KCNJ16*		THIK-1	*KCNK13*	
Kir6 Subfamily			THIK-2	*KCNK12*	
Kir6.1	*KCNJ8*	I_{KATP} ??	*TALK Subfamily*		
Kir6.2	*KCNJ11*	I_{KATP}	TALK-1	*KCNK16*	
			TALK-2	*KCNK17*	

Note: Bold type indicates proteins expressed in mammalian heart.

Diversity of Myocardial Voltage-Gated K^+ (Kv) Currents

Depolarization-activated Kv currents influence action potential amplitudes and durations and, in most cells, two broad classes of Kv currents have been distinguished: transient outward K^+ currents (I_{to}) and delayed, outwardly rectifying K^+ currents (I_K) (see Table 28-1). The transient currents (I_{to}) activate rapidly and underlie early (phase 1) repolarization, whereas the delayed rectifiers (I_K) determine the latter phase (phase 3) of action potential repolarization (see Fig. 28-1). These are broad classifications, however, and there are actually multiple types of transient (I_{to}) and delayed rectifier (I_K) Kv currents (see Table 28-1) expressed in cardiac cells.[3,6,7] Electrophysiologic and pharmacologic studies, for example, have clearly demonstrated that there are two types of transient outward K^+ currents, now referred to as I_{to} fast ($I_{to,f}$) and I_{to} slow ($I_{to,s}$), and that these currents are differentially distributed.[3,7] The rapidly activating and inactivating transient outward K^+ current, $I_{to,f}$, is also characterized by rapid recovery from steady-state inactivation, whereas $I_{to,s}$ recovers slowly from inactivation.[3,6,7] In addition, $I_{to,f}$ is readily distinguished from other Kv currents (including $I_{to,s}$) using *Heteropoda* toxin-2 or -3.[3,7]

Although originally identified in Purkinje fibers, $I_{to,f}$ is a prominent repolarizing Kv current in atrial and ventricular myocytes, as well as in nodal cells, in most species.[7] There are, however, marked regional differences in $I_{to,f}$ densities, with the highest densities typically in atrial myocytes.[3,7] In mammalian ventricles, $I_{to,f}$ and $I_{to,s}$ are differentially distributed.[3,7] In canine left ventricle (LV), for example, $I_{to,f}$ density is five- to sixfold higher in epicardial (Epi) and midmyocardial (M) cells than in endocardial (Endo) cells (Fig. 28-2).[2] There are also marked regional differences in $I_{to,f}$ densities in adult mouse ventricles.[7-9] Specifically, $I_{to,f}$ density is higher in right ventricle (RV) than in LV myocytes and, within the LV, $I_{to,f}$ densities are higher in apex than in base myocytes.[7-9] In the mouse, even greater Kv current heterogeneity is seen in cells isolated from the septum: All ventricular septum cells express $I_{to,s}$, and most (~80%) also express $I_{to,f}$.[8] When present, however, $I_{to,f}$ density is significantly

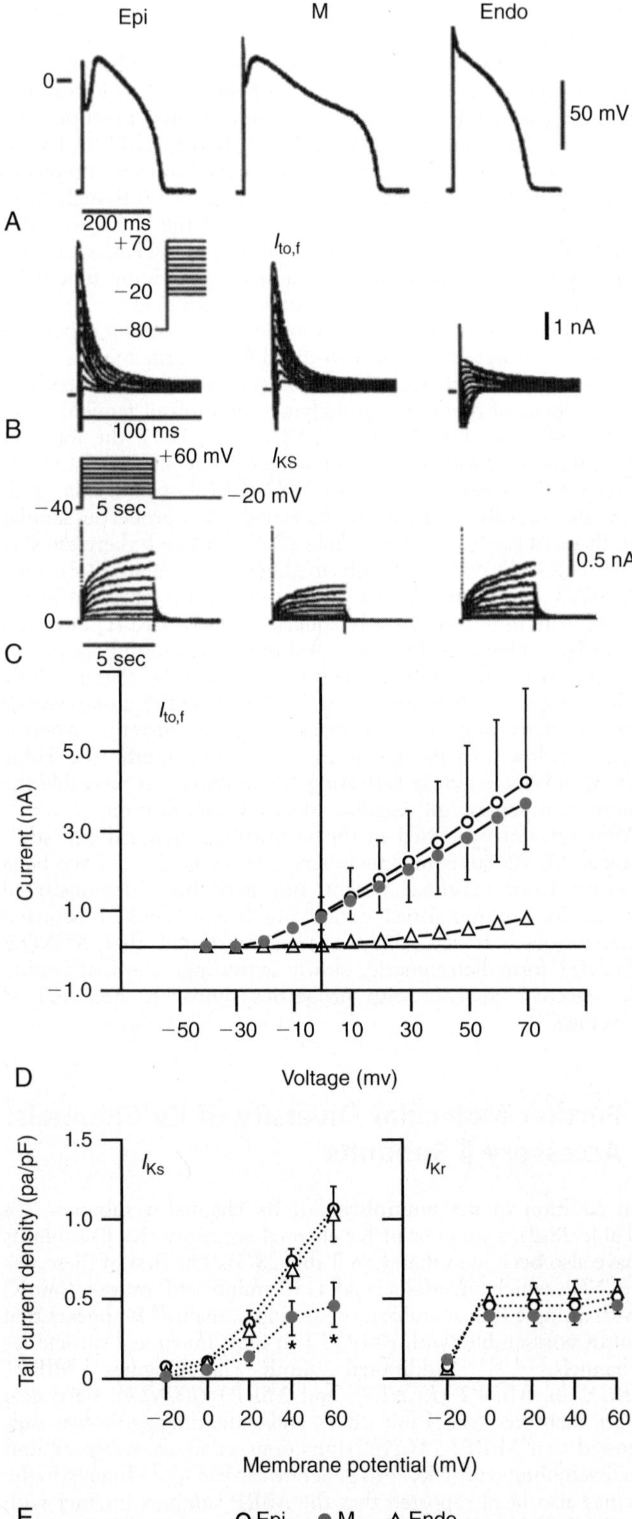

Figure 28-2 Transmural differences in action potential waveforms and Kv currents in canine ventricular myocytes. **A,** Representative action potentials recorded from epicardial (Epi), midmyocardial (M), and endocardial (Endo) canine left ventricular (LV) myocytes. Transient outward (I_{to}) **(B)** and slow delayed rectifier (I_{Ks}) **(C)** Kv current waveforms recorded in canine Epi, M, and Endo LV cells. **D,** Average peak current–voltage relation for I_{to} in Epi, M, and Endo LV cells; values are means plus or minus standard deviation. **E,** The density of I_{Ks} (defined as the E-4031–insensitive component of the outward current tails), but not I_{Kr}, is significantly (*$P < .05$) lower in M than in either Epi or Endo LV cells; values are means plus or minus the standard error of the mean. (Adapted with permission from Antzelevitch C, Dumaine R: Electrical heterogeneity in the heart: Physiological, pharmacological and clinical implications. In Page E, Fozzard HA, Solaro RJ (eds): Handbook of Physiology, Section 2: The Cardiovascular System, vol 1. New York, Oxford, 2002, pp 654-692.)

($P < .001$) lower in septum cells than in RV or LV cells.[8] $I_{to,f}$ and $I_{to,s}$ are also differentially expressed in ferret LV, and $I_{to,s}$ is only detected in Endo LV cells.[10] In spite of heterogeneities in functional expression, the properties of $I_{to,f}$ and $I_{to,s}$ in different cardiac cell types (and species) are remarkably similar, leading to suggestions that the molecular compositions of the underlying ($I_{to,f}$ and $I_{to,s}$) channels are also similar.[7]

Electrophysiologic and pharmacologic studies have also distinguished multiple types of cardiac delayed rectifier K^+ currents, I_K (see Table 28-1), and revealed that these currents are also differentially expressed. In atrial myocytes, for example, the dominant repolarizing K^+ current is a very rapidly activating, non-inactivating K^+ current, I_{Kur} (ultrarapid I_K), which is not prominent (and typically not detected) in ventricular or nodal cells.[3,7] In most ventricular myocytes, in contrast, there are two prominent components of delayed rectification, I_{Kr} (rapid I_K) and I_{Ks} (slow I_K), that are quite different from I_{Kur} in terms of time- and voltage-dependent properties.[3,7] The biophysical properties of I_{Kr} and I_{Ks}, for example, are distinct: I_{Kr} activates and inactivates rapidly, displays marked inward rectification, and is selectively blocked by class III antiarrhythmics, including dofetilide and sotalol.[11] In contrast, no inward rectification is evident for I_{Ks}, and this current activates very slowly. It is now clear that the molecular correlates of these (I_{Kr} and I_{Ks}) K^+ channels are also distinct.[3,7,12]

Similar to the transient outward K^+ currents, there are also marked regional differences in the functional expression of I_{Ks} and I_{Kr} in mammalian ventricular myocytes.[1,2,7] As illustrated in Figure 28-2, for example, I_{Ks} density in canine LV is higher in Epi and Endo cells than in M cells.[13] There are also regional differences in the functional expression of I_{Kr} and I_{Ks} channels in guinea pig LV.[13] In cells isolated from the LV free wall, for example, the density of I_{Kr} is higher in subepi myocytes than in M or subendo myocytes.[13] At the base of the LV, in contrast, I_{Kr} and I_{Ks} densities are significantly lower in endo LV cells than in either M or epi LV cells.[13] These differences in functional Kv current densities contribute to the variations in action-potential waveforms recorded in different regions (atria and ventricles, right and left ventricles, apex and base of the ventricles) of the heart, as well as in different layers (epi, M, and endo) of the LV and RV walls.[1-3,6-9,12,13]

In rodent ventricles, there are additional components of I_K with properties distinct from I_{Ks} and I_{Kr} (see Table 28-1). In mouse and rat ventricular myocytes, for example, there are novel delayed rectifier voltage-gated K^+ currents that have been referred to as I_K, $I_{K,slow}$ and I_{ss} (sustained) (see Table 28-1).[3,7] Mouse ventricular $I_{K,slow}$ was first identified as a rapidly activating and slowly inactivating K^+ current with properties distinct from $I_{to,f}$, $I_{to,s}$, and I_{ss} expressed in the same cells.[14] $I_{K,slow}$ was shown to be blocked selectively by micromolar concentrations of 4-aminopyridine (4-AP), which does not affect $I_{to,f}$ or $I_{to,s}$.[14] Subsequent work, however, revealed the presence of two distinct components of mouse ventricular $I_{K,slow}$: $I_{K,slow1}$, which is blocked by micromolar 4-AP, and, $I_{K,slow2}$, which is blocked selectively by tetraethylammonium (TEA).[15-18] It has also been demonstrated that $I_{K,slow1}$ and $I_{K,slow2}$ reflect the expression of distinct molecular entities.[15-18] In contrast to the differential distribution of $I_{to,f}$ and $I_{to,s}$, however, $I_{K,slow1}$, $I_{K,slow2}$ and I_{ss} appear to be uniformly expressed in mouse atrial and ventricular myocytes.[7,15-19]

Other Myocardial K^+ Currents Contributing to Repolarization

In addition to the Kv currents, inwardly rectifying K^+ (Kir) currents, specifically the cardiac Kir current, I_{K1}, and the adenosine triphosphate (ATP)-dependent K^+ current, I_{KATP}, also contribute to shaping myocardial action potential waveforms.[20-22] Similar to the Kv Kir currents, the densities of the Kir currents vary in different regions (the atria, ventricles, and conducting tissue) of the heart.[3,7] In contrast to the Kv currents, however, myocardial Kir currents appear to be uniformly (or nearly so) expressed in mammalian ventricles.[3,7]

In atrial and ventricular myocytes, I_{K1} plays a role in establishing the resting membrane potential and the plateau potential and contributes to phase 3 repolarization (see Fig. 28-1). The fact that the conductances of I_{K1} channels are high at negative membrane potentials underlies the contribution of I_{K1} to atrial and ventricular resting membrane potentials.[20] Although the voltage-dependent properties of I_{K1} channels are such that conductances are very low at potentials positive to approximately −40 mV, these channels nevertheless do contribute outward K^+ currents during the plateau phase of the action potential in ventricular cells,[20] as well as during phase 3 repolarization (see Fig. 28-1), because the driving force on K^+ is high at depolarized membrane potentials.

Myocardial ATP-dependent potassium channels are weakly inwardly rectifying channels that are inhibited by (elevated) intracellular ATP and activated by nucleotide diphosphates.[21] In ventricular myocytes, activation of I_{KATP} channels during periods of hypoxia and ischemia is reflected in the shortening of action potential durations, suggesting that these channels provide a link between cellular metabolism and membrane potential.[21,22] The opening of I_{KATP} channels appears to contribute to the cardioprotection resulting from ischemic preconditioning.[22] Unlike ventricular Kv channels, I_{KATP} channels appear to be distributed uniformly in the right and left ventricles and through the thickness of the (right or left) ventricular walls. Interestingly, however, I_{KATP} channels are expressed at much higher densities than other sarcolemmal myocardial potassium channels,[21] suggesting that action potentials will be shortened markedly when only a few I_{KATP} channels are activated.

Molecular Diversity of Voltage-Gated K^+ (Kv) Channel Pore-Forming α Subunits

Kv channel pore-forming (α) subunits are proteins spanning six transmembrane domains (Fig. 28-3), with a region between the fifth and sixth transmembrane domains that contributes to the K^+-selective pore.[4] The positively charged fourth transmembrane domain in the Kv α subunits (see Fig. 28-3) is homologous to the corresponding regions in voltage-gated Na^+ and voltage-gated Ca^{2+} channel α subunits, placing them in the S4 superfamily of voltage-gated channels.[3,4] In contrast to voltage-gated Na^+ and Ca^{2+} channels, in which only a single α subunit is required to form a channel, functional Kv channels comprise four α subunits (see Fig. 28-3). Similar to the diversity of functional myocardial Kv channels (see Table 28-1), however, several Kv α subunits have been identified. There are several homologous Kv α subunit subfamilies (Kv1.x, Kv2.x, Kv3.x, Kv4.x, Kv10.x, Kv11.x; see Table 28-2), and many members of these Kv α subunit subfamilies are expressed in the mammalian heart (see Table 28-2). In addition, further functional Kv channel diversity could arise through alternative splicing of transcripts, as well as through the formation of heteromultimeric channels between two or more Kv α subunit proteins in the same Kv α subunit subfamily.[3-7]

In contrast to most of the Kv α subunit subfamilies, heterologous expression of Kv α subunits of the Kv5.x to Kv9.x subfamilies (see Table 28-2) alone does not produce functional Kv channels.[3,4] Coinjection of these (Kv5.1, Kv6.1, Kv8.1, or Kv9.1) α subunits with Kv2.x subfamily members, however, attenuates the amplitudes of the Kv2.x-induced currents.[7] Although these observations suggest that Kv α subunits of the Kv5.x to Kv9.x subfamilies function as regulatory subunits of the Kv2.x subfamily, the role(s) of these silent subunits in generating functional myocardial Kv channels remains to be determined.[7]

Additional subfamilies of mammalian Kv α subunit genes (see Table 28-2) were revealed with the cloning of the human ether-a-go-go–related (HERG) gene, *KCNH2*, subsequently identified as the locus of mutations underlying one form of familial long-QT syndrome, LQT2, and *KCNQ1* (KvLQT1), the locus of mutations in another inherited long-QT syndrome, LQT1.[12] Heterologous expression of *KCNH2* (ERG1) (see Table 28-2) reveals inwardly rectifying Kv currents[12] with properties similar to those of cardiac I_{Kr} (see Table 28-1). Although there are several ERG (*KCNH*) subfamily members (see Table 28-2), only *KCNH2* (which encodes ERG1) appears to be expressed in the myocardium.[3,7] Alternatively spliced forms of ERG1, however, have been identified in mouse and human heart and are postulated to play roles in the generation of cardiac I_{Kr} channels.[3,7,12] Heterologous expression of *KCNQ1* (KvLQT1) alone reveals rapidly activating and non-inactivating Kv currents, whereas coexpression with the Kv accessory subunit, minK (see Table 28-3), produces slowly activating Kv currents that resemble the slow component of cardiac delayed rectification, I_{Ks}.[3,7,12] Although not expressed in the mammalian myocardium, additional *KCNQ* subfamily members (see Table 28-2) have been cloned from neuronal tissues and have been demonstrated to be loci of mutations underlying benign familial neonatal convulsions.[7] It has also been demonstrated that *KCNQ2*/*KCNQ3* form heteromeric, slowly activating, non-inactivating K^+-selective currents with properties similar to neuronal M channels.[23]

Further Molecular Diversity of Kv Channels: Accessory β Subunits

In addition to the multiplicity of Kv channel α subunits (see Table 28-2), a number of Kv channel accessory (Kv β) subunits have also been identified (see Table 28-3). The first of these was *KCNE1*, which encodes a small (130 amino acid) protein (minK) with a single transmembrane-spanning domain.[24] It appears that minK coassembles with KvLQT1 to form functional cardiac I_{Ks} channels.[3,7,12,24] Additional minK homologues, MiRP1 (*KCNE2*), MiRP2 (*KCNE3*), and MiRP3 (*KCNE4*), have also been identified (see Table 28-3), and some time ago it was suggested that MiRP1 (*KCNE2*) functions as an accessory subunit coassembling with ERG1 to generate cardiac I_{Kr}.[25] Interestingly, it has also been reported that the MiRP subunits interact with multiple Kv channel α subunit subfamilies and modify the properties of the resulting Kv channels.[24] MiRP2, for example, coassembles with Kv3.4 in mammalian skeletal muscle,[26] and MiRP1 coassembles with Kv4.x α subunits when coexpressed in heterologous cells.[27] These observations suggest the interesting possibility that the MiRP (*KCNE*) accessory Kv subunits can assemble with a variety of Kv channel α subunits and contribute to the formation of multiple types of myocardial Kv channels. Direct experimental support for this hypothesis, however, has not been provided, and the roles of the various *KCNE* subunits

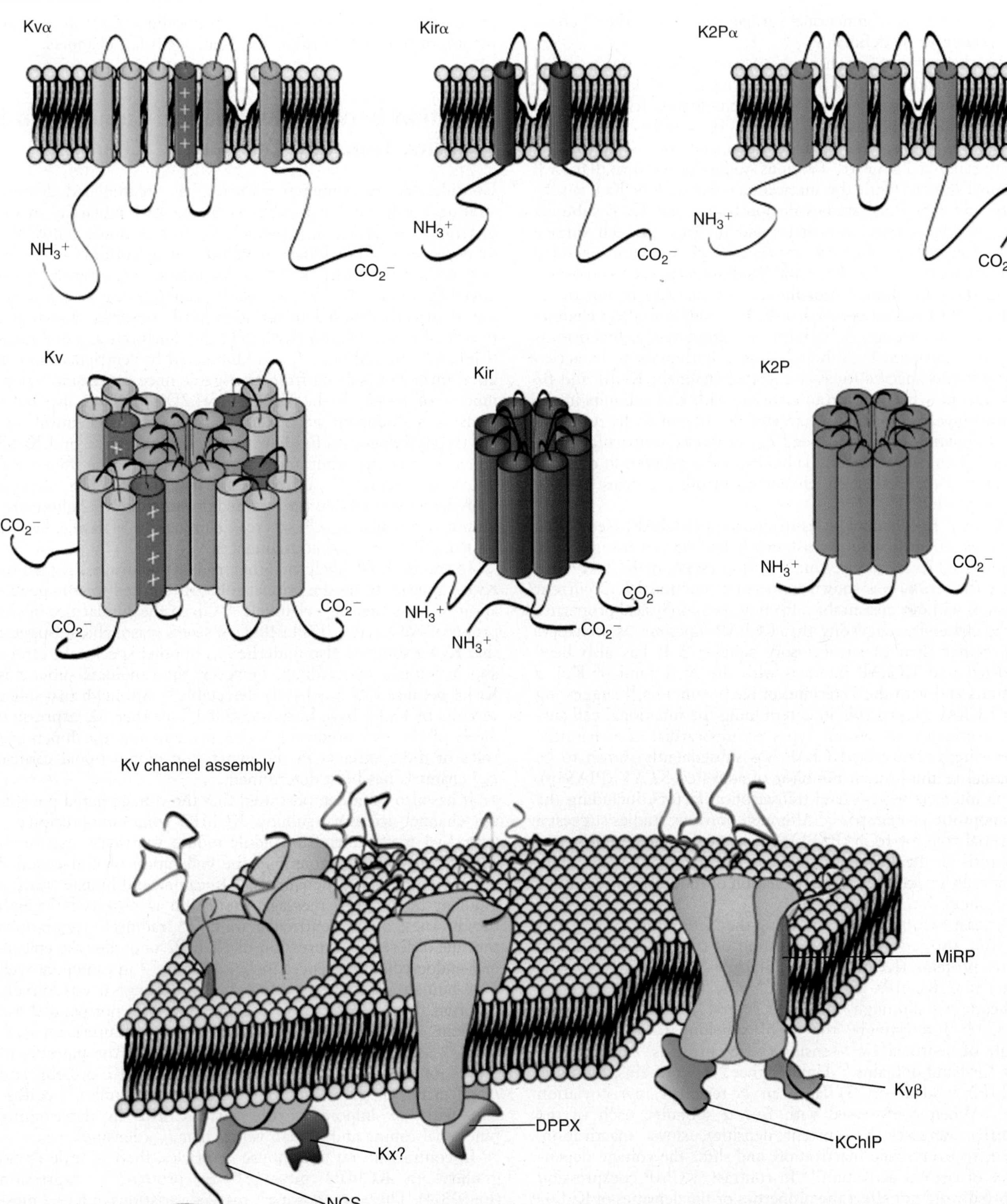

Figure 28-3 Pore-forming (α) subunits and assembly of functional cardiac K^+ channels. *Top*, Linear sequences and transmembrane topologies of the α subunits encoding voltage-gated (Kv), inwardly rectifying (Kir), and two-pore domain (K2P) K^+ channels are illustrated. The tetrameric assembly of Kv and Kir subunits and the dimeric assembly of K2P subunits are illustrated below the primary sequences. *Bottom*, Schematic illustrating functional myocardial Kv channels, composed of pore-forming Kv α and accessory Kv subunits, including KChIP2 (K^+ channel interacting proteins), Kv β, MiRP (minK-related peptide) subunits. DPPX, dipeptidyl-aminopeptidase-like protein; and NCS, neuronal Ca^{2+}-sensing protein.

in the generation of functional cardiac Kv[26,27] or other[28] channels remain to be defined.

Another type of Kv channel accessory subunit was revealed with the isolation of low molecular weight (~45 kD) cytosolic (Kv β) subunits from brain.[5] Three homologous Kv β subunits, Kv β1, Kv β2, and Kv β3 (see Table 28-3), as well as alternatively spliced transcripts, have been identified, and both Kv β1 and Kv β2 are expressed in heart.[7] Previous studies have shown that Kv β subunits interact with the intracellular domains of Kv1 α subunits, and functional studies demonstrated that Kv β subunits affect the biophysical properties and increase the cell surface expression of heterologously expressed Kv1 α subunit-encoded Kv currents.[5,7] Because Kv α and β subunits appear to coassemble in the endoplasmic reticulum,[29] the increase in functional channel expression suggests that the Kv β subunits affect channel assembly, processing, or stability or, alternatively, function as chaperone proteins.[5,7] Although originally thought to be accessory subunits specific for Kv1-encoded channels, Kv β1 and β2 have also now been shown to associate with Kv4 subunits in the mouse myocardium, and the targeted deletion of Kv β1 results in the attenuation of Kv4-encoded $I_{to,f}$ in mouse ventricular myocytes.[30] The role(s) of Kv β subunits in the generation of myocardial $I_{to,f}$ (and other Kv channels?) in other species has not been explored.

A novel Kv channel accessory protein (KChAP) (see Table 28-3) was identified in a yeast two-hybrid screen using the N terminus of Kv2.1 as the bait.[31] Coexpression of KChAP with Kv2.1 (or Kv2.2) was shown to increase functional Kv2 current densities without measurably affecting the biophysical properties of the channels, suggesting that KChAP functions as a chaperone, rather than as an accessory subunit.[31] It has also been reported that KChAP interacts with the N termini of Kv1 α subunits and with the C termini of Kv β_1 subunits,[31] suggesting that KChAP plays a role in determining the functional cell surface expression of several types of myocardial Kv channels. Interestingly, however, KChAP was subsequently shown to be identical to the protein inhibitor of activated STAT (PIAS3β), which interacts with several transcription factors, including the proapoptotic protein p53.[32] Although previous studies suggest a potential role for KChAP (PIAS3β) in mediating K^+ efflux and apoptosis in dividing cells (perhaps in cancer), no clear functional role for KChAP in the regulation or modulation of cardiac Kv channels has been defined.

A yeast two-hybrid screen, using the N terminus of Kv4.2 as the bait, also led to the identification of the Kv channel interacting proteins (KChIPs) (see Table 28-3) in brain.[33] Of the (now) four KChIPs identified,[33,34] only KChIP2 is expressed in heart,[33,35] although there are several KChIP2 splice variants.[36-38] Interestingly, the KChIPs belong to the recoverin family of neuronal Ca^{2+}-sensing (NCS) proteins[39] and contain four EF-hand domains.[33] Unlike other NCS proteins, however, KChIP2 (and KChIP3) lacks an N-terminal myristoylation site.[33] When coexpressed with Kv4 α subunits, each of the KChIPs increases K^+ current densities, slows inactivation, speeds recovery from inactivation, and shifts the voltage-dependence of current activation.[33] In contrast, KChIP coexpression reportedly did not affect the properties or the densities of Kv1.4- or Kv2.1-encoded K^+ currents, consistent with the suggestion that the modulatory effects of the KChIPs are specific for Kv4 α subunit-encoded Kv channels.[33] More recent experimental evidence, however, suggests that the KChIPs can, at least in heterologous expression systems, modulate the functional cell surface expression of Kv1.5-encoded Kv channels.[40] Although KChIP binding to Kv4 α subunits is not Ca^{2+}-dependent, mutations in EF-hand domains 2, 3, and 4 were reported to eliminate the modulatory effects of KChIP1 on Kv4- and Kv1.5-encoded Kv currents,[33,40] suggesting a role for intracellular Ca^{2+} in the regulation of functional cardiac (Kv4-encoded) $I_{to,f}$ channels.

Relation between Kv Channel Subunits and Cardiac Transient Outward K^+ Channels

Considerable experimental evidence has accumulated demonstrating a role for Kv α subunits of the Kv4 subfamily in the generation of cardiac $I_{to,f}$ channels. In rat and mouse ventricular myocytes exposed to antisense oligodeoxynucleotides (AsODNs) targeted against Kv4.2 or Kv4.3, for example, $I_{to,f}$ density is reduced by about 50%.[41,42] Rat ventricular $I_{to,f}$ density is also reduced in cells exposed to an adenoviral construct encoding a truncated Kv4.2 subunit (Kv4.2ST) that functions as a dominant negative.[43] In addition, $I_{to,f}$ is eliminated in ventricular and in atrial myocytes isolated from transgenic mice expressing a pore mutant of Kv4.2, Kv4.2W362F (Kv4.2DN), which also functions as a dominant negative.[44,45] Although biochemical and electrophysiologic studies have suggested that Kv4.2 and Kv4.3 are associated in adult mouse ventricles and that functional mouse ventricular $I_{to,f}$ channels are heteromeric,[42] it has now been demonstrated that the targeted deletion of Kv4.2 eliminates mouse ventricular $I_{to,f}$,[46] whereas elimination of Kv4.3 has no measurable functional consequences.[47]

In mouse (and likely in other rodent) ventricles, therefore, Kv4.2 appears to be the critical subunit required for the generation of functional $I_{to,f}$ channels.[46] Given the similarities in the properties of $I_{to,f}$ (see Table 28-1), it seems reasonable to suggest that Kv4 α subunits also underlie $I_{to,f}$ in other species. In canine and in human myocardium, however, the candidate subunit is Kv4.3 because Kv4.2 is barely detectable.[48] Although two splice variants of Kv4.3 have been identified,[49] neither the expression levels of the two predicted Kv4.3 proteins nor the functional roles of these variants in the generation of functional cardiac $I_{to,f}$ channels has been determined.

It has also been demonstrated that the voltage-gated potassium channel accessory subunit KChIP2 coimmunoprecipitates with Kv4 α subunits from adult mouse ventricles, consistent with a role for this subunit in the generation of Kv4-encoded mouse ventricular $I_{to,f}$ channels.[41] In canine and human heart, a gradient in KChIP2 message expression is observed through the thickness of the ventricular wall,[35,36] leading to suggestions that the differential expression of KChIP2 underlies the epicardial-endocardial differences in $I_{to,f}$ densities[2,3] in canine (as well as in human) ventricles (see Fig. 28-2). Although it was initially reported that KChIP2 protein expression does not parallel the gradient in KChIP2 message expression in canine myocardium,[36] subsequent studies have revealed that the patterns of expression of the KChIP2 message, the KChIP2 protein, and $I_{to,f}$ densities in canine ventricles are, indeed, similar,[50] consistent with an important role for KChIP2 in determining functional canine and human ventricular $I_{to,f}$ densities.

In contrast, in rat and mouse ventricles, there is little or no gradient in KChIP2 message[46] or protein[42,51] expression (Fig. 28-4). There are, however, marked variations in Kv4.2 message[52] and protein[42] expression (see Fig. 28-4), and it appears that the regional differences in Kv4.2 expression underlie the observed heterogeneities in $I_{to,f}$ densities in rodent ventricles.[42,46,48,51] Molecular insights into the regulation of the observed regional variations in the expression of the Kv4.2 transcripts were provided with the demonstrations that the expression levels of the transcription factors, Irx5 and NFAT, are positively and negatively (respectively) correlated with the differences in Kv4.2 expression and $I_{to,f}$ densities.[53,54] Interestingly, a

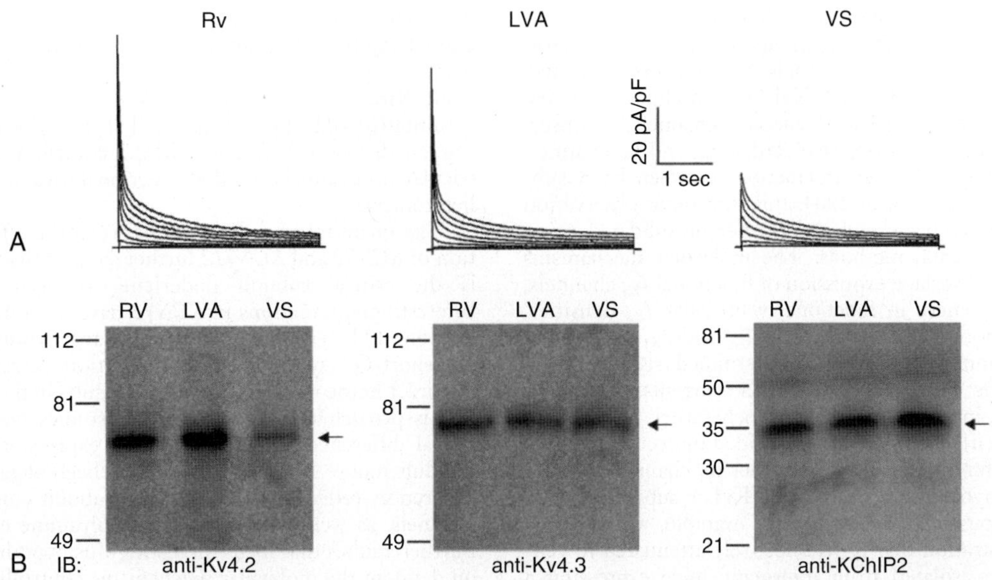

Figure 28-4 Molecular basis of heterogeneities in mouse ventricular fast transient outward current ($I_{to,f}$) expression. **A,** Whole-cell voltage clamp recordings from isolated adult mouse ventricular myocytes reveal that peak outward Kv current and $I_{to,f}$ densities are higher in right ventricular (RV) than in left ventricular apex (LVA) myocytes and that peak outward Kv and $I_{to,f}$ densities are substantially lower in cells isolated from the interventricular septum (VS). **B,** Western blot analyses of Kv4.2, Kv4.3, and KChIP2 expression in adult mouse ventricles. Equal amounts of membrane proteins (50 μg in each lane) obtained from the RV, LVA, and VS of adult C57BL6 mice were fractionated on 8% sodium dodecyl sulfate polyacrylamide (SDS-PAGE) gels, transferred to polyvinylidine fluoride (PVDF) membranes, and immunoblotted with specific anti-Kv4.2, anti-Kv4.3, and anti-KChIP2 antibodies. A single specific band at about 70 kDa *(arrow)* was recognized by anti-Kv4.2 *(left)*, a single band at about 75 kDa was detected by anti-Kv4.3 *(middle)*, and a single band at about 35 kDa was identified with the anti-KChIP2 *(right)* antibody. Kv4.3 and KChIP2 expression appear to be uniformly high in adult mouse ventricles, whereas there is a gradient in Kv4.2 protein expression that parallels the regional heterogeneities in functional $I_{to,f}$ expression *(upper panel)*. (Adapted with permission from Brunet S, Aimond, F, Li H, et al: Heterogeneous expression of repolarizing voltage-gated K^+ currents in adult mouse ventricles. J Physiol 559: 103-120, 2004; and Guo W, Li H, Aimond F, et al: Role of heteromultimers in the generation of myocardial transient outward K^+ currents. Circ Res 90:586-593, 2002.)

number (~25) of transcription factors were subsequently shown to be differentially expressed in the ventricles,[55] although the functional impact of these findings remains to be determined.

A role for the KChIP2 splice variant, KChIP2b, in determining regional differences in ferret ventricular $I_{to,f}$ densities has also been proposed.[37] The KChIP-related (NCS family) protein NCS-1 appears to be uniformly expressed in adult mouse ventricles and, in addition, coimmunoprecipitates with Kv4 α subunits.[56] The protein expression pattern of this putative Kv4 channel accessory subunit has not been examined in canine or human heart, and a role for NCS-1 in controlling functional myocardial $I_{to,f}$ densities has not been determined directly. The functional roles of additional voltage-gated potassium accessory subunits, including members of the *KCNE*[27,57] and *DPPX*[58,59] subfamilies, in the generation of cardiac $I_{to,f}$ channels or in determining regional differences in myocardial $I_{to,f}$ densities remain to be defined.

The kinetic and pharmacologic properties of the slow transient outward K^+ currents, $I_{to,s}$, in ventricular myocytes are quite different from $I_{to,f}$ (see Table 28-1), observations interpreted as suggesting that the molecular correlates of ventricular $I_{to,s}$ and $I_{to,f}$ channels are also distinct. Direct experimental support for this hypothesis was provided in electrophysiologic experiments on myocytes isolated from mice with a targeted deletion of the Kv1.4 gene, Kv1.4$^{-/-}$,[60] demonstrating that $I_{to,s}$ is undetectable in septum cells.[61] The properties and the densities of $I_{to,f}$, I_{Ks1}, I_{Ks2}, and I_{ss} in Kv1.4$^{-/-}$ left and right ventricular (and atrial) myocytes, however, are indistinguishable from those measured in wild-type cells.[60,61] Interestingly, up-regulation of $I_{to,s}$ (and the Kv1.4 protein) has been shown to underlie the electrical remodeling evident in the ventricles of Kv4.2DN-expressing mice in which $I_{to,f}$ is eliminated.[62] Given the similarities in the time- and voltage-dependent properties of the slow transient outward K^+ currents in other species with mouse $I_{to,s}$,[3] it seems reasonable to suggest that Kv1.4 likely also encodes $I_{to,s}$ in ferret, rabbit, human, and canine ventricular myocytes.

Relation between Kv Channel Subunits and Cardiac Delayed Rectifier K^+ Channels

As noted earlier, ERG1 is the locus of mutations in *LQT2*, and heterologous expression of ERG1 reveals voltage-gated inwardly rectifying K^+-selective channels that are similar to cardiac I_{Kr}.[12] Alternatively processed forms of ERG1, with unique N- and C-termini, have also been identified in mouse and human heart, although the role(s) of these variants in the generation of functional I_{Kr} channels has not been clarified.[63-65] It has also been suggested that functional cardiac I_{Kr} channels are multimeric, comprising ERG1 and minK, and biochemical studies have demonstrated co-immunoprecipitation of ERG1 and minK from equine ventricles.[66] It is not clear if ERG1 and minK or other members of the *KCNE* family are also found in association in other species.

Although heterologous expression of *KCNQ1*, the locus of mutations in LQT1, reveals rapidly activating, non-inactivating Kv currents, coexpression with minK produces slowly activating Kv currents similar to cardiac I_{Ks}.[12] These observations, together with biochemical data demonstrating that heterologously expressed KvLQT1 and minK associate, were interpreted as suggesting that minK coassembles with KvLQT1 to form functional cardiac I_{Ks} channels.[7,12] Direct biochemical evidence for the *in situ* coassembly of KvLQT1 and minK was provided in studies on equine ventricles.[66] Similar data for human ventricular I_{Ks} has yet to be provided, however, even in equine heart, and the stoichiometry of functional I_{Ks} channels has not been defined. Interestingly, it was reported that KvLQT1 modulates the distribution and properties of ERG1-encoded channels, an observation interpreted as suggesting that cardiac I_{Ks} and I_{Kr} channels are regulated directly through interactions between Kv α subunits.[67] Although reported in 2004, this intriguing observation appears not to have been explored further or validated using alternative experimental methods. The molecular mechanisms controlling the cell surface expression of functional I_{Ks} channels, the regional differences in functional ventricular I_{Ks} densities, and the interaction(s) between cardiac I_{Ks} and I_{Kr} (as well as other cardiac channels?) remain to be determined (see Fig. 28-2).

Similar to the transient outward Kv currents, molecular genetic methods, in combination with biochemistry and electrophysiology, primarily in mice, have provided molecular insights into the basis of functional delayed rectifier Kv channel diversity in the murine myocardium. A role for Kv1 α subunits in the generation of mouse ventricular I_{Ks}, for example, was revealed with the demonstration that I_{Ks} is selectively attenuated in ventricular myocytes isolated from transgenic mice expressing a truncated, dominant negative Kv1 α subunit, Kv1.1DN.[14] It was subsequently shown, however, that I_{Ks} is also reduced in ventricular myocytes expressing a dominant negative Kv2.1 mutant, Kv2.1DN.[15] The simplest interpretation of these results is that there are two distinct components of wild-type mouse ventricular I_{Ks}: one, now referred to as $I_{K,slow1}$, that is sensitive to micromolar concentrations of 4-AP and encoded by Kv1 α subunits; and the other, now referred to as $I_{K,slow2}$, that is sensitive to TEA and encoded by Kv2 α subunits.[15]

Subsequent studies revealed that $I_{K,slow1}$ is eliminated in ventricular myocytes isolated from mice harboring the targeted disruption of the *KCNA5* (Kv1.5) locus, revealing that Kv1.5 encodes $I_{K,slow1}$.[16] These findings, together with the previous studies completed on cells from Kv1.4$^{-/-}$ animals,[60] in which $I_{to,s}$ is eliminated,[61] reveal that, in contrast to the Kv4 α subunits (Kv4.2 and Kv4.3[42]), the Kv1 α subunits (Kv1.4 and Kv1.5) do not associate in adult mouse ventricles *in situ*. Rather, functional Kv1 α subunit-encoded Kv channels in mouse ventricular myocytes are homomeric, composed of Kv1.4 α subunits ($I_{to,s}$)[61] or Kv1.5 α subunits (I_{Ks1}).[16] The role(s) of Kv channel accessory subunits in the generation of functional $I_{to,s}$, $I_{K,slow1}$ and $I_{K,slow2}$ channels and the molecular mechanisms controlling the differential expression patterns of these channels, however, remain to be determined.

Molecular Correlates of Other Cardiac K$^+$ Currents

In cardiac and other cells, inwardly rectifying K$^+$ (I_{K1}) channels are encoded by a large and diverse subfamily of inward rectifier K$^+$ (Kir) channel pore-forming α subunit genes (see Table 28-4), each of which encodes a protein with two transmembrane domains that assemble as tetramers to form K$^+$-selective pores (see Fig. 28-3). Based on the properties of the currents produced in heterologous expression systems, Kir2 α subunits were long thought to encode the strongly inwardly rectifying cardiac I_{K1} channels,[20] and several members of the Kir2 subfamily (see Table 28-4) are expressed in the myocardium.[68]

Direct insights into the role(s) of Kir2 α subunits in the generation of cardiac I_{K1} channels were provided in studies completed on myocytes isolated from mice lacking *KCNJ2* (Kir2.1$^{-/-}$) or *KCNJ12* (Kir2.2$^{-/-}$).[69] Although the Kir2.1$^{-/-}$ mice have cleft palate and die shortly after birth, precluding electrophysiologic studies on myocytes from adult animals, voltage-clamp recordings from isolated newborn Kir2.1$^{-/-}$ ventricular myocytes revealed that I_{K1} is absent.[69] Recordings from adult Kir2.2$^{-/-}$ ventricular myocytes, in contrast, revealed a quantitative reduction in I_{K1}.[69] Taken together, these results suggest that both Kir2.1 and Kir2.2 contribute to (mouse) ventricular I_{K1} channels and that functional cardiac I_{K1} channels are heteromeric.

The quantitative differences between the effects of the deletion of *KCNJ2* and *KCNJ12* further suggest that Kir2.1 (*KCNJ2*) is the critical subunit underlying (mouse) I_{K1} channels.[69] Interestingly, mutations in *KCNJ2* have been linked to congenital long-QT syndrome (Andersen-Tawil syndrome, or LQT7) and short-QT syndrome.[70,71] In addition, increasing expression of Kir2.1 in the mouse heart, which results in the upregulation of I_{K1}, is proarrhythmic.[72,73] Previous studies have identified regional differences in myocardial I_{K1} expression and properties in adult mouse heart,[74,75] and it has been suggested that these differences reflect variability in the subunit composition of the channels, as well as differences in polyamine concentrations.[76] Further studies that focus on testing this hypothesis directly and on defining the molecular mechanisms controlling the observed regional differences in the expression of functional I_{K1} channels in species other than mice are also clearly warranted.

In the mammalian heart, I_{KATP} channels appear not to play a prominent role in action potential repolarization, but rather are thought to be important in myocardial ischemia and preconditioning.[21,22] In heterologous systems, I_{KATP} channels can be reconstituted by coexpression of Kir6.x subunits with one or more ATP-binding cassette proteins that encode sulfonylurea receptors (SURs).[77] Although pharmacologic and mRNA expression studies suggested that cardiac sarcolemmal I_{KATP} channels are likely encoded by Kir6.2 and SUR2A, the essential role of Kir6.2 was demonstrated in experiments showing that I_{KATP} channels are undetectable in ventricular myocytes isolated from Kir6.2$^{-/-}$ animals.[78] In addition, cardiac I_{KATP} channel activity is reduced in SUR2$^{-/-}$ myocytes[79] and unaffected in SUR1$^{-/-}$ myocytes,[80] suggesting an important role for SUR2. Interestingly, the properties of the residual I_{KATP} channels in SUR2$^{-/-}$ myocytes are similar to those produced in heterologous cells on coexpression of Kir6.2 and SUR1,[79] suggesting the interesting possibility that SUR1 also contributes to the generation of functional cardiac I_{KATP} channels by coassembling with Kir6.2 α subunits alone or with SUR2A. Biochemical and molecular genetic strategies will need to be combined to explore the molecular components of functional I_{KATP} channels.

Although action potential waveforms in Kir6.2$^{-/-}$ and wild-type ventricular myocytes are indistinguishable, the action potential shortening observed in wild-type cells during ischemia or metabolic blockade is abolished in the Kir6.2$^{-/-}$ cells,[78] consistent with the hypothesis that cardiac I_{KATP} channels play an important role under pathophysiologic conditions, particularly those involving metabolic stress. Interestingly, action potential durations are largely unaffected in transgenic animals expressing mutant I_{KATP} channels with markedly (40-fold) reduced ATP sensitivity, suggesting that additional inhibitory mechanisms regulate cardiac I_{KATP} channel activity *in vivo*.[81] Similar to the strongly inwardly rectifying myocardial Kir currents (I_{K1}), further studies are needed to provide molecular insights into the mechanisms controlling regional differences in the functional expression of myocardial I_{KATP} channels.

Two-Pore Domain K$^+$ Channels

In addition to the Kv (see Table 28-2) and Kir (see Table 28-4) channel pore-forming (α) subunits that assemble as tetramers (see Fig. 28-3), a novel type of K^+ channel α subunit with four transmembrane-spanning regions and two pore domains (see Fig. 28-3) was identified with the cloning of *TWIK-1*.[82] Both pore domains contribute to the formation of the K^+-selective pore, and *TWIK-1* subunits assemble as dimers.[83] A large number of two-pore domain K^+ (K2P) channel α subunit genes have been identified, and several are expressed in the mammalian myocardium (see Table 28-4). Heterologous expression of K2P subunits reveals currents with distinct biophysical properties and sensitivities to several potential intracellular and extracellular modulators, including anesthetics, pH, and fatty acids.[82]

The multiplicity of K2P α subunits (see Table 28-4), the widespread distribution of expressed subunits, and the finding that the properties of the channels encoded by K2P subunits are regulated by a variety of physiologically (and pathophysiologically) relevant stimuli[82] suggest that K2P channels likely subserve a variety of important functions. As in other cell types, the physiologic roles of these subunits and channels in the myocardium are just beginning to be explored.[82] TREK-1 and TASK-1 are detected in heart, and heterologous expression of these subunits gives rise to instantaneous non-inactivating K^+ currents that display little or no voltage dependence.[82] These properties suggest that K2P subunits might contribute to background or leak K^+ channels, i.e., channels with properties similar to the steady-state non-inactivating K^+ current (I_{ss}) that is robustly expressed and well-characterized in rodent myocytes.[8,9,82-87] In recent studies completed on rat atrial and ventricular myocytes, roles for both the TASK1[85-87] and TREK1[83,84] subunits in the generation of I_{ss} have been suggested. Clearly, experiments focused on testing these hypotheses directly are needed to provide clear insights into the molecular basis of I_{ss} and to allow further studies that focus on defining the mechanisms controlling the physiologic and the pathophysiologic regulation of I_{ss} channels.

Summary and Conclusions

Cellular electrophysiologic studies have distinguished multiple types of voltage-gated inward and outward currents that contribute to action potential repolarization in mammalian cardiac cells (see Table 28-1). The outward (K^+) currents are more numerous and more diverse than the inward (Na^+, Ca^{2+}) currents, and most cardiac cells express a repertoire of Kv and Kir channels (see Table 28-1). In addition, several of these (K^+) are expressed differentially in different myocardial cell types, as well as through the thickness of the ventricular walls. Molecular cloning has led to the identification of several voltage-gated (Kv), nonvoltage-gated, inwardly rectifying (Kir), and weakly rectifying non-inactivating (K2P) K^+ channel pore-forming α subunits (Tables 28-2 and 28-4) and an increasing number of channel accessory (β) subunits (see Table 28-3) that contribute to the formation of the various cardiac K^+ currents that have been distinguished electrophysiologically (see Table 28-1).

Considerable progress has also been made in identifying the pore-forming Kir and Kv α subunits that contribute to the formation of most of the K^+ channels expressed in mammalian cardiac myocytes (Tables 28-2 and 28-4). Biochemical studies have also provided some insights into the molecular mechanisms underlying the observed heterogeneities in the expression of myocardial Kv and Kir currents. For cardiac $I_{to,f}$, for example, regional differences in current densities are correlated with differences in Kv4.2 protein expression in adult mouse ventricles,[42] whereas variable expression of the KChIP2 accessory channel protein appears to underlie the transmural gradient in $I_{to,f}$ densities in canine and several human ventricles.[35,50] For cardiac I_{K1} channels, in contrast, several studies suggest that differences in Kir channel α subunit composition or differences in the concentrations of the intracellular polyamines, previously shown to regulate the rectification properties of cardiac I_{K1} channels, play a role in the diversity of these channels.[75]

In contrast to the progress made in defining the Kv and the Kir α subunits encoding functional and myocardial Kv and Kir channels and currents, however, much less is known about the functional roles of most of the Kv channel accessory subunits (see Table 28-3) and K2P subunits (see Table 28-4). It seems certain that a major focus of future work will be on defining the roles of the various Kv β and the K2P α subunits in the generation of functional myocardial K^+ channels and on exploring the molecular mechanisms controlling the properties and the cell-surface expression of myocardial K^+ channels encoded by Kv α and β, Kir α, and K2P α subunits.

Numerous studies have documented changes in functional K^+ channel expression in a variety of myocardial disease states, changes that could reflect modifications in channel properties, as well as alterations in the molecular compositions of the channels or the processing of the underlying channel subunits. There are numerous possible (transcriptional, translational, and post-translational) molecular mechanisms involved in regulating the functional expression and the properties of myocardial K^+ channels in the normal, as well as in the damaged or diseased, myocardium. It seems certain that a major focus of future work will be on exploring these mechanisms in detail.

References

1. Nerbonne JM, Guo W: Heterogeneous expression of voltage-gated potassium channels in the heart: Roles in normal excitation and arrhythmias. J Cardiovasc Electrophysiol 13:406-409, 2002.
2. Antzelevitch C, Dumaine R: Electrical heterogeneity in the heart: Physiological, pharmacological and clinical implications. In Page E, Fozzard HA, Solaro RJ (eds): Handbook of Physiology, Section 2: The Cardiovascular System, vol 1. New York, Oxford, 2002, pp 654-692.
3. Nerbonne JM, Kass RS: Molecular physiology of cardiac repolarization. Physiol Rev 85:1205-1253, 2005.
4. Coetzee WA, Amarillo Y, Chiu J, et al: Molecular diversity of K^+ channels. Ann N Y Acad Sci 868:233-285, 1999.
5. Pongs O, Leicher T, Berger M, et al: Functional and molecular aspects of voltage-gated K^+ channel β subunits. Ann N Y Acad Sci 868:344-355, 1999.
6. Oudit GY, Kassiri Z, Sah R, et al: The molecular physiology of the cardiac transient outward potassium current (I_{to}) in normal and diseased myocardium. J Mol Cell Cardiol 33:851-872, 2001.
7. Nerbonne JM: Molecular analysis of voltage-gated K^+ channel diversity and functioning in the mammalian heart. In Page E, Fozzard HA, Solaro RJ, (eds): Handbook of Physiology, Section 2: The Cardiovascular System, vol 1. New York, Oxford, 2002, pp 568-594.
8. Xu H, Guo W, Nerbonne JM: Four kinetically distinct depolarization-activated K+ currents in adult mouse ventricular myocytes. J Gen Physiol 113:661-678, 1999.
9. Brunet S, Aimond F, Li H, et al: Heterogeneous expression of repolarizing voltage-gated K^+ currents in adult mouse ventricles. J Physiol 559:103-120, 2004.
10. Brahmajothi MV, Campbell DL, Rasmussen RL, et al: Distinct transient outward potassium current (I_{to}) phenotypes and distribution of fast-inactivating potassium channel alpha subunits in ferret left ventricular myocytes. J Gen Physiol 113:581-600, 1999.
11. Jurkiewicz NK, Sanguinetti MC: Rate-dependent prolongation of cardiac action potentials by a methanesulfonanilide class III antiarrhythmic agent. Specific block of

rapidly activating delayed rectifier K^+ current by dofetilide. Circ Res 72:75-83, 1993.

12. Keating MT, Sanguinetti MC: Molecular and cellular mechanisms of cardiac arrhythmias. Cell 104:569-580, 2001.
13. Bryant SM, Wan X, Shipsey SJ, Hart G: Regional differences in the delayed rectifier current (I_{Kr} and I_{Ks}) contribute to the differences in action potential duration in basal left ventricular myocytes in guinea-pig. Cardiovasc Res 40:322-331, 1998.
14. London B, Jeron A, Zhou J, et al: Long QT and ventricular arrhythmias in transgenic mice expressing the N terminus and first transmembrane segment of a voltage-gated potassium channel. Proc Natl Acad Sci U S A 95:2926-2931, 1998.
15. Xu H, Barry DM, Li H, et al: Attenuation of the slow component of delayed rectification, action potential prolongation, and triggered activity in mice expressing a dominant-negative K_V2 α subunit. Circ Res 85:623-633, 1999.
16. London B, Guo W, Pan XH, et al: Targeted replacement of $K_V1.5$ in the mouse leads to loss of the 4-aminopyridine–sensitive component of $I_{K,slow}$ and resistance to drug-induced QT prolongation. Circ Res 88:940-946, 2001.
17. Zhou J, Kodirov S, Murata M, et al: Regional upregulation of $K_V2.1$-encoded current, $I_{K,slow2}$, in K_V1DN mice is abolished by crossbreeding with K_V2DN mice. Am J Physiol Heart Circ Physiol 284:H491-H500, 2003.
18. Li H, Guo W, Yamada KA, Nerbonne JM: Selective elimination of $I_{K,slow1}$ in mouse ventricular myocytes expressing a dominant negative $K_V1.5\alpha$ subunit. Am J Physiol Heart Circ Physiol 286:H319-H328, 2004.
19. Bou-Abboud E, Li H, Nerbonne JM: Molecular diversity of the repolarizing voltage-gated K^+ currents in mouse atrial cells. J Physiol 529:345-358, 2000.
20. Lopatin AN, Nichols CG: Inward rectifiers in the heart: An update on I_{K1}. J Mol Cell Cardiol 33:625-638, 2001.
21. Flagg TP, Nichols CG: Sarcolemmal K_{ATP} channels: What do we really know? J Mol Cell Cardiol 39:61-70, 2005.
22. Grover GJ, Garlid KD: ATP-sensitive potassium channels: A review of their cardioprotective pharmacology. J Mol Cell Cardiol 32:677-695, 2000.
23. Wang HS, Pan Z, Shi W, et al: KCNQ2 and KCNQ3 potassium channel subunits: Molecular correlates of the M-channel. Science 282:1890-1893, 1998.
24. Abbott GW, Goldstein SA: A superfamily of small potassium channel subunits: Form and function of the MinK-related peptides (MiRPs). Q Rev Biophys 31:357-398, 1998.
25. Abbott GW, Sesti F, Splawski I, et al: MiRP1 forms I_{Kr} potassium channels with HERG and is associated with cardiac arrhythmia. Cell 97:175-187, 1999.
26. Abbott GW, Butler MH, Bendahhou S, et al: MiRP2 forms potassium channels in skeletal muscle with $K_V3.4$ and is associated with periodic paralysis. Cell 104:217-231, 2001.
27. Zhang M, Jiang M, Tseng GN: minK-related peptide 1 associates with $K_V4.2$ and modulates its gating function: Potential role as beta subunit of cardiac transient outward channel? Circ Res 88:1012-1019, 2001.
28. Yu H, Wu J, Potapova I, et al: MinK-related peptide. 1: A beta subunit for the HCN ion channel subunit family enhances expression and speeds activation. Circ Res 88:E84-E87, 2001.
29. Nagaya N, Papazian DM: Potassium channel alpha and beta subunits assemble in the endoplasmic reticulum. J Biol Chem 272:3022-3027, 1997.
30. Aimond F, Kwak SP, Rhodes KJ, Nerbonne JM: Accessory K_V β_1 subunits differentially modulate the functional expression of voltage-gated K^+ channels in mouse ventricular myoctyes. Circ Res 96:451-458, 2005.
31. Wible BA, Yang Q, Kuryshev YA, et al: Cloning and expression of a novel K^+ channel regulatory protein, KChAP. J Biol Chem 273:11745-11751, 1998.
32. Wible BA, Wang L, Kuryshev YA, et al: Increased K^+ efflux and apoptosis induced by the potassium channel modulatory protein KChAP/PIAS3beta in prostate cancer cells. J Biol Chem 277:17852-17862, 2002.
33. An WF, Bowlby MR, Betty M, Cao J, et al: Modulation of A-type potassium channels by a family of calcium sensors. Nature 403:553-556, 2000.
34. Morohashi Y, Hatano N, Ohya S, Takikawa R, et al: Molecular cloning and characterization of CALP/KChIP4, a novel EF-hand protein interacting with presenilin 2 and voltage-gated potassium channel subunit K_V4. J Biol Chem 277:14965-14975, 2002.
35. Rosati B, Pan Z, Lypen S, et al: Regulation of KChIP2 potassium channel beta subunit gene expression underlies the gradient of transient outward current in canine and human ventricle. J Physiol 533:119-125, 2001.
36. Deschenes I, DiSilvestre D, Juang GJ, et al: Regulation of $K_V4.3$ current by KChIP2 splice variants: A component of native cardiac I_{to}? Circulation 106:423-429, 2002.
37. Patel S, Campbell DL, Morales MJ, Strauss HC: Heterogenous expression of KChIP2 isoforms in the ferret heart. J Physiol 539:649-656, 2002.
38. Decher N, Barth AS, Gonzalez T, et al: Novel KChIP2 isoforms increase functional diversity of transient outward potassium currents. J Physiol 557:761-772, 2004.
39. Burgoyne RD, Weiss JL: The neuronal calcium sensor family of Ca^{2+}-binding proteins. Biochem J 353:1-12, 2001.
40. Li H, Guo W, Mellor RL, Nerbonne JM: KChIP2 modulates the cell surface expression of $K_V1.5$-encoded K^+ channels. J Mol Cell Cardiol 39:121-132, 2005.
41. Fiset C, Clark RB, Shimoni Y, Giles WR: Shal-type channels contribute to the Ca^{2+}-independent transient outward K^+ current in rat ventricle. J Physiol 500:51-64, 1997.
42. Guo W, Li H, Aimond F, et al: Role of heteromultimers in the generation of myocardial transient outward K^+ currents. Circ Res 90:586-593, 2002.
43. Johns DC, Nuss HB, Marban E: Suppression of neuronal and cardiac transient outward currents by viral gene transfer of dominant-negative $K_V4.2$ constructs. J Biol Chem 272:31598-31603, 1997.
44. Barry DM, Xu H, Schuessler RB, Nerbonne JM: Functional knockout of the transient outward current, long-QT syndrome, and cardiac modeling in mice expressing a dominant-negative K_V4 α subunit. Circ Res 83:560-567, 1998.
45. Xu H, Li H, Nerbonne JM: Elimination of the transient outward current and action potential prolongation in mouse atrial myocytes expressing a dominant negative K_V4 α subunit. J Physiol 519:11-21, 1999.
46. Guo W, Jung WE, Marionneau C, et al: Targeted deletion of $K_V4.2$ eliminates I_{to},f and results in electrical and molecular remodeling, with no evidence of ventricular hypertrophy or myocardial dysfunction. Circ Res 97:1342-1350, 2005.
47. Niwa N, Wang W, Sha Q, et al: $K_V4.3$ is not required for the generation of functional I_{to},f channels in adult mouse ventricles. J Mol Cell Cardiol 44:95-104, 2008.
48. Dixon JE, Shi W, Wang HS, et al: Role of the $K_V4.3$ K^+ channel in ventricular muscle. A molecular correlate for the transient outward current. Circ Res 79:659-668, 1996.
49. Kong W, Po S, Yamagishi T, et al: Isolation and characterization of the human gene encoding I_{to}: Further diversity by alternative mRNA splicing. Am J Physiol 275:H1963-H1970, 1998.
50. Rosati B, Grau F, Rodriguez S, et al: Concordant expression of KChIP2 mRNA, protein and transient outward current throughout the canine ventricle. J Physiol 548(Pt 3):815-822, 2003.
51. Teutsch C, Kondo RP, Dederko DA, et al: Spatial distributions of K_V4 channels and KChIP2 isoforms in the murine heart based on laser capture microdissection. Cardiovasc Res 73:739-749, 2007.
52. Dixon JE, McKinnon D: Quantitative analysis of potassium channel mRNA expression in atrial and ventricular muscle of rats. Circ Res 75:252-260, 1994.
53. Costantini DL, Arruda EP, Agarwal P, et al: The homeodomain transcription factor Irx5 establishes the mouse cardiac ventricular repolarization gradient. Cell 123:347-358, 2005.
54. Rossow CF, Dilly KW, Santana LF: Differential calcineurin/NFATc3 activity contributes to the I_{to} transmural gradient in the mouse heart. Circ Res 98:1306-1313, 2006.
55. Rosati B, Grau F, McKinnon D: Regional variation in mRNA transcript abundance within the ventricular wall. J Mol Cell Cardiol 40:295-302, 2006.
56. Guo W, Malin SA, Johns DC, et al: Modulation of K_V4-encoded K^+ currents in the mammalian myocardium by neuronal calcium sensor-1. J Biol Chem 277:26436-26443, 2002.
57. Radicke S, Cotella D, Graf EM, et al: Functional modulation of the transient outward current I_{to} by KCNE beta-subunits and regional distribution in human non-failing and failing hearts. Cardiovasc Res 71:695-703, 2006.

58. Nadal MS, Ozaita A, Amarillo Y, et al: The CD26-related dipeptidyl aminopeptidase-like protein DPPX is a critical component of neuronal A-type K^+ channels. Neuron 37:449-461, 2003.
59. Radicke W, Cotella D, Graf EM, et al: Expression and function of dipeptidyl-aminopeptidase-like protein 6 as a putative beta-subunit of human cardiac transient outward current encoded by $K_V4.3$. J Physiol 565:751-756, 2005.
60. London B, Wang DW, Hill JA, Bennett PB: The transient outward current in mice lacking the potassium channel gene $K_V1.4$. J Physiol 509:171-182, 1998.
61. Guo W, Xu H, London B, Nerbonne JM: Molecular basis of transient outward K^+ current diversity in mouse ventricular myocytes. J Physiol 521:587-599, 1999.
62. Guo W, Li H, London B, Nerbonne JM: Functional consequences of elimination of $I_{to,f}$ and $I_{to,s}$: early afterdepolarizations, atrioventricular block, and ventricular arrhythmias in mice lacking $K_V1.4$ and expressing a dominant-negative K_V4 α subunit. Circ Res 87:73-79, 2000.
63. Pond AL, Scheve BK, Benedict AT, et al: Expression of distinct ERG proteins in rat, mouse, and human heart. Relation to functional I_{Kr} channels. J Biol Chem 275:5997-6006, 2000.
64. Jones EM, Roti Roti EC, Wang J, et al: Cardiac I_{Kr} channels minimally comprise hERG 1a and 1b subunits. J Biol Chem 279:44690-44694, 2004.
65. Phartiyal P, Jones EM, Robertson GA: Heteromeric assembly of human ether-a-go-go–related gene (hERG) 1a/1b channels occurs cotranslationally via N-terminal interactions. J Biol Chem 282:9874-9882, 2007.
66. Finley MR, Li Y, Hua F, et al: Expression and coassociation of ERG1, KCNQ1, and KCNE1 potassium channel proteins in horse heart. Am J Physiol 283:H126-H138, 2002.
67. Ehrlich JR, Pourrier M, Weerapura M, et al: K_VLQT1 modulates the distribution and biophysical properties of HERG. A novel alpha-subunit interaction between delayed rectifier currents. J Biol Chem 279:1233-1241, 2004.
68. Liu GX, Derst C, Schlichthorl G, et al: Comparison of cloned Kir2 channels with native inward rectifier K^+ channels from guinea-pig cardiomyocytes. J Physiol 532:115-126, 2001.
69. Zaritsky JJ, Redell JB, Tempel BL, Schwarz TL: The consequences of disrupting cardiac inwardly rectifying K^+ current (I_{K1}) as revealed by the targeted deletion of the murine Kir2.1 and Kir2.2 genes. J Physiol 533:697-710, 2001.
70. Tristani-Firouzi M, Jensen JL, Donaldson MR, et al: Functional and clinical characterization of *KCNJ2* mutations associated with LQT7 (Andersen syndrome). J Clin Invest 110:381-388, 2002.
71. Priori SG, Pandit SV, Rivolta I, et al: A novel form of short QT syndrome (SQT3) is caused by a mutation in the *KCNJ2* gene. Circ Res 96:800-807, 2005.
72. Noujaim SF, Pandit SV, Berenfeld O, et al: Up-regulation of the inward rectifier K^+ current (I_{K1}) in the mouse heart accelerates and stabilizes rotors. J Physiol 578:315-326, 2007.
73. Piao L, Li J, McLerie M, Lopatin AN: Transgenic upregulation of I_{K1} in the mouse heart is proarrhythmic. Basic Res Cardiol 102:416-428, 2007.
74. Dhamoon AS, Pandit SV, Sarmast F, et al: Unique Kir2.x properties determine regional and species differences in the cardiac inward rectifier K^+ current. Circ Res 94:1332-1339, 2004.
75. Panama BK, McLerie M, Lopatin AN: Heterogeneity of I_{K1} in the mouse heart. Am J Physiol Heart Circ Physiol 293:H3558-H3567, 2007.
76. Panama BK, Lopatin AN: Differential polyamine sensitivity in inwardly rectifying Kir2 potassium channels. J Physiol 571:287-302, 2006.
77. Babenko AP, Aguilar-Bryan L, Bryan J: A view of SUR/KIR6.X, KATP channels. Ann Rev Physiol 60:667-687, 1998.
78. Suzuki M, Li RA, Miki T, et al: Functional roles of cardiac and vascular ATP-sensitive potassium channels clarified by Kir6.2-knockout mice. Circ Res 88:570-577, 2001.
79. Pu J, Wada T, Valdivia C, et al: Evidence of KATP channels in native cardiac cells without SUR. Biophys J 80:625-626, 2001.
80. Seghers V, Nakazaki M, DeMayo F, et al: SUR1 knockout mice. A model for K_{ATP} channel-independent regulation of insulin secretion. J Biol Chem 275:9270-9277, 2000.
81. Koster JC, Knopp A, Flagg TP, et al: Tolerance for ATP-insensitive K_{ATP} channels in transgenic mice. Circ Res 89:1022-1029, 2001.
82. Lesage F, Lazdunski M: Molecular and functional properties of two-pore-domain potassium channels. Am J Physiol Renal Physiol 279:F793-F801, 2000.
83. Goldstein SA, Bockenhauer D, O'Kelly I, Zilberberg N: Potassium leak channels and the KCNK family of two-P-domain subunits. Nat Rev Neurosci 2:175-184, 2001.
84. Terrenoire C, Lauritzen I, Lesage F, et al: A TREK-1-like potassium channel in atrial cells inhibited by beta-adrenergic stimulation and activated by volatile anesthetics. Circ Res 89:336-342, 2001.
85. Barbuti A, Ishii S, Shimizu T, et al: Block of the background K^+ channel TASK-1 contributes to arrhythmogenic effects of platelet-activating factor. Am J Physiol Heart Circ Physiol 282:H2024-H2030, 2002.
86. Besana A, Barbuti A, Tateyama MA, et al: Activation of protein kinase C epsilon inhibits the two-pore domain K^+ channel, TASK-1, inducing repolarization abnormalities in cardiac ventricular myocytes. J Biol Chem 279:33154-33160, 2004.
87. Putzke C, Wemhoner K, Sachse FB, et al: The acid-sensitive potassium channel TASK-1 in rat cardiac muscle. Cardiovasc Res 75:59-68, 2007.

Gap Junction Distribution and Regulation in the Heart 29

Paul D. Lampe and Glenn I. Fishman

CHAPTER OUTLINE

More than half a century ago, Weidmann demonstrated that cardiac cells must be electrically coupled with one another.[1] The anatomic basis for this behavior gradually unfolded over subsequent decades with the identification of arrays of intercellular channels, known as gap junction channels, clustered at the intercalated disks that bounded adjacent cells.[2,3] Since the molecular cloning of the first gap junction channel gene, or connexin, in the 1980s,[4] there has been an explosion in our knowledge of the diversity of genes encoding gap junction channels, the distribution of gap junction channel proteins in the heart, and the regulation of gap junction channels during development, under normal physiologic conditions, and in response to various pathologic conditions. In this chapter, we briefly review gap junction expression patterns in the heart, a topic which has previously been covered in great detail,[5-7] then focus on the state of our knowledge with respect to regulation of connexin transcription and the gap junction life cycle in normal hearts and in response to pathologic stressors. Additional information on gap junction channel molecular structure and biophysical properties can be found elsewhere in this book.

Gap Junction Expression in the Heart

Gap junctional proteins are encoded by the connexin multigene family. In the human genome there are 20 unique family members, and a comparable number is found in the mouse.[8,9] Within the hearts of most mammalian species studied to date, three connexin isoforms predominate, connexin (Cx)43, Cx40 and Cx45,[10,11] although other connexin proteins have been described in specific compartments of the heart including nodal tissue and other components of the specialized conduction system.[12] Biophysical properties of channels assembled from individual connexins display unique characteristics and regulatory properties, including unitary conductances, sensitivity to transjunctional and transmembrane voltage, and permselectivity.[13] Inasmuch as individual cardiomyocytes can express multiple connexins, an additional level of complexity arises from the potential for assembly of multiple isoforms into heteromeric and heterotypic channels.[14,15] This diversity of expression is presumably designed to optimize the tightly orchestrated temporal excitation of the multichambered heart, including the requisite slowing of conduction within the atrioventricular (AV) node and rapid excitation along the Purkinje fibers within the ventricular myocardium.

Connexin43

Cx43 is widely expressed in numerous tissues, and it is the predominant gap junctional protein detected in many cell types within the cardiovascular system. Cx43 is abundant in the working cardiomyocytes of the adult ventricle and atria. Cx43 is also found in the His bundle, bundle branches, and Purkinje fibers in human hearts.[10,11] Genetic engineering in the mouse has been exploited to identify specific functional roles for many of the individual connexin isoforms that are expressed in the heart. Inasmuch as some of the connexin genes are expressed in multiple lineages, these strategies may be accompanied by a host of developmental defects, complicating analyses of the electrophysiologic sequelae. In fact, germline deletion of Cx43 is associated with a broad range of congenital defects, including some affecting the cardiovascular system, such as perturbation of right ventricular outflow tract maturation and coronary artery anomalies, resulting in perinatal death.[16] However, these defects have been circumvented by cardiomyocyte-restricted knockout of Cx43, clarifying the critical role for this isoform in ventricular impulse propagation.[17] Indeed, loss of function of Cx43 in the heart leads to a highly penetrant and dramatic phenotype of spontaneous ventricular tachyarrhythmias and death (Fig. 29-1).

Mutations in Cx43 have been identified as a cause of the dominantly inherited syndrome of oculodentodigital dysplasia.[18] To date, one Cx43 mutant mouse identified in an unbiased chemical mutagenesis screen and two additional site-specific genetically engineered mouse knock-in models of oculodentodigital dysplasia have been reported.[19-21] Although there is some phenotypic variability among these models, in all cases posttranslational phosphorylation of Cx43 is affected, gap junction formation is diminished, and impulse propagation is abnormal (Fig. 29-2). Another strain of Cx43 mutant mice, harboring one null allele and a second that encodes a tailless Cx43 mutant protein (missing the cytoplasmic carboxy terminus) has also been described.[22] These mice have alterations in the number and size of cardiac gap junctional plaques but otherwise appear functionally relatively normal. In addition, in an effort to discriminate between shared and unique connexin functions, mice

Our research is supported by grants from the National Institutes of Health.

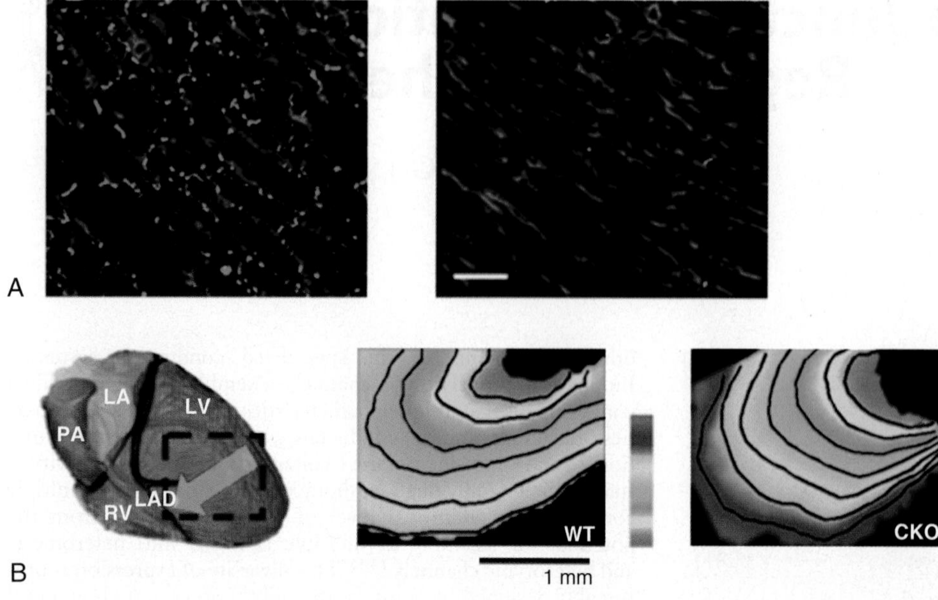

Figure 29-1 **A,** Immunohistochemical staining for Cx43 *(green)* in the ventricles of wild-type *(left)* and Cx43 conditional knockout mice *(right)* demonstrating absence of immunoreactive gap junctional protein in the mutant heart. Staining for wheat germ agglutinin *(red)* visualizes cell borders. Bar = 50 μm. **B,** Impulse propagation over the epicardial surface of the heart *(left)* visualized with voltage-sensitive dyes demonstrate normal conduction in a wild-type heart *(middle)* and slow conduction in a mutant heart *(right)*. Color scale bar indicates 0 *(red)* to 4 ms *(purple)*. **C,** Telemetric recording from Cx43 conditional knockout mice demonstrating spontaneous onset of ventricular tachycardia. CKO, conditional knockout; LA, left atrium; LAD, left anterior descending artery; LV, left ventricle; PA, pulmonary artery; RV, right ventricle; WT, wild type. (Adapted from Gutstein DE, Morley GE, Tamaddon H, et al: Conduction slowing and sudden arrhythmic death in mice with cardiac-restricted inactivation of connexin43. Circ Res 88:333-339, 2001.)

in which the Cx43 gene has been replaced by other individual isoforms including Cx26, Cx31, Cx32 and Cx40 have also been described.[23-25] These studies demonstrate that a subset of Cx43 functions can be subserved by alternative connexins, but there is not complete redundancy among individual isoforms.

Connexin40

Cx40 is abundant and is coexpressed with Cx43 in atrial myocardium, the His bundle, bundle branches, and Purkinje fibers.[10,26,27] Loss of function of Cx40 in the mouse is associated with slowing of impulse propagation characterized by first-degree AV block and right bundle branch block.[28-30] Recent human genetic studies suggest that somatic mutations in the Cx40 coding region might predispose to idiopathic atrial fibrillation and that specific polymorphisms in the promoter are associated with increased risk of atrial fibrillation.[31,32]

Connexin45

Cx45 appears to be primarily expressed in nodal tissue, including the sinoatrial node and the compact zone of the AV node, and more weakly in the atrium, His bundle, bundle branches, and Purkinje fibers.[12,33] Conditional loss of Cx45 only in cardiomyocytes results in death of the embryo with conduction block, indicating a requirement for this gap junctional protein in the developing heart.[34]

Connexin30.2

Cx30.2 is expressed primarily in the sinoatrial and AV nodes of the mouse.[35] Channels formed from Cx30.2 exhibit low unitary conductance values, and loss of function of this isoform leads to accelerated AV nodal conduction. These data suggest that Cx30.2 interacts with other connexin isoforms in nodal tissue and dominantly reduces junctional conductance. Whether these results can be extended to the human orthologue, Cx31.9, and human AV nodal conduction is uncertain.[36]

Transcriptional Regulation of Cardiac Connexins

The abundance of connexin proteins and assembled gap junction channels is regulated in part through transcriptional control mechanisms. Numerous descriptive but relatively few detailed mechanistic studies of connexin gene expression have been reported. The genomic organization of all of the major connexins expressed in heart have been described,[8,37] and the common structure includes a small 5′-untranslated exon 1 and a larger exon 2 that includes the entire protein-coding region. There are, however, some examples of alternative splicing involving the 5′-untranslated regions.[38] Many of these transcriptional studies have been performed in cultured cell model systems, and

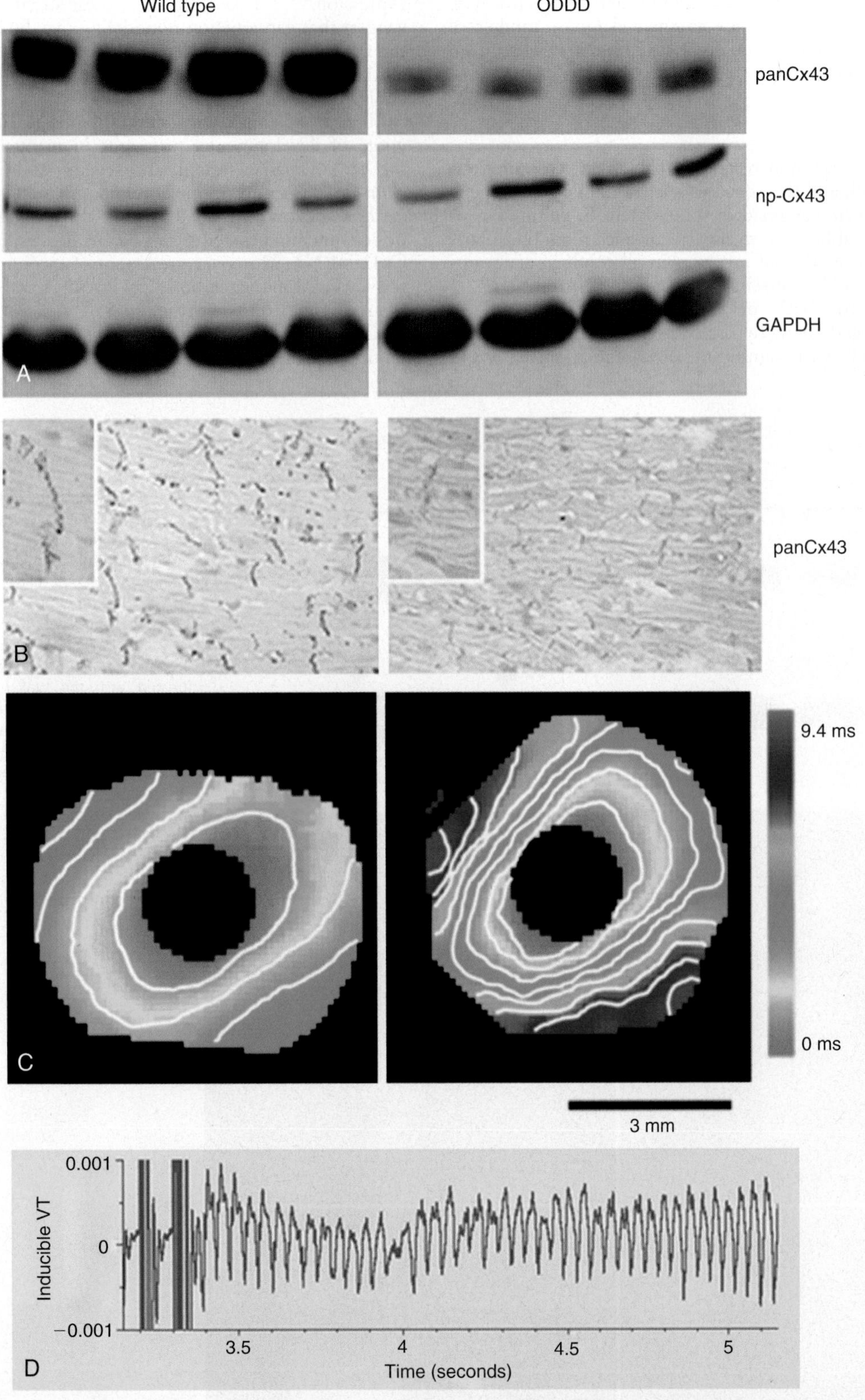

Figure 29-2 **A,** Western blot analysis of wild-type and ODDD mutant (ODDD) hearts using rabbit antibody 18B, which reacts with all forms of connexin43 (Cx43) (panCx43), and mouse monoclonal CX1B1, which preferentially reacts with the P0 form of Cx43 (np-Cx43) and GAPDH. Phosphorylated forms of Cx43 are specifically reduced in mutant hearts. **B,** Immunohistochemical staining of wild-type and ODDD mutant hearts with antibodies recognizing all forms of Cx43 (panCx43). Gap-junctional plaques are markedly reduced in ODDD mutant hearts. **C,** Impulse propagation over the epicardial surface of the heart visualized with voltage-sensitive dyes demonstrates normal conduction in a wild-type heart and slow conduction in a mutant heart. Color scale bar indicates 0 *(red)* to 9.4 ms *(purple)*. **D,** Programmed electrical stimulation showing induction of sustained VT in an ODDD heart. GAPDH, glyceraldehyde 3-phosphate dehydrogenase; np-Cx43, nonphosphorylated connexin43; VT, ventricular tachycardia. (Adapted from 20. Kalcheva N, Qu J, Sandeep N, et al: Gap junction remodeling and cardiac arrhythmogenesis in a murine model of oculodentodigital dysplasia. Proc Natl Acad Sci U S A 104(51):20512-20516, 2007.)

their relevance to in vivo gene regulation is uncertain. However, with the explosion in genetically engineered mouse models of cardiovascular development and disease, additional insights from in vivo studies are beginning to accumulate.

Connexin43

Hypertrophy is a common response of the heart to numerous pathologic stimuli, and the effects of such stimuli on Cx43 gene expression has been examined in some detail. In cultured neonatal myocytes, dibutyryl cyclic adenosine monophosphate (cAMP), angiotensin II, and myotrophin all result in acute upregulation of Cx43 messenger RNA (mRNA) levels.[39-41] However, in vivo, both in experimental animals and in humans, prolonged hemodynamic overload is more commonly associated with significant downregulation of Cx43 expression.[42-45] Taken together, these in vitro and in vivo data suggest that gap junction remodeling may be biphasic, although the second phase, characterized by reduced expression and concordant diminished density of junctional channels, may be more clinically relevant.

The *Wnt* signal transduction pathway influences a broad range of developmental processes in many lineages including the cardiovascular system, and several studies have implicated *Wnts* in the transcriptional regulation of Cx43. Neonatal rat cardiomyocytes responded to Li^+ (which mimics *Wnt* signaling) by accumulating the effector protein β-catenin and induction of Cx43 mRNA. Moreover, treatment of cardiomyocytes with bioactive Wnt-1 increased both Cx43 mRNA and a Cx43 promoter-reporter gene construct (Fig. 29-3).[46]

Gender differences in connexin abundance have been reported,[47] and indeed there is also some evidence that the

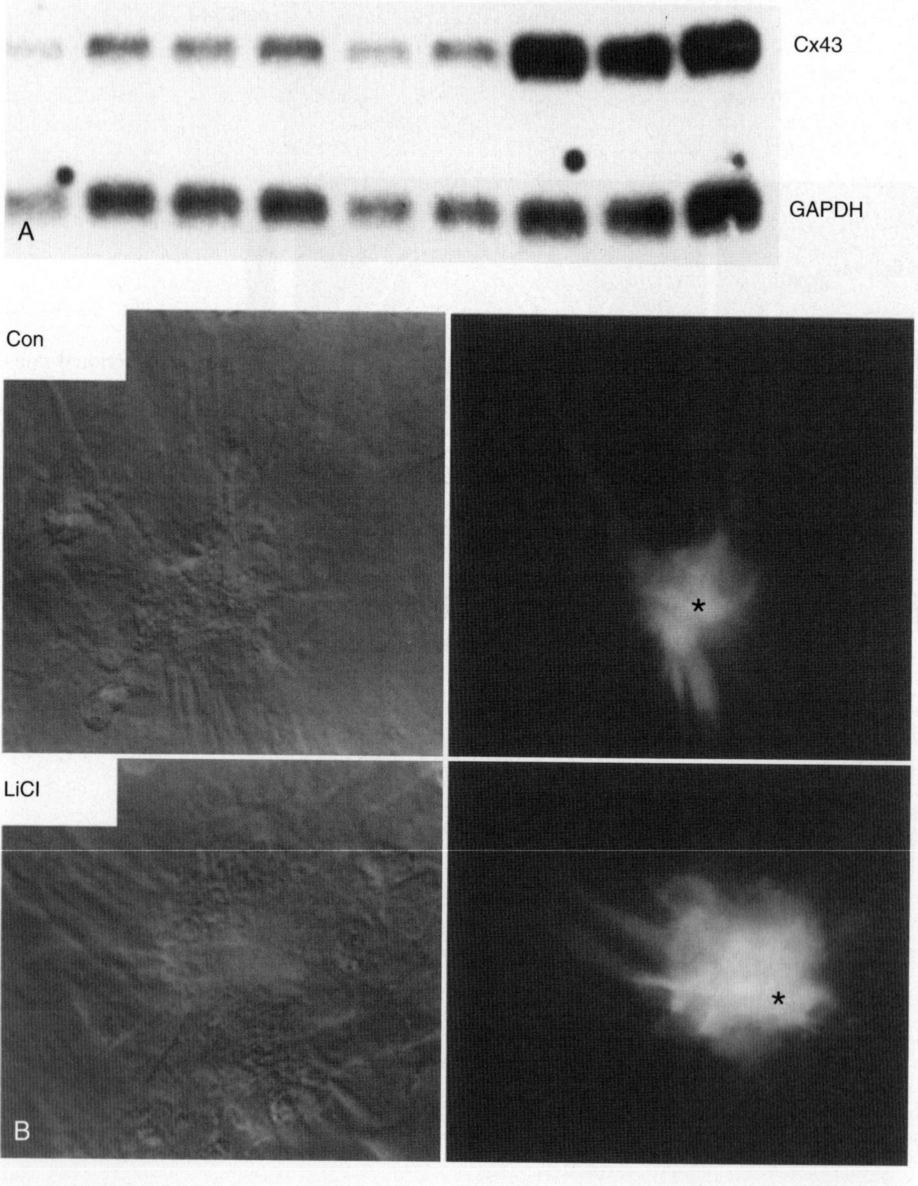

Figure 29-3 **A,** Northern blot analysis of neonatal rat cardiomyocytes co-cultured with Rat-2 fibroblasts transduced with retroviral vectors expressing Wnt-4, empty vector (Con), or Wnt-1. Connexin43 (Cx43) mRNA is specifically induced in response to Wnt-1. Glyceraldehyde 3-phosphate dehydrogenase (GAPDH) is shown to demonstrate loading. **B,** Dye coupling in cardiac myocytes treated with vehicle alone (Con) or treated with the Wnt mimetic LiCl. In each panel, paired phase contrast micrographs *(left)* and fluorescence micrographs (using fluorescein isothiocyanate [FITC] excitation and emission filters) are shown *(right)*. Photographs were taken at 1 minute after dye injection. Injected cardiac myocytes are indicated by asterisks. Note that LiCl significantly increases dye coupling among cardiac myocytes. (Adapted from Ai Z, Fischer A, Spray DC, et al: Wnt-1 regulation of connexin43 in cardiac myocytes. J Clin Invest 105:161-171, 2000.)

Cx43 gene is sensitive to sex hormones. Studies in a heterologous expression system (HeLa cells), demonstrated that the Cx43 promoter was estrogen responsive,[48] whereas in cultured cardiac myocytes, estradiol-17β upregulated Cx43.[49] Interestingly, external heavy ion–beam irradiation has been shown to induce Cx43 mRNA expression in control hearts and in experimentally infarcted hearts, although the mechanisms responsible for this effect are obscure.[50] Conversely, several factors that repress Cx43 expression have been described, including lipopolysaccharide (LPS) and tumor necrosis factor α.[51] In addition, activation of c-Jun N-terminal kinase (JNK) signaling appears to potently repress Cx43 expression at the mRNA level, and this pathway might play a role in pathologic gap junction remodeling associated with various myopathic stimuli.[52]

Connexin40

Several transcription factors have been shown to influence expression of Cx40 in the heart, often associated with functional conduction defects localized to the specialized cardiac conduction system. For example, targeted inactivation of *HF-1b*, an Sp1-related transcription factor, has been reported to result in perturbed Cx40 expression in the ventricular specialized conduction system and enhanced arrhythmogenesis.[53] Mutations in *Tbx5* are responsible for Holt-Oram syndrome. Studies of *Tbx5* heterozygous mice have suggested that *Tbx5* and *Nkx2.5* cooperatively transactivate the Cx40 promoter, and reduced cell-cell coupling might account in part for the heart block seen in patients with these mutations.[54-56] In fact, disruption of *Nkx2.5* alone results in downregulation of multiple connexins, including Cx43, Cx45, and Cx40.[57]

Loss of function of the *Shox2* gene has been shown to result in hypoplasia of the sinus venosus myocardium, including the sinoatrial nodal region and venous valves, associated with aberrant expression of both Cx40 and Cx43, which may be operating through *Nkx2.5*, which is also reduced.[58] The small homeodomain-only protein (Hop) has been implicated in Cx43 as well, and loss of function of Hop results in downregulation of Cx40 expression and infranodal conduction defects.[59] Neuregulin-1 has been implicated in conduction system differentiation in vivo,[60] and several studies using embryonic cardiomyocytes indicate that neuregulin treatment results in upregulation of Cx40 and Cx45 mRNA.[61,62]

Connexin Life Cycle: Half-life, Export to the Plasma Membrane, and Degradation

When examining fixed intercalated disk structures of cardiac tissue via light- or electron-microscopic methods, it is easy to come away with the impression that the structure and its constituents are static and unchanging. In fact, the structures are dynamic, with rapid changes in protein content. For example, the half-life of Cx43 in heart tissue has been calculated to be 1.3 hours[63] and thus must have a highly controlled life cycle. As integral membrane proteins, connexins are synthesized in the endoplasmic reticulum, are transported through the Golgi apparatus and are exported to the plasma membrane, where they assemble into gap junction structures.

However, connexins are not typical integral membrane proteins in many ways. First, they do not have a classic cleaved leader sequence. Second, at least several family members do not oligomerize into their hexameric structure (termed a connexon) until after they leave the endoplasmic reticulum.[64] Third, microtubule-dependent targeting to the whole plasma membrane has been clearly documented,[65-67] and connexins might even be directed to cell-cell junctional structures in certain cases.[68] Fourth, connexins can potentially form two types of channels: Connexons can, under specific conditions, function as a hemichannel or they can dock with a connexon in an adjacent cell membrane and form the canonical cell-to-cell channel. Fifth, the rapid 1- to 3-hour half-life of connexins is much shorter than the typical integral membrane protein ($t_{1/2}$ ranges from 15 to 90 hours).[69] Sixth, both proteasomal and lysosomal machinery have been implicated in connexin degradation. Misfolded connexins can be degraded via the proteasome (i.e., endoplasmic reticulum–associated degradation [ERAD]).[70] Disease-associated Cx32 mutants[71] or Cx43 from cells that are unable to assemble junctions[72,73] are targeted for degradation early in the secretory pathway in response to quality control checkpoints. Seventh, plasma membrane Cx43 can be degraded via a modified form of endocytosis that involves formation of double membrane annular junctions or connexosomes that are degraded via fusion with a lysosome.[74] Several reports have indicated that Cx43 can be ubiquitinylated under specific conditions or particular cell types. However, the role of the proteasome in degradation of plasma membrane Cx43 is more controversial.

Cx43 is highly phosphorylated, with more than 10 serines and two tyrosines being reported as substrates under different conditions. Phosphorylation has been implicated in the control of Cx43 export to the plasma membrane, assembly into a gap junctional structure, and internalization.[75,76] Increases in the levels of cAMP have been shown to upregulate gap junctional communication in cells expressing Cx43,[77,78] Cx40,[79,80] and Cx32,[81] but they downregulate Cx36 and Cx45[82] channels. In Cx43–expressing cells, cAMP trafficking from intracellular locations to plasma membrane increases.[77,78,83] Casein kinase 1 activity and phosphorylation of Cx43 at serine 325, 328, and 330 has been implicated in the regulation of gap junction assembly. Activation of protein kinase C via phorbol esters has been shown to decrease the half-life of Cx43.[84] Therefore, phosphorylation of connexins can affect connexin localization, gap junctional conductance properties, and turnover.

Analysis of Connexin43 Phosphorylation

Cx40, Cx43, and Cx45 are phosphoproteins and separate as multiple isoforms when analyzed by sodium dodecyl sulfate polyacrylamide gel electrophoresis. Phosphorylated species migrate more slowly, and dephosphorylated connexins migrate faster (2-6 kD apparent difference). When tissue or cellular lysates that express Cx43 are subjected to immunoblotting with anti-Cx43 antibodies, several bands are observed, including a faster migrating form that includes nonphosphorylated and potentially some phosphorylated isoforms, termed P0, and at least two slower migrating forms, commonly termed P1 and P2.[85,86] Pulse chase analysis indicates that the Cx43 isoforms progress from P0 to P1 to P2, and the P2 isoform is associated with gap junctional structures.[72] These phosphorylation events also occur in vivo because the slower migrating phosphorylated isoforms predominate when cardiac tissue is immunoblotted for Cx43.

In the past, most studies on connexin phosphorylation were performed via the addition of kinase activators and inhibitors to cells in culture, and in most cases, the specific residues affected by these pharmacologic agents were not identified. Treatment of cells with various stimuli can result in a shift of Cx43 to slower migrating forms and is often associated with downregulation of gap junctional intercellular communication. Several studies have focused on using growth factors and phorbol esters in combination with mitogen-activated protein kinase (MAPK) and protein kinase C (PKC) inhibitors to correlate changes in Cx43 isoform migration with shutdown of gap junctional intercellular communication. The sites where extracellular signal–regulated kinase 1/2 (ERK1/2) phosphorylates Cx43 have been determined to be S255, S279, and S282,[87] and when wild-type Cx43 or S279, S282, or S255A mutant Cx43 were expressed in HeLa cells, treatment with epidermal growth factor (EGF) led to a migration shift in both wild-type and mutant expressing cells, although inhibition of communication was only observed in wild-type Cx43-expressing cells.[87,88] Inhibition of ERK1/2 reversed both of these effects. Advances in mass spectrometric techniques, the use of site-directed mutations of connexin proteins in specific assays, and the development of phosphospecific antibodies that only recognize a connexin when it is phosphorylated at a specific site have led to a better understanding of the role specific kinases and phosphorylation events play in connexin regulation.

Connexin43 Conformation: The Utility of Phosphorylation Status–Specific Antibodies

The gap junction plaque–associated, Triton X-100–insoluble P2 isoform of Cx43 has been shown to be phosphorylated at S325, S328, or S330 (or some combination) using an antibody phosphospecific for these sites in cell lines and heart tissue.[89] Cells expressing site-directed mutants, in which these serines were converted to alanines, do not assemble gap junctions efficiently, nor do they make the P2 isoform of Cx43.[89] These data indicate that phosphorylation on S325, S328, or S330 is required for formation of the gap junction plaque–associated P2 isoform of Cx43. Because casein kinase 1 (CK1) has been shown to be important for gap junction assembly and to be able to phosphorylate some combination of these residues,[90] these data are consistent with the idea that phosphorylation on some combination of S325, 328, and 330 by CK1 results in a conformational change resulting in the P2 isoform and inclusion in a gap-junction plaque.

Similarly, antibody reagents and site-directed mutants have also been used to gain insights into formation of the P1 electrophoretic isoform. Use of a monoclonal antibody that has been epitope mapped and shown to be specific for Cx43 *not* phosphorylated on S364 or S365 did not react with the P1 isoform.[91] Immunofluoresence with this antibody indicated that it primarily labeled Cx43 in cytoplasmic membranes of heart tissue only after treatments leading to dephosphorylation.[91] Generation of an antibody phosphospecific for Cx43 phosphorylated at S365 only reacted with P1 and P2 (not P0), and only labeled control but not hypoxic heart tissue.[92]

Connexin Interacting Proteins: Zona Occludens-1 and Src Crosstalk

Many connexin-interacting proteins have been discovered that range from kinases and scaffolding proteins to molecules of unknown function. For example, Cx43 has been reported to interact with zona occludens-1 (ZO-1), ZO-2, and Src; protein kinase A (PKA), PKC, and protein kinase G (PKG); MAPK; the cyclin-dependent kinase cdc2; CK1; dystrophia myotonica protein kinase (DMPK); receptor protein tyrosine phosphatase μ (RPTPμ); β-catenin, α-catenin, and p120-catenin; cadherin; cysteine-rich 61; connective tissue growth factor; nephroblastoma-overexpressed family of growth regulators (NOV/CNN3); caveolin-1; CIP85; 14-3-3; α/β-tubulin; and drebrin.[93-95]

The first-identified and most widely studied Cx43-interacting protein, ZO-1, is a scaffold protein containing several protein-protein interaction domains: three PSD95/Dlg/ZO-1 (PDZ) domains, a Src homology 3 (SH3) domain, and a guanylate kinase domain. A region near the carboxyl-terminus of Cx43 has been shown to interact with the second PDZ domain of ZO-1.[96] Microscopy-based analyses examining colocalization of ZO-1 and Cx43 in the plasma membrane indicate that ZO-1 is found predominantly at the outer edges of gap junction plaques.[97-99] When interaction between these two proteins is inhibited, plaque size increased.[97,99] Hunter and colleagues proposed that ZO-1 interaction at the periphery of the plaque limits the rate of free hemichannel addition, resulting in smaller plaques. Consistent with this concept are data indicating that cells in G0 phase of the cell cycle have increased interaction with ZO-1 and smaller gap junctions than S phase cells.[100] However, these studies manipulated the ZO-1-Cx43 interaction by interfering with the Cx43 PDZ binding domain, which could be interacting with other PDZ domain–containing proteins in addition to ZO-1.

The viral-Src (v-Src) oncogene[101] and the cellular-Src (c-Src) proto-oncogene[102,103] have been shown to interact with Cx43 and mediate phosphorylation of S247 and S265. These interactions occur via binding of the Src homology 2 and 3 (SH2 and SH3) domains. Pull-down experiments using lysates from cells expressing v-Src or Cx43 mutants indicate that the proline-rich segment $P_{253}LSP_{256}$ of Cx43 is critical for SH3 binding. Phosphorylation on S265 could create a potential SH2 binding site, allowing phosphorylation on S247 and culminating in channel closure.[104] Src binding to Cx43 has also been shown to inhibit the ability of ZO-1 and Cx43 to interact.[103,105] Structural studies indicate that Src binding to Cx43 could displace ZO-1, even though the binding sites for these domains are quite distant.[106] Consistent with this, in cardiac myocytes, expression of constitutively active c-Src inhibited the interaction between ZO-1 and wild-type Cx43 but not the Cx43 mutant, Y265F.[103] Additionally, Cx43 from cultured astrocytes exposed to chemical ischemia had an increased association with c-Src, ERK1/2, and MAPK phosphatase-1[107] and a decreased association with ZO-1.[108]

Gap Junction Remodeling

Alterations in the abundance and subcellular localization of gap junctional proteins are observed in response to diverse acute and chronic pathologic stressors.[44,45] This process has been termed *gap junction remodeling*, akin to the electrical remodeling associated with alterations in the expression and function of sarcolemmal ion channels. Using immunohistochemical techniques (primarily for Cx43), gap junction remodeling is often associated with redistribution of the channel protein away from the intercalated disc at the ends of cells and toward the lateral borders; increased cytoplasmic immunoreactivity is also often observed. These observations are consistent with either aberrant targeting of connexins to the junctional membrane or other defects in the connexin life cycle. Post-translational phosphorylation of Cx43 is typically deranged in response to cardiovascular stressors, often as an early and persistent abnormality, suggesting that the alterations in phosphorylation may be mechanistically linked to the remodeling process. The precise molecular mechanisms responsible for gap junction remodeling remain elusive; however, amelioration or reversal of the remodeling

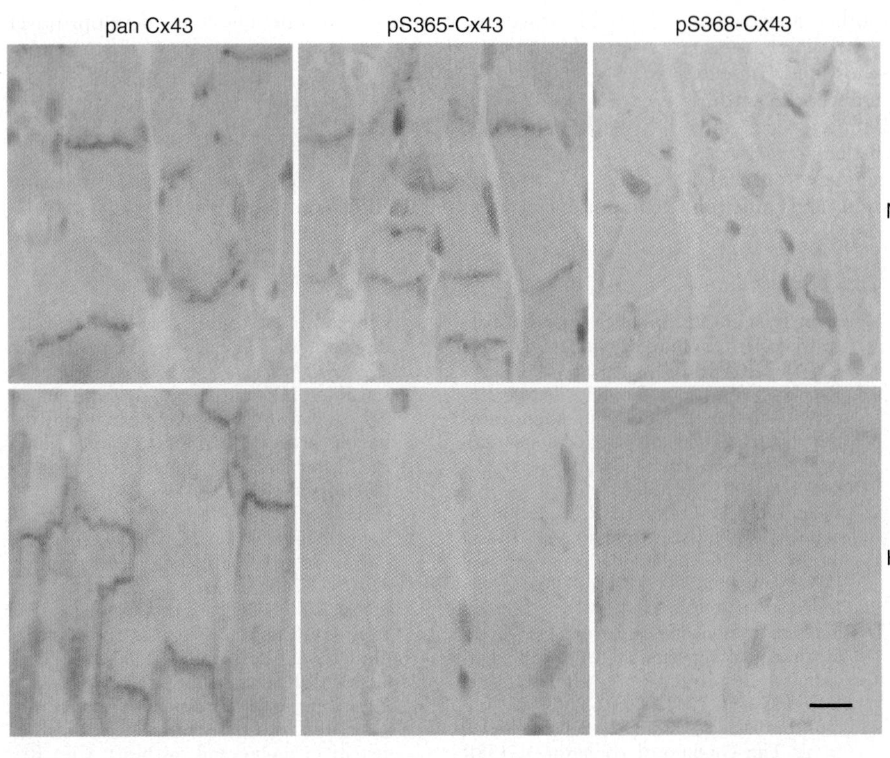

Figure 29-4 Phosphorylation of connexin43 (Cx43) localized at intercalated disks versus lateral edges of myocytes in the normoxic and ischemic heart. Total Cx43 and pS365-Cx43 antibodies stain primarily intercalated disk Cx43 in control tissue. pS365-Cx43 is lost and pS368-Cx43 increases in hypoxic hearts, but total Cx43 staining occurs at both intercalated disk and lateral edge regions of myocytes. Nuclei are stained with hematoxylin (bar = 10 μm). (Adapted from Solan JL, Marquez-Rosado L, Sorgen PL, et al: Phosphorylation at S365 is a gatekeeper event that changes the structure of Cx43 and prevents down-regulation by PKC. 179(6):1301-1309, 2007.)

process is considered an important potential antiarrhythmia target. Some examples of these findings are discussed more fully next.

Ischemia and Hypoxia Regulate Cx43 Localization and Function

Many investigators have shown that myocardial ischemia leads to Cx43 dephosphorylation (i.e., the loss of P1, P2, etc., and gain of P0) and loss of localization from the intercalated disk, which likely contributes to contractile failure and arrhythmias.[109,110] Cx43 localized to intercalated disks is phosphorylated at S365[92] and S325, S328, or S330[89] (or some combination), and ischemia leads to loss of these phosphorylation events and relocalization of the protein. Ischemic preconditioning (exposure of the heart to a brief period of ischemia (e.g., 2-5 min) followed by reperfusion) before a more prolonged ischemic period (i.e., $\geq$30 min) protects the heart against necrosis and fatal arrhythmias.[110-112] PKC is activated during preconditioning and appears to be necessary for protection against injury during the subsequent prolonged ischemic period. Cardiac ischemia and hypoxia also causes PKC activation, unidentified Cx43 dephosphorylation events, Cx43 relocalization,[109,110] and PKC-dependent phosphorylation of Cx43 at S368 (Fig. 29-4).[113] Because phosphorylation at S365 occurs in control heart tissue but not in hypoxic heart (see Fig 29-4) and phosphorylation at S365 prevents phosphorylation at S368,[92] the interrelationship of Cx43 phosphorylation at S365 and S368 could likely prove to be important in ischemia and preconditioning. Furthermore, because phosphorylation of Cx43 at S368 is increased by tumor-promoting agents, is controlled during the cell cycle, and is developmentally regulated,[114-116] this gatekeeper role for S365 phosphorylation may be critical for growth control.

Chronic Pressure-Overload Hypertrophy and Gap Junction Remodeling

Whereas acute hypertrophic stimuli are often associated with increased Cx43 abundance, persistent hemodynamic overload typically results in gap junction remodeling and slowing of impulse propagation, despite the increase in cell size, which would favor enhanced conduction velocity.[117] For example, in mice subjected to transverse aortic constriction, progressive cardiac hypertrophy is associated with demonstrable alterations in Cx43 phosphorylation patterns and diminution in overall Cx43 abundance (according to our unpublished observations). These molecular changes are associated with significant slowing of impulse propagation, as determined by optical mapping of isolated-perfused hearts using voltage-sensitive fluorescent dyes. Gap junction remodeling is also observed in the hearts of rats overexpressing angiotensin II, in spontaneous and L-NAME (N^{ω}-nitro-L-arginine methylester) murine models of hypertension, and in the right ventricles of rats with monocrataline-induced pulmonary hypertension.[118-120] These studies underscore the mechanistic role that gap junction remodeling might play in the increased arrhythmic risk associated with cardiac hypertrophy.

Summary

The regulation of connexin gene transcription and the life cycle of gap junctional proteins are highly dynamic processes that greatly influence the electrophysiologic behavior of the heart.Although our understanding of the regulatory processes remains incomplete, particularly the mechanisms responsible for gap junction remodeling in the setting of acute and chronic disease processes, there are compelling reasons to believe that amelioration of the remodeling process or other approaches toward normalizing cell-cell coupling in the heart might prove salutary with respect to arrhythmic syndromes. Indeed, recent work suggests that introduction of embryonic cardiomyocytes or even Cx43-expressing skeletal muscle cells into infarct zones protects against inducible ventricular tachycardia.[121] Clearly, elucidation of the genetic and environmental factors that influence gap junction expression and function should prove most fruitful in our quest to develop novel antiarrhythmic strategies.

Acknowledgements

Due to space limitations, we were not able to cite many important original publications and for this we apologize.

References

1. Weidmann S: The electrical constants of Purkinje fibres. J Physiol 118:348-360, 1952.
2. Revel JP, Karnovsk MJ: Hexagonal array of subunits in intercellular junctions of the mouse heart and liver. J Cell Biol 33: C7-C12, 1967.
3. Unwin PN, Zampighi G: Structure of the junction between communicating cells. Nature 283:545-549, 1980.
4. Paul DL: Molecular cloning of cDNA for rat liver gap junction protein. J Cell Biol 103:123-134, 1986.
5. Vozzi C, Dupont E, Coppen SR: Chamber-related differences in connexin expression in the human heart. J Mol Cell Cardiol 31:991-1003, 1999.
6. Kanno S, Saffitz JE: The role of myocardial gap junctions in electrical conduction and arrhythmogenesis. Cardiovasc Pathol 10:169-177, 2001.
7. Desplantez T, Dupont E, Severs NJ, Weingart R: Gap Junction Channels and Cardiac Impulse Propagation. J Membr Biol 218(1-3):13-28, 2007.
8. Sohl G, Willecke K: Gap junctions and the connexin protein family. Cardiovasc Res 62:228-232, 2004.
9. Cruciani V, Mikalsen SO: Evolutionary selection pressure and family relationships among connexin genes. Biol Chem 388:253-264, 2007.
10. Davis LM, Kanter HL, Beyer EC, Saffitz JE: Distinct gap junction protein phenotypes in cardiac tissues with disparate conduction properties. J Am Coll Cardiol 24:1124-1132, 1994.
11. Davis LM, Rodefeld ME, Green K, et al: Gap junction protein phenotypes of the human heart and conduction system. J Cardiovasc Electrophysiol 6:813-822, 1995.
12. Boyett MR, Inada S, Yoo S, et al: Connexins in the sinoatrial and atrioventricular nodes. Adv Cardiol 42:175-197, 2006.
13. Harris AL: Connexin channel permeability to cytoplasmic molecules. Prog Biophys Mol Biol 94:120-143, 2007.
14. Kanter HL, Saffitz JE, Beyer EC: Cardiac myocytes express multiple gap junction proteins. Circ Res 70:438-444, 1992.
15. Moreno AP: Biophysical properties of homomeric and heteromultimeric channels formed by cardiac connexins. Cardiovasc Res 62:276-286, 2004.
16. Reaume AG, de Sousa PA, Kulkarni S, et al: Cardiac malformation in neonatal mice lacking connexin43. Science 267:1831-1834, 1995.
17. Gutstein DE, Morley GE, Tamaddon H, et al: Conduction slowing and sudden arrhythmic death in mice with cardiac-restricted inactivation of connexin43. Circ Res 88:333-339, 2001.
18. Paznekas WA, Boyadjiev SA, Shapiro RE, et al: Connexin 43 *(GJA1)* mutations cause the pleiotropic phenotype of oculodentodigital dysplasia. Am J Hum Genet 72: 408-418, 2003.
19. Flenniken AM, Osborne LR, Anderson N, et al: A *GJA1* missense mutation in a mouse model of oculodentodigital dysplasia. Development 132:4375-4386, 2005.
20. Kalcheva N, Qu J, Sandeep N, et al: Gap junction remodeling and cardiac arrhythmogenesis in a murine model of oculodentodigital dysplasia. Proc Natl Acad Sci U S A 104(51):20512-20516, 2007.
21. Dobrowolski R, Sasse P, Schrickel JW, et al: The conditional connexin43G138R mouse mutant represents a new model of hereditary oculodentodigital dysplasia in humans. Hum Mol Genet 17(4):539-554, 2007.
22. Maass K, Shibayama J, Chase SE, et al: C-terminal truncation of connexin43 changes number, size, and localization of cardiac gap junction plaques. Circ Res 101(12):11283-11291, 2007.
23. Winterhager E, Pielensticker N, Freyer J, et al: Replacement of connexin43 by connexin26 in transgenic mice leads to dysfunctional reproductive organs and slowed ventricular conduction in the heart. BMC Dev Biol 7:26, 2007.
24. Zheng-Fischhofer Q, Ghanem A, Kim JS, et al: Connexin31 cannot functionally replace connexin43 during cardiac morphogenesis in mice. J Cell Sci 119:693-701, 2006.
25. Plum A, Hallas G, Magin T, et al: Unique and shared functions of different connexins in mice. Curr Biol 10:1083-1091, 2000.
26. Gros D, Jarry-Guichard T, Ten Velde I, et al: Restricted distribution of connexin40, a gap junctional protein, in mammalian heart. Circ Res 74:839-851, 1994.
27. Gourdie RG, Severs NJ, Green CR, et al: The spatial distribution and relative abundance of gap-junctional connexin40 and connexin43 correlate to functional properties of components of the cardiac atrioventricular conduction system. J Cell Sci 105(Pt 4):985-991, 1993.
28. Simon AM, Goodenough DA, Paul DL: Mice lacking connexin40 have cardiac conduction abnormalities characteristic of atrioventricular block and bundle branch block. Curr Biol 8:295-298, 1998.
29. Tamaddon HS, Vaidya D, Simon AM, et al: High-resolution optical mapping of the right bundle branch in connexin40 knockout mice reveals slow conduction in the specialized conduction system. Circ Res 87:929-936, 2000.
30. van Rijen HV, van Veen TA, van Kempen MJ, et al: Impaired conduction in the bundle branches of mouse hearts lacking the gap junction protein connexin40. Circulation 103:1591-1598, 2001.
31. Gollob MH, Jones DL, Krahn AD, et al: Somatic mutations in the connexin 40 gene *(GJA5)* in atrial fibrillation. N Engl J Med 354:2677-2688, 2006.
32. Hauer RN, Groenewegen WA, Firouzi M, et al: Cx40 polymorphism in human atrial fibrillation. Adv Cardiol 42:284-291, 2006.
33. Coppen SR, Dupont E, Rothery S, Severs NJ: Connexin45 expression is preferentially associated with the ventricular conduction system in mouse and rat heart. Circ Res 82:232-243, 1998.
34. Nishii K, Kumai M, Egashira K, et al: Mice lacking connexin45 conditionally in cardiac myocytes display embryonic lethality similar to that of germline knockout mice without endocardial cushion defect. Cell Commun Adhes 10:365-369, 2003.
35. Kreuzberg MM, Schrickel JW, Ghanem A, et al: Connexin30.2 containing gap junction channels decelerate impulse propagation through the atrioventricular node. Proc Natl Acad Sci U S A 103:5959-5964, 2006.
36. Bukauskas FF, Kreuzberg MM, Rackauskas M, et al: Properties of mouse connexin 30.2 and human connexin 31.9 hemichannels: Implications for atrioventricular conduction in the heart. Proc Natl Acad Sci U S A 103:9726-9731, 2006.
37. Teunissen BE, Bierhuizen MF: Transcriptional control of myocardial connexins. Cardiovasc Res 62:246-255, 2004.
38. Willecke K, Eiberger J, Degen J, et al: Structural and functional diversity of connexin genes in the mouse and human genome. Biol Chem 383:725-737, 2002.
39. Darrow BJ, Fast VG, Kleber AG, et al: Functional and structural assessment of intercellular communication. Increased conduction velocity and enhanced connexin expression in dibutyryl cAMP–treated cultured cardiac myocytes. Circ Res 79: 174-183, 1996.
40. Dodge SM, Beardslee MA, Darrow BJ, et al: Effects of angiotensin II on expression of the gap junction channel protein connexin43 in neonatal rat ventricular myocytes. J Am Coll Cardiol 32:800-807, 1998.
41. Mukherjee DP, McTiernan CF, Sen S: Myotrophin induces early response genes and enhances cardiac gene expression. Hypertension 21:142-148, 1993.

42. Uzzaman M, Honjo H, Takagishi Y, et al: Remodeling of gap junctional coupling in hypertrophied right ventricles of rats with monocrotaline-induced pulmonary hypertension. Circ Res 86:871-878, 2000.
43. Emdad L, Uzzaman M, Takagishi Y, et al: Gap junction remodeling in hypertrophied left ventricles of aortic-banded rats: Prevention by angiotensin II type 1 receptor blockade. J Mol Cell Cardiol 33: 219-231, 2001.
44. Severs NJ, Coppen SR, Dupont E, et al: Gap junction alterations in human cardiac disease. Cardiovasc Res 62:368-377, 2004.
45. Severs NJ, Dupont E, Thomas N, et al: Alterations in cardiac connexin expression in cardiomyopathies. Adv Cardiol 42: 228-242, 2006.
46. Ai Z, Fischer A, Spray DC, et al: Wnt-1 regulation of connexin43 in cardiac myocytes. J Clin Invest 105:161-171, 2000.
47. Rosenkranz-Weiss P, Tomek RJ, Mathew J, Eghbali M: Gender-specific differences in expression of mRNAs for functional and structural proteins in rat ventricular myocardium. J Mol Cell Cardiol 26: 261-270, 1994.
48. Yu W, Dahl G, Werner R: The connexin43 gene is responsive to oestrogen. Proc Biol Sci 255:125-132, 1994.
49. Grohe C, Kahlert S, Lobbert K: Cardiac myocytes and fibroblasts contain functional estrogen receptors. FEBS Lett 416: 107-112, 1997.
50. Amino M, Yoshioka K, Tanabe T, et al: Heavy ion radiation up-regulates Cx43 and ameliorates arrhythmogenic substrates in hearts after myocardial infarction. Cardiovasc Res 72:412-421, 2006.
51. Fernandez-Cobo M, Gingalewski C, Drujan D, De Maio A: Downregulation of connexin 43 gene expression in rat heart during inflammation. The role of tumour necrosis factor. Cytokine 11:216-224, 1999.
52. Petrich BG, Gong X, Lerner DL, et al: c-Jun N-terminal kinase activation mediates downregulation of connexin43 in cardiomyocytes. Circ Res 91:640-647, 2002.
53. Nguyen-Tran VT, Kubalak SW, Minamisawa S, et al: A novel genetic pathway for sudden cardiac death via defects in the transition between ventricular and conduction system cell lineages. Cell 102: 671-682, 2000.
54. Bruneau BG, Nemer G, Schmitt JP, et al: A murine model of Holt-Oram syndrome defines roles of the T-box transcription factor Tbx5 in cardiogenesis and disease. Cell 106:709-721, 2001.
55. Kasahara H, Wakimoto H, Liu M, et al: Progressive atrioventricular conduction defects and heart failure in mice expressing a mutant Csx/Nkx2.5 homeoprotein. J Clin Invest 108:189-201, 2001.
56. Pizard A, Burgon PG, Paul DL, et al: Connexin 40, a target of transcription factor Tbx5, patterns wrist, digits, and sternum. Mol Cell Biol 25:5073-5083, 2005.
57. Dupays L, Jarry-Guichard T, Mazurais D, et al: Dysregulation of connexins and inactivation of NFATc1 in the cardiovascular system of Nkx2-5 null mutants. J Mol Cell Cardiol 38:787-798, 2005.
58. Blaschke RJ, Hahurij ND, Kuijper S, et al: Targeted mutation reveals essential functions of the homeodomain transcription factor Shox2 in sinoatrial and pacemaking development. Circulation 115:1830-1838, 2007.
59. Ismat FA, Zhang M, Kook H, et al: Homeobox protein Hop functions in the adult cardiac conduction system. Circ Res 96:898-903, 2005.
60. Rentschler S, Zander J, Meyers K, et al: Neuregulin-1 promotes formation of the murine cardiac conduction system. Proc Natl Acad Sci U S A 99:10464-10469, 2002.
61. Patel R, Kos L: Endothelin-1 and neuregulin-1 convert embryonic cardiomyocytes into cells of the conduction system in the mouse. Dev Dyn 233:20-28, 2005.
62. Ruhparwar A, Er F, Martin U, et al: Enrichment of cardiac pacemaker-like cells: Neuregulin-1 and cyclic AMP increase I_f-current density and connexin 40 mRNA levels in fetal cardiomyocytes. Med Biol Eng Comput 45:221-227, 2007.
63. Beardslee MA, Laing JG, Beyer EC, Saffitz JE: Rapid turnover of connexin43 in the adult rat heart. Circ Res 83:629-635, 1998.
64. Musil LS, Goodenough DA: Multisubunit assembly of an integral plasma membrane channel protein, gap junction connexin43, occurs after exit from the ER. Cell 74:1065-1077, 1993.
65. Gaietta G, Deerinck TJ, Adams SR, et al: Multicolor and electron microscopic imaging of connexin trafficking. Science 296:503-507, 2002.
66. Johnson RG, Meyer RA, Li XR, et al: Gap junctions assemble in the presence of cytoskeletal inhibitors, but enhanced assembly requires microtubules. Exp Cell Res 275:67-80, 2002.
67. Lauf U, Giepmans BN, Lopez P, et al: Dynamic trafficking and delivery of connexons to the plasma membrane and accretion to gap junctions in living cells. Proc Natl Acad Sci U S A 99:10446-10451, 2002.
68. Shaw RM, Fay AJ, Puthenveedu MA, et al: Microtubule plus-end-tracking proteins target gap junctions directly from the cell interior to adherens junctions. Cell 128:547-560, 2007.
69. Chu FF, Doyle D: Turnover of plasma membrane proteins in rat hepatoma cells and primary cultures of rat hepatocytes. J Biol Chem 260:3097-3107, 1985.
70. VanSlyke JK, Musil LS: Dislocation and degradation from the ER are regulated by cytosolic stress. J Cell Biol 157:381-394, 2002.
71. VanSlyke JK, Deschenes SM, Musil LS: Intracellular transport, assembly, and degradation of wild-type and disease-linked mutant gap junction proteins. Mol Biol Cell 11:1933-1946, 2000.
72. Musil LS, Goodenough DA: Biochemical analysis of connexin43 intracellular transport, phosphorylation, and assembly into gap junctional plaques. J Cell Biol 115:1357-1374, 1991.
73. VanSlyke JK, Musil LS: Cytosolic stress reduces degradation of connexin43 internalized from the cell surface and enhances gap junction formation and function. Mol Biol Cell 16:5247-5257, 2005.
74. Laird DW: Life cycle of connexins in health and disease. Biochem J 394:527-543, 2006.
75. Laird DW: Connexin phosphorylation as a regulatory event linked to gap junction internalization and degradation. Biochim Biophys Acta 1711:172-182, 2005.
76. Solan JL, Lampe PD: Connexin phosphorylation as a regulatory event linked to gap junction channel assembly. Biochim Biophys Acta 1711:154-163, 2005.
77. Atkinson MM, Lampe PD, Lin HH, et al: Cyclic AMP modifies the cellular distribution of connexin43 and induces a persistent increase in the junctional permeability of mouse mammary tumor cells. J Cell Sci 108(Pt 9):3079-3090, 1995.
78. Burghardt RC, Barhoumi R, Sewall TC, Bowen JA: Cyclic AMP induces rapid increases in gap junction permeability and changes in the cellular distribution of connexin43. J Membr Biol 148:243-253, 1995.
79. Bolon ML, Kidder GM, Simon AM, Tyml K: Lipopolysaccharide reduces electrical coupling in microvascular endothelial cells by targeting connexin40 in a tyrosine-, ERK1/2-, PKA-, and PKC-dependent manner. J Cell Physiol 211:159-166, 2007.
80. Bolon ML, Ouellette Y, Li F, Tyml K: Abrupt reoxygenation following hypoxia reduces electrical coupling between endothelial cells of wild-type but not connexin40 null mice in oxidant- and PKA-dependent manner. FASEB J 19: 1725-1727, 2005.
81. Chanson M, White MM, Garber SS: cAMP promotes gap junctional coupling in T84 cells. Am J Physiol 271:C533-C539, 1996.
82. van Veen TA, van Rijen HV, Jongsma HJ: Electrical conductance of mouse connexin45 gap junction channels is modulated by phosphorylation. Cardiovasc Res 46:496-510, 2000.
83. Paulson AF, Lampe PD, Meyer RA, et al: Cyclic AMP and LDL trigger a rapid enhancement in gap junction assembly through a stimulation of connexin trafficking. J Cell Sci 113(Pt 17):3037-3049, 2000.
84. Lampe PD: Analyzing phorbol ester effects on gap junctional communication: A dramatic inhibition of assembly. J Cell Biol 127:1895-1905, 1994.
85. Musil LS, Cunningham BA., Edelman GM, Goodenough DA: Differential phosphorylation of the gap junction protein connexin43 in junctional communication-competent and -deficient cell lines. J Cell Biol 111:2077-2088, 1990.
86. Crow DS, Beyer EC, Paul DL, et al: Phosphorylation of connexin43 gap junction protein in uninfected and Rous sarcoma virus–transformed mammalian fibroblasts. Mol Cell Biol 10:1754-1763, 1990.
87. Warn-Cramer BJ, Lampe PD, Kurata WE, et al: Characterization of the mitogen-activated protein kinase phosphorylation sites on the connexin-43 gap junction protein. J Biol Chem 271:3779-3786, 1996.
88. Warn-Cramer BJ, Cottrell GT, Burt JM, Lau AF: Regulation of connexin-43 gap junctional intercellular communication by

mitogen-activated protein kinase. J Biol Chem 273:9188-9196, 1998.

89. Lampe PD, Cooper CD, King TJ, Burt JM: Analysis of connexin43 phosphorylated at S325, S328 and S330 in normoxic and ischemic heart. J Cell Sci 119:3435-3442, 2006.
90. Cooper CD, Lampe PD: Casein kinase 1 regulates connexin-43 gap junction assembly. J Biol Chem 277:44962-44968, 2002.
91. Sosinsky GE, Giepmans BN, Deerinck TJ, et al: Markers for correlated light and electron microscopy. Methods Cell Biol 79:575-591, 2007.
92. Solan JL, Marquez-Rosado L, Sorgen PL, et al: Phosphorylation at S365 is a gatekeeper event that changes the structure of Cx43 and prevents down-regulation by PKC. 179(6):1301-1309, 2007.
93. Giepmans BN: Gap junctions and connexin-interacting proteins. Cardiovasc Res 62:233-245, 2004.
94. Giepmans BN: Role of connexin43-interacting proteins at gap junctions. Adv Cardiol 42:41-56, 2006.
95. Herve JC, Bourmeyster N, Sarrouilhe D: Diversity in protein-protein interactions of connexins: Emerging roles. Biochim Biophys Acta 1662:22-41, 2004.
96. Giepmans BN, Moolenaar WH: The gap junction protein connexin43 interacts with the second PDZ domain of the zona occludens-1 protein. Curr Biol 8:931-934, 1998.
97. Hunter AW, Barker RJ, Zhu C, Gourdie RG: Zonula occludens-1 alters connexin43 gap junction size and organization by influencing channel accretion. Mol Biol Cell 16:5686-5698, 2005.
98. Zhu C, Barker RJ, Hunter AW, et al: Quantitative analysis of ZO-1 colocalization with Cx43 gap junction plaques in cultures of rat neonatal cardiomyocytes. Microsc Microanal 11:244-248, 2005.
99. Akoyev V, Takemoto DJ: ZO-1 is required for protein kinase C gamma-driven disassembly of connexin 43. Cell Signal 19:958-967, 2007.
100. Singh D, Solan JL, Taffet SM, et al: Connexin 43 interacts with zona occludens-1 and -2 proteins in a cell cycle stage-specific manner. J Biol Chem 280:30416-30421, 2005.
101. Loo LW, Kanemitsu MY, Lau AF: In vivo association of pp60v-Src and the gap-junction protein connexin 43 in v-Src-transformed fibroblasts. Mol Carcinog 25:187-195, 1999.
102. Giepmans BN, Hengeveld T, Postma FR, Moolenaar WH: Interaction of c-Src with gap junction protein connexin-43. Role in the regulation of cell-cell communication. J Biol Chem 276:8544-8549, 2001.
103. Toyofuku T, Akamatsu Y, Zhang H, et al: c-Src regulates the interaction between connexin-43 and ZO-1 in cardiac myocytes. J Biol Chem 276:1780-1788, 2001.
104. Lin R, Warn-Cramer BJ, Kurata WE, Lau AF: v-Src phosphorylation of connexin 43 on Tyr247 and Tyr265 disrupts gap junctional communication. J Cell Biol 154:815-827, 2001.
105. Giepmans BN, Verlaan I, Moolenaar WH: Connexin-43 interactions with ZO-1 and alpha- and beta-tubulin. Cell Commun Adhes 8:219-223, 2001.
106. Sorgen PL, Duffy HS, Sahoo P, et al: Structural changes in the carboxyl terminus of the gap junction protein connexin43 indicates signaling between binding domains for c-Src and zonula occludens-1. J Biol Chem 279:54695-54701, 2004.
107. Li WE, Nagy JI: Connexin43 phosphorylation state and intercellular communication in cultured astrocytes following hypoxia and protein phosphatase inhibition. Eur J Neurosci 12:2644-2650, 2000.
108. Duffy HS, Ashton AW, O'Donnell P, et al: Regulation of connexin43 protein complexes by intracellular acidification. Circ Res 94:215-222, 2004.
109. Beardslee MA, Lerner DL, Tadros PN, et al: Dephosphorylation and intracellular redistribution of ventricular connexin43 during electrical uncoupling induced by ischemia. Circ Res 87:656-662, 2000.
110. Schulz R, Gres P, Skyschally A, et al: Ischemic preconditioning preserves connexin 43 phosphorylation during sustained ischemia in pig hearts in vivo. FASEB J 17:1355-1357, 2003.
111. Cohen MV, Baines CP, Downey JM: Ischemic preconditioning: From adenosine receptor to KATP channel. Annu Rev Physiol 62:79-109, 2000.
112. Jain SK, Schuessler RB, Saffitz JE: Mechanisms of delayed electrical uncoupling induced by ischemic preconditioning. Circ Res 92:1138-1144, 2003.
113. Ek-Vitorin JF, King TJ, Heyman NS, et al: Selectivity of connexin 43 channels is regulated through protein kinase C—dependent phosphorylation. Circ Res 98:1498-1505, 2006.
114. King TJ, Lampe PD: Temporal regulation of connexin phosphorylation in embryonic and adult tissues. Biochim Biophys Acta 1719:24-35, 2005.
115. Lampe PD, Lau AF: Regulation of gap junctions by phosphorylation of connexins. Arch Biochem Biophys 384:205-215, 2000.
116. Solan JL, Fry MD, TenBroek EM, Lampe PD: Connexin43 phosphorylation at S368 is acute during S and G2/M and in response to protein kinase C activation. J Cell Sci 116:2203-2211, 2003.
117. Spach MS, Heidlage JF, Dolber PC, Barr RC: Electrophysiological effects of remodeling cardiac gap junctions and cell size: experimental and model studies of normal cardiac growth. Circ Res 86:302-311, 2000.
118. Fischer R, Dechend R, Gapelyuk A, et al: Angiotensin II–induced sudden arrhythmic death and electrical remodeling. Am J Physiol Heart Circ Physiol 293:H1242-H1253, 2007.
119. Fialova M, Dlugosova K, Okruhlicova L, et al: Adaptation of the heart to hypertension is associated with maladaptive gap junction connexin-43 remodelling. Physiol Res 57(1):7-11, 2008.
120. Sasano C, Honjo H, Takagishi Y, et al: Internalization and dephosphorylation of connexin43 in hypertrophied right ventricles of rats with pulmonary hypertension. Circ J 71:382-389, 2007.
121. Roell W, Lewalter T, Sasse P, et al: Engraftment of connexin 43-expressing cells prevents post-infarct arrhythmia. Nature 450:819-824, 2007.

Ionic Mechanisms of Ventricular Action Potential Excitation 30

JONATHAN SILVA AND YORAM RUDY

CHAPTER OUTLINE

Genetic mutations or adverse drug interactions that affect any of the major ionic currents that shape the action potential can predispose patients to cardiac arrhythmia through many different mechanisms.[1] Successful prevention of arrhythmia in these situations is therefore aided by understanding the mechanism whereby affected channels alter the whole-cell electrophysiology. Unfortunately, this is a daunting task that defies intuition in most cases, because each channel can influence other channels through its effects on the transmembrane potential (V_m) and cellular ionic environment, resulting in a highly nonlinear system. The advent of computational action potential models has greatly facilitated these studies because of their ability to quantitatively reproduce these nonlinear interactions.

Computer models of the action potential are typically formulated by starting from equations that reproduce the response of individual ionic currents to a voltage input, a response that can be measured experimentally in native cells or an expression system.[2] Formulation of the membrane conductance for each current is modeled to be in series with a driving force, typically specified by the Nernst equation.[3] Each of these current models is then set in parallel with a capacitor, which represents the charge-separating effect of the membrane. The resulting model can then be used to predict the cellular consequences of changing the gating or conductance of an ion channel and also to examine the mechanism whereby channel alteration due to mutation, disease, or drug binding causes pathology (Fig. 30-1).

The Luo-Rudy[4] and Hund-Rudy[5] dynamic models of the ventricular action potential (Fig. 30-2) have been widely used to study channel interactions in mammalian ventricular myocytes. Studies have involved simulating mutations that cause the long QT syndrome,[6-11] which is so named because the QT interval on the electrocardiogram (ECG), reflecting ventricular repolarization, is prolonged. Although rare, these mutations have proved to be important, because the resultant pathology provides insight into the function of the affected channel. For example, *LQT1* mutations affect the slow delayed rectifier potassium current, I_{Ks}, and patients with this type of mutation are typically predisposed to arrhythmia when β-adrenergic tone is elevated.[12] Therefore, one would expect that I_{Ks} plays a primary role in action potential shortening during exercise or heightened emotional state and is less important under control conditions. By simulating mutation effects in an action potential model, one gains insight not only into the mechanism of the pathology but also into the role of ion channels in action potential formation and its dependence on rate.

The first long QT mutation to be studied in detail with the Luo-Rudy dynamic model was the Δ-KPQ mutation to the *SCN5A* gene that encodes the cardiac sodium channel. Δ-KPQ mutant channels generate late sodium current due to failure of inactivation.[11] Normally, in wild-type channels, the inactivation process keeps the channel closed throughout the latter portion of the action potential. To simulate the mutation accurately, it was necessary to use a Markov-type model that allowed explicit representation of the ion-channel gating transitions and their interdependence. This formulation had the additional benefit of enabling easy tracking of the channel state occupancy (closed, open, or inactivated) throughout the action potential.[13] By examining the state-to-state transitions of each channel during the action potential, we can evaluate the importance of specific channel conformational changes in generating the action potential under control and disease conditions. Here, we present simulation results from detailed Markov models of four major currents that underlie the action potential: the fast sodium current (I_{Na}), the L-type calcium current (I_{CaL}), and the rapid delayed rectifier (I_{Kr}) and the slow delayed rectifier (I_{Ks}) potassium currents to examine the role of their gating transitions in action potential formation. The work presented in this chapter updates and summarizes material from previous publications.[13,14]

Fast Sodium Current

I_{Na} causes the rapid upstroke that initiates the action potential and ensures excitation and conduction[15,16] of the action potential by the large current (300 μA/μF) that it carries (Fig. 30-3).

Studies in this chapter were supported by NIH-NHLBI Merit Award R37-HL33343, grant R01-HL49054 (to Yoram Ruby) and fellowship F31-HL68318 (to Jonathan Silva).

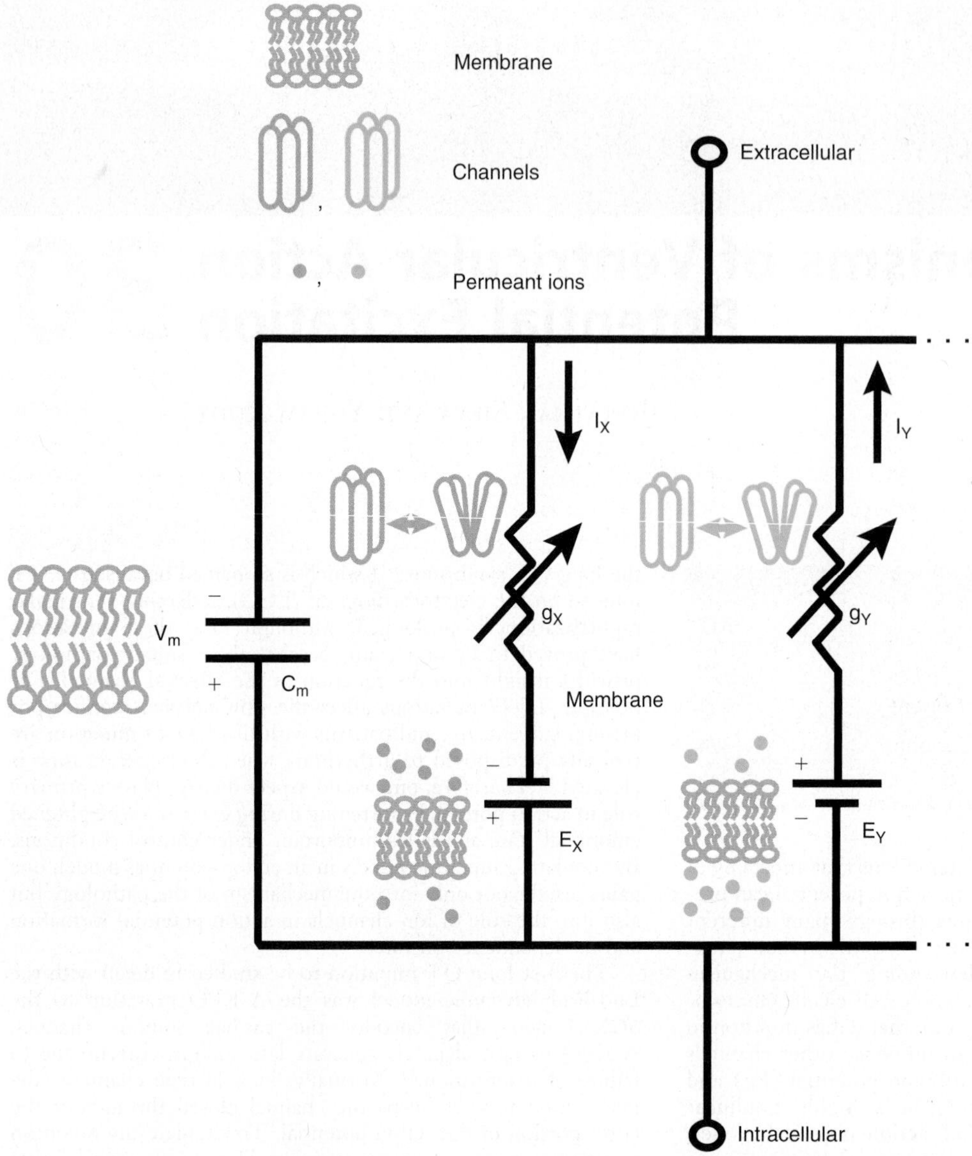

Figure 30-1 Generic circuit model for excitable tissue. Channel opening and closing is modeled by resistors with variable conductance (g_X and g_Y). These are positioned in series with the reversal potential (E_X and E_Y) typically calculated via the Nernst equation,[3] which depends on the difference between intracellular and extracellular ion concentrations. The currents in each of the branches (I_X and I_Y) are in parallel with a capacitor C_m, which represents charge separation by the membrane. Because the conductance of many channels is voltage dependent, a highly nonlinear system arises, namely, varying transmembrane potential (V_m) affects channel conductances, which leads to further changes in V_m.

Following fast activation, a rapid decline is caused by a fast inactivation process that suppresses the I_{Na} inward current by channel transitions into a fast inactivated state. The sustained depolarization of V_m then causes I_{Na} channels to transition into an intermediate inactivated state that has a longer time constant of recovery. This transition ensures I_{Na} suppression for the entire action potential duration; it is also required to reproduce the restitution and rate-dependent properties of the action potential.

The importance of the inactivation mechanism is highlighted by long-QT syndrome mutations that cause I_{Na} inactivation to fail.[11,17] Failure of inactivation generates an inward current throughout the action potential and prolongs action potential duration (APD). Cardiac I_{Na} channels are formed by the α-subunit $Na_V1.5$, which is genetically encoded by *SCN5A*.[18] Association of several modulatory β-subunits (β_1-β_4) has also been detected. $Na_V1.5$ has four homologous domains (DI-DIV), each with six transmembrane-spanning segments (S1-S6) and a pore-forming P-loop between S5 and S6. Positively charged residues in S4 of each domain link channel activation to changes in V_m.[19] A conserved phenylalanine residue in the III-IV linker of heart and brain I_{Na} channels has been linked to fast inactivation[20,21] and is part of three hydrophobic amino acids (isoleucine-phenylalanine-methionine [IFM]) that have been shown to block the open pore.[22-24] Docking sites for this inactivation gate have been identified on the S4-S5 linkers in domains III and IV.[25] Recently, the C-terminus has been shown to participate in fast inactivation by interacting with the III-IV linker and stabilizing the inactivated state.[26]

Each of these processes is represented in the Markov model shown in Figure 30-3A.[9] Because I_{Na} activation is a cooperative process[27] (activation of a voltage sensor in one domain influences activation in the other domains), three closed states are included in the model, each representing a possible conformation of all four voltage sensors, rather than modeling the activation of the voltage sensor in each domain separately. In the model, fast inactivation takes place preferentially from the open state, reflecting its dependence on channel activation.[28,29]

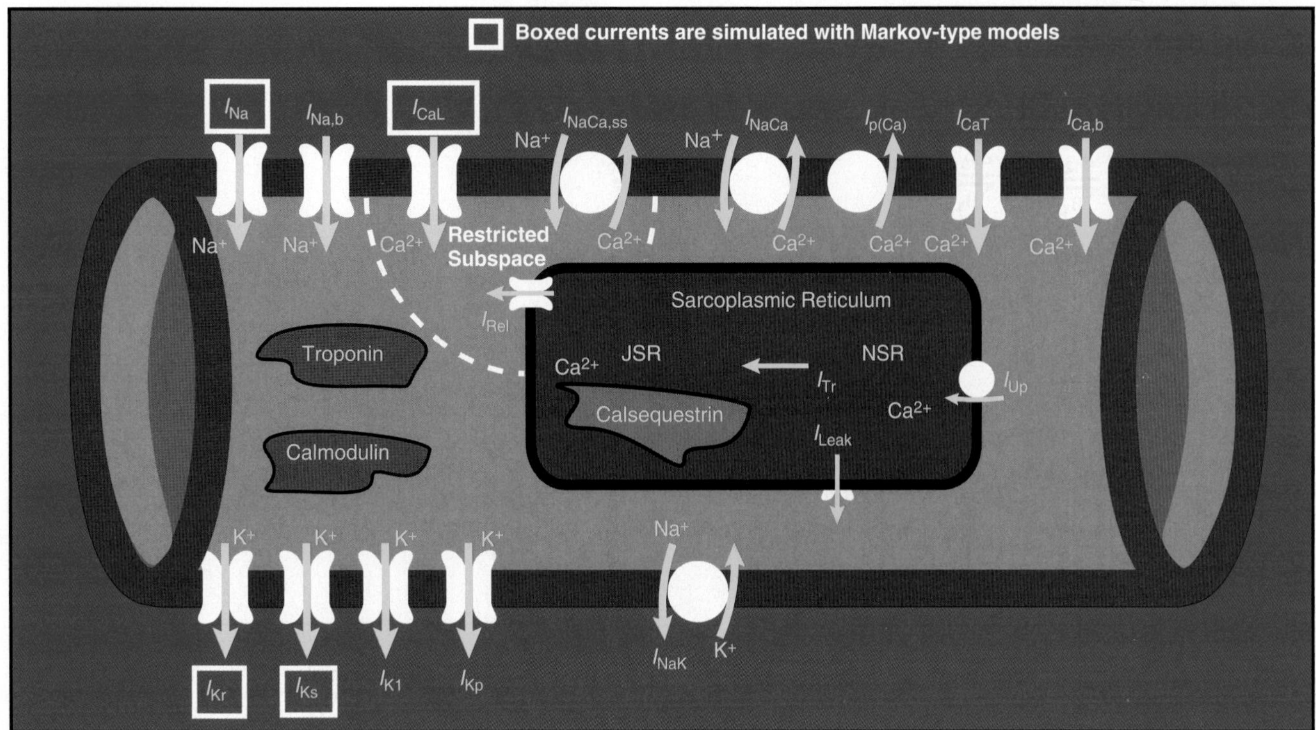

Figure 30-2 Schematic of the ventricular cell model.[4,7,16,47,83-87] Dynamics of intracellular Na^+, K^+, and Ca^{2+} are accounted for in the model. Dynamic changes of intracellular Ca^{2+} are determined by transmembrane fluxes, release and uptake by a two-compartment sarcoplasmic reticulum (SR) and by Ca^{2+} interactions with buffers. Boxed ionic currents are simulated with recently published Markov formulations (other currents follow the Hodgkin-Huxley formulation). The restricted subspace ($[Ca^{2+}]_{ss}$ in the text) represents a small volume near the interface of the I_{CaL} channels and the ryanodine receptors that generate I_{Rel}.[37,45] A fraction of the Na^+-Ca^{2+} exchange current ($I_{NaCa,ss}$) can also enter this space through exchangers that are localized to the area. Calmodulin and troponin represent calcium buffers in the myoplasm. Calsequestrin is a calcium buffer in the JSR. I_{Na}, fast sodium current; I_{CaL}, calcium current through L-type calcium channels; I_{CaT}, calcium current through T-type calcium channels[73-75]; I_{Kr}, rapid delayed rectifier potassium current[10,55]; I_{Ks}, slow delayed rectifier potassium current[55]; I_{K1}, inward rectifier potassium current[76]; I_{Kp}, plateau potassium current[77,78]; $I_{Na,b}$, sodium background current; $I_{Ca,b}$, calcium background current; I_{NaK}, sodium-potassium pump current; $I_{NaCa,ss}$ sodium-calcium exchange current in the restricted space; I_{NaCa}, sodium-calcium exchange current outside the restricted space; $I_{p(Ca)}$ calcium pump in the sarcolemma[79]; I_{up}, calcium uptake from the myoplasm to network sarcoplasmic reticulum (NSR)[80]; I_{rel}, calcium release from junctional sarcoplasmic reticulum[81]; I_{leak}, calcium leakage from NSR to myoplasm; I_{tr}, calcium translocation from NSR to JSR[82]; JSR, junctional sarcoplasmic reticulum. Details can be found at http://rudylab.wustl.edu, where the model code is also provided.

Inactivation can then be stabilized by a transition from IF to an intermediate inactivated state IM_1, which reflects participation of the C-terminus,[30] and channels that have been slowly inactivated reside in IM_2. Closed-state inactivation has been included by movement from C_3 and C_2 into the inactivated tier (IC_3 and IC_2) to correctly simulate channel availability.[9]

I_{Na} is strongly dependent on APD and the diastolic interval, the time between repolarization of one action potential and the initiation of the next. These properties make I_{Na} highly rate dependent. Following the initial upstroke, channels continually transition to stable inactivated states IM_1 and IM_2 for the duration of the action potential. The number of channels that remain in these states between beats determines channel availability for the subsequent action potential. At slow rates, there is practically no accumulation of channels in IM_1 and IM_2 (see Fig. 30-3B). Because V_m is depolarized for a greater percentage of the time at fast rate, more channels transition to IM_1 and IM_2 with less time to recover. At a pacing cycle length of 300 ms, 20% of channels remain in these unavailable states between beats, and I_{Na} magnitude is noticeably reduced (see Fig. 30-3C). This reduced depolarizing current results in a lower peak V_m, which affects the activation of other channels that are important determinants of APD, such as I_{CaL}, I_{Kr}, and I_{Ks}.[13] I_{Na} magnitude also affects the rate of action potential upstroke, dV_m/dt_{max}, which in turn affects the velocity of action potential propagation.[15] Therefore, the model predicts slowing of conduction at fast pacing rates compared to slow rates, as observed experimentally.[31]

L-type Calcium Current

The ventricular action potential's primary role is to signal contraction. Signal transduction is achieved by entry of Ca^{2+} ions through L-type calcium channels, which induces release of large intracellular Ca^{2+} stores from the sarcoplasmic reticulum (SR) to further increase intracellular Ca^{2+} concentration, $[Ca^{2+}]_i$. Functional L-type channels are composed from a minimum of four subunits. The primary subunit α_1 contains the pore, voltage sensor, and gates and is tightly bound—in functional channels—to three accessory subunits α_2/δ and β. The α subunit of the ventricular L-type channel (α_{1C}) is encoded by $Ca_V1.2$, which produces a protein with four domains (DI-DIV) each with six transmembrane spanning segments (S1-S6), similar to

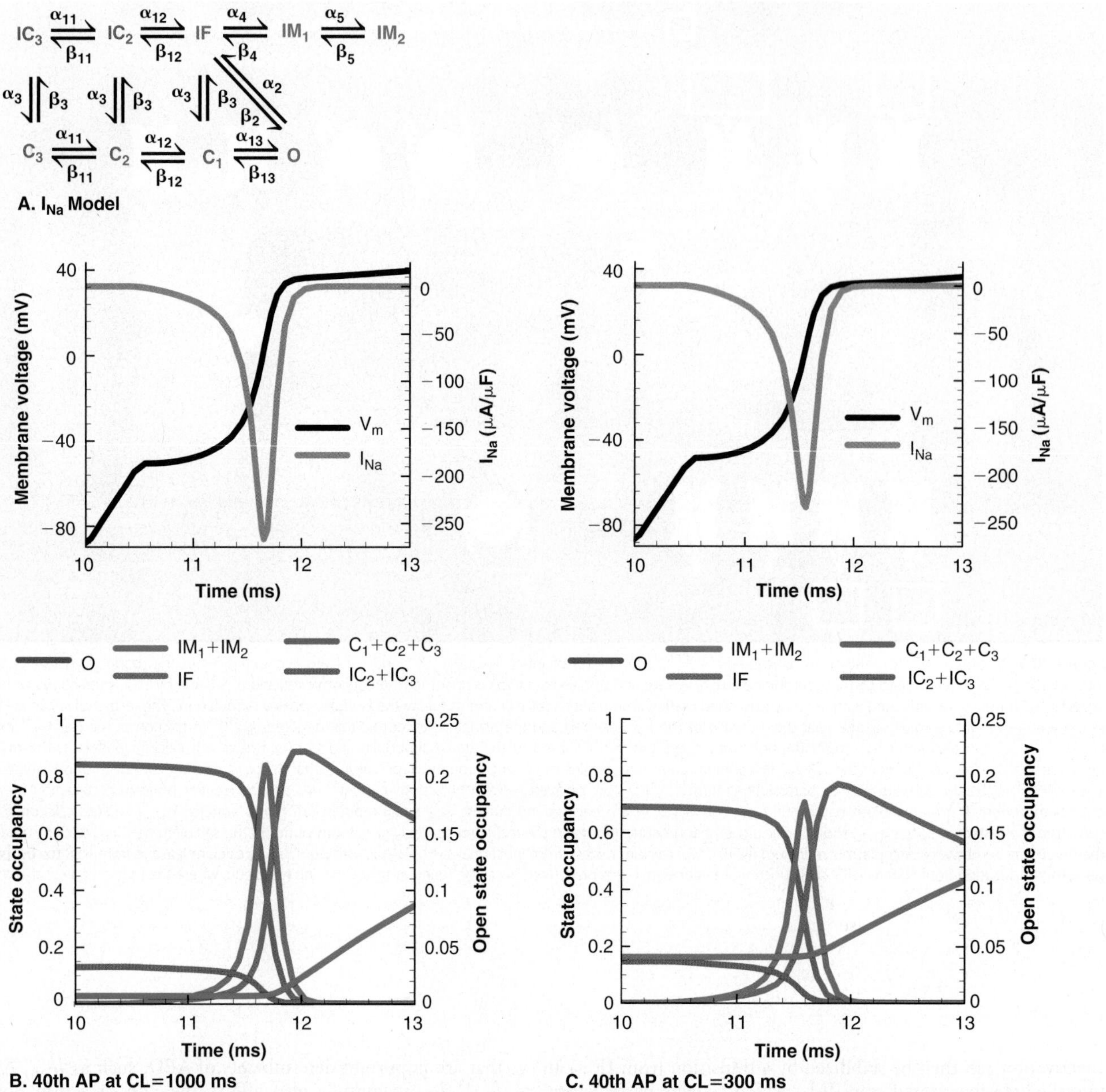

Figure 30-3 Kinetic transitions of sodium channels during the action potential (AP) at slow and fast rate. **A,** Markov model of the sodium channel.[9] States are color coded according to their type: closed-inactivated (I_C, *gray*), fast-inactivated (I_F, *purple*), intermediate *(slower)* inactivated (I_{M1}, I_{M2}, *green*), closed (C, *blue*), open (O, *red*). **B,** fast sodium current (I_{Na}), transmembrane potential (V_m), and channel state occupancies during the first 3 ms of the 40th action potential at slow rate, cycle length (CL) = 1000 ms. The channel state occupancies during this time period *(bottom)* show a rapid transition out of the closed states into the open state (rapid activation). The time course of fast inactivation after channel opening determines peak $I_{Na} = -270$ μA/μF. While V_m remains at depolarized potentials, channels enter the intermediate (slower) inactivated states. At slow rate, few channels are inactivated at the initiation of the AP. C. I_{Na}, V_m, and channel state occupancies during the first 3 ms of the 40th AP at fast rate, CL = 300 ms. Accumulation of channels in the intermediate inactivated states *(green)* at fast rate results in reduction of I_{Na} during the upstroke and consequently a slower dV_m/dt_{max}. (Modified from reference 13. Rudy Y, Silva JR: Computational biology in the study of cardiac ion channels and cell electrophysiology. Q Rev Biophys 39:57-116, 2006.)

Na$_V$1.5. A membrane-penetrating stretch between S5 and S6 (P-loop) encodes the channel pore, and positive charges on S4 are thought to confer voltage dependence of activation (see Bodi and colleagues[32] for a review).

The α_2 subunit, which resides entirely on the extracellular side, is linked intracellularly to α_1 through interaction with the δ subunit that has a single transmembrane-spanning domain. The most probable role for the α_2/δ complex is to facilitate proper membrane insertion.[32] The third subunit, β, is contained entirely on the intracellular face of the channel and interacts with a stretch of amino acids in the linker between domains I and II, the α-interaction domain. The I-II linker also contains an endoplasmic reticulum (ER) retention signal, which is blocked by interaction with the β subunit, suggesting a role in channel trafficking. The I-II linker has also been implicated in channel inactivation, and this might explain why the β-subunit has also been linked to I_{CaL} inactivation. The β subunit contains a phosphorylation site for PKA, which confers interaction with the β-adrenergic signaling cascade.[32]

In addition to β-adrenergic regulation, I_{CaL} is also regulated by changes in $[Ca^{2+}]_i$. The two primary regulators of this interaction are calmodulin and the calcium/calmodulin-dependent protein kinase II (CaMKII), both of which sense Ca^{2+} and interact with the C-terminus of the α_1 subunit. CaMKII activation causes downstream I_{CaL} facilitation (longer and more frequent openings),[33,34] through interaction with calmodulin and the α_{1C} and β subunits.[35]

Recent ventricular myocyte models have included CaMKII as a regulator of I_{CaL} among other processes, and they have demonstrated CaMKII involvement in alternans generation and in maintaining a positive relationship between force and frequency.[5,36,37] A Timothy syndrome (LQT8)[38] mutation that affects I_{CaL} has also been linked to a defect in CaMKII regulation of the α_{1C} subunit. This mutation, G406R, resides on the cytoplasmic side of S6 in DI and is near S409, which is thought to be a serine that is targeted by CaMKII for phosphorylation. Recordings of current from rabbit ventricular myocytes carrying a homologous mutation indicate that the mutation results in an abundance of current that seems to result from overphosphorylation of α_{1C} by CaMKII.[33] The implication of a role for the CaMKII pathway in Timothy syndrome further supports its involvement in regulation of ventricular electrophysiology.

I_{CaL} can be inactivated due to changes in V_m (VDI) as revealed by experiments where the charge carrier is $[Ba^{2+}]$,[39] and this process has been linked to binding of the I-II linker[40] to a region near the pore. The downstream consequence of the I-II linker motion is facilitation of an inactivating conformational change in the channel pore.[41,42] In addition to VDI, calcium channels can also be inactivated via a calmodulin-mediated response to changes in Ca^{2+} (CDI) in a restricted subspace, $[Ca^{2+}]_{ss}$, which is a small region of the cell containing the interface of the I_{CaL} channel and the ryanodine receptor (RyR), the SR calcium-release channel responsible for I_{Rel}, (see Fig. 30-2). Calmodulin is activated via Ca^{2+} binding to four distinct sites on the molecule, which enhance its sensitivity to changes in $[Ca^{2+}]_{ss}$[43] (multiple binding sites result in a steeper slope of activation in response to Ca^{2+}). Once calmodulin is activated, it can reduce I_{CaL} by accelerating the rate of channel inactivation caused by I-II linker–mediated occlusion of the pore.[40] Because the presence of Ca^{2+} has also been linked to a predisposition of the pore to the inactivated state, CDI has often been modeled with two processes. The first, more rapid process depends on the rate of ions traveling through the pore, and the second process depends directly on the Ca^{2+} concentration near the intracellular face of the channel ($[Ca^{2+}]_{ss}$).[5,44]

The magnitude of the current is affected by the concentration difference between the extracellular space and the local area near the intracellular face of the channel (the restricted subspace), in addition to channel conductance and expression. Whereas for most channels this relationship can be described by the Nernst equation (see Fig. 30-1), the vast difference in concentrations across the cell membrane ($[Ca^{2+}]_o$ = 2.0 mM, $[Ca^{2+}]_{ss} = 10^{-4}$ to 10^{-3} mM) and the channel permeability to Na^+ and K^+ has led to application of the more rigorous Goldman-Hodgkin-Katz equation for describing the driving force for current through the channel.[4] Faber and Ruby have proposed that Ca^{2+} ions near the pore dehydrate the region, disallowing Na^+ and K^+ fluxes, which led to the use of a simpler equation that only accounts for Ca^{2+} permeation.[45]

The model presented here[14,46] (Fig. 30-4A) explicitly represents the activation of each of the four protein domains, with each closed state corresponding to a permutation of subunit activation (i.e., C_0 represents channels where all the voltage sensors in the four domains are in the resting position, C_1 is where one has been activated and three are resting, and so forth). Once a channel nears the open conformation (at least 3 voltage sensors are activated, C_3 or O), channels can begin transitioning into the voltage-inactivated states. These states were hypothesized based on the two components of voltage-dependent inactivation observed in native guinea pig currents.[39] Voltage-dependent inactivated states can be thought of as representing inactivation by the I-II linker. CDI in the model is assumed to be independent of channel activation and VDI (as in previous models).[4,47] Thus, this model does not reflect the proposal of a common inactivation pathway mediated by the I-II linker. Still, the CDI states (lower tier in Fig. 30-4A) can be thought of as representing channels that have gone through accelerated inactivation facilitated by activated calmodulin binding to α_{1C}.

Once I_{Na} has successfully raised the membrane potential to −40 mV, I_{CaL} activates and contributes additional depolarizing current to the action potential upstroke. This initial spike in Ca^{2+} entry results in a large amount of Ca^{2+} release from the SR, which leads to rapid reduction in I_{CaL} magnitude (see Fig. 30-4B) via calmodulin-mediated CDI. As the action potential continues, $[Ca^{2+}]_i$ decreases because of Ca^{2+} uptake through the sarcoplasmic Ca^{2+}-ATPase (SERCA) into the network SR. Consequently, continued maintenance of I_{CaL} inactivation is a result of VDI, which recovers as the action potential repolarizes. As can be seen in the state diagrams at cycle lengths of 300 and 1000 ms (see Fig. 30-4B and 4C), during action potential repolarization, channels transition from VDI to closed states. However, if the repolarization slope of V_m (dV_m/dt) is too shallow, then channels can move from VDI to the open state and cause a secondary depolarization (early afterdepolarization).[48] Shallow slopes of repolarization are often caused by reduction in repolarizing currents such as I_{Kr} and I_{Ks}.

Rapid Delayed Rectifier Potassium Current

In large mammals, I_{Kr} is the primary repolarizing current, a role that is highlighted by the severity of long QT syndrome mutations that affect it (LQT2) compared to those that affect I_{Ks} (LQT1).[1] Patients taking drugs that reduce I_{Kr} are also predisposed to arrhythmia (drug-induced LQT).[49] In contrast to I_{Na} and I_{CaL}, functional homomeric channels are formed by four α-subunits (HERG), each containing six transmembrane-spanning domains (S1-S6). In expression systems, HERG has been shown to interact with minK-related peptide (MiRP1), a single transmembrane-spanning domain protein that affects channel gating.[50] MiRP1 expression is detected in atrial and Purkinje cells, but expression in ventricle is negligible. HERG is also able to interact with minK (aka KCNE1),[51,52] which is a critical part of the I_{Ks} channel structure. However, the physiologic role of HERG and minK interaction is still unclear.

As is typical for potassium channels, I_{Kr} activation is a consequence of the movement of S4 in response to change in V_m. Voltage-dependent inactivation is caused by conformational changes in the outer mouth of the channel that mechanistically resemble C-type inactivation in *Shaker* channels.[53] While it is plausible that charges in S4 could be involved in the voltage dependence of inactivation, mutation of these charges does not affect the amount of gating charge transfer during inactivation.[54] An alternative possibility is that voltage dependence is conferred

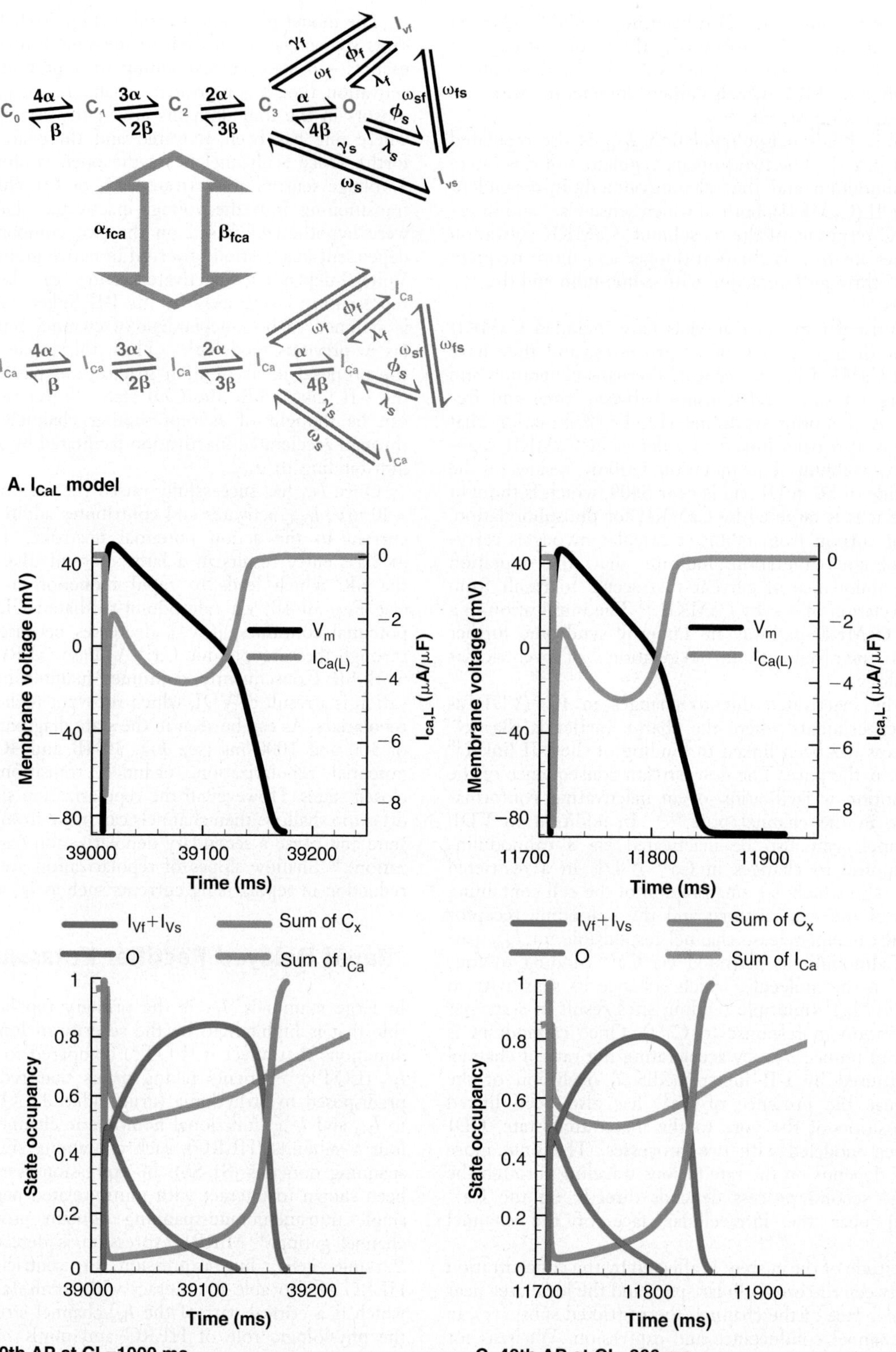

Figure 30-4 Kinetic transitions of L-type calcium channels (I_{CaL}) during the action potential (AP) at slow and fast rate. **A**, Markov model of the L-type calcium channel.[14,46] States are color coded according to their type: closed, C *(blue)*; open, O *(red)*; voltage-inactivated I_{Vf}, I_{Vs} *(green)*; Ca^{2+}-inactivated, I_{Ca} *(purple)*. **B**, I_{CaL}, V_m, and channel state occupancies of the 40th AP at slow rate, cycle length (CL) = 1000 ms. The channel state occupancies show that after rapid activation into the open state *(red)*, channels transition quickly into Ca^{2+}-dependent inactivated states *(purple)*. As the $[Ca^{2+}]_i$ transient decreases during the course of the AP, so does the level of Ca^{2+}-dependent inactivation (CDI) *(purple)*. As CDI diminishes, transmembrane potential (V_m)-dependent inactivation (VDI) *(green)* is required for I_{CaL} to remain inactivated until channels deactivate at repolarized potentials at the end of the AP (*blue*, channels transitioning back to the closed state). **C**, I_{CaL}, V_m, and channel state occupancies of the 40th AP at fast rate, CL = 300 ms. As can be seen by the similarity of the state occupancies and the I_{CaL} current trace to those at slow rate, adaptation of I_{CaL} does not play a significant role in AP duration rate-dependent adaptation in the guinea pig.

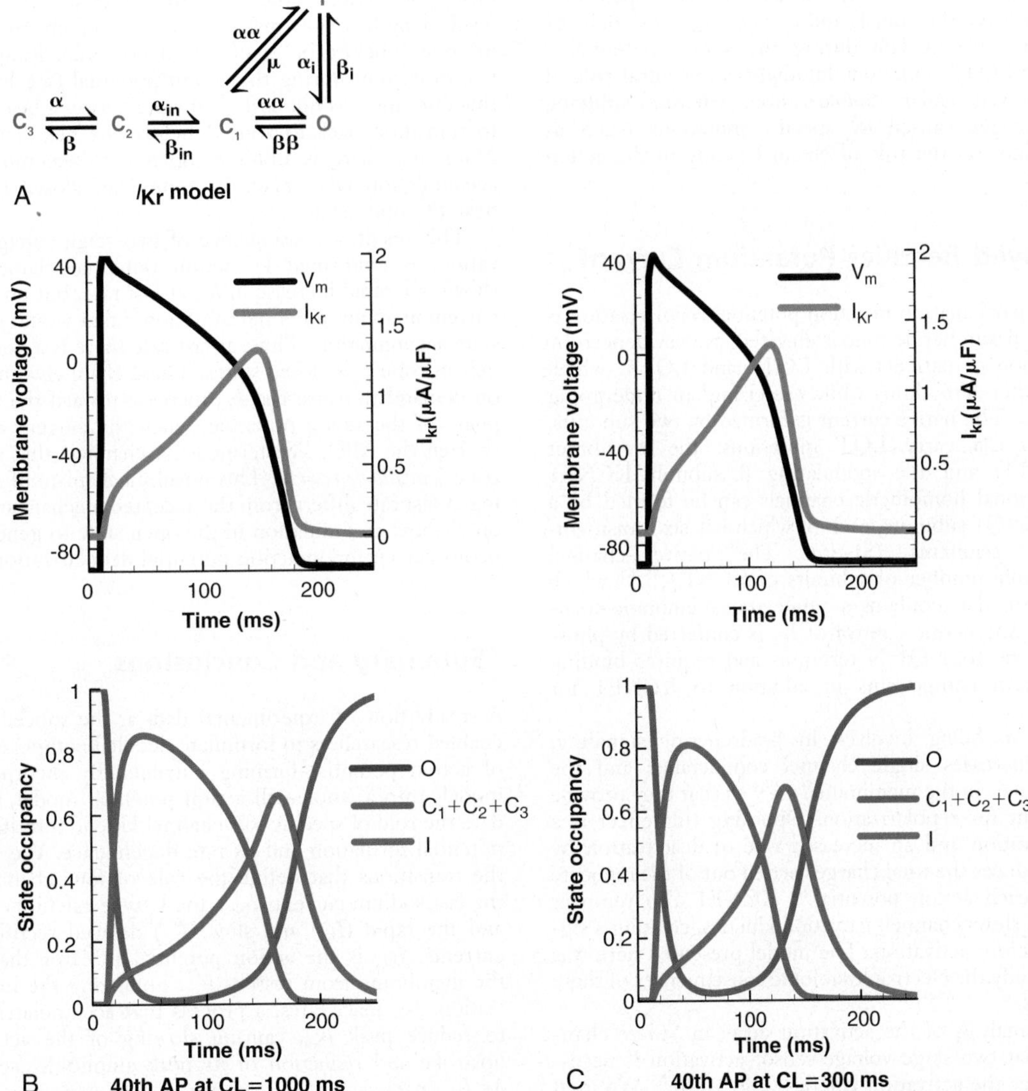

Figure 30-5 Kinetic transitions of rapid delayed rectifier potassium current (I_{Kr}) channels during the action potential (AP) at slow and fast rate. **A,** Markov model of the I_{Kr} channel.[10,55] States are color coded according to their type: closed, C *(blue)*; inactivated, I *(purple)*; open, O *(red)*. **B,** I_{Kr}, transmembrane potential (V_m), and channel state occupancies during the 40th AP at slow rate, cycle length (CL) = 1000 ms. Even though I_{Kr} activates nearly instantaneously, few channels move into the open state because of rapid inactivation. Then, as V_m decreases, channels begin to recover from inactivation, generating a pronounced peak of open-state occupancy and peak current during the late phase of the AP. **C,** I_{Kr}, V_m, and channel state occupancies during the 40th AP at fast rate, CL = 300 ms. Surprisingly, peak I_{Kr} is not changed significantly at fast rate. Examination of the state occupancies *(bottom)* reveals that conditions at AP initiation are identical at fast and slow rates, preventing any current accumulation. However, faster increase of I_{Kr} at fast rate during the AP contributes to shortening of the AP duration. (Modified from Rudy Y, Silva JR: Computational biology in the study of cardiac ion channels and cell electrophysiology. Q Rev Biophys 39:57-116, 2006.)

by the P-helix (positions 614-621 of the NH_2-terminal half of the P-loop).[54]

I_{Kr} activation is modeled using cooperative transitions,[10] and inactivation occurs preferentially from the open state (Fig. 30-5A).[10,55] Some inactivation can also occur from the closed state nearest to the open state (C_1), as demonstrated by single channel recordings.[56] During most of the action potential, the balance between I_{Kr} activation and inactivation favors inactivation (see Fig. 30-5B and C), preventing the development of a large current. As V_m repolarizes and reaches levels where significant channel recovery from inactivation occurs, open-state occupancy rises to a maximum and I_{Kr} intensifies, reaching a peak late during the action potential (see Fig. 30-5B and C). Consequently, I_{Kr} participates mostly late during the action potential, where it can significantly influence repolarization due to the delicate balance between inward and outward currents at this stage. Because voltage dependence of recovery is much stronger than time dependence during the action potential, peak I_{Kr} is similar at slow and fast rates (compare Fig. 30-5B and C), making I_{Kr} secondary to I_{Ks} in underlying rate-dependent adaptation of APD (shortening of APD at fast rate) in guinea pig ventricular myocytes.

An LQT2 mutation to HERG, R56Q, illustrates the role of the timing of I_{Kr} deactivation.[57] The mutation increases the rate of I_{Kr} deactivation dramatically, which reduces open-state occupancy of recovered channels and prevents I_{Kr} from delivering repolarizing current late during the action potential.[10] The severity of LQT2 mutations highlights the central role of I_{Kr} in human ventricular repolarization, whereas studying the kinetic changes caused by specific mutations (such as R56Q) sheds light on the role of channel gating in the action potential.

Slow Delayed Rectifier Potassium Current

In humans, I_{Ks} participation in action potential repolarization is increased when β-adrenergic tone is elevated, as is evidenced by the predisposition of patients with LQT1 and LQT5, which affect I_{Ks}, to suffer arrhythmia while exercising[1] or undergoing emotional stress. The native current is formed by two subunits, both of which can carry LQT mutations: the α subunit KCNQ1 (LQT1) and the modulating β subunit KCNE1 (LQT5). Functional homomeric channels can be formed by a tetramer of KCNQ1 subunits, each of which has six transmembrane-spanning segments (S1-S6). The native channel includes a variable number of subunits of KCNE1,[58-61] which is a short protein that contains a single transmembrane-spanning α-helix. β-Adrenergic control of I_{Ks} is conferred by phosphorylation of the KCNQ1 N terminus and requires binding of several protein components in addition to KCNE1 for transduction.

In addition to being involved in β-adrenergic signaling, KCNE1 also increases single channel conductance and the number of channels in the membrane[59,62,63] so that they provide sufficient current for repolarization. Opposing this effect is a slowing of activation and an increased rate of deactivation by KCNE1 that reduces the total charge carried out of the myocyte by I_{Ks} during each action potential.[64] KCNE1 also removes inactivation and slows channel-activation kinetics, creating a significant delay before activation. The model presented here was formulated to study the electrophysiologic consequences of these opposing effects.

Biophysical analysis of the activation delay in *Shaker* channels suggests that two-stage voltage-sensor activation is necessary to reproduce the activation kinetics (Fig. 30-6).[65] We used a similar model for I_{Ks}, where each closed state represents a possible combination of voltage-sensor positions.[55] We added a cooperative, voltage-independent transition before opening so as to reproduce steady-state activation measurements.[66] Application of phosphatidylinositol-4,5-bisphosphate (PIP_2) to excised patches containing I_{Ks} channels strongly affects their open probability, but it does not change the voltage-dependent properties of the channel,[67] indicating that PIP_2 interaction is with this voltage-independent transition (observed in *Shaker* K^+ channels as well).[68] A second open state, also included in the model, is evident when the channel is probed with rubidium and is responsible for two exponential components of deactivation observed experimentally.[69] The complete I_{Ks} model is shown in Figure 30-7A; details can be found in Silva and Rudy's paper.[55]

Closed states in the model are divided into two zones: Zone 2 (green) contains channels where at least one subunit still has to make a first slower transition to the intermediate state R_2, and zone 1 (blue) contains channels with voltage sensors that only need to make more rapid second transitions into the activated state A. As shown in Figure 30-7B, at the slow rate (cycle length = 1000 ms), 60% of I_{Ks} channels reside in zone 2 before action potential depolarization and must make a slow transition into zone 1 before opening. At this rate, only 40% of channels reside in zone 1 before onset of action potential. In contrast, at the fast rate (cycle length = 300 ms), nearly 75% of channels accumulate in zone 1 before onset of action potential, leading to a rapid rise in current during the action potential (see Fig. 30-7C). At this rate, there is not sufficient time between beats for channels to transition back to zone 2 before the next action potential. Note that there is minimal open-state accumulation; rather, accumulation takes place in zone 1 of closed states that are near the open state.

This result, a consequence of two-stage voltage-sensor activation, is confirmed by action potential clamp experiments showing a rapid increase in I_{Ks} at fast rate, but no instantaneous current at action potential initiation[70] that would indicate open-state accumulation. Thus, at fast rate there is a buildup of channels in zone 1 of closed states. These channels can open quickly on demand to cause fast I_{Ks} increase toward the repolarization phase of the action potential, when the current can effectively shorten the APD. We termed the channels that accumulate in zone 1 *available reserve*. This novel mechanism of APD shortening at fast rate differs from the accepted mechanism, which relies on channel accumulation in the open state to generate instantaneous current upon action potential depolarization.

Summary and Conclusions

A steady flow of experimental data at the subcellular level has enabled researchers to formulate detailed computational models of action potential–forming currents. By incorporating these models into a whole-cell action potential model, we can elucidate the role of specific ion-channel kinetic transitions in action potential formation and its rate dependence. We have describe the transitions that define the role of four channels in detail: the fast sodium current (I_{Na}), the L-type calcium current (I_{CaL}), and the rapid (I_{Kr}) and slow (I_{Ks}) delayed rectifier potassium currents. I_{Na} is the action potential initiator that depolarizes the membrane from resting V_m. Following the initial depolarization, I_{Na} inactivates, a process that accumulates at fast rates to reduce peak I_{Na}, causing slowing of the action potential upstroke and reduction of its peak amplitude (see Fig. 30-3). As I_{Na} inactivates, I_{CaL} activates and sustains the action potential plateau.

During this phase, I_{CaL} is determined by two inactivation processes, CDI and VDI. Initially the presence of Ca^{2+} (CDI) is required to maintain inactivation, but as time progresses elevated V_m (VDI) is responsible for $I_{Ca,L}$ inactivation (see Fig. 30-4). In the guinea pig, I_{CaL} does not contribute to action potential rate dependence, but its interaction with the transient outward current, I_{to}, in higher species can affect APD significantly.[5,71] The end of the action potential occurs when the outward K^+ fluxes, I_{Kr} and I_{Ks}, overcome inward I_{CaL} and return V_m to the resting state. I_{Kr} increases during the action potential plateau as V_m repolarizes and channels recover from inactivation (see Fig. 30-5). In contrast, I_{Ks} activates slowly and peaks toward the end of the action potential as channels continually move out of the deep closed states (see Fig. 30-7). Although there is no change in I_{Kr} at fast rate compared to slow rate (see Fig. 30-5), I_{Ks} increases significantly at fast rate due to accumulation of channels in closed states near the open states, from which they can open rapidly (see Fig. 30-7). In higher species, the population of I_{Ks} channels in these states is likely to be increased in the presence of β-adrenergic tone, a situation that occurs even at basal levels of activity.

Experiments showing long-QT syndrome mutation effects on various action potential currents have been especially helpful in demonstrating the role of specific channel transitions in the

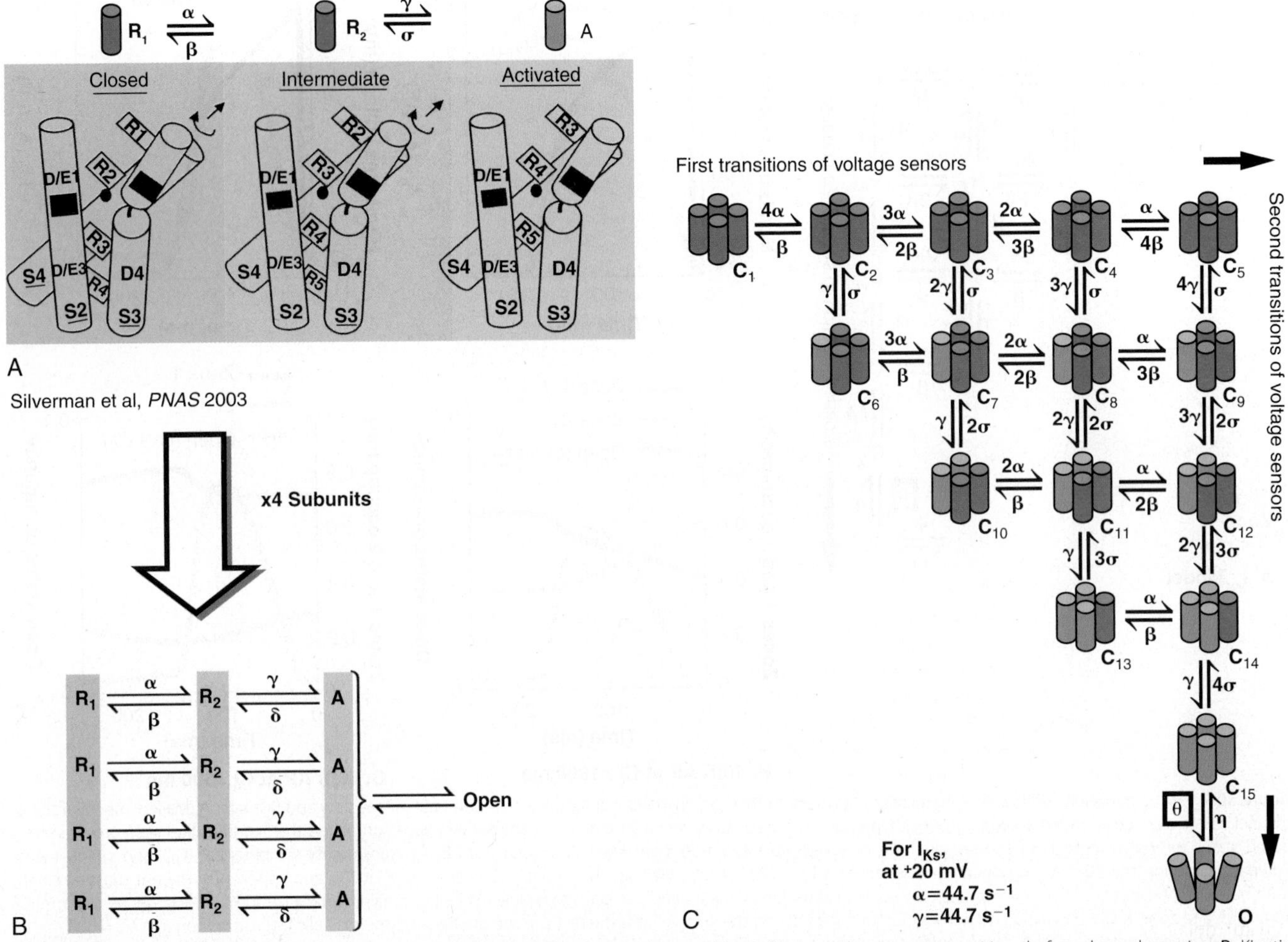

Figure 30-6 Conformational changes of potassium channels during activation. **A,** Structural basis for two voltage-sensor transitions before channel opening. **B,** Kinetic representation of the two voltage-sensor transitions in **A**. All four α subunits that form the channel undergo a first transition from a resting state (R_1) to an intermediate state (R_2) and a second transition from R_2 to an activated state (A). Once all voltage sensors are in the activated state, the channel can open. **C,** Total number of combinations of voltage-sensor positions in the four subunits is 15 and can be represented by 15 closed states before channel opening. *Blue, red,* and *green* indicate a voltage sensor in position R_1, R_2, or A, respectively. (**A** is based on data from ether-a-go-go and *Shaker* K^+ channels and is adapted from Silverman WR, Roux B, Papazian DM: Structural basis of two-stage voltage-dependent activation in K^+ channels. Proc Natl Acad Sci U S A 100:2935-2940, 2003. **C** is from Rudy Y: Modelling and imaging cardiac repolarization abnormalities. J Intern Med 259:91-106, 2006.)

action potential. As examples, we have described the modeling of two mutations, LQT2 mutation R56Q and LQT3 mutation Δ-KPQ. The R56Q model demonstrates that the timing of I_{Kr} deactivating transitions during the action potential plays a role in determining APD. Δ-KPQ shows the importance of voltage-dependent maintenance of I_{Na} inactivation in maintaining action potential stability. That these mutations result in long QT-syndrome in patients, a consequence of the APD prolongation predicted by the models, further supports the suggested role of the simulated channel transitions in shaping the action potential.

Genetic mutations can also affect electrophysiology by altering the response of an affected channel to intracellular signaling molecules. An example of such a mutation is the LQT1 mutation G589D, which disrupts KCNQ1 phosphorylation by PKA. A recent modeling study showed that this loss of repolarizing current coupled with PKA enhancement of I_{CaL} can result in triggered activity.[72] The Timothy syndrome mutation G406R, described earlier, causes an augmentation of I_{CaL} due to over-phosphorylation by CaMKII, a clear indication of CaMKII participation in action potential regulation. The existence of these mutations that predispose patients to arrhythmia and are directly linked to intracellular regulation of the channels points to a critical role for these molecules (CaMKII and PKA) in the formation of the action potential.

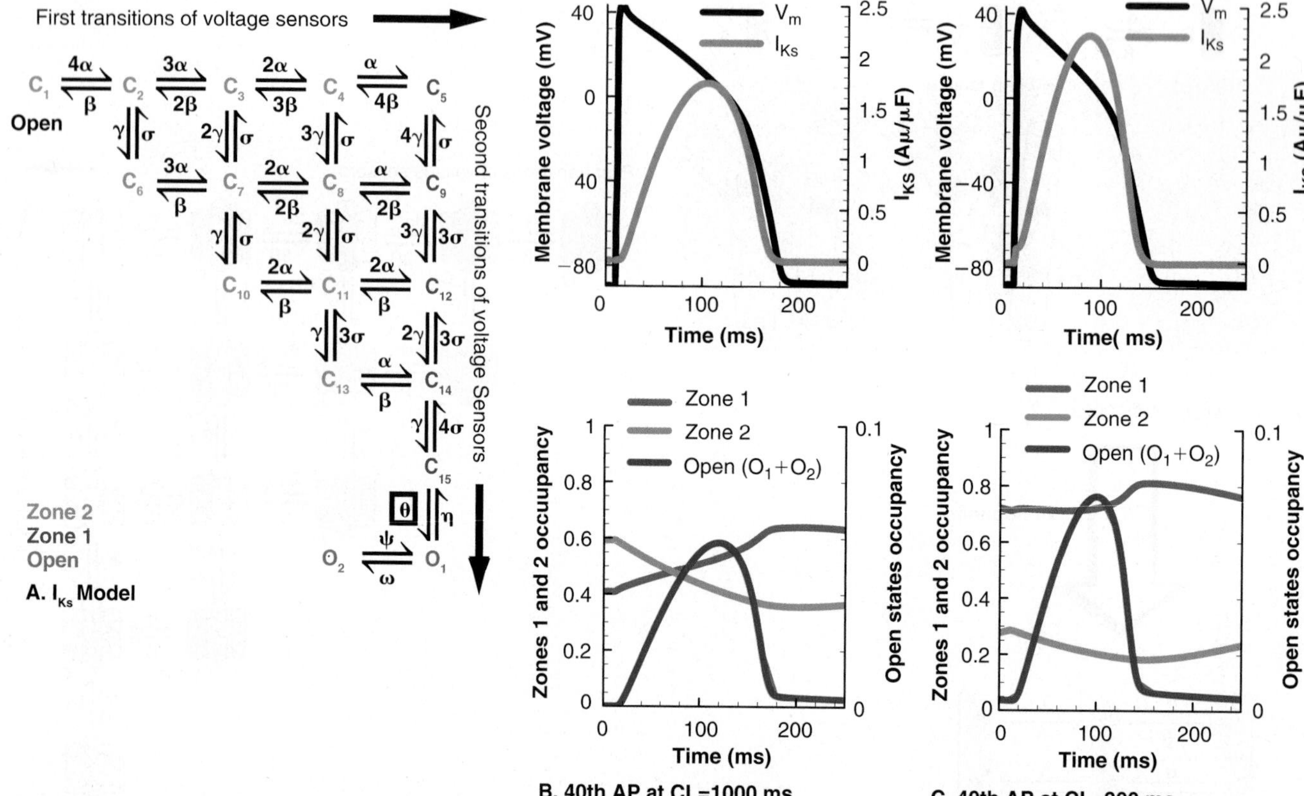

Figure 30-7 Kinetic transitions of slow delayed rectifier potassium current (I_{Ks}) channels during the action potential (AP) at slow and fast rate. **A,** Markov model of the I_{Ks} channel.[55] States are color coded according to their type: zone 2, closed states for which not all voltage sensors have completed the first transition *(light green)*; zone 1, closed states for which all four voltage sensors have completed the first transition *(blue)*; and open *(red)*. **B,** I_{Ks}, transmembrane potential (V_m), and channel state occupancies during the 40th AP at slow rate, cycle length (CL) = 1000 ms. I_{Ks} rises slowly, resulting in peak current at the end of the AP, where it most efficiently contributes to repolarization. Only 40% of channels reside in zone 1 at AP onset and can activate rapidly. While V_m remains depolarized, channels continue to transition from zone 2 to zone 1. **C,** I_{Ks}, V_m, and channel state occupancies during the 40th AP at fast rate, CL = 300 ms. Because the diastolic interval is shorter at CL = 300 ms, V_m stays at depolarized potentials for a greater percentage of time, which causes channel accumulation in zone 1 of closed states. At AP onset, 75% of channels reside in zone 1, facilitating rapid transitions to the open state. This results in increased I_{Ks} late during the AP and shortening of the AP duration. Note that the mechanism for I_{Ks} increase is accumulation in closed states near the open state (zone 1) as opposed to open state accumulation. The accumulation in zone 1 creates a reserve of channels that are ready to open rapidly, on demand, to generate a greater repolarizing current; we call this pool of channels *available reserve*. (Modified from Rudy Y, Silva JR: Computational biology in the study of cardiac ion channels and cell electrophysiology. Q Rev Biophys 39:57-116, 2006.)

References

1. Shimizu W, Aiba T, Antzelevitch C: Specific therapy based on the genotype and cellular mechanism in inherited cardiac arrhythmias. Long QT syndrome and Brugada syndrome. Curr Pharm Des 11:1561-1572, 2005.
2. Hille B: Ion Channels of Excitable Membranes, 3rd ed. Sunderland, MA: Sinauer, 2001.
3. Hodgkin AL, Huxley AF: A quantitative description of membrane current and its application to conduction and excitation in nerve. J Physiol 117:500-544, 1952.
4. Luo CH, Rudy Y: A dynamic model of the cardiac ventricular action potential. I. Simulations of ionic currents and concentration changes. Circ Res 74:1071-1096, 1994.
5. Hund TJ, Rudy Y: Rate dependence and regulation of action potential and calcium transient in a canine cardiac ventricular cell model. Circulation 110:3168-3174, 2004.
6. Viswanathan PC, Rudy Y: Cellular arrhythmogenic effects of congenital and acquired long-QT syndrome in the heterogeneous myocardium. Circulation 101:1192-1198, 2000.
7. Viswanathan PC, Rudy Y: Pause induced early afterdepolarizations in the long QT syndrome: A simulation study. Cardiovasc Res 42:530-542, 1999.
8. Gima K, Rudy Y: Ionic current basis of electrocardiographic waveforms: a model study. Circ Res 90:889-896, 2002.
9. Clancy CE, Rudy Y: Na^+ channel mutation that causes both Brugada and long-QT syndrome phenotypes: A simulation study of mechanism. Circulation 105:1208-1213, 2002.
10. Clancy CE, Rudy Y: Cellular consequences of HERG mutations in the long QT syndrome: Precursors to sudden cardiac death. Cardiovasc Res 50:301-313, 2001.
11. Clancy CE, Rudy Y: Linking a genetic defect to its cellular phenotype in a cardiac arrhythmia. Nature 400:566-569, 1999.
12. Schwartz PJ: The congenital long QT syndromes from genotype to phenotype: Clinical implications. J Intern Med 259:39-47, 2006.
13. Rudy Y, Silva JR: Computational biology in the study of cardiac ion channels and cell electrophysiology. Q Rev Biophys 39: 57-116, 2006.
14. Faber GM, Silva J, Livshitz L, Rudy Y: Kinetic properties of the cardiac L-type Ca^{2+} channel and its role in myocyte electrophysiology: A theoretical investigation. Biophys J 92:1522-1543, 2007.
15. Kléber AG, Rudy Y: Basic mechanisms of cardiac impulse propagation and associated arrhythmias. Physiol Rev 84:431-488, 2004.

16. Shaw RM, Rudy Y: Ionic mechanisms of propagation in cardiac tissue. Roles of the sodium and L-type calcium currents during reduced excitability and decreased gap junction coupling. Circ Res 81:727-741, 1997.
17. Dumaine R, Wang Q, Keating MT, et al: Multiple mechanisms of Na^+ channel–linked long-QT syndrome. Circ Res 78:916-924, 1996.
18. George AL Jr, Varkony TA, Drabkin HA, et al: Assignment of the human heart tetrodotoxin-resistant voltage-gated Na^+ channel alpha-subunit gene (SCN5A) to band 3p21. Cytogenet Cell Genet 68:67-70, 1995.
19. Grant AO: Molecular biology of sodium channels and their role in cardiac arrhythmias. Am J Med 110:296-305, 2001.
20. Hartmann HA, Tiedeman AA, Chen SF, et al: Effects of III-IV linker mutations on human heart Na^+ channel inactivation gating. Circ Res 75:114-122, 1994.
21. Moorman JR, Kirsch GE, Brown AM, Joho RH: Changes in sodium channel gating produced by point mutations in a cytoplasmic linker. Science 250:688-691, 1990.
22. McPhee JC, Ragsdale DS, Scheuer T, Catterall WA: A critical role for the S4-S5 intracellular loop in domain IV of the sodium channel alpha-subunit in fast inactivation. J Biol Chem 273:1121-1129, 1998.
23. McPhee JC, Ragsdale DS, Scheuer T, Catterall WA: A critical role for transmembrane segment IVS6 of the sodium channel alpha subunit in fast inactivation. J Biol Chem 270:12025-12034, 1995.
24. McPhee JC, Ragsdale DS, Scheuer T, Catterall WA: A mutation in segment IVS6 disrupts fast inactivation of sodium channels. Proc Natl Acad Sci U S A 91:12346-12350, 1994.
25. Balser JR: Structure and function of the cardiac sodium channels. Cardiovasc Res 42:327-338, 1999.
26. Motoike HK, Liu H, Glaaser IW, et al: The Na^+ channel inactivation gate is a molecular complex: A novel role of the COOH-terminal domain. J Gen Physiol 123:155-165, 2004.
27. Chanda B, Asamoah OK, Bezanilla F: Coupling interactions between voltage sensors of the sodium channel as revealed by site-specific measurements. J Gen Physiol 123:217-230, 2004.
28. Armstrong CM, Bezanilla F: Inactivation of the sodium channel. II. Gating current experiments. J Gen Physiol 70:567-590, 1977.
29. Bezanilla F, Armstrong CM: Inactivation of the sodium channel. I. Sodium current experiments. J Gen Physiol 70:549-566, 1977.
30. Veldkamp MW, Viswanathan PC, Bezzina C, et al: Two distinct congenital arrhythmias evoked by a multidysfunctional Na^+ channel. Circ Res 86:E91-E97, 2000.
31. Restivo M, Yin H, Caref EB, et al: Reentrant arrhythmias in the subacute infarction period. The proarrhythmic effect of flecainide acetate on functional reentrant circuits. Circulation 91:1236-1246, 1995.
32. Bodi I, Mikala G, Koch SE, et al: The L-type calcium channel in the heart: The beat goes on. J Clin Invest 115:3306-3317, 2005.
33. Erxleben C, Liao Y, Gentile S, et al: Cyclosporin and Timothy syndrome increase mode 2 gating of $Ca_V1.2$ calcium channels through aberrant phosphorylation of S6 helices. Proc Natl Acad Sci U S A 103:3932-3937, 2006.
34. Dzhura I, Wu Y, Colbran RJ, et al: Calmodulin kinase determines calcium-dependent facilitation of L-type calcium channels. Nat Cell Biol 2:173-177, 2000.
35. Pitt GS: Calmodulin and CaMKII as molecular switches for cardiac ion channels. Cardiovasc Res 73:641-647, 2007.
36. Livshitz LM, Rudy Y: Regulation of Ca^{2+} and electrical alternans in cardiac myocytes: Role of CAMKII and repolarizing currents. Am J Physiol Heart Circ Physiol 292:H2854-H2866, 2007.
37. Hund TJ, Rudy Y: A Role for calcium/calmodulin-dependent protein kinase II in cardiac disease and arrhythmia. In Kass RS, Clancy CE (eds): Basis and Treatment of Cardiac Arrhythmias (Handbook of Experimental Pharmacology). Heidelberg, Springer-Verlag, 2006, pp 201-220.
38. Splawski I, Timothy KW, Decher N, et al: Severe arrhythmia disorder caused by cardiac L-type calcium channel mutations. Proc Natl Acad Sci U S A 102:8089-8096, 2005.
39. Findlay I: Voltage-dependent inactivation of L-type Ca^{2+} currents in guinea-pig ventricular myocytes. J Physiol 545:389-397, 2002.
40. Kim J, Ghosh S, Nunziato DA, Pitt GS: Identification of the components controlling inactivation of voltage-gated Ca^{2+} channels. Neuron 41:745-754, 2004.
41. Babich O, Reeves J, Shirokov R: Block of $Ca_V1.2$ channels by Gd^{3+} reveals preopening transitions in the selectivity filter. J Gen Physiol 129:461-475, 2007.
42. Babich O, Matveev V, Harris AL, Shirokov R: Ca^{2+}-dependent inactivation of $Ca_V1.2$ channels prevents Gd^{3+} block: does Ca^{2+} block the pore of inactivated channels? J Gen Physiol 129:477-483, 2007.
43. Kandel ER, Schwartz JH, Jessell TM: Principles of Neural Science, 4th ed. New York, McGraw-Hill, 2000.
44. Hirano Y, Hiraoka M: Ca^{2+} entry-dependent inactivation of L-type Ca current: A novel formulation for cardiac action potential models. Biophys J 84:696-708, 2003.
45. Rice JJ, Jafri MS, Winslow RL: Modeling gain and gradedness of Ca^{2+} release in the functional unit of the cardiac diadic space. Biophys J 77:1871-1884, 1999.
46. Faber GM, Rudy Y: Calsequestrin mutation and catecholaminergic polymorphic ventricular tachycardia: A simulation study of cellular mechanism. Cardiovasc Res 75:79-88, 2007.
47. Faber GM, Rudy Y: Action potential and contractility changes in $[Na^+]_i$ overloaded cardiac myocytes: A simulation study. Biophys J 78:2392-2404, 2000.
48. Luo CH, Rudy Y: A dynamic model of the cardiac ventricular action potential. II. Afterdepolarizations, triggered activity, and potentiation. Circ Res 74:1097-1113, 1994.
49. Roden DM: Drug-induced prolongation of the QT interval. N Engl J Med 350:1013-1022, 2004.
50. Abbott GW, Sesti F, Splawski I, et al: MiRP1 forms I_{Kr} potassium channels with HERG and is associated with cardiac arrhythmia. Cell 97:175-187, 1999.
51. Ohyama H, Kajita H, Omori K, et al: Inhibition of cardiac delayed rectifier K^+ currents by an antisense oligodeoxynucleotide against I_{sK} (minK) and over-expression of I_{sK} mutant D77N in neonatal mouse hearts. Pflugers Arch 442:329-335, 2001.
52. Yang T, Kupershmidt S, Roden DM: Anti-minK antisense decreases the amplitude of the rapidly activating cardiac delayed rectifier K^+ current. Circ Res 77:1246-1253, 1995.
53. Smith PL, Baukrowitz T, Yellen G: The inward rectification mechanism of the HERG cardiac potassium channel. Nature 379:833-836, 1996.
54. Zhang M, Liu J, Tseng GN: Gating charges in the activation and inactivation processes of the HERG channel. J Gen Physiol 124:703-718, 2004.
55. Silva J, Rudy Y: Subunit interaction determines I_{Ks} participation in cardiac repolarization and repolarization reserve. Circulation 112:1384-1391, 2005.
56. Kiehn J, Lacerda AE, Brown AM: Pathways of HERG inactivation. Am J Physiol 277:H199-H210, 1999.
57. Chen J, Zou A, Splawski I, et al: Long QT syndrome–associated mutations in the Per-Arnt-Sim (PAS) domain of HERG potassium channels accelerate channel deactivation. J Biol Chem 274:10113-10118, 1999.
58. Wang W, Xia J, Kass RS: MinK-K_VLQT1 fusion proteins, evidence for multiple stoichiometries of the assembled I_{sK} channel. J Biol Chem 273:34069-34074, 1998.
59. Sesti F, Goldstein SA: Single-channel characteristics of wild-type I_{Ks} channels and channels formed with two minK mutants that cause long QT syndrome. J Gen Physiol 112:651-663, 1998.
60. Chen H, Kim LA, Rajan S, Xu S, Goldstein SA: Charybdotoxin binding in the I_{Ks} pore demonstrates two minK subunits in each channel complex. Neuron 40:15-23, 2003.
61. Cui J, Kline RP, Pennefather P, Cohen IS: Gating of I_{sK} expressed in Xenopus oocytes depends on the amount of mRNA injected. J Gen Physiol 104:87-105, 1994.
62. Pusch M: Increase of the single-channel conductance of K_VLQT1 potassium channels induced by the association with minK. Pflugers Arch 437:172-174, 1998.
63. Yang Y, Sigworth FJ: Single-channel properties of I_{Ks} potassium channels. J Gen Physiol 112:665-678, 1998.
64. Tristani-Firouzi M, Sanguinetti MC: Voltage-dependent inactivation of the human K^+ channel K_VLQT1 is eliminated by association with minimal K^+ channel (minK) subunits. J Physiol 510(Pt 1): 37-45, 1998.
65. Zagotta WN, Hoshi T, Dittman J, Aldrich RW: Shaker potassium channel gating. II: Transitions in the activation pathway. J Gen Physiol 103:279-319, 1994.

66. Lu Z, Kamiya K, Opthof T, et al: Density and kinetics of I_{Kr} and I_{Ks} in guinea pig and rabbit ventricular myocytes explain different efficacy of I_{Ks} blockade at high heart rate in guinea pig and rabbit: Implications for arrhythmogenesis in humans. Circulation 104:951-956, 2001.
67. Loussouarn G, Park KH, Bellocq C, et al: Phosphatidylinositol-4,5-bisphosphate, PIP2, controls KCNQ1/KCNE1 voltage-gated potassium channels: A functional homology between voltage-gated and inward rectifier K^+ channels. Embo J 22:5412-5421, 2003.
68. Koren G, Liman ER, Logothetis DE, et al: Gating mechanism of a cloned potassium channel expressed in frog oocytes and mammalian cells. Neuron 4:39-51, 1990.
69. Pusch M, Bertorello L, Conti F: Gating and flickery block differentially affected by rubidium in homomeric KCNQ1 and heteromeric KCNQ1/KCNE1 potassium channels. Biophys J 78:211-226, 2000.
70. Rocchetti M, Besana A, Gurrola GB, et al: Rate dependency of delayed rectifier currents during the guinea-pig ventricular action potential. J Physiol 534:721-732, 2001.
71. Greenstein JL, Wu R, Po S, et al: Role of the calcium-independent transient outward current I_{to1} in shaping action potential morphology and duration. Circ Res 87:1026-1033, 2000.
72. Saucerman JJ, Healy SN, Belik ME, et al: Proarrhythmic consequences of a KCNQ1 AKAP-binding domain mutation: Computational models of whole cells and heterogeneous tissue. Circ Res 95:1216-1224, 2004.
73. Balke CW, Rose WC, Marban E, Wier WG: Macroscopic and unitary properties of physiological ion flux through T-type Ca^{2+} channels in guinea-pig heart cells. J Physiol 456:247-265, 1992.
74. Droogmans G, Nilius B: Kinetic properties of the cardiac T-type calcium channel in the guinea-pig. J Physiol 419:627-650, 1989.
75. Vassort G, Alvarez J: Cardiac T-type calcium current: Pharmacology and roles in cardiac tissues. J Cardiovasc Electrophysiol 5:376-393, 1994.
76. Kurachi Y: Voltage-dependent activation of the inward-rectifier potassium channel in the ventricular cell membrane of guinea-pig heart. J Physiol 366:365-385, 1985.
77. Yue DT, Marban E: A novel cardiac potassium channel that is active and conductive at depolarized potentials. Pflugers Arch 413:127-133, 1988.
78. Backx PH, Marban E: Background potassium current active during the plateau of the action potential in guinea pig ventricular myocytes. Circ Res 72:890-900, 1993.
79. Caroni P, Zurini M, Clark A, Carafoli E: Further characterization and reconstitution of the purified Ca^{2+}-pumping ATPase of heart sarcolemma. J Biol Chem 258:7305-7310, 1983.
80. Tada M, Shigekawa M, Kadoma M, Nimura Y: Uptake of calcium by sarcoplasmic reticulum and its regulation and functional consequences. In Sperelakis N (ed): Physiology and pathophysiology of the heart, 2nd ed. Boston, Kluwer Academic Publishers, 1989, pp 267-290.
81. Meissner G: Sarcoplasmic reticulum ion channels. In Zipes DP, Jalife J (eds): Cardiac electrophysiology: From cell to bedside, 2nd ed. Philadelphia, Saunders, 1995, pp 51-58.
82. Yue DT, Burkhoff D, Franz MR, et al: Postextrasystolic potentiation of the isolated canine left ventricle. Relationship to mechanical restitution. Circ Res 56:340-350, 1985.
83. Zeng J, Laurita KR, Rosenbaum DS, Rudy Y: Two components of the delayed rectifier K^+ current in ventricular myocytes of the guinea pig type. Theoretical formulation and their role in repolarization. Circ Res 77:140-152, 1995.
84. Viswanathan PC, Shaw RM, Rudy Y: Effects of I_{Kr} and I_{Ks} heterogeneity on action potential duration and its rate dependence: A simulation study. Circulation 99:2466-2474, 1999.
85. Luo CH, Rudy Y: A model of the ventricular cardiac action potential. Depolarization, repolarization, and their interaction. Circ Res 68:1501-1526, 1991.
86. Hund TJ, Kucera JP, Otani NF, Rudy Y: Ionic charge conservation and long-term steady state in the Luo-Rudy dynamic cell model. Biophys J 81:3324-3331, 2001.
87. Rudy Y: The cardiac ventricular action potential. In Page E, Fozzard HA, Solaro RJ (eds): The Cardiovascular System. vol 1: The Heart. New York, Oxford University Press, 2002, pp 531-547.
88. Silverman WR, Roux B, Papazian DM: Structural basis of two-stage voltage-dependent activation in K^+ channels. Proc Natl Acad Sci U S A 100:2935-2940, 2003.
89. Rudy Y: Modelling and imaging cardiac repolarization abnormalities. J Intern Med 259:91-106, 2006.

Theory of Reentry 31

Alexander V. Panfilov

CHAPTER OUTLINE

The largest cause of death in the Western world is sudden cardiac death caused by cardiac arrhythmias.[1] Cardiac arrhythmias are driven by abnormal sources of excitation, which in most cases occur as a result of phenomena of circus movement and reentry. The idea of reentrant circulation has been known in cardiology since the beginning of the 19th century. This is how it was described by G. R. Mines in 1913[2]: "If a closed circuit of muscle is provided of considerably greater length than the wave of excitation, it is possible to start a wave in this circuit which will continue to propagate itself round and round the circuit for an indefinite number of times."

Figure 31-1A illustrates such circular movement in a ring of cardiac tissue: The direction of rotation is shown by an arrow, and the refractory period is depicted by various levels of blue. Rotation is possible if the ring is longer than the refractory tail of the wave or, in other words, if the wavelength $\Lambda = v \times R$ is longer than the ring size (here v is the wave velocity and R is the refractory period). Let us consider similar rotation around a circular obstacle in a two-dimensional (2D) sheet of cardiac cells (see Fig. 31-1B to D). In this case, a tip of the wave (point O) will follow the boundary of the obstacle; the rest of the wave will propagate upward (in accordance with Huygens' principle). As a result we will obtain a formation of a spiral wave rotating around an obstacle. Such 2D rotation was studied in 1946 by Wiener and Rosenblueth[3] in application to atrial arrhythmias. Two years later, Selfridge[4] demonstrated that such spiral wave rotation is also possible without any obstacles. His main idea was that the wave can circle around its own refractory tail, which serves as a functional obstacle for wave propagation. Hence spiral waves rotating in tissue without obstacles are often called *functional reentry*, and rotation around an obstacle is usually referred to as *anatomic reentry*. The rotation period in anatomic reentry (see Fig. 31-1B to D) is determined by the obstacle size and may be long for a large obstacle. The rotation period of functional reentry is short and usually close to the refractory period of the tissue; in this case, the front of the wave closely follows its refractory tail.

Rotation of spiral waves causes periodic excitation of cardiac cells and cardiac arrhythmias. Spiral waves in many aspects are similar to other, more usual excitation sources, such as the firing of ectopic foci or the excitations generated by an external stimulation electrode. Figure 31-2 presents typical wave patterns of a spiral wave rotating at the center of a tissue and a pattern produced by periodic stimulation of the same tissue. Although we can see some differences in overall excitation patterns (see Fig. 31-2A and B), such differences disappear if only a part of the tissue is available for observation (compare Fig. 31-2C and D). However, there is a major difference between a point source and a spiral: The point source can be eliminated by ablation of the firing region, whereas similar ablation at the spiral core does not remove the spiral, as the wave continues rotation around the ablated region.

Spiral waves have been studied extensively using various theoretical approaches. Some results of these theoretical studies were confirmed in experimental and clinical research. Some of them are still awaiting verification. In this chapter I review some aspects of the theory of reentry, in particular the properties and dynamics of stable spiral waves, including spiral wave meandering and its relation to excitability, drift of spiral waves in heterogeneous tissue, mechanisms of initiation of spiral waves, and some ideas on eliminating spiral waves using overdrive pacing and resonant drift. Where possible, I illustrate mechanisms of these effects using a simple geometric approach similar to the kinematic theory of spiral waves.[5] Several important theoretical results on spiral waves are beyond the scope of this chapter. In particular, I do not cover the phenomenon of spiral breakup,[6] which is considered now one of possible mechanisms of ventricular fibrillation, the restitution hypothesis of ventricular fibrillation.[7-11] In addition to previously published results, the chapter contains a few new simulations made for illustrative purposes using the FitzHugh-Nagumo model for cardiac tissue. Technical details of these simulations are given at the end of the chapter.

Geometry of the Spiral Wave

A spiral wave acquires its spiral shape at some distance from the center of rotation. It is possible to show that in an idealized isotropic tissue, the shape of the wave far from the center will be just an Archimedean spiral, which in the polar coordinates (r,f) is given by $r \cong \lambda\phi/2\pi$, where $\lambda = v(T)T$ is the wavelength, T is the rotation period, and $v(T)$ is the velocity of wave propagation at this period. For anisotropic tissue, this expression should be modified to account for different wave velocities and wavelengths in different directions. It turns out that for cardiac tissue this asymptotic shape cannot be normally seen in experiments. This is because the size of the heart is small and comparable with the wavelength of the spiral. More important are the structure and dynamics of a spiral wave closer to its center, the core of the spiral wave.

Unfortunately, we still do not know all factors determining the core of a spiral wave. It is currently impossible to predict the

This work was supported by a grant from the Netherlands Organization for Scientific Research (NWO grants 620061351 and 814.02.014).

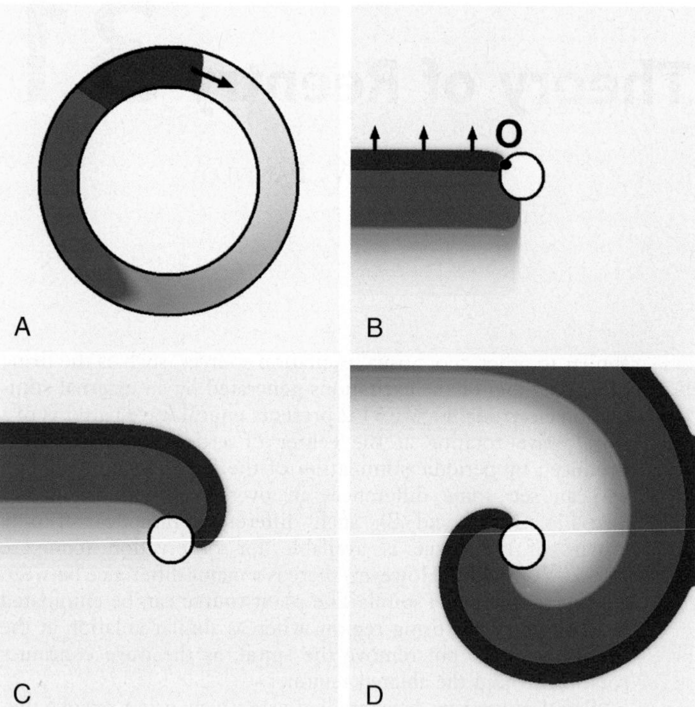

Figure 31-1 Schematic representation of reentry in one dimension (**A**) and two dimensions (**B to D**). *Arrows* show direction of wave propagation. *Dark blue* represents the excited state of the tissue, and different levels of *light blue* represent different extents of recovery. For further explanation, see text.

shape or size of the core or the dynamics of spiral wave rotation from the measurable characteristics of cardiac tissue, such as shape of the action potential, conduction velocity, and restitution. However, we can get some insights from the following simple geometric consideration.

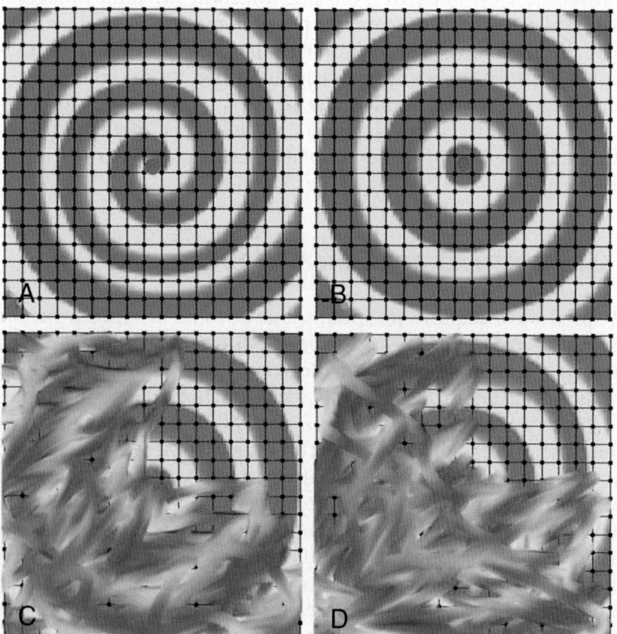

Figure 31-2 Overall (**A, B**) and regional wave patterns generated by a spiral wave (**A, D**) and induced by periodic stimulation at the center (**B, C**) with a period close to the period of the spiral wave.

Let us consider evolution of a straight wave break from Figure 31-3A into a spiral wave. Note that points A and O of the wave break are in quite different conditions. Due to symmetry, the local current supporting wave propagation at and around point A is directed upward, but at point O the current diverges in many directions, reducing the local current density. As a result, the velocity of wave propagation at point A will be higher than at point O, and, as was shown theoretically,[12] in extreme cases of low excitability, the wave at tip O will not be able to extend itself further in cardiac tissue. Instead it will shrink and finally disappear at the left boundary (see Fig. 31-3B).[12] Thus, at very low excitability we cannot obtain a spiral wave in two dimensions, although one-dimensional propagation of the wave would still be possible.[12] At some intermediate excitability, the wave tip will be able to extend to the right, but its velocity will be small and the wave will make a rotation only along a circle with a large radius. If motion along this circle takes longer than the refractory period of the tissue, we obtain a spiral wave with a circular core, with no interactions between the wave front and the wave tail, as shown in Figure 31-3C.

Now let us consider the opposite case: cardiac tissue with high excitability and long refractory period. In this case the wave tip will be able to extend easily to all nonrefractory regions adjacent to point O. As a result, the wave tip will follow its own refractory tail (see Fig. 31-3D), thus moving along a straight line until the tissue to the left from the wave break recovers. After that, it will be able to make another turn (see Fig. 31-3D), and, continuing in this fashion, we will get a rotation along a linear core with a period close to the refractory period of the medium.

It turns out that between the cases of low and high excitability there exist regimes of complex front-and-tail interactions causing meandering of spiral waves.[13] The meandering patterns are studied in various models of cardiac tissue, and it is established that with increasing excitability they change from epicycloidal rotation (inward petals) to hypocycloidal rotation (outward petals).[13,14,15] Figure 31-3E shows the overall patterns of spiral

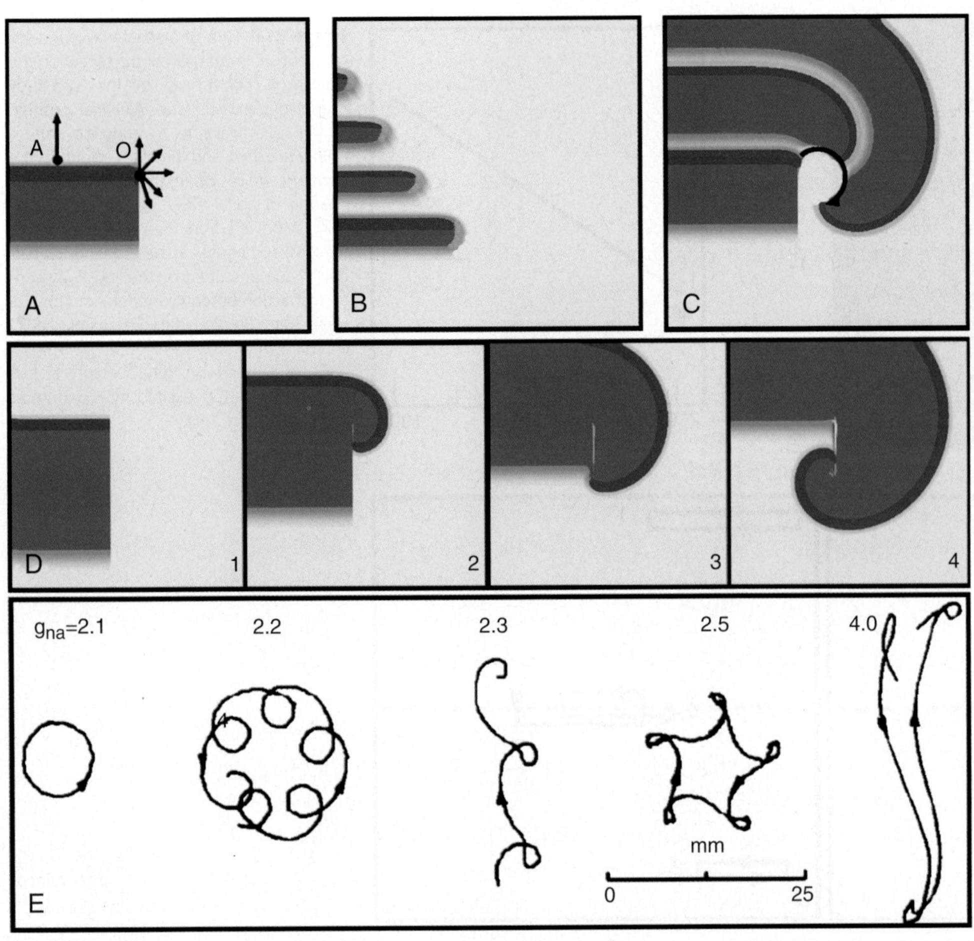

Figure 31-3 Evolution of a wave break and the core of a spiral wave at different levels of tissue excitability. **A,** Initial wave break. **B,** Shrinking of a wave break at low excitability.[12] **C,** Circular core at intermediate excitability. **D,** Linear core at high excitability. The pictures were obtained from integration of equation 3 with a = 0.235 for B, a = 0.21 for C, and a = 0.13 for D. Further details on the model can be found at the end of the chapter. **E,** Different types of meandering of spiral waves, depending on cardiac tissue excitability. Tip trajectories are at different g_{Na}. Excitability is increased by increasing the maximal conductance of the sodium current g_{Na}. Simulation is performed in the Beeler-Reuter model. (From Efimov I, Krinsky VI, Jalife J: Dynamics of rotating vortices in the Beeler-Reuter model of cardiac tissue. Chaos 5:513-526, 1995.)

wave dynamics at different levels of excitability obtained in the Beeler-Reuter model of cardiac tissue,[16] where the excitability was increased by increasing conductance of the sodium current. We see a successive transition from circular to inward meandering, then to outward meandering, and finally to the linear core, when the conductance of sodium current is increased.

Meandering patterns can be more complex than those shown in Figure 31-3E. For example, in hypermeandering regimes, the spiral wave tip undergoes complex chaotic displacement analogous to that of a Brownian particle.[14,17,18] One hypothesis relates different types of spiral wave dynamics to different arrhythmia types; monomorphic tachycardia is related to a rigid rotation of the spiral wave, and meandering or drift of spiral waves is related to polymorphic ventricular tachycardia.[19,20,21,22]

Spiral Waves in Heterogeneous Tissue

There are many types of heterogeneity in the heart. Properties of cardiac cells differ between the basal and apical regions; between endocardial, epicardial and midmyocardial regions[23,24,25]; between left and right ventricles[26]; and so on. The heterogeneity can be abrupt, stepwise,[27] or in the form of a gradient.[25] Heterogeneity is an important factor for initiation of spiral waves (see next section), as well as for dynamics of spiral wave rotation.

Effects of gradient heterogeneity on spirals were studied in FitzHugh Nagumo models[28,29] and later in the ionic Luo-Rudy model of cardiac cells[30]; in both types of model, heterogeneity induced drift of spiral waves. Figure 31-4A and B shows a typical example of such dynamics. The spiral wave was placed at the lower part of the tissue (see Fig. 31-4A), and the dynamics of its rotation was hypocycloidal meandering. In time, the average position of the tip gradually shifted to the direction shown by the white arrow. Drift occurred at some angle to the heterogeneity gradient, which in this figure was directed along the vertical axis. Let us decompose it into two components: the longitudinal component, along the direction of the gradient, and the transverse component, orthogonal to the gradient direction. Now let us consider how the components of drift depend on properties of both the spiral wave and the cardiac tissue.

In Figure 31-4A we increased parameter G_K along the vertical axis (from the bottom to the top of the medium). Increase in G_K also increases the period of spiral wave rotation. The direction of drift was upward, along the gradient of heterogeneity, and thus it increased the period of the spiral wave. This is further illustrated in Figure 31-4B, which depicts the change of the rotation period during its drift. It turns out that drift in the direction of longer period is a general result that has been demonstrated in various models of cardiac tissue and for different parameter gradients.[28,29,30] The transverse component of the drift depends on several factors. First, it obviously depends on the direction of spiral wave rotation. Indeed, if one were to observe the drift of the spiral in Figure 31-4A on a mirror placed at the right side of the medium, one would find that the rotation of the spiral wave changes from clockwise to

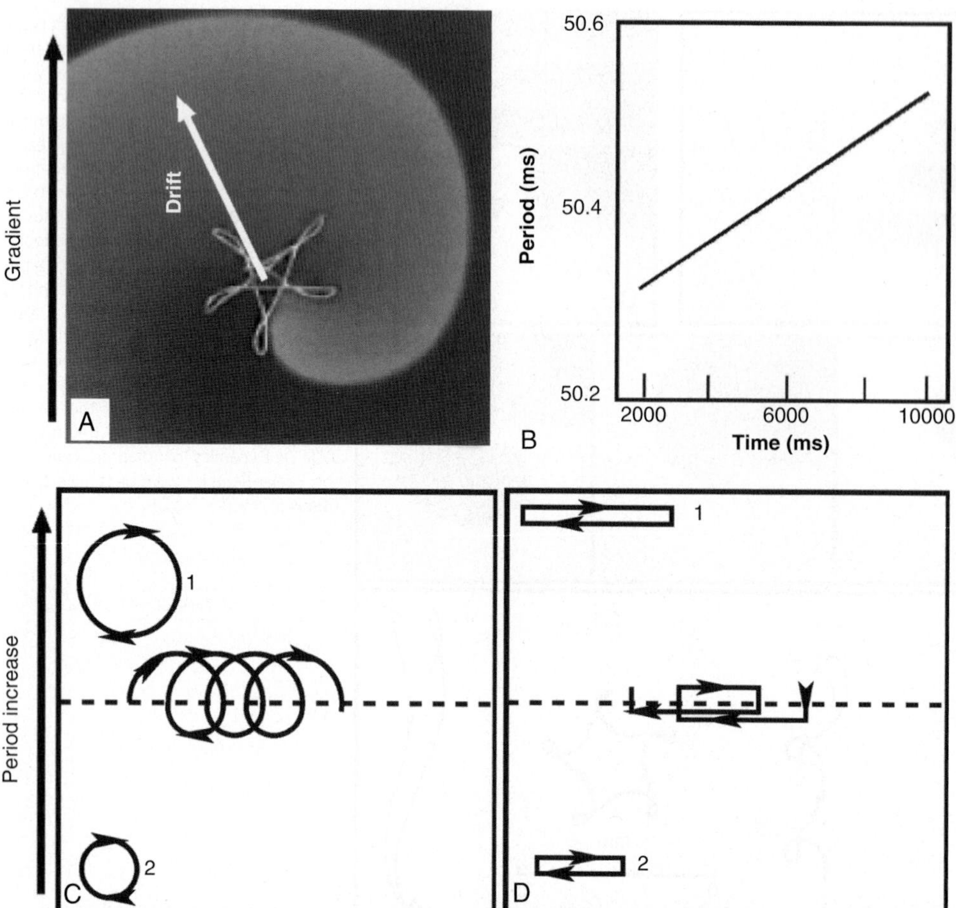

Figure 31-4 Drift of a spiral wave under a gradient of maximal conductance of the potassium current g_K in the Luo-Rudy model of cardiac tissue. **A,** Initial position of the spiral wave, its meandering pattern *(thin while line)*, and direction of drift in the medium *(thick white arrow)*. **B,** Average change of spiral wave period during the drift. (Modified from Ten Tusscher KHWJ, Panfilov A: Reentry in heterogeneous cardiac tissue described by the Luo-Rudy ventricular action potential model. Am J Physiol Heart Circ Physiol 284:H542-H548, 2003.) Mechanism of transverse drift of a spiral wave at a step-wise heterogeneity at low **(C)** and high **(D)** excitability. For further explanation, see text.

counterclockwise, and the direction of the transversal drift will also be opposite: The spiral will move toward the left boundary. (The direction of longitudinal drift, of course, will remain the same, along the gradient.) For the case of Figure 31-4A, this relation of the transverse and longitudinal drift with the rotation direction can be expressed by the following equation:

$$t = l \times w \qquad [1]$$

where t and l are unit vectors along the transverse and longitudinal drift components, respectively, and w is the unit vector of the angular velocity of the spiral wave.[28,30]

In addition to rotation direction, the transverse component is also determined by the excitability of the tissue. This could be understood from the following simple geometric consideration[29] for stepwise heterogeneity in a medium consisting of two layers (1 and 2 in Fig. 31-4C and D). If we assume that the spiral in layer 1 has a longer rotation period than the spiral in layer 2, then for tissue with low excitability, where the spiral wave has a circular core with no interactions between the wave front and wave tail (see Fig. 31-3C), the size of the core in medium 1 will be larger than in medium 2 (see Fig. 31-4C). Thus a spiral wave rotating at the boundary of this heterogeneity will spend approximately half its time in medium 1 rotating along a larger circle and half its time in medium 2 rotating around the smaller circle. As a result, the spiral will drift to the right.

If we project this result to the case of a heterogeneity gradient (see Fig. 31-4A) and represent it as a relation of longitudinal and transverse drifts to each other in the form of equation 1, we find that the transverse drift will be given as $t = -l \times w$, thus opposite to equation 1 and Figure 31-4A. Indeed if we compare the spirals in Figure 31-4C and Figure 31-4A, we find that the direction of the gradient of period (thus l) and the direction of spiral rotation (thus w) is the same in both, but the directions of the transverse drift are opposite. For the case of high excitability (e.g., linear core), a similar situation is depicted in Figure 31-4D. Here also medium 1 has a longer period of rotation, that is, a longer core. However, for high excitability, the core size is determined by the refractory period (see Fig. 31-3D), and thus medium 1 is assumed to have substantially longer refractoriness than medium 2.

As in Figure 31-4C, a spiral wave rotating at the boundary will spend part of its time in medium 1 and part of its time in medium 2, but the transition between the layers will be different. The wave will be able to exit from medium 2 to medium 1 only after medium 1 is recovered, and during that waiting time the wave tip will be traveling to the left. Similarly the wave from medium 1 has to travel to the right, waiting for the recovery of medium 2. Overall, because the recovery of medium 1 is longer, the wave on average will travel longer to the left than to the right, resulting in drift to the left.[31,29] Therefore, the transverse drift direction in this case coincides with that given by equation 1 and Figure 31-4A. The dependency of direction of the transverse drift on tissue excitability considered earlier was confirmed numerically in several models of cardiac tissue.[29,30]

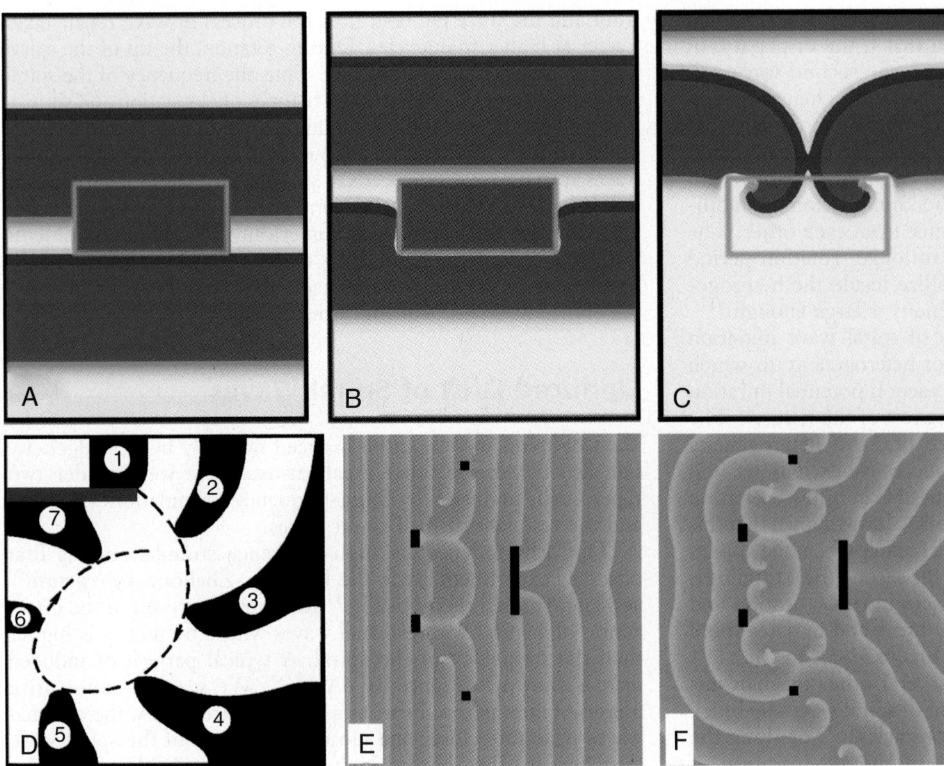

Figure 31-5 A to C, Generation of a spiral wave in heterogeneous cardiac tissue. The refractory period inside the *orange rectangle* is longer than in the rest of the tissue. The second wave breaks at the heterogeneity **(B)** and forms two counter-rotating spiral waves **(C)**. The pictures were obtained from integration of equation 3 with a = 0.195 to increase the refractory period in the orange rectangle. The value of ϵ for $e < 0.05$, $g = 1.2$ was decreased two-fold (ϵ (e,g) = 0.005 for $e < 0.05$, $g = 1.2$). **D,** Formation of spiral wave at a barrier. Numbers *1* to *7* show subsequent positions of the wave break. (From Panfilov AV, Pertsov AM: [Mechanism of spiral wave initiation in active media connected with critical curvature phenomenon.] Biofizika 27:886-888, 1982. Wave propagation around anatomic obstacles is shown at low frequency **(E)** and at high frequency **(F)**. (Modified from Agladze KI, Keener JP, Müller SC, Panfilov AV: Rotating spiral waves created by geometry. Science 264:1746-1748, 1994.)

The transverse drift direction is important for understanding interactions of spirals in heterogeneous tissue. If we consider a figure-of-eight reentry—that is, the reentry composed of two interconnected counter-rotating spirals—then the interaction of spiral waves in a gradient heterogeneity will be different for different regimes of the transverse drift.[28,29,30] As a result, the two spirals in a figure-of-eight reentry can diverge from each other and eventually form two separate spiral waves, or they can converge and even mutually annihilate in some cases.

As mentioned earlier, the longitudinal component of spiral wave drift does not depend on the direction of spiral wave rotation and is always directed to the region of longer rotation period. Although this effect is very robust and reproducible, we still do not know its mechanism. There is only a simplified one-dimensional theory for drift of reentry rotating on two electrically coupled heterogeneous cardiac fibers.[32] However, it remains unclear how this theory can be applied for the case of two-dimensional spiral waves. Equations for tip trajectory of drifting spiral waves can be derived phenomenologically[33] or by using the kinematic approach (see the review by Mikhailov and colleagues[5]).

Initiation of Spiral Waves

The mechanisms of spiral wave initiation are crucial for understanding the mechanisms of onset of reentrant cardiac arrhythmias. Two classic ways of initiating spiral waves are with the S1S2 stimulation protocol and as a result of the inherent heterogeneity of cardiac tissue with respect to refractoriness.

In the S1S2 mechanism, the spiral waves are induced by two stimuli, S1 and S2, applied at different locations, with the S2 stimulus timed during the local relatively refractory period.[3,34,19] The S2 stimulus initiates a wave that propagates in some directions and is blocked in other directions. As a result wave breaks occur that can evolve into two counter-rotating spiral waves. Such a mechanism has been demonstrated experimentally[37] and has been further studied theoretically in bidomain models of cardiac tissue and for the case of three-dimensional propagation.[35,36]

The S1S2 mechanisms do not necessarily require external electrical stimulation of the heart. It can occur, for example, as a result of early or late afterdepolatizations.[38] It has also been assumed that a similar mechanism might explain the mechanical induction of heart rhythm disturbances in commotio cordis, which occurs as a result of a critically timed mechanical impact. It was suggested that the impact acts as S2 (mechanical) stimulation, which triggers a spiral wave arrhythmia (see the review by Li and colleagues[39]).

Another classic mechanism of spiral wave initiation is the result of heterogeneity with respect to refractoriness, which was originally introduced by Krinsky in 1966 (Fig. 31-5A to C).[40] Assume that cardiac tissue with refractory period R_n contains a region with a prolonged refractory period R_h, (marked by the orange rectangle in Fig. 31-5A to C). Let us apply two stimuli with coupling interval T_s such that

$$R_n < T_s < R_h \qquad [2]$$

The second wave will not be able to penetrate into the heterogeneity R_h, as this region will not recover ($T_S < R_h$) and form two wave breaks as shown in Figure 31-5B. The wave breaks will follow the side boundary of the heterogeneity, then the upper boundary, and will enter the region of heterogeneity when the tissue there is recovered (see Fig. 31-5C). As a result, two spiral waves will be formed.

This mechanism of spiral wave initiation was further studied by Panfilov and Vasiev.[41] It was shown that if the dispersion of wave velocity is taken into consideration, the second wave will propagate slower and the wave break can enter the heterogeneity not only at the upper boundary but also at the side boundaries. It was also shown that the counter-rotating spiral waves that occur at the heterogeneity drift toward each other (in accordance with equation 1). This drift can result in either annihilation or stabilization of the spiral waves at some distance from each other. The spiral waves also drift in the direction of longer rotation period (see the previous section) and can stabilize inside the heterogeneous region if the size of the heterogeneity is large enough.[41]

More recently, similar mechanisms of spiral wave initiation were studied for a more general type of heterogeneity in which the heterogeneous region has a different action potential duration (APD) restitution curve compared to the rest of the tissue.[42] The interesting aspect here is that the size of APD heterogeneity depends on the time interval between successive excitations, and the heterogeneity may be completely invisible at a low excitation frequency but pronounced at high frequency. It was shown that this type of heterogeneity induces spiral wave reentry when one applies three stimuli (S1S2S3) instead of two. If the second (S2) stimulus is premature, it produces regional differences in repolarization and the next stimulus (S3) then creates wave break and initiates spiral waves in a way similar to that shown in Figure 31-5A to C.

In addition to those listed above, several other mechanisms were proposed that explain the initiation of spiral waves by block of wave propagation around anatomic obstacles[43,44] or along the barriers formed, for example, by lines of lateral separation of cells.[45] These mechanisms do not require any heterogeneity with respect to refractory period or even a carefully timed stimulus application.

Figure 31-5D shows a process of spiral wave formation at a barrier studied by Panfilov and Pertsov.[45] We see that at the end of the barrier (position 1) the wave tip cannot make an instantaneous rotation to follow the other barrier boundary. As a result, the wave tip detaches from the boundary and forms a spiral wave. This mechanism was confirmed in simulations using detailed ionic models for cardiac cells[46,47] and in experiments.[48,47] The formation of a spiral wave here requires the wave tip not to undergo a fast rotation at the end of the barrier, which, as shown in Figure 31-3B, occurs at low levels of excitability of the cardiac tissue. Theoretical and experimental studies[46,47] have confirmed that the initiation of spiral waves via this mechanism requires low excitability.

Spiral waves can be initiated also by high-frequency stimulation around small anatomic obstacles.[43,44] Under normal conditions, anatomic obstacles do not cause problems for wave propagation. Figure 31-5E shows the propagation of a wave-train around several anatomic obstacles at relatively low wave frequency. Here the waves temporarily split at the obstacles into two parts, which meet again at some distance behind the obstacle. However, if the frequency of the external forcing increases, the breaks approach each other at lower speed and the distance of their re-encounter behind the obstacle increases progressively.[49,43,44] At some high frequency of forcing, this results in the formation of substantially separated wave breaks, and when the external stimulation is stopped, these breaks form spiral waves (see Fig. 31-5F).[43,44]

It is possible to determine the qualitative conditions of stimulation frequency necessary to initiate spiral waves on this mechanism. As discussed earlier for Figure 31-3B and C, the velocity of break elongation, which is the process that repairs the waves propagating around obstacles, decreases with a decrease in tissue excitability. Increasing the frequency of stimulation is qualitatively equivalent to decreasing the excitability, due to interactions between the wave front and the wave tail, and thus the process of wave repair takes longer at higher frequencies. During rotation, the tip of the spiral wave does not elongate or shrink. Thus the frequency of the spiral wave approximately separates the regimes of elongation and shrinking of a wave tip and thus it should separate the repair and lack-of-repair regimes. It therefore follows that in order to obtain spiral waves at an obstacle, one needs to stimulate the tissue at a frequency that is higher than that of the spiral wave itself. This simple qualitative idea has been confirmed numerically[43,44] and in experiments using the Belousov-Zhabotinsky reaction.[44] The formation of a spiral wave at an anatomic obstacle in a slightly different setup was shown in experiments in cardiac tissue.[48,47]

Induced Drift of Spiral Waves

Drift of spiral waves can be induced not only by heterogeneity but also by several other mechanisms. Here we consider two types: drift induced by high-frequency stimulation of tissue and the resonant drift of spiral waves.

The drift induced by high-frequency stimulation was first observed experimentally in the Belousov-Zhabotinsky reaction[50] and later studied theoretically.[51] It occurs as a result of the interaction of a spiral with external waves whose frequency is higher than the frequency of the spiral. A typical pattern of induced drift is shown in Figure 31-6A to C. We see two consecutive phases of interaction. First, as seen in Figure 31-6A, the external waves penetrate closer and closer to the core of the spiral wave (just because they have a higher frequency). At this stage, the rotation of the spiral wave is unaffected and its location remains intact. During the second stage, the external waves penetrate all the way to the core of the spiral and directly interact with the spiral tip. Such an interaction induces drift of the tip away from the source of external stimulation (see Fig. 31-6B and C), and finally the spiral is eliminated at the boundary.

A detailed theoretical analysis of the induced drift performed by Ermakova and colleagues[51] shows that in addition to the drift shown in Figure 31-6A to C, there are other regimes of interaction of spiral waves with an external high-frequency source. For stimulation frequencies slightly higher than the frequency of the spiral, the velocity of the induced drift can be zero (synchronization), or even negative; that is, the tip of the spiral wave will not be pushed away, but will drift toward the external high frequency source. The induced spiral wave drift may be a mechanism whereby overdrive pacing eliminates functional reentrant sources in the heart. Further understanding of this phenomenon might improve the efficiency of this method.

Another type of induced spiral wave drift occurs as a result of periodic temporal modulation of the properties of tissue, the resonant drift. Figure 31-6D to F shows an example of such drift by Panfilov and colleagues.[52] Here the whole tissue is periodically stimulated by electrical subthreshold current, which does not result in initiation of new excitations but periodically alters the tissue properties. The frequency of such stimulation is synchronized with the frequency of the spiral wave via the ECG pattern. As a result, the spiral wave shifts to the right and eventually disappears at the boundary.

The mechanism of resonant drift can also be explained via a simple geometric consideration. Let us assume that a parameter P affects the excitability of cardiac tissue and for some value denoted by *1* the spiral wave has a larger core than for a parameter value denoted by *2* (Fig. 31-7A). If we start changing parameter P between these two values and we do it with the period of the spiral wave (see Fig. 31-7B), the spiral wave will undergo one half of the rotation along the larger circle *1* and the other half along the smaller circle *2*. As a result, the spiral wave will drift to the

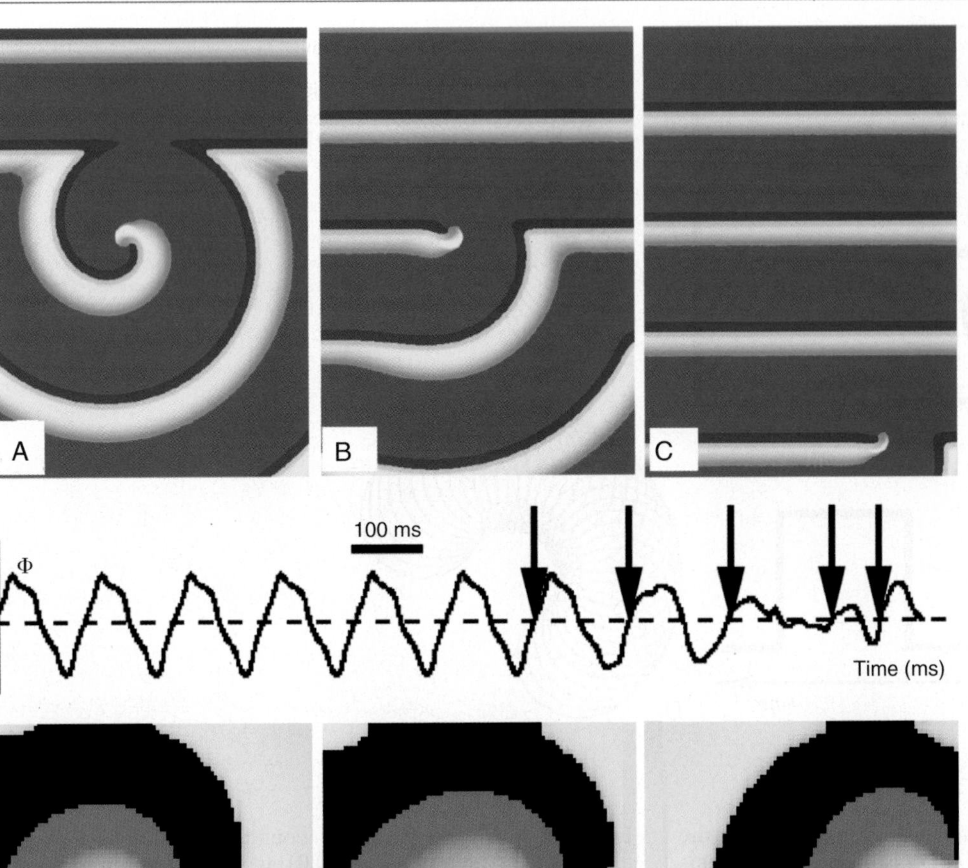

Figure 31-6 **A** to **C,** Induction of spiral wave drift at high frequency external forcing after 10 **(A),** 20 **(B),** and 35 **(C)** external stimulations at a period that is 0.9 of the period of the spiral wave. The pictures were obtained from integration of equation 3 with a = 0.195. Graph in the *middle panel* shows a simulated electrocardiogram before and during stimulation. Moments of time when the stimuli were applied are marked by *arrows.* **D** to **F,** Elimination of spiral wave due to resonant drift. **D,** Pattern of excitation just before application of the first stimulus. **E,** Pattern after two stimuli. **F,** Pattern after four stimuli. (From Panfilov AV, Müller SC, Zykov VS, Keener J: Elimination of spiral waves in cardiac tissue by multiple electrical shocks. Phys Rev E 61:4644-4647, 2000.)

right, as schematically shown in Figure 31-7A. If the period of the parameter change does not coincide with the period of the spiral, such a stimulation will induce a cycloidal motion of the tip similar to spiral wave meandering (see the review by Mikhailov and colleagues[5]). The type of cycloidal motion (epicycloid or hypocycloid) depends on the model parameters and on the relation between the frequency of the external forcing and the frequency of the spiral wave. Figure 31-7C and D shows that forcing below the frequency of the spiral and forcing above the frequency of spiral results in different types of cycloidal motion.[5]

Resonant drift was predicted theoretically from the kinematic theory of spiral waves (see the review by Mikhailov and colleagues[5]) and was observed experimentally in the Belousov-Zhabotinsky reaction.[53] In recent years, the possibility of spiral wave control using resonance was extensively studied theoretically. It was shown that the result of the control procedure depends on the method of measuring the period of the spiral. For a local measurement, the spiral wave can be attracted to that measuring point if it is located sufficiently close to it.[54] If the initial distance is too large, the tip of spiral wave will approach a stable cycloidal trajectory with its center at the measuring point.[54] The drift pattern of a spiral wave is also affected by the delay in the control loop.[54,55]

Another way of determining the period is using global characteristics of the wave pattern,[56] for example the ECG.[52] An elegant graphical method for description of spiral wave drift under global feedback has been developed.[57,58,59] Using this method it is possible to find all the attractors that exist in the medium for different delays in the feedback loop.

It was proposed that resonant drift could be used for low-voltage cardiac defibrillation.[55] The existence of resonant drift was confirmed in detailed models of cardiac tissue.[60,61] It remains to be seen if the resonant drift can be applied in the management of arrhythmias in experimental and clinical studies.

Model Used for Illustrations

Figures 31-1, 31-3, 31-5, and 31-6 were obtained using numerical integration of the following FitzHugh Nagumo type system of differential equations:

$$de/dt = \Delta e - 8e(e - a)(e - 1) - eg \qquad [3]$$

$$dg/dt = \epsilon(e, g)(8e - g) \qquad [4]$$

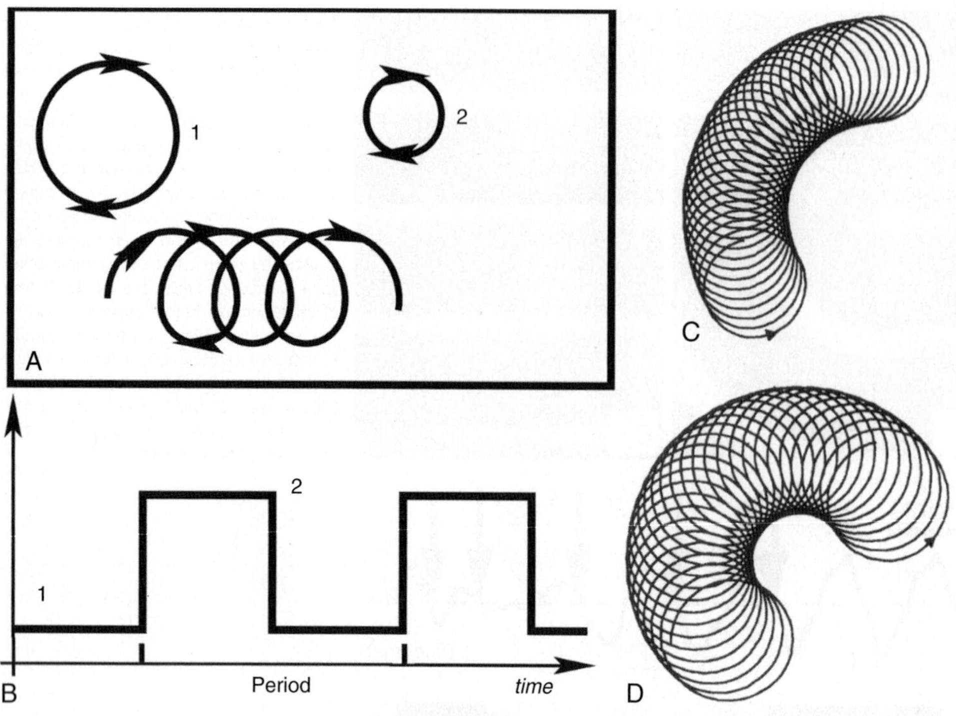

Figure 31-7 Mechanisms of resonant drift. **A,** Core shapes for two values of parameter *P*. **B,** Drift of the spiral wave tip for parameter change with the period equal to the period of the spiral wave. Trajectories of the spiral wave tip when the frequency of the parameter change is lower **(C)** and higher **(D)** than the frequency of the spiral wave. (From Mikhailov AS, Davydov VA, Zykov V: Complex dynamics of spiral waves and motion of curves. Physica D 70:1-39, 1994.)

where e is the transmembrane potential with values scaled to the interval (0,1), and $-8e(e-a)(e-1)-eg$ is the total transmembrane ionic current per unit area.[62] This description reproduces many characteristics of cardiac tissue such as refractoriness, dispersion relation, and rate-duration properties, for example, $\epsilon(e, g) = \epsilon_1 = 0.1$ for $e > 0.6$; $\epsilon(e, g) = \epsilon_2 = 0.01$ for $e = 0.6$; $\epsilon(e, g) = \epsilon_3 = 0.5$ for $e < 0.05$ and $g < 1.2$. Equations 3 and 4 were numerically integrated on a square domain using the Euler method with Neumann boundary conditions with the dimensionless time step up to 0.01 and space step up to 0.3.

Acknowledgments

The author thanks V. N. Biktashev and R. Clayton for valuable comments on the manuscript.

References

1. Zheng Z, Croft J, Giles W, Mensah G: Sudden cardiac death in the United States, 1989 to 1998. Circulation 104:2158-2163, 2001.
2. Mines GR: On dynamic equilibrium of the heart. J Physiol 46:349-482, 1913.
3. Wiener N, Rosenblueth A: The mathematical formulation of the problem of conduction of impulses in a network of connected excitable elements, specifically in cardiac muscle. Arch Inst Cardiol Mex 16:205-265, 1946.
4. Selfridge O: Studies on flutter and fibrillation. Some notes on the theory of flutter. Arch Inst Cardiol Mex 18:177-187, 1948.
5. Mikhailov AS, Davydov VA, Zykov V: Complex dynamics of spiral waves and motion of curves. Physica D 70:1-39, 1994.
6. Panfilov AV, Holden AV: Self-generation of turbulent vortices in a two-dimensional model of cardiac tissue. Phys Lett A 147:463-466, 1990.
7. Qu Z, Weiss J, Garfinkel A: Cardiac electrical restitution properties and stability of reentrant spiral waves: A simulation study. Am J Physiol 276:H269-H283, 1999.
8. Weiss J, Garfinkel A, Karagueuzian H, et al: Chaos and transition to ventricular fibrillation. Circulation 99:2819-2826, 1999.
9. Panfilov AV: Spiral breakup as a model of ventricular fibrillation. Chaos 8:57-64, 1998.
10. Panfilov AV, Pertsov AM: Ventricular fibrillation: Evolution of the multiple wavelet hypothesis. Phil Trans R Soc Lond A 359:1315-1325, 2001.
11. Weiss J, Qu Z, Chen P, et al: The dynamics of cardiac fibrillation. Circulation 112: 1232-1240, 2005.
12. Pertsov AM, Panfilov AV, Medvedeva F: Instabilities of autowaves in excitable media associated with critical curvature phenomena. Biofizika 28:100-102, 1983.
13. Zykov VS: Simulation of Wave Processes in Excitable Media. Manchester, Manchester University Press, 1987.
14. Winfree AT: Varieties of spiral wave behavior: An experimental approach to the theory of excitable media. Chaos 1: 303-334, 1990.
15. Barkley D: Euclidean symmetry and the dynamics of rotating spiral waves. Phys Rev Lett 72:164-167, 1994.
16. Efimov I, Krinsky VI, Jalife J: Dynamics of rotating vortices in the Beeler-Reuter model of cardiac tissue. Chaos 5:513-526, 1995.
17. Biktashev VN, Holden AV: Deterministic brownian motion in the hypermeander of spiral waves. Physica D 116:342-354, 1998.
18. Qu Z, Xie F, Garfinkel A, Weiss J: Origins of spiral wave meander and breakup in a two-dimensional cardiac tissue model. Ann Biomed Eng 28:755-771, 2000.
19. Winfree AT: Electrical instability in cardiac muscle: Phase singularities and rotors. J Theor Biol 138:353-405, 1989.
20. Abildskov JA, Lux RL: The mechanism of simulated torsades de pointes in a computer model of propagated excitation. J Cardiovasc Electrophysiol 2:224-237, 1991.
21. Gray RA, Jalife J, Panfilov A, et al: Nonstationary vortex-like reentrant activity as a mechanism of polymorphic ventricular tachycardia in the isolated rabbit heart. Circulation 91:2454-2469, 1995.
22. Garfinkel A, Qu Z: Nonlinear dynamics of excitation and propagation in cardiac tissue. In Zipes DP, Jalife J (eds): Cardiac Electrophysiology: From Cell to Bedside, 3rd ed. Philadelphia, Saunders, 1999, pp 315-320.
23. Burton FL, Cobbe SM: Dispersion of ventricular repolarization and refractory period. Cardiovasc Res 50:10-23, 2001.

24. Liu DW, Antzelevitch C: Characteristics of the delayed rectifier current (I_{Kr} and I_{Ks}) in canine ventricular epicardial, midmyocardial, and endocardial myocytes. A weaker I_{Ks} contributes to the longer action potential of the M cell. Circ Res 76:351-365, 1995.
25. Schram G, Pourrier M, Melnyk P, Nattel S: Differential distribution of cardiac ion channel expression as a basis for regional specialization in electrical function. Circ Res 90:939-950, 2002.
26. Samie FH, Berenfeld O, Anumonwo J, et al: Rectification of the background potassium current: a determinant of rotor dynamics in ventricular fibrillation. Circ Res 89:1216-1223, 2001.
27. Fast VG, Pertsov AM: Drift of a vortex in the myocardium. Biophysics 35:489-494, 1990.
28. Rudenko AN, Panfilov AV: Drift and interaction of vortices in two-dimensional heterogeneous active medium. Studia Biophysica 98:183-188, 1983.
29. Ivanitsky G, Krinsky V, Panfilov AV, Tsiganov M: Two regimes of the drift of reverberators in nonhomogeneous active media. Biofizika 34:297-299, 1989.
30. Ten Tusscher KHWJ, Panfilov A: Reentry in heterogeneous cardiac tissue described by the Luo-Rudy ventricular action potential model. Am J Physiol Heart Circ Physiol 284:H542-H548, 2003.
31. Krinsky VI: Fibrillation in excitable media. Problemy Kibernetiki 2:59-80, 1968.
32. Khramov R, Rudenko AN, Panfilov AV, Krinsky VI: Drift of vortices in heterogeneous active medium (simplified analysis). Studia Biophysica 102:69-74, 1984.
33. Pertsov AM, Yermakova Y: Mechanism of drift of a helical wave in an inhomogeneous medium. Biofizica 33:318-323, 1988.
34. Winfree AT: When Time Breaks Down. Princeton, Princeton University Press, 1987.
35. Roth BJ: The pinwheel experiment revisited. J Theor Biol 190:389-393, 1998.
36. Sambelashvili A, Efimov I: The pinwheel experiment re-revisited. J Theor Biol 214:147-153, 2002.
37. Chen PS, Wolf P, Dixon EG, et al: Mechanism of ventricular vulnerability to single premature stimuli in open-chest dogs. Circ Res 62:1191-1209, 1988.
38. Starmer CF, Romashko DN, Reddy R, et al: Proarrhythmic response to potassium channel blockade. Circulation 92:595-605, 1995.
39. Li W, Kohl P, Trayanova N: Induction of ventricular arrhythmias following mechanical impact: A simulation study in 3D. J Mol Histol 35(7):679-686, 2004.
40. Krinsky VI: Spread of excitation in an inhomogeneous medium (state similar to cardiac fibrillation). Biophysics 11: 676-683, 1966.
41. Panfilov AV, Vasiev BN: Vortex initiation in a heterogeneous excitable medium. Physica D 49:107-113, 1991.
42. Clayton R, Taggart P: Regional differences in APD restitution can initiate wavebreak and re-entry in cardiac tissue: A computational study. Biomed Eng Online 4:54, 2005.
43. Panfilov AV, Keener JP: Effects of high frequency stimulation in excitable medium with obstacle. J Theor Biol 163:439-448, 1993.
44. Agladze KI, Keener JP, Müller SC, Panfilov AV: Rotating spiral waves created by geometry. Science 264:1746-1748, 1994.
45. Panfilov AV, Pertsov AM: [Mechanism of spiral wave initiation in active media connected with critical curvature phenomenon.]. Biofizika 27:886-888, 1982.
46. Fast VG, Kleber AG: Role of wavefront curvature in propagation of cardiac impulse. Cardiovasc Res 33(2):258-271, 1997.
47. Cabo C, Pertsov AM, Davidenko J, Jalife J: Electrical turbulence as a result of the critical curvature for propagation in cardiac tissue. Chaos 8(1):116-126, 1998.
48. Cabo C, Pertsov AM, Davidenko J, et al: Vortex shedding as a precursor of turbulent electrical activity in cardiac muscle. Biophys J 70:1105-1111, 1996.
49. Pertsov AM, Ermakova E, Shnol E: On the diffraction of autowaves. Physica D 44:178-199, 1990.
50. Krinsky VI, Agladze KI: Interaction of rotating waves in an active chemical medium. Physica D 8:50-56, 1983.
51. Ermakova E, Krinskii V, Panfilov AV, Pertsov AM: Interaction of spiral and flat periodic autowaves in an active medium. Biofizica 31:318-323, 1986.
52. Panfilov AV, Müller SC, Zykov VS, Keener J: Elimination of spiral waves in cardiac tissue by multiple electrical shocks. Phys Rev E 61:4644-4647, 2000.
53. Agladze KI, Davydov VA, Mikhailov AS: An observation of resonance of spiral waves in distributed excitable medium. JETP Lett 45:767-769, 1987.
54. Grill S, Zykov VS, Müller SC: Feedback-controlled dynamics of meandering spiral waves. Phys Rev Lett 75:3368-3371, 1995.
55. Biktashev VN, Holden AV: Design principles of a low voltage cardiac defibrillator based on the effect of feedback resonant drift. J Theor Biol 169:101-112, 1994.
56. Zykov VS, Mikhailov AS, Müller SC: Controlling spiral waves in confined geometries by global feedback. Phys Rev Lett 78:3398-3401, 1997.
57. Zykov VS, Bordiougov G, Brandtstadter H, et al: Global control of spiral wave dynamics in an excitable domain of circular and elliptical shape. Phys Rev Lett 92(1):018304, 2004.
58. Zykov VS, Engel H: Dynamics of spiral waves under global feedback in excitable domains of different shapes. Phys Rev E Stat Nonlin Soft Matter Phys 70(1 Pt 2): 016201, 2004.
59. Zykov VS, Engel H: Feedback-mediated control of spiral wave. Physica D 199:243-263, 2004.
60. Biktashev VN, Holden AV: Control of re-entrant activity in a model of mammalian atrial tissue. Proc Roy Soc Lond B 260: 211-217, 1995.
61. Biktashev VN, Holden AV: Re-entrant activity and its control by resonant drift in a two-dimensional model of isotropic homogeneous ventricular tissue. Proc Roy Soc Lond B 263:1373-1382, 1996.
62. Aliev RR, Panfilov AV: A simple two-variable model of cardiac excitation. Chaos Solitons Fractals 7:293-301, 1996.

Nonlinear Dynamics of Excitation and Propagation in Cardiac Muscle 32

ZHILIN QU AND JAMES N. WEISS

CHAPTER OUTLINE

Over the past several decades, great progress has been made in understanding the mechanisms of cardiac fibrillation, characterized by multiple wavelets coursing through the heart. Fibrillation typically arises from an initial single or a figure-of-eight reentrant circuit, and it is maintained by either spiral wave breakup caused by dynamic instabilities (multiple wavelets hypothesis)[1,2] or fibrillatory conduction block caused by a high-frequency source such as a mother rotor (mother-rotor hypothesis).[3,4]

There are several distinct transitions leading to fibrillation (Fig. 32-1A). The first transition is the initiation of single or figure-of-eight reentry by one or more premature extrasystoles (see Fig. 32-1B), leading to tachycardia. Tachycardia may be sustained if the reentry is stable, or it can undergo the second transition in which the single or figure-of-eight reentrant circuit degenerates into multiple turbulent reentrant wavelets (see Fig. 32-1C), leading to fibrillation. Depending on tissue properties and dynamic stabilities of reentrant waves, fibrillation can be maintained, leading to sudden cardiac death, or it can self-terminate (though rarely) to resume sinus rhythm (see Fig.32-1A).

Cardiac arrhythmias are traditionally attributed to intrinsic tissue heterogeneities, which are usually amplified in diseased hearts due to electrical and structural remodeling.[5,6] However, theoretical and experimental studies since the 1980s have shown that dynamic instabilities of membrane voltage (V_m) and intracellular calcium (Ca^{2+}) cycling are also important for generating and maintaining cardiac arrhythmias.[7,8] In fact, heterogeneities, dynamic instabilities, and cardiac arrhythmias interact to regulate stability and maintenance of arrhythmias. Tissue heterogeneities include both electrical and structural heterogeneities, such as transmural and apex-to-base gradients in action potential and intracellular Ca^{2+} transients, fiber orientation, fibrosis, and nonuniform anatomical structure, among others. Electrical heterogeneities can be induced due to dynamic instabilities. Dynamic instabilities originate mainly from V_m and intracellular Ca^{2+} cycling and their couplings, but they can also be caused or modulated by tissue heterogeneities.

Tissue heterogeneities and dynamic instabilities regulate the wave dynamics in tissue during both normal and abnormal heart rhythms. However, the heart rate also prominently affects tissue heterogeneities and cellular dynamic factors, because contraction activates the mechanosensitive channels that alter action potential features; faster heart rates cause Ca^{2+} accumulation and other ionic changes that affect action potential features, including inducing afterdepolarizations; arrhythmias can cause global ischemia, changing both tissue and cellular properties and the dynamics of arrhythmias; and long-lasting arrhythmias or fast heart rates cause both electrical and structural remodeling of the myocardium.

This research is supported by NIH/NHLBI grant P01 HL078931 and by the Laubisch and Kawata Endowments.

Voltage and Calcium Dynamics in Isolated Cardiac Myocytes

Nonlinear Dynamics of Spontaneous and Triggered Activities

The cardiac myocyte is an excitable system in which a small suprathreshold stimulus can cause a large transient excursion in membrane potential V_m and the intracellular Ca^{2+} transient (Fig. 32-2A). Spontaneous oscillatory activity (see Fig. 32-2B) can originate in either the V_m subsystem[9] or the Ca^{2+} subsystem due to Ca^{2+}-induced Ca^{2+} release.[10] The bifurcation from the excitable regime to spontaneous oscillatory regime is a generic feature of excitable systems, specifically a bifurcation from a stable steady state to limit cycle oscillations through a Hopf bifurcation.[11] In the normal heart, both the ventricles and the atria are in the excitable regime, except for pacemaking tissues such as the sinoatrial node, atrioventricular junction, and His-Purkinje system, which are in limit-cycle regimes.

Abnormal excitations can also arise due to triggered activity, which includes early afterdepolarizations (EADs, see Fig. 32-2C) and delayed afterdepolarizations (DADs, see Fig. 32-2D). EADs are depolarizations occurring during the repolarizing phase of the action potential, usually caused by the L-type Ca^{2+} window current in the setting of reduced repolarization reserve (i.e., reduced net outward currents). Although the detailed nonlinear dynamics is not well understood, an analogy is found in the bursting dynamics of neurons, in which a homoclinic bifurcation leads to the bursting behavior.[11] It is likely that EADs can be caused by dynamic instabilities arising purely from the V_m system or from its interactions with Ca^{2+} cycling. DADs are transient depolarizations that occur after the action potential has repolarized, and if they are sufficiently large can trigger additional action potentials. DADs originate from intracellular Ca^{2+} cycling dynamics, undergoing a transient limit cycle phase. Currently, however, the nonlinear dynamics of EADs and DADs are not well understood and await further investigation.

Nonlinear Dynamics of Voltage and Ca^{2+} During Periodic Pacing

Dynamics Due to Restitution of Action Potential Duration

The cardiac action potential results from the coordinated opening and closing of thousands of individual membrane ion

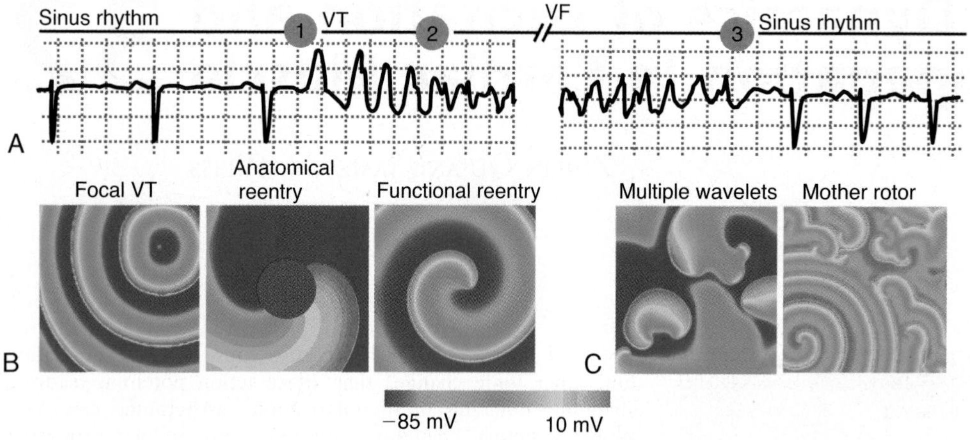

Figure 32-1 The transition to fibrillation. **A**, A typical electrocardiogram from a patient[4] illustrating distinct transitions from *1*, sinus rhythm to ventricular tachycardia (VT); *2*, VT to ventricular fibrillation (VF); and *3*, self-termination of VF back to sinus rhythm. **B** and **C**, Snapshots of membrane voltage (*red* most depolarized, *blue* most repolarized) during various forms of VT and VF in simulated two-dimensional tissue.

channels with different conductances, ion selectivity, and kinetic properties. Because of the time it takes for certain ion channels to recover from inactivation or to deactivate, the action potential duration (APD) of a premature beat (S2) following a sinus beat (S1) depends on the diastolic interval preceding the premature stimulus (Fig. 32-3A). The dependence of APD on diastolic interval is called *APD restitution* and is usually denoted as $APD_{n+1} = f(DI_n)$, where APD is the action potential duration and DI is the diastolic interval. APD restitution is usually a monotonic function of diastolic interval: APD decreases monotonically as diastolic interval decreases (see Fig. 32-3B).[12,13] However, nonmonotonic curves have also been observed (see Fig. 32-3C).[14,15] The detailed physiologic mechanisms for different types of APD restitution curve are still not very clear.

The relationship between APD restitution and dynamic instability was first elucidated in 1968 by Nolasco and Dahlen,[16] who studied strips of in vitro frog ventricular muscle subjected to electrical stimulation. They showed that when the slope of the APD restitution curve exceeded 1, periodic beating gave way to APD alternans (a *long-short-long-short* alternating pattern of APD). Later studies[17-19] showed that in addition to alternans, more complex dynamics can be elicited by periodic pacing. From these pioneering studies, the APD restitution equation was reformulated in terms of an iterated map as:

$$APD_{n+1} = f(DI_n) = f(mT - APD_n) \quad [1]$$

where m is chosen so that $(m - 1)T < APD_n + DI_{min} < mT$ and DI_{min} is the minimum diastolic interval eliciting an action potential.

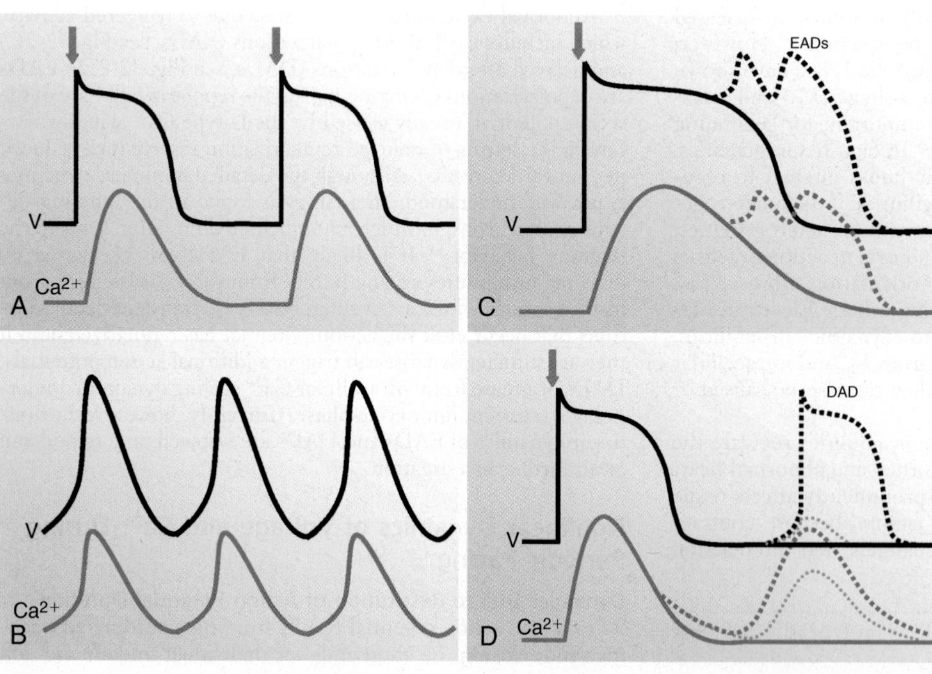

Figure 32-2 Illustrative traces of voltage and intracellular Ca^{2+} during a normal action potential (**A**), spontaneous oscillations (**B**), early afterdepolarizations (EADs) (**C**), and delayed afterdepolarization (DAD) (**D**). Arrows indicate stimulation.

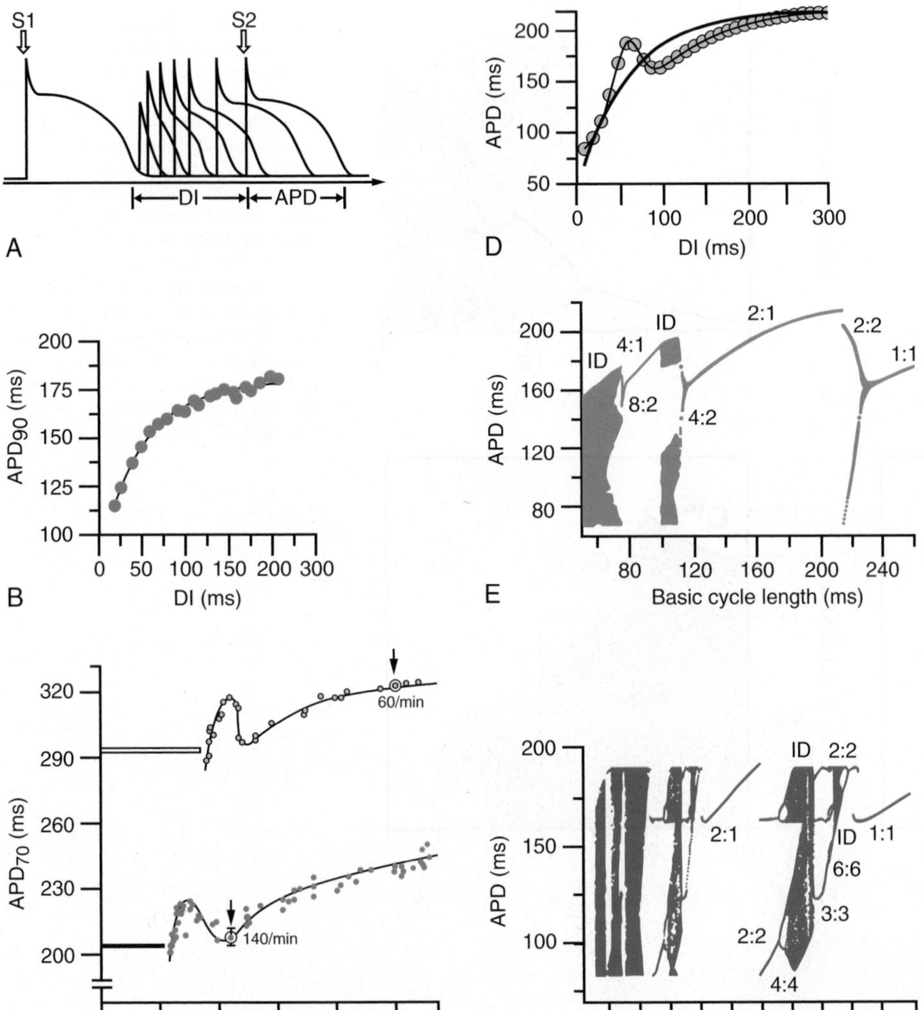

Figure 32-3 **A,** Protocol for measuring S1S2 restitution of action potential duration (APD) by progressively shortening the diastolic interval of the S2 beat. **B,** APD restitution from a rabbit showing a monotonic curve.[13] **C,** APD restitution from a human showing a nonmonotonic curve.[14] **D,** Two theoretical APD restitution functions used to generate the bifurcation diagrams in **E** (for the curve indicated by the *thick line*) and **F** (from the curve indicated by *colored circles*). DI, diastolic interval.

If the slope of the APD restitution curve is smaller than 1 everywhere ($f' = df/dDI < 1$ for all diastolic intervals), the equilibrium state is always stable; that is, a stable 1:1 response occurs for all pacing rates until 2:1 block occurs. When $f' < 1$ for all diastolic intervals is not satisfied, then complex nonlinear dynamics can occur. If $f(DI)$ is a monotonically increasing function (line in Fig. 32-3D), as the pacing cycle length decreases, bifurcations from the stable equilibrium state (1:1) to alternans (2:2), from 2:2 alternans to 2:1 block and 4:2 alternans, and then to beat-to-beat irregular (or chaotic) APD patterns occur (see Fig. 32-3E).

To understand the onset of APD alternans—that is, loss of stability of the equilibrium state—one can perform a linear stability analysis. Assume a small perturbation ΔDI_n ($=-\Delta APD_n$) is given to the equilibrium state (APD_{ss}, DI_{ss}), then inserting $DI_n = DI_{ss} + \Delta DI_n$ into equation 1 gives us:

$$\begin{aligned} APD_{ss} + \Delta APD_{n+1} &= f(DI_{ss}) + f'\Delta DI_n \\ &= f(T - APD_{ss}) - f'\Delta APD_n \end{aligned} \quad [2]$$

where f' is the slope of APD restitution at the equilibrium state.

Because at the equilibrium state, $APD_{ss} = f(DI_{ss}) = f(T - APD_{ss})$, then from equation 2, we have $\Delta APD_{n+1} = f'\Delta DI_n = -f'\Delta APD_n$. For the next beat, the perturbation becomes $\Delta APD_{n+2} = (-f')^2 \Delta APD_n$, and for the mth beat after the perturbation, it becomes $\Delta APD_{n+m} = (-f')^m \Delta APD_n$. Therefore, if $f' < 1$, APD alternans is progressively attenuated, eventually approaching the steady state APD_{ss}, because $(f')^m \to 0$ as $m \to \infty$. If $f' > 1$, however, APD alternans progressively expands, because $(f')^m \to \infty$ as $m \to \infty$]. However, this expansion may be suppressed due to the nonlinearity of the APD restitution curve, eventually resulting in (2:2) stable alternans, or, if alternans becomes too large, 2:1 block and other complex dynamics, as in Figure 32-3E. In this case, chaos always occurs after 2:1 block, because stimulation failure + $f' > 1$ is required for the genesis of chaos, equivalent to a shift map mechanism of chaos.[19,20] If $f(DI)$ is a nonmonotonic function (symbols in Fig. 32-3D), chaos can occur before stimulation failure (see Fig. 32-3F). In this case, chaos occurs due to a unimodal map mechanism,[20] such as the logistic map.

The bifurcation sequences shown in Figure 32-3E are very similar to bifurcation sequences in experiments in cardiac Purkinje fibers observed by Chialvo and colleagues,[18] in which the sequence was 1:1 → 2:2 → 2:1 → 4:2 → 3:1 → 6:2 → 4:1 → 8:2 → ID, whereas in Figure32-3E, it is 1:1 → 2:2 → 2:1 → 4:2 → ID → 4:1 → 8:2 → ID. Another experiment by Watanabe

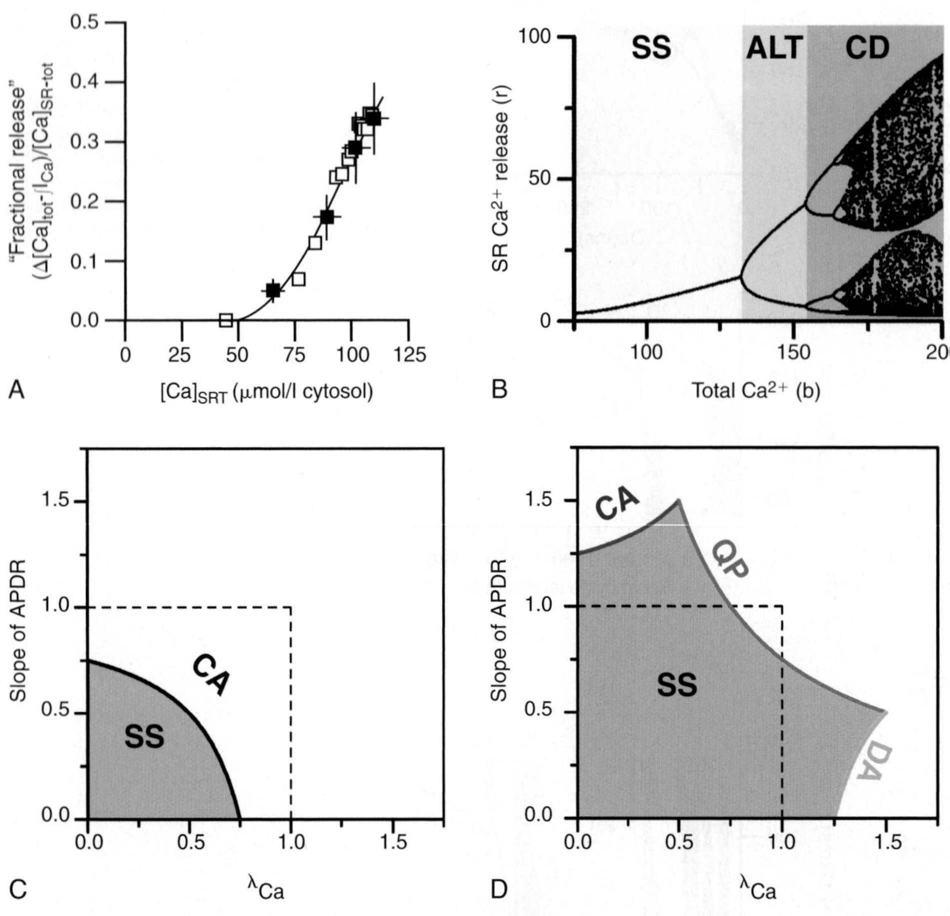

Figure 32-4 A, Experimentally measured sarcoplasmic reticulum (SR) Ca^{2+} release curve, plotting the fraction of SR Ca^{2+} released versus the SR Ca^{2+} load. **B,** Bifurcation diagram using the curve in **A. C** and **D,** Phase diagrams when Ca^{2+}-to-APD coupling is positive and negative, respectively. *Dashed lines* show the thresholds for alternans caused by steep APD restitution slope (*y* axis) and Ca^{2+} cycling dynamics (*x* axis), respectively, when V_m and Ca^{2+} are not coupled. ALT, alternans (2:2); APD, action potential duration; CA, electromechanically concordant alternans; CD, complex dynamics; DA, electromechanically discordant alternans; QP, quasiperiodicity; SS, stable steady state.

and coworkers[15] demonstrated an APD restitution curve that was nonmonotonic in sheep epicardial muscle. The bifurcation sequence observed was 1:1 → ID → 8:8 → 4:4 → ID → 2:2 → 2:1 as the basic cycle length decreased from 200 ms to 109 ms. In Figure 32-3F, the bifurcation sequence is 1:1 → 2:2 → ID → 6:6 → 3:3 → ID → 4:4 → 2:2 → 2:1, which qualitatively agrees with the experimentally observed bifurcation sequence.

Dynamics Due to Intracellular Ca^{2+} Cycling

V_m and intracellular Ca^{2+} are bidirectionally coupled in cardiac myocytes, mainly through Ca^{2+}-sensitive ionic currents such as the L-type calcium current and the Na^+-Ca^{2+} exchange current. Ca^{2+} entry through L-type calcium channels triggers release of Ca^{2+} from the sarcoplasmic reticulum (SR) into the cytoplasm by activating SR Ca^{2+}-release channels. Therefore, if APD alternates or varies chaotically due to APD restitution, the Ca^{2+} transient amplitude will also follow secondarily in response to the changing L-type Ca^{2+} current amplitude. A larger L-type Ca^{2+} current causes a larger Ca^{2+} transient. On the other hand, Ca^{2+} is negatively coupled to the L-type Ca^{2+} channel, causing it to inactivate more quickly, but also positively coupled to electrogenic Na^+-Ca^{2+} exchange. Due to this competition, a larger Ca^{2+} transient can either increase or decrease the inward current during repolarization, thus either prolonging or shortening APD. Therefore, if a dynamic instability causes the Ca^{2+} transient to alternate or vary chaotically, then the APD will passively follow suit and also begin to alternate or change chaotically.

Voltage clamp experiments[21,22] have documented that Ca^{2+} transients in isolated myocytes can exhibit profound alternans despite a constant V_m waveform. Experiments with free-running action potentials in intact tissue[23] and in isolated ventricular myocytes[13] indicate that the onset of APD alternans is primarily generated by an instability in intracellular Ca^{2+} cycling dynamics, rather than steep APD restitution, because the onset of APD alternans occurred at a pacing cycle length at which APD restitution slope was still considerably smaller than 1.

Several studies[20,24-26] have investigated the factors causing dynamic instabilities in Ca^{2+} cycling leading to Ca^{2+} transient alternans and irregular dynamics. Eisner and coworkers[24] first proposed a steep dependence of SR Ca^{2+} release on SR Ca^{2+} load as the cause of alternans, which was treated theoretically by Shiferaw and colleagues.[25] Similar to the APD restitution case, an iterated map equation can be developed by assuming that the SR Ca^{2+} load for the $(n+1)$th beat (l_{n+1}) equals the SR Ca^{2+} load of the nth beat (l_n) less the amount released on the same beat (r_{n+1}) plus the Ca^{2+} reuptake (u_{n+1}) by the SR, namely:

$$l_{n+1} = l_n - r_{n+1} + u_{n+1} \qquad [3]$$

According to the experimental measurements,[27] the fraction of Ca^{2+} released from the SR is a function of the SR Ca^{2+} load (Fig. 32-4A), that is, $r_{n+1} = g(l_n)$. For Ca^{2+} reuptake, experimental data[28] suggest a sigmoidal function of intracellular Ca^{2+}. Assuming that it is a function of the peak cytoplasmic Ca^{2+}, namely, $u_{n+1} = h(c^p_{n+1})$, then peak cytosolic Ca^{2+} equals total Ca^{2+} (b) less the SR Ca^{2+} load (l_n) plus the SR Ca^{2+} release (r_{n+1}), that is, $c^p_{n+1} = b - l_n + r_{n+1}$. Then equation 3 becomes:

$$l_{n+1} = l_n - g(l_n) + h[b - l_n + g(l_n)] \quad [4]$$

Similar to the APD case, inserting $l_n = l_{ss} + \Delta l_n$ into equation 4, one obtains the iterated equation for the perturbation as (see Qu and colleagues[20] for details):

$$\Delta l_{n+1} = (1 - g' - h' + g'h')\Delta l_n = -\lambda_{Ca}\Delta l_n \quad [5]$$

where $g' = dg/dl_n$ is the slope of the release curve at the equilibrium state, and $h' = dh/dc^p_{n+1}$ is the slope of the uptake curve at the equilibrium state. For this perturbation to grow requires $1 - g' - h' + g'h' > 1$, which leads to $(2-h')/(1-h') < g' < h'/(h'-1)$. When this equation is satisfied, the equilibrium state is unstable; otherwise it is stable. For Ca^{2+} alternans to occur, $-\lambda_{Ca} = 1 - g' - h' + g'h' < -1$ is required, namely, $(2-h')/(1-h')$. Therefore, for a certain slope h' of the uptake curve, the slope of the release curve has to reach a critical value for alternans to occur. Besides the dynamics of alternans, more complex dynamics such as chaos can occur due to a steep SR Ca^{2+} release curve, as shown by the bifurcation diagram in Figure 32-4B.

Effects of Voltage and Calcium Couplings

Because the coupling between APD and the Ca^{2+} transient is bidirectional, an important question is how the V_m dynamics and Ca^{2+} dynamics interact with each other to affect the onset and pattern of cellular alternans. This issue has been studied theoretically by Shiferaw and colleagues[29] and Qu and colleagues.[20] When Ca^{2+}-to-APD coupling is positive—that is, a larger Ca^{2+} transient promotes a longer APD—instability is promoted such that the onset of the alternans instability occurs sooner (see Fig. 32-4C). For example, the onset of APD and Ca^{2+} alternans can occur when both $f'<1$ and $\lambda_{Ca} <1$. When Ca^{2+}-to-APD coupling is negative—that is, a larger Ca^{2+} transient promotes a shorter APD and vice versa—then the two dynamic instabilities oppose each other, each inhibiting the other's ability to cause alternans (see Fig. 32-4D).

For example, alternans might not occur even when $f'>1$. When alternans does occur, its pattern depends on which instability predominates. If alternans is primarily from V_m dynamics by steep APD restitution slope, APD and Ca^{2+} transient alternans is electromechanically concordant (long APD associated with large Ca^{2+} transient), as is often seen in the experiments.[21] When alternans is from Ca^{2+} cycling dynamics, it is electromechanically discordant (long APD associated with small Ca^{2+} transient), which is also shown in experiments.[22] When the V_m and Ca^{2+} cycling instabilities are more equally balanced, the pattern of alternans becomes quasiperiodic (i.e., APD and Ca^{2+} transient alternans fluctuate in both their amplitudes and degree of electromechanical concordance and discordance). This might provide a mechanistic explanation to the quasiperiodic behavior observed by Otani and Gilmour.[30]

Wave Dynamics in Cardiac Tissue

Spatially Discordant Alternans and Dynamically Induced Electrical Heterogeneities

For wave propagation in cardiac tissue, new dynamics and patterns emerge, among which spatially discordant APD alternans is the best studied. Spatially discordant alternans was observed first in experiments[31,32] and then mechanistically explained by theoretical studies.[32-34] Figures 32-5A and B show the optical mapping of concordant and discordant APD alternans in guinea pig hearts by Pastore and colleagues.[31] As pacing rate increases, APD first alternates in the same *long-short-long-short* pattern everywhere in the mapping area, which is spatially concordant. At faster pacing, however, APD begins to alternate out of phase in space, with one region exhibiting a *long-short-long-short* pattern while the adjacent tissue alternates in a *short-long-short-long* pattern, which is spatially discordant.

The same phenomenon was demonstrated in computer simulations (see Fig. 32-5C)[33,34] and shown to depend either on a premature beat that locally resets the phase of alternans or on the combination of APD alternans due to steep APD restitution or intracellular Ca^{2+} cycling dynamics coupled to engagement of conduction velocity restitution. Similar to APD restitution, conduction velocity restitution describes the functional relationship between the conduction velocity of a propagating action potential and its preceding diastolic interval (see Fig. 32-5D). When no conduction velocity restitution is engaged, spatially concordant alternans occurs. When conduction velocity restitution is engaged, so that the conduction velocity of the wavefront varies as it propagates through the tissue, APD alternans becomes spatially discordant. One interesting observation is that when alternans is spatially concordant, only T-wave alternans occurs in the electrocardiogram (ECG), but when alternans is spatially discordant, both T-wave alternans and QRS complex alternans occur (see Fig. 32-5E).[31,33] Because QRS is the reflection of the wavefront conduction, QRS alternans indicates the engagement of conduction velocity restitution in spatially discordant alternans.

A novel dynamic mechanism of inducing dispersion of refractoriness was investigated by Xie and colleagues,[35] who demonstrated that loss of chaos synchronization in cardiac tissue can induce macroscopic dispersion of refractoriness both transverse and longitudinal to the direction of propagation. Due to sensitivity to initial conditions, identical chaotic systems tend to diverge. However, diffusive coupling can cause them to remain synchronized over a characteristic length scale. Synchronization fails when the tissue exceeds a critical size, causing irregular macroscopic heterogeneity in refractoriness to develop. In this case, tiny amounts of noise can lead to reentry in homogeneous tissue, without the requirement of preexisting heterogeneities or different locations of stimulation.

Vulnerability to Spiral Wave Reentry

Reentry can be initiated based on Winfree's pinwheel experiment,[36] even in homogeneous tissue, if a critical amount of tissue is depolarized in the refractory wake of a previous excitation (Fig. 32-6), either by a very high strength stimulus (e.g., as in fibrillation threshold testing) or by stimulation of a large region (e.g., as with a mechanical stimulus in commotio cordis). Reentry can also be induced by a modestly suprathreshold point stimulus in heterogeneous tissue if the gradient of refractoriness and area of the heterogeneity are sufficiently large.[37,38] Critical gradients in refractoriness for unidirectional conduction block leading to reentrant arrhythmias have been measured in animal experiments. In normal guinea pig hearts, Laurita and Rosenbaum[39] found that a minimum repolarization gradient of 3.2 ms/mm was required for unidirectional conduction block. In a one-dimensional (1D) cable of cardiac cells, it has been shown theoretically[38] that if the premature beat propagates in the same direction as the sinus beat, the critical gradient (σ) in refractoriness for conduction block of a premature extrasystole is a function of conduction velocity of the sinus beat (θ_1) and the minimum conduction velocity (θ_c) at which a premature beat can conduct, that is, $\sigma = 1/\theta c - 1/\theta_1$

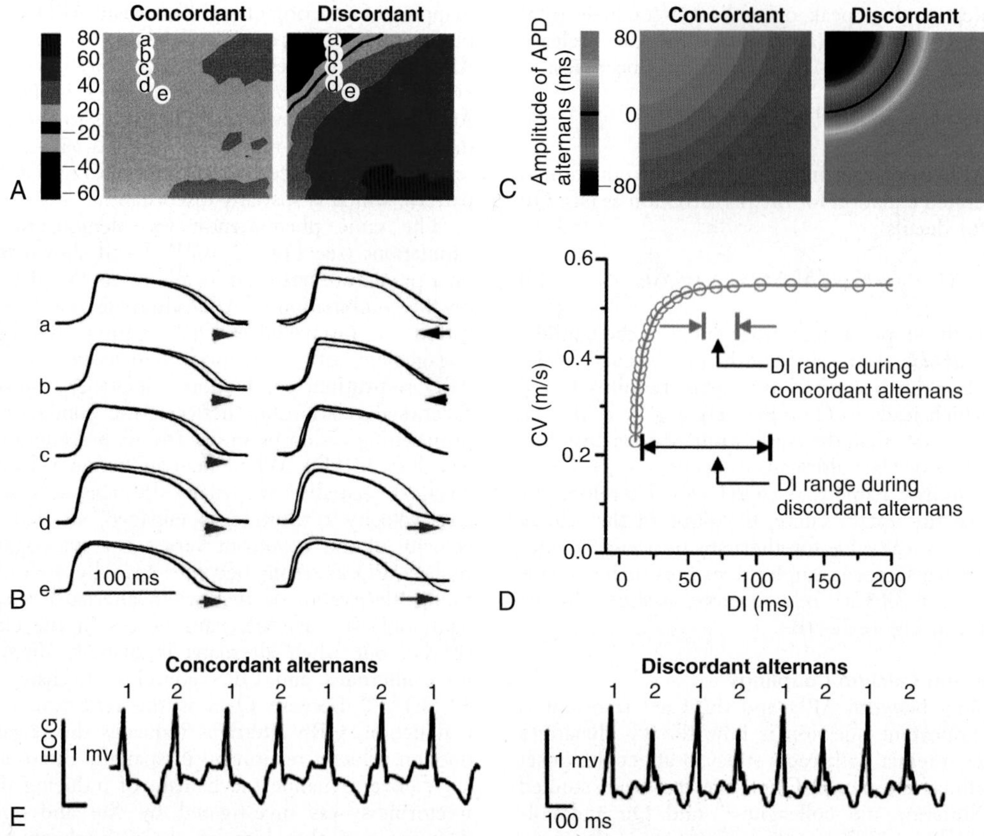

Figure 32-5 The transition from spatially concordant to discordant alternans. **A,** Action potential duration (APD) alternans amplitude (i.e., the APD difference between two consecutive beats) distribution obtained from optical mapping in guinea pig heart by Pastore and colleagues.[31] During pacing at 285 beats per minute (*left*), the alternans amplitude is positive everywhere over the mapped area, indicating spatially concordant alternans. At faster pacing at 315 beats per minute (*right*), however, the alternans amplitude is negative in one area but positive in the adjacent area, indicating spatially discordant alternans. The *black line* in the *right panel* is the nodal line at which alternans amplitude is zero: the APDs are the same for two consecutive beats. **B,** Optical action potential tracings recorded from selected ventricular sites (*a* through *e*) for the spatially concordant and discordant APD alternans shown in **A.** Action potentials recorded from two consecutive beats *(thick* and *thin tracings)* are superimposed to demonstrate alternation in transmembrane potential. **C,** APD alternans amplitude in space obtained from a computer simulation in *homogeneous* two-dimensional tissue, showing spatially concordant APD alternans at 315 beats per minute *(left,)* and spatially discordant APD alternans at 342 beats per minute *(right)*. **D,** Conduction velocity (CV) restitution curves, constructed by plotting the CV of the S2 beat versus the preceding diastolic interval (DI) in a one-dimensional cable of coupled cardiac cells. The DI ranges over the entire tissue during spatially concordant and discordant alternans are indicated. During concordant alternans, the DI varied in a range over which CV was almost constant, but during discordant alternans, DI varied in a larger range in which CV also varied markedly, i.e., CV restitution is engaged. **E.** Pseudoelectrocardiogram (ECG) recorded from experiments[31] during spatially concordant and discordant alternans. Spatially concordant APD alternans produces T-wave alternans alone, whereas spatially discordant alternans produces both QRS and T-wave alternans.

(note that this relation is different if two beats propagate in opposite directions.[38]

For normal cardiac conduction where θ_l = 0.5 mm/ms and θ_c = 0.2 mm/ms, a gradient $\sigma > 3$ ms/mm is predicted, which is close to that measured experimentally in normal tissue.[39] In 1D cable, once the critical gradient is reached, the vulnerable window of conduction block increases in proportion to the refractory barrier, that is, the difference in APD.[38] However, in 2D tissue, the vulnerable window of reentry increases first in proportion to the refractory barrier, but it then decreases as the barrier becomes higher.[40]

Whether the gradient of refractoriness is preexisting or induced by premature extrasystoles or rapid pacing,[33] once it reaches the critical value, unidirectional conduction block can occur. Figure 32-7 illustrates the induction of reentry by a premature stimulation in a tissue with induced spatially discordant APD alternans.

Spiral and Scroll Wave Stabilities

Once reentry forms, it might remain stable as tachycardia, or it might degenerate into turbulent multiple wavelets underlying fibrillation (the second transition in Fig. 32-1A). Two major hypotheses of fibrillation have been proposed and validated experimentally in animal models: the *mother rotor hypothesis* and the *multiple wavelet hypothesis*. In the mother rotor hypothesis, preexisting heterogeneities (dispersion of refractoriness) cause fibrillatory conduction block of waves from a stable high-frequency focal source or a mother rotor, accounting for the multiple wavelets observed during fibrillation.[3,4] In the multiple wavelet hypothesis,[1] however, preexisting heterogeneities are not necessary, because fibrillation is maintained by spontaneous spiral wave breakup due to dynamic instabilities.

Computer simulations[41,42] have shown that APD restitution is a critical parameter that controls the stability of the spiral wave. As the APD restitution slope increases, the induced

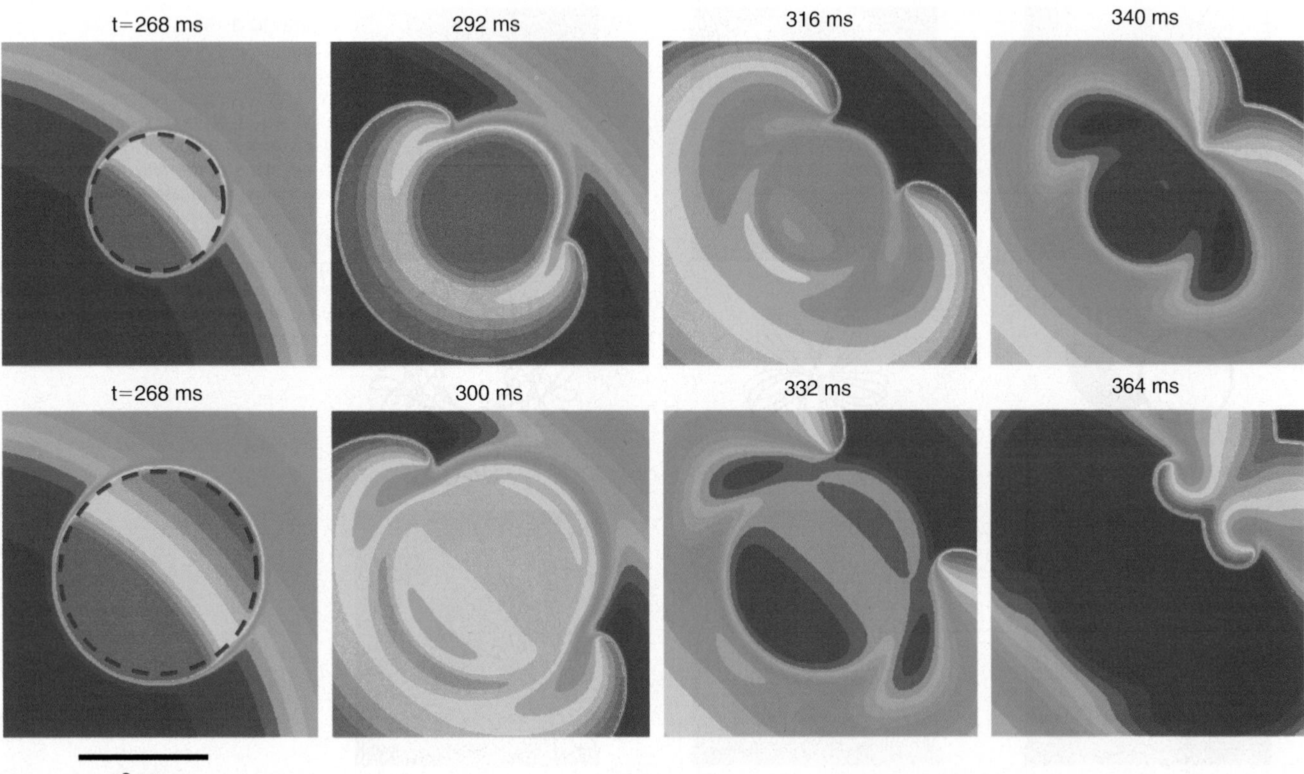

Figure 32-6 Induction of spiral wave reentry by a premature stimulus. Voltage snapshots showing a premature stimulus depolarizing an area (*dashed circle*, 2 cm in diameter) smaller than the critical area *(upper panels)*, in which reentry was not induced, compared to a premature stimulus depolarizing an area (*dashed circle*, 3 cm in diameter) larger than the critical area *(lower panels)*, in which figure-of-eight reentry was initiated. *Red* indicates most depolarized, *blue* indicates most repolarized.

spiral wave becomes more and more unstable (Fig. 32-8A to C). When APD restitution becomes steep enough, the induced spiral wave is so unstable that it breaks up spontaneously into multiple small reentrant waves, resembling fibrillation (see Fig. 32-8D). Note that the computer simulations shown in Figure 32-8 were performed in completely homogeneous tissue models, yet a large dispersion of refractoriness resulted purely from the dynamic instability of the spiral waves. In this case, reentrant waves are constantly created and disappear in an irregular or chaotic manner, as shown by the recording of the spiral tips versus time in Figure 32-8D. Experimental studies[43,44] have shown that pharmacologic agents that reduce the slope of

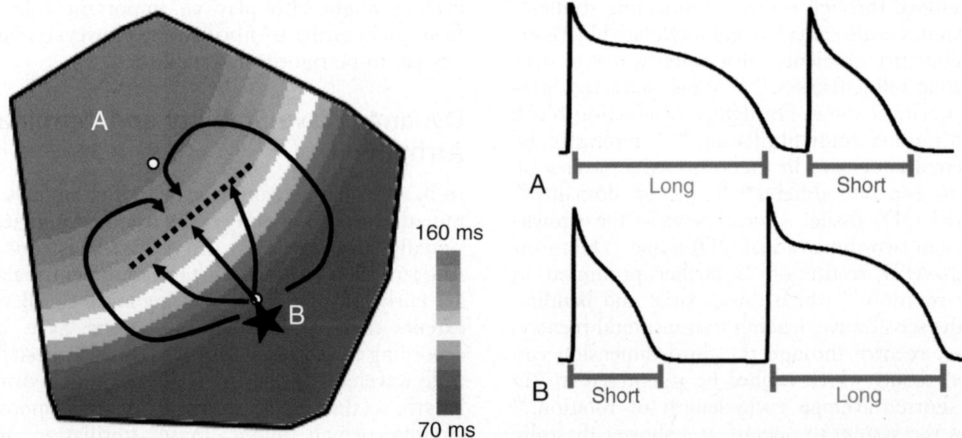

Figure 32-7 Mechanism of initiation of reentry by a premature ectopic beat during spatially discordant action potential duration (APD) alternans. A premature ectopic beat (S2) occurring in the region of short APD blocks as it propagates across the nodal line into the region with long APD. Meanwhile, the ectopic beat successfully propagates laterally, waiting for the long APD region to repolarize, and then reenters the blocked region to initiate figure-of-eight reentry.

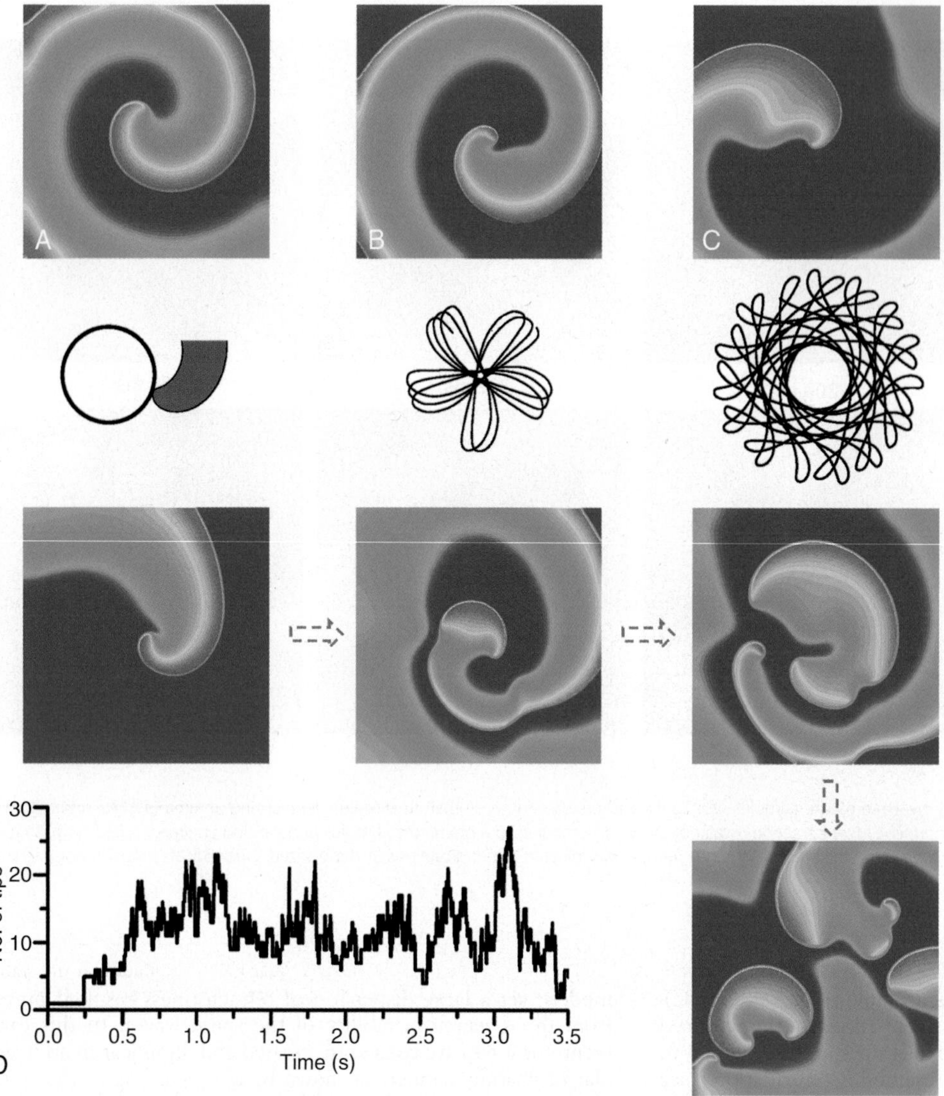

Figure 32-8 Effects of action potential duration (APD) restitution slope on spiral wave tip dynamics in two-dimensional tissue. **A** to **C**, Stationary and meandering spiral waves. Voltage snapshots of spiral waves and corresponding tip trajectories as the slope of the APD restitution curve progressively increases from **A** to **C**. **D**, Spiral wave breakup. Voltage snapshots at successive times (indicated by the *arrows*) show spiral wave breakup in the case of even steeper APD restitution. Graph shows the number of spiral wave tips versus time.

APD restitution converted fibrillation into tachycardia, supporting the theory developed through computer-modeling studies.

Spiral wave dynamics is also affected and modulated by tissue heterogeneities. Refractory gradients cause spiral waves to drift toward regions of long refractoriness.[45,46] When refractory gradients increase to a critical value, fibrillatory conduction block occurs, resulting in mother rotor fibrillation.[46,47] Interestingly, to maintain different frequencies in the same tissue, a chaotic zone must form to separate different frequency domains.[48] In three-dimensional (3D) tissue, a scroll wave is the equivalent of a spiral wave in two-dimensional (2D) tissue. The instability due to steep APD restitution is further promoted in 3D tissue by fiber rotation,[49] which causes twist and bending of the filament of the scroll wave, leading to transmural reentry. Unlike the 2D case, reentry through the third dimension can enter the recovered tissue, which cannot be re-entered in 2D tissue, causing a shorter average cycle length of rotation.[49] This in turn causes the system to operate at a shorter diastolic interval, in a steeper region of the APD restitution curve, facilitating scroll wave breakup. New dynamic instabilities can also occur due to tissue thickness,[49,50] especially under conditions of low excitability.[51] Instabilities caused by intracellular Ca^{2+} cycling might also play an important role in the transition from tachycardia to fibrillation. However, the theoretical basis has yet to be rigorously established.

Dynamic Wave Stability and Termination of Arrhythmias

In hearts of large mammals, including humans, spontaneous termination of fibrillation occurs frequently in atria but only occasionally in ventricles (Fig. 32-1A is one such example). Antiarrhythmic drugs can terminate ventricular fibrillation and are fairly effective at terminating atrial fibrillation.[52,53] To some extent, their antifibrillatory actions have been rationalized according to Garrey's critical mass hypothesis[54] and Moe's multiple wavelet hypothesis.[1] Class IA and III drugs prolong wavelength, so that the same-size tissue can support fewer reentrant circuits, which might cause fibrillation to self-terminate. However, this mechanism has been challenged by experimental studies[55,56] that showed that these drugs had limited effects on wavelength and refractory period. Recent computer modeling studies[46,57,58] showed that dynamic wave stability plays an important role in the termination of fibrillation.

Dynamic instability due to steep APD restitution promotes wave breaks maintaining fibrillation, but it also enhances the probability of wave extinction by promoting wave meandering and collision with tissue borders, facilitating spontaneous termination of fibrillation. The latter effect predominates as dynamic instability or the steepness of the APD restitution increases, so that fibrillation is more likely to self-terminate in a finite size tissue. The likelihood of spontaneous termination of fibrillation decreases exponentially as tissue size increases.[57]

Class I or III antiarrhythmic drugs can terminate fibrillation through their effects on electrical restitution as well as wavelength. The reverse-use dependence of potassium-channel blockers prolongs APD at slow rates, but much less at fast rates, which makes APD restitution steeper. This steepening causes the reentrant waves to become more unstable, enhancing their probability of colliding with other waves or tissue borders and thus promoting self-termination. In mother rotor fibrillation, these effects can also destabilize the mother rotor, promoting its self-termination by drifting and colliding with a tissue border.

An experimental study[59] in rabbit ventricles showed that the I_{Kr} blocker nifekalant destabilized a stable rotor, promoting meander, which facilitated termination of the rotor by this mechanism. In another study, Banville and Gray[60] showed that under control conditions, fibrillation was sustained, but after treatment with the excitation-contraction uncoupled diacetyl monoxime, which shortens APD and flattens APD restitution, reentry was stabilized. Conversely, the uncoupler cyto-D, which steepens APD restitution, caused fibrillation to become nonsustained. In the atrium, APD restitution might also be important in self-termination of fibrillation, because electrical remodeling due to long period of fibrillation causes APD to shorten and APD restitution to become flatter.[61]

These effects might play a role in the atrial fibrillation–begets–atrial fibrillation scenario, in which nonsustained fibrillation becomes sustained as its duration increases.[62]

Conclusions and Perspectives

Normal and abnormal cardiac conduction results from a complex system that involves many levels of regulation, from the molecule to the organ. The development of cardiac arrhythmias requires triggers, such as the premature extrasystoles, with proper timing and spatial location to interact with a dynamically changing substrate to facilitate the transitions shown in Figure 32-1. The ideal antiarrhythmic drug should be able to *simultaneously* suppress triggers, reduce the vulnerable window of reentry, prevent the transition to fibrillation, and promote self-termination of fibrillation. The minimum effective drug must be effective in at least one step without worsening the others. A major challenge in the new era of arrhythmia biology is to integrate the nonlinear dynamics illuminated by computer simulations with animal experiments and clinical observations in order to develop a systems biology approach that can transform the resulting knowledge into practical strategies to prevent fibrillation and sudden cardiac death.

References

1. Moe GK: On the multiple wavelet hypothesis of atrial fibrillation. Arch Int Pharmacodyn Ther 14:183-188, 1982.
2. Weiss JN, Chen PS, Qu Z, et al: Ventricular fibrillation: How do we stop the waves from breaking? Circ Res 87:1103-1107, 2000.
3. Jalife J, Berenfeld O, Mansour M: Mother rotors and fibrillatory conduction: A mechanism of atrial fibrillation. Cardiovasc Res 54:204-216, 2002.
4. Chen PS, Wu TJ, Ting CT, et al: A tale of two fibrillations. Circulation 108:2298-2303, 2003.
5. Janse MJ, Wit AL: Electrophysiological mechanisms of ventricular arrhythmias resulting from myocardial ischemia and infarction. Physiol Rev 69:1046-1169, 1989.
6. Peters NS, Wit AL: Myocardial architecture and ventricular arrhythmogenesis. Circulation 97:1746-1754, 1998.
7. Weiss JN, Qu Z, Chen PS, et al: The dynamics of cardiac fibrillation. Circulation 112:12321240, 2005.
8. Qu Z, Weiss JN: Dynamics and cardiac arrhythmias. J Cardiovasc Electrophysiol 17:1042-1049, 2006.
9. Noble D: A modification of the Hodgkin-Huxley equations applicable to Purkinje fibre action and pace-maker potentials. J Physiol 160:317-352, 1962.
10. Keizer J, Levine L: Ryanodine receptor adaptation and Ca^{2+}-induced Ca^{2+} release-dependent Ca^{2+} oscillations. Biophys J 71:3477-3487, 1996.
11. Izhikevich EM: Dynamic Systems in Neuroscience. Cambridge, MIT Press, 2007.
12. Koller ML, Riccio ML, Gilmour RF Jr: Dynamic restitution of action potential duration during electrical alternans and ventricular fibrillation. Am J Physiol 275:H1635-H1642, 1998.
13. Goldhaber JI, Xie LH, Duong T, et al: Action potential duration restitution and alternans in rabbit ventricular myocytes: The key role of intracellular calcium cycling. Circ Res 96:459-466, 2005.
14. Franz MR, Swerdlow CD, Liem LB, et al: Cycle length dependence of human action potential duration in vivo: Effects of single extrastimuli, sudden sustained rate acceleration and deceleration, and different steady-state frequencies. J Clin Invest 82:972-979, 1988.
15. Watanabe M, Otani NF, Gilmour RF: Biphasic restitution of action potential duration and complex dynamics in ventricular myocardium. Circ Res 76:915-921, 1995.
16. Nolasco JB, Dahlen RW: A graphic method for the study of alternation in cardiac action potentials. J Appl Physiol 25:191-196, 1968.
17. Guevara MR, Ward G, Shrier A, et al: Electrical alternans and period doubling bifurcations. IEEE Comp Cardiol 562:167-170, 1984.
18. Chialvo DR, Gilmour RF, Jalife J: Low dimensional chaos in cardiac tissue. Nature 343:653-657, 1998.
19. Lewis TJ, Guevara MR: Chaotic dynamics in an ionic model of the propagated cardiac action potential. J Theor Biol 146:407-432, 1990.
20. Qu Z, Shiferaw Y, Weiss JN: Nonlinear dynamics of cardiac excitation-contraction coupling: An iterated map study. Phys Rev E Stat Nonlin Soft Matter Phys 75:011927, 2007.
21. Chudin E, Goldhaber J, Garfinkel A, et al: Intracellular Ca^{2+} dynamics and the stability of ventricular tachycardia. Biophys J 77:2930-2941, 1999.
22. Huser J, Wang YG, Sheehan KA, et al: Functional coupling between glycolysis and excitation-contraction coupling underlies alternans in cat heart cells. J Physiol 524:795-806, 2000.
23. Pruvot E, Katra RP, Rosenbaum DS, et al: Calcium cycling as mechanism of repolarization alternans onset in the intact heart. Circulation 106:191-192, 2002.
24. Eisner DA, Choi HS, Diaz ME, et al: Integrative analysis of calcium cycling in cardiac muscle. Circ Res 87:1087-1094, 2000.
25. Shiferaw Y, Watanabe MA, Garfinkel A, et al: Model of intracellular calcium cycling in ventricular myocytes. Biophys J 85:3666-3686, 2003.
26. Weiss JN, Karma A, Shiferaw Y, et al: From pulsus to pulseless: The saga of cardiac alternans. Circ Res 98:1244-1253, 2006.
27. Shannon TR, Ginsburg KS, Bers DM: Potentiation of fractional sarcoplasmic reticulum calcium release by total and free intra-sarcoplasmic reticulum calcium concentration. Biophys J 78:334-343, 2000.
28. Bers DM: Excitation-Contraction Coupling and Cardiac Contractile Force. 2nd ed. Dordrecht, Kluwer Academic Publishers, 2001.
29. Shiferaw Y, Sato D, Karma A: Coupled dynamics of voltage and calcium in paced

cardiac cells. Phys Rev E Stat Nonlin Soft Matter Phys 71(2 Pt 1):021903, 2005.
30. Otani NF, Gilmour RF: Memory models for the electrical properties of local cardiac systems. J Theor Biol 187:409-436, 1997.
31. Pastore JM, Girouard SD, Laurita KR, et al: Mechanism linking T-wave alternans to the genesis of cardiac fibrillation. Circulation 99:1385-1394, 1999.
32. Cao JM, Qu Z, Kim YH, et al: Spatiotemporal heterogeneity in the induction of ventricular fibrillation by rapid pacing: Importance of cardiac restitution properties. Circ Res 84:1318-1331, 1999.
33. Qu Z, Garfinkel A, Chen PS, et al: Mechanisms of discordant alternans and induction of reentry in simulated cardiac tissue. Circulation 102:1664-1670, 2000.
34. Watanabe MA, Fenton FH, Evans SJ, et al: Mechanisms for discordant alternans. J Cardiovasc Electrophysiol 12:196-206, 2001.
35. Xie Y, Hu G, Sato D, et al: Dispersion of refractoriness and induction of reentry due to chaos synchronization in a model of cardiac tissue. Phys Rev Lett 99:118101, 2007.
36. Winfree AT: Electrical instability in cardiac muscle: Phase singularities and rotors. J Theor Biol 138:353-405, 1989.
37. Clayton RH, Holden AV: Dispersion of cardiac action potential duration and the initiation of reentry: A computational study. Biomed Eng Online 4:11, 2005.
38. Qu Z, Garfinkel A, Weiss JN: Vulnerable window for conduction block in a one-dimensional cable of cardiac cells, 1: Single extrasystoles. Biophys J 91:793-804, 2006.
39. Laurita KR, Rosenbaum DS: Interdependence of modulated dispersion and tissue structure in the mechanism of unidirectional block. Circ Res 87:922-928, 2000.
40. Tran DX, Yang M-J, Weiss JN, et al: Vulnerability to reentry in simulated two-dimensional cardiac tissue: Effects of electrical restitution and stimulation sequence. Chaos 7(4):043115, 2007.
41. Courtemanche M: Complex spiral wave dynamics in a spatially distributed ionic model of cardiac electrical activity. Chaos 6:579-600, 1996.
42. Qu Z, Xie F, Garfinkel A, et al: Origins of spiral wave meander and breakup in a two-dimensional cardiac tissue model. Ann Biomed Eng 28:755-771, 2000.
43. Garfinkel A, Kim YH, Voroshilovsky O, et al: Preventing ventricular fibrillation by flattening cardiac restitution. Proc Natl Acad Sci U S A 97:6061-6066, 2000.
44. Riccio ML, Koller ML, Gilmour RF Jr: Electrical restitution and spatiotemporal organization during ventricular fibrillation. Circ Res 84:955-963, 1999.
45. Ten Tusscher KH, Panfilov AV: Reentry in heterogeneous cardiac tissue described by the Luo-Rudy ventricular action potential model. Am J Physiol Heart Circ Physiol 284:H542-H548, 2003.
46. Qu Z, Weiss JN: Effects of Na^+ and K^+ channel blockade on vulnerability to and termination of fibrillation in simulated normal cardiac tissue. Am J Physiol Heart Circ Physiol 289:H1692-H1701, 2005.
47. Xie F, Qu Z, Garfinkel A, et al: Electrophysiological heterogeneity and stability of reentry in simulated cardiac tissue. Am J Physiol Heart Circ Physiol 280:H535-H545, 2001.
48. Xie FG, Qu ZL, Weiss JN, et al: Coexistence of multiple spiral waves with independent frequencies in a heterogeneous excitable medium. Phys Rev E 63:031905, 2001.
49. Qu Z, Kil J, Xie F, et al: Scroll wave dynamics in a three-dimensional cardiac tissue model: Roles of restitution, thickness, and fiber rotation. Biophys J 78:2761-2775, 2000.
50. Qu Z, Xie F, Garfinkel A: Diffusion-induced 3-dimensional vortex filament instability in excitable media. Phys Rev Lett 83:2668-2671, 1999.
51. Alonso S, Panfilov AV: Negative filament tension in the Luo-Rudy model of cardiac tissue. Chaos 17:015102, 2007.
52. Manoach M, Varon D, Neuman M, et al: Spontaneous termination and initiation of ventricular fibrillation as a function of heart size, age, autonomic autoregulation, and drugs: A comparative study on different species of different age. Heart Vessels Suppl 2:56-68, 1987.
53. Naccarelli GV, Wolbrette DL, Khan M, et al: Old and new antiarrhythmic drugs for converting and maintaining sinus rhythm in atrial fibrillation: Comparative efficacy and results of trials. Am J Cardiol 91:15D-26D, 2003.
54. Garrey W: The nature of fibrillatory contraction of the heart: Its relation to tissue mass and form. Am J Physiol 33:397-414, 1914.
55. Goy JJ, Maendly R, Grbic M, et al: Cardioversion with flecainide in patients with atrial fibrillation of recent onset. Eur J Clin Pharmacol 27:737-738, 1985.
56. Wijffels M, Dorland R, Mast F, et al: Widening of the excitable gap during pharmacological cardioversion of atrial fibrillation in the goat—effects of cibenzoline, hydroquinidine, flecainide, and D-sotalol. Circulation 102:260-267, 2000.
57. Qu Z: Critical mass hypothesis revisited: Role of dynamic wave stability in spontaneous termination of cardiac fibrillation. Am J Physiol Heart Circ Physiol 290:H255-H263, 2006.
58. Kneller J, Kalifa J, Zou R, et al: Mechanisms of AF termination by pure sodium channel blockade in an ionically-realistic mathematical model. Circ Res 96:e35-e47, 2005.
59. Yamazaki M, Honjo H, Nakagawa H, et al: Mechanisms of destabilization and early termination of spiral wave reentry in the ventricle by a class III antiarrhythmic agent, nifekalant. Am J Physiol Heart Circ Physiol 292:H539-H548, 2007.
60. Banville I, Gray RA: Effect of action potential duration and conduction velocity restitution and their spatial dispersion on alternans and the stability of arrhythmias. J Cardiovasc Electrophysiol 13:1141-1149, 2002.
61. Allessie M, Ausma J, Schotten U: Electrical, contractile and structural remodeling during atrial fibrillation. Cardiovasc Res 54:230-246, 2002.
62. Wijffels M, Kirchhof C, Dorland R, et al: Atrial fibrillation begets atrial fibrillation—a study in awake chronically instrumented goats. Circulation 92:1954-1968, 1995.

Rotors and Spiral Waves in the Heart 33

RICHARD A. GRAY

CHAPTER OUTLINE

The study of the mechanisms underlying cardiac arrhythmias has a long history. In this chapter I provide a review and comparison of some of this research, focusing on data collected directly from experimental models involving whole hearts during sustained, unstable, ventricular tachyarrhythmias, most notably ventricular fibrillation (VF). Simultaneous recordings from many sites are required to capture the spatiotemporal complexity of these unstable tachyarrhythmias; therefore, I concentrate on recordings from extracellular electrode arrays and from optical mapping systems using voltage-sensitive dyes. I do not review the extensive data collected from isolated cells, cardiac monolayers, or isolated ventricular or septum preparations; torsades de points; the extensive literature of the theory of wave propagation and spiral waves; or the numerous relevant numerical simulations, which are discussed elsewhere in the book. This chapter begins with an explanation of Wiggers stages of VF and a discussion of phase mapping and rotors, followed by a review of the literature of the spatial patterns of electrical activity in the heart during tachyarrhythmias from a variety of experimental models in mouse, guinea pig, rabbit, dog, pig, and human.

Stages of Ventricular Fibrillation

The first detailed spatiotemporal description of the events occurring in the intact heart during VF was presented in the landmark paper by Carl Wiggers in 1930.[1] Moving pictures from the surface of hearts in open-chest dogs illuminated by three 1000-watt lamps were taken using a Bell-Howell camera on 16-mm film at a rate of 32 exposures per second. Wiggers performed the first meticulous, in depth optical-mapping study by repeated visualization of the reflections from the glistening epicardial surface resulting from mechanical contractions evident in the slow-motion replays of the VF movies. He found that VF induction caused a decrease in aortic pressure accompanied by an immediate cessation of oscillations and that VF lasted an average of 24 minutes before complete standstill. Wiggers characterized his observations into temporal phases and introduced the now-classic four stages of fibrillation.[1]

Wiggers called stage 1 the *initial tachysystolic phenomena*, which lasts less than 1 second and is characterized by 2 to 8 peristaltic waves that sweep rapidly over the entire heart surface. These waves are accompanied by large electrocardiogram (ECG) deflections whose amplitude decreases beat to beat while the rate increases (cycle length [CL] is 80-100 ms). These beats are accompanied by oscillations of left ventricle (LV) pressure of decreasing magnitude.

Stage 2, *convulsive incoordination*, is 15 to 40 seconds in duration. The global sequence of contraction is much less regular, and the frequency of contraction increases locally. Sequential contraction waves follow different paths and involve different regions of the heart, and the frequencies vary spatially and bear no relation to each other. The ECG is characterized by large oscillations that vary considerably in amplitude, period, and shape with cycle length between 90 and 100 ms, although sometimes much more rapid deflections are observed (but do not correlate to observed contractions).

Stage 3, *tremulous incoordination*, lasts 2 to 3 minutes, and contraction waves spread rapidly and only over short distances. Wiggers provides a particularly vivid description of this stage: "Reflected light beams from the epicardium give the impression of darting wriggling worms of contraction waves chasing each other in circles." The ECG oscillations in stage 3 decrease in magnitude and increase in frequency, although the frequency of contractions on the heart surface is about the same as in stage 2.

In Stage 4, *progressive atonic incoordination*, the visible waves become coarser and slower and spread only over a small area of epicardium. Regions begin to stop moving until only areas near coronary vessels are contracting. The ECG oscillations actually increase (CL, ~110 ms) before decreasing in amplitude and frequency (CL, ~160ms), eventually leading to flatline.

Phase Mapping, Phase Singularities, and Rotors

Wiggers's high spatial and temporal recordings (i.e., movies) of the *mechanical* contractions from the heart surface using the Bell-Howell camera led to the pioneering insights and classifications of the stages of VF. Similarly, voltage-sensitive dyes and fluorescence imaging with high-speed video charge coupled device (CCD) cameras has allowed the visualization of the complex spatiotemporal *electrical* events during VF.

Gray and colleagues recorded transmembrane activity from 20,000 sites on the surface of isolated rabbit and sheep hearts during sustained VF using a CCD camera running at 120 frames per second.[2] Fluorescence recordings from the heart surface during VF exhibited action potentials of irregular shape, duration, and interval. The frequency content of these signals computed using the Fourier transform exhibited a narrow-banded spectrum centered near 8 Hz (CL, 125 ms). Gray developed a novel approach to visualize and analyze these data using the fact that "transmembrane signals (F) recorded from the surface of rabbit and sheep hearts during fibrillation exhibited attractors in reconstructed two-dimensional phase space, when $F(t)$ was plotted against $F(t+\tau)$ where t is time and τ is the embedding delay."[2] A unique *phase* variable (θ) was computed at each site (x,y) based on state space encoding, defined as:

$$\theta(x, y, t) = arctan(F(t + \tau) - F^*, F(t) - F^*) \quad [1]$$

where F^* loosely represents a threshold. In this study, F^* was the mean value of 4 seconds of VF and was computed at each site.

State space encoding (as opposed to temporal encoding) was necessary because VF intervals vary over space and time, making a global interpretation of the relative *time* differences meaningless. In state space encoding, each suprathreshold action potential (presumably corresponding to a propagating impulse) circulates around the state space origin (F^*, F^*) and exhibits a phase change equal to 2π, independent of the value of the VF interval as shown in Figure 33-1. In contrast, subthreshold activations (presumably corresponding to nonpropagating waves) do not circulate around the origin and thus do not undergo a full range of phase ($<2\pi$). This state space representation of phase at each site is critical to the interpretation and analysis of the spatial patterns of phase during VF.

Gray's phase-mapping approach (i.e., transforming spatiotemporal movies of fluorescence amplitude to phase) provides the ability to identify the tips of reentrant waves as phase singularities (Fig. 33-2). "A spatial phase singularity is a site in an excitable medium at which the phase of the site is arbitrary; the neighboring elements exhibit a continuous progression of phase that is equal to $\pm 2\pi$ around this site."[2] A phase singularity is defined mathematically as the line integral of the change in phase around the singularity point equal to $\pm 2\pi$ (i.e., $\int d\theta = \pm 2\pi$); at all other sites this line integral is equal to zero (i.e., $\int d\theta = 0$).

One major advantage of analyzing phase singularities dynamics (e.g., formation, termination, movement) using this approach is that it allows the study of these phenomena on a time scale much less than the VF interval, allowing Gray's group to elucidate the mechanism of rotor formation and termination by analyzing successive frames of $\theta(x,y,t)$. It is very important to keep in mind that a phase singularity is a necessary but not sufficient condition for a rotor: only a fraction of phase singularities last for more than one rotation and become the organizing center for a rotor. The following description and the schematic in Figure 33-3 illustrating the formation of a pair of counter-rotating rotors should help clarify this issue.

Figure 33-3 shows a wave front (black solid line) propagating from right to left into a region of nonuniform recovery. The wave encounters refractory tissue in the center and blocks, instantly giving rise to two phase singularities around which the wave continues to propagate. The upper portion of the wave propagates counterclockwise around the phase singularity of negative charge ($\int d\theta = -2\pi$), and the lower portion of the wave propagates clockwise around the phase singularity of positive charge ($\int d\theta = +2\pi$). As the central isthmus area recovers, both the upper and lower wave fragments merge together and continue to propagate to the left. If the source-sink relationship in the isthmus between the two singularities does favor regenerative propagation in the retrograde direction (from left to right in this case) then two new rotors are formed. However, if the source-sink relationship in the isthmus between the two singularities does not favor regenerative propagation in the retrograde direction, then no rotors are formed. That is, there is a wave break resulting from regional conduction block associated with two phase singularities of opposite chirality (i.e., rotation direction), but this event by itself is not proarrhythmic, specifically, no new reentrant waves are generated.

The critical event for rotor (not phase singularity) initiation occurs within the isthmus in the form of a newly generated wave propagating in the retrograde direction. That is, a new wave has been introduced into the heart and connects the two opposite chirality phase singularities through the isthmus, resulting in a counter-rotating rotor pair. Rotor termination is similar and "occurs when rotors of opposite chirality merge or when a single rotor collides with a boundary (both of these occurrences are topologically equivalent for a non-flux boundary). Specifically, rotor pairs are mutually annihilated if the phase gradient between the rotors, perpendicular to the line connecting the phase singularities, is sufficiently large to stop propagation."[2] In fact, every time the wave connecting the rotors travels through the corresponding isthmus (which can move and change shape considerably) the source-sink relationship must favor regenerative propagation for this rotor pair to survive. Therefore, it is rotors (not phase singularities) that are the elements sustaining functional reentry and thus, presumably, driving VF.

Gray and colleagues state, "Lifespan histograms for both rabbits and sheep indicate that the majority (80% for rabbit and 84% for sheep) of phase singularities lasted <100 ms, which is less than one rotation. Therefore, only ~20% of phase singularities formed rotors."[2] They computed the density of rotors (not phase singularities) on the epicardial surface as one rotor per 12 ± 4 cm^2 and thus estimated the number of epicardial rotors in fibrillation as one or two in rabbits, about five in sheep, and about 15 in humans.

Animal Models

Protocols and Definitions

The specific experiments reviewed here result from a variety of animal preparations, and protocol specifics are important to keep in mind.[3-6] Some of the details are provided in the text below, and more details regarding the specific methodology are contained in the original manuscripts. All data are from the epicardium unless stated otherwise. The optical mapping data were recorded from either a photo-diode-array or a CCD camera, and the fluorescence dye, di-4-ANEPPS was used unless stated otherwise.

Wavelength has been defined two ways: as the product of action potential duration (APD) and conduction velocity (CV) and as the product of CL and CV (technically, CV is a vector, and the direction is included if published; wave speed is also used if originally used by the authors). I identify the particular wavelength definition in each case and convert all frequencies to CL for comparison purposes. I use the terms "rotor," "reentry," and "reentrant wave" interchangeably in this chapter, although they can be considered synonymous with "spiral wave" or "scroll wave" (specifically, a three-dimensional spiral wave).

Mouse

Optical mapping from the isolated Langendorff-perfused mouse heart model has provided insight into the mechanisms of tachyarrhythmias in very small hearts. Vaidya and coworkers showed that polymorphic ventricular tachycardia (PVT) and VF could be initiated by burst pacing in four of seven hearts, two without diacetyl monoxime (BDM) and two with BDM in which limited mapping did not demonstrate any rotors.[7] They also found that monomorphic ventricular tachycardia (MVT) with cycle length about 70 ms could be initiated by burst pacing in all hearts, and mapping always revealed rotors.

One major advantage of the mouse model is the ability for gene manipulation. Vaidya and colleagues showed that neonatal connexin43 knockout hearts were arrhythmic in vivo as well as ex vivo; during PVT, a transient rotor of three rotations was

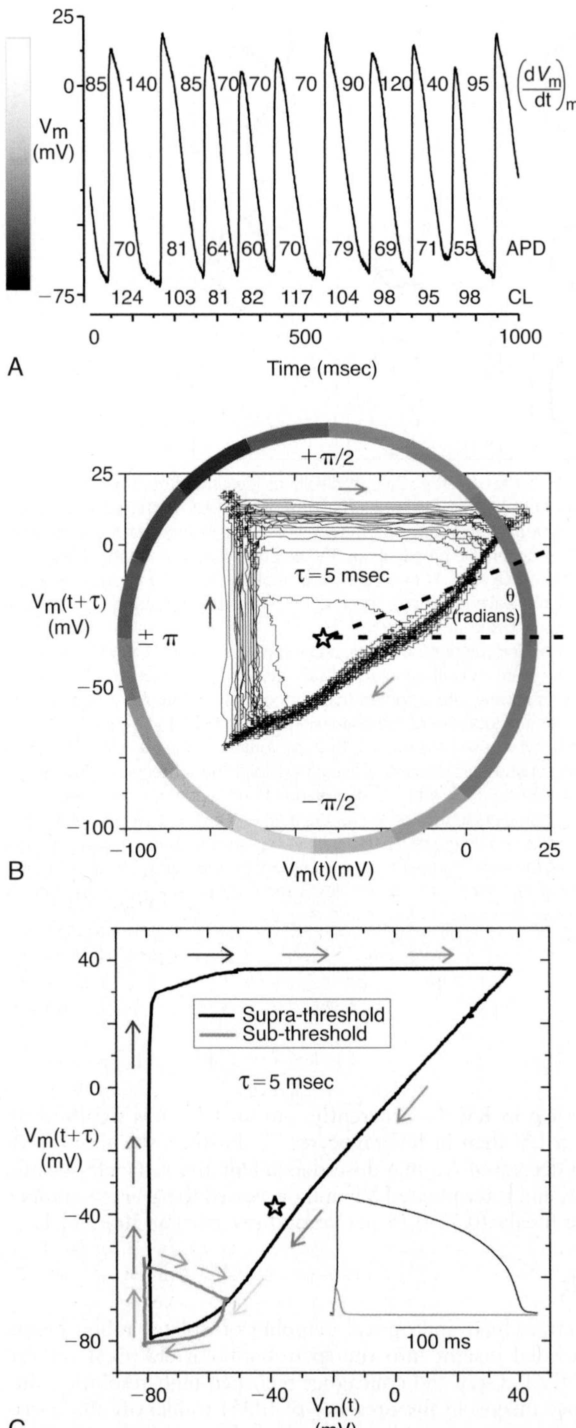

Figure 33-1 Microelectrode recordings: amplitude and phase. **A,** Transmembrane potential (V_m) recording in mV from the surface of an isolated rabbit heart during ventricular fibrillation. The cycle length, action potential duration, and $(dV_m/dt)_{max}$ values are shown for each beat in milliseconds. The grayscale bar to the *left* is the color scale for amplitude (see Fig. 33-2). **B,** The signal in **A** plotted in reconstructed state space, i.e. $V_m(t+\tau)$ versus $V_m(t)$. The phase variable θ is computed as $\arctan[V_m(t+\tau) - V^*, V_m(t) - V^*]$. The *star* in **B** and **C** represents (V^*,V^*), and τ represents the embedding delay, which here is equal to 5 ms. The *ring* represents the color scale for phase and is circular due to the periodic nature of the arctan function. The *arrows* (colored according to phase) indicate the flow of time and the direction of the state space trajectories; i.e., depolarization (upstroke) lies above the 45-degree line passing through (V^*,V^*) because $V_m(t+\tau) > V_m(t)$, and repolarization occurs below the same 45-degree line because $V_m(t+\tau) < V_m(t)$. **C,** V_m recording from an isolated cardiac myocyte at stimuli of 1.1 times threshold (suprathreshold, *black lines*) and 0.9 times threshold (subthreshold, *magenta lines*) plotted in reconstructed state space; the *inset* shows the corresponding time series traces.

observed.[8] Noujaim's group used optical mapping in isolated transgenic mice overexpressing the rectifying potassium current I_{K1}.[9] They showed that these mice were able to sustain stable VT or VF for an average of 5.8 minutes with cycle length of 23 ms, whereas tachyarrhythmias in wild-type hearts were short-lived (3 sec) with cycle length of 38 ms.

Cerrone and colleagues used epicardial and endocardial optical mapping in a ryanodine receptor (RyR2) knockin mouse model to investigate the mechanisms of catecholaminergic PVT.[10] During perfusion with high calcium and isoproterenol, spontaneous ventricular arrhythmias occurred in seven of 13 RyR2 hearts but only one of 11 wild-type hearts; in hearts perfused with caffeine and epinephrine, eight of 12 RyR hearts and two of 10 wild-type hearts showed spontaneous arrhythmias. "Epicardial mapping showed that monomorphic VT, bidirectional VT, and polymorphic VT manifested as concentric epicardial breakthrough patterns, suggesting a focal origin in the His-Purkinje networks of either or both ventricles."[10] PVT eventually became reentrant on the epicardium and degenerated into ventricular fibrillation. Endocardial mapping demonstrated the origin of the focal arrhythmias as Purkinje fibers and chemical ablation of the right ventricular endocardium induced complete right bundle branch block.

Guinea Pig

The isolated perfused guinea pig heart model has also been used extensively to study tachyarrhythmias via optical mapping. Pastore and coworkers showed rate-dependent APD alternans that were spatially discordant at rapid rates and that "in the presence of discordant alternans, a small acceleration of pacing cycle length produced a characteristic sequence of events: unidirectional block of an impulse propagating against steep gradients of repolarization, reentrant propagation, and the initiation of ventricular fibrillation."[11] In hearts perfused with the dye

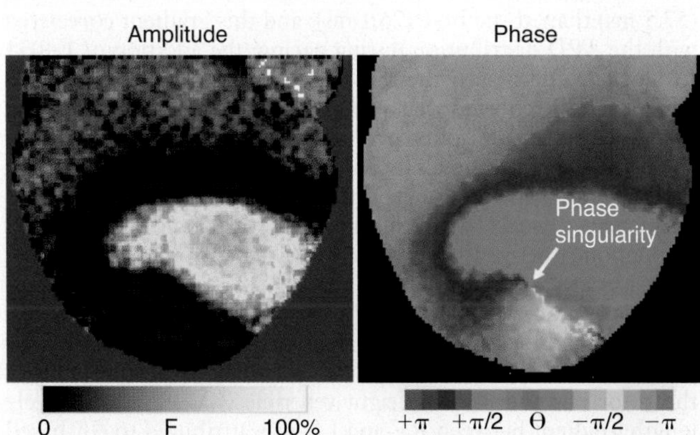

Figure 33-2 Rotor: amplitude and phase. The epicardial spatial pattern of fluorescence amplitude, F(x,y,), is shown in grayscale *(left)* and phase $\theta(x,y)$ in color *(right)* during reentry in the isolated rabbit heart.

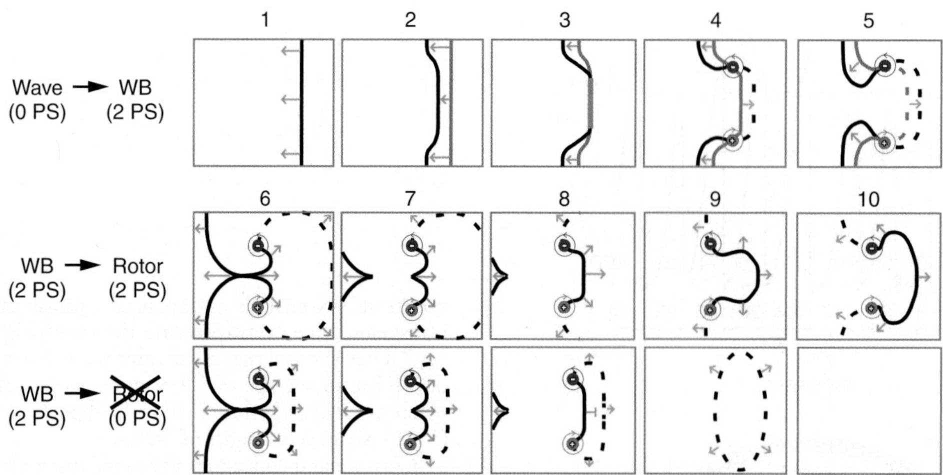

Figure 33-3 Rotor formation (schematic). *Top,* The sequence of events during wave break (WB) formation. The wave is initially propagating from right to left. The numbers above each panel represent time (t), the *thick lines* represent the isopotential line at threshold (V*), the solid portion represents depolarization (specifically $dV_m/dt > 0$ at $V_m = V^*$), and the *dashed portion* represents repolarization ($dV_m/dt < 0$ at $V_m = V^*$). The *gray thick lines* represent the position of the isopotential at the previous time. The *cyan arrows* indicate the conduction vector of the wave front (active depolarization and regenerative propagation). The *orange arrows* indicate the direction of repolarization. PS stands for phase singularity. At t = 1, only the uniformly propagating wave front can be seen. At t = 2, the wave front encounters a partially refractory region near the center slowing down propagation, but only in the middle of the wave. At t = 3, the wave front splits (breaks), propagating at the top and bottom as before but being blocked in the central region as this portion of the wave front encounters refractory tissue; at this instant, $dV_m/dt = 0$ at $V_m = V^*$ in this central line of block *(magenta).* At this time, repolarization ($dV_m/dt < 0$) begins creating a significant V_m gradient behind the previously propagating wave front, and the V* isopotential moves to the right either by passive diffusion or active repolarization. Previous to time t = 3, no sites were repolarizating, specifically $dV_m/dt \geq 0$ everywhere. At t = 4 the V* isopotential is made up of two parts, the depolarization portion ($dV_m/dt > 0$), shown as a *solid black line,* and a portion that is repolarization ($dV_m/dt < 0$), shown as *dashed black line.* At two sites at either end of the line of block, $dV_m/dt = 0$ at $V_m = V^*$, and these are the locations of the phase singularities, indicated by a *plus sign* and *minus sign* inside a *red* or *blue circle* corresponding to the wave front rotation direction (phase chirality). At t = 5, the top and bottom portions of the wave front continue propagating to the left but also curl inward due to the lower V_m in the center, and repolarization continues as before to the right. *Bottom,* The subsequent sequence of events (t = 6 to 10) for the case of rotor formation in the upper row and for no rotor formation in the bottom row. At t = 6, the top and bottom portions of the wave front *(black solid lines)* merge at the center (same for *upper* and *bottom panels*), resulting in a wave front propagating to the left (antegrade) and a wave fragment moving to the right (retrograde). More tissue has recovered in the *upper panel* (compared to the *bottom*) as indicated by the distance between the wave front *(black solid line, cyan arrows)* and tail *(black dashed line, orange arrows)* in the *right half* of the panel. In the upper row, the wave fragment actively propagates (due to the large recovered region) to the right through the central isthmus (original line of block, *magenta*), generating a pair of rotors (t = 7 to 10). See Figs. 3 and 4 in Gray et al[2] for an example of rotor pair formation and corresponding phase maps during ventricular fibrillation. In the *bottom row,* rotors are not formed because the wave dies out due to the small recovered region (t = 7 to 10).

RH-421, Salama and colleagues found that activation patterns during VT were similar to patterns recorded during direct pacing of the ventricles and that during VT, at a cycle length of 100 ms, APD was 60 to 105 ms with no diastolic interval (DI), and CV decreased by 68% compared to pacing.[12]

During VF in guinea pig hearts stained with di-4-ANEPPS, Choi's group found that VF cycle length was shorter at the apex (57.5 ms) than at the base (76.1 ms), and this gradient correlated with the APD distribution during pacing; the addition of E4031 to block I_{Kr} decreased the VF rate.[13] In the same preparation, Choi's group reported that wave breaks during VF occurred at a frequency of 5.8 splits per second per cm^2 and found no correlation of wave break location and coronary vessels.[14]

Samie and coworkers reported that during VF, "dominant frequencies (peak with maximal power) were distributed throughout the ventricles in clearly demarcated domains."[15] The average VF cycle length was 38 ms on the anterior left LV wall and was the result of persistent rotor activity. Intermittent block and wave breaks occurred at the periphery of rotors, and the VF cycle length was longer (66 ms) outside the rotor periphery in the right ventricle (RV). This VF cycle length gradient between RV and LV was attributed to I_{K1} based on patch-clamp data from ventricular myocytes.[15]

A follow-up study by Jalife's group also found that "mRNA levels for Kir2.1 and Kir2.3 were significantly larger in LV than in RV. Concurrently, outward I_{K1} was significantly larger in LV than in RV myocytes."[16] Further, the addition of barium decreased I_{K1} in a dose-dependent and ventricle-specific manner, and it terminated VF and decreased the average number of wave breaks (0.52-0.25 per second per cm^2) at 50 μmol/L.

Rabbit

Both extracellular and optical mapping of isolated rabbit hearts has provided insight into the spatiotemporal electrical activity during PVT. Gray and colleagues recorded high-resolution fluorescence images in the presence of BDM to identify the transmembrane patterns on the epicardium during MVT and PVT. "We identified the organizing centers of the reentrant circuits on the epicardial surface during polymorphic tachycardia, and these centers moved during the episodes. In addition, the arrhythmias that showed the greatest movement of the reentrant centers displayed the largest changes in QRS morphology."[17] They found that MVT and PVT in the healthy, isolated rabbit heart was the result of either a single or paired (figure-of-eight) rotor. Cycle length in the majority of episodes was about 150 ms, and one episode revealed 2:1 block at base with reentry near apex.

Banville and Gray found that stable reentry (CL, 139 ms; APD, 87 ms) resulted when the perfusate contained BDM (>20 mM) whereas nonstable nonsustained reentry (CL, 157 ms; APD, 109 ms) occurred in the presence of cytochalsin D.[18] Allessie's group has performed extracellular mapping in isolated rabbit hearts before and after a cyroabalation procedure that resulted in a surviving rim of epicardial tissue. Schalij and colleagues found that only VF could be induced in the intact hearts and only MVT with cycle length of 130 ms could be initiated after cyroablation.[19]

Boersma and colleagues state "During regional cooling, episodes of polymorphic VT with a maximum duration of 35 seconds could be induced in all hearts. High-resolution mapping (229 electrodes) of epicardial activation revealed that polymorphic VT was caused by a functional reentrant circuit located partially within the region of prolonged refractoriness. The reentrant wavefront was continuously shifting along the border of the cooled region, resulting in beat-to-beat changes in the excitation pattern."[20] The cycle length of these PVT episodes was approximately 150 ms.

Kodama and coworkers studied rotor behavior via optical mapping on the surviving epicardial rim of the rabbit heart in the presence of BDM (15 mM); rotors were observed with cycle length of 152 ms in control hearts.[21] They found that pilsicainide (5 μM) increased cycle length by 24%, decreased CV by 35%, and increased the functional line of block (similar results were obtained with disopyramide and cibenzoline). Nifekalant (0.1 μM) increased rotor cycle length to 172 ms, increased APD (up to 25%), and destabilized reentry because of an increase in wave front-tail interactions. Amiodarone (5 μM) increased rotor cycle length by 25%, reduced CV and increased APD by about 10%, and dramatically decreased VT duration.

The high spatial resolution of CCD video imaging has been instrumental in elucidating the patterns on the heart surface during VF. Gray and colleagues provided a novel mechanism for VF by demonstrating that a single rotor could give rise to the initial stages of fibrillation if it was moving rapidly throughout the heart.[22] They observed rotors moving at speeds greater than 30% of the wave speed, and the ratio of the rotor and wave speeds is related in a nonlinear fashion to the range of periods (therefore frequencies) throughout the heart during VF; this relationship is expressed mathematically via the Doppler effect. We concluded that "our data demonstrate that the Doppler phenomenon provides a robust mechanistic explanation for the narrow-banded frequency spectra characteristic of fibrillation that has perplexed investigators for many years."[22]

Kwaku and Dillon mapped VF optically with the dye WW781 and found that VF cycle length was 66 ms and increased slightly with D600 to 74 ms. During VF, propagation never occurred for activations occurring at less than 50% VF cycle length, about half propagated at 60% VF cycle length, and about 90% propagated at VF cycle length of 75% and above.[23]

Chen and colleagues mapped VF without uncouplers and observed rotors (CL, 80 ms) on the epicardial surface in only 3 of 24 episodes.[24] They found that the average lifespan of wave breaks was very short (14.7 ms), and only 2% lasted for at least one rotation.

A variety of manipulations during VF have been performed in an effort to better understand VF mechanisms. Mandapati and coworkers studied VF activation patterns during global ischemia and during perfusion with tetrodotoxin (TTX) without any uncoupling drugs.[25] VF cycle length during control was 73 ms; it increased to 108 ms after 5 minutes of global ischemia and increased to 143 ms after 2 min of TTX infusion. They found that the rotor period observed on the epicardium strongly correlated with the inverse of the dominant frequency of the simultaneously acquired global ECG. The rotor core area was measured as 0.053 cm^2 during control and increased during both global ischemia (0.136 cm^2) and TTX perfusion (0.168 cm^2). In addition, the density of wave fronts decreased during both global ischemia and TTX perfusion compared with control. They concluded that "similar findings in the TTX protocol suggest that reduced excitability during ischemia is an important underlying mechanism for the changes seen."[25]

Chorro and colleagues electrically mapped VF and the effects of perfusion with flecainide, sotalol, and verapamil.[26] They found that VF cycle length ranged from 64 to 80 ms in control and increased with flecainide and sotalol but decreased with verapamil; CV during VF was about 45 cm/sec and decreased with flecainide and sotalol but did not change with verapamil. They showed that the functional refractory period during VF was 41 to 47 ms and increased with flecainide and sotalol but decreased with verapamil, and wavelength (computed as the product of CV and the functional refractory period) during VF was about 2 cm and increased with flecainide and sotalol but decreased with verapamil. In addition, they demonstrated that "flecainide and sotalol increased the circuit size of the reentrant activations, whereas verapamil decreased it. The 3 drugs significantly reduced the percentages of more complex activation maps during VF."[26]

Samie's group[27] recorded VF optically with no uncouplers during verapamil (1 mg/L) infusion. The addition of verapamil to the perfusate during sustained VF (CL, 62 ms) always resulted in the conversion to reentrant MVT (CL, 74 ms) with a concomitant decrease in wave break density from 1.04/cm^2 to 0.32/cm^2 and increase in core size from 0.045 cm^2 to 0.092 cm^2.

Wu and colleagues confirmed these findings (and those of Mandapati with TTX)[25] but also found that even higher concentrations of verapamil (2-5 mg/L) converted VT to slow VF (CL, 84 ms).[28] A follow-up study showed that this slow VF resulted from a single rotor that "either slowly drifted or intermittently anchored on the papillary muscle of the left ventricle" or from an epicardial breakthrough pattern.[29]

Choi and coworkers demonstrated that nifedipine organized VF by reducing the number of wave fronts.[30]

Chorro and colleagues studied the effect of compartmentalizing the ventricles with radiofrequency (RF) lesions "comprising: (1) the posterior zone of the septum and of the walls of both ventricles (n = 10); (2) the anterior zone of the septum and of the walls of both ventricles (n = 11); and (3) the midseptal zone (n = 10)." For complete isolation of the zones, VF could not be induced from within the zone in one of 16, but it could be induced from outside the zone in 15 of 16 with similar results for partial isolation.[31] Reentry was observed in 11% of their VF activation maps.

Dog

Studies in Normal Dogs

Numerous electrical mapping studies have been performed in open-chest normal dogs in which VF initiation halts blood flow so VF is accompanied by a decrease in tissue function as it progresses. Early studies with only sparse epicardial coverage suggested that the first few beats during VF initiation (resulting from strong premature stimuli) appeared to be reentrant,[32,33] and dispersion of refractory periods provides a substrate for the initiation of tachyarrhythmias.[34,35] The development of extracellular arrays with hundreds of electrodes as exemplified by Ideker's group has led to many insights into the spatiotemporal patterns on the heart during tachyarrhythmias. Because the dynamics of VF in the healthy open-chest dogs change dramatically within the first minute of VF, the specifics of exactly when the data were collected is presented.[1]

Cao's group found that the induction of VF was associated with oscillations of cycle length response to pacing that exhibited spatial variation (the pacing cycle length that induced VF was 174 ms).[36] A critical increase in conduction time of 20 ms was required for VF, implicating the importance of CV restitution as well as APD restitution.

Cha and colleagues looked at the first seconds of VF initiated via a strong premature stimulus and found that reentry with a cycle length of 118 ms was observed. Eight of 60 episodes had more than 10 cycles, and the other episodes had an average of 3.2 cycles, conduction block occurred across fibers, and the refractory period was about 60 ms, but there were normally 91 ms between activations, demonstrating strong evidence for an excitable gap.[37] They showed similar results after endocardial ablation via Lugol solution, for which reentry cycle length was 124 ms: 10 of 57 episodes had more than 10 cycles, others averaged 3.1 cycles.

During the first 3 seconds of VF, Ohara and coworkers found that VF cycle length was 131 to 134 ms, longitudinal CV was 53 cm/sec, and transverse CV was 37 cm/sec. Rotors were observed eight to 10 times in each 3-second episode, rotor core perimeter was 3 cm, and rotor period was 100 to 105 ms.[38] In the epicardial border zone of healed infarcts, the numbers of waves increased, CV decreased, VF cycle length was unchanged, and rotor incidence increased (rotor incidence also increased outside the border zone).

Lee and colleagues recorded episodes of 3 to 5 seconds' duration starting 2.5 sec after VF initiation and found rotors with cycle length of 107 ms in 12 of 45 runs that had core size of 2.9 cm and average life spans of 3.2 cycles. Similar results were found following endocardial ablation.[39] Kwan's group also recorded episodes of 3 to 5 seconds' duration starting 2.5 sec after VF initiation and found VF cycle length of 101 ms, CV of 93 cm/sec, refractory period of 54 ms, wavelength (refractory period × CV) of 5.1 cm, and wave density of 7.25/cm^2 per second.[40] They found that procainamide altered these values: VF cycle length was 125 ms, CV was 42 cm/sec, refractory period was 119 ms, wavelength was 5 cm, and wave density was 4.45/cm^2 per second.

Damle and colleagues recorded during the first 10 sec of VF and studied the ability of spatial and temporal information to predict future VF patterns. Patterns were organized with spatial information being more predictive than temporal information, and predictability decreased from r = 0.75 initially to r = 0.62 after 6 to 7 seconds of VF.[41]

Huang and coworkers recorded data from the first 20 seconds of VF and found that VF cycle length was 122 ms, wave speed was 54 cm/sec, rotor core perimeter was 4.2 cm, wavelength (CV × CL) was 6.6 cm. They demonstrated that both acute and chronic amiodarone decreased VF cycle length to 172 ms and wave speed to 42 cm/sec.[42] "In the mapped region, acute and chronic amiodarone decreased the number of VF wavefronts by 42% and 60%. Acute amiodarone decreased conduction block by 22%, while chronic amiodarone increased block by 41% but decreased wave fractionation by 50%. Both chronic and acute amiodarone increased the size of the core of reentrant circuits and decreased the incidence of reentry by 44% and 57%; however, chronic amiodarone increased wavelength, while acute amiodarone did not."[42]

Zhou and colleagues recorded from floating microelectrodes during the first 20 seconds of VF and found that VF cycle length was 86 ms and APD_{50} (APD at 50% of repolarization) was 64 ms.[43] Chen's group reported VF cycle length of 92 ms after 20 seconds of VF.[44]

At 1 minute after VF initiation, Cha and colleagues found that VF cycle length for LV (127 ms) was longer than for RV (123 ms) and the endocardial cycle length was significantly shorter for both ventricles (LV, 102 ms; RV, 114 ms) compared to the epicardium. Endocardial ablation eliminated the epicardial-endocardial gradient on the RV but not the LV.[45]

Newton and coworkers used plunge needles to study the transmural activation gradient during VF and found that VF cycle length was shortest at the epicardium and longest at the endocardium for the first 70 seconds but reversed by 2 minutes.[46]

Opthof and colleagues found during VF on cardiopulmonary bypass that VF cycle length was 86 ms more than 10 minutes after VF initiation and that VF cycle length was altered by stellate ganglion stimulation with spatial variability in effects.[47] They also found a significant relationship between VF cycle length and refractory periods during pacing.

Effects of Ischemia and Infarction

A number of investigators have studied the effects of ischemia and infarctions on VF in the dog heart. Ideker and coworkers studied activation patters in open-chest dogs following 15 minutes of occlusion of the proximal circumflex artery. VF occurred in eight of 10 episodes during reperfusion, and analysis of the first few seconds indicated a period of organized wave propagation originating in the border zone, followed by a decrease in CV and increase in rate, eventually resulting in more than one wave on the heart surface at one instant.[48]

Kavanagh and colleagues studied VF initiation in the open-chest dog 4 days after occlusion-reperfusion of the left anterior descending coronary artery (LAD) using an S1-S2 protocol. VT and VF were induced. The cycle length of the first six beats was 152 ms and 115 ms, respectively.[49] VT occurred if the spared myocardial layer was thin, and VF resulted if most of the wall was intact. Figure-of-eight reentrant patterns were observed in early beats for both VT and VF.

Tweddell and coworkers recorded from open-chest dogs on cardiopulmonary bypass 3 to 6 days after a myocardial infarction using epicardial and endocardial foam rubber molds. they observed sustained VT with cycle length of 156 ms that did not deteriorate to VF. The earliest activation site was on endocardium in 12 of 13 dogs.[50] In a later study in the same model, they observed sustained VT with cycle length of 184 ms. Patterns were consistent with LV endocardial reentry in seven of 15 VTs, albeit with an isoelectric gap accompanied by concentric wave propagation on the LV epicardium;[51]

Pogwizd and colleagues used transmural needle electrodes to record from open-chest dogs with ischemic cardiomyopathy. They observed MVT and PVT resulting from subendocardial focal activity lasting 3 to 12 beats, with a VT cycle length of about 300 ms.[52]

Rankovic's group studied VF before and during ischemia 10 minutes after LAD ligation. They found that VF cycle length increased from 113 ms in control to 150 ms in the ischemic zone, with an accompanying 10-fold increase in the percentage of conduction block. No changes of these variables were observed outside the ischemic region.[53]

At 4 seconds after VF initiation, Taneja and colleagues reported VF cycle length of 102 ms. After 18 seconds, the VF cycle length increased to 116 ms. VF cycle length in subacute and chronic infarction models at 4 seconds was 149 ms and 129 ms, respectively, and was 153 ms and 126 ms, respectively, at 18 seconds.[54] They found a poor correlation of VF cycle length and effective refractory period during pacing for the 112 sites. Rotors were more common in control (22.4% of cycles) compared to the subacute (5.3%) and chronic (7.5%) models.

Akiyama recorded from microelectrodes during VF in open-chest dogs after reperfusion following 30 minutes of LAD occlusion and found VF cycle length was 200 to 350 ms and APD was 134 ms.[55]

Studies in Isolated Hearts

A few studies have been carried out in isolated dog hearts. Witkowski and coworkers used blood perfusion and optically mapped from 30% of the epicardium with no uncouplers.

They found that a strong premature stimulus produced figure-of-eight reentry with peak correlation of spatial patterns of 0.5. After 10 minutes, no reentry was observed, with peak correlation of 0.28.[56] Tabereaux and colleagues perfused hearts with Tyrode solution but did not perfuse during VF to study the temporal dynamics of the first 10 minutes of VF. They found that "Purkinje activations occurred in >84% of activation wave fronts throughout the 10 minutes of VF".[57] Janse recorded from Langendorff-perfused hearts with a blood-Tyrode mixture during regional ischemia induced by clamping the LAD. Spontaneous premature ventricular contractions occurred after 73% of ligations. In 55% of these hearts, VT (>5 beats) was initiated, with half these VTs degenerating into VF.[58]

Pig

Studies in Normal Pigs

Many VF studies have been carried out in open-chest normal swine hearts. Hillsley's group recorded from 5% of the epicardium and found that VF cycle length was 133 ms during the first 30 seconds of VF, which was about 40% of the mean number of activation fronts per second. Reentry occurred completely in the recording array in only 5% of activation waves.[59]

Huang and colleagues mapped 20% of epicardium in 500 ms epochs at 0, 10, 20, 30, and 40 sec after VF initiation. VF cycle length was 119 ms initially, 142 ms at 10 sec, 147 ms at 20 sec, and 158 ms at 30 sec. Wave speed during pacing was 80 cm/sec and decreased during VF to about 45 cm/sec initially, then leveled out at about 38 cm/sec. The number of wave fronts increased from 0 to 10 seconds, then decreased.[60]

Rogers and coworkers found that 2.3% of activation pathways were reentrant, although "from scaling analysis, an additional 28% of the pathways may also have been reentrant."[61] Rotors were short-lived (1.5 cycles). The core perimeter was 4 cm and core area was 0.83 cm^2. Rotor cycle length was 93 ms. The number of rotor cycles, core area, core perimeter, cycle length, and rotor incidence increased from 1 to 40 seconds. Rogers also showed that VF is more organized in the RV compared to the LV with fewer, larger wave fronts and less conduction block.[62] Rotor lifetime in the RV was greater than 2 beats and longer than in the LV (~1.5 cycles). Activation rate was significantly less in RV (RV:VF CL = 119 ms; LV:VF CL = 109 ms). There was no RV-LV difference in rotor cycle length (~95 ms) or core area (2.5-3 cm^2).

Newton and colleagues also found a VF cycle length gradient during the first 25 seconds of VF. The longest was in the RV base (118 ms) and the shortest was in the LV base (109 ms).[63]

Nanthakumar's group found that VF cycle length was shorter in the posterior (100 ms) than the anterior (108 ms) LV, more wave fronts blocked in the anterior LV, the anterior LV had a higher incidence of rotors, and waves on the LV propagated from the posterior to the anterior LV.[64]

Rogers and colleagues recorded VF while cardiac perfusion was maintained, with two epicardial arrays separated by a row of transmural needles. They found that VF cycle length was 100 ms and "in 3 of the 6 animals, sustained epicardial reentry (i.e., reentry persisting for more than a few cycles) was consistently present, often lasting for several seconds." However, intramural reentry was only "sporadically present" and was short lived.[65]

Huang and coworkers reported a lower incidence of rotors (1% of waves) and longer VF cycle length (116 ms) in the septum compared to the LV (2% of waves; VF CL = 96 ms). In addition, they found no difference in parameters during the first 20 seconds of VF before and after cardiopulmonary bypass.[66]

Newton and colleagues used plunge needles to study the transmural activation gradient and found that VF cycle length was shortest at the epicardium and longest at the endocardium for the first 70 seconds of VF and did not change much during the first 3 minutes.[46]

Huang and colleagues recorded from floating microelectrodes during VF and found that DI was a poor predictor of APD during VF. APD_{60} was 97.3 ms during the first 20 seconds and decreased to 89.7 ms after 20 to 40 seconds and to 89.6 ms 40 to 60 seconds after VF induction. The mean VF cycle length did not change significantly over the 60 seconds of VF, ranging from 119 to 125 ms.[67]

Studies in Isolated Hearts

Both extracellular and optical mapping studies have been performed in isolated pig hearts. Qin and colleagues studied the effects of heart isolation (Tyrode perfusion), BDM, and di-4-ANEPPS during the first 30 sec of VF using an electrode plaque. They found that all factors affected VF dynamics, in general, as to slow VF rate and organize patterns (consistent with losing excitability).[6]

Janse and coworkers recorded after 30 sec of VF initiated by burst pacing before and after cyroablation, leaving a surviving rim on the LV but completely destroying the RV. They found that the corresponding unipolar electrograms were indistinguishable; however, the epicardial patterns after cryoablation were more organized and had fewer waves.[68]

Chattipakorn and colleagues recorded VF 10 seconds after initiation via optical mapping with BDM (Tyrode perfusion) and found the VF cycle length was 92 ms and APD was 50 ms.[69]

Banville's group, using the same model, found that during sustained VF the VF cycle length was 106 ms and APD was 57 ms. The DI-APD pairs during VF fell significantly below the steady state restitution data.[70] They did not observe alternans before conduction block or during rapid pacing. In some episodes, transient VT (CL, 186 ms; APD, 107 ms) resulted after defibrillation shocks. In the same model, Kay's group demonstrated that 12 rotors with lifetime longer than 200 ms were visible on the epicardium at any given instant.[71] and Rogers and colleagues found that "complete reentrant pathways were always present on the epicardial surface and therefore, that wavefront infusion from nonepicardial sources was not strictly necessary for VF maintenance."[72]

Janse and coworkers studied isolated hearts perfused with a blood-Tyrode's mixture and induced regional ischemia by clamping the LAD. Spontaneous premature ventricular contractions occurred between 2 and 8 minutes after occlusion in 72% of ligations. In 62% of these hearts, VT (>5 beats) resulted, and 71% of these degenerated into VF.[58] The activity emerged from the border zone in the initial beats. Conduction slowed during successive beats with islands of conduction block, followed by circus movement with diameter of 1 to 2 cm.

Zaitsev and colleagues optically mapped isolated perfused hearts (blood-Tyrode mixture) and found VF cycle length was 93 to 106 ms, with a uniform distribution of phase singularities during control.[73] Ischemia following LAD occlusion resulted in a decrease of wave breaks in the ischemic zone and an increase of wave breaks in the border zone without a significant change in the nonischemic region. They also recorded from microelectrodes within the ischemic region and found that cycle length increased to about 160 ms, with a significant increase in DI compared to control hearts. In the same model, Huizar and colleagues induced VF and recorded the first 10 minutes following global ischemia. They concluded "1) at least three distinct phases of VF dynamics are present in our model, and 2) the newly described aperiodic phase is related to ischemia-specific dynamic instability of the action potential shape, which underlies broadening of the ECG spectrum during VF evolution."[74]

Human

Despite the inherent complexities involved (including the varied patient population), a number of investigators have performed extracellular mapping from human hearts on cardiopulmonary bypass in the operating room. Downar and colleagues used an endocardial balloon and epicardial sock in patients with chronic ischemic heart disease and found that "the recordings suggested an extensive sheet of surviving myocardial fibers with multiple entry and exit points allowing for different reentrant paths at different times all in the same heart," with accompanying epicardial breakthrough patterns that generated waves propagating over the entire heart.[75] Hood and coworkers used a sock electrode and plunge needles to record from patients with healed infarctions undergoing surgery for sustained MVT and revealed the VT mechanism to be focal in five patients and macroreentrant in five patients.[76]

Pogwizd and colleagues used a similar mapping strategy to record from patients with healed infarctions and refractory VT. They found that 50% of episodes began as intramural reentry with marked conduction delay inside the wall and 50% were initiated via a focal mechanism.[77] Pogwizd's group also studied spontaneous and electrically induced nonsustained (3-7 beats) VT in patients with idiopathic dilated cardiomyopathy undergoing cardiac transplantation and found that arrhythmias were initiated in the subendocardium or subepicardium by a focal mechanism. In addition, they demonstrated progressive slowing of conduction during programmed stimulation; the cycle length of the subsequent VT beats was 252 ms.[78]

Misier and colleagues used an epicardial plaque in the noninfarcted part of the LV in patients undergoing surgery for refractory tachyarrhythmias.[79] They found that VF cycle length was not significantly different in patients with hemodynamically tolerable sustained VT and in patients with documented sudden cardiac death (136 vs 129 ms). However, the spatial dispersion of VF cycle length was significantly larger in the sudden cardiac death group.

Nanthakumar and coworkers used an epicardial plaque to record from patients undergoing aortocoronary bypass surgery 5 to 30 sec after the initiation of VF and found VF cycle length was 172 ms. They also found large organized wave fronts, and rotors (always lasting <2 cycles) were identified in 62% of 2-second segments.[80]

Nash and coworkers studied 10 patients (six with coronary artery disease, four with aortic valve disease) by recording the first 20 to 40 seconds of VF using an epicardial sock array. They took their recordings before bypass in seven patients and after bypass in three patients. "Early human VF was sustained by large coherent wavefronts punctuated by periods of disorganized wavelet behavior."[81] They found the initial VF cycle length to be 196 ms, which continuously decreased as VF progressed. "Epicardial reentry was present in all fibrillating hearts, typically with low numbers of phase singularities. In some cases, persistent phase singularities interacted with multiple complex wavelets; in other cases, VF was driven at times by a single reentrant wave that swept the entire epicardium for several cycles."[81]

Masse and colleagues have provided the most comprehensive view of human VF yet by using an epicardial sock array in conjunction with endocardial balloon arrays in the RV and LV in 5 patients with cardiomyopathy.[82] By analyzing data 1 second after VF initiation, they found rotors in all hearts. The rotors lasted an average of 3.2 seconds, and the endocardial rotors were faster (CL, 192 ms) than the epicardial rotors (CL, 220 ms). "These rotors frequently localized to border regions of myocardium with bipolar electrogram amplitude of <0.5 mV. The organization of electrical activity during early VF in myopathic human hearts is characterized by wavefronts emanating from a few rotors."[82]

Walcott and colleagues inserted a 36-site (4-mm spacing) electrode catheter to record from the LV endocardium during VF in 16 patients undergoing implantation of an internal cardioverter-defibrillator.[83] Ejection fraction was 33%; 10 patients had coronary artery disease. Data collected 6 to 8 seconds after VF initiation revealed a long correlation length of 9 cm, 9.2 waves per second, and VF cycle length of 218 ms.

A few studies have been carried out in explanted Langendorff-perfused isolated human hearts. Wu and colleagues recorded sustained VF in five isolated hearts (perfused with blood-Tyrode mixture) from patients with dilated cardiomyopathy. They found that rotors lasted 1 to 4 cycles with a average period of 172 ms in 55 of 75 episodes. Lines of conduction block were associated with increased fibrosis. Most waves were non-reentrant, and many patterns were characterized as breakthroughs followed by conduction block and incomplete reentry.[84] Nanthakumar and coworkers studied five explanted hearts from cardiomyopathy patients perfused with Tyrode solution and during VF identified large waves, rotors, and reduced CV (25 cm/sec compared to 41-87 cm/sec during pacing).[85]

Table 33-1 Minimum Wavelengths for Various Species

Species	Minimum Wavelength*	$VFCL_{min}$	Source of Measurement	Comments
Mouse	1.3 cm	38 ms	Noujaim et al[9]	Transverse CV = 34 cm/sec during pacing at 80 ms CL[7]
Guinea pig	1.14 cm	38 ms	Samie et al[15]	There is much spatial variability Transverse CV = 30 cm/sec during VT with CL = 100 ms[12]
Rabbit	2.8 cm	62 ms	Samie et al[27]	CV = 45 cm/sec during VF[26]
Dog	3.2 cm	86 ms	Zhou et al[43] Opthof et al[47]	Transverse CV = 37 cm/sec during VF[38]
Pig	4.1 cm	92 ms	Chen et al[44] Chattipakorn et al[69]	Transverse CV = 45 cm/sec during VF[60]
Human	3.2 cm	129 ms	Misier et al[79]	CV = 25 cm/sec during VF[85]

CL, cycle length; CV, conduction velocity; $VFCL_{min}$, ventricular fibrillation cycle length.
*$VFCL_{min} \times CV$.

Summary

How do we make sense of all these data? First, let us review the data on normal hearts, keeping in mind that experiments involving field shocks and VF initiation, body-surface mapping, and noncontact electrodes were not reviewed here.

There is ample evidence that rotors occur in the first seconds of VF initiated by electrical stimuli. Obviously, a rotor requires some space to propagate and rotate, and even more tissue is required if the rotor is to move or break up (hallmarks of VF). This is the basis for the critical mass hypothesis of VF.[86] Unstable tachyarrhythmias have been observed in all species reviewed here, and these heart sizes span a wide range. A more detailed look at VF maintenance requires the relevant parameters regarding heart size and rotor size. Clearly, the surface area, wall thickness, and volume are all different and useful measures of heart size. The relevant parameters for the size of a rotor are thought to be its wavelength, that is cycle length, CV, and APD (e.g., cycle length cannot be shorter than APD).[87,88] The minimum wavelength ($VFCL_{min}$ × CV) for the species reviewed here are shown in Table 33-1.

Of course there are no data available from normal human hearts during VF, and relevant animal models of human disease are rare due to the variety and complexity of patients experiencing VF and difficulty in comparison between species. Therefore, it is essential to remember that manipulations to animal models to mimic disease tend to increase VF cycle length and often organize VF (this occurs even in normal hearts during prolonged VF). Rotors have been observed in all the species reviewed here, but there is an enormous range (and various definitions) in the values of rotor lifetime, size, density, and other parameters. Although the mother rotor hypothesis is particularly difficult to disprove,[89] more detailed and comprehensive tracking of phase singularities throughout the heart (e.g., see Rogers and colleagues[72]) is warranted.

Acknowledgements

I want to extend my sincere thanks to Dr. Venya Y. Sidorov and Dr. John Wikswo at Vanderbilt University for providing the rabbit ventricular fibrillation microelectrode data in Figure 33-1A, Deliliah J. Huelsing for providing the rabbit action potential microelectrode recordings in Figure 33-1C, and Kate M. Sreenan for editorial assistance in manuscript preparation.

References

1. Wiggers CJ, Bell JR, Paine M: Studies of ventricular fibrillation caused by electric shock: II Cinematographic and electrocardiographic observations of the natural process in the dog's heart: Its inhibition by potassium and the revival of coordinated beats by calcium. Am Heart J 5:351-365, 1930.
2. Gray RA, Pertsov AM, Jalife J: Spatial and temporal organization during cardiac fibrillation. Nature 392(6671):75-78, 1998.
3. Gillis AM, Kulisz E, Mathison HJ: Cardiac electrophysiological variables in blood-perfused and buffer-perfused, isolated, working rabbit heart. Am J Physiol 271 (2 Pt 2):H784-H789, 1996.
4. Girouard SD, Laurita KR, Rosenbaum DS: Unique properties of cardiac action potentials recorded with voltage-sensitive dyes. J Cardiovasc Electrophysiol 7(11):1024-1038, 1996.
5. Gray RA: What exactly are optically recorded "action potentials"? J Cardiovasc Electrophysiol 10(11):1463-1466, 1999.
6. Qin H, Kay MW, Chattipakorn N, et al: Effects of heart isolation, voltage-sensitive dye, and electromechanical uncoupling agents on ventricular fibrillation. Am J Physiol 284(5):H1818-H1826, 2003.
7. Vaidya D, Morley GE, Samie FH, Jalife J: Reentry and fibrillation in the mouse heart. A challenge to the critical mass hypothesis. Circ Res 85(2):174-181, 1999.
8. Vaidya D, Tamaddon HS, Lo CW, et al: Null mutation of connexin43 causes slow propagation of ventricular activation in the late stages of mouse embryonic development. Circ Res 88(11):1196-1202, 2001.
9. Noujaim SF, Pandit SV, Berenfeld O, et al: Up-regulation of the inward rectifier K^+ current (I_{K1}) in the mouse heart accelerates and stabilizes rotors. J Physiol 578(Pt 1): 315-326, 2007.
10. Cerrone M, Noujaim SF, Tolkacheva EG, et al: Arrhythmogenic mechanisms in a mouse model of catecholaminergic polymorphic ventricular tachycardia. Circ Res 101(10):1039-1048, 2007.
11. Pastore JM, Girouard SD, Laurita KR, et al: Mechanism linking T-wave alternans to the genesis of cardiac fibrillation. Circulation 99(10):1385-1394, 1999.
12. Salama G, Kanai A, Efimov IR: Subthreshold stimulation of Purkinje fibers interrupts ventricular tachycardia in intact hearts. Experimental study with voltage-sensitive dyes and imaging techniques. Circ Res 74(4):604-619, 1994.
13. Choi BR, Liu T, Salama G: The distribution of refractory periods influences the dynamics of ventricular fibrillation. Circ Res 88(5):E49-E58, 2001.
14. Choi BR, Jang W, Salama G: Spatially discordant voltage alternans cause wavebreaks in ventricular fibrillation. Heart Rhythm 4(8):1057-1068, 2007.
15. Samie FH, Berenfeld O, Anumonwo J, et al: Rectification of the background potassium current: A determinant of rotor dynamics in ventricular fibrillation. Circ Res 89(12):1216-1223, 2001.
16. Warren M, Guha PK, Berenfeld O, et al: Blockade of the inward rectifying potassium current terminates ventricular fibrillation in the guinea pig heart. J Cardiovasc Electrophysiol 14(6):621-631, 2003.
17. Gray RA, Jalife J, Panfilov A, et al: Nonstationary vortexlike reentrant activity as a mechanism of polymorphic ventricular tachycardia in the isolated rabbit heart. Circulation 91(9):2454-2469, 1995.
18. Banville I, Gray RA: Effect of action potential duration and conduction velocity restitution and their spatial dispersion on alternans and the stability of arrhythmias. J Cardiovasc Electrophysiol 13:1141-1149, 2002.
19. Schalij MJ, Boersma L, Huijberts M, Allessie MA: Anisotropic reentry in a perfused 2-dimensional layer of rabbit ventricular myocardium. Circulation 102(21):2650-2658, 2000.
20. Boersma L, Zetelaki Z, Brugada J, Allessie M: Polymorphic reentrant ventricular tachycardia in the isolated rabbit heart studied by high-density mapping. Circulation 105(25):3053-3061, 2002.
21. Kodama I, Honjo H, Yamazaki M, et al: Optical imaging of spiral waves: pharmacological modification of spiral-type excitations in a 2-dimensional layer of ventricular myocardium. J Electrocardiol 38(4 Suppl):126-130, 2005.
22. Gray RA, Jalife J, Panfilov AV, et al: Mechanisms of cardiac fibrillation. Science 270(5239):1222-1223, 1995.
23. Kwaku KF, Dillon SM: Shock-induced depolarization of refractory myocardium prevents wave-front propagation in defibrillation. Circ Res 79(5):957-973, 1996.
24. Chen J, Mandapati R, Berenfeld O, et al: High-frequency periodic sources underlie ventricular fibrillation in the isolated rabbit heart. Circ Res 86(1):86-93, 2000.
25. Mandapati R, Asano Y, Baxter WT, et al: Quantification of effects of global ischemia on dynamics of ventricular fibrillation in isolated rabbit heart. Circulation 98(16):1688-1696, 1998.
26. Chorro FJ, Cánoves J, Guerrero J, et al: Alteration of ventricular fibrillation by flecainide, verapamil, and sotalol: An experimental study. Circulation 101(13):1606-1615, 2000.
27. Samie FH, Jalife J: Mechanisms underlying ventricular tachycardia and its transition to ventricular fibrillation in the structurally normal heart. Cardiovasc Res 50(2):242-250, 2001.

28. Wu TJ, Lin SF, Weiss JN, et al: Two types of ventricular fibrillation in isolated rabbit hearts: Importance of excitability and action potential duration restitution. Circulation 106(14):1859-1866, 2002.
29. Wu TJ, Lin SF, Baher A, et al: Mother rotors and the mechanisms of D600-induced type 2 ventricular fibrillation. Circulation 110(15):2110-2118, 2004.
30. Choi BR, Nho W, Liu T, Salama G: Life span of ventricular fibrillation frequencies. Circ Res 91(4):339-345, 2002.
31. Chorro FJ, Blasco E, Trapero I, et al: Selective myocardial isolation and ventricular fibrillation. Pacing Clin Electrophysiol 30(3):359-370, 2007.
32. Moe GK, Harris AS, Wiggers CJ: Analysis of the initiation of fibrillation by electrographic studies. Am J Physiol 134: 473-492, 1941.
33. Harumi K, Smith GR, Abildskov JA, et al: Detailed activation sequence in the region of electrically induced ventricular fibrillation in dogs. Jpn Heart J 21(4):533-544, 1980.
34. Kuo CS, Munakata K, Reddy CP, Surawicz B: Characteristics and possible mechanism of ventricular arrhythmia dependent on the dispersion of action potential durations. Circulation 67(6):1356-1367, 1983.
35. Han J, Moe GK: Nonuniform recovery of excitability in ventricular muscle. Circ Res 14:44-60, 1964.
36. Cao JM, Qu Z, Kim YH, et al: Spatiotemporal heterogeneity in the induction of ventricular fibrillation by rapid pacing: Importance of cardiac restitution properties. Circ Res 84(11):1318-1331, 1999.
37. Cha YM, Birgersdotter-Green U, Wolf PL, et al: The mechanism of termination of reentrant activity in ventricular fibrillation. Circ Res 74(3):495-506, 1994.
38. Ohara T, Ohara K, Cao JM, et al: Increased wave break during ventricular fibrillation in the epicardial border zone of hearts with healed myocardial infarction. Circulation 103(10):1465-1472, 2001.
39. Lee JJ, Kamjkoo K, Hough D, et al: Reentrant wave fronts in Wiggers' stage II ventricular fibrillation. Characteristics and mechanisms of termination and spontaneous regeneration. Circ Res 78(4):660-675, 1996.
40. Kwan YY, Van W, Hough D, et al: Effects of procainamide on wave-front dynamics during ventricular fibrillation in open-chest dogs. Circulation 97(18):1828-1836, 1998.
41. Damle RS, Kanaan NM, robinson NS, et al: Spatial and temporal linking of epicardial activation directions during ventricular fibrillation in dogs. Evidence for underlying organization. Circulation 86(5):1547-1558, 1992.
42. Huang J, Skinner JL, Rogers JM, et al: The effects of acute and chronic amiodarone on activation patterns and defibrillation threshold during ventricular fibrillation in dogs. J Am Coll Cardiol 40(2):375-383, 2002.
43. Zhou X, Wolf PD, Rollins DL, et al: Effects of monophasic and biphasic shocks on action potentials during ventricular fibrillation in dogs. Circ Res 73(2):325-334, 1993.
44. Chen PS, Wolf PD, Melnick SD, et al: Comparison of activation during ventricular fibrillation and following unsuccessful defibrillation shocks in open-chest dogs. Circ Res 66(6):1544-1560, 1990.
45. Cha YM, Uchida T, Wolf PL, et al: Effects of chemical subendocardial ablation on activation rate gradient during ventricular fibrillation. Am J Physiol 269(6 Pt 2): H1998-H2009, 1995.
46. Newton JC, Smith WM, Ideker RE: Estimated global transmural distribution of activation rate and conduction block during porcine and canine ventricular fibrillation. Circ Res 94(6):836-842, 2004.
47. Opthof T, Misier AR, Coronel R, et al: Dispersion of refractoriness in canine ventricular myocardium. Effects of sympathetic stimulation. Circ Res 68(5):1204-1215, 1991.
48. Ideker RE, Klein GJ, Harrison L, et al: The transition to ventricular fibrillation induced by reperfusion after acute ischemia in the dog: a period of organized epicardial activation. Circulation 63(6):1371-1379, 1981.
49. Kavanagh KM, Kabas JS, Rolins DL, et al: High-current stimuli to the spared epicardium of a large infarct induce ventricular tachycardia. Circulation 85(2):680-698, 1992.
50. Tweddell JS, Branham BH, Harada A, et al: Potential mapping in septal tachycardia. Evaluation of a new intraoperative mapping technique. Circulation 80(3 Pt 1):I97-I108, 1989.
51. Tweddell JS, Rokkas CK, Harada A, et al: Anterior septal coronary artery infarction in the canine: A model of ventricular tachycardia with a subendocardial origin. Ablation and activation sequence mapping. Circulation 90(6):2982-2992, 1994.
52. Pogwizd SM: Focal mechanisms underlying ventricular tachycardia during prolonged ischemic cardiomyopathy. Circulation 90(3):1441-1458, 1994.
53. Rankovic V, Patel N, Jain S, et al: Characteristics of ischemic and periischemic regions during ventricular fibrillation in the canine heart. J Cardiovasc Electrophysiol 10(8):1090-1100, 1999.
54. Taneja T, Horvath G, Racker DK, et al: Is there a correlation between ventricular fibrillation cycle length and electrophysiological and anatomic properties of the canine left ventricle? Am J Physiol 287(2):H823-H832, 2004.
55. Akiyama T: Intracellular recording of in situ ventricular cells during ventricular fibrillation. Am J Physiol 240(4):H465-H471, 1981.
56. Witkowski FX, Leon LJ, Penkoske PA, et al: Spatiotemporal evolution of ventricular fibrillation. Nature 392(6671):78-82, 1998.
57. Tabereaux PB, Walcott GP, rogers JM, et al: Activation patterns of Purkinje fibers during long-duration ventricular fibrillation in an isolated canine heart model. Circulation 116(10):1113-1119, 2007.
58. Janse MJ, van Capelle FJ, Morsink H, et al: Flow of "injury" current and patterns of excitation during early ventricular arrhythmias in acute regional myocardial ischemia in isolated porcine and canine hearts. Evidence for two different arrhythmogenic mechanisms. Circ Res 47(2):151-165, 1980.
59. Hillsley RE, Bollacker KD, Simpson EV, et al: Alteration of ventricular fibrillation by propranolol and isoproterenol detected by epicardial mapping with 506 electrodes. J Cardiovasc Electrophysiol 6(6):471-485, 1995.
60. Huang J, Rogers JM, Kenknight BH, et al: Evolution of the organization of epicardial activation patterns during ventricular fibrillation. J Cardiovasc Electrophysiol 9(12):1291-1304, 1998.
61. Rogers JM, Huang J, Smith WM, Ideker RE: Incidence, evolution, and spatial distribution of functional reentry during ventricular fibrillation in pigs. Circ Res 84(8): 945-954, 1999.
62. Rogers JM, Huang J, Pedoto RW, et al: Fibrillation is more complex in the left ventricle than in the right ventricle. J Cardiovasc Electrophysiol 11(12):1364-1371, 2000.
63. Newton JC, Johnson PL, Justice RK, et al: Estimated global epicardial distribution of activation rate and conduction block during porcine ventricular fibrillation. J Cardiovasc Electrophysiol 13(10):1035-1041, 2002.
64. Nanthakumar K, Huang J, Rogers JM, et al: Regional differences in ventricular fibrillation in the open-chest porcine left ventricle. Circ Res 91(8):733-740, 2002.
65. Rogers JM, Huang J, Melnick SB, Ideker RE: Sustained reentry in the left ventricle of fibrillating pig hearts. Circ Res 92(5):539-545, 2003.
66. Huang J, Walcott GP, Killingsworth CR, et al: Quantification of activation patterns during ventricular fibrillation in open-chest porcine left ventricle and septum. Heart Rhythm 2(7):720-728, 2005.
67. Huang J, Zhou X, Smith WM, Ideker RE: Restitution properties during ventricular fibrillation in the in situ swine heart. Circulation 110(20):3161-3167, 2004.
68. Janse MJ, Wilms-Schopman FJ, Coronel R: Ventricular fibrillation is not always due to multiple wavelet reentry. J Cardiovasc Electrophysiol 6(7):512-521, 1995.
69. Chattipakorn N, Banville J, Gray RA, Ideker RE: Mechanism of ventricular defibrillation for near-defibrillation threshold shocks: A whole-heart optical mapping study in swine. Circulation 104(11):1313-1319, 2001.
70. Banville I, Chattipakorn N, Gray RA: Restitution dynamics during pacing and arrhythmias in isolated pig hearts. J Cardiovasc Electrophysiol 15(4):455-463, 2004.
71. Kay MW, Walcott GP, Gladden JD, et al: Lifetimes of epicardial rotors in panoramic optical maps of fibrillating swine ventricles. Am J Physiol 291(4):H1935-1941, 2006.
72. Rogers JM, Walcot GP, Gladden JD, et al: Panoramic optical mapping reveals continuous epicardial reentry during ventricular fibrillation in the isolated swine heart. Biophys J 92(3):1090-1095, 2007.
73. Zaitsev AV, Guha PK, Sarmast F, et al: Wavebreak formation during ventricular fibrillation in the isolated, regionally

ischemic pig heart. Circ Res 92(5):546-553, 2003.

74. Huizar JF, Warren MD, Shevedko AG, et al: Three distinct phases of VF during global ischemia in the isolated blood-perfused pig heart. Am J Physiol 293(3): H1617-H1628, 2007.
75. Downar E, Kimber S, Harris L, et al: Endocardial mapping of ventricular tachycardia in the intact human heart. II. Evidence for multiuse reentry in a functional sheet of surviving myocardium. J Am Coll Cardiol 20(4):869-878, 1992.
76. Hood MA, Pogwizd SM, Peirick J, Cain ME: Contribution of myocardium responsible for ventricular tachycardia to abnormalities detected by analysis of signal-averaged ECGs. Circulation 86(6):1888-1901, 1992.
77. Pogwizd SM, Hoyt RH, Saffitz JE, et al: Reentrant and focal mechanisms underlying ventricular tachycardia in the human heart. Circulation 86(6):1872-1887, 1992.
78. Pogwizd SM, McKenzie JP, Cain ME: Mechanisms underlying spontaneous and induced ventricular arrhythmias in patients with idiopathic dilated cardiomyopathy. Circulation 98(22):2404-2414, 1998.
79. Misier AR, Opthof T, van Hemel NM, et al: Dispersion of "refractoriness" in noninfarcted myocardium of patients with ventricular tachycardia or ventricular fibrillation after myocardial infarction. Circulation 91(10):2566-2572, 1995.
80. Nanthakumar K, Wlacott GP, Melnick S, et al: Epicardial organization of human ventricular fibrillation. Heart Rhythm 1(1):14-23, 2004.
81. Nash MP, Mourad A, Clayton RH, et al: Evidence for multiple mechanisms in human ventricular fibrillation. Circulation 114(6):536-542, 2006.
82. Massé S, Downar E, Chauhan V, et al: Ventricular fibrillation in myopathic human hearts: Mechanistic insights from in vivo global endocardial and epicardial mapping. Am J Physiol 292(6):H2589-H2597, 2007.
83. Walcott GP, Kay GN, Plumb VJ, et al: Endocardial wave front organization during ventricular fibrillation in humans. J Am Coll Cardiol 39(1):109-115, 2002.
84. Wu TJ, Ong JJ, Hwang C, et al: Characteristics of wave fronts during ventricular fibrillation in human hearts with dilated cardiomyopathy: Role of increased fibrosis in the generation of reentry. J Am Coll Cardiol 32(1):187-196, 1998.
85. Nanthakumar K, Jalife J, Massé S, et al: Optical mapping of Langendorff-perfused human hearts: Establishing a model for the study of ventricular fibrillation in humans. Am J Physiol 293(1):H875-H1880, 2007.
86. Zipes DP, Fischer J, King RM, et al: Termination of ventricular fibrillation in dogs by depolarizing a critical amount of myocardium. Am J Cardiol 36(1):37-44, 1975.
87. Winfree AT: Electrical turbulence in three-dimensional heart muscle. Science 266(5187):1003-1006, 1994.
88. Panfilov AV, Keldermann RH, Nash MP: Drift and breakup of spiral waves in reaction-diffusion-mechanics systems. Proc Natl Acad Sci U S A 104(19):7922-7926, 2007.
89. Ideker RE, Rogers JM: Human ventricular fibrillation: Wandering wavelets, mother rotors, or both? Circulation 114(6):530-532, 2006.

Modeling Cardiac Defibrillation 34

Natalia A. Trayanova and Gernot Plank

CHAPTER OUTLINE

Cardiac fibrillation is the breakdown of the organized cardiac electrical activity, driving the heart's periodic pumping, into disorganized self-sustained activation patterns. A fibrillation episode results in the loss of cardiac output, and unless timely intervention is administered, death quickly ensues. The only known effective therapy for lethal disturbances in cardiac rhythm is defibrillation, the delivery of a strong electric shock to the heart. This technique, as accomplished nowadays by automatic implantable cardioverter defibrillators (ICDs), constitutes the most important means of combating sudden cardiac death.

Over the years, defibrillation devices have become smaller and their batteries longer-lasting, but defibrillation remains a traumatic experience, and thousands of patients are affected by high-voltage-component ICD malfunctions and experience severe psychological trauma.[1] A significant reduction in shock energy can only be achieved by fully appreciating the mechanisms by which a shock interacts with the heart and then exploiting these mechanisms to devise novel low-voltage therapeutic approaches. However, elucidating the mechanisms by which electric shocks halt life-threatening arrhythmias has been a long and arduous process.

Recent developments in experimental methodology have provided new characterizations of tissue responses to shocks, but mechanistic inquiry into the success and failure of defibrillation has been hampered by the inability of currently available experimental techniques to resolve, with sufficient accuracy, electrical behavior confined to the depth of the ventricles during and after the shock. Mapping the entire epicardial surface of the ventricles, the current state of the art in optical imaging,[2] does not reveal the global three-dimensional (3D) activity that follows the shock because activations can propagate intramurally, without a signature on the epicardial surface. Realistic 3D simulations of the ventricular defibrillation process in close conjunction with experimental observations have proved to be an invaluable tool in the pursuit of understanding the electrical events that ensue from the interaction between fibrillating myocardium and applied shock. This chapter examines the contributions of and the insights provided by realistic 3D simulations of the process of defibrillation.

Brief Historical Overview of Defibrillation Mechanisms

The initial understanding of the events taking place in the process of defibrillation was established during the 1980s and 1990s. It was based on the concept of reentry induction by the shock, with series of theoretical studies promoting the critical point hypothesis.[3] The critical point hypothesis centers around the idea that an electrical shock generates an extracellular potential gradient that falls off with the distance from the shock electrode.[4] When an electrical shock is delivered prematurely to a propagating action potential wave front, the intersection of a critical extracellular potential gradient isoline of the shock and a critical recovery isoline of the propagating wave is the critical point around which a rotor is formed.[3,4] Assuming that the extracellular potential gradient is directly proportional to the induced transmembrane potential,[5] then the elevation in transmembrane potential in the wake of a propagating wave front caused by the stimulus (shock) creates a unidirectional block and thus creates conditions for reentrant activity. So long as the critical point remains within the boundaries of the myocardium, the tissue is vulnerable to reentry. The upper limit of vulnerability (ULV) would be reached when the shock is so strong that the critical potential gradient isoline is at or beyond the borders of the myocardium.[6] Above the ULV, an electric shock cannot initiate reentry. Thus, a successful defibrillation shock must not only prevent propagation of pre-existing activity but also must be above the ULV so it will not initiate new reentrant activations.[7]

These mechanisms were conjectured from experimental recordings of extracellular potentials following the defibrillation shock. In these studies, overwhelming electrical artifacts had prevented researchers from recording during and shortly after the shock; thus there was no direct evidence of some of these mechanistic concepts. A breakthrough in mapping cardiac activity associated with defibrillation occurred with the introduction of potentiometric dyes, which allowed recording, with high spatiotemporal resolution, of activity before, during, and after the shock. At the same time, the theoretical electrophysiology community adopted a novel modeling methodology, termed the *bidomain model.* The bidomain model is a continuum representation of the myocardium that takes into consideration current distribution resulting from a particular characteristic of cardiac tissue: the fact that the two spaces composing the myocardium—the intra- and extracellular—are both anisotropic but to a different degree; the myocardium is thus characterized with unequal anisotropy ratios. The bidomain model instantly became a powerful modeling tool in the study of stimulation of cardiac tissue.

Early Insights Provided by the Bidomain Model

The first significant achievement of the new bidomain approach was the study of the passive (i.e., the ionic currents are not accounted for) shock-induced change in transmembrane potential, ΔV_m, following a strong unipolar stimulus (near-field effects). Bidomain simulations by Sepulveda and colleagues[8] demonstrated that the tissue response in the vicinity of a strong unipolar stimulus involved simultaneous occurrence of positive (depolarizing) and negative (hyperpolarizing) effects in close proximity. This finding of virtual electrodes was in stark contrast to the established view that tissue responses should only be depolarizing if the stimulus was cathodal and should only be hyperpolarizing if the stimulus was anodal. Optical mapping studies that followed convincingly confirmed these theoretical predictions.[9-12]

The next big contribution of passive bidomain modeling was the detailed analysis of virtual electrode polarization (VEP) etiology and its dependence on cardiac tissue structure and the configuration of the applied field; both were shown to be major determinants of the shape, location, polarity, and intensity of the shock-induced polarization.[11,13-15] In particular, theoretical considerations led to the recognition of two types of VEP: *surface VEP*, which penetrates the ventricular wall over a few cell layers, due to current redistribution near the boundaries separating myocardium from blood cavity or surrounding bath, and *bulk VEP* throughout the ventricular wall.[14-16] Analysis of the bidomain equations revealed that a necessary condition for the existence of the bulk VEP is the unequal anisotropy in the myocardium. Sufficient conditions include either spatial nonuniformity in applied electric field[11] or nonuniformity in tissue architecture, such as fiber curvature,[17] fiber rotation,[16] fiber branching and anastomosis, and local changes in tissue conductivity due to resistive heterogeneities.[18-20]

These findings provided the background for the development of a comprehensive set of mechanisms explaining the success or failure of a defibrillation shock based on the application of the bidomain model. This set of mechanisms includes the generation of VEP in the 3D ventricles by the defibrillation electrodes (far-field effects); the initiation of postshock activations, whose origin depends on shock strength and waveform; the formation of an isoelectric window (a period of electrical quiescence) following the shock; and the breakdown of the postshock activations into (re)fibrillation. Developing this comprehensive understanding required large-scale simulations of defibrillation in the whole heart.

Three-Dimensional Models of Defibrillation

To model defibrillation realistically in the 3D organ, myocardial geometry and fiber architecture needs to be acquired. All 3D realistic models of defibrillation have been based on the University of California at San Diego (UCSD) model of rabbit ventricular geometry and fiber orientation (Fig. 34-1).[21] Other geometries now being used are based on reconstructions of cardiac structure from high-resolution imaging modalities. Figure 34-2 presents an example of an left ventricle (LV) rabbit wedge geometry reconstructed from high-resolution (isotropic 25 μm) MRI scans[22] and the corresponding computational mesh. We applied an octree-based meshing technique to produce this boundary-fitted, locally refined, and conformal multielement mesh.[23]

For defibrillation studies, all membrane models need to be modified to ensure stability during the shock, when a dramatic change in transmembrane potential takes place. Furthermore, defibrillation shocks induce complex changes in transmembrane potential, which have been consistently observed in experiments but never reproduced by membrane models. In the study by Ashihara and Trayanova,[24] the authors demonstrated that the experimentally observed responses to shocks could only be reproduced by the addition of electroporation and an outward current activated upon strong shock-induced depolarization, I_a, where I_a was assumed to be part of the K^+ flow through the L-type Ca^+ channel.

In the realistic 3D model of defibrillation, shock electrodes are represented as 3D isocurrent density or isovoltage surfaces within the 3D computational grid (ventricles plus perfusing bath and blood in cavities); these are typically chosen to mimic geometry and location of electrodes in optical mapping experiments (far-field). The examples in this chapter include external plate (at the boundaries of the perfusing chamber) and ICD defibrillation electrode configurations (see Fig. 34-1); cuff electrodes have also been implemented in previous studies.[25] The shock waveforms include square waves as well as truncated-exponential (62% tilt) monophasic and biphasic shocks[26-31] of different polarities and durations.

Most of the studies on the 3D mechanisms of defibrillation in entire ventricles actually examined vulnerability to electric shocks;[27-31] studies by Tryanova and colleagues[25] and by Aguel and colleagues[32] are the exceptions. The reason for the focus on the effect of shocks given to paced activations rather than fibrillatory activity rests with the strong link between cardiac vulnerability and defibrillation. Research has demonstrated that an electric shock can induce ventricular arrhythmias if it is given during the vulnerable window within the normal cardiac cycle.[33] Fabiato and coworkers were the first to suggest that the mechanisms of induction and termination of ventricular fibrillation (VF) might be similar.[34] This suggestion is supported by the correlation between ULV and defibrillation threshold (DFT).[7] For a defibrillation shock to succeed, it must extinguish existing VF activations throughout the myocardium (or in a critical mass of it), and it must not initiate fibrillation anew. Therefore, understanding cardiac vulnerability to electric shocks is a route to understanding defibrillation and arrhythmogenesis by failed shocks.

Virtual Electrode Polarization Induced by the Shock in the Three-Dimensional Volume of the Ventricles

The pattern of VEP established in the 3D organ strongly depends on gross geometry and fiber orientation as well as on spatial nonuniformity of the applied field.[14] Here we present examples of large-scale VEP established in the rabbit ventricles following external and ICD shocks of different waveforms.

Figure 34-3A illustrates VEP at the end of 4-ms-long square-wave shocks of different strengths, applied at a coupling interval of 105 ms through a set of external defibrillation electrodes. VEP on the surfaces exhibits two main areas of opposite polarization: the right ventricle (RV) epicardium, which is near the cathode, is depolarized, and the LV epicardium is de-excited (postshock excitable area). A zone of intermediate voltage levels (green and yellow colored areas) is created between oppositely polarized

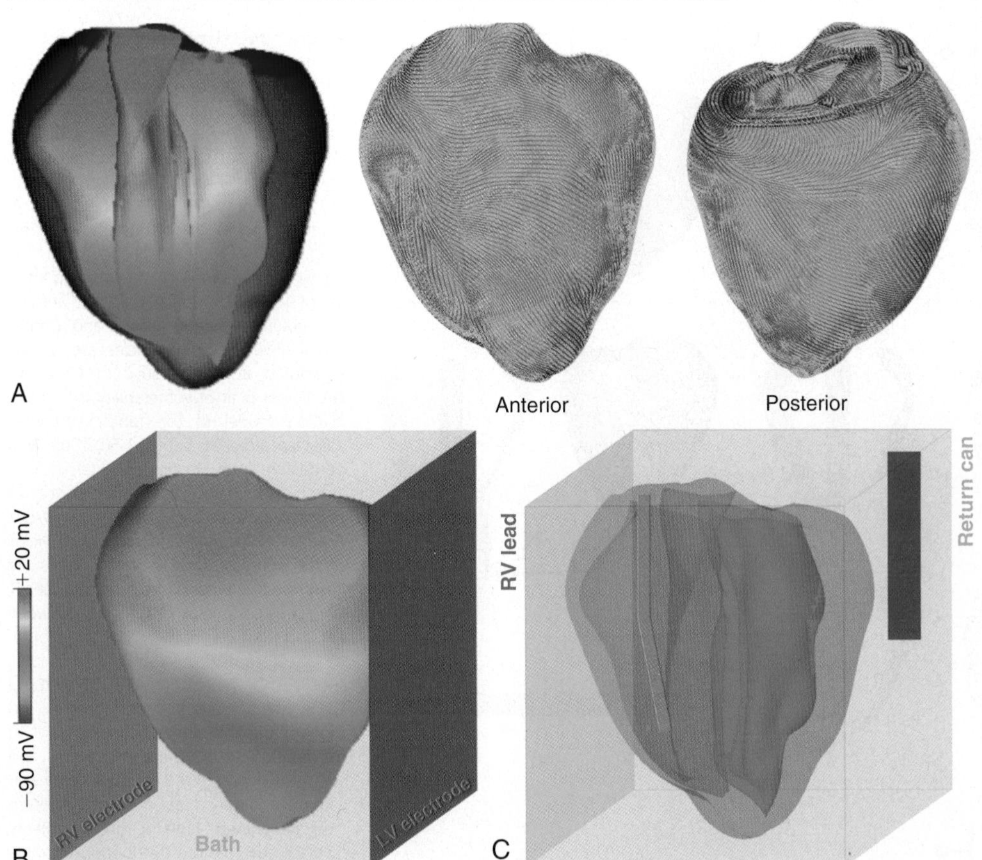

Figure 34-1 **A,** Geometry (semitransparent rendering) and posterior and anterior views of epicardial fiber orientation *(short white lines)* in the rabbit ventricular model. **B,** Configuration of the perfusing chamber (3.92 cm wide) and external shock electrodes. The ventricles are paced at the apex, and the colors represent the distribution of transmembrane potential during a paced beat. **C,** Configuration of the same perfusing chamber with implanted cardioverter defibrillator–like shock electrodes.

areas; increasing shock strength reduces the width of this zone, resulting in larger spatial gradients between areas of opposite membrane polarity.

In contrast to the surface VEP, transmural views present a more complex distribution of transmembrane potential throughout the midmyocardium. In all cases, the LV freewall exhibits a wide excitable area that extends toward the base with the increase in shock strength. In contrast, the RV freewall and the septum are mostly depolarized at shock end. As determined by simulation studies,[14,16] differences in VEP between ventricular surfaces and midmyocardium emanate from the different mechanisms that govern surface polarization and polarization in the tissue bulk and result in different postshock electrophysiologic behavior on the surfaces and in depth, as demonstrated later. For weak shocks such as 1.0 V/cm, the electric field is unable to reset the preshock state of the tissue, and dispersion of refractoriness in the apex-base direction resulting from the preshock beat can still be observed. However, with increasing shock strength, the remnants of the paced beat in the shock-end transmembrane potential distribution disappear.

The fact that strong shock-induced hyperpolarization can abolish the action potential means that a new excitable area is created during the shock. For very strong shocks, this excitable area depends only on the shape and location of the virtual anodes in the myocardium and is practically independent of preshock activity. Overall, pre-existing activity and shock-induced depolarization and hyperpolarization combine to create the shock-end distribution of transmembrane potential: Certain regions are depolarized, but excitability is restored in others. The outcome of the shock depends on this shock-end distribution and, more importantly, on the interaction between the oppositely polarized areas.

The effect of polarity reversal on VEP induced by external shocks is illustrated in Figure 34-3B, where the more clinically relevant truncated-exponential waveform is used. For left-to-right direction of the applied field, regardless of shock strength and coupling interval of shock application, the main postshock excitable area is always within the LV wall (5 V/cm shock episode illustrated in Fig. 34-3B). At shock end, the septum is either mildly or strongly positively (depending on shock strength)

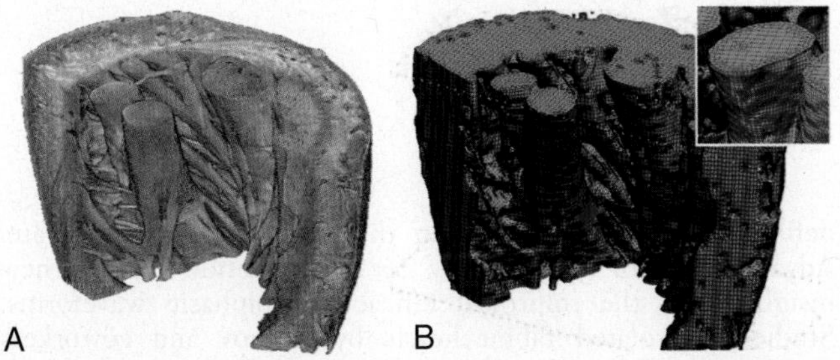

Figure 34-2 Reconstruction of a left ventricular wedge from the rabbit heart. **A,** Segmented magnetic resonance imaging stack. **B,** Computational mesh. (Modified from Trayanova NA, Plank G, Rodriguez B: What have we learned from mathematical models of defibrillation and postshock arrhythmogenesis? Application of bidomain simulations. Heart Rhythm 3:1232-1235, 2006.)

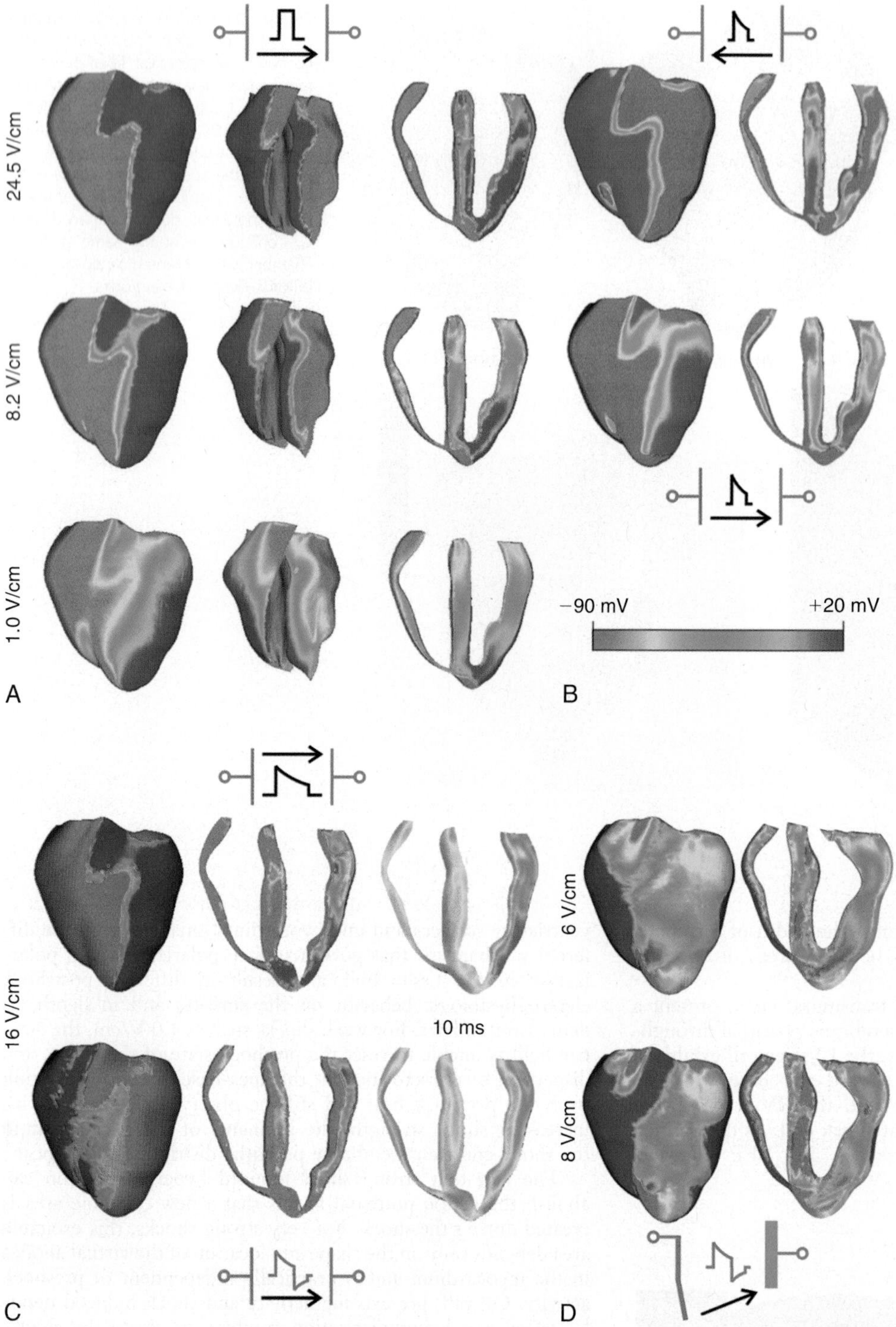

Figure 34-3 Transmembrane potential distribution at shock-end for various shock electrode configurations, waveforms, strengths, and polarities as indicated within each panel. The color scale is saturated; that is, the transmembrane potentials above 20 mV and below 90 mV appear as 20 mV and 90 mV, respectively. **A,** External shocks are monophasic, 4 ms long, and of strengths shown in the figure; they are applied at a coupling interval of 105 ms. For each case, the anterior epicardium and endocardium and a transmural view of the ventricles are shown. (Reprinted from Rodriguez B, Trayanova NA: Upper limit of vulnerability in a defibrillation model of the rabbit ventricles. J Electrocardiol 36 Suppl:51-56, 2003, with permission from Elsevier.) **B,** External truncated exponential monophasic shocks of reversed polarity and strength ~5 V/cm. Anterior epicardium and transmural views of the ventricles are shown. (Images are based on figures published in Rodriguez B, Li L, Eason JC, et al: Differences between left and right ventricular chamber geometry affect cardiac vulnerability to electric shocks. Circ Res 97:168-175, 2005.) **C,** External truncated-exponential (62% tilt) monophasic and biphasic shocks are of 10 ms duration, coupling interval 220 ms, and strengths shown in the figure. Anterior epicardium and transmural views of the ventricles are shown. Biphasic shock polarity reverses at 6 ms. The distribution of transmembrane potential 10 ms after shock-end is shown in a transmural view. **D,** Implanted cardioverter defibrillator–like electrode configuration delivers truncated-exponential (62% tilt) biphasic shocks of 10 ms duration at coupling interval 140 ms and of strengths shown in the figure.

polarized and is not an avenue for postshock propagation. The shock-end negative polarization in the RV is a thin stripe in a thin wall; thus, the RV is not a major structure for postshock propagation (discussed more later).

Reversal of shock polarity, such as in biphasic shock waveforms, has been found to improve defibrillation efficacy in humans[35,36] and in animal models,[37,38] and it is the current standard in clinical defibrillation. The mechanisms underlying the superiority of biphasic shock waveforms in achieving defibrillation success has been the subject of much debate. Advancement of VEP theory for defibrillation offered new insights into the improved efficacy of biphasic waveforms. Studies of isolated rabbit hearts by Efimov and coworkers demonstrated that the second phase of the biphasic shock reversed positive and negative polarization asymmetrically.[39] The latter is owed to the rectification properties of the voltage-dependent ionic channels; an appropriate (optimal) countershock, whose energy is found to be 20% to 70% that of the first shock,[37,39] reverses the negative VEP while partially preserving the positive, and an overall depolarization is achieved throughout the ventricles.

Figure 34-3C compares the response of the ventricles to mono- and biphasic truncated exponential shocks of strength 16 V/cm and 10 ms duration (6 ms/4 ms biphasic pulse duration). For the biphasic shock, VEP induced by the 6-ms-long first pulse reversed sign following the 4-ms-long second pulse. In this case, transmembrane potential gradient between virtual anodes and cathodes at shock end was markedly lower than at the end of the monophasic shock, indicating decreased likelihood that new activations will originate at the end of the shock. Furthermore, the intramural excitable area in the LV was significantly diminished, being located only near the base. Ten ms after the shock, there is still a significant excitable area within the LV following the monophasic shock episode, whereas following the biphasic shock the excitable area has nearly disappeared.

In Figure 34-3D the VEP distributions at shock-end are the result of two biphasic shocks; however, the shock is now delivered through the ICD configuration shown in Figure 34-1C. Although the distribution on the epicardial surface is more nonuniform in this case, the cross-sectional images demonstrate that for this defibrillation electrode configuration, the main intramural postshock excitable area is again located in the thick LV, providing an excitable pathway for postshock propagation.

Synthesizing Fluorescent Imaging Maps of Virtual Electrode Polarization in the Ventricles

Optical mapping is a powerful tool that can provide high-resolution recordings of wave-front dynamics during arrhythmia and defibrillation. The technique has, however, an important limitation: signal distortion due to scattering of fluorescent photons from a 3D volume of tissue beneath the recording site. A consequence of fluorescent scattering is that information regarding transmembrane potentials within the mid-myocardium is transduced through the ventricular wall by scattered photons and is manifested in the optical signal. There is a significant disparity in the magnitude of the optically recorded and simulated VEP induced by a defibrillation-strength shock. A recent simulation study by our group[40] demonstrated that this disparity is due to 3D scattering of photons, the latter originating from midmyocardial regions of significantly weaker VEP relative to those on the epicardium.

To generate simulated optical maps from our 3D transmembrane potential (V_m) maps, we based our approach on the photon diffusion equation for highly scattering media adapted to the 3D geometry and fiber orientation of the rabbit ventricles.[41] A 3D finite element model of epicardial optical signals was constructed by combining the bidomain representation of electrical activity with finite element solutions to the photon diffusion equation, simulating both the excitation and emission processes. Physically realistic boundary conditions were implemented on the epicardium, which allow simulation of different experimental setups.

Figure 34-4A presents shock-end anterior epicardial VEP maps of calculated transmembrane (V_m, left), synthesized optical (V_{opt}, center), and experimental optical (V_{exp}, right) potentials for a shock of 16 V/cm delivered at two coupling intervals. For comparison between simulations and experiments, the white outline over the simulated epicardial maps shows the optical field of view in the experiments. The experimental measurements were conducted on excised rabbit hearts under conditions identical to those used in the simulations.[40] Figure 34-4A shows that photon scattering results in differences between V_m and V_{opt} maps, with V_{opt} maps being a significantly better match to the V_{exp} maps than to the V_m maps. These differences are also highlighted by the action potential traces shown in Figure 34-4A, taken from a location where the cells were undergoing an action potential plateau at the time of shock delivery. Although in the V_m maps, the majority of the epicardium has strong positive and negative VEP, both V_{opt} and V_{exp} maps contain large areas of intermediate polarization. The paper by Bishop and colleagues[40] demonstrated that 3D photon scattering accounts for this discrepancy. Indeed, because VEP of diminishing magnitude is distributed, at the time of shock termination, within a scattering volume beneath an epicardial recording site, the optical signal at that instant, which represents a weighted-average of VEP values within that volume, has a lower resultant value as compared to the VEP value at the actual epicardial site.

What is the contribution of small-scale resistive heterogeneities to the overall VEP pattern in the ventricles and is it reflected in the optical maps? Fast and coworkers[42,43] attempted to address this question experimentally by recording intramural VEP using isolated coronary-perfused LV wall preparations excised from pigs' hearts. The effect of a uniform-field shock was examined on the transmural surface of the wedge preparation. The studies found surprising results, namely that for strong shocks (around 28 V/cm and greater), the entire transmural surface was negatively polarized, regardless of shock polarity or boundary conditions. It was suggested[42,43] that heterogeneities in the myocardium, such as intercellular clefts and collagen septa, combined with the negative bias in shock-induced transmembrane potential transient,[24] could underlie the overwhelming negative polarization observed in the optical map from the surface of an LV wedge.

To assess the effect of small-scale resistive heterogeneities inherent in myocardial structure on surface VEP, and to determine whether their presence could lead to the formation of a predominantly negative polarization on that surface as observed in the optical maps in the 3D bidomain simulation paper by Plank and coworkers,[44] stochastic fluctuations in the conductivity values at each element in the computational mesh were incorporated in a model of a wedge preparation with a layer of conductive fluid above the imaged surface; the wedge was subjected to uniform-field shocks. The results of the simulations for a field strength of 28 V/cm are shown in Figure 34-4B. VEP patterns are characterized with small-scale fluctuations in transmembrane potential superimposed over the large-scale VEP (top and bottom left panels) arising from the geometry of the preparation; such small-scale fluctuations have been documented by Fast and colleagues[42] using very high magnification in the optical mapping system. However, comparison with the respective optical signals with and without small-scale heterogeneities in Figure 34-4B revealed no significant change in the overall appearance of VEP. These results demonstrate that despite the negative bias in shock-induced V_m, small-scale heterogeneities could not be responsible per se for the appearance of predominantly negative polarization on the cut surface following strong shocks, even when the distortion in the optical signal is taken into account. Thus, whether small heterogeneities contribute in a major way to VEP and ultimately to the success or failure of the defibrillation shock remains to be determined.

Activity Originating from the Virtual Electrode Polarization Established by the Shock

How do cells respond to externally imposed changes in their transmembrane potential, such as those described in the

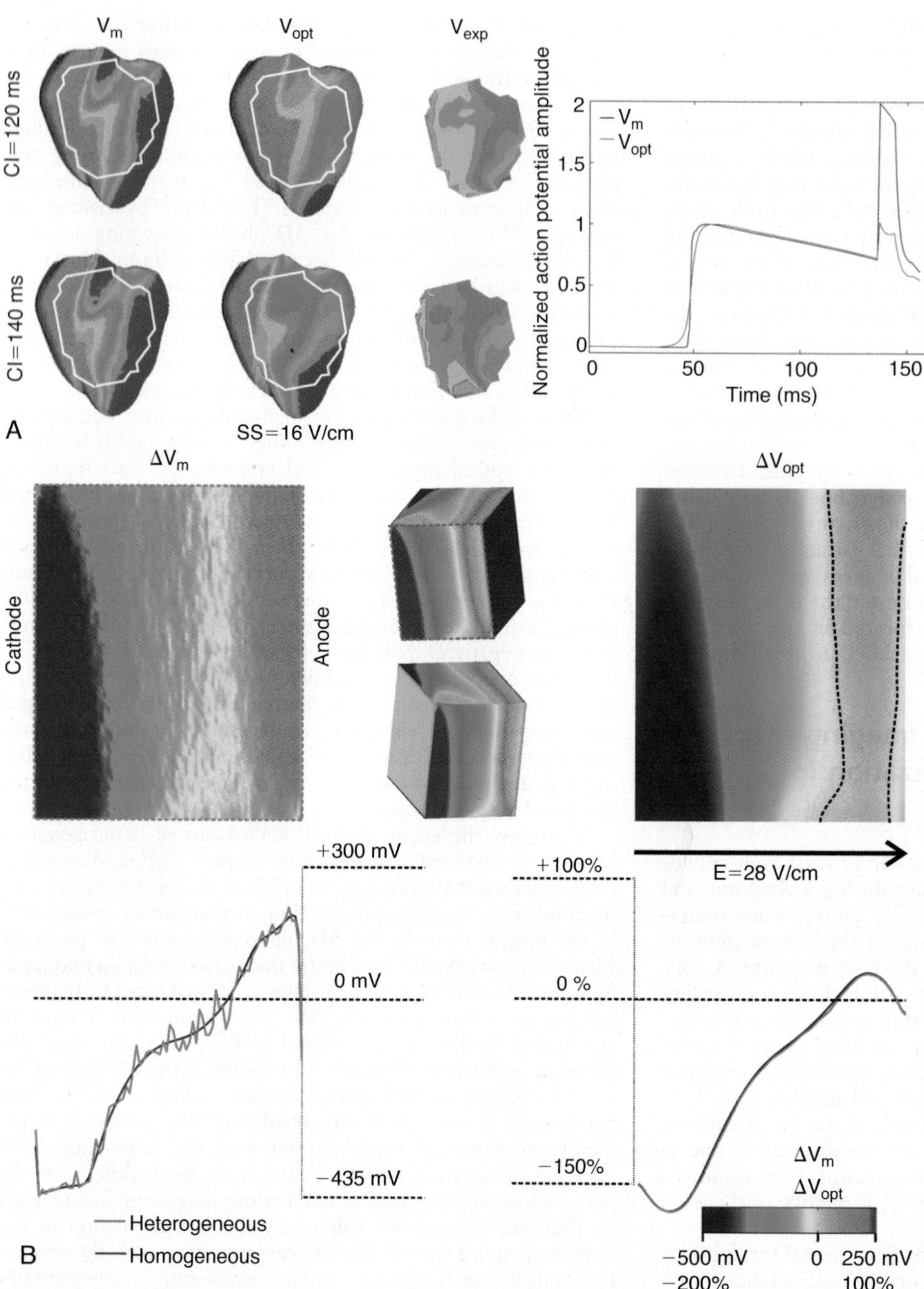

Figure 34-4 **A,** Shock-end virtual electrode polarization (VEP) maps from simulations and experiments for a shock of 16 V/cm given at two coupling intervals. Simulated maps include distributions of transmembrane potential (V_m, *left*) and optical signals (V_{opt}, *center*). Experimental maps (rabbit epicardial surface), V_{exp}, are normalized between −85 and 15 mV. V_m and V_{opt} maps are presented with color scale limits between 0 and 1 (normalized limits of the paced action potential). White outline in the simulated maps shows experimental optical field of view. V_m and V_{opt} action potential traces from a site in plateau before the shock are shown on the *right*. CI, coupling interval. (Based on figures published in Bishop M, Rodriguez B, Eason J, et al: Synthesis of voltage-sensitive optical signals: Application to panoramic optical mapping. Biophys J 90:2938-2945, 2006.) **B,** *Left, Top panel* shows the effect of small-scale resistive heterogeneities on the shock-induced distribution on the cut surface of a wedge preparation with a 2-mm conductive layer over the surface. *Bottom panel* shows a plot of profiles, with and without small-scale heterogeneities, along the centrally located horizontal line (endocardium to epicardium) in the middle of the map. Numbers indicate peak voltage. *Right, Top panel* shows the optical map of ΔV_{opt} on the wedge surface. *Dotted lines* in the map are zero isofluorescence lines. *Bottom panels* show a plot of ΔV_{opt} profiles, with and without small-scale heterogeneities, along the centrally located horizontal line (endocardium to epicardium) in the middle of the ΔV_{opt} map. Optical potentials are normalized as percentage of normal action potential magnitude. Shock strength is 28 V/cm; fiber orientation is rotational (120 degrees). (Based on figures published in Plank G, Prassl A, Hofer E, Trayanova NA: Evaluating intramural virtual electrodes in the myocardial wedge preparation: Simulations of experimental conditions. Biophys J 94(5):1904-1915, 2008.)

previous sections? The cellular response to shock-induced VEP depends on its magnitude and polarity as well as on the electrophysiologic state of the cell at the time of shock delivery. Positive VEP can result in regenerative depolarization in regions where tissue is at or near diastole; such activation is termed *make* because it takes place at the onset (make) of the shock. Action potential duration can be either extended (by positive VEP) or shortened (by negative VEP) to a degree that depends on VEP magnitude and shock timing. Finally, strong negative VEP can completely abolish (de-excite) the action potential (i.e., regenerative repolarization), thus creating postshock excitable areas in the virtual anode regions, as demonstrated in Figure 34-3.

Analyzing results of two-dimensional (2D) bidomain simulations of near-field behavior (behavior in the vicinity of a stimulus), Roth[45] demonstrated that the close proximity of a de-excited region and a virtual cathode could result in an excitation at shock end, termed *break excitation* (i.e., at the break of the shock); the virtual cathode serves as an electrical stimulus, eliciting a regenerative depolarization and a propagating wave in the newly created excitable area. Break excitations were documented to arise at the borders between oppositely polarized regions provided that the transmembrane potential gradient across the border spans the threshold for regenerative depolarization.[46] The finding of break excitations, combined with the fact that positive VEP can result in regenerative depolarization in regions where tissue is near rest, resulted in a novel understanding of how a strong stimulus can result in the development of new postshock activations.

A shock succeeds in extinguishing fibrillatory wave fronts and not initiating new re-entry if make and break excitations manage to traverse the shock-induced excitable gaps before the rest of the myocardium recovers from shock-induced depolarization.[28,39,47] This is illustrated in Figure 34-5. Panel A portrays the distribution of transmembrane potential in the ventricles 30 ms after shock end for the same set of shock strengths (square-wave shock) as in Figure 34-3A. The three views of V_m distribution show that for shock strength of 24.5 V/cm, the

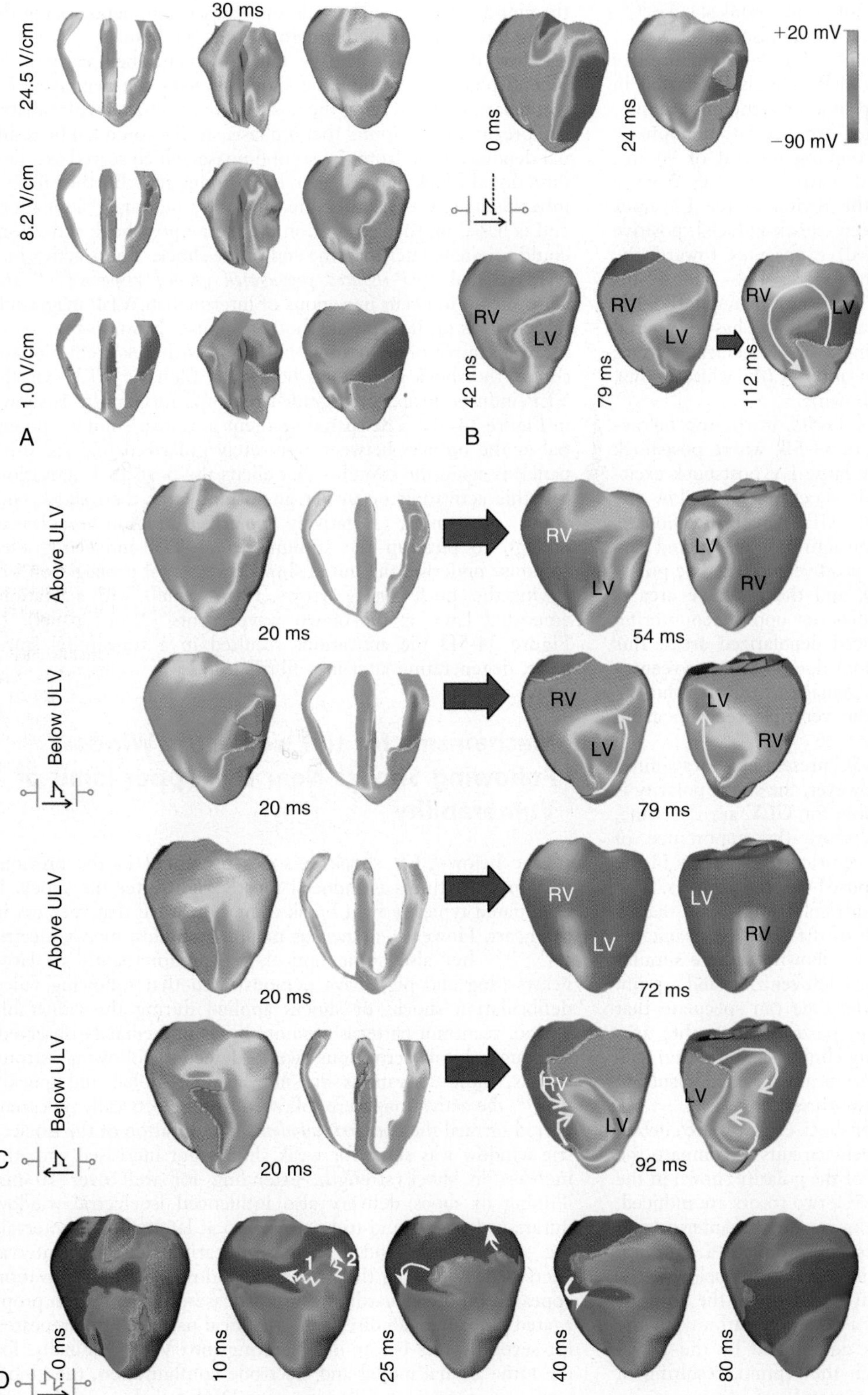

Figure 34-5 Postshock activations. **A,** Transmembrane potential distributions 30 ms after the shock end. The episodes correspond to those shown in Figure 34-4A. (Images are based on figures published in Rodriguez B, Trayanova NA: Upper limit of vulnerability in a defibrillation model of the rabbit ventricles. J Electrocardiol 36 Suppl:51-56, 2003.) **B,** Evolution of activity from shock-end until the end of the first cycle of a figure-of-eight reentry with the isthmus located at the apex. The shock is external 3.2 V/cm truncated exponential of 8 ms duration, and is applied at a coupling interval of 96 ms. Transmembrane potential distribution on the anterior epicardium is shown. The *arrow* indicates direction of propagation of the stable reentrant circuit. LV, left ventricle; RV, right ventricle. (Based on figures published in Rodriguez B, Li L, Eason JC, et al: Differences between left and right ventricular chamber geometry affect cardiac vulnerability to electric shocks. Circ Res 97:168-175, 2005.) **C,** Mechanisms for the existence of upper limit of vulnerability (ULV) demonstrated through the evolution of postshock activity for shocks of reversed polarity. Anterior epicardial and transmural views of transmembrane potential distribution are shown on the *left*, and anterior and posterior views are rendered on the *right*. For the *top panel* polarity, the ULV is 9.6 V/cm; for the bottom panel polarity, ULV is 12.7 V/cm. *White arrows* represent direction of propagation. (Based on figures published in Rodriguez B, Li L, Eason JC, et al: Differences between left and right ventricular chamber geometry affect cardiac vulnerability to electric shocks. Circ Res 97:168-175, 2005.) **D,** Induction of a postshock arrhythmia with a biphasic shock of strength 4 V/cm and duration 6/4 ms. Anterior epicardial views of transmembrane potential distribution are shown. *Zigzag arrows* 1 and 2 denote propagated graded responses induced by virtual electrode polarization (VEP). *White arrows* represent direction of propagation. (Based on figures from. Ashihara T, Constantino J. Trayanova NA: Tunnel propagation of postshock activations as a hypothesis for fibrillation induction and isoelectric window. Circ Res 102(6):737-745, 2008.)

ventricles are completely depolarized. This is because when the shock is turned off, the large voltage gradients at the boundaries between oppositely polarized areas quickly result in break excitations at multiple sites within the LV free wall and the septum. These new wave fronts rapidly depolarize the shock-induced excitable areas. The latency in the onset of these excitations, their propagation velocity in excitable areas, and shock-induced extension of refractoriness in depolarized areas (blocking propagation; see Fig. 34-5C, above-ULV panels) determine how quickly postshock activity subsides after successful shocks,[46,47] as shown in Figure 34-5A for the 8.2 V/cm episode.

Vulnerability to electric shocks and defibrillation failure can also stem from the shock-induced VEP. This is illustrated in Figure 34-5B, which presents an episode of arrhythmia induction following an external truncated-exponential monophasic shock of 3.2 V/cm applied at a coupling interval of 96 ms. Following the shock, a transmural wave emanating from a break excitation at shock end in the region of the LV apex (where the largest gradient between shock-induced positive and negative polarization is formed) propagates toward the base through the remaining excitable area (24- and 42-ms panels). The wave returns toward the apex through the RV wall and the septum, and once tissue there has recovered (79-ms panel), it reenters, establishing a stable reentrant circuit (112 ms), with one spiral wave on the anterior (the white arrow), and another on the posterior (not shown).

The episode presented in Figure 34-5C, in the top below-ULV panel, is the same as in Figure 34-5B, where postshock propagation takes place through the large LV postshock excitable area, initiating arrhythmia; this shock is thus below the ULV. In the Figure 34-5C top above-ULV panel, the shock is stronger (9.6 V/cm) and therefore the activation is initiated earlier due to larger gradients between positive and negative polarization at the apex (20-ms panels), and the excitable area is quickly traversed. The wave front dies out upon encountering refractory tissue in the shock-induced depolarized areas; this episode is thus above the ULV. A shock does not initiate reentry if break excitations are elicited that manage to traverse the LV excitable area before the rest of the ventricle recovers from shock-induced depolarization.

The bottom panels of Figure 34-5C present episodes similar to those shown in the top panels, however, the shock polarity is reversed. The mechanisms responsible for ULV are the same, but these simulation results underscore the importance of accounting for the geometry of the ventricular chambers in the quest to understand generation of postshock arrhythmias. The difference in the thickness of the ventricular walls is ultimately manifested as a preferential location of the postshock excitable area; the postshock excitable areas are shown by these simulations[28] to be always located in the thick left ventricle and septum and never in the thin right ventricle. One can speculate that identifying the location of the main postshock excitable area could be very important for improving clinical defibrillation efficacy because its eradication can be specifically targeted, resulting in a dramatic decrease in defibrillation threshold.

In addition, the location of the postshock excitable area determines the types of postshock reentrant circuits[30] (compare the below-ULV panels in Fig. 34-5C). For the polarity shown in the top below-ULV panel of Figure 34-5C, two rotors are induced, one counterclockwise and one clockwise, on the anterior and posterior sides of the ventricles, respectively, with a common pathway in the apex. In contrast, in the bottom below-ULV panel, the reentrant circuit is a figure-of-eight on the anterior and another on the posterior, with a common pathway in the LV. The pattern of the reentry is determined by the initial postshock propagation, here through the septum, resulting in subsequent activation through both free walls.

Vulnerability also has a lower limit (LLV), the lowest shock strength below which arrhythmia is not induced. The failure to induce reentry in the paced ventricles with shocks of strength below the LLV is due to the absence of unidirectional block. In this case (for instance 1 V/cm shock; episode not shown; refer to Rodriguez and Trayanova[29]), shock-induced depolarization is weak and the myocardium there is refractory only for the first few milliseconds following the shock. As a consequence of this, the wave front initiated at the apex propagates simultaneously through both ventricular walls and the septum, depolarizing the entire heart and ultimately dying out at the base.

How do biphasic shocks fail? As mentioned earlier, the second phase of the biphasic shock reverses the negative VEP while partially preserving the positive. Experiments with isolated RV preparations[48] found that biphasic shocks could fail by residual depolarization from the second phase, which served as a unidirectional block and led to reentry induction. Further insight into this issue was also obtained from 3D bidomain simulations and is based on the recognition that some postshock activations could originate later than the end of the shock. These activations were termed *VEP-induced propagated graded responses*[49,50] and were shown to occur in regions of intermediate VEP magnitude (green areas in the biphasic shock response shown in Fig. 34-3).

An example of arrhythmia induction with a 4 V/cm biphasic shock (the shock strength is below the biphasic ULV) via the VEP-induced propagated graded response mechanism is shown in Figure 34-5D. The spatial gradient in transmembrane potential at the borders between oppositely polarized regions (0-ms panel) is again the stimulus that elicits the postshock activation, but this activation occurs at an instant later than shock end, when the mildly negatively polarized region repolarizes enough to pick up the stimulus. The VEP-induced graded response underlies the initial slow decremental propagation following the shock (zigzag arrows, 10-ms panel), with activations emerging later as full-blown wave fronts (25-ms panel). In Figure 34-5D the activations resulted in a transmural spiral wave, degenerating later into fibrillation.

Mechanisms for the Isoelectric Window Following Shocks Near the Upper Limit of Vulnerability

In the below-ULV shock episodes presented in the previous section, arrhythmia is induced mostly right after the shock. It is initiated typically by a break excitation wave that reenters in the heart. However, numerous mapping studies, mostly electrical[11,51-53] but also some optical,[54,55] predominantly of large hearts (dog and pig), have demonstrated that following failed defibrillation shocks or shocks applied during the vulnerable period, reentrant patterns are not always immediately observed. Although local activations were detected following strong shocks, these activations did not become global and quickly died[56]; the activations were followed by an electrically quiescent period termed the *isoelectric window*. The duration of the isoelectric window was short for weak shocks but increased with the increase in shock strength, extending for well over 50 ms. Timing of shock delivery also influenced isoelectric window duration: It was found to be near zero at late coupling intervals (i.e., near diastole) and to increase linearly as coupling interval decreased. Following the isolectric window pause, an activation appeared on the epicardium. In most cases, this activation propagated globally in all directions as a focal pattern, often repeated for several cycles before degenerating into VF.[53,54] Finally, for the same animal model and electrode configuration, the global propagation patterns following near-DFT failed or shocks were

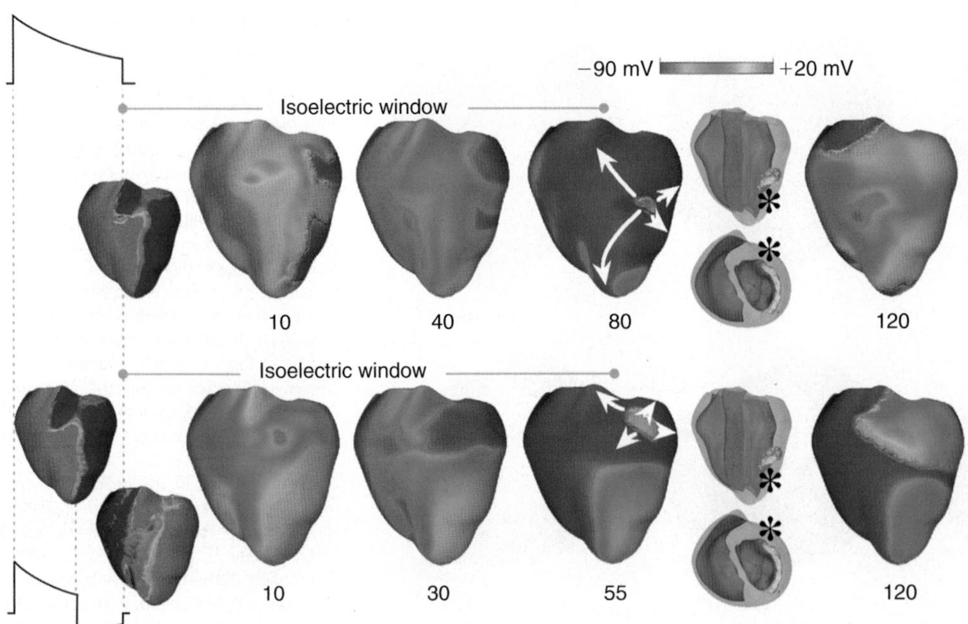

Figure 34-6 Monophasic *(top)* and biphasic *(bottom)* shock episodes resulting in isoelectric window and arrhythmia initiation. Progression of activity from virtual electrode polarization through intramural activation (marked by * in transparent views) to epicardial breakthrough, followed by focal activation pattern and reentry. Shocks are external, of 10 ms duration (6/4 ms for the biphasic shock) and of strengths 16 (monophasic) and 12 (biphasic) V/cm and are delivered at 220 ms coupling interval. (Based on figures from Ashihara T, Constantino J. Trayanova NA: Tunnel propagation of postshock activations as a hypothesis for fibrillation induction and isoelectric window. Circ Res 102(6):737-745, 2008.)

very similar to the patterns following shocks applied during the vulnerable period and slightly weaker than the ULV.[52-54]

The mechanisms underlying the origin of the first global postshock activations following the isoelectric window have also been the topic of much discussion and debate. Research has suggested that the focal or breakthrough pattern following the isoelectric window is a manifestation of transmural reentry; however, endocardial and transmural mapping studies do not support this conjecture. Micro-reentry has also been considered but is difficult to establish without closely spaced transmural recordings. Yet another hypothesis claims that slow propagation of depolarizing cellular graded responses preceding the initiation of a regenerative activation underlies the existence of the isoelectric window.[57] However, such mechanism appears to pertain only to activity in the vicinity of localized bipolar stimuli rather than to defibrillation shocks where anode and cathode are widely spaced. Simulations of defibrillation in ventricular slices by our group[58] have suggested that a transmural breakthrough could also underlie the isoelectric window and the focal appearance of the first global postshock activation. Early afterdepolarizations resulting from reactivation of the sodium current have also been considered[59] as well as ionic fluxes through electroporated cell membranes.[60]

Hwang and coworkers[61] have demonstrated that the heterogeneous distribution of intracellular calcium concentration during the isoelectric window plays a key role in the defibrillation outcome for near-DFT shocks. Another study[62] proved that the Purkinje system could be another source of the first postshock activations, because Purkinje activations were recorded before local postshock myocardial activation during the first postshock activation cycle.

A 3D simulation study from our group recently proposed a new mechanism for the existence of the isoelectric window.[63] Figure 34-6 (top) presents an episode of earliest postshock activation following an isoelectric window in a 16 V/cm monophasic shock. Formation of VEP, quick re-excitation, and synchronous repolarization take place sequentially. However, a wave front, which originated at a location deep within the wall, remained submerged (transparent panels, wave front indicated by *) until it made a breakthrough onto the epicardium, and then propagated, resulting in intramural reentry. In this example, the isoelectric window was nearly 80 ms. Figure 34-6, bottom presents an example of a postshock activation following an isoelectric window induced by 12 V/cm biphasic shock. Here again, the wave front originating 20 ms after shock-end (* in transparent views), which remained submerged for another 35 ms, made a breakthrough onto the epicardium, resulting in an intramural scroll wave. In this case the isoelectric window was approximately 55 ms.

The simulations showed that the isoelectric window duration following monophasic and biphasic shocks increased as shock strength increased, with duration similar to that obtained in the experiment.[52,53] The existence of the isoelectric window is explained by propagation of the postshock activations through intramural excitable areas (as shown in Fig. 34-3), bounded by the long-lasting postshock depolarization of the surfaces. Such intramural postshock propagation is consistent with transmural plunge electrode recordings, demonstrating that the site of origin of the postshock activation was within the myocardium rather than on the surface.[53] Furthermore, the study demonstrated that for near-ULV biphasic shocks, activations originated in the midmyocardium with a certain delay (~20 ms, Fig. 34-6B); this delay occurred because intramural VEP following biphasic shocks are weaker than following monophasic shocks, and thus the origin of the intramural activation is via VEP-induced graded responses.

Shock-Induced Phase Singularities and Filaments

Shock-induced arrhythmias are often examined in terms of the dynamics of the phase singularities, the organizing centers of reentry. The onset of a break excitation is associated with the formation of a (VEP-induced) phase singularity[64]; it forms at a point along the boundary between shock-induced depolarization and deexcitation[39,64] and is independent of the pre-shock state of

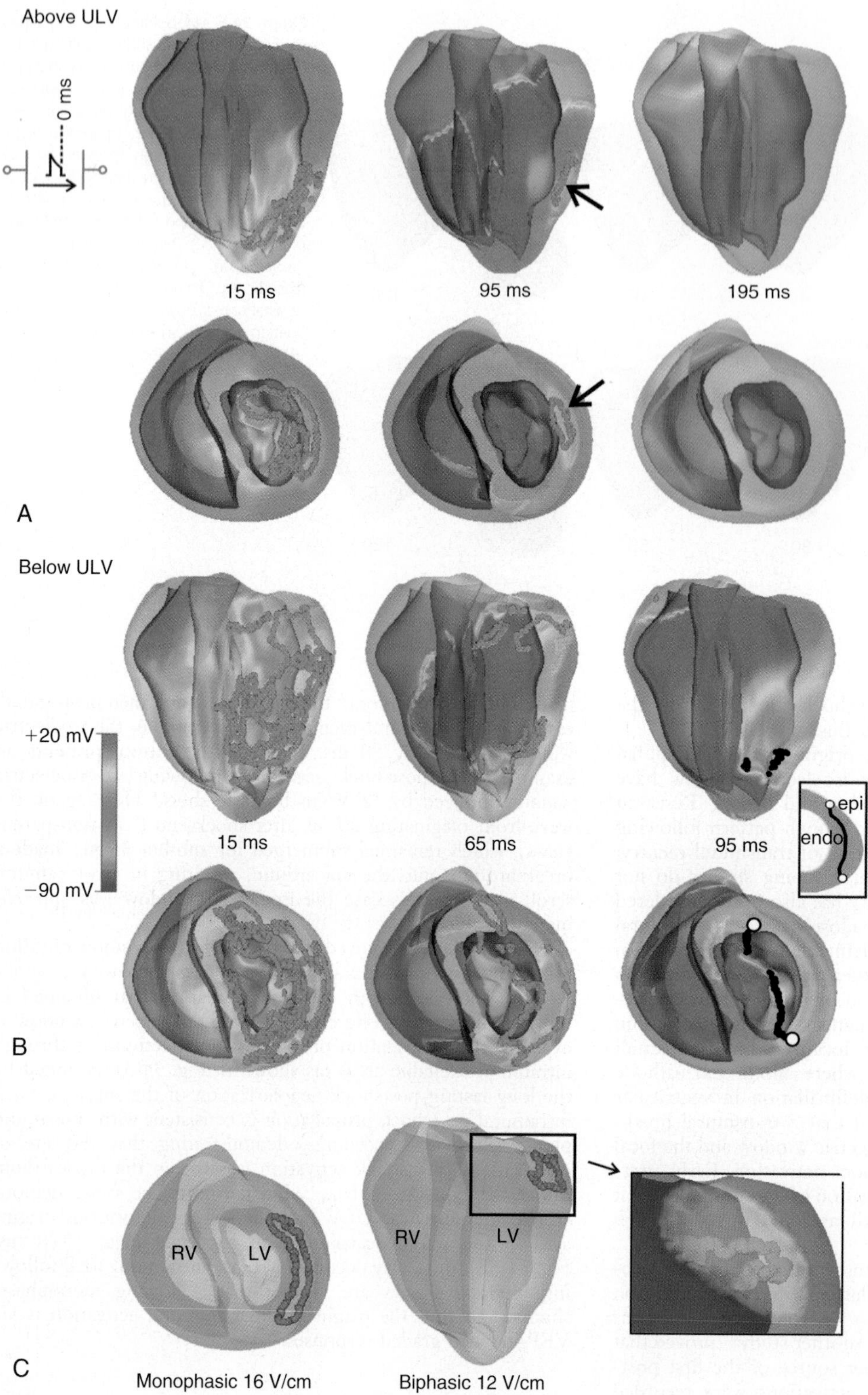

Figure 34-7 **A** and **B,** Evolution of postshock activity and filament dynamics for shocks above the upper limit of vulnerability (ULV) (**A**) and below the ULV (**B**). Transmembrane potential distributions are shown in anterior epicardial (*top rows* in each panel) and apex-to-base (*bottom rows* in each panel) views, with the ventricles rendered semitransparent. Scroll-wave filaments are shown in *pink/purple*, and the filament corresponding to the sustained reentrant circuit is depicted in *black. Inset* in **B** shows that the filament is attached with both ends *(small white circles)* to the epicardial surface (U-shape filament). *Black arrows* in **A** point toward the O-shaped filament. endo, endocardium; epi, epicardium. (Images are based on figures in Arevalo H, Rodriguez B, Trayanova NA: Arrhythmogenesis in the heart: Multiscale modeling of the effects of defibrillation shocks and the role of electrophysiological heterogeneity. Chaos 17:015103, 2007.) **C,** O-shape filaments following shocks of strengths just below the respective ULVs; in both cases the postshock activity exhibits an isolelectric window. *Inset* shows origin of focal activity associated with the O-shaped filament. LV, left ventricle; RV, right ventricle. (Based on figures from Ashihara T, Constantino J. Trayanova NA: Tunnel propagation of postshock activations as a hypothesis for fibrillation induction and isoelectric window. Circ Res 102(6):737-745, 2008.)

the myocardium. If these phase singularities survive allowing a spiraling wave front to develop, the shock results in the (re)initiation of reentrant arrhythmia. A phase singularity is typically observed on the ventricular surface (epicardium) because reentrant activity (spiral waves) is imaged there. However, in the context of the 3D geometry of the ventricles, a phase singularity represents the intersection of a scroll-wave filament, the 3D organizing center of reentry, with the ventricular surface. 3D bidomain simulations of postshock behavior have provided important insight in elucidating the dynamics of the postshock filaments.

Figure 34-7A presents two monophasic shock episodes, one above the ULV (top) and one below it (bottom). In both cases, the shock induces a large number of filaments of complex geometry. At 15 ms after shock, there are fewer and smaller filaments following the stronger shock. In both cases, the number of the filaments decreases with time following the shock (middle panels). In the stronger shock episode, at 95 ms the remaining filament has an O-shape (see black arrow). O-shaped filaments are unstable and collapse on themselves, such as in the case shown in the figure, leading to termination of the reentrant activity. In contrast, in the weaker shock episode, a single filament persists, causing the establishment of a sustained ventricular tachycardia. This is a U-shaped filament (a U-shaped filament is a filament both ends of which are in contact with the same, endocardial or epicardial, surface) with both ends attached to the epicardium, and it underlies the same reentrant circuit as in Figure 34-5B.

Results from bidomain simulations have also provided important insights into how the 3D postshock reentrant circuits established soon after a failed shock can further degrade into ventricular fibrillation.[65] The mechanisms underlying the superiority of biphasic shock waveforms in achieving defibrillation success as well as of the lower biphasic-waveform ULV can also be explained in terms of phase singularities: Because the biphasic shock reverses the negative VEP while partially preserving the positive, phase singularities that might be generated by the first shock phase are erased by the second.

Monophasic and biphasic shocks associated with an isoelectric window also result in the development of O-shaped filaments. This is illustrated in Figure 34-7B. The O-shaped filament ensuing from the monophasic shock was typically long and followed the contour of the ventricular wall, whereas that originating from the biphasic shock was much smaller. In both cases, activity was mushroom-like, consistent with a scroll wave rotating around a filament ring,[3] and therefore the earliest epicardial activation exhibited a focal pattern consistent with experimental data.

Conclusions

The information and examples presented in this chapter regarding the development, achievements, and mechanistic insight provided by the 3D models of shock-induced arrhythmogenesis and defibrillation underscore the power of realistic simulations. Simulations are particularly useful in revealing electrical behavior hidden within the cardiac wall. Insights into vulnerability and defibrillation, such as those presented here, cannot be achieved with experimental methodology alone. When supported by experimental observations of behavior during and after the shock over the cardiac surfaces, realistic whole-organ simulations become invaluable in providing mechanistic insight. In general, such models can be successfully employed to study any aspect of arrhythmogenesis and serve as a testbed for new potential antiarrhythmia therapies.

References

1. Maisel W: Pacemaker and ICD generator reliability: Meta-analysis of device registries. JAMA 95:1929-1934, 2006.
2. Qu F, Nikolski VP, Grimm C, Efimov IR: Three dimensional panoramic fast fluorescence imaging of cardiac arrhythmias in the rabbit heart. J Biomed Opt 12:044019, 2007.
3. Winfree AT: When Time Breaks Down. Princeton: Princeton University Press, 1987.
4. Frazier DW, Wolf PD, Wharton JM, et al: Stimulus induced critical point: Mechanism for electrical initiation of reentry in normal canine myocardium. J Clin Invest 83:1039-1052, 1989.
5. Krassowska W, Pilkington TC, Ideker RE: Periodic conductivity as a mechanism for cardiac stimulation and defibrillation. IEEE Trans Biomed Eng 34:555-560, 1987.
6. Chen PS, Wolf PD, Ideker RE: Mechanism of cardiac defibrillation: A different point of view. Circulation 84:913-919, 1991.
7. Chen PS, Shibata N, Dixon EG, et al: Comparison of the defibrillation threshold and the upper limit of ventricular vulnerability. Circulation 73:1022-1028, 1986.
8. Sepulveda NG, Roth BJ, Wikswo JP Jr: Current injection into a two-dimensional anistropic bidomain. Biophys J 55:987-999, 1989.
9. Wikswo JP Jr, Lin SF, Abbas RA: Virtual electrodes in cardiac tissue: A common mechanism for anodal and cathodal stimulation. Biophys J 69:2195-2210, 1995.
10. Efimov IR, Cheng Y, Biermann M, et al: Transmembrane voltage changes produced by real and virtual electrodes during monophasic defibrillation shock delivered by an implantable electrode. J Cardiovasc Electrophysiol 8:1031-1045, 1997.
11. Knisley SB, Trayanova NA, Aguel F: Roles of electric field and fiber structure in cardiac electric stimulation. Biophys J 77:1404-1417, 1999.
12. Efimov IR, Aguel F, Cheng Y, et al: Virtual electrode polarization in the far field: Implications for external defibrillation. Am J Physiol 279:H1055-H1070, 2000.
13. Sobie EA, Susil RC, Tung L: A generalized activating function for predicting virtual electrodes in cardiac tissue. Biophys J 73:1410-1423, 1997.
14. Trayanova NA, Skouibine K, Aguel F: The role of cardiac tissue structure in defibrillation. Chaos 8:221-233, 1998.
15. Trayanova NA: Concepts of defibrillation. Phil Trans Roy Soc London A 359:1327-1337, 2001.
16. Entcheva E, Trayanova NA, Claydon F: Patterns of and mechanisms for shock induced polarization in the heart: A bidomain analysis. IEEE Trans Biomed Eng 46:260-270, 1999.
17. Trayanova NA, Roth BJ, Malden LJ: The response of a spherical heart to a uniform electric field: A bidomain analysis of cardiac stimulation. IEEE Trans Biomed Eng 40:899-908, 1993.
18. Fast VG, Rohr S, Gillis AM, Kleber AG: Activation of cardiac tissue by extracellular electrical shocks: Formation of "secondary sources" at intercellular clefts in monolayers of cultured myocytes. Circ Res 82:375-385, 1998.
19. Fishler MG: Syncytial heterogeneity as a mechanism underlying cardiac far-field stimulation during defibrillation-level shocks. J Cardiovasc Electrophysiol 9:384-394, 1998.
20. Hooks DA, Tomlinson KA, Marsden SG, et al: Cardiac microstructure: Implications for electrical propagation and defibrillation in the heart. Circ Res 91:331-338, 2002.
21. Vetter FJ, McCulloch AD: Three-dimensional analysis of regional cardiac function: A model of rabbit ventricular anatomy. Prog Biophys Mol Biol 69:157-183, 1998.
22. Burton RA, Plank G, Schneider JE, et al: Three-dimensional models of individual cardiac histoanatomy: Tools and challenges. Ann N Y Acad Sci 1080:301-319, 2006.
23. Trayanova NA, Plank G, Rodriguez B: What have we learned from mathematical models of defibrillation and postshock arrhythmogenesis? Application of bidomain simulations. Heart Rhythm 3:1232-1235, 2006.
24. Ashihara T, Trayanova NA: Asymmetry in membrane responses to electrical shocks: Insight from bidomain simulations. Biophys J 87:2271-2282, 2004.
25. Trayanova NA, Eason JC, Aguel F: Computer simulations of cardiac defibrillation: A look inside the heart. Comp Visual Sc 4:259-270, 2002.
26. Anderson C, Trayanova NA, Skouibine K: Termination of spiral waves with biphasic shocks: The role of virtual electrode polarization. J Cardiovasc Electrophysiol 11:1386-1396, 2000.
27. Rodriguez B, Tice B, Eason J, et al: Cardiac vulnerability to electric shocks during phase 1a of acute global ischemia. Heart Rhythm 6:695-703, 2004.
28. Rodriguez B, Li L, Eason JC, et al: Differences between left and right ventricular chamber geometry affect cardiac vulnerability to electric shocks. Circ Res 97:168-175, 2005.

29. Rodriguez B, Trayanova NA: Upper limit of vulnerability in a defibrillation model of the rabbit ventricles. J Electrocardiol 36 Suppl:51-56, 2003.
30. Rodriguez B, Eason JC, Trayanova NA: Differences between left and right ventricular anatomy determine the types of reentrant circuits induced by an external electric shock. A rabbit heart simulation study. Prog Biophys Mol Biol 90:399-413, 2006.
31. Arevalo H, Rodriguez B, Trayanova NA: Arrhythmogenesis in the heart: Multiscale modeling of the effects of defibrillation shocks and the role of electrophysiological heterogeneity. Chaos 17:015103, 2007.
32. Aguel F, Eason J, Trayanova NA: Advances in modeling cardiac defibrillation. Int J Bifurcation Chaos 13:3791-3805, 2003.
33. Moe GK, Harris AS, Wiggers CJ: Analysis of the initiation of fibrillation by electrographic studies. Am J Physiol 134:473-492, 1941.
34. Fabiato A, Coumel P, Gourgon R, Saumont R: [The threshold of synchronous response of the myocardial fibers. Application to the experimental comparison of the efficacy of different forms of electroshock defibrillation]. Arch Mal Cur 60:527-544, 1967.
35. Bardy GH, Ivey TD, Allen MD, et al: A prospective randomized evaluation of biphasic versus monophasic waveform pulses on defibrillation efficacy in humans. J Am Coll Cardiol 14:728-733, 1989.
36. Saksena S, An H, Mehra R, et al: Prospective comparison of biphasic and monophasic shocks for implantable cardioverter-defibrillators using endocardial leads. Am J Cardiol 70:304-310, 1992.
37. Feeser SA, Tang ASL, Kavanagh KM, et al: Strength-duration and probability of success curves for defibrillation with biphasic waveforms. Circulation 82:2128-2141, 1990.
38. Kavanagh KM, Tang ASL, Rollins DL, et al: Comparison of the internal defibrillation thresholds for monophasic and double and single capacitor biphasic waveforms. J Am Coll Cardiol 14:1343-1349, 1989.
39. Efimov IR, Cheng Y, Yamanouchi Y, Tchou PJ: Direct evidence of the role of virtual electrode–induced phase singularity in success and failure of defibrillation. J Cardiovasc Electrophysiol 11:861-868, 2000.
40. Bishop M, Rodriguez B, Qu F, et al: The role of photon scattering in optical signal distortion during arrhythmia and defibrillation. Biophys J 93:3714-3726, 2007.
41. Bishop M, Rodriguez B, Eason J, et al: Synthesis of voltage-sensitive optical signals: Application to panoramic optical mapping. Biophys J 90:2938-2945, 2006.
42. Sharifov OF, Ideker RE, Fast VG: High-resolution optical mapping of intramural virtual electrodes in porcine left ventricular wall. Cardiovasc Res 64:448-456, 2004.
43. Sharifov OF, Fast VG: Intramural virtual electrodes in ventricular wall: Effects on epicardial polarizations. Circulation 109:2349-2356, 2004.
44. Plank G, Prassl A, Hofer E, Trayanova NA: Evaluating intramural virtual electrodes in the myocardial wedge preparation: Simulations of experimental conditions. Biophys J 94(5):1904-1915, 2008.
45. Roth BJ: A mathematical model of make and break electrical stimulation of cardiac tissue by a unipolar anode or cathode. IEEE Trans Biomed Eng 42:1174-1184, 1995.
46. Cheng Y, Mowrey KA, Van Wagoner DR, et al: Virtual electrode induced re-excitation: A mechanism of defibrillation. Circ Res 85:1056-1066, 1999.
47. Skouibine K, Trayanova NA, Moore P: Success and failure of the defibrillation shock: Insights from a simulation study. J Cardiovasc Electrophysiol 11:785-796, 2000.
48. Evans FG, Gray R: Shock-induced epicardial and endocardial virtual electrodes leading to ventricular fibrillation via reentry, graded responses and transmural activation. J Cardiovasc Electrophysiol 15:79-87, 2004.
49. Bourn DW, Gray RA, Trayanova NA: Characterization of the relationship between preshock state and virtual electrode polarization–induced propagated graded responses resulting in arrhythmia induction. Heart Rhythm 3:583-595, 2006.
50. Trayanova NA, Gray RA, Bourn DW, Eason JC: Virtual electrode induced positive and negative graded responses: New insights into fibrillation induction in defibrillation. J Cardiovasc Electrophysiol 14:756-763, 2003.
51. Chen PS, Shibata N, Dixon EG, et al: Activation during ventricular defibrillation in open-chest dogs: Evidence of complete cessation and regeneration of ventricular fibrillation after unsuccessful shocks. J Clin Invest 77:810-823, 1986.
52. Shibata N, Chen PS, Dixon EG, et al: Epicardial activation after unsuccessful defibrillation shocks in dogs. Am J Physiol 255:H902-H909, 1988.
53. Chattipakorn N, Rogers J, Ideker RE: Influence of postshock epicardial activation patterns on initiation of ventricular fibrillation by upper limit of vulnerability shocks. Circulation 101:1329-1336, 2000.
54. Chattipakorn N, Banville I, Gray RA, Ideker RE: Mechanism of ventricular defibrillation for near-defibrillation threshold shocks: A whole-heart optical mapping study in swine. Circulation 104:1515-1525, 2001.
55. Wang NC, Lee MH, Ohara T, et al: Optical mapping of ventricular defibrillation in isolated swine ventricles: Demonstration of a postshock isoelectric window after near-threshold defibrillation shocks. Circulation 104:227-233, 2001.
56. Chattipakorn N, KenKnight BH, Rogers JM, et al: Locally propagated activation immediately after internal defibrillation. Circulation 97:1401-1410, 1998.
57. Karagueuzian HS, Chen PS: Cellular mechanism of reentry induced by a strong electrical stimulus: Implications for fibrillation and defibrillation. Cardiovasc Res 50:251-262, 2001.
58. Hillebrenner MG, Eason JC, Trayanova NA: Mechanistic inquiry into decrease in probability of defibrillation success with increase in complexity of preshock reentrant activity. Am J Physiol 286:H909-H917, 2004.
59. Kodama IN, Shibata N, Sakuma I, et al: Aftereffects of high-intensity DC stimulation on the electromechanical performance of ventricular muscle. Am J Physiol 267:H248-H258, 1994.
60. Ohuchi K, Fukui Y, Sakuma I, et al: A dynamic action potential model analysis of shock-induced aftereffects in ventricular muscle by reversible breakdown of cell membrane. IEEE Trans Biomed Eng 49:18-30, 2002.
61. Hwang GS, Hayashi H, Tang L, Ogawa M, et al: Intracellular calcium and vulnerability to fibrillation and defibrillation in Langendorff-perfused rabbit ventricles. Circulation 114:2595-2603, 2006.
62. Dosdall DJ, Cheng KA, Huang J, et al: Transmural and endocardial Purkinje activation in pigs before local myocardial activation after defibrillation shocks. Heart Rhythm 4:758-765, 2007.
63. Ashihara T, Constantino J, Trayanova NA: Tunnel propagation of postshock activations as a hypothesis for fibrillation induction and isoelectric window. Circ Res 102(6):737-745, 2008.
64. Efimov IR, Cheng Y, Van Wagoner DR, et al: Virtual electrode–induced phase singularity: A basic mechanism of defibrillation failure. Circ Res 82:918-925, 1998.
65. Trayanova NA, Aguel F, Larson C, Haro C: Modeling cardiac defibrillation: An inquiry into post-shock dynamics. In Zipes D, Jalife J (eds): Cardiac Electrophysiology: From Cell to Bedside, 4th ed. Philadelphia, WB Saunders, 2004, pp 282-291.

Adrenergic Signaling and Cardiac Ion Channels 35

RONALD A. LI AND NIPAVAN CHIAMVIMONVAT

CHAPTER OUTLINE

Overview of the Adrenergic Signaling in the Heart

Adrenergic receptors belong to a conserved family of seven transmembrane proteins known as *guanine nucleotide-binding regulatory protein-coupled receptors* (GPCRs). GPCRs have a wide distribution throughout the body and play important functional roles in diverse cellular regulatory processes, and as such, they represent one of the largest classes of receptors for drug targets. Indeed, drugs targeting adrenergic and angiotensin GPCR signaling pathways account for the majority of cardiovascular drugs used clinically.

Heart rate (chronotropy) and cardiac contractility (inotropy) are regulated on a beat-to-beat basis to meet the demand of physical activity and emotional stress as needed for fight-or-flight responses. This fundamental function of the heart is achieved by fine tuning cardiac excitability via the regulation of cardiac ion channels by the autonomic nervous system. This modulation of cardiac excitability requires an exquisite control and precise integration of the signaling components in a dynamic fashion. Indeed, abnormalities in the autonomic regulation can result in life-threatening cardiac arrhythmias.[1]

Cardiac myocytes and pacemaking tissues are highly innervated. Various subtypes of adrenergic receptors are expressed in mammalian hearts and are responsible for transmitting the activation of sympathetic nervous system from neurotransmitter norepinephrine and the adrenal medullary hormone epinephrine into changes in heart rate and contractility. They are also responsible for regulating blood pressure and hypertrophic responses. Studies have shown that different subtypes of adrenergic receptors are remodeled during pathologic processes. This chapter reviews the vast amount of literature on the adrenergic signaling and cardiac ion channels. Specifically, we concentrate on Na^+, K^+, Ca^{2+} and hyperpolarization-activated cyclic nucleotide gated (HCN) channels. Other aspects of neural control of cardiac excitability are covered in other chapters. The reader is referred elsewhere for more general reviews of GPCR and adrenergic receptor signaling.[2-5]

G-Protein Coupled Receptors

GPCRs represent the largest and most diverse superfamily of receptors in the human genome, and they share a conserved protein structure with extracellular amino termini, intracellular carboxyl termini, and seven transmembrane α helices, which are connected by three extracellular and three intracellular loops. It has been estimated that about 200 different GPCRs are expressed in various cardiac cell types and up to 1000 different such receptors exist in mammals.[2,6] Structure-function analyses of GPCRs have revealed that the receptor proteins are activated by ligand binding to an extracellular active site, resulting in a conformational change in the protein followed by the coupling of the receptor to heterotrimeric G proteins.[2,7,8] Studies have reported the crystal structure of a human β_2-adrenergic receptor at about 0.2-nm resolution.[9-11] These studies provided a high-resolution structure of a human GPCR bound to a diffusible ligand. It was observed from the crystal structure that the ligand-binding site accessibility is enabled by the second extracellular loop of the GPCR, which is maintained out of the binding cavity by a pair of disulfide bonds and a short helical segment within the loop (Fig. 35-1A).

Heterotrimeric G proteins consist of three different subunits: α, β, and γ. Upon activation by GPCRs, the G protein converts guanosine triphosphate (GTP) to guanosine diphosphate (GDP) on the α subunit, leading to the dissociation of the G_α subunit from the $G_{\beta\gamma}$ subunits.[2,4,5] There are four primary families of G_α subunits ($G_{\alpha s}$ (stimulatory G protein), $G_{\alpha i}$ (inhibitory or pertussis toxin–sensitive G protein), $G_{\alpha q}$, and $G_{\alpha 11/12}$). Apart from the large number of GPCR subtypes expressed in the cells, diversity in the downstream signaling pathways is further brought about by interaction of GPCRs with a specific subset of heterotrimeric G proteins. Dissociated G_α subunits can interact with downstream effectors to inhibit or activate various enzymes such as adenylyl cyclase and phospholipase Cβ (PLC_β), or an ion channel.[2,4,5] Dissociated $G_{\beta\gamma}$ subunits can target various signaling pathways involved in desensitization and down-regulation of the receptor proteins, apoptosis, and ion channel activation ($I_{K,ACh}$).[2,4,5]

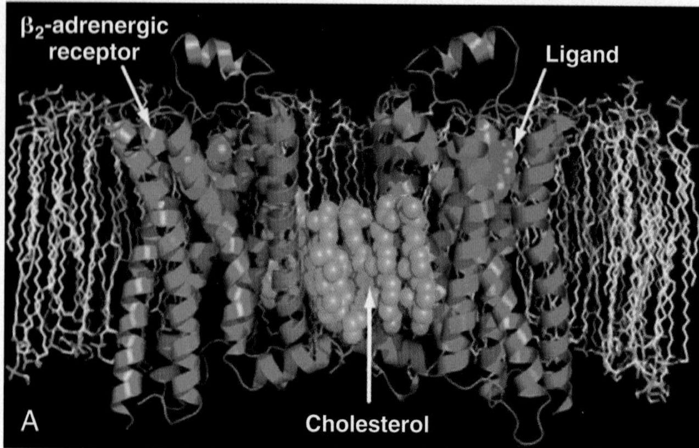

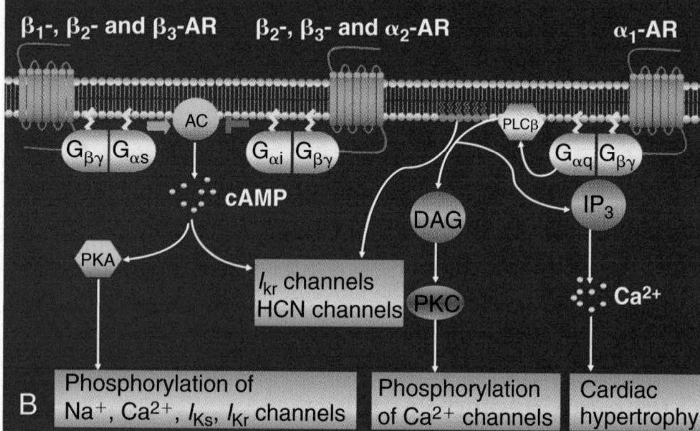

Figure 35-1 Overview of α- and β-adrenergic signaling. **A,** Structure of a human G-protein coupled receptor (GPCR) bound to a diffusible ligand. (Taken from Cherezov V, Rosenbaum DM, Hanson MA, et al: High-resolution crystal structure of an engineered human beta2-adrenergic G protein-coupled receptor. Science 318:1258-1265, 2007 with permission.) **B,** Agonist binding to adrenergic receptors (ARs) results in the coupling to heterotrimeric G proteins and the conversion of guanosine triphosphate (GTP) to guanosine diphosphate (GDP) and the dissociation of $G_{\alpha i}$ and $G_{\beta\gamma}$ subunits. β_1-ARs couple primarily to stimulatory $G_{\alpha s}$ and initiates the activation of a membrane-bound effector molecule, adenylyl cyclase (AC), to produce second messenger, cyclic adenosine 3′,5′ monophosphate (cAMP), and activation of protein kinase A (PKA). Downstream effectors of PKA include sodium, calcium, and potassium channels. cAMP also directly modulates I_f (HCN) and I_{Kr} channels. β_2- and β_3-ARs signal through both $G_{\alpha s}$- and $G_{\alpha i}$-proteins, and α_2-ARs couple primarily to $G_{\alpha i}$-protein. $G_{\alpha s}$ stimulates AC, and activation of $G_{\alpha i}$ inhibits AC, reducing the accumulation of cAMP. α_1-ARs, on the other hand, predominantly couple through $G_{\alpha q}$-protein. Activated $G_{\alpha q}$ protein in turn leads to downstream activation of the membrane-bound effector molecule, phospholipase C β (PLCβ) to produce second messengers, diacylglycerol (DAG) and inositol 1,4,5-triphosphate (IP_3), which activate a variety of downstream signals involved in the regulation of contractility, hypertrophy, and apoptosis. The substrate for PLCβ is phosphatidyl-4,5-bisphosphate (PIP_2), a membrane phospholipid. DAG is the physiologic activator of protein kinase C (PKC). (Adapted from Salazar NC, Chen J, Rockman HA: Cardiac GPCRs: GPCR signaling in healthy and failing hearts. Biochim Biophys Acta 1768:1006-1018, 2007.)

Adrenergic Receptors in the Heart

Adrenergic receptors are composed of two main subtypes: α-adrenergic receptors and β-adrenergic receptors. Three β-adrenergic receptor subtypes are found in mammalian hearts, and all are activated by catecholamine, norepinephrine, and epinephrine. The β_1-receptor subtype predominates in the heart and accounts for about 80% of the β-adrenergic receptors; β_3-adrenergic receptors are the least abundant.[4] Apart from differences in the level of expression among the three subtypes, they couple to distinct G proteins to activate the various effector functions. β_1-Adrenergic receptors couple primarily to stimulatory $G_{\alpha s}$ to regulate heart rate and contractility via activation of adenylyl cyclase–cyclic adenosine monophosphate–protein kinase A (AC-cAMP-PKA). β_2-Adrenergic receptors were originally thought to signal exclusively through $G_{\alpha s}$. Like the β_1-adrenergic receptor, $G_{\alpha s}$ signaling leads to regulation of heart rate and contractility. β_2-Adrenergic receptors differ importantly from β_1-adrenergic receptors in that they can also couple to the $G_{\alpha i}$ protein after receptor phosphorylation by PKA.[12] β_3-adrenergic receptors can couple to both $G_{\alpha s}$ and $G_{\alpha i}$ proteins (see Fig. 35-1B).

α-Adrenergic receptors can be divided into two main subtypes, α_1 and α_2. α_1-Adrenergic receptors predominantly couple through $G_{\alpha q}$ protein in response to sympathetic nervous system stimulation, specifically α_{1A}, α_{1B}, and α_{1D} subtypes. Activation of heterotrimeric G proteins results in the dissociation of $G_{\alpha q}$ subunits from $G_{\beta\gamma}$ subunits. Activated $G_{\alpha q}$ protein in turn leads to downstream activation of PLC_β. The substrate for PLC_β is phosphatidyl-4,5-bisphosphate (PIP_2), a membrane phospholipid, which is hydrolyzed into intracellular second messengers, 1,4,5-inositol-triphosphate (IP_3), and diacyl glycerol (DAG). IP_3 leads to the mobilization of Ca^{2+} entry into intracellular compartments, inducing hypertrophic response. DAG is the physiologic activator of protein kinase C (PKC), a serine- and threonine-dependent protein kinase. Thus, activation of α_1-adrenergic receptor leads to an increase in the concentrations of second messengers IP_3 and DAG, with a concomitant reduction of PIP_2 within the plasma membrane. α_2-Adrenergic receptors, on the other hand, couple to $G_{\alpha i}$-protein, leading to inhibitory effects on the enzyme adenylyl cyclase, thereby reducing the intracellular concentration of the second messenger cAMP (see Fig. 35-1B). Finally, remodeling of adrenergic receptors occurs during pathologic conditions, such as heart failure, with varying consequences from each adrenergic receptor subtype.

Specificity and Integration of Adrenergic Signaling via Compartmentalization

Cardiac excitability and propagation are often regulated with millisecond precision. A multitude of signaling cascades and associated molecules are involved in this regulation. This raises a fundamental question: Is it possible for this diverse group of proteins and second messengers to work together and yet provide the needed specificity and efficiency within the required time scale?

A common theme has emerged that supports the notion that exquisite specificity and integration of membrane excitability are achieved via compartmentalization of the signaling networks in membrane microdomains in which relevant proteins are maintained within the same physical space.[13,14] Specifically, certain features of the adrenergic signaling in cardiomyocytes are inconsistent with traditional models that assume receptors, G proteins, and effectors freely mobile on the surface of the membranes. Rather, there is physical compartmentalization of the signaling complexes to allow a fast, effective, and precise integration of the networks. For example, within a cardiac myocyte, there is subcellular compartmentalization of AC-cAMP-PKA signaling complexes such that cAMP can gain access only to a subset of cAMP-dependent PKA, and PKA can only interact with a subset of relevant cellular substrates.

The molecular mechanisms responsible for the selective interactions of the signaling complexes include localization of receptors, G proteins, multiple isoforms of adenylyl cyclase, protein kinases, and phosphatases within discrete membrane microdomains. Membrane microdomains such as caveolae or lipid rafts are sites that differentially localize individual β-adrenergic receptor subtypes together with the downstream signaling complexes. Caveolae are omega-shaped membrane invaginations enriched in cholesterol and sphingolipids and are defined by their principal structural protein, caveolin. β_1-Adrenergic receptors reside in both caveolar and noncaveolar membranes, however, β_2-adrenergic receptors appear to be confined mainly to caveolae.

In contrast, muscarinic acetyl choline receptors (M_2Rs) are excluded from caveolae. In this context, parasympathetic modulation of the β_1-adrenergic response is facilitated but not the β_2-adrenergic response. It has been documented that ion channels form multiprotein complexes with adaptor proteins such as A-kinase anchoring proteins (AKAP) that specifically target PKA, phosphodiesterase (PDE) isoforms, and phosphoprotein phosphatases within discrete subcellular regions. Several types of cardiac ion channels and transporters, including voltage-gated sodium and calcium channels, voltage-gated potassium channels (K_V1.5), the Na^+-Ca^{2+} exchanger, and HCN channels have been localized to caveolar membranes.[15-18] Taken together, the colocalization of ion channels with specific subtypes of GPCRs and downstream molecules provides the necessary compartmentalization of signaling networks, enabling rapid and precise regulation of the channel function. This physical arrangement has important implications for the adrenergic signaling of cardiac excitation and impulse propagation.

Finally, studies have provided evidence that signal integration of the adrenergic receptors might further arise from heterodimerization of members of distinct subfamilies of GPCRs. Such receptor heterodimerization helps to expand the functional diversity and characteristics of the receptors involved.[19] For example, heterodimerization of β_1- and β_2-adrenergic receptors in intact cardiac myocytes has been reported to give rise to a new population of β-adrenergic receptors with enhanced signaling properties.[20]

Voltage-Gated Sodium Channels

Voltage-gated sodium channels are responsible for generating the rapid upstroke of action potentials in cardiac myocytes, and hence they are important in generating and propagating impulses. Previous studies have provided evidence to support the notion that cardiac sodium channels can be modulated by β-adrenergic receptor stimulation via dual G protein pathways, which include indirect pathway through G protein–regulated second messenger cascades and direct pathway by a membrane-delimited modulation of the channel (Fig. 35-2A).[21-24] The indirect pathway occurs via phosphorylation of the pore-forming α subunit of the sodium channels by PKA at serine residues, resulting in changes in current amplitude as well as time- and voltage-dependent kinetics of the channel proteins. The α subunits of rat and human cardiac sodium channels have been shown to contain multiple PKA consensus sites.[25,26] More-recent work provides evidence for the PKA-dependent modulation of the trafficking of the sodium-channel proteins.[27-29] Specifically, these studies demonstrate that both α-subunit phosphorylation and the presence of putative endoplasmic reticulum (ER) retention signals are required for the PKA-mediated increase in cardiac sodium current. Moreover, the increase in Na_V1.5 current by PKA can be prevented by inhibitors of cell membrane recycling, suggesting that PKA activation promotes trafficking of channels to the plasma membrane.

In contrast to the PKA-dependent pathway, the direct membrane-delimited β-adrenergic signaling on the sodium channel is PKA-independent, but is dependent upon direct stimulation by $G_{\alpha s}$ and results from a change in the number of functional channels.[30] More-recent data further suggest the localization of a fraction of cardiac sodium channel in caveolae.[15] Stimulation of β-adrenergic receptors by activating $G_{\alpha s}$ promotes the presentation of cardiac sodium channels associated with caveolar membranes to the sarcolemma, resulting in the increase in the number of functional channels.[15] Indeed, membrane microdomains including caveolae and lipid rafts have been shown to play critical roles in the compartmentalization of β-adrenergic signaling by differential colocalization of β-adrenergic receptor subtypes as well as downstream signaling molecules.[13]

On the other hand, controversy exists regarding the directionality of the current modulation by PKA stimulation. β-Adrenergic stimulation on sodium currents was found to be inhibitory in some studies[21] and stimulatory in others.[22,24,26] The conflicting results might stem directly from differences in the model systems used in these studies. Moreover, the β-adrenergic receptor could switch its coupling to different G proteins[12] further suggesting the complexity of β-adrenergic modulation of cardiac ion channels.

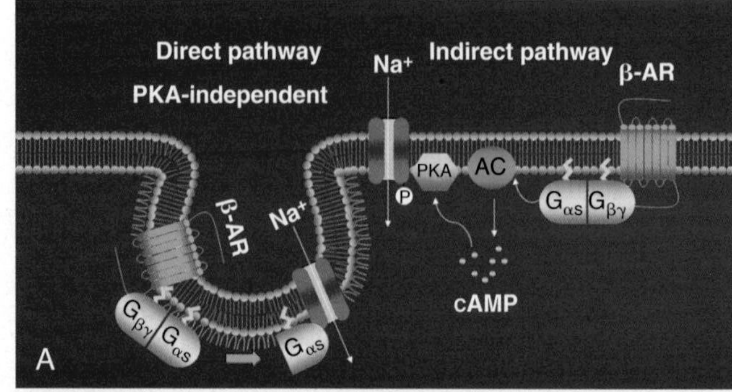

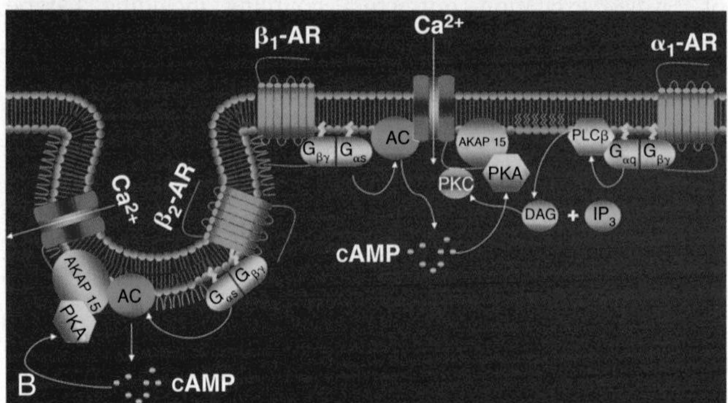

Figure 35-2 Adrenergic modulation of cardiac sodium and calcium channels. **A,** Modulation of cardiac sodium channels by β-adrenergic receptor (β-AR) stimulation via dual G protein pathways, which include indirect pathway through G protein–regulated second messenger cascades and direct pathway by a membrane-delimited modulation of the channel. The indirect pathway occurs via phosphorylation of the sodium channels by protein kinase A (PKA). On the other hand, the direct membrane-delimited β-adrenergic signaling on the sodium channel is PKA-independent, but it is dependent upon direct stimulation by $G_{\alpha s}$. The diagram depicts a subpopulation of sodium channels within caveolae structures, which are cave-like indentations of the sarcolemma coated with caveolin. β-AR stimulation, by activating $G_{\alpha s}$, promotes the presentation of cardiac sodium channels associated with caveolar membranes to the sarcolemma, resulting in the increase in the number of functional channels. **B,** Activation and consequent phosphorylation by β_1-ARs of the Ca_V1.2 channel by cyclic adenosine monophosphate (cAMP)-dependent PKA. Ca_V1.2 channels form complexes with A-kinase anchoring protein (AKAP)15, which colocalizes Ca_V1.2 channels with PKA. A subpopulation of CaV1.2 channels are localized to the caveolar membranes and mediate β_2-AR but not β_1-AR signaling. α_1-AR activation leads to stimulation of PKC isoforms through activation of phospholipase C (PLC) and production of IP_3 and diacylglycerol (DAG). PKC is shown to form a macromolecular complex with the Ca_V1.2 channel and phosphorylates the channel upon activation. AC, adenylyl cyclase. (Adapted from Steinberg SF, Brunton LL: Compartmentation of G protein–coupled signaling pathways in cardiac myocytes. Annu Rev Pharmacol Toxicol 41:751-773, 2001. Reprinted with permission from the *Annual Review of Pharmacology and Toxicology,* Volume 41, ©2001 by Annual Review www.annualreviews.org.)

Voltage-Gated Calcium Channels

The main isoform of the L-type calcium channels in the heart is $Ca_V1.2$; $Ca_V1.3$ is also expressed in atria and pacemaking tissues.[31,32] Activation of L-type calcium channels in cardiac myocytes initiates excitation-contraction coupling, which is central to the function of the heart as a pump. Intracellular Ca^{2+} is intimately involved in a large number of cellular processes including gene regulation, termed *excitation-transcription coupling*.[33] In response to sympathetic nervous system activation, there is an increase in cardiac contractility, a result of the modulation of catecholamine on several key elements of cardiac excitation-contraction coupling including L-type calcium channels, ryanodine receptor, and phospholamban. See Chapter 6 for a detailed discussion of sarcoplasmic reticulum ion channels.

In response to activation of β-adrenergic receptors and consequent phosphorylation of $Ca_V1.2$ by cAMP-dependent PKA, there is a significant increase in the L-type calcium current through $Ca_V1.2$ channels in cardiac myocytes. Previous studies using site-directed mutagenesis have demonstrated that A kinase–anchoring protein 15 (AKAP15) directly interacts with the C terminus of cardiac $Ca_V1.2$ via a conserved leucine zipper motif and colocalizes with $Ca_V1.2$ channels and PKA in the transverse tubules of ventricular myocytes to ensure rapid and efficient regulation of L-type calcium currents in response to β-adrenergic stimulation and local increases in cAMP. Disruption of PKA anchoring to $Ca_V1.2$ channels via AKAP15 markedly inhibits the β-adrenergic regulation of $Ca_V1.2$ channels by the PKA pathway.[34,35]

Although both β_1 and β_2-adrenergic receptor subtypes stimulate L-type calcium channels via adenylyl cyclase and $G_{\alpha s}$ protein, significant differences exist. Specifically, stimulation via the β_1-adrenergic receptor activates L-type calcium channels throughout cardiac myocytes, while the β_2-adrenergic receptor only activates L-type calcium channels in close proximity to the receptor.[16,36] Similar to those for cardiac sodium channels, previous studies have demonstrated that a subpopulation of L-type calcium channels are localized to the caveolar membranes in ventricular myocytes.[16] Indeed, intact caveolae are required for β_2-adrenergic receptor but not β_1-adrenergic receptor signaling of the calcium channels (see Fig. 35-2B). L-type calcium channels within caveolae exist as part of a macromolecular complex composed of β_2-adrenergic receptor, adenylyl cyclase, $G_{\alpha s}$, PKA regulatory subunit II (RII), protein phosphatase (PP2A), and caveolar resident protein caveolin-3.[16] Therefore, localization of $Ca_V1.2$ channels to caveolar macromolecular signaling complexes is necessary for the regulation of these channels by β_2-adrenergic receptor signaling pathways.[16]

PKC has also been shown to form a macromolecular complex with the $Ca_V1.2$ subunit of the calcium channel through direct interaction with the C terminus. In response to activators of PKC, the channel is phosphorylated at specific serine residues, resulting in an increase of the calcium current.[37] Activation of angiotensin II, α_1-adrenergic receptor, and endothelin-1 receptors leads to stimulation of PKC isoforms through activation of PLC and production of IP_3 and DAG. α_1-Adrenergic receptor stimulation has also been shown to potentiate calcium channel through activation of Ca^{2+}-calmodulin–dependent protein kinase II (CaMKII) in rat ventricular myocytes. Specifically, α_1-adrenergic receptor activation results in phosphorylation of CaMKII, which is localized near the transverse tubules; CaMKII activation directly potentiates the L-type calcium channel.[38]

Voltage-Gated Potassium Channels

Cardiac excitability is controlled on a beat-to-beat basis by the autonomic nervous system via direct modulation of cardiac ion channels responsible for the depolarization, impulse propagation, and cardiac excitation-contraction coupling. Cardiac repolarization by voltage-gated potassium channels is also dynamically controlled to ensure adequate diastolic filling during chronotropic response by sympathetic activation. Indeed, several voltage-gated potassium channels are under complex control by α- and β-adrenergic stimulation. Two voltage-gated potassium channels are examined in detail here.

Slowly Activating Delayed-Rectifier Potassium Channel

The slowly activating delayed-rectifier potassium current (I_{Ks}) activates slowly in response to changes in the membrane potential and contributes to repolarization during the later phase of cardiac action potentials. I_{Ks} has been considered the potassium current most responsible for adrenergic- and cAMP-mediated changes in cardiac repolarization during stress.[39,40] The I_{Ks} channel is formed by the coassembly of α (KCNQ1) and β (KCNE1) subunits.[41,42] Mutations of the *KCNQ1* gene cause long-QT syndrome (LQTS) type 1 (LQT1), the most common form of LQTS; mutations in the *KCNE1* gene cause LQT5. β-Adrenergic stimulation enhances I_{Ks} current amplitude and changes its kinetics, resulting in the shortening of the cardiac action potential that is necessary to ensure adequate diastolic filling between beats in the phase of an increase in heart rate that accompanies sympathetic nerve stimulation. Clinical studies have shown that LQT1 appears to be the most adrenaline-sensitive among the different LQTS subtypes because episodes (fainting, aborted cardiac arrest, or sudden death) often occur during exercise, swimming, or with strong emotion.[24] These patients generally exhibit a failure of the QT interval to shorten during exercise. β-Adrenergic receptor blockers (which decrease adrenaline's effects on the heart) have been shown to be effective in reducing episodes in LQT1.[25]

Key molecules involved in the β-adrenergic modulation of I_{Ks} channels have been extensively investigated (Fig. 35-3A). Studies have shown that I_{Ks} channel forms a macromolecular complex with the A kinase anchoring protein (AKAP) yotiao, a 200-kD protein, and that β-adrenergic modulation of I_{Ks} requires targeting of cAMP-dependent PKA and protein phosphatase 1 (PP1) to the channel protein through the adaptor protein yotiao. Specifically, yotiao binds to the α subunit of the channel protein via a leucine zipper motif.[43] These studies support the role of yotiao as the anchoring protein that brings together the key regulators involved in phosphorylation (PKA) and dephosphorylation (PP1) and the channel protein to ensure high efficiency and specificity of the channel phosphorylation state. Additional studies have shown that yotiao itself can be phosphorylated and that the phosphorylation of the anchoring protein further contributes to the PKA regulation of channel protein.[44,45]

Rapidly Activating Delayed-Rectifier Potassium Channel

The human *ether-a-go-go related* gene (*HERG*: *KCNH2*) encodes the channel pore-forming α subunit that carries the rapidly activating delayed rectifier potassium current (I_{Kr}). MiRP1 (minK-related protein 1), encoded by *KCNE2*, has been shown to coassemble with HERG to form the functional I_{Kr} channel.[46] I_{Kr} plays a unique role during cardiac repolarization in that the

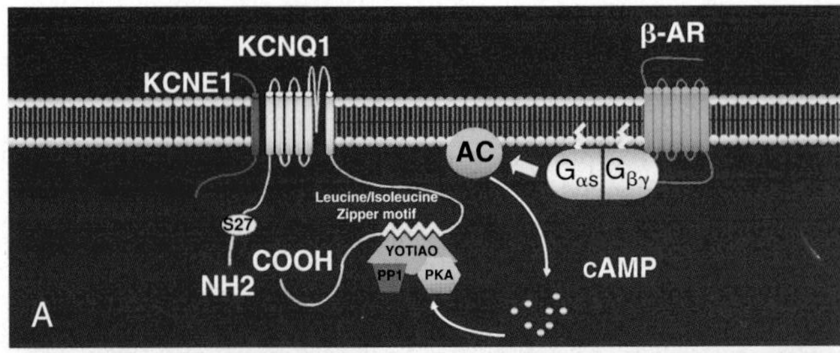

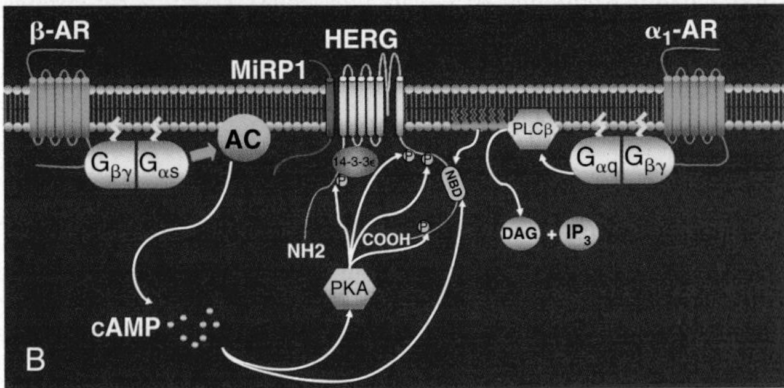

Figure 35-3 Adrenergic modulation of I_{Ks} and I_{Kr} channels. **A,** A schematic diagram of I_{Ks} macromolecular complexes. I_{Ks} channels are composed of α subunits (KCNQ1) and β subunits (KCNE1). The A-kinase anchoring protein yotiao interacts with the KCNQ1 C-terminus via a leucine/isoleucine zipper motif. Yotiao recruits key enzymes, including protein kinase A (PKA) and protein phosphatase 1 (PP1) to the channel complex. S27 is a PKA phosphorylation site on the KCNQ1 N-terminus. **B,** A schematic model of the cyclic adenosine monophosphate (cAMP) regulation of I_{Kr} channel protein using two distinct pathways. I_{Kr} channels are composed of α subunits (HERG) and β subunits (MiRP1). Stimulation of the β-adrenergic receptor (AR) results in the activation of $G_{\alpha s}$-protein, adenyl cyclase (AC)/cAMP and PKA phosphorylation of the channel protein. cAMP also binds directly to the nucleotide-binding domain (NBD) in the C-terminus of the α subunit. Finally, I_{Kr} channel is regulated by changes in PIP_2 concentrations by direct interaction of phosphatidyl-4,5-bisphosphate (PIP_2) with the C-terminus of the channel. Stimulation of cardiac α-AR-coupled $G_{\alpha q}$ results in the activation of phospholipase C (PLC), the consumption of endogenous PIP_2, and a reduction in I_{Kr}. (Adapted from Kass RS, Kurokawa J, Marx SO, Marks AR: Leucine/isoleucine zipper coordination of ion channel macromolecular signaling complexes in the heart: Roles in inherited arrhythmias. Treds Cardiovasc Med 13:52-56, 2003, and Cui J, Melman Y, Palma E, et al: Cyclic AMP regulates the HERG K^+ channel by dual pathways. Curr Biol 10:671-674, 2000.)

channels are inactivated during the major portion of the plateau potential but becomes reactivated and contributes importantly to the repolarization during the late phase of cardiac action potentials. Mutations in *KCNH2* gene have been linked to LQT2[47] and represent about 45% of the known LQTS defects; mutations in *KCNE2* have been associated with LQT6.[46] The vast majority of drugs associated with drug-induced LQTS are HERG-channel blockers. Even though there is some uncertainty regarding the exact partners of MiRP1 subunits, it is reasonable to conclude that *KCNE2* is functionally important in regulating cardiac excitability, as evidenced by the fact that *KCNE2* mutations are associated with LQTS and drug-induced LQTS.[46,48]

Sympathetic signaling modulates I_{Kr} in a highly complex manner via multiple G proteins, including $G_{\alpha s}$ and $G_{\alpha q}$ (see Fig. 35-3B). The regulation might provide an additional link among cardiovascular stresses, autonomic nervous system stimulation, and arrhythmias (both hereditary and acquired). Specifically, recent reports demonstrate that cAMP can regulate HERG channels via two distinct pathways: through PKA-dependent phosphorylation and by direct interaction of cAMP with the channel protein.[49,50] Activation of cAMP-dependent PKA causes phosphorylation of channel proteins, leading to a reduction in current amplitude, acceleration of channel deactivation, and depolarizing shift in voltage-dependent activation. cAMP also binds directly to the channel protein with the opposing effect of a hyperpolarizing shift in voltage-dependent activation. Hence, sympathetic activation during stress and exercise modulates I_{Kr} via a single second messenger exerting through two distinct pathways.

Additional evidence further suggests that phosphorylation of the channel by PKA is more complex than originally envisioned. HERG channels can interact with a newly identified adaptor protein 14-3-3ε via specific interaction sites on both N- and C-termini on the channel protein.[51] The interaction requires phosphorylation of the channel by PKA, leading to an acceleration and augmentation of current activation, in contrast to the depression of current with phosphorylation alone. When sufficient 14-3-3 is available, the phosphorylation state of the channel is stabilized and prolonged. Thus, 14-3-3 interactions add an additional layer of complexity to the dynamic regulation of the HERG channel by the autonomic control of cardiac membrane excitability.[51]

More-recent studies have documented another mechanism of HERG-channel regulation by autonomic nervous system. HERG is one of the first voltage-gated channels shown to be regulated by changes in the concentration of PIP_2 (see Fig. 35-3B).[52] The polycationic region in the carboxyl terminus of HERG represents the interaction site for PIP_2. Stimulation of cardiac α-adrenergic receptor–coupled $G_{\alpha q}$ results in activation of PLC, consumption of endogenous PIP_2, and a reduction in I_{Kr}. The regulation of HERG by changes in PIP_2 might have significant impact on cardiac repolarization, particularly during periods of extreme stress and autonomic stimuli. On the other hand, the effect of PKC on I_{Kr} remains controversial. Some studies documented the enhancement, and others showed an inhibitory effect on I_{Kr} by PKC activation. The variable findings might result from differences in the tissues used for these studies.

Sinoatrial and Atrioventricular Nodes

Pacemaker Current

Pacemaker current, also known as the funny current (I_f), was first described in 1979 in cardiac pacemaker cells and found to be an inward current that slowly activates upon hyperpolarization.[53] A similar current, termed I_h, was later shown in different types of neurons. Subsequent work has further substantiated the role of I_f in the spontaneous diastolic depolarization of the sinoatrial and atrioventricular nodes. On the other hand, alternative mechanisms exist for initiating spontaneous depolarization in the pacemaking cells.[54] Specifically, data suggest that the spontaneous rhythm is initiated and regulated by oscillatory Ca^{2+} releases from the sarcoplasmic reticulum in sinoatrial node cells. The Ca^{2+} releases, in turn, activate the forward mode of the Na^+-Ca^{2+} exchanger, resulting in inward membrane current, which initiates the spontaneous diastolic depolarization. Studies using specific blockers of I_f provide supports for the notion that I_f is responsible, at least in part, for the spontaneous firing of the pacemaking tissues in the heart.[55,56]

Significant progress in the field was made in the late 1990s by the discovery of the hyperpolarization-activated cyclic nucleotide–gated (HCN) family of channels.[57-59] HCN channels are nonselective cation channels with sequence homology to potassium and cyclic nucleotide–gated (CNG) channels and represent

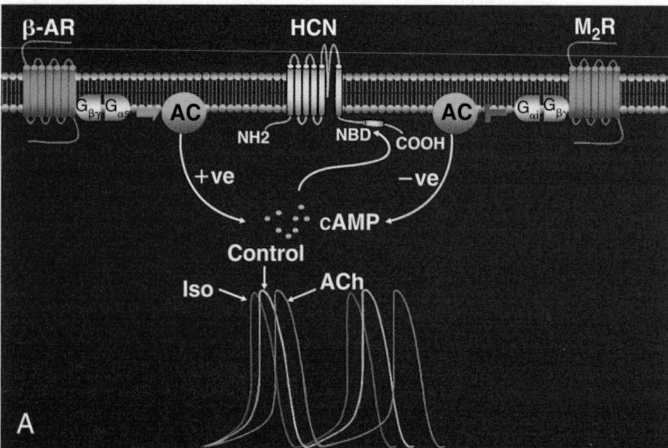

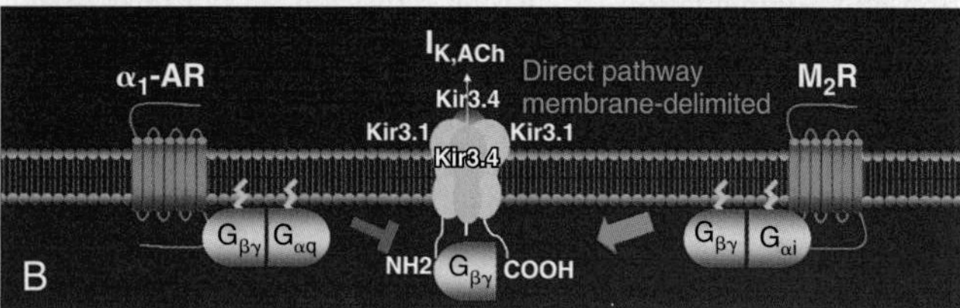

Figure 35-4 Adrenergic modulation of I_f and $I_{K,ACh}$ channels. **A,** A schematic diagram of cyclic adenosine monophosphate (cAMP) regulation of the hyperpolarization-activated cyclic nucleotide gated (HCN) channel via direct binding of cAMP on the nucleotide-binding domain (NBD) in the C-terminus of the HCN channels. Stimulation of β-adrenergic receptor (β-AR) and coupling of the receptor to the stimulatory $G_{\alpha s}$, followed by activation of adenylyl cyclase (AC), increases the production of cAMP. cAMP binding to the channels causes a positive shift in the voltage-dependent of activation of I_f and the increase in the spontaneous action potentials of the pacemaker cells, e.g., by isoproterenol (Iso). Conversely, stimulation of muscarinic receptors (M_2R) results in $G_{\alpha i}$-dependent inhibition of cAMP synthesis and a decrease in the firing frequency of the spontaneous action potential, e.g., by acetylcholine (ACh). **B,** A schematic diagram illustrating direct membrane-delimited activation of $I_{K,ACh}$ channels by M_2R activation. $I_{K,ACh}$ channel in the heart is formed by Kir3.1 and Kir3.4 proteins in heterotetrameric complexes. Upon activation of the M_2R receptors by acetylcholine (ACh), the receptors catalyze the conversion of GTP to GDP on the G_α subunit, the freed $G_{\beta\gamma}$ subunit directly activates $I_{K,ACh}$ channel. Conversely, α_1-AR stimulation directly disrupts the Kir channel–$G_{\beta\gamma}$ interactions, leading to a reduction in the probability of $G_{\beta\gamma}$ binding to the channel. (**A** (lower panel) adapted from Accili EA, Robinson RB, DiFrancesco D: Properties and modulation of I_f in newborn versus adult cardiac SA nodes. Am J Physiol Heart Circ Physiol 272:H1549-H1552, 1997.)

the molecular correlates for I_f in the heart and I_h currents in nerve cells. The functional channels are formed by four homologous subunits arranged around a centrally located pore, with a cyclic nucleotide-binding domain located in the intracellular C-terminal region of each subunit.[60] In mammals, four isoforms have been cloned (HCN1-4), and the four isoforms differ quantitatively in their modulation and voltage-dependent kinetics. The HCN channels are modulated by the binding of cyclic nucleotides such as cAMP and cGMP.[61] The binding of cAMP to the nucleotide-binding domain accelerates the activation kinetics and shifts the voltage dependence of activation to more positive voltages (Fig. 35-4A).

Sinoatrial and atrioventricular nodes are richly innervated by the autonomic nervous system. In this regard, I_f is directly responsible for the sympathetic and parasympathetic modulation of heart rate. Sympathetic stimulation accelerates the heart rate and parasympathetic stimulation decelerates it by acting through β-adrenergic and muscarinic receptors (M_2R) to increase and decrease, respectively, intracellular cAMP concentrations and hence the degree of activation of I_f.

Specifically, previous work has shown that sympathetic activity increases I_f via activation of β-adrenergic receptor and coupling of the receptor to the stimulatory $G_{\alpha s}$, followed by activation of adenylyl cyclase and production of cAMP. cAMP binds directly to HCN channels and causes a positive shift in the voltage-dependent activation of I_f without changes in single-channel conductances.[62,63] The extent of current activation then determines the slope of diastolic depolarization and hence of the firing frequency of pacemaker cells. These early studies using excised patches provided evidence that cAMP modulates I_f by direct binding of cAMP molecules to the channels and not by phosphorylation.[64] This was the first evidence that the activation of I_f is gated not only by voltage but also by cyclic nucleotide, similar to CNG channels in sensory neurons.

Conversely, I_f is inhibited by acetylcholine (see Fig. 35-4A).[65-68] The stimulation of muscarinic receptors by parasympathetic activation shifts the I_f activation curve to more-negative voltages without changes in the channel conductances by a process involving $G_{\alpha i}$-dependent inhibition of cAMP synthesis.[66-68] Previous work has also identified an acetylcholine-activated potassium current ($I_{K,ACh}$) as a possible regulator of heart rate.[69] However, it was demonstrated that inhibition of I_f requires a 20-fold lower concentration of acetylcholine compared to concentrations required for $I_{K,ACh}$ activation.[65]

Acetylcholine-Sensitive Inward Rectifier Potassium Channel

Acetylcholine-sensitive inward-rectifier potassium current ($I_{K,ACh}$) channels are expressed in sinoatrial and atrioventricular nodes and in atrial and Purkinje cells. The channels are formed by Kir3.1 (G protein–linked inwardly rectifying potassium channel 1 [GIRK1]) and Kir3.4 (GIRK4) proteins in heterotetrameric complexes with a stoichiometric ratio of 1:1. The channels are directly coupled to M_2 muscarinic acetylcholine receptors (M_2R) through a pertussis toxin–sensitive G protein.[70] Upon activation by acetylcholine released by the vagus nerve, the receptors catalyze the conversion of GTP to GDP on the G_α subunit; the freed $G_{\beta\gamma}$ subunit directly binds to multiple domains on the intracellular surface of the channels and activates the $I_{K,ACh}$ channel (see Fig. 35-4B).[70] These channels were thought to play a role in pacemaking tissues by generating membrane hyperpolarization to oppose the slow depolarization of I_f.

Data using a mouse model with targeted deletion of one of the Kir subunits, Kir3.4, suggests that $I_{K,ACh}$ is a critical effector of the parasympathetic branch of the heart rate regulatory system. Specifically, in this mouse model, $I_{K,ACh}$ accounts for approximately half of the bradycardia induced by vagal stimulation and is necessary for fast regulation (<2 sec) of the heart rate, both at rest and during baroreflex stimulation.[71] Kir3.4 null mice were resistant to the development of atrial fibrillation upon exposure to the acetylcholine receptor agonist carbachol, suggesting that $I_{K,ACh}$ channels may be involved in the cholinergic induction of atrial fibrillation.[72]

Cholinergic and α-adrenergic signals differentially affect $I_{K,ACh}$. Activation of α-adrenergic receptor–coupled $G_{\alpha q}$ leads to an inhibitory effect on $I_{K,ACh}$[73] by directly disrupting the Kir channel–$G_{\beta\gamma}$ interactions, leading to a reduction in the probability of $G_{\beta\gamma}$ binding to the channel and, hence, a diminished parasympathetic effect on $I_{K,ACh}$. Previous studies have shown that $I_{K,ACh}$ channels exist as macromolecular complexes with association of Kir channels with GPCR, $G_{\beta\gamma}$, GPCR kinase, adenylyl cyclase, cAMP-dependent protein kinase, protein phosphatases, PP1 and PP2A, and actin.[74] In this microenvironment, $I_{K,ACh}$ provides a dynamic integration and coordination of the adrenergic and cholinergic signals in the regulation of heart rate.[75] I_{KACh} channel activity is also modulated by levels of intracellular Na^+, ATP, and fatty acids.[70,76,77]

Conclusions

Cardiac excitability is tightly regulated with millisecond precision via the fine tuning of the repertoire of ion channel proteins that govern the excitability and conduction throughout the heart. Indeed, abnormalities in autonomic regulation can result in life-threatening cardiac arrhythmias. A multitude of interconnecting signaling cascades is involved in this regulation. To achieve the needed diversity and yet provide the specificity, a common theme has emerged. The exquisite specificity and integration of membrane excitability is achieved via compartmentalization of the signaling networks in membrane microdomains in which relevant proteins are maintained within the same physical space. Ion channel proteins have been shown to form macromolecular complexes with adaptor proteins (e.g., A kinase–anchoring protein) that target protein kinases and protein phosphatases to the channel proteins to ensure a high degree of efficiency and specificity.

References

1. Kass RS, Kurokawa J, Marx SO, Marks AR: Leucine/isoleucine zipper coordination of ion channel macromolecular signaling complexes in the heart. Roles in inherited arrhythmias. Trends Cardiovasc Med 13:52-56, 2003.
2. Wess J: G-protein-coupled receptors: Molecular mechanisms involved in receptor activation and selectivity of G-protein recognition. FASEB J 11:346-354, 1997.
3. Insel PA, Tang CM, Hahntow I, Michel MC: Impact of GPCRs in clinical medicine: Monogenic diseases, genetic variants and drug targets. Biochim Biophys Acta 1768:994-1005, 2007.
4. Salazar NC, Chen J, Rockman HA: Cardiac GPCRs: GPCR signaling in healthy and failing hearts. Biochim Biophys Acta 1768:1006-1018, 2007.
5. Lefkowitz RJ: Seven transmembrane receptors: Something old, something new. Acta Physiol (Oxf) 190:9-19, 2007.
6. Tang CM, Insel PA: GPCR expression in the heart: "New" receptors in myocytes and fibroblasts. Trends Cardiovasc Med 14:94-99, 2004.
7. Farrens DL, Altenbach C, Yang K, et al: Requirement of rigid-body motion of transmembrane helices for light activation of rhodopsin. Science 274:768-770, 1996.
8. Ballesteros JA, Jensen AD, Liapakis G, et al: Activation of the β_2-adrenergic receptor involves disruption of an ionic lock between the cytoplasmic ends of transmembrane segments 3 and 6. J Biol Chem 276:29171-29177, 2001.
9. Cherezov V, Rosenbaum DM, Hanson MA, et al: High-resolution crystal structure of an engineered human β_2-adrenergic G protein–coupled receptor. Science 318:1258-1265, 2007.
10. Rasmussen SG, Choi HJ, Rosenbaum DM, et al: Crystal structure of the human β_2 adrenergic G-protein–coupled receptor. Nature 450:383-387, 2007.
11. Rosenbaum DM, Cherezov V, Hanson MA, et al: GPCR engineering yields high-resolution structural insights into β_2-adrenergic receptor function. Science 318:1266-1273, 2007.
12. Daaka Y, Luttrell LM, Lefkowitz RJ: Switching of the coupling of the β_2-adrenergic receptor to different G proteins by protein kinase A. Nature 390:88-91, 1997.
13. Steinberg SF: β_2-Adrenergic receptor signaling complexes in cardiomyocyte caveolae/lipid rafts. J Mol Cell Cardiol 37:407-415, 2004.
14. Steinberg SF, Brunton LL: Compartmentation of G protein–coupled signaling pathways in cardiac myocytes. Annu Rev Pharmacol Toxicol 41:751-773, 2001.
15. Yarbrough TL, Lu T, Lee HC, Shibata EF: Localization of cardiac sodium channels in caveolin-rich membrane domains: Regulation of sodium current amplitude. Circ Res 90:443-449, 2002.
16. Balijepalli RC, Foell JD, Hall DD, et al: Localization of cardiac L-type Ca^{2+} channels to a caveolar macromolecular signaling complex is required for β_2-adrenergic regulation. Proc Natl Acad Sci U S A 103:7500-7505, 2006.
17. Barbuti A, Terragni B, Brioschi C, DiFrancesco D: Localization of f-channels to caveolae mediates specific β_2-adrenergic receptor modulation of rate in sinoatrial myocytes. J Mol Cell Cardiol 42:71-78, 2007.
18. Bossuyt J, Taylor BE, James-Kracke M, Hale CC: The cardiac sodium-calcium exchanger associates with caveolin-3. Ann N Y Acad Sci 976:197-204, 2002.
19. Prinster SC, Hague C, Hall RA: Heterodimerization of G protein–coupled receptors: Specificity and functional significance. Pharmacol Rev 57:289-298, 2005.
20. Zhu WZ, Chakir K, Zhang S, et al: Heterodimerization of β_1- and β_2-adrenergic receptor subtypes optimizes beta-adrenergic modulation of cardiac contractility. Circ Res 97:244-251, 2005.
21. Schubert B, VanDongen AM, Kirsch GE, Brown AM: Beta-adrenergic inhibition of cardiac sodium channels by dual G-protein pathways. Science 245:516-519, 1989.
22. Matsuda JJ, Lee H, Shibata EF: Enhancement of rabbit cardiac sodium channels by beta-adrenergic stimulation. Circ Res 70:199-207, 1992.
23. Cukierman S: Regulation of voltage-dependent sodium channels. J Membr Biol 151:203-214, 1996.
24. Frohnwieser B, Chen LQ, Schreibmayer W, Kallen RG: Modulation of the human cardiac sodium channel alpha-subunit by cAMP-dependent protein kinase and the responsible sequence domain. J Physiol 498(Pt 2):309-318, 1997.
25. Fozzard HA, Hanck DA: Structure and function of voltage-dependent sodium channels: Comparison of brain II and cardiac isoforms. Physiol Rev 76:887-926, 1996.
26. Schreibmayer W, Frohnwieser B, Dascal N, et al: Beta-adrenergic modulation of currents produced by rat cardiac Na^+ channels expressed in *Xenopus laevis* oocytes. Receptors Channels 2:339-350, 1994.
27. Hallaq H, Yang Z, Viswanathan PC, et al: Quantitation of protein kinase A–mediated trafficking of cardiac sodium channels in living cells. Cardiovasc Res 72:250-261, 2006.
28. Zhou J, Shin HG, Yi J, et al: Phosphorylation and putative ER retention signals are required for protein kinase A–mediated potentiation of cardiac sodium current. Circ Res 91:540-546, 2002.
29. Zhou J, Yi J, Hu N, et al: Activation of protein kinase A modulates trafficking of the human cardiac sodium channel in *Xenopus oocytes*. Circ Res 87:33-38, 2000.
30. Lu T, Lee HC, Kabat JA, Shibata EF: Modulation of rat cardiac sodium channel by the stimulatory G protein alpha subunit. J Physiol 518(Pt 2):371-384, 1999.
31. Zhang Z, He Y, Tuteja D, et al: Functional roles of $Ca_V1.3$ (α_{1D}) calcium channels in atria: Insights gained from gene-targeted null mutant mice. Circulation 112:1936-1944, 2005.
32. Zhang Z, Xu Y, Song H, et al: Functional roles of $Ca_V1.3$ (α_{1D}) calcium channel in sinoatrial nodes: Insight gained using gene-targeted null mutant mice. Circ Res 90:981-987, 2002.
33. Dolmetsch R: Excitation-transcription coupling: Signaling by ion channels to the nucleus. Sci STKE 2003(166):PE4, 2003.
34. Hulme JT, Scheuer T, Catterall WA: Regulation of cardiac ion channels by signaling complexes: Role of modified leucine zipper motifs. J Mol Cell Cardiol 37:625-631, 2004.
35. Catterall WA, Hulme JT, Jiang X, Few WP: Regulation of sodium and calcium channels by signaling complexes. J Recept Signal Transduct Res 26:577-598, 2006.
36. Zheng M, Zhang SJ, Zhu WZ, et al: β_2-Adrenergic receptor–induced p38 MAPK activation is mediated by protein kinase A rather than by G_i or $G_{\beta\gamma}$ in adult mouse cardiomyocytes. J Biol Chem 275:40635-40640, 2000.
37. Yang L, Liu G, Zakharov SI, et al: Ser1928 is a common site for $Ca_V1.2$ phosphorylation by protein kinase C isoforms. J Biol Chem 280:207-214, 2005.
38. O-Uchi J, Komukai K, Kusakari Y, et al: α_1-Adrenoceptor stimulation potentiates

L-type Ca^{2+} current through Ca^{2+}/calmodulin-dependent PK II (CaMKII) activation in rat ventricular myocytes. Proc Natl Acad Sci U S A 102:9400-9405, 2005.
39. Walsh KB, Kass RS: Regulation of a heart potassium channel by protein kinase A and C. Science 242:67-69, 1988.
40. Lo CF, Numann R: Independent and exclusive modulation of cardiac delayed rectifying K^+ current by protein kinase C and protein kinase A. Circ Res 83: 995-1002, 1998.
41. Barhanin J, Lesage F, Guillemare E, et al: K_VLQT1 and lsK (minK) proteins associate to form the I_{Ks} cardiac potassium current. Nature 384:78-80, 1996.
42. Sanguinetti MC, Curran ME, Zou A, et al: Coassembly of K_VLQT1 and minK (IsK) proteins to form cardiac I_{Ks} potassium channel. Nature 384:80-83, 1996.
43. Marx SO, Kurokawa J, Reiken S, et al: Requirement of a macromolecular signaling complex for beta adrenergic receptor modulation of the KCNQ1-KCNE1 potassium channel. Science 295:496-499, 2002.
44. Chen L, Kurokawa J, Kass RS: Phosphorylation of the A-kinase-anchoring protein yotiao contributes to protein kinase A regulation of a heart potassium channel. J Biol Chem 280:31347-31352, 2005.
45. Chen L, Kass RS: Dual roles of the A kinase-anchoring protein yotiao in the modulation of a cardiac potassium channel: A passive adaptor versus an active regulator. Eur J Cell Biol 85:623-626, 2006.
46. Abbott GW, Sesti F, Splawski I, et al: MiRP1 forms I_{Kr} potassium channels with HERG and is associated with cardiac arrhythmia. Cell 97:175-187, 1999.
47. Curran ME, Splawski I, Timothy KW, et al: A molecular basis for cardiac arrhythmia: HERG mutations cause long QT syndrome. Cell 80:795-803, 1995.
48. Splawski I, Shen J, Timothy KW, et al: Spectrum of mutations in long-QT syndrome genes. *KVLQT1, HERG, SCN5A, KCNE1,* and *KCNE2.* Circulation 102:1178-1185, 2000.
49. Thomas D, Zhang W, Karle CA, et al: Deletion of protein kinase A phosphorylation sites in the HERG potassium channel inhibits activation shift by protein kinase A. J Biol Chem 274:27457-27462, 1999.
50. Cui J, Melman Y, Palma E, et al: Cyclic AMP regulates the HERG K^+ channel by dual pathways. Curr Biol 10:671-674, 2000.
51. Kagan A, McDonald TV: Dynamic control of hERG/I_{Kr} by PKA-mediated interactions with 14-3-3. Novartis Found Symp 266:75-89, 2005.
52. Bian JS, McDonald TV: Phosphatidylinositol 4,5-bisphosphate interactions with the HERG K^+ channel. Pflugers Arch 455:105-113, 2007.
53. Brown HF, DiFrancesco D, Noble SJ: How does adrenaline accelerate the heart? Nature 280:235-236, 1979.
54. Maltsev VA, Lakatta EG: Normal heart rhythm is initiated and regulated by an intracellular calcium clock within pacemaker cells. Heart Lung Circ 16(5): 335-348, 2007.
55. Bucchi A, Barbuti A, Baruscotti M, DiFrancesco D: Heart rate reduction via selective 'funny' channel blockers. Curr Opin Pharmacol 7:208-213, 2007.
56. DiFrancesco D: Funny channels in the control of cardiac rhythm and mode of action of selective blockers. Pharmacol Res 53:399-406, 2006.
57. Santoro B, Grant SG, Bartsch D, Kandel ER: Interactive cloning with the SH3 domain of N-src identifies a new brain specific ion channel protein, with homology to eag and cyclic nucleotide-gated channels. Proc Natl Acad Sci U S A 94:14815-14820, 1997.
58. Santoro B, Liu DT, Yao H, et al: Identification of a gene encoding a hyperpolarization-activated pacemaker channel of brain. Cell 93:717-729, 1998.
59. Zagotta WN, Olivier NB, Black KD, et al: Structural basis for modulation and agonist specificity of HCN pacemaker channels. Nature 425:200-205, 2003.
60. Siu CW, Lieu DK, Li RA.HCN-encoded pacemaker channels: From physiology and biophysics to bioengineering. J Membr Biol 214:115-122, 2006.
61. Biel M, Schneider A, Wahl C: Cardiac HCN channels: Structure, function, and modulation. Trends Cardiovasc Med 12:206-212, 2002.
62. DiFrancesco D, Ferroni A, Mazzanti M, Tromba C: Properties of the hyperpolarizing-activated current (I_f) in cells isolated from the rabbit sino-atrial node. J Physiol 377:61-88, 1986.
63. DiFrancesco D, Mangoni M: Modulation of single hyperpolarization-activated channels (I_f) by cAMP in the rabbit sino-atrial node. J Physiol 474:473-482, 2006.
64. DiFrancesco D, Tortora P: Direct activation of cardiac pacemaker channels by intracellular cyclic AMP. Nature 351:145-147, 1991.
65. DiFrancesco D, Ducouret P, Robinson RB: Muscarinic modulation of cardiac rate at low acetylcholine concentrations. Science 243:669-671, 1989.
66. DiFrancesco D, Tromba C: Acetylcholine inhibits activation of the cardiac hyperpolarizing-activated current, I_f. Pflugers Arch 410:139-142, 1987.
67. DiFrancesco D, Tromba C: Inhibition of the hyperpolarization-activated current (I_f) induced by acetylcholine in rabbit sino-atrial node myocytes. J Physiol 405: 477-491, 1988.
68. DiFrancesco D, Tromba C: Muscarinic control of the hyperpolarization-activated current (I_f) in rabbit sino-atrial node myocytes. J Physiol 405:493-510, 1988.
69. Sakmann B, Noma A, Trautwein W: Acetylcholine activation of single muscarinic K^+ channels in isolated pacemaker cells of the mammalian heart. Nature 303:250-253, 1983.
70. Kurachi Y: G protein regulation of cardiac muscarinic potassium channel. Am J Physiol 269:C821-C830, 1995.
71. Wickman K, Nemec J, Gendler SJ, Clapham DE: Abnormal heart rate regulation in GIRK4 knockout mice. Neuron 20:103-114, 1998.
72. Kovoor P, Wickman K, Maguire CT, et al: Evaluation of the role of I_{KACh} in atrial fibrillation using a mouse knockout model. J Am Coll Cardiol 37:2136-2143, 2001.
73. Braun AP, Fedida D, Giles WR: Activation of α_1-adrenoceptors modulates the inwardly rectifying potassium currents of mammalian atrial myocytes. Pflugers Arch 421:431-439, 1992.
74. Nikolov EN, Ivanova-Nikolova TT: Coordination of membrane excitability through a GIRK1 signaling complex in the atria. J Biol Chem 279:23630-23636, 2004.
75. Nikolov EN, Ivanova-Nikolova TT: Dynamic integration of α-adrenergic and cholinergic signals in the atria: Role of G protein–regulated inward rectifying K^+ channels. J Biol Chem 282:28669-28682, 2007.
76. Lavine N, Ethier N, Oak JN, et al: G protein-coupled receptors form stable complexes with inwardly rectifying potassium channels and adenylyl cyclase. J Biol Chem 277:46010-46019, 2002.
77. Yamada M, Inanobe A, Kurachi Y: G protein regulation of potassium ion channels. Pharmacol Rev 50:723-760, 1998.

Nerve Sprouting and Cardiac Arrhythmias 36

LAN S. CHEN AND PENG-SHENG CHEN

CHAPTER OUTLINE

Following division, crushing, interference of blood supply, or other means of injury, the peripheral nerves undergo Wallerian degeneration and axonal regeneration. This regenerative process, namely nerve sprouting, is well described, both in the central nervous system and in the peripheral nervous system. If the nerve sprouts form synapses, they can result in permanent changes of local innervation leading to functional consequences. Myocardial infarction causes nerve injury and regional sympathetic denervation. Afterwards, nerve sprouting occurs and results in regional increase of sympathetic hyperinnervation.[1] Although the magnitude of nerve sprouting varies from person to person, there is a correlation between the density of sympathetic nerve and occurrence of cardiac arrhythmia.[2-3] In this chapter, we review the relationship between sympathetic nerve sprouting and cardiac arrhythmia.

Cardiac Nerves

The preganglionic sympathetic nerves that innervate the heart arise in the upper four or five segments of thoracic spinal cord. These preganglionic sympathetic nerves pass through white rami communicates, enter the sympathetic trunk, and terminate in the superior cervical ganglion, the middle cervical ganglion (if present), and the cervicothoracic (stellate) ganglion. These ganglia give off cardiac nerves that join with the cardiac branches of the vagus nerve and form the cardiac plexus. The cardiac plexus, which is divided into the superficial (ventral) and deep (dorsal) cardiac plexus, then give branches of the coronary and atrial plexuses to innervate the heart. The sympathetic nerves are distributed in the superficial epicardial layer throughout most surfaces and penetrate into myocardium along coronary arterial pathways. Sympathetic nerves are located primarily around blood vessels and between myocytes. The nerve fibers are oriented along the long axis of myocytes.

The parasympathetic innervation to the heart comes from the vagus nerve. The cardiac branches of the vagus nerve, which are preganglionic fibers, make synaptic connections with ganglion cells in the cardiac plexus or intracardiac ganglia. In addition to parasympathetic nerves, the vagal nerves also contain some sympathetic (adrenergic) nerve fibers.[4] The coexistence of both sympathetic and parasympathetic nerves within the vagal nerve suggest that stimulating vagal nerves might activate both sympathetic and parasympathetic branches of the autonomic nervous system.

Cardiac nerves can be demonstrated by labeling nerve-specific markers such as S100 protein (marker of Schwann cells), neurofilament, synaptophysin, protein gene product 9.5, and various regulatory neuropeptides (e.g., neuropeptide-Y) using immunohistochemistry techniques.[5,6] Sympathetic nerves can be identified by immunolabeling tyrosine hydroxylase and parasympathetic nerves by acetylcholinesterase or cholineacetyltransferase. Like other peripheral nerves, cardiac nerves include both myelinated and unmyelinated nerve fibers. The former can be identified by immunostaining of myelin marker, such as basic myelin protein. Using immunohistochemistry on whole-mount cardiac tissues with confocal microscopy techniques, Marron and colleagues[5] demonstrated that all nerve terminals in the epicardium were immunoreactive to tyrosine hydroxylase (sympathetic), and the endocardium was also predominantly innervated by myelinated sympathetic nerves. Nerve terminals that display acetylcholinesterase immunoreactivity (parasympathetic) are nonexistent in the epicardium and account for less than 5% of nerve fibers in the endocardium. However, parasympathetic nerves are dominant in the conduction system, representing 60% to 70% of innervation in the nodal tissues and penetrating atrioventricular bundle.[7] Tan and colleagues[8] studied autonomic innervation at the human pulmonary vein–left atrial junction. They found that adrenergic and cholinergic nerves have highest densities within 5 mm from the junction but are highly colocated, indicating that it is impossible to selectively target either vagal or sympathetic nerves during ablation procedures. There are more sympathetic than parasympathetic nerves at those locations.

These data indicate that sympathetic nerves, which are far more abundant than parasympathetic nerves, are widely distributed in the human heart.[5,9] In this chapter, discussion is focused on the relationship between sympathetic nerve sprouting and the development of cardiac arrhythmia. Whether or not the density of parasympathetic nerves also increases after myocardial infarction (MI) remains a subject of investigation.

This study was supported by a Medtronic-Zipes Endowment, P01 HL78931, R01s HL78932, 66389 and 71140.

Imaging Evidence of Sympathetic Neural Remodeling

Clinically, cardiac sympathetic innervation can be measured in vivo by ^{123}I-metaiodobenzylguanidine (MIBG, a norepinephrine analogue taken up by sympathetic nerve terminals) scanning or by ^{11}C-hydroxyephedrine (HED) positron emission tomography (PET) imaging.[10,11] A regional defect of MIBG uptake (denervation) in the ventricle was demonstrated in subjects after MI. There is also regional reduction of myocardial innervation for 2 months after the development of hibernating myocardium. This inhomogeneous reduction of sympathetic innervation might be a source of cardiac arrhythmia.[11] The uptake defect in the infarct myocardium persisted up to 30 months.[12,13] However, an increase of MIBG uptake (reinnervation) was reported in peri-infarct zone between 3 to 12 months after MI.[14] The MIBG defect was also seen in subjects with coronary artery disease but without previous MI. The size of the uptake defect was correlated with severity of coronary stenoses.[15] The uptake was also observed in subjects who had coronary spastic angina, and the defects lasted for 2 months in 85% subjects and for 6 months in 32% subjects.[16] Chronic sympathetic nerve denervation was demonstrated in dogs with transient coronary occlusion.[17] These data suggest that cardiac sympathetic nerves are vulnerable to ischemic injury, sympathetic denervation persisted in infarct myocardium, and reinnervation can occur in the peri-infarct area.

Histologic Evidence of Sympathetic Neural Remodeling

After Myocardial Injury

The presence of nerve sprouting in human hearts is supported by several histologic studies. Vracko and coworkers[18] reported that in the left ventricular scars, there are higher densities of nerve fibers than in adjacent intact myocardium. The nerve fibers aggregate irregularly along the periphery of lesions. These nerve fibers appeared to be oriented predominantly in the long axis of myocytes located at the edges of the lesions. The authors concluded that human myocardial nerve fibers regenerate after necrotizing injuries and that at least some of the resulting scar-associated fibers have structural features differing from those in uninjured myocardium. They also hypothesized that these structural differences might be associated with functional alterations that could be a mechanism of ventricular arrhythmias.

Cao and colleagues[2] showed an inhomogeneous distribution of nerve fibers in ventricular myocardium obtained from native hearts of cardiac transplant recipients with diagnosis of either coronary artery disease or idiopathic cardiomyopathy. Nerve structures, which were identified by S100 immunoreactivity (for Schwann cells) or tyrosine hydroxylase (for sympathetic nerves), were most abundant at the periphery of necrotic tissues or in the perivascular regions (Figs. 36-1 and 36-2). In contrast, the central necrotic zone of infarct and areas with dense fibrotic tissues were devoid of nerve fibers. There was a twofold increase in the density of nerves, which was immunoreactive to S100, in the ventricular myocardium of the explanted hearts as compared to the hearts obtained at autopsy from cadavers with no history of cardiac disease (Table 36-1).

Abundant nerve fibers are found from the origin of ventricular tachycardia in human patients (see Fig. 36-2). Because sympathetic nerves are far more abundant than parasympathetic nerves and tyrosine hydroxylase is colocalized with S100 in most nerve fibers, these data most likely represent an increase of sympathetic innervation in the injured myocardium, indicating the existence of sympathetic nerve sprouting in human hearts. Therefore, MI-induced nerve sprouting can eventually cause highly heterogeneous distribution of sympathetic innervation in the heart with areas of denervation, hyperinnervation, and relatively normal nerve fiber density.

After Orthotopic Cardiac Transplantation

Cardiac transplantation procedure completely disconnects the cardiac nerves from their extrinsic sources. Afterward, some patients have nuclear imaging evidence of sympathetic reinnervation and others are persistently denervated.[19] Patients with successful cardiac sympathetic reinnervation have increased peak oxygen uptake, heart rate, and contraction during exercise stress testing.[20,21] To document post-transplant reinnervation, Kim and colleagues[22] performed immunostaining of the tissues from transplanted human hearts that were subsequently explanted. Abundant growth-associated protein (GAP) 43-positive and tyrosine hydroxylase–positive nerves were found in these hearts. Heterogeneous sympathetic nerve sprouting and reinnervation occurred around blood vessels in the allografts. The magnitude of nerve sprouting increased with time and varied greatly from patient to patient. Patients with ischemic heart diseases had greater nerve sprouting and reinnervation than did those with dilated cardiomyopathy.

Mechanisms of Sympathetic Neural Remodeling

Figure 36-1 is a schematic illustration of nerve regeneration after nerve injury. The regenerating axon splits into many fine strands that reach Schwann tubes of degenerating stumps. Some of regenerating axonal sprouts become completely surrounded by plasma membrane of Schwann cells. Many axonal sprouts exist in the early phase of regeneration. However, only those that make synaptic contacts with receptors or effector endings persist. The elimination of excess nonfunctional sprouts can take considerable time. The axonal regeneration is initially slow, but it accelerates to reach a constant rate by the third day after injury.[23] However, the rate varies depending on the injury type, age, or species. Estimates of the rate of regeneration vary between 1 and 3 mm/day.[23] In unconditioned rat sciatic nerve, for example, the regeneration rate is 3.2 mm/day.

The mechanisms underlying cardiac nerve regeneration are not entirely clear. In mice, MI results in denervation in the infarcted myocardium and induces diffuse nerve sprouting evident by an increased density of nerve fibers immunopositive for GAP43.[24] The density of sympathetic nerve fiber was persistently increased up to 1 month after MI in the peri-infarct area. Oh and coworkers[24] also observed that gene expression of nerve growth factor (NGF), insulin-like growth factor (IGF), leukemia inhibitory factor (LIF), transforming growth factor-β3 (TGF-β3) and interleukin-1α (IL-1α) was increased up to 2 months after MI as compared to normal controls. The expression of these growth factors was more pronounced and persistent in the peri-infarct area than the area remote to infarction.

Zhou and colleagues[25] reported similar findings of nerve sprouting and NGF level in a canine model of MI. Acute MI elicited immediate elevation of transcardiac (difference between coronary sinus and aorta) NGF level within 3.5 hours, followed by up-regulation of NGF and GAP43 expression. The nerve-sprouting activity peaked earlier with a significantly greater level of GAP43 immunopositive nerve fiber density in the MI dogs than the control (normal) dogs. NGF protein level was increased

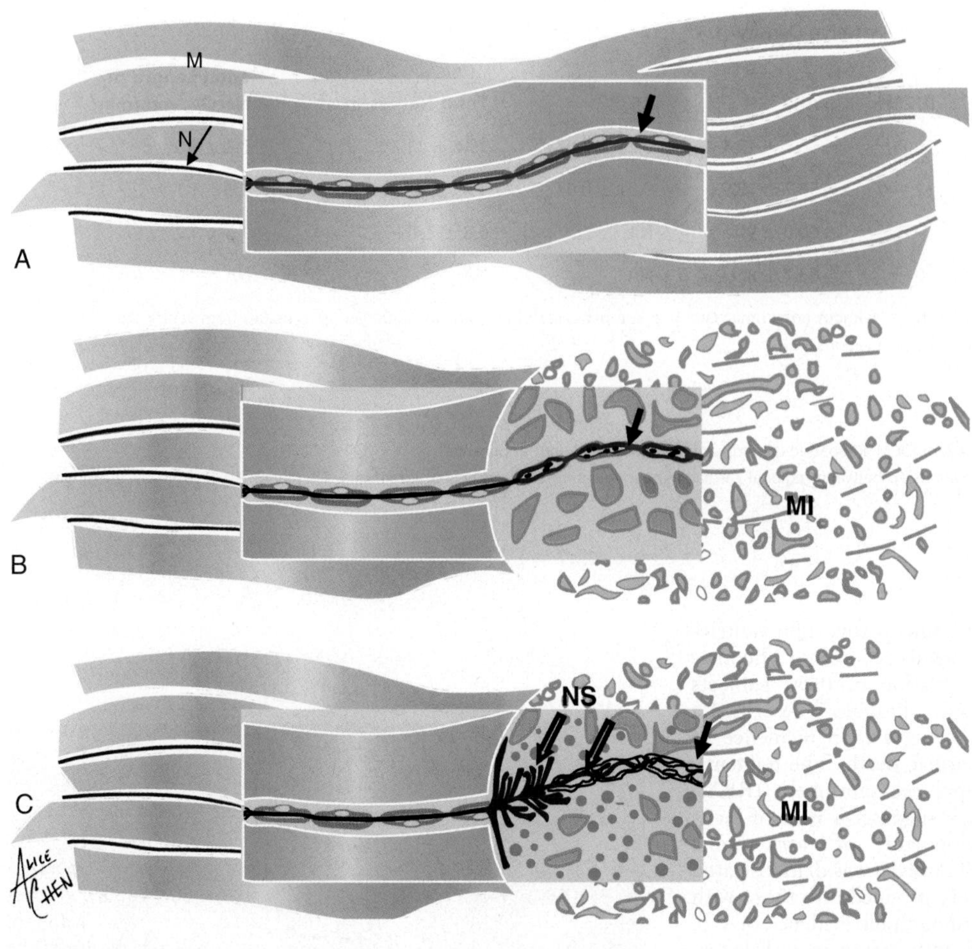

Figure 36-1 Nerve sprouting after myocardial infarction (MI). **A,** Sympathetic nerves are distributed in perivascular areas and between myocytes. Nerve fibers, along with the Schwann cells, are oriented along the long axis of myocytes *(solid arrow)*. **B,** After MI, nerve fibers in the infarcted area are injured. The distal stumps undergo wallerian degeneration (*solid arrows* in **B** and **C**). **C,** The regeneration of axonal sprouts occurs in nerve fibers proximal to the injury *(open arrows)*. There is also Schwann cell proliferation along with the axonal nerve sprouting. M, myocytes; N, nerve fiber; NS: nerve sprouts.

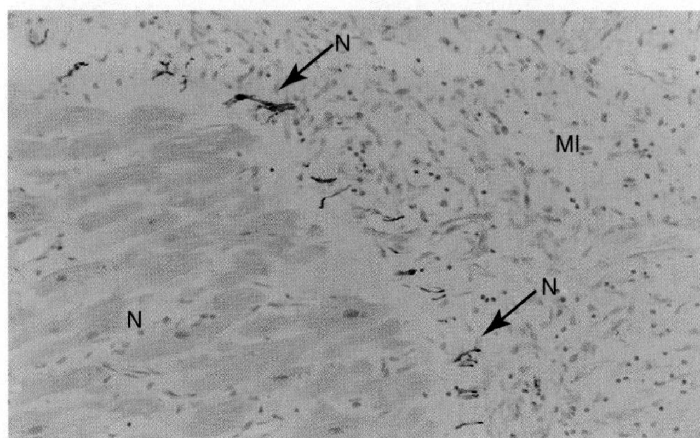

Figure 36-2 Regional hyperinnervation 2 weeks after acute myocardial infarction (MI). Immunostaining for S100 protein identified Schwann cells *(arrows)* at the periphery of infarct. In contrast, the necrotic and fibrotic zone of infarct is devoid of Schwann cells, implying denervation. The denervation and nerve sprouting after MI result in an inhomogeneous distribution of cardiac sympathetic nerves. N, Normal surviving myocardium. (From Chen P-S, Chen LS, Cao JM, et al: Sympathetic nerve sprouting, electrical remodeling and the mechanisms of sudden cardiac death. Cardiovasc Res 50(2):409-416, 2001, with permission.)

in the left stellate ganglion from 3 days after MI without concomitant increased NGF mRNA. These data from both mouse and canine models of MI indicate that MI induces a diffuse up-regulation of growth factors in the myocardium. These growth factors, NGF in particular, are up-regulated more in the area adjacent to the injury. NGF is not only produced locally in the myocardium, but it is also increased in the stellate ganglion, probably via retrograde axonal transport mechanism.[26]

It is also possible that NGF is produced outside the heart as a response to MI. An increase of NGF level in the SG and serum can facilitate nerve sprouting in both peri-infarct and noninfarct areas. The normal synaptic network between sympathetic nerve terminals and target myocytes is likely better preserved in the area remote from infarct. Therefore, fewer sprouting nerve terminals might form mature synapses. The lack of mature synapses leads to the eventual regression of sprouted nerves in the remote area. MI-induced nerve sprouting can eventually cause highly heterogeneous distribution of sympathetic innervation in the heart with areas of denervation, hyperinnervation, and relatively normal nerve fiber density.

Alteration of Sympathetic Innervation and Cardiac Arrhythmia

Many studies have demonstrated regional reduction of MIBG uptakes in subjects with various electrophysiologic diagnoses, including idiopathic ventricular tachycardia (VT),

Table 36-1 Clinical Characteristics and Ventricular Nerve Density

Group	Number	CAD	IDCM	Age	EF	Total Nerves/mm^2	Total Length of Nerves, mm/mm^2
1A	30	14	16	56.7 ± 12.1	0.22 ± 0.07	19.6 ± 11.2*	3.3 ± 3.0‡
1B	23	11	12	56.7 ± 12.9	0.21 ± 0.07	13.5 ± 6.1	2.0 ± 1.1
2	5	-	-	60.0 ± 9.7	NA	6.8 ± 2.4§	1.6 ± 1.2
3	7	7	0	63.7 ± 8.9	NA	NA	NA

Group 1A: subjects with arrhythmia; Group 1B: subjects without arrhythmia; Group 2: autopsy cases of noncardiac death; Group 3: tissues from ventricular tachycardia origin in subjects who underwent surgical ablations.

*Group 1A vs Group 1B: $P < 0.05$.

‡Group 1A vs Group 1B: $P < 0.01$.

§Group 2 vs Group 1A: $P < 0.01$.

CAD, coronary artery disease; EF, ejection fraction; IDCM, idiopathic dilated cardiomyopathy; NA, not applicable.

From Cao J-M, Fishbein MC, Han JB, et al: Relationship between regional cardiac hyperinnervation and ventricular arrhythmia. Circulation 101:1960-1969, 2000, with permission.

arrhythmogenic right ventricular cardiomyopathy, right ventricular outflow tract tachycardia, and Brugada syndrome. The incidence of regional sympathetic denervation in these subjects ranged from 33% to 88%. Moise and colleagues[27] described a colony of German shepherd dogs having a high incidence of spontaneous VT and even sudden cardiac death. The tendency of arrhythmia occurring during rapid eye movement (REM) sleep or after exercise in these dogs suggests a role of sympathetic activity in the development of arrhythmia. Inhomogeneous distribution of MIBG uptake was demonstrated in these dogs.[28] When these dogs were grouped into those with (n = 6) and without (n = 5) electrocardiographic evidence of VT, the group with VT showed a significantly larger area of denervation as compared to the group without VT (35% ± 16.5% vs12% ± 5.6%, P <0.02). The region with decreased MIBG uptake was associated with a paucity of sympathetic fibers on immunohistochemical study confirming the sympathetic denervation. These data suggest that regional sympathetic denervation may be causally related to the development of VT. Denervation supersensitivity has been proposed to be the mechanism of denervation-induced arrhythmogenesis.[29]

In the study of Cao and coworkers,[2] ventricular tissues of explanted hearts from transplant recipients were classified into two groups according to each subject's history: group 1 with documented sustained VT or nonsustained VT (>3 beats) or sudden cardiac death and group 2 without history of cardiac arrhythmia. There was no difference in the density of nerve fibers immunoreactive to S-100 between patients with ischemic versus nonischemic cardiomyopathy. However, the ventricular nerve density was significantly higher in group 1 than in group 2, suggesting an association of ventricular sympathetic nerve density and history of VT and sudden cardiac death (see Table 36-1). Ventricular tissues resected from the origin of VT were also characterized by areas of fibrosis and normal-appearing myocytes mixed with abundant nerve fibers (Figs. 36-2 and 36-3). The association of higher sympathetic nerve density has also been demonstrated in patients with a diagnosis of atrial fibrillation.[30] These clinical and histologic data indicate the regional sympathetic hyperinnervation after myocardial injury is associated with the occurrence of cardiac arrhythmia in humans.

Data from MIBG studies and histologic observations seem to generate opposite hypotheses in explaining how an alteration of sympathetic innervation might cause ventricular arrhythmia, namely regional denervation versus regional hyperinnevation as

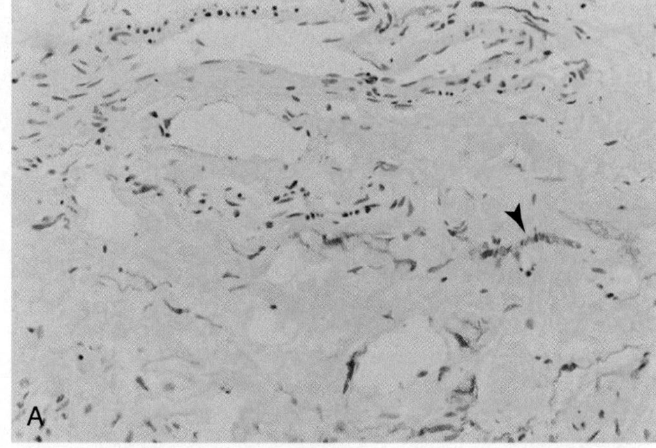

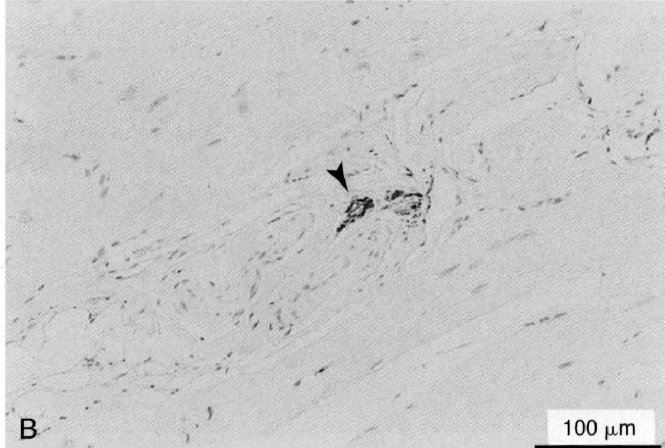

Figure 36-3 S100- and TH- positive nerve fibers from the origin of ventricular tachycardia (VT) in patients with coronary artery diseases who underwent surgical ablation of VT. **A,** S100 immunopositive nerve fibers located in perivascular area and areas with fibrosis *(arrowhead)*. **B,** TH-positive nerve fibers around coronary artery *(arrowhead)*. (From Chen P-S, Chen LS, Cao JM, et al: Sympathetic nerve sprouting, electrical remodeling and the mechanisms of sudden cardiac death. Cardiovasc Res 50(2):409-416, 2001, with permission.)

the arrhythmogenic mechanism. However, these hypotheses are not mutually exclusive. A regional decrease of MIBG uptake does not rule out the presence of sympathetic regeneration. A twofold increase of nerve terminals scattered in the myocardium adjacent to infarct zone as shown in Cao's[2] study might be below the sensitivity of MIBG. In fact, the area of decreased MIBG uptake is often associated with an increase of washout, suggesting an enhanced catecholamine turnover and a possibility of increased sympathetic activity in the denervated area. Both the denervation-induced adrenergic supersensitivity and sympathetic hyperinnervation may be synergic in altering electrophysiologic properties of injured myocardium. Furthermore, the heterogeneity of sympathetic nerve distribution, due to denervation in the injured myocardium, can be enhanced by scattered hyperinnervation. The inhomogeneity of sympathetic innervation might also be important in the development of cardiac arrhythmia.

Sympathetic Neural Remodeling and Cardiac Arrhythmia

To elucidate the arrhythmogenic role of sympathetic hyperinnervation in infarcted myocardium, two canine experiments were conducted to facilitate sympathetic nerve sprouting and augment sympathetic hyperinnervation in the heart with MI and complete atrioventricular (AV) block. Complete AV block was induced by radiofrequency catheter ablation of the AV junction. MI was caused by ligating the left anterior descending coronary artery below the first diagonal branch. Sympathetic nerve sprouting was induced by either chronic NGF infusion into the left stellate ganglion or chronic electrical stimulation to the left stellate ganglion. An implantable cardioverter-defibrillator (ICD) was implanted to detect VT and ventricular fibrillation (VF). As compared to control dogs (with MI and AV block only), NGF infusion increased sympathetic nerve density by twofold and increased the incidence of VT by 10-fold.[3] Four of nine dogs died from documented VF. Long-term subthreshold electrical stimulation to the left stellate ganglion induced fourfold increase of sympathetic nerve density (93 ± 42 μm/mm^2 vs 26 ± 16 μm/mm^2) and a much higher incidence of VT (36 ± 6 per day). Four of six dogs in that study died of sudden cardiac death.

To further prove a causal relationship between sympathetic hyperinnervation and ventricular arrhythmia, we studied the temporal relationship of sympathetic activity and occurrence of arrhythmia in these canine models of sudden cardiac death. Jardine and colleagues[31,32] have recorded cardiac sympathetic nerve activity from sheep by multiple electrodes glued to the left cardiothoracic nerves; wires were exteriorized through incisions. This in vivo recording demonstrated an increase of burst frequencies of cardiac sympathetic nerve activity up to 7 days after MI and also documented a spontaneous VF episode preceded immediately by a paroxysm of increased cardiac sympathetic nerve activity in one sheep with acute MI.[33]

Using implanted radiotransmitters, Jung and coworkers[34] performed long-term simultaneous continuous (24 hours a day, 7 days a week) recording of stellate ganglion nerve activity in six dogs. The authors found that the stellate ganglion nerve activity was followed immediately (<1 sec) by heart rate and blood pressure elevation. Heart rate correlated significantly with stellate ganglion nerve activity. Both heart rate and stellate ganglion nerve activity showed statistically significant ($P < .01$) circadian variation. The data imply the feasibility of continuous monitoring cardiac of sympathetic activity in ambulatory animals by recording stellate ganglion activity.

Zhou and colleagues[35] and Ogawa and coauthors[4] have successfully applied this long-term stellate ganglion recording technique in a canine model of sudden cardiac death and heart failure (Fig. 36-4). Nerve activity recorded from the left stellate ganglion included low-amplitude burst discharge activity and high-amplitude spike discharge activity. Both low-amplitude burst discharge activity and high-amplitude spike discharge activity accelerated heart rate. In dogs with MI, complete AV block and NGF infusion to the left stellate ganglion, most ventricular tachycardia (86.3%) and sudden cardiac death were preceded within 15 seconds by either low-amplitude burst discharge activity or high-amplitude spike discharge activity; the closer to the onset of ventricular tachycardia, the higher the nerve activity became. Most instances of high-amplitude spike discharge activity were followed immediately by either ventricular arrhythmia (21%) or QRS morphology changes (65%). The data provide direct evidence of temporal correlation of ventricular arrhythmia and sympathetic activity in dogs with cardiac sympathetic hyperinnervation.

Other groups have also successfully developed large animal models of sudden cardiac death.[36,37] In the model reported by Issa and colleagues,[38] the investigators created MI in dogs by percutaneous transcatheter embolization. The dogs were then rapidly paced for 3 weeks to induce heart failure. Dogs with healing MI and heart failure were highly susceptible to ventricular arrhythmia. Acute transient ischemia induced sustained VT or VF in 21 of 29 (72%) dogs that survived the surgery. Killingsworth and coworkers[39] reported a sheep model of sudden cardiac death. In that model, sheep had either AV block alone or combined AV block and MI. The frequency of phase-2 VT (from day 8 to day 42) was 20-fold higher in the group of sheep with both MI and AV block than in the group with AV block alone (a total of 482 episodes vs 23 episodes). Three animals in the MI and AV block group experienced sudden cardiac death resulting from ventricular tachyarrhythmia. Although the nerve densities were not determined in either study, we speculate that MI and rapid pacing likely have induced heterogeneous sympathetic hyperinnervation and contributed to the increased susceptibility to ventricular arrhythmia.[40,41,42]

Sympathetic hyperinnervation might also play an important mechanistic role in atrial fibrillation. Long-term rapid pacing to the right atrium induced sustained atrial fibrillation in dogs. Chang and colleagues demonstrated a three-fold to five-fold increase of sympathetic nerve density in the atrium in the dogs with atrial fibrillation.[41] Using the same canine model of atrial fibrillation, Jayachandran and coauthors demonstrated a heterogeneous increase of sympathetic innervation in the atrium.[43] Swissa and colleagues also observed high incidence of spontaneous paroxysmal atrial fibrillation (1.3 ± 1.6 episodes per day) and paroxysmal atrial tachycardia (2.5 ± 2.2 episodes per day) in dogs with MI, complete AV block, and sympathetic hyperinnervation induced by either NGF infusion or electrical stimulation to the left stellate ganglion.[44] Direct nerve recordings in two different models showed a temporal association between sympathetic nerve activity and the onset of atrial arrhythmias, including atrial tachycardia and atrial fibrillation.[4,45]

Arrhythmogenic Mechanism of Sympathetic Nerve Sprouting after MI

Because most sudden cardiac deaths occur in subjects with histories of coronary artery disease or MI, the electrical and anatomic remodeling created by infarction must be crucial factors in the pathogenesis of VT and sudden cardiac death. We propose that the interaction of neural remodeling and electrical remodeling is the mechanism underlying the ventricular arrhythmia after MI. Neural remodeling resulting from sympathetic nerve

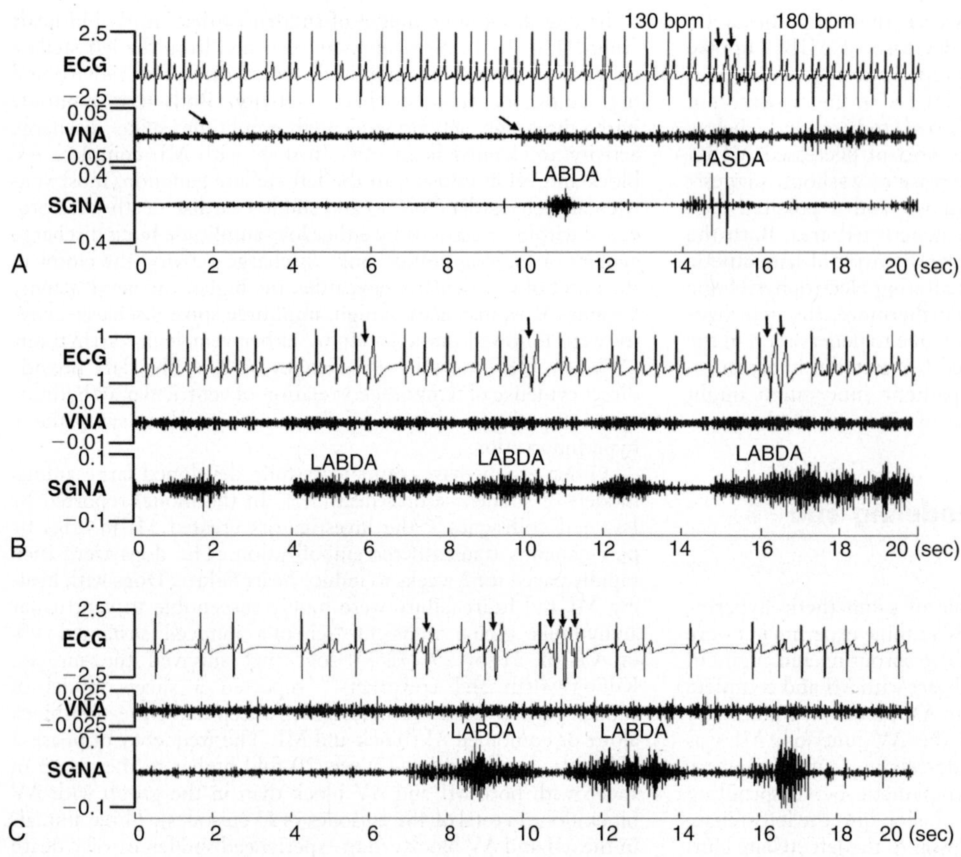

Figure 36-4 Low-amplitude burst discharge activity (LABDA) and high-amplitude spike discharge activity (HASDA). **A,** HASDA-induced couplets and abruptly increased heart rate 6 days after cessation of rapid pacing in dog 2. **B,** LABDA episodes associated with isolated premature ventricular contraction and couplets 1 day after cessation of rapid pacing in dog 3. **C,** LABDA episodes associated with isolated premature ventricular contraction and triplets (ventricular tachycardia) 1 day after cessation of rapid pacing in dog 2. (From Ogawa M, Zhou S, Tan AY, et al: Left stellate ganglion and vagal nerve activity and cardiac arrhythmias in ambulatory dogs with pacing-induced congestive heart failure. J Am Coll Cardiol 50:335-343, 2007, with permission. Reprinted with permission from the *Annual Review of Pharmacology and Toxicology*, Volume 41, ©2001 by Annual Review www.annualreviews.org.)

sprouting might serve as a trigger, and an electrically remolded myocardium serves as a substrate for inducing VT.

Electrical Remodeling after Myocardial Infarction

In experimental models, permanent occlusion of left anterior descending artery causes transmural anteroseptal myocardial infarction. The surviving rim of myocardial fibers (a few cells to several hundred cells thick) on the epicardial surface of a transmural infarct is known as the epicardial border zone (EBZ).[46] The EBZ is the frequent site of origin of inducible VT or VF 1 week after occlusion of the left anterior descending artery (healing phase of MI). In the first week after occlusion of the left anterior descending artery, myocardial remodeling leads to increased connective tissue and edema between the epicardial muscle bundles, resulting in nonuniform anisotropy. Active membrane properties of EBZ are altered. Peak L-type inward Ca^{2+} current is reduced in myocytes isolated from the EBZ,[47] and the recovery of the fast inward sodium current is delayed.[48] The changes of membrane properties alter the excitability and post-repolarization refractoriness in the EBZ, promoting conduction block and reentry either during premature stimulation or during rapid pacing.[48]

Electrical remodeling is not limited to the EBZ. Significant changes can also occur in noninfarcted myocardium. Qin and coworkers[49] demonstrated that MI might result in prolongation of action potential duration (APD) and marked heterogeneity of the time course of repolarization in the noninfarcted myocardium. These changes could be explained by the reduction of transient outward K^+ currents. Aimond and colleagues[50] subjected young rats to left coronary ligature. After 4 to 6 months, they studied enzymatically dissociated ventricular cells. They found that long-term coronary ligation resulted in a significantly altered L-type calcium current, including reduced peak amplitude and a slower inactivation. They also found a significantly altered K^+ current in post-MI cells. These findings indicate that MI results in significant electrical remodeling in the EBZ and in other noninfarcted myocardium.[51]

Interaction between Sympathetic Neural Remodeling and Electrical Remodeling

β-Adrenergic stimulation is known to increase ionic current through L-type calcium currents (I_{CaL}), I_{Ks}, and chloride channels ($I_{Cl,Ca}$ and $I_{Cl\text{-}cAMP}$). The increased I_{Ks} tends to shorten APD and the increased I_{Ca} tends to prolong APD. In normal canine ventricles in vivo, sympathetic stimulation results in shortening of APD and decreasing dispersion of refractoriness,[52] implying that there is a net increase of outward repolarizing I_{Ks} and I_{Cl} versus the inward I_{Ca}. However, the same is not true when I_{Ks} is suppressed or downregulated after MI.[53] In the perfused canine tissues, chromanol 293B (a specific I_{Ks} blocker) prolongs the QT interval and APD at 90% repolarization (APD_{90}) of all myocardial cells but does not widen the T wave or induce torsades de pointes. Isoproterenol in the continued presence of chromanol 293B abbreviated the APD_{90} of epicardial and endocardial cells but not that of the M cells, resulting in widening of the T wave and a dramatic accentuation of dispersion of repolarization. Spontaneous an programmed electrical stimulation–induced torsades de pointes was observed only after exposure to the I_{Ks} blocker and isoproterenol. The I_{Ks} was also abnormal in patients with type I congenital long-QT syndrome (LQT1).[54,55] During exercise testing, these subjects had diminished chronotropic response and paradoxical prolongation of QT interval.[56] Epinephrine might induce torsades de pointes, and β-blocker therapy and left sympathectomy are antiarrhythmic in subjects with LQT1. The left sympathectomy can also result in shortening of QT interval in patients with LQT syndrome.[57]

These data suggest that sympathetic stimulation is arrhythmogenic if the I_{Ks} is genetically abnormal (such as in the congenital long-QT syndrome), inhibited by pharmacologic agents, or down-regulated (such as in MI). Sympathetic stimulation in these ventricles can increase the dispersion of repolarization and the torsades de pointes arrhythmia. The mechanism is most likely related to a large augmentation of residual I_{Ks} in epicardial and endocardial cells but not in M cells, in which I_{Ks} is intrinsically weak.[53]

In addition to prolongation of QT interval, sympathetic stimulation can increase the sarcoplasmic calcium release through the ryanodine receptor. Mutation of the type 2 ryanodine receptor is known to be arrhythmogenic in humans, especially during exercise, when sympathetic tone is greatly increased.[58] The mechanisms of arrhythmogenesis in mice with abnormal ryanodine receptors could be due to the development of delayed afterdepolarizations and triggered activity from the subendocardial Purkinje fibers.[59] In addition to ventricular fibrillation, one study expanded the spectrum of ryanodine receptor–related diseases to other cardiac arrhythmias, such as sinus node dysfunction and atrial fibrillation.[60]

If sympathetic stimulation is important in arrhythmogenesis and sudden cardiac death, then left sympathectomy should be effective in preventing cardiac arrhythmia. Compatible with this hypothesis, left cardiac sympathetic denervation in general has been shown to be antiarrhythmic. In human subjects and in animals, left cardiac sympathetic denervation is effective in preventing sudden cardiac death after MI that had acquired abnormalities of potassium channels due to electrical remodeling.[61,62] In congenital LQT1, the abnormal potassium channel activity was genetic rather than acquired. However, left stellectomy was also useful (although not 100% effective) in preventing the recurrence of cardiac arrhythmia.[63] These results show that an interaction between abnormal electrophysiologic substrate and sympathetic stimulation is important in cardiac arrhythmogenesis.

One interesting finding of our canine model of sudden cardiac death, created by NGF infusion to left stellate ganglia in dogs with MI and AV block, is that NGF infusion to the left stellate ganglion in normal dogs caused nerve sprouting but did not result in ventricular arrhythmia or sudden cardiac death. In the control group, electrical remodeling induced by MI and complete AV block also failed to increase sudden cardiac death. An interaction between nerve sprouting (neural remodeling) and electrical remodeling is needed to cause high incidence of VT, VF, or sudden cardiac death.

Conclusions

Sympathetic nerve sprouting might occur in some (but not all) subjects after myocardial injury. There is an association between the density of myocardial sympathetic nerves and ventricular arrhythmia. NGF infusion to the left stellate ganglion in dogs with chronic MI and complete AV block augments sympathetic nerve sprouting and results in high incidence of spontaneous VT, VF, and sudden cardiac death. The magnitude of sympathetic nerve sprouting may be an important determinant of VT or sudden cardiac death in chronic MI. We propose the nerve-sprouting hypothesis of sudden cardiac death as follows: Neural remodeling resulting from sympathetic nerve sprouting can occur after cardiac injury, such as MI. The heterogeneously increased sympathetic innervation might serve as a trigger for cardiac arrhythmias and sudden cardiac death in the electrically remodeled myocardium.

The nerve-sprouting hypothesis explains the efficacy of β-blockers in preventing sudden cardiac death after MI.[64] It might also explain the results of some clinical trials. For example, sotalol, a drug with β-blocking effects, is known to be effective in preventing ventricular arrhythmias in subjects with chronic MI. If the β-blocking activity is removed (such as in D-sotalol), then the drug increases mortality in subjects with MI.[65] It is also known that left cardiac sympathetic denervation is effective in preventing sudden cardiac death after MI both in animal models and in humans. All these observations are compatible with the nerve-sprouting hypothesis of sudden cardiac death.

Acknowledgment

We thank Alice Shinyi Chen for her artwork.

References

1. Chen P-S, Chen LS, Cao JM, Sharifi B, et al: Sympathetic nerve sprouting, electrical remodeling and the mechanisms of sudden cardiac death. Cardiovasc Res 50(2): 409-416, 2001.
2. Cao J-M, Fishbein MC, Han JB, et al: Relationship between regional cardiac hyperinnervation and ventricular arrhythmia. Circulation 101:1960-1969, 2000.
3. Cao J-M, Chen LS, KenKnight BH, et al: Nerve sprouting and sudden cardiac death. Circ Res 86:816-821, 2000.
4. Ogawa M, Zhou S, Tan AY, et al: Left stellate ganglion and vagal nerve activity and cardiac arrhythmias in ambulatory dogs with pacing-induced congestive heart failure. J Am Coll Cardiol 50:335-343, 2007.
5. Marron K, Wharton J, Sheppard MN, et al: Distribution, morphology, and neurochemistry of endocardial and epicardial nerve terminal arborizations in the human heart. Circulation 92(8):2343-2351, 1995.
6. Chow LT, Chow WH, Lee JC, et al: Postmortem changes in the immunohistochemical demonstration of nerves in human ventricular myocardium. J Anat 192 (Pt 1):73-80, 1998.
7. Crick SJ, Sheppard MN, Ho SY, Anderson RH: Localisation and quantitation of autonomic innervation in the porcine heart I: Conduction system. J Anat 195 (Pt 3): 341-357, 1999.
8. Tan AY, Li H, Wachsmann-Hogiu S, et al: Autonomic innervation and segmental muscular disconnections at the human pulmonary vein–atrial junction: Implications for catheter ablation of atrial-pulmonary vein junction. J Am Coll Cardiol 48: 132-143, 2006.
9. Chow LT, Chow SS, Anderson RH, Gosling JA: The innervation of the human myocardium at birth. J Anat 187 (Pt 1): 107-114, 1995.
10. Bulow HP, Stahl F, Lauer B, et al: Alterations of myocardial presynaptic sympathetic innervation in patients with multi-vessel coronary artery disease but without history of myocardial infarction. Nucl Med Commun 24(3):233-239, 2003.
11. Luisi AJ Jr, Suzuki G, Dekemp R, et al: Regional ^{11}C-hydroxyephedrine retention in hibernating myocardium: chronic inhomogeneity of sympathetic innervation in the absence of infarction. J Nucl Med 46(8):1368-1374, 2005.
12. Bengel FM, Barthel P, Matsunari I, et al: Kinetics of ^{123}I-MIBG after acute myocardial infarction and reperfusion therapy. J Nucl Med 40(6):904-910, 1999.
13. Podio V, Spinnler MT, Spandonari T, et al: Regional sympathetic denervation after myocardial infarction: a follow-up study using ^{123}I-MIBG. Q J Nucl Med 39 (4 Suppl 1):40-43, 1995.
14. Hartikainen J, Kuikka J, Mantysaari M, et al: Sympathetic reinnervation after acute myocardial infarction. Am J Cardiol 77:5-9, 1996.
15. Hartikainen J, Mustonen J, Kuikka J, et al: Cardiac sympathetic denervation in patients with coronary artery disease

without previous myocardial infarction. Am J Cardiol 80:273-277, 1997.

16. Inobe Y, Kugiyama K, Miyagi H, et al: Long-lasting abnormalities in cardiac sympathetic nervous system in patients with coronary spastic angina: quantitative analysis with iodine 123 metaiodobenzylguanidine myocardial scintigraphy. Am Heart J 134(1):112-118, 1997.
17. Dae MW, O'Connell JW, Botvinick EH, Chin MC: Acute and chronic effects of transient myocardial ischemia on sympathetic nerve activity, density, and norepinephrine content. Cardiovasc Res 30: 270-280, 1995.
18. Vracko R, Thorning D, Frederickson RG: Nerve fibers in human myocardial scars. Hum Pathol 22:138-146, 1991.
19. Wilson RF, Christensen BV, Olivari MT, et al: Evidence for structural sympathetic reinnervation after orthotopic cardiac transplantation in humans. Circulation 83(4):1210-1220, 1991.
20. Schwaiblmair M, von Scheidt W, Uberfuhr P, et al: Functional significance of cardiac reinnervation in heart transplant recipients. J Heart Lung Transplant 18:838-845, 1999.
21. Bengel FM, Ueberfuhr P, Schiepel N, et al: Effect of sympathetic reinnervation on cardiac performance after heart transplantation. N Engl J Med 345(10):731-738, 2001.
22. Kim DT, Luthringer DJ, Lai AC, et al: Sympathetic nerve sprouting after orthotopic heart transplantation. J Heart Lung Transplant 23(12):1349-1358, 2004.
23. Fu SY, Gordon T: The cellular and molecular basis of peripheral nerve regeneration. Mol Neurobiol 14:67-116, 1997.
24. Oh Y-S, Jong AY, Kim DT, et al: Spatial distribution of nerve sprouting after myocardial infarction in mice. Heart Rhythm 3:728-736, 2006.
25. Zhou S, Chen LS, Miyauchi Y, et al: Mechanisms of cardiac nerve sprouting after myocardial infarction in dogs. Circ Res 95:76-83, 2004.
26. Ginty DD, Segal RA: Retrograde neurotrophin signaling: Trk-ing along the axon. Curr Opin Neurobiol 12(3):268-274, 2002.
27. Moise NS, Gilmour RF Jr, Riccio ML: An animal model of spontaneous arrhythmic death. J Cardiovasc Electrophysiol 8: 98-103, 1997.
28. Dae MW, Lee RJ, Ursell PC, et al: Heterogeneous sympathetic innervation in German shepherd dogs with inherited ventricular arrhythmia and sudden cardiac death. Circulation 96:1337-1342, 1997.
29. Inoue H, Zipes DP: Results of sympathetic denervation in the canine heart: Supersensitivity that may be arrhythmogenic. Circulation 75:877-887, 1987.
30. Gould PA, Yii M, McLean C, et al: Evidence for increased atrial sympathetic innervation in persistent human atrial fibrillation. Pacing Clin Electrophysiol 29(8):821-829, 2006.
31. Jardine DL, Charles CJ, Melton IC, et al: Continual recordings of cardiac sympathetic nerve activity in conscious sheep. Am J Physiol Heart Circ Physiol 282(1):H93-H99, 2002.
32. Jardine DL, Charles CJ, Ashton RK, et al: Increased cardiac sympathetic nerve activity following acute myocardial infarction in a sheep model. J Physiol 565:325-333, 2005.
33. Jardine DL, Charles CJ, Forrester MD, et al: A neural mechanism for sudden death after myocardial infarction. Clin Auton Res 13(5):339-341, 2003.
34. Jung B-C, Dave AS, Tan AY, et al: Circadian variations of stellate ganglion nerve activity in ambulatory dogs. Heart Rhythm 3:78-85, 2005.
35. Zhou S, Jung B-C, Tan AY, et al: Spontaneous stellate ganglion nerve activity and ventricular arrhythmia in a canine model of sudden death [abstract]. Heart Rhythm 3(1S):S106, 2006.
36. Moise NS, Meyers-Wallen V, Flahive WJ, et al: Inherited ventricular arrhythmias and sudden death in German shepherd dogs. J Am Coll Cardiol 24(1):233-243, 1994.
37. Canty JM Jr, Suzuki G, Banas MD, et al: Hibernating myocardium: Chronically adapted to ischemia but vulnerable to sudden death. Circ Res 94(8):1142-1149, 2004.
38. Issa ZF, Rosenberger J, Groh WJ, et al: Ischemic ventricular arrhythmias during heart failure: A canine model to replicate clinical events. Heart Rhythm 2(9):979-983, 2005.
39. Killingsworth CR, Walcott GP, Gamblin TL, et al: Chronic myocardial infarction is a substrate for bradycardia-induced spontaneous tachyarrhythmias and sudden death in conscious animals. J Cardiovasc Electrophysiol 17(2):189-197, 2006.
40. Hamabe A, Chang C-M, Zhou S, et al: Induction of atrial fibrillation and nerve sprouting by prolonged left atrial pacing in dogs. Pacing Clin Electrophysiol 26:2247-2252, 2003.
41. Chang C-M, Wu T-J, Zhou S-M, et al: Nerve sprouting and sympathetic hyperinnervation in a canine model of atrial fibrillation produced by prolonged right atrial pacing. Circulation 103:22-25, 2001.
42. Cha YM, Redfield MM, Shah S, et al: Effects of omapatrilat on cardiac nerve sprouting and structural remodeling in experimental congestive heart failure. Heart Rhythm 2(9):984-990, 2005.
43. Jayachandran JV, Sih HJ, Winkle W, et al: Atrial fibrillation produced by prolonged rapid atrial pacing is associated with heterogeneous changes in atrial sympathetic innervation. Circulation 101:1185-11891, 2000.
44. Swissa M, Zhou S, Paz O, et al: A canine model of paroxysmal atrial fibrillation and paroxysmal atrial tachycardia. Am J Physiol Heart Circ Physiol 289(5):H1851-H1857, 2005.
45. Tan AY, Zhou S, Gholmieh G, et al: Spontaneous autonomic nerve activity and paroxysmal atrial tachyarrhythmias [abstract]. Heart Rhythm 3(1S):184, 2006.
46. Ursell PC, Gardner PI, Albala A, et al: Structural and electrophysiological changes in the epicardial border zone and canine myocardial infarcts during infarct healing. Circ Res 56:436-451, 1985.
47. Aggarwal R, Boyden PA: Diminished Ca^{2+} and Ba^{2+} currents in myocytes surviving in the epicardial border zone of the 5-day infarcted canine heart. Circ Res 77: 1180-1191, 1995.
48. Pu J, Boyden PA: Alterations of Na^+ currents in myocytes from epicardial border zone of the infarcted heart. A possible ionic mechanism for reduced excitability and postrepolarization refractoriness. Circ Res 81:110-119, 1997.
49. Qin D, Zhang ZH, Caref EB, et al: Cellular and ionic basis of arrhythmias in postinfarction remodeled ventricular myocardium. Circ Res 79:461-473, 1996.
50. Aimond F, Alvarez JL, Rauzier JM, et al: Ionic basis of ventricular arrhythmias in remodeled rat heart during long-term myocardial infarction. Cardiovasc Res 42: 402-415, 1999.
51. Pinto JM, Boyden PA: Electrical remodeling in ischemia and infarction. Cardiovasc Res 42:284-297, 1999.
52. Takei M, Sasaki Y, Yonezawa T, et al: The autonomic control of the transmural dispersion of ventricular repolarization in anesthetized dogs. J Cardiovasc Electrophysiol 10:981-989, 1999.
53. Shimizu W, Antzelevitch C: Cellular basis for the ECG features of the LQT1 form of the long-QT syndrome: Effects of beta-adrenergic agonists and antagonists and sodium channel blockers on transmural dispersion of repolarization and torsades de pointes. Circulation 98:2314-2322, 1998.
54. Sanguinetti MC, Curran ME, Zou A, et al: Coassembly of K_VLQT1 and minK (IsK) proteins to form cardiac I_{Ks} potassium channel. Nature 384:80-83, 1996.
55. Barhanin J, Lesage F, Guillemare E, et al: K_VLQT1 and IsK (minK) proteins associate to form the I_{Ks} cardiac potassium current. Nature 384:78-80, 1996.
56. Swan H, Viitasalo M, Piippo K, et al: Sinus node function and ventricular repolarization during exercise stress test in long QT syndrome patients with K_VLQT1 and HERG potassium channel defects. J Am Coll Cardiol 34:823-829, 1999.
57. Moss AJ, McDonald J: Unilateral cervicothoracic sympathetic ganglionectomy for the treatment of long QT interval syndrome. N Engl J Med 285(16):903-904, 1971.
58. Priori SG, Napolitano C, Tiso N, et al: Mutations in the cardiac ryanodine receptor gene (hRyR2) underlie catecholaminergic polymorphic ventricular tachycardia. Circulation 103(2):196-200, 2001.
59. Cerrone M, Noujaim SF, Tolkacheva EG, et al: Arrhythmogenic mechanisms in a mouse model of catecholaminergic polymorphic ventricular tachycardia. Circ Res 101(10):1039-1048, 2007.
60. Bhuiyan ZA, Van Den Berg MP, van Tintelen JP, et al: Expanding spectrum of human RYR2-related disease: New electrocardiographic, structural, and genetic features. Circulation 116(14):1569-1576, 2007.
61. Schwartz PJ, Motolese M, Pollavini G, et al; Italian Sudden Death Prevention Group: Prevention of sudden cardiac death after a first myocardial infarction by pharmacologic or surgical antiadrenergic

interventions. J Cardiovasc Electrophysiol 3:2-16, 1992.

62. Schwartz PJ, La Rovere MT, Vanoli E: Autonomic nervous system and sudden cardiac death. Experimental basis and clinical observations for post-myocardial intarction risk stratification. Circulation 85:I-77-I-91, 1992.
63. Schwartz PJ, Priori SG, Cerrone M, et al: Left cardiac sympathetic denervation in the management of high-risk patients affected by the long-QT syndrome. Circulation 109(15):1826-1833, 2004.
64. Rarnaot M: Nicotine patches may not be safe. BMJ 310:663-664, 1995.
65. Waldo AL, Camm AJ, deRuyter H, et al: Effect of D-sotalol on mortality in patients with left ventricular dysfunction after recent and remote myocardial infarction. The SWORD Investigators. Survival With Oral D-Sotalol. Lancet 348:7-12, 1996.

Neurocardiac Imaging 37

Gary D. Hutchins, Michael A. Miller, and Douglas P. Zipes

CHAPTER OUTLINE

The autonomic nervous system (ANS) plays a crucial role in maintaining cardiovascular performance under diverse physiologic conditions encountered in daily activity. Disruption of the excitatory and inhibitory mechanisms of the ANS may be at least partially responsible for the degradation of cardiovascular performance and rhythm disturbances found in a variety of cardiac disorders, including coronary artery disease, hypertrophy, and cardiomyopathy, as well as electrophysiologic abnormalities observed in otherwise apparently normal hearts.

The in vivo evaluation of the cardiac ANS has been limited by a lack of adequate assessment tools. Direct venous plasma blood sampling techniques enable evaluation of sympathetic tone on a global basis but cannot provide regional information.[1,2] Invasive sampling techniques that directly assess catecholamine kinetics also provide valuable information about the function of the cardiac ANS.[3] Unfortunately, these techniques require long cardiac catheterization sessions and do not permit regional assessment of ANS function. Monitoring cardiovascular system responses to the administration of pharmacologic agents that affect the physiology of the heart represents another approach used to study the ANS. Once again, however, these techniques do not enable evaluation of regional alterations caused by cardiovascular disorders, nor do they permit the characterization of an unperturbed system.

Radiopharmaceuticals developed for conventional nuclear medicine and positron emission tomography (PET) provide unique imaging approaches for the regional in vivo assessment of the cardiac ANS.[4,5] These imaging-based techniques enabling the characterization of physiologic processes in vivo are the product of collaborative activities between investigators from diverse scientific disciplines, including cardiology, radiology, medicinal chemistry, medical physics, pharmacology, biochemistry, and physiology. Using imaging-based techniques, it has become possible to examine regional alterations in ANS neuron distribution and function.

This chapter is an update of Chapter 92 of the fourth edition of this book. It reviews the techniques that are used to image the cardiac ANS and some of the experimental and clinical observations to date. We have added a summary of some of the more recently developed tracers and of relevant review articles.

Autonomic Nervous System

The ANS regulates heart rate, contractile force, and conduction velocity through two main subdivisions, the sympathetic and parasympathetic nervous systems.[6] The sympathetic system provides excitatory stimulation, resulting in an increase in heart rate, an increase in the force of ventricular contraction, and an increase in the conduction velocity of several fiber types.[7] In contrast, the parasympathetic system is inhibitory and tends to oppose the effects of the sympathetic system. Both of these systems affect control of the myocardium through the release of neurotransmitters that interact with receptor sites on cardiomyocytes and neurons. The principal neurotransmitters of these systems are norepinephrine and acetylcholine for the sympathetic and parasympathetic systems, respectively.[8] These neurotransmitters exert their effects on the heart by either activating (norepinephrine) or inhibiting (acetylcholine) adenylate cyclase through receptor-mediated processes. The processes of neurotransmitter synthesis, release, and binding to membrane protein receptor sites, neurotransmitter inactivation through metabolic degradation, and presynaptic neurotransmitter uptake and storage all provide potential targets for radiopharmaceuticals to characterize the ANS using imaging techniques. A schematic representation of these processes is diagrammed in Figure 37-1.

It has been shown that the sympathetic nerve fibers travel along the vasculature on the epicardial surface of the heart and penetrate into the ventricular myocardium in a pattern that appears similar to the coronary artery distribution (Fig. 37-2).[9] In contrast, parasympathetic nerve fibers enter the ventricles at the epicardial surface and quickly penetrate the myocardial tissue, distributing along the endocardial surface (see Fig. 37-2).[10-12] Sympathetic innervation, as assessed on the basis of norepinephrine content, shows a high density of innervation throughout the left ventricle, with a small gradient extending from the base to the apex.[9] The sympathetic innervation density also appears to be greater in the endocardial wall than in the epicardial wall of the left venticle.[9] The primary receptor sites for norepinephrine (β-adrenergic receptors) have a distribution pattern that is inversely related to the presynaptic neuronal density pattern, with greater receptor densities in the subepicardial layer than in the subendocardial layer of the heart and a small receptor density gradient extending from the apex to the base.[10-12] Parasympathetic innervation, as assessed on the basis of choline acetyltransferase levels, is highest in the atria and appears to be sparse in the ventricles.[13-15] Acting through muscarinic

This work was supported in part by National Institutes of Health grant NIH HL 52323 and the Indiana Genomics Initiative. The Indiana Genomics Initiative is supported in part by the Lilly Endowment.

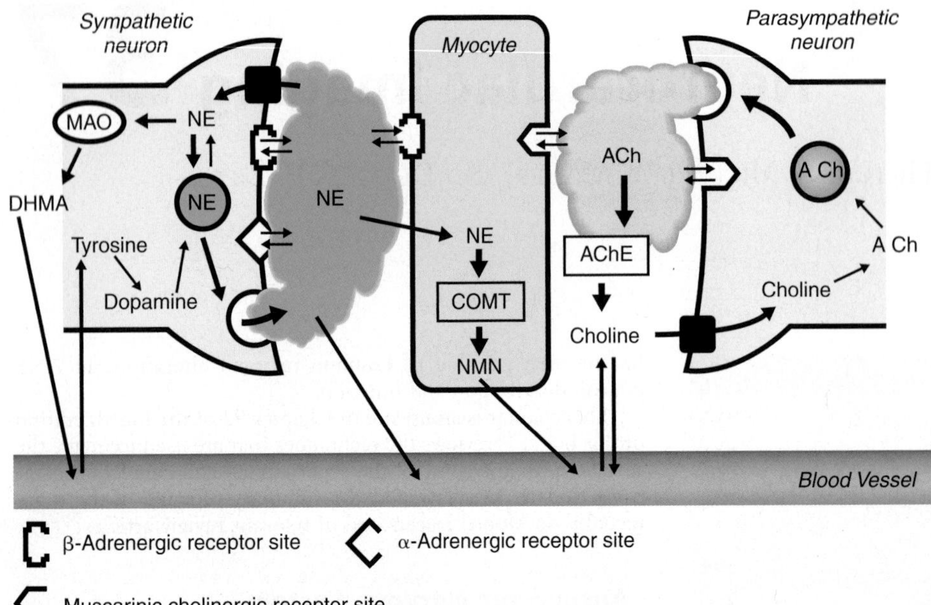

Figure 37-1 The mechanism involved in the synthesis, release, and reuptake of the primary neurotransmitters of the autonomic nervous system is shown in this sketch. Control of heart rate, contractility, and conduction is maintained in part through this system. All processes diagrammed in the figure represent potential targets for radiopharmaceutical probes. ACh, acetylcholine; AChE, acetylcholinesterase; COMT, catechol-*O*-methyltransferase; DBH, dopamine-β-hydroxylase; DHMA, 3,4-dihydroxymandelic acid; MAO, monoamine oxidase; NE, norepinephrine; NMN, normetanephrine.

cholinergic receptors, acetylcholine has an inhibitory effect on the chronotropic and inotropic properties of the heart. The muscarinic receptors in the ventricle of the heart are located in the sarcolemma.[16]

Radiopharmaceuticals

Radiopharmaceuticals used to image the ANS target specific processes associated with either presynaptic neurotransmitter uptake and storage mechanisms or postsynaptic receptor site interactions. In either case, the radiopharmaceutical must be administered intravenously and delivered to the tissue by blood flow. Once these tracers are delivered to the target organ, they must be capable of moving across the capillary membrane, either by diffusion or by specific transport mechanisms. On crossing the capillary membrane, the tracer should interact specifically and with relatively high affinity for the target protein site. General criteria required for a radiopharmaceutical to isolate specific protein site densities and distributions successfully within tissue using imaging techniques include saturability, specificity, stereoselectivity, affinity, biodistribution, correlation with biologic effect, resistance to metabolism, pharmacokinetics, and toxicity.[17-20]

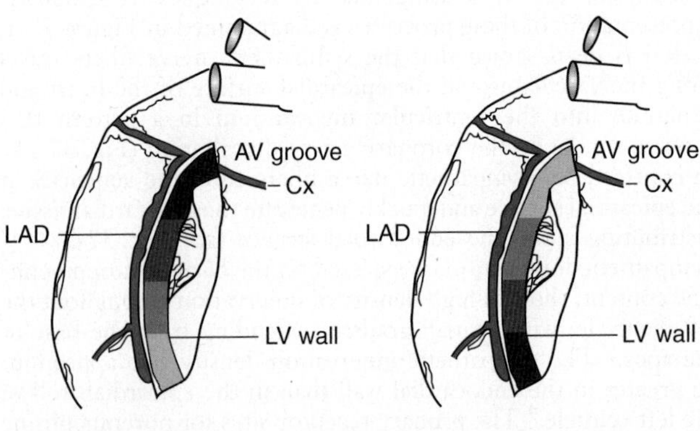

Figure 37-2 Sagittal view of the left ventricle schematically demonstrating the sympathetic neuron and β-adrenergic receptor density gradients. The sympathetic neuron density is highest in the base of the left ventricle and decreases slightly moving toward the apex. The β-receptor density shows an inverse relationship, with higher densities in the apex than in the base of the left ventricle. AV, atrioventricular; Cx, circumflex artery; LAD, left anterior descending artery; LV, left ventricle.

Criteria for Radiopharmaceuticals

Saturability

The number of protein sites for either uptake transport systems or receptor sites is finite. Therefore, the processes associated with these proteins should be saturable when large concentrations of the specific pharmaceutical are administered. If saturability cannot be demonstrated, the tracer accumulation likely does not reflect interaction with the specific protein site.[21]

Specificity

Ideally, the radiopharmaceutical will interact with only a single protein site. If interaction occurs with multiple protein sites, isolation and quantification of each type of interaction become extremely difficult.

Stereoselectivity

The interaction of neurotransmitters with protein uptake transport or receptor sites typically is specific and displays some level of stereoselectivity. In contrast, nonspecific radiopharmaceutical binding or interactions tend to occur independent of the conformational orientation of the molecule.[22,23]

Affinity

Radioligands used for imaging purposes typically interact with high affinity for the protein site(s) of interest. High affinities for the protein site help ensure that adequate contrast can be achieved between the accumulation of specifically bound or stored radiopharmaceutical and nonspecific accumulations in the tissue.[24]

Biodistribution

The regional biodistribution of the radiopharmaceutical in tissue must permit the delineation of accumulation within the target organ from surrounding tissues. For example, when imaging the heart, the blood pool should clear rapidly relative to the radiopharmaceutical kinetics in the myocardium. Adjacent organs such as the lungs and liver should have minimal levels of tracer accumulation to minimize the background signal that spills over into the heart when imaged on systems with limited spatial resolution, contaminating the signal of interest.[25]

Correlation with Biologic Effect

Correlation between radiopharmaceutical binding and a specific physiologic response becomes an essential criterion to validate the specificity of the chosen agent. Differentiation of an agent that demonstrates saturable and displaceable binding to a nonspecific binding site from an agent that binds to the protein site of interest becomes extremely difficult without this criterion.[5]

Resistance to Metabolism

Endogenous neurotransmitters are typically inactivated quickly through degradation by endogenous enzymes. Generally it is preferable that imaging radiopharmaceuticals show minimal metabolic degradation to simplify the interpretation of measured radionuclide concentrations. However, when the radiolabeled metabolites do not accumulate in the target organ to appreciable levels, successful imaging studies can still be performed. In some instances, metabolism of imaging radiopharmaceuticals is used to help delineate biologic processes of interest.

Pharmacokinetics

To be successfully used as an imaging agent, the kinetic properties of tracer uptake and washout must be rate limited by interaction with the specific protein site of interest. Many promising radiopharmaceuticals fail to meet expectations because the interaction of the tracer with a specific protein site is so rapid that blood flow or tracer delivery becomes the dominant rate-limiting step in the tracer kinetics. Unfortunately, low-affinity radiopharmaceuticals also fail because the specificity of tracer accumulation is inadequate to isolate the specific interaction between the tracer and the protein site. Hence, tracers must be identified with sufficiently high affinities to overcome the specificity limitations, but affinities must not be so high that the kinetics of tracer uptake and washout become rate limited by blood flow.

Toxicity

Agonists or antagonists used as imaging agents must not be toxic at the low levels typically administered for imaging studies.

Development of Radiopharmaceuticals

Radiopharmaceuticals that meet most or all of these characteristics have been successfully developed for in vivo imaging of the cardiac ANS. At present, more success has been achieved in the development of radiopharmaceuticals for assessing presynaptic function of the adrenergic system than for the postsynaptic sites. The compounds that have been evaluated include radiolabeled forms of the endogenous neurotransmitters, or closely related derivatives, and a class of compounds called *false neurotransmitters*. Compounds that have been developed and evaluated as probes of presynaptic function in sympathetic neurons include ^{123}I-metaiodobenzylguanidine (MIBG),[26-29] ^{11}C-m-hydroxyephedrine (HED),[30-32] ^{18}F-metaraminol,[33,34] ^{18}F-fluorodopamine,[35,36] ^{18}F-fluoronorepinephrine,[37] ^{11}C-phenylephrine,[38,39] [11C]-(-)-α-α-dideutero-phyneylephrine, ^{18}F-fluorobenzylguanidine,[40] ^{18}F-para-fluorobenzylguanidine, 4-[18F]-fluoro-3-iodobenzylguanidine and ^{76}Br-bromobenzylguanidine,[41] ^{11}C-epinephrine, ^{11}C-norepinephrine, ^{11}C-nitromethane, ^{11}C-dopamine, ^{11}C-metariminol, and more recently ^{11}C-labeled phenethylguanidine analogues.[42]

Of these compounds, MIBG, HED, fluorodopamine, and epinephrine have been used in human trials. All four of these radiopharmaceuticals produce excellent high-contrast images of the myocardium.[28,31,42] The commercial availability of [^{123}I]MIBG in Japan and Europe, and to a lesser extent of [^{121}I]MIBG in the United States, has led to a large number of studies of the application of MIBG in cardiac imaging.[85] The efforts devoted to developing presynaptic markers of the parasympathetic system have not resulted in any agents that have been successfully validated and translated into trials in human subjects. Animal studies using radiolabeled forms of vesamicol and benzovesamicol show some potential for imaging this system.[43-47]

The lack of success in developing the presynaptic parasympathetic markers is due in part to the very high selectivity and metabolic steps involved in the transport of choline, metabolism to acetylcholine, and vesicular storage.[5] In addition, the sparse parasympathetic innervation of the left ventricle is difficult to differentiate from the proportionately large nonspecific accumulation of these tracers.

The development of compounds for postsynaptic receptor sites has been focused primarily on antagonists, which tend to exhibit higher binding affinities than observed for agonists. Compounds that have been developed and tested for PET imaging include ^{11}C- and ^{18}F-labeled forms of practolol,[48] propanolol,[49] fluorocarazolol,[50,51] ^{11}C-CGP 12177,[52,53] ^{11}C-CGP 12388[54] and ^{11}C-GB67.[55] More recently, efforts have been devoted to the synthesis of ^{123}I-labeled β-adrenergic receptor antagonist.[56] Unfortunately, the ^{123}I-labeled compounds have yet to meet a sufficient number of the criteria to be moved into preclinical trials. Of the PET compounds, only ^{11}C-CGP 12177 has been used routinely in human studies. Several radiolabeled antagonists have also been developed to study the muscarinic cholinergic receptor sites of the parasympathetic system.[5] The only agent used routinely in human studies is the hydrophilic ligand ^{11}C-*N*-methyl quinuclidinylbenzylate (MQNB).[57,58]

Principles of Tomographic Imaging

Current state-of-the-art nuclear medicine imaging techniques enable the noninvasive assessment of the function and distribution of the cardiac ANS by measuring the temporal characteristics of regional radiopharmaceutical concentrations using single photon emission tomographic (SPECT) and PET imaging techniques. Each of these techniques produces three-dimensional images of radionuclide distribution in the heart based on a series of projection images of the body. In SPECT imaging, projection images of gamma-ray–emitting radionuclides are typically formed using conventional collimated gamma cameras to define individual ray-sums that form the projection image (Fig. 37-3). The gamma camera is rotated around the patient to acquire projection images through angles of either 180 or 360 degrees, enabling the mathematical reconstruction of tomographic or cross-sectional images of the body (see Fig. 37-3). Modern SPECT systems employ unique geometrical designs that enable simultaneous measurement of multiple projections to minimize data acquisition times.

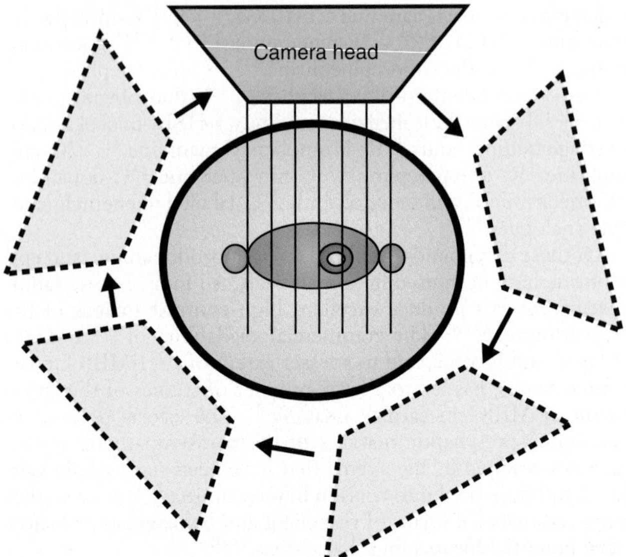

Figure 37-3 Geometry of SPECT imaging systems. Gamma camera imaging systems are rotated around the subject, acquiring a series of projection images. The data from the individual projection images are used to generate tomographic slices of the body.

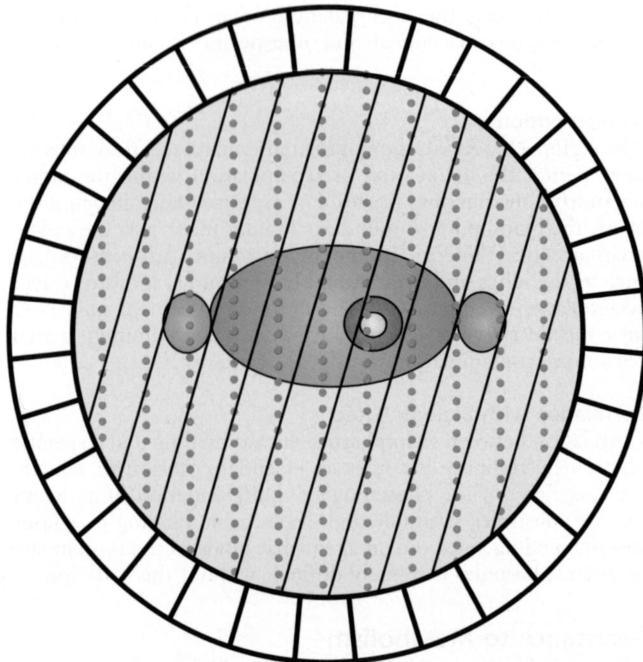

Figure 37-5 Geometry of PET imaging systems. Rings of detectors are used to detect coincident photons from positron-electron annihilations. Electronic collimation in these systems enable the simultaneous acquisition of all projection data sets needed to reconstruct the tomographic images.

In PET-based techniques, electronic collimation is achieved as a result of the physical characteristics of the pair of 511-keV photons formed in the process of positron-electron annihilation (Fig. 37-4). When a positron-emitting radionuclide decays, a proton within the nucleus is converted to a neutron, and the excess positive charge is emitted as a positron (a particle with the same rest mass and spin as an electron, but with a positive rather than a negative charge). Positron-emitting radionuclides emit positrons with a continuous distribution of energies that cover a range up to a maximum end-point energy. This end-point energy is characteristic of each radionuclide and determines the average distance the positrons travel in tissue. The positrons typically travel through distances up to several millimeters in tissue, losing energy through electrostatic interactions with the electrons and protons associated with the chemical composition of the tissue. As the positrons lose energy, the probability that they will combine with an electron increases, and a hydrogen-like entity called positronium (positron-electron pair) is formed.

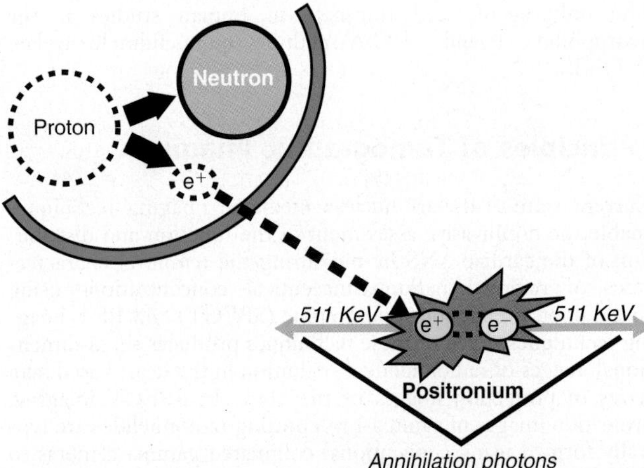

Figure 37-4 Positron-emitting radionuclide decay process. Positron-emitting radionuclides are unstable due to excess positive charge in the nucleus (i.e., the proton/neutron mix is not balanced). One mode of decay for these radionuclides is the conversion of a proton into a neutron with the emission of the positive charge as a positron (e^+). The positron will combine with an electron, forming positronium. Positronium quickly annihilates, and the mass of the particles is converted into energy in the form of two 180-degree opposed 511 KeV photons.

Positronium is very unstable and decays within tens of nanoseconds through a process called *annihilation* (complete conversion of mass into energy). In positronium annihilation, conservation of energy and momentum dictates that two 511-keV photons are emitted in directions 180 degrees opposed. In PET, the projection images are formed using rings of detectors that surround the subject, and the individual ray-sums are formed electronically though the simultaneous or coincident detection of both photons (Fig. 37-5). A unique advantage of PET is the capability to simultaneously measure all projection angles, without the use of lead collimators, which are required to calculate tomographic images. Through the development of techniques to estimate the distribution of photons scattered or absorbed in the tissue, SPECT and PET imaging enables the noninvasive generation of quantitative images of radionuclide concentrations in tissue.

Quantification of Autonomic Nervous System Function

Isolation of interactions between specific radiopharmaceutical and protein sites for identification of protein densities and

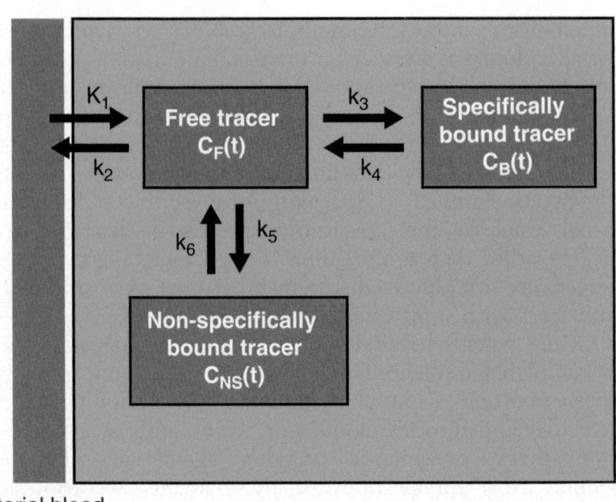

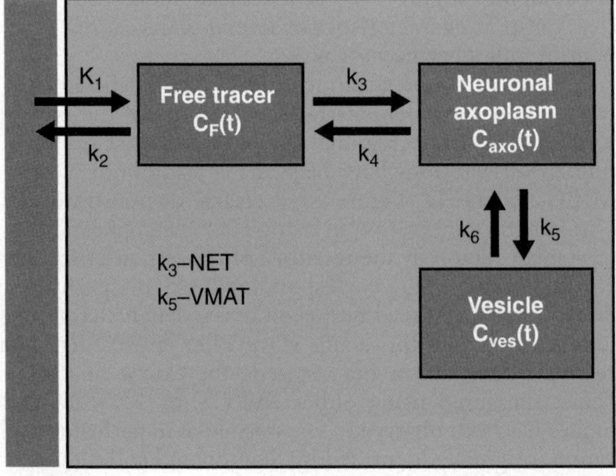

Figure 37-6 General compartmental models used in neurocardiac imaging applications. **A,** Three-tissue compartment model used to assess neuroreceptor site expression and distribution. These compartments represent the free unbound tracer in the tissue, the tracer that has bound specifically to the protein site of interest, and the tracer that is bound to nonspecific sites. The rate constants k_1 to k_6 are used to describe the transfer of tracer between each compartment. The rate constant k_3 is referred to as the binding potential for receptor studies and is proportional to the product of the association rate constant for the ligand binding to the receptor site and the number of available receptor sites. **B,** Three-tissue compartment model used to assess neurotransmitter uptake and release from the presynaptic side of cardiac neurons. In this model, k_3 represents the norepinephrine transporter (NET) and k_5 represents the vesicular monoamine transporter (MVAT). These models are often simplified in practice. $C_{axo}(t)$, neuronal axoplasm tracer concentration; $C_B(t)$, bound tracer concentration; $C_F(t)$ free tracer concentration; $C_{NS}(t)$, non-specifically bound tracer concentration; $C_{ves}(t)$, vesicle tracer concentration.

binding affinities, or the functional assessment of the neurotransmission system, requires the use of mathematical models.[59-61,156] Approaches that have been used to isolate these interactions include the assessment of the level of accumulation of the tracer in tissue at a specified point in time after administration (often referred to as *tracer retention* or *retention fraction*) and fitting parameterized models describing radiopharmaceutical kinetics, isolating the parameters that represent the

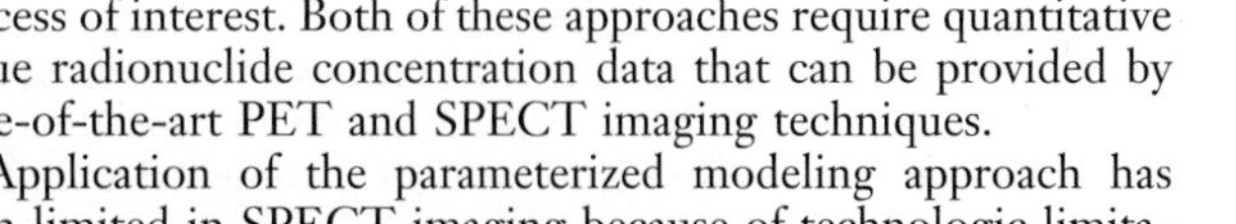

process of interest. Both of these approaches require quantitative tissue radionuclide concentration data that can be provided by state-of-the-art PET and SPECT imaging techniques.

Application of the parameterized modeling approach has been limited in SPECT imaging because of technologic limitations prohibiting the measurement of rapidly changing radionuclide concentrations in tissue in many SPECT systems. The two general classes of parameterized models used to analyze kinetics measured in PET studies are compartmental models[62] and distributed models.[63-65] Distributed models describe the kinetics of the radiopharmaceutical in terms of a series of linear or nonlinear processes. Typically, the distributed models consist of a large number of parameters that are often difficult to estimate reliably because of the high level of statistical noise in the temporal data series measured with tomographic systems. To overcome these limitations, the models often are simplified to represent a small number of tracer compartments, with linear first-order kinetics describing the transfer of tracer between the compartments.

General compartmental models typical of those used in neurocardiac imaging are shown in Figure 37-6.[60,66-69,42] These models consist of one compartment representing the tracer concentration in the blood being delivered to the tissue ($C_A[t]$) and several compartments representing localization of the tracer within the tissue. $C_F(t)$ is free tracer in the tissue extracellular space, $C_B(t)$ is tracer bound to a protein site, $C_{axo}(t)$ is tracer in the neuronal axoplasm, $C_{ves}(t)$ is tracer in the vesicles, and $C_{NS}(t)$ is a compartment to describe the nonspecifically bound tracer concentration. The equations describing these models are fit to regional tissue radionuclide concentration versus time curves to identify specific parameters of interest. In the general model for neuroreceptor imaging shown in Figure 37-6, the parameter k_3 is the product of the tracer affinity for the receptor site and the concentration of free receptor sites in the tissue. This parameter is often referred to as the *binding potential* in receptor imaging studies.[67,68] In situations where the binding potential does not provide sufficient information, the tracer affinity and receptor site concentrations can be isolated using multiple tracer injections under varying levels of receptor occupancy in a fashion that is conceptually analogous to a Scatchard plot analysis.[58]

Experimental and Clinical Observations

Presynaptic Radiotracer Studies

Radiopharmaceuticals used to study the cardiac ANS have been based primarily on radiolabeled analogues of the false neurotransmitter guanethidine. Initially, bretylium and guanethidine were shown selectively to interfere with the function of adrenergic neurons.[26] Based on these observations, medicinal chemists developed related compounds with even higher potencies for adrenergic system interactions. This in turn led to development of radioiodinated forms of substituted aralkylguanidines for human imaging studies.[27-29] These compounds share the same transport, storage, and release mechanisms used by norepinephrine. However, these compounds have a dramatically diminished ability to stimulate postsynaptic responses through receptor-mediated interactions, and hence they have been categorized as false neurotransmitters. The most common radiopharmaceutical used for imaging applications from this class of compounds is MIBG with radioiodine incorporated into the phenyl ring.[29] This compound has been used in both planar nuclear medicine and SPECT imaging studies.

Numerous studies have been performed to validate the capability of MIBG to map the function and distribution of the presynaptic sympathetic neurons. These studies include the comparison of MIBG and endogenous catecholamine biodistribution,[29,70-73] pharmacologic blocking studies of the cellular and vesicular uptake mechanisms to demonstrate the specificity of tracer uptake,[70,71,74-77] studies following experimental and pharmacologic sympathectomies,[76,78,79] studies of tracer turnover rates as a function of sympathetic tone,[76,80,81] correlation of regional uptake abnormalities with alterations in cardiac electrophysiology,[82-84] and studies in experimental models of cardiac disease.[80,83-92] Collectively, these validation studies demonstrate that the uptake and retention of MIBG closely parallels regional norepinephrine levels throughout the left ventricle after the administration of pharmacologic blocking agents and after chemical or surgical sympathetic denervation. However, subtle differences between the behavior of MIBG and norepinephrine exist, and the mechanisms responsible for these differences have yet to be elucidated.[4] Nonetheless, the similarities between MIBG and norepinephrine outweigh the differences, and MIBG has been reliably used noninvasively to image the integrity and function of the presynaptic sympathetic nervous system in vivo.

Other false neurotransmitters have been labeled with positron-emitting radionuclides for use in PET imaging studies. The first PET radioligand developed from the false neurotransmitter class of compounds was 6-^{18}F-fluorometaraminol.[33,34] This tracer exhibited excellent imaging characteristics in preliminary animal studies, demonstrating pharmacokinetic properties that enabled the differentiation of specific neuronal tracer transport rates from other physiologic processes such as blood flow. Unfortunately, the synthetic approach used to make 6-^{18}F-fluorometaraminol resulted in a relatively large mass of unlabeled fluorometaraminol that was too close to pharmacologically active levels to be used safely in human applications.

This limitation led to the investigation of N-methyl sympathomimetic amines and the synthesis of metahydroxyephedrine (HED) labeled with carbon-11.[30,31] The specific activity of HED ranged from 500 to 2000 Ci/mmol and was suitable for use in human subjects. Unfortunately, HED did not exhibit the ideal characteristics observed with fluorometaraminol. Studies examining the metabolism of HED in guinea pigs demonstrate that only unmetabolized HED accumulates in myocardial tissue. However, two metabolites (α-methylepinephrine and the 3-*O*-methyl derivative of α-methylepinephrine) were observed in the blood.[31]

Accumulation of HED in presynaptic sympathetic neurons has also been shown to be less dependent on the vesicular storage system than storage of norepinephrine.[32] Two specific studies demonstrate this behavior. In the first study, it was shown that pretreatment of the heart with reserpine (a vesicular uptake inhibitor) reduced the accumulation of HED only by 50% compared with control. In the second study, the administration of desipramine after the accumulation of HED in sympathetic neurons significantly increased the washout rate of HED from the tissue. These studies suggest that HED accumulation in myocardial tissue is driven primarily by an intact uptake-1 mechanism. Because HED is resistant to metabolism by mitochondrial monoamine oxidase, it can remain in the cytoplasm of the cell undisrupted, unlike norepinephrine. These studies also demonstrate that release of HED from presynaptic sympathetic nerve terminals occurs, at least in part, independently from the rate of catecholamine release associated with sympathetic tone. Even given these limitations, HED has been successfully used to image sympathetic denervation and dysfunction associated with cardiac disease.

Two compounds related to HED have more recently been investigated: [^{11}C]epinephrine and [^{11}C]phenylephrine. HED cycles in and out of neurons, but [^{11}C]epinephrine is rapidly sequestered within neuronal vesicles, resulting in a slowed metabolism into [^{11}C]methylamine.[85,86] [^{11}C]Phenylephrine was developed as a tracer for neuronal monoamine oxidase activity.[143] Studies of clearance of [^{11}C]phenylephrine indicate that [^{11}C]phenylephrine is also quickly stored in vesicles but that it subsequently leaks in to the neuronal cytoplasm where it is metabolized by monoamine oxidase and released as [^{11}C]methylamine.[85] The leaking of these tracers from the neuronal vesicles is the rate-limiting process in clearance from the heart, rather than monoamine oxidase metabolism. Thus these tracers are not able to distinguish between areas of denervation and areas with suppressed vesicular function.

More recently, Raffel and colleagues have developed a series of radiolabeled phenethylguanidines for imaging cardiac sympathetic neurons.[42] The phenethylguanidine radiopharmaceuticals were developed to overcome a principal limitation shared by the sympathetic presynaptic imaging agents described earlier, namely, the uptake rates of these agents are too rapid to enable reliable compartmental modeling that can differentiate the transport rates of the norepinephrine transporter and the vesicular monoamine transporter from tracer delivery via blood flow. These tracers are still in the very early stages of evaluation, but results from small-animal PET imaging studies are very encouraging. Figure 37-7 schematically demonstrates the relative transport characteristics of several of the cardiac sympathetic neuron radiopharmaceuticals.

Studies of the presynaptic uptake of radiolabeled false neurotransmitters have demonstrated the ability of these compounds to clearly delineate regional sympathetic denervation.[73,78,87-102] Similar observations have been made using both radioiodinated MIBG and HED. Figure 37-8 clearly demonstrates a zone of sympathetic denervation in a dog after the application of phenol to a small region in the territory of the left anterior descending coronary artery. The corresponding ammonia perfusion images demonstrate preserved perfusion in the denervated region of the left ventricle. In the acute stage after myocardial infarction, regional denervation that exceeds the extent of the perfusion defect measured using either SPECT or PET imaging techniques has been observed. The mismatch in perfusion and innervation, originally identified by Stanton and colleagues,[103] is well demonstrated in Figure 37-9.

Both MIBG and HED imaging techniques have shown evidence of recovery or partial reinnervation of the sympathetic system. In studies of patients in the chronic stage after myocardial infarction, paired MIBG-perfusion SPECT studies have shown partial reinnervation and enhanced catecholamine

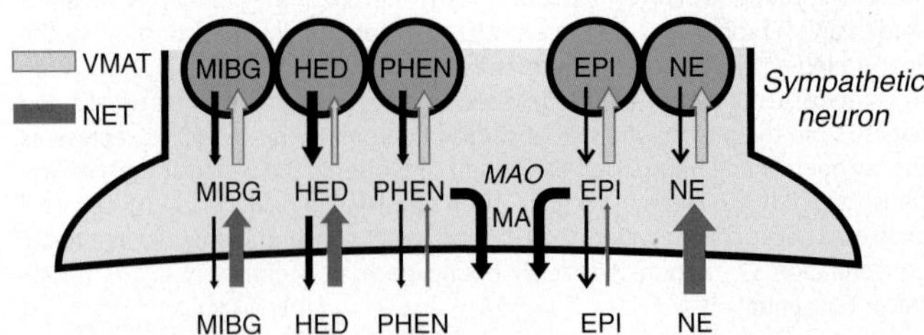

Figure 37-7 Relative magnitude of sympathetic presynaptic radiopharmaceutical transport rates. The thickness of the *arrows* approximately represent the magnitude of the transport rates for several tracers. The *red arrows* in the figure represent transport by the norepinephrine transporter (NET) and the *green arrows* represent transport by the vesicular monoamine transporter (MVAT). EPI, epinephrine; HED, ^{11}C-m-hydroxyephedrine; MAO, monoamine oxidase; MA, methylamine; MIBG, ^{123}I-metaiodobenzylguanidine; NE, norepinephrine; PHEN, phenylephrine. (Adapted from Raffel DM, Wieland DM: Assessment of cardiac sympathetic nerve integrity with positron emission tomography. Nucl Med Biol 28:541-559, 2001, figure 6, with permission from Elsevier.)

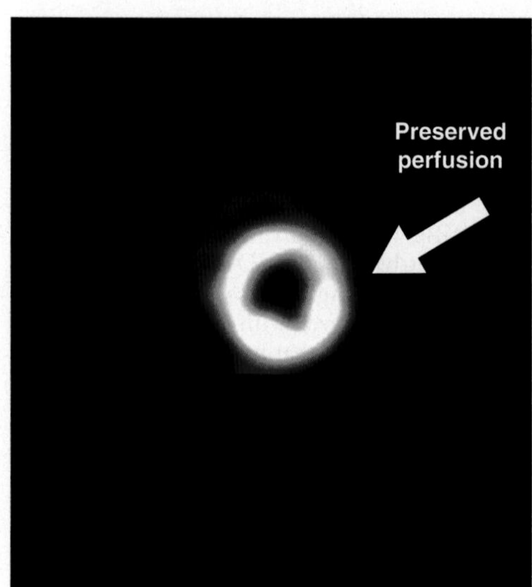

Figure 37-8 Sympathetic denervation in a dog. The images show a midventricle short axis view of ^{13}N-ammonia ($^{13}N-NH_3$) (perfusion) and ^{11}C-m-hydroxyephedrine (^{11}C-HED) (sympathetic innervation) in a dog following regional sympathetic denervation using phenol.

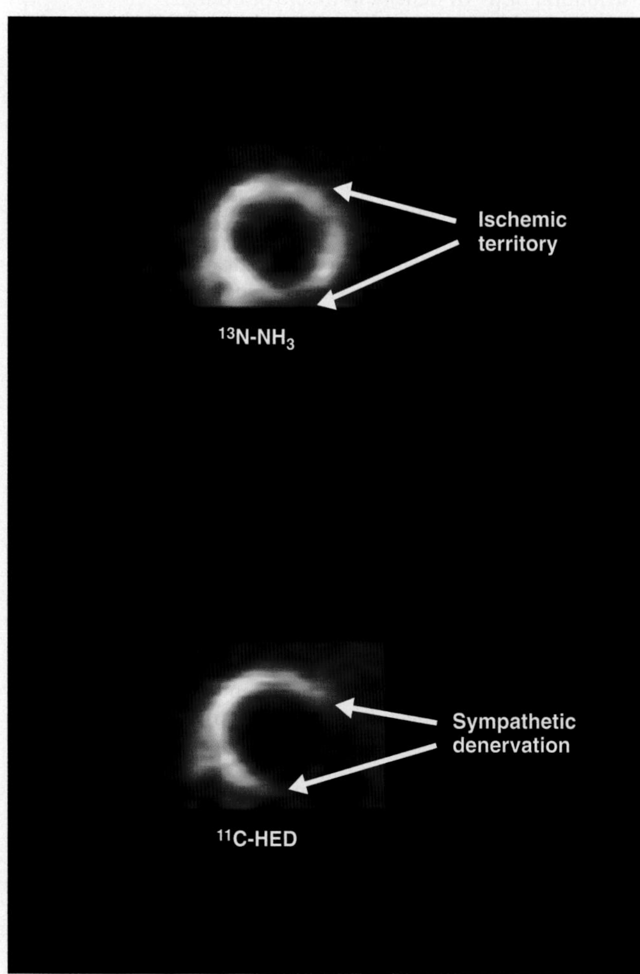

Figure 37-9 Sympathetic denervation in a human subject with coronary artery disease. The images show myocardial perfusion *(top)* and sympathetic innervation *(bottom)*. The lateral wall of the left ventricle shows a relatively large area with a mild reduction in perfusion. The corresponding HED image demonstrates that the function of the sympathetic system is impaired in the region of the left ventricle. ^{11}C-HED, ^{11}C-m-hydroxyephedrine; $^{13}N-NH_3$, ^{13}N-ammonia.

uptake in the period 2 to 6 months after myocardial infarction.[103-121] Interestingly, the time frame of sympathetic system recovery or reinnervation is consistent with the time frame for heightened risk of lethal arrhythmias after myocardial infarction.[113] A small number of studies provide some evidence to suggest that the sympathetic system dysfunction is located in peri-infarct regions of the left ventricle that are ischemic. Terada and colleagues[118] observed that studies performed under exercise converted mismatched myocardial segments at rest into matched perfusion-MIBG uptake defects with exercise. Although exercise did not produce this effect in all patients, these studies still permit the hypothesis that the ischemic thresholds for sympathetic neurons and cardiomyocytes differ.

A number of studies have been performed to evaluate the function of the sympathetic nervous system in heart failure. Studies have been performed in patients with ischemic and idiopathic cardiomyopathy,[122-127] left and right ventricular hypertrophy,[128] diabetic neuropathy,[129,130] and chemotherapeutic cardiotoxicity.[131,132] Across this heterogeneous population of patients, consistent patterns of normal or only slightly reduced levels of MIBG uptake were observed, followed by significantly increased rates of MIBG washout from the tissue. Similar observations were also obtained using PET studies of HED uptake and washout in patients with cardiomyopathy suffering from heart failure.[133]

Transection of the cardiac nerves associated with removing the heart for transplantation results in global denervation. In studies of cardiac transplant recipients, partial reinnervation as assessed by both MIBG and HED imaging of the left ventricle is observed after much longer periods than were required for recovery of catecholamine uptake in patients with myocardial infarction. Imaging studies performed shortly after cardiac transplantation showed dramatically reduced levels of MIBG and HED accumulation in myocardial tissue.[78,97-100] Increased regional uptake of MIBG and HED was observed in the period from 13 to 24 months after transplantation. In both of these studies, the pattern of reinnervation was confined to the anterior and basal segments of the left ventricle.[99,100] It has been shown by DiCarli and coworkers[133] that the zones of reinnervation in the cardiac transplant recipients are functional and produce increased regional myocardial perfusion during cold pressor testing. Bengel and coworkers[134,135] have shown with

HED that the reinnervation process progresses slowly and even after 15 years following transplant surgery the process has not restored the innervation back to the level observed in a healthy heart. Bengel and coworkers have also demonstrated that several additional factors including duration of surgery, donor and recipient age, and frequency of rejection impact the reinervation observed with HED imaging.

Several studies have also been performed to examine the relationship between electrophysiologic abnormalities in patients and their patterns of sympathetic innervation. In studies performed in heterogeneous populations of patients with electrophysiologic abnormalities, consistently heterogeneous patterns of MIBG accumulation were observed. These patient populations included subjects with long QT syndrome, ventricular tachycardia in structurally normal hearts, cardiomyopathy, left ventricular hypertrophy, valvular disease, right ventricular disease, and myocardial infarction.[4] When evaluating this heterogeneous population of patients, it becomes evident that in subjects who have a region of sympathetic denervation with apparently preserved perfusion, the propensity for electrophysiologic abnormalities is increased. It is also apparent that as the regions of mismatch between sympathetic innervation and perfusion increase, the likelihood that the patient will experience electrophysiologic abnormalities is increased.

MIBG SPECT imaging studies of patients with ischemic cardiomyopathies and of patients with idiopathic cardiomyopathies have been performed to determine the prognostic value of MIBG imaging relative to clinical cardiac function indices (New York Heart Association function class, LV dimension at end-diastole and end-systole, LV ejection fraction).[136] Of the cardiac function and quantitative imaging indices considered, suppressed [^{123}I]MIBG activity (heart-to-mediastinum ratio) was found to be the most powerful long-term predictor of cardiac death for both groups. Assessment of MIBG activity and of cardiac function is more likely to identify increased risk in both groups. Kinetics was evaluated by measuring relative change between early and late MIBG activity. Patients who had idiopathic cardiomyopathies and who died from cardiac conditions had a significantly greater washout rate than those who survived. No difference in washout rate was observed between surviving ischemic patients and those who died.

Another study[137] investigated the level of cardiac adrenergic innervation in patients in the very early stage of coronary artery disease. SPECT studies, MIBG for innervation and [^{99m}Tc]sestamibi (MIBI) for perfusion, and quantitative coronary angiography were performed in 30 asymptomatic volunteers with high familial risk of coronary artery disease. In each case, the degree of stenosis was considered not hemodynamically significant. MIBI uptake was not correlated with degree of stenosis. Degree of stenosis in the LAD was significantly correlated with late MIBG activity and anticorrelated with MIBG washout rate. This suggests that even very mild coronary artery disease affects myocardial adrenergic function before any ischemia or denervation occurs.

PET HED imaging has been used to examine the diabetic heart. These studies have shown reduced HED uptake in the apical, inferior, and lateral walls in patients who have diabetic neuropathy[138] and that the severity of the HED reduction depended on the neuropathic severity.[139]

The studies of presynaptic innervation previously described have shown that cardiac neuroimaging can play a valuable prognostic role. A logical subsequent question is what is the capability of cardiac neuroimaging to assess the effectiveness of treatment strategies to restore neuronal function in disease. A study has been carried out to see if abnormal cardiac presynaptic innervation is reversible by exercise and if it is accompanied by changes in functional measures.[140] Baseline PET images were acquired with [^{11}C]HED, $C^{15}O$ and $H_2{}^{15}O$. The scans were repeated following a 6-month exercise training period. Mean myocardial blood flow (MBF) was calculated from the $C^{15}O$ and $H_2{}^{15}O$ images and a single compartment model. Mean HED retention indices were calculated from the [^{11}C]HED images. Mean blood flow values were used to arrive at blood flow-corrected HED retention values. The exercise training did not affect global MBF, but it did cause increases in areas with locally reduced flow at baseline. HED retention increased significantly with exercise training. These improvements in image-derived measures correlates well with functional measures of the autonomic system, indicating that imaging of presynaptic innervation may be useful as a tool to monitor and possibly individualize therapy for patients with chronic heart failure.

The role of PET imaging in the study of myocardial β-adrenoceptor receptors has been summarized by de Jong and colleagues.[141] In the half century since the existence of the β-adrenoceptor (β-AR) was first postulated, much has been learned about the role it plays in the regulation of cardiac function. Changes in β-AR density are associated with a number of cardiac diseases, but clinical investigations have been hampered by the lack of a noninvasive, in vivo measurement technique. Graphical methods and kinetic modeling of PET imaging data with β-AR tracers might provide a noninvasive method for measuring the spatial distribution of β-AR density in the myocardium.

Several β-blockers have been labeled with PET isotopes, but many of them do not meet the requirements enumerated. The radioligand [^{11}C]CGP 12177 has been successfully used for PET studies, but its usefulness is limited by the difficulty of synthesizing it. Clinical studies of β-AR density have been carried out only at two centers.

The radiologand [^{11}C]CCP 12388 has been synthesized using a simpler method. The lack of β subtype specificity limits remains a limitation of both CGP-12177 and CGP-12388. Tracers with subtype selectivity for the β_1 and β_2 receptors are being investigated, but successful subtype-selective ligands are yet to be developed. As ligands are developed and synthesized at multiple centers, the role of PET will increase, both in pathophysiologic research and in the clinical management in patients.

Postsynaptic Radiotracer Studies

Radiopharmaceuticals that have been developed for the in vivo study of cardiac receptors have predominantly been antagonists of either β-adrenergic or muscarinic acetylcholine receptors. Although they have similar structures, these compounds differ in their affinity for the receptor sites, lipophilicity, and subtype selectivity.[5] To date, the only compounds that meet most of the criteria for imaging ligand–protein site interactions and that have been used routinely in human studies are ^{11}C-CGP 12177[25,142,143] for the β-adrenergic receptors and ^{11}C-MQNB for the muscarinic acetylcholine receptors.[58] Imaging the β-adrenergic receptors using SPECT techniques has been limited by the availability of radiopharmaceuticals that meet the specific criteria for good imaging agents. Radiolabeled forms of the β-adrenergic antagonists pindolol[144] and iodocyanopindolol[145] have been evaluated as imaging agents. Unfortunately, these compounds have either high levels of nonspecific binding (pindolol) or demonstrate significant pulmonary uptake (iodocyanopindolol), limiting the utility of both as SPECT imaging agents.

More promising results have been obtained using the β-adrenergic antagonists CGP 12177 labeled with carbon-11 and imaged with PET techniques.[25,142] CGP has been shown to have low levels of nonspecific binding, has met the criteria defined earlier for an imaging agent, and has been validated as a tracer for measuring β-adrenergic receptor densities in vivo. ^{11}C-CGP 12177 is a potent β-blocker with a high affinity for the receptor site and low levels of nonspecific binding or accumulation in the tissue. Validation of the specificity of ^{11}C-CGP 12177 for β-adrenergic sites has been demonstrated using displacement and blocking studies. In addition, a correlation was observed between the decreases in heart rate and the level of displacement achieved through competition at the receptor site, demonstrating a biologic effect coinciding with the displacement of the compound.[57,146,147]

In subsequent studies, validation of the use of ^{11}C-CGP 12177 for the quantitative measurement of receptor densities in both animals and humans has been demonstrated by comparing in vivo measurements with biopsy samples assayed using in vitro binding assay techniques.[59,148] Clinical PET imaging studies with ^{11}C-CGP 12177 have shown diffuse reductions in myocardial β-adrenergic receptors in patients with primary hypertrophic cardiomyopathy and elevated plasma catecholamine levels.[149]

N-Methyl quinuclidinylbenzylate demonstrates most of the criteria required for an imaging agent to assess receptor densities quantitatively in vivo.[58] It is a potent hydrophilic antagonist that displays a high affinity for muscarinic cholinergic receptors. The kinetic characteristics of MQNB are well suited for imaging studies, with minimal lung uptake and rapid blood pool clearance creating good contrast between myocardial tissue and background sources of radiotracer contamination. In displacement studies, the antagonist AF-DX 116 displaced 25% of MQNB in myocardial tissue, whereas no displacement was observed after pirenzepine administration.[5] Atropine administration after bolus administration displaced approximately 94% of the accumulated MQNB in dog studies, demonstrating low levels of nonspecific binding of MQNB in the myocardium.[57] Stereospecificity was also demonstrated. It was shown that dexetimide but not levetimide can displace MQNB from its binding sites.[57] Physiologic studies have also shown that MQNB binding in the septum of the human left ventricle appears to be inversely related to heart rate during the study.[150]

These observations support the hypothesis that muscarinic cholinergic receptors can exist in two active states: a high-affinity agonist–low-affinity antagonist state and a low-affinity agonist–high-affinity antagonist state.[151] With increased parasympathetic tone, binding of the endogenous neurotransmitter to a high-affinity agonist state converts the receptor site to a low-affinity agonist–high-affinity antagonist state, increasing the accumulation of MQNB in the tissue. Although parasympathetic tone was not directly measured in these studies, the results suggest that MQNB imaging might allow the identification of the physiologically active conformation of the muscarinic receptor. Using mathematical models similar to those used for quantification of β-adrenergic receptor densities, it has also been shown that the kinetic characteristics of MQNB permit the quantification of muscarinic receptor densities in vivo.[152]

To date, the in vivo assessment of muscarinic cholinergic receptor density and affinity using MQNB and PET imaging have not documented any changes except in a recent study of patients with increased receptor density in idiopathic dilated cardiomyopathy.[153] Careful study of ANS denervation in animal models and human transplant recipients also did not show any changes in either density or affinity of the muscarinic receptors.[154] As a result, the value of in vivo imaging of muscarinic receptor density in the left ventricle is unclear at present.

Additional Reading

Several review articles on the subject of cardiac neuroimaging have been published. Raffel and Wieland review the assessment of sympathetic innervation with PET.[85] Carrió presents a review with more detail on applications of SPECT.[155] DeGrado and colleagues have published a review of tracer kinetic modeling as applied to nuclear cardiology.[156] More recent reviews of PET and SPECT cardiac neuroimaging by Lautamaki and colleagues[157] and Yamashina and Yamazaki[158] delineate applications in patient populations.

Conclusion

PET and SPECT imaging techniques are the only noninvasive methods available for visualizing presynaptic and postsynaptic aspects of the ANS. Although the optimal radiopharmaceuticals for completely characterizing the ANS have not yet been fully developed and validated, the utility of these methods as a research tool to study the function of the ANS in the development of arrhythmias and sudden cardiac death is clear. To obtain a precise understanding of the relationship between the distribution and volume of ANS denervation and function, a complete assessment of both presynaptic and postsynaptic function for the sympathetic and parasympathetic systems will be necessary. At present, the clinical application of these imaging techniques is unclear. When the physiologic substrates responsible for electrophysiologic abnormalities in patients with cardiac disease are more clearly understood, the role of these noninvasive in vivo imaging techniques in aiding in the diagnosis and therapy of patients will be better delineated. Nonetheless, it is clear that neurocardiac imaging represents an important component of the arsenal of methodologies available to evaluate and understand the function of the ANS.

References

1. Goldstein DS: Plasma norepinephrine as an indicator of sympathetic neural activity. Am J Cardiol 48:1147-1154, 1981.
2. Schwaiger M, Allman K, Hutchins G, et al: Neurocardiology: Is there a future for imaging? In Zarat B (ed): Nuclear Cardiology: State of the Art and Future Directions, 1st ed. St. Louis, Mosby–Year Book, 1993, pp 314-322.
3. Goldstein DS, Brush JE Jr, Eisenhofer G, et al: In vivo measurement of neuronal uptake of norepinephrine in the human heart. Circulation 78:41-48, 1988.
4. Hutchins GD, Zipes D: Imaging the cardiac autonomic nervous system. In Skorton DJ, Schelbert HR, Wolf GL, et al (eds): Marcus Cardiac Imaging: A Companion to Braunwald's Heart Disease. Philadelphia, WB Saunders, 1996, pp 1052-1061.
5. Syrota A: Positron emission tomography: Evaluation of cardiac receptors and neuronal function. In Skorton DJ, Schelbert HR, Wolf GL, et al (eds): Marcus Cardiac Imaging: A Companion to Braunwald's Heart Disease. Philadelphia, WB Saunders, 1996, pp 1186-1203.
6. Rossi L: Neuroanatomopathology of the cardiovascular system. In Kulbertus HE, Franck G (eds): Neurocardiology. Mt. Kisco, NY, Futura, 1988, pp 22-55.
7. Levy MN: Sympathetic-parasympathetic interactions in the heart. In Kulbertus HE, Franck G (eds): Neurocardiology, Mt. Kisco, NY, Futura, 1988, pp 85-98.
8. Randell WC, Ardell JL: Functional anatomy of the cardiac efferent innervation. In Kulbertus HE, Franck G (eds): Neurocar-diology, Mt. Kisco, NY, Futura, 1988, pp 3-24.
9. Zipes D: Autonomic modulation and cardiac arrhythmias. In Zipes D, Jalife J (eds): Cardiac Electrophysiology: From Cell to Bedside, 2nd ed. Philadelphia, WB Saunders, 1995, p 1612.
10. Lathers CM, Levin RM, Spivey WH: Regional distribution of myocardial beta-adrenoceptors in the cat. Eur J Pharmacol 130:111-117, 1986.

11. Wei J-W, Sulakhe PV: Regional and subcellular distribution of beta- and alpha-adrenergic receptors in the myocardium of different species. Gen Pharmacol 10:263-267, 1979.
12. Murphree SS, Saftitz JE: Distribution of adrenergic receptors in failing human heart: Implications for mechanisms of down regulation. Circulation 79:1214-1225, 1989.
13. Schmid PG, Greif BJ, Lund DD, Roskoski R Jr: Regional choline acetyltransferase activity in the guinea pig heart. Circ Res 42:657-660, 1978.
14. Stanley R, Conaster J, Dettbarn WD: Acetylcholine, choline acetyltransferase and cholinesterases in the rat heart. Biochem Pharmacol 27:2409-2411, 1987.
15. Takahashi N, Barber MJ, Zipes D: Efferent vagal innervation of canine ventricle. Am Physiol Soc 246:H89-H97, 1985.
16. Manalan AS, Werth DK, Jones LR, et al: Enrichment, solubilization, and partial characterization of digitonin-solubilized muscarinic receptors derived from canine ventricular myocardium. Circ Res 52:664-676, 1983.
17. Elsinga PH, van Waarde A, Visser TJ, Vaalberg W: Visualization of β-adrenoceptors using PET. Clin Positron Imaging 1:81-94, 1998.
18. Laduron PM: Criteria for receptor sites in binding studies. Biochem Pharmacol 33:833-839, 1984.
19. Eckelman WC: The application of receptor theory to receptor-binding and enzyme binding oncologic pharmaceuticals. Nucl Med Biol 21:759-769, 1994.
20. Van Waarde A, Elsinga PH, Anthonio RL, et al: Study of cardiac receptor ligands by positron emission tomography. In van der Wall EE, Niemeyer MG, Paans AMJ (eds): Cardiac Positron Emission Tomography. Dordrecht, Kluwer Academic, 1995, pp 171-182.
21. Law MP: Demonstration of the suitability of CGP 12177 for in vivo studies of β-adrenoceptors. Br J Pharmacol 109:1101-1109, 1993.
22. Laduron PM: Stereospecificity in binding studies: A useful criterion though insufficient to prove the presence of receptors. Biochem Pharmacol 37:37-40, 1988.
23. Krawietz W, Erdmann E: Specific and unspecific binding of [3H](-)dihydroalprenolol to cardiac tissue. Biochem Pharmacol 28:1283-1288, 1979.
24. Gibson RE, Eckelman WC, Rzeszotarski WJ, et al: Radiotracer localization by receptor-ligand interactions. In C LG (ed): Principles of Radiopharmacology, vol 2. West Palm Beach, FL, CRC Press, 1979, pp 7-40.
25. Staehelin, M, Simons P, Jaeggi K, Wigger N: CGP-12177: A hydrophilic beta-adrenergic receptor radioligand reveals high affinity binding of agonists to intact cells. J Biol Chem 258:3496-3502, 1983.
26. Nickerson M, Collier B: Drugs inhibiting adrenergic nerves and structures innervated by them. In Gilman A, Goodman LS (eds): The Pharmacological Basis of Therapeutics, 5th ed. New York, Macmillan, 1975, pp 533-564.
27. Short JH, Darby DT: Sympathetic nervous system blocking agents: III. Derivatives of benzylguanidine. J Med Chem 10:833-840, 1967.
28. Wieland D, Swanson DP, Brown LE, Beierwaltes WH: Imaging the adrenal medulla with an I-131-labeled antiadrenergic agent. J Nucl Med 20:155-158, 1979.
29. Wieland DM, Brown LE, et al: Radiolabeled adrenergic neuron-blacking agents: Adrenomedullary imaging with [^{131}I]iodobenzylguanidine. J Nucl Med 21:349-353, 1980.
30. Van Dort ME, Gildersleeve DL, Wieland DM: Synthesis of ^{3}H-labeled sympathomimetic amines for neuronal mapping. J Label Compounds Radiopharmacol 28:831-840, 1990.
31. Rosenspire K, Haka MS, Van Dort ME, et al: Synthesis and preliminary evaluation of ^{11}C-meta-hydroxyephedrine: A false transmitter agent for neuronal imaging. J Nucl Med 31:1328-1334, 1990.
32. Wieland DM: Heart neuronal imaging with 11C- and fluorine-18-labeled tracers. In van der Wall EE, Righetti A, Sochor H, Niemeyer MG (eds): What's New in Cardiac Imaging? Amsterdam, Kluwer, 1992, pp 413-426.
33. Mislankar SG, Gildersleeve DL, Wieland DM, et al: 6-[18F]Fluorometaraminol: A radiotracer for in vivo mapping of adrenergic nerves of the heart. J Med Chem 31:362-366, 1988.
34. Wieland DM, rosenspire KC, Hutchins GD, et al: Neuronal mapping of the heart with 6-[18F]fluorometaraminol. J Med Chem 33:956-964, 1990.
35. Eisenhofer G, Hovevey-Sion D, Kopin IJ, et al: Neuronal uptake and metabolism of 2- and 6-fluorodopamine: False neurotransmitters for position emission tomographic imaging of sympathetically innervated tissues. J Pharmacol Exp Ther 248:419-427, 1989.
36. Ding Y-S, Fowler JS, Gatley SJ, et al: Synthesis of high specific activity of 6-18F-fluorodopamine for positron emission tomography studies of sympathetic nervous tissue. J Med Chem 34:861-863, 1991.
37. Ding Y-S, Fowler JS, Gatley SJ, et al: Synthesis of high specific activity (+)- and (-)- 6-18F-fluoronorepinephrine via the nucleophilic aromatic substitution reaction. J Med Chem 34:767-771, 1991.
38. Raffel DM, del Rosario RB, et al: Clinical evaluation of carbon-11-phenylephrine: MAO-sensitive marker of cardiac sympathetic neurons. J Nucl Med 37:1923-1931, 1996.
39. Del Rosario RB, Jung YW, Caraher J, et al: Synthesis and preliminary evaluation of [11C]-(-)-phenylephrine as a functional heart neuronal PET agent. Nucl Med Biol 23:611-616, 1996.
40. Vaidyanathan G, Affleck DJ, Zalutsky MR: et al: (4-[18F]fluoro-3-iodobenzyl)guanidine, a potential MIBG analogue for positron emission tomography. J Med Chem 37:3655-3662, 1994.
41. Loc'h C, Mardon K, Valette H, et al: Preparation and pharmacological characterization of 76-meta-bromobenzylguanidine (76-MBBG). Nucl Med Biol 21: 49-55, 1994.
42. Raffel DM, Jung YW, Gildersleeve DL, et al: Radiolabeled phenethylguanidines: novel imaging agents for cardiac sympathetic neurons and adrenergic tumors. J Med Chem 50:2078-2088, 2007.
43. Kilbourn MR, Jung YW, Haka MS, et al: Mouse brain distribution of a carbon-11 labeled vesamicol derivative: Presynaptic marker of cholinergic neurons. Life Sci 47:1955-1963, 1990.
44. Mulholland GK, Buck F, Sherman PS, et al: 4-18F-Fluorobenzyl-ABV: A new potential marker for central cholinergic presynaptic sites (abstract). J Nucl Med 32:994, 1991.
45. Mulholland GK: Improved synthesis of 11C-methyl-aminobenzovesamicol. J Label Compounds Radiopharmacol 31:253-259, 1992.
46. Mulholland GK, Yong-Moon J, Wieland DM, et al: Synthesis of 18F-fluoroethoxybenzovesamicol, a radiotrace for cholinergic neurons. J Label Compounds Radiopharmacol 33:583-591, 1993.
47. Rogers GA, Stone-Elander S, Ingvar M, et al: 18F-Labelled vesamicol derivatives: Syntheses and preliminary in vivo small animals positron emission tomography evaluation. Nucl Med Biol 21:219-230, 1994.
48. Berger G, Prenant C, Sastre J, et al: Synthesis of a beta-blocker for heart visualization: 11C-practolol. Int J Appl Radiat Isot 34:1556-1557, 1983.
49. Berger G, Maziere M, Prenant C, et al: Synthesis of 11C-propranolol. J Radioanal Chem 74:301-306, 1982.
50. Berridge MS, Cassidy EH, Terris AH, Vesselle JM: Preparation and in vivo binding of [11C]carazolol, a radiotracer for the beta-adrenergic receptor. Int J Radiat Appl Instrum B 19:563-569, 1992.
51. Zheng LB, Berridge MS, Ernsberger P: Synthesis, binding properties, and ^{18}F labeling of fluorocarazolol, a high-affinity β-adrenergic receptor antagonist. Nucl Med Biol 37:3219-3230, 1994.
52. Boullais C, Crouzel C, Syrota A: Synthesis of 4-(3-t-butylamino-2-hydroxypropoxy-benzamidazol-2-11C) one (CGP 12177). J Label Compounds Radiopharmacol 23:565-567, 1986.
53. Hammadi A, Crouzel C: Asymmetric synthesis of (2S) and (2R)-4-(butylamino-2-hydroxypropoxy-benzamidazol-2-11C) one (S) and (R) (11C CGP 12177) from optically active precursors. J Label Compounds Radiopharmacol 29:681-690, 1991.
54. Elsinga PH, van Waarde A, Jaeggi KA, et al: Synthesis and evaluation of (S)-4-(3-(2′-[11C] isopropylamino)-2-hydroxy-proproxy)-^{2}H-benzimidazol-2-one (S-[11C]CGP 12388) and S-4-(3-((1′-[18F]-fluoroisopropyl) amino) -2-hydroxypropoxy)-^{2}H-benzimidazol-2-one ((S)-[18F] fluoro-CGP 12388) for visualization of β-adrenoceptors with positron emission tomography. J Med Chem 40:3829-3835, 1997.
55. Law MP, Osman S, Pike VW, et al: Evaluation of [11C]GB67, a novel radioligand for imaging myocardial alpha 1-adrenoceptors with positron emission tomography. Eur J Nucl Med 27:7-17, 2000.
56. Dubois EA, van den Bos JC, Janssen AG, et al: Development of radioligands for the

imaging of cardiac beta-adrenoceptors using SPECT: Part II. Pharmacological characterization in vitro and in vivo of new 123I-labeled beta-adrenoceptor antagonists. Nucl Med Biol 24:9-13, 1997.

57. Maziere M, Coman D, Godot JM, et al: In vivo characterization of myocardium muscarinic receptors by positron emission tomography. Life Sci 29:2391-2397, 1981.
58. Syrota A, Paillotin G, Davy JM, Aumont MC: Kinetics of in vivo binding of antagonist to muscarinic cholinergic receptor in the human heart studied by positron emission tomography. Life Sci 35:937-945, 1984.
59. Delforge J, Syrota A, Cançon JP, et al: Cardiac β-adrenergic receptor density measured in vivo using PET, CGP 12177 and a new graphical method. J Nucl Med 32:739-748, 1991.
60. Farde L, Hall H, Ehrin E, Sedvall G: Quantitative analysis of D2 dopamine receptor binding in the living human brain by PET. Science 231:258-261, 1986.
61. Fowler J, Wolf AP, Christman DR, et al: Carrier-free 11C labeled catecholamines. In Subramanian G (ed): Radiopharmaceuticals. New York, Society of Nuclear Medicine, 1975, pp 196-204.
62. Huang S-C, Phelps ME: Principles of tracer kinetic modeling in positron emission tomography and autoradiography. In Phelps ME, Schelbert HR (eds): Positron Emission Tomography and Autoradio-graphy. New York, Raven Press, 1986, pp 287-346.
63. Bassingthwaighte JB: Modeling in the analysis of solute and water exchange in the microvasculature. In Renkin EM (ed): Handbook of Physiology: The Cardiovascular System. New York, American Physiology Society, 1984, pp 549-626.
64. Kuikka J, Levin M, Bassingthwaighte JB: Multiple tracer dilution estimates of D- and 2-deoxy-D-glucose uptake by the heart. Am J Physiol 250:H29-H42, 1986.
65. Caldwell JH, Kroll K, Li Z, et al: Quantitation of presynaptic cardiac sympathetic function with carbon-11-meta-hydroxyephedrine. J Nucl Med 39:1327-1334, 1998.
66. Delforge J, Syrota A, Mazoyer BM: Experimental design optimisation: Theory and application to estimation of receptor model parameters using dynamic positron emission tomography. Phys Med Biol 34:419-435, 1989.
67. Mintun MA, Raichle ME, Kilbourn MR, et al: A quantitative model for the in vivo assessment of drug binding sites with positron emission tomography. Ann Neurol 15:217-227, 1984.
68. Perlmutter JS, Larson KB, Raichle ME, et al: Strategies for in vivo measurement of receptor binding using positron emission tomography. J Cereb Blood Flow Metab 6:154-169, 1986.
69. Wong D, Gjedde A, Wagner HN, et al: Quantification of neuroreceptors in the living human brain: II. Inhibition studies of receptor density and affinity. J Cereb Blood Flow Metab 6:147-153, 1986.
70. Matsunari I, Bunko H, Taki J, et al: Regional uptake of iodine-125-metaiodobenzylguanidine in the rat heart. Eur J Nucl Med 20:1104-1107, 1993.
71. Glowniak JV, Kilty JE, Amara SG, et al: Evaluation of metaiodobenzylguanidine uptake by the norepinephrine, dopamine and serotonin transporters. J Nucl Med 34:1140-1146, 1993.
72. Shiga K, Sasano H, Inoue T, et al: The distribution and kinetics of 123I-MIBG in normal human hearts. Jpn J Nucl Med 30:1359-1367, 1993.
73. Gill JS: Heterogeneity of the human myocardial sympathetic innervation: In vivo demonstration by iodine 123–labeled metaiodobenzylguanidine scintigraphy. Am Heart J 126:390-398, 1993.
74. Glowniak JV, Wilson RA, Joyce ME, turner FE: Evaluation of metaiodobenzylguanidine heart and lung extraction fraction by first-pass analysis in pigs. J Nucl Med 33:716-723, 1992.
75. Wieland DM, Brown LE, rogers WL, et al: Myocardial imaging with a radioiodinated norepinephrine storage analog. J Nucl Med 22:22-31, 1981.
76. Sisson JC, Wieland DM, Sherman P, et al: Metaiodobenzylguanidine as an index of the adrenergic nervous system integrity and function. J Nucl Med 28:1620-1624, 1987.
77. Wafelman AR, Hoefnagel CA, Maes RA, Beijnen JH: Radioiodinated metaiodobenzylguanidine: A review of its biodistribution and pharmacokinetics, drug interactions, cytotoxicity and dosimetry. Eur J Nucl Med 21:545-559, 1994.
78. Dae MW, De Marco T, Bovinick EH, et al: Scintigraphic assessment of MiBG uptake in globally denervated human and canine hearts—implications for clinical studies. J Nucl Med 33:1444-1450, 1992.
79. Dae MW, O'Connell JW, Botvinick EH, et al: Scintigraphic assessment of regional cardiac adrenergic innervation. Circulation 79:634-644, 1989.
80. Sisson JC, Shapiro B, Meyers L, et al: Metaiodobenzylguanidine to map scintigraphically the adrenergic nervous system in man. J Nucl Med 28:1625-1636, 1987.
81. Sisson JC, Bolgos G, Johnson J: Measuring acute changes in adrenergic nerve activity of the heart in the living animal. Am Heart J 121:1119-1123, 1991.
82. Minardo JD, Tuli MM, Mock BH, et al: Scintigraphic and electrophysiological evidence of canine myocardial sympathetic denervation and reinnervation produced by myocardial infarction or phenol application. Circulation 78:1008-1019, 1988.
83. Mori H, Pisarri TE, Aldea GS, et al: Usefulness and limitations of regional cardiac sympathectomy by phenol. Am J Physiol 257:H1523-H1533, 1989.
84. Newman D, Munoz L, Chin M, et al: Effects of canine myocardial infarction on sympathetic efferent neuronal function: Scintigraphic and electrophysiologic correlates. Am Heart J 126:1106-1112, 1993.
85. Raffel DM, Wieland DM: Assessment of cardiac sympathetic nerve integrity with positron emission tomography. Nucl Med Biol 28:541-559, 2001.
86. Nguyen NT, DeGrado TR, Chakraborty P, et al: Myocardial kinetics of C-11 epinephrine in the isolated working rat heart. J Nucl Med 38:780-785, 1997.
87. Sisson JC, Johnson J, Bolgos G, et al: Portrayal of adrenergic denervation in the presence of myocardial infarction: A feasibility study. Am J Physiol Imaging 5:151-166, 1990.
88. Barber MJ, Mueller TM, Henry DP, et al: Transmural myocardial infarction in the dog produces sympathectomy in noninfarcted myocardium. Circulation 67:787-796, 1983.
89. Nishimura T, Oka H, Sago M, et al: Serial assessment of denervated but viable myocardium following acute myocardial infarction in dogs using iodine-123 metaiodobenzylguanidine and thallium-201 chloride myocardial single photon emission tomography. Eur J Nucl Med 19:25-29, 1992.
90. Inoue H, Zipes DP: Time course of denervation of efferent sympathetic and vagal nerves after occlusion of the coronary artery in the canine heart. Circ Res 62:1111-1120, 1988.
91. Dae MW, De Marco T, Botvinick EH, et al: Scintigraphic assessment of sympathetic innervation after transmural versus nontransmural myocardial infarction. J Am Coll Cardiol 17:1416-1423, 1991.
92. Miyazaki T, Zipes DP: Protection against autonomic denervation following acute myocardial infarction by preconditioning ischemia. Circ Res 64:437-448, 1989.
93. Nohara R, Kambara H, Okuda K, et al: Effects of cardiac sympathetic nervous system on the stunned myocardium: Experimental study with ^{123}I-metaiodobenzylguanidine. Jpn Circ J 55:893-899, 1991.
94. Wakasugi S, Wada A, Hasegawa Y, et al: Detection of abnormal cardiac adrenergic neuron activity in adriamycin-induced cardiomyopathy with iodine-125-metaiodobenzylguanidine. J Nucl Med 33:208-214, 1992.
95. Wakasugi S, Fischman AJ, Babich JW, et al: Metaiodobenzylguanidine: Evaluation of its potential as a tracer for monitoring doxorubicin cardiomyopathy. J Nucl Med 34:1283-1286, 1993.
96. Ito M, Pride HP, Zipes DP: Defibrillating shocks delivered to the heart impair efferent sympathetic responses. Circulation 88:2661-2673, 1993.
97. Rabinovitch MA, Rose CP, Schwab AJ, et al: A method of dynamic analysis of iodine-123-metaiodobenzylguanidine scintigrams in cardiac mechanical overload hypertrophy and failure. J Nucl Med 34:589-600, 1993.
98. Fagret D, Wolfe JE, Vanzetto G, Borrel E: Myocardial uptake of metaiodobenzylguanidine in patients with left ventricular hypertrophy secondary to valvular aortic stenosis. J Nucl Med 34:57-60, 1993.
99. Dae MW, De Marco T, Botvinick EH, et al: MIBG uptake at one year post cardiac transplant: Evidence for partial reinnervation in man [abstract]. J Nucl Med 33:896, 1992.
100. Schwaiger M, Hutchins GD, Kalff V, et al: Evidence for regional catecholamine uptake and storage sites in the transplanted human heart by positron emission

tomography. J Clin Invest 87:1681-1690, 1991.
101. Allman K, Wolfe E, Sitomer J, et al: C-11-Hydroxyephedrine assessment of regional myocardial sympathetic neuronal function following acute myocardial infarction in man [abstract]. J Nucl Med 32:1040, 1991.
102. Allman KC, Wieland Dm, Muzik O, et al: Carbon-11 hydroxyephedrine with positron emission tomography for serial assessment of cardiac adrenergic neuronal function after acute myocardial infarction in human. J Am Coll Cardiol 22:368-375, 1993.
103. Stanton MS, Tuli MM, Radtke NL, et al: Regional sympathetic denervation after myocardial infarction in humans detected noninvasively using I-123-metaiodobenzylguanidine. J Am Coll Cardiol 14:1519-1526, 1989.
104. Tulli MM, Stanton MS, Mock BH, et al: Comparative SPECT 123I-metaio-dobenzylguanidine (MIBG) and 201thallium (TL) cardiac imaging following myocardial infarction [abstract]. J Nucl Med 29:840, 1989.
105. McGhie AL, Corbett JR, Akers MS, et al: Regional cardiac adrenergic function using ^{123}I-metaiodobenzylguanidine tomographic imaging after acute myocardial infarction. Am J Cardiol 67:236-242, 1991.
106. Nishimura T, Uehara T, Hayashida K, et al: Newly developed myocardial imaging by using single photon emission computed tomography (SPECT). Jpn Circ J 54:328-332, 1990.
107. Satoh K, Katoh K, Murata, et al: [Assessment of ischemic damage of the cardiac sympathetic nerve function by semi-quantitative analysis using ^{123}I-MIBG (metaiodobenzylguanidine)-SPECT: Comparison with 201Tl-Cl-SPECT]. Kaku Igaku 27:821-831, 1990.
108. Morozumi T, Ishida Y, Tani A, et al: [Myocardial adrenergic derangement due to myocardial ischemia: Decreased myocardial uptake of I-123 metaiodobenzylguanidine after PTCA in a patient with effort angina]. Kaku Igaku 27:735-740, 1990.
109. Hirosawa K, Tanaka T, Hisada K, Bunko H: [Clinical evaluation of ^{123}I-MIBG for assessment of the sympathetic nervous system in the heart (multi-center clinical trial)]. Kaku Igaku 28:461-476, 1991.
110. Tanaka T, Aizawa T, Katou K, et al: [Interesting PYP, 201Tl, MIBG, AM and BMIPP myocardial SPECT images in a patient under successful reperfusion therapy]. Kokyu To Junkan 40:609-614, 1992.
111. Tahara Y, Taya M, Nishimura T, et al: [Assessment of denervated but viable myocardium in patients with myocardial infarction by myocardial imaging with 201Tl and 123I-MIBG]. Kokyu To Junkan 39:795-799, 1991.
112. Wharton JM, Friedman IM, Greenfield RA, et al: Quantitative perfusion and sympathetic nerve defect size after myocardial infarction in humans [abstract]. J Am Coll Cardiol 19:264A, 1992.
113. Mitrani R, Burt RW, Klein LS, et al: Regional cardiac sympathetic denervation and reinnervation following myocardial infarction in humans [abstract]. Circulation 86(suppl 4):247, 1992.
114. Nishimura T, Uehara T, Shimonagata T, et al: Assessment of myocardial viability by using newly developed myocardial SPECT imaging. Jpn Circ J 56:603-607, 1992.
115. Tanaka T, Aizawa T, Kato K, et al: [Interesting PYP, Tl-201, MIBG and AM myocardial SPECT images in a patient under successful reperfusion therapy]. Kaku Igaku 28:1099-1103, 1991.
116. Guertner C, Klepzig H Jr, Maul FD, et al: Noradrenaline depletion in patients with coronary artery disease before and after percutaneous transluminal coronary angioplasty with iodine-123 metaiodobenzylguanidine and single-photon emission tomography. Eur J Nucl Med 20:776-782, 1993.
117. Spinnler MT, Lombardi F, Moretti C, et al: Evidence of functional alterations in sympathetic activity after a myocardial infarction. Eur Heart J 14:1334-1343, 1993.
118. Terada K, Sugihara H, Taniguchi Y, et al: [A case of acute coronary syndrome followed by 201Tl, 123I-BMIPP and 123I-MIBG myocardial imaging before and after PTCA]. Kaku Igaku 30:1459-1463, 1993.
119. Lekakis J, Antoniou A, Vassilopoulos N, et al: I-123 metaiodobenzylguanidine-thallium-201 mismatch following myocardial infarction. Clin Cardiol 17:21-25, 1994.
120. Tanaka T, Aizawa T, Kato K, et al: [Study of sympathetic nervous function under effort induced ischemia in patients with angina pectoris with I-123 metaiodobenzylguanidine (MIBG) myocardial SPECT images]. Kaku Igaku 27:143-147, 1990.
121. Katoh K, Nishimura S, Nakanishi S, et al: Stunned myocardium and sympathetic denervation: Clinical assessment using MIBG scintigraphy. Jpn Circ J 55:919-922, 1991.
122. Yamakado K, Takeda K, Kitano T, et al: Serial change of iodine-123 metaiodobenzylguanidine (MIBG) myocardial concentration with dilated cardiomyopathy. Eur J Nucl Med 19:265-270, 1992.
123. Morozumi T, Ishida Y, Tani A, et al: [Clinical significance of I-123 MIBG myocardial scintigraphy for evaluating the severity of congestive heart failure]. Kaku Igaku 28:271-280, 1991.
124. Schofer J, Spielmann R, Schuchert A, et al: Iodine-123 meta-iodobenzylguanidine scintigraphy: A noninvasive method to demonstrate myocardial adrenergic nervous system disintegrity in patients with idiopathic dilated cardiomyopathy. J Am Coll Cardiol 12:1252-1258, 1988.
125. Merlet P, Valette H, Dubois-Randé JL, et al: Prognostic value of cardiac metaiodobenzylguanidine imaging in patients with heart failure. J Nucl Med 33:471-477, 1992.
126. Maeno M, Ishida Y, Shimonagata T, et al: [The significance of 201Tl/123I MIBG (metaiodobenzylguanidine) mismatched myocardial regions for predicting ventricular tachycardia in patients with idiopathic dilated cardiomyopathy]. Kaku Igaku 30:1221-1229, 1993.
127. Shimizu M, Sugihara N, Kita Y, et al: Long-term course and cardiac sympathetic nerve activity in patients with hypertrophic cardiomyopathy. Br Heart J 67:155-160, 1992.
128. Nakajima K, Bunko H, Taki J, et al: Quantitative analysis of 123I-meta-iodobenzylguanidine (MIBG) uptake in hypertrophic cardiomyopathy. Am Heart J 119:1329-1337, 1990.
129. Mantysaari M, Kuikka J, Mustonen J, et al: Noninvasive detection of cardiac sympathetic nervous dysfunction in diabetic patients using [123I]metaiodobenzylguanidine. Diabetes 41:1069-1075, 1992.
130. Katono E, Owada K, Takeda H, et al: [Usefulness of myocardial imaging by 123I-MIBG in assessment of diabetic neuropathy]. Kaku Igaku 30:1235-1239, 1993.
131. Morozumi T, Ishida Y, Tani A, et al: [Gallium-67 myocardial imaging for the detection of Adriamycin cardiomyopathy]. Kaku Igaku 27:477-484, 1990.
132. Valdes Olmos R, ten Bokkel Huinink WW, Greve J, et al: I-123 MIBG and serial radionuclide angiocardiography in doxorubicin-related cardiotoxicity. Clin Nucl Med 17:163-167, 1992.
133. Di Carli MF, Tobes MC, Mangner T, et al: Effects of cardiac sympathetic innervation on coronary blood flow. N Engl J Med 336:1208-1215, 1997.
134. Bengel FM, Ueberfuhr P, Ziegler SI, et al: Serial assessment of sympathetic reinnervation after orthotopic heart transplation. A longitudinal study usning PET and C-11 hydroxyephedrine. Circulation, 99(14):1866-1871, 1999.
135. Bengel FM, Ueberfuhr P, Hesse T, et al: Clinical determinants of ventricular sympathetic reinnervation after orthotopic heart transplantation. Circulation 106(7):831-835, 2002.
136. Wakabayashi T, Nakata T, Hashimoto A, et al: Assessment of underlying etiology and cardiac sympathetic innervation to identify patients at high risk of cardiac death. J Nucl Med 42:1757-1767, 2001.
137. Simula S, Vanninen E, Viltanen L, et al: Cardiac adrenergic innervation is affected in asymptomatic subjects with very early stage of coronary artery disease. J Nucl Med 43:1-7, 2002.
138. Allman KC, Stevens, MJ, Wieland DM, et al: Noninvasive assessment of cardiac diabetic neuropathy by carbon-11 hydroxyephedrine and positron emission tomography. J Am Coll Cardiol 22(5):1425-1432, 1993.
139. Stevens MJ, Raffel DM, Allman KC, et al: Cardiac sympathetic dysinnervation in diabetes: Implications for enhanced cardiovascular risk. Circulation 98(10): 961-968, 1998.
140. Pietilä M, Malminiemi K, Vesalainen R, et al: Exercise training in chronic heart failure: Beneficial effects on cardiac ^{11}C-hydroxyephedrine PET, autonomic nervous control and repolarization. J Nucl Med 43:733-779, 2002.
141. de Jong RM, Blanksma PK, van Waarde A, van Veldhuisen DJ: Measurement of myocardial β-adrenoceptor density in clinical studies: A role for positron

emission tomography? Eur J Nucl Med Mol Imaging 29:88-97, 2002.
142. Staehelin M, Hertel C: [3H]CGP-12177, a beta-adrenergic ligand suitable for measuring cell surface receptors. J Recept Res 3(1-2):35-43, 1983.
143. Hertel C, Müller P, Portenier M, Staehelin M: Determination of the desensitization of beta-adrenergic receptors by 3H-CGP-12177. Biochem J 216:669-674, 1983.
144. Hughes B, Marshall DR, Sobel BE, Bergmann SR: Characterization of beta-adrenoreceptors in vivo with iodine-131 pindolol and gamma scintigraphy. J Nucl Med 27:660-667, 1986.
145. Sisson J, Wieland DM, Johnson J, et al: Portrayal of cardiac beta receptors in living animals. J Am Coll Cardiol 13:64A, 1989.
146. Syrota A, Dormont D, Berger G, et al: C-11 ligand binding to adrenergic and muscarinic receptors in the human heart studied in vivo by PET [abstract]. J Nucl Med 24:P20, 1983.
147. Seto M, Crouzel C, et al: Beta adrenergic receptors in the dog heart characterized by 11C-CGP 12 177 and PET [abstract]. J Nucl Med 27:949-000, 1986.
148. Merlet P, Delforge J, Syrota A, et al: Positron emission tomography with 11C CGP-12177 to assess β-adrenergic receptor concentration in idiopathic dilated cardiomyopathy. Circulation 87:1169-1178, 1993.
149. Lefroy DM, de Silva R, Choudhury L, et al: Diffuse reduction in myocardial beta-adrenoceptors in hypertrophic cardiomyopathy: A study with positron emission tomography. J Am Coll Cardiol 22:1653-1660, 1993.
150. Syrota A, Comar D, Paillotin G, et al: Muscarinic cholinergic receptor in the human heart evidenced under physiological conditions by positron emission tomography. Proc Natl Acad Sci U S A 82:584-588, 1985.
151. Burgisser E, Lefkowitz RJ: Reciprocal modulation of agonist and antagonist binding to muscarinic cholinergic receptor by guanine nucleotide. Proc Natl Acad Sci U S A 79:1732-1736, 1985.
152. Delforge J, Janier M, Syrota A, et al: Noninvasive quantification of muscarinic receptors in vivo with positron emission tomography in the dog heart. Circulation 82:1494-1504, 1990.
153. Le Guludec D, Cohen-Solal A, Delforge J, et al: Increased myocardial muscarinic receptor density in idiopathic dilated cardiomyopathy: An in vivo PET study. Circulation 96:3416-3422, 1997.
154. Le Guludec D, Delforge J, Syrota A, et al: In vivo quantification of myocardial muscarinic receptors in heart transplant patients. Circulation 909:172-178, 1994.
155. Carrió I: Cardiac neurotransmission imaging. J Nucl Med 42:1062-1076, 2001.
156. DeGrado TR, Bergmann SR, Ng CK, Raffel DM: Tracer kinetic modeling in nuclear cardiology. J Nucl Cardiol 7:686-700, 2000.
157. Lautamaki, R, Tipre D, Bengel M: Cardiac sympathetic neuronal imaging using PET. Eur J Nucl Med Mol Imaging 34:S74-S85, 2007.
158. Yamashina S, Yamazaki J: Neuronal imaging using SPECT. Eur J Nucl Med Mol Imaging 34:S62-S73, 2007.

Neural Mechanisms Initiating and Maintaining Arrhythmias: Summarizing Data from Animal Models and Human Diseases

38

JAMES B. MARTINS

CHAPTER OUTLINE

The autonomic nervous system modulates cardiac arrhythmias, especially when additional abnormal structure or function occurs in the heart. We review reflex control of the heart and vessels and then human and animal models of arrhythmias studied recently.[1]

Autonomic Neural Mechanisms

Numerous reflexes can promote arrhythmias. The parasympathetic transmitter is acetylcholine and the sympathetic transmitter is norepinephrine. Other transmitters have not been shown to participate in arrhythmias. Many redundant interactions promote balance, including presynaptic inhibition of one limb versus the other as well as interactions at the heart cell on receptors and intracellular messenger interactions.[2,3] However, this yin-yang of parasympathetic and sympathetic is too simplistic a view.

Myocardial ischemia is the best-described entity, with simultaneous increases in activity of both limbs.[4] Also, excess sympathetic humeral and neural influences impair high-pressure baroreflexes, which are restored by sympathectomy in ischemic models of heart failure.[5] Restoration of more normal sympathetic influence by β-adrenergic receptor–blocking drugs reverses these abnormalities, providing rationale for preventing arrhythmia.

Investigators have begun to study higher-center reduction of sympathetic efferents. Spinal cord stimulation at C8-T4 ameliorates oxygen supply/demand relationships in patients with coronary artery disease and heart failure without eliminating pain of myocardial infarction.[6] Spinal cord stimulation prolongs sinus cycle and atrio-His interval in dogs, which was totally blocked by cervical vagotomy, therefore mediated by parasympathetic activation.[7] Spinal cord stimulation also modifies intrinsic cardiac neurons[8]; right atrial (RA) fat pad (ganglionated plexi) recordings fell to one third of their original with spinal cord stimulation, and the increase in ganglionated plexi recordings with myocardial infarction was dramatically prevented by spinal cord stimulation, which was blocked by stellate ganglionectomy. Thus spinal cord stimulation reduces pain by activating multiple efferent reflexes.[6]

In the brain, parasympathetic activity in nucleus tractus solitaris is selectively modified by substance P, but sympathetic regulation by the baroreflex is not.[9] Central sympathetic control by dorsal raphe serotoninergic neurons is restored in days by selective serotonin reuptake inhibitors,[10] enhancing baroreflex sensitivity (BRS) in a model of hind limb unloading. Thus, central mechanisms regulate reflex function modifiable by a clinically available therapy.

Efferent denervation and resultant supersensitivity (no nerves to take up norepinephrine and stop its effects on receptors in the synaptic cleft) produces cardiac electrophysiologic effects described by several laboratories. However, central or local denervation ultimately results in reinnervation, because axons of passage rapidly reinnervate from remaining cell bodies.[4] Permanent denervation results when all cell bodies innervating the heart are destroyed.

Developmental sympathetic defects influence several ionic currents.[11] German shepherd dogs with such abnormalities might undergo inadequate cellular ionic development and have a tendency to ventricular fibrillation (VF). Whether this occurs in humans is unclear. However, there is little evidence that acquired cardiac denervation or reinnervation changes regulation of ionic channels to cause arrhythmias independent from associated disease states such as myocardial scarring.

The high-pressure baroreflex is the defense against extreme pressures damaging the brain. Its powerful effects are used clinically to stop, modify, or diagnose supraventricular tachycardia (SVT) and ventricular tachycardia (VT). With afferents in the carotid sinus and aortic arch, the reflex increases sympathetics and decreases parasympathetics in patients with heart disease when hypotension results. Although this reflex maintains blood pressure during arrhythmias, it can result in continued or recurrent arrhythmia.

The cardiopulmonary or low-pressure baroreflex involves stretch-responsive and chemoresponsive receptors that are found in the lungs, bronchi, and all heart chambers. Cardiopulmonary reflexes mainly originate from the heart, with only small changes in efferents modified by pulmonary reflexes alone. Cardiac afferents can regulate neural input to the same myocardial site, but the efferent area influenced is much larger, with beat-to-beat regulation from many sites.[4] Afferents involve the nodose ganglion, the dorsal root ganglion, and intrathoracic nerves. In general these are more chemosensitive than mechanosensitive nerves responding to adenosine, adenosine triphosphate (ATP), bradykinin, substance P, and others. Ischemia differentially affects afferents,[4] with the nodose ganglion recording low frequencies (0.2-2 Hz) and the dorsal root ganglia recording higher frequencies (2-8 Hz), thus producing more rapid and detailed control. Adenosine mediates coronary pain proven by intracoronary injection in patients with symptoms mimicking angina.

The chemoreflex is a powerful stimulant of simultaneous parasympathetic and sympathetic nervous modulation of the heart.[13] It is activated by hypoxia (see Chapter 95).

The somatic reflexes involve pain and also stretch of skin to cause an increase in both parasympathetic and sympathetic outflow to the heart. In animal models, stimulating the somatic nociceptive reflex by pinch inhibits parasympathetic but not sympathetic modulation by the baroreflexes.[14] Thus at least tachycardia with pain may be due to parasympathetic withdrawal.

Temperature stimulates sympathetic nerves. Cold decreases parasympathetic drive unrelated to baroreflex mechanisms,[15] but with Valsalva (diving reflex) both parasympathetic and sympathetic increases result in VT with long-QT syndromes.[13]

Many studies to be reviewed do not physiologically modulate a reflex but only do efferent stimulation, which might nonphysiologically affect arrhythmias. Thus, work needs to be done to study reflex modulation of arrhythmic and antiarrhythmic effects.

Sinus Bradycardia and Tachycardia (Patient Studies)

Patients and physicians alike think of vasovagal syncope or neurocardiogenic syncope (NCS) and related orthostatic disorders as a defect in the autonomic nervous system. Two reviews summarize our knowledge[16,17] of these poorly understood and therefore poorly treated patients.

Heart rate variability (HRV) measures sinus node function, indicating at least vagal neural influence as the high-frequency power component (0.15-0.4 Hz) or root mean square of successive differences (RMSSD) of the time domain analysis. The low-frequency power (0.06-0.1 Hz) and the ratio of low to high frequency might indicate neural or humoral sympathetic influences. Parasympathetic and sympathetic effects on the heart are otherwise unmeasurable in humans. Muscle sympathetic nerve activity provides useful mechanistic results in patients; however, selective output to various organs depending on the reflex makes the assumption of cardiac versus peripheral sympathetic tenuous.

Studies have attempted to clarify the abnormalities in NCS. BRS, measured in various ways, is always abnormal. In 18 NCS patients compared with 17 controls, the initial response to tilt testing was to appropriately increase peroneal muscle sympathetic activity and low power HRV to maintain blood pressure. Syncope was associated with abrupt blood pressure drop correlated with a drop in sympathetic nerve activity, the other most common finding in this disorder. Interestingly, high-frequency HRV did not increase more than in the control group. The cause of initial blood pressure drop was also investigated in patients with recurrent NCS[18] divided into tilt-resistant and tilt-sensitive groups, measuring cardiac output serially with two rapid methods. The sensitive group had a significant drop in cardiac output brought on by venous dilatation and inadequate cardiac filling, possibly mediated by sympathetic neural withdrawal. Although BRS was abnormal, the further abrupt drop in sympathetic activity was unexplained.

In a study of patients with NCS compared to controls during lower-body negative pressure, eliminating positional change,[19] BRS was depressed. Because β-adrenergic blockade can restore BRS, some patients may benefit from aggressive β-blocker therapy.

Kamiya[20] studied normal subjects after days of bed rest to investigate orthostatic hypotension. Abrupt sympathetic withdrawal was found only in subjects with syncope on tilt, but all had equivalent impairment of BRS. The investigators speculated that central sympathetic withdrawal was the major reason for orthostasis. In a study of normal subjects undergoing lower-body negative pressure to syncope,[21] those who fainted had a greater impairment of BRS compared to resistant subjects. Thus normal subjects with orthostasis are as complicated as patients with NCS.

To confirm abnormal BRS, patients with syncope and controls were studied with neck pressure to load and unload baroreflexes, measuring time to response of forearm vascular resistance.[22] BRS was no different but latency was slower (14 seconds compared to 9 seconds in resistant fainters and 10 seconds in controls). Again, abnormal BRS underlies NCS in most patients.

Donadio[23] reported that phobic NCS patients have a greater inhibitory sympathetic response to arousal compared to healthy controls. The patients had lower and prolonged inhibition of nerve activity than controls provoked by somatosensory stimuli to a finger. Thus psychological factors inhibit sympathetic activity, which is the neural component of NCS.

In general, peripheral sympathetic augmentation works to prevent symptoms in patients with NCS; thus midodrine and yohimbine improve sympathetic response, as does increased volume and salt intake or mineralocorticoids. Directly addressing BRS, glomectony[24] was performed in 40 patients with recurrent NCS; all patients became asymptomatic whether their arrhythmia was cardioinhibitory or vasodepressor in origin. Even though baroreflexes can recover after surgical interruption, patients might stay hypertensive. Thus the major player in NCS is an altered baroreflex, which needs to be thoughtfully addressed by new therapies. The vagus nerve does not mediate the bradycardia.

Inappropriate sinus tachycardia may be due to abnormal sinus node function. Leon[25] studied HRV and baroreflex gain in eight patients compared with nine controls. Baroreflex gain was 50% of that measured in controls in the patients at rest and during tilt. Consistent with this finding was an increased arterial pressure. Although HRV measures, including RMSSD, suggested impaired parasympathetic input, intrinsic sinus rate was abnormal after autonomic blockade as previously reported. Although the findings are consistent with prior measures of HRV, abnormal sinus node function might not allow accurate reflex assessment.

Inappropriate sinus tachycardia does occur after radiofrequency (RF) ablation of the AVN area, suggesting neural connections are altered. In 30 patients undergoing slow-pathway RF ablation (cumulative duration was 107 seconds) for AVN reentry, significant reductions in high-frequency HRV occurred immediately but returned to normal 1 day later.[26] Similarly, no difference in HRV was reported[27] in patients 1 month after RF ablation of AVN, septal, or free-wall accessory pathways, despite one quarter showing heart rates of greater than 100 beats per minute on the day after RF ablation. A 1-year follow-up of RF ablation in AVN and septal sites versus free-wall sites showed impaired parasympathetic function.[28] Clearly, the amount of possible neural damage plays a role. In fact, patients receiving almost 10,000 J for atrial tachycardia originating from the AVN area[29] were compared to patients receiving RF ablation in areas away from the AVN. Parasympathetic impairment of HRV was observed only in patients with AVN ablation. Thus nerves in the atrial septum may be interrupted depending on the site and dose of RF ablation. Transient inappropriate sinus tachycardia suggests limited denervation reversed by reinnervation.

Postural orthostatic tachycardia syndrome (POTS) is considered a mild form of autonomic failure. However, a study of nine patients and 12 controls[30] showed twice the sympathetic nerve activity in response to Valsalva maneuver and head-up tilt in POTS patients, and sympathetic BRS tended to be higher.

This finding was confirmed by increased norepinephrine turnover observed in POTS patients compared to controls.[31] Therefore, POTS has a different autonomic mechanism, perhaps involving peripheral response to sympathetic activation. Patients do poorly with β-adrenergic blockers simply because their sinus node is responding to baroreflex adjustments to make up for inadequate peripheral vascular response.

Atrial Fibrillation (Animal Studies)

Several reviews have detailed the pathophysiology of atrial fibrillation (AF),[3,32,33] the specifics of cholinergic AF,[34] and detailed insights from animal models.[35] In the normal atrium, parasympathetic excess is often responsible for AF, and animal models using vagal nerve stimulation (VNS) to test antiarrhythmics correlate with clinical results. A greater density of acetylcholine-activated potassium current (I_{KACh}) in the left atrium (LA) might explain why it is the dominant chamber in AF.[35] Influencing components of I_{KACh} or regulatory G proteins may be a more effective strategy to treat AF rather than interrupting neural components, which activate it.[36]

Nattel[35] examined the possibility that shortening of refractoriness and conduction velocity by sympathetic stimulation could initiate AF in dogs, as does parasympathetic stimulation. Despite similar electrophysiology, the duration of AF was eight times longer with VNS. The rate of AF was also greater with VNS (730 compared to 550 activations per minute). Mapping showed VNS facilitated 3.3 reentrant circuits as opposed to 1.8 with sympathetic stimulation. These data suggest that greater heterogeneity of atrial refractoriness and conduction properties accounts for the AF with parasympathetic effects.

Various investigations tested the hypothesis that autonomic effects promote atrial electrical remodeling.[32] Parasympathetic effects might prevent remodeling unless tachypacing results in sustained AF; this correlates with the paroxysmal nature of parasympathetically mediated lone AF. More consistently sympathetic effects in combination with tachypacing promote remodeling and long-lasting AF. Thus sympathetic neural increases mediated by the high-pressure baroreflex, while promoting hemodynamic stability, might maintain AF chronically. Over time BRS may be impaired with development of tachycardia-mediated cardiomyopathy.

Sympathetic innervation of the ligament of Marshall has been thought to be its major contribution to atrial arrhythmias. Data[37] suggest a richer (10 times the sympathetic) parasympathetic innervation in the dog, the ablation of which almost entirely eliminates refractory period shortening in adjacent appendage, pulmonary vein, and coronary sinus produced by left vagus stimulation. The authors did not assess the effect of the ablation on AF.

The octopus hypothesis of remote initiation of AF produced by transatrial 100 Hz stimulation[38] was suggested by pacing an electrode positioned near the ganglionated plexi and recording onset of AF with noncontact mapping. A window of vulnerability for AF induction with single premature stimuli widened in proportion to the voltage for stimulation of ganglionated plexi and as the distance from the ganglionated plexi. Additionally, AF initiation occurred at a RA appendage pacing site centimeters away from the ganglionated plexi; this apparent conduction velocity of 4 m/s is greater than atrial muscle velocity. Thus, cell bodies of neurons may be activated to release acetylcholine in the vicinity but also at a distance where axons innervate other atrial sites (legs of the octopus). Activation of the axon peripherally—namely, the appendage—might also trigger acetylcholine release in greater amount near the cell body. Thus the intrinsic cardiac neural network might importantly contribute to the complexity of atrial heterogeneity by facilitating focal initiation of AF.

Sachauerte[39] reported that ganglionated plexi stimulation (200 Hz) induced AF from the pulmonary veins or superior vena cava, preventable partly by β blockade and totally by atropine. Thus stimulation of ganglionated plexi activates both autonomic limbs, causing focal AF in the pulmonary veins in normal and coronary-occluded dogs.[40] Action potentials recorded in pulmonary veins provided direct evidence of early afterdepolarizations (EADs) in a study of isolated dog pulmonary vein, LA, or RA preparations exposed to stimulation at 100 Hz with various voltages synchronized to tissue pacing.[41] Incremental stimulation produced hyperpolarization and action potential shortening, which preceded AF originating from 22 of 28 pulmonary veins (not RA or LA) with rates of 782 ± 158 beats per minute appearing to be triggered by EADs. There was no AF if pacing was not performed, confirming triggering. If action potential shortening was not observed after atropine, AF either did not occur in six of eight subjects or was slowed in two of eight subjects; in the latter, atenolol blocked the remaining. Atenolol alone blocked AF in all eight subjects. The pulmonary vein arrhythmias were also blocked by ryanodine and high $[Ca^{2+}]_o$. These results present a plausible alternative—EAD and triggering—to the classic AF explanation by reentry.

The possibility was tested of facilitating AF by transatrial ablation of autonomic innervation traveling in ganglionated plexi of dogs.[39,42] Ganglionated plexi were identified by high-frequency stimulation, and RF ablation was performed, preventing the ability of cervical VNS to produce AF and shorten effective refractory period (ERP). Standard pulmonary vein isolation for AF ablation might also prevent short-term ERP response to VNS and AF induction in dogs.[43] However, evidence of parasympathetic denervation produced by surgical ablation of two of the three ganglionated plexi in the dog with right VNS was reversed in 4 weeks[44] and AF was induced as easily as before ablation. Although the left vagus and a third ganglionated plexus were left intact, allowing reinnervation, these results dampen enthusiasm for a limited transatrial ablation.

Optical mapping of RA tissue[45] during stimulation of the ganglionated plexi showed that action potentials shortened less, but heterogeneously, compared with acetylcholine superfusion. Mechanisms of AF with stimulation were likely macroreentrant in 64% and focal in 36%, compared to nearly all focal with acetylcholine. Using intact dogs, RF ablation of the ganglionated plexi at the junction of the right pulmonary vein and the right atrium prevented ERP shortening of the high RA but facilitated induction of AF, suggesting that incomplete denervation might worsen AF by heterogeneity with parasympathetic stimulation.[46]

Atrial three-dimensional mapping in dogs during VNS showed common foci of spontaneously occurring AF (always starting after VNS-induced bradycardia) to originate from RA free wall or Bachmann's bundle.[47] AF was blocked with atropine and only modified by β-blockers. These sites are typical subsidiary automatic sites occurring during VNS, suggesting possible mechanistic relationships with normal escape mechanisms, although AF cycle lengths were in the 40- to 70-ms range. This reproducible AF could be prevented by spinal cord stimulation in 60% of cases but not in animals with stellate ganglionectomy.[48] Bradycardia during VNS was also minimized.

In summary, parasympathetic and, to a lesser extent, sympathetic neural influences facilitate AF; some models suggest both are needed for pulmonary vein or RA atrial foci. Neural effects might importantly influence atrial remodeling. Transatrial stimulation and ablation of ganglionated plexi might prevent AF, but provocation of AF might occur if results are heterogeneous. Inhibition of spinal neural effects may be an effective preventive.

Supraventricular Tachycardia and Atrial Fibrillation (Patient Studies)

HRV measured in patients prior to an arrhythmia may suggest autonomic mechanisms initiating it. In the 6 minutes preceding atrial flutter, HRV favored sympathetic increase[33]; unfortunately, no autonomic interruptions are reported that prevent atrial flutter. HRV studies performed 1 hour before onset of lone AF show evidence of increased (50% increase in low-frequency power) sympathetic influence in 75% versus increased (doubled high-frequency power) parasympathetic influences in one quarter of 28 patients.[49] These patients with no heart disease were taking no medications. There was no clustering of episodes with increased high-frequency power at night, although others studying a similar group found nocturnal clustering.[50] Others studying uncontrolled groups of patients taking medications show mixed results.[51] Patients studied after coronary bypass[52] operations had higher heart rates and increased high-frequency power, suggesting superimposed parasympathetic and sympathetic input to sinus node. These studies give no greater insight to AF occurrence, but they present a possible testable hypothesis that autonomic influences on the sinus node may be separated from initiation of AF.

In 133 patients without structural heart disease, atrioventricular (AV) reentry SVT responded more often to vagal maneuvers than AV nodal reentry did (53% vs 33%), corresponding with lower BRS (also compared to controls) in the latter.[33] Functional conduction properties in the limbs of each SVT also predicted responses. Isoproterenol doses to increase sinus rate were lower in the AVN group, perhaps explaining the weaker BRS because of less-accentuated antagonism (less background sympathetic effect, modulated by parasympathetic influences). However, differences in ventricular filling during SVT might produce greater sympathetic stimulation. AV sequential pacemakers were programmed at varying AV relationships to heart rate of 175 beats per minute, showing arterial and venous pressure changes that were significantly less, as was sympathetic nerve activity with long RP tachycardia than with short or simultaneous RP tachycardia.[53] These results suggest the baroreflex-mediated sympathetic outflow maintains blood pressure and promotes AVN reentry, also explaining the resistance to vagal maneuvers.

AF commonly occurs with SVT. Tai studied patients with SVT with and without AF. Those with AF had larger atria, more dispersion of atrial refractoriness, and higher BRS determined by phenylephrine bolus.[54] HRV was no different between groups. The authors speculated that greater parasympathetic influence activated during SVT might contribute to AF. However, phenylephrine (parasympathetic activation and sympathetic inactivation), which slowed sinus cycle length from 708 ± 91 to 927 ± 174 ms, reduced or stopped AF episodes mapped to pulmonary vein foci.[54] Thus pulmonary vein foci of AF may be inhibited by sympathetic withdrawal via the high-pressure baroreflex and might not be worsened by parasympathetic activation.

One report showed carotid sinus massage induced AF in a 51-year-old man with a normal heart and electrophysiologic study for syncope.[55] The onset occurred within 3 seconds of marked massage-induced bradycardia (atrial rate <40 beats per minute) and after an escape P wave without an intervening QRS, but it stopped in 5 minutes and was not observed on implanted recorder in the following 10 months. Carotid massage therefore produced AF by direct vagal excess or by bradycardia-induced heterogeneity of refractoriness.

Basket-catheter mapping studies[56] in patients and in in vitro studies in canine sleeves suggest that triggered activity due to EADs caused most AF of the pulmonary vein origin. AF foci typically centimeters inside the pulmonary vein, without evidence of reentry, mostly occurred after tachycardia pause pacing. Study of canine sleeves with tachycardia pause pacing and stimulation of ganglionated plexi showed repetitive triggering preceded by EADs in one third of preparations. As before,[41] either atropine or atenolol blocked the EADs. These data together suggest a focal triggered mechanism in pulmonary veins, dependent on both parasympathetic and sympathetic effects.

Several groups have performed ganglionated plexi stimulation (20 Hz) before and after RF ablation. Lemery[57] showed that about four sites in the LA resulted in bradycardia consistent with stimulation of ganglionated plexi; ablation was performed in these areas, and wide encircling RF ablation lesions were also made. After ablation, bradycardia with ganglionated plexi stimulation was blocked in 88%. Verma[58] also reported results of two groups of patients undergoing antral RF ablation without knowledge of the site where ganglionated plexi stimulation was observed. Prevention of bradycardia during ganglionated plexi stimulation was seen in 18, and blunting was seen in 2. An additional 20 patients undergoing repeat ablation also showed no bradycardia with ganglionated plexi stimulation. Thus, wide-encircling RF ablation might also produce short-term and long-term ganglionated plexi block. The latter suggests that ganglionated plexi may be abated but might not contribute to AF recurrence.

Clinical studies of patients undergoing various RF ablation procedures for AF have suggested variable results. Oral[59] reported patients undergoing pulmonary vein ostial disconnection versus likely autonomic etiology; those with nocturnal onset, suggesting parasympathetic etiology, were less likely (50% vs 69% or 83%) to have freedom from AF compared to patients with random occurrence or exercise-mediated AF. Conversely, Pappone,[60] using a wide-encircling RF ablation procedure, reported that patients with RF ablation–mediated bradycardia with continued RF ablation until the presumed parasympathetic stimulation was ablated did better than others in his experience with similar clinical characteristics of AF. However, HRV indices indicating vagal interruption were normalized after a 1-year follow-up.[60] Finally,[61] studies of HRV including deceleration and acceleration capacity after pulmonary vein disconnection versus wide-encircling RF ablation showed acute autonomic interruption in both groups. After 1 year, only the encircling RF ablation showed persistent autonomic impairment, but this did not correlate with AF prevention. Thus, parasympathetic changes are variable with various RF ablation procedures, and their relation to AF prevention is unclear.

Endovascular ganglionated plexi stimulation techniques in patients might guide standard ablations, targeting pulmonary veins to greater than 90% success.[42] It was noted that sites of complex fractionated activity in both atria, which were successfully ablated previously and prevented AF,[62] were sites where ganglionated plexi were thought to be located. Performing only primary ablation of ganglionated plexi in lone-AF in patients prevented short-term recurrence of AF in more than 90%.[63] Another laboratory recorded less success in preventing AF, with epicardial ablation of only sites with bradycardia during ganglionated plexi stimulation in three of seven patients.[64] Additional studies and follow-up will be needed to know whether catheter ablation of ganglionated plexi alone will prevent lone AF.

Intraoperative high-frequency stimulation and ablation of ganglionated plexi was performed as a stand-alone, limited thoracotomy procedure[65] in 41 patients with an average of 5 ganglionated plexi on the right and 2 on the left. Common sites were along the interatrial groove and along the ligament of Marshall. RF ablation was applied to each site with prevention of heart rate slowing; 6-month follow-up in 15 patients showed freedom from AF in 14, many with continuous ECG monitoring.

Patients undergoing coronary bypass surgery for ischemic heart disease have undergone ganglionated plexi denervation by several groups with varying results. Davis[66] hypothesized that denervation induced by interruption of the aortic ganglionated plexi (on the ascending aorta, anterior to the pulmonary artery, which normally may be interrupted by bypass procedures) would make postoperative AF more frequent. Although a pilot study randomizing patients suggested that ganglionated plexi dissection (denervation) made postoperative AF more frequent (N = 131), addition of an extended patient group (n = 189) made the entire experience of AF equivalent. Melo[67] proposed the reverse hypothesis that denervation of the aortic ganglionated plexi would prevent postoperative AF. Results suggested a decrease in AF occurrence compared with randomized controls. However, Alex,[68] in a similarly randomized study with wider denervation procedures around the aorta, pulmonary artery, and superior vena cava, found no difference.

In summary, HRV data confirm the parasympathetic and sympathetic etiology of AF; studies should be done to manipulate autonomic function to determine effects on AF occurrence. Pulmonary vein origin by triggering may be facilitated by both. RF ablation of ganglionated plexi alone or with standard ablation procedures can achieve short-term success preventing AF in patients with normal atria. Surgical interruption of ganglionated plexi without testing does not prevent postoperative AF. Pathologic states such as fibrosis might play more important roles than autonomic nerves.

Ventricular Tachycardia and Ventricular Fibrillation (Animal Studies)

A clinically relevant model results from dogs taught to run on a treadmill that have prior anterior myocardial infarction and then during the last minute of exercise undergo circumflex coronary occlusion resulting in additional acute ischemia that is maintained for 1 more minute after exercise. This model has resulted in important observations,[69] particularly in the area of reproducibility of VF in susceptible animals during coronary occlusion and less than 2% of VF occurring during reperfusion. The dogs resistant to VF never have occurrence of VF on multiple repeat tests. Dogs susceptible to VF have larger anterior infarction sizes of 18% versus the resistant group at 13%.

In this model, left stellate ganglionectomy was most effective in preventing VF in all of 11 susceptible animals. This effect is due to β_1 and β_2 blockade because both propranolol and ICI, a β_2 antagonist, but not α_1 blockade prevents VF. Efferent VNS also prevented VF in 27 of 30 susceptible animals, of which only five of nine were protected when atrial pacing prevented slower heart rate during exercise. BRS and HRV predict VF susceptibility when increased sympathetic and decreased parasympathetic influences predominate. Endurance training normalizes BRS and HRV and prevents VF. These studies support clinical observations and therapies in patients with coronary artery disease such as β-blockade and exercise training. Although it is clear that myocardial scar with superimposed ischemia and autonomic influence are required, three-dimensional initiating and maintaining mechanisms of the VF are unknown.

We have identified focal endocardial and Purkinje-mediated VT and VF induced in dogs with acute ischemia due to triggered activity[70]; in vitro triggered activity was inducible from endocardium excised from sites of focal VT (about 60%) much more often than from ischemic sites not at the origin of VT or VF (about 30%) or normal sites (about 5%). Isoproterenol superfusion was required to see triggered activity 75% of the time.[70] Because the endocardium and Purkinje are clearly innervated as demonstrated by studies with epicardial phenol denervation, it remains for us to document reflex modulation of sympathetic neural influences on this focal VT as we did previously in spontaneous VT 24 hours after coronary occlusion. This focal Purkinje VT occurs in patients with acute coronary syndromes.

That sympathetic neural activity directly gives rise to VT and VF has been shown by several studies. VF occurred in an anesthetized sheep with acute coronary occlusion from which central sympathetic nerve activity was being recorded.[71] Hemodynamics were intact until central sympathetic nerve activity dramatically increased prior to the development of VF. BRS relating blood pressure to RR interval was not changed in the immediate minutes before VF. During stellate ganglion stimulation,[72] a rat model of heart failure produced by myocardial infarction scar developed VT (37%) and VF (36%). This study found no VT or VF during stellate ganglion stimulation when myocardial infarction was not produced or small. Thus, the initiating effects of sympathetic stimulation occurred mainly in the presence of large infarction, a clinical predictor of VT and VF. Pacing and norepinephrine to the same levels produced by left stellate ganglion stimulation did not induce VT or VF. This model of heart failure is an important one because it does not require acute ischemia, as other models do. Thus sympathetic neural activation might trigger VT or VF, but the presence of severe structural heart disease is necessary.

Many laboratories have demonstrated at least transient malfunction of sympathetic effects in ventricle. Recent data suggest that this effect may be produced by endogenous adenosine inhibiting exocytotic norepinephrine release from nerve terminals.[73] When nerves do become damaged as a result of ischemia, denervation supersensitivity can occur.[1] However, the impact of supersensitivity on arrhythmogenesis in animal or human VT and VF is not clear. Although a halo of denervation surrounds animal and clinical infarcts, response to β-blockers and the specific characteristics of the arrhythmia in response to β-agonists do not clearly indicate that denervation supersensitivity plays a mechanistic role in the VT.

Spinal cord stimulation might also prevent VT and VF. In dogs with old anterior myocardial infarction, heart failure produced by pacing and a new circumflex coronary occlusion, spinal cord stimulation decreased blood pressure by 10 mm Hg and heart rate by 7.5 beats per minute. Spontaneous VF during repeat occlusion was significantly decreased from 59% to 23%.[74] The same model was used to show that clonidine at a dose of 100 to 250 μg injected intrathecally in the C8 to T4 region slowed heart rate after 21 minutes and decreased VF occurrence from nine of 12 to three of 12 dogs.[75] The latter might well be a central effect, but we have shown electrophysiologic responsiveness of α_2-adrenergic receptors located on Purkinje but not on ventricular muscle.[76] Clonidine given systemically prevents induction of focal endocardial VT in vivo and triggered activity in vitro, the latter at concentrations of 10^{-7} M. Thus clonidine has multiple antiarrhythmic effects both centrally and peripherally. Spinal cord stimulation may be an effective way to interrupt ischemic VT and VF.

Li[77] demonstrated a beneficial effect of VNS in rats after myocardial infarction with heart failure. VNS decreased heart rate by 25 beats per minute, left ventricular filling pressure from 24 to 17 mm Hg, and norepinephrine circulating levels from 1250 to 500 μg/mL. VNS improved survival from 50% without VNS to 90% by preventing VT and VF. These findings suggest that effects of VNS decrease norepinephrine release and prevent VF and improve survival in a heart-failure model.

Ando[78] studied rats with VNS, decreasing heart rate, during an acute coronary occlusion showing a reduction of VF compared with controls. However, rats preconditioned with VNS before occlusion also showed freedom from VT and VF without heart rate slowing. VNS preserved phosphorylated connexin43 in the ischemic zone, suggesting that gap junctional function was improved. We suggest that VNS prevented reentrant VT and VF, considering our data in acute myocardial infarction and reproducibly inducible VT given a drug that phosphorylates gap junctions, blocking only reentrant[79] but not triggered VT.[80] Future studies should confirm this effect of more physiologic parasympathetic stimulation.

In summary, increased sympathetic effects promote occurrence of VT and VF but clearly require damaged ventricles to operate. Triggered activity might account for VT and VF occurring with acute or ongoing ischemia, which might respond to autonomic interventions or ablation procedures targeted to the damaged area. Even reentry produced by coronary occlusion can be interrupted by improvements in connexin43, which can result from VNS. Physical training might also be helpful in reducing the likelihood of recurrent VT or VF by augmenting parasympathetic restraint on sympathetic neural influences as well as improving gap junction function. Stellate ganglionectomy and spinal cord stimulation are intriguing therapies that might substantially reduce VT and VF. However, short-term animal models might never truly mimic human VT and VF.

Ventricular Tachycardia and Ventricular Fibrillation (Patient Studies)

Coronary artery disease with or without myocardial infarction is the most common cause of VT in the West; mechanisms underlying these arrhythmias are reviewed in Chapter 62, and VTs occurring in diseased ventricles with no occluded vessels are reviewed in Chapters 63 and 66. Recent reviews have summarized present knowledge.[81]

HRV recorded before initiation of VT or VF can give insight in a role for the autonomics. Electrophysiologic Study Versus Electrocardiographic Monitoring (ESVEM) investigators showed heart rate increased prior to VT in all. Two subgroups were identified: those with a decrease in low-frequency power in the 2-hour period before VT and those with no change or increase. The first group also had a total decreased HRV via decreased parasympathetic effect, explaining the increase in heart rate. In the other group, patients had increased low-frequency power immediately prior to the episode, suggesting an increase in sympathetic effect. The autonomic effect on the ventricles was unknown, but the results suggest VT can occur by either decreased parasympathetic or increased sympathetic neural influences. Another report from the same trial also suggested multiple mechanisms that depended on whether VT was initiated by a morphologically distinct ventricular premature complex versus a premature complex with the same VT morphology. HRV before the different morphology group had no change, suggesting no autonomic alteration in initiation of VT. However, the same morphology group had an autonomic contribution as based on the HRV change before VT. Thus autonomic mechanisms might play a role when VT initiates at its origin.

Several but not all studies have suggested accuracy of HRV or BRS (studied by phenylephrine infusion) in predicting major arrhythmic events in patients with heart disease. Nevertheless, in a very well studied group of 263 patients with idiopathic disease[82] followed for 52 months, malignant VT or VF or sudden death occurred in 14%. There was no difference in HRV or BRS in patients who survived versus those who had malignant arrhythmias. Undoubtedly autonomic effects play a role in initiating some VT and VF; however, electrical abnormalities in diseased tissue can initiate other VT or VF.

Yet another case report of VF produced by left carotid sinus massage emphasized the possibility of neural mediation without a change in heart rate from 60 beats per minute or QT.[83] The patient was being evaluated for syncope and was not taking digitalis. Normal work-up included signal averaged ECG, repeated massage, and electrophysiology study with intravenous flecainide. An ICD was implanted without recorded VT or VF for 2 years. Thus a transient parasympathetic discharge, reflexly initiated, can produce enough electrophysiologic abnormality to fibrillate the heart.

Lampert[84] showed that patients with coronary disease undergoing noninvasive programmed stimulation via an ICD could have VT induced much easier with the recall of anger, associated with an increase in norepinephrine levels by 50%, proving neural release. The mental stress increased heart rate and blood pressure, shortened ventricular refractoriness, and importantly shortened the cycle length of the induced VT or VF, requiring ICD shock for therapy instead of previously successful pace termination. These findings show that an increase in sympathetic neural input to the ventricle promotes VT requiring ICD therapy.

Forty-two patients with ICD for secondary prevention were followed for ICD shocks. Chemoreflex[85] sensitivity was calculated by dividing the difference in heart rate produced by inhalation of 100% oxygen for 5 minutes, by the change in venous Po_2 with oxygen. Lower chemoreflex sensitivity (1.6 ± 1.1 vs 3.5 ± 2.3 ms/mm Hg) and ejection fraction (33% ± 16% vs 48% ± 18%), but not BRS, HRV, or abnormal signal-averaged ECG predicted ICD therapy for VT or VF. These data suggest an important initiating role for the chemoreflex; more studies of this index are warranted.

Simões[86] studied 67 patients with thallium perfusion scans as well as MIBG scans indicating sympathetic neural innervation in patients after myocardial infarction (see Chapter 37). The size of the perfusion defect was approximately one third of the MIBG defect (19 ± 15 vs 39 ± 22). The mismatch, which was uniform throughout the group in 60 of 67 patients, was not correlated with abnormal QTC or signal-averaged ECG. Only two cardiac deaths unrelated to the size of the denervated area occurred on follow-up. How the denervation measured by MIBG scan can influence inducibility of VT or VF in patients with ICD placed for secondary prophylaxis in patients of various etiologies was studied by repeated inductions for more than 2 years[87]; those with variable inducibility of VT or VF had more denervation than those with reproducible induction. Nearly all patients took a β-blocker or amiodarone, or both. However, denervation did not predict occurrence of spontaneous VT. Thus, we question whether denervation that results from myocardial infarction in fact plays any major mechanistic role in VT/VF.

In sum, sympathetic neural influence promotes occurrence of VT or VF in heart disease, often documented by HRV immediately preceding it; β-blockers are useful in preventing sudden cardiac death and ICD shock. However, β-blockers are competitive inhibitors, which can be overridden; approaches like spinal cord stimulation might provide more effective and continuous sympathetic suppression to reduce VT and VF. Population studies simply cannot use approaches such as HRV or BRS to predict who will have VT or VF because other electrophysiologic factors including scar size, additional ischemia, and heart failure influence ultimate occurrence of VT and VF.

Long-QT syndrome has perhaps been the best-studied nonstructural heart disease–mediated malignant arrhythmic syndrome producing VF in patients (Chapters 50 and 51). Although the primary defect in this heterogeneity of ion channel defects is not affected, sympathetic innervation has been studied, showing more heterogeneous sympathetic innervation by ^{11}C-hydroxyephedrine in persistently symptomatic patients of both defects in *KCNQ1* (LQT1) and LQT2 (HERG).[88] However, sympathetic neural denervation by stellate ganglionectomy has consistently been shown to protect against frequent symptomatic VT or VF,[89] especially for patients in whom effective β-blockade does not eliminate symptoms. This is particularly important when a patient is treated with an ICD, which produces sympathetic activation when a first shock treats an episode, setting up a possible storm of VT or VF. Improvements in the ganglionectomy surgery have shown effectiveness in suppressing VF and VT without producing Horner's syndrome.[90] Modern understanding of cardiac ionic channels notwithstanding, stellate ganglionectomy should be considered for continually symptomatic patients, ineffectively treated with β-blockers. A similar situation occurs in the catecholaminergic polymorphic VT associated with abnormalities of the ryanodine receptor (see Chapter 52). Nevertheless, stellate ganglionectomy has been quite effective in preventing VT, as indicated by initial reports.[91]

Takotsubo (ampula cardiomyopathy) is a possibly autonomically mediated large LV denervation problem. It has fewer spontaneous VTs on monitoring than age- and gender-matched patients with ST segment elevation myocardial infarction have despite longer QT but flatter, more normal, QT-RR relationships.[92] It occurs predominantly in menopausal women undergoing psychological or physical stress or even catheter ablation[93] accompanied by diffuse ECG T-wave inversions and large apical reversible dyskinesis. Serial imaging of sympathetic nerves without perfusion abnormalities demonstrated resolution toward normal over 1 year.[94]

Coronary vasospastic disease (ST segment elevation), also associated with denervation[95] is typically not observed.[93,94,96] However, 19 patients with the syndrome had blood epinephrine two to four times and norepinephrine two times that of patients with Killip class III acute myocardial infarction. Cardiac biopsy showed contraction necrosis indicating catecholamine damage. These findings suggest a pathophysiologic mechanism, perhaps originating in the brain.[96] However, no patient had VT or VF. Literature review produced only one episode of torsades de pointes[97]; given the frequency of reports, it would seem that sympathetic excess alone seems limited in production VT or VF in absence of heart disease.

The latter argument affects the hypothesis of voodoo death, proposed to be due to catecholamine excess and contraction band necrosis.[98] Because the latter does not have to be arrhythmogenic, voodoo death may be an example of two true statements without causation.

Depression either alone[99] or accompanying stroke[100] or MI may be an important risk factor for sudden death independent of other factors. These data correspond with observational studies suggesting depression is a risk factor for appropriate ICD shocks.[101] An animal model of depression, anhedonia, showed decreased HRV and facilitation of VT or VF with intravenous aconitine.[102] The risk of increased mortality is blocked by administration of antidepressant medication after the index event.[100] Given the connection of nerves in the dorsal raphe with the medullary autonomic centers, therapy with selective serotonin reuptake blockers makes sense. Taken together, these data, at least in stroke, suggest a direct brain involvement in provocation of VT and VF. It is not clear whether unknown structural heart disease is also producing the VT or VF.

Conclusion

We emphasize the highly organized regulation of the heart and vascular system by autonomic nerves. NCS can cause bradycardia, but syncope is produced by a vasodilation, mediated via sympathetic withdrawal associated with reduced BRS. Rarely, autonomic activation, either reflex or centrally driven, causes arrhythmias in isolation. Vagal parasympathetic effects might underlie lone AF both in initiating and possibly maintaining AF. EAD-mediated triggering might underlie pulmonary vein foci produced by both parasympathetic and sympathetic stimulation. Ablation of ganglionated plexi guided by high-frequency stimulation might alone or combined with other procedures prevent lone AF. Sympathetic neural effects clearly predominate in the ventricle initiating and perhaps maintaining VT or VF, whereas vagal parasympathetic effects antagonize the sympathetic.

However, almost all VT or VF depends on other disease states in the myocardium. Best studied in ischemic heart disease, triggered activity and reentry may be arrhythmia mechanisms by which autonomic effects involving α_2-adrenergic receptor activation and changes in connexin43 act, respectively. Physical training can physiologically improve vagal antagonism of adrenergic effects in heart failure and ischemic heart disease. As an adjuctive intervention, spinal cord stimulation may be a new, effective means to control arrhythmia occurrence in all heart chambers.

References

1. Schwartz PJ, Zipes DP: Autonomic modulation of cardiac arrhythmias. In Zipes DP, Jalife J (eds): Cardiac Electrophysiology: From Cell to Bedside, 3rd ed. Philadelphia, WB Saunders, 2000, pp 300-314.
2. Steinberg SF, Robinson RB, Rosen MR: Molecular and cellular bases of β-adrenergic and α-adrenergic modulation of cardiac rhythm. In Zipes DP, Jalife J (eds): Cardiac Electrophysiology: From Cell to Bedside, 4th ed. Philadelphia, WB Saunders, 2005, pp 291-297.
3. Olshansky B: Interrelationships between the autonomic nervous system and atrial fibrillation. Prog Cardiovasc Dis 48:57-78, 2005.
4. Armour JA: Cardiac neuronal hierarchy in health and disease. Am J Physiol 287:R262-R271, 2004.
5. Mircoli L, Fedele L, Betetti M, et al: Preservation of the baroreceptor heart rate reflex by chemical sympathectomy in experimental heart failure. Circulation 106: 866-872, 2002.
6. Foreman RD: Neurological mechanisms of chest pain and cardiac disease. Cleve Clin J Med 74:S30-S42, 2007.
7. Olgin JE, Takahashi T, Wilson E, et al: Effects of thoracic spinal cord stimulation on cardiac autonomic regulation of the sinus and atrioventicular nodes. J Cardiovasc Electrophysiol 13:475-481, 2002.
8. Foreman RD, Linderoth B, Ardell JL, et al: Modulation of intrinsic cardiac neurons by spinal cord stimulation: Implications from its therapeutic use in angina pectoris. Cardiovasc Res 47:367-375, 2000.
9. Pickering AE, Boscan P, Paton JFR: Nociception attenuates parasympathetic but not sympathetic baroreflex via NK_1 receptors in the rat nucleus tractus solitarii. J Physiol 551:589-599, 2003.
10. Moffitt JA, Johnson AK: Short-term fluoxetine treatment enhances baroreflex control of sympathetic nerve system activity after hindlimb unloading. Am J Physiol 286: R584-R590, 2004.
11. Qu J, Robinson RB: Cardiac ion channel expression and regulation: The role of innervation. J Mol Cell Cardiol 37:439-448, 2004.
12. Konidala S, Gutterman DD: Coronary vasospasm and the regulation of coronary blood flow. Prog Cardiovasc Dis 46: 349-373, 2004.
13. Paton JFR, Nalivaiko E, Boscan P, et al: Reflexly evoked coactivation of cardiac

vagal and sympathetic motor outflows: Observations and functional implications. Clin Exp Pharmacol Physiol 33:1245-1250, 2006.
14. Pickering AE, Boscan P, Paton JFR: Nociception attenuates parasympathetic but not sympathetic baroreflex via NK_1 receptors in the rat nucleus tractus solitarii. J Physiol 551:589-599, 2003.
15. Khurana RK, Wu, R: The cold face test: A non-baroreflex mediated test of cardiac vagal function. Clin Auto Res 16:202-207, 2006.
16. Mathias CJ, Young TM: Water drinking in the management of orthostatic intolerance due to orthostatic hypotension, vasovagal syncope and the postural tachycardia syndrome. Eur J Neurol 11:613-619, 2004.
17. Grubb BP: Neurocardiogenic syncope and related disorders of orthostatic intolerance. Circulation 111:2997-3006, 2005.
18. Jardine DL, Melton IC, Crozier IG, et al: Decrease in cardiac output and muscle sympathetic activity during vasovagal syncope. Am J Physiol 282:H1804-H1809, 2002.
19. Béchir M, Binggeli C, Corti R, et al: Dysfunctional baroreflex regulation of sympathetic nerve activity in patients with vasovagal syncope. Circulation 107:1620-1625, 2003.
20. Kamiya A, Michikami D, Fu Q, et al: Pathophysiology of orthostatic hypotension after bed rest: Paradoxical sympathetic withdrawal. Am J Physiol 285: H1158-H1167, 2003.
21. Ichinose M, Saito M, Fujii N, et al: Modulation of the control of muscle sympathetic nerve activity during severe orthostatic stress. J Physiol 576:947-958, 2006.
22. Gulli G, Cooper VL, Claydon VE, et al: Prolonged latency in the baroreflex mediated vascular resistance response in subjects with postural related syncope. Clin Auton Res 15:207-212, 2005.
23. Donadio V, Liguori R, Elam M, et al: Arousal elicits exaggerated inhibition of sympathetic nerve activity in phobic syncope patients. Brain 130:1653-1662, 2007.
24. Streian CG, Socoteanu I, Cozma D: Glomectomy in carotid sinus syncope and associated arrhythmias: Symptomatic bradycardia, atrial flutter and atrial fibrillation. Rom J Intern Med 44(2):153-163, 2006.
25. Leon H, Guzman JC, Kuusela T, et al: Impaired baroreflex gain in patients with inappropriate sinus tachycardia. J Cardiovasc Electrophysiol 16:64-68, 2005.
26. Markowitz SM, Christini DJ, Stein KM, et al: Time course and predictors of autonomic dysfunction after ablation of the slow atrioventricular nodal pathway. Pacing Clin Electrophysiol 27:1638-1643, 2004.
27. Emkanjoo Z, Alasti M, Haghjoo AM, et al: Heart rate variability: Does it change after RF ablation of reentrant supraventricular tachycardia? Int J Cardiol 14:147-151, 2005.
28. Guo H, Wang P, Xing Y, et al: Delayed injury of autonomic nerve induced by radiofrequency catheter ablation. J Electrocardiol 40:355.e1-355.e4, 2007.
29. Kongo M, Fujii E, Matsuoka K, et al: Changes in autonomic nervous activity after catheter ablation of atrial tachycardia arising from the atrioventricular annulus. Pacing Clin Electrophysiol 28:S237-S241, 2005.
30. Swift NM, Charkoudian N, Dotson RM, et al: Baroreflex control of muscle sympathetic nerve activity in postural orthostatic tachycardia syndrome. Am J Physiol 289:H1226-H1233, 2005.
31. Goldstein DS, Holmes C, Frank SM, et al: Cardiac sympathetic dysautonomia in chronic orthostatic intolerance syndromes. Circulation 106:2358-2365, 2002.
32. Chen J, Wasmund SL, Hamdan MH: Back to the future: The role of the autonomic nervous system in atrial fibrillation. Pacing Clin Electrophysiol 29:413-421, 2006.
33. Tai CT, Chiou CW, Chen SA: Interaction between the autonomic nervous system and atrial tachyarrhythmias. J Cardiovasc Electrophysiol 13:83-87, 2002.
34. Rosenshtraukh LV, Fedorov VV, Sharifov OF: Cholinergic atrial fibrillation. In Zipes DP, Jalife J (eds): Cardiac Electrophysiology: From Cell to Bedside, 4th ed. Philadelphia, WB Saunders, 2005, pp 291-297.
35. Nattel S, Shiroshita-Takeshita A, Brundel BJJM, et al: Mechanisms of atrial fibrillation: Lessons from animal models. Prog Cardiovasc Dis 48:9-28, 2005.
36. Arora R, Villuendas R, Ng J, et al: Targeted G-protein inhibition in the posterior left atrium: A novel method to selectively inhibit parasympathetic signaling in the left atrium. Heart Rhythm 4:S9, 2007.
37. Ulphani JS, Arora R, Cain JH, et al: The ligament of Marshall as a parasympathetic conduit. Am J Physiol 293:H1629-H1635, 2007.
38. Zhou J, Scherlag BJ, Edwards J, et al: Gradients of atrial refractoriness and inducibility of atrial fibrillation due to stimulation of ganglionated plexi. J Cardiovasc Electrophysiol 18:83-90, 2007.
39. Schauerte P, Scherlag BJ, Pitha J, et al: Catheter ablation of cardiac autonomic nerves for prevention of vagal atrial fibrillation. Circulation 102:2774-2780, 2000.
40. Patterson E, Yu X, Huang S, et al: Suppression of autonomic-mediated triggered firing in pulmonary vein preparations, 24 hours postcoronary artery ligation in dogs. J Cardiovasc Electrophysiol 17:763-770, 2006.
41. Patterson E, Po SS, Scherlag BJ, et al: Triggered firing in pulmonary veins initiated by in vitro autonomic nerve stimulation. Heart Rhythm 2(6):624-631, 2005.
42. Scherlag BJ, Nakagawa H, Jackman WM, et al: Electrical stimulation to identify neural elements on the heart: Their role in atrial fibrillation. J Interv Card Electrophysiol 13:37-42, 2005.
43. Razavi M, Zhang S, Yang D, et al: Effects of pulmonary vein ablation on regional vagal innervation and vulnerability to atrial fibrillation in dogs. J Cardiovasc Electrophysiol 16:879-884, 2005.
44. Oh S, Zhang Y, Bibevski S, et al: Vagal denervation and atrial fibrillation inducibility: Epicardial fat pad ablation does not have long-term effects. Heart Rhythm 3:701-708, 2006.
45. Hirose M, Carlson MD, Laurita KR: Cellular mechanisms of vagally mediated atrial tachyarrhythmias in isolated arterially perfused canine right atria. J Cardiovasc Electrophysiol 13:918-926, 2002.
46. Hirose M, Leatmanoratn Z, Laurita KR, et al: Partial vagal denervation increases vulnerability to vagally induced atrial fibrillation. J Cardiovasc Electrophysiol 13:1272-1279, 2002.
47. Armour JA, Richer LP, Pagé P, et al: Origin and pharmacological responses of atrial tachyarrhythmias induced by activation of mediastinal nerves in canines. Auton Neurosci 118:68-78, 2005.
48. Cardinal R, Pagé P, Vermeulen M, et al: Spinal cord stimulation suppresses bradycardias and atrial tachyarrhymias induced by mediastinal nerve stimulation in dogs. Am J Physiol 291:R1369-R1375, 2006.
49. Fioranelli M, Piccoli M, Mileto GM, et al: Analysis of heart rate variability five minutes before the onset of paroxysmal atrial fibrillation. Pacing Clin Electrophysiol 22:743-749, 1999.
50. Tomita T, Takei M, Saikawa Y, et al: Role of autonomic tone in the initiation and termination of paroxysmal atrial fibrillation in patients without structural heart disease. J Cardiovasc Electrophysiol 14:559-564, 2003.
51. Dimmer C, Szili-Torok T, Tavernier R, et al: Initiating mechanisms of paroxysmal atrial fibrillation. Europace 5:1-9, 2003.
52. Amar D, Zhang H, Miodownik S, et al: Competing autonomic mechanisms precede the onset of postoperative atrial fibrillation. J Am Coll Cardiol 42:1262-1268, 2003.
53. Hamdan MH, Zagrodzky JD, Page RL, et al: Effect of P-wave timing during supraventricular tachycardia on the hemodynamic and sympathetic neural responses. Circulation 103:96-101, 2001.
54. Tai CT, Chiou CW, Wen ZH, et al: Effect of phenylephrine on focal atrial fibrillation originating in the pulmonary veins and superior vena cava. J Am Coll Cardiol 36:788-793, 2000.
55. Manolis A, Giotopoulou A, Koutouzis M, et al: Atrial fibrillation induced by carotid sinus massage (Letter to the Editor). Int J Cardiol 114:e103-e104, 2007.
56. Patterson E, Jackman WM, Beckman KJ, et al: Spontaneous pulmonary vein firing in man: Relationship to tachycardia-pause early afterdepolarizations and triggered arrhythmia in canine pulmonary veins in vitro. J Cardiovasc Electrophysiol 18:1067-1075, 2007.
57. Lemery R, Birnie D, Tang ASL, et al: Feasibility study of endocardial mapping of ganglionated plexuses during catheter ablation of atrial fibrillation. Heart Rhythm 3:387-396, 2006.
58. Verma A, Saliba WI, Lakkireddy D, et al: Vagal responses induced by endocardial left atrial autonomic ganglion stimulation before and after pulmonary vein antrum isolation for atrial fibrillation. Heart Rhythm 4:1177-1182, 2007.
59. Oral H, Chugh A, Scharf C, et al: Pulmonary vein isolation for vagotonic, adrenergic and random episodes of

paroxysmal atrial fibrillation. J Cardiovasc Electrophysiol 15:402-405, 2004.

60. Pappone C, Santinelli V, Manguso F, et al: Pulmonary vein denervation enhances long-term benefit after circumferential ablation for paroxysmal atrial fibrillation. Circulation 109:327-334, 2004.
61. Bauer A, Deisenhofer I, Schneider R, et al: Effects of circumferential or segmental pulmonary vein ablation for paroxysmal atrial fibrillation on cardiac autonomic function. Heart Rhythm 3:1428-1435, 2006.
62. Nademanee K, McKenzie J, Kosar E, et al: A new approach for catheter ablation of atrial fibrillation: Mapping of the electrophysiologic substrate. J Am Coll Cardiol 43:2054-2056, 2004.
63. Scherlag BJ, Patterson E, Po SS: The neural basis of atrial fibrillation. J Electrocardiol 39:S180-S183, 2006.
64. Scanavacca M, Pisani CF, Hachul D, et al: Selective atrial vagal denervation guided by evoked vagal reflex to treat patients with paroxysmal atrial fibrillation. Circulation 114:876-885, 2006.
65. Mehall JR, Kohut RM, Schneeberger EW, et al: Intraoperative epicardial electrophysiologic mapping and isolation and autonomic ganglionic plexi. Ann Thorac Surg 83:538-541, 2007.
66. Davis Z, Jacobs KH: Aortic fat pad destruction and postoperative atrial fibrillation. Card Electrophysiol Rev 7:185-1188, 2003.
67. Melo J, Voigt P, Sonmez B, et al: Ventral cardiac denervation reduced the incidence of atrial fibrillation after coronary artery bypass grafting. J Thorac Cardiovasc Surg 127:511-516, 2004.
68. Alex J, Guvendik L: Evaluation of ventral cardiac denervation as a prophylaxis against atrial fibrillation after coronary artery bypass grafting. Ann Thorac Surg 79:517-20, 2005.
69. Billman GE: A comprehensive review and analysis of 25 years of data from an in vivo canine model of sudden cardiac death: Implications for future anti-arrhythmic drug development. Pharmacology & Therapeutics 111:808-835, 2006.
70. Xing D, Martins JB: Triggered activity due to delayed afterdepolarizations in sites of focal origin of ischemic ventricular tachycardia. Am J Physiol 287:H2078-H2084, 2004.
71. Jardine DI, Charles CJ, Forrester MDE, et al: A neural mechanism for sudden death after myocardial infarction. Clin Auton Res 13:339-341, 2003.
72. Du XJ, Cox HS, Dart AM, et al: Sympathetic activation triggers ventricular arrhythmias in rat heart with chronic infarction and failure. Cardiovasc Res 43:919-929, 1999.
73. Burgdorf C, Richardt D, Kurz T, et al: Adenosine inhibits norepinephrine release in the postischemic rat heart: The mechanism of neuronal stunning. Cardiovasc Res 49:713-720, 2001.
74. Issa ZF, Zhou X, Ujhelyi MR, et al: Thoracic spinal cord stimulation reduces the risk of ischemic ventricular arrhythmias in a postinfarction heart failure canine model. Circulation 111:3217-3220, 2005.
75. Issa ZF, Ujhelyi MR, Hildebrand KR, et al: Intrathecal clonidine reduces the incidence of ischemia-provoked ventricular arrhythmias in a canine post-infarction heart failure model. Heart Rhythm 2:1122-1127, 2005.
76. Arnar DO, Xing D, Lee HC, et al: Prevention of ischemic ventricular tachycardia of purkinje origin: A role for α-2 adrenoceptors in purkinje? Am J Physiol 280:H1182-H1190, 2001.
77. Li M, Zheng C, Sato T, et al: Vagal nerve stimulation markedly improves long-term survival after chronic heart failure in rats. Circulation 109:120-124, 2004.
78. Ando M, Katare RG, Kakinuma Y, et al: Efferent vagal nerve stimulation protects heart against ischemia-induced arrhythmias by preserving connexin43 protein. Circulation 112:164-170, 2005.
79. Xing D, Kjølbye AL, Nielsen MS, et al: ZP123 increases gap junctional conductance and prevents reentrant ventricular tachycardia during myocardial ischemia in open chest dogs. J Cardiovasc Electrophysiol 14:510-520, 2003.
80. Xing D, Kjølbye AL, Petersen JS, et al: Pharmacological stimulation of cardiac gap junction coupling does not affect ischemia-induced focal ventricular tachycardia or triggered activity in dogs. Am J Physiol 288:H511-H516, 2005.
81. Verrier RL, Antzelevitch C: Autonomic aspects of arrhythmogenesis: The enduring and the new. Curr Opin Cardiol 19:2-11, 2004.
82. Grimm W, Christ M, Sharkova J, et al: Arrhythmia risk prediction in idiopathic dilated cardiomyopathy based on heart rate variability and baroreflex sensitivity. Pacing Clin Electrophysiol 28:S202-S206, 2005.
83. Deepak SM, Jenkins NP, Davidson NC, et al: Ventricular fibrillation induced by carotid sinus massage without preceding bradycardia. Europace 7:638-640, 2005.
84. Lampert R, Jain D, Burg MM, et al: Destabilizing effects of mental stress on ventricular arrhythmias in patients with implantable cardioverter-defibrillators. Circulation 101:158-164, 2000.
85. Hennersdorf MG, Niebch V, Perings C, et al: Chemoreflex sensitivity as a predictor of arrhythmias relapse in ICD recipients. Int J Cardiol 86:169-175, 2002.
86. Simões MV, Barthel P, Matsunari I, et al: Presence of sympathetically denervated but viable myocardium and its electrophysiologic correlates after early revascularized, acute myocardial infarction. Eur Heart J 25:551-557, 2004.
87. Hayashi M, Kobayashi Y, Morita N, et al: Clinical significance and contributing factors of long-term variability in induced ventricular tachyarrhythmias. J Cardiovasc Electrophysiol 14:1049-1056, 2003.
88. Mazzadi AN, André-Fouët X, Duisit J, et al: Cardiac retention of [^{11}C]HED in genotyped long QT patients: A potential amplifier role for severity of the disease. Am J Physiol 385:H1286-H1293, 2003.
89. Schwartz PJ, Priori SG, Cerrone M, et al: Left cardiac sympathetic denervation in the management of high-risk patients affected by the long-QT syndrome. Circulation 109:1826-1833, 2004.
90. Li C, Hu D, Shang L, et al: Surgical left cardiac sympathetic denervation for long QT syndrome: Effects on QT interval and heart rate. Heart Vessels 20:137-141, 2005.
91. Facchini M, Crotti L, Ferrandi C, et al: Left cardiac sympathetic denervation for catecholaminergic polymorphic ventricular tachycardia. Heart Rhythm 4:S48, 2007.
92. Bonnemeier H, Ortak J, Bode F, et al: Modulation of ventricular repolarization in patients with transient left ventricular apical ballooning: A case control study. J Cardiovasc Electrophysiol 17:1340-1347, 2006.
93. Davis DR, Lemery R, Green M, et al: Transient left ventricular apical ballooning following a prolonged ablation. J Interv Card Electrophysiol 17:47-49, 2006.
94. Owa M, Aizawa K, Urasawa N, et al: Emotional stress-induced "ampulla cardiomyopathy"—discrepancy between the metabolic an sympathetic innervation imaging performed during the recovery course. Jpn Circ J 65:349-352, 2001.
95. Watanabe K, Takahashi T, Miyajima S, et al: Myocardial sympathetic denervation, fatty acid metabolism, and left ventricular wall motion in vasospastic angina. J Nucl Med 43:1476-1481, 2002.
96. Wittstein IS, Thiemann DR, Lima JAC, et al: Neurohumoral features of myocardial stunning due to sudden emotional stress. N Engl J Med 352:539-548, 2005.
97. Nault MA, Baranchuk A, Simpson CS, et al: Takotsubo cardiomyopathy: A novel "proarrhythmic" disease. Anatol J Cardiol 7 Suppl 1:101-103, 2007.
98. Samuels MA: Voodoo death revisited: The modern lessons of neurocardiology. Cleveland Clinical J Med 74:S8-S14, 2007.
99. Empana JP, Jouven X, Lemaitre RN, et al: Clinical depression and risk of out-of-hospital cardiac arrest. Arch Intern Med 166:195-200, 2006.
100. Jorge RE, Robinson RG, Arndt S, et al: Mortality and poststroke depression: A placebo-controlled trial of antidepressants. Am J Psychiatry 160:1823-1829, 2003.
101. Whang W, Albert CM, Sears SF Jr, et al, for the TOVA Study Investigators: Depression as a predictor for appropriate shocks among patients with implantable cardioverter-defibrillators. J Am Coll Cardiol 45:1090-1095, 2005.
102. Grippo AJ, Santos CM, Johnson RF, et al: Increased susceptibility to ventricular arrhythmias in a rodent model of experimental depression. Am J Physiol 286:H619-H626, 2004.

Role of Cardiac and Thoracic Veins in Arrhythmogenesis 39

Méléze Hocini, Prashanthan Sanders, Pierre Jaïs, Jacques Clémenty, and Michel Haïssaguerre

CHAPTER OUTLINE

Atrial fibrillation (AF) is the most common sustained cardiac arrhythmia affecting humans.[1] Although several theories have been advanced for the mechanisms maintaining AF, the importance of the interaction among triggers, perpetuators, and substrate in initiating and maintaining AF is increasingly recognized.[2] Recent evidence has demonstrated an important role for rapid and repetitive activity originating from the thoracic veins in this process. More than 90% of triggers initiating AF have been observed to originate from the pulmonary veins,[3] and the remainder originate from the superior vena cava (SVC), coronary sinus, ligament of Marshall, left superior vena cava (SVC), and scattered other atrial sites (crista terminalis, atrial myocardium, and atrioventricular valves). These thoracic veins appended to the atria have atrial muscle sleeves that extend a variable distance into these structures and have been implicated in the mechanisms of atrial tachycardia (AT) and also AF.[3-7] This chapter reviews the evidence that focal sources from the pulmonary and thoracic veins are involved in the initiation and maintenance of AF.

Role of the Pulmonary Veins

Pulmonary Vein Tachycardia and Triggers Initiating Atrial Fibrillation

The pulmonary veins are implicated in focal AT and in the initiation and maintenance of AF. In a large series of patients at a single center, focal AT originating from the pulmonary veins accounted for 16% of all focal ATs and 78% of all left atrial ATs.[8] Clinical studies have demonstrated that up to 94% of triggers initiating AF originate within the pulmonary veins.[3] These triggers interact with the atrial substrate by using discrete or wide fascicles connecting the pulmonary veins to the left atrium (LA); ablation of these connections electrically isolates the pulmonary veins. However, even after electrical isolation, the pulmonary veins have been observed to have spontaneous dissociated slow rhythms in up to 33% of pulmonary veins (see Fig. 39-2) and can sustain spontaneous or induced tachycardia within the pulmonary vein, further highlighting their arrhythmogenic potential.[9]

Several factors suggest that the mechanisms of arrhythmogenicity in these arrhythmias may be different. Patients with paroxysmal AF originating from the pulmonary veins often demonstrate a wide spectrum of atrial arrhythmias that coexist; these include isolated ectopy, bursts of AT, atrial flutter, and AF. At electrophysiologic evaluation, patients with AF might have multiple pulmonary vein foci in multiple veins, and many of these foci originate distally in those veins. These features have mandated a strategy of electrical isolation of the pulmonary veins. In contrast, patients with focal AT originating from the pulmonary veins demonstrate largely a focal process, without evidence of a more progressive and diffuse process as observed in the AF population and without a tendency to develop further atrial arrhythmias during long-term follow-up.[8] In the vast majority of these cases, the focus originated from the ostium of the vein (or within 1 cm of the designated ostium) rather than from further distally (2 to 4 cm) and was curable by focal ablation.

Mechanisms of Arrhythmogenicity of Pulmonary Veins

Several mechanisms have been postulated and observed for pulmonary vein arrhythmogenicity. Studies have suggested that the pulmonary veins are capable of sustaining automaticity. Blom and colleagues, studying the human embryo using monoclonal antibodies to stain conducting tissue, demonstrated the presence of cardiac conduction tissue within the pulmonary vein during embryonic development.[10] However, although node-like cells have been observed in the pulmonary veins of rats, detailed histology of the atrial myocardial sleeves in human hearts has thus far failed to reveal any node-like structures. Cheung found spontaneous activity from the pulmonary vein in the guinea pig with digitalis.[11] Other experiments have demonstrated early and delayed afterdepolarization and automatic high-frequency irregular rhythms related to calcium-sensitive inward currents following infusion of ryanodine, atrial distention, rapid atrial pacing, or congestive heart failure, but most groups have not observed these in normal pulmonary vein cardiomyocytes.[12-14]

A possible role for reentry has also been implicated in the genesis of spontaneous activity from the pulmonary vein. Conduction delay and block have been associated with changing myocardial fiber orientation, producing nonuniform anisotropy and fractionated electrograms in pulmonary veins and at the pulmonary vein–left atrial junction.[15] Arora and coworkers, performing optical mapping studies of normal canine pulmonary vein, demonstrated that these structures possess both anisotropic conduction and repolarization heterogeneity. With extrastimulus testing they observed regions of unidirectional conduction block and slowed conduction that then initiated leading circle reentry, becoming sustained with the use of isoproterenol. Focal sources of activity were observed to occur more proximally.

In the clinical setting, ectopy initiating episodes of AF has been largely localized to the distal pulmonary vein musculature, from multiple pulmonary veins or from multiple sites within a given pulmonary vein. Chen and colleagues demonstrated that the distal pulmonary vein had significantly shorter refractory periods than the adjacent LA.[16] Jaïs and coauthors demonstrated distinctive electrophysiologic properties in the pulmonary veins in patients with AF (compared to controls), with shorter pulmonary vein refractory periods, more frequent and greater degree of decremental conduction to the LA, and a propensity for pulmonary vein extrastimuli to initiate AF.[17] At shorter coupling intervals there was increased complexity of the circumferential activation sequence, with fractionation, double potentials and change in the LA breakthrough. Sanders and colleagues have demonstrated that these observations are accentuated in the setting of atrial stretch, a frequent substrate predisposing to AF.[18]

Several mechanisms have been implied in pulmonary vein arrhythmogenicity. In a large series of patients, Arentz and coworkers used a high-density 64-pole basket catheter to investigate the activation pattern of spontaneous pulmonary vein ectopic beats and the initial 2 seconds of AF. They demonstrated that, in the majority of cases, there was centrifugal activation favoring a focal mechanism. Kumagai and colleagues have provided further evidence supporting a reentrant mechanism for arrhythmia originating from the pulmonary veins by demonstrating directional conduction delay within the pulmonary vein, with regions of preferential conduction within the pulmonary vein, with exit and entry of the activation front at the pulmonary vein–left atrial junction during short bursts of repetitive activity.[19]

Pulmonary Veins in the Maintenance of Atrial Fibrillation

The pulmonary veins have also been implicated in the maintenance of paroxysmal AF in some patients. Jaïs and coauthors have observed rapid focal discharges sustained sometimes for hours, days, or even longer that drive sustained AF, representing the true focal or focally driven AF. Focal ablation eliminated the arrhythmia, demonstrating that pulmonary veins formed not only the trigger but also the substrate maintaining AF. Wu and colleagues performed high-density mapping at the time of surgery in patients with chronic AF and identified rapid activity emanating from the pulmonary vein region (corners of the mapping plaque) continuously, intermittently, or alternately.[20]

Pulmonary vein isolation performed during ongoing AF has given a novel insight into the machanisms of AF. We performed pulmonary vein ablation in patients with long-duration spontaneous or induced AF while monitoring the AF cycle length (AFCL) at a site remote to ablation (coronary sinus or left atrial appendage).[21] Pulmonary vein isolation produced a progressive prolongation of the AFCL, varying in extent from vein to vein and between patients, culminating in AF termination in 75% of patients, after a significant cumulative increase in the AFCL. This decline in AF frequency was less in patients without AF termination. There was a significant relationship between the number of pulmonary veins requiring isolation to achieve termination and the initial duration of AF, but there was no correlation with the amount of radiofrequency (RF) energy delivery. Strikingly, in several series it has been demonstrated that following isolation of the pulmonary veins, AF is no longer inducible in 50% to 60% of patients despite repetitive and aggressive burst pacing. Indeed, noninducibility in this setting has been demonstrated to predict a better long-term outcome from pulmonary vein isolation.[21-23]

The global frequency of fibrillatory activity progressively declines with pulmonary vein ablation, providing evidence for the direct participation of pulmonary vein activity in the maintenance of paroxysmal AF. pulmonary vein isolation produced not only prolongation of AFCL but also termination of AF. This strongly suggests that at least for paroxysmal AF, the arrhythmia mechanism is not one that is random (wandering wavelets widely distributed) but rather one with organization (sources confined) whereby the pulmonary vein–left atrial junction has a critical role (the venous wave hypothesis).[24]

Pulmonary Veins in Permanent Atrial Fibrillation

In a selected group of patients we have previously observed that the pulmonary veins may have a crucial role in persistent and permanent AF.[25] In this study, following cardioversion of persistent AF, triggers reinitiating AF were targeted at the pulmonary vein and resulted in a modest long-term suppression of arrhythmia. More recently we have extended these observations in a nonselected group of patients with persistent and permanent AF. In this study, we have demonstrated that AF can be terminated by catheter ablation in 87% of patients using a randomized stepwise approach, initially converting AF to AT and then subsequently up to sinus rhythm.[26,27]

During such a staged procedure, we evaluated the impact of the ablation at various sites on the basis of prolongation of the AF cycle length (at a remote site), and conversion to AT and to sinus rhythm. In so doing, three sites were identified as critical regions contributing to the maintenance of persistent and permanent AF: the pulmonary veins, the coronary sinus, and the base of the left atrial appendage. Although prior studies have not consistently demonstrated an effect on the AF process by pulmonary vein ablation being performed as a first step in this subset of patients,[28,29] using a randomized order of ablation, we observed a mean increase in AFCL (7.52 ± 8.87 ms), with a significant prolongation of AFCL observed in 56% by pulmonary vein ablation.

These observations argue in favor of the pulmonary veins being an important perpetuator or substrate in persistent or permanent AF. Nevertheless, in our experience, in this subset of patients, pulmonary vein isolation as a sole strategy is of limited use, implicating additional atrial or venous sites in the mechanisms of AF.

Catheter Ablation of the Pulmonary Veins

With the significant evidence for the role of the pulmonary vein in all forms of AF, either as triggers or as part of the perpetuators or substrate for AF, and given the frequent occurrence of multiple sites within a certain pulmonary vein and also involvement of multiple pulmonary veins, we have included empirical electrical isolation of these structures in all patients undergoing ablation of AF without any attempt to identify arrhythmogenic veins. Isolation is routinely performed and confirmed using a

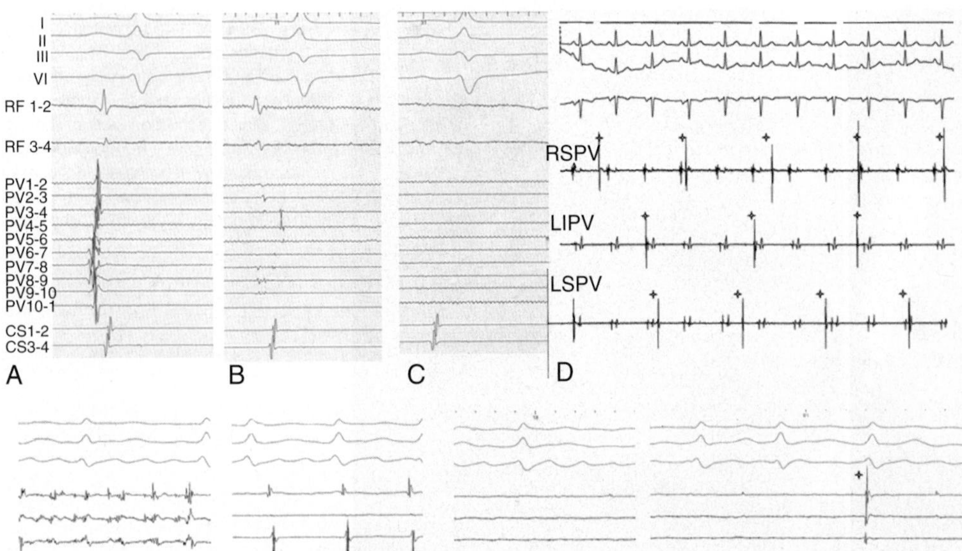

Figure 39-1 Electrical isolation of the pulmonary vein during sinus rhythm. **A,** The initial target for this patient was the site of earliest activity located at the bottom of the right superior pulmonary vein. **B,** This led to a change in pulmonary vein activation. **C,** Ablation at top anterior results in electrical isolation. **D,** Dissociation (+) of pulmonary vein electrical activity. Demonstrated is the circumferential mapping signals at the right and left superior pulmonary vein and inferior left pulmonary vein in sinus rhythm. **E** to **G,** Electrical isolation of right superior pulmonary vein during atrial fibrillation. **H,** Dissociation of pulmonary vein electrical activity.

circumferential mapping catheter positioned at the venous ostium (Lasso catheter). As isolation of pulmonary veins is performed in the vast majority of patients during atrial fibrillation, ablation is deployed circumferentially individually or as ipsilateral pairs. The power is limited to 30 W for the right veins and 25 W for the anterior aspect of the left veins, where infringement within the proximal portion of the veins is often necessary to achieve isolation. Temperature is limited to 48°C, with a target tissue temperature of 42°C achieved by manual titration of the irrigation rate between 5 and 20 mL/min (0.9% saline via Cool Flow [Biosense Webster, Waterloo, Belgium]).

The endpoint of ablation is the elimination or dissociation of all pulmonary vein potentials (Figs. 39-1, 39-2, and 39-3). This procedural endpoint is achieved in 100% of patients with a cooled-tip catheter. Data from our institution demonstrate that pulmonary vein isolation can be performed using 35 ± 15 minutes of RF energy application and takes 70 ± 21 minutes to perform. The success of ablation when pulmonary vein isolation is used as an endpoint has been remarkably similar from a number of groups. In our experience, at 10 ± 5 months of follow-up, 69% of patients with paroxysmal AF have remained in sinus rhythm without antiarrhythmic drugs.

Superior Vena Cava

Mechanisms of Superior Vena Cava Arrhythmogenicity

Of the other thoracic veins, the SVC is probably the most common cause of AF. Previous studies have shown that myocardial fibers connect the right atrium (RA) to the SVC, and electrical activity within these fibers could trigger arrhythmias in a manner similar to the pulmonary veins. Electrically active myocardial tissue has been recorded up to 5 cm within the SVC. Chen and coworkers have demonstrated heterogeneity in this myocardial sleeve and also that isolated cardiomyocytes from this muscle are capable of spontaneous depolarization.[30] The origin of the SVC from the right sinus horn probably provides the embryologic basis for the arrhythmogenic activity of SVC cardiomyocytes in AF induction and maintenance.

Superior Vena Cava in Initiating and Maintaining Atrial Fibrillation

Although electrical activity had been described from the atrial myocardial extensions within the SVC, their role in the initiation of AF was only described in 1994. We demonstrated a focal source at the junction of the SVC and the RA in a patient with paroxysmal AF.[31] Ino and colleagues reported a case of focal AF confined to the SVC where successful ablation was performed at the earliest site, 3 cm within the SVC.[32] Tsai and coauthors have demonstrated that in a consecutive series of patients undergoing paroxysmal AF ablation, 7% had triggering activity from the SVC.[6] These ectopic events had electrophysiologic similarities to those arising from the pulmonary veins in the initiation of AF, but they were distinctly recognizable by their P wave morphology, which was similar to sinus rhythm, with significantly higher amplitude in the inferior leads, by virtue of their anatomic origin at the top of the heart. Several clinical studies have reported that AF or AT could originate in the SVC and demonstrated the safety and efficacy of ablation within this structure.[6,33] Lin and colleagues have reported that 37% of the non–pulmonary vein triggers were from the SVC.[34] During repeated procedures, 20% of AF recurrences were initiated by SVC triggers.[35]

Although it has been suggested that there may be significant ethnic differences to account for these observations, recently others have made similar observations. Arruda and coworkers

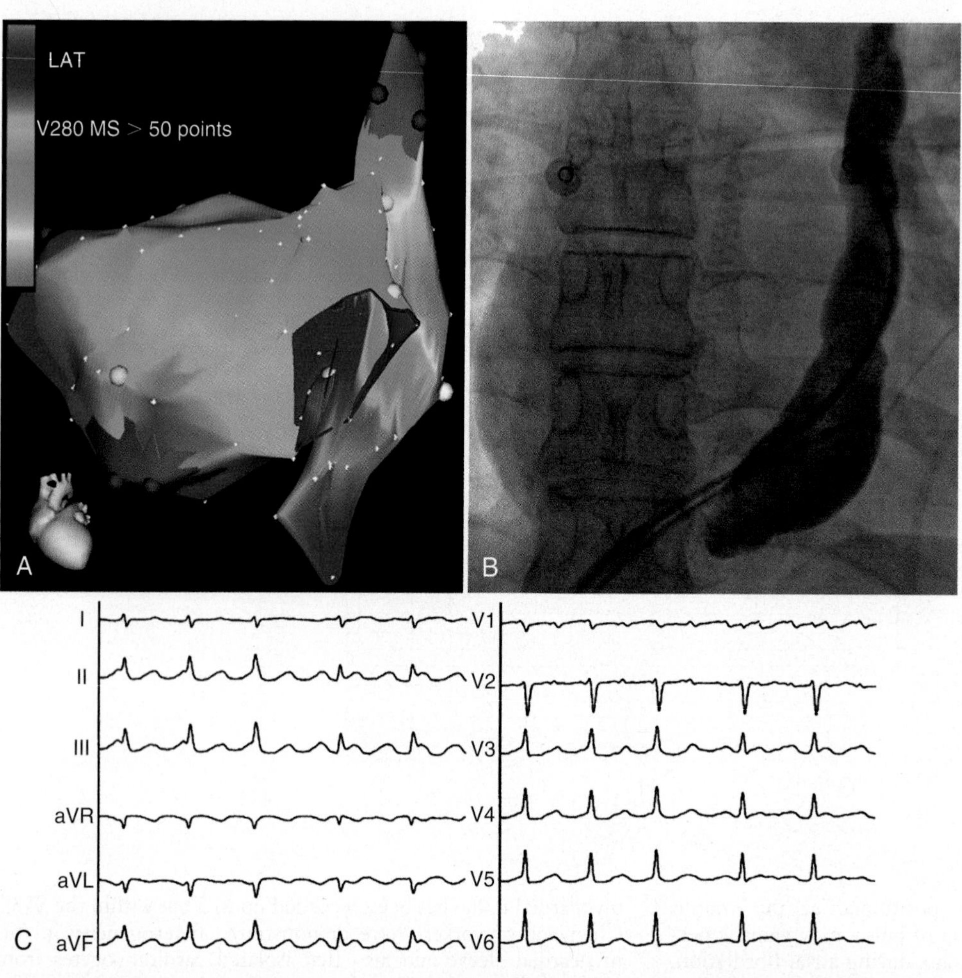

Figure 39-2 A, Electroanatomic map (left anterior oblique view) during atrial tachycardia of the left atrium and the persistent left superior vena cava showing the site of earliest activation within the left superior vena cava. **B,** Corresponding fluoroscopic view (left anterior oblique) of the left superior vena cava. **C,** A 12-lead electrocardiogram of the atrial tachycardia.

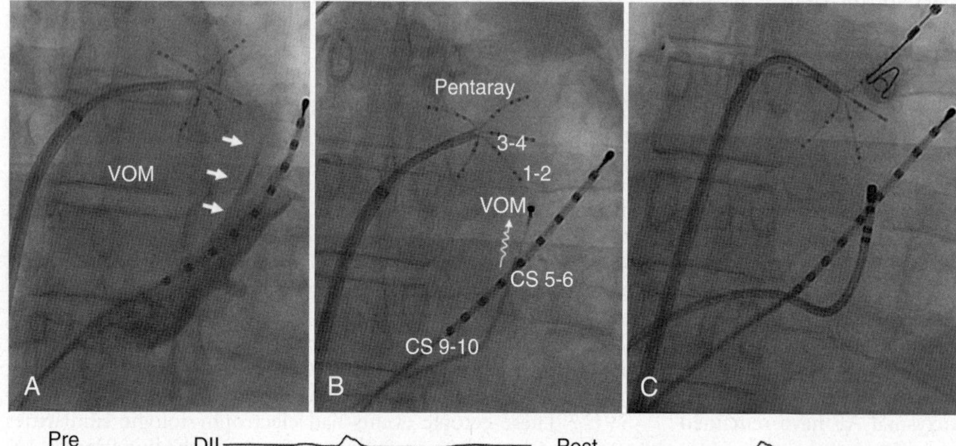

Figure 39-3 A, Venogram of the coronary sinus (CS) and the vein of Marshall (VOM) *(arrows)*. **B** and **D,** Late potential activation sequence spanning inferosuperiorly from distal CS (CS 5-6, *s) to the inferior arm of the Pentaray catheter (PR) placed in the lateral left atrium (PR 1-2, PR 3-4). On this latter catheter, the activation is inferosuperior, i.e., from distal (PR 1-2) to proximal (PR 3-4). A bipolar catheter is inserted inside the VOM. Continuous activity is seen bridging inferior and superior activity of the Marshall potential. **C** and **E,** Ablation catheter placed at the ostium of the VOM, facing CS 5-6. The Marshall potential disappears on the CS 5-6 and lateral left atrium.

evaluated the incidence of SVC triggers of AF and the role of empirical SCV isolation.[36] In a consecutive series of 190 patients undergoing pulmonary vein antral isolation (PVAI), mapping was performed of spontaneous or induced non–pulmonary vein ectopic atrial activity. SVC triggers were seen in 12.6% (24 of 190). All these patients also exhibited triggers arising from the adjacent right superior pulmonary vein. However, pulmonary vein ablation alone had failed to eliminate AT or AF and was successfully abolished by SVC isolation. Based on these observations, they undertook empirical SVC as an adjunct to PVAI in the subsequent 217 patients presenting for AF ablation, which resulted in a higher long-term success rate (16% recurrence rate). However, to date there have been no randomized studies that have suggested a better outcome from empirical adjuvant SVC isolation.

Endpoint of Catheter Ablation of the Superior Vena Cava

The ideal strategy for SVC ablation—focal ablation or isolation—remains unclear. The ablation of this structure has to date been variably included in AF ablation strategies. Initial attempts at focal ablation at the site of earliest activity suggest that although it is more effective than focal ablation within the pulmonary veins, several patients could develop triggers from other sites within the SVC.

Goya and colleagues performed detailed electroanatomic mapping of the connections between the right atrium and the SVC.[7] In this study, SVC potentials were found over a large amount of the circumference, suggesting widespread muscle coverage of the SVC with 1.4 ± 0.5 RA-to-SVC breakthroughs per patient. These breakthroughs could be eliminated with 3.1 ± 1.7 RF applications per breakthrough. Arruda and coauthors observed that 96% of SVCs exhibited potentials as recorded by the circular catheter, and nine (4%) had a silent SVC-RA junction.[36] Complete SVC-RA electrical isolation (abolishing all high-frequency SVC potentials) could be achieved by segmental ablation (50% ± 12% of the SVC circumference) in 59% of patients. Ablation along the entire SVC circumference was required in 19%. In this study, complete SVC-RA disconnection was not possible in 18% due to phrenic nerve stimulation.

Phrenic nerve injury, SVC stenosis, and injury to the sinus node remain potential complications of ablation in this region. However, centers performing such ablation often suggest that the risks associated with isolation may be minimal especially by localizing phrenic nerve trajectory by pacing. Hsieh and colleagues suggest that in more than 100 patients undergoing such ablation, only one patient developed sinus node injury after three procedures for SVC isolation and no other patients had any SVC stenosis or phrenic nerve injury.[37] They suggest that especially when ablation is guided by a three-dimensional mapping system, with a detailed geometry of the SVC and accurate identification of the sinus node location and phrenic nerve route, SVC isolation can be performed safely in most patients.

Left Superior Vena Cava

A persistent left SVC is the most common thoracic venous anomaly (incidence is 0.3%-2%). In the embryonic heart, bilateral pacemaker areas are present near the sinus horns of the cardinal veins. The right side develops to take over sinus pacemaker function, and the presence of a left common cardinal vein or left SVC may be associated with the presence of pacemaker tissue and hence ectopic activity. The presence of electrically viable myocardium within the left SVC is well recognized. Venous potentials are observed circumferentially at the proximal left SVC near its junction with the coronary sinus, but at the mid level they are only recorded in part of this vein.

Left Superior Vena Cava in Atrial Fibrillation

Hsu and coworkers described five patients in whom ectopy and repetitive bursts of activity from the left SVC resulted in AF after pulmonary vein ablation.[38] The incidence of AF initiated from this site was described as 0.4%. These ectopic beats were observed to precede P wave onset by 67 ± 13 ms. Indeed, the left SVC was observed to be connected both to the lateral LA (1.6 ± 0.5 connections) and via the coronary sinus to the RA (4.1 ± 2.3 connections). In these patients ablation required isolation of this structure, in some cases necessitating ablation at both ends. We have also reported a patient with an AT originating from left SVC that was terminated by ablation (see Fig. 39-2).

Elayi and coworkers have presented a similar series of six patients.[39] In this series, most patients had undergone prior pulmonary vein ablation and had recurrence of arrhythmia with persistent isolation of the pulmonary veins. Circumferential mapping–guided isolation of the left SVC was performed using 10.3 ± 1.6 minutes of RF energy and with no complications. After follow-up of 13 ± 7.4 months, all patients were in sinus rhythm and free from AF without antiarrhythmic drugs.

Endpoint of Catheter Ablation of the Left Superior Vena Cava

The relative ease with which left SVC isolation can be performed argues in favor of electrical isolation compared to ablation at the earliest site. However, both these series have shown this structure is connected to the atria at the proximal and distal ends, requiring ablation at both sites to effectively achieve electrical isolation.

Ligament of Marshall

The vein of Marshall is located within a vestigial fold of pericardium, the ligament of Marshall, which is the developmental remnant of the embryonic left SVC. This structure typically runs in a superior-to-inferior direction immediately anterior to the left pulmonary veins. The vein of Marshall typically undergoes atrophic transition to the ligament of Marshall during the course of development. However, in some patients, a persistent vein of Marshall may be observed and runs in the lateral left atrial groove on the epicardial surface. In 1972, Scherlag and colleagues observed electrical activity emanating from this structure.[40] Interest has been renewed in the arrhythmogenic potential of this structure as a source of focal firing in AF.[41-44] The muscle fibers from the Marshall bundle are directly connected to the coronary sinus and might extend up to the left pulmonary veins.

Vein of Marshall as an Arrhythmogenic Structure

Doshi and coauthors have demonstrated that the vein of Marshall, in dogs subjected to long-term rapid pacing, can serve as a source of rapid and repetitive activity that could induce AF in vitro.[44] Wu and colleagues, in a canine model of AF, observed the shortest cycle length activity and the highest dominant frequency activity occurred in the pulmonary veins or the vein of Marshall.[13] Hwang and coworkers have used small-diameter catheters to cannulate the vein of Marshall through the coronary sinus and demonstrated the presence of Marshall vein potentials in up to half the patients.[41] In a canine model, these investigators demonstrated that these potentials were distinct from coronary artery and left atrial activity. Patients with AF originating from the ligament of Marshall have predominantly been healthy young men with adrenergic AF. These patients often describe arrhythmia in the early morning when sympathetic tone is present and during exercise.

Ablation of Triggers from the Vein of Marshall

In keeping with the association with adrenergic AF, isoproterenol is often useful to induce arrhythmia in the laboratory. The P wave morphology of the ectopy has been variable and depends to a degree on the predominant connection between the ligament of Marshall and the atria. However, the most common pattern is of a negative or biphasic P wave in the inferior leads. Experience from mapping connections in patients with AF originating from persistent left SVCs has implications for ablation of the more common ligament of Marshall. Myocardial tracts inserting into the coronary sinus and left atrial free wall have been described in the ligament of Marshall.[43]

On the basis of anatomic studies of the ligament of Marshall, two possible techniques can be used for ablation of this structure. The most commonly used technique is to perform endocardial ablation in the region of the lateral LA to sever both its LA and coronary sinus connections.[41] This was performed by Hwang and colleagues, guided by cannulation of the vein of Marshall, and resulted in AF termination in four of six patients, but it did not completely eliminate all signals from the ligament of Marshall. In a different study, combined endocardial and distal coronary sinus ablation, resulting in abolition of all ligament of Marshall signals, was associated with better clinical outcome than endocardial ablation alone (see Fig. 39-3).[45] The second method of ablation of the vein of Marshall is the epicardial approach, which requires a percutaneous pericardial approach. This provides direct access to the ligament of Marshall, but there is limited experience using this technique.

In a series of 21 patients in whom mapping confirmed triggers from the ligament of Marshall, ablation was performed to achieve total elimination of all Marshall bundle potentials.[46] A single broad connection was identified in 15 patients, and six patients had two connections. Such ablation resulted in one patient developing a 40% left inferior pulmonary vein stenosis. More recently, these investigators have aimed at eliminating these potentials endocardially by wide encircling pulmonary vein ablation just outside the left pulmonary vein ostia. Indeed there are some early experimental suggestions that in some cases the ligament of Marshall inserts to the LA through the left pulmonary veins.[47]

Coronary Sinus

Mechanisms of Coronary Sinus Arrhythmogenicity

The extent of the coronary sinus musculature has been characterized and ranges from 2 to 11 mm into the great cardiac vein. In parts, this muscle demonstrated variable thickness and has been postulated to function in a sphincter-like fashion. The valve of Vieussens was found in 87% of cases, whereas the ostium of the oblique vein was a more constant marker for determining the beginning of the coronary sinus. Chauvin and coauthors demonstrated histologic continuity between the right and left atria through the coronary sinus musculature in all hearts that were evaluated.[48] Striated muscle connecting the coronary sinus to the adjacent atria were observed in two distinct parts: A muscular cuff (circumferential) surrounded the coronary sinus wall along 25 to 51 mm of its length, and other fibers emerged from this cuff to join the LA myocardium (oblique); these fibers had anatomic characteristics that varied from a few discrete fascicles to widely interconnecting plexus. Antz and colleagues have also demonstrated the existence of coronary sinus–to–left atrial connections in an experimental study in isolated dog hearts.[49] They demonstrated centrifugal activation of the LA from discrete inputs originating from the coronary sinus musculature.

Coronary Sinus in Arrhythmogenesis

Previous studies have supported the role of the coronary sinus region as a wide arrhythmogenic complex by exhibiting focal or reentrant local mechanisms as well as its involvement as a conducting pathway for macro-reentrant arrhythmias. Olgin and coworkers described a case of atrial macro-reentry that involved the coronary sinus musculature and used a coronary sinus–to–left atrial breakthrough to complete the circuit.[50] A critical isthmus was identified within the coronary sinus by entrainment mapping and confirmed by ablation. In this case, ablation resulted in bidirectional conduction block to the RA. Kasai and colleagues observed an abrupt change in activation sequence during delivery of decremented extrastimuli from the distal coronary sinus, suggesting block between the coronary sinus and the LA.[51] This phenomenon was more common in patients with a history of AF or atrial flutter. Ndrepepa and coauthors observed left atrial–to–coronary sinus conduction block during atrial arrhythmia by simultaneous mapping of the left and right atria and the coronary sinus in nine patients with AF or atrial flutter.[52]

Increased automaticity has been observed within the musculature of the coronary sinus or surrounding nonatrial structures with spontaneous focal tachycardia[53] and accessory pathway automaticity following ablation.[54] Our understanding of the complex relationship of the coronary sinus musculature to its surrounding structures was expanded in a study in patients with posteroseptal or left posterior accessory pathways.[55] This study provides evidence that in some accessory pathways, the ventricular end is formed by extensions of the coronary sinus musculature along the adjacent cardiac vein to the epicardial surface of the ventricle. Thus, cure of these arrhythmias required careful definition of the coronary sinus anatomy or an epicardial approach.

The role of triggers in the development of AF is now well established. Although AF has been considered a random and chaotic process, Jaïs and colleagues reported a small series of patients in whom irregular rapid focal discharges from the pulmonary vein or coronary sinus, persisting sometimes for hours, days, or even longer, could drive sustained AF, the true focal AF.[56] Arrhythmia in these patients was cured by focal ablation, suggesting that in these cases, the pulmonary vein or coronary sinus formed not only the trigger but also the substrate maintaining AF. Sanders and coworkers performed ablation to electrically disconnect the coronary sinus from the left and right atria in a patient in whom triggers from this structure recurrently induced AF.[57] In this case, extensive ablation was required endocardially along the mitral annulus and at the coronary sinus ostium to achieve electrical isolation. Following isolation of the coronary sinus as part of AF ablation, focal ectopy and rapid bursts of AT and AF have been observed within the isolated coronary sinus.[58,59]

More recently, our group has demonstrated the role of the coronary sinus in the maintenance of organized AF in a series of patients by activation mapping where AF is driven by sources centrifugally spreading from the coronary sinus region (earliest discrete activity recorded at the rim of coronary sinus os or within the coronary sinus or from the initial 3 cm of coronary sinus).[60] Coronary sinus activity could fire in episodic bursts of varying cycle lengths or in sustained fashion (Fig. 39-4).

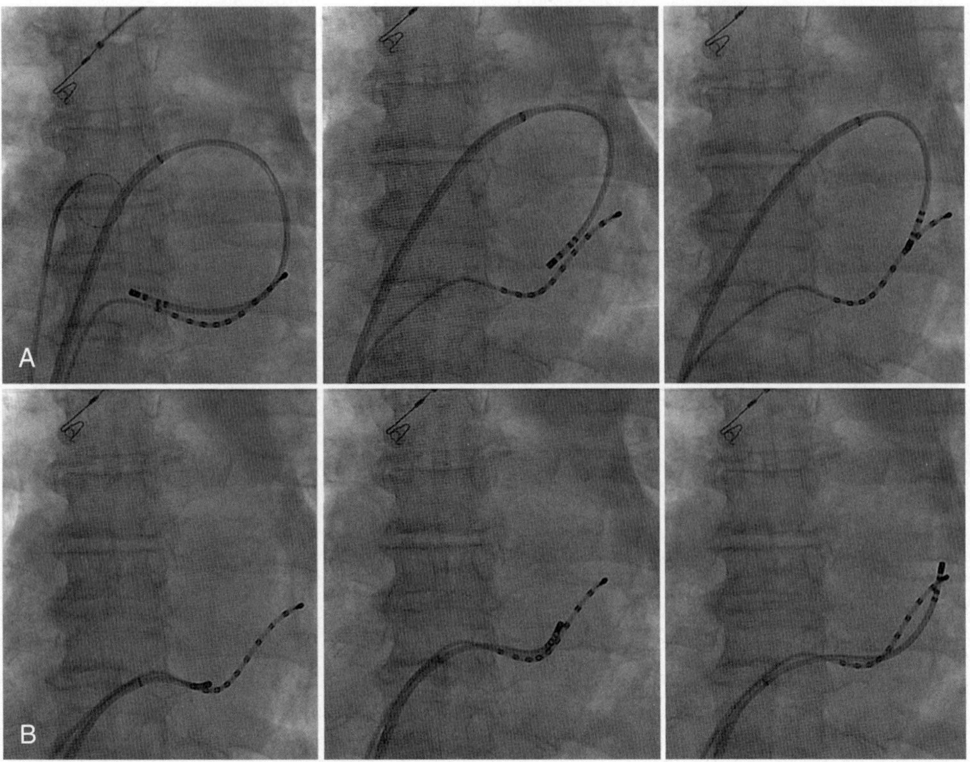

Figure 39-4 Anteroposterior fluoroscopic visualization of the catheter position during ablation of the inferior left atrium **(A)** and coronary sinus **(B)**. **A,** After looping the catheter into the left atrium facing the coronary sinus ostium *(left)*, the catheter is then gradually withdrawn parallel to the coronary sinus along the posterior mitral annulus toward the lateral left atrium *(center* and *right)*. **B,** Corresponding catheter position at the ostial *(left)*, middle *(center)*, and distal *(right)* segments within the coronary sinus.

In a study using a stepwise approach for the ablation of long-lasting persistent AF, the coronary sinus region appeared to be a major site perpetuating persistent AF.[26] Ablation of the coronary sinus region from the endocardial and epicardial aspect during AF prolongs the mean AFCL by 8.95 ± 9.7 ms, with a significant prolongation of AFCL observed in 57% of patients. In this region, endocardial ablation of the inferior LA (i.e., along the mitral annulus) produced a significant prolongation of AFCL in 46% of patients, and epicardial ablation within the coronary sinus prolonged AFCL in an additional group of 11% (total with an effect, 57%). In addition, focal AT following termination of AF originated at any part of the coronary sinus connection (circumferential or longitudinal) with LA.

We further evaluated the impact of catheter ablation of the coronary sinus in paroxysmal and permanent AF in a series of 45 patients.[61] Ablation of the coronary sinus starting endocardially significantly prolonged the cycle length by 17 ± 5 ms and organized the coronary sinus activation sequence. Additional epicardial ablation further increased local cycle length. Coronary sinus ablation was associated with AF termination in 16 (35%) patients (46% of paroxysmal and 30% of persistent AF). There are several potential mechanisms of arrhythmogenicity from the inferior left atrial–coronary sinus region as inferred from these observations. It is feasible that endocardial ablation might suppress or inhibit continuous interaction or exchange of activity between these two contiguous structures, which may be a mechanism perpetuating AF in these patients.

Endpoint of Catheter Ablation of the Coronary Sinus

Ablation of the coronary sinus musculature and LA connections is commenced along the endocardial aspect of the mitral annulus and completed from within the vessel (epicardial) as required. The ablation catheter is dragged along the endocardium of the inferior LA after looping the catheter in such a way as to position it parallel to the coronary sinus catheter. After achieving a loop in the LA, the catheter then is gradually withdrawn from the septal area and ablation commenced along the posterior mitral annulus, from a site adjacent to the coronary sinus ostium and progressing to the lateral LA (4 o'clock in the left anterior oblique projection) (Fig. 39-5). The endpoint is elimination of local endocardial electrograms bordering the mitral annulus.

Ablation within the coronary sinus is performed at all sites showing persistent rapid potentials with a cycle length shorter than in the left atrial ablation. Ablation is started distally (4 o'clock in left anterior oblique position) and pursued along the vein up to the ostium; additional RF applications are continued around the coronary sinus orifice from the RA. The endpoint is slowing of coronary sinus potentials (below the LA appendage cycle length) rather than abolition, based on a prior study, which demonstrated little additional benefit with total disconnection compared to mere coronary sinus slowing.[27]

RF energy is delivered endocardially with a power of 30 to 35 W using irrigation rates of 20 to 60 mL/min (0.9% saline via a Cool Flow pump) to achieve the desired power delivery. However, inside the coronary sinus, power is limited to 20 W distally. often associated with local high impedance requiring the maximal irrigation flow (60 mL/min); 25 to 30 W is delivered at the coronary sinus ostium. Temperature is limited to 50°C.

Inferior Vena Cava

In general, the inferior vena cava (IVC) is considered to lack an investiture of atrial myocardium. In keeping with this, only isolated studies have reported triggers or drivers of AF from this site.[62] Triggers from this site demonstrate a negative polarity of the P wave morphology in the inferior leads and in V1.

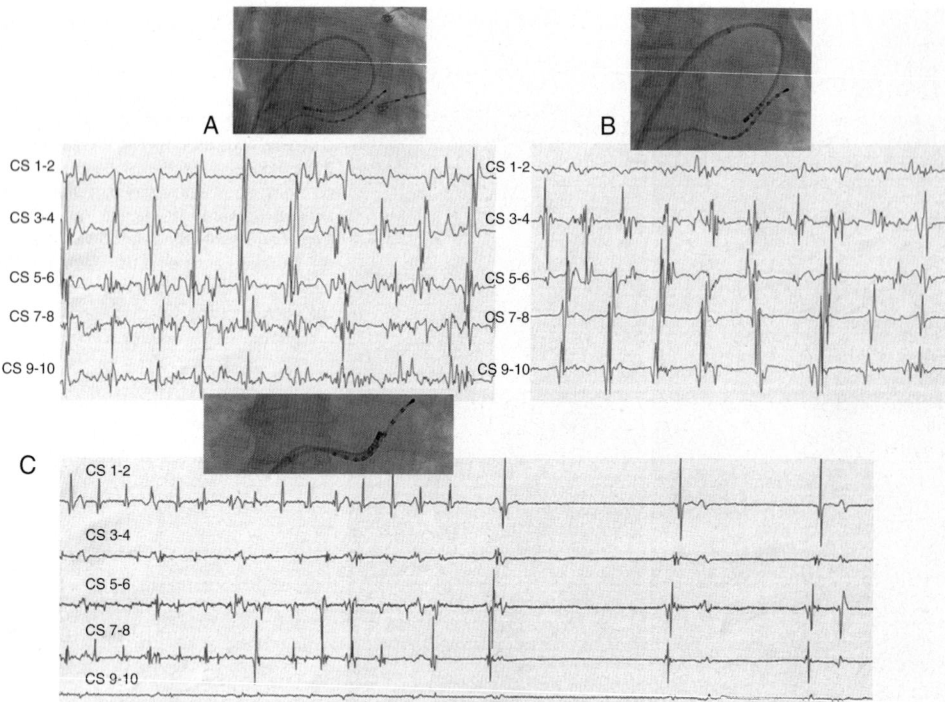

Figure 39-5 **A,** Impact of endocardial ablation along the inferior left atrium on coronary sinus activation. Before ablation, coronary sinus activation is inconsistent with short cycle length in CS 7-8 and 9-10. **B,** During ablation, the coronary sinus becomes organized with slowing and pause. **C,** Termination of atrial fibrillation with ablation inside the coronary sinus.

Mansour and colleagues described two cases of ectopic beats originating from the posterolateral ostium of the IVC initiating AF.[63] In contrast, in the case described by Scavee and coauthors, the trigger site was identified relatively deep in the IVC rather than at the ostia.[62] Mizobuchi and colleagues have described a further case of paroxysmal AF originating from IVC.[64] This site served not only as trigger but also as driver for maintenance of AF. They observed that during AF, the IVC demonstrated the rapid and fractionated potentials that exit into both atria with conduction block. In all cases to date, ablation at this site has been targeted by focal ablation at the site of earliest activity, presumably a reflection of the paucity of myocardial extensions into this structure.

Conclusion

The thoracic veins have an important role in atrial arrhythmogenesis. These structures are annexed to the atria, and the atrial myocardium invades, providing an electrical connection. This tissue is capable of generating and maintaining spontaneous or reentrant electrical activity that manifests as AT or AF. Why these structures are able to cause AF and AT in some patients but not others remains to be elucidated. At the moment, the most effective strategy is to electrically disconnect the veins from the atria.

References

1. Kannel WB, Abbott RD, Savage DD, McNamara PM: Epidemiologic features of chronic atrial fibrillation: The Framingham study. N Engl J Med 306:1018-1022, 1982.
2. Allessie MA, Boyden PA, Camm AJ, et al: Pathophysiology and prevention of atrial fibrillation. Circulation 103:769-777, 2001.
3. Haissaguerre M, Jais P, Shah DC, et al: Spontaneous initiation of atrial fibrillation by ectopic beats originating in the pulmonary veins. N Engl J Med 339:659-666, 1998.
4. Hocini M, Haissaguerre M, Shah D, et al: Multiple sources initiating atrial fibrillation from a single pulmonary vein identified by a circumferential catheter. Pacing Clin Electrophysiol 23:1828-1831, 2000.
5. Haissaguerre M, Shah DC, Jais P, et al: Electrophysiological breakthroughs from the left atrium to the pulmonary veins. Circulation 102:2463-2465, 2000.
6. Tsai CF, Tai CT, Hsieh MH, et al: Initiation of atrial fibrillation by ectopic beats originating from the superior vena cava: Electrophysiological characteristics and results of radiofrequency ablation. Circulation 102:67-74, 2000.
7. Goya M, Ouyang F, Ernst S, et al: Electroanatomic mapping and catheter ablation of breakthroughs from the right atrium to the superior vena cava in patients with atrial fibrillation. Circulation 106: 1317-1320, 2002.
8. Kistler PM, Sanders P, Fynn SP, et al: Electrophysiological and electrocardiographic characteristics of focal atrial tachycardia originating from the pulmonary veins: Acute and long-term outcomes of radiofrequency ablation. Circulation 108:1968-1975, 2003.
9. Takahashi Y, Iesaka Y, Takahashi A, et al: Reentrant tachycardia in pulmonary veins of patients with paroxysmal atrial fibrillation. J Cardiovasc Electrophysiol 14:927-932, 2003.
10. Blom NA, Gittenberger-de Groot AC, et al: Development of the cardiac conduction tissue in human embryos using HNK-1 antigen expression: Possible relevance for understanding of abnormal atrial automaticity. Circulation 99:800-806, 1999.
11. Cheung DW: Electrical activity of the pulmonary vein and its interaction with the right atrium in the guinea-pig. J Physiol 314:445-456, 1981.
12. Chen YJ, Chen SA, Chen YC, et al: Effects of rapid atrial pacing on the arrhythmogenic activity of single cardiomyocytes from pulmonary veins: implication in initiation of atrial fibrillation. Circulation 104:2849-5284, 2001.
13. Wu TJ, Ong JJ, Chang CM, et al: Pulmonary veins and ligament of Marshall

as sources of rapid activations in a canine model of sustained atrial fibrillation. Circulation 103:1157-1163, 2001.

14. Honjo H, Boyett MR, Niwa R, et al: Pacing-induced spontaneous activity in myocardial sleeves of pulmonary veins after treatment with ryanodine. Circulation 107:1937-1943, 2003.
15. Hocini M, Ho SY, Kawara T, et al: Electrical conduction in canine pulmonary veins: Electrophysiological and anatomic correlation. Circulation 105:2442-2448, 2002.
16. Chen SA, Hsieh MH, Tai CT, et al: Initiation of atrial fibrillation by ectopic beats originating from the pulmonary veins: Electrophysiological characteristics, pharmacological responses, and effects of radiofrequency ablation. Circulation 100:1879-1886, 1999.
17. Jais P, Hocini M, Macle L, et al: Distinctive electrophysiological properties of pulmonary veins in patients with atrial fibrillation. Circulation 106:2479-2485, 2002.
18. Sanders P, Sacher F, Jais P, et al: Stretch induced pulmonary vein electrical remodeling in humans. Heart Rhythm 3:S84, 2006.
19. Kumagai K, Ogawa M, Noguchi H, et al: Electrophysiologic properties of pulmonary veins assessed using a multielectrode basket catheter. J Am Coll Cardiol 43:2281-2289, 2004.
20. Wu TJ, Doshi RN, Huang HL, et al: Simultaneous biatrial computerized mapping during permanent atrial fibrillation in patients with organic heart disease. J Cardiovasc Electrophysiol 13:571-577, 2002.
21. Haissaguerre M, Sanders P, Hocini M, et al: Changes in atrial fibrillation cycle length and inducibility during catheter ablation and their relation to outcome. Circulation 109:3007-3013, 2004.
22. Essebag V, Baldessin F, Reynolds MR, et al: Non-inducibility post–pulmonary vein isolation achieving exit block predicts freedom from atrial fibrillation. Eur Heart J 26:2550-2555, 2005.
23. Jais P, Hocini M, Sanders P, et al: Long-term evaluation of atrial fibrillation ablation guided by noninducibility. Heart Rhythm 3:140-145, 2006.
24. Haissaguerre M, Sanders P, Hocini M, et al: Pulmonary veins in the substrate for atrial fibrillation: the "venous wave" hypothesis. J Am Coll Cardiol 43:2290-2292, 2004.
25. Haissaguerre M, Jais P, Shah DC, et al: Catheter ablation of chronic atrial fibrillation targeting the reinitiating triggers. J Cardiovasc Electrophysiol 11:2-10, 2000.
26. Haissaguerre M, Sanders P, Hocini M, et al: Catheter ablation of long-lasting persistent atrial fibrillation: Critical structures for termination. J Cardiovasc Electrophysiol 16:1125-1137, 2005.
27. Haissaguerre M, Hocini M, Sanders P, et al: Catheter ablation of long-lasting persistent atrial fibrillation: Clinical outcome and mechanisms of subsequent arrhythmias. J Cardiovasc Electrophysiol 16: 1138-1147, 2005.
28. Oral H, Knight BP, Tada H, et al: Pulmonary vein isolation for paroxysmal and persistent atrial fibrillation. Circulation 105:1077-1081, 2002.
29. Sanders P, Nalliah CJ, Dubois R, et al: Frequency mapping of the pulmonary veins in paroxysmal versus permanent atrial fibrillation. J Cardiovasc Electrophysiol 17:965-972, 2006.
30. Chen YJ, Chen YC, Yeh HI, et al: Electrophysiology and arrhythmogenic activity of single cardiomyocytes from canine superior vena cava. Circulation 105:2679-2685, 2002.
31. Haissaguerre M, Gencel L, Fischer B, et al: Successful catheter ablation of atrial fibrillation. J Cardiovasc Electrophysiol 5:1045-1052, 1994.
32. Ino T, Miyamoto S, Ohno T, Tadera T: Exit block of focal repetitive activity in the superior vena cava masquerading as a high right atrial tachycardia. J Cardiovasc Electrophysiol 11:480-483, 2000.
33. Shah DC, Haissaguerre M, Jais P, Clementy J: High-resolution mapping of tachycardia originating from the superior vena cava: Evidence of electrical heterogeneity, slow conduction, and possible circus movement reentry. J Cardiovasc Electrophysiol 13:388-392, 2002.
34. Lin WS, Tai CT, Hsieh MH, et al: Catheter ablation of paroxysmal atrial fibrillation initiated by non-pulmonary vein ectopy. Circulation 107:3176-3183, 2003.
35. Hsieh MH, Tai CT, Lee SH, et al: The different mechanisms between late and very late recurrences of atrial fibrillation in patients undergoing a repeated catheter ablation. J Cardiovasc Electrophysiol 17:231-235, 2006.
36. Arruda M, Mlcochova H, Prasad SK, et al: Electrical isolation of the superior vena cava: An adjunctive strategy to pulmonary vein antrum isolation improving the outcome of AF ablation. J Cardiovasc Electrophysiol 18(12):1261-1266, 2007.
37. Hsieh MH, Chen SA: Is it necessary to routinely perform isolation of the superior vena cava in every atrial fibrillation patient? J Cardiovasc Electrophysiol 18:1267-1268, 2007.
38. Hsu LF, Jais P, Keane D, et al: Atrial fibrillation originating from persistent left superior vena cava. Circulation 109:828-832, 2004.
39. Elayi CS, Fahmy TS, Wazni OM, et al: Left superior vena cava isolation in patients undergoing pulmonary vein antrum isolation: Impact on atrial fibrillation recurrence. Heart Rhythm 3:1019-1023, 2006.
40. Scherlag BJ, Yeh BK, Robinson MJ: Inferior interatrial pathway in the dog. Circ Res 31:18-35, 1972.
41. Hwang C, Wu TJ, Doshi RN, et al: Vein of Marshall cannulation for the analysis of electrical activity in patients with focal atrial fibrillation. Circulation 101:1503-1505, 2000.
42. Hwang C, Karagueuzian HS, Chen PS: Idiopathic paroxysmal atrial fibrillation induced by a focal discharge mechanism in the left superior pulmonary vein: Possible roles of the ligament of Marshall. J Cardiovasc Electrophysiol 10:636-648, 1999.
43. Kim DT, Lai AC, Hwang C, et al: The ligament of Marshall: A structural analysis in human hearts with implications for atrial arrhythmias. J Am Coll Cardiol 36: 1324-1327, 2000.
44. Doshi RN, Wu TJ, Yashima M, et al: Relation between ligament of Marshall and adrenergic atrial tachyarrhythmia. Circulation 100:876-883, 1999.
45. Katritsis D, Ioannidis JP, Anagnostopoulos CE, et al: Identification and catheter ablation of extracardiac and intracardiac components of ligament of Marshall tissue for treatment of paroxysmal atrial fibrillation. J Cardiovasc Electrophysiol 12:750-758, 2001.
46. Hwang C, Chen PS: Clinical electrophysiology and catheter ablation of atrial fibrillation from the ligament of Marshall. In Chen SA, Haissaguerre M, Zipes DP (eds): Thoracic Vein Arrhythmias: Mechanisms and Treatment. Malden, MA, Blackwell Publishing, 2004, pp 276-284.
47. Tan AY, Chou CC, Zhou S, et al: Electrical connections between left superior pulmonary vein, left atrium, and ligament of Marshall: Implications for mechanisms of atrial fibrillation. Am J Physiol Heart Circ Physiol 290:H312-H322, 2006.
48. Chauvin M, Shah DC, Haissaguerre M, et al: The anatomic basis of connections between the coronary sinus musculature and the left atrium in humans. Circulation 101:647-652, 2000.
49. Antz M, Otomo K, Arruda M, et al: Electrical conduction between the right atrium and the left atrium via the musculature of the coronary sinus. Circulation 98:1790-1795, 1998.
50. Olgin JE, Jayachandran JV, Engesstein E, et al: Atrial macroreentry involving the myocardium of the coronary sinus: A unique mechanism for atypical flutter. J Cardiovasc Electrophysiol 9:1094-1099, 1998.
51. Kasai A, Anselme F, Saoudi N: Myocardial connections between left atrial myocardium and coronary sinus musculature in man. J Cardiovasc Electrophysiol 12:981-985, 2001.
52. Ndrepepa G, Zrenner B, Schneider MA, et al: Dissociation between coronary sinus and left atrial conduction in patients with atrial fibrillation and flutter. J Cardiovasc Electrophysiol 12:623-628, 2001.
53. Volkmer M, Antz M, Hebe J, Kuck KH: Focal atrial tachycardia originating from the musculature of the coronary sinus. J Cardiovasc Electrophysiol 13:68-71, 2002.
54. Macle L, Shah DC, Jais P, Haissaguerre M: Accessory pathway automaticity after radiofrequency ablation. J Cardiovasc Electrophysiol 13:285-287, 2002.
55. Sun Y, Arruda M, Otomo K, et al: Coronary sinus–ventricular accessory connections producing posteroseptal and left posterior accessory pathways: Incidence and electrophysiological identification. Circulation 106:1362-1367, 2002.
56. Jais P, Haissaguerre M, Shah DC, et al: A focal source of atrial fibrillation treated by discrete radiofrequency ablation. Circulation 95:572-576, 1997.

57. Sanders P, Jais P, Hocini M, Haissaguerre M: Electrical disconnection of the coronary sinus by radiofrequency catheter ablation to isolate a trigger of atrial fibrillation. J Cardiovasc Electrophysiol 15:364-368, 2004.
58. Rotter M, Sanders P, Takahashi Y, et al: Images in cardiovascular medicine. Coronary sinus tachycardia driving atrial fibrillation. Circulation 110:e59-e60, 2004.
59. Oral H, Ozaydin M, Chugh A, et al: Role of the coronary sinus in maintenance of atrial fibrillation. J Cardiovasc Electrophysiol 14:1329-1336, 2003.
60. Haissaguerre M, Hocini M, Sanders P, et al: Localized sources maintaining atrial fibrillation organized by prior ablation. Circulation 113:616-625, 2006.
61. Haissaguerre M, Hocini M, Takahashi Y, et al: Impact of catheter ablation of the coronary sinus on paroxysmal or persistent atrial fibrillation. J Cardiovasc Electrophysiol 18:378-386, 2007.
62. Scavee C, Jais P, Weerasooriya R, Haissaguerre M: The inferior vena cava: An exceptional source of atrial fibrillation. J Cardiovasc Electrophysiol 14:659-662, 2003.
63. Mansour M, Ruskin J, Keane D: Initiation of atrial fibrillation by ectopic beats originating from the ostium of the inferior vena cava. J Cardiovasc Electrophysiol 13: 1292-1295, 2002.
64. Mizobuchi M, Enjoji Y, Shibata K, et al: Case report: Focal ablation for atrial fibrillation originating from the inferior vena cava and the posterior left atrium. J Interv Card Electrophysiol 16:131-134, 2006.

Dominant Frequency and the Mechanisms of Maintenance of Atrial Fibrillation 40

Omer Berenfeld

CHAPTER OUTLINE

About 2.3 million people in the United States are currently afflicted with atrial fibrillation (AF), the most common sustained cardiac arrhythmia in humans, and many more cases are predicted in the near future.[1] Antiarrhythmic drugs are only partially effective in treating AF, and they have potential serious side effects, including life-threatening proarrhythmia. On the other hand, it has been demonstrated that paroxysmal AF in patients is initiated by focal triggers localized usually to one of the pulmonary veins[2] and can be cured by a catheter-based ablation procedure.[3] However, in persistent AF, the prevailing theory is that multiple random wavelets of activation coexist to create a chaotic cardiac rhythm,[4] and therapy is more challenging.[5]

To enhance our understanding of AF, early studies on regional differences in activation cycle length during AF[6,7] were followed by an increased interest in the analysis of the frequency spectrum as a measure of the activation rate in animal models.[8-11] Furthermore, works demonstrating how measurements of AF cycle length in patients can contribute to its treatment[12,13] motivated my collaborators and me to translate experimental knowledge and methods into analysis of human AF in the frequency domain.[14] As suggested by our recent studies,[15,16] high-resolution analysis of the Fourier power spectrum with its dominant frequency (DF) offers the unique opportunity of being able to systematically correlate the spatial distribution of excitation frequency with cardiac anatomy and ablation procedures and to provide mechanistic insight into different types of AF.

The central objectives of this chapter are to discuss recent experimental and clinical data from our laboratory supporting the hypothesis that acute AF in the sheep and some groups of human patients is not a totally random phenomenon. As will be demonstrated, the spatiotemporal organization of waves in the normally structured isolated sheep heart suggests that maintenance of acute AF depends on localized reentrant sources in the left atrium (LA) and fibrillatory conduction in its periphery. In human patients, on the other hand, DF-based analysis reveals that the suggested reentrant sources are localized primarily to the pulmonary veins in the case of paroxysmal AF but elsewhere in the case of chronic AF.[14]

The research reported in this chapter was supported in part by grants PO1 HL039707 and RO1 HL060843 from the National Institutes of Health and the Scientist Development Grant 0230311N from the American Heart Association.

Relation between Activity in the Left and Right Atria

The notion that the spatiotemporal complexity of wave propagation during AF is reflected in the local activation rate dispersion led us to characterize dominant frequencies in the power spectrum throughout both atria; we found them to be organized in discrete domains.[9] Most notably, during the arrhythmia the activation frequencies in certain areas of the LA were consistently faster than those in any other areas.[8-10] In a search for the mechanism underlying such frequency distribution in space, a subsequent study demonstrated the way interatrial pathways mediate fibrillatory conduction and the establishment of frequency gradients between the LA and right atrium (RA)[11] along Bachmann's bundle and the inferoposterior interatrial pathway that underlies the coronary sinus, both of which are well-known routes of interatrial electrical communication.[17,18]

An example of LA-to-RA frequency gradient is illustrated in Figure 40-1A, which shows a color map of DFs obtained from optical mapping of both atria in combination with electrograms from the left and right sides of Bachmann's bundle and the inferoposterior interatrial pathway. The DF map was constructed from a 3-second episode during AF in the presence of acetylcholine (ACh; see Mansour and coworkers[11] for a detailed discussion). The map shows a high degree of organization, with discrete frequency domains and a LA-to-RA frequency gradient.[8-11] For the most part, the DF in the LA was highest at 18.8 Hz. The left side of Bachmann's bundle shows a DF of 18.7 Hz, whereas the inferoposterior interatrial pathway on the same side was activated at 14.8 Hz. Moving farther to the right, the DF at the right end of Bachmann's bundle was 14.5 Hz; in the inferoposterior interatrial pathway it was 14.1 Hz. Finally, the RA shows a DF of 9.8 Hz. The same pattern of discrete DF domain distribution persisted for several minutes in all hearts, with less than about 20% temporal variability during sustained AF.[9] The average area of the domains was 2.99 ± 1.49 and 1.17 ± 1.57 cm^2 in the LA and RA, respectively.[9]

Both the stability of the spatial distribution of DFs and the significant differences in activation frequency and organization between LA and RA strongly suggest that the underlying electrophysiologic properties of the former somehow enable it to support greater activation frequencies than the latter. Moreover, the results indicated that the largest decay in frequency occurred at the junction between Bachmann's bundle

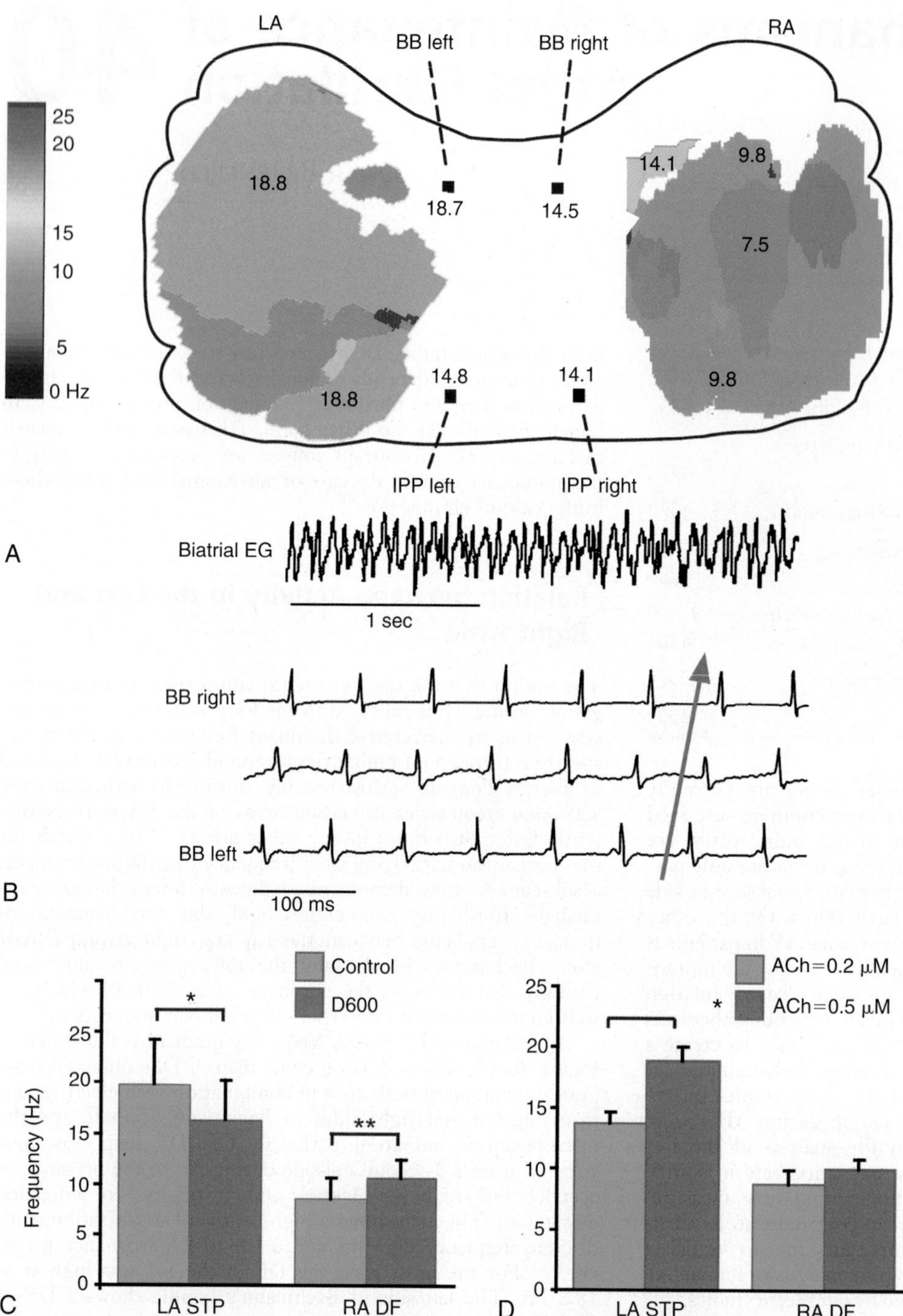

Figure 40-1 Relation between activity in the left atrium (LA) and the right atrium (RA). **A,** LA-to-RA gradient in dominant frequency (DF). DF maps of the epicardial surfaces of LA and RA, with values of DF along Bachmann's bundle (BB) and inferoposterior pathway (IPP). Numbers are expressed in Hertz. The areas of the frequency maps indicate the optical mapping field. **B,** Left-to-right directionality of impulse propagation during atrial fibrillation. Recordings are from a biatrial electrogram (EG, *top trace*) and three bipolar electrodes along Bachmann's bundle, the tracing in the bottom being most leftward. **C,** Effect of D600 and acetylcholine on the LA and RA frequencies. ACh, acetylcholine; LA STP, frequencies of LA spatiotemporal periodicity; RA DF, right atrial dominant frequency. (From Mansour M, Mandapati R, Berenfeld O, et al: Left-to-right gradient of atrial frequencies during acute atrial fibrillation in the isolated sheep heart. Circulation 103:2631-2636, 2001.)

and the RA, where significant pectinate muscle branching occurs, suggesting that the intricate three-dimensional architecture of the pectinate muscle network might have been the substrate for fibrillatory propagation on the RA free wall.[11,19]

Further support for this hypothesis was sought by monitoring the direction of conduction along Bachmann's bundle and inferoposterior interatrial pathway over a distance covered by a minimum of three consecutive bipolar electrodes located on each pathway—that is, 2 cm over Bachmann's bundle and 2.6 cm over the inferoposterior interatrial pathway.[11] Figure 40-1B illustrates an example of left-to-right propagation along Bachmann's bundle during an episode of AF. The top trace is a biatrial electrogram of AF in a 3-sec episode. The bottom three traces are electrograms from the right, middle, and left of Bachmann's bundle during the same episode. Propagation along this pathway was organized and occurred from left to right in the direction of decrease in DF value. Quantification of this finding revealed that wave fronts propagated from left to right in 81% and 80% of the analyzed activations along Bachmann's bundle and inferoposterior interatrial pathway, respectively. Conversely, right-to-left propagation occurred in a significantly smaller percentage of cases.[11]

The data presented in Figure 40-1A and B suggest that in our model, AF results from impulses generated at high frequency by sources in the LA. Such impulses propagate along interatrial pathways to activate the RA in a spatially complex manner. Because the conditions are suggested to be those of fibrillatory propagation, one would expect the existence of LA-to-RA frequency gradients that would be directly related to the source frequency (greatest local frequency observed in the AF episode), with greater degrees of intermittent block at faster rates. To this end, we used D600 (a methoxy derivative of verapamil) to decrease the frequencies (n = 4). Verapamil analogues have been shown to increase organization of ventricular fibrillation (VF) that is also accompanied by a decrease in the VF DF.[20]

In another set of experiments, we increased ACh concentration to increase the AF frequency (n = 4). As shown in Figure 40-1C, D600 decreased the fastest LA frequency from 19.7 ± 4.4 Hz to 16.2 ± 3.9 Hz ($P < 0.01$) and paradoxically increased RA DF from 8.6 ± 2.0 Hz to 10.7 ± 1.8 Hz ($P < 0.05$). In contrast, increasing the ACh concentration from 0.2 to 0.5 μM increased the LA-to-RA frequency gradient from 4.9 ± 1.8 Hz to 8.9 ± 1.8 Hz ($P = 0.02$), as shown in Figure 40-1D. Thus it becomes evident that the LA-to-RA frequency gradient and the RA frequency are determined by the LA frequency. Such a result is incompatible with the multiple wavelet hypothesis or with an independent RA and could only be explained by frequency-dependent change in fibrillatory propagation away from a source in the LA, allowing a greater number of waves to reach the RA at lower source frequencies. In fact, a greater source frequency would result in intermittent blockade because of sink-to-source mismatch between the interatrial pathways and the RA components. When the source frequency was reduced, RA DF increased (remaining lower than the DF of the LA), which indicates lesser mismatch at lower frequencies and explains the experimental findings with D600. Moreover, the increase of the DF induced by ACh in the LA also suggests that the underlying mechanism sustaining AF is unlikely to be a pacemaker or triggered activity.

In sum, we found a clear difference between mean LA and RA DFs, and left-to-right impulse propagation was present in about 80% of cases along Bachmann's bundle and the inferoposterior interatrial pathway.[11] As suggested by more-recent studies, repetitive activation might also originate from the septum[21] or the pulmonary veins.[2,21] Altogether, the data support the contention that AF, as seen on the electrocardiogram (ECG), results from rapidly successive wave fronts emanating from fast sources localized in the LA. The wave fronts propagating through both atria interact with anatomic or functional obstacles (or both), leading to fragmentation and wavelet formation.[8,10,11,22]

Reentrant Activity during Acute Atrial Fibrillation in the Isolated Sheep Heart

The general working hypothesis that acute AF results from activity of a small number of high-frequency reentrant sources localized in one atrium, with fibrillatory conduction to the other atrium, is based primarily on results obtained in the isolated, Langendorff-perfused, sheep heart.[10] We localized the sources that maintain AF by a combined use of optical mapping and frequency analysis. Figure 40-2 shows data from an AF episode in which the site of the high-frequency periodic activity was localized.[10] In Figure 40-2A, an isochrone map from the LA shows one cycle of a vortex that rotated clockwise at a period of 68.6 ± 8.9 ms (~14.7 Hz) and persisted for the entire length of the episode (25 min). The fact that the frequency of this reentrant source (rotor) was equal to the highest and narrowest DF peak (most regular signal) recorded from all sites (optical and electrical recordings; see Mandapati et al[10] for details) provides direct evidence that it was the mechanism underlying AF in this episode.[23] The summation of the activity throughout the field of view (LA pseudo-electrocardiogram in Fig. 40-2B) demonstrates that the entire LA was being activated at 14.7 Hz.

To assess the exact role of a given reentrant activity in determining the global DF of an episode, we collected 14 identified LA vortices with completed rotations. Figure 40-2C shows the relation between the rotation period and the inverse of the global DF obtained from the power spectrum of the corresponding LA pseudo-ECG. The slope of the linear fitted curve was 0.93 ($R = 0.91$), which strongly suggested that the periodicity of rotating spiral waves is the main contributor to the DF in the optically mapped region. Measurements of the dimensions of the core of these rotating waves revealed minuscule cores; the mean core perimeter and area were 10.4 ± 2.8 mm and 3.8 ± 2.8 mm^2, respectively.

Many studies have suggested that AF is characterized by incomplete reentry and multiple unstable reentrant circuits,[8,19,21,24-26] which seems to be consistent with the multiple wavelet hypothesis.[4,26] Thus, for many years interest shifted away from the hypothesis, originally put forth by Lewis[27] and later by Scherf,[28] that a single high-frequency source of stable reentry may be an underlying mechanism that maintains AF.[23] According to the latter concept, despite the presence of a unique and periodic source at any given time, the electrical activity elsewhere could still present as incomplete or as short-lived and unstable reentrant circuits because of fibrillatory conduction.[22] For instance, Schuessler and colleagues[29] found that in an isolated canine right atrial preparation, increasing concentrations of ACh converted multiple reentrant circuits into a single, relatively stable high-frequency reentry that generated fibrillatory conduction. Thus, it seems that the results of the ACh-induced AF presented in Figure 40-2 are in agreement with those of Schuessler's group,[29] and both support the hypothesis that a single or a small number of sources of ongoing reentrant activity is the mechanism underlying AF in this setting.

Frequency-Dependent Breakdown of Propagation

What evidence supports the prediction that a spectral transformation from a periodic source to slower peripheral regions, as expected in fibrillatory conduction (see Figs. 40-1 and 40-2) actually occurs in the atria during high-frequency excitation? Does such a transformation depend on the input frequency? It is well known that during atrial flutter both atria are excited in a 1:1 manner at frequencies as high as 300 beats per minute (5 Hz). On the other hand, data obtained from experimentally induced AF in the sheep heart do show that stationary reentrant sources in the LA can rotate at frequencies greater than 7 Hz and generate impulses that propagate toward the RA.[10,11] Yet the RA is usually not activated at such high frequencies. This suggests that there must be a critical frequency at which the 1:1 input-output relation between the LA and RA breaks down.

In Figure 40-3, I show results of optical mapping experiments and DF analysis in the isolated RA of a sheep heart that demonstrate the principle of frequency-dependent breakdown in conduction.[22] The preparation was subjected to periodic pacing through a bipolar electrode at Bachmann's bundle to simulate activity arriving from a periodic LA source across Bachmann's bundle into the RA.[22] As shown in panel A, stimulation at 5.0 Hz resulted in 1:1 activation of the entire RA, and thus the output DF was also 5.0 Hz everywhere on the

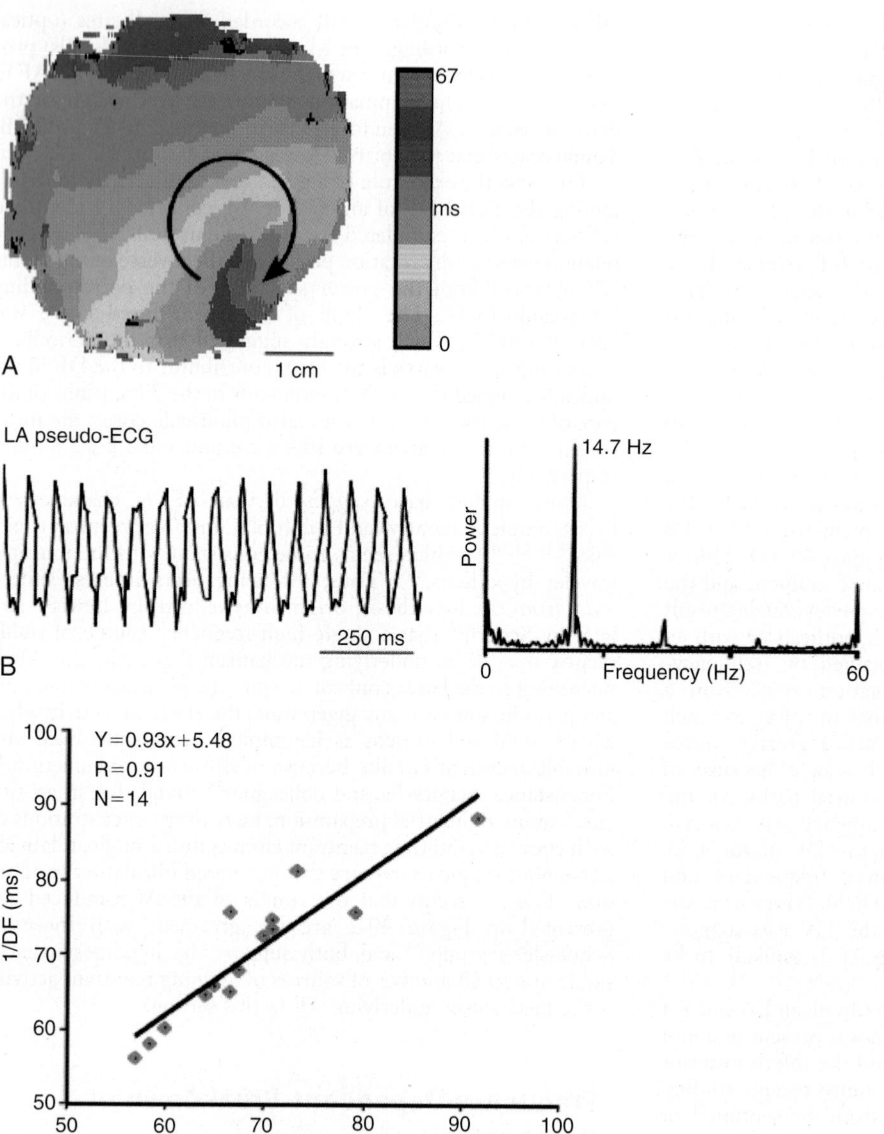

Figure 40-2 Reentrant sources of atrial fibrillation (AF). **A,** Isochrone map of optical activity from the free wall of the left atrium (LA) during sustained AF showing a clockwise reentry. **B,** Optical pseudo-electrocardiogram (ECG) of the LA during the same episode of AF, with its corresponding power spectrum. **C,** Correlation between inverse dominant frequency (DF) from pseudo-ECGs of entire movies (~3 sec long) and rotation period of rotors found within an episode of AF. (From Mandapati R, Skanes A, Chen J, et al: Stable microreentrant sources as a mechanism of atrial fibrillation in the isolated sheep heart. Circulation 101:194-199, 2000.)

endocardial and epicardial surfaces. However, at 7.7 Hz, propagation into the RA was no longer 1:1. Instead, a heterogeneous distribution of DF domains was established in both the endocardium and the epicardium, with frequencies ranging between 3.5 and 7.7 Hz.

Composite data from five experiments are presented in graphic form in panel B. The DFs measured on the endocardium are plotted as a function of the pacing frequency. Clearly, below 6.7 Hz the response DF showed no dispersion in any of the experiments, which meant that activation was 1:1 everywhere in the RA. Above the breakdown frequency of 6.7 Hz, there was a large DF dispersion manifest as multiple domains whose individual frequencies were either equal to or lower than the pacing frequency. In addition, we found that intermittent block resulted in a significant loss of consistency in the beat-to-beat direction of wavefront propagation, which provided a direct explanation for the difficulty in finding an origin of the activation during fibrillatory conduction.[22] We also found that the distribution of action potential duration at a low pacing rate of 3.3 Hz did not correspond to the distribution of DF domains, which led us to suggest that dispersion of refractoriness at normal frequencies is a poor predictor of the spatial distribution of intermittent block patterns that characterize AF outside the source region.[22]

Spatial Distribution of Dominant Frequencies during Atrial Fibrillation in Patients

Several studies have characterized the spatial distribution of DF during AF in patients.[15,30,31] Using the CARTO electroanatomic mapping system, Sanders and colleagues[15] sequentially acquired 5-second-long bipolar recordings from about 120 points throughout both atria and the coronary sinus (CS) in 32 patients during sustained AF. The recorded signals were rectified[32] and 3- to 15-Hz band-pass filtered, then fast Fourier transform was used to determine the DF of each of 120 segments lasting 4.096 sec

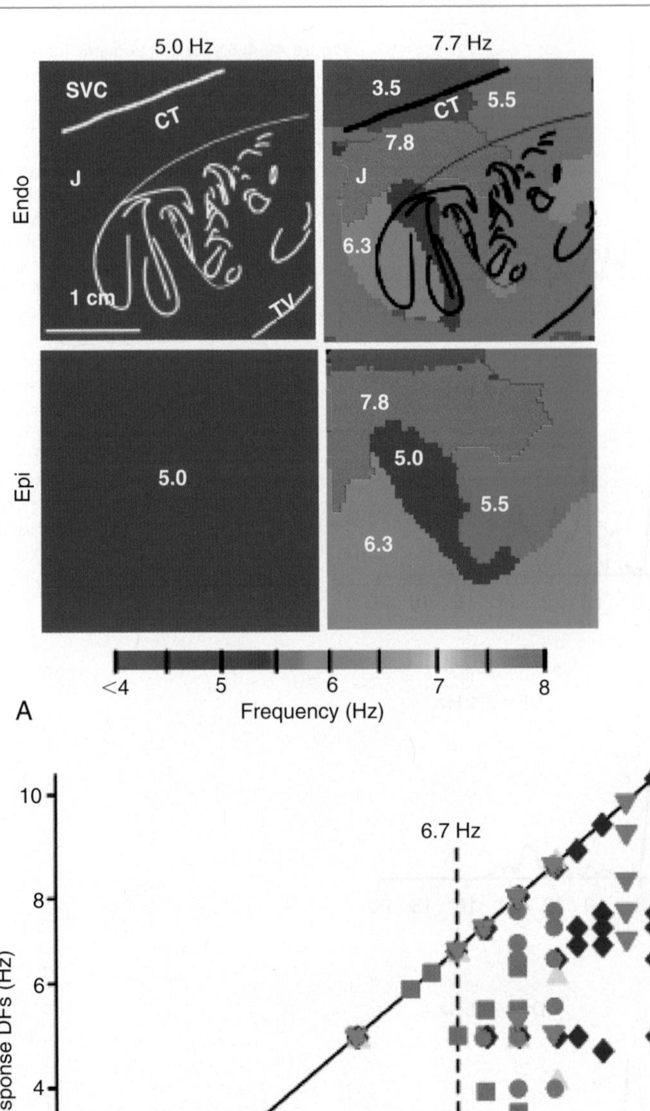

Figure 40-3 The breakdown frequency in a sheep heart. A, Endocardial (Endo) and epicardial (Epi) dominant frequency (DF) maps of the same isolated right atrial preparation paced at 5.0 and 7.7 Hz. B, the appearance of heterogeneous DF domains at 7.7 Hz. B, Response DFs versus the pacing rate (n = 5). Each symbol represents one experiment. Pacing Bachmann's bundle at rates below ~6.7 Hz results in 1:1 activation. At higher rates, the number of domains increases but the DFs' values decrease. (From Berenfeld O, Zaitsev AV, Mironov SF, et al: Frequency-dependent breakdown of wave propagation into fibrillatory conduction across the pectinate muscle network in the isolated sheep right atrium. Circ Res 90:1173-1180, 2002.)

with a resolution of 0.24 Hz.[33] Patients with paroxysmal AF and patients with permanent AF demonstrated dominant frequency gradients from LA to RA to CS. However, compared to patients with paroxysmal AF, patients with permanent AF demonstrated significantly higher average frequencies of activity.[15,16,31,34]

Figure 40-4 shows four sample bipolar electrograms with their respective power spectra acquired from endocardial sites in the LA and RA of a patient with paroxysmal AF of spontaneous onset.[15] On the left are typical AF recordings with variable amplitudes and interbeat intervals, which do not enable accurate cycle length analysis, particularly in the top recording. However, the spectra on the right show relatively narrow bands in the 3- to 15-Hz range, with distinct peaks of DFs approximately corresponding to the activation rate and the inverse of the average cycle length in the electrograms.[33,35]

In all patients, electrograms were collected from multiple sites (typically 120 in both atria), and their corresponding DFs were superimposed on the atrial geometry to generate color DF maps,[15] as illustrated in Figure 40-5. On each DF map, sites that demonstrated high-frequency activity with a gradient of 20% or more relative to the surrounding atrial tissue were defined as high-DF sites. In this study, most high-DF sites involved a single point, but in some the high-DF site extended over two or three adjacent points.

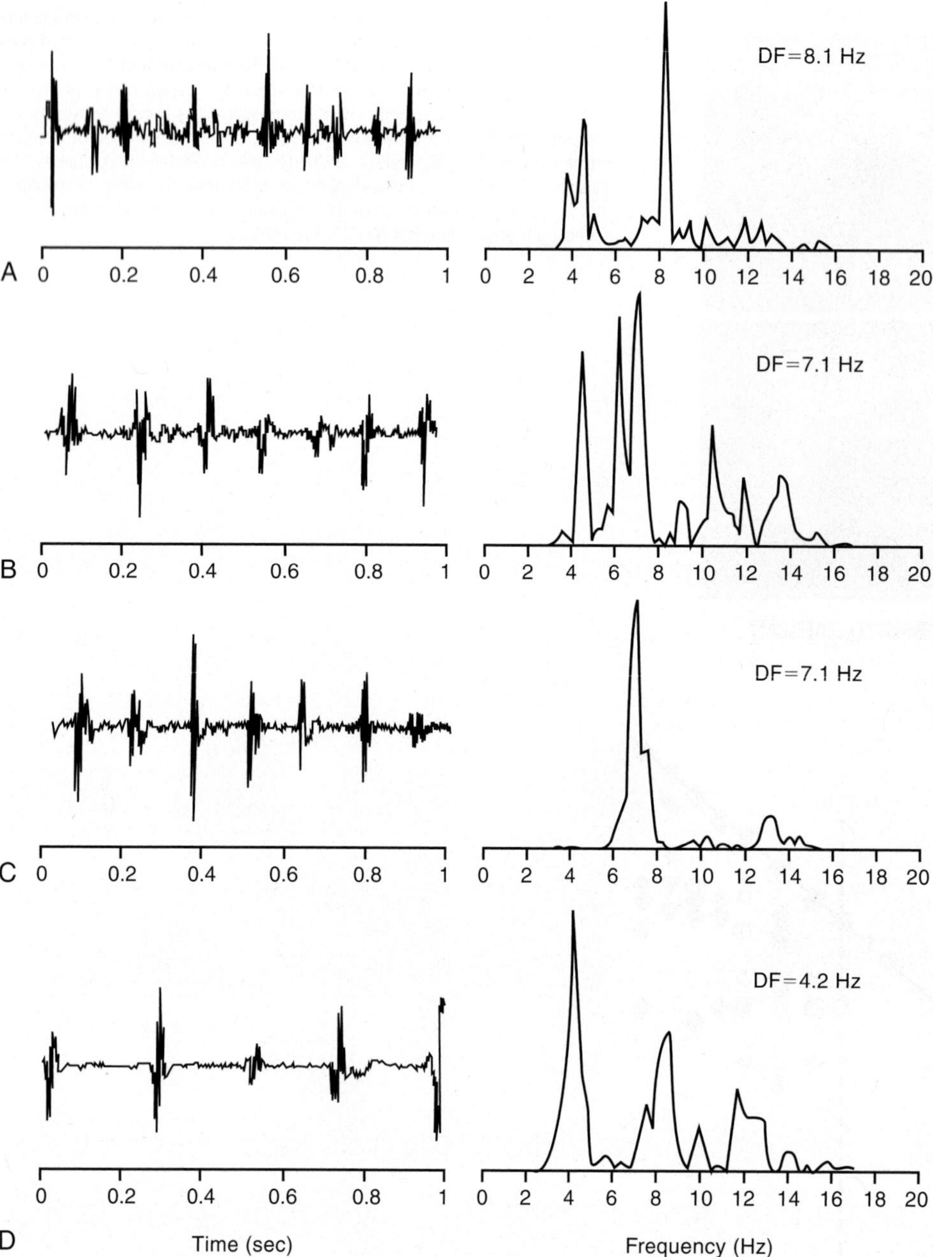

Figure 40-4 Bipolar electrograms and corresponding power spectra obtained from four points in a patient with spontaneous paroxysmal atrial fibrillation. Each site shows distinct dominant frequency (DF) and regularity index (RI) values. **A,** This tracing clearly demonstrates the utility of spectral analysis. The bipolar recording shows low-amplitude complex signals that make accurate determination of frequency of activation difficult. The power spectrum clearly demonstrates the DF at 8.1 Hz. The DF map of this patient is shown in Figure 41-5A. This tracing is from the site of maximal DF at the right inferior pulmonary vein. **B** and **C,** Tracings from other high-DF sites in the right superior pulmonary vein and left superior pulmonary vein. **D,** Tracing from the posterior right atrium. (From Sanders P, Berenfeld O, Hocini M, et al: Spectral analysis identifies sites of high-frequency activity maintaining atrial fibrillation in humans. Circulation 112:789-797, 2005.)

Figure 40-5A reproduces left anterior oblique (left) and posteroanterior (right) views[15] of the same map showing fibrillatory activity at mean DF of about 4.8 Hz in the paroxysmal AF patient whose electrograms are shown in Figure 40-4. Although frequency in the majority of the atria and CS was relatively slow (5 Hz), the posterior wall of the LA was activated at faster rates (7-8 Hz), with notable high-DF sites at each of the pulmonary veins. In this patient, focal radiofrequency ablation applied to the high-DF site near the right inferior pulmonary vein (RIPV) effectively terminated AF. Figure 40-5B shows a DF map from a patient with permanent AF. Compared with the patient with paroxysmal AF, this patient had a higher frequency at the maximal high-DF site (13.7 Hz), and both atria demonstrated higher global frequency of activity, and many of the high-DF sites were located in the atria rather in the pulmonary vein region.[15,16]

We concluded that in the cohort of patients studied, paroxysmal AF was characterized by the hierarchical spatial distribution of DFs where the LA and pulmonary veins were always the fastest regions. By contrast, in persistent AF, a more uniform distribution of higher DF values was observed, where the highest DFs could rarely be found in the pulmonary vein region.[15,16]

High Dominant Frequency Sites and Maintenance of Atrial Fibrillation

AF mapping studies have recognized the presence of temporally and spatially periodic activity[10,36-38] emanating from the pulmonary vein region with regularity,[8] suggesting that these

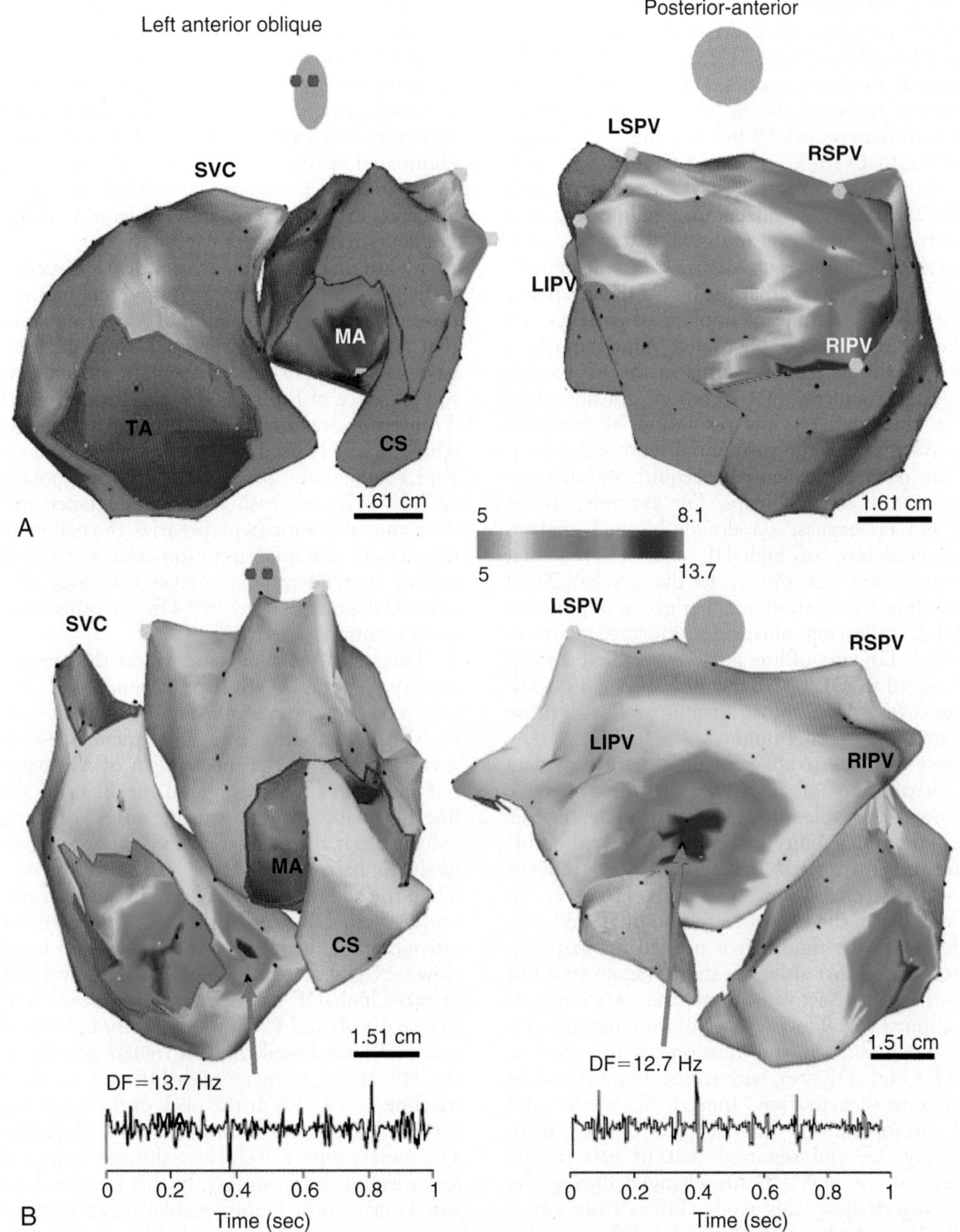

Figure 40-5 Dominant frequency (DF) maps of human atrial fibrillation (AF). **A,** DF map in a patient with paroxysmal AF (6 hours). Note high-DF sites in each of the pulmonary veins. Ablation sequence in this patient was left superior pulmonary vein (LSPV), left inferior pulmonary vein (LIPV), right superior pulmonary vein (RSPV), and right inferior pulmonary vein (RIPV) (site of AF termination); AF cycle length increased by 10 ms, 25 ms, 9 ms, and 75 ms, respectively, before termination. **B,** DF map in a patient with permanent AF (24 months). The maximal DF and atrial frequency are higher than those of the patient in **A**. In addition, many of the high-DF sites are located outside the pulmonary veins. Ablation sequence in this patient was RIPV, RSPV, LSPV, and LIPV; AF cycle length increased by 5 ms, 2 ms, 0 ms, and 5 ms, respectively. The electrograms of the sites of maximal DF in the left atrium and right atrium are presented showing significant fractionation. Color-bar, scale in Hz. MA, mitral annulus; SVC, superior vena cava; TA, tricuspid annulus. (From Sanders P, Berenfeld O, Hocini M, et al: Spectral analysis identifies sites of high-frequency activity maintaining atrial fibrillation in humans. Circulation 112:789-797, 2005.)

structures might have a role in maintaining AF[10] by harboring either localized short cycle length reentrant sources or focal automatic activity.[39,40] A recent study using a morphologically accurate computer model of the atria has demonstrated that the pulmonary vein region is a preferential site for anchoring rotors.[41] In the clinic, paroxysms of short cycle length activity have been observed in the pulmonary veins of patients undergoing AF ablation.[42-44] Sequential ablation of sites showing the shortest cycle length has been associated with a progressive slowing of AF frequency, culminating in termination in 75% of patients with paroxysmal AF.[13]

Using a blind correlation between atrial DF distribution and ablation, without any attempt at identifying potentially arrhythmogenic sites at the time of the procedure, Sanders and coworkers[15] found that ablation at pulmonary veins harboring high-DF sites resulted in an increase in AF cycle length (AFCL) (≥5 ms) within the CS in 89% of cases. This was true in patients with either paroxysmal or permanent AF. However, eventual arrhythmia termination occurred during ablation in 15 (88%) out of 17 patients with paroxysmal AF but in none with permanent AF ($P < 0.0001$). In 13 (87%) of the 15 patients with paroxysmal AF, arrhythmia termination was associated with ablation at a high-DF site; 11 localized to a pulmonary vein and two to the LA roof and the fossa ovalis.

These data together with those of Atienza and colleagues[16] and Lazar's group[45] clearly indicate that the high-DF sites play a role in maintaining AF in a significant number of patients. To what extent one should expect to be able to determine the role of the high-DF sites in maintaining arrhythmia in the AF patient population at large? To address that question, consideration should be given to the relatively low resolution of currently available mapping systems and the substantial temporal limitation imposed by the need to sequentially acquire the electrograms needed to generate the DF maps. For example, in the study of Sanders and colleagues,[15] a double-blinded analysis showed that the percentage of high-DF sites ablated that resulted in AF termination was similar to the percentage of sites that did not result in termination in either group of patients. On the other hand, following ablation performed without knowledge of the high-DF site, offline analysis revealed significantly shorter RF duration (21.9 ± 18.6 minutes) per high-DF site ablated in patients with AF termination compared with those in whom AF persisted (42.4 ± 26.4 minutes; $P = 0.008$).

Such data suggest that due to the sequential nature of data acquisition, the distribution of high-DF sites might have changed by the time the ablation was performed. In this regard, studies on temporal stability of DFs at or near the pulmonary veins[30] and the entire atria[15] have found no significant change over periods between 10 and 20 seconds. However, an assessment of the stability in the CS over a period of 50 minutes, which is more relevant to the time that is needed for mapping and ablation, demonstrated that although there was no trend of acceleration or slowing of the activation rate, the instantaneous rate fluctuated by about 1 Hz. The presence of such fluctuations possibly reflected spatial shifts in the locations of the discrete drivers responsible for high-DF sites, with concomitant transient alterations in local rate of activation. Indeed, Schuessler and coworkers[34] used intraoperatively bipolar electrograms from epicardial sites during AF and reported that in half of the patients the location of the high-DF site changed during the recording period. Nevertheless, this study differs from other studies by the finding that the location of the high-DF was independent of the type of AF, which raises the possibility that it might not reflect the location of the actual high-DF site. The obvious conclusion here is that efficient use of DF mapping as a clinical electrophysiologic tool to localize and terminate AF drivers by RF ablation in many patients will require higher resolution mapping, with multiple simultaneous electrograms and online power spectral analysis.

Activation Frequency and Driver Mechanisms

Overall, it seems that the dynamic nature of AF keeps the spatiotemporal variability of the DF within a limit that allows consistent identification of high-DF sites as discrete AF drivers despite the mapping limitations. Morillo and colleagues targeted ablation to sites of short cycle length activity in the posterior LA and observed the termination of arrhythmia in a canine model of AF.[6] Using a sterile pericarditis model, Kumagai's group identified in the septum dominant unstable reentrant circuits of very short CL that maintained AF and could be successfully terminated by focal ablation.[21,46] Others have reported that in some patients, sustained focal activity at the pulmonary veins, CS, or superior vena cava initiated and maintained AF and could be eliminated by discrete ablation.[47] However, to this date, whether such sites are automatic, triggered, or reentrant and whether changes in the driver activity would alter spatial frequency gradients remains unresolved.

Identifying rotors as drivers of AF directly in patients is very difficult with the existing mapping techniques.[48,49] Yet, the ACh dose-dependent acceleration of rotor frequency[50] offered an idea that enabled translating animal experiments to the patient and gave us the opportunity to obtain evidence, albeit indirect, for the presence of rotors as drivers through pharmacologic means. Translation was made possible also by the fact that adenosine, which is widely used in the clinic, is known to activate the same Kir3.x subfamily of inward rectifier potassium channels as ACh.[51-53] By increasing K^+ conductance in the atrium, both ACh and adenosine hyperpolarize the cell membrane, abbreviate the action potential duration and the refractory period, and inhibit spontaneous pacemaker discharge as well as early and delayed depolarizations.[51,52] On the other hand they both accelerate reentrant activity.[50]

Thus, we used adenosine to test the hypothesis that localized reentry maintains AF also in humans.[16] We determined the effects of adenosine infusion on DF at varying locations of both atria with the idea that adenosine-induced acceleration reveals reentry as the mechanism of AF maintenance and rules out an automatic or triggered mechanism. We generated baseline DF maps of the LA using novel real-time spectral analysis software that allowed determination of the specific high-DF sites likely to harbor the AF drivers[15] in paroxysmal AF patients. Then the adenosine effect was measured at the primary and secondary high-DF sites in the LA. Figure 40-6 shows a representative example where the AF frequency at baseline was relatively slow (<5 Hz) and three high-DF sites were identified, with the primary high-DF site being located near the RIPV (red arrow). Figure 40-6B and C shows that although the adenosine infusion practically abolished the ventricular activity as detected by V5, the DF at the primary high-DF site accelerated from 4.64 at baseline to 6.35 Hz at the peak of the adenosine effect. An additional adenosine infusion performed while measuring activity at a secondary high-DF site also showed an increase in DF, but to a lesser extent. Interestingly, in this patient the arrhythmia terminated during post-mapping ablation at the primary high-DF site, supporting again the critical role of such sites as AF drivers.[15] Compared to baseline, adenosine significantly accelerated the primary and secondary high-DF sites in these patients from about 5 to 6.7 Hz,[16] demonstrating that the sites involved in the maintenance of AF are clearly affected by adenosine.

In a larger cohort of paroxysmal and persistent AF patients, Atienza and colleagues[16] analyzed the effect of adenosine on the activation rate in specific regions at the junction of the pulmonary vein and the LA, the roof of the RA, and the CS. In general, patients with persistent AF demonstrated significantly higher maximal baseline DFs than patients with paroxysmal AF ($P < 0.001$). However, adenosine infusion in patients with persistent AF increased local DFs only in the roof of the RA. The increase in the pulmonary vein–left atrial junction was not statistically significant, and there was no change in the CS DF.

In sum, adenosine infusion increased frequency primarily at sites that activated at the highest rate at baseline. In patients with paroxysmal AF, adenosine increased activation frequency in the pulmonary vein–left atrial junction. In patients with persistent AF, the highest-frequency sources accelerated by adenosine were

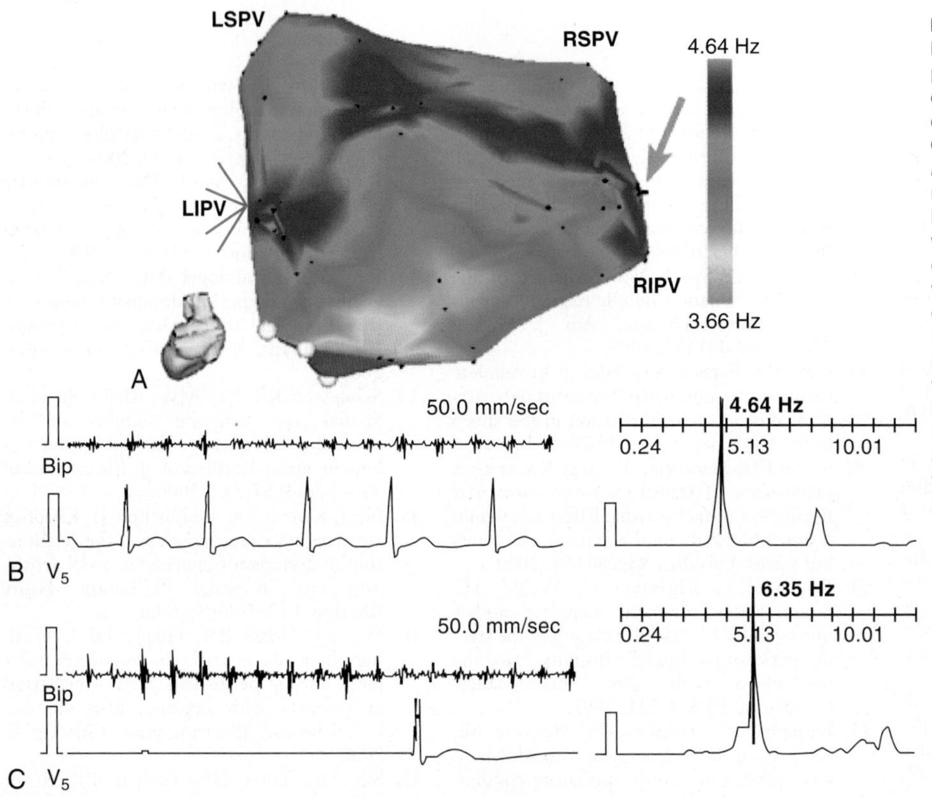

Figure 40-6 Accelerating effect of adenosine on high–dominant frequency (DF) site. **A,** Left atrium posterior view DF map from a patient with paroxysmal atrial fibrillation. The DF map was produced by the real-time frequency-mapping CARTO system before infusion of adenosine. The *red arrow* indicates the primary high-DF site near the right inferior pulmonary vein (RIPV). **B,** Baseline recording at the primary high-DF site with its power spectrum and simultaneous V_5 reference. **C,** Recording at the primary high-DF site with power spectrum and simultaneous V_5 reference during peak adenosine effect showing increase of DF. Bip, bipolar catheter; LIPV, left inferior pulmonary vein; LSPV, left superior pulmonary vein; RSPV, right superior pulmonary vein. (From Atienza F, Almendral J, Moreno J, et al: Activation of inward rectifier potassium channels accelerates atrial fibrillation in humans: evidence for a reentrant mechanism. Circulation 114:2434-2442, 2006.)

located in either atrium but not at pulmonary vein sites. Thus, the response to adenosine is consistent with reentrant drivers maintaining AF that have different locations in patients with paroxysmal compared with persistent AF.[16]

Summary and Future Directions

Experimental studies of cholinergic AF in the isolated sheep heart[54] demonstrated that high-frequency sources in the LA drive the fibrillatory activity throughout both atria. Following those results and based on a large body of work investigating how measurements of the cycle length of activity in patients during AF can contribute to its treatment,[12,13,15,16] we focused our analysis on the organization of DF of the activity during AF in humans. Using electroanatomic mapping and Fourier methods, we generated three-dimensional, whole-atrial DF maps in patients undergoing AF ablation procedures and identified relatively small high-DF sites. In patients with paroxysmal AF, the high-DF sites are often localized to the posterior LA near the ostia of the pulmonary veins. In contrast, patients with permanent AF demonstrate high-DF sites that are more often localized to either atrium than to the junction of the posterior LA and pulmonary vein. In our study, ablation at high-DF sites resulted in significant slowing of the arrhythmia and termination of sustained AF in 87% of patients with paroxysmal AF.[15] The response of the arrhythmia to adenosine is consistent with the mechanistic hypothesis that reentry in those high-DF sites maintains human AF and that reentrant drivers have different locations in patients with paroxysmal AF compared with patients with persistent AF.

In the future, the combined use of time and frequency domain measures, including electrogram fractionation[55] and DF mapping, should help elucidate AF mechanism, mainly in two specific areas. The first is the broad range of chronic conditions that are responsible for remodeling the atria, either electrically or structurally. Experimental data from our laboratory[56] and others[57] indicate that the spatiotemporal organization of fibrillatory waves depends on the type of remodeling. It is envisioned that the use of advanced analysis methods will allow better correlation of arrhythmia dynamics with the remodeled atria and facilitate the translation of knowledge into the clinical setting,[16] where chronic conditions underlying AF currently pose the greatest therapeutic challenge.[5,15] The clinical application of frequency spectrum analysis is therefore the second major area of interest. The ability to determine whether AF is maintained by discrete high-frequency sources and to identify their location might help improve the efficacy of ablation procedures. Indeed, DF analysis of bipolar recordings obtained during AF ablation strongly suggests that specific high-DF sites are the drivers that maintain AF in certain groups of patients.[15] Identification of the drivers and characterization of their dynamics might provide an efficient means of developing more patient-specific ablation procedures[58] with increased efficacy and safety.[59,60]

References

1. Chen LY, Shen WK: Epidemiology of atrial fibrillation: A current perspective. Heart Rhythm 4:S1-S6, 2007.
2. Haissaguerre M, Jais P, Shah DC, et al: Spontaneous initiation of atrial fibrillation by ectopic beats originating in the pulmonary veins. N Engl J Med 339:659-666, 1998.
3. Haissaguerre M, Shah DC, Jais P, et al: Mapping-guided ablation of pulmonary veins to cure atrial fibrillation. Am J Cardiol 86:9K-19K, 2000.
4. Moe GK, Abildskov JA: Atrial fibrillation as a self-sustaining arrhythmia independent of focal discharges. Am Heart J 58:59-70, 1959.
5. Oral H, Pappone C, Chugh A, et al: Circumferential pulmonary-vein ablation for chronic atrial fibrillation. N Engl J Med 354:934-941, 2006.
6. Morillo CA, Klein GJ, Jones DL, Guiraudon CM: Chronic rapid atrial pacing: Structural, functional, and electrophysiological characteristics of a new model of sustained atrial fibrillation. Circulation 91:1588-1595, 1995.
7. Harada A, Sasaki K, Fukushima T, et al: Atrial activation during chronic atrial fibrillation in patients with isolated mitral valve disease. Ann Thorac Surg 61:104-112, 1996.
8. Skanes AC, Mandapati R, Berenfeld O, et al: Spatiotemporal periodicity during atrial fibrillation in the isolated sheep heart. Circulation 98:1236-1248, 1998.
9. Berenfeld O, Mandapati R, Dixit S, et al: Spatially distributed dominant excitation frequencies reveal hidden organization in atrial fibrillation in the Langendorff-perfused sheep heart. J Cardiovasc Electrophysiol 11:869-879, 2000.
10. Mandapati R, Skanes A, Chen J, et al: Stable microreentrant sources as a mechanism of atrial fibrillation in the isolated sheep heart. Circulation 101:194-199, 2000.
11. Mansour M, Mandapati R, Berenfeld O, et al: Left-to-right gradient of atrial frequencies during acute atrial fibrillation in the isolated sheep heart. Circulation 103:2631-2636, 2001.
12. Pappone C, Rosanio S: Pulmonary vein isolation for atrial fibrillation. In Zipes DP, Jalife J (eds): Cardiac Electrophysiology: From Cell to Bedside. Philadelphia, Saunders, 2004, pp 1039-1052.
13. Haissaguerre M, Sanders P, Hocini M, et al: Changes in atrial fibrillation cycle length and inducibility during catheter ablation and their relation to outcome. Circulation 109:3007-3013, 2004.
14. Berenfeld O: Quantifying activation frequency in atrial fibrillation to establish underlying mechanisms and ablation guidance. Heart Rhythm 4:1225-1234, 2007.
15. Sanders P, Berenfeld O, Hocini M, et al: Spectral analysis identifies sites of high-frequency activity maintaining atrial fibrillation in humans. Circulation 112:789-797, 2005.
16. Atienza F, Almendral J, Moreno J, et al: Activation of inward rectifier potassium channels accelerates atrial fibrillation in humans: evidence for a reentrant mechanism. Circulation 114:2434-2442, 2006.
17. Antz M, Otomo K, Arruda M, et al: Electrical connections between the right atrium and the left atrium via the musculature of the coronary sinus. Circulation 98:1790-1795, 1998.
18. Dolber PC, Spach MS: Structure of the canine Bachmann's bundle related to propagation of excitation. Am J Physiol 257:H1446-H1457, 1989.
19. Gray RA, Pertsov AM, Jalife J: Incomplete reentry and epicardial breakthrough patterns during atrial fibrillation in the sheep heart. Circulation 94:2649-2661, 1996.
20. Samie FH, Mandapati R, Gray RA, et al: A mechanism of transition from ventricular fibrillation to tachycardia: Effect of calcium channel blockade on the dynamics of rotating waves. Circ Res 86:684-691, 2000.
21. Kumagai K, Khrestian C, Waldo AL: Simultaneous multisite mapping studies during induced atrial fibrillation in the sterile pericarditis model. Insights into the mechanisms of its maintenance. Circulation 95:511-521, 1997.
22. Berenfeld O, Zaitsev AV, Mironov SF, et al: Frequency-dependent breakdown of wave propagation into fibrillatory conduction across the pectinate muscle network in the isolated sheep right atrium. Circ Res 90:1173-1180, 2002.
23. Jalife J, Berenfeld O, Skanes A, Mandapati R: Mechanisms of atrial fibrillation: Mother rotors or multiple daughter wavelets, or both? J Cardiovasc Electrophysiol 9:S2-S12, 1998.
24. Ortiz J, Niwano S, Abe H, et al: Mapping the conversion of atrial flutter to atrial fibrillation and atrial fibrillation to atrial flutter. Insights into mechanisms. Circ Res 74:882-894, 1994.
25. Ikeda T, Wu TJ, Uchida T, et al: Meandering and unstable reentrant wave fronts induced by acetylcholine in isolated canine right atrium. Am J Physiol 273:H356-H370, 1997.
26. Allessie MA, Lammers WJEP, Bonke FIM, Hollen J: Experimental evaluation of Moe's wavelet hypothesis of atrial fibrillation. In Zipes DP, Jalife J (eds): Cardiac Electrophysiology and Arrhythmias. Orlando, Grune & Stratton, 1985, pp 265-275.
27. Lewis T: The Mechanism and Graphic Registration of the Heart Beat. London, Shaw & Sons, 1925.
28. Scherf D: Studies on auricular tachycardia caused by aconitine administration. Proc Soc Exp Biol Med 64:233-239, 1947.
29. Schuessler RB, Grayson TM, Bromberg BI, et al: Cholinergically mediated tachyarrhythmias induced by a single extrastimulus in the isolated canine right atrium. Circ Res 71:1254-1267, 1992.
30. Lazar S, Dixit S, Marchlinski FE, et al: Presence of left-to-right atrial frequency gradient in paroxysmal but not persistent atrial fibrillation in humans. Circulation 110:3181-3186, 2004.
31. Sahadevan J, Ryu K, Peltz L, et al: Epicardial mapping of chronic atrial fibrillation in patients: Preliminary observations. Circulation 110:3293-3299, 2004.
32. Botteron GW, Smith JM: Quantitative assessment of the spatial organization of atrial fibrillation in the intact human heart. Circulation 93:513-518, 1996.
33. Fischer G, Stuhlinger MC, Nowak CN, et al: On computing dominant frequency from bipolar intracardiac electrograms. IEEE Trans Biomed Eng 54:165-169, 2007.
34. Schuessler RB, Kay MW, Melby SJ, et al: Spatial and temporal stability of the dominant frequency of activation in human atrial fibrillation. J Electrocardiol 39(4 Suppl):S7-S12, 2006.
35. Ng J, Kadish AH, Goldberger JJ: Effect of electrogram characteristics on the relationship of dominant frequency to atrial activation rate in atrial fibrillation. Heart Rhythm 3:1295-1305, 2006.
36. Wu TJ, Doshi RN, Huang HLA, et al: Simultaneous biatrial computerized mapping during permanent atrial fibrillation in patients with organic heart disease. J Cardiovasc Electrophysiol 13:571-577, 2002.
37. Sih HJ, Zipes DP, Berbari EJ, et al: Differences in organization between acute and chronic atrial fibrillation in dogs. J Am Coll Cardiol 36:924-931, 2000.
38. Wu TJ, Ong JJC, Chang CM, et al: Pulmonary veins and ligament of Marshall as sources of rapid activations in a canine model of sustained atrial fibrillation. Circulation 103:1157-1163, 2001.
39. Arora R, Verheule S, Scott L, et al: Arrhythmogenic substrate of the pulmonary veins assessed by high-resolution optical mapping. Circulation 107:1816-1821, 2003.
40. Kalifa J, Jalife J, Zaitsev AV, et al: Intra-atrial pressure increases rate and organization of waves emanating from the superior pulmonary veins during atrial fibrillation. Circulation 108:668-671, 2003.
41. Vigmond EJ, Tsoi V, Kuo S, et al: The effect of vagally induced dispersion of action potential duration on atrial arrhythmogenesis. Heart Rhythm 1:334-344, 2004.
42. Kumagai K, Yasuda T, Tojo H, et al: Role of rapid focal activation in the maintenance of atrial fibrillation originating from the pulmonary veins. Pacing Clin Electrophysiol 23:1823-1827, 2000.
43. O'Donnell D, Furniss SS, Bourke JP: Paroxysmal cycle length shortening in the pulmonary veins during atrial fibrillation correlates with arrhythmogenic triggering foci in sinus. Rhythm J Cardiovasc Electrophysiol 13:124-128, 2002.
44. Oral H, Ozaydin M, Tada H, et al: Mechanistic significance of intermittent pulmonary vein tachycardia in patients with atrial fibrillation. J Cardiovasc Electrophysiol 13:645-650, 2002.
45. Lazar S, Dixit S, Callans DJ, et al: Effect of pulmonary vein isolation on the left-to-right atrial dominant frequency gradient

in human atrial fibrillation. Heart Rhythm 3:889-895, 2006.

46. Kumagai K, Uno K, Khrestian C, Waldo AL: Single site radiofrequency catheter ablation of atrial fibrillation: Studies guided by simultaneous multisite mapping in the canine sterile pericarditis model. J Am Coll Cardiol 36:917-923, 2000.
47. Jais P, Haissaguerre M, Shah DC, et al: A focal source of atrial fibrillation treated by discrete radiofrequency ablation. Circulation 95:572-576, 1997.
48. Sanders P, Hocini M, Jais P, et al: Characterization of focal atrial tachycardia using high-density mapping. J Am Coll Cardiol 46:2088-2099, 2005.
49. Hsu LF, Jais P, Hocini M, et al: High-density circumferential pulmonary vein mapping with a 20-pole expandable circular mapping catheter. Pacing Clin Electrophysiol 28(Suppl 1):S94-S98, 2005.
50. Sarmast F, Kolli A, Zaitsev A, et al: Cholinergic atrial fibrillation: $I_{K,ACh}$ gradients determine unequal left/right atrial frequencies and rotor dynamics. Cardiovasc Res 59:863-873, 2003.
51. Kabell G, Buchanan LV, Gibson JK, Belardinelli L: Effects of adenosine on atrial refractoriness and arrhythmias. Cardiovasc Res 28:1385-1389, 1994.
52. Belardinelli L, Shryock JC, Song Y, et al: Ionic basis of the electrophysiological actions of adenosine on cardiomyocytes. FASEB J 9:359-365, 1995.
53. Khositseth A, Clapham DE, Ackerman MJ: Intracellular signaling and regulation of cardiac ion channels. In Zipes DP, Jalife J (eds): Cardiac Electrophysiology: From Cell to Bedside. Philadelphia, Saunders, 2004, pp 33-41.
54. Jalife J, Berenfeld O, Mansour M: Mother rotors and fibrillatory conduction: A mechanism of atrial fibrillation. Cardiovasc Res 54:204-216, 2002.
55. Nademanee K, McKenzie J, Kosar E, et al: A new approach for catheter ablation of atrial fibrillation: Mapping of the electrophysiologic substrate. J Am Coll Cardiol 43:2044-2053, 2004.
56. Tanaka K, Zlochiver S, Vikstrom KL, et al: Spatial distribution of fibrosis governs fibrillation wave dynamics in the posterior left atrium during heart failure. Circ Res 101:839-847, 2007.
57. Everett TH, Wilson EE, Verheule S, et al: Structural atrial remodeling alters the substrate and spatiotemporal organization of AF: A comparison in canine models of structural and electrical atrial remodeling. Am J Physiol Heart Circ Physiol 291(6):H2911-H2923, 2006.
58. Oral H, Chugh A, Good E, et al: A tailored approach to catheter ablation of paroxysmal atrial fibrillation. Circulation 113:1824-1831, 2006.
59. Bertaglia E, Zoppo F, Tondo C, et al: Early complications of pulmonary vein catheter ablation for atrial fibrillation: A multicenter prospective registry on procedural safety. Heart Rhythm 4:1265-1271, 2007.
60. Cappato R, Calkins H, Chen SA, et al: Worldwide survey on the methods, efficacy, and safety of catheter ablation for human atrial fibrillation. Circulation 111:1100-1105, 2005.

Electrophysiologic Basis of Electrogram Fragmentation in Atrial Fibrillation 41

Jérôme Kalifa

CHAPTER OUTLINE

Catheter ablation targeting fractionated electrograms during atrial fibrillation (AF) has been proposed as a standalone technique or in association with other approaches.[1-4] Although several variants exist, in general, the approach consists of delivering radio-frequency energy to areas in the atria that have complex fractionated atrial electrograms (CFAEs). As originally defined, CFAEs are electrograms with highly fractionated potentials; a very short cycle length (<120 ms) or low voltage (0.06-0.25 mV), or both; and multiple potentials.[5]

During AF ablation, identification and elimination of the areas with CFAEs has been implemented by several centers with variable success.[1-4] Although the exact indications of this technique are still debated, the basic understanding of the electrophysiologic mechanisms of electrogram fractionation is critical to improving the definition, the software-detection algorithms, the interpretation of electrogram fractionation, and ultimately the use of CFAE ablation to terminate AF. Various experimental models as well as data in patients have provided mechanistic insight into atrial electrogram fractionation.

Atrial fractionation can be found in strictly normal atria[6-8] or can indicate the presence of a pathophysiologic process potentially leading to AF.[9,10] Numerical simulations and optical mapping techniques, as well as data in patients, have suggested the possibility of localizing AF sources by means of combined dominant frequency and fractionation measurements.[2,11] This chapter summarizes some of these studies.

Complex Fractionated Atrial Electrograms

The definition of CFAEs published in the expert consensus statement of the Heart Rhythm Society, the European Heart Rhythm Association, and the European Cardiac Arrhythmias Society (HRS/EHRA/ECAS)[5] includes several parameters that are commonly reported.[1,2,12] An AF atrial electrogram is classified as fractionated if it includes multiple deflections (at least two) or continuous electrical activity at low voltage. In practice, this definition is difficult to implement in the electrophysiology laboratory, and most investigators use an eyeball evaluation instead. This rough estimate, however, has proved challenging when attempting to retrospectively determine mechanisms underlying CFAEs.

We have demonstrated that during stable AF in the isolated sheep heart, electrograms obtained from the areas that harbor the highest-frequency activity (maximum dominant frequency [DF_{max}] domain) in the posterior left atrium (LA) are regular and highly organized, whereas electrograms recorded at the outer limit of the DF_{max} domains are highly variable and fractionated.[11] These results introduced a new perspective for the combined use of dominant-frequency mapping and CFAE analysis in both paroxysmal and chronic AF to precisely localize and target AF sources at the posterior LA and elsewhere. Unfortunately, the idea has not found widespread use in the clinic, in part because some influential opinion leaders erroneously believe that mapping high dominant-frequency areas is ineffective in chronic AF patients, even in the presence of CFAEs.[13]

Yet, contrary to this idea, it has been independently demonstrated by several laboratories that DF mapping is a highly effective tool to investigate the AF substrate and differentiate between paroxysmal and chronic AF patients in terms of the number of AF sources and their localization in the atria.[14-16] Moreover, as detailed later, high dominant-frequency and electrogram fractionation are correlated both spatially[11] and temporally.[2] On the other hand, caution should be exercised because quantification of fractionation cannot be entirely reduced to electrogram frequency measurement because fractionated electrograms can be recorded during sinus rhythm and also in areas activated at a slow frequency of excitation during AF and other atrial arrhythmias. Finally, it is an oversimplification to associate fractionation of electrograms with a unique type of AF atrial substrate or heterogeneity of impulse propagation.

Experience over many years by a number of laboratories has led to the conclusion that electrogram fractionation can accompany a variety of impulse-propagation abnormalities related to alterations in the anatomy or function of the atria, or both. Various experimental models, as well as data in patients, have shown that CFAEs can be found in strictly normal atria,[6-8] but they can also indicate the presence of a pathophysiologic process potentially leading to AF.[9,10] This chapter is framed on an account of selected experimental and clinical studies found in the literature as well as recent experimental results. It is aimed at understanding the pathophysiologic relationship between high-frequency excitation and CFAEs.

Fractionation of Atrial Electrograms: General Mechanism

In theory, any heterogeneity responsible for an increased variability in the velocity or directionality of the atrial electrical impulse can translate into electrogram fractionation (Fig. 41-1). In turn, changes in impulse direction and velocity are likely to be associated with delays, intermittent block, wave breaks, and reentry. Various types of heterogeneities—anatomic, functional,

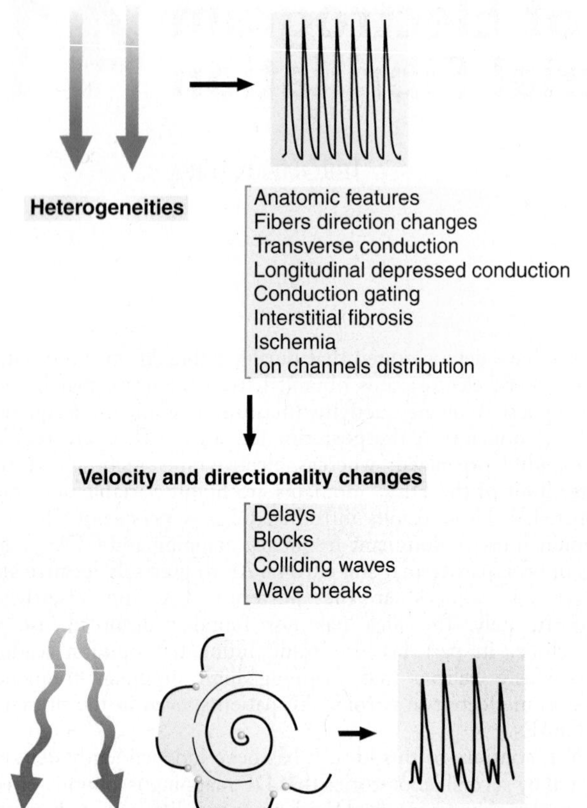

Figure 41-1 General mechanism of atrial electrogram fractionation.

macroscopic, or microscopic—can underlie fractionated electrograms. Most commonly, anisotropy of conduction, anatomic barriers, and interstitial fibrosis have been shown to generate electrogram fractionation in healthy atria but also in pathophysiologic conditions that often lead to AF persistence, such as heart failure or aging.[17]

Transverse, Longitudinal, and Zigzag Conduction

In their pioneering work in isolated atrial tissue, but also in Purkinje fibers and ventricular preparations, Spach and colleagues demonstrated that extracellular electrograms are fractionated at the limits of the atrial free walls in the vicinity of the atrial appendages,[6] as a result of colliding impulses in the His-Purkinje network,[18] or because of anisotropy-related discontinuous propagation. For example, Figure 41-2 shows extracellular waveforms recorded in an isolated dog atrial bundle after premature stimulation. Depressed conduction resulted in multiple-deflection electrograms that occurred first in the transverse direction and subsequently in the longitudinal direction, called *dissociated zigzag longitudinal propagation*.[19]

In the healed infarcted ventricles, a variation of this definition of zigzag conduction was given by de Bakker and coworkers.[20] Slow conduction perpendicular to the fiber direction was shown to be caused by a zigzag path of activation at high conduction speed throughout a web of branched myocyte bundles.[20] Although the identical mechanism was not described for the atria, it is likely to occur, especially in diseased hearts. Importantly, it was established that depressed conduction is not sufficient to generate electrogram fractionation but that heterogeneous activation is needed to record fractionated

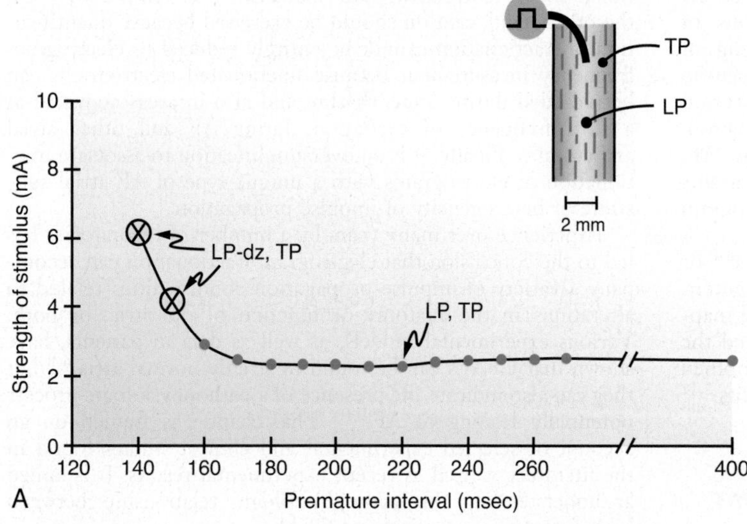

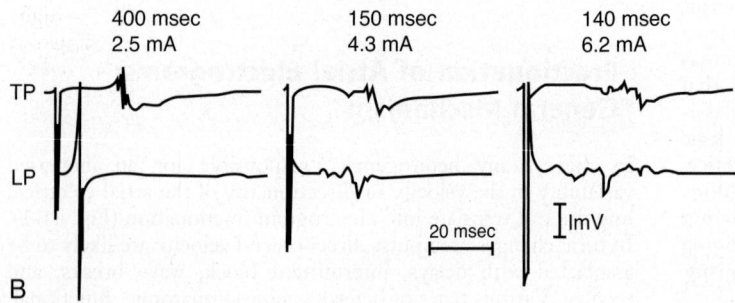

Figure 41-2 Strength-interval curve and extracellular waveforms in nonuniform anisotropic atrial crista terminalis. Extracellular waveforms were monitored at four sites, two sites along each of the major axes with respect to fiber orientation. Constant duration pulses (1 ms) were delivered at variable premature intervals after every 10th beat at a basic cycle length of 400 ms. **A,** Each point on the curve represents the minimum current required to produce longitudinal propagation (LP) and transverse propagation (TP). There was no propagation in either direction at premature intervals of ≤138 ms. **B,** Waveforms (measured at sites indicated in the *upper drawing*) show development of dissociated zigzag longitudinal propagation (LPdz) at the minimal current strength necessary to induce propagation at short premature intervals (140-150 ms). (Modified from Spach MS, Dolber PC, Heidlage JF: Influence of the passive anisotropic properties on directional differences in propagation following modification of the sodium conductance in human atrial muscle. A model of reentry based on anisotropic discontinuous propagation. Circ Res 62:811-832, 1988, with permission.)

electrograms.[21] Interestingly, this heterogeneity was shown to be possible during both transverse and longitudinal propagation.

Numerical simulations in a two-dimensional multicellular model demonstrated that the difference of side-to-side versus longitudinal coupling is the substrate of a velocity that is overall slower transversely than longitudinally but with a *maximal* velocity that is larger in side-to-side coupling. Thus, normal propagation in the transverse direction, which provides a basis for physiologic fractionated electrograms, could be described as inhomogeneous, hesitant, or pseudosaltatory.[22] At the microscopic level, such a heterogeneous conduction might in fact have a protective effect by maintaining the overall wavefront shape and preventing unidirectional block.[22]

In the longitudinal direction, a phenomenon responsible for electrogram fractionation, named *conduction gating*, was described in aged atrial bundles. It consisted of decremental followed by incremental conduction along myocardial fibers and was shown to be a prelude for reentry.[10]

Atrial Fibrosis

Interstitial fibrosis is well known to be associated with the aging process and various other conditions leading to atrial fibrillation.[23] For instance, discrete regions of fibrosis were shown to be responsible of conduction disturbances in the atria of failing hearts.[24] Spach and colleagues have indicated that microfibrosis, by creating interbundle septa, amplifies the physiologic transverse conduction delays and generates extracellular waveform fractionation.[19] As detailed earlier, the same group had also shown depressed longitudinal conduction in fibrotic aged atrial bundles.[10]

My laboratory has explored the role of fibrosis distribution in AF dynamics at the posterior left atrium.[17] We demonstrated that an increased percentage of fibrosis with patchy distribution can be responsible for an increase in electrogram complexity. We investigated the mechanism of AF associated with heart failure in isolated sheep hearts exposed to chronic ventricular tachypacing.[17] Fibrillatory wave propagation was recorded on the posterior left atrium using optical mapping techniques. We observed an overall slower frequency of activation[17] and increased beat-to-beat variability of directionality in failing hearts (Fig. 41-3). Also, in experiments and in numerical simulations, fibrotic patches—located in the vicinity of the pulmonary veins, and significantly larger in failing hearts—could create unstable anchoring points for microanatomic reentry. We observed that after short periods, an atrial reentry could shift to different anchoring sites formed by other fibrotic patches or even anatomic obstacles like the pulmonary vein ostia. As an example, Figure 41-4 shows that a reentry initially anchored to a large fibrotic obstacle terminated while a persistent anatomical reentry around the pulmonary vein ostium ensued. Thus, in the presence of fibrosis at the posterior left atrium, the mechanism of increased fractionation is the increased complexity of AF dynamics due to major delays, spatially distributed intermittent block processes, changes in wave directionality, and unstable anchoring sites.[17]

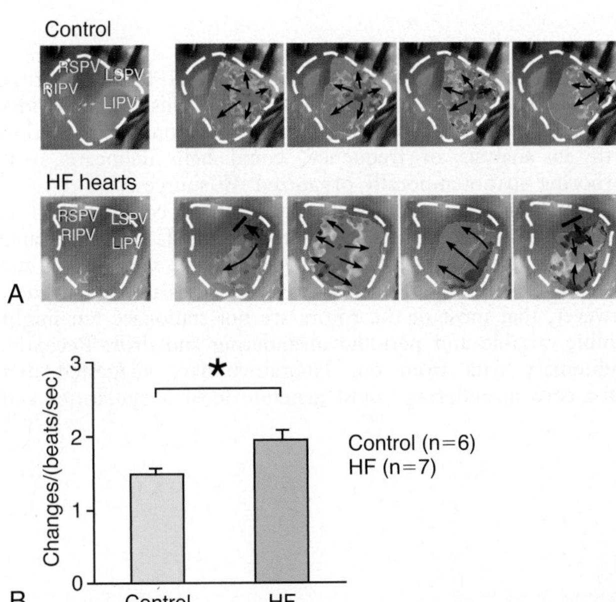

Figure 41-3 **A,** Activation maps of four consecutive atrial fibrillation (AF) waves at the posterior left atrium in heart failure (HF) and control groups. The maps are superimposed on a color picture of the preparation. The mapped area includes the four pulmonary vein ostia: right superior pulmonary vein (RSPV), left inferior pulmonary vein (LIPV), left superior pulmonary vein (LSPV), and right inferior pulmonary vein (RIPV). The patterns of propagation are highly recurrent in control hearts *(top)* in comparison to HF hearts *(bottom)*. **B,** Number of changes (normalized to the frequency) of wave pattern during AF waves in control and HF hearts. $*P < 0.05$. (Modified from Tanaka K, Zlochiver S, Vikstrom KL, et al: The spatial distribution of fibrosis governs fibrillation wave dynamics in the posterior left atrium during heart failure. Circ Res 101(8):839-47,2007. with permission.)

Relation between Frequency and Fractionation: Boundary of the High-Frequency Domains

As shown earlier, fractionated electrograms are the hallmark of impaired impulse conduction or of specific atrial areas particularly prone to delays, intermittent block, or wave break. Further, it could be postulated that areas harboring fractionated electrograms could help delineate areas prone to initiate or maintain the fibrillatory activity. The demonstration that AF in animals and in patients can be maintained by a discrete number of localized left atrial reentrant sources[15,16,25] opens the possibility of being able to use rapid fractionated electrograms as a beacon to help locate rotors or any other type of high-frequency spatiotemporally organized sources. The areas harboring AF sources, generally in the left atrium, were shown to exhibit fast and highly organized activity both in space and time,[15,16,26] whereas more-complex patterns of propagation were found in other atrial areas.[27]

By employing an experimental model in which AF is maintained by left atrial microreentrant activity,[25] we analyzed the relationship among spatiotemporal organization, frequency, and fractionation of AF waves. AF was initiated in the presence of 0.5μM acetylcholine in isolated sheep hearts, and the atria were mapped at high resolution using optical mapping. After fast Fourier transformation of the fluorescent signal, dominant frequency (DF) maps were constructed and areas with the highest frequency of excitation (DF_{max}) were localized. As shown in Figures 41-5 and 41-6, DF_{max} areas (activated at the highest frequency of excitation) were found to be those with the highest regularity, or the least fractionation. For example, Figure 41-5 shows a DF map during AF. A single-pixel recording from location 1 indicates that the fastest area corresponded to the most regular activity, and other atrial areas (locations 2 and 3) exhibited increased fractionation.

To further illustrate the mechanisms of fractionation at the boundary of the DF_{max} domain, Figure 41-6 shows a two-dimensional numerical simulation of AF implementing a

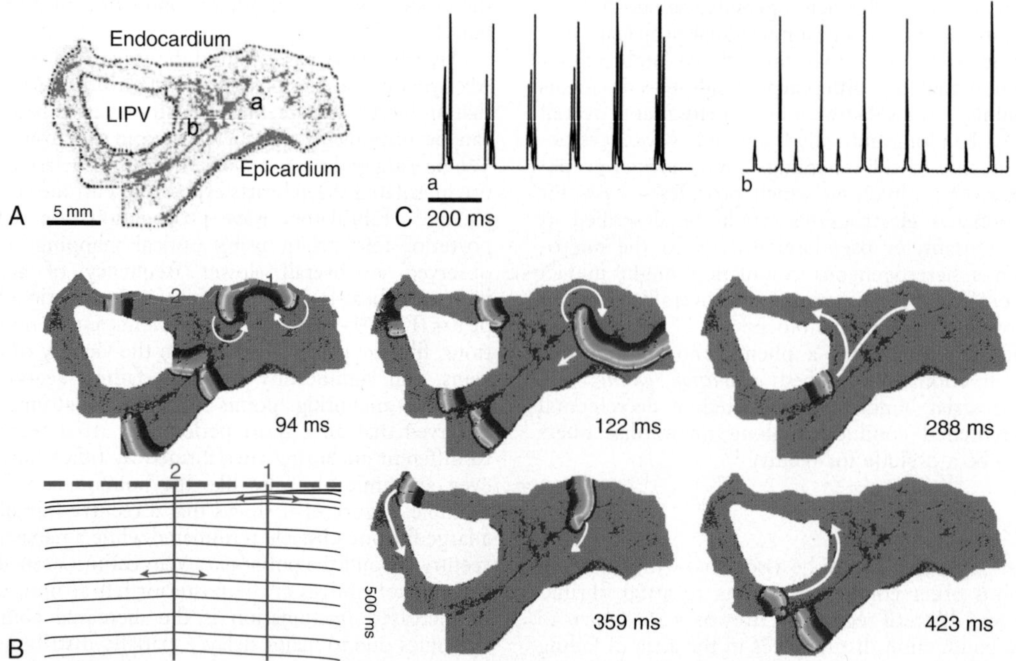

Figure 41-4 Computer simulation implementing a periosteal left inferior pulmonary vein (LIPV) topographic map of fibrosis from a transmural slice of the posterior left atrium in a failing heart. **A,** Transmural 4-μm thick slice. *Red areas* indicate fibrosis. **B,** Snapshots of electrical activity at several timeframes: 94, 122, 288, 359, and 423 ms. Reentry was initiated using S1-S2 stimulation, and spatiotemporal endocardial activity is given as a time-space plot along the *dashed red profile* marked on the snapshot at 94 ms. **C,** Two representative electrograms measured at locations *a* and *b* (as marked in **A**) show that the shift of reentry anchoring site introduced additional complexity. (Modified from Tanaka K, Zlochiver S, Vikstrom KL, et al: The spatial distribution of fibrosis governs fibrillation wave dynamics in the posterior left atrium during heart failure. Circ Res 101(8):839-47,2007. with permission.)

human atrial model.[28] The 5 × 5 cm sheet is divided into two areas, the upper one having twice the density of acetylcholine-activated K^+ current, $I_{K,ACh}$, than the lower one. Having initiated a rotor by cross-field stimulation, we observed that AF waves were breaking at the boundary between the two hemisheets (see Fig. 41-6 A and B). Interestingly, a single-pixel recording at the boundary of the DF_{max} area (between the two hemisheets) was markedly fractionated in comparison with recordings from the DF_{max} area or the low-frequency area. Figure 41-6C shows that the boundary of the DF_{max} area is also a line of increased conduction velocity variability and accentuated beat-to-beat directionality changes (see Fig 41-6E). Both phenomena are the common mechanistic features of any type of electrogram fractionation (see Fig. 41-1) because they lead to delays, block and wave breaks. Thus this study provides an example of how atrial electrogram fractionation, together with an analysis of frequency, could help delineate areas harboring spatiotemporally organized AF sources.

We therefore propose that under those conditions, it is expected that AF sources yield regular and fast electrograms and that fractionated electrograms would be recorded in the immediate periphery of those sources. One has also to consider, however, that most of the rotors are not stationary but might exhibit variable and periodic meandering and drift. Recently, preliminary data from our laboratory have suggested that rotor core meandering could generate local irregularities and

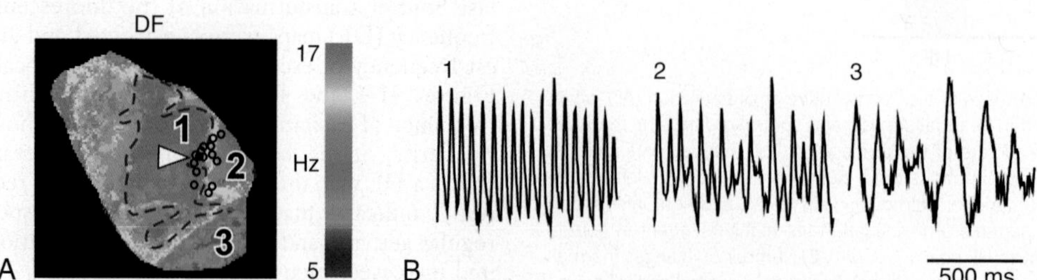

Figure 41-5 **A,** Posterior left atrial dominant frequency (DF) map during atrial fibrillation. The DF_{max} area is delimited by *dashed lines*. The predominant direction of impulse propagation that appeared as endocardial breakthroughs is indicated by the *white arrowhead*. *Open circles* are sites of wave break. **B,** Representative pixel recordings at location 1, 2, and 3 (left to right) indicating that the signal from the boundary of the DF_{max} domain is the most fractionated.

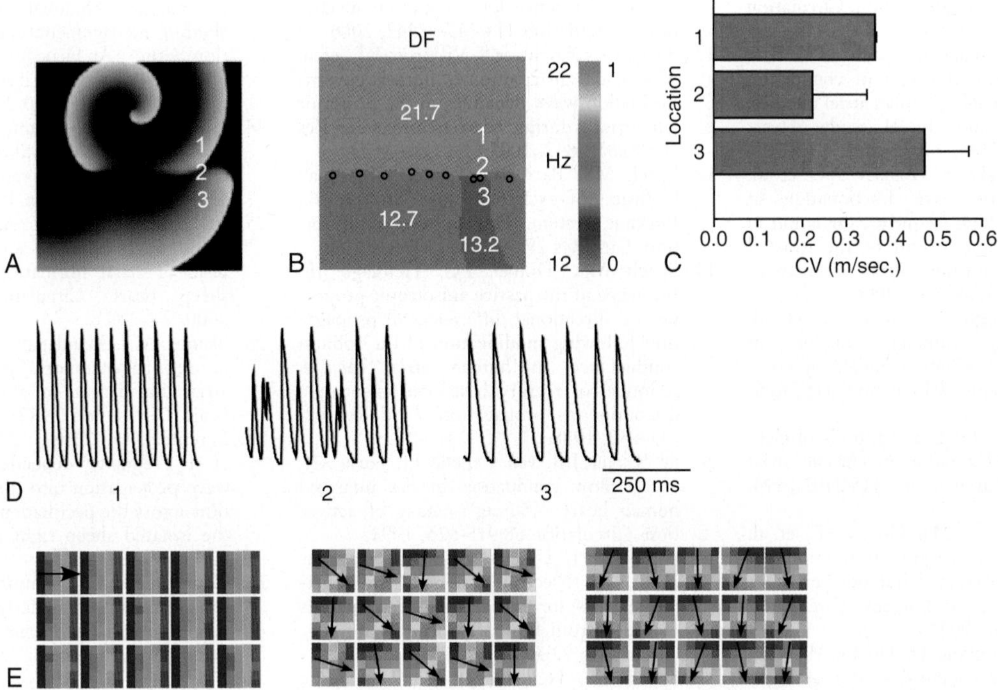

Figure 41-6 Numerical simulation. **A,** Snapshot of a fast and stable reentry in the upper half (high $I_{K,ACh}$) sending waves that block intermittently at the interface with the bottom half (low $I_{K,ACh}$). **B,** Dominant frequency (DF) map. At the border of the DF_{max} domain, a band of highly fractionated signal is present. *Circles* indicate sites of wave break. **C,** Average conduction velocity (CV) values at locations 1, 2, and 3. **D,** Vectoral best-fit analysis shows direction of propagation for 15 sequential (left to right, top to bottom) activations at pixels 1, 2, and 3. **E,** *Pixel 1:* No variability in directionality or conduction velocity (corresponding to the area of highest DF). *Pixel 2,* Maximum variability of directionality and conduction velocity (boundary of the DF_{max} domain) *Pixel 3,* Slightly reduced variability in conduction velocity and directionality. Color scale is the normalized activation time from blue to red. (Modified from Kalifa J, Tanaka K, Zaitsev AV, et al: Mechanisms of wave fractionation at boundaries of high frequency excitation in the posterior left atrium of the isolated sheep heart during atrial fibrillation. Circulation 113:626-633, 2006, with permission.)

fractionation, which in turn could be detectable by analyzing the frequencies associated with the meandering of the rotor tip.[29]

Summary

CFAEs are a valuable marker of conduction impairment during AF. As such, they can represent a spatial or temporal indicator of areas critical for initiating and maintaining AF. During stable AF, the electrograms obtained from the areas that harbor the DF_{max} are regular and highly organized, whereas those at the outer limit of the DF_{max} domains are highly variable and fractionated; this discovery opens a new perspective for the combined use in the clinical electrophysiology laboratory of DF mapping and CFAE analysis to precisely localize sources of AF at the posterior LA and elsewhere. This approach could greatly improve the recognition and differentiation of the various mechanisms or atrial substrates underlying CFAEs. In the future, the combination of DF mapping with specific means of fractionation measurements, as well as their appropriate interpretation in the context of multimodality atrial imaging, should lead to a refinement of the definition, interpretation, and diagnostic value of CFAEs for the treatment of patients with paroxysmal or persistent AF.

References

1. Nademanee K, McKenzie J, Kosar E, et al: A new approach for catheter ablation of atrial fibrillation: Mapping of the electrophysiologic substrate. J Am Coll Cardiol 43: 2044-2053, 2004.
2. Rostock T, Rotter M, Sanders P, et al: High-density activation mapping of fractionated electrograms in the atria of patients with paroxysmal atrial fibrillation. Heart Rhythm 3:27-34, 2006.
3. Oral H, Chugh A, Good E, et al: A tailored approach to catheter ablation of paroxysmal atrial fibrillation. Circulation 113: 1824-1831, 2006.
4. Kanj M, Wazni O, Natale A: Pulmonary vein antrum isolation. Heart Rhythm 4:S73-S79, 2007.
5. Calkins H, Brugada J, Packer DL, et al: HRS/EHRA/ECAS expert Consensus Statement on catheter and surgical ablation of atrial fibrillation: Recommendations for personnel, policy, procedures and follow-up. A report of the Heart Rhythm Society (HRS) Task Force on catheter and surgical ablation of atrial fibrillation. Heart Rhythm 4:816-861, 2007.
6. Spach MS, King TD, Barr RC, et al: Electrical potential distribution surrounding the atria during depolarization and repolarization in the dog. Circ Res 24:857-873, 1969.
7. Jais P, Haissaguerre M, Shah DC, et al: Regional disparities of endocardial atrial activation in paroxysmal atrial fibrillation. Pacing Clin Electrophysiol 19:1998-2003, 1996.
8. Konings KT, Smeets JL, Penn OC, et al: Configuration of unipolar atrial electrograms during electrically induced atrial fibrillation in humans. Circulation 95:1231-1241, 1997.
9. Oral H, Knight BP, Tada H, et al: Pulmonary vein isolation for paroxysmal

and persistent atrial fibrillation. Circulation 105:1077-1081, 2002.
10. Spach MS, Heidlage JF, Dolber PC, Barr RC: Mechanism of origin of conduction disturbances in aging human atrial bundles: Experimental and model study. Heart Rhythm 4:175-185, 2007.
11. Kalifa J, Tanaka K, Zaitsev AV, et al: Mechanisms of wave fractionation at boundaries of high frequency excitation in the posterior left atrium of the isolated sheep heart during atrial fibrillation. Circulation 113:626-633, 2006.
12. Oral H, Chugh A, Good E, et al: Radiofrequency catheter ablation of chronic atrial fibrillation guided by complex electrograms. Circulation 115:2606-2612, 2007.
13. Nademanee K: Trials and travails of electrogram-guided ablation of chronic atrial fibrillation. Circulation 115:2592-2594, 2007.
14. Lazar S, Dixit S, Marchlinski FE, et al: Presence of left-to-right atrial frequency gradient in paroxysmal but not persistent atrial fibrillation in humans. Circulation 110:3181-3186, 2004.
15. Sanders P, Berenfeld O, Hocini M, et al: Spectral analysis identifies sites of high-frequency activity maintaining atrial fibrillation in humans. Circulation 112:789-797, 2005.
16. Atienza F, Almendral J, Moreno J, et al: Activation of inward rectifier potassium channels accelerates atrial fibrillation in humans: Evidence for a reentrant mechanism. Circulation 114:2434-2442, 2006.
17. Tanaka K, Zlochiver S, Vikstrom KL, et al: The spatial distribution of fibrosis governs fibrillation wave dynamics in the posterior left atrium during heart failure. Circ Res 101(8):839-847, 2007.
18. Spach MS, Barr RC, Serwer GS, et al: Collision of excitation waves in the dog Purkinje system. Extracellular identification. Circ Res 29:499-511, 1971.
19. Spach MS, Dolber PC, Heidlage JF: Influence of the passive anisotropic properties on directional differences in propagation following modification of the sodium conductance in human atrial muscle. A model of reentry based on anisotropic discontinuous propagation. Circ Res 62: 811-832, 1988.
20. de Bakker JM, van Capelle FJ, Janse MJ, et al: Slow conduction in the infarcted human heart. "Zigzag" course of activation. Circulation 88:915-926, 1993.
21. Gardner PI, Ursell PC, Fenoglio JJ Jr, Wit AL: Electrophysiologic and anatomic basis for fractionated electrograms recorded from healed myocardial infarcts. Circulation 72:596-611, 1985.
22. Spach MS, Heidlage JF: The stochastic nature of cardiac propagation at a microscopic level. Electrical description of myocardial architecture and its application to conduction. Circ Res 76:366-380, 1995.
23. Go AS, Hylek EM, Phillips KA, et al: Prevalence of diagnosed atrial fibrillation in adults: National implications for rhythm management and stroke prevention: the AnTicoagulation and Risk Factors in Atrial Fibrillation (ATRIA) Study. JAMA 285:2370-2375, 2001.
24. Li D, Fareh S, Leung TK, Nattel S: Promotion of atrial fibrillation by heart failure in dogs: Atrial remodeling of a different sort. Circulation 100:87-95, 1999.
25. Mandapati R, Skanes A, Chen J, et al: Stable microreentrant sources as a mechanism of atrial fibrillation in the isolated sheep heart. Circulation 101:194-199, 2000.
26. Skanes AC, Mandapati R, Berenfeld O, et al: Spatiotemporal periodicity during atrial fibrillation in the isolated sheep heart. Circulation 98:1236-1248, 1998.
27. Berenfeld O, Zaitsev AV, Mironov SF, et al: Frequency-dependent breakdown of wave propagation into fibrillatory conduction across the pectinate muscle network in the isolated sheep right atrium. Circ Res 90:1173-1180, 2002.
28. Courtemanche M, Ramirez RJ, Nattel S: Ionic mechanisms underlying human atrial action potential properties: Insights from a mathematical model. Am J Physiol 275:H301-H321, 1998.
29. Zlochiver S, Yamazaki M, Kalifa J, Berenfeld O: Rotor meandering contributes to irregularity in electrograms during atrial fibrillation. Heart Rhythm 5:846-854, 2008.

Structural Atrial Remodeling Alters the Substrate and Spatiotemporal Organization of Atrial Fibrillation 42

THOMAS H. EVERETT IV AND JEFFREY E. OLGIN

CHAPTER OUTLINE

Atrial fibrillation (AF) is a common arrhythmia that is associated with varied underlying structural heart diseases or can be idiopathic. Several animal models have been developed in order to study the pathophysiology of AF, many of which have relevant correlates to the variety of clinical settings in which AF occurs.[1-8] Although AF occurs in each of the animal models, the atrial substrate of the AF appears to be different among the animal models. For example, the rapid atrial pacing (RAP) and methylcholine models have been shown to be dominated by atrial electrical remodeling, which includes a shortening of the atrial refractoriness without atrial structural changes or alterations in conduction.[4,6,9] In contrast, the mitral regurgitation (MR) and congestive heart failure (CHF) models do not appear to have significant decreases in refractoriness; these are dominated by changes that result in alterations of conduction produced by atrial fibrosis in the CHF model and myocyte architecture disruption and inflammation in the MR model.[3,7,9]

Several different signal-analysis techniques have been used to study the spatiotemporal organization of AF to gain insights into its mechanism, including cross-correlation,[10] wavelet analysis,[11] sample entropy,[12,13] chaos theory,[14,15] signal linearity,[16] and frequency-domain analysis using the fast Fourier transform (FFT).[17-19] These are described in Chapter 40. These analyses can be used to describe the characteristics of fibrillation and to quantitate organization within a seemingly chaotic rhythm, for which activation mapping is limited. These different types of signal analysis can be used to analyze AF signals to investigate the spatiotemporal organization of AF and they can be used to study the characteristics of AF in the different models of structural and electrical remodeling. These differences in substrate (structural or electrical) and conduction in turn lead to differences in the characteristic and spatiotemporal organization of the AF in each model. In addition to using these signal-processing tools to identify mechanisms of AF, these analysis tools may be developed for identifying ablation sites[20,21] and to time defibrillation and pacing for AF termination.[22,23]

Substrate Differences among Models of Atrial Fibrillation

Several animal models of AF have been developed with distinct features. The most widely studied animal models include CHF, MR, RAP, a cholinergically mediated model induced with acetylcholine, an atrial ischemic model, and a sterile pericarditis model. The structural and electrical characteristics of each of these models is outlined in this section.

Congestive Heart Failure

A study by Li and colleagues was the first to show that CHF in dogs—created by ventricular tachypacing—produced atrial interstitial fibrosis, which in turn produced disrupted conduction throughout the atria (Fig. 42-1) and an increased vulnerability to AF.[3] Along with atrial structural remodeling, atrial ionic remodeling was also seen and characterized as a decrease in transient outward current (I_{to}), slow delayed rectifier K^+ current (I_{Ks}), and calcium current (I_{Ca}) and an upregulation of the Na^+-Ca^{2+} exchange current.[24] These ionic changes have been shown to cause an increase in atrial effective refractory period (AERP). When tachypacing was terminated and CHF resolved, AF vulnerability continued even after a 5-week recovery period[25] and with complete recovery of ionic remodeling.[26] These studies showed that the electrical properties of the atria did not contribute to the increased AF vulnerability and that the structural changes that occurred during tachycardia pacing played a key role in the AF substrate.

Mitral Regurgitation

Similar to the CHF model, structural changes dominate the substrate in the MR model, but they have different features (similar degrees of LA enlargement, but minimal amounts of fibrosis) than in the CHF model over the same time period of model development.[7] Despite this difference, vulnerability to AF is similar in this model compared to the CHF model.[27] In the MR model, enlargement of the left atrium (LA) is seen along with signs of chronic inflammation, fiber separation, and a small increase in interstitial fibrosis. The electrical properties of the atria showed a small increase in the AERP over that of controls, and despite this there was an increase in AF inducibility.[7] Similar to the CHF model, these results supported the hypothesis that the structural changes that occurred in the atria in this model were responsible for the increase in AF vulnerability rather than any electrical remodeling. Figures 42-2 and 42-3 show that when conduction mapping was studied with high-resolution optical mapping, the LA showed an increase in conduction heterogeneity and anisotropy but no change in action potential duration or other action potential properties.[9]

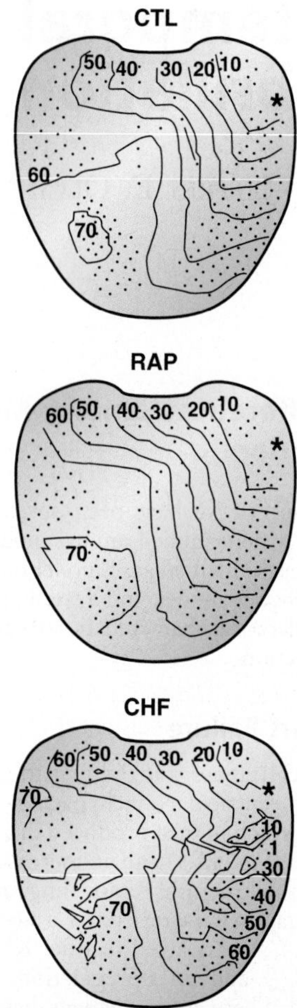

Figure 42-1 Isochronal activation maps for control (CTL), rapid atrial pacing (RAP), and congestive heart failure (CHF). The CHF model, which is associated with structural atrial remodeling, had an increase in conduction heterogeneity as compared to the other models. The RAP model, which is associated with electrical atrial remodeling, had homogeneous conduction that was similar to control. (From Li D, Fareh S, Leung TK, Nattel S: Promotion of atrial fibrillation by heart failure in dogs: Atrial remodeling of a different sort. Circulation 100:87-95, 1999.)

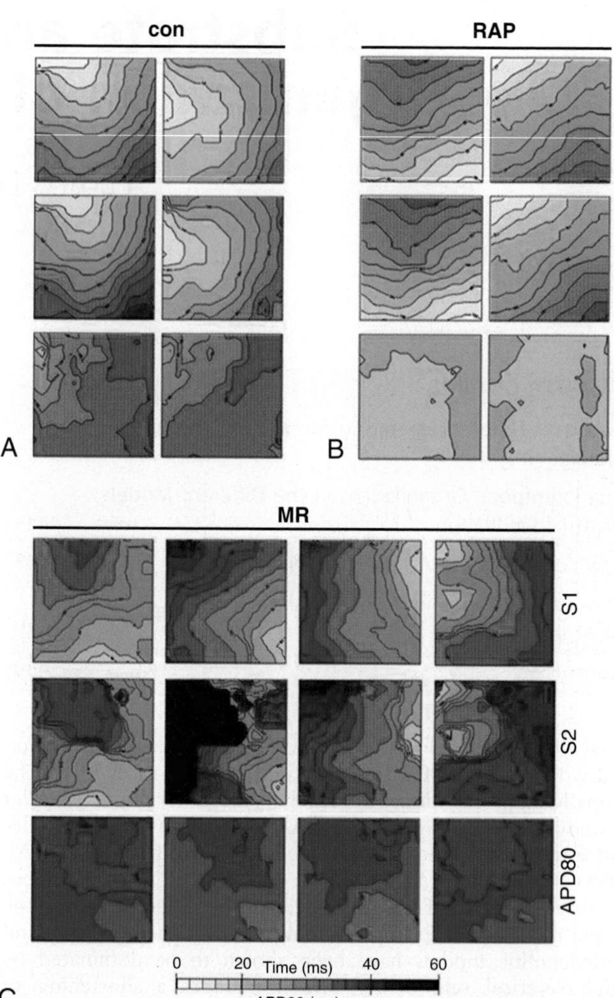

Figure 42-2 Conduction patterns recorded with optical mapping during pacing at 350 ms (S1) and with an extra stimulus (S2) in the left atrium along with the action potential duration at 80% (APD80) during the S1. For the control (con) **(A)** and rapid atrial pacing (RAP) **(B)**, two stimulus sites are shown, and similar conduction is seen at each site. For the mitral regurgitation (MR) group **(C)**, four stimulus sites are shown because the conduction was more variable and depended on the stimulation site. The MR model, which is associated with structural atrial remodeling, had an increase in conduction heterogeneity as compared to the other models. The RAP model, which is associated with electrical atrial remodeling, had homogeneous conduction that was similar to control. (From Verheule S, Wilson E, Banthia S, et al: Direction-dependent conduction abnormalities in a canine model of atrial fibrillation due to chronic atrial dilatation. Am J Physiol Heart Circ Physiol 287:H634-H644, 2004.)

Acute Atrial Ischemia

Sinno and coworkers developed another model of structural remodeling,[28] in which the branch of the right coronary artery that perfuses the free wall of the right atrium (RA) was ligated for up to 5 hours. Structural changes were seen in the form of patchy necrosis in the RA. The development of necrosis over time corresponded to altered conduction in the RA and an increase in AF vulnerability. The electrical properties of the atria showed no change in the AERP from that at baseline. This followed the theme of the CHF and MR models in that structural atrial remodeling leads to altered atrial conduction patterns, which then leads to an increase in AF vulnerability.

The CHF, MR, and acute ischemia models are characterized by atrial structural remodeling that results in alterations in conduction properties. However, the type and degree of structural remodeling is different in these models because the CHF model has extensive atrial fibrosis, the MR model has only a minimal amount, and the acute ischemia model is characterized by necrosis, but the degree of conduction heterogeneities is similar. To study the effects of these conduction abnormalities in the vulnerability to AF and to determine the extent to which these are due to alterations in gap junction function, studies by Guerra and colleagues and Takeshita and coauthors analyzed the effects of rotigaptide (ZP123), a compound that enhances gap junction conductance. In these two studies, ZP123 was studied in the three different canine models of AF that have abnormal atrial conduction as the substrate for AF.[27,29]

In a canine model of MR, which produces LA enlargement with little atrial fibrosis, and the canine model of acute ischemia, which produces necrosis with no LA enlargement, ZP123 significantly reduced AF vulnerability in these models. However, the compound had no effect on reducing AF vulnerability in a canine model of CHF in both studies.[27,29] Although these

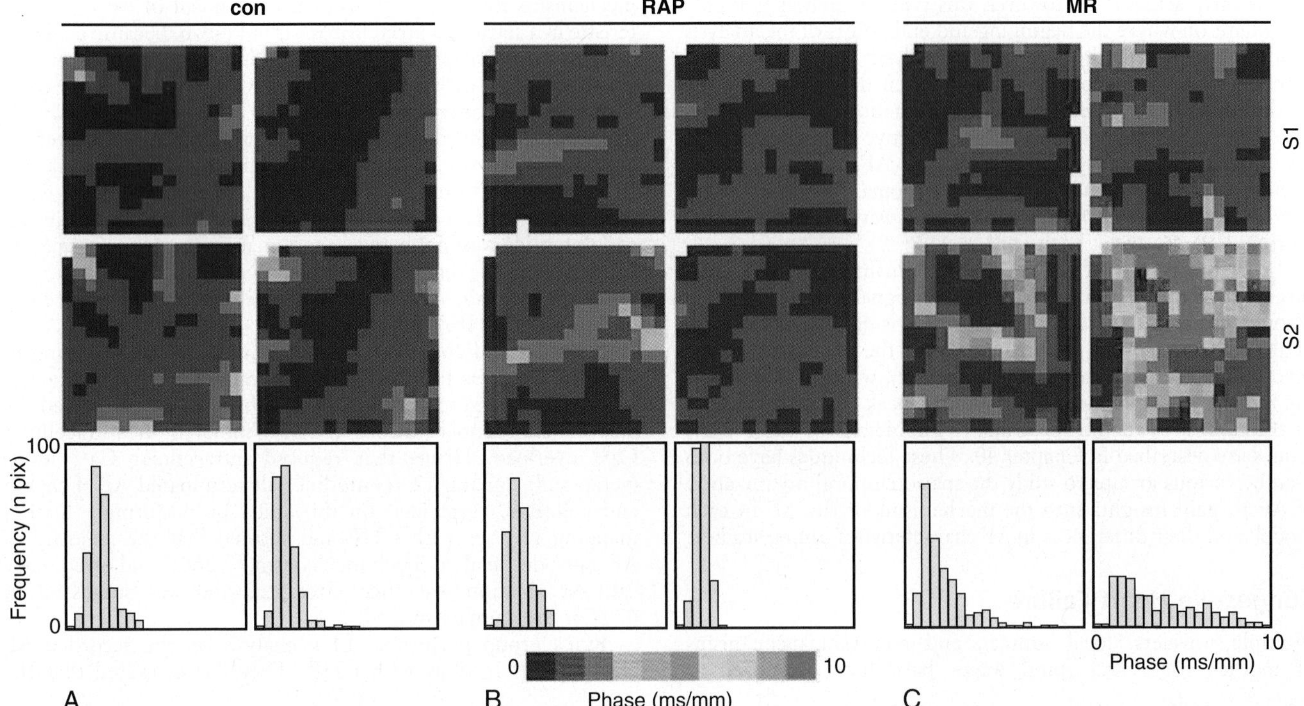

Figure 42-3 Examples of phase difference distributions in the left atria of the models of control (con) **(A)**, rapid atrial pacing (RAP) **(B)**, and mitral regurgitation (MR) **(C)**. These maps were derived from the activation maps that are shown in Figure 42-2 to quantify the differences in conduction heterogeneity. High phase differences (*yellow* to *red*) indicate more heterogeneous conduction. During pacing at 350 ms, each model shows little difference in phase. During extrastimulation (S2), the phase differences were low in the control and RAP models. This was in contrast to the MR model, in which high phase differences were evident during the extra stimulus. (From Verheule S, Wilson E, Banthia S, et al: Direction-dependent conduction abnormalities in a canine model of atrial fibrillation due to chronic atrial dilatation. Am J Physiol Heart Circ Physiol 287:H634-H644, 2004.)

models demonstrate abnormal atrial conduction and a high degree of AF vulnerability,[3,7] ZP123 was only effective in the MR and the acute ischemia models. This suggests that alterations in conduction in the MR and acute ischemia models may be due at least in part to functional changes in gap junctions, whereas alterations in the CHF model are due to irreversible structural derangements (fibrosis).

Rapid Atrial Pacing

The most recognizable model of AF is the RAP model, which is characterized by a decrease in the AERP[4,8] and action potential duration (APD)[30] along with an increase in the dispersion of refractoriness.[31] This type of remodeling, or atrial electrical remodeling, has been shown to increase AF vulnerability and has been used to demonstrate the phenomenon of AF begets AF.[4,8] However, as shown in Figures 42-1 and 42-2, the RAP model shows homogeneous conduction similar to that of a control atrium and shows no difference in conduction heterogeneity and the degree of anisotropy as compared to control.[9] In goat and canine RAP models, studies on myocardial ultrastructure have shown severe loss of myofibrillar structure, glycogen accumulation, changes in mitochondrial morphology, and cellular hypertrophy.[4,32] However, this model develops AF before any significant fibrosis[33-35] and conduction abnormalities occur.[9]

Methylcholine

The oldest model of AF is an acute model that is created through vagal stimulation or cholinergic agonists, such as methylcholine.[6] With the infusion of methylcholine, there is a dose-dependent decrease in the AERP and a concomitant increase in AF vulnerability. This is because of the primary effects of activating the potassium acetylcholine channel, which shortens the action potential in the atrium. This is an acute model in structurally normal hearts, and thus no structural atrial remodeling is necessary for AF in this model. Previous studies have shown that acetylcholine has little or no effect on the conduction in the atrium.[36,37]

The RAP and methylcholine models are characterized primarily by atrial electrical changes. However, how this remodeling is achieved is different for each model. The RAP model uses 6 weeks of RAP to achieve the desired effects. During this time, some cellular changes occur. However, in both whole heart and optical mapping studies, no conduction abnormalities are observed. For the methylcholine model, the remodeling occurs acutely on the ionic level with no other cellular changes.

Spatiotemporal Organization in the Different Models of Atrial Fibrillation

Several parameters have been used to measure the spatiotemporal organization of AF in different animal models to aid in understanding of the different characteristics and mechanisms of the AF. One simple method is either endocardial or epicardial activation mapping of the AF. For each atrial activation, the time at which the maximum first derivative (dV/dT) occurs is determined and isochronal maps are constructed. From these maps, several behavior characteristics of the AF can be determined. These characteristics include wavefront direction and propagation, the number of wavefronts, and the number of sites that exhibit early activation. However, this type of analysis is highly dependant on where the beginning and end points of the analysis window are placed, the size of the analysis window, and the accuracy of marking local activation (often determined by the maximum dV/dT).[38] Because of these limitations, other analyses have been developed that are more objective measurements of the spatiotemporal organization of the AF. These analyses include cross-correlation,[10] frequency domain analysis using the FFT,[17-19] measuring the linking of wavefronts,[39] sample entropy,[13] and wavelet analysis.[11]

From the results of the frequency domain analysis, a measurement of the organization of the AF signal can be obtained through either the regularity index, which is defined as the ratio of the area under the dominant peak to the total area of the spectrum,[40] or the organization index (OI), which is defined as the ratio of the area under the dominant peak *and* its harmonics to the total area of the spectrum.[17] The details of these techniques are described in Chapter 40. These techniques have been used by various groups to study the spatiotemporal organization of AF to gain insights into the mechanisms of the AF in each model, and their differences in AF characteristics can be studied.

Congestive Heart Failure

Multiple wavelets, focal sources, and reentrant mechanisms of mother rotor and spiral waves have been proposed as mechanisms for AF.[18,41-44] Which mechanism of AF is characteristic in a setting of atrial fibrosis is unknown, because evidence exists for both reentry and discrete, stable foci as an AF mechanism in dogs with pacing induced CHF. Li and colleagues showed a mechanism of macroreentry with conduction abnormalities providing the milieu for AF propagation before termination with dofetilide, a rapid K^+ current (I_{Kr}) channel blocker.[45] In contrast, this study also showed that in a model of RAP, multiple wavelets was demonstrated to be the likely mechanism, and dofetilide was ineffective in terminating the AF. In a separate study comparing endocardial versus epicardial activation, this same group again showed an AF mechanism of macroreentry in dogs with CHF.[47]

Stambler and coworkers suggested that AF in the setting of CHF in dogs was focal in origin and caused by triggered activity.[48] This triggered activity was shown to be produced by delayed afterdepolarizations (DADs) initiated by intracellular Ca^{2+} overload. Drugs that reduced intracellular Ca^{2+} levels (verapamil, flunarazine, ryanodine) all terminated AF. Fenelon and colleagues expanded on this study by performing biatrial mapping in dogs with CHF and showed that the majority of AF episodes had a focal mechanism.[49] Focal radiofrequency catheter ablation was then attempted and was successful in 67% of the animals studied.

Ryu's group performed FFT analysis on the recorded AF electrograms in dogs with CHF. They demonstrated that the

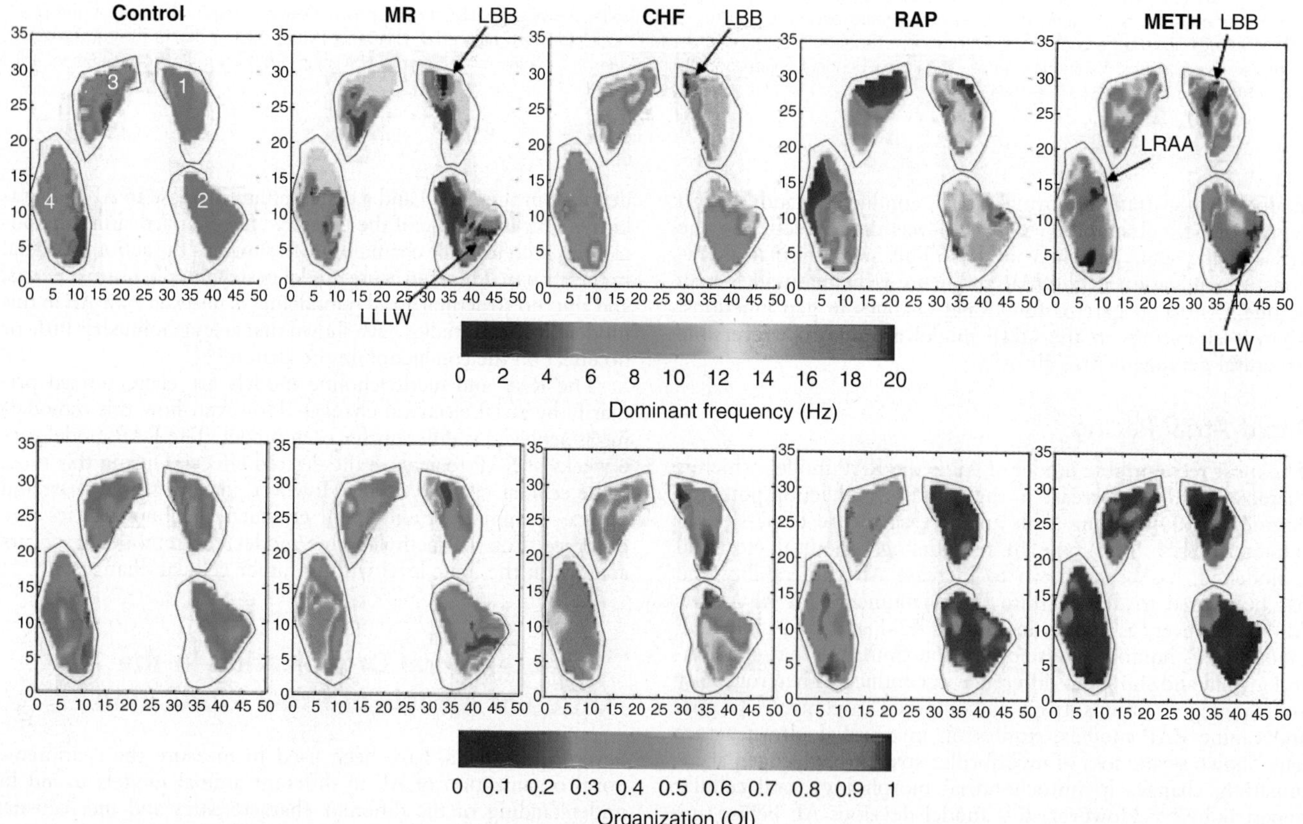

Figure 42-4 Examples of static dominant frequency maps *(top)* and organization maps *(bottom)* for canine models of both structural atrial remodeling (congestive heart failure [CHF] and mitral regurgitation [MR]) and electrical atrial remodeling (rapid atrial pacing [RAP] and methylcholine [METH]) along with control. Dominant frequency (DF) and organization index (OI) are shown from a fast Fourier transform (FFT) performed on a 2-second window of atrial fibrillation. The stable, discrete high-DF areas are identified in the MR and CHF dogs, along with their atrial location. For the methylcholine dogs, the representative DF map shows the stable, discrete high-DF areas in both the RA and LA. *Arrows* indicate locations of discrete, stable high-frequency areas. LBB, left atrial Bachman's bundle; LLLW, left atrial low lateral wall; LRAA, lateral right atrial appendage. (From Everett TH, Wilson EE, Verheule S, et al: Structural atrial remodeling alters the substrate and spatiotemporal organization of AF: A comparison in canine models of structural and electrical atrial remodeling. Am J Physiol Heart Circ Physiol 291:H2911-H2923, 2006.)

AF had stable drivers in both the LA and RA, and they confirmed this with activation mapping.[50] In seven of 12 dogs studied, two distinct foci were seen: one in the RA and one in the LA, with different frequencies and fibrillatory conduction emanating out from the driver region. Discrete stable high-frequency areas were also seen during AF in a CHF dog model in a study by Everett and colleagues.[33] Using frequency domain analysis, stable high-frequency areas were seen as the characteristic of AF in dogs with pacing-induced heart failure. Whereas Ryu and coworkers showed multiple drivers during the same episode of AF, these high-frequency areas were seen in either the RA or the LA in Everett's study, and there was a steep frequency gradient away from these sites.

Figure 42-4 shows an example of the DF maps during AF in a dog with CHF. A high-DF area is seen in the LA. Upon further inspection of unipolar electrograms at this site, fractionated electrograms were seen with low organization levels. In this study, it was also shown that these high-frequency areas could occur in either the RA or LA. In contrast, no discrete high-frequency areas were seen in a model of RAP. It has also been suggested that the focal sources could be originating from the pulmonary veins in this CHF dog model of AF.[51] Chen and colleagues performed high-density mapping of the pulmonary veins during AF in dogs with CHF. In half of the AF episodes recorded in the CHF model, focal activation was seen from within the vein independent of the LA. This type of activation was not seen in any of the AF in controls because the pulmonary veins were activated passively from wavefronts originating from the LA.

Mitral Regurgitation

Several studies have looked at the mechanisms of AF in the CHF model, but currently, there are significantly less data published on the mechanisms of AF in the MR model. Similar to the CHF model, the MR model is one that is dominated by conduction abnormalities.[7] Also, similar to the CHF model, stable high-frequency areas have been reported in the MR model.[33] Everett and coauthors performed two studies that included open chest epicardial mapping of MR dogs. In one study, four of nine dogs had a stable high-frequency area (three LA, one RA),[33] and in the second study two of five dogs had this type of frequency pattern.[52] The MR model had a similar frequency distribution and a similar amount of linked beats within both the RA and LA as the CHF model. As shown in Figures 42-5 and 42-6, when high-density optical mapping was used, stable

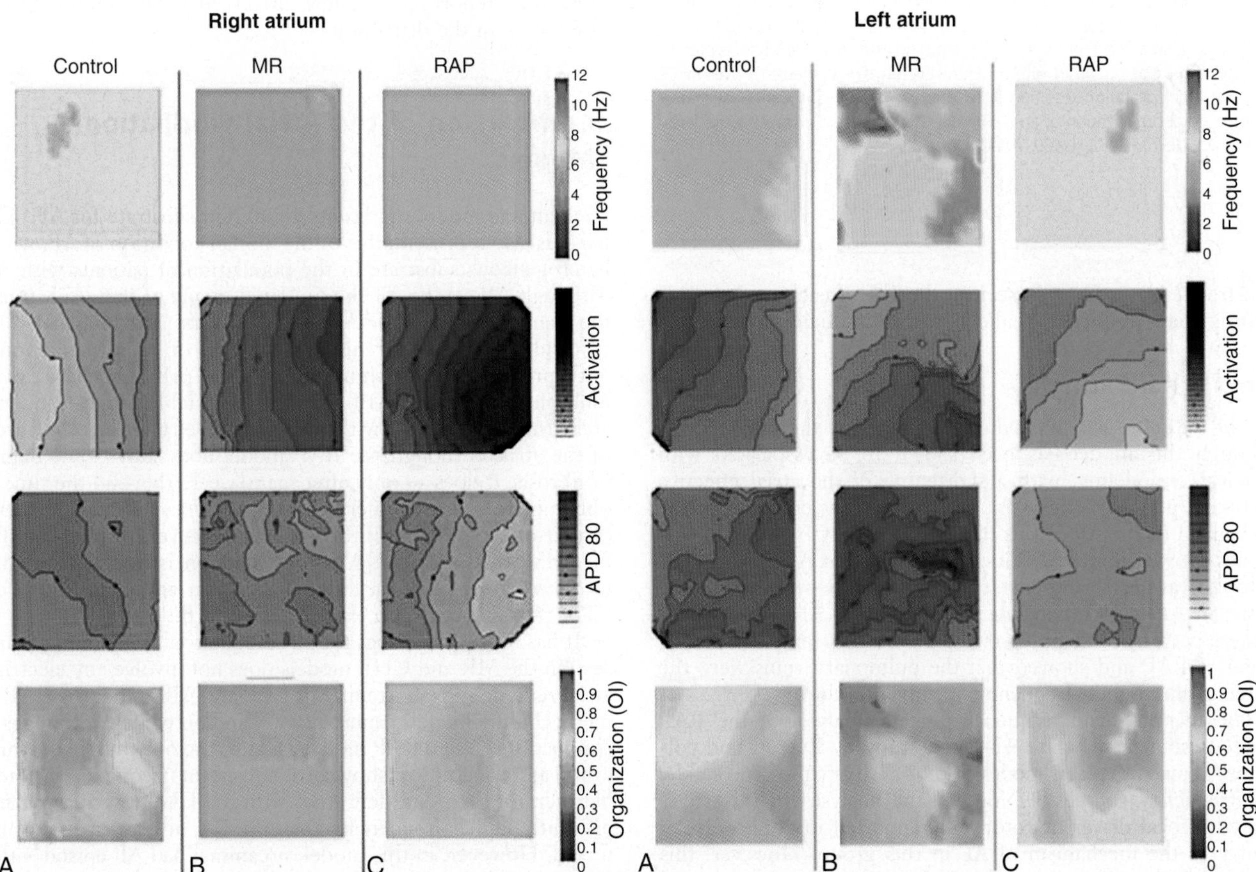

Figure 42-5 Dominant frequency (row 1), activation patterns (row 2), action potential duration at 80% (APD80) (row 3), and organization (row 4) maps in the right and left atria for control **(A)**, mitral regurgitation (MR) **(B)**, and rapid atrial pacing (RAP) **(C)**. All scales are shown to the right for their corresponding panels. As these figures demonstrate, the atrial fibrillation (AF) in the right atrium (RA) was very similar for each of the models because the majority of each dominant frequency map is composed of a single frequency, and the organization maps are composed of large areas of higher organization index (OI) values. In contrast, the AF in the left atrium (LA) of the MR model was significantly different from the AF in the other models. The MR dominant frequency map shows several discrete areas of different frequencies, including an area composed of the highest frequencies. This frequency pattern was not observed in the frequency maps from the other AF models. The MR organization map shows large areas of lower OI values than is shown in the organization maps for the other models. In both the RA and LA, it is shown that the dominant frequencies followed conduction patterns and not the distribution of APD80. (From Everett TH, Verheule S, Wilson EE, et al: Left atrial dilatation resulting from chronic mitral regurgitation decreases spatiotemporal organization of atrial fibrillation in left atrium. Am J Physiol Heart Circ Physiol 286(6):H2452-H2460, 2004.)

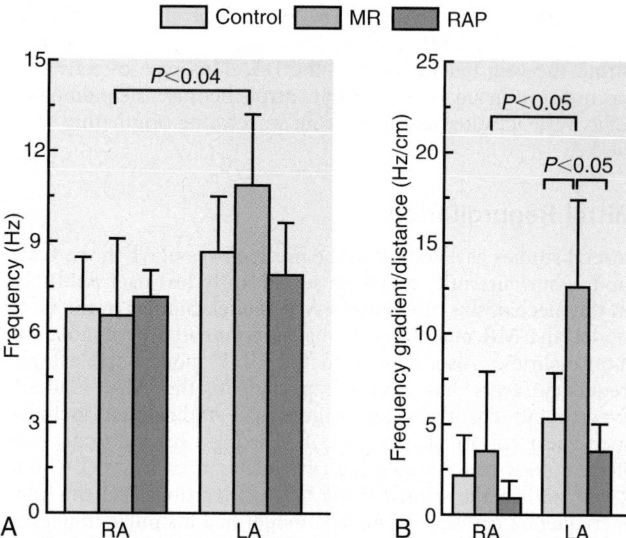

Figure 42-6 Quantification of dominant frequency (DF). **A,** The highest DF that was calculated for each DF map. In the mitral regurgitation (MR) group, atrial fibrillation (AF) in the left atrium (LA) had a significantly higher measured DF than that in the right atrium (RA) of the same group. **B,** The largest measured frequency gradient over the distance that the gradient occurs. AF in the LA of the MR model had significantly higher ratios than that of the RA MR and the LA of the other models. For all panels, the *light gray bars* represent the control group, the *light blue bars* represent the MR group, and the *dark gray bars* represent the rapid atrial pacing (RAP) group. (From Everett TH, Verheule S, Wilson EE, et al: Left atrial dilatation resulting from chronic mitral regurgitation decreases spatiotemporal organization of atrial fibrillation in left atrium. Am J Physiol Heart Circ Physiol 286(6):H2452-H2460, 2004.)

high-frequency areas were seen in the LA of each preparation, creating steep frequency gradients within the field of view.[53]

Rapid Atrial Pacing

One of the more widely studied AF models is the RAP model. Although this model has been shown to be associated with electrical remodeling, with a shortening of the atrial effective refractory period,[4,8] there is still controversy concerning the mechanism of the AF in this model. One study by Sih and colleagues showed that a RAP model of persistent AF consisted of multiple wavelets[54] and that there were more wavelets in the persistent AF model than in a model of acute AF. Wu and coworkers performed mapping of the pulmonary veins in a canine model of RAP and showed that the pulmonary veins were the source of the highest frequency of activation during AF.[55]

The mapping and frequency domain analysis of the RAP model as shown in Figure 42-4 in a study by Everett and colleagues showed that this model did not have any discrete, stable, high-frequency sources.[56] None of the analyses in this study favored a focal driver or rotor and supported multiple-wavelet reentry as the mechanism of AF in this group. However, this model did show large, transient higher-frequency areas, and the LA had consistently higher frequencies than the RA, but there were no discrete LA-LA gradients or stable high-frequency areas. The LA was likely activated at a higher frequency overall related to differences in refractoriness[57] and more fibrillatory conduction in the RA, leading to lower frequency of activation in the RA.[58] When optical mapping was performed on hearts from this model, the results of FFTs calculated from the AF signals (see Figs. 42-5 and 42-6) showed homogeneous frequency maps with an average of one frequency domain per square centimeter and no stable high-frequency regions within the field of view.[53]

Methylcholine

Studies characterizing AF induced with acetylcholine in a Langendorff-perfused isolated sheep heart first demonstrated the existence of stable, high-frequency sources during the AF.[18] These high-frequency sources were demonstrated to be a vortex rotating at a frequency higher than any other recorded in the atrium,[43] and thus it was considered to be driving the AF. In this sheep model, it was shown that all of the high-frequency sources existed in the LA, and that at a critical frequency, a gradient developed between the LA and RA.[59] However, this finding may be species specific.[6] In a study by Everett's group, AF was also induced with methylcholine in a canine heart, and in this group, as shown in Figure 42-4, high-frequency sources were seen in the RA as well as the LA, and no frequency gradient was seen.[56] Additionally, when the highest DF was plotted against frequency dispersion, the result was a linear relationship, which supports what has been previously shown in the sheep acetylcholine model: The faster the driving source, the greater the degree of fibrillatory conduction.[43] This difference between these data showing several high-frequency drivers and those previously reporting a single driver may be due to species differences in the distribution of I_{kAch}.[60]

Comparison of the Atrial Fibrillation Models

Each animal model represents a different substrate for AF. This likely is also representative of the human condition of AF, with a heterogeneous substrate in the population of patients with AF. Although AF can be reliably initiated in any of these substrates, the characteristics of the AF in each differs. The models known to result in electrical remodeling (RAP) or vagal mediation—both producing ERP shortening[4,8]—had AF characteristics of multiple wavelets (RAP) or multiple stable, high-frequency areas (methylcholine), with multiple wavefronts in other areas of the atria. Although the RAP model does show some degree of fibrosis, it does so only after many weeks (beyond the time to obtain increased AF vulnerability), and it does not reach the level of that of the MR or CHF models. Moreover, in many studies involving this model, if AV node ablation is not performed, a tachycardia-mediated cardiomyopathy can ensue similar to the CHF model (but over a longer period of time).

It has been shown that the structural atrial remodeling that is seen in the MR and CHF models does not involve any electrical atrial remodeling (shortening of ERP and APD) that the RAP or methycholine models experience[3,7,9] and only involve changes in conduction.[3,9] The RAP model was also the only model in which every animal studied showed a consistent frequency gradient between the right and left atria, with the LA always having significantly higher frequencies than the RA, at least in the canine model. However, in this model, no animal had AF episodes that had stable, discrete high-frequency areas or frequency gradients within the LA. This could be due to the smaller degree of structural changes and lack of remodeling that affects conduction in the RAP model, so that the entire LA is activated at a similar frequency, masking a potential high-frequency site.

In the case of the methylcholine model, multiple stable, high-frequency areas were seen that also corresponded to lower organization levels, lower correlation coefficients, and higher temporal and spatial variances in frequency and organization. This supports the hypothesis that the methylcholine model had an AF mechanism of multiple rotors spinning off several daughter wavelets that were colliding with each other, creating varying frequency patterns away from the rotors.

The models that experienced structural remodeling known to result in alterations in conduction[3,7,9] had stable, discrete high-frequency areas in the DF maps. Steep frequency gradients and large areas of similar frequencies were seen away from the high-frequency areas. The frequency characteristics remained stable from epoch to epoch. This resulted in lower spatial and temporal frequency and organization variances and higher correlation coefficient values. This would suggest a stable rotor in these models, with highly organized wavefronts in the other areas of the atria, which would correlate with the mother-rotor theory as an AF mechanism in these models.

These discrete, stable high-frequency areas seen in the MR, CHF, and methylcholine models were not always confined to the LA. In the methylcholine AF model, discrete, stable high-frequency areas were observed in both the RA and LA simultaneously, whereas in the MR and CHF models these stable areas were singular. Interestingly, in each animal with stable high-frequency areas, the areas remained consistently spatially located from episode to episode. Based on data from other studies, these high-DF areas likely represent either mother rotors or triggered activity that is driving the AF.[43] Also, the data presented by Everett and colleagues show that these high-frequency areas correlated with fractionated electrograms and lower organization levels. A study by Kalifa and colleagues showed that these high-frequency areas do have an area of fast, highly-organized activity with high-frequency fractionated electrograms surrounding this area.[40] The high-DF organized area was found to have a diameter of about 2 mm.

The spatial resolution of the plaque electrodes used in the study by Everett and colleagues is not adequate to record this size of an area. What is likely being recorded is the larger area of high-frequency, fractionated electrograms that surround the smaller area of highly-organized, high-DF electrograms. The exit block from the high-frequency source results in other peaks within the FFT between the harmonics and is influenced by the relative size of the driver and electrode spacing. It has been shown that block causes other peaks to appear near the dominant peak.[61,62] This causees the OI to decrease. A similar scenario occurs with fractionated electrograms, which have been shown to occur near regions of conduction block.[63] This study also supported this finding because the high-frequency areas corresponded to fractionated electrograms. The relative size of the high-frequency driver to the recording electrode must be considered when interpreting the meaning of fractionated electrograms in human mapping studies of AF, as these experiments demonstrate. The structural changes seen in the MR and CHF models likely contribute to the frequency gradient that occurs outward from the high-frequency area as the structural remodeling promotes conduction delay and block as well as wave break.

Other Applications with the Different Models of Atrial Fibrillation

Defibrillation Thresholds

Frequency domain analysis has shown that AF has regions of high and low organization (see earlier discussion) and that globally, AF has periods of both high and low organization.[23] These temporal changes in organization may be important in timing of successful defibrillation, or they might even provide brief moments where the AF is susceptible to pace termination. It has been shown that the period of AF just before a successful shock is more organized than the period of AF before an unsuccessful shock.[17] If one times defibrillation shocks to periods of increased global AF organization (empirically defined as an OI of 0.5), the 50% defibrillation success voltage is reduced from a mean of 183 volts to 142 volts.[23] Similar to the defibrillation studies, burst pace termination for AF is more efficacious when pacing is timed to periods of higher organization.[22]

A similar atrial defibrillation threshold ($ADFT_{50}$) protocol was applied in cardioverting AF in the canine models of CHF, MR, RAP, methylcholine, and control.[52] As shown in Figure 42-7, control, MR, and CHF models all had similar defibrillation energy levels (160 ± 30 V, 120 ± 50 V, and 132 ± 20 V). The RAP and methylcholine models had significantly higher defibrillation energy levels than the other models (668 ± 205 V and 593 ± 128 V; analysis of variance [ANOVA] $P < 0.0001$). Interestingly, the MR and CHF had significantly more atrial enlargement than the RAP and methylcholine, yet they had lower defibrillation thresholds, suggesting that the mechanism of AF in these models (single stable high-frequency sources in CHF and MR and multiple wavelets or drivers in RAP and methylcholine) might play more of a role in determining defibrillation efficacy than atrial mass does.

Clinical Data

FFT analysis is now being applied to AF in the clinical setting as a research tool to understand mechanisms of AF and for its potential as a mapping tool to target ablation. Sanders and coworkers performed FFT analysis on AF signals from patients with paroxysmal AF and from patients with permanent AF.[21] High-frequency areas were seen within the pulmonary vein region in both types of patients. However, each of the points that composed these maps was a short duration of signal recorded on a point-by-point basis over time. Sahadevan and colleagues recorded simultaneous epicardial electrograms from both the RA and LA in nine patients with chronic AF. Seven of the nine patients had areas of higher dominant frequencies that might have been driving the AF.[64] However, in both of these studies, in the clinical setting, it is not known if these frequencies are stable. As was seen in the canine models of AF, stable, high-frequency areas were model specific,[56] and the stability of the frequency components of AF signals in humans has only been studied on a limited basis.

Lazar and coauthors[65] and Sanders and colleagues[21] both analyzed the temporal stability of the dominant frequencies of AF over time. In the first study, intracardiac bipolar signals of AF were recorded for up to 2 minutes from five different sites.[65] Each site showed a range of frequencies between the start of the recording and the end, but there was no significant difference in the measured DFs. In the second study, Sanders and coworkers took 10-second AF recordings from different sites and broke the signals down into two 5-second intervals and showed that there was no difference in the DFs between the first 5 seconds as opposed to the second 5-second interval.[21] Similar to the first study, each recording site did show a range of frequencies with repeated recordings, but the differences in frequencies over time was not significant. In a final look at temporal stability of DFs, AF signals were recorded within the coronary sinus for 35 to 48 minutes. There was a 1.1 ± 0.5 Hz range in the frequencies that were recorded during this time period.

Schuessler and colleagues performed frequency domain analysis on epicardial bipolar electrograms from 250 sites in patients with AF.[66] A discrete, high-frequency area was seen in 91% of the patients, and in 48% of the patients this high-frequency area

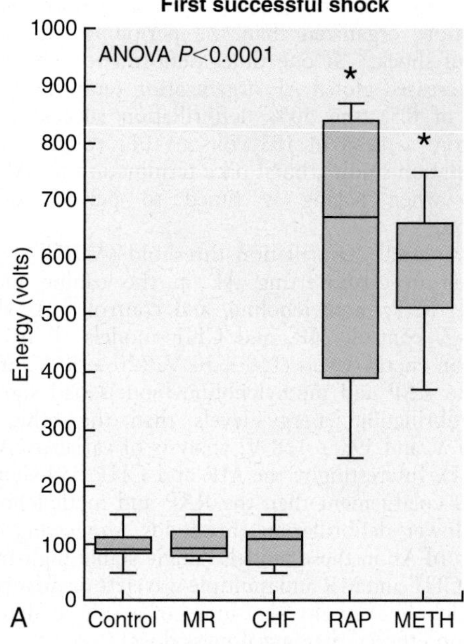

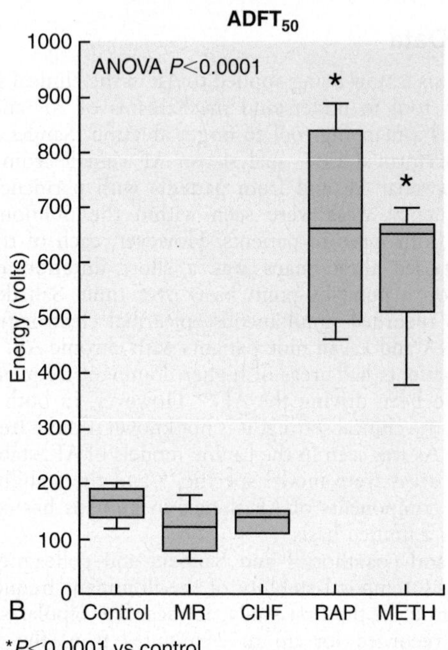

Figure 42-7 Summary data for voltage levels of the first successful shock (A) and atrial defibrillation threshold at 50% ($ADFT_{50}$) (B) for the canine models of control, mitral regurgitation (MR), congestive heart failure (CHF), rapid atrial pacing (RAP), and methylcholine (METH). The models that were associated with electrical atrial remodeling (RAP and METH) had significantly higher defibrillation energy levels than those of the models associated with structural atrial remodeling (CHF and MR). ANOVA, analysis of variance. (From Everett TH, Wilson EE, Olgin JE: Effects of atrial fibrillation substrate and spatiotemporal organization on atrial defibrillation thresholds. Heart Rhythm 4:1048-1056, 2007.)

changed locations. Targeting the sites of discrete high frequencies was shown to be successful in patients with paroxysmal AF when Sanders and colleagues reported AF termination in 17 of 19 patients.[21] However, with this protocol, there was no AF termination in patients with permanent AF.

In addition to searching for discrete, high-frequency areas, frequency domain analysis is now being used in the clinical setting to study the characteristics of different types of AF and how different atrial substrates and altering the substrate through catheter ablation can alter the characteristics of the AF. Lin and colleagues used FFTs to study the spatial distribution of frequencies during different types of paroxysmal AF.[67] The location of the initiating foci was determined, and the area from which the AF originated had the highest DF. When the AF originated from the pulmonary veins, a LA-to-RA frequency gradient existed. A gradient was not seen when the AF originated from the SVC. In a study by Lazar and coworkers, recordings were made in both the RA and LA in patients with paroxysmal and persistant AF.[65] A LA-to-RA frequency gradient was observed, but this gradient was only seen in patients with paroxysmal AF and not those with persistent AF. Sanders and colleagues also looked at the effects of pulmonary vein isolation on the AF frequencies.[68] Pulmonary vein isolation resulted in a significant decrease in the dominant frequencies in patients with paroxysmal AF but not those with permanent AF. In another study by Lazar and coauthors, it was shown that a LA-to-RA frequency gradient disappears with pulmonary vein isolation.[69] Takahashi and colleagues used signal processing techniques to show that the organization of AF increases after catheter ablation of the pulmonary veins.[70] It was also shown that a high OI value was associated with AF termination.

Another approach to spectral mapping of AF signals is to use FFTs to locate fractionated electrograms or AF nests.[20] Any sort of fractionation within the atrial activation sequence will add other peaks, with the magnitude spectrum other than the dominant peak. Normal conduction produces an electrogram with no extra peaks within it. Heterogeneous depolarization produces extra peaks in the activation sequence, which then produces extra peaks in the magnitude spectrum. A recording electrode can exhibit a fractionated electrogram if the signal is subject to block, fibrillatory conduction, or multiple waves. Targeting the sites with fractionated electrograms for ablation has been shown to decrease the incidence of AF,[20] but it remains unclear if these approaches will prove to be any more effective than simply taking an anatomic approach to ablation of AF.

These studies suggest that spectral mapping of AF may be useful to define mechanisms of AF in patients and that ablation can affect the AF frequency. However, many questions remain unanswered—such as the temporal stability, the impact of a large recording electrode that exists on an ablation catheter to resolve potentially small drivers, and appropriate interpretation of data—before it can be routinely used as a mapping tool to guide ablation.

Conclusion

Several different canine models have been developed to study AF. Even though each model shows an increase in AF vulnerability, the substrate that is created in each model that allows the AF to occur is different. These differences in substrate lead to different characteristics of the AF organization and likely to different mechanisms of AF.

References

1. Everett TH, Li H, Mangrum JM, et al: Electrical, morphological, and ultrastructural remodeling and reverse remodeling in a canine model of chronic atrial fibrillation. Circulation 102(12):1454-1460, 2000.
2. Kumagai K, Khrestian C, Waldo AL: Simultaneous multisite mapping studies during induced atrial fibrillation in the sterile pericarditis model. Insights into the mechanism of its maintenance. Circulation 95(2):511-521, 1997.
3. Li D, Fareh S, Leung TK, Nattel S: Promotion of atrial fibrillation by heart failure in dogs: Atrial remodeling of a different sort. Circulation 100(1):87-95, 1999.
4. Morillo CA, Klein GJ, Jones DL, Guiraudon CM: Chronic rapid atrial pacing. Structural, functional, and electrophysiological characteristics of a new model of sustained atrial fibrillation. Circulation 91(5):1588-1595, 1995.
5. Neuberger HR, Schotten U, Blaauw Y, et al: Chronic atrial dilation, electrical remodeling, and atrial fibrillation in the goat. J Am Coll Cardiol 47(3):644-653, 2006.
6. Schuessler RB, Grayson TM, Bromberg BI, et al: Cholinergically mediated tachyarrhythmias induced by a single extrastimulus in the isolated canine right atrium. Circ Res 71(5):1254-1267, 1992.
7. Verheule S, Wilson E, Everett T, et al: Alterations in atrial electrophysiology and tissue structure in a canine model of chronic atrial dilatation due to mitral regurgitation. Circulation 107(20):2615-2622, 2003.
8. Wijffels MC, Kirchhof CJ, Dorland R, Allessie MA: Atrial fibrillation begets atrial fibrillation. A study in awake chronically instrumented goats. Circulation 92(7):1954-1968, 1995.
9. Verheule S, Wilson E, Banthia S, et al: Direction-dependent conduction abnormalities in a canine model of atrial fibrillation due to chronic atrial dilatation. Am J Physiol Heart Circ Physiol 287(2):H634-H644, 2004.
10. Botteron GW, Smith JM: A technique for measurement of the extent of spatial organization of atrial activation during atrial fibrillation in the intact human heart. IEEE Trans Biomed Eng 42(6):579-586, 1995.
11. Lee KW, Everett TH, Ilhan HT, et al: Feature extraction of the atrial fibrillation signal using the continuous wavelet transform. Presented at the 26th Annual International Conference of the Institute of Electrical and Electronics Engineers Engineering in Medicine and Biology Society, San Francisco, CA, September 1-5, 2004.
12. Akar JG, Everett TH, Kok LC, et al: Effect of electrical and structural remodeling on spatiotemporal organization in acute and persistent atrial fibrillation. J Cardiovasc Electrophysiol 13(10):1027-1034, 2002.
13. Richman JS, Moorman JR: Physiological time-series analysis using approximate entropy and sample entropy. Am J Physiol Heart Circ Physiol 278(6):H2039-H2049, 2000.
14. Garfinkel A, Chen PS, Walter DO, et al: Quasiperiodicity and chaos in cardiac fibrillation. J Clin Invest 99(2):305-314, 1997.
15. Gray RA, Jalife J: Ventricular fibrillation and atrial fibrillation are two different beasts. Chaos 8(1):65-78, 1998.
16. Sih HJ, Zipes DP, Berbari EJ, Olgin JE: A high-temporal resolution algorithm for quantifying organization during atrial fibrillation. IEEE Trans Biomed Eng 46(4):440-450, 1999.
17. Everett TH, Kok LC, Vaughn RH, et al: Frequency domain algorithm for quantifying atrial fibrillation organization to increase defibrillation efficacy. IEEE Trans Biomed Eng 48(9):969-978, 2001.
18. Skanes AC, Mandapati R, Berenfeld O, et al: Spatiotemporal periodicity during atrial fibrillation in the isolated sheep heart. Circulation 98(12):1236-1248, 1998.
19. Ryu K, Sahadevan J, Khrestian CM, et al: Use of fast Fourier transform analysis of atrial electrograms for rapid characterization of atrial activation—implications for delineating possible mechanisms of atrial tachyarrhythmias. J Cardiovasc Electrophysiol 17(2):198-206, 2006.
20. Pachon MJ, Pachon ME, Pachon MJ, et al: A new treatment for atrial fibrillation based on spectral analysis to guide the catheter RF-ablation. Europace 6(6):590-601, 2004.
21. Sanders P, Berenfeld O, Hocini M, et al: Spectral analysis identifies sites of high-frequency activity maintaining atrial fibrillation in humans. Circulation 112(6): 789-797, 2005.
22. Everett TH, Akar JG, Kok LC, et al: Use of global atrial fibrillation organization to optimize the success of burst pace termination. J Am Coll Cardiol 40(10):1831-1840, 2002.
23. Everett TH, Moorman JR, Kok LC, et al: Assessment of global atrial fibrillation organization to optimize timing of atrial defibrillation. Circulation 103(23):2857-2861, 2001.
24. Cha TJ, Ehrlich JR, Zhang L, Nattel S: Atrial ionic remodeling induced by atrial tachycardia in the presence of congestive heart failure. Circulation 110(12):1520-1526, 2004.
25. Shinagawa K, Shi YF, Tardif JC, et al: Dynamic nature of atrial fibrillation substrate during development and reversal of heart failure in dogs. Circulation 105(22):2672-2678, 2002.
26. Cha TJ, Ehrlich JR, Zhang L, et al: Dissociation between ionic remodeling and ability to sustain atrial fibrillation during recovery from experimental congestive heart failure. Circulation 109(3):412-418, 2004.
27. Guerra JM, Everett TH, Lee KW, et al: Effects of the gap junction modifier rotigaptide (ZP123) on atrial conduction and vulnerability to atrial fibrillation. Circulation 114(2):110-118, 2006.
28. Sinno H, Derakhchan K, Libersan D, et al: Atrial ischemia promotes atrial fibrillation in dogs. Circulation 107(14):1930-1936, 2003.
29. Shiroshita-Takeshita A, Sakabe M, Haugan K, et al: Model-dependent effects of the gap junction conduction-enhancing antiarrhythmic peptide rotigaptide (ZP123) on experimental atrial fibrillation in dogs. Circulation 115(3):310-318, 2007.
30. Yue L, Feng J, Gaspo R, et al: Ionic remodeling underlying action potential changes in a canine model of atrial fibrillation. Circ Res 81(4):512-525, 1997.
31. Fareh S, Villemaire C, Nattel S: Importance of refractoriness heterogeneity in the enhanced vulnerability to atrial fibrillation induction caused by tachycardia-induced atrial electrical remodeling. Circulation 98(20):2202-2209, 1998.
32. Ausma J, Wijffels M, Thone F, et al: Structural changes of atrial myocardium due to sustained atrial fibrillation in the goat. Circulation 96(9):3157-3163, 1997.
33. Everett TH, Wilson EE, Verheule S, et al: Structural atrial remodeling alters the substrate and spatiotemporal organization of AF: A comparison in canine models of structural and electrical atrial remodeling. Am J Physiol Heart Circ Physiol 291(6):H2911-H2923, 2006.
34. Allessie M, Ausma J, Schotten U: Electrical, contractile and structural remodeling during atrial fibrillation. Cardiovasc Res 54(2):230-246, 2002.
35. Ausma J, Litjens N, Lenders MH, et al: Time course of atrial fibrillation–induced cellular structural remodeling in atria of the goat. J Mol Cell Cardiol 33(12):2083-2094, 2001.
36. Schuessler RB, Bromberg BI, Boineau JP: Effect of neurotransmitters on the activation sequence of the isolated atrium. Am J Physiol 258(6 Pt 2):H1632-H1641, 1990.
37. Rensma PL, Allessie MA, Lammers WJ, et al: Length of excitation wave and susceptibility to reentrant atrial arrhythmias in normal conscious dogs. Circ Res 62(2):395-410, 1988.
38. Ideker RE, Smith WM, Blanchard SM, et al: The assumptions of isochronal cardiac mapping. Pacing Clin Electrophysiol 12(3):456-478, 1989.
39. Gerstenfeld EP, Sahakian AV, Swiryn S: Evidence for transient linking of atrial excitation during atrial fibrillation in humans. Circulation 86(2):375-382, 1992.
40. Kalifa J, Tanaka K, Zaitsev AV, et al: Mechanisms of wave fractionation at boundaries of high-frequency excitation in the posterior left atrium of the isolated sheep heart during atrial fibrillation. Circulation 113(5):626-633, 2006.
41. Allessie M, Lammers WJEP, Bonke FIM, Hollen J: Experimental evaluation of Moe's multiple wavelet hypothesis of atrial fibrillation. In Zipes DP, Jalife J (eds): Cardiac Electrophysiology and Arrhythmias. Orlando, FL, Grune and Straton, 1985, pp 265-275.
42. Haissaguerre M, Jais P, Shah DC, et al: Spontaneous initiation of atrial fibrillation by ectopic beats originating in the pulmonary veins. N Engl J Med 339(10):659-666, 1998.

43. Mandapati R, Skanes A, Chen J, et al: Stable microreentrant sources as a mechanism of atrial fibrillation in the isolated sheep heart. Circulation 101(2):194-199, 2000.
44. Moe GK, Rheinboldt WC, Abildskov JA: A computer model of atrial fibrillation. Am Heart J 67:200-220, 1964.
45. Li D, Benardeau A, Nattel S: Contrasting efficacy of dofetilide in differing experimental models of atrial fibrillation. Circulation 102(1):104-112, 2000.
46. Lee KW, Everett TH, Rahmutula D, et al: Pirfenidone prevents the development of a vulnerable substrate for atrial fibrillation in a canine model of heart failure. Circulation 114(16):1703-1712, 2006.
47. Derakhchan K, Li D, Courtemanche M, et al: Method for simultaneous epicardial and endocardial mapping of in vivo canine heart: Application to atrial conduction properties and arrhythmia mechanisms. J Cardiovasc Electrophysiol 12(5):548-555, 2001.
48. Stambler BS, Fenelon G, Shepard RK, et al: Characterization of sustained atrial tachycardia in dogs with rapid ventricular pacing–induced heart failure. J Cardiovasc Electrophysiol 14(5):499-507, 2003.
49. Fenelon G, Shepard RK, Stambler BS: Focal origin of atrial tachycardia in dogs with rapid ventricular pacing–induced heart failure. J Cardiovasc Electrophysiol 14(10):1093-1102, 2003.
50. Ryu K, Shroff SC, Sahadevan J, et al: Mapping of atrial activation during sustained atrial fibrillation in dogs with rapid ventricular pacing induced heart failure: Evidence for a role of driver regions. J Cardiovasc Electrophysiol 16(12):1348-1358, 2005.
51. Okuyama Y, Miyauchi Y, Park AM, et al: High resolution mapping of the pulmonary vein and the vein of Marshall during induced atrial fibrillation and atrial tachycardia in a canine model of pacing-induced congestive heart failure. J Am Coll Cardiol 42(2):348-360, 2003.
52. Everett TH, Wilson EE, Olgin JE: Effects of atrial fibrillation substrate and spatiotemporal organization on atrial defibrillation thresholds. Heart Rhythm 4(8):1048-1056, 2007.
53. Everett TH, Verheule S, Wilson EE, Foreman S, Olgin JE: Left atrial dilatation resulting from chronic mitral regurgitation decreases spatiotemporal organization of atrial fibrillation in left atrium. Am J Physiol Heart Circ Physiol 286(6):H2452-H2460, 2004.
54. Sih HJ, Zipes DP, Berbari EJ, et al: Differences in organization between acute and chronic atrial fibrillation in dogs. J Am Coll Cardiol 36(3):924-931, 2000.
55. Wu TJ, Ong JJ, Chang CM, et al: Pulmonary veins and ligament of Marshall as sources of rapid activations in a canine model of sustained atrial fibrillation. Circulation 103(8):1157-1163, 2001.
56. Everett TH, Wilson EE, Verheule S, et al: Structural atrial remodeling alters the substrate and spatiotemporal organization of atrial fibrillation: A comparison in canine models of structural and electrical atrial remodeling. Am J Physiol Heart Circ Physiol 291(6):H2911-H2923, 2006.
57. Moriguchi M, Niwano S, Yoshizawa N, et al: Inhomogeneity in the appearance of electrical remodeling during chronic rapid atrial pacing: Evaluation of the dispersion of atrial effective refractoriness. Jpn Circ J 65(4):335-340, 2001.
58. Berenfeld O, Zaitsev AV, Mironov SF, et al: Frequency-dependent breakdown of wave propagation into fibrillatory conduction across the pectinate muscle network in the isolated sheep right atrium. Circ Res 90(11):1173-1180, 2002.
59. Mansour M, Mandapati R, Berenfeld O, et al: Left-to-right gradient of atrial frequencies during acute atrial fibrillation in the isolated sheep heart. Circulation 103(21):2631-2636, 2001.
60. Sarmast F, Kolli A, Zaitsev A, et al: Cholinergic atrial fibrillation: $I_{K,ACh}$ gradients determine unequal left/right atrial frequencies and rotor dynamics. Cardiovasc Res 59(4):863-873, 2003.
61. Newton JC, Johnson PL, Justice RK, et al: Estimated global epicardial distribution of activation rate and conduction block during porcine ventricular fibrillation. J Cardiovasc Electrophysiol 13(10):1035-1041, 2002.
62. Evans FG, Rogers JM, Smith WM, Ideker RE: Automatic detection of conduction block based on time-frequency analysis of unipolar electrograms. IEEE Trans Biomed Eng 46(9):1090-1097, 1999.
63. de Bakker JM, van Capelle FJ, Janse MJ, et al: Fractionated electrograms in dilated cardiomyopathy: Origin and relation to abnormal conduction. J Am Coll Cardiol 27(5):1071-1078, 1996.
64. Sahadevan J, Ryu K, Peltz L, et al: Epicardial mapping of chronic atrial fibrillation in patients: Preliminary observations. Circulation 110(21):3293-3299, 2004.
65. Lazar S, Dixit S, Marchlinski FE, et al: Presence of left-to-right atrial frequency gradient in paroxysmal but not persistent atrial fibrillation in humans. Circulation 110(20):3181-3186, 2004.
66. Schuessler RB, Kay MW, Melby SJ, et al: Spatial and temporal stability of the dominant frequency of activation in human atrial fibrillation. J Electrocardiol 39 (4 Suppl):S7-S12, 2006.
67. Lin YJ, Tai CT, Kao T, et al: Frequency analysis in different types of paroxysmal atrial fibrillation. J Am Coll Cardiol 47(7):1401-1407, 2006.
68. Sanders P, Nalliah CJ, Dubois R, et al: Frequency mapping of the pulmonary veins in paroxysmal versus permanent atrial fibrillation. J Cardiovasc Electrophysiol 17(9):965-972, 2006.
69. Lazar S, Dixit S, Callans DJ, et al: Effect of pulmonary vein isolation on the left-to-right atrial dominant frequency gradient in human atrial fibrillation. Heart Rhythm 3(8):889-895, 2006.
70. Takahashi Y, Sanders P, Jais P, et al: Organization of frequency spectra of atrial fibrillation: Relevance to radiofrequency catheter ablation. J Cardiovasc Electrophysiol 17(4):382-388, 2006.

Molecular Remodeling and Chronic Atrial Fibrillation 43

Stanley Nattel, Brett Burstein, and Dobromir Dobrev

CHAPTER OUTLINE

When atrial fibrillation (AF) is induced (for example by electrical burst pacing) in a normal person or experimental animal, it rarely persists. Typically, the induced AF self-terminates within about a minute. However, a variety of changes in atrial structure or electrical function can change atrial properties to produce a substrate in which AF becomes spontaneously sustained, a process called *atrial remodeling*. The pathologic molecular mechanisms that produce atrial remodeling and result in a stable AF substrate, producing chronic AF, are the subject of this chapter.

Features of the Atrial Fibrillation–Maintaining Substrate

The functional substrates leading to AF persistence are illustrated in Figure 43-1 (for a detailed description of the underlying mechanisms, see Nattel[1]). The mechanisms that can maintain AF include rapid local activity from an ectopic focus, single-circuit reentry, and multiple-circuit reentry. Ectopic activity can contribute either by acting as a trigger to initiate reentry in a vulnerable substrate or by acting as a rapid atrial driver that maintains fibrillatory activity. Single-circuit reentry can also maintain AF by acting as a rapid regional driver. Rapid single local drivers, whether due to spontaneous ectopic activity or to a single stable reentry circuit, cause fibrillation rather than atrial tachycardia or flutter when they produce fibrillatory conduction in atrial regions that are unable to follow 1:1, either because of heterogeneous refractory properties or by virtue of conduction complexities.[2] Multiple-circuit reentry involves multiple coexisting functional reentry circuits that maintain fibrillatory activity because the rate of formation of new circuits balances the rate of functional circuit extinction, so that a sufficient number of circuits to maintain AF remains at all times.

The molecular processes that lead to AF persistence alter underlying electrophysiologic function in a way that enhances the likelihood of one or more of the three fundamental AF-maintaining mechanisms illustrated in Figure 43-1. According to classic leading-circle theory, the maintenance of reentry requires a reentering impulse to traverse the entire potential reentry circuit in a period long enough for the initially activated tissue zone to regain excitability. The wavelength, the distance traveled by the electrical impulse in one refractory period (given by the product of the refractory period and conduction velocity), gives the minimum size of a functional reentrant circuit and has to be longer than the available circuit length for reentry to persist. The conditions favoring reentry maintenance therefore include slow conduction and abbreviated refractoriness (which reduce the wavelength) and atrial dilation (which increases potential circuit sizes).[1]

The refractory period depends primarily on the duration of the cardiac action potential (APD). APD can be reduced by an enhancement of outward repolarizing K^+ currents or a reduction in the primary inward current ($I_{Ca,L}$) that maintains the action potential plateau. Atrial conduction impairment can result from tissue fibrosis, resulting in physical separation of muscle fibers; dysfunction of the primary source current for atrial conduction, sodium current (I_{Na}); and abnormalities in the specialized connexin proteins that couple cardiac cells to each other. Ectopic activity can result from an enhancement of intrinsic pacemaker mechanisms, such as via an increase in the pacemaker current known as the *funny current* (I_f). Ectopic activity can also result from triggered activity, the most important cause of which is abnormalities in Ca^{2+} handling that cause spontaneous diastolic Ca^{2+} release events that induce delayed afterdepolarizations (DADs).[1,3] Ectopic activity can also result from excessive APD prolongation, which produces early afterdepolarizations (EADs).[1]

Paradigms of Atrial Fibrillation Maintenance

The factors favoring AF maintenance have been elucidated on the basis of animal models mimicking clinical paradigms of sustained AF. Two well-characterized types of animal models allow induction of AF that persists for prolonged periods. These are atrial tachycardia remodeling and atrial structural remodeling. Both of these produce alterations that favor reentrant arrhythmias. We first briefly review their pathophysiology and then discuss in detail the underlying molecular mechanisms. In addition, there is evidence for ectopic firing underlying AF in specific clinical and experimental paradigms. We review this evidence and then present the potential molecular basis.

This research is supported by the Canadian Institutes of Health Research (MGP 6957, MOP 44365), the Quebec Heart and Stroke Foundation, the Mathematics of Information Technology and Complex Systems (MITACS) Network of Centers of Excellence, the German Federal Ministry of Education and Research (Atrial Fibrillation Competence Network grant 01Gi0204), and a network grant (European-North American Atrial Fibrillation Research Alliance ENAFRA) from Fondation Leducq.

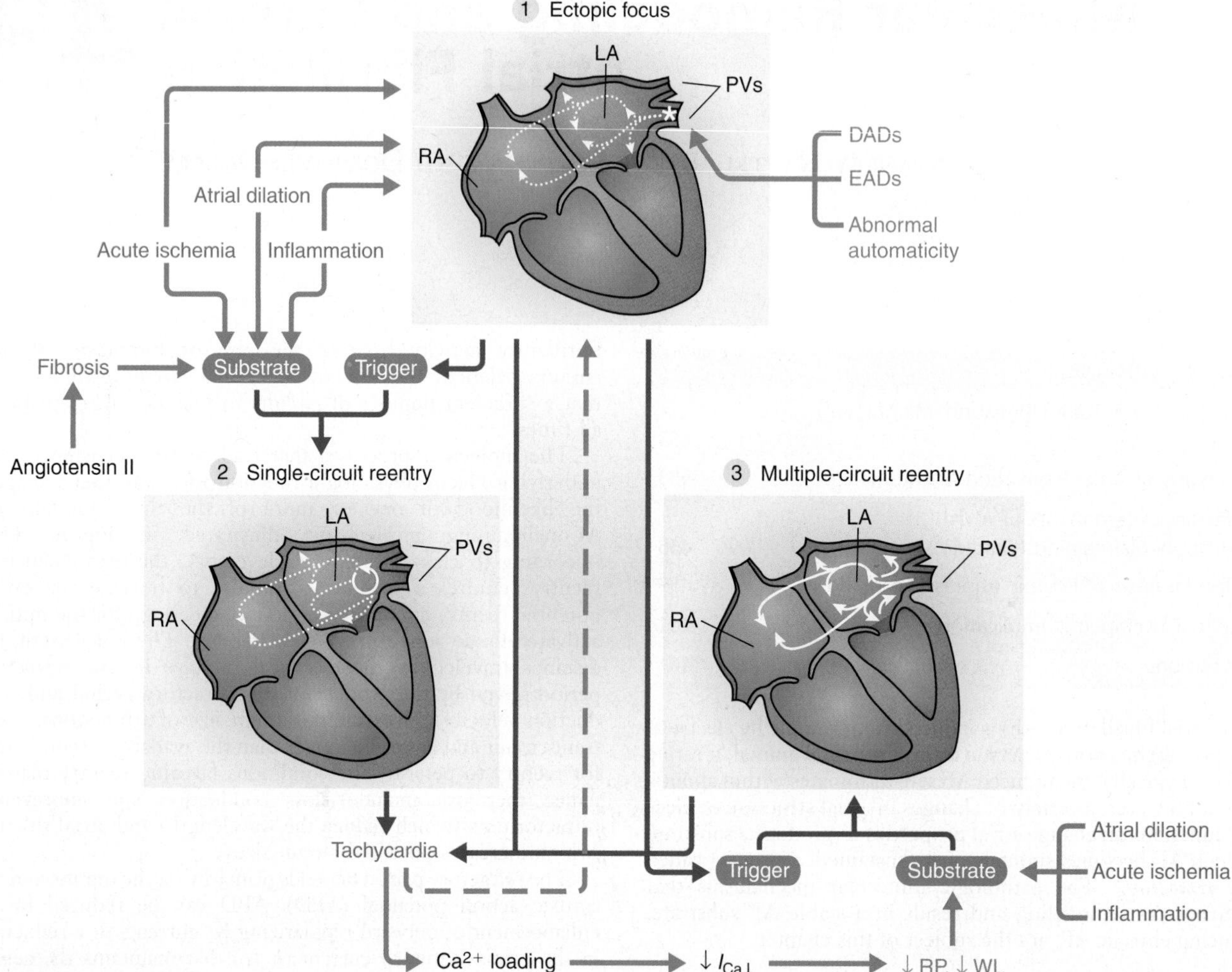

Figure 43-1 Three primary mechanisms are believed to be able to maintain atrial fibrillation: Rapidly discharging ectopic foci, single-circuit reentry, and multiple-circuit reentry. Reentry mechanisms require a vulnerable substrate, which is acted on by a trigger (usually from an ectopic activation) to produce reentry. Vulnerable substrates usually require some change in atrial properties (typically abbreviated refractoriness or slowed conduction) that can be caused by atrial fibrosis, dilation, ischemia or inflammation. Ectopic foci can arise as a result of delayed afterdepolarizations (DADs), early afterdepolarizations (EADs), or abnormal automaticity. Atrial tachycardias that arise from any of the three mechanisms cause tachycardia-induced remodeling, primarily via decreased calcium current ($I_{Ca,L}$) which reduces the refractory period (RP) and wavelength (WL). LA, left atrium; PV, pulmonary vein; RA, right atrium.

Atrial Tachycardia Remodeling

The recognition that AF alters atrial electrophysiologic properties in a way that promotes AF induction and maintenance was an important advance in understanding AF pathophysiology. The phenomenon was initially called *electrical remodeling* and descriptively termed "AF begets AF,"[4] but subsequent evidence for other forms of electrical remodeling and an awareness that AF induces electrical remodeling owing to its very rapid rate led to the widespread use of the term *atrial tachycardia remodeling* (ATR).

The mechanisms by which ATR promotes AF are illustrated in Figure 43-2. ATR abbreviates atrial refractoriness (thereby decreasing the wavelength) and reduces the rate dependence of the refractory period,[4] changes that are due to corresponding APD alterations.[5] These alterations are primarily caused by $I_{Ca,L}$ downregulation,[5] but increased inward-rectifier potassium current function also plays a role.[6-8] ATR can also interfere with atrial conduction by affecting connexins, gap-junction proteins that connect cardiomyocytes, in particular by causing spatially heterogeneous downregulation of the primarily atrial connexin40.[9] The reduced wavelength caused by APD, in conjunction with conduction abnormalities caused by connexin suppression, decreases the size of functional atrial reentry circuits and promotes multiple circuit reentry. In addition, ATR impairs atrial contractility, principally by causing Ca^{2+}-handling abnormalities,[10] thereby producing atrial dilation that further promotes reentry (see Fig. 43-2).

Atrial Structural Remodeling

Congestive heart failure (CHF) is a very important cause of AF, and AF implies a poorer prognosis in CHF.[11] Dogs with experimental CHF often show prolonged AF when the arrhythmia is induced by atrial burst pacing.[12] CHF tends to increase atrial refractoriness and does not reduce the wavelength. Rather, CHF-induced AF promotion is related to the development of prominent atrial fibrosis, which causes localized regions of

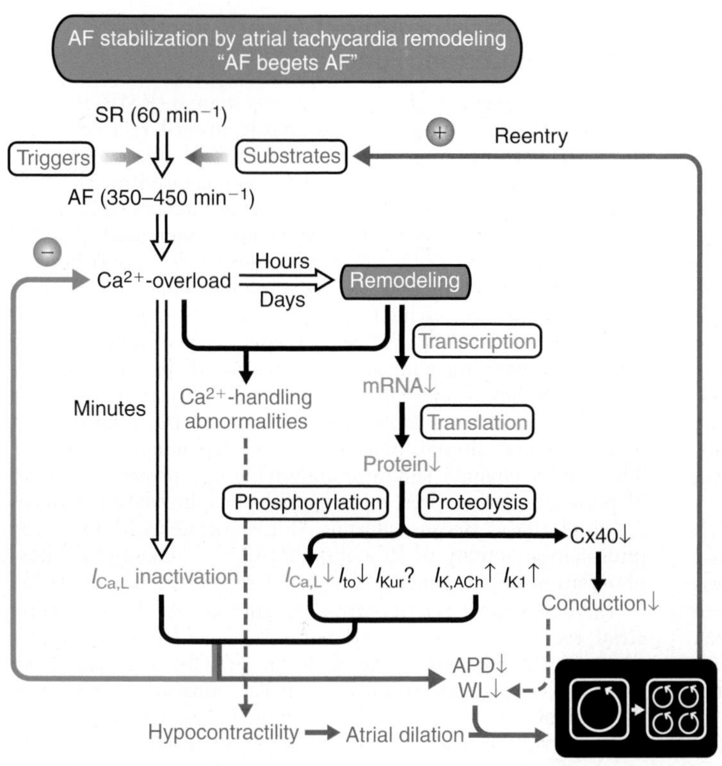

Figure 43-2 Mechanisms underlying atrial tachycardia remodeling. The rapid atrial rate increases Ca^{2+} loading, which can be cytotoxic. Cells protect themselves by reducing L-type calcium current ($I_{Ca,L}$), by rapidly acting functional mechanisms (current inactivation) and by more slowly developing changes in gene expression and altered protein regulation (proteolysis and phosphorylation changes). Processes with cell-protecting functions are indicated in *green;* arrhythmogenic mechanisms are indicated in *red.* Reduced $I_{Ca,L}$ protects the cell from Ca^{2+} overload by decreasing Ca^{2+} entry during each action potential, but because of the reduced plateau inward (depolarizing) $I_{Ca,L}$, action potential duration (APD) is reduced. Decreased APD abbreviates refractoriness and decreases the wavelength (WL), allowing smaller reentry circuits, a larger number of which can now be accommodated. Atrial fibrillation (AF) is much less likely to terminate in atria that can accommodate a large number of circuits, because termination would require all circuits to stop at the same time, which is statistically improbable. In addition to decreased $I_{Ca,L}$, atrial tachycardia also changes K^+ currents, with increases in the inward rectifier currents I_{K1} and constitutive $I_{K,ACh,c}$, contributing to APD shortening and AF promotion. Cx40, connexin40; mRNA, messenger RNA; SR, sarcoplasmic reticulum.

conduction slowing, presumably by physically separating muscle bundles and interfering with impulse propagation. The importance of atrial fibrosis, a prominent feature of atrial structural remodeling (ASR), is illustrated by the fact that when dogs are allowed to fully recover from ventricular tachycardiomyopathy, their ventricular function, ion-channel remodeling, and chamber dimensions virtually normalize, and yet atrial fibrosis remains and prolonged AF can still be induced.[13,14]

Paradigms of Atrial Fibrillation Maintained by Atrial Ectopic Firing

Patients with paroxysmal AF often appear to have important focal tachyarrhythmic activity originating in the pulmonary veins. Ablation of the originating site can prevent occurrence and maintenance of the arrhythmia.[15,16] There is evidence that focal drivers contribute to AF in dogs with CHF,[17,18] probably on the basis of DAD-related triggered activity.[19] There is also evidence of focal activity in the pulmonary vein region in dogs with both CHF and ATR,[20,21] although the basis of this pulmonary vein activity and its precise role in maintaining AF are still unclear.

Molecular Determinants of Atrial Fibrillation–Maintaining Paradigms

AF maintenance is determined by the fundamental factors governing the occurrence of reentry and formation of ectopic impulses. The likelihood of reentry is primarily established by the tissue properties of conduction and refractoriness, whereas formation of ectopic impulse is governed by the factors controlling the occurrence of afterdepolarizations (primarily Ca^{2+} handling for DADs and APD prolongation for EADs) and of spontaneous automaticity (particularly the pacemaker current I_f).

Signal Transduction of Atrial Repolarization Abnormalities

The molecular mechanisms leading to the repolarization changes in ATR are incompletely understood. Increased atrial rate causes cellular Ca^{2+} loading,[22] which induces important changes in cellular signaling and Ca^{2+} handling, triggering a series of processes that cause ATR (see Fig. 43-2). A very rapid shortening of APD and ERP because of functional $I_{Ca,L}$ inactivation attenuates initial Ca^{2+} overload. Persistent AF produces sustained Ca^{2+} loading that is offset by decreased expression and function of L-type calcium-channel subunit proteins, causing reduced $I_{Ca,L}$, and by increased Ca^{2+} extrusion via Na^+-Ca^{2+} exchanger. These compensatory changes limit cytotoxic Ca^{2+} influx but cause further ERP abbreviation that decreases wavelength, favoring multiple circuit reentry.[1,9,23]

The increase in intracellular Ca^{2+} ($[Ca^{2+}]_i$) is likely a primary signal for altered gene expression and regulation of ion channels. In a mouse atrial HL-1 cell line, rapid pacing reduces protein levels of calcium channels by activating Ca^{2+}-dependent calpain proteases,[24] and calpain activity is increased in AF.[25] However, generalized proteolysis is not consistent with preserved protein levels of ryanodine receptor channels[26] or increased protein amounts of I_{K1},[27] suggesting that multiple mechanisms of ion-channel adaptation to high-rate related Ca^{2+} overload are operative.

Molecular Determinants of Alterations to L-type Calcium Current

Ca^{2+} enters the cell with each action potential, so that an abrupt increase in atrial rate (about eight-fold) causes substantial increases in Ca^{2+} flux into the cell. Atrial cardiomyocytes respond to reduce Ca^{2+} influx and prevent potentially cytotoxic Ca^{2+} overload (see Fig. 43-2), initially by a combination of Ca^{2+}-dependent $I_{Ca,L}$ inactivation and incomplete recovery from voltage- and time-dependent $I_{Ca,L}$ inactivation. With time, longer-term adaptive mechanisms come into play, causing sustained decreases in $I_{Ca,L}$.[9] In agreement with this notion, reduced $I_{Ca,L}$ density is a consistent finding in animal models and patients with AF.[5,9,28] In control cardiomyocytes, inhibition of $I_{Ca,L}$ with calcium-channel blockers mimics the APD shortening and loss of rate adaptation in ATR and AF;[5] therefore, reduced $I_{Ca,L}$ was initially considered to be the only determinant of abbreviation of APD or refractoriness in ATR and AF. Subsequent studies, however, indicated important contributions of increased I_{K1} along with constitutively active acetylcholine-activated potassium current ($I_{K,ACh}$). In addition, altered Ca^{2+} handling likely contributes to loss of APD rate dependence and might promote reentry-facilitating alternans behavior in ATR.[29]

The molecular basis of decreased $I_{Ca,L}$ in ATR and AF is complex and likely depends partly on underlying heart disease. Transcriptional downregulation of the $Ca_V1.2$ α subunit was initially considered to be the only molecular mechanism of decreased $I_{Ca,L}$.[30,31] Some subsequent studies at the mRNA and protein level confirmed the reductions in $Ca_V1.2$ α subunit abundance,[27,32] whereas other reports found no change in protein amount or dihydropyridine receptor density in AF.[33-35]. Some, but not all, investigations detected reduced expression of accessory β_1, β_{2a}, β_{2b}, β_3 and $\alpha_2\delta_2$ that might also contribute to the reduction of $I_{Ca,L}$.[27,28,33,34]

The mechanisms of reduced $Ca_V1.2$ α subunit mRNA expression are not fully understood. Chronic exposure to transforming growth factor β_1 (TGF-β_1), a critical contributor to atrial structural remodeling,[36] reduces atrial, but not ventricular, $Ca_V1.2$ α subunit mRNA and decreases $I_{Ca,L}$.[37] Thus, increased TGF-β_1 levels[38] might participate in the transcriptional downregulation of $I_{Ca,L}$ in AF. Direct measurements confirm that AF quickly increases cardiomyocyte $[Ca^{2+}]_i$.[22] In vitro studies of tachypaced canine atrial cardiomyocytes suggest that Ca^{2+} influx via $I_{Ca,L}$ and the related Ca^{2+} overload are major determinants of the transcriptional downregulation of $I_{Ca,L}$ and I_{to} and implicate mechanisms related to calmodulin, Ca^{2+}-dependent protein kinase II (CaMKII), and calcineurin in modification of transcription.[39] Ca^{2+} overload-related increases in calpain activity and increased breakdown of the $Ca_V1.2$ α subunit might also contribute to $I_{Ca,L}$ downregulation,[40] because calpains can degrade $Ca_V1.2$ α subunits and calpain inhibitors prevent $Ca_V1.2$ protein degradation in an in vitro tachypaced HL-1 atrial-cardiomyocyte system.[24]

There is evidence for increased calcium-channel dephosphorylation by increased activity of serine/threonine protein phosphatase type 1 (PP1) and type 2A (PP2A) in AF.[34,35,41] Defective regulation of $I_{Ca,L}$ by src-type tyrosine kinases also participate in $I_{Ca,L}$ dysregulation.[35] Drugs with antioxidant properties (e.g., statins) prevent the ATR-induced downregulation of $Ca_V1.2$ α subunit protein expression and the associated abbreviation of refractoriness and promotion of AF.[42] Decreased expression of the endogenous antioxidant glutathione, the major cellular reducing agent, correlates inversely with the extent of *S*-nitrosylation.[43] *S*-nitrosylation of the $Ca_V1.2$ α subunit is increased in AF, and exogenously applied glutathione partially restores the AF-related $I_{Ca,L}$ reduction.[43] Thus, oxidative stress could play an important role in $I_{Ca,L}$ changes. Finally, recent findings suggest increased atrial levels of ZnT-1, a protein normally involved in zinc homeostasis, in both ATR and AF.[44,45] The increase of ZnT-1 is associated with reduced $I_{Ca,L}$ amplitude, possibly by limiting Ca^{2+} influx through the channel pore.[44]

Molecular Basis of Altered Inward Rectifier Potassium-Current Function

The cardiomyocyte resting membrane potential (RMP) is set by background K^+ conductances, primarily inward rectifiers, and the RMP becomes more negative in AF.[7,46-48] The background inward rectifier potassium current I_{K1} is increased in AF.[7,46-48] The first study in dogs with ATR detected unchanged I_{K1},[5] but subsequent work showed consistently increased I_{K1}.[8,49] Increased Kir2.1 mRNA[27,46] and protein levels[27] contribute to enhanced I_{K1} in clinical AF, whereas in dogs with ATR of up to 6 weeks' duration, Kir2.1 remains stable,[30] suggesting that increased Kir2.1 mRNA is likely a consequence of long-standing ATR or underlying clinical conditions in AF patients. Single-channel studies show that I_{K1} open probability is increased in AF.[7] The underlying molecular mechanisms are unknown but might involve altered phosphorylation-dependent regulation. The Kir2.x channel subunits underlying I_{K1} possess a variety of phosphorylation sites, and channel phosphorylation reduces I_{K1} amplitude.[50] Because chronic AF is associated with increased phosphatase activity of PP1 and PP2A,[34,35,41] channel dephosphorylation might contribute to the increased I_{K1} activity in AF.

Increased vagal activity strongly promotes AF by stabilizing atrial reentrant rotors,[51] and clinical AF often begins under vagotonic conditions.[52] Acetylcholine (ACh) released from vagal nerve endings stimulates cardiac muscarinic receptors that activate the inward-rectifier current $I_{K,ACh}$, which produces highly arrhythmogenic, spatially heterogeneous decreases in atrial refractoriness. In knockout mice lacking $I_{K,ACh}$, stimulation of muscarinic receptors does not induce AF.[53] ATR and AF reduce the activation of $I_{K,ACh}$ in response to stimulation of muscarinic receptors.[6,46,47] Recent work suggests that the reduced $I_{K,ACh}$ activation by muscarinic agonists is related to a change in coupling, with increased agonist-independent constitutive $I_{K,ACh}$ ($I_{K,ACh.c}$) in canine ATR[6,8,54] and in patients with chronic, but not paroxysmal, AF.[7,48] Blockade of $I_{K,ACh.c}$ suppresses abbreviation of APD and promotion of AF in ATR preparations,[8] indicating that $I_{K,ACh.c}$ contributes to ATR-induced atrial arrhythmogenesis.

Agonist-independent $I_{K,ACh.c}$ results from increased channel open probability due to a reduction in closing rate.[7,54] Messenger RNA and protein expression of Kir3.1 and Kir3.4 subunits are unchanged in experimental ATR,[54] whereas in patients with AF, mRNA and protein levels of both subunits are decreased.[27,31,46,55] In atrial myocardium, $I_{K,ACh}$ is localized in a macromolecular complex including catalytic subunits of PKA, PKC, CaMKII, PP1, and PP2A.[56] Altered composition of this complex in AF can lead to abnormal phosphorylation-dependent $I_{K,ACh}$ regulation. Blockade of PKC reduces $I_{K,ACh.c}$ activity, and the abundance of PKCε protein is enhanced in AF.[48] Thus, $I_{K,ACh}$ PKC hyperphosphorylation can contribute to the AF-related development of agonist-independent constitutive activity.

ATP-sensitive inward rectifier potassium currents are important contributors to ischemia-induced changes in cardiac electrophysiology, and relative ischemia is a potential contributor to ATR. $I_{K,ATP}$ amplitude is increased under ischemic conditions in cells of patients with AF,[57] whereas $I_{K,ATP}$ enhancement by agonists such as rilmakalim is reduced.[58] Variable expression changes of the pore-forming Kir6.2 subunit[31,55] have been reported and underscore the complexity of $I_{K,ATP}$ regulation in AF.

Mechanisms of Altered Voltage-Gated Potassium Currents

I_{to} is consistently decreased in animal ATR and in patients with AF.[5,9,28,30,59] The functional consequences of reduced I_{to} are unclear, but its downregulation might facilitate wave propagation by indirectly increasing the amplitude of the action potential. In ATR and AF, decreases in I_{to} are paralleled by reductions in mRNA and protein expression of the pore-forming $K_V4.3$ subunit.[30,59] Increased calpain-mediated proteolysis might also contribute to reduced $K_V4.3$ proteins.[25,40] CaMKII activity is higher in AF and CaMKII accelerates I_{to} inactivation, but the increased PP1 and PP2A phosphatase expression in AF[34,35,41] might offset the effect of CaMKII enhancement. PP1 also inactivates transcription factors and represses protein translation.[60] Thus, increased phosphatase activity can contribute to AF-related expression changes.[27,61,62] Ca^{2+}-dependent protein phosphatases such as calcineurin can suppress $K_V4.3$ gene transcription by a mechanism dependent on nuclear factor of activated T cells (NFAT),[39,63] and calcineurin activity is increased in AF.[64]

Results concerning the ultra-rapid delayed-rectifier I_{Kur} are inconsistent, showing either unchanged or reduced I_{Kur} amplitude in AF.[59] Because the role of I_{Kur} in atrial repolarization depends strongly on action potential morphology and is increased with short-duration triangular action potentials as occur in AF, I_{Kur} might contribute more strongly to atrial repolarization in AF cardiomyocytes.[65,66] The inconsistent results regarding I_{Kur} function likely result from variations in expression and post-translational modifications of the principal channel α subunit $K_V1.5$. $K_V1.5$ protein degradation might result from increased proteolysis by calpains.[25] The intracellular redox state is likely altered by increased oxidant production in ATR and AF,[67,68] and $K_V1.5$ currents are inhibited by *S*-nitrosylation.[69] Variations in underlying cardiac diseases[27] or concomitant medication can contribute to some of the inconsistencies in various clinical studies.[59]

The delayed-rectifier currents I_{Kr} and I_{Ks} are not changed in experimental ATR,[5] and information from AF patients is lacking, likely because of difficulties in recording I_{Kr} and I_{Ks} in human atrial cardiomyocytes isolated with the chunk method. Molecular studies in AF patients have reported varying I_{Ks} α subunit (K_VLQT1) expression changes, along with increased mRNA and protein abundance of the β subunit minK, and decreased mRNA and protein abundance of the I_{Kr} HERG subunit.[27,55,59] However, in the absence of functional data, the clinical relevance of these alterations remains unclear.

Signal Transduction of Atrial Conduction Abnormalities

Structural Remodeling and Fibrosis

Extensive evidence indicates that structural remodeling, particularly interstitial fibrosis, is an important contributor to the AF substrate.[70] Fibrosis is thought to increase AF vulnerability by causing local conduction slowing and predisposing to reentry.[1] Atrial fibrosis can result from a variety of cardiac insults sharing common dysregulated fibroproliferative signaling pathways. The regulatory mechanisms underlying atrial extracellular matrix (ECM) remodeling remain incompletely understood, and the precise signaling pathways involved might depend on the specific AF paradigm. Several individual secreted factors are known to be profibrotic and often act synergistically.[71,72] Angiotensin II and TGF-β_1 are among the best-established profibrotic molecules, and evidence also suggests a significant role for platelet-derived growth factor (PDGF) and connective tissue growth factor (CTGF). Figure 43-3 depicts the interplay of these signaling systems.

Angiotensin II Angiotensin II is implicated in myocardial fibrosis for a variety of cardiac pathologies including hypertensive heart disease, CHF, myocardial infarction, and cardiomyopathy. Transgenic mice with cardiac-restricted angiotensin-converting enzyme (ACE) overexpression show marked atrial dilation with focal fibrosis and AF.[73] Circulating or locally produced angiotensin II acts by binding to either angiotensin type I (AT1) or type II (AT2) receptors, the actions of which initiate opposing signaling cascades. AT1 binding is generally thought to be responsible for angiotensin II profibrotic actions, stimulating fibroblast proliferation, cardiomyocyte hypertrophy, and apoptosis.[70,74]

Signaling occurs through the Shc/Grb2/SOS adapter protein complex to activate the small guanosine triphosphatase (GTPase) Ras, which in turn initiates mitogen-activated protein kinase (MAPK) phosphorylation cascades.[75] Downstream phosphorylation by the MAPKs extracellular signal-related kinase-1 and -2 (ERK1/2), p38, and c-Jun N-terminal kinase (JNK) activates Elk-1, c-Jun and c-Fos transcription factors, which then modulate gene expression. In addition, AT1 activation stimulates phospholipase C (PLC), with downstream effects related to diacylglycerol (DAG) activation of PKC and inositol 1,4,5-triphosphate (IP3)-mediated intracellular calcium release. Additionally, signal transduction through the JAK/STAT pathway activates transcription factors such as AP-1 and nuclear factor κB (NFκB). Angiotensin II binding to AT2 is thought to mediate MAPK inhibitory actions[75] through the dephosphorylating actions of phosphotyrosine phosphatase (PTP) and PP2A, leading to antiproliferative and survival-promoting effects. The balance between the actions of these counterregulatory angiotensin II receptor subtypes might have important therapeutic implications for atrial fibrosis.

Transforming Growth Factor β_1 TGF-β_1 is a cytokine that acts as a primary downstream mediator of angiotensin II effects in an autocrine-paracrine manner.[76] Angiotensin II induces TGF-β_1 synthesis, which potently stimulates fibroblast activity, while in turn reciprocally enhancing the production of angiotensin II and additional profibrotic factors,[76,77] to create positive feedback. TGF- β_1 acts primarily through the SMAD signaling pathway (SMAD proteins are homologues of both the *Caenorhabditis elegans* protein [SMA] and the *Drosophila* protein mothers against decapentaplegic [MAD]) to stimulate fibroblast activation and collagen deposition.[78] Type 1 and type 2 TGF-β_1 receptors (TGFβR1 and TGFβR2) form a complex upon ligand binding, causing a unidirectional phosphorylation event in which TGFβR2 phosphorylates TGFβR1, activating its kinase domain. Activated TGFβR1 directly phosphorylates Smad2/3, stimulating release from the receptor complex, association with Smad4, and translocation to the nucleus to interact with DNA binding proteins to regulate gene expression.[78] Crosstalk with other signaling cascades provides an additional level of complexity, because MAPKs have been found to directly phosphorylate SMAD proteins[79] and TGF-β_1 also activates ERK1/2, p38, and JNK through upstream kinase activators such as TGF-β activated kinase 1 (TAK1) and protein kinase B (PKB).[78] It is notable that cardiac overexpression of constitutively active TGF-β_1 causes selective atrial fibrosis, conduction heterogeneity, and AF.[36]

Platelet-Derived Growth Factor PDGF is a member of the PDGF–vascular endothelial growth factor family that stimulates fibroblast proliferation and differentiation to promote fibrosis.[80] Occupation or dimerization of the PDGF tyrosine kinase receptor results in autophosphorylation of the intercellular domain, which initiates signaling through MAPK, JAK/STAT, and PLC pathways shared with both TGF-β_1 and angiotensin II signaling. Not surprisingly, PDGF has been shown to work in concert with these profibrotic molecules.[80] Transgenic mice with cardiac overexpression of PDGF exhibit cardiac fibrosis followed by dilated cardiomyopathy and cardiac failure.[81,82]

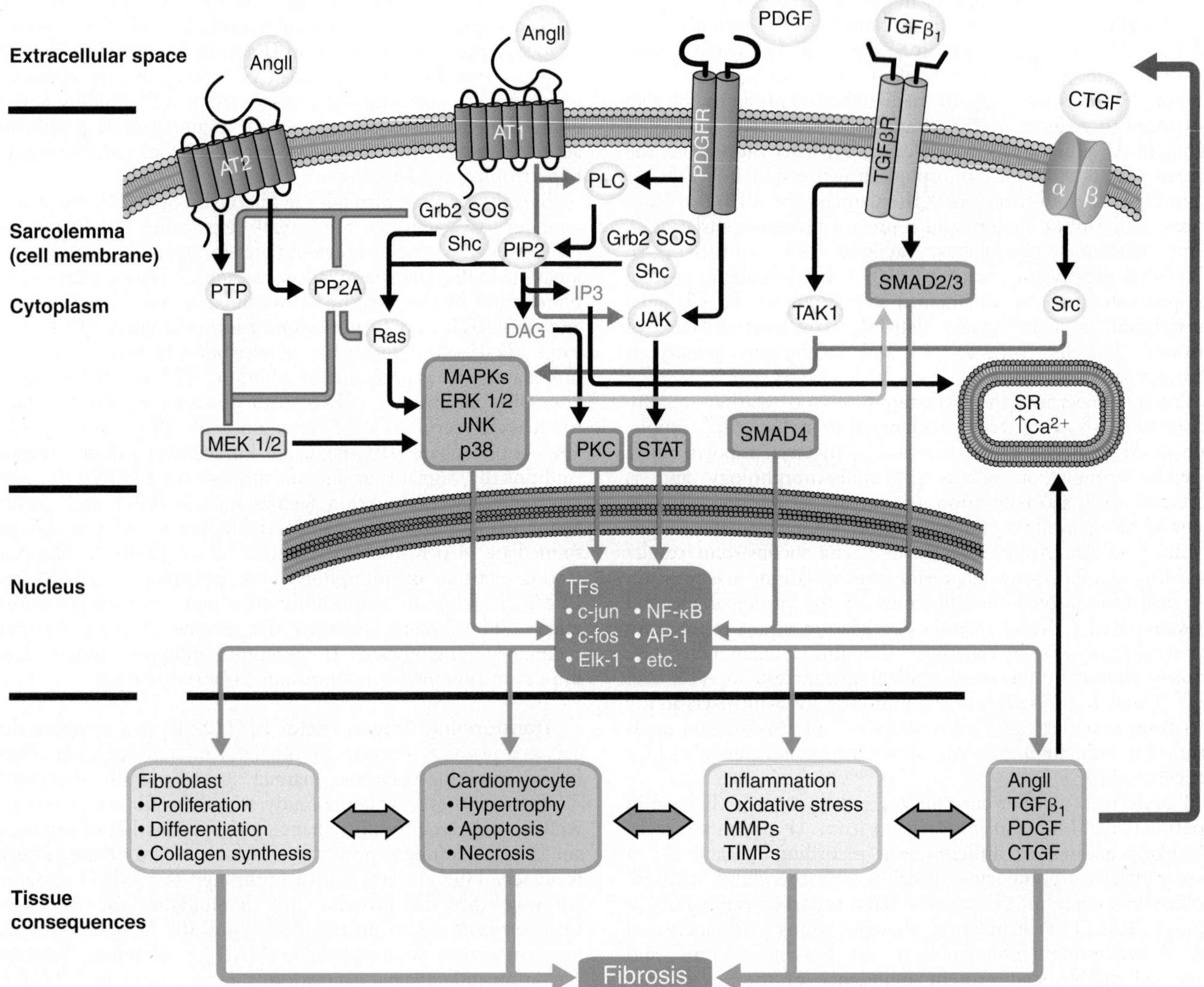

Figure 43-3 Schematic of major profibrotic signaling pathways, illustrating how crosstalk between pathways results in positive feedback and leads to atrial fibrotic remodeling. A schematic cell is shown, with the cytoplasm and nuclear space delimited by schematic representations of the sarcolemma and nuclear envelope, respectively. Sarcolemmal membrane receptors are shown in the *dark blue* cell membrane, factors affecting gene transcription are indicated in *beige*. Tissue consequences of the signaling indicated are summarized at the bottom. αβ, integrin receptor α and β subunits; AngII, angiotensin II; AP-1, activator protein-1; AT1, angiotensin type I receptor; AT2, angiotensin type II receptor; CTGF, connective tissue growth factor; DAG, diacylglycerol; ERK1/2, extracellular signal-related kinase 1/2; Grb2, growth factor receptor binding protein 2; IP3, inositol 1,4,5-trisphosphate; JAK, Janus kinase; JNK, c-Jun N-terminal kinase; MAPK, mitogen-activated protein kinase; MEK 1/2, mitogen-activated/ERK kinase 1/2; MMP, matrix metalloproteinase; NFκB, nuclear factor κB; PKC, protein kinase C; PDGF, platelet-derived growth factor; PDGFR, platelet-derived growth factor receptor; PIP2, phosphatidylinositol bisphosphate; PLC, phospholipase C; PP2A, protein serine/threonine phosphatase 2A; PTP, phosphotyrosine phosphatase; SR, sarcoplasmic reticulum; Shc, src homologous and collagen protein; SMAD, sma- and mad-related proteins; SOS, son of sevenless protein; STAT, signal transducers and activators of transcription; TAK1, TGF-β_1-activated kinase 1; TF, transcription factor; TGFβ_1, transforming growth factor-β; TGFβR, transforming growth factor-β receptor; TIMP, tissue inhibitor of matrix metalloproteinase.

Connective Tissue Growth Factor CTGF, an important mediator in fibrotic conditions,[83] is a member of the CCN (cyr61, ctgf, nov) protein family of matricellular regulatory factors and a major downstream effector of the profibrotic actions of TGF-β_1. In regions of active myocardial remodeling, CTGF is coordinately expressed with TGF-β_1.[84] CTGF is upregulated by both angiotensin II[85,86] and TGF-β_1[77] and directly stimulates fibroblast activation in vitro.[83,85] Signaling mechanisms are not well elucidated, but they appear to act mainly through integrins, because binding occurs at the cell surface with subsequent crosstalk with MAPK pathways.[79,83,87]

Profibrotic Signaling in Various Atrial Fibrillation Paradigms The atrial renin-angiotensin system is strongly activated in experimental tachycardiomyopathic CHF, with atrial angiotensin II expression increasing rapidly after the onset of ventricular tachypacing.[88] Inhibition of the renin-angiotensin-aldosterone system by ACE inhibitors,[89] angiotensin-receptor blockers,[90] or aldosterone antagonists[91] prevents atrial fibrosis and associated promotion of AF. ACE inhibition attenuates activation of ERK but not p38-kinase or JNK.[89] Rapid and sustained increases of atrial TGF-β_1 activation occur during tachypacing-induced CHF,[92] and TGF-β_1 inhibition by pirfenidone attenuates remodeling and AF.[93]

A genomic study comparing the ATR and ASR paradigms revealed prominent time-dependent alterations in genes controlling ECM proteins in experimental CHF.[62] After 2 weeks of ventricular tachypacing, coincident with the development of extensive fibrosis, prominent ECM gene changes included eight collagen genes upregulated more than 10-fold, fibrillin-1 upregulated 8-fold, and matrix metalloproteinase (MMP2) upregulated 4.5-fold, whereas no significant changes were seen in these genes at 24 hours, when no significant fibrosis had occurred. Other ECM genes (e.g., fibronectin, lysine oxidase–like 2, and tissue inhibitor of matrix metalloproteinase-1 [TIMP-1]) increased at both time points (~10-fold, ~5-fold, and ~6-fold, respectively). Pathway analysis implicated CTGF as a potentially important mediator. There is a delicate balance between MMPs and their inhibitors (TIMPs) in ECM degradation, and important changes in the TIMP-MMP system are seen in AF patients.[94,95]

Infiltration by inflammatory cells and increased cell death via both apoptotic and necrotic pathways are seen in CHF-induced ASR.[92] There is also evidence for oxidant-stress activation in AF,[67,68,96] principally via enhanced nicotinamide adenine dinucleotide phosphate (NADPH) and xanthine oxidase function, which can promote fibrosis via cell-death and inflammatory pathways. The small G-protein Rac1-GTPase regulates NADPH-oxidase function, is upregulated in human AF, and produces atrial fibrosis and an AF substrate upon targeted overexpression in mice.[97] This pathway thus might play an important role in AF development, particularly because statins, which suppress Rac1 GTPase, are effective in preventing atrial remodeling.[42,98]

It is clear that atrial fibrosis produces a reentry-promoting substrate that can maintain AF, but whether long-standing AF per se can lead to atrial fibrosis remains controversial. Recent studies have shown ECM-gene upregulation and tissue fibrosis in a porcine model of sustained AF induced by atrial tachypacing[99,100] and have implicated angiotensin II signaling as playing a key role. ECM volume is similarly increased in a canine model of atrial tachypacing-induced AF,[101] and ECM-gene upregulation can be shown after 1 week of sustained ATR with a controlled ventricular rate.[74] Qualitatively similar changes occur as early as 24 hours after the onset of atrial tachypacing.[62] In vitro studies suggest that rapidly firing atrial (HL-1) cardiomyocytes secrete factors that alter fibroblast function, decreasing their proliferation but increasing ECM-gene expression.[74]

Remodeling of Ion Channels Involved in Atrial Conduction

Remodeling of Gap Junctions Ventricular expression and function of the major cardiac connexin, connexin43 (Cx43), is altered by structural remodeling, with changes that correlate with proarrhythmic slowing of conduction.[102] Dephosphorylation and redistribution to lateral cell borders are prominent and important.[102,103] Relatively little is known about remodeling of gap junctions in the atria, and results in the literature disagree.[9] The specific alteration might depend on time course and the underlying cardiac pathology.[104] Spatially heterogeneous Cx40 remodeling is observed in the well-controlled goat AF-remodeling system,[105] consistent with the extensive clinical evidence pointing to disturbances in Cx40 as a basis for genetic AF predisposition.[106-108]

Remodeling of Sodium Channels I_{Na} density is reduced in the canine ATR model, with corresponding decreases in channel mRNA and protein expression.[30] Such changes could contribute to the atrial conduction slowing seen in AF. However, Gaborit and colleagues did not find evidence of atrial I_{Na} changes at the genomic level in AF patients.[27]

Molecular Basis of Ectopic Impulse Formation

Ionic Determinants of Ectopic Firing in Conditions That Produce Chronic Atrial Fibrillation

Ectopic firing can be caused by afterdepolarization-induced triggered activity or by enhanced automatic mechanisms. Changes in Ca^{2+} handling (particularly I_{Ca} downregulation) occur in ATR and participate in AF promotion. However, disease-related Ca^{2+}-handling abnormalities also lead to triggered activity and can contribute to both structural remodeling and reentry promotion by favoring alternans behavior. The interplay among these various factors, with altered cellular Ca^{2+} homeostasis as a common underlying theme, is illustrated in Figure 43-4. Defective Ca^{2+} handling has emerged as a potentially important candidate to explain the spontaneous atrial activity, particularly in the pulmonary veins, which underlies AF in many patients.[15] This activity likely involves

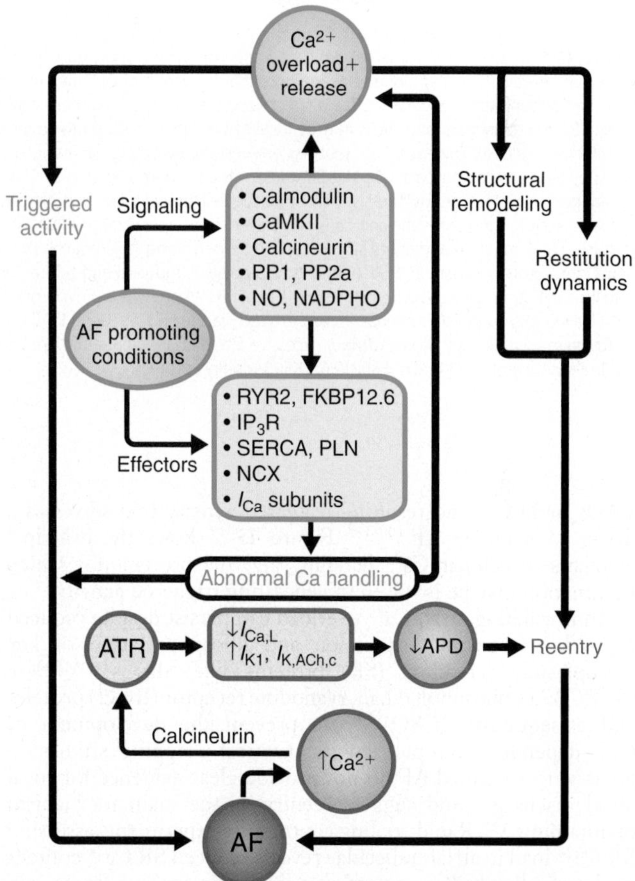

Figure 43-4 Processes related to Ca^{2+} homeostasis abnormalities that participate in promotion of atrial fibrillation. Arrhythmogenic changes in proteins that mediate or target Ca^{2+} handling are indicated in *green*. Processes involved in atrial tachycardia remodeling (ATR), believed to be initiated by Ca^{2+}-loading, are indicated in *red*. AF, atrial fibrillation; APD, action potential duration; CaMKII, Ca^{2+}-dependent protein kinase II; FKBP12.6, FK506 binding protein; I_{Ca}, calcium current; $I_{Ca,L}$, L-type calcium current; $I_{K,ACh,c}$, constitutive acetylcholine-activated potassium current; IP_3R, inositol 1,4,5-trisphosphate receptor; NADPH, nicotinamide adenine dinucleotide phosphate; NCX, Na^+-Ca^{2+}-exchanger; NO, nitric oxide; PLN, phospholamban; PP1, protein phosphatase type 1; PP2a, protein phosphatase type 2A; RYR2, ryanodine receptor; SERCA, sarcoplasmic reticulum-Ca^{2+}-ATPase.

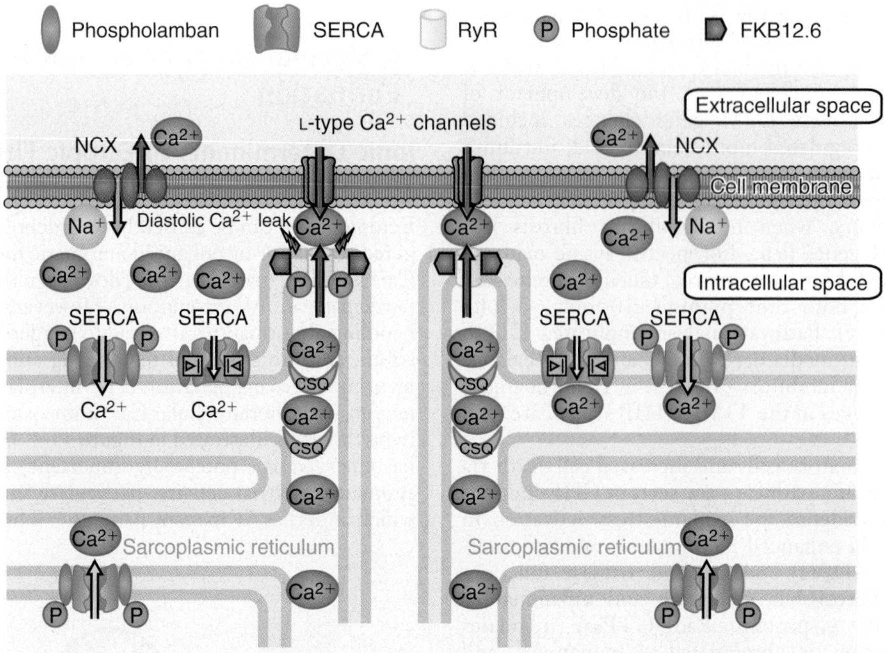

Figure 43-5 A schematic of the cellular Ca^{2+}-handling system, showing the principal factors involved in regulating cytoplasmic Ca^{2+} concentrations over the cardiac cycle. Ca^{2+} enters the cell during the action potential as a result of Ca^{2+} flux through L-type Ca^{2+}-channels ($I_{Ca,L}$). The Ca^{2+} that enters triggers Ca^{2+}-induced Ca^{2+} release from the sarcoplasmic reticulum (SR) via specialized Ca^{2+}-release channels, called ryanodine receptors (RyRs) because they were first identified based on their strong affinity for the toxin ryanodine. RyRs may be localized in close physical proximity to $I_{Ca,L}$s (although less so in the atria than ventricles) to optimize coupling of Ca^{2+} entry with SR Ca^{2+} release. The extra Ca^{2+} that has entered the cytoplasm during electrical systole (the depolarized phase of the action potential) is handled in two principal ways: by active pumping back into the SR via the SR Ca^{2+} pump, known as SR Ca^{2+}-ATPase (or SERCA), and by extrusion across the membrane through the Na^+-Ca^{2+}-exchanger (NCX). NCX brings three Na^+ ions into the cell for every Ca^{2+} ion extruded and therefore carries a net inward (depolarizing) current. When there is diastolic Ca^{2+} excess, the NCX depolarizes the cell, causing delayed afterdepolarizations (DADs). SERCA is regulated by an accessory protein, phospholamban. Phospholamban normally inhibits SERCA function and limits SR Ca^{2+} uptake. When phospholamban is phosphorylated (e.g., by adrenergically stimulated protein kinase A or by Ca^{2+}/calmodulin-dependent protein kinase) its SERCA-inhibitory capacity is reduced and SR Ca^{2+} uptake is enhanced. RyRs also have an accessory protein, known as FKBP12.6. FKBP12.6 stabilizes RyR function and prevents diastolic Ca^{2+}-leak. When RyRs are hyperphosphorylated, FKBP12.6 dissociates from them, promoting diastolic Ca^{2+} leak from the SR. Ca^{2+} leaked out during diastole has to be extruded via the NCX, favoring DAD generation. Calsequestrin (CSQ) is the principal SR Ca^{2+}-binding protein, and it allows the SR to maintain large Ca^{2+} stores without excessive free SR Ca^{2+} concentration. Calsequestrin (CSQ) deficiency renders SR Ca^{2+} handling unstable and promotes abnormal Ca^{2+}-release events and DADs. FKBP12.6, FK506 binding protein.

EADs or DADs and resulting triggered activity that serves as a driver to maintain AF.[109-113] Figure 43-5 shows the principal elements of cellular Ca^{2+} handling and the proteins for which dysfunction may be involved in generating triggered activity.

In fibrillating atria, Ca^{2+} overload can persist despite reduced $I_{Ca,L}$, but preserved expression and phosphorylation of key sarcoplasmic reticulum (SR) proteins like SR-Ca^{2+}-ATPase (SERCA2a), phospholamban, ryanodine receptor (RyR2) protein, and calsequestrin (CSQ)[114] can prevent the development of Ca^{2+}-dependent ectopic activity. Optical mapping studies in goats with sustained AF do not provide clear evidence for focal atrial discharges and suggest reentry as the main mechanism maintaining AF. Rapid cooling contracture experiments assessing SR Ca^{2+} load in atrial trabeculae reveals reduced SR Ca^{2+} content in chronically fibrillating goat atria,[115] consistent with findings in ATR dogs.[10] On the other hand, in dogs and in patients with sustained AF, RYR2 is hyperphosphorylated, causing FKBP12.6 dissociation and increased SR Ca^{2+} leak under diastolic conditions.[26] FKBP12.6-deficient mice show an increased incidence of spontaneous SR Ca^{2+} release events and a greater prevalence of inducible AF.[116] Thus, at late stages of AF progression, diastolic SR Ca^{2+} leak can lead to Ca^{2+}-dependent DADs and triggered activity that might help to maintain AF.

Both reentry and focal-driver mechanisms related to triggered activity appear to underlie CHF-induced AF.[17-19,117] Atrial Ca^{2+} handling is significantly disturbed in myocytes from dogs with CHF. SR Ca^{2+} load and diastolic $[Ca^{2+}]_i$ are substantially increased.[118] These changes predispose to spontaneous Ca^{2+}-release events, DADs, and triggered activity.[118] Although atrial expression of the HCN4 subunit underlying pacemaker current (I_f) increases in CHF,[119] DADs and triggered activity are prevented by blockade of RYR2, but not of I_f, suggesting abnormal SR Ca^{2+}-releases through defective RYR2 channels as the primary underlying mechanism.[118]

In patients with long-term AF and accompanying heart diseases, it is quite possible that the combined influences of atrial tachycardia and heart disease–based remodeling disturb atrial Ca^{2+} handling to produce Ca^{2+}-induced triggered activity and focal sources driving AF,[120] although other evidence points toward reentrant pulmonary vein activity.[121] During Ca^{2+}-overload conditions in vivo, reduced inhibition of SERCA2a by hyperphosphorylated (inactivated) phospholamban[41] helps to maintain a normal SR Ca^{2+} load despite increased spontaneous Ca^{2+}-release events (sparks) and Ca^{2+} waves through potentially leaky (hyperphosphorylated) RYR2 channels.[26,122] Increased spontaneous Ca^{2+}-release and Ca^{2+} waves can induce DADs and triggered activity that induces or maintains

AF. Although it is very possible that Ca^{2+}-dependent focal sources contribute to maintenance of AF,[120] direct experimental proof of the relationship between local Ca^{2+} release events and focal activity in fibrillating atria is lacking.

Molecular Basis of Calcium-Handling Abnormalities and Related Triggered Activity in Atrial Fibrillation

Relatively little is known about upstream signaling mechanisms causing impaired atrial Ca^{2+} handling in AF. The expression levels of calsequestrin, RyR2, and phospholamban appear to be preserved in AF.[26,27,34,41,123] PKA phosphorylation of RyR2 is increased in chronic AF,[26] potentially increasing RyR2-channel Ca^{2+}-release activity and promoting spontaneous diastolic SR Ca^{2+}-release events.[122] Increased Na^+-Ca^{2+}-exchange (NCX1) expression has been noted in some studies,[27,41,123] which would favor accelerated Ca^{2+} removal (preventing Ca^{2+} overload) but at the expense of a larger inward current produced by electrogenic Ca^{2+} extrusion that might generate DADs. PKA- and CaMKII-mediated hyperphosphorylation of phospholamban at Ser16 and Thr17, respectively, together with the reduced abundance of sarcolipin,[41,124] another endogenous SERCA2a inhibitor, might enhance SERCA2a function to compensate for the diastolic SR Ca^{2+} leak through RyR2-channels.

Observations of phospholamban hyperphosphorylation by CaMKII in AF are in agreement with evidence for enhanced CAMKII stimulation at increased heart rates.[125] High stimulation frequencies do not affect PKA phosphorylation at Ser16 of PLB or at Ser2809 of RYR2[125] and β-adrenoceptor density, and G_s protein abundance and adenylyl cyclase activity are preserved in AF.[123] Increased phosphorylation of phospholamban and RyR2 can result from reduced dephosphorylating function of PP1 caused by enhanced activity of the phosphatase inhibitor protein-1 (I-1), a regulator of PP1 activity that functions exclusively in the SR compartment.[126] Ten-fold greater PKA (Thr35)-phosphorylation (activation) of I-1 has been observed in AF[41] and is sufficient to completely suppress SR-bound PP1 activity, substantially increasing phospholamban and RYR2 phosphorylation.[127] The mechanism underlying increased PKA phosphorylation of I-1 in AF is not known. Mice that overexpress the PKA catalytic subunit exhibit hyperphosphorylation of phospholamban and RyR2 and develop AF,[128] supporting the arrhythmogenic potential of hyperphosphorylated phospholamban and RyR2 in AF.

Recent reports have emphasized the importance of inositol 1,4,5-trisphosphate receptor (IP_3R2)-channel-dependent SR Ca^{2+} release in the generation of EADs and DADs in atrial cardiomyocytes.[129,130] IP_3R2 channel protein expression increases in ATR.[131] IP_3Rs co-localize with RYR2[129] and can therefore amplify Ca^{2+}-induced Ca^{2+} release.[132] Abnormal IP_3R2 function might therefore contribute to Ca^{2+} overload and Ca^{2+}-dependent triggered activity in fibrillating atria.

Autonomic Nervous System and Ectopic Activity

Sympathovagal discharge can trigger AF, and experimental evidence points to sources in the pulmonary veins.[111,112,133,134] Autonomic nerve system (ANS) stimulation can promote EADs or DADs and triggered activity by simultaneous prolongation of intracellular Ca^{2+} transients (sympathetic affects) and abbreviation of APD (parasympathetic effect). Although vagal activation generally induces AF by reentrant mechanisms, acetylcholine infusion can also induce late-phase EADs and triggered activity in normal canine atria[110] if acetylcholine-induced APD abbreviation is coupled with increased Ca^{2+} transients (Ca^{2+}-transient triggering). It is presumed that this mechanism involves an increase in $[Ca^{2+}]_i$ during final action potential repolarization at voltages negative to the equilibrium potential for Na^+-Ca^{2+} exchange. This combination of changes is postulated to lead to increased inward Na^+-Ca^{2+}-exchange current that generates EADs and triggered activity.[112,121,133]

Stimuli facilitating SR Ca^{2+} release, such as low ryanodine concentrations, can cause spontaneous Ca^{2+}-release events that facilitate the development of pacemaker activity in rabbit pulmonary veins.[109] In pulmonary vein–left atrium preparations of normal dogs, sympathetic stimulation and low-dose ryanodine infusion have been shown to induce spontaneous cellular Ca^{2+} concentration rises that precede focal-discharge action potential upstrokes during triggered activity,[111] suggesting a primary role of Ca^{2+}-dependent mechanisms. During experimental ANS imbalance in canine pulmonary veins, spontaneous Ca^{2+} release and DADs occur simultaneously after the termination of rapid pacing, suggesting that ANS discharge-mediated pulmonary vein ectopy might also involve DAD-mediated triggered activity.[113] These finding are consistent with the idea that ANS discharge might promote pulmonary vein EAD- and DAD-related ectopic activity that can then initiate or maintain AF. However, the precise role of the pulmonary veins in animal models of AF is unclear, particularly in view of demonstrations that pulmonary vein isolation fails to suppress AF in canine models of vagal-, ATR-, and ASR-related AF.[135,136]

Potential Therapeutic Implications

Extensive evidence indicates the importance of atrial remodeling in the pathophysiology of AF.[9,59] It is therefore logical to investigate the possibility that preventing atrial remodeling may be a useful approach to AF prevention and therapy. There is experimental evidence for the potential value of agents targeting T-type calcium channels, tissue inflammation, and oxidation in the prevention of ATR and for drugs targeting renin-angiotensin-aldosterone, TGF-β, and inflammation or oxidation in the prevention of ASR (for reviews, see Nattel and Carlsson[137] and Burstein and Nattel[70]). Preliminary clinical data have been promising, but definitive assessment of the value of this approach requires detailed prospective clinical trials, some of which are ongoing. The clinical heterogeneity of the AF population, which points to a variety of underlying mechanisms and pathophysiologic bases, will require careful consideration in developing a mechanistically based approach to AF treatment.

Conclusions

Considerable progress has been made in understanding the molecular mechanisms underlying atrial arrhythmogenic remodeling. The resulting insights have provided important new knowledge about the molecular basis of the arrhythmia and have opened the door to potential new treatment approaches. However, much more work needs to be done, particularly in order to understand in more detail the links between pathologic inducers, signaling systems, and arrhythmogenic biophysical consequences. In addition, there is a great need for mechanistic clinical research that will allow the detailed results of experimental studies to be translated into the clinical setting. There is, nevertheless, hope that the recent advances in understanding the molecular pathophysiology of AF-related atrial remodeling will lead to improved management of this challenging arrhythmia.

References

1. Nattel S: New ideas about atrial fibrillation 50 years on. Nature 415:219-226, 2002.
2. Berenfeld O, Zaitsev AV, Mironov SF, et al: Frequency-dependent breakdown of wave propagation into fibrillatory conduction across the pectinate muscle network in the isolated sheep right atrium. Circ Res 90:1173-1180, 2002.
3. Pogwizd SM, Bers DM: Cellular basis of triggered arrhythmias in heart failure. Trends Cardiovasc Med 14:61-66, 2004.
4. Wijffels MC, Kirchhof CJ, Dorland R, et al: Atrial fibrillation begets atrial fibrillation. A study in awake chronically instrumented goats. Circulation 92:1954-1968, 1995.
5. Yue L, Feng J, Gaspo R, et al: Ionic remodeling underlying action potential changes in a canine model of atrial fibrillation. Circ Res 81:512-525, 1997.
6. Ehrlich JR, Cha TJ, Zhang L, et al: Characterization of a hyperpolarization-activated time-dependent potassium current in canine cardiomyocytes from pulmonary vein myocardial sleeves and left atrium. J Physiol 557:583-597, 2004.
7. Dobrev D, Friedrich A, Voigt N, et al: The G-protein gated potassium current $I_{K,ACh}$ is constitutively active in patients with chronic atrial fibrillation. Circulation 112:3697-3706, 2005.
8. Cha TJ, Ehrlich JR, Chartier D, et al: $K_{ir}3$-based inward rectifier potassium current: potential role in atrial tachycardia remodeling effects on atrial repolarization and arrhythmias. Circulation 113:1730-1737, 2006.
9. Nattel S, Maguy A, Le Bouter S, et al: Arrhythmogenic ion-channel remodeling in the heart: Heart failure, myocardial infarction, and atrial fibrillation. Physiol Rev 87:425-456, 2007.
10. Sun H, Gaspo R, Leblanc N, et al: Cellular mechanisms of atrial contractile dysfunction caused by sustained atrial tachycardia. Circulation 98:719-727, 1998.
11. Ehrlich JR, Nattel S, Hohnloser SH: Atrial fibrillation and congestive heart failure: Specific considerations at the intersection of two common and important cardiac disease sets. J Cardiovasc Electrophysiol 13:399-405, 2002.
12. Li D, Fareh S, Leung TK, et al: Promotion of atrial fibrillation by heart failure in dogs: Atrial remodeling of a different sort. Circulation 100:87-95, 1999.
13. Shinagawa K, Shi YF, Tardif JC, et al: Dynamic nature of atrial fibrillation substrate during development and reversal of heart failure in dogs. Circulation 105:2672-2678, 2002.
14. Cha TJ, Ehrlich JR, Zhang L, et al: Dissociation between ionic remodeling and ability to sustain atrial fibrillation during recovery from experimental congestive heart failure. Circulation 109:412-418, 2004.
15. Haïssaguerre M, Jaïs P, Shah DC, et al: Spontaneous initiation of atrial fibrillation by ectopic beats originating in the pulmonary veins. N Engl J Med 339:659-666, 1998.
16. Oral H: Catheter ablation for chronic atrial fibrillation. Heart Rhythm 4:691-694, 2007.
17. Fenelon G, Shepard RK, Stambler BS: Focal origin of atrial tachycardia in dogs with rapid ventricular pacing-induced heart failure. J Cardiovasc Electrophysiol 14:1093-1102, 2003.
18. Ryu K, Shroff SC, Sahadevan J, et al: Mapping of atrial activation during sustained atrial fibrillation in dogs with rapid ventricular pacing induced heart failure: evidence for a role of driver regions. J Cardiovasc Electrophysiol 16:1348-1358, 2005.
19. Stambler BS, Fenelon G, Shepard RK, et al: Characterization of sustained atrial tachycardia in dogs with rapid ventricular pacing-induced heart failure. J Cardiovasc Electrophysiol 14:499-507, 2003.
20. Okuyama Y, Miyauchi Y, Park AM, et al: High resolution mapping of the pulmonary vein and the vein of Marshall during induced atrial fibrillation and atrial tachycardia in a canine model of pacing-induced congestive heart failure. J Am Coll Cardiol 42:348-360, 2003.
21. Zhou S, Chang CM, Wu TJ, et al: Nonreentrant focal activations in pulmonary veins in canine model of sustained atrial fibrillation. Am J Physiol Heart Circ Physiol 283:H1244-H1252, 2002.
22. Sun H, Chartier D, Leblanc N, et al: Intracellular calcium changes and tachycardia-induced contractile dysfunction in canine atrial myocytes. Cardiovasc Res 49:751-761, 2001.
23. Nattel S, Shiroshita-Takeshita A, Brundel BJ, et al: Mechanisms of atrial fibrillation: Lessons from animal models. Prog Cardiovasc Dis 48:9-28, 2005.
24. Brundel BJ, Kampinga HH, Henning RH: Calpain inhibition prevents pacing-induced cellular remodeling in a HL-1 myocyte model for atrial fibrillation. Cardiovasc Res 62:521-528, 2004.
25. Goette A, Arndt M, Rocken C, et al: Calpains and cytokines in fibrillating human atria. Am J Physiol Heart Circ Physiol 283:H264-H272, 2002.
26. Vest JA, Reiken SR, Wehrens XHT, et al: Defective cardiac ryanodine receptor regulation during atrial fibrillation. Circulation 111:2025-2032, 2005.
27. Gaborit N, Steenman M, Lamirault G, et al: Human atrial ion channel and transporter subunit gene-expression remodeling associated with valvular heart disease and atrial fibrillation. Circulation 112:471-481, 2005.
28. Bosch RF, Scherer CR, Rüb N, et al: Molecular mechanisms of early electrical remodeling: Transcriptional downregulation of ion channel subunits reduces $I_{Ca,L}$ and I_{to} in rapid atrial pacing in rabbits. J Am Coll Cardiol 41:858-869, 2003.
29. Kneller J, Sun H, Leblanc N, et al: Remodeling of Ca^{2+}-handling by atrial tachycardia: Evidence for a role in loss of rate-adaptation. Cardiovasc Res 54:416-426, 2002.
30. Yue L, Melnyk P, Gaspo R, et al: Molecular mechanisms underlying ionic remodeling in a dog model of atrial fibrillation. Circ Res 84:776-784, 1999.
31. Brundel BJ, Van Gelder IC, Henning RH, et al: Ion channel remodelling is related to intraoperative atrial effective refractory periods in patients with paroxysmal and persistent atrial fibrillation. Circulation 103:684-690, 2001.
32. Klein G, Schröder F, Vogler D, et al: Increased open probability of single cardiac L-type calcium channels in patients with chronic atrial fibrillation. Role of phosphatase 2A. Cardiovasc Res 59:37-45, 2003.
33. Schotten U, Haase H, Frechen D, et al: The L-type Ca^{2+}-channel subunits α_{1C} and β_2 are not downregulated in atrial myocardium of patients with chronic atrial fibrillation. J Mol Cell Cardiol 35:437-443, 2003.
34. Christ T, Boknik P, Wöhrl S, et al: Reduced L-type Ca^{2+} current density in chronic human atrial fibrillation is associated with increased activity of protein phosphatases. Circulation 110:2651-2657, 2004.
35. Greiser M, Halaszovich CR, Frechen D, et al: Pharmacological evidence for altered Src-kinase regulation of $I_{Ca,L}$ in patients with chronic atrial fibrillation. Naunyn Schmiedebergs Arch Pharmacol 375:383-392, 2007.
36. Verheule S, Sato T, Everett T 4th, et al: Increased vulnerability to atrial fibrillation in transgenic mice with selective atrial fibrosis caused by overexpression of TGF-β1. Circ Res 94:1458-1465, 2004.
37. Avila G, Medina IM, Jiménez E, et al: Transforming growth factor-β1 decreases cardiac muscle L-type Ca^{2+} current and charge movement by acting on the $Ca_V1.2$ mRNA. Am J Physiol Heart Circ Physiol 292:H622-H631, 2007.
38. Chen CL, Lin JL, Lai LP, et al: Altered expression of FHL1, CARP, TSC-22 and P311 provide insights into complex transcriptional regulation in pacing-induced atrial fibrillation. Biochim Biophys Acta 1772:317-329, 2007.
39. Qi XY, Yeh YH, Xiao L, et al: Cellular signalling underlying atrial tachycardia remodeling of L-type calcium-current. Cir Res 103:845-854, 2008.
40. Brundel BJ, Ausma J, Van Gelder IC, et al: Activation of proteolysis by calpains and structural changes in human paroxysmal and persistent atrial fibrillation. Cardiovasc Res 54:380-389, 2002.
41. El-Armouche A, Boknik P, Eschenhagen T, et al: Molecular determinants of altered Ca^{2+} handling in human chronic atrial fibrillation. Circulation 114:670-680, 2006.
42. Shiroshita-Takeshita A, Schram G, Lavoie J, et al: Effect of simvastatin and antioxidant vitamins on atrial fibrillation promotion by atrial-tachycardia remodeling in dogs. Circulation 110:2313-2319, 2004.
43. Carnes CA, Janssen PM, Ruehr ML, et al: Atrial glutathione content, calcium current,

and contractility. J Biol Chem 282:28063-28073, 2007.
44. Beharier O, Etzion Y, Katz A, et al: Crosstalk between L-type calcium channels and ZnT-1, a new player in rate-dependent cardiac electrical remodeling. Cell Calcium 42:71-82, 2007.
45. Etzion Y, Ganiel A, Beharier O, et al: Correlation between atrial ZnT-1 expression and atrial fibrillation in humans: A pilot study. J Cardiovasc Electrophysiol 19(2):157-164, 2008.
46. Dobrev D, Graf E, Wettwer E, et al: Molecular basis of down-regulation of G-protein–coupled inward rectifying K^+ current ($I_{K,ACh}$) in chronic human atrial fibrillation. Decrease in GIRK4 mRNA correlates with reduced $I_{K,ACh}$ and muscarinic receptor–mediated shortening of action potentials. Circulation 104:2551-2557, 2001.
47. Dobrev D, Wettwer E, Kortner A, et al: Human inward rectifier potassium channels in chronic and postoperative atrial fibrillation. Cardiovasc Res 54:397-404, 2002.
48. Voigt N, Friedrich A, Bock M, et al: Differential phosphorylation-dependent regulation of constitutively active and muscarinic receptor–activated $I_{K,ACh}$ channels in patients with chronic atrial fibrillation. Cardiovasc Res 74:426-437, 2007.
49. Cha TJ, Ehrlich JR, Zhang L, et al: Tachycardia remodeling of pulmonary vein cardiomyocytes: Comparison with left atrium and potential relation to arrhythmogenesis. Circulation 111:728-735, 2005.
50. Karle CA, Zitron E, Zhang W, et al: Human cardiac inwardly-rectifying K^+ channel $K_{ir}2.1b$ is inhibited by direct protein kinase C-dependent regulation in human isolated cardiomyocytes and in an expression system. Circulation 106:1493-1499, 2002.
51. Kneller J, Zou R, Vigmond EJ, et al: Cholinergic atrial fibrillation in a computer model of a two-dimensional sheet of canine atrial cells with realistic ionic properties. Circ Res 90:E73-E87, 2002.
52. Yeh Y-H, Lemola K, Nattel S: Vagal atrial fibrillation. Acta Cardiol Sin 23:1-12, 2007.
53. Kovoor P, Wickman K, Maguire CT, et al: Evaluation of the role of I_{KACh} in atrial fibrillation using a mouse knockout model. J Am Coll Cardiol 37:2136-2143, 2001.
54. Voigt N, Maguy A, Yeh YH, et al: Changes in $I_{K,ACh}$ single channel activity with atrial tachycardia remodeling in canine atrial cardiomyocytes. Cardiovasc Res 77(1):35-43, 2008.
55. Brundel BJ, Van Gelder IC, Henning RH, et al: Alterations in potassium channel gene expression in atria of patients with persistent and paroxysmal atrial fibrillation: differential regulation of protein and mRNA levels for K^+ channels. J Am Coll Cardiol 37:926-932, 2001.
56. Nikolov EN, Ivanova-Nikolova TT: Coordination of membrane excitability through a GIRK1 signaling complex in the atria. J Biol Chem 279:23630-23636, 2004.
57. Wu G, Huang CX, Tang YH, et al: Changes of $I_{K,ATP}$ current density and allosteric modulation during chronic atrial fibrillation. Chin Med J 118:1161-1166, 2005.
58. Balana B, Dobrev D, Wettwer E, et al: Decreased ATP-sensitive K^+ current density during chronic human atrial fibrillation. J Mol Cell Cardiol 35:1399-1405, 2003.
59. Dobrev D, Ravens U: Remodeling of cardiomyocyte ion channels in human atrial fibrillation. Basic Res Cardiol 98:137-148, 2003.
60. Ceulemans H, Bollen M: Functional diversity of protein phosphatase-1, a cellular economizer and reset button. Physiol Rev 84:1-39, 2004.
61. Barth AS, Merk S, Arnoldi E, et al: Reprogramming of the human atrial transcriptome in permanent atrial fibrillation: Expression of a ventricular-like genomic signature. Circ Res 96:1022-1029, 2005.
62. Cardin S, Libby E, Pelletier P, et al: Contrasting gene expression profiles in two canine models of atrial fibrillation. Circ Res 100:425-433, 2007.
63. Rossow CF, Dilly KW, Santana LF: Differential calcineurin/*NFATc3* activity contributes to the I_{to} transmural gradient in the mouse heart. Circ Res 98:1306-1313, 2006.
64. Bukowska A, Lendeckel U, Hirte D, et al: Activation of the calcineurin signaling pathway induces atrial hypertrophy during atrial fibrillation. Cell Mol Life Sci 63:333-342, 2006.
65. Courtemanche M, Ramirez RJ, Nattel S: Ionic targets for drug therapy and atrial fibrillation-induced electrical remodeling: Insights from a mathematical model. Cardiovasc Res 42:477-489, 1999.
66. Wettwer E, Hála O, Christ T, et al: Role of I_{Kur} in controlling action potential shape and contractility in the human atrium: Influence of chronic atrial fibrillation. Circulation 110:2299-2306, 2004.
67. Kim YM, Guzik TJ, Zhang YH, et al: A myocardial Nox2 containing NAD(P)H oxidase contributes to oxidative stress in human atrial fibrillation. Circ Res 97:629-636, 2005.
68. Dudley SC Jr, Hoch NE, McCann LA, et al: Atrial fibrillation increases production of superoxide by the left atrium and left atrial appendage: Role of the NADPH and xanthine oxidases. Circulation 112:1266-1273, 2005.
69. Núnez L, Vaquero M, Gómez R, et al: Nitric oxide blocks $hK_V1.5$ channels by S-nitrosylation and by a cyclic GMP-dependent mechanism. Cardiovasc Res 72: 80-89, 2006.
70. Burstein B, Nattel S: Atrial fibrosis: Mechanisms and clinical relevance for atrial fibrillation. J Am Coll Cardiol 51(8):802-809, 2008.
71. Katz AM: Proliferative signaling and disease progression in heart failure. Circ J 66:225-231, 2002.
72. Aharinejad S, Krenn K, Paulus P, et al: Differential role of TGF-β_1/bFGF and ET-1 in graft fibrosis in heart failure patients. Am J Transplant 5:2185-2192, 2005.
73. Xiao HD, Fuchs S, Campbell DJ, et al: Mice with cardiac-restricted angiotensin-converting enzyme (ACE) have atrial enlargement, cardiac arrhythmia, and sudden death. Am J Pathol 165:1019-1032, 2004.
74. Burstein B, Qi XY, Yeh YH, et al: Atrial cardiomyocyte tachycardia alters cardiac fibroblast function: A novel consideration in atrial remodeling. Cardiovasc Res 76: 442-452, 2007.
75. Hunyady L, Catt KJ: Pleiotropic AT1 receptor signaling pathways mediating physiological and pathogenic actions of angiotensin II. Mol Endocrinol 20:953-970, 2006.
76. Rosenkranz S: TGF-β1 and angiotensin networking in cardiac remodeling. Cardiovasc Res 63:423-432, 2004.
77. Chen MM, Lam A, Abraham JA, et al: CTGF expression is induced by TGF-β in cardiac fibroblasts and cardiac myocytes: A potential role in heart fibrosis. J Mol Cell Cardiol 32:1805-1819, 2000.
78. Attisano L, Wrana JL: Signal transduction by the TGF-β superfamily. Science 296:1646-1647, 2002.
79. Leask A, Abraham DJ: TGF-β signaling and the fibrotic response. FASEB J 18:816-827, 2004.
80. Bonner JC: Regulation of PDGF and its receptors in fibrotic diseases. Cytokine Growth Factor Rev 15:255-273, 2004.
81. Ponten A, Li X, Thoren P, et al: Transgenic overexpression of platelet-derived growth factor–C in the mouse heart induces cardiac fibrosis, hypertrophy, and dilated cardiomyopathy. Am J Pathol 163:673-682, 2003.
82. Ponten A, Folestad EB, Pietras K, et al: Platelet-derived growth factor D induces cardiac fibrosis and proliferation of vascular smooth muscle cells in heart-specific transgenic mice. Circ Res 97:1036-1045, 2005.
83. Leask A, Abraham DJ: The role of connective tissue growth factor, a multifunctional matricellular protein, in fibroblast biology. Biochem Cell Biol 81:355-363, 2003.
84. Chuva de Sousa Lopes SM, Feijen A, Korving J, et al: Connective tissue growth factor expression and Smad signaling during mouse heart development and myocardial infarction. Dev Dyn 231:542-550, 2004.
85. Ahmed MS, Oie E, Vinge LE, et al: Connective tissue growth factor—a novel mediator of angiotensin II–stimulated cardiac fibroblast activation in heart failure in rats. J Mol Cell Cardiol 36:393-404, 2004.
86. Iwanciw D, Rehm M, Porst M, et al: Induction of connective tissue growth factor by angiotensin II: Integration of signaling pathways. Arterioscler Thromb Vasc Biol 23:1782-1787, 2003.
87. Crean JK, Finlay D, Murphy M, et al: The role of p42/44 MAPK and protein kinase B in connective tissue growth factor induced extracellular matrix protein production, cell migration, and actin cytoskeletal rearrangement in human mesangial cells. J Biol Chem 277:44187-44194, 2002.
88. Cardin S, Li D, Thorin-Trescases N, et al: Evolution of the atrial fibrillation substrate in experimental congestive heart failure: Angiotensin-dependent and -independent

pathways. Cardiovasc Res 60:315-325, 2003.
89. Li D, Shinagawa K, Pang L, et al: Effects of angiotensin-converting enzyme inhibition on the development of the atrial fibrillation substrate in dogs with ventricular tachypacing-induced congestive heart failure. Circulation 104:2608-2614, 2001.
90. Kumagai K, Nakashima H, Urata H, et al: Effects of angiotensin II type 1 receptor antagonist on electrical and structural remodeling in atrial fibrillation. J Am Coll Cardiol 41:2197-2204, 2003.
91. Shroff SC, Ryu K, Martovitz NL, et al: Selective aldosterone blockade suppresses atrial tachyarrhythmias in heart failure. J Cardiovasc Electrophysiol 17:534-541, 2006.
92. Hanna N, Cardin S, Leung TK, et al: Differences in atrial versus ventricular remodeling in dogs with ventricular tachypacing-induced congestive heart failure. Cardiovasc Res 63:236-244, 2004.
93. Lee KW, Everett TH, Rahmutula D, et al: Pirfenidone prevents the development of a vulnerable substrate for atrial fibrillation in a canine model of heart failure. Circulation 114:1703-1712, 2006.
94. Nakano Y, Niida S, Dote K, et al: Matrix metalloproteinase-9 contributes to human atrial remodeling during atrial fibrillation. J Am Coll Cardiol 43:818-825, 2004.
95. Mukherjee R, Herron AR, Lowry AS, et al: Selective induction of matrix metalloproteinases and tissue inhibitor of metalloproteinases in atrial and ventricular myocardium in patients with atrial fibrillation. Am J Cardiol 97:532-537, 2006.
96. Cai H, Li Z, Goette A, et al: Downregulation of endocardial nitric oxide synthase expression and nitric oxide production in atrial fibrillation: Potential mechanisms for atrial thrombosis and stroke. Circulation 106:2854-2858, 2002.
97. Adam O, Frost G, Custodis F, et al: Role of Rac1 GTPase activation in atrial fibrillation. J Am Coll Cardiol 50:359-367, 2007.
98. Shiroshita-Takeshita A, Brundel BJ, Burstein B, et al: Effects of simvastatin on the development of the atrial fibrillation substrate in dogs with congestive heart failure. Cardiovasc Res 74:75-84, 2007.
99. Lin CS, Lai LP, Lin JL, et al: Increased expression of extracellular matrix proteins in rapid atrial pacing–induced atrial fibrillation. Heart Rhythm 4:938-949, 2007.
100. Pan CH, Lin JL, Lai LP, et al: Downregulation of angiotensin converting enzyme II is associated with pacing-induced sustained atrial fibrillation. FEBS Lett 581:526-534, 2007.
101. Chiu YT, Wu TJ, Wei HJ, et al: Increased extracellular collagen matrix in myocardial sleeves of pulmonary veins: An additional mechanism facilitating repetitive rapid activities in chronic pacing–induced sustained atrial fibrillation. J Cardiovasc Electrophysiol 16:753-759, 2005.
102. Akar FG, Spragg DD, Tunin RS, et al: Mechanisms underlying conduction slowing and arrhythmogenesis in nonischemic dilated cardiomyopathy. Circ Res 95:717-725, 2004.
103. Akar FG, Nass RD, Hahn S, et al: Dynamic changes in conduction velocity and gap junction properties during development of pacing induced heart failure. Am J Physiol Heart Circ Physiol 293:H1223-H1230, 2007.
104. Wetzel U, Boldt A, Lauschke J, et al: Expression of connexins 40 and 43 in human left atrium in atrial fibrillation of different aetiologies. Heart 91:166-170, 2005.
105. Ausma J, van der Velden HM, Lenders MH, et al: Reverse structural and gap-junctional remodeling after prolonged atrial fibrillation in the goat. Circulation 107:2051-2058, 2003.
106. Firouzi M, Ramanna H, Kok B, et al: Association of human connexin40 gene polymorphisms with atrial vulnerability as a risk factor for idiopathic atrial fibrillation. Circ Res 95:e29-e33, 2004.
107. Juang JM, Chern YR, Tsai CT, et al: The association of human connexin 40 genetic polymorphisms with atrial fibrillation. Int J Cardiol 116:107-112, 2007.
108. Gollob MH, Jones DL, Krahn AD, et al: Somatic mutations in the connexin 40 gene (*GJA5*) in atrial fibrillation. N Engl J Med 354:2677-2688, 2006.
109. Honjo H, Boyett MR, Niwa R, et al: Pacing-induced spontaneous activity in myocardial sleeves of pulmonary veins after treatment with ryanodine. Circulation 107:1937-4193, 2003.
110. Burashnikov A, Antzelevitch C: Reinduction of atrial fibrillation immediately after termination of the arrhythmia is mediated by late phase 3 early afterdepolarization–induced triggered activity. Circulation 107:2355-2360, 2003.
111. Chou CC, Nihei M, Zhou S, et al: Intracellular calcium dynamics and anisotropic reentry in isolated canine pulmonary veins and left atrium. Circulation 111:2889-2897, 2005.
112. Patterson E, Lazzara R, Szabo B, et al: Sodium-calcium exchange initiated by the Ca^{2+} transient: An arrhythmia trigger within pulmonary veins. J Am Coll Cardiol 47:1196-1206, 2006.
113. Hirose M, Laurita KR: Calcium-mediated triggered activity is an underlying cellular mechanism of ectopy originating from the pulmonary vein in dogs. Am J Physiol Heart Circ Physiol 292:H1861-H1867, 2007.
114. Wakili R, Yeh HY, Kääb S, et al: Molecular determinants of defective calcium handling in atrial tachycardia and congestive heart failure models of atrial fibrillation. Heart Rhythm 4:155 (abstract PO2-40), 2007.
115. Greiser M, Neuberger HR, Harks E, et al: Molecular determinants of Ca^{2+}-handling abnormalities underlying contractile dysfunction in dilated versus fibrillating goat atria. Circulation 116(Suppl II):II-84-II-85, 2007.
116. Sood S, Ghelu MG, Santonastasi M, et al: Increased sarcoplasmic reticulum calcium leak in FKBP12.6 mice associated with atrial fibrillation. Circulation 116 (Suppl II):II-276, 2007.
117. Tanaka K, Zlochiver S, Vikstrom KL, et al: Spatial distribution of fibrosis governs fibrillation wave dynamics in the posterior left atrium during heart failure. Circ Res 101:839-847, 2007.
118. Yeh Y-H, Wakili R, Qi XY, et al: Calcium handling abnormalities underlying atrial arrhythmogenesis and contractile dysfunction in dogs with congestive heart failure. Circulation: Arrhythmia and Electrophysiology 1:93-102, 2008.
119. Zicha S, Fernández-Velasco M, Lonardo G, et al: Sinus node dysfunction and hyperpolarization-activated (HCN) channel subunit remodeling in a canine heart failure model. Cardiovasc Res 66:472-481, 2005.
120. Patterson E, Jackman WM, Beckman KJ, et al: Spontaneous pulmonary vein firing in man: Relationship to tachycardia-pause early afterdepolarizations and triggered arrhythmia in canine pulmonary veins in vitro. J Cardiovasc Electrophysiol 18:1067-1075, 2007.
121. Atienza F, Almendral J, Moreno J, et al: Activation of inward rectifier potassium channels accelerates atrial fibrillation in humans: evidence for a reentrant mechanism. Circulation 114:2434-2442, 2006.
122. Hove-Madsen L, Llach A, Bayes-Genís A, et al: Atrial fibrillation is associated with increased spontaneous calcium release from the sarcoplasmic reticulum in human atrial myocytes. Circulation 110:1358-1363, 2004.
123. Schotten U, Greiser M, Benke D, et al: Atrial fibrillation–induced atrial contractile dysfunction: A tachycardiomyopathy of a different sort. Cardiovasc Res 53:192-201, 2002.
124. Uemura N, Ohkusa T, Hamano K, et al: Down-regulation of sarcolipin mRNA expression in chronic atrial fibrillation. Eur J Clin Invest 34:723-730, 2004.
125. Wehrens XH, Lehnart SE, Reiken SR, et al: Ca^{2+}/calmodulin–dependent protein kinase II phosphorylation regulates the cardiac ryanodine receptor. Circ Res 94:e61-e370, 2004.
126. Pathak A, del Monte F, Zhao W, et al: Enhancement of cardiac function and suppression of heart failure progression by inhibition of protein phosphatase 1. Circ Res 96:756-766, 2005.
127. Herzig S, Neumann J: Effects of serine/threonine protein phosphatases on ion channels in excitable membranes. Physiol Rev 80:173-210, 2000.
128. Antos CL, Fey N, Marx SO, et al: Dilated cardiomyopathy and sudden death resulting from constitutive activation of protein kinase A. Circ Res 89:997-1004, 2001.
129. Mackenzie L, Bootman MD, Laine M, et al: The role of inositol 1,4,5-trisphosphate receptors in Ca^{2+} signalling and the generation of arrhythmias in rat atrial myocytes. J Physiol 541:395-409, 2002.
130. Li X, Zima AV, Sheikh F, et al: Endothelin-1-induced arrhythmogenic Ca^{2+} signaling is abolished in atrial myocytes of inositol-1,4,5-trisphosphate (IP3)-receptor type 2–deficient mice. Circ Res 96:1274-1281, 2005.

131. Zhao ZH, Zhang HC, Xu Y, et al: Inositol-1,4,5-trisphosphate and ryanodine-dependent Ca^{2+} signaling in a chronic dog model of atrial fibrillation. Cardiology 107:269-276, 2007.
132. Zima AV, Blatter LA: Inositol-1,4,5-trisphosphate–dependent Ca^{2+} signalling in cat atrial excitation-contraction coupling and arrhythmias. J Physiol 555:607-615, 2004.
133. Patterson E, Po SS, Scherlag BJ, et al: Triggered firing in pulmonary veins initiated by in vitro autonomic nerve stimulation. Heart Rhythm 2:624-631, 2005.
134. Ogawa M, Zhou S, Tan AY, et al: Left stellate ganglion and vagal nerve activity and cardiac arrhythmias in ambulatory dogs with pacing-induced congestive heart failure. J Am Coll Cardiol 50:335-343, 2007.
135. Lemola K, Chartier D, Yeh YH, et al: Pulmonary vein region ablation in experimental vagal atrial fibrillation: Role of pulmonary veins versus autonomic ganglia. Circulation 117(4):470-477, 2008.
136. Sakabe M, Lemola K, Chiba K, et al: Role of the pulmonary veins in experimental paradigms of remodeling-associated atrial fibrillation. Circulation 116(Suppl II): II-139, 2007.
137. Nattel S, Carlsson L: Innovative approaches to anti-arrhythmic drug therapy. Nat Rev Drug Discov 5:1034-1149, 2006.

Noninvasive Electrocardiographic Imaging: Methodology and Excitation of the Normal Human Heart 44

YORAM RUDY, CHARULATHA RAMANATHAN, AND SUBHAM GHOSH

CHAPTER OUTLINE

Despite the reliance of modern medicine on noninvasive imaging modalities such as computed tomography (CT), magnetic resonance imaging (MRI), and ultrasound for diagnosis and guidance of therapy, an equivalent noninvasive modality for imaging cardiac electrophysiology (EP) and arrhythmias is not yet available in clinical practice. Noninvasive diagnosis of arrhythmias is still based on the standard electrocardiogram (ECG), which records electrical activity from only a few sites on the body surface, far away from the heart. The ECG has been a most useful clinical tool over more than 100 years. However, by measuring the reflection of cardiac electrical activity at only few locations remote from the heart it lacks specificity (can fail to classify the arrhythmia or determine its location) and sensitivity (can fail to detect abnormal electrophysiologic substrate or abnormal cardiac activity). It is clear that a noninvasive imaging modality for cardiac arrhythmias that can reconstruct details of the excitatory process on the heart itself is much needed. It could be used not only for clinical diagnosis and treatment but also as a research tool for studying the properties and mechanisms of arrhythmias in humans, where the EP substrate can be very different from that in animal models.

Computation of cardiac electrical activity from body-surface potential measurements constitutes the "inverse problem of electrocardiography."[1] Several mathematical and computational approaches have been introduced to solve this problem. Some approaches have used bidomain models or uniform dipole-layer models to compute activation times (isochrones) in the heart.[2-4] Another approach computes potentials on the epicardial surface of the heart,[1, 5-7] from which epicardial electrograms (potential over time at a given epicardial site), activation isochrones, and repolarization patterns can be constructed.

In this chapter we describe the latter, potential-based approach and its implementation in a novel noninvasive imaging modality for cardiac electrophysiology and arrhythmia called *electrocardiographic imaging* (ECGI). We also provide ECGI images of activation and repolarization of the normal intact human heart under complete physiologic conditions.

Yoram Rudy chairs the scientific advisory board and holds equity in CardioInsight Technologies (CIT). CIT does not support any research conducted by Yoram Rudy, including that presented here. Charulatha Ramanathan is an equity holder and a paid employee of CIT. Studies presented in this chapter were supported by NIH-NHLBI Merit Award R37-HL-33343 and Grant R01-HL-49054 to Yoram Rudy.

Application of ECGI in the clinical setting to image abnormal cardiac activity is described in Chapter 89.

Electrocardiographic Imaging Methodology

The physical basis for ECGI is the property that the electric potential field, ϕ, generated by cardiac excitation in the passive (source-free) torso volume conductor (between the epicardium and the body surface) obeys Laplace's equation:

$$\nabla^2\phi = 0 \quad [1]$$

subject to the following boundary conditions on the torso surface:

$$\frac{\partial\phi}{\partial n} = 0 \quad [2]$$

where n is normal to the surface; this condition states that no current can leave the torso into the surrounding air, an insulating medium that cannot support current flow; and

$$\phi = \phi_T \quad [3]$$

where ϕ_T is the known (recorded) electrocardiographic potential distribution on the body surface. This mathematical formulation is known as a *Cauchy problem*. ECGI seeks to compute ϕ on the epicardial surface of the heart, ϕ_E, from the measured ϕ_T on the body surface.

Because the heart and torso surfaces are irregular, the problem must be solved numerically. The first step in this procedure is the discretization of the relationship between the epicardial potentials and the torso surface potentials. We have employed two methods to discretize the problem: the boundary element method (BEM)[1] and the method of fundamental solutions (MFS).[8]

BEM is derived from Green's second theorem,[1] which relates the potential in a volume to the potential on its bounding surfaces:

$$\int_v \left[\phi\nabla^2\left[\frac{1}{r}\right] - \frac{1}{r}\nabla^2\phi\right]dv = \int_s \left[\phi\frac{\partial(\frac{1}{r})}{\partial n} - \frac{1}{r}\frac{\partial\phi}{\partial n}\right]ds \quad [4]$$

where the surface S includes the epicardial surface S_E and the torso surface S_T, and V is the torso volume enclosed by these surfaces; r is the Euclidian distance in three-dimensional space.

Manipulation of equation (4) considering that $\nabla^2\phi = 0$ in V, and discretization of S_E and S_T into triangular elements, leads to the following matrix equation relating ϕ_T to ϕ_E:

$$\phi_T = A\phi_E \quad [5]$$

where ϕ_T is a vector of torso potentials and ϕ_E is a vector of epicardial potentials. A is a transfer matrix that contains the geometric relationship between the heart surface and torso surface.

The potential over each triangular element can be assumed to be constant or to vary as a linear or higher-order function of the intrinsic element coordinates.

MFS is a meshless method that does not require meshing (discretizing) the heart and torso surfaces, as required by BEM. This provides several advantages: The application is faster, because the meshing and mesh-optimization procedures are time consuming and constitute the time-limiting step in ECGI; there is no need for mesh-optimization (a procedure requiring manual editing), which enhances automation of ECGI in the clinical application; mesh-induced artifacts are eliminated, especially for complex geometries such as the atria; complex singular integrals are eliminated. It was shown[8] that BEM and MFS achieve similar accuracy in ECGI computations. In MFS, an approximate solution to the Cauchy problem is represented as a linear superposition of source functions located on auxiliary surfaces that enclose the heart and torso surfaces. Because these virtual (fictitious) sources are placed outside the torso volume, this representation satisfies Laplace's equation (equation [1]) in this (source-free) volume. In addition, the boundary conditions (equations [2] and [3]) are imposed on a set of collocation points on the actual torso surface. MFS is then applied to express each boundary condition as a discrete summation over the virtual source points on the fictitious auxiliary surface.

Equation (5) can be used to compute ϕ_T from a known ϕ_E in a given heart-torso geometry (provided by matrix A). This formulation constitutes the forward problem of electrocardiography. The objective of ECGI is to compute ϕ_E from a known ϕ_T, a formulation that constitutes the inverse problem. This problem is ill posed in the sense that even low-level noise in the measured data (torso potentials) can cause unbounded errors in the solution (epicardial potentials). In equation (5), this property makes A an ill-conditioned matrix, which prevents direct inversion of A to compute ϕ_E from ϕ_T. To overcome this difficulty, we have applied two different computational schemes in the ECGI application: Tikhonov regularization (TR)[1] and the generalized minimal residual (GMRes) method.[9]

TR stabilizes the computation by imposing constraints on the solution through the following objective function:

$$\min_{\phi_E} \left[\|\phi_T - A\phi_E\|^2 + t\|R\phi_E\|^2 \right] \qquad [6]$$

By minimizing this function with respect to ϕ_E, one finds the ϕ_E that best approximates (in the least-square sense) a solution to equation (5) subject to a given constraint. The first term in equation (6) represents the solution, and the second term is the regularization term that imposes bounds on ϕ_E (for R = I, the unit matrix), its steepness (for R = G, the surface gradient operator), or its curvature (for R = L, the surface Laplacian operator); *t* is a regularization parameter that controls the weight of the imposed constraint.

The GMRes method is an iterative scheme that does not apply constraints. As such it is an independent approach, unrelated to TR. It does not require a priori knowledge of solution properties for imposing appropriate constraints, nor does it involve determination of an optimal regularization parameter as required in TR. Application of the GMRes method to ECGI has been formulated and evaluated by Ramanathan and colleagues.[9] Overall, the accuracy of the GMRes and TR ECGI solutions is very similar, although in certain cases GMRes reconstructed localized epicardial potential features (e.g., multiple potential minima) that were lost in TR reconstructions due to the smoothing effect of the imposed constraint. The complementary application of these two independent methods in clinical ECGI ensures reliability and maximal extraction of diagnostic information even in the absence of a priori information about a patient's condition.

Equation (6) computes ϕ_E from ϕ_T at one time instant during the cardiac cycle. By repeating the computation at a given time interval (typically every millisecond), the entire set of epicardial potential maps during the cardiac cycle (or many consecutive cycles) is obtained. From this set of epicardial maps, one can construct an electrogram (potential as function of time) at any given epicardial point (we typically compute 600 epicardial electrograms). Once electrograms are constructed, activation time at each epicardial site is determined as the time of maximum negative derivative on the electrogram. Isochrone maps showing the sequence of epicardial activation are constructed by connecting all sites with the same activation time. Repolarization time is determined as the time of maximum derivative on the electrogram T wave. Activation recovery intervals are computed by subtracting the activation time from the recovery time at each epicardial site; activation recovery interval was shown to be a surrogate of the local action potential duration (APD).[10]

The A matrix in equations (5) and (6) provides the geometric relationship between the heart surface and the torso surface. It can be readily expanded to include other torso compartments such as the lungs, spine, or skeletal muscle. A previous study[10a] showed that exclusion of these compartments from the computation does not cause significant deterioration of accuracy. Importantly, epicardial potential patterns, electrograms, and isochrones and locations of pacing sites were reconstructed with comparable accuracy when the torso was approximated as a homogeneous volume. This property simplifies the clinical application of ECGI.

ECGI requires two sets of data: electrocardiographic potentials over the entire torso (ϕ_T in equations [5] and [6]) and the geometric relationship between the heart and torso surfaces (matrix A in equations [5] and [6]). The torso electrocardiographic data are recorded using a computerized mapping system with either 224 Ag/AgCl body-surface electrodes embedded in a vest or 250 conductive carbon electrodes organized in strips (the carbon electrodes are x-ray transparent and do not interfere with fluoroscopy when ECGI is conducted interactively in the EP laboratory). The geometric information is obtained using CT with scans usually set to axial resolution between 0.6 and 1 mm and gated to the ECG. From the transverse slices, the geometry of the heart and torso surfaces is assembled in a common coordinate system to provide the A matrix. Figure 44-1 shows a schematic description of the ECGI procedure.[11]

Activation and Repolarization of the Normal Human Heart

Our knowledge of normal human cardiac electrical excitation is derived from invasive intraoperative epicardial mapping[12] and from studies of isolated human hearts.[13] These studies were conducted under nonphysiologic conditions (e.g., effects of isolation and absence of neural inputs and mechanical loading in isolated hearts; anesthesia effects and heart exposure during intraoperative mapping). Knowledge of normal excitation provides a necessary baseline for understanding abnormal cardiac activity and arrhythmia. In this section we describe normal activation and repolarization of the human heart based on in vivo noninvasive ECGI images from seven (four male and three female) healthy adults under complete physiologic conditions.[14]

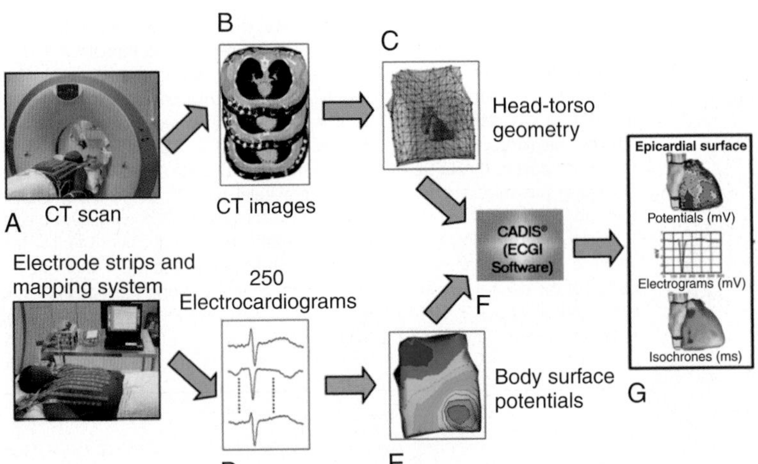

Figure 44-1 Block diagram of the electrocardiographic imaging (ECGI) procedure. **A,** Multielectrode (224 or 250) mapping system is used to obtain electrocardiograms over the entire torso surface *(bottom)*. Computed tomography (CT) scan, conducted during application of the electrodes, provides the heart-torso geometrical relationship *(top)*. **B,** Transverse CT slices showing the epicardial contour *(red)* and torso electrodes *(shiny dots)*. **C,** Three-dimensional heart-torso geometry constructed from the CT slices. **D,** Sample ECG signals from the mapping system. **E,** Body surface potential map obtained from the ECGs in **D** for one instance during the cardiac cycle. **F,** ECGI software package reconstructs epicardial data from the data in **C** and **E. G,** Examples of noninvasive ECGI images, including (top to bottom) epicardial potentials, electrograms, and isochrones. (Adapted by permission from Macmillan Publishers, Ltd. From Ramanathan C, Ghanem RN, Jia P, et al: Noninvasive electrocardiographic imaging for cardiac electrophysiology and arrhythmia. Nat Med 10(4):422-428, 2004.)

Atrial Activation

ECGI imaged atrial activation sequences (isochrones) from two hearts are shown in Figure 44-2, bottom panels. Earliest activation (dark red) starts in the right atrium (RA) near the attachment of the superior vena cava, at the anatomic location of the sinoatrial (SA) node where the impulse originates. It then propagates radially to the rest of the RA and the left atrium (LA). The LA appendage is the last area to activate. This noninvasively imaged sequence is consistent with isochrones recorded directly from isolated human hearts (see Fig. 44-2, top panel). Note that the anatomic location of impulse generation (earliest activation, dark red) varies between the two hearts in Figure 44-2, bottom; in the left panel the earliest activation occurs inferior to that in the right panel. This observation is consistent with the complex spatial organization of the SA node, which extends inferiorly towards the atrioventricular (AV) node.

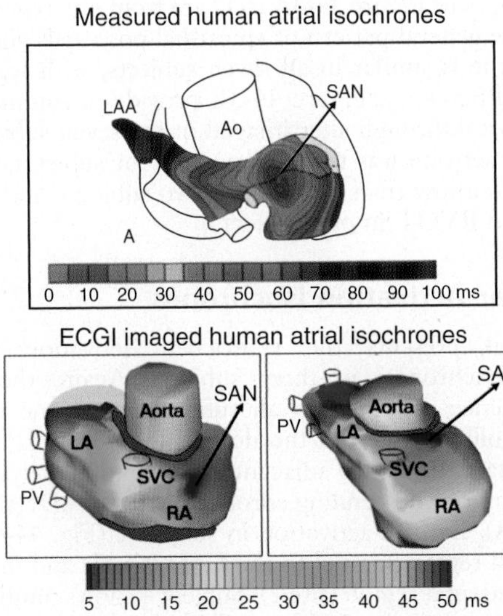

Figure 44-2 Isochrones for normal atrial activation. *Top*, Isochrones recorded directly from an isolated human heart (from Durrer D, van Dam RT, Freud GE, et al: Total excitation of the isolated human heart. Circulation 41:899-912, 1970, with permission). *Bottom*, Noninvasively imaged atrial isochrones in two hearts using electrocardiographic imaging (ECGI). (Adapted by permission from Macmillan Publishers, Ltd. Compiled from Ramanathan C, Ghanem RN, Jia P, et al: Noninvasive electrocardiographic imaging for cardiac electrophysiology and arrhythmia. Nat Med 10(4):422-428, 2004; and Ramanathan C, Jia P, Ghanem RN, et al: Activation and repolarization of the normal human heart under complete physiological conditions. Proc Natl Acad Sci U S A 103(16):6309-6314, 2006, with permission. Copyright 2006 National Academy of Sciences, U.S.A.). SAN, sinoatrial node; RA, right atrium; LA, left atrium; LAA, left atrial appendage; SVC, superior vena cava; Ao, aorta; PV, pulmonary veins.

Ventricular Activation

Following conduction through the AV node and left and right bundle branches of the specialized conduction system, the cardiac impulse establishes broad activation fronts that propagate transmurally from endocardium to epicardium in the walls of both ventricles.[13] These broad wave fronts, which are parallel to the blood cavities, are established by the Purkinje network and the anisotropic fiber architecture. Epicardial breakthrough occurs when the wavefront arrives at the epicardium and breaks through the epicardial surface. The locations and timing of breakthrough events provide important information on the sequence of ventricular activation.

Epicardial Potentials During Ventricular Activation

Prior to epicardial breakthrough, the activation front, which can be represented electrically as a dipole layer approaching the epicardium (cartoon in Fig. 44-3A, right panel), generates a positive potential region (red + sign in the cartoon). Upon breakthrough, the dipoles diverge and generate negative potentials at the breakthrough site (cartoon in Fig. 44-3B, right panel). The first epicardial breakthrough occurs in the right ventricular (RV) anterior-paraseptal region during early QRS and is termed *RV breakthrough*. Figure 44-3A and B, left, show ECGI images of this RV breakthrough sequence in one normal subject. At 13 ms after QRS onset (see Fig 44-3A), RV epicardium is covered with positive potentials (red + signs). Upon breakthrough at 18 ms (see Fig 44-3B), this positive region is invaded by a local potential minimum (blue − sign) at the breakthrough site. This RV breakthrough sequence was imaged in all seven subjects.[14] Among these subjects, the earliest RV breakthrough occurred at 18 ms and the latest at 24 ms, with average RV breakthrough time of 20.7 ms from QRS onset.

Following RV breakthrough, breakthrough minima appear on RV and left ventricular (LV) epicardium. During mid-QRS (see Fig 44-3C, left), additional breakthroughs occur in the left-anterior paraseptal region (site 2), right inferior RV (site 3), and apical RV region (site 4). At this time, the RV breakthrough minimum (site 1) has enlarged and spread in all directions. The breakthrough at site 2 is attributed to an activation front

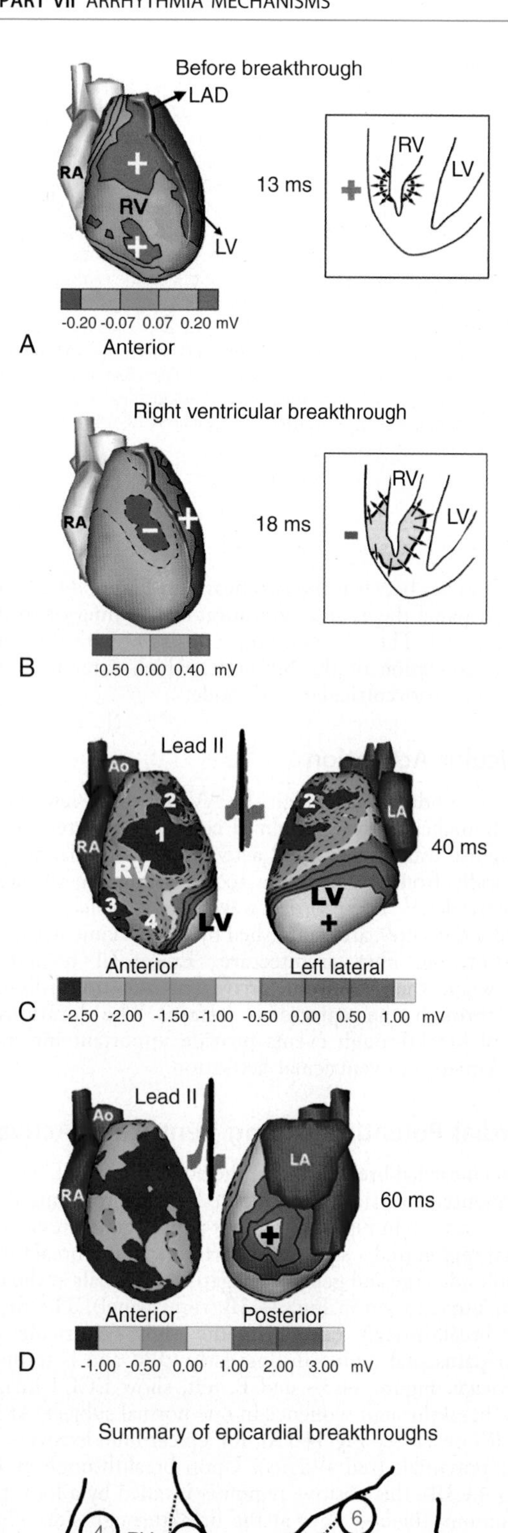

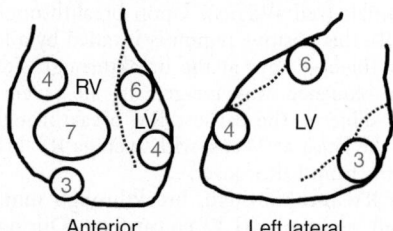

Figure 44-3 Epicardial potentials during normal ventricular activation. Data shown in **A** to **D** are from one representative subject. **A,** At 5 ms before epicardial breakthrough. Cartoon *(right)* shows the activation wavefront, represented by a dipole-layer, approaching the RV epicardium and generating positive potentials (+). At this time, positive potentials cover the RV epicardium *(left)*. **B,** Right ventricular breakthrough: The cartoon *(right)* shows the wavefront breaking through the RV epicardial surface, generating negative potentials *(−)*. The imaged epicardial potentials *(left)* show an intense local negative potential minimum at the breakthrough site *(dark blue)*. **C,** Epicardial potential maps during mid-QRS (40 ms after QRS onset; electrocardiogram (ECG) lead II provides timing). Multiple breakthrough minima *(dark blue,* marked 1-4) are observed. A broad maximum covers the LV apex (left lateral view). **D,** Late QRS (60 ms). Apical maximum has migrated toward LV posterolateral base. **E,** Summary of breakthrough locations for all seven subjects. Numbers indicate in how many subjects a breakthrough minimum was imaged at each site. RV, right ventricle; LV, left ventricle. (From Ramanathan C, Jia P, Ghanem RN, et al: Activation and repolarization of the normal human heart under complete physiological conditions. Proc Natl Acad Sci U S A 103(16):6309-6314, 2006, with permission. Copyright 2006, National Academy of Sciences, U.S.A.)

initiated by the left-anterior fascicular branch of the left bundle branch of the specialized conduction system. At the end of QRS (panel D), the RV minima from the various breakthrough sites coalesce and cover the entire RV epicardium with negative potentials (left panel). RV epicardial activation in the normal human heart occurs through coalescence of multiple breakthrough events, as also demonstrated by direct high-resolution mapping in the canine.[15]

LV epicardial potentials during mid-QRS (see Fig. 44-3C, right) display an extensive positive maximum over the lateral-apical region as a consequence of endocardium-to-epicardium wavefront propagation in the LV free wall. As QRS progresses, this maximum migrates superiorly, from lateral LV apex toward the posterolateral LV base, as seen in Figure 44-3D, right. In the subject shown, this was the last area to activate.

The images of Figure 44-3A to D are from one representative subject. The general pattern of epicardial potentials and its evolution in time is similar in all seven subjects, with some inter-individual differences. Figure 44-3E provides a summary of all epicardial breakthrough sites imaged in the seven subjects. The last area to activate was the LV base in four subjects, the right ventricular outflow tract (RVOT) in two subjects, and both the LV base and RVOT in one subject.

Ventricular Activation Isochrones

Figure 44-4 presents the ventricular activation sequence (temporal isochrones) in three subjects. Again, the general global sequence is similar in all subjects, but some interindividual variability is seen in the details. In subject 1, epicardial activation starts from two adjacent sites on a line perpendicular to the left anterior descending coronary artery (LAD) (sites 1 and 2 in panel A). Earliest activation in subject 2 (Fig. 44-4B) is on an elongated region parallel to the LAD (site 1) and in the left-anterior paraseptal region (site 2). Subject 4 shows multiple areas of early activation: the RV breakthrough region (site 1), left paraseptal (site 2), left apical (site 3), and posterior LV (site 4). In the three subjects shown, the LV base is last to activate (blue), and epicardial slow conduction is seen in the RVOT (as manifested in crowded isochrones there).

Ventricular Repolarization

Unlike the dynamic, fast-changing potential patterns during activation that reflect wavefront propagation (see Fig. 44-3), the potential pattern associated with repolarization is relatively static and only intensifies in amplitude from early

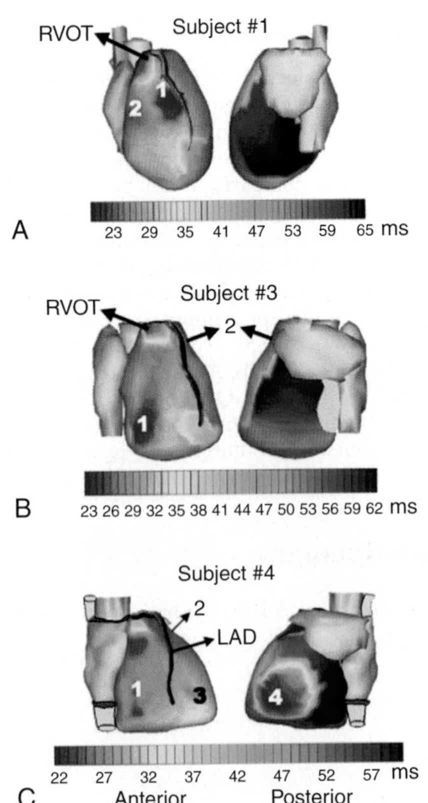

Figure 44-4 Ventricular isochrones of normal activation. Data from three subjects are shown. Numbers indicate locations of early activation sites. LAD, left anterior descending coronary artery; RVOT, right ventricular outflow tract. (From Ramanathan C, Jia P, Ghanem RN, et al: Activation and repolarization of the normal human heart under complete physiological conditions. Proc Natl Acad Sci U S A 103(16):6309-6314, 2006, with permission. Copyright 2006, National Academy of Sciences, U.S.A.)

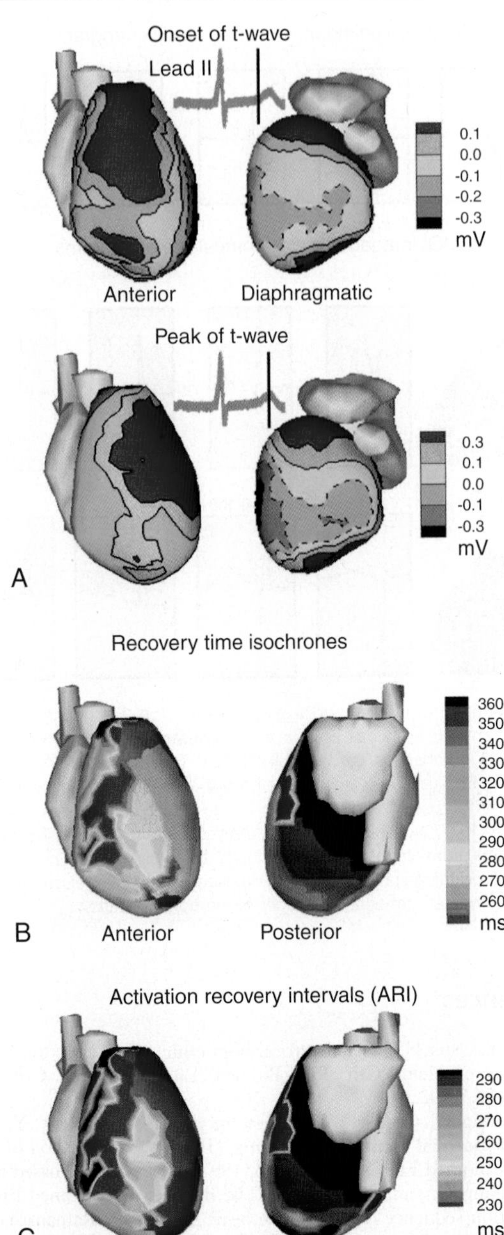

Figure 44-5 Normal ventricular repolarization. Representative data from one subject are shown. **A,** Epicardial potentials during T-wave onset *(upper)* and peak *(lower)*. **B,** Epicardial recovery time isochrones. **C,** Epicardial activation recovery interval map. (From Ramanathan C, Jia P, Ghanem RN, et al: Activation and repolarization of the normal human heart under complete physiological conditions. Proc Natl Acad Sci U S A 103(16):6309-6314, 2006, with permission. Copyright 2006, National Academy of Sciences, U.S.A.)

to peak T wave (Fig. 44-5A). This is consistent with the large spatial extent of the repolarization process that engulfs the ventricles and does not involve a dynamically propagating wavefront. Figure 44-5B shows recovery time isochrones (recovery times take into account the time of arrival of the activation front and is the sum of the local activation time plus the duration of local activity to complete repolarization).

Figure 44-5C shows activation-recovery intervals (ARIs) where activation times are subtracted. ARI indicates local repolarization only, without the contribution of the activation sequence; it reflects the local action potential duration (APD).[10] There is a striking similarity between the recovery isochrones (see Fig 44-5B) and the ARIs (see Fig 44-5C), indicating that in the normal heart the effect of the activation sequence on repolarization is very small, and repolarization is determined mostly by local repolarization properties (local APD). This is so because normal activation via the Purkinje system is fast, and spatial differences in activation times are much smaller than in repolarization times. Thus, to a good approximation, differences in activation times can be ignored and local APD determines the sequence of repolarization.

Mean imaged ARIs among all subjects was 235 ms, in the range of measured human ventricular APD. ECGI also imaged ARI gradients (APD dispersion) between RV and LV; in subject 1 (see Fig. 44-5C), average LV ARI is longer by 32 ms than RV ARI, and ARI at LV base is longer by 30 ms than at LV apex (average apex to base dispersion for all subjects is 42 ms).

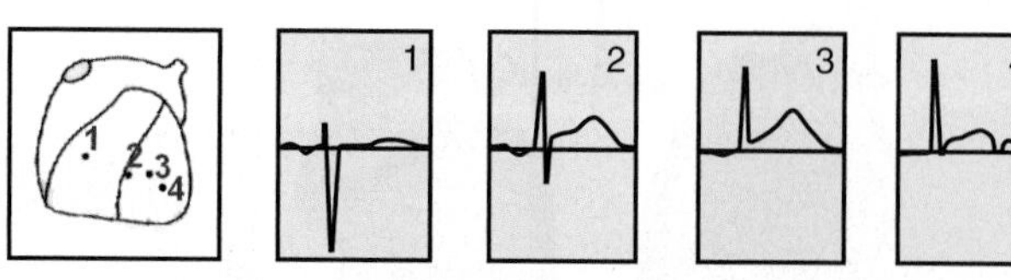

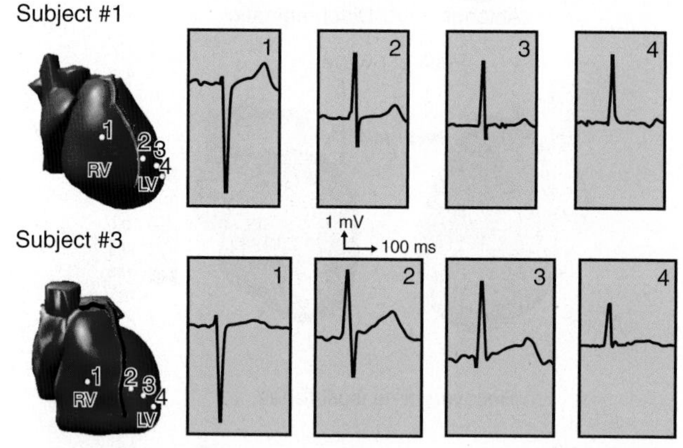

Figure 44-6 Ventricular epicardial electrograms. *Top*, Electrograms recorded directly from four epicardial sites in a chimpanzee. Electrogram locations are indicated by numbers on the heart sketch *(left)*. (Adapted from Spach MS, Barr RC, Lanning CF, Tucek PC: Origin of the body surface QRS and T wave potentials from epicardial potential distributions in the intact chimpanzee. Circulation 55:268-278, 1977, with permission.) *Middle* and *bottom*, Noninvasively imaged electrograms from corresponding anatomic locations in two human hearts using electrocardiographic imaging (ECGI). Numbers identify electrogram locations on computed tomography images of the human hearts.

Ventricular Electrograms

Figure 44-6 shows selected ECGI-imaged epicardial electrograms from two subjects (bottom two panels). The four anatomic locations of the electrograms were chosen to correspond to those recorded directly from the chimpanzee heart (top panel)[16] so that comparison can be made. Electrograms from the entire epicardium and an extensive discussion of their origin are provided in a paper by Ramanathan and colleagues.[14] Electrogram 1 has an rS morphology, as expected for the RV breakthrough site; the small positive r-wave reflects wavefront propagation toward the epicardium (see Fig. 44-3A), and the large negative S wave reflects occurrence and expansion of the breakthrough (see Fig. 44-3B). As the electrogram sites progress from 1 to 4 (RV to LV), the QRS becomes biphasic (negative-positive at site 2) and then mostly positive (sites 3 and 4). This progression is seen in all subjects and is very similar to that recorded in the chimpanzee (top panel).[16]

Acknowledgement

Special thanks to Debra Adams for her expert help in preparing the manuscript.

References

1. Rudy Y, Oster HS: The electrocardiographic inverse problem. Crit Rev Biomed Eng 20:25-46, 1992.
2. Huiskamp G, Greensite F: A new method for myocardial activation imaging. IEEE Trans Biomed Eng 44(6):433-446, 1997.
3. Huiskamp G, van Oosterom A: The depolarization sequence of the human heart surface computed from measured body surface potentials. IEEE Trans Biomed Eng 35(12):1047-1058, 1988.
4. Fischer G, Pfeifer B, Seger M, et al: Computationally efficient noninvasive cardiac activation time imaging. Methods Inf Med 44(5):674-686, 2005.
5. Barr RC, Spach MS: Inverse solutions directly in terms of potentials. In Nelson CV, Geselowitz DB (eds): The Theoretical Basis of Electrocardiography. Oxford, Carendon Press, 1976, pp 294-304.
6. Franzone P, Taccardi B, Viganotti C: An approach to inverse calculation of epicardial potentials from body surface maps. Adv Cardiol 21:50-54, 1978.
7. Rudy Y, Messinger-Rapport BJ: The inverse problem in electrocardiography: Solutions in terms of epicardial potentials. Crit Rev Biomed Eng 16(3):215-268, 1988.
8. Wang Y, Rudy Y: Application of the method of fundamental solutions to potential-based inverse electrocardiography. Ann Biomed Eng 34(8):1272-1288, 2006.
9. Ramanathan C, Jia P, Ghanem R, et al: Noninvasive electrocardiographic imaging (ECGI): Application of the generalized minimal residual (GMRes) method. Ann Biomed Eng 31(8):981-994, 2003.
10. Lux RL, Green LS, MacLeod RS, Taccardi B: Assessment of spatial and temporal characteristics of ventricular repolarization. J Electrocardiol 27:100-105, 1994.
10a. Ramanathan C, Rudy Y: Electrocardiographic imaging: II. Effect of torso inhomogeneities on noninvasive reconstruction of epicardial potentials, electrograms, and isochrones. J Cardiovasc Electrophysiol 12: 241-252, 2001.
11. Ramanathan C, Ghanem RN, Jia P, et al: Noninvasive electrocardiographic imaging for cardiac electrophysiology and arrhythmia. Nat Med 10(4):422-428, 2004.
12. Wyndham CR., Meeran MK, Smith T, et al: Epicardial activation of the intact human heart without conduction defect. Circulation 59:161-168, 1979.
13. Durrer D, van Dam RT, Freud GE, et al: Total excitation of the isolated human heart. Circulation 41:899-912, 1970.
14. Ramanathan C, Jia P, Ghanem RN, et al: Activation and repolarization of the normal human heart under complete physiological conditions. Proc Natl Acad Sci U S A 103(16):6309-6314, 2006.
15. Arisi G, Macchi E, Baruffi S, et al: Potential fields on the ventricular surface of the exposed dog heart during normal excitation. Circ Res 52:706-715, 1983.
16. Spach MS, Barr RC, Lanning CF, Tucek PC: Origin of the body surface QRS and T wave potentials from epicardial potential distributions in the intact chimpanzee. Circulation 55:268-278, 1977.

Dynamics and Molecular Mechanisms of Ventricular Tachycardia and Fibrillation in Normal Hearts 45

Viviana Muñoz, Sami F. Noujaim, and José Jalife

CHAPTER OUTLINE

Turbulent flows seem almost "alive."

A. T. Winfree

Ventricular fibrillation (VF) is by far the most important immediate cause of sudden cardiac death. Every year, VF is responsible for an estimated 300,000 deaths in the United States alone.[1,2] Because of its highly complex electrocardiographic (ECG) appearance,[3] VF is commonly thought of as an exceptionally complex and disorganized cardiac activation, in which electrical waves propagate through the ventricles chaotically and unpredictably. In fact, during VF, the ventricular activation sequence is profoundly abnormal; electrical wavefronts do not follow the usual paths. The heart rate accelerates to the extreme, and the electrical waves assume a complex vortex-like behavior that looks a lot like eddy formation and turbulence in water. Such turmoil renders the heart unable to pump blood. Thus the blood pressure drops and immediate loss of consciousness follows. Unfortunately, despite many years of research and speculation, the mechanism underlying VF continues to be a matter of speculation and debate.

Evidence has accumulated supporting the idea that although VF is indeed complex, it is in fact deterministic, quantifiable, and in theory, mechanistically understandable. In this regard, it seems reasonable to suggest that achieving a comprehensive knowledge of VF mechanisms will require a clear familiarity with the underlying bases of cardiac excitation and its frequency dependence, in which cardiac ion channels play important roles. More specifically, it is our contention that advances in VF understanding will require thorough quantitative knowledge of the ionic mechanisms of the extremely complex phenomena that underlie the initiation and maintenance of VF, including wavebreak and rotor formation, rotor stabilization, and spiral wave behavior. In this chapter, we briefly review the most salient aspects related to the dynamics of VF in structurally normal hearts, as well as current knowledge, however incomplete, of the role played by inward rectifying and delayed rectifier potassium channels in the molecular mechanisms of VF initiation and maintenance.

This research is supported by grants PO1 HL039707, RO1 HL070074, and RO1 HL060843 from the National Heart, Lung, and Blood Institute.

Functional Reentry and Spiral Waves

Thoeretical[4,5] and experimental[6] studies that began to appear in the relevant literature in the 1950s have established that the heart can sustain electrical activity that rotates about a functional obstacle. In this regard, the experimental work of Allessie and collaborators in the 1970s that gave birth to the leading-circle concept was an essential initial step toward our current understanding of the phenomenon of functional reentry in cardiac tissue; that is, reentry without the involvement of an anatomic obstacle (Fig. 45-1A-B).[6] At about the same time, work conducted by Soviet scientists using the Belousov-Zhabotinski reaction and its numerical counterparts led to the idea that two-dimensional spiral autowaves (see Fig. 45-1C) could be a possible mechanism of cardiac arrhythmias.[7] Subsequently, the notion of spiral autowaves was brilliantly expanded into the third dimension (see Fig. 45-1D) by the late Arthur T. Winfree,[8] who in fact coined the term *rotor* to signify the actual vortex that generates the spiral (scroll) wave activity, and led to the virtual abandonment of the use of the term *leading circle*. Thereafter, much work has focused on rotors as the underlying mechanism of ventricular tachycardia and VF.

Rotors and Their Breakup

Life-threatening, complex cardiac tachyarrhythmias can be due to the activity of a reentrant electrical source, namely, a rotor of characteristic size and angular velocity from which spiral waves radiate at a high frequency.[8,9] The basic components of the rotor are a curved wave front, a curved wave tail, and a core around which the wave front and tail rotate (see Fig. 45-1C). The rotor might drift and travel along complex paths, or it may be completely stationary, with spiral waves emanating from it and propagating through the ventricles.[3,10] The waves might undergo a variety of behavior; for example, they may be highly stable and spiral periodically around their generating rotor to activate the ventricles at extremely high frequencies, or they might undergo breakup in the rotor's periphery and result in fibrillatory conduction, the net result being complex spatial and temporal patterns of ventricular activation.[11] In other words, the behavior of the rotor, and that of the waves generated by it, may be reflected on ECG as monomorphic or polymorphic ventricular tachycardias[12] or even VF.[3]

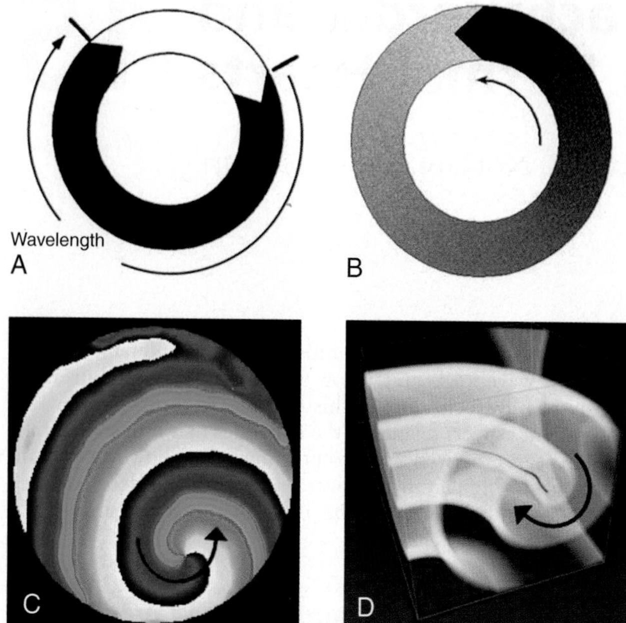

Figure 45-1 Four different concepts of reentry. **A,** Reentry around a ring-like anatomical obstacle. Successful reentry occurs when wavelength *(black)* is smaller than pathlength and allows a fully excitable gap *(white)*. **B,** Leading circle reentry around a functional obstacle. Partially excitable gap allows wave front to bite its wavetail of refractoriness. **C,** Two-dimensional spiral wave rotating around an unexcited but excitable core in a neonatal rat ventricular myocyte monolayer. **D,** Diagrammatic representation of a three-dimensional scroll wave.

Rotors and Ventricular Fibrillation in the Human Heart

During VF, there may be a wide spectrum of rotor behavior.[3,13,14] Under appropriate conditions, even in the structurally normal heart of small animals, rotors may be long lasting and result in a high degree of spatial and temporal organization.[14] Consequently, a question may be raised as to whether the same applies to the ventricles of larger animals such as dogs, pigs, and humans. Studies[15-18] suggest that even in large hearts such as that of the pig, the dynamics of wave propagation during VF are not as complex as might occur if the mechanism were spiral breakup or as random as would be expected from the multiple wavelet hypothesis.[15,16,19] In fact, Rogers and coworkers[15] were unable to rule out the possibility that mother rotors located in unmapped regions in their swine heart experiments maintained the fibrillatory activity. Additionally, a study has proposed that the mother rotor and the multiple wavelets are both mechanisms of VF in the human heart.[19,20] Yet another study, in which the epicardium of the human left ventricle was mapped, concluded that there is significant organization of human VF.[21]

The results described in the previous paragraph are consistent with data of Thomas and colleagues,[22] who investigated the way activation is organized during VF induced in the presence of an old anterior left ventricular wall infarct. By using 20 needles carrying multiple monopolar electrodes to record the transmural activity of the left ventricle of the sheep heart, Thomas and colleagues demonstrated that the regions with the highest activation frequency displayed less-variable cycle lengths and were generally hidden within the ventricular myocardium. In some experiments they were able to reveal regions deep in the myocardium whose activity was stable and extremely rapid but highly regular. In other words, although the characteristics of VF in the epicardium were constantly changing in space and time, the activity within the myocardium had a higher frequency and was also highly periodic and organized.[22] Such findings are clearly compatible with the hypothesis that in that experimental model, fibrillatory activity is maintained by only one or two three-dimensional rotors.

Nanthakumar and colleagues[19] have investigated whether human VF is the result of wave breaks and singularity point formation and is maintained by high-frequency rotors and fibrillatory conduction. They used explanted hearts from five cardiomyopathic patients who underwent transplantation. The hearts were Langendorff-perfused with Tyrode's solution (95% O_2 and 5% CO_2), and di-4-ANEPPS was injected as a bolus into the coronary circulation. High-resolution activation and phase maps demonstrated phase singularity points, wave breaks, and rotor formation in human VF, with fractionation of wave fronts resulting in fibrillatory conduction. On many occasions the VF wave fronts were as large as the entire vertical length (8 cm) of the mapping field, suggesting that there are a limited number of wave fronts on the human heart during VF.

Potassium Channels and Cardiac Excitation

In the heart, potassium currents are diverse in that their individual properties depend not only on the membrane potential and their dissimilar activation and recovery kinetics but also on the activation frequency. Diffusion of potassium ions through the inward rectifier potassium channels gives rise to the inward rectifier potassium current (I_{K1}) and maintains the resting membrane potential in all cardiac cells. In most mammals, upon action potential depolarization (phase 0), the transient outward current (I_{to}) is rapidly activated to mediate the initial phase of repolarization (phase 1), followed by rapid inactivation. The more slowly activating delayed rectifier currents (I_{Ks} and I_{Kr}), contribute to the slow repolarization that characterizes the action potential plateau (phase 2). During the terminal phase of repolarization (phase 3), I_{K1} predominates, rapidly restoring the membrane potential to resting values (phase 4). During tachyarrhythmias, probably all potassium currents involved in cardiac repolarization participate to various degrees in helping to establish the dynamics of cardiac excitation and propagation. Here we focus our attention on the specific role played by I_{K1} in the mechanisms of rotor formation and maintenance and the way I_{Ks} contributes to post-repolarization refractoriness and fibrillatory conduction.

Inwardly Rectifying Potassium Current Controls Ventricular Fibrillation Frequency

I_{K1} flows through membrane channels formed by members of the strong inward rectifier (Kir2.x) subfamily of proteins. Inward rectifier potassium channels are part of a large family of membrane-spanning proteins that have a conserved GYG sequence in the domain responsible for K^+ selectivity. Each protein spans the membrane twice, and both N and C termini are intracellular.[23,24] Four homomeric or heteromeric subunits can form a channel.[25] These channels are termed *inward rectifiers* because their permeability to potassium is greater in the inward than in the outward directions. Rectification is due to a voltage-dependent blockade of the channel of positively charged molecules such as polyamines and Mg^{2+} that move from the intracellular space into the pore.[25,26] Spermine and spermidine

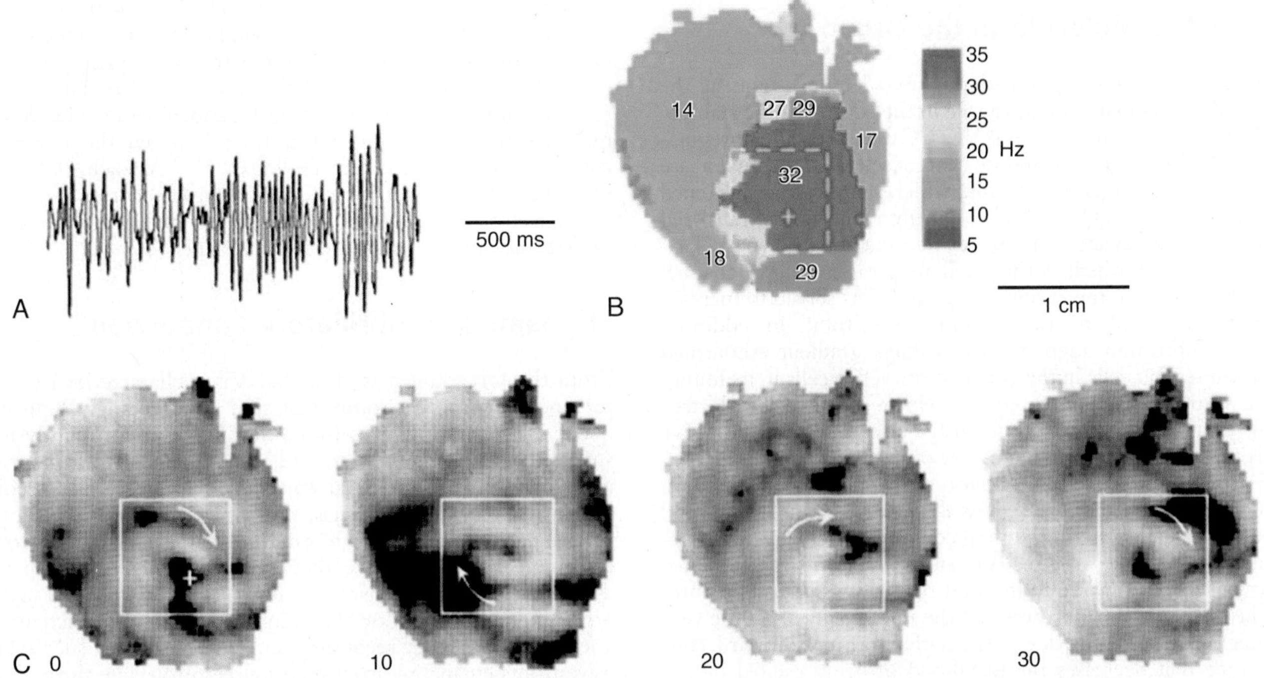

Figure 45-2 High-frequency rotor in an isolated, Langendorff-perfused guinea pig heart. **A,** Electrocardiogram (ECG) trace of ventricular fibrillation (VF). **B,** Dominant frequency map showing the LV-RV gradient in frequencies. **C,** Snapshots of a long-lasting rotor on the anterior LV wall at four different times during one rotation. Numbers in **B** are in Hertz; numbers in **C** are in milliseconds. LV, left ventricle; RV, right ventricle. (Reproduced from Samie FH, Berenfeld O, Anumonwo J, et al: Rectification of the background potassium current: A determinant of rotor dynamics in ventricular fibrillation. Circ Res 89:1216-223, 2001, with permission from Circulation Research.)

are the most potent polyamine blockers of I_{K1}.[27] At voltages positive to the resting membrane potential, polyamines and Mg^{2+} are drawn to the pore. They block it, reducing the outflow of potassium ions, resulting in a smaller outward current relative to the inward component.[26] Increasing the density of I_{K1} abbreviates the action potential duration (APD). Decreasing its density has the reciprocal effect.[24]

The role of I_{K1} in rotor behavior has been investigated in computer simulations and in experiments. In the guinea pig heart, VF is manifested by a stable, high-frequency sustained rotor anchored in the left ventricle (LV), as illustrated in Figure 45-2.[13] This causes the frequency of activation of the LV (see Fig 45-2B, 32 Hz) to be higher than the right ventricle (RV, 14 Hz). The anchoring of the rotor in the LV and the subsequent regional difference in frequency between the LV and RV have been attributed to differences in I_{K1} density between the two chambers.[13] As shown in Figure 45-3, incorporation of the characteristics demonstrated for I_{K1} in the LV and RV into a computer-based ionic model of the cardiac ventricular myocytes[13] reproduced a stable rotor with a rotation frequency of 35 Hz in the region with larger I_{K1}. Fibrillatory conduction characterized the region of the model with right ventricular I_{K1}.

Further experimentation explored the effect of I_{K1} blockade on the dynamics of VF in this model. Ba^{2+} was used at relatively low concentrations (1-50 μM) to selectively block I_{K1} in the isolated, Langendorff-perfused guinea pig heart.[26] The major finding was that Ba^{2+} perfusion resulted in a dose-dependent decrease in the frequency of reentry. At 50 μM, Ba^{2+} perfusion terminated VF.[26] It was shown as well that Ba^{2+} caused a proportional decrease in the density of I_{K1} in isolated myocytes. Those experiments indicated that I_{K1} affected the stability and duration of reentry.

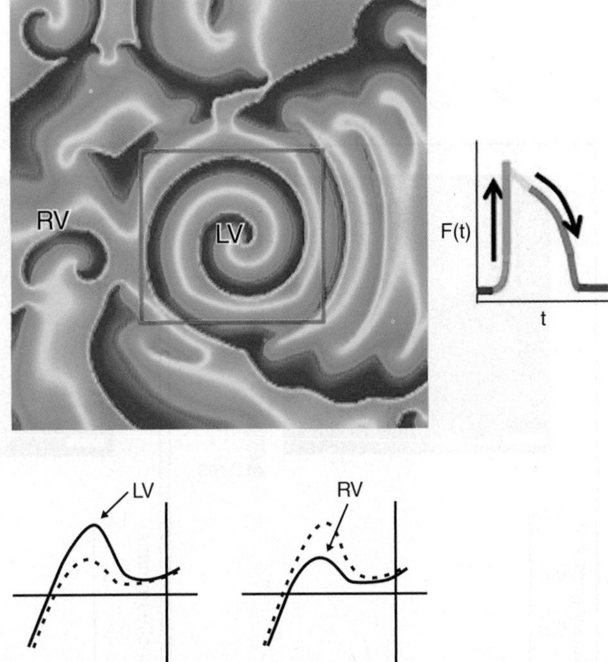

Figure 45-3 Role of I_{K1} density in ventricular fibrillation (VF) dynamics in a two-dimensional model (6 × 6 cm^2) of the guinea pig ventricles consisting of >200,000 excitable elements (cells). The simulated left ventricle (LV, center) is surrounded by the right ventricle (RV, periphery). *Top*, phase map of VF maintained by a stable rotor in the LV, with fibrillatory conduction to RV. *Red square* shows the perimeter of the LV model (area, 2 × 2 cm^2). As illustrated by the inset on the right, each color represents a different phase of the action potential in each cell. *Bottom*, Current-voltage (IV) relations of I_{K1} used for LV *(left)* and RV *(right)*. Note the larger I_{K1} density in LV. Broken curve is I_{K1} with nominal density. For further explanation see text and Samie et al.[13]

From the Molecule to the Organ

A more-recent study provided the first demonstration at the molecular level that I_{K1} plays a role in the control of the stability and frequency of rotors and of VF.[28] Cardiac-specific upregulation of I_{K1} in a transgenic mouse heart accelerated the final phase of action potential repolarization, which significantly shortened the APD and the QT interval.[27] During reentry, this translated into a shorter wavelength and relative membrane hyperpolarization, both of which contributed to greater sodium channel availability during the excitable gap, and thus served to increase excitability ahead of the rotating wavefront. In addition, I_{K1} overexpression augments the voltage gradient established between resting cells in the core and the active cells in its immediate surroundings. These effects help to enhance the electrotonic currents that flow continuously between resting and active cells, which further contributes not only to hastening the repolarization of the active cells but also to reducing the propagation velocity very near the core.[28,29] As shown in Figure 45-4, the end result is a steeper rise in the local conduction velocity as a function of the distance from the core and a faster, more stable rotor in transgenic, compared to the wild-type, hearts. During reentry in the hearts that overexpress I_{K1}, the unexcited cells at the very center of the core provide a larger-than-normal outward conductance that decreases the likelihood of being excited by the depolarizing influence of their immediate, actively depolarized neighbors (sink-to-source mismatch), helping to reduce core size and meandering and to stabilize the rotor.

Taken together, experimental data in isolated guinea pig and transgenic mouse hearts and in computer simulations strongly argue that I_{K1} is a stabilizer of reentry because of its ability to shorten APD and reduce conduction velocity near the center of rotation.[10,13,28,29] Increased I_{K1} should hamper interactions between the wave front and wavetail and consequently prevent destabilization and breakup of the rotor.[10,13,29] In this regard, I_{K1} is an important current during functional reentry because it mediates the electrotonic interactions between the unexcited core and its immediate surroundings.[10,13,29] As such, the interplay between I_{K1} and the rapid sodium inward current (I_{Na}) is a major factor in the control of cardiac excitability and therefore the stability and frequency of reentry[28] and VF.

Dynamics of Fibrillatory Conduction

From the foregoing it is clear that VF is characterized by the presence of electrical rotors that spin at exceedingly high frequencies, generating wave fronts that block intermittently in a spatially distributed manner, with consequent wave front fragmentation (wave break), and wavelet formation. In fact, studies in hearts from several species, ranging in size from the mouse to the pig,[13,15,30] have demonstrated that even a single rotor can result in ECG patterns that are indistinguishable from VF. This suggests that at least some forms of fibrillation are highly organized and depend on the uninterrupted periodic activity of a few high-frequency reentrant sources. The rapidly succeeding wave fronts emanating from such sources propagate throughout the ventricles and interact with tissue heterogeneities, both functional and anatomic, leading to fragmentation and wavelet formation,[13,26] the end result being fibrillatory conduction. A wave break occurs if the stimulatory efficacy of a wave front does not suffice to excite the tissue downstream. The newly formed wavelets can undergo decremental conduction or they

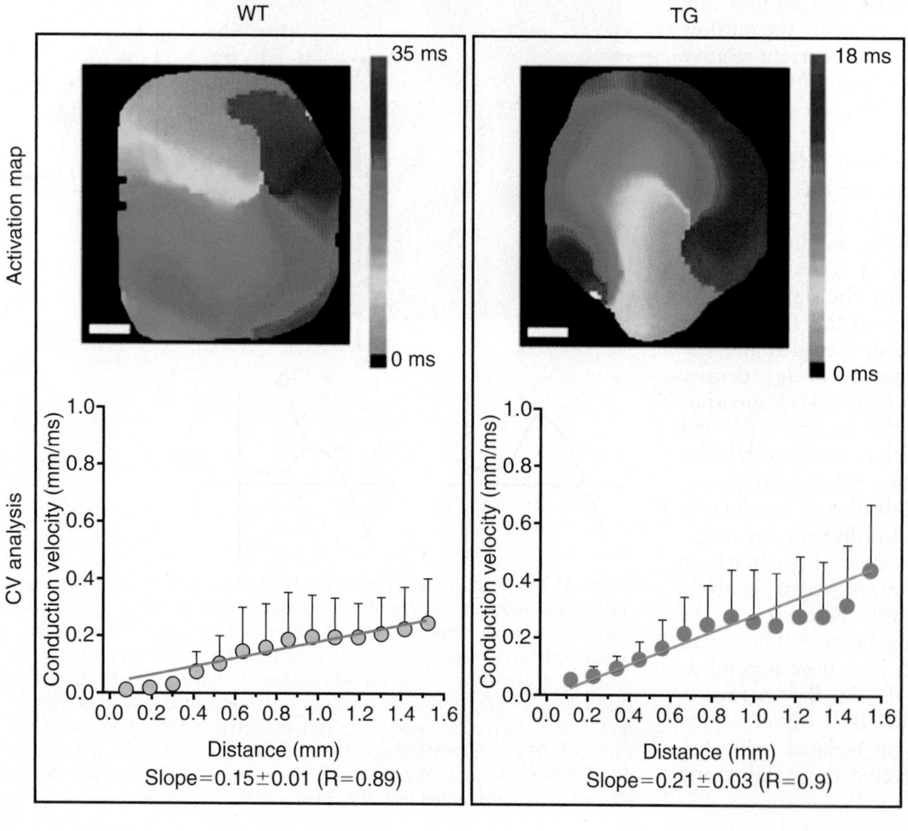

Figure 45-4 Distance-velocity relationships in wild-type (WT) mice compared with transgenic (TG) mice overexpressing Kir2.1 channels. *Top*, Color activation maps. *Bottom*, Conduction velocity (CV) as a function of radial distance from the rotor's core. Note the significantly steeper slope in TG (right) than WT (left) and the faster rotor in TG. (Modified from Noujaim SF, Pandit SV, Berenfeld O, et al: Up-regulation of the inward rectifier K$^+$ current (I_{K1}) in the mouse heart accelerates and stabilizes rotors. J Physiol 578:315-326, 2007, with permission from the *Journal of Physiology*.)

may be annihilated by collision with another wavelet or a boundary, and still others can curl and give rise to new sustained rotors. The result would be never-ending fibrillatory conduction, or the frequency-dependent fragmentation of wave fronts into what appears to be multiple independent wavelets.[13,26]

I_{Ks} Overexpression and Fibrillatory Conduction

To date, the molecular mechanisms of wave breaks leading to fibrillatory conduction remain poorly understood. Previous studies have shown that the gating kinetics of the delayed rectifier potassium current (I_K) contribute to postrepolarization refractoriness leading to frequency-dependent intermittent excitation failure in isolated cardiomyocytes.[31] However, the impact of such kinetics on arrhythmogenesis, particularly VF, remains unknown.

We have used neonatal cardiomyocyte monolayers as a two-dimensional biologic excitable medium to investigate the consequences of the overexpression of the slow component of I_K, I_{Ks}, on excitation, propagation, and the dynamics of reentrant activation.[32] We hypothesized that expression of I_{Ks} in rat cardiomyocyte monolayers contributes to wave break formation and facilitates fibrillatory conduction by promoting post-repolarization refractoriness. Consequently, we performed optical mapping experiments using rat ventricular myocyte monolayers infected with an adenovirus carrying the genomic sequences of K_VLQT1 and minK (molecular correlates of I_{Ks}) and littermate controls infected with a GFP adenovirus. As shown in Figure 45-5, APD was significantly shorter in I_{Ks} than in control monolayers at all rotation frequencies. Moreover, as shown in Figure 45-6A during reentry, conduction velocity as a function of distance from the core had a significantly less pronounced increase in the I_{Ks} monolayers consistent with a less-excitable preparation.[32] As a result, wavelengths in

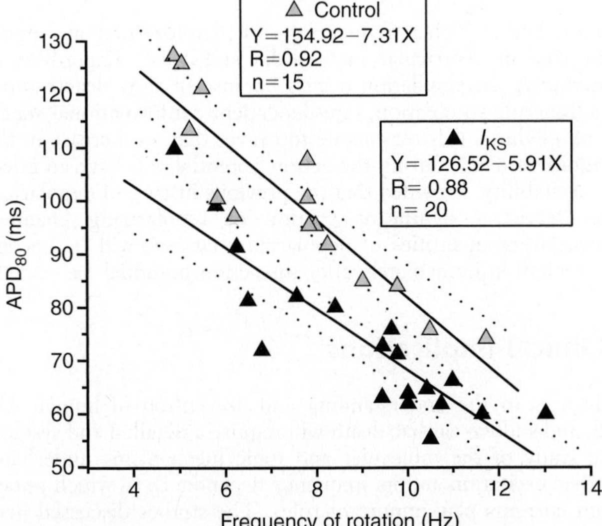

Figure 45-5 Action potential duration at 80% (APD_{80}) as a function of frequency of rotation in control versus I_{Ks} monolayers. Each symbol represents one monolayer. (Modified from Muñoz V, Grzeda KR, Desplantez T, et al: Adenoviral expression of I_{Ks} contributes to wavebreak and fibrillatory conduction in neonatal rat ventricular cardiomyocyte monolayers. Circ Res 101:475-483, 2007, with permission from Circulation Research.)

the latter were significantly shorter than in littermate controls at all rotation frequencies (see Fig. 45-6B). Consequently, stable rotors occurred in both groups, with significantly higher rotation frequencies, lower conduction velocities, and shorter action potentials in the I_{Ks} group.

Another important difference was that unlike control monolayers, the waves emanating from rotors in the I_{Ks} preparations frequently underwent wave break, fibrillatory conduction, and formation of new, short-lived rotors in a time-dependent fashion. Figure 45-7 illustrates the contrasting evolution of the two groups. In Figure 45-7A, the top frames show individual phase maps of a control monolayer obtained at 0, 120, 240, and 360 seconds of the onset of the experiment. The bottom frames show similar phase maps of littermate monolayers infected with I_{Ks} at 0, 90, 180, and 270 seconds after the onset of the experiment. In both cases, waves were generated by a single reentrant source rotating at 8.2 Hz (control) and 9.4 Hz (I_{Ks}). It is clear from these examples that whereas in the control there was a single rotor giving rise to well-organized wave fronts are at all times, I_{Ks} overexpression resulted in a time-dependent increase in the density of wave breaks and the complexity of the fibrillatory conduction pattern. As shown in Figure 45-7B, the number of wave breaks increased progressively. Moreover, the density of wave breaks increased with time as long as a stable source sustained the fibrillatory activity. None of the controls showed any wave breaks other than the original rotor giving rise to sustained reentrant activity.

Apparently chaotic waves often recorded optically during VF in intact hearts and attributed to fibrillatory conduction may be generated by sources outside the field of view. In monolayers, however, the area recorded corresponded to the entire preparation, allowing the strong conclusion that all the episodes of fibrillatory conduction were sustained by at least one stable rotor. In summary, during sustained reentry, I_{Ks} overexpression decreases APD, conduction velocity, and wavelength at frequencies ranging between 4.9 and 13 Hz. However, despite inducing such a significant wavelength shortening, I_{Ks} overexpression results in a history-dependent sink-to-source mismatch during diastole that leads to wave break and fibrillatory conduction, particularly at high frequencies of reentry.

I_{Ks} and Postrepolarization Refractoriness

Recovery of excitability after an action potential can be a slow process that greatly outlasts the APD.[33] Previous studies in isolated guinea pig ventricular myocytes have shown that activation failure can occur at diastolic potentials, even if the sodium current, I_{Na}, has had sufficient time to recover completely from inactivation, because of the slow gating kinetics of I_K.[31] This phenomenon is called *post-repolarization refractoriness*. However, it was uncertain whether the results observed at the single cell level could be extrapolated to allow inferences related to the propagation of the electrical impulse where, in addition to cellular excitability, one has to consider electrical coupling and wavefront curvature,[34] as well as structural heterogeneities, as potential contributors to the success or failure of propagation of the action potential.

We found that I_{Ks} significantly shortens the wavelength while slightly but significantly increasing the frequency of reentry in the monolayers. Yet in this model, waves emanating from a stable source more readily encounter tissue that is repolarized but not yet excitable, leading to wave fragmentation. Such an apparent paradox was explained by results obtained in HEK293 (human embryonic kidney) cells showing that in the presence of full repolarization, the slow deactivation kinetics of I_{Ks} significantly impair the recovery of excitability at early diastolic

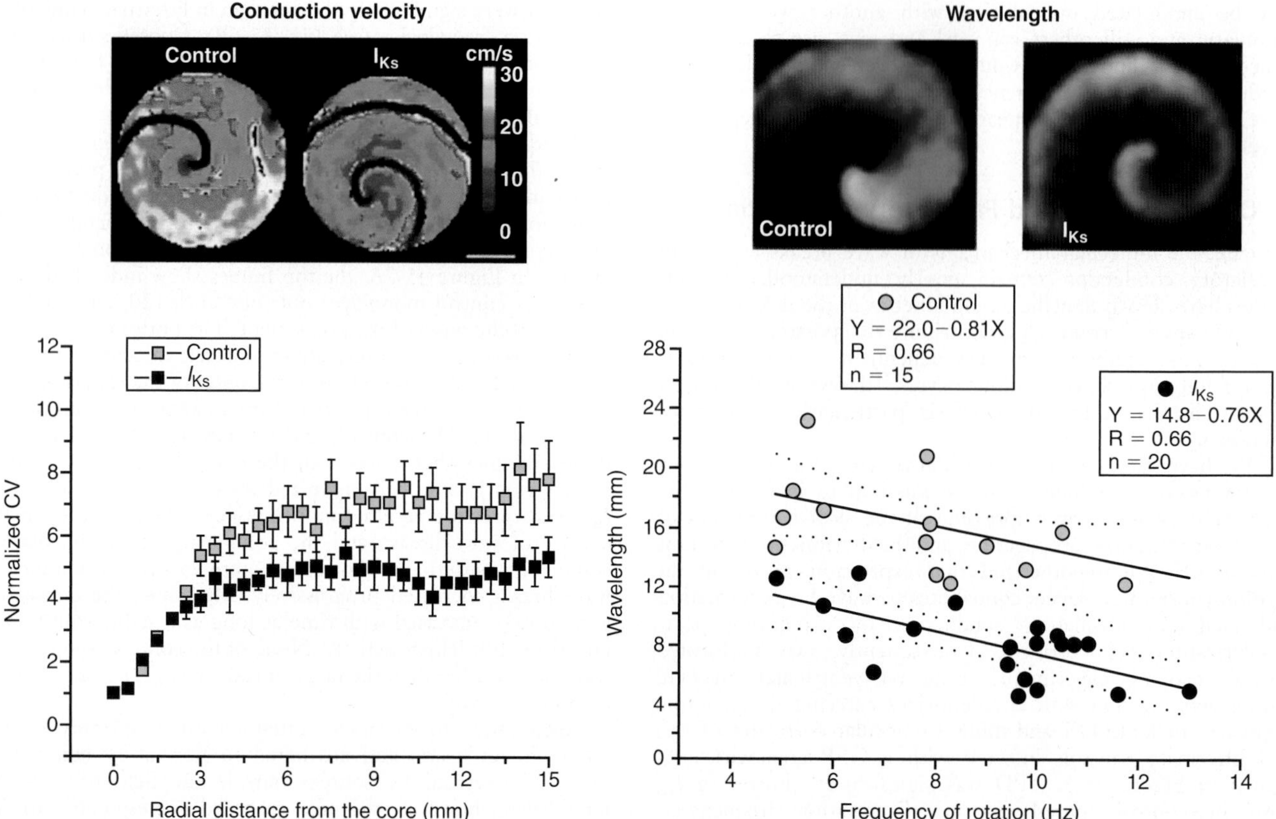

Figure 45-6 Conduction velocity (CV) and wavelength during reentry in cardiomyocyte monolayers. **A,** *top,* CV maps. Note greater velocities in the core periphery of control *(left)* than slow K^+ current (I_{Ks}) *(right)* monolayer; *bottom,* normalized CV as a function of radial distance from the core. **B,** *top,* Snapshots of electrical spirals in control (8.3 Hz; *left*) and I_{Ks} (10.1 Hz; *right*) monolayers. Wavelength, defined as the spatial extension of the excited state, was greater in control than I_{Ks}; *bottom,* wavelength, measured 5 mm from the core was significantly larger in control than I_{Ks} at all rotation frequencies. (Modified from Muñoz V, Grzeda KR, Desplantez T, et al: Adenoviral expression of I_{Ks} contributes to wavebreak and fibrillatory conduction in neonatal rat ventricular cardiomyocyte monolayers. Circ Res 101:475-483, 2007, with permission from Circulation Research.)

intervals (Fig. 45-8). This is not to say that the I_{Na} threshold, or the rate of recovery of I_{Na} and I_{Ca}, are not critical for cell excitability; however, under conditions in which these parameters are fully recovered at any given location, an increase in the number of I_{Ks} channels that remain open during diastole will act to oppose any depolarizing current. Thus, the approach to threshold would be delayed, with the possible occurrence of wave break.

Computer simulations aided in establishing that a spatial dispersion in the conformational state of the I_{Ks} channel, or spatially inhomogeneous recovery kinetics during diastole, may be sufficient to allow formation of wave break and reentry at specific locations. Therefore, the simplified nature of the monolayer, together with the results of simulations, allows us to postulate that the spatially distributed wave breaks and intermittent block processes that are often observed during VF result in part from inherent spatial heterogeneities in I_{Ks} distribution and of its slow gating kinetics.

Role of I_{Ks} Accumulation

I_{Ks} activates more slowly than any other known potassium current and requires membrane depolarization on the order of seconds to reach a steady state,[35] conditions that are not achieved in vivo. Moreover, the slow deactivation kinetics of I_{Ks} allow it to accumulate at higher frequencies and therefore play an important role in ventricular tachycardia and VF.[36] Regardless of whether I_{Ks} accumulation occurs because of slow deactivation, β-adrenergic stimulation, rate-dependent conformational states, or all of these, it is reasonable to expect that an increase in the magnitude of I_{Ks} during the action potential will have an effect on excitability. Provided that the previous history of depolarization leaves a significant portion of repolarizing channels open, larger quantities of depolarizing current will be needed for excitation immediately after the action potential has ended.

Clinical Implications

Advances in the understanding and prevention of human AF, VF, and sudden cardiac death will require a detailed and systematic study of the molecular and ionic mechanisms underlying cardiac excitation and its frequency dependence in which potassium currents play important roles. The studies discussed here focus specifically on such mechanisms and are highly relevant to the understanding of clinical arrhythmias. They represent a systematic approach at the molecular level to investigate the way potassium channels contribute to the control of wave propagation under conditions of high-frequency excitation that are germane to atrial and ventricular fibrillation. The clinical

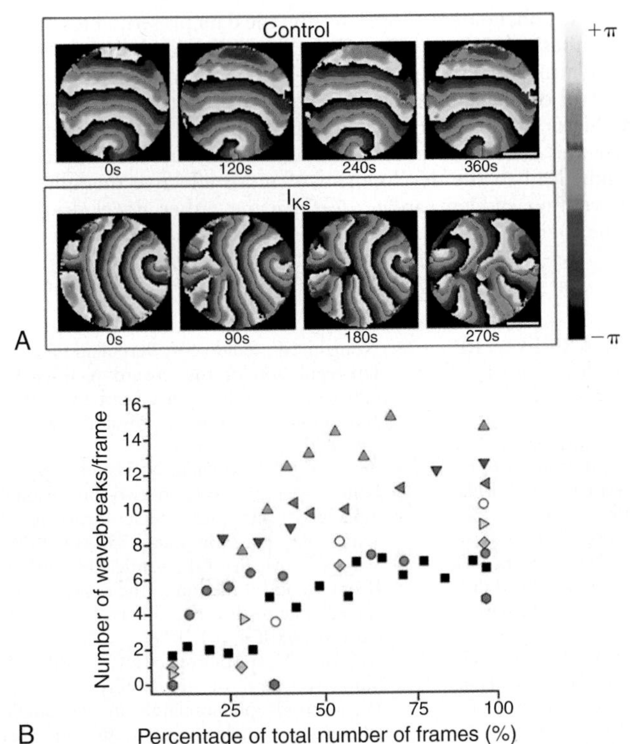

Figure 45-7 I_{Ks} overexpression results in fibrillatory conduction **A,** *Top,* Sequential phase maps of a control monolayer; *bottom,* phase maps of littermate monolayers infected with I_{Ks}. Waves are generated by a single reentrant source rotating at 8.2 and 9.4 Hz for *top* and *bottom,* respectively. Scale bars = 10 mm; numbers indicate time in seconds. **B,** The number of wave breaks increased progressively in the I_{Ks} monolayers that developed fibrillatory conduction. (Reproduced from Muñoz V, Grzeda KR, Desplantez T, et al: Adenoviral expression of I_{Ks} contributes to wavebreak and fibrillatory conduction in neonatal rat ventricular cardiomyocyte monolayers. Circ Res 101:475-483, 2007, with permission from Circulation Research.)

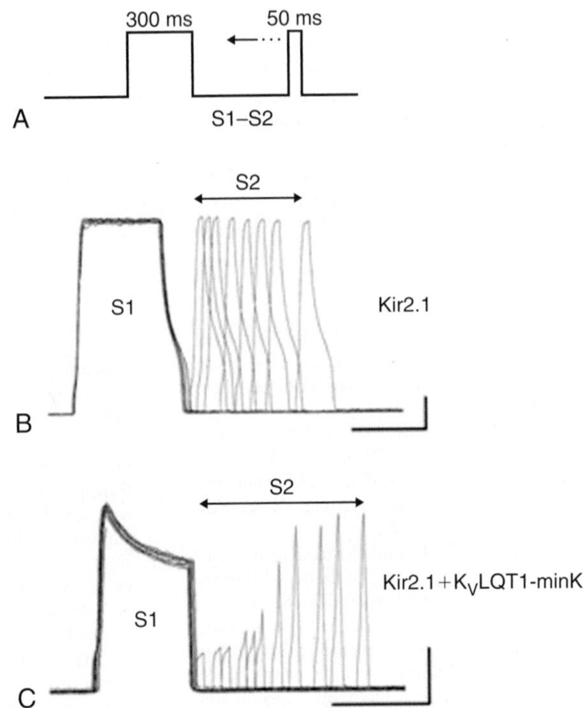

Figure 45-8 Current-clamp data in HEK293 cells. **A,** S1-S2 protocol. **B,** Responses of a representative cell transfected with Kir2.1. **C,** Response of a representative cell cotransfected with Kir2.1 and K$_V$LQT1-minK. Scale bars: horizontal = 250 ms, vertical = 25 mV. (Reproduced from Muñoz V, Grzeda KR, Desplantez T, et al: Adenoviral expression of I_{Ks} contributes to wavebreak and fibrillatory conduction in neonatal rat ventricular cardiomyocyte monolayers. Circ Res 101:475-483, 2007, with permission from Circulation Research.)

applicability of this work is highlighted by the demonstration that persistent AF in patients is associated with upregulation of different potassium channel genes[37-39] and also by the recent discovery of the short QT syndrome (SQTS) as a novel inherited disorder that occurs in persons who have a structurally intact heart but increased susceptibility to cardiac arrhythmias and sudden death.[40]

On ECG, SQTS is manifested by a remarkably accelerated repolarization that is reflected in a shorter-than-normal QTc interval. Clinical manifestations of SQTS range from syncopal events to cardiac arrest; affected and asymptomatic persons have also been identified.[40,41] Importantly, even if only few families with SQTS have been reported to date, three different genetic loci (SQT1, SQT2, and SQT3) have already been linked to the disease. SQTS1 is caused by a mutation in the *KCNH2* gene,[42] leading to a gain-of-function substitution (N588K) in the α subunit of the HERG (I_{Kr}) channel; loss-of-function mutations in this gene cause the second genetic form of LQTS, LQT2. SQT2 is caused by a mutation in the *KCNQ1* gene,[43] which leads to a gain-of-function substitution (V307L) in the α subunit of the K$_V$LQT1 (I_{Ks}) channel; loss-of-function mutations in this gene cause the first genetic form of LQTS (LQT1).

Priori and colleagues[44] have identified a new variant, SQTS3, which is characterized by asymmetrical T waves, and a defect in the *KCNJ2* gene that causes a significant increase in the outward component of the I-V relation of I_{K1}. The ECG pattern in the two affected family members was clearly different from those previously reported in patients affected by SQTS.[41-43] In addition, the screening of the *KCNJ2* gene encoding the cardiac inward rectifier Kir2.1 channel disclosed the presence of a single base-pair mutation, resulting in a D172N substitution located in the second transmembrane region of the channel.

The identification of the short QT syndrome has highlighted the concept that genetic abnormalities leading to gain-of-function mutations in specific potassium channels might predispose to the development of tachyarrhythmias and sudden cardiac death. The studies discussed here provide novel and useful insights into the molecular mechanisms of arrhythmias in SQTS patients and possibly also in large numbers of patients affected by unexplained idiopathic VF.[40,44]

Conclusions

The experiments discussed in this chapter were designed to identify the mechanism of cardiac fibrillation, which is a major cause of morbidity and mortality in the United States. Evidence is presented in support of the idea that understanding the mechanisms of wave break and wavelet formation in cardiac fibrillation requires detailed knowledge of the molecular and ionic mechanisms underlying cardiac cell excitation and its frequency dependence, in which membrane potassium channels play important roles. In the nonischemic ventricles, the interplay between the inward-rectifying properties of I_{K1}, the slow-gating kinetics of I_{Ks}, and the activation and inactivation properties of the sodium inward current and the L-type calcium current provides the necessary foundation for such frequency dependence as well as for wave break formation.

We have focused on the effects of separately changing the levels of expression of I_{K1} and I_{Ks} in two different experimental models as an initial approach to providing insight into such a complex phenomenon. Specifically, the data presented tested the hypothesis that I_{K1} and I_{Ks} are key mediators and modulators of fibrillation. The results demonstrate the importance of I_{K1} in the control of the stability and frequency of reentry and of I_{Ks} as a mediator of fibrillatory conduction. Validation of this hypothesis provides the framework for an ionic basis of fibrillation that might lead to the development of more effective therapies for preventing sudden cardiac death, using either novel drugs or gene therapy.

References

1. Myerburg RJ, Spooner PM: Opportunities for sudden death prevention: Directions for new clinical and basic research. Cardiovasc Res 50:177-185, 2001.
2. Zipes DP, Wellens HJ: Sudden cardiac death. Circulation 98:2334-2351, 1998.
3. Jalife J: Ventricular fibrillation: Mechanisms of initiation and maintenance. Annu Rev Physiol 62:25-50, 2000.
4. Selfridge O: Studies on flutter and fibrillation. V. Some notes on the theory of flutter. Arch Inst Cardiol Mex 18:177-187, 1948.
5. Wiener N, Rosenblueth A: The mathematical formulation of the problem of conduction of impulses in a network of connected excitable elements, specifically in cardiac muscle. Arch Inst Cardiol 16: 1-61, 1946.
6. Allessie MA, Bonke FI, Schopman FJ: Circus movement in rabbit atrial muscle as a mechanism of tachycardia. III. The "leading circle" concept: A new model of circus movement in cardiac tissue without the involvement of an anatomical obstacle. Circ Res 41:9-18, 1977.
7. Krinsky VI, Biktashev VN, Pertsov AM: Autowave approaches to cessation of reentrant arrhythmias. Ann N Y Acad Sci 591:232-246, 1990.
8. Winfree AT: Electrical instability in cardiac muscle: phase singularities and rotors. J Theor Biol 138:353-405, 1989.
9. Jalife J, Berenfeld O: Molecular mechanisms and global dynamics of fibrillation: An integrative approach to the underlying basis of vortex-like reentry. J Theor Biol 230:475-487, 2004.
10. Beaumont J, Jalife J: Rotors and spiral waves in 2 dimensions. In Zipes D, Jalife J (eds): Cardiac Electrophysiology: From Cell to Bedside, 3rd ed. Philadelphia, Saunders, 2000, pp 327-335.
11. Chen J, Mandapati R, Berenfeld O, et al: Dynamics of wavelets and their role in atrial fibrillation in the isolated sheep heart. Cardiovasc Res 48:220-32, 2000.
12. Garfinkel A, Qu Z: Nonlinear dynamics, spirals, and heart rhythms. In Zipes D, Jalife J (eds): Cardiac Electrophysiology: From Cell to Bedside, 3rd ed. Philadelphia, Saunders, 2000, pp 315-327.
13. Samie FH, Berenfeld O, Anumonwo J, et al: Rectification of the background potassium current: A determinant of rotor dynamics in ventricular fibrillation. Circ Res 89:1216-223, 2001.
14. Davidenko JM, Pertsov AV, Salomonsz R, et al: Stationary and drifting spiral waves of excitation in isolated cardiac muscle. Nature 355:349-351, 1992.
15. Rogers JM, Huang J, Melnick SB, Ideker RE: Sustained reentry in the left ventricle of fibrillating pig hearts. Circ Res 92:539-545, 2003.
16. Huang J, Rogers JM, Killingsworth CR, et al: Evolution of activation patterns during long-duration ventricular fibrillation in dogs. Am J Physiol Heart Circ Physiol 286:H1193-H1200, 2004.
17. Bayly PV, KenKnight BH, Rogers JM, et al: Spatial organization, predictability, and determinism in ventricular fibrillation. Chaos 8:103-115, 1998.
18. Huang J, Zhou X, Smith WM, Ideker RE: Restitution properties during ventricular fibrillation in the in situ swine heart. Circulation 110:3161-3167, 2004.
19. Nanthakumar K, Jalife J, Masse S, et al: Optical mapping of Langendorff perfused human hearts: Establishing a model for the study of ventricular fibrillation in humans. Am J Physiol Heart Circ Physiol 293(1):H875-H880, 2007.
20. Nash MP, Mourad A, Clayton RH, et al: Evidence for multiple mechanisms in human ventricular fibrillation. Circulation 114:536-542, 2006.
21. Nanthakumar K, Walcott GP, Melnick S, et al: Epicardial organization of human ventricular fibrillation. Heart Rhythm. 1:14-23, 2004.
22. Thomas SP, Thiagalingam A, Wallace E, et al: Organization of myocardial activation during ventricular fibrillation after myocardial infarction: Evidence for sustained high-frequency sources. Circulation 112: 157-63, 2005.
23. Kubo Y, Reuveny E, Slesinger PA, et al: Primary structure and functional expression of a rat G-protein–coupled muscarinic potassium channel. Nature 364:802-806, 1993.
24. Lopatin AN, Nichols CG: Inward rectifiers in the heart: An update on I_{K1}. J Mol Cell Cardiol 33:625-638, 2001.
25. Dhamoon AS, Pandit SV, Sarmast F, et al: Unique $K_{ir}2.x$ properties determine regional and species differences in the cardiac inward rectifier K^+ current. Circ Res 94:1332-1339, 2004.
26. Warren M, Guha PK, Berenfeld O, et al: Blockade of the inward rectifying potassium current terminates ventricular fibrillation in the guinea pig heart. J Cardiovasc Electrophysiol 14:621-631, 2003.
27. Li J, McLerie M, Lopatin AN: Transgenic up-regulation of I_{K1} in the mouse heart leads to multiple abnormalities of cardiac excitability. Am J Physiol Heart Circ Physiol 287(6):H2790-H2802, 2004.
28. Noujaim SF, Pandit SV, Berenfeld O, et al: Up-regulation of the inward rectifier K^+ current (I_{K1}) in the mouse heart accelerates and stabilizes rotors. J Physiol 578:315-326, 2007.
29. Beaumont J, Davidenko N, Davidenko JM, Jalife J: Spiral waves in two-dimensional models of ventricular muscle: formation of a stationary core. Biophys J 75:1-14, 1998.
30. Vaidya D, Morley GE, Samie FH, Jalife J: Reentry and fibrillation in the mouse heart. A challenge to the critical mass hypothesis. Circ Res 85:174-181, 1999.
31. Delmar M, Michaels DC, Jalife J: Slow recovery of excitability and the Wenckebach phenomenon in the single guinea pig ventricular myocyte. Circ Res 65:761-774, 1989.
32. Muñoz V, Grzeda KR, Desplantez T, et al: Adenoviral expression of I_{Ks} contributes to wavebreak and fibrillatory conduction in neonatal rat ventricular cardiomyocyte monolayers. Circ Res 101:475-483, 2007.
33. Delmar M, Glass L, Michaels DC, Jalife J: Ionic basis and analytical solution of the Wenckebach phenomenon in guinea pig ventricular myocytes. Circ Res 65:775-88, 1989.
34. Cabo C, Pertsov AM, Baxter WT, et al: Wave-front curvature as a cause of slow conduction and block in isolated cardiac muscle. Circ Res 75:1014-1028, 1994.
35. Sanguinetti MC, Jurkiewicz NK: Two components of cardiac delayed rectifier K^+ current. Differential sensitivity to block by class III antiarrhythmic agents. J Gen Physiol 96:195-215, 1990.
36. Stengl M, Volders PG, Thomsen MB, et al: Accumulation of slowly activating delayed rectifier potassium current (I_{Ks}) in canine ventricular myocytes. J Physiol 551:777-86, 2003.
37. Dobrev D, Graf E, Wettwer E, et al: Molecular basis of downregulation of G-protein-coupled inward rectifying K^+ current ($I_{K,ACh}$) in chronic human atrial fibrillation: Decrease in GIRK4 mRNA correlates with reduced IK,ACh and muscarinic receptor–mediated shortening of action potentials. Circulation 104:2551-2557, 2001.
38. Bosch RF, Zeng X, Grammer JB, et al: Ionic mechanisms of electrical remodeling in human atrial fibrillation. Cardiovasc Res 44:121-31, 1999.
39. Van Wagoner DR, Pond AL, McCarthy PM, et al: Outward K^+ current densities and Kv1.5 expression are reduced in chronic human atrial fibrillation. Circ Res 80:772-781, 1997.

40. Viskin S, Zeltser D, Ish-Shalom M, et al: Is idiopathic ventricular fibrillation a short QT syndrome? Comparison of QT interval of patients with idiopathic ventricular fibrillation and healthy controls. Heart Rhythm 1:587-591, 2004.
41. Gaita F, Giustetto C, Bianchi F, et al: Short QT syndrome: Pharmacological treatment. J Am Coll Cardiol 43:1494-1499, 2004.
42. Brugada R, Hong K, Dumaine R, et al: Sudden death associated with short-QT syndrome linked to mutations in HERG. Circulation 109:30-35, 2004.
43. Bellocq C, van Ginneken AC, Bezzina CR, et al: Mutation in the KCNQ1 gene leading to the short QT-interval syndrome. Circulation 109:2394-2397, 2004.
44. Priori SG, Pandit SV, Rivolta I, et al: A novel form of short QT syndrome (SQT3) is caused by a mutation in the KCNJ2 gene. Circ Res 96:800-807, 2005.

Mechanisms of Ischemic Ventricular Fibrillation 46

Alexey V. Zaitsev and Mark D. Warren

CHAPTER OUTLINE

Sudden cardiac death is a major cause of mortality in the rapidly expanding industrialized world. A common scenario of sudden cardiac death involves a coronary event leading to regional myocardial ischemia that precipitates ventricular fibrillation (VF). The onset of VF results in immediate collapse of the coronary circulation, leading to global myocardial ischemia. Global ischemia alters the dynamics of fibrillatory waves, culminating in asystole. Thus, sudden cardiac death is a *process* extended in time in which ischemic changes set the stage for the formation of ectopic triggers and reentrant ventricular tachycardia (VT), degeneration of VT into VF, and subsequent maintenance and evolution of VF dynamics. In this chapter we address critical mechanisms operative at each stage of VF, highlighting the most recent advancements in the context of more established knowledge and offering speculations where knowledge is still far from complete.

Ventricular Fibrillation Associated with Acute Regional Ischemia

Clinical Connection

Sudden cardiac death is the most common and often the first manifestation of coronary artery disease.[1] In a large fraction of cases, sudden cardiac death is caused by primary VF; that is, VF in the setting of acute ischemia and in the absence of heart failure.[1] In one study, more than 90% of cases of primary VF developed within 2 hours after onset of complaints.[2] However, these data were obtained in VF survivors who represented about 10% of the total primary VF population; 90% of sudden cardiac death victims do not reach the hospital alive.[3] In animal experiments, VF occurs in distinct phases (Ia, Ib, and II, reviewed by Janse and Wit[4]), and the majority of VF episodes occur within the first 30 minutes after coronary occlusion. The temporal distribution of VF with respect to the onset of ischemia in humans is not known. However, the earliest phases could have been missed in clinical studies.

Thus, in the majority of cases the prelude to VF is short, providing little opportunity for planned intervention. It is highly desirable to identify risk factors specific for primary VF during acute myocardial infarction (MI). Unfortunately, conventional cardiovascular risk factors, the infarct size and localization, or the general medical history do not predict primary VF.[2,5] Recent studies indicate that the risk of primary VF is determined by the magnitude of changes in the ST segment (cumulative ST deviation[2] or ST elevation[5]) and familial history of sudden cardiac death.[2] Although the familial history is a clinically valuable tool for individualized risk stratification, it offers little help for identifying the immediate precipitating event[6] that triggers VF. On the other hand, changes in the ST segment are directly linked to electrical heterogeneities in acute ischemia, which therefore remain the major factor of ischemic arrhythmogenesis and are discussed later.

Pathophysiologic Factors

Border Zones of Ischemia and Associated Heterogeneities

The largest heterogeneities in the regionally ischemic heart are associated with the border zone separating ischemic and nonischemic zones; these are partly determined by the presence or absence of collateral circulation.[4] The subendocardial border zone is possibly the main provider of electrical triggers largely due to the presence of a thin viable layer of Purkinje cells between the partially uncoupled and depolarized ischemic zone and well-oxygenated volume of intracavitary blood (see more about triggering mechanisms later). The epicardial border zone shows transient depression and subsequent recovery of excitability and conduction during the first 10 to 20 minutes of ischemia, which may be related to non-monotonic time courses of extracellular potassium ($[K^+]_o$) accumulation,[7] release of catecholamines,[4] or eventual uncoupling of the epicardial border zone from the ischemic core.[8] The partial and nonuniform uncoupling of the epicardial border zone is a potential substrate for reentry and VF during phase 1b (15-40 min) of acute ischemia.[8] The time course of electrophysiologic changes and the onset of inexcitability in the epicardial border zone, the most accessible and therefore most studied with all mapping modalities, vary between different studies, which may in part be related to varying experimental conditions on the epicardial surface (such as temperature and concentration of O_2 and CO_2 in the gaseous or fluid environment[9]).

The border zone gradients of $[K^+]_o$ and pH are the most relevant to VF. Hyperkalemia causes depolarization of the resting membrane potential, decrease in the conduction velocity, and shortening of the action potential duration (APD) but not of the effective refractory period, which is prolonged and extends beyond APD due to postrepolarization refractoriness.[10] Reduction of the resting membrane potential and delayed activation caused by increased $[K^+]_o$ in the ischemic zone provide conditions for the flow of injury current between the ischemic zone and nonischemic zone,[4] which might induce or promote spontaneous cellular activity, especially in Purkinje fibers (see more later). A sufficiently large volume of ischemic tissue with intermediate (8-13 mmol) levels of $[K^+]_o$ is necessary for induction of VF with premature electrical stimuli in phase Ia (2-10 min) of acute regional ischemia.[11]

Low pH (or high $[H^+]_i$) in the ischemic zone exaggerates many of the effects of high $[K^+]_o$ on the action potential, including depolarization, decrease in action potential amplitude, and slowing the action potential upstroke.[7] There is an intriguing and not yet fully understood link between CO_2 accumulation and elevation of $[K^+]_o$ early in ischemia,[9] which might be mediated through changes in $[H^+]_i$. This is especially relevant for the epicardial and the endocardial border zones, where diffusion of CO_2 through the surfaces can attenuate potassium accumulation, preserving excitability in the border zone while enhancing heterogeneity between the border zone and the ischemic zone. The extrusion of CO_2 may be especially efficient in papillary muscles having a larger surface per volume ratio than flat areas of the endocardial surface. This might explain the distinct activation patterns of papillary muscles during VF in the globally ischemic heart (see more later).[12]

Abnormalities of Calcium Handling

Alterations of intracellular calcium handling are commonly implicated in ischemic arrhythmias,[6] but this link has yet to be experimentally demonstrated. Triggered activity related to spontaneous Ca^{2+} releases from the sarcoplasmic reticulum (SR) depends on the degree of SR Ca^{2+} overload. The SR content is determined by the dynamic balance between Ca^{2+} release through ryanodine receptor (RyR) channels and reuptake via the SR Ca^{2+} adenosine triphosphatase (ATPase) (SERCA). During metabolic inhibition, both such processes are suppressed,[13] which can result in either increased or decreased SR load. However, even with increased SR load, the frequency of spontaneous Ca^{2+} releases is reduced in metabolic inhibition.[13] As ischemia progresses, inhibition of Ca^{2+} reuptake should invariably lead to reduced SR content, making spontaneous Ca^{2+} releases even less likely in the ischemic core.

On the other hand, appropriate conditions for spontaneous Ca^{2+} events can exist in the border zone. Tsujii and colleagues[14] imaged Ca^{2+}-sensitive fluorescence in border zone cardiomyocytes 2 hours after coronary occlusion using a high-resolution confocal system. In this study, cells adjacent to the infarcted area showed high static level of fluorescence without any Ca^{2+} transients, indicating severe Ca^{2+} overload with completely halted SR Ca^{2+} cycling. Cells surrounding the Ca^{2+} overloaded cells exhibited slow Ca^{2+} waves asynchronous with the ventricular complexes observed in the electrocardiogram (ECG), which, however, rarely crossed cell boundaries. Further toward the normal myocardium there was a mixture of cells showing spontaneous Ca^{2+} waves and those showing normal Ca^{2+} transients. Thus, within a thin rim of the border zone, there is a large heterogeneity of the Ca^{2+} response at the spatial scale of individual cells. Sharp differences in Ca^{2+} response across the border zone may be determined in part by a gradient in pH. Acidosis alters Ca^{2+} transient as a net result of complex interactions between protons and a variety of intracellular processes.[15] Due to low H^+_i mobility in ventricular myocytes, the pH gradient across the border zone may be very steep, which can create a substrate for induction of large and stable spatial heterogeneities in Ca^{2+} transients.[16]

The pioneering study by Tsujii and colleagues[14] leaves many important questions unanswered, however. First, it would be important to know whether the cells exhibiting spontaneous Ca^{2+} waves are electrically excitable and how the spontaneous Ca^{2+} waves in these cells affect the action potential. Second, it would be important to study earlier, more arrhythmogenic phases of ischemia.[4] A crucial question is whether at the earlier stages of ischemia Ca^{2+} waves at the border zone can cross cell boundaries and bring a critical number of cells to the excitation threshold, leading to a propagated response. These unanswered questions should motivate further studies in this direction.

Cellular Electrical Uncoupling

Several mechanisms have been implicated to explain cellular uncoupling during ischemia, including increased levels of intracellular Ca^{2+} and H^+, accumulation of lipid metabolites that might act as uncoupling agents, and dephosphorylation of the gap junction protein connexin43 (Cx43).[17] There is a temporal association among Cx43 dephosphorylation, the rapid phase of cellular uncoupling (as indicated by an increase in the tissue impedance), and outburst of VF incidence during phase 1b.[8,17] Reduced expression of Cx43 in mice accelerates the onset and increases the incidence, frequency, and duration of ventricular tachyarrhythmias after coronary artery occlusion.[17]

It has been shown that Cx43 dephosphorylation is directly linked to cellular adenosine triphosphate (ATP) levels in confluent monolayers of rat neonatal cariomyocytes.[18] Importantly, Cx43 dephosphorylation was not a passive consequence of high-energy phosphate depletion, because phosphorylation of the extracellular signal-regulated kinase (ERK) increased under the same conditions.[18] While the direct ATP sensor remains to be identified, it is intriguing that cellular uncoupling may be linked to the same metabolic signal as the opening of ATP-sensitive potassium channel ($I_{K,ATP}$). This might explain the correlation between the second phase of $[K^+]_o$ rise and cellular uncoupling[7] and implies that ATP depletion may be a direct precursor of enhanced arrhythmogenesis during this phase.[8]

Dynamics of Electrical Waves

Triggers

The most complete and direct information about the localization of initial ectopic excitations during acute regional ischemia has been obtained using three-dimensional mapping using multipolar plunge needle electrodes.[4,19,20] In dogs, the common observation is the predominance of focal origin of the first arrhythmic excitation in all types of arrhythmias (premature beats, nonsustained and sustained VT, and VF). Moreover, the majority of the premature excitations triggering VT and VF in the regionally ischemic canine heart emerge either from the subendocardium or more specifically from the subendocardial Purkinje network.[4,19,20]

A unique combination of conditions at the endocardium makes the subendocardial Purkinje network highly conducive to spontaneous activity during ischemia. Even under normal conditions, electrical coupling between the Purkinje network and the working myocardium is limited to discrete Purkinje-muscle junctions where the junctional resistivity is relatively high.[21] The Purkinje-muscle junction resistance further increases as the ischemia progresses concomitant with depolarization of the ischemic core. However, a thin (~500 μm) subendocardial layer of Purkinje and muscle cells remains relatively unaffected[4] due to the volume of well-oxygenated blood overflowing the endocardium. A large depolarizing injury current[4] can therefore develop between Purkinje and ventricular myocytes. A study using an isolated rabbit Purkinje cell coupled to an electronic cell showed that weak coupling to a moderately depolarized (−60 to −50 mV) myocyte *alone* was sufficient to induce spontaneous activity in the Purkinje cell.[22]

Although both Purkinje and working ventricular cardiomyocytes can develop early and delayed afterdepolarizations (EADs and DADs) when subjected to catecholamines and depolarizing injury current in the critical range of coupling resistances,[22-25] the relatively large membrane resistance of the Purkinje cells[22] makes them more conducive to development of triggered activity as well as spontaneous automaticity even under less severe conditions.[22,23] In any case, a critical role of partial uncoupling between the normal and ischemic zone in facilitation of ectopic activity at the border zone has been demonstrated in numerous experimental and numerical simulations of ischemic conditions,[25-27] which agrees well with the correlation between the phase of rapid uncoupling and the increased arrhythmogenesis during phase 1b of acute ischemia.[8]

The specific geometry of the endocardial border zone might also explain why triggers occurring there seem to be especially important for initiating VF. There is new evidence for a role of subendocardial ectopic activity in the *maintenance* of VF in a globally ischemic heart.[28]

Formation of Reentry and Wave Breaks

The classic paradigm of functional reentry involves a heterogeneous spatial distribution of the duration of refractory periods to set the conditions for unidirectional block and reentry. Clearly, the ischemic zone provides ample opportunity for this scenario (Fig. 46-1A), given that the refractory period is much prolonged in the ischemic region due to postrepolarization refractoriness. However, in order to initiate VF, a single reentrant wave front has to split into multiple wavelets. The role of the ischemic zone in this latter process may be limited, because reentrant circuits involving ischemic zone have a relatively long revolution time due to long refractory periods. As a result, the wave fronts emanating from reentrant circuits anchored in the ischemic zone activate the nonischemic zone at intervals that permit safe propagation of waves without breaking. It is possible that for a reentrant circuit to initiate VF, it has to detach from the ischemic zone and reside entirely in the nonischemic zone (see Fig. 46-1B). For example, in the study of Zhang and colleagues,[20] four out of five episodes of VF followed relatively long periods of VT initiated in the ischemic zone, yet the last two cycles preceding VF were due to intramural reentry in the nonischemic zone. During established VF, the sources with fastest frequency of excitation are located in the nonischemic zone, with a predominant direction of wave propagation from nonischemic zone to ischemic zone (see Fig. 46-1C left and center).[29]

The dynamics of spiral wave reentry in the ischemic zone and border zone remain far from understood. It is very difficult to simulate these conditions realistically given the multitude of different factors and the complex interplay between them, including the geometry of the ischemic zone and border zone. In general, spiral waves drift along the gradient of electrophysiologic properties toward the area with longer rotation period.[30] Because longer rotation periods occur within the ischemic

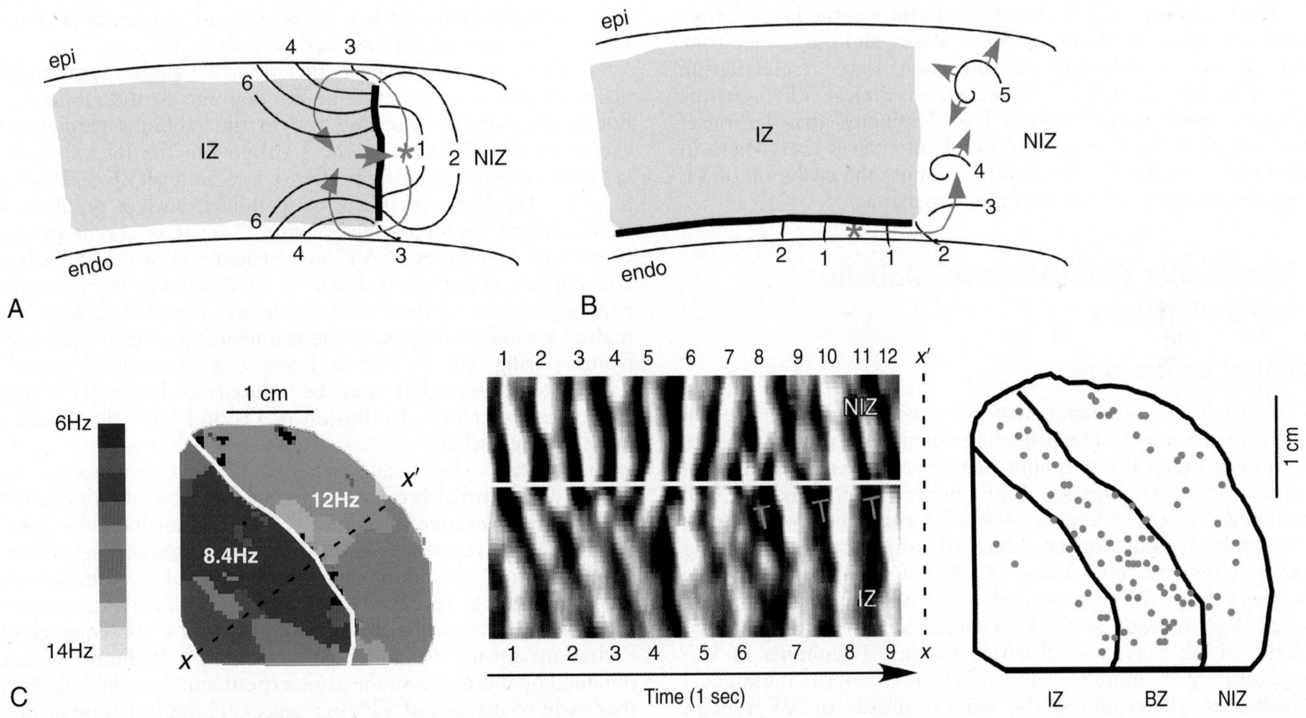

Figure 46-1 Mechanisms of reentry and wave fragmentation in regional ischemia. In **A** and **B,** *thin lines with numbers* represent consecutive positions of the wavefront (isochrones) at arbitrary time intervals. Thick lines indicate conduction block. **A,** A simplified diagram of functional reentry due to unidirectional block at the border zone (BZ). A premature ectopic impulse (*) occurring in the nonischemic zone (NIZ) is blocked at the BZ and invades the ischemic zone (IZ) only after the IZ recovers from prolonged refractoriness. The impulse then propagates slowly inside the IZ and reenters the NIZ when the NIZ recovers from refractoriness of normal duration. **B,** A diagram of a hypothetical mechanism for detachment of a wavefront from the IZ and subsequent formation of a spiral wave in the NIZ. Premature ectopic impulse formed at the endocardial BZ (*) propagates through the Purkinje network and does not invade the electrically uncoupled or unexcitable IZ. The ectopic wave experiences an abrupt increase in the electrical load as it expands into the bulk of the NIZ, leading to detachment of the wavefront[31,32] (isochrone 3) and formation of a spiral wave in the NIZ (isochrones 4-5). **C,** During ventricular fibrillation (VF), the sources remain in the NIZ, and the BZ provides a substrate for increased wave break. *Left,* A dominant frequency (DF) map during VF induced at 15 minutes of ischemia. The *white line* indicates the ischemic border. *Center,* A time-space plot constructed for the line *x-′′* perpendicular to the borderline. There are more activations per second in the NIZ than the IZ (ratio, 12/9), and the wave fragmentation occurs more frequently close to the borderline. *Right,* Points of wavebreak observed during 1.65 seconds of VF. (**C** is reproduced with modifications from Zaitsev AV, Guha PK, Sarmast F, et al: Wavebreak formation during ventricular fibrillation in the isolated, regionally ischemic pig heart. Circ Res 92:546-553, 2003).

region, this mechanism cannot account for eventual migration of a spiral wave into the nonischemic zone.

An interesting mechanism was offered by Xu and Guevara.[31] In their numerical study, pacing with increasingly short coupling intervals outside the simulated ischemic zone, rendered unexcitable due to high $[K^+]_o$, led to eventual detachment of the wave tip from the ischemic zone and a subsequent curling and formation of a spiral wave entirely in the nonischemic zone.[31] In the experimental study by Zhang and colleagues[20] the cycles immediately preceding the transition of VT into VF showed a reentrant circuit in the nonischemic zone, but the ischemic zone remained silent. The mechanism responsible for such a detachment may be conceptually similar to vortex shedding demonstrated by Cabo and coworkers in two-dimensional ventricular slices.[32]

One can speculate that premature excitations emerging in the subendicardial Purkinje network amid unexcitable or uncoupled ischemic core could propagate in the plane of the relatively unaffected Purkinje network with a high margin of safety, until it reaches the corner of the ischemic zone, where the wave front would suddenly experience a large increase in electrical load as it invades the full thickness of the nonischemic zone (see Fig. 46-1B). Such an expansion, hypothetically, could lead to the source-to-sink mismatch and detachment of the wave front with subsequent formation of a spiral wave[32] in the nonischemic zone, as shown schematically in Figure 46-1B. Unfortunately, this mechanism remains highly speculative. Clearly, more work has to be done to fully understand why only a fraction of abundant ectopic excitations occurring during acute ischemia[20] provide a proper trigger for VF.

Once a fast spiral wave reentry is formed in the nonischemic zone it tends to break into multiple waves, and the border zone can provide a substrate for increased wave fragmentation (see Fig. 46-1C, right).[29] However, in clinical VF, ischemic changes occur globally within 1 to 2 minutes after VF onset and will alter the dynamics of fibrillatory waves everywhere in the heart. The rest of this chapter examines the evolution of VF organization in the context of global ischemia.

Ventricular Fibrillation in Globally Ischemic Heart

Clinical Connection

Less than 5% of patients survive out-of-hospital cardiac arrest in the United States.[33] The probability of survival rapidly declines with time after VF onset, approaching zero after 10 minutes of cardiac arrest. The impact of VF duration on treatment is well recognized in the emergency-medicine community. For example, results of a randomized clinical trial suggest that performing cardiopulmonary resuscitation (CPR) before defibrillation may be more effective, as compared with immediate defibrillation, when VF duration exceeds 4 minutes.[33] Accordingly, two phases of VF were defined within the first 10 minutes of VF: electrical (0–4 minutes) and circulatory (4-10 minutes).[33] Mechanisms determining the clinical phases of VF remain virtually unknown.

Evolution of the Dynamics of Ventricular Fibrillation in Globally Ischemic Heart

The dynamics of electrical activity during VF undergo rapid changes with time after onset of VF. Using high-speed cinematography, Wiggers[34] described four different stages of VF: undulatory or tachysystolic, lasting for a second or two; convulsive incoordination, which lasts from 15 to 40 seconds; tremulous incoordination, lasting 2 to 3 minutes; and atonic fibrillation, which usually develops 2 to 5 min after the onset of VF. Wiggers's classification was revisited by several groups based on information obtained with high-resolution electrical or optical mapping.

Huang and colleagues[35] distinguished five phases (i-v) during the first 10 minutes of VF, based on quantitative analysis of the spatiotemporal dynamics of wave fronts extracted from multielectrode epicardial maps in open-chest dogs. Notably, they found a nonmonotonic evolution of activation patterns during long-duration VF, with a transient phase of increased periodicity and organization between 63 and 86 seconds after VF onset and a rapid decrease in organization in later phases of VF.[35] Huizar and coworkers[36] found similarly nonmonotonic evolution of VF in globally ischemic isolated porcine hearts and defined three phases of VF: relatively periodic (<1 min), highly periodic (1-2 min) and aperiodic (>3 min). They emphasized markedly increased beat-to-beat fluctuations of the action potential amplitude and duration during the aperiodic phase of VF. The onset of the action potential instability was recognizable in the ECG as broadening of the ECG frequency spectrum.[36]

Continuous ECG recordings during long-duration VF in patients are expectedly scarce, but the one example we found[37] shows an evolution of the ECG spectrum qualitatively similar to the one recorded in the Huizar group's study, namely, the ECG spectrum was relatively narrow up to about 2 to 3 minutes of VF, at which point it suddenly became very broad. Thus, the onset of the aperiodic phase, the broadening of the ECG spectrum, and the onset of clinically defined circulatory phase of VF[33] occur approximately at the same time and might have a common cellular or metabolic mechanism relevant to worsening of resuscitation outcome after prolonged periods of VF.

The three-dimensional organization of VF changes dramatically with time of ischemia in the dog and in the rabbit, but not in the pig.[38] In the dog and in the rabbit, a gradient of excitation rate develops in the LV between the (faster) endocardium and the epicardium after 3 to 5 min of VF and ischemia.[38,39] However, in the porcine model, such a gradient is small and of the opposite direction,[38] or it is absent for up to at least 5 minutes of VF and ischemia (Warren, Shvedko, and Zaitsev, unpublished data). As an exception, the posterior papillary muscle in the left ventricle was reported to have the highest excitation frequency and the majority of reentrant wave fronts during VF in canine heart and in porcine heart.[12] The latter observation may be related to lower $[H^+]_i$ and $[K^+]_o$ due to facilitated diffusion of O_2 and CO_2[9] in papillary muscles (see earlier).

In the rabbit heart, late ischemic VF was characterized by repetitive epicardial breakthroughs, which most often occurred near the interventricular septum.[39] The highest local dominant frequency of repetitive epicardial breakthroughs correlated strongly with the dominant frequency of simultaneously recorded sites of endocardial temporal periodicity, suggesting that repetitive epicardial breakthroughs were a consequence of excitations arising from the endocardium.[39] Preliminary data obtained by this group in the same experimental model indicated that early recurrence of VF after successful defibrillation during global ischemia was associated with reactivation of repetitive epicardial breakthroughs after 1 to 3 ventricular escape beats, which suggests that the substrate of repetitive epicardial breakthroughs is resistant to defibrillation shocks.[40]

Cellular Factors in the Evolution of Ventricular Fibrillation

The mechanisms linking primary ischemic syndromes and VF evolution are largely unexplored and we can only provide speculations here, which we hope will motivate further investigations of this subject. In the further discussion, substantial interspecies differences should be kept in mind, because they complicate generalization of individual observations.

A transient increase in the organization of VF and stabilization of reentrant sources observed in the epicardial activation maps obtained in the dog[35] and in the pig[36] after 1 to 2 minutes of VF and ischemia may be explained by a rapid accumulation of extracellular K^+. Increased $[K^+]_o$ per se stabilizes rotors and might convert VF into monomorphic VT.[41] The endocardial and epicardial gradients of excitation rate in the dog and in the rabbit may be related to O_2, CO_2, $[K^+]_o$ and pH gradients across the endocardial border zone[4] and also to transmural gradients in the density of ionic currents (e.g., I_{to}, $I_{K,ATP}$) or intrinsic gradients related to the metabolic state[42] (e.g., the rate of anaerobic glycolysis or ATP levels, mitochondrial depolarization,[43] degree of $I_{K,ATP}$ channel activation). A gradient of metabolic properties could lead to a higher $[K^+]_o$ on the epicardium and could explain a transmural dispersion in tissue excitability and localization of VF sources to the endocardium in the dog and in the rabbit.[12,39]

Detailed mapping of extracellular potentials generated by Purkinje fibers and working ventricular myocardium on the endocardium indicated that under conditions of VF and prolonged ischemia, focal activity can arise from either Purkinje fibers or working ventricular myocardium and contribute to VF maintenance.[28] We can only speculate here that these focal activations reflect abnormal automaticity or triggered activity due to the same mechanisms (injury current, partial cellular uncoupling, catecholamines) that are operative in the endocardial border zone of regionally ischemic heart (see earlier), but reentry within the Purkinje fibers network or between the Purkinje fibers and the working ventricular myocardium cannot be ruled out.

However, in the porcine heart there is no indication that the endocardium harbors the dominant sources of VF, because the transmural gradient of excitation rate is insignificant (see earlier). In the porcine model, VF after 3 minutes of global ischemia is characterized by destabilization of the action potential, leading to a secondary decrease in spatiotemporal organization (Fig. 46-2).[36] Such destabilization may be related to the intrinsic

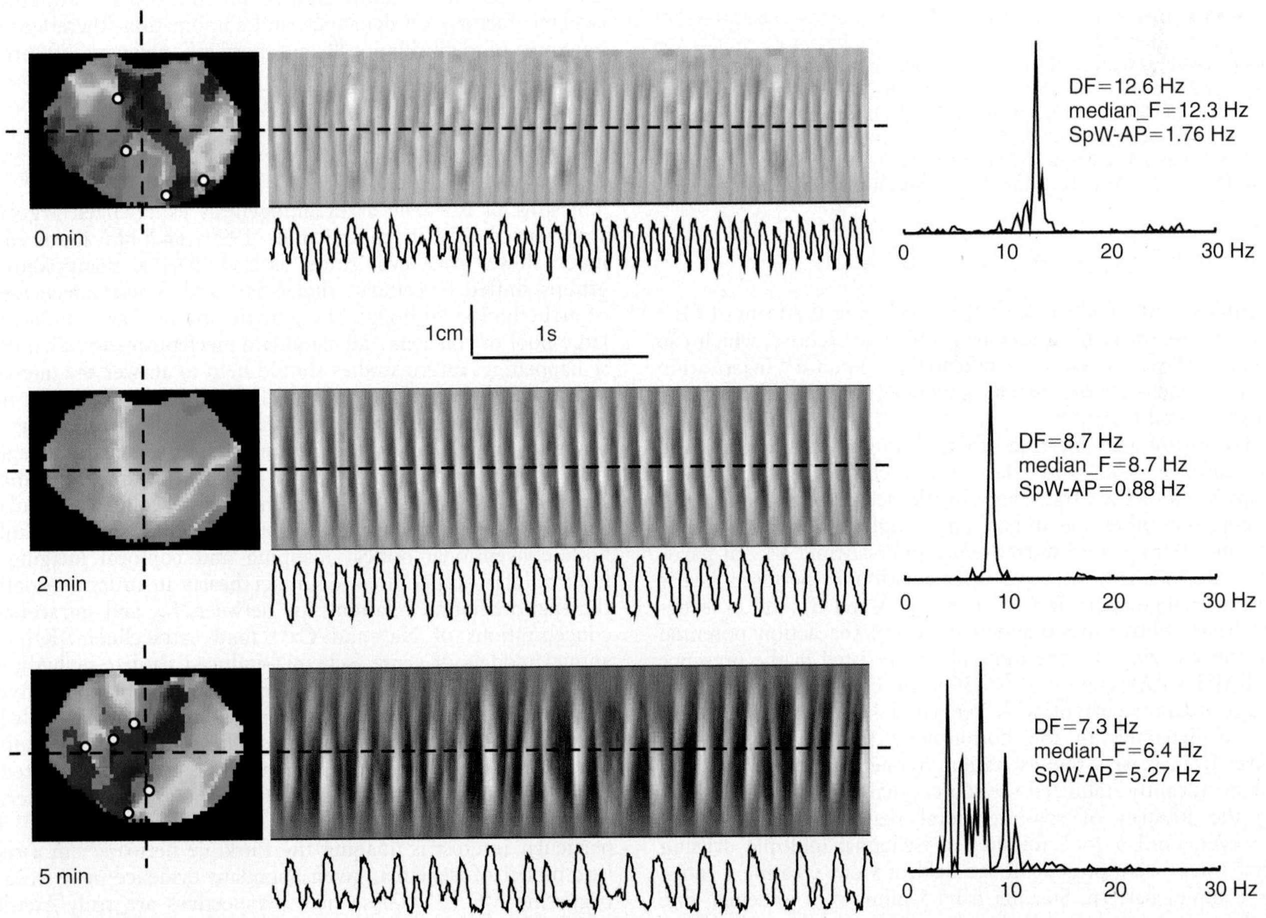

Figure 46-2 Spatiotemporal organization of ventricular fibrillation at different stages of global ischemia. *Top* to *bottom*, results obtained at 0, 2, and 5 minutes of ischemia. For each time point, we show the following data representations: *Left*, a snapshot of the action potential phase distribution. *White circles* indicate location of singularity points (wave breaks). *Top center*, A time-space plot constructed for the vertical line across the center of the mapped area *(vertical dashed line)*. *Bottm center*, The signal recorded from the central pixel. (*dashed line* in time-space plot). *Right*, the power spectrum for the signal recorded from the central pixel. (Reproduced with permission from Huizar, JF, Warren MD, Shvedko SG, et al: Three distinct phases of VF during global ischemia in the isolated blood-perfused pig heart. Am J Physiol Heart Circ Physiol 293:H1617-H1628, 2007.)

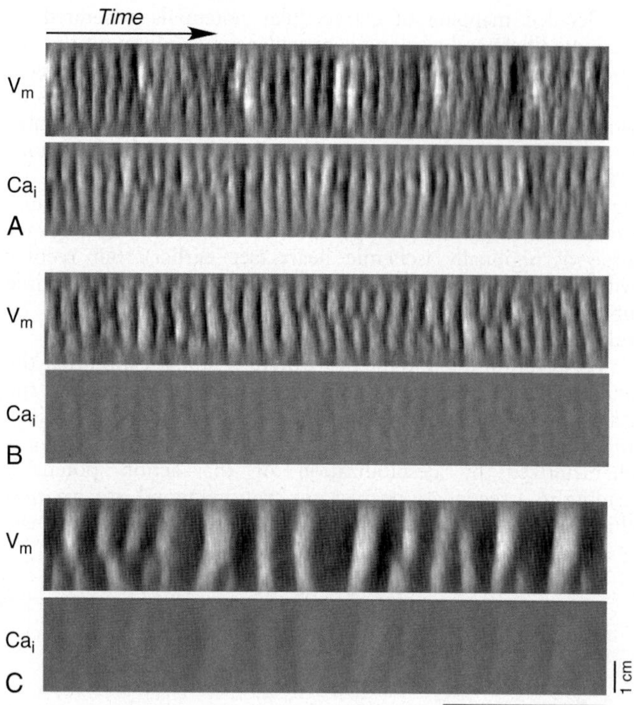

Figure 46-3 Effects of buffering Ca_i by BAPTA-AM on ventricular fibrillation (VF) dynamics in oxygenated and globally ischemic heart. Time-space plots of voltage-sensitive (RH237, V_m) and Ca-sensitive (Rhod2, Ca_i) fluorescence intensity in a selected line of pixels during VF in the absence of BAPTA-AM (**A**), in the presence of BAPTA-AM and normal perfusion (**B**), and in the presence of BAPTA-AM after 5 minutes of global ischemia (**C**). Note that suppression of Ca_i transient with BAPTA-AM does not prevent wave fragmentation either in normoxemic or in ischemic heart. Ca_i, intracellular Ca^{2+}; V_m, transmembrane potential.

dynamics of intracellular Ca^{2+} (Ca_i) cycling in the form of Ca^{2+} transient alternans and spontaneous SR Ca^{2+} release, which can influence the transmembrane potential (V_m) via Ca^{2+} inactivation of $I_{Ca,L}$ and inward current generated by the electrogenic Na^+-Ca^{2+} exchanger.[44]

To test the possible role of Ca_i cycling in the ischemic VF, we buffered Ca_i with fast Ca^{2+} chelator BAPTA-AM. Suppression of Ca^{2+} transients slightly decreased excitation frequency, but otherwise it had surprisingly little effect on V_m dynamics during both normoxemic and ischemic VF. In particular, the intensity of wave fragmentation in perfused hearts did not change appreciably[45] (Fig. 46-3A and B), and in ischemic hearts both wave fragmentation and the action potential instability during the aperiodic phase persisted in the presence of BAPTA-AM (see Fig. 46-3C). In contrast, blockade of L-type calcium current with verapamil had a dramatic effect on VF dynamics in the normoxemic and in the ischemic heart. It increased the excitation frequency almost two-fold and significantly stabilized the sources maintaining VF, increasing the lifespan of spatiotemporal periodicity (Fig. 46-4). However, until 5 to 7 minutes of ischemia, multiple drifting spiral waves were present in the field of view, creating a globally complex pattern. Starting from 5 minutes of ischemia, one of the sources stabilized, giving rise to a mother rotor pattern,[46] with fibrillatory propagation away from the source (see Fig. 4B and D). These results emphasize an important role of $I_{Ca,L}$ in the spiral wave dynamics, especially in ischemia, where blockade of $I_{Ca,L}$ abolishes the aperiodic phase[36] and stabilizes the dominant rotor. On the other hand, intracellular Ca^{2+} dynamics do not seem to influence VF dynamics either in normoxemic or in ischemic porcine heart. The BAPTA test also speaks against a significant contribution of DADs[47] in the maintenance of VF in the porcine model.

In general, the possibility of a contribution from triggered endocardial activity to the maintenance of VF may depend on the ability of the bulk of the ischemic myocardium to sustain fast reentrant circuits. As long as the tissue is viable enough to support rapid reentrant activations, the ectopic activity arising from the Purkinje network will probably be overridden by reentrant waves, making the Purkinje system a bystander during VF.[48] Conversely, if reentrant circuits become very slow or nonsustainable, then the ectopic activity will get the chance to spread into the midmyocardium, where it will undergo fragmentation and intermittent conduction block as it propagates toward the epicardium.

These conjectures await experimental support. For one thing, it would be interesting to see how focal activations arising endocardially during VF in globally ischemic canine ventricle[28] respond to the pharmacologic interventions described earlier. In any case, an important conclusion from this analysis is that VF in the ischemic heart is different from VF in normoxemic heart and may be driven by different mechanisms (both reentrant and non-reentrant). Future studies should investigate the role of ischemic factors, VF dynamics, and combinations thereof in the outcome of defibrillation[40] and post-VF recovery of cardiac function.

Future Directions

The area of ischemic arrhythmogenesis experienced a golden age from the 1970s to the mid- 1990s and has advanced at much slower pace ever since, as the focus of many research groups shifted to cellular, molecular, and genetic mechanisms of arrhythmias. Although the genetic studies have produced a large pool of concepts and candidate mechanisms for what *could be* happening, future studies should help to answer the question what *is really* happening at the cellular level in the stages preceding VF in acutely ischemic heart, as well as following VF onset in the globally ischemic heart. In this regard, imaging studies at various spatial scales in intact heart preparations can provide a missing links among the subcellular-, cellular-, and tissue-level mechanisms. Future studies should employ both conventional optical mapping and confocal imaging in multicellular preparations or intact hearts in order "to define the spatiotemporal relationships between V_m and intracellular concentrations of Na^+ and Ca^{2+} (and extracellular $[K^+]_o$) in animal models of acute ischemia–induced cardiac arrhythmias and sudden cardiac death by simultaneously mapping transmembrane voltage and ion concentrations."[6] To that wish list we should add monitoring of metabolic state including indicators of mitochondrial inner membrane potential and redox state,[43,49] in lieu of the emerging role of mitochondrial criticality[49] in early ischemic changes and arrhythmogenesis.[43] Of particular interest is imaging the Purkinje network[50] in a realistic model of ischemia, given abundant evidence of its role in triggering VF.[19,28] These new perspectives are truly exciting and we hope that the next edition of this book will feature a chapter with the intriguing title "Cardiac Death Under the Microscope".

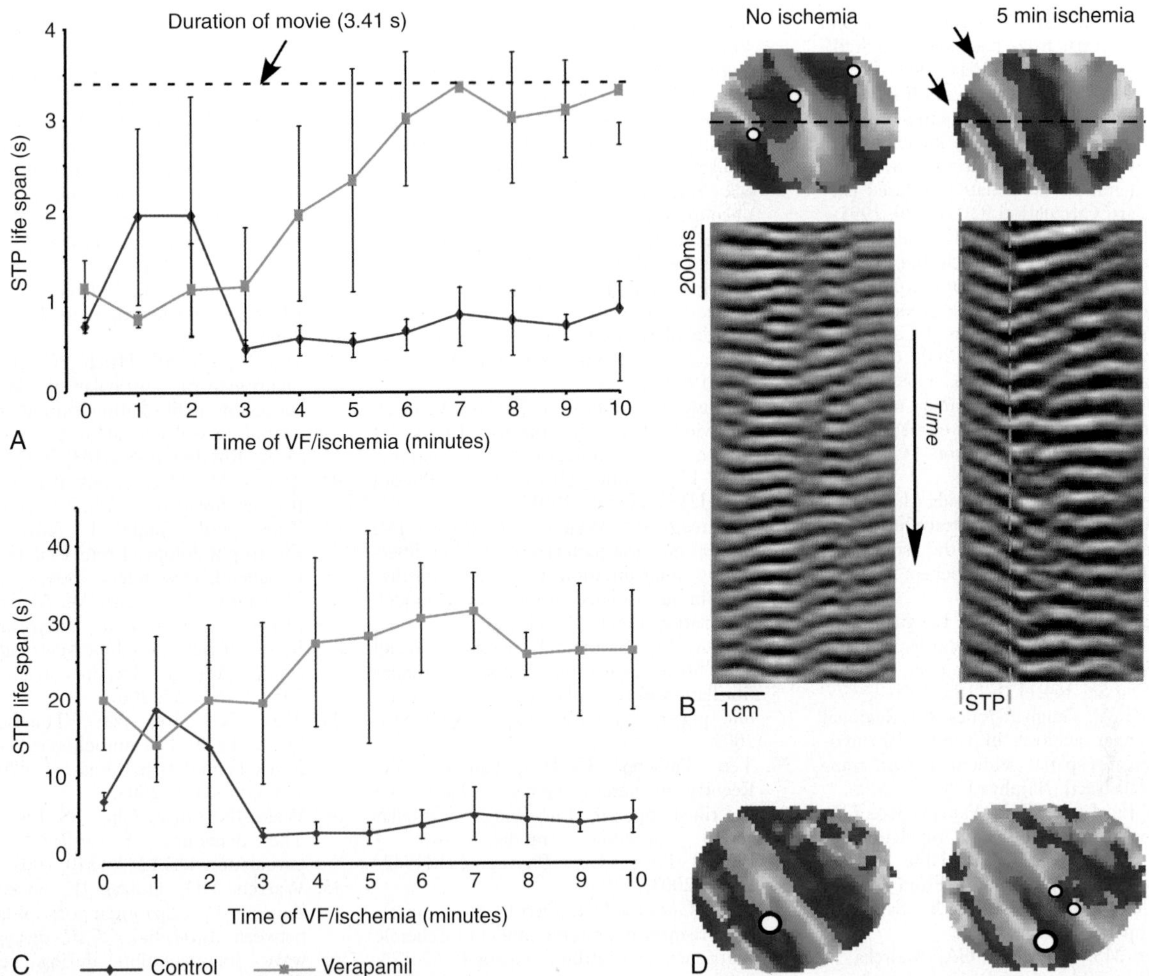

Figure 46-4 Effects of blockade of L-type Ca^{2+} current ($I_{Ca,L}$) by verapamil on ventricular fibrillation (VF) dynamics in perfused versus globally ischemic heart. **A**, The life span of spatiotemporal periodicity (STP) during VF as a function of ischemia duration in the absence *(blue)* and the presence *(red)* of verapamil. **B**, Snapshots of the action potential phase distribution (*top*) and time-space plots (*bottom*) constructed for the centermost row of pixels indicated by a *dashed line* in the phase maps. These data are shown for normal perfusion (*right*) and 5 minutes of global ischemia (*left*). During normal perfusion, multiple drifting spiral waves are present in the phase map *(white circles)*, but there are no fixed STP sites. In contrast, at 5 minutes of ischemia there is a fixed area of STP on the left side of the field, which sheds trains of waves *(short arrows)* undergoing fragmentation on the right side of the field. The area of STP is demarcated with *red dashed lines* in the time-space plot. **C**, Same as **A**, but expressed in number of activation cycles. Verapamil dramatically increases the life span of STP during ischemia and establishes a stable dominant source of VF after 5 to 7 minutes of ischemia. **D**, Two phase snapshots (25 ms apart) from a different experiment showing a stable spiral wave source *(large white circle)* in the middle of the field in the presence of verapamil (5 minutes of ischemia). The *right* snapshot shows the emergence of two wave breaks *(small circles)* on the arm of the spiral wave. Such wave breaks gave rise to short-living daughter wavelets, but the mother rotor persisted throughout the entire movie (~65 cycles).

References

1. Zipes DP, Wellens HJ: Sudden cardiac death. Circulation 98:2234-2251, 1998.
2. Dekker LRC, Bezzina CR, Henriques JPS, et al: Familial sudden death is an important risk factor for primary ventricular fibrillation: A case-control study in acute myocardial infarction patients. Circulation 114:1140-1145, 2006.
3. de Vreede-Swagemakers JJ, Gorgels APM, van Ree JW, et al: Out-of-hospital cardiac arrest in the 1990's: A population-based study in the Maastricht area on incidence, characteristics and survival. J Am Coll Cardiol 30:1500-1505, 1997.
4. Janse MJ, Wit AL: Electrophysiological mechanisms of ventricular arrhythmias resulting from myocardial ischemia and infarction. Phys Rev 69:1049-1169, 1989.
5. Gheeraert PJ, De Buyzere ML, Taeymans YM, et al: Risk factors for primary ventricular fibrillation during acute myocardial infarction: A systematic review and meta-analysis. Eur Heart J 27:2499-2510, 2006.
6. Rubart M, Zipes DP: Mechanisms of sudden cardiac death. J Clin Invest 115:2305-2315, 2005.
7. Cascio WE, Johnson TA, Gettes LS: Electrophysiologic changes in ischemic ventricular myocardium: I. Influence of ionic, metabolic and energetic changes. J Cardiovasc Electrophysiol. 6:1039-1062, 1995.
8. de Groot JR, Coronel R: Acute ischemia-induced gap junctional uncoupling and arrhythmogenesis. Cardiovasc Res 62:323-334, 2004.
9. Cascio WE, Yan GX, Kleber AG: Early changes in extracellular potassium in ischemic rabbit myocardium. The role of extracellular carbon dioxide accumulation and diffusion. Circ Res 70:409-422, 1992.

10. Carmeliet E: Cardiac ionic currents and acute ischemia: from channels to arrhythmias. Phys Rev 79:917-1017, 1999.
11. Coronel R, Wilms-Schopman FJG, Dekker LRC, Janse MJ: Heterogeneities in $[K^+]_o$ and TQ potential and the inducibility of ventricular fibrillation during acute regional ischemia in the isolated perfused porcine heart. Circulation 92:120-129, 1995.
12. Pak HN, Kim YH, Lim HE, et al: Role of the posterior papillary muscle and Purkinje potentials in the mechanism of ventricular fibrillation in open chest dogs and swine: Effects of catheter ablation. J Cardiovasc Electrophysiol 17:777-783, 2006.
13. Overend CL, Eisner DA, O'Neill SC: Altered cardiac sarcoplasmic reticulum function of intact myocytes of rat ventricle during metabolic inhibition. Circ Res 88:181-187, 2001.
14. Tsujii E, Tanaka H, Oyamada M, et al: In situ visualization of the intracellular Ca^{2+} dynamics at the border of the acute myocardial infarct. Mol Cell Biochem 248:135-139, 2003.
15. Crampin EJ, Smith NP, Langham AE, et al: Acidosis in models of cardiac ventricular myocytes. Philos Transact A Math Phys Eng Sci 364:1171-1186, 2006.
16. Spitzer KW, Vaughan-Jones RD: Regional intracellular acidosis in ventricular myocytes creates spatial gradients in Ca^{2+} transients [abstract]. Biophys J 90:73a, 2006.
17. Saffitz JE, Lerner DL, Yamada KA: Gap junction distribution and regulation in the heart. In Zipes DP, Jalife J (eds): Cardiac Electrophysiology: From Cell to Bedside. Philadelphia, WB Saunders, 2004, pp 181-191.
18. Turner MS, Haywood GA, Andreka P, et al: Reversible connexin 43 dephosphorylation during hypoxia and reoxygenation is linked to cellular ATP levels. Circ Res 95:726-733, 2004.
19. Arnar DO, Bullinga JR, Martins JB: Role of the Purkinje system in spontaneous ventricular tachycardia during acute ischemia in a canine model. Circulation 96:2421-2429, 1997.
20. Zhang S, Skinner JL, Sims AL, et al: Three-dimensional mapping of spontaneous ventricular arrhythmias in a canine thrombotic coronary occlusion model. J Cardiovasc Electrophysiol 11:762-772, 2000.
21. Rawling DA, Joyner RW, Overholt ED: Variations in the functional electrical coupling between the subendocardial Purkinje and ventricular layers of the canine left ventricle. Circ Res 57:252-261, 1985.
22. Huelsing DG, Spitzer KW, Pollard AE: Spontaneous activity induced in rabbit Purkinje myocytes during coupling to a depolarized model cell. Cardiovasc Res 59:620-627, 2003.
23. Huelsing DJ, Spitzer KW, Pollard AE: Electrotonic suppression of early afterdepolarizations in isolated rabbit Purkinje myocytes. Am J Physiol Heart Circ Physiol 279:H250-H259, 2000.
24. Verkerk AO, Veldkamp MW, de Jonge N, et al: Injury current modulates afterdepolarizations in single human ventricular cells. Cardiovasc Res 47:124-132, 2000.
25. Pollard AE, Cascio WE, Fast VG, Knisley SB: Modulation of triggered activity by uncoupling in the ischemic border A model study with phase 1b–like conditions. Cardiovasc Res 56:381-392, 2002.
26. Saiz J, Ferrero JM Jr, Monserrat M, et al: Influence of electrical coupling on early afterdepolarizations in ventricular myocytes. IEEE Trans Biomed Eng 46:138-147, 1999.
27. Arutunyan A, Pumir A, Krinsky V, et al: Behavior of ectopic surface: Effects of β-adrenergic stimulation and uncoupling. Am J Physiol Heart Circ Physiol 285:H2531-H2542, 2003.
28. Tabereaux PB, Walcott GP, Rogers JM, et al: Activation patterns of Purkinje fibers during long-duration ventricular fibrillation in an isolated canine heart model. Circulation 116:1113-1119, 2007.
29. Zaitsev AV, Sarmast F, Kolli A, et al: Wavebreak formation during ventricular fibrillation in the isolated, regionally ischemic pig heart. Circ Res 92(5):546-553, 2003.
30. Ten Tusscher KHWJ, Panfilov AV: Reentry in heterogeneous cardiac tissue described by the Luo-Rudy ventricular action potential model. Am J Physiol Heart Circ Physiol 284:H542-H548, 2003.
31. Xu A, Guevara MR: Two forms of spiral-wave reentry in an ionic model of ischemic ventricular myocardium. Chaos 8:157-174, 1998.
32. Cabo C, Pertsov AM, Davidenko JM, et al: Vortex shedding as a precursor of turbulent electrical activity in cardiac muscle. Biophys J 70:1105-1111, 1996.
33. Hong MF, Dorian P: Update on advanced life support and resuscitation techniques. Arrhythmias. Curr Opin Cardiol 20:1-6, 2005.
34. Wiggers CJ, Bell JR, Paine M: Studies of ventricular fibrillation caused by electric shock. II. Cinematographic and electrocardiographic observations of the natural process in the dog's heart: Its inhibition by potassium and the revival of coordinated beats by calcium. Am Heart J 5:351-365, 1930.
35. Huang J, Rogers JM, Killingsworth CR, et al: Evolution of activation patterns during long-duration ventricular fibrillation in dogs. Am J Physiol Heart Circ Physiol 286:H1193-H1200, 2004.
36. Huizar JF, Warren MD, Shvedko AG: Three distinct phases of VF during global ischemia in the isolated blood-perfused pig heart. Am J Physiol Heart Circ Physiol 293:H1617-H1628, 2007.
37. Martin DR, Brown CG, Dzwonczyk R: Frequency analysis of the human and swine electrocardiogram during ventricular fibrillation. Resuscitation 22:85-91, 1991.
38. Newton JC, Smith WM, Ideker RE: Estimated global transmural distribution of activation rate and conduction block during porcine and canine ventricular fibrillation. Circ Res 94:836-842, 2004.
39. Wu TJ, Lin SF, Hsieh YC, et al: Ventricular fibrillation during no-flow global ischemia in isolated rabbit hearts. J Cardiovasc Electrophysiol 17:1112-1120, 2006.
40. Wu TJ, Lin SF, Hsieh YC, et al: Early recurrence of ventricular fibrillation after successful defibrillation during global ischemia in isolated rabbit hearts [abstract]. Heart Rhythm 4(5S):S163, 2007.
41. Zaitsev AV: Mechanisms of ischemic ventricular fibrillation: Who's the killer? In Zipes DP, Jalife J (eds): Cardiac Electrophysiology: From Cell to Bedside. Philadelphia, Saunders, 2004.
42. Michailova A, Lorentz W, McCulloch A: Modeling transmural heterogeneity of K_{ATP} current in rabbit ventricular myocytes. Am J Physiol Cell Physiol 293:C542-C557, 2007.
43. Akar FG, Aon MA, Tomaselli GF, O'Rourke B: The mitochondrial origin of postischemic arrhythmias. J Clin Invest 115:3527-3535, 2005.
44. Weiss JN, Qu Z, Chen PS, Lin SF, et al: The dynamics of cardiac fibrillation. Circulation 112:1232-1240, 2005.
45. Warren MD, Huizar JF, Shvedko AG, Zaitsev AV: Spatiotemporal relationship between intracellular Ca^{2+} dynamics and wave fragmentation during ventricular fibrillation in isolated blood-perfused pig hearts. Circ Res 101:E90-E101, 2007.
46. Jalife J, Berenfeld O: Molecular mechanisms and global dynamics of fibrillation: An integrative approach to the underlying basis of vortex-like reentry. J Theor Biol 21:475-487, 2004.
47. Marban E, Robinson SW, Wier WG: Mechanisms of arrhythmogenic delayed and early afterdepolarizations in ferret ventricular muscle. J Clin Invest 78:1185-1192, 1986.
48. Berenfeld O, Jalife J: Purkinje-muscle reentry as a mechanism of polymorphic ventricular arrhythmias in a 3-dimensional model of the ventricles. Circ Res 82:1063-1077, 1998.
49. Aon MA, Cortassa S, Akar FG, O'Rourke B: Mitochondrial criticality: A new concept at the turning point of life or death. Biochim Biophys Acta 1762:232-240, 2006.
50. Hamamoto T, Tanaka H, Mani H, et al: In situ Ca^{2+} dynamics of Purkinje fibers and its interconnection with subjacent ventricular myocytes. J Mol Cell Cardiol 38:561-569, 2005.

Insight into Mechanisms of Ventricular Tachycardia from Isolated Wedge Preparations

47

JIASHIN WU, HIROSHI MORITA, AND DOUGLAS P. ZIPES

CHAPTER OUTLINE

Although it is well known that ventricular tachycardia (VT) can be initiated and maintained by rapid repetitive focal activation (e.g., early afterdepolarizations [EADs] and delayed afterdepolarizations [DADs]) and reentrant excitation, their triggering by acute events and interactions with proarrhythmic substrates in diseased ventricle are less clear. We have investigated the mechanisms of VT in isolated canine ventricular tissue models of ischemia and reperfusion, long QT, Brugada, and Andersen-Tawil syndromes. This chapter summarizes the mechanistic insights gained from these experimental studies.

Ventricles have electrophysiologic heterogeneity in the membrane densities of ion currents and in the shapes of action potentials (APs).[1] Compared to endocardial cells, epicardial cells have a greater transient outward K^+ current, I_{to}, a stronger ATP-sensitive K^+ current, I_{KATP}, and APs having a deeper phase-1 notch and larger phase-2 dome and a larger ischemia-induced shortening. The canine left ventricle has a lower density of the slow delayed rectifier K^+ current, I_{Ks}, in the midmyocardium than in the epicardium and endocardium, and the density of the rapid delayed rectifier K^+ current, I_{Kr}, is similar transmurally. The heterogeneic ion currents cause dispersion of AP and of repolarization, which normally serves physiologic functions of the heart. However, excessively large dispersion of repolarization in a diseased heart contributes to the occurrence of VT by promoting both spontaneous focal activations and reentry. Premature focal activations, which are commonly seen in diseased heart, can also interact with a conducting wavefront to cause reentry and VT without requiring a large dispersion of repolarization.

Ventricular Tachycardia Caused by Focal Activation in Proarrhythmic Substrates

A diseased ventricle (e.g., by gene mutations, coronary disease, or cardiomyopathies) can provide a proarrhythmic substrate with abnormalities in the function, density, or distribution of ion channels or in cellular and interstitial concentrations of ions, leading to abnormalities in ion currents, in AP, in tissue excitability, or in conduction. In a proarrhythmic substrate, acute events can easily induce focal activations, causing VT and ventricular fibrillation (VF). A net inward current during or after repolarization (e.g., in long-QT and Andersen-Tawil syndromes and when a cytosolic Ca^{2+} transient is longer than the repolarization of AP) can promote spontaneous ventricular activation in the form of EADs and DADs. Minor downregulation of the net repolarization current might not have identifiable effects on the duration of the AP, but it can reduce repolarization reserve, providing a proarrhythmic substrate in which an acute additional reduction of the net repolarization current can cause excessive delay of repolarization and focal activation. Severe abnormalities in ion currents can cause spontaneous focal activation in ventricular tissue in the absence of a clear trigger.

Ventricular Tachycardia Triggered by Acute Delay of Repolarization in a Proarrhythmic Substrate

We carried out two studies to explore the mechanisms of VT triggered by acute events that stressed repolarization but, by themselves, might not initiate arrhythmias.

It is well known that myocardial ischemia can induce persistent proarrhythmic remodeling even after sufficient reperfusion. In the first study, we created a proarrhythmic substrate by inducing 40 minutes of ischemia followed by reperfusion and mapped APs on the cut-exposed transmural surfaces of 10 isolated wedge samples of canine left ventricular free wall and compared them with ischemia-free wedge samples.[2] Eight wedges recovered well from ischemia, with return of both duration of AP and velocity of conduction back to normal values after 60 minutes of reperfusion. Subsequent perfusion with anemone toxin II (ATX-II, 20 nmol/L), a drug that delays the inactivation of Na^+ current (reduces the net repolarization current), prolonged AP durations significantly and induced EADs in all and spontaneous VTs in seven of the eight wedges. Focal EADs and reentry were responsible for 73% and 18% of the activations in the VTs (e.g., Fig. 47-1). Changes in the EAD foci and conduction pathways altered the contour of the transmural electrocardiogram (ECG) during VT. In comparison, all eight ischemia-free control wedges had less-prolonged duration of AP, less dispersion of repolarization, and no EADs or VT after the same ATX-II exposure. The exaggerated prolongation of AP duration by the ATX-II treatment indicated the presence of a low repolarization reserve in the postischemia wedges, which provided a proarrhythmic substrate for the observed EADs and VTs. Therefore, a brief episode of ischemia, even after apparent reperfusion recovery of AP and of conduction velocity, can cause long-lasting reduction of repolarization reserve with arrhythmic consequences.

In the second study,[3] we created a proarrhythmic substrate by continuous ATX-II (20 nmol/L) perfusion, which induced type 3 long QT syndrome (LQTS), and mapped APs on the transmural

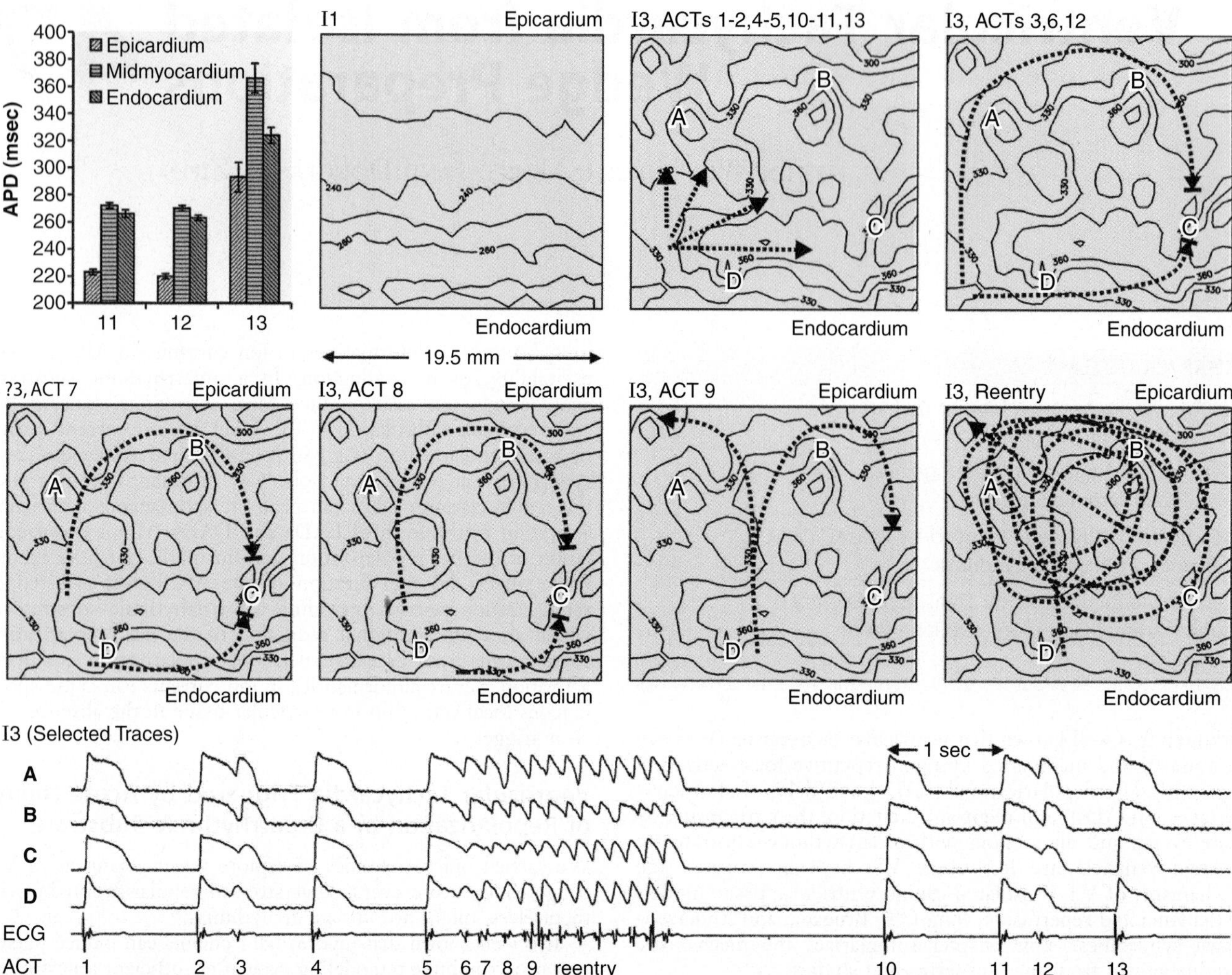

Figure 47-1 Prior ischemia promoted spontaneous early afterdepolarizations (EADs) and ventricular tachyarrhythmia (VT) in a canine left ventricular tissue having ATX-II-induced long-QT syndrome. The mean epicardial, midmyocardial, and endocardial action potential durations (APDs) before ischemia (I1), after ischemia (I2), and after ATX-II (I3) are displayed at *upper left*. The APD contour maps (I1 and I3s) show the transmural distributions of APD (in ms). Action potentials (I3, from the sites A-D) and the transmural electrocardiogram (ECG) are shown at the *bottom*, with activations (ACTs 1-9) and reentry indicated below. The APDs in the I3 contour maps are measured from ACT 4. ACTs 3 and 12 are EADs. ACTs 6 to 9 are focal EADs that triggered VT. The first I3 map shows the paced activations (ACTs 1, 2, 4, 5, 10, 11, and 13). The other I3 maps show the conductions of focal EADs and reentry (6 loops) (From Ueda N, Zipes DP, Wu J: Prior ischemia enhances arrhythmogenicity in isolated canine ventricular wedge model of long QT 3. Cardiovasc Res 63:69-76, 2004, with permission.)

surface of isolated wedge samples of canine left ventricular free wall before, during, and after 40 minutes of ischemia (LQTS-ischemia wedges). Controls were wedges having ATX-II perfusion only (LQTS-only wedges) or ischemia only (ischemia-only wedges). Ischemia initially prolonged (during the first 4 minutes) and then abbreviated APs. EADs occurred during the initial 4 minutes of ischemia in four of the 10 LQTS-ischemia wedges at a cycle length of 2000 ms but not in the LQTS-only and ischemia-only wedges or in any wedges at a cycle length of 1000 ms. Sixty minutes of reperfusion restored a normal duration of AP in the ischemia-only wedges but caused AP duration to overshoot its original duration, with increased dispersion in the LQTS-ischemia wedges. Reperfusion arrhythmia was sustained after 60 minutes of reperfusion in seven and six of the 10 LQTS-ischemia wedges but only in two and one of the 10 ischemia-only and in none of the LQTS-only wedges, at the cycle lengths of 1000 and 2000 ms, respectively. Therefore, additional prolonged AP duration during the initial minutes of ischemia can be sufficient for arrhythmogenesis in ventricles having LQTS, and an episode of ischemia is highly arrhythmogeneic in LQTS even after sufficient reperfusion due to cumulative suppression of repolarization reserve.

Clinical implications of these studies are that patients with reduced repolarization reserve due to drugs, inherited ion-channel abnormalities, or diseases might be at increased risk for arrhythmic episodes during or after periods of ischemia.

Proarrhythmic Substrate in Andersen-Tawil Syndrome

Andersen-Tawil syndrome is a channelopathy affecting the inward rectifier K^+ current, I_{K1}, and is associated with mild QT prolongation, large U waves, and frequent VT.[4,5] We investigated the mechanism of VT in isolated left ventricular free wall

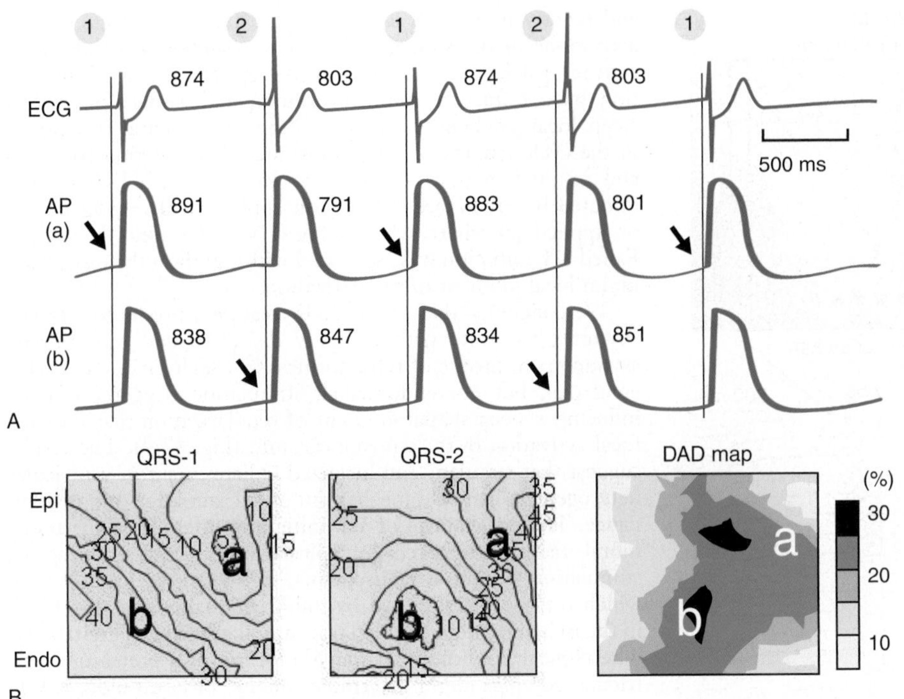

Figure 47-2 Examples of bidirectional ventricular tachycardia in an isolated wedge of canine left ventricular free wall having CsCl-induced (10 mmol/L) Andersen-Tawil syndrome. **A,** Traces of electrocardiogram (ECG) and action potential (AP) (at the foci) are shown. The numbers in the ECG and AP traces indicate the cycle length in milliseconds. The *arrows* in the AP traces indicate the earliest activations of each beat. **B,** Maps of activation isochrone (in ms) and of delayed afterdepolarization (DAD) amplitude (in percentage of the phase 0 of local AP) are shown. Alternating DADs from two endocardial foci (*a* and *b*) generated QRS alternans and triggered bidirectional ventricular tachycardia. $[K^+]_o$: 2.5 mmol/L. Endo, endocardium; Epi, epicardium. (From Morita H, Zipes DP, Morita ST, Wu J: Mechanism of U wave and polymorphic ventricular tachycardia in a canine tissue model of Andersen-Tawil syndrome. Cardiovasc Res 75:510-518, 2007, with permission.)

wedges that had Andersen-Tawil syndrome induced by I_{K1} blockade with CsCl (5-10 mmol/L).[6] We mapped APs on the transmural surface of the wedges at control, after CsCl, and after additional 0.15 μmol/L isoproterenol. I_{K1} blockade delayed late phase 3 repolarization and prolonged the AP, more so during low $[K^+]_o$ perfusion. Rapid pacing induced DADs in all low $[K^+]_o$ and in 71% of normal $[K^+]_o$ preparations after I_{K1} blockade. In all preparations, addition of isoproterenol caused DADs originating in the mid to endocardium that initiated VT. Migration of DAD foci resulted in multifocal VT. Alternating DADs at two foci resulted in bidirectional VT (Fig. 47-2). Delayed late phase 3 repolarization and DADs generated U waves. The clinical implication is that multifoci DADs may be responsible for VT in Andersen-Tawil syndrome.

Dynamics of Ventricular Heterogeneity As a Proarrhythmic Substrate

Differences in the distribution of ion channels cause heterogeneity of ion currents and, consequently, heterogeneity in APs and in their responses to modulating factors. In addition, nonuniform dynamic factors, such as focal activation, collision of activation wavefronts, and differences in refractory periods can further enhance the heterogeneity of APs, leading to transient and localized steep gradients of repolarization and conduction disturbances. New focal activations can occur when a transiently formed steep local gradient of repolarization supplies sufficient intercellular current to reactivate postrefractory cells downstream to the gradient. A dynamically changing pattern of repolarization also provides functional conduction block for initiating reentry. Repetitive focal activations and reentry in association with constantly changing pathways of conduction and instability in the wavefront can lead to polymorphic VT and VF.

Proarrhythmic Substrate with Functional Exaggeration of Heterogeneity

A distinct group of midmyocardial M cells in the ventricular wall, which have exceedingly long duration of AP during long cycle length activations,[1,7] have been reported to contribute to the T and U waves in ECG, to the dispersion of repolarization, and to the initiation of VT. However, M cells were not found in some studies.[7,8] We recently attempted to reconcile these different observations by demonstrating that the M cell behavior is a functional expression of ventricular repolarization heterogeneity.[9]

We mapped AP durations on the transmural surfaces of left ventricular free wall wedges during Na^+ current modification with ATX-II. Before ATX-II, the layer of cells having the longest mean AP duration (APD_L layer) was in the (sub)endocardium. ATX-II prolonged the AP duration heterogeneously (mid-myocardium > endocardium > epicardium) and moved the APD_L layer progressively from the endocardium deeper into the midmyocardium (e.g., Fig. 47-3). We detected M cells (statistically significant longer durations of AP in the APD_L layer than in the endocardium and epicardium) in 18 wedges exposed to at least 5 nmol/L ATX-II but not in 18 wedges having up to 2.5 nmol/L ATX-II. Therefore, the occurrence and location of M cells changed, depending on experimental conditions.

We also evaluated the presence of M cells in canine ventricular septum.[10] In contrast to ventricular free wall, none of the 22 tested septum wedges showed preferential midmyocardial prolongation of AP duration under the same experimental conditions, although there was transseptal gradient of AP duration, with the longest in the left ventricular endocardium and shortest in the right ventricular endocardium. Therefore, in contrast to the left ventricular free wall, we were not able to demonstrate the M cell phenotype in the canine ventricular septum.

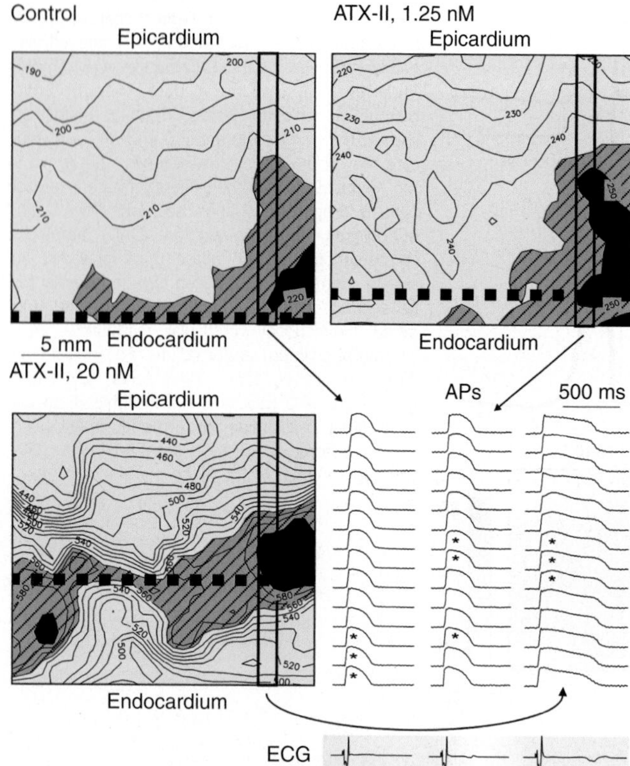

Figure 47-3 Functional M cell behavior in canine left ventricular free wall. The longest action potential durations (APDs) have moved to deeper positions with increasing concentrations of anemone toxin II (ATX-II) (0, 1.25, and 20 nmol/L). The isochronal maps show the transmural distributions of APDs (in ms) with the diagonal hatch lines and solid black highlighting the regions of longer and longest APDs. The *thick dashed lines* indicate the APD_L (longest mean-APD) layer. Selected columns of action potentials (APs) are displayed at *lower right;* *s indicate the longest three APDs. Endocardial pacing cycle length, 1000 ms. Mapping area: 19.5 × 17.0 mm^2. The longest APDs are mostly in the (sub)endocardium during control and appeared as islands in the midmyocardium after 20 nmol/L ATX-II. ECG, electorcardiogram. (From Ueda N, Zipes DP, Wu J: Functional and transmural modulation of M cell behavior in canine ventricular wall. Am J Physiol Heart Circ Physiol 287:H2569-H2574, 2004, with permission.)

Ventricular Tachycardia Triggered by Transient Steep Local Gradient of Repolarization

Premature activation in the epicardium is more likely to initiate R-on-T extrasystoles causing VT than similar endocardial activation, especially in ventricular tissue with prolonged duration of AP.[11] To explore the mechanism, we tested the hypothesis that premature epicardial stimulation transiently increased the dispersion of repolarization, leading to VT.[12] We mapped APs on the transmural surfaces of isolated canine ventricular tissue models of LQTS (created with ATX-II).

These LQTS wedges had asymmetrical transmural profiles of repolarization, earliest in the epicardium and latest in the deep subendocardium. Earliest excitable epicardial stimulation activated the epicardium, delayed repolarization in the still refractory midmyocardium, and caused steep local gradient of repolarization (between the midmyocardium and subendocardium). VT occurred 197 ± 72 ms (10 wedges) after epicardial stimulation from foci in the earliest repolarizing subendocardial region downstream to the steepest local spatial gradients of repolarization, and it was maintained by new focal activations and reentry in 5 of 18 tested wedges. The focal origin of new activations in the subendocardium was supported by the long activation delay, separation from the epicardial site of stimulation by a refractory midmyocardium, and association with a steep local gradient of repolarization. Transmural differences in the cycle lengths of activations altered conduction pathways and resulted in polymorphic VT. In contrast, VTs were not initiated by premature stimulation applied to the endocardium or applied anywhere when ATX-II was 2.5 nmol/L or less. Failed VT initiation was associated with significantly lower maximum local gradient of repolarization.

We concluded that the ATX-II treatment produced a proarrhythmic substrate with a highly dispersed and transmurally asymmetrical profile of refractoriness in which earliest excitable epicardial, but not endocardial, stimulation triggered VT by inducing a steep spatial gradient of repolarization that initiated focal activation in the subendocardium (Fig. 47-4). The results suggest that transient and localized enhancement of ventricular heterogeneity can be a mechanism of VT initiation and maintenance. This mechanism of VT initiation differs from the transmural reentry triggered by epicardial, but not endocardial, stimulation during acute ischemia, as shown on page 496, in which reentry was initiated by unidirectional conduction block in the ischemia-induced steep transmural gradient of excitability. The clinical implication is that the origin of a premature ventricular complex might determine whether or not it induces VT.

Ventricular Tachycardia Induced by Phase 2 Reentry in Brugada Syndrome

Phase 2 reentry, caused by conduction of the phase 2 dome of APs from regions having a dome to regions without a dome, can lead to VT. Phase 2 reentry occurs in ventricular substrates having significant dispersion of repolarization. We have recently investigated phase 2 reentry and VT in isolated canine tissue models of Brugada syndrome.

Brugada syndrome has multiple origins. Mutations in the sodium channel gene (SCN5A) [13] that hamper its opening have been identified in 18% to 30% of Brugada syndrome patients.[14] Reduction in sodium current contributes to VT in Brugada syndrome.[15] Mutations in the calcium channel gene were also found in some Brugada syndrome patients.[16] The absence of gene mutations in the majority of Brugada syndrome patients suggests that either unknown mutations or nongenetic remodeling also causes similar abnormalities in ion currents.

We reproduced the major electrophysiologic characteristics of Brugada syndrome in isolated right ventricular outflow tract (RVOT) tissues with pilsicainide, a sodium-channel blocker; pinacidil, a potassium-channel opener; and terfenadine, a combined sodium- and calcium-channel blocker, and investigated the mechanisms of VT in Brugada syndrome. Both pilsicainide and terfenadine reduce I_{Na}, simulating the sodium-channel dysfunction in Brugada syndrome. Terfenadine also reduces $I_{Ca,L}$, mimicking a mutated calcium-channel gene observed in some patients with Brugada syndrome and also an effect of testosterone. Pinacidil deepened the phase 1 notch of the AP, a characteristic of Brugada syndrome that is normally related to the sex hormones and thus represented the male predominance of Brugada syndrome.

We demonstrated the critical role of RVOT heterogeneity in the arrhythmogenesis in Brugada syndrome.[17] We mapped APs on the epicardium of 14 RVOT tissues and on the transmural surfaces of 15 pairs of RVOT and right ventricular anteroinferior (RVAI) tissues. Compared to the paired RVAI tissues, RVOT tissues have a deeper phase 1 notch of AP (especially

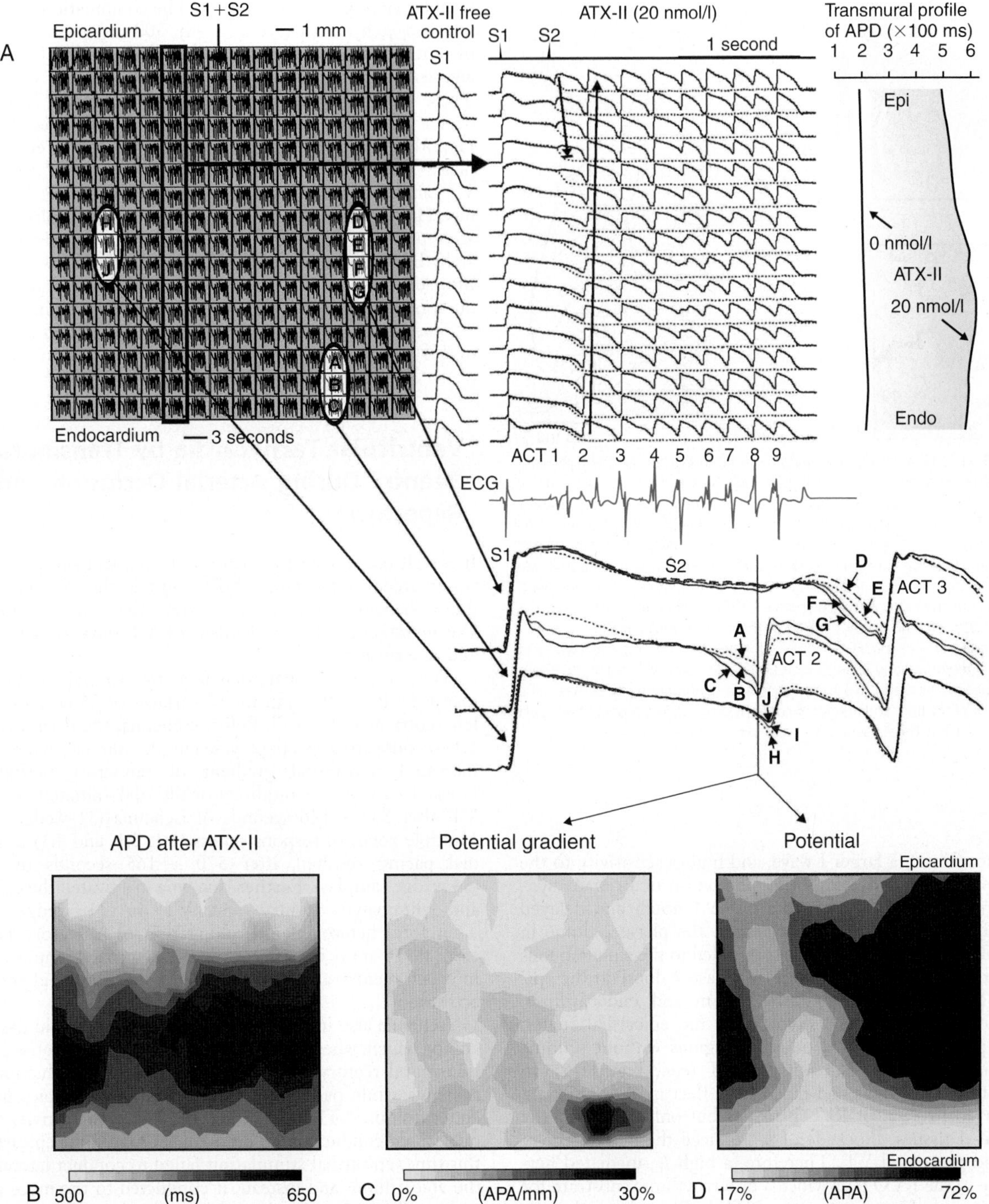

Figure 47-4 An example of ventricular tachycardia (VT) triggered by premature epicardial stimulation (S1-S1: 1000 ms, S1-S2: 400 ms) in a wedge of canine left ventricular free wall treated with anemone toxin II (ATX-II) (20 nmol/L). **A,** The mosaic shows VT activities at all recording sites (separated by the grids). Stimuli were applied to either the endocardium (S1, control) or epicardium (S1+S2, ATX-II). The framed column in the mosaic is expanded under ATX-II, with *solid lines* for VT and *dashed lines* for the S1-only action potentials (APs), and under ATX-II-free for the control APs. The transmural profiles of APD in the framed column are show at the *right*. The activations (ACTs 1-9) in VT are indicated beneath the ATX-II traces, along with the transmural ECG. Initial sections of selected traces (A-J, circled in the AP mosaic) are expanded at the *bottom*. **B,** Transmural distribution of APD (in ms) after ATX-II (same S1 activation as the dashed traces under ATX-II in A). **C** and **D,** Distributions of spatial gradient of membrane potential (percentage of the action potential amplitude (APA) per millimeter **(C)** and membrane potential (percentage of APA, **D**) immediately before (the vertical line under ATX-II in **A**) the first activation (ACT 2) in the VT. ATX-II prolonged APD and created a highly dispersed asymmetrical transmural profile of repolarization (**A** and **B**). Although the S2 activation (ACT 1) was blocked in the midmyocardium, it delayed the midmyocardial repolarization **(A)** and initiated new focal activation (ACT 2) in the subendocardial region of earliest repolarization **(D)** next to the steepest gradient of repolarization potential **(C).** ACT 2 conducted transmurally to the midmyocardium and epicardium (the *arrow line* in the APs under ATX-II in **A**) following the post-S2 sequence of repolarization. The next activation (ACT 3) arose from the midmyocardial region (*D-G* in the AP mosaic in **A**) with a similar mechanism. In contrast, nonfocal regions were associated with much smaller local dispersion of repolarization potential (**A** and **C**) or later repolarization **(D)**. The mapping area is 19.5 × 19.5 mm^2. (From Ueda N, Zipes DP, Wu J: Epicardial but not endocardial premature stimulation initiates ventricular tachyarrhythmia in canine in vitro model of Long QT syndrome. Heart Rhythm 1:684-694, 2004, with permission.)

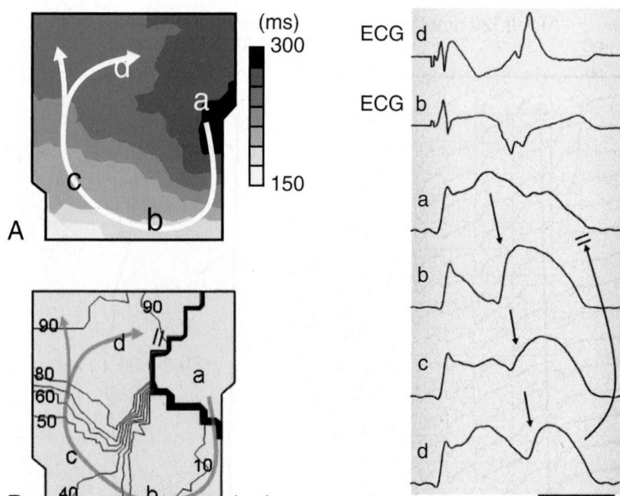

Figure 47-5 Phase-2 reentry in the epicardium of an isolated canine right ventricular outflow tract preparation having Brugada type electorcardiogram (ECG) (pilsicainide 12.5 μmol/L, pinacidil 10 μmol/L, terfenadine 2.0 μmol/L). **A,** Epicardial isochronal map of action potential duration (APD). Long APD region *(upper)* had a deep phase-1 notch and large phase-2 dome. **B,** Isochronal activation time map of a premature ventricular activation (PVA) beat. Phase-2 dome conducted (along the *arrow line*) from the region with long APDs *(a)* to the regions having shorter APDs *(b* and *c)*, then reentered the long APD region *(d)*, and finally blocked at the original region *(a)*. **C,** ECG and action potentials at sites *a-d*. ECG showed ST elevation with negative T wave in the long APD region *(d)* and large ST elevation in the short APD region *(b)* (From Morita H, Zipes DP, Morita ST, Wu J: Differences in arrhythmogenicity between the canine right outflow tract and anteroinferior right ventricle in a model of Brugada syndrome. Heart Rhythm 4:66-74, 2007, with permission.)

in the epicardium), a larger J wave, and higher sensitivity to the Brugada syndrome–inducing drugs. Induction of Brugada syndrome progressively deepened the phase 1 notch and delayed and enhanced initially, then abbreviated, the phase 2 dome in the RVOT epicardial AP. These changes led to the simultaneous presence of APs with and without the phase 2 dome in the epicardium but not in the midmyocardium and endocardium. Conduction of the phase 2 dome from the epicardial region having a prominent phase 2 dome to regions without a dome led to phase 2 reentry and initiated VT (e.g., Fig. 47-5). In contrast, the same drugs had much less effect in RVAI tissues. VT occurred in 47% of RVOT tissues but only in 7% of the paired RVAI tissues. Blockade of I_{to} reduced the heterogeneity of APs and prevented VT. Therefore, a high I_{to}-mediated heterogeneity in the RVOT provided a proarrhythmic substrate for the initiation of phase 2 reentry and VT in Brugada syndrome.

T-wave alternans can be a precursor of VT because it indicates repolarization instability. In the isolated RVOT tissue models of Brugada syndrome, bradycardia (cycle length, 2632 ± 496 ms, 19 tissues) induced adjacent regions having APs with alternating domes, with constant domes, and without domes in the epicardium and caused T-wave alternans.[18] The dynamic and heterogeneic APs during T-wave alternans augmented the dispersion of repolarization both within the epicardium and across the ventricular wall, leading to phase-2 reentry and VT.

Ventricular tachycardia in Brugada syndrome is temperature sensitive.[13,14] We investigated the mechanisms of temperature sensitivity of VT in isolated RVOT models of Brugada syndrome.[19] Compared to normal temperature (36.5° C), hyperthermia (40° C) facilitated the maintenance of reentry and VT by abbreviating the AP duration. The combination of hyperthermia and tachycardia (cycle length, 500 ms) promoted the loss-of-dome type AP in the epicardium,[13] along with J-ST elevation and without deep negative T waves in the transmural ECG. These changes resembled the ECG changes in Brugada syndrome patients who have sinus tachycardia induced by fever. Hypothemia (32°C) prolonged AP duration, enhanced the phase-1 notch of epicardial APs, promoted phase 2 reentry and VT, and elevated J-ST during bradycardia (cycle length, 2000 ms). However, the prolonged AP duration often blocked reentry attempts. I_{to} blockade eliminated the temperature-related arrhythmias. Therefore, the temperature sensitivity of VT in Brugada syndrome is caused by temperature modulations of duration of AP and of dispersion of repolarization.

The clinical implication of these studies is that a mechanism of VT in Brugada syndrome might result from spontaneous phase 2 reentry in the epicardium of the RVOT.

Ventricular Tachycardia by Transmural Reentry During Arterial Occlusion and Reperfusion

It is well recognized that acute ischemia and subsequent reperfusion are strong triggers of VT and that the ventricular epicardium becomes inexcitable faster than the endocardium. We investigated the mechanism of VT during acute ischemia and reperfusion.[20, 21]

We induced global ischemia by arterial occlusion and mapped APs on the transmural surfaces of 36 wedges of canine left ventricular free wall. Before ischemia, the tissues responded 1:1 to endocardial pacing (cycle length, 300 ms). Acute ischemia increased transmural gradient of refractory period, which blocked conduction unidirectionally and initiated reentry and VT after 535 ± 146 seconds of ischemia (31 wedge samples). Multiple zones of responsiveness (1:1, 2:1, and 4:1) to endocardial pacing resulted after 570 ± 165 seconds of ischemia (34 wedge samples). Further ischemia inactivated the epicardium and eliminated reentry and VT in 24 wedge samples. Therefore, heterogeneic prolongation of refractory period by early (9-15 min) ischemia provided a proarrhythmic substrate in which reentry and VT could be induced by rapid endocardial activations.

Ischemia also increased transmural differences in tissue excitability, which, when combined with epicardial activation, initiated transmural reentry. We mapped transmural conduction during ischemia while pacing alternately between the epicardium and endocardium.[21] The transmural gradient of sensitivity to ischemia caused conduction failure to occur first in the epicardium. At this time, epicardial stimulation failed to conduct laterally along the epicardium, and instead, it conducted to the more excitable endocardium, then conducted laterally along the endocardium, and finally reentered the subepicardium (in 9 of 18 wedge samples after 719 ± 399 sec of ischemia). Endocardial stimulation, immediately before or after the epicardial-initiated reentry, spread along the endocardium and then transmurally toward the epicardium without reentry in these wedges.

During the first minute of reperfusion, reappearance of AP was associated with significant prolongation of AP, EADs, and DADs in the epicardium but not in the endocardium, leading to reentry, VT, and fibrillation. Further reperfusion reduced transmural dispersion of AP and eliminated arrhythmias.

Acute ischemia provides a proarrhythmic substrate that has steep transmural gradients of excitability and refractory period, leading to unidirectional block and reentry. Transmural differences in the reperfusion recovery can trigger reperfusion VT by providing a steep transmural gradient of AP duration and by promoting focal activation. The clinical implication is that reentry appears to be the predominant mechanism of ventricular arrhythmias during and after global ischemia.

Summary

The wedge preparations have illustrated several mechanisms of VT: focal activation triggered by acute delay of repolarization in a proarrhythmic substrate having reduced repolarization reserve (e.g., post-ischemia, LQTS), focal activation in an arrhythmogenic substrate having unstable resting membrane (Adersen-Tawil syndrome), focal activation in a proarrhythmic substrate having excessive heterogeneity of repolarization (e.g., LQTS) and with transient functional enhancement of repolarization heterogeneity (e.g., by earliest excitable epicardial stimulation), phase 2 reentry in a proarrhythmic substrate having adjacent regions with and without a phase 2 dome in the AP (in the RVOT epicardium in Brugada syndrome), and unidirectional block of conduction at the steep transmural gradients of excitability and refractory period during acute ischemia and reperfusion. The wedge studies showed that a minor reduction in the net repolarization current that is normally insufficient to initiate an arrhythmia can do so when another event also contributes to impairing repolarization. The wedge models also demonstrated a common mechanism of the polymorphism in VT, caused by sequential shifting of foci sites or reentrant routes, or both, due to the electrophysiologic heterogeneity and functional dynamics in ventricular tissue.

References

1. Antzelevitch C, Oliva A: Amplification of spatial dispersion of repolarization underlies sudden cardiac death associated with catecholaminergic polymorphic VT, long QT, short QT and Brugada syndromes. J Intern Med 259:48-58, 2006.
2. Ueda N, Zipes DP, Wu J: Prior ischemia enhances arrhythmogenicity in isolated canine ventricular wedge model of long QT 3. Cardiovasc Res 63:69-76, 2004.
3. Ueda N, Zipes DP, Wu J: Coronary occlusion and reperfusion promote early afterdepolarizations and ventricular tachycardia in a canine tissue model of long QT 3. Am J Physiol Heart Circ Physiol 290:H607-H612, 2006.
4. Dhamoon A, Jalife J: The inward rectifier current (I_{K1}) controls cardiac excitability and is involved in arrhythmogenesis. Heart Rhythm. 2:316-324, 2005.
5. Tsuboi M, Antzelevitch C: Cellular basis for electrocardiographic and arrhythmic manifestations of Andersen-Tawil syndrome (LQT7). Heart Rhythm 3:328-335, 2006.
6. Morita H, Zipes DP, Morita ST, Wu J: Mechanism of U wave and polymorphic ventricular tachycardia in a canine tissue model of Andersen-Tawil syndrome. Cardiovasc Res 75:510-518, 2007.
7. Anyukhovsky EP, Sosunov EA, Gainullin RZ, Rosen MR: The controversial M cell. J Cardiovasc Electrophysiol 10:244-260, 1999.
8. Taggart P, Sutton P, Opthof T, et al. Electrotonic cancellation of transmural electrical gradients in the left ventricle in man. Prog Biophys Mol Biol 82:243-244, 2003.
9. Ueda N, Zipes DP, Wu J: Functional and transmural modulation of M cell behavior in canine ventricular wall. Am J Physiol Heart Circ Physiol 287:H2569-H2574, 2004.
10. Morita ST, Zipes DP, Morita H, Wu J: Analysis of action potentials in the canine ventricular septum: No phenotypic expression of M cells. Cardiovasc Res 74:96-103, 2007.
11. Medina-Ravell VA, Lankipalli RS, Yan G-X, et al: Effect of epicardial or biventricular pacing to prolong QT interval and increase transmural dispersion of repolarization—does resynchronization therapy pose a risk for patients predisposed to long QT or torsade de pointes? Circ 107:740-746, 2003.
12. Ueda N, Zipes DP, Wu J: Epicardial but not endocardial premature stimulation initiates ventricular tachyarrhythmia in canine in vitro model of Long QT syndrome. Heart Rhythm 1:684-694, 2004.
13. Keller DI, Rougier JS, Kucera JP, et al: Brugada syndrome and fever: Genetic and molecular characterization of patients carrying SCN5A mutations. Cardiovasc Res 67:510-519, 2005.
14. Antzelevitch C, Brugada P, Borggrefe M, et al: Brugada syndrome: Report of the second consensus conference. Heart Rhythm. 2:429-440, 2005.
15. Morita H, Morita ST, Nagase S, et al: Ventricular arrhythmia induced by sodium channel blocker in patients with Brugada syndrome. J Am Coll Cardiol 42:1624-1631, 2003.
16. Antzelevitch C, Pollevick GD, Cordeiro JM, et al: Loss-of-function mutations in the cardiac calcium channel underlie a new clinical entity characterized by ST-segment elevation, short QT intervals, and sudden cardiac death. Circulation 115:442-449, 2007.
17. Morita H, Zipes DP, Morita ST, Wu J: Differences in arrhythmogenicity between the canine right outflow tract and anteroinferior right ventricle in a model of Brugada syndrome. Heart Rhythm 4:66-74, 2007.
18. Morita H, Zipes DP, Lopshire J, et al: T wave alternans in an in vitro canine tissue model of Brugada syndrome. Am J Physiol Heart Circ Physiol 291:421-428, 2006.
19. Morita H, Zipes DP, Morita ST, Wu J: Temperature modulation of ventricular arrhythmogenicity in a canine tissue model of Brugada syndrome. Heart Rhythm 4:188-197, 2007.
20. Wu J, Zipes DP: Transmural reentry during global acute ischemia and reperfusion in canine ventricular muscle. Am J Physiol Heart Circ Physiol 280:H2717-H2725, 2001.
21. Wu J, Zipes DP: Transmural reentry triggered by epicardial stimulation during acute ischemia in canine ventricular muscle. Am J Physiol Heart Circ Physiol 283:H2004-H2011, 2002.

Mechanisms of Defibrillation 48

Derek J. Dosdall, Vladimir G. Fast, and Raymond E. Ideker

CHAPTER OUTLINE

While the ability of an electric shock to halt ventricular fibrillation (VF) has been known for more than a century and defibrillation has saved countless lives over the last half century, it has only been since the 1980s that electrical and optical mapping experiments and computer simulations have begun to provide information about the mechanisms by which electric shocks succeed or fail in halting VF. This chapter reviews the more recent of the experimental studies; the computer simulation studies are reviewed in Chapter 34. This chapter discusses the mechanisms by which defibrillation shocks alter the transmembrane potential to create virtual electrodes; the ionic currents responsible for this alteration in transmembrane potential, including the role of electroporation; the mechanisms by which a shock, while halting the VF activation fronts, can reinitiate reentry and VF, causing the shock to fail by producing two kinds of critical points; the mechanisms by which a shock defibrillates, including the possible cause for the isoelectric window (i.e., the sizeable pause between the shock and the first recorded postshock activation fronts); and the future research needed to answer questions dealing with the mechanism of defibrillation, about which there is not yet universal agreement.

This work has in part been supported by National Institutes of Health Research grants HL42760 and HL85370.

Mechanisms by Which Defibrillation Shocks Alter the Transmembrane Potential

To defibrillate, a shock must alter the transmembrane potential in such a way that it halts the VF wave fronts but does not create new wave fronts that immediately reinduce VF.[1] To understand

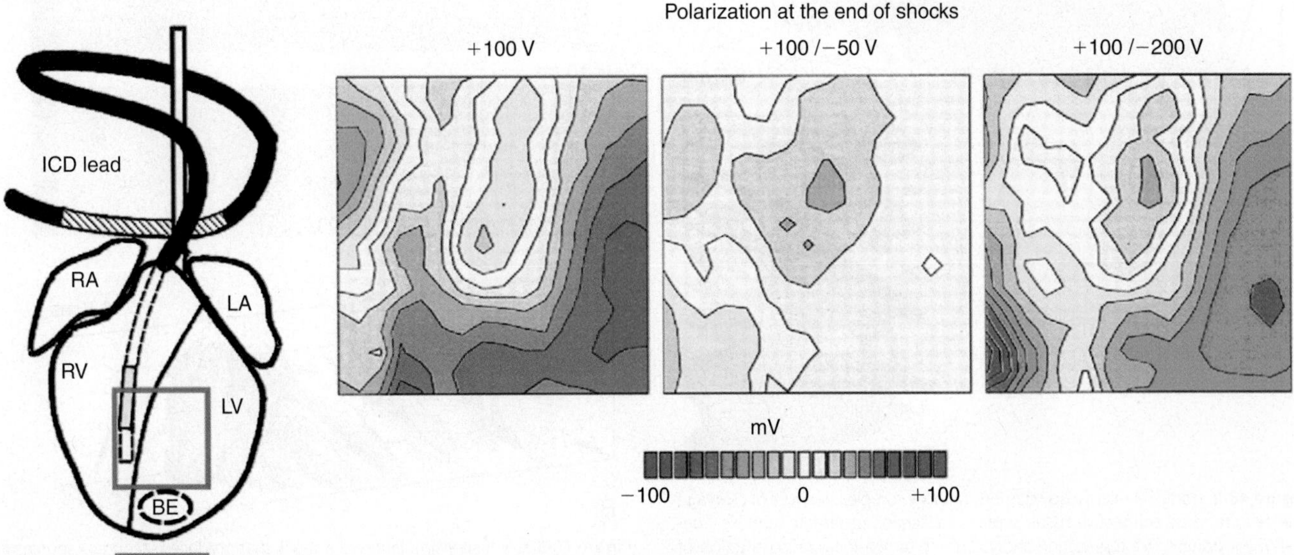

Figure 48-1 The spatial pattern of polarization at the end of the shock produced by a monophasic shock (+100 V, 7th ms of an 8-ms shock), optimal biphasic shock with more charge in the first than the second phase (+100/−50 V, 15th ms of a 16-ms shock), and nonoptimal biphasic shock with less charge in the first than the second phase (+100/−200 V, 15th ms of a 16-ms shock). The shocking electrodes were in the RV and above the right atrium, labeled *ICD lead*. The area from which the optical recordings were made is shown by the *red box* on the rabbit heart diagram. Values of polarization are shown relative to the preshock transmembrane voltage, with various colors assigned to positive and negative polarization, and white to areas of no polarization. BE, bipolar electrode; ICD, implantable cardioverter defibrillator; LA, left atrium; LV, left ventricle; RA, right atrium; RV, right ventricle. (Used with permission from Efimov IR, Cheng Y, Van Wagoner DR, et al: Virtual electrode-induced phase singularity: A basic mechanism of defibrillation failure. Circ Res 82:918-925, 1998.)

the mechanism of defibrillation, it is necessary first of all to understand the mechanism by which electrical stimuli alter the transmembrane potential.

The relationship between the stimulus electric field and the change it creates in the transmembrane potential has been quantified by the generalized activating function derived by Sobie and Tung.[2] The generalized activating function contains two factors. One factor is based on the spatial derivative of the potential gradient created in the heart by the stimulus, and the second factor is based on the potential gradient itself and variations in intracellular resistivity. The effect of both factors of the generalized activating function is to create virtual electrodes, also known as secondary sources, at sites in the tissue away from the real stimulating electrodes. For example, as shown in the left map of membrane polarization in Figure 48-1, an anodal electrode in the right ventricular (RV) cavity not only hyperpolarizes the membrane in the tissue on the epicardium overlying the real electrode, but it also depolarizes the nearby tissue in the left ventricle (LV), creating a virtual cathode in this region.

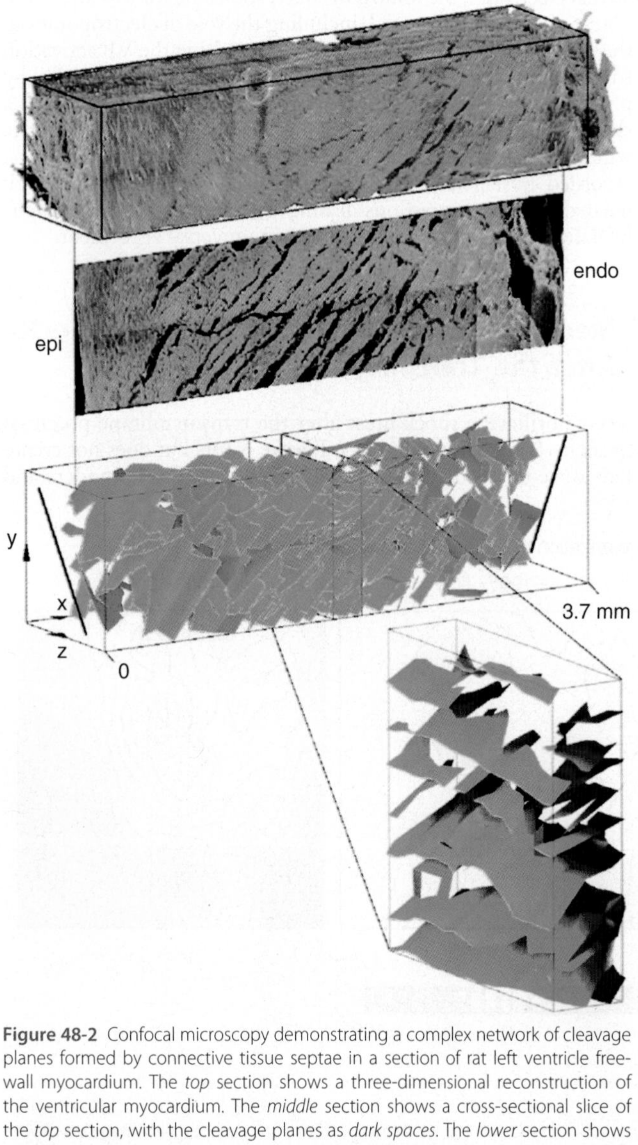

Figure 48-2 Confocal microscopy demonstrating a complex network of cleavage planes formed by connective tissue septae in a section of rat left ventricle free-wall myocardium. The *top* section shows a three-dimensional reconstruction of the ventricular myocardium. The *middle* section shows a cross-sectional slice of the *top* section, with the cleavage planes as *dark spaces*. The *lower* section shows a finite element geometric model of the cleavage planes shown in *green* with a smaller subsection magnified *below*. The cleavage planes are about 80 μm in thickness and might play an important role in the creation of secondary sources in defibrillation. (Used with permission from Hooks DA, Tomlinson KA, Marsden SG, et al: Cardiac microstructure: Implications for electrical propagation and defibrillation in the heart. Circ Res 91:331-338, 2002.)

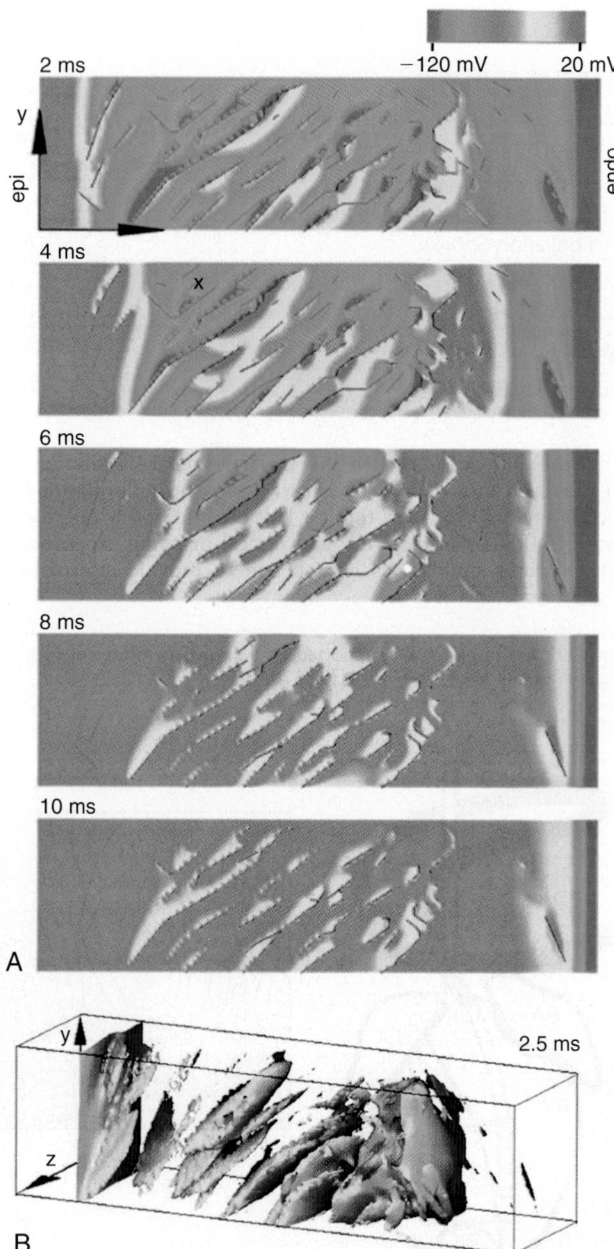

Figure 48-3 Computer simulation of a shock that produces secondary sources in a model based on the confocal microscopic image of ventricular rat tissue shown in Figure 48-2. **A,** Progression of activation during a 10-ms shock. Transmembrane potentials of a single midvolume plane are shown according to the color scale at the *top*. **B,** A three-dimensional view of secondary sources with transmembrane potentials greater than −60 mV at 2.5 ms into the shock. (Used with permission from Hooks DA, Tomlinson KA, Marsden SG, et al: Cardiac microstructure: Implications for electrical propagation and defibrillation in the heart. Circ Res 91:331-338, 2002.)

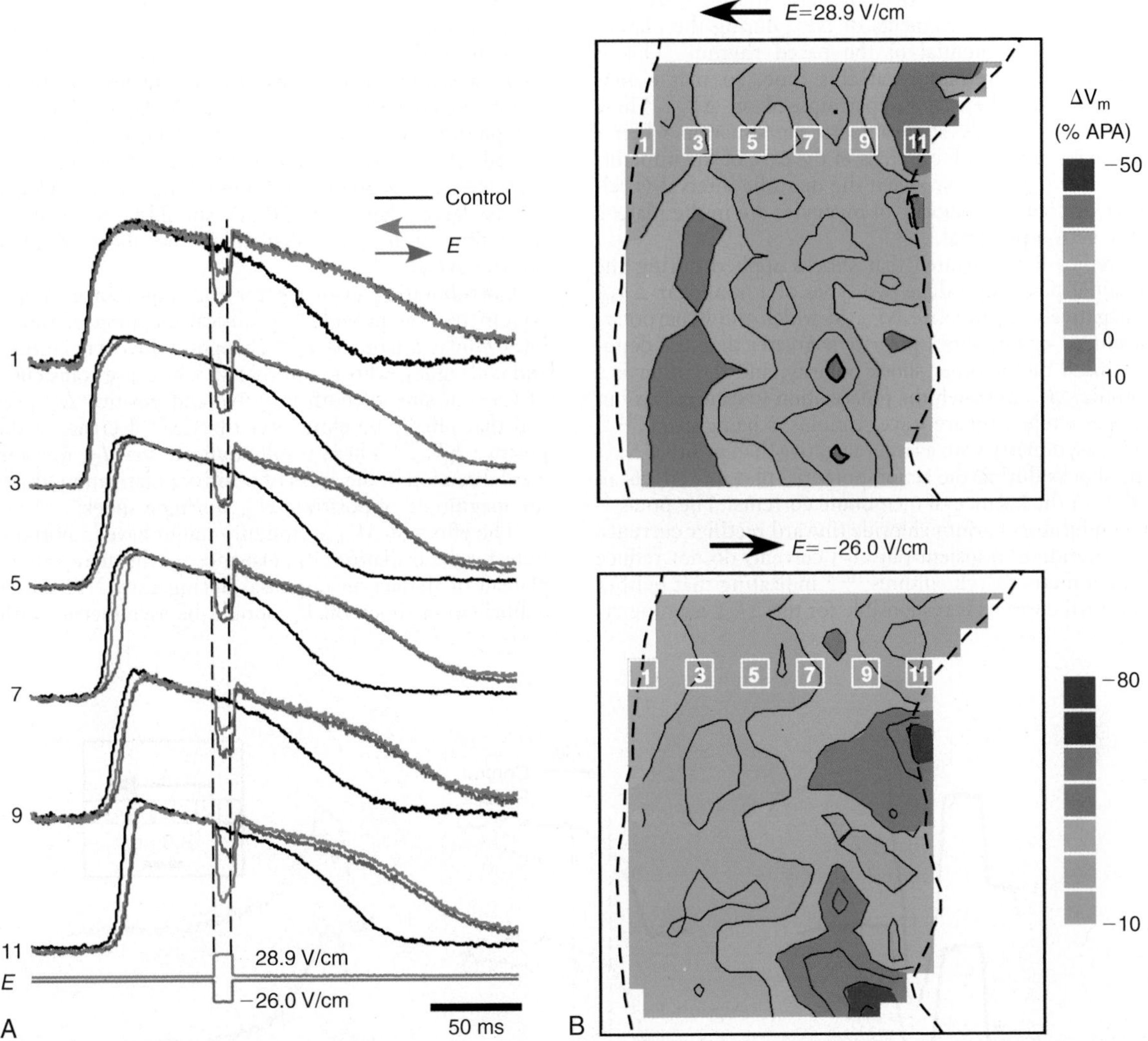

Figure 48-4 Effects of shocks on intramural transmembrane potential in a porcine left ventricle wedge preparation. **A,** Optical recordings of transmembrane potential in control action potentials and during shock application. *E*, shock strength. The numbers correspond to the photodiodes indicated in **B. B,** Isopotential maps of shock-induced changes in the transmembrane potential distribution measured 9 ms after shock onset. (Used with permission from Fast VG, Sharifov OF, Cheek ER, et al: Intramural virtual electrodes during defibrillation shocks in left ventricular wall assessed by optical mapping of membrane potential. Circulation 106:1007-1014, 2002.)

Changes in intracellular resistivity that contribute to virtual electrodes by the second factor in the generalized activating function can occur by several different mechanisms. Examples of some of these mechanisms include increases in resistance between cells at intercalated disks, curvature of the myofibers, variation in cell shape, alteration in the surface-to-volume ratio of the myofibers, and separation of bundles of myofibers by connective tissue sheaths and septae (Fig. 48-2). Although the exact mechanism responsible for virtual electrodes is not known, available theoretical and experimental data indicate that the last mechanism may be particularly important in causing the formation of virtual electrodes in the intramural bulk of the myocardium. Computer simulation indicates that these interruptions of the intracellular space cause a virtual anode of hyperpolarization to be formed on the side of each intracellular interruption closest to the anode and a virtual cathode of depolarization to be formed on the side closest to the real cathode (Fig. 48-3).[4] Fast and colleagues and Windisch and coworkers have shown experimentally that virtual electrodes are created throughout most of the myocardium by a shock (Fig. 48-4) and that some of the membrane polarizations created by these virtual electrodes are sufficiently large to stimulate the tissue at the virtual electrode.[5,6] The reason these numerous virtual electrodes are not seen in the epicardial recordings shown in Figure 48-1 is probably that the connective tissue septae shown in Figures 48-2 and 48-3 do not extend all the way to the epicardium.

Ionic Currents Responsible for the Changes of Transmembrane Potential During Defibrillation Shocks

In addition to understanding the changes in transmembrane potential (V_m) during a shock, it is also important to understand the cause of these V_m changes. Although early theoretical studies in mathematical models indicated that shock-induced changes in V_m (ΔV_m) were linear, experimental studies demonstrated that

ΔV_m are strongly nonlinear. Most of these studies were performed using optical measurements of ΔV_m during the plateau phase of the action potential of the paced rhythm. This is because the cells are refractory at this time, so that a new action potential upstroke is not superimposed on ΔV_m. These measurements are directly applicable to the situation when a shock is given soon after VF onset, as in the case of the implantable cardioverter defibrillator, when the diastolic interval is relatively short, so that the majority of myocytes are in the plateau phase of the action potential.[7]

These studies demonstrated that shocks applied during the action potential plateau produce two types of a nonlinear ΔV_m: One is a negatively asymmetric ΔV_m in which the hyperpolarization produced by one shock polarity is greater than the depolarization caused by the other shock polarity, and the other is a nonmonotonic ΔV_m in which the polarization first increases but then decreases while a square wave stimulus is being given.[8,9]

The ΔV_m asymmetry with a larger negative than positive ΔV_m induced by shocks during the action potential plateau reflects an outward shift in the balance of membrane currents. The potassium channel inhibitors barium chloride (inward rectifier current), and 4-aminopyridine (transient outward current) do not reduce this ΔV_m asymmetry in cell cultures,[10,11] indicating that neither of these outward currents is responsible for the ΔV_m asymmetry. However, the asymmetric behavior of ΔV_m is reversed by the calcium channel blocker nifedipine in the cultured cell strands.[11] This effect of nifedipine on ΔV_m suggests that the ΔV_m asymmetry is caused by the outward flow of calcium current (I_{Ca}) in the depolarized portions of the cell strands. Although I_{Ca} is inward in the physiologic range of V_m, it changes direction when V_m exceeds the reversal potential for I_{Ca}, which in rat and rabbit myocytes is 45 to 50 mV.[12,13] Therefore, positive ΔV_m with magnitudes larger than 45 to 50 mV should be reduced by the outward flow of I_{Ca}, thus explaining the effect of nifedipine on positive ΔV_m.

Corroborating evidence for the importance of I_{Ca} in ΔV_m asymmetry was provided by optical mapping of shock-induced intracellular calcium (Ca_i^{2+}) changes in myocyte cultures by Fast and colleagues, who found that shocks cause transient decreases of Ca_i^{2+} at sites of both negative and positive ΔV_m (Fig. 48-5) and that nifedipine eliminates the Ca_i^{2+} decrease at the sites of positive ΔV_m.[14] These results indicate that I_{Ca} flows in an outward direction in the areas of positive polarization, thus reducing the magnitude of positive ΔV_m during a shock.

The effect of ΔV_m asymmetry might have important implications for defibrillation. Because most of the myocardium is in the plateau of the action potential during early VF, the effect of a defibrillation shock on V_m should be asymmetric, with a larger

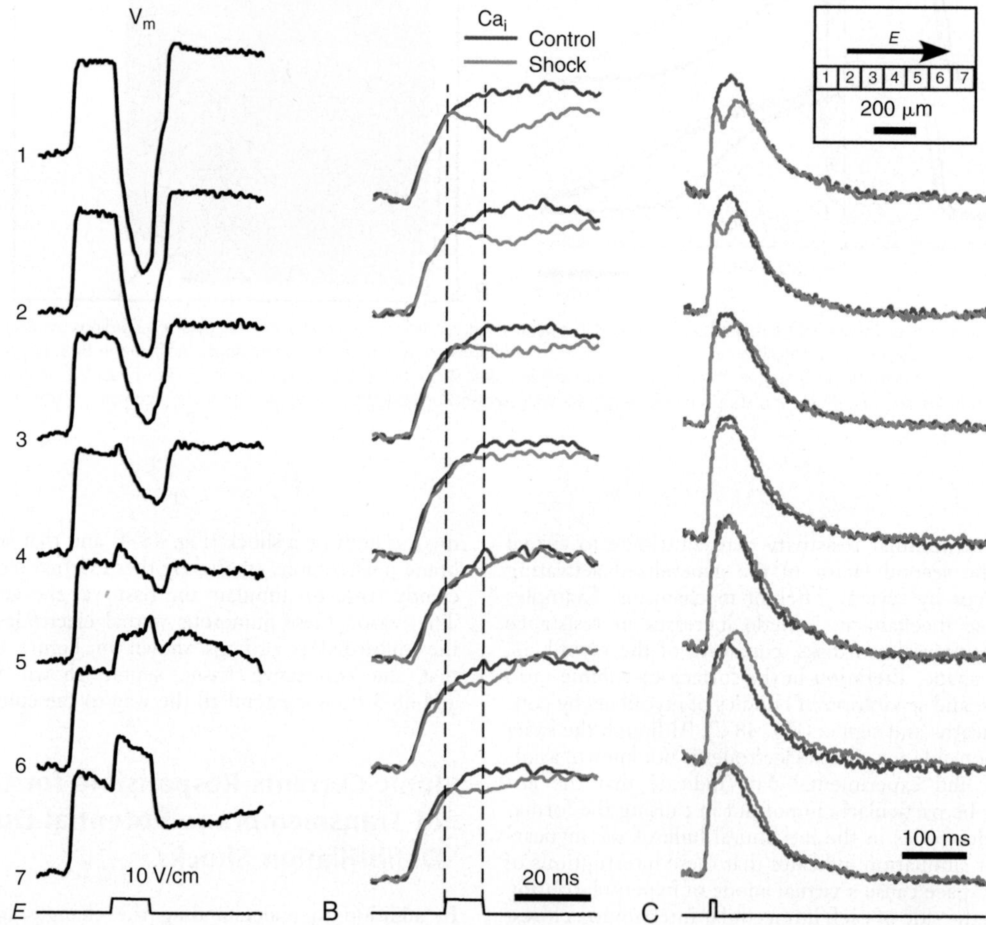

Figure 48-5 Shock-induced changes in Ca_i^{+2} associated with an asymmetric ΔV_m in the hyperpolarized and depolarized regions of a cell strand in response to a square wave shock. **A,** Changes in transmembrane potential induced by the shock. Locations of the recordings are shown in the *inset* in **C. B,** Changes in Ca_i^{+2} during the shock in comparison to control recordings. **C,** Longer recordings of Ca_i^{+2} transients. (Used with permission from Fast VG, Cheek ER, et al: Effects of electrical shocks on Ca_i^{+2} and V_m in myocyte cultures. Circ Res 94:1589-1597, 2004.)

portion of myocardium undergoing a negative rather than a positive V_m change. As discussed later in this chapter, interaction between areas of hyperpolarization and depolarization can lead to the formation of a reentrant circuit reinitiating VF immediately after the shock, causing defibrillation failure.[15] Because the asymmetry in (I_p),[16] ΔV_m affects the size and the shape of the areas of hyperpolarization and depolarization, it could affect the outcome of a defibrillation shock.

The other type of nonlinear shock-induced polarization, nonmonotonic negative ΔV_m, could be caused by two mechanisms: activation of a hyperpolarization-induced inward ionic current or flow of a nonspecific inward current caused by membrane electroporation. Two ionic inward currents operate at large negative V_m: the inward rectifier current, I_{K1}, and the hyperpolarization-induced funny current (I_p),[16] which might play a role in anodal break excitation.[17] However, application of either cesium chloride (I_f blocker) or barium chloride (I_{K1} blocker) does not change the negative ΔV_m caused by shocks in cell cultures, indicating that these currents are not responsible for the nonmonotonic V_m response.[18]

A method to determine if electroporation is responsible for the nonmonotonic ΔV_m is to expose cells to a membrane-impermeable dye and to measure any cell uptake of the dye caused by shocks. This method was applied in cell cultures[10] and rabbit hearts[9] using the fluorescent dye propidium iodide. In cell cultures, application of a series of shocks of a strength similar to those inducing a nonmonotonic ΔV_m in hyperpolarized regions causes cell uptake of propidium iodide in the hyperpolarized region at the anodal side of cell strands but not in the cathodal region.[18] Weaker shocks cause neither nonmonotonic ΔV_m nor dye uptake. Similar findings were obtained in rabbit hearts, where strong shocks of either polarity cause increased staining of subepicardial tissue with propidium iodide lasting several minutes but weaker shocks do not (Fig. 48-6).[9] These findings indicate that nonmonotonic ΔV_m is caused by membrane electroporation rather than the passage of a particular type of ion through ion channels.

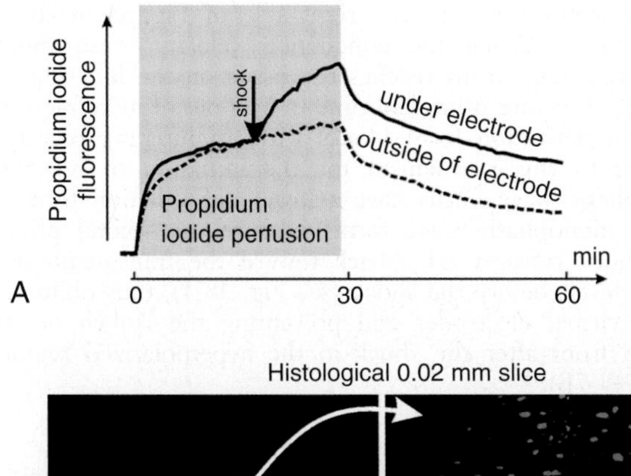

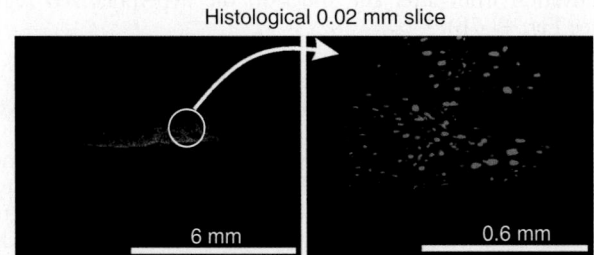

Figure 48-6 Uptake of membrane-impermeable propidium iodide after a strong shock showing evidence of electroporation. **A,** Propidium iodide fluorescence increased after a strong shock (1.6 A/cm^2, 20 ms). **B,** Fluorescence images made in the stimulation area shows propidium iodide–stained nuclei. (Used with permission from Nikolski VP, Sambelashvili AT, Krinsky VI, et al: Effects of electroporation on optically recorded transmembrane potential responses to high-intensity electrical shocks. Am J Physiol Heart Circ Physiol 286:H412-H418, 2004.)

Mechanisms by Which Defibrillation Shocks Reinitiate Reentry and Ventricular Fibrillation

For a shock to defibrillate, the virtual electrodes created by the shock field must be of sufficient amplitude to halt the activation fronts of VF. However, this is not sufficient to ensure successful defibrillation, because these virtual electrodes can themselves initiate new activation fronts that reinitiate VF. Therefore, to completely understand the mechanism of defibrillation, it is necessary to also understand the mechanism by which shocks can initiate VF. For this reason, many studies have investigated the mechanisms by which shocks given during the vulnerable period of a regular rhythm (rather than during VF) initiate VF. Some of the earliest of these studies found that there is an upper limit to the strength of shocks given during the vulnerable period that could induce VF,[19] which is called the *upper limit of vulnerability*.[20] If there were no upper limit of vulnerability, it might not be possible to defibrillate, because VF is so complex that some portions of the myocardium are probably in their vulnerable period no matter when the shock is given and, if there were no upper limit of vulnerability, the shock field should reinduce VF in these regions.

Two mechanisms have been proposed by which a shock can induce VF. The first of these was predicted based on theoretical considerations by Winfree[21] and observed experimentally by electrical mapping.[22] As shown in Figure 48-7A, reentry is formed about a point called the *critical point*, where a critical degree of refractoriness of the tissue during the vulnerable period intersected a critical value of potential gradient created by the shock field. The critical value of the potential gradient about which reentry forms during the vulnerable period of regular rhythm is approximately the same as the minimum potential gradient required throughout the ventricles for defibrillation.[23] This finding is consistent with the fact that the shock strength at the upper limit of vulnerability is approximately equal to the shock strength needed to defibrillate and supports the hypothesis that the mechanism by which a shock induces VF when given during the vulnerable period of regular rhythm is similar to that by which a shock fails to defibrillate during VF.[24] The importance of the potential gradient, both in the initiation of VF during the vulnerable period and in defibrillation, suggests that the second factor in the generalized activation function discussed previously has an important effect on membrane polarization.

According to the mechanism of reentry induction by the interaction of the shock potential gradient and the degree of refractoriness during the vulnerable period, an upper limit of vulnerability exists because certain shocks do not create critical points within the ventricles so that reentry does not occur. These are shocks that are sufficiently large that their potential gradient exceeds the critical potential gradient level for the induction of reentry throughout the myocardium. According to this concept, the smallest shock in which the critical potential gradient is not present within the ventricles is the upper limit of vulnerability strength. According to this critical-point mechanism, some biphasic wave forms have a lower defibrillation threshold than monophasic wave forms because the critical potential gradient for reentry induction is less for the biphasic than for the monophasic wave forms.[23,25] Because it takes a smaller shock to create a potential gradient field that exceeds this smaller potential gradient throughout the ventricular myocardium for the biphasic wave form than for the monophasic wave form, the biphasic wave form has a lower defibrillation threshold.

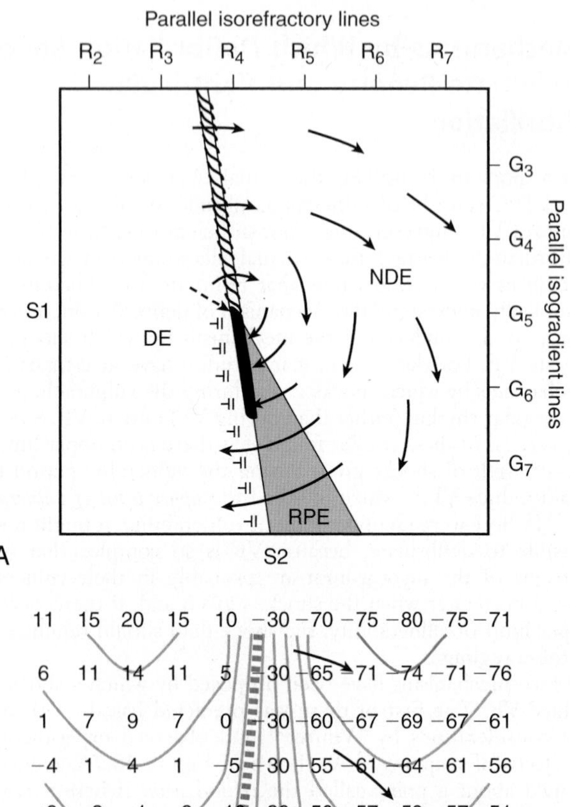

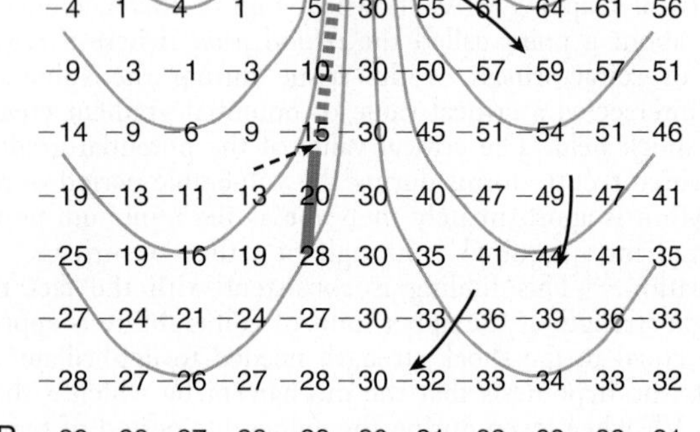

Figure 48-7 Two types of critical points created by a shock initiating reentry. **A,** An idealized diagram is shown with a critical point *(dashed arrow)* formed at the intersection of a critical shock potential gradient of G5 and a critical tissue refractoriness of R4. S1 pacing is performed from the left to cause a dispersion of refractoriness at the time of the S2 shock, with R2 representing less and R7 more refractoriness. The S2 shock is given during the vulnerable period from the bottom of the region with large gradient G7 at the *bottom* and small gradient G3 at the *top*. The area on the *left* is sufficiently recovered so that it is directly excited (DE) by the shock potential gradient field. The *shaded region*, although exposed to a higher gradient, is more refractory and undergoes refractory period extension (RPE), such that unidirectional block occurs from DE to RPE and activation in the DE tissue cannot propagate through this region. The region on the *right* is too refractory to be affected even with a large gradient and is not directly excited (NDE). Thus, propagation conducts unidirectionally from the DE to the NDE region at the *top*, encircling the critical point in a clockwise direction and reentering the DE region to create a reentrant circuit. **B,** An idealized diagram is shown of a critical point *(dashed arrow)* caused by adjacent regions of depolarized and hyperpolarized transmembrane potential changes caused by the shock. Numbers represent transmembrane potentials at the end of the shock, with isolines spaced every 10 mV beginning at −45 mV. The depolarized region *(upper left)* and the hyperpolarized region *(upper right)* are separated by a zone with a large spatial gradient of membrane polarization as indicated by the closely spaced isolines. The depolarized tissue in this zone is able to activate the adjacent hyperpolarized tissue to launch an activation front *(dashed line)* that propagates through the hyperpolarized region *(arrows)*. Below, where the spatial gradient in transmembrane potential is smaller, propagation cannot occur. A critical point is formed at the intersection of the frame and block lines where one end of the propagating activation front terminates in both panels. In both panels, the *solid line* represents the site of conduction block and the *dashed line* indicates the location from which an activation front is launched after the shock. (Used with permission from Chattipakorn N, Ideker RE: Mechanism of defibrillation. In Aliot E, Clémenty J, Prystowsky EN (eds): Fighting Sudden Cardiac Death: A Worldwide Challenge. Armonk, NY, Futura Publishing, 2000, pp 593-615.)

The second mechanism by which a shock can induce reentry and VF was discovered by computer bidomain simulations as discussed in Chapter 34 and by optical mapping experiments. This mechanism also involves reentry around a critical point. However, the critical point is the pattern of the virtual electrodes of hyperpolarization and depolarization caused by a shock given during the action potential plateau, not the strength of the shock potential gradient field or the degree of refractoriness, as in the first type of critical point.[15,26] Even though the shock is given during the plateau of the action potential when the tissue is in its absolute refractory period, the myocardium is de-excited within the hyperpolarized region so that its action potential is truncated and excitability is restored. This restoration of excitability allows the adjacent depolarized region to activate the hyperpolarized tissue, giving rise to an activation front that forms a rotor around a critical point formed where the adjacent hyperpolarization and depolarization decrease to the point that a postshock activation front is not initiated (see Fig. 48-7B). Thus, although the virtual electrodes are necessary to halt the VF activation fronts present at the time of the shock, the activation front formed in the de-excited region after the shock can lead to the reinitiation of reentry and VF so that the shock fails to defibrillate.[15,26]

According to this mechanism of reentry induction, an upper limit of vulnerability exists because, as the degree of hyperpolarization and depolarization increases in magnitude as the shock strength is increased, the conduction velocity of the activation front propagating around the right side of Figure 48-7B is also increased. When the conduction velocity is so rapid that the activation front reaches the tissue on the left side of Figure 48-7B before it has had time to pass out of its refractory period, the activation front blocks without initiating reentry. According to this mechanism for the initiation of reentry, some biphasic wave forms have a lower defibrillation threshold than monophasic wave forms because the second phase of the shock restores ΔV_m back toward the transmembrane potential levels before the shock (see Fig. 48-1), thus obliterating the virtual electrodes and preventing the launch of an activation front after the shock in the hyperpolarized region (see Fig. 48-7B).[15]

Mechanisms by Which a Shock Defibrillates

The two mechanisms for the induction of reentry by shocks discussed in the previous section each invoke a different type of critical point, and they both predict two findings that should be observed if they are the mechanisms by which a shock given during VF fails to defibrillate: An activation front should arise immediately after the shock, and this activation front should immediately form a reentrant circuit. However, with one exception,[15] epicardial and intramural electrical and optical mapping studies in which shocks of a strength near the defibrillation threshold were given during VF did not observe either of the types of critical points described above, the immediate appearance after the shock of an activation front, or the

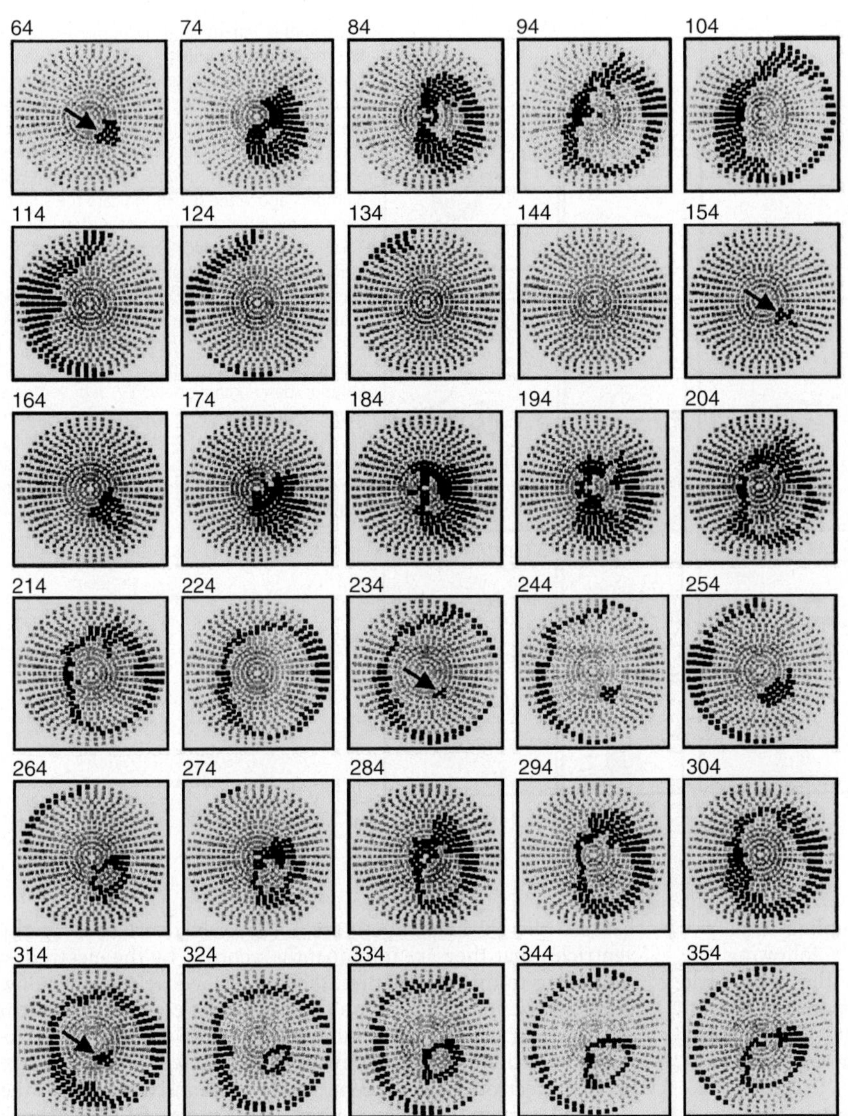

Figure 48-8 Example of the first postshock cycles after a failed shock of a strength near the defibrillation threshold. The shock was delivered during ventricular fibrillation from electrodes in the right ventricular apex and the superior vena cava. Recordings were made simultaneously from 504 electrodes distributed globally over the ventricular epicardium of a pig. Electrode sites are indicated in *gray* on a polar projection, with the atrioventricular groove at the *periphery* and the left ventricle (LV) apex in the *center*. Anterior is at the *bottom* of the projection and the LV is to the *right*. Each panel shows in *black* the electrode sites at which an activation occurred at any time during a 10-ms interval. Numbers above the panels indicate the start of each 10 ms interval in milliseconds relative to the shock onset. *Arrows* indicate the site of earliest recorded activation from each cycle. The first cycle appeared on the epicardium 64 ms after the shock at the anteroapical LV. The second cycle (154 ms) arose on the epicardium in the same region as the first cycle and also propagated away in a focal pattern. The third (235 ms) and fourth (315 ms) cycles arose before the activation front from the previous cycle disappeared. (Used with permission from Chattipakorn N, Fotuhi PC, Ideker RE: Prediction of defibrillation outcome by epicardial activation patterns following shocks near the defibrillation threshold. J Cardiovasc Electrophysiol 11:1014-1021, 2000.)

consistent finding of reentry once an activation front first appears following the shock.[20,27-31]

Instead, activation is not recorded for an interval of 50 to 90 ms following a shock near the defibrillation threshold strength—the isoelectric window—after which activation often arises focally and spreads away in all directions to activate the entire myocardium (Fig. 48-8).[28,32] If the shock fails to defibrillate, these foci arise rapidly and repetitively for four or more cycles, after which activation fronts degenerate back into VF. If the shock successfully defibrillates, either no foci are observed (a type A defibrillation success) or the focal activation pattern only lasts 1 or 2 cycles before it stops spontaneously (a type B defibrillation success).[20] In addition to electrical mapping, these findings have also been observed in optical mapping, which is not subject to saturation of the electrical recordings by the shock, as is electrical mapping.[30,31]

To determine if, during the isoelectric window observed in the epicardial recordings as in Figure 48-8, intramural activation fronts were present and if intramural reentry was present formed by one of the two types of critical point mechanisms discussed previously, transmural activation was mapped following near-defibrillation threshold strength shocks.[29,33] An isoelectric window of 58 ± 23 ms (mean plus or minus standard deviation) was present in the intramural recordings and the activation front propagating away from the earliest activating site after the shock frequently formed a focal activation pattern (Fig. 48-9).[29] All of these studies taken together indicate that the postshock isoelectric window observed following shocks that are near the defibrillation threshold in strength is real and not an artifact of the recording technique or of not recording from the appropriate site.

One possible explanation for the isoelectric window is that the shock halts all VF activation fronts without generating new activation fronts and that the earliest activation following the isoelectric window arises by triggered activity. However, neither pinacidil (an early afterdepolarization inhibitor) nor flunarizine (a delayed afterdepolarization inhibitor) significantly alters the defibrillation threshold, the length of the isoelectric window, or the ventricular location of earliest postshock activation.[34] Another possibility raised by the simultaneous optical recording of V_m and Ca_i^{2+} is that earliest postshock activation

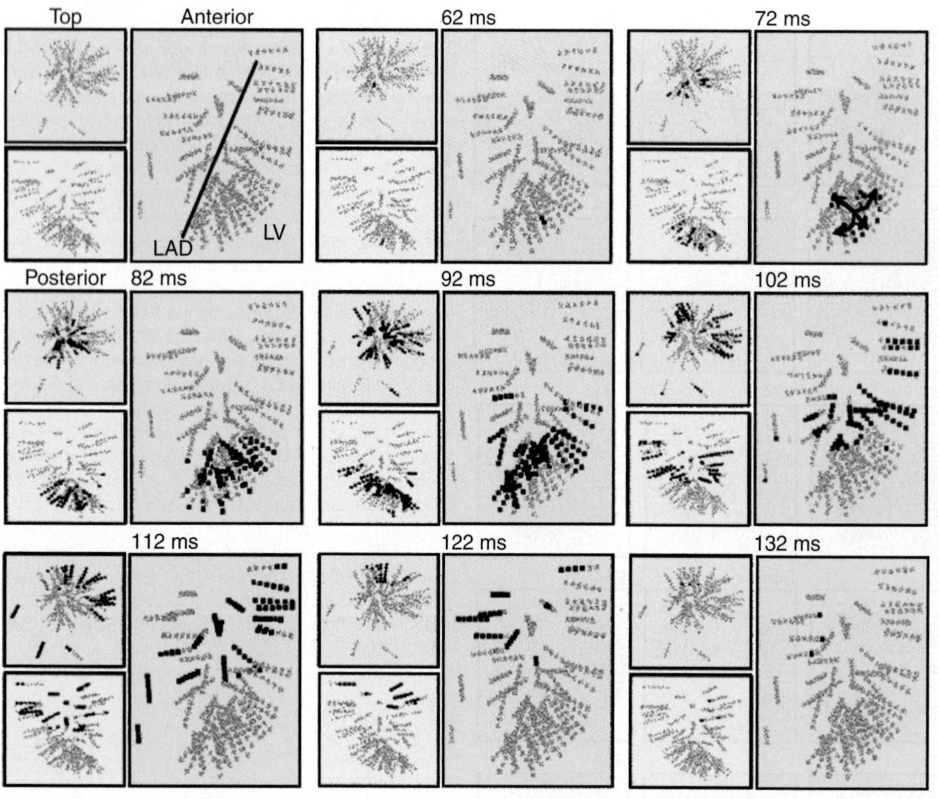

Figure 48-9 Intramural activation maps of the first postshock activation cycle after a failed shock of near defibrillation threshold strength in a pig. Plunge needles with 4 to 6 electrodes were inserted around the heart. Each panel shows in *black* the electrode sites at which an activation occurred during a 10-ms interval. Numbers above the panels indicate the start of each 10-ms interval relative to the shock onset. There was an isoelectric window of 62 ms before the first activation, after which activation spread away from a focal site to activate the remainder of the ventricles. There was no evidence of intramural activation or reentry during the postshock isoelectric window. LAD, left anterior descending artery; LV, left ventricle. (From Chattipakorn N, Fotuhi PC, Chattipakorn SC, et al: Three-dimensional mapping of earliest activation after near-threshold ventricular defibrillation shocks. J Cardiovasc Electrophysiol 14:65-69, 2003.)

arises from reverse excitation-contraction coupling at a site where low Ca_i^{2+} is surrounded by high Ca_i^{2+} following the shock.[35] A third possible explanation for the isoelectric window is that a slowly propagated graded response is present intramurally during the isoelectric window, and this response that is too small to be recorded by electrical plunge-needle recordings.[36,37]

A fourth possible explanation for the isoelectric window is that activation is present in the specialized conduction system during this time but is undetected in the intramural recordings because the Purkinje fibers are so sparsely distributed in the ventricles that they are infrequently recorded by the electrodes. According to this explanation, the end of the isoelectric window occurs when activation within the specialized conduction system propagates through the Purkinje-muscle junction into the working myocardium, where activation is detected by the plunge needle electrodes. A recent study demonstrated that the Purkinje system is indeed active during the first postshock cycle (Fig. 48-10), but there were too few Purkinje recordings to determine if activation initiated within the specialized

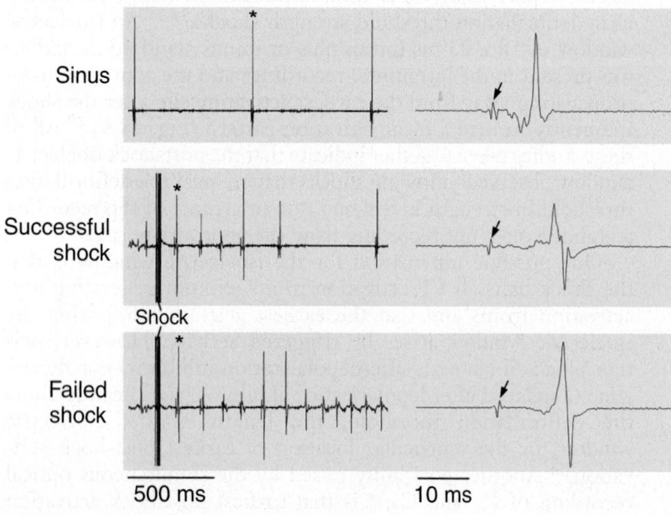

Figure 48-10 Temporal derivatives of plunge-needle electrograms from a single bipolar electrode during normal sinus rhythm, after a successful defibrillation shock, and after a failed defibrillation shock in a pig. The activations marked with *asterisks* are enlarged on the *right*. Purkinje fiber activations are marked with *arrows*.

conduction system or if it propagated retrogradely into it from the working myocardium.[38]

Future Research

Much has been learned about the mechanisms of defibrillation, but additional research is needed to determine the relative importance of the two factors in the general activating function in causing ΔV_m by a defibrillation shock, the relative importance of the two types of critical point mechanisms for initiating reentry by a shock, and the cause of the isoelectric postshock window.

Most studies of the mechanism of defibrillation have been performed in early VF when the diastolic interval is relatively short, which is appropriate for defibrillation with an implantable cardioverter defibrillator. However, during sudden cardiac arrest, defibrillation is typically not performed until after VF has been present for several minutes, by which time the tissue is ischemic and the diastolic interval is much larger.[39] This raises the possibility that the mechanism of defibrillation is different after long-duration VF than short-duration VF. Therefore, additional research is needed to investigate the mechanism of defibrillation following long-duration VF.[35,40]

References

1. Ideker RE: Ventricular fibrillation: How do we put the genie back in the bottle? Heart Rhythm 4:665-674, 2007.
2. Sobie EA, Susil RC, Tung L: A generalized activating function for predicting virtual electrodes in cardiac tissue. Biophys J 73:1410-1423, 1997.
3. Clerc L: Directional differences of impulse spread in trabecular muscle from mammalian heart. J Physiol 255:335-346, 1976.
4. Hooks DA, Tomlinson KA, Marsden SG, et al: Cardiac microstructure: Implications for electrical propagation and defibrillation in the heart. Circ Res 91:331-338, 2002.
5. Fast VG, Sharifov OF, Cheek ER, et al: Intramural virtual electrodes during defibrillation shocks in left ventricular wall assessed by optical mapping of membrane potential. Circulation 106:1007-1014, 2002.
6. Windisch H, Platzer D, Bilgici E: Quantification of shock-induced microscopic virtual electrodes assessed by subcellular resolution optical potential map-ping in guinea pig papillary muscle. J Cardiovasc Electrophysiol 18:1086-1094, 2007.
7. Huizar JF, Warren MD, Shvedko AG, et al: Three distinct phases of VF during global ischemia in the isolated blood-perfused pig heart. Am J Physiol Heart Circ Physiol 293:H1617-H1628, 2007.
8. Fast VG, Rohr S, Ideker RE: Nonlinear changes of transmembrane potential caused by defibrillation shocks in strands of cultured myocytes. Am J Physiol Heart Circ Physiol 278:H688-H697, 2000.
9. Nikolski VP, Sambelashvili AT, Krinsky VI, et al: Effects of electroporation on optically recorded transmembrane potential responses to high-intensity electrical shocks. Am J Physiol Heart Circ Physiol 286:H412-H418, 2004.
10. Fast VG, Cheek ER: Optical mapping of arrhythmias induced by strong electrical shocks in myocyte cultures. Circ Res 90:664-670, 2002.
11. Cheek ER, Ideker RE, Fast VG: Nonlinear changes of transmembrane potential during defibrillation shocks: Role of Ca^{2+} current. Circ Res 87:453-459, 2000.
12. Yuan W, Ginsburg KS, Bers DM: Comparison of sarcolemmal calcium channel current in rabbit and rat ventricular myocytes. J Physiol 493(Pt 3):733-746, 1996.
13. Gomez JP, Potreau D, Branka JE, et al: Developmental changes in Ca^{2+} currents from newborn rat cardiomyocytes in primary culture. Pflugers Arch 428:241-249, 1994.
14. Fast VG, Cheek ER, Pollard AE, et al: Effects of electrical shocks on Ca_i^{2+} and V_m in myocyte cultures. Circ Res 94:1589-1597, 2004.
15. Efimov IR, Cheng Y, Van Wagoner DR, et al: Virtual electrode-induced phase singularity: A basic mechanism of defibrillation failure. Circ Res 82:918-925, 1998.
16. Yu H, Chang F, Cohen IS: Pacemaker current I_f in adult canine cardiac ventricular myocytes. J Physiol 485(Pt 2):469-483, 1995.
17. Ranjan R, Chiamvimonvat N, Thakor NV, et al: Mechanism of anode break stimulation in the heart. Biophys J 74:1850-1863, 1998.
18. Cheek ER, Fast VG: Nonlinear changes of transmembrane potential during electrical shocks: Role of membrane electroporation. Circ Res 94:208-214, 2004.
19. Lesigne C, Levy B, Saumont R, et al: An energy-time analysis of ventricular fibrillation and defibrillation thresholds with internal electrodes. Med Biol Eng 14:617-622, 1976.
20. Chen P-S, Shibata N, Dixon EG, et al: Comparison of the defibrillation threshold and the upper limit of ventricular vulnerability. Circulation 73:1022-1028, 1986.
21. Winfree AT: When Time Breaks Down: The Three-Dimensional Dynamics of Electrochemical Waves and Cardiac Arrhythmias. Princeton: Princeton University Press, 1987.
22. Frazier DW, Wolf PD, Wharton JM, et al: Stimulus-induced critical point: Mechanism for electrical initiation of reentry in normal canine myocardium. J Clin Invest 83:1039-1052, 1989.
23. Zhou X, Daubert JP, Wolf PD, et al: Epicardial mapping of ventricular defibrillation with monophasic and biphasic shocks in dogs. Circ Res 72:145-160, 1993.
24. Chen P-S, Feld GK, Kriett JM, et al: Relation between upper limit of vulnerability and defibrillation threshold in humans. Circulation 88:186-192, 1993.
25. Ideker RE, Alferness C, Melnick S, et al: Reentry site during fibrillation induction in relation to defibrillation efficacy for different shock waveforms. J Cardiovasc Electrophysiol 12:581-591, 2001.
26. Efimov IR, Cheng YN, Biermann M, et al: Transmembrane voltage changes produced by real and virtual electrodes during monophasic defibrillation shocks delivered by an implantable electrode. J Cardiovasc Electrophysiol 8:1031-1045, 1997.
27. Usui M, Callihan RL, Walker RG, et al: Epicardial shock mapping following monophasic and biphasic shocks of equal voltage with an endocardial lead system. J Cardiovasc Electrophysiol 7:322-334, 1996.
28. Chattipakorn N, Fotuhi PC, Ideker RE: Prediction of defibrillation outcome by epicardial activation patterns following shocks near the defibrillation threshold. J Cardiovasc Electrophysiol 11:1014-1021, 2000.
29. Chattipakorn N, Fotuhi PC, Chattipakorn SC, et al: Three-dimensional mapping of earliest activation after near-threshold ventricular defibrillation shocks. J Cardiovasc Electrophysiol 14:65-69, 2003.
30. Chattipakorn N, Banville I, Gray RA, et al: Mechanism of ventricular defibrillation for near-defibrillation threshold shocks: A whole heart optical mapping study in swine. Circulation 104:1313-1319, 2001.
31. Wang NC, Lee MH, Ohara T, et al: Optical mapping of ventricular defibrillation in isolated swine right ventricles: Demonstration of a postshock isoelectric window after near- threshold defibrillation shocks. Circulation 104:227-233, 2001.
32. Chattipakorn N, Banville I, Gray RA, et al: Mechanisms of VF reinitiation after failed defibrillation shocks: An optical mapping study in isolated swine hearts. J Am Coll Cardiol 37:135A, 2001.
33. Chen PS, Shibata N, Dixon EG, et al: Activation during ventricular defibrillation in open-chest dogs. Evidence of complete cessation and regeneration of ventricular fibrillation after unsuccessful shocks. J Clin Invest 77:810-823, 1986.
34. Zheng X, Walcott GP, Smith WM, et al: Evidence that activation following failed defibrillation is not caused by triggered activity. J Cardiovasc Electrophysiol 16:1200-1205, 2005.
35. Hwang GS, Hayashi H, Tang L, et al: Intracellular calcium and vulnerability to fibrillation and defibrillation in Langendorff-perfused rabbit ventricles. Circulation 114:2595-2603, 2006.
36. Gotoh M, Uchida T, Mandel WJ, et al: Cellular graded responses and ventricular vulnerability to reentry by a premature stimulus in isolated canine ventricle. Circulation 95:2141-2154, 1997.

37. Ashihara T, Constantino J, Trayanova NA: Tunnel propagation of postshock activations as a hypothesis for fibrillation induction and isoelectric window. Circ Res 102:737-745, 2008.
38. Dosdall DJ, Cheng KA, Huang J, et al: Transmural and endocardial Purkinje activation in pigs before local myocardial activation after defibrillation shocks. Heart Rhythm 4:758-765, 2007.
39. Tovar OH, Jones JL: Electrophysiological deterioration during long-duration ventricular fibrillation. Circulation 102:2886-2891, 2000.
40. Wu TJ, Lin S-F, Hsieh YC, et al: Early recurrence of ventricular fibrillation after successful defibrillation during prolonged global ischemia in isolated rabbit hearts. J Cardiovasc Electrophysiol 19(2):203-210, 2008.

Single Nucleotide Polymorphisms and Cardiac Arrhythmias 49

David J. Tester and Michael J. Ackerman

CHAPTER OUTLINE

Within the field of molecular cardiac electrophysiology, research since the 1980s has elucidated the fundamental genetic substrates underlying many arrhythmogenic cardiac channelopathic disorders associated with sudden cardiac death including long QT syndrome (LQTS), catecholaminergic polymorphic ventricular tachycardia (CPVT), Brugada syndrome, short-QT syndrome (SQTS), Andersen-Tawil syndrome (ATS), progressive cardiac conduction disease, familial atrial fibrillation, idiopathic ventricular fibrillation, and some cases of autopsy-negative sudden unexplained death during infancy, childhood, adolescence, and beyond.

The fundamental pathogenic mechanisms responsible for these disorders have been partially elucidated, and marked genetic and clinical heterogeneity is a common and now recurrent theme; several genes and allelic variants are now known to be responsible for disease pathogenesis. Hundreds of disease-causing or contributing mutations at the single-nucleotide level have been identified in nearly 20 channelopathy-susceptibility genes: 12 LQTS-susceptibility genes, three SQTS-susceptibility genes, three CPVT-susceptibility genes, and six Brugada syndrome–susceptibility genes. Most represent primary pathogenic disease-causing mutations only discovered in disease cohorts, but others represent common or rare genetic polymorphisms identified in disease and in health that might or might not confer an increased risk for arrhythmias in certain settings.

This chapter focuses primarily on the proarrhythmic contributions (disease gene-modifier effects) associated with specific common polymorphisms within the known channelopathy-susceptibility genes. We begin with a brief primer on molecular genetics and single nucleotide polymorphisms (SNPs), followed by sections on the role of functional, common polymorphisms within the genes that encode for either potassium, sodium, or calcium-release channel α and β subunits. The chapter concludes with an examination of the role of common arrhythmia-associated polymorphisms occurring in non–ion channel genes thought to influence either the cardiac action potential duration or autonomic response to sympathetic activation.

Dr. Ackerman is a consultant for PGxHealth with respect to the FAMILION genetic test for cardiac ion channel mutations.

Primer on Molecular Genetics and Single Nucleotide Polymorphisms

In 1953, Watson and Crick described the basic structure of the molecular essence of life, the DNA molecule.[1] DNA is a polymeric nucleic acid macromolecule composed of building blocks called *deoxyribonucleotides*, of which there are four: adenine (A), guanine (G), thymine (T), and cytosine (C). The DNA molecule is essentially nucleotides that are polymerized into long polynucleotide chains. DNA segments that store genetic information in the form of a genetic code are called *genes*. Genes are composed of protein encoding segments (exons) and intervening DNA sequences (introns) that are not a part of the genetic code. Usually 20 to 100 (sometimes several hundred) base pairs upstream from the first translated exon is a regulatory element (promoter) that controls transcription of the hereditary message as defined by the gene sequence. Assembly of a polypeptide or protein is governed by a triplet genetic code, or codon (three consecutive bases), of which there are 64 types that encode for 20 unique amino acids. Each codon is decoded sequentially to give a specific sequence of amino acids that are covalently linked through peptide bonds and ultimately constitute a protein.[2]

Inherited variation in the genome is the foundation of human and medical genetics. Reciprocal forms of genetic information at a precise locus (location) along the genome are called *alleles*. Technically, *allele* can refer to a particular gene, a particular segment of DNA, or even a particular nucleotide. The normal version of genetic information is often referred to as the *wild-type* or *normal* allele. A large majority of the human genome is essentially a clone, being identical at more than 98% of the 3 billion pairs of nucleotides. However, there are many small sections of

DNA sequences or even single nucleotides that differ from one person to another. These normal variations at particular loci in the DNA sequence are called *polymorphisms*.

Some polymorphisms are quite common, and others represent rare forms of the genetic information. In medical genetics, *disease-causing mutation* refers to a variation in DNA sequence that represents an abnormal allele and is not found in the normal population but exists only in the disease population. If a person has a pair of identical alleles, one maternal and one paternal, that person is said to be homozygous for that allele. When the alleles are different, then that person is heterozygous for that particular allele. The terms *genotype* and *phenotype* refer to a person's genetic or DNA sequence makeup at a particular locus or at a collective body of loci (genotype) and to a person's observed clinical expression of disease (phenotype) in terms of a morphologic, biochemical, or molecular trait.

Single-gene mutations can involve alterations at the nucleotide level and can disrupt the normal function of a single gene product. The most common type of single-gene mutation is a single nucleotide substitution (SNP). If a single nucleotide substitution occurs in the coding region (exon), the consequence may be either a synonymous (silent) mutation whereby a different codon still specifies the same amino acid (because of the redundancy of 64 codons for 20 amino acids) or a nonsynonymous mutation whereby the altered codon dictates a different amino acid (mis-sense mutation) or terminates further protein assembly (introduces a premature stop codon or nonsense mutation). Importantly, a mis-sense mutation can result in a functionally perturbed protein or can exhibit a wild-type, or normal, phenotype. The functional consequence of a mis-sense mutation often depends on the differences in biochemical properties between the amino acids that are being exchanged or the location in the protein at which a particular exchange of amino acids occurs.

Base substitutions occurring in the intron can result in an altered gene product as well. The normal process by which intronic sequences are cleaved from newly transcribed RNA to give a mature messenger RNA (mRNA) product relies on specific nucleotide sequences located at the intron-exon (acceptor site) and exon-intron (donor site) boundaries. Base substitutions within these highly conserved regions can result in inappropriate splicing of the immature RNA. In some cases, entire exons can be deleted or entire introns can be included in the mature mRNA. Single-nucleotide substitutions within the promoter region of a gene can influence the overall expression of that gene, leading to either an increase or reduction in copy number of the gene transcript and its transcribed product (protein).[2]

Not all nucleotide substitutions (mutations) create a new gene product that causes a clinical disease state. A DNA sequence variation that might (nonsynonymous) or might not (synonymous) alter the encoded protein is called a *common polymorphism* if it is present in at least 1% of the normal population. Although not pathogenic or disease causing, nonsynonymous single-nucleotide polymorphisms can indeed be *functional* polymorphisms and exert a significant effect on how endogenous and exogenous triggers are handled. That is, under certain endogenous or exogenous stressors, the variant form of the protein (other then wild-type) might exude an abnormal function or phenotype. Rare gene variations (allelic frequency <1%) might also be functionally relevant genetic determinants. Functional polymorphisms are sought to explain the human variation observed with therapeutic and side-effect profiles of pharmaceutical agents (pharmacogenomics) or to rationalize (modifier genes) the heterogeneous expression of disease in families harboring the same presumptive disease-causing mutation.

Prevalence of Channel Variants in LQTS-Associated Genes Among Healthy Subjects

In contrast to rare, pathogenic LQTS-causing channel mutations present in an estimated 1 in 2500 persons, comprehensive genetic testing of the open reading frames (all translated exons) for *KCNQ1*, *KCNH2*, *SCN5A*, *KCNE1*, and *KCNE2* for nearly 1000 healthy volunteers has revealed that approximately 3% to 5% of whites and a similar proportion of blacks, Asians, and Hispanics host rare nonsynonymous genetic variants (<0.5% allelic frequency), yielding a background rate of amino acid substitutions of uncertain significance.[3,4] In fact, a total of 65 distinct nonsynonymous channel variants were detected among these healthy subjects including 20 variants in the *KCNH2*-encoded HERG channel.[3,4] Most of these rare variants are seemingly ethnic-specific, with roughly 10% represented in more than one ethnic group and half found only among blacks. Whether any of these 65 variants are either functionally or clinically relevant requires further examination. In the meantime, their existence serves as an important reminder that genetic testing ultimately is probabilistic in nature, not binary, and that there is the potential for a false-positive genetic test result.

Besides this background rate (3%-5%) of rare variants, 16 common polymorphisms (allelic frequency >0.5% in at least one ethnic group) have been identified in the four potassium-channel subunit genes,[3] and eight common polymorphisms in the sodium channel have been discovered (Fig. 49-1).[4] Several studies indicate that some of these common polymorphisms may be clinically informative and relevant to the identification of those at risk for cardiac arrhythmias.

Functional Common Polymorphisms within Channelopathy-Susceptibility Genes

Extremes of electrocardiographic QT interval, as a measure of cardiac repolarization and action potential duration is associated with an increased risk for sudden cardiac death in the general population, specifically among those being administered potential QT-prolonging drugs. Both rare and common genetic cardiac channel variants and environmental factors (drug-induced acquired LQTS) can influence the QT interval and subsequently increase risk for cardiac arrhythmias and sudden cardiac death. Electrophysiologic and association studies of common genetic determinates (polymorphisms) in genes encoding proteins that orchestrate the cardiac action potential have been performed (Table 49-1).

Clinical Relevance of Common Potassium Channel Single Nucleotide Polymorphisms

Among the common polymorphisms of the *KCNH2*-encoding I_{Kr} potassium channel (also known as HERG), the K897T and R1047L polymorphisms have received the most attention. K897T-HERG is a result of a single nucleotide substitution of an adenine (A) for a cytosine (C) at nucleotide position 2690 (designated 2690 A>C) of the *KCNH2* gene, which alters the 897th codon, resulting in the replacement of the wild-type amino acid, lysine (K) for a threonine (T) in the mature protein. Thus the only difference in liner topology between a K897-HERG channel and a T897-HERG channel is the exchange of these two amino acids at this exact position in the protein. The K897T-HERG is the most common HERG

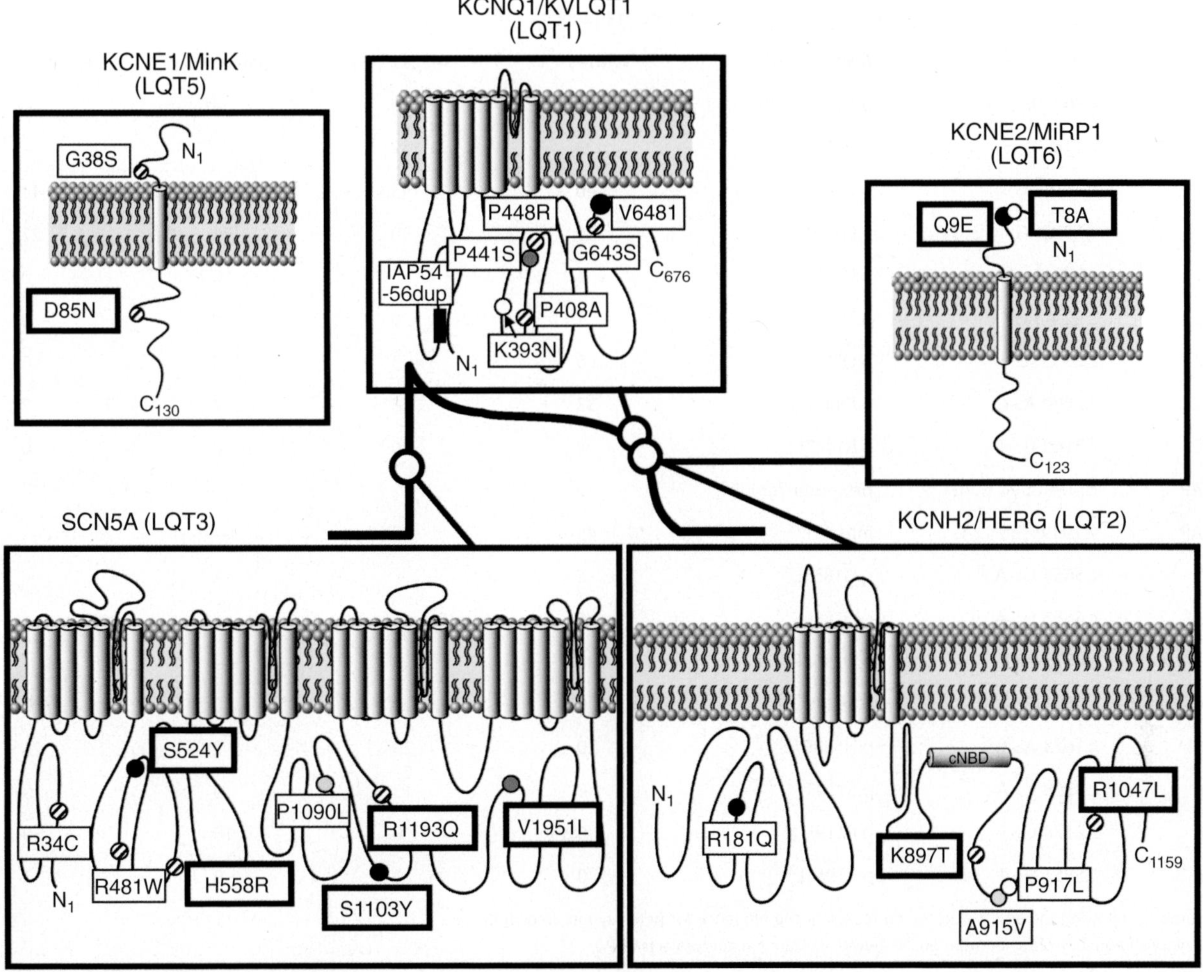

Figure 49-1 Summary of common long-QT syndrome (LQTS)-associated channel polymorphisms. Linear topologies of five LQTS-associated cardiac channel α and β subunits with localization of the 24 unique common nonsynonymous single nucleotide polymorphisms (SNPs) (allelic frequency >0.5% in at least one ethnic group) identified among healthy subjects. Polymorphisms shown in *bold boxes* represent functionally characterized polymorphisms with the potential for increased risk of cardiac arrhythmias. Ethnic-specific polymorphisms are indicated as: *white circle*, white; *black circle*, black; *light-gray circle*, Asian; *dark-gray circle*, Hispanic; *hatched circle*, multiple ethnicities. The *rectangle* designates an in-frame deletion.

polymorphism, with approximately 33% of whites, 8% of blacks, 7.5% of Asians, and 6.8% of Hispanics being heterozygous (see Table 49-1).[5]

Several association studies have attempted to demonstrate a QT-interval duration effect by K897T-HERG. In a 2002 Finnish cohort study, female subjects who were heterozygous (K897T) or homozygous (TT897) for the T897-encoding minor allele had longer QT intervals compared to wild-type subjects.[6] However, four much larger independent population-based studies (more than 5000 subjects collectively) have now provided the opposite, yet definitive conclusion that the minor allele is associated with a shorter QT duration, particularly among female subjects.[7-10]

Similarly, previous expression studies performed to determine the functional sequelae of K897T have been inconsistent. One study reported altered channel kinetics and a 10% to 30% decrease in current density that might cause a subtle increase in action potential duration in T897-HERG channels compared with wild-type (K897) channels.[11] This observation would be consistent with the initial Finnish clinical study but at polar-opposite variance with the rendered conclusions from the larger studies that suggest a modest QT-attenuating effect by T897 containing HERG channels.

A second study observed a smaller current density with reduced cell surface expression of T897-HERG channels and slower activation kinetics with a higher degree of inactivation. These alterations would decrease channel function and perhaps alter drug sensitivity, because several commonly used drugs inhibiting HERG channel function bind preferentially to the inactivated state of the channel.[12] Taken together, these cellular studies suggest that T897 channels may be associated with a reduced repolarization reserve, a longer QT interval, and a pro-arrhythmic response, which may be enhanced in the setting of HERG channel blocking drugs compared with the wild-type K897 channels. In fact, K897T appears to affect the QTc response to ibutilide in a gender-specific manner.[13] In contrast, a third study, using computer-based simulation based on their own electrophysiology data, concluded that T897 might decrease the action potential duration and lead to hastened cardiac repolarization and shorter QT intervals.[7]

Table 49-1 Summary of Common Polymorphisms with Heterozygote Frequencies

Gene	Nucleotide	Amino Acid	Whites (%)	Blacks (%)	Asians (%)	Hispanics (%)
ADRA2C	c.967_978del	p.Del322-325[47]	4	49	—	—
ADRB1	c.1165 C>G	p.G389R[47]	32	57	—	—
ADRB2	c.46 A>G	p.G16R*	40	43.5	16	41
ADRB2	c.79 C>G	p.Q27E*	50	30	21	27
KCNE1	c.253 G>A	p.D85N[1]	1	0.7	0.7	0
KCNE2	c.22 A>G	p.T8A[1]	1	0	0	0
KCNE2	c.25 C>G	p.Q9E[1]	0	3	0	0
KCNH2	c.2690 A>C	p.K897T[1]	33	8	7.5	7
KCNH2	c.3140 G>T	p.R1047L[1]	4	0.3	0	0
NOS1AP	rs10918594 C>G	promoter region[43]	42	32	—	—
NOS1AP	rs10494366 T>G	intron 1[43]	45	45	—	—
RYR2	c.5654 G>A	p.G1885E[39]	8	—	—	—
RYR2	c.5656 G>A	p.G1886S[39]	6	—	—	—
RYR2	c.8873 A>G	p.Q2958R[40]	38	8	—	—
SCN5A	c.1571 C>A	p.S524Y[2]	0	6	0	0
SCN5A	c.1673 A>G	p.H558R[2]	20	29	9	23
SCN5A	c.3308 C>A	p.S1103Y[2]	0	13	0	0
SCN5A	c.3578 G>A	p.R1193Q[2]	0.3	0	16	0
SCN5A	c.5851 G>T	p.V1951L[2]	0	0	0	7

Note: Numbers following the amino acid coding represent the reference for heterozygote frequency.
*Heterozygote frequency obtained from dbSNP (www.ncbi.nlm.nih.gov/projects/SNP/).

Although its modifying effect might not be clear on a population-based scale or an otherwise normal host, the proarrhythmic, disease-modifying effect of K897T has been demonstrated in a vulnerable host, that is a patient already hosting a putative LQT2-causing mutation on the other *KCNH2* allele (Fig. 49-2).[14] The coexistence of K897T and the A1116V-KCNH2 mutation (on opposite alleles) led to a more-severe clinical course in a single Italian LQTS family. The A1116V mutation by itself produced a subclinical phenotype of mild QT prolongation and an asymptomatic course, whereas the proband hosting both variants had clinically overt disease consisting of a diagnostic QT prolongation, presyncopal episodes, and cardiac arrest.[14] Recall that the HERG potassium channel involves post-translational assembly of the *KCNH2*-encoded monomeric subunits into a tetramer. Consequently, I_{Kr} whole-cell current is a summation of 1/16 exclusively maternally derived channels, 1/16 exclusively paternally derived channels, and admixtures in between, with approximately 50% of the channels resulting from the assembly of two maternally and two paternally derived monomers. Consistent with the pedigree analysis, coexpression cellular electrophysiology studies of equimolar amounts of K897T-HERG and A1116V-HERG constructs (mimicking the proband's genomic state) revealed a significantly greater reduction in channel current as compared to either individual variant or wild-type channel.[14]

R1047L-KCNH2 is the second most common nonsynonymous polymorphism in *KCNH2* and is predominantly found in whites, with a prevalence of approximately 4%.[15] This polymorphism appears to confer increased risk for dofetilide-induced torsades de pointes. Among 105 *KCNH2* genotyped patients treated with dofetilide for atrial fibrillation, two of the seven (29%) who developed dofetilide-induced torsades de pointes were identified as R1047L carriers compared with only five of 98 (5%) patients who were free of torsades de pointes.[16] However, as with the K897T story, expression studies have yielded conflicting results here also: One suggested a positive shift in steady-state activation of the channel, and the other found L1047-containing HERG channels to be electrophysiologically indistinguishable from wild-type (R1047) channels.[11,16]

Besides these common potassium channel α-subunit polymorphisms, three common polymorphisms (D85N-KCNE1, T8A-KCNE2, and Q9E-KCNE2) involving auxiliary β subunits have been implicated in drug-induced arrhythmia susceptibility.[17,18] D85N-KCNE1 (also annotated as minK) has a prevalence of 1% to 2% in the general population,[5] is associated with increased risk for drug-induced LQT and arrhythmias, and electrophysiologically exhibits altered kinetic properties of the I_{Ks} potassium current (concomitant expression of KCNQ1 and KCNE1 channel subunits) resulting from slower KCNQ1 channel activation and accelerated deactivation, compared with

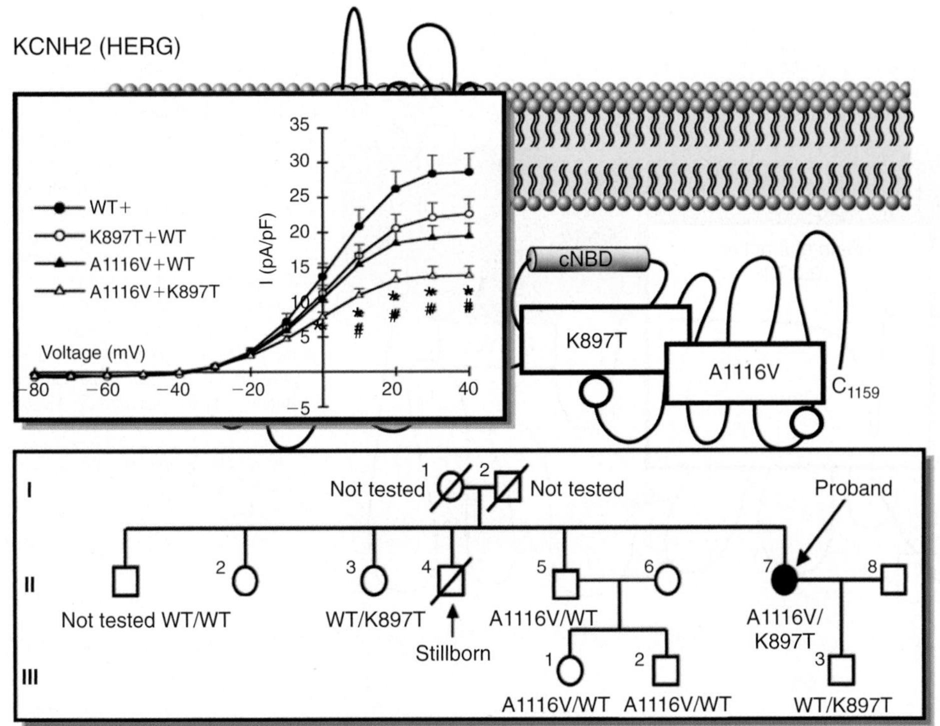

Figure 49-2 Illustrated is the modifying affect of the common polymorphism K897T-KCNH2 on the clinical and molecular phenotype for a family with a putative type 2 long-QT syndrome (LQT2)-associated mutation in *KCNH2* (A1116V). Pedigree analysis demonstrated that only the proband, carrying both the K897T and A1116V variants (inferred to be on opposite alleles), has clinically overt disease. Coexpression studies revealed a significantly lower tail current density in cells expressing both K897T-containing and A1116V-containing HERG channels compared to wild-type only, K897T/wild-type, and A1116V/wild-type. *Significant difference between K897T + A1116V and WT; #significant difference between K897T + A1116V and A1116V + WT. (Adapted from Crotti L, Lundquist AL, Insolia R, et al: KCNH2-K897T is a genetic modifier of latent congenital long-QT syndrome. Circulation 112:1251-1258, 2005.)

wild-type channels.[17] Similarly, T8A-KCNE2 is a 1% prevalent polymorphism among whites and appears overrepresented among patients with quinidine-induced arrhythmias.[18]

Q9E-KCNE2 (also annotated MiRP1, for minK-related peptide-1) was initially discovered in a 76-year-old black woman being treated for pneumonia with clarithromycin, an antibiotic with known potential for an unwanted QT-prolonging side effect.[18] Following only two doses, her baseline QTc increased from 460 to 560 ms and she developed drug-induced torsades de pointes and ventricular fibrillation that required external cardioversion. Genetic testing revealed Q9E, and functional studies demonstrated that Q9E-MiRP1–containing channels were considerably more sensitive to clarithromycin-induced HERG block then wild-type channels, thus providing a functional mechanism for the patient's torsadogenic drug reaction.[18] Notably, Q9E was concluded to represent a rare pathogenic LQT6-associated mutation by virtue of its absence in more than 1000 controls.[18] However, the critical importance of using ethnic-matched controls was demonstrated subsequently by showing that in fact, Q9E was not a rare variant but an ethnic-specific common polymorphism present in approximately 3% of blacks.[3] The extent to which Q9E might confer increased risk for drug-induced arrhythmias in the setting of exposure to QT-prolonging medications among blacks has not been investigated further.

Clinical Relevance of Common Sodium Channel Single-Nucleotide Polymorphisms

Common polymorphisms of the *SCN5A*-encoded cardiac sodium channel have been proposed to confer increased risk for cardiac arrhythmias and serve as genetic modifiers of cardiac sodium channel–mediated LQTS (LQT3), Brugada syndrome (BrS1), or progressive conduction disease. Of the eight nonsynonymous common *SCN5A* SNPs discovered in various ethnic populations, five (S524Y, H558R, S1103Y, R1193Q, and V1951L) have been examined for their contribution to cardiac disease (see Fig. 49-1 and Table 49-1).

H558R (wild-type histidine [H] at amino acid 558 exchanged for an arginine [R]) is the most common sodium channel SNP and the only polymorphism present in all ethnicities previously studied, with a minor allelic frequency of approximately 29% in blacks, 20% in whites, 23% in Hispanics, and 9% in Asians.[19] The electrophysiologic functional signature of R558-SCN5A channels is indistinguishable from wild-type H558-containing channels. However, H558R has been shown to be a genetic modifier of sodium channel disease through intrageneic complementation of other SCN5A mutations (Fig. 49-3).[20]

In the setting of the sporadic, spontaneous germline pathogenic mutation, M1766L, that was discovered postmortem in a 16-month-old boy previously manifesting only a prolonged QT interval (QTc 480-530 ms),[21] H558R had a profound influence on the expression of the mutant L1766-SCN5A channel.[20] In the context of H558, L1766-containing sodium channels displayed BrS1-like loss of function pursuant to defective ion-channel trafficking. However, in the context of R558, the L1766-containing sodium channels were processed properly and localized to the plasma membrane, but they displayed a 10-fold increase in persistent late sodium current consistent with type 3 LQTS (LQT3). Besides establishing the pathogenic mechanisms and the modifying effect of this common polymorphism, these observations illustrate the need for channel expression studies to be performed in the context of the proper channel background.[20]

In contrast to the need for post-translational assembly of the monomeric potassium channel subunits, the *SCN5A* gene already contains the architectural blueprints for the entire pore-forming α subunit. As such, the sodium current is a 50:50 composite of wholly maternally derived and wholly paternally

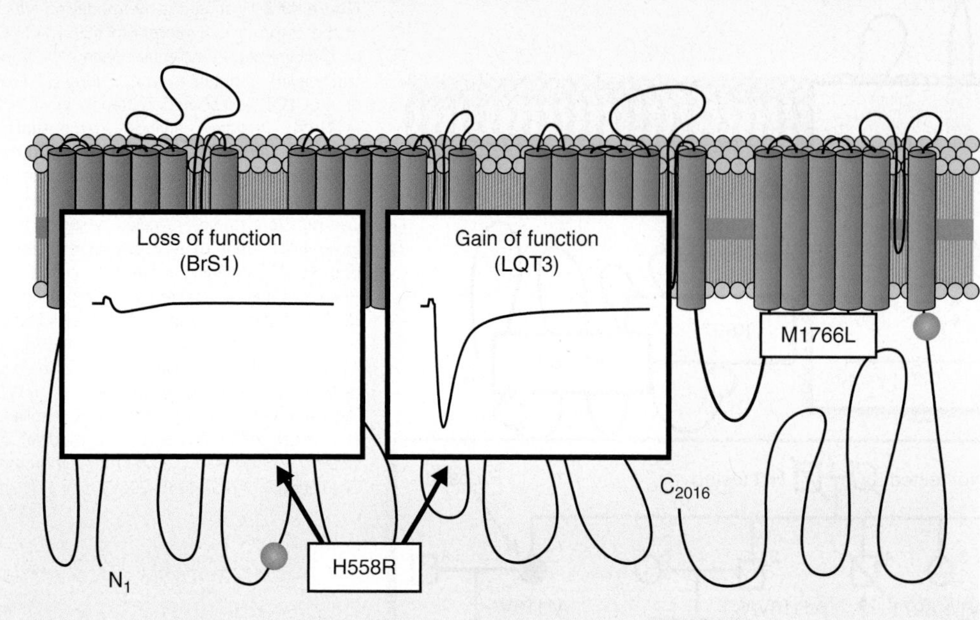

Figure 49-3 Intragenic complementation H558R modifying effect on the M1766L SCN5A mutation. In the context of H558, L1766 channels displayed loss-of-function phenotype BrS1 pursuant to defective ion-channel trafficking. However, in the context of R558, L1766 channels were processed properly and localized to the plasma membrane, but they displayed a 10-fold increase in persistent late sodium current consistent with type 3 long-QT syndrome (LQT3). (Adapted from Ye B, Valdivia CR, Ackerman MJ, Makielski JC: A common human SCN5A polymorphism modifies expression of an arrhythmia causing mutation. Physiol Genomics 12:187-193, 2003.)

derived sodium channels. Because the patient manifested QT prolongation and not a Brugada ECG pattern, it is assumed that both R558 and L1766 resided on the same allele, resulting in rescued sodium current with increased late current. Similarly, H558R has been shown to alter the kinetics of the T512I cardiac conduction disorder mutation.[22] To what extent H558R is involved as a genetic modifier in the expression of other SCN5A mutations or even rare polymorphisms remains to be seen.

An interesting aspect to the cardiac sodium channel is the universal presence of two alternatively spliced transcripts of *SCN5A* in human heart, resulting in the expression of two distinct cardiac sodium channels: one comprising 2016 amino acids and containing a glutamine at position 1077 (Q1077) and one having only 2015 amino acid residues and lacking the glutamine at this position (Q1077del).[23] These two transcripts differing only by either the inclusion or exclusion of a single amino acid are present in all hearts examined in an approximate 2:1 ratio. Nearly two thirds (65%) of the total *SCN5A* transcript is made up of the 2015 amino-acid variant lacking Q1077 (Q1077del) and one third (35%) is the full-length, Q1077-containing sodium channel.[23] Thus, any mutation or polymorphism at any site in *SCN5A* would be expressed in the context of both alternatively spliced transcripts, and the expression can be profoundly different between the two transcripts.

For example, R558 expressed in the context of the major transcript (Q1077del) yields a channel of normal function, but R558 expressed in the setting of the minor transcript (Q1077) produces a normal trafficking channel but with profoundly reduced current density to less than 5% of that of the wild-type, resulting in a nonfunctional channel (Fig. 49-4).[23] Accordingly, an estimated 9% of blacks and 5% of whites who are homozygous for the minor R558-encoding allele theoretically would have an estimated 30% reduction in peak sodium current. Similarly, S524Y, a relatively ethnic-specific polymorphism with a prevalence of 6% among blacks, displayed a pronounced 75% loss-of-function phenotype when expressed in the Q1077 background.[24] Whether this genetically derived reduced depolarization capacity is arrhythmogenic and a potential risk factor for drug-induced torsades de pointes remains to be determined. Rare pathogenic SCN5A mutations leading to a 50% reduction in peak sodium current provide the pathogenic substrate for approximately 20% to 30% of Brugada syndrome.[25] In this regard, R558 was significantly over-represented (26% vs 10%) in 48 Chinese Brugada patients compared with 120 control patients.[26] In addition, the R558-encoding minor allele was over-represented (30% vs 21%) among 157 white patients with early-onset lone atrial fibrillation compared with 314 matched controls.[27]

The most prominent common SNP to confer arrhythmia susceptibility in an ethnic-specific manner is S1103Y-SCN5A (originally annotated as the Y1102 variant).[28] Notably, most carriers of this polymorphism never have an arrhythmia, but evidence suggests that potential lethal arrhythmias associated with this variant might occur in the setting of common endogenous factors such as exposure to QT-prolonging drugs, hypokalemia, structural heart disease, and conditions of acidosis.[29,30] S1103Y, seen in 13% of blacks, but not observed in any white or Asian controls (>1000 subjects), was over-represented in arrhythmia cases,[29,] among black adolescent and adult cases of autopsy-negative sudden unexplained death (SUD)[31] and sudden infant death syndrome (SIDS).[30,32] S1103Y has very subtle alterations in channel kinetics in heterologous expression studies when studied under basal conditions.[29] However, functional and modeling studies supported the potential for QT prolongation, reactivation of calcium channels, early afterdepolarizations, and arrhythmias, particularly in the setting of concomitant exposure to HERG-blocking drugs.[29] Further, under conditions mimicking cellular acidosis, Y1103-SCN5A channels exhibited significant persistent late sodium current, a signature phenotype of LQT3 (Fig. 49-5).[30]

R1193Q and V1951L are two common SCN5A polymorphisms among Asians (16% prevalence) and Hispanics (7%prevalence)[19] that were initially reported as BrS1-causing

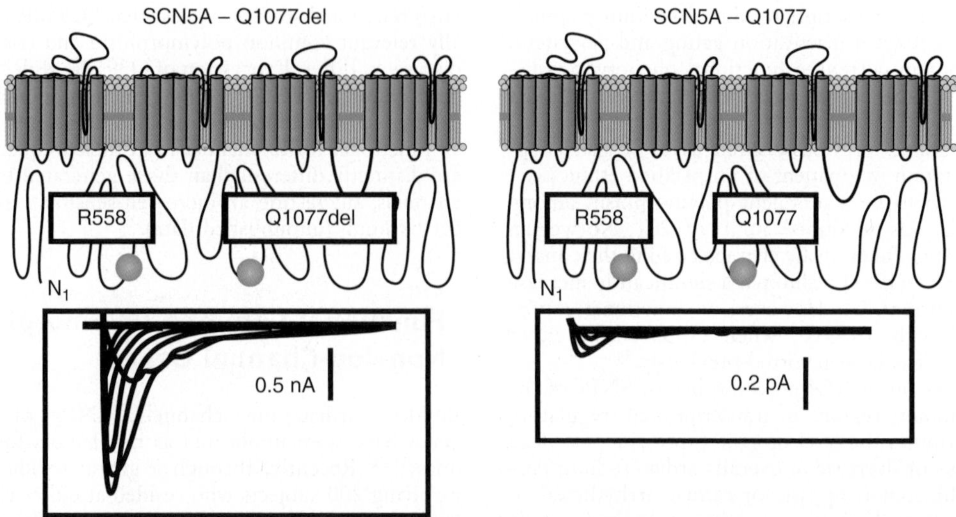

Figure 49-4 R558 and the ubiquitous Q1077 splice variant. The linear topology of two alternatively spliced transcripts of SCN5A resulting in the expression of two distinct cardiac sodium channels: one having 2016 amino acids and containing a glutamine at position 1077 (Q1077), and one having only 2015 amino acid residues and lacking the glutamine at this position (Q1077del). Nearly two thirds (65%) of the total SCN5A transcript is made up of Q1077del and a third (35%) is made up of Q1077. In the context of the major transcript (Q1077del), the common polymorphism, R558, yields a normal functioning channel, whereas R558/Q1077-SCN5A results in a trafficking-defective, nonfunctional channel. Accordingly, an estimated 9% of blacks and 5% of whites who are homozygous for R558 theoretically would have an estimated 30% reduction in peak sodium current. (Adapted from Fitzgerald PT, Ackerman MJ: Drug-induced torsades de pointes: The evolving role of pharmacogenetics. Heart Rhythm 2:S30-S37, 2005.)

mutations.[33,34] Depending on the *SCN5A* transcript (Q1077 or Q1077del) used in expression studies, R1193Q has been characterized functionally as either a loss-of-function (BrS1-like) or gain-of-function (LQT3-like) sodium channel. R1193Q (previously denoted R1192Q) was described originally in a Japanese family with sudden unexplained nocturnal death syndrome (SUNDS), a phenocopy of Brugada syndrome.[34] When expressed in *Xenopus* oocytes, presumably in the context of Q1077del (the major *SCN5A* transcript), the R1193Q mutation accelerated fast inactivation of the sodium channel and resulted in reduced sodium current consistent with a Brugada syndrome phenotype.[34] Another study identified R1193Q in one of seven patients with acquired LQTS, an 82-year-old white man with a normal baseline QTc of 442 ms who developed marked QT prolongation following administration of both sotalol and quinidine.[35] Here, R1193Q expressed in the context of Q1077

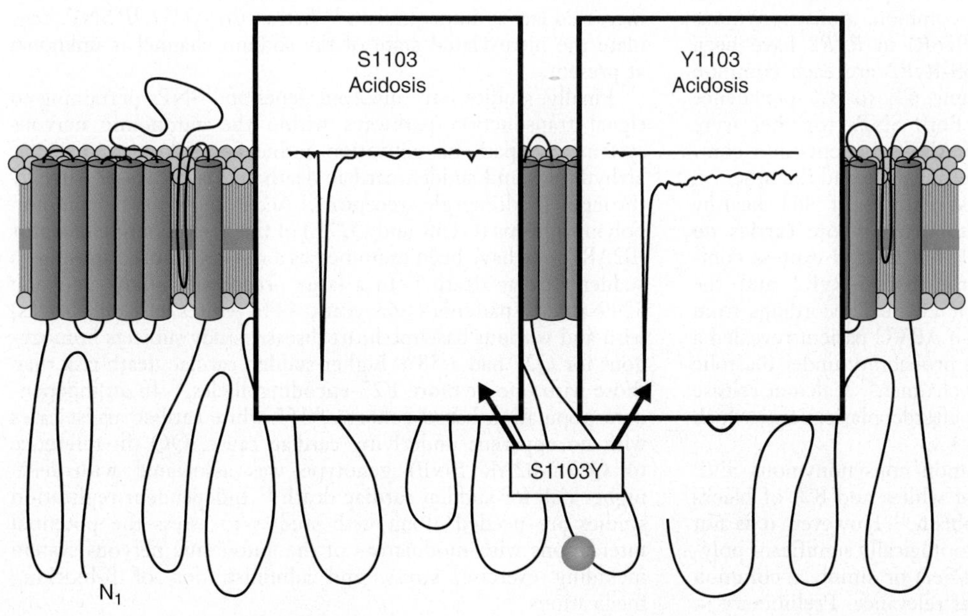

Figure 49-5 Depicted is the ethnic-specific common polymorphism, S1103Y, present in 13% of healthy blacks, but over-represented among cases of sudden unexplained death (SUD) and sudden infant death syndrome (SIDS). Under conditions of acidosis, Y1103-SCN5A channels yield significant persistent late sodium current, a signature phenotype of LQT3. (Adapted from Plant LD, Bowers PN, Liu QY, et al: A common cardiac sodium channel variant associated with sudden infant death in African Americans, SCN5A S1103Y. J Clin Invest 116:430-435, 2006.)

(i.e., the minor *SCN5A* transcript) produced sodium channels characterized by destabilized inactivation gating and persistent, non-inactivating sodium current, a functional phenotype indistinguishable from other previously characterized LQT3 mutations.[35]

The V1951L variant, previously cited as a Brugada syndrome–causing mutation in a patient of unspecified ethnicity,[33] has now been shown to be a prevalent polymorphism among Hispanics. V1951L was identified in 1 of 201 Norwegian SIDS victims, and when functionally characterized in the context of Q1077del-SCN5A, V1951L exhibited a significantly increase persistent sodium current.[36,37] However, no functional abnormalities associated with V1951L, when expressed in either SCN5A background, has been reported previously.[24]

Besides coding region *SCN5A* polymorphisms, SNPs of the *SCN5A* core promoter region, a transcriptional regulatory sequence that determines the level of gene expression, can lead to either an increase or decrease in overall cardiac sodium current density, thereby conferring risk for cardiac arrhythmias or modulate sodium channel disease phenotype. A single study identified a set of six *SCN5A* promoter polymorphisms and a haplotype denoted as HapB with an allelic frequency of 22% in Asians, having a significant impact on sodium channel expression, variance in ECG conduction parameters, including PR and QRS durations, and predicting variable pharmacologic drug response of sodium channel blockers.[38] The *SCN5A* HapB variant, which as a result of reduced sodium channel current, slowed cardiac conduction in normal persons and exacerbated conduction slowing in Brugada patients. In addition, further depression of sodium channel function through administration of sodium channel–blocking drugs further exacerbated conduction slowing in a gene- and dose-dependent manner.[38] The extent to which regulatory region polymorphisms influence the risk for arrhythmias and sudden cardiac death remain to be investigated.

Clinical Relevance of Common Calcium Release Channel (Ryanodine Receptor) Single Nucleotide Polymorphisms

Catecholaminergic polymorphic ventricular tachycardia (CPVT) and arrhythmogenic right ventricular cardiomyopathy (ARVC), two potentially fatal disorders, result in part from perturbations of the *RYR2*-encoded cardiac ryanodine receptor/calcium release channel.[39-41] To date, only three common, nonsynonymous SNPs (G1885E, G1886S, and Q2958R) in *RYR2* have been reported.[41-43] G1885E- and G1886S-RyR2 are each common polymorphisms with an approximately 6% to 8% prevalence among healthy control subjects.[42] Both SNPs together were found exclusively in three out of 85 ARVC patients in a composite heterozygote (one on the maternal allele and the other on the paternal allele) form compared with 0 of 463 healthy German blood donors.[42] Composite heterozygote carries do not express wild-type RyR2 channels but instead express composite channels containing both the E1885-RyR2 and the S1886-RyR2 channel subunits. Single channel recordings from native RyR2 isolated from heart of an ARVC patient revealed a channel with greatly enhanced open probability under diastolic conditions, indicating a leaky RyR2 channel.[42] Calcium release during diastole can provoke delayed afterdepolarizations, which can initiate fatal arrhythmias.

Q2958R-RyR2 is the most common nonsynonymous SNP in *RYR2*, and approximately 38% of whites and 8% of blacks are heterozygous for this polymorphism.[43] However, it is not known whether or not Q2958R is a biologically significant polymorphism (i.e., a disease gene modifier) or simply a common variant with no functional or clinical relevance. Preliminary in vitro functional studies suggest that Q2958R may be a functionally relevant common polymorphism and consequently a novel disease modifier. Expression of Q2958R-RyR2 in human embryonic kidney (HEK293) cells generates spontaneous Ca^{2+}- and caffeine-sensitive intracellular Ca^{2+} transients, as expected from all functional RyR2 channels, but their frequency and amplitude are distinctly different than those generated by wild-type RyR2 channels, suggesting an increased sensitivity to luminal or high Ca^{2+} stimuli (unpublished data).

Functional Common Polymorphisms within Non–Ion-Channel Genes

Besides cardiac ion channels, SNPs of non–ion-channel genes have been implicated as risk factors for cardiac arrhythmias.[44-48] Recently, through a genome-wide association study involving 200 subjects who resided at either extreme of a population-based QT-interval distribution derived from nearly 4000 subjects[44] and several large replication studies,[44-46] investigators showed that two SNPs (rs10918594 C>G, located in the promoter region, heterozygote frequency of 42%; and rs10494366 T>G, located in intron 1, heterozygote frequency of 45%) of *NOS1AP* (the gene encoding the nitric oxide synthase 1 adapter protein) were associated with QT interval duration and accounted for less than 2% of the individual variability in QT interval duration. The minor allele (G) for each SNP was associated independently with an increase in QT duration (ranging from 3.8 to 9.3 ms for rs10494366 and from 3.6 ms to 12.5 ms for rs10918594, depending on the study).[45,46]

Although these variants account for only a small portion of the total variation in QT duration, identification of a gene not previously known to be involved in cardiac repolarization reveals a novel biologic pathway to be investigated for potential determinants of risk for arrhythmia and sudden cardiac death. Convergence between disease-susceptibility genes for uncommon heritable arrhythmia syndromes and commonly occurring proarrhythmic SNPs is occurring with respect to this biologic pathway as well, with the recent identification of mutations in *SNTA1*-encoded syntrophin alpha as a novel pathogenic mechanism for LQTS.[49] Here, perturbations in syntrophin alpha culminated in dysregulation of nNOS, increased *S*-nitrosylation of the sodium channel, and consequently, increased late sodium current. Whether the *NOS1AP* SNPs regulate the nitrosylated state of the sodium channel is unknown at present.

Finally, studies have involved genes and SNPs pertaining to signal transduction pathways within the autonomic nervous system. Sympathetic activation influences risk of ventricular arrhythmias and sudden cardiac death and is mediated partially through β-adrenergic receptors. Accordingly, two common polymorphisms (G16R and Q27E) of the β_2-adrenergic receptor (B2AR) gene have been examined as a risk factor predisposing to sudden cardiac death.[47] In a large prospective study involving 5249 elderly patients ($\geq$65 years, 4441 whites and 808 blacks) with and without baseline heart disease, study subjects homozygous for Q27 had a 58% higher sudden cardiac death risk than those with one or more E27-encoding alleles.[47] In an independent population-based cohort of 155 white cardiac arrest cases with no apparent underlying cardiac cause, QQ (in reference to Q27E-B2AR SNP) genotype was associated with 64% higher risk for sudden cardiac death.[47] Independent replication studies are needed along with studies to assess the potential interactions with modulators of the autonomic nervous system including exercise, stress, and administration of β-blocking medications.

Differences in autonomic response might influence the clinical severity observed in LQTS, specifically patients with type 1 LQTS (LQT1) in whom the main arrhythmic triggers involve sympathetic activation. Among a South African LQT1 founder population with A341V-KCNQ1, there was a strong correlation between major cardiac events and resting heart rate and baroreflex sensitivity (BRS).[48] Specifically, lower resting heart rate and relatively low BRS appeared to be protective factors among patients carrying the A341V mutation. In other words, lower BRS values were associated with a lower probability of being symptomatic for cardiac events including syncope or cardiac arrest.[48] BRS, a quantitative marker of autonomic responses, is thought to be partly under genetic control.[50] As such, genetic polymorphisms of the adrenergic cascade known to modify norepinepherine release or adrenergic receptor sensitivity to catecholamines were assessed. Interestingly, two common polymorphisms (del322-325-ADRA2C and G389R-ADRB1) influenced BRS within this LQT1 founder population.[51] Specifically, BRS values increased with the presence of the R389 allele alone. Patients homozygous for R389-ADRB1 and heterozygous carriers of Del322-325-ADRA2C had the highest BRS values and the greatest risk for cardiac events, suggesting that these two polymorphisms could act synergistically to modify BRS.[48]

Since the sentinel discovery of rare pathogenic mutations in genes that encode critical cardiac channel α subunits as the pathogenic basis for LQTS in 1995, a decade of investigations from bench to bedside and back again were necessary before genetic testing transcended research laboratories, maturing into clinically available diagnostic tests to assist in the diagnostic evaluation and management of patients and families with a suspected cardiac channelopathy. Although the present compendium of proarrhythmic common SNPs is much smaller than the myriad of rare pathogenic mutations, the extent of their disease modification still requires far greater scrutiny before any proarrhythmic SNP departs from the research laboratory into a clinically relevant, informative, and actionable biomarker.

References

1. Watson JD, Crick FH: Molecular structure of nucleic acids: A structure for deoxyribose nucleic acid. Nature 171:737-738, 1953.
2. Ensenauer RE, Reinke SS, Ackerman MJ, et al: Primer on medical genomics part VIII: Essentials of medical genetics for the practicing physician. Mayo Clin Proc 78:846-857, 2003.
3. Ackerman MJ, Tester DJ, Jones GS, et al: Ethnic differences in cardiac potassium channel variants: Implications for genetic susceptibility to sudden cardiac death and genetic testing for congenital long QT syndrome. Mayo Clin Proc 78:1479-1487, 2003.
4. Ackerman MJ, Splawski I, Makielski J, et al: Spectrum and prevalence of cardiac sodium channel variants among black, white, Asian, and Hispanic individuals: Implications for arrythmogenic susceptibility and Brugada/long QT syndrome genetic testing. Heart Rhythm 1:600-607, 2004.
5. Ackerman MJ, Tester DJ, Jones GS, et al: Ethnic differences in cardiac potassium channel variants: Implications for genetic susceptibility to sudden cardiac death and genetic testing for congenital long QT syndrome. Mayo Clin Proc 78:1479-1487, 2003.
6. Pietila E, Fodstad H, Niskasaari E, et al: Association between HERG K897T polymorphism and QT interval in middle-aged Finnish women. J Am Coll Cardiol 40:511-514, 2002.
7. Bezinna CR, Verkerk AO, Busjahn A, et al: A common polymorphism in KCNH2 (HERG) hastens cardiac repolarization. Cardiovasc Res 59:27-36, 2003.
8. Gouas L, Nicaud V, Berthet M, et al; Group DESIRS: Association of *KCNQ1*, *KCNE1*, *KCNH2* and *SCN5A* polymorphisms with QTc interval length in a healthy population. Eur J Hum Genet 13:1213-1222, 2005.
9. Pfeufer A, Jalilzadeh S, Perz S, et al: Common variants in myocardial ion channel genes modify the QT interval in the general population: results from the KORA study. Circulation Research 96:693-701, 2005.
10. Newton-Cheh C, Guo CY, Larson MG, et al: Common genetic variation in *KCNH2* is associated with QT interval duration: The Framingham Heart Study. Circulation 116:1128-1136, 2007.
11. Anson BD, Ackerman MJ, Tester DJ, et al: Molecular and functional characterization of common polymorphisms in HERG (KCNH2) potassium channels. Am J Physiol Heart Circ Physiol 286:H2434-H2441, 2004.
12. Paavonen KJ, Chapman H, Laitenen PJ, et al: Functional characterization of the common amino acid 897 polymorphism of the cardiac potassium channel KCNH2 (HERG). Cardiovasc Res 59:603-611, 2003.
13. Kannankeril PJ, Norris KJ, Gillani MS, et al: A common polymorphism in *KCNH2* (HERG) eliminates gender differences in drug-induced QT prolongation. Heart Rhythm abstract supplement P2-P34, 2005.
14. Crotti L, Lundquist AL, Pedrazzini M, et al: Common *KCNH2* polymorphism (K897T) as a genetic modifier of congenital long QT syndrome. Heart Rhythm abstract supplement P1-P19, 2005.
15. Ackerman MJ, Tester DJ, Jones G, et al: Ethnic differences in cardiac potassium channel variants: Implications for genetic susceptibility to sudden cardiac death and genetic testing for congenital long QT syndrome. Mayo Clin Proc 78:1479-1487, 2003.
16. Sun Z, Milos PM, Thompson JF, et al: Role of KCNH2 polymorphism (R1047L) in dofetilide-induced torsades de pointes. J Mol Cell Cardiol 37:1031-1039, 2004.
17. Wei J, Yang IC, Tapper AR: KCNE1 polymorphism confers risk of drug-induced long QT syndrome by altering properties of I_{Ks} potassium channels. Circulation (supplement I):I-495, 1999.
18. Abbott GW, Sesti F, Splawski I, et al: MiRP1 forms I_{Kr} potassium channels with HERG and is associated with cardiac arrhythmia. Cell 97:175-187, 1999.
19. Ackerman MJ, Splawski I, Makielski JC, et al: Spectrum and prevalence of cardiac sodium channel variants among black, white, Asian, and Hispanic individuals: Implications for arrhythmogenic susceptibility and Brugada/long QT syndrome genetic testing. Heart Rhythm 1:600-607, 2004.
20. Ye B, Valdivia CR, Ackerman MJ, Makielski JC: A common human SCN5A polymorphism modifies expression of an arrhythmia causing mutation. Physiol Genomics 12:187-193, 2003.
21. Valdivia CR, Ackerman MJ, Tester DJ, et al: A novel SCN5A arrhythmia mutation, M1766L, with expression defect rescued by mexiletine. Cardiovasc Res 55:279-289, 2002.
22. Viswanathan PC, Benson DW, Balser JR: A common SCN5A polymorphism modulates the biophysical effects of an SCN5A mutation. J Clin Invest 111:341-346, 2003.
23. Makielski JC, Ye B, Valdivia CR, et al: A ubiquitous splice variant and a common polymorphism affect heterologous expression of recombinant human SCN5A heart sodium channels. Circ Res 93:821-828, 2003.
24. Tan B-H, Valdivia CR, Rok BA, et al: Common human *SCN5A* polymorphisms have altered electrophysiology when expressed in Q1077 splice variants. Heart Rhythm 2:741-747, 2005.
25. Ackerman MJ. Cardiac channelopathies: It's in the genes. Nat Med 10:463-464, 2004.
26. Chen JZ, Xie XD, Wang XX, et al: Single nucleotide polymorphisms of the *SCN5A* gene in Han Chinese and their relation with Brugada syndrome. Chin Med J 117:652-656, 2004.
27. Chen LY, Ballew JD, Herron KJ, et al: A common polymorphism in SCN5A is associated with lone atrial fibrillation. Clin Pharmacol Ther 81:35-41, 2007.
28. Splawski I, Timothy KW, Tateyama M, et al: Variant of SCN5A sodium channel implicated in risk of cardiac arrhythmia. Science 297:1333-1336, 2002.
29. Splawski I, Timothy KW, Tateyama M, et al: Variant of SCN5A sodium channel implicated in risk of cardiac arrhythmia. Science 297:1333-1336, 2002.
30. Plant LD, Bowers PN, Liu QY, et al: A common cardiac sodium channel variant

associated with sudden infant death in blacks, SCN5A S1103Y. J Clin Invest 116:430-435, 2006.
31. Burke A, Creighton W, Mont E, et al: Role of SCN5A Y1102 polymorphism in sudden cardiac death in blacks. Circulation 112:798-802, 2005.
32. Van Norstrand DW, Tester DJ, Ackerman MJ: Overrepresentation of the proarrhythmic, sudden death predisposing sodium channel polymorphism S1103Y in a population-based cohort of African-American sudden infant death syndrome. Heart Rhythm 5:712-715, 2008.
33. Priori SG, Napolitano C, Gasparini M, et al: Natural history of Brugada syndrome: Insights for risk stratification and management. Circulation 105:1342-1347, 2002.
34. Vatta M, Dumaine R, Varghese G, et al: Genetic and biophysical basis of sudden unexplained nocturnal death syndrome (SUNDS), a disease allelic to Brugada syndrome. Hum Mol Genet 11:337-345, 2002.
35. Wang Q, Chen S, Chen Q, et al: The common *SCN5A* mutation R1193Q causes LQTS-type electrophysiological alterations of the cardiac sodium channel. J Med Genet 41:e66, 2004.
36. Arnestad M, Crotti L, Rognum TO, et al: Prevalence of long-QT syndrome gene variants in sudden infant death syndrome. Circulation 115:361-367, 2007.
37. Wang DW, Desai RR, Crotti L, et al: Cardiac sodium channel dysfunction in sudden infant death syndrome. Circulation 115:368-376, 2007.
38. Bezzina CR, Shimizu W, Yang P, et al: Common sodium channel promoter haplotype in asian subjects underlies variability in cardiac conduction. Circulation 113:338-344, 2006.
39. Laitinen PJ, Brown KM, Piippo K, et al: Mutations of the cardiac ryanodine receptor (RyR2) gene in familial polymorphic ventricular tachycardia. Circulation 103:485-490, 2001.
40. Priori SG, Napolitano C, Tiso N, et al: Mutations in the cardiac ryanodine receptor gene (hRyR2) underlie catecholaminergic polymorphic ventricular tachycardia. Circulation 103:196-200, 2001.
41. Tiso N, Stephan DA, Nava A, et al: Identification of mutations in the cardiac ryanodine receptor gene in families affected with arrhythmogenic right ventricular cardiomyopathy type 2 (ARVD2). Hum Mol Genet 10:189-194, 2001.
42. Milting H, Lukas N, Klauke B, et al: Composite polymorphisms in the ryanodine receptor 2 gene associated with arrhythmogenic right ventricular cardiomyopathy. Cardiovasc Res 71:496-505, 2006.
43. Tester DJ, Salisbury BA, Judson RS, et al: Spectrum and prevalence of genetic variants in the RyR2-encoded cardiac ryanodine receptor-calcium release channel in healthy subjects (Abstract 2464). Circulation 112(17 Suppl):II-516, 2005.
44. Arking DE, Pfeufer A, Post W, et al: A common genetic variant in the NOS1 regulator NOS1AP modulates cardiac repolarization. Nat Genet 38:644-651, 2006.
45. Aarnoudse AJ, Newton-Cheh C, de Bakker PI, et al: Common NOS1AP variants are associated with a prolonged QTc interval in the Rotterdam Study. Circulation 116:10-16, 2007.
46. Lehtinen AB, Newton-Cheh C, Ziegler JT, et al: Association of NOS1AP genetic variants with QT interval duration in families from the Diabetes Heart Study. Diabetes 57:1108-1114, 2008.
47. Sotoodehnia N, Siscovick DS, Vatta M, et al: β_2-Adrenergic receptor genetic variants and risk of sudden cardiac death. Circulation 113:1842-1848, 2006.
48. Schwartz PJ, Vanoli E, Crotti L, et al: Neural control of heart rate is an arrhythmia risk modifier in long QT syndrome. J Am Coll Cardiol 51:920-929, 2008.
49. Ueda K, Valdivia C, Medeiros-Domingo A, et al: Syntrophin mutation associated with long QT syndrome through activation of the nNOS-SCN5A macromolecular complex. Proc Natl Acad Sci U S A 105:9355-9360, 2008.
50. Tank J, Jordan J, Diedrich A, et al: Genetic influences on baroreflex function in normal twins. Hypertension 37:907-910, 2001.
51. Small KM, Wagoner LE, Levin AM, et al: Synergistic polymorphisms of β_1- and α_2C-adrenergic receptors and the risk of congestive heart failure. N Engl J Med 347:1135-1142, 2002.

Inheritable Sodium Channel Diseases 50

ALFRED L. GEORGE, JR.

CHAPTER OUTLINE

More than a decade ago, the discovery and characterization of a mutation in the gene encoding a human cardiac voltage-gated sodium channel gene (*SCN5A*) began a new era in our understanding of the molecular and genetic basis of arrhythmias. Subsequent work has revealed an unexpectedly large number of pathophysiologically diverse conditions associated with an ever-growing number of mutations in this gene (Box 50-1). The diversity of clinical disorders (phenotypes) associated with *SCN5A* is explained in part by corresponding heterogeneity in mutant channel dysfunction. These discoveries have helped reshape the diagnostic paradigm and clinical management of familial arrhythmia syndromes to include genetic testing, gene-specific considerations in therapy, and increased awareness of the need to assess disease risk in family members.

This chapter focuses primarily on molecular genetic and pathophysiologic aspects of the inheritable cardiac sodium-channel diseases. As an organizational framework, these disorders have been grouped into categories based upon their predominant clinical manifestations: ventricular arrhythmia and increased risk of sudden death, impaired cardiac conduction (progressive cardiac conduction disease, familial heart block) syndromes having mixed phenotypes, and other arrhythmic disorders of special interest. However, there is extensive clinical overlap among these broad categorizations, and this is emphasized where appropriate. In the last section of this chapter, special diagnostic and therapeutic challenges in the management of patients with sodium channel disorders are discussed, with particular emphasis on their recognition, proper use and interpretation of genetic tests, identification and management of at-risk family members, and gene-specific treatment strategies. Chapters 1, 9, and 16 provide complementary information about the structure, function, and pharmacology of sodium channels, and references to other chapters are made where appropriate when discussing specific diseases.

Cardiac Sodium Channel Gene

The cardiac sodium channel gene *(SCN5A)* encodes the major voltage-gated sodium channel expressed in human heart. This gene spans approximately 100 kb on the short arm of chromosome 3 (3p21)[1] and is composed of 28 exons ranging in size from 53 (exon 24) to 3257 (exon 28) base pairs (Fig. 50-1).[2] The full-length product of *SCN5A* is a 2016–amino acid protein designated $Na_V1.5$, but other nomenclature (hH1) is also used to describe recombinant forms.[3,4] Alternatively spliced messenger RNAs (mRNAs) transcribed from *SCN5A* have also been detected in heart. One particularly common splice variant is generated by alternative use of splice acceptor sequences at the junction between intron 17 and exon 18, resulting in either inclusion or exclusion of glutamine at position 1077.[5] Approximately half of mature *SCN5A* mRNA in heart encodes the 2015–amino acid alternative form of the protein that arises from this alternative splicing event, and this affects the function of certain variants.[6,7]

Transcription of human *SCN5A* is under the control of a promoter that flanks the first exon, and other determinants of transcription reside in the first intron.[8] Common polymorphisms in the *SCN5A* promoter influence the level of gene expression and are clinically relevant. In particular, a combination of polymorphisms constituting a common haplotype within the promoter has been associated with longer duration of PR and QRS and with the extent of QRS widening during challenge with sodium channel–blocking drugs in Asian subjects.[9] These observations suggest that unequal transcription from the two copies of *SCN5A* (allelic imbalance) could influence the clinical expression of heterozygous mutations in this gene.

Disorders with Ventricular Arrhythmia and Sudden Death

Congenital Long-QT Syndrome

Congenital long-QT syndrome (LQTS) is an inherited condition of abnormal myocardial repolarization. This disorder is characterized clinically by increased risk of potentially fatal ventricular arrhythmias, especially torsades de pointes, manifesting as syncope, cardiac arrest, and sudden unexplained death in otherwise healthy young adults and children. The syndrome is most often transmitted in families as an autosomal dominant trait (Romano-Ward syndrome). Additional information related to this disorder can be found in Chapter 69.

Molecular Genetics

Genetic linkage analysis initially localized an LQTS gene to a region on chromosome 3p (LQT3 locus) in a small number of multigenerational LQTS pedigrees, and this prompted a mutation survey of *SCN5A*, a logical candidate gene mapped previously to this genetic interval.[1] Approximately 10% of autosomal-dominant LQTS can be attributed to mutations at LQT3, but most patients with this inheritable arrhythmia syndrome carry mutations in cardiac potassium-channel genes, mainly *KCNQ1* (LQT1) and *KCNH2* (LQT2).[10,11] Recessive LQTS with congenital deafness has not been attributed to sodium-channel defects. The first *SCN5A* mutation described

Box 50-1 Disorders of the Cardiac Sodium-Channel Gene, *SCN5A*

VENTRICULAR ARRHYTHMIA AND SUDDEN DEATH

Congenital long-QT syndrome type 3
Brugada syndrome type 1
Idiopathic ventricular fibrillation
Sudden unexplained nocturnal death syndrome
Sudden infant death syndrome

IMPAIRED CARDIAC CONDUCTION

Progressive cardiac conduction system disease (Lenègre)
Familial atrioventricular block
Congenital sick sinus syndrome
Atrial standstill

LATENT ARRHYTHMIA SUSCEPTIBILITY

Drug-induced long-QT syndrome
Arrhythmia susceptibility in African Americans (S1103Y)

OTHER

Mixed phenotypes or overlap syndromes
Dilated cardiomyopathy with arrhythmia
Atrial fibrillation

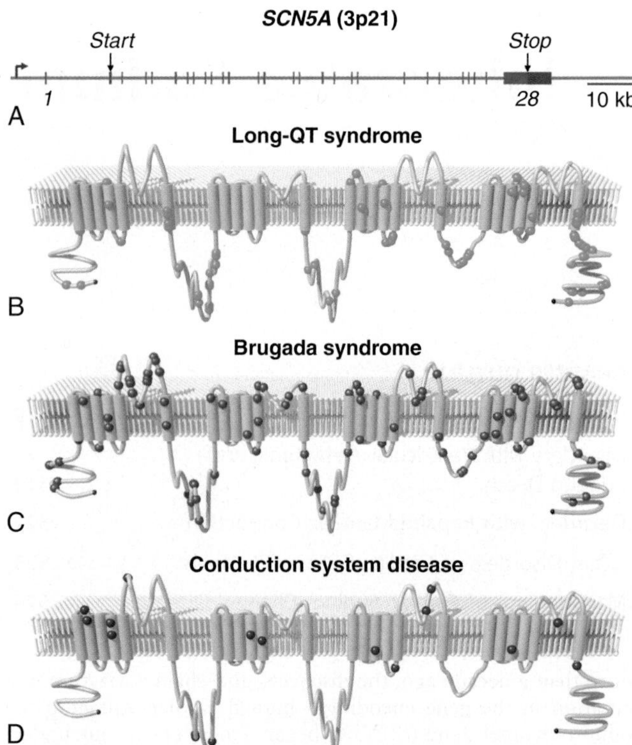

Figure 50-1 *SCN5A* gene structure and mutations. **A,** Schematic of the *SCN5A* gene illustrating relative positions of the 28 exons (vertical lines; *red* for coding exons and *dark gray* for noncoding exons). The *arrow* indicates the approximate location of the gene promoter. Locations of the translation start and stop codons are indicated. **B** to **D,** Location of mutations associated with LQT3 (**B**), Brugada syndrome (**C**), and disorders of cardiac conduction (**D**) superimposed on a two-dimensional membrane topology map of the cardiac sodium channel protein. (Images were prepared by Dr. Robert Abraham of Vanderbilt University using software generously supplied by Dr. Andrel Linnenbank of the University of Amsterdam. Mutation data were obtained from the online Inherited Arrhythmias database http://www.fsm.it/cardmoc/).

was an in-frame deletion of three highly conserved amino acid residues (delKPQ 1505-1507) located within the cytoplasmic loop connecting domains 3 and 4 of $Na_V1.5$,[12] a structural domain responsible for fast inactivation of the channel.

Since discovery of the first *SCN5A* mutation, more than 70 distinct mostly missense mutations have been identified in families with LQT3 (see Fig. 50-1). Although mutations are found throughout the channel sequence, there are a few structural regions where multiple mutations are clustered. One of these regions is the S4 segment of domain 4, a critical structural determinant of voltage sensing and inactivation. Another interesting cluster of mutations can be found in the proximal carboxyl-terminus, a region also implicated in inactivation.[13]

In addition to *SCN5A* mutations, there are reports of rare forms of LQTS that clinically resemble the LQT3 subtype but that have mutations in other genes. Missense mutations in *SCN4B* encoding the β_4 accessory sodium channel subunit[14] and mutations in the gene encoding caveolin-3 (*CAV3*),[15] a protein involved in vesicular trafficking, might exert their pathologic effects by disturbing normal $Na_V1.5$ function.

Genotype-Phenotype Correlation

Carriers of *SCN5A* mutations associated with LQTS often present with distinct clinical features including sinus bradycardia and a tendency for cardiac events to occur during sleep or rest.[16,17] In addition to bradycardia, certain features of the surface electrocardiogram (ECG), such as T-wave morphology, can offer additional clues to the presence of an *SCN5A* mutation in the setting of LQTS. In particular, narrow and late-onset peaked or biphasic T waves occur in approximately half of subjects with genotype-proven LQT3.[18] Cardiac events are less common in carriers of *SCN5A* mutations than they are in LQT1 and LQT2 patients.[19-21] However, in children and adults, the risk of dying after a cardiac event is greater with LQT3 than with LQT1 or LQT2. There is conflicting evidence supporting an influence of sex on risk of cardiac events in LQT3.[20,21]

SCN5A mutations can cause severe LQTS in neonates and infants.[22] Mutations can occur de novo in affected children of asymptomatic parents. Abnormal cardiac conduction (2:1 atrioventricular [AV] block, or atrial standstill) might also be present,[23,24] further emphasizing that LQTS producing cardiac events during the first months of life is a more severe form of the disease. Recurrent third-trimester fetal loss due to inheritance of an *SCN5A* mutation (R1623Q) from a mother who was mosaic for the mutant allele has been reported.[25]

Relationship of LQT3 with Sudden Infant Death Syndrome

There is evidence that occult LQTS can clinically manifest as the sudden infant death syndrome (SIDS) (see Chapter 76). Cardiac mechanisms, including life-threatening arrhythmias, have been suspected as risk factors for SIDS, and mutations in genes responsible for LQTS, especially *SCN5A*, have been identified in 5% to 10% of cases.[26,27] *SCN5A* mutations have accounted for approximately 50% of all LQTS mutations identified in SIDS. Common LQTS gene variants might also increase arrhythmia risk in infants. One study suggested that African-American SIDS victims are more often homozygous for a common *SCN5A* nonsynonymous variant (S1103Y) when compared with non-SIDS infant deaths.[28]

Drug-Induced LQTS

Acquired or drug-induced LQTS is most commonly associated with drugs that block the rapid delayed rectifier current (I_{Kr}). In rare cases, a subclinical *SCN5A* mutation may be a predisposing genetic factor.[29,30] A novel mechanism has been described in which the provocative drug (cisapride) rescues a trafficking defective *SCN5A* mutation (L1825P) to the plasma membrane, where it exhibits abnormal functional properties and evokes LQTS.[31]

Pathophysiology

In LQT3, most *SCN5A* mutations exhibit a dominant gain-of-function phenotype at the molecular level characterized by impairment of inactivation leading to increased persistent inward sodium current (Fig. 50-2).[32-34] A more-severe slowing of inactivation may be present in mutations associated with clinically severe LQTS,[35] and a few mutations alter voltage dependence of activation or inactivation but do not affect the level of persistent current.[36] *SCN5A* mutations associated with SIDS also exhibit this functional abnormality overtly or under certain conditions (acidosis, context of common splice variant).[26,28,37,38]

Increased persistent sodium current provides an explanation for abnormal myocardial repolarization in LQTS.[39] Cardiac action potentials last several hundred milliseconds due to a prolonged depolarization phase (plateau), the result of opposing inward (mainly Na^+ and Ca^{2+}) and outward (K^+) ionic currents. Repolarization occurs when net outward current exceeds net inward current. Increased persistent sodium current shifts this balance toward inward current and delays onset of repolarization, thus lengthening the action potential duration and the corresponding QT interval. Delayed repolarization predisposes to ventricular arrhythmias by exaggerating the dispersion of refractoriness throughout the myocardium and increasing the probability of early afterdepolarization (EAD).[40] Both of these phenomena create conditions that allow electrical signals from depolarized regions of the heart to prematurely re-excite adjacent myocardium that has already repolarized, the basis for a reentrant arrhythmia.

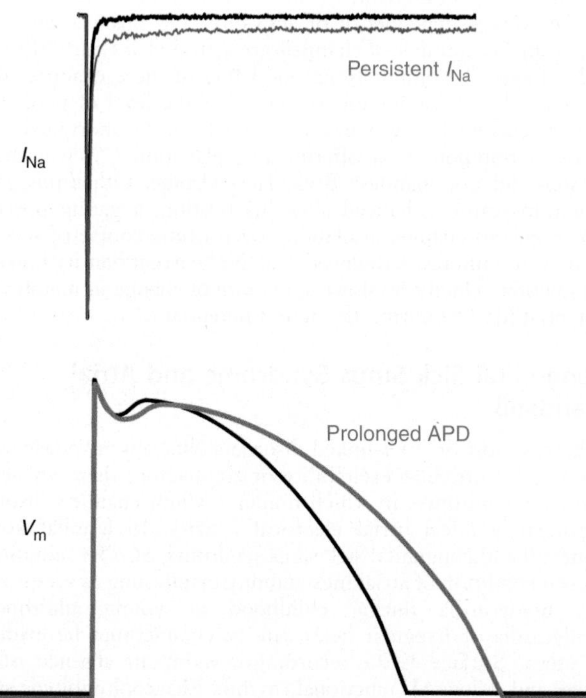

Figure 50-2 Increased persistent sodium current (I_{Na}) in LQT3. *Top,* A representative current recording from a cell expressing wild-type cardiac sodium channels *(black trace)* and a mutation associated with LQT3 *(red trace)* illustrating increased persistent I_{Na}. *Bottom,* A normal ventricular action potential waveform *(black line)* and an illustration of prolonged action potential duration (APD; *red line*) as occurs in LQTS. V_m, transmembrane potential.

Mice engineered to carry the delKPQ mutation exhibit spontaneous life-threatening ventricular arrhythmias and an increased persistent sodium current in cardiac myocytes.[41] There is further evidence from the delKPQ mouse that delayed afterdepolarization (DAD) caused by a Ca^{2+}-dependent diastolic transient inward current, possibly evoked by abnormal Na^+ entry through mutant channels, also contributes to arrhythmia susceptibility and might account for the greater lethality of this LQTS subtype.[42]

Brugada Syndrome

Mutations in *SCN5A* have been associated with Brugada syndrome, an inheritable form of idiopathic ventricular fibrillation.[43,44] Persons with Brugada syndrome have increased risk of potentially fatal ventricular arrhythmias (polymorphic ventricular tachycardia or fibrillation) typically during sleep, but in the absence of myocardial ischemia, electrolyte abnormalities, or structural heart disease. Increased risk of atrial fibrillation and intraventricular conduction abnormalities can also occur in Brugada syndrome. Persons with the disease might exhibit a characteristic baseline ECG pattern consisting of ST elevation in the right precordial leads, apparent right bundle branch block, and normal QT intervals.[45] Administration of sodium channel–blocking agents (procainamide, flecainide, ajmaline) and fever might expose this ECG pattern in latent cases.[46,47] Inheritance is autosomal dominant with incomplete, often low, penetrance and a substantial male predominance. A family history of unexplained sudden death is typical. The sudden unexplained death syndrome (SUDS) is clinically similar to Brugada syndrome and causes sudden death, typically during sleep, in young and middle-aged men in Southeast Asian countries.[48-50] Additional information about Brugada syndrome can be found in Chapter 68.

Molecular Genetics

Chen and colleagues first identified three distinct *SCN5A* mutations in two unrelated Brugada syndrome families and in a third sporadic case.[43] One mutation was missense (T1620M), and the other alleles included a frameshift caused by a single nucleotide deletion and a putative splice site defect. The missense mutation occurred in a proband who was also heterozygous for a second rare variant (R1232W) on the same chromosome, and although this amino acid substitution did not affect function of the sodium channel, it might have contributed to the final dysfunction of the compound mutant allele.[51] This first report of *SCN5A* mutations in Brugada syndrome was followed by several other reports culminating in the discovery of more than 90 alleles (see Fig. 50-1). *SCN5A* mutations have also been identified in subjects with SUDS. By contrast with LQT3, many mutations in Brugada syndrome are predicted to cause truncated proteins by introduction of a frameshift, by a premature stop codon (nonsense mutations), or by predicted splicing errors. These observations suggested that *SCN5A* loss of function is responsible for the disorder.

Genotype-Phenotype Correlation

Mutations in *SCN5A* account for 18% to 30% of Brugada syndrome cases. Certain ECG features can help distinguish between *SCN5A* mutation-positive and mutation-negative patients.

A prolonged PQ interval (≥210 ms) and a correspondingly longer His-ventricle interval (≥60 ms) are more common in Brugada syndrome patients with *SCN5A* mutations than in mutation-negative patients.[52] The QRS duration can also be prolonged in Brugada syndrome caused by *SCN5A* mutations.[53,54] Age-related progression of intraventricular conduction defects occurs in a subset of patients with Brugada syndrome. This phenotypic overlap is further illustrated by a large French family segregating a single *SCN5A* mutation that caused Brugada syndrome or isolated conduction defects in different members.[55]

Most *SCN5A* mutation–positive Brugada syndrome subjects are heterozygous, but there have been a few reports of homozygosity or persons who carry two different mutations inherited from each parent (compound heterozygosity).[56,57] Most *SCN5A* mutation–positive Brugada syndrome families exhibit low penetrance (low concordance between genotype and clinical disease). There are many potential explanations for this phenomenon but very little data supporting any single mechanism. One attractive hypothesis to explain incomplete penetrance in Brugada syndrome is the existence of genetic modifiers, and preliminary evidence supporting a role for intragenic modifiers in Brugada syndrome has been reported. In one Brugada syndrome family segregating a trafficking defective missense mutation (R282H), one asymptomatic mutation carrier had a common variant (H558R) on the opposite allele.[58] In vitro experiments suggested that H558R rescues the trafficking defect through interactions between the two variant $Na_V1.5$ proteins.

Pathophysiology

Reduced sodium current is the primary pathophysiologic event in Brugada syndrome, and this is consistent with *SCN5A* mutations predicted to encode nonfunctional channels (e.g., frameshift mutations, splice-site defects, premature stop codons).[43,59] Furthermore, some missense mutations are nonfunctional either because of impaired protein trafficking to the cell membrane or because of disrupted ion conductance.[51,60,61] Other missense mutations are functional but have biophysical defects predicted to reduce channel availability, such as altered voltage dependence of activation, more rapid fast inactivation, and enhanced slow inactivation.[62-64] One mutation (E1053K) disrupts binding of the channel to ankyrin-G, and this alters membrane trafficking and localization in cardiac myocytes.[65]

Two proposed mechanisms explain the cellular basis of Brugada syndrome.[66] In one mechanism, a reduction in myocardial sodium current exaggerates differences in action potential duration between endocardium and epicardium.[40,67,68] These differences occur because of unequal distribution of transient outward current (I_{to}), a repolarizing current more prominent in the epicardial layer that contributes to the characteristic spike-and-dome shape of the cardiac action potential. Reduced myocardial sodium current causes disproportionate shortening of epicardial action potentials because of unopposed I_{to}, leading to an exaggerated transmural voltage gradient, dispersion of repolarization, and a substrate promoting reentrant arrhythmias. The second hypothesis suggests that the main effect of reduced myocardial sodium current is conduction slowing and delayed activation in the right ventricle and right ventricular outflow tract.[66,69-71] It is not clear whether these two hypotheses are mutually exclusive.

Disorders with Impaired Cardiac Conduction

Mutations in *SCN5A* have also been associated with a heterogeneous group of familial disorders characterized by impaired cardiac conduction manifest as abnormal AV conduction (AV block), slowed intraventricular conduction, or atrial inexcitability (atrial standstill).[72-75] The degree of impaired cardiac conduction can progress with advancing age. Inheritance may be autosomal dominant or autosomal recessive, but in rare cases, digenic inheritance of a heterozygous *SCN5A* mutation with a promoter variant in the connexin40 gene has been described.[74,76]

Familial Progressive Cardiac Conduction System Disease

Age-related defects in conduction along the His-Purkinje system have been referred to as Lenègre or Lev disease and may be caused by progressive fibrosis of the specialized conducting tissues in heart.[77] However, clinically similar conditions may be inherited and are sometimes associated with *SCN5A* mutations (see Chapter 75).[78] A variety of names have been applied to this genetic subtype, including *progressive cardiac conduction disease*, *familial AV block*, and *hereditary Lenègre disease*. The clinical phenotype is quite heterogeneous, with presentation in either early childhood or adulthood. In children, progressive AV block is most typical, whereas adults with these disorders usually have intraventricular conduction abnormalities such as right or left bundle branch block.

Approximately 15 *SCN5A* mutations have been reported in association with cardiac conduction disease (see Fig. 50-1). The first mutations described by Schott and colleagues were predicted to be complete loss-of-function alleles (premature stop codon or splice-site error).[72] Several missense mutations have since been characterized in vitro, and these alleles are either nonfunctional or exhibit complex biophysical abnormalities that are generally predicted to reduce peak sodium current density at physiologic voltages.[73,79] In the case of G514C, a missense mutation segregating with conduction disease in a Dutch family, the mutant sodium channel exhibits unequal depolarizing shifts in the voltage dependence of activation and inactivation such that a smaller number of channels are activated at typical threshold voltages.[79] Computational modeling of these changes supported reduced conduction velocity, but the level of predicted sodium current loss was not sufficient to evoke shortened epicardial action potentials, offering an explanation as to why these persons did not manifest Brugada syndrome. Other missense mutations cause enhanced slow inactivation, a gating process that regulates channel availability over a time course of several seconds to minutes.[73] Reduced peak Na^+ current density impairs conduction velocity by slowing the rate of change in membrane potential (dV/dt) during the action potential.

Congenital Sick Sinus Syndrome and Atrial Standstill

Whereas most *SCN5A*-linked disorders clinically manifest with abnormal ventricular excitability or conduction, there are less-common syndromes in which mutant sodium channels disproportionately affect atrial electrical activity. In familial atrial standstill and congenital sick sinus syndrome, *SCN5A* mutations cause a condition of atrial inexcitability manifesting as symptomatic bradycardia during childhood or young adulthood. Bradycardia or irregular heart rate may sometimes be evident in utero. Surface ECG recordings exhibit an absence of P waves and a slow AV junctional rhythm. Electrophysiologic studies might reveal prolonged His-ventricular conduction, indicating a more generalized defect in cardiac conduction. The atria, but not ventricles, are refractory to electrical pacing.

Familial atrial standstill has been associated with heterozygous *SCN5A* mutations coinherited with a common variant in the connexin40 gene promoter that is predicted to reduce transcriptional activity and expression.[74,76] In these families, inheritance of the sodium channel mutation alone was not sufficient to evoke a clinical phenotype, and this supported the notion of digenic inheritance with the connexin40 variant. Congenital sick sinus syndrome has been associated with recessive *SCN5A* mutations in which affected persons inherited a nonfunctional or severely dysfunctional mutation from one parent and a less severely impaired allele from the other parent.[75] The parents, who are carriers of single mutations, were asymptomatic or had subclinical first-degree AV block. The predominant atrial phenotype in these cases might stem from differences in sodium-channel density between atrial and ventricular myocardium or other chamber-specific factors.

Other Disorders of Cardiac Sodium Channels

Mixed Phenotypes and Overlap Syndromes

Mutations in *SCN5A* have also been associated with more-complex phenotypes representing combinations of LQTS, Brugada syndrome, and conduction system disease. Initially, there was a suggestion that these more-complex disorders represented overlap syndromes. However, with evolution in recognizing phenotype complexity among LQTS and Brugada syndrome cases, there has been greater appreciation for overlapping clinical features observed in many patients. For example, severe LQT3 can manifest with conduction disturbances such as 2:1 AV block,[23,80] and some patients with Brugada syndrome exhibit prolonged PQ and QRS intervals as well as progressive conduction system disease.[55] Certain mutations might have different clinical manifestations in different families (e.g., D1275N)[74,81-83] or even among members of the same family,[55] perhaps because of host-specific factors such as modifier genes that influence the final clinical expression. Nonetheless, there are perplexing cases such as LQTS combined with Brugada syndrome[84] that may be pathophysiologically distinct and represent true overlap syndromes.

Mutant cardiac sodium channels associated with mixed clinical phenotypes exhibit more complex functional properties as compared with pure LQTS and Brugada syndrome mutations. The in-frame insertion mutation (1795insD) identified in a family segregating both LQTS and Brugada syndrome causes an inactivation defect resulting in increased persistent Na^+ current typical of LQT3, but it also confers enhanced slow inactivation with reduced channel availability that is more characteristic of Brugada syndrome.[84] These distinct biophysical abnormalities are predicted to predispose to ventricular arrhythmia by different mechanisms at opposite extremes of heart rate.[85] Whereas increased persistent current prolongs action potentials, especially at slow heart rates, enhanced slow inactivation predisposes to activity-dependent loss of sodium channel availability at fast rates. These findings were confirmed in a mouse model genetically engineered with this mutation.[86] In another unusual case, deletion of lysine 1500 in *SCN5A* was associated with the unique combination of LQTS, Brugada syndrome, and impaired cardiac conduction in the same family.[87] This mutation impairs inactivation, causing increased persistent sodium current, but it also reduces sodium channel availability by opposite shifts in voltage dependence of inactivation and activation.

Dilated Cardiomyopathy with Arrhythmia

Mutations affecting cardiac ion channels primarily predispose to disorders of heart rhythm, whereas familial cardiomyopathy is typically associated with mutations in genes encoding sarcomeric or contractile proteins. An exception to this paradigm was implied by discovery of *SCN5A* mutations associated with familial dilated cardiomyopathy. In 2004, McNair and colleagues[81] reported a missense mutation, *SCN5A*-D1275N, segregated with a phenotype including dilated cardiomyopathy of variable expression, abnormal atrioventricular conduction, sinus node dysfunction, and atrial and ventricular arrhythmias in a four-generation kindred. A subsequent survey of 156 unrelated dilated cardiomyopathy patients for *SCN5A* variants led to discovery of other mutations, including one frameshift (2 bp insertion) and three missense alleles (T220I, R814W, D1595H).[82] Most of these mutations segregated in families with a heterogeneous phenotype characterized by variable expression of dilated cardiomyopathy, sick sinus syndrome, atrial and ventricular arrhythmias. Transmission was autosomal dominant with incomplete penetrance. In those families, 43% of carriers exhibited early-onset atrial fibrillation (AF) or atrial flutter. Characterization of two *SCN5A* mutations associated with this syndrome (R814W, D1595H) indicated that a unique combination of biophysical defects most likely predispose myocytes to disordered intracellular Na^+ and Ca^{2+} homeostasis, leading to myocardial dysfunction.[88]

Atrial Fibrillation

SCN5A has been considered as a candidate gene for lone and familial AF. This idea was based on the observed association of atrial arrhythmias with dilated cardiomyopathy (see earlier) and the increased prevalence of AF in patients with Brugada syndrome. In a cohort of 157 white subjects with early-onset AF (mean age at diagnosis, 44.5 ± 10.3 years) who did not have traditional risk factors for the arrhythmia, there was a significant association with the minor allele of the common *SCN5A* variant, H558R.[89] No other coding sequence variants were identified in that study. However, in a subsequent survey for *SCN5A* mutations in 257 persons with AF, including 118 cases without known risk factors, mutations were identified in 5.9%.[90] Among the mutations identified, eight were novel and 11 had been previously associated with either LQTS or Brugada syndrome. Segregation of the *SCN5A* mutations with AF followed a pattern consistent with autosomal-dominant inheritance in six families, further suggesting that mutations in this gene might predispose to familial AF.

Clinical Significance of Common *SCN5A* Variants

Common variants within the *SCN5A* coding region have been identified in certain populations, and some of these might confer increased risk of cardiac arrhythmia or influence the efficacy of antiarrhythmic drugs. One common variant carried by approximately 13% of African Americans (S1103Y, also reported as S1102Y) has been associated with an eight-fold increased risk for ventricular arrhythmia.[91] The functional consequences of S1103Y include increased transient and persistent current sufficient to evoke early afterdepolarizations in a computational model of cardiac action potentials. Another variant found in approximately 3% African Americans (S524Y) does not affect baseline sodium channel function but does enhance use-dependent block by certain class Ia (quinidine) and Ic (flecainide) antiarrhythmic agents.[92]

Other common *SCN5A* variants have less clear significance. Approximately 7% of presumed healthy Latin Americans carry V1951L,[93] but this variant has also been associated with SIDS in white Norwegians[2,7] possibly suggesting that ethnic background influences the clinical impact of this polymorphism. This variant might have a latent functional defect that occurs only in the presence of a common *SCN5A* splice variant (deletion of Q1077).[38] R1193Q is common in Asians but is a rare variant (0.3%) in whites.[93] This variant has been reported in subjects with acquired and with congenital LQTS[94,95] and in SUDS.[50] In one study, this variant exhibited increased persistent sodium current,[94] whereas another analysis demonstrated faster inactivation.[50]

Management of Cardiac Sodium Channel Diseases

Clinical Recognition

Recognizing patients who might have an underlying sodium channel mutation is a critical first step in managing the disorders discussed in this chapter. Specific clinical scenarios should raise suspicion for *SCN5A* mutations: LQTS associated with an unexpected degree of bradycardia or torsades de pointes occurring during rest or sleep, LQTS associated with heart block, an ECG pattern suggesting Brugada syndrome, or severe perinatal ventricular arrhythmias associated with bradycardia or congenital heart block. These scenarios are not specific for *SCN5A* mutations, but recognizing the potential for an inherited arrhythmia will prompt further inquiry related to the familial nature of the problem and further diagnostic testing.

Special Diagnostic and Therapeutic Challenges

Ascertaining the family history of cardiac arrhythmias and unexpected death is of utmost importance when considering a sodium-channel disorder. In performing a detailed family history, the clinician should pay special attention to the sudden unexpected death, especially among young adults and children in the family, and should identify relatives with implanted cardiac devices. A pedigree drawing helps in the recognition of an inheritance pattern (e.g., autosomal dominant) compatible with a familial disorder, but keep in mind the possibility that there may be incomplete penetrance. Information about the patient and close relatives is helpful in making final decisions about the use of genetic testing to confirm suspicions about an inheritable sodium-channel disorder.

Genetic Testing

Genetic testing is a specialized diagnostic procedure that is available for LQTS, Brugada syndrome, and disorders associated with *SCN5A* mutations through commercial and large academic laboratories.[96] Unlike more commonly used laboratory tests, genetic testing requires additional discussions with the patient regarding the potential risks, benefits, and limitations of the tests. Methods to identify *SCN5A* mutations are not 100% sensitive, and therefore a negative test does not completely exclude a sodium channel disorder. Certain detectable DNA sequence variants might not have a clear causal role in the patient's condition either because they are rare polymorphisms that have been detected previously in presumed healthy persons[93] or are located in regions of the sodium channel that do not have known functional importance. Nonetheless, genetic testing can identify mutations that help confirm clinical suspicions and offer opportunities to direct specific testing of at-risk relatives.

Genotype-Specific Treatment Strategies

Mexiletine and other sodium channel–blocking drugs can reduce persistent sodium current and shorten the QT interval in LQT3 patients,[97-100] although there are no data indicating that this therapeutic strategy reduces mortality. In LQT3 mouse models, mexiletine shortens the myocyte action potential and prevents arrhythmias.[101,102] Selective suppression of persistent current by the antianginal drug ranolazine has also been demonstrated in vitro for various LQT3 mutations.[103] In addition to correcting the functional defect of mutant sodium channels, mexiletine has been demonstrated to rescue trafficking defective *SCN5A* mutants in vitro.[104]

References

1. George AL, Varkony TA, Drabkin HA, et al: Assignment of the human heart tetrodotoxin-resistant voltage-gated Na$^+$ channel α-subunit gene *(SCN5A)* to band 3p21. Cytogenet Cell Genet 68:67-70, 1995.
2. Wang Q, Li ZZ, Shen JX, et al: Genomic organization of the human *SCN5A* gene encoding the cardiac sodium channel. Genomics 34:9-16, 1996.
3. Gellens ME, George AL, Chen L, et al: Primary structure and functional expression of the human cardiac tetrodotoxin-insensitive voltage-dependent sodium channel. Proc Natl Acad Sci U S A 89:554-558, 1992.
4. Ye B, Valdivia CR, Ackerman MJ, et al: A common human *SCN5A* polymorphism modifies expression of an arrhythmia causing mutation. Physiol Genomics 12:187-193, 2003.
5. Makielski JC, Ye B, Valdivia CR, et al: A ubiquitous splice variant and a common polymorphism affect heterologous expression of recombinant human *SCN5A* heart sodium channels. Circ Res 93:821-828, 2003.
6. Tan BH, Valdivia CR, Rok BA, et al: Common human *SCN5A* polymorphisms have altered electrophysiology when expressed in Q1077 splice variants. Heart Rhythm 2:741-747, 2005.
7. Tan BH, Valdivia CR, Song C, et al: Partial expression defect for the *SCN5A* missense mutation G1406R depends upon splice variant background Q1077 and rescue by mexiletine. Am J Physiol Heart Circ Physiol 291:H1822-H1828, 2006.
8. Yang P, Kupershmidt S, Roden DM: Cloning and initial characterization of the human cardiac sodium channel *(SCN5A)* promoter. Cardiovasc Res 61:56-65, 2004.
9. Bezzina CR, Shimizu W, Yang P, et al: Common sodium channel promoter haplotype in Asian subjects underlies variability in cardiac conduction. Circulation 113:338-344, 2006.
10. Curran ME, Splawski I, Timothy KW, et al: A molecular basis for cardiac arrhythmia: *HERG* mutations cause long QT syndrome. Cell 80:795-803, 1995.
11. Wang Q, Curran ME, Splawski I, et al: Positional cloning of a novel potassium channel gene: *KVLQT1* mutations cause cardiac arrhythmias. Nature Genet 12:17-23, 1996.
12. Wang Q, Shen J, Splawski I, et al: *SCN5A* mutations associated with an inherited cardiac arrhythmia, long QT syndrome. Cell 80:805-811, 1995.
13. Motoike HK, Liu H, Glaaser IW, et al: The Na$^+$ channel inactivation gate is a molecular complex: A novel role of the COOH-terminal domain. J Gen Physiol 123:155-165, 2004.
14. Medeiros-Domingo A, Kaku T, Tester DJ, et al: *SCN4B*-encoded sodium channel β4 subunit in congenital long-QT syndrome. Circulation 116:134-142, 2007.
15. Vatta M, Ackerman MJ, Ye B, et al: Mutant caveolin-3 induces persistent late sodium current and is associated with long-QT syndrome. Circulation 114:2104-2112, 2006.
16. Schwartz PJ, Priori SG, Spazzolini C, et al: Genotype-phenotype correlation in the long-QT syndrome: Gene-specific triggers for life-threatening arrhythmias. Circulation 103:89-95, 2001.
17. Schwartz PJ, Priori SG, Locati EH, et al: Long QT syndrome patients with mutations of the *SCN5A* and *HERG* genes have differential responses to Na$^+$ channel blockade and to increases in heart rate. Implications for gene-specific therapy. Circulation 92:3381-3386, 1995.
18. Zhang L, Timothy KW, Vincent GM, et al: Spectrum of ST-T–wave patterns and repolarization parameters in congenital long-QT syndrome: ECG findings identify genotypes. Circulation 102:2849-2855, 2000.
19. Zareba W, Moss AJ, Schwartz PJ, et al: Influence of genotype on the clinical course

of the long-QT syndrome. International Long-QT Syndrome Registry Research Group. N Engl J Med 339:960-965, 1998.

20. Zareba W, Moss AJ, Locati EH, et al: Modulating effects of age and gender on the clinical course of long QT syndrome by genotype. J Am Coll Cardiol 42:103-109, 2003.
21. Priori SG, Schwartz PJ, Napolitano C, et al: Risk stratification in the long-QT syndrome. N Engl J Med 348:1866-1874, 2003.
22. Berul CI: Neonatal long QT syndrome and sudden cardiac death. Prog Pediatr Cardiol 11:47-54, 2000.
23. Lupoglazoff JM, Cheav T, Baroudi G, et al: Homozygous *SCN5A* mutation in long-QT syndrome with functional two-to-one atrioventricular block. Circ Res 89:E16-E21, 2001.
24. Miura M, Yamagishi H, Morikawa Y, et al: Congenital long QT syndrome and 2:1 atrioventricular block with a mutation of the *SCN5A* gene. Pediatr Cardiol 24:70-72, 2003.
25. Miller TE, Estrella E, Myerburg RJ, et al: Recurrent third-trimester fetal loss and maternal mosaicism for long-QT syndrome. Circulation 109:3029-3034, 2004.
26. Ackerman MJ, Siu BL, Sturner WQ, et al: Postmortem molecular analysis of *SCN5A* defects in sudden infant death syndrome. JAMA 286:2264-2269, 2001.
27. Arnestad M, Crotti L, Rognum TO, et al: Prevalence of long-QT syndrome gene variants in sudden infant death syndrome. Circulation 115:361-367, 2007.
28. Plant LD, Bowers PN, Liu Q, et al: A common cardiac sodium channel variant associated with sudden infant death in African Americans, *SCN5A* S1103Y. J Clin Invest 116:430-435, 2006.
29. Makita N, Horie M, Nakamura T, et al: Drug-induced long-QT syndrome associated with a subclinical *SCN5A* mutation. Circulation 106:1269-1274, 2002.
30. Piippo K, Holmstrom S, Swan H, et al: Effect of the antimalarial drug halofantrine in the long QT syndrome due to a mutation of the cardiac sodium channel gene *SCN5A*. Am J Cardiol 87:909-911, 2001.
31. Liu K, Yang T, Viswanathan PC, et al: New mechanism contributing to drug-induced arrhythmia: Rescue of a misprocessed LQT3 mutant. Circulation 112:3239-3246, 2005.
32. Bennett PB, Yazawa K, Makita N, et al: Molecular mechanism for an inherited cardiac arrhythmia. Nature 376:683-685, 1995.
33. Dumaine R, Wang Q, Keating MT, et al: Multiple mechanisms of Na^+ channel–linked long-QT syndrome. Circ Res 78:916-924, 1996.
34. Wang DW, Yazawa K, George AL Jr, et al: Characterization of human cardiac Na^+ channel mutations in the congenital long QT syndrome. Proc Natl Acad Sci U S A 93:13200-13205, 1996.
35. Kambouris NG, Nuss HB, Johns DC, et al: Phenotypic characterization of a novel long-QT syndrome mutation (R1623Q) in the cardiac sodium channel. Circulation 97:640-644, 1998.
36. Abriel H, Cabo C, Wehrens XH, et al: Novel arrhythmogenic mechanism revealed by a long-QT syndrome mutation in the cardiac Na^+ channel. Circ Res 88:740-745, 2001.
37. Schwartz PJ, Priori SG, Dumaine R, et al: A molecular link between the sudden infant death syndrome and the long-QT syndrome. N Engl J Med 343:262-267, 2000.
38. Wang DW, Desai RR, Crotti L, et al: Cardiac sodium channel dysfunction in sudden infant death syndrome. Circulation 115:368-376, 2007.
39. Clancy CE, Rudy Y: Linking a genetic defect to its cellular phenotype in a cardiac arrhythmia. Nature 400:566-569, 1999.
40. Antzelevitch C, Yan GX, Shimizu W: Transmural dispersion of repolarization and arrhythmogenicity: The Brugada syndrome versus the long QT syndrome. J Electrocardiol 32 Suppl:158-165, 1999.
41. Nuyens D, Stengl M, Dugarmaa S, et al: Abrupt rate accelerations or premature beats cause life-threatening arrhythmias in mice with long-QT3 syndrome. Nature Med 7:1021-1027, 2001.
42. Fredj S, Lindegger N, Sampson KJ, et al: Altered Na^+ channels promote pause-induced spontaneous diastolic activity in long QT syndrome type 3 myocytes. Circ Res 99:1225-1232, 2006.
43. Chen Q, Kirsch GE, Zhang D, et al: Genetic basis and molecular mechanism for idiopathic ventricular fibrillation. Nature 392:293-296, 1998.
44. Akai J, Makita N, Sakurada H, et al: A novel *SCN5A* mutation associated with idiopathic ventricular fibrillation without typical ECG findings of Brugada syndrome. FEBS Lett 479:29-34, 2000.
45. Brugada J, Brugada P: Further characterization of the syndrome of right bundle branch block, ST segment elevation, and sudden cardiac death. J Cardiovasc Electrophysiol 8:325-331, 1997.
46. Brugada R, Brugada J, Antzelevitch C, et al: Sodium channel blockers identify risk for sudden death in patients with ST-segment elevation and right bundle branch block but structurally normal hearts. Circulation 101:510-515, 2000.
47. Keller DI, Huang H, Zhao J, et al: A novel *SCN5A* mutation, F1344S, identified in a patient with Brugada syndrome and fever-induced ventricular fibrillation. Cardiovasc Res 70:521-529, 2006.
48. Baron RC, Thacker SB, Gorelkin L, et al: Sudden death among Southeast Asian refugees. An unexplained nocturnal phenomenon. JAMA 250:2947-2951, 1983.
49. Nademanee K, Veerakul G, Nimmannit S, et al: Arrhythmogenic marker for the sudden unexplained death syndrome in Thai men. Circulation 96:2595-2600, 1997.
50. Vatta M, Dumaine R, Varghese G, et al: Genetic and biophysical basis of sudden unexplained nocturnal death syndrome (SUNDS), a disease allelic to Brugada syndrome. Hum Mol Genet 11:337-345, 2002.
51. Baroudi G, Acharfi S, Larouche C, et al: Expression and intracellular localization of an *SCN5A* double mutant R1232W/T1620M implicated in Brugada syndrome. Circ Res 90:E11-E16, 2002.
52. Smits JP, Eckardt L, Probst V, et al: Genotype-phenotype relationship in Brugada syndrome: Electrocardiographic features differentiate *SCN5A*-related patients from non–*SCN5A*-related patients. J Am Coll Cardiol 40:350-356, 2002.
53. Yokokawa M, Noda T, Okamura H, et al: Comparison of long-term follow-up of electrocardiographic features in Brugada syndrome between the *SCN5A*-positive probands and the *SCN5A*-negative probands. Am J Cardiol 100:649-655, 2007.
54. Probst V, Allouis M, Sacher F, et al: Progressive cardiac conduction defect is the prevailing phenotype in carriers of a Brugada syndrome *SCN5A* mutation. J Cardiovasc Electrophysiol 17:270-275, 2006.
55. Kyndt F, Probst V, Potet F, et al: Novel *SCN5A* mutation leading either to isolated cardiac conduction defect or Brugada syndrome in a large French family. Circulation 104:3081-3086, 2001.
56. Cordeiro JM, Barajas-Martinez H, Hong K, et al: Compound heterozygous mutations P336L and I1660V in the human cardiac sodium channel associated with the Brugada syndrome. Circulation 114:2026-2033, 2006.
57. Frigo G, Rampazzo A, Bauce B, et al: Homozygous *SCN5A* mutation in Brugada syndrome with monomorphic ventricular tachycardia and structural heart abnormalities. Europace 9:391-397, 2007.
58. Poelzing S, Forleo C, Samodell M, et al: *SCN5A* polymorphism restores trafficking of a Brugada syndrome mutation on a separate gene. Circulation 114:368-376, 2006.
59. Schulze-Bahr E, Eckardt L, Breithardt G, et al: Sodium channel gene *(SCN5A)* mutations in 44 index patients with Brugada syndrome: Different incidences in familial and sporadic disease. Hum Mutat 21:651-652, 2003.
60. Baroudi G, Pouliot V, Denjoy I, et al: Novel mechanism for Brugada syndrome: Defective surface localization of an *SCN5A* mutant (R1432G). Circ Res 88:E78-E83, 2001.
61. Valdivia CR, Tester DJ, Rok BA, et al: A trafficking defective, Brugada syndrome-causing *SCN5A* mutation rescued by drugs. Cardiovasc Res 62:53-62, 2004.
62. Dumaine R, Towbin JA, Brugada P, et al: Ionic mechanisms responsible for the electrocardiographic phenotype of the Brugada syndrome are temperature dependent. Circ Res 85:803-809, 1999.
63. Wang DW, Makita N, Kitabatake A, et al: Enhanced Na^+ channel intermediate inactivation in Brugada syndrome. Circ Res 87:E37-E43, 2000.
64. Rook MB, Alshinawi CB, Groenewegen WA, et al: Human *SCN5A* gene mutations alter cardiac sodium channel kinetics and are associated with the Brugada syndrome. Cardiovasc Res 44:507-517, 1999.
65. Mohler PJ, Rivolta I, Napolitano C, et al: $Na_V1.5$ E1053K mutation causing Brugada syndrome blocks binding to ankyrin-G and expression of $Na_V1.5$ on the surface of cardiomyocytes. Proc Natl Acad Sci U S A 101:17533-17538, 2004.

66. Meregalli PG, Wilde AA, Tan HL: Pathophysiological mechanisms of Brugada syndrome: Depolarization disorder, repolarization disorder, or more? Cardiovasc Res 67:367-378, 2005.
67. Yan GX, Antzelevitch C: Cellular basis for the Brugada syndrome and other mechanisms of arrhythmogenesis associated with ST-segment elevation. Circulation 100:1660-1666, 1999.
68. Antzelevitch C: Ion channels and ventricular arrhythmias: Cellular and ionic mechanisms underlying the Brugada syndrome. Curr Opin Cardiol 14:274-279, 1999.
69. Tukkie R, Sogaard P, Vleugels J, et al: Delay in right ventricular activation contributes to Brugada syndrome. Circulation 109:1272-1277, 2004.
70. Zhang ZS, Tranquillo J, Neplioueva V, et al: Sodium channel kinetic changes that produce Brugada syndrome or progressive cardiac conduction system disease. Am J Physiol Heart Circ Physiol 292:H399-H407, 2007.
71. Coronel R, Casini S, Koopmann TT, et al: Right ventricular fibrosis and conduction delay in a patient with clinical signs of Brugada syndrome: A combined electrophysiological, genetic, histopathologic, and computational study. Circulation 112:2769-2777, 2005.
72. Schott JJ, Alshinawi C, Kyndt F, et al: Cardiac conduction defects associate with mutations in *SCN5A*. Nature Genet 23:20-21, 1999.
73. Wang DW, Viswanathan PC, Balser JR, et al: Clinical, genetic, and biophysical characterization of *SCN5A* mutations associated with atrioventricular conduction block. Circulation 105:341-346, 2002.
74. Groenewegen WA, Firouzi M, Bezzina CR, et al: A cardiac sodium channel mutation cosegregates with a rare connexin40 genotype in familial atrial standstill. Circ Res 92:14-22, 2003.
75. Benson DW, Wang DW, Dyment M, et al: Congenital sick sinus syndrome caused by recessive mutations in the cardiac sodium channel gene *(SCN5A)*. J Clin Invest 112:1019-1028, 2003.
76. Makita N, Sasaki K, Groenewegen WA, et al: Congenital atrial standstill associated with coinheritance of a novel *SCN5A* mutation and connexin 40 polymorphisms. Heart Rhythm 2:1128-1134, 2005.
77. Lenègre J: Etiology and pathology of bilateral bundle branch block in relation to complete heart block. Prog Cardiovasc Dis 6:409-444, 1964.
78. Wolf CM, Berul CI: Inherited conduction system abnormalities—one group of diseases, many genes. J Cardiovasc Electrophysiol 17:446-455, 2006.
79. Tan HL, Bink-Boelkens MT, Bezzina CR, et al: A sodium-channel mutation causes isolated cardiac conduction disease. Nature 409:1043-1047, 2001.
80. Chang CC, Acharfi S, Wu MH, et al: A novel *SCN5A* mutation manifests as a malignant form of long QT syndrome with perinatal onset of tachycardia/bradycardia. Cardiovasc Res 64:268-278, 2004.
81. McNair WP, Ku L, Taylor MR, et al: *SCN5A* mutation associated with dilated cardiomyopathy, conduction disorder, and arrhythmia. Circulation 110:2163-2167, 2004.
82. Olson TM, Michels VV, Ballew JD, et al: Sodium channel mutations and susceptibility to heart failure and atrial fibrillation. JAMA 293:447-454, 2005.
83. Laitinen-Forsblom PJ, Makynen P, Makynen H, et al: *SCN5A* mutation associated with cardiac conduction defect and atrial arrhythmias. J Cardiovasc Electrophysiol 17:480-485, 2006.
84. Bezzina C, Veldkamp MW, van Den Berg MP, et al: A single Na^+ channel mutation causing both long-QT and Brugada syndromes. Circ Res 85:1206-1213, 1999.
85. Clancy CE, Rudy Y: Na^+ channel mutation that causes both Brugada and long-QT syndrome phenotypes: A simulation study of mechanism. Circulation 105:1208-1213, 2002.
86. Remme CA, Verkerk AO, Nuyens D, et al: Overlap syndrome of cardiac sodium channel disease in mice carrying the equivalent mutation of human *SCN5A*-1795insD. Circulation 114:2584-2594, 2006.
87. Grant AO, Carboni MP, Neplioueva V, et al: Long QT syndrome, Brugada syndrome, and conduction system disease are linked to a single sodium channel mutation. J Clin Invest 110:1201-1209, 2002.
88. Nguyen TP, Wang DW, Rhodes TH, et al: Divergent biophysical defects caused by mutant sodium channels in dilated cardiomyopathy with arrhythmia. Circ Rec 102:364-371, 2008.
89. Chen LY, Ballew JD, Herron KJ, et al: A common polymorphism in *SCN5A* is associated with lone atrial fibrillation. Clin Pharmacol Ther 81:35-41, 2007.
90. Darbar D, Kannankeril PJ, Donahue BS, et al: Cardiac sodium channel (SCN5A) variants associated with atrial fibrillation. Circulation 117:1927, 1988.
91. Splawski I, Timothy KW, Tateyama M, et al: Variant of *SCN5A* sodium channel implicated in risk of cardiac arrhythmia. Science 297:1333-1336, 2002.
92. Shuraih M, Ai T, Vatta M, et al: A common *SCN5A* variant alters the responsiveness of human sodium channels to class I antiarrhythmic agents. J Cardiovasc Electrophysiol 18:434-440, 2007.
93. Ackerman MJ, Splawski I, Makielski JC, et al: Spectrum and prevalence of cardiac sodium channel variants among black, white, Asian, and Hispanic individuals: Implications for arrhythmogenic susceptibility and Brugada/long QT syndrome genetic testing. Heart Rhythm 1:600-607, 2004.
94. Wang Q, Chen S, Chen Q, et al: The common *SCN5A* mutation R1193Q causes LQTS-type electrophysiological alterations of the cardiac sodium channel. J Med Genet 41:e66, 2004.
95. Hwang HW, Chen JJ, Lin YJ, et al: R1193Q of *SCN5A*, a Brugada and long QT mutation, is a common polymorphism in Han Chinese. J Med Genet 42:e7, 2005.
96. Tester DJ, Will ML, Haglund CM, et al: Compendium of cardiac channel mutations in 541 consecutive unrelated patients referred for long QT syndrome genetic testing. Heart Rhythm 2:507-517, 2005.
97. Schwartz PJ, Priori SG, Locati EH, et al: Long QT syndrome patients with mutations of the *SCN5A* and *HERG* genes have differential responses to Na^+ channel blockade and to increases in heart rate—implications for gene-specific therapy. Circulation 92:3381-3386, 1995.
98. Wang DW, Yazawa K, Makita N, et al: Pharmacological targeting of long QT mutant sodium channels. J Clin Invest 99:1714-1720, 1997.
99. Windle JR, Geletka RC, Moss AJ, et al: Normalization of ventricular repolarization with flecainide in long QT syndrome patients with *SCN5A*: ΔKPQ mutation. Ann Noninvasive Electrocardiol 6:153-158, 2001.
100. Abriel H, Wehrens XH, Benhorin J, et al: Molecular pharmacology of the sodium channel mutation D1790G linked to the long-QT syndrome. Circulation 102:921-925, 2000.
101. Fabritz L, Kirchhof P, Franz MR, et al: Effect of pacing and mexiletine on dispersion of repolarisation and arrhythmias in ΔKPQ *SCN5A* (long QT3) mice. Cardiovasc Res 57:1085-1093, 2003.
102. Tian XL, Yong SL, Wan X, et al: Mechanisms by which *SCN5A* mutation N1325S causes cardiac arrhythmias and sudden death in vivo. Cardiovasc Res 61:256-267, 2004.
103. Fredj S, Sampson KJ, Liu H, et al: Molecular basis of ranolazine block of LQT-3 mutant sodium channels: evidence for site of action. Br J Pharmacol 148:16-24, 2006.
104. Valdivia CR, Ackerman MJ, Tester DJ, et al: A novel *SCN5A* arrhythmia mutation, M1766L, with expression defect rescued by mexiletine. Cardiovasc Res 55:279-289, 2002.

Inheritable Potassium Channel Diseases 51

Arthur A. M. Wilde and Hanno L. Tan

CHAPTER OUTLINE

Potassium channels are instrumental for proper functioning of many cell types, including cardiac myocytes. A comprehensive discussion of the physiology of various potassium channels is provided elsewhere in this book. This chapter focuses on the pathophysiology of potassium channel–related inherited cardiac disorders.

Among the first genes that were implicated in inherited arrhythmia syndromes in the mid-1990s was a potassium channel encoded by the human ether-a-go-go–related gene *(HERG)*, now referred to as *KCNH2*.[1,2]

In later years, other potassium channel–encoding genes were identified in the etiology of various inherited arrhythmia syndromes, including the long-QT syndromes (LQTSs), the short QT syndromes (SQTSs), and familial atrial fibrillation. These include *KCNQ1* (previously annotated as K_VLQT1), *KCNJ2*, and the potassium channel β-subunits *KCNE1*, and *KCNE2*. The identification of all these causally involved genes has led to a subdivision of the LQTSs and SQTSs into different subtypes according to the affected gene with different clinical and electrocardiogram (ECG) characteristics. This subdivision is based on the chronological order in which the subtypes were reported (LQT1, LQT2, LQT3, etc.). This subdivision, although not ideal, is followed in this chapter.

Long-QT Syndromes

Among the 10 currently described subtypes, long QT syndrome types 1 and 2, based on the potassium channel–encoding genes *KCNQ1* and *KCNH2*, respectively, are the most prevalent. Types 5, 6, and 7 are also based on variants in potassium channel (α or β) subunits (*KCNE1*, *KCNE2*, and *KCNJ2*, respectively), but are rare. Type 3 is a sodium channelopathy (with an estimated prevalence of 5%-8%); it is discussed in Chapter 50. Type 4 is based on mutations in ankyrin-B, an anchoring protein that binds proteins involved in cardiac electrophysiology and cellular calcium homeostasis.[3] Type 8 is based on mutations in the α-subunit of the slow calcium channel (*CACNA1C*, Timothy syndrome),[4] and types 9 and 10, both very rare, are based on mutations in *CAV3* (which encodes caveolin-3, the predominant proteins in membrane caveolae in striated muscle,[5] and *SCN4B* (which encodes $Na_{v\beta}4$, a α_4-subunit that is believed to coassemble with the α-subunit of the cardiac sodium channel to form $Na_V1.5$.[6] Secondary alterations probably underlie QT interval prolongation in LQT4, LQT9, and LQT10. Thus, intracellular calcium homeostasis is disrupted and afterdepolarizations occur in ankyrin-B mutants, whereas the persistent sodium current is increased and action potential duration is prolonged in the presence of *CAV3* or *SCN4B* mutants.

Pathophysiology of QT Interval Prolongation and Arrhythmias

A delicate balance between inward and outward ion currents determines the plateau phase of the ventricular action potential, which is represented by the QT interval on the surface ECG. During this phase of the cardiac cycle, an increase in depolarizing (Na^+ or Ca^{2+}) current or a decrease in repolarizing (K^+) current delays repolarization, thereby prolonging the QT interval. Accordingly, mutations in *KCNQ1*, *KCNH2*, *KCNE1*, or *KCNE2* that result in loss of function of the potassium channel protein (i.e., decreased repolarizing K^+ current during the action potential plateau) prolong the action potential plateau phase.[7-10] This allows recovery from inactivation and reactivation of L-type calcium channels, resulting in early afterdepolarizations (EADs) that can trigger torsades de pointes (TdP) ventricular tachycardia, the signature tachyarrhythmia of LQTS.[11] In contrast, the K^+ current encoded by *KCNJ2* is active during the terminal phase of the action potential. Loss-of-function mutations in this gene, as found in LQT7, are predicted to prolong the final repolarization phase of the action potential rather than its plateau phase. This can evoke arrhythmias by a different mechanism, namely, by EADs carried by the Na^+-Ca^{2+} exchanger.[12] LQTS-associated mutations in *SCN5A* and *CACNA1C* increase the Na^+ and Ca^{2+} currents, respectively, also shifting the balance into the direction of delayed repolarization.

Biophysical characterization of mutant channels expressed in heterologous systems such as *Xenopus* oocytes or mammalian cell lines has unequivocally demonstrated that channels encoded by mutant *KCNQ1*, *KCNH2*, *KCNE1*, *KCNE2*, and *KCNJ2* that are associated with LQTS exhibit a loss of function.[7-10] In general, current magnitude may be reduced by a reduction in the number of functional ion channels in the sarcolemma or by biophysical disruptions of the ion channel, that is, changes in the speed or extent to which these channels transit from various ion-conducting and non–ion-conducting conformations (gating).[13] Reduced K^+ current is observed when mutant subunits are coexpressed with wild-type subunits, reflecting the situation where both normal (wild-type) and mutant subunits coexist, as in the case of a person who inherits a normal allele from one parent and a mutant allele from the other parent.

Because α subunits of the family of Kv channels (which includes *KCNQ1* and *KCNH2*) assemble as tetramers to form ion channels (see Chapter 28), the ratio of normally and abnormally functioning channels is predicted to result from the stochastic distribution of normal and mutant subunits. When mutant subunits assemble with normal subunits, they can act as poison peptides, exerting dominant-negative effects and disturbing the biophysical properties of the resultant ion channel, thereby reducing potassium current. If it is assumed that the presence of one mutant subunit alone is sufficient to disrupt channel function, only 6.25% (1/16) of channels, in theory, will function normally, because it is this small portion that is fully composed of four normal subunits.[7] Thus, the overall loss of current carried by the affected potassium channel will exceed 50%.

In contrast, when mutant subunits do not participate in tetramer assembly, haploinsufficiency results, and a 50% reduction of current magnitude is anticipated. This situation can arise from defective intracellular processing, which leads to impaired transport of mutant subunits to the sarcolemma,[14] which seems to be of particular importance in *KCNH2*-related LQTS.[15] In accordance with this concept, dominant-negative mutations in *KCNQ1* have a worse clinical outcome than mutations that cause haploinsufficiency and a predicted 50% reduction in channel function.[16]

For cardiac I_{Kr} channels, a complicating issue is the presence of HERG1a and HERG1b subunits that together form functional HERG channels.[17] In one small family with a severe arrhythmia phenotype, including intrauterine fetal death, it was demonstrated that complete lack of the subunit HERG1a led to a severe cardiac phenotype but to normal development otherwise.[18] It has been postulated that an important molecular mechanism that accounts for reduced I_{Kr} current in patients is permeation and degradation of mutant mRNA by the nonsense-mediated mRNA decay (NMD) pathway.[19]

The proteins encoded by the genes *KCNE1* and *KCNE2* appear to play a major role in modulation of the function of *KCNQ1*- and *KCNH2*-encoded potassium channels. Thus, abnormal function of either protein also might give rise to a clinical phenotype. The four α subunits encoded by *KCNQ1* assemble with the β subunit encoded by *KCNE1* to form the channel that conducts the slowly activating delayed rectifier K^+ current, I_{Ks}.[7,8] Similarly, four α-subunits encoded by *KCNH2* are thought to assemble with the β subunit encoded by *KCNE2* to form the channel that conducts the rapidly activating delayed rectifier K^+ current, I_{Kr}.[10] Whether the interaction between *KCNH2* and *KCNE2* is relevant for ventricular repolarization is, however, unclear, because the level of expression of *KCNE2* in ventricle is very low.[20,21]

Clinical Phenotype

The first description of the long-QT syndrome was provided by Jervell and Lange-Nielsen in 1957.[22] They described a family with sudden death at a young age and congenital deafness (JLN syndrome). A few years later, Romano and Ward described, in independent reports, the same electrocardiographic and clinical entity, but without deafness.[23,24] This phenotype turned out to be far more prevalent than JLN syndrome and is now recognized as the Romano-Ward syndrome.

Romano-Ward syndrome is inherited in an autosomal-dominant fashion and is estimated to affect 1 per 5000 persons, although estimates as high as 1 in 2000 have been made.[25] The JLN syndrome is inherited in an autosomal-recessive fashion and is associated with sensorineural deafness. JLN syndrome is based on homozygous carriership of mutations in *KCNQ1*[26] or *KCNE1*,[9] explaining its recessive nature. Parents of JLN patients (who are both heterozygous carriers of either JLN-associated mutation of their child) have, in general, a less-severe clinical phenotype (normal or near-normal QT interval) than *KCNQ1*-related Romano-Ward syndrome patients (LQT1), who are also heterozygous mutation carriers. This is in agreement with the finding that most JLN-associated *KCNQ1* mutants do not participate in tetramer formation to produce the I_{Ks}-generating ion channel, because they are nonsense, deletion, or frameshift mutations (although mis-sense mutations have also been described in a minority). Thus, they do not exert dominant-negative effects, and the overall loss of function does not exceed 50%.[27] In rare instances, QT interval prolongation forms part of a multisystem disorder that affects other organs besides the heart. Two such disorders, Andersen syndrome[28-30] (LQT7) and Timothy syndrome[31] (LQT8) have been recognized.

The number of patients affected by one of the first three LQTS subtypes (LQT1, LQT2, and LQT3) is sufficiently high to accurately describe and compare the clinical phenotypes. Other subtypes have only been identified in single patients or small families. A systematic analysis of genetic testing for five ion channel–encoding genes in 262 patients revealed that 42% of patients had a mutation in *KCNQ1*, 45% in *KCNH2*, 8% in *SCN5A* (LQT3), 3% in *KCNE1*, and 2% in *KCNE2*.[32] The number of different mutants in the various genes is enormous, in particular, in the most common genes, *KCNQ1* and *KCNH2*.[33] Yet it is estimated that in 30% to 40% of patients with a clear phenotype, the genotype cannot be established at present.

Shortly after the first genes causing LQTS were identified, attempts to define a genotype-phenotype relationship were made. Indeed, gene-specific clinical and electrophysiologic phenotypes are present. This includes gene-specific triggers for arrhythmic events, differential ages at which the first symptoms occur, specific ST-T segment morphologies, and modes of onset of arrhythmias.[34-36] Most importantly, therapy also exhibits gene-specific elements.[36,37] Recognizing gene-specific features can also be used to direct genetic screening to the most likely culprit gene. When ECG and clinical signs in the patient or family are taken into account, the yield of mutation detection in the first gene tested was as high as 90% in patients in whom the genotype could be established.[38]

Triggers for LQTS-related symptoms, namely syncope or cardiac arrest, differ between the various LQTS subtypes. Whereas triggers associated with increased adrenergic stimulation are most prevalent in LQT1 patients[34,36] and less so in LQT2 patients, LQT3 patients are, conversely, at greatest risk at rest or during sleep.[36] Specific triggers, such as diving or swimming in LQT1 patients, and acoustic stimuli and arousal-related stimuli in LQT2 patients, are of clinical relevance.[34-36] The age at which cardiac events occur for the first time is generally lowest in LQT1 patients.[39] At age 10 years, 40% of LQT1 patients have become symptomatic, but only 10% of LQT2 patients and even fewer LQT3 patients show symptoms at this age.

It has not been determined whether this information can be used to guide treatment, specifically, whether or not one can safely delay treatment in LQT2 and LQT3 patients until they have reached puberty. Still, Kaplan-Meyer event-free survival analysis suggests that one could. This idea is attractive, particularly in the case of LQT3 patients in whom an ICD might be the only beneficial treatment (see later).

The same analysis also suggests that the number of patients who develop symptoms for the first time after 20 years of age is very limited in LQT1,[40,41] whereas the cumulative rate of first events continues to increase slowly with increasing age in LQT2 patients. Due to the very limited number of LQT3 patients, no conclusions can be drawn on this subtype. More-recent studies in relatively large cohorts of LQT1 patients seem to confirm these observations.[41,37] Thus, asymptomatic adult patients with newly identified LQT1 seem to be at low risk.

The genotype affects the ECG, in particular, T-wave morphology and the ST-T-wave patterns.[42,43] Typically, in LQT1, the T waves are broad-based with a high amplitude (Fig. 51-1A), whereas in LQT2, the ST-T segment has a low amplitude in the limb leads and a biphasic pattern in the precordial leads (see Fig. 51-1B). In LQT3, the T-wave is peaked (narrow-based) and preceded by a long isoelectric ST-T segment.

Exercise elicits a gene-specific response. I_{Ks} is the most important current to abbreviate the cardiac action potential at fast heart rates (e.g., exercise) because, due to its slow kinetics,

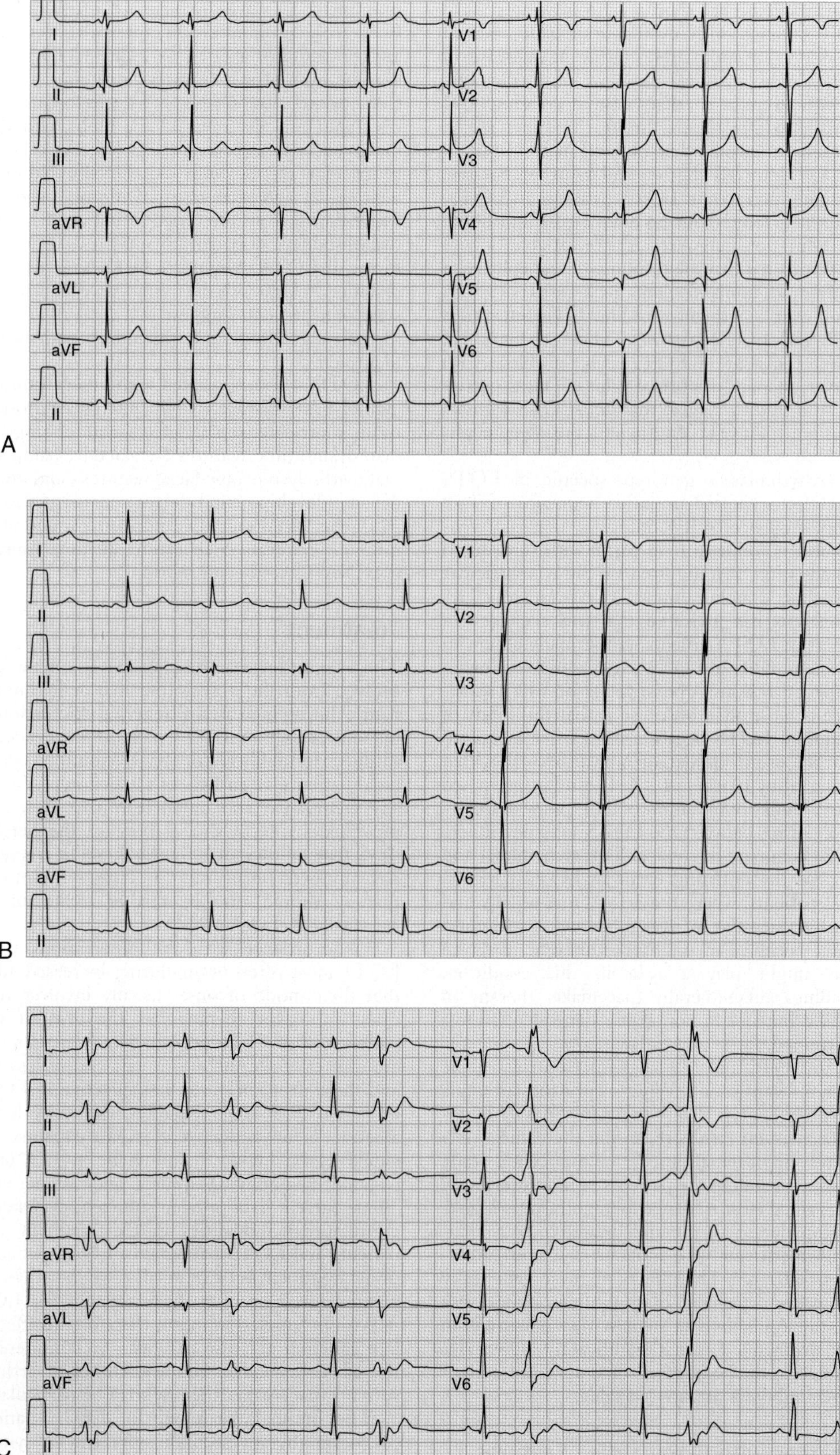

Figure 51-1 Electrocardiograms (ECGs) of long-QT syndrome (LQTS) patients. In both cases the QTc interval is 548 ms. **A,** ECG from a patient with a type 1 LQTS (LQT1). Typical wide-based T-waves with a large amplitude are observed. **B,** ECG from an LQT2 patient. The T-wave has a low amplitude in the extremity leads and a notch in some of the precordial leads. Both features are characteristic for LQT2. **C,** ECG of an LQT7 patient. Characteristic features are the bigeminy of ventricular extrasystoles, which might be present most of the day, and the large amplitude U-waves. The ventricular extrasystoles originate from these U-waves. In this case, the patient is using β-blocker therapy, which probably explains the slow sinus rate.

deactivation is incomplete at short diastolic intervals.[44] Accordingly, LQT1 patients with dysfunctioning I_{Ks} fail to shorten their QT interval appropriately during an increase in heart rate, and QTc might actually lengthen[45] (normally, QT intervals shorten with exercise so that, with decreasing R-R intervals, QTc remains within normal limits). The increase in heart rate during exercise is somewhat blunted in LQT1.[45] In contrast to LQT1, QT intervals shorten and can even become normal when heart rate increases in LQT3 patients. In LQT3, the QT interval is actually longest during bradycardia. In LQT2, the changes in QTc duration upon exercise are variable.[45]

It has also been postulated that the response to epinephrine, a recommended method to unmask silent gene-carriers,[46-49] is gene specific. Significant lengthening of the QTc interval is observed in LQT1 and LQT2 patients. These changes are stable in LQT1 but transient in LQT2. The problem with these tests is, however, the lack of normal values. This is particularly relevant, because studies suggest that non-LQTS patients might also develop significant QTc lengthening during epinephrine infusion.[50]

The onset of arrhythmias is genotype-specific in LQTS patients. The most-often reported initiation sequence of TdP is a short-long-short sequence of R-R intervals, that is, a ventricular premature beat is followed by a pause with subsequent excessive QT prolongation that is attended by a ventricular extrasystole (with a short coupling interval) that initiates TdP. However, recent analysis has indicated that this sequence of events is only present in LQT2 patients and virtually absent in LQT1 patients.[51] The number of LQT3 patients was too low to draw any meaningful conclusions. A possible reason why a short-long-short sequence is most often observed is that this mode of onset occurs in acquired LQTS because, most often, acquired LQTS results from the use of cardiac or noncardiac drugs that prolong the QT interval by blocking I_{Kr}.[52] It can be speculated whether the different modes of initiation of TdP point to different arrhythmia mechanisms between the LQTS subtypes. There is consensus that EADs initiate the typical TdP arrhythmia, and EADs are likely to be the initiating event in LQT2 patients. However, in LQT1 patients, where the arrhythmia usually and predictably (see earlier) starts at increased heart rate without a preceding pause, the mechanism might be different. Delayed afterdepolarizations might play a role in this condition. Whether these findings affect therapy (pacemaker therapy in pause-dependent TdP but not in non–pause-dependent forms) remains to be determined.

Emerging data in LQT1 and LQT2 point to a role of the genetic findings in risk stratification. Whereas previous attempts to identify a genotype-phenotype relationship for *KCNQ1* mutations did not yield consistent results regarding the clinical outcome of the type and site of mutations,[53,54] a multicenter study of 600 LQT1 patients (including the patients in both previously reported studies) provided clear evidence for significantly higher cardiac event rates in patients with mutants located in transmembrane segments and in patients with mutants that exert dominant-negative effects on I_{Ks}.[16] The effects of these genetically determined factors are independent of traditional clinical risk factors. In LQT2, the available data suggest that mutations in the transmembrane segments confer a significantly higher risk than mutations located in the N-terminal or C-terminal ends.[55] Similar data on other subtypes are not available.

Long-QT Syndromes with Extracardiac Features

Prolongation of the QT interval also occurs in conjunction with other (extracardiac) manifestations. Andersen-Tawil syndrome, also referred to as LQT7,[28-30] manifests with ECG features that include abnormal T-wave morphology, often with very prominent U waves (which are often difficult to distinguish from truly prolonged QT intervals), ventricular arrhythmias, and potassium-sensitive periodic paralysis. In addition, there may be dysmorphic features, including short stature, scoliosis, cleft palate, low-set ears, hypertelorism, micrognathia, and developmental disorders in the limbs (clinodactyly, syndactyly, brachydactyly). A typical ECG (see Fig. 51-1C) shows frequent ventricular ectopy with occasionally bidirectional ventricular tachycardia and recurrent polymorphic ventricular tachycardia, which can give rise to syncope and cardiac arrest. However, the risk of sudden cardiac death appears to be low compared to other forms of LQTS. Mutations in *KCNJ2* have been linked to this disorder.[30] Although the dysmorphic features in Andersen-Tawil syndrome patients suggest that *KCNJ2* is involved in developmental signalling, no signalling pathways have yet been identified.

LQT8 is also associated with other disorders, including congenital heart disease (patent ductus arteriosus, patent foramen ovale, ventricular septal defects, and tetralogy of Fallot), noncardiac dysmorphic features (syndactyly, baldness at birth, abnormal teeth, dysmorphic facial features), and noncardiac functional defects (developmental delays consistent with language, motor, and generalized cognitive impairment and abnormalities in the immune system). A recurrent de novo mutation (G406R) in CACNA1C has been reported.[31]

Treatment

The suggestion that therapy may be gene specific has mainly evolved from the observation that arrhythmias occur predominantly during increased adrenergic stimulation in LQT1 patients but only rarely in LQT3 patients. Either way, an implantable cardioverter defibrillator (ICD) should be considered in resuscitated patients, regardless of the genotype. In general, ICD therapy seems safe, and initial fears that electrical storms may be provoked by ICD shocks because the heightened adrenergic drive that follows an ICD shock might trigger new arrhythmias have not been borne out.[56,57] Thus, symptoms that recur despite therapy should prompt further treatment steps that might eventually include an ICD.

In accordance with the observations that arrhythmias in LQT1 most often occur during increased adrenergic tone and that their mode of onset usually involves relatively fast heart rates, β-blocker therapy has the greatest efficacy in LQT1 patients (Fig. 51-2, pooled data[36,37]). Conversely, β-blockers are also effective in LQT2, but clearly less so than in LQT1, and these drugs are even less effective in LQT3.[36,37] Similarly, other antiadrenergic therapies, especially left stellate ganglion ablation, is most effective in LQT1 patients,[58] although, in individual cases, highly symptomatic LQT3 patients might also respond favorably (Schwartz and Wilde, unpublished data). Thus, current data provide sufficient evidence that antiadrenergic treatment modalities are the treatment of choice in LQT1 patients and LQT2 patients. In LQT2 patients, however, additional treatment is often needed. Higher-than-normal serum potassium levels seem to be of benefit for LQT2 patients, and potassium suppletion might therefore be effective.[59,60] Left stellate ganglion ablation may also be considered[58] and, based on the pause-dependent mode of onset of arrhythmias in LQT2 patients, pacemaker therapy may be particularly effective.

The optimal treatment for LQT3 patients is less clear. β-Blocker therapy seems insufficient for symptomatic patients, and ICD implantation may be considered. Based on the pathophysiologic basis of LQT3 (i.e., persistent inward sodium current during the plateau phase of the action potential), sodium channel blockade has been tried. Although the initial results showed significant abbreviation of the QT interval,[61] it should

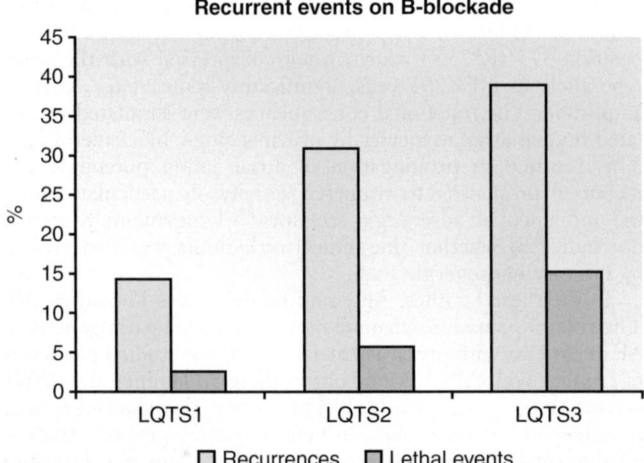

Figure 51-2 Recurrent events on β-adrenoceptor blocking therapy in LQT patients with different genotypes. The data are pooled from the two studies with 271 and 335 patients.[36,37] Mean follow-up is up to 5 years in the second study and not indicated in the first study. It is clear that the β-blockade is most effective in LQT1, followed by LQT2. In LQT3, almost 40% of patients experience a recurrent event, 15% of which are fatal. These data question the efficacy of β-adrenoceptor blockade in LQT3.

be realized that long-term results on outcome are not available and that, in the meantime, failures on sodium channel blockade have been described.[62] It is clear that the choice of treatment is even more difficult in asymptomatic LQT3 patients.

Short-QT Syndromes

In recent years, shorter-than-normal QT intervals have attracted interest. The clinical entity associated with this is, predictably, referred to as short-QT syndrome (SQTS). The number of patients that has been decribed so far is still very limited. Gussak and colleagues introduced the term *short QT syndrome* after the first description of a family with atrial arrhythmias.[63] In 2004, Gaita and coworkers[64] linked the disease to malignant ventricular arrhythmias (including sudden cardiac death at a young age) and, shortly thereafter, the first causal gene was described (*KCNH2*, i.e., SQTS1).[65] In the meantime, more families have been described with different genotypes,[66,67] but the total number is still limited.[68] In a Finnish population study, the prevalence of short-QT intervals was studied along with its impact on survival. QTc intervals shorter than 320 and 340 ms were observed in 0.1% and 0.4% of the population, respectively. All-cause or cardiovascular mortality of these patients did not differ compared to persons with normal QTc intervals.[69]

Pathophysiology of QT Interval Shortening

In a short time, three subtypes of SQTS have been recognized (SQT1, SQT2, and SQT3). These SQTSs are associated with mutations in genes encoding the potassium channel: *KCNH2*, *KCNQ1*, and *KCNJ2*, respectively.[65-67] All mutations so far analyzed biophysically exhibited gain of function of their respective gene product, secondary to gating changes.

In SQTS1, two mis-sense mutations were found that are predicted to result in the same amino acid change, N588K.[65] This residue is located in the S5-pore loop region at the outer mouth of the channel. This mutation caused reduction in inactivation. Because inactivation is responsible for inward rectification (decrease in outward current at sustained depolarization), this resulted in removal of rectification and an increase in outward current at early stages of the action potential, including its plateau phase. The net result is QT interval shortening. It was proposed that spatially inhomogeneous QT shortening (due to the spatial inhomogeneity of ion channel expression) would contribute to reentrant excitation, thereby facilitating tachyarrhythmias. The biophysical changes of this outer pore–located mutation are in good agreement with the notion that residues in the outer pore of the channel are responsible for C-type inactivation.[70]

In SQTS2, two KCNQ1 mutations were reported, V307L[66] and V141M.[71] The V307L mutant accelerated the rate of activation, and voltage-dependent activation of V307L was shifted to hyperpolarized potentials, thereby facilitating channel activation. These changes were predicted to increase I_{Ks}. It was proposed that the preservation of time-dependence of channel opening (faster, but not instantaneous opening) explained why this mutant was not associated with atrial fibrillation (see later), where gain-of-function *KCNQ1* mutations produced instantaneous (time-independent) I_{Ks}. It was hypothesized that constitutive repolarizing current in the atrium might result in atrial fibrillation. In accordance with this hypothesis, the V141M mutant, which did produce constitutively active I_{Ks}, caused both SQTS and atrial fibrillation.[71]

In SQT3, the D172N mutation in *KCNJ2* was reported.[67] This mutation exhibited reduced inward rectification at depolarized potentials, specifically, larger amplitude of outward current and a shift of this peak to more depolarized potentials. The prediction that these changes would speed up repolarzation of the terminal phase of the action potential (as the membrane potential returns from depolarized levels to hyperpolarized levels) was supported by modeling studies, which indicated that abbreviation of the action potential was solely due to abbreviation of its terminal phase. These findings compare well with the characteristic shape of the T wave of affected persons, which exhibits an abrupt return of its terminal portion (descending limb) to baseline levels.[67]

Atrial Fibrillation

Atrial fibrillation (AF) is the most common clinically relevant arrhythmia. AF is most often associated with structural heart disease and, in this setting in particular, associated with an unfavorable prognosis. Heritability has long been proposed, but only recently have causal genes been identified. The number of identified genes is rapidly increasing and involve various genes that encode potassium channel (sub)units (for review see Fatkin and colleagues[72]). All reported cases still relate to only isolated patients or families.

KCNQ1 was identified as the causal gene in 2003 in a large Chinese family with permanent AF.[73] The mutation S140G led to a gain of function of I_{Ks}, putatively leading to abbreviation of the atrial action potential and refractory period and promoting reentrant arrhythmias in the atrium. A paradoxical finding in this family is that QT prolongation was observed in carriers of the mutant gene (in nine of 16 persons, the QT interval was between 460 and 530 ms). Gain-of-function mutations in *KCNQ1* have been associated with SQTS (see earlier), and the observed QT prolongation is therefore not fully explained. It was proposed that this unexpected finding was explained by the fact that cardiac repolarization is a complex process that involves many different proteins, and these proteins may be differentially expressed in atrium and ventricle, thereby imposing disparate electrophysiologic phenotypes in both cardiac compartments. In any case, the role of *KCNQ1* seems to be limited, because several studies failed to identify aberrancies in KCNQ1 in other AF families,[73-75] with the exception of a *KCNQ1* mutation in one small family.[75]

Because I_{Ks} results from an interaction between the potassium channel α-subunit *KCNQ1* and the β-subunits *KCNE1* and *KCNE2*, mutation screening was performed in *KCNE1*, *KCNE2*, and other KCNE isoforms. These efforts have resulted in the identification of a *KCNE2* mutation (R27C) in one family[76] and a *KCNE3* mutation (R53H) in another.[77] Although the R27C mutant resulted in increased I_{Ks} amplitude, the R53H mutant did not alter I_{Ks} amplitude, casting doubts on a possible causal role. Moreover, other studies have not supported the notion that the KCNE family plays a major role, because no other gene aberrancies were found.[75,78]

KCNH2 mutations have also been associated with familial AF, but only in families with significant QT-interval shortening (SQTS).[79] The N588K *KCNH2* variant was also associated with a gain of function, putatively leading to abbreviation of action potentials in atrium and ventricle and comfortably explaining the associated short-QT interval. In only one of the three described families with this mutation, the phenotype included AF at a young age. One gain-of-function *KCNJ2* mutation was identified in a series of 30 probands.[80]

Finally, the *KCNA5* gene that encodes Kv1.5, a component of the atrial-specific ultrarapid component of the delayed rectifier potassium current, I_{Kur}, hosted a sequence variant in one family out of a series of 154 persons.[81] The heterozygous nonsense mutation (1123G>T) was predicted to cause a stop codon at position 375 (E375X) which, when coexpressed with the wild-type allele in HEK293 cells, significantly reduced I_{Kur} current amplitude. The functional consequences were simulated in isolated human atrial myocytes by pharmacologic blockade of I_{Kur}. This resulted in prolongation of atrial action potentials and increased propensity to triggered activity, in particular, under the influence of adrenergic stressors.[81] Unfortunately, it was not indicated whether the clinical arrhythmia was also evoked by increased adrenergic tone.

In the these families, AF could be defined as idiopathic AF. The role of potassium-channel mutations in the pathogenesis of AF in patients with presumed atrial stretch was studied in a series of families with AF.[75] In one out of these 50 families, a *KCNQ1* variant (R14C) was observed. This family also showed a high prevalence of hypertension. In heterologous expression studies, no abnormal current was observed at baseline, but after exposure to hypotonic solution (to mimic atrial stretch, as a consequence of hypertension), a gain of function was observed, putatively leading to abbreviated action potential durations and an increased likelihood of reentrant atrial arhythmias.[75] This latter finding can be regarded as a proof of principle, but it is clear that more studies will be needed to explore the role of genetic variants in establishing AF in the setting of structural heart disease.

References

1. Jiang C, Atkinson D, Towbin JA, et al: Two long QT syndrome loci map to chromosomes 3 and 7 with evidence for further heterogeneity. Nat Genet 8:141-147, 1994.
2. Sanguinetti MC, Curran ME, Spector PS, Keating MT: Spectrum of HERG K^+-channel dysfunction in an inherited cardiac arrhythmia. Proc Natl Acad Sci U S A 93:2208-2212, 1996.
3. Mohler PJ, Schott J-J, Gramolini AO, et al: Ankyrin-B mutation causes type 4 long-QT cardiac arrhytmia and sudden cardiac death. Nature 421:634-639, 2003.
4. Splawski I, Timothy KW, Sharpe LM, et al: $Ca_V1.2$ calcium channel dysfunction causes a multisystem disorder including arrhythmia and autism. Cell 119:19-31, 2004.
5. Vatta M, Ackerman MJ, Ye B, et al: Mutant caveolin-3 induces persistent late sodium current and is associated with long-QT syndrome. Circulation 114:2104-2112, 2006.
6. Medeiros-Domingo A, Kaku T, Tester DJ, et al: SCN4B-encoded sodium channel β4 subunit in congenital long-QT syndrome. Circulation 116:134-142, 2007.
7. Sanguinetti MC, Curran ME, Zou A, et al: Coassembly of KvLQT1 and minK (IsK) proteins to form cardiac I_{Ks} potassium channel. Nature 384:80-83, 1996.
8. Barhanin J, Lesage F, Guillemare E: KvLQT1 and IsK (minK) proteins associate to form the I_{Ks} cardiac potassium current. Nature 384:78-80, 1996.
9. Splawski I, Tristani-Firouzi M, Lehmann MH, et al: Mutations in the *hminK* gene cause long QT syndrome and suppress I_{Ks} function. Nat Genet 17:338-340, 1997.
10. Abbott GW, Sesti F, Splawski I, et al: MiRP1 forms I_{kr} potassium channels with *HERG* and is associated with cardiac arrhythmia. Cell 97:175-187, 1999.
11. January CT, Riddle JM: Early afterdepolarizations: Mechanisms of induction and block a role for L-type Ca^{2+} current. Circ Res 64:977-990, 1989.
12. Tristani-Firouzi M, Jensen JL, Donaldson MR, et al: Functional and clinical characterization of *KCNJ2* mutations associated with LQT7 (Andersen syndrome). J Clin Invest 110:381-388, 2002.
13. Clancy CE, Kass RS: Inherited and acquired vulnerability to ventricular arrhythmias: Cardiac Na^+ and K^+ channels. Physiol Rev 85:33-47, 2005.
14. Zhou Z, Gong Q, Epstein ML, January CT: HERG channel dysfunction in human long QT syndrome. Intracellular transport and functional defects. J Biol Chem 273:21061-21066, 1998.
15. Anderson CL, Delisle BP, Anson BD, et al: Most *LQT2* mutations reduce $K_V11.1$ (hERG) current by a class 2 (trafficking-deficient) mechanism. Circulation 113: 365-373, 2006.
16. Moss AJ, Shimizu W, Wilde AAM, et al: Genotype-phenotype aspects of type-1 long-QT syndrome. Circulation 115: 2481-2489, 2007.
17. Jones EM, Roti Roti EC, Wang J, et al: Cardiac I_{Kr} channels minimally comprise *hERG* 1a and 1b subunits. J Biol Chem 279:44690-44694, 2004.
18. Hoorntje ThM, Alders M, van Tintelen PJ, et al: Homozygous premature truncation of the HERG protein: The human HERG knockout. Circulation 100:1264-1267, 1999.
19. Gong Q, Zhang L, Vincent GM, et al: Nonsense mutations in *hERG* cause a decrease in mutant mRNA transcripts by nonsense-mediated mRNA decay in human long QT syndrome. Circulation 116:17-24, 2007.
20. Lundquist AL, Manderfield LJ, Vanoye CG, et al: Expression of multiple *KCNE* genes in human heart may enable variable modulation of I_{Ks}. J Mol Cell Cardiol 38:277-287, 2005.
21. Pourrier M, Zicha S, Ehrlich J, et al: Canine ventricular KCNE2 expression resides predominantly in Purkinje fibers. Circ Res 93:189-191, 2003.
22. Jervell A, Lange-Nielsen F: Congenital deaf-mutism, functional heart disease with prolongation of Q-T interval and sudden death. Am Heart J 54:59-68, 1957.
23. Romano C, Gemme G, Pongiglione R: Aritmie cardiache rare dell'eta pediatrica. II. Accessi sincopali per fibrillazione ventricuolare parossistica. (Presentazione del primo caso della letteratura pediatrica Italiana). Clin Pediatr 45:656-683, 1963.
24. Ward OC: A new familial cardiac syndrome in children. J Irish Med Assoc 54:103-106, 1964.
25. Crotti L, Stramba-Badiale M, Pedrazzini M, et al: Prevalence of long QT syndrome. Circulation 112(suppl II):II-660, 2005.
26. Chen QY, Zhang DM, Gingell RL, et al: Homozygous deletion in *KVLQT1* associated with Jervell and Lange-Nielsen syndrome. Circulation 99:1344-1347, 1999.
27. Wilde AAM, Escande D: LQT genotype-phenotype relationships: patients and patches. Cardiovasc Res 51:627-629, 2001.
28. Andersen ED, Krasilnikoff PA, Overvad H: Intermittent muscular weakness, extrasystoles, and multiple developmental anomalies. A new syndrome? Acta Paediatr Scand 60:559-564, 1971.
29. Tawil R, Ptacek LJ, Pavlakis SG, et al: Andersen's syndrome: Potassium-sensitive periodic paralysis, ventricular ectopy, and

dysmorphic features. Ann Neurol 35:326-330, 1994.

30. Tristani-Firouzi M, Jensen JL, Donaldson MR, S, et al: Functional and clinical characterization of *KCMJ2* mutations associated with LQT7 (Andersen syndrome). J Clin Invest 110:381-388, 2002.
31. Splawski I, Timothy KW, Sharpe LM, et al: $Ca_V1.2$ calcium channel dysfunction causes a multisystem disorder including arrhythmia and autism. Cell 119:19-31, 2004.
32. Splawski I, Shen J, Timothy KW, et al: Spectrum of mutations in long-QT syndromes. *KVLQT1, HERG, SCN5A, KCNE1,* and *KCNE2*. Circulation 102:1178-1185, 2000.
33. Fondazione Salvatore Maugeri: Gene connection for the heart. Available at http://www.fsm.it/cardmoc/. Accessed September 15, 2008.
34. Wilde AAM, Jongbloed RJE, Doevendans PA, et al: Auditory stimuli as a trigger for arrhythmic events differentiate HERG-related (LQTS2) patients from KVLQT1-related patients (LQTS1). J Am Coll Cardiol 33:327-332, 1999.
35. Moss AJ, Robinson JL, Gessman L, et al: Comparison of clinical and genetic variables of cardiac events associated with loud noise versus swimming among subjects with the long QT syndrome. Am J Cardiol 84:876-879, 1999.
36. Schwartz PJ, Priori SG, Spazzolini C, et al: Genotype-phenotype correlation in the long-QT syndrome: Gene specific triggers for-life threatening arrhythmias. Circulation 103:89-95, 2001.
37. Priori SG, Napolitano C, Schwartz PJ, et al: Association of long QT syndrome loci and cardiac events among patients treated with β-blockers. JAMA 292: 1341-1344, 2004.
38. Van Langen I, BirnieE, AldersM, et al: The use of genotype-phenotype correlations in mutation analysis for the long QT syndrome. J Med Genet 40:141-145, 2003.
39. Zareba W, Moss AJ, Schwartz PJ, et al: Influence of genotype on the clinical course of the long-QT syndrome. International Long-QT Syndrome Registry Research Group. N Engl J Med 339:960-965, 1998.
40. Hobbs JB, Peterson DR, Moss AJ, et al: Risk of aborted cardiac arrest or sudden cardiac death during adolescence in the long-QT syndrome. JAMA 296:1249-1254, 2006.
41. Moss AJ, Shimizu W, Wilde AAM, et al: Genotype-phenotype aspects of type-1 long-QT syndrome. Circulation 115:2481-2489, 2007.
42. Moss AJ, Zareba W, Benhorin J, et al: ECG T-wave patterns in genetically distinct forms of the hereditary long QT syndrome. Circulation 92:2929-2934, 1995.
43. Zhang L, Timothy KW, Vincent GM, et al: Spectrum of ST-T–wave patterns and repolarization parameters in congenital long-QT syndrome: ECG findings identify genotypes. Circulation 102:2849-2855, 2000.
44. Faber GM, Rudy Y: Action potential and contractility changes in $[Na^+_i$ overloaded cardiac myocytes: A simulation study. Biophys J 78:2392-2404, 2000.
45. Swan H, Viitasalo M, Piippo K, et al: Sinus node function and ventricular repolarization during exercise stress test in long QT syndrome patients with KvLQT1 and HERG potassium channel defects. J Am Coll Cardiol 34:823-829, 1999.
46. Ackerman MJ, Khositseth A, Tester DJ, et al: Epinephrine-induced QT interval prolongation: A gene-specific paradoxical response in congenital long QT syndrome. Mayo Clin Proc 77:413-421, 2002.
47. Noda T, Takaki H, Kurita T, et al: Gene-specific response of dynamic ventricular repolarization to sympathetic stimulation in LQT1, LQT2 and LQT3 forms of congenital long QT syndrome. Eur Heart J 23:975-983, 2002.
48. Shimizu W, Tanabe Y, Aiba T, et al: Differential effects of beta-blockade on dispersion of repolarization in the absence and presence of sympathetic stimulation between the LQT1 and LQT2 forms of congenital long QT syndrome. J Am Coll Cardiol 39:1984-1991, 2002.
49. Shimizu W, Noda T, Takaki H, et al: Diagnostic value of epinephrine test for genotyping LQT1, LQT2, and LQT3 forms of congenital long QT syndrome. Heart Rhythm 3:276-283, 2004.
50. Magnano AR, Talathoti N, Hallur R, et al: Sympathomimetic infusion and cardiac repolarization: The normative effects of epinephrine and isoproterenol in healthy subjects. J Cardiovasc Electrophysiol 17:983-989, 2006.
51. Tan HL, Bardai A, Shimizu W, et al: Genotype-specific onset of arrhythmias in congenital long QT syndrome: Possible therapy implications. Circulation 114: 2096-2103, 2006.
52. Roden DM: Drug-induced prolongation of the QT interval. N Engl J Med 350:1013-1022, 2004.
53. Zareba W, Moss AJ, Sheu G, et al: Location of mutation in the *KCNQ1* and phenotypic presentation of long QT syndrome. J Cardiovasc Electrophysiol 14:1149-1153, 2003.
54. Shimizu W, Horie M, Ohno S, et al: Mutation site-specific differences in arrhythmic risk and sensitivity to sympathetic stimulation in the LQT1 form of congenital long QT syndrome: Multicenter study in Japan. J Am Coll Cardiol 44:117-125, 2004.
55. Moss AJ, Zareba W, Kaufman ES, et al: Increased risk of arrhythmic events in long QT-syndrome with mutations in the pore region of the human ether-a-go-go–related gene potassium channel. Circulation 105:794-799, 2002.
56. Wilde AAM: Is there a role for implantable cardioverter defibrillator therapy in the long QT syndrome. J Cardiovasc Electrophysiol 13:S110-S113, 2002.
57. Zareba W, Moss AJ, Daubert JP, et al: Implantable cardioverter defibrillator in high-risk long QT syndrome patients. J Cardiovasc Electrophysiol 14:337-341, 2003.
58. Schwartz PJ, Priori SG, Cerrone M, et al: Left cardiac sympathetic denervation in the management of high-risk patients affected by the long-QT syndrome. Circulation 109:1826-1833, 2004.
59. Tan HL, Alings AMW, van Olden R, Wilde AAM: Chronic potassium treatment in congenital *HERG*-related long QT syndrome. J Cardiovasc Electrophysiol 10:229-233, 1999.
60. Etheridge SP, Compton SJ, Tristani-Firouzi M, Mason JW: A new oral therapy for long QT syndrome: Long-term oral potassium improves repolarization in patients with *HERG* mutations. J Am Coll Cardiol 42:1777-1782, 2003.
61. Moss AJ, Windle JR, Hall WJ, et al: Safety and efficacy of flecainide in subjects with long QT3 syndrome (ΔKPQ mutation): A randomized double-blind, placebo-controlled clinical trial. Ann Noninvasive Electrophysiol 10:Suppl 59-66, 2005.
62. Ten Harkel AD, Witsenburg M, de Jong PL, et al: Efficacy of an implantable cardioverter-defibrillator in a neonate with LQT3 associated arrhythmias. Europace 7:77-84, 2005.
63. Gussak I, Brugada P, Brugada J, et al: Idiopathic short QT interval: A new clinical syndrome? Cardiology 94:99-102, 2000.
64. Gaíta F, Giustetto C, Bianchi F, et al: Short QT syndrome: A familial cause of sudden death. Circulation 108:965-970, 2003.
65. Brugada R, Hong K, Dumaine R, et al: Sudden death associated with short-QT syndrome linked to mutations in *HERG*. Circulation 109:r151-r156, 2004.
66. Bellocq C, van Ginneken ACG, Bezzina CR, et al: Mutation in the *KCNQ1* gene leading to the short QT interval syndrome. Circulation 109:2394-2397, 2004.
67. Priori SG, Pandit SV, Rivolta I, et al: A novel form of short QT syndrome (SQT3) is caused by a mutation in the *KCNJ2* gene. Circulation 96:800-807, 2005.
68. Giustetto C, Di Monte F, Wolpert C, et al: Short QT syndrome: Clinical findings and diagnostic-therapeutic implications. Eur Heart J 27:2440-2447, 2006.
69. Anttonen O, Junttila MJ, Rissanen H, et al: Prevalence and prognostic significance of short QT interval in a middle-aged Finnish popultion. Circulation 116:714-720, 2007.
70. Spector PS, Curran ME, Zou A, et al: Fast inactivation causes rectification of the I_{Kr} channel. J Gen Physiol 107:611-619, 1996.
71. Hong K, Piper DR, Diaz-Valdecantos A, et al: De novo *KCNQ1* mutation responsible for atrial fibrillation and short QT syndrome in utero. Cardiovasc Res 68: 433-440, 2005.
72. Fatkin D, Otway R, Vandenberg JI: Genes and atrial fibrillation: A new look at an old problem. Circulation 116:782-792, 2007.
73. Chen Y-H, Xu S-J, Bendahhou S, et al: *KCNQ1* gain-of-function mutation in familial atrial fibrillation. Science 299:251-254, 2003.
74. Ellinor PT, Moore RK, Patton KK, et al: Mutations in the long QT gene, *KCNQ1*, are an uncommon cause of atrial fibrillation. Heart 90:1487-1488, 2004.
75. Otway R, Vandenberg JI, Guanglan G, et al: Stretch-sensitive *KCNQ1* mutation: A link between genetic and environmental

factors in the pathogenesis of atrial fibrillation? J Am Coll Cardiol 49:578-586, 2007.
76. Yang Y, Xia M, Qingfeng J, et al: Identification of a *KCNE2* gain-of-function mutation in patients with familial fibrillation. Am J Hum Genet 75:899-905, 2004.
77. Zhang DF, Liang B, Lin J, et al: *KCNE3* R53H substitution in familial atrial fibrillation. Chin Med J 118:1735-1738, 2005.
78. Ellinor PT, Petrov-Kondratov VI, Zakharova E, et al: Potassium channel gene mutations rarely cause atrial fibrillation. BMC Med Genet 7:70, 2006.
79. Hong K, Bjerregaard P, Gussak I, Brugada R: Short QT syndrome and atrial fibrillation caused by mutation in *KCNH2*. J Cardiovasc Electrophysiol 16:394-396, 2005.
80. Xia M, Jin Q, Bendahhou S, et al: A $K_{ir}2.1$ gain of function mutation underlies familial atrial fibrillation. Biochem Biophys Res Commun 332:1012-1019, 2005.
81. Olson TM, Alekseev AE, Liu XK, et al: Kv1.5 channelopathy due to *KCNA5* loss-of-function mutation causes human atrial fibrillation. Hum Mol Genet 15:2185-2191, 2006.

Inheritable Disease of Intracellular Calcium Regulation 52

NIAN LIU, CARLO NAPOLITANO, AND SILVIA G. PRIORI

CHAPTER OUTLINE

Intracellular calcium homeostasis plays a crucial role in many physiologic processes in cells. In cardiac myocytes, the delicate balance of calcium fluxes between the intracellular compartment and the extracellular space is a prerequisite for normal heart rhythm and normal contractile function. A large body of evidence from clinical and experimental data has demonstrated that dysfunction of calcium handling underlies the pathophysiology of heart failure and of heart failure–related arrhythmias.[1] It is therefore plausible that the understanding of calcium-handling disorders in the heart might lead to the identification of new targets for therapy.[2,3]

Mutations in genes encoding the cardiac ryanodine receptor *(RyR2)* and cardiac calsequestrin *(CASQ2)*, two proteins implicated in the regulation of intracellular calcium, have been identified in an inherited arrhythmogenic disease called *catecholaminergic polymorphic ventricular tachycardia* (CPVT).[4,5] Analogous to what the long-QT syndrome has represented for the understanding of arrhythmogenesis related to dysfunction of voltage-dependent channels, CPVT has become a paradigm to the study of calcium-mediated arrhythmogenesis. In the last few years, thanks to major genotyping efforts, several *RyR2* and *CASQ2* mutations have been identified and functionally characterized in vitro, and several CPVT transgenic mouse models have been engineered, thus providing a window for the understanding of the role of ryanodine receptor and calsequestrin in calcium-mediated arrhythmogenesis. In this chapter we review the current knowledge about basic mechanisms for arrhythmias in CPVT. The clinical aspects of the disease are addressed in Chapter 70.

Genetics

Catecholaminergic Polymorphic Ventricular Tachycardia Causing Mutations in the *RyR2* Gene

The *RyR2* gene is one of the largest in the human genome; it comprises 105 exons[6] and encodes for a protein composed of 4967 amino acids. The ryanodine receptor is a tetrameric intracellular calcium-release channel located in sarcoplasmic reticulum (SR) and is required for cardiac excitation-contraction coupling. Each RyR2 monomer is composed of two major structural regions. The carboxy terminus (spanning approximately from amino acid 4500 to the end of the protein) represents the transmembrane domain of the protein and is the pore-forming region of the channel. Although this portion is relatively small, it is most important, because it represents the functional calcium-release channel and the site of interaction with important luminal regulatory proteins such as calsequestrin, triadin, and junctin. The second portion of RyR2, which represents nine-tenths of the protein and includes the central domain and the N terminus of the protein (Fig. 52-1), corresponds to the large cytoplasmic domain that binds numerous cytoplasmic proteins, forming a massive calcium-release complex that directly or indirectly regulates RyR2 activity.[7]

In 2001, Priori and colleagues[5] identified *RyR2* mutations in four families with the diagnosis of CPVT, thus demonstrating that *RyR2* is the gene for autosomal dominant CPVT; shortly after, Laitinen and coworkers[8] confirmed this finding. Based on the observations established in the cohort of patients enrolled in our CPVT database, which is the world's largest repository of data on the disease, *RyR2* mutations can be identified in approximately 60% to 70% of patients and have mean penetrance of 80%.[9] To date, 71 *RyR2* mutations have been reported (more information is available online at http://www.fsm.it/cardmoc/). Seventy *RyR2* mutations identified so far in CPVT are single-base-pair substitutions leading to the replacement of highly conserved amino acids; only one mutation, a duplication of nucleotides 13967 to 13972, causes the in-frame insertion of two amino acids.[10] Most *RyR2* mutations cluster in three regions: the N-terminal region, the central region, and the C-terminal region. A similar clustering is observed in mutations identified in the *RyR1* gene (encoding the ryanodine receptor present in skeletal muscles) that cause malignant hyperthermia and central core disease.

No *RyR2* mutations have been identified in the calcium pore-forming structure (P-loop) and in the extreme C-terminal region, which is involved in channel stability, and no mutations leading to stop codons and no in-frame insertions or deletions leading to protein truncation have been identified. These observations are consistent with the evidence that the development of the CPVT phenotype requires the presence of a structurally integrated ryanodine receptor harboring minor structural changes located in regions that are not critical for the function of the protein. Given that RyR2 serves such a vital function in the heart, the presence of major abnormalities is likely to abolish its function,[11] resulting in a lethal condition. This hypothesis is supported by the evidence that RyR2 homozygous knockout mice die during embryonic life.[12]

Danieli's group reported that selected *RyR2* mutations (A77V, R176Q/T2504M, R420W, L433P, N2386I and Y2392C) are associated with the clinical phenotype of a mild form of arrhythmogenic right ventricular cardiomyopathy (ARVC2) that combines minor or nearly absent macroscopic structural abnormalities of the right ventricle with typical stress-induced polymorphic ventricular tachycardia (VT).[6,13] After the initial report, however, only one group from Japan confirmed the association between *RyR2* mutations and ARVC2 (*RyR2* R420W mutation),[14] and other authors failed to support this hypothesis. For example, in a relatively large cohort

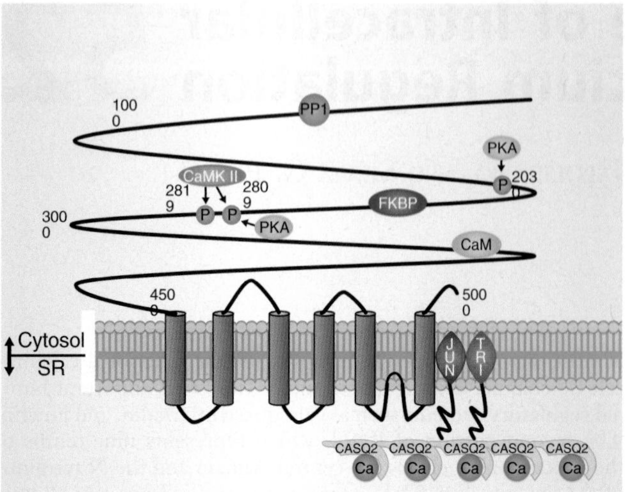

Figure 52-1 Schematic cartoon showing the predicted structure of the cardiac ryanodine receptor, RyR2, including the sites of interaction with key ancillary proteins and the phosphorylation sites. Calsequestrin (CASQ2), junction (JUN), and triadin (TRI), proteins interacting with ryanodine receptor in the sarcoplasmic reticulum (SR) are also depicted. CaM, calmodulin; CaMKII, calmodulin-dependent protein kinase II; P, phosphorylation sites; PKA, protein kinase A; PP1, protein phosphatase.

of 85 ARVC patients, Milting and colleagues[15] failed to identify carriers of mutations in the *RyR2* gene. Overall, considering that even in the original report from the group of Padua[6] the structural abnormalities typical of ARVC failed to cosegregate with the *RyR2* mutations, and considering the growing evidence that ARVC is a disease of desmosomes,[16] we favor the view that heterozygous *RyR2* mis-sense mutations do not cause the phenotype of ARVC.

Catecholaminergic Polymorphic Ventricular Tachycardia Causing Mutations in the *CASQ2* Gene

The CASQ2 protein serves as the major calcium reservoir within the SR of cardiac myocytes and as a luminal modulator of RyR2.[4] CASQ2 exists in monomeric and polymeric forms; CASQ2 polymerization occurs at high SR calcium contents. Polymeric CASQ2 has a high calcium-binding capacity. Evidence has been gathered supporting the view that calsequestrin is not only a calcium buffer, but, more importantly it is a RyR2 modulator. CASQ2 controls RyR2 opening (directly or via protein-protein interactions possibly involving triadin and junctin) in a manner that depends on the amount of calcium within the SR lumen (the CASQ2-dependent luminal RyR2 calcium regulatory mechanism).[17] This mechanism is an important feedback mechanism that is activated whenever luminal calcium is low and therefore CASQ2 inhibits RyR2 channel opening by reducing its cytosolic calcium sensitivity, thus terminating the SR calcium release process. Whenever luminal calcium increases, this inhibition is removed and the cytosolic calcium sensitivity of the channel returns to its resting condition.

In 2001, Lahat and coworkers identified the first mis-sense mutation (D307H) in a highly conserved region of the *CASQ2* gene in a family affected by an autosomal-recessive form of CPVT in whom they had previously shown linkage to chromosome 1p13-21.[4] As expected for a recessive disease, *CASQ2*-related CPVT is an uncommon variant of CPVT, and in our experience it represents only 7% (4 out of 60) of all the probands in our CPVT registry.[9] To date, five homozygous *CASQ2* mutations have been reported in the literature: a one-base-pair deletion, a 16-base-pair deletion, one splicing junction mutation, and two mis-sense mutations. We have reported the first CPVT patient carrier of two distinct *CASQ2* mutations, thus demonstrating that the compound heterozygous mutations can also lead to the CPVT phenotype.[18] Postma and colleagues[19] reported the identification of one heterozygous nonsense mutation (R33X) in one symptomatic CPVT patient, but they could not conclusively demonstrate that haploinsufficiency of CASQ2 protein is sufficient to produce the phenotype.

The issue of whether a single loss of function mutation in *CASQ2* can predispose to arrhythmias remains open. Analysis of the clinical literature suggests that in most instances heterozygous carriers do not have the disease phenotype. In the family harbouring the heterozygous $CASQ2^{R33X}$ mutation, only the proband presented typical CPVT during adrenergic stimulation, two of five heterozygous carriers displayed a milder CPVT phenotype detectable during exercise tests, and the remaining three heterozygous carriers did not manifest any symptoms of CPVT.[19] In a recessive CPVT family that we identified as carriers of the G112+5X *CASQ2* deletion, none of 11 carriers of the heterozygous truncation presented an arrhythmogenic phenotype either at rest or during exercise.

Chopra and colleagues[20] reported increased susceptibility to ventricular tachycardia in heterozygous $CASQ2^{+/-}$ transgenic mice, in which 25% reduction of CASQ2 protein was observed. These authors claimed that even modest reductions in CASQ2 can increase SR calcium leak, and persons with only one functional *CASQ2* allele may be at increased risk for ventricular arrhythmias and sudden death. At present, the issue remains open, and more data are required to fully characterize the arrhythmic risk of carriers of heterozygous truncations of the CASQ2 protein.

New Loci for Catecholaminergic Polymorphic Ventricular Tachycardia

Because not all persons with CPVT phenotype carry either *RyR2* or *CASQ2* mutations, it is likely that new genes for CPVT are still to be identified. Recently, Bhuiyan and colleagues[21] identified a novel highly malignant autosomal-recessive form of CPVT in a consanguineous family in which no mutations in *RYR2* or *CASQ2* gene could be identified. The authors mapped this disorder to a 25-megabase interval on chromosome 7p14-22. The screening of several candidate genes in that region (*SP4*, *NPY*, *FKBP9*, *FKBP14*, *PDE1C*, and *TBX20*) failed to reveal a disease-causing mutation, and thus the proof that this family is affected by a novel genetic form of CPVT remains to be conclusively demonstrated.

Pathophysiology

After the identification of mutations in *RYR2* and *CASQ2* in CPVT patients, many investigations were initiated aiming at their functional characterization. Several approaches have been undertaken to link DNA abnormalities to functional derangement of calcium-controlling proteins spanning from in vitro heterogeneous expression of mutant proteins (Table 52-1) to the engineering of knockin animals (Table 52-2). Overall, these studies have advanced the understanding of intracellular calcium handling and have provided new information on structure and function relationships in RyR2 and in CASQ2.

Table 52-1 In Vitro Characterization of Catecholaminergic Polymorphic Ventricular Tachycardia–Related *RyR2* and *CASQ2* Mutations

Amino Acid Change	Mutation Type	Phenotype	Protein Domain	Experiment Types	In Vitro Characterizations	Reference
RyR2						
R176Q	Mis-sense	CPVT and ARVD	Cytoplasmatic loop	HEK cell	Increased calcium release upon caffeine activation	Thomas[51]
R176Q/T2504M	Mis-sense	CPVT and ARVD	Cytoplasmatic loop	HEK and HL-1 cell, planar lipid bilayer	Increased luminal calcium sensitivity (enhanced SOICR) and increased calcium leak	Jiang[27]
R176Q/T2504M	Mis-sense	CPVT and ARVD	Cytoplasmatic loop	HEK cell	Increased cytosolic calcium sensitivity and increased calcium release upon caffeine activation	Thomas[51]
L433P	Mis-sense	ARVD	Cytoplasmatic loop	HEK and HL-1 cell, planar lipid bilayer	Increased luminal calcium sensitivity (enhanced SOICR) and increased calcium leak	Jiang[27]
L433P	Mis-sense	ARVD	Cytoplasmatic loop	HEK cell	Decreased calcium release upon caffeine activation	Thomas[51]
S2246L	Mis-sense	CPVT	Cytoplasmatic loop	HL-1 cell	Increased calcium leak upon adrenergic stimulation	George[29]
S2246L	Mis-sense	CPVT	Cytoplasmatic loop	HEK and HL-1 cell, planar lipid bilayer	Increased luminal calcium sensitivity (enhanced SOICR) and increased calcium leak	Jiang[27]
S2246L	Mis-sense	CPVT	Cytoplasmatic loop	Planar lipid bilayer, biochemical assays	Decreased FKBP12.6 binding affinity; PKA phosphorylation aggravates this defect; increased channel activity	Wehrens[23]
R2267H	Mis-sense	SIDS	Cytoplasmatic loop	Planar lipid bilayer	Increased channel activity upon PKA activation	Tester[52]
P2328S	Mis-sense	CPVT	FKBP binding domain	HEK cell	Increased calcium release upon adrenergic activation	Paavola[43]
P2328S	Mis-sense	CPVT	FKBP binding domain	HEK and HL-1 cell, planar lipid bilayer	Decreased FKBP12.6 binding affinity; PKA phosphorylation aggravates this defect; increased calcium leak	Lehnart[22]
N2386I	Mis-sense	ARVD	FKBP binding domain	HEK cell	Increased cytosolic calcium sensitivity Increased calcium release upon caffeine activation	Thomas[31]
R2474S	Mis-sense	CPVT	FKBP binding domain	Planar lipid bilayer, biochemical assays	Decreased FKBP12.6 binding affinity; PKA phosphorylation aggravates this defect; increased channel activity	Wehrens[23]
R2474S	Mis-sense	CPVT	FKBP binding domain	HEK and HL-1 cell, planar lipid bilayer	Increased luminal calcium sensitivity (enhanced SOICR) and increased calcium leak	Jiang[27]
T2504M	Mis-sense	CPVT/ARVD	FKBP binding domain	HEK cell	Increased calcium release upon caffeine activation	Thomas[51]
N4104K	Mis-sense	CPVT	Transmembrane domain	HEK cell, planar lipid bilayer	Increased luminal calcium sensitivity (enhanced SOICR) and increased calcium leak	Jiang[30]
N4104K	Mis-sense	CPVT	Transmembrane domain	HL-1 cell	Increased calcium leak upon adrenergic stimulation	George[29]

Continued

Table 52-1 In Vitro Characterization of Catecholaminergic Polymorphic Ventricular Tachycardia–Related *RyR2* and *CASQ2* Mutations—cont'd

Amino Acid Change	Mutation Type	Phenotype	Protein Domain	Experiment Types	In Vitro Characterizations	Reference
Q4201R	Mis-sense	CPVT	Transmembrane domain	Planar lipid bilayer, biochemical assays	Decreased FKBP12.6 binding affinity; PKA phosphorylation aggravates this defect; increased channel activity	Lehnart[22]
Q4201R	Mis-sense	CPVT	Transmembrane domain	HEK cell, planar lipid bilayer	Increased luminal calcium sensitivity (enhanced SOICR) and increased calcium leak	Jiang[27]
R4496C (mouse)	Mis-sense	CPVT	Transmembrane domain	HEK cell, lipid bilayer	Increased basal channel activity, increased channel sensitivity by calcium and caffeine, increased calcium leak	Jiang[42]
R4497C	Mis-sense	CPVT	Transmembrane domain	Planar lipid bilayer, biochemical assays	Decreased FKBP12.6 binding affinity; PKA phosphorylation aggravates this defect; increased channel activity	Wehrens[23]
R4497C	Mis-sense	CPVT	Transmembrane domain	HL-1 cell	Increased calcium leak upon adrenergic stimulation	George[29]
S4565R	Mis-sense	SIDS	Transmembrane domain	Planar lipid bilayer	Increased channel activity upon PKA activation	Tester[52]
V4653F	Mis-sense	CPVT	Transmembrane domain	Planar lipid bilayer, biochemical assays	Decreased FKBP12.6 binding affinity; PKA phosphorylation aggravates this defect; increased channel activity	Lehnart[22]
V4653F	Mis-sense	CPVT	Transmembrane domain	HEK cell	Increased calcium release upon adrenergic activation	Paavola[43]
I4867M	Mis-sense	CPVT	C-terminus	HEK and HL-1 cell, planar lipid bilayer	Increased luminal calcium sensitivity (enhanced SOICR) and increased calcium leak	Jiang[27]
N4895D	Mis-sense	CPVT	C-terminus	HEK cell, planar lipid bilayer	Increased luminal calcium sensitivity (enhanced SOICR) and increased calcium leak	Jiang[30]
CASQ2						
R33Q	Mis-sense	CPVT		Infected cardiac myocytes, planar lipid bilayer	Disrupted interactions with RyR2, increased spontaneous calcium release, and exhibited DAD	Terentyev[47]
G112+5X	Deletion/ frameshift	CPVT	Domain I	Infected cardiac myocytes	Loss of calcium binding capacity, increased spontaneous calcium release, and exhibited DAD	di Barletta[18]
L167H	Mis-sense	CPVT		Infected cardiac myocytes	Disrupted interactions with RyR2, increased spontaneous calcium release, and exhibited DAD	di Barletta[18]
D307H	Mis-sense	CPVT	Interdomain space	Infected cardiac myocytes	Decreased calcium buffering capacity, increased spontaneous calcium release and exhibited DAD.	Viatchenko and Karpinski[46]

ARVD, arrhythmogenic right ventricular cardiomyopathy; CPVT, catecholaminergic polymorphic ventricular tachycardia; DAD, delayed afterdepolarization; FKBP, FK506 binding protein; HEK, human embryonic kidney; PKA, protein kinase A; SIDS, sudden infant death syndrome; SOICR, store-overload-induced Ca2+ release.

Table 52-2 Transgenic Catecholaminergic Polymorphic Ventricular Tachycardia Mouse Models

Mutation	Clinical Phenotypes	Transgenic Methods	Phenotypes In Vivo	Phenotypes in Isolated Myocytes	Cardiac Structure	Reference
RyR2						
R4496C	CPVT	Knockin	No spontaneous arrhythmias, bidirectional and/or multiple VT induced by adrenergic and caffeine stimulation in heterozygous mice	DADs and TA developed in resting condition, increased TA upon adrenergic stimulation	Normal	Cerrone,[35] Liu[28]
R176Q	ARVD and CPVT	Knockin	No spontaneous arrhythmias, bidirectional and/or multiple VT induced by adrenergic and/or caffeine stimulation in heterozygous mice	Spontaneous calcium oscillations in resting condition and increased nonevoked calcium transients upon adrenergic stimulation	Normal	Kannankeril[40]
CASQ						
D307H	CPVT	Overexpression	No spontaneous arrhythmias, VT induced by adrenergic and caffeine stimulation, normal cardiac structure	Spontaneous calcium transient and TA upon adrenergic and caffeine stimulation	Normal	Dirksen[53]
		Knockout (homozygous)	No spontaneous arrhythmias, VT induced by adrenergic stimulation in homozygous mice	Decreased SR calcium contents, spontaneous calcium release and TA upon adrenergic stimulation	Cardiac hypertrophy	Knollmann[48]
		Knock-out (heterozygous)	No spontaneous arrhythmias, ventricular ectopy and VT induced by adrenergic stimulation and programmed stimulation respectively in heterozygous mice	Normal SR calcium contents in resting condition, increased calcium leak and triggered beats upon adrenergic stimulation	Normal	Chopra[20]
D307H	CPVT	Knockin	Spontaneous arrhythmias in unstressed homozygous mice; adrenergic stress aggravates arrhythmias further	Decreased SR calcium contents, spontaneous calcium release and TA upon adrenergic stimulation	Normal in young mice, cardiac hypertrophy in aged mice	Song[49]
ΔE9		Knockin	Spontaneous arrhythmias in unstressed homozygous mice; adrenergic stress aggravates arrhythmias further	Decreased SR calcium contents, spontaneous calcium release, and TA upon adrenergic stimulation	Normal in young mice, cardiac hypertrophy in aged mice	Song[49]
R33Q	CPVT	Knockin	Spontaneous arrhythmias in unstressed homozygous mice; adrenergic stress aggravates arrhythmias further	Decreased SR calcium contents, spontaneous calcium release, and TA upon adrenergic stimulation	Normal	Rizzi[50]

ARVD, arrhythmogenic right ventricular cardiomyopathy; CPVT, catecholaminergic polymorphic ventricular tachycardia; DAD, delayed afterdepolarization; SR, sarcoplasmic reticulum; TA, tachyarrhythmia; VT, ventricular tachycardia.

In Vitro Studies of *RYR2* Mutations

Because *RyR2* is one of the largest genes in the genome, it has been technically challenging to express mutant *RyR2* in native cardiac myocytes. As a consequence, in vitro characterizations of *RyR2* mutations have been performed in planar lipid bilayer and in transfected cell lines (see Table 52-1). Most *RyR2* mutations cause a gain of function and present an increased channel-open probability upon adrenergic stimulation or administration of caffeine; some of the mutants show abnormally enhanced channel activity even in unstimulated conditions. Despite intensive investigations, the mechanisms by which mutations induce

RyR2-mediated diastolic calcium leakage from the SR during adrenergic stimulation remain highly controversial.

Marks and coworkers first proposed a unifying hypothesis suggesting that all *RyR2* mutations are characterized by an impairment in the binding of the regulatory protein FKBP12.6.[22,23] FKBP12.6 is one of the several proteins of the *RyR2* macromolecular complex that acts as a stabilizer that preserves the RyR2 channel closed during diastole. According to Marks and coworkers, CPVT-related mutations in *RyR2* reduce the binding affinity of ryanodine receptor to FKBP12.6 under basal conditions, and such a reduced binding is further exaggerated after protein kkinase A (PKA) phosphorylation of RyR2, as happens during adrenergic activation. These authors supported their theory by showing that the benzothiazepine derivative compound K201 (formerly called JTV519), which enhances the binding of FKBP12.6 to mutant RyR2, can rescue the function of CPVT mutant RyR2 channels.[22] The same authors[24] engineered an FKBP12.6 knockout heterozygous mouse model that develops polymorphic VT upon adrenergic stimulation and showed that administration of the K201 drug prevents arrhythmias, thus supporting their view that by enhancing FKBP12.6 binding to RyR2 it is possible to reduce calcium leakage from the SR. Although we agree on the fact that lack of FKBP12.6 predisposes to adrenergically mediated arrhythmias, we disagree on the interpretation that the FKBP12.6 knockout mouse model is a model of CPVT, and we believe that more robust data are needed to prove that in humans, lack of FKBP12.6 causes CPVT. So far, despite intensive screening, none of the clinical groups has been able to find mutations in the *FKBP12.6* gene in CPVT patients.

It has also been suggested that FKBP12.6 dissociation from the RyR2 complex is a pivotal mechanism for arrhythmogenesis in acquired diseases such as heart failure[25] and in atrial fibrillation,[26] thus supporting the view that adrenergically mediated triggered arrhythmias in a variety of diseases are all caused by abnormal calcium leakage triggered by augmented unbinding of FKBP12.6 from PKA-phosphorylated RyR2. Although this unifying hypothesis is attractive, several groups performed biochemical studies from in vitro expression and from native protein from transgenic mice and showed that the interaction between mutant RyR2 and FKBP12.6 is normal not only in the resting condition but also under adrenergic stimulation.[27,28,29]

A pathogenetic hypothesis for *RyR2*-related CPVT, independent from FKBP12.6, has been put forward by Wayne Chen's group. These authors suggest that mutations in *RyR2* reduce the threshold for the occurrence of spontaneous calcium release from SR, and they call this the store overload–induced calcium release (SOICR) model that accounts for abnormal RyR2 and CASQ2 regulation in CPVT. These authors demonstrated that most RyR2 mutations increase the channel sensitivity to luminal calcium but not its sensitivity to cytosolic calcium.[27,30] Given that most CPVT mutations are located in the cytoplasmic domain of RyR2, the mechanism by which these mutations confer hypersensitivity to calcium within the SR remains unclear. At variance with Chen and coworkers, Thomas and colleagues[31] reported that *RyR2* mutations increase RyR2 activation by cytosolic (rather than luminal) calcium. The reasons for the discrepant results of the two groups on whether *RyR2* mutations modify the control of RyR2 mediated by luminal or cytosolic calcium remain unclear.

The third hypothesis advanced to explain the pathophysiology of *RyR2*-mediated CPVT comes from George and colleagues,[32] who provided evidence that RyR2 mutations impair the interdomain interactions. It is known that intramolecular interaction between discrete RyR2 domains is necessary for the proper folding of the channel, and it is an important mode of channel self-regulation. The role of defective interdomain interactions in determining RyR dysfunction has also been advocated by Yamamoto and colleagues[33] who proposed that N-terminal and central domains interact with each other and work as the regulatory element that controls channel gating. They also suggested that a tight zipping of the two domains is associated with channel stability and an unzipping of the two domains leads to calcium leakage. The same authors also suggested that mutations in the central or in the N-terminal domain might cause unzipping of domains and facilitate abnormal calcium release (Fig. 52-2).[34]

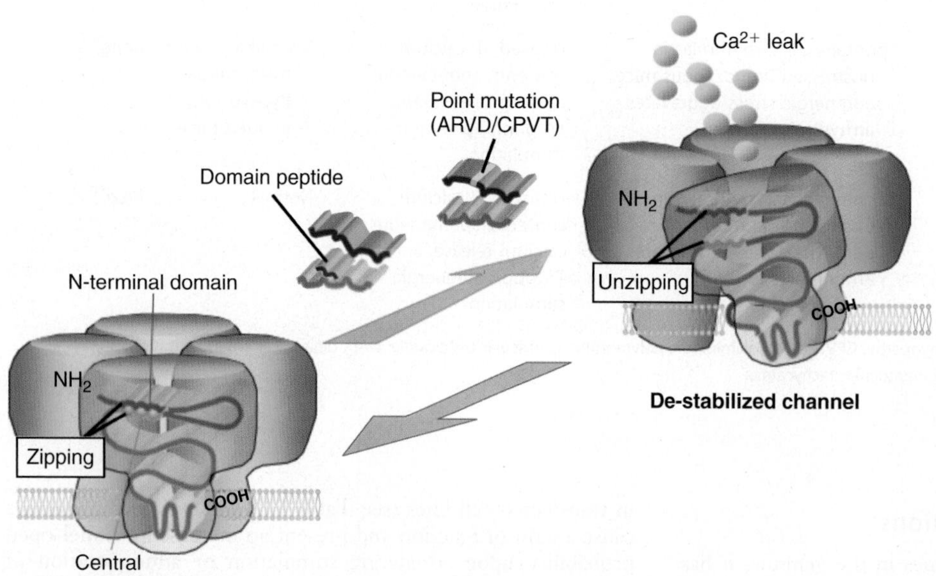

Figure 52-2 Schematic diagram of domain-domain interaction within the ryanodine receptor RyR2, a new therapeutic target. The N-terminal and central domain interact with each other to function as a regulatory switch for channel gating, with a tight zipping of the interacting domains serving to stabilize the channel. A mutation in either domain weakens the interdomain interaction (unzipping), which causes activation and leakiness of the calcium ion channel. Synthetic domain peptides corresponding to key subdomains of the RyR2 are capable of mimicking diseased conditions of the RyR2 channel by interfering with the interactions between domains. ARVD, arrhythmogenic right ventricular cardiomyopathy; CPVT, catecholaminergic polymorphic ventricular tachycardia. (Adapted from Yano M, Yamamoto T, Ikeda Y, et al: Mechanisms of disease: Ryanodine receptor defects in heart failure and fatal arrhythmia. Nat Clin Pract Cardiovasc Med 3:43-52, 2006, by permission from Macmillan Publishers Ltd.)

RyR2 Knockin Mouse Models

The development of knockin animal models is an important tool in the understanding of pathophysiology of genetic diseases. The use of mice to replicate cardiac channelopathies, however, presents a special challenge given the differences existing in the electrophysiologic properties of the heart between humans and mice. The likelihood to observe in a murine model a phenotype similar to that observed in patients is therefore unpredictable.

In 2005, we developed the first conditional knockin mouse model carrier of the *RyR2* R4496C mutation,[35] the mouse equivalent to the R4497C mutations identified in one of our CPVT families.[5] The in vivo characterization of this model showed that in resting condition, no RyR2$^{R4496C+/-}$ mice exhibit spontaneous arrhythmia but upon epinephrine and caffeine administration, at variance with wild-type mice and in striking analogy with patients, 50% of RyR2$^{R4496C+/-}$ mice develop bidirectional VT or polymorphic VT, or both. Histologic examination of the heart of RyR2$^{R4496C+/-}$ mice did not show any cardiac structural abnormality. In this CPVT model we tested whether K201 can prevent polymorphic VT induced in the setting of sympathetic stimulation and caffeine administration and, in contrast with the expectations raised by the results reported by Wherens and colleagues,[24] we failed to document an antiarrhythmic activity of this drug both in vivo and in vitro.[28] The fact that in our RyR2$^{R4496C+/-}$ knockin mouse model K201 fails to prevent the arrhythmias provides an even more compelling evidence that FKBP12.6 dissociation is not the unique arrhythmogenic mechanism[28] and that, as suggested by some authors,[36,37] the ability of K201 of suppressing diastolic calcium release may be independent from FKBP12.6.

More recently Yano and coworkers found that K201 can correct the defective function of *RyR2* mutations positioned in the central domain but not of those located in the C-terminal (cytoplasmic) region.[38] This observation raises the interesting possibility that, analogous to SCN5A mutations that present variable response to mexiletine treatment,[39] based on their localization, *RyR2* mutations might have differential response to therapeutic agents. It will be interesting to see if knockin mice carriers of mutations in the central domain show suppression of polymorphic VT with K201.

So far, the only other mouse model with *RyR2* mutations has been reported by Kannankeril and colleagues. These authors developed a knockin carrier of the *RyR2* R176Q mutation,[40] which had been associated with the phenotype of ARVC2. Interestingly, the family with the *RyR2* R176Q mutation also harbors a second *RyR2* mutation that is not present in the murine model.[13]

In RyR2$^{R176Q+/-}$ mice, polymorphic VT can be observed after caffeine and epinephrine administration, but histologic analysis of hearts reveals no evidence of fibrofatty infiltration or structural abnormalities characteristic of ARVC, thus concurring with the questioning of the link between *RyR2* mutations and right ventricular cardiomyopathy. Taken together, the data from the two *RyR2* knockin mouse models reinforce the concept that the presence of a heterozygous *RyR2* mis-sense mutation predisposes the murine heart to bidirectional and polymorphic VT in response to adrenergic stimulation and that it fails to induce structural abnormalities of the heart.

Electrophysiologic Mechanisms in Autosomal-Dominant Catecholaminergic Polymorphic Ventricular Tachycardia

Bidirectional VT is the trademark arrhythmia of CPVT. Because the electrocardiographic pattern of this form of ventricular tachycardia closely resembles the arrhythmias associated with digitalis toxicity, researchers have speculated that the two conditions might share the same electrophysiologic mechanism. Digitalis is known to induce intracellular calcium overload, leading to delayed afterdepolarizations (DADs),[41] thus suggesting that bidirectional VT in CPVT might also be initiated and possibly sustained by triggered activity. In vitro characterization of *RyR2* mutations identified in CPVT patients further supports this view, showing that the gain of function of *RyR2* mutations upon catecholamine administration causes calcium leak from the SR, which in turn leads to intracellular calcium overload, thus setting the stage for development of DADs and triggered activity.

Studying our *RyR2*^{R4496C} knockin mouse model,[35] we were able to provide more conclusive data on the role of triggered activity in CPVT. Upon recording of action potential in isolated RyR2$^{R4496C+/-}$ myocytes, our data showed that administration of isoproterenol fosters development of DADs and triggered activity (Fig. 52-3).[28] DADs were observed under resting conditions in 63%, and triggered activity was observed under resting conditions in 12% of RyR2$^{R4496C+/-}$ myocytes but not in wild-type myocytes (Fig. 52-4),[28] this observation is in agreement with the finding of Jiang and colleagues,[42] suggesting that RyR2 mutations enhance abnormal calcium release even in unstimulated subjects. These findings were subsequently confirmed in RyR2$^{R176Q+/-}$ myocytes.[40]

Paavola and colleagues,[43] using monophasic action potentials recoding, documented the presence of delayed afterdepolarizations in CPVT patients who were carriers of *RyR2* mutations, thus providing evidence that observations made in CPVT mice are relevant to the clinical setting.

One of the most intriguing aspect of CPVT is the typical electrocardiographic aspect of bidirectional VT manifesting with QRS axis rotation by 180 degrees on a beat-by-beat basis.

In a collaborative study with Jalife and coworkers, the mechanisms underlying this peculiar TV morphology were investigated. The study[44] was conducted in our RyR2$^{R4496C+/-}$ knockin mouse model, and optical mapping with voltage-sensitive dyes was used to locate the origin of ventricular tachycardia elicited by catecholamine administration. Data showed that the beats with the bidirectional morphology originated alternatively from the right and left apical portion of the heart, a pattern compatible with the hypothesis of alternating firing from the right and left branches of the Purkinje fibers (Fig. 52-5). The observation that arrhythmias might originate from Purkinje fibers is consistent with data showing that fibers are more susceptible than ventricular myocytes to calcium overload,[45] possibly because of their greater sodium load and longer action potential duration. It is known that Purkinje fibers become intoxicated by digitalis at a time when ventricular myocardial fibers still show normal action potentials. Additional data from our knockin mouse model demonstrated that isolated Purkinje fibers$^{R4496C+/-}$ develop DAD-induced triggered activity at lower pacing frequency and at lower concentrations of adrenergic agonists than wild-type fibers and that selective chemical ablation of the right ventricular Purkinje network changed the bidirectional VT into monophasic VT with wide QRS. Overall it is proposed that bidirectional VT is generated by beat-to-beat alternating firing from Purkinje fibers in the right and left ventricle.

In Vitro Studies of *CASQ2* Mutations

CASQ2 is a relatively small gene, and therefore it has been possible to express *CASQ2* mutations in infected cardiac myocytes (see Table 52-1). Viatchenko-Karpinski and colleagues[46] were the first to investigate the *CASQ2* D397H mutation in vitro, and they demonstrated that overexpression of *CASQ2* D397H in cardiac myocytes reduces the SR calcium contents, supporting the view that the mutation might reduce the calcium-binding properties of calsequestrin. *CASQ2* D397H myocytes exposed

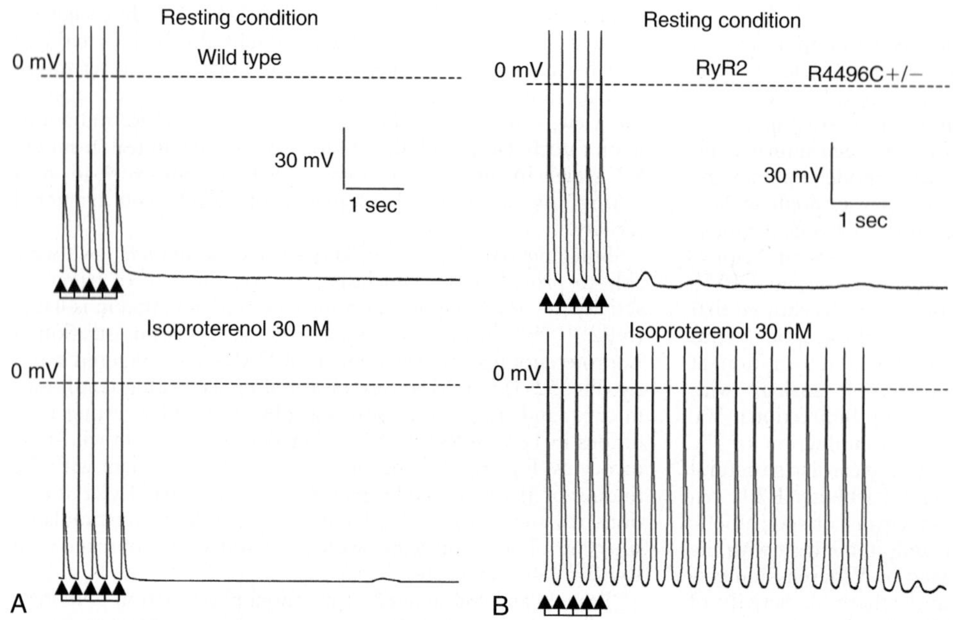

Figure 52-3 Action potential recording from a wild-type myocyte **(A)** and a *RyR2* R4496C$^{+/-}$ myocyte **(B)** in the absence *(top)* and in the presence *(bottom)* of isoproterenol (30 nM). *Arrows* indicate the last five paced action potentials.

to adrenergic stimulation were more prone to manifest spontaneous calcium release and to develop DADs. Normal rhythmic activity was restored in *CASQ2* D397H myocytes by loading the SR with the low-affinity calcium buffer, citrate, thus highlighting the importance of the calcium-buffering properties of *CASQ2* in maintaining normal excitability in cardiac myocytes.

Terentyev and coworkers investigated the properties of the *CASQ2* R33Q mutation[47] and demonstrated that myocytes overexpressing the R33Q mutation exhibit spontaneous calcium release upon adrenergic stimulation but, at variance with the

1 Hz 2 Hz 3 Hz 4 Hz
5 Hz
0 mV
A
B 1 Hz
C 2 Hz
D 3 Hz
E 4 Hz
40 mV
F 5 Hz

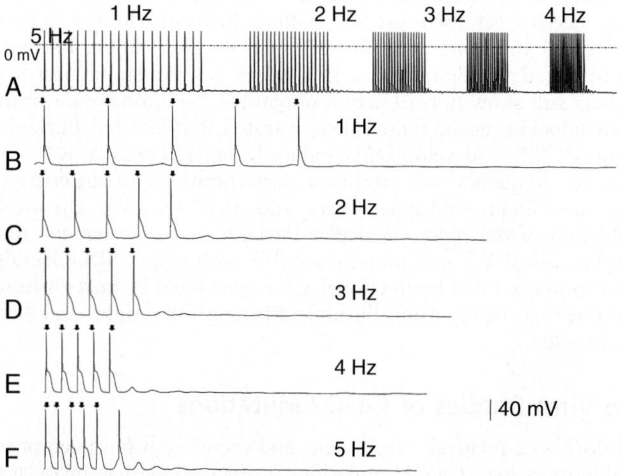

Figure 52-4 **A,** Action potentials recorded from *RyR2* R4496C$^{+/-}$ myocytes stimulated at 1 to 5 Hz are shown. Delayed afterdepolarizations (DADs) develop when pacing is interrupted. **B** to **F,** The last five driven action potentials at each pacing frequency and DADs and triggered activity developing when pacing is discontinued. DAD amplitude increases and DAD coupling interval decreases at faster pacing frequencies. At 5 Hz **(F)**, one triggered beat develops. Arrows indicate stimulated beats.

D397H mutation, no change in the SR calcium content was observed, suggesting that the calcium-binding capacity of R33Q was not different from that of wild-type *CASQ2*. The authors demonstrated that R33Q lacks the ability to inhibit RyR2 activity at low luminal calcium levels, leading to the speculation that this mutation causes CPVT mainly by disrupting the interaction between *CASQ2* and RyR2.

In collaboration with Gyorke's group, we investigated the two *CASQ2* mutations identified in the first CPVT patient with compound heterozygous *CASQ2* mutations. The two mutations were a deletion (G112-5X) and a point mutation (L167H).[18] In vitro, both mutants decreased the SR calcium-storing capacity, reduced the amplitude of I_{Ca}-induced calcium transients, and increased spontaneous calcium sparks in permeabilized myocytes.

Overall, it is possible to conclude that *CASQ2* mutations cause CPVT through two molecular mechanisms: The first is the impairment of calcium-binding properties and the second is the abnormal interaction with the RyR2 complex.

CASQ2 Knockout and Knockin Mouse Models

The identification of patients carriers of homozygous truncation of the *CASQ2* (like our patient homozygous carrier of the G112-5X *CASQ2* mutation) is the proof of the concept that the lack of *CASQ2* is compatible with life and that the phenotypical manifestation of the absence of cardiac calsequestrin is CPVT. The latter observation led Knollmann and colleagues to engineer a *CASQ2* knockout mouse model[48] and to demonstrate that *CASQ2*$^{-/-}$ mice develop polymorphic VT in response to catecholamines, thus mimicking a CVPT phenotype. Despite the complete loss of *CASQ2*, the myocytes isolated from the heart of knockout mice showed a modest (11%) decrease of SR calcium content. Interestingly, in parallel with lack of *CASQ2*, the authors reported that *CASQ2*$^{-/-}$ myocytes present an increase of the SR volume and a downregulation of triadin and junctin that might help maintain SR calcium storage. Surprisingly, *CASQ2*$^{-/-}$ mice also displayed a modest increase in ventricular wall thickness, although left ventricular contractility and cavity size were unchanged.

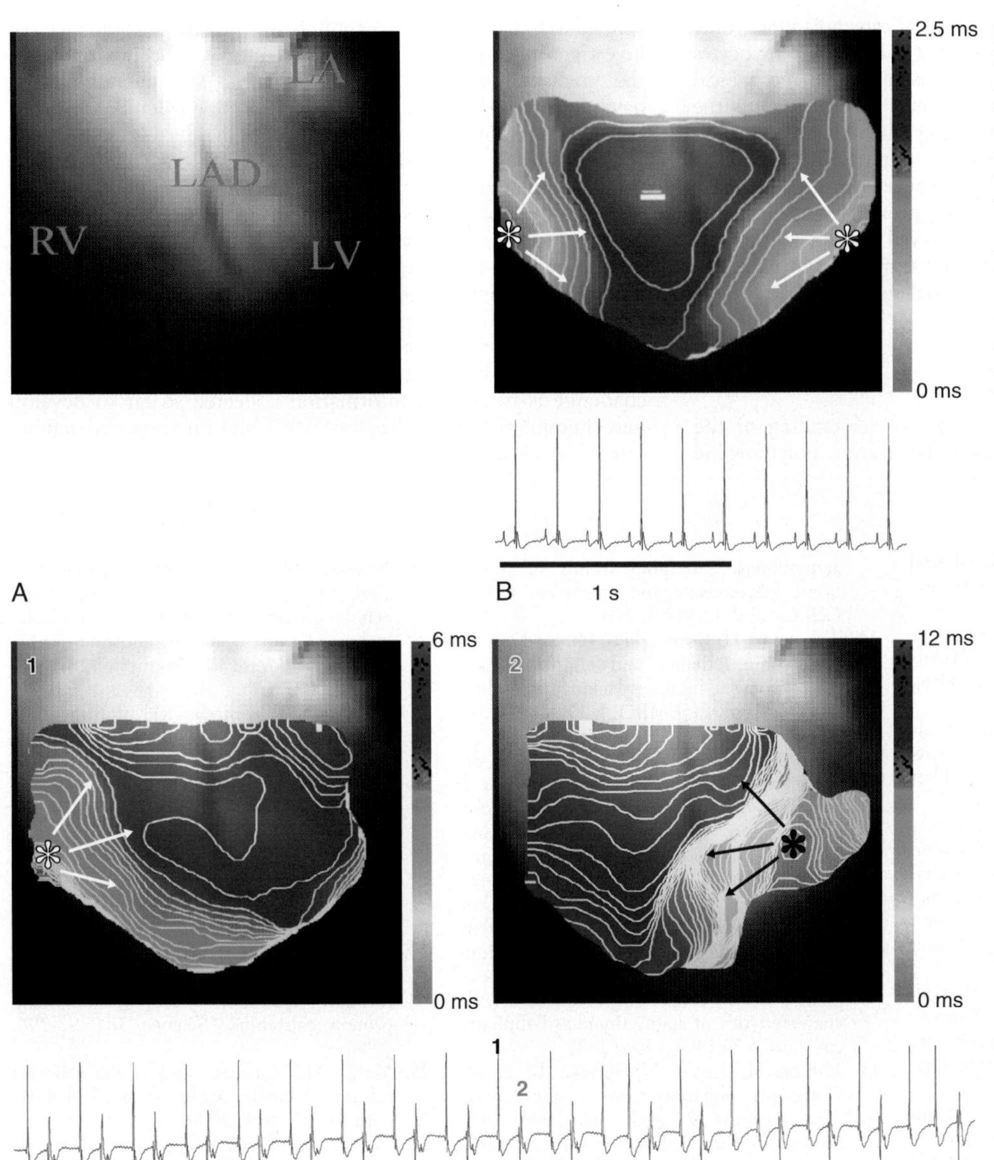

Figure 52-5 Bidirectional VT in *RyR2* R4496C$^{+/-}$ heart. **A,** Heart image. **B,** Epicardial activation map and electrocardiogram (ECG) in sinus rhythm. **C,** Epicardial activation maps of two consecutive ventricular beats with an origin that changed from right ventricle (beat1) to left ventricle (beat 2). *Bottom*, ECG in bidirectional ventricular tachycardia (2.7 mM Ca^{2+}; 100 nM isoproterenol). LA, left atrium; LAD, left anterior descending coronary artery; LV, left ventricle; RV, right ventricle. Asterisks indicate activation epicardial breakthroughs and arrows indicate the epicardial spreading of activation waves.

Song and coworkers[49] developed two knockin mouse models carriers of the *CASQ2* D307H and of the *CASQ2* ΔE9 mutations. Both strains of mice manifested CPVT and responded to adrenergic stimulation with the development of polymorphic and bidirectional VT. Both mutations also caused structural abnormalities, such as cardiac hypertrophy, mild left ventricular dysfunction, and atrial enlargement that became more pronounced in aging mice (35 weeks). The *CASQ2* D307H$^{+/+}$ knockin mice showed a 90% reduction of the levels of CASQ2 despite mRNA unmodified RNA levels. These data suggest that the D307H mutant, despite manifesting reduced calcium-binding properties as identified in the in vitro studies,[46] produces the clinical phenotype of CPVT by unknown post-transcriptional mechanisms that suppress CASQ2 levels. Interestingly, protein levels of calreticulin and RyR2 increased in *CASQ2* D307H$^{+/+}$ and *CASQ2* ΔE9$^{+/+}$ myocytes.

We developed a knockin mouse model carrier of the *CASQ2* R33Q mutation.[50] *CASQ2* R33Q$^{+/+}$ mice presented normal cardiac structure at 8 weeks, spontaneous ventricular arrhythmias in unstressed condition, and typical development of polymorphic VT and bidirectional VT in response to adrenergic stimulation. Biochemical studies from *CASQ2* R33Q$^{+/+}$ myocytes revealed that *CASQ2* mRNA level were normal even though CASQ2 protein decreased by 40%. Trypsin digestion showed that *CASQ2* R33Q protein was more susceptible to proteolysis than the wild-type protein, suggesting that this enhanced response to proteolysis may be the mechanism of decreased CASQ2 protein in *CASQ2* R33Q$^{+/+}$ myocytes.

Electrophysiologic Mechanisms in Autosomal Recessive Catecholaminergic Polymorphic Ventricular Tachycardia

Knollmann and colleagues[48] described enhanced spontaneous calcium release in CASQ2$^{-/-}$ myocytes in resting condition compared with wild-type myocytes. In the presence of catecholamines, only the *CASQ2*$^{-/-}$, *CASQ2* $\Delta E9^{+/+}$, and *CASQ2* D307H$^{+/+}$ myocytes developed aftercontractions that are considered the mechanical equivalent of DADs.[48,49] We have isolated myocytes from the heart of *CASQ2* R33Q$^{+/+}$ mice, and using patch clamp recording we demonstrated that 56% of cardiac myocytes R33Q$^{+/+}$ develop DADs. This response is substantially enhanced during adrenergic stimulation.[50] Overall, these observations provide compelling evidence that, analogous to what is observed in the autosomal-dominant form of CPVT, DAD-induced triggered activity is the electrophysiologic mechanism in autosomal-recessive CPVT.

Conclusions

Major advances have been made in the understanding of the clinical and genetic profile of catecholaminergic polymorphic ventricular tachycardia. Although the primary objective of investigators in gathering this information has been to improve the management of affected patients, the data collected have provided novel insights into calcium-mediated arrhythmogenesis.

The interest in expressing in vitro *RYR2* and *CASQ2* mutations, originated by the challenge of treating carriers of these molecular abnormalities, has also advanced the understanding of the function of the two proteins in the heart and highlighted novel structure-function relationships within the two proteins. The development of transgenic mouse models has allowed identification of novel factors that facilitate development of intracellular calcium abnormalities and has established new links between physiology of the SR and arrhythmogenesis. The next challenge is to use the information collected so far to develop new therapeutic approaches for CPVT and for triggered activity caused by abnormal calcium handling.

References

1. Yano M, Ikeda Y, Matsuzaki M: Altered intracellular Ca^{2+} handling in heart failure. J Clin Invest 115:556-564, 2005.
2. Wehrens XH, Marks AR: Novel therapeutic approaches for heart failure by normalizing calcium cycling. Nat Rev Drug Discov 3:565-573, 2004.
3. Hoshijima M: Gene therapy targeted at calcium handling as an approach to the treatment of heart failure. Pharmacol Ther 105:211-228, 2005.
4. Lahat H, Pras E, Olender T, et al: A missense mutation in a highly conserved region of CASQ2 is associated with autosomal recessive catecholamine-induced polymorphic ventricular tachycardia in Bedouin families from Israel. Am J Hum Genet 69:1378-1384, 2001.
5. Priori SG, Napolitano C, Tiso N, et al: Mutations in the cardiac ryanodine receptor gene (hRyR2) underlie catecholaminergic polymorphic ventricular tachycardia. Circulation 103:196-200, 2001.
6. Tiso N, Stephan DA, Nava A, et al: Identification of mutations in the cardiac ryanodine receptor gene in families affected with arrhythmogenic right ventricular cardiomyopathy type 2 (ARVD2). Hum Mol Genet 10:189-194, 2001.
7. Priori SG, Napolitano C: Cardiac and skeletal muscle disorders caused by mutations in the intracellular Ca^{2+} release channels. J Clin Invest 115:2033-2038, 2005.
8. Laitinen PJ, Brown KM, Piippo K, et al: Mutations of the cardiac ryanodine receptor (RyR2) gene in familial polymorphic ventricular tachycardia. Circulation 103:485-490, 2001.
9. Cerrone M, Colombi B, Bloise R, et al: Clinical and molecular characterization of a large cohort of patients affected with catecholaminergic polymorphic ventricular tachycardia. Circulation 110:II-552, 2004.
10. Tester DJ, Arya P, Will M, et al: Genotypic heterogeneity and phenotypic mimicry among unrelated patients referred for catecholaminergic polymorphic ventricular tachycardia genetic testing. Heart Rhythm 3:800-805, 2006.
11. George CH, Jundi H, Thomas NL, et al: Ryanodine receptors and ventricular arrhythmias: Emerging trends in mutations, mechanisms and therapies. J Mol Cell Cardiol 42:34-50, 2007.
12. Takeshima H, Komazaki S, Hirose K, et al: Embryonic lethality and abnormal cardiac myocytes in mice lacking ryanodine receptor type 2. EMBO J 17:3309-3316, 1998.
13. Bauce B, Rampazzo A, Basso C, et al: Screening for ryanodine receptor type 2 mutations in families with effort-induced polymorphic ventricular arrhythmias and sudden death: Early diagnosis of asymptomatic carriers. J Am Coll Cardiol 40:341-349, 2002.
14. Nishio H, Iwata M, Suzuki K: Postmortem molecular screening for cardiac ryanodine receptor type 2 mutations in sudden unexplained death: R420W mutated case with characteristics of status thymico-lymphaticus. Circ J 70:1402-1406, 2006.
15. Milting H, Lukas N, Klauke B, et al: Composite polymorphisms in the ryanodine receptor 2 gene associated with arrhythmogenic right ventricular cardiomyopathy. Cardiovasc Res 71:496-505, 2006.
16. Corrado D, Thiene G: Arrhythmogenic right ventricular cardiomyopathy/dysplasia: Clinical impact of molecular genetic studies. Circulation 113:1634-1637, 2007.
17. Gyorke S, Hagen BM, Terentyev D, et al: Chain-reaction Ca^{2+} signaling in the heart. J Clin Invest 117:1758-1762, 2007.
18. di Barletta MR, Viatchenko-Karpinski S, Nori A, et al: Clinical phenotype and functional characterization of CASQ2 mutations associated with catecholaminergic polymorphic ventricular tachycardia. Circulation 114:1012-1019, 2006.
19. Postma AV, Denjoy I, Hoorntje TM, et al: Absence of calsequestrin 2 causes severe forms of catecholaminergic polymorphic ventricular tachycardia. Circ Res 91:e21-e26, 2002.
20. Chopra N, Kannankeril PJ, Yang T, et al: Modest reductions of cardiac calsequestrin increase sarcoplasmic reticulum Ca^{2+} leak independent of luminal Ca^{2+} and trigger ventricular arrhythmias in mice. Circ Res 101:617-626, 2007.
21. Bhuiyan ZA, Hamdan MA, Shamsi ET, et al: A novel early onset lethal form of catecholaminergic polymorphic ventricular tachycardia maps to chromosome 7p14-p22. J Cardiovasc Electrophysiol 18:1060-1066, 2007.
22. Lehnart SE, Wehrens XH, Laitinen PJ, et al: Sudden death in familial polymorphic ventricular tachycardia associated with calcium release channel (ryanodine receptor) leak. Circulation 109:3208-3214, 2004.
23. Wehrens XH, Lehnart SE, Huang F, et al: FKBP12.6 deficiency and defective calcium release channel (ryanodine receptor) function linked to exercise-induced sudden cardiac death. Cell 113:829-840, 2003.
24. Wehrens XH, Lehnart SE, Reiken SR, et al: Protection from cardiac arrhythmia through ryanodine receptor–stabilizing protein calstabin2. Science 304:292-296, 2004.
25. Marks AR: Cardiac intracellular calcium release channels: Role in heart failure. Circ Res 87:8-11, 2000.
26. Vest JA, Wehrens XH, Reiken SR, et al: Defective cardiac ryanodine receptor regulation during atrial fibrillation. Circulation 111:2025-2032, 2005.
27. Jiang D, Wang R, Xiao B, et al: Enhanced store overload-induced Ca^{2+} release and channel sensitivity to luminal Ca^{2+} activation are common defects of RyR2 mutations linked to ventricular tachycardia and sudden death. Circ Res 97:1173-1181, 2005.
28. Liu N, Colombi B, Memmi M, et al: Arrhythmogenesis in catecholaminergic polymorphic ventricular tachycardia: Insights from a RyR2 R4496C knock-in mouse model. Circ Res 99:292-298, 2006.
29. George CH, Higgs GV, Lai FA: Ryanodine receptor mutations associated with stress-induced ventricular tachycardia mediate increased calcium release in stimulated cardiomyocytes. Circ Res 93:531-540, 2003.
30. Jiang D, Xiao B, Yang D, et al: RyR2 mutations linked to ventricular tachycardia and sudden death reduce the threshold for store-overload-induced Ca^{2+} release (SOICR). Proc Natl Acad Sci U S A 101:13062-13067, 2004.

31. Thomas NL, Lai FA, George CH: Differential Ca^{2+} sensitivity of RyR2 mutations reveals distinct mechanisms of channel dysfunction in sudden cardiac death. Biochem Biophys Res Commun 331:231-238, 2005.
32. George CH, Jundi H, Walters N, et al: Arrhythmogenic mutation-linked defects in ryanodine receptor autoregulation reveal a novel mechanism of Ca^{2+} release channel dysfunction. Circ Res 98:88-97, 2006.
33. Yamamoto T, El-Hayek R, Ikemoto N: Postulated role of interdomain interaction within the ryanodine receptor in Ca^{2+} channel regulation. J Biol Chem 275:11618-11625, 2000.
34. Yano M, Yamamoto T, Ikeda Y, et al: Mechanisms of disease: Ryanodine receptor defects in heart failure and fatal arrhythmia. Nat Clin Pract Cardiovasc Med 3:43-52, 2006.
35. Cerrone M, Colombi B, Santoro M, et al: Bidirectional ventricular tachycardia and fibrillation elicited in a knock-in mouse model carrier of a mutation in the cardiac ryanodine receptor. Circ Res 96:e77-e82, 2005.
36. Hunt DJ, Jones PP, Wang R, et al: K201 (JTV519) suppresses spontaneous Ca^{2+} release and [^{3}H]ryanodine binding to RyR2 irrespective of FKBP12.6 association. Biochem J 404:431-438, 2007.
37. Loughrey CM, Otani N, Seidler T, et al: K201 modulates excitation-contraction coupling and spontaneous Ca^{2+} release in normal adult rabbit ventricular cardiomyocytes. Cardiovasc Res 76:236-246, 2007.
38. Tateishi H, Yano M, Ohno M, et al: Potential treatment of mutation-linked lethal arrhythmia by correcting defective inter-domain interaction within the cardiac ryanodine receptor. Circulation 116:II-478, 2007.
39. Ruan Y, Liu N, Bloise R, et al: Gating properties of SCN5A mutations and the response to mexiletine in long-QT syndrome type 3 patients. Circulation 116:1137-1144, 2007.
40. Kannankeril PJ, Mitchell BM, Goonasekera SA, et al: Mice with the R176Q cardiac ryanodine receptor mutation exhibit catecholamine-induced ventricular tachycardia and cardiomyopathy. Proc Natl Acad Sci U S A 103:12179-12184, 2006.
41. Binah H, Cohen I, Rosen M: The effects of adriamycin on normal and ouabain-toxic canine Purkinje and ventricular muscle fibers. Circ Res 53:655-662, 1983.
42. Jiang D, Xiao B, Zhang L, et al: Enhanced basal activity of a cardiac Ca^{2+} release channel (ryanodine receptor) mutant associated with ventricular tachycardia and sudden death. Circ Res 91:218-225, 2002.
43. Paavola J, Viitasalo M, Laitinen-Forsblom PJ, et al: Mutant ryanodine receptors in catecholaminergic polymorphic ventricular tachycardia generate delayed afterdepolarizations due to increased propensity to Ca^{2+} waves. Eur Heart J 28:1135-1142, 2007.
44. Cerrone M, Noujaim SF, Tolkacheva EG, et al: Arrhythmogenic mechanisms in a mouse model of catecholaminergic polymorphic ventricular tachycardia. Circ Res 101:1039-1048, 2007.
45. Vassalle M, Lin CI: Calcium overload and cardiac function. J Biomed Sci 11:542-565, 2004.
46. Viatchenko-Karpinski S, Terentyev D, Gyorke I, et al: Abnormal calcium signaling and sudden cardiac death associated with mutation of calsequestrin. Circ Res 94:471-477, 2004.
47. Terentyev D, Nori A, Santoro M, et al: Abnormal interactions of calsequestrin with the ryanodine receptor calcium release channel complex linked to exercise-induced sudden cardiac death. Circ Res 98:1151-1158, 2006.
48. Knollmann BC, Chopra N, Hlaing T, et al: CASQ2 deletion causes sarcoplasmic reticulum volume increase, premature Ca^{2+} release, and catecholaminergic polymorphic ventricular tachycardia. J Clin Invest 116:2510-2520, 2006.
49. Song L, Alcalai R, Arad M, et al: Calsequestrin 2 (CASQ2) mutations increase expression of calreticulin and ryanodine receptors, causing catecholaminergic polymorphic ventricular tachycardia. J Clin Invest 117:1814-1823, 2007.
50. Rizzi N, Liu N, Arcelli D, et al: Novel insights in arrhythmogenesis of catecholaminergic ventricular tachycardia from the first knock in model of homozygous calsequestrin mutation. Circulation 116:II-255, 2007.
51. Thomas NL, George CH, Lai FA: Functional heterogeneity of ryanodine receptor mutations associated with sudden cardiac death. Cardiovasc Res 64:52-60, 2004.
52. Tester DJ, Dura M, Carturan E, et al: A mechanism for sudden infant death syndrome (SIDS): Stress-induced leak via ryanodine receptors. Heart Rhythm 4:733-739, 2006.
53. Dirksen WP, Lacombe VA, Chi M, et al: A mutation in calsequestrin, CASQ2D307H, impairs Sarcoplasmic Reticulum Ca^{2+} handling and causes complex ventricular arrhythmias in mice. Cardiovasc Res 75:69-78, 2007.

52

Pharmacogenomics of Cardiac Arrhythmias and Effect on Drug Therapy 53

DAN M. RODEN

CHAPTER OUTLINE

Individuals vary widely in their responses to therapy with most drugs. Indeed, response to antiarrhythmic drug therapy is so highly variable that study of the underlying mechanisms has elucidated important lessons for understanding variable responses to drug therapy in general.

There are two key steps in the long series of events that take place between administration of a drug and manifestation of its effects. First, drug must be delivered to its molecular site of action (e.g., receptor, ion channel). The magnitude of the effect at the target is determined by drug concentration, and the study of the relationship of drug dose and concentration of drug (and metabolites) achieved in plasma, tissue, or other sites such as urine or bile is termed *pharmacokinetics*. The second major process that determines drug action has been termed *pharmacodynamics* and broadly includes the processes that must occur between a drug interacting with a specific molecular target and manifestation of drug action at the molecular, cellular, whole organ, and whole patient levels. Because drugs act in a complex (and often abnormal) biologic milieu, considerable intersubject variability in drug effects can arise from pharmacodynamic mechanisms.

Although these principles of pharmacokinetics and pharmacodynamics have been recognized for decades, it is now apparent that they are manifestations of the highly regulated function of individual molecules. Thus metabolism of a drug in the liver can be conceptualized as an interaction of the drug with specific hepatic enzymes whose function and expression is regulated by a host of genetic and environmental factors. Similarly, variability in the biologic milieu in which drugs act can be conceptualized as variability in the function of multiple molecules whose integrated behavior determines normal and abnormal cellular and whole-organ function.

Genes whose expression underlies these variable drug effects have been identified and characterized, opening the way to studies of the way variants in these genes affect pharmacokinetics and pharmacodynamics. Some variants are rare, cause specific diseases like the long QT syndrome, and are termed *mutations*. More common variants are termed *polymorphisms*, and might or might not alter function or expression of the encoded protein. Protein function can be altered if a polymorphism results in a change in primary amino acid sequence (a *nonsynonymous polymorphism*) or if it changes the rate of mRNA transcription from the gene, and thus the amount of protein generated. A change in a single nucleotide, a *single nucleotide polymorphism* (SNP), is the most common type. One emerging view is that polymorphisms may be physiologically silent until an environmental stressor, such as adrenergic stress, acute myocardial ischemia, or administration of a drug, is superimposed; it is under these conditions that DNA polymorphisms determine highly individual responses to such pathophysiologic conditions.

The idea that some variability in response to drug therapy is determined by genetic factors is actually more than a century old. Isolated examples of unusual drug responses, segregating in families and usually resulting from specific mutations, have been recognized for several decades and initiated the field of *pharmacogenetics*. The newer term *pharmacogenomics* is often used to describe the way multiple common DNA variants across the genome modulate drug responses.[1-3]

This research is supported in part by grants from the United States Public Health Service (HL65962, GM54724).

Pharmacokinetics

Presystemic Clearance

Consideration of the relationship between drug dose and concentration achieved is traditionally broken down into four components: absorption, distribution, metabolism, and elimination, whose collective effect is termed *drug disposition*. When a drug is not administered intravenously, the amount entering the systemic circulation may be less than 100%. *Bioavailability* is the amount of drug entering the systemic circulation, compared to that with the same dose administered intravenously. For orally administered drugs, reduced bioavailability can have two major mechanisms: a drug may be incompletely soluble and thus not cross the intestinal mucosa; or a drug can undergo presystemic clearance, as illustrated in Figure 53-1. Both enterocytes and hepatocytes (to which drug is exposed before entering the systemic circulation) express drug-uptake molecules, drug-metabolizing enzymes, and drug-efflux molecules. Thus, the amount of a drug entering the systemic circulation may be limited by drug metabolism at either site or by drug excretion into the intestinal lumen or into the bile before entering the systemic circulation.

Drug Transport Is an Active Process

Drug entry into and efflux from cellular sites can be either passive (diffusional) or regulated; that is, it can reflect normal function and expression of specific energy-dependent drug transport molecules.[4,5] In hepatocytes and enterocytes, drug-uptake and drug-efflux transporters are expressed in a domain-specific fashion, that is, concentrated on apical or basolateral cell surfaces.

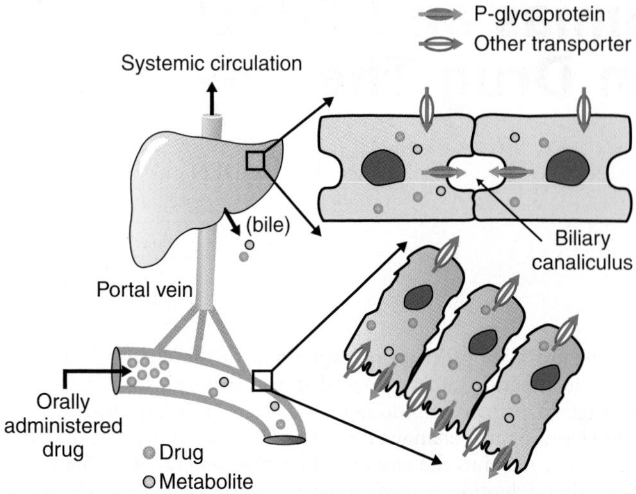

Figure 53-1 A contemporary view of presystemic clearance. An orally administered drug must first cross the intestinal epithelium. As shown in the *lower inset*, enterocytes express drug transporters on both apical and basal surfaces; these cells also express cytochrome P-450s (CYPs) responsible for drug metabolism. Efflux back into the intestine (accomplished by P-glycoprotein), limits systemic availability. Once a drug has traversed the intestinal barrier, it is exposed to the hepatocytes, where further drug metabolism and drug efflux into the bile occur.

As with drug metabolism, specific drugs are substrates for a limited number of transport molecules. The most studied drug transporter is P-glycoprotein, the product of the expression of the *ABCB1* (also termed *MDR1*) gene. P-glycoprotein is an efflux pump extensively expressed on the apical lumen of the enterocyte, the biliary aspect of the hepatocyte, and the capillary endothelium of the brain. At each of these sites, P-glycoprotein–mediated efflux reduces intracellular and thus tissue drug concentrations. In the enterocyte, P-glycoprotein re-excretes drug into the lumen, limiting bioavailability; in the hepatocyte, P-glycoprotein excretes drugs into the bile (see Fig. 53-1). In the brain capillary endothelium, P-glycoprotein serves to limit access of drug to the central nervous system, and thus forms an important component of the blood-brain barrier. Expression of drug uptake and efflux transporters has now been identified in heart, so it seems likely that drug access to the intramyocyte space (and this includes the site of action of virtually all antiarrhythmic drugs) can be regulated by transporter function or expression.[6,7]

Molecules Mediating Drug Metabolism

Most drug metabolism occurs in the hepatocyte, where drugs are biotransformed to one or more metabolites, usually by oxidation.[8,9] Drug metabolites are generally more polar than the parent drug and are themselves excreted or conjugated (most commonly as glucuronides) before renal or biliary excretion. As with drug transport, each drug is a substrate for one or more specific drug-metabolizing enzymes. Oxidation is usually accomplished by members of the cytochrome P-450 (CYP) superfamily, the most important members of which for drug metabolism are the CYP 3A family (CYP 3A4 and CYP 3A5), CYP 2D6, CYP 2C9, and CYP 2C19; the major drug-metabolizing enzyme in intestine is CYP 3A5. Conjugation is accomplished by uridine glucuronyl transferase,[10] *N*-acetyltransferase, or a group of methyltransferases.[11]

Modeling Drug Disposition

The processes of drug absorption, distribution, metabolism, and elimination can be studied mathematically, using either compartmental or noncompartmental approaches. Compartmental approaches model the body as a series of compartments, with drug being transferred into and out of compartments via rate constants that almost always behave in a first-order fashion; that is, the rate of the process depends on the amount of substrate driving the process. By contrast, zero-order kinetics refers to a process whose rate is constant, regardless of the substrate. The metabolism of aspirin and of propafenone follow zero order, rather than first-order, elimination; as a result, small increases in dosage can lead to disproportionate increases in plasma concentrations and effects.

Using this approach, common parameters describing drug disposition can be derived; examples include various volumes of distribution (central volume, total volume, volume at steady state) and the first-order rate constants describing intercompartment drug transfer. Noncompartmental approaches use time-concentration data (without making any assumptions about compartments) to derive a series of different parameters, such as clearance and elimination half-life, to describe drug disposition.

Half-Lives

The most important measures used to describe drug disposition are bioavailability, distribution and elimination half-lives, clearance, and central volume of distribution. After a single drug dose, plasma concentration peaks and then declines (as drug is eliminated) by 50% after one elimination half-life, by 75% after two elimination half lives, by 87.5% after three, and by 93.75%, after four. For practical purposes, elimination is complete after four or five elimination half-lives. During chronic drug therapy, a steady state is achieved under which the amount of drug eliminated per unit time is equal to the amount drug administered per unit time. Whenever drug therapy is started, the drug dosage changed, or drug therapy stopped, the time required to achieve the new steady state plasma concentration is 4 or 5 elimination half-lives (Fig. 53-2).

Rapid intravenous administration of a drug may be followed by an initial precipitous decline in drug concentration followed by a slower decline, and disappearance from plasma can then be modeled as a biexponential function. The initial rapid phase generally reflects distribution out of plasma into tissues, and the slower phase reflects elimination. Thus, lidocaine disappears after an intravenous bolus with a distribution half-life of 8 minutes and an elimination half-life of 120 minutes; during an infusion, steady state concentrations are thus achieved in 8 to 10 hours (4 or 5 elimination half lives). When a drug is administered orally, concentrations rise as drug enters the systemic circulation, and a distinct drug distribution phase is not usually observed.

Loading Doses

Steady state is not synonymous with a stable plasma concentration. Under some conditions, a near–steady-state drug concentration can be achieved rapidly by using a loading dose (see Fig. 53-2). This has the disadvantage of potentially conferring drug-related side effects, especially if the selected loading dose is too great, and unless therapeutic plasma concentrations are required urgently (e.g., to suppress an arrhythmia), a loading regimen has only the risk of side-effects without any benefit of accelerating the time to true steady state.

Clearance refers to a volume (generally of plasma) cleared of a drug per unit time. In addition to total body clearance, organ-specific clearances (e.g., renal clearance, hepatic clearance) can be calculated to provide indices of organ-specific excretory function.

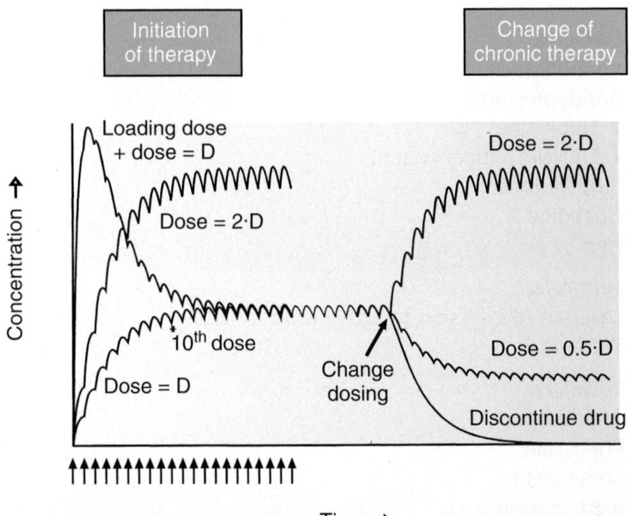

Figure 53-2 Simulated time-concentration plots during initiation of oral therapy *(left)* and during a change in a stable oral dosing regimen *(right)*. In this simulation, doses administered during the approach to steady state are depicted as *arrows* under the abscissa. The dosing interval in this simulation is 50% of the elimination half-life. Steady state is approximated after about five elimination half lives, or the 10th dose *(*)* in this case. If the dose were doubled, the concentration achieved would also be doubled, assuming the common case of first-order elimination. Administration of a loading dose results in higher initial concentrations but the same steady state. A change in the dosing regimen (increasing or decreasing the dose or stopping the drug altogether) results in a new steady state in about 5 elimination half lives.

Mechanisms of Drug Interactions

High-Risk Pharmacokinetics

Drug interactions due to interference with normal metabolism or excretory pathways assumes the greatest clinical importance with a drug that has a narrow margin between effective dose and toxic dose and that has a single predominant route of elimination. One spectacular example has been drug interactions involving substrates of CYP 3A4, notably the antihistamine terfenadine and the promotility agent cisapride. These compounds are high-potency I_{Kr} blockers that ordinarily undergo very extensive presystemic metabolism by CYP 3A (and no other major pathway) to non–I_{Kr}-blocking metabolites. When drugs that inhibit CYP 3A are coadministered, presystemic metabolism is inhibited, concentrations of terfenadine or cisapride entering the systemic circulation can rise several orders of magnitude, and torsades de pointes due to I_{Kr} block becomes a real risk. This risk led to withdrawal of these drugs from the market.[12]

Another widely used drug that is eliminated largely by a single molecular mechanism is digoxin, whose hepatic and renal excretion is mediated by P-glycoprotein.[13] The well-recognized effect of quinidine, amiodarone, verapamil, and numerous other drugs (erythromycin, itraconazole, cyclosporine) to elevate digoxin concentrations likely reflects interference with this P-glycoprotein elimination pathway. Similarly, sotalol and dofetilide are eliminated largely by renal excretion of unchanged drug, so marked QT prolongation is a real risk in patients with renal dysfunction given usual drug dosages. Flecainide is a CYP 2D6 substrate, but because it also undergoes renal excretion, loss of CYP 2D6 activity (on a genetic basis or through drug interactions) is not usually a problem. However, CYP 2D6 becomes the major determinant of flecainide elimination in patients with renal failure, and this is one setting in which flecainide toxicity can occur.[14]

Some drugs increase the rate of drug metabolism or transport molecules by inducing, or increasing transcription of, the responsible genes (Box 53-1). These interactions then result in decreased plasma concentrations of parent drug and generally reduced effect. Under some circumstances, drug metabolism results not in bioinactivation but in generation of more-active metabolites. Active metabolites can have elimination characteristics and pharmacologic properties that are similar to or different from those of the parent drug.

Pharmacodynamic Drug Interactions

Drug interactions can also occur through pharmacodynamic mechanisms. Drugs can interact at the same effector site; the marked increase in isoproterenol dosage required to increase heart rate in the presence of a β-blocker is a trivial example of both an agonist and an antagonist interacting with the same target molecule (the β_1-adrenergic receptor). Drugs can also interact at the same receptor to produce synergistic effects (e.g., two different sodium blockers with different dissociation characteristics) or to allow additive pharmacologic effects while minimizing the risk of non-cardiac adverse effects present with high doses of a single drug.

More commonly, drugs interact through pharmacodynamic mechanisms by acting at different molecular targets, both of which modulate the end-organ drug response. An I_{Kr} blocker and a sympathomimetic drug do not act at the same target site, yet both independently and synergistically increase the risk of long-QT–related arrhythmias because they both act on the action potential to promote arrhythmogenic behavior. Low extracellular potassium increases the potency of I_{Kr} blockers;[15] thus K^+-wasting diuretics act synergistically with I_{Kr} blockers to prolong QT interval (same site). In addition, some diuretics also block I_{Ks} to further prolong QT.[16]

Role of Genetics in Pharmacokinetics and Pharmacodynamics

Mutations

Single nucleotide changes can, by disrupting gene product function, produce dramatic changes in physiology: The long QT syndromes and the inherited errors of metabolism such as alkaptonuria are examples. Indeed, the recognition that inborn errors of metabolism arose from defective biotransformation of endogenous substrates led to the suggestion more than a century ago that exogenous substrates (drugs) might similarly be aberrantly metabolized and produce unusual actions in affected patients.[1] This paradigm been validated by the recognition of individual patients and families with defects in the genes encoding specific drug-metabolizing enzymes. As with drug interactions, these defects become most prominent when other pathways for drug elimination are absent and accumulation of parent drug leads to major adverse effects. Some of these are rare (e.g., prolonged paralysis after succinylcholine in pseudocholinesterase deficiency), and others are quite common and thus are best termed polymorphisms. Persons homozygous for loss-of-function alleles in CYP 2D6 (5%-10% of European and African populations) display markedly enhanced β-blocking action, including bronchospasm and bradyarrhythmias, during propafenone therapy because of accumulation of the parent drug.[9,17] Further examples are listed in Box 53-1.

Box 53-1 Interactions Based on Drug Metabolism

CYP 3A4

Substrates
Cyclosporine
Many Ca^{2+} channel blockers
Many HMG CoA reductase inhibitors (statins; exception: pravastatin)
Quinidine
Sildenafil

Inhibitors
Amiodarone
Diltiazem
Erythromycin, clarithromycin (not azithromycin)
Grapefruit juice (large quantities)
Itraconazole
Ketoconazole
Verapamil

Inducers
Phenobarbital
Phenytoin
Rifampin

CYP 2D6

Substrates
β-Blockers
- Carvedilol
- Metoprolol
- Propranolol
- Timolol

Codeine (conversion to active metabolite by 2D6)
Propafenone
Flecainide

Inhibitors
Amiodarone
Antidepressants
- Fluoxetine
- Tricyclic antidepressants

Propafenone
Quinidine

CYP 2C9

Substrates
Losartan (conversion to active drug by 2C9)
Warfarin

Inhibitors
Amiodarone
Phenytoin
Some statins

P-GLYCOPROTEIN

Substrates
Digoxin
Many antineoplastic agents

Inhibitors
Amiodarone
Cyclosporine
Erythromycin
Itraconazole
Ketoconazole
Quinidine
Verapamil

Inducers
Rifampin

Major cardiovascular drugs are presented here. For a more complete listing, see http://medicine.iupui.edu/flockhart/

Polymorphisms

A polymorphism, according to one definition, is a variant that occurs in more than 1% of a given study population. The distinction between polymorphism and mutation is blurred, because common polymorphisms can modulate variable human phenotypes, polymorphisms may be common in one ethnic group but absent in others, and rare DNA variants that apparently have no functional significance are increasingly recognized. The vast majority of polymorphisms across human genomes are in noncoding regions and so have no function or modulate gene transcription. Such regulation can arise because of polymorphisms in the promoter (the region that directly controls gene transcription, usually directly upstream of exon 1) or in more distant genomic regions. Proving that a common DNA variant contributes to a specific clinical phenotype (such as an unusual drug response) requires compelling statistical arguments and replication in multiple datasets; demonstration that a variant produces altered biologic properties in vitro can also be a supporting argument. The rapid proliferation of polymorphism databases has led to a very large number of false-positive associations between polymorphisms and variable human phenotypes, associations that are subsequently not reproduced.[18]

Despite these challenges, there are excellent data that common polymorphisms contribute to variable drug response[1,2,19-21] and other phenotypes such as susceptibility to disease. The ultimate hope is that such studies will usher in a new era of personalized medicine in which an individual patient's polymorphism set will be used to efficiently diagnose disease, determine disease susceptibility, and select optimal therapies. The challenges in developing such an approach are considerable and include ethical issues[22] and the size of trials needed to identify, validate, and establish cost-effectiveness of genetic associations.[18,23] DNA variants can affect drug responses through three broad mechanisms: changes in pharmacokinetics, changes in the molecule that a drug targets to effect its action, and changes in the broad biologic context in which the drug–target molecule interaction occurs.

Polymorphisms and Pharmacokinetics

The exaggerated effects of drugs in patients with defective cytochrome P450 systems are discussed earlier and listed in Box 53-1. Although the activity of CYP 3A4, the most important enzyme mediating drug disposition, varies among individual patients, the reasons are not completely understood[24] because there are no important polymorphisms that alter the primary amino acid sequence of the protein. However, there are potentially important polymorphisms in the promoter and there are functionally important polymorphisms in the coding region of the very closely related gene for CYP 3A5, expressed in enterocytes and hepatocytes. Loss-of-function alleles are more common in African American patients than in white patients.

Patients with entirely defective P-glycoprotein have not been described, although mice in which the gene is disrupted have no manifest baseline phenotype.[25] However, because of the very prominent role of P-glycoprotein in maintenance of an effective blood-brain barrier, these mice display striking accumulation in the central nervous system and resulting toxicity when exposed to certain drugs, including digoxin. Polymorphisms have been described that modulate function of drug transport molecules in vitro, and these have been linked to variability in plasma and tissue concentrations and effects of digoxin[26-28] and many other drugs.[4,5,29]

Polymorphisms and Drug Targets

DNA polymorphisms can result in important functional changes in drug-target molecules. One example is the common R389G (substitution of glycine for arginine at position 389) variant in the gene encoding the β_1-adrenergic receptor. The R389 variant demonstrated two-fold to four-fold greater increase in myocyte contractility during exposure to β-agonists and predicted a beneficial response of patients with heart failure receiving bucindolol; in fact, clinical response in G389 carriers was no different from response to placebo.[30] Another example may be polymorphisms in the *KCNE2* gene. Some, but not all, studies suggest that *KCNE2* can partner with and modify the function of HERG, the protein whose expression results in I_{Kr}.[31] A *KCNE2* polymorphism resulting in T8A increases sensitivity to I_{Kr} blockers approximately three-fold and has been linked to susceptibility to drug-induced torsades de pointes.[32]

Polymorphisms and the Biologic Milieu of Drug Action

The rapidly increasing identification and characterization of polymorphisms across the genome is being paralleled by an increasing number of markers for variable drug responses, in multiple disciplines, that arise from variability in the biologic context in which drugs act. Studies of mechanisms in torsades de pointes highlight these approaches. Virtually all drugs that cause torsades de pointes are I_{Kr} blockers.[12] The biologic context in which I_{Kr} blockers act includes other elements of the action potential (e.g., I_{Kr}, I_{Na}, I_{Ca}) as well as mechanisms that control normal autonomic function and serum potassium. Thus, variants in any of the genes modulating these processes could in theory modulate the extent to which I_{Kr} blockers prolong QT interval and generate torsades de pointes. Multiple reports support this concept by describing individuals in which mutations associated with long-QT syndrome were not manifest at baseline but were exposed on challenge with a QT-prolonging drug.[33-35] In addition, a common nonsynonymous SNP in the cardiac sodium channel gene resulting in S1103Y is detected only in African Americans and has been reported to modulate the risk of a range of arrhythmias[36] as well as the sudden infant death syndrome.[37] These findings are consistent with the notion that the mechanisms that maintain a short QT interval vary among individual patients, and patients with reduced repolarization reserve[38] due to genetic or environmental factors are at increased risk for developing torsades de pointes on challenge with an I_{Kr} blocker. Variable I_{Ks} appears to play an important role in maintaining this reserve.[39-41]

Another field in which this intersection among monogenic disease, DNA polymorphisms, and environmental stressors can occur is in sudden death risk. Multiple lines of evidence demonstrate that loss of sodium channel function, through genetic mechanisms (the Brugada syndrome)[42] or through pharmacologic challenge (e.g. the result of the Cardiac Arrhythmia Suppression Trial[43]), is arrhythmogenic. Similarly, evidence from large clinical databases and from in vitro studies support the idea that acute myocardial ischemia potentiates the arrhythmogenic effects of reduced sodium channel function.[44] Thus it is tempting to speculate that subtle variations in the amount of sodium channel protein present at the cell surface may be an important modulator of baseline electrophysiologic characteristics and of the likelihood of precipitating fatal arrhythmias on challenge with acute myocardial ischemia: reduced antifibrillatory reserve. Indeed, a variant in the sodium channel promoter has been described that reduces promoter activity and is associated with longer QRS duration (slower conduction) at baseline and with greater QRS prolongation with sodium channel–blocking drug challenge.[45]

Emerging Approaches in Genomic Medicine

The idea that genetics might play a role in variable drug responses saw its first confirmation with identification of rare mutations, with very large pathologic consequences. The field then progressed to the understanding that commoner polymorphisms could also mediate variable drug effects. An emerging trend in genome science is the concept that individual variability in important traits, such as disease susceptibility or response to exogenous stressors such as drugs or myocardial ischemia reflects variability in function or expression of multiple genes.

Sometimes, single or multiple responsible genes can be inferred from an understanding of pathophysiology. Variable responses to warfarin provide an example of a drug in which two genes play an important role. One is *CYP2C9*, responsible for the bioinactivation of S-warfarin, the active enantiomer of the drug. Patients with *CYP2C9* variants that result in loss of function have higher plasma drug levels, increased drug effect, excess risk of bleeding at ordinary doses, and decreased steady state dose requirements.[46,47] A second is *VKORC1*, encoding an important component of the warfarin drug target (the vitamin K complex). Very rare patients have *VKORC1* coding region mutations, resulting in warfarin resistance.[48] In addition, however, common variation in the promoter clearly modulates VKOC1 hepatic mRNA and can be related to warfarin sensitivity.[49] In fact, initial warfarin dose requirement appears more dependent on *VKORC1* variants than on those in *CYP2C9*.

The mapping of millions of SNPs[50] has enabled the technique of genome-wide association to identify, in an unbiased fashion, new genes and pathways mediating human physiology. The concept is that comparing the frequencies of many (at least hundreds of thousands) common SNPs across the genome in well-defined cases and controls will identify regions mediating variable and common human traits.[23] False positives are an inevitable problem, but studies in common diseases such as diabetes or coronary disease[51] have identified and replicated such findings. The technique is very new, and in most cases the function of the implicated genomic region is unknown.

Genome-wide association was used to identify *NOS1AP*, encoding a nitric oxide synthase subunit, as a modulator of QT interval duration.[52-54] The contribution of *NOS1AP* variants to QTc variability is small ($<$10 ms) in normal populations, but it is reasonable to think that variants could contribute to phenotypes like variability in risk for drug-induced QT prolongation. The physiologic function of *NOS1AP* in control of repolarization is not yet determined; establishing that function will further illuminate QT control and may well define new physiologic pathways that would have been inaccessible using other methods. Similarly, a genome-wide approach has implicated a locus on chromosome 4 in atrial fibrillation risk.[55] The role of this locus in AF is unknown, and validating this finding and elucidating the underlying mechanisms may be important steps in creating individualized therapeutic approaches in affected patients.

Summary

Appreciation of individual variability in response to drug treatment has been followed by clinical, cellular, and molecular studies of mechanisms underlying that variability. These studies coupled with dramatic advances in our understanding of the diversity of the human genome now offer unparalleled opportunities not only for improving drug therapy but also for more generally understanding the way humans vary in their response to exogenous stressors.

References

1. Roden DM, Altman RB, Benowitz NL, et al: Pharmacogenomics: Challenges and opportunities. Ann Intern Med 145:749-757, 2006.
2. Giacomini KM, Brett CM, Altman RB, et al: The pharmacogenetics research network: From SNP discovery to clinical drug response. Clin Pharmacol Ther 81:328-345, 2007.
3. Giacomini KM, Krauss RM, Roden DM, et al: When good drugs go bad. Nature 446:975-977, 2007.
4. Ho RH, Kim RB: Transporters and drug therapy: Implications for drug disposition and disease. Clin Pharmacol Ther 78:260-277, 2005.
5. Kim RB: Transporters and drug discovery: Why, when, and how. Mol Pharm 3:26-32, 2006.
6. Grube M, Meyer Zu Schwabedissen HE, et al: Uptake of cardiovascular drugs into the human heart: Expression, regulation, and function of the carnitine transporter OCTN2 (SLC22A5). Circulation 113:1114-1122, 2006.
7. McBride BF, Yang T, Liu K, et al: Potentiation of drug actions by drug uptake transporter expression in heart. Circulation 112:II-494, 2005.
8. Guengerich FP: Cytochrome P-450 3A4: Regulation and role in drug metabolism. Annu Rev Pharmacol Toxicol 39:1-17, 1999.
9. Meyer UA, Zanger UM: Molecular mechanisms of genetic polymorphisms of drug metabolism. Ann Rev Pharmacol Toxicol 37:269-296, 1997.
10. Ratain MJ: From bedside to bench to bedside to clinical practice: An odyssey with irinotecan. Clin Cancer Res 12:1658-1660, 2006.
11. Weinshilboum RM: Pharmacogenomics: Catechol *O*-methyltransferase to thiopurine *S*-methyltransferase. Cell Mol Neurobiol 26:539-561, 2006.
12. Roden DM: Drug-induced prolongation of the QT interval. N Engl J Med 350:1013-1022, 2004.
13. Fromm MF, Kim RB, Stein CM, et al: Inhibition of P-glycoprotein–mediated drug transport: A unifying mechanism to explain the interaction between digoxin and quinidine. Circulation 99:552-557, 1999.
14. Evers J, Eichelbaum M, Kroemer HK: Unpredictability of flecainide plasma concentrations in patients with renal failure: Relation to side effects and sudden death? Ther Drug Monit 16:349-351, 1994.
15. Yang T, Roden DM: Extracellular potassium modulation of drug block of I_{Kr}: Implications for torsades de pointes and reverse use-dependence. Circulation 93:407-411, 1996.
16. Fiset C, Drolet B, Hamelin BA, Turgeon J: Block Of I_{Ks} by the diuretic agent indapamide modulates cardiac electrophysiological effects of the class III antiarrhythmic drug DL-sotalol. J Pharmacol Exp Ther 283:148-156, 1997.
17. Lee JT, Kroemer HK, Silberstein DJ, et al: The role of genetically determined polymorphic drug metabolism in the beta-blockade produced by propafenone. N Engl J Med 322:1764-1768, 1990.
18. Hirschhorn JN, Lohmueller K, Byrne E, Hirschhorn K: A comprehensive review of genetic association studies. Genet Med 4:45-61, 2002.
19. Evans WE, McLeod HL: Pharmacogenomics—drug disposition, drug targets, and side effects. N Engl J Med 348:538-549, 2003.
20. Evans WE, Relling MV: Moving towards individualized medicine with pharmacogenomics. Nature 429:464-468, 2004.
21. Eichelbaum M, Ingelman-Sundberg M, Evans WE: Pharmacogenomics and individualized drug therapy. Annu Rev Med 57:119-137, 2006.
22. Clayton EW: Ethical, legal, and social implications of genomic medicine. N Engl J Med 349:562-569, 2003.
23. Hirschhorn JN, Daly MJ: Genome-wide association studies for common diseases and complex traits. Nat Rev Genet 6:95-108, 2005.
24. Wojnowski L, Kamdem LK: Clinical implications of CYP3A polymorphisms. Expert Opin Drug Metab Toxicol 2:171-182, 2006.
25. Schinkel AH, Smit JJM, van Tellingen O, et al: Disruption of the mouse *mdr1a* P-glycoprotein gene leads to a deficiency in the blood-brain barrier and to increased sensitivity to drugs. Cell 77:491-502, 1994.
26. Hoffmeyer S, Burk O, von Richter O, et al: Functional polymorphisms of the human multidrug-resistance gene: Multiple sequence variations and correlation of one allele with P- glycoprotein expression and activity in vivo. Proc Natl Acad Sci U S A 97:3473-3478, 2000.
27. Kim RB: Drugs as P-glycoprotein substrates, inhibitors, and inducers. Drug Metab Rev 34:47-54, 2002.
28. Kim RB, Leake BF, Choo EF, et al: Identification of functionally variant MDR1 alleles among European Americans and African Americans. Clin Pharmacol Ther 70:189-199, 2001.
29. Shu Y, Leabman MK, Feng B, et al: Evolutionary conservation predicts function of variants of the human organic cation transporter, OCT1. Proc Natl Acad Sci U S A 100:5902-5907, 2003.
30. Liggett SB, Mialet-Perez J, Thaneemit-Chen S, et al: A polymorphism within a conserved β_1-adrenergic receptor motif alters cardiac function and β-blocker response in human heart failure. Proc Natl Acad Sci U S A 103:11288-11293, 2006.
31. Abbott GW, Sesti F, Splawski I, et al: MiRP1 forms I_{Kr} potassium channels with HERG and is associated with cardiac arrhythmia. Cell 97:175-187, 1999.
32. Sesti F, Abbott GW, Wei J, et al: A common polymorphism associated with antibiotic-induced cardiac arrhythmia. Proc Natl Acad Sci U S A 97:10613-10618, 2000.
33. Yang P, Kanki H, Drolet B, et al: Allelic variants in Long QT disease genes in patients with drug-associated torsades de pointes. Circulation 105:1943-1948, 2002.
34. Paulussen AD, Gilissen RA, Armstrong M, et al: Genetic variations of KCNQ1, KCNH2, SCN5A, KCNE1, and KCNE2 in drug-induced long QT syndrome patients. J Mol Med 82:182-188, 2004.
35. Lehtonen A, Fodstad H, Laitinen-Forsblom P, et al: Further evidence of inherited long QT syndrome gene mutations in antiarrhythmic drug–associated torsades de pointes. Heart Rhythm 4:603-607, 2007.
36. Splawski I, Timothy KW, Tateyama M, et al: Variant of SCN5A sodium channel implicated in risk of cardiac arrhythmia. Science 297:1333-1336, 2002.
37. Plant LD, Bowers PN, Liu Q, et al: A common cardiac sodium channel variant associated with sudden infant death in African Americans, SCN5A S1103Y. J Clin Invest 116:430-435, 2006.
38. Roden DM: Taking the idio out of idiosyncratic—predicting torsades de pointes. Pacing Clin Electrophysiol 21:1029-1034, 1998.
39. Silva J, Rudy Y: Subunit interaction determines I_{Ks} participation in cardiac repolarization and repolarization reserve. Circulation 112:1384-1391, 2005.
40. Jost N, Virag L, Bitay M, et al: Restricting excessive cardiac action potential and QT

prolongation: A vital role for I_{Ks} in human ventricular muscle. Circulation 112:1392-1399, 2005.

41. Roden DM, Yang T: Protecting the heart against arrhythmias: Potassium current physiology and repolarization reserve. Circulation 112:1376-1378, 2005.
42. Alings M, Wilde A: "Brugada" syndrome: Clinical data and suggested pathophysiological mechanism. Circulation 99:666-673, 1999.
43. The CAST Investigators: Preliminary report: Effect of encainide and flecainide on mortality in a randomized trial of arrhythmia suppression after myocardial infarction. N Engl J Med 321:406-412, 1989.
44. Akiyama T, Pawitan Y, Greenberg H, et al; The CAST Investigators: Increased risk of death and cardiac arrest from encainide and flecainide in patients after non–Q-wave acute myocardial infarction in the Cardiac Arrhythmia Suppression Trial. Am J Cardiol 68:1551-1555, 1991.
45. Bezzina CR, Shimizu W, Yang P, et al: Common sodium channel promoter haplotype in Asian subjects underlies variability in cardiac conduction. Circulation 113:338-344, 2006.
46. Aithal GP, Day CP, Kesteven PJ, Daly AK: Association of polymorphisms in the cytochrome P450 CYP2C9 with warfarin dose requirement and risk of bleeding complications. Lancet 353:717-719, 1999.
47. Taube J, Halsall D, Baglin T: Influence of cytochrome P-450 CYP2C9 polymorphisms on warfarin sensitivity and risk of over-anticoagulation in patients on long-term treatment. Blood 96:1816-1819, 2000.
48. Rost S, Fregin A, Ivaskevicius V, et al: Mutations in VKORC1 cause warfarin resistance and multiple coagulation factor deficiency type 2. Nature 427:537-541, 2004.
49. Rieder MJ, Reiner AP, Gage BF, et al: Effect of VKORC1 haplotypes on transcriptional regulation and warfarin dose. N Engl J Med 352:2285-2293, 2005.
50. The International HapMap Consortium: A haplotype map of the human genome. Nature 437:1299-1320, 2005.
51. The Wellcome Trust Case Control Consortium: Genome-wide association study of 14,000 cases of seven common diseases and 3,000 shared controls. Nature 447:661-678, 2007.
52. Arking DE, Pfeufer A, Post W, et al: A common genetic variant in the NOS1 regulator NOS1AP modulates cardiac repolarization. Nat Genet 38:644-651, 2006.
53. Post W, Shen H, Damcott C, et al: Associations between genetic variants in the NOS1AP (CAPON) gene and cardiac repolarization in the Old Order Amish. Hum Hered 64:214-219, 2007.
54. Aarnoudse AJ, Newton-Cheh C, et al: Common NOS1AP variants are associated with a prolonged QTc interval in the Rotterdam study. Circulation 116:10-16, 2007.
55. Gudbjartsson DF, Arnar DO, Helgadottir A, et al: Variants conferring risk of atrial fibrillation on chromosome 4q25. Nature 448:353-357, 2007.

Supraventricular Arrhythmias: Mechanisms, Features, and Management

PART IX

Morphologic Correlates of Atrial Arrhythmias

54

Siew Yen Ho

CHAPTER OUTLINE

Advances in electrophysiologic mapping have provided a crucial insight into atrial arrhythmias. A better understanding of atrial anatomy is essential to make further progress, especially in fine-tuning interventional techniques and developing computer models. The atrial walls have functional roles in the dynamics of the cardiac chambers and atrioventricular valves, as well as serving as the substrate for conduction of the cardiac impulse. Although cellular, molecular, and physiologic aspects of the tissues that make up the atrial walls are extremely important, the gross structure of the chambers themselves cannot be neglected. In particular, the arrangement of the myofibers that make up the muscular wall can provide a morphologic basis for atrial conduction. The term *myofibers* is used to represent the macroscopic appearance of strands of myocytes that are aligned with their long axis in similar orientation.[1] These strands are not surrounded by thick insulating fibrous tissue sheaths, and they are not specialized tracts for conduction. Rather, studying their arrangements transmurally, through the atrial walls, helps us to gain a better understanding of the preferential routes of conduction from one part of the atrium to the other and between the atria. Because conduction along the length of myocytes is more rapid than conduction occurring transversely, myofiber arrangements have implications for impulse propagation. Activation maps on mammalian hearts have shown correlations with arrangement of atrial myofibers in recent studies.[2] Complex arrangements may suggest intercellular electrical uncoupling with nonuniform anisotropy that may play an important role in setting up microreentry.[3,4]

At the outlets of the atria, the myocardium of the distal parts of the vestibule overlap the atrial surface of the leaflets of the tricuspid and mitral valves to a greater or lesser degree, albeit for distances of only a millimeter or so. The atrial myocardium, however, is electrically isolated from ventricular myocardium owing to the insulation provided by fibrofatty tissues at the hingelines (annuli) of the valves. It is well recognized that for normal conduction of the cardiac impulse from atria to ventricles, only one pathway of muscular continuity exists, and this is through the specialized myocytes of the atrioventricular conduction system originally described by Tawara in 1906.[5] This chapter presents features of cardiac morphology pertinent to atrial arrhythmias.

Siew Yen Ho receives funding support from The Royal Brompton and Harefield Hospital Charitable Fund for her research.

The Heart in the Chest and the Atria

The right border of the heart is formed exclusively by the right atrium, with the superior and inferior caval veins joining at its upper and lower margins. On the frontal silhouette, the left atrium is barely seen; only its appendage curling round the edge of the pulmonary trunk is visible. Thus, the left atrium is the most posteriorly situated cardiac chamber. When the heart is viewed in situ, the proximity of the esophagus to the posterior wall of the left atrium is clear (Fig. 54-1). This spatial relationship is crucial to ablationists in order to reduce the risk of the postprocedural complication of atrioesophageal fistula formation.[6,7]

The heart itself is enclosed in a fibrous sac, the pericardium, which separates the surface of the heart from adjacent structures. On the surface of the pericardial sac descend the phrenic nerves and their accompanying pericardiophrenic arteries, which are branches from the internal mammary artery. The right phrenic nerve descends vertically along the right anterolateral surface of the superior caval vein to be related to the right aspect of the right atrial wall, and in front of the root of the lung, to reach the diaphragm adjacent to the lateral border of the entrance of the inferior caval vein.[8] Along the way, the right phrenic nerve can be less than 2 mm from the anterior wall of the right superior pulmonary vein (Fig. 54-2). The left phrenic nerve descends on the left side, close to the aortic arch, and onto the pericardium

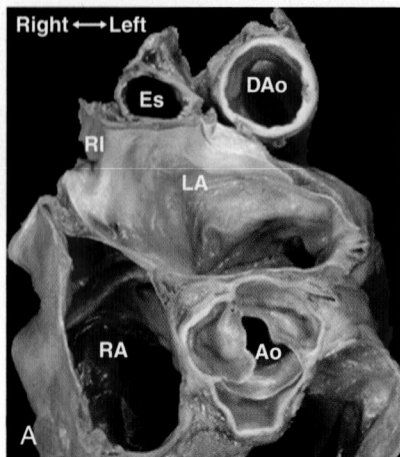

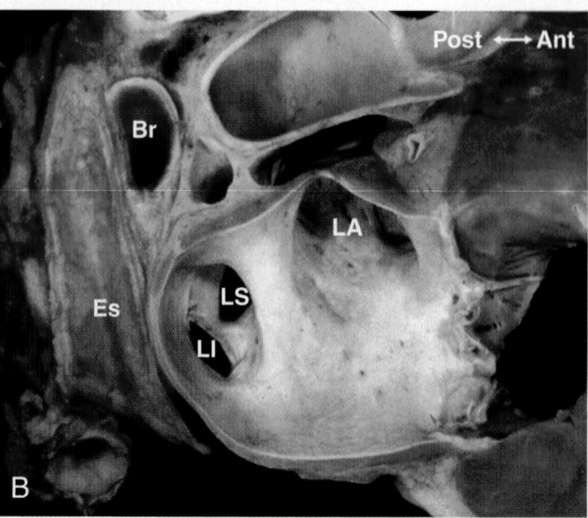

Figure 54-1 These short axis (**A**) and long axis (**B**) cuts show the esophagus descending immediately behind the left atrium. The *arrow* indicates the atrial septum. Ao, aortic valve; Br, bronchus; DAo, descending aorta; Es, esophagus; LA, left atrium; LI, left inferior pulmonary vein; LS, left superior pulmonary vein; RA, right atrium; RI, right inferior pulmonary vein.

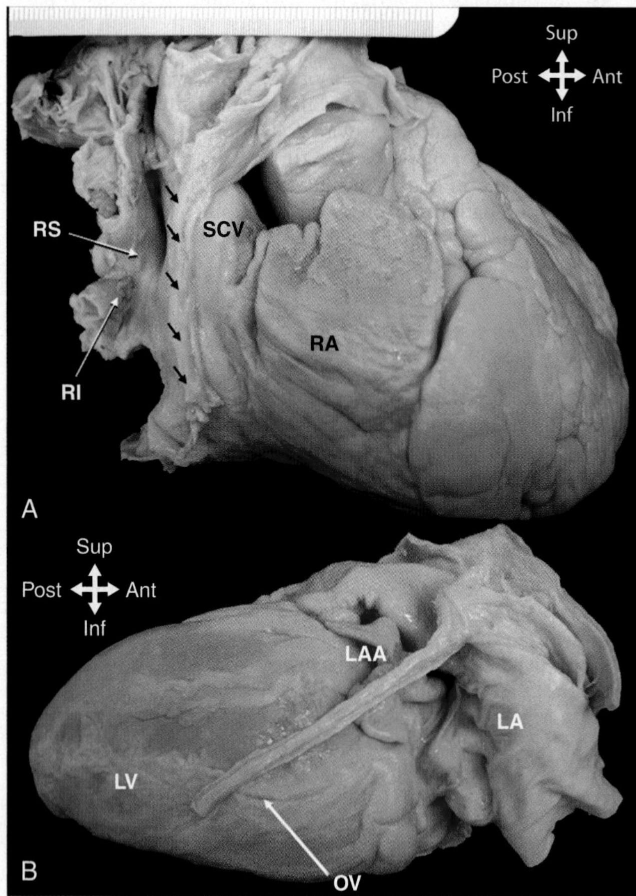

Figure 54-2 Right (**A**) and left (**B**) views of a heart specimen after the pericardial sac has been dissected open. The right and left phrenic nerves are kept in place. Note the proximity of the right phrenic nerve (*black arrows* on **A**) to the right pulmonary veins. The left phrenic nerve passes over the left atrial appendage (LAA) and the obtuse marginal vein (OV). LA, left atrium; LV, left ventricle; RA, right atrium; RI, right inferior pulmonary vein; RS, right superior pulmonary vein; SCV, superior caval vein.

overlying the left atrial appendage and the left ventricle. It takes one of two courses over the left ventricle: either over the anterior surface or leftward over the obtuse margin. The latter course is close to the lateral vein or left obtuse marginal vein.

Viewed from the front, the cavity of the right atrium is right and anterior, and the left atrium is situated to the left and mainly posteriorly. The front of the left atrium lies just behind the transverse pericardial sinus. In humans, the right superior pulmonary vein passes posterior to the superior caval vein, with the right inferior vein posterior to the venous component of the right atrium.

The atrial septum, best appreciated in transverse section, runs obliquely from the front extending backwards and to the right (see Fig. 54-1). Related posteriorly and inferiorly to the left atrium is the coronary sinus, which is the continuation of the great cardiac vein (Fig. 54-3). The oblique vein (of Marshall) passes from superiorly, between the left atrial appendage and the left superior pulmonary vein, along the posterior atrial wall to join the coronary sinus, which is located inferiorly. This vein is obliterated in a majority of people, although it may remain patent as an isolated malformation, with the persistent left superior caval vein draining into the coronary sinus.

Structure of the Right Atrium

The right atrium is best considered in terms of three anatomic components—the appendage, the venous part, and the vestibule. A fourth component, the septum, is shared by the two atria. The dominant feature of the right atrium is the large, triangle-shaped appendage, which is located anterior and laterally (Fig. 54-4). A muscular ridge, the terminal crest ("crista terminalis"), separates the appendage from the venous component. The crest corresponds on the epicardial aspect to the terminal groove, a landmark for the location of the the sinus node which lies close to the superior cavoatrial junction. Right atrial musculature often extends a short distance into the superior caval vein externally (see Fig. 54-4). Muscular sleeves have come under scrutiny among cardiac electrophysiologists in recent years owing to their association with focal activity initiating atrial arrhythmias.[9] The inferior caval vein usually lacks a muscular sleeve. The atrial wall at the intercaval area also may be lacking in myocardium near the entrance of the inferior caval vein.

An extensive array of pectinate muscles is characteristic of the right atrium. Arising from the terminal crest, these muscles spread throughout the entire wall of the appendage, extending

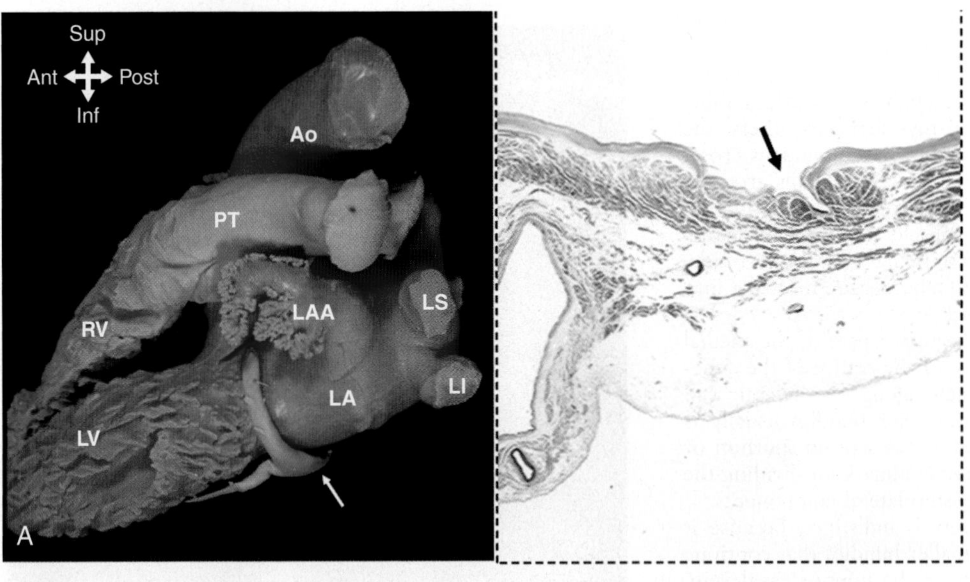

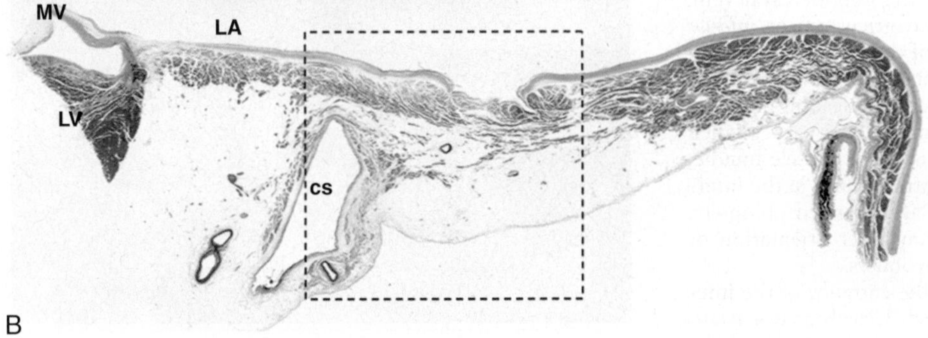

Figure 54-3 **A,** The endocast viewed from the left shows the course of the coronary sinus *(arrow)* inferior to the left atrium. **B,** This histologic section through the region of the "mitral isthmus" is stained to show fibrous tissue in *green* and myocardium in *red.* Note the muscular continuity between the wall of the coronary sinus and the left atrium. The *enlarged box* shows a pit *(arrow)* on the endocardial surface. Ao, aorta; cs, coronary sinus; LA, left atrium; LAA, left atrial appendage; LI, left inferior pulmonary vein; LS, left superior pulmonary veins; LV, left ventricle; MV, mitral valve; PT, pulmonary trunk; RV, right ventricle.

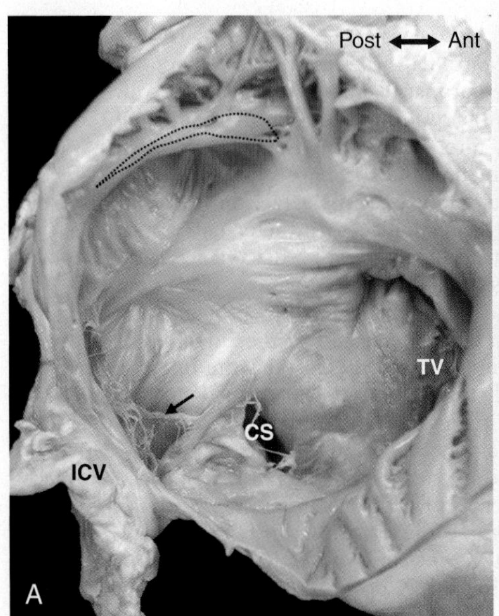

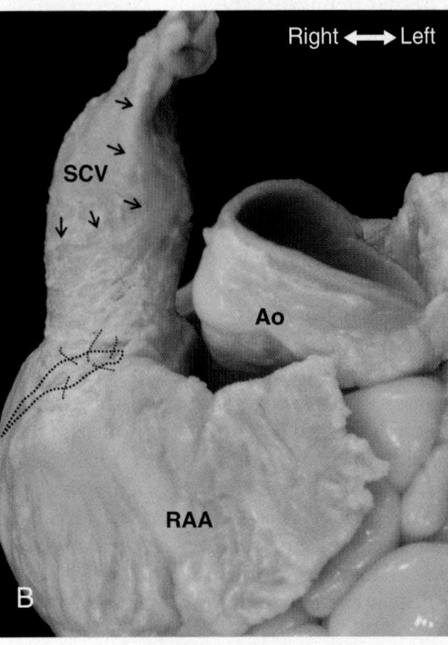

Figure 54-4 **A,** The right atrium is opened and displayed in simulated right anterior oblique projection. The *dotted shape* marks the site of the sinus node in the musculature of the terminal crest. Note the array of pectinate muscles arising from the terminal crest. The eustachian valve in this heart is a fenestrated Chiari network *(arrow).* **B,** This heart, viewed from the front, shows muscular extensions over the wall of the superior caval vein. The distal margins are irregular *(arrows).* The *dotted shape* depicts the location of the sinus node and its prongs of nodal extensions. Ao, aorta; CS, coronary sinus; ICV, inferior caval vein; RAA, right atrial appendage; SCV, superior caval vein; TV, tricuspid valve.

to the lateral and inferior walls of the atrium (see Fig. 54-4). In between the ridges of pectinate muscles, the wall is very thin, almost parchment-like in some instances. In some hearts, the ridges along the parietal wall are aligned in nearly parallel fashion with longitudinally arranged myofibers. In others, the ridges are not as uniformly arranged but have abundant cross-overs with thin interlacing strands in between.[10] This arrangement may play a role in initiating intra-atrial reentry. Although present in abundance, the pectinate muscles never reach the orifice of the tricuspid valve. A smooth muscular rim, the vestibule, surrounds the valvar orifice, with the musculature inserting into the atrial surface of the valvar leaflets.

The terminal crest begins on the upper part of the medial wall and then turns laterally in front of the orifice of the superior caval vein to descend obliquely along the lateral wall (see Fig. 54-4). One of the anterosuperior bundles usually is more prominent, and it is described as the septum spurium or *sagittal muscle bundle*. It is a convenient landmark for dividing the appendage into anteromedial and posterolateral components.

The terminal portion of the crest is indistinct, because it divides into a variable number of smaller bundles that continue toward the vestibule and the orifice of the inferior caval vein, feeding into the area of the "flutter"(cavotricuspid) or *inferior isthmus*. The nonuniform arrangement of the terminal ramifications of the crest may account for delay and discontinuities in the spread of the excitatory wavefront, potentially leading to atrial reentry.[10-12] Myocytes within the terminal crest are aligned mainly longitudinally along the long axis of the muscle bundle, favoring preferential conduction. By contrast, those in the intercaval area adjoining the terminal crest are arranged obliquely, producing either an abrupt change in myofiber orientation or intermingling of irregularly arranged myofibers.

The eustachian valve, which guards the entrance of the inferior caval vein, also is variably developed. Usually it is a triangular flap of fibrous or fibromuscular tissue that inserts medially to the eustachian ridge, or "sinus septum." The so-called sinus septum is not septal but is simply the atrial wall between the oval fossa and the coronary sinus. In some cases, the valve is particularly large and muscular, posing an obstacle to passage of catheters from the inferior caval vein to the inferior part of the right atrium. Occasionally, the valve is perforated or even takes the form of a delicate filigree described as a Chiari network (see Fig. 54-4). The free border of the eustachian valve continues as a tendon that runs in the musculature of the sinus septum. It is the posterior border of the triangle (of Koch) that delineates the location of the atrioventricular node (Fig. 54-5). The anterior border is marked by the hinge of the septal leaflet of the tricuspid valve. Superiorly, at the apex of the triangle, the central fibrous body is the landmark for the penetrating bundle of His. The inferior border of the triangle is the orifice of the coronary sinus, together with the vestibule immediately anterior to it. This vestibular portion, also known as the *septal isthmus* (Fig. 54-6), is the area often targeted for ablation of the slow pathway in atrioventricular nodal reentrant tachycardia. To describe this isthmus as septal is misleading because it is only a thin layer of vestibular myocardium and separated from ventricular myocardium by epicardial fibroareolar tissue of the inferior pyramidal space. In fact, it is paraseptal in location and occasionally contains the inferior extensions of the atrioventricular node. When present, the nodal extensions are 1 to 3 mm beneath the endocardium. On the epicardial side there are often collections of parasympathetic ganglia or fibers of autonomic nerves. The so-called fast pathway in atrioventricular nodal reentrant tachycardia corresponds to the area of musculature close to the apex of the triangle of Koch. Ablating in this region increases the risk of direct damage to the atrioventricular node (see Fig. 54-5).

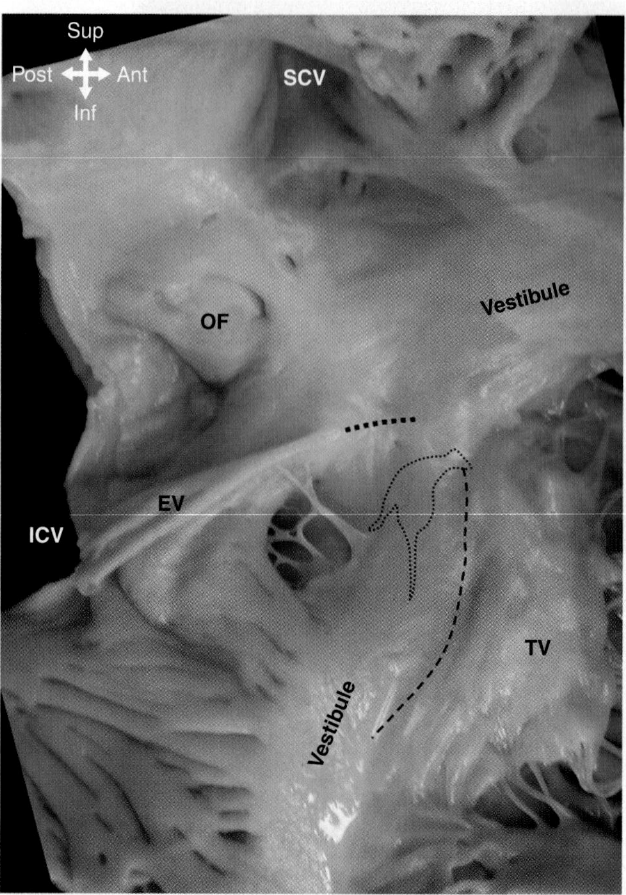

Figure 54-5 This right atrium is opened to show the landmarks of the triangle of Koch. The projection of the eustachian valve (EV) traced in the sinus septum *(dotted line)* marks the posterior border of the triangle. The anterior border *(dashed line)* is the hingeline of the septal leaflet of the tricuspid valve. At the apex between the anterior and posterior borders lies the central fibrous body with the membranous septum *(pale color)*. The *dotted shape* marks the compact atrioventricular node with its inferior prongs. The Thebesian valve is fenestrated. ICV, inferior caval vein; SCV, superior caval vein; TV, tricuspid valve

A small crescentic flap, the Thebesian valve, usually guards the orifice of the coronary sinus. Frequently, the valve is fenestrated (see Fig. 54-5). An imperforate valve completely covering the orifice is very rare. In 80% to 90% of hearts, a flimsy valve is present in the lumen of the coronary sinus, marking its junction with the great cardiac vein. This valve, the valve of Vieussens, can provide a little resistance to catheter entry. Once past the valve, an acute bend in the great cardiac vein can cause further obstruction, as is found in approximately 20% of patients. The atrial wall inferior to the orifice of the coronary sinus usually is pouch-like and often is described as the sinus of Keith, or the sub-eustachian sinus. The area between the inferior caval vein and the tricuspid valve (see Fig.54-6) corresponds to the critical isthmus in the circuit of common (typical) atrial flutter.[13,14] It often includes the pouch-like sinus, but its profile also can be flat or concave, requiring an individually tailored approach to delivery of ablation energy.[15] This isthmus, the central isthmus or *cavotricuspid isthmus*, is the most inferiorly situated isthmus when the right atrium is viewed in attitudinal orientation with the heart in situ. It has three morphologic components of variable thickness and is bordered anteriorly by the hinge of the tricuspid

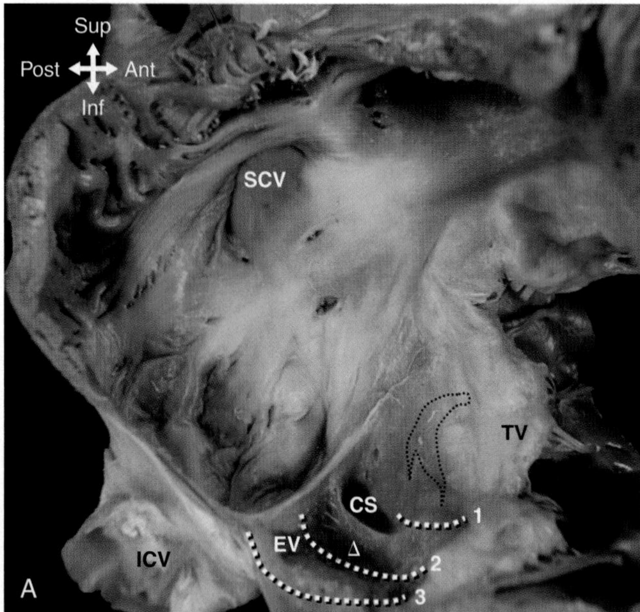

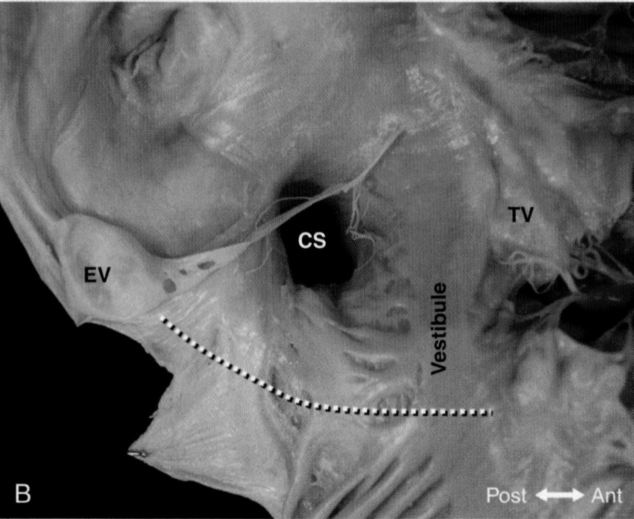

Figure 54-6 **A,** The right atrium is displayed in simulated right anterior oblique projection to show the terminal crest and the three lines of isthmus (numbered 1 to 3) across the inferior wall. The paraseptal isthmus (1) is at the base of the triangle of Koch between the orifice of the coronary sinus (CS) and the attachment of the tricuspid valve (TV). The cavotricuspid isthmus (2) is the most inferiorly situated. It often traverses through a "sub-eustachian" pouch *(triangle)*. The inferolateral isthmus (3) is the longest and the farthest away from the compact atrioventricular node *(dotted shape)*. **B,** This magnified view of the cavotricuspid isthmus *(dotted line)* shows a membrane-like wall posteriorly, a combination of muscle bundles and membranes in the middle, and smooth muscular wall of the vestibule anteriorly. EV, eustachian valve; ICV, inferior caval vein; SCV, superior caval vein.

valve and posteriorly by the eustachian valve guarding the orifice of the inferior caval vein[12] (see Fig. 54-6). The posterior component is mainly fibrous, whereas the anterior component is the musculature of the atrial vestibule and has a smooth endocardial surface. In the middle is a zone of muscular trabeculations representing the distal ramifications of the terminal crest which are separated by variable extents of thin atrial wall composed mainly of fibrous and fatty tissue. The myofibers of the trabeculations continue into the eustachian ridge to surround the mouth of the coronary sinus and into the sinus wall. Often, the arrangement of the myofibers in the isthmus is nonuniform, with many intersecting bundles and branches. Variations in morphology of this zone are common. In some hearts, muscular trabeculations dominate while in others this zone is represented by a thin, membrane-like wall.

A further isthmus is recognized in the right atrium. This is the *inferolateral isthmus*, which, as its name suggests, separates the lateral aspect of the entrance of the inferior caval vein from the tricuspid valve (see Fig. 54-6). It is the widest of the three isthmus lines and at closest proximity to the right coronary artery which passes at less than 4 mm away from the endocardium in half of the heart specimens examined.[12] Compared with the inferolateral and paraseptal isthmuses, the inferior isthmus (also called the central isthmus) appears most appropriate for ablationists to target on account of its thicker wall, shorter length and distance from the atrioventricular node.

The Atrial Septum

Accessing the left atrium from the right requires an appreciation of the extent of the true atrial septum. From the right atrial aspect, the septum is marked by the valve of the oval fossa and a raised muscular rim immediately superior, posterior, and inferior to it (see Fig. 54-5). The musculature that gives the impression of an extensive anterior septal wall is the anteromedial wall of the right atrium lying behind the aorta through the transverse pericardial sinus. The muscular rim superiorly is the infolded wall between the superior caval vein and the right pulmonary veins, the embryonic "septum secundum." Although belonging to the right atrium, the leftward part of the muscular fold apposing the fossa valve continues into the musculature of the left atrial wall. Significantly, the folded rim is not a septal area. The valve of the oval fossa is the true septal structure that can be perforated with a catheter without risk of exiting the heart or damaging the arterial supply to the sinus node. The left aspect of the atrial septum lacks the crater-like feature of the right side. The valve itself, the embryonic "septum primum," usually is thin, comprising of a bilaminar arrngement of orthogonally arranged myocytes intespersed with fibrous tissue. It has been suggested that this arrangement may contribute to maintenance of left septal atrial flutter.[16]

Structure of the Left Atrium

As with the right atrium, the left atrium has three anatomic components and shares its septum. Its components are joined by the atrial body, which makes up the larger part of the atrial wall between the pulmonary venous portion and the vestibule. The atrial appendage is characteristically small and finger-like, forming a cul-de-sac in which thrombi may lodge. The pectinate muscles within the appendage are whorl-like, interlacing networks with membrane-like walls in between. Owing to its tubular shape, its junction with the left atrium is narrow and fairly well defined. The tip of the appendage can be directed anteriorly overlying the pulmonary trunk, superiorly behind the arterial pedicle, or posteriorly. When its tip is directed anteriorly, the body of the appendage usually also overlies the main stem of the left coronary artery.[17]

The remnant of the vein of Marshall runs in a fold on the lateral epicardial aspect of the neck of the appendage, anterior to the left pulmonary veins. On the endocardial aspect, the fold of atrial wall appears like a ridge that is commonly called the left atrial ridge (left lateral ridge) (Fig. 54-7). In a majority of heart

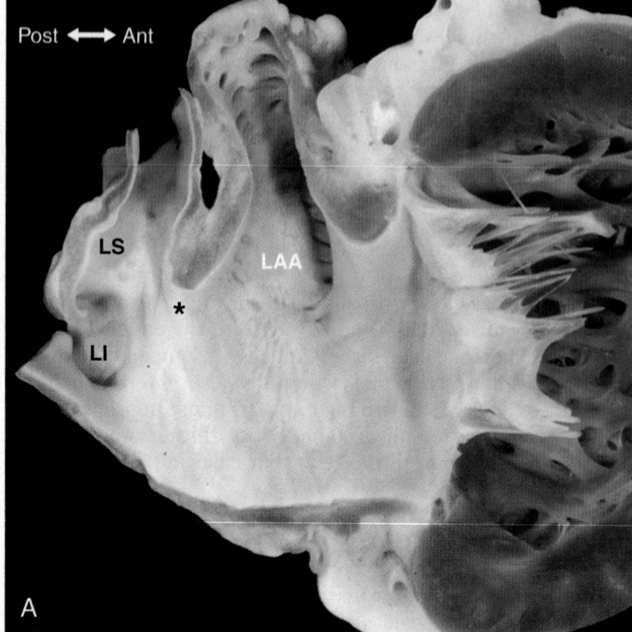

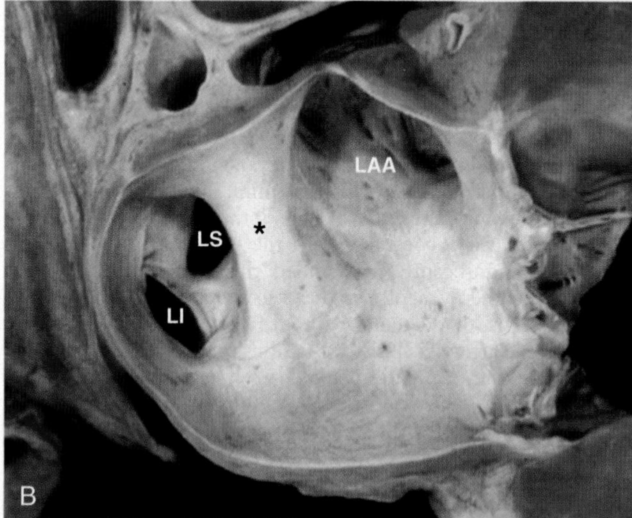

Figure 54-7 A and B are views of the left atrial "ridge" *(asterisks)* showing the range in widths. The ridge is an infolding of the atrial wall between the orifice of the left superior pulmonary vein (LS) and the left atrial appendage (LAA). LI, left inferior pulmonary vein.

specimens, the ridge is less than 5 mm wide, making it tricky to achieve stability of the ablating catheter.[18] The ligament of Marshall and its adjacent epicardium are richly innervated by autonomic nerve fibers.[18,19] Experimental studies have shown predominance of cholinergic nerve fibers in the region of the ligament of Marshall, as well as muscular bridges with the left atrium or left pulmonary veins, suggesting that these features may be important in genesis or maintenance of atrial fibrillation.[20,21]

In contrast with the right atrium, virtually all of the pectinate muscles in the left atrium are confined within the appendage. The major portion of the atrium, including the septal component, is smooth-walled. Nevertheless, areas of exceptionally thin atrial wall commonly are seen in the vicinity of the os of the appendage, and pits and troughs may be observed in the inferior wall of the atrial body leading to the vestibule.[17,22] The pits and troughs may be arranged in a row, giving the region a ladder-like appearance of muscular trabeculations separated by thin walls. This region traverses the so-called mitral isthmus, or left atrial isthmus (see Fig. 54-3).[22]

The vestibule that leads to the mitral orifice has the smoothest wall. Its proximal margin is indistinguishable from the wall of the atrial body. The inferior quadrant of the vestibule overlies the course of the coronary sinus and its continuation into the great cardiac vein. The venous channel usually is sited 6 to 10 mm proximal to the plane of the mitral "annulus" (see Fig. 54-3).[23] The coronary sinus has its own muscular wall, which often has myocardial connections with the atrial wall. In this region, the site of the mitral isthmus, the thicker wall may require additional "burns" to be carried out inside the coronary sinus to achieve transmural isolation.

On the endocardial surface, the smoothest parts are the superior and posterior walls, which make up the pulmonary venous component, and the vestibule. The walls are composed of one to three, or more, overlapping "layers" of differently aligned myocardial fibers (see later on), with marked regional variations in thickness. The area of the anterior wall just behind the aorta usually is thin, whereas the superior wall, or dome, is thicker but tends to thin out nearer to the left pulmonary veins. The posterior wall in patients with atrial fibrillation tends to be thinner than normal.[24]

The venous component receives the pulmonary veins. Large clinical series using magnetic resonance imaging and computed tomography have demonstrated considerable variability in number, anatomy, and size of the pulmonary venous orifices.[25-27] The juncture between atrium and vein is smooth. On looking at the inside of the atrium, it often is difficult to define precisely the venoatrial junction, especially when the entrances of the veins are funnel-shaped. It is not uncommon to find adjacent veins coming together and sharing a short common vestibule (antrum) with the atrial chamber.

Muscular continuity of left atrial myocardium into the wall of the pulmonary veins has long been recognized, as have recordings of electrical activity in the veins. It is only in recent decades, however, that the muscular sleeves have been shown to play a role in initiating or maintaining atrial fibrillation. The venous wall is composed of an innermost lining of endothelium that is wrapped by a media layer (tunica media) containing connective tissue and smooth muscle cells and an outermost layer of adventitia composed of fibrous tissue, fat, nerves, and small blood vessels. At the venoatrial junction, the endothelium of the left atrium continues into the venous endothelium, and the venous media is overlapped by the continuation of left atrial muscle (Fig. 54-8). Although sandwiched between the media and the adventitia, a fibrofatty tissue plane usually separates the muscular sleeve from the venous wall. Muscular sleeves are common, especially around the superior pulmonary veins. They also tend to be longer and more extensive in the superior veins than in the inferior veins. The sleeves are thickest and most complete around the venoatrial junctions. Encirclement is less complete distally as they become thinner toward the lung hilum.[28] The distal margins of the sleeves are highly variable. Some parts end abruptly; still other parts, on the same vein, taper in finger-like fashion and become isolated in the fibrous adventitia (see Fig. 54-8). Extensive fibrosis has been observed in the tips of the sleeves. The arrangement of the myofibers that make up the sleeves is variable, but these myofibers are mostly circumferential around the veins, pierced by longitudinal or oblique bundles in a complex fashion (see Fig. 54-8).[28] Nonuniform anisotropy, together with fibrosis, may play a role in electrical instability. An experimental study has revealed that abnormal conduction, as shown

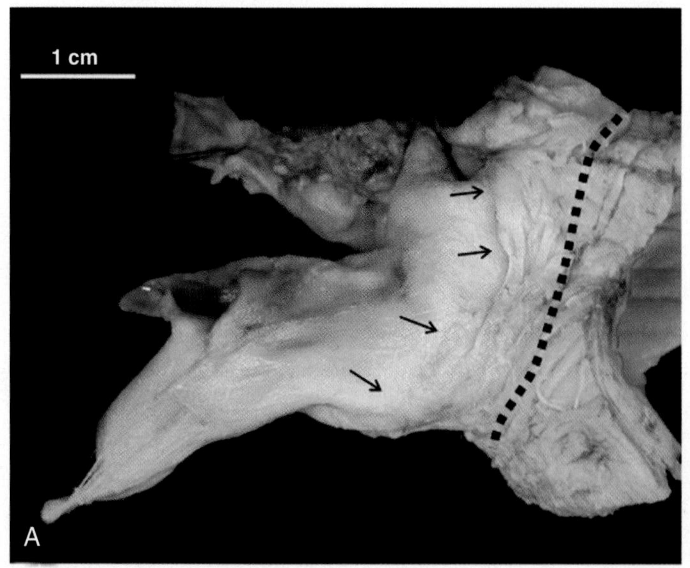

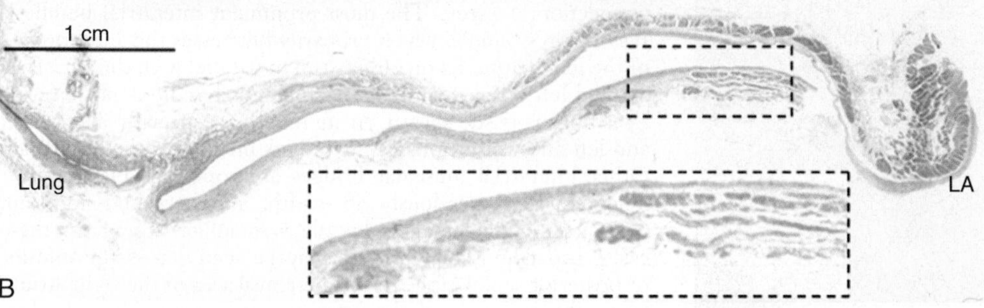

Figure 54-8 **A,** This dissection shows the muscular sleeve *(arrows)* of a right superior pulmonary vein terminating abruptly *(upper portion)* or fading out gradually *(lower portion)*. The *dotted line* indicates the junction between vein and atrium. **B,** This histologic section shows a venous sleeve extending more than 3 cm toward the lung hilum. The *magnified view* shows circularly arranged myofibers (stained *red*) sandwiching longitudinally arranged myofibers. A gap is present in the sleeve, and the distal part of the sleeve is fibrotic. The stain shows fibrous tissue as green and muscle as red. LA, left atrium.

by fractionated electrograms, is related to sites of complex myofiber arrangement.[3] Node-like specialized cells producing automaticity have been reported in experimental studies but have not been demonstrated physiologically in human pulmonary veins.

Myoarchitecture and Interatrial Connections

The elegant dissections of Papez[29] demonstrated the complex arrangement of bundles of similarly aligned myocytes, myofibers, in the atrial walls. Changes in orientation transmurally may be gradual or abrupt. The orientations are described as *circular* when the myofibers approximate to the plane of the atrioventricular junction and *longitudinal* when they are perpendicular to this plane. Oblique myofibers are those in an *intermediate* orientation. *Myoarchitecture* refers to the generalized arrangement of the myofibers in so-called layers of changes in orientation but, of importace, does not imply fibrous separation or insulation of layers. Moreover, changes in myofiber orientation often are not discrete but there are interconnections between bundles and layers.

In the right atrium, the terminal crest is well recognized as a bundle of longitudinally aligned fibers that favors preferential conduction. To either side of the terminal crest, nonuniform arrangement of myofibers is seen. On the appendage side, pectinate muscles arise nearly perpendicularly (see Figs. 54-4 and 54-6). The adjoining intercaval musculature on the venous side also changes direction at the juncture with the crest and, potentially, is a substrate for slowing conduction. At the apex of the crest, in the subepicardium, is the right atrial origin of the upper bifurcation of the interatrial bundle commonly known as *Bachmann's bundle*. The atrial appendage is embraced between the bifurcation.

Pectinate muscles insert at an angle into the circularly arranged myofibers that make up the right atrial vestibule. As noted previously, the cavotricuspid isthmus includes a fibromuscular portion, often with disarray of muscle bundles. In the subepicardium, the vestibule is continuous with the lower bifurcation from the rightward extension of Bachmann's bundle.

Myofibers encircle the prominent muscular rim around the oval foramen. Myofibers in the posterior rim extend posterolaterally to blend into the obliquely aligned myofibers of the intercaval wall. The myofibers in the anterior and anterosuperior rim also combine with fibers in the respective regions of the atria.

Apart from its appendage, the wall of the left atrium is deceptively uniform-looking. It is composed of overlapping myofibers of differing orientations combined with marked variations in wall thickness. In the subendocardium, the vestibular myofibers tend to be circular but blend in with fibers from the septal, posterior, and lateral walls.[1,29] The subendocardium of the anterior wall is made up of a myofiber bundle described by Papez[29] as the septoatrial bundle. This ascends obliquely from the anterior septal raphe and then fans out as it sweeps superiorly toward the right and left pulmonary venous orifices, where it combines

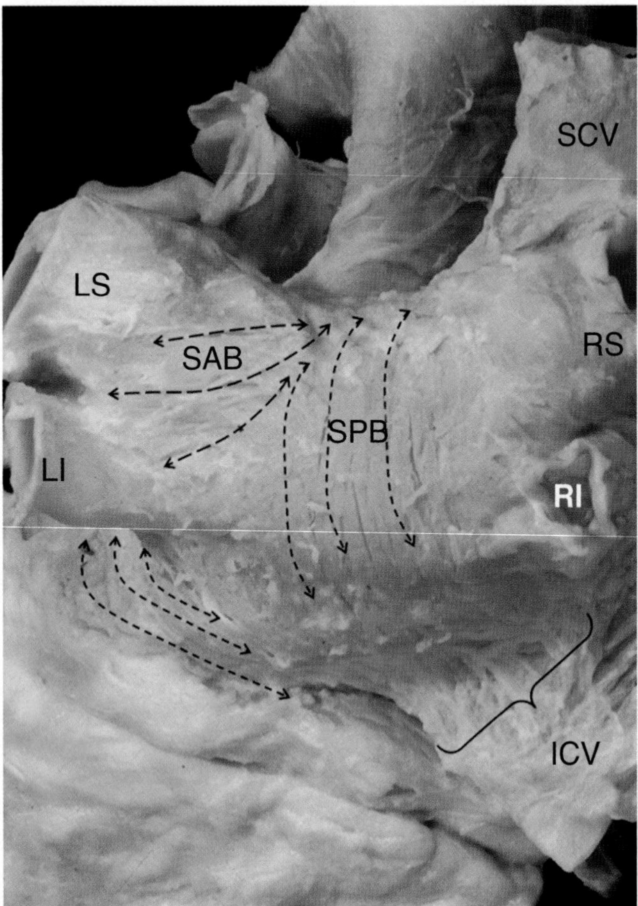

Figure 54-9 This left atrium, viewed from behind has been dissected to display the arrangement of the subepicardial myofibers *(dashed lines)* of the septopulmonary bundle (SPB) and septoatrial bundle (SAB). In this heart, a broad band of interatrial connection *(brace)* is evident in the posteroinferior wall. ICV, inferior caval vein; LI, left inferior pulmonary vein; LS, left superior pulmonary vein; RI, right inferior pulmonary vein; RS, right superior pulmonary vein; SCV, superior caval vein.

with myofibers from a more superficial bundle known as the *septopulmonary bundle*.[1,29] At the crossovers, abrupt changes in fiber orientations are seen. Another branch from the septoatrial bundle turns leftward to surround the os of the appendage. The septopulmonary bundle, superficial to the septoatrial bundle, arises from the anterosuperior part of the septal raphe and passes superiorly mainly in longitudinal orientation and descends in the posterior wall between the left and right pulmonary venous orifices (Fig. 54-9). Branches from this bundle fan out to pass around the venous insertions, continuing as the muscular sleeves. Overlying the septopulmonary bundle, circularly oriented myofibers dominate toward the atrioventricular groove. Arising from the septal raphe, these pass leftward, blending with fibers from Bachmann's bundle, to either side of the entrance of the appendage, to continue into the lateral wall. The structural heterogeneities and discontinuities in fiber orientations through the thickness of the atrial wall, together with regional variations in wall thickness, must be considered among factors that can affect anisotropic conduction. Abrupt changes in orientation of the major bundles may produce functional lines of conduction block.[30]

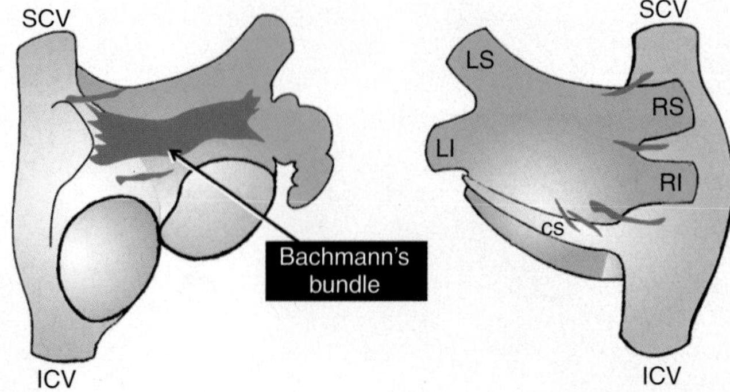

Figure 54-10 Anterior *(left panel)* and posterior *(right panel)* views of the aorta. Muscular interatrial connections *(blue bands)* other than Bachmann's bundle are very common. Cs, coronary sinus; ICV, inferior caval vein; LI, left inferior pulmonary vein; LS, left superior pulmonary vein; RI, right inferior pulmonary vein; RS, right superior pulmonary vein.

Apart from the true septum, other sites of muscular interatrial connection are seen. The most prominent interatrial bundle is Bachmann's bundle, which primarily buttresses the anterior wall of the left atrium. Its myofibers run in parallel with the circularly aligned left atrial myofibers. Bachmann's bundle is not encased by a fibrous tissue sheath. At its margins, especially at its right and left atrial insertions, its myofibers blend into the atrial wall. Other interatrial muscular bridges are common (Fig. 54-10).[1] They vary tremendously in width, number, and location. Occasionally, Bachmann's bundle is small or absent. In these cases, broad muscular bridges may be seen across the inferior or posterior septal raphe to the intercaval area of the right atrium or to the insertion of the inferior caval vein.[1] These bridges provide the potential for inferior breakthrough of sinus impulse.[31,32]

Smaller muscle bridges connecting the right pulmonary veins, or the left atrial wall between the veins, with the right atrium or the muscular sleeve of the superior caval vein are common.[33] Interatrial muscular connections may play a role in perpetuation of atrial fibrillation or give the potential for macroreentry. Targeting these with endocardial ablation may be difficult because they may be located subepicardially and cross the septal raphe some distance away from the true septum. As discussed previously, further bridges connect the musculature of the coronary sinus and vein/ligament of Marshall with the left atrium, providing the potential for interatrial conduction.

Cardiac Conduction System: Sinus Node and Atrioventricular Node

The cardiac conduction tissues in the human heart are composed of specialized myocytes that can be differentiated from ordinary working myocardium with routine histologic staining. Both cardiac nodes are sited in the atria, with ordinary atrial myocardium in between. Atrial myocardium is separated from ventricular myocardium by fibrofatty tissues at the atrioventricular junction, except at the site of the penetrating bundle of His.

The *sinus node* is shaped like a tadpole, with a head section situated anterosuperiorly and a tapering tail that extends for a variable distance inferiorly toward the entrance of the inferior caval vein.[34] In the subepicardium, the long axis of the node runs parallel to the terminal groove. Thus, the fatty tissue of the terminal groove serves as the epicardial landmark, whereas the terminal crest in the anterolateral quadrant of the entrance of the superior caval vein is the endocardial landmark for the nodal head (see Fig. 54-4). The nodal body and tail lie in the terminal crest, at various depths from the endocardium. In the adult, the length of the nodal body is approximately 1 to 2 cm, but the tail portion can be considerably longer.[34]

The sinus node is composed mainly of small, interlacing myocytes. The nodal margins may be discrete, with fibrous separation from atrial myocardium, or, as commonly seen, interdigitate through a transitional zone. In the latter arrangement, prongs of nodal and transitional cells extend into the myocardium of the terminal crest and atrial wall, giving multiple sites of entry and exit (see Fig. 54-4).[34] Occasional prongs can be found extending toward the wall of the superior caval vein. In some hearts, the distal part of the nodal tail appears as clusters of specialized myocytes among fibrofatty tissues and ordinary atrial myocytes in the subendocardium. These may be substrates for ectopic activity, giving rise to inappropriate sinus tachycardia, or they may persist as subsidiary pacemakers even after the sinus node is modified with ablation.

The pioneering work of Tawara[5] a century ago recognized a collection of histologically distinct cells (*knoten*) at the base of the atrial septum. This has subsequently become known as the *atrioventricular node*. As described earlier, the anatomic landmark for the atrioventricular node is the apex of the triangle of Koch. The node comprises a compact portion and a zone of transitional cells that forms the interface between atrial myocardium and compact portion. Thus, the compact node, approximately 5 mm long, 5 mm wide, and 0.8 mm thick in adults, is adjacent to the central fibrous body on one side but is uninsulated on its other sides, allowing contiguity with atrial myocardium. Transitional cells from the left and right sides of the atrial septum reach the left and right margins of the compact node. Further transitional cells approach the compact node from inferiorly and posteriorly from the mouth of the coronary sinus and the eustachian ridge. The right margin of the compact node faces the vestibule of the right atrium. Here, in the subendocardium, an overlay of ordinary myocytes from the atrial wall in front of the oval fossa streams over the layer of transitional cells.

Inferiorly, toward the base of Koch's triangle, the compact area separates into two prongs, usually with the artery supplying the node running in between. The prongs bifurcate toward the tricuspid and mitral annuli, respectively, with variable length. They have been implicated in so-called slow pathway conduction in atrioventricular nodal reentrant tachycardia.[35]

Accessory Atrioventricular Pathways

Any aberrant muscle bundles breaching the tissue plane outside of the regular atrioventricular conduction system are potential substrates for ventricular preexcitation. Accessory atrioventricular pathways most often are found in the parietal atrioventricular junctional areas, including the paraseptal areas. They are hardly ever found in the area of fibrous continuity between the aortic and mitral valves. On the left parietal side, the accessory pathways tend to pass close to the hingeline of the mitral valve. In the right atrioventicular junction, the atrioventricular groove is much deeper than on the left side, allowing the accessory muscle bundles to traverse at any depth. Most of the pathways identified on microscopy have been ordinary myocardium, with only a few reported to contain histologically specialized cells. These threads of musculature are thicker at their atrial origins but branch into finer strands at the ventricular insertions. They are up to 3 mm in width but may be 10 mm or more in length. The pathways may occur singly, or several may be present.

Other types of accessory atrioventricular pathways found in certain circumstances are well recognized. Those located close to the acute margin of the tricuspid orifice may be composed of specialized cells, with the atrial insertion into a node-like structure, forming an "atriofascicular tract." Accessory pathways related to coronary veins usually are in the form of extensive myocardial cuffs around the veins crossing the atrioventricular junction or are expanded as diverticula into the ventricular mass. Others are related to the atrial appendages overlying ventricular masses. Multiple pathways can occur in the setting of so-called Purkinje cell tumors, often found with additional tumors within the ventricles.

Innervation

Recent years have seen increasing interest in the role of the autonomic system in initiation and perpetuation of atrial fibrillation. Vagal denervation procedures have been performed experimentally and in patients with atrial fibrillation.[36] Anatomically, epicardial fat pads containing ganglionated plexuses are present in the vicinity of the insertions of the caval veins and pulmonary vein.[37,38] They are located in five atrial regions described by Armour and colleagues[37] as superior left atrial plexus, posterolateral left atrial plexus, right superior atrial plexus, right posterior atrial plexus, and posteromedial plexus. The last two plexuses fuse medially and extend into the interatrial raphe to innervate the atrioventricular node. The right superior plexus innervates the sinus node. It is thought that extensive lesions created by circumferential ablations not only isolate areas capable of maintaining reentry wavelets or rotors but also affect innervation and vascularization of the atrial tissues to a greater extent.[36,39,40]

Remodeling

With age and with disease, the atrial wall remodels.[41,42-44] Aging is associated with electrophysiologic remodeling with regions of conduction delay, areas of low voltage and changes in biatrial electrophysiology.[45] Atrial dilatation may be the consequence of disorganized contractility, in turn leading to alterations in electrophysiologic properties of the tissues. Structural remodeling often involves remodeling of the extracellar matrix, resulting in increased fibrosis.[42,43] However, increased fibrosis also may be due to replacement fibrosis caused by ischaemic damage resulting from occlusive disease of atrial arteries, a neglected entity.

Dilation of the pulmonary veins may in itself initiate ectopy.[46] The extent of pulmonary venous sleeves is comparable between patients with atrial fibrillation and control subjects. The sleeves in patients with atrial fibrillation, however, more often are discontinuous, with the myocytes hypertrophied and surrounded by more fibrosis.[41,43,46,47]

Conclusions

The structure of the walls and the atrial septum confers a three-dimensional arrangement of muscle bundles and myoarchitecture that allows preferential conduction of electrical activity without the need for tracts of specialized myocytes to link the sinus and atrioventricular nodes. The orifices of the systemic and pulmonary veins, together with the atrioventricular valves and the oval fossa, form the obstacles that separate bands (isthmuses) of atrial walls made of ordinary myocardium. Nevertheless, in bundles of atrial myocardium such as the terminal crest and Bachmann's bundle, the well-aligned arrangement of the myofibers almost certainly facilitates preferential conduction. On the other hand, marked changes in orientation—for example, in subendocardial myofibers—may account for functional lines of block observed during endocardial activation.[30] The heterogeneous transmural myoarchitecture and interatrial connections should not be neglected in developing computer models to study atrial arrhythmias. Added to these factors must be the effect of aging on remodeling of cellular connectivity.[48]

References

1. Ho SY, Anderson RH, Sánchez-Quintana D: Atrial structure and fibres: Morphological basis of atrial conduction. Cardovasc Res 54:325-336, 2002.
2. Betts TR, Ho SY, Sanchez-Quintana D, et al: Characteristics of right atrial activation during coronary sinus pacing. J Cardiovasc Electrophysiol 13:794-800, 2002.
3. Hocini M, Ho SY, Kawara T, et al: Electrical conduction in the canine pulmonary veins: Electrophysiologic and anatomic correlations. Circulation 105: 2442-2448, 2002.
4. Chung CY, Bien H, Entcheva E: The role of cardiac tissue alignment in modulating electrical function. J Cardiovasc Electrophysiol 18:1323-1329, 2007.
5. Tawara S: Das Reizleitungssystem des Säugetierherzens. Jena, Gustav Fischer, 1906. Translated by Suma K, Shimada M: The Conduction System of the Mammalian Heart. Imperial College Press, 2000, pp 1-209.
6. Pappone C, Oral H, Santinelli V, et al: Atrio-esophageal fistula as a complication of percutaneous transcatheter ablation of atrial fibrillation. Circulation 109:2724-2726, 2004.
7. Sánchez-Quintana D, Cabrera JA, Climent V, et al: Anatomic relations between the esophagus and left atrium and relevance for ablation of atrial fibrillation. Circulation 112:1400-1405, 2005.
8. Sánchez-Quintana D, Cabrera JA, Climent V, et al: How close are the phrenic nerves to cardiac structures? Implications for cardiac interventionalists. J Cardiovasc Electrophysiol 16:309-313, 2005.
9. Kholová I, Kautzner J: Morphology of atrial myocardial extensions into human caval veins: A postmortem study in patients with and without atrial fibrillation. Circulation 110:483-488, 2004.
10. Sánchez-Quintana D, Anderson RH, Cabrera JA, et al: The terminal crest: Morphological features relevant to electrophysiology. Heart 88:406-411, 2002.
11. Redfearn DP, Skanes AC, Gula LJ, et al: Cavotricuspid isthmus conduction is dependent on underlying anatomic bundle architecture: Observations using a maximum voltage-guided ablation technique. J Cardiovasc Electrophysiol 17:832-838, 2006.
12. Cabrera JA, Sánchez-Quintana D, Farré J, et al: The inferior right atrial isthmus: Further architectural insights for current and coming ablation technologies. J Cardiovasc Electrophysiol 16:402-408, 2005.
13. Tai CT, Huang JL, Lee PC, et al: High-resolution mapping around the crista terminalis during typical atrial flutter: New insights into mechanisms. J Cardiovasc Electrophysiol 15:406-414, 2004.
14. Liu TY, Tai CT, Huang BH, et al: Functional characterization of the crista terminalis in patients with atrial flutter: Implications for radiofrequency ablation. J Am Coll Cardiol 43:1639-1645, 2004.
15. Chang SL, Tai CT, Lin YJ, et al: The electroanatomic characteristics of the cavotricuspid isthmus: implications for the catheter ablation of atrial flutter. J Cardiovasc Electrophysiol 18:18-22, 2007.
16. Marrouche NF, Natale A, Wazni OM, et al: Left septal atrial flutter: Electrophysiology, anatomy and results of ablation. Circulation 108:2440-2447, 2004.
17. Su P, McCarthy KP, Ho SY: Occluding the left atrial appendage: Anatomical considerations. Heart 2007 May 8 [ePub ahead of print] doi:10.1136/hrt.2006.111989.
18. Cabrera JA, Ho SY, Climent V, et al: The architecture of the left lateral atrial wall: A particular anatomic region with implications for ablation of atrial fibrillation. Eur Heart J 29:356-362, 2008.
19. Makino M, Inoue S, Matsuyama TA, et al: Diverse myocardial extension and autonomic innervation on ligament of Marshall in humans. J Cardiovasc Electrophysiol 17:594-599, 2006.
20. Ulphani JS, Arora R, Cain JH, et al: The ligament of Marshall as a parasympathetic conduit. Am J Physiol Heart Circ Physiol 293:H1629-H1635, 2007.
21. Tan AY, Chou CC, Zhou S, et al: Electrical connections between left superior pulmonary vein, left atrium, and ligament of Marshall: Implications for mechanisms of atrial fibrillation. Am J Physiol Heart Circ Physiol 290:H312-H322, 2006.
22. Wittkampf FHM, van Oosterhout MF, Loh P, et al: Where to draw the mitral isthmus line in catheter ablation of atrial fibrillation: Histological analysis. Eur Heart J 26:689-695, 2005.
23. Maselli D, Guarracino F, Chiaramonti F, et al: Percutaneous mitral annuloplasty: An anatomic study of human coronary sinus and its relation with mitral valve annulus and coronary arteries. Circulation 114:377-380, 2006.
24. Platonov PG, Ivanov V, Ho SY, et al: Left atrial posterior wall thickness in patients with and without atrial fibrillation: Data from 298 consecutive autopsies. J Cardiovasc Electrophysiol 1-4, 2008.
25. Kato R, Lickfett L, Meininger G, et al: Pulmonary vein anatomy in patients undergoing catheter ablation of atrial fibrillation. Lesson learned by use of magnetic resonance imaging. Circulation 107:2004-2010, 2003.
26. Mansour M, Holmvang G, Sosnovik D, et al: Assessment of pulmonary vein anatomic variability by magnetic resonance imaging: Implication for catheter ablation techniques for atrial fibrillation. J Cardiovasc Electrophysiol 15:387-393, 2004.
27. Ahmed J, Sohal S, Malchano ZJ, et al: Three-dimensional analysis of pulmonary venous ostial and antral anatomy: Implications for balloon catheter–based pulmonary vein isolation. J Cardiovasc Electrophysiol 17:251-255, 2006.
28. Ho SY, Cabrera JA, Tran VH, et al: Architecture of the pulmonary veins: Relevance to radiofrequency ablation. Heart 86:265-270, 2001.
29. Papez JW: Heart musculature of the atria. Am J Anat 27:255-277, 1920-21.
30. Markides V, Schilling RJ, Ho SY, et al: Characterization of left atrial activation in the intact human heart. Circulation 107:733-739, 2003.
31. De Ponti R, Ho SY, Salerno-Uriarte JA, et al: Electroanatomic analysis of sinus impulse propagation in normal human atria. J Cardiovasc Electrophysiol 13:1-10, 2002.
32. Platonov PG, Mitrofanova LB, Chireikin LV, et al: Morphology of inter-atrial conduction routes in patients with atrial fibrillation. Europace 4:183-192, 2002.
33. Ho SY: Overview of cardiac anatomy relevant to catheter ablation. In Wilbur D, Packer D, Stevenson W (eds): Catheter Ablation of Cardiac Arrhythmias: Basic Concepts and Clinical Applications, 3rd ed. Blackwell Futura, 2008, pp 3-19.
34. Sánchez-Quintana D, Cabrera JA, Farré J, et al: Sinus node revisited in the era of electroanatomical mapping and catheter ablation. Heart 91:189-194, 2005.
35. Katritsis DG, Becker A: The atrioventricular nodal reentrant tachycardia circuit: A proposal. Heart Rhythm 4:1354-1360, 2007.
36. Chen J, Wasmund SL, Hamdan MH: Back to the future: The role of the autonomic nervous system in atrial fibrillation. Pacing Clin Electrophysiol 29:413-421, 2006.
37. Armour JA, Murphy DA, Yuan BX, et al: Gross and microscopic anatomy of the human intrinsic cardiac nervous system. Anat Rec 247:289-298, 1997.
38. Pauza DH, Skripka V, Pauziene N: Morphology of the intrinsic cardiac nervous system in the dog: A whole-mount study employing histochemical staining with acetylcholinesterase. Cells Tissues Organs 172:297-320, 2002.
39. Mehall JR, Kohut RM Jr, Schneeberger EW, et al: Intraoperative epicardial electrophysiologic mapping and isolation of autonomic ganglionic plexi. Ann Thorac Surg 83:538-541, 2007.
40. Scherlag BJ, Po S: The intrinsic cardiac nervous system and atrial fibrillation. Curr Opin Cardiol 21:51-54, 2006.

41. Becker AE: How structurally normal are human atria in patients with atrial fibrillation? Heart Rhythm 1:627-631, 2004.
42. Anné W, Willems R, Roskams T, et al: Matrix metalloproteinases and atrial remodelling in patients with mitral valve disease and atrial fibrillation. Cardiovasc Res 67:655-666, 2005.
43. Everett TH 4th, Olgin JE: Atrial fibrosis and the mechanisms of atrial fibrillation. Heart Rhythm 4(3 Suppl):S24-S27, 2007.
44. Burstein B, Nattel S: Atrial fibrosis: Mechanisms and clinical relevance in atrial fibrillation. J Am Coll Cardiol 51:802-809, 2008.
45. Kistler PM, Sanders P, Fynn SP, et al: Electrophysiologic and electroanatomic changes in the human atrium associated with age. J Am Coll Cardiol 44:109-116, 2004.
46. Pan NH, Tsao HM, Chang NC, et al: Aging dilates atrium and pulmonary veins: Implications for the genesis of atrial fibrillation. Chest 133:190-196, 2008.
47. Tanaka K, Zlochiver S, Vikstrom KL, et al: Spatial distribution of fibrosis governs fibrillation wave dynamics in the posterior left atrium during heart failure. Cardiovasc Res 101:839-847, 2007.
48. Spach MS, Heidlage JF, Dolber PC, et al: Mechanism of origin of conduction disturbances in aging human atrial bundles: Experimental and model study. Heart Rhythm 4:175-185, 2007.

54

Atrial Flutter 55

ALBERT L. WALDO AND FELIPE ATIENZA

CHAPTER OUTLINE

Atrial flutter was described by Jolly and Ritchie in 1911.[1] It was not until recent decades, however, that major advances were made concerning its mechanism, diagnosis, and management. As a result of these advances, a sophisticated understanding of the mechanisms of atrial flutter has now been achieved, new techniques to diagnose atrial flutter have evolved, and significant improvements in acute and long-term therapy of atrial flutter have become available. This chapter reviews these subjects.

Mechanism of Atrial Flutter

For a long time, a controversy existed regarding whether atrial flutter was caused by rapid firing of a single focus or by some sort of reentrant excitation; when triggered activity was recognized, it was thought that perhaps this rhythm might be caused by either early or delayed afterdepolarizations. The overwhelming evidence now indicates that atrial flutter results from reentry located primarily in the right atrium.

Insights from Animal Models of Atrial Flutter

Several animal models of atrial flutter have been developed over the years. In the first studies by Lewis and coworkers,[1] stable atrial flutter was infrequently induced in the normal canine heart by applying faradic current. Then atrial electrograms were recorded sequentially from a few selected sites. On the basis of these studies and on vector analysis of electrocardiograms (ECGs) in patients, these investigators concluded that atrial flutter was caused by reentry, in which the reentrant wavefront circulated around both the superior and the inferior venae cavae, presumably (although not specifically mentioned) with an area of block between them. It was clear, however, that induction of "stable" atrial flutter in the normal canine heart usually was not possible.

Subsequently, Rosenbleuth and Garcia-Ramos,[1] apparently recognizing that stable conduction block between the venae cavae was necessary to permit reliable induction of sustained atrial flutter in the normal canine heart, created a crush lesion between the superior and the inferior vena cava. Then atrial flutter was readily induced, and data from limited, sequential site mapping studies were interpreted as showing that the induced atrial flutter resulted from reentry around the venae cavae and the obstacle created by the intercaval crush lesion. More recent studies by Frame and associates[1] included not only an intercaval surgical lesion but also a surgical lesion extending toward the right atrial appendage to form a Y-shaped lesion. Then, reliably induced, stable atrial flutter was shown to be caused by clockwise or counterclockwise circus movement around the tricuspid valve annulus.

Several other experimental canine models of atrial flutter that result from right atrial free-wall lesions have been described.[1] In these instances, the reentrant excitation wavefront was shown always to circulate around the central area of block created by the lesion, although a limitation was that no maps of the atrial septum were obtained. These models are of interest for several reasons, but in particular because of the demonstrated or likely presence of clinical counterparts in patients who have undergone open heart surgical correction of congenital lesions and perhaps even some acquired lesions. For instance, it is well recognized that the postoperative incidence of chronic atrial flutter is very high among patients who have had a Mustard, Senning, or Fontan procedure.[1,2] Several groups of investigators[3-6] have now shown that although the reentrant circuit may travel around a lesion (lesion reentry) caused by an incision or a suture line, in a majority of instances of intra-atrial reentrant tachycardia after surgical repair of congenital heart lesions, the reentrant circuit includes the critical isthmus (so-called flutter isthmus) between the tricuspid valve annulus, the inferior vena cava, the eustachian ridge, and the coronary sinus ostium, much like that during classic atrial flutter.

Of importance, Tomita and colleagues[7] have shown that in the normal canine heart, a sufficiently long incision in the right atrial free wall may develop a functional extension of the line of fixed block to one or both of the venae cavae. When such extension occurs, the atrial flutter mechanism is that of typical or reverse typical atrial flutter—that is, the reentrant wavefront travels up the septum and down the right atrial free wall, or vice versa. This seems to explain how the surgical atriotomy or placement of suture lines that is a part of the surgical procedure creates a line of block between the venae cavae such that the substrate for classical atrial flutter is produced. Of course, reentry around a surgical incision or suture line also is possible (lesion reentry).

Most recently, Cox's group showed that atrial flutter may be induced in a canine model[8] or may develop spontaneously in patients[9] after a procedure in which the pulmonary veins are detached en bloc and then reanastomosed. In these instances, the atrial flutter reentrant circuit circulates in the left atrium around the created surgical lesion. Atrial flutter also is a well-recognized complication of the surgical maze procedure to treat atrial fibrillation when a line or lines of block created as part of the procedure are not continuous or do not extend to a boundary.[10] Reentry around an incomplete line of block is then possible. With the advent of radiofrequency ablation of atrial fibrillation, one of the consequences has been an incidence of lesion reentry atrial flutter, principally in the left atrium, as a result of inadvertent creation of gaps in otherwise contiguous lesions made to isolate the pulmonary veins, the most common location of the triggers that induce and can even maintain atrial fibrillation.[11,12] Another relatively common location of left atrial flutter secondary to ablative lesions created in an effort to prevent atrial fibrillation is the mitral valve annulus.[11,13] In such instances, atrial flutter is more likely to be the result of ablation lines in the left atrium made in addition to those for pulmonary vein isolation. The reported incidence of left atrial flutter after ablation of atrial fibrillation is at least 10% and may be as high as 40%.[11,13]

Models that do not require primary atrial lesions also have been described. The acetylcholine model studies of Allessie and coworkers in the canine heart[1] have shown that atrial flutter caused by atrial reentry can occur at numerous places in either atrium and can occur in the absence of an anatomic obstacle. Of note, the cycle length of the reentrant circuit in this model was uniformly short, most often 100 ms or less, so it was suggested that this model may represent type II atrial flutter. Perhaps even more important, this also would provide an explanation for the observation that atrial flutter of very short cycle length may serve as a driver that then generates atrial fibrillation in patients,[14,15] the fibrillation resulting because large parts of the atria cannot respond 1 for 1 (i.e., 1:1) to the short cycle length of the driver.[15] Studies in several other models of atrial flutter in the canine heart[1,16] have indicated that the reentrant circuit is confined to the right atrium and principally to the right atrial free wall. Studies in the sterile pericarditis model, which included systematic mapping of the atrial septum,[1] point to the septum as a critical component of the reentrant circuit characterized by a single loop reentry (activation up the septum and down the right atrial free wall or vice versa) or a figure-of-eight reentry (presence of the just-described reentrant circuit along with a functionally determined reentrant circuit confined to the right atrial free wall). During figure-of-eight reentry, each reentrant circuit shares in common activation of the pectinate muscle region, so that the right atrial free-wall circuit demonstrates clockwise or counterclockwise activation, depending on the direction of activation of the pectinate muscle region.

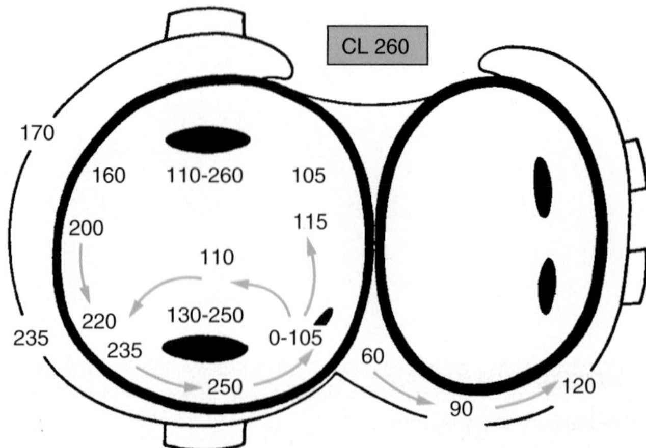

Figure 55-1 Typical atrial flutter activation map. *Arrows* indicate the general direction of the circuit. CL, cycle length (in ms). (From Cosio FG, Lopez-Gil M, Goicolea A, et al: Radiofrequency ablation of the inferior vena cava–tricuspid valve isthmus in common atrial flutter. Am J Cardiol 71:705-709, 1993.)

Atrial Flutter in Humans

For a long time, only limited mapping studies of atrial flutter in humans were available.[1] Even so, studies by Puech and colleagues[1] suggested that the entire duration of the atrial flutter cycle length could be explained by reentrant activation in the right atrium alone, including activation of the atrial septum and the right atrial free wall. The subsequent demonstration in humans of transient entrainment and interruption of atrial flutter[1] provided strong evidence that atrial flutter is an intra-atrial reentrant rhythm with an excitable gap. Subsequently, more detailed mapping studies[1] demonstrated that the reentrant circuit in atrial flutter in humans usually involves reentrant excitation in the right atrium, with the impulse traveling in a caudocranial direction in the interatrial septum and a craniocaudal direction in the right atrial free wall (Fig. 55-1), much as originally suggested by Puech and colleagues.[1] The studies of Cosio and coworkers[1] and Olshansky and colleagues[1] also provided evidence that an area of slow conduction is present in the posteroinferior aspect of the reentrant circuit, and that the central area of block around which the reentrant wavefront circulates includes an anatomic component, the venae cavae, and a functional component between the venae cavae in the region of the crista terminalis. Further studies by Cosio and coworkers[1] have shown that this reentrant circuit can be operative in a reverse direction, producing reverse typical atrial flutter.[17]

Subsequent studies[18-20] using entrainment mapping techniques and mapping with intracavitary echocardiography techniques have further refined the reentrant circuit. Thus, it is now recognized that the tricuspid valve ring serves as one boundary of the atrial flutter reentrant circuit, and the venae cavae with a line of block between them serves as another boundary of the reentrant circuit. Friedman and colleagues[21] suggested that this line of block was in the sinus venosus region. Regardless, in the atrial flutter reentrant circuit, a critical isthmus exists bounded by the tricuspid valve annulus, the inferior vena caval orifice, the eustachian ridge, and the coronary sinus ostium.[18-20,22] It is this flutter isthmus that is the target of ablation techniques to cure typical and reverse typical atrial flutter. Of note, studies by Kinder and colleagues[23] suggest that this flutter isthmus was not an area of slow conduction. Furthermore, studies from investigators in Bordeaux, France, using three-dimensional mapping techniques, have confirmed the course of the atrial flutter reentrant circuit and refined it still further, demonstrating that the superior turnaround or pivot point involves the superior vena cava.[24]

It also is well established that in some patients in whom persistent or recurrent atrial flutter is noted long after open heart surgery, atrial flutter is caused by reentrant excitation around a surgical incision (lesion reentry) created to permit the surgical repair by the surgeon.[2] Alternatively, if a long enough lesion is made at the time of surgery in the right atrial free wall so that it provides a sufficient line of block between the superior and inferior venae cavae, it will permit development of atrial flutter of the classic type—that is, reentrant activation up the atrial septum and down the right atrial free wall, or vice versa.[3-6] Heart transplantation constitutes another interesting model of surgically induced typical atrial flutter. In this model, the suture line of the atrioatrial anastomosis forms the posterior barrier of the reentrant circuit, whereas the tricuspid annulus represents the anterior boundary, enabling either counterclockwise or clockwise activation of the donor-derived portion of the right atrium (Fig. 55-2). Ablation in the donor-derived portion of the isthmus between the tricuspid valve and the atrial anastomosis near the inferior vena cava creates bidirectional conduction block and can successfully cure this arrhythmia.[25]

Figure-of-eight reentry in the atria also has been demonstrated in patients, especially after cardiac surgery, congenital heart disease repair, and atrial fibrillation ablation.[26-30] It is likely to affect more patients than is currently appreciated, largely because conventional catheter mapping techniques have not had the resolution to demonstrate it. Today, however,

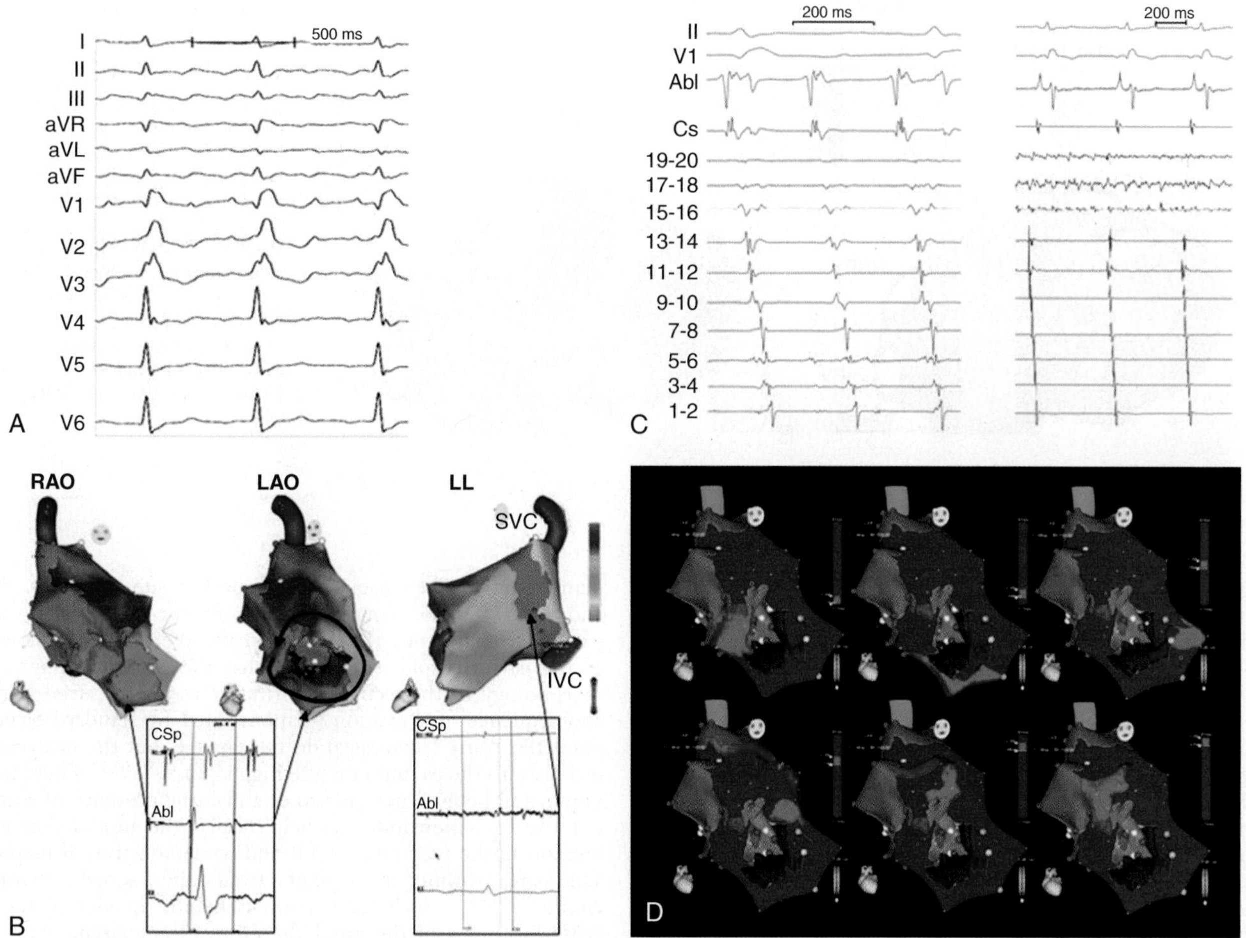

Figure 55-2 Electroanatomic mapping of typical atrial flutter in the transplanted heart. **A,** Surface electrocardiogram shows a characteristic "sawtooth" atrial activation pattern in leads II, III, and aVF. **B,** The activation map shows counterclockwise wavefront propagation around a reentrant circuit bounded anteriorly by the tricuspid annulus and posteriorly by extensive areas of scar in the connection with the recipient atrium; *red* is the arbitrary zone of earliest activation, and purple is the latest. *Dark gray areas* represent zones of low voltage (less than 0.1 mV), which correspond to the connecting orifice scar, and *light gray area* corresponds to the recipient atrium. **C,** *Left*: The sequence of intracardiac electrograms recorded along the tricuspid annulus of the right donor atrium supports this observation. *Right*, intracardiac recordings from bipoles 15 to 20 demonstrate atrial fibrillation in the recipient atrium. **D,** The temporal sequence of atrial activation, in which *blue* represents unactivated regions and *red* represents the advancing activation front. The advancing wavefront shows counterclockwise propagation around the reentrant circuit, with craniocaudal activation of the lateral wall, followed by that of the cavo–tricuspid isthmus, and caudocranial septal activation that proceeds anterior to the recipient superior vena cava to descend again toward the lateral wall. A radiofrequency ablation line of block at the cavo–tricuspid isthmus level interrupted the typical atrial flutter in the donor right atrium, whereas the recipient atrium remained in atrial fibrillation (**C,** *right panel*).

comprehensive three-dimensional electroanatomic mapping enables the identification of complex reentrant circuits in an increasing number of patients. Characteristically, in double-loop figure-of-eight reentry associated with a right atriotomy, one loop travels by way of the cavotricuspid isthmus up the atrial septum and then down the right atrial free wall anterior to the atriotomy (counterclockwise reentry), whereas the other loop travels around the atriotomy (clockwise reentry), with both loops sharing the pathway anterior to the atriotomy.[26] Other figure-of-eight reentrant circuit locations are possible, either in the left atrium (Fig. 55-3) or even involving both atria.[28-30] Moreover, multiple coexisting loops also have been described.[28]

Variations of atrial flutter, including atypical atrial flutter and left atrial flutter, have now been identified and variously characterized in patients.[17,26,27,31-35] They include double-wave reentry (two wavefronts traveling simultaneously around the typical atrial flutter reentrant circuit), lower loop reentry (the reentrant wavefront uses the atrial flutter isthmus, activates the posterior right atrium, and then skirts the inferior vena cava, so that it is in essence reentry using the lower portion of the typical atrial flutter reentrant circuit), atrial septal reentry, upper loop reentry (flutter isthmus–independent reentry involving the upper right atrium), and reentry around a functional line of block in the right atrial free wall.

Finally, an interesting point is that the onset of atrial flutter is almost always through a transitional rhythm of atrial fibrillation.[1,14,15] As indicated by mapping studies,[1,15] it is during the atrial fibrillation that the functional components required to complete the reentrant circuit form. In particular, it is the development of a functional line of block between the inferior and superior venae cavae that seems most critical.[15]

Entrainment of Atrial Flutter

Transient entrainment of a tachycardia was first described during the study of atrial flutter in patients after open heart

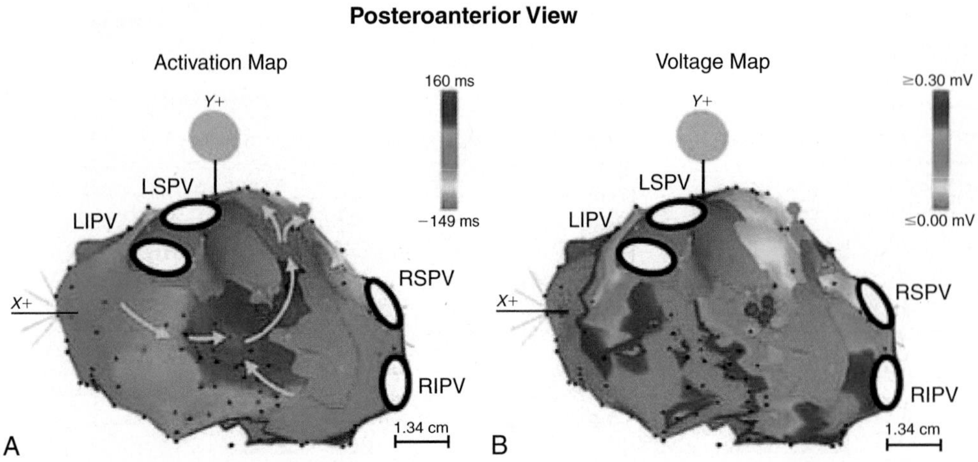

Figure 55-3 Illustration of dual-loop left atrial circuit in a patient with prior mitral valve repair. **A** and **B,** Demonstration of a protected isthmus between two posterior electrically silent areas (in *gray*) around the pulmonary veins, and a low-amplitude area within the isthmus. Radiofrequency pulses (*brown tags*) terminated the arrhythmia and blocked the isthmus. LIPV, left inferior pulmonary vein; LSPV, left superior pulmonary vein; RIPV, right inferior pulmonary vein; RSPV, right superior pulmonary vein. (**A** and **B,** From Ouyang F, Ernst S, Vogtmann T, et al: Characterization of reentrant circuits in left atrial macroreentrant tachycardia. Circulation 105:1934-1942, 2002.)

surgery.[1] As summarized recently,[36] during transient entrainment of a reentrant tachycardia, the wavefront from each pacing impulse enters into the excitable gap of the reentry circuit and travels bidirectionally (Figs. 55-4 to 55-6). One wavefront travels antidromically—that is, in the opposite direction of the circulating wavefront of the spontaneous tachycardia—where it collides with the orthodromic wavefront of the preceding beat. The other travels orthodromically—that is, in the same direction as the circulating wavefront of the spontaneous tachycardia. The orthodromic wavefront both continues the tachycardia and resets it to the pacing rate. This explanation, universal for transient entrainment of any tachycardia caused by reentry with an excitable gap, has now been confirmed in studies using in vivo mapping techniques during ventricular tachycardia and atrial flutter in canine models.[1]

The demonstration of any one of four criteria, presented in Table 55-1, establishes the presence of transient entrainment and thus the presence of reentry with an excitable gap. Transient entrainment of a tachycardia may occur, however, but it may not be possible to demonstrate any of the transient entrainment criteria. This is *concealed* entrainment.[1,36] This can result when pacing is performed from a site that is orthodromically distal to the area of slow conduction in the reentry circuit, but then one must also show that transient entrainment can be demonstrated when pacing from another site (see Figs. 55-4 and 55-5).[1] Also, concealed entrainment may occur with pacing directly from an isthmus in the reentrant circuit, such as the cavotricuspid isthmus, so that the electrocardiographic morphology of the tachycardia (flutter waves for atrial flutter) and sequence of activation (demonstrated by standard electrogram recording techniques) do not change, but the tachycardia increases to the pacing rate (see Fig. 55-6).[18,20,36,37] These techniques can be used not only to establish the presence of reentry but also to demonstrate and help localize the area of slow conduction in the reentrant circuit and to demonstrate if mapping sites are within or distant from the actual reentrant circuit.[18,20,36,37] Such localization is helpful in identifying the critical isthmus in the atrial flutter reentrant circuit with use of ablation techniques to cure atrial flutter.[1,18,20,36,37]

Clinical Features of Atrial Flutter

Incidence and Clinical Setting

The incidence of atrial flutter is uncertain. It is said to be more common in men than in women, with a reported male-to-female ratio of 4.7:1.[1] Atrial flutter usually is paroxysmal, lasting for

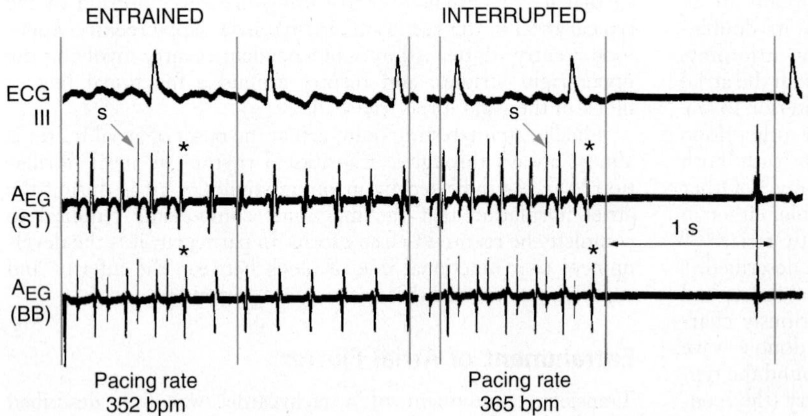

Figure 55-4 Demonstration of concealed entrainment of atrial flutter. Electrocardiogram lead III recorded simultaneously with bipolar atrial electrograms (A_{EG}) from the sulcus terminalis (ST) and Bachmann bundle (BB) recording sites at the termination of 30 seconds of rapid atrial pacing (*left*, 352 beats per minute; *right*, 365 beats per minute) from the posteroinferior left atrium in a patient with spontaneous atrial flutter rate of 320 beats per minute. Comparison of events during rapid pacing and its termination at each rate fails to show any evident transient entrainment criteria, despite that the atrial flutter was interrupted by rapid pacing at 365 beats per minute. *Asterisks* indicate the last captured beat at each recording site. S, stimulus artifact. Time lines are at 1-second intervals.

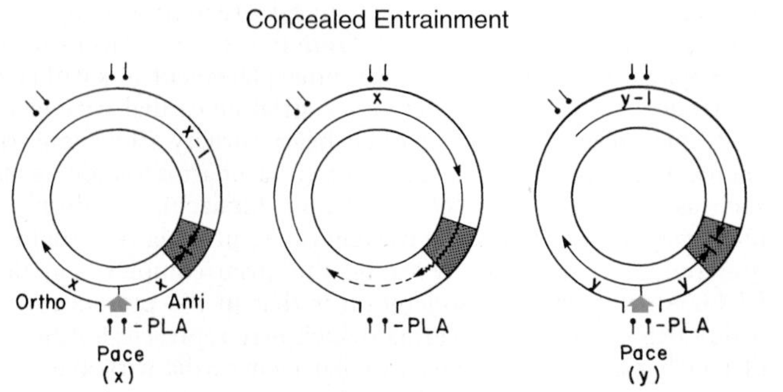

Figure 55-5 Diagrammatic representation of concealed entrainment of atrial flutter. *Left*, The *large arrow* indicates the pacing impulse (x) (e.g., at a rate of 352 beats per minute, as in Fig. 55-4) from the atrial pacing site (the posteroinferior left atrium [PLA]) entering into the reentry circuit, where it is conducted orthodromically (Ortho) and antidromically (Anti). The antidromic wavefront blocks, presumably in the area of slow conduction. The orthodromic wavefront of the preceding beat (x−1) also blocks in the area of slow conduction because it encounters the refractoriness created by the antidromic wavefront from pacing impulse (x). The orthodromic wavefront from the pacing impulse (x) continues the tachycardia, resetting it to the pacing rate. *Center*, The orthodromic wavefront from the last pacing impulse (x) (e.g., at a rate of 352 beats per minute, as in Fig. 55-4) is conducted completely around the reentry circuit, resulting in resumption of the atrial flutter. This occurs because the latter wavefront now conducts through the area of slow conduction because it is not blocked by the refractoriness created by the antidromic wavefront of a subsequent pacing impulse. No criteria of transient entrainment are demonstrable. *Right*, The *large arrow* indicates the pacing impulse (y) (e.g., at a rate of 365 beats per minute, as in Fig. 55-4) from the same atrial pacing site entering into the reentry circuit, where it is conducted orthodromically and antidromically. As expected, the antidromic wavefront blocks in the area of slow conduction. However, the orthodromic wavefront from the previous paced beat (y − 1) also blocks, presumably in the area of slow conduction, but this occurs independently of either collision with or refractoriness secondary to the previous antidromic wavefront. Because both the antidromic and orthodromic wavefronts of the same beat are blocked, the atrial flutter is interrupted. This is not appreciable from the electrocardiogram, however, because none of the transient entrainment criteria have been evident (predictable because pacing has been performed from a site orthodromically distal to the area of slow conduction). Only termination of pacing will permit knowledge of whether interruption of the atrial flutter has occurred (see Fig. 55-4).

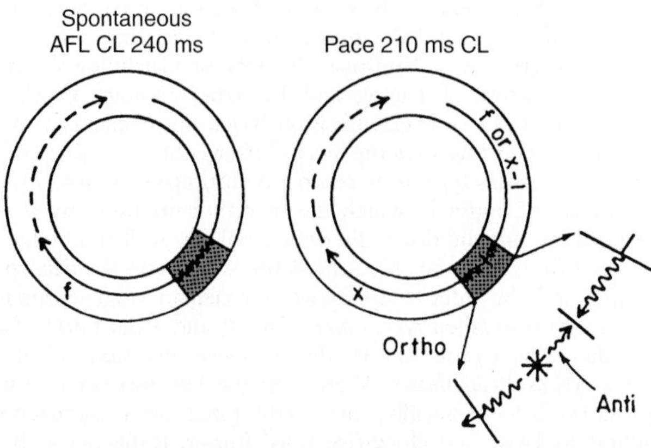

Figure 55-6 Concealed entrainment of atrial flutter when pacing from a site in the reentrant circuit, which is both an isthmus and an area of slow conduction. *Left*, Diagram shows the reentrant circuit during spontaneous type I atrial flutter (AFL) at a cycle length (CL) of 240 ms. The f represents the circulating wavefront of the atrial flutter. *Right*, Diagram shows pacing at a CL of 210 ms from a site *(asterisk)* in the area of slow conduction. An enlargement of the area of slow conduction is shown at *lower right*. Note that the antidromic (Anti) wavefront from the pacing impulse blocks in the area of slow conduction. The orthodromic (Ortho) wavefront (x) from the pacing impulse activates the atria exactly as during spontaneous atrial flutter. The orthodromic wavefront from the previous beat, either a spontaneous atrial flutter beat (f) or the previous atrial paced beat (x−1), blocks in the area of slow conduction. Alternatively, the orthodromic wavefront of the previous beat may collide with the antidromic wavefront of the paced beat. Because the antidromic wavefront from the pacing impulse activates only a small area and therefore has no effect on the electrocardiogram, and because the atria are activated at the pacing CL by the orthodromic wavefront of the pacing impulse just as during spontaneous atrial flutter, concealed entrainment has occurred. (From Waldo AL: Atrial flutter: Entrainment characteristics. J Cardiovasc Electrophysiol 8:337-352, 1997.)

Table 55-1 Criteria to Establish the Presence of Transient Entrainment

1. The demonstration of constant fusion beats in the electrocardiogram (ECG) during the period of rapid pacing at a constant rate except for the last captured beat, which is entrained but not fused (i.e., the last entrained beat demonstrates the electrocardiographic morphology of the spontaneous tachycardia)
2. The demonstration of *progressive fusion*—that is, constant fusion beats in the ECG during rapid pacing at any constant rate, but with different degrees of constant fusion at different rapid rates
3. The demonstration that interruption of the tachycardia is associated with localized conduction block to a site or sites for one beat, followed by subsequent activation of that site or sites from a different direction, manifested by a change in morphology of the electrogram at the blocked sites, and with a shorter conduction time
4. The demonstration of a change in conduction time and electrogram morphology at one recording site during pacing from another site at two different constant pacing rates, each of which is faster than the spontaneous rate of the tachycardia but fails to interrupt it (electrogram equivalent of progressive fusion)

variable periods of time. It rarely is a persistent rhythm, because it usually evolves to atrial fibrillation if it lasts for any prolonged period. A unique population in which atrial flutter commonly occurs consists of those patients in the first week after open heart surgery. In this population, an approximately 30% incidence of supraventricular tachyarrhythmias has been reported; approximately one third of these cases are atrial flutter.[1] Moreover, atrial flutter is commonly associated with atrial fibrillation.[1,14,15,38] In fact, the two rhythms often are noted to occur in the same patient, and the rhythm disturbance may even be seen to go back and forth between the two. It is also seen in association with chronic obstructive pulmonary disease, mitral or tricuspid valve disease, thyrotoxicosis, and after repair of congenital cardiac lesions in which the atria, most often the right atrium, are incised to a considerable extent, such as with the Mustard, Senning, or Fontan procedure.[1-6] It also is associated with enlargement of the atria for any reason, especially the right atrium.[1,8] Lesion-related atrial flutter, such as that secondary to cardiac surgery, either congenital or acquired, and atrial fibrillation ablation is becoming remarkably common.[11,12,25,26,28-30]

Types of Atrial Flutter

Atrial flutter is a rapid, regular atrial rhythm, with a rate range from approximately 240 to 340 or 350 beats per minute, and is caused by atrial reentry.[1] In view of all of the new information about atrial flutter and the profusion of terms that have been used to describe it, a European Society of Cardiology/North American Society of Pacing and Electrophysiology Working Group[17] offered a new classification based on mechanism. Any reentrant circuit that uses the atrial flutter isthmus as part of its circuit constitutes typical or reverse typical atrial flutter. Thus, classical atrial flutter in which the reentrant impulse travels up the atrial septum and down the right atrial free wall and includes the atrial flutter isthmus (i.e., the isthmus between the tricuspid annulus and the inferior vena cava–eustachian ridge–coronary sinus ostium) is called *typical atrial flutter*, and atrial flutter that uses the same circuit but in the opposite direction is called *reverse typical atrial flutter*. Viewed in the left anterior oblique projection fluoroscopically, these arrhythmias are recognized as counterclockwise and clockwise atrial flutter, respectively. It is thought that 90% of atrial flutters fall into the typical or reverse typical category. Atrial flutter in which the reentrant circuit is confined to the left atrium is called *left atrial flutter*. Reentry around an incisional line of block in the rate range of atrial flutter is called *lesion atrial reentry*. All other forms of reentrant atrial tachycardia in the rate range of atrial flutter that are not described by the above are called *atypical atrial flutter*.

Management of Atrial Flutter

Diagnosis

Whenever atrial flutter is suspected, the diagnosis should be clearly established before initiation of therapy, unless the tachycardia is clinically life-threatening. Atrial flutter usually can be diagnosed from the ECG by identifying flutter waves in the ECG, principally in leads II, III, A_{VF}, and V_1. Flutter waves are atrial complexes of constant morphology, polarity, and cycle length in a rate range from 240 to 340 beats per minute.[1,17] In typical atrial flutter, in the inferior leads (II, III, and A_{VF}), the flutter waves usually are primarily negative and have the morphologic appearance of a picket fence (see Figs. 55-2 and 55-4). In reverse typical atrial flutter, the flutter waves usually are positive in the inferior leads.[1]

Atrioventricular (AV) conduction during atrial flutter commonly is 2:1 or 4:1, but it may be irregular and, rarely, may even be 1:1. The 1:1 ratio most commonly is seen in patients with Wolff-Parkinson-White syndrome, in which the accessory AV connection has a short antegrade effective refractory period. However, 1:1 AV conduction also may be present in patients with a short PR interval (less than 0.12 second) during sinus rhythm. In addition, it may become 1:1 during exertion or in the presence of therapy with catecholamines, sympathomimetic amines, or phenytoin administered as therapy for another clinical problem. Both the atrial flutter rate and ventricular response rate may be affected by the presence of antiarrhythmic drug therapy. Thus, if the patient is taking a class I antiarrhythmic agent, the atrial flutter rate may slow considerably, especially if the drug is a class IC antiarrhythmic agent, in which case the atrial rate may be as slow as 180 to 200 beats per minute. With the slower atrial flutter rate, AV conduction is more likely to be 1:1, resulting in a faster ventricular rate than before drug administration.

If the diagnosis of atrial flutter is not clear from a standard ECG and if circumstances permit, any of a number of vagal maneuvers (carotid sinus pressure, Valsalva maneuver, invoking the diving reflex) can be used to produce transient increased AV block while the ECG is recorded. This approach should reveal the atrial flutter complexes if present. Then, if the diagnosis remains unclear, either of the following diagnostic maneuvers may be used if permitted by the clinical situation: (1) An electrogram may be recorded directly from the atria by placement of an esophageal electrode, by transvenous placement of a catheter electrode, or by use of a temporary atrial epicardial wire electrode placed at the time of open heart surgery (the mode of choice after open heart surgery); or (2) a pharmacologic agent such as adenosine, esmolol, verapamil, diltiazem, or edrophonium may be administered intravenously to prolong AV conduction transiently, thereby revealing the atrial complexes in the ECG. An important consideration is that in the presence of a wide QRS complex tachycardia (which may represent a ventricular tachycardia or a supraventricular tachycardia with aberrant ventricular conduction or AV conduction over an accessory AV connection), drug intervention to establish the diagnosis of atrial flutter is fraught with danger, and usually it is contraindicated; rather, direct current cardioversion usually is indicated.

Treatment of Acute Atrial Flutter

When the diagnosis of atrial flutter is made, three choices are available to restore sinus rhythm: (1) antiarrhythmic drug therapy (intravenous ibutilide[1,39]), (2) direct current cardioversion, or (3) rapid atrial pacing to interrupt atrial flutter.[1] In large measure, the treatment depends on the clinical status of the patient, as well as both the clinical availability and ease of applying the therapy. Direct current cardioversion requires administration of an anesthetic agent, making this choice undesirable in the patient who presents with atrial flutter after having recently eaten or the patient who has severe chronic obstructive lung disease. In such patients, treatment with an antiarrhythmic agent or rapid atrial pacing to interrupt atrial flutter, or with agents to slow the ventricular response rate, is appropriate. For the patient in whom atrial flutter develops after open heart surgery, use of the temporary atrial epicardial wire electrodes to perform rapid atrial pacing to restore sinus rhythm is the treatment of choice.[1]

Whenever rapid control of the ventricular response rate to atrial flutter is desirable, it usually can be readily accomplished using either an intravenous calcium channel–blocking agent (verapamil or diltiazem) or an intravenous beta-blocker (esmolol). If prompt conversion to sinus rhythm is required, either direct current cardioversion or rapid atrial pacing must be used, because conversion with antiarrhythmic drug therapy usually takes time (up to 1 or 2 hours with ibutilide and up to twice that with the oral agents). Several caveats are in order regarding the use of ibutilide: (1) Serum potassium should be normal, preferably 4 mEq/L or more; (2) the QTc interval should be 440 ms or less; (3) its use in patients with ventricular dysfunction is not advised; and (4) torsade de pointes, usually brief and of no clinical consequence, may occur, but occasionally cardioversion or defibrillation and even intravenous administration of magnesium may be required.[39] Antiarrhythmic drug therapy also may be initiated before the performance of either direct current cardioversion or rapid atrial pacing (1) to enhance the efficacy of rapid atrial pacing in restoring sinus rhythm (use of quinidine, procainamide, disopyramide, or ibutilide[1,40]) or (2) to suppress recurrent atrial flutter after effective direct current cardioversion (use of a class IA, IC, or III antiarrhythmic agent).

Techniques of Rapid Atrial Pacing to Interrupt Atrial Flutter

Several atrial pacing techniques are available and effective.[1] Whenever possible, pacing should be performed from the high right atrium, because the appearance of positive atrial complexes (flutter waves) in ECG lead II is the hallmark of interruption of atrial flutter.[1] One can use either the ramp atrial pacing technique (Fig. 55-7) (bipolar atrial pacing is initiated at a rate about 10 beats per minute faster than the spontaneous atrial rate, and

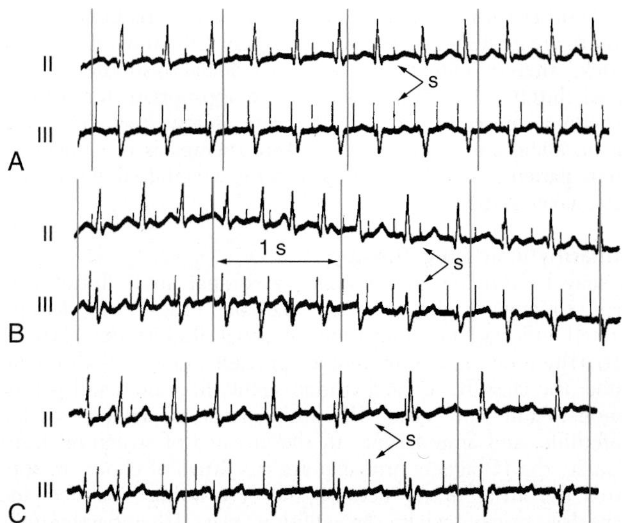

Figure 55-7 A to C, Continuous traces of electrocardiogram leads II and III during the period of overdrive pacing of type I atrial flutter in a patient whose spontaneous atrial rate was 294 beats per minute (cycle length of 204 ms). In this patient, overdrive atrial pacing was initiated at a cycle length of 194 ms, and then the ramp pacing technique (in which the pacing rate is gradually increased until the atrial complexes become positive and then is decreased) was used. As the pacing cycle length was decreased from 171 to 157 ms (**A**), the atrial complexes became positive in both leads. The atrial pacing cycle length then was increased; that is, the pacing rate was decreased (**B**, **C**). Note that as the pacing cycle length became longer than that of the spontaneous atrial flutter (end of **B**), the atrial complexes remained positive. As the atrial pacing cycle length was further increased (**C**), the atrial flutter did not recur. In fact, atrial capture was maintained as the pacing cycle length was increased to 545 ms, a pacing rate of 110 beats per minute *(not shown)*. Thus, using the ramp atrial pacing technique, the atrial flutter initially was transiently entrained and finally was interrupted by rapid pacing. Time lines are at 1-second intervals. S, stimulus artifact. (**A** to **C**, Modified from Waldo AL, MacLean WAH, Karp RB, et al: Entrainment and interruption of atrial flutter with atrial pacing: Studies in man following open heart surgery. Circulation 56:737-745, 1977.)

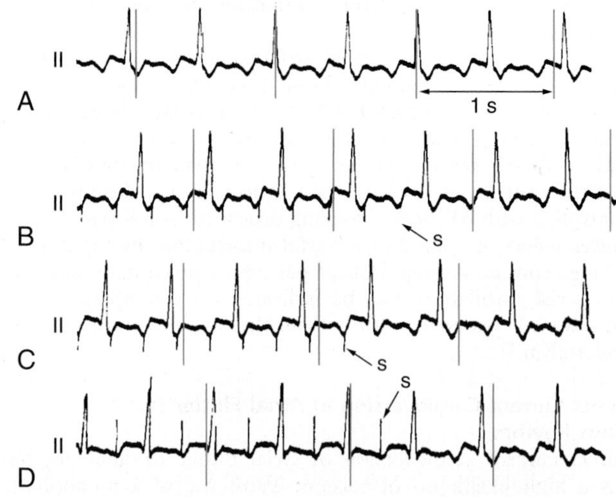

Figure 55-8 Electrocardiogram lead II recorded from a patient with classical (type I) atrial flutter (atrial cycle length of 264 ms) (**A**) and at the end of 30 seconds of rapid atrial pacing from a high right atrial site at a cycle length of 254 ms (**B**), at a cycle length of 242 ms (**C**), and at a cycle length of 232 ms (**D**). The atrial flutter was transiently entrained at each pacing rate. Note that in comparing the morphology of the atrial complexes during atrial pacing at each cycle length, especially comparing the atrial complexes during atrial pacing in **D** with those in **A** and **B**, progressive fusion has occurred. S, stimulus artifact. Time lines are at 1-second intervals. (**A** to **D**, Modified from Waldo AL, MacLean WAH, Karp RB, et al: Entrainment and interruption of atrial flutter with atrial pacing: Studies in man following open heart surgery. Circulation 56:737-745, 1977.)

then is gradually increased; when the atrial complexes in ECG lead II become positive, either atrial pacing may be abruptly terminated or the pacing rate may be rapidly slowed to a desirable atrial pacing rate) or the constant rate pacing technique (Figs. 55-8 and 55-9) (rapid atrial pacing is generally best initiated at a rate 120% to 130% of the spontaneous atrial flutter rate and continued for 15 to 30 seconds, or until the atrial complexes in ECG lead II become positive; then, pacing is either abruptly terminated or rapidly slowed to a desirable atrial pacing rate; this is repeated, increasing the atrial pacing rate in increments of 5 to 10 beats per minute until atrial flutter is successfully interrupted).

Several caveats are, in order of importance, as follows: (1) Occasionally, atrial pacing rates higher than 400 beats per minute may be required to interrupt atrial flutter, because slower rates only entrain the atrial flutter[1]; (2) a critical duration of pacing (recommend a minimum of 10 seconds) at the critical pacing rate is required[1]; and (3) the stimulus strength required for atrial capture at the rapid rates necessary to interrupt atrial flutter is usually high[1]; it is recommended that pacing be initiated with a stimulus strength of at least 10 mA, but it is not unusual to require an even stronger stimulus[1]; (4) when esophageal pacing is used to interrupt atrial flutter, to capture the atria the stimulus must be at least 9 to 10 ms in duration and up to 30 mA in stimulus strength; (5) pacing through the esophagus tends to be somewhat painful, so pacing should be as brief as possible; and (6) before initiation of rapid pacing of any sort, pacing should be initiated at a relatively slow rate to demonstrate that no ventricular capture is inadvertently produced.

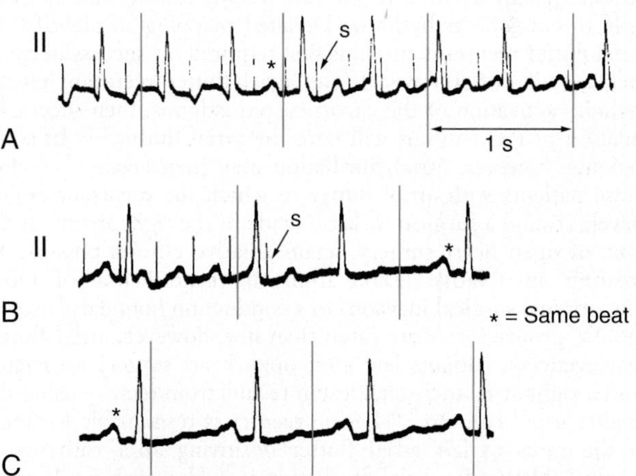

Figure 55-9 **A,** Electrocardiogram (ECG) lead II recorded in the same patient as in Figure 55-8 during high right atrial pacing from the same site at a cycle length of 224 ms. Note that with the seventh atrial beat in this tracing, and after 22 seconds of atrial pacing at a constant rate, the atrial complexes suddenly became positive *(asterisk)*. **B,** ECG lead II recorded at the termination of atrial pacing in the same patient. Note that with abrupt termination of pacing, sinus rhythm occurs. **C,** The first beat in this trace *(asterisk)* is identical with the last beat in **B** *(asterisk)*. S, Stimulus artifact. Time lines are at 1-second intervals. (**A** to **C**, Modified from Waldo AL, MacLean WAH, Karp RB, et al: Entrainment and interruption of atrial flutter with atrial pacing: Studies in man following open heart surgery. Circulation 56:737-745, 1977.)

Pacing Precipitation of Atrial Fibrillation (Inadvertent and Deliberate)

Despite appropriate care, rapid atrial pacing will provoke atrial fibrillation in some patients. Most often, the atrial fibrillation lasts seconds to minutes before spontaneously converting to sinus rhythm. When it persists, it almost always is associated with a slower ventricular response rate than in atrial flutter, and the ventricular response rate almost always is more easily controlled with AV node–blocking drugs. In fact, if type I atrial flutter recurs, despite its successful interruption by rapid atrial pacing, continuous rapid atrial pacing to precipitate and sustain atrial fibrillation may be indicated on a temporary basis in selected patients until other therapeutic strategies are undertaken.[1]

Direct Current Cardioversion of Atrial Flutter to Sinus Rhythm

Direct current cardioversion of atrial flutter to sinus rhythm has a high likelihood of success. With use of a monophasic shock, it also requires as little as 25 J, although at least 50 J generally is recommended because it is more often successful. Because 100 J is virtually always successful and virtually never harmful, it should be considered as the initial shock. Even less energy is required in using a biphasic shock to achieve cardioversion.

Treatment of Chronic Atrial Flutter

Medical therapy for atrial flutter often fails to control the arrhythmia and can be associated with tachycardias, bradycardias, and other troublesome adverse effects, particularly in the elderly. Catheter ablation usually is effective, especially in cavotricuspid isthmus–dependent atrial flutter and, in general, is considered the treatment of choice. In many if not most (82%)[15,41] patients, however, atrial fibrillation will develop later despite successful ablation of flutter. This is because of the interrelationship of atrial flutter and atrial fibrillation.[15]

Catheter Ablation Therapy

For any patient in whom atrial flutter is a recurring problem, radiofrequency ablation techniques usually can be used successfully to cure the arrhythmia. Detailed mapping to identify the atrial flutter reentrant circuit is first required for successful treatment of all flutter types. If the atrial flutter reentrant circuit includes activation of the cavotricuspid isthmus, then successful ablation of this isthmus will cure the atrial flutter.[1,22] In some patients, however, atrial fibrillation may then ensue.[1,15,22] For those patients with atrial flutter in which the reentrant circuit travels around a surgical incision made in the right atrium at the time of open heart surgery, again ablative cure is possible by creating an ablative lesion from the central line of block (the original surgical incision) to a conduction boundary, usually the AV groove.[2,26] More often than not, however, atrial flutter that occurs in patients late after open heart surgery associated with a right atrial incisional lesion results from reentry using the cavotricuspid isthmus.[3-6] Lesion reentry is responsible for most of the cases of left atrial flutter occurring after catheter or surgical ablation for atrial fibrillation.[12,30] However, scar formation due to atrial fibrosis caused by several cardiomyopathies (hypertrophic or dilated) or coronary artery disease, and even in aging without structural heart disease, also may be the substrate for left atrial flutter.[30] Advanced mapping techniques and navigation systems are required for adequate characterization and successful ablation of atypical atrial flutters. They usually are best treated with catheter ablation, sometimes necessitating only a single radiofrequency application to close a conduction gap between previously placed lesions or scars.[12,26,28-30]

Another form of catheter ablation involves His bundle ablation to create high-degree AV block (generally, third-degree AV block), thereby eliminating rapid ventricular response rates to atrial flutter.[1] This technique may be appropriate for patients in whom cure of the atrial flutter with ablative techniques was unsuccessful and antiarrhythmic drug therapy is not tolerated. Such patients are then managed with a standard permanent pacemaker system.

Antiarrhythmic Drug Therapy

It may be difficult to suppress paroxysmal atrial flutter with drug therapy. Eight currently available drugs have demonstrated efficacy in suppression of atrial flutter: the class IA antiarrhythmic agents quinidine, procainamide, and disopyramide; the class IC antiarrhythmic agents flecainide and propafenone; and the class III antiarrhythmic agents sotalol, dofetilide, and amiodarone. In the absence of structural heart disease, the IC agents probably are the drugs of choice to suppress the atrial flutter because they are better tolerated and have less organ toxicity. In addition, class III antiarrhythmic agents (e.g., amiodarone, dofetilide, or sotalol) likewise may be effective. If a patient requires therapy for atrial flutter, however, radiofrequency ablation rather than drug therapy is primarily indicated. Long-term drug therapy should be reserved for unusual circumstances, because of its low efficacy and frequent association with bradyarrhythmias and other adverse side effects. A randomized prospective trial has compared catheter ablation with electric cardioversion followed by long-term amiodarone therapy in elderly patients.[41] Compared with medical therapy with amiodarone, catheter ablation was followed by fewer recurrences of atrial flutter and less antiarrhythmic drug side effects, but similar risk of subsequent atrial fibrillation. These findings support the use of catheter ablation as first-line therapy, even after the first episode of symptomatic atrial flutter, in elderly patients.[42]

Anticoagulation Therapy

Although one study found neither atrial clot formation nor stroke associated with atrial flutter in a relatively small cohort of patients after open heart surgery,[1] other studies indicate that the incidence of stroke associated with atrial flutter approaches that in atrial fibrillation.[1,38,43-45] Furthermore, the fact that atrial flutter and atrial fibrillation often coexist in patients simply adds clinical weight to this consideration.[43] In addition, in studies[43-47] that have used transesophageal echocardiography in patients with atrial flutter, a high incidence of spontaneous echo contrast and atrial thrombi has been documented, along with striking abnormalities in the left atrial appendage. In short, in patients with atrial flutter, daily warfarin therapy to achieve an international normalized ratio (INR) between 2 and 3 (target INR of 2.5) is recommended, using the same criteria as for atrial fibrillation.[48]

Summary

Atrial flutter is caused by a reentrant circuit located principally in the right atrium. The diagnosis of all atrial flutter types should always be possible using classical mapping techniques, but navigation systems are extremely helpful to better characterize atypical flutter circuits. The interruption of atrial flutter should always be possible using atrial pacing, or direct current cardioversion, or antiarrhythmic drug therapy, alone or in combination. Long-term antiarrhythmic drug therapy to suppress recurrent atrial flutter is rarely indicated. Atrial flutter may be cured with catheter ablation techniques applied to a critical portion of the atrial flutter reentry circuit.

References

1. Waldo AL: Atrial flutter: From mechanism to treatment. In Camm AJ (ed): Clinical Approaches to Tachyarrhythmias, Armonk, NY, Futura Publishing, 2001, pp 1-56.
2. VanHare GF, Lesh MD, Ross BA, et al: Mapping and radiofrequency ablation of intraatrial reentrant tachycardia after the Senning or Mustard procedure for transposition of the great arteries. Am J Cardiol 77:985-991, 1996.
3. Chan DP, Van Hare GF, Mackall JA, et al: Importance of atrial flutter isthmus in postoperative intra-atrial reentrant tachycardia. Circulation 102:1283-1289, 2000.
4. Kanter RJ, Papagiannis J, Carboni MP, et al: Radiofrequency catheter ablation of supraventricular tachycardia substrates after Mustard and Senning operations for *d*-transposition of the great arteries. J Am Coll Cardiol 35:428-441, 2000.
5. Collins KK, Love BA, Walsh EP, et al: Location of acutely successful radiofrequency catheter ablation of intraatrial reentrant tachycardia in patients with congenital heart disease. Am J Cardiol 86:969-974, 2000.
6. Anne W, van Rensburg H, Adams J, et al: Ablation of post-surgical intra-atrial tachycardia. Predilection target sites and mapping approach. Eur Heart J 23:1609-1616, 2002.
7. Tomita Y, Matsuo K, Sahadevan J, et al: Role of functional block extension in lesion related to atrial flutter. Circulation 102:1025-1030, 2001.
8. Gandhi SK, Bromberg BI, Schuessler RB, et al: Left-sided atrial flutter: Characterization of a novel complication of pediatric lung transplantation in an acute canine model. J Thorac Cardiovasc Surg 112:992-1001, 1996.
9. Gandhi SK, Bromberg BI, Mallory GB, Huddleston CB: Atrial flutter: A newly recognized complication of pediatric lung transplantation. J Thorac Cardiovasc Surg 112:984-991, 1996.
10. Gillinov AM, Blackstone EH, McCarthy PM: Atrial fibrillation: Current surgical options and their assessment. Ann Thorac Surg 74:2210-2217, 2002.
11. Calkins H, Brugada J, Packer DL, et al. HRS/EHRA/ECAS expert Consensus Statement on catheter and surgical ablation of atrial fibrillation; recommendations for personnel, policy, procedures and follow-up. A report of the Heart Rhythm Society (HRS) Task Force on catheter and surgical ablation of atrial fibrillation. Heart Rhythm 4:816-861, 2007.
12. Gerstenfeld EP, Marchlinski FE. Mapping and ablation of left atrial tachycardias occurring after atrial fibrillation ablation. Heart Rhythm 4:S65-S72, 2007.
13. Jaïs P, Hocini M, Hsu LF, et al. Technique and results of linear ablation at the mitral isthmus. Circulation 110:2996-3002, 2004.
14. Waldo AL, Cooper TB: Spontaneous onset of Type I atrial flutter in patients. J Am Coll Cardiol 28:707-712, 1996.
15. Waldo AL, Feld GK: Interrelationships of atrial fibrillation and atrial flutter. Mechanisms and clinical implications. J Am Coll Cardiol 51:779-86, 2008.
16. Uno K, Kumagai K, Khrestian C, Waldo AL: New insights regarding the atrial flutter reentrant circuit: Studies in the canine sterile pericarditis model. Circulation 100:1354-1360, 1999.
17. Saoudi N, Cosio F, Waldo A, et al: Classification of atrial flutter and regular atrial tachycardia according to electrophysiologic mechanism and anatomical bases. A statement from a joint expert group from the Working Group of Arrhythmias of the European Society of Cardiology and the North American Society of Pacing and Electrophysiology. Eur Heart J 22: 1162-1182, 2001; and J Cardiovasc Electrophysiol, 12:852-866, 2001.
18. Olgin J, Kalman J, Fitzpatrick A, et al: The role of right atrial endocardial structures as barriers to conduction during human Type I atrial flutter: Activation and entrainment mapping guided by intracardiac echocardiography. Circulation 92:1831-1848, 1995.
19. Olgin JE, Kalman JM, Lesh MD: Conduction barriers in human atrial flutter: Correlation of electrophysiology and anatomy. J Cardiovasc Electrophysiol 7:1112-1126, 1996.
20. Nakagawa H, Lazzara R, Khastgir T, et al: Role of the tricuspid annulus and the Eustachian valve/ridge on atrial flutter. Relevance to catheter ablation of the septal isthmus and a new technique for rapid identification of ablation success. Circulation 94:407-424, 1996.
21. Friedman PA, Luria D, Fenton AM, et al: Global right atrial mapping of human atrial flutter: The presence of posteromedial (sinus venosa region) functional block and double potentials. Circulation 101:1568-1577, 2000.
22. Cosio FG, Lopez-Gil M, Giocolea A, et al: Radiofrequency ablation of the inferior vena cava-tricuspid valve isthmus in common atrial flutter. Am J Cardiol 71:705-709, 1993.
23. Kinder C, Kall J, Kopp D, et al: Conduction properties of the inferior vena cava-tricuspid annular isthmus in patients with typical atrial flutter. J Cardiovasc Electrophysiol 8:727-737, 1997.
24. Shah DC, Jais P, Haissaguerre M, et al: Three-dimensional mapping of the common atrial flutter circuit in the right atrium. Circulation 96:3904-3912, 1997.
25. Heist EK, Doshi SK, Singh JP, Di Salvo T, Semigran MJ, Reddy VY, Keane D, Ruskin JN, Mansour M. Catheter ablation of atrial flutter after orthotopic heart transplantation. J Cardiovasc Electrophysiol 15:1366-70, 2004.
26. Shah D, Jais P, Takahashi A, et al: Dual-loop intra-atrial reentry in humans. Circulation 101:631-639, 2000.
27. Kall JG, Rubenstein DS, Kopp DE, et al: Atypical atrial flutter originating in the right atrial free wall. Circulation 101:270-279, 2000.
28. Nakagawa H, Shah N, Matsudaira K, et al: Characterization of reentrant circuit in macroreentrant right atrial tachycardia after surgical repair of congenital heart disease. Circulation 103:699-709, 2001.
29. Jais P, Shah DC, Haissaguerre M, et al: Mapping and ablation of left atrial flutters. Circulation 101:2928-2934, 2000.
30. Ouyang F, Ernst S, Vogtmann T, et al: Characterization of reentrant circuits in left atrial macroreentrant tachycardia. Circulation 105:1934-1942, 2002.
31. Olgin JE, Jayachandran JV, Engelstein E, et al: Atrial macroreentry involving the myocardium of the coronary sinus: A unique mechanism for atypical atrial flutter. J Cardiovasc Electrophysiol 9:1094-1099, 1998.
32. Cheng J, Scheinman MM: Acceleration of typical atrial flutter due to double wave reentry induced by programmed electrical stimulation. Circulation 97:1589-1596, 1998.
33. Cheng J, Cabeen WR Jr, Scheinman MM: Right atrial flutter due to lower loop reentry: Mechanism and anatomic substrates. Circulation 99:1700-1705, 1999.
34. Scheinman MM, Cheng J, Yang Y: Mechanisms and clinical implications of atypical atrial flutter. J Cardiovasc Electrophysiol 10:1153-1157, 1999.
35. Yang J, Cheng J, Bochoeyer A, et al: Atypical right atrial flutter patterns. Circulation 103:3092-3098, 2001.
36. Waldo AL: From bedside to bench: Entrainment and other stories. Heart Rhythm 1:94-106, 2004.
37. Van Hare G, Waldo AL: The atrial flutter reentrant circuit: Additional pieces of the puzzle. Circulation 94:244-246, 1996.
38. Biblo AL, Yuan Z, Quan KJ, et al: Risk of stroke in patients with atrial flutter. Am J Cardiol 87:346-349, 2001.
39. Ellenbogen KA, Stambler BS, Wood MA, et al: Efficacy of intravenous ibutilide for rapid termination of atrial fibrillation and atrial flutter: A dose-response study. J Am Coll Cardiol 28:130-136, 1996.
40. Stambler BS, Wood MA, Ellenbogen KA: Comparative efficacy of intravenous ibutilide versus procainamide for enhancing termination of atrial flutter by atrial overdrive pacing. Am J Cardiol 77:960-966, 1996.
41. Ellis K, WazbiO, Marrouche N, et al: Incidence of atrial fibrillation post–cavotricuspid isthmus ablation in patients with typical atrial flutter: Left atrial size as an independent predictor of atrial fibrillation recurrence. J Cardiovasc Electrophysiol 18:799-802, 2007.
42. Da Costa A, Thévenin J, Roche F, et al: Results from the Loire-Ardèche-Drôme-Isère-Puy-de-Dôme (LADIP) Trial on atrial flutter, a multicentric prospective randomized study comparing amiodarone and radiofrequency ablation after the first episode of symptomatic atrial flutter. Circulation 114:1676-1681, 2006.
43. Wood KA, Eisenberg SJ, Kalman JM, et al: Risk of thromboembolism in chronic atrial flutter. Am J Cardiol 79:1043-1047, 1997.
44. Weiss R, Marcovitz P, Knight BP, et al: Acute changes in spontaneous echo

contrast and atrial function after cardioversion of persistent atrial flutter. Am J Cardiol 82:1052-1055, 1998.
45. Seidl K, Haver B, Schwick NG, et al: Risk of thromboembolic events in patients with atrial flutter. Am J Cardiol 82:580-584, 1998.
46. Grimm RA, Stewart WJ, Arheart KL, et al: Left atrial appendage "stunning" after electrical cardioversion of atrial flutter: An attenuated response compared with atrial fibrillation as the mechanism for lower susceptibility to thromboembolic events. J Am Coll Cardiol 29:582-589, 1997.
47. Irani WN, Grayburn PA, Afridi I: Prevalence of thrombus, spontaneous echo contrast, and atrial stunning in patients undergoing cardioversion of atrial flutter: A prospective study using transesophageal echocardiography. J Am Coll Cardiol 29:582-589, 1997.
48. Fuster V, Ryden LE, Cannon DS, et al: ACC/AHA/ESC 2006 Guidelines for the management of patients with atrial fibrillation: Executive summary. J Am Coll Cardiol 48:854-906, 2006.

Atrial Fibrillation: Mechanisms, Features, and Management 56

HAKAN ORAL

CHAPTER OUTLINE

Atrial fibrillation (AF) is a common supraventricular arrhythmia characterized by disorganized atrial activity. An overview of the recent advances in elucidating its mechanisms, features, and management is presented in this chapter.

Epidemiologic Aspects

The prevalence of AF increases with age and is estimated at 0.4% to 1%.[1] AF is more prevalent among men than among women when data are adjusted for age. The incidence of AF is less than 0.1% per year in patients younger than 40 years of age and greater than 1.5% to 2% in patients older than 80 years, respectively. Approximately 2.2 million patients in the United States and 4.5 million in the European Union are affected by AF.[1] A 12.6% increase in the age- and gender-adjusted risk of AF has been documented.[2] The number of patients with AF in the United States is estimated to reach greater than 12 million by 2050 (Fig. 56-1).

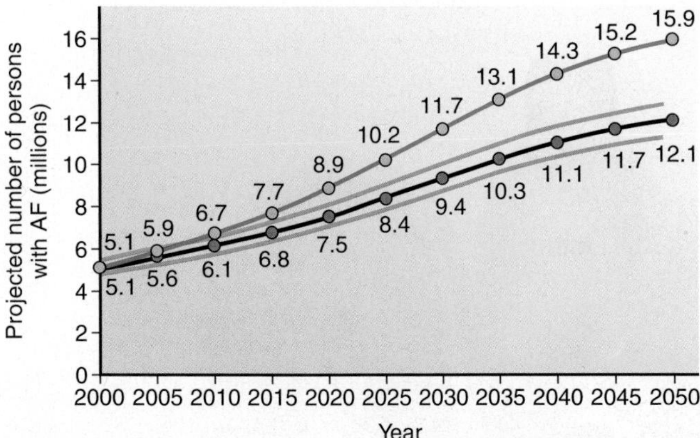

Figure 56-1 Secular trends in the incidence of atrial fibrillation (AF). Projected number of persons with AF in the United States between 2000 and 2050, assuming no further increase in age-adjusted AF incidence *(black curve)* and assuming a continued increase in incidence rate as evident in 1980 to 2000 *(blue curve)*. (From Miyasaka Y, Barnes ME, Gersh BJ, et al: Secular trends in incidence of atrial fibrillation in Olmsted County, Minnesota, 1980 to 2000, and implications on the projections for future prevalence. Circulation 114:119-125, 2006.)

Classification

According to a recent consensus statement based on the clinical presentation,[1,3] *paroxysmal AF* refers to recurrent episodes of AF (two or more) that terminate spontaneously within 7 days of the onset of AF. *Persistent AF* indicates episodes of AF that last for more than 7 days or require cardioversion regardless of the duration of the episode. *Long-standing persistent AF* refers to continuous episodes of persistent AF for longer than 1 year. *Permanent AF* implies that restoration and maintenance of sinus rhythm either has failed or has not been attempted. An episode must last for longer than 30 seconds to be considered to represent clinical AF.

Pathophysiology

The mechanisms of AF are multifactorial. These mechanisms may not be mutually exclusive (Fig. 56-2).

Multiple-Wavelet Hypothesis

Reentry forms the basis of the multiple-wavelet hypothesis of AF pathogenesis.[4] Atrial substrate should be able to accommodate the wavelength (i.e., conduction velocity × effective refractory period [ERP]). It is possible that multiple wavelets and reentry with fibrillatory conduction play a role in perpetuation of AF, particularly in patients with atrial electroanatomic remodeling.[5]

Pulmonary Veins

The seminal observation that premature depolarizations from the PVs initiate AF led to the development of novel mechanistic and therapeutic paradigms.[6] Automaticity, triggered activity, and reentry have been implicated in PV arrhythmogenesis. The mechanisms by which PVs become arrhythmogenic and initiate AF in some patients and remain dormant in others are not clear. Genetic predisposition, stretch, neurohormonal milieu, and changes in autonomic tone have been implicated in PV arrhythmogenesis.

During embryonic development, the common PV is incorporated into the left atrium. An immunohistochemical study demonstrated that the composition of the PV and the smooth-walled portion of the left atrium are identical[7] (Fig. 56-3), explaining why the antral regions of the PVs and the posterior left atrium also are arrhythmogenic.

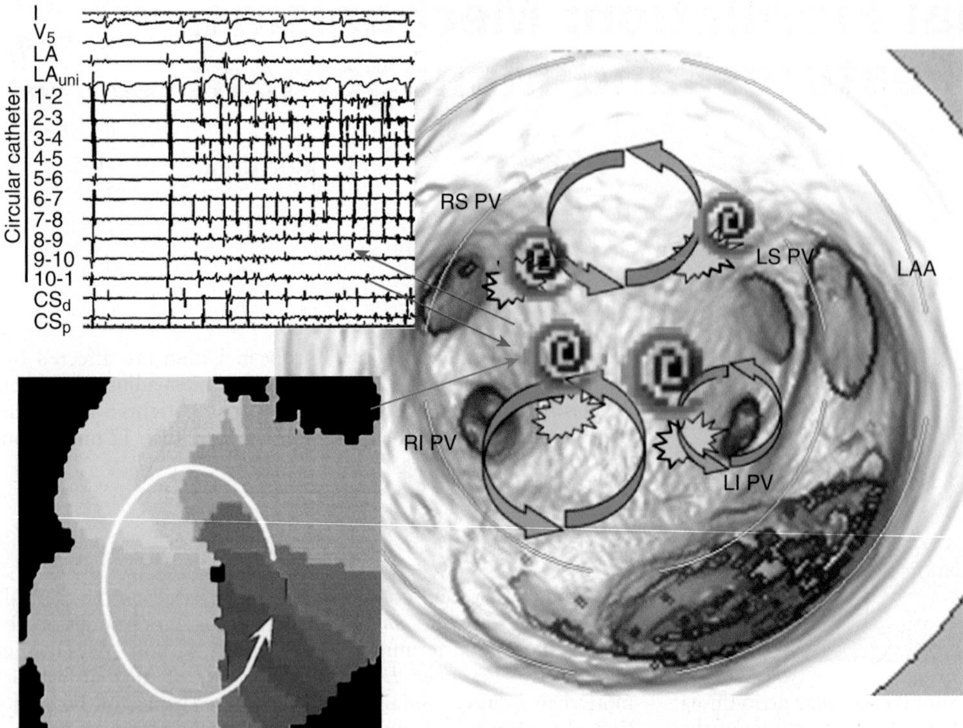

Figure 56-2 Multifactorial nature of the genesis of atrial fibrillation (AF). A three-dimensional computed tomographic image of the left atrium, endoscopic view *(right)*. Potential mechanisms of AF include PV tachycardias that initiate and perpetuate AF *(upper left)*, rotors *(blue spirals*; a magnified phase map is at *lower left*), multiple reentrant circuits *(green arrow circles)* and autonomic modulation through ganglionated plexi *(yellow patches)*. A dynamic interplay occurs between the PVs and other drivers of AF such that they continually activate and perpetuate each other. LAA, left atrial appendage; LI PV, left inferior pulmonary vein; LS PV, left superior pulmonary vein; RI PV, right inferior pulmonary vein; RS PV, right superior pulmonary vein. (Adapted from Jalife J: Rotors and spiral waves in atrial fibrillation. J Cardiovasc Electrophysiol 14:776-780, 2003.)

Intermittent PV tachycardias that occur as burst of rapid repetitive PV depolarizations may play a critical role in initiation and perpetuation of AF.[8,9] Moreover, there appears to be a dynamic interplay between the PVs and the adjacent left atrium, as the site of rapid electrical activity alternates between the PVs and the left atrium (Fig. 56-4; see also Fig. 56-2). It is possible that PV tachycardias and other drivers of AF may continually activate each other and perpetuate AF.

High-Frequency Sources or Rotors

Animal and computer models of AF suggest that high-frequency sources or rotors due to anisotropic reentry may perpetuate AF.[10] Wavebreak and fibrillatory conduction occur at the periphery of a rotor possibly at anatomic barriers. There appears to be a frequency gradient from the PVs to the left and to the right atrium.[11] Elimination of PV tachycardias and ablation of complex fractionated atrial electrograms (CFAEs) result

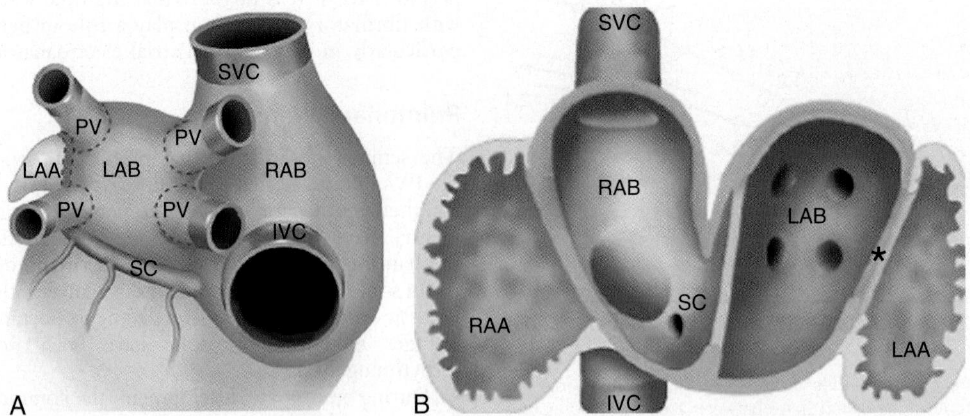

Figure 56-3 A, Schematic depiction of outer side of atrial chambers with pulmonary veins (PVs) and systemic veins. Left atrial body (LAB) and right atrial body (RAB) covered by myocardium with smooth-walled inner aspect *(blue)*, which stretches out over extracardiac segments of PV and over small peripheral part of systemic veins *(blue area* above and below *dotted line)*. Left atrial appendage (LAA) and right atrial appendage (RAA) consist of trabeculated myocardium *(brown)*. IVC, inferior vena cava; SVC, superior vena cava. **B,** Schematic depiction of tissue types found in left and right atria seen from inside of atria. Vessel wall tissue is shown in *red*; myocardial tissue with smooth-walled inner aspect, in *blue*; primary atrial segment tissue, in *brown*; left-sided sinus venosus tissue is indicated by the *asterisk*. (From Douglas YL, Jongbloed MR, Gittenberger-de Groot AC, et al: Histology of vascular myocardial wall of left atrial body after pulmonary venous incorporation. Am J Cardiol 97:662-670, 2006.)

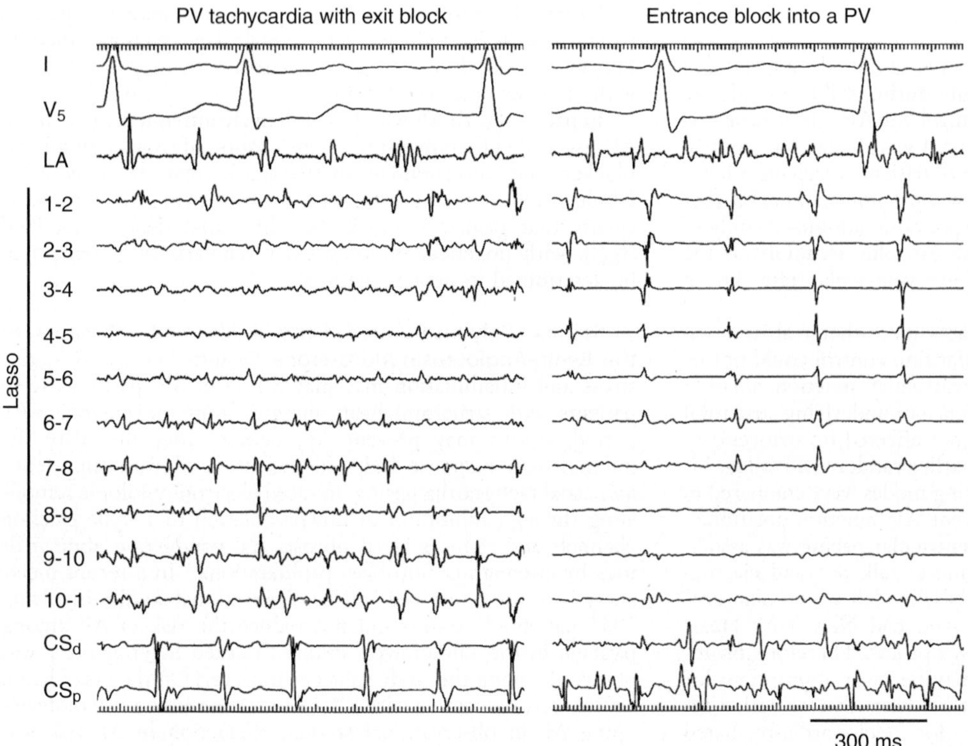

Figure 56-4 Alternation in the site of shortest cycle length between a pulmonary vein (PV) and the adjacent left atrium. Shown are leads I and V5 and intracardiac electrograms recorded from the left atrial (LA), Lasso, and coronary sinus (CS) catheters. (From Oral H, Ozaydin M, Tada H, et al: Mechanistic significance of intermittent pulmonary vein tachycardia in patients with atrial fibrillation. J Cardiovasc Electrophysiol 13:645-650, 2002.)

in a decrease in the frequency content.[12,13] In patients with persistent AF, the amount of reduction in dominant frequency after electrogram-guided ablation predicts a higher probability of maintaining sinus rhythm.[13] Anchor points of rotors may be more prevalent at the antral regions of the PVs. A shorter effective refractory period at sites of autonomic innervation within the PV antrum may promote development of rotors.

Autonomic Innervation

The heart has an intrinsic nervous system and an interactive atrial neural network.[14] An increase in parasympathetic tone may promote AF by shortening the ERP or facilitating premature depolarizations.[15] Stimulation of ganglionated plexi promotes PV arrhythmogenicity and inducibility of AF.[16] In animal models, ablation of ganglionated plexi was demonstrated to prevent vagal AF.[17] In an earlier study, parasympathetic denervation after circumferential PV ablation was associated with a higher probability of maintaining sinus rhythm in patients with paroxysmal AF.[18] The effects of cardiac denervation by surgical dissection of ganglionated fat pads have been conflicting, however.[19,20] The role of ablation of ganglionated plexi either as a stand-alone ablation strategy or in conjunction with PV isolation remains to be determined.

Treatment

Rate versus Rhythm Control

Several studies attempted to address whether rate vs rhythm control should be the primary therapeutic strategy in patients with AF. In the Atrial Fibrillation Follow-up Investigation of Rhythm Management (AFFIRM) study, 4060 patients with AF and aged 66 years and older or who had other risk factors for stroke or death were randomized to receive therapy using either a rate or a rhythm control strategy, which consisted of antiarrhythmic drug therapy and cardioversion as necessary.[21] In an intention-to-treat analysis, a trend toward higher overall mortality was observed in the rhythm control group (P = .08). Subsequent post hoc analyses suggested that potential adverse effects of antiarrhythmic drug therapy may have negated any beneficial effects.[22] An on-treatment analysis demonstrated that maintenance of sinus rhythm and warfarin use was associated with a decrease in mortality, whereas antiarrhythmic drug use was associated with an increase in mortality.[23] In the Rate Control Versus Electrical Cardioversion for Persistent Atrial Fibrillation (RACE) trial, no significant difference was found in the primary composite endpoint of cardiovascular mortality, heart failure, thromboembolic complications, bleeding, need for a pacemaker, and severe adverse antiarrhythmic drug effects among the 522 patients who were randomized to receive therapy using a rhythm or a rate control strategy.[24] As in the AFFIRM study, the study subjects were older, with one or more risk factors for stroke in more than 90%.

The findings of the AFFIRM and RACE trials suggest that rate control strategy may be an acceptable approach in older patients with baseline risk factors who have no or minimal symptoms attributable to AF. It remains to be determined whether a rhythm control strategy, particularly in the context of catheter ablation, will be associated with a decrease in long-term morbidity and mortality compared with a rate control strategy. In a registry of 1171 consecutive patients with AF, a significant decrease in all-cause mortality, improvement in quality of life, and reduction in incidence of heart failure and cerebrovascular ischemic events were reported after catheter ablation during a mean follow-up period of 900 days.[25]

Rate Control

A ventricular rate less than 100 beats per minute during rest and between 90 and 115 beats per minute during mild to moderate exertion is targeted during rate control for AF.[1] In a post hoc analysis of the AFFIRM study, optimal ventricular rate control was achieved in a higher proportion of patients receiving a beta-blocker (70%) than in those receiving a calcium channel blocker (54%) or digoxin (58%).[26] In a prospective randomized study of digoxin, atenolol, and diltiazem, digoxin plus atenolol was the most effective regimen in controlling ventricular rate during daily activities.

In patients who are not candidates for catheter ablation to eliminate AF and in whom ventricular rate control could not be achieved pharmacologically, atrioventricular junction ablation has been highly effective. In the absence of underlying structural heart disease, long-term survival is not affected by atrioventricular (AV) junction ablation. In an earlier randomized study, biventricular and right ventricular pacing modes were compared in 184 patients with AF who underwent AV junction ablation.[27] At 6 months after the ablation, biventricular pacing was associated with an improvement in 6-minute walk test and ejection fraction only in patients who had a baseline left ventricular ejection fraction of 45% or lower or who had New York Heart Association (NYHA) class II or III symptoms. Therefore, biventricular pacing after AV junction may be most appropriate for patients who have underlying structural heart disease with a reduced ejection fraction, except for tachycardia-mediated cardiomyopathy.

Rhythm Control

Maintenance of sinus rhythm has been associated with an improvement in quality of life and with an increase in left ventricular ejection fraction and decrease in left atrial size.

Pharmacologic Therapy

Antiarrhythmic Drug Therapy Once a decision for rhythm control is made, a trial of one or more antiarrhythmic drugs usually is warranted unless the patient is unwilling, the long-term risk-to-benefit ratio is not favorable, or presence of comorbid conditions limits the choice of therapeutic agents. In patients with preserved left ventricular ejection fraction, no inducible ischemia, and no significant left ventricular hypertrophy, a class IC antiarrhythmic drug usually is the initial choice. Owing to potential risk of proarrhythmia, class IA agents are being used less often. However, disopyramide may be helpful in patients with vagotonic variety of AF because of its anticholinergic effects.

In a recent randomized study, time to recurrence of AF was longer among patients who received amiodarone, (487 days) than among those receiving sotalol (74 days) or placebo (6 days).[28] In a subgroup analysis of patients with ischemic heart disease, time to recurrence of AF was similar in the amiodarone and sotalol treatment groups. Amiodarone is the antiarrhythmic agent least likely to cause proarrhythmia in patients with structural heart disease and can be used in patients with renal insufficiency. Careful monitoring for its potential cumulative systemic side effects is indicated, however.

Dronedarone has electrophysiologic effects similar to those of amiodarone, except for a shorter half life of 1 to 2 days. In a recent trial, time to recurrence of AF was longer in the dronedarone group in than in the placebo group.[29] However, AF recurred in 64% and 75% of the patients who received dronedarone and placebo, respectively. The risk of thyroid, liver, and pulmonary toxicity was not increased. Unlike amiodarone, dronedarone is associated with increased mortality in patients with congestive heart failure.

Dofetilide, another class III agent, also may be used in patients with a reduced left ventricular ejection fraction. However, dofetilide has a very narrow therapeutic window with complex pharmacokinetics.

In patients with AF who have relatively infrequent episodes of AF, as-needed therapy using a combination of short-acting beta-blocker and propafenone or flecainide may be effective.[30] Clinical efficacy and safety of atrioselective antiarrhythmic agents that primarily block the ultra-rapid delayed rectified (I_{Kur}), with no effect on ventricular repolarization, remain to be determined in patients with AF.

Statins, Polyunsaturated Fatty Acids, and Inhibitors of the Renin-Angiotensin-Aldosterone System Because oxidative stress and inflammation may play a role in AF, particularly in patients with structural heart disease or in the postoperative period, statins may prevent AF, because they modulate the inflammatory response and oxidative stress. Simvastatin attenuates atrial tachycardia pacing–induced electrophysiologic remodeling through inhibition of downregulation of L-type calcium channels and reduces atrial fibrosis and conduction abnormalities by attenuating fibroblast proliferation.[31] In a recent meta-analysis of 6 randomized and 10 observational studies involving 7041 patients,[32] statins did not reduce the risk of AF among patients in the randomized studies. Marked heterogeneity was observed among the study subjects, however. On the other hand, statins were associated with a 23% reduction in the risk of developing AF in observational studies. Reduction in AF risk was most apparent in patients with postoperative AF.

Omega(n)-3-polyunsaturated fatty acids (PUFAs) have antioxidant, anti-inflammatory, and lipid-lowering effects. PUFAs also block sodium and L-type calcium channels and modulate membrane fluidity.[33] In an animal model of vagally induced AF, pretreatment with fish oil reduced the expression of connexins Cx40 and Cx43 by 50% and decreased the inducibility of AF.[34] In an observational, prospective study of 4815 adults older than 65 years, fish consumption was associated with a 30% reduction in the incidence of AF during a 12-year follow-up period.[35] However, a beneficial association between fish intake and incidence of AF could not be demonstrated in two other observational studies.[36,37] In a randomized study, treatment with PUFAs reduced postoperative AF by 50% after coronary artery bypass surgery.[38] Taken together, these observations suggest that statins and PUFAs are likely to have a beneficial effect in a subset of patients with AF in whom oxidative stress or inflammation plays a major role.

Activation of the renin-angiotensin-aldosterone axis results in fibrosis and promotes electroanatomic remodeling.[39] Renin-angiotensin gene polymorphisms are associated with an increased risk of AF.[40] Local expression of angiotensin-converting enzyme (ACE) is increased in patients with chronic AF. Inhibition of renin-angiotensin system may prevent AF by improving left ventricular remodeling and hemodynamics and decreasing left atrial stretch, by attenuating angiotensin-induced fibrosis, and by direct effects on ion channels.[39]

In a meta-analysis of data from 11 studies involving 56,308 patients, treatment with an ACE inhibitor (ACEI) or adrenergic receptor blocker (ARB) was associated with a 28% decrease in the relative risk of AF in patients with congestive heart failure, hypertension, or myocardial infarction.[41] The reduction in AF was similar with an ACEI and with an ARB and was most pronounced in patients with congestive heart failure. Except among patients with left ventricular hypertrophy, a similar reduction in AF risk was not observed in patients with hypertension. Enalapril and irbesartan reduced the probability of recurrent AF after cardioversion by approximately 50% when used in combination with amiodarone.[42,43]

Aldosterone also promotes inflammation and fibrosis. In an animal model of pacing-induced congestive heart failure, selective blockade of aldosterone was associated with a decrease in inducibility of atrial arrhythmias and a prolongation in atrial ERP.[44] The role of ACEIs, ARBs, and aldosterone blockers for primary therapy of AF in the absence of other comorbid conditions remains to be determined.

Catheter Ablation

Based on the current understanding of the mechanisms of AF, either of two major strategies may be considered for catheter ablation of AF alone or in combination; anatomic ablation and tailored, stepwise, electrogram-guided ablation.

Anatomic Ablation The premise of anatomic ablation is that mechanisms of AF use same or similar sites in patients with AF, so empirical ablation at these sites should be effective in eliminating AF. Because PVs play a critical role both in initiation and in perpetuation of AF,[6,8,9] they often are routinely targeted using a variety of techniques, including PV isolation by segmental ostial ablation, circumferential PV ablation, wide-area circumferential ablation, and antral PV isolation.[45-49]

Unlike segmental ostial PV isolation, antral PV isolation or wide-area circumferential ablation has been effective for both patients with paroxysmal AF and those with persistent AF.[46] In an earlier randomized study, circumferential PV ablation resulted in maintenance of sinus rhythm in 74% of patients with chronic AF (Fig. 56-5).[45] Maintenance of sinus rhythm was associated with a significant improvement in quality of life, left ventricular ejection fraction and left atrial size. Wide-area or antral PV isolation may result in (1) elimination of arrhythmogenic sites within the PVs and their antra; (2) debulking of the left atrium by 25% to 30%; (3) elimination of anchor points of rotors; (4) ablation of ganglionated plexi; and (5) possibly ablation of the ligament of Marshall.

Linear ablation also has been performed using anatomic landmarks either as a stand-alone ablation strategy or in conjunction with PV isolation or circumferential ablation. The rationale for use of linear ablation is to interrupt reentrant circuits that may perpetuate AF. Left atrial roof, mitral isthmus, posterior mitral annulus, inferoposterior wall of the left atrium, septal aspect of the left atrium, and anterior wall are frequently targeted sites. Conduction gaps along the lines may facilitate macroreentrant atrial flutters.

Tailored, Stepwise, Electrogram-Guided Ablation Tailored or stepwise ablation performed until AF terminates and becomes noninducible (in patients with paroxysmal AF), guided by local electrograms either as a standalone strategy or in conjunction with PV isolation, has been proposed as a novel strategy to eliminate AF.[50-54] The rationale for an electrogram-guided ablation strategy includes the following points:

- Empirical ablation guided by anatomic landmarks may be more than necessary in some patients and insufficient in others. Unnecessary applications of radiofrequency energy may result in inadvertent collateral injury and thromboembolic

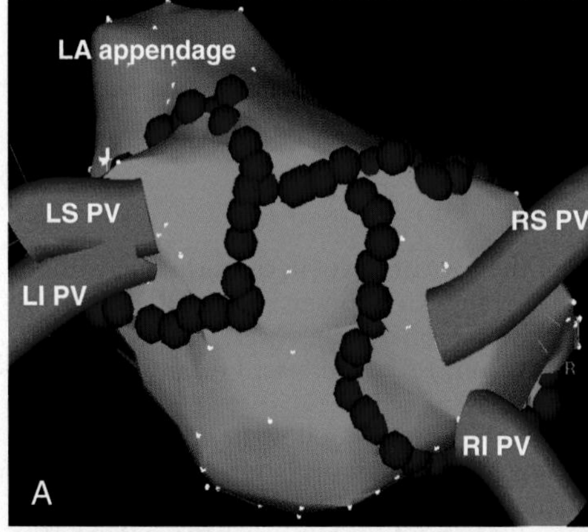

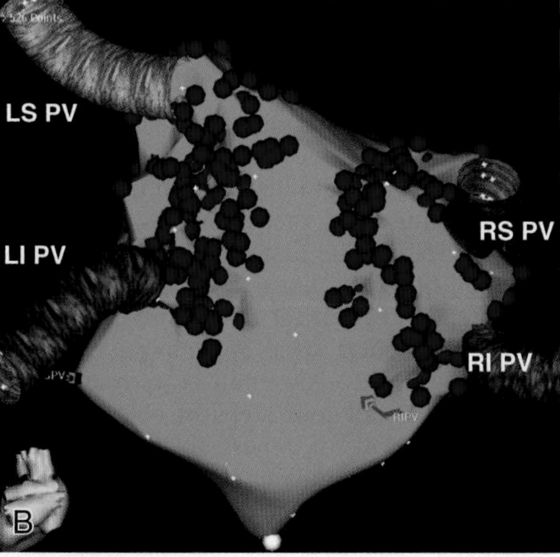

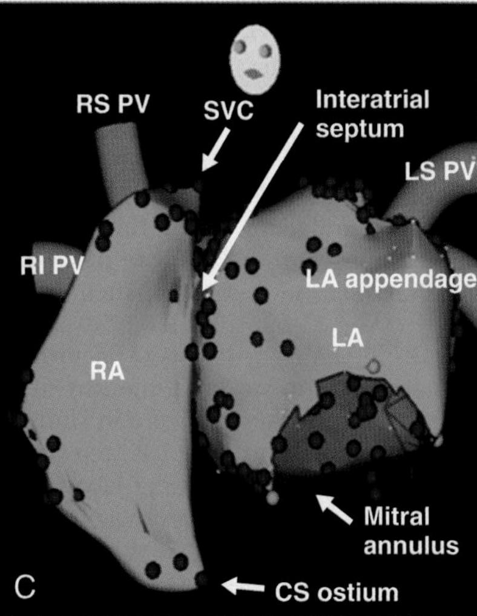

Figure 56-5 Examples of catheter ablation for atrial fibrillation (AF). Shown is electroanatomic depiction of the left atrium. Circumferential pulmonary vein (PV) ablation (**A**), antral PV isolation (**B**), and left and right atrial electrogram-guided ablation (**C**) are shown. *Red tags* indicate ablation sites. CPVA, circumferential pulmonary vein ablation; CS, coronary sinus; LA, left atrium; LI PV, left inferior pulmonary vein; LS (PV), left superior pulmonary vein; RA, right atrium; RS PV, right superior pulmonary vein; RI PV, right inferior pulmonary vein; SVC, superior vena cava. (Adapted from Oral H, Pappone C, Chugh A, et al: Circumferential pulmonary-vein ablation for chronic atrial fibrillation. N Engl J Med 354:934-941, 2006; and Oral H, Chugh A, Good E, et al: Radiofrequency catheter ablation of chronic atrial fibrillation guided by complex electrograms. Circulation 115:2606-2612, 2007.)

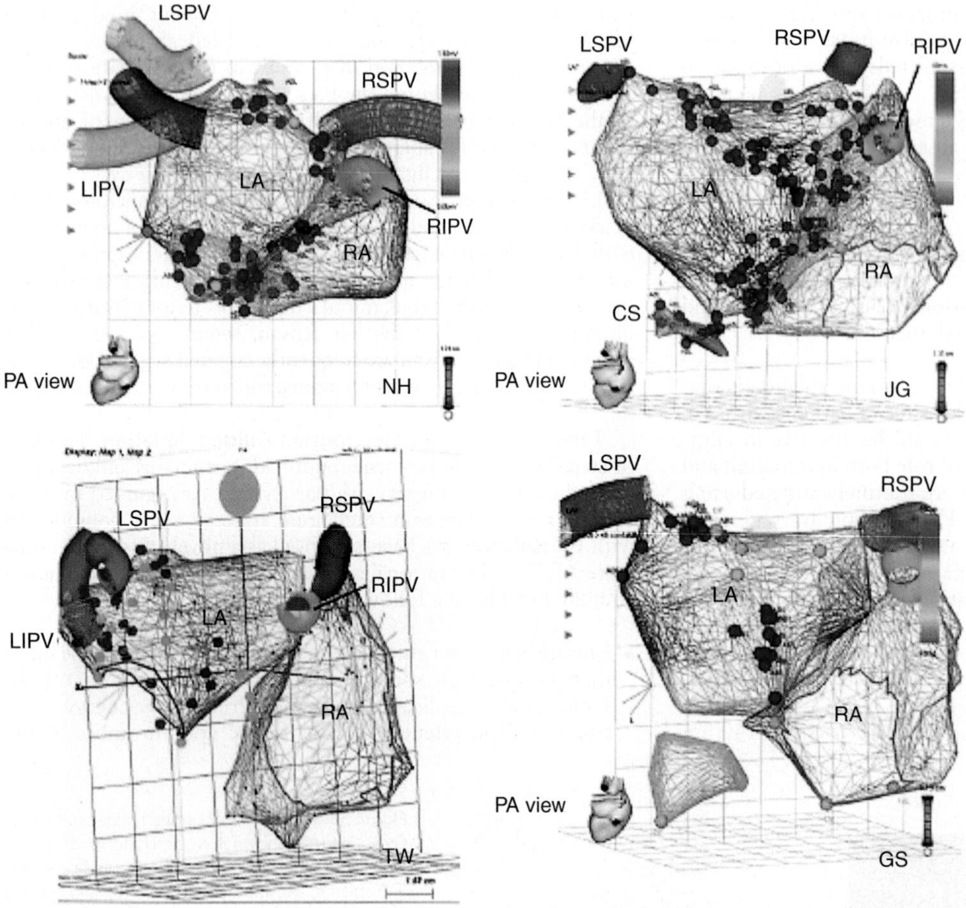

Figure 56-6 Electrogram-guided ablation. Shown are posteroanterior (PA) views of four maps from two patients with paroxysmal atrial fibrillation (AF) *(left panels)* and two patients with chronic AF *(right panels)*. Ablation sites are indicated by *red tags*. CS, coronary sinus; LA, left atrium; LIPV, left inferior pulmonary vein; LSPV, left superior pulmonary vein; RA, right atrium; RIPV, right inferior pulmonary vein; RSPV, right superior pulmonary vein. (Reproduced with permission from Nademanee K, McKenzie J, Kosar E, et al: A new approach for catheter ablation of atrial fibrillation: Mapping of the electrophysiologic substrate. J Am Coll Cardiol 43:2044-2053, 2004.)

complications, facilitate proarrhythmia, impair left atrial transport function, and prolong the procedure.

- Triggers and drivers of AF can be identified by analysis of electrograms.
- Termination and noninducibility of AF (for paroxysmal AF) indicates effective elimination of all mechanism of AF and identifies patients who are more likely to remain in sinus rhythm than patients who still are in AF or inducible after ablation.

Electrogram-guided ablation often is guided by CFAEs characterized by a short cycle length (less than 120 ms), fractionation, or continuous electrical activity. CFAEs may indicate sites of slow conduction, pivot points for reentrant circuits, wavefront collision, and conduction block. Therefore, reentry may be facilitated at these sites. CFAEs may be recorded at sites of overlapping tissue layers.[55] A shortening in ERP at sites of autonomic innervation also may facilitate development of CFAEs.[56]

In an earlier study that targeted CFAEs in the PVs, left and right atria, and the coronary sinus, AF terminated in 95% of the patients during ablation (with ibutilide in 28%)[51] (Fig. 56-6). At 1-year follow-up evaluation, 91% of the 121 patients with paroxysmal or persistent AF were free from recurrent arrhythmias, including 8 patients receiving amiodarone. Repeat ablation was performed in 24% of the patients.

In 153 patients with paroxysmal AF, ablation was tailored to target CFAEs in the PVs, left atrium, coronary sinus, and the superior vena cava until AF terminated and became noninducible.[52] A repeat ablation was performed in 18% of the patients. At 11 months, 77% of the patients were in sinus rhythm without antiarrhythmic drug therapy. In another study, CFAEs in the PVs, left atrium, and the coronary sinus were targeted in 100 patients with chronic AF until AF terminated or all identifiable CFAEs were eliminated.[53] AF could be terminated in only 16% of the patients during ablation. At follow-up evaluation at a mean of 14 ± 7 months after a single ablation procedure, 33% of patients were in sinus rhythm without antiarrhythmic drugs. A repeat ablation was performed in 44%, and PV tachycardias were identified in all patients during repeat ablation. At 13 ± 7 months after the last ablation procedure, 57% of patients were in sinus rhythm without antiarrhythmic drugs.

A stepwise ablation strategy was described in 60 patients with long-lasting persistent AF.[50,54] The steps of the ablation strategy were isolation of the PVs, the superior vena cava, and the coronary sinus; ablation at atrial sites with complex electrogram, short cycle length, or an activation gradient; and linear ablation along the roof, mitral isthmus, and the cavotricuspid isthmus until AF terminated (Fig. 56-7). The first three steps were performed in random order, however, linear ablation always was performed as the last step. Sites critical to termination of AF included the PVs, base of the left atrial appendage, coronary sinus, the roof and mitral isthmus. AF could be terminated in 87% of the patients; however, all four steps of ablation were necessary in a majority of patients. A repeat ablation was performed in 50% of the patients to eliminate recurrent AF or atrial tachycardia. At 11 months of follow-up, 95% of the patients remained in sinus rhythm.

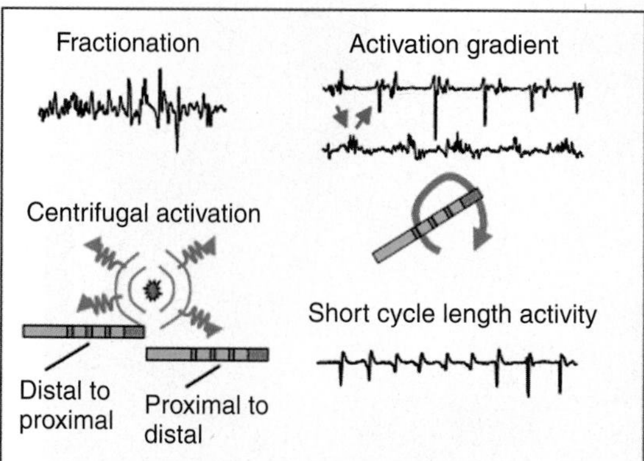

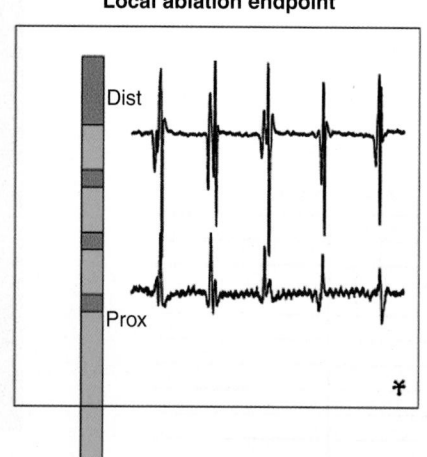

Figure 56-7 Ablation targets and endpoint of atrial ablation. **Left,** The targets for atrial ablation: areas of continuous fractionated electrograms *(left, top)*; sites with an activation gradient between distal and proximal electrodes *(right, top)*; sites with centrifugal activity suggesting the presence of a localized source *(left, bottom)*; and regions with a short cycle length *(right, bottom)*. **Right,** The endpoint of local ablation with organization of the electrograms, slowing of the local activity, and synchronous activation of the distal and proximal bipoles. (From Haissaguerre M, Sanders P, Hocini M, et al: Catheter ablation of long-lasting persistent atrial fibrillation: Critical structures for termination. J Cardiovasc Electrophysiol 16:1125-1137, 2005.)

Endpoints for Catheter Ablation During PV (and antrum) isolation, the optimal endpoint is complete electrical isolation, confirmed by elimination of all PV potentials, entrance block into the PVs, and exit block during pacing at multiple sites within the PV. Complete isolation may also be assessed after isoproterenol or adenosine infusion. Endpoints for individual applications of radiofrequency energy include elimination of target potentials, voltage abatement by greater than 80%,[46] impedance decrease, slowing of the AF cycle length, and elimination of local activation gradients.[50]

Termination and noninducibility of AF during catheter ablation predict freedom from recurrent AF[8,52,54,57,58] (Fig. 56-8). *Termination* of AF indicates effective elimination of all triggers and drivers of AF active at a specific point in time, whereas *noninducibility* suggests absence of any residual triggers and drivers that may initiate and perpetuate AF. In patients with paroxysmal AF, termination may more frequently be random than in persistent AF. Therefore, termination alone is not a reliable predictor of freedom from recurrent AF in patients with paroxysmal AF, whereas noninducibility identifies patients who are likely to remain in sinus rhythm. In an earlier study, rendering AF noninducible by linear ablation at sites of CFAEs after circumferential PV ablation resulted in higher probability of maintaining sinus rhythm (see Fig. 56-8).[58]

Noninducibility has been assessed by rapid atrial pacing.[8,57] Although rapid atrial pacing is very sensitive for induction of AF, it may lack specificity.[8,57] In a recent study, isoproterenol infusion up to 20 μg/minute was demonstrated to have a high specificity and sensitivity to assess PV arrhythmogenicity in patients with AF.[59] Whether assessment of noninducibility by rapid atrial pacing after infusion of high-dose isoproterenol will improve diagnostic accuracy of noninducibility remains to be determined.

Owing to extensive electroanatomic remodeling in patients with persistent AF, rapid atrial pacing often results in reinduction of AF. Because AF rarely terminates spontaneously in patients with persistent AF, termination during ablation has been demonstrated to be a predictor of freedom from recurrent AF.[54,60]

Related Structures of Thoracic Veins, Coronary Sinus, Superior Vena Cava, and the Ligament of Marshall and Right Atrium Thoracic veins and related structures other than the PVs—the superior and inferior venae cavae, coronary sinus, and the ligament of Marshall—have been reported to possess arrhythmogenic activity similar to, although less frequent than, that of the PVs.[61-64] Because the superior vena cava and the ligament of Marshall may initiate AF in less than 5% to 10% of patients with AF, it may be preferable to target arrhythmogenic foci in these structures only when they are confirmed to induce AF.

On the other hand, the coronary sinus may play a more complex role in the initiation and perpetuation of AF. Foci at the ostium and body of the coronary sinus have been reported to initiate AF.[62,63,65] Reentrant circuits involving left atrium may use parts of the coronary sinus.[66] In an earlier study, bursts of focal rapid repetitive activity were identified in the coronary sinus in 3% of 144 patients with paroxysmal or persistent AF.[65] Complex multilayered structure of the coronary sinus and adjacent left atrial myocardium with resultant anisotropy may facilitate reentry.

Another study suggested that the site of the fastest electrical activity alternates between the coronary sinus and left atrium during AF, in a manner similar to that of the dynamic interplay occurring between the PVs and the left atrium.[67] In that study, systematic disconnection of the coronary sinus from the left atrium rendered AF to be less inducible after PV isolation in patients with paroxysmal AF. In a recent study, epicardial and endocardial ablation along and in the coronary sinus was performed in 45 patients with paroxysmal or persistent AF who remained in AF after PV isolation.[68] Coronary sinus ablation was associated with a prolongation in AF cycle length and termination of AF in 35% of the patients (46% in paroxysmal and 30% in persistent AF). Taken together, these findings suggest that the coronary sinus may play a mechanistic role in the initiation and perpetuation of AF.

The right atrium also may be important in the genesis of AF. Focal triggers originating from the crista terminalis and ostium of the coronary sinus, in addition to venae cavae, have been reported to initiate AF.[62] Conduction gaps along the crista terminalis also have been reported to facilitate localized reentry, thereby perpetuating AF.[69]

In a study of stepwise ablation in patients with persistent AF, termination occurred during right atrial ablation in only 3% of the patients.[50] In a recent study, 85 patients with persistent AF who still remained in AF after ablation of CFAEs in the PVs, left atrium, and coronary sinus were randomized to undergo no further ablation or additional ablation in the right atrium (see Fig. 56-5).[60] AF terminated in 3% of the aptients during right atrial ablation. During a mean follow-up period of

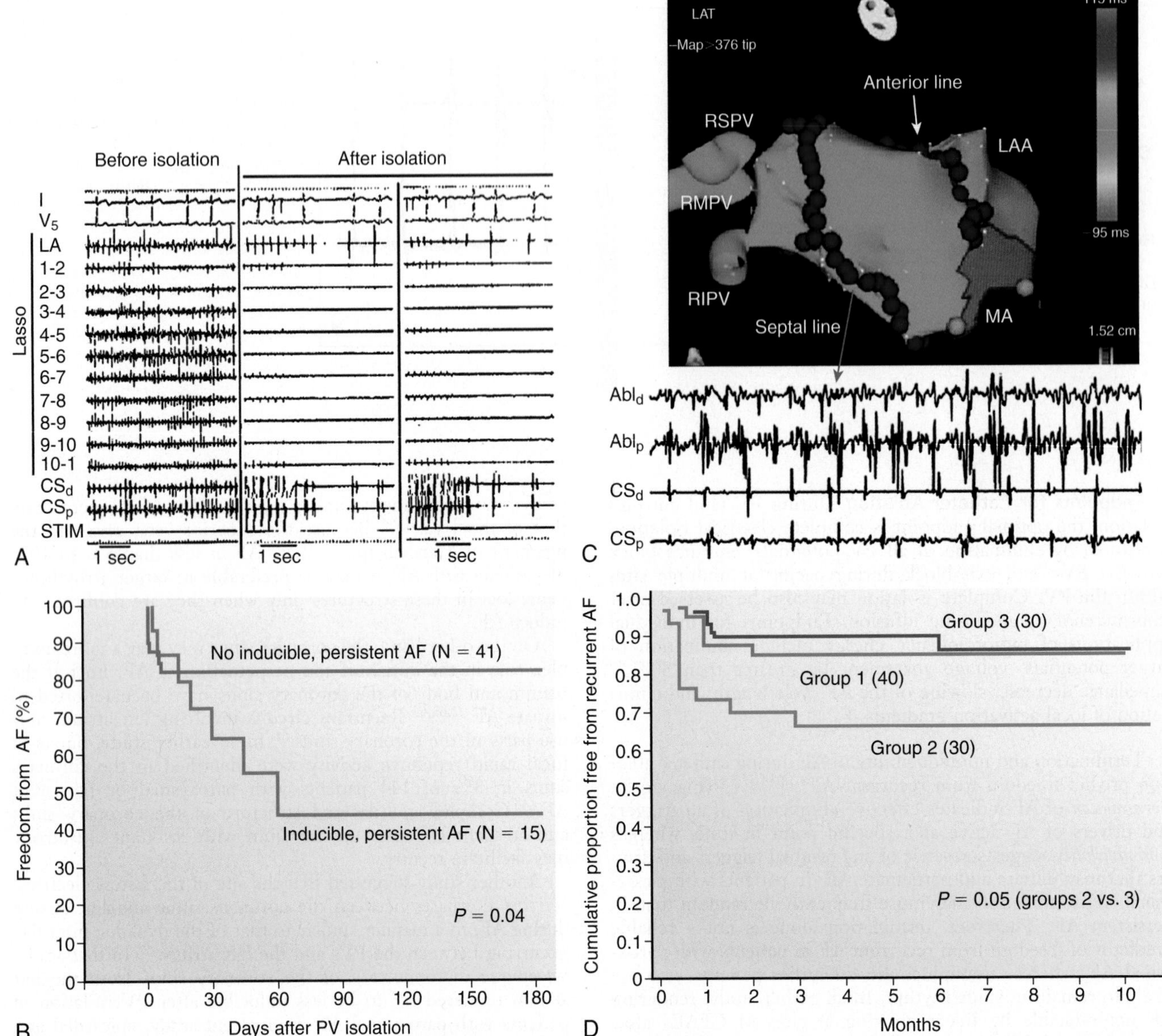

Figure 56-8 Inducibility of atrial fibrillation (AF) before and after pulmonary vein (PV) isolation. **A,** Before vein isolation, persistent AF was inducible by atrial pacing at a cycle length of 200 ms. After isolation of the left superior, left inferior, and right superior PVs, persistent AF was no longer inducible. **B,** Graph showing freedom from recurrence of AF in patients who did and those who did not have inducible persistent AF after PV isolation. **C,** In another study, left atrial electrograms guided placement of additional ablation lines after circumferential ablation (Abl). CS, coronary sinus. **D,** Graph showing freedom from symptomatic AF in the absence of antiarrhythmic drug therapy in patients who no longer had inducible AF after circumferential PV ablation (*green line*, Group 1), who still had inducible or spontaneous AF and did not undergo additional ablation (*blue line*, Group 2), and who still had inducible AF and underwent additional left atrial ablation (*red line*, Group 3). (Adapted from Oral H, Ozaydin M, Tada H, et al: Mechanistic significance of intermittent pulmonary vein tachycardia in patients with atrial fibrillation. J Cardiovasc Electrophysiol 13:645-650, 2002; and Oral H, Chugh A, Lemola K, et al: Noninducibility of atrial fibrillation as an end point of left atrial circumferential ablation for paroxysmal atrial fibrillation: A randomized study. Circulation 110:2797-2801, 2004.)

16 months, sinus rhythm was maintained in 58% and 52% of the patients who were randomized to additional right atrial ablation and to no further ablation, respectively.

These observations suggest that the right atrium may play a role in a small proportion of patients with AF. It will be important to better identify and selectively target right atrial mechanisms that contribute to AF, rather than to rely on empirical routine right atrial ablation.

Surgical Ablation

The classic surgical maze procedure with the cut-and-sew technique has been highly effective in eliminating AF.[70,71] Because of the technical complexity of the surgery, so-called mini-maze procedures have been performed more frequently[71-73] (Fig. 56-9). No studies have been conducted to compare the efficacy of surgical and catheter ablation techniques for correcting AF. In a recent meta-analysis of 48 studies involving

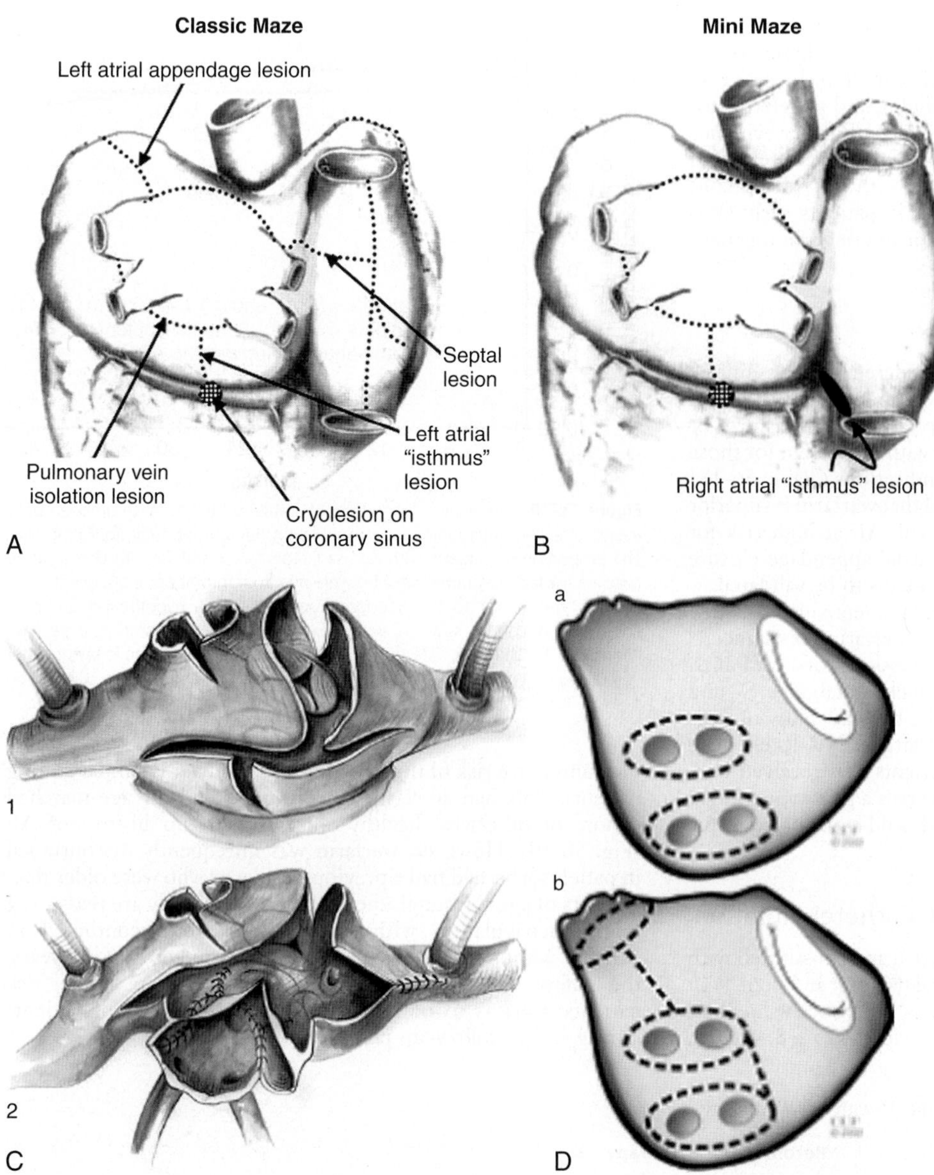

Figure 56-9 Examples of surgical classic and mini-maze procedures. Classic maze procedure is shown in **A** and **C**. Mini-maze procedure with slight modifications in technique is shown in **B** and **D**. (Data from published studies by Cox,[70,71] Ballaux,[72] and Gillinov and McCarthy.[73])

3832 patients, sinus rhythm was maintained in 83% of the patients who underwent the classic maze procedure with cut-and-sew technique and in 78% of the patients in whom ablation using alternative energy sources was performed (P = .03).[74] Of note, however, alternative energy sources were more often used in older patients with comorbid conditions and during concomitant cardiac surgery. After adjustment for these variables, a significant difference in efficacy was no longer observed.

Patient Selection

Catheter ablation for AF usually is considered for symptomatic patients with AF in whom therapy with one or more antiarrhythmic agents has failed.[1,3] Age, functional and symptomatic status, long-term thromboembolic risk and structural remodeling associated with AF, long-term risks associated with pharmacologic and anticoagulant therapy, presence of structural heart disease, presence of tachycardia-mediated cardiomyopathy, left atrial size, duration of AF, and availability of effective and tolerable pharmacologic therapy should be carefully weighed against the long-term efficacy and risk of complications associated with catheter ablation.

Surgical ablation may be most appropriate for patients who require concomitant cardiac surgery. Whether surgical ablation also may be preferred in patients in whom multiple attempts at catheter ablation have failed or who have massive enlargement of the left atrium, or in patients who have persistent left atrial appendage thrombus, remains to be validated in future studies.

Thromboembolism and Anticoagulation in Atrial Fibrillation

Thromboembolic Risk

The risk of thromboembolic events is increased five-fold in patients with AF. Left atrial mechanical dysfunction and stasis promote thrombus formation in the left atrial appendage. However, approximately 25% of all strokes in patients with AF are due to intrinsic cerebrovascular disease and atherosclerotic aortic disease.[75] AF also may be associated with a hypercoagulable state, and platelet and endothelial dysfunction. Increases in fibrinogen, D-dimer levels, thromboglobulin, and platelet factor 4 levels have been reported in patients with AF. Further evidence of the presence of a systemic involvement has been elevated C-reactive protein (CRP) levels in patients with AF.[76] It remains unclear whether the thromboembolic risk in patients with AF is due primarily to a hypercoaguable state or to left atrial mechanical dysfunction, or to both.

Anticoagulation

The risk of thromboembolism is considered similar among patients with paroxysmal, persistent, or permanent AF and those with atrial flutter. Antithrombotic therapy with aspirin or warfarin is recommended for all patients with AF, except for those with lone AF or those who have contraindications (Table 56-1).[1] A recent randomized study demonstrated that warfarin is superior to aspirin plus clopidogrel in patients with AF at high risk for stroke.[77] The role of percutaneous left atrial appendage closure in preventing thromboembolic events remains to be validated.

Functional abnormalities of the vitamin K–epoxide reductase complex (VKORC1) gene results in warfarin resistance.[78] Genetic polymorphisms in the expression of CYP2C9, CYP3A4, CYP31A2, and CYP31A1, which metabolize S- and R-enantiomers of warfarin, may affect the bioavailability of warfarin.[79] In a recent randomized trial,[80] target INR levels were maintained in a similar proportion of patients who received warfarin according to conventional dosing versus a genotype-guided algorithm, except in patients who had wild-type or multiple genetic variants.

Long-Term Anticogulation after Catheter Ablation

In a recent study, warfarin was discontinued and substituted with aspirin in 79% of the patients without risk factors, and in 68% of the patients with one or more risk factor(s) after successful ablation of AF.[81] During a mean follow-up period of 25 ± 8 months, the cumulative risk of thromboembolic events was similar among patients who had warfarin discontinued and an age-matched cohort of otherwise healthy subjects with no history of AF (Fig. 56-10). However, warfarin was infrequently discontinued in patients who had had a previous stroke or who were older than 65 years of age. Although the findings of this study are reassuring that anticoagulation with warfarin can be discontinued in patients without a history of stroke and younger than 65 years, the safety of discontinuing anticoagulation in higher-risk patients remains to be determined in larger series of patients during longer follow-up periods.

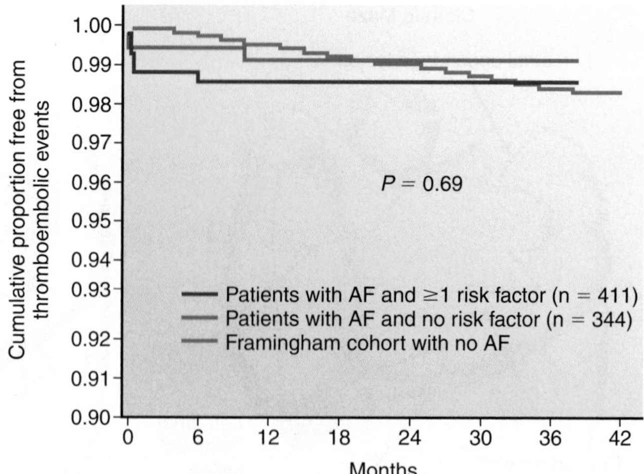

Figure 56-10 Cumulative proportion of patients free from thromboembolic events after left atrial radiofrequency ablation (LARFA) for atrial fibrillation (AF). The proportion of patients with no risk factors *(green line)* or with one or more baseline risk factors *(purple line)* who were free from thromboembolic events after ablation was similar to the freedom from stroke in a hypothetical group of age-matched control subjects with no history of atrial fibrillation *(blue line)*. (From Oral H, Chugh A, Ozaydin M, et al: Risk of thromboembolic events after percutaneous left atrial radiofrequency ablation of atrial fibrillation. Circulation 114:759-765, 2006.)

Table 56-1 Antithrombotic Therapy for Patients with Atrial Fibrillation

Risk Category	Recommended Therapy	
No risk factors	Aspirin, 81 to 325 mg daily	
One moderate-risk factor	Aspirin, 81 to 325 mg daily, or warfarin (INR 2.0 to 3.0, target 2.5)	
Any high-risk factor OR more than one moderate-risk factor	Warfarin (INR 2.0 to 3.0, target 2.5)*	
Less Validated or Weaker Risk Factors	**Moderate-Risk Factors**	**High-Risk Factors**
Female gender	Age 75 years or older	Previous stroke, TIA, or embolism
Age 65 to 74 years	Hypertension	Mitral stenosis
Coronary artery disease	Heart failure	Prosthetic heart valve*
Thyrotoxicosis	LV ejection fraction 35% or less	
	Diabetes mellitus	

*If patient has a mechanical valve, target INR is greater than 2.5.

INR, international normalized ratio; LV, left ventricular; TIA, transient ischemic attack.

(From Fuster V, Ryden LE, Cannom DS, et al: ACC/AHA/ESC 2006 guidelines for the management of patients with atrial fibrillation: Full text: A report of the American College of Cardiology/American Heart Association Task Force on practice guidelines and the European Society of Cardiology Committee for Practice Guidelines (Writing Committee to Revise the 2001 Guidelines for the Management of Patients with Atrial Fibrillation) developed in collaboration with the European Heart Rhythm Association and the Heart Rhythm Society. Europace 8:651-745, 2006.)

Conclusions and Future Directions

Recognition of the role of PVs and their antral regions play in the genesis of AF has resulted in substantial progress in the understanding and treatment of AF over the past decade. However, important challenges remain. A better understanding of the mechanisms of AF is needed. It will be critical to accurately identify and eliminate specific drivers of AF, particularly those beyond the PVs, to further improve clinical efficacy of ablation. Refinements in the techniques and advances in mapping and ablation technology should result in improvements in the safety and efficiency of ablative therapy. Novel atrioselective pharmacologic agents that are safe and effective also should be helpful. Finally, long-term efficacy, morbidity, thromboembolic risk, and potential survival benefits after ablation need to be determined in large long-term studies.

References

1. Fuster V, Ryden LE, Cannom DS, et al: ACC/AHA/ESC 2006 guidelines for the management of patients with atrial fibrillation: Full text: A report of the American College of Cardiology/American Heart Association Task Force on practice guidelines and the European Society of Cardiology Committee for Practice Guidelines (Writing Committee to Revise the 2001 Guidelines for the Management of Patients with Atrial Fibrillation) developed in collaboration with the European Heart Rhythm Association and the Heart Rhythm Society. Europace 8:651-745, 2006.
2. Miyasaka Y, Barnes ME, Gersh BJ, et al: Secular trends in incidence of atrial fibrillation in Olmsted County, Minnesota, 1980 to 2000, and implications on the projections for future prevalence. Circulation 114:119-125, 2006.
3. Calkins H, Brugada J, Packer DL, et al: HRS/EHRA/ECAS expert Consensus Statement on catheter and surgical ablation of atrial fibrillation: Recommendations for personnel, policy, procedures and follow-up. A report of the Heart Rhythm Society (HRS) Task Force on catheter and surgical ablation of atrial fibrillation. Heart Rhythm 4:816-861, 2007.
4. Moe GK: A conceptual model of atrial fibrillation. J Electrocardiol 1:145-146, 1968.
5. Sahadevan J, Ryu K, Peltz L, et al: Epicardial mapping of chronic atrial fibrillation in patients: Preliminary observations. Circulation 110:3293-3299, 2004.
6. Haissaguerre M, Jais P, Shah DC, et al: Spontaneous initiation of atrial fibrillation by ectopic beats originating in the pulmonary veins. N Engl J Med 339:659-666, 1998.
7. Douglas YL, Jongbloed MR, Gittenberger-de Groot AC, et al: Histology of vascular myocardial wall of left atrial body after pulmonary venous incorporation. Am J Cardiol 97:662-670, 2006.
8. Oral H, Ozaydin M, Tada H, et al: Mechanistic significance of intermittent pulmonary vein tachycardia in patients with atrial fibrillation. J Cardiovasc Electrophysiol 13:645-650, 2002.
9. Oral H, Knight BP, Ozaydin M, et al: Segmental ostial ablation to isolate the pulmonary veins during atrial fibrillation: Feasibility and mechanistic insights. Circulation 106:1256-1262, 2002.
10. Jalife J: Rotors and spiral waves in atrial fibrillation. J Cardiovasc Electrophysiol 14:776-780, 2003.
11. Lazar S, Dixit S, Marchlinski FE, et al: Presence of left-to-right atrial frequency gradient in paroxysmal but not persistent atrial fibrillation in humans. Circulation 110:3181-3186, 2004.
12. Sanders P, Berenfeld O, Hocini M, et al: Spectral analysis identifies sites of high-frequency activity maintaining atrial fibrillation in humans. Circulation 112:789-797, 2005.
13. Lemola K, Ting M, Gupta P, et al: Effects of two different catheter ablation techniques on spectral characteristics of atrial fibrillation. J Am Coll Cardiol 48:340-348, 2006.
14. Hou Y, Scherlag BJ, Lin J, et al: Interactive atrial neural network: Determining the connections between ganglionated plexi. Heart Rhythm 4:56-63, 2007.
15. Bettoni M, Zimmermann M: Autonomic tone variations before the onset of paroxysmal atrial fibrillation. Circulation 105:2753-2759, 2002.
16. Po SS, Scherlag BJ, Yamanashi WS, et al: Experimental model for paroxysmal atrial fibrillation arising at the pulmonary vein-atrial junctions. Heart Rhythm 3:201-208, 2006.
17. Lemola K, Chartier D, Yeh YH, et al: Pulmonary vein region ablation in experimental vagal atrial fibrillation. Role of pulmonary veins versus autonomic ganglia. Circulation 117:470-477, 2008.
18. Pappone C, Santinelli V, Manguso F, et al: Pulmonary vein denervation enhances long-term benefit after circumferential ablation for paroxysmal atrial fibrillation. Circulation 109:327-334, 2004.
19. Cummings JE, Gill I, Akhrass R, et al: Preservation of the anterior fat pad paradoxically decreases the incidence of postoperative atrial fibrillation in humans. J Am Coll Cardiol 43:994-1000, 2004.
20. Melo J, Voigt P, Sonmez B, et al: Ventral cardiac denervation reduces the incidence of atrial fibrillation after coronary artery bypass grafting. J Thorac Cardiovasc Surg 127:511-516, 2004.
21. Wyse DG, Waldo AL, DiMarco JP, et al: A comparison of rate control and rhythm control in patients with atrial fibrillation. N Engl J Med 347:1825-1833, 2002.
22. Steinberg JS, Sadaniantz A, Kron J, et al: Analysis of cause-specific mortality in the Atrial Fibrillation Follow-up Investigation of Rhythm Management (AFFIRM) study. Circulation 109:1973-1980, 2004.
23. Corley SD, Epstein AE, DiMarco JP, et al: Relationships between sinus rhythm, treatment, and survival in the Atrial Fibrillation Follow-Up Investigation of Rhythm Management (AFFIRM) Study. Circulation 109:1509-1513, 2004.
24. Van Gelder IC, Hagens VE, Bosker HA, et al: A comparison of rate control and rhythm control in patients with recurrent persistent atrial fibrillation. N Engl J Med 347:1834-1840, 2002.
25. Pappone C, Rosanio S, Augello G, et al: Mortality, morbidity, and quality of life after circumferential pulmonary vein ablation for atrial fibrillation: outcomes from a controlled nonrandomized long-term study. J Am Coll Cardiol 42:185-197, 2003.
26. Olshansky B, Rosenfeld LE, Warner AL, et al: The Atrial Fibrillation Follow-up Investigation of Rhythm Management (AFFIRM) study: Approaches to control rate in atrial fibrillation. J Am Coll Cardiol 43:1201-1208, 2004.
27. Doshi RN, Daoud EG, Fellows C, et al: Left ventricular-based cardiac stimulation post AV nodal ablation evaluation (the PAVE study). J Cardiovasc Electrophysiol 16:1160-1165, 2005.
28. Singh BN, Singh SN, Reda DJ, et al: Amiodarone versus sotalol for atrial fibrillation. N Engl J Med 352:1861-1872, 2005.
29. Singh BN, Connolly SJ, Crijns HJ, et al: Dronedarone for maintenance of sinus rhythm in atrial fibrillation or flutter. N Engl J Med 357:987-999, 2007.
30. Alboni P, Botto GL, Baldi N, et al: Outpatient treatment of recent-onset atrial fibrillation with the "pill-in-the-pocket" approach. N Engl J Med 351:2384-2391, 2004.
31. Shiroshita-Takeshita A, Schram G, Lavoie J, et al: Effect of simvastatin and antioxidant vitamins on atrial fibrillation promotion by atrial-tachycardia remodeling in dogs. Circulation 110:2313-2319, 2004.
32. Liu T, Li L, Korantzopoulos P, et al: Statin use and development of atrial fibrillation: A systematic review and meta-analysis of randomized clinical trials and observational studies. Int J Cardiol 126:160-170, 2008.
33. Reiffel JA, McDonald A: Antiarrhythmic effects of omega-3 fatty acids. Am J Cardiol 98:50i-60i, 2006.
34. Sarrazin JF, Comeau G, Daleau P, et al: Reduced incidence of vagally induced atrial fibrillation and expression levels of connexins by *n*-3 polyunsaturated fatty acids in dogs. J Am Coll Cardiol 50:1505-1512, 2007.
35. Mozaffarian D, Psaty BM, Rimm EB, et al: Fish intake and risk of incident atrial fibrillation. Circulation 110:368-373, 2004.
36. Frost L, Vestergaard P: *n*-3 Fatty acids consumed from fish and risk of atrial

fibrillation or flutter: The Danish Diet, Cancer, and Health Study. Am J Clin Nutr 81:50-54, 2005.

37. Brouwer IA, Heeringa J, Geleijnse JM, et al: Intake of very long-chain *n*-3 fatty acids from fish and incidence of atrial fibrillation. The Rotterdam Study. Am Heart J 151:857-862, 2006.
38. Calo L, Bianconi L, Colivicchi F, et al: N-3 Fatty acids for the prevention of atrial fibrillation after coronary artery bypass surgery: A randomized, controlled trial. J Am Coll Cardiol 45:1723-1728, 2005.
39. Ehrlich JR, Hohnloser SH, Nattel S: Role of angiotensin system and effects of its inhibition in atrial fibrillation: Clinical and experimental evidence. Eur Heart J 27:512-518, 2006.
40. Tsai CT, Lai LP, Lin JL, et al: Renin-angiotensin system gene polymorphisms and atrial fibrillation. Circulation 109:1640-1646, 2004.
41. Healey JS, Baranchuk A, Crystal E, et al: Prevention of atrial fibrillation with angiotensin-converting enzyme inhibitors and angiotensin receptor blockers: A meta-analysis. J Am Coll Cardiol 45:1832-1839, 2005.
42. Ueng KC, Tsai TP, Yu WC, et al: Use of enalapril to facilitate sinus rhythm maintenance after external cardioversion of long-standing persistent atrial fibrillation. Results of a prospective and controlled study. Eur Heart J 24:2090-2098, 2003.
43. Madrid AH, Bueno MG, Rebollo JM, et al: Use of irbesartan to maintain sinus rhythm in patients with long-lasting persistent atrial fibrillation: A prospective and randomized study. Circulation 106:331-336, 2002.
44. Shroff SC, Ryu K, Martovitz NL, et al: Selective aldosterone blockade suppresses atrial tachyarrhythmias in heart failure. J Cardiovasc Electrophysiol 17:534-541, 2006.
45. Oral H, Pappone C, Chugh A, et al: Circumferential pulmonary-vein ablation for chronic atrial fibrillation. N Engl J Med 354:934-941, 2006.
46. Oral H, Scharf C, Chugh A, et al: Catheter ablation for paroxysmal atrial fibrillation: Segmental pulmonary vein ostial ablation versus left atrial ablation. Circulation 108:2355-2360, 2003.
47. Pappone C, Oreto G, Rosanio S, et al: Atrial electroanatomic remodeling after circumferential radiofrequency pulmonary vein ablation: Efficacy of an anatomic approach in a large cohort of patients with atrial fibrillation. Circulation 104:2539-2544, 2001.
48. Verma A, Marrouche NF, Natale A: Pulmonary vein antrum isolation: Intracardiac echocardiography–guided technique. J Cardiovasc Electrophysiol 15:1335-1340, 2004.
49. Ouyang F, Bansch D, Ernst S, et al: Complete isolation of left atrium surrounding the pulmonary veins: New insights from the double-Lasso technique in paroxysmal atrial fibrillation. Circulation 110:2090-2096, 2004.
50. Haissaguerre M, Sanders P, Hocini M, et al: Catheter ablation of long-lasting persistent atrial fibrillation: Critical structures for termination. J Cardiovasc Electrophysiol 16:1125-1137, 2005.
51. Nademanee K, McKenzie J, Kosar E, et al: A new approach for catheter ablation of atrial fibrillation: Mapping of the electrophysiologic substrate. J Am Coll Cardiol 43:2044-2053, 2004.
52. Oral H, Chugh A, Good E, et al: A tailored approach to catheter ablation of paroxysmal atrial fibrillation. Circulation 113:1824-1831, 2006.
53. Oral H, Chugh A, Good E, et al: Radiofrequency catheter ablation of chronic atrial fibrillation guided by complex electrograms. Circulation 115:2606-2612, 2007.
54. Haissaguerre M, Hocini M, Sanders P, et al: Catheter ablation of long-lasting persistent atrial fibrillation: Clinical outcome and mechanisms of subsequent arrhythmias. J Cardiovasc Electrophysiol 16:1138-1147, 2005.
55. Jacquemet V, Virag N, Ihara Z, et al: Study of unipolar electrogram morphology in a computer model of atrial fibrillation. J Cardiovasc Electrophysiol 14(10 Suppl): S172-S179, 2003.
56. Lin J, Scherlag BJ, Zhou J, et al: Autonomic mechanism to explain complex fractionated atrial electrograms (CFAE). J Cardiovasc Electrophysiol 18:1197-1205, 2007.
57. Haissaguerre M, Sanders P, Hocini M, et al: Changes in atrial fibrillation cycle length and inducibility during catheter ablation and their relation to outcome. Circulation 109:3007-3013, 2004.
58. Oral H, Chugh A, Lemola K, et al: Noninducibility of atrial fibrillation as an end point of left atrial circumferential ablation for paroxysmal atrial fibrillation: A randomized study. Circulation 110: 2797-2801, 2004.
59. Oral H, Crawford T, Frederick M, et al: Inducibility of paroyxsmal atrial fibrillation by isoproterenol and its relation to the mode of onset of atrial fibrillation. J Cardiovasc Electrophysiol 19:466-470, 2008.
60. Oral H, Chugh A, Good E, et al: Radiofrequency catheter ablation of chronic atrial fibrillation guided by complex electrograms. Circulation 115:2606-2612, 2007.
61. Chen PS, Wu TJ, Hwang C, et al: Thoracic veins and the mechanisms of non-paroxysmal atrial fibrillation. Cardiovasc Res 54:295-301, 2002.
62. Lin WS, Tai CT, Hsieh MH, et al: Catheter ablation of paroxysmal atrial fibrillation initiated by non-pulmonary vein ectopy. Circulation 107:3176-3183, 2003.
63. Chen PS, Chou CC: Coronary sinus as an arrhythmogenic structure. J Cardiovasc Electrophysiol 13:863-864, 2002.
64. Scavee C, Jais P, Weerasooriya R, et al: The inferior vena cava: An exceptional source of atrial fibrillation. J Cardiovasc Electrophysiol 14:659-662, 2003.
65. Knecht S, O'Neill MD, Matsuo S, et al: Focal arrhythmia confined within the coronary sinus and maintaining atrial fibrillation. J Cardiovasc Electrophysiol 18: 1140-1146, 2007.
66. Chugh A, Oral H, Good E, et al: Catheter ablation of atypical atrial flutter and atrial tachycardia within the coronary sinus after left atrial ablation for atrial fibrillation. J Am Coll Cardiol 46:83-91, 2005.
67. Oral H, Ozaydin M, Chugh A, et al: Role of the coronary sinus in maintenance of atrial fibrillation. J Cardiovasc Electrophysiol 14:1329-1336, 2003.
68. Haissaguerre M, Hocini M, Takahashi Y, et al: Impact of catheter ablation of the coronary sinus on paroxysmal or persistent atrial fibrillation. J Cardiovasc Electrophysiol 18:378-386, 2007.
69. Liu TY, Tai CT, Chen SA: Treatment of atrial fibrillation by catheter ablation of conduction gaps in the crista terminalis and cavotricuspid isthmus of the right atrium. J Cardiovasc Electrophysiol 13:1044-1046, 2002.
70. Cox JL: Cardiac surgery for arrhythmias. J Cardiovasc Electrophysiol 15:250-262, 2004.
71. Cox JL: Atrial fibrillation II: Rationale for surgical treatment. J Thorac Cardiovasc Surg 126:1693-1699, 2003.
72. Ballaux PK, Geuzebroek GS, van Hemel NM, et al: Freedom from atrial arrhythmias after classic maze III surgery: A 10-year experience. J Thorac Cardiovasc Surg 132:1433-1440, 2006.
73. Gillinov AM, McCarthy PM: Advances in the surgical treatment of atrial fibrillation. Cardiol Clin 22:147-157, 2004.
74. Khargi K, Hutten BA, Lemke B, et al: Surgical treatment of atrial fibrillation; a systematic review. Eur J Cardiothorac Surg 2005; 27:258-265, 2005.
75. Miller VT, Rothrock JF, Pearce LA, et al: Ischemic stroke in patients with atrial fibrillation: effect of aspirin according to stroke mechanism. Stroke Prevention in Atrial Fibrillation Investigators. Neurology 43:32-36, 1993.
76. Aviles RJ, Martin DO, Apperson-Hansen C, et al: Inflammation as a risk factor for atrial fibrillation. Circulation 108:3006-3010, 2003.
77. Connolly S, Pogue J, Hart R, et al: Clopidogrel plus aspirin versus oral anticoagulation for atrial fibrillation in the Atrial Fibrillation Clopidogrel Trial with Irbesartan for Prevention of Vascular Events (ACTIVE W): A randomised controlled trial. Lancet 367:1903-1912, 2006.
78. Rost S, Fregin A, Ivaskevicius V, et al: Mutations in VKORC1 cause warfarin resistance and multiple coagulation factor deficiency type 2. Nature 427:537-541, 2004.
79. Yin T, Miyata T: Warfarin dose and the pharmacogenomics of CYP2C9 and VKORC1—rationale and perspectives. Thromb Res 120:1-10, 2007.
80. Anderson JL, Horne BD, Stevens SM, et al: Randomized trial of genotype-guided versus standard warfarin dosing in patients initiating oral anticoagulation. Circulation 116:2563-2570, 2007.
81. Oral H, Chugh A, Ozaydin M, et al: Risk of thromboembolic events after percutaneous left atrial radiofrequency ablation of atrial fibrillation. Circulation 114:759-765, 2006.

Atrial Tachycardia 57

Kenneth A. Ellenbogen, Bruce S. Stambler, and Mark A. Wood

CHAPTER OUTLINE

Atrial tachycardias constitute an uncommon cause of supraventricular tachycardia. In most clinical series, atrial tachycardias account for approximately 5% of all supraventricular arrhythmias for which adult patients undergo electrophysiology studies. In the pediatric population, atrial tachycardias occur more frequently, generally in the 10% to 15% range in children without congenital heart disease, and in a much higher percentage of children who have undergone surgical correction of congenital heart disease.

This chapter reviews new information about the classification, mechanisms, electrocardiographic localization, and electrophysiologic characterization of atrial tachycardias.

Classification and Mechanisms

An expert consensus group from the European Society of Cardiology and the North American Society of Pacing and Electrophysiology published a classification of atrial flutter and regular atrial tachycardias based on mechanism and anatomy.[1] Atrial tachycardias were classified as tachycardias with a regular atrial rate arising from the atrium and were further categorized as either focal or macro-reentrant. *Focal* atrial tachycardia may be caused by automatic, triggered, or micro-reentrant mechanisms. Focal atrial tachycardias are characterized by radial, circular, or centrifugal spread of activation from a single focus or point source and lack of electrical activation spanning the tachycardia cycle length. *Macro-reentrant* atrial tachycardias are due to reentry through relatively large, potentially well-characterized circuits. Macro-reentrant atrial tachycardias are characterized by a repetitive pattern of electrical activation encompassing the entire cardiac cycle. Patterns that have been described include a single loop (such as common isthmus-dependent flutter), two reentrant loops creating a figure of eight, and reentry through narrow channels adjacent to scars or natural anatomic barriers, such as the tricuspid annulus. Typical atrial flutter, lower loop reentry, double loop reentry, left atrial macro-reentrant atrial tachycardia, scar atrial tachycardia, reverse typical atrial flutter, and right atrial free-wall macro-reentry all are classified as macro-reentrant atrial tachycardias. Atrial tachycardias occurring in the setting of congenital heart disease are described in Chapter 60, and those occurring after atrial fibrillation ablation in Chapter 56, 105, and 106. Atrial tachycardias occurring after atrial fibrillation ablation may be extremely complex, involving multiple loops, and often are related to gaps in the previously created ablation lines.

Under this classification scheme, some atrial tachycardias are left unclassified. For example, inappropriate sinus tachycardia and sinus node reentry cannot be easily classified. Despite the limitations of this classification scheme and the fact that most clinical arrhythmias are not classified by mechanism, it is useful to think of atrial tachycardias as being either focal or macro-reentrant. This differentiation has important implications for ablation therapy, because macro-reentrant atrial tachycardias often require mapping of large segments of the circuit using techniques of "entrainment mapping" or "scar mapping" and delivery of multiple radiofrequency ablation lesions for termination of tachycardia.

Focal Atrial Tachycardias

The three potential mechanisms of focal atrial tachycardia are automaticity, triggered activity, and micro-reentry. Chen and colleagues[2] studied 36 patients with atrial tachycardia using a variety of pacing and pharmacologic maneuvers. Structural heart disease was absent in 70% of the patients. These investigators classified the atrial tachycardias into one of the three mechanistic categories based on the following groups of findings.

Automatic atrial tachycardia was identified by the presence of one or more of the following characteristics: (1) Atrial tachycardia could be initiated only by isoproterenol infusion; (2) programmed electrical stimulation could not initiate or terminate atrial tachycardia; (3) atrial tachycardia could be transiently suppressed with overdrive pacing, but subsequently resumed with a gradual increase in atrial rate; (4) termination could be achieved with propranolol; (5) a "warm-up" or "cool-down" phenomenon, or both, could be demonstrated; and (6) the rhythm showed adenosine insensitivity. Seven of the 36 patients had this mechanism identified as the predominant mechanism of their atrial tachycardia.

Atrial tachycardia attributed to *triggered activity* was found in 9 of 36 patients. Triggered activity was characterized by one or more of the following: (1) Initiation of tachycardia occurred with rapid atrial pacing or atrial extrastimuli, typically dependent on reaching a certain range of atrial pacing cycle lengths; (2) entrainment of atrial tachycardia was not demonstrated, but overdrive suppression or termination was noted; (3) delayed afterdepolarizations were recorded from a monophasic action potential catheter at the tachycardia site of origin, but not

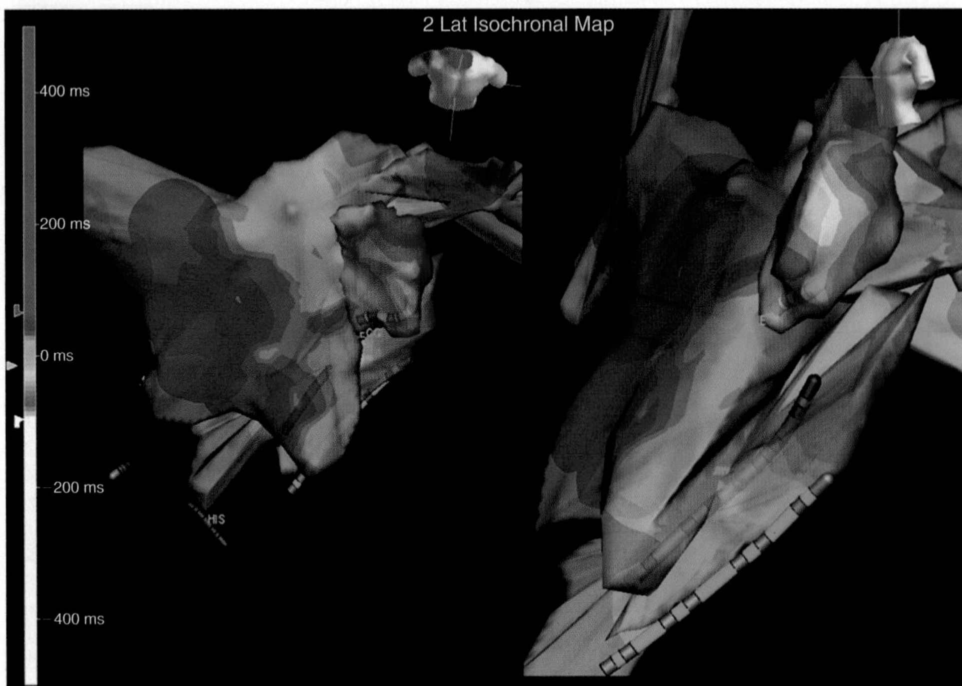

Figure 57-1 Computerized mapping from a patient with a focal (left) atrial tachycardia arising from the epicardial surface of the left atrial appendage. Structural heart disease was absent, but the patient had an incessant tachycardia. The site of origin is focal, with rapid radial spread of atrial activation from the earliest site of activation.

recorded from areas remote from the tachycardia; (4) adenosine terminated the tachycardia; (5) isoproterenol was rarely required to induce tachycardia; and (6) dipyridamole, propranolol, verapamil, edrophonium, Valsalva maneuvers, and carotid sinus pressure terminated tachycardia in all patients.

Atrial tachycardia attributed to *micro-reentry* was found in 20 patients. Micro-reentry was characterized by the following: (1) Atrial tachycardia was reproducibly initiated and terminated by atrial pacing and extrastimuli; (2) delayed afterdepolarizations were not found on monophasic action potential catheter recordings; (3) pacing during tachycardia fulfilled criteria for manifest and concealed entrainment; (4) frequent termination by verapamil and adenosine was observed; and (5) the interval between the initiating premature beat and the first beat of tachycardia were inversely related.

The major limitation to this careful analysis is the observation of some overlap in the electrophysiologic and pharmacologic characterization of mechanisms. For example, verapamil and adenosine both terminate atrial tachycardias caused by micro-reentry and triggered activity. Additionally, programmed stimulation may initiate and terminate both atrial tachycardias caused by triggered activity and micro-reentry. The clinical significance of the different mechanisms is unknown. For example, verapamil-sensitive atrial tachycardias originate from both the atrioventricular (AV) nodal vicinity and the atrioventricular annulus.[3] This observation emphasizes the fact that the localization of the anatomic site of origin of a focal atrial tachycardia is not an accurate predictor of the mechanism or of ablation outcome.

Extensive activation sequence mapping also has been used to define the mechanism of atrial tachycardia. In one study, electroanatomic mapping (CARTO, Biosense, Webster, California) of the right atrium was performed during 13 tachycardia episodes in 10 patients who had had previous cardiac surgery.[4] Focal atrial tachycardias were defined in 3 patients, and macro-reentrant circuits were found in 7 patients. The mapping system allowed rapid distinction between a focal atrial tachycardia and a macro-reentrant mechanism. In the patients with focal mechanisms, a radial spread of activation was noted from the site of earliest activation in all directions on an isochronal map (Fig. 57-1). The right atrial activation time was markedly shorter than the tachycardia cycle length, accounting for, on average, 14% of the tachycardia cycle length. In patients with a macro-reentrant mechanism, isochronal maps showed a continuous progression of activation around the right or left atrium, with close proximity of earliest and latest local activation (Fig. 57-2). The right atrial activation time was in a range similar to that of tachycardia cycle length, occupying 70% or more of the tachycardia cycle length.

The effects of adenosine on atrial tachycardia have been carefully studied by Markowitz and associates,[5] who examined the mechanism-specific effects of adenosine on 85 atrial tachycardias in 82 patients. In response to adenosine, termination occurred in 67 cases (84%), 2 exhibited a nonspecific response, and 6 were insensitive (8%). Adenosine-insensitive atrial tachycardias arose near the pulmonary veins and in the right atrium, whereas adenosine-sensitive atrial tachycardias arose from a wide distribution of sites in both atria. These sites included the tricuspid annulus (n = 45), mitral annulus (n = 8), crista terminalis (n = 15), and other sites (posteroseptal right atrium, atrial appendage, and interatrial septum). Electrograms at the site of origin of adenosine-insensitive atrial tachycardia typically were highly fractionated and had longer durations and lower amplitudes compared with atrial tachycardias that were terminated or transiently suppressed. Similar observations were made by De Groot and Schalij, who showed that the site of origin of focal atrial tachycardias was characterized by double potentials and fractionated and low-voltage, long-duration electrograms—findings attributed to poor cell-to-cell coupling.[6]

Sanders and colleagues reported on the use of high-density mapping of focal atrial tachycardia. They used a high-density mapping catheter (PentaRay, Biosense) to characterize a group of patients in whom prior attempts at atria tachycardia ablation or atrial fibrillation ablation had failed.[7] They noted that a localized focus was found in 70%, whereas 30% had evidence of localized

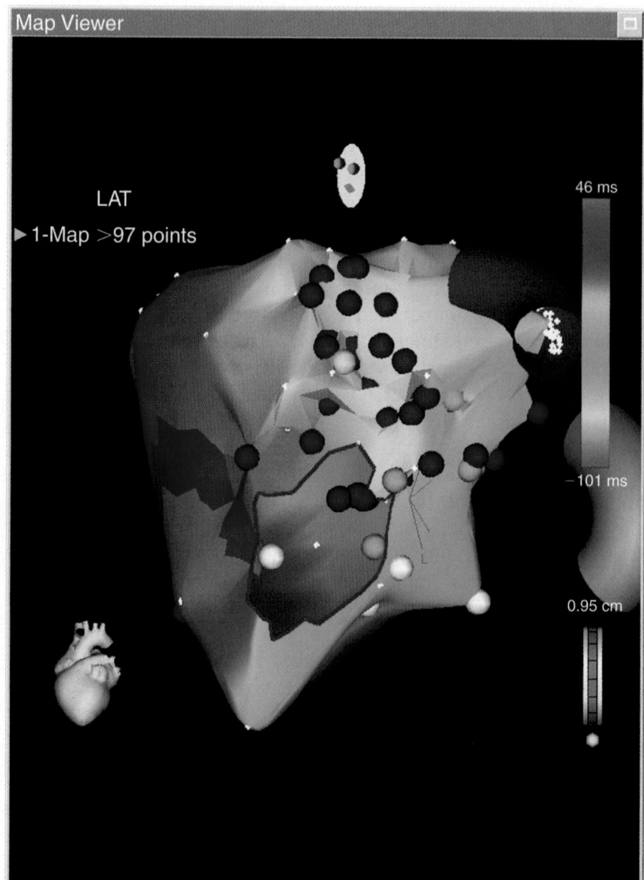

Figure 57-2 Left atrial electroanatomic map of a macro-reentrant atrial tachycardia. This electroanatomic map shows a mitral isthmus reentrant tachycardia. More than 90 points were mapped, and the map shows an "earliest meets latest" or "head meets tail" on the lateral mitral valve isthmus. The postpacing interval minus the tachycardia cycle length (PPI − TCL) was less than 10 ms from the distal coronary sinus; see Figure 57-5. This patient previously had undergone minimally invasive surgical atrial fibrillation ablation.

reentry characterized by the ability to record electrograms during 95% of the tachycardia cycle length. They demonstrated that with high-density mapping, it was possible to define regions of preferential conduction and intra-atrial conduction delay. Higa and associates made similar observations using the technique of noncontact mapping.[8] These investigators demonstrated that focal atrial tachycardia originates from a small area of tissue but spreads through the atrium by way of regions of preferential conduction. These investigators made several additional important observations: Most atrial tachycardias originate from near a border of a low-voltage zone or an area of anisotropic conduction, and the site of successful ablation is near the site of tachycardia origin or the proximal portion of the preferential conduction pathway, rather than at the "breakout" point.

The autonomic nervous system may play a role in initiating or triggering some atrial tachycardias. The precise mechanism for this effect is unknown, and the autonomic effects may be modulated by changes in atrial volume. Reports of atrial tachycardia triggered by changes in posture, belching, swallowing, and inspiration, as well as termination of tachycardia by the Valsalva maneuver, edrophonium, or β-adrenergic blockers, all confirm the probable role of the authonomic nervous system in some patients.

Electrocardiographic Localization of Focal Atrial Tachycardia

Generally, focal atrial tachycardia is characterized by P waves separated by an isoelectric interval in all electrocardiographic leads. There is extensive literature on P wave morphology and the site of the atrial focus. This literature dates back to early studies of differential pacing during electrophysiology studies or during open heart surgery. These algorithms are useful, despite considerable overlap in P wave morphology, because most atrial tachycardias originate from relatively few sites. The overlap in P wave morphology reflects the limited spatial resolution of the P wave of at best 2 cm, based on discrimination between two different atrial pacing sites from mapping studies. Additionally, the P wave often is obscured by the T wave or QRS complex during tachycardia. Finally, the algorithms for differentiation of atrial tachycardias have been based largely on analysis of tracings from patients without structural heart disease and atrial dilatation. Recently published algorithms help to determine the localization of atrial tachycardia site of origin[9-13] (Figs. 57-3 and 57-4).

The predominant areas of origin of focal atrial tachycardia include the area along the crista terminalis, near or inside the four pulmonary veins (superior veins more commonly), around or inside the coronary sinus os, superior vena cava, atrial septum, and Koch's triangle. Tang and coworkers constructed an algorithm to help localize the site of atrial tachycardia.[9] They studied 12-lead electrocardiograms (ECGs) from 31 patients with focal atrial tachycardia who underwent mapping and successful ablation and proposed an algorithm that distinguished right atrial from left atrial foci with a sensitivity of 88% to 93% and a specificity of 79% to 88%. The P wave configurations in leads aVL and V_1 were most helpful in differentiating right atrial from left atrial foci. A positive or biphasic P wave in aVL predicted a right atrial focus, whereas a positive P wave in V_1 predicted a left

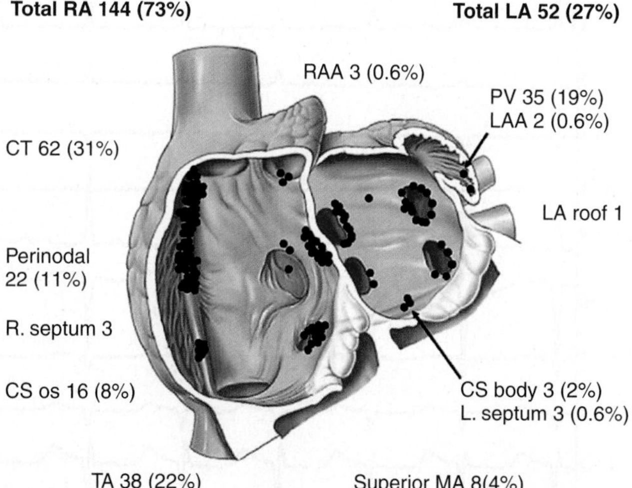

Figure 57-3 A schematic representation of the anatomic distribution of focal atrial tachycardias. The atrioventricular valvular annuli have been removed. CS, coronary sinus; CT, crista terminalis; LA, left atrium; LAA, left atrial appendage; MA, mitral annulus; PV, pulmonary vein; RA, right atrium; RAA, right atrial appendage; TA, tricuspid annulus. (From Kistler PM, Roberts-Thompson KC, Haqqani HM, et al: P-wave morphology in focal atrial tachycardia: Development of an algorithm to predict the anatomic site of origin. J Am Coll Cardiol 48:1010-1017, 2006.)

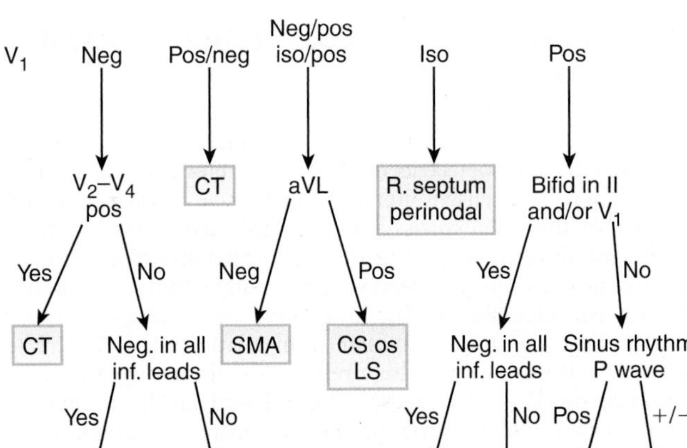

Figure 57-4 Algorithm for localizing the site of origin for focal atrial tachycardias. The algorithm, constructed on the basis of findings from 130 atrial tachycardias, correctly localized the focus in 93%. CS, coronary sinus; CT, crista terminalis; inf., inferior; iso, isoelectric; LA, left atrium; LAA, left atrial appendage; MA, mitral annulus; PV, pulmonary vein; RA, right atrium; RAA, right atrial appendage; SMA, superior mitral annulus; TA, tricuspid annulus. (From Kistler PM, Roberts-Thompson KC, Haqqani HM, et al: P-wave morphology in focal atrial tachycardia: Development of an algorithm to predict the anatomic site of origin. J Am Coll Cardiol 48:1010-1017, 2006.)

atrial focus. The algorithm incorrectly predicted the location of atrial tachycardia in patients with a right superior pulmonary vein focus, showing a positive P wave in aVL instead of the expected negative P wave, probably because of the close location of the right superior pulmonary vein to the high lateral right atrium. In these patients, close inspection of the P wave morphology during sinus rhythm and during atrial tachycardia showed the change in P wave morphology in V_1 from biphasic to a positive P wave with a right superior pulmonary vein tachycardia.

This algorithm was further refined for right atrial tachycardias by Tada and associates.[10] Based on the left anterior oblique view of the right atrium, tachycardias were classified as occurring at superolateral, inferolateral, and inferomedial locations at the time of ablation. A negative P wave in lead aVR identified an atrial tachycardia lying on the crista terminalis with a 100% sensitivity and 93% specificity. A positive P wave in the inferior leads differentiated superolateral atrial tachycardias from inferolateral atrial tachycardias with a sensitivity of 86% and a specificity of 100%. In any atrial tachycardia with inferomedial or inferolateral foci, the P wave in at least one of the inferior leads was negative. Negative P waves in leads V_5 and V_6 identified inferomedial atrial tachycardias with a sensitivity of 92% and a specificity of 100%. In atrial tachycardias coming from the Koch's triangle, the P wave duration in the inferior leads was shorter than during sinus rhythm (see Fig. 55-4). Foci from the right atrial appendage are uncommon and have a characteristic P wave morphology, a negative P wave in lead V_1 becoming progressively positive across the precordial leads, and low-amplitude positive P waves in the inferior leads in a majority of patients (Fig. 57-5). Irrigated radiofrequency energy typically is required to achieve adequate power for successful ablation at this site.

Another refinement of the algorithm for pulmonary vein foci was reported by Haissaguerre and colleagues.[11] Based on analysis of data from 30 patients, three criteria were devised to distinguish right from left pulmonary vein sites: A positive and relatively flat P wave in lead aVL and a positive P wave in lead I of greater than 50 μV indicated a right pulmonary vein origin with a specificity of 100% and 97% and a sensitivity of 38% and

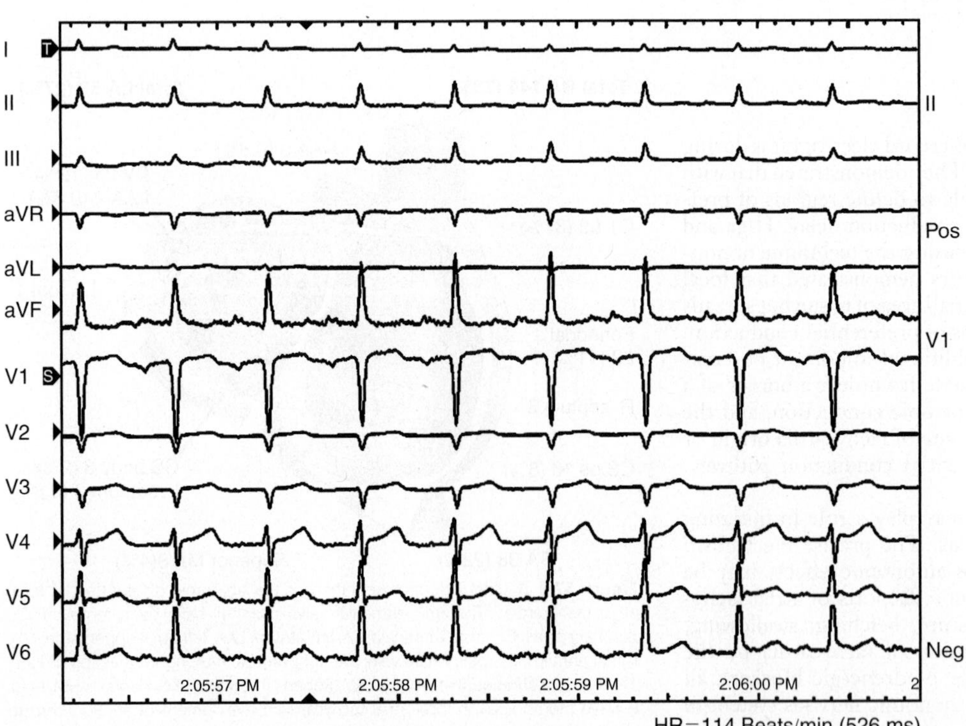

Figure 57-5 A 12-lead electrocardiogram from a patient referred for treatment of inappropriate sinus tachycardia. Electrophysiology studies and computerized mapping showed a focal atrial tachycardia from the right atrial appendage.

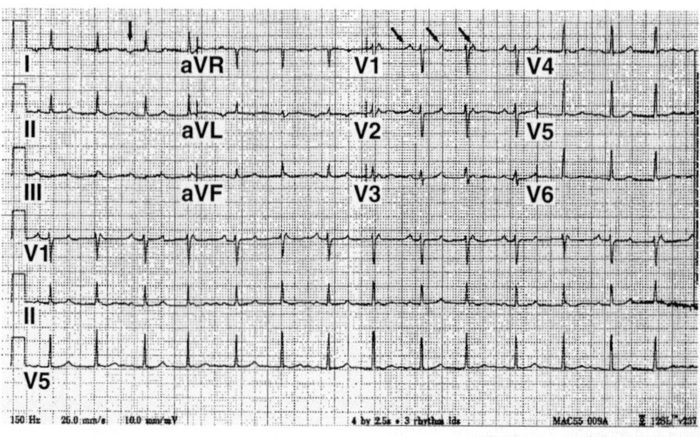

Figure 57-6 A 12-lead electrocardiogram from a patient with an epicardial atrial tachycardia originating in the left atrial appendage. The electroanatomic map for this patient is shown in Figure 57-1.

72%, respectively. The positive predictive value of these two criteria were 100% and 98%. A notched P wave in lead II was a predictor of left pulmonary vein origin with a specificity of 95% and sensitivity of 39%. An amplitude ratio of lead III/II of 0.8 or greater and the duration of positivity in lead V_1 (longer than 80 ms) also were helpful in differentiating left from right pulmonary vein origin. These two criteria had specificity of 75% and 73%, sensitivity of 96% and 85%, and positive predictive value for left pulmonary vein sites of 79% and 76%, respectively. Left pulmonary vein sites were characterized by low-amplitude and flat P waves in lead I, negative polarity in lead aVL, similar amplitudes in both limb leads III and II, and longer duration of positivity in lead V_1. Superior pulmonary veins were distinguished from inferior pulmonary veins on the basis of P wave amplitude for superior pulmonary vein origin in lead II of 100 μV or greater. This value differentiated superior from inferior P waves with specificity of 74%, sensitivity of 81%, and positive predictive value of 86%. Focal atrial tachycardias arising from the left atrial appendage can be distinguished from left or right pulmonary vein tachycardias by a deeply negative P wave in lead I. In addition, LAA atrial tachycardias also have a P wave that is upright or biphasic in lead V_1 and highly positive in the inferior leads (Fig. 57-6).

More recently, Hachiya and associates refined and simplified the algorithm for left atrial tachycardia. Their algorithm involves two steps: A positive P wave in V_1 localizes the site of origin to the pulmonary veins, and a biphasic or negative P wave in V_1, to the septal or superior mitral annulus or left atrial appendage.[12] Kistler and coworkers, building on all of these algorithms and using data from a series of 126 patients with 130 atrial tachycardias, devised an algorithm that identifies tachycardia site of origin.[13] This algorithm is presented as Figure 55-5. In their series, once again V_1 was critical. They found a negative or a positive-negative P wave in V_1 demonstrated a specificty of 100% for a right atrial focus and a positive or negative-positive P wave in V_1 demonstrated a sensitivity of 100% for a left atrial focus.

A new observation that may be useful to localize focal atrial tachycardia was made by Mohamed and associates.[14] These investigators performed atrial overdrive pacing during atrial tachycardia at a rate slighter faster than the tachycardia rate. Measurement of the postpacing interval minus the tachycardia cycle length (PPI-TCL) from various sites in the right and left atrium localized the tachycardia focus when the PPI-TCL was minimized (e.g., for the successful ablation site, 11 ± 8 ms). The investigators explained this observation by hypothesizing that the difference between the PPI and the TCL was proportional to the distance of the pacing site to the tachycardia focus and conduction time through the surrounding or perifocal tissue. In this study, overdrive suppression of the atrial tachycardia focus was not apparent. The PPI-TCL was never greater than 20 ms at a successful ablation site, suggesting minimal slowing by tissue near the atrial focus.

Atrial Tachycardia Arising from the Crista Terminalis

Intracardiac echocardiography may be particularly useful to demonstrate the close anatomic proximity of the tachycardia focus to the crista. Atrial tachycardias may be located all along the crista terminalis, which has been described as a "ring of fire" because it is a common location for atrial tachycardias in patients without structural heart disease, accounting for two thirds of right atrial tachycardias in one study. One physiologic factor contributing to the clustering of atrial tachycardias in this area is that the crista terminalis demonstrates marked anisotropy due to poor transverse cell-to-cell coupling, which could contribute to slow conduction and micro-reentry. Another contributory factor is that the crista terminalis contains clusters of cells with automaticity. The ECG characteristics of these tachycardias are described earlier and depend on site of origin from the crista terminalis (e.g., superior versus inferior).

Atrial Tachycardia Arising from the Atrioventricular Annulus

Atrial tachycardias originating from the tricuspid annulus are relatively uncommon, accounting for up to 20% of atrial tachycardias in one series.[13] The typical P wave morphology is negative in the precordial and inferior leads. Atrial tachycardias also may arise from the mitral annulus, in which case the P waves are negative in aVL and positive in V_1. In one study, 5 of 6 patients experienced termination of atrial tachycardia with doses of adenosine less than one half of those used to terminate AV nodal reentry. Recent attention has focused on the origin of focal atrial tachycardia from the superior region of the mitral annulus, or the mitral-aortic continuity. The P wave morhpology in the precordial leads typically shows a biphasic pattern, with an inverted component followed by an upright component or positive throughout the precordium.[15,16] Earliest endocardial activation is recorded on the His bundle catheter. The sensitivity of these tachycardias to adenosine and the demonstration of cells with AV nodal electrophysiologic properties lacking connexin43 (Cx43) near the annulus has led some researchers to postulate that the mechanism of these atrial tachycardias is micro-reentry involving these nodal-type cells.

Atrial Tachycardia Arising from the Coronary Sinus

Focal atrial tachycardias were reported to arise from the coronary sinus area in up to 10% of patients in one study.[13] Most patients had tachycardia arising from outside the coronary sinus or just inside the os. Atrial tachycardia arose from deep within the coronary sinus, presumably from the coronary sinus musculature, based on the observation that the tachycardia could not be ablated from the left atrial endocardium but could be ablated from within the coronary sinus.[17] A discrete potential is noted after the coronary sinus electrogram in sinus rhythm and preceding the surface P wave by 30 to 50 ms during tachycardia. The arrhythmogenic substrate is believed to be the muscular

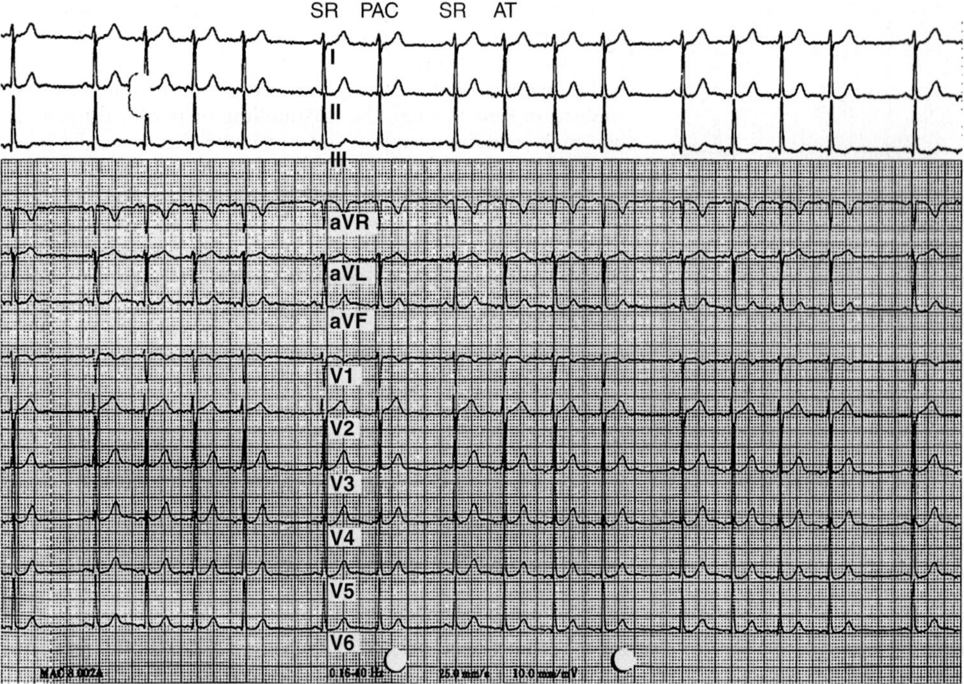

Figure 57-7 A 12-lead electrocardiogram from a patient with atrial tachycardia from the left side of the atrial septum. AT, atrial tachycardia; PAC, premature atrial contraction; SR, sinus rhythm.

sleeves surrounding the coronary sinus extending from the epicardial atrial surface. The electrocardiographic pattern is fairly typical, with negative P waves in the inferior leads and positive P waves in V_1 and aVR, as well as a transition to negative P waves in V_4 to V_6. Both atrial tachycardias and atypical atrial flutters involving the coronary sinus musculature have been reported after left atrial ablation. Atrial tachycardias also may arise from the ostium of the coronary sinus, and in these cases the P wave in V_1 may be isoelectric, negative/positive, and positive in aVL. The successful site typically has an activation 20 ms before the onset of the P wave.[18] Macro-reentrant atrial tachycardias also may involve the coronary sinus and require ablation on the left atrial endocardial surface as well as the coronary sinus.

Atrial Tachycardia Arising from the Atrial Septum

Focal atrial tachycardias in the area of the atrial septum include atrial tachycardia arising from the anterior septum, mid-septum, and posterior septum areas and from Koch's triangle.[19-22] These tachycardias, like the ones arising from near the tricuspid annulus, tend to be more sensitive to lower doses of adenosine than atrial tachycardias arising from the crista terminalis. Additionally, in one study, 45% of patients with a septal tachycardia required isoproterenol for tachycardia induction, compared with 32% of patients with atrial tachycardia originating in the right atrial free wall. Anteroseptal and midseptal right atrial tachycardias have a biphasic or negative P wave morphology in lead V_1. The combination of a negative or biphasic P wave in V_1 and a positive or biphasic P wave in all inferior leads favors an anteroseptal atrial tachycardia; presence of a negative or biphasic P wave in V_1 and a negative P wave in at least two of the three inferior leads favors a midseptal atrial tachycardia. Presence of a positive P wave in V_1 and a negative P wave in all three inferior leads favors a posteroseptal atrial tachycardia. The electrophysiology study is critical for differentiating these tachycardias from atypical AV node reentry or a septal accessory pathway. In several series, 27% to 35% of patients had tachycardias originating from this region.

Atrial tachycardias may originate from near the apex of Koch's triangle (region of AV nodal transitional cells) in up to 10% of patients with tachycardias arising from the right atrium (Fig. 57-7). It must be emphasized that these tachycardias also are adenosine-sensitive and may require isoproterenol for induction. In most patients, these tachycardias can be ablated without damage to AV nodal conduction. The P wave duration during tachycardia is, on average, 20 ms shorter than during sinus rhythm. In patients without structural heart disease, it is important to map the left atrial septum as well (Fig. 57-8). Atrial activation mapping on the right side alone will not differentiate between a right and left atrial site of tachycardia origin, implying rapid direct transseptal conduction by way of Bachmann's bundle, which results in an early right-sided breakthrough. In patients with a left-sided origin, P waves in V_1 were always positive in one series, but not in another.[21,22] In one series of 16 patients with the earliest atrial activation in the triangle of Koch, a left atrial focus was found in nearly 40% of patients. Recently, a series of patients with atrial tachycardia mapping to the para-Hisian region has been reported. Localization of tachycardia to this region revealed a suprising insensitivity to adenosine, with P waves that were upright or biphasic in lead I and aVL and a variety of P wave morphologies in the inferior leads. Low radiofrequency energies were used in ablating in this region, and no junctional rhythm was observed during ablation.[23]

A recent report showed that some focal atrial tachycardias could be mapped and ablated from the noncoronary aortic cusp, and most of these patients had undergone multiple previous failed ablation procedures. The P wave morphology was positive in leads I and aVL and positive or negative in V_1 and V_2. The P waves in leads II, II, and aVF were positive or negative in most patients as well.[24] In summary, tachycardias located in this region present a risk of heart block during ablation and careful mapping of both sides of the septum, and in some

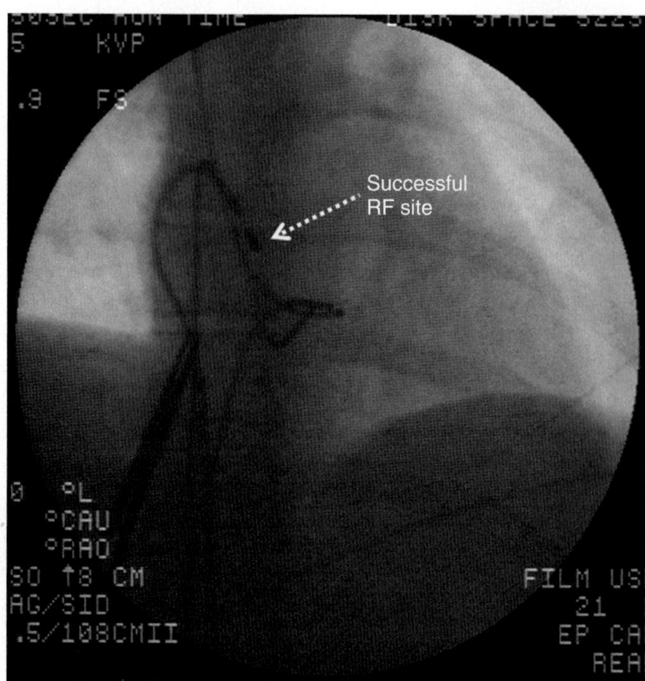

Figure 57-8 Right anterior oblique fluoroscopic view of successful radiofrequency (RF) ablation site for the patient whose 12-lead electrocardiogram is shown in Figure 57-7.

cases, mapping and ablation in the aortic root is necessary. The aortic root occupies a central location between the tricuspid and mitral annulus and in close vicinity to the His bundle.

Sinus Node Reentrant Tachycardia

Atrial tachycardias arising from this region are presumed to be due to micro-reentry in tissue near the sinus node or perinodal region (superior crista terminalis). The P wave morphology during tachycardia should be identical to that seen during sinus rhythm. Focal atrial tachycardias may also arise from the superior vena cava. Atrial tachycardia arising from the area of the superior vena cava may conduct to the right atrium. Fibrillatory conduction from a focus in the superior vena cava with exit block to the right atrium masquerading as a focal right atrial tachycardia occasionally has been reported. Conduction delay in the superior vena cava–right atrial junction may contribute to tachycardia initiation.

Left Atrial Tachycardia

The pulmonary veins and the mitral valve annulus are the main source of focal left atrial tachycardias. A majority of pulmonary vein tachycardias originate from the ostium of the pulmonary veins, rather than from deep inside the pulmonary veins. Additionally, it is rare for atrial tachycardias to recur from different sites in the pulmonary veins or for atrial fibrillation to develop after a pulmonary vein focal atrial tachycardia ablation.[25,26] Superior (Bachmann's bundle), inferior (coronary sinus), and septal (fossa ovalis) interatrial electrical connections exist between the right and left atrium. Additional posterior electrical connections between the right sided pulmonary veins and right atrial posterior walls exist in human hearts. This may compound the difficulty differentiating between an atrial tachycardia originating from the pulmonary veins and one arising from the posterior right atrium. P wave configuration in V_1 may be helpful; the posterior right atrial sites had a biphasic P wave in V_1 with a positive-negative configuration, and the right superior pulmonary vein sites had a positive P wave in V_1 (see Fig. 57-4). A second differentiating feature is that P waves from the right superior pulmonary vein show notching in lead II in 80%, but are smooth with those coming from the region of the superior vena cava (see Fig. 57-4). Finally, double potentials may be recorded from a posterior right atrial catheter and when the amplitude of the first component (near field electrogram, a sharper electrogram) is higher than that of the second component, the atrial tachycardia originates from the right atrium. Atrial tachycardia may also occur from the left atrial appendage and tends to be localized to the base of the left atrial appendage, primarily on the medial side. The atrial activation sequence typically shows activation in the distal coronary sinus earlier than the P wave, and a negative P wave in leads I and aVL, which has a sensitivity of 92% and a positive predictive accuracy of 92% with a specificity of 97% (see Fig. 57-4).[27] Rarely, a left atrial appendage tachycardia will need to be ablated epicardially.

Inappropriate Sinus Tachycardia

The uncommon, poorly characterized entity of inappropriate sinus tachycardia is probably a heterogeneous disorder. The hallmark feature of this syndrome is a consistently elevated resting heart rate (higher than 95 beats per minute) and an exaggerated heart rate response to low levels of physical activity. The average sinus rate during during 24-hour Holter monitoring usually is greater than 90 beats per minute and a persistent increase of at least 25 beats per minute occurs on arising from supine to upright position, in the absence of orthostatic arterial hypotension. Some affected patients have an elevated intrinsic heart rate, and others have increased responsiveness to infusions of isoproterenol. The ECG characteristics of this tachycardia include an identical P wave configuration in tachycardia and sinus rhythm. It is likely that some patients have primary autonomic abnormalities, including postural orthostatic tachycardia syndrome in some. Some patients may have primary abnormalities of the sinus node. A recent analysis of 18 patients with inappropriate sinus tachycardia receiving intravenous adenosine (0.1 to 0.15 mg/kg) showed that these patients demonstrated a blunted response with less sinus cycle length prolongation than age-matched control subjects undergoing electrophysiology studies.[28] The blunted response was seen after pharmacologic autonomic blockade as well. These observations suggested that structural abnormalities of the sinus node are responsible for this syndrome. A recent report[29] suggested that β-adrenergic receptor autoantibodies may be involved in the mechanism of inappropriate sinus tachycardia. In the electrophysiology laboratory, distinction should be made between inappropriate sinus tachycardia and a focal automatic, atrial tachycardia with an origin close to the superior crista terminalis.[29]

Electrophysiologic Differential Diagnosis of Focal Atrial Tachycardia

Atrial tachycardias, particularly those originating from the septal region, must be differentiated from concealed septal bypass tract–mediated tachycardia (i.e., orthodromic reciprocating tachycardia [ORT]), AV node reentry tachycardia (AVNRT) and its variants, and other rare entities including concealed nodoventricular or nodofascicular pathways. One of the most

Table 57-1 Prevalence and Diagnostic Value of Baseline Observations and Tachycardia Features

Baseline Observation/ Feature	Prevalence (%)	Sensitivity (%)			Specificity (%)			PPV (%)			NPV (%)		
		AVNRT	ORT	AT	AVNRT	ORT	AT	AVNRT	ORT	AT	AVNRT	ORT	AT
Baseline Observation													
Preexcitation present during sinus rhythm	15	3	41	4	69	97	83	10	86	3	46	78	86
Dual AV nodal physiology	55	86	10	36	83	24	42	86	6	8	82	36	82
VA block CL >600 ms at baseline	11	8	2	50	84	84	84	41	5	55	41	66	93
Extranodal response to para-hisian pacing	18	5	47	0	67	96	80	17	83	0	36	80	85
Tachycardia Features													
Induction dependent on a critical AH interval	55	90	16	4	88	26	36	91	8	1	87	42	71
Isoproterenol required to sustain tachycardia	39	47	23	57	68	51	62	65	18	17	56	58	91
Tachycardia CL ≥500 ms	3	4	2	0	99	96	97	83	17	0	44	69	87
Septal VA interval >70 ms	53	16	100	100	0	69	54	17	59	24	0	100	100
Eccentric atrial activation	31	0	74	61	30	89	74	0	76	24	19	88	93
Spontaneous AV block during tachycardia	10	11	0	33	91	85	93	60	0	40	44	65	91
Spontaneous termination with AV block	28	33	31	0	78	73	67	66	34	0	48	70	82
Development of RBBB	32	31	36	30	66	69	67	54	35	11	42	71	82
Development of LBBB	12	1	36	4	73	99	87	4	92	4	36	81	87
Increase in VA interval >20 ms with BBB	7	0	35	0	69	100	80	0	100	0	51	57	92

From Knight BP, Ebinger M, Oral H, et al: Diagnostic value of tachycardia features and pacing maneuvers during paroxysmal supraventricular tachycardia. J Am Coll Cardiol 36:574-582, 2000.

AH, atrial His bundle; AT, atrial tachycardia; AVNRT, atrioventricular nodal reentry tachycardia; BBB, bundle branch block; CL, cycle length; LBBB, left bundle branch block; NPV, negative predictive value; ORT, orthodromic reciprocating tachycardia; PPV, positive predictive value; RBBB, right bundle branch block; SVT, supraventricular tachycardia; VA, ventriculoatrial.

useful electrocardiographic or electrophysiologic findings is AV block during tachycardia; when it occurs, a concealed bypass tract is eliminated as a diagnostic possibility.

Adenosine has been advocated as being a useful diagnostic tool in patients with supraventricular tachycardia.[30] In a report from Scheinman and coworkers, 229 patients with supraventricular tachycardia during an electrophysiology study received intravenous boluses of 6 to 18 mg of adenosine. For patients with atrial tachycardia (n = 53), no correlation was found between the response to adenosine and the location of the atrial focus. Termination or suppression of tachycardia with adenosine was observed in 56% of patients but was not helpful for differentiating automatic tachycardias from triggered or reentrant tachycardias. Only patients with atrial tachycardias demonstrated atrial cycle length oscillations (23%) before suppression with adenosine. AV block after adenosine was observed only in patients with atrial tachycardia, but it occurred uncommonly, being noted in only 27% of patients. Termination of atrial tachycardia makes it highly unlikely that a macro-reentrant atrial tachycardia is present.

A variety of pacing maneuvers have been reported to be useful for differentiation of atrial tachycardia from other forms of supraventricular tachycardia[31,32] (Tables 57-1 and 57-2). Ventricular pacing may be useful for differentiating atrial tachycardia from AV nodal reentry tachycardia and AV reentry tachycardia. Ventricular burst pacing for at least 3 to 6 beats at a cycle length generally much faster than tachycardia results in tachycardia termination, entrainment of the tachycardia, or dissociation of the ventricle from the tachycardia. If the ventricle is dissociated from the tachycardia, a bypass tract is excluded. If burst pacing reproducibly terminates tachycardia without conduction to the atrium, atrial tachycardia is excluded as the mechanism.

Burst pacing sometimes can be performed from the right ventricle for longer periods of time at a cycle length just shorter than the tachycardia cycle length. When atrial activation is

Table 57-2 Diagnostic Value of Pacing Maneuvers during Supraventricular Tachycardia

Pacing Maneuver/ Result	% Tachycardias with Maneuver Attempted	% Able to Entrain	Frequency of Results (%)	Sensitivity (%)			Specificity (%)			PPV (%)			NPV (%)		
				AVNRT	ORT	AT	AVNRT	ORT	AT	AVNRT	ORT	AT	AVNRT	ORT	AT
Pace atrium at 10-40 ms <SVT CL to entrain ventricle	89	87													
Fixed VA interval			87	97	98	5	27	18	3	64	35	1	87	96	17
Pace atrium at the AV block CL	69	NA													
Termination dependent on AH			80	96	76	8	44	20	11	69	30	1	88	65	47
Pace ventricle at 10-40 ms <SVT CL to entrain atrium	97	78													
Atrial activation same as SVT			92	100	100	0	20	13	0	64	36	0	100	100	0
AV response after pacing			94	100	100	0	14	89	0	63	37	0	100	100	0
VA block CL >SVT CL			7	3	0	48	86	89	98	20	0	80	41	66	93
Ventricular pacing CL 200-250 ms	91	NA													
Termination without affecting atrium			27	27	37	0	74	78	69	57	43	0	44	73	83
Ventricle dissociated from SVT			16	11	0	16	95	88	93	75	0	25	45	66	89
Ventricular extrastimulus during diastole	80	NA													
SVT terminates, atrium not affected, His bundle refractory			3	0	8	0	94	100	97	0	100	0	42	71	87
SVT terminates, atrium affected, His bundle refractory			10	0	27	0	80	100	92	0	100	0	38	75	86
SVT does not terminate, atrium affected, His bundle refractory			12	0	34	0	76	100	88	0	100	0	37	77	86

From Knight BP, Ebinger M, Oral H, et al: Diagnostic value of tachycardia features and pacing maneuvers during paroxysmal supraventricular tachycardia. J Am Coll Cardiol 36:574-582, 2000.

AT, atrial tachycardia; AV, atrioventricular; AVNRT, atrioventricular nodal reentry tachycardia; CL, cycle length; NA, not applicable; NPV, negative predictive value; ORT, orthodromic reciprocating tachycardia; PPV, positive predictive value; SVT, supraventricular tachycardia; VA, ventriculoatrial.

57

accelerated to the pacing rate with 1:1 ventriculoatrial conduction, and if the atrial activation sequence during pacing is different from that during tachycardia, then either an atrial tachycardia or a bystander accessory pathway is present. When ventricular pacing is stopped and the electrogram sequence following the last paced ventricular beat demonstrates a V-A-A-V response (i.e., the last atrial complex accelerated to the pacing rate is followed by another atrial complex before the next ventricular complex), an atrial tachycardia is present. A "pseudo" V-A-A-V response may be seen in patients with slowly conducting septal accessory pathways or AV node reentry, particularly of the fast-slow or slow-slow types. A "V-A-A-H-V" sequence also may be seen with AV nodal reentry.

Atrial pacing maneuvers also can be helpful to differentiate the various forms of supraventricular tachycardia. Overdrive pacing of the right atrium during tachycardia at a cycle length slightly shorter than the tachycardia cycle length can result in tachycardia termination (diagnostic maneuver not helpful) or tachycardia continuation upon cessation of pacing. If the V-A interval of the return cycle is within 10 ms of the V-A interval during the tachycardia, then the tachycardia is due to AV nodal reentry or a bypass tract. If the V-A interval is variable or different after pacing ceases, then atrial tachycardia is present. A second maneuver is atrial overdrive pacing during tachycardia at the longest cycle length that results in AV block. The last paced atrial-His bundle (A-H) interval upon cessation of pacing is evaluated. If termination of the tachycardia is associated with a relatively short A-H interval compared with the A-H intervals that resulted in continuation of the tachycardia, then the tachycardia is considered to be AV node–dependent and cannot be an atrial tachycardia. Another useful maneuver is to compare the A-H interval during tachycardia and during atrial pacing from the high right atrium at or near the tachycardia cycle length. If the A-H interval during atrial pacing at the tachycardia cycle length is more than 40 ms longer than the A-H interval during tachycardia, atypical AV nodal reentry is much more likely. The A-H intervals during atrial pacing and tachycardia will be within 20 ms for atrial tachycardias and concealed bypass tracts.

Atrial pacing should be performed as soon as possible after tachycardia termination.Tachycardia cycle length variability of 15 ms or more associated with a change in atrial cycle length that predicts a change in ventricular cycle length favors either atrial tachycardia or atypical AVNRT. A change in atrial cycle length that is preceded by the change in the preceding cycle length or H-H interval is suggestive of AVNRT or ORT.[33]

Impact of Mapping Technologies

Technologies for mapping arrhythmias include basket mapping, electroanatomic mapping, and noncontact mapping systems. The mapping technologies have definite advantages over point-by-point catheter mapping, including the ability to map unstable, poorly reproducible, and nonsustained arrhythmias. With these technologies, short episodes of arrhythmias can be mapped with one or several beats, or the arrhythmia substrate can be mapped for areas of low voltage or double potentials. Many series describing the use of each of these new technologies to map and ablate atrial tachycardias have been reported.[34,35] These technologies typically are accompanied by decreased fluoroscopic exposure for the operator, more precise localization of tachycardia, and a better appreciation of atrial anatomy.

These advanced mapping systems have been found to facilitate identification and ablation of atrial tachycardias arising from either atrial chamber, the atrial septum, pulmonary veins, superior vena cava, or coronary sinus. Color-coded display of activation timing is very useful in demonstrating the site of origin of focal atrial tachycardias. The color-coded display of chamber geometry within three-dimensional space provided by these mapping systems helps to visualize the complex anatomy and relationships between cardiac structures that cannot be fully appreciated with use of fluoroscopic imaging. The three-dimensional anatomic display is very useful in defining the left atrial anatomy along with the locations of pulmonary veins. The variable projections of the electroanatomic system allow individually optimized views of the target area, display of the tip and distal shaft of the ablation catheter, and the potential for precise re-navigation to predetermined sites. Furthermore, newer mapping technologies can overcome some of the difficulties of traditional point-to-point catheter mapping of activation sequence, which is burdensome and compounded by the lack of accurate reproducibility of catheter location based on fluoroscopic projection alone. The ability to collect a large number of points with high spatial resolution (at the level of 1 to 2 mm) enables the construction of a detailed activation map that is combined with the three-dimensional anatomy of the relevant chamber. This information provides valuable insight into the mechanism of tachycardia, the anatomic origin, and relationship to other cardiac and extracardiac structures that are useful to guide ablation. Color-coded maps of myocardial voltage at each point also can provide a map of the cardiac chamber voltage, which is helpful for identifying areas of scar and substrate abnormalities and may provide insight into the underlying disease process or pathophysiology. The ability to navigate the catheter in three-dimensional space without exposure to ionizing radiation is a valuable benefit for both patient and operator. Furthermore, use of these systems may reduce procedural time and promote success and safety. Finally, the ability to register the location of individual ablative lesions within the heart offers a significant advantage in successful ablation of complex arrhythmias.

A limitation of these systems that must be recognized and is important in studying focal atrial tachycardias is that the earliest activation within a given chamber will be recorded as the "site of origin" (that is, earliest activation within that chamber), even if the arrhythmia arises from another chamber. This is especially important to recognize in performing electroanatomic mapping of the right atrium when the tachyardia originates from the left atrium or pulmonary veins. Not infrequently, unsuccessful prolonged attempts are made to ablate focal tachycardias from the right atrium before performance of detailed left-sided mapping and ultimately successful ablation.

Macro-reentrant Atrial Tachycardia

Classification

Macro-reentrant atrial tachycardias can be divided into those that are isthmus-dependent (dependent on conduction through the tricuspid annulus–inferior vena cava isthmus) and non–isthmus-dependent.[1] A majority of macro-reentrant atrial tachycardias in the adult population are isthmus dependent. A majority of non–isthmus-dependent macro-reentrant atrial tachycardias are related to an area of scar, often from a previous surgical incision. Some examples of macro-reentrant atrial tachycardias include typical atrial flutter, lower loop reentry, double-wave reentry, macro-reentrant atrial tachycardia from the right atrial free wall, and macro-reentrant atrial tachycardias occurring in the right or left atrium related to previous surgery, including atriotomy, surgical scarring, and presence of septal prosthetic patches, suture lines, or other anatomic obstacles. Recently an increasing awareness of macro-reentrant atrial tachycardias arising from scarring in patients who have not undergone previous atrial surgery. Such "spontaneous" scarring has been described in the posterior wall of the left atrium, as well as in the posterolateral and lateral right atrium.[36] An increasing frequency of macro-reentrant left atrial tachycardias is now being seen after atrial fibrillation ablation. Some unusual causes of macro-reentrant tachycardia include reentry at sites of donor recipient anastomosis from either orthotopic heart transplantation or lung transplantation.[37]

Recently, a new technique has been proposed to differentiate between focal and macro-reentrant atrial tachycardias. Using computerized signal-averaging techniques, the study investigators used quantitative ECG metrics using the short atrial activation time relative to the tachycardia cycle length to differentiate focal atrial tachycardias from macro-reentrant atrial tachycardias, which have activation throughout the cycle length. The investigators were able to develop algorithms to quantify P or F wave duration with overlying T waves by transitions in slope or dV/dT relative to the expected T waves generated from scaling of the sinus rate T wave. Electrocardiographic P wave duration correlated with the duration of intra-atrial activation. Focal atrial tachycardias had shorter P wave durations and smaller ratios of P wave to cycle length.[38] Some of these tachycardias are discussed in detail in other chapters (see Chapters 55-57).

Diagnostic Maneuvers

Electrophysiologic characterization, mapping, and ablation of macro-reentrant atrial tachycardia were described by several groups of investigators in the early 1990s. These investigators used standard electrophysiologic techniques to demonstrate entrainment by recording diastolic atrial potentials from an area of slow conduction. They extrapolated data from animal studies showing that anatomic barriers resulting from residual atrial scars provide the substrate for atrial reentry. Multiple endocardial recordings were made to define the "protected zone of slow conduction," generally using standard techniques of entrainment. For example, potential target sites for ablation were defined by determining whether pacing from that site was associated with concealed entrainment. Specifically, these investigators applied the pacing techniques developed for ablation of ventricular tachycardia. They performed atrial mapping and looked for the first postpacing interval within 10 to 30 ms of the tachycardia cycle length (Fig. 57-9). When a postsurgical structural abnormality was present or a natural anatomic barrier (e.g., a venous orifice or a valve annulus) was nearby, mapping was more detailed in that region. In contrast with focal atrial tachycardia ablation, in which a single site of origin may be ablated to terminate tachycardia, macro-reentrant atrial tachycardia usually requires ablation performed over a larger region, often defined by anatomic barriers, or by adjacent scars separated by an isthmus of tissue that serves as a critical area of slow conduction. Often these sites are characterized by double potentials or areas with low-voltage, longer-duration, more fractionated electrograms. Cycle length variability (greater than 15%) is rarely seen with macro-reentrant atrial tachycardia but is not uncommon with focal atrial tachycardia. Atrial macro-reentrant tachycardias also may less commonly occur in patients without previous cardiac surgery, catheter ablation, or obvious structural heart disease. In these patients, electrically silent areas act as barriers for tachycardia. Like focal atrial tachycardias, macro-reentrant atrial tachycardias generally incorporate several "typical" areas as part of the reentrant circuit. For example, the most common site involved in the right atrium is the isthmus between the tricuspid valve and the inferior vena cava and in the left atrium the mitral isthmus, roof, or atrial septum.

The advent of computer mapping techniques has allowed a more precise and rapid identification of arrhythmia mechanisms. A second approach to studying the mechanism of macro-reentrant atrial tachycardias has focused on the concept of macro-reentry around a scar or previous surgical incision. These new technologies have allowed anatomic reconstruction of the cardiac chambers with recording of local activation times and identification of atrial scar tissue, allowing for construction of isochronal maps of a substantial portion or the entire tachycardia circuit in many patients. Nakagawa and colleagues[39] made a fundamental contribution in this area with a study of 16 patients who had had congenital heart disease surgery and underwent mapping and ablation of right atrial macro-reentrant tachycardias. These workers mapped 15 macro-reentrant atrial tachycardias in 13 patients using the CARTO electroanatomic mapping system. First, they noted that all macro-reentrant atrial tachycardias propagated through narrow channels (less than 2.7 cm) defined by the mapping system as an area of decreased electrogram voltage between two close dense or thin scars. These workers coined the phrase "no channel–no macro-reentry." In their study, electrogram morphology, electrogram amplitude, and electrogram timing did not differentiate between sites within and those outside a narrow channel. Entrainment mapping failed to differentiate sites within the circuit but outside the channel ("outer loop" sites) from sites within the circuit and within the channel. Entrainment pacing was not done in many of the patients because it often resulted in induction of a new tachycardia or in termination of the original tachycardia. Additional limitations to entrainment mapping include difficulty measuring postpacing intervals due to low amplitude or absence of atrial potentials in scarred atria or inability to pace the tissue. Entrainment mapping also can induce atrial fibrillation. Finally, the investigators were able to record double potentials during atrial pacing at slow rates, suggesting fixed sites of anatomic block. In general, it appears that the size and location of the scars or associated natural anatomic barriers (e.g., valve annulus, superior vena cava, pulmonary veins, or inferior vena cava) determine the size and properties of the tachycardia circuit.

The sensitivity and specificity of classical criteria for concealed entrainment for identification of a critical isthmus are based on studies performed during ventricular tachycardia. The sensitivity and specificity of these criteria for defining entrainment in the atrium were examined by Morton and coworkers.[40] They used the model of typical atrial flutter and performed entrainment mapping from seven sites at four different cycle lengths. Concealed entrainment identified any isthmus site with 100% sensitivity with the flutter cycle length −10 ms but with a specificity of only 54%. Specificity increased to 98% with pacing at flutter cycle length −40 ms, but the sensitivity was decreased to 65%. At the flutter cycle length −30 ms, sensitivity and specificity were 85% and 90%, respectively. Concealed entrainment was seen from a nonisthmus site in 5 of 10 patients. Thse findings highlights the observation by Nakagawa and associates[39] that targeting sites for ablation based solely on entrainment will result in a less than ideal success rate. These findings underscore the difficulties of relying on any one criterion for defining sites of ablation of these complex macro-reentrant tachycardias. In general, current approaches that combine definition of anatomy with electrophysiologic mapping data are warranted for attempted ablation of these complex arrhythmias.

Electrocardiographic Characterization of Macro-reentrant Atrial Tachycardia

Electrocardiographic localization of macro-reentrant atrial tachycardias is much more complex than localization of focal atrial tachycardias. Electrocardiographic localization of the macro-reentrant tachycardia circuit is influenced by altered atrial anatomy, previous surgical incisions, and conduction of

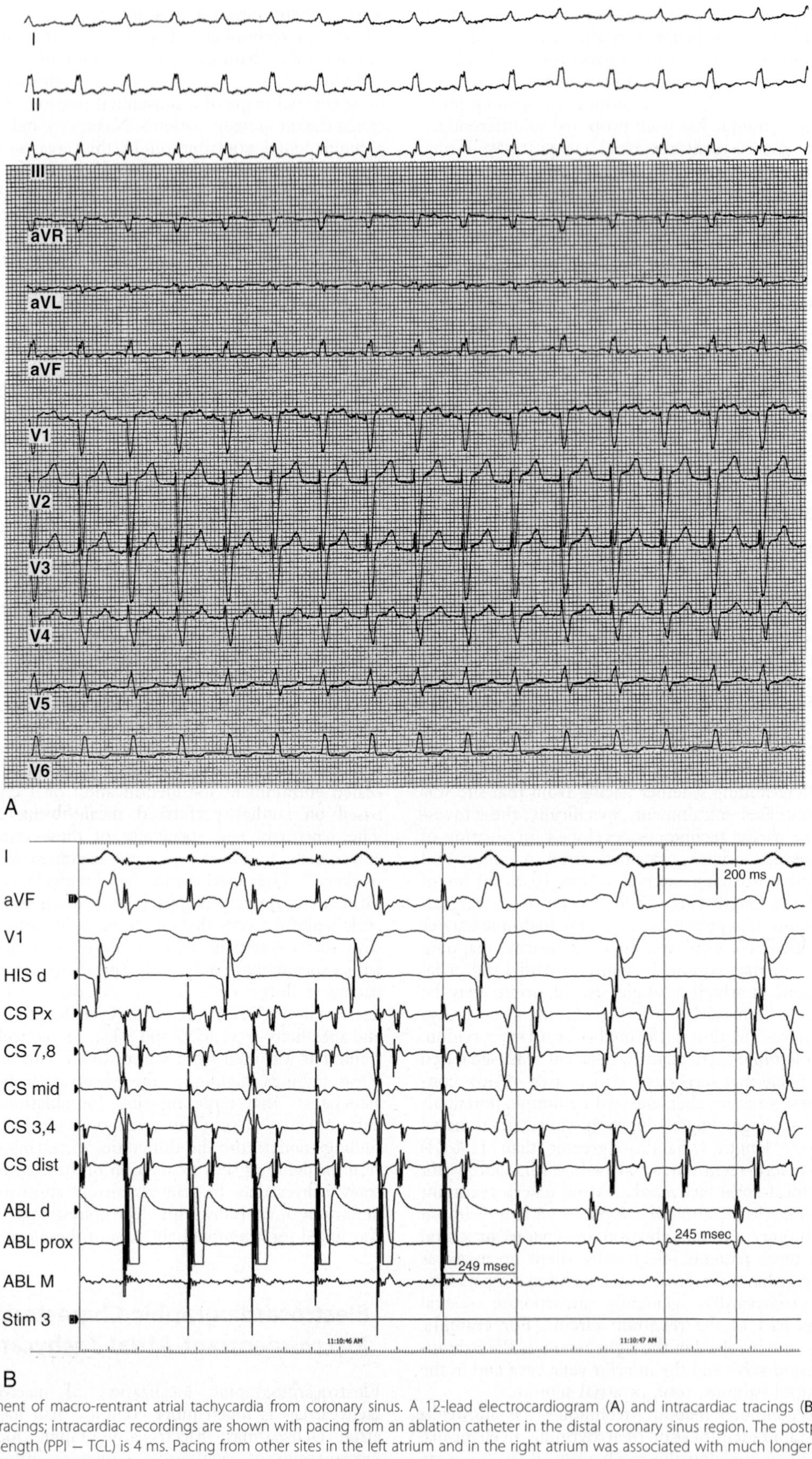

Figure 57-9 Entrainment of macro-rentrant atrial tachycardia from coronary sinus. A 12-lead electrocardiogram (A) and intracardiac tracings (B) are shown. Surface electrocardiographic tracings; intracardiac recordings are shown with pacing from an ablation catheter in the distal coronary sinus region. The postpacing interval minus the tachycardia cycle length (PPI − TCL) is 4 ms. Pacing from other sites in the left atrium and in the right atrium was associated with much longer postpacing intervals.

the atrial wavefront. For example, clockwise and counterclockwise atrial flutter are characterized by P waves of opposite polarity in the inferior leads. The tachycardia circuit encompassed by these two flutters is the same, but the P wave polarity is affected by the direction in which the atrial wavefront travels (e.g., craniocaudal or reverse direction). Macro-reentrant circuits near the subeustachian isthmus may result in P wave morphology similar or identical to that seen with typical atrial flutter.[40] Left-sided atrial flutter originating from the posterior or lateral wall of the left atrium and involving the left pulmonary veins is characterized by coronary sinus activation that usually proceeds from the distal or mid coronary sinus to the proximal coronary sinus and usually demonstrates craniocaudal activation, with flat or positive flutter waves in lead V_1 and often upright P waves in leads II, III, and aVF.[41,42] A negative component in lead I, when present, is the most useful electrocardiographic feature for differentiating counterclockwise mitral annular flutter from left pulmonary vein atrial tachycardias, whereas a positive F wave in lead I was best for differentiating clockwise mitral annular flutters from counterclockwise right atrial flutter. An important point is that once the patient has had a previous ablation, the electrocardiographic appearance of the P wave morphology may be altered. A focal atrial tachycardia that arises near an area of previous ablation may appear electrocardiographically like a flutter because of the altered atrial activation sequence caused by the line of block.

Recently, Miyazaki and colleagues described a simplified approach to the rapid differentiation of left and right atrial tachycardias.[43] Entrainment was performed at three sites: the high right atrium, proximal coronary sinus, and distal coronary sinus. PPI-TCL less than or greater than 50 ms at the high RA distinguished RA from LA reentrant circuits. PPI-TCL was less than 50 ms for right atrial circuits and greater than 50 ms from the high lateral right atrium for left atrial circuits. For left atrial circuits, the PPI-TCL difference at the proximal and distal coronary sinus greater than or less than 50 ms differentiated perimitral reentry, from reentry involving the right pulmonary veins and septum. If the PPI-TCL difference was less than 50 ms from the proximal coronary sinus but greater than 50 ms at the distal coronary sinus, then the tachycardia was likely to involve the right pulmonary veins and septum (see Fig. 55-9). The predictive accuracy for determining the successful ablation region was 93%.

Specific Types of Macro-reentrant Atrial Tachycardia

Several recent studies from three different laboratories have characterized left atrial macro-reentrant circuits, or "left atrial flutters." Lerman and colleagues[44] described a series of 10 patients with macroreentrant tachycardias after mitral valve surgery. Six tachycardias originated from the right atrium, four originated from the left atrium, and one was biatrial. In 80% of patients, the tachycardia circuits were defined by surgical atrial lesions or surgical cannulation sites. Three macro-reentrant tachycardias were mapped involving the left atrial septum and the right pulmonary veins, with the tachycardia making a single reentrant loop in two patients and a figure-of-eight reentry in one patient involving a clockwise loop around an area of low voltage in the posterior wall and a counterclockwise loop around the mitral annulus with a central isthmus between two areas of low voltage. Of interest, in three patients the tachycardia had a focal origin.

In two other studies, macro-reentrant left atrial flutters were mapped with the CARTO electroanatomic mapping system and were successfully ablated in more than 70% of patients.[45,46] Most patients had structural heart disease, and 14% to 32% had mitral valve disease. The investigators described macro-reentrant atrial tachycardias as having a continuous sequence of atrial activation, with adjacent earliest and latest activation and the range of activation times occupying 90% or more of the tachycardia cycle length. Entrainment mapping was done in some patients to locate a critical isthmus of slow conduction. A right atrial macro-reentrant circuit was excluded by showing that the postpacing interval in the right atrium was longer than the tachycardia cycle length by 40 ms or longer from three or more sites in the right atrium including the cavotricuspid isthmus and right atrial free wall; spontaneous variation of greater than 100 ms was seen in the right atrium, with concomitant variations in the left atrium of less than 20 ms; and right atrial activation accounted for less than 50% of the arrhythmia cycle length from more than eight points during sequential catheter mapping. The left atrial flutters typically were characterized by large reentrant circuits that rotated around the mitral annulus, electrically silent areas, and lines of double potentials near acquired or natural anatomic barriers such as the pulmonary veins (Fig. 57-10). Electrically silent areas were defined as those with no recordable electrogram or an electrogram amplitude of less than 0.05 mV. A dual-loop reentrant circuit was defined for 74% of tachycardias and a single-loop circuit in the remaining 26% of tachycardias in one series of patients. In some studies, the mapping can be very complex and involve up to four loops rotating simultaneously. Much as with the observations of Nakagawa and other investigators in patients with right atrial tachycardias, the isthmuses described for left atrial tachycardias were relatively narrow, with low-amplitude electrograms in many patients.

Atrial macro-reentrant tachycardias after atrial fibrillation (catheter or surgical) ablation may be complex and are discussed in more detail in Chapters 105 and 106. These tachycardias typically are micro-reentrant or macro-reentrant. Briefly, the type of tachycardia observed after atrial fibrillation ablation depends significantly on the previous atrial fibrillation ablation strategy.[47-49] Recurrent organized left atrial tachycardias may be seen in 5% to 30% of patients, and are more likely to be focal in patients with pulmonary vein isolation procedures and more likely to be macro-reentrant in patients with linear lesions.

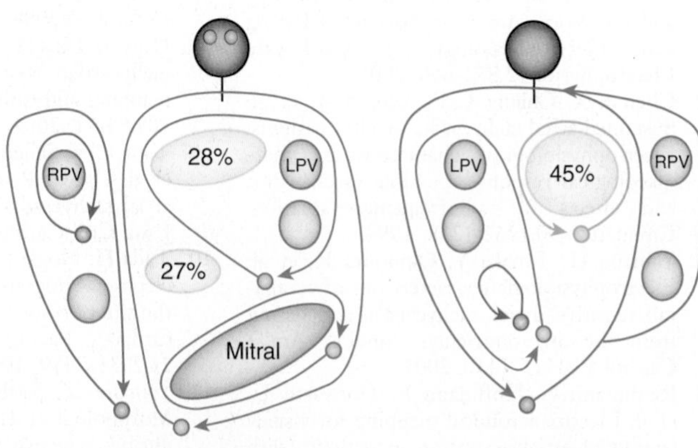

Figure 57-10 Schematic diagram of left atrial flutter circuits showing the location of silent areas and the percentage with circuits encountered in the left atrium. Nearly half of the silent areas were located in the posterior left atrium. LPV, left pulmonary vein; RPV, right pulmonary vein. (From Jais P, Shah DC, Haissaguerre M, et al: Mapping and ablation of left atrial flutters. Circulation 101:2928-2934, 2000.)

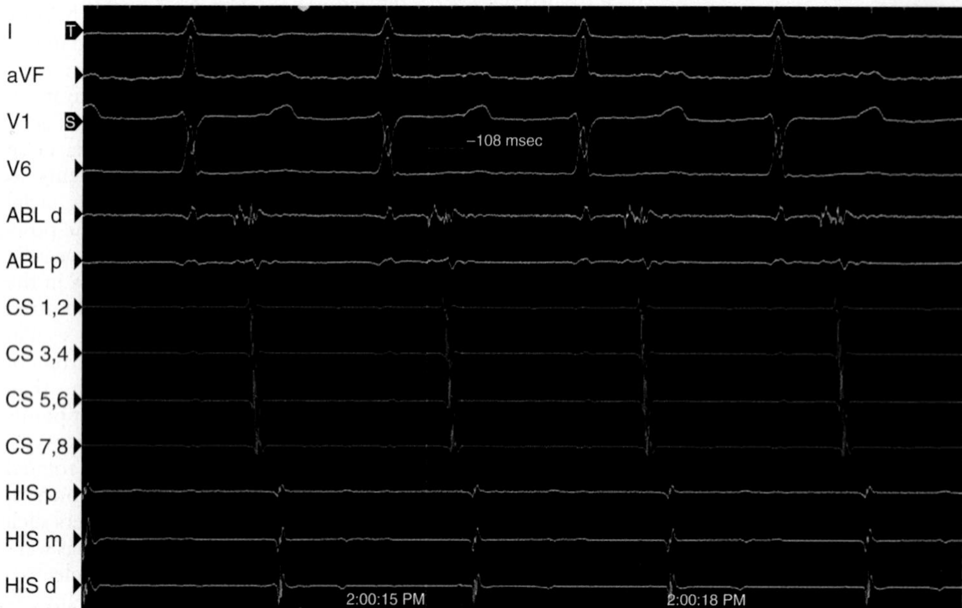

Figure 57-11 Surface *(top)* and intracardiac *(bottom)* recordings from a patient with a focal left atrial tachycardia at the base of the left atrial appendage who previously had undergone atrial fibrillation ablation. Note the complex fractionated atrial electrogram recorded at the site of successful ablation.

Most patients with a focal origin for their tachycardia will have a site mapped to or near a reconnected pulmonary vein, while others have "small loop" micro-reentry due to a focally ablatable small isthmus near a pulmonary vein. Typically, these patients will have fragmented, long-duration and low-voltage electrograms, presumable owing to incomplete ablation of atrial tissue (e.g., gap-related) in their previous procedure (Fig. 57-11). Others have been noted to have a macro-reentrant tachycardia, which most commonly involves conduction across the mitral isthmus, the posterior wall, or gaps from previous ablation. The explanation for this abnormal atrial electrogram is believed to be altered intra-atrial conduction and decreased left atrial voltage.[50] Unusual forms of atrial macro-reentry may occur after atrial fibrillation ablation, including circuits that incorporate the coronary sinus and its musculature, necessitating ablation inside the coronary sinus.[51]

References

1. Saoudi N, Cosio F, Waldo A, et al: Classification of atrial flutter and regular atrial tachycardia according to electrophysiologic mechanism and anatomic bases: A statement from a joint expert group from the Working Group of Arrhythmias of the European Society of Cardiology and the North American Society of Pacing and Electrophysiology. J Cardiovasc Electrophysiol 12:852-866, 2001.
2. Chen S-A, Chiang C-E, Yang C-J, et al: Sustained atrial tachycardia in adult patients: Electrophysiological characteristics, pharmacological response, possible mechanisms and effects of radiofrequency ablation. Circulation 90:1262-1278, 1994.
3. Yamabe H, Tanaka Y, Okumura K, et al: Electrophysiologic characteristics of verapamil-sensitive atrial tachycardia originating from the atrioventricular annulus. Am J Cardiol 95:1425-1430, 2005.
4. Reithmann C, Hoffmann E, Dorwarth U, et al: Electroanatomical mapping for visualization of atrial activation in patients with incisional atrial tachycardias. Eur Heart J 22:237-246, 2001.
5. Markowitz SM, Nemirovksy D, Stein KM, et al: Adenosine-insensitive focal atrial tachycardia. J Am Coll Cardiol 49:1324-1333, 2007.
6. De Groot NMS, Schalij MJ: Fragmented, long-duration, low-amplitude electrograms characterize the origin of focal atrial tachycardia. J Cardiovasc Electrophysiol 17:1-7, 2006.
7. Sanders P, Hocini M, Jais P, et al: Characterization of focal atrial tachycardia using high-density mapping. J Am Coll Cardiol 46:2088-2099, 2005.
8. Higa S, Tai CT, Lin YJ, et al: Focal atrial tachycardia: New insight from noncontact mapping and catheter ablation. Circulation 109:84-91, 2004.
9. Tang CW, Scheinman MM, Van Hare GF, et al: Use of P wave configuration during atrial tachycardia to predict site of origin. J Am Coll Cardiol 26:1315-1324, 1995.
10. Tada H, Nogami A, Naito S, et al: Simple electrocardiographic criteria for identifying the site of origin of focal right atrial tachycardia. Pacing Clin Electrophysiol 21:2431-2439, 1998.
11. Yamane T, Shah DC, Peng J-T, et al: Morphological characteristics of P waves during selective pulmonary vein pacing. J Am Coll Cardiol 38:1505-1510, 2001.
12. Hachiya H, Ernst S, Ouyang F, et al: Topographic distribution of focal left atrial tachycardias defined by electrocardiographic and electrophysiologic data. Circ J 69:205-210, 2005.
13. Kistler PM, Roberts-Thompson KC, Haqqani HM, et al: P-wave morphology in focal atrial tachycardia: Development of an algorithm to predict the anatomic site of origin. J Am Coll Cardiol 48:1010-1017, 2006.
14. Mohamed U, Skanes AC, Gula LJ, et al: A novel pacing maneuver to localize focal atrial tachycardia. J Cardiovasc Electrophysiol 8:1-6, 2007.
15. Gonzalez MD, Contreras LJ, Jongbloed MRM, et al: Left atrial tachycardia originating from the mitral annulus-aorta junction. Circulation 110:3187-3192, 2004.
16. Kistler PM, Sanders P, Hussin A, et al: Focal atrial tachycardia arising from the mitral annulus. Electrocardiographic and electrophysiologic characterization. J Am Coll Cardiol 41:2212-2219, 2003.
17. Badhar N, Kalman JM, Sparks PB, et al: Atrial tachycardia arising from the coronary sinus musculature. Electrophysiological characteristics and long-term outcome after radiofrequency ablation. J Am Coll Cardiol 46:1921-1930, 2005.
18. Kistler PM, Synn SP, Haqqani H, et al: Focal atrial tachycardia from the ostium of the coronary sinus. Electrocardiographic and electrophysiological characterization and radiofrequency ablation. J Am Coll Cardiol 45:1488-1493, 2005.

19. Lai LP, Lin JL, Chen T-F, et al: Clinical, electrophysiological characteristics, and radiofrequency catheter ablation of atrial tachycardia near the apex of Koch's triangle. Pacing Clin Electrophysiol 21:367-374, 1998.
20. Connors SP, Vora A, Green MS, Tang ASL: Radiofrequency ablation of atrial tachycardia originating from the triangle of Koch. Can J Cardiol 16:39-43, 2000.
21. Frey B, Kreiner G, Gwechenberger M, Gossinger HD: Ablation of atrial tachycardia originating from the vicinity of the atrioventricular node: Significance of mapping both sides of the interatrial septum. J Am Coll Cardiol 38:394-400, 2001.
22. Marrouche NF, Sippens Groenewegen A, Yang Y, et al: Clinical and electrophysiologic characteristics of left septal atrial tachycardia. J Am Coll Cardiol 40:1133-1139, 2002.
23. Zhou Y, Guo J, Xu Y, et al: Electrophysiologic characteristics and radiofrequency ablation of focal atrial tachycardia arising from para-Hisian region. Int J Clin Pract 61:385-391, 2007.
24. Ouyang F, Ma J, Ho SY, et al: Focal atrial tachycardia originating from the non-coronary aortic sinus. Electrophysiological characteristics and catheter ablation. J Am Coll Cardiol 48:122-131, 2006.
25. Dong J, Zrenner B, Schreieck J, et al: Catheter ablation of left atrial focal tachycardia guided by electroanatomic mapping and new insights into interatrial electrical conduction. Heart Rhythm 2:578-591, 2005.
26. Kistler PM, Sanders P, Fynn SP, et al: Electrophysiological and electrocardiographic characteristics of focal atrial tachycardia originating from the pulmonary veins. Acute and long-term outcomes of radiofrequency ablation. Circulation 108:1968-1975, 2003.
27. Yamada T, Murakami Y, Yoshida Y, et al: Electrophysiological and electrocardiographic characteristics and radiofrequency catheter ablation of focal atrial tachycardia originationg from the left atrial appendage. Heart Rhythm 4:1284-1291, 2007.
28. Still A-M, Huikuri HV, Juhani KE, et al: Impaired negative chronotropic response to adenosine in patients with inappropriate sinus tachycardia. J Cardiovasc Electrophysiol 13:557-562, 2002.
29. Chiale PA, Garro HA, Schmidberg J, et al: Inappropriate sinus tachycardia may be related to an immunologic disorder involving cardiac beta andrenergic receptors. Heart Rhythm 3:1182-1186, 2006.
30. Glatter KA, Cheng J, Dorostkar P, et al: Electrophysiologic effects of adenosine in patients with supraventricular tachycardia. Circulation 99:1034-1040, 1999.
31. Knight BP, Ebinger M, Oral H, et al: Diagnostic value of tachycardia features and pacing maneuvers during paroxysmal supraventricular tachycardia. J Am Coll Cardiol 35:574-582, 2000.
32. Knight BP, Zivin A, Souza J, et al: A technique for the rapid diagnosis of atrial tachycardia in the electrophysiology laboratory. J Am Coll Cardiol 33:775-781, 1999.
33. Crawford TC, Mukerji S, Good E, et al: Utility of atrial and ventricular cycle length variability in determining the mechanism of paroxysmal supraventricular tachycardia. J Cardiovasc Electrophysiol 18:698-703, 2007.
34. Wetzel U, Hindricks G, Schirdewahn P, et al: A stepwise mapping approach for localization and ablation of ectopic right, left, and septal atrial foci using electroanatomic mapping. Eur Heart J 23:1387-1393, 2002.
35. Schmitt H, Weber S, Schwab JO, et al: Diagnosis and ablation of focal right atrial tachycardia using a new high-resolution, non-contact mapping system. Am J Cardiol 87:1017-1021, 2001.
36. Stevenson IH, Kistler PM, Spence SJ, et al: Scar-related right atrial macroreentrant tachycardia in patients without prior atrial surgery: Electroanatomic characterization and ablation outcomes. Heart Rhythm 2:594-601, 2005.
37. Sacher F, Vest J, Raymond JM, Stevenson WG: Incessant donor-to-recipient atrial tachycardia after bilateral lung transplantation. Heart Rhythm 5:149-151, 2008.
38. Brown JP, Krummen DE, Feld GK, Narayan SM: Using electrocardiographic activation time and diastolic intervals to separate focal from macro-reentrant atrial tachycardias. J Am Coll Cardiol 49:1965-1973, 2007.
39. Nakagawa H, Shah N, Matsudaira K, et al: Characterization of reentrant circuit in macroreentrant right atrial tachycardia after surgical repair of congenital heart disease: Isolated channels between scars allow "focal" ablation. Circulation 103:699-709, 2001.
40. Morton JB, Sanders P, Deen V, et al: Sensitivity and specificity of concealed entrainment for the identification of a critical isthmus in the atrium: Relationship to rate, anatomic location and antidromic penetration. J Am Coll Cardiol 39:896-906, 2002.
41. Gerstenfeld EP, Dixit S, Bala R, et al: Surface electrocardiogram characteristics of atrial tachycardias occurring after pulmonary vein isolation. Heart Rhythm 4:1136-1143, 2007.
42. Della Bella P, Fraticelli A, Tonod C, et al: Atypical atrial flutter: Clinical features, electrophysiological characteristics and response to radiofrequency catheter ablation. Europace 4:241-253, 2002.
43. Miyazaki H, Stevenson WG, Stephenson K, et al: Entrainment mapping for rapid distinction of left and right atrial tachycardias. Heart Rhythm 3:516-523, 2006.
44. Markowitz SM, Brodman RF, Stein KM, et al: Lesional tachycardias related to mitral valve surgery. J Am Coll Cardiol 39:1973-1983, 2002.
45. Jais P, Shah DC, Haissaguerre M, et al: Mapping and ablation of left atrial flutters. Circulation 101:2928-2934, 2000.
46. Ouyang F, Ernst S, Vogtmann T, et al: Characterization of reentrant circuits in left atrial macroreentrant tachycardia: Critical isthmus block can prevent atrial tachycardia recurrence. Circulation 105:1934-1942, 2002.
47. Gerstenfeld EP, Marchlinski FE: Mapping and ablation of left atrial tachycardias occurring after atrial fibrillation ablation. Heart Rhythm 4:S65-S72, 2007.
48. Deisenhofer I, Estner H, Zrenner B, et al: Left atrial tachycardia after circumferential pulmonary vein ablation for atrial fibrillation: Incidence, electrophysiological characteristics, and results of radiofrequency ablation. Europace 8:573-582, 2006.
49. Wazni O, Saliba W, Fahmy T, et al: Atrial arrhythmias after surgical maze. Findings during catheter ablation. J Am Coll Cardiol 48:1405-1409, 2006.
50. Chugh A, Latchamsetty R, Oral H, et al: Characteristics of cavotricuspid isthmus–dependent atrial flutter after left atrial ablation of atrial fibrillation. Circulation 113:609-615, 2006.
51. Chugh A, Oral H, Good E, et al: Catheter ablation of atypical atrial flutter and atrial tachycardia within the coronary sinus after left atrial ablation for atrial fibrillation. J Am Coll Cardiol 45:83-91, 2005.

Atrioventricular Reentry and Variants 58

Aman Chugh and Fred Morady

CHAPTER OUTLINE

Definitions

Atrioventricular (AV) reentry accounts for approximately one third of the cases of paroxysmal supraventricular tachycardia among patients referred for catheter ablation. It is a macro-reentrant tachycardia that uses both the normal conduction system and an accessory pathway. The vast majority of instances of AV reentrant tachycardia (AVRT) involve the AV node and the accessory pathway for anterograde and retrograde conduction, respectively. The result is a regular, narrow complex rhythm referred to as *orthodromic reciprocating tachycardia* (ORT). Less commonly, a wide-complex rhythm may be observed when anterograde conduction occurs over the accessory pathway and retrograde conduction occurs over the AV node, referred to as *antidromic reciprocating tachycardia* (ART).

If the accessory pathway is capable of anterograde conduction, the resting electrocardiogram demonstrates a short PR interval and a slurred upstroke of the QRS complex that constitutes the delta wave—the hallmarks of ventricular preexcitation. The accessory pathway is thus termed *manifest* (Fig. 58-1). In approximately 50% of patients with AVRT, the accessory pathway is capable of only retrograde conduction. The electrocardiogram during sinus rhythm shows a normal QRS complex because the accessory connection is *concealed*. Patients with evidence of preexcitation on the resting electrocardiogram and documented tachycardia are said to have the Wolff-Parkinson-White (WPW) syndrome. A WPW pattern describes an electrocardiogram with evidence of preexcitation in a patient with no arrhythmic symptoms.

Anatomic Substrate for Atrioventricular Reentry

Accessory pathways are anomalous bypass tracts that typically are composed of working myocardial cells. The vast majority of accessory pathways insert along the mitral or tricuspid valve and are referred to as AV pathways. Approximately 60% of accessory pathways insert along the mitral valve and are referred to as left free-wall pathways. Approximately one fourth insert along the septal aspect of the tricuspid or mitral valve and are classified as septal pathways. The remaining 15% are right free-wall pathways.

Occasionally one may encounter accessory pathways that do not insert along the AV valves. Examples are atriofascicular, nodoventricular, nodofascicular, and atrionodal pathways. Atriofascicular pathways connect the right atrium to the distal ramifications of the right bundle and are capable of only anterograde conduction. Nodoventricular and nodofascicular pathways connect the AV node to the right ventricular myocardium and to the specialized conduction system, respectively. Atriofascicular and nodoventricular connections also are notable for decremental conduction. Atrionodal pathways are rare and connect the right atrial myocardium to the AV node. The fact that these unusual pathways do not insert along the AV annulus calls for a mapping approach different from that for typical AV pathways. Another unusual variety of accessory pathway inserts at the right or left atrial appendage instead of the tricuspid or mitral annulus.

Clinical Presentation

The presentation of patients with AVRT is clinically indistinguishable from that in patients with other causes of paroxysmal supraventricular tachycardia. Symptoms commonly include rapid palpitations, chest discomfort, dizziness or lightheadedness, dyspnea, weakness, neck pulsations, and presyncope. Syncope is an uncommon symptom of AVRT. Occasionally, patients with AVRT develop atrial fibrillation (AF) that may lead to hemodynamic deterioration owing to rapid anterograde conduction over the accessory pathway (Fig. 58-2). This may cause syncope, aborted cardiac arrest, or even sudden death.

Although AVRT may occur at any age, it usually occurs in young patients without evidence of structural heart disease. Accordingly, patients typically do not require an extensive cardiac workup. Rarely, AVRT may be associated with other cardiac conditions, such as hypertrophic cardiomyopathy or Ebstein's anomaly. The physical examination and the resting electrocardiogram are helpful in screening for these unusual associations. Although the electrocardiogram during AVRT (or other causes of supraventricular tachycardia) may reveal ST segment abnormalities, such changes usually are not indicative of myocardial ischemia. Thus, coronary angiography is usually not required. Among patients with paroxysmal supraventricular tachycardia, male gender and onset at a younger age are more likely to be associated with AVRT than atrioventricular nodal reentrant tachycardia or atrial tachycardia.

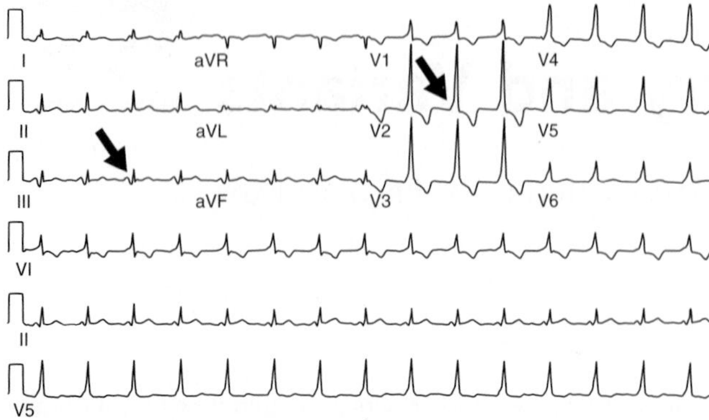

Figure 58-1 An example of ventricular preexcitation in a patient with a history of supraventricular tachycardia. The electrocardiogram during sinus rhythm shows a short PR interval and delta waves *(arrows)*. The positive delta wave in lead V_1 and the negative delta wave in the inferior leads are compatible with a left free-wall accessory pathway inserting at the posterior or posterolateral mitral annulus. The accessory pathway was successfully ablated at the posterior mitral annulus.

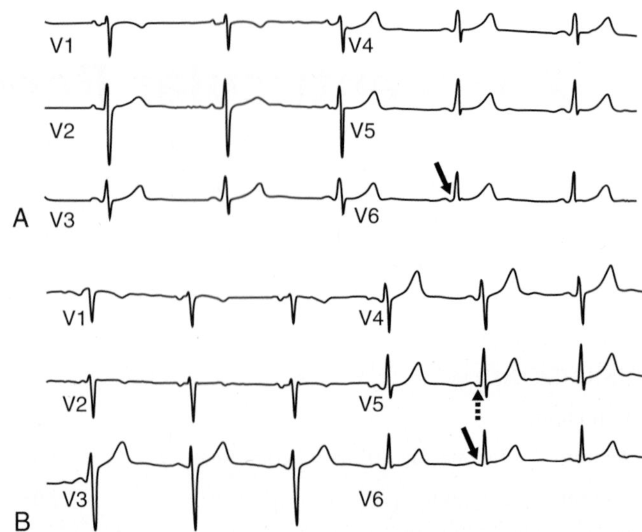

Figure 58-3 **A,** An example of subtle ventricular preexcitation. This electrocardiogram was recorded from a patient with documented supraventricular tachycardia. Slight slurring of the QRS complex upstroke *(arrow)*, along with a short PR interval, can be seen, suggestive of ventricular preexcitation. Also note that the QRS complex in the lateral precordial leads lacks a "septal" q wave. Paper speed = 25 mm/second. **B,** A post-ablation electrocardiogram from the same patient as in Figure 58-3A. The patient was found to have a manifest left lateral accessory pathway that was successfully ablated. Note that after elimination of the accessory pathway, a longer PR interval (*dashed arrow*) and a small q wave in lead V_6 *(solid arrow)* are apparent, reflecting normal septal activation. Paper speed = 25 mm/second.

Electrocardiographic Characterization

The electrocardiogram during sinus rhythm and during tachycardia may be helpful in formulating a differential diagnosis regarding the mechanism of the tachycardia. Evidence of preexcitation during sinus rhythm in a patient with a history of tachycardia makes AVRT very likely. The degree of preexcitation may be subtle, especially in patients with a left free-wall accessory pathway and in those with a slowly conducting accessory pathway. In the former, it is helpful to analyze the QRS morphology in the lateral precordial leads. In patients with subtle preexcitation due to a left free-wall accessory pathway, a "septal" q wave should not be present in the lateral precordial leads. (Fig. 58-3A and B). The remote location of the pathway allows ventricular activation to proceed more so over the AV node than would be possible with right-sided pathways. As a result, right-sided accessory pathways are associated with a greater degree of ventricular preexcitation. In patients with an equivocal electrocardiogram, administration of adenosine is helpful in unmasking preexcitation.

In most patients with ORT, the electrocardiogram shows a regular, narrow QRS complex tachycardia. The timing of the P wave with respect to the QRS is a useful clue. During ORT, since atrial activation can only occur following ventricular activation, the P wave is inscribed after the QRS complex, frequently within the ST segment (Fig. 58-4). It should be mentioned that this feature is suggestive but not diagnostic of ORT as it may be

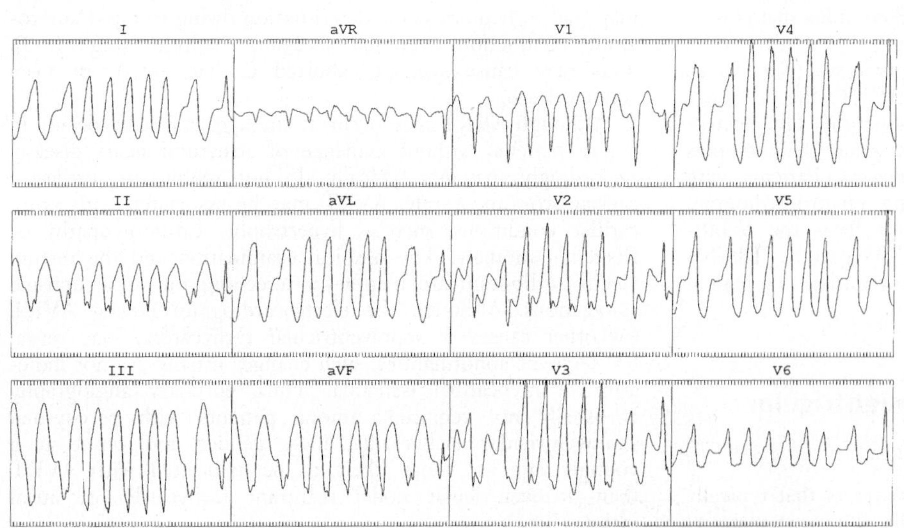

Figure 58-2 Example of atrial fibrillation (AF) with rapid conduction over a posteroseptal accessory pathway. Note the extremely rapid (up to 300 beats per minute) and irregular ventricular rate and the variable degree of fusion due to ventricular activation by way of the atrioventricular node and the accessory pathway. The pathway was successfully ablated outside the os of the coronary sinus.

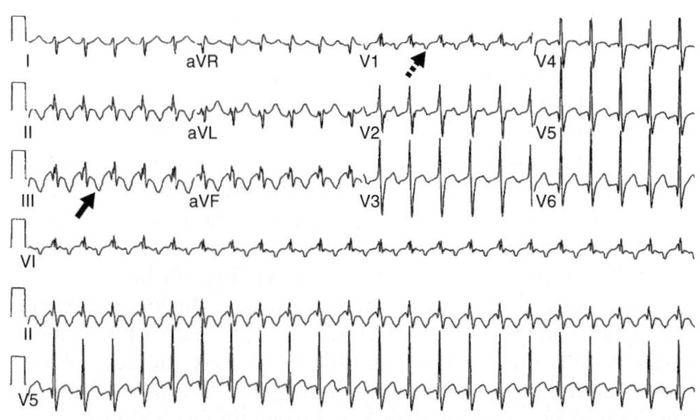

Figure 58-4 An example of orthodromic reciprocating tachycardia (ORT). The patient had a history of Ebstein's anomaly and had undergone implantation of a dual-chamber pacemaker for sinus node dysfunction. Ventricular pacing using the right ventricular lead during supraventricular tachycardia yielded an atrioventricular (AV) response, along with a short postpacing interval, consistent with a diagnosis of ORT. The electrocardiogram during ORT shows relatively wide, negative P waves in the ST segment *(solid arrow)* in the inferior leads, consistent with caudocranial activation. The P wave in lead V_1 is predominantly negative (*dashed arrow*), consistent with a right-sided accessory pathway. Electrophysiologic testing demonstrated ORT using a concealed, right posterior accessory pathway that was successfully ablated.

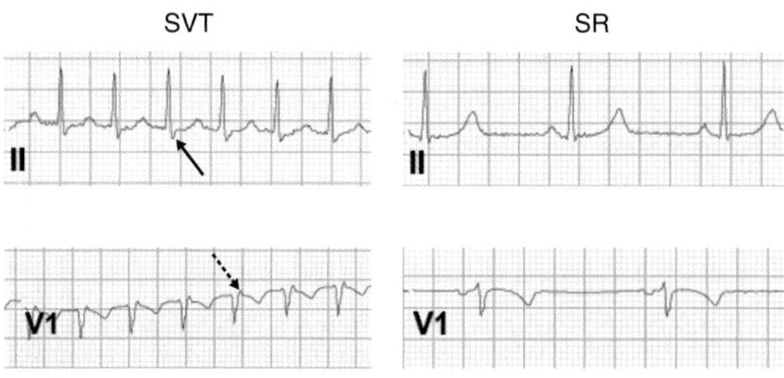

Figure 58-5 Example of typical AV nodal reentrant tachycardia. **Left,** A pseudo S wave (*arrow* in lead II) and a pseudo R′ (*dashed arrow* in lead V_1). **Right,** These electrocardiographic features are not seen during sinus rhythm (SR), indicating that atrial activation is nearly coincident with ventricular activation during SVT. These findings also rule out orthodromic reciprocating tachycardia. SVT, supraventricular tachycardia.

seen with AV nodal reentrant tachycardia or atrial tachycardia. During typical ("slow-fast") AV nodal reentrant tachycardia, the atrium and ventricle usually are activated nearly simultaneously. The P wave is inscribed within or at the end of the QRS complex, resulting in a pseudo R′ in lead V_1 and a pseudo S-wave in lead II (Fig. 58-5). These features are diagnostic of AV nodal reentrant tachycardia and hence help rule out ORT as the mechanism.

The mode of tachycardia initiation and termination may be very helpful in discerning the mechanism of the tachycardia. If the tachycardia is initiated with anterograde block in the accessory pathway, the mechanism is very likely to be due to ORT (Fig. 58-6). If the tachycardia persists despite AV block, ORT is ruled out because the ventricle is an obligatory component of the reentrant circuit. If the tachycardia terminates with AV block, atrial tachycardia is unlikely.

Beat-to-beat alternation of the QRS amplitude may be more commonly seen in ORT as opposed to AV nodal reentrant tachycardia and atrial tachycardia. QRS alternans is not specific for ORT, however, and probably is related to the faster heart rate during ORT. Although the electrocardiogram is a helpful guide, it often does not provide unambiguous diagnostic features. In fact, approximately 20% of tachycardias are misclassified when the diagnosis is based on only the electrocardiogram.

Analysis of the P wave morphology during ORT may be helpful in localizing the accessory pathway (see Fig. 58-4). For example, negative P waves in the inferior leads are consistent with an atrial insertion at the inferoposterior aspect of the AV valves. Upright P waves in the inferior leads are associated with craniocaudal activation from the anterosuperior aspect of the AV valves. Relatively narrow P waves typically are inscribed during ORT utilizing a septal accessory pathway, whereas broad P waves are consistent with activation over a free-wall accessory pathway. It should be noted that the P waves may be obscured by the ST segment during tachycardia, making it difficult to discern their morphology.

The electrocardiogram in patients with an atriofascicular accessory pathway is notable for several reasons. During sinus rhythm, the electrocardiogram usually does not reveal

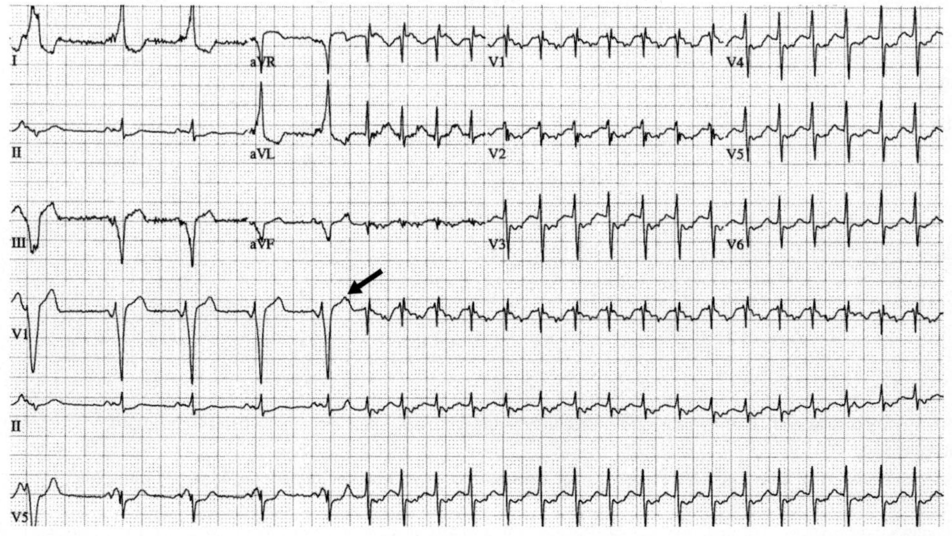

Figure 58-6 Example of spontaneous initiation of orthodromic reciprocating tachycardia (ORT). The electrocardiogram was recorded from a patient who presented to the emergency room with palpitations. The first five beats are consistent with sinus arrhythmia with evidence of preexcitation, consistent with a right-sided accessory pathway. An atrial premature depolarization *(arrow)* results in anterograde block in the accessory pathway and initiates supraventricular tachycardia. Tachycardia that initiates with block in the accessory pathway is very likely to be due to ORT. The paper speed is 25 mm/s.

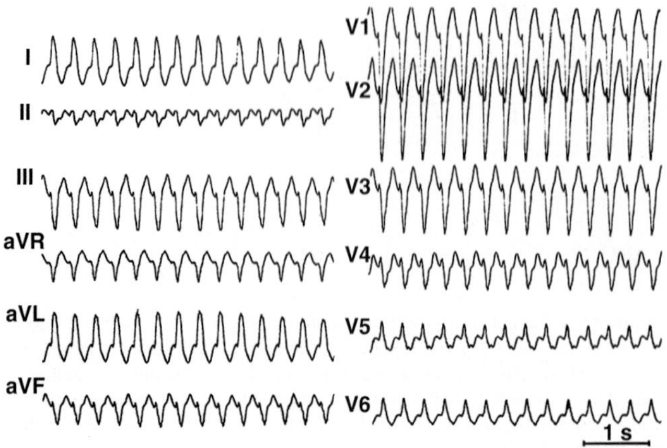

Figure 58-7 Example of antidromic reciprocating tachycardia using an atriofascicular pathway. Note the late precordial transition at lead V_5.

preexcitation since conduction preferentially occurs over the AV node owing to the long conduction time over the accessory pathway. The electrocardiogram during ART shows a wide-complex tachycardia that resembles a typical left bundle branch block pattern. Also, the precordial transition occurs relatively late, typically at lead V_5 (Fig. 58-7).

Electrophysiologic Characterization

Findings during Sinus Rhythm

In the electrophysiologic laboratory, several features may be observed during sinus rhythm that support the diagnosis of AVRT (Table 58-1). Evidence of preexcitation (His-ventricular [H-V] interval less than 35 ms) strongly suggests that the mechanism of the tachycardia is ORT. If preexcitation is subtle, as in the case of a slowly conducting or left free-wall accessory pathway, atrial pacing is helpful in unmasking preexcitation. In a patient with an atriofascicular or a nodoventricular connection, atrial pacing results in decremental conduction over the accessory pathway. During atrial pacing, a gradual increase in preexcitation is accompanied by a progressive increase in stimulus-delta wave and atrial-His (A-H) intervals, hallmarks of decrementally conducting accessory pathways (Fig. 58-8).

Evidence of eccentric atrial activation during ventricular pacing also supports the diagnosis of ORT. Lack of ventriculoatrial (VA) conduction makes ORT extremely unlikely. Rarely, isoproterenol may bring out retrograde accessory pathway conduction in a patient with VA dissociation at baseline.

Para-Hisian pacing is very helpful in determining whether retrograde conduction is occurring over the AV node versus a septal accessory pathway.[1] A minimum of two catheters are required, one at the His position and another in the right atrium. High-output pacing is performed and the stimulus-atrial time is analyzed with and without His capture. During His capture, both the specialized conduction system and the basal right ventricular myocardium are captured, resulting in a relatively narrow QRS (Fig. 58-9A and 9B). At lower output, only the ventricular myocardium is captured, due to the higher capture threshold of the His bundle, yielding a wide QRS. If the stimulus-atrial time is the same irrespective of His capture, this indicates retrograde conduction over a septal accessory pathway. During an "AV nodal" response to para-Hisian pacing, the stimulus-atrial interval is shorter when the His is captured. Such a response suggests that retrograde activation depends upon capture of the specialized conduction system. The reason that the stimulus-atrial time is longer when the His bundle is not captured is that the atria can only be activated after depolarization of the right ventricular myocardium, followed by engagement of distal ramifications of the His-Purkinje system, the His bundle, and the AV node. During His bundle capture, however, the atrial

Table 58-1 Positive Predictive Value and Prevalence of Baseline Observations and Tachycardia Features for the Tachycardia Mechanism during an Electrophysiology Study for Evaluation of Paroxysmal Supraventricular Tachycardia

		Positive Predictive Value (%)		
Baseline Observation/Tachycardia Feature	**Prevalence (%)**	**AVNRT**	**ORT**	**AT**
Preexcitation present during sinus rhythm	15	10	86	3
Extranodal response to para-Hisian pacing	18	17	83	0
VA block cycle length >600 ms at baseline	11	41	5	55
Septal VA interval >70 ms	53	17	59	24
Eccentric atrial activation	31	0	76	24
Spontaneous AV block during tachycardia	10	60	0	40
Spontaneous termination with AV block	28	66	34	0
Development of LBBB	12	4	92	4
Increase in VA interval >20 ms with BBB	7	0	100	0

AV, atrioventricular; AT, atrial tachycardia; AVNRT, atrioventricular nodal reentry tachycardia; BBB, bundle branch block; LBBB, left bundle branch block; ORT, orthodromic reciprocating tachycardia; VA, ventriculoatrial.

From Knight BP, Morady F: Atrioventricular reentry and variants. In Zipes DP, Jalife J (eds): Cardiac Electrophysiology: From Cell to Bedside, 4th ed. Philadelphia, Saunders, 2004, p 530.

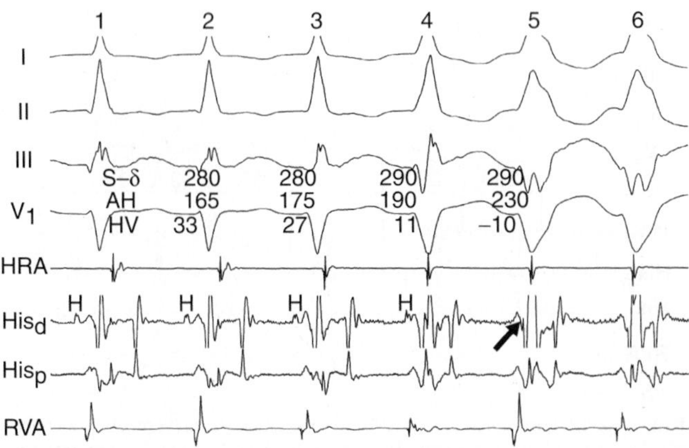

Figure 58-8 Example of decremental conduction properties of an atriofascicular accessory pathway. During right atrial pacing at 330 ms, evidence of progressive prolongation in the stimulus-delta (S-δ) and atrial-His (AH) intervals can be seen. Concomitantly, a gradual increase in the degree of ventricular preexcitation occurs, as evidenced by widening of the QRS complex and a decrease in the His-ventricular (H-V) interval. The third and fourth QRS complexes are generated as result of fusion between activation over the AV node and the accessory pathway. The fifth and sixth QRS complexes are fully preexcited. The *arrow* refers to the His (H) depolarization. HRA, high right atrium; RVA, right ventricular apex.

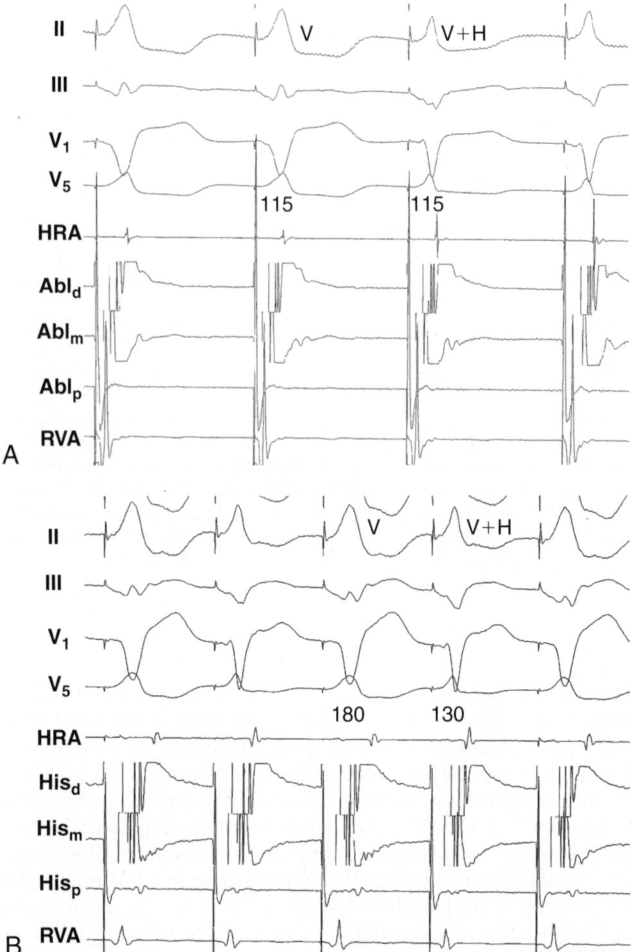

Figure 58-9 **A,** The response to para-Hisian pacing in a patient with a concealed anteroseptal accessory pathway. The stimulus-atrial time at the high right atrium (HRA) is 115 ms, irrespective of whether ventricle (V) or ventricle plus His bundle (V+H) is captured. Thus, atrial activation depends only on ventricular capture, consistent with retrograde activation over an accessory pathway. Note that His capture results in a narrower QRS complex than during ventricular capture alone. **B,** An atrioventricular nodal response to para-Hisian pacing in the same patient as in **A** after successful ablation of the anteroseptal accessory pathway. The stimulus-atrial time at the high right atrium during ventricular plus His bundle (V+H) capture is 130 ms, which is shorter than with ventricular (V) capture alone (180 ms). This observation is consistent with retrograde conduction over the atrioventricular node and confirms that retrograde accessory pathway conduction has been eliminated. d, distal; m, mid; p, proximal; RVA, right ventricular apex.

activation occurs earlier, because the impulse needs to conduct only from the very proximal aspect of the specialized conduction system. Para-Hisian pacing also is helpful in determining whether a septal accessory pathway has been successfully ablated (see Fig. 58-9A and B).

Findings during Tachycardia

A helpful maneuver during supraventricular tachycardia is observing the response upon cessation of ventricular overdrive pacing that entrains the tachycardia.[2] An AV response after cessation of pacing rules out atrial tachycardia, leaving AV nodal reentrant tachycardia and ORT as the most likely possibilities. Thereafter, a number of other maneuvers and observations can be used to distinguish between these two possibilities. If the high right atrial electrogram is recorded within or at the end of the QRS complex, ORT may be ruled out, because atrial activation can occur only following ventricular activation during ORT. More precisely, a VA time less than 70 ms as measured on the His bundle electrogram is extremely specific for AV nodal reentrant tachycardia and rules out ORT.[3] If atrial activation is not simultaneous with ventricular activation, a His-synchronous ventricular extrastimulus is delivered during tachycardia. If the timing of the atrial electrogram following the extrastimulus is altered, an extranodal accessory pathway is present, supporting the diagnosis of ORT. A number of responses are possible. The atrial electrogram may be advanced (Fig. 58-10) or delayed, or the tachycardia may be terminated in the retrograde limb without affecting the atrial electrogram. The latter finding is diagnostic of ORT. Failure to affect the tachycardia with a His-synchronous ventricular extrastimulus does not rule out ORT if the accessory pathway is located remote from the right ventricular pacing site, for example, in the case of left free-wall pathways.

An intermittent bundle branch block during supraventricular tachycardia may provide important clues to the mechanism of the tachycardia. Prolongation of the V-A interval during bundle branch block is diagnostic of ORT using an accessory pathway ipsilateral to the affected bundle. Specifically, if the V-A time prolongs by more than 30 ms, the tachycardia is using a free-wall accessory pathway. Prolongation of the V-A interval by less than 30 ms is consistent with a left posteroseptal accessory pathway when a left bundle branch block is present and with an anteroseptal accessory pathway when a right bundle branch block is present (Figs. 58-11 and 58-12).

Several clues are helpful in making the diagnosis of ART. First, the electrocardiogram during tachycardia shows a wide-complex rhythm in which the QRS does not resemble a typical left or right bundle branch block pattern and is identical to the maximally preexcited QRS during atrial pacing. Second, the His bundle electrogram lacks a His potential before ventricular activation, suggestive of anterograde activation over an accessory pathway. The most helpful maneuver is to insert an atrial

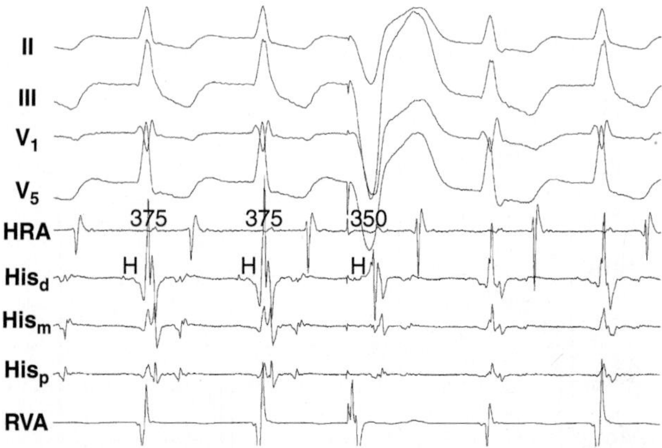

Figure 58-10 The response to introduction of a His–synchronous ventricular extrastimulus during supraventricular tachycardia. The atrial electrogram after the ventricular extrastimulus is advanced by 25 ms, consistent with the presence of an accessory pathway. This response proves that an extranodal accessory pathway is present but does not necessarily prove that the tachycardia is orthodromic reciprocating tachycardia. H, bundle of His potential; HRA, high right atrium; RVA, right ventricular apex; V+H, ventricular plus His bundle.

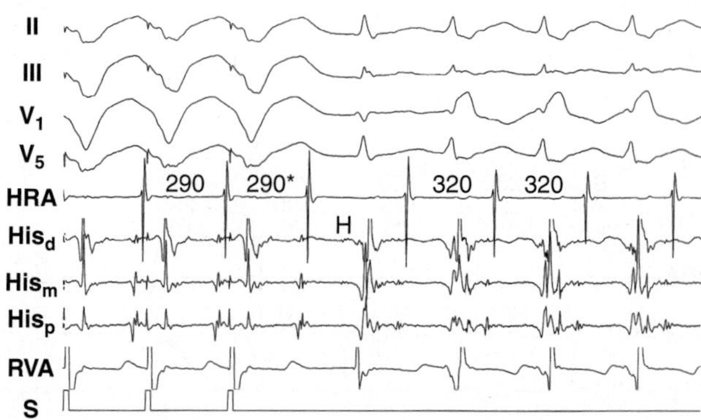

Figure 58-12 Response to ventricular pacing during supraventricular tachycardia. The tachycardia is accelerated to the pacing rate (290 ms). The last entrained atrial electrogram *(asterisk)* is followed by a ventricular electrogram, constituting an atrioventricular response and ruling out atrial tachycardia. Further maneuvers confirmed the diagnosis of orthodromic reciprocating tachycardia. Note that ventriculoatrial time does not change with development of right bundle branch block pattern, ruling out a right free-wall accessory pathway. Successful ablation was performed at the lateral mitral annulus. H, bundle of His potential; HRA, high right atrium; RVA, right ventricular apex; S, stimulus.

extrastimulus at the time when the AV node should be refractory. If the subsequent ventricular electrogram is advanced with a morphology identical to that during tachycardia, anterograde conduction over an accessory pathway is assured (Fig. 58-13).

In distinguishing atypical AV nodal reentrant tachycardia ("fast-slow") from ORT using a slow-conducting septal accessory pathway, the postpacing interval after cessation of ventricular pacing is very helpful. If the postpacing interval minus the tachycardia cycle length is less than 115 ms, the diagnosis is ORT.[4] Because the ventricle is a part of the reentry circuit in ORT, the return cycle during ventricular pacing should be shorter than that during AV nodal reentrant tachycardia. Alternatively, if the postpacing interval minus the tachycardia cycle length is greater than 115 ms, the diagnosis is atypical AV nodal reentrant tachycardia (Fig. 58-14).

If the tachycardia consistently terminates during ventricular overdrive pacing, the operator must rely on various other maneuvers to elucidate the mechanism. Comparison of A-H intervals during tachycardia and atrial pacing (i.e., ΔA-H) is helpful in distinguishing among various causes of a long RP interval tachycardia. If the A-H interval during atrial pacing at the tachycardia cycle length exceeds that during tachycardia by more than 40 ms, atypical AV nodal reentrant tachycardia is much more likely than ORT using a slowly-conducting accessory pathway or atrial tachycardia. By contrast, a ΔA-H of 10 to 20 ms is consistent with either ORT or atrial tachycardia.

Ventricular burst pacing during tachycardia may provide some insight into the mechanism of the tachycardia. Dissociation of the atrial electrograms during ventricular pacing rules out ORT. Termination of the tachycardia without affecting the atrial electrogram makes atrial tachycardia very unlikely. However, ventricular pacing may rarely terminate an atrial tachycardia without influencing the atrial electrogram, possibly as a result of atrial stretch or activation of a vagal reflex.

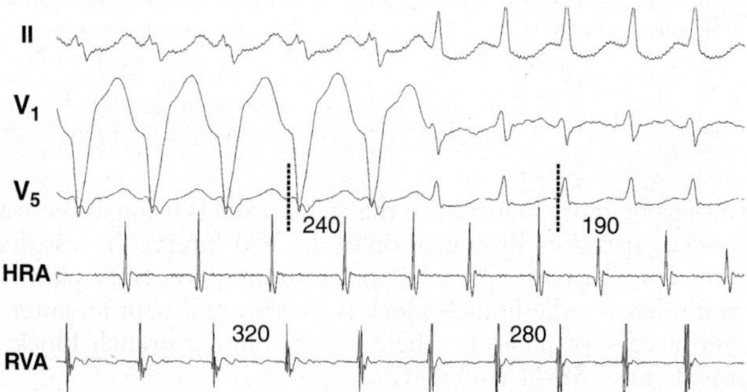

Figure 58-11 Change in ventriculoatrial (VA) time with left bundle branch block (LBBB). This tachycardia occurred during catheter placement in a patient undergoing electrophysiologic testing. The V-A interval during LBBB (240 ms) is longer than when the QRS complex is narrow (190 ms), which is diagnostic of orthodromic reciprocating tachycardia using a left free-wall accessory pathway. Mapping confirmed the presence of a concealed left lateral accessory pathway that was successfully ablated. Dotted lines refer to onset of ventricular activation. HRA, high right atrium; RVA, right ventricular apex.

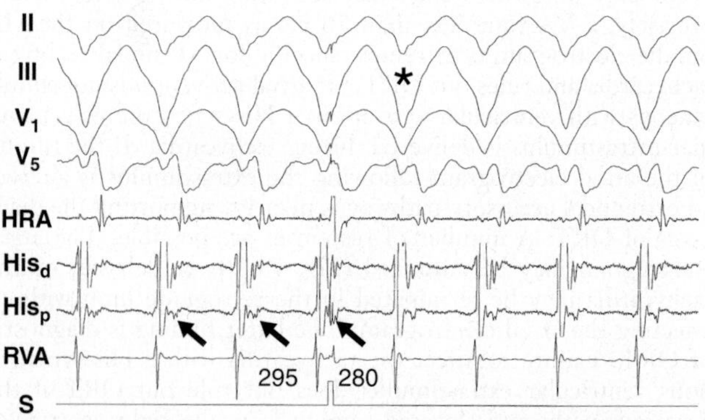

Figure 58-13 An example of antidromic reciprocating tachycardia (ART). An atrial extrastimulus is introduced coincident with the septal atrial electrogram *(arrows)*, at a time when the atrioventricular node should be refractory. The following QRS complex *(asterisk)* is advanced with no change in QRS morphology and with resetting of the tachycardia, consistent with anterograde conduction over the accessory pathway and the diagnosis of ART. H, bundle of His potential; HRA, high right atrium; RVA, right ventricular apex.

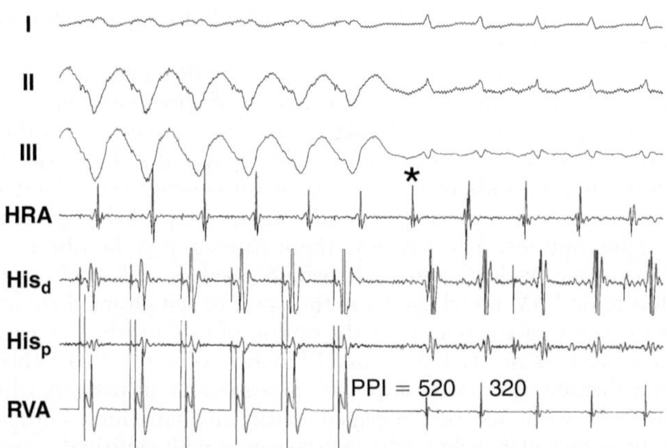

Figure 58-14 Diagnosis of a long ventriculoatrial interval tachycardia with a single pacing maneuver. The tachycardia is accelerated to 300 ms during entrainment from the right ventricular apex (RVA). An atrioventricular (AV) response is seen on cessation of pacing, ruling out atrial tachycardia. The postpacing interval (PPI) is 520 ms, which exceeds the tachycardia cycle length (320 ms) by 200 ms. Because the PPI minus the tachycardia cycle length is greater than 115 ms, the diagnosis is atypical AV nodal reentrant tachycardia, as opposed to orthodromic reciprocating tachycardia using a slowly conducting, septal accessory pathway. HRA, high right atrium.

Mapping and Ablation of Accessory Pathways

Mapping in patients with a concealed accessory pathway is best performed during ORT. It also is possible to map the accessory pathway during ventricular pacing. Ventricular pacing in a patient with a septal accessory pathway is not helpful, however, because the operator is unable to distinguish between retrograde AV nodal and accessory pathway conduction. Even in patients with free-wall accessory pathways, ventricular pacing may yield inconsistent findings since atrial activation may occur as a result of fusion between AV nodal and accessory pathway conduction. In patients with a manifest accessory pathway, mapping may be performed either in sinus rhythm or ORT.

It is essential to be aware of the fact that many accessory pathways insert obliquely along the AV annulus (Fig. 58-15A to C).[1] In other words, the earliest atrial activation during ORT or ventricular pacing and the earliest ventricular activation during sinus rhythm may not occur at the same point along the AV annulus. Confusion is avoided in most cases by targeting the earliest atrial activation when the mapping catheter is on the atrial side of the annulus, and by mapping for earliest ventricular activation when the ablation catheter is on the ventricular side of the annulus.

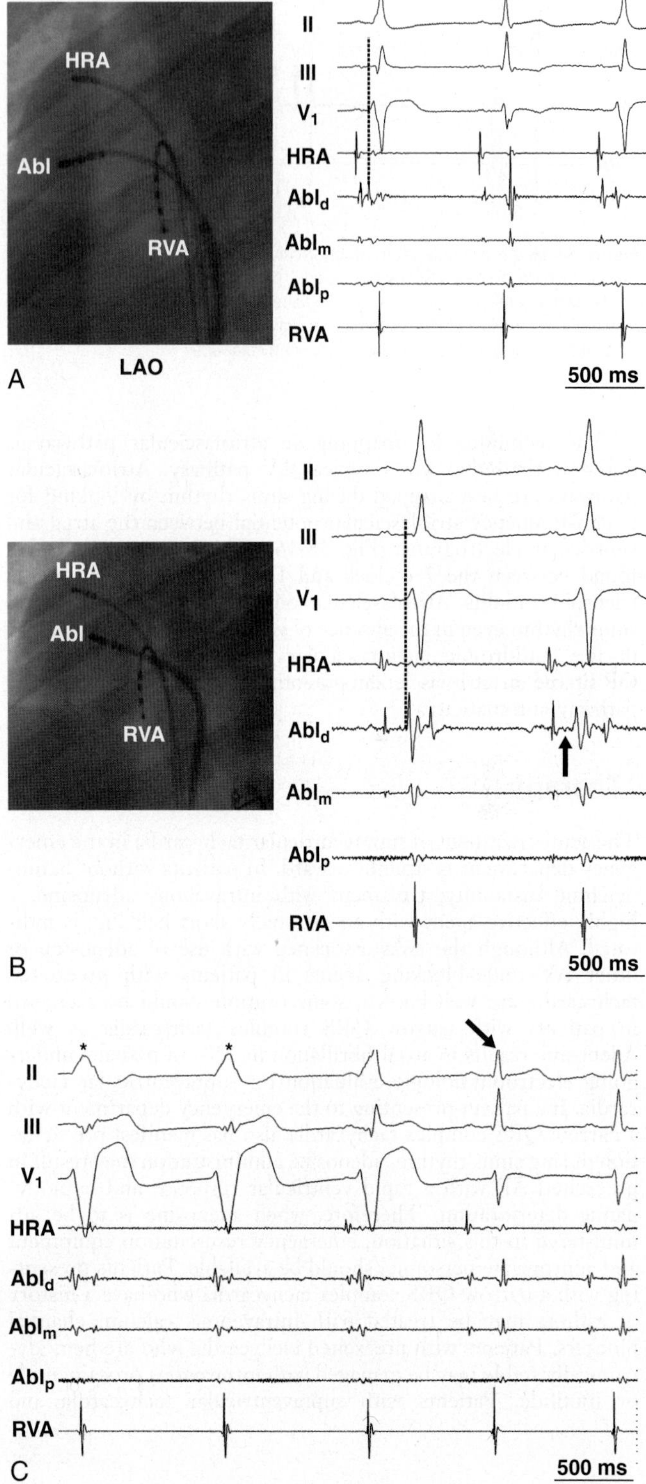

Figure 58-15 A, An example of an oblique accessory pathway. Mapping demonstrated a manifest right free-wall accessory pathway with decremental conduction properties. "Bump" mapping at the lateral tricuspid isthmus *(left)* resulted in transient loss of preexcitation *(arrow, right)*. However, radiofrequency energy delivery at this site only transiently abolished preexcitation. Note that local ventricular activation recorded by the distal bipole of the ablation catheter (Abl$_d$) precedes the delta wave *(dashed line)* by 10 ms. **B,** Further mapping at the anterolateral tricuspid annulus *(left)* revealed the electrogram shown here. Even though the local ventricular activation does not precede the delta wave *(dashed line)*, radiofrequency energy delivery was successful in permanently eliminating preexcitation (see Fig. 58-15C), probably owing to the presence of a possible accessory pathway potential *(arrow)*. The earliest ventricular activation occurred at approximately 9 o'clock on the tricuspid annulus, whereas the successful ablation site was found at 10 o'clock, consistent with an oblique course along the tricuspid annulus. **C,** Energy delivery at the site noted in Figure 58-15B resulted in thermally induced automatic activity *(asterisks)* followed by loss of preexcitation *(arrow)*. Note that the third QRS complex is a result of fusion. HRA, high right atrium; LAO, left anterior oblique (projection); RVA, right ventricular apex.

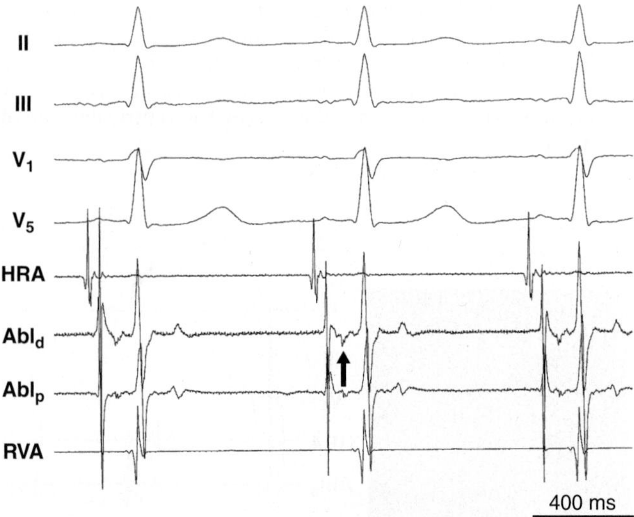

Figure 58-16 An example of an atriofascicular potential in a patient with antidromic tachycardia. Note the high-frequency potential *(arrow)* that was recorded at the posterolateral tricuspid annulus. Radiofrequency energy delivery at this site resulted in thermally induced automatic activity followed by elimination of preexcitation. HRA, high right atrium; RVA, right ventricular apex.

The technique for mapping an atriofascicular pathway is different than that for a typical AV pathway. Atriofascicular pathways are best mapped during sinus rhythm by looking for a high-frequency atriofascicular potential between the atrial and ventricular electrograms (Fig. 58-16). These sites typically are found between the 7 o'clock and 11 o'clock positions on the tricuspid annulus. Atriofascicular potentials are present during sinus rhythm even in the absence of ventricular preexcitation and during antidromic atriofascicular tachycardia. Ablation at the site of an atriofascicular potential may be accompanied by pathway automaticity.

Therapy

The acute treatment of supraventricular tachycardia in the emergency department is straightforward. In patients without hemodynamic instability, treatment with intravenous adenosine, a highly effective agent with an extremely short half-life, is indicated. Although the risks associated with use of adenosine or other AV node–blocking agents in patients with preexcited tachycardia are well known, some caution should be exercised in patients with narrow QRS complex tachycardia as well. Adenosine results in atrial fibrillation in 12% of patients undergoing electrophysiologic evaluation for supraventricular tachycardia. If a patient presenting to the emergency department with a narrow QRS complex tachycardia also has manifest preexcitation during sinus rhythm, adenosine administration may result in preexcited AF with a rapid ventricular response and hemodynamic deterioration. Therefore, when adenosine is to be administered in this situation, emergency resuscitation equipment and appropriate personnel should be available. Patients presenting with a narrow QRS complex tachycardia who have a history of asthma may be treated with intravenous calcium channel blockers. Patients with preexcited tachycardia who are hemodynamically stable may be managed with intravenous procainamide or ibutilide. Patients with supraventricular tachycardia and severe hypotension or other serious symptoms should undergo direct current cardioversion.

The chronic treatment of patients with ORT must be individualized. Patients without evidence of preexcitation may be managed in a fashion similar to that for patients with other types of paroxysmal supraventricular tachycardia. In a patient with a first episode of tachycardia or infrequent, well-tolerated episodes, abortive maneuvers and reassurance probably are reasonable options. Alternatively, these patients may be offered a "pill-in-the-pocket" approach, which involves self-administration of oral AV-nodal agents at the onset of symptoms. Patients with recurrent episodes have the option of medical therapy with beta-blockers or calcium channel blockers versus catheter ablation therapy. A curative approach is reasonable in patients who do not wish to be managed with antiarrhythmic drugs. Supraventricular tachycardia in association with ventricular preexcitation is considered a class I indication for an electrophysiologic evaluation and catheter ablation.[5] Catheter ablation is highly effective in eliminating accessory pathway conduction, thus eliminating the symptoms caused by supraventricular tachycardia and the small risk of sudden death associated with the WPW syndrome. Patients with the WPW syndrome who are not candidates for catheter ablation or in whom ablation would be very likely to result in high-grade AV block should receive pharmacologic therapy with an AV-nodal blocking agent and an antiarrhythmic agent capable of blocking conduction over the accessory pathway, such as propafenone, flecainide, sotalol, or amiodarone.

Most asymptomatic patients in whom the electrocardiogram incidentally shows evidence of preexcitation do not require an electrophysiologic evaluation, because their risk of sudden death is relatively low.[5] Some evidence, however, suggests that catheter ablation in this group reduces the risk of arrhythmic events.[6] The decision to perform catheter ablation in asymptomatic patients with "high-risk" occupations (such as pilots and bus drivers) should be individualized.

Catheter ablation of accessory pathways has been shown to be highly effective and is associated with a low risk of complications. A few years ago, results of catheter ablation of accessory pathways were pooled from several electrophysiology laboratories. Among 6065 patients, catheter ablation resulted in a successful long-term outcome in 98% of the patients.[7] A repeat procedure was required in approximately 2% of patients. A serious complication—tamponade, AV block, coronary artery injury, retroperitoneal hemorrhage, or stroke—occurred in 0.6% of patients. One fatality (0.02%) was reported in this series. Therefore, the one-time risk of an ablation procedure compares favorably with the cumulative risk of sudden death in patients with the WPW syndrome.

Summary

Atrioventricular reentry is the most common arrhythmia in patients with the WPW syndrome. It is also the second most common arrhythmia mechanism in patients presenting for an electrophysiologic evaluation for paroxysmal supraventricular tachycardia. AVRT uses both the specialized conduction system and the accessory pathway, which typically inserts at the AV annulus. Catheter ablation of accessory pathways participating in AVRT is highly effective and associated with a very low risk of complications. Catheter ablation is the treatment of choice in patients with the WPW syndrome and in those patients with recurrent paroxysmal supraventricular tachycardia mediated by a concealed accessory pathway.

References

1. Nakagawa H, Jackman WM: Catheter ablation of paroxysmal supraventricular tachycardia. Circulation 116:2465-2478, 2007.
2. Knight BP, Morady F: Atrioventricular reentry and variants. In Zipes DP, Jalife J (eds): Cardiac Electrophysiology: From Cell to Bedside, 4th ed. Philadelphia, Saunders, 2004, pp 528-536.
3. Knight BP, Ebinger M, Oral H, et al: Diagnostic value of tachycardia features and pacing maneuvers during paroxysmal supraventricular tachycardia. J Am Coll Cardiol 36:574-582, 2000.
4. Michaud GF, Tada H, Chough S, et al: Differentiation of atypical atrioventricular node re-entrant tachycardia from orthodromic reciprocating tachycardia using a septal accessory pathway by the response to ventricular pacing. J Am Coll Cardiol 38:1163-1167, 2001.
5. Blomstrom-Lundqvist C, Scheinman MM, Aliot EM, et al: ACC/AHA/ESC guidelines for the management of patients with supraventricular arrhythmias—Executive Summary: A report of the American College of Cardiology/American Heart Association Task Force on Practice Guidelines and the European Society of Cardiology Committee for Practice Guidelines (Writing Committee to Develop Guidelines for the Management of Patients With Supraventricular Arrhythmias). Circulation 108:1871-1909, 2003.
6. Pappone C, Santinelli V, Manguso F, et al: A randomized study of prophylactic catheter ablation in asymptomatic patients with the Wolff-Parkinson-White syndrome. N Engl J Med 349:1803-1811, 2002.
7. Morady F: Catheter ablation of supraventricular arrhythmias: State of the art. J Cardiovasc Electrophysiol 15:124-139, 2004.

Electrophysiologic Characteristics of Atrioventricular Nodal Reentrant Tachycardia: Implications for Reentrant Circuits

59

Deborah Lockwood, Hiroshi Nakagawa, and Warren M. Jackman

CHAPTER OUTLINE

Atrioventricular nodal reentrant tachycardia (AVNRT), the most common form of paroxysmal supraventricular tachycardia, is a fascinating complex of arrhythmias. AVNRT originally was proposed to result from reentry totally confined within the compact atrioventricular (AV) node.[1] Today, however, the so-called typical form of AVNRT—"Slow/Fast AVNRT"—is thought to involve a component of atrial myocardium, at least two atrionodal connections, and the AV node.[2-10] Much of the current understanding about the components of the reentrant circuit has evolved from the development of ablation procedures in which one of the atrionodal connections, remote from the compact AV node, is destroyed, eliminating AVNRT without producing AV block.[2-7,11]

AVNRT is more common in women than in men.[2-4] Of 557 consecutive patients referred to the Heart Rhythm Institute at the University of Oklahoma Health Sciences Center for catheter ablation for treatment of AVNRT, 436 (78%) were female. This arrhythmia is thought to be uncommon in children, but 72 of these patients (13%) were 16 years of age or younger, including 10 (1.8%) patients aged 2 to 5 years, 8 (1.4%) patients aged 6 to 10 years, 16 (2.9%) patients aged 11 to 13 years, and 38 (6.8%) patients aged 14 to 16 years.

Dual–Atrioventricular Nodal Pathway Physiology

Early investigators proposed that AVNRT resulted from reentry within the compact AV node as a result of functional longitudinal dissociation within the AV node into a fast and a slow pathway.[1] This hypothesis was based on the absence of any potentials recorded between the timing of atrial activation and His bundle activation, and the observation that dual–AV nodal pathway physiology usually was present (up to 85%) in patients with AVNRT and initially was thought to be absent in most patients without AVNRT.[16] It also was thought that atrial activation could be dissociated from the tachycardia. Such cases of atrial dissociation are surprisingly rare, but suggest that at least in some patients, the reentrant circuit is contained within a "protected" region.[1] The inability to dissociate the atrium from Slow/Fast AVNRT in most patients supports the involvement of atrial tissue outside the triangle of Koch and the coronary sinus myocardium in the reentrant circuit. Furthermore, the small size and irregular orientation of the fibers in the compact AV node make functional longitudinal dissociation into two pathways with fixed conduction times unlikely.

Dual–AV nodal pathway physiology was defined by atrial extrastimulus testing, using the arbitrary criterion of an increase of 50 ms or greater in the interval between the local atrial potential and the His bundle potential (A_2-H_2) after a 10-ms decrease in the local atrial coupling interval (A_1-A_2).[13] Dual-pathway physiology also was defined during decremental atrial pacing by an increase of 50 ms or greater in the atrial activation–His bundle activation (A-H) interval after a 10-ms decrease in the atrial pacing cycle length.[14,15] The abrupt increase in AV nodal conduction time was interpreted to represent conduction block in the fast pathway with selective conduction over the slow pathway. When the conduction time over the slow pathway became sufficiently long to allow recovery of the presumed region of the AV node comprising the fast pathway, retrograde conduction to the atrium occurred over the fast pathway, resulting in an atrial echo complex or AVNRT.

More recent studies suggest that the fast and slow pathways involved in the reentrant circuit of AVNRT represent conduction over different atrio-nodal connections, rather than being formed by functional longitudinal dissociation within the compact AV node.[2-10,16-28] These observations include (1) differences in the site of earliest atrial activation between retrograde conduction over the fast and slow pathways[2,6,8,9,16] (originally described by Sung and coworkers[16]); (2) resetting of the tachycardia by a late atrial extrastimulus delivered outside the compact AV node to the inferior aspect of the triangle of Koch or coronary sinus[6,8,10,17,18]; (3) microelectrode and extracellular recordings and optical mapping of AV nodal conduction in dogs and rabbits[24,27,28]; and (4) selective elimination of fast or slow pathway conduction by ablation in the atrium remote from the compact AV node.[2-6,11,19-21,29,30]

Fast Atrioventricular Nodal Pathway

The atrial connections of the fast and slow pathways can be identified by locating the site of earliest atrial activation during selective retrograde conduction over these pathways.[2,16,31,32] Recent detailed histologic examination of the AV junction (Fig. 59-1) has identified anatomic counterparts of the functional activation patterns discussed here. During retrograde fast pathway conduction, conventional widely spaced bipolar electrodes (5- to 10-mm interelectrode spacing) record earliest atrial activation at the same site recording the His bundle potential (the "His bundle electrogram"). However, the wide bipolar electrode

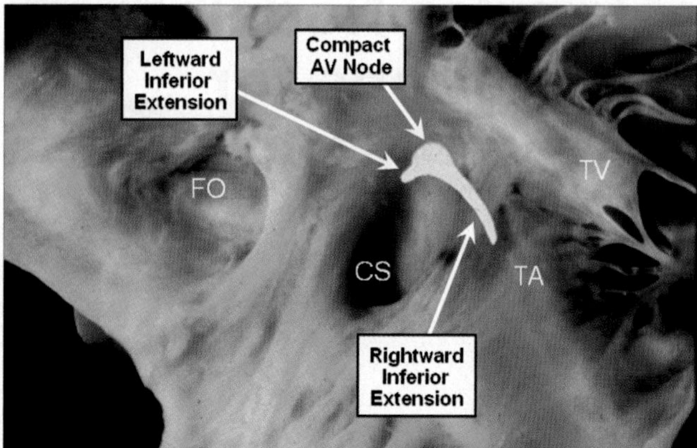

Figure 59-1 Representation of the locations of the rightward and leftward inferior extensions. This photograph (right-sided view) of the atrioventricular (AV) septal junction of a human heart shows the locations of the rightward and leftward inferior extensions of the AV node and the compact node as identified from detailed histologic study. The locations of the inferior extensions correlate with the sites of earliest retrograde activation during retrograde conduction over two slow AV nodal pathways. CS, coronary sinus; FO, fossa ovalis; TA, tricuspid annulus; TV, tricuspid valve. (Modified from Inoue S, Becker AE: Posterior extensions of the human compact atrioventricular node: A neglected anatomic feature of potential clinical significance. Circulation 97:188-193, 1998.)

records activity spanning a relatively long distance, from the region posterior to (behind) the tendon of Todaro (outside the triangle of Koch) to the proximal right bundle branch. Right atrial mapping using closely spaced electrodes (1 mm edge to edge) in 48 patients identified earliest right atrial activation at a site located a mean of 5 ± 3 mm inferior and 8 ± 3 mm posterior to the site recording the proximal His bundle potential[32] (Figs. 59-2 to 59-4). In 47 of the 48 patients, the catheter recording earliest retrograde atrial activation was located leftward of the His bundle catheter as seen in the left anterior oblique projection, indicating that the mapping catheter was not constrained by the tricuspid annulus and tendon of Todaro (unlike the His bundle catheter) and that the site of earliest atrial activation was located posterior to (behind) the tendon of Todaro, outside the triangle of Koch (see Figs. 59-3 and 59-4).[32] If the mapping catheter had been positioned across the tendon of Todaro, close to the tricuspid annulus (within the triangle of Koch), the catheter would have been oriented parallel to the His bundle catheter as seen in the left anterior oblique projection, rather than being oriented leftward.

During retrograde fast pathway conduction, right atrial activation beginning behind the tendon of Todaro (outside the triangle of Koch) propagates away in the posterior, superior, and inferior directions (Fig. 59-5, green arrows #2). Activation propagating inferiorly along the posterior aspect of the eustachian ridge produces an early far-field atrial potential recorded from the inferior aspect of the triangle of Koch (Fig. 59-6, A_{far}, Inf ToK electrogram). Atrial activation within the triangle of Koch (adjacent to the tricuspid annulus) occurs relatively late and proceeds in the inferior-to-superior direction, beginning just outside the coronary sinus ostium (Fig. 59-7B, left beat; see also

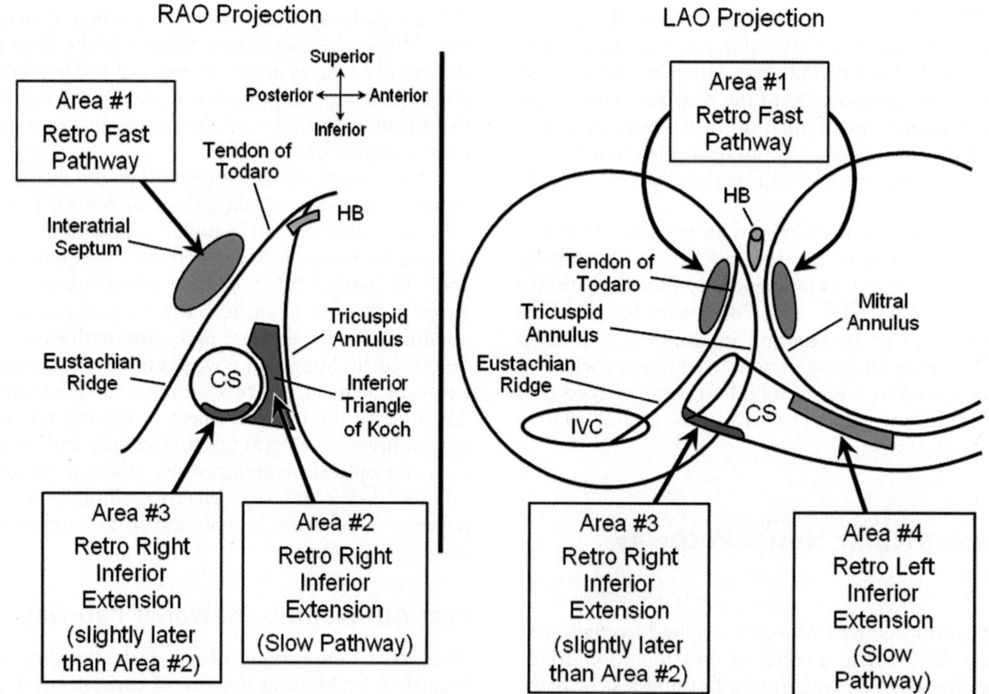

Figure 59-2 Schematic representation of the sites of earliest retrograde atrial activation during retrograde conduction over the fast and slow atrioventricular (AV) nodal pathways. Earliest atrial activation during retrograde conduction over the fast pathway (Retro fast pathway, Area #1, *red*) is recorded at the true interatrial septum, posterior to the tendon of Todaro and inferior to the site recording the His bundle potential. Activation can be recorded at least as early from the left side of the septum as from the right. Retrograde conduction over a slow AV nodal pathway may be conducted in retrograde fashion over the rightward inferior extension or the leftward inferior extension. For retrograde slow pathway conduction over the rightward inferior extension (Retro right inferior extension), earliest activation is recorded at the inferior triangle of Koch (Area #2, *blue*), followed by activation at the floor of the coronary sinus ostium (Area #3, *blue*). For retrograde slow pathway conduction over the leftward inferior extension (Retro left inferior extension), earliest activation is recorded at the roof of the coronary sinus, 1 to 4 cm from the ostium (Area #4, *purple*). CS, coronary sinus; HB, His bundle; IVC, inferior vena cava; LAO, left anterior oblique; RAO, right anterior oblique.

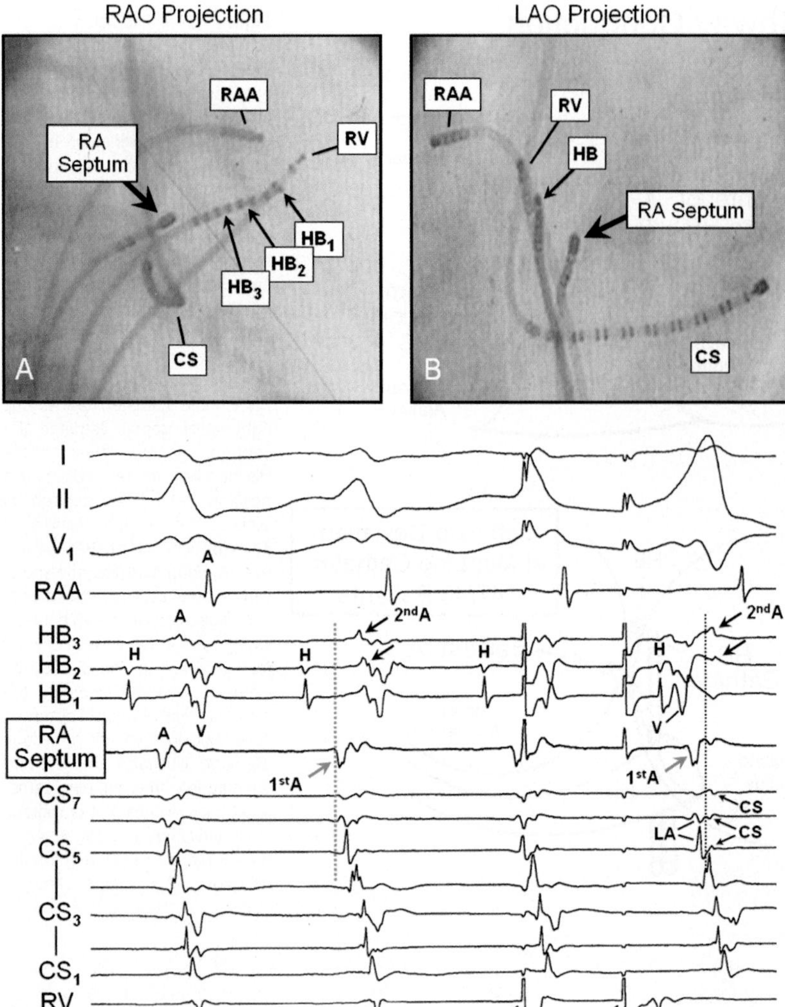

Figure 59-3 Pattern of atrial activation during Slow/Fast atrioventricular nodal reentrant tachycardia (AVNRT). **A** and **B**, Radiographs in the right anterior oblique (RAO) and left anterior oblique (LAO) projections, showing catheter positions. The octapolar His bundle catheter (HB) was positioned across the tendon of Todaro and tricuspid annulus. The angle for the LAO projection was selected to be parallel with the His bundle catheter (on looking straight at the tip). The mapping catheter at the right atrial septum (RA septum) was positioned at the site of earliest retrograde right atrial activation during Slow/Fast AVNRT, approximately 1.5 cm posterior and inferior to the site recording most proximal His bundle activation (HB_2). In the LAO projection (**B**), the mapping (RA septum) catheter is deviated leftward of the His bundle catheter, confirming a location behind the tendon of Todaro. **C**, Bipolar electrograms (filter 30 to 500 Hz) recorded with closely spaced electrodes, during Slow/Fast AVNRT from the catheters shown in **A** and **B**. Two distinct sets of potentials were recorded from the His bundle–right atrial septum region. The first potential (1st A, *red arrows, dotted red line*) was recorded behind the tendon of Todaro by the electrode at the right atrial septum (RA Sept). This was the site of earliest activation found during mapping of the right atrium and coronary sinus. The second potential (2nd A) was recorded near the apex of the triangle of Koch (electrograms HB_3 and HB_2). Note that propagation is in the inferior-to-superior direction (HB_3, then HB_2) (*black arrows*) and the potential is recorded after coronary sinus myocardial activation (electrograms CS_5 to CS_7, *black arrows, dotted black line*) and 40 ms after earliest atrial activation recorded behind the tendon of Todaro (1st A). LA, left atrial activation; RAA, right atrial appendage; V, ventricular electrogram.

Fig. 59-5, blue arrow #6, and Fig. 59-6, A_{SP} potential) and propagates toward the apex of the triangle (see Fig. 59-3, *arrows*, 2nd A inside triangle of Koch). High-resolution electroanatomic mapping in a small number of patients confirmed late activation within the triangle of Koch, with latest activation at the apex of the triangle occurring at a median of 50 ms after earliest activation.[31] The two sets of potentials propagating in opposite directions suggest conduction block across the tendon of Todaro (see Fig. 59-5, green arrow #2 and blue arrow #6). Both sets of potentials (outside and inside the triangle of Koch) often are recorded together, at or just inferior to the site recording the proximal His bundle electrogram (Fig. 59-8). The timing of the second atrial potential near the apex of the triangle of Koch is later than the timing of atrial activation in the inferior triangle of Koch (between the coronary sinus ostium and the tricuspid annulus), which is later than the timing of activation within the proximal coronary sinus. This finding suggests that the tissue within the triangle of Koch is activated by the coronary sinus myocardium (see Fig. 59-5, brown arrows).

The presence of two potentials during retrograde fast pathway activation may lead to an incorrect diagnosis. If only the second potential (near the apex of the triangle) is recorded on the His bundle electrogram during Slow/Fast AVNRT, this may lead to the erroneous impression that activation is earliest in the inferior triangle of Koch or in the coronary sinus. Accordingly, retrograde conduction would then seem to be occurring over a slow pathway—leading to the incorrect diagnosis of Slow/Slow AVNRT. This error can be avoided by mapping behind the tendon of Todaro as well as along the tricuspid annulus and coronary sinus to identify the true site of earliest activation (see Fig. 59-3).

At the site of earliest right atrial activation during Slow/Fast AVNRT, the filtered (30- to 250-Hz) bipolar atrial potential usually exhibits two components: a rounded, negative initial component followed, approximately 10 ms later, by a sharper, predominantly positive component (Fig. 59-9, RA_{Sept} electrogram).[32] Because this location (behind the tendon of Todaro) is at the true interatrial septum, the initial low-frequency component of the atrial potential may represent the far-field recording of activation originating at the left side of the septum. Right and left atrial mapping in a few patients with patent foramen ovale revealed a sharp (near-field) potential on the left side of the atrial septum, simultaneous with the initial low-frequency component recorded on the right side of the septum, consistent with earlier activation of the left side of the atrial septum (see Fig. 59-9).[32,33] Early activation of the left side of the septum accounts for the relatively early activation recorded in the proximal coronary sinus.

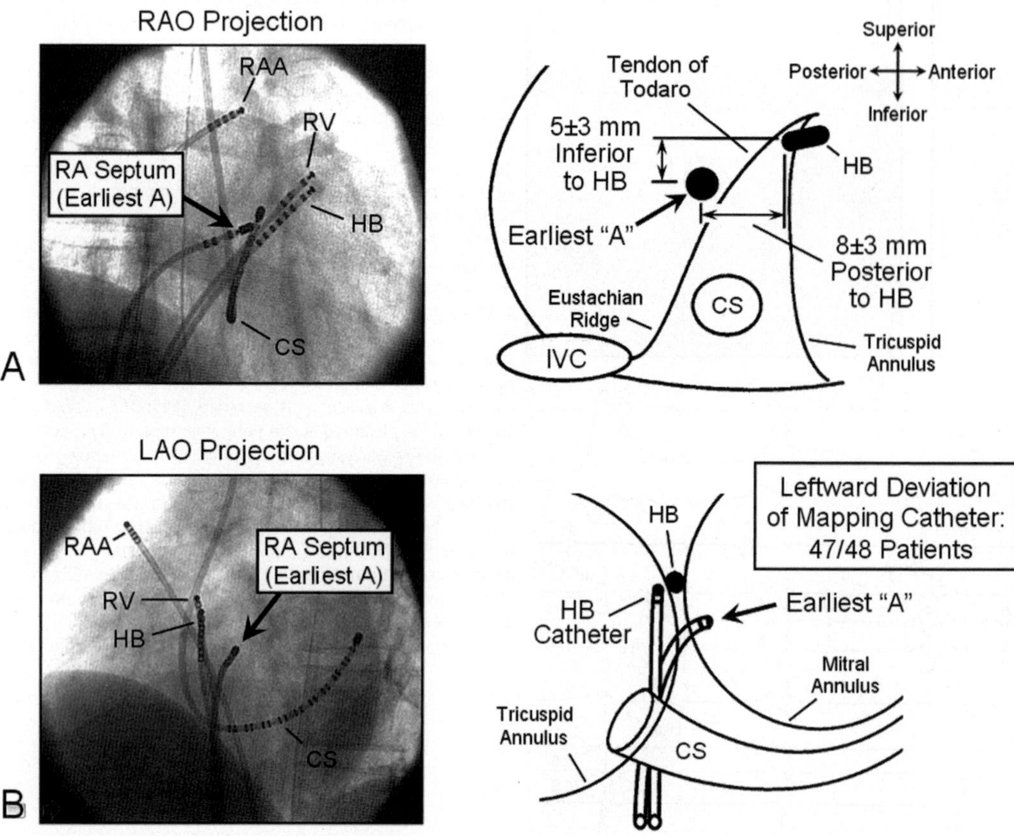

Figure 59-4 Radiographic and schematic representation, showing the site of earliest retrograde atrial activation during Slow/Fast atrioventricular nodal reentrant tachycardia in a series of 48 consecutive patients. **A** and **B**, Radiographs (*left*) showing the relationship between the His bundle catheter (HB) and the catheter on the right side of the interatrial septum (RA Septum) at the site recording earliest retrograde atrial activation (Earliest A). The LAO radiograph (with angle selected to be parallel with the His bundle catheter) shows the right atrial septal catheter (RA Septum) oriented leftward of the His bundle catheter, indicating a position behind the tendon of Todaro, outside the triangle of Koch (**B**). Schematic in RAO projection (**A,** *right*) illustrates the site of earliest atrial activation (*solid circle* and *large arrow*) in the 48 patients, which was located a mean of 8 ± 3 mm posterior to and 5 ± 3 mm inferior to the site recording the proximal His bundle potential. Schematic in the LAO projection (**B,** *right*) illustrates the leftward orientation of the mapping catheter at the site of earliest retrograde atrial activation, present in 47 of the 48 patients. LAO, left anterior oblique; RAO, right anterior oblique.

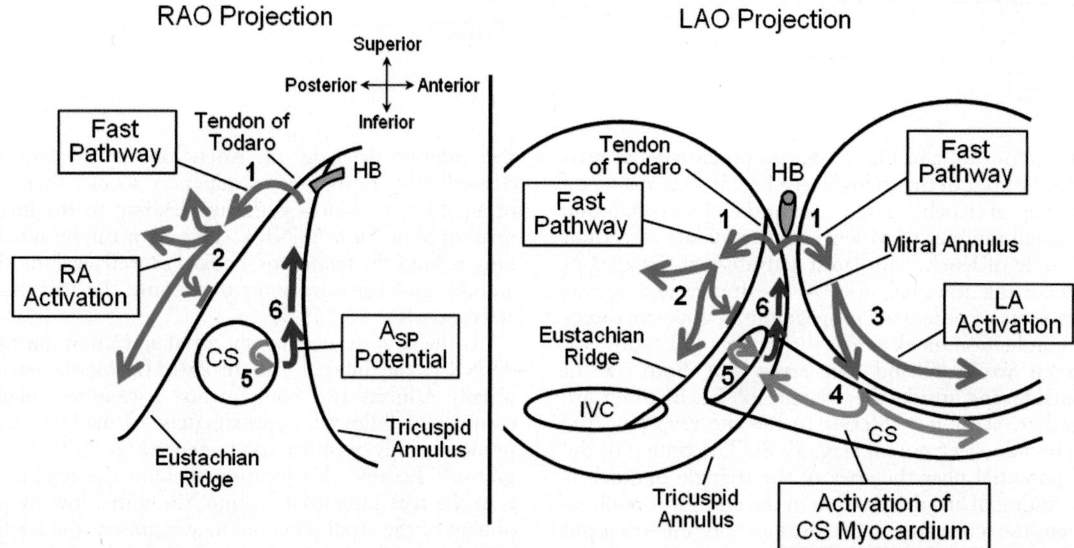

Figure 59-5 Proposed pattern of atrial activation during retrograde conduction over the fast pathway. After emerging (Fast pathway, *red arrow*, #1) behind the tendon of Todaro (outside the triangle of Koch) at the interatrial septum, right atrial activation propagates away in the posterior, superior, and inferior directions (RA activation, *green arrows*, #2). This results in superior-to-inferior right atrial activation along the eustachian ridge, outside the triangle of Koch. This right atrial wavefront is unable to cross the eustachian ridge and tendon of Todaro to enter the triangle of Koch, presumably owing to conduction block at the eustachian ridge (*short perpendicular green arrow*). Retrograde conduction over the fast pathway also activates the left atrial septum (*red arrow*, #1 in LAO projection). Propagation occurring inferiorly from the left side of the interatrial septum (*green arrows*, #3 in LAO projection) activates the coronary sinus (CS) myocardium, approximately 1 to 3 cm from the ostium (*brown arrows*, #4 in LAO projection). The reentrant impulse propagates along the coronary sinus myocardium to the coronary sinus ostium (*brown arrows*, #4), from where it activates the inferior triangle of Koch (*brown arrow*, #5), producing the A_{SP} potential, with activation proceeding in the inferior-to-superior direction within the triangle of Koch (*blue arrows*, #6). HB, His bundle; LAO, left anterior oblique; RAO, right anterior oblique.

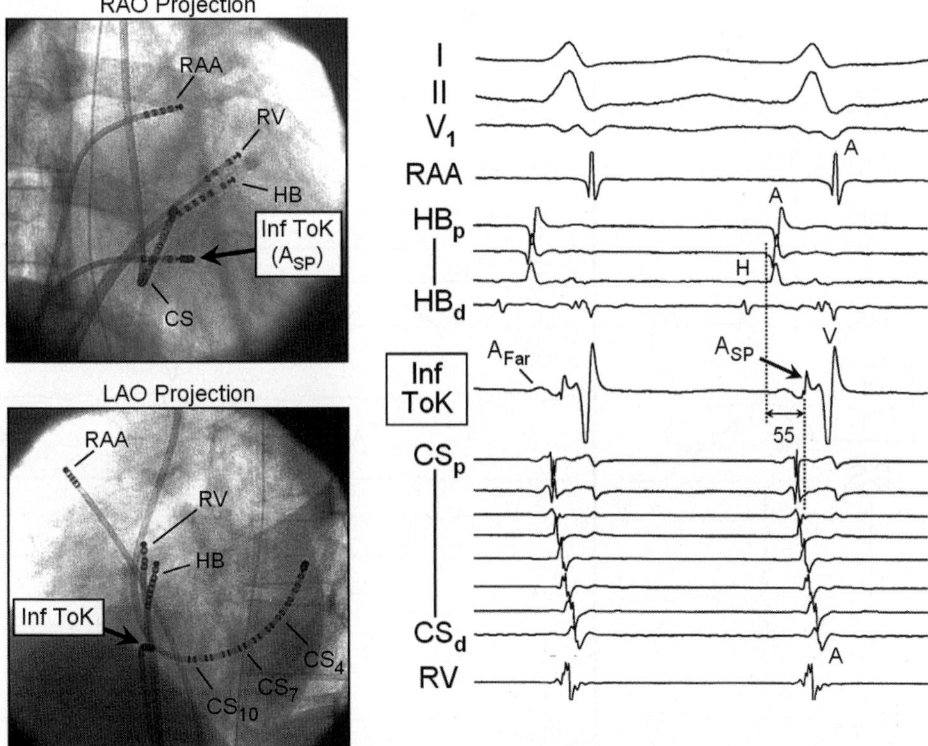

Figure 59-6 Timing of atrial activation at the inferior triangle of Koch during Slow/Fast atrioventricular nodal reentrant tachycardia (AVNRT). The radiographs, in right and left anterior oblique (RAO and LAO) projections, show the positions of the catheters for the electrograms presented. Catheters are positioned in the right atrial appendage (RAA), para-Hisian right ventricular pacing site (RV), and coronary sinus (CS) and at the inferior triangle of Koch (Inf ToK), between the mid–coronary sinus ostium and the tricuspid annulus. The His bundle catheter (HB) has been positioned across the tendon of Todaro, with a His bundle potential recorded only on the distal and second HB electrograms, such that the early atrial potentials (A, HB electrogram) are recorded from behind the tendon of Todaro. Right atrial activation propagating inferiorly along the posterior aspect of the eustachian ridge produces an early far-field atrial potential recorded from the inferior aspect of the triangle of Koch (A_{far}, Inf ToK electrogram); local activation (within the triangle of Koch) is represented as a much later sharp potential (A_{SP}). During Slow/Fast AVNRT in this patient, activation at the inferior triangle of Koch (A_{SP} potential) was recorded 55 ms after earliest atrial activation. V, ventricular electrogram. (Modified from Jackman WM, Lockwood D, Nakagawa H, et al: Catheter ablation of atrioventricular nodal reentrant tachycardia. In Wilber DJ, Packer DL, Stevenson WG [eds]: Catheter Ablation of Cardiac Arrhythmias: Basic Concepts and Clinical Applications, 3rd ed. Blackwell Futura, 2008, pp 120-148.)

Earliest attempts at selective ablation of Slow/Fast AVNRT targeted the right side of the septum at the site of earliest retrograde atrial activation, just posterior to the tendon of Todaro. This strategy was found to selectively eliminate conduction over the fast pathway and to eliminate Slow/Fast AVNRT in approximately 90% of patients.[4] Studies in intact and isolated perfused canine hearts (Langendorff preparation) have shown that radiofrequency current applied posterior to the tendon of Todaro selectively eliminates anterograde fast AV nodal pathway conduction. Histology confirmed that the lesions were limited to the region posterior to the tendon of Todaro and did not involve tissue within the triangle of Koch.[21] This area includes transitional cells, as verified by microelectrode recordings demonstrating action potentials with features intermediate between those of atrial cells and AV nodal cells. The transitional cells cross the tendon of Todaro, toward the AV node.[21,34] Microelectrode studies in rabbit hearts suggest that these anterior transitional cells insert into the AV bundle relatively close to the central fibrous body (i.e., His bundle).[35] These observations suggest that the right atrial component of the fast AV nodal pathway begins in the region of the anterior limbus of the fossa ovalis as atrial cells, becoming transitional cells as the connection approaches the tendon of Todaro and inserts into the common AV bundle, distal to most of the compact AV node.[35] This distal insertion may explain why the fast pathway, compared with the slow pathway, exhibits less decremental conduction properties, less response to typical AV node–blocking agents (β-adrenergic blockers, calcium channel blockers), and a greater response to sodium channel–blocking agents.

A study in isolated perfused canine hearts found that anterograde conduction block in the fast pathway occurred posterior to the tendon of Todaro. As the atrial pacing rate was increased, block occurred at progressively more proximal locations, that is, closer to the anterior limbus of the fossa ovalis and further from the tendon of Todaro.[21] The site of anterograde block in the fast pathway, outside the triangle of Koch, may prevent retrograde invasion of the slow pathway, and this may facilitate initiation of "AV nodal" reentry.

Slow Atrioventricular Nodal Pathway

During ventricular pacing or programmed ventricular stimulation, a shift from retrograde conduction over the fast pathway to retrograde conduction over the slow pathway is associated with a shift in the site of earliest atrial activation from the interatrial septum (outside the triangle of Koch) to a site within the triangle of Koch or within the proximal coronary sinus (see Fig. 59-2). In most patients, the earliest retrograde high-frequency potential (A_{SP} potential), is recorded between the tricuspid annulus and the coronary sinus ostium[2,16] (Fig. 59-10, blue arrow, #2; see also Fig. 59-7B).

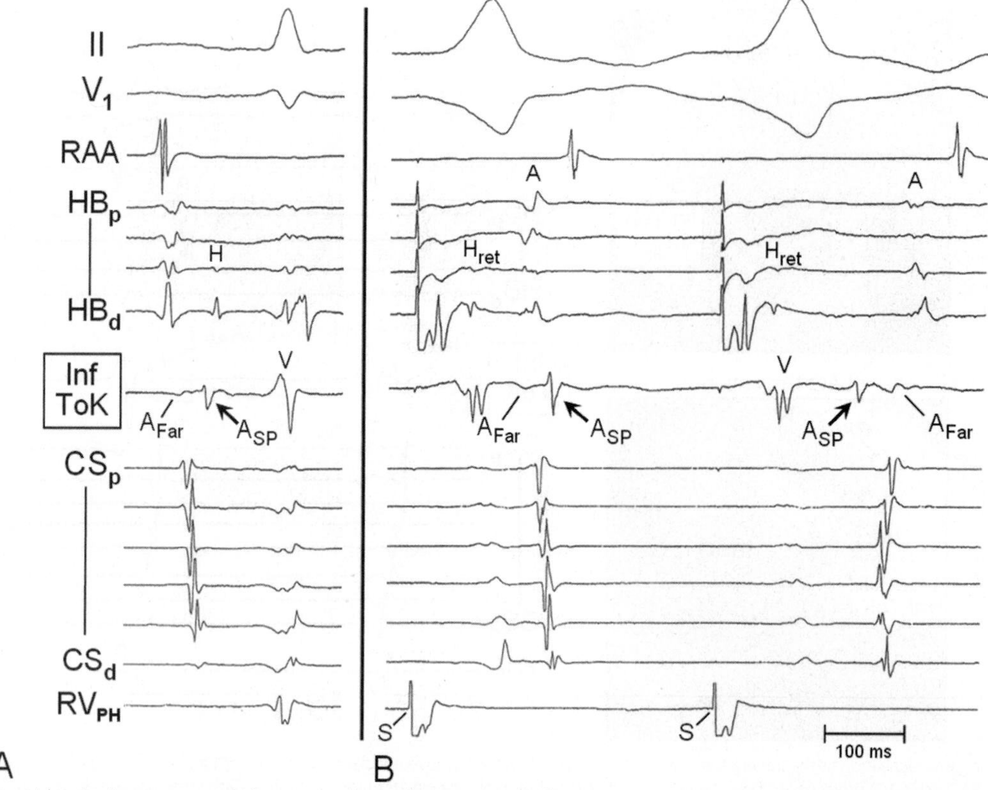

Figure 59-7 Different atrial activation sequence during retrograde conduction over the fast and slow atrioventricular nodal pathways. The catheters are in similar position to those in Figure 59-6. **A,** During sinus rhythm, the anterograde A_{SP} potential was recorded after activation in the proximal coronary sinus (CS_p) and long after septal activation recorded in the His bundle electrogram. **B,** Ventricular pacing (S) from the para-Hisian right ventricle (RV_{PH}). During retrograde conduction over the fast pathway (first beat), early atrial activation (A) is appreciated in the His bundle electrograms recorded from behind the tendon of Todaro. Activation propagates inferiorly behind the eustachian ridge to produce a far-field potential (A_{Far}) in the inferior triangle of Koch (Inf ToK). Relatively late activation of the inferior triangle of Koch itself is represented by the sharper A_{SP} potential. Note that the A_{SP} potential is recorded after the timing of activation of the proximal coronary sinus myocardium, suggesting that the inferior triangle of Koch may be activated from the coronary sinus. A similar pattern of activation is seen in the inferior triangle of Koch (Inf ToK) during sinus rhythm (**A**), with an early far-field atrial potential (A_{Far}) followed by a later A_{SP} potential. During retrograde conduction over the slow pathway (rightward inferior extension, second beat in **B**), the A_{SP} potential is earliest, with later activation behind the eustachian ridge (A_{Far}) and behind the tendon of Todaro (potential A in the HB electrogram). Combined with closely spaced bipolar electrodes on the His bundle catheter, pacing from the para-Hisian position results in early completion of the local ventricular potential recorded in the His bundle electrograms, allowing visualization of retrograde His bundle activation (H_r).

This is consistent with retrograde conduction over the rightward inferior extension of the AV node (see Fig. 59-1).[33,36] With this retrograde slow pathway, the next earliest activation is recorded at the floor of the coronary sinus ostium (Fig. 59-11B; see also Fig. 59-10, brown arrow, #3). The coronary sinus myocardium propagates the impulse leftward and superiorly and activates the left atrial myocardium approximately 2 to 3 cm from the coronary sinus ostium (see Fig. 59-10, green arrows #4 and #5). Left atrial activation proceeds leftward and rightward to the septum and propagates across the interatrial septum to activate the right atrium behind the tendon of Todaro (see Fig. 59-10, green arrows #5 to #7). Right atrial activation proceeds inferiorly, behind the eustachian ridge and coronary sinus ostium (A_{far}, Inf ToK electrogram in the second complex in Figs. 59-7B and 59-11B) and superiorly behind the tendon of Todaro, creating the atrial potentials recorded in the His bundle electrogram.

Evidence for this pattern of activation during retrograde slow pathway conduction is supported by at least two observations. First, the coronary sinus myocardium forms an electrical connection between the triangle of Koch at the coronary sinus ostium and the left atrium.[37,38] Second, the eustachian valve and tendon of Todaro form a complete line of block[31,39] that may confine the retrograde slow pathway impulse within the triangle of Koch. This line of conduction block may account for the ability to dissociate the retrograde A_{SP} potential from right atrial activation (Fig. 59-12C) and also may account for the late timing of the anterograde A_{SP} potential during sinus rhythm. The A_{SP} potential during sinus rhythm, representing the timing of activation between the inferoseptal tricuspid annulus and the coronary sinus ostium, is recorded after activation in the proximal coronary sinus and long after atrial activation in the His bundle electrogram (see Figs. 59-7A and 59-11A), even though there is a relatively small distance between the electrodes recording the His bundle electrogram and the A_{SP} potential. It is likely that the atrial potential recorded in the His bundle electrogram is generated behind the tendon of Todaro (outside the triangle of Koch). Although the right atrial impulse propagates across the tendon of Todaro along the transitional cells forming the fast pathway, these cells may not be able to activate the atrial myocardium within the triangle of Koch[39] (Fig. 59-13, red arrows). The anterograde A_{SP} potential during sinus rhythm probably represents activation in the inferior-to-superior direction (based on the response to ablation as described below). The A_{SP} potential during sinus rhythm may result from activation of

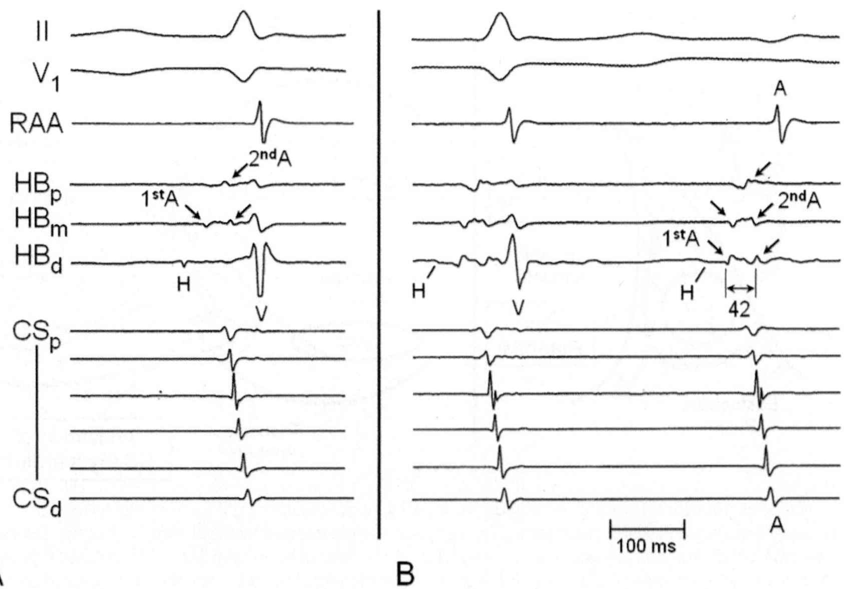

Figure 59-8 Two distinct sets of atrial potentials recorded in the proximal His bundle electrograms during Slow/Fast atrioventricular nodal reentrant tachycardia (AVNRT). **A,** The His bundle catheter was positioned to record the proximal His bundle potential from the distal pair of electrodes (HB_d electrogram). Two distinct sets of atrial potentials were recorded in the HB_m and HB_p electrograms. The first set of potentials originate posterior to the tendon of Todaro, outside the triangle of Koch (1st A). The second set (2nd A) are generated close to the tricuspid annulus, inside the triangle of Koch. **B,** The His bundle catheter was withdrawn proximally, such that only a tiny, far-field His bundle potential was recorded in the first complex (H). AV block occurred during the second complex, allowing clear identification of the two sets of atrial potentials in the absence of the ventricular potential. The first set of potentials (1st A) was activated in the distal-to-proximal direction (inferior-to-superior, *left arrows* in HB_d and HB_m electrograms). The second set of potentials (2nd A) propagated in the proximal to distal direction (superior-to-inferior, *right arrows* in HB_p to HB_d electrograms). The time between the first and second atrial potentials in HB_d was 42 ms. This delay supports the concept of conduction block across the eustachian ridge and tendon of Todaro.

the inferior aspect of the triangle of Koch either by the coronary sinus musculature, which is activated from the left atrium (see Fig. 59-13A), or by the crista terminalis (see Fig 59-13B).

The response to ablation provides strong evidence that the A_{SP} potential represents activation at the atrial connection of the slow pathway (rightward inferior extension of the AV node). Delivery of radiofrequency current to the inferior aspect of the triangle of Koch, between the tricuspid annulus and the coronary sinus ostium (at the level of the middle of the coronary sinus ostium or even lower), at a site recording a large, sharp A_{SP}

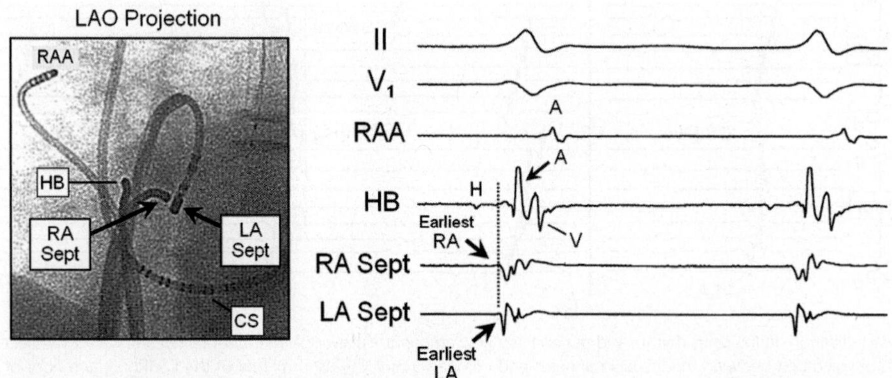

Figure 59-9 Recording earliest retrograde atrial activation on the right and left sides of the interatrial septum simultaneously during Slow/Fast atrioventricular nodal reentrant tachycardia (AVNRT). **Left,** The radiograph, in left anterior oblique (LAO) projection, shows two mapping catheters positioned to record earliest retrograde atrial activation from the right (RA Sept) and left (LA Sept) sides of the interatrial septum. The angle for the LAO projection was selected to be parallel with the His bundle catheter (HB). The catheter recording earliest right atrial activation (RA Sept) was positioned on the right atrial septum, leftward of the His bundle (HB) catheter (indicating a location posterior to the tendon of Todaro). Left atrial mapping was performed via a patent foramen ovale. Earliest left atrial activation was recorded on the septum (LA Sept), directly opposite the right atrial mapping catheter. **Right,** The right and left interatrial septum electrograms recorded during Slow/Fast AVNRT show nearly simultaneous onset of the downstroke of the bipolar atrial potentials (*arrows*, Earliest RA and Earliest LA). These potentials precede atrial activation in the His bundle electrogram (*arrow*, A) by more than 10 ms. The steeper downstroke in the LA Sept recording may suggest earlier activation at this side of the septum. H, His bundle potential; V, ventricular electrogram.

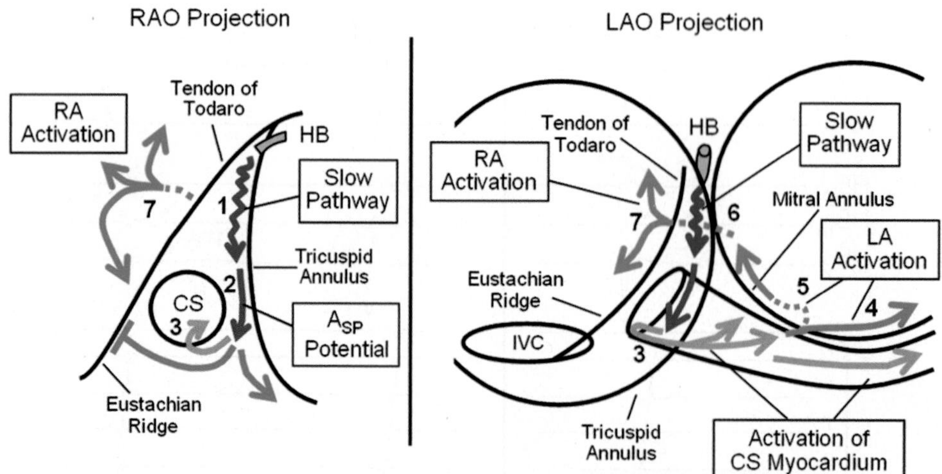

Figure 59-10 Postulated atrial activation sequence following retrograde slow pathway conduction (rightward inferior extension). Retrograde conduction over the rightward inferior extension (#1, *upper blue arrow*) activates the myocardium between the inferoseptal tricuspid annulus and the coronary sinus ostium to produce the retrograde A_{SP} potential (#2, *lower blue arrow*) and then activates the coronary sinus at the floor of the ostium (#3, *brown arrows*). Activation in the triangle of Koch does not cross the eustachian ridge to the right atrium (*perpendicular green line*) but proceeds leftward along the coronary sinus myocardium (*brown arrows* in LAO projection) to activate the left atrium. Left atrial activation propagates rapidly in the leftward direction (#4, solid green arrow in LAO projection) but first must reverse direction to propagate in the septal direction (#5, *dashed green line*). The reversal of direction produces late left atrial activation at the inferoseptal region and a second potential in proximal CS electrograms (recorded from the CS roof). This septal left atrial wavefront activates the interatrial septum (#6, *dashed green line*), which is followed by activation of the right atrium posterior to the tendon of Todaro and eustachian ridge (#7, *green arrows* in both projections). HB, His bundle; LAO, left anterior oblique; RAO, right anterior oblique.

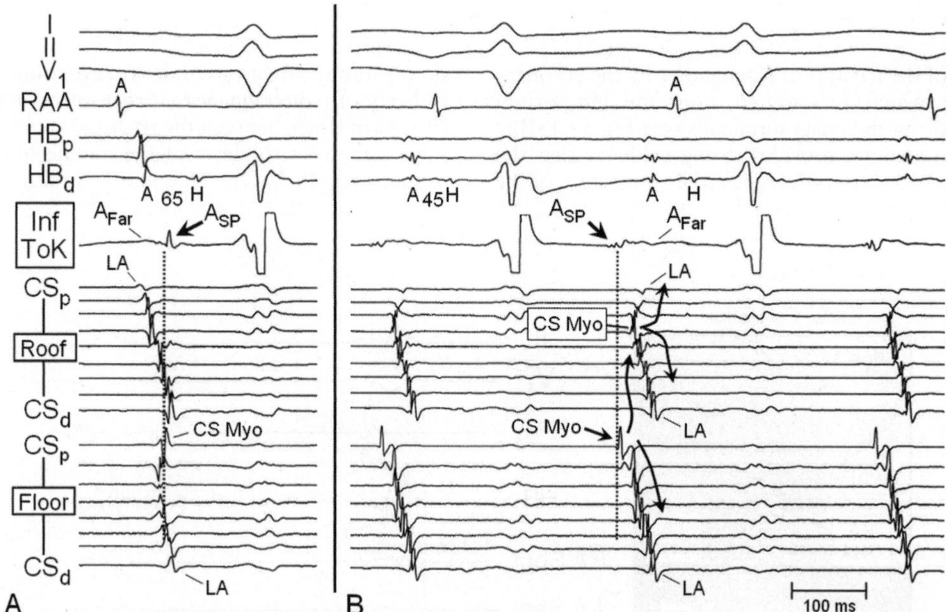

Figure 59-11 Pattern of atrial activation during sinus rhythm and during Fast/Slow atrioventricular nodal reentrant tachycardia (AVNRT). Electrograms recorded from the inferior triangle of Koch (Inf ToK, recorded between the tricuspid annulus and coronary sinus [CS] ostium), roof of the CS (Roof), and floor of the CS (Floor) during sinus rhythm and during Fast/Slow AVNRT. **A,** During sinus rhythm, atrial activation recorded at the inferior triangle of Koch (A_{SP} potential, *arrow*) is later than atrial activation in the His bundle electrograms and the roof of the proximal coronary sinus (*dotted vertical line*). **B,** During Fast/Slow AVNRT, earliest retrograde atrial activation (A_{SP}) is recorded at the Inf ToK region, followed by activation of the floor of the CS ostium (*dotted line, arrow*, CS myo in Floor CS_p electrogram). Activation propagates laterally along the CS myocardium (Floor CS_p to Floor CS_d), whereas the left atrium is activated by the CS myocardium (CS myo in the Roof CS electrograms, *curved arrows*). Left atrial activation (LA) then propagates septally and laterally (*curved arrows*). The late far-field potential (A_{Far}) following the A_{SP} potential in the Inf ToK electrograms is probably the recording of right atrial activation, posterior to the eustachian ridge, with timing similar to atrial activation recorded in the His bundle electrograms (**A**). We believe that this pattern of activation represents retrograde conduction over the rightward inferior extension of the AV node. Note that the atrial-His interval in the HBd electrogram is shorter during Fast/Slow AVNRT (45 ms) than during sinus rhythm (65 ms). (Modified from Jackman WM, Lockwood D, Nakagawa H, et al: Catheter ablation of atrioventricular nodal reentrant tachycardia. In Wilber DJ, Packer DL, Stevenson WG [eds]: Catheter Ablation of Cardiac Arrhythmias: Basic Concepts and Clinical Applications, 3rd ed. Blackwell Futura, 2008, pp 120-148.)

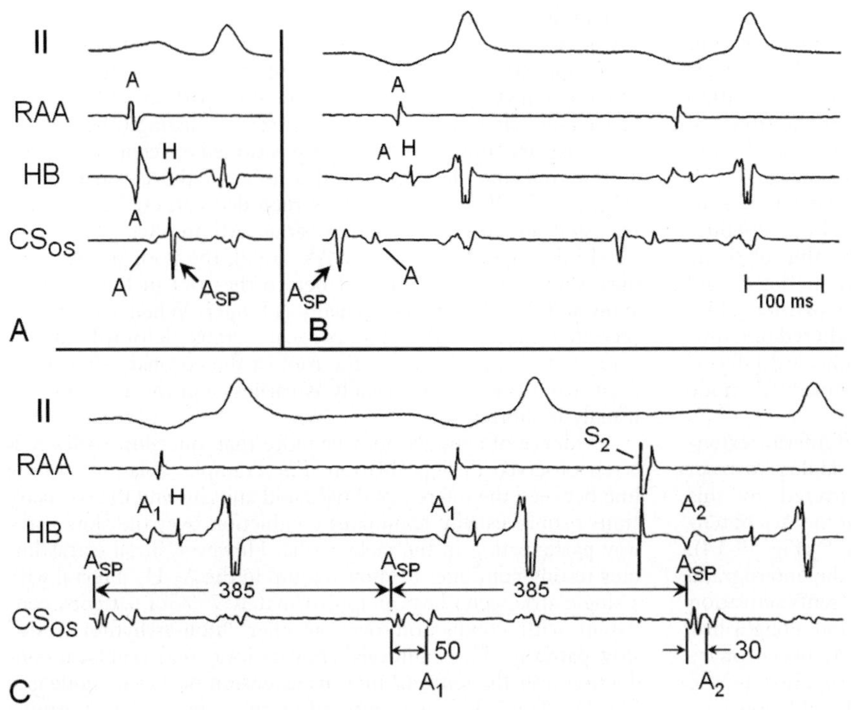

Figure 59-12 Dissociation of the retrograde A_{SP} potential from right atrial activation. **A,** During sinus rhythm, a large sharp A_{SP} potential is recorded just outside the coronary sinus ostium (CS_{OS} electrogram), 40 ms after the timing of atrial activation in the His bundle electrogram (A in HB electrogram). **B,** Fast/Slow AVNRT, cycle length 385 ms, showing the A_{SP} potential preceding right atrial activation. **C,** An atrial extrastimulus delivered to the right atrial appendage (S_2 in RAA electrogram) advances atrial activation outside the triangle of Koch (A_2) by 46 ms in the HB electrogram and by 20 ms in the CS_{OS} electrogram ($A_{SP} - A_2 = 30$ ms, compared with $A_{SP} - A_1 = 50$ ms) without altering the timing or morphology of the A_{SP} potential inside the triangle of Koch. The failure to advance the A_{SP} potential suggests right atrial activation was blocked from entering the triangle of Koch.

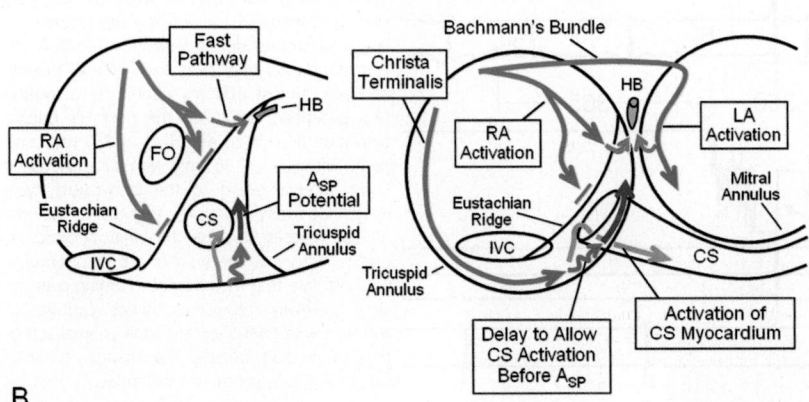

Figure 59-13 Schematic representation of two possible patterns of activation during sinus rhythm that may explain the late A_{SP} potential in the triangle of Koch. **A,** Postulate #1: Right atrial (RA) activation does not penetrate the triangle of Koch owing to conduction block across the eustachian ridge (*green arrows* and *short perpendicular green lines*). The left atrium is activated rapidly over Bachmann's bundle (*horizontal green arrow* in LAO projection). Left atrial (LA) activation proceeds inferiorly and laterally (*green arrows* in LAO projection), activating the CS myocardium (*brown arrows*). CS myocardial activation propagates in the septal direction along the CS myocardium to the CS ostium (*brown arrows*) and activates the inferior region of the triangle of Koch between the CS ostium and tricuspid annulus to generate the late A_{SP} potential (*blue arrows*). **B,** Postulate #2: Septal right atrial (RA) activation does not cross the eustachian ridge to activate the triangle of Koch (similar to Postulate #1). Activation inferiorly along the crista terminalis activates the region between the tricuspid annulus and eustachian ridge (sub-eustachian isthmus, *long green arrow* in LAO prejection). Continued right atrial activation in the septal direction (*short squiggly green arrows*) activates the inferior region of the triangle of Koch to generate the late A_{SP} potential (*blue arrows*) and the CS ostium (*brown arrows*). This postulate does not easily explain the usual finding that the A_{SP} potential is later than activation at the roof of the proximal CS during sinus rhythm. CS, coronary sinus; FO, fossa ovalis; HB, His bundle; IVC, inferior vena cava; LAO, left anterior oblique; RAO, right anterior oblique.

potential (on the unipolar electrogram), results in an immediate accelerated junctional rhythm with retrograde conduction over the fast pathway.[40] In some patients, the junctional rhythm is preceded by one to three atrial extrasystoles with an activation pattern consistent with retrograde activation over the slow AV nodal pathway. The occurrence of accelerated junctional rhythm during the radiofrequency application usually is associated with modification or elimination of anterograde and retrograde slow pathway conduction, without depressing fast pathway conduction.[2,3] The junctional automaticity indicates heating of tissue connected to the slow pathway. Histologic studies in dogs[41] and in a patient with AVNRT[42] who underwent slow pathway ablation showed that the radiofrequency lesions that altered or eliminated slow pathway conduction involved the rightward inferior extension of the AV node, while leaving the compact AV node intact.

Further evidence for the role of the rightward inferior extension of the AV node as a slow pathway is the ability to reset Slow/Fast AVNRT by an extrastimulus delivered to this region long after local atrial activation (including the A_{SP} potential), indicating direct capture of the slow pathway[18] (Fig. 59-14).

The response to ablation also suggests that the anterograde A_{SP} potential recorded during sinus rhythm represents activation in the inferior-to-superior direction. After ablation along a line between the inferoseptal tricuspid annulus and the coronary sinus ostium, the A_{SP} potential is eliminated superior to the ablation site, but remains present inferior to the ablation site. If radiofrequency current is then applied superior to the initial ablation line, junctional rhythm results (slow pathway automaticity), whereas if radiofrequency current is applied inferior to the ablation line, junctional rhythm usually does not occur. These observations are in contrast to the hypothesis that the A_{SP} potential results from anisotropic propagation across the triangle of Koch in the posterior to-anterior direction, perpendicular to the longitudinal direction of the fibers.[39]

Strong evidence indicates that the slow AV nodal pathway is not a single entity. Patients with multiple, abrupt increases of 50 ms or more ("jumps") in the A_2-H_2 interval during atrial extrastimulus testing have long been recognized.[43] In some patients, programmed ventricular stimulation demonstrates two distinct retrograde atrial activation sequences with different His bundle activation–atrial activation (H-A) intervals, representing retrograde conduction over two separate slow pathways.[44] The two retrograde slow pathways can best be distinguished using two coronary sinus catheters, one positioned to record activation at the roof and the other at the floor of the coronary sinus (Fig. 59-15). When activation is recorded earliest between the tricuspid annulus and coronary sinus ostium (A_{SP} site—rightward inferior extension of the AV node), the floor of the coronary sinus ostium is activated before the roof of the coronary sinus and the H-A interval usually is longer. When activation is recorded earlier within the coronary sinus (leftward inferior extension of the AV node), the roof of the coronary sinus (1 to 3 cm from the ostium) usually is earliest and the H-A interval usually is shorter.[44]

Evidence of conduction over more than one slow pathway is often observed during ablation. For example, ablation along a line between the inferoseptal tricuspid annulus and the coronary sinus ostium usually eliminates conduction over the slow pathway participating in the tachycardia. However, atrial extrastimulus testing continues to show a jump in the A_2-H_2 interval with a single atrial echo beat in approximately 75% of patients, consistent with conduction over another "non-arrhythmogenic" slow pathway. This additional slow pathway may represent conduction over the leftward inferior extension of the AV node (see Fig. 59-1).[34,36] This is supported by mapping studies in canine and rabbit hearts, showing that this additional "slow pathway" enters the region of the triangle of Koch superior to the coronary sinus ostium.[22,45]

The superior and inferior atrial inputs to the AV node, which form the fast pathway and slow pathways, respectively, are present in normal hearts.[24,34,36] This observation suggests that conduction over the fast pathway and slow pathways (dual-pathway physiology) should be demonstrable in most people. In a series of 200 consecutive patients who underwent radiofrequency catheter ablation of an accessory pathway (without a history of AVNRT or inducible AVNRT during the procedure), evidence of dual-pathway physiology in either the anterograde or

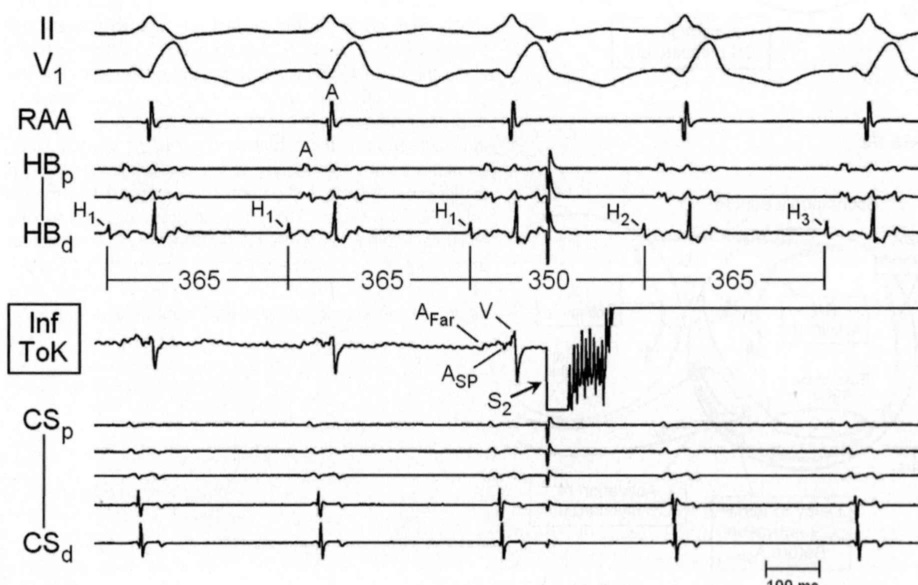

Figure 59-14 Resetting of Slow/Fast atrioventricular nodal reentrant tachycardia (AVNRT) by an extrastimulus delivered at the inferior triangle of Koch after local atrial activation, suggesting direct capture of the rightward inferior extension. The mapping catheter (Inf ToK) is positioned in the inferior triangle of Koch, between the coronary sinus and tricuspid annulus at a site recording a late A_{SP} potential during Slow/Fast AVNRT. A late extrastimulus (S_2) delivered to the inferior triangle of Koch, almost 100 ms after local activation (A_{SP} potential), advanced the next His bundle activation (H_2) by 15 ms (H_1-H_2 = 350 ms, compared with H_1-H_1 = 365 ms), with the subsequent H_2-H_3 interval equal to the tachycardia cycle length (365 ms), confirming that the tachycardia has been reset. Because the atrial myocardium was refractory at the time of the extrastimulus, we postulate that the advance in timing over the slow pathway represents direct capture of the rightward inferior extension. A_{Far}, atrial activation originating outside the triangle of Koch (i.e., far-field); V, ventricular potential.

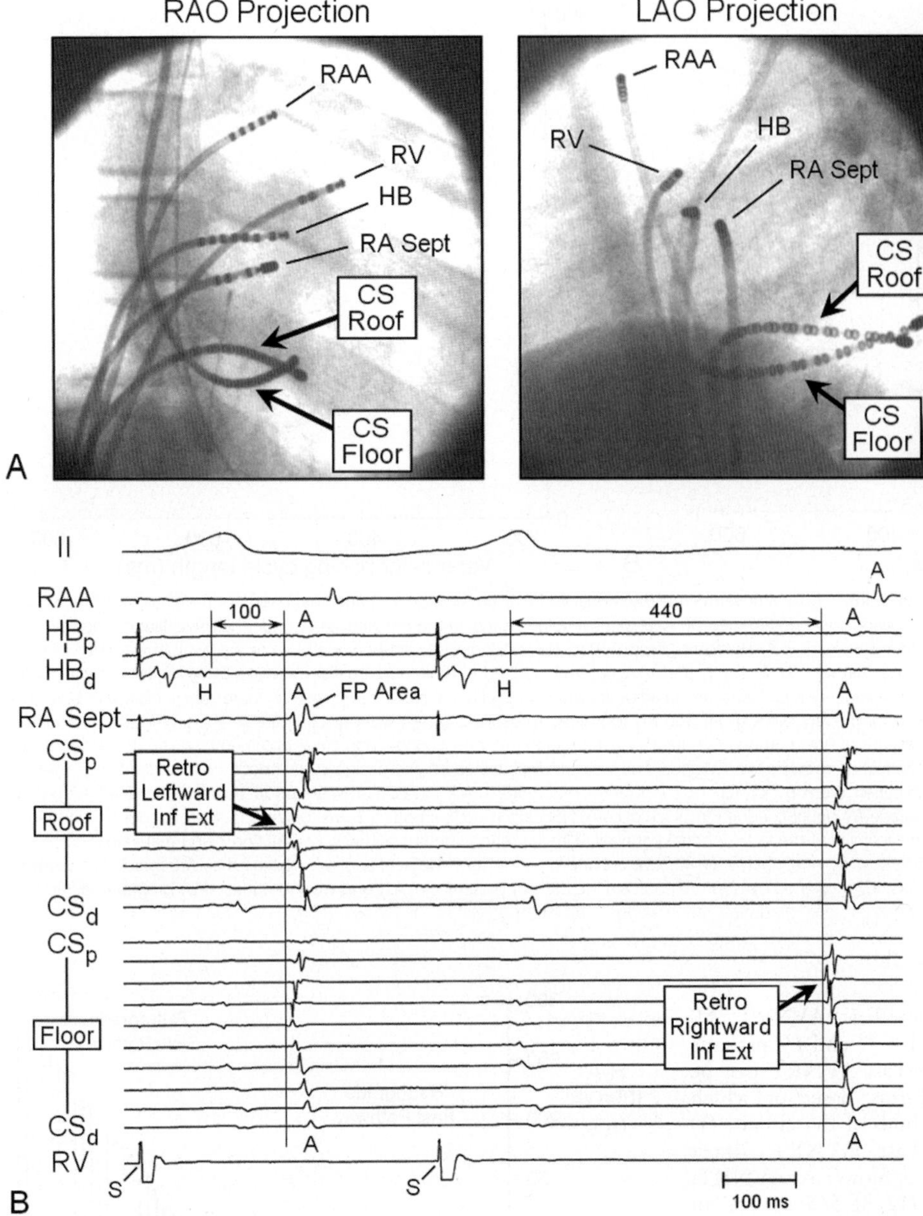

Figure 59-15 Two distinct retrograde atrial activation sequences following retrograde conduction over two different slow atrioventricular (AV) nodal pathways. **A,** Radiographs in the RAO and LAO projections show the catheter positions. Two catheters are positioned in the coronary sinus (CS): one inserted by way of the right subclavian vein and positioned along the floor of the CS and one inserted by way of the right femoral vein and positioned along the roof of the CS. A mapping catheter (RA Sept) is positioned on the right atrial septum, posterior to the tendon of Todaro where earliest right atrial activation had been previously recorded during retrograde fast pathway conduction. **B,** Electrograms recorded after two paced ventricular complexes. Retrograde atrial activation following the first ventricular complex has a His-atrial (H-A) interval of 100 ms, measured from the end of the retrograde His bundle potential to earliest atrial activation which was recorded from the roof of the CS (*arrow* in Roof CS electrograms), approximately 3 cm from the CS ostium consistent with retrograde activation over the leftward inferior extension (Retro Leftward Inf Ext). Activation of the right atrial septum (RA Sept) in the fast pathway area (FP area) is recorded later, excluding retrograde conduction over the fast pathway. Atrial activation following the second ventricular complex has a longer H-A interval (440 ms) and different retrograde atrial activation sequence. Earliest CS activation was recorded at the floor of the CS ostium (*arrow* in Floor CS electrograms). This pattern may represent retrograde conduction over the rightward inferior extension of the AV node (Retro Rightward Inf Ext). HB, His bundle; LAO, left anterior oblique; RAO, right anterior oblique.

retrograde direction was present in 168 (84%).[14,15] The ability to demonstrate dual-pathway physiology in a high percentage of patients probably was related to heavy sedation or general anesthesia, which depressed anterograde and retrograde fast pathway conduction, allowing the demonstration of slow pathway conduction. Small doses of isoproterenol (0.25 to 0.5 μg/min) enhanced fast pathway conduction to a greater extent than slow pathway conduction, often completely obscuring anterograde and retrograde slow pathway conduction (Fig. 59-16). These low doses of isoproterenol in heavily sedated or anesthetized patients probably have effects that mimic normal resting sympathetic tone, which explains the low incidence of dual-pathway physiology observed previously in non-sedated patients without AVNRT.[12] Other possible reasons for the low incidence of anterograde dual-pathway physiology (jump in A_2-H_2 interval) are a similar conduction time over the fast and slow pathways just before block in the fast pathway[46] and conduction over an intermediate pathway (possibly the leftward inferior extension of the AV node).[24] In most patients, however, A-H or A_2-H_2 intervals greater than 200 ms correspond to anterograde conduction over the slow AV nodal pathway.[14]

A smooth transition from fast pathway conduction to slow pathway conduction may also be seen in the retrograde direction. Significant overlap is seen in H-A interval for the fast and slow pathways in some patients (Fig. 59-17).[15] Therefore, no specific value of H-A interval identifies retrograde slow pathway conduction. However, the transition from retrograde fast pathway conduction to retrograde slow pathway conduction is easy to recognize because of the shift in retrograde atrial activation sequence (see Fig. 59-7).

At least five distinct forms of AVNRT can be identified. In our experience with 734 patients referred for catheter ablation of

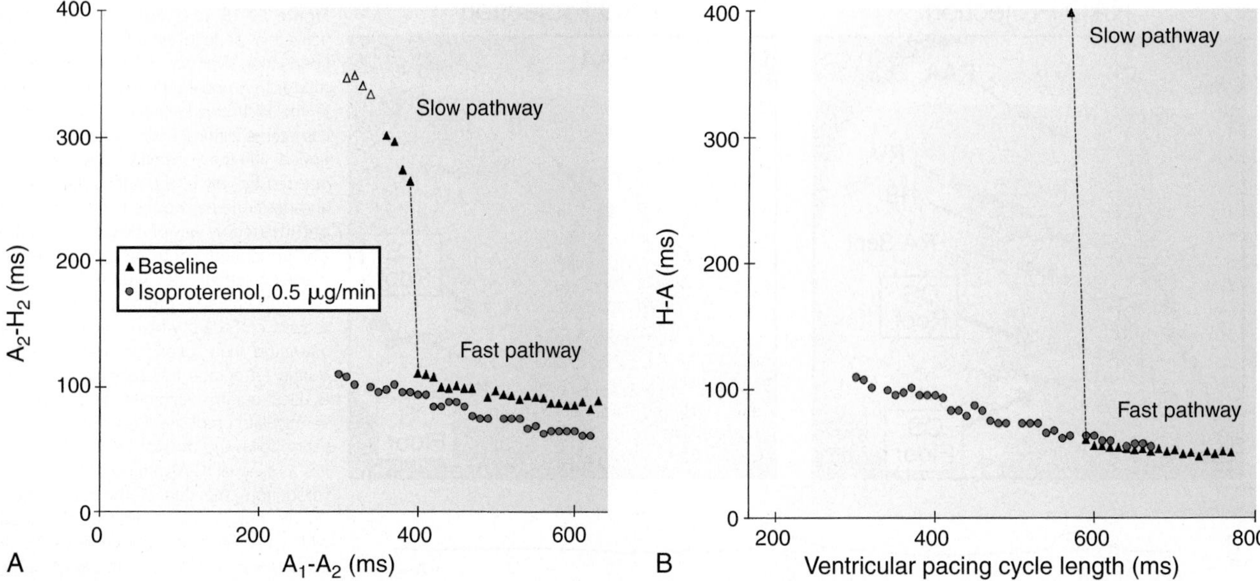

Figure 59-16 Effects of low-dose isoproterenol (0.5 μg/min) on dual–atrioventricular (AV) nodal pathway physiology in a patient who did not have atrioventricular nodal reentrant tachycardia (AVNRT). **A,** AV nodal refractory period curve determined by atrial extrastimulus testing. In the baseline state (under heavy sedation), shortening of the A_1-A_2 interval from 400 to 390 ms resulted in a 155-ms increase in A_2-H_2 interval (from 110 to 265 ms), indicating anterograde block in the fast pathway with selective conduction over the slow AV nodal pathway *(triangles)*. Further shortening of the A_1-A_2 interval resulted in additional smaller increases in A_2-H_2 interval with single reentrant atrial echo complexes (slow pathway anterograde–fast pathway retrograde) occurring at A_2-H_2 intervals of 335 ms or more *(open triangles)*. Low-dose isoproterenol shortened the effective refractory period of the fast pathway by 100 ms (from 390 to 290 ms, *circles*) without comparable shortening of the refractory period of the slow pathway, totally obscuring the presence of slow pathway conduction. **B,** Retrograde AV nodal conduction curve obtained by decremental ventricular pacing. In the baseline state *(triangles)*, retrograde conduction over the fast AV nodal pathway was maintained only to pacing cycle length 590 ms. At pacing cycle 580 ms, a 335-ms increase in His-atrial (H-A) interval occurred (from 65 to 400 ms), indicating retrograde block in fast pathway conduction with selective retrograde conduction over the slow AV nodal pathway. Retrograde AV nodal conduction block occurred at pacing cycle length 570 ms. Low-dose isoproterenol administration *(circles)* greatly enhanced the retrograde conduction capability of the fast AV nodal pathway, with 1:1 retrograde fast pathway conduction being maintained to pacing cycle length 300 ms. Retrograde conduction over the slow AV nodal pathway was not enhanced to the same degree, and was obscured by retrograde fast pathway conduction. Note that the H-A interval was not significantly shortened by isoproterenol. AVNRT was not present clinically and was not induced by programmed atrial or ventricular stimulation, in the baseline state, or during isoproterenol administration at doses up to 4 μg/min.

AVNRT, 515 patients (77%) had Slow/Fast AVNRT, 80 patients (11%) had Slow/Slow AVNRT,[47,48] and 89 patients (12%) had Fast/Slow AVNRT.[4,48] Slow/Fast AVNRT can be further subdivided into at least three forms, based on which slow pathway provides the anterograde limb of the circuit: (1) Rightward Inferior Extension Slow/Fast AVNRT (most common); (2) Leftward Inferior Extension Slow/Fast AVNRT; and (3) left atrial Slow/Fast AVNRT (12 of 565 or 2% of patients with Slow/Fast AVNRT).

Slow/Fast Atrioventricular Nodal Reentrant Tachycardia

Rightward Inferior Extension Slow/Fast Atrioventricular Nodal Reentrant Tachycardia

Slow/Fast AVNRT, also referred to as "common type" or "typical" AVNRT, is thought to use the slow AV nodal pathway (usually the rightward inferior extension of the AV node) for anterograde conduction and the fast AV nodal pathway for retrograde conduction. The induction of this form of AVNRT by programmed atrial stimulation typically occurs with an abrupt (greater than 50 ms) increase in the A-H interval, suggesting that anterograde conduction occurs over the slow pathway.[13] In some patients, however, the induction of tachycardia may occur after a smooth increase in the A-H interval (without a "jump") because of similar conduction times over the two pathways at the time of

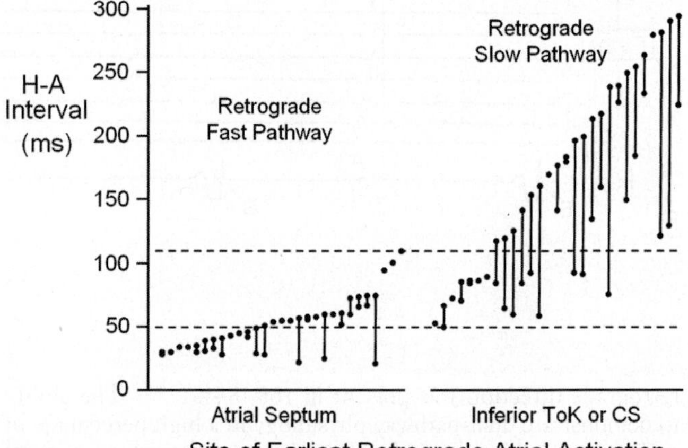

Figure 59-17 Overlap in His-atrial (H-A) intervals during retrograde conduction over fast and slow atrioventricular (AV) nodal pathways. H-A intervals were measured during decremental ventricular pacing in 29 patients demonstrating retrograde conduction over both fast and slow AV nodal pathways. Retrograde conduction was considered to be over the fast pathway when earliest activation was recorded at the interatrial septum (behind the tendon of Todaro) and over a slow pathway when earliest retrograde conduction was recorded at the inferior triangle of Koch or in the coronary sinus. The shortest and longest H-A interval for each patient over each pathway is represented by two *vertical dots* connected by a *vertical line*. Significant overlap between patterns in H-A intervals over the fast and slow pathways is evident. When the H-A interval was between 50 and 110 ms (*horizontal dashed lines*), retrograde conduction could be over either fast or slow pathway, showing that the H-A interval alone cannot be used to distinguish between the two.

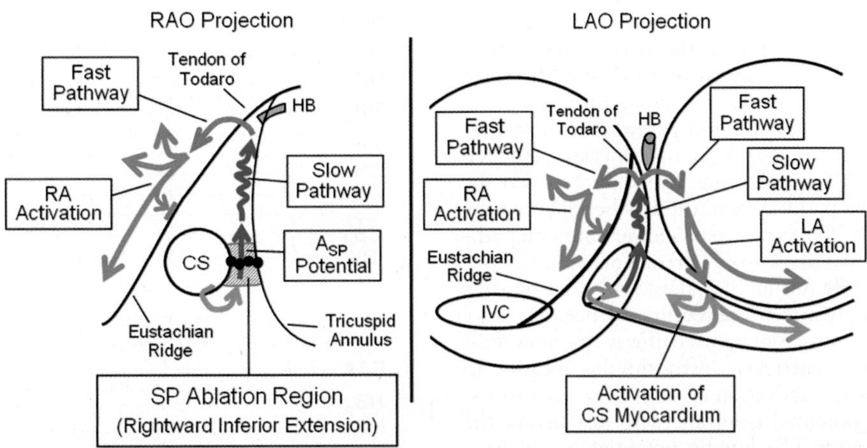

Figure 59-18 Schematic representation of the circuit and ablation sites for Slow/Fast atrioventricular nodal reentrant tachycardia (AVNRT) using the rightward inferior extension of the atrioventricular (AV) node for the anterograde slow pathway. The right (RA) and left (LA) atrial activation pattern (*red* and *green arrows*) is the same as that in Figure 59-5. The coronary sinus (CS) myocardium (*brown arrows*) activates the floor of the CS ostium, followed by activation of the inferior triangle of Koch, generating the A_{SP} potential (*blue line*) and then conducting in the anterograde direction over the rightward inferior extension (*squiggly blue arrow*, slow pathway). Ablation between the inferoseptal tricuspid annulus and the anterior (apical) margin of the coronary sinus ostium (*red striped area* and *black dots*) interrupts anterograde conduction over the rightward inferior extension and eliminates Rightward Inferior Extension Slow/Fast AVNRT. HB, His bundle; IVC, inferior vena cava; LAO, left anterior oblique; RAO, right anterior oblique.

transition.[13,46] The A-H interval during Slow/Fast AVNRT is relatively long (usually more than 200 ms) and, in our experience, has been as long as 550 ms (median, 290 ms). The H-A interval measured in the His bundle electrogram is relatively short, usually 25 to 90 ms (median, 50 ms). Mapping of the right atrium and coronary sinus differentiates this tachycardia from Slow/Slow AVNRT by recording earliest retrograde atrial activation behind the tendon of Todaro, outside the triangle of Koch. In the left anterior oblique projection the tip of the mapping catheter (recording earliest activation during retrograde fast pathway activation) is oriented leftward of the His bundle catheter (see Figs. 59-3 and 59-4).

The short H-A interval during Slow/Fast AVNRT usually results in superimposition of the P wave onto the QRS complex in the electrocardiogram, obscuring most of the P wave. However, the terminal portion of the P wave may be distinguishable at the end of the QRS complex, producing a characteristic late positive component in lead V_1 (pseudo-r′) or negative component in the inferior leads (pseudo-S wave).

The distance between the atrial connections of the fast and slow pathways suggests that the reentrant circuit in Slow/Fast AVNRT may contain a relatively large atrial component, in which the re-entrant impulse propagates from the atrial end of the fast pathway to the atrial end of the slow pathway. One technique that can be used to identify parts of the atria close to (or involved in) the reentrant circuit is resetting by an atrial extrastimulus. The extrastimulus must be delivered sufficiently late to prevent the paced atrial impulse from reaching the site of earliest atrial activation before retrograde activation of this area by the fast pathway.[8,10,17] If an atrial site is located close to or within the atrial component of the reentrant circuit, a late atrial extrastimulus delivered to that site should advance the timing of the next His bundle potential and reset the tachycardia. In theory, at sites within the reentrant circuit, the postpacing interval (extrastimulus to next local atrial potential) should closely approximate the tachycardia cycle length. However, additional delay of the paced impulse within the AV node may lead to a lengthening of the postpacing interval (greater than the tachycardia cycle length) at pacing sites within the circuit, making it difficult to differentiate between sites within and near the reentrant circuit. Sites of resetting with shortest postpacing intervals include the inferior triangle of Koch between the tricuspid annulus and the coronary sinus ostium at sites generating the A_{SP} potential (see Fig. 59-14) and the proximal coronary sinus (1 to 2 cm from the ostium).[8,10,17] Conversely, atrial extrastimuli delivered behind the eustachian ridge, at the level of the middle of the coronary sinus ostium, fail to reset the tachycardia without first advancing the timing of the atrial potential in the His bundle electrogram, dissociating this region from the re-entrant circuit.[17] These observations, combined with the timing of activation (earliest outside and latest inside the triangle of Koch; see Figs. 59-3 and 59-6 to 59-9) suggest the hypothesis for the reentrant circuit in Slow/Fast AVNRT shown in Figure 59-18. In this hypothesis, retrograde activation over the fast pathway activates both the right and left sides of the interatrial septum, but it is only the left-sided activation that participates in the reentrant circuit. Propagation from the left side of the interatrial septum activates the coronary sinus myocardium, approximately 1 to 3 cm from the ostium. The reentrant impulse propagates along the coronary sinus myocardium to the coronary sinus ostium. Activation at the floor of the coronary sinus ostium activates fibers which connect with the rightward inferior extension of the AV node, initiating propagation along the slow pathway. One study[49] reported that earliest coronary sinus activation during Slow/Fast AVNRT was recorded distal to the coronary sinus ostium in 47% of patients studied, confirming that, at least in this subgroup, the coronary sinus myocardium is activated from the left atrium.

The traditional hypothesis, in which the reentrant circuit is confined within the triangle of Koch, does not explain the ability to reset the tachycardia by late atrial extrastimuli delivered to the coronary sinus or successful ablation of the atrial connection to the slow pathway by radiofrequency current delivered between the tricuspid annulus and the coronary sinus ostium.

The distal junction of the fast and slow pathways in Slow/Fast AVNRT has traditionally been considered to be located in the AV node, with a region of AV nodal tissue extending between the distal junction of the two pathways and the His bundle (i.e., the lower common pathway). The presence of a lower common pathway comprised of AV nodal tissue would predict occasional block proximal to the His bundle during Slow/Fast AVNRT, but this phenomenon is exceedingly rare. More recent evidence suggests a very short or minimal lower common pathway in Slow/Fast AVNRT.[47,50-55] A late ventricular extrastimulus begins to advance the timing of atrial activation as soon as the *end* of the retrograde His bundle potential is advanced to just before the time when the anterograde His bundle potential would have begun without the extrastimulus[52] (Fig. 59-19). A linear relationship generally exists between the degree of advance in timing of the retrograde His bundle potential (H_1-H_2 interval) and the advance in timing of atrial activation (A_1-A_2 interval; see Fig. 59-19C), suggesting relatively little decremental conduction in the lower common pathway and the retrograde fast pathway.

Similar evidence of minimal lower common pathway is obtained by comparing the H-A intervals during Slow/Fast AVNRT and during ventricular pacing at the same cycle length. The H-A interval during tachycardia should be equal to the conduction time over the retrograde fast pathway *minus* the anterograde conduction time over the lower common pathway (from the distal junction of the two pathways to the His bundle) (Fig. 59-20). The H-A interval during ventricular pacing, measured from the end of the retrograde His bundle potential to the onset of atrial activation, should be equal to the retrograde conduction time over the fast pathway *plus* the retrograde conduction time over the lower common pathway (from the His bundle to the fast pathway). Given the assumption that the retrograde fast pathway is the same anatomically during tachycardia and during ventricular pacing and has the same retrograde conduction time, then subtracting the H-A interval during tachycardia from the H-A interval during ventricular pacing would equal the sum of the anterograde and retrograde conduction times over the lower common pathway (see Fig. 59-20).[54-57] Of importance, the most proximal His bundle potential must be recorded, because recording more distally will erroneously increase the H-A interval during ventricular pacing and shorten the H-A interval during tachycardia (Fig. 59-21), incorrectly suggesting a longer lower common pathway. To record the end of the most proximal retrograde His bundle potential, ventricular pacing must be performed at a site that separates the activation times of the His bundle and the local ventricular myocardium. This can be accomplished by pacing at the superior basal right ventricular septum, very close to the proximal right bundle branch, but not capturing the proximal right bundle branch (para-Hisian pacing).[53] This results in retrograde activation of the His bundle long after completion of the local ventricular potential (see Figs. 59-7 and 59-21). The most accurate comparison is obtained when a sustained episode of Slow/Fast AVNRT (greater than 3 minutes) is terminated by a 3- to 4-beat burst of rapid atrial pacing, and ventricular pacing at the tachycardia cycle length is initiated immediately after termination of the tachycardia (Fig. 59-22). This technique minimizes any change in autonomic tone between pacing and tachycardia.

Using this methodology, the H-A interval during pacing (measured from the *end* of the retrograde His bundle potential) is a mean of 9 ms *shorter* than the H-A interval during Slow/Fast AVNRT (Figs. 59-23A and 59-24).[54-56] This seemingly paradoxical finding (H-A interval longer during tachycardia than during ventricular pacing), implying minimal lower common pathway in Slow/Fast AVNRT, has several possible explanations. One is that the retrograde fast pathway arises from the His bundle (i.e., no

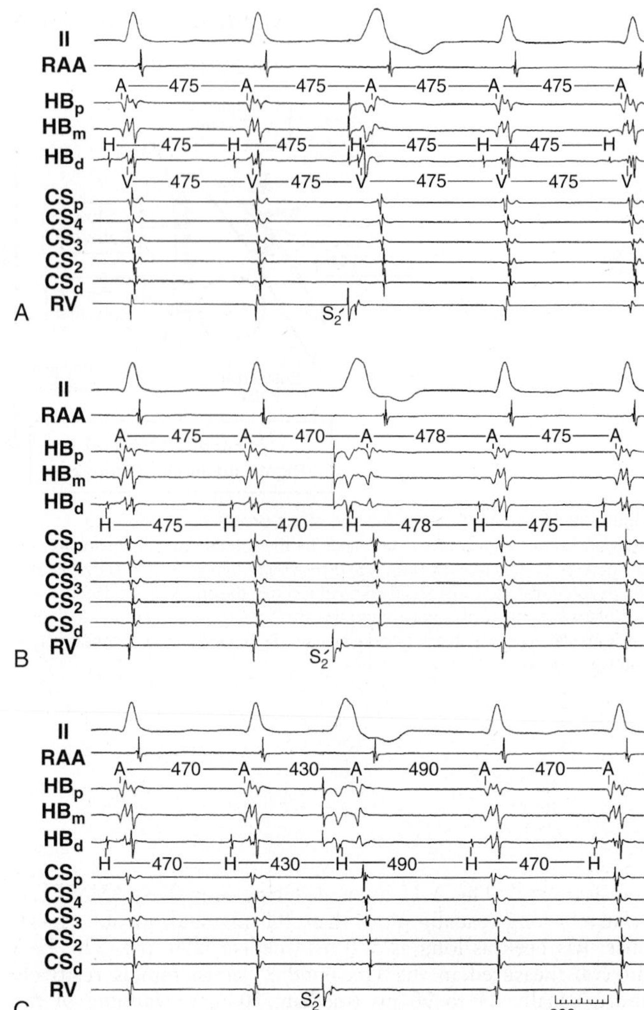

Figure 59-19 Use of ventricular extrastimuli to verify the diagnosis of Slow/Fast atrioventricular nodal reentrant tachycardia (AVNRT). **A,** During tachycardia, a single extrastimulus (S_2) was delivered to the superior-basal right ventricular septum (para-Hisian region), close to the site of earliest atrial activation. This advanced the timing of ventricular activation in the electrograms recording earliest atrial activation (His bundle [HB] electrograms) by 60 ms (V-V = 415 ms, compared with 475 ms). S_2 did not advance the timing of His bundle activation (H) or the timing of retrograde atrial activation (A-A interval remained 475 ms). This indicates that atrial activation during tachycardia is independent of the timing of local ventricular activation, excluding retrograde conduction over an accessory pathway and orthodromic AV reentrant tachycardia. **B,** Earlier ventricular extrastimulus (S_2) resulted in retrograde activation of the His bundle. The end of the retrograde His bundle potential occurred 5 ms before anterograde His bundle activation would have occurred (H-H = 470 ms, compared with 475 ms). This was associated with a 5 ms advance in the timing of the retrograde atrial activation (A-A = 470 ms, compared with 475 ms) without a change in the atrial activation sequence, indicating that atrial activation was dependent on retrograde His bundle activation, excluding an atrial tachycardia and confirming the diagnosis of AVNRT. **C,** Further shortening of the extrastimulus coupling interval resulted in earlier retrograde activation of the His bundle. This was associated with an identical advance in the timing of retrograde atrial activation (H-H = A-A = 430 ms). RAA, right atrial appendage; RV, right ventricle.

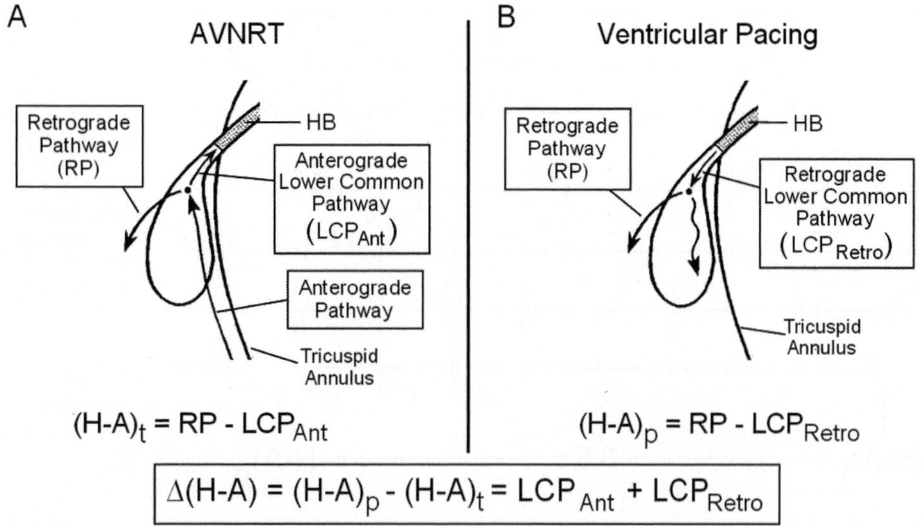

Figure 59-20 Schematic representation of measurements used to estimate the combined anterograde and retrograde conduction time over the lower common pathway during atrioventricular nodal reentrant tachycardia (AVNRT), by comparing the His-atrial (H-A) interval during AVNRT and during ventricular pacing at the same cycle length. **A,** The H-A interval during tachycardia, $(H\text{-}A)_t$, measured from the onset of the most proximal His bundle (HB) potential to the onset of retrograde atrial activation, is comprised of the conduction time over the retrograde pathway (RP) minus the anterograde conduction time over the lower common pathway (LCP_{Ant}). **B,** The H-A interval during ventricular pacing, $(H\text{-}A)_p$, measured from the end of the most proximal His bundle potential to the onset of atrial activation, is comprised of the conduction time over the retrograde pathway (RP) plus the retrograde conduction time over the lower common pathway (LCP_{Retro}). Assuming the retrograde pathway is the same anatomically and has the same conduction time during tachycardia and during ventricular pacing, the difference in H-A interval Δ(H-A), i.e., subtracting $(H\text{-}A)_t$ from $(H\text{-}A)_P$, should be roughly equivalent to the combined anterograde and retrograde conduction times over the lower common pathway (LCP_{Ant} + LCP_{Retro}).

lower common pathway) (Fig.59-25A). This is unlikely, however, because histologic examination in a small number of explanted human hearts with documented dual-pathway physiology revealed no atrio-Hisian pathway, and no evident anatomic differences from "normal" hearts.[58] In addition, a histologic study of 687 autopsy hearts identified a true atrio-Hisian connection in only 2 (0.3%) hearts.[59] Because we now believe that dual–AV nodal pathway physiology results from the multiple atrial inputs into the AV node and is present in all hearts,[15] atrio-Hisian pathways would have to be present in a large number of people to explain dual-pathway physiology. Other possible explanations for a longer H-A interval during tachycardia than pacing include (1) the recording of activation of the AV bundle proximal to the central fibrous body (before the junction of the fast and slow

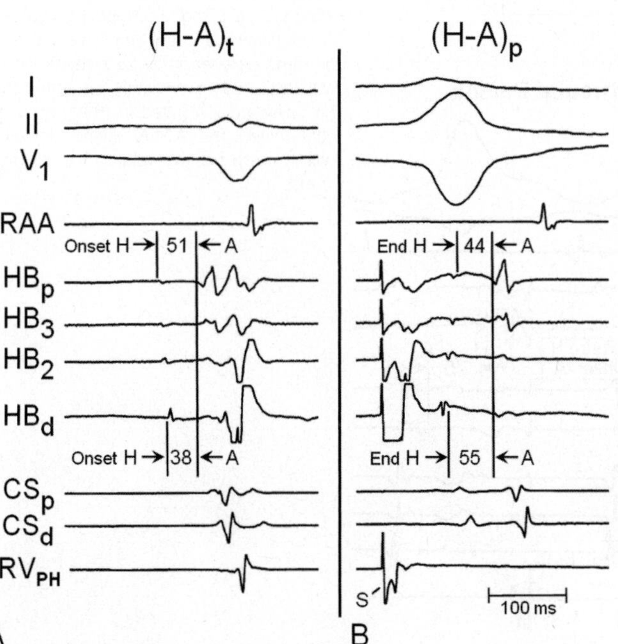

Figure 59-21 Differences in measurement technique greatly affect estimates of the conduction time over the lower common pathway. **A,** During Slow/Fast atrioventricular nodal reentrant tachycardia (AVNRT), the most proximal His bundle potential was recorded on the proximal His bundle electrogram (HB_P). His bundle and right bundle branch potentials are recorded at progressively later intervals on the HB_3, HB_2, and HB_d electrograms, respectively. $(H\text{-}A)_t$, measured from the onset of the most proximal His bundle potential (HB_P electrogram), is 51 ms. $(H\text{-}A)_t$, measured from the onset of the sharp His bundle or right bundle branch potential in the HB_d electrogram, is only 38 ms (13 ms less than HB_P). **B,** Right ventricular pacing from the para-Hisian region (S in RV_{PH} electrogram) at the same cycle length as the tachycardia. Note the separation of the His bundle (and right bundle branch) potentials from the local ventricular potential, allowing identification of the end of the His bundle potentials (H). $(H\text{-}A)_P$, measured from the end of the most proximal His bundle potential (HB_P electrogram) is only 44 ms. $(H\text{-}A)_P$, measured from the end of the sharp His bundle or right bundle branch in HB_d electrogram is 55 ms, 11 ms longer. Δ(H-A), $(H\text{-}A)_P - (H\text{-}A)_t$, measured from the most proximal His bundle potential, is a negative value, −7 ms (44 − 51 ms). Δ(H-A), measured incorrectly from the distal His bundle (or right bundle branch) potential, is a positive value, 17 ms (55 − 38 ms). This error, caused by recording too distally, results from an artificial shortening of $(H\text{-}A)_t$ and lengthening of $(H\text{-}A)_P$. In effect, this approach adds the His bundle (and proximal right bundle branch) to the lower common pathway.

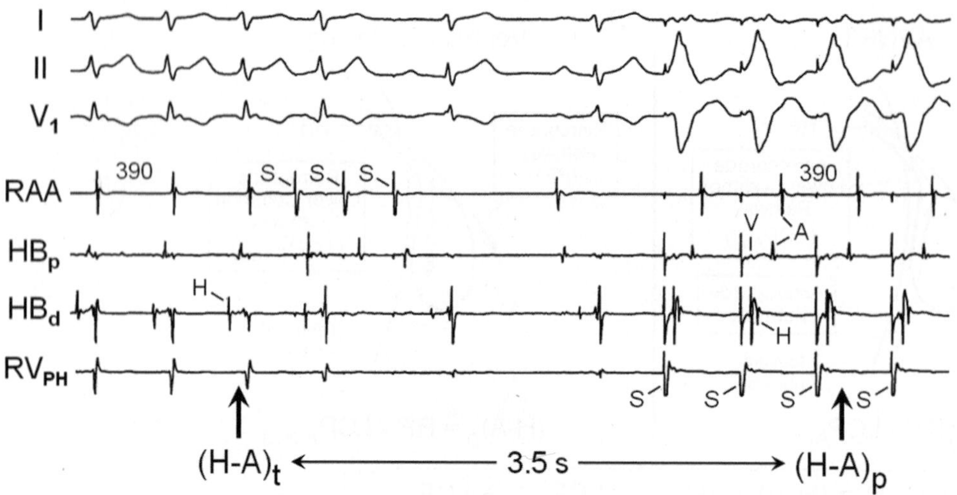

Figure 59-22 Technique for measuring His-atrial (H-A) intervals during atrioventricular nodal reentrant tachycardia and ventricular pacing under the same autonomic conditions. A sustained (stabilized) episode of tachycardia (greater than 3 minutes duration) is terminated by 3 to 4 beats of rapid atrial pacing (S, RAA electrogram) followed immediately by para-Hisian right ventricular pacing (S, RV_{PH} electrogram) at the tachycardia cycle length (390 ms). The H-A interval during tachycardia $(H\text{-}A)_t$ is measured just before termination *(first arrow)*, and the H-A interval during ventricular pacing $(H\text{-}A)_p$ is measured as soon as the interval stabilizes *(second arrow)*, only 3.5 seconds later, under the same autonomic conditions to allow accurate assessment of the lower common pathway.

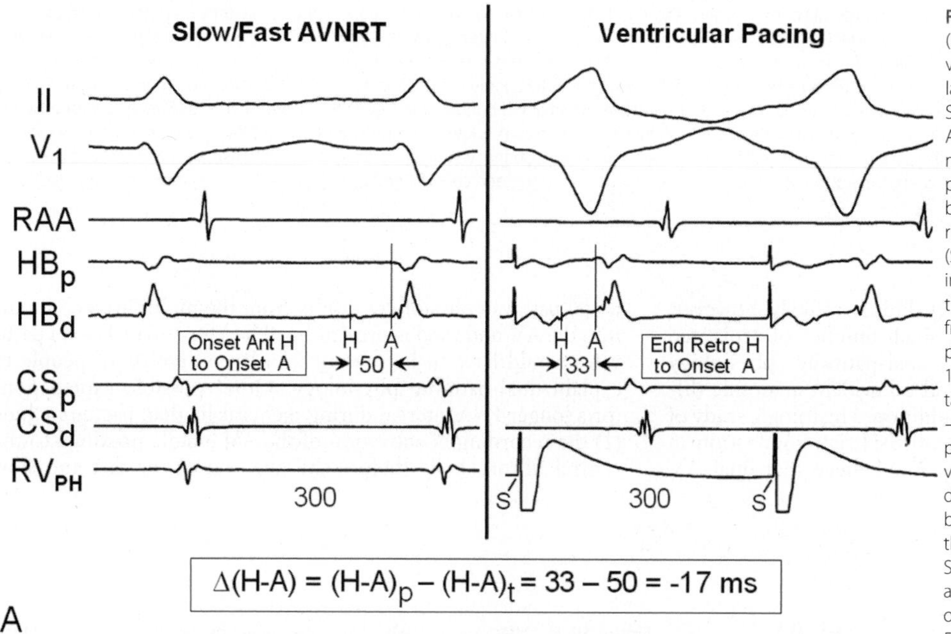

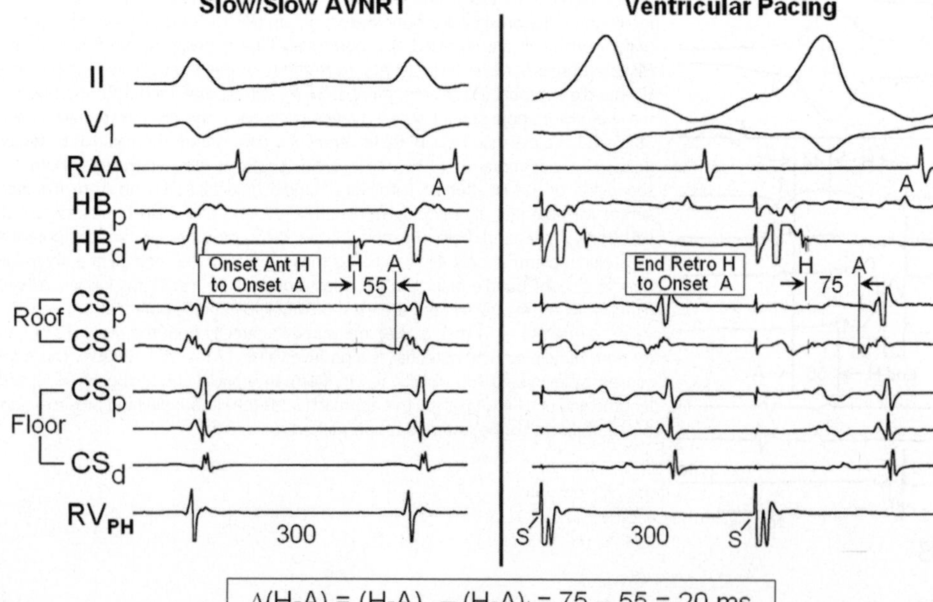

Figure 59-23 Comparison of the His-atrial (H-A) intervals during tachycardia and during ventricular pacing for Slow/Fast atrioventricular nodal reentrant tachycardia (AVNRT) and Slow/Slow AVNRT. **A,** During Slow/Fast AVNRT at cycle length 300 ms, $(H\text{-}A)_t$ was 50 ms, measured from the onset of the most proximal anterograde (Onset Ant H) His bundle (HB) potential *(left panel)*. Para-Hisian right ventricular pacing at cycle length 300 ms (S in RV_{PH} electrogram, *right panel*) was initiated immediately after termination of the tachycardia. The H-A interval measured from the end of the retrograde His bundle potential, (End Retro A) $(H\text{-}A)_p$, was 33 ms, 17 ms shorter than the H-A interval during tachycardia, resulting in a negative $\Delta(H\text{-}A)$ of −17 ms. Note that para-Hisian ventricular pacing resulted in very early ventricular activation in the His bundle electrogram and delayed retrograde activation of the His bundle, allowing identification of the end of the retrograde His bundle potential. **B,** During Slow/Slow AVNRT *(left panel)*, earliest atrial activation was recorded at the roof of the coronary sinus (CS Roof electrogram). $(H\text{-}A)_t$ was 55 ms. Para-Hisian right ventricular pacing at the same cycle length as for tachycardia (300 ms), instituted immediately on terminating the tachycardia, resulted in $(H\text{-}A)_p$ of 75 ms *(right panel)*. The $\Delta(H\text{-}A)$ during Slow/Slow AVNRT was a positive value: 75 − 55 ms = 20 ms.

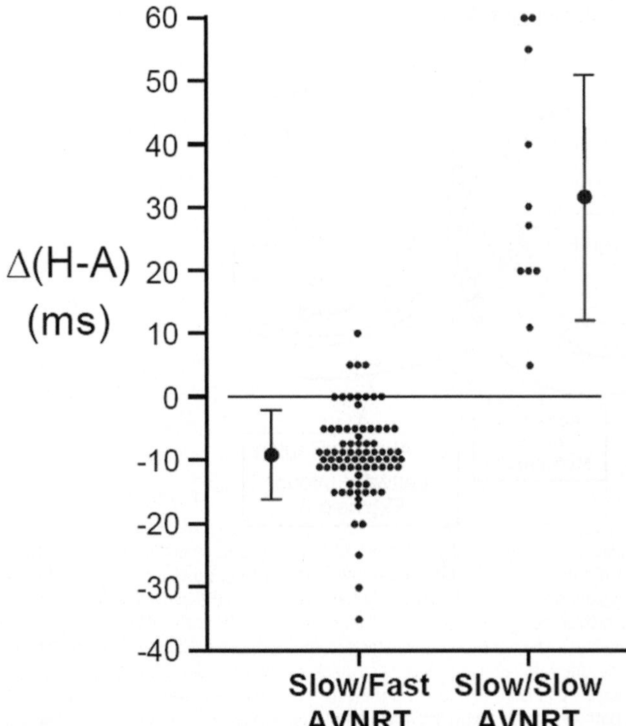

Figure 59-24 Plot of Δ(H-A), the difference between His-atrial (H-A) interval during tachycardia $(H\text{-}A)_t$ and that during ventricular pacing at the tachycardia cycle length $(H\text{-}A)_p$, in 79 patients with Slow/Fast atrioventricular nodal reentrant tachycardia (AVNRT) (mean Δ(H-A) = −9 ms) and 11 patients with Slow/Slow AVNRT (mean Δ(H-A) = 32 ms). The Δ(H-A) was positive in all 11 patients with Slow/Slow AVNRT, consistent with a significant lower common pathway. By contrast, the Δ(H-A) was negative in all but 11 of the 79 patients with Slow/Fast AVNRT, suggesting a much smaller (or absent) lower common pathway.

pathways, stippled area in Fig. 59-25B) and misinterpreting this as activation of the His bundle, which would artificially increase the H-A interval during tachycardia; (2) a true increase in the H-A interval during tachycardia produced by a delay associated with the change in direction of the wavefront at the junction of the two pathways (squiggly line in Fig. 59-25C),[39] thereby decreasing the amount of current available to activate the fast pathway and lengthening the conduction time over the fast pathway; and (3) different routes of retrograde conduction during AVNRT and during ventricular pacing.

The minimal lower common pathway may be explained anatomically by studies in rabbit hearts suggesting that the transitional cell fibers forming the fast pathway cross the tendon of Todaro and insert into the AV node close to the central fibrous body (i.e., close to the His bundle).[35]

The high success rate for eliminating Slow/Fast AVNRT by ablation procedures exclusively targeting tissue in the inferior triangle of Koch, outside the coronary sinus, provides the best evidence that a majority of these tachycardias use the rightward inferior extension in the anterograde slow pathway limb of the tachycardia. However, the failure to eliminate Slow/Fast AVNRT by ablation of the rightward inferior extension in a small percentage of patients supports the role of other anatomic substrates for the slow pathway in these patients.

Leftward Inferior Extension Slow/Fast Atrioventricular Nodal Reentrant Tachycardia

In approximately 5% of patients with Slow/Fast AVNRT, the anterograde limb of the circuit (slow pathway) appears to be formed by the leftward inferior extension of the AV node (Fig. 59-26). This can be identified by testing the resetting response within the coronary sinus and inferior triangle of Koch. In these patients, the His bundle potential is advanced (and the tachycardia reset) by a later extrastimulus delivered at the roof of the proximal coronary sinus than at the inferior triangle of Koch (between the tricuspid annulus and the coronary sinus ostium) or at the floor of the coronary sinus.

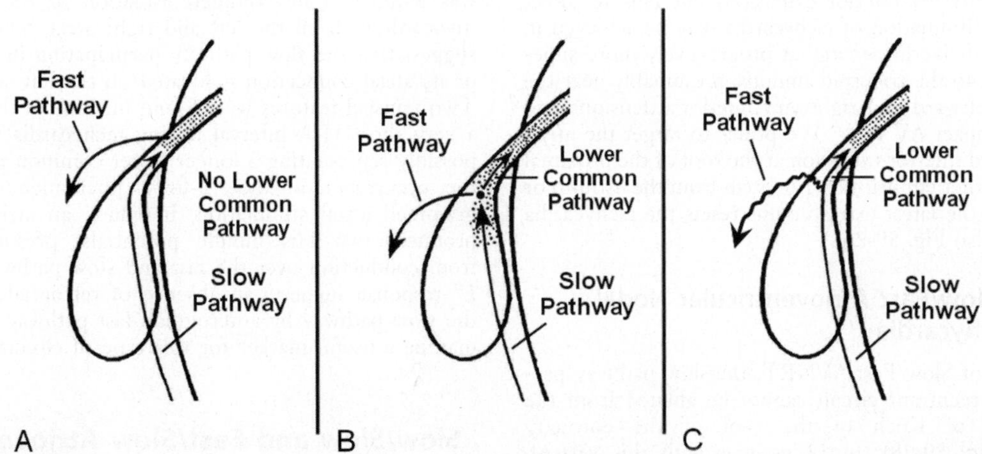

Figure 59-25 Schematic representation of three possible explanations for an $(H\text{-}A)_t$ longer than $(H\text{-}A)_P$ in Slow/Fast atrioventricular nodal reentrant tachycardia. **A,** Fast pathway connects directly with the His bundle (*stippled area*)—that is, an atrio-Hisian connection. This anatomy would have no lower common pathway. **B,** Activation of the AV bundle before penetration into the central fibrous body (pre-penetrating bundle) is recorded as the proximal His bundle potential (*lower region* of the *stippled area*). This would appear as though His bundle activation begins before activation of the lower common pathway (*arrow*), falsely lengthening $(H\text{-}A)_t$ and falsely shortening $(H\text{-}A)_P$, because the proximal retrograde His bundle potential will be generated after activation of the fast pathway. **C,** Conduction velocity over the fast pathway is reduced during tachycardia owing to the reversal in the direction of activation from the slow pathway. The delay during reversal (*beginning of squiggly line*) results in reduced current available to activate the remainder of the fast pathway, further lengthening conduction time over the fast pathway. During ventricular pacing, rapid conduction over the His bundle may activate the fast pathway with greater current, resulting in shorter conduction time over the fast pathway, mimicking an atrio-Hisian connection.

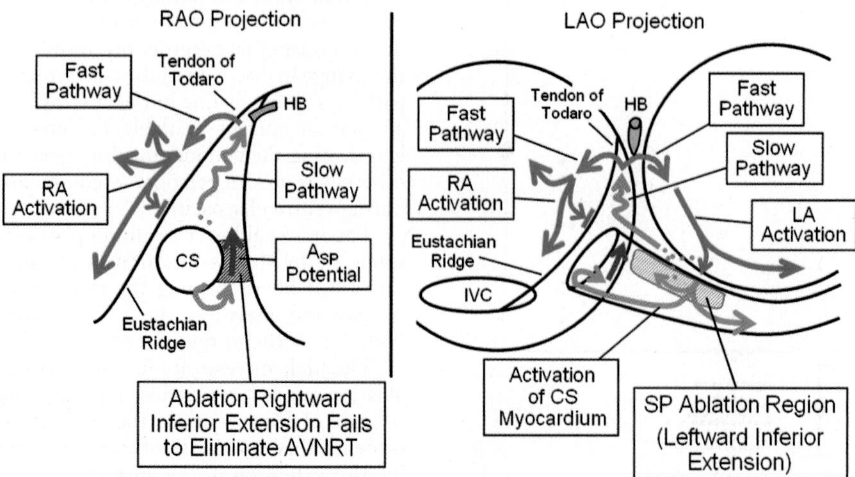

Figure 59-26 Schematic representation of the postulated circuit and ablation sites postulated for Leftward Inferior Extension Slow/Fast atrioventricular nodal reentrant tachycardia (AVNRT). Retrograde conduction over the fast pathway (*red arrows*) activates the right and left sides of the interatrial septum, posterior to the tendon of Todaro, at a level slightly inferior to that of the His bundle (HB). Just as in Rightward Inferior Extension Slow/Fast AVNRT, right atrial activation (RA activation, *green arrows*) fails to reenter the triangle of Koch, presumably as a result of conduction block at the eustachian ridge (*short perpendicular green lines*). Left atrial activation propagates from the septum, around the mitral annulus (LA activation, *green arrows* in the LAO projection). The left atrium activates the coronary sinus (CS) myocardium (*brown arrows*) and the atrial end of the leftward inferior extension of the atrioventricular (AV) node (*short dotted purple lines*). Activation propagates along the leftward inferior extension of the AV node in the anterograde direction towards the compact AV node (*squiggly purple arrows*) forming the slow pathway and completing the reentrant circuit. For ablation of the atrial end of the leftward inferior extension, (anterograde slow pathway in this tachycardia) we empirically target the roof of the proximal CS, beginning the ablation 2 to 4 cm from the CS ostium and continuing proximally toward the superior-anterior edge of the CS ostium (*red cross-hatched area*). The *gray cross-hatched area* indicates failure of ablation of the rightward inferior extension to eliminate the tachycardia. IVC, inferior vena cava; LAO, left anterior oblique; RAO, right anterior oblique.

However, a circuit using the leftward inferior extension for the slow pathway is most often identified by the response to ablation.[29,60] Ablation across the inferior triangle of Koch, between the tricuspid annulus (at the level of the middle of the coronary sinus ostium) and the apical edge of the coronary sinus ostium produces vigorous accelerated junctional rhythm (indicating injury to the rightward inferior extension) but fails to affect the tachycardia. Elimination of tachycardia may be achieved in one approach by delivering energy at progressively more superior sites adjacent to the tricuspid annulus, presumably near the junction of the leftward and rightward inferior extensions and closer to the compact AV node. We prefer to target the atrial end of the leftward inferior extension at the roof of the proximal coronary sinus, either empirically (1 to 3 cm from the ostium) or at the site where the latest extrastimulus resets the tachycardia (Fig. 59-27; see also Fig. 59-26).

Left Variant Slow/Fast Atrioventricular Nodal Reentrant Tachycardia

In a rare variant of Slow/Fast AVNRT, the slow pathway participating in the reentrant circuit cannot be ablated from the inferior triangle of Koch or the roof of the coronary sinus[19,20,25,26] (Fig. 59-28). In 12 patients with this variant, the tachycardia could be reset by a late left atrial extrastimulus delivered close to the inferolateral mitral annulus (Fig. 59-29A to C). In 9 of these 12 patients, the slow pathway was eliminated by ablation at the inferolateral mitral annulus, at the site of resetting.[19] Radiofrequency current at these sites produced accelerated junctional rhythm (with 1:1 retrograde fast pathway conduction) identical to that observed during radiofrequency current delivered to the inferior triangle of Koch (see Fig. 59-29D) in patients with Rightward Inferior Extension Slow/Fast AVNRT, indicating heating of the slow pathway. In one other patient, ablation was empirically targeted septal to the site of resetting at the inferoseptal mitral annulus and selectively eliminated retrograde (but not anterograde) fast pathway conduction. In the remaining two patients, AVNRT was eliminated by complete isolation of the coronary sinus myocardium from the left and right atria. These observations suggest that the slow pathway participating in this tachycardia or its atrial connection is located on the left side of the heart. Two unusual features were found in some of these patients: (1) a very short H-A interval during tachycardia (15 ms or less), possibly representing a longer lower common pathway; and (2) the occurrence of the "2-for-1 phenomenon" during programmed atrial stimulation, in which an atrial extrastimulus produces two His bundle potentials, presumably resulting from conduction over the fast and slow pathways. The "2 for 1" response suggests an absence of retrograde penetration of the slow pathway by anterograde fast pathway conduction and may be a useful marker for this type of circuit.

Slow/Slow and Fast/Slow Atrioventricular Nodal Reentrant Tachycardia

Slow/Slow AVNRT and Fast/Slow AVNRT are distinguished from Slow/Fast AVNRT by recognition of earliest retrograde activation at the inferior triangle of Koch or coronary sinus rather than at the interatrial septum behind the tendon of Todaro. Slow/Slow and Fast/Slow AVNRT are then differentiated by the relative duration of the H-A and A-H intervals.

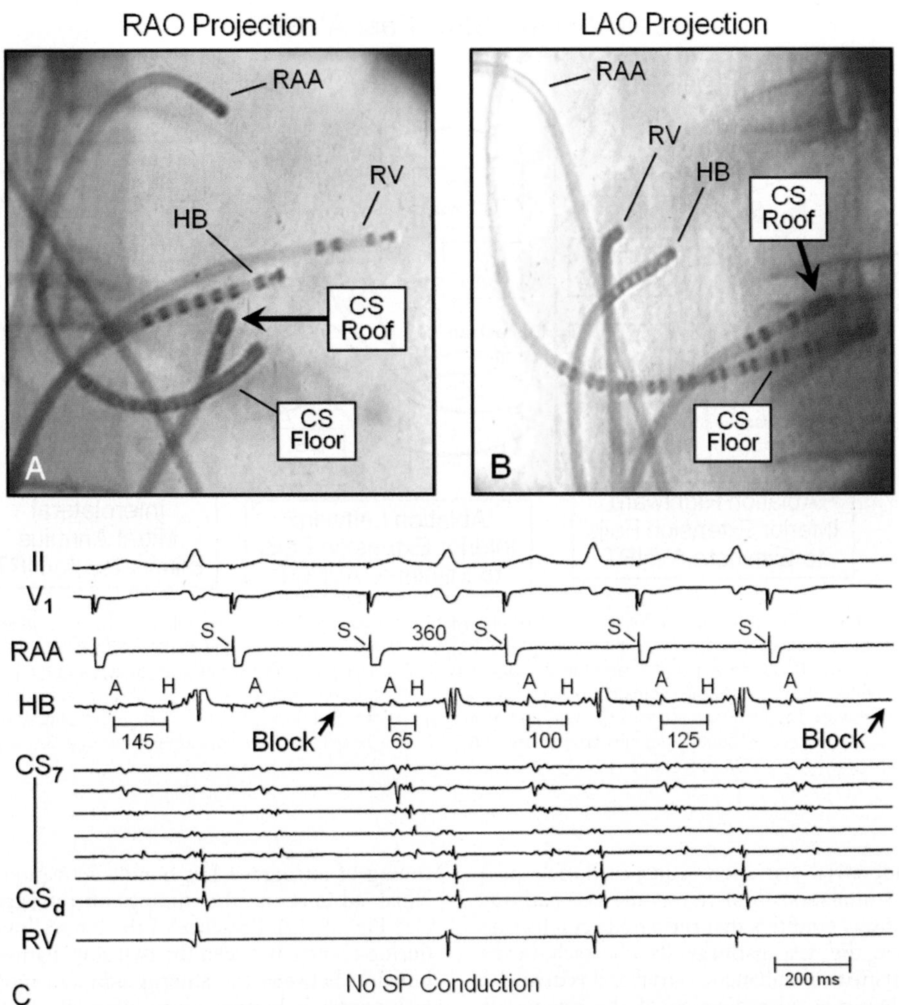

Figure 59-27 Catheter ablation of Leftward Inferior Extension Slow/Fast atrioventricular nodal reentrant tachycardia (AVNRT) by radiofrequency (RF) ablation at the roof of the proximal coronary sinus (CS). The first three RF applications were delivered between the inferoseptal tricuspid annulus and CS ostium at the level of the middle of the CS ostium (inferior triangle of Koch). These produced vigorous accelerated junctional rhythm, but sustained Slow/Fast AVNRT remained inducible by programmed atrial stimulation. Two RF applications were then delivered between the tricuspid annulus (at the level of the superior margin of the CS ostium) and the anterior-superior CS ostium. These RF applications again produced an accelerated junctional rhythm, but sustained Slow/Fast AVNRT remained inducible (with unchanged cycle length). Two RF applications were then delivered along the roof of the proximal coronary sinus. **A** and **B,** Radiographs in the RAO and LAO projections show the position of the ablation catheter (CS Roof) for the second of these two RF applications (the seventh application), which eliminated all residual anterograde slow pathway conduction and the inducibility of AVNRT. **C,** Recordings during decremental atrial pacing from the right atrial appendage (RAA) (pacing stimuli, S, in RAA electrogram) after delivery of the seventh RF application along the roof of the proximal coronary sinus. A decrease in atrial pacing cycle length to 360 ms was associated with Wenckebach block in fast pathway conduction with longest atrial-His (A-H) interval of only 145 ms, suggesting complete absence of anterograde conduction over any slow pathway (SP). It is likely that ablation at the inferior triangle of Koch eliminated conduction over the rightward inferior extension, and that ablation at the roof of the proximal CS eliminated conduction over the leftward inferior extension of the AV node, eliminating all slow pathway conduction. HB, His bundle; LAO, left anterior oblique; RAO, right anterior oblique; RV, right ventricle.

Slow/Slow Atrioventricular Nodal Reentrant Tachycardia

Slow/Slow AVNRT, like Slow/Fast AVNRT, uses a slow pathway for anterograde conduction, reflected by a long A-H interval (up to 485 ms in our experience; median, 240 ms). When induced by programmed atrial stimulation, the initiation is associated with an abrupt increase in the A-H interval. These patients often exhibit multiple jumps in the A_2-H_2 interval during atrial extrastimulus testing, consistent with multiple slow pathways. Retrograde conduction over a slow pathway is confirmed by identifying earliest retrograde activation at the roof of the coronary sinus (leftward inferior extension) (Fig. 59-30) or less commonly in the inferior triangle of Koch (rightward inferior extension).

Compared with Slow/Fast AVNRT, Slow/Slow AVNRT has a much wider range of H-A interval—in our experience, ranging from −30 to 260 ms (median, 120 ms).[56,57,61] The H-A interval often is short, resulting in simultaneous atrial and ventricular activation, mimicking Slow/Fast AVNRT (Fig. 59-31). Because of the short H-A interval, this tachycardia often is not differentiated from Slow/Fast AVNRT or is considered to be a variant of Slow/Fast AVNRT with an inferior exit for the retrograde fast pathway (formerly described as "posterior type" AVNRT).[6,7] Approximately half of the patients with Slow/Slow AVNRT, however, also have retrograde conduction over the fast pathway.

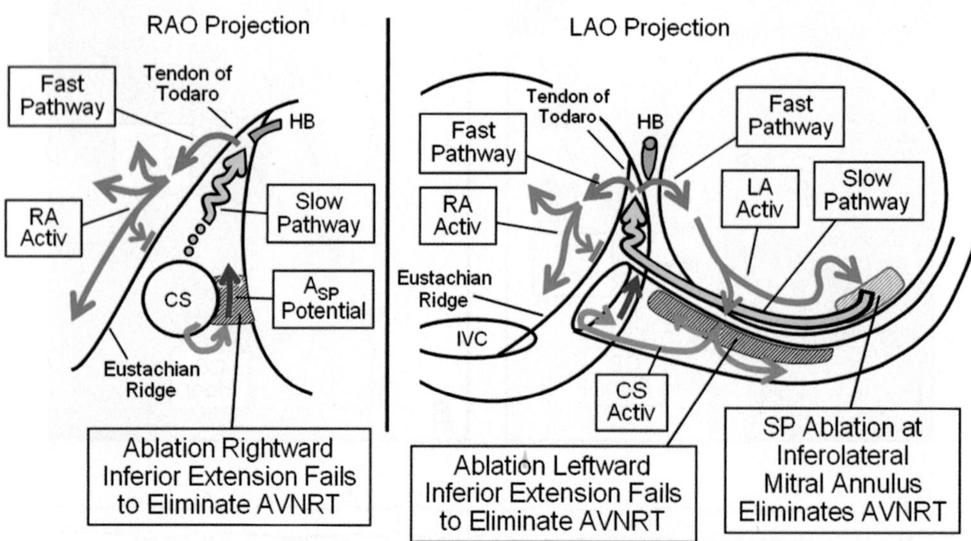

Figure 59-28 Postulated circuit and ablation site for Left Variant Slow/Fast atrioventricular nodal reentrant tachycardia (AVNRT). Retrograde conduction over the fast pathway (*red arrows*) activates the interatrial septum. Right atrial activation (RA Activ, *green arrows*) fails to reenter the triangle of Koch (*short perpendicular green lines*). Left atrial activation (LA Activ, *green arrows* in LAO projection) activates the coronary sinus (CS) myocardium (*brown arrows*), which activates the inferior triangle of Koch (*blue arrows*), generating an A_{SP} potential. Ablation at the inferior triangle of Koch (*gray area in RAO, cross-hatched*) and at the roof of the proximal CS (*gray cross-hatched area in LAO*) fails to eliminate the tachycardia. The left atrium activates the atrial end of an as-yet unidentified slow pathway (*yellow arrows*) originating close to the inferolateral mitral annulus (*red cross-hatched area*). HB, His bundle; IVC, inferior vena cava; LAO, left anterior oblique; RAO, right anterior oblique; SP, Slow pathway.

The shift in retrograde atrial activation sequence during programmed ventricular stimulation from retrograde fast pathway to retrograde slow pathway confirms that retrograde conduction is not occurring over the fast pathway during tachycardia (Fig. 59-32). In patients with simultaneous atrial and ventricular activation during tachycardia, identification of the retrograde atrial activation sequence is facilitated by the use of late para-Hisian ventricular extrastimuli, which separate the atrial and ventricular potentials (see Fig. 59-31).

During Slow/Slow AVNRT, the H-A interval usually is consistently shorter (by a mean of 30 ms) than during ventricular pacing at the tachycardia cycle length (see Figs. 59-23B and 59-24), whereas in Slow/Fast AVNRT, the H-A interval usually is slightly shorter during ventricular pacing (see Fig. 59-23A).[54,55] In patients with AVNRT exhibiting a short H-A interval (Slow/Fast or Slow/Slow AVNRT), an H-A interval during ventricular pacing exceeding the H-A interval during tachycardia (ΔHA) by 15 ms or longer probably is diagnostic of Slow/Slow AVNRT (see Fig. 59-24).[56] Because the H-A interval represents the conduction time over the retrograde slow pathway *minus* the anterograde conduction time over the lower common pathway (see Fig. 59-20A), lengthening of the conduction time over the lower common pathway results in shortening of the H-A interval. The long conduction time over the lower common pathway probably explains the frequent occurrence of a short H-A interval in Slow/Slow AVNRT and even the occasional negative H-A interval (atrial activation recorded before His bundle activation; see Fig. 59-32).

The longer lower common pathway also can be demonstrated by ventricular extrastimuli during tachycardia. In Slow/Slow AVNRT, atrial activation is not advanced until the extrastimulus retrogradely advances the end of the His bundle by 30 to 60 ms compared with the expected timing of the beginning of the anterograde His bundle activation (Fig. 59-33). This is in contrast with Slow/Fast AVNRT, in which any advance in the timing of retrograde His bundle activation usually results in an equal advance in the timing of retrograde atrial activation (see Fig. 59-19). Presence of the longer lower common pathway during reentry between the two slow pathways suggests that the junction between the anterograde and retrograde limbs of this tachycardia is located more inferiorly in the triangle of Koch than during Slow/Fast AVNRT.

It is important to differentiate Slow/Slow AVNRT from Slow/Fast AVNRT for at least two reasons. First, the technique of fast pathway ablation, now only rarely used for ablation of Slow/Fast AVNRT, does not eliminate Slow/Slow AVNRT. In fact, Slow/Slow AVNRT with a short H-A interval, mimicking Slow/Fast AVNRT, probably accounts for the 5% to 10% incidence of "atypical AVNRT" reported after fast pathway ablation in patients *thought to have* Slow/Fast AVNRT.[48] Second, in our experience, the recurrence rate after slow pathway ablation is greater for Slow/Slow AVNRT than for Slow/Fast AVNRT (8.3% versus 0.5%, respectively); therefore, more extensive ablation in the inferior triangle of Koch and roof of the coronary sinus (targeting both rightward and leftward inferior extensions) may be justified in patients with Slow/Slow AVNRT. Of 650 consecutive patients with AVNRT exhibiting a short H-A interval (less than 120 ms) referred for ablation in our laboratory, earliest retrograde activation was recorded behind the tendon of Todaro (Slow/Fast AVNRT) in 541 (83%), whereas 109 (17%) had Slow/Slow AVNRT.

Fast/Slow Atrioventricular Nodal Reentrant Tachycardia

When the H-A interval is longer than the A-H interval, AVNRT is classified as Fast/Slow.[4,48] Consistent with retrograde conduction over a slow pathway, earliest retrograde activation is most often recorded at the inferior triangle of Koch (retrograde A_{SP} potential—retrograde conduction over the rightward inferior

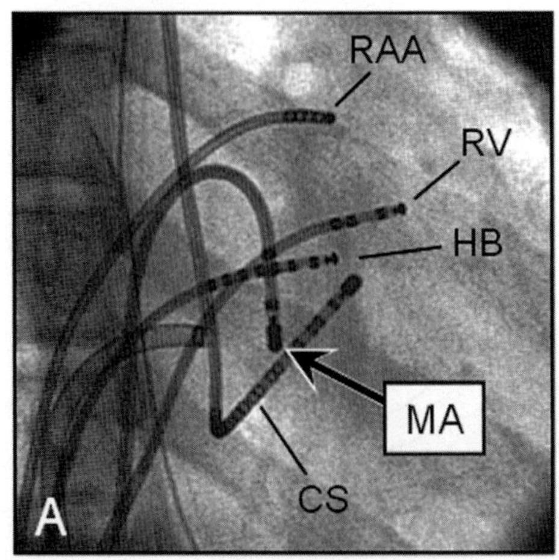

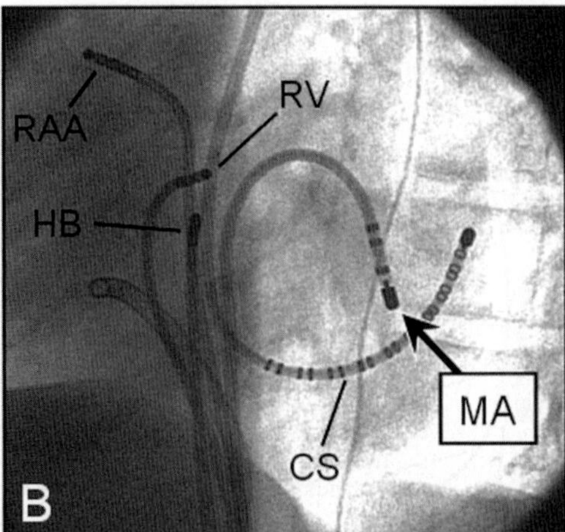

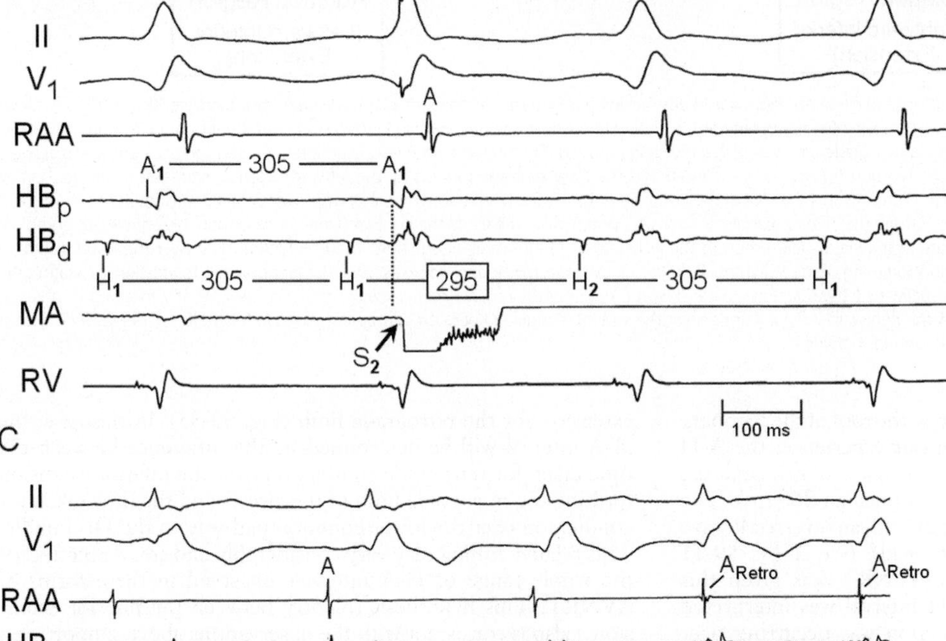

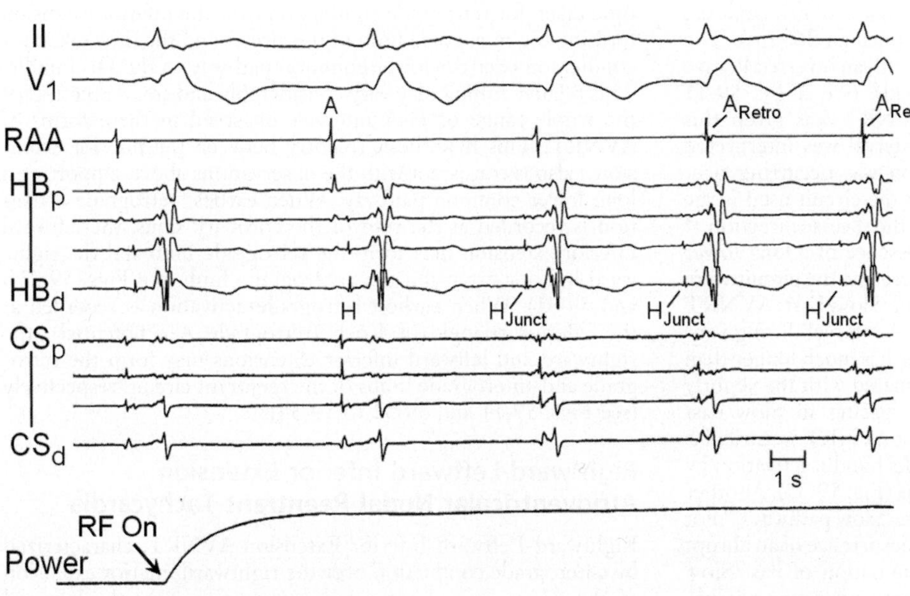

Figure 59-29 Localization of the slow pathway using the resetting technique followed by catheter ablation of left variant Slow/Fast atrioventricular nodal reentrant tachycardia (AVNRT) close to the inferolateral mitral annulus. **A** and **B,** Radiographs in the RAO and LAO projections show catheter positions, including the mapping catheter in the left atrium (transseptal technique), positioned close to the inferolateral mitral annulus (MA). **C,** During Slow/Fast AVNRT with constant cycle length of 305 ms, an atrial extrastimulus was delivered to the mapping catheter in the left atrium close to the inferolateral mitral annulus (*arrow,* S_2 in MA electrogram) after retrograde atrial activation had occurred (A_1-A_1 = 305 ms in the HB_p electrogram). The atrial extrastimulus advanced the next His bundle potential by 10 ms (H_1-H_2 = 295 ms). The advanced His bundle potential (H_2) was followed by an interval equal to the tachycardia cycle length (305 ms, resetting response). The resetting of the tachycardia suggests the site where the left atrial extrastimulus was delivered was located close to an atrial connection of the slow pathway forming the anterograde limb of the reentrant circuit. **D,** An application of radiofrquency (RF) current to the resetting site in the left atrium (*arrow,* RF On, in the Power tracing) produced an immediate accelerated junctional rhythm. Each His bundle potential of the accelerated junctional rhythm (H_{Junct}) was followed by retrograde conduction over the fast AV nodal pathway (A_{Retro}), consistent with heating-induced automaticity of the slow pathway. CS, coronary sinus; HB, His bundle; RAA, right atrial appendage; RV, right ventricle; RAO, right anterior oblique; LAO, left anterior oblique.

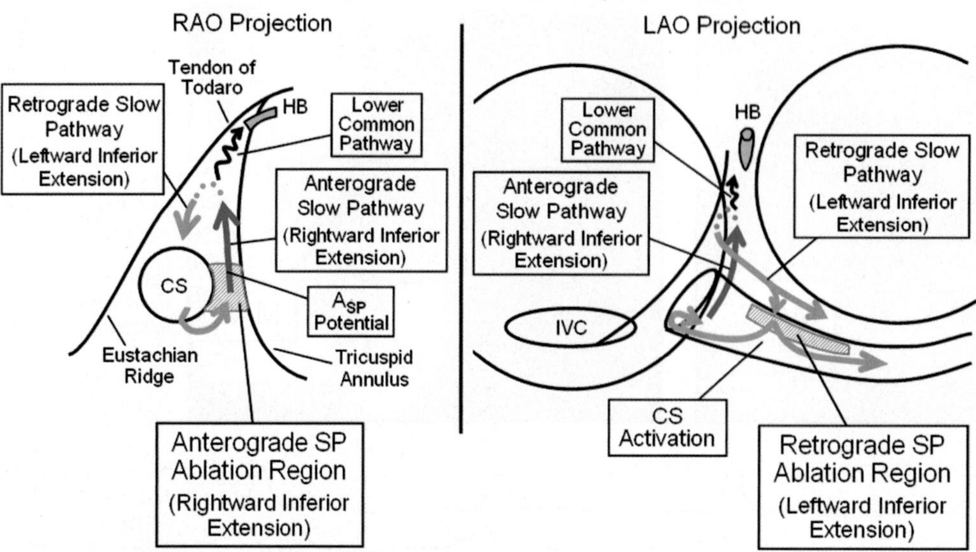

Figure 59-30 Schematic representation of the proposed circuit for Rightward-Leftward Inferior Extension atrioventricular nodal reentrant tachycardia (AVNRT) (i.e., Slow/Slow AVNRT). We postulate reentry between the rightward inferior and leftward inferior extensions of the atrioventricular (AV) node as the reentrant circuit in most cases of Slow/Slow AVNRT. Activation propagates in the anterograde direction along the slow pathway (SP) formed by the rightward inferior extension (*blue arrows*) to activate the lower common pathway in the anterograde direction (*squiggly black arrows*) and the slow pathway formed by the leftward inferior extension in the retrograde direction (*purple arrows*). The leftward inferior extension activates the roof of the coronary sinus myocardium (*brown arrows*), which propagates the impulse to the floor of the coronary sinus (CS) ostium (*brown arrows*) to activate the inferior triangle of Koch (A_{SP} potential) and back to the rightward inferior extension (*blue arrows*) to complete the circuit. The fast pathway does not participate in the circuit, even though the His-atrial (H-A) interval is often short. The conduction time over the lower common pathway delays His bundle activation, resulting in shortening of the H-A interval during tachycardia, mimicking Slow/Fast AVNRT. Our approach to ablation is to target the atrial end of the retrograde limb of the circuit (usually the leftward inferior extension at the roof of the coronary sinus, *red crosshatched area in LAO*), followed by ablation of the atrial end of the anterograde limb (usually the rightward inferior extension at the inferior triangle of Koch, *red crosshatched area in RAO*). HB, His bundle; IVC, inferior vena cava; LAO, left anterior oblique; RAO, right anterior oblique.

extension) and less commonly recorded at the roof of the coronary sinus (leftward inferior extension). In our experience, the A-H interval ranges from 30 to 185 ms (median 80 ms) and the H-A interval ranges from 135 to 435 ms (median 260 ms). The RP interval is longer than the PR interval, with an inverted P wave in the inferior electrocardiographic leads (see Figs. 59-11 and 59-12). Traditionally, Fast/Slow AVNRT was given this label because the relatively short A-H interval was interpreted as indicating that anterograde conduction was occurring over the fast pathway. This label suggests that the circuit used is the same as that in Slow/Fast AVNRT, but in the reverse direction.[24] Several findings, however, suggest the presence of a long lower common pathway, which would not be present if the circuit were using the same anatomic substrate as in Slow/Fast AVNRT (i.e., using the fast pathway). First, the H-A interval during ventricular pacing at the tachycardia cycle length is much longer than the H-A interval during tachycardia (compared with the slightly shorter H-A interval during ventricular pacing in Slow/Fast AVNRT).[54,55] Second, unlike in Slow/Fast AVNRT, ventricular extrastimuli during tachycardia advance His bundle activation by 30 to 60 ms before resetting the tachycardia (Fig. 59-34). Another observation supporting reentry between the "slow pathways," not involving the fast pathway, is the frequent occurrence of an abrupt increase in the A-H interval during the initiation of Fast/Slow AVNRT by programmed atrial stimulation, suggesting anterograde conduction over one slow pathway, followed by retrograde conduction over another slow pathway.

We have hypothesized (as in the previous edition of this book) that the circuits in both Slow/Slow and Fast/Slow AVNRT use one of the inferior extensions of the AV node (rightward or leftward) for the anterograde limb and the other extension for the retrograde limb (Fig. 59-35). In this case, the H-A interval will be determined by the difference between the time taken for retrograde conduction over the inferior extension forming the retrograde limb of the circuit and the time taken for conduction over the lower common pathway to the His bundle. This relative timing may vary considerably and could account for the whole range of H-A intervals observed in these forms of AVNRT. This hypothesis (reentry between the inferior extensions) also is consistent with the observations above supporting a long lower common pathway. When earliest retrograde activation is recorded at the roof of the coronary sinus, the leftward inferior extension may form the retrograde limb and the rightward inferior extension the anterograde limb (see Figs. 59-23B and 59-31). When earliest retrograde activation is recorded at the inferior triangle of Koch (retrograde A_{SP} potential), the rightward and leftward inferior extensions may form the retrograde and anterograde limbs of the reentrant circuit, respectively (see Figs. 59-11 and 59-32 to 59-34).

Rightward-Leftward Inferior Extension Atrioventricular Nodal Reentrant Tachycardia

Rightward-Leftward Inferior Extension AVNRT, characterized by anterograde conduction over the rightward inferior extension of the AV node and retrograde conduction over the leftward inferior extension, typically has a relatively long A-H interval and short H-A interval, with earliest retrograde activation recorded at the roof of the coronary sinus (1 to 3 cm from the ostium) (see Figs. 59-23B and 59-31). This circuit accounts for a majority of tachycardias traditionally referred to as Slow/Slow AVNRT.

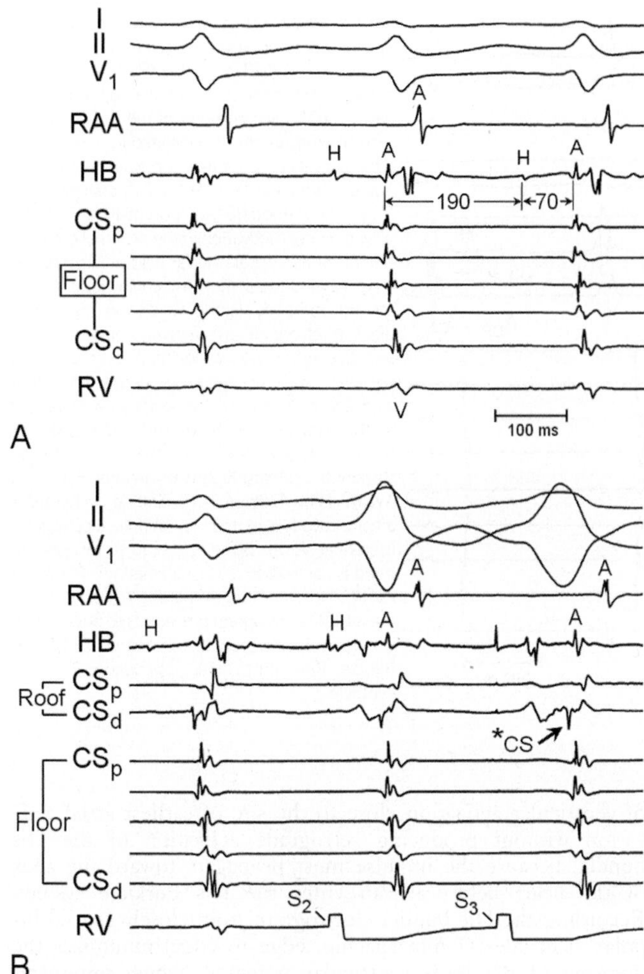

Figure 59-31 Rightward-Leftward Inferior Extension atrioventricular nodal reentrant tachycardia (AVNRT) (i.e., Slow/Slow AVNRT) with a short His-atrial (H-A) interval, mimicking Slow/Fast AVNRT. **A,** During Slow/Slow AVNRT, a short H-A interval (70 ms in HB electrogram) resulted in simultaneous atrial and ventricular activation, which obscures the retrograde atrial activation sequence and mimics Slow/Fast AVNRT. **B,** Two right ventricular (RV) extrastimuli (S_2 and S_3) were delivered to the para-Hisian right ventricular septum. The second ventricular extrastimulus (S_3) advanced the timing of local ventricular activation, revealing the retrograde atrial activation sequence with earliest activation recorded at the roof of the proximal CS (*asterisk* in CS $Roof_d$ electrogram), consistent with retrograde conduction over the slow pathway formed by the leftward inferior extension, with activation propagating away in both directions in the CS electrograms. CS, coronary sinus; HB, His bundle; RAA, right atrial appendage.

Leftward-Rightward Inferior Extension Atrioventricular Nodal Reentrant Tachycardia

This tachycardia, with anterograde conduction over the leftward inferior extension and retrograde conduction over the rightward inferior extension usually produces a relatively short A-H interval and long H-A interval, with earliest retrograde activation recorded at the inferior triangle of Koch (see Fig. 59-11). This circuit probably accounts for almost all of the tachycardias traditionally classified as Fast/Slow AVNRT but occasionally accounts for tachycardias traditionally classified as Slow/Slow AVNRT (see Figs. 59-32 and 59-33).

In the more usual manifestation of this tachycardia (long H-A), the short A-H interval may be even shorter than during sinus rhythm (see Figs. 59-11 and 59-12). The short A-H (and PR) interval may be explained by the following mechanism: Retrograde activation of the rightward inferior extension (Fig. 59-36, *blue arrows*) activates the coronary sinus myocardium (see Fig. 59-36, *brown arrows*), which activates the left atrium (see Fig. 59-36, *green arrow* in LAO projection). Conduction along the left atrium to the interatrial septum (see Fig. 59-36, *dotted green line* and *short green arrows*) may result in anterograde activation of the fast pathway (see Fig. 59-36, *red arrows*), producing a short A-H interval. In this mechanism, the fast pathway activates the His bundle but does not participate in the reentrant circuit (bystander). This pattern of activation is supported by closely spaced bipolar electrograms recorded at the inferior triangle of Koch and along the floor of the coronary sinus (Fig. 59-37). Shortly after earliest retrograde activation is recorded at the inferior triangle of Koch (A_{SP}) (see Fig. 59-37), two separate potentials are recorded from the proximal coronary sinus. The first potential begins at the ostium and propagates into the coronary sinus (CS myo) (see Fig. 59-37). The second potential begins 5 to 10 mm from the ostium and propagates back toward the right. Mapping of the left atrium shows that the timing of the second potential corresponds to activation of the left atrium at the inferoseptal mitral annulus, such that the first potential probably represents activation of the coronary sinus myocardium. These recordings suggest that activation proceeds from the A_{SP} site to the floor of the coronary sinus ostium, then into the coronary sinus, with subsequent activation of the left atrium at the inferior mitral annulus. Atrial activation then propagates back towards the interatrial septum. A single potential is seen in the more distal coronary sinus electrograms due to simultaneous propagation laterally in the distal coronary sinus myocardium and the left atrium (see Fig. 59-37, *long brown* and *green arrow* in LAO projection). The need for the coronary sinus myocardium to be activated in order to reach the left atrium, and from there the fast pathway in Leftward-Rightward Inferior Extension AVNRT is demonstrated by the finding of block at the inferior triangle of Koch (after retrograde conduction over the rightward inferior extension), resulting in the failure to activate the coronary sinus, the atria, or AV node (Fig. 59-38). The failure to reach the right atrium also supports the concept that activation cannot cross the eustachian ridge or tendon of Todaro.

Differential Diagnosis and Management of Atrioventricular Nodal Reentrant Tachycardia

Differentiating Atrioventricular Nodal Reentrant Tachycardia from Orthodromic Atrioventricular Reentrant Tachycardia and Atrial Tachycardia

The atrial activation sequence of the various forms of AVNRT may be indistinguishable from the atrial activation sequence of either orthodromic AV reentrant tachycardia (using an anteroseptal, inferoseptal, or left posterior accessory pathway) or atrial tachycardia arising from the septum or region surrounding the coronary sinus. AVNRT with a short H-A interval can often be distinguished from orthodromic AV reentrant tachycardia and atrial tachycardia by the timing of atrial activation. In orthodromic AV reentrant tachycardia, the reentrant impulse activates the ventricles (through the His-Purkinje system) before reaching the accessory pathway and then the atrium. This results in a ventriculoatrial (VA) conduction time (measured from the onset of ventricular activation to the onset of retrograde atrial activation) of at least 50 ms, and usually more than 60 ms.[62] The retrograde P wave begins near the end of the QRS complex or within the ST segment. By contrast, the reentrant circuit in

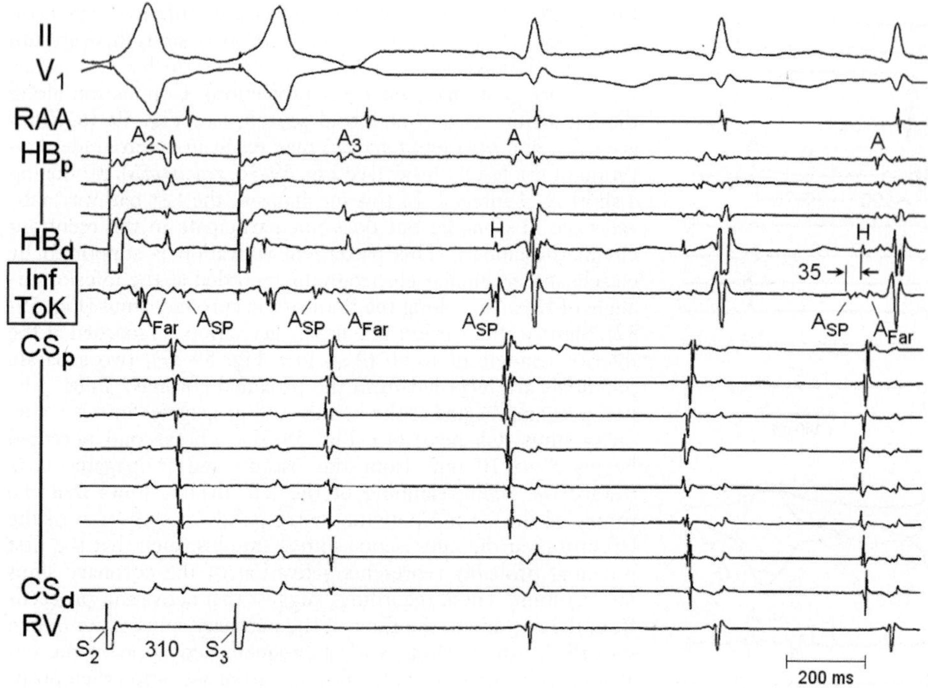

Figure 59-32 Induction of Leftward-Rightward inferior extension atrioventricular nodal reentrant tachycardia (AVNRT) (i.e., Slow/Slow AVNRT) with negative His-atrial (H-A) interval by ventricular pacing. In the first complex of the tracing, a ventricular extrastimulus (S_2) resulted in a retrograde atrial activation sequence consistent with retrograde conduction over the fast AV nodal pathway. Note the retrograde A_{SP} potential follows the timing of atrial activation in the proximal coronary sinus (CS) as well as the far field atrial potential (A_{Far}) from behind the eustachian ridge. In the second complex, ventricular pacing resulted in block in retrograde fast pathway conduction and selective retrograde conduction over the slow pathway, with activation sequence consistent with conduction over the slow pathway formed by the rightward inferior extension (A_{SP} potential precedes atrial activation at other sites), initiating sustained Leftward-Rightward Inferior Extension AVNRT (Slow/Slow AVNRT). During tachycardia, atrial activation in the His bundle electrogram (potential A in HB electrograms) follows His bundle activation (H), simulating Slow/Fast AVNRT. However, the retrograde A_{SP} potential in the Inf ToK electrogram preceded His bundle activation by 35 ms (negative H-A interval). HB, His bundle; RAA, right atrial appendage; RV, right ventricle.

AVNRT does not use the ventricles. The ventricle activation–atrial activation (V-A) interval is less than 50 ms in most patients with Slow/Fast AVNRT and some patients with Slow/Slow AVNRT, excluding orthodromic AV reentrant tachycardia (see Figs. 59-3, 59-6, 59-8, 59-9, 59-14, 59-19, 59-21, 59-23, 59-29, 59-31, and 59-32).

Any form of AVNRT can be differentiated from orthodromic AV reentrant tachycardia and atrial tachycardia by the use of single or double late ventricular extrastimuli, which establishes whether the reentrant circuit incorporates ventricular myocardium. The extrastimuli are best delivered to the base of the ventricle, close to the site of earliest retrograde atrial activation. Beginning approximately 50 ms after the onset of the His bundle potential, the extrastimuli are advanced in 5 to 10 ms increments. An advance in the timing of atrial activation without first retrogradely activating the His bundle establishes the presence of an accessory AV pathway. If the atrial activation sequence of the advanced complex is identical to the other tachycardia complexes and if a slight advance in the timing of atrial activation results in a change in the timing of the next His bundle activation (resetting the tachycardia), then an accessory pathway is being activated during the tachycardia and it forms part of the reentrant circuit, respectively. Conversely, an accessory AV pathway is unlikely to be present if the timing and sequence of retrograde atrial activation are unchanged by a ventricular extrastimulus that advances the timing of ventricular activation close to the site of earliest retrograde atrial activation by 50 ms or more (see Figs. 59-19A, 59-31, 59-33A, and 59-34A). For tachycardias with earliest atrial activation at the superior septum, ventricular pacing is best performed adjacent to (but not capturing) the proximal right bundle branch (para-Hisian pacing site[53]). For tachycardias with earliest atrial activation recorded at the inferoseptal tricuspid annulus or proximal coronary sinus, ventricular pacing can be performed at the inferobasal right ventricular septum, close to the tricuspid annulus at the level of the coronary sinus. These pacing sites allow the greatest advance in the timing of ventricular activation close to the site of earliest atrial activation without producing retrograde activation of the His bundle, because the impulse must propagate toward the apex of the heart before it can enter the His Purkinje system. Recording the His bundle electrogram from closely spaced bipolar electrodes (1-mm spacing, edge to edge) minimizes the duration of the local ventricular potential, which minimizes overlapping of the local ventricular and His bundle potentials, allowing verification of anterograde or retrograde His bundle activation (see Figs. 59-3, 59-7, 59-15, 59-19, 59-21, 59-23, 59-31, and 59-33).

AVNRT can be differentiated from atrial tachycardia by the use of earlier ventricular extrastimuli. Ventricular extrastimuli that significantly advance the timing of retrograde His bundle activation (30 to 60 ms or more) will alter the timing of atrial activation (without a change in atrial activation sequence), or produce VA block and terminate tachycardia in AVNRT (see Figs. 59-19B and C, 59-33C, and 59-34C), but will have no effect on the timing of earliest atrial activation in atrial tachycardia. This degree of advance in His bundle activation often requires the use of multiple ventricular extrastimuli or continuous ventricular pacing at a cycle length slightly shorter than tachycardia cycle length. Atrial tachycardia is diagnosed if ventricular extrastimuli or ventricular pacing during tachycardia retrogradely advances His bundle activation by more than 60 to 80 ms without changing the timing or sequence of atrial activation. The long advance in His bundle activation is required due to the long lower common pathway in reentry between the rightward and leftward inferior extensions. AVNRT can also be excluded by the administration of adenosine during tachycardia. A period of complete AV block (more than 2 to 3 beats) without altering the timing or morphology of atrial activation strongly supports atrial tachycardia.

Para-Hisian pacing with intermittent His bundle capture can be used to differentiate retrograde conduction over the fast or slow AV nodal pathway from retrograde conduction over an anteroseptal or inferoseptal accessory pathway, respectively.[53]

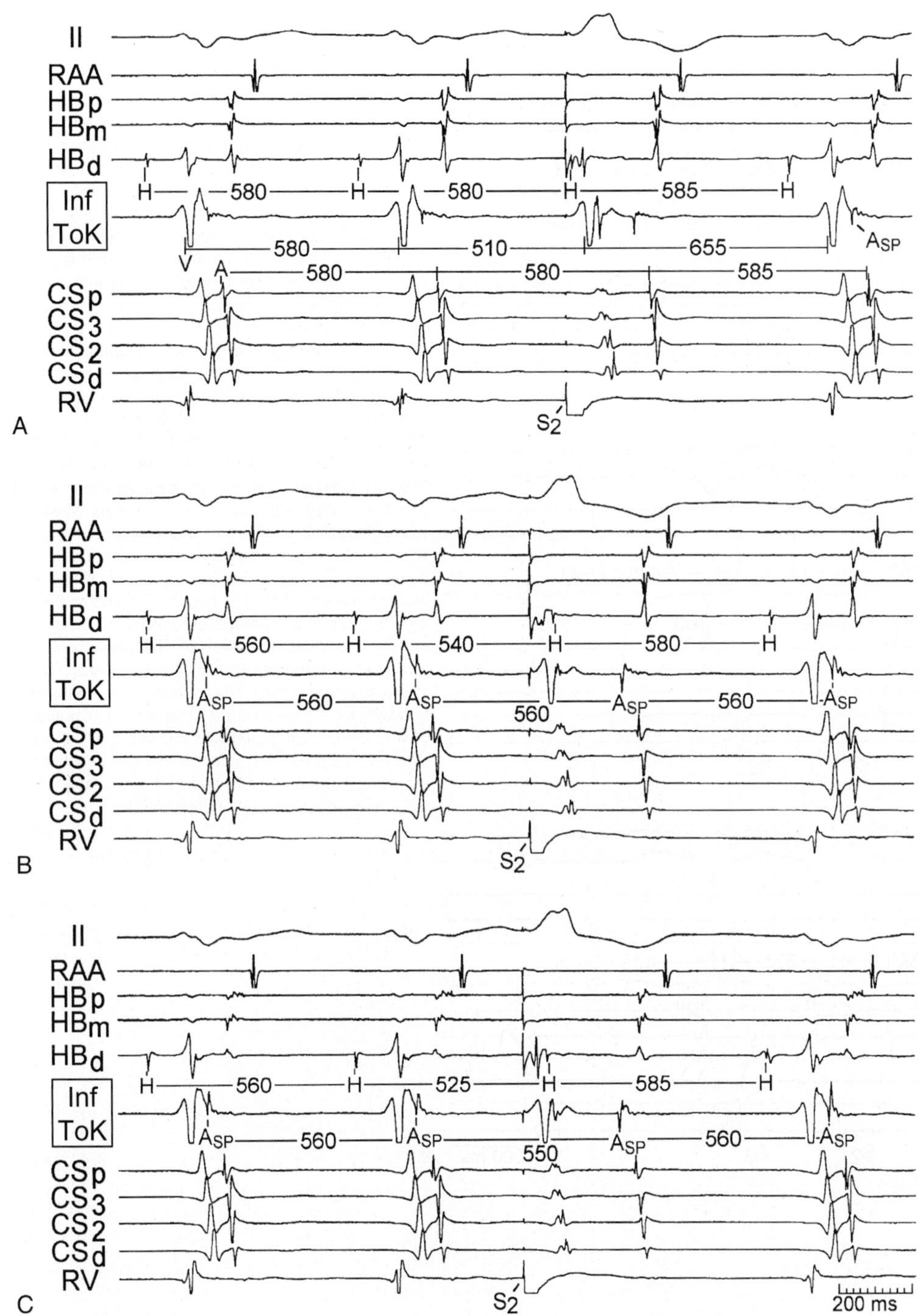

Figure 59-33 Use of ventricular extrastimuli to verify the diagnosis of Leftward-Rightward Inferior Extension atrioventricular nodal reentrant tachycardia (AVNRT) (i.e., Slow/Slow AVNRT). **A,** During tachycardia, a single extrastimulus (S_2) was delivered to the para-Hisian right ventricular septum. This advanced the timing of local ventricular activation in the inferior triangle of Koch (Inf ToK) electrogram (which recorded earliest retrograde activation, A_{SP}) by 70 ms (V-V = 510 ms, compared with 580 ms). However, S_2 did not advance the timing of His bundle (HB) activation (H) or atrial activation, excluding retrograde conduction over an inferoseptal accessory pathway and orthodromic atrioventricular (AV) reentrant tachycardia. Note that the ventricular extrastimulus provided further separation of the ventricular and atrial potentials allowing clear identification of the retrograde atrial activation sequence, including the early retrograde A_{SP} potential. **B,** An earlier ventricular extrastimulus resulted in retrograde activation of the His bundle. The end of the retrograde His bundle potential occurred 20 ms before anterograde His bundle activation would have occurred (H-H = 540 ms, compared with 560 ms). However, this did not advance the timing of retrograde atrial activation (A_{SP}-A_{SP} = 560 ms), consistent with either AVNRT with a long lower common pathway or atrial tachycardia. **C,** Further shortening of the extrastimulus coupling interval resulted in earlier retrograde activation of the His bundle. The end of the retrograde His bundle potential occurred 35 ms before the anterograde His bundle potential would have occurred (H-H = 525 ms, compared with 560 ms). This resulted in a 10-ms advance in the timing of retrograde atrial activation without a change in the atrial activation sequence (A_{SP}-A_{SP} = 550 ms, compared with 560 ms), indicating that the timing of atrial activation was dependent on the timing of His bundle activation, excluding an atrial tachycardia and confirming AVNRT. RAA, right atrial appendage; RV, right ventricle.

Ventricular pacing is initiated during sinus rhythm at the superior basal right ventricular septum, 3 to 5 mm superior and apical to the site recording activation of the His bundle or proximal right bundle branch, such that at a high pacing output the QRS complex narrows and the His bundle potential is advanced, indicating direct capture of the His bundle or proximal right bundle branch (HB-RB capture). Small variations in electrode position with respiration result in intermittent HB-RB capture. Alternatively, the pacing output can be increased and decreased to gain and lose HB-RB capture, respectively, whereas local ventricular capture is maintained throughout. With the loss of HB-RB capture, a delay in the timing of atrial activation (equal to the delay in the timing of His bundle activation) without a change in the atrial activation sequence identifies retrograde conduction over the AV node (Fig. 59-39A). With the loss of HB-RB capture, the absence of change in the timing and sequence of atrial activation identifies retrograde conduction occurring exclusively over an accessory pathway (see Fig. 59-9B). A partial delay (less than the delay in the timing of His bundle activation) combined with a shift in the atrial activation sequence identifies retrograde conduction occurring over both an accessory pathway and the AV node (see Fig. 59-39C).

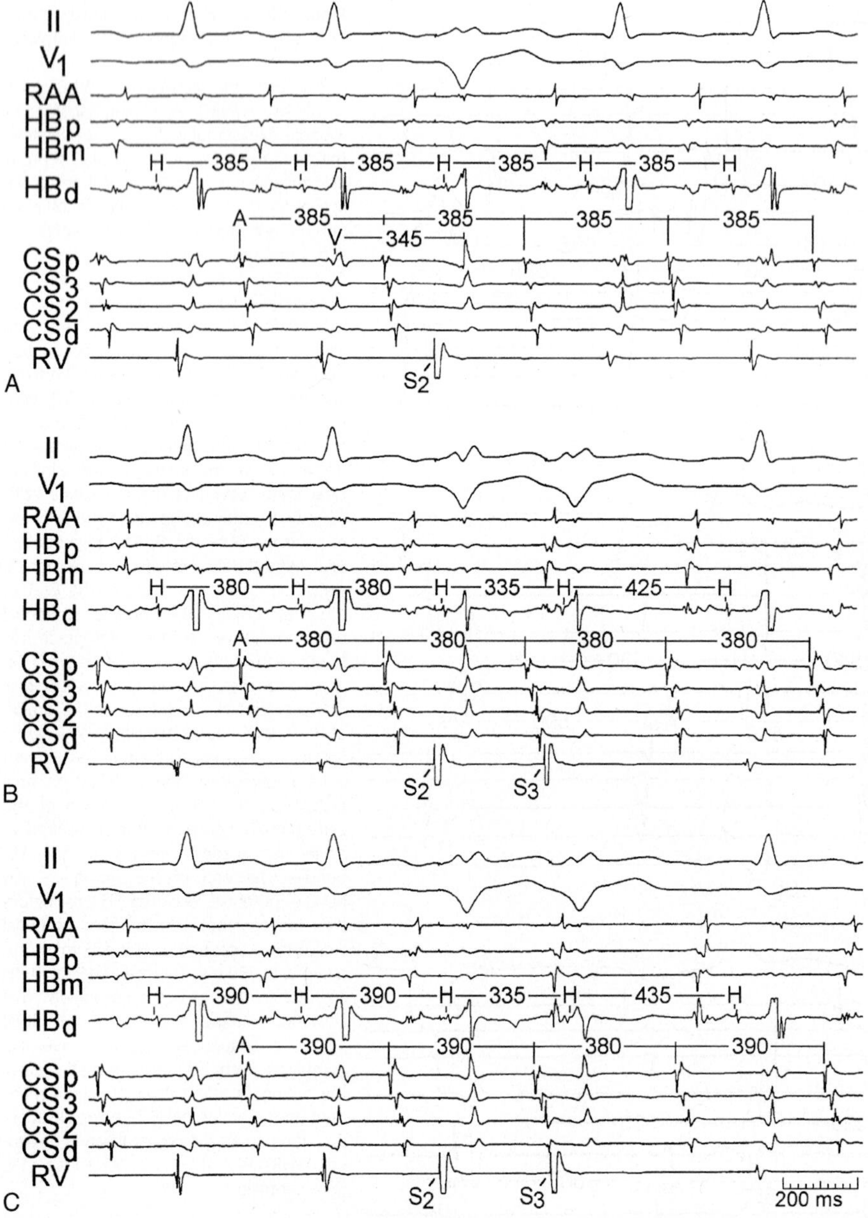

Figure 59-34 Use of ventricular extrastimuli to verify the diagnosis of Leftward-Rightward Inferior Extension atrioventricular nodal reentrant tachycardia (AVNRT) (i.e., Fast/Slow AVNRT). **A,** During tachycardia, a single ventricular extrastimulus (S_2) advanced the timing of ventricular activation in the proximal coronary sinus electrogram (CS_p), near the site of earliest retrograde activation, by 40 ms (V-V = 345 ms, compared with 385 ms). This did not advance the timing of His bundle (HB) activation or retrograde atrial activation. This indicates that atrial activation during this tachycardia is independent of local ventricular activation, excluding retrograde conduction over an Inferoseptal accessory pathway and orthodromic atrioventricular (AV) reentrant tachycardia. **B,** Two ventricular extrastimuli were delivered. The second ventricular extrastimulus (S_3) resulted in retrograde activation of the His bundle. The end of the retrograde His bundle potential occurred 45 ms before the anterograde His bundle activation would have occurred (H-H = 335 ms, compared with 380 ms). However, this did not advance the timing of retrograde atrial activation (A-A = 380 ms), consistent with either AVNRT with a very long lower common pathway or atrial tachycardia. **C,** Further shortening of the extrastimulus coupling intervals resulted in earlier retrograde activation of the His bundle. The end of the retrograde His bundle potential occurred 55 ms before the anterograde His bundle potential would have begun (H-H = 335 ms, compared with 390 ms). This resulted in a 10-ms advance in the timing of retrograde atrial activation without a change in the atrial activation sequence (A-A = 380 ms, compared with 390 ms), indicating that atrial activation was dependent on His bundle activation, excluding atrial tachycardia and confirming AVNRT. RAA, right atrial appendage; RV, right ventricle.

Management of Atrioventricular Nodal Reentrant Tachycardia

Termination of a sustained episode of AVNRT is accomplished by producing transient block in the AV node. Vagal maneuvers such as carotid sinus massage, the Valsalva maneuver, or the dive reflex usually are used as the first step and generally work by terminating the tachycardia with conduction block in the slow pathway. If vagal maneuvers are unsuccessful in terminating tachycardia, the tachycardia usually can be terminated by administration of adenosine. If the tachycardia quickly resumes, success is likely with either a calcium channel blocker (verapamil or diltiazem) or pretreatment with a β-adrenergic blocker (esmolol, propranolol, or metoprolol) followed by adenosine.

Ablation of the slow AV nodal pathway involved in the reentrant circuit has become first-line therapy for all forms of AVNRT. This procedure is highly effective (95% to 99% success rate),[2,3,29] with a low risk of AV block (less than 1%). For patients in whom ablation therapy is not desirable or available, long-term pharmacologic therapy may be effective. β-Adrenergic blockers and calcium channel blockers often are used first because of their safety and availability, targeting primarily conduction over the slow pathway. Efficacy usually is greater with class I antiarrhythmic agents such as flecainide and propafenone, which depress retrograde fast pathway conduction. Class III agents such as sotalol and amiodarone also may be effective but are less frequently used for AVNRT.

Hypothesis for Slow/Slow and Fast/Slow AVNRT

Rightward/Leftward Inferior Extension AVNRT (Usually Slow/Slow AVNRT)

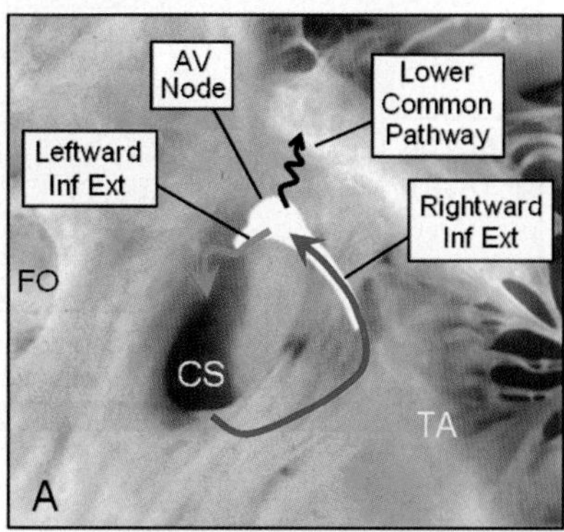

Leftward/Rightward Inferior Extension AVNRT (Usually Fast/Slow AVNRT)

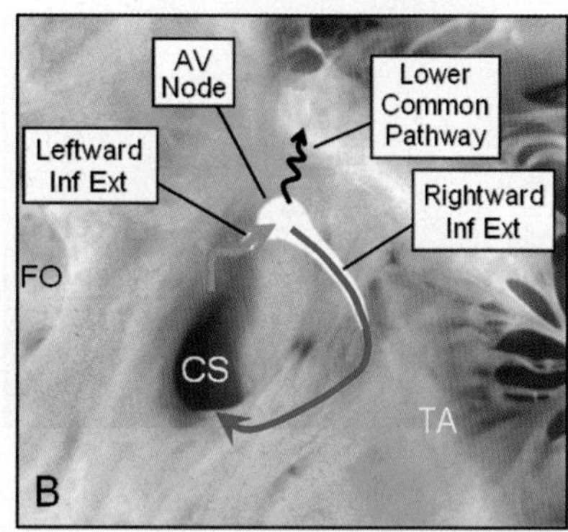

Figure 59-35 Hypothesis that Slow/Slow atrioventricular nodal reentrant tachycardia (AVNRT) and Fast/Slow AVNRT result from reentry between the rightward and leftward inferior extensions of the atrioventricular (AV) node. **A,** Reentry using rightward inferior extension (Rightward Inf Ext) in the anterograde direction (*blue arrow*) and the leftward inferior extension (Leftward Inf Ext) in the retrograde direction (*purple arrow*) most often produces a long atrial–His bundle (A-H) interval, shorter H-A interval, and sequence of atrial activation (earliest activation in the roof of the proximal coronary sinus [CS]) typical of Slow/Slow AVNRT. **B,** Reentry using leftward inferior extension for anterograde conduction (*purple arrow*) and the rightward inferior extension for retrograde conduction (*blue arrow*) produces a short A-H (left atrium activates the fast pathway), long H-A interval, and earliest activation at the inferior triangle of Koch (A_{SP} potential), typical of Fast/Slow AVNRT. FO, fossa ovalis; TA, tricuspid annulus. (Modified from Inoue S, Becker AE: Posterior extensions of the human compact atrioventricular node: A neglected anatomic feature of potential clinical significance. Circulation 97:188-193, 1998.)

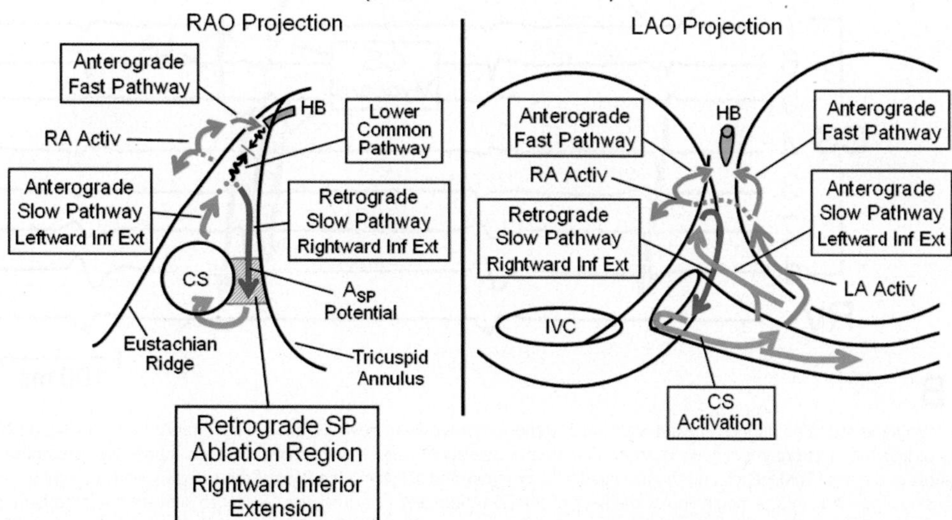

Figure 59-36 Schematic representation of the proposed circuit for Leftward Rightward Inferior Extension AVNRT (accounting for a majority of episodes of Fast/Slow AVNRT). Activation propagates in the anterograde direction along the slow pathway formed by the leftward inferior extension (Leftward Inf Ext, *purple arrows*) to activate the lower common pathway in the anterograde direction (*lower squiggly black arrow* in RAO projection) and the retrograde slow pathway formed by the rightward inferior extension in the retrograde direction (Rightward Inf Ext, *blue arrows*). The rightward inferior extension activates the floor of the coronary sinus (CS) ostium (*brown arrows*). The CS myocardium propagates the impulse laterally (*brown arrow*) to activate the left atrium (LA Activ, *green arrow*) and the leftward inferior extension in the anterograde direction (*purple arrows*) to complete the circuit. Left atrial activation propagates rapidly (*green arrow* in LAO projection) to the atrial septum (*dotted green lines*) to activate the fast pathway (*red arrows*), producing a short atrial-His (A-H) interval. The fast pathway serves as a bystander. Ablation is targeted to the atrial end of the retrograde slow pathway at the inferior triangle of Koch, at a site recording a sharp retrograde A_{SP} potential (*red cross-hatched area*, Retrograde SP Ablation Region, Rightward Inf Ext). HB, His bundle; IVC, inferior vena cava; LAO, left anterior oblique; RAO, right anterior oblique; TA, tricuspid annulus.

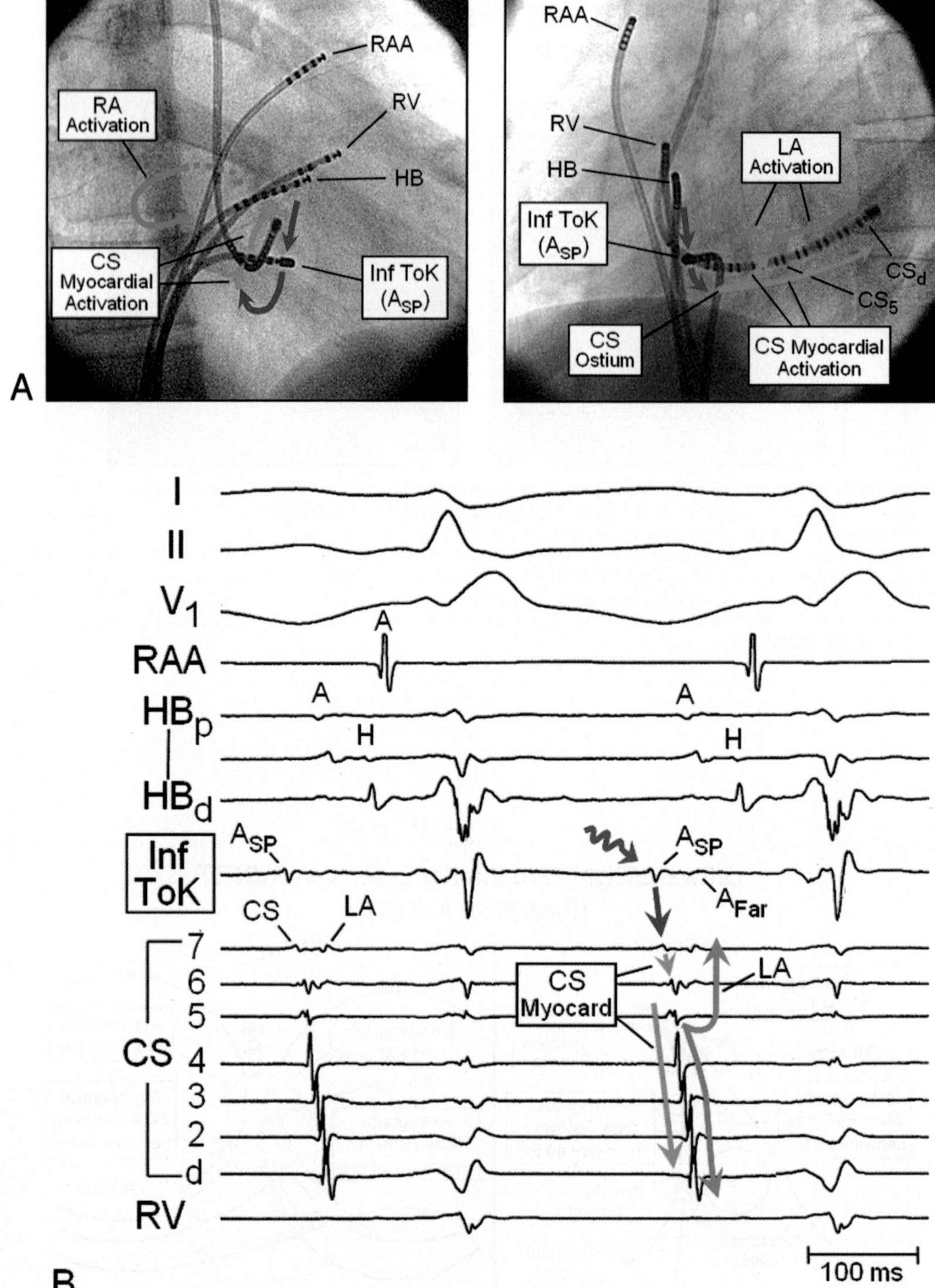

Figure 59-37 Pattern of retrograde activation during Leftward-Rightward Inferior Extension (Fast/Slow) AVNRT. **A,** Radiographs in the RAO and LAO projections showing the catheter positions recording the electrograms. *Arrows* illustrate direction of activation: *Blue arrows*: retrograde conduction over the rightward inferior extension, activating the inferior triangle of Koch (Inf ToK), generating the retrograde A_{SP} potential and activating the floor of the coronary sinus (CS) ostium. *Brown arrows*: leftward activation of the coronary sinus myocardium (CS), beginning at the floor of the CS ostium and activating the CS roof to activate the left atrium. *Solid green arrow*, LAO projection: rapid left atrial activation (LA activation), propagating laterally (same direction as for CS myocardial activation). *Dotted green arrow*, LAO projection: reversal in direction of left atrial activation toward the septum and then superiorly to the interatrial septum. *Dotted green line*, RAO projection: activation across the interatrial septum from left atrium to right atrium. *Solid green arrow*, RAO projection: right atrial activation (RA Activation) beginning at the septum. **B,** Electrograms show long His-atrial (H-A) and short A-H intervals typical of Fast/Slow AVNRT. Retrograde conduction over the rightward inferior extension (*squiggly blue arrow*) results in earliest activation at the inferior triangle of Koch (A_{SP} potential in the Inf ToK electrogram) with propagation to the floor of the coronary sinus ostium (*solid blue arrow*). Activation enters the coronary sinus at the floor of the CS ostium (*short brown arrow*) and propagates leftwards along the coronary sinus myocardium (*long brown arrow*, CS Myocard). The coronary sinus myocardium activates the left atrium in the region of the CS_5-CS_6 electrograms (*green arrows*). Left atrial activation propagates rapidly in the lateral direction, simultaneous with the coronary sinus myocardium (*lower green and brown arrows*), resulting in a single (fused) potential in electrograms CS_5 to CS_d. Turning of the atrial wave front towards the septum (*upper green arrow*), produces conduction delay, resulting in two distinct potentials in the proximal CS electrograms (CS myocardial potential followed by left atrial potential). Left atrial activation propagates to the interatrial septum to activate the right atrium and produce the atrial potential recorded in the His bundle (HB) electrograms (labeled A) and the far-field atrial potential recorded from the inferior triangle of Koch (labeled A_{Far}). The A_{Far} potential is generated from the right atrium posterior to the eustachian ridge. HB, His bundle; RAO, right anterior oblique; RAA, right atrial appendage; LAO, left anterior oblique; RV, right ventricle.

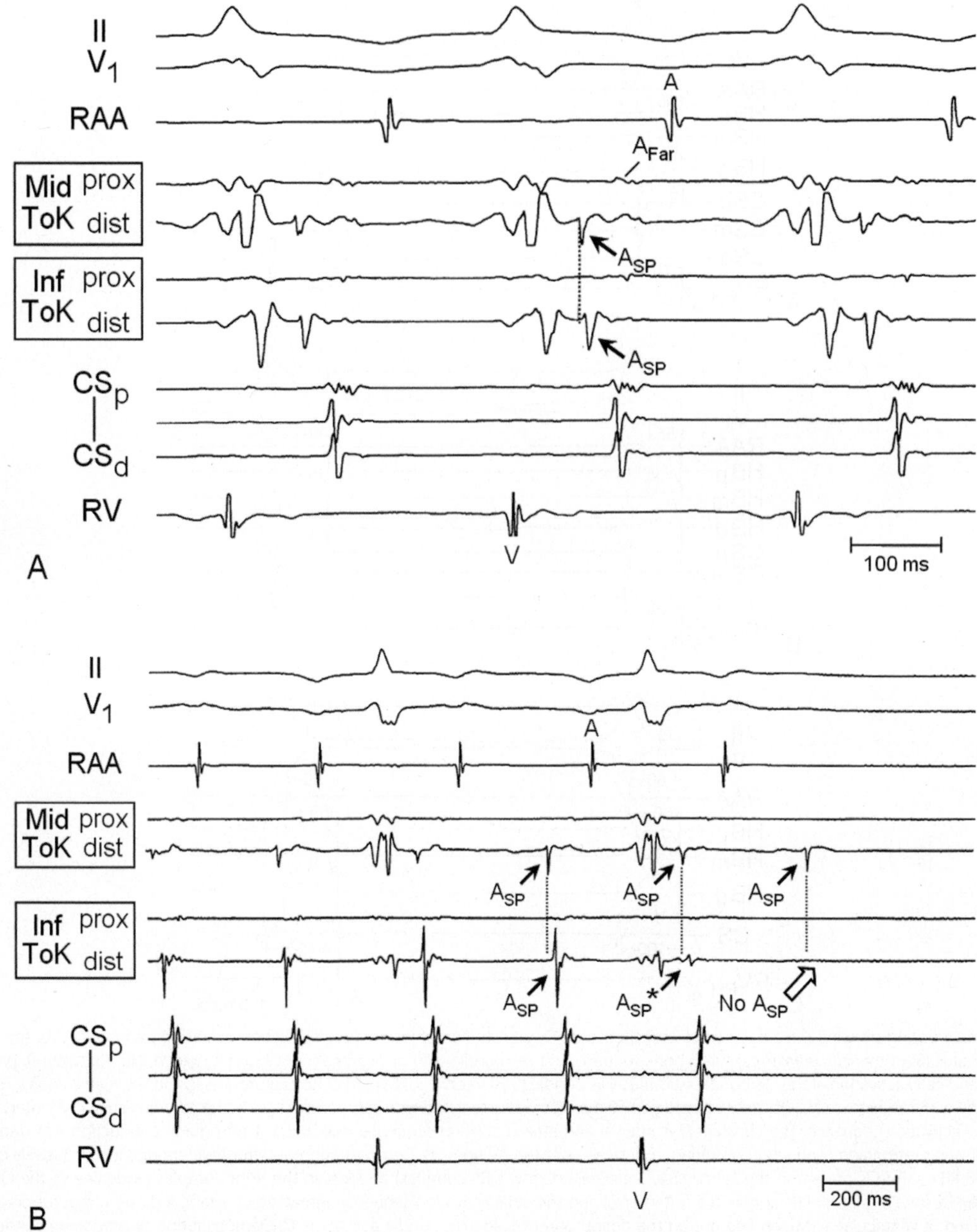

Figure 59-38 Evidence during Leftward-Rightward Inferior Extension atrioventricular nodal reentrant tachycardia (AVNRT) (i.e., Fast/Slow AVNRT) that retrograde slow pathway activation must reach the coronary sinus for the left and right atria to be activated. **A,** During Fast/Slow AVNRT, the electrogram recorded from the inferior triangle of Koch (Inf ToK) at the level of the mid–coronary sinus (CS) ostium exhibits a large, sharp retrograde A_{SP} potential (*arrow*, A_{SP}) preceding activation in the coronary sinus. The electrogram recorded superior to this site, at the mid-septal tricuspid annulus (between the level of the His bundle and CS, Mid ToK electrogram), shows a retrograde A_{SP} potential (*top arrow*, A_{SP}), recorded 9 ms earlier than the A_{SP} potential recorded in the Inf ToK electrogram. The order of the retrograde A_{SP} potentials suggests conduction in the triangle of Koch in the superior-to-inferior direction. **B,** Continuation of the episode of Fast/Slow AVNRT with 2:1 atrioventricular block. The A_{SP} potential is unchanged in the Mid ToK electrogram. However, the A_{SP} potential in the Inf ToK electrogram becomes smaller in amplitude, delayed, and then absent (*open arrow*, No A_{SP}), indicating block inferior to the Mid ToK region and superior to the Inf ToK region. Loss of the A_{SP} potential in the Inf ToK electrogram is associated with loss of activation in the coronary sinus, left atrium, and right atrium and termination of the tachycardia. This suggests that activation within the triangle of Koch may not be able to activate the right atrium directly owing to block across the eustachian ridge. RAA, right atrial appendage; RV, right ventricle. (Modified from Jackman WM, Lockwood D, Nakagawa H, et al: Catheter ablation of atrioventricular nodal reentrant tachycardia. In Wilber DJ, Packer DL, Stevenson WG [eds]: Catheter Ablation of Cardiac Arrhythmias: Basic Concepts and Clinical Applications, 3rd ed. Blackwell Futura, 2008, pp 120-148.)

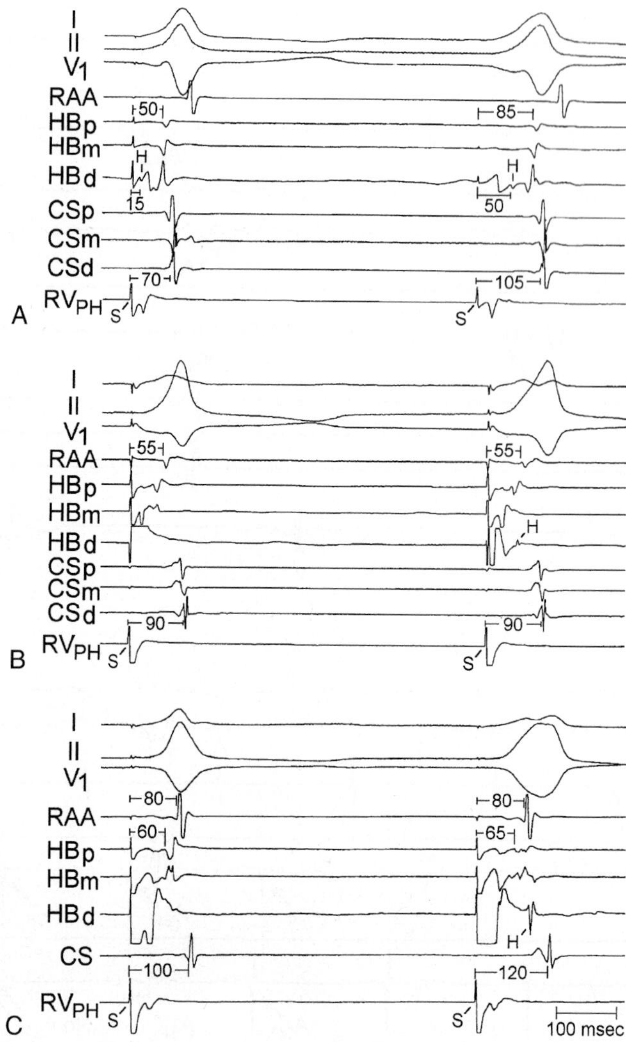

Figure 59-39 Para-Hisian pacing showing three basic types of response. **A,** Demonstration of retrograde conduction occurring exclusively over the atrioventricular (AV) node. The pacing stimulus (S) in the *left complex* captured both ventricle and His bundle (HB) or proximal right bundle branch (HB-RB capture), producing a relatively narrow QRS complex and early activation of the His bundle (stimulus–His bundle [S-H] interval = 15 ms). HB-RB capture was lost in the *right complex*, resulting in widening of the QRS complex and a 35-ms increase in S-H interval from 15 to 50 ms. This was associated with a 35-ms increase in the stimulus-atrial (S-A) interval without a change in the retrograde atrial activation sequence. The constant H-A interval and atrial activation sequence indicate that retrograde conduction was dependent only on His bundle activation, indicating retrograde conduction occurring exclusively over the AV node. **B,** Demonstration of retrograde conduction exclusively over an anteroseptal accessory pathway. HB-RB capture is present in the *left complex* (relatively narrow QRS complex) and lost in the right complex (widening of the QRS complex and an increase in S-H interval). Despite loss of HB-RB capture, the S-A interval and the atrial activation sequence remained constant, indicating that retrograde conduction was dependent on the timing of ventricular activation and not on the timing of retrograde His bundle activation. **C,** Demonstration of retrograde conduction over both an anteroseptal accessory pathway and the AV node. With loss of HB-RB capture (*right complex*), the atrial activation sequence changed, indicating the presence of retrograde conduction over both an accessory pathway and the AV node (different amount of atria being activated by the accessory pathway and the AV node between HB-RB capture and HB-RB noncapture). The S-A interval recorded from the right atrial appendage (RAA) remained constant (80 ms) with loss of HB-RB capture (*right complex*), indicating that this region of the atria was activated by the accessory pathway during HB-RB capture and HB-RB noncapture. With loss of HB-RB capture, the S-A interval lengthened by 5 ms in the HB electrogram and 20 ms in the CS electrogram, which represented smaller increments than the amount of increase in S-H interval, indicating that these regions of atria were activated by the AV node during HB-RB capture and by the accessory pathway during HB-RB noncapture. RV_{PH}, para-Hisian right ventricle.

References

1. Josephson ME, Kastor JA: Paroxysmal supraventricular tachycardia: Is the atrium a necessary link? Circulation 54:430-435, 1976.
2. Jackman WM, Beckman KJ, McClelland JH, et al: Treatment of supraventricular tachycardia due to atrioventricular nodal reentry, by radiofrequency catheter ablation of slow-pathway conduction. N Engl J Med 327:313-318, 1992.
3. Haissaguerre M, Gaita F, Fischer B, et al: Elimination of atrioventricular nodal reentrant tachycardia using discrete slow potentials to guide application of radiofrequency energy. Circulation 85:2162-2175, 1992.
4. Lee MA, Morady F, Kadish A, et al: Catheter modification of the atrioventricular junction with radiofrequency energy for control of atrioventricular nodal reentry tachycardia. Circulation 83:827-835, 1991.
5. Lo HM, Lin FY, Tseng CD, et al: Selective surgical ablation of the slow atrioventricular

nodal pathway by posterior perinodal dissection. Am J Cardiol 71:1457-1459, 1993.

6. McGuire MA, Lau KC, Johnson DC, et al: Patients with two types of atrioventricular junctional (AV nodal) reentrant tachycardia: Evidence that a common pathway of nodal tissue is not present above the reentrant circuit. Circulation 83:1232-1246, 1991.
7. Ross DL, Johnson DC, Denniss AR, et al: Curative surgery for atrioventricular junctional ("AV nodal") reentrant tachycardia. J Am Coll Cardiol 6:1383-1392, 1985.
8. Jackman WM, Beckman KJ, McClelland JH, et al: Participation of atrial myocardium (posterior septum) in AV nodal reentrant tachycardia: Evidence from resetting by atrial extrastimuli [abstract]. Pacing Clin Electrophysiol 14:646, 1991.
9. McGuire M, Bourke J, Robotin M, et al: High resolution mapping of Koch's triangle using sixty electrodes in humans with atrioventricular junctional (AV nodal) reentrant tachycardia. Circulation 88:2315-2328, 1993.
10. Yamabe H, Misumi I, Fukushima H, et al: Electrophysiological delineation of the tachycardia circuit in atrioventricular nodal reentrant tachycardia. Circulation 100:621-627, 1999.
11. Oglin JE, Ursell P, Kao AK, Lesh MD: Pathological findings following slow pathway ablation for AV nodal reentrant tachycardia. J Cardiovasc Electrophysiol 7:625-631, 1996.
12. Denes P, Wu D, Dhingra R, et al: Dual atrioventricular nodal pathways: A common electrophysiological response. Br Heart J 37:1069-1076, 1975.
13. Denes P, Wu D, Dhingra RC, et al: Demonstration of dual A-V nodal pathways in patients with paroxysmal supraventricular tachycardia. Circulation 48:549-555, 1973.
14. Moulton KP, Wang X, Xu Y, et al: High incidence of dual AV nodal pathway physiology in patients undergoing radiofrequency ablation of accessory pathways [abstract]. Circulation 82:iii-319, 1990.
15. Hazlitt HA, Beckman KJ, McClelland JH, et al: Prevalence of slow AV nodal pathway potentials in patients without AV nodal reentrant tachycardia [abstract]. J Am Coll Cardiol 21:281A, 1993.
16. Sung RJ, Waxman HL, Saksena S, Juma Z: Sequence of retrograde atrial activation in patients with dual atrioventricular nodal pathways. Circulation 64:1059-1067, 1981.
17. Otomo K, Beckman KJ, McClelland JH, et al: Resetting response suggests the absence of an upper common pathway in Slow/Fast and presence in Slow/Slow atrioventricular nodal reentrant tachycardia [abstract]. Pacing Clin Electrophysiol 19:730, 1996.
18. Lockwood DJ, Po SS, Beckman KJ, et al: Late extrastimuli (after atrial activation) captures rightward inferior extension of AV node (slow pathway) resetting slow/fast AV nodal reentrant tachycardia in 5 patients [abstract]. Heart Rhythm 5:S165, 2008.
19. Tondo C, Otomo K, McClelland J, et al: Atrioventricular nodal reentrant tachycardia: Is the reentrant circuit always confined in the right atrium? [abstract]. J Am Coll Cardiol 27:159A, 1996.
20. Tondo C, Beckman KJ, McClelland JH, et al: Response to radiofrequency catheter ablation suggests that the coronary sinus forms part of the reentrant circuit in some patients with atrioventricular nodal reentrant tachycardia [abstract]. Circulation 94:i-380, 1996.
21. Antz M, Scherlag BJ, Patterson E, et al: Electrophysiology of the right anterior approach to the atrioventricular node: Studies in vivo and in the isolated perfused dog heart. J Cardiovasc Electrophysiol 8:47-61, 1997.
22. Tchou P, Cheng Y, Mowrey K, et al: Relation of the atrial input sites to the dual atrioventricular nodal pathways: Crossing of conduction curves generated with posterior and anterior pacing. J Cardiovasc Electrophysiol 8:1133-1144, 1997.
23. Medkour D, Becker AE, Khalife K, Billette J: Anatomic and functional characteristics of a slow posterior AV nodal pathway: Role in dual-pathway physiology and reentry. Circulation 98:164-174, 1998.
24. Wu J, Wu J, Olgin J, et al: Mechanisms underlying the reentrant circuit of atrioventricular nodal reentrant tachycardia in isolated canine atrioventricular nodal preparation using optical mapping. Circ Res 88:1189-1195, 2001.
25. Altemose GT, Scott LR, Miller JM: Atrioventricular nodal reentrant tachycardia requiring ablation on the mitral annulus. J Cardiovasc Electrophysiol 11: 1281-1284, 2000.
26. Sorbera C, Cohen M, Woolfe P, Kalapatapu SR: Atrioventricular nodal reentry tachycardia: Slow pathway ablation using the transeptal approach. PACE 23:1343-1349, 2000.
27. Scherlag BJ, Patterson E, Jackman WM, Lazzara R: The elusive extracellular AV nodal potential: Studies from the canine heart, ex vivo. J Intervent Cardiac Electrophysiol 7:39-52, 2002.
28. Patterson E, Scherlag BJ: Decremental conduction in the posterior and anterior AV nodal inputs. J Intervent Cardiac Electrophysiol 7:137-148, 2002.
29. Jackman WM, Lockwood D, Nakagawa H, et al: Catheter ablation of atrioventricular nodal reentrant tachycardia. In Wilber DJ, Packer DL, Stevenson WG (eds): Catheter Ablation of Cardiac Arrythmias: Basic Concepts and Clinical Applications, 3rd ed. Blackwell Futura, 2008, pp 120-148.
30. Patterson E, Scherlag BJ: Delineation of AV conduction properties by selective transection: Effects on antegrade and retrograde transmission. J Intervent Cardiac Electrophysiol 13:95-105, 2005.
31. Ashar MS, Otomo K, Wang Z, et al: Late activation in the triangle of Koch suggests block at the tendon of Todaro in Slow/Fast AVNRT [abstract]. Pace Clin Electrophysiol 25:II-542, 2002.
32. Otomo K, Antz M, Beckman KJ, et al: Left atrial activation precedes right atrial activation in Slow/Fast atrioventricular nodal reentrant tachycardia [abstract]. Circulation 94:i-683, 1996.
33. Katritsis DG, Ellenbogen KA, Becker AE. Atrial activation during atrioventricular nodal reentrant tachycardia: Studies on retrograde fast pathway conduction. Heart Rhythm 3:993-1000, 2006.
34. Becker AE, Anderson RH: Morphology of the human atrioventricular junction area. In Wellens HJJ, Lie KI, Janse MJ (eds): The Conduction System of the Heart: Structure, Function and Clinical Implications. Philadelphia, Lea & Febiger, 1976, pp 263-286.
35. Patterson E, Scherlag BJ: Fast pathway–His bundle connections in the rabbit heart. J Intervent Cardiac Electrophysiol 10:121-129, 2004.
36. Inoue S, Becker AE: Posterior extensions of the human compact atrioventricular node: A neglected anatomic feature of potential clinical significance. Circulation 97:188-193, 1998.
37. Antz M, Otomo K, Arruda M, et al: Electrical conduction between the right atrium and the left atrium via the musculature of the coronary sinus. Circulation 98:1790-1795, 1998.
38. Sun y, Arruda MS, Otomo K, et al: Coronary sinus–ventricular accessory connections producing posteroseptal and left posterior accessory pathways: Incidence and electrophysiological identification. Circulation 106:1362-1367; 2002.
39. Spach MS, Josephson ME: Initiating reentry: The role of nonuniform anisotropy in small circuits. J Cardiovasc Electrophysiol 5:182-209, 1994.
40. Jentzer JH, Goyal R, Williamson BD, et al: Analysis of junctional ectopy during radiofrequency ablation of the slow pathway in patients with atrioventricular nodal reentrant tachycardia. Circulation 90:2820-2826, 1994.
41. Racker DK: Atrioventricular node and input pathways: A correlated gross anatomical and histological study of the canine atrioventricular junctional region. Anat Rec 224:336-354, 1989.
42. Inoue S, Becker AE, Gaita F: Interruption of the posterior extension of the compact atrioventricular node underlies successful radiofrequency ablation of atrioventricular nodal reentrant tachycardia [abstract]. Pacing Clin Electrophysiol 21:796, 1998.
43. Kuck KH, Kuch B, Bleifeld W: Multiple antegrade and retrograde AV nodal pathways: Demonstration by multiple discontinuities in the AV nodal conduction curves and echo time intervals. Pacing Clin Electrophysiol 7:656-662, 1984.
44. Foresti S, Lockwood DJ, Po SS, et al: Two distinct retrograde slow pathways are consistent with rightward and leftward posterior extensions of the AV node [abstract]. Heart Rhythm 1:S45, 2004.
45. Antz M, Scherlag BJ, Otomo K, et al: Evidence for multiple atrio-AV nodal inputs in the normal dog heart. J Cardiovasc Electrophysiol 9:395-408, 1998.
46. Sheahan RG, Klein GJ, Yee R, et al: Atrioventricular node reentry with "smooth" AV node function curves: A different arrhythmia substrate? Circulation 93:969-972, 1996.

47. Baerman J, Wang X, Jackman WM: Atrioventricular nodal reentry with an antegrade slow pathway and retrograde slow pathway: Clinical and electrophysiologic properties [abstract]. J Am Coll Cardiol 17:338A, 1991.
48. Goldberger J, Brooks R, Kadish A: Physiology of "atypical" atrioventricular junctional reentrant tachycardia occurring following radiofrequency catheter modification of the atrioventricular node. Pacing Clin Electrophysiol 15:2270-2282, 1992.
49. Anselme F, Papageorgiou P, Monahan K, et al: Presence and significance of the left atrionodal connection during atrioventricular nodal reentrant tachycardia. Am J Cardiol 83:1530-1536, 1999.
50. Li YG, Bender B, Bogun F, et al: Location of the lower turnaround point in typical AV nodal reentrant tachycardia: A quantitative model. J Cardiovasc Electrophysiol 11:34-40, 2000.
51. A, Josephson ME, Saoudi N: Entrainment of typical AV nodal reentrant tachycardia using para-Hisian pacing: Evidence for a lower common pathway within the AV node. J Cardiovasc Electrophysiol 10:655-661, 1999.
52. Thibault B, Beckman K, McClelland J, et al: Use of ventricular stimuli to examine lower common pathway in S/F AVNRT [abstract]. Circulation 90:i-214, 1994.
53. Hirao K, Otomo K, Wang X, et al: Para-Hisian pacing: A new method for differentiating retrograde conduction over an accessory AV pathway from conduction over the AV node. Circulation 94:1027-1035, 1996.
54. Heidbüchel H, Beckman K, McClelland J, et al: Presence or absence of a lower common pathway differentiates Slow/Slow from Slow/Fast AV nodal reentrant tachycardia [abstract]. Pacing Clin Electrophysiol 17:759, 1994.
55. Heidbüchel H, Ector H, De Were FV: Prospective evaluation of the length of the lower common pathway in the different diagnosis of various forms of AV nodal reentrant tachycardia. Pacing Clin Electrophysiol 21:209-216, 1998.
56. Heidbuchel H, Jackman WM: Characterization of subforms of AV nodal reentrant tachycardia. Europace 6:316-329, 2004.
57. Heidbuchel H, Jackman WM: Catheter ablation of atypical atrioventricular nodal reentrant tachycardia. In Zipes DP, Haissaguerre M (eds): Catheter Ablation of Arrhythmias. Armonk, NY, Futura, 2002, pp 249-276.
58. Ho SW, McComb JM, Scott CD, Anderson RH: Morphology of the cardiac conduction system in patients with electrophysiologically proven dual atrioventricular nodal pathways. J Cardiovasc Electrophysiol 4:504-512, 1993.
59. Brechenmacher C: Atrio-His bundle tracts. Br Heart J 37:853-855, 1975.
60. Otomo K, Okamura H, Noda T, et al. "Left variant" atypical atrioventricular nodal reentrant tachycardia: Electrophysiological characteristics and effect of slow pathway ablation within coronary sinus. J Cardiovasc Electrophysiol 17:1177-1183, 2006.
61. Thibault B, Beckman K, McClelland J, et al: Variation in H-A interval suggests a lower common pathway in Slow/Slow AVNRT [abstract]. Pacing Clin Electrophysiol 17:840, 1994.
62. Benditt DG, Pritchett EL, Smith WM, Gallagher JJ: Ventriculoatrial intervals: Diagnostic use in paroxysmal supraventricular tachycardia. Ann Intern Med 91:161-166, 1979.

Atrial Arrhythmias in Congenital Heart Disease 60

John K. Triedman

CHAPTER OUTLINE

General Considerations

The development of advanced surgical techniques for congenital heart disease (CHD) has created a burgeoning population of children and young adults with significant cardiac disease. Approximately 1 million people have some form of CHD in the United States, with 15% to 20% requiring surgical intervention. Atrial arrhythmias are prevalent among patients with CHD, particularly long-term survivors who have undergone extensive atrial surgeries. Atypical atrial reentrant tachycardias and bradycardia secondary to sinus node dysfunction are particularly common. These arrhythmias, which are rarely seen in young, anatomically normal hearts, appear to be associated with the myocardial hypertrophy and fibrosis caused by cyanosis and chronic hemodynamic overload, and superimposed surgical scarring. The natural history and management of these arrhythmias have emerged as a major focus of interest for physicians working with these patients.

The concomitant presence of CHD in a patient with an arrhythmia significantly alters the clinical interpretation of arrhythmia symptoms, assessment of the potential severity of the arrhythmia, and the safety and feasibility of various therapies. Thus, in addition to analyzing a patient's arrhythmia complaint, the physician must obtain complete and specific knowledge of the patient's cardiovascular anatomy, as well as the consequences of that anatomy and associated surgical interventions on cardiovascular function.

This chapter reviews the pathophysiology, natural history, evaluation, and management of atrial arrhythmias in patients with CHD.

Clinical Background

In adult patients with acquired heart disease, precise and clinically useful assessment of the risk of cardiac sudden death has been made possible by large, prospective clinical studies. These patients can be segregated into large, relatively homogeneous groups with similarly elevated risks (e.g., patients in the first year after myocardial infarction, or with depressed ejection fraction). By contrast, CHD populations are small, anatomically diverse, and subject to continually evolving surgical therapies and have relatively low rates of sudden death, with mortality rates less than 2% per year in even "high-risk" groups.[1] As a result, it is difficult to identify similarly specific risk factors in CHD and to measure the effect of interventions on unambiguous endpoints, such as survival. Although the natural history of arrhythmia and death in older patients with CHD remains incompletely understood, it nevertheless is clear that arrhythmia is prevalent and sudden death is a major contributor to their overall mortality.[2] Anatomic classification of congenital heart defects is complex, but three major categories, as characterized in Table 60-1, constitute a large percentage of patients with CHD and concomitant arrhythmia, owing to their frequency in the population and high incidence of arrhythmia. Certain clinical findings also have been associated with adverse outcomes for a variety of anatomic defects, including the presence of residual hemodynamic defects, performance of surgical repair later in life, and longer duration of follow-up.

Intra-atrial Reentrant Tachycardia

Overview

Various names have been proposed for the atrial reentrant tachycardias common to patients with CHD, including atrial flutter, atypical atrial flutter, intra-atrial reentrant tachycardia, macroreentrant atrial tachycardia, and incisional atrial tachycardia. This varied terminology reflects provisional attempts by different investigators to clarify the clinical and electrophysiologic manifestations of this problem by careful description. In this chapter, the term *intra-atrial reentrant tachycardia* (IART) is used, which specifically excludes the diagnosis of atrial fibrillation.

Although uncommon in normal hearts, IART is a common late complication of many types of CHD. Like atrial flutter, IART has a stable cycle length and P wave morphology, suggesting that it is organized by a fixed myocardial substrate. A typical, ambulatory electrocardiographic example is shown in Figure 60-1, demonstrating the frequent association of sinus node dysfunction and variable AV conduction. IART usually is considered to be a right atrial arrhythmia, whereas atrial fibrillation is more commonly a manifestation of left atrial disease. Comparison of the postoperative abnormalities of the right atrium seen in patients with CHD with the abnormalities of left atrial size and function seen in patients with acquired heart disease would suggest that this is a credible generalization. Organized atrial reentry arising from the left atrium has been described,[3] however, and the right atrium also has now been implicated in the generation and maintenance of some types of atrial fibrillation. The occurrence of this CHD-associated "tachy-brady" syndrome results in a clinical spectrum of arrhythmia presentations that ranges from occult, asymptomatic arrhythmia to sudden death. Incessant or recurrent arrhythmia

Table 60-1 Congenital Heart Defects Associated with Arrhythmia

Mustard and Senning procedures	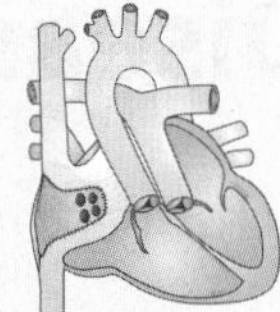	Patients born with transposition of the great vessels in the 1970s through the early 1990s received palliative surgical treatment consisting of the construction of intra-atrial baffles either using synthetic material (the *Mustard procedure*) or by folding and augmentation of the atrial wall (the *Senning procedure*). With both approaches, caval and pulmonary venous blood is redirected to correct cyanosis, and the right ventricle is used as the systemic ventricle.
Fontan procedure	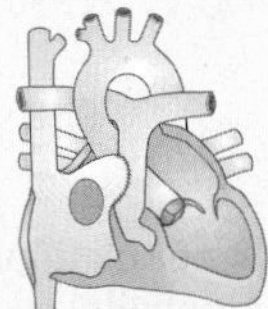	Many congenital heart defects have common anatomic features that preclude surgical septation of the ventricles, resulting in univentricular physiology. The common endpoint of staged surgical palliation is the *Fontan procedure*, which uses the single ventricle as the systemic ventricle and directs systemic venous return to the pulmonary arteries. Several variants have been devised; currently, an anastomosis between superior vena cava and pulmonary artery is created and an intercaval connection is made by tube graft or intra-atrial baffle.
Repaired tetralogy of Fallot	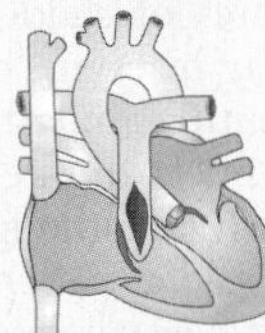	The prevalence of tetralogy of Fallot, the relatively high survival rate through childhood without operation, and the early date at which reparative surgery became available have resulted in a large group of patients with relatively homogeneous clinical experience. Repair involves closure of the ventricular septal defect and relief of right ventricular obstruction, often requiring both ventriculotomy and atriotomy.

Adapted from Triedman JK: Arrhythmias in adults with congenital heart disease. Heart 87:383-389, 2002.

may cause gradual hemodynamic deterioration, and vice versa, often resulting in a vicious circle of clinical decompensation. Thrombosis and thromboembolic events also are associated with IART. Symptoms, frequent need for hospitalization, and the management of cardiac devices and antiarrhythmic drugs constitute a significant burden on quality of life.

Pathogenic processes that underlie IART have now been characterized by observational and experimental studies. Its prevalence among patients who have undergone surgical procedures involving extensive atrial dissection and repair indicates a particular correlation with surgical injury, and animal models explicitly patterned after surgical procedures associated with IART result in tachycardias similar to those observed clinically.

Epidemiology and Natural History

IART is common among patients with CHD. An early, retrospective multicenter study of young patients with "atrial flutter" showed that more than 80% had associated repaired or unrepaired CHD, whereas only 8% had anatomically and functionally normal hearts.[4] Although IART has been described as a long-term complication after almost every form of cardiac surgery, certain combinations of CHD and surgical procedures are associated with a considerably increased prevalence. These include procedures involving an atriotomy or other significant surgical manipulation of the atrium, such as atrial septal defect (ASD) repair, Mustard and Senning palliations of transposition of the great arteries, construction of Fontan anastomoses for palliation

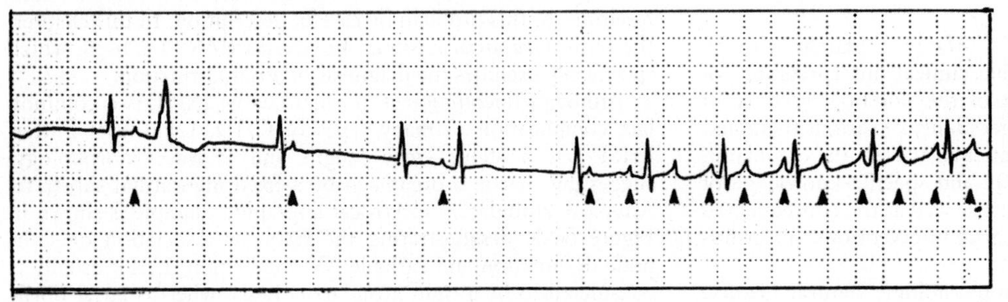

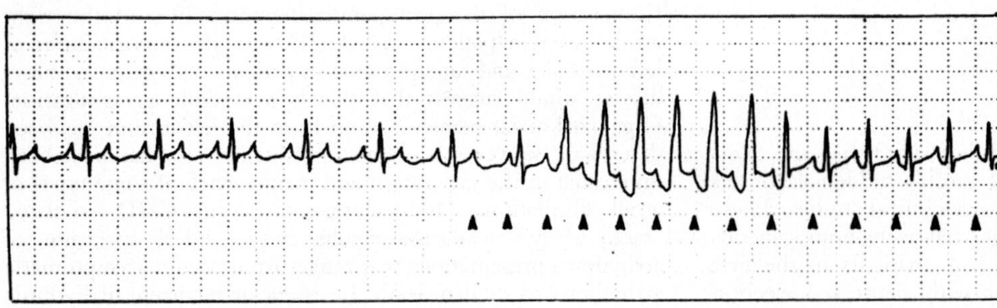

Figure 60-1 A typical, ambulatory electrocardiographic record of the onset of intra-atrial reentrant tachycardia in a patient with concomitant sinus node dysfunction and junctional escape rhythm. Atrioventricular conduction is variable, and transient QRS aberration mimicking ventricular tachycardia occurs in this case, with sudden increase in conducted rate.

Table 60-2 Occurrence of Intra-atrial Reentrant Tachycardia after Fontan Procedure

Study	No. of Patients	Conduit*	APC	TCPC		Follow-up
Gelatt et al, 1994[9]	269	11%	30%	17%	S	3.8 y
Cecchin et al, 1995[10]	132	—	42%	26%	S	3.2 y
Durongpisitkul et al, 1996[8]	499	—	17%	22%	NS	5.0 y
Fishberger et al, 1997[7]	278	38%	28%	5%	NS	5.1 y
Weipert et al, 2004[11]	162	17%	20%	—	NS	12.4 y

*Right atrial–right ventricular or right atrial–pulmonary artery conduit.

APC, atriopulmonary connection; S/NS, statistically significant/no statistically significant difference in frequency between surgical approaches; TCPC, total cavopulmonary connection.

of single-ventricle physiology, correction of tetralogy of Fallot, and repair of anomalous pulmonary venous connection.

Between one fourth and one third of patients who have undergone the Fontan and Mustard procedures have inducible sustained atrial tachycardia,[5] a proportion similar to that in patients in whom atrial tachycardias develop spontaneously years after those operations. A study of nearly 500 early survivors of the Mustard procedure identified an IART prevalence of 27% at 20 years of follow-up, and 60% had sinus node dysfunction, frequently in association with IART. Sudden death occurred in 6.5% of patients over a mean follow-up period of 11.6 years.[1] Among patients with single-ventricle physiology and the Fontan procedure, the natural history of atrial arrhythmia is described by retrospective studies from several large cardiac surgical centers totaling approximately 1400 patients. These data indicate that between 25% and 50% of patients who have undergone the Fontan procedure will have clinical documentation of IART by 10 years of follow-up (Table 60-2).[6-10] Risk factors for IART include older age at operation and longer follow-up. Patients who have undergone the lateral tunnel variant of the Fontan with cavopulmonary anastomosis appear to be less prone to the development of atrial tachycardia than those who had the older variants of the Fontan procedure (connection of the entire right atrium to the pulmonary artery or vestigial right ventricle by anastomosis or conduit).[6,11] The notion that these tachycardias are a by-product of surgical scarring has been put forward as one rationale for the extracardiac Fontan, performed using an intercaval tube graft and minimizing atrial manipulation. Although the incidence of atrial tachycardia may be reduced using this approach,[12,13] it does not appear to be eliminated. Finally, a retrospective study on the occurrence of atrial flutter in 53 patients with tetralogy of Fallot was performed by Roos-Hesselink and coworkers. They found that sinus node dysfunction and IART each were present in approximately one third of the population after a mean follow-up period of 18 years, more prevalent than ventricular tachycardia, and more likely to be associated with symptoms.[14]

A retrospective follow-up study of IART after CHD surgery revealed a sudden-death mortality rate of 10% over a period of 6.5 years.[4] Although clearly associating IART occurrence with congestive heart failure and thrombosis, a more recent study did not identify IART as a specific risk factor for death in multivariate analyses.[2] Reports of stroke after cardioversion of IART in CHD patients are rare; nevertheless, intravascular and intracardiac thromboses often are associated with the Fontan procedure. Co-occurrence of IART may further promote thrombosis, and a prevalence of intracardiac thrombi in 42% of patients undergoing echocardiography before cardioversion has been reported[15] (Fig. 60-2). It is not clear whether atrial tachycardias promote such events or are simply a common comorbid condition in these sick patients.

The natural history of intra-atrial reentrant tachycardia is characterized by increasingly frequent recurrences of tachycardia. A group of patients with IART from Children's Hospital Boston was retrospectively examined for response to treatment with a variety of antiarrhythmic medications. In those unpublished data, recurrence rates of 60% to 80% were noted at 2-year follow-up evaluation in all patients, regardless of therapy. Among patients undergoing ablative procedures in an attempt to control their arrhythmias, a pattern of gradually increasing frequency of arrhythmia recurrence over a period of 12 to 24 months before ablation attempt was noted.

Electrocardiographic Manifestations

Intra-atrial reentrant tachycardias occurring in patients with CHD may sometimes share the electrocardiographic characteristics of common type I atrial flutter—a sawtooth baseline

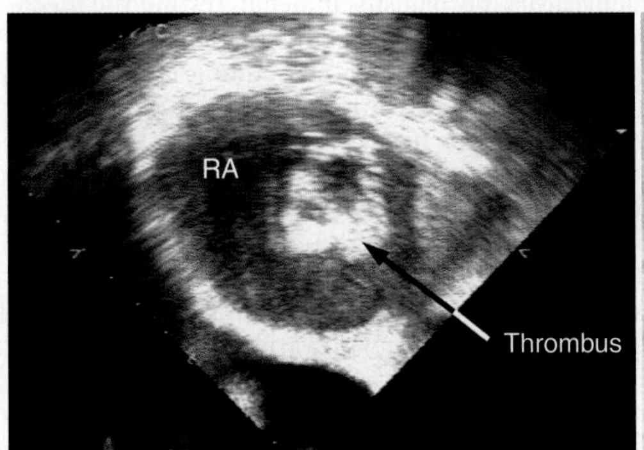

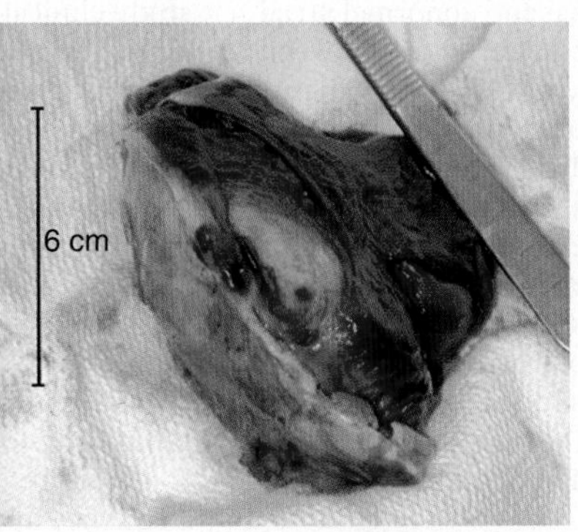

Figure 60-2 Giant right atrial thrombi may be observed at late follow-up evaluation in patients who underwent a Fontan procedure and subsequently acquire chronic, recurrent intra-atrial reentrant tachycardia. **Left panel,** Echocardiographic identification of floating thrombus in the right atrium (RA). **Right panel,** Large thrombus adherent to right atrial wall was removed at the time of Fontan revision surgery.

Table 60-3 Electrocardiographic Manifestations of Intra-atrial Reentrant Tachycardia

- Aberrant but uniform P wave or flutter morphology
- Constant cycle length, but often longer than common atrial flutter
- Multiple ECG morphologies in an individual patient
- Variable AV block, may conduct 1:1
- Sudden onset and offset
- Initiated and terminated by pacing, entrainable

AV, atrioventricular; ECG, electrocardiogram.

of cycle length 200 to 250 ms with 2:1 or higher degree of AV block. Atypical electrocardiographic morphologies are common, however, being seen in approximately 70% of ECG records of IART. P waves are frequently discernible, with long periods of isoelectric electrocardiographic baseline. Cycle length typically is significantly longer than that in atrial flutter, especially in patients with a previous Fontan procedure, and often long enough to permit 1:1 AV conduction (Table 60-3). Examination of P wave axes during tachycardia in patients with a variety of congenital diagnoses and reveals that among patients with previous Fontan procedures, P wave axis is more likely to have a leftward axis, whereas patients with previous Mustard and Senning procedures are more likely to have frontal plane P wave axes oriented either superiorly or inferiorly.

Although a specific occurrence of IART generally is electrocardiographically stable, it is common to record multiple, different IART electrocardiograms from a single patient, distinct with regard to cycle length or P wave axis and morphology.[16] Such variability represents different atrial activation patterns based on reversal of activation of a given IART circuit, use of an alternate circuit, or changes in passive activation of the atrium outside the arrhythmia circuit itself.

Schoels and coworkers performed high-density epicardial mapping on animal preparations of a variety of atypical atrial flutters induced using a sterile pericarditis model. After classifying these as either "flutter wave" or P wave tachycardias, they demonstrated that periods of isoelectric atrial diastole were correlated with activation of narrow corridors of slowly conducting atrial tissue, whereas maps of flutter wave tachycardias were less likely to display such features.[17] This electrocardiographic discrimination between flutter wave and P wave morphologies may be practically useful with respect to designing ablation strategies in these patients.

Mechanism of Intra-atrial Reentrant Tachycardia

Detailed understanding of the surgical procedures used for correction of CHD and their relation to normal and abnormal atrial anatomy allows for speculation about the correlations between cardiac anatomy and the electrophysiology of IART. In patients with CHD, the atrial myocardium is subjected to a variety of stresses from birth. In addition to underlying abnormalities of atrial and valvar anatomy, surgical scars are created by atriotomy and baffling, resulting in either complete conduction block or abnormal conduction. New discontinuities of the atrial surface (e.g., atrial septal defects, right atrial to pulmonary artery anastomosis and pulmonary vein reimplantation, bypass cannulation sites) are created in the course of many surgical procedures to address CHD. The resulting geometry of nonconductive structures may be complex and capable of supporting a variety of reentrant circuits.

The importance and sufficiency of surgically created barriers to conduction for maintenance of these IARTs are well established (see later), but the significance of other variables such as fibrosis due to hypertrophy or inflammation, the effects of changes in cardiac autonomic function after congenital heart surgery[18] and bradycardia-mediated alterations in dispersion of refractoriness are less well understood. Although IART most often is a postoperative rhythm, it is also seen in those who have not yet undergone atrial surgery. The atrial myocardium may be subject in CHD to chronic cyanosis and increased atrial wall stress from birth or even fetal life, as well as periodic pericardial inflammation associated with surgical manipulation. Resulting fibrosis and myocyte hypertrophy are likely to affect cell-to-cell conduction in the atrium and may constitute important features of the arrhythmia substrate. Additionally, acquired sinus node dysfunction is common. Bradycardia and the effects of autonomic denervation of the heart associated with surgery may further contribute to arrhythmogenesis by their effects on the dispersion of atrial refractoriness.

Animal Models of Intra-atrial Reentrant Tachycardia

Canine surgical models of atrial reentry have been developed to mimic the surgical anatomy associated with CHD and are particularly relevant to furthering current understanding of postoperative atrial reentrant tachycardias (Fig. 60-3). A sham Mustard procedure for transposition of the great vessels suggested that extensive atrial suture lines are in themselves arrhythmogenic, providing several possible conductive boundaries that may potentially constrain the arrhythmia circuits. A common pathway for most of the observed tachycardias was identified in the free wall of the right atrium, and an incision connecting the atriotomy to the tricuspid valve annulus uniformly resulted in termination of tachycardia. Acute and chronic models of the classic and "lateral tunnel" varieties of the Fontan procedure also have been studied. In these carefully mapped and highly arrhythmogenic preparations, the long, encircling suture line associated with the baffle appeared to serve as the primary determinant of the arrhythmia circuit. Inclusion of the crista terminalis in the suture line further increased vulnerability to arrhythmia. As with the Mustard procedure model, the arrhythmogenic substrate could be eliminated by creating a "blocking" lesion anchoring the suture line to the nonconductive boundary of the tricuspid annulus. The antiarrhythmic effect of such lesions was maximal when the crista terminalis, the sham suture line, and the atriotomy all were incorporated, thus eliminating their negating potential to act as conduction barriers.[19,20]

Studies of Clinical Mechanism

Intra-atrial reentrant tachycardia often is hemodynamically well tolerated. This has allowed the use of mapping technologies to study clinical tachycardia mechanisms in detail, testing the mechanistic hypotheses based on animal models and electrocardiographic observations described earlier, and adding to the current understanding of the specific correlations between atrial anatomic features and electrophysiologic mechanisms. Figure 60-4 presents two examples of IART characterized by electroanatomic mapping. In turn, empirical anatomic approaches to the treatment and prophylaxis of IART based on these observations are being developed and tested. These techniques may use either linear ablative techniques in the catheterization laboratory or application of linear cryolesions in the operating room, with various degrees of direct electrophysiologic guidance.

Acute interruption of an atrial tachycardia circuit by radiofrequency application is strong evidence that the site of ablation

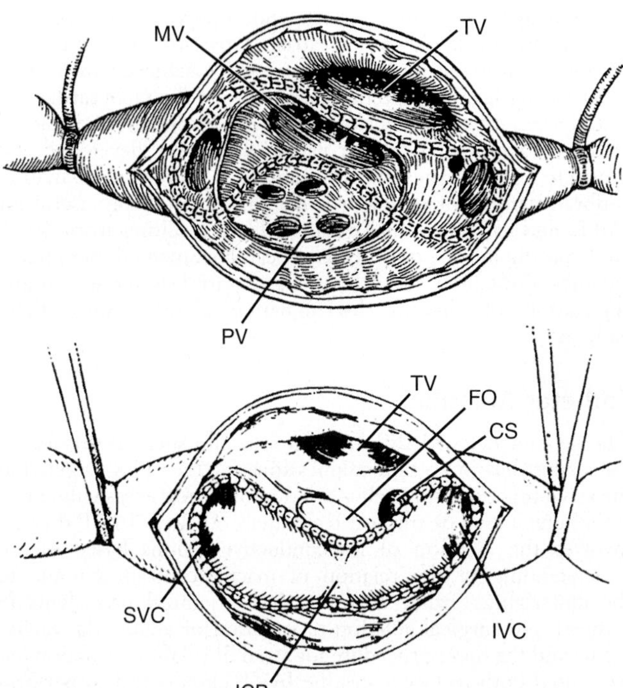

Figure 60-3 Surgeon's view of canine models of postoperative intra-atrial reentrant tachycardia. **Upper panel,** Sham suture line and atriotomy used to model the effect of the Mustard procedure, in which an internal atrial baffle is created to direct caval blood flow across the atrial septum (excised) to the mitral valve, and pulmonary venous return to the tricuspid valve. MV, mitral valve; PV, pulmonary veins; TV, tricuspid valve. **Lower panel,** Sham suture line and atriotomy used to model the effect of the commonly performed "lateral tunnel" variant of Fontan procedure, in which an atrial baffle directs inferior caval blood flow to the superior vena cava, and subsequently to the pulmonary arteries by way of a cavopulmonary anastomosis *(not shown)*. CS, coronary sinus; FO, foramen ovale; ICB, intracardiac baffle; IVC, inferior vena cava; SVC, superior vena cava. (From Gandhi SK, Bromberg BI, Schuessler RB, et al: Characterization and surgical ablation of atrial flutter after the classic Fontan repair. Ann Thorac Surg 61:1666-1678, 1996.)

is a critical component of the tachycardia circuit. Initial evaluation of successful ablation sites in patients with CHD and IART allowed some preliminary grouping of successful sites, demonstrating that critical sites for circuit interruption are dependent to some degree on the primary congenital heart lesion.[21] Patients who have a right-sided AV valve (e.g., those who have had biventricular repairs or previous Mustard and Senning procedures) are most likely to have an IART circuit that is isthmus-dependent, as in patients with the common form of atrial flutter.[22,23] Reentrant circuits using the isthmus but anchored to the ostium of the inferior vena cava ("pericaval reentry") also have been described.[24] Although the AV valve may be either mitral or tricuspid and located in either the systemic or the pulmonary venous atrium, successful ablation for these IART circuits targets the area anterior to the Eustachian ridge. By contrast, patients with a previous Fontan repair have been noted to have sites widely distributed throughout the atrium, but clustered to some extent along the lateral wall of the right atrium.

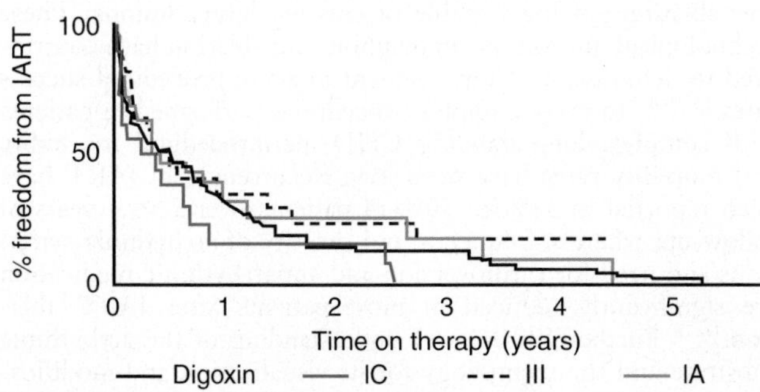

Figure 60-4 Time to recurrence of intra-atrial reentrant tachycardia (IART) in patients receiving digoxin and other classes (IA, IC, III) of antiarrhythmic agents.

Careful analysis of successful ablation sites along the lateral right atrial wall also has highlighted the importance of conduction block caused by right atriotomy incisions in the genesis of "incisional" atrial tachycardias.[23,25] Such incisions may result in tachycardias arising from the free wall or as dual-loop tachycardias in conjunction with an isthmus-dependent circuit. Although the notion that the underlying conduction block is fixed in the atrial myocardium by previous surgical scar seems reasonable, the exact location of atrial scar is at present difficult to predict by imaging. One approach to defining their location is to identify lines of "split" or "double" potentials, which indicate simultaneous recording of multiple discrete activation events at a single location. This model proposes that clusters of double potentials represent a continuous atrial scar that serves as a conduction barrier or "central obstacle" defining the IART circuit, and which can be functionally eliminated by using ablation to extend the scar to a nonconductive boundary. Love and colleagues characterized a variety of anatomic and electrophysiologic central obstacles that served to anchor IART circuits, including the right AV valve (when present), atrial septal defects, and surgical scars located on the free wall of the right atrium.[26] Examples of such IART circuits have been characterized in their entirety in a number of cases by anatomic mapping of the response to entrainment pacing.

The critical role of the crista terminalis and the eustachian ridge in determining the mechanism of common atrial flutter has been well established. Slow transverse conduction across the crista terminalis may be detectable using careful intracardiac mapping techniques, but during atrial flutter, conduction across the crista is effectively blocked, separating the anterior and posterior aspects of the right atrial free wall in a manner that facilitates a long, stable macro-reentrant circuit. Many patients with IART and CHD have activation patterns that are indistinguishable from that of common atrial flutter, so it is likely that the crista terminalis plays a similar role in these tachycardia circuits. Its role in other forms of IART has not been clearly delineated, however.

Accordingly, a relatively small number of corridors or isthmuses are responsible for most or all of the potential IART circuits clinically observed in the right atrium. These include the isthmus of tissue between the inferior vena cava and the right AV valve, the limbic band running between the superior aspect of the fossa ovalis and the superior vena cava, and corridors existing between atrial free wall scars and either the right AV valve annulus or the more posteriorly located crista terminalis. The overall electrical amplitude of endocardial signals measured from the right atrium are markedly decreased in patients with CHD,[27] particularly in the area surrounding the crista and at nearby sites of surgical intervention. Critical channels of active myocardium, coursing amid complex islands of atrial "scar" defined by arbitrary voltage criteria, also have been successfully targeted for ablation. Focal atrial tachycardias, triggered by pacing and arising predominantly from right atrial tissue, also have been observed to occur at low frequency among these patients.[28] Careful mapping studies by de Groot and colleagues suggest that these IARTs represent areas of atrial micro-reentry occurring in circumscribed areas of diseased tissue.[29] Finally, circuits have been anecdotally described that relate anatomically to repair of either atrial septal defect or to the left atrium, as in anomalous pulmonary venous connection or patients with recurrent IART after a maze procedure.

Therapy of Intra-atrial Reentrant Tachycardia

Atrial tachycardias in congenital heart patients often are transient phenomena, symptoms may vary widely from episode to episode, and decisions to intervene therapeutically are a matter of clinical judgment. It is difficult to measure and compare the outcomes of various treatment modalities for IART, especially because the available outcome data have been collected primarily retrospectively in relatively small series of patients with various degrees of illness. Prospective studies will need to involve more structured monitoring for transient atrial events, such as those applied to the study of interventions for atrial fibrillation. Scales incorporating arrhythmia frequency, severity of associated symptoms, and the risk of associated morbidity are being developed[30] but must still be validated.

Cardioversion

The mainstay of acute therapy of IART is cardioversion, typically performed by synchronous direct current shock. Liberman and coworkers have recently showed that minimum successful biphasic shock energies for these atrial reentrant arrhythmias ranged from 0.25 to 0.5 J/kg.[31] Alternative modes of cardioversion are available, including pacing by means of an implanted pacemaker or the transesophageal route and use of ibutilide. In the case of the latter, similar efficacy rates and risk profile for ventricular proarrhythmia as for adult patients have been described.[32] Although thromboembolism complicating cardioversion is rare, echocardiographic observation of atrial thrombi is not infrequent,[16] and echocardiographic screening generally is performed for patients who have been in tachycardia without anticoagulation for more than 48 to 72 hours.

Drug Therapy

Antiarrhythmic drugs generally have been the first line of prophylaxis for IART. Drugs of all classes have been used, but no prospective studies have demonstrated their efficacy or safety. Retrospective and anecdotal evidence from small case series indicates that certain agents such as sotalol and amiodarone may decrease the frequency of tachycardia recurrence. However, although symptomatic arrhythmias can sometimes be suppressed in individual patients using these agents, other data suggest that no antiarrhythmic drug prolongs time to IART recurrence in patients with CHD (see Fig. 60-4).

The occurrence of thrombosis in adult patients with CHD is rare but potentially catastrophic. Recent studies have estimated the rate of stroke in patients with a previous Fontan repair to be 2 per 1000 to 3 per 1000 patient-years, and the rate of all thromboses to be approximately four times that.[33-35] It is uncertain, however, whether the use of anticoagulant regimens alters this risk. Although most clinicians believe that atrial tachycardia increases this risk further in these patients and that anticoagulant therapy is warranted, the value of such therapy remains unproved.

Pacemaker Therapy

Atrial pacemakers have been an important adjunct to the therapy of IART and, in some cases, used as primary therapy. In patients with sinus node dysfunction, atrial antibradycardia pacing alone sometimes results in symptomatic improvement and decreased tachycardia frequency. The relative contributions of heart rate, favorable atrial activation pattern, and improved hemodynamics due to appropriately timed atrial activation are unknown. Because conversion of IART often can be achieved with rapid atrial pacing leading to temporary block of the tachycardia circuit, devices capable of performing this type of automatic tachycardia recognition and burst pacing have been developed and shown to be efficacious in many patients.[36] Nevertheless, neither antibradycardia nor antitachycardia pacing is reliably useful for IART, and cases of lethal proarrhythmia resulting from AAIT mode pacing in such patients have been documented. Significant technical difficulties also are associated with lead placement and application of rhythm discrimination algorithms in these patients.

Catheter Ablation

The dependence of IART on anatomic and surgical features of the atrium has important implications for therapies targeted at the atrial myocardium itself—ablation of critical areas vulnerable to catheter-based or surgical techniques. Ablative IART therapy involves the creation of nonconductive lesions based on an understanding of the relation of macro-reentrant circuits to the underlying cardiac anatomy. It has clinical precedents in catheter and surgical ablation procedures for ventricular tachycardia and the maze procedure for atrial fibrillation. Ablation has been used both to target specific IART circuits and to perform empirical, anatomically based modification of the atrial myocardium.

Catheter ablation procedures usually target individual macro-reentrant circuits, seeking a vulnerable site for application of radiofrequency lesions. In patients with a right AV valve, as is the case with previous Mustard and Senning procedures, tetralogy of Fallot repair, and other biventricular repairs, as well as surgical correction of some more complex lesions, the isthmus between that valve and the inferior vena cava commonly supports IART, as it does with common atrial flutter. The observation of multiple IART circuits is common, however. Although mapping of clinical IART circuits has shown that most are located in the anatomic right atrium, other anatomic or surgical features relevant to ablation may be difficult to locate. It also may be difficult to generate the large, confluent and transmural lesions that appear to be needed in some cases to interrupt these circuits.

Despite these difficulties, catheter ablation has been applied to IART with increasing success. Recent reports of acute ablation success have ranged from 72% to 94%, using both standard and advanced mapping and ablative technologies.[10,21,25,30,37,38] Advanced technologies include precise, three-dimensional mapping and navigational systems, capable of defining the anatomy of IART circuits, characterizing the electrical potentials and response to entrainment of the underlying atrial tissue, integrating preablative three-dimensional cardiac imaging, and guiding the placement of ablation lesions (Fig. 60-5), and irrigated catheter ablation systems capable of creating larger lesions. These technological innovations in mapping and ablation have contributed to demonstrable improvement in acute procedural success rates.[16,30,37] In these complex procedures, performed in patients with complex, long-standing CHD, periprocedural morbidity and mortality rates have been low. Recurrences of IART have been reported in 35% to 50% of patients over 2 to 4 years of follow-up, whereas frequency and severity of arrhythmia symptoms and need for cardioversion and antiarrhythmic medication are significantly reduced in most patients after IART ablation.[16,38] Further advances in understanding of the arrhythmia substrate and the technology for its visualization and modification it will be necessary to improve these important clinical outcomes.

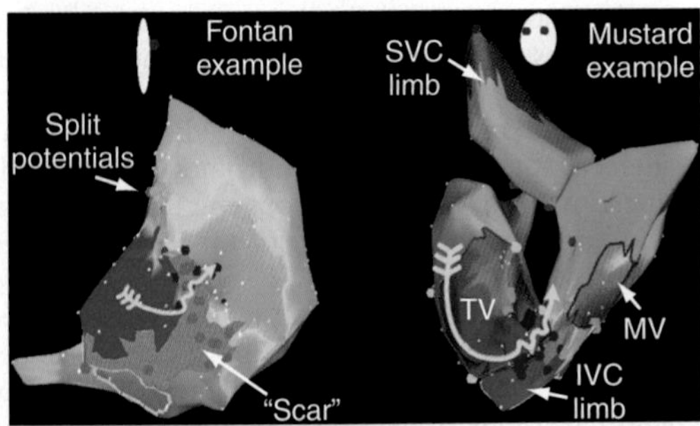

Figure 60-5 Case examples of electroanatomic mapping of intra-atrial reentrant tachycardia (IART) in patients with congenital heart disease. Color mapping represents latency of bipolar electrograms measured at endocardial surface; successful radiofrequency ablation sites are indicated by *dark red dots*. *Yellow arrows* represent the direction of the activation wavefront through protected corridors. **Left image,** Right lateral view of the atrial free wall of a patient who has undergone the Fontan procedure. IART is dependent on conduction through a narrow corridor of tissue located on the inferior right atrial (RA) surface, bounded below by an area of electrically silent tissue (presumed to represent scarring) and above by a line of double potentials (*pink dots*), which identify a line of conduction block secondary to anisotropic properties of the crista terminalis or the effects of surgical scarring. **Right image,** Left anterior oblique view of the right and left atria of a patient who has undergone the Mustard procedure. The unusual anatomy of the superior and inferior vena caval (SVC and IVC) "limbs" of the surgical baffle and the connection of the more posterior pulmonary venous atrium to the tricuspid valve (TV) around the lateral margin of the "crotch" of the baffle legs are demonstrated. IART is dependent on the cavotricuspid isthmus, with counterclockwise rotation about the tricuspid valve as with common atrial flutter, and termination was accomplished with ablation on the pulmonary venous aspect of the baffle, adjacent to the tricuspid annulus. MV, mitral valve.

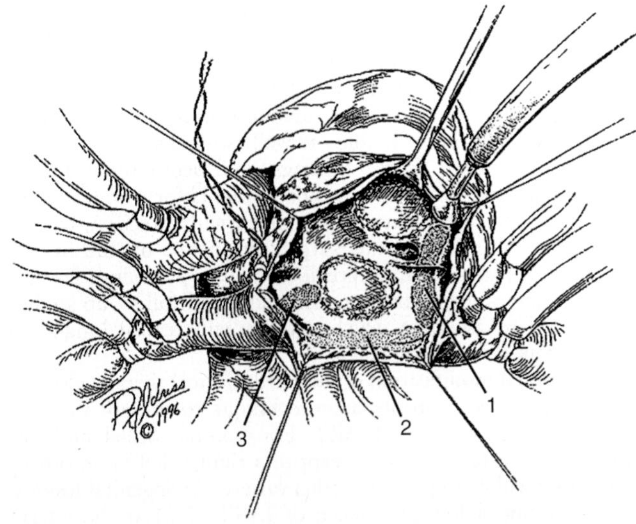

Figure 60-6 Empirical cryoablative right atrial maze procedure used by Mavroudis and associates, in association with Fontan revision surgery, for prophylaxis against recurrence of intra-atrial reentrant tachycardia postoperatively. Lesion set includes intercaval ablation and lines connecting superior vena cava to atrial septal defect (region 3) and intercaval region (region 2), and inferior vena cava to coronary sinus and right atrioventricular valve annulus (region 1), if present. In patients who have established atrial fibrillation, lesions also include isolation of the pulmonary veins, amputation of the left atrial appendage, and additional anchoring lesions in the left atrium as with the maze procedure for atrial fibrillation. (Reprinted with permission from Mavroudis C, Deal BJ, Backer CL, Johnsrude CL: Fontan conversion to cavopulmonary connection and arrhythmia circuit cryoablation. J Thorac Cardiovasc Surg 115:547-556, 1998.)

Surgical Therapy

Patients with older variants of the Fontan procedure may require surgical revision to cavopulmonary-type connections for several hemodynamic reasons. However, even though primary performance of a lateral tunnel or extracardiac repair may be associated with a lower incidence of atrial arrhythmias later in life, simple surgical revision later in life does not prevent IART recurrence in patients with established arrhythmia.[39] Several clinical centers have thus attempted to adapt the adult cardiac surgical experience with the atrial maze procedure to those patients with Fontan connections who have IART. These centers have used surgical or cryoablative techniques, or both, to apply both targeted and empirical lesions to the right and, in some cases, left atrium to prevent postoperative IART (Fig. 60-6). The combined experience of these series shows that these patients achieve symptomatic relief and measurable functional benefit, but at the cost of associated morbidity. The combined perioperative and early follow-up mortality rate for larger series of Fontan revisions is approximately 9%, and recurrence rates of atrial tachycardia (including both simple revisions and those with associated maze procedures) are reported as between 8% and 40% over the relatively short follow-up available (Table 60-4).[40-45]

Table 60-4 Outcomes of Surgical Revision of Fontan Procedure

Study	No. of Patients	Mortality*	Transplant	Failure Rate	Arrhythmia Recurrence†	Follow-up (mo)
Morales et al, 2005[41]	35	2	0	6%	23%	29
Backer et al, 2006[42]	82	5	4	11%	NR	NR
Sheikh et al, 2004[43]	15	0	0	0%	33%	43
Weinstein and Chan, 2005[44]	15	2	0	13%	8%	38
Takahashi et al, 2008[45]	40	5	1	15%	40%	50
Kim et al, 2005[46]	16	0	0	0%	13%	27

*Number of deaths reported during the follow-up period.
†Arrhythmia recurrence figures include both patients who did and those who did not undergo a partial or full maze procedure in conjunction with Fontan revision.
NR, not reported.

Subgroup analyses of these series demonstrate the specific value of inclusion of a maze procedure among patients with established IART.[45] Studies of patients without atrial fibrillation and with surgical revision limited to right atrial lesions also showed lower recurrence rates, demonstrating the importance of intercaval and limbic lesions, as well as blocking of the cavotricuspid isthmus.[46] These findings underscore the value of including a maze procedure in those patients for whom Fontan revision is indicated, particularly those with preoperative arrhythmia. The effect of this surgical sequence on the overall longevity of patients with a previous Fontan procedure has not yet been determined, however, and additional follow-up studies are needed to ascertain which patients will realize long-term benefit from this approach.

Intentional modification of standard surgical therapy also has been proposed as a prophylactic technique to prevent the late, spontaneous occurrence of IART. For example, Stulak and colleagues have extended the concept of a right-sided maze procedure more widely to patients with a variety of congenital lesions, demonstrating a low prevalence of IART (7%) at short-term follow-up of 2.7 years.[47] More subtle surgical modifications also have been proposed, based on observations made in animal models that placement of atriotomy incisions is predictive of propensity to arrhythmia.[20] Attempts to place the atriotomy off the crista terminalis and to "anchor" it to nonconducting anatomic features have been shown to be feasible and to result in measurable early changes in atrial activation and arrhythmia inducibility, but the time course of natural evolution of clinical arrhythmia in these patients has made the efficacy of such modifications difficult to study.[5,48]

Atrial Fibrillation

Atrial fibrillation is less prevalent than IART in CHD but may occur in as many as 25% to 30% of patients with atrial tachycardia, more commonly among those with residual left-sided obstructive lesions or unrepaired heart disease.[49] This relative preference suggests that the chronic hemodynamic overload experienced by the right atrium, and the superimposition of surgical scars on top of this challenge promotes right atrial arrhythmias in patients with CHD, and dilation of the left ventricle and left atrium promotes atrial fibrillation in patients with acquired ventricular dysfunction. Principles of management are drawn from those applicable in the general adult population, including anticoagulation and rate control. Patients with CHD often do not tolerate loss of AV synchrony well, and cardioversion, prophylactic antiarrhythmic drugs, and atrial pacing are used to prevent the establishment of permanent atrial fibrillation if possible. The occurrence of in patients who also have IART reduces the likelihood that therapy targeted at the individual arrhythmia will be beneficial, and may prompt consideration of more empirical therapies, such as the use of antiarrhythmic medications or surgical or catheter-based maze procedures.

Bradycardia

Early perioperative sinus node dysfunction is common after surgery for CHD, as is gradual, progressive loss of sinus rhythm seen at late clinical follow-up evaluation. This problem is particularly prevalent in patients undergoing procedures involving extensive dissection and modification of the right atrium, and surgical procedures have evolved in an attempt to minimize this complication.[50,51] With respect to current practice of the Fontan procedure, the extracardiac conduit variant appears to result in a somewhat lower incidence of sinus node dysfunction than that observed with the lateral tunnel approach in most recent studies.[12,52,53] Patients with sinus venosus defects or heterotaxy syndromes, particularly left atrial isomerism, also may have congenital abnormalities of the sinus node that are independent of the effects of their surgical procedures.

Paroxysmal atrial tachycardias frequently are associated with sinus node dysfunction, and loss of sinus rhythm appears to increase risk of sudden death. Electrophysiologic study of patients who have undergone older variants of the Fontan procedure have identified abnormalities of atrial electrophysiology, including prolonged sinus node recovery times and intra-atrial conduction times and atrial refractoriness. Direct surgical injury to the sinus node has been proposed as a cause of observed abnormalities of sinus node function in patients with a previous Mustard procedure. The progressive loss of sinus rhythm observed over extended follow-up, however, implies additional ongoing pathophysiologic processes, perhaps related to chronic hemodynamic abnormality.

Third-degree and high-grade second-degree heart block are clear indications for permanent cardiac pacing in CHD. In the absence of clearly documented symptomatic bradycardia, however, insufficient data are available to guide the determination of appropriate indications for atrial pacing for isolated sinus bradycardia or junctional escape rhythm, and published guidelines for class II and III indications reflect expert consensus rather than evidence-based conclusions. Although chronic bradycardia often is tolerated, pacing may sometimes alleviate signs of congestive heart failure and symptoms such as fatigue, exercise intolerance, dizziness, or syncope in patients with junctional escape rhythms, severe resting bradycardia, chronotropic incompetence, or prolonged pauses. Pacing also may be necessary to permit therapy with antiarrhythmic medications.

Clinical experience demonstrates the value of AV synchrony and favors implantation of a system capable of providing a physiologic heart rate response. However, the specific value of rate-responsive and dual-chambered pacing as compared with simpler pacing modalities is not well established in CHD. Long-term clinical outcomes seem to be improved in patients who have undergone Fontan procedures and are maintained with AV synchronous pacing, as opposed to ventricular pacing alone,[54] and a recent clinical study showed that VOO mode pacing in perioperative Fontans caused acute, significant hemodynamic deterioration in comparison with AOO or DOO modes.[55]

Practical limitations often require that the choice of system be adapted to patient-specific problems related to lead placement and maintenance, and many of the benefits that may potentially be derived from atrial pacing may be offset by the difficulties encountered in positioning an effective pacing lead. In patients who have experienced multiple operations and are left with a fibrous atrial wall that is adherent to surrounding pericardium, the isolation of atrial muscle that provides both a suitable pacing threshold and capability of sensing an atrial electrogram reliably is challenging and sometimes impossible. Congenital and acquired cardiovascular abnormalities and intracardiac shunts may limit opportunities for endocardial lead placement, necessitating an epicardial or even a hybrid approach.[56] Occasionally, such systems can be implanted on the left atrial epicardial surface through a left thoracotomy. A review of lead function in adults with CHD showed lead complications to be not significantly different for endocardial and epicardial systems, but with a trend to increased survival with endocardial leads.[57] A more general recent study of lead utility and survival in pediatric patients with acquired cardiac disease and those with congenital heart problems by Fortescue and associates showed a relatively high rate of lead failure (23%) in this population, with risk factors for failure including CHD, small patient size, and epicardial lead placement; a subsequent study comparing transvenous and steroid-eluting epicardial leads, however, showed these two technologies to be roughly equivalent in terms of performance and survival.[58,59]

Although the feasibility of transvenous pacing in congenital patients is established, even in the setting of intracardiac septation,[60] anecdotal experience shows that finding adequate pacing sites on the endocardial surface can be equally difficult, and that the proclivity of some patients for the development of right atrial thrombi may be further enhanced by the presence of a pacemaker lead functioning as a foreign body. A multicenter study reported by Khairy and colleagues showed that patients with CHD who have an endocardial pacing lead and any intracardiac shunt had greater than double the risk for a thromboembolic event, regardless of whether anticoagulants were used.[61]

Conclusions

Atrial arrhythmias have emerged as major long-term sequelae for patients with CHD. These patients have poor outcomes, but the small size of and anatomic diversity within this group make it difficult to determine whether arrhythmia control in and of itself will lead to measurable gains in longevity and health. Understanding of these arrhythmias has increased owing to an improved understanding of the extended natural history of these disorders in patients who have survived many years beyond their initial surgeries, and through the innovative application of technologies for diagnosis and therapy that are designed for and tested in patients without CHD. Animal models, modifications of surgical procedures, and the application of evolving interventional techniques have provided with valuable insights into the anatomic substrates of arrhythmia in patients with CHD. Development of a more comprehensive picture of the pathophysiologic changes in the myocardium underlying these arrhythmias will continue to assist in the development of strategies and therapeutic procedures to prevent their occurrence.

References

1. Gelatt M, Hamilton RM, McCrindle BW, et al: Arrhythmia and mortality after the Mustard procedure: A 30-year single-center experience. J Am Coll Cardiol 29:194-201, 1997.
2. Ghai A, Harris L, Harrison DA, et al: Outcomes of late atrial tachyarrhythmias in adults after the Fontan operation. J Am Coll Cardiol 37:585-592, 2001.
3. Jais P, Shah DC, Haissaguerre M, et al: Mapping and ablation of left atrial flutters. Circulation 101:2928-2934, 2000.
4. Garson A Jr, Bink-Boelkens MTE, Hesslein PS, et al: Atrial flutter in the young: A collaborative study in 380 cases. J Am Coll Cardiol 6:871-878, 1985.
5. Law IH, Fischbach PS, Goldberg C, et al: Inducibility of intra-atrial reentrant tachycardia after the first two stages of the Fontan sequence. J Am Coll Cardiol 37:231-237, 2001.
6. Fishberger SB, Wernovsky G, Gentles TL, et al: Factors that influence the development of atrial flutter after the Fontan operation. J Thorac Cardiovasc Surg 113:80-86, 1997.
7. Durongpisitkul K, Porter CJ, Cetta F, et al: Predictors of early- and late-onset supraventricular tachyarrhythmias after Fontan operation. Circulation 98:1099-1107, 1998.
8. Gelatt M, Hamilton RM, McCrindle BW, et al: Risk factors for atrial tachyarrhythmias after the Fontan operation. J Am Coll Cardiol 24:1735-1741, 1994.
9. Cecchin F, Johnsrude CL, Perry JC, Friedman RA: Effect of age and surgical technique on symptomatic arrhythmias after the Fontan procedure. Am J Cardiol 76:386-391, 1995.
10. Weipert J, Noebauer C, Schreiber C, et al: Occurrence and management of atrial arrhythmia after long-term Fontan circulation. J Thorac Cardiovasc Surg 127:457-464, 2004.
11. Stamm C, Triedman JK, Mayer JE, et al: Long-term results of the lateral tunnel Fontan operation. J Thorac Cardiovasc Surg 121:28-41, 2000.
12. Nurnberg JH, Ovroutski S, Alexi-Meskishvili V, et al: New onset arrhythmias after the extracardiac conduit Fontan operation compared with the intraatrial lateral tunnel procedure: Early and midterm results. Ann Thorac Surg 78:1979-1988, 2004.
13. Amodeo A, Galletti L, Marianeschi S, et al: Extracardiac Fontan operation for complex cardiac anomalies: Seven years' experience. J Thorac Cardiovasc Surg 114:1020-1030, 1997.
14. Roos-Hesselink J, Perlroth MG, McGhie J, Spitaels S: Atrial arrhythmias in adults after repair of tetralogy of Fallot. Correlations with clinical, exercise, and echocardiographic findings. Circulation 91:2214-2219, 1995.
15. Hoernstein MS, Karpawich PP, Epstein ML, Singh TP: Transthoracic echocardiography for precardioversion screeing during atrial flutter/fibrillation in young patients. Clin Cardiol 27:413-416, 2004.
16. Triedman JK, Alexander ME, Love BA, et al: Influence of patient factors and ablative technologies on outcomes of radiofrequency ablation of intra-atrial re-entrant tachycardia in patients with congenital heart disease. J Am Coll Cardiol 39:1827-1835, 2002.
17. Schoels W, Offner B, Brachmann J, et al: Circus movement atrial flutter in the canine sterile pericarditis model: Relation of characteristics of the surface electrocardiogram and conduction properties of the reentrant pathway. J Am Coll Cardiol 23:799-808, 1994.
18. Davos CH, Francis DP, Leenarts MFE, et al: Global impairment of cardiac autonomic nervous activity late after Fontan operation. Circulation 108(Suppl II): II-180-II-185, 2003.
19. Gandhi SK, Bromberg BI, Schuessler RB, et al: Characterization and surgical ablation of atrial flutter after the classic Fontan repair. Ann Thorac Surg 61:1666-1678, 1996.
20. Gandhi SK, Bromberg BI, Rodefeld MD, et al: Lateral tunnel suture line variation reduces atrial flutter after the modified Fontan operation. Ann Thorac Surg 61:1299-1309, 1996.
21. Collins KK, Love BA, Walsh EP, et al: Location of acutely successful radiofrequency catheter ablation of intraatrial reentrant tachycardia in patients with congenital heart disease. Am J Cardiol 86:969-974, 2000.
22. Magnin-Poull I, De Chillou C, Miljoen H, et al: Mechanisms of right atrial tachycardia occurring late after surgical closure of atrial septal defects. J Cardiovasc Electrophysiol 16:681-687, 2005.
23. Lukac P, Pedersen AK, Mortensen PT, et al: Ablation of atrial tachycardia after surgery for congenital and acquired heart disease using an electroanatomic mapping system: Which circuits to expect in which substrate. Heart Rhythm 2:65-72, 2005.
24. Mandapati R, Walsh EP, Triedman JK: Pericaval and periannular intraatrial reentrant tachycardias among patients with congenital heart disease. J Cardiovasc Electrophysiol 14:119-125, 2003.
25. Seiler J, Schmid DK, Irtel TA, et al: Dual-loop circuits in postoperative atrial macro re-entrant tachycardias. Heart 93:325-330, 2007.
26. Love BA, Collins KK, Walsh EP, Triedman JK: Electroanatomic characterization of conduction barriers in sinus/atrially paced rhythm and association with intra-atrial reentrant tachycardia circuits following congenital heart disease surgery. J Cardiovasc Electrophysiol 12:17-25, 2001.
27. De Groot NM, Kuijper AF, Blom NA, et al: Three-dimensional distribution of bipolar atrial electrogram voltages in patients with congenital heart disease. PACE 24:1334-1342, 2001.

28. Seslar SP, Alexander ME, Berul CI, et al: Ablation of nonautomatic focal atrial tachycardia in children and adults with congenital heart disease. J Cardiovasc Electrophysiol 17:359-365, 2006.
29. De Groot NMS, Zeppenfeld K, Wijffels MC, et al: Ablation of focal atrial arrhythmia in patients with congenital heart defects after surgery: Role of circumscribed areas with heterogeneous conduction. Heart Rhythm 3:526-535, 2006.
30. Triedman JK, DeLucca JM, Alexander ME, et al: Prospective trial of electroanatomically guided, irrigated catheter ablation of atrial tachycardia in patients with congenital heart disease. Heart Rhythm 2:700-705, 2005.
31. Liberman L, Hordof AJ, Altmann K, Pass RH: Low energy biphasic waveform cardioversion of atrial arrhythmias in pediatric patients and young adults. PACE 29:1383-1386, 2006.
32. Hoyer AW, Balaji S: The safety and efficacy of ibutilide in children and in patients with congenital heart disease. PACE 30:1003-1008, 2007.
33. Mahnke CB, Boyle GJ, Janosky JE, et al: Anticoagulation and incidence of late cerebrovascular accidents following the Fontan procedure. Pediatr Cardiol 26: 56-61, 2005.
34. Kaulitz R, Ziemer G, Rauch R, et al: Prophylaxis of thromboembolic complications after the Fontan operation (total cavopulmonary anastomosis). J Thorac Cardiovasc Surg 129:569-575, 2005.
35. Seipelt RG, Franke A, Vazquez-Jimenez JF, et al: Thromboembolic complications after Fontan procedures: Comparison of different therapeutic approaches. Ann Thorac Surg 74:556-562, 2002.
36. Stephenson EA, Casavant D, Tuzi J, et al: Efficacy of atrial antitachycardia pacing using the Medtronic AT500 pacemaker in patients with congenital heart disease. Am J Cardiol 92:871-876, 2003.
37. Tanner H, Lukac P, Schwick N, et al: Irrigated-tip catheter ablation of intraatrial reentrant tachycardia in patients late after surgery of congenital heart disease. Heart Rhythm 3:268-275, 2004.
38. Kannankeril PJ, Anderson ME, Rottman JN, et al: Frequency of late recurrence of intra-atrial reentry tachycardia after radiofrequency catheter ablation in patients with congenital heart disease. Am J Cardiol 92:879-881, 2003.
39. Deal BJ, Mavroudis C, Backer CL, et al: Impact of arrhythmia circuit cryoablation during Fontan conversion for refractory atrial tachycardia. Am J Cardiol 83:563-568, 1999.
40. Morales DLS, Dibardino DJ, Braud BE, et al: Salvaging the failing Fontan: Lateral tunnel versus extracardiac conduit. Ann Thorac Surg 80:1445-1452, 2005.
41. Backer CL, Deal BJ, Mavroudis C, et al: Conversion of the failed Fontan circulation. Cardiol Young 16(Suppl 1):85-91, 2006.
42. Sheikh AM, Tang ATM, Roman K, et al: The failing Fontan: Successful conversion of atriopulmonary connections. J Thorac Cardiovac Surg 128:60-66, 2004.
43. Weinstein S, Chan D: Extracardiac Fontan conversion, cryoablation, and pacemaker placement for patients with a failed Fontan. Semin Thorac Cardiovasc Surg 17:170-178, 2005.
44. Takahashi K, Fynn-Thompson F, Cecchin F, et al: Clinical outcomes of Fontan revision surgery with and without associated arrhythmia intervention. Int J Cardiol 2008 Aug. 13, doi:10.1016/j.ijcard.2008.06.074.
45. Kim WH, Lim HG, Lee JR, et al: Fontan conversion with arrhythmia surgery. Eur J Cardiothorac Surg 27:250-257, 2005.
46. Deal BJ, Mavroudis C, Backer CL, et al: Comparison of anatomic isthmus block with the modified right atrial maze procedure for late atrial tachycardia in Fontan patients. Circulation 106:575-579, 2002.
47. Stulak JM, Dearani JA, Puga FJ, et al: Right-sided maze procedure for atrial tachycarrythmias in congenital heart disease. Ann Thorac Surg 81:1780-1785, 2006.
48. Collins KK, Rhee EK, Delucca JM, et al: Modification to the Fontan procedure for the prophylaxis of intra-atrial reentrant tachycardia: Short-term results of a prospective randomized blinded trial. J Thorac Cardiovasc Surg 127:721-729, 2004.
49. Kirsh JA, Walsh, Triedman JK: Prevalence of and risk factors for atrial fibrillation and intraatrial reentrant tachycardia among patients with congenital heart disease. Am J Cardiol 90:40-43, 2002.
50. Cohen MI, Bridges ND, Gaynor JW, et al: Modifications to the cavopulmonary anastomosis do not eliminate early sinus node dysfunction. J Thorac Cardiovasc Surg 120:891-900, 2000.
51. Kirjavainen M, Happonen JM, Louhimo I: Late results of Senning operation. J Thorac Cardiovasc Surg 117:488-495, 1999.
52. Dilawar M, Bradley SM, Saul JP, et al: Sinus node dysfunction after intraatrial lateral tunnel and extracardiac Fontan procedures. Pediatr Cardiol 24:284-288, 2003.
53. Lee JR, Kwak J, Kim KC, et al: Comparison of lateral tunnel and extracardiac conduit Fontan procedure. Interact Cardiovasc Thorac Surg 6:328-330, 2007.
54. Dodge-Khatami A, Rahn M, Pretre R, Bauersfeld U: Dual chamber epicardial pacing for the failing atriopulmonary Fontan patient. Ann Thorac Surg 80:1440-1444, 2005.
55. Barber BJ, Batra AS, Burch GH, et al: Acute hemodynamic effects of pacing in patients with Fontan physiology. J Am Coll Cardiol 46:1937-1942, 2005.
56. Hansky B, Blanz U, Peuster M, et al: Edocardial pacing after Fontan-type procedures. PACE 28:140-148, 2005.
57. Walker F, Siu SC, Woods S, et al: Long-term outcomes of cardiac pacing in adults with congenital heart disease. J Am Coll Cardiol 43:1894-1901, 2004.
58. Fortescue EB, Berul CI, Cecchin F, et al: Patient, procedural and hardware factors associated with pacemaker lead failures in pediatrics and congenital heart disease. Heart Rhythm 1:150-159, 2004.
59. Fortescue EB, Berul CI, Cecchin F, et al: Comparison of modern steroid-eluting epicardial and thin transvenous pacemaker leads in pediatric and congenital heart disease patients. J Intervent Card Electrophysiol 14:27-36, 2005.
60. Shah MJ, Nehgme R, Carboni M, Murphy JD: Endocardial atrial pacing lead implantation and midterm follow-up in young patients with sinus node dysfunction after the Fontan procedure. PACE 27:949-954, 2004.
61. Khairy P, Landzberg MJ, Gatzoulis MA, et al: Transvenous pacing leads and systemic thromboemboli in patients with intracardiac shunts: A multicenter study. Circulation 113:2391-2397, 2006.

Ventricular Tachycardia in Patients with Structurally Normal Hearts 61

BRUCE B. LERMAN

CHAPTER OUTLINE

Idiopathic ventricular tachycardia is a generic term that refers to ventricular arrhythmias that originate in hearts without structural disease. Several discrete forms of idiopathic monomorphic ventricular tachycardia have been identified, and electropharmacologic data suggest that multiple arrhythmogenic mechanisms may account for these arrhythmias.[1,2] Idiopathic ventricular tachycardia has been classified with respect to the ventricle of origin, the response to pharmacologic agents, evidence for catecholamine dependence, the morphologic features of the arrhythmia (QRS configuration and axis), and the clinical pattern of the tachycardia—repetitive, nonsustained, or sustained. In general, the response of the arrhythmia to programmed stimulation and to adenosine, verapamil, and propranolol differentiates among nearly all forms of idiopathic ventricular tachycardia.

Adenosine-Sensitive Ventricular Tachycardia

Mechanism

The most common form of idiopathic ventricular tachycardia originates from the ventricular outflow tract (OT), with approximately 80% of cases occurring from the the right ventricular outflow tract (RVOT) and the remainder from the left ventricular outflow tract (LVOT).[3] Idiopathic OT arrhythmias usually exhibit one of three phenotypes: repetitive monomorphic premature ventricular complexes (PVCs); nonsustained, repetitive monomorphic ventricular tachycardia (RMVT); or paroxysmal, exercise-induced sustained ventricular tachycardia. The signature characteristic of sustained RVOT and LVOT tachycardia is termination by adenosine[3-5] (Fig. 61-1). Sensitivity of ventricular tachycardia to blockade of the L-type calcium channel current ($I_{Ca,L}$) with verapamil is another distinguishing feature (see Fig. 61-1).

Considerable overlap may be observed among the three phenotypes of outflow tract arrhythmias. For example, patients who present with exercise-induced ventricular tachycardia may demonstrate spontaneous or catecholamine facilitated progression of uniform PVCs to salvos of nonsustained ventricular tachycardia and finally to sustained ventricular tachycardia[6] (Fig. 61-2). Conversely, patients with only repetitive PVCs may have sustained ventricular tachycardia induced during programmed stimulation[6] (Fig. 61-3). The observation that ablating one phenotype at a discrete site eliminates the other two phenotypes of arrhythmia suggests that that the three phenotypes are a continuum of the same focal cellular process.

Most evidence to date supports the hypothesis that adenosine-sensitive OT tachycardia is caused by triggered activity, which is mediated by catecholamine-induced delayed afterdepolarizations (DADs).[4,7,8] Catecholamine stimulation of the β-adrenergic receptor results in an increase in intracellular cyclic adenosine monophosphate (cAMP), and in $I_{Ca,L}$, and a spontaneous oscillatory release of Ca^{2+} from the sarcoplasmic reticulum that activates a transient inward current (I_{ti}), giving rise to a DAD. I_{ti} is generated by activation of the Na^+-Ca^{2+} exchanger (NCX).[9] Because activation of adenylyl cyclase and $I_{Ca,L}$ is critical for the development of cAMP-mediated triggered activity, the triggered arrhythmia is sensitive to a constellation of electropharmacologic perturbations: beta-blockade, calcium channel blockade (verapamil), vagal maneuvers, and adenosine[10,11] (Fig. 61-4).

Adenosine's effects on ventricular tachycardia, with rare exceptions, are mechanism-specific, terminating only ventricular tachycardia that is due to cAMP-mediated triggered activity. In the absence of β-adrenergic stimulation, adenosine has no effect on ventricular resting membrane potential, action potential amplitude and duration, or levels of intracellular cAMP. Cyclic AMP–mediated effects on the action potential, however, are attenuated or completely reversed by adenosine. Because adenosine abolishes DADs and I_{ti} induced by isoproterenol and forskolin (an adenylyl cyclase activator) but not those induced by dibutyryl cAMP, adenosine's antiadrenergic effects are thought

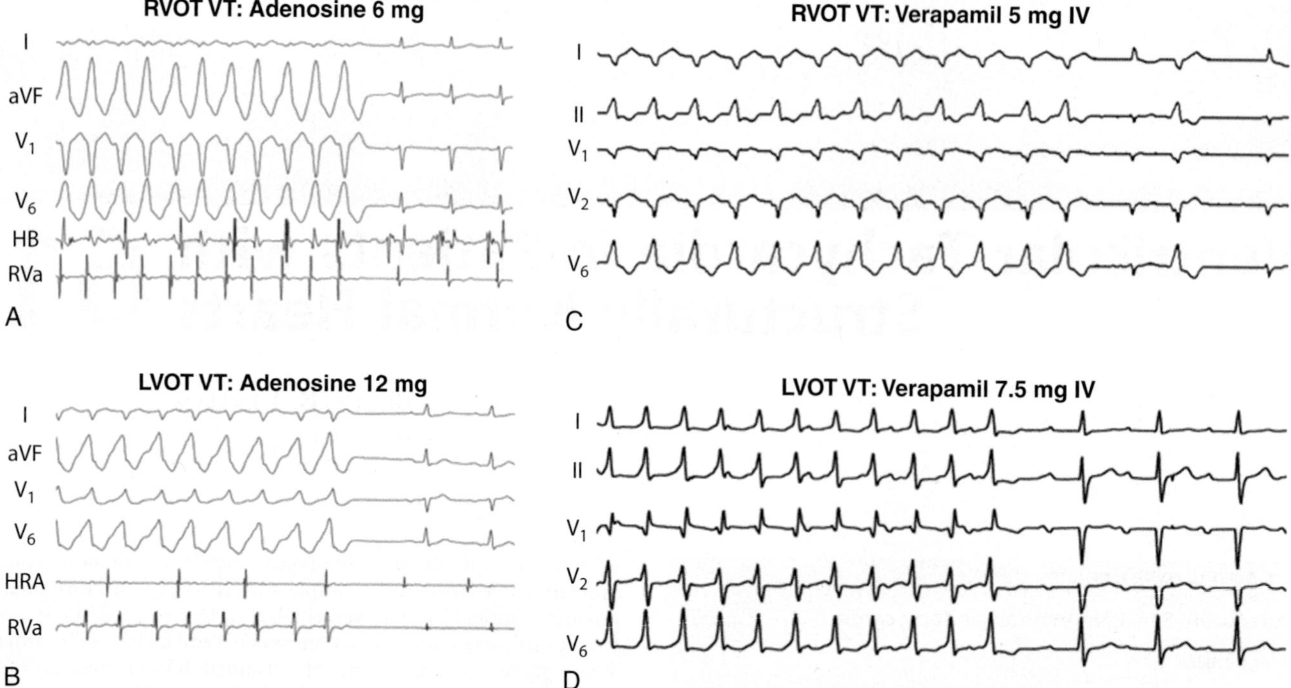

Figure 61-1 Sensitivity of right ventricular and left ventricular outflow tract tachycardia (LVOT) to adenosine and verapamil. **A,** Termination of sustained right ventricular outflow tract (RVOT) tachycardia 6 seconds after administration of adenosine. Electrocardiographic leads I, aVF, V_1, and V_6 are displayed, along with intracardiac electrograms from the His bundle (HB) and right ventricular apex (RVa). **B,** Termination of sustained LVOT tachycardia 15 seconds after administration of adenosine. **C,** Termination of sustained RVOT tachycardia after intravenous infusion of verapamil, with a single premature ventricular complex after termination of sustained ventricular tachycardia (VT). **D,** Termination of sustained LVOT tachycardia after intravenous infusion of verapamil. Electrocardiographic leads are displayed, along with intracardiac electrograms from the high right atrium (HRA) and RVa. (From Iwai S, Cantillon DJ, Kim RJ, et al: Right and left ventricular outflow tract tachycardias: Evidence for a common electrophysiologic mechanism. J Cardiovasc Electrophysiol 17:1052-1058, 2006. Copyright 2006, Blackwell Publishing Co.)

to be mediated at a level proximal to cAMP, that is, at the level of adenylyl cyclase.[8] Specifically, adenosine's electrophysiologic effects are mediated by a pertussis toxin–sensitive inhibitory G protein (G_i), which couples the A_1 receptor to adenylyl cyclase, thereby decreasing stimulated levels of intracellular cAMP.

Adenosine's effects are also specific with regard to the etiology of the DAD because it is ineffective in attenuating DADs and I_{ti} induced by cAMP-independent mechanisms (e.g., digitalis-induced inhibition of Na^+,K^+-ATPase).[8] Furthermore, adenosine has no effect on phase 2 early afterdepolarizations (EADs) induced by quinidine or the calcium channel activator Bay K 8644.[8] Of particular significance is that adenosine has no effect on catecholamine-facilitated reentry due to structural heart disease.[12] Consistent with this finding, adenosine has only a minimal antiadrenergic effect on depressed action potentials in infarcted Purkinje fibers or in partially depolarized ventricular or Purkinje cells. The mechanism for adenosine's desensitization in these tissues is unknown, but possibilities include downregulation of the A_1-adenosine receptor or uncoupling of the receptor from its G protein. Although agents such as verapamil, flunarizine and nicorandil also can terminate DAD-triggered arrhythmias, they lack the mechanism specificity of adenosine.

An important but unresolved issue regarding ventricular tachycardia due to cAMP-mediated triggered activity centers on the biochemical or molecular substrate for this arrhythmia. Nearly all clinical forms of monomorphic ventricular tachycardia are due to an anatomic substrate. However, this arrhythmia occurs in the absence of anatomic abnormalities and originates from a discrete focus (smaller than 1 cm diameter) in the OT. It has been hypothesized that mutations in the various signal transduction pathways involving cAMP may be the etiology for ventricular tachycardia in some of these patients. To this end, a somatic cell mutation has been identified in the inhibitory G protein $G_\alpha i2$ in a patient with a variant form (adenosine-insensitive) of adrenergically mediated idiopathic RVOT tachycardia.[13] A point mutation (F200L) in the guanosine triphosphate (GTP)-binding domain of $G_\alpha i2$ has been detected in biopsy samples from the arrhythmogenic focus. This mutation increases intracellular cAMP in response to β-adrenergic stimulation (presumably potentiating ventricular tachycardia) and inhibits suppression of cAMP by adenosine. The mutation in $G_\alpha i2$ was not identified in myocardial tissue obtained from regions remote from the site of tachycardia origin or from peripheral lymphocytes. These results demonstrate that a somatic cell mutation in the cAMP-dependent signal transduction pathway, occurring during myocardial development, may be an etiologic factor in some forms of OT tachycardia.

Clinical Characteristics and Evaluation

Outflow tract tachycardia occurs with equal frequency in men and women. The mean age at diagnosis is 50 ± 15 years (range, 6 to 80 years).[3,6] A benign course is observed in most patients, suggesting that the underlying pathophysiologic process is not progressive and that the tachycardia does not represent an early manifestation of an occult cardiomyopathy. These findings have

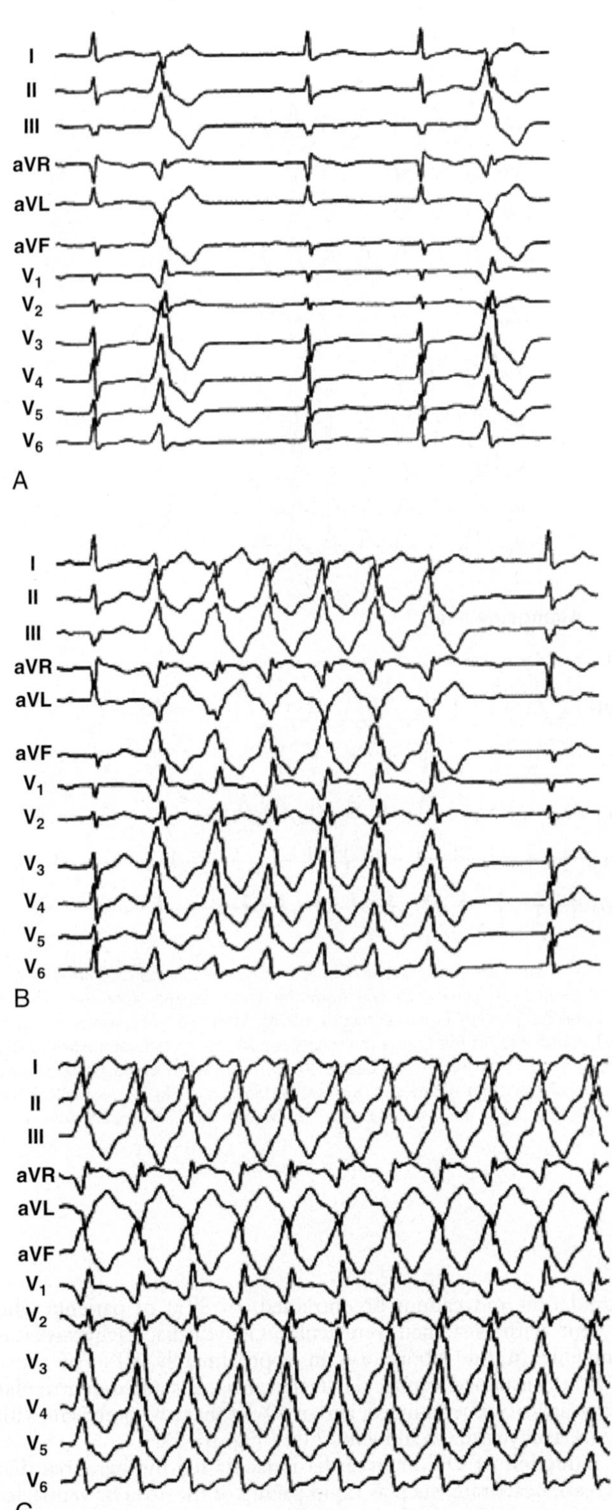

Figure 61-2 Identical morphologic patterns for premature ventricular complexes (PVCs), nonsustained ventricular tachycardia (NSVT), and sustained ventricular tachycardia (VT) from a patient with exercise-induced VT. These three sets of 12-lead surface electrocardiographic recordings demonstrate identical morphologic patterns for repetitive monomorphic PVCs (**A**), a 6-beat run of NSVT (**B**), and sustained VT (**C**), all of which occurred consecutively during infusion of isoproterenol. Ablation at the earliest site of activation of the PVC from the left ventricular outflow tract (LVOT) eliminated all three forms of arrhythmia. (From Kim RJ, Iwai S, Markowitz SM, et al: Clinical and electrophysiological spectrum of idiopathic ventricular outflow tract arrhythmias. J Am Coll Cardiol 49:2035-2043, 2007. Copyright 2007, American College of Cardiology.)

also been confirmed during long-term follow-up of patients with frequent RVOT ectopic beats.[14] In a small subset of patients with incessant repetitive monomorphic RVOT tachycardia, however, secondary cardiomyopathy can develop,[15] and in those with frequent uniform ventricular ectopy, a PVC-induced cardiomyopathy can develop.[16,17] Typically, the PVCs comprise between 5% and 40% of all beats in affected persons and can originate from either the RVOT or the LVOT. Ablation of the PVC focus reverses the cardiomyopathy and restores normal left ventricular function within 3 to 6 months. Therefore, not all outflow tract PVCs are benign. Accordingly, patients diagnosed with "idiopathic cardiomyopathy" should undergo ambulatory monitoring to assess their degree of PVC burden. In those with frequent uniform ectopy, ablation may be warranted. Other data suggest that RVOT PVCs infrequently can trigger idiopathic ventricular fibrillation or polymorphic ventricular tachycardia.[18] These beats also can trigger ventricular fibrillation in patients with the long QT and Brugada syndromes.[19] Ablation of the arrhythmogenic focus appears to eliminate recurrent episodes of the malignant arrhythmia.

The electrocardiogram (ECG) during sinus rhythm usually is unremarkable. Approximately 15% of patients with OT tachycardia have a ventricular conduction delay or bundle branch block, and 5% have precordial T wave inversions in two or more leads.[6] Echocardiographic findings are normal in 90% of patients. Slight enlargement of the right ventricle is rarely noted.

Exercise testing induces ventricular tachycardia in approximately 70% of patients who present with sustained ventricular tachycardia and in 10% of those who present with either NSVT or PVCs.[6] Two general positive response patterns are seen: (1) initiation of ventricular tachycardia during the exercise test and (2) onset of ventricular tachycardia during the recovery phase.[20]

Change in sympathovagal balance preceding OT tachycardia may be due to withdrawal of parasympathetic tone or to an increase in sympathetic tone. Consistent with the latter is a progressive decrease in the RR interval preceding ventricular couplets and runs in the absence of parasympathetic withdrawal.[7] Ventricular runs (2 to 4 beats) and ventricular tachycardia also show a circadian variation, with two prominent peaks, one at 7 AM and the other between 5 and 6 PM, both of which are eliminated by β-adrenergic blockade.[21]

Time-domain analysis of signal-averaged electrocardiograms (SAECGs) typically is unremarkable in patients with OT tachycardia. Late potentials, if present, usually are identified by an abnormal root-mean-square (RMS) voltage during the last 40 ms of the filtered QRS or abnormal duration of the low-amplitude signal (LAS). The filtered QRS duration usually is normal. Findings on microvolt T wave alternans (TWA) testing also are unremarkable in these patients; in approximately 40%, an indeterminate result is obtained, frequently owing to ventricular ectopy.[6]

Magnetic resonance imaging (MRI) studies have reported structural defects in patients with idiopathic RVOT tachycardia, including focal wall thinning, abnormal systolic wall motion, and focal fatty infiltration, findings not appreciated with echocardiography or right ventricular angiography.[22,23] The most common site of abnormality was the right ventricular free wall. In general, however, these abnormal findings did not correspond to the site of origin of ventricular tachycardia, and 30% of patients had no defects at all. More recent studies using newer technology have found a considerably lower prevalence of abnormalities (10%).[3,6,24]

Right ventricular biopsy samples from patients with RVOT tachycardia have shown a wide spectrum of findings, ranging from normal to nonspecific cardiomyopathy. Pathologic findings

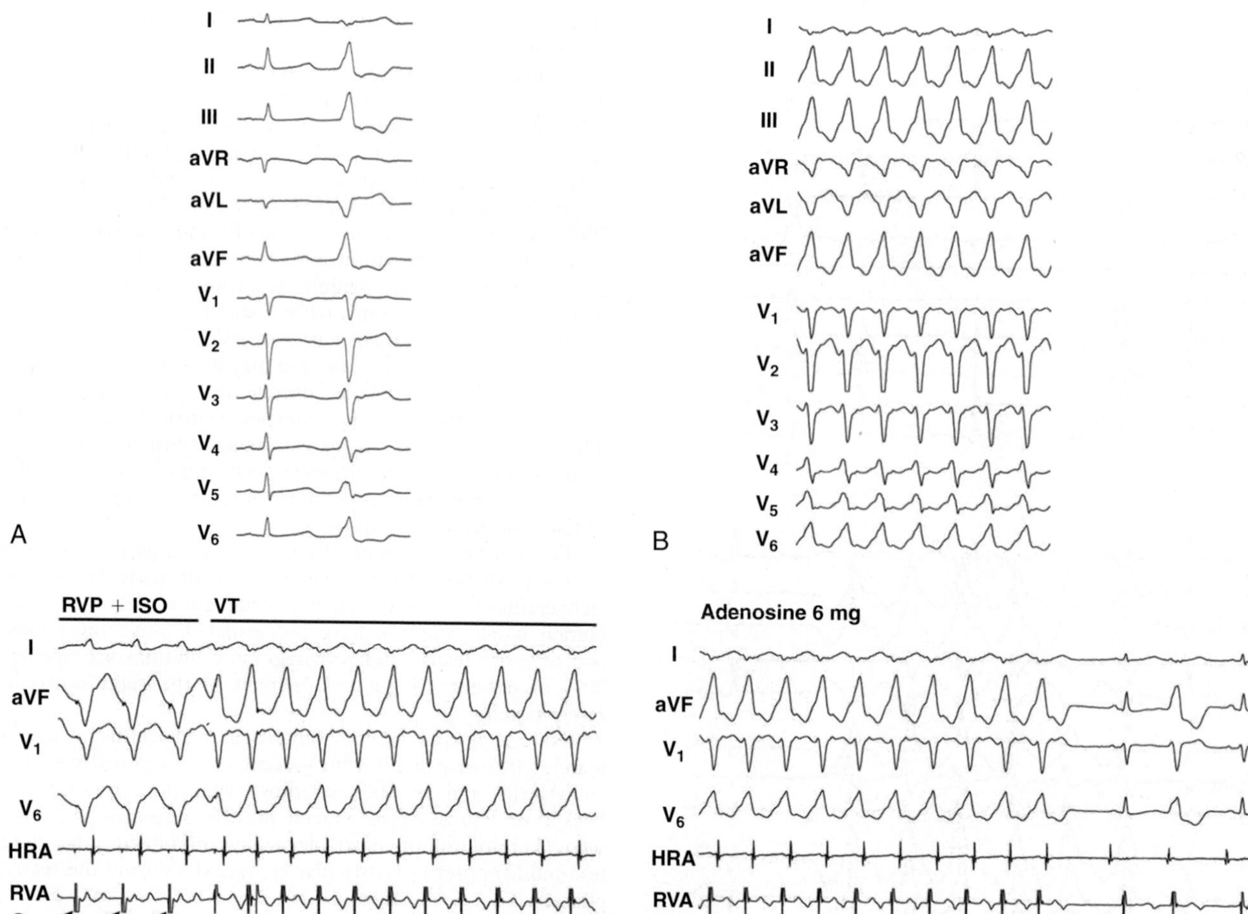

Figure 61-3 Electrophysiologic profile of a patient who presented with repetitive premature ventricular complexes (PVCs). **A,** A 12-lead electrocardiogram showing a sinus beat followed by a PVC. **B,** A 12-lead electrocardiogram of induced sustained ventricular tachycardia (VT) from the same patient. Note the identical morphologic patterns for induced VT and for the spontaneous PVC. **C,** Induction of sustained VT with rapid ventricular pacing from the right ventricular apex (*arrows*) during concomitant infusion of isoproterenol (ISO). Note that the first beat of VT (*fourth beat* in the figure) represents pseudo-fusion between a ventricular pacing spike and the first beat of VT and that the fifth ventricular pacing spike (noncapture) occurs after the second beat of VT. **D,** Termination of induced sustained VT with adenosine. HRA, high right atrium; RVA, right ventricular apex; RVP, right ventricular pacing. (From Kim RJ, Iwai S, Markowitz SM, et al: Clinical and electrophysiological spectrum of idiopathic ventricular outflow tract arrhythmias. J Am Coll Cardiol 49:2035-2043, 2007. Copyright 2007, American College of Cardiology.)

have included myocellular hypertrophy and interstitial and perivascular fibrosis, myocarditis, and small-vessel disease, characterized by intimal and medial sclerosis and luminal narrowing. Several points are worth noting: (1) The association of a nonspecific histologic abnormality on endomyocardial biopsy in patients with RVOT tachycardia does not prove causality; (2) the diagnosis of ARVD should be carefully considered in examining biopsy samples from patients with suspected RVOT tachycardia; and (3) the presence of some fat may be a normal finding in the right ventricle.

Electrophysiologic Diagnosis

The clinical diagnosis of cAMP-mediated triggered activity is supported by sensitivity of ventricular tachycardia to adenosine, Valsalva maneuvers, carotid sinus pressure, edrophonium, verapamil, and beta-blockers (see Figs. 61-1 and 61-4). The tachycardia also is initiated and terminated with programmed stimulation and cannot be entrained. In 80% of patients who present with sustained ventricular tachycardia, tachycardia is inducible in the laboratory; in approximately 50% of those with nonsustained ventricular tachycardia, sustained ventricular tachycardia can be induced; and in 5% of those who present with PVCs, tachycardia is inducible[6] (see Fig. 61-3).

Induction of OT tachycardia is facilitated by measures that increase heart rate, such as rapid pacing of the atria or ventricles or infusion of a catecholamine alone or in combination with pacing. The ability to induce triggered activity is dependent on the immediate autonomic status of the patient: Induction is less likely in a heavily sedated patient. The vagaries of autonomic status on inducibility in this form of tachycardia often are highlighted by the observation that strenuous but unsuccessful efforts to induce tachycardia during one study can be contrasted with ready inducibility of ventricular tachycardia during a subsequent study. Therefore, noninducibility during a single study does not provide sufficient evidence to attribute the arrhythmia to an automatic or nontriggered mechanism.

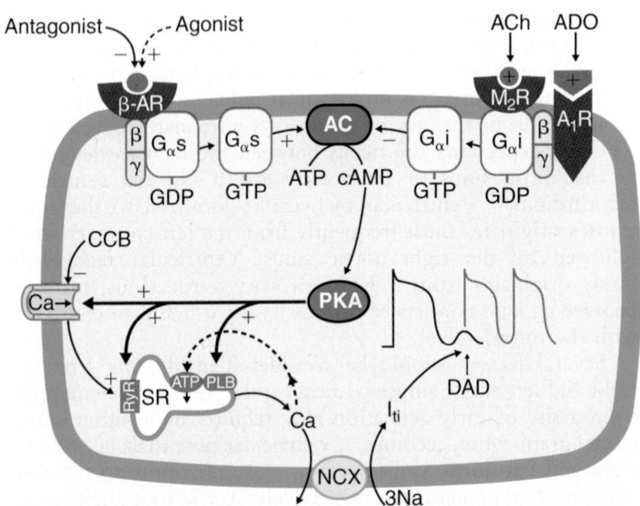

Figure 61-4 Signal transduction schema for initiation and termination of cAMP-mediated triggered activity. AC, adenylyl cyclase; ACh, acetylcholine; ADO, adenosine; A_1R, A_1-adenosine receptor; B-AR, β-adrenergic receptor; cAMP, cyclic adenosine monophosphate; CCB, calcium channel blocker; DAD, delayed afterdepolarization; $G_{\alpha}i$, inhibitory G protein; $G_{\alpha}s$, stimulatory G protein; GDP, guanosine diphosphate; GTP, guanosine triphosphate; NCX, Na^+-Ca^{2+} exchanger; PLB, phospholamban; PKA, protein kinase A; RyR, ryanodine receptor; SR, sarcoplasmic recticulum. (From Lerman BB: Mechanism of outflow tract tachycardia. Heart Rhythm 4:973-976, 2007. Copyright 2007, Heart Rhythm Society.)

Treatment

The decision to treat OT tachycardia depends on the frequency and severity of symptoms. If symptoms are infrequent and relatively mild, treatment may be conservative. Alternatively, if symptoms associated with ventricular tachycardia include presyncope or syncope, or if frequent ventricular extrasystoles are debilitating, then radiofrequency catheter ablation of the arrhythmogenic focus is the treatment of choice. The symptom complex for most patients falls between these ends of the spectrum. In these patients, viable therapeutic options include medical and ablative approaches.

The evaluation of antiarrhythmic efficacy usually relies on the results of Holter monitoring, exercise stress testing, and programmed stimulation. Significant limitations to these modalities are recognized, however, based on the sensitivity of OT tachycardia to autonomic influences, resulting in poor day-to-day reproducibility of the arrhythmia. Fortunately, however, the response to antiarrhythmic therapy is far more favorable for OT tachycardia than for ventricular tachycardia secondary to structural heart disease (most data are derived from patients with RVOT tachycardia). Also noteworthy is that OT tachycardia is responsive to all classes of antiarrhythmic agents.

The initial drug of choice for antiarrhythmic therapy usually is a beta-blocker. Calcium channel blockers, such as verapamil and diltiazem, also may be considered and can be synergistic with beta-blockers. Class I (IA and IC) antiarrhythmic drugs also are effective in OT tachycardia, as are class III drugs, such as sotalol and amiodarone.

Acute termination of OT tachycardia can be achieved by several means. The initial step is to increase vagal tone by Valsalva maneuvers or applying carotid sinus pressure. If these strategies are ineffective, adenosine can be given (6 to 24 mg). Another option is intravenous verapamil (10 mg), given over 60 seconds, which is effective in approximately 75% of patients within 1 to 2 minutes after administration of the bolus. Lidocaine (1-1.5 mg/kg) also is an effective agent.

Several electrophysiologic characteristics of RVOT tachycardia make this form of arrhythmia readily amenable to ablation. The tachycardia focus is discrete, well-circumscribed, and located in an accessible region. The 12-lead ECG during ventricular tachycardia provides a first approximation of the RVOT origin.[25] Inspection of the precordial QRS transition usually is informative in determining whether the RVOT tachycardia origin is septal or free wall. A free-wall site is associated with a later transition (V_4 or later) than a septal site (V_3 or later). The QRS duration during ventricular tachycardia usually is greater than 140 ms if the arrhythmia originates from the free-wall aspect of the RVOT, and 140 ms or less if it originates from the septal aspect of the RVOT. The latter probably results from activation of the ventricles through the septal Purkinje network. Notching and a relatively large R wave amplitude may be observed in the inferior leads in ventricular tachycardia with a free-wall origin. The anterior position of the free wall relative to the septum also accounts for the deeper S wave inscribed in lead V_2 than that with ventricular tachycardia originating from the RVOT septum. A septal site also is associated with a Q/q wave in lead I, whereas a free-wall site inscribes an R/r wave.

Ventricular tachycardia that originates from within the pulmonary artery (approximately 1 cm above the pulmonic valve) is associated with a precordial transition in leads V_3 or V_4. Because the pulmonary artery is located leftward of and anterior to the RVOT, ventricular tachycardia from this region frequently has a qR configuration in lead I and a larger Q wave in lead aVL than in aVR; its location superior to the RVOT results in a relatively greater R wave amplitude in the inferior leads.[26,27] PVCs or ventricular tachycardia also may originate from the right ventricular inflow tract along region of the the tricuspid annulus.[28,29] Although multiple periannular sites have been identified, the most common site of origin is para-Hisian.[29] Characteristic ECG findings for para-Hisian ventricular tachycardia include inscription of an R wave in leads I and aVL, relatively small R waves in the inferior leads, a QS wave in V_1, and a precordial transition in V_2 to V_4.[28] Sites of successful ablation record an atrial and a ventricular potential.

Techniques to identify the earliest site of activation have relied primarily on bipolar activation mapping and pace mapping. Other useful modalities include the deployment of three-dimensional electroanatomic and noncontact mapping systems. In general, successful ablation sites are associated with activation times 10 to 45 ms before the onset of earliest surface QRS but are not substantially different from those at unsuccessful sites. Unipolar recordings also have proved to be effective for localizing the earliest site of activation: A characteristic initial negative deflection is recorded on a unipolar tracing at a site of early activation (as a result of movement of the dipole away from the recording electrode). To eliminate far-field stimulation effects, pace mapping is evaluated during either unipolar or closely spaced bipolar pacing at twice the diastolic threshold. Although pace mapping has proved useful in identifying the successful ablation site, it has limitations with regard to resolution. Identical pace maps can be observed up to 8 mm from a tachycardia focus.[30]

Most successful ablation sites are located within the septal region of the RVOT, usually immediately inferior to the pulmonic valve. Delivery of radiofrequency energy at a successful site can result in a rapid ventricular response (with a QRS morphology identical to that of ventricular tachycardia) followed by gradual slowing and complete resolution, a finding associated with a relatively high specificity but low sensitivity.[31] Subtle variations in QRS morphology may be observed in some patients during ventricular tachycardia. This variability is associated with slight changes in ECG morphology and activation time recorded by the mapping catheter. Such changes have been attributed to multiple exit sites from either a discrete focus or a more diffuse focus. The latter is identified by the requirement for several radiofrequency lesions at contiguous sites in order to eliminate the arrhythmogenic focus.[32] Ablation success is achieved in approximately 90% of patients, and ablation also has been performed safely in children and adolescents.[6] Recurrence rates are approximately 10%. Although complications are rare, a new right bundle branch block (RBBB) block develops in 2% of patients, and at least one death has been reported, secondary to complications from RVOT perforation.

Left Ventricular Outflow Tract Tachycardia

Although adenosine-sensitive ventricular tachycardia most commonly originates from the RVOT, the site of origin in approximately 20% of patients is from the LVOT.[2,3] LVOT tachycardia can originate from several sites, including the superior basal region of the left interventricular septum, the aortomitral continuity, mitral annulus, aortic coronary cusps, and epicardial sites in the region of the great cardiac and anterior interventricular veins. A basal left interventricular or septal origin is suggested by a left bundle branch block (LBBB) morphology in association with an early precordial transition in lead V_2 or V_3, an S wave in lead V_6 (due to activation of the left bundle Purkinje system), and a relatively narrow QRS complex,[33] whereas ventricular tachycardia from the region of the left fibrous trigone (aortomitral valve continuity) is associated with an RBBB ventricular tachycardia morphology in lead V_1 and broad monophasic R-waves across the precordium. Regardless of where along the circumference of the mitral annulus ventricular tachycardia originates, the ECG shows an RBBB pattern across the precordium and an S wave in lead V_6.[34,35] The more lateral the site, the more likely is the presence of an S wave in lead I and of notching in the inferior leads. In contrast with the other mitral annular sites, a posterior focus will have a superior axis.

Ablation of mitral annular ventricular tachycardia can be performed using a retrograde endocardial approach and recording an atrial and ventricular potential at the successful ablation site. If this strategy proves unsuccessful, it may be because the epicardial focus requires more direct delivery of energy. This can be achieved by delivering radiofrequency energy or cryoablating through a catheter advanced into the great cardiac vein or, alternatively, by accessing the pericardial space through a percutaneous subxiphoid puncture.[36,37] Limitations in ablating within the great cardiac vein as well as other tributaries of the coronary sinus include rupture, thrombosis, stenosis, and injury to an adjacent coronary artery. If this approach is used, coronary arteriography should be performed before and after ablation to confirm patency.

Because the aortic valve lies to the right of and posterior to the RVOT, ventricular tachycardia originating from the sinuses of Valsalva has a longer R wave duration and greater amplitude in leads V_1 or V_2 than RVOT tachycardia (R/QRS duration greater than 50% and R/S amplitude greater than 30%).[38] Other findings include relatively large R waves inscribed in the inferior leads owing to the subepicardial location of the focus. The substrate of this arrhythmia probably originates from crescents of ventricular myocardium present at the bases of the right and left aortic sinuses.[39] At successful ablation sites, late potentials following the local ventricular electrogram sometimes are recorded during sinus rhythm. During tachycardia, a reversal of activation sequence is seen, with the late potential becoming a presystolic signal that precedes the earliest ventricular electrogram.[38,40] An analogous phenomenon has been described for ventricular tachycardia originating from the pulmonary artery.[26] The exact electrophysiologic substrate of the "prepotential" is unknown. It is likely that the potential originates from the site of origin of ventricular tachycardia or PVCs or represents the nexus between the tachycardia source in the aortic sinus or pulmonary artery and the ventricular myocardium.[41] Ventricular tachycardia localized to the aortic sinuses originates most frequently from the left coronary sinus, followed by the right aortic sinus. Ventricular tachycardia rarely originates from the noncoronary aortic sinus, probably because its base consists of fibrous tissue, which is in continuity with the mitral valve.

Several factors should be considered in ablating from the right and left aortic sinuses. Local capture during pace mapping from a site of early activation may require high output. Atrial electrograms often accompany ventricular potentials because the right and left aortic sinuses are in close proximity to the right and left atrial appendages, respectively. Aortic root angiography identifies the ostia of the right coronary artery and left main coronary artery. For ablation of the left aortic sinus, the left main coronary artery can be cannulated and serve as a landmark. The successful catheter position is usually located 10 mm or more below the ostium. Radiofrequency energy is targeted to achieve a temperature of 55° C by delivering 15 to 30 W. Ablation is performed during continuous fluoroscopy to observe for catheter dislodgment. Coronary angiography is often performed immediately after the ablative procedure to rule out spasm, dissection, or thrombus.

Rarely, epicardial adenosine-sensitive LVOT tachycardia also can occur along the course of the anterior interventricular vein and at its junction with the great cardiac vein. Findings suggestive of an epicardial site of origin include suboptimal pace maps acquired from the ventricular endocardial surface, low-amplitude far-field potentials at the earliest endocardial sites, a delayed intrinsicoid deflection, and large R waves in the inferior leads. Other findings that may suggest an epicardial site remote from the left sinus of Valsalva include a deep S wave in V_1 and a large aVL-to-aVR Q wave ratio. In contrast with left venticular endocardial ventricular tachycardia, no S wave is present in lead V_6.

Verapamil-Sensitive Fascicular Tachycardia

Clinical Characteristics

Two predominant forms of idiopathic left ventricular tachycardia are recognized: LVOT tachycardia and verapamil-sensitive fascicular tachycardia. The latter usually originates in the region of the left posterior fascicle and has a characteristic RBBB, left superior axis morphology. Fascicular tachycardia usually manifests between the ages of 15 and 40 years. Approximately 60% to 80% of patients are male. The resting ECG in most cases is unremarkable, but nonspecific transient inferolateral T wave changes may be present after cessation of tachycardia. Coronary arteriography findings and left ventricular function typically are normal. Fascicular ventricular tachycardia can be incessant and may cause a reversible tachycardia-related cardiomyopathy. Sudden cardiac death usually is not associated with this form of ventricular tachycardia.

Fascicular ventricular tachycardia originally was described as occurring primarily at rest, but sensitivity of tachycardia initiation to catecholamine stimulation (e.g., exercise or post-exercise) or emotional distress also is a prominent characteristic.[2,42] The tachycardia is characterized by an RBBB, left superior axis morphology in 90% to 95% of patients, suggesting an exit site in the region of the left posterior fascicle, near the inferoposterior left ventricular septum. Ventricular tachycardia exiting from the inferoapical region may demonstrate a right superior axis. The remainder of patients have ventricular tachycardia with an RBBB, right inferior axis morphology that exits in the region of the left anterior fascicle, near the anterosuperior left ventricular septum. SAECGs analyzed in the time domain are normal.

Anatomic Substrate

The anatomic basis for this arrhythmia has provoked considerable interest. Endocardial mapping during ventricular tachycardia initially identified the earliest site of activation in the region of the inferoposterior left ventricular septum. This finding, along with the tachycardia's characteristic QRS morphology during ventricular tachycardia and short retrograde ventricular His-bundle (V-H) interval, suggested a left posterior fascicular origin. Other evidence also pointed to an origin within the Purkinje fiber network of the left posterior fascicle, including the recording of high-frequency potentials preceding the site of earliest ventricular activation during ventricular tachycardia and sinus rhythm.[42] These potentials are thought to represent activation of Purkinje fibers and are recorded from the posterior one third of the left ventricular septum. Successful ablation is achieved at sites where the Purkinje potential is recorded 30 to 40 ms before the ventricular tachycardia QRS complex, suggesting that the tachycardia originates from this site or contiguous tissue. Other observations suggest that the tachycardia circuit may comprise a macro-reentrant circuit, with the posterior fascicle serving as one limb and abnormal decremental Purkinje tissue serving as the other.[43-46]

A portion of the tachycardia circuit may originate from a false tendon or fibromuscular band that extends from the posteroinferior left ventricle to the basal septum. Surgical extirpation of the false tendon with either laser photocoagulation, resection, or cryoablation of the myocardial attachment, or radiofrequency catheter ablation at the septal insertion of the false tendon, reportedly eliminates tachycardia. Histologic examination of a resected false tendon from one such patient disclosed abundant Purkinje fibers that were oriented parallel to the long axis of the tendon and inserted into the endocardium.[47]

False tendons are present in a high percentage of patients with left posterior fascicular tachycardia,[48] although the specificity of this finding has been disputed.[49] It is possible that a false tendon either constitutes part of the tachycardia circuit, or that the tendon elicits stretch on Purkinje fibers in the left ventricular septum and thereby initiates tachycardia.

Mechanism

Fascicular tachycardia is due to a reentrant mechanism. In support of this inference is the demonstration that criteria for entrainment are fulfilled.[50] Of note, during orthodromic capture, activation of the earliest site occurs through a region associated with slow, decremental conduction. The entrance site to the zone of slow conduction is thought to be near the base of the left interventricular septum,[46] providing a possible explanation for the observation that manifest entrainment more frequently is achieved with pacing from the RVOT than from the right ventricular apex. The putative entrance and exit sites are further delineated during concealed entrainment (Fig. 61-5).

The precise substrate of the reentrant circuit has not been unequivocally established, but compelling data suggest that one limb involves the posterior fascicle, whereas the other limb is dependent on slowly conducting Purkinje tissue. The electrophysiologic relationship between the two limbs is illustrated in Figures 61-6 and 61-7. As shown in Figure 61-6A, Purkinje potentials from the left posterior fascicle are activated in anterograde fashion (proximal to distal sequence) during sinus rhythm and precede ventricular activation. After ventricular depolarization, fusion of diastolic ascending and descending potentials occurs. These findings are consistent with anterograde conduction proceeding simultaneously over two pathways, with rapid conduction advancing over the posterior fascicle and slow conduction traversing the abnormal Purkinje tissue. Conduction in the abnormal Purkinje tissue blocks in a proximal segment, allowing for retrograde activation of this pathway to proceed by propagation from the distal posterior fascicle. A reversal of

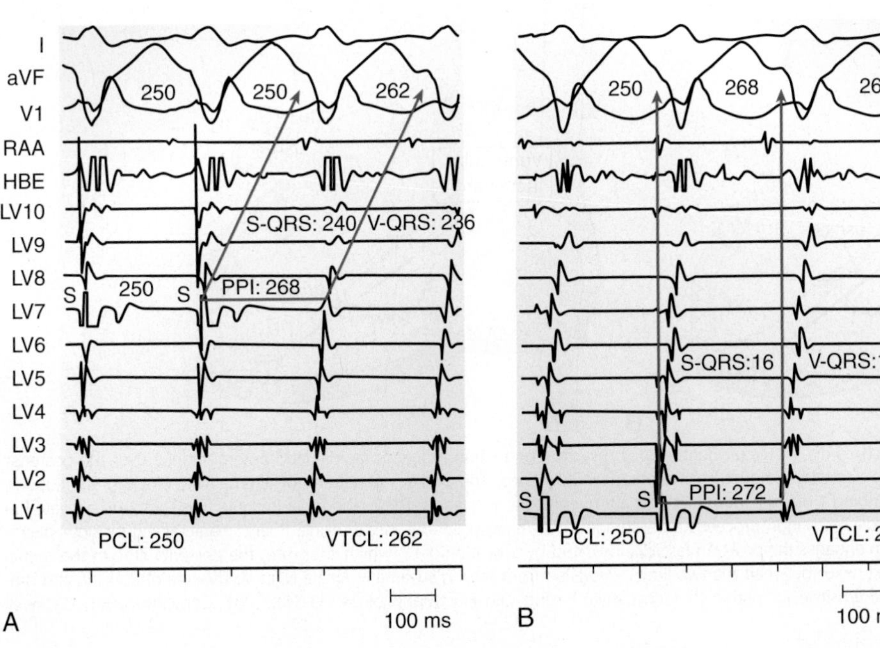

Figure 61-5 Concealed entrainment of fascicular tachycardia from a site near the entrance of the slow conduction zone (**A**) and near the exit site of the slow conduction zone (**B**). The left ventricular (LV) catheter was positioned across the area of slow conduction in the ventricular septum. Pacing at the entrance site was performed from the midseptum of the left ventricle, and pacing at the exit site was delivered from the apical septum. All values are given in ms. PCL, pacing cycle length; PPI, postpacing interval measured at the pacing lead; RAA, right atrial appendage; S-QRS, interval from the stimulus to onset of the QRS complex; V-QRS, interval from the local myocardial potential to onset of the QRS complex; VTCL, ventricular tachycardia cycle length. (From Maruyama M, Tadera T, Miyamoto S, et al: Demonstration of the reentrant circuit of verapamil-sensitive idiopathic left ventricular tachycardia: Direct evidence for macroreentry as the underlying mechanism. J Cardiovasc Electrophysiol 12:968-972, 2001. Copyright 2001, Blackwell Publishing Co.)

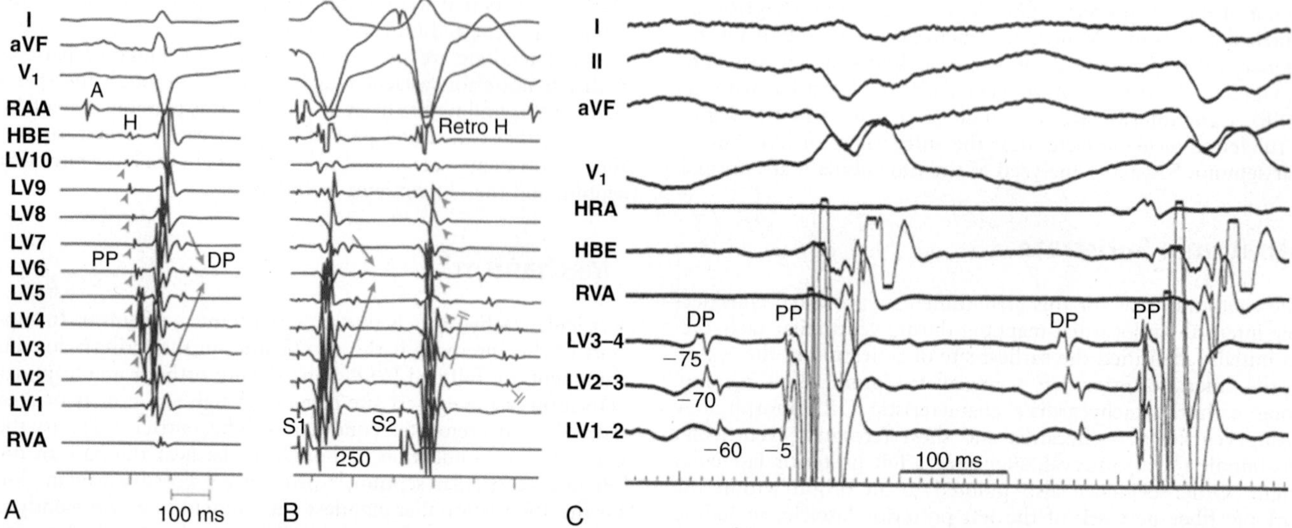

Figure 61-6 The relationship between Purkinje potentials (PPs) and diastolic potentials (DPs) during sinus rhythm, ventricular pacing and ventricular tachycardia in posterior fascicular tachycardia. **A,** Sequential high-frequency PPs, thought to originate from the left posterior fascicle (*arrowheads*), were recorded along the left ventricular septum during sinus rhythm (proximal to distal). Low-frequency anterograde and retrograde DPs also were observed after ventricular activation (*long arrows*). **B,** During the basic ventricular drive (S_1), low-frequency DPs were recorded after ventricular activation. At a coupling interval of 250 ms (S_2), the ascending DPs blocked, which allowed the descending impulse to conduct to the apical septum before conduction ultimately failed. Surface leads I, aVF, and V_1, and intracardiac bipolar electrograms were recorded from the right atrial appendage (RAA), His bundle electrogram (HBE), left ventricular septal electrograms (LV1 to LV10), and right ventricular apex (RVA). **C,** Relationship between PPs and DPs during posterior fascicular tachycardia. Recordings from a left ventricular (LV) midseptal catheter are proximal to distal. Note that activation of DP is proximal to distal and that of PP, distal to proximal. HRA, high right atrium. (From Maruyama M, Tadera T, Miyamoto S, et al: Demonstration of the reentrant circuit of verapamil-sensitive idiopathic left ventricular tachycardia: Direct evidence for macroreentry as the underlying mechanism. J Cardiovasc Electrophysiol 12:968-972, 2001. Copyright 2001, Blackwell Publishing Co.; and from Nogami A, Naito S, Toda H, et al: Demonstration of diastolic and presystolic Purkinje potentials as critical potentials in a macroreentry circuit of verapamil-sensitive idiopathic left ventricular tachycardia. J Am Coll Cardiol 36:811-823, 2000. Copyright 2000, American College of Cardiology.)

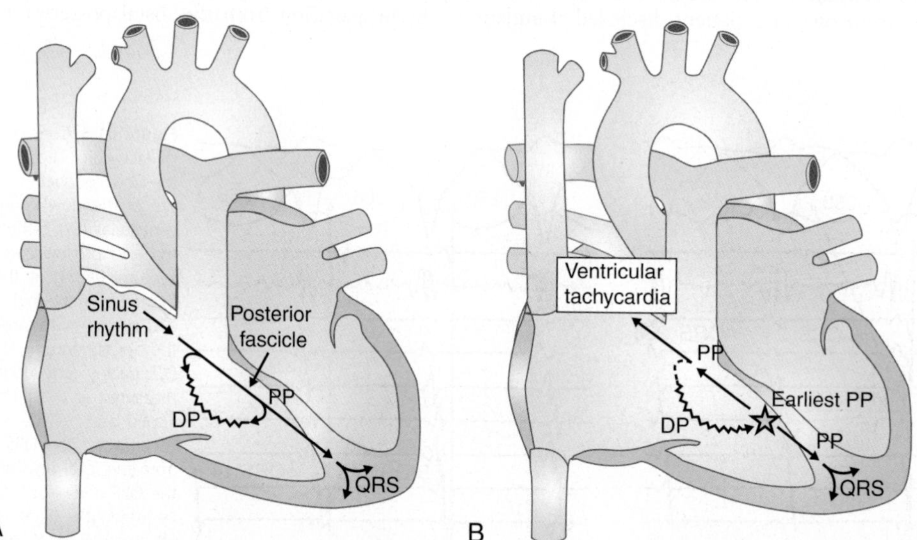

Figure 61-7 Proposed circuit for posterior fascicular tachycardia. **A,** Circuit during sinus rhythm. Conduction proceeds rapidly (and anterogradely) over the posterior fascicle, inscribing a Purkinje potential (PP). The impulse also may conduct in anterograde fashion over and partially penetrate (or alternatively block in) contiguous, diseased Purkinje fibers (drawn as a parallel circuit), inscribing a diastolic potential (DP) after ventricular activation. These abnormal Purkinje fibers also are activated in retrograde fashion. **B,** Circuit during ventricular tachycardia. Activation proceeds anterogradely over a region of diseased Purkinje fibers, characterized by slow, decremental conduction, which inscribes DP. The impulse then engages the posterior fascicle, indicated by activation of PP, which consitutes the posterior limb of the circuit. The ventricular myocardium may or may not serve as the nexus between the two limbs. (Modified from Aiba T, Suyama K, Aihara N, et al: The role of Purkinje and pre-Purkinje potentials in the reentrant circuit of verapamil-sensitive idiopathic LV tachycardia. Pacing Clin Electrophysiol 24:333-344, 2001. Copyright 2001, Blackwell Publishing Co.)

this sequence occurs during ventricular pacing and initiation of ventricular tachycardia. For example, after ventricular pacing, retrograde activation of Purkinje potentials and the His bundle occurs, presumably by way of the posterior fascicle (see Fig. 61-6B). During the drive train (i.e., stimulus 1 [S_1]), bidirectional activation of diastolic potentials is again observed. Retrograde activation of diastolic potentials occurs in parallel, with activation of Purkinje potentials in the distal posterior fascicle, whereas anterograde activation of diastolic potentials occurs after, being activated by the proximal segment of the left posterior fascicle. During a ventricular extrastimulus (S_2), block of the diastolic potential in the retrograde limb of the abnormal Purkinje tissue, allows activation of the retrograde posterior fascicle (or Purkinje potential) to be followed by unimpeded anterograde conduction over the abnormal Purkinje tissue. An earlier extrastimulus results in additional conduction delay in the anterograde limb, allowing the diastolic potential (DP) to then activate the Purkinje potentials (PPs) retrogradely and initiate ventricular tachycardia (see Fig. 61-6C). Therefore, DP activation during ventricular tachycardia is anterograde, whereas PP activation is retrograde, resulting in earliest activation of the most distal PP within the circuit. The anterograde limb thus appears to be composed of abnormal Purkinje tissue, which exhibits slow, decremental conduction, is verapamil-sensitive and gives rise to DPs along the midseptum (see Fig. 61-7B). The retrograde limb consists of Purkinje system tissue from the left posterior fascicle (or contiguous to it), giving rise to PPs. A schematic of the proposed circuit during sinus rhythm (which is a reversal of the circuit during ventricular tachycardia) is shown in Figure 61-7A.

The zone of slow conduction appears to depend on the slow-inward calcium current, because the degree of slowing of ventricular tachycardia cycle length in response to verapamil is largely attributable to its negative dromotropic effects on the area of slow conduction. A lesser degree of slowing is observed with lidocaine.[51] These data suggest that Purkinje fibers composing the reentrant circuit have partially depolarized resting membrane potentials, with the depolarizing currents relatively more dependent on the slow-inward calcium current than on depressed fast sodium channels.

Fascicular reentrant tachycardia has a characteristic electropharmacologic profile. Like other forms of idiopathic ventricular tachycardia, it is responsive to verapamil, but in contrast with ventricular tachycardia originating from the outflow tract, adenosine and Valsalva maneuvers usually have no effect on this form of ventricular tachycardia.[52] These responses are useful for clinical and mechanistic distinctions between these two forms of idiopathic ventricular tachycardia. They suggest that although the substrates for both tachycardias are calcium-dependent, the reentrant tissue in fascicular tachycardia appears to be dependent primarily on the basal slow inward calcium current in partially depolarized Purkinje fibers. By contrast, outflow tract tachycardia, due to triggered activity, is dependent on intracellular calcium overload that is achieved through cAMP stimulation and increased calcium channel conductance.

Therapy

Although it is well-established that acute treatment of fascicular tachycardia with intravenous verapamil is effective, available data regarding efficacy of chronic antiarrhythmic therapy are relatively scarce. Verapamil (160 to 320 mg/day) ameliorates symptoms in patients who are moderately impaired by tachycardia but has little effect in patients who are significantly debilitated.

Patients with fascicular ventricular tachycardia associated with presyncope or syncope, those with recurrent sustained tachycardia, and patients who are intolerant or resistant to antiarrhythmic therapy are appropriate candidates for ablative therapy. The results of radiofrequency ablation in this group of patients are excellent, with outcomes similar to those achieved with radiofrequency ablation for OT tachycardia. Aggregate data from studies in which the ablative approach, long-term results, and complications are well described report success rates of approximately 90%.[42-46]

Multiple strategies have been deployed to identify the appropriate site for ablation. Initial approaches used pace mapping and activation mapping and sought concordance between the QRS morphology of the 12-lead ECG during ventricular tachycardia and pace mapping, as well as local ventricular activation that preceded the surface QRS complex by at least 30 ms. Another mapping approach targets high-frequency Purkinje potentials or PPs that precede earliest ventricular activation in the region of the left posterior fascicle.[42]

Other approaches focus on the identification of diastolic potentials or DPs during ventricular tachycardia. These potentials may be recorded along a span of 25 mm of the mid-left interventricular septum and precede PPs during tachycardia. Successful ablation sites are often associated with progressive prolongation of the DP-PP interval, with termination of ventricular tachycardia coincident with conduction block between the two potentials.[43,44] Success is not necessarily predicated on targeting the earliest (most proximal) DP. Success may be achieved by ablating a DP slightly distal to the earliest potential, which also reduces the potential for damaging the trunk of the left bundle. An alternative strategy is to ablate sharp, high-frequency late potentials recorded during sinus rhythm. Late potentials occur approximately 150 to 450 ms after the PP and have been observed only in patients with fascicular tachycardia.[53] These potentials are recorded in the midinferior septum, in the region of the posterior fascicle. As described above, these sinus rhythm potentials correspond to DPs observed during ventricular tachycardia and probably represent activation of abnormal Purkinje tissue. Targeting these late potentials during sinus rhythm is associated with ablation success, a useful approach in those patients in whom tachycardia cannot be induced (Fig. 61-8). Another approach for ablating patients who are noninducible is to create a linear lesion equidistant between the base and apex, beginning at the level of the mid-inferior septum and continuing the line to the the point where the septum joins the inferior wall.[54]

Although electrophysiologically distinct but anatomically related to fascicular tachycardia, interfascicular tachycardia confined to the left ventricle should be considered in the differential diagnosis of idiopathic left ventricular tachycardia.[55] Insufficient data are available at present to determine whether, as with bundle branch reentry, conduction disease and dilated cardiomyopathy are associated conditions, although RBBB and anterior or posterior fascicular block are often present during sinus rhythm. The reentrant tachycardia circuit involves anterograde conduction over the left anterior or left posterior fascicle, with the retrograde limb consisting of the alternative fascicle. Therefore, tachycardia with an RBBB, left posterior fascicular block morphology would indicate anterograde conduction over the left anterior fascicle with retrograde conduction over the left posterior fascicle. Criteria required to diagnose left interfascicular tachycardia include (1) RBBB morphology during tachycardia which is similar to that recorded in sinus rhythm, (2) reversal in activation sequence of the His and left bundle potentials during tachycardia, (3) an H-V interval shorter during ventricular tachycardia than sinus rhythm, (4) spontaneous oscillations of tachycardia cycle length due to

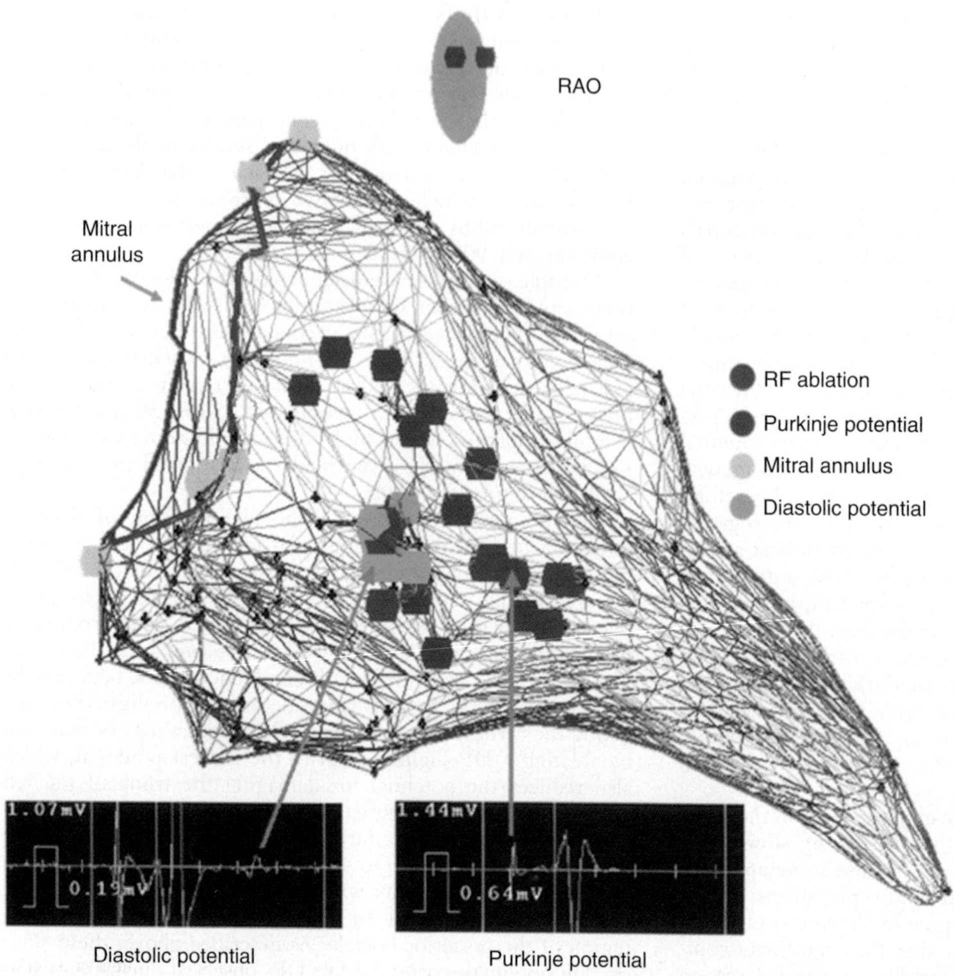

Figure 61-8 Sinus rhythm map of Purkinje potentials (PPs) in a patient with fascicular ventricular tachycardia. The *green tags* identify PPs recorded from the region of the left posterior fascicle. The *right inset* shows the electrogram recorded from this region. The first spike represents the PP, and the second signal is the ventricular electrogram. The *pink tags* correspond to the area in which retrograde delayed/diastolic potentials (DPs) were recorded. The *left inset* shows an electrogram from this region. The first signal is a PP, followed by a ventricular electrogram and then a low-amplitude retrograde DP. This site, which recorded the earliest DP during sinus rhythm, was the site of successful ablation. RF, radiofrquency; RAO, right anterior oblique (projection).

changes in the left bundle–left bundle interval that precede and drive the ventricular cycle length, and (5) termination of tachycardia with ventricular extrastimuli or radiofrequency ablation that produces block in either of the two fascicles.

References

1. Lerman BB, Stein KM, Markowitz SM: Adenosine-sensitive ventricular tachycardia: A conceptual approach. J Cardiovasc Electrophysiol 7:559-569, 1996.
2. Lerman BB, Stein KM, Markowitz SM: Mechanisms of idiopathic left ventricular tachycardia. J Cardiovasc Electrophysiol 8:571-583, 1997.
3. Iwai S, Cantillon DJ, Kim RJ, et al: Right and left ventricular outflow tract tachycardias: Evidence for a common electrophysiologic mechanism. J Cardiovasc Electrophysiol 17:1052-1058, 2006.
4. Lerman BB, Belardinelli L, West GA, et al: Adenosine-sensitive ventricular tachycardia: Evidence suggesting cyclic AMP-mediated triggered activity. Circulation 74:270-280, 1986.
5. Lerman BB: Response of nonreentrant catecholamine and mediated ventricular tachycardia to endogenous adenosine and acetylcholine: Evidence for receptor mediated effects. Circulation 87:382-390, 1993.
6. Kim RJ, Iwai S, Markowitz SM, et al: Clinical and electrophysiological spectrum of idiopathic ventricular outflow tract arrhythmias. J Am Coll Cardiol 49:2035-2043, 2007.
7. Lerman BB, Stein K, Engelstein ED, et al: Mechanism of repetitive monomorphic ventricular tachycardia. Circulation 92:421-429, 1995.
8. Song Y, Thedford S, Lerman BB, Belardinelli L: Adenosine-sensitive afterdepolarizations and triggered activity in guinea pig ventricular myocytes. Circ Res 70:743-753, 1992.
9. Han X, Ferrier GR: Contribution of Na^+-Ca^{2+} exchange to stimulation of transient inward current by isoproterenol in rabbit cardiac Purkinje fibers. Circ Res 76:664-674, 1995.
10. Lerman BB, Wesley RC, DiMarco JP, et al: Antiadrenergic effects of adenosine on His-Purkinje automaticity: Evidence for accentuated antagonism. J Clin Invest 82:2127-2135, 1988.
11. Lerman BB: Mechanism of outflow tract tachycardia. Heart Rhythm 4:973-976, 2007.
12. Lerman BB, Stein KM, Markowitz SM, et al: Catecholamine facilitated reentrant ventricular tachycardia: Uncoupling of adenosine's antiadrenergic effects. J Cardiovasc Electrophysiol 10:17-26, 1999.
13. Lerman BB, Dong B, Stein KM, et al: Right ventricular outflow tract tachycardia due to a somatic cell mutation in G protein subunit αi_2. J Clin Invest 101:2862-2868, 1998.
14. Gaita F, Giustetto C, DiDonna P, et al: Long-term follow-up of right ventricular monomorphic extrasystoles. J Am Coll Cardiol 38:364-370, 2001.
15. Grimm W, Menz V, Hoffman J, et al: Reversal of tachycardia induced cardiomyopathy following ablation of repetitive monomorphic ventricular outflow tract tachycardia. Pacing Clin Electrophysiol 24:166-171, 2001.
16. Yarlagadda RK, Iwai S, Stein KM, et al: Reversal of cardiomyopathy in patients

with repetitive monomorphic ventricular ectopy originating from the right ventricular outflow tract. Circulation 112:1092-1097, 2005.
17. Takemoto M, Yoshimura H, Ohba Y, et al: Radiofrequency catheter ablation of premature ventricular complexes from right ventricular outflow tract improves left ventricular dilation and clinical status in patients without structural heart disease. J Am Coll Cardiol 45:1259-1265, 2005.
18. Haissaguerre M, Shoda M, Jais P, et al: Mapping and ablation of idiopathic ventricular fibrillation. Circulation 106:962-967, 2002.
19. Haissaguerre M, Extramiana F, Hocini M, et al: Mapping and ablation of ventricular fibrillation associated with long-QT and Brugada syndromes. Circulation 108:925-928, 2003.
20. Gill JS, Prasad K, Blaszyk K, et al: Initiating sequences in exercise induced idiopathic ventricular tachycardia of left bundle branch-like morphology. Pacing Clin Electrophysiol 21:1873-1880, 1998.
21. Hayashi H, Fujiki A, Tani M, et al: Circadian variation of idiopathic ventricular tachycardia originating from right ventricular outflow tract. Am J Cardiol 84:99-101, 1999.
22. Carlson MD, White RD, Trohman RG, et al: Right ventricular outflow tract ventricular tachycardia: Detection of previously unrecognized anatomic abnormalities using cine magnetic resonance imaging. J Am Coll Cardiol 24:720-727, 1994.
23. Markowitz SM, Litvak BL, Ramirez de Arellano EA, et al: Adenosine-sensitive ventricular tachycardia: Right ventricular abnormalities delineated by magnetic resonance imaging. Circulation 96:1192-1200, 1997.
24. Tandri H, Bluemke DA, Ferrari VA, et al: Findings on magnetic resonance imaging of idiopathic right ventricular outflow tachycardia. Am J Cardiol 94:1441-1445, 2004.
25. Kamakura S, Shimizu W, Matsuo K, et al: Localization of optimal ablation site of idiopathic ventricular tachycardia from right and left ventricular outflow tract by body surface ECG. Circulation 98:1525-1533, 1998.
26. Timmermans C, Rodriquez LM, Crijins HJG, et al: Idiopathic left bundle-branch block-shaped ventricular tachycardia may originate above the pulmonary valve. Circulation 108:1960-1967, 2003.
27. Sekiguchi Y, Aonuma K, Takahashi A, et al: Electrocardiographic and electrophysiologic characteristics of ventricualr tachycardia originating within the pulmonary artery. J Am Coll Cardiol 45:887-895, 2005.
28. Yamauchi Y, Aonuma K, Takahashi A, et al: Electrocardiographic characteristics of repetitive monomorphic right ventricular tachycardia originating near the His-bundle. J Cardiovasc Electrophysiol 16:1041-1048, 2005.
29. Tada H, Tadokoro K, Ito S, et al: Idiopathic ventricular arrhythmia originating from the tricuspid annulus: Prevalence, electrocardiographic characteristics, and results of radiofrequency catheter ablation. Heart Rhythm 4:7-16, 2007.
30. Green LS, Lux RL, Ershler PR, et al: Resolution of pace mapping stimulus site separation using body surface potentials. Circulation 90:462-468, 1994.
31. Chinushi M, Aizawa Y, Ohhira K, et al: Repetitive ventricular responses induced by radiofrequency ablation for idiopathic ventricular tachycardia originating from the outflow tract of the right ventricle. Pacing Clin Electrophysiol 21:669-678, 1998.
32. Chinushi M, Aizawa Y, Takahashi K, et al: Morphological variation of nonreentrant idiopathic ventricular tachycardia originating from the right ventricular outflow tract and effect of radiofrequency lesion. Pacing Clin Electrophysiol 20:325-336, 1997.
33. Ito S, Tada H, Naito S, et al: Development and validation of an ECG algorithm for identifying the optimal ablation site for idiopathic ventricular outflow tract tachycardia. J Cardiovasc Electrophysiol 14:1280-1286, 2003.
34. Kumagai K, Yamuchi Y, Takahashi A, et al: Idiopathic left ventricular tachycardia originating from the mitral annulus. J Cardiovasc Electrophysiol 16:1029-1036, 2005.
35. Tada H, Ito S, Naito S, et al: Idiopathic ventricular arrhythmia arising from the mitral annulus. A distinct subgroup of idiopathic ventricular arrhythmias. J Am Coll Cardiol 45:877-886, 2005.
36. Obel OA, d'Avila A, Neuzil P, et al: Ablation of left ventricular epicardial outflow tract tachycardia from the distal great cardiac vein. J Am Coll Cardiol 48:1813-1817, 2006.
37. Daniels DV, Lu YY, Morton JB, et al: Idiopathic epicardial left ventricalr tachycardia originating remote from the sinus of Valsalva. Electropjysiological characteristics, catheter ablation, and identification from the 12-lead electrecardiogram. Circulation 113:1659-1666, 2006.
38. Ouyang F, Fotuhi P, Ho SY, et al: Repetitive monomorphic ventricular tachycardia originating from the aortic sinus cusp: Electrocardiographic characterization for guiding catheter ablation. J Am Coll Cardiol 39:500-508, 2002.
39. Anderson RH: Clinical anatomy of the aortic root. Heart 24:670-673, 2000.
40. Tada H, Naito S, Ito S, et al: Significance of two potentials for predicting successful catheter ablation from the left sinus of Valsalva for left ventricular epicardial tachycardia. Pacing Clin Electrophysiol 27:1053-1059, 2004.
41. Lerman BB: Ablating left ventricular outflow tract tachycardia: In search of Ockham's razor. Pacing Clin Electrophysiol 27:1051-1052, 2004.
42. Nakagawa H, Beckman KJ, McClelland JH, et al: Radiofrequency catheter ablation of idiopathic left ventricular tachycardia guided by a Purkinje potential. Circulation 88:2607-2617, 1993.
43. Tsuchiya T, Okumura K, Honda T, et al: Significance of late diastolic potential preceding Purkinje potential in verapamil-sensitive idiopathic left ventricular tachycardia. Circulation 99:2408-2413, 1999.
44. Nogami A, Naito S, Tada H, et al: Demonstration of diastolic and presystolic Purkinje potentials as critical potentials in a macroeentry circuit of verapamil-sensitive idiopathic left ventricular tachycardia. J Am Coll Cardiol 36:811-823, 2000.
45. Aiba T, Suyama K, Aihara N, et al: The role of Purkinje and pre-Purkinje potentials in the reentrant circuit of verapamil-sensitive idiopathic LV tachycardia. Pacing Clin Electrophysiol 24:333-344, 2001.
46. Maruyama M, Tadera T, Miyamoto S, Ino T: Demonstration of the reentrant circuit of verapamil-sensitive idiopathic left ventricular tachycardia: Direct evidence for macroreentry as the underlying mechanism. J Cardiovasc Electrophysiol 12:968-972, 2001.
47. Suwa M, Yoneda Y, Nagao H, et al: Surgical correction of idiopathic paroxysmal ventricular tachycardia possibly related to left ventricular false tendon. Am J Cardiol 64:1217-1220, 1989.
48. Thakur RK, Klein GJ, Sivaram CA, et al: Anatomic substrate for idiopathic left ventricular tachycardia. Circulation 93:497-501, 1996.
49. Lin FC, Wen MS, Wang CC, et al: Left ventricular fibromuscular band is not a specific substrate for idiopathic left ventricular tachycardia. Circulation 93:525-528, 1996.
50. Okumura K, Yamabe H, Tsuchiya T, et al: Characteristics of slow conduction zone demonstrated during entrainment of idiopathic ventricular tachycardia of left ventricular origin. Am J Cardiol 77:379-383, 1996.
51. Tsuchiya T, Okumura K, Honda T, et al: Effects of verapamil and lidocaine on two components of the re-entry circuit of verapamil-sensitive idiopathic left ventricular tachycardia. Am J Cardiol 37:1415-1421, 2001.
52. Griffith MJ, Garratt CJ, Rowland E, et al: Effects of intravenous adenosine on verapamil-sensitive "idiopathic" ventricular tachycardia. Am J Cardiol 73:759-764, 1994.
53. Ouyang F, Cappato R, Ernst S, et al: Electroanatomic substrate of idiopathic left ventricular tachycardia. Circulation 105:462-469, 2002.
54. Lin D, Hsia HH, Gerstenfeld EP, et al: Idiopathic fascicular left ventricular tachycardia: Linear ablation lesion strategy for noninducible or nonsustained tachycardia. Heart Rhythm 2:934-939, 2005.
55. Crijns HJ, Smeets JL, Rodriguez LM, et al: Cure of interfascicular reentrant ventricular tachycardia by ablation of the anterior fascicle of the left bundle branch. J Cardiovasc Electrophysiol 6:486-492, 1995.

Ventricular Tachycardia in Patients with Coronary Artery Disease 62

DAVID CALLANS

CHAPTER OUTLINE

Healed myocardial infarction is the most frequent clinical setting for the development of sustained ventricular tachycardia (VT). The first episode of VT can occur years after infarct healing, often without apparent intercurrent changes in the clinical course. The range of clinical presentation is broad, from tolerated sustained VT to sudden cardiac death. With the increased use of defibrillator devices for primary prevention, the most frequent presentation is that of recurrent defibrillator shocks in a patient with an implantable cardioverter-defibrillator (ICD). Current understanding of both the anatomic substrate and the triggers that produce individual episodes is far from complete. To date, this lack of understanding has defied attempts to identify those patients in whom ventricular arrhythmias will develop after infarction.

Pathophysiologic Substrate

Classic studies have demonstrated that sustained, monomorphic VT generally arises from an anatomic substrate of extensive, healed myocardial infarction. The extent of myocardial necrosis, presence of septal involvement and the degree of left ventricular dysfunction are the most important determinants of arrhythmia risk after infarction. Patients with tolerated VT have more extensive infarction, more frequent incidence of discrete left ventricular aneurysm, and more pronounced left ventricular dysfunction than patients with nonsustained ventricular tachycardia or sudden cardiac death.[1] Traditionally, the incidence of sustained, monomorphic VT after infarction was approximately 3%. Contemporary therapy has led to smaller infarcts and less frequent aneurysm formation, with a reduction in the incidence of VT to less than 1% in patients with successful infarct revascularization.[2] Despite this reduction, the population risk for ventricular arrhythmias and sudden cardiac death has been fairly stable, owing to an aging population with a greater number of surviving patients at risk.

Many researchers have wondered if more aggressive revascularization and improved pharmacologic therapy to prevent infarct remodeling have fundamentally changed the pathophysiology of ventricular arrhythmias after myocardial infarction. It generally is assumed that the resulting smaller, and perhaps more mottled, infarcts may lead to more poorly tolerated polymorphic arrhythmias, rather than relatively slow, well-tolerated VT. In patients referred for ablation therapy for frequent VT episodes (albeit a population with recognizably skewed characteristics), however, underlying disease processes appear to be comparable to those reported in the classic studies (Fig. 62-1). Post–myocardial infarction patients referred for VT ablation at the University of Pennsylvania in 2004 and 2005 had lower ejection fractions and more frequently received amiodarone and ICD therapy, compared with patients referred from 1993 to 1997.

VT consistently arises from surviving myocytes within extensive areas of infarction.[2] Although normal sodium-dependent action potentials are recorded from cells within this border zone after infarct healing, conduction is slow and discontinuous, owing to fibrosis and abnormalities in gap junction distribution and function. Extracellular recordings from sites of VT origin during sinus rhythm consistently demonstrate low-amplitude, prolonged, multicomponent potentials (Fig. 62-2). The individual components of these fractionated electrograms appear to be generated by individual "islets" of isolated myocyte groups. The duration of the local electrogram represents the abnormally slow, fractionated conduction that results in delayed activation of individual sites within the electrode field of view.

The electrophysiologic substrate for VT gradually develops in the first 2 weeks after myocardial infarction and, once established, appears to remain indefinitely. Although the relationship between inducible VT and spontaneous VT is poorly understood, inducible monomorphic VT signifies the presence of an anatomic VT substrate and confirms increased susceptibility for arrhythmic events. Arrhythmia triggers, such as acute ischemia, surges in autonomic tone, or the onset of clinical heart failure, provide the link between susceptibility and spontaneous VT. It is important to recognize the preeminent importance of the anatomic substrate, even when VT episodes are precipitated by such potentially reversible clinical situations.[3] Once sustained monomorphic VT occurs, the risk for arrhythmia continues indefinitely, even if acute ischemia and heart failure are adequately controlled.

The obligate relationship of the VT circuit to the anatomy of the infarct was established with the development of effective surgical therapy for post–myocardial infarction ventricular arrhythmias. Recent developments in how to "visualize" the infarct anatomy with endocardial voltage mapping during sinus rhythm have led to a number of insights regarding the nature of VT circuits. The "protected isthmus" of the VT circuit is consistently contained within the dense infarct (bipolar voltage values of less than 0.5 mV); the circuit exit sites consistently exit at the border zone, which is defined by electrogram voltage between 0.5 and 1.5 mV (Fig. 62-3). This realization led to the concept that individual VT morphologic patterns could be regionalized in accordance with findings on pace mapping at the infarct border zone.[4] Furthermore, strategies to identify "channels" of apparent preferential conduction through the infarct, as indicated by relatively preserved voltage, presence of

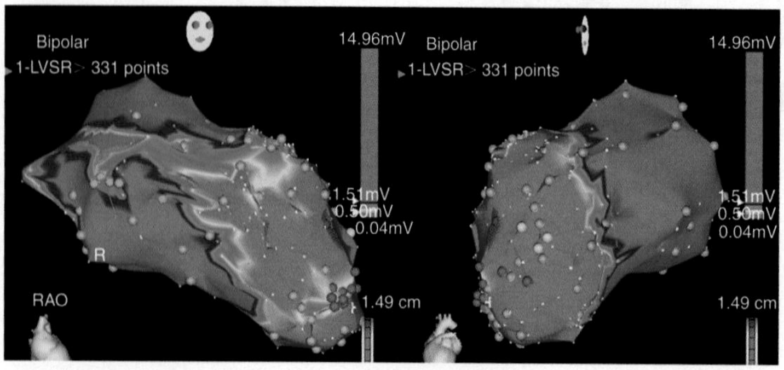

Figure 62-1 Sinus rhythm mapping in a patient with VT in the setting of extensive healed anterior infarction. The map is color-coded to represent bipolar electrogram voltage: *red* (representing dense scar) denotes = 0.5 mV, *purple* = 1.5 mV, and the *intervening colors* represent voltage values in between. The large area of anterior apical scar was calcified and aneurysmal. Multiple inducible VTs of varied morphology were localized to circuits within the scar. LAO, left anterior oblique; RAO, right anterior oblique.

long stimulus to QRS time with pacing during sinus rhythm, or the presence of isolated late potentials in sinus rhythm, have increased the ability of investigators to recognize potential protected isthmus sites without prolonged mapping during VT.[5-10] In addition to the implications these findings have for guiding ablation (discussed more completely in Chapters 108 and 109), this experience has increased current understanding of the relatively large dimension (1 to 2 cm across) of the protected zone in sustained VT in this setting.

Again, based initially on the experience with surgical ablation, the major portion of the present catheter mapping investigation has focused on the endocardial aspect of the VT circuit in healed infarction. Although in some cases of well-tolerated VT, a major portion of the reentrant circuit can be identified on the endocardial surface, it would be difficult to believe that VT represents two-dimensional reentry on the endocardium. Although catheter ablation from the epicardium in this clinical setting has a lower likelihood of success, that is not to say that the epicardial and transmural layers cannot contribute to the substrate of the circuit. Epicardial ablation may provide unique advantages in selected cases, particularly in inferior infarction.

Mechanism of Sustained Ventricular Tachycardia

The available evidence strongly suggests that reentry is the mechanism for a majority of cases of sustained VT in healed myocardial infarction.[1] The ability to reproducibly initiate and terminate VT with programmed ventricular extrastimuli is considered the sine qua non of reentry. Arrhythmias caused by normal or abnormal automaticity cannot be induced with programmed stimulation, and triggered rhythms caused by delayed afterdepolarizations are more easily induced with overdrive pacing and often require catecholamine infusion. In our experience, 95% of patients with healed myocardial infarction and spontaneous sustained VT have inducible VT with programmed stimulation.

Other characteristics of VT in coronary disease support a reentrant mechanism. Induction of VT in coronary disease is stimulation site–specific; 22% of tachycardias are initiated from the right ventricular outflow tract after aggressive stimulation at the apex fails. Site specificity has not been demonstrated in triggered rhythms. An inverse relationship of the

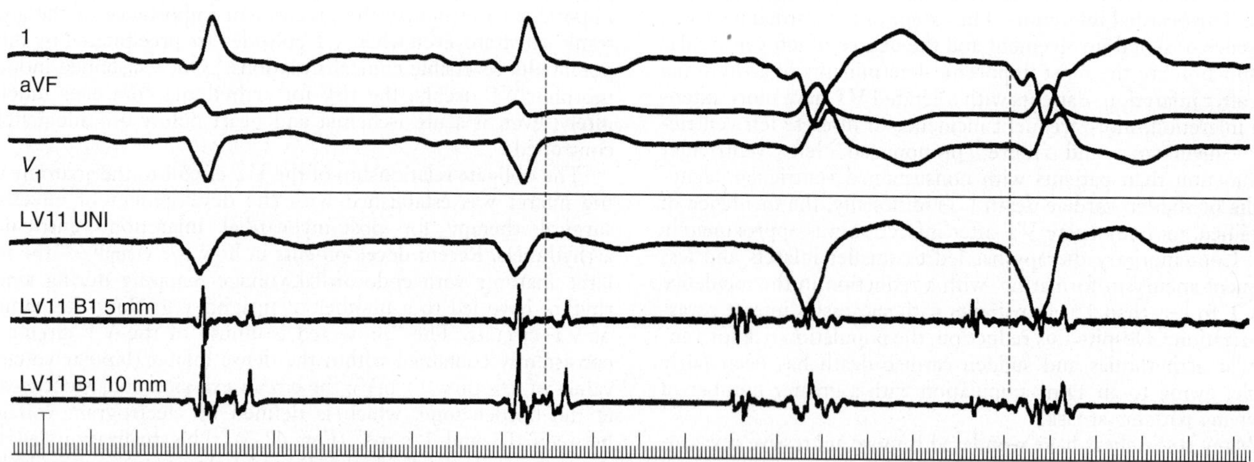

Figure 62-2 Electrogram abnormalities during sinus rhythm and ventricular tachycardia (VT). Three surface electrocardiogram (ECG) leads are shown with three intracardiac recordings from a catheter placed from the left ventricular (LV) anterior wall. During sinus rhythm, a fractionated, multicomponent signal is recorded; the final component of this electrogram is recorded after the end of the surface QRS complex. During VT (*final two beats* of the tracing), the electrogram at this site precedes the QRS complex by 90 ms. (From Josephson ME: Clinical Cardiac Electrophysiology: Techniques and Interpretations, 3rd ed. Philadelphia, Lippincott Williams & Wilkins, 2002.)

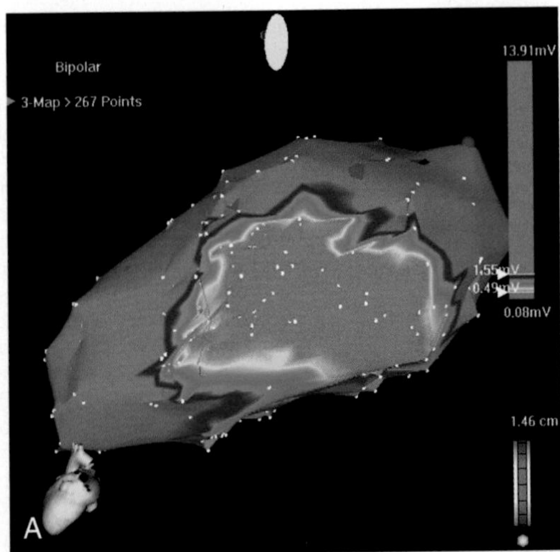

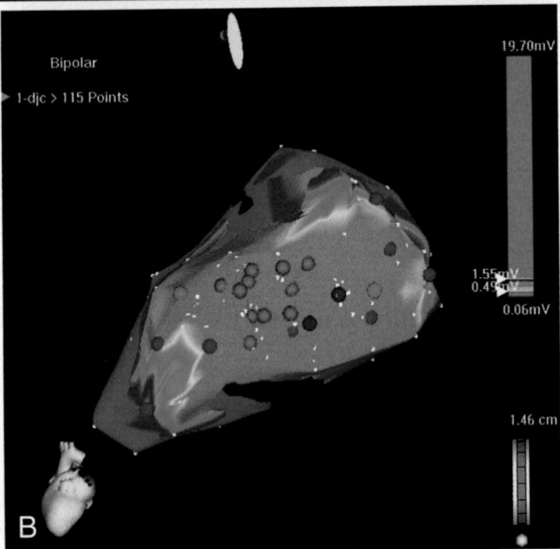

Figure 62-3 The relationship of the ventricular tachycardia (VT) circuit to the infarct anatomy as determined by sinus rhythm voltage mapping. **A,** An electroanatomic voltage map of the left ventricle in a patient with an inferior infarction is shown (left lateral view). The color representation of bipolar voltage is as described in the legend to Figure 62-1. **B,** Colored icons are placed on the context of the sinus voltage map, indicating the response to entrainment during a right bundle right inferior axis VT. The *pink* icon represents the circuit exit site. *Teal, blue,* and *green* icons represent isthmus, entrance, and inner loop sites, respectively. The *purple* sites are not within the circuit—demonstrating that the exit site often corresponds to the border zone of the infarct, and that the physical size of the circuit within the dense infarct often is quite large.

extrastimulus coupling interval to the onset of the first tachycardia beat is observed in many VTs. This observation suggests that slow conduction, a major prerequisite for reentry, which is more pronounced at closer coupling intervals, is necessary for initiation of VT. The identification of mid-diastolic potentials at the arrhythmia site of origin or markedly presystolic electrograms is inconsistent with focal arrhythmia mechanisms. The demonstration that initiation and maintenance of a tachycardia depend on development of a critical degree of slow conduction manifested by continuous electrical activity throughout diastole is consistent with a reentrant mechanism.

Nonetheless, the impact of non-reentrant rhythms in patients with myocardial infarction may be substantial. The sudden death risk implied by the presence of ventricular arrhythmias in this setting assumed reentry as a mechanism. Particularly as enthusiasm for pre-ICD electrophysiology studies has waned, it is not clear how often other mechanisms of VT (e.g., triggered activity) come into play. Both stable reentry involving the fascicular system and focal "triggers" of polymorphic VT from peri-infarct areas have been identified; again, the incidence of these phenomena is not clear. Although both diseased myocardium and Purkinje system activity have been the source of these triggers,[11,12] the role of the Purkinje system in the spread of activity and the maintenance of ventricular fibrillation may be more important.

Response to Programmed Stimulation

The most convincing evidence for reentry in the absense of documentation of the entire reentrant circuit with mapping (an uncommon event) is the response of VT to programmed stimulation–induced resetting and entrainment. In addition to clarifying the mechanism for VT, these stimulation techniques have been used to study the response to antiarrhythmic drug and pacing interventions, for VT mapping, and to investigate the electrophysiologic properties of the VT circuit. A significant limitation is that these techniques can be applied only in hemodynamically tolerated sustained VT.

Entrainment and resetting both are manifestations of the same physiologic events: Paced stimuli enter the VT circuit, block with the existing tachycardia wavefront in the antidromic direction, and conduct through the circuit orthodromically to produce the return cycle beat. The return cycle beat occurs earlier in time (i.e., is reset) because the last stimulated beat does not traverse the entire circuit in the orthodromic direction; rather, it traverses only the distance between the entrance and the exit. One important difference is that, with resetting, only one stimulus interacts with the tachycardia circuit (even when double extrastimuli are used). During entrainment, the first beat of the pacing drive that interacts with the circuit foreshortens the excitable gap to the extent that it arrives prematurely. Subsequent paced beats in the drive interact with the previously reset tachycardia circuit, which may lead to the development of progressive orthodromic conduction delay at coupling intervals that result in a flat resetting curve. This leads to early interpretation of this delay as decremental conduction during VT. Resetting demonstrating a flat response curve over a long zone of coupling intervals suggests that most monomorphic VTs have a fully excitable gap.

Entrainment techniques are used extensively for mapping VT during ablation procedures. Pacing at sites in a protected isthmus within the circuit demonstrate concealed entrainment (entrainment without evidence of surface or intracardiac fusion) with a return cycle approximating the VT cycle length (Fig. 62-4). This finding is useful in identifying targets that are vulnerable sites for ablation techniques, as described in greater detail in Chapter 118.

The response to stimulation has several implications about the physiology of reentry in this setting. Resetting or entrainment with fusion implies the presence of a relatively large circuit with a separate entrance and exit. The demonstration of a substantial excitable gap and the finding of concealed entrainment with long stimulation to QRS times implies circuit barriers imposed by the structure of the infarct that are fairly permanent, or anatomically determined. By contrast, in the canine subacute infarction model, stimuli delivered from areas within or adjacent to the circuit may temporarily alter the circuit barriers, which are functional in nature. The barriers in human VT appear to be less malleable, presumably because they are at least partially fixed by the anatomy of the more extensive infarct scar. To this end, pacing during sinus

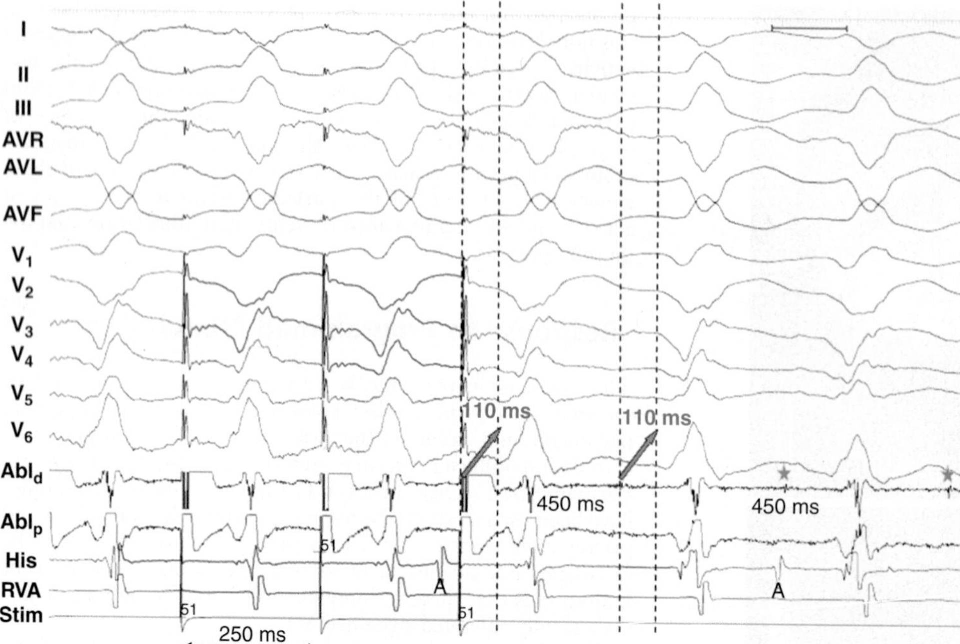

Figure 62-4 Concealed entrainment of ventricular tachycardia. Surface electrocardiogram (ECG) leads are shown with intracardiac electrograms from the left ventricular ablation catheter, right ventricular apex (RVA), and His bundle region. Entrainment pacing from a protected isthmus within the scar is recognized by the following characteristics: (1) exact duplication of the QRS morphology (and orthodromic entrained intracardiac recordings) during entrainment compared with ventricular tachycardia (VT); (2) a stimulus to QRS equal to the electrogram to QRS duration during VT; and (3) a post-pacing interval equal to the VT cycle length. Often these sites are located several centimeters from the scar border and are marked by isolated mid-diastolic potentials (*stars*).

rhythm at sites within of the VT circuit that have isolated late potentials often produces a QRS that matches an inducible VT morphology. This finding implies that the circuit may be almost entirely anatomic in these VTs, because the conduction barriers that form circuit boundaries are always present, even in slow-paced rhythm. However, circuit barriers in human VTs also may be changed by interaction with stimuli in a direction-dependent fashion.[13] These studies indicate a variable contribution of anatomic and functionally determined characteristics in VT circuit barriers.

Clinical Presentation and Management

VT in the setting of chronic coronary artery disease results in a wide spectrum of clinical presentations, ranging from incidental detection to cardiac arrest. The key determinant of hemodynamic tolerance of a VT episode is the tachycardia rate; other factors include baseline left ventricular function, the development of ischemia, and mitral insufficiency. The degree of hemodynamic tolerance should dictate the initial therapeutic strategy. Despite the persistent belief that lidocaine is the drug of choice for treatment of VT in the setting of remote myocardial infarction, intravenous procainamide, sotalol, and amiodarone have been demonstrated to have superior efficacy. VT causing severe symptoms of angina or hemodynamic collapse almost invariably responds to synchronous cardioversion.

A majority of patients who present with sustained VT have infrequent episodes and typically do not require acute treatment with antiarrhythmic drugs. In patients who present with "VT storm" or who experience frequent episodes of or incessant, often poorly tolerated VT, an increasing focus is placed on reducing sympathetic tone, rather than on antiarrhythmic therapy per se. Acute ischemia is not a frequent cause of this presentation but needs to be considered. Intravenous amiodarone (which acts primarily as a postsynaptic β-antagonist), sedation, stellate ganglion injection, and intrathecal administration of sympatholytic agents have been used for refractory arrhythmias. Urgent catheter ablation is necessary when pharmacologic therapy is unsuccessful.

Long-Term Management

In the United States, the vast majority of patients with coronary heart disease and VT are managed with ICD therapy. This approach stems from progressive distrust in available pharmacologic therapy and is based largely on the findings of secondary prevention ICD trials demonstrating benefit in patients with life-threatening arrhythmias. Several controversies remain in the interpretation of these studies, however: In view of the high cost of this therapy, an optimal strategy would be to identify subsets of patients likely to benefit the most, thereby saving the expense and morbidity of ICD therapy in those less likely to benefit. In most models, the highest-risk patients have demonstrated the greatest benefit of ICD therapy. However, this logic may be flawed in two ways. First, despite the incremental benefit that the sickest patients derive, their residual risk may be too high to reap meaningful clinical benefits. In such patients, appropriate ICD shocks greatly increase the short-term mortality rate, again suggesting the concept of competing modes of death. Second, the short duration of randomized trials focuses the outcome events on the highest risk populations. Over the lifetime of the ICD generator, given the progressive nature of ischemic myopathy, patients who were less sick at enrollment will may well begin to accumulate endpoint events.[14]

The secondary prevention trials have focused exclusively on patients with poorly tolerated VT or those who experience cardiac arrest. The optimal management of patients with hemodynamically tolerated VT is less certain.[15,16] Although classic studies demonstrated a low risk of drug therapy guided by programmed stimulation in these patients, more recent data suggest that patients with tolerated VT may remain at risk for sudden cardiac death on arrhythmia recurrence. Ablative therapy has been proposed as an alternative to ICD therapy in this setting;

however, the outcome of primary catheter ablation for treatment of tolerated VT is largely untested. On the other hand, recent studies have focused some attention on possible detrimental effects of ICD therapy, such as an increase in the incidence of heart failure (with and without relationship to right ventricular pacing) and an increase in the incidence of VT episodes (device proarrhythmia).[17-19]

Despite these considerations, most patients receive ICDs after initial presentation, and the most difficult decisions involve the management of recurrent VT causing ICD shocks. Although it initially was thought that sotalol may significantly reduce the need for ICD therapy, the recent Optimal Pharmacological Therapy in Cardioverter Defibrillator Patients (OPTIC) trial provided a more discouraging view of the benefit of pharmacologic therapy to prevent recurrent VT.[20] On the basis of observational studies, many centers express great enthusiasm for catheter ablation in this setting, but randomized data are not available. In a recent multicenter study, catheter ablation of post-infarction VT was associated with major complications in approximately 8% of patients, with a 2.7% procedural mortality rate.[21] An important recent randomized study in patients after myocardial infarction with previous cardiac arrest demonstrated that prophylactic catheter ablation, using primarily substrate-based strategies, reduced the need for ICD therapy in follow-up, with a reduction of recurrent events by greater than 60%.[22]

Future Directions

A number of frontiers merit exploration for continued progress. Prevention of VT episodes may prove feasible, particularly if the electrical and physical circumstances that precipitate VT can be defined. ICD technology will continue to advance and be increasingly useful for primary prevention in high-risk subgroups; this will further depend on the development of risk stratification methods beyond left ventricular function. A deeper understanding of the relationship of the VT circuit and infarct anatomy will improve the use of catheter ablation, potentially advancing its application as the primary therapy. Most important, our ability to recognize patient subgroups that are likely to respond to a given therapeutic modality will improve, allowing tailored, specific therapy.

References

1. Josephson ME: Clinical Cardiac Electrophysiology: Techniques and Interpretations, 4th ed. Philadelphia, Lippincott Williams & Wilkins, 2008.
2. de Bakker JM, Janse MJ: Pathophysiological correlates of ventricular tachycardia in hearts with a healed infarct. In Zipes DP, Jalife J (eds): Cardiac Electrophysiology: From Cell to Bedside, 3rd ed. Philadelphia, WB Saunders, 2000, pp 415-421.
3. Wyse DG, Friedman PL, Brodsky MA, et al: Life-threatening ventricular arrhythmias due to transient or correctable causes: High risk for death in follow-up. J Am Coll Cardiol 38:1718-1724, 2001.
4. Marchlinski FE, Callans DJ, Gottlieb CD, Zado E: Linear ablation lesions for control of unmappable ventricular tachycardia in patients with ischemic and nonischemic cardiomyopathy. Circulation 101:1288-1296, 2000.
5. Soejima K, Stevenson WG, Sapp JL, et al: Endocardial and epicardial radiofrequency ablation of ventricular tachycardia associated with dilated cardiomyopathy: the importance of low-voltage scars. J Am Coll Cardiol 43:1834-1842, 2004.
6. Arenal A, Glez-Torrecilla E, Ortiz M, et al: Ablation of electrograms with an isolated, delayed component as treatment of unmappable monomorphic ventricular tachycardia in patients with structural heart disease. J Am Coll Cardiol 41:81-92, 2003.
7. Brunckhorst CB, Delacretaz E, Soejima K, et al: Identification of ventricular tachycardia isthmus after infarction by pace mapping. Circulation 110:652-659, 2004.
8. Arenal A, del Castillo S, Gonzalez-Torrecilla E, et al: Tachycardia related channel in the scar tissue in patients with sustained monomorphic ventricular tachycardias. Influence of the voltage scar definition. Circulation 110:2568-2574, 2004.
9. Hsia HH, Lin D, Sauer WH, et al: Anatomical characterization of endocardial substrate for hemodynamically stable reentrant ventricular tachycardia: Identification of endocardial conducting channels. Heart Rhythm 3:503-512, 2006.
10. Jacobson JT, Afonso VX, Eisenman G, et al: Characterization of the infarct substrate and ventricular tachycardia circuits with noncontact unipolar mapping in a porcine model of myocardial infarction. Heart Rhythm 3:189-197, 2006.
11. Szumowski L, Sanders P, Walczak F, et al: Mapping and ablation of polymorphic ventricular tachycardia after myocardial infarction. J Am Coll Cardiol 44:1700-1706, 2004.
12. Marrouche NF, Verma A, Wazni O, et al: Mode of initiation and ablation of ventricular fibrillation storms in patients with ischemic cardiomyopathy. J Am Coll Cardiol 44:1715-1720, 2004.
13. Segal OR, Chow AW, Markides V, et al: Characterization of the effects of single ventricular extrastimuli on endocardial activation in human infarct-related ventricular tachycardia. J Am Coll Cardiol 49:1315-1323, 2007.
14. Salukhe TV, Dimopoulos K, Sutton R, et al: Life-years gained from defibrillator implantation: Markedly nonlinear increase during 3 years of follow-up and its implications. Circulation 109:1848-1853, 2004.
15. Callans DJ: Patients with hemodynamically tolerated ventricular tachycardia require implantable cardioverter-defibrillators. Circulation 116:1196-1203, 2007.
16. Almendral J, Josephson ME: All patients with hemodynamically tolerated postinfarction ventricular tachycardia do not require an implantable cardioverter-defibrillator. Circulation 116:1204-1212, 2007.
17. Hohnloser SH, Kuck KH, Dorian P, et al: Prophylactic use of an implantable cardioverter-defibrillator after acute myocardial infarction. N Engl J Med 351:2481-2488, 2004.
18. Moss AJ, Greenberg H, Case RB, et al: Long-term clinical course of patients after termination of ventricular tachyarrhythmias by an implanted defibrillator. Circulation 110:3760-3765, 2004.
19. Germano JJ, Reynolds M, Essebag V, et al: Frequency and causes of implantable cardioverter-defibrillator therapies: Is device therapy proarrhythmic? Am J Cardiol 97:1255-1261, 2006.
20. Connolly SJ, Dorian P, Roberts RS, et al: Comparison of beta-blockers, amiodarone plus beta-blockers, or sotalol for prevention of shocks from implantable cardioverter defibrillators: The OPTIC study: A randomized trial. JAMA 295:211-213, 2006.
21. Calkins H, Epstein A, Packer D, et al: Catheter ablation of ventricular tachycardia in patients with structural heart disease using cooled radiofrequency energy: Results of a prospective multicenter study. Cooled RF Multi Center Investigators Group. J Am Coll Cardiol 35:1905-1914, 2000.
22. Reddy VY, Reynolds MR, Neuzil P, et al: Prophylactic catheter ablation for the prevention of defibrillator therapy. N Eng J Med 357:2657-2665, 2007.

Ventricular Tachycardia in Patients with Dilated Cardiomyopathy

63

Joseph M. Galvin and Jeremy N. Ruskin

CHAPTER OUTLINE

Dilated cardiomyopathy (DCM) is a syndrome characterized by left or biventricular dilatation and impaired systolic function (Fig. 63-1). Coronary artery disease, valvular heart disease, ethanol ingestion, hypertension, pregnancy, and infections are the most common etiologic factors. In idiopathic dilated cardiomyopathy, by definition, the etiology has not been determined, although genetic, autoimmune, viral, and metabolic causes have been implicated. A common feature of DCM irrespective of the underlying cause is a propensity to the development of ventricular arrhythmias and sudden death. This chapter focuses on incidence and survival, mechanisms of arrhythmogenesis, predictors of sudden death, and management of ventricular arrhythmias in DCM. In this chapter, DCM is *idiopathic* unless otherwise stated.

Incidence and Survival

Congestive heart failure (CHF) afflicts approximately 4 million persons in the United States and is responsible for more than 200,000 deaths per year. More than 10,000 deaths are attributed to DCM each year. The incidence of DCM varies, ranging from 4 to 8 cases per 100,000 population, depending on diagnostic criteria, case ascertainment, and geographic location. The overall sex- and age-adjusted annual incidence rate from 1975 through 1984 in Olmsted County, Minnesota, was 6.0 per 100,000 person-years, and the prevalence in 1985 was 36.5 per 100,000 population, almost twice that of hypertrophic cardiomyopathy, reflecting either a true increase in incidence or improved case ascertainment.

Most commonly, DCM manifests in patients between 18 and 50 years of age, but children of all ages and the elderly also can be affected. It occurs more frequently in men than in women (in a ratio of 2.5:1), and in African Americans than in whites (in a 2.5:1 ratio), but the causes of these differences are not understood. Survival rates in DCM generally are poor but are determined principally by the severity of symptoms and the degree of left ventricular dysfunction in the cohort being examined, ranging from 46% at 1 year in a subgroup of mildly symptomatic patients with left ventricular ejection fractions of less than 25% who were refused transplantation to 95% at 1 year in a population-based analysis (Fig. 63-2). When ischemic and nonischemic cardiomyopathies are considered collectively, survival rates range from 48% to 95% at 1 year and from 19% to 66% at 2 years. Longer survival rates have been achieved with improvements in medical therapy such as with angiotensin-converting enzyme (ACE) inhibitors and beta-blockers and with interventions such as use of implantable cardioverter-defibrillators (ICDs) and biventricular pacing.

Genetics

Approximately 35% of patients with DCM have familial disease, which in most cases appears to be inherited in an autosomal dominant fashion, although X-linked, autosomal recessive, and mitochondrial modes of inheritance also are seen. Major advances have been made in the past 10 years in the identification of candidate genes responsible for DCM[1] (Fig. 63-3). The more common autosomal dominant form of familial DCM is of two main types: "pure" DCM and DCM associated with cardiac conduction system disease. Mitochondrial inheritance is seen most often in childhood forms of familial DCM, whereas cases with X-linked and autosomal recessive inheritance seem to be evenly distributed between childhood and adult forms of the disease. With X-linked forms of DCM, two disorders have been well characterized: X-linked cardiomyopathy, which presents in adolescents and young adults, and Barth syndrome, which is most frequently identified in infancy.

In the case of pure DCM, linkage analysis has identified a number of candidate genes in which mutations have subsequently been found, including those that code for actin (chromosomal locus 15q14),[1] desmin (2q35),[2] β-sarcoglycan (4q12),[3] δ-sarcoglycan (5q33),[4] cardiac troponin T (1q32),[5] α-tropomyosin (15q2),[6] and β-myosin heavy chain (14q11)[5] (see Fig. 63-1). So far, DCM with conduction system disease candidate genes have included the lamin A/C gene (chromosomal locus 1q21.2-3)[7] and the sodium channel gene *SCN5A* (3p22-25).[8] The mechanisms responsible for the development of DCM and conduction system abnormalities are currently unknown. First described in 1987 as a form of DCM occurring in teenage boys and men in their early 20s, with rapid progression from CHF to death or transplantation, *X-linked cardiomyopathy* is distinguished by increased amounts of serum creatine kinase muscle isoforms,[9] a sign of underlying skeletal muscle disease. Among female carriers, a tendency to develop mild to moderate DCM in the sixth decade of life has been noted, and the disease is slowly progressive. Towbin and colleagues[10] identified a disease-causing gene that codes for dystrophin, a cytoskeletal protein. The relationship between individual genotypes and arrhythmogenicity is poorly understood. It is likely, however, that as more putative genes are identified, genotyping will become an important tool in confirming the presence

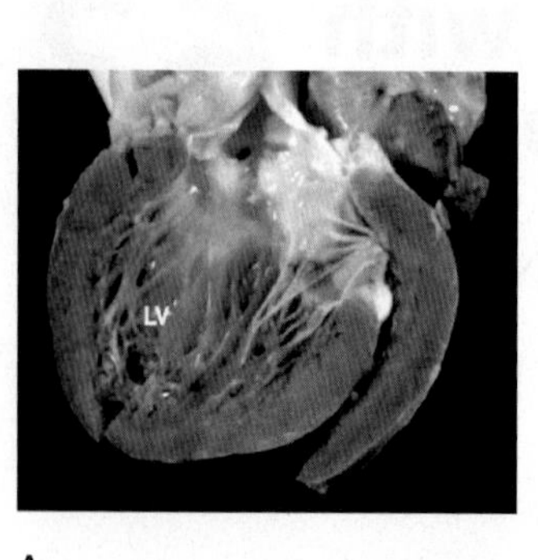

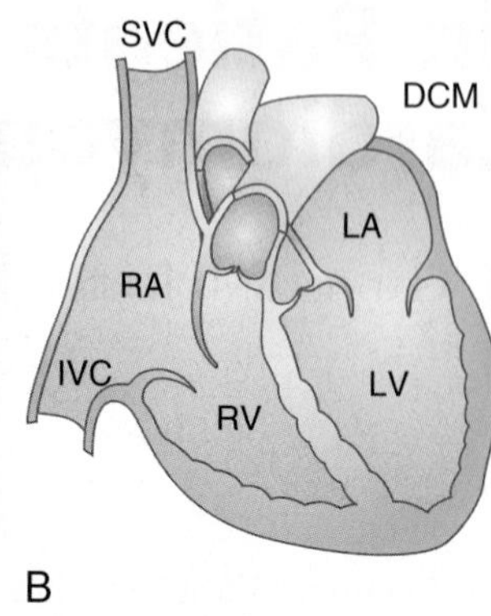

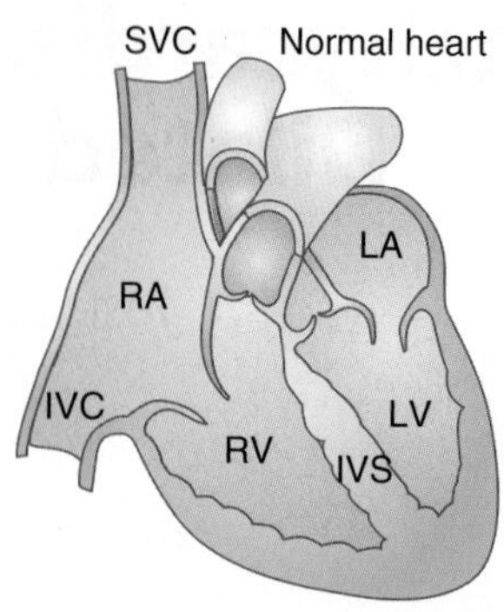

A B

Figure 63-1 Dilated cardiomyopathy. A, Post-mortem specimen of advanced DCM with severe LV dilatation. B, Schematic diagram showing LV dilatation in DCM. IVC, inferior vena cava; IVS, intraventricular septum; LA, left atrium; LV, left ventricle; RA, right atrium; RV, right ventricle; SVC, superior vena cava.

or absence of disease in family members of patients with DCM and potentially in determining the risk for ventricular arrhythmias in affected persons.

Pathophysiology

Arrhythmogenesis

No single mechanism is responsible for ventricular arrhythmias in DCM; rather, multiple factors clearly contribute (Table 63-1). At autopsy, extensive subendocardial scarring in the left ventricle has been described in 33% of patients and multiple patchy areas of replacement fibrosis have been noted in 57% of patients with DCM. These areas may act as sites for reentry. Ischemia, through smaller coronary artery thrombi or emboli, and electrolyte imbalances, especially hypokalemia and hypomagnesemia, also may precipitate arrhythmias. Alterations in ventricular mechanics and geometry may predispose affected patients to reentrant arrhythmias through variable wall tension and stretch-dependent shortening of the ventricular refractory period or by resulting in abnormal automaticity or triggered activity. Increased circulating catecholamines may cause arrhythmias indirectly by driving potassium intracellularly or directly through triggered activity. Finally, antiarrhythmic drugs may exert a proarrhythmic effect.

Mechanisms of Ventricular Tachycardia

Although other mechanisms of ventricular tachycardia are common in patients with DCM, bundle branch reentry ventricular tachycardia (BBRVT) is perhaps the most characteristic. Bundle branch reentry produces ventricular tachycardia through a macro-reentrant circuit involving the His-Purkinje system, usually with antegrade conduction over the right bundle branch and retrograde conduction over the left bundle branch. In one series, it was the mechanism responsible for ventricular tachycardia in up to 6% of all patients and in up to 41% of patients with DCM. In another series, 45% of all patients in whom BBRVT could be induced had underlying DCM.

BBRVT usually is rapid, with a mean cycle length of 280 ms. Syncope occurs in a majority of patients. Degeneration to ventricular fibrillation can occur. Baseline electrocardiography typically shows a nonspecific intraventricular conduction delay or left bundle branch block. His-ventricular (H-V) intervals recorded during sinus rhythm are characteristically prolonged. Tachycardias induced by right ventricular stimulation show left bundle branch block morphology. A short-to-long change in cycle length before the extrastimulus has been reported to be more successful at initiating tachycardia, although this claim has been disputed. Myocardial ventricular tachycardia can be excluded by the QRS morphology and the presence of a His signal before the ventricular signal, with an H-V interval

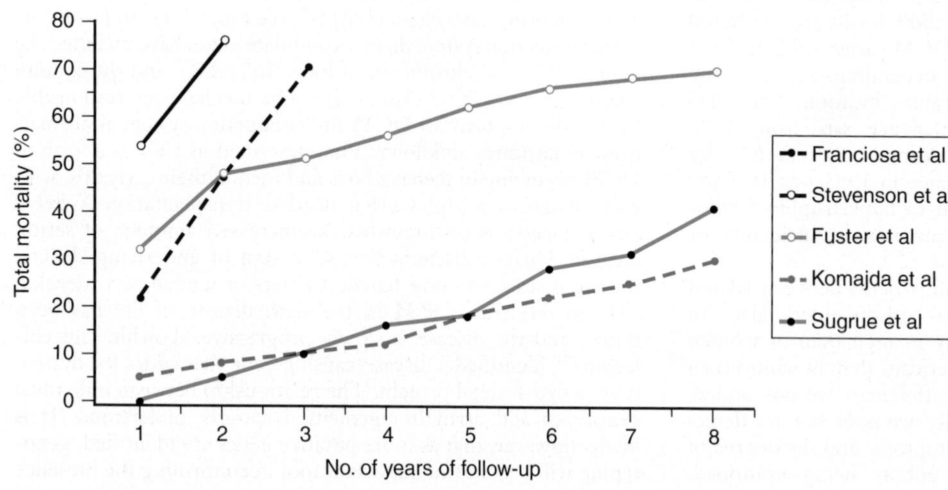

Figure 63-2 Cumulative total mortality in reported series of patients with dilated cardiomyopathy between 1978 and 1996. (Adapted from Tamburro P, Wilber D: Sudden death in idiopathic dilated cardiomyopathy. Am Heart J 124:1035-1045, 1992.) (Data from references 30-35).

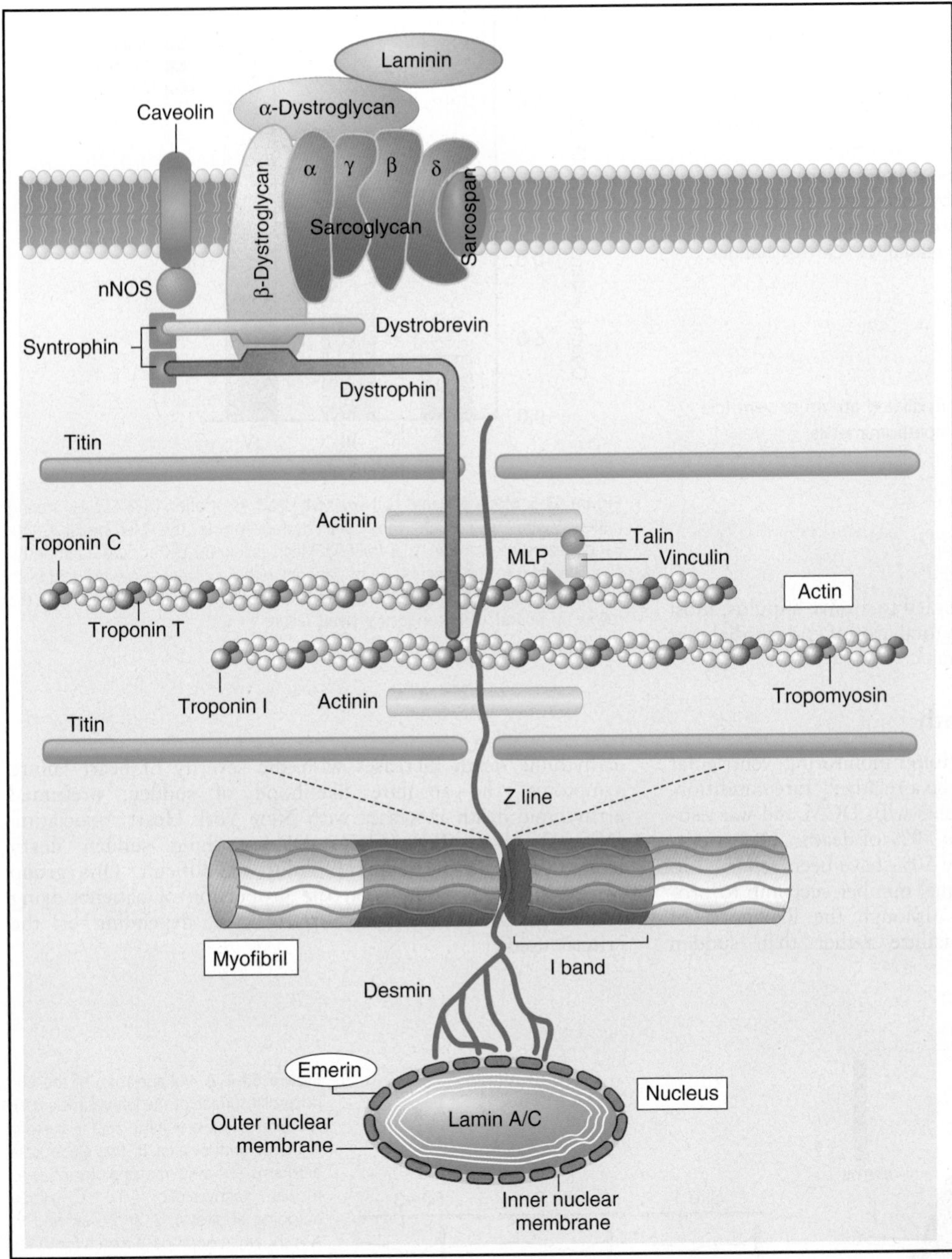

Figure 63-3 Schematic diagram of proteins implicated in the pathogenesis of dilated cardiomyopathy.[1] Identified genes that result in dilated cardiomyopathy include those coding for the cytoskeletal proteins β- and δ-sarcoglycan in the sarcolemma, dystrophin, and the intermediate filament protein–encoding genes desmin and lamin A/C. Sarcomeric protein–encoding genes actin, β-myosin heavy chain, α-tropomyosin, and cardiac troponin T cause either dilated cardiomyopathy or hypertrophic cardiomyopathy, whereas cardiac troponin I, titin, and the myosin light chains cause hypertrophic cardiomyopathy. Mutations in dystrobrevin cause the intermediate phenotype, left ventricular noncompaction. MLP, muscle LIM protein; nNOS, neuronal nitric oxide.

that usually is slightly longer than that in sinus rhythm, owing to rate-related reduction in conduction velocity. BBRVT is an important arrhythmia to recognize because catheter ablation of the right bundle branch is curative. Some patients will require dual-chamber pacing after right bundle branch ablation, particularly those with a preceding wide left bundle branch block. Depending on the severity of left ventricular dysfunction, placement of a dual-chamber ICD may be warranted.

Insights from Electroanatomic Mapping

Electroanatomic mapping has allowed new insights into the basis of structural abnormalities in the genesis of ventricular arrhythmias in DCM through the creation of voltage maps of the endocardium and epicardium. Peak-to-peak electrogram voltages less than 1.5 mV generally are associated with the presence of scar if catheter contact with the myocardium is good. These "scar maps" may be color-coded so that all areas of viable myocardium are given the same color code and the scar may be further differentiated into different zones according to the local voltage at multiple points within the scar (Fig. 63-4). This approach facilitates design of empirical ablation lines. Soejima and coworkers[11] characterized ventricular tachycardia using electroanatomic mapping and found macro-reentry to be the dominant mechanism. A critical isthmus was found in 12 patients during endocardial mapping and in 7 patients during epicardial mapping. All patients who underwent endocardial mapping had at least one area of scar, with an average of 2 scars per patient.

Table 63-1 Factors Contributing to Arrhythmogenesis in Dilated Cardiomyopathys

- Hypokalemia, hypomagnesemia (often related to diuretic use)
- Sustained stretch-induced shortening of refractory period and action potential duration, predisposing to reentry
- Short, pulsatile, stretch-induced after depolarizations
- Diastolic calcium overload caused by decreased sacrcoplasmic reticulum Ca^{2+}–adenosine triphosphatase pump
- Afterdepolarizations induced by increased Na^{+}-Ca^{2+} exchanger activity
- Increased circulating catecholamines
- Increased sympathetic tone
- Myocardial fibrosis/scar
- Purkinje system conduction delay
- Increased endocardial surface area in dilated atrium or ventricle
- Drugs (antiarrhythmics, digoxin, sympathomimetics, phosphodiesterase inhibitors)

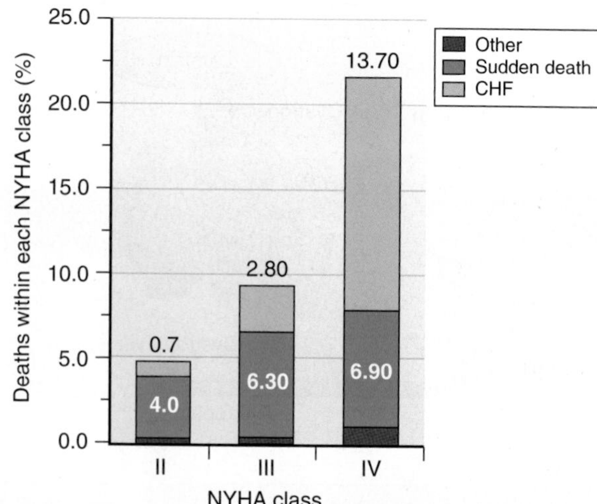

Figure 63-5 Mode of death by New York Heart Association (NYHA) class among patients with severe left ventricular dysfunction in the Metoprolol CR/XL Randomized Intervention Trial (MERIT). Mean follow-up period was 12 months. *Numbers* refer to the percentage of patients within a given class who died from sudden arrhythmic or progressive pump failure, or from another cause, within the follow-up period. CHF, congestive heart failure.

More than half of the 32 scars extended to a valve annulus, most commonly the mitral annulus. The total area of endocardial scar per patient was approximately 16 cm^2.

Mechanisms of Sudden Death

With the advent of telemetry and Holter monitoring, ventricular tachycardia, previously thought to be a relatively rare condition, was noted in 50% to 60% of patients with DCM and was estimated to be responsible for 8% to 50% of deaths. Of patients with all-cause CHF, approximately 50% have been reported to die suddenly. An approximately equal number succumb to progressive ventricular dysfunction. Although the likelihood of death from progressive pump failure rather than sudden arrhythmic death increases with the severity of heart failure symptoms, the absolute likelihood of sudden, presumed arrhythmic death increases with New York Heart Association (NYHA) class (Fig. 63-5). Distinguishing sudden death from death caused by pump failure is difficult. One group of investigators[12] found that the proportion of patients dying suddenly varied from 31% up to 55%, depending on the criteria used.

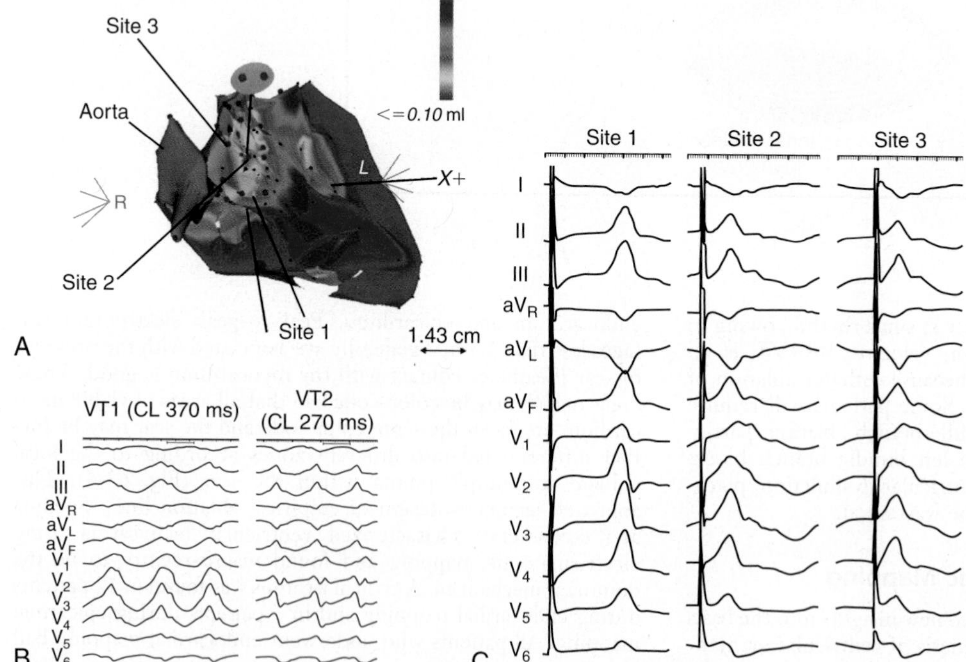

Figure 63-4 **A,** Voltage map of the endocardial surface of the left ventricle (LV). An extensive low-voltage area is present in the LV outflow area. **B,** Two electrocardiograms showing morphology of ventricular tachycardia (VT). **C,** Pace mapping at sites 1, 2, and 3 labeled in **A** is shown. A good pace match for VT1 is observed at sites 2 and 3, and a long S-QRS delay (200 ms), consistent with slow conduction away from the pacing site, is observed during pace mapping at site 1. A series of radiofrequency lesions *(red dots)* across this region from the aortic annulus to the dense scar above the mitral annulus abolished both VTs. (From Soejima K, Stevenson WG, Sapp JL, et al: Endocardial and epicardial radiofrequency ablation of ventricular tachycardia associated with dilated cardiomyopathy: The importance of low-voltage scars. J Am Coll Cardiol 43:1834-1842, 2004.)

Despite their common occurrence, ventricular arrhythmias are not the only cause of sudden death in patients with DCM. Luu and associates[13] reviewed data for 21 episodes of cardiac arrest in 20 hospitalized, monitored patients with end-stage heart failure caused by ischemic or nonischemic cardiomyopathy. Primary ventricular tachyarrhythmias occurred in only 38% of arrests. Bradycardia or electromechanical dissociation was the initial event in 62% of all patients and in every patient with DCM. First- and second-degree forms of atrioventricular (AV) block have been identified as markers of poor prognosis in patients with DCM. Ischemia, secondary to acute coronary artery thrombi or emboli, also may lead to sudden death in a small number of patients. Pulmonary emboli and hyperkalemia are other significant precipitants of sudden death in patients with heart failure.

Imaging

Both echocardiography and left ventriculography provide important information on the degree of overall left ventricular dysfunction and dilatation, regional wall motion, the presence of scar, and the severity of associated mitral regurgitation. These factors are important in determining prognosis, optimizing pharmacologic therapy, identifying the need for biventricular pacing or an ICD, and in planning ablation procedures for patients with drug-refractory ventricular tachycardia. Noninvasive or, more usually, invasive coronary angiography is required to establish the absence of significant coronary artery disease and to confirm the diagnosis of a nonischemic DCM.

A more detailed examination of the presence, extent, and transmurality of myocardial scar is possible with cardiac magnetic resonance imaging (MRI). Initially described in patients by McCrohon and colleagues, who found longitudinal striae of midwall enhancement consistent with fibrosis in 28% of patients with DCM.[14] MRI can be used to quantitate the extent of scar and define its location. Nazarian and associates[15] demonstrated a propensity for scarring in the basal mid-myocardial layers of the left ventricle in DCM patients and found that the amount of nontransmural scar (26% to 75% wall thickness) was an independent predictor of the inducibility of ventricular tachycardia by programmed ventricular stimulation. In several cases, location of scar could be correlated with the origin of the clinical ventricular tachycardia (Fig. 63-6). It is likely that imaging of the structural abnormalities underlying ventricular tachycardia in DCM, such as the location and extent of myocardial scar, and integration of these images with mapping systems will play an increasing role in catheter ablation of ventricular tachycardia in DCM.

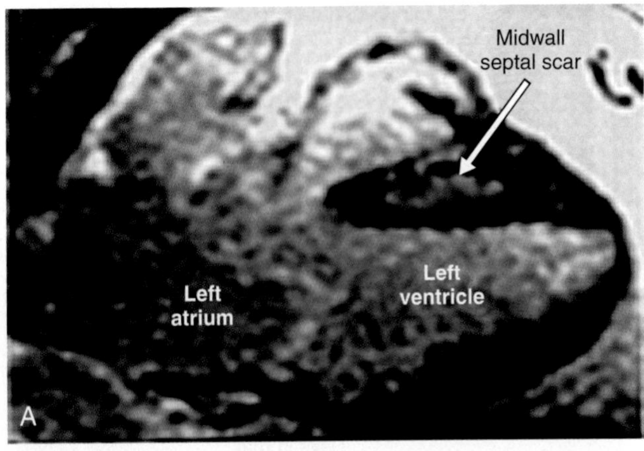

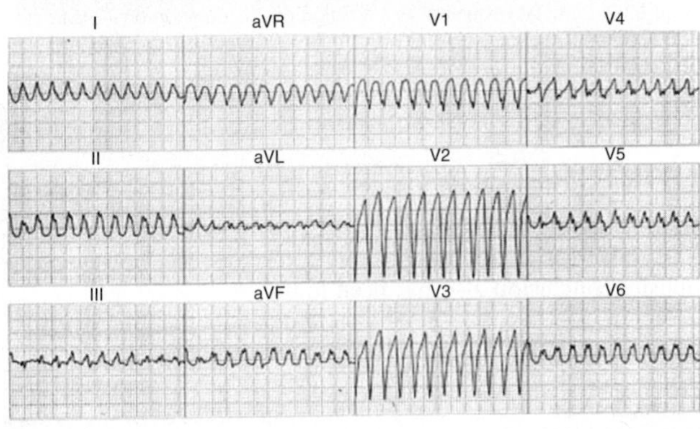

Figure 63-6 Example of the relation between scar location on delayed enhancement images and morphology of ventricular tachycardia on 12-lead electrocardiogram (ECG). **A,** A four-chamber image of the heart, with the right atrium and ventricle at the *top* of the image and left atrium and ventricle at the *bottom*. **B,** The left bundle branch–like configuration in lead V_1 of the ventricular tachycardia ECG suggests an exit site in the right ventricle or interventricular septum and is compatible with the scar location in **A**. (From Nazarian S, Bluemke D, Lardo A, et al: Magnetic resonance assessment of the substrate for inducible ventricular tachycardia in nonischemic cardiomyopathy. Circulation 112:2821-2825, 2005.)

Predictors of Mortality and Ventricular Arrhythmias

Perhaps the greatest challenge facing the clinician managing the patient with DCM and ventricular arrhythmias is the assessment of the relative risk for sudden death compared with the risk for any death and the determination of likely life expectancy with only the relatively crude predictors currently available.

Clinical Predictors of Mortality

The severity of left ventricular dysfunction is the most powerful predictor of mortality in patients with DCM and CHF. A reduced left ventricular ejection fraction has been shown to correlate strongly with poor survival. In one such study, 84% of patients with idiopathic cardiomyopathy and an ejection fractions less than 35% died over a mean of 39 months, compared with 46% of patients with ejection fractions greater than 35%. Although ejection fraction is used most frequently, other indices of left and right ventricular function including pulmonary capillary wedge pressure, cardiac index, stroke work index, stroke volume, and right atrial pressure also predict mortality in patients with cardiomyopathy.

On account of the subjective nature of the data, clinical observations and heart failure classification are not as strong predictors of mortality as indices of left ventricular function. Nevertheless, both NYHA classification and the presence of a third heart sound correlate with survival in DCM and other causes of CHF. In DCM, the incidence of sudden death is significantly greater in patients with syncope. Laboratory values found to be predictive of mortality include low serum sodium and increased plasma norepinephrine, renin, and both atrial and brain natriuretic peptide levels. Exact morphometric analysis of biopsy specimens has not found histologic findings to be predictive of survival. Left ventricular dimensions, independent of ventricular function, do not predict survival. Most studies that have included patients with ischemic and nonischemic

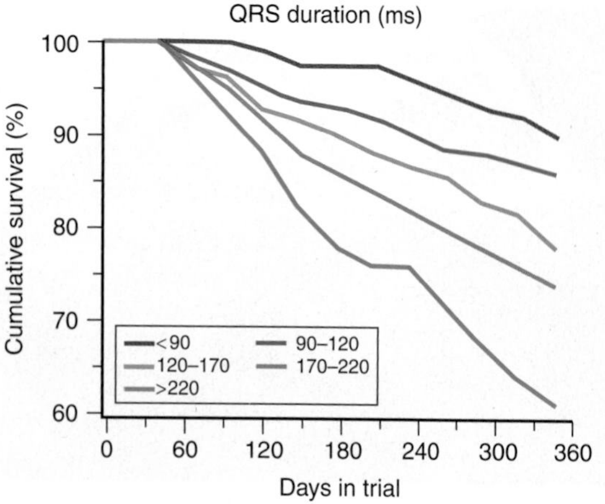

Figure 63-7 Cumulative survival as a function of QRS duration on 12-lead electrocardiogram at trial entry in the vesnarinone trial (VesT) study. (Adapted from Gottipaty V, Krelis SP, Lu F, et al: [Abstract 847-4]. J Am Coll Cardiol 33:145A, 1999.)

cardiomyopathy have demonstrated a marginally worse prognosis in those patients with coronary artery disease; however, the opposite conclusion also has been found.

Electrophysiologic Predictors of Arrhythmias and Death

Electrocardiogram

The presence of left bundle branch block and of first- and second-degree AV block has been associated with poor outcome in DCM. Data from the Vesnarinone Trial (VEST) have confirmed a significant association between the degree of QRS prolongation and mortality (Fig. 63-7). The development of atrial fibrillation appears to portend a poorer prognosis, although some workers disagree. In the largest study to date, 19% of 390 patients with advanced heart failure, including 191 patients with DCM, developed paroxysmal or chronic atrial fibrillation. One-year actuarial survival of patients with atrial fibrillation compared with patients in sinus rhythm was 52% versus 71% (P = .001). However, the difference did not remain significant when data were corrected for an increased pulmonary wedge pressure. Atrial fibrillation may reduce survival by increasing thromboembolic events or ventricular arrhythmias, the latter through long-short cycle lengths increasing the dispersion of refractoriness in the ventricle. Alternatively, atrial fibrillation may merely be a marker of severe left ventricular dysfunction.

Spontaneous Ventricular Arrhythmias

Multiform premature ventricular contractions, ventricular pairs, and nonsustained ventricular tachycardia are present in 80% to 95% of patients with DCM. In one study using 24-hour Holter monitoring, 53% of patients demonstrated more than 500 premature ventricular contractions, 54% had ventricular pairs, and 31% experienced episodes of nonsustained ventricular tachycardia. In CHF, ventricular arrhythmias become more frequent and more complex as left ventricular function deteriorates. The prevalence rate of nonsustained ventricular tachycardia has been shown to increase from 15% to 20% in patients with class I or II CHF to 50% to 70% in patients with class IV CHF. Despite the frequency of high-grade ventricular ectopic activity, these arrhythmias usually are not associated with symptoms. Although their ubiquity makes their significance difficult to assess, ventricular arrhythmias have been reported as independent predictors of total cardiac mortality or sudden cardiac death, or both, by some investigators but not by others. Arrhythmic complexity was a major predictor of survival in 218 patients studied by De Maria,[16] although not as strong as left ventricular ejection fraction or stroke work index. By contrast, Romeo[17] found Lown grade 4 or greater arrhythmias to be independent predictors of sudden death in 104 patients with DCM.

Programmed Ventricular Stimulation

Programmed electrical stimulation has not been shown to be an accurate predictor of sudden death in patients with nonischemic DCM. In most patients with nonischemic cardiomyopathy, electrophysiologic studies are unreliable in the induction of sustained monomorphic ventricular tachycardia, making serial drug testing and thus drug therapy problematic. Sustained monomorphic ventricular tachycardia is uncommonly inducible in patients with DCM. Polymorphic ventricular arrhythmias can be induced in up to 86% of patients with DCM, but these are nonspecific endpoints that are not useful for serial drug testing and are without prognostic significance.

When it does occur, sustained monomorphic ventricular tachycardia is predominantly induced in patients with this arrhythmia. As in patients with coronary artery disease, sustained monomorphic ventricular tachycardia is induced much less frequently in patients with cardiac arrest or nonsustained ventricular tachycardia than in those with sustained monomorphic ventricular tachycardia. Sustained monomorphic ventricular tachycardia is rarely induced in patients with no or low-grade ectopy.

The inducibility of ventricular tachycardia is much less predictive of arrhythmia recurrence and sudden death in patients with nonischemic cardiomyopathy than in patients with coronary artery disease (Table 63-2). Analysis of pooled data shows that, of patients with inducible ventricular tachycardia suppressed by drug therapy, 28% who initially presented with ventricular tachycardia experienced recurrence, whereas 43% who presented with cardiac arrest later died suddenly. Failure to induce sustained monomorphic ventricular tachycardia during programmed electrical stimulation is associated with high rates of arrhythmia recurrence and sudden death, although these rates are lower than in patients with inducible ventricular tachycardia. Therefore, programmed ventricular stimulation should not be used for risk stratification in patients with DCM.

Noninvasive Electrocardiographic Predictors

A number of noninvasive electrocardiogram (ECG) features have shown promise in small series as predictors of clinical and inducible ventricular tachycardia as well as sudden death in patients with DCM. In the largest trial to date, the Marburg Cardiomyopathy study, Grimm and associates[18] examined the predictive value of echocardiography, 24-hour Holter monitoring, signal-averaged electocardiography (SAECG), heart rate variability, QT dispersion, microvolt T wave alternans, and baroreflex sensitivity in 343 patients with DCM. After an average follow-up period of 52 months, 13% of patients had a sustained ventricular arrhythmia or died suddenly. The relative risk of ventricular tachycardia and sudden cardiac death was increased 2.3-fold for each 10% reduction in ejection fraction and 1.7-fold when ventricular tachycardia was present on a Holter monitor trace and reduced by 40% when patients received beta-blockers. However, none of the other five noninvasive measures proved useful in predicting events.

In the asymptomatic patient with DCM, ejection fraction and the presence of ventricular tachycardia on Holter monitoring remain the only clinically useful predictors of sudden cardiac

Table 63-2 Programmed Stimulation in Patients with Dilated Cardiomyopathy and No History of Sustained Ventricular Arrhythmias

		Inducible Arrhythmia				Follow-up	Arrhythmic Events during Follow-up		
Study*	**No. of Patients**	**NSVT**	**VES**	**SMVT**	**PMVT/VF**	**(mo)**	**MMVT Inducible**	**PMVT/VF Inducible**	**Noninducible†**
Meinertz et al, 1985	42	35%	1-2	0 (0%)	1 (2%)	16	0 (0%)	0 (0%)	2 (5%)
Stamato et al, 1986	15	93%	1-2	0 (0%)	0 (0%)	19	0 (0%)	0 (0%)	2 (13%)
Poll et al, 1986	20	100%	1-3	2 (10%)	4 (20%)	17	0 (0%)	2 (50%)	5 (36%)
Das et al, 1986	24	NA	1-3	1 (4%)	4 (17%)	12		1 (100%)	1 (25%)
Gossinger et al, 1990	32	100%	1-3	4 (13%)	0 (0%)	21	1 (25%)	0 (0%)	2 (7%)
Brembilla-Perrot, 1991	92	46%	1-3	3 (3%)	5 (5%)	24	2 (67%)	2 (40%)	3 (4%)
Kadish et al, 1993	43	100%	1-3	6 (14%)	NA	20	1 (17%)	NA	6 (16%)
Turrito et al, 1994	80	100%	1-3	10 (13%)	7 (9%)	22	3 (30%)	0 (0%)	6 (10%)
Grimm et al, 1997	34	100%	1-3	3 (9%)	10 (29%)	24	1 (33%)	3 (30%)	5 (24%)

*Full publication information on these studies is found in the original source as given below.

†No sustained ventricular arrhythmia inducible.

MMVT, monomorphic ventricular tachycardia; NA, not available; NSVT, nonsustained ventricular tachycardia at baseline; PMVT/VF, polymorphic ventricular tachycardia or ventricular tachycardia; VES, ventricular extrastimuli (number used).

Modified slightly from Grimm W, Hoffmann J, Menz V, et al: Programmed ventricular stimulation for arrhythmia risk prediction in patients with idiopathic dilated cardiomyopathy and nonsustained ventricular tachycardia. J Am Coll Cardiol 32:739-745, 1998.

death. Ongoing work examining the association between the presence and extent of myocardial fibrosis on cardiac MRI and subsequent fatal or nonfatal ventricular arrhythmias in DCM may lead to identification of additional risk predictors in this population.

Drug Therapy

Vasodilator Therapy

Vasodilators improve survival in patients with CHF by lessening the progression of left ventricular dysfunction. ACE inhibitors, in contrast with other vasodilators, may be unique in reducing sudden death in such patients. In Veterans Heart Failure Trial II (VHeFT-II), the reduction in mortality rates (18% versus 28%) with enalapril was attributed to a reduction in the incidence of sudden death (37% versus 46%) in the enalapril group. Ventricular tachycardia was less frequent at 3 months, and new ventricular tachycardia developed less frequently at 1 year and 2 years in the enalapril group. In the Evaluation of Losartan in the Elderly (ELITE) trial, an angiotensin II receptor antagonist, losartan, was shown to reduce overall mortality rates by 46% and sudden death by 64% compared with captopril in an elderly group of patients with symptomatic heart failure and left ventricular systolic dysfunction.[19] These results were not confirmed in the subsequent ELITE II trial, which showed no difference in mortality rates, total or sudden, between an ACE inhibitor and an angiotensin II receptor blocker.[20]

Adrenergic Receptor–Blocking Agents

In 1975, Waagstein and associates[21] first reported an improvement in ventricular function and exercise tolerance in seven patients with DCM treated with β-adrenergic receptor–blocking agents. Since then, several studies have shown symptomatic improvement in patients with nonischemic dilated cardiomyopathies treated with beta-blockers. Pooled data from 9 studies involving 144 patients over 2 to 19 months show that symptoms were decreased in 66% and unchanged in 19%; in 15%, symptoms worsened or the patient died. The rationale for therapy with beta-blockers in patients with DCM is to counteract the deleterious effects of heightened sympathetic tone and circulating catecholamines such as cytosolic calcium overload mediated through ryanodine receptor hyperphosphorylation (Fig. 63-8) or decreased synthesis of contractile proteins.[22]

The largest reported trials of beta-blockers in CHF included mainly patients with ischemic cardiomyopathy. Carvedilol, a nonselective beta-blocker that also is an α-adrenergic receptor antagonist and antioxidant, was associated with a remarkable 65% reduction in mortality rates among 1094 patients with class III or IV heart failure and ejection fraction of less than 35% who could tolerate the drug and were randomized to receive it or placebo in addition to conventional therapy. The Metoprolol CR/XL Randomized Intervention Trial in Congestive Heart Failure (MERIT-HF) study randomized 3991 patients with ejection fraction of 0.40 or less and NYHA class II to IV heart failure to receive metoprolol or placebo in addition to conventional therapy. Overall mortality rate was reduced 34% at 21 months among the patients receiving metoprolol, with significant reductions noted in patients with and without coronary artery disease (40% and 30%, respectively). Outcomes included a 49% reduction in heart failure–related deaths and a 41% reduction in sudden cardiac deaths. In the Cardiac Insufficiency Bisoprolol Study II (CIBIS II) trial, 2647 patients with NYHA III or IV symptoms and ejection fraction less than 0.35 were randomized to receive bisoprolol or placebo in addition to an ACE inhibitor and diuretic. A highly significant 34% reduction was observed in total mortality rate at 1.3 years, mainly because of a 44% reduction in sudden-death mortality

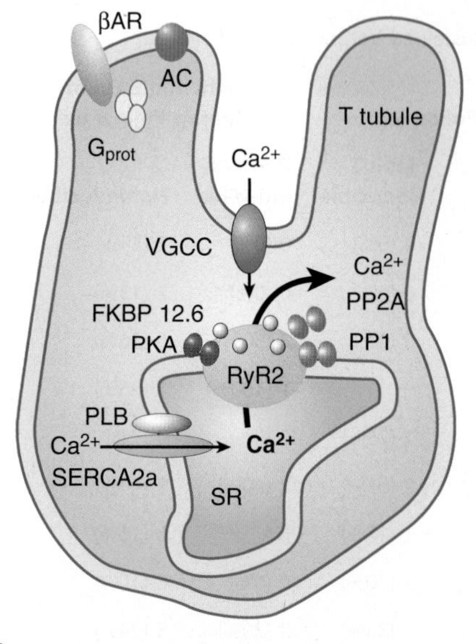

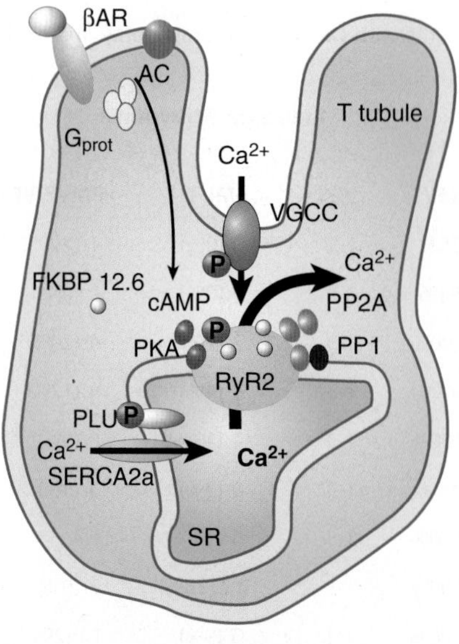

Figure 63-8 Catecholamine-induced polymorphic ventricular tachycardia. Constant adrenergic stimulation through β-adrenergic receptors (β-ARs) causes a positive shift in ryanodine receptor 2 (RyR2) kinetics, and Ca^{2+} leaks back into the cytosol in diastole, causing early afterdepolarizations (EADs) and premature ventricular contractions (PVCs). These Ca^{2+} leaks can be reduced by beta-blockade through inhibition of adenylate cyclase (AC)-mediated cyclic adenosine monophosphate (cAMP) production and less RyR2 activation. Identified mutations include: P2328S, Q4201R, V4653F in the calsequestrin 2 gene (Calsq2). FKBP, FK-506 binding protein; G_{prot}, G proteins; PLB, phospholamban; PKA, protein kinase A; PP1, protein phosphatase 1; PP2A, protein phosphatase 2A; SERCA2a, sarcoplasmic reticulum calcium ATPase; SR, sarcoplasmic reticulum; VGCC, voltage-gated calcium channel.

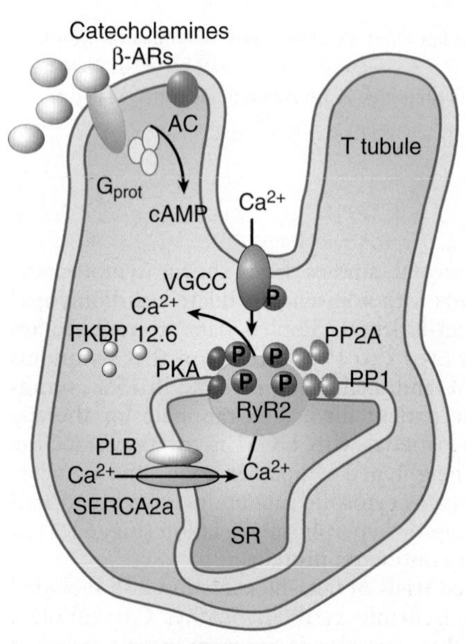

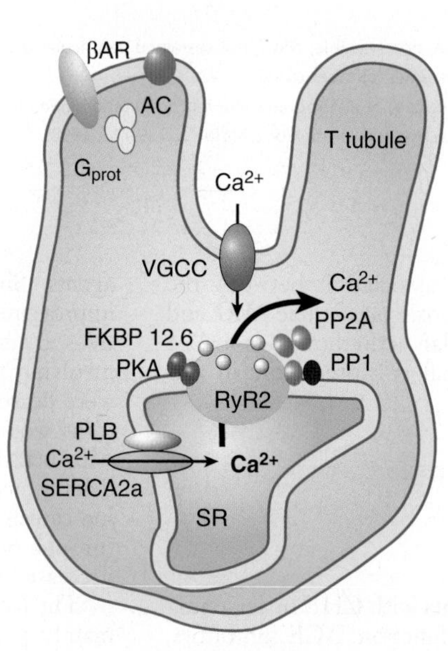

rates after 1.3 years, which led to the trial's being halted prematurely.

The striking similarities in the outcomes of these three trials indicate that the large reductions in mortality rates seen with carvedilol are likely to represent a class effect, rather than being isolated to a single agent, thereby adding to the burden of evidence that all patients with CHF should receive both ACE inhibitors and beta-blockers unless a specific contraindication exists (Table 63-3).

Antiarrhythmic Drug Therapy

Antiarrhythmic drugs may be used for the treatment of ventricular tachycardia or atrial arrhythmias in DCM. They also have been used in an attempt to reduce mortality in DCM in patients without any arrhythmias. Most conventional antiarrhythmic agents can exacerbate left ventricular dysfunction, particularly disopyramide and flecainide. Life-threatening complications, including CHF and proarrhythmia, occur far more frequently in patients with lower baseline ventricular function.

Amiodarone, a vasodilator with antiadrenergic effects, is the most frequently used antiarrhythmic drug in DCM. Neri and colleagues found that amiodarone significantly reduced the incidence of complex ventricular arrhythmias and sudden death among 64 patients with DCM and ventricular tachycardia. Side effects developed in slightly more than one half of the patients, but termination of therapy was necessary in only 9.8%. In another study, among 232 patients with DCM

Table 63-3 Results of the Three Largest Prospective, Randomized Trials of Beta-Blockers in Congestive Heart Failure[22,23]

Trial with Total No. of Patients/No. with DCM	Inclusion	Drug	Relative Risk Reduction (%) TD	SD	CHFD
Carvedilol HFSG: 1094/570	NYHA class II-IV, (52%); EF ≤0.35	Carvedilol 3.125-50 mg twice daily	65%	55%	79%
CIBIS II: 2647/317	NYHA class III, IV (12%); EF ≤0.35	Bisoprolol 1.25-10 mg/d	34%	44%	26%
MERIT-HF: 3991/1385	NYHA class II-IV, (35%); EF ≤0.4	Metoprolol 12.5-25 mg/d	34%	41%	49%

Carvedilol HFSG, Carvedilol Heart Failure Study Group; CHFD, congestive heart failure death; CIBIS II, Cardiac Insufficiency Bisoprolol Study II; DCM, dilated cardiomyopathy; EF, ejection fraction; MERIT-HF, Metoprolol CR/XL Randomized Intervention Trial in Congestive Heart Failure; NYHA, New York Heart Association; SD, sudden death; TD, total deaths.

Data from Saxon L, Bristow M, Boehmer J, et al: Predictors of sudden cardiac death and appropriate shock in the Comparison of Medical Therapy, Pacing, and Defibrillation in Heart Failure (COMPANION) trial. Circulation 114:2766-2772, 2006; and Bänsch D, Antz M, Boczor S, et al for the CAT Investigators: Primary prevention of sudden cardiac death in idiopathic dilated cardiomyopathy. The Cardiomyopathy Trial (CAT). Circulation 105:1453-1457, 2002.

being evaluated for cardiac transplantation, treatment with amiodarone was not found to prolong survival, although randomization was not a feature of the study. As with conventional antiarrhythmic agents, the efficacy and tolerance of amiodarone decrease with deteriorating ventricular function. De Paola and coworkers found that efficacy and tolerance were 80% in patients with left ventricular ejection fractions of 0.30 or greater and 60% in patients with ejection fractions less than 0.30.

In the largest trial to date, the Sudden Cardiac Death in Heart Failure Trial (SCD-HeFT),[23] 2521 patients with an ejection fraction less than 0.35 with coronary artery disease (52%) and nonischemic DCM (48%) with NYHA class II or III CHF but no arrhythmia requiring amiodarone therapy were randomized to receive placebo, amiodarone, or an ICD. No difference in mortality was observed for the amiodarone and placebo treatment groups of patients with nonischemic cardiomyopathy. On the basis of this trial, it has been recommended that amiodarone not be used routinely in patients with DCM unless a specific arrhythmic indication exists. When used to treat ventricular tachycardia in the setting of DCM, antiarrhythmic drug therapy is most commonly used as an adjunct to ICD therapy. Both sotalol and amiodarone have been shown to lengthen ventricular tachycardia cycle length and to reduce ICD shock frequency without significantly worsening heart failure symptoms.

Device Therapy

Biventricular Pacing

Between 30% and 50% of patients with DCM have intraventricular conduction disturbances resulting in a QRS duration greater than 120 ms, most commonly with a left bundle branch block. Delayed activation of the left ventricular free wall can result in dyssynchronous free-wall contraction relative to the septum, with resulting reduction in left ventricular stroke volume and cardiac output and increased mitral regurgitation. In addition, delayed activation can result in delayed relaxation, so that passive filling of the left ventricle can be almost simultaneous with atrial contraction, particularly at faster heart rates. It has been shown that earlier activation of the left ventricular free wall by pacing will (1) improve systolic function by shortening the duration of mechanical systole and increasing dP/dt, (2) improve diastolic function by prolonging diastolic filling time, and (3) reduce presystolic mitral regurgitation by earlier activation of the lateral papillary muscle without the adverse effect on the sympathetic nervous system seen with inotropic agents. The results from prospective randomized trials published to date have consistently demonstrated an improvement in acute hemodynamics, left ventricular dP/dt, left ventricular ejection fraction, NYHA class, and 6-minute walk duration, as well as a reduction in hospitalization for heart failure and, in one study, significant cost reduction at 1 year after implantation with biventricular pacing. In addition, among those patients randomized to undergo biventricular ICD implantation, a reduction in frequency of ICD shocks, number of therapies required, and number of episodes of nonsustained ventricular tachycardia was found.

Two large trials assessing the effects of biventricular pacing on mortality have included patients with DCM. The Cardiac Resynchronization–Heart Failure (CARE-HF) study followed 813 patients (46% with nonischemic DCM) who had NYHA class III or IV heart failure despite receiving standard pharmacologic therapy, with a left ventricular ejection fraction of no more than 35% and a QRS interval of at least 120 ms on the electrocardiogram.[24] Patients with a QRS interval of 120 to 149 ms were required to meet two of three additional criteria for dyssynchrony: an aortic preejection delay of more than 140 ms, an interventricular mechanical delay of more than 40 ms, or delayed activation of the posterolateral left ventricular wall. After 2.5 years of follow-up, they found a 36% reduction in mortality rate from 30% to 20% and a 37% reduction from 55% to 39% in death or hospitalization among those randomized to management with biventricular pacing. As compared with medical therapy, cardiac resynchronization reduced the interventricular mechanical delay, the end-systolic volume index, and the area of the mitral regurgitant jet; increased the left ventricular ejection fraction; and improved symptoms and the quality of life ($P < .01$ for all comparisons).

In the Comparison of Medical Therapy, Pacing, and Defibrillation in Heart Failure (COMPANION) study,[25] 1520 patients with NYHA class III or IV QRS duration longer than

120 ms, PR interval longer than 150 ms, and left ventricular ejection fraction less than 35% were randomized in a 1:2:2 ratio to receive optimal medical therapy, biventricular pacing alone, or biventricular pacing–ICD therapy therapy. Of note, 44% of the patients had nonischemic cardiomyopathy. Biventricular pacing and biventricular pacing–ICD therapy reduced the combined end-point of mortality and hospitalization by 34% and 40%, respectively, compared with optimal medical therapy alone. Mortality was reduced by 24% and 36% respectively with the larger rediction in the biventricular pacing–ICD reaching statistical significance. NYHA class IV heart failure has been considered a contraindication to ICD implantation (except as a bridge to transplant) because of the high likelihood of pump failure death within 1 year. Therefore, biventricular pacemakers would seem to be the most appropriate therapy in patients with severe (NYHA IV) heart failure who are too old to be considered for transplantation, whereas biventricular ICDs may be more appropriate for younger patients. However, this approach may need to be revised in those cases in which biventricular pacing results in marked improvement in heart failure symptoms to NYHA class II or III and prevents pump failure death. Although some 30% of patients fail to respond biventricular pacing, it has proved difficult to identify nonresponders before device implantation.

Implantable Cardioverter-Defibrillators

A number of recent trials have examined the role of prophylycatic ICDs in the treatment of DCM. The Cardiomyopathy Trial randomized 104 patients with DCM and an ejection fraction less than 30% to receive an ICD or no ICD in addition to conventional therapy. The study population size was determined on the basis of an estimated annual mortality rate of 30% and an estimated 1348 patients were to be included in the study. After enrolling 104 patients over a 6 year period, the actual mortality rate at 1 year was just 6%, with no arrhythmic deaths. The study was stopped prematurely on the basis that the anticipated sample size was too small and enrollment too slow to show significant differences between the two groups.[26]

In the Defibrillators in Non-Ischemic Cardiomyopathy Treatment Evaluation (DEFINITE) trial, Kadish and associates[27] randomized 458 subjects with DCM and ejection fraction less than 36% to receive standard or ICD therapy. More than 90% were already on best medical therapy with a beta-blocker and an ACE inhibitor or adrenergic receptor (AR) blocker. Mean left ventricular ejection fraction was 21%, and 90% of patients had nonsustained ventricular tachycardia. Symptom class was NYHA class I in 22%, II in 57%, and III in 21%. The primary endpoint was total mortality. After 2 years, 14.1% of the standard therapy group and 7.9% of the ICD therapy group had died, giving 6.2% absolute and 35% relative risk reduction. This did not reach statistical significance (P = .08) because of sample size and a lower-than-expected death rate in the standard therapy group. Arrhythmic mortality, a secondary endpoint, was reduced by 80% (P = .006). Mortality reduction was greater in NYHA class III than in class II patients.

In the Amiodarone versus Implantable Cardioverter-Defibrillator Trial (AMIOVIRT),[28] Strickberger and colleagues randomized 103 patients with DCM, NSVT, and ejection fraction less than 35% to receive either amiodarone or an ICD. Mortality rates at 1 and 2 years were similar (10% versus 4% and 12% versus 13%, respectively; P was not significant). No difference in quality of life between groups was observed.

In the largest trial to date, the Sudden Cardiac Death Heart Failure (SCD-HeFT) trial, Bardy and colleagues[23] randomized 2521 patients with both coronary artery disease and DCM with class II or III CHF and ejection fraction less than 35% to receive placebo, weight-adjusted amiodarone therapy, or an ICD. At 5 years of follow-up, absolute and relative mortality reduction rates in the ICD group compared with placebo were 7.2% and 23%, respectively (P = .007). Mortality benefits were similar in the ischemic and nonischemic groups, (see Fig. 63-7), but improvement was limited to those with class II rather than class III failure (Fig. 63-9). Together, these trials show similar significant reductions in total mortality among patients with DCM who are implanted with an ICD rather than treated with standard medical therapy or the addition of amiodarone and support the empirical use of prophylactic ICDs in patients with DCM and severely reduced left ventricular function in the absence of NYHA class IV CHF.

Left Ventricular Assist Devices

Ventricular assist devices are a recent advance in the management of patients with end-stage heart failure. Although such devices previously were used solely as an in-hospital bridge to transplantation, many patients have now been discharged from the hospital as part of ongoing clinical trials of the HeartMate (Thoratec, Pleasanton, California) and AbioCor (AbioMed, Danvers, Massachusetts) and other vented electrical implantable devices.[29] Anecdotally, some patients with assist devices appear to tolerate ventricular arrhythmias remarkably well, because cardiac output is device- rather than ventricle-dependent. In patients with poor right ventricular function and those with ventricular fibrillation, however, significant hemodynamic compromise may develop with left ventricular assist devices. Use of these devices is limited by their cost, the risk for infection related to the percutaneous power or drive cable, and the risk for systemic thromboembolism. However, their increasing use as destination therapy or a bridge to recovery, rather than as a bridge to transplantation, is an indication of their success in end-stage DCM.

Catheter Ablation

Although ICDs have reduced the likelihood of arrhythmic death, they do not prevent the recurrence of symptomatic ventricular tachycardia. Pharmacologic control of ventricular tachycardia is successful in approximately 40% of cases, leaving a significant proportion of patients with symptomatic ventricular tachycardia or ICD shocks. Experience with catheter ablation of ventricular tachycardia in DCM has been limited and has been associated with lower success rates than ventricular tachycardia ablation in the setting of coronary disease and post–myocardial infarction scar. However, the advent of electroanatomic mapping systems, irrigated tip ablation catheters, and epicardial mapping and ablation has been associated with significant improvement in success rates.

Ablation of ventricular tachycardia in DCM usually is performed with one or more of a number of mapping modailities including pace mapping, entrainment mapping and electroanatomically guided voltage and activation sequence mapping. The use of integrated mapping systems, which permit merging of three-dimensional CT or MRI Dicom images with real-time electroanatomic mapping, has been a significant advance. Re-creation of both the endocardial and epicardial surfaces of the ventricle permits creation of a virtual three-dimensional myocardium (Fig. 63-10). Voltage mapping using electroanatomic mapping systems allows rapid identification of the presence of scar particularly on the endocardium. The presence of low voltage on the epicardium may represent either scar or

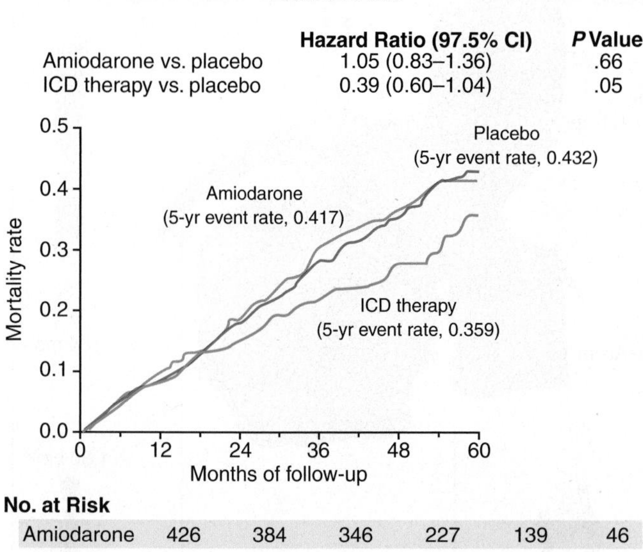

No. at Risk

Amiodarone	426	384	346	227	139	46
Placebo	453	415	370	244	152	48
ICD therapy	431	395	365	244	144	48

A

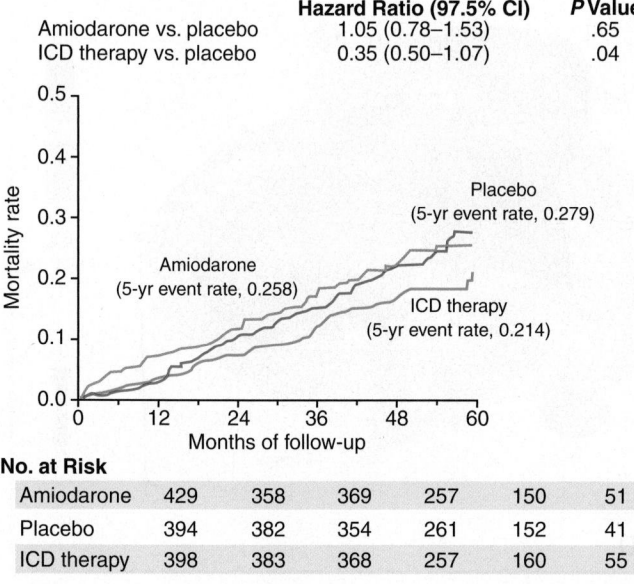

Nonischemic CHF

	Hazard Ratio (97.5% CI)	P Value
Amiodarone vs. placebo	1.05 (0.78–1.53)	.65
ICD therapy vs. placebo	0.35 (0.50–1.07)	.04

Placebo (5-yr event rate, 0.279)

Amiodarone (5-yr event rate, 0.258)

ICD therapy (5-yr event rate, 0.214)

Mortality rate: 0.0, 0.1, 0.2, 0.3, 0.4, 0.5

Months of follow-up: 0, 12, 24, 36, 48, 60

No. at Risk

Amiodarone	429	358	369	257	150	51
Placebo	394	382	354	261	152	41
ICD therapy	398	383	368	257	160	55

B

Figure 63-9 Kaplan-Meier analysis of freedom from death among patients with ischemic and nonischemic dilated cardiomyopathy (congestive heart failure [CHF]) randomized to receive placebo, implantable defibrillators, or amiodarone in the Sudden Cardiac Death in Heart Failure Trial (SCD-HeFT). Mortality reduction rates with ICD therapy compared with placebo were similar in the ischemic and nonischemic groups. Amiodarone failed to reduce mortality in either group. ICD, implantable cardioverter-defibrillator. (From Bardy GH, Lee KL, Mark DB, et al: Amiodarone or an implantable cardioverter-defibrillator for congestive heart failure. N Engl J Med 352:225-37, 2005.)

epicardial fat. These systems can create helpful road maps in identifying reentrant circuits which may be re-created using three-dimensional activation sequence mapping and in then designing ablation targets or linear lesions. Soejima and coworkers[11] demonstrated myocardial reentry as the dominant mechanism, responsible for ventricular tachycardia in 75% of patients. Other mechanisms were focal and bundle branch reentry (17% and 7%, respectively). In 19 of 22 patients, a critical reentry isthmus was identified—endocardial in 12 patients and epicardial in 7. Elimination of the ventricular tachycardia circuit was possible in 12 patients, and modification was possible in another 4 patients, resulting in no further ventricular tachycardia at 11 months of follow-up despite frequent ventricular tachycardia and ICD shocks before ablation. Animal models of myocardial CT imaging have demonstrated the feasability of color coding of different tissue characteristics such as scar to allow clearer labelling of scar based on tissue characteristics rather than just local voltage.[30] This should provide additional information to help in creation of the best strategic approach to ablation of ventricular tachycardia in a patient based on the global presence and location of left ventricular scar, rather than just the circuit of one inducible ventricular tachycardia. Failure to ablate ventricular tachycardia from the epicardium or endocardium may be due to a midmyocardial source or critical isthmus or inability to reach an epicardial source due to the presence of epicardial fat. Novel catheter designs including needle-tipped catheters are being developed to address these issues.

Irrigated tip catheters have proved useful both in increasing lesion depth toward the mid-myocardial layers, where myocardial fibrosis has been frequently identified in patients with DCM, and in reducing the likelihood of endocardial charring and thrombus formation. The increasing use of percutaneous epicardial catheter ablation is a result of moderate success rates only with endocardial approaches. In patients with DCM, approximately one third of ventricular tachycardias are ablated epicardially rather than endocardially. Challenges of epicardial catheter ablation include (1) difficulties accessing the posterior left ventricle and diaphragmatic aspects of both ventricles, (2) the need to keep catheter irrigation at low rates to avoid tamponade, (3) the need for concomitant coronary angiography to avoid arterial injury during ablation, and (4) the presence of epicardial fat, which can prevent access to target sites.

Conclusions

The goals in management of patients with nonischemic DCM and ventricular arrhythmias are to reduce the risk for sudden death and to minimize symptomatic ventricular tachycardia. As left ventricular function deteriorates in DCM, the incidence of both sudden death and heart failure–related death increases. Discriminating from this population a subgroup of patients who, despite being at increased risk for terminal pump failure, die an arrhythmic death has proved difficult. The use of beta-blockers and ACE inhibitors, biventricular pacing, and ICDs has led to an improvement in overall survival and consequently an increasing prevalence of DCM and associated ventricular arrhythmias. Recent advances in catheter ablation technology have led to improved succcess rates and an increase in the use of catheter ablation in this growing population.

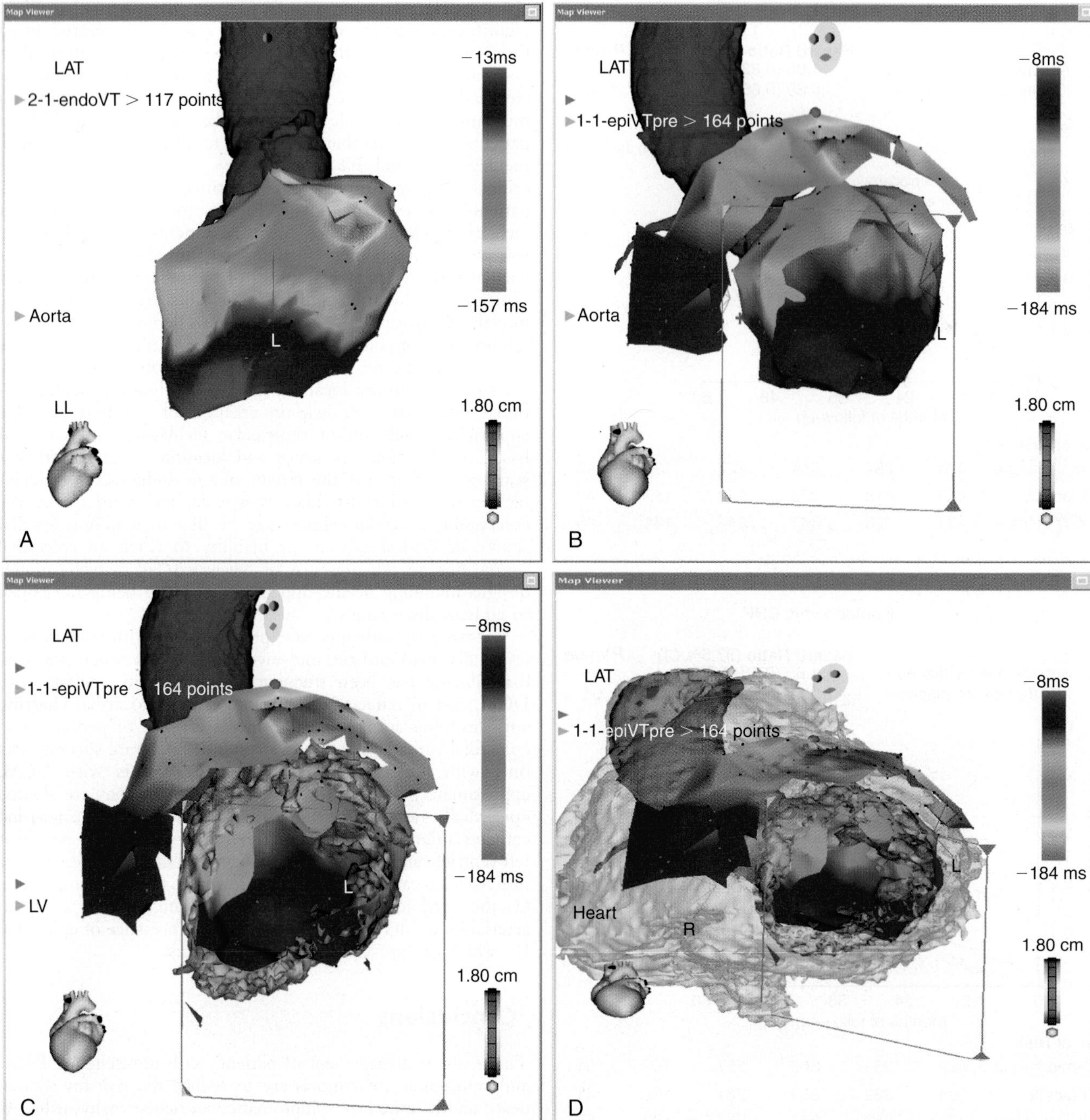

Figure 63-10 CARTO electroanatomic mapping activation of the left ventricle (LV) during ventricular tachycardia in a patient with dilated cardiomyopathy and conduction system disease. **A,** Endocardial activation map showing earliest activation in anterobasal area. **B,** Combined endocardial and epicardial map demonstrating earlier activation on the epicardial than the endocardial surface. **C,** CARTO map merged with computed tomography (CT) rendering of the endocardial surface of the LV. **D,** CARTO map merged with CT renderings of both endocardial and epicardial surfaces of the LV. LL, left lateral view.

References

1. Olson TM, Michels VV, Thibodeau SN, et al: Actin mutations in dilated cardiomyopathy, a heritable form of heart failure. Science 280:750-752, 1998.
2. Li D, Tapscoft T, Gonzalez O, et al: Desmin mutations responsible for idiopathic dilated cardiomyopathy. Circulation 100: 461-464, 1999.
3. Barresi R, Di Blasi C, Negri T, et al: Disruption of heart sarcoglycan complex and severe cardiomyopathy caused by β-sarcoglycan mutations. J Med Genet 37:102-107, 2000.
4. Tsubata S, Bowles KR, Vatta M, et al: Mutations in the human δ-sarcoglycan gene in familial and sporadic dilated cardiomyopathy. J Clin Invest 106:655-662, 2000.
5. Kamisago M, Sharma SD, DePalma SR, et al: Mutations in sarcomeric protein genes as a cause of dilated cardiomyopathy. N Engl J Med 343:1688-1696, 2000.
6. Olson TM, Kishimoto NY, Whitby FG, Michels VV: Mutations that alter the surface

change of α-tropomyosin are associated with dilated cardiomyopathy. J Mol Cell Cardiol 33:723-732, 2001.
7. Brodsky GL, Muntoni F, Miocic S, et al: Lamin A/C gene mutation associated with dilated cardiomyopathy with variable skeletal muscle involvement. Circulation 101:473-476, 2000.
8. Olson TM, Keating MT: Mapping a cardiomyopathy locus to chromosome 3p22-p25. J Clin Invest 97:528-532, 1996.
9. Berko BA, Swift M: X-linked dilated cardiomyopathy. N Engl J Med 316:1186-1191, 1987.
10. Towbin JA, Hejtmancik JF, Brink P, et al: X-linked dilated cardiomyopathy (XLCM): Molecular genetic evidence of linkage to the Duchenne muscular dystrophy gene at the Xp21 locus. Circulation 87:1854-1865, 1993.
11. Soejima K, Stevenson WG, Sapp JL, et al: Endocardial and epicardial radiofrequency ablation of ventricular tachycardia associated with dilated cardiomyopathy: The importance of low-voltage scars. J Am Coll Cardiol 43:1834-1842, 2004.
12. Leier CV: The cardiomyopathies: mortality, sudden death, and ventricular arrhythmias. Cardiovasc Clin 22:275-306, 1992.
13. Luu M, Stevenson WG, Stephenson LW, et al: Diverse mechanisms of unexpected cardiac arrest in advanced heart failure. Circulation 80:1675-1680, 1989.
14. McCrohon JA, Moon JC, Prasad SK, et al: Differentiation of heart failure related to dilated cardiomyopathy and coronary artery disease using gadolinium-enhanced cardiovascular magnetic resonance. Circulation 108:54-59, 2003.
15. Nazarian S, Bluemke D, Lardo A, et al: Magnetic resonance assessment of the substrate for inducible ventricular tachycardia in nonischemic cardiomyopathy. Circulation 112:2821-2825, 2005.
16. De Maria R, Gavazzi A, Caroli A, et al: Ventricular arrhythmias in dilated cardiomyopathy as an independent prognostic hallmark. Am J Cardiol 69:1451-1457, 1992.
17. Romeo F, Pelliccia F, Cianfrocca C, et al: Predictors of sudden death in idiopathic dilated cardiomyopathy. Am J Cardiol 63:138-140, 1989.
18. Grimm W, Christ M, Bach J, et al: Noninvasive arrhythmia risk stratification in idiopathic dilated cardiomyopathy: Results of the Marburg Cardiomyopathy Study. Circulation 108:2883-2891, 2003.
19. Pitt B, Segal R, Martinez FA, et al: Randomised trial of losartan versus captopril in patients over 65 with heart failure (Evaluation of Losartan in the Elderly Study, ELITE). Lancet 349:747-752, 1997.
20. Pitt B, Poole-Wilson PA, Segal Rfor the ELITE II Investigators: Effect of losartan compared with captopril on mortality in patients with symptomatic heart failure: Randomised trial-the Losartan Heart Failure Survival Study ELITE II. Lancet 355:1582-1587, 2000.
21. Waagstein F, Hjalmarson A, Varnauskas E, Wallentin F: Effect of chronic beta adrenergic receptor blockade in congestive cardiomyopathy. Br Heart J 37:1022-1036, 1975.
22. Marks AR, Reiken S, Marx SO: Progression of heart failure: Is protein kinase a hyperphosphorylation of the ryanodine receptor a contributing factor? Circulation 105:272-275, 2002.
23. Bardy G, Lee K, Mark D, et al for the SCD-HeFT Investigators: Amiodarone or an implantable cardioverter-defibrillator for congestive heart failure. N Engl J Med 352:225-237, 2005.
24. Cleland J, Daubert JC, Erdmann E, et al for the Cardiac Resynchronization–Heart Failure (CARE-HF) Study Investigators: The effect of cardiac resynchronization on morbidity and mortality in heart failure. N Engl J Med 352:1539-1549, 2005.
25. Saxon L, Bristow M, Boehmer J, et al: Predictors of sudden cardiac death and appropriate shock in the Comparison of Medical Therapy, Pacing, and Defibrillation in Heart Failure (COMPANION) trial. Circulation 114:2766-2772, 2006.
26. Bänsch D, Antz M, Boczor S, et al for the CAT Investigators: Primary prevention of sudden cardiac death in idiopathic dilated cardiomyopathy. The Cardiomyopathy Trial (CAT). Circulation 105:1453-1457, 2002.
27. Kadish A, Dyer A, Daubert JP, et al: Prophylactic defibrillator implantation in patients with nonischemic dilated cardiomyopathy. N Engl J Med 350:2151-2158, 2004.
28. Strickberger SA, Hummel J, Bartlett T, et al: Amiodarone Versus Implantable Cardioverter Defibrillator Trial: Randomized trial in patients with nonischemic dilated cardiomyopathy and asymptomatic nonsustained ventricular tachycardia. AMIOVIRT. J Am Coll Cardiol 41:1707-1712, 2003.
29. Poirier VL: The HeartMate left ventricular assist system: Worldwide clinical results. Eur J Cardiothorac Surg 11:S39-S44, 1997.
30. Dong J, Calkins H, Solomon S, et al: Integrated electroanatomic mapping with three-dimensional computed tomographic images for real-time guided ablations. Circulation 113:186-194, 2006.
31. Franciosa JA, Wilen M, Ziesche S, Cohn JN: Survival in men with severe chronic left ventricular failure due to either coronary artery disease or idiopathic dilated cardiomyopathy. Am J Cardiol 51:831-836, 1983.
32. Stevenson LW, Fowler MB, Schroder JS, et al: Poor survival of patients with idiopathic dilated cardiomyopathy considered too well for transplantation. Am J Med 83:871-876, 1987.
33. Fuster V, Gersh BL, Giuliani ER, et al: The natural history of idiopathic dilated cardiomyopathy. Am J Cardiol 47:525-531, 1981.
34. Komajda M, Jais JP, Reeves F, et al: Factors predicting mortality in idiopathic dilated cardiomyopathy. Eur Heart J 11:824-831, 1990.
35. Sugrue DD, Rodeheffer RJ, Codd MB, et al: The clinical course of idiopathic dilated cardiomyopathy: A population-based study. Ann Intern Med 117:117-123, 1992.

63

Arrhythmogenic Right Ventricular Cardiomyopathies 64

Guy Fontaine and Philippe Charron

CHAPTER OUTLINE

Terminology

The most frequently encountered form of arrhythmogenic right ventricular cardiomyopathy (ARVC) is arrhythmogenic right ventricular dysplasia (ARVD). The designation *dysplasia* is appropriate because this pathologic component has been defined as a "disturbance in development." A striking example of such disturbance is seen in Uhl's anomaly, first reported at Johns Hopkins, with total absence of right ventricular myocardium and apposition of epicardium against endocardium.

Of note, the classic Marcus paper included a case of the adult form of Uhl's anomaly in the absence of cardiac arrhythmia. On pathologic examination of a typical ARVD fetus (at 27 weeks), shown to be arrhythmic in utero, the findings of right ventricular aneurysm and fibrofatty replacement limited to the right ventricular myocardium demonstrated that the abnormalities associated with the disease may start in the embryonic stage (Fig. 64-1). However, clinical evidence and histologic features suggest that in ARVD, focal signs of inflammation or major fibrosis, generally considered to be the result of a wide spectrum of presentation, are due to myocarditis, which seems superimposed on the genetic background of ARVD. The updated classification of ARVCs presented in this chapter is based on our clinical experience at the La Salpêtrière hôpital in Paris in more than 300 patients, our examination of histologic material from more than 100 patients, and recent data from genetics and molecular biology studies.

Advances in Cellular and Molecular Biology and in the Understanding of Arrhythmogenic Right Ventricular Cardiomyopathies

Advances in cellular and molecular biology have been instrumental in elucidating the genetics, clinical features, and mechanisms of ARVCs. An overview of these advances is presented in this section.

Cell-Cell Adhesion Proteins and Apoptosis

A major advance in the study of right ventricular cardiomyopathies has been the discovery of the role played by cell-cell adhesion proteins (Fig. 64-2) and apoptosis. In 1989 Guiraudon noted the distortion of desmosomes on electron microscopic studies in patients with typical ARVD (Fig. 64-3).[1] In 1996 apoptosis was demonstrated for the first time in the human heart in patients with ARVD.[2] Major apoptosis can initiate the process of fibrosis.[3]

However, elucidation of the genetic basis of ARVCs came after the discovery of plakoglobin gene mutation. This was the result of my encouraging McKenna to investigate the genetics of Naxos disease. It was obvious that a study of this disease should be able to identify a genetic mechanism, based on readily identifiable diagnostic features on echocardiograms (ECGs) and histologic studies of surgical biopsy specimens in all of the affected patients with palmoplantar keratoderma and woolly hair (Fig. 64-4).

The first locus for Naxos disease was identified on chromosome 17 in 1998, and 2 years later the first mutated gene implicated in ARVCs was discovered.[4] The protein encoded by the mutated gene, called plakoglobin, located in the desmosomes, was found to be truncated on its carboxyl (C) terminus. Because plakoglobin is a ubiquitous protein located in all desmosomes, especially in the skin and in the cardiac tissue, it was possible that this unique abnormal protein could be the key to an explanation of the pathogenic mechanism of Naxos disease. Later it was proved that all of the patients with the typical form of the syndromic Naxos pattern were homozygous for the mutation. This finding is in accordance with the recessive transmission observed in the families. In the heterozygous form, it was discovered that some affected persons demonstrated a phenotypic pattern of outflow tract ventricular tachycardia.

Identification of abnormal plakoglobin opened new vistas to investigate other proteins located in the desmosomes. It was therefore possible to pursue the discovery of other abnormal proteins producing the general phenotypic pattern of ARVCs. Identification of desmoplakin was reported in 2002,[5] of plakophilin-2 in 2004,[6] and of desmoglein-2 and desmocollin-2 in 2006 (Fig. 64-5).[7,8]

To clarify the importance of these major components of the cell-cell junction, it is necessary to review the location and relevant cellular structure of these proteins and their role in myocardial function, which is unique in comparison with that of molecules functioning in skeletal muscle.

Cardiac contraction is the result of the complex interplay of two main molecules, actin and myosin, contained inside each cardiomyocyte. However, transmission of the mechanical forces elaborated inside the myocardial cells from one cell to the adjacent cell is produced by two structures, the desmosomes

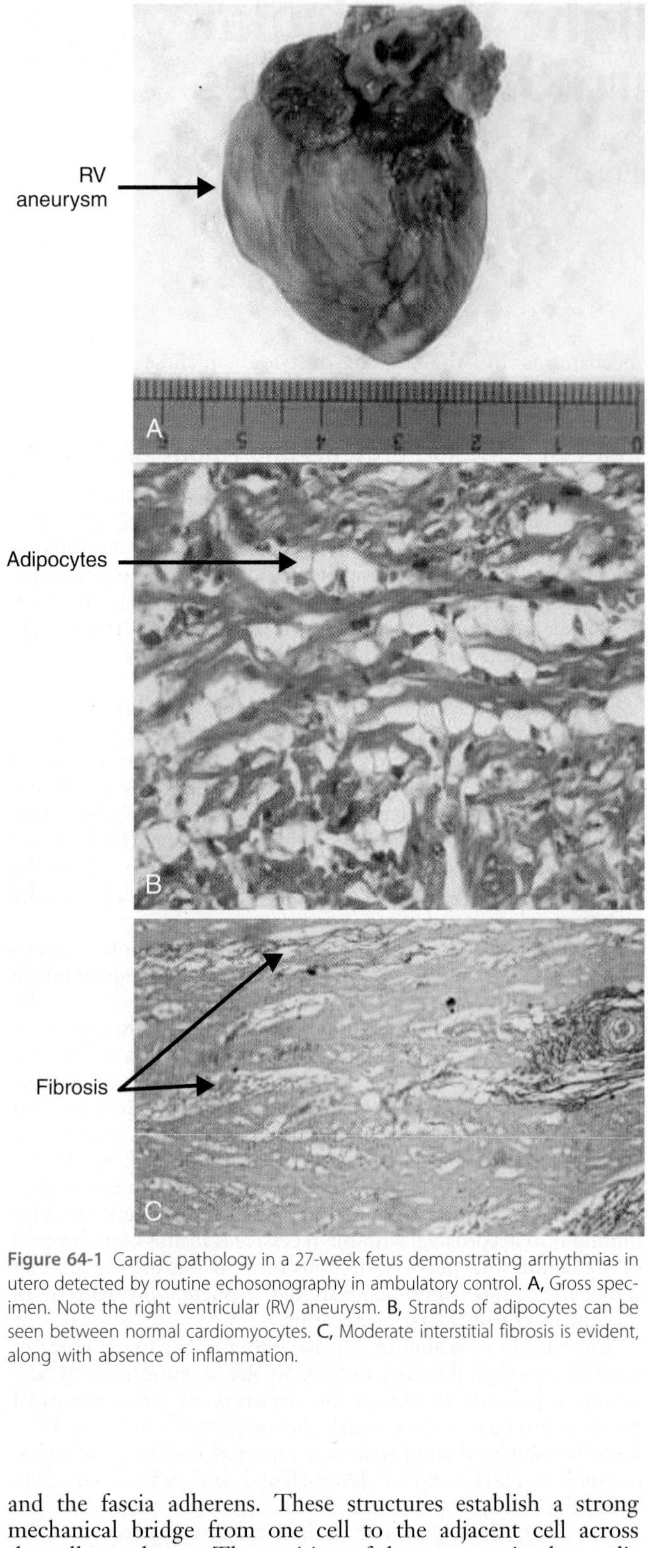

Figure 64-1 Cardiac pathology in a 27-week fetus demonstrating arrhythmias in utero detected by routine echosonography in ambulatory control. A, Gross specimen. Note the right ventricular (RV) aneurysm. B, Strands of adipocytes can be seen between normal cardiomyocytes. C, Moderate interstitial fibrosis is evident, along with absence of inflammation.

and the fascia adherens. These structures establish a strong mechanical bridge from one cell to the adjacent cell across the cell membrane. The position of desmosomes in the cardiomyocytes and a similar but smaller structure, the fascia adherens, is represented in Figure 64-2. A more detailed depiction showing the position of extracellular and intracellular components of the desmosomal proteins is shown in Figure 64-5.

Most of the proteins presented in this schematic representation have been identified to be involved in some forms of ARVC. At present, however, mutations in these desmosomal genes are found in only 50% of the cases. In several reports, and in our own experience, most mutations are found in the plakophilin-2 gene.

Gap Junctions

If plakoglobin is impaired and desmosomes are subsequently distorted in Naxos disease, it may be inferred that gap junctions, which are a fragile structure of cell-cell electrical conduction, also are modified. Gap junctions have no mechanical properties. They consist of two holes bordered by the connexin Cx43, located on the opposite parts of two adjacent cardiac cells. These gap junctions are mostly observed on the lateral portions of the intercalated disks, as represented in Figure 64-6.

The first demonstration of altered gap junctions—underexpression of Cx 43—in ARVC was made by Saffitz and colleagues.[9] The heart specimen from a patient who died suddenly with Naxos disease was studied in our laboratory for confirmation of the histologic pattern of typical ARVD. In this patient, underexpression of gap junctions was noted in the left ventricle, but severe underexpression of this protein was evident in the right ventricular myocardium (Fig. 64-7).

In a recent experimental study, the silencing of rat cardiomyocytes induced profound remodeling of Cx43 and also alteration of functional coupling, supporting the notion of molecular crosstalk between desmosomal and gap-junction proteins.[10] The distortion of desmosomes also may be a new mechanism of abnormal cell-to-cell conduction. This abnormality can be a pathogenic factor, in addition to the marked replacement of cardiac cells by fat and fibrosis. Underexpression of specific gap junction proteins may prove to be useful in diagnosis of right ventricular cardiomyopathies.

Wnt Family Signaling Pathway

An important parameter to explain the pathogenesis of adipocytes in ARVCs was provided by the study of a group of proteins called Wnt.[11] These proteins also are part of the Armadillo family, which plays a role in the structure of the proteins of the desmosomes.

Plakoglobin, also known as γ-catenin, has structural and functional similarities to β-catenin, which is the effector for canonical Wnt signaling. Plakoglobin is known to compete with β-catenin, with a net negative effect on the canonical Wnt–β-catenin signaling pathway through T cell–lymphoid–enhancing binding (Lef-Tcf4) transcription factors. The Wnt–β-catenin signaling pathway is a key regulator of the transcriptional switch from myogenesis to adipogenesis. Activation of the Wnt pathway favors the cardiomyocyte phenotype, and the adipocyte phenotype is inhibited; suppression of the pathway results in a switch to adipogenesis and fibrogenesis.

Mutation of desmosomal protein by impairing desmosome assembly may free plakoglobin from the desmosomes. The plakoglobin mathen translocate into the nucleus and, by competition with β-catenin, suppress signaling through the canonical Wnt–β-catenin Lef-Tcf4 pathway. Suppression of Wnt–β-catenin signaling provokes adipogenesis, fibrogenesis, and apoptosis.

Suppression of expression of desmoplakin in cardiomyocyte cells, and also in engineered mice, recently was found to result to nuclear translocation of plakoglobin, reduced canonical Wnt signaling, enhanced myocyte apoptosis, and excess fibrogenesis and adipogenesis, supporting the previous hypothesis. Taken together, these findings provide a new mechanism for the pathogenesis of ARVC, which eventually may lead to myocardial dysfunction and ventricular arrhythmias.

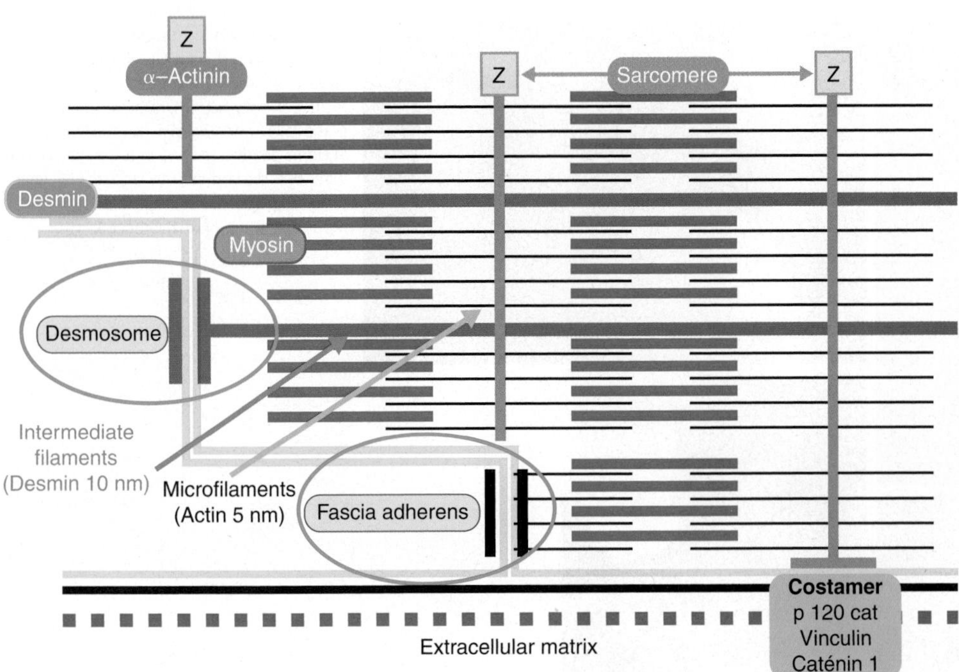

Figure 64-2 Junction of two cardiomyocytes illustrating the role of desmosome and fascia adherens, the two zones of cell-cell adhesion proteins.

Fibrogenesis

Four possible explanations have been advanced for the presence of fibrosis in ARVD:

- Role of Wnt signaling pathway during embryogenesis (some zones of interstitial fibrosis were observed in our fetal heart) (see Fig. 64-1)
- Presence of massive abnormal apoptosis by phagocytosis of apoptotic bodies,[2,3] also observed during embryogenesis and during the disease progression
- Ischemia produced by distal coronary spasms of the distal coronary arteries (small-vessel disease)
- Replacement fibrosis in case of superimposed myocarditis, as discussed later in the chapter

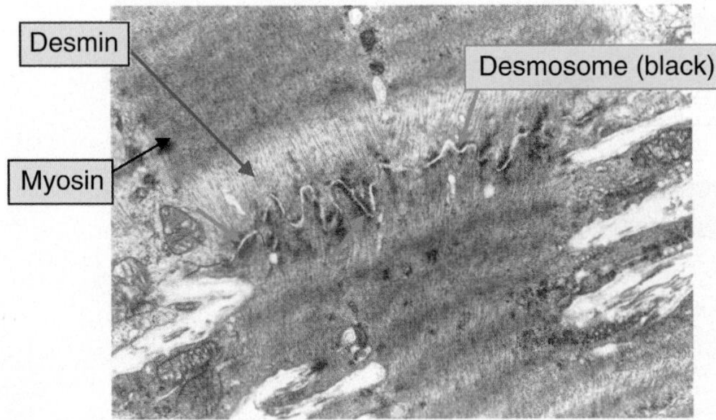

Figure 64-3 Distorsion of desmosomes.

Classification of Arrhythmogenic Right Ventricular Cardiomyopathies

Arrhythmogenic Right Ventricular Dysplasia

Phenotype Arrhythmogenic right ventricular dysplasia is an inherited condition transmitted in a dominant form, with variable expression and penetrance among affected family members. It is generally discovered during adolescence with recognition of symptoms due to ventricular arrhythmias originating in the right ventricle. It is a progressive condition.

Histology The epicardial and frequently mediomural layers of right ventricular myocardium are replaced by fat and fibrosis. Some aspects suggest that the pathologic process starts in the mediomural layers, mostly extending toward the epicardium, which may be replaced entirely by fat and fibrotic tissue, suggesting that the disease progresses from epicardium to endocardium. Fibrosis generally borders or embeds surviving fibers. Full-thickness examination of the right ventricular myocardium is necessary to depict the typical topographic features of the lesions. Therefore, histologic examination showing atrophy of remaining cardiomyocytes and presence of diffuse fatty and fibrous tissue (better seen with HPS staining) in the right ventricular free wall is the standard method to ascertain the diagnosis (Fig. 64-8).

Involvement of the left ventricle is frequently observed, mostly at the apex, which looks covered by fat on gross pathologic examination. However, some focal zones of fibrosis and fatty tissue can be found on light microscopy over the entire left ventricular myocardium. This may explain the decrease in left ventricular function found even in the mild forms of the disease (Fig. 64-9).

Genotype In addition to all of the desmosomal proteins that have been identified thus far in this form of ARVC, the

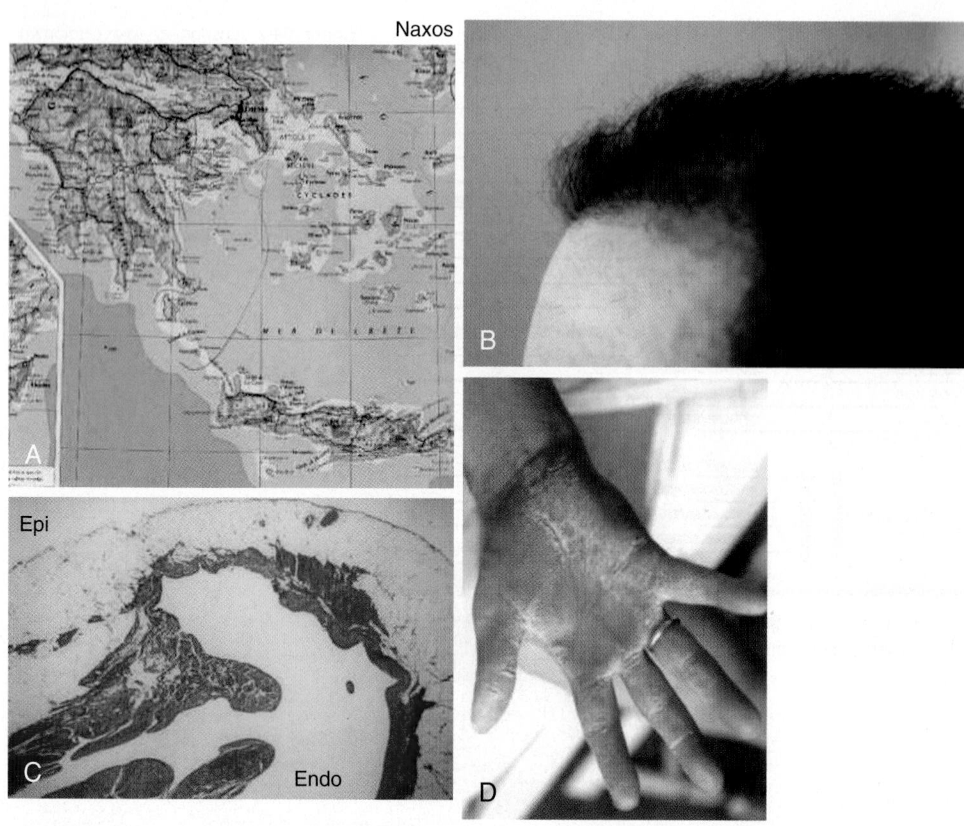

Figure 64-4 Manifestations of Naxos disease, discovered on a Greek island (**A**), the largest of the Cyclades. Typical features include woolly hair (**B**), right ventricular dysplasia (**C**), and palmar keratoderma (**D**). Sudden death occurred in a female patient with the disease at the age of 16 years. (Courtesy of Dr. Protonotarios, Naxos Medical Center, Naxos, Greece.)

transforming growth factor have been mentioned. However, the transforming growth factor-β (TGF-β3) gene is a new gene related to the phenotypic presentation of classic ARVD.[12]

In most of the literature reports, no differences in presentation have been found between plakophilin-positive and plakophilin-negative cases. It has been suggested that the familial forms may have a more severe or earlier presentation as compared with the isolated cases. The penetrance in family members varies, ranging from 20% to 70%. Precise natural history and phenotype-genotype correlations remain, however, to be studied in well-characterized populations.

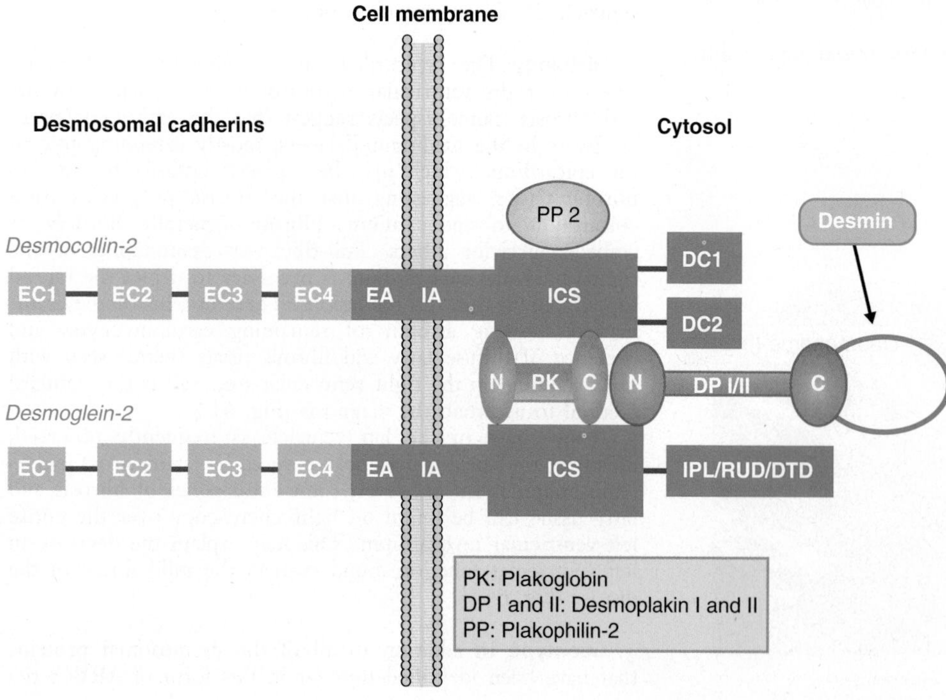

Figure 64-5 Molecules of desmosomes: desmoplakin (DP), plakoglobin (PK), and plakophilin-2 (PP2). Naxos disease is related to truncation of the C terminus of plakoglobin, distorting its connection with desmoplakin.

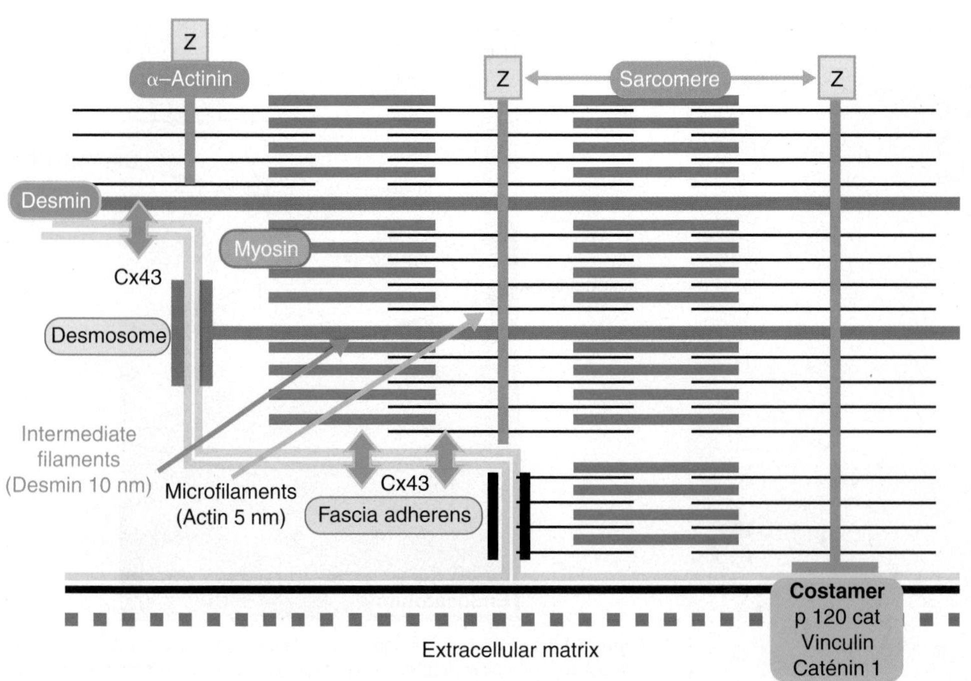

Figure 64-6 Location of proteins Cx43 responsible for transmission of electrical activation in the intercalated disks.

Biventricular Dysplasia

Phenotype Because of loss of myocardial tissue of the left ventricle, biventricular dysplasia frequently leads to congestive heart failure.

Histology In biventricular dysplasia, the same fibrofatty replacement of myocardium is observed in both ventricles. The disease seems to progress from epicardium to endocardium, however, as opposed to classic ARVD, in which fibrofatty replacement seems to start in the mediomural layers.

Right Ventricular Dysplasia without Arrhythmia

Quiescent Form

Phenotype In the quiescent form of right ventricular dysplasia without arrhythmia, by definition, no obvious arrhythmias are detected. This may be related to total electrical silence of the arrhythmogenic substrate or to the presence of minor arrhythmias that are not severe enough to be symptomatic.

Histology In the quiescent form, observed in 3.7% of the general population (Fig. 64-10), the typical histologic pattern of ARVD is observed in the right ventricular free wall. The arrhythmogenic substrate is dormant, however. This can be explained by the absence of all of the necessary critical electrophysiologic parameters necessary to induce the reentrant mechanism or, possibly, by the absence of neutrophil activation.

Right Ventricular Dysplasia with Congestive Heart Failure

Phenotype Congestive heart failure can be the result of two different mechanisms. In the first mechanism, rapid progression of the dysplastic process continuously replaces myocardium by fat and fibrosis in the right ventricle, leading to subsequent involvement of the left ventricle. The second possibility is that the congestive heart failure is due to a superimposed myocarditis (discussed next). Because no or only minor arrhythmias may be present, these cases can mimic idiopathic dilated cardiomyopathy.

Arrhythmogenic Right Ventricular Dysplasia with Superimposed Myocarditis

Clinical as well as histologic data indicate that various forms of myocarditis can be superimposed on ARVD, suggesting a susceptibility of dysplastic myocardium to viral or bacterial factors of inflammation. This concept was deduced from the analysis of left ventricular ejection fraction observed in our population of patients, as well as from data published in the literature (see Fig. 64-9). The bimodal nature of this parameter also has been confirmed in a recent series (see Fig. 19-2 in the publication by Coronel, et al).[13] It is a general concept that can be extended to other forms of cardiomyopathy. Presence of coxsackievirus as well as adenoviruses has been reported in the myocardium of patients with ARVD.[14] In most cases, myocarditis involves both right and left ventricles. Both the severity of left ventricular involvement and the rate of myocarditis progression are the determinants of prognosis.

Quiescent Form

Phenotype By definition, the quiescent form of ARVD with superimposed myocarditis is asymptomatic.

Histology Presence of lymphocytes is common in the general population (being seen with a frequency of.1% to 5.5%). This finding appears to be more common in patients with ARVD.

Hyperacute Form

Phenotype Features include fever, asthenia, dyspnea, hypotension, and fulminant heart failure, with death occurring within a few days.[15]

Histology Histologic findings include diffuse round cell infiltration, polymorphonuclear macrophages, and eosinophils.

Acute Form

Phenotype Phenotypic features include fever, chest pain, and atrioventricular (AV) conduction disorder ranging from

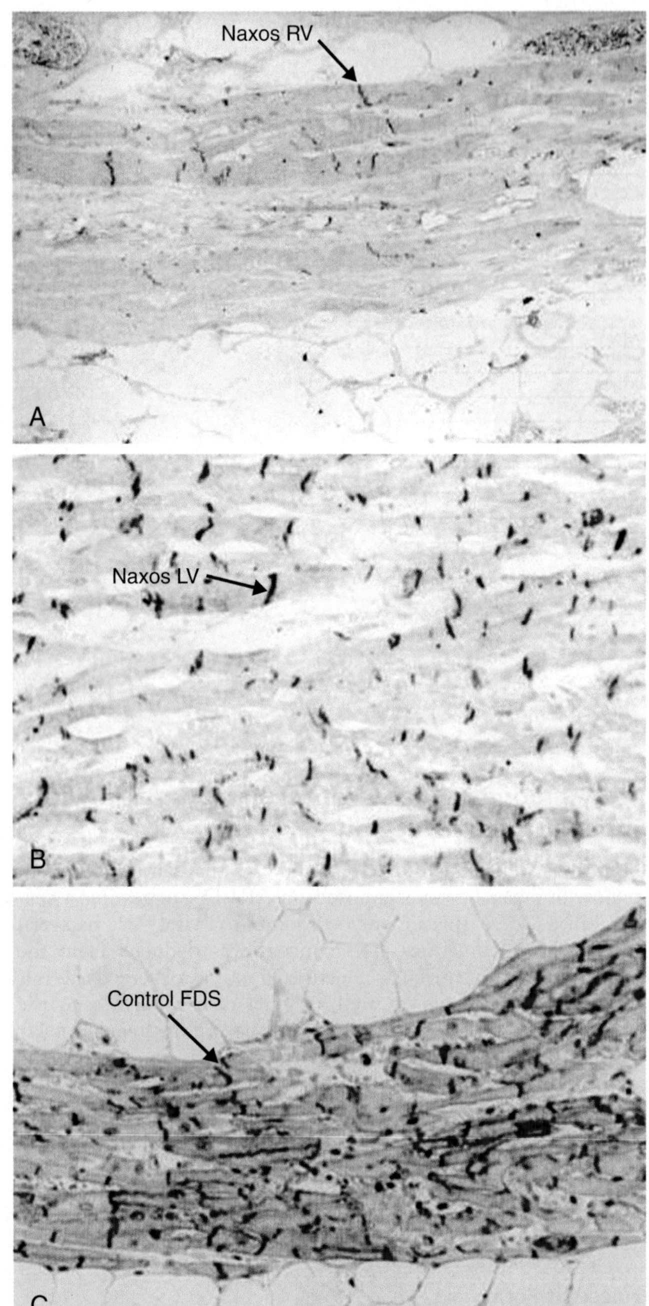

Figure 64-7 Underexpression of connexin43 (Cx43) in Naxos disease involving both the left ventricle (LV) (**B**) and the right ventricle (RV), but more marked in the RV (**A**). Note the presence of normal expression of Cx43 in a case of focal fat dissociation syndrome (FDS) serving as control (**C**). (Courtesy of Dr. Jeff Saffitz, St. Louis, Missouri.)

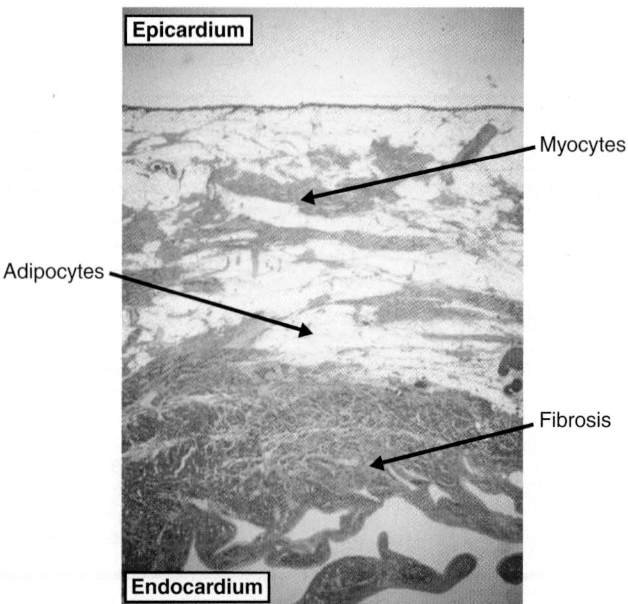

Figure 64-8 Full thickness of right ventricular free wall, showing all of the basic components of typical dysplasia, except for signs of inflammation, not visible at this magnification.

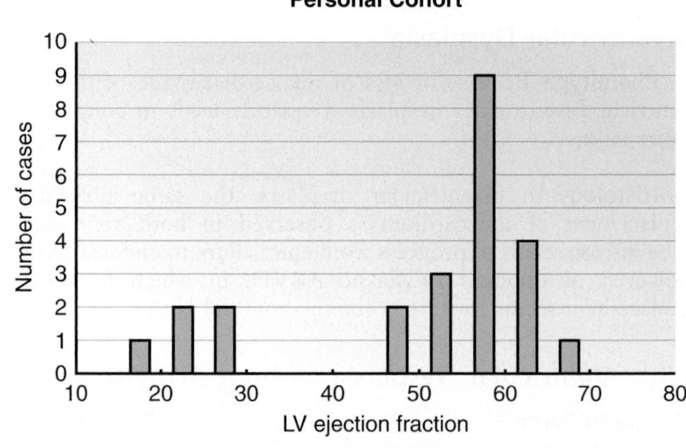

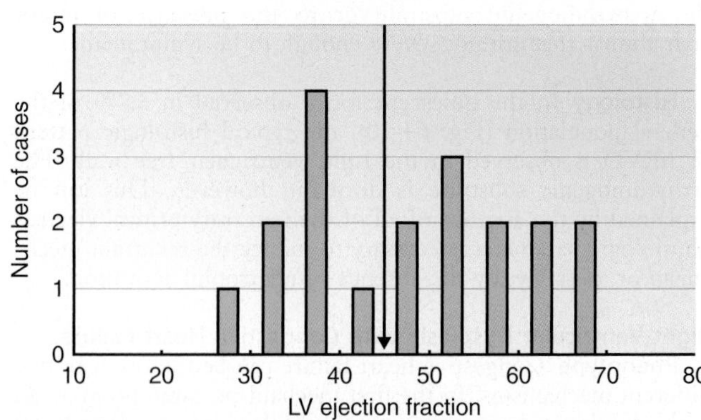

Figure 64-9 Distribution of left ventricular (LV) ejection fraction in patients with arrhythmogenic right ventricular dysplasia from our clinical experience and in data from the literature. Note the bimodal pattern suggesting the implication of two different phenomena. All of the patients with the lower ejection fraction (EF) had histologic signs of major inflammation and fibrosis.

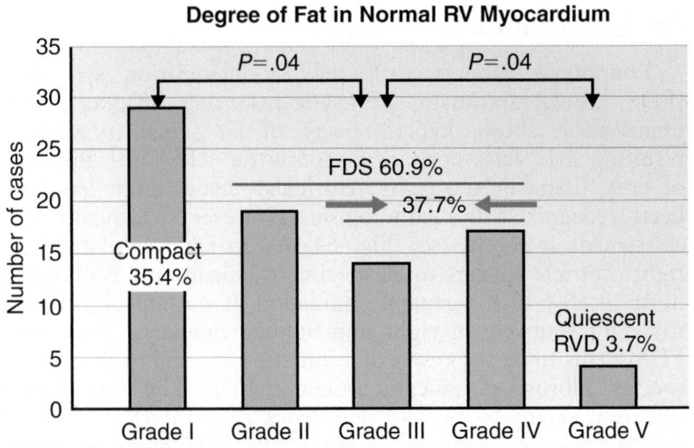

Degree of Fat in Normal RV Myocardium

Figure 64-10 Grades of fat in the right ventricular (RV) free wall in a control group of 85 patients who died in a general hospital of a noncardiac cause. Severity increases from *left* (normal) to *right* (quiescent dysplasia). Fat dissociation syndrome (FDS) is seen from grade II to grade IV in 40% to 60% of the cases. This is a significant difference from normal subjects or patients with right ventricular dysplasia (RVD).

PR prolongation to complete AV block. The acute disease may last from a few days to several weeks and may be associated with release of cardiac enzymes (troponin 1C).

Histology Round cells (lymphocytes) are seen on histologic examination.

Chronic Form

Phenotype Clinical signs of heart failure, asthenia, and dyspnea are characteristic.

Histology Healed myocarditis results in areas of replacement fibrosis. Lymphocytes have disappeared or remain in small quantities.

Chronic-Active Form

Phenotype Clinical signs are of moderate severity and include heart failure, asthenia, dyspnea increasing with time, palpitations, and syncope.

Histology Myocarditis gradually replaces additionale myocardium by fibrosis. Lymphocytes are present.

Variability

These multiple forms of ARVD associated with superimposed myocarditis explain the varied clinical presentations. Gene mutations explaining viral susceptibility have not been proved.

Naxos Disease

Phenotype This phenotype is identical to that of classic ARVD associated with wooly hair and keratoderma. Inheritance is autosomal recessive.

Histology As in typical ARVD, association with signs of myocarditis and arrhythmias is frequent.

Genotype Homozygous plakoglobin mutations are responsible for Naxos disease.

Israelian Desmoplakin-Recessive Right Ventricular Dysplasia

Phenotype An ARVD syndrome associated with wooly hair, keratoderma, and right ventricular dysplasia, similar to that in Naxos disease, has been observed in the Arabic population of Israel.

Genotype Desmoplakin truncation is the monogenic factor producing the disease.[16]

Venetian Desmoplakin-Dominant Right Ventricular Dysplasia

Phenotype The phenotype of Venetian desmoplakin-dominant ARVD seems similar to that in the typical form of the disease.

Histology Histologic features are typical for ARVD.

Genotype Inheritance is autosomal dominant.[17]

Uhl's Anomaly

Uhl's anomaly is an extremely rare anomaly.

Phenotype Two forms are recognized:
Pediatric form: Affects newborns (differential diagnosis should rule out Ebstein disease) with congestive heart failure
Adult form: Features arrhythmias, congestive heart failure, or both; frequently confused with ARVD

Histology Findings on pathologic examination are pathognomonic and unmistakable. Myocardium is totally absent on most of the right ventricular free wall (myocardium is preserved at the base), consisting, in the most severely affected areas, of epicardium and endocardium separated only by a thin layer of adipocytes occupied by coronary vessels, which may exhibit abnormal proliferation of the media. In these areas the wall is, properly speaking, transparent.[18]

Arrhythmogenic Right Ventricular Dysplasia Mimicking Uhl's Anomaly

Phenotype In an unpublished case, a patient with ARVD was found to have a markedly enlarged right ventricle. The extremely thin right ventricular free wall, seen with all imaging techniques, gave the appearance of Uhl's anomaly.

Histology In the aforementioned case, after heart transplantation for terminal heart failure, a thin layer of myocardium was found to be present. The wall was translucent but not transparent. This entity is therefore different from the typical adult form of Uhl's anomaly.

Biventricular Spongy Dysplasia

Phenotype Slowly progressive congestive heart failure is characteristic of biventricular spongy dysplasia. Only one case from Portugal has been reported.[18]

Histology Total absence of myocardium in the right ventricle, with thick endocardium and epicardium, is characteristic. Interstitial fat may be present in the left ventricle, along with minor fibrosis, suggesting major apoptosis.

Catecholaminergic Ventricular Tachycardias

Phenotype Episodes of polymorphic ventricular tachycardias may be triggered by effort or psychological stress. A high risk of sudden death is associated with this disorder.

Histology Two presentations are recognized:
With structural heart disease: Histologic features are similar to those in classic ARVD.
Without structural heart disease: This form is classified as a borderline syndrome.

Genotype Mutation of the gene coding for the ryanodine receptor RyR2 on sarcoplasmic reticulum is the underlying defect.[19]

Brugada Syndrome

Phenotype Brugada syndrome is characterized by ST segment elevation in the right precordial leads (V_1 to V_3), incomplete or complete right bundle branch block, with susceptibility to ventricular tachyarrhythmia and sudden cardiac death at rest or during sleep. This syndrome was reported originally in the French literature in 1988 and then in the succeeding year in the English literature by the group of Padua. The prevalence of Brugada syndrome in the general population ranges from 5 per 1000 in Europe and the United States; the syndrome is three times more frequent in Japan. Syncope, frequently misconstrued as being of vasovagal origin, is a common presentation in adolescents. In some cases, ventricular fibrillation may lead to sudden death. The implantable cardioverter-defibrillator (ICD) has proved to be effective for the treatment of cardiac arrest in this condition. The identification of high-risk subjects by ECG and its electrophysiologic features is the subject of ongoing debate. Some cases may be characterized by overlap in the clinical pattern with ARVD (see earlier). Nevertheless, the effectiveness of isoprenaline for preventing ventricular arrhythmias in Brugada syndrome is in sharp contrast with its effect in ARVD, in which it is used to induce the arrhythmia. Quinidine has been reported as a promising treatment for patients at high risk and may reduce the number of ICD shocks in the case of frequent recurrences of ventricular tachycardia and ventricular fibrillation.

Histology In some patients with Brugada syndrome who died suddenly, the pathologic examination showed structural heart disease typical of ARVD.[20]

Genotype Inheritance is autosomal dominant. Multiple mutations in *SCN5A* have been described, but this gene is observed in less than 15% of the cases. In addition, in some families, *SCN5A* mutations are considered rather as cofactors and no longer the main determinant of Brugada syndrome.

Right Ventricular Outflow Tract Tachycardia

Phenotype Extrasystoles, runs of repetitive short runs of ventricular tachycardia, can be highly symptomatic. In some patients, progression can be observed from isolated extrasystoles to couplets, triplets, and short runs of nonsustained ventricular tachycardia to sustained or incessant ventricular tachycardia. A structural heart disease has been identified by imaging techniques in some patients.

Histology A typical pattern of dysplasia, including small-vessel disease and signs of inflammation, has been reported in some cases.[18]

Fat Dissociation Syndrome

Phenotype Patients with the fat dissociation syndrome (FDS) are asymptomatic. Magnetic resonance imaging (MRI) examination shows hyperintensity of fat signal (potentially resulting in a false-positive diagnosis for ARVD).[21] Presence of fatty tissue in the right ventricular myocardium has long been recognized by pathologists. However, its quantitative assessment is recent (see Fig. 64-10). In addition, fat in the right ventricle appears to be specific to humans and is observed in up to 60% of the general population. It was not observed in the right ventricle of eight non-Bonobo monkeys. Therefore, FDS seems to be the result of a mutation specific to the human species. Fibrosis is basically absent in FDS. The clinical presentation seems to be less dangerous than in ARVD.[21] Our own experience, however, suggests that FDS also may occur in other settings, as in unexpected right ventricular failure, seen in the postoperative period of a successful heart transplantation; this observation has been confirmed by a group of investigators in Boston.[22]

Borderline Syndromes

Mitral valve prolapse is more frequent in cases with predominant fatty transformation similar to that in fat dissociation syndrome. *Carvajal-Huerta disease* is characterized by a recessive form of transmission, associated with the same clinical presentation as in Naxos syndrome. Typically, however, it mostly affects the left ventricle, with extensive involvement by fibrosis without fatty transformation. *Desmoplakin arrhythmogenic left ventricular cardiomyopathy* has been reported but is controversial because it can be interpreted as ARVD associated with severe replacement of left ventricular myocardium by a chronic form of myocarditis, producing massive replacement fibrosis.[23]

Differential Diagnosis

The following entities should be ruled out in the differential diagnosis:

- Right ventricular outflow tract (RVOT) ventricular tachycardia with no structural heart disease
- Catecholaminergic ventricular tachycardia with no structural heart disease
- Brugada syndrome caused by nonstructural heart disease
- Myocarditis, in which replacement fibrosis is associated with clusters of adipocytes, which can mimic ARVD, except that the transmural pattern is absent
- Idiopathic dilated cardiomyopathy with ventricular tachycardia involving the right ventricle and preservation of left ventricular function
- Sarcoidosis, which can mimic ARVD, although the concomitant presence of the two diseases has been reported

Animal Models

ARVD patterns have been observed in both cats and dogs.[24]

Summary

ARVCs have emerged as a global cardiomyopathy mostly involving the right ventricle. This cardiomyopathy generally is progressive, leading to severe right ventricular involvement and heart failure. However, both ventricles can be involved from the onset, leading to biventricular failure as a result of loss of left ventricular myocardium replaced by fat and fibrotic tissue.

Molecular biology studies have provided a better understanding of pathogenesis of the disease. ARVCs appear to be the result of a distortion in biomolecular features localized to the molecules responsible for cell-cell adhesion proteins, as well as in transcriptional switching to produce fat, fibrosis, and apoptosis.

After a concealed phase, the first most obvious clinical manifestations are cardiac arrhythmias and sudden death. These arrhythmias are facilitated by environmental factors such as the practice of competitive sports and superimposed inflammatory factors.

Acknowledgments

We extend our gratitude to Ziad Mallat, MD (Paris), for his contribution to the mechanism of apoptosis and fibrosis, and to Patrick Bruneval, MD (Paris), and Paul Fornès, MD (Reims), for their histologic expertise in the analysis of the fetal heart.

We also are indebted to Drs. Jean Louis Hébert, Véronique Fressart, Francoise Hidden-Lucet, Jérome Lacotte, and Robert Frank, who also have made a significant contribution to the preparation of this chapter.

References

1. Guiraudon CM: Histological diagnosis of right ventricular dysplasia: A role for electron microscopy? Eur Heart J 10:Suppl D, 95-96, 1989.
2. Mallat Z, Tedgui A, Fontaliran F, et al: Evidence of apoptosis in arrhythmogenic right ventricular dysplasia. N Engl J Med 335:1190-1196, 1966.
3. Zhan SS, Jiang JX, Wu J, et al: Phagocytosis of apoptotic bodies by hepatic stellate cells induces NADPH oxidase and is associated with liver fibrosis in vivo. Hepatology 43:435-443, 2006.
4. McKoy G, Protonotarios N, Crosby A, et al: Identification of a deletion in plakoglobin in arrhythmogenic right ventricular cardiomyopathy with palmoplantar keratoderma and woolly hair (Naxos disease). Lancet 355:2119-2124, 2000.
5. Rampazzo A, Nava A, Malacrida S, et al: Mutation in human desmoplakin domain binding to plakoglobin causes a dominant form of arrhythmogenic right ventricular cardiomyopathy. Am J Hum Genet 71:1200-1206, 2002.
6. Gerull B, Heuser A, Wichter T, et al: Mutations in the desmosomal protein plakophilin-2 are common in arrhythmogenic right ventricular cardiomyopathy. Nat Genet 36:1162-1164, 2004.
7. Pilichou K, Nava A, Basso C, et al: Mutations in desmoglein-2 gene are associated with arrhythmogenic right ventricular cardiomyopathy. Circulation 113:1171-1179, 2006.
8. Syrris P, Ward D, Evans A, et al: Arrhythmogenic right ventricular dysplasia/cardiomyopathy associated with mutations in the desmosomal gene desmocollin-2. Am J Hum Genet 79:978-984, 2006.
9. Kaplan SR, Gard JJ, Protonotarios N, et al: Remodeling of myocyte gap junctions in arrhythmogenic right ventricular cardiomyopathy due to a deletion in plakoglobin (Naxos disease). Heart Rhythm 1:3-11, 2004.
10. Oxford EM, Musa H, Maass K, et al: Connexin43 remodeling caused by inhibition of plakophilin-2 expression in cardiac cells. Circ Res 101:703-711, 2007.
11. Garcia-Gras E, Lombardi R, Giocondo MJ, et al: Suppression of canonical Wnt/beta-catenin signaling by nuclear plakoglobin recapitulates phenotype of arrhythmogenic right ventricular cardiomyopathy. J Clin Invest 116:2012-2021, 2006.
12. Beffagna G, Occhi G, Nava A, et al: Regulatory mutations in transforming growth factor-beta3 gene cause arrhythmogenic right ventricular cardiomyopathy type 1. Cardiovasc Res 65:366-373, 2005.
13. Fontaine G, Lacotte J, Hidden-Lucet FR: Catheter ablation of ventricular tachycardia. In Marcus FI, Nava A, Thiene G (eds): Arrhythmogenic RV Cardiomyopathy/Dysplasia, Milan, Springer-Verlag, 2007, pp 181-188.
14. Bowles NE, Ni J, Marcus FI, Towbin JA: The detection of cardiotropics viruses in the myocardium of patients with arrhythmogenic right ventricular dysplasia/cardiomyopathy. J Am Coll Cardiol 39:892-895, 2002.
15. Carniel E, Sinagra G, Bussani R, et al: Fatal myocarditis: Morphologic and clinical features. Ital Heart J 5:702-706, 2004.
16. Alcalai R, Metzger S, Rosenheck S, et al: A recessive mutation in desmoplakin causes arrhythmogenic right ventricular dysplasia, skin disorder, and woolly hair. J Am Coll Cardiol 42:319-327, 2003.
17. Bauce B, Basso C, Rampazzo A, et al: Clinical profile of four families with arrhythmogenic right ventricular cardiomyopathy caused by dominant desmoplakin mutations. Eur Heart J 26:1666-1675, 2005.
18. Fontaine G, Fornes P, Hebert JL, et al: Ventricular tachycardia in arrhythmogenic right ventricular cardiomyopathies. In Zipes DP, Jalife J (eds): Cardiac Electrophysiology: From Cell to Bedside, 4th ed. Philadelphia, Saunders, 2004, pp 588-600.
19. Tiso N, Bauce B, Rampazzo A, et al: Gene symbol: *RYR2*. Disease: Arrhythmogenic right ventricular cardiomyopathy type 2. Hum Genet 114:405, 2004.
20. Coronel R, Casini S, Koopmann TT, et al: Right ventricular fibrosis and conduction delay in a patient with clinical signs of Brugada syndrome: A combined electrophysiological, genetic, histopathologic and computational study. Circulation 112: 2769-2777, 2005.
21. Macedo R, Prakasa K, Tichnell C, et al: Marked lipomatous infiltration of the right ventricle: MRI findings in relation to arrhythmogenic right ventricular dysplasia. Am J Roentgenol 188:W423-W427, 2007.
22. Krishnamani R, Nawgiri RS, Konstam MA, et al: Fatty infiltration of right ventricle (adipositas cordis): An unrecognized cause of early graft failure after cardiac transplantation. J Heart Lung Transplant 24:1143-1145, 2005.
23. Norman M, Simpson M, Mogensen J, et al: Novel mutation in desmoplakin causes arrhythmogenic left ventricular cardiomyopathy. Circulation 112:636-642, 2005.
24. Basso C, Fox PR, Meurs KM, et al: Arrhythmogenic right ventricular cardiomyopathy causing sudden cardiac death in boxer dogs: A new animal model of human disease. Circulation 109:1180-1185, 2004.

Note: A more extensive version of this chapter, including historical background and quoting 56 references, is available on the website www.guyfontaine.com

Ventricular Arrhythmias in Hypertrophic Cardiomyopathy 65

Barry J. Maron

CHAPTER OUTLINE

Hypertrophic cardiomyopathy (HCM) is a genetic cardiac disease with heterogeneous clinical presentation.[1,2] Although the clinical course is diverse and compatible with normal longevity, unexpected sudden cardiac death (SCD) has been recognized as a devastating consequence of HCM since the initial description of this disease 50 years ago.[3] Occurrences of ventricular tachyarrhythmias have always been regarded as a prominent feature and source of concern in this disease, primarily because of the perceived causal relationship between such arrhythmias and SCD.[4-9] This chapter presents a contemporary accounting of the profile of ventricular tachyarrhythmias, the linkage with SCD, and the role of contemporary preventive interventions in HCM.

Historical Context

Since Teare's original pathologic report of HCM,[3] recognition that a small but critically important subgroup of patients with this disease are at increased risk for SCD has generated considerable interest and investigative work on the role of arrhythmias and the process of risk stratification, as well as evolving strategies for effective prevention of these unpredictable catastrophes.[1,2,4-16] Many authors have emphasized that SCD in HCM is not rare in young asymptomatic patients,[1-16] with annual mortality rates of approximately 1% reported for the general population with this disease.[2]

Identification of ventricular tachyarrhythmias has been regarded as a priority in HCM because of the association with SCD risk. On routine 24-hour ambulatory (Holter) electrocardiographic monitoring, 90% of patients with HCM demonstrate ventricular arrhythmias, which not uncommonly are frequent and complex, including premature ventricular depolarizations (200 or more in 24 hours in more than 20% of patients).[9,12] Also common are ventricular couplets (in more than 40% of patients) and, most important, bursts of nonsustained ventricular tachycardia (NSVT) (in 20% to 30% of patients) [4,8,9,12] (Fig. 65-1). Approximately 10% of patients show particularly substantial ectopy, including (in combination) 200 or more premature ventricular depolarizations, 5 or more couplets, and 1 or more runs of NSVT in a single 24-hour monitoring period (see Fig. 65-1). This frequency of ventricular ectopy in HCM is disproportionate to the relatively low prevalence of SCD in this patient population.[1,2,16]

Ventricular Tachycardia

In the early 1980s, short and infrequent bursts of NSVT (usually 3 to 6 beats) were identified as markers of sudden death in two studies from tertiary HCM centers.[4,8] Furthermore, sustained monomorphic ventricular tachycardia is regarded as a high-risk marker in HCM,[1,6,13-15] often associated with left ventricular apical aneurysm.[17] Taken together, these initial clinical observations focused attention on the importance of ventricular tachyarrhythmias in HCM and stimulated considerable interest in ambulatory Holter monitoring as a means of stratifying the risk for SCD in these patients.[4,8,16,18,19]

Ventricular tachyarrhythmias identified on ambulatory electrocardiographic monitoring in HCM generally are clinically occult, and inconsistently associated with palpitations, lightheadedness or other cardiac events.[1,4,8,16] Nevertheless, short bursts of NSVT identified the on Holter electrocardiogram (ECG) have been linked to an eight-fold enhanced risk for SCD—that is, 8% per year, compared with less than 1% per year in the absence of NSVT. Similar to other risk markers in HCM, NSVT is associated with high negative predictive value (i.e., 95%) and relatively low positive predictive value (i.e., aproximately 20%),[4,8,9,12,16] owing largely to a low event rate and clinical heterogeneity.[1,2,15]

Despite these limitations, screening by ambulatory (Holter) monitoring for NSVT has proved to be a useful and widely practiced noninvasive risk stratification strategy in adult patients with HCM for determining sudden death risk. For example, the absence of NSVT on Holter monitoring in patients with HCM can support a no- or low-risk clinical profile, allowing a large measure of reassurance to be conveyed to patients (i.e., high negative predictive value). However, identification of NSVT on ambulatory monitoring may place patients in a potentially high-risk subgroup for which further risk evaluation is justified, including serial ambulatory recordings to better judge the arrhythmia profile over more extended periods of time. For those few individual patients with multiple and repetitive NSVTs persistently evident on serial Holter ECGs, this pattern of arrhythmias can be considered as evidence of increased risk, a manifestation of the primary arrhythmogenic substrate in HCM, and a possible trigger mechanism for SCD. Although specific evidence is lacking, prolonged isolated episodes of NSVT on Holter ECG (i.e., more than 10 beats) have been regarded (as a matter of clinical practice) as a marker of high risk in selected patients.

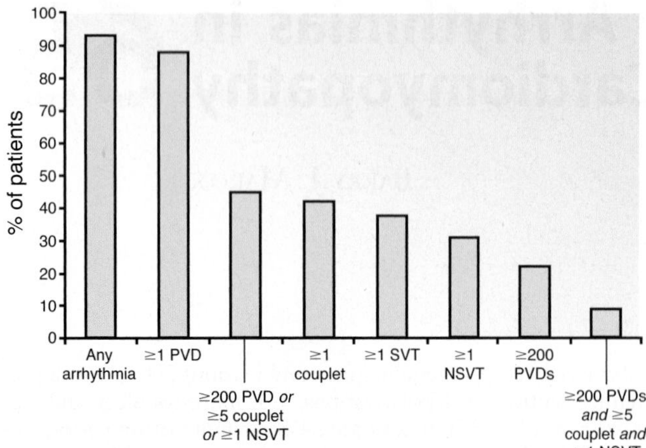

Figure 65-1 Prevalence of ventricular and supraventricular arrhythmias on 24-hour ambulatory (Holter) electrocardiographic recording in 178 patients from a community-based population of patients with hypertrophic cardiomyopathy (HCM). NSVT, nonsustained ventricular tachycardia; PVD, premature ventricular depolarization; SVT, supraventricular tachycardia. (From Adabag AS, Casey SA, Kuskowski MA, et al: Spectrum and prognostic significance of arrhythmias on ambulatory Holter electrocardiogram in hypertrophic cardiomyopathy. J Am Coll Cardiol 45:697-704, 2005. Reproduced with permission of the American College of Cardiology.)

Mechanisms of Sudden Death

Although the pathogenesis of SCD in HCM probably is a complex and multifactorial process, these events ultimately result from primary ventricular tachyarrhythmias.[4,6,8,14] Arrhythmia sequences documented by analysis of stored electrocardiographic recordings in patients with HCM implanted with cardioverter-defibrillators (ICDs) and experiencing appropriate device interventions (Fig. 65-2) offer a unique window through which those mechanisms responsible for SCD in HCM can be examined.[6,14]

In a large multicenter ICD registry of high-risk patients with HCM,[6] appropriate device activations were triggered in each case by rapid ventricular tachycardia or ventricular fibrillation, thereby supporting the long-standing hypothesis that these primary arrhythmias are responsible for the unexpected and unpredictable catastrophes in this disease (see Fig. 65-2).[1,2] Bradyarrhythmias do not appear to play a major role in the pathogenesis of SCD in HCM, although bradycardia-mediated events cannot be absolutely excluded, owing to the back-up pacing capability of the ICD. In one study, sinus tachycardia often was a triggering arrhythmia, suggesting that high sympathetic drive can be proarrhythmic in the presence of a susceptible substrate.[20] It also is possible that other, more diverse arrhythmia mechanisms will prove to be involved in these events.

Device activations occurring in patients with HCM are not uncommonly triggered by rapid ventricular tachycardia. Some investigators have suggested that when the ICD automatically intervenes for nonsustained bursts of ventricular tachycardia (within approximately 10 seconds after sensing of a potentially lethal arrhythmia), the device is in effect merely aborting arrhythmias that otherwise would have resolved spontaneously had the device not been present (i.e., self-termination). It is a relevant consideration, however, that such long runs of ventricular tachycardia far exceed those evident on Holter recordings in this disease (in which bursts of even 10 to 15 beats are regarded as highly unusual) and suggest increased clinical risk.

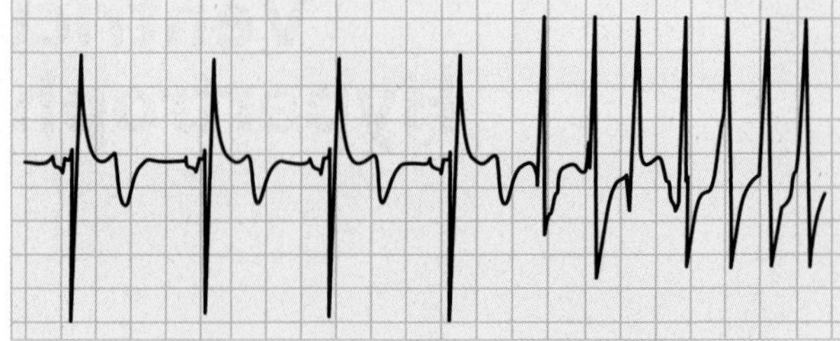

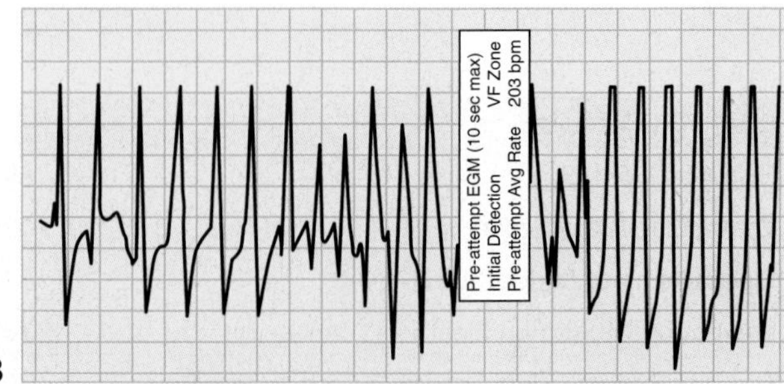

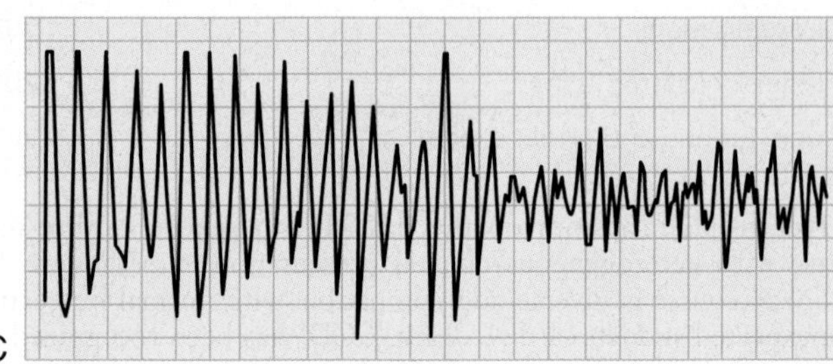

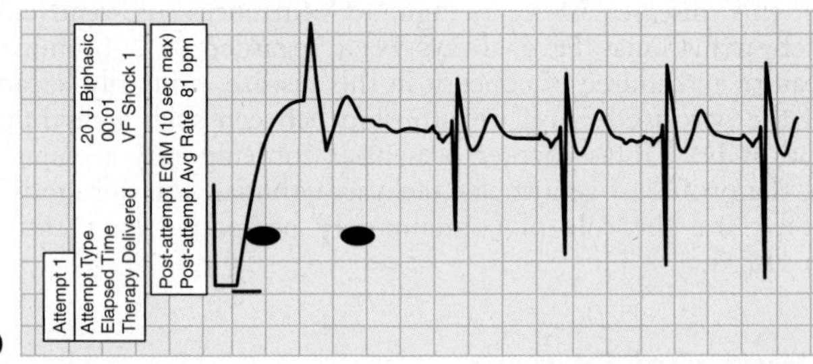

Figure 65-2 Primary prevention of sudden cardiac death in HCM. Stored ventricular electrogram from an asymptomatic 35-year-old man who received an ICD prophylactically, due to a family history of HCM-related sudden death and marked ventricular septal hypertrophy (i.e., wall thickness, 31 mm). Intracardiac electrogram was triggered 4 years and 8 months after the defibrillator implant (at 1:20 AM during sleep). Continuous recording at 25 mm/s, shown in four contiguous panels, with the tracing recorded continuously left-to-right in each segment. **A,** Starts with 4 beats of sinus rhythm and, thereafter, ventricular tachycardia begins abruptly (at 200 beats per minute). **B,** Device senses ventricular tachycardia and charges. **C,** Ventricular tachycardia deteriorates into ventricular fibrillation. **D,** Defibrillator discharges appropriately (20-J shock) during ventricular fibrillation and restores sinus rhythm. (From Maron BJ, Shen W-K, Link MS, et al: Efficacy of implantable cardioverter-defibrillators for the prevention of sudden death in patients with hypertrophic cardiomyopathy. N Engl J Med 342:365-373, 2000. With permission of the Massachusetts Medical Society.)

Consequently, ventricular tachycardia episodes that trigger the ICD in HCM are unlikely to be innocent in this disease which is characterized by greatly increased left ventricular mass and wall thickening, microvascular ischemia, impaired left ventricular compliance, and often outflow obstruction.[1,2]

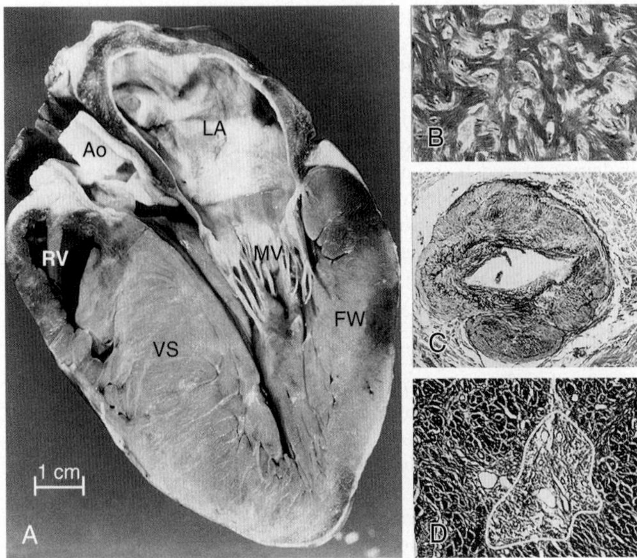

Figure 65-3 Morphologic substrate for electrical instability and sudden death in HCM. **A,** Gross heart specimen sectioned in a cross-sectional plane similar to that of the echocardiographic (parasternal) long axis; left ventricular wall thickening shows an asymmetrical pattern and is confined primarily to the ventricular septum (VS), which bulges prominently into the left ventricular outflow tract. Left ventricular cavity appears reduced in size. FW, left ventricular free wall. **B** to **D,** Histologic features characteristic of left ventricular myocardium and representative of the arrhythmogenic substrate in HCM. **B,** Markedly disordered architecture with adjacent hypertrophied cardiac muscle cells arranged at perpendicular and oblique angles. **C,** intramural coronary artery with thickened wall, due primarily to medial hypertrophy and an apparently narrowed lumen. **D,** replacement fibrosis (after myocyte death) in an area of ventricular myocardium adjacent to an abnormal intramural coronary artery. Ao, aorta; LA, left atrium; RV, right ventricle. (Reprinted from The Lancet, from Maron BJ: Hypertrophic cardiomyopathy. Lancet 350:127-133, 1997; with permission from Elsevier.)

In HCM, ventricular tachyarrhythmias probably emanate primarily from a substrate of electrical instability and distorted electrophysiologic transmission created by the disorganized left ventricular myocardial architecture,[1-3] or "bursts" of myocardial ischemia (probably due to structurally abnormal and narrowed intramural arterioles), thereby leading to myocyte necrosis and repair in the form of replacement fibrosis and scarring[21] (Fig. 65-3). This myocardial substrate may be vulnerable to a variety of triggers, either intrinsic (related to the HCM disease process, such as abrupt increase in outflow obstruction) or extrinsic, environmental factors such as intense physical exertion (e.g., in trained athletes). Of note, however, a component of individual susceptibility undoubtedly also plays a role in determining which patients with HCM will experience life-threatening events at particular moments in the natural history of their disease.

Prevention of Sudden Death

Pharmacologic Treatment

Historically, in the pre-ICD era, the management of high-risk patients with HCM was limited to prophylactic pharmacologic treatment strategies with beta-blockers, verapamil, antiarrhythmic agents such as procainamide and quinidine, and later amiodarone.[1,2,18,19] Retrospective data are very limited, however, and no controlled studies in HCM supporting the efficacy of prophylactic drug treatment for SCD have been performed.[11,22] Type IA antiarrhythmic agents (such as procainamide and quinidine) were abandoned several years ago as treatment modalities for patients with HCM experiencing NSVT on ambulatory (Holter) ECG, because of the proarrhythmic potential of these drugs.[1,2]

One report, from more than 20 years ago, proposed that amiodarone was protective against the risk for SCD in symptomatic or mildly symptomatic patients with HCM-related NSVT on Holter ECG in a retrospective study with only historical controls.[18] Claims that amiodarone is absolutely protective against SCD in HCM[18] no longer seem credible in light of more recent observations. For example, in studies using the ICD in high-risk patients with HCM,[6,14] approximately 50% of those experiencing an appropriate device discharge for ventricular tachycardia–ventricular fibrillation had been taking amiodarone concomitantly; also, in a high-risk cohort in which only medications were used for arrhythmia protection, an important proportion of the patients died suddenly (including more than 25% of those on amiodarone).[22] Finally, the possibility of severe pulmonary and other side effects associated with chronic administration of amiodarone severely limits its application to SCD prevention in young patients with HCM, who characteristically harbor long periods of risk over many decades.[1,2,6,14,15] Therefore, it is no longer customary to recommend prophylactic long-term treatment with low-dose amiodarone (200 mg per day) or other antiarrhythmic drugs for perceived high-risk status in the ICD era.

Implantable Defibrillator

Since its introduction into clinical practice by Mirowski and colleagues[23] more than 25 years ago, the ICD has achieved widespread acceptance as a treatment for SCD prevention by automatically terminating life-threatening ventricular tachyarrhythmias and prolonging life, principally in high-risk patients with advanced coronary heart disease.[24-27] In such patient populations, superiority of the ICD over antiarrhythmic drug treatment has been documented in prospective, randomized trials for secondary and primary prevention.[24-27] Not until 2000, however, was there any impetus for systematic application of prophylactic device therapy in HCM, or in other genetic cardiac diseases associated with increased SCD risk, such as long QT and Brugada syndromes, and arrhythmogenic right ventricular cardiomyopathy.[28-36] Undoubtedly, when initially designing and promoting the ICD, Mirowski and colleagues[23] did not consider or envision such device effectiveness in the context of the extraordinary pathology often encountered in HCM, a disease often associated with marked increase in left ventricular mass[7] and dynamic obstruction to left ventricular outflow.[37]

Other than evidence from a few early and relatively small studies,[38-40] most of the data concerning the efficacy of the ICD in HCM comes from a large multicenter international registry of patients considered to be at high risk for SCD, based on the clinical judgment of the responsible cardiologists and electrophysiologists (Fig. 65-4).[6,14] This prospectively and retrospectively studied cohort of 506 patients with HCM was followed for an average period of 3.7 years after an ICD was implanted for either primary or secondary prevention of sudden death. Appropriate device discharges (either defibrillation shocks or antitachycardia pacing), triggered by ventricular tachycardia–ventricular fibrillation, occurred in 20% of patients, with an average discharge rate of 5.5% per year (Fig. 65-5; see also Fig. 65-4). Furthermore, 45% of those patients who received effective defibrillator therapy experienced multiple appropriate interventions.

Not unexpectedly, life-saving defibrillator interventions are most frequent in those patients implanted specifically for secondary prevention—i.e., following fortuitous resuscitation from

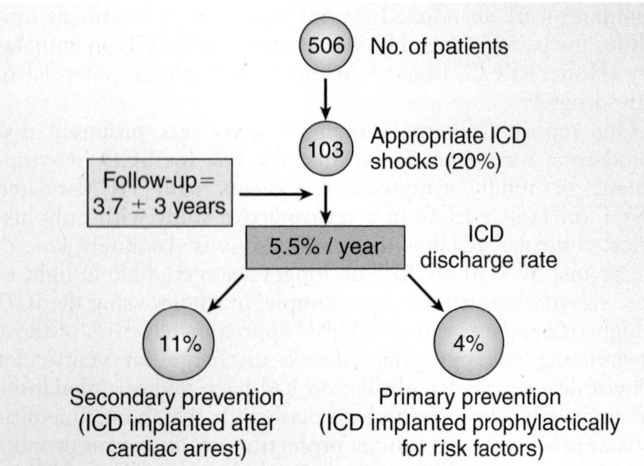

Figure 65-4 Flow diagram showing outcome for 506 high-risk patients with HCM who had received implantable cardioveter-defibrillators (ICDs) for primary prevention (based on one or more risk factors) or secondary prevention (in those who had experienced cardiac arrest or sustained ventricular tachycardia). Two patients *(not included here)* died of HCM with refractory end-stage heart failure and systolic dysfunction (despite the ICD).

cardiac arrest (with documented ventricular fibrillation) or after an overt episode of spontaneous and sustained ventricular tachycardia. Over 40% of such patients received appropriate shocks during a relatively short follow-up period (11% per year) (see Figs. 65-4 and 65-5).

Of note, patients treated with ICDs for primary prevention also show a substantial appropriate intervention rate reported to be 4% per year (see Figs. 65-4 and 65-5). Prophylactic implants due to high-risk status were based on clinical profiles in which one or more of the acknowledged sudden death risk factors were present: (1) family history of premature HCM-related death, particularly if sudden, in a close relative, or multiple in occurrence; (2) unexplained syncope, particularly in young patients, or if demonstrated to be arrhythmia-based; (3) frequent, multiple, or prolonged episodes of NSVT documented on serial ambulatory (Holter) ECG monitoring; (4) hypotensive or attenuated blood pressure response to exercise; and (5) extreme left ventricular hypertrophy with maximum wall thickness of 30 mm or greater, particularly in young patients. In clinical practice, however, it is rare for a patient with HCM to be regarded as high risk solely on the basis of an abnormal blood pressure response to exercise. Presence or magnitude of left ventricular outflow tract obstruction has not proved to be a consistently strong independent risk factor for SCD in HCM and therefore does not constitute a sole justification for prophylactic ICD implantation.[37,41]

A measure of controversy has arisen regarding the precise selection of HCM patients for primary prevention ICD strategies.[1,2,6,10,11,14] Much of the European cardiovascular community subscribes to a criterion of two or more risk factors for a recommendation of a prophylactic defibrillator.[10,11] Certainly, the presence of multiple risk factors creates a clinical environment in which ICD decision making becomes more intuitive. Nevertheless, in the largest available HCM cohort managed with ICDs ($n = 506$ patients),[6] 35% of the primary prevention patients who received appropriate device interventions for potentially lethal ventricular arrhythmias had in fact been selected for ICD implantation on the basis of only one risk factor. In addition, no significant difference was observed among patients with one, two, or three or more high-risk markers with respect to the likelihood of appropriate ICD discharges (Fig. 65-6).

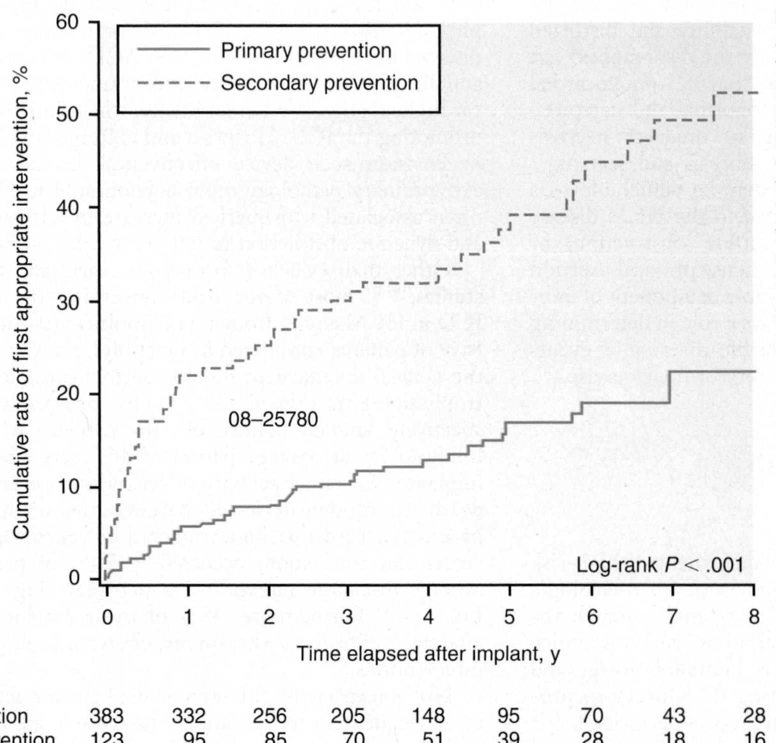

Figure 65-5 Estimated cumulative rates of first appropriate discharges, calculated separately for those patients with HCM who received implantable cardioverter-defibrillators (ICDs) for primary prevention because of risk factors, and for those patients in whom ICDs were implanted for secondary prevention after cardiac arrest or for sustained ventricular tachycardia. (From Maron BJ, Spirito P, Shen W-K, et al: Implantable cardioverter-defibrillators and prevention of sudden cardiac death in hypertrophic cardiomyopathy. JAMA 298:405-412, 2007. With permission of the American Medical Association.)

Nevertheless, it would be imprudent to promote universal ICD implantation for all patients with HCM in whom one risk factor has been identified. Indeed, although one risk factor can often be sufficient to intervene with an ICD, not all one-risk-factor patients merit consideration for an ICD. In a heterogeneous genetic disease such as HCM, numerous complex clinical scenarios involving ambiguous "gray areas" with respect to the presence, strength, or number of risk factors, and ultimately decisions regarding prophylactic ICDs, are inevitable. One such example is that of the elderly patient with syncope as a single risk factor. Such patients may not be candidates for primary prevention, for several reasons: HCM-related sudden death is uncommon in this age group; survival to advanced age itself declares lower risk status in this disease; and syncope is common in the elderly.

Also, it should be underscored that primary SCD prevention, as practiced with the ICD in HCM, represents a novel strategy: It is based solely on noninvasive risk factors identified in asymptomatic (or only mildly symptomatic) patients, typically in the absence of a previous major cardiovascular event, and often without evidence of spontaneous ventricular tachyarrhythmias.[6,14,15,42]

Electrophysiologic testing with programmed ventricular stimulation to identify the substrate for SCD has been largely abandoned as a strategy.[1,15] In view of the inherent risks and inconvenience of the electrophysiologic procedure (as well as its time-consuming nature), the considerable uncertainty surrounding the significance of the induced arrhythmias, and the fact that most high-risk patients can be identified using noninvasive clinical markers,[6,42] the routine use of such laboratory-based testing to replicate clinical arrhythmias now appears to have little practical role for stratifying SCD risk in patients with HCM.

The Risk Period in Hypertrophic Cardiomyopathy

Crucial to understanding the role of the ICD within the broad HCM disease spectrum is an appreciation of the demographic distinctions from device therapy in coronary artery disease. Patients with coronary artery disease are of relatively advanced age at the time of implantation (average, about 65 years), often with severe and progressive heart failure as a consequence of previous myocardial infarction and left ventricular dysfunction.[24-27] In sharp contrast, ICDs usually are implanted in high-risk patients with HCM at much younger ages and also with few or no symptoms; mean age at implantation (and also at appropriate device intervention) is only approximately 40 years, with 30% of the patients aged 30 years or younger. Hence, in HCM an extended risk period for SCD has been noted in patients into mid-life and even beyond.[1,2,6,43] Therefore, although annual event and appropriate intervention rates for HCM are lower than in those reported with coronary artery disease, they are nevertheless significant because of the much younger patient population usually free of significant heart failure and noncardiac disease. Protected by the ICD, these patients could potentially survive many decades of productive life with few or no symptoms, achieving near-normal or even normal longevity if not encumbered by other major HCM-related disease complications such as severe heart failure or stroke.[43]

By extrapolating the reported appropriate primary prevention appropriate shock rate for HCM over time,[6] it can be estimated that within 10 years, more than one third of the defibrillators implanted prophylactically in young patients could intervene to abort an SCD event. Indeed, the 5% annual appropriate discharge rate reported in high-risk patients with HCM implanted with an ICD is remarkably similar to the SCD rate previously reported in the highly selected at-risk HCM cohorts of patients evaluated at tertiary referral centers between 1960 and 1990.[1]

Of particular note, the time interval from recognition of high-risk status and implantation to the first appropriate ICD intervention may be quite variable and in fact can be considerable, with particularly long time delays of up to 10 years documented for the first life-saving intervention,[6,14] or as long as 30 years after cardiac arrest with or without the aid of a defibrillator[43] (Fig. 65-7). These observations underscore the unpredictable timing of lethal tachyarrhythmias and SCD in HCM, for which the ICD may remain dormant for substantial periods of time before it is ultimately required to intervene and interrupt the arrhythmia. This principle of unpredictability for potentially lethal events in HCM also is underscored by the not-uncommon occurrence of appropriate shocks for ventricular tachycardia or fibrillation relatively early after implantation (often in the first 12 months).[6,44] The explanation for a shift toward earlier appropriate ICD interventions, as well as the mechanisms underlying the timing of these events, is unresolved at present.

Also, decisions to prophylactically implant ICDs in patients with HCM often are dictated fortuitously by the precise time at which risk stratification is undertaken and evidence of increased risk is recognized. For example, a patient identified as being at high risk at age 15 years (and implanted at that time) will still be young and presumably at increased risk 15 years later at age 30, even if the ICD has not yet discharged appropriately. Consequently, once the decision is made to implant an ICD in a high-risk patient with HCM, this intervention is likely to represent a life-long preventive measure and should be presented to patients in this context.

Finally, physician and patient attitudes toward ICDs (and access to devices within respective health care systems) can vary considerably among countries and cultures[45] (Fig. 65-8), thereby affecting clinical decision making and specifically the threshold for primary prevention implantation in patients with HCM. For example, ICD use relative to population size is significantly higher in the United States—several times greater than in European countries, particularly the United Kingdom (see Fig. 65-8). Such disparities in implantation rates suggest that patients with HCM at equivalent risk levels are subject to different thresholds for primary prevention of SCD, depending on their country of residence.

Complications

Potential complications of ICD therapy are well documented and represent an important consideration in any decision to proceed with implantation.[42,46,49-51] Approximately 25% of patients with HCM may experience one or more inappropriate shocks due to sinus tachycardia, atrial fibrillation, lead malfunction or oversensing.[6] Overall, these events have been reported with similar frequencies among those patients with versus those without appropriate shocks, in patients implanted for primary versus secondary prevention, and in patients 30 years of age or younger versus those older than 30 years. Recently, the popular Sprint Fidelis small-diameter high-voltage defibrillator lead (Medtronic, Inc., Minneapolis, Minnesota) has been removed from the market place owing to its susceptibility to fractures and failure, often heralded by inappropriate shocks and high or variable impedance, particularly in young active patients with vigorous left ventricular contractility (such as those with HCM).[46] Reduced lead survival appears to be caused by early fracture of the pace-sense conductor and coil and the high-voltage conductor.

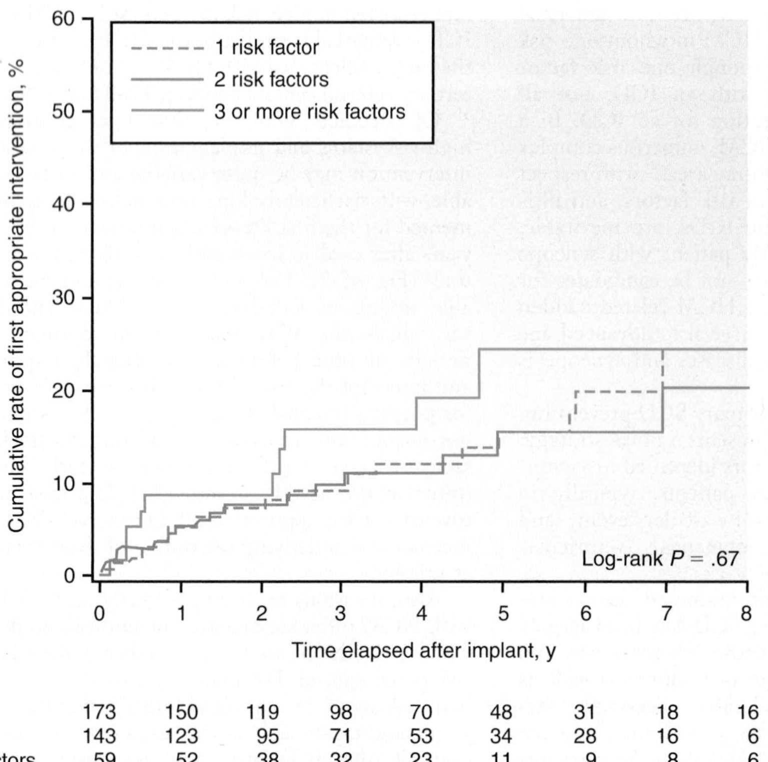

Figure 65-6 Cumulative rates for first appropriate implantable cardioverter-defibrillator (ICD) intervention in HCM patients with 1, 2, or 3 or more risk factors who had received devices for primary prevention. (Maron BJ, Spirito P, Shen W-K, et al: Implantable cardioverter-defibrillators and prevention of sudden cardiac death in hypertrophic cardiomyopathy. JAMA 298:405-412, 2007. With permission of the American Medical Association.)

Other major complications reported in a small number of patients include infection, hemorrhage or thrombosis, and lead fracture or dislodgment. It should be emphasized, however, that ICD-related problems do not arise with equal frequency at all electrophysiology centers, and careful attention to technique and device maintenance can minimize the likelihood of many adverse events.

The possibility of inappropriate shocks and other device-related complications, as well as occasional loss of employment opportunities along with some limitations to quality of life, underscore the importance of balancing these concerns against the potential ICD benefit—that is, protection from sudden death as well as the psychological reassurance offered to many adult patients by the presence of the ICD.[6] Also, of note, ICD therapy

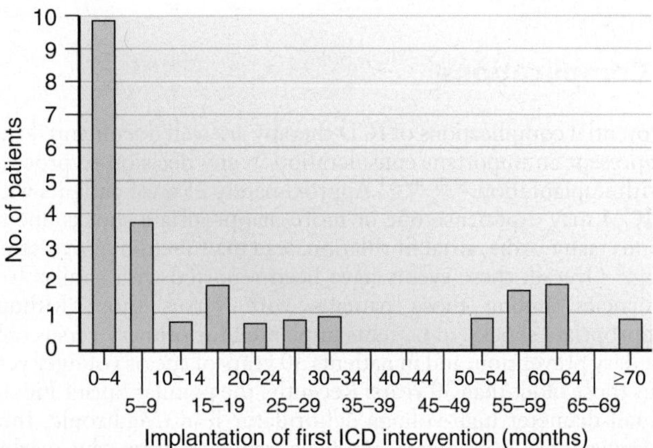

Figure 65-7 Interval between implantation of the implantable cardioverter-defibrillator (ICD) and the first appropriate device discharge. Note that a substantial proportion of patients experienced their initial appropriate defibrillation shock 5 to 10 years after implantation. (From Maron BJ, Spirito P, Shen W-K, et al: Implantable cardioverter-defibrillators and prevention of sudden cardiac death in hypertrophic cardiomyopathy. JAMA 298:405-412, 2007. With permission of the American Medical Association.)

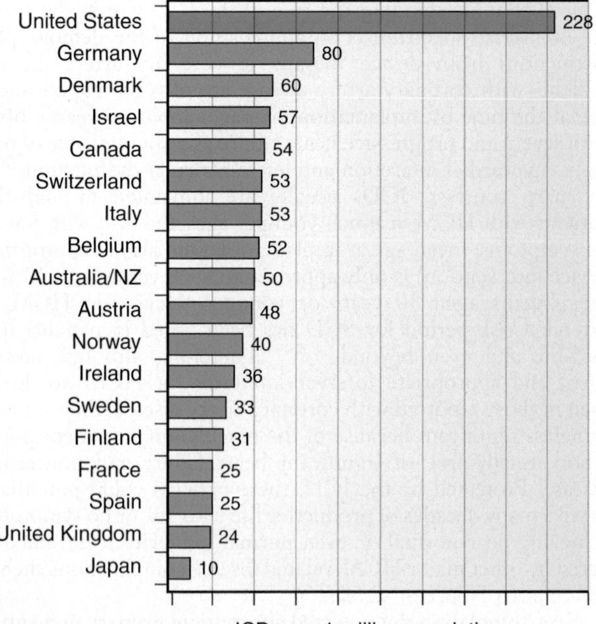

Figure 65-8 Implantable cardioverter-defibrillators (ICDs) in use worldwide in the year 2006, shown by country (per 1 million population). The rates shown are for all ICD indications but, largely represent implants in patients with coronary artery disease. NZ, New Zealand.

in young, high-risk patients with HCM also has been shown to be a cost-effective (and even cost-saving) strategy, owing to the additional years of productive life made possible by appropriate device interventions. This advantage calculates to an estimated $20,000 gained per quality-adjusted life-year saved.[47]

Implantation of the defibrillator is itself a safe procedure in both children and adults with HCM. However, in a few selected patients with unique clinical findings, such as particularly massive left ventricular hypertrophy or previous administration of amiodarone, transvenous defibrillation has proved to be problematic, necessitating epicardial lead placement and selection of high-energy ICDs.[48]

Industry-Related Issues

As indicated by a reasonably large published experience, ICDs have proved to be remarkably effective in preventing sudden death in virtually every patient incurring potentially lethal ventricular tachyarrythmia associated with the typical clinical and phenotypic expression of HCM (i.e., absent progressive heart failure with systolic dysfunction, or embolic stroke).[6] One notable exception is the reported case of a 21-year-old college student with nonobstructive HCM, extreme left ventricular hypertrophy, preserved systolic function, and a history of syncope, who died suddenly when his mechanically defective ICD (Prizm2DR, 1861, Guidant, Minneapolis, MN) failed to deliver an appropriate shock because of massive electrical overstress resulting from short-circuiting,[49-51] which in turn was due to inadequate insulation between the backfill tube and feedthrough wire in the pulse generator.

Six other deaths and more than 75 other device failures were documented from defective Prizm defibrillators, ultimately triggering a cascade of events known as the Guidant Affair in which a series of voluntary and nonvoluntary recalls and advisories ensued, involving 300,000 defibrillators and pacemakers (approximately 80% of the Guidant–Boston Scientific product line).[50,51] Public disclosure revealed that Guidant (now Boston Scientific) had been aware of this manufacturing defect but failed to inform physicians, patients, or the general public while continuing to market and sell potentially defective defibrillators to patients.

A number of insights have resulted from the Guidant Affair. Certainly, far greater recognition has emerged within the industry and the physician community of the fundamental principle concerning the autonomous rights of patients to full disclosure of all relevant medical information related to therapeutic options that may potentially impact their health, safety, and risk for death or injury, and access to active participation in treatment decisions that potentially dictate their medical destiny. In addition, several proposals have been advanced to improve communication and the safety of implantable devices from the U.S. Food and Drug Administration (FDA) and other governmental agencies, including the formulation of guidelines for the promotion and marketing of ICDs in the United States. The Heart Rhythm Society has called for more formalized and detailed disclosure of defibrillator- and pacemaker-related safety issues and has promoted an industry-wide independent advisory and safety panel composed of outside consultative medical experts responsible for postmarketing monitoring of device performance (using data from the FDA and the manufacturers).

Conclusions and Implications

Primary ventricular tachyarrhythmias arising from an electrically unstable myocardial substrate constitute the basis for sudden and unexpected death in susceptible patients with HCM, who can be identified in large measure by the risk stratification profiles currently in use. The ICD represents an important treatment advance in HCM that has proved effective in preventing SCD and in altering the natural history of this disease for many patients, and which now has an established role for both secondary and primary prevention of SCD. Prevention of SCD in HCM may well allow patients to achieve normal or near-normal longevity, a reasonable aspiration for many young high-risk patients, in view of the substantial experience with ICDs available in this genetic heart disease.

References

1. Maron BJ, McKenna WJ, Danielson GK, et al: American College of Cardiology/European Society of Cardiology Clinical Expert Consensus Document on Hypertrophic Cardiomyopathy. A report of the American College of Cardiology Task Force on Clinical Expert Consensus Documents and the European Society of Cardiology Committee for Practice Guidelines Committee to Develop an Expert Consensus Document on Hypertrophic Cardiomyopathy. J Am Coll Cardiol 42:1687-1713, 2003.
2. Maron BJ: Hypertrophic cardiomyopathy. A systematic review. JAMA 287:1308-1320, 2002.
3. Teare D: Asymmetrical hypertrophy of the heart in young patients. Br Heart J 20:1-8, 1958.
4. Maron BJ, Savage DD, Wolfson JK, Epstein SE: Prognostic significance of 24-hour ambulatory electrocardiographic monitoring in patients with hypertrophic cardiomyopathy: A prospective study. Am J Cardiol 48:252-257, 1981.
5. Saumarez RC, Grace AA: Paced ventricular electrogram fractionation and sudden death in hypertrophic cardiomyopathy and other non-coronary heart diseases. Cardiovasc Res 47P:11-22, 2000.
6. Maron BJ, Spirito P, Shen W-K, et al: Implantable cardioverter-defibrillators and prevention of sudden cardiac death in hypertrophic cardiomyopathy. JAMA 298:405-412, 2007.
7. Spirito P, Bellone P, Harris KM, et al: Magnitude of left ventricular hypertrophy predicts the risk of sudden death in hypertrophic cardiomyopathy. N Engl J Med 324:1778-1785, 2000.
8. McKenna WJ, England D, Doi YL, et al: Arrhythmia in hypertrophic cardiomyopathy: I—influence on prognosis. Br Heart J 46:168-172, 1981.
9. Adabag AS, Casey SA, Kuskowski MA, et al: Spectrum and prognostic significance of arrhythmias on ambulatory Holter electrocardiogram in hypertrophic cardiomyopathy. J Am Coll Cardiol 45:697-704, 2005.
10. Elliott PM, Gimeno JR, Mahon NG, et al: Relation between severity of left-ventricular hypertrophy and prognosis in patients with hypertrophic cardiomyopathy. Lancet 357:420-424, 2001.
11. Elliott PM, Poloniecki J, Dickie S, et al: Sudden death in hypertrophic cardiomyopathy: Identification of high risk patients. J Am Coll Cardiol 36:2212-2218, 2000.
12. Adabag AS, Maron BJ: Implications of arrhythmias and prevention of sudden death in hypertrophic cardiomyopathy. Ann Noninvas Electrocardiol 12:171-180, 2007.
13. Spirito P, Autore C: Management of hypertrophic cardiomyopathy. BMJ 332:1251-1255, 2006.
14. Maron BJ, Shen W-K, Link MS, et al: Efficacy of implantable cardioverter-defibrillators for the prevention of sudden death in patients with hypertrophic cardiomyopathy. N Engl J Med 342:365-373, 2000.
15. Maron BJ, Estes NAM III, Maron MS, et al: Primary prevention of sudden death as a novel treatment strategy in hypertrophic cardiomyopathy. Circulation 107: 2872-2875, 2003.
16. Monserrat L, Elliott PM, Gimeno JR, McKenna WJ: Non-sustained ventricular tachycardia in hypertrophic cardiomyopathy: An independent marker of sudden

death risk in young patients. J Am Coll Cardiol 42:873-879, 2003.
17. Maron MS, Finley JJ, Bos JM, et al: Prevalence, clinical significance, and natural history of left ventricular apical aneurysms in hypertrophic cardiomyopathy. Circulation 118:1541-1549, 2008.
18. McKenna WJ, Oakley CM, Krikler DM, Goodwin JF: Improved survival with amiodarone in patients with hypertrophic cardiomyopathy and ventricular tachycardia. Br Heart J 53:412-416, 1985.
19. Cecchi F, Olivotto I, Montereggi A, et al: Prognostic value of non-sustained ventricular tachycardia and the potential role of amiodarone treatment in hypertrophic cardiomyopathy: Assessment in an unselected non-referral based patient population. Heart 79:331-336, 1998.
20. Cha Y-M, Gersh BJ, Maron BJ, et al: Electrophysiologic manifestations of ventricular tachyarrhythmias provoking appropriate defibrillator interventions in high-risk patients with hypertrophic cardiomyopathy. J Cardiovasc Electrophysiol 18:1-5, 2007.
21. Maron BJ, Wolfson JK, Epstein SE, Roberts WC: Intramural ("small vessel") coronary artery disease in hypertrophic cardiomyopathy. J Am Coll Cardiol 8:545-557, 1986.
22. Melacini P, Maron BJ, Bobbo F, et al: Evidence that pharmacological strategies lack efficacy for the prevention of sudden death in hypertrophic cardiomyopathy. Heart 93:708-710, 2007.
23. Mirowski M, Reid PR, Mower MM, et al: Termination of malignant ventricular arrhythmias with an implanted automatic defibrillator in human beings. N Engl J Med 303:322-324, 1980.
24. The Antiarrhythmics Versus Implantable Defibrillators (AVID) Investigators: A comparison of anitarrhythmic-drug therapy with implantable defibrillators in patients resuscitated from near-fatal ventricular arrhythmias. N Engl J Med 337:1576-1583, 1997.
25. Moss AJ, Zareba W, Hall WJ, et al: Prophylactic implantation of a defibrillator in patients with myocardial infarction and reduced ejection fraction. N Engl J Med 346:877-883, 2002.
26. Bardy GH, Lee KL, Mark DB, et al for the Sudden Cardiac Death in Heart Failure Trial (SCD-HeFT) Investigators: Amiodarone or an implantable cardioverter-defibrillator for congestive heart failure. N Engl J Med 352:225-237, 2005.
27. Kadish A, Dyer A, Daubert JP, et al for the Defibrillators in Non-Ischemic Cardiomyopathy Treatment Evaluation (DEFINITE) Investigators:N Engl J Med 350:2151-2158, 2004.
28. Wichter T, Paul M, Wollmann C, et al: Implantable cardioverter-defibrillator therapy in arrhythmogenic right ventricular cardiomyopathy. Single-center experience of long-term follow-up and complications in 60 patients. Circulation 109:1503-1508, 2004.
29. Sarkozy A, Boussy T, Kourginnides G, et al: Long-term follow-up of primary prophylactic implantable cardioverter-defibrillator therapy in Brugada syndrome. Eur Heart J 28:334-344, 2007.
30. Roguin A, Bomma CS, Nasir K, et al: Implantable cardioverter-defibrillators in patients with arrhythmogenic right ventricular dysplasia/cardiomyopathy. J Am Coll Cardiol 43:1843-1852, 2004.
31. Piccini JP, Dalal D, Roguin A, et al: Predictors of appropriate implantable defibrillator therapies in patients with arrhythmogenic right ventricular dysplasia. Heart Rhythm 2:1188-1194, 2005.
32. Corrado D, Leoni L, Link MS, et al: Implantable cardioverter-defibrillator therapy for prevention of sudden death in patients with arrhythmogenic right ventricular cardiomyopathy/dysplasia. Circulation 108:3084-3091, 2003.
33. Zareba W, Moss AJ, Daubert JP, et al: Implantable cardioverter defibrillator in high-risk long QT syndrome patients. J Cardiovasc Electrophysiol 14:337-341, 2003.
34. Sacher F, Probst V, Iesaka Y, et al: Outcome after implantation of a cardioverter-defibrillator in patients with Brugada syndrome. A multicenter study. Circulation 114:2317-2324, 2006.
35. Nademanee K, Veerakul G, Mower M, et al: Defibrillator versus β-blockers for unexplained death in Thailand (DEBUT). A randomized clinical trial. Circulation 107:2221-2226, 2003.
36. Stephenson EA, Berul CI: Electrophysiologic interventions for inherited arrhythmia syndromes. Circulation 116:1062-1080, 2007.
37. Maron MS, Olivotto I, Betocchi S, et al: Effect of left ventricular outflow tract obstruction on clinical outcome in hypertrophic cardiomyopathy. N Engl J Med 2003; 348:295-303, 2003.
38. Jayatilleke I, Doolan A, Ingles J, et al: Long-term follow-up of implantable cardioverter-defibrillator therapy for hypertrophic cardiomyopathy. Am J Cardiol 93:1192-1194, 2004.
39. Pablo Kaski J, Tomé Esteban MT, Lowe M, et al: Outcomes after implantable cardioverter-defibrillator treatment in children with hypertrophic cardiomyopathy. Heart 93:372-374, 2007.
40. Woo A, Monakier D, Harris L, et al: Determinants of implantable defibrillator discharges in high risk patients with hypertrophic cardiomyopathy. Heart 93:1044-1045, 2007.
41. Maron BJ, Olivotto I, Maron MS: The dilemma of left ventricular outflow tract obstruction in hypertrophic cardiomyopathy: Do patients with gradients really deserve prophylactic defibrillators? [editorial]. Eur Heart J 27:1895-1897, 2006.
42. Nishimura RA, Ommen SR: Hypertrophic cardiomyopathy, sudden death and implantable cardiac defibrillators. How low the bar? [editorial]. JAMA 298:452-454, 2007.
43. Maron BJ, Haas TS: Unanticipated long-term survival after cardiac arrest in hypertrophic cardiomyopathy [abstract]. Circulation 116(Suppl II):II-766, 2007.
44. Almquist AK, Hanna CA, Haas TS, Maron BJ: Significance of appropriate defibrillator shock 3 hours and 20 minutes following implantation in a patient with hypertrophic cardiomyopathy. J Cardiovasc Electrophysiol 19:319-322, 2008.
45. Camm AJ, Nisam S: The utilization of the implantable defibrillator—a European enigma. Eur Heart J 21:1998-2004, 2000.
46. Hauser RG, Kallinen LM, Almquist AK, et al: Early failure of a small diameter high-voltage implantable cardioverter-defibrillator lead. Heart Rhythm 4:892-896, 2007.
47. Goldenberg I, Moss AJ, Maron BJ, et al: Cost effectiveness of implanted defibrillators in young people with inherited cardiac arrhythmias. Ann Noninvas Electrocardiol 10(Suppl 4):67-83, 2005.
48. Almquist AK, Montgomery JV, Haas TS, Maron BJ: Cardioverter-defibrillator implantation in high-risk patients with hypertrophic cardiomyopathy. Heart Rhythm 2:814-819, 2005.
49. Gornick CC, Hauser RG, Almquist AK, Maron BJ: Unpredictable implantable cardioverter-defibrillator pulse generator failure due to electrical overstress causing sudden death in a young high-risk patient with hypertrophic cardiomyopathy. Heart Rhythm 2:681-683, 2005.
50. Hauser RG, Maron BJ: Lessons from the failure and recall of an implantable cardioverter defibrillator. Circulation 112:2040-2042, 2005.
51. Maron BJ, Hauser RG: Past and future perspectives on the failure of pharmaceutical and medical device industries to protect the public health interests. Am J Cardiol 100:147-151, 2007.

Ventricular Tachycardia in Patients with Heart Failure 66

MARK E. ANDERSON AND DENICE M. HODGSON-ZINGMAN

CHAPTER OUTLINE

Overview

Sudden cardiac death due to ventricular arrhythmias is a major public health problem. Approximately one half of patients diagnosed with heart failure will die suddenly, and a majority of these deaths are from ventricular tachyarrhythmias.[1] On the other hand, arrhythmias can contribute to heart failure by reducing pumping efficiency and by directly causing cardiomyopathy. The overall clinical impact of these latter effects is unknown, and the mechanisms for arrhythmogenic causes of heart failure are not discussed here. Instead, this chapter considers cellular and tissue substrate contributions to arrhythmias in heart failure and discusses some of the biologic signals that contribute to the clinical phenotypes of heart failure and arrhythmias. One overarching theme of this analysis is that heart failure and arrhythmias occur together because they are both due to dysfunction of myocardial excitation-contraction coupling. Cellular disorders are superimposed on a tissue substrate with abnormal conduction and repolarization properties. A combination of cellular and tissue changes in heart failure conspires to favor arrhythmias while at the same time reducing the mechanical efficiency of contraction and relaxation to cause heart failure.

Electrical Remodeling

The general electrical phenotype of heart failure consists of slowed or nonuniform conduction, heterogeneous reduction of depolarizing and repolarizing currents (i.e., loss of repolarization reserve leading to action potential prolongation), triggered activity, dispersion of refractoriness, slowed *intrinsic* heart rate, disordered calcium handling, and altered β-adrenergic receptor responsiveness (extensive reviews have been published on this subject[2-4]). This phenotype is the result of perturbations in current generation, syncytial conductive or resistive properties, and extrinsic modulators (e.g., innervation, neuroendocrine, reactive oxygen species) (Fig. 66-1). These changes probably are initially adaptive and preserve cardiac function; however, they ultimately produce a proarrhythmic substrate.

A tremendous reservoir of data is available on electrical remodeling in heart failure. Heart failure is neither etiologically nor temporally a discrete entity, however. Numerous causes and types of heart failure (e.g., ischemic versus genetic versus tachycardia-induced) are recognized, each with unique electrophysiologic features. In addition, the electrical remodeling response also varies according to the stage and duration of heart failure.[5] Animal studies are invaluable in determining mechanisms that cannot be studied in patients or in human heart tissue, but direct correlations to patients can be complicated owing to the great variations in normal cardiac electrical physiology in animal species, as well as to the array of heart failure models used (including ischemic, pacing-induced, toxin-induced, genetic modification, pressure overload, and volume overload models).[2] Accordingly, the electrical properties of heart failure discussed in this section are generalized, incorporating the most consistent data, but may not hold for all forms or time points of human cardiomyopathy.

Conduction Properties

Conduction abnormalities can manifest as both slowed conduction velocity (affects the excitable gap necessary for initiation and maintenance of reentry) and nonuniform anisotropy (affects the generation of divergent wavefronts, excitable gaps, and functional lines of block). In a simplistic view, conduction velocity in ventricular myocytes is determined by the upstroke velocity of the action potential that reflects inward sodium current. A more sophisticated and complete understanding of conduction velocity, however, recognizes the contributions of cell coupling, down-stream resistive and capacitive tissue properties, as well as the physics of wavefront shape (i.e., concave versus convex). Thus, action potential propagation is affected by structural and functional variations in myocyte shape, gap junction location and distribution, extracellular matrix, and fiber orientation. These factors contribute to smooth conduction patterns along favored axes and resistance to conduction or discontinuities along unfavored axes, the phenomenon known as *anisotropy*. In normal ventricular myocardium, anisotropy is considered to be uniform because the advancing wavefront is smooth and the difference between longitudinal and transverse conduction velocities is large. In heart failure, abnormalities in conduction of the cardiac impulse arising from changes in ion channels, cell-cell coupling, and tissue impedance result in slowed conduction and nonuniform anisotropy that support the generation and maintenance of arrhythmias by disrupting the balance among conduction pattern and velocity, path length, and recovery of excitability (excitable gap). Specific changes in heart failure that lead to disrupted conduction include altered sodium current; perturbations in gap junction location and expression; changes in myocyte size, shape, and orientation; variation in the distribution and volume of extracellular connective tissue (fibrosis); and

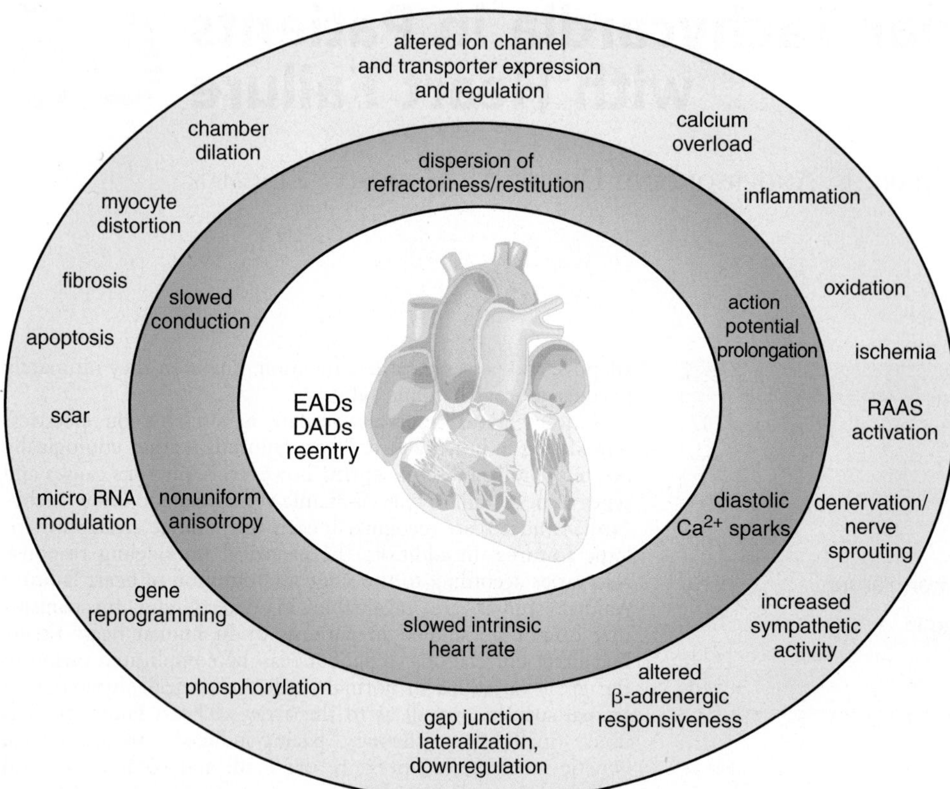

Figure 66-1 Pathogenesis of proarrhythmia in heart failure. Pathogenic alterations in heart failure *(outer ring)* produce the electrophysiologic manifestations *(middle ring)* that promote arrhythmia mechanisms *(inner ring)*—early afterdepolarizations (EADs), delayed afterdepolarizations (DADs), and reentry. RAAS, renin-angiotensin-aldosterone system.

modifications in gross architecture (ventricular size). Some of these changes are examined individually in the following paragraphs.

Sodium Current

Reductions in myocyte sodium current (I_{Na}) are associated with reduced conduction velocity and ventricular arrhythmias such as seen in Brugada syndrome or proarrhythmic actions of class I antiarrhythmic drugs. I_{Na} is decreased in the epicardial border zone of infarcted canine hearts[6] and in failing human hearts,[7,8] although this effect is not seen in all models. Recent evidence from explanted failing human hearts indicates that altered transcription of the sodium channel gene *SCN5A* results in increased expression of truncated, nonfunctional splice variants and decreased expression of the full-length protein.[8] Functional decrease in I_{Na} also appears to occur as a result of prolonged repolarization in heart failure, leading to delayed recovery from inactivation of sodium channels.[6,9] Slowed recovery from inactivation particularly affects premature beats, resulting in conduction slowing and functional block that has been shown to promote reentry in a murine model of heart failure.[9]

Gap Junctions and Connexins

Cardiac ventricular gap junctions are arrays of *inter*cellular channels that are composed primarily of the 43-kD protein subunit connexin43 (Cx43). Connexins Cx40 and Cx45 also are represented in some subsets of cardiomyocytes. In normal hearts, gap junction proteins predominantly localize at the intercalated disks, forming chemical and electrical conduits between adjacent cells in the longitudinal direction, contributing to uniform anisotropic conduction. Connexin expression is dynamic, with increases in response to increased physiologic demands, and rapid uncoupling as a protective cellular response to injury.[10] In both acute and chronic heart failure of various forms, studies have shown changes in expression and localization of gap junction proteins. Both overall Cx43 expression reduction[11-13] and lateralization[12,13] are consistently seen, with increased proportions of the proteins found in the transverse plane between cells. In human dilated cardiomyopathy, Cx43 reduction in right ventricular biopsies was associated with sustained ventricular tachycardia,[14] whereas mathematical simulations confirm development of spatial asymmetry of conduction as a consequence of gap junction uncoupling.[15] Lateralization would be expected to contribute to the fractionated conduction characteristic of failing hearts and is shown to coincide with marked reduction in conduction velocities in later stages of heart failure development.[13] Of interest, dephosphorylation of Cx43 appears to correlate better with decreased conduction velocity than does overall Cx43 expression.[13] Indeed, gap junction dephosphorylation by PP1 and PP2A results in cellular uncoupling. An increased proportion of dephosphorylated Cx43 has been demonstrated in animal and human heart failure.[11,12] Additionally, PP1 and PP2A expression is increased in failing hearts, as is co-localization of PP2A with Cx43,[11] suggesting that post-translational changes in intercellular coupling are important for proarrhythmic electrical remodeling in heart failure.

Fibrosis/Matrix

Fibrosis occurs in both ischemic and some forms of nonischemic cardiomyopathies.[16-19] Poorly conducting fibrotic tissue interspersed between cardiomyocytes predisposes to discontinuities in conduction velocities, conduction block, and reentry.[20] In a small study of explanted failing human hearts in which failure was due to various causes, the pattern of fibrosis has been shown to affect conduction patterns with dense, patchy fibrosis and long, fibrotic strands associated with the greatest degree of nonuniform anisotropy and longest activation delay.[20]

Myocyte Size and Shape

Distortions of cell size and shape characterize the failing heart, whereas myocyte size is a critical determinant of the properties of anisotropic conduction in the ventricle.[21] In heart failure, changes in myocyte shape correlate with alterations in the cytoskeletal composition.[16,18,19] In experiments using the cytoskeletal disrupters cytochalasin-D and phalloidin, actin has been implicated in modulation of myocyte ion currents including $I_{Ca,L}$, I_{Na}, I_{KATP}, and stretch-activated currents,[22] suggesting that alterations in the cytoskeleton in heart failure may have a direct impact on ion channel gating. Structural changes in failing myocytes also could heighten barriers to nucleotide and ion diffusion that could directly (in the case of K_{ATP} channels[23,24]) or indirectly affect ion channel and transporter function.[22]

Ischemia

In ischemic or infarcted myocardium, the impact of structural factors on arrhythmogenesis is often at an extreme, with large areas of both functional and anatomic barriers to conduction providing a substrate for reentry, as well as unique properties of ischemic tissue that favor abnormal impulse generation. Even in the absence of overt coronary artery disease in "nonischemic" dilated cardiomyopathy, global or regional ischemia may occur as a consequence of supply and demand imbalance, resulting in an arrhythmogenic substrate. Key arrhythmogenic features of ischemic myocardium include prolonged action potential duration,[25] abnormal calcium handling, and altered localization of connexins.[26] Other tissue changes in the ischemic heart further contribute to arrhythmogenesis, such as apoptosis with compensatory hypertrophy in nonischemic regions and increased interstitial connective tissue.[27] Systemic effects including increased adrenergic stimulation, increased inflammatory mediators[28] and altered or inhomogeneous cardiac innervation[29] further predispose the vulnerable substrate to arrhythmia.

Heart Rate

Heart failure is characterized by increased sympathetic nerve activity and decreased parasympathetic activity,[30,31] resulting in decreased heart rate variability, which is associated with increased risk of sudden death.[32] Electrical remodeling of the sinus node itself also occurs, resulting in a decrease in *intrinsic* heart rate (heart rate in the presence of autonomic blockade).[33]

HCN

The intrinsic sinus rate is slowed in heart failure—potentially as a protective response in an attempt to compensate for increased sympathetic activity in this disease state. Sinoatrial nodal cell depolarization and thus sinus rate are determined in part by the "funny current" (I_f) generated by hyperpolarization-activated cyclic nucleotide–gated (HCN) channels. In animal models, I_f is significantly reduced in the setting of pressure overload– and volume overload–induced heart failure,[33] whereas sinus node HCN expression of both messenger RNA (mRNA) and protein is significantly reduced in a canine pacing-induced model of heart failure.[34]

Repolarization

Heart failure is characterized by increased action potential duration and loss of repolarization reserve, which promotes both triggered and reentrant arrhythmias. Furthermore, remodeling of repolarization is heterogeneous, leading to accentuated dispersion of refractoriness and restitution that further promotes reentry. Alterations in a number of repolarizing potassium currents have been described in failing hearts. However, the contributions of various potassium channels to repolarization vary among animal models and human hearts, and the degree to which porassium currents are altered is in some cases dependent on the etiology of congestive heart failure (CHF). Effects of abnormal Ca^{2+} handling are defined and discussed in further detail in later sections of this chapter.

Transient Outward Current

Downregulation of the transient outward current (I_{to}) is the most consistent ion channel alteration in animal and human heart failure of various causes,[35-39] with a few exceptions (a detailed review is available[2]). I_{to} forms phase 1 of the action potential and determines the level of the action potential plateau and, as such, influences later repolarizing currents. I_{to} also contributes significantly to the transmural heterogeneity of repolarization, with greater current density in epicardium than in endocardium, an effect that is preserved after I_{to} downregulation in both canine and human heart failure.[40] I_{to} is composed of various α and β subunit combinations, with the downregulation of current associated with variable decrease in mRNA for different subunits, suggesting that regulatory pathways preferentially act through specific subunits.[39,40]

Delayed Rectifier Currents

Animal models of cardiomyopathy and human heart failure indicate variable reduction in one or both of the delayed rectifier currents—the rapid (I_{Kr}) and slow (I_{Ks}) components of the delayed rectifier—with reduction in I_{Ks} more consistently reported.[35-38,41] Of interest, examination of mRNA and channel protein expression (in contrast with currents) in canine pacing-induced cardiomyopathy revealed no significant decrease in proteins underlying either current,[39] suggesting that regulation of these currents occurs predominantly by means of post-translational modification of channel components.

ATP-Gated Potassium Channels

Cardiac sarcolemmal K_{ATP} channels are potassium channels with an ATP-catalyzing regulatory subunit that adjust action potential duration and membrane excitability according to the metabolic status of the myocyte, through coupling with intracellular energetic cascades (e.g., creatine kinase and adenylate kinase phosphotransfer, mitochondrial respiration).[42-48] K_{ATP} channel–dependent action potential shortening under metabolic stress has a protective effect by limiting calcium entry and the potential for injury due to calcium overload, as well as reducing the substantial cellular energetic resources required for diastolic calcium resequestration.[49-52] An association between loss of sarcolemmal K_{ATP} channel ATP responsiveness and hypertrophy has been recognized.[53,54] More recently, loss of K_{ATP} channel function has been demonstrated to be a contributor[55-58] and also a consequence[23] of heart failure. Indeed, genetic deletion of cardiac K_{ATP} channels results in inappropriately long action potentials and predisposes to intracellular calcium overload, triggered activity, and ventricular arrhythmias,[52,59] as well as progressive contractile dysfunction and death in response to acute and chronic stressors.[52,55-57]

In a subset of patients with dilated cardiomyopathy, mutations were uncovered in the gene encoding the regulatory subunit of the K_{ATP} channel that result in reduced K_{ATP} channel ATPase activity and altered reaction kinetics, translating into a channel phenotype with impaired metabolic signal decoding.[58] Alternately, in a murine model of dilated cardiomyopathy and heart failure, intrinsic gating properties of cardiac sarcolemmal K_{ATP} channels are unchanged; however, coupling of the channel to the cardiac metabolic status is disrupted, presumably through a variety of mechanisms including alteration of creatine kinase phosphotransfer, myocyte structural effects on intracellular compartmentalization and diffusion barriers, mitochondrial location and respiration, and possibly K_{ATP} channel expression and localization.[23] As a result, cardiac K_{ATP} channels in this model display a lack of appropriate action potential shortening under stress, leading to excessive vulnerability of cardiomyocytes to calcium loading and necrosis.[23] Thus, the loss of K_{ATP} channel–dependent protective action potential shortening under acute and chronic metabolic stresses in heart failure, due to genetic disruption of the channel proteins affecting gating or disease-related alterations in metabolic signal generation and delivery to the channel, contributes to proarrhythmia, as well as to further cellular injury and progression of heart failure.

The Inward Rectifier

The inward rectifier (I_{K1}) is responsible for maintaining the cardiomyocyte resting potential, as well as contributing to the terminal phase of repolarization. In animal models of heart failure, reported changes in I_{K1} densities are inconsistent, but most studies report a decrease in I_{K1}.[36-39] In human heart failure, decrease in I_{K1} current of variable degree has been reported and appears to be dependent on heart failure etiology.[60] Of note, however, no clear decrease has been seen in mRNA for the pore-forming protein Kir2.1[39] or of the Kir2.1 protein itself[39] in canine pacing-induced heart failure, suggesting post-translational modification of I_{K1}.

Sodium Current

A late component of the dominant cardiac sodium current (I_{NaL}) has been described that may affect action potential duration and arrhythmogenesis in both human and canine heart failure. Specifically, chronic heart failure leads to larger and slower I_{NaL}, contributing to greater sodium influx and action potential duration variability.[61] The I_{NaL} has been shown to be markedly increased by the activity of the multifunctional Ca^{2+}- and calmodulin-dependent protein kinase II (CaMKII), which itself is increased in heart failure.[62] Slowed recovery from inactivation of I_{Na} also has been described in the epicardial border zone of infarcted hearts.[6]

Calcium and Arrhythmogenesis in Heart Failure

Cardiac Action Potentials Grade Intracellular Ca^{2+} Release

Intracellular Ca^{2+} concentration rises within milliseconds of action potential activation and then declines to baseline diastolic levels during action potential repolarization. These rhythmic changes in intracellular Ca^{2+} are central to the physiology of excitation-coupling and help determine myofilament contraction and relaxation. Cell membrane depolarization leads to activation (opening) of voltage-gated calcium channels (predominantly the L-type calcium channel, $Ca_V1.2$ in ventricular myocytes). The duration of the intracellular Ca^{2+} transient is linked to the duration of the action potential plateau, because I_{Ca} inactivation is partly voltage dependent and because the Na^+-Ca^+ exchanger (NCX) is electrogenic. Most I_{Ca} studies are performed using voltage clamp commands with square waveforms (see Chapters 9 and 17) to simplify analysis and reduce capacitative current artifacts. However, when physiologic action potential waveforms are used in voltage clamp experiments with healthy ventricular myocytes, the resulting I_{Ca} inactivates more slowly than with square wave commands, and with long *versus* short action potential waveforms. Pathologically prolonged action potentials elicit markedly prolonged I_{Ca},[63] contributing to intracellular Ca^{2+} overload and activation of afterdepolarization-initiating inward currents.[64] The electrical remodeling that occurs in heart failure and results in action potential prolongation can contribute to prolongation of the intracellular calcium transient, in part by slowing I_{Ca} inactivation.

I_{Ca} Is Amplified to Produce Physiologic Intracellular Calcium Transients

The calcium current (I_{Ca}) is amplified in the cell by a process termed *calcium-induced Ca^{2+} release* (CICR). The $Ca_V1.2$ protein is located in the sarcolemma, where it is predominantly present in T tubule invaginations and resides in close apposition to intracellular Ca^{2+} release channel ryanodine receptors (RyR). I_{Ca} triggers opening of RyR that allows extrusion of Ca^{2+} from the sarcoplasmic reticulum to the cytoplasm for myofilament activation and cell shortening. In diastole, most cytoplasmic Ca^{2+} is actively pumped back into the sarcoplasmic reticulum lumen by a Ca^{2+}-ATPase, the *sarcoplasmic-endoplasmic reticulum Ca^{2+}-ATPase* (SERCA), and a smaller amount is extruded to the extracellular space by NCX. Phospholamban is a small sarcoplasmic reticulum membrane–spanning protein that inhibits SERCA. The low-capacity, high-affinity sarcolemmal Ca^{2+}-ATPase contributes only a minor fraction to resolution of the cytosolic calcium transient. The kinetic properties of I_{Ca}, RyR, and SERCA are enhanced by protein kinase A (PKA) and CaMKII during catecholamine stimulation. CaMKII activity is recruited during catecholamine stimulation,[65] and PKA and CaMKII appear to target distinct sites on $Ca_V1.2$,[66,67] RyR,[68] and phospholamban.[69] The effects of protein kinases on these excitation-contraction coupling proteins are central to classic "fight or flight" properties of myocardium (i.e., to heart rate increases and increased inotropy) but are now recognized to contribute arrhythmias in heart failure.

Remodeling of Ca^{2+} Dynamics in Heart Failure

Disturbance of intracellular Ca^{2+} concentration is the central proarrhythmic feature of failing myocardium. In general, the sarcoplasmic reticulum Ca^{2+} content is reduced,[70] and the intracellular calcium transient is diminished in amplitude and prolonged in failing cardiomyocytes from animal models and from patients.[71] The reduction in sarcoplasmic reticulum Ca^{2+} content may play a central role in reducing inotropy.[72] Multiple mechanisms underlie prolongation of the intracellular calcium transient in heart failure. One cause is action potential prolongation due to electrical remodeling (see earlier), but failing cardiomyocytes also are marked by transcriptional and post-transcriptional changes in the key calcium-homeostatic proteins that make up the cellular machinery for excitation-contraction coupling. These changes in calcium-homeostatic proteins can vary between models and in accordance with a variety of other factors such as the predominance of systolic or diastolic failure,[73] but general features of failing human cardiomyocytes are discussed briefly in the following paragraphs.

L-Type Calcium Channels

The expression of the $Ca_V1.2$ pore-forming α subunit does not markedly change in failing hearts, but heart failure can result in a change in the predominant auxiliary β subunit isoform from β1 to β2.[74] L-type calcium channels display increased activity, manifested as increased opening probability.[75] Increased $Ca_V1.2$ opening probability is a likely mechanism underlying early afterdepolarizations (EADs) (see later on).[76] The increased duration of the intracellular calcium transient may stimulate various calcium-activated signaling molecules. The best-understood example in this regard is CaMKII: because of its multimeric structure, CaMKII undergoes a series of activating intersubunit phosphorylation events that increase total enzyme activity and convert CaMKII into a longer-lasting, calcium-independent species.[77] CaMKII activity and expression are increased in failing human hearts,[78] and CaMKII induces $Ca_V1.2$ channels to become highly active,[79] resembling the effects of catecholamine stimulation and PKA. These findings provide a molecular rationale for increased arrhythmias in heart failure.[80]

Na^+-Ca^{2+} Exchanger

In heart failure, NCX assumes increased prominence, whereas the velocity of cytoplasmic Ca^{2+} uptake to the sarcoplasmic reticulum by SERCA is relatively reduced.[81] Both of these effects are due at least partly to transcriptional reprogramming in heart failure, because expression of both mRNA and protein for NCX and SERCA is reduced.[82] The increased importance of NCX contributes to prolongation of the intracellular calcium transient and favors arrhythmia-initiating delayed afterdepolarizations (DADs).[83] Failing hearts show elevated intracellular Na^+ concentration over that in healthy hearts.[84] The increase in intracellular Na^+ concentration reduces the ability of NCX to extrude Ca^{2+} and enhances the probability of DADs.[85] The increase in intracellular Na^+ in failing hearts may be due partly to an increased noninactivating component of the voltage activated Na^+ current that results from elevated CaMKII activity.[62]

Ryanodine Receptors

RyR dysfunction is now widely accepted to be a key factor leading to arrhythmias in heart failure. RyR dysfunction is manifested as increased channel opening probability and uncoordinated opening of RyR cluster ("sparks"); both of these behaviors may contribute to pathologic "waves" of intracellular Ca^{2+}, disordered myofilament activation, and generation of arrhythmia-initiating afterdepolarizations. Although RyR expression is reduced in some reports, increased phosphorylation by PKA[86] and CaMKII[87] appears to be an important arbiter of RyR dysfunction in failing heart. RyR hyperphosphorylation in structural heart disease and heart failure occurs in overlapping RyR regions that are targets of a genetic arrhythmia syndrome (catecholaminergic polymorphic ventricular tachycardia, Chapter 70).[88,89] Therapeutic interventions such as ventricular assist devices and β-adrenergic receptor antagonist regimens result in improved mechanical performance, reduced arrhythmias, and normalization of RyR phosphorylation.[90] RyR function is critically dependent on a highly ordered cellular ultrastructure wherein RyRs are arrayed against the cytoplasmic face of $Ca_V1.2$ across a narrow span of cytoplasm. This highly ordered ultrastructure is distorted in failing hearts, leaving RyRs "orphaned" from normally apposing $Ca_V1.2$.[91] Orphaned RyRs are more likely to open asynchronously, a situation that leads to disordered sarcoplasmic reticulum Ca^{2+} release events (i.e., sparks and waves), resulting in mechanical dyssynchrony and arrhythmia-initiating afterdepolarizations.

Remodeling of Cellular Signaling Molecules in Heart Failure

The activity and expression of a wide variety of protein kinases and phosphatases are altered in failing hearts.[92] The net phosphorylation of target proteins reflects the relative activity of the kinase and phosphatase. Remodeling of signaling in heart failure provides a potential molecular rationale for the close clinical association between heart failure and sudden death due to arrhythmias. For example, hyperphosphorylation by PKA and CaMKII can increase RyR[87] and $Ca_V1.2$[75,93] opening probability, which contributes to cellular Ca^{2+} overload. Protein kinases also can activate transcription factors to activate heart failure gene programs that govern myofilament isoform switching and pathologic expression changes in excitation-contraction coupling proteins that cause mechanical dysfunction in heart failure.[94] Of particular interest as targets for future therapies are calcium-activated kinases and phosphatases, which have the potential to amplify initial distortions of cellular calcium homeostasis that are present before the development of overt heart failure.[95]

Mechanisms of Electrical Remodeling in Heart Failure

Protein Expression and Modification

Electrical remodeling in heart failure occurs at the levels of transcription, translation, and post-translational modification of ion channel, transporter, and gap junction proteins. Furthermore, the altered cytokine and neurohumoral environment results in the generation of transcription factors that modify the gene program of the myocyte. Specifically, heart failure has been associated with reinitiation of the fetal gene program.[96] As noted earlier, human heart failure is associated with altered transcription of the sodium channel gene *SCN5A*. Also, as discussed elsewhere in this chapter, evidence from specific cases points to post-translational modification of channel proteins or other electrophysiologically active cellular components, such as hyperphosphorylation of the ryanodine receptor by PKA and CAMKII, leading to dysregulated calcium transients, and increased dephosphorylation of gap junction Cx43, leading to cellular uncoupling.

Particularly intriguing as a mechanism for electrical remodeling in heart failure is the recent implication of post-transcriptional modulation of protein expression by microRNA. MicroRNAs are recently discovered endogenous small, approximately 22-base, single-stranded noncoding RNA sequences that can bind in an antisense direction to mRNA targets to suppress or silence protein translation or enhance mRNA degradation. MicroRNAs also can have a net result of increased protein expression through negative modulation of inhibitory genes. The effects of microRNAs are best described in developmental regulation and oncogenesis but recently have been associated with heart failure of varied etiology,[97-103] as well as contributors to ion channel remodeling and proarrhythmia in post–myocardial infarction hearts.[104] The muscle-specific microRNA miR-1 was found to be upregulated in post-infarction, remodeled human heart tissue as well as in the infarct border zone in rat hearts. Overexpression of miR-1 in an experimental model reduced the expression of Cx43 as well as Kir2.1, the principal pore-forming subunit for the repolarizing potassium channel current I_{K1}. As discussed elsewhere in this chapter, these changes would be expected to promote arrhythmia; as such, overexpression or injection of miR-1 in rat heart also recapitulates phenotypic components of postinfarct electrical remodeling, including action potential prolongation and slowed conduction. Overexpression of miR-1 results in susceptibility to premature ventricular contractions and arrhythmias, whereas blockade of miR-1 normalizes these effects. Muscle-specific microRNA has also been shown to post-translationally regulate expression of genes encoding I_{Ks} (*KCNQ1* and *KCNE1*), with demonstrated spatial heterogeneity of *miR-1/miR-133* implicated as a contributor to regional differences and disparity between mRNA content and protein expression of I_{Ks} components.[105]

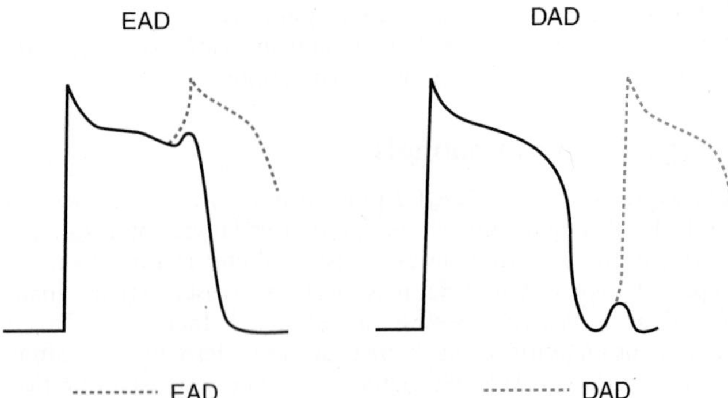

Figure 66-2 Afterdepolarizations. Oscillatory changes in cell membrane voltage are produced by abnormal Ca^{2+} handling and may result in repetitive depolarization. Such afterdepolarizations are classified as *early afterdepolarizations* (EADs) when they occur during phase 2 or 3 of action potential repolarization and *delayed afterdepolarizations* (DADs) if they occur during phase 4.

Oxidation/Inflammation

In addition to the effect of inflammation on atherosclerotic plaque formation, rupture, and thrombosis, which can lead to acute ischemia or infarction, predisposing the patient to ventricular arrhythmias, as well as ischemia-independent effects in the pathogenesis of heart failure, cytokines and other inflammatory mediators upregulated in heart failure have direct effects on ion channels that can be proarrhythmic.[106,107] Indeed, the circulating stress-induced inflammatory cytokine tumor necrosis factor-α (TNF- α) has recently been associated with a downregulation of I_{to}, apparently through induction of iNOS.[108] Oxidative stress, mediated through free radical–generating systems, also has been shown to reduce L-type calcium current in nonfailing ventricular myocytes[109] and heterologous expression systems[110]—effects that also may occur in heart failure. Oxidation also can contribute to activation of kinase signaling by inactivating phosphatases[111] and by directly activating kinases.[112]

Neurohumoral Activation and Cardiac Innervation

Proarrhythmia in heart failure can be attributed to the exposure of the susceptible substrate, as thus far described, to a malignant environment extrinsic to the myocardium. As with cytokines, other inflammatory mediators, and oxidative stress, increased catecholamines and upregulation of the renin-angiotensin-aldosterone system (RAAS) can be indirectly proarrhythmic through effects on heart failure pathogenesis and progression. Furthermore, β-adrenergic receptor agonists and RAAS components can directly affect ion channel function. Catecholamines affect Ca^{2+} handling as discussed in previous sections, whereas angiotensin II inhibits I_{to}[113] and delayed rectifiers[114] and decreases Na^+,K^+-ATPase activity.[115] Altered cardiac sympathetic innervation is found in both ischemic and nonischemic cardiomyopathy.[116] Although sympathetic denervation in infarcted hearts is associated with exaggerated action potential shortening and vulnerability to arrhythmia in the face of catecholamine challenge,[117] an increase in nerve regeneration (sprouting) also is associated with malignant ventricular arrhythmias in patients with structural heart disease.[116]

Mechanisms for Triggered Activity

Early and Delayed Afterdepolarizations

Afterdepolarizations are oscillatory changes in cell membrane voltage (Fig. 66-2). Afterdepolarizations are classified as *early* (i.e., EADs) when they occur during the action potential plateau. Sometimes EADs are further subclassified as phase 2 or 3, to denote their association with phase 2 or 3 of action potential repolarization. Afterdepolarizations that occur during diastole, after completion of action potential repolarization, are designated *delayed* (i.e., DADs). Afterdepolarizations can occur with a net increase in inward current. Such an increase may be small, particularly for EADs, because the sarcolemmal resistivity is highest during the action potential plateau. Multiple candidate inward currents underlying EADs and DADs have been proposed, but the best evidence suggests that EADs are due primarily to increased L-type calcium current,[118] and that increased NCX, operating in "forward mode" in which 1 Ca^{2+} is exchanged for 3 Na^+, resulting in net inward current (historically called the transient inward current), underlies DADs.[64]

Both EADs and DADs are favored by changes associated with heart failure—namely, electrical remodeling, remodeling of Ca^{2+} dynamics, molecular signaling remodeling, and ultrastructural remodeling. Electrical remodeling leads to action potential prolongation, which favors EADs by lengthening the action potential plateau phase, with increased opportunities for $Ca_V1.2$ reopening in the "window current" voltage range.[76] Action potential prolongation also leads to increased cellular Ca^{2+} loading by voltage-gated calcium channels (mostly $Ca_V1.2$), with reduced efficacy of NCX to extrude cytoplasmic Ca^{2+} to the extracellular space (forward mode) and increased electrochemical driving force for NCX, thereby increasing cytoplasmic Ca^{2+} uptake (reverse mode).[64]

The prolonged cellular calcium transient in failing ventricular myocytes is a powerful stimulus for activating the multifunctional Ca^{2+}- and calmodulin-dependent protein kinase II (CaMKII).[77,119] CaMKII is increased in failing hearts,[78] and CaMKII inhibition prevents EADs,[63] the transient inward current,[64] and ventricular tachycardia in normal[120] and structurally diseased (hypertrophic[93] or failing[121]) hearts with QT interval prolongation. The mechanism for proarrhythmic actions of CaMKII appears to be multifactorial but is targeted to key excitation-contraction proteins. CaMKII induces $Ca_V1.2$ into a high-activity gating mode[79] (so-called mode 2 gating) by a mechanism that requires phosphorylation of the auxiliary β subunit.[66] CaMKII increases sarcoplasmic reticulum Ca^{2+} release from RyR2[68,87] and reduces the inhibitory action of phospholamban on SERCA-dependent sarcoplasmic reticulum Ca^{2+} uptake.[122] CaMKII inhibition reduces sarcoplasmic reticulum Ca^{2+} content and prevents sarcoplasmic reticulum Ca^{2+} overload from catecholamine stimulation, primarily by reducing phospholamban phosphorylation.[123]

An intriguing finding is that CaMKII also participates in transcriptional reprogramming that leads to cardiac hypertrophy and heart failure.[124] CaMKII inhibition reduces mechanical dysfunction, structural and electrical remodeling after pathologic stress[65] and CaMKII inhibition can improve myocardial function in a severe heart failure model due to overexpression of calcineurin.[121] CaMKII is recruited during catecholamine stimulation, and catecholamine stimulation favors afterdepolarization.[65] Protein kinase A (PKA) also is generated by β-adrenergic receptor stimulation. PKA phosphorylates the same key excitation-contraction coupling proteins as those handled by CaMKII, albeit at differing sites. Improved understanding of the interplay between CaMKII and PKA signaling is an important goal for arrhythmia science. Taken together, these findings suggest that "remodeling" of signaling molecules may provide an explanation of why arrhythmias and heart failure occur together. Finally, the ultrastructural changes that orphan RyR lead to loss of local control, dyssynchronous Ca^{2+} release, and DADs.[91]

Certain cells may be particularly vulnerable to EADs and DADs. So-called M cells are electrophenotypically distinct from endocardium and epicardium in that they have relatively prolonged repolarization at baseline.[125] M cells have less repolarization reserve than that typical of other ventricular cardiomyocytes and therefore show exaggerated action potential prolongation with stress that reduces repolarizing currents.[86] Purkinje fibers also are highly vulnerable to afterdepolarizations as a result of basal action potential prolongation.[126] Inducible and spontaneous ventricular arrhythmias in failing human hearts frequently are due to a focal mechanism[127] that may be afterdepolarization. The specific cell type that serves as the apparent focus for these arrhythmias is unknown, however.

References

1. Zipes DP, Camm AJ, Borggrefe M, et al for the American College of Cardiology/American Heart Association Task Force, European Society of Cardiology Committee for Practice Guidelines, European Heart Rhythm Association, Heart Rhythm Society: ACC/AHA/ESC 2006 guidelines for management of patients with ventricular arrhythmias and the prevention of sudden cardiac death. Circulation 114:e385-e484, 2006.
2. Tomaselli GF, Marban E: Electrophysiological remodeling in hypertrophy and heart failure. Cardiovasc Res 42:270-283, 1999.
3. Tomaselli GF, Zipes DP: What causes sudden death in heart failure? Circ Res 95:754-763, 2004.
4. Janse MJ: Electrophysiological changes in heart failure and their relationship to arrhythmogenesis. Cardiovasc Res 61:208-217, 2004.
5. Hoshijima M, Chien KR: Mixed signals in heart failure: Cancer rules. J Clin Invest 109:849-855, 2002.
6. Pu J, Boyden PA: Alterations of Na^+ currents in myocytes from epicardial border zone of the infarcted heart. A possible ionic mechanism for reduced excitability and postrepolarization refractoriness. Circ Res 81:110-119, 1997.
7. Valdivia CR, Chu WW, Pu J, et al: Increased late sodium current in myocytes from a canine heart failure model and from failing human heart. J Mol Cell Cardiol 38:475-483, 2005.
8. Shang LL, Pfahnl AE, Sanyal S, et al: Human heart failure is associated with abnormal C-terminal splicing variants in the cardiac sodium channel. Circ Res 101:1146-1154, 2007. Epub 2007 Sep 27.
9. London B, Baker LC, Lee JS, et al: Calcium-dependent arrhythmias in transgenic mice with heart failure. Am J Physiol Heart Circ Physiol 284:H431-H441, 2003.
10. Beardslee MA, Lerner DL, Tadros PN, et al: Dephosphorylation and intracellular redistribution of ventricular connexin43 during electrical uncoupling induced by ischemia. Circ Res 87:656-662, 2000.
11. Ai X, Pogwizd SM: Connexin 43 downregulation and dephosphorylation in nonischemic heart failure is associated with enhanced colocalized protein phosphatase type 2A. Circ Res 96:54-63, 2005.
12. Akar FG, Spragg DD, Tunin RS, et al: Mechanisms underlying conduction slowing and arrhythmogenesis in nonischemic dilated cardiomyopathy. Circ Res 95:717-725, 2004.
13. Akar FG, Nass RD, Hahn S, et al: Dynamic changes in conduction velocity and gap junction properties during development of pacing-induced heart failure. Am J Physiol Heart Circ Physiol 293:H1223-H1230, 2007.
14. Kitamura H, Ohnishi Y, Yoshida A, et al: Heterogeneous loss of connexin43 protein in nonischemic dilated cardiomyopathy with ventricular tachycardia. J Cardiovasc Electrophysiol 13:865-870, 2002.
15. Rudy Y, Shaw RM: Cardiac excitation: An interactive process of ion channels and gap junctions. Adv Exp Med Biol 430:269-279, 1997.
16. Hein S, Kostin S, Heling A, et al: The role of the cytoskeleton in heart failure. Cardiovasc Res 45:273-278, 2000.
17. Kostin S, Hein S, Arnon E, et al: The cytoskeleton and related proteins in the human failing heart. Heart Fail Rev 5:271-280, 2000.
18. Chien KR: Stress pathways and heart failure. Cell 98:555-558, 1999.
19. Bradham WS, Bozkurt B, Gunasinghe H, et al: Tumor necrosis factor-alpha and myocardial remodeling in progression of heart failure: A current perspective. Cardiovasc Res 53:822-830, 2002.
20. Kawara T, Derksen R, de Groot JR, et al: Activation delay after premature stimulation in chronically diseased human myocardium relates to the architecture of interstitial fibrosis. Circulation 104:3069-3075, 2001.
21. Spach MS, Heidlage JF, Dolber PC, Barr RC: Electrophysiological effects of remodeling cardiac gap junctions and cell size: Experimental and model studies of normal cardiac growth. Circ Res 86:302-311, 2000.
22. Calaghan SC, Le Guennec JY, White E: Cytoskeletal modulation of electrical and mechanical activity in cardiac myocytes. Prog Biophys Mol Biol 84:29-59, 2004.
23. Hodgson DM, Zingman LV, Kane GC, et al: Cellular remodeling in heart failure disrupts K(ATP) channel-dependent stress tolerance. EMBO J 22:1732-1742, 2003.
24. Selivanov VA, Alekseev AE, Hodgson DM, et al: Nucleotide-gated K_{ATP} channels integrated with creatine and adenylate kinases: Amplification, tuning and sensing of energetic signals in the compartmentalized cellular environment. Mol Cell Biochem 256-257:243-256, 2004.
25. Bito V, Heinzel FR, Weidemann F, et al: Cellular mechanisms of contractile dysfunction in hibernating myocardium. Circ Res 94:794-801, 2004.
26. Saffitz JE, Hames KY, Kanno S: Remodeling of gap junctions in ischemic and nonischemic forms of heart disease. J Membr Biol 218:65-71, 2007. Epub 2007 Jun 22.
27. Lim H, Fallavollita JA, Hard R, et al: Profound apoptosis-mediated regional myocyte loss and compensatory hypertrophy in pigs with hibernating myocardium. Circulation 100:2380-2386, 1999.
28. Kalra D, Baumgarten G, Dibbs Z, et al: Nitric oxide provokes tumor necrosis factor-alpha expression in adult feline myocardium through a cGMP-dependent pathway. Circulation 102:1302-1307, 2000.
29. Barber MJ, Mueller TM, Davies BG, et al: Interruption of sympathetic and vagal-mediated afferent responses by transmural myocardial infarction. Circulation 72:623-631, 1985.
30. Porter TR, Eckberg DL, Fritsch JM, et al: Autonomic pathophysiology in heart failure patients. Sympathetic-cholinergic interrelations. J Clin Invest 85:1362-1371, 1990.
31. Binkley PF, Nunziata E, Haas GJ, Nelson SD, Cody RJ. Parasympathetic withdrawal is an integral component of autonomic imbalance in congestive heart failure: Demonstration in human subjects and verification in a paced canine model of ventricular failure. J Am Coll Cardiol 18:464-472, 1991.
32. Odemuyiwa O, Malik M, Farrell T, et al: Comparison of the predictive characteristics of heart rate variability index and left ventricular ejection fraction for all-cause mortality, arrhythmic events and sudden death after acute myocardial infarction. Am J Cardiol 68:434-439, 1991.
33. Verkerk AO, Wilders R, Coronel R, et al: Ionic remodeling of sinoatrial node cells by heart failure. Circulation 108:760-766, 2003.

34. Zicha S, Fernandez-Velasco M, Lonardo G, et al: Sinus node dysfunction and hyperpolarization-activated (HCN) channel subunit remodeling in a canine heart failure model. Cardiovasc Res 66:472-481, 2005.
35. Li GR, Lau CP, Leung TK, Nattel S: Ionic current abnormalities associated with prolonged action potentials in cardiomyocytes from diseased human right ventricles. Heart Rhythm 1:460-468, 2004.
36. Li GR, Lau CP, Ducharme A, et al: Transmural action potential and ionic current remodeling in ventricles of failing canine hearts. Am J Physiol Heart Circ Physiol 283:H1031-H1041, 2002.
37. Tsuji Y, Opthof T, Kamiya K, et al: Pacing-induced heart failure causes a reduction of delayed rectifier potassium currents along with decreases in calcium and transient outward currents in rabbit ventricle. Cardiovasc Res 48:300-309, 2000.
38. Rose J, Armoundas AA, Tian Y, et al: Molecular correlates of altered expression of potassium currents in failing rabbit myocardium. Am J Physiol Heart Circ Physiol 288:H2077-H2087, 2005.
39. Akar FG, Wu RC, Juang GJ, et al: Molecular mechanisms underlying K^+ current downregulation in canine tachycardia-induced heart failure. Am J Physiol Heart Circ Physiol 288:H2887-H2896, 2005.
40. Zicha S, Xiao L, Stafford S, et al: Transmural expression of transient outward potassium current subunits in normal and failing canine and human hearts. J Physiol 561:735-748, 2004.
41. Petkova-Kirova PS, Gursoy E, Mehdi H, et al: Electrical remodeling of cardiac myocytes from mice with heart failure due to the overexpression of tumor necrosis factor-alpha. Am J Physiol Heart Circ Physiol 290:H2098-H2107, 2006.
42. Inagaki N, Gonoi T, Clement JP, et al: A family of sulfonylurea receptors determines the pharmacological properties of ATP-sensitive K^+ channels. Neuron 16:1011-1017, 1996.
43. Zingman LV, Alekseev AE, Bienengraeber M, et al: Signaling in channel/enzyme multimers: ATPase transitions in SUR module gate ATP-sensitive K^+ conductance. Neuron 31:233-245, 2001.
44. Bienengraeber M, Alekseev AE, Abraham MR, et al: ATPase activity of the sulfonylurea receptor: A catalytic function for the KATP channel complex. FASEB J 14:1943-1952, 2000.
45. Abraham MR, Selivanov VA, Hodgson DM, et al: Coupling of cell energetics with membrane metabolic sensing. Integrative signaling through creatine kinase phosphotransfer disrupted by M-CK gene knock-out. J Biol Chem 277:24427-2434, 2002.
46. Carrasco AJ, Dzeja PP, Alekseev AE, et al: Adenylate kinase phosphotransfer communicates cellular energetic signals to ATP-sensitive potassium channels. Proc Natl Acad Sci U S A 98:7623-7628, 2001.
47. Dzeja PP, Terzic A: Phosphotransfer reactions in the regulation of ATP-sensitive K^+ channels. FASEB J 12:523-529, 1998.
48. Crawford RM, Ranki HJ, Botting CH, et al: Creatine kinase is physically associated with the cardiac ATP-sensitive K^+ channel in vivo. FASEB J 16:102-104, 2002.
49. Nichols CG, Ripoll C, Lederer WJ: ATP-sensitive potassium channel modulation of the guinea pig ventricular action potential and contraction. Circ Res 68:280-287, 1991.
50. Rajashree R, Koster JC, Markova KP, et al: Contractility and ischemic response of hearts from transgenic mice with altered sarcolemmal K(ATP) channels. Am J Physiol Heart Circ Physiol 283:H584-H590, 2002.
51. Suzuki M, Sasaki N, Miki T, et al: Role of sarcolemmal K(ATP) channels in cardioprotection against ischemia/reperfusion injury in mice. J Clin Invest 109:509-516, 2002.
52. Zingman LV, Hodgson DM, Bast PH, et al: Kir6.2 is required for adaptation to stress. Proc Natl Acad Sci U S A 99:13278-13283, 2002.
53. Cameron JS, Kimura S, Jackson-Burns DA, et al: ATP-sensitive K^+ channels are altered in hypertrophied ventricular myocytes. Am J Physiol 255:H1254-H1258, 1988.
54. Yuan F, Brandt NR, Pinto JM, et al: Hypertrophy decreases cardiac KATP channel responsiveness to exogenous and locally generated (glycolytic) ATP. J Mol Cell Cardiol 29:2837-2848, 1997.
55. Kane GC, Behfar A, Dyer RB, et al: *KCNJ11* gene knockout of the Kir6.2 KATP channel causes maladaptive remodeling and heart failure in hypertension. Hum Mol Genet 15:2285-2297, 2006.
56. Kane GC, Behfar A, Yamada S, et al: ATP-sensitive K^+ channel knockout compromises the metabolic benefit of exercise training, resulting in cardiac deficits. Diabetes 53(Suppl 3):S169-S175, 2004.
57. Yamada S, Kane GC, Behfar A, et al: Protection conferred by myocardial ATP-sensitive K^+ channels in pressure overload-induced congestive heart failure revealed in KCNJ11 Kir6.2-null mutant. J Physiol 577:1053-1065, 2006.
58. Bienengraeber M, Olson TM, Selivanov VA, et al: ABCC9 mutations identified in human dilated cardiomyopathy disrupt catalytic KATP channel gating. Nat Genet 36:382-387, 2004.
59. Liu XK, Yamada S, Kane GC, et al: Genetic disruption of Kir6.2, the pore-forming subunit of ATP-sensitive K^+ channel, predisposes to catecholamine-induced ventricular dysrhythmia. Diabetes 53(Suppl 3):S165-S168, 2004.
60. Koumi S, Backer CL, Arentzen CE: Characterization of inwardly rectifying K^+ channel in human cardiac myocytes. Alterations in channel behavior in myocytes isolated from patients with idiopathic dilated cardiomyopathy. Circulation 92:164-174, 1995.
61. Maltsev VA, Silverman N, Sabbah HN, Undrovinas AI: Chronic heart failure slows late sodium current in human and canine ventricular myocytes: Implications for repolarization variability. Eur J Heart Fail 9:219-227, 2007.
62. Wagner S, Dybkova N, Rasenack EC, et al: Ca^{2+}/calmodulin-dependent protein kinase II regulates cardiac Na^+ channels. J Clin Invest 116:3127-3138, 2006.
63. Wu Y, MacMillan LB, McNeill RB, et al: CaM kinase augments cardiac L-type Ca^{2+} current: A cellular mechanism for long Q-T arrhythmias. Am J Physiol 276: H2168-H2178, 1999.
64. Wu Y, Roden DM, Anderson ME: Calmodulin kinase inhibition prevents development of the arrhythmogenic transient inward current. Circ Res 84:906-912, 1999.
65. Zhang R, Khoo MS, Wu Y, et al: Calmodulin kinase II inhibition protects against structural heart disease. Nat Med 11:409-417, 2005.
66. Grueter CE, Abiria SA, Dzhura I, et al: L-type Ca^{2+} channel facilitation mediated by phosphorylation of the beta subunit by CaMKII. Mol Cell 23:641-650, 2006.
67. Ganesan AN, Maack C, Johns DC, et al: Beta-adrenergic stimulation of L-type Ca^{2+} channels in cardiac myocytes requires the distal carboxyl terminus of alpha1C but not serine 1928. Circ Res 98:e11-e18, 2006.
68. Wehrens XH, Lehnart SE, Reiken SR, Marks AR: Ca^{2+}/calmodulin-dependent protein kinase II phosphorylation regulates the cardiac ryanodine receptor. Circ Res 94:e61-e70, 2004.
69. Chu G, Lester JW, Young KB, et al: A single site (Ser16) phosphorylation in phospholamban is sufficient in mediating its maximal cardiac responses to beta-agonists. J Biol Chem 275:38938-38943, 2000.
70. Piacentino V 3rd, Weber CR, Chen X, et al: Cellular basis of abnormal calcium transients of failing human ventricular myocytes. Circ Res 92:651-658, 2003.
71. Gwathmey JK, Copelas L, MacKinnon R, et al: Abnormal intracellular calcium handling in myocardium from patients with end-stage heart failure. Circ Res 61:70-76, 1987.
72. Pieske B, Sutterlin M, Schmidt-Schweda S, et al: Diminished post-rest potentiation of contractile force in human dilated cardiomyopathy. Functional evidence for alterations in intracellular Ca^{2+} handling. J Clin Invest 98:764-776, 1996.
73. Hasenfuss G, Schillinger W, Lehnart SE, et al: Relationship between Na^+-Ca^{2+}-exchanger protein levels and diastolic function of failing human myocardium. Circulation 99:641-648, 1999.
74. Hullin R, Matthes J, von Vietinghoff S, et al: Increased expression of the auxiliary beta2-subunit of ventricular L-type Ca^{2+} channels leads to single-channel activity characteristic of heart failure. PLoS ONE 2007 2:e292, 2007.
75. Handrock R, Schroder F, Hirt S, et al: Single-channel properties of L-type calcium channels from failing human ventricle. Cardiovasc Res 37:445-455, 1998.
76. January CT, Riddle JM, Salata JJ: A model for early afterdepolarizations: Induction with the Ca^{2+} channel agonist Bay K 8644. Circ Res 62:563-571, 1988.
77. De Koninck P, Schulman H: Sensitivity of CaM kinase II to the frequency of Ca^{2+} oscillations. Science 279:227-230, 1998.
78. Zhang T, Brown JH: Role of Ca^{2+}/calmodulin-dependent protein kinase II in

cardiac hypertrophy and heart failure. Cardiovasc Res 63:476-486, 2004.
79. Dzhura I, Wu Y, Colbran RJ, et al: Calmodulin kinase determines calcium-dependent facilitation of L-type calcium channels. Nat Cell Biol 2:173-177, 2000.
80. Anderson ME: Calmodulin kinase and L-type calcium channels: A recipe for arrhythmias? Trends Cardiovasc Med 14: 152-161, 2004.
81. Gaughan JP, Furukawa S, Jeevanandam V, et al: Sodium/calcium exchange contributes to contraction and relaxation in failed human ventricular myocytes. Am J Physiol 277:H714-H724, 1999.
82. Hasenfuss G, Reinecke H, Studer R, et al: Calcium cycling proteins and force-frequency relationship in heart failure. Basic Res Cardiol 91(Suppl)2:17-22, 1996.
83. Pogwizd SM: Increased Na(+)-Ca(2+) exchanger in the failing heart. Circ Res 87:641-643, 2000.
84. Despa S, Islam MA, Weber CR, et al: Intracellular Na(+) concentration is elevated in heart failure but Na/K pump function is unchanged. Circulation 105: 2543-2548, 2002.
85. Pogwizd SM, Bers DM: Cellular basis of triggered arrhythmias in heart failure. Trends Cardiovasc Med 14:61-66, 2004.
86. Marx SO, Reiken S, Hisamatsu Y, et al: PKA phosphorylation dissociates FKBP12.6 from the calcium release channel (ryanodine receptor): Defective regulation in failing hearts. Cell 101:365-376, 2000.
87. Ai X, Curran JW, Shannon TR, et al: Ca^{2+}/calmodulin-dependent protein kinase modulates cardiac ryanodine receptor phosphorylation and sarcoplasmic reticulum Ca^{2+} leak in heart failure. Circ Res 97:1314-1322, 2005.
88. Lehnart SE, Wehrens XH, Laitinen PJ, et al: Sudden death in familial polymorphic ventricular tachycardia associated with calcium release channel (ryanodine receptor) leak. Circulation 109:3208-3214, 2004.
89. Cerrone M, Colombi B, Santoro M, et al: Bidirectional ventricular tachycardia and fibrillation elicited in a knock-in mouse model carrier of a mutation in the cardiac ryanodine receptor. Circ Res 96:e77-e82, 2005.
90. Reiken S, Wehrens XH, Vest JA, et al: Beta-blockers restore calcium release channel function and improve cardiac muscle performance in human heart failure. Circulation 107:2459-2466, 2003.
91. Song LS, Sobie EA, McCulle S, et al: Orphaned ryanodine receptors in the failing heart. Proc Natl Acad Sci U S A 103:4305-4310, 2006.
92. Anderson ME, Higgins LS, Schulman H: Disease mechanisms and emerging therapies: Protein kinases and their inhibitors in myocardial disease. Nat Clin Pract Cardiovasc Med 3:437-445, 2006.
93. Wu Y, Temple J, Zhang R, et al: Calmodulin kinase II and arrhythmias in a mouse model of cardiac hypertrophy. Circulation 106:1288-1293, 2002.
94. McKinsey TA: Derepression of pathological cardiac genes by members of the CaM kinase superfamily. Cardiovasc Res 73:667-677, 2007.
95. Maier LS, Zhang T, Chen L, et al: Transgenic CaMKIIdeltaC overexpression uniquely alters cardiac myocyte Ca^{2+} handling: Reduced SR Ca^{2+} load and activated SR Ca^{2+} release. Circ Res 92:904-911, 2003.
96. Chien KR, Zhu H, Knowlton KU, et al: Transcriptional regulation during cardiac growth and development. Annu Rev Physiol 55:77-95, 1993.
97. Care A, Catalucci D, Felicetti F, et al: MicroRNA-133 controls cardiac hypertrophy. Nat Med 13:613-668, 2007.
98. Cheng Y, Ji R, Yue J, et al: MicroRNAs are aberrantly expressed in hypertrophic heart: Do they play a role in cardiac hypertrophy? Am J Pathol 170:1831-1840, 2007.
99. Sayed D, Hong C, Chen IY, et al: MicroRNAs play an essential role in the development of cardiac hypertrophy. Circ Res 100:416-424, 2007.
100. Tatsuguchi M, Seok HY, Callis TE, et al: Expression of microRNAs is dynamically regulated during cardiomyocyte hypertrophy. J Mol Cell Cardiol 42:1137-1141, 2007.
101. Thum T, Galuppo P, Wolf C, et al: MicroRNAs in the human heart: A clue to fetal gene reprogramming in heart failure. Circulation 116:258-267, 2007.
102. van Rooij E, Sutherland LB, Liu N, et al: A signature pattern of stress-responsive microRNAs that can evoke cardiac hypertrophy and heart failure. Proc Natl Acad Sci U S A 103:18255-18260, 2006.
103. Ikeda S, Kong SW, Lu J, et al: Altered microRNA expression in human heart disease. Physiol Genomics 31:367-373, 2007. Epub 2007 Aug 21.
104. Yang B, Lin H, Xiao J, et al: The muscle-specific microRNA miR-1 regulates cardiac arrhythmogenic potential by targeting GJA1 and KCNJ2. Nat Med 13: 486-491, 2007.
105. Luo X, Xiao J, Lin H, et al: Transcriptional activation by stimulating protein 1 and post-transcriptional repression by muscle-specific microRNAs of I_{Ks}-encoding genes and potential implications in regional heterogeneity of their expressions. J Cell Physiol 212:358-367, 2007.
106. Hoffman BF, Guo SD, Feinmark SJ: Arrhythmias caused by platelet activating factor. J Cardiovasc Electrophysiol 7:120-133, 1996.
107. Hoffman BF, Feinmark SJ, Guo SD: Electrophysiologic effects of interactions between activated canine neutrophils and cardiac myocytes. J Cardiovasc Electrophysiol 8:679-687, 1997.
108. Fernandez-Velasco M, Ruiz-Hurtado G, Hurtado O, et al: TNF-alpha downregulates transient outward potassium current in rat ventricular myocytes through iNOS overexpression and oxidant species generation. Am J Physiol Heart Circ Physiol 293:H238-H245, 2007.
109. Hammerschmidt S, Wahn H: The effect of the oxidant hypochlorous acid on the L-type calcium current in isolated ventricular cardiomyocytes. J Mol Cell Cardiol 30:1855-1867, 1998.
110. Fearon IM, Palmer AC, Balmforth AJ, et al: Modulation of recombinant human cardiac L-type Ca^{2+} channel alpha1C subunits by redox agents and hypoxia. J Physiol 514:629-637, 1999.
111. Meng TC, Fukada T, Tonks NK: Reversible oxidation and inactivation of protein tyrosine phosphatases in vivo. Mol Cell 9:387-399, 2002.
112. Cross JV, Templeton DJ: Oxidative stress inhibits MEKK1 by site-specific glutathionylation in the ATP-binding domain. Biochem J 381:675-683, 2004.
113. Yu H, Gao J, Wang H, et al: Effects of the renin-angiotensin system on the current I(to) in epicardial and endocardial ventricular myocytes from the canine heart. Circ Res 86:1062-1068, 2000.
114. Clement-Chomienne O, Walsh MP, Cole WC: Angiotensin II activation of protein kinase C decreases delayed rectifier K^+ current in rabbit vascular myocytes. J Physiol 495:689-700, 1996.
115. Hool LC, Whalley DW, Doohan MM, Rasmussen HH: Angiotensin-converting enzyme inhibition, intracellular Na^+, and Na^+-K^+ pumping in cardiac myocytes. Am J Physiol 268:C366-C375, 1995.
116. Cao JM, Fishbein MC, Han JB, et al: Relationship between regional cardiac hyperinnervation and ventricular arrhythmia. Circulation 101:1960-1969, 2000.
117. Inoue H, Zipes DP: Results of sympathetic denervation in the canine heart: Supersensitivity that may be arrhythmogenic. Circulation 75:877-887, 1987.
118. January CT, Riddle JM: Early afterdepolarizations: Mechanism of induction and block. A role for L-type Ca^{2+} current. Circ Res 64:977-990, 1989.
119. Anderson ME, Braun AP, Wu Y, et al: KN-93, an inhibitor of multifunctional Ca^{++}/calmodulin-dependent protein kinase, decreases early afterdepolarizations in rabbit heart. J Pharmacol Exp Ther 287:996-1006, 1998.
120. Mazur A, Roden DM, Anderson ME: Systemic administration of calmodulin antagonist W-7 or protein kinase A inhibitor H-8 prevents torsade de pointes in rabbits. Circulation 100:2437-2442, 1999.
121. Khoo MS, Li J, Singh MV, et al: Death, cardiac dysfunction, and arrhythmias are increased by calmodulin kinase II in calcineurin cardiomyopathy. Circulation 114:1352-1359, 2006.
122. Kranias EG, Gupta RC, Jakab G, et al: The role of protein kinases and protein phosphatases in the regulation of cardiac sarcoplasmic reticulum function. Mol Cell Biochem 82:37-44, 1988.
123. Wu Y, Shintani A, Grueter C, et al: Suppression of dynamic Ca(2+) transient responses to pacing in ventricular myocytes from mice with genetic calmodulin kinase II inhibition. J Mol Cell Cardiol 40:213-223, 2006.
124. Zhang T, Maier LS, Dalton ND, et al: The deltaC isoform of CaMKII is activated in cardiac hypertrophy and induces dilated cardiomyopathy and heart failure. Circ Res 92:912-919, 2003.

125. Sicouri S, Antzelevitch C: Electrophysiologic characteristics of M cells in the canine left ventricular free wall. J Cardiovasc Electrophysiol 6:591-603, 1995.

126. Boyden PA, Pu J, Pinto J, Keurs HE: Ca(2+) transients and Ca(2+) waves in Purkinje cells: Role in action potential initiation. Circ Res 86:448-455, 2000.

127. Pogwizd SM, McKenzie JP, Cain ME: Mechanisms underlying spontaneous and induced ventricular arrhythmias in patients with idiopathic dilated cardiomyopathy. Circulation 98:2404-2414, 1998.

Ventricular Tachycardia in Patients after Surgery for Congenital Heart Disease 67

George F. Van Hare

CHAPTER OUTLINE

Background

Ventricular tachycardia and sudden cardiac death remain difficult management issues in patients who have undergone surgical repair of congenital heart defects. For the most part, the presenting life-threatening anatomic and hemodynamic abnormalities in these patients have been successfully managed by surgery, often years or decades before the occurrence of a fatal arrhythmia. In patients who have undergone major atrial surgery, such as the Mustard or Senning repair for transposition of the great vessels, atrial flutter with rapid conduction is certainly involved in the etiology of sudden death. Because of the frequent occurrence of premature ventricular contractions, however, nonsustained and sustained ventricular in patients who have undergone complete repair of tetralogy of Fallot and related defects such as double-outlet right ventricle, ventricular tachycardia has been implicated in the etiology of sudden death in this patient group. Postoperative tetralogy of Fallot is the most common condition seen in young patients with previous congenital heart disease who have experienced sudden death.

By far the most information concerning patients with ventricular tachycardia and congenital heart disease pertains to tetralogy of Fallot, as compared with other forms of congenital heart disease. Ventricular arrhythmias occur much more rarely in patients with other lesions.[1] For the purposes of management, however, tetralogy of Fallot can be viewed as a model for other lesions when patients with such lesions present with ventricular arrhythmias associated with previous ventriculotomy or in the setting of right ventricular dysfunction.

Controversy still exists regarding the relationship between ventricular arrhythmias and sudden death and the role of electrophysiologic testing and other procedures for risk stratification. Fundamentally, the correct management of postoperative patients with ventricular tachycardia is unclear. Unfortunately, as Bricker has pointed out, sufficient numbers of operated patients may not be available to permit an adequately powered cohort study to sort out the various likely predictors of sudden death.[2]

Anatomy and Surgical Technique

An appreciation of the changes in surgical technique that have taken place over the years is essential to an understanding of how patient age, age at repair, and method of repair may interact to increase the risk of arrhythmias. Complete repair of tetralogy of Fallot became quite common in older patients starting in the 1960s, and primary repair in infancy is now the current practice everywhere.

Tetralogy of Fallot is characterized by a ventricular septal defect with significant right ventricular outflow tract obstruction, leading to chronic cyanosis in the patient with an unrepaired defect. The placement of a systemic-to-pulmonary artery shunt as a palliative procedure causes some left ventricular volume overload. Correction of tetralogy of Fallot involves patch closure of the ventricular septal defect, with relief of right ventricular obstruction. In nearly all patients, this requires resection of a large amount of right ventricular muscle, often with a right ventriculotomy. The pulmonary annulus usually is small, and placement of a transannular patch leads to chronic pulmonic insufficiency, which may be very severe, particularly if it is associated with distal obstruction due to pulmonary arterial stenosis. It is likely that ventricular arrhythmias in these patients are due to the effect of years of chronic cyanosis, the presence of a ventriculotomy, elevation of right ventricular pressures due to inadequate relief of obstruction, and severe pulmonic regurgitation with right ventricular dysfunction. Over time, these factors are likely to lead to myocardial fibrosis, resulting in creation of the substrate for reentrant ventricular arrhythmias. This hypothesis is supported by the observation that fractionated electrograms and mid-diastolic potentials may be recorded from the right ventricle on electrophysiology studies, suggesting the presence of slow conduction. Although coronary artery abnormalities are present in 5% of cases of tetralogy of Fallot, putting the left anterior descending coronary artery or other large branches at risk at the time of complete repair, coronary artery injury has not been implicated in the etiology of ventricular arrhythmias or of sudden death.

Recent studies involving a porcine model of ventricular tachycardia may shed some light on mechanisms. Zeltser and associates showed that of the various factors involved in tetralogy of Fallot repair—ventriculotomy, right ventricular volume overload, and right ventricular pressure overload—volume overload is the most important as a predictor for inducible ventricular arrhythmias.[3] In their model, noncontact mapping shows that the right ventriculotomy supports the macro-reentrant circuit, with diastolic activation demonstrable along the margin.[4]

Invasive electrophysiology studies in patients with clinically occurring ventricular tachycardia after tetralogy repair have found that the mechanism of ventricular tachycardia is reentry involving the right ventricular outflow tract, either at the site of anterior right ventriculotomy or at the site of a ventricular septal defect patch. Transient entrainment can be documented, with constant fusion at the paced cycle length and progressive fusion at decreasing cycle lengths, and the evaluation of postpacing intervals strongly suggests that sites in the right ventricular outflow tract are part of a macro-reentrant circuit.

Spontaneous Occurrence of Ventricular Arrhythmias

Early reports noted the frequent occurrence of premature ventricular contractions in patients who had previously undergone repair of tetralogy of Fallot. With Holter monitoring, frequency is reported to be as high as 48%.[5] In approximately one half of these patients, ventricular ectopy is complex, defined as multiform beats, couplets, or ventricular tachycardia. In the great majority of patients, this ventricular ectopy is entirely asymptomatic.

Many investigators have tried to correlate the incidence of ventricular ectopy with various factors, including age at presentation, age at time of repair, and various hemodynamic features. Four factors seem most important: age at initial repair, time since repair, presence of residual right ventricular obstruction, and presence of significant pulmonic insufficiency. Older age at time of operation, especially beyond 10 years of age, has been associated with nearly a 100% incidence of ventricular arrhythmias, regardless of follow-up interval. Garson and colleagues, in a study of 488 patients with repaired tetralogy of Fallot, showed that the incidence of ventricular arrhythmias was closely related to right ventricular hemodynamics.[6] The incidence of ventricular arrhythmias was significantly higher in patients with right ventricular systolic pressure greater than 60 mm Hg and in those with a right ventricular end-diastolic pressure greater than 8 mm Hg, suggesting that residual right ventricular outflow tract obstruction, as well as pulmonic insufficiency, negatively influences outcome. These investigators also found a relationship to age at surgery, but this was not as important as the follow-up interval. Their observations have been confirmed in other, subsequent studies, which have emphasized the importance of pulmonic insufficiency.

The observation of the importance of right ventricular dysfunction in the etiology of sudden death after tetralogy repair highlights the need for a good assessment tool. The evaluation of right ventricular function by echocardiography has always been problematic, and a more reproducible method of right ventricular functional assessment is desirable. Recently, much progress has been made in the use of cardiac magnetic resonance imaging (MRI) for the evaluation of right ventricular function in such patients.[7,8] At present, most large congenital heart centers use this modality for postoperative follow-up assessment. In a large study by Knauth and associates, a right ventricular ejection fraction measured by cardiac MRI was a predictor for long-term adverse outcomes, including ventricular tachycardia.[9] A closer correlation between MRI findings and actual arrhythmia risk is lacking to date, however, and the increasingly frequent use of pacemakers and implantable cardioverter-defibrillators (ICDs) in this population precludes the use of MRI in some patients.

As a subset of ventricular arrhythmias, spontaneously occurring sustained ventricular tachycardia is, in fact, fairly uncommon among patients who have undergone surgical repair of their tetralogy defects. The best data in this regard come from a report by Harrison and associates of patients with repaired tetralogy of Fallot attending an adult congenital heart disease clinic.[10] Eighteen of 210 patients (8.6%) had either documented sustained ventricular tachycardia or syncope or near-syncope with palpitations and inducible sustained monomorphic ventricular tachycardia on electrophysiologic testing. Ventricular tachycardia was closely related to right ventricular hemodynamics—in particular, to right ventricular outflow tract aneurysms and pulmonic insufficiency.

Inducible Ventricular Tachycardia and Sudden Death

The occasional but persistent observation of sudden unexpected death in this group of patients with repaired congenital heart disease, along with the high incidence of spontaneously occurring ventricular arrhythmias, both simple and complex, has lead to the hypothesis that sudden death in such patients is due to ventricular tachycardia. In some patients, this dysrhythmia has been observed to quickly progress to ventricular fibrillation. Furthermore, the residual hemodynamic abnormalities in congenital heart disease patients, and especiallly those with tetralogy of Fallot, are important because they make any given ventricular tachycardida less well tolerated.[11] In the past, attempts to prevent the occurrence of sudden death have logically been directed at suppressing ventricular arrhythmias, either ventricular ectopy occurring spontaneously or ventricular tachycardia inducible on electrophysiologic testing. A standard practice was to perform such studies in a large proportion of patients who had undergone repair of tetralogy of Fallot or related congenital defects, in an attempt to identify inducible sustained monomorphic ventricular tachycardia. Nearly all such patients were asymptomatic in terms of arrhythmias. Antiarrhythmic drug therapy often was prescribed on the basis of results of such studies. This approach has, for the most part, fallen out of favor, owing to the lack of strong evidence supporting the proposition that sudden death can be prevented with this strategy. Furthermore, the possibility of a proarrhythmic effect of the antiarrhythmic medications chosen for treatment has not been adequately evaluated.

The results of invasive electrophysiologic testing in a large number of patients with repaired tetralogy of Fallot are disturbing in that ventricular tachycardia can be induced in a large proportion, nearly all of who have never had a clinical episode of ventricular tachycardia. Early reports, coupled with the data of Garson and colleagues suggesting a direct link between ventricular arrhythmias and sudden death, lead to the widespread use of invasive electrophysiologic testing in largely asymptomatic patients, with subsequent antiarrhythmic treatment, often with repeated electrophysiology studies to guide therapy. Subsequent examination of the results of this approach have not supported its utility, however. In a large multicenter review, Chandar and coworkers reported the experience with 359 postoperative tetralogy of Fallot patients who underwent invasive electrophysiologic testing.[5] Ventricular tachycardia could be induced in 17% of patients, but not in any patient who was asymptomatic and had normal findings on a 24-hour electrocardiogram. Although late sudden death occurred in 5 patients, none of these patients had inducible ventricular tachycardia on electrophysiologic testing.

Subsequently, Kairy and colleagues reported the results of a multicenter study of patients with repaired tetralogy of Fallot who underwent programmed stimulation.[12] These results, in a group of pediatric and adult patients whose surgical repair was performed in a later era compared with those in the report of Chandar and coworkers, are somewhat more promising. In this later study, the positive predictive value of inducibility of ventricular tachycardia on electrophysiologic testing was 55% for predicting clinical ventricular tachycardia or sudden cardiac death. The negative predictive value was 91.5%. The findings

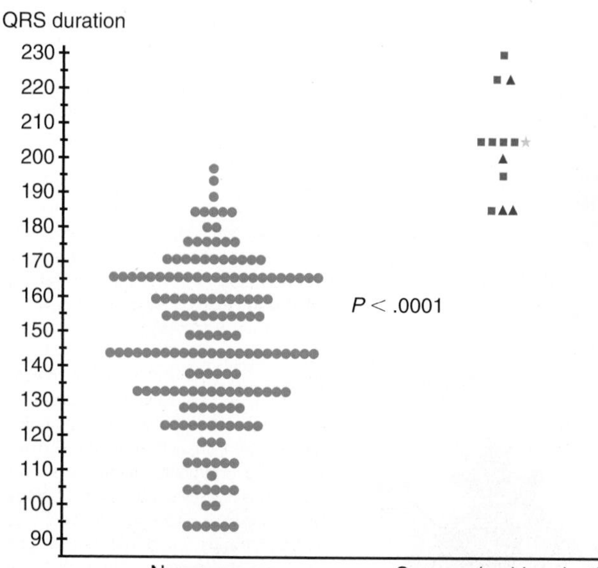

Figure 67-1 Plot of QRS duration in 182 patients with previously repaired tetralogy of Fallot. Those with syncope and ventricular tachycardia (*squares*), sudden death (*triangles*), and syncope with atrial flutter (*star*) are plotted separately. (From Gatzoulis MA, Till JA, Redington AN: Depolarization-repolarization inhomogeneity after repair of tetralogy of Fallot. The substrate for malignant ventricular tachycardia? Circulation 95:401-404, 1997.)

of both of these large multicenter studies question the rationale behind aggressive diagnostic investigation in patients who are asymptomatic, although the study by Khairy and colleagues suggests that negative results on electrophsiologic testing may be reassuring.

It is now clear that the risk of ventricular tachycardia can be assessed from the surface electrocardiogram QRS duration. Gatzoulis and associates found that in a group of 48 well-studied postoperative tetralogy patients, those with a QRS duration longer than 180 ms had a greatly increased risk of spontaneous ventricular tachycardia or sudden death[13] (Fig. 67-1). The mechanism underlying this correlation is uncertain. Certainly, patients with corrected tetralogy of Fallot usually have a right bundle branch block, with resulting QRS prolongation. Excessive QRS prolongation in such patients may be a marker for the degree of pulmonic insufficiency and right ventricular volume overload, as has been established by studies of the effect of pulmonary valve replacement in patients with prolonged QRS duration.[14]

The incidence of sudden death is in fact much lower than was previously feared and may in fact be falling, owing to earlier age at surgery and improvements in surgical technique. As indicated by some evidence, however, it may increase at late follow-up. In a careful study of 490 survivors of tetralogy of Fallot repair at a single center, Nollert and coworkers constructed actuarial survival curves out to 36 years after surgery.[15] They found that the yearly actuarial mortality rate during the first 25 years was 0.24% per year but increased dramatically after 25 years to 0.94% per year. Mortality in most cases was related to sudden death. Mortality also was related to date of operation (highest rates were observed for series from before 1970), the degree of preoperative polycythemia (highest with hematocrit greater than 48), and the use of a right ventricular outflow tract patch (highest with a patch). The last factor certainly is related to the presence of pulmonic insufficiency, as noted earlier.

The importance of pulmonic insufficiency as a risk factor has led to some interest in a more aggressive strategy for reoperation to correct the insufficiency.[16] Certainly, such a strategy will reduce right ventricular volume overload and halt the progression of QRS prolongation, but it is not yet certain whether this approach will have an effect on the incidence of serious ventricular arrhythmias.[17]

Treatment of Ventricular Tachycardia in the Postoperative Patient

The treatment decision in patients with ventricular ectopy after correction of congenital heart disease may be directed at one or both of two goals: the prevention of sudden death and the suppression or termination of symptomatic episodes of ventricular tachycardia. Treatment may involve antiarrhythmic medication, radiofrequency catheter ablation, surgical cryoablation, or implantation of a tiered-therapy device providing antitachycardia pacing and cardioversion-defibrillation.

It is difficult to know which patients merit electrophysiologic study or treatment, or both. In view of the fact that no prospective studies have been performed demonstrating that sudden death can be prevented in any group of postoperative patients by treatment of any type, routine electrophysiologic study and treatment of a majority of asymptomatic patients with ventricular ectopy cannot be recommmended. Although it is possible that certain subgroups exist in which carefully chosen antiarrhythmic therapy may exert a beneficial effect in lowering mortality, another possibility is the existence of subgroups for which the proarrhythmic potential of antiarrhythmic medications more than counters any beneficial effect. Until such prospective, controlled trials are performed, therapy with drugs such as flecainide, quinidine, and sotalol cannot be recommended for most asymptomatic patients.

If ventricular tachycardia is easily inducible and well tolerated hemodynamically, radiofrequency ablation may be considered. Because most evidence supports the concept of macro-reentry as the mechanism of such well-tolerated ventricular tachycardia, the use of entrainment pacing and mapping techniques is indicated. A number of investigators have reported successful procedures using radiofrequency energy in the setting of well-tolerated inducible monomorphic ventricular trachycardia.[18] Many patients have more poorly tolerated arrhythmias, however, and are not candidates for this approach. At least one group of investigators has addressed this problem by targeting areas of delayed electrogram activity, reasoning that these areas of mid-diastolic activity are likely to be involved in the macro-reentrant circuit.[19]

A more involved method is the use of dynamic substrate mapping to define the anatomic and electrophysiologic substrate without the need for mapping during tachycardia. Zeppenfield and colleagues in particular have reported the utility of electroanatomic voltage mapping, combined with unipolar high-output pacing, to identify areas of scar in the right ventricle[20] (Fig. 67-2). These investigators showed that in patients with tetralogy of Fallot, congenital and surgical anatomy combine to create a number of predictable ventricular tachycardia circuits, in which surgically created lines of block serve as barriers to constrain conduction (Fig. 67-3)—a situation similar to that seen in patients with postoperative atrial tachycardia. This finding is exciting because it supports an approach to mapping and ablation that does not require mapping during ventricular tachycardia and further suggests a

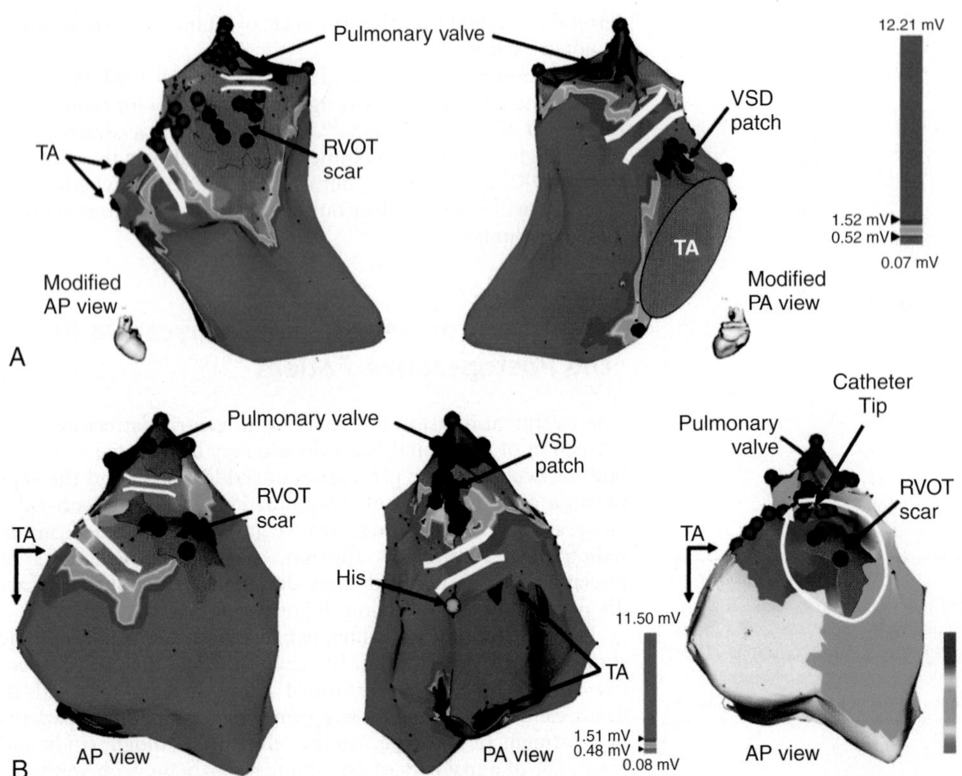

Figure 67-2 **A,** Voltage maps of right ventricle (RV) in a modified anteroposterior (AP) view and a modified posteroanterior (PA) view in a patient with tetralogy of Fallot. Three anatomic isthmuses were delineated (*white lines*). In this patient, isthmus 1 is bordered by the pulmonary valve and right ventricular outflow tract (RVOT) scar. No muscular rim is present between the ventricular septal defect (VSD) patch and the tricuspid annulus (TA). Linear ablation lesions (*red tags*) transect anatomic isthmus 1. **B,** Voltage maps of RV in an AP view (*left*) and a PA view (*center*) in another patient with tetralogy of Fallot. In contrast with **A,** a muscular rim is present between the VSD patch and the TA. An activation map of VT3 is seen in an AP view (*right*). Activation time is color-coded; the activation time (270 ms) equals the ventricular tachycardia cycle length. The macro-reentrant circuit propagates clockwise around the RVOT scar through isthmus 2 and inferiorly to superiorly through isthmus 1. The catheter tip indicates the termination site. (From Zeppenfeld K, Schalij MJ, Bartelings MM, et al: Catheter ablation of ventricular tachycardia after repair of congenital heart disease: Electroanatomic identification of the critical right ventricular isthmus. Circulation 116:2241-2252, 2007.)

means of preventing the creation of such circuits at the time of initial surgical repair.

Using a similar dynamic substrate mapping approach but applying noncontact mapping technology (EnSite system, St. Jude medical, St. Paul, MN), Kriebel and associates reported their experience with 10 repaired-tetralogy patients with ventricular tachycardia.[21] Mapping unipolar voltage in sinus rhythm, the anatomic features are first outlined, and areas of low voltage can be defined, suggesting channels between areas of low-voltage patch or scar that may potentially support macro-reentry (Fig. 67-4). Noncontact mapping during ventricular tachycardia is then used to confirm the target for subsequent ablation, which in this series was performed with standard radiofrequency ablation catheters, with a high success rate.

Several investigators have reported on intraoperative mapping. In particular, Downer and coworkers have performed intraoperative mapping of the right ventricular outflow tract in the beating heart, using an endocardial electrode balloon and a simultaneous epicardial electrode sock array.[22] Ablation was carried out by cryotherapy lesioning during normothermic cardiopulmonary bypass with the heart beating, or during anoxic arrest, with good success in three patients. Other investigators

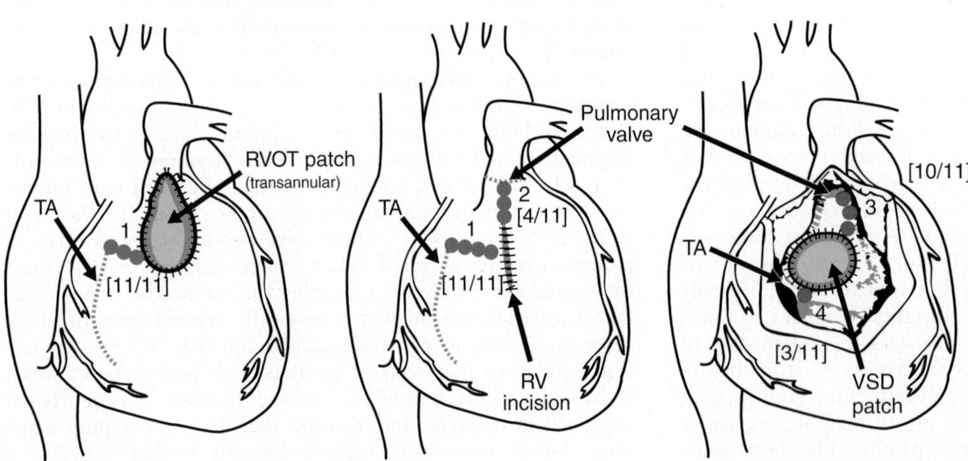

Figure 67-3 Schematic of the localization of anatomic boundaries for ventricular tachycardia after repair of congenital heart disease and the resulting anatomic isthmuses. Frequencies of the distinct isthmuses in 11 patients are shown in *brackets*. RV, right ventricular; RVOT, right ventricular outflow tract; TA, tricuspid annulus; VSD, ventricular septal defect. (From Zeppenfeld K, Schalij MJ, Bartelings MM, et al: Catheter ablation of ventricular tachycardia after repair of congenital heart disease: Electroanatomic identification of the critical right ventricular isthmus. Circulation 116:2241-2252, 2007.)

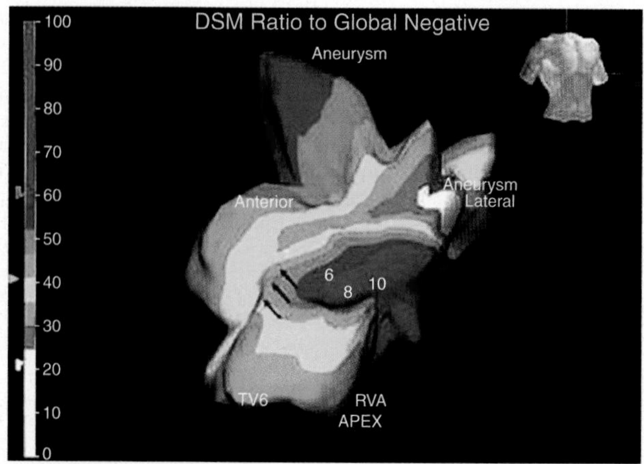

Figure 67-4 Dynamic substrate map (DSM) of the right ventricle in a patient with tetralogy of Fallot, during sinus rhythm. Geometry of the right ventricle has been reconstructed (30-degree right anterior oblique view). The scale on the *left* shows the ratio of the peak negative voltage through the cardiac cycle. Negative voltage is displayed on the endocardial surface, with *white* illustrating low peak negative voltage (less than 25% of the largest unipolar deflection) and *purple* the most negative peak voltage (greater than 57.5%). Two areas of low peak negative voltage (less than 35%) are identified: between the right anterior wall and the right ventricular outflow tract and between the tricuspid valve annulus and the right ventricular apex. The presence of a critical channel of electrical conduction can be suspected between the two low-voltage areas (*arrows*). Aneurysm, right ventricular outflow tract aneurysm; anterior, anterior right ventricular free wall; Lateral, right ventricular lateral wall; RVA/Apex, right ventricular apex; TV6, tricuspid valve annulus at 6 o'clock position; 6 to 10, localization of virtual catheter electrograms. (From Kriebel T, Saul JP, Schneider H, et al: Noncontact mapping and radiofrequency catheter ablation of fast and hemodynamically unstable ventricular tachycardia after surgical repair of tetralogy of Fallot. J Am Coll Cardiol 50:2162-2168, 2007.)

also have reported success with similar techniques,[23] particularly when the surgery takes place at centers with a great deal of experience in arrhythmia surgery for all forms of congenital heart disease.[24]

Implantable cardioverter-defibrillators (ICDs) are becoming first-line treatment for patients with ventricular tachycardia after repair of congenital heart disease, for both secondary and primary prevention indications. Apart from the technical issues regarding implantation of ICDs in such patients relating to venous access and venous anomalies, the issue of patient selection for this therapy is controversial. Clearly, patients who meet the usual criteria (e.g., cardiac arrest due to ventricular arrhythmia, recurrent poorly tolerated sustained ventricular tachycardia) are candidates for ICD implantation for secondary prevention. Whether other patients are candidates for primary prevention is less clear. For example, should patients with some risk factors for sudden death but without clinically documented cardiac arrest or poorly tolerated ventricular tachycardia be considered for this strategy? A case can be made for use of this approach in certain types of patients. One hypothetical example is that of a patient who has undergone repair for tetralogy of Fallot and postoperatively has pulmonic insufficiency, poor right ventricular function, and frequent ventricular ectopy, and who has experienced syncope but has had a negative result on electrophysiology studies. In many centers, such a patient will be offered an ICD as primary prevention. In the multicenter study of Khairy and colleagues,[25] nearly half of all ICDs in patients with tetralogy of Fallot were implanted for primary prevention, and the annual actuarial rate of appropriate shock was as high in the primary prevention group (7.7%) as in the secondary prevention group (9.8%). This finding suggests that the currently accepted risk factors for sudden death in patients with tetralogy of Fallot are likely to be appropriate.

References

1. Vetter VL, Horowitz LN: Electrophysiologic residua and sequelae of surgery for congenital heart defects. Am J Cardiol 50:588-604, 1982.
2. Bricker JT: Sudden death and tetralogy of Fallot. Risks, markers, and causes. Circulation 92:158-159, 1995.
3. Zeltser I, Gaynor JW, Petko M, et al: The roles of chronic pressure and volume overload states in induction of arrhythmias: An animal model of physiologic sequelae after repair of tetralogy of Fallot. J Thorac Cardiovasc Surg 130:1542-1548, 2005.
4. Kaltman JR, Gillespie MJ, Seymour T, et al: Substrate characterization of ventricular tachycardia in a porcine model of tetralogy of Fallot using noncontact mapping. Pacing Clin Electrophysiol 30:1316-1322, 2007.
5. Chandar JS, Wolff GS, Garson A Jr, et al: Ventricular arrhythmias in postoperative tetralogy of Fallot. Am J Cardiol 65:655-661, 1990.
6. Garson A Jr, Randall DC, Gillette PC, et al: Prevention of sudden death after repair of tetralogy of Fallot: Treatment of ventricular arrhythmias. J Am Coll Cardiol 6:221-227, 1985.
7. Norton KI, Tong C, Glass RB, Nielsen JC: Cardiac MR imaging assessment following tetralogy of Fallot repair. Radiographics 26:197-211, 2006.
8. van Straten A, Vliegen HW, Hazekamp MG, de Roos A: Right ventricular function late after total repair of tetralogy of Fallot. Eur Radiol 15:702-707, 2005.
9. Knauth AL, Gauvreau K, Powell AJ, et al: Ventricular size and function assessed by cardiac MRI predict major adverse clinical outcomes late after tetralogy of Fallot repair. Heart 94:211-216, 2008.
10. Harrison DA, Harris L, Siu SC, et al: Sustained ventricular tachycardia in adult patients late after repair of tetralogy of Fallot. J Am Coll Cardiol 30:1368-1373, 1997.
11. Ohuchi H, Ohashi H, Watanabe K, et al: Blood pressure dynamics during simulated ventricular tachycardia in patients after right ventricular outflow tract reconstruction mainly for tetralogy of Fallot compared with patients after ventricular septal defect closure. Am J Cardiol 93:1445-1448, A1412, 2004.
12. Khairy P, Landzberg MJ, Gatzoulis MA, et al: Value of programmed ventricular stimulation after tetralogy of Fallot repair: A multicenter study. Circulation 109:1994-2000, 2004.
13. Gatzoulis MA, Till JA, Somerville J, Redington AN: Mechanoelectrical interaction in tetralogy of Fallot. QRS prolongation relates to right ventricular size and predicts malignant ventricular arrhythmias and sudden death. Circulation 92:231-237, 1995.
14. Oosterhof T, Vliegen HW, Meijboom FJ, et al: Long-term effect of pulmonary valve replacement on QRS duration in patients with corrected tetralogy of Fallot. Heart 93:506-509, 2007.
15. Nollert G, Fischlein T, Bouterwek S, et al: Long-term survival in patients with repair of tetralogy of Fallot: 36-year follow-up of 490 survivors of the first year after surgical repair. J Am Coll Cardiol 30:1374-1383, 1997.
16. Gengsakul A, Harris L, Bradley TJ, et al: The impact of pulmonary valve replacement after tetralogy of Fallot repair: A matched comparison. Eur J Cardiothorac Surg 32:462-468, 2007.
17. Warner KG, O'Brien PK, Rhodes J, et al: Expanding the indications for pulmonary valve replacement after repair of tetralogy of Fallot. Ann Thorac Surg 76:1066-1071, 2003.
18. Rostock T, Willems S, Ventura R, et al: Radiofrequency catheter ablation of a macroreentrant ventricular tachycardia late after surgical repair of tetralogy of Fallot using the electroanatomic mapping (CARTO). Pacing Clin Electrophysiol 27:801-804, 2004.

19. Arenal A, Glez-Torrecilla E, Ortiz M, et al: Ablation of electrograms with an isolated, delayed component as treatment of unmappable monomorphic ventricular tachycardias in patients with structural heart disease. J Am Coll Cardiol 41:81-92, 2003.
20. Zeppenfeld K, Schalij MJ, Bartelings MM, et al: Catheter ablation of ventricular tachycardia after repair of congenital heart disease: Electroanatomic identification of the critical right ventricular isthmus. Circulation 116:2241-2252, 2007.
21. Kriebel T, Saul JP, Schneider H, et al: Noncontact mapping and radiofrequency catheter ablation of fast and hemodynamically unstable ventricular tachycardia after surgical repair of tetralogy of Fallot. J Am Coll Cardiol 50:2162-2168, 2007.
22. Downar E, Harris L, Kimber S, et al: Ventricular tachycardia after surgical repair of tetralogy of Fallot: Results of intraoperative mapping studies. J Am Coll Cardiol 20:648-655, 1992.
23. Karamlou T, Silber I, Lao R, et al: Outcomes after late reoperation in patients with repaired tetralogy of Fallot: The impact of arrhythmia and arrhythmia surgery. Ann Thorac Surg 81:1786-1793, 2006.
24. Deal BJ, Mavroudis C, Backer CL: Beyond Fontan conversion: Surgical therapy of arrhythmias including patients with associated complex congenital heart disease. Ann Thorac Surg 76:542-553, 2003.
25. Khairy P, Harris L, Landzberg MJ, et al: Implantable cardioverter-defibrillators in tetralogy of Fallot. Circulation 117:363-370, 2008. Epub 2008 Jan 2.

The Brugada Syndrome 68

Tim Boussy, Ramon Brugada, Josep Brugada, and Pedro Brugada

CHAPTER OUTLINE

Overview

In 1992, Brugada syndrome was introduced as a new clinical entity linking typical, but variable, ST segment changes in the right precordial electrocardiographic leads to an increased vulnerability for lethal ventricular arrhythmias. In the affected patients, no structural heart disease could be identified despite thorough invasive and noninvasive investigation. Brugada syndrome is a genetically transmissible disease manifesting as an autosomal dominant and age-dependent trait.

Multiple cohorts of patients with the disorder have been reported throughout the world. In the Asian cohorts, patients in whom the arrhythmias proved to be fatal previously had been thought to have *sudden unexplained death syndrome* (SUDS). Being one of the major causes of sudden cardiac death in young persons, Brugada syndrome has gained much international interest. In particular, the search for reliable predictors of arrhythmic events has been at the center of attention. By general agreement, symptomatic patients with Brugada syndrome should receive protection by surgical placement of an implantable cardioverter-defibrillator (ICD). Patients presenting with a diagnostic Brugada syndrome electrocardiogram (ECG) at baseline conditions have an increased risk for sudden death and need further assessment. The role of electrophysiology studies in further risk stratification of asymptomatic patients with Brugada syndrome remains controversial.

Up till now, more than 80 causative gene mutations have been identified, mostly located on the *SCN5A* gene, encoding the pore-forming α subunit of the cardiac sodium channel. The tremendous phenotypic variations within families and the overlap with other channelopathies illustrate the complex genetic heterogeneity underlying this syndrome.

Diagnosis

The diagnosis of Brugada syndrome is based on clinical and electrocardiographic features. Patients present with syncope or (aborted) sudden cardiac death due to malignant ventricular arrhythmias. No apparent structural heart disease can be found. The hallmark of Brugada syndrome is the transient appearance of typical ECG changes in the right precordial leads. The second Brugada Syndrome Consensus Report of 2005 (endorsed by the Heart Rhythm Society and the European Heart Rhythm Association)[1] stated the current recommendations regarding the diagnostic criteria. Three different ECG patterns (Fig. 68-1), all featuring ST segment elevation in the right precordial leads, have been recognized: Type I is the only pattern that is diagnostic for Brugada syndrome. It consists of a coved-type ST segment elevation greater than 2 mm, followed by a descending negative T wave in at least one right precordial lead (V_1 to V_3). Type II and type IIII are saddleback-shaped patterns, with a high initial augmentation followed by an ST elevation greater than 2 mm for type II and less than 2 mm for type III. Both patterns are suggestive of but not diagnostic for Brugada syndrome.

Recent studies illustrate the dynamic character of these ECG patterns.[2,3] Whenever a large number of baseline ECGs were available during follow-up, the diagnostic pattern could be documented in only approximately 25% of the tracings. Because the presence of the spontaneous coved-type (type I) ECG pattern is thought to be a useful predictor of future arrhythmic events in asymptomatic patients, these findings are of great clinical importance. The class IC antiarrhythmic drug test provided a tool to unmask these concealed forms.[4] Intravenous administration of ajmaline, flecainide, or procainamide was able to elicit the diagnostic coved-type Brugada syndrome ECG pattern (Fig. 68-2). On the basis of the results of comparative studies[5] and clinical experience, ajmaline, in a dose of 1 mg/kg, is considered to be the preferred drug. Recently, the full stomach drug test was proposed as an alternative tool in diagnosing Brugada syndrome.[6] Here, the ST segment changes appear to be provoked by an enhanced vagal tone. Adrenergic stimulation decreases the ST segment elevation, whereas vagal stimulation worsens it. Obviously, it is important to exclude other causes of ST segment elevation before making the diagnosis of Brugada syndrome. These other causes are shown in Table 68-1.

The episodes of syncope and sudden death (aborted or not) are caused by fast polymorphic ventricular tachycardia or ventricular fibrillation. These arrhythmias appear with no warning. Only a very few cases manifest alternation of long-short sequences before the onset of polymorphic ventricular tachycardia, a finding common in other arrhythmias, such as torsade de pointes in the long QT syndrome. Also absent is any preceding acceleration of the heart rate, as occurs in the case of catecholamine-dependent polymorphic ventricular tachycardia (Chapter 70), an arrhythmia caused by mutations in the ryanodine receptor.

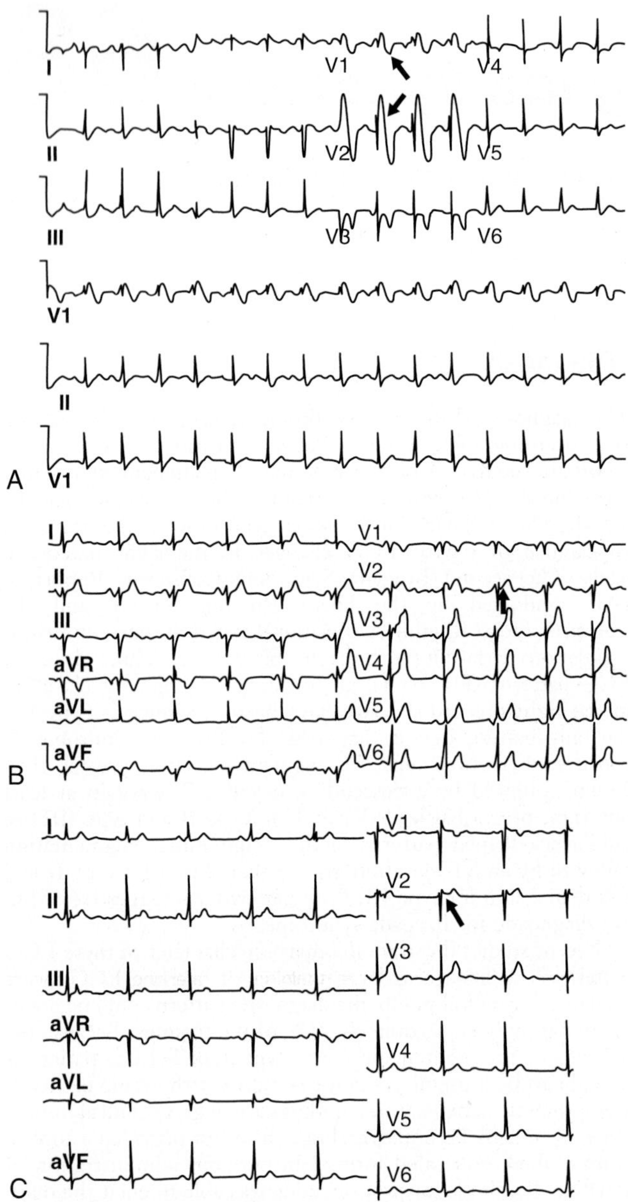

Figure 68-1 Brugada electrocardiogram (ECG) patterns. **A,** A diagnostic coved-type (type I) Brugada ECG pattern documented in a 9-year-old girl who presented with syncope and positive family history of Brugada syndrome. Note the pattern resembling a right bundle branch block *(arrows)* in leads V_1 and V_2, with typical ST elevation. **B,** Baseline ECG of a 58-year-old asymptomatic man with positive family history of Brugada syndrome. Example of a type II saddleback Brugada ECG pattern. Genetic analysis revealed a mutation in the *SCN5A* gene. Note the saddleback-shaped patterns, with a high initial augmentation followed by an ST elevation greater than 2 mm in lead V_2. **C,** Example of a baseline type III saddleback Brugada ECG pattern *(arrow)* documented in a 61-year-old asymptomatic man who was diagnosed on the basis of a positive result on class IC antiarrhythmic drug testing.

Historical Background

The first patient with Brugada syndrome was seen in 1986. This patient, a 3-year-old Polish boy, had been resuscitated multiple times by his father. Of interest, many of the episodes occurred during febrile illness. His sister had died suddenly at age 2 years after multiple episodes of aborted sudden death. The ECGs of the two siblings were very similar and abnormal. The identification of two additional patients allowed presentation of the preliminary data at the meeting of the North American Society of Pacing and Electrophysiology (NASPE) in 1991. The first paper, including 8 patients, was published in 1992.[7] Since then, an exponential increase has occurred in the number of patients recognized all over the world. Other investigators reported ECG patterns similar to the one presented in Figure 68-1. These were, however, considered to represent variants of the normal ECG, and no definitive link to sudden death was established.

Indigenous populations of Asia knew about the problem for many decades. In the Philippines, the problem was known as *bangungut* (scream followed by sudden death during sleep) and, in Japan, as *pokkuri* (unexpected sudden death at night). In Thailand, this form of death is known as *lai tai* (death during sleep), or SUDS.[8] In 1997 it was discovered that these patients suffer from a syndrome identical to Brugada syndrome. Mutations identified in these Thai men with SUDS are the same as in Brugada syndrome.

Incidence and Distribution

Because the syndrome has been identified only recently, it is difficult to ascertain its incidence and distribution worldwide. On analysis of the data from the various published studies, the disease is seen to be responsible for 4% to 12% of unexpected sudden deaths and for up to 50% of all sudden deaths in patients with an apparently normal heart.

With present data, the disease seems to be spread all over the world, which is not surprising in view of the high mobility of the population and the genetic basis of the disease. In the future, a sizable increase in the number of identified cases may be expected as recognition of the disease grows. A prospective study[9] of an adult Japanese population (22,027 subjects) showed an incidence of 0.05% of ECG patterns compatible with the syndrome (12 subjects). A second study of adults in Awa[10] (Japan) showed an incidence of 0.6% (66 cases in 10,420). However, a third study of children from Japan showed an incidence of ECG patterns compatible with the syndrome of only 0.0006% (1 case in 63,110).[11] These results suggest that the syndrome manifests primarily during adulthood, which is in concordance with the mean age of victims of sudden death (35 to 40 years).

Etiology and Genetics

In the past decade, an enormous amount of data has been gathered concerning the genetic aspects of Brugada syndrome. Brugada syndrome is inherited as an autosomal dominant trait with variable and probably age-dependent expression. In 1998, the first identified gene mutation was located on the *SCN5A* gene,[12] encoding the pore-forming α subunit of the cardiac sodium channel (Fig. 68-3). Currently, more than 70 *SCN5A* mutations have been linked to Brugada syndrome, all creating an impaired sodium influx. This is caused by alteration of the trafficking or gating function of the cardiac sodium channel. In 2002, Weiss and coworkers[13] located a second locus on chromosome 3. These same investigators reported mutations in the glycerol-3-phosphate dehydrogenase 1-like (GDP1-L) gene[14] causing a decreased expression of *SCN5A* products in the cardiac cell membrane. Furthermore, loss-of-function mutations in genes encoding the cardiac L-type calcium channel have been linked to Brugada syndrome phenotypes combined with shorter-than-normal QT intervals.[15]

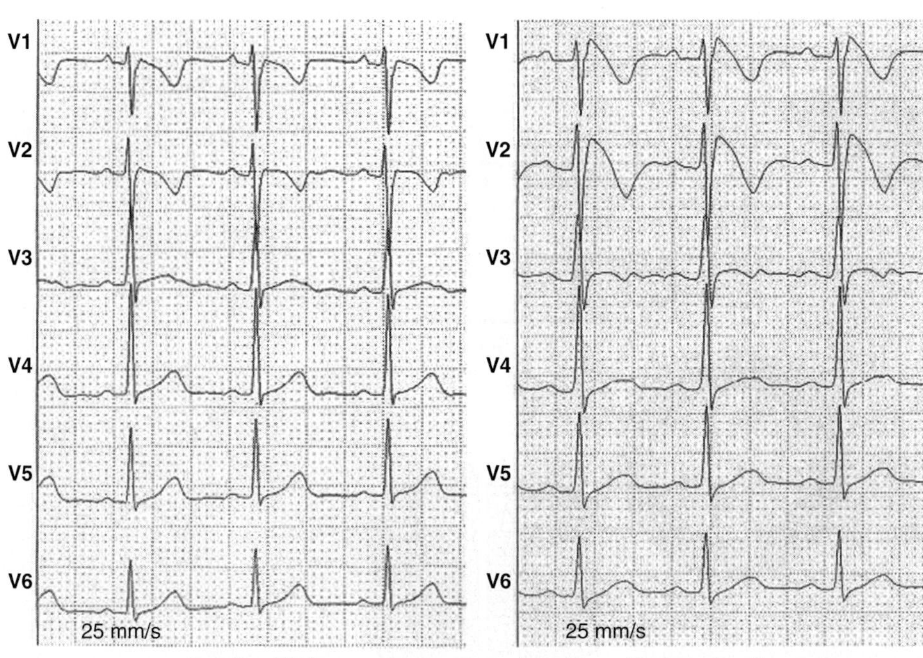

Figure 68-2 Induction of a diagnostic coved-type (type I) electrocardiogram (ECG) by administration of a sodium channel–blocking agent. See text for details of the ajmaline test.

Table 68-1 Acquired Brugada Syndrome: Differential Diagnosis of ST Segment Elevation in Electrocardiogram Leads V_1 and V_2

Drugs	Antiarrhythmic drugs	• Class 1C sodium channel blockers (e.g., flecainide, pilsicainide, propafenone) • Class 1A sodium channel blockers (e.g., procainamide, disopyramide, cibenzoline) • Verapamil (L-type calcium channel blocker) • Beta-blockers (inhibit $I_{Ca,L}$)
	Antianginal drugs	• Nitrates • Calcium channel blockers (e.g., nifedipine, diltiazem)
	Psychotropic agents	• Tricyclic antidepressants (e.g., amitriptiline, desipramine, clomipramine, nortriptyline) • Tetracyclic antidepressants (e.g., maprotiline) • Phenothiazines (e.g., perphenazine, cyamemazine) • Selective serotonine uptake inhibitors (e.g., fluoxetine) • Cocaine intoxication
	Antiallergic agents	• Histamine H1 antihistaminics. First-generation (dimenhydrinate)
Acute ischemia in RVOT		
Electrolyte disturbances	Hyperkalemia Hypercalcemia	
Hyperthermia and hypothermia		
Elevated insulin level		
Mechanical compression of RVOT		

RVOT, right ventricular outflow tract.

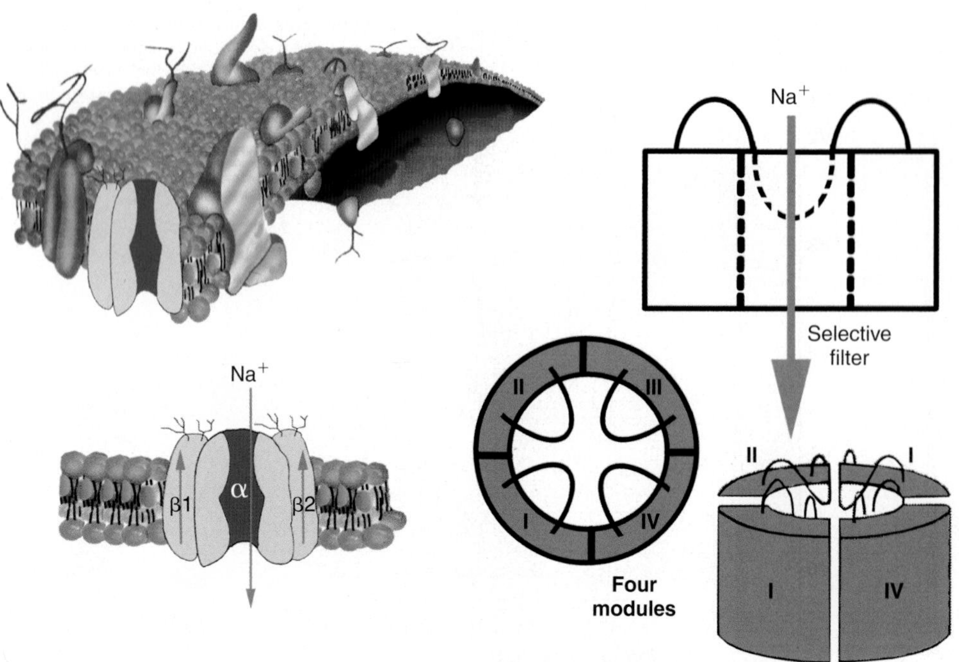

Figure 68-3 The cardiac sodium channel. *Upper and lower left*, Tridimensional illustration of sodium channels incorporated in the bilipid cardiac celmembrane; *upper right*, transmembrane segment with selective filtering; *lower right*, clockwise arrangement of four internal domains. The trafficking properties in this pore-forming unit are deficient in patients with Brugada syndrome.

The loss of function *SCN5A* mutations also have been described as being responsible for Lev-Lenègre disease, or progressive cardiac conduction defect. This phenotypic overlap is illustrated by the frequent occurrence of conduction abnormalities in patients with Brugada syndrome. Probst and associates studied these conduction abnormalities in a cohort of 78 patients with *SCN5A*-positive Brugada syndrome.[16] These workers observed significant PR and QRS prolongation in a majority of gene carriers, in comparison with the *SCN5A*-negative family members. *SCN5A* previously was shown to be the cause of LQT3, a form of Romano-Ward long QT syndrome. The differences in the clinical findings between LQT3 and Brugada syndrome are due to the different biophysical features dictated by the position of the mutations within the gene. Unlike the Brugada syndrome, LQT3 occurs as a result of an augmentation of late I_{Na} carried by *SCN5A* channels.

Despite the differences between long QT syndrome and Brugada syndrome, important similarities should be noted. In particular, both of these disorders in which life-threatening ventricular tachyarrhythmias (tachycardias) occur are due to mutations in genes encoding ion channels. Nowadays, these inherited primary electrical disorders are called *channelopathies*. This group also includes the recently discovered short QT syndrome and catecholaminergic polymorphic ventricular tachycardia, which affect the cardiac potassium channels and ryanodine receptors, respectively. Recently, interesting data were published[17] regarding the importance of single-nucleotide polymorphisms that may possibly elucidate the difference in clinical phenotype or in incidence of Brugada syndrome observed in various geographic regions. Bezzina and colleagues described ethnic-specific single-nucleotide polymorphism distribution[18] in the *SCN5A* promoter region. A certain combination of six single-nucleotide polymorphisms occurred only in Asian subjects and was absent in the other ethnic groups. This genotype variant resulted in decreased sodium channel expression and function. It neither caused Brugada phenotype nor was more frequent in the Brugada syndrome population, but it did visibly influence conduction velocities and was responsible for longer PR and QRS intervals.

Pathophysiology

Several pathophysiologic models have been proposed to explain the Brugada syndrome ECG abnormalities. The most strongly supported is the repolarization disorder theory of Yan and Antzelevitch.[19] This model is based on unequal expression of I_{to} current in the different transmural layers of the heart. It seems that I_{to} expression is more profound in the epicardium than in the endocardium. The impaired Brugada syndrome sodium channels in the epicardial cells are subject to stronger I_{to} defects, which results in an altered "spike and dome" morphology of the epicardial action potential. The differences in action potential morphology create a transmural gradient between the endocardium and the epicardium. This gradient manifests on the surface ECG as the typical coved-type ST elevation and increases dispersion of the cardiac repolarization (Fig. 68-4). It is this dispersion that creates the vulnerable window in which cardiac cells are more susceptible to malignant arrhythmias.

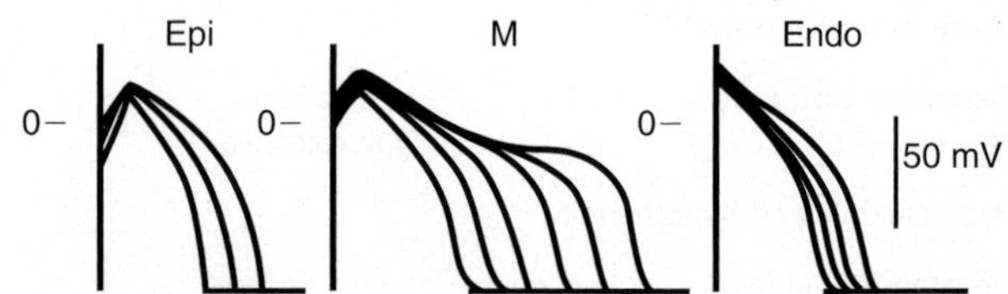

Figure 68-4 Dispersion of cardiac repolarization due to an impaired sodium influx. Because I_{to} channels are predominantly expressed in the epicardium (Epi), the alteration in action potential morphology is most prominent epicardially. See text for details. Endo, endocardium.

Electrophysiologic Substrate

Patients with Brugada syndrome ECG patterns clearly have a proclivity to develop rapid polymorphic ventricular tachycardia–ventricular fibrillation. Before the episode, the patients have a regular sinus rhythm (with no changes in the QT interval). In some rare cases, it seems that the ST segment elevation increases just before the onset of polymorphic ventricular tachycardia. We have observed the triggering of the arrhythmia after a short-long-short cycle in only two cases. It is clear that these patients have an electrophysiologic substrate for ventricular tachycardia–ventricular fibrillation, as evidenced by- the fact that a majority of patients who have the syndrome have inducible polymorphic ventricular tachycardia–ventricular fibrillation. Patients with the syndrome frequently have a prolonged His bundle–ventricle conduction time (H-V interval).

Differential Diagnosis

Initially, several investigators believed that Brugada syndrome was a forme fruste of arrhythmogenic right ventricular dysplasia orcardiomyopathy. It should, however, be emphasized that despite many efforts to prove otherwise, no macroscopic structural heart disease is present in patients with Brugada syndrome. Definitive diagnosis of Brugada syndrome can be made only after thorough invasive ("left-right" heart catheterization, endocardial biopsy) and noninvasive (echocardiography, cardiac imaging) investigation excluding all possible structural abnormalities. Recent studies, however, suggest that microscopic alterations could be present.

Frustaci and associates performed histologic analysis of biventricular biopsy specimens in 18 consecutive probands who were clinically diagnosed with Brugada syndrome.[20] Angiography documented morphologic abnormalities in 7 patients. Of interest, all non-*SCN5A* mutation carriers showed histologic changes (myocarditis, fibrofatty infiltrations). These investigators concluded that environmental factors such as viral infections and inflammation can cause myocardial damage underlying the ECG changes in Brugada syndrome. The most likely explanation for these results is that myocarditis can sometimes simulate Brugada syndrome.

Coronel and coworkers[21] electrophysiologically and histopathologically studied the prelevated heart of a patient clinically diagnosed with the syndrome. Transplantation was performed because of intolerable numbers of implantable cardioverter-defibrillator (ICD) discharges. The postmortem analysis identified discrete interstitial changes (mainly fibrosis) in the RV causing RV conduction delay. In this particular case, transmural repolarization gradient was not found and the underlying mechanism supports the previously described "conduction delay theory" rather than the repolarization theory.

Multiple case reports of ECG patterns that mimic those of Brugada syndrome have been published. A overview of possible causes of ST segment elevation in the right precordial leads is presented in Table 68-1.

Clinical Manifestations

The complete syndrome is characterized by episodes of rapid polymorphic ventricular tachycardia in patients with an ECG pattern of right bundle branch block (BBB) and ST segment elevation in leads V_1 to V_3. It predominantly affects males, with a mean age at onset of 40 years. When the episodes terminate spontaneously, the patient develops syncopal attacks. When the episodes are sustained, full blown cardiac arrest and eventually sudden death occur. Thus, these manifestations can range widely: At one end of the spectrum are asymptomatic persons; at the other end are those who die suddenly. Other signs and symptoms include seizures, agonal respiration, and, in patients who suffer an episode at night during sleep, labored respiration, agitation, loss of urinary bladder control, and recent memory loss, which is not uncommon (perhaps owing to brain anoxia). Many patients who have the disease can appear to be otherwise very healthy and active, vigorously engaging in exertional activity or exercise. Findings on physical examination are almost always normal. Physicians who first work with these patients have a strong tendency to believe that the syncopal attacks are benign and of vasovagal origin. Many patients who underwent a tilt-table test with a positive result received treatment in accordance with these findings but subsequently died suddenly. As seen in other clinical-electrocardiographic syndromes, different presentations of the disease are common.

Asymptomatic persons may be recognized when the atypical ECG pattern is detected during routine examination. This ECG pattern cannot be distinguished from that in symptomatic patients. In other patients, the characteristic ECG pattern is recorded during screening after the sudden death of a family member with the disease. On the other hand, another group of symptomatic patients have been diagnosed as suffering syncopal episodes of unknown cause or vasovagal origin or who have a diagnosis of idiopathic ventricular fibrillation. Subsequently, some of these patients are correctly diagnosed at follow-up when the ECG pattern changes spontaneously from normal to the typical pattern of the syndrome. This is also the case for those persons in whom the disease is unmasked by the administration of an antiarrhythmic drug given for other arrhythmias—for instance, atrial fibrillation.

Prognosis and Risk Stratification

In the past decade, risk stratification in Brugada syndrome has become the subject of intense interest owing to the fact that early recognition of patients at increased future risk of sudden death can save many lives. Nevertheless, active research in this area by several study groups revealed that risk stratification in Brugada syndrome is difficult and leads to quite a few controversial issues. The principal goal of risk stratification is the prediction of future arrhythmic events at any time during life. This is particularly difficult in adult patients who have never had any symptoms and in whom the diagnosis is incidental. General agreement exists that reanimated patients with Brugada syndrome have an increased risk of recurrent life-threatening events (17% to 62% in the ensuing 4 to 7 years) and therefore should receive an internal defibrillator[23] (Fig. 68-5). On the other hand, considerable controversy[22] is ongoing regarding what to do in the absence of an aborted sudden death. The three most important arrhythmia predictors that have been studied are syncope, a baseline coved-pattern type I ECG, and response to programmed ventricular stimulation.

Syncope

Currently, three large registries of patients with Brugada syndrome who had a history of syncope have been reported. During a follow-up period of 24 to 39 months, 6% to 19% of these patients suffered an arrhythmic event. The general consensus is that patients with a history of syncope who did not suffer a cardiac arrest do have an increased risk for future arrhythmic events. Our registry[23] (comprising 547 patients, 124 with

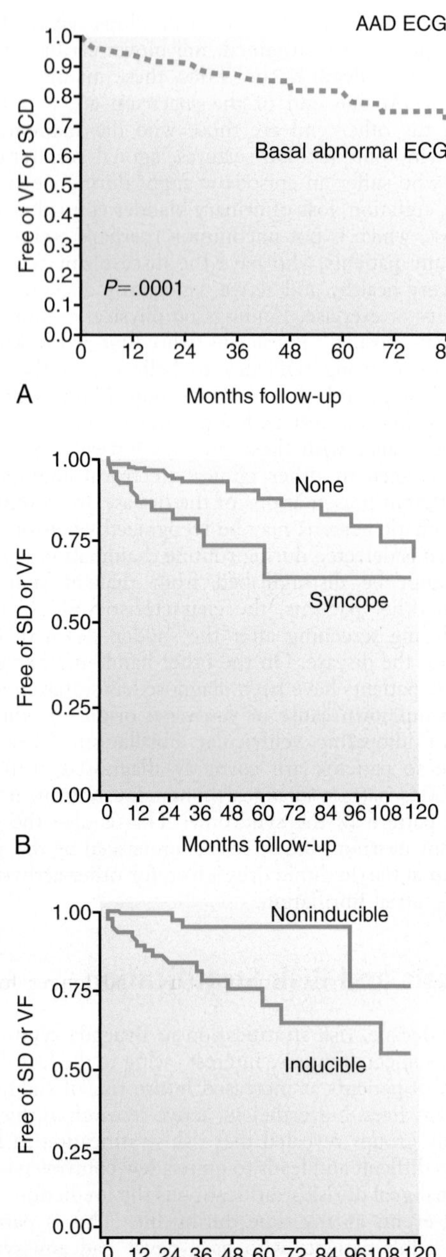

Figure 68-5 **A**, Kaplan-Meier analysis of life-threatening arrhythmic events during follow-up, depending on the presence of spontaneously abnormal electrocardiogram (ECG) pattern in patients in our international registry. **B**, Kaplan-Meier analysis of life-threatening arrhythmic events during follow-up, depending on the presence of syncope in patients in our international registry. **C**, Kaplan-Meier analysis of life-threatening arrhythmic events during follow-up, depending on inducibility during the electrophysiology study in patients in our registry. AAD, antiarrhythmic drugs; SD, sudden death; SCD, sudden cardiac death; VF, ventricular fibrillation.

syncope) and a second European multicenter registry (comprising 212 patients, 65 with syncope) recommend ICD implantation in all patients with a history of syncope of unknown origin. A third, Italian registry (comprising 200 patients, 34 with syncope) provided treatment only for those patients who had syncope and a documented baseline coved-type (type I) ECG pattern.

Spontaneous Coved-Type (Type I) Electrocardiographic Pattern

The predictive value of the presence of a baseline coved-type ECG pattern also has been investigated by the three registry study groups. In our registry of 547 patients with or without syncope but without previous aborted sudden cardiac death, univariate analysis identified the baseline diagnostic ECG pattern as a significant predictor of future events. On multivariate analysis, a spontaneously abnormal ECG pattern no longer was an independent predictor. On logistic regression analysis, in the presence of a baseline diagnostic ECG pattern, the 2-year probability of arrhythmic events ranged between 1.8% and 27%, whereas in the absence of a spontaneous type I ECG pattern, it ranged between 0.5% and 9.7%. In the registry from Eckhart and colleagues[25] (comprising 212 patients), the presence of a spontaneous type I ECG pattern tended to be a predictor of future arrhythmic events only on univariate analysis.[40] Finally, in the Italian registry[24] (200 patients with a type I or type II ECG pattern), life-table method analysis also recognized baseline spontaneous ST segment elevation as a valid predictor of future events. All groups seemed to agree that patients with a spontaneous Brugada syndrome ECG pattern belong to a subgroup with higher risk of future arrhythmic events.

Programmed Ventricular Stimulation

At present, the most controversial issue in risk stratification of patients with Brugada syndrome is the value of programmed ventricular stimulation (PVS). Our group has continually analyzed the registry data in general and in different subpopulations (symptomatic, asymptomatic), with consistent results. In 547 patients without previous cardiac arrest inducibility of a sustained ventricular arrhythmia was a strong predictor of arrhythmia-free survival.[39] The Eckhardt registry, comprising 212 patients with or without ASCD, in the presence of low statistical power due to low event rates, stated that inducibility during PVS could not predict future arrhythmic events. Here, all asymptomatic noninducible patients remained asymptomatic.[40] The Priori registry, comprising 200 patients with saddleback- or coved-type ECG patterns, also could not assign any predictive value to PVS.

A possible explanation for the different outcomes for the three registries is the higher event rate in our registry as compared with the other two registries. Furthermore, patients included in our database were subject to a selection bias, in that more severely affected patients and families were included, especially in the early 1990s. Use of different stimulation protocols also may have contributed to the discrepancies. In our study population, stimulation was applied from only one site (right ventricular apex), with a maximum of three basic cycle lengths and three extrasystoles and a minimum coupling interval of 200 ms. Finally, different inclusion criteria and different statistical methods between the three registries also may have played a role.

Recently, these findings were incorporated in a new risk stratification protocol for patients diagnosed with Brugada syndrome: All symptomatic patients receive an implantable defibrillator. In asymptomatic patients with a normal baseline ECG pattern, reassurance is adequate management, because their risk for future arrhythmic events is similar to that in the general population. Asymptomatic patients with a baseline coved-type ECG pattern have an elevated risk that justifies further exploration by means of PVS. Low-risk patients not receiving any treatment are advised to contact us immediately in case of syncope, to avoid all drugs that can worsen Brugada syndrome, and to aggressively treat all fever episodes.

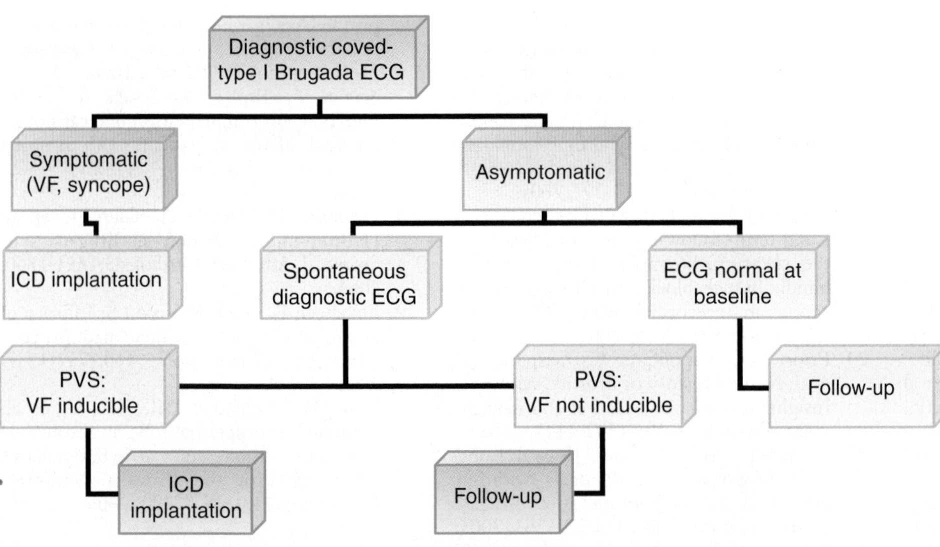

Figure 68-6 Current risk stratification scheme used at the Heart Rhythm Management Centre, UZ Brussel, Brussels, Belgium. ICD, implantable cardioverter-defibrillator; ECG, electrocardiogram; PVS, programmed ventricular stimulation; VF, ventricular fibrillation.

On the basis of these results, we recently created a new risk stratification scheme for patients diagnosed with Brugada syndrome. This is presented in Figure 68-6.

Treatment

The first long-term follow-up studies conducted in patients with Brugada syndrome who received an ICD have only recently been published.

Our center reported the results for 47 patients with ICDs during a 4-year follow-up period.[26] Documentation of a spontaneously abnormal ECG pattern and the occurrence of nonsustained ventricular tachycardias increased the probability of delivery of appropriate shocks. The inappropriate shock-free interval was considerably shorter in younger patients and in patients with episodes of atrial fibrillation.

The Eckhardt group reported similar results: Of 220 patients with ICDs, 8% had appropriate therapy, whereas 28% received inappropriate shocks, mostly as a result of inadequate programming of the device.[27]

Today, extensive research is ongoing to find alternative pharmacologic options for patients with Brugada syndrome for whom ICD implantation is contraindicated for various reasons. Quinidine[28,29] and dimethyl lithospermate B (Danshen's extract[30]) have been suggested as drugs that reduce the tendency for ventricular arrhythmias. Larger patient groups and longer follow-up periods are necessary to evaluate these products, however.

References

1. Antzelevitch C, Brugada P, Borggrefe M, et al: Brugada syndrome: Report of the Second Consensus Conference. Circulation 111: 659-670, 2005.
2. Veltmann C, Schimpf R, Echternach C, et al: A prospective study on spontaneous fluctuations between diagnostic and non-diagnostic ECGs in Brugada syndrome: Implications for correct phenotyping and risk stratification. Eur Heart J 27:2544-2552, 2006.
3. Richter S, Sarkozy A, Chierchia GB, et al: Variability of the diagnostic coved-type ECG during long-term follow-up of patients with Brugada syndrome and primary prophylactic ICD implantation. Eur Heart J 27(S1):2008.
4. Hong K, Brugada J, Oliva A, et al: Value of electrocardiographic parameters and ajmaline test in the diagnosis of Brugada syndrome caused by *SCN5A* mutations. Circulation 110:3023-3027, 2004.
5. Wolpert C, Echternach C, Veltmann C, et al: Intravenous drug challenge using flecainide and ajmaline in patients with Brugada syndrome. Heart Rhythm 2:254-260, 2005.
6. Ikeda T, Abe A, Yusu S, et al: The full stomach test as a novel diagnostic technique for identifying patients at risk of Brugada syndrome. J Cardiovasc Electrophysiol 17:602-607, 2006.
7. Brugada P, Brugada J: Right bundle branch block, persistent ST-segment elevation and sudden cardiac death: A distinct clinical and electrocardiographic syndrome. A multicenter report. J Am Coll Cardiol 20:1391-1396, 1992.
8. Vatta M, Dumaine R, Varghese G, et al: Genetic and biophysical basis of sudden unexplained nocturnal death syndrome (SUNDS), a disease allelic to Brugada syndrome. Hum Mol Genet 11:337-345, 2002.
9. Tohyou Y, Nakazawa K, Ozawa A, et al: A survey in the incidence of right bundle branch block with ST segment elevation among normal population. Jpn J Electrocardiol 15:223-226, 1995.
10. Namiki T, Ogura T, Kuwabara Y, et al: Five-year mortality and clinical characteristics of adult subjects with right bundle branch block and ST elevation. Circulation 93:334, 1995.
11. Hata Y, Chiba N, Hotta K, et al: Incidence and clinical significance of right bundle branch block and ST segment elevation in V1-V3 in 6- to 18-year-old school children in Japan. Circulation 20:2310, 1997.
12. Chen Q, Kirsch GE, Zhang D, et al: Genetic basis and molecular mechanism for idiopathic ventricular fibrillation. Nature 392:293-296, 1998.
13. Weiss R, Barmada MM, Nguyen T, et al: Clinical and molecular heterogeneity in the Brugada syndrome: A novel gene locus on chromosome 3. Circulation 105:707-713, 2002.
14. London B, Sanyal S, Michalec M, et al: A mutation in the glycerol-3-phosphate dehydrogenase 1-like gene (*GPD1L*) causes Brugada syndrome. Heart Rhythm 3:S32, 2006.
15. Antzelevitch C, Poolevick G, Cordeiro JM, et al: Loss-of-function mutations in the cardiac sodium channel underlie a new clinical entity characterized by ST-segment elevation, short QT-intervals and sudden cardiac death. Circulation 115:442-449, 2007. Epub 2007 Jan 15.
16. Probst V, Allouis M, Sacher F, et al: Progressive cardiac conduction defect is the prevailing phenotype in carriers of a Brugada syndrome *SCN5A* mutation. J Cardiovasc Electrophysiol 17:270-275, 2006.
17. Poelzing S, Forleo C, Samodell M, et al: *SCN5A* polymorphism restores trafficking

of a Brugada syndrome mutation on a separate gene. Circulation 114:368-376, 2006.
18. Bezzina CR, Shimizu W, Yang P, et al: Common sodium channel promoter haplotype in asian subjects underlies variability in cardiac conduction. Circulation 113:338-344, 2006.
19. Antzelevitch C: The Brugada syndrome: Ionic basis and arrhythmia mechanisms. J Cardiovasc Electrophysiol 12:268-272, 2001.
20. Frustaci A, Priori SG, Pieroni M, et al: Cardiac histological substrate in patients with clinical phenotype of Brugada syndrome. Circulation 112:3680-3687, 2005.
21. Coronel R, Casini S, Koopmann T, et al: Right ventricular fibrosis and conduction delay in a patient with clinical signs of Brugada syndrome. Circulation 112:2769-2777, 2005.
22. Controversies in Cardiovascular Medicine: Should patients with an asymptomatic Brugada electrocardiogram undergo pharmacological and electrophysiological testing? Part 1: Brugada P, Brugada R, Brugada J: Patients with an asymptomatic Brugada electrocardiogram should undergo pharmacological and electrophysiological testing. Part II: Priori SG, Napolitano C. Management of patients with Brugada syndrome should not be based on programmed electrical stimulation. Circulation 112:279-292, 2005.
23. Brugada J, Brugada R, Antzelevitch C, et al: Long-term follow-up of individuals with the electrocardiographic pattern of right bundle-branch block and ST-segment elevation in precordial leads V1 to V3. Circulation 105:73-78, 2002.
24. Priori SG, Napolitano C, Gasparini M, et al: Natural history of Brugada syndrome: Insights for risk stratification and management. Circulation 105:1342-1347, 2002.
25. Eckardt L, Probst V, Smits JP et al: Long-term prognosis of individuals withright precordial ST-segment-elevation Brugada syndrome. Circulation 111:257-263, 2005.
26. Sarkozy A, Boussy T, Kourgianiddes G, et al: Long term follow up of primary prophylactic cardioverter-defibrillator therapy in Brugada syndrome. J Cardiovasc Electrophysiol 17:902-906, 2006.
27. Sacher F, Probst V, Iesaka Y, et al: Outcome after implantation of a cardioverter-defibrillator in patients with Brugada syndrome. Circulation 114:2317-2324, 2006.
28. Hermida JS, Denjoy I, Clerc J, et al: Hydroquinidine therapy in Brugada syndrome. J Am Coll Cardiol 43:1853-1860, 2004.
29. Belhassen B, Glick A, Viskin S: Efficacy of quinidine in high risk patients with Brugada syndrome. Circulation 110:1731-1737, 2004.
30. Fish JM, Welchons DR, Kim Y, et al: Dimethyl lithospermate B, an extract of Danshen, suppresses arrhythmogenesis associated with the Brugada syndrome. Circulation 113:1393-1400, 2006.

Long QT and Short QT Syndromes 69

Peter J. Schwartz and Lia Crotti

CHAPTER OUTLINE

Long QT Syndrome

Overview

The congenital *long QT syndrome* is a relatively uncommon but important clinical disorder. Since 1975,[1] two hereditary variants of the long QT syndrome have been recognized: The *Jervell and Lange-Nielsen syndrome* is associated with deafness,[2] whereas the *Romano-Ward syndrome* is not.[3]

The clinical manifestations of the disease are rather dramatic as they involve syncopal episodes that often result in cardiac arrest and sudden death and usually occur in conditions of either physical or emotional stress in otherwise healthy young persons, mostly children and teenagers. The high mortality rate among symptomatic patients not receiving appropriate treatment, in the face of ready availability of very effective therapies, renders unacceptable the existence of undiagnosed cases in this patient population. The genetic findings of the last 15 years or so have made long QT syndrome a unique paradigm for genetically mediated sudden cardiac death that allows correlation of genotype and phenotype and provides a direct bridge between molecular biology and clinical cardiology.

Molecular Genetics of Long QT Syndrome

After the identification in 1995 and 1996 of the first three long QT syndrome genes[4] associated with the most frequent variants—LQT1, LQT2, and LQT3—several other genes were identified. Unfortunately, haste or enthusiasm has created a terminology problem because some of these genes cannot be regarded as truly being responsible for long QT syndrome. What have been called LQT4 and LQT7 (Andersen-Tawil syndrome) are complex clinical disorders in which a modest prolongation of the QT interval[4] is only a secondary epiphenomenon and should not be regarded as part of the long QT syndrome. LQT5, LQT6, and LQT8, although rare, are additional variants of long QT syndrome. For LQT9, LQT10, LQT11, and LQT12 only preliminary descriptions are available.

The main characteristic of all of the long QT syndrome genes identified so far is to encode cardiac ion channel subunits or to modulate ionic currents (e.g., CAV3).

KCNQ1 (LQT1) and *KCNE1* (LQT5)

The delayed rectifier current (I_K) is a major determinant of phase 3 of the cardiac action potential. It comprises two independent components: one rapid (I_{Kr}) and one slow (I_{Ks}).

The *KCNQ1* gene and the *KCNE1* gene encode, respectively, the α subunit (KvLQT1) and the β subunit (MinK) of the potassium channel conducting the I_{Ks} current. KCNQ1 mutations are found in the LQT1 variant of long QT syndrome, which also is the most prevalent. LQT5 is an uncommon (2% to 3%) variant caused by mutations in the *KCNE1* gene.

Homozygous or compound heterozygous mutations of *KCNQ1* and of *KCNE1* have been associated with the recessive Jervell and Lange-Nielsen form of long QT syndrome (JLN1 and JLN2).

Expression studies of mutated proteins have suggested multiple mechanisms of functional failure. Defective proteins may coassemble with wild-type protein and exert a dominant negative effect. Other mutations lead to defective proteins that do not assemble with wild-type peptides, resulting in a loss of function that reduces the I_{Ks} current by 50% or less (haploinsufficiency). Finally, defective peptides may not even reach the membrane of the cardiac cell because the mutations interfere with intracellular protein trafficking.[4]

In 600 patients with LQT1, Moss and associates demonstrated that both the transmembrane location of the mutations and their dominant-negative effect are independent risk factors for cardiac events[5]; however, neither the localization of a mutation nor the cellular electrophysiologic studies are always sufficient to predict the clinical phenotype.[6] Indeed, in a population of patients with long QT syndrome from several countries and all carrying the A341V mutation, a well-known "hot spot," the clinical severity was significantly greater than that of patients with long QT syndrome involving either transmembrane mutations or mutations with a dominant-negative effect. This finding suggests that the current biophysical assessments of the electrophysiologic effects of long QT syndrome–causing mutation do not provide the whole gamut of information necessary to make a complete genotype-phenotype correlation.[6]

The I_{Ks} current is increased by sympathetic activation and by heart rate increases and is essential for QT adaptation. If I_{Ks} is defective, the QT interval will fail to shorten appropriately during tachycardia; this creates a highly arrhythmogenic condition.

KCNH2 (LQT2) and *KCNE2* (LQT6)

The *KCNH2* gene and the *KCNE2* gene encode, respectively, the α subunit (i.e., the HERG [human ether-à-go-go–related gene] protein) and the β subunit (i.e., MiRP [MinK-related peptide]) of the potassium channel conducting the I_{Kr} current. This is the second most common variant of long QT syndrome, accounting for 35% to 40% of mutations in long QT syndrome–genotyped patients. Mutations in *KCNH2* cause a reduction of I_{Kr} current. Defective proteins either may cause a dominant negative effect on the wild-type subunits or may not interfere with the function of the normal subunits, thereby resulting in haploinsufficiency. Trafficking abnormalities constitute another consequence of *KCNH2* mutations.[7]

Mutations in the *KCNE2* gene are found in the LQT6 variant of long QT syndrome. This gene encodes MiRP1, a small peptide that coassembles with the HERG protein to form the I_{Kr} channel. Few examples of *KCNE2* mutations associated with long QT syndrome have been reported.

SCN5A (LQT3) and *SCN4B* (LQT10)

The *SCN5A* gene encodes the protein of the cardiac sodium channel. In vitro expression studies[8] showed that long QT syndrome *SCN5A* mutations produce the long QT syndrome phenotype by inducing a "gain of function" leading to increase in the sodium inward current, which prolongs action potential duration. The prevalence of LQT3 among patients with long QT syndrome is 10% to 15%. Recently, mutations in the sodium channel subunit $Na_V\beta4$ were suggested to represent LQT10.

CACNA1C (LQT8—Timothy Syndrome)

LQT8, often referred to as *Timothy syndrome*, is a rare variant characterized by marked QT interval prolongation, often presenting with 2:1 functional atrioventricular block and macroscopic T wave alternans, and syndactyly. LQT8 is highly malignant, and 10 of 17 (59%) of the children in the series reported by Splawski and colleagues[9] died at a mean age of 2.5 years. Some children with Timothy syndrome also had congenital heart diseases, immune deficiency, intermittent hypoglycemia, cognitive abnormalities, and autism.

Molecular screening identified a missense mutation (G406R) in the voltage-gated calcium channel gene (*CACNA1C*), in all probands analyzed.[9] G406R produces sustained inward calcium currents by causing nearly complete loss of voltage-dependent inactivation.[9] In the heart, prolonged calcium current delays cardiomyocyte repolarization and increases risk of arrhythmia.

CAV3 (LQT9)

The *CAV3* gene encodes caveolin-3, a protein component of caveolae and an integral membrane protein in trans-Golgi–derived vesicles. Caveolins participate in many important cellular processes, including vesicular transport and signal transduction.

Four missense mutations in *CAV3*-encoded caveolin-3 were recently identified in four long QT syndrome probands and in none of the 400 reference alleles.[10] They all produced a gain-of-function, LQT3-like molecular-cellular phenotype. *CAV3* mutations also were implicated in a few cases of SIDS.[11]

Prevalence

Already in 1975[1] it was suggested that LQTS "could be more unrecognized than rare." However, the prevalence was assumed to be anywhere between 1/5,000 and 1/20,000. None of these estimates was based on actual data.

The first data-driven indication of the prevalence of LQTS comes from the largest prospective study of neonatal electrocardiography ever performed[12] and involving 44,596 infants of 3-4 weeks of age. Among them, 0.47% had a QTc between 451 and 470 ms and 0.7/1,000 had a QTc greater than 470 ms, regarded as markedly prolonged by the European Task Force on Neonatal Electrocardiography.[13] Molecular screening was initiated from the infants with the longer QTc values. So far, among genotyped infants disease-causing mutations were found in 13/28 (46%) with a QTc greater than 470 ms and in 13/28 (33%) with a QTc between 461 and 470 ms. One genotype-negative infant was diagnosed as affected by LQTS on established clinical grounds. In total, 18/44,596 infants were affected by LQTS demonstrating a prevalence of at least 1:2,478 live births (95% C.I. 1:1,568-1:4,810). Furthermore, logical inferences based on the not yet genotyped infants with QTc between 451 and 470 ms strongly suggest that this prevalence is close to 1:2,000. This is the first time that the prevalence of a cardiac disease of genetic origin has been quantified based on actual data.

Clinical Presentation of the Romano-Ward Syndrome

The typical clinical presentation in long QT syndrome has been regarded as the occurrence of syncope or cardiac arrest, precipitated by emotional or physical stress, in a young person with a prolonged QT interval on the electrocardiogram (ECG). If these symptomatic patients received no treatment, the syncopal episodes would recur and eventually prove fatal in most cases. This concept reflected the fact that the patients diagnosed in the early days were those most severely affected. Today, however, numerous cases and families with a very benign course also have been recognized.

The clinical history of repeated episodes of loss of consciousness under emotional or physical stress is so typical and unique to be almost unmistakable, provided that the physician is aware of long QT syndrome. The clinical presentation is not always so clear, however, and the diagnosis sometimes may require clinical experience.

The two cardinal manifestations of long QT syndrome are syncope and electrocardiographic abnormalities.

Cardiac Events and Their Relation to Genotype

The syncopal episodes are due to torsade de pointes, often degenerating into ventricular fibrillation. It was well known for some time that in most patients, the symptoms develop under stress; it also was known that these life-threatening cardiac events occasionally occur at rest. The reason(s) for these different patterns remained obscure until molecular biology allowed researchers to distinguish among different genotypes. The unexpected observation in 1995[14] that among a tiny group of genotyped patients, those with LQT2 appeared to be at higher risk during emotional stress, whereas those with LQT3 suffered their events mostly at rest or during sleep, fostered a large and

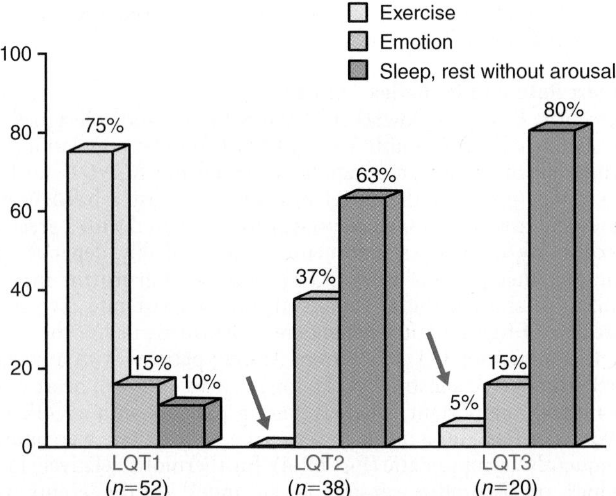

Figure 69-1 Frequency of lethal cardiac events by triggers and genotype for long QT syndrome variants LQT1, LQT2, and LQT3. *Numbers in parentheses* are patients. (Modified from Schwartz PJ, Priori SG, Spazzolini C, et al: Genotype-phenotype correlation in the long-QT syndrome: Gene-specific triggers for life-threatening arrhythmias. Circulation 103:89-95, 2001.)

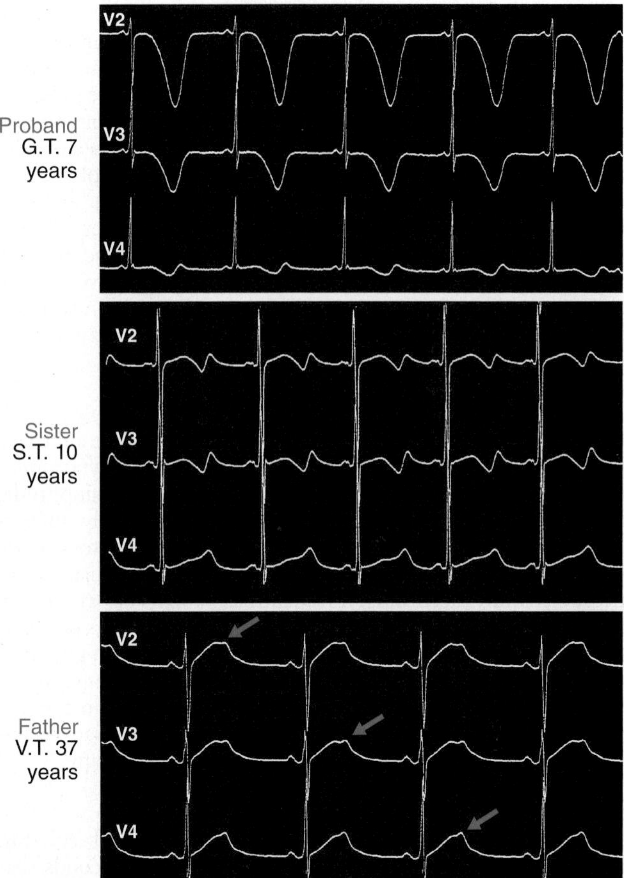

Figure 69-2 Different T wave morphologies in affected members of the same family. The electrocardiogram (ECG) of the proband, with cardiac arrest as his first clinical manifestation, shows deep negative T waves in the precordial leads and a very prolonged QTc. The ECG of his asymptomatic sister shows biphasic T waves. His father, whose ECG shows notched T waves and a QTc of 584 ms, had two syncopal episodes. The *arrows* point to examples of notched T waves. (From Schwartz PJ, Priori SG, Napolitano C: The long QT syndrome. In Zipes DP, Jalife J [eds]: Cardiac Electrophysiology: From Cell to Bedside, 3rd ed. Philadelphia, Saunders, 2000, pp 597-615.)

targeted study[15] that shed light on this issue of major clinical relevance.

In 670 patients with long QT syndrome of known genotype who all had suffered symptoms (syncope, cardiac arrest, or sudden death), Schwartz and colleagues examined possible relations between genotype and the conditions ("triggers") associated with the events.[15] As predicted by the observed impairment in I_{Ks} current (essential for QT shortening during increases in heart rate), most of the events in patients with LQT1 occurred during exercise or stress. Many of the events (including the fatal ones) in patients with LQT2 occurred during emotional stress, such as from auditory stimuli (sudden noises and telephone ringing, especially occurring while the person is at rest), and most of the events in patients with LQT3 occurred while they were asleep or at rest (Fig. 69-1).

LQT2 and LQT3 patients are at low risk for life-threatening arrhythmias during exercise because they have a well-preserved I_{Ks} current, allowing appropriate shortening of the QT interval whenever heart rate increases. The practical implication is that youngsters with LQT2 and LQT3 should be allowed to play rather freely (although participation in competitive sports is contraindicated), with significant psychological benefit.

Even in the postpartum period, genotype is important, because risk is higher for patients with LQT2 than for those with LQT1.[16,17] The higher risk for women with LQT2 is probably related partly to sleep disruption; accordingly, we recommend that their husbands take on the responsibility of night-time feedings for the infant, thereby allowing a fair amount of uninterrupted sleep for their LQT2-affected wives.

Electrocardiographic Aspects

The bizarre electrocardiogram of many patients with long QT syndrome should be easily recognized (Fig. 69-2). Besides QT prolongation, the T wave has several morphologic patterns, easily recognizable with clinical experience, that are difficult to quantify but useful for diagnosis.

QT Interval Duration

The Bazett's correction for heart rate remains very useful, despite unrelenting criticism, although hypercorrection and undercorrection occur at slow and fast rates. QTc values greater than 440 ms are considered prolonged; however, values up to 460 ms may still be normal among females. Despite exceptions, the longer the QT, greater is the risk for malignant arrhythmias, and when QTc exceeds 500 to 550 ms, risk definitely increases.

The initial and understandable concept that QT prolongation was the essential cornerstone of long QT syndrome was challenged by Schwartz and colleagues, who in 1980 and 1985[3,18] proposed that some patients may be affected by long QT syndrome and nonetheless have a normal QT interval on the surface ECG. The validity of this unorthodox concept was proved by the existence of mutation carriers with a normal QT interval,[4] as a consequence of low penetrance. This concept has important practical and medicolegal implications because, for example, it no longer allows a cardiologist to state that a sibling of an affected patient with a normal QTc "is definitely not affected by long QT syndrome."

T Wave Morphology

The T wave often is biphasic or notched (see Fig. 69-2). These abnormalities are particularly evident in the precordial leads and contribute to the diagnosis of long QT syndrome; they often are more immediately striking than is the sheer prolongation of the

QT interval. After cessation of exercise, major repolarization changes often appear, and they are useful for the diagnosis.

Notched T waves are more frequent in symptomatic patients (81% versus 19%, $P < .005$).[3] They probably reflect the presence of subthreshold early afterdepolarizations (EADs). Their appearance after exercise is markedly more frequent (85% versus 3%, $P < .0001$) among patients than among healthy controls.

Gene-specific ECG patterns have been identified.[7] Patients with LQT1 tend to have smooth, broad-based T waves whereas patients with LQT2 frequently have low-amplitude and notched T waves; patients with LQT3 have a more distinctive pattern characterized by a late onset of the T wave. Even within families, however, extreme heterogeneity of T wave morphology may be observed (see Fig. 69-2).

T Wave Alternans

In 1975 Schwartz and colleagues proposed that T wave alternans represents a characteristic ECG feature of long QT syndrome.[3] Beat-to-beat alternation of the T wave, in polarity or amplitude, may be present at rest for brief moments but usually appears during emotional or physical stress and may precede torsade de pointes (Fig. 69-3). T wave alternans is a marker of major electrical instability; accordingly, it identifies patients at particularly high risk. Its transient nature limits the possibility of its observation. This is a rather gross phenomenon that should not go unnoticed when present. The presence of T wave alternans on the ECG tracing of a patient with long QT syndrome on therapy strongly suggests the presence of a high degree of cardiac electrical instability and should prompt reassessment of therapy.

Sinus Pauses

Several patients with long QT syndrome have been observed to have sudden pauses in sinus rhythm exceeding 1.2 seconds that are unrelated to sinus arrhythmia,[3] and which may contribute to the initiation of torsade de pointes. These pauses often are followed by the appearance of a notch on the T wave, and it is mostly from these notches that repetitive ventricular beats take off.[3] Their occurrence in patients with LQT3 represents an important warning signal that requires upping safety measures.

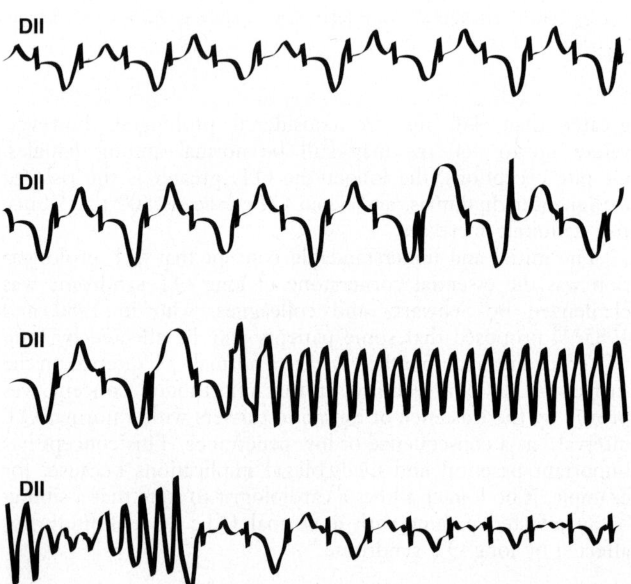

Figure 69-3 Tracing recorded from a 5-year-old patient with Jervell and Lange-Nielsen syndrome during a syncopal episode. T wave alternans precedes the onset of torsade de pointes; the torsade event is not preceded by a pause. (From Pernot C: Le syndrome cardio-auditif de Jervell et Lange-Nielsen. Aspects electrocardiographiques. Proc Assoc Europ Paediatr Cardiol 8:28-36, 1972.)

Heart Rate and Its Reflex Control

Recently, Brink and coworkers[19] and Schwartz and colleagues,[20] in a study of a large South African LQT1 founder population, in which all of the affected members carried the *KCNQ1* A341V mutation, provided the novel evidence that faster basal heart rates and brisk autonomic responses are associated with a greater probability of being symptomatic. This probably depends on the fact that patients with LQT1 have an impairment in the ability to shorten the QT interval during heart rate increases because of the mutation-dependent impairment in I_{Ks}, the current essential for QT adaptation. Among patients with a major arrhythmogenic substrate (QTc longer than 500 ms), heart rate is rather unimportant, whereas among patients with a QTc of 500 ms or less, those in the lower tertile of heart rate were more frequently asymptomatic (Fig. 69-4). Furthermore, relatively low values of baroreflex sensitivity—an index of the ability to respond with brisk increases in either vagal or sympathetic activity—were associated with a reduced probability of being symptomatic. The lack of QT shortening during sudden heart rate increases favors the R-on-T phenomenon and initiation of ventricular tachycardia–ventricular fibrillation, whereas sudden pauses elicit early afterdepolarizations in patients with long QT syndrome, which can trigger torsade de pointes. Blunted autonomic responses, revealed by relatively low values of baroreflex sensitivity, imply a reduced ability to change heart rate suddenly, which appears to be a protective mechanism for patients with LQT1.

An intriguing twist in the search for mechanisms contributing to the differing clinical severity often observed among persons carrying the same mutation is the preliminary finding that in the *KCNQ1* A341V South African population just described, the presence of two polymorphisms predicting increased adrenergic responses

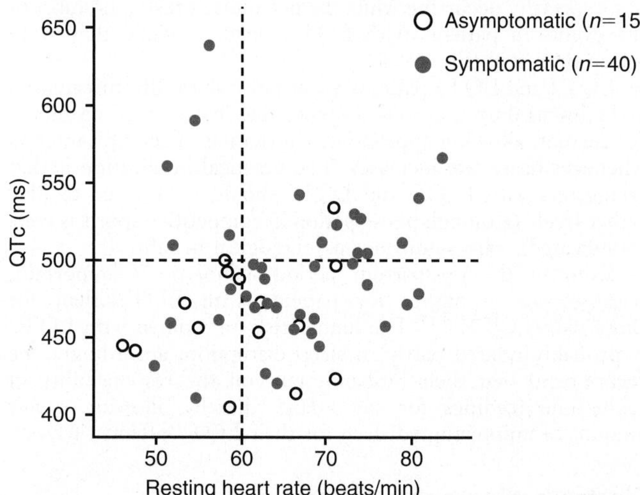

Figure 69-4 Differential risk for arrhythmic events among mutation carriers (MCs) according to resting heart rate and QTc in absence of β-blocker therapy. The *dashed horizontal line* represents the predefined cut-off for QTc (500 ms) whereas the *dashed vertical line* corresponds to the first tertile (60 beats per minute) of the heart rate values distribution. In the group of patients with a QTc ≤ 500 ms, those in the first tertile (heart rate ≤ 60 beats per minute) were less frequently symptomatic than MCs in the other two tertiles (odds ratio 0.19, 95% confidence interval, 0.04 to 0.79, $P = 0.023$). A QTc greater than 500 ms clearly represents a more severe arrhythmogenic substrate as 15 of 16 (94%) MCs with a QTc greater than 500 ms were symptomatic. (From Schwartz PJ, Vanoli E, Crotti L, et al: Neural control of heart rate modifies arrhythmia risk in congenital long QT syndrome. J Am Coll Cardiol 51:920-929, 2008.)

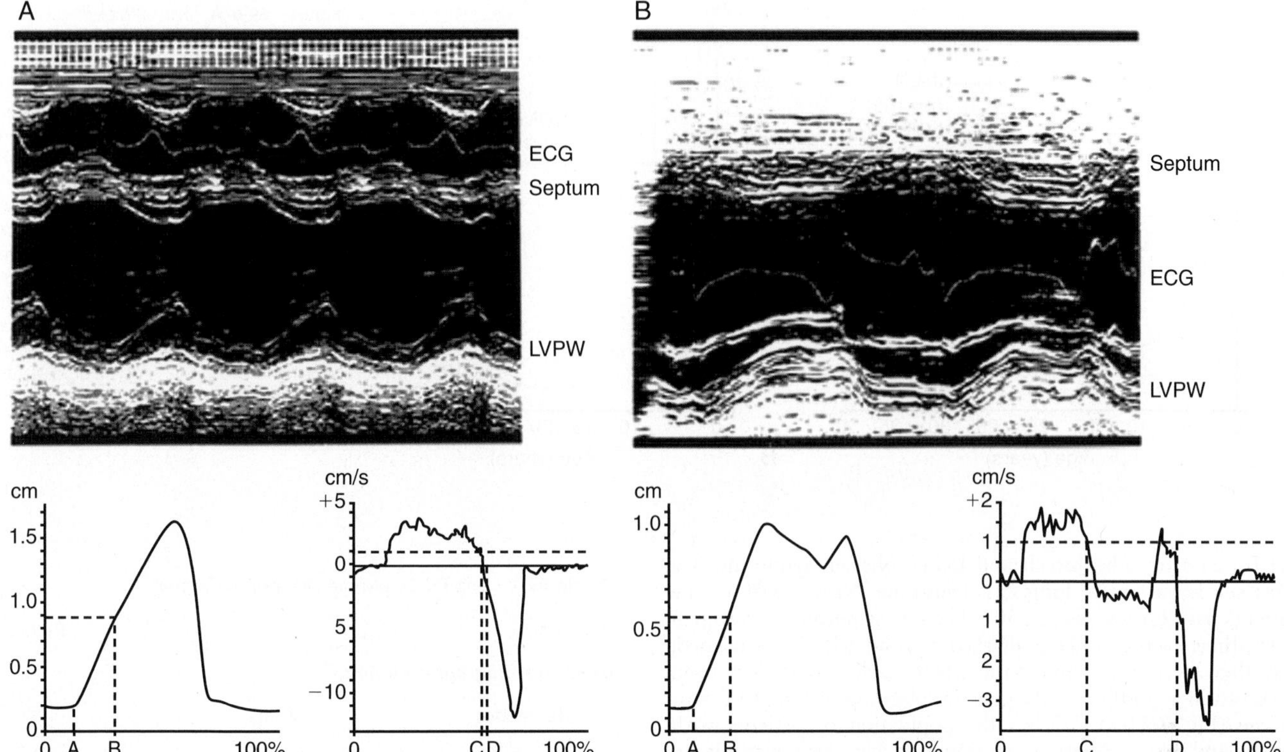

Figure 69-5 Echocardiographic appearance in long QT syndrome, with graphed curves for relevant functions. **A,** M-mode ultrasound examination from the long-axis parasternal view of the heart in a female control subject 16 years of age. *Upper panel* shows the echocardiographic tracing and the electrocardiogram at a paper speed of 100 mm/second. *Lower left panel* reproduces the endocardial contour of the movement of the left ventricular posterior wall (LVPW). *Lower right panel* shows the first derivative of wall thickening. Segment A-B indicates the time to reach half-maximal systolic contraction as percent of cardiac cycle (Th1/Th2). Segment C-D indicates the time spent during the late thickening phase, before rapid relaxation, at a rate less than 1 cm/second (TSTh). **B,** M-mode ultrasound examination from the long-axis parasternal view in a 10-year-old girl with long QT syndrome. The main abnormality is a major prolongation of the time spent in the late thickening phase and especially the occurrence of a dip followed by a second anterior movement of the endocardium, resulting in a double-peak morphology. (From Nador F, Beria G, De Ferrari GM, et al: Unsuspected echocardiographic abnormality in the long QT syndrome: Diagnostic, prognostic, and pathogenetic implications. Circulation 84:1530-1542, 1991.)

was associated with higher baroreflex sensitivity, faster heart rates, and a trend for more cardiac events.[20] The coexistence of an LQT1 mutation with a polymorphism creating a genetic propensity toward brisk autonomic reflexes, a combination apparently associated with increased risk for life-threatening arrhythmias, is simply the play of chance but contributes to explain the major clinical heterogeneity present in long QT syndrome.

Echocardiographic Abnormalities

LQTS is regarded as a purely electrical disease without any mechanical alteration. Contrary to this view a case-control study demonstrated the frequent presence of highly unusual echocardiographic abnormalities among the patients.[21] These abnormalities included an increased rate of thickening in the early phase of contraction (Th1/Th2) and the presence of a slow movement in the late thickening phase with a plateau morphology (TSTh) sometimes accompanied by a second peak. These quantitative measurements are shown in Figure 69-5 as they appear in normal individuals and in one of the most impressive LQTS patients. Thus, LQTS is not a purely electrical disease. Very recently, strong and independent confirmation of our original findings has been published, thus providing final evidence for the presence of mechanical alterations in LQTS patients.[22,23]

These abnormalities were more frequent in symptomatic than in asymptomatic patients, thus suggesting that they may reflect the presence of an arrhythmogenic mechanism. The subsequent evidence that the calcium-entry blocker verapamil completely normalizes the contraction pattern[3] suggests that symptomatic LQTS patients may have an abnormal increase in the intracellular calcium concentration before relaxation has completed and that this may be related to an early afterdepolarization: the contraction abnormality would be the mechanical equivalent of an EAD. The inward flux of calcium linked to the EAD may cause a small but rapid increase in intracellular calcium which may be sufficient to trigger the calcium-induced release of calcium from the sarcoplasmic reticulum, causing a much greater increase in cytosolic calcium and the occurrence of a second contraction or the prolongation of the contraction itself.

Clinical Presentation of the Jervell and Lange-Nielsen Syndrome

The Jervell and Lange-Nielsen syndrome,[2] characterized by congenital deafness, is due to the presence of two homozygous or compound heterozygous mutations on either the *KCNQ1* or *KCNE1* genes.[2]

Data on 187 patients with Jervell and Lange-Nielsen syndrome have shown clear differences from the other types of long QT syndrome, including LQT1, the variant that shares with Jervell and Lange-Nielsen syndrome an impairment in

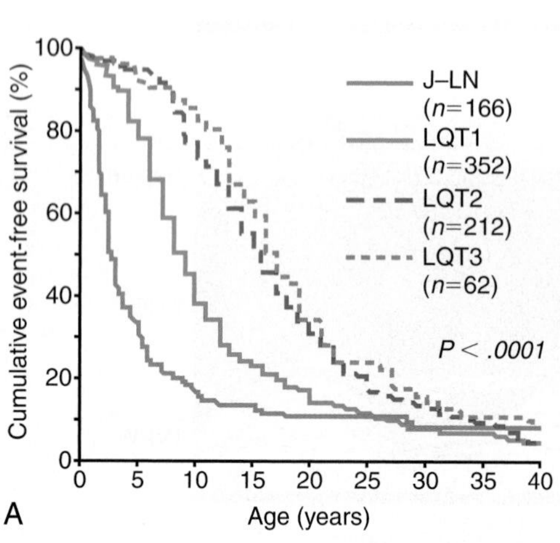

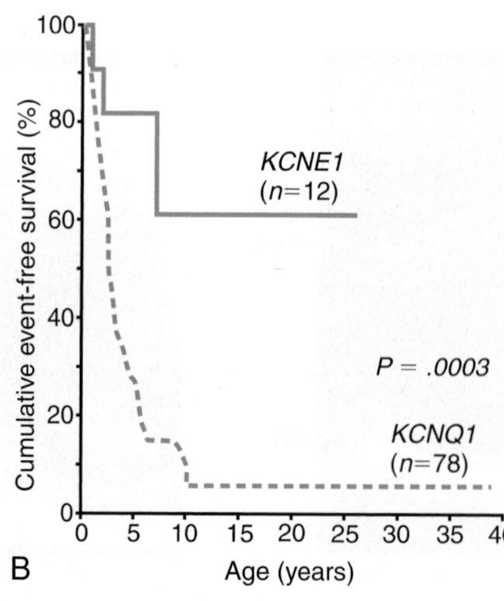

Figure 69-6 **A,** Kaplan-Meier curves of event-free survival comparing patients with Jervell and Lange-Nielsen syndrome (J-LN) and those with symptomatic LQT1, LQT2 and LQT3. **B,** Kaplan-Meier curve of event-free survival in patients with Jervell and Lange-Nielsen syndrome and those with mutations in *KCNQ1* or *KCNE1* genes. (Color-coding for plotted curves is the same as in **A.**) (**A,** Modified from Schwartz PJ, Priori SG, Spazzolini C, et al: Genotype-phenotype correlation in the long-QT syndrome: Gene-specific triggers for life-threatening arrhythmias. Circulation 103:89-95, 2001; **B,** from Schwartz PJ, Spazzolini C, Crotti L, et al: The Jervell and Lange-Nielsen syndrome. Natural history, molecular basis, and clinical outcome. Circulation 113:783-790, 2006.)

the I_{Ks} current. The Jervell and Lange-Nielsen syndrome is a most severe variant of long QT syndrome. Nearly 90% of the patients have cardiac events, 50% become symptomatic by age 3 years, their average QTc is markedly prolonged (557 ± 65 ms), and they become symptomatic much earlier than has been observed in any other major genetic subgroup of long QT syndrome (Fig. 69-6A). Within the population of patients with Jervell and Lange-Nielsen syndrome, it has been possible to identify subgroups at lower risk—namely, those with a QTc shorter than 500 ms and those without syncope in the first year of life.[2] Even though the clinical diagnosis of Jervell and Lange-Nielsen syndrome is rather straightforward, it is important to genotype all of these patients, because those in the smaller group with *KCNE1* mutations exhibit a markedly less severe clinical course than that typical for patients with mutations on *KCNQ1* (see Fig. 69-6B).

The therapeutic approach to patients with Jervell and Lange-Nielsen syndrome is made complex by the early age at which most of them become symptomatic, and especially by the fact that beta-blockers appear to have limited efficacy. Left cardiac sympathetic denervation may be less effective than in other patients with long QT syndrome. Thus, for many patients with Jervell and Lange-Nielsen syndrome, an implantable cardioverter-defibrillator (ICD) should be seriously considered, in addition to the traditional therapies. For the subgroups at lower risk,[2] it may be reasonable to postpone a decision about ICD implantation until the patient reaches the age of 8 to 10 years.

Clinical Diagnosis

In view of the characteristic features of long QT syndrome, the typical cases present no diagnostic difficulty for physicians aware of the disease. Borderline cases are more complex, however, and require the evaluation of multiple variables besides clinical history and ECG. Diagnostic criteria were proposed in 1985[18] and subsequently updated in 1993[24] and in 2006.[25]

The new diagnostic criteria are listed in Table 69-1. On the basis of our experience, we have arbitrarily divided the point score into three probability categories: (1) a score of 1 point or less indicates a low probability of long QT syndrome; (2) more than 1 to 3.0 points, an intermediate probability of long QT syndrome; and (3) 3.5 points or more, a high probability of long QT syndrome. Whenever a patient receives a score of 2 to 3 points, serial ECGs and especially several 24-hour Holter recordings should be obtained because the QTc value in patients

Table 69-1 Long QT Syndrome Diagnostic Criteria*

Criteria		Points
Electrocardiographic Findings†		
A. QTc interval‡	≥480 ms	3
	460-479 ms	2
	450-459 ms (in males)	1
B. Torsades de pointes§		2
C. T wave alternans		1
D. Notched T waves in three leads		1
E. Low heart rate for age‖		0.5
Clinical History		
A. Syncope§	With stress	2
	Without stress	1
B. Congenital deafness		0.5
Family History¶		
A. Family members with definite long QT syndrome		1
B. Unexplained sudden cardiac death below age 30 among immediate family members		0.5

Scoring

≤1 point = low probability of long QT syndrome
>1 to 3 points = intermediate probability of long QT syndrome
≥3.5 points = high probability of long QT syndrome

*1993-2006.
†In the absence of medications or disorders known to affect these electrocardiographic features.
‡QTc calculated by Bazett's formula, where $QTc = QT/\sqrt{RR}$.
§Mutually exclusive.
‖Resting heart rate below the second percentile for age.
¶The same family member cannot be counted in both A and B.

with long QT syndrome may vary from time to time and from day to night. In this group with intermediate probability of long QT syndrome, the presence of additional morphologic abnormalities may help in diagnostic decisions. The use of precordial leads often is more informative. Symptoms and signs often appear in the first few years of life, and the clinical manifestions may resemble epileptic convulsions.[3]

These diagnostic criteria were conceived in the pre-molecular era and should be applied with common sense. Obviously, they cannot be of value in identifying the so-called silent mutation carriers who have a normal QT interval. For such persons, molecular screening is essential. The main value of these clinical criteria is during a first contact with a patient and in clinical studies when uniformity in diagnosis is essential.

Molecular Diagnosis

Who Should Be Screened for Long QT Syndrome and Medicolegal Implications

Molecular diagnosis should always be attempted whenever the diagnosis of long QT syndrome either has been made or is suspected on sound clinical grounds. When successful (70% to 80% of cases in our laboratory), it allows the rapid screening of all family members and the identification of all silent mutation carriers (i.e., individuals with a disease-causing mutation and a QTc interval shorter than 440 ms), whose prevalence increases from 10% in LQT3 to 37% in LQT1. To increase the number of genotyped-positive patients it is important to consider that also intronic substitutions could be disease-causing, interfering with Per-mRNA processing.[26]

The possibility of silent mutation carrier status has major clinical and medicolegal implications. Imagine a family with a boy and a girl, the boy and one parent being clearly affected (with syncope and prolonged QTc). If the girl has a normal QT interval and is incorrectly assumed to be unaffected, she might later on be given one of the many drugs that block the I_{Kr} current, leading to the development of fatal torsade de pointes. This would not be bad luck; it would be the direct responsibility of the physician who had not attempted molecular screening in the boy, who was clearly affected. Identification of the disease-causing mutation would have allowed rapid determination of whether the girl was or not a mutation carrier—and this would have saved her life. Physicians who do not attempt to genotype their long QT syndrome–affected probands are willfully choosing to ignore the possibility that other family members may potentially be mutation carriers at risk for sudden death.

Molecular Genetics and Risk Stratification

Molecular genetics contribute importantly to risk stratification. In 1998,[7] based on 38 families, Zareba and coworkers suggested that patients with LQT1 and LQT2 had more events but that events in patients with LQT3 had greater lethality. In 2003,[27] data on 647 patients of known genotype and from 193 families indicated that the incidence of life-threatening events was lower among patients with LQT1, partly because of the high prevalence of silent mutation carriers (QTc less than 440 ms); the risk was higher among LQT2 females than among LQT2 males and in LQT3 males than in LQT3 females. Independent of genotype, the risk of becoming symptomatic was strongly correlated with QTc and was markedly greater with QTc longer than 500 ms. A majority of patients with LQT1 go through life without ever suffering cardiac events; moreover, in the LQT2 and LQT3 populations, almost half of the patients remain asymptomatic. This fact often is forgotten, as dramatically shown by the growing inclination to implant ICDs in asymptomatic persons just because they have been diagnosed as affected by long QT syndrome.

Following the reports by Donger and associates[6] and Piippo and colleagues[6] that mutations located in the carboxyl (C)-terminal region were associated with a less severe clinical phenotype, in 2002 Moss and coworkers[28] indicated that patients affected with LQT2 with mutations in the pore region were at higher risk compared with patients also with LQT2 with mutations in different regions of the same gene. In 2007 Moss and coworkers[5] demonstrated in 600 patients with LQT1 that both the transmembrane location of the mutations and their dominant-negative effect are independent risk factors for cardiac events. Shortly afterwards, Crotti and colleagues[6] focused on the "hot spot" *KCNQ1* A341V, a common mutation responsible for a founder effect in 25 South African families, and demonstrated that the unusually high clinical severity already reported by Brink and coworkers[19] for the South African families also is present among patients with LQT1 from different ethnic backgrounds but carrying the same A341V mutation. Moreover, because *KCNQ1* A341V has a mild dominant-negative effect (the current loss barely exceeds 50%), its striking clinically severe phenotype is explained neither by the location (transmembrane) nor by the functionally consequence of the mutation (dominant-negative). This implies that the current biophysical assessments of the electrophysiological effects of long QT syndrome–causing mutations do not provide all of the information necessary to make a complete genotype-phenotype correlation. In this regard, the study by Crotti's group[6] paves the way for mutation-specific risk stratification.

The risk stratification process is complicated by the presence of additional genetic variants that may modify clinical severity, as demonstrated in an LQT2 family with the C-terminal A1116V mutation, wherein the risk for life-threatening events was increased by the presence of the very common *KCNH2* K897T polymorphism. Electrophysiologic evidence did show that K897T produces an accentuation of the mutation-dependent I_{Kr} current loss, resulting in the unmasking of a clinically latent C-terminal LQT2 mutation.[29,30]

Drug-Induced Torsades de Pointes as a Manifestation of a Forme Fruste of Long QT Syndrome

The incomplete penetrance of long QT syndrome gene mutations explains a number of cases of drug-induced torsades de pointes. Several reports have followed the first evidence[31] of a disease-causing mutation in a patient with normal QTc and torsades de pointes–ventricular fibrillation while on therapy with cisapride. These observations confirmed the hypothesis proposed by Moss and Schwartz[3] in 1982 that a significant number of cases of drug-induced long QT syndrome may occur in patients with a forme fruste of long QT syndrome.

Epidemiology

The International Registry

In 1979, the International Long QT Syndrome Registry was established by Moss and Schwartz, with the main goals to define the natural and clinical history of long QT syndrome during a 25-year follow-up period.[32] In their words:

The value of the International Registry exceeded the expectations we had in 1979. At that time it did not escape us that this truly long-term project was bound to contribute to a better understanding and management of LQTS [long QT syndrome] but we could not anticipate the explosion of knowledge produced by the genetic and molecular findings from 1995 onward and the central role that the Registry, with its well-defined clinical phenotypes and family pedigrees without which molecular biology would be a toothless tool, would play in unmasking the secrets of LQTS. Neither could we have imagined the now clear evidence that LQTS represents indeed a paradigm for the understanding of the mechanisms underlying sudden cardiac death in more common cardiac diseases.[32]

Relation of Long QT Syndrome with Sudden Infant Death

Sudden infant death syndrome (SIDS) remains the leading cause of sudden death during the first year of life in the western world, but its causes remain largely unknown. In 1976 Schwartz proposed that an undefined number of SIDS victims might die because of an arrhythmic death favored by a prolongation of the QT interval with a mechanism similar to that of long QT syndrome.[33] This hypothesis was tested by prospectively measuring the QT interval during the first week of life in more than 33,000 infants and by following them for a possible occurrence of SIDS. The study[33] showed that 12 of the 24 SIDS victims but none of the other infants who died had a prolonged QTc. A QTc longer than 440 ms increased the risk for SIDS 41-fold.

Subsequently, two proof-of-concept studies identifying long QT syndrome–causing mutations in victims of SIDS or a typical episode or near-miss episode with documented ventricular fibrillation[34,35] paved the way to cohort studies. One of the two studies found long QT syndrome–causing mutations in 5.2% of 68 white infants.[36] The second,[11] based on 201 SIDS victims and 187 control subjects, all from Norway, identified functional[37,38] mutations in long QT syndrome genes in 9.5% (95% confidence intervals, 5.8 to 14.4) of the victims and in none of the controls. Considering that in 30% of unequivocal cases of long QT syndrome, it is likely that 11% to 13% of cases currently labeled as SIDS are actually due to long QT syndrome. Accordingly, these are preventable deaths.

These data obviously support the controversial concept of neonatal ECG screening[39,40] according to the guidelines proposed by the Task Force of the European Society of Cardiology.[13] The aim is the prevention of those sudden deaths due to unrecognized long QT syndrome, which may occur during the first few months of life or later on in life. Such screening is markedly cost-effective in Europe.[41]

Therapy

The trigger for most of the episodes of life-threatening arrhythmias of long QT syndrome is a sudden increase in sympathetic activity, largely mediated by the quantitatively dominant left cardiac sympathetic nerves.[18] Indeed, antiadrenergic therapies provide the greatest degree of protection.

Antiadrenergic Interventions

Despite the passage of time, the most significant information on therapy still comes from a 1985 study.[18] That analysis included 233 symptomatic patients and demonstrated the dramatic change in survival produced by pharmacologic or surgical antiadrenergic therapy when compared with any other therapy or no treatment. Such a large group of severely affected patients left without treatment is obviously no longer available.

β-Adrenergic Blockade

β-Adrenergic receptor blockade represents first-line therapy in symptomatic patients with long QT syndrome, barring specific contraindications.

Propranolol still is the most widely used β-adrenergic–blocking drug, at 2 to 3 mg/kg per day; sometimes the dosage is increased to 4 mg/kg. Nowadays, nadolol is used very often because its longer half-life allows twice-a-day administration, usually at 1 to 1.5 mg/kg per day. Atenolol has been associated to clinical failures more often than propranolol or nadolol. Seldom, beta-blockers result in excessive bradycardia, especially if the dosage is very gradually increased over several weeks.

In a large number of patients of unknown genotype, the mortality rate during beta-blocker therapy was 2%, and it was 1.6% for patients with syncope (no cardiac arrest) and without events in the first year of life.[42] Clear evidence demonstrates that beta-blockers are extremely effective in patients with LQT1. Data from two large studies[43,44] indicate an overall mortality rate of approximately 0.5%, and the rate of sudden death combined with cardiac arrest reaches 1%. The impairment in the I_{Ks} current makes these patients particularly sensitive to catecholamines and quite responsive to beta-blockade. These patients seldom need more than antiadrenergic therapy.

Compared with patients with LQT1, patients with LQT2 have more life-threatening events despite beta-blocker therapy, but most of these events are resuscitated cardiac arrest (6% to 7%).[15,43] Among patients with LQT3, major events occur more frequently (10% to 15%) despite beta-blocker therapy,[15,43] and some patients may require additional therapies (see later on). Also, many patients with Jervell and Lange-Nielsen syndrome are not adequately protected by beta-blockers.[2]

Strict adherence to the prescribed drug regimen is essential for patients with long QT syndrome treated with beta-blockers. Most of the so-called failures of beta-blocker therapy are due to incomplete compliance.[44]

Left Cardiac Sympathetic Denervation

After a small incision is made in the left subclavicular region, left cardiac sympathetic denervation (LCSD) is performed by an extrapleural approach, making thoracotomy unnecessary. The average time for surgery is 35 to 40 minutes.[45] LCSD requires removal of the first four thoracic ganglia. The cephalic portion of the left stellate ganglion is left intact, to avoid Horner's syndrome.[45] In nearly 30% of patients, a very modest (1- to 2-mm) ptosis results, which can be noted only on close examination but fully escapes notice in normal social interaction.

The latest data, published in 2004, include 147 patients with long QT syndrome who underwent LCSD during the previous 35 years.[45] They represent a very high-risk group, for several reasons: 99% were symptomatic; their mean QTc was very long (563 ± 65 ms); 48% had a cardiac arrest; and, especially, 75% continued to experience syncope despite full-dose beta-blocker therapy. The evidence most relevant to current clinical decisions is that obtained in patients without cardiac arrest who suffer syncope despite receiving full-dose beta-blocker therapy—and therefore should receive an ICD. During a mean follow-up period of 8 years, a 91% reduction in cardiac events was seen. LCSD produced a mean QTc shortening of 39 ms, pointing to an action on the substrate as well as on the trigger. The mortality rate was 3% in this high-risk group. A post-surgery QTc less than 500 ms predicted a very favorable outcome. Of importance, this series included 5 patients who underwent LCSD owing to multiple ICD shocks and electrical storms. In this group, over a 4-year follow-up period, a 95% decrease occurred in the number of shocks (from an average of

29 shocks per year), with a dramatic improvement in quality of life for both patients and their families.

The major antifibrillatory efficacy of LCSD has been demonstrated previously in high-risk post–myocardial infarction patients,[46] and very recently in patients with catecholaminergic polymorphic ventricular tachycardia (CPVT) not protected by beta-blockers and receiving multiple appropriate shocks by the ICD.[47]

Whenever syncopal episodes recur despite full-dose beta-blocker therapy, LCSD should be considered and implemented when possible. It is unfortunate that, despite its relative simplicity, LCSD is not performed in many high-risk patients, because cardiovascular surgeons are no longer familiar with the procedure, in contrast with the 1950s and 1960s, when LCSD frequently was used for the management of angina pectoris until it was superseded by the advent of beta-blockers. The consequence is that too often the choice goes to the easiest approach—namely, ICD implantation—even when this approach is not the best option for the patient. Before any therapeutic decision regarding a young patient with breakthrough syncope despite beta-blocker therapy, both patient and family members have the right to be informed about the long-term benefits and limitations of both LCSD and ICD.

Cardiac Pacing

Patients with long QT syndrome for whom cardiac pacing is indicated are very few. In infants or young children with 2:1 atrioventricular block and pause-dependent torsades, this remains a reasonable choice as a bridge to ICD implantation. The fact that onset of torsade de pointes often is preceded by a pause[3] justifies consideration for a pacemaker as an adjunct to therapy in selected patients with long QT syndrome. If a pacemaker is being considered, however, it may be more logical to implant an ICD with pacing modes.

Implantable Cardioverter Defibrillators

A major increase, largely unjustified, has been documented in the number of ICDs implanted in patients with long QT syndrome. There is consensus for immediate ICD implantation in case of a documented cardiac arrest, either on or off therapy. By contrast, opinions differ strongly regarding the use of ICDs in patients without cardiac arrest.

The U.S.[48] and the European[49] ICD–long QT syndrome registries provide the disquieting information that a majority of patients undergoing ICD implantation had not suffered a cardiac arrest and, moreover, that many had not even failed beta-blocker therapy. A recent multicenter study went so far as to identify the mere presence of a *SCN5A* mutation, even in a totally asymptomatic person, as sufficient indication for immediate ICD implantation.[50] There are actual data that contradict this attitude.[51]

It should not be forgotten that ICDs do not prevent occurrence of malignant arrhythmias and that torsade de pointes frequently is self-terminating in patients with long QT syndrome. The recurrence of electrical storms has led to suicide attempts in teenagers, and its high incidence (more than 10%) in children has been considered by a large group of experienced pediatric cardiologists to be "devastating."[52] The massive release of catecholamines, triggered by pain and fear, that follows an ICD discharge in a conscious patient—especially a young one—leads to further arrhythmias and consequent further discharges, producing a dramatic vicious circle.

Special caution is necessary regarding the decision for ICD implantation in a child with long QT syndrome. Such a decision is seldom justified before a proper trial with combined antiadrenergic therapy, that is, full-dose beta-blockade and LCSD, which prevents sudden death in 96% to 97% of symptomatic and high-risk patients[45] and which still allows for ICD implantation in case of a new syncope or cardiac arrest. On the other hand, the nature of the disease is such that cardiac arrests may recur, with potentially fatal consequences. Thus, the dilemma of concern for the life of the patient in the face of medicolegal considerations represents a reality. The risk-benefit ratio for an ICD should be clearly explained to the patient or to his or her parents, together with information on the pros and cons of LCSD, to allow them the possibility of a choice. Paradoxically, the decision to implant an ICD as an additional precaution even in a patient who appears to do well with combined antiadrenergic therapy, has a certain logic because such a patient has a low but not zero risk of cardiac arrest. Cardioversions are therefore unlikely to occur, but the presence of the ICD may provide a means of survival against the unexpected episode of an otherwise lethal arrhythmia. The need for several battery and lead replacements remains a major problem with young patients.

Our current policy is always to implant an ICD after a cardiac arrest, always when requested by the patient, when syncope recurs despite beta-blockade and LCSD, and whenever our clinical sense detects imminent danger despite therapy.

Gene-Specific Therapy and Management

Patients with LQT1 are at higher risk for life-threatening arrhythmias during sympathetic activation, such as during exercise and emotions. They should not participate in competitive sports. Swimming is particularly dangerous, as 99% of the arrhythmic episodes associated with swimming occur in these patients.[15]

In patients with LQT2, some of whom have a tendency to lose potassium, it is essential to maintain adequate potassium levels. Use of oral potassium supplements in combination with potassium-sparing agents constitutes a reasonable approach. Because these patients are at higher risk, especially when aroused from sleep or rest by a sudden noise,[4,15] we recommend that telephones and alarm clocks be removed from their bedrooms and that, especially with children, awakening them from sleep in the morning be done gently, and without yelling.

The realization that *SCN5A* mutations producing LQT3 have a "gain-of-function" effect[8] lends support to our early suggestion[14] to test sodium channel blockers, especially mexiletine, as possible adjuvants in the management of patients with this variant.[25,53] We test the effectiveness of mexiletine in all LQT3 patients by the acute oral drug test technique (half the daily dose during continuous ECG monitoring). Within 90 minutes, the peak plasma concentration is reached, and if the QTc is shortened by more than 40 ms, then we add mexiletine to the beta-blocker therapy. As a matter of fact, in most LQT3 patients treated with mexiletine, QTc shortens by more than 70 to 80 ms (Fig. 69-7). Even though conclusive evidence is lacking for a beneficial effect and definite failures have occurred, evidence also is increasing for significant benefit in a number of individual cases. In certain highly malignant forms manifesting in infancy due to mutations causing extremely severe electrophysiologic dysfunction, the functional defect can be corrected by the combination of mexiletine and propranolol.[53]

During heart rate increases, QTc shortens more in patients with LQT3 than among healthy controls,[14] and indeed, normal physical activity may not need to be restricted in these patients. They are, however, at higher risk for death at rest and especially at nighttime. When these patients sleep and are in a horizontal position, the onset of torsade de pointes produces a progressive but slow fall in blood pressure that leads to a noisy gasping preceding death. In some reported cases, in both LQT2

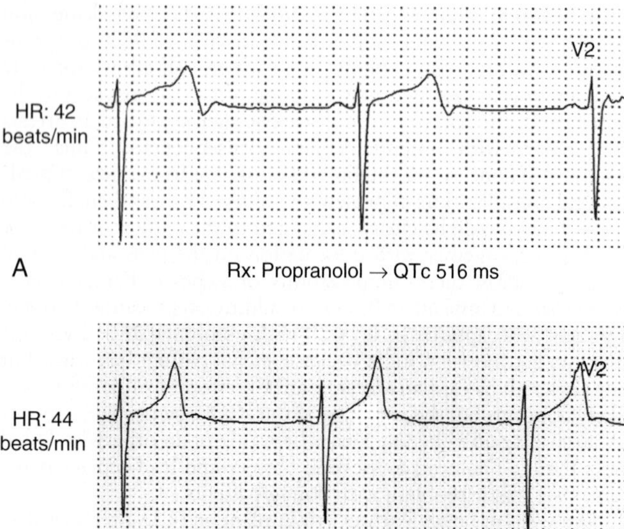

Figure 69-7 **A,** Major QTc prolongation (QTc of 516 ms) in a 17-year-old boy with LQT3 was not modified by beta-blocker therapy. **B,** The addition of oral chronic therapy with mexiletine (200 mg twice daily) produced a major shortening of QTc by more than 100 ms, persisting over time.

(also associated with risk for death during sleep or rest) and LQT3, a family member, such as the spouse sleeping in the same bed, was alerted by the noisy breathing and was able to save the patient. Accordingly, we recommend that patients with these two variants have an intercom system in their bedrooms and—if young—in their parents' bedrooms.

Finally, QT interval shortening, albeit encouraging, cannot be assumed automatically to imply protection from life-threatening arrhythmias. It is essential to keep in mind the tragic failures of earlier attempts to shorten QT by digitalis.[1] The use of novel and experimental therapies should not deprive symptomatic patients of therapies with established protective effect.

Asymptomatic Patients with Long QT Syndrome and Patients with a Normal QTc

Because the first manifestation of long QT syndrome in approximately 12% of cases is sudden death, beta-blocker treatment should be initiated in all patients, including those who are still asymptomatic. Among those without symptoms, reasonable exceptions appear to be men with LQT1 who are older than 20 to 25 years of age, because very seldom does a first event occur any later in this patient population, and adults with a QTc less than 500 ms. Women with LQT2 seem to remain at risk throughout life, and we recommend that these patients always receive treatment. Patients with a normal QTc (less than 440 ms) appear to be at very low risk for life-threatening arrhythmias. In absence of clear follow-up data, treatment for this patient subgroup is optional; the characterization of the mutation and the age of the patient could influence this choice.

Cardiac and noncardiac drugs that block the I_{Kr} current and thereby prolong the QT interval should always be avoided in patients with long QT syndrome. A drug list is published at www.torsades.org. Such a list, updated every year, should be given to all patients, because their physicians may not be aware of these electrophysiologic actions.

Overview of Therapy

The sound data available, and decades of clinical experience, dictate the therapeutic approach to the patient affected by long QT syndrome *who already has had a syncopal episode*. Treatment should always begin with beta-blockers, unless valid contraindications are known. If the patient has one more syncopal episode despite full-dose beta-blockade, LCSD should be performed without hesitation, and ICD implantation should be considered, with the final decision based on individual patient characteristics (age, gender, previous history, genetic subgroup including certain mutation-specific features, and presence of signs indicating high electrical instability on the ECG, including 24-hour Holter recordings). In the end, there is no substitute for careful clinical judgment,[51] accompanied by a thorough knowledge of the several variants of this unique life-threatening cardiac disorder, when the goal is to protect these patients and at the same time to ensure their quality of life.

Short QT Syndrome

Although the association between the QT interval and sudden death has been known for more than 50 years, only recently it has become evident that not only a long but also a short QT interval could be associated with an increased risk of life-threatening ventricular arrhythmias.[54,55]

Molecular Genetics of Short QT Syndrome

Three main genetic variants have been described so far in the short QT syndrome, and they all involve potassium channel genes. Although mutations on the potassium channel genes causing long QT syndrome are loss-of-function mutations, those observed in short QT syndrome are gain-of-function mutations that shorten action potential duration.

Genetic screening in the first two kindreds with short QT syndrome and familial sudden cardiac death[54] identified two different missense mutations on *KCNH2* resulting in the same amino acid change of the cardiac I_{Kr} channel (*KCNH2* N588K).[7] Expression studies in human embryonic kidney cells by Brugada and colleagues demonstrated that N558K causes a loss of the normal rectification of the current at plateau voltages, which results in a significant increase of I_{Kr} during the action potential plateau and leads to an abbreviation of the action potential and refractory period.[7] Thus, *KCNH2* is the gene responsible for SQTS1.

Bellocq and coworkers,[7] in a 70-year-old patient with a QTc of 302 ms and aborted sudden cardiac death, identified a mutation in the *KCNQ1* gene (V307L), causing a gain of function of I_{Ks}, resulting in an abbreviation of the action potential duration and shortening of the QT interval. Another mutation (V141M) in *KCNQ1* was identified[56] in an infant born with atrial fibrillation with slow ventricular response and short QT interval. Computer modeling of V141M suggests that it would shorten ventricular action potential duration and abolish pacemaker activity of the sinoatrial node. *KCNQ1* is therefore responsible not only for LQT1 but also for SQTS2.

SQTS3 is associated with a gain-of-function mutation (G514A) in the *KCNJ2* gene, encoding the strong inwardly rectifying channel protein Kir2.1 involved in the Andersen-Tawil syndrome. Functional characterization by Priori and associates demonstrated a significant increase in the outward I_{K1} current.[7]

Antzelevitch and coworkers described three patients in whom the Brugada syndrome phenotype and a family history for sudden cardiac death were associated with QTc of 360 ms or less.[57] Mutations in genes encoding the α1 or β2b subunit of the cardiac L-type calcium channel were identified and found to be associated with a major loss of function in calcium channel activity. The QTc in these patients and of affected family members ranged between 330 and 370 ms, values greater than those in typical families with this variant. It seems premature to consider *CACNB2B* and *CACNA1C* as short QT syndrome genes. These cases may represent a new clinical entity with overlapping phenotypes.

Molecular screening is not yet a diagnostic tool for short QT syndrome but may help identify silent mutation carriers, whose arrhythmic risk is unknown.

Clinical Presentation

The very few reported cases of short QT syndrome limit the possibility of a generalized clinical picture because the initial cases of rare diseases are always the most severe. Thus far, all patients have a QTc less than 320 ms, without structural heart disease. They appear to be at high risk for syncope or sudden cardiac death due to ventricular tachyarrhythmias, and atrial fibrillation has been documented frequently, even in children. Cardiac arrest has occurred both at rest and under stress.

In 2000 Gussak and colleagues made a first report focused on a 17-year-old female patient with atrial fibrillation and QTc of 300 ms.[54] Her brother and mother had episodes of atrial fibrillation and a QTc less than 300 ms. Neither syncope nor sudden death occurred in this family. Also mentioned was a 37-year-old female patient with syncope and very short QTc (266 ms) who died suddenly at home.

In 2003 Gaita and associates reported their findings for seven more patients. All of their patients had a QTc less than 300 ms and a family history positive for sudden death (including that of a 3-month-old infant).[55] Electrophysiologic studies performed in four of the seven patients documented short atrial and ventricular refractory periods, as well as increased ventricular vulnerability to fibrillation in three of them. Molecular screening identified *KCNH2* as the first disease-causing gene of short QT syndrome.[7]

Clinical heterogeneity is clearly present in short QT syndrome, with reported first manifestations occurring from intrauterine period to the age of 70 years and presenting with either atrial or ventricular fibrillation and sometimes appearing as SIDS.[38]

Diagnosis

Diagnostic criteria for short QT syndrome are not available. In most reported cases, the QTc was less than 320 ms, but the lower limit of QTc is not fully established, and its significance is uncertain. Two large studies in normal populations (both including more than 10,000 subjects) addressed this issue, with the following conclusions: (1) A QTc of 330 ms or less is extremely rare in healthy persons, but the presence of a QT interval in the lowest half-percentile of the normal distribution does not imply a significant risk of sudden death;[58] and (2) no sudden deaths occurred among persons with QTc less than 340 ms.[59] It follows that the mere presence of a short QT interval is not sufficient to make a diagnosis of short QT syndrome.

Affected patients also demonstrate shortening or absence of the ST segment, with the T wave initiating immediately from the S wave. In patients with SQT1, the T waves in precordial leads often are tall, narrow, and symmetrical, with a relatively prolonged T_{peak}-T_{end} interval[51] (Fig. 69-8), suggesting augmented transmural dispersion of repolarization. In patients with SQT2, the T waves appear to be symmetrical, but not so tall and narrow.[7] The only two patients with SQT3 show an asymmetrical pattern, with a less steep ascending section of the T wave followed by a rapid descending terminal phase.[7]

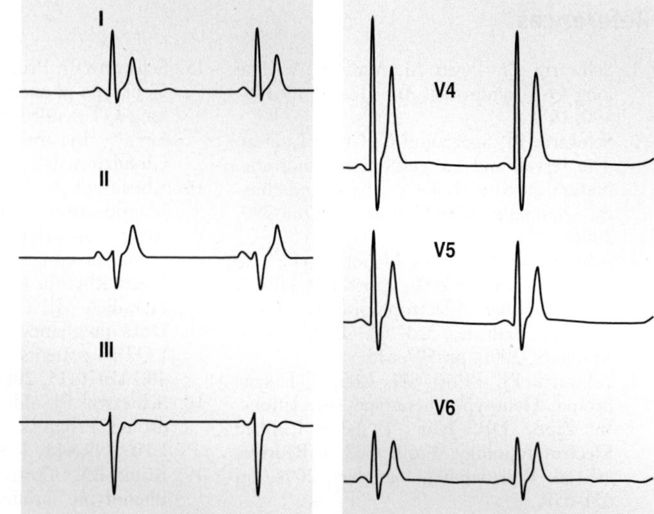

Figure 69-8 Example of short QT syndrome. This 12-lead electrocardiogram of a patient in sinus rhythm shows a heart rate of 52 beats per minute, left axis deviation, and QTc of 280 ms. Paper speed, 25 mm/second. (Modified from Gaita F, Giustetto C, Bianchi F, et al: Short QT syndrome: A familial cause of sudden death. Circulation 108:965-970, 2003.)

An additional feature in patients with short QT syndrome is the lack of QT adaptation to heart rate changes.

In a recently reported series, 11 patients with short QT syndrome, all carrying the *KCNH2* N588K mutation, underwent electrophysiology studies. Both atrial and ventricular effective refractory periods were found to be extremely short (141 ± 18 ms and 147 ± 18 ms for atrial and ventricular effective refractory periods, respectively).[56] Moreover, in 10 of the 11 patients (91%), ventricular tachyarrhythmias were found to be inducible.

Therapy

Uncertainty exists about the therapy for short QT syndrome. Gaita and associates,[60] in six patients with SQT1, tried flecainide, ibutilide, sotalol, and quinidine. Only quinidine normalized the QT interval, the T wave morphology, and the ventricular effective refractory period and made ventricular fibrillation noninducible. Indeed, the N558R mutation produces only a 5.8-fold decrease in the I_{Kr} channel–blocking effect of quinidine, in contrast with the 20-fold decrease in the effect of sotalol.[56] In vitro studies of the N588K *HERG* mutation and data in two patients with SQT1 suggested high efficacy of disopyramide for normalizing ECG features.[61] These investigations are limited by the small number of patients, the homogeneous genetic background (only patients with SQT1 and the N588K mutation), and the lack of evidence for a reduction in spontaneous arrhythmic events.

The high mortality rate observed in the approximately 30 cases of short QT syndrome reported so far makes reasonable the consideration of ICD implantation as the therapy of choice. When more patients will have been described and the actual clinical picture will have been clarified, with the likely emergence of a number of asymptomatic patients, it will become possible to refine the therapeutic recommendations.

In very young asymptomatic patients, the suggestion to use and test oral quinidine as a bridge to ICD implantation later in life is not unreasonable. In patients who already have an ICD, the addition of oral quinidine could provide useful data on its efficacy (or lack thereof), with the safety net provided by the ICD.

References

1. Schwartz PJ, Periti M, Malliani A: The long Q-T syndrome. Am Heart J 89:378-390, 1975.
2. Schwartz PJ, Spazzolini C, Crotti L, et al: The Jervell and Lange-Nielsen syndrome. Natural history, molecular basis, and clinical outcome. Circulation 113:783-790, 2006.
3. Schwartz PJ, Priori SG, Napolitano C: The long QT syndrome. In Zipes DP, Jalife J (eds): Cardiac Electrophysiology: From Cell to Bedside, 3rd ed. Philadelphia, Saunders, 2000, pp 597-615.
4. Schwartz PJ, Priori SG: Long QT syndrome: Genotype-phenotype correlations. In Zipes DP, Jalife J (eds): Cardiac Electrophysiology: From Cell to Bedside, 4th ed. Philadelphia, Saunders, 2004, pp 651-659.
5. Moss AJ, Shimizu W, Wilde AA, et al: Clinical aspects of type-1 long-QT syndrome by location, coding type, and biophysical function of mutations involving the *KCNQ1* gene. Circulation 115:2481-2489, 2007.
6. Crotti L, Spazzolini C, Schwartz PJ, et al: The common long QT syndrome mutation KCNQ1/A341V causes unusually severe clinical manifestations in patients with different ethnic backgrounds: Toward a mutation-specific risk stratification. Circulation 116:2366-2375, 2007.
7. Priori SG, Napolitano C, Schwartz PJ: Genetics of cardiac arrhythmias. In Libby P, Bonow RO, Mann DL, Zipes DP (eds): Braunwald's Heart Disease, 8th ed. Philadelphia, Saunders, 2008, pp 101-109.
8. Bennett PB, Yazawa K, Makita N, George AL Jr: Molecular mechanism for an inherited cardiac arrhythmia. Nature 376:683-685, 1995.
9. Splawski I, Timothy KW, Sharpe LM, et al: $Ca_V1.2$ calcium channel dysfunction causes a multisystem disorder including arrhythmia and autism. Cell 119:19-31, 2004.
10. Ye B, Tester DJ, Vatta M, et al: Molecular and functional characterization of novel CAV3-encoded caveolin-3 mutations in congenital long QT syndrome. Heart Rhythm 3(Suppl):S1, 2006.
11. Arnestad M, Crotti L, Rognum TO, et al: Prevalence of long QT syndrome gene variants in sudden infant death syndrome. Circulation 115:361-367, 2007.
12. Stramba-Badiale M, Crotti L, Goulene K, et al: Electrocardiographic and genetic screening for long QT syndrome: results from a prospective study on 44,596 neonates. Circulation 116(Abstr Suppl):II-377, 2007.
13. Schwartz PJ, Garson A Jr, Paul T, et al: Guidelines for the interpretation of the neonatal electrocardiogram. Eur Heart J 23:1329-1344, 2002.
14. Schwartz PJ, Priori SG, Locati EH, et al: Long QT syndrome patients with mutations of the *SCN5A* and *HERG* genes have differential responses to Na^+ channel blockade and to increases in heart rate. Implications for gene-specific therapy. Circulation 92:3381-3386, 1995.
15. Schwartz PJ, Priori SG, Spazzolini C, et al: Genotype-phenotype correlation in the long-QT syndrome: Gene-specific triggers for life-threatening arrhythmias. Circulation 103:89-95, 2001.
16. Khositseth A, Tester DJ, Will ML, et al: Identification of a common genetic substrate underlying postpartum cardiac events in congenital long QT syndrome. Heart Rhythm 1:60-64, 2004.
17. Heradien MJ, Goosen A, Crotti L, et al: Does pregnancy increase cardiac risk for LQT1 patients? J Am Coll Cardiol 48:1410-1415, 2006.
18. Schwartz PJ: Idiopathic long QT syndrome: Progress and questions. Am Heart J 109:399-411, 1985.
19. Brink PA, Crotti L, Corfield V, et al: Phenotypic variability and unusual clinical severity of congenital long QT syndrome in a founder population. Circulation 112:2602-2610, 2005.
20. Schwartz PJ, Vanoli E, Crotti L, et al: Neural control of heart rate modifies arrhythmia risk in congenital long QT syndrome. J Am Coll Cardiol 51:920-929, 2008.
21. Nador F, Beria G, De Ferrari GM, et al: Unsuspected echocardiographic abnormality in the long QT syndrome: Diagnostic, prognostic, and pathogenetic implications. Circulation 84:1530-1542, 1991.
22. Haugaa KH, Edvardsen T, Leren TP, et al: Left ventricular mechanical dispersion by tissue Doppler imaging: a novel approach for identifying high-risk individuals with long QT syndrome. Eur Heart J 30:330-337, 2009.
23. De Ferrari GM, Schwartz PJ: Long QT syndrome, a purely electrical disease? Not anymore. Eur Heart J 30:253-255, 2009.
24. Schwartz PJ, Moss AJ, Vincent GM, Crampton RS: Diagnostic criteria for the long QT syndrome: an update. Circulation 88:782-784, 1993.
25. Schwartz PJ: The congenital long QT syndromes from genotype to phenotype: Clinical implications. J Intern Med 259:39-47, 2006.
26. Crotti L, Lewandowska MA, Schwartz PJ, et al: A KCNH2 branch point mutation causing aberrant splicing contributes to an explanation of genotype-negative long QT syndrome. Heart Rhythm 6:212-218, 2009.
27. Priori SG, Schwartz PJ, Napolitano C, et al: Risk stratification in the long-QT syndrome. N Engl J Med 348:1866-1874, 2003.
28. Moss AJ, Zareba W, Kaufman ES, et al: Increased risk of arrhythmic events in long-QT syndrome with mutations in the pore region of the human ether-à-go-go–related gene potassium channel. Circulation 105:794-799, 2002.
29. Crotti L, Lundquist AL, Insolia R, et al: KCNH2-K897T is a genetic modifier of latent congenital long QT syndrome. Circulation 112;1251-1258, 2005. Corrections in Circulation 112:e295, 2005.
30. Rubart M, Zipes DP: Genes and cardiac repolarization. The challenge ahead. Circulation 112:1242-1244, 2005.
31. Napolitano C, Schwartz PJ, Brown AM, et al: Evidence for a cardiac ion channel mutation underlying drug-induced QT prolongation and life-threatening arrhythmias. J Cardiovasc Electrophysiol 11:691-696, 2000.
32. Moss AJ, Schwartz PJ: 25th anniversary of the International Long QT Syndrome Registry: An ongoing quest to uncover the secrets of LQTS. Circulation 111:1199-1201, 2005.
33. Schwartz PJ, Stramba-Badiale M: Prolonged repolarization and sudden infant death syndrome. In Zipes DP, Jalife J (eds): Cardiac Electrophysiology: From Cell to Bedside, 4th ed. Philadelphia, Saunders, 2004, pp 711-719.
34. Schwartz PJ, Priori SG, Dumaine R, et al: A molecular link between the sudden infant death syndrome and the long QT syndrome. N Engl J Med 343:262-267, 2000.
35. Schwartz PJ, Priori SG, Bloise R, et al: Molecular diagnosis in a child with sudden infant death syndrome. Lancet 358:1342-1343, 2001.
36. Ackerman MJ, Siu BL, Sturner WQ, et al: Postmortem molecular analysis of *SCN5A* defects in sudden infant death syndrome. JAMA 286:2264-2269, 2001.
37. Wang DW, Desai RR, Crotti L, et al: Cardiac sodium channel dysfunction in sudden infant death syndrome: Is it time to consider newborn electrocardiographic screening? Circulation 115:368-376, 2007.
38. Rhodes TE, Abraham RL, Welch RC, et al: Cardiac potassium channel dysfunction in sudden infant death syndrome. J Mol Cell Cardiol 44:571-581, 2008.
39. Schwartz PJ: Newborn ECG screening to prevent sudden cardiac death. Heart Rhythm 11:1353-1355, 2006.
40. van Langen IM, Wilde AA: Newborn screening to prevent sudden cardiac death? Heart Rhythm 3:1356-1359, 2006.
41. Quaglini S, Rognoni C, Spazzolini C, et al: Cost-effectiveness of neonatal ECG screening for the long QT-syndrome. Eur Heart J 15:1824-1832, 2006.
42. Moss AJ, Zareba W, Hall WJ, et al: Effectiveness and limitations of beta-blocker therapy in congenital long-QT syndrome. Circulation 101:616-623, 2000.
43. Priori SG, Napolitano C, Schwartz PJ, et al: Association of long QT syndrome loci and cardiac events among patients treated with beta-blockers. JAMA 292: 1341-1344, 2004.
44. Vincent GM, Schwartz PJ, Denjoy I, et al: High efficacy of beta-blockers in long QT syndrome type 1: contribution of non-compliance and QT prolonging drugs to the occurrence of beta-blocker treatment "failures". Circulation 119:215-221, 2009.
45. Schwartz PJ, Priori SG, Cerrone M, et al: Left cardiac sympathetic denervation in the management of high-risk patients affected by the long QT syndrome. Circulation 109:1826-1833, 2004.
46. Schwartz PJ, Motolese M, Pollavini G, et al, for the Italian Sudden Death Prevention Group: Prevention of sudden

cardiac death after a first myocardial infarction by pharmacologic or surgical antiadrenergic interventions. J Cardiovasc Electrophysiol 3:2-16, 1992.

47. Wilde AAM, Bhuiyan ZA, Crotti L, et al: Left cardiac sympathetic denervation for catecholaminergic polymorphic ventricular tachycardia. N Engl J Med 358:2024-2029, 2008.
48. Zareba W, Moss AJ, Daubert JP, et al: Implantable cardioverter defibrillator in high-risk long QT syndrome patients. J Cardiovasc Electrophysiol 14:337-341, 2003.
49. Crotti L, Spazzolini C, De Ferrari GM, et al: Is the implantable defibrillator appropriately used in the long QT syndrome? Data from the European Registry. Heart Rhythm 1(Suppl):582, 2004.
50. Etheridge SP, Sanatani S, Cohen MI, et al: Long QT syndrome in children in the era of implantable defibrillators. J Am Coll Cardiol 50:1335-1340, 2007.
51. Schwartz PJ, Spazzolini C, Crotti L: All LQT3 patients need an ICD. True or false? Heart Rhythm 6:113-120, 2009.
52. Wolf MJ, Zeltser IJ, Salerno J, et al: Electrical storm in children with an implantable cardioverter defibrillator: Clinical features and outcome. Heart Rhythm 4(Suppl):S43, 2007.
53. Wang DW, Crotti L, Shimizu W, et al: Malignant perinatal variant of long QT syndrome caused by a profoundly dysfunctional cardiac sodium channel. Circulation Arrhythmia and Electrophysiology 1:370-378, 2008.
54. Gussak I, Brugada P, Brugada J, et al: Idiopathic short QT interval: A new clinical syndrome? Cardiology 94:99-102, 2000.
55. Gaita F, Giustetto C, Bianchi F, et al: Short QT syndrome: A familial cause of sudden death. Circulation 108:965-970, 2003.
56. Hong K, Piper DR, Diaz-Valdecantos A, et al: De novo *KCNQ1* mutation responsible for atrial fibrillation and short QT syndrome in utero. Cardiovasc Res 68:433-440, 2005.
57. Antzelevitch C, Pollevick GD, Cordeiro JM, et al: Loss-of-function mutations in the cardiac calcium channel underlie a new clinical entity characterized by ST-segment elevation, short QT intervals, and sudden cardiac death. Circulation 115:442-449, 2007.
58. Gallagher MM, Magliano G, Yap YG, et al: Distribution and prognostic significance of QT intervals in the lowest half centile in 12,012 apparently healthy persons. Am J Cardiol 98:933-935, 2006.
59. Anttonen O, Junttila MJ, Rissanen H, et al: Prevalence and prognostic significance of short QT interval in a middle-aged Finnish population. Circulation 116:714-720, 2007.
60. Gaita F, Giustetto C, Bianchi F, et al: Short QT syndrome: pharmacological treatment. J Am Coll Cardiol 43:1494-1499, 2004.
61. Schimpf R, Veltmann C, Giustetto C, et al: In vivo effects of mutant HERG K^+ channel inhibition by disopyramide in patients with a short QT-1 syndrome: A pilot study. J Cardiovasc Electrophysiol 18:1157-1160, 2007.

Catecholaminergic Polymorphic Ventricular Tachycardia 70

CARLO NAPOLITANO, YANFEI RUAN, AND SILVIA G. PRIORI

CHAPTER OUTLINE

Definition

Catecholaminergic polymorphic ventricular tachycardia (CPVT) is an inherited disorder associated with syncope and sudden death that manifests predominantly in children and teenagers[1,2] with structurally normal hearts. CPVT is characterized by the presence of a normal pattern on the resting electrocardiogram (ECG) and a typical pattern of onset and offset of adrenergically induced ventricular and supraventricular arrhythmias.[3,4]

Since its initial description,[1] CPVT (identification number 604772 in the Online Mendelian Inheritance in Man [OMIM] database) was recognized as a genetically determined disease. In parallel with elucidation of the molecular bases of the disease, its pathophysiologic mechanisms are being progressively unveiled. This chapter focuses on the clinical presentation and genetics of CPVT; the pathophysiologic mechanisms are described in Chapter 52.

Clinical Phenotype and Diagnosis

Electrocardiographic Characteristics

Resting Electrocardiogram

Patients with CPVT present with an unremarkable pattern on the resting ECG. Only subtle abnormalities such as prominent U waves and lower-than-normal resting heart rate are reported.[4-6]

The presence of a prominent U wave is a frequent finding, although it cannot be considered to be a diagnostic indicator of CPVT. Aizawa and colleagues[5] observed U wave beat-to-beat variability (U wave alternans) in the recovery phase of exercise when ventricular tachycardia was induced. Combination of clinical and experimental data may provide hints to the origin of this phenomenon. In a transgenic model of CPVT,[7] delayed afterdepolarizations (DADs), possibly arising from the Purkinje network,[8] were demonstrated to be the electrophysiologic mechanisms of arrhythmias' onset. Paavola and coworkers investigated the origin of U wave using monophasic action potential recordings[9] from the right ventricular septum. The presence of DADs was detected in 3 of 15 patients with CPVT (20%) in resting conditions and in 27% during epinephrine infusion. Of interest, DAD–QRS coupling paralleled U wave–QRS coupling, suggesting that U wave in patients with CPVT could be the result of the occurrence of DADs.

Diagnostic Value of Exercise Stress Testing

The typical patient with CPVT seeks medical advice during childhood or early adolescence for recurrence of syncopal events elicited by physical or emotional stress. In such cases, findings on cardiac evaluation by ECG and echocardiogram are unremarkable. Accordingly, symptoms may be attributed to neurologic disorders, with consequent delayed diagnosis. In our series, the mean time to diagnosis after the first manifestation was 2 years.[3] Such delay in diagnosis may be life-threatening.

Exercise stress testing often is the most useful procedure to establish the diagnosis of CPVT. Unfortunately, reluctance to consider this study as a first-line examination in children with syncope is common. However, at variance with findings in long QT syndrome, in which patients experience exercise-related syncope but arrhythmias do not develop during exercise stress testing, patients with CPVT very often experience progressive worsening of supraventricular and ventricular arrhythmias that parallels the increase in workload during such testing.

Isolated supraventricular and ventricular ectopies usually start at a heart rate threshold of 100 to 110 beats per minute. The complexity and frequency of arrhythmia progressively worsen from isolated premature beats to bigeminy, couplets and to runs of ventricular and supraventricular tachycardias (Fig. 70-1). If exercise is not promptly discontinued, ventricular tachycardia may become faster and progressively more disorganized until it degenerates into ventricular fibrillation. Usually arrhythmias promptly recede during recovery.

The distinguishing ventricular tachycardia pattern that is suggestive of CPVT is called *bidirectional ventricular tachycardia* and is characterized by a 180-degree alternating QRS axis on a beat-to-beat basis; a minority of patients show irregular polymorphic ventricular tachycardia.[3,10] Sumitomo and coworkers investigated the site of origin of ventricular tachycardia by analyzing the morphology of the initiating beat on surface ECG.[11] They showed that nearly 90% of episodes originated from the right ventricular outflow tract, whereas the second most-represented site of origin was the left ventricular outflow tract. Of interest, approximately 80% of the patients with multiple episodes of ventricular tachycardia showed reproducible morphology of the first beat of the dysrhythmia. The variable ventricular tachycardia origin suggests that the bidirectional pattern is not always detectable from the same ECG lead.

Supraventricular arrhythmias also are frequently elicited in patients with CPVT during exercise. Isolated atrial ectopic beats, nonsustained supraventricular tachycardia, and (less frequently) short runs of atrial fibrillation may be observed during exercise.[3,4,11]

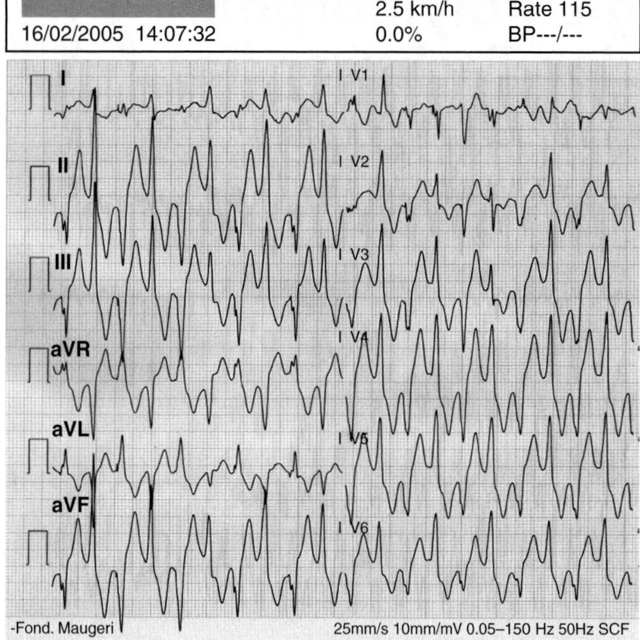

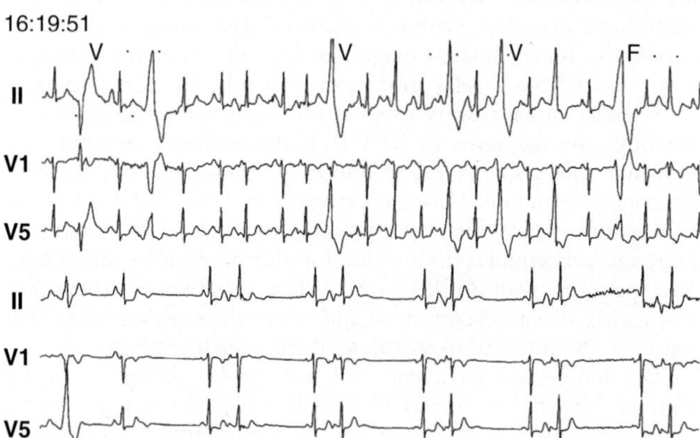

Figure 70-1 Electrocardiographic strips showing the typical bidirectional ventricular tachycardia in a patient with catecholaminergic polymorphic ventricular tachycardia during exercise stress testing *(upper panel)* and supraventricular arrhythmias detected at Holter monitoring during acute emotion (response to an alarm bell) *(lower panel)*.

Cardiac Events and Natural History

CPVT is a potentially fatal disorder with high incidence of symptomatic arrhythmic events and high mortality rate among patients who do not receive appropriate treatment. The available data on the natural history consistently show that the vast majority (60% to 80%) of patients experience syncope or cardiac arrest before the age of 40 years.[3,4,6,11,12]

In the series of Leenhardt and colleagues,[4] the mean age at first event was 7.8 ± 4 years—very similar to that reported by Priori and associates (8 ± 2 years)[3] and by Sumitomo and coworkers (10 years).[11] Occasionally the first manifestation may be during adulthood.[13]

Cardiac arrest may be the first manifestation of CPVT. CPVT patients have a structurally intact heart and a normal ECG pattern; therefore the underlying disorder may be diagnosed as *idiopathic ventricular fibrillation*. In 2002 our group[3] was the first to report CPVT mutations in two patients with IVF; other workers[14] subsequently confirmed this finding. Khran and colleagues[15] showed that 56% of patients resuscitated from an unexplained cardiac arrest with normal coronary arteries, normal ventricular function, and normal ECG can be clinically diagnosed with CPVT.

Data from our CPVT registry show that approximately 30% of patients experience a resuscitated cardiac arrest or sudden death by age 40, and that in one half of them, the cardiac arrest is the first manifestation of the disease.[12] Patients with CPVT very often have a very strong family history of juvenile sudden death. In our series, up to 30% of probands had a family history of at least one sudden death before the age of 40 years.[3,4]

As a consequence, it seems logical to suggest that family history of juvenile sudden death occurring during adrenergic activation should prompt the consideration of CPVT as a likely diagnosis in a family member evaluated for syncope occurring during exercise or emotion.

It is reasonable to assume that as a cause of cardiac death during childhood, CPVT may account for a fraction of sudden infant death syndrome (SIDS) cases. Indeed, some researchers have attempted to quantify the percentage of CPVT in a SIDS cohort by genotyping 137 SIDS victims,[16] in which they identified two *RYR2* mutations. Although they provided proof of the concept that CPVT may be a cause of SIDS, the yield of the analysis was too low to justify routine *RYR2* screening for SIDS.

Genetic Features and Genotype-Phenotype Correlations

Growing knowledge on the genetic determinants of CPVT has been gathered over the last few years. It is now clear that CPVT is a genetically heterogeneous disorder of intracellular calcium handling (see Table 70-1). Of interest, genetic mutations that may give raise to CPVT phenocopies have been reported in the context of other inherited arrhythmia syndromes (see Table 70-1), and they are discussed next because of the potential implications for clinical management.

Autosomal Dominant Catecholaminergic Polymorphic Ventricular Tachycardia: CPVT1

Mutations in the Cardiac Ryanodine Receptor

Autosomal dominant transmission of the CPVT phenotype and familial sudden death have been reported since the initial description of the disease.[1,4,17] In 1999, Swan and coworkers performed genome-wide linkage analysis of the dominant CPVT phenotype and mapped the disease to chromosomal locus 1q42-43, with a logarithm of the odds ratio (LOD) score of 4.74.[10]

The human cardiac ryanodine receptor (RyR2) appeared to be the strongest candidate in the critical region.[18] We therefore performed molecular screening and first reported RyR2 mutations in four families with CPVT, thereby demonstrating that *RYR2* is the gene for autosomal dominant CPVT.[19] The involvement of the cardiac ryanodine receptor as the cause of CPVT was subsequently confirmed by Laitinen and associates[20] and by several other investigators in the past several years (www.fsm.it/cardmoc).

RyR2 is a large tetrameric protein (4967 amino acids, 564 kD) spanning the membrane of the sarcoplasmic reticulum, and it releases Ca^{2+} ions from the sarcoplasmic reticulum in response to Ca^{2+} entry through the L-type channels during

Table 70-1 Genetics of Catecholaminergic Polymorphic Ventricular Tachycardia (CPVT)

Variant	Chromosomal Locus	Gene	Inheritance	Phenotype
CPVT1	1q42-43	*RYR2*	AD	CPVT, IVF
CPVT2	1p23-21	*CASQ2*	AR	CPVT
CPVT3	7p14-22	Unknown	AR	CPVT, QT interval prolongation
CPVT-Related Phenotypes				
LQT4	4q25-26	*ANK2*	AD	IVF, QT prolongation (atypical), stress-induced bidirectional VT
ATS	17q23.1-q24.2	*KCNJ2*	AD	U waves, bidirectional VT, periodic paralysis, facial dysmorphisms
CPVT/DCM	1q42-43	*RYR2*	AD	Stress-induced VT, sinus node dysfunction, dilated cardiomyopathy

AD, autosomal dominant; AR, autosomal recessive; ATS, Andersen-Tawil syndrome; DCM, dilated cardiomyopathy; IVF, idiopathic ventricular fibrillation; VT, ventricular tachycardia.

phase 2 of the action potential. The RyR2 structure, the biophysical consequences of mutations, and their link to arrhythmogenesis are discussed in Chapter 52; here we simply state that the final common consequence of *RYR2* mutations is to cause abnormal diastolic Ca^{2+} release from the sarcoplasmic reticulum, thereby facilitating the development of afterdepolarizations and triggered arrhythmias.[21]

A recent analysis of published *RYR2* mutations showed that they tend to cluster in 25 exons encoding four discrete domains of the RyR2 protein: domain I (amino acids 77 to 466), II (amino acids 2246 to 2534), III (3778 to 4201), and IV (4497 to 4959)[22] (Fig. 70-2) (see http://www.fsm.it/cardmoc). These clusters are made by amino acid sequences highly conserved throughout species and among RyR isoforms[22] and are thought to be functionally important.

Only few recurrent RyR2 mutations have been identified in unrelated CPVT families. The most frequent *RYR2* CPVT mutations are R176Q, S2246L, R4497C and G3946S; however, because the absolute number of carriers of this recurrent mutations is low, it has been impossible to establish a relationship between clinical presentation (arrhythmia pattern, mortality, age at onset, and so on) and specific mutations. Approximately 19% of *RYR2* mutations arise de novo. Preliminary evidence suggests that de novo mutations may be associated with a severe phenotype with significantly lower age at onset of symptoms.[22]

Because *RYR2* is one of the largest genes in the human genome (105 exons on more than 800 kilobases), CPVT genetic testing is time-consuming and expensive. We believe that despite mutation of *RYR2* tend to cluster in specific regions, in the clinical setting the genetic testing should be performed by screening the entire coding region of the gene. Indeed, the yield of targeted screening is approximately 40%,[23] whereas complete screening allows successful genotyping in up to 50% to 60% of patients with definite clinical diagnosis.[21] A recent analysis of data from our CPVT-RyR2 screening program showed that 17% of mutations localize outside the clusters.[24]

When a clinical diagnosis of CPVT is established, genetic testing is indicated to allow presymptomatic diagnosis among family members whenever the *RYR2* mutation is identified in the proband. This step is important because early identification of affected persons allows implementation of pharmacologic therapy that may be life-saving.[25]

Autosomal Recessive Catecholaminergic Polymorphic Ventricular Tachycardia: CPVT2

Mutations in Cardiac Calsequestrin: *CASQ2*

In 2001 Lahat and coworkers[26] mapped a recessive variant of CPVT in a 16-centimorgans interval at chromosomal locus 1p23-21, with an LOD score of 8.24. Subsequently the same group identified one cardiac calsequestrin mutation (*CASQ2*), thus demonstrating that *CASQ2* is the gene for this variant of

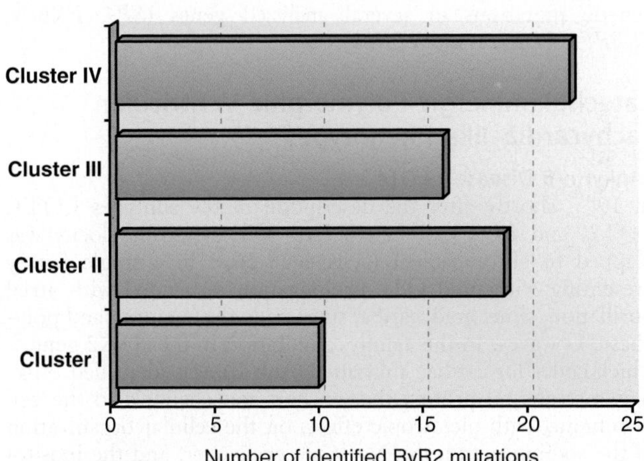

Function:
- **Cluster I**: domain–domain interaction; oxidoreductase-like; excitation-contraction coupling.
- **Cluster II**: FKBP12.6-binding domain; agonist sensitivity; Ca^{2+}-dependent regulation; excitation-contraction coupling; domain–domain interaction; protein kinase A regulation contraction coupling
- **Cluster III**: calmodulin-like domain; Ca^{2+} binding; agonist sensitivity; channel modulation; Ca^{2+} sensor; calmodulin
  Kinase regulation; FKBP12.6 interaction; Ca^{2+} sensitivity; domain interaction; protein kinase A regulation
- **Cluster IV**: transmembrane segments; pore-forming loop; excitation-contraction coupling; endoplasmic reticulum retention signal; Ca^{2+} regulation; domain interactions; oligomerization signal.

Figure 70-2 Mutation clustering in the RyR2-related autosomal dominant catecholaminergic polymorphic ventricular tachycardia. *Colored bars* show the number of mutations for each functional cluster.[21] Known functions for clusters I to IV are listed at the *bottom* of the figure. (Reported mutations are from www.fsm.it/cardmoc.)

CPVT.[27] The *CASQ2* gene product is the cardiac-specific isoform of calsequestrin; it serves as a major calcium-binding protein localized in the terminal cisternae of the sarcoplasmic reticulum. Calsequestrin, together with triadin and junctin, belongs to the RyR2 macromolecular complex that regulates sarcoplasmic reticulum Ca^{2+} release in cardiac muscle.[28]

CPVT2 is an infrequent form of the disease. In our experience, this variant represents 3% of CPVT mutants.[12] Whereas homozygote carriers of the *CASQ2* mutation present with full-blown phenotype, heterozygous carriers usually are asymptomatic.[29,30] Whether heterozygote carriers have an increased susceptibility to cardiac arrhythmias is still debated. Only one clinical study[31] supports this possibility: One of six heterozygous carriers of the R33X mutation were reported to have a typical CPVT phenotype. This aspect also is discussed in Chapter 52, because some interesting data on the phenotype of partial loss of calsequestrin has been derived from experimental studies

Despite recessive inheritance, *CASQ2* molecular screening should be performed in RyR2-negative sporadic cases not only when consanguinity is present. Indeed, the existence of compound heterozygous mutation carriers (i.e., persons who inherited two independent mutations from nonconsanguineous parents) has been documented.[29]

A Novel Locus for Catecholaminergic Polymorphic Ventricular Tachycardia?

A novel recessive CPVT locus recently was mapped to the short arm of chromosome 7 (7p14-22), with a maximal multipoint LOD score of 3.17 at marker D7S493.[32] The study was carried out in a single kindred with a high level of consanguinity, three cases of sudden death at young age (10 years), and confirmation of stress-induced ventricular arrhythmias in one living subject. Of interest, the available clinical evidence suggests that this CPVT variant may be associated with QT interval prolongation (480 to 490 ms). Unfortunately, candidate gene screening in the 25-cM critical region did not lead to the identification of pathogenetic mutations in several analyzed genes (*SP4*, *FKBP9*, *FKBP14*, *PDE1C*, and *TBX20*).

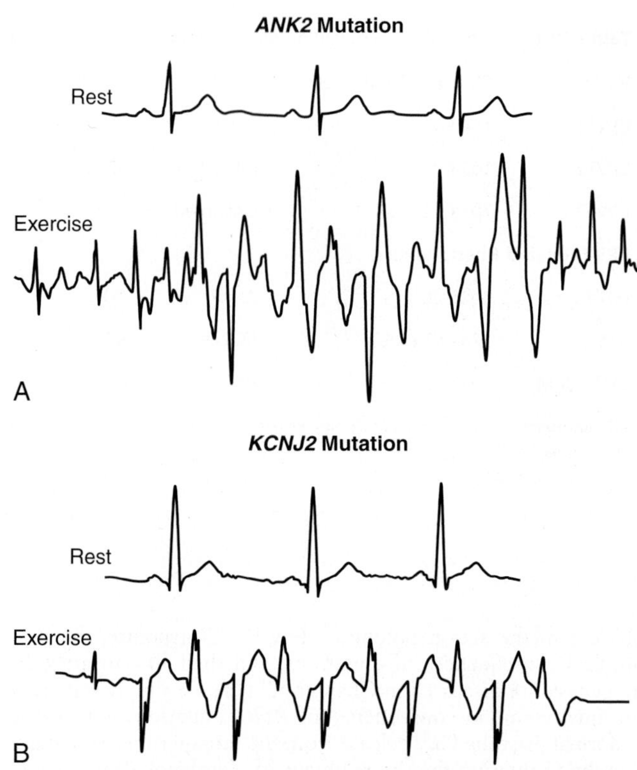

Figure 70-3 Electrocardiogram (ECG) features in catecholaminergic polymorphic ventricular tachycardia phenocopies. **A,** An ECG recorded during exercise stress testing in a patient with *ANK2* mutation shows bidirectional ventricular tachycardia. **B,** A resting electrocardiogram recorded in a patient with *KCNJ2* mutation also shows bidirectional ventricular tachycardia. (**A,** from Sherman J, Tester DJ, Ackerman MJ: Targeted mutational analysis of ankyrin-B in 541 consecutive, unrelated patients referred for long QT syndrome genetic testing and 200 healthy subjects. Heart Rhythm 2:1218-1223, 2005.)

Catecholaminergic Polymorphic Ventricular Tachycardia–like Phenotypes

"Ankyrin-B Disease": LQT4

In 1995, shortly after the description of the subtypes LQT1, LQT2, and LQT3, a fourth long QT syndrome locus was mapped to chromosomal locus 4q25-26,[33] in a single family presenting with mild QTc prolongation associated with atrial fibrillation, sinus bradycardia, sinus node dysfunction, and polyphasic U waves. In this family, a mutation in the *ANK2* gene,[34] which codes for cardiac ankyrin-B (Ank-B), was identified. Ank-B is a structural protein that anchors ion channels to the cell membrane, with pleiotropic effects on the cellular organization of the sodium pump, the Na^+-Ca^{2+} exchanger, and the inositol 1,4,5-trisphosphate receptors. Screening of 269 patients with long QT syndrome resulted in identification of a mutation in *ANK2*[35] in 3%. Of interest, all carriers of *ANK2* mutations had been diagnosed as having "atypical" or "borderline" long QT syndrome. Subsequently a group of patients characterized by a broad range of "adrenergically mediated arrhythmias" were screened for *ANK2*, including patients who had CPVT without mutations on *RYR2* or *CASQ2*. In one of our patients presenting with adrenergically mediated bidirectional ventricular tachycardia[36] (Fig. 70-3A), an ankyrin mutation was identified. Functional assay showed that the mutation causes a loss of expression and mislocalization of the Na^+,K^+-ATPase, the Na^+-Ca^{2+} exchanger, and the inositol 3-phosphate ($InsP_3$) receptors.[36]

The yield of *ANK2* screening in patients with CPVT is still undefined (but is likely to be very low); therefore, the clinical applicability of such testing is unknown. At present, *ANK2* cannot be considered a CPVT gene, but it is important to keep in mind that *ANK2* mutations may induce a clinical phenotype resembling CPVT (Table 70-1).

KCNJ2 Disease: Andersen-Tawil Syndrome

A possible phenotypic overlap also may exist between CPVT and Andersen-Tawil syndrome (see Table 70-1). The latter, also defined as LQT7, is an inherited arrhythmogenic disorder caused by mutations in the *KCNJ2* gene. Andersen-Tawil syndrome is characterized by cardiac (QT prolongation, prominent U waves) and extracardiac (facial dysmorphisms, periodic paralysis) phenotypes.[37] Some affected patients, however, may present with atypical manifestations including mild (or no) QT interval prolongation[38] and bidirectional ventricular tachycardia with evidence of an adrenergic trigger (see Fig. 70-3B).[39,40]

It is unclear at present whether patients with clinical manifestations that overlap with CPVT also have a highly unfavorable prognosis, such as that for *RYR2*- and *CASQ2*-genotyped patients with CPVT, or whether they have the more benign outcome typical of patients with Andersen-Tawil syndrome.[41,42]

70

Table 70-2 Clinical Management of Catecholaminergic Polymorphic Ventricular Tachycardia (CPVT) According to ACC/AHA/ESC Guidelines

Indication	Recommendation
Class I	Beta-blockers are indicated for patients who are clinically diagnosed with CPVT on the basis of presence of spontaneous or documented stress-induced ventricular arrhythmias.
	ICD with beta-blockers is indicated for patients with CPVT surviving cardiac arrest.
Class IIa	Beta-blockers can be effective in patients without clinical manifestations when the diagnosis of CPVT is established during childhood based on genetic analysis.
	ICD with the use of beta-blockers can be effective with CPVT with syncope and/or documented ventricular tachycardia during beta-blocker therapy.
Class IIb	Beta-blockers may be considered for patients with CPVT who were genetically diagnosed in adulthood and never manifested clinical symptoms.

ACC, American College of Cardiology; AHA, American Heart Association; ESC, European Society of Cardiology; ICD, implantable cardioverter-defibrillator.

CPVT and Structural Abnormalities

Whether or not cardiac ryanodine receptor mutations also may cause structural abnormalities typical of right ventricular cardiomyopathy disease or other forms of dilated cardiomyopathy has been the focus of active scientific discussion since the initial identification of RyR2 mutations. This aspect of cardiomyopathy is discussed in Chapter 52.

Clinical Management: Risk Stratification and Specific Therapy

Clinical management of CPVT according to current guidelines[43] is summarized in Table 70-2. Preliminary evidence shows that cardiac events occur at a younger age in patients with RyR2 mutations have than in patients with non RyR2-CPVT, and that male gender is a risk factor for syncope in RyR2-type CPVT (relative risk, 4.2).[3] The lack of large study populations in the epidemiologic registries, however, has thus far prevented robust genotype-phenotype correlation. Therefore, risk stratification is based entirely on clinical considerations.

Regular follow-up visits with exercise stress testing constitute an effective approach for beta-blocker dose titration and monitoring of susceptibility to arrhythmias. Holter monitoring also may have a role, because in some patients, the onset of ventricular arrhythmias can be triggered more easily by acute emotions that by graded exercise. On the other hand, programmed electrical stimulation is not useful either for diagnosis or for risk stratification.[3,4]

Beta-blockers have been proposed as the mainstay of CPVT therapy since the earlier reports.[1,4,19] Leenhardt and colleagues[4] and Postma and associates[6] suggested that beta-blockers achieve a 100% success rate in the prevention of arrhythmic episodes, provided that patients are compliant with therapy. Other workers (including those in our own group),[3,11] however, have observed that despite adequate compliance, cardiac events recur in approximately 40% of patients receiving with the maximally tolerated dose of the drug; in such instances, ICD implantation has been recommended. Despite the possibility of recurrence of arrhythmic events on long-term follow-up, in view of the overall efficacy of beta-blockers in prolonging the arrhythmia-free interval and tolerability of therapy, these agents have a class I indication in CPVT (see Table 70-2).[43]

When arrhythmia control is unsatisfactory, the use of an ICD is indicated (class IIa),[43] as supported by evidence showing that appropriate interventions of the device occur in one half of the patients after a mean follow-up period of 2 years after implantation.[3] According to guidelines, an ICD also is indicated for secondary prevention of cardiac arrest with a class I indication.[43]

Additional pharmacologic therapies could be considered for patients who are not adequately protected by beta-blockers. Sodium channel blockers[11] and amiodarone[4] have been reported to be of little help in controlling arrhythmias in CPVT. On the other hand, preliminary evidences suggest that calcium channel blockers may afford adjunctive protection.[11,44,45]

Summary and Conclusions

The epidemiologic data collected so far clearly show that CPVT is a potentially fatal disorder. Unfortunately, possibly because of the low level of awareness on the disease, patients may still have delayed diagnosis, with increased exposure time to risk of life-threatening events. On the other hand, CPVT can be readily diagnosed in a majority of patients with noninvasive clinical tests (exercise stress test and Holter monitoring), and therapy with beta-blockers often is effective. Therefore, early diagnosis is critically important. Genetic testing has a high success rate (comparable with that achievable in long QT syndrome), and it is relevant in order to identify susceptible persons in CPVT families and for reproductive risk assessment.

With the exception of beta-blockers, no pharmacologic therapy of proven effectiveness is available. Thus, patients with CPVT who still experience arrhythmias despite chronic therapy with maximally tolerated dosage are candidates for ICD implantation.

The identification of robust genotype-phenotype correlation and novel therapies for CPVT is still curbed by the limited availability of large cohorts of patients collected in the epidemiologic registries. On the other hand, at present, many investigators are involved in basic research studies aimed at elucidation of CPVT pathophysiology and at identifying novel therapeutic strategies. This research will surely lead to substantial advances in the future.

References

1. Coumel P, Fidelle J, Lucet V, et al: Catecholaminergic-induced severe ventricular arrhythmias with Adams-Stokes syndrome in children: Report of four cases. Br Heart J 40:28-37, 1978.
2. Reid DS, Tynan M, Braidwood L, et al: Bidirectional tachycardia in a child. A study using His bundle electrography. Br Heart J 37:339-344, 1975.
3. Priori SG, Napolitano C, Memmi M, et al: Clinical and molecular characterization of patients with catecholaminergic polymorphic ventricular tachycardia. Circulation 106:69-74, 2002.

4. Leenhardt A, Lucet V, Denjoy I, et al: Catecholaminergic polymorphic ventricular tachycardia in children. A 7-year follow-up of 21 patients. Circulation 91:1512-1519, 1995.
5. Aizawa Y, Komura S, Okada S, et al: Distinct U wave changes in patients with catecholaminergic polymorphic ventricular tachycardia (CPVT). Int Heart J 47:381-389, 2006.
6. Postma AV, Denjoy I, Kamblock J, et al: Catecholaminergic polymorphic ventricular tachycardia: RYR2 mutations, bradycardia, and follow up of the patients. J Med Genet 42:863-870, 2005.
7. Liu N, Colombi B, Memmi M, et al: Arrhythmogenesis in catecholaminergic polymorphic ventricular tachycardia. Insights from a RyR2 R4496C knock-in mouse model. Circ Res 99:292-298, 2006.
8. Cerrone M, Noujaim SF, Tolkacheva EG, et al: Arrhythmogenic mechanisms in a mouse model of catecholaminergic polymorphic ventricular tachycardia. Circ Res 11:1039-1048, 2007.
9. Paavola J, Viitasalo M, Laitinen-Forsblom PJ, et al: Mutant ryanodine receptors in catecholaminergic polymorphic ventricular tachycardia generate delayed afterdepolarizations due to increased propensity to Ca^{2+} waves. Eur Heart J 28:1135-1142, 2007.
10. Swan H, Piippo K, Viitasalo M, et al: Arrhythmic disorder mapped to chromosome 1q42-q43 causes malignant polymorphic ventricular tachycardia in structurally normal hearts. J Am Coll Cardiol 34:2035-2042, 1999.
11. Sumitomo N, Harada K, Nagashima M, et al: Catecholaminergic polymorphic ventricular tachycardia: Electrocardiographic characteristics and optimal therapeutic strategies to prevent sudden death. Heart 89:66-70, 2003.
12. Cerrone M, Colombi B, Bloise R, et al: Clinical and molecular characterization of a large cohort of patients affected with catecholaminergic polymorphic ventricular tachycardia. Circulation 110:552(Suppl II), 2004.
13. Martini B, Buja GF, Canciani B, et al: Bidirectional tachycardia. A sustained form, not related to digitalis intoxication, in an adult without apparent cardiac disease. Jpn Heart J 29:381-387, 1988.
14. Tester DJ, Spoon DB, Valdivia HH, et al: Targeted mutational analysis of the RyR2-encoded cardiac ryanodine receptor in sudden unexplained death: A molecular autopsy of 49 medical examiner/coroner's cases. Mayo Clin Proc 79:1380-1384, 2004.
15. Krahn AD, Gollob M, Yee R, et al: Diagnosis of unexplained cardiac arrest: Role of adrenaline and procainamide infusion. Circulation 112:2228-2234, 2005.
16. Tester DJ, Dura M, Carturan E, et al: A mechanism for sudden infant death syndrome (SIDS): Stress-induced leak via ryanodine receptors. Heart Rhythm 4:733-739, 2007.
17. Fisher JD, Krikler D, Hallidie-Smith KA: Familial polymorphic ventricular arrhythmias: A quarter century of successful medical treatment based on serial exercise-pharmacologic testing. J Am Coll Cardiol 34:2015-2022, 1999.
18. Otsu K, Fujii J, Periasamy M, et al: Chromosome mapping of five human cardiac and skeletal muscle sarcoplasmic reticulum protein genes. Genomics 17:507-509, 1993.
19. Priori SG, Napolitano C, Tiso N, et al: Mutations in the cardiac ryanodine receptor gene (hRyR2) underlie catecholaminergic polymorphic ventricular tachycardia. Circulation 103:196-200, 2001.
20. Laitinen PJ, Brown KM, Piippo K, et al: Mutations of the cardiac ryanodine receptor (RyR2) gene in familial polymorphic ventricular tachycardia. Circulation 103:485-490, 2001.
21. Priori SG, Napolitano C: Cardiac and skeletal muscle disorders caused by mutations in the intracellular Ca^{2+} release channels. J Clin Invest 115:2033-2038, 2005.
22. George CH, Jundi H, Thomas NL, et al: Ryanodine receptors and ventricular arrhythmias: Emerging trends in mutations, mechanisms and therapies. J Mol Cell Cardiol 42:34-50, 2007.
23. Tester DJ, Arya P, Will M, et al: Genotypic heterogeneity and phenotypic mimicry among unrelated patients referred for catecholaminergic polymorphic ventricular tachycardia genetic testing. Heart Rhythm 3:800-805, 2006.
24. Rossenbacker T, Bloise R, De Giuli L, et al: Catecholaminergic polymorphic ventricular tachycardia: Genetics, natural history and response to therapy. Circulation 116:II-179 (abs), 2007.
25. Priori SG, Napolitano C: Role of genetic analyses in cardiology: Part I: Mendelian diseases: Cardiac channelopathies. Circulation 113:1130-1135, 2006.
26. Lahat H, Eldar M, Levy-Nissenbaum E, et al: Autosomal recessive catecholamine- or exercise-induced polymorphic ventricular tachycardia: Clinical features and assignment of the disease gene to chromosome 1p13-21. Circulation 103:2822-2827, 2001.
27. Eldar M, Pras E, Lahat H: A missense mutation in the *CASQ2* gene is associated with autosomal-recessive catecholamine-induced polymorphic ventricular tachycardia. Trends Cardiovasc Med 13:148-151, 2003.
28. Zhang L, Kelley J, Schmeisser G, et al: Complex formation between junctin, triadin, calsequestrin, and the ryanodine receptor. Proteins of the cardiac junctional sarcoplasmic reticulum membrane. J Biol Chem 272:23389-23397, 1997.
29. Raffale di Barletta M, Viatchenko-Karpinski S, Nori A, et al: Clinical phenotype and functional characterization of CASQ2 mutations associated with catecholaminergic polymorphic ventricular tachycardia. Circulation 114:1012-1019, 2006.
30. Terentyev D, Nori A, Santoro M, et al: Abnormal interactions of calsequestrin with the ryanodine receptor calcium release channel complex linked to exercise-induced sudden cardiac death. Circ Res 98:1151-1158, 2006.
31. Postma AV, Denjoy I, Hoorntje TM, et al: Absence of calsequestrin 2 causes severe forms of catecholaminergic polymorphic ventricular tachycardia. Circ Res 91:e21-e26, 2002.
32. Bhuiyan ZA, Hamdan MA, Shamsi ET, et al: A novel early onset lethal form of catecholaminergic polymorphic ventricular tachycardia maps to chromosome 7p14-p22. J Cardiovasc Electrophysiol 18:1060-1066, 2007.
33. Schott JJ, Charpentier F, Peltier S, et al: Mapping of a gene for long QT syndrome to chromosome 4q25-27. Am J Hum Genet 57:1114-1122, 1995.
34. Mohler PJ, Schott JJ, Gramolini AO, et al: Ankyrin-B mutation causes type 4 long-QT cardiac arrhythmia and sudden cardiac death. Nature 421:634-639, 2003.
35. Sherman J, Tester DJ, Ackerman MJ: Targeted mutational analysis of ankyrin-B in 541 consecutive, unrelated patients referred for long QT syndrome genetic testing and 200 healthy subjects. Heart Rhythm 2:1218-1223, 2005.
36. Mohler PJ, Splawski I, Napolitano C, et al: A cardiac arrhythmia syndrome caused by loss of ankyrin-B function. Proc Natl Acad Sci U S A 101:9137-9142, 2004.
37. Andersen ED, Krasilnikoff PA, Overvad H: Intermittent muscular weakness, extrasystoles, and multiple developmental anomalies. A new syndrome? Acta Paediatr Scand 60:559-564, 1971.
38. Plaster NM, Tawil R, Tristani-Firouzi M, et al: Mutations in Kir2.1 cause the developmental and episodic electrical phenotypes of Andersen's syndrome. Cell 105:511-519, 2001.
39. Ruan Y, Theiade J, Memmi M, et al: *KCNJ2* mutations in patients referred for catecholaminergic polymorphic ventricular tachycardia gene screening. Circulation 118:S-252 (abs), 2007.
40. Tristani-Firouzi M, Jensen JL, Donaldson MR, et al: Functional and clinical characterization of *KCNJ2* mutations associated with LQT7 (Andersen syndrome). J Clin Invest 110:381-388, 2002.
41. Sansone V, Griggs RC, Meola G, et al: Andersen's syndrome: A distinct periodic paralysis. Ann Neurol 42:305-312, 1997.
42. Peters S, Schulze-Bahr E, Etheridge SP, et al: Sudden cardiac death in Andersen-Tawil syndrome. Europace 9:162-166, 2007.
43. Zipes DP, Camm AJ, Borggrefe M, et al: ACC/AHA/ESC 2006 guidelines for management of patients with ventricular arrhythmias and the prevention of sudden cardiac death: A report of the American College of Cardiology/American Heart Association Task Force and the European Society of Cardiology Committee for Practice Guidelines (Writing Committee to Develop Guidelines for Management of Patients with Ventricular Arrhythmias and the Prevention of Sudden Cardiac Death). Developed in collaboration with the European Heart Rhythm Association and the Heart Rhythm Society. Europace 8:746-837, 2006.

44. Swan H, Laitinen P, Kontula K, et al: Calcium channel antagonism reduces exercise-induced ventricular arrhythmias in catecholaminergic polymorphic ventricular tachycardia patients with RyR2 mutations. J Cardiovasc Electrophysiol 16:162-166, 2005.
45. Rosso R, Kalman JM, Rogowski O, et al: Calcium channel blockers and beta-blockers versus beta-blockers alone for preventing exercise-induced arrhythmias in catecholaminergic polymorphic ventricular tachycardia. Heart Rhythm 4:1149-1154, 2007.

Andersen-Tawil Syndrome 71

MARTIN TRISTANI-FIROUZI AND SUSAN P. ETHERIDGE

CHAPTER OUTLINE

This chapter summarizes a relatively new ion channelopathy, the Andersen-Tawil syndrome. This clinically pleiotropic disorder results from mutations in an ion channel gene that modulates the most terminal portion of cardiac repolarization. Andersen-Tawil syndrome is fundamentally a disorder of ventricular repolarization, although the clinical manifestations are distinct from those of classic long QT syndrome. The degree of repolarization derangement observed in this entity is directly related to the contribution of the disordered ion channel to the repolarization phase of the cardiac action potential. This chapter discusses the most recent genetic, cellular, and clinical data underlying this unique ion channelopathy.

Background

In 1971, Andersen and colleagues reported their observations in a series of patients with periodic skeletal muscle paralysis, ventricular ectopy, and dysmorphic features—the triad of clinical manifestations initially known as Andersen's syndrome.[1] Prolongation of the QT interval was incorporated as an important cardiac manifestation in subsequent larger studies of this disorder.[2] The syndrome was renamed *Andersen-Tawil syndrome* in recognition of the exceptional contributions of the clinical neurologist Rabi Tawil. Within the cardiovascular field, this disorder remained obscure until mutations in the potassium channel gene *KCNJ2* were identified as a cause of the syndrome.[3] *KCNJ2* encodes the inward rectifier potassium channel Kir2.1, a component of the inward rectifier current, I_{K1}. I_{K1} provides substantial repolarizing current during the most terminal repolarization phase of the cardiac action potential and is the primary conductance controlling the diastolic membrane potential.[4]

Clinical Manifestations

The clinical features of Andersen-Tawil syndrome represent a spectrum of phenotypic manifestations encompassing the skeletal muscle and cardiac systems, in addition to craniofacial and skeletal anomalies (Fig. 71-1). A major obstacle to clinical diagnosis of the syndrome is the high degree of phenotypic variability and nonpenetrance. The full triad of clinical features (ventricular arrhythmias, periodic paralysis, and characteristic dysmorphic features) is present in 58% to 78% of mutation-positive patients[5]; between 32% and 81% manifest involvement of two of the three affected organ systems.[3,5,6] Nonpenetrance ranges from 6% to 20% among mutation-positive persons.[5,6] In an interesting report, a large family affected with Andersen-Tawil syndrome presented with sex-specific clinical manifestations. In this kindred, females manifested ventricular arrhythmias, whereas affected males had periodic paralysis. None of 41 mutation carriers expressed the complete triad of syndrome features.[6] These sex-specific clinical findings, however, appear to be unique to this particular family in that the same mutation was reported in other persons who manifested the typical triad of features.[7] Recently, the Andersen-Tawil syndrome phenotype was expanded to include several consistent craniofacial features and dental and skeletal anomalies that were observed in all members of a small cohort, irrespective of cardiac or neuromuscular findings.[8] These new findings help to clinch the clinical diagnosis when cardiac or skeletal muscle findings are absent.

Andersen-Tawil syndrome is an autosomal dominant or sporadic disorder of ventricular repolarization manifested by mild QTc interval prolongation but marked prolongation of the QUc interval[5,9] (Fig. 71-2). Prominent U waves are commonly described. Zhang and colleagues recently reported distinct electrocardiographic findings unique to this syndrome that included prolongation of the T wave downslope, wide T-U junction, and high-amplitude, broad U waves.[9] Arrhythmias in these patients include frequent premature ventricular contractions (PVCs), bigeminy, and polymorphic ventricular tachycardia.[5] Typically, ventricular tachycardia is nonsustained and bidirectional in nature, with heart rates in the range of 130 to 150 beats per minute. The degree of ventricular ectopy is quite variable between subjects, but up to 50% of all beats may be ventricular in origin.[8] Although tachycardia burden often is high in these patients,[10] degeneration into lethal ventricular arrhythmias is relatively uncommon.[11] For example, torsades de pointes was documented in only 3 of 96 *KCNJ2* mutation–positive patients.[9]

Molecular Correlate of I_{K1}

The inward rectifier potassium current I_{K1} is the major determinant of the resting membrane potential in the heart and participates in the most terminal phase of action potential repolarization.[4] I_{K1} is conducted by homotetrameric or heterotetrameric channels (or both) formed by coassembly of the Kir2.x subfamily of proteins: Kir2.1, Kir2.2, and Kir2.3. Message and protein expression studies indicate that Kir2.1 is the most abundant subfamily member in ventricular tissue.[12,13] The finding that mutations in *KNCJ2* cause human disease (but not the genes encoding Kir2.2 and Kir2.3) further underscores the pivotal role of Kir2.1 as a primary component of I_{K1}.

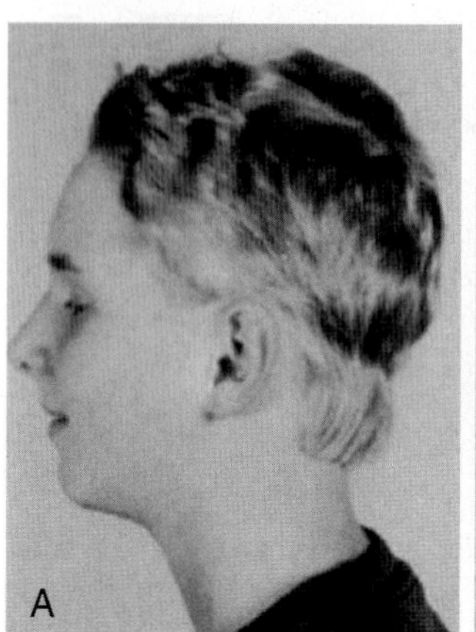

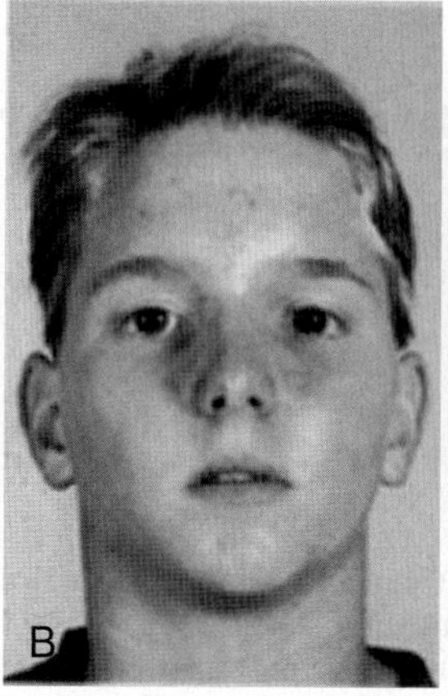

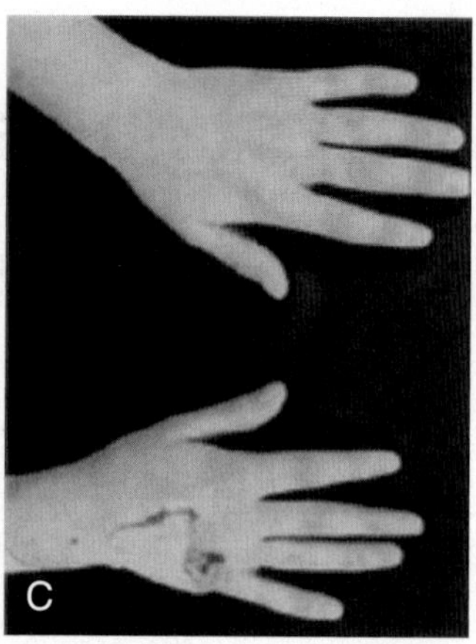

Figure 71-1 Typical dysmorphic features in a subject with Andersen-Tawil syndrome. Note the low-set ears, hypertelorism (wide interpupillary distance), micrognathia (small jaw) (**A** and **B**), and clinodactyly of the fifth digits (**C**). (From Plaster NM, Tawil R, Tristani-Firouzi M, et al: Mutations in Kir2.1 cause the developmental and episodic electrical phenotypes of Andersen's syndrome. Cell 105:511-519, 2001.)

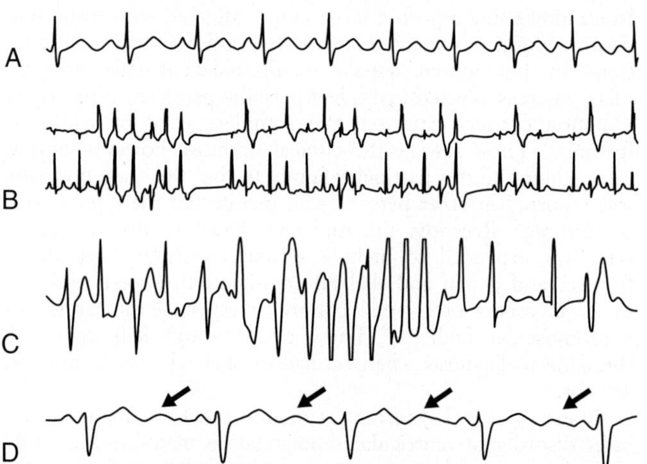

Figure 71-2 Representative electrocardiograms (ECGs) from patients with Andersen-Tawil syndrome. **A,** ECG demonstrating prolongation of the QT interval. **B,** ECG traces demonstrating a short run of nonsustained polymorphic ventricular tachycardia (VT) followed by bigeminy. **C,** Bidirectional VT (note alternating QRS axis polarity) degenerating into a rapid run of polymorphic VT. **D,** ECG trace demonstrating prominent U wave (indicated by *arrows*). (From Tristani-Firouzi M, Jensen JL, Donaldson MR, et al: Functional and clinical characterization of *KCNJ2* mutations associated with LQT7 (Andersen syndrome). J Clin Invest 110:381-388, 2002.)

Cellular Basis for the Clinical Syndrome

Nearly all of the *KCNJ2* mutations described to date in patients with Andersen-Tawil syndrome cause dominant-negative suppression of Kir2.1 channel function (Fig. 71-3). A minority of mutations alter channel assembly and trafficking, with resultant accumulation of subunits within the endoplasmic reticulum and Golgi apparatus.[14] Most mutant subunits coassemble with wild-type subunits and traffic appropriately to the cell surface but then fail to function normally. The mechanism underlying this abnormal function is an altered sensitivity of the mutant channel to the membrane-delimited second messenger phosphatidylinositol 4,5-biphosphate (PIP_2), an essential activator of most inward rectifier potassium channels.[15] Nearly one half of all reported *KCNJ2* mutations occur at residues known to be important for PIP_2-channel interaction, supporting the idea that reduced PIP_2 binding is critical to the pathogenesis of Andersen-Tawil syndrome.[7] Recently, the effects of Andersen-Tawil syndrome mutations were studied at the atomic level by crystallizing the amino-terminal (N-terminal) and carboxyl-terminal (C-terminal) cytoplasmic domains of Kir2.1. Arg218 and Glu303 in the C terminus form charged and polar interactions with neighboring residues Thr309

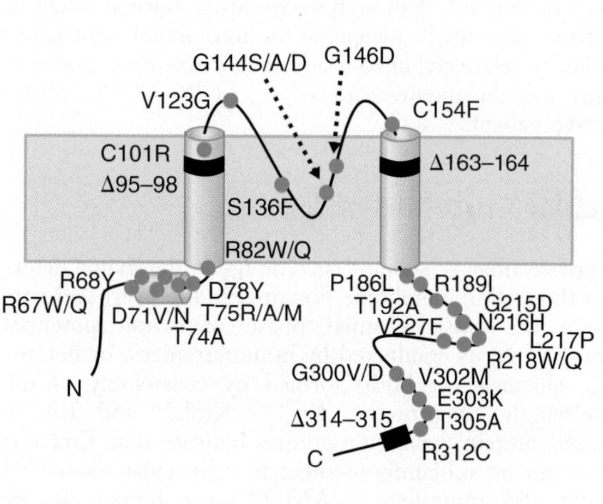

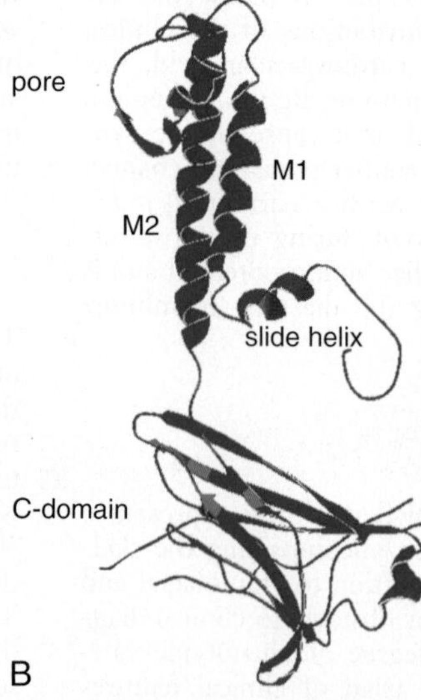

Figure 71-3 Locations of Andersen-Tawil syndrome (ATS) mutations published to date. **A,** Topology of Kir2.1 channel subunit demonstrating position of ATS-associated mutations in *KCNJ2*. **B,** Homology model of Kir2.1 channel subunit based on the crystal structure of the bacterial inward rectifier KirBac1.1.[27] Amino acids associated with ATS missense mutations are depicted in *red*. A majority of ATS mutations are located on the amino (N)-terminal slide helix and the carboxyl (C)-terminal cytoplasmic domain (C-domain).

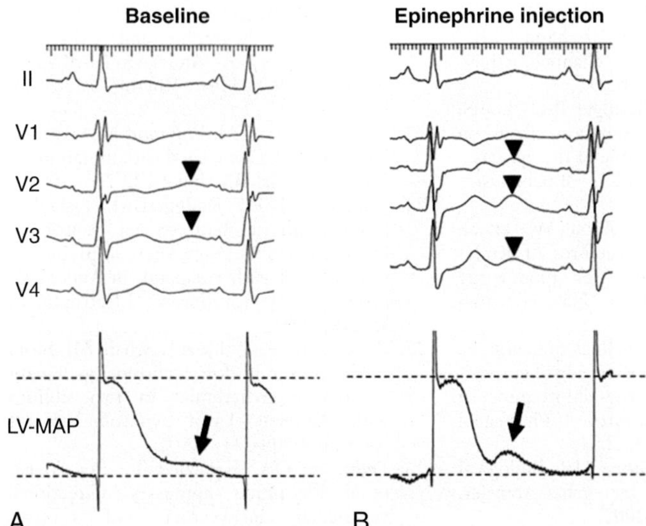

Figure 71-4 Comparison of surface electrocardiogram (ECG) leads and monophasic action potentials recorded from the left ventricle (LV-MAP) in a patient with Andersen-Tawil syndrome. **A,** LV-MAP recording demonstrates prolongation of the most terminal portion of the MAP, resulting in a small secondary depolarization or "hump" *(large arrow)*. The position of the hump corresponds to the position of the U wave on the surface ECG leads *(arrowheads)*. **B,** Epinephrine infusion accentuates the secondary depolarization as well as the magnitude of U waves on surface ECGs. In silico simulations suggest that the secondary depolarization is due to depolarizing current generated by the Na^+-Ca^{2+} exchanger.[5] (From Nagase S, Kusano KF, Yoshida M, Ohe T: Electrophysiologic characteristics of an Andersen syndrome patient with *KCNJ2* mutation. Heart Rhythm 4:512-515, 2007.)

and Arg312.[16,17] Andersen-Tawil syndrome mutations at Arg218 and Glu303 destabilize these interactions and probably render the channel insensitive to the activating effects of PIP_2.[16,17] To date, no clear genotype-phenotype correlation in Andersen-Tawil syndrome has been found. No single mutation described to date is associated with a higher likelihood of unstable arrhythmias.

How does reduced Kir2.1 channel function lead to arrhythmia susceptibility? Selective I_{K1} blockade in feline Purkinje fibers results in action potential prolongation and an increased frequency of spontaneous action potentials.[18] In an elegant in vivo study, gene transfer of a Kir2.1 dominant-negative construct resulted in QT prolongation in adenovirus-transfected guinea pigs, as well as spontaneous action potentials in isolated ventricular myocytes.[19] Both studies support the idea that a reduction in I_{K1} leads to the generation of spontaneous ventricular activity. The cellular consequences of reduced I_{K1} have been studied using *in silico* approaches. Reductions in I_{K1} initially cause mild prolongation of the most terminal foot of the cardiac action potential.[20] Greater reductions in I_{K1} result in the generation of spontaneous action potentials that are triggered by the Na^+-Ca^{2+} exchanger.[5,20,21] This is unlike in the traditional forms of long QT syndrome, in which prolongation of the plateau phase results in L-type calcium channel–triggered early afterdepolarizations.

Computer simulations of reduced I_{K1} in virtual left ventricular tissue reveal an increase in action potential duration across the ventricular wall, without an increase in transmural dispersion of repolarization[20] (Fig. 71-4). Thus, the low frequency of torsades de pointes arrhythmia in patients with Andersen-Tawil syndrome may be a consequence of the lack of transmural dispersion of repolarization in the setting of reduced I_{K1}, despite the fact that action potential duration is prolonged. The in silico data are consistent with data from the isolated canine wedge preparation using $BaCl_2$ as a model of Andersen-Tawil syndrome.[22] Of interest, the contribution of I_{Kr} to phase 3 repolarization increased dramatically in the setting of computer-simulated I_{K1} reductions.[20] The consequences of this observation are that patients with Andersen-Tawil syndrome may be particularly susceptible to arrhythmias in the setting of reduced I_{Kr} (such as with HERG channel blockers or decreased extracellular K^+ concentration), because of the baseline reduced repolarization reserve and the dependence on I_{Kr} as a substitute for reduced I_{K1}.

Treatment Options

The frequent ventricular ectopy typical of Andersen-Tawil syndrome is notoriously difficult to suppress with pharmacologic therapy.[10,23] In the University of California-San Francisco International ATS Registry, a majority of subjects are prescribed beta-blocking agents, but in most cases, the frequency of ventricular ectopy does not change (unpublished data). A single case report documented the efficacy of verapamil in suppressing bidirectional ventricular tachycardia in a patient with Andersen-Tawil syndrome.[24] In a subsequent report, however, verapamil was documented to induce runs of torsades de pointes arrhythmia and syncope.[25] Recently, the efficacy of flecainide therapy in suppressing ventricular arrhythmias in these patients has been reported.[25,26]

Because many patients with frequent ventricular ectopy are entirely asymptomatic, the question arises as to whether therapy is indicated in most patients. Although therapy may be debatable, there remains the difficult task of identifying the subset of patients with Andersen-Tawil syndrome at risk for life-threatening arrhythmias.[10,23] In light of the absence of published criteria for therapy, any patient with runs of rapid polymorphic ventricular tachycardia or symptoms such as syncope should be considered a candidate for placement of an implantable cardioverter-defibrillator (ICD).

References

1. Andersen ED, Krasilnikoff PA, Overvad H: Intermittent muscular weakness, extrasystoles, and multiple developmental anomalies. A new syndrome? Acta Paediatr Scand 60:559-564, 1971.
2. Sansone V, Griggs RC, Meola G, et al: Andersen's syndrome: A distinct periodic paralysis. Ann Neurol 42:305-312, 1997.
3. Plaster NM, Tawil R, Tristani-Firouzi M, et al: Mutations in Kir2.1 cause the developmental and episodic electrical phenotypes of Andersen's syndrome. Cell 105:511-519, 2001.
4. Sanguinetti MC, Tristani-Firouzi M: Delayed and inward rectifier potassium channels. In Zipes DP, Jalife J (eds): Cardiac Electrophysiology: From Cell to Bedside, 3rd ed. Philadelphia, Saunders, 2000, pp 79-86.
5. Tristani-Firouzi M, Jensen JL, Donaldson MR, et al: Functional and clinical characterization of KCNJ2 mutations associated with LQT7 (Andersen syndrome). J Clin Invest 110:381-388, 2002.
6. Andelfinger G, Tapper AR, Welch RC, et al: KCNJ2 mutation results in Andersen syndrome with sex-specific cardiac and skeletal muscle phenotypes. Am J Hum Genet 71:663-668, 2002.
7. Donaldson MR, Jensen JL, Tristani-Firouzi M, et al: PIP(2) binding residues of Kir2.1 are common targets of mutations causing Andersen syndrome. Neurology 60:1811-1816, 2003.
8. Yoon G, Oberoi S, Tristani-Firouzi M, et al: Andersen-Tawil syndrome: Prospective cohort analysis and expansion of the phenotype. Am J Med Genet A 140:312-321, 2006.

9. Zhang L, Benson DW, Tristani-Firouzi M, et al: Electrocardiographic features in Andersen-Tawil syndrome patients with KCNJ2 mutations: Characteristic T-U-wave patterns predict the KCNJ2 genotype. Circulation 111:2720-2726, 2005.
10. Chun TU, Epstein MR, Dick M 2nd, et al: Polymorphic ventricular tachycardia and KCNJ2 mutations. Heart Rhythm 1:235-241, 2004.
11. Venance SL, Cannon SC, Fialho D, et al: The primary periodic paralyses: Diagnosis, pathogenesis and treatment. Brain 129:8-17, 2006.
12. Wang Z, Yue L, White M, et al: Differential distribution of inward rectifier potassium channel transcripts in human atrium versus ventricle. Circulation 98:2422-2428, 1998.
13. Zobel C, Cho HC, Nguyen TT, et al: Molecular dissection of the inward rectifier potassium current (IK1) in rabbit cardiomyocytes: Evidence for heteromeric co-assembly of Kir2.1 and Kir2.2. J Physiol 550:365-372, 2003.
14. Bendahhou S, Donaldson MR, Plaster NM, et al: Defective potassium channel Kir2.1 trafficking underlies Andersen-Tawil syndrome. J Biol Chem 278:51779-51785, 2003.
15. Lopes CM, Zhang H, Rohacs T, et al: Alterations in conserved Kir channel-PIP2 interactions underlie channelopathies. Neuron 34:933-944, 2002.
16. Pegan S, Arrabit C, Slesinger PA, Choe S: Andersen's syndrome mutation effects on the structure and assembly of the cytoplasmic domains of Kir2.1. Biochemistry 45:8599-8606, 2006.
17. Pegan S, Arrabit C, Zhou W, et al: Cytoplasmic domain structures of Kir2.1 and Kir3.1 show sites for modulating gating and rectification. Nat Neurosci 8:279-287, 2005.
18. Sanchez-Chapula JA, Salinas-Stefanon E, Torres-Jacome J, et al: Blockade of currents by the antimalarial drug chloroquine in feline ventricular myocytes. J Pharmacol Exp Ther 297:437-445, 2001.
19. Miake J, Marban E, Nuss HB: Biological pacemaker created by gene transfer. Nature 419:132-133, 2002.
20. Seemann G, Sachse FB, Weiss DL, et al: Modeling of I_{K1} mutations in human left ventricular myocytes and tissue. Am J Physiol Heart Circ Physiol 292:H549-H559, 2007. Epub 2006 Aug 25.
21. Silva J, Rudy Y: Mechanism of pacemaking in I(K1)-downregulated myocytes. Circ Res 92:261-263, 2003.
22. Tsuboi M, Antzelevitch C: Cellular basis for electrocardiographic and arrhythmic manifestations of Andersen-Tawil syndrome (LQT7). Heart Rhythm 3:328-335, 2006.
23. Tristani-Firouzi M: Polymorphic ventricular tachycardia associated with mutations in KCNJ2. Heart Rhythm 1:242-243, 2004.
24. Kannankeril PJ, Roden DM, Fish FA: Suppression of bidirectional ventricular tachycardia and unmasking of prolonged QT interval with verapamil in Andersen's syndrome. J Cardiovasc Electrophysiol 15:119, 2004.
25. Bokenkamp R, Wilde AA, Schalij MJ, Blom NA: Flecainide for recurrent malignant ventricular arrhythmias in two siblings with Andersen-Tawil syndrome. Heart Rhythm 4:508-511, 2007.
26. Pellizzón OA, Kalaizich L, Ptacek LJ, et al: Flecainide suppresses bidirectional ventricular tachycardia and reverses tachycardia-induced cardiomyopathy in Andersen-Tawil syndrome. J Cardiovasc Electrophysiol 19:95-97, 2008. Epub 2007 Jul 27.
27. Kuo A, Gulbis JM, Antcliff JF, et al: Crystal structure of the potassium channel KirBac1.1 in the closed state. Science 300:1922-1926, 2003.

Timothy Syndrome 72

Silvia G. Priori, Igor Splawski, Raffaella Bloise, and Carlo Napolitano

CHAPTER OUTLINE

Timothy syndrome is a rare but highly malignant inherited disorder characterized by cardiac and extracardiac abnormalities. Since its description, Timothy syndrome has been classified as a variant of the long QT syndrome (LQT8), but its complex phenotype, involving central nervous system and metabolic abnormalities, may justify a separate classification. The phenotypic abnormalities in Timothy syndrome are extremely severe, with a high mortality rate. Accordingly, the prevalence of the disease is low, and only a few cases have been reported. Timothy syndrome is caused by mutations in the *CACNA1C* gene, encoding the voltage-dependent L-type calcium channel $Ca_V1.2$. This chapter reviews the clinical presentation and the pathophysiology of this disorder.

Historical Notes

In 1992, Reichenbach and associates reported a case of intrauterine bradycardia followed by evidence of pronounced QT interval prolongation and a second-degree atrioventricular block after birth.[1] The affected infant, a boy, also was found to have hand and foot syndactyly. He died suddenly at 5 months of age, and the investigators concluded that the phenotype could represent a novel clinical entity. A few other anecdotal cases were reported thereafter,[2] all sharing the presence of a severe phenotype, high mortality rate, and lack of familial recurrence. Only recently have the clinical features of this disorder, defined as Timothy syndrome, been analyzed in deeper detail.[3]

Phenotype and Natural History

Fetal bradycardia often is the initial manifestation of the disease. Soon after birth, the evidence of markedly prolonged ventricular repolarization, 2:1 functional atrioventricular conduction block, and soft tissue syndactyly of hands and feet allows the diagnosis to be made (Fig. 72-1). The overall clinical presentation of Timothy syndrome is complex and encompasses several cardiac and extracardiac abnormalities (Tables 72-1 and 72-2; see also Fig. 72-1).

The QT interval is remarkably prolonged and often exceeds 550 to 600 ms.[3] Besides the abnormal duration of repolarization, the morphology of the T wave is characterized by a set of abnormalities ranging from straight ST segment with small T wave (LQT3-type pattern) (Fig. 72-2) to giant negative T waves and macroscopic T wave alternans (see Fig. 72-2).

Cardiac structural abnormalities also are observed in patients with Timothy syndrome (see Table 72-1). Congenital cardiac defects are present in approximately 60% of the patients; cardiac hypertrophy and ventricular dilatation are reported less frequently.[3-5]

Cardiac Events and Mortality in Timothy Syndrome

A mortality rate of 58%, with a mean age at death of 2.5 years, has been reported for Timothy syndrome.[3] Ventricular tachyarrhythmias (ventricular tachycardia or ventricular fibrillation), which occur in approximately 80% of patients, are a common manifestation of the disease and constitute the most frequent cause of death.

Non–arrhythmia-related deaths also may occur in Timothy syndrome. Among the 21 patients followed at Molecular Cardiology of the Maugeri Foundation in Pavia, Italy, one died of sepsis and two of intractable hypoglycemia.[4] Of interest, functional atrioventricular (AV) block leading to bradycardia has been documented in 85% of patients with this syndrome. However, bradyarrhythmias have not played a role in cardiac-related deaths in these patients.

No specific trigger for cardiac arrhythmias has been reported. Anecdotal reports have described the occurrence of life-threatening arrhythmias during anesthesia,[4] but no information is available on specific anesthetics that may be dangerous to these patients.[6]

Genetics of Timothy Syndrome

The ST-T wave morphology in patients with Timothy syndrome often resembles that in patients with long QT syndrome with sodium channel mutations (the LQT3 variant) (see Chapter 69). This resemblance in morphology of the QT interval suggested the involvement of an inward current active during the plateau phase of the cardiac action potential. Because no mutations were identified in the *SCN5A* gene, we considered the cardiac calcium channel gene (*CACNA1C*) on chromosome 12 to be a plausible candidate gene for Timothy syndrome.

CACNA1C encodes the α subunit of the voltage-dependent L-type calcium channel (Fig. 72-3). This gene undergoes complex tissue-specific splicing.[7] As reported in 2004, the G1216A transition in exon 8A (an alternatively spliced exon), which causes G406R amino acid transition in transmembrane segment 6 in domain I (see later on), was identified in patients with

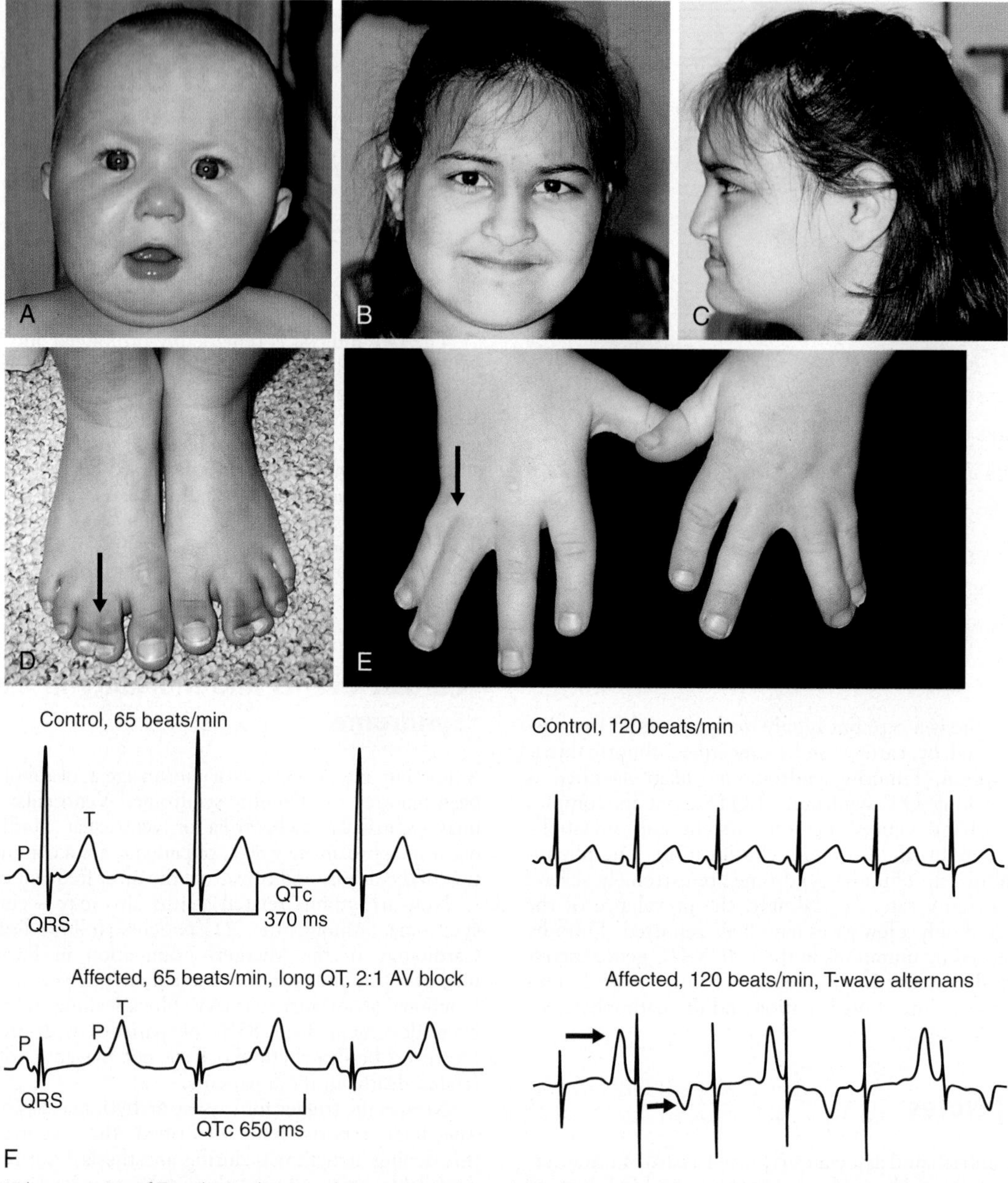

Figure 72-1 Clinical presentation of Timothy syndrome: multisystem anomalies and developmental defects. **A** to **C**, The dysmorphic facial features typically include round face, flat nasal bridge, receding upper jaw, and thin upper lip. **D** and **E**, Webbing of the toes and fingers (syndactyly) is also a feature. **F**, *Left*, The electrocardiogram shows severe QT interval prolongation, causing 2:1 atrioventricular (AV) block, seen as two atrial beats (P waves) for each ventricular beat (QRS complex). *Right*, Another electrocardiogram shows alternating T wave polarity (*arrows*), indicating severe cardiac repolarization abnormality.

Timothy syndrome.[3] Of interest, the same nucleotide variation was detected in all affected patients, suggesting an unusual molecular homogeneity in Timothy syndrome compared with other long QT syndrome entities. In 2005, Splawski and coworkers reported two additional mutations (G406R and G402S) in exon 8, which undergoes alternative splicing with exon 8A. Both of the affected patients presented with typical multifaceted Timothy syndrome but without syndactyly.[8]

In 2007, Antzelevitch and colleagues reported a *CACNA1C* mutation in an inherited arrhythmogenic disease characterized by ST segment elevation and abnormally short QT interval.[9] This disorder suggested that multiple phenotypes may be caused by calcium channel mutations, as with the plethora of phenotypes associated with *SCN5A* (the cardiac sodium channel gene) mutations.

The high malignancy of Timothy syndrome prevents a majority of affected patients from reaching reproductive age. Thus, Timothy syndrome usually is seen in sporadic cases, and genetic testing shows de novo mutations in most probands. Parent-to-offspring transmission of the clinical phenotype has never been reported. However, familial recurrence in the offspring of normal parents has been described in three families in which it was attributed to parental mosaicism.[3] Of interest, in the original report by Reichenbach and associates,[1] the

Table 72-1 Cardiac Phenotype of Timothy Syndrome

Clinical Manifestation	Prevalence (%)
Electrical Abnormalities	
QT prolongation	100
T wave alternans	63
AV block/bradycardia	82
Structural Abnormalities	
Patent ductus arteriosus Patent foramen ovale, ventricular septal defect, tetralogy of Fallot	58
Hypertrophy/cardiomegaly	26

AV, atrioventricular.

Table 72-2 Extracardiac Phenotype of Timothy Syndrome

Affected System/ Structure	Clinical Manifestation	Prevalence (%)
Skin/dysmorphisms	Syndactyly	98*
	Bald at birth, flat nasal bridge, small upper jaw	94
CNS	Autism,† autism spectrum disorders, language delay	83
Others	Recurrent infections	53
	Hypoglycemia	20

*Two cases without syndactyly have been reported.[8]

†Overt autism is present in approximately 30% of cases.

CNS, central nervous system.

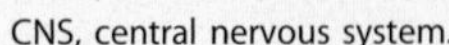

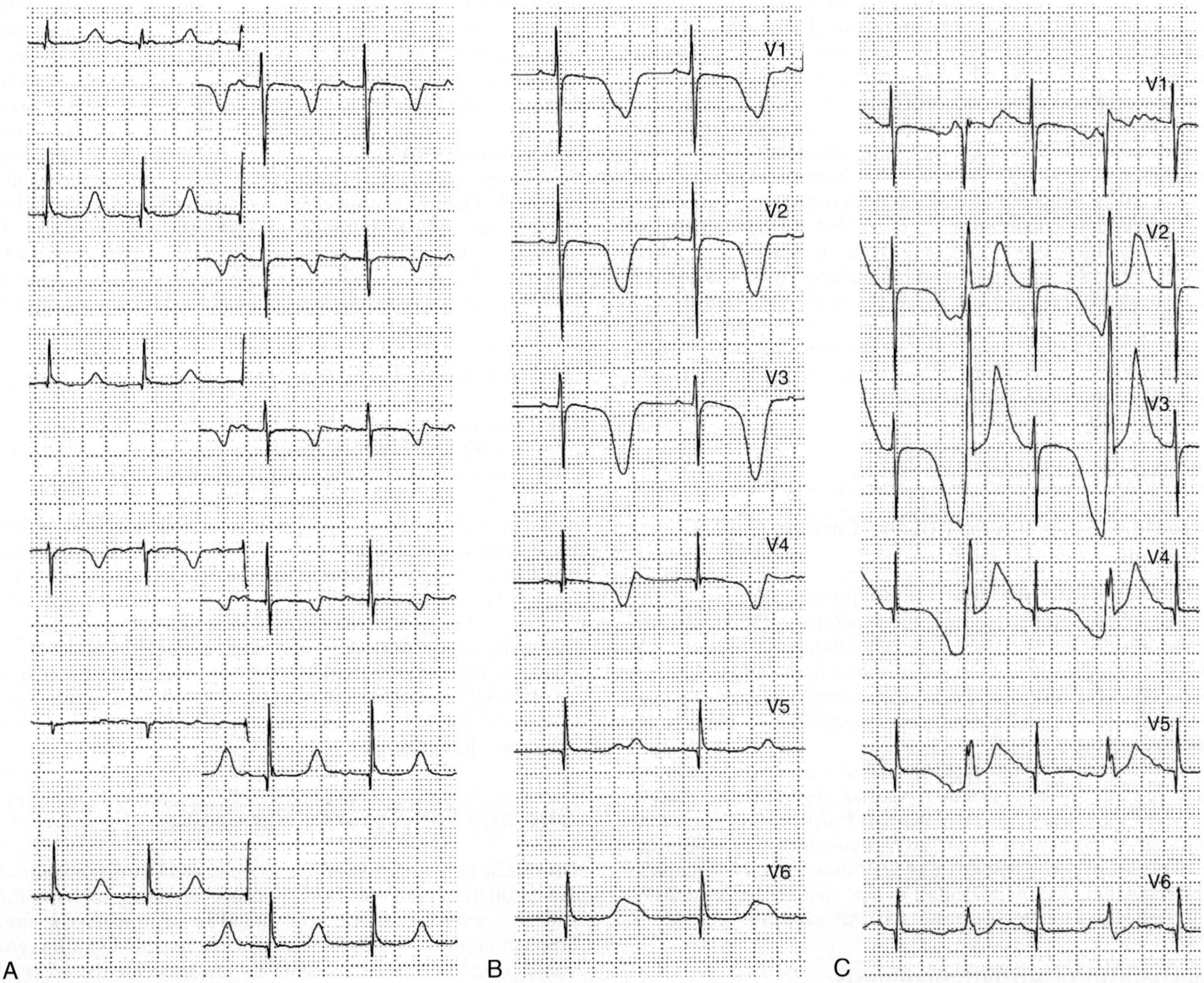

Figure 72-2 Electrocardiographic manifestations of Timothy syndrome. **A,** LQT3-type morphology of repolarization with straight ST segment and small T waves. **B,** Giant negative T waves on precordial leads with notches. **C,** Macroscopic T wave alternans with extremely prolonged ventricular repolarization, causing intraventricular conduction delay on a beat-to-beat basis.

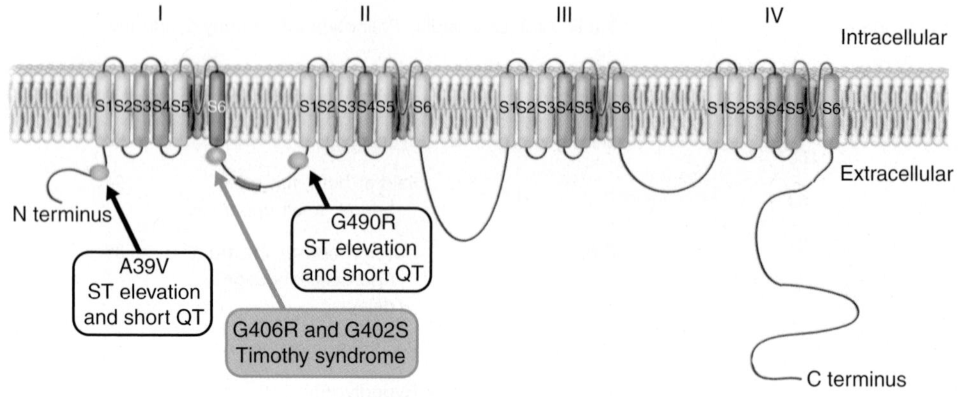

Figure 72-3 Schematic diagram of the predicted transmembrane topology of the calcium channel, showing the location of the Timothy syndrome mutations as well as of the mutations identified in short QT and ST elevation syndrome.[8]

proband's father presented with mild QT prolongation and carpal synostosis. The study authors suggested an autosomal dominant mode of transmission, but in view of the father's mild phenotype (as compared with the usual Timothy syndrome presentation), the presence of parental mosaicism was possible. Mosaicism was first documented in an Italian family by Splawski and coworkers in 2005.[8] Because of the technical limitations in detecting mosaicism, its frequency may be higher than previously reported. Therefore, mosaicism should be carefully considered in all apparently sporadic cases because its presence can have a crucial impact on genetic and reproductive counseling.

Finally, it is important to consider that the combination of syndactyly and QT prolongation may occur in a different inherited arrhythmogenic disorder, the Andersen-Tawil syndrome.[10] This disorder, also defined as LQT7, is characterized by QT prolongation, ventricular arrhythmias, periodic paralysis, and facial dysmorphisms. This aspect of the differential diagnosis is important because Andersen-Tawil syndrome is a benign condition that rarely causes sudden death.[11]

Pathophysiology

Structure and Function of the Cardiac $Ca_V1.2$ Channel

$Ca_V1.2$ constitutes the pore-forming protein, the α1 subunit, responsible for the L-type voltage-dependent calcium channel in the heart. The structure of the α 1 subunit is similar to that of the sodium channel and consists of four homologous domains (I to IV), each one formed by transmembrane-spanning segments (S1 to S6), and a membrane-associated loop between S5 and S6 (see Fig. 72-3).[12]

$Ca_V1.2$ is the calcium channel conducting the voltage-dependent inward calcium current (I_{Ca}) that maintains the plateau phase of the cardiac action potential. Furthermore, Ca^{2+} ions play an important role in excitation-contraction coupling, because I_{Ca} triggers the release of Ca^{2+} ions from the sarcoplasmic reticulum. Any perturbation of this channel has significant potential to create an electrically unstable substrate.

Mechanism of Arrhythmogenesis

The most striking biophysical consequence of the G406R mutation is the impaired control of I_{Ca} macroscopic current, with a loss of voltage dependence of inactivation.[3] In a mathematical model of a human ventricular myocyte,[8] such loss of voltage dependence of inactivation led to significant action potential prolongation. The prolongation was associated with the onset of delayed afterdepolarizations and triggered activity. In another study, single-channel recordings of Timothy syndrome mutant channels showed decreased unitary conductance but an increase in spontaneous so-called mode 2 gating, with increased open probability and longer channel activations.[13] Such mode 2 gating could produce the apparent loss of macroscopic current inactivation at the whole-cell level. Finally, an increased sensitivity to phosphorylation through the calcium-calmodulin–dependent protein kinase II pathway, with reduced tendency to dephosphorylation, was observed. This effect is consistent with an increased sensitivity of calcium cannels to adrenergic stimulation in Timothy syndrome.

Extracardiac Phenotype

The calcium channel is a crucial protein in several organs. In keeping with the complex phenotype of Timothy syndrome, *CACNA1C* undergoes tissue-specific alternative splicing.

Exon 8A (the Timothy syndrome exon) is expressed in all of the central nervous system structures implicated in autism (hippocampus, cerebellum, and amygdala), supporting the concept that patients with Timothy syndrome have a genetic predisposition to behavioral disorders. Exon 8A of *CACNA1C* also is expressed throughout the heart and the vascular system, and in developing digits and teeth, and abnormalities in all of these systems are found in the syndrome phenotype.[3] The association of *CACNA1C* mutations and congenital defects in Timothy syndrome also suggests an important role of this gene during embryonic development.

Therapy for Timothy Syndrome

Ventricular tachyarrhythmias (ventricular tachycardia or ventricular fibrillation) are the leading cause of death in Timothy syndrome, and their prevention should be of primary concern. Although no data are specifically available for the Timothy syndrome patient cohort, beta-blockers are used on the basis of evidence that they are effective in persons with long QT syndrome.[14] Additional pharmacologic therapies, with mexiletine or calcium channel blockers, have been proposed to shorten ventricular repolarization, restore 1:1 AV conduction, and reduce the risk of arrhythmias. The use of these agents must be considered investigational, however. The administration of verapamil allowed control of arrhythmias or implantable cardioverter-defibrillator (ICD) discharges and improvement in mood, cognition, and social capabilities (in the autism-like disorders) in one mosaic 21-year-old patient who suffered from multiple cardiac arrests beginning at the age of 6 years.[15]

Despite the very young age of affected patients, implantation of an ICD is the most important approach to the prevention of sudden cardiac death in persons with Timothy syndrome. The implant should be considered in all patients with confirmed diagnosis.

Cardiac arrhythmia prevention is the primary goal for therapy. Also of importance, however, is careful monitoring for recurrent infections (secondary to altered immune responses) and blood glucose levels, because deaths due to sepsis (despite aggressive antibiotic therapy) and intractable hypoglycemia have been reported. Close monitoring of glucose levels, especially in patients receiving beta-blockers, is essential, because these drugs may mask the symptoms of hypoglycemia.

Summary

Timothy syndrome is considered a rare but malignant variant of long QT syndrome with peculiar manifestations and multiorgan involvement. The research studies directed at Timothy syndrome are contributing to the understanding of the complex and crucial physiologic role of the L-type calcium channel, not only for cardiac excitability but also in the central nervous system, in immune responses, and in embryonic development.

Unfortunately, therapeutic options for affected patients are still limited and should be targeted to aggressive prevention of sudden death with an ICD. The unusual genetic homogeneity of this disorder makes the diagnosis relatively easy. Reproductive counseling should always take into account the possibility of parental mosaicism.

References

1. Reichenbach H, Meister EM, Theile H: The heart-hand syndrome. A new variant of disorders of heart conduction and syndactylia including osseous changes in hands and feet. Kinderarztl Prax 60:54-56, 1992.
2. Marks ML, Trippel DL, Keating MT: Long QT syndrome associated with syndactyly identified in females. Am J Cardiol 76:744-745, 1995.
3. Splawski I, Timothy KW, Sharpe LM, et al: Ca(V)1.2 calcium channel dysfunction causes a multisystem disorder including arrhythmia and autism. Cell 119:19-31, 2004.
4. Bloise R, Napolitano C, Timothy KW, et al: Clinical profile and risk of sudden death in children with Timothy syndrome. Circulation 114(Suppl II):502, 2007.
5. Lo ANS, Wilde AA, van Erven L, Blom NA: Syndactyly and long QT syndrome ($Ca_V1.2$ missense mutation G406R) is associated with hypertrophic cardiomyopathy. Heart Rhythm 2:1365-1368, 2005.
6. Joseph-Reynolds AM, Auden SM, Sobczyzk WL: Perioperative considerations in a newly described subtype of congenital long QT syndrome. Paediatr Anaesth 7:237-241, 1997.
7. Wang D, Papp AC, Binkley PF, et al: Highly variable mRNA expression and splicing of L-type voltage-dependent calcium channel alpha subunit 1C in human heart tissues. Pharmacogenet Genomics 16:735-745, 2006.
8. Splawski I, Timothy KW, Decher N, et al: Severe arrhythmia disorder caused by cardiac L-type calcium channel mutations. Proc Natl Acad Sci U S A 102:8089-8096, 2005.
9. Antzelevitch C, Pollevick GD, Cordeiro JM, et al: Loss-of-function mutations in the cardiac calcium channel underlie a new clinical entity characterized by ST-segment elevation, short QT intervals, and sudden cardiac death. Circulation 115:442-449, 2007.
10. Andelfinger G, Tapper AR, Welch RC Jr, Benson DW: *KCNJ2* mutation results in Andersen syndrome with sex-specific cardiac and skeletal muscle phenotypes. Am J Hum Genet 71:663-668, 2002.
11. Peters S, Schulze-Bahr E, Etheridge SP, Tristani-Firouzi M: Sudden cardiac death in Andersen-Tawil syndrome. Europace 9:162-166, 2007.
12. Catterall WA: Structure and regulation of voltage-gated Ca^{2+} channels. Annu Rev Cell Dev Biol 16:521-555, 2000.
13. Erxleben C, Liao Y, Gentile S, et al: Cyclosporin and Timothy syndrome increase mode 2 gating of $Ca_V1.2$ calcium channels through aberrant phosphorylation of S6 helices. Proc Natl Acad Sci U S A 103:3932-3937, 2006.
14. Priori SG, Napolitano C, Schwartz PJ, et al: Association of long QT syndrome loci and cardiac events among patients treated with beta-blockers. JAMA 292:1341-1344, 2004.
15. Jacobs A, Knight BP, McDonald KT, Burke MC: Verapamil decreases ventricular tachyarrhythmias in a patient with Timothy syndrome (LQT8). Heart Rhythm 3:967-970, 2006.

Idiopathic Ventricular Fibrillation 73

Rainer Schimpf, Christian Wolpert, and Martin Borggrefe

CHAPTER OUTLINE

Sudden cardiac death (SCD) occurs predominantly in patients with known or previously unrecognized underlying heart disease, in most cases caused by sustained ventricular tachyarrhythmias. Coronary artery disease is the leading cause for approximately 80% of patients who experience SCD.[1] Furthermore, structural cardiac abnormalities in idiopathic, hypertrophic, and arrhythmogenic right (or left) ventricular cardiomyopathies account for the second largest number of sudden death of cardiac origin (10% to 15%). In 5% to 10% of the victims, however, evidence of structural heart disease is lacking. Patients without underlying heart disease who succumb to SCD usually are younger than 40 years of age.

Overview

The diagnosis of *idiopathic ventricular fibrillation* (IVF) is based mainly on exclusion of an underlying heart disease. Over the years, however, distinct groups of patients surviving ventricular fibrillation have been found to present with characteristic electrocardiographic patterns revealing ion channelopathies such as the long QT syndrome, Brugada syndrome, catecholaminergic polymorphic ventricular tachycardia (CPVT), or the short QT syndrome. In the meantime, molecular genetic studies revealed a variety of underlying mutations in ion channel genes or cellular structural proteins contributing to the risk of developing IVF. Thus, the number of patients with "true" IVF has substantially decreased. Several patients with IVF have been described, however, in whom the underlying mechanism remains unknown. In addition, transient factors such as ischemia, electrolyte disturbances, and unknown drug interactions may contribute to the occurrence of ventricular tachyarrhythmias. Data collected from large series of victims of cardiac arrest demonstrate that IVF occurs in approximately 1% of survivors of cardiac arrest and in up to 8% of victims of SCD.[2]

Diagnostic Evaluation

Prerequisite for the diagnosis of IVF is a complete cardiologic workup that excludes any evidence of structural or primary electrical abnormalities (Table 73-1). A comprehensive document on natural history, risk prediction, evaluation, and prevention of SCD was given by the Task Force on Sudden Cardiac Death of the European Society of Cardiology.[2] Because coronary artery disease accounts for the largest number of sudden deaths of cardiac etiology, ischemia must be excluded in the workup for IVF. After the exclusion of acute myocardial infarction or reversible triggers of arrhythmias such as electrolyte imbalance, intoxication, or myocarditis, systematic noninvasive and invasive examinations are mandatory. Impairment of left ventricular function, valve disease, regional wall motion abnormalities, and right ventricular enlargement of different origin have to be excluded. Echocardiography should be repeated during follow-up evaluation because cardiopulmonary resuscitation often leads to temporary impairment of left ventricular function, which may be misdiagnosed as structural disease in some cases. Ventricular tachyarrhythmias and ventricular fibrillation have been reported in left apical ballooning (Tako-Tsubo cardiomyopathy) as a newly recognized form of cardiomyopathy.[3] Cardiac magnetic resonance imaging may be applied to examine diagnostic criteria of arrhythmogenic right ventricular cardiomyopathy (ARVC). Evidence of intramyocardial enhancement with contrast media (late enhancement) may point to a scar caused by either coronary artery disease or myocarditis, ARVC, or hypertrophic cardiomyopathy. Extracardiac diseases with potential cardiac involvement, such as sarcoidosis, Fabry disease, and neurodegenerative disorders, should be excluded as well (see Table 73-1).

Invasive evaluation must be performed in every patient to exclude coronary artery disease or coronary artery malformations. Electrophysiology studies may provide some additional information about underlying electrophysiologic abnormalities such as reduced effective refractory periods associated with short QT syndromes, sinus node recovery time, and AV node conduction parameters associated with conduction disorders or Brugada syndrome. Furthermore, Wolff-Parkinson-White (WPW) syndrome with short effective refractory periods of the accessory pathways has to be excluded.

Pharmacologic drug challenge should be considered for exclusion of Brugada syndrome[4-6] (Fig. 73-1). Exercise testing is indicated if the arrhythmic event was related to physical activity. Especially in children and patients younger than 40 years of age, induction of polymorphic or bidirectional tachycardias during exercise facilitates the diagnosis of CPVT.

Patients with dilated cardiomyopathy caused by lamin A/C defects, for example, may demonstrate only a mild phenotype, with a subtle PR prolongation and a narrow QRS complex. The disease is associated with a high risk of SCD before changes in left ventricular contraction and dilatation become detectable.[7]

Detailed family history may reveal a familial origin and should initiate further diagnostic work-up. Examination of relatives of young SCD victims has a high diagnostic yield. Tan and coworkers could demonstrate in 43 families with a history of more than one sudden cardiac death that 40% could be diagnosed with an underlying familial disease: CVPT (n = 5 families); long QT syndrome (n = 4 families); Brugada syndrome (n = 2); long QT syndrome or Brugada syndrome (n = 1);

Table 73-1 Differential Diagnosis in Aborted Sudden Cardiac Death

Disease	Manifestation
Coronary artery disease	Acute myocardial infarction
Cardiomyopathy	Chronic coronary artery disease (scar, reduced left ventricular function)
	Coronary malformations
	Dilated cardiomyopathy
	Hypertrophic cardiomyopathies
	Arrhythmogenic right ventricular cardiomyopathy
	Acute/chronic myocarditis
	Tako-Tsubo cardiomyopathy
	Valve disease
	Cardiac involvement of extracardiac diseases
Primary electrical disease	Long QT syndrome
	Short QT syndrome
	Brugada syndrome
	Catecholaminergic polymorphic ventricular tachycardia
	Wolff-Parkinson-White syndrome

arrhythmogenic right ventricular cardiomyopathy (ARVC) (*n* = 3); hypertrophic cardiomyopathy (*n* = 1); and familial hypercholesterolemia (*n* = 1).[8]

In the past years, significant advances in molecular genetic screening revealed a broad spectrum of mutations responsible for ion channelopathies of the heart such as long QT syndrome, Brugada syndrome, CPVT, and short QT syndrome. Therefore, progress in revealing further mechanisms for IVF and molecular genetic defects is to be expected. However, molecular genetic screening is at present not part of a routine workup in patients with IVF unless prompted by an obvious family history.

Electrocardiographic Features

General Findings

IVF is observed in patients without obvious structural heart disease. After exclusion of structural abnormalities, several ion channelopathies such as long QT syndrome, Brugada syndrome, or short QT syndrome have to be ruled out. Thus, a complete and repetitive analysis of the electrocardiogram (ECG) is mandatory before establishing the diagnosis of IVF. Serial ECG evaluations are required because primary electrical diseases may manifest with either minor abnormalities or fluctuating repolarization patterns, or even with completely normal baseline findings. Prolongation of the QT interval (QTc longer than 440 ms in men and longer than 460 ms in women) and characteristic T wave patterns suggesting specific long QT syndrome subtypes have to be excluded. Several baseline ECGs and Holter ECGs are recommended to detect possible transitional prolongations of the QT interval. In genetic long QT syndrome, approximately 20% of affected persons present with normal QT intervals.[9]

Repolarization abnormalities in the precordial leads as seen in Brugada syndrome type I or nondiagnostic types II and III ECG patterns have to be analyzed (see Fig. 73-1).[6,10] Recording of modified right precordial leads at the third and second intercostal spaces at baseline ECG and during drug challenge is recommended.[4]

Identification of a QT interval shorter than 330 ms (QTc) after exclusion of a secondary QT interval shortening makes the diagnosis of a short QT syndrome likely.[11-14] The frequency of a short QT interval in the population of 0.1% for a QTc shorter than 320 ms and 0.4% for a QTc shorter than 340 ms is very low and not necessarily associated with an increased arryhthmogenic risk.[15] However, in patients with a history of atrial fibrillation, especially at young age, syncope, or ventricular tachyarrhythmias, a congenital short QT syndrome is suspected.[11-14] Additional features pointing to a short QT syndrome are the morphology of the T waves which appear often tall and symmetrical.[16] Furthermore, a reduced QT interval adaptation to increases in heart rate during exercise is present in patients

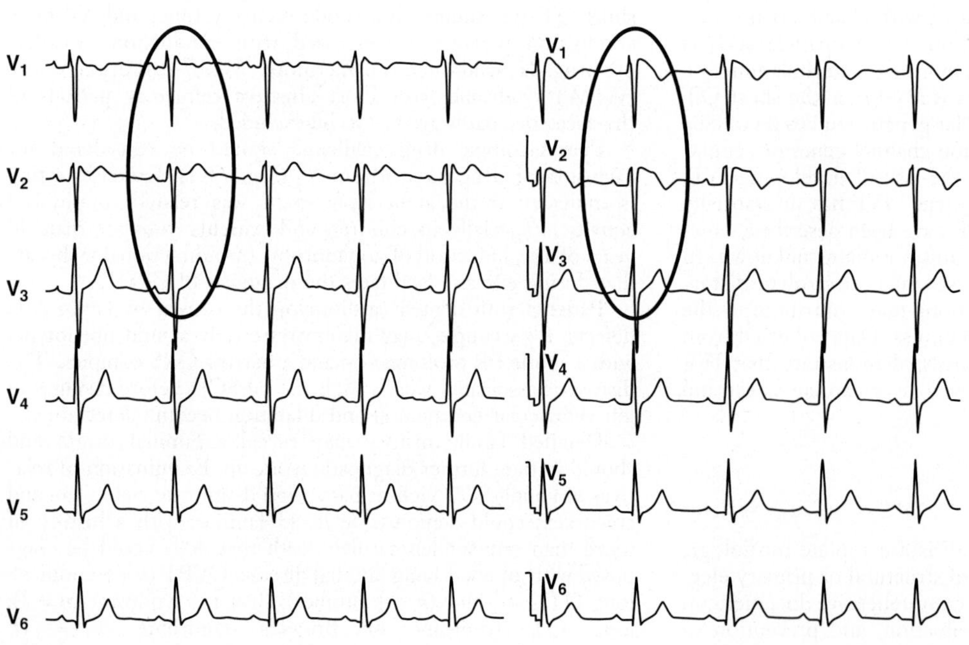

Figure 73-1 Electrocardiogram (ECG) of a 26-year-old man with a history of aborted sudden cardiac death before and after intravenous drug challenge (chest leads). The precordial leads *(encircled)* demonstrate change of type II ECG pattern *(left)* to a diagnostic type I Brugada ECG pattern after application of 70 mg of ajmaline *(right)*. Paper speed, 25 mm/second.

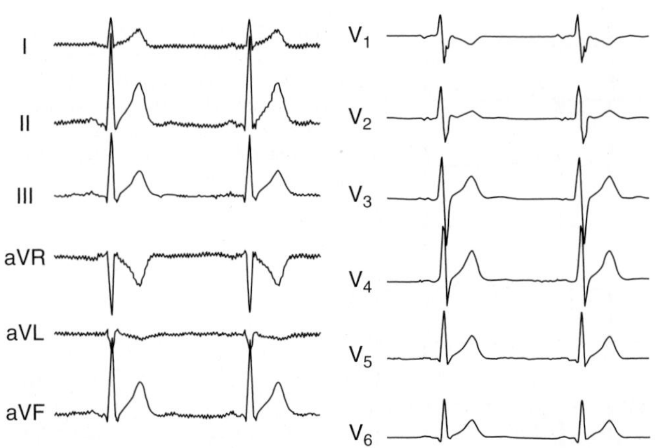

Figure 73-2 Electrocardiogram of a 21-year-old man with a history of aborted sudden cardiac death during swimming. Elevated ST segment in lead V_2 is suggestive of a Brugada type III electrocardiographic pattern. QT interval, 320 ms (QTc, 340 ms). Paper speed, 50 mm/second.

with a short QT syndrome in comparison with normal controls (−0.2 to 0.6 ms/beats per minute versus −1.3 ms/beats per minute in control subjects).[17,18]

In one retrospective analysis by Viskin and coworkers, it could be demonstrated that 35% of men who were classified as patients with IVF presented with QTc intervals shorter than 360 ms, versus only 10% of men in a comparable group of asymptomatic healthy subjects.[19] Further data showed QTc intervals ranging from 330 to 370 ms, together with a Brugada-type ECG pattern, in patients with a history of familial IVF. Genetic screening revealed loss-of-function mutations of the cardiac L-type calcium channels in these patients, representing a further primary electrical abnormality[20] (Fig. 73-2). However, prediction of an arrhythmogenic risk in patients with a borderline shortened QT interval remains unclear at present.

J Wave

Notching of the terminal QRS complex recently has been reported to be associated with IVF.[21] Traditionally, the prominent elevated notch in the inferior and mid-to-lateral precordial leads mostly described as J wave or as *early repolarization* has long been regarded as a benign ECG pattern.[22] The prevalence of the ECG phenomenon of early repolarization has been found in 1% to 2% of healthy young adult men.[23] Furthermore, it is observed during hypothermia (Osborne wave), with cocaine abuse, and in patients with hypertrophic cardiomyopathy. However, several reports on patients with IVF raised the possibility that the presentation of early repolarization may not be as benign as has been generally believed.[24-28]

In a recent multicenter study, Haissaguerre and coworkers compared a group of 155 patients and IVF with a control group of 155 healthy age- and sex-matched subjects.[29] The ECG pattern of early repolarization, defined as the presence of a J wave deviating from baseline by greater than 0.1 mV in the inferior or lateral leads (or both), could be identified significantly more often in the IVF group than in the control group (in 31% of 48 patients, versus 4% of 6 normal subjects; $P = .002$). The circumstances of SCD were reported during rest or normal physical activities in 45 patients. Intravenous drug challenge or electrophysiologic testing had a low diagnostic yield. Furthermore, the investigators reported a recurrence of ventricular fibrillation in 21 patients (14%) during a follow-up period of 57 ± 46 months.

The J wave represents a deflection that appears in the ECG as delta wave–like or as a second R wave (Ŕ) usually visible in the inferior leads II, III, aVR, and aVF and the mid- to lateral precordial leads V_2 to V_4. Furthermore, an upward-oriented concavity of the ST segment can be noted, with a reciprocal ST segment depression in lead aVR. A lowering of the ST segment with age, circadian variations, and increase in the J wave deflection at bradycardia have been reported. For the first time, Yan and Antzelevitch could show, in canine ventricular wedge preparations, underlying mechanisms for the generation of the J wave. A more prominent I_{to}-mediated spike-and-dome action potential notch in epicardium but not endocardium provides a voltage gradient that manifests the J wave or J point elevation.[30,31]

A failure of a development of the action potential notch at some sites compared with others with normal action potentials may induce a dispersion of repolarization. Propagation of the action potential dome from the sites where it is maintained to the sites where it is lost may result in reexcitation of local tissue. This phase 2 reentry could induce closely coupled ventricular extraystole, thereby creating the possibility to induce a reentrant arrhythmia.[31] Evidence of the role of a phase 2 reentry in the initiation of PVCs and tachyarrhythmias could be demonstrated in patients.[32]

Owing to a 1% to 2% prevalence of early repolarization in the general population, however, it remains unclear how to identify at present those persons who are at increased risk of sudden death.

Triggers

Extensive studies on the mechanisms of IVF have been performed that at present favor two major mechanisms: One mechanism postulates multiple self-sustaining reentry wavelets propagating through the ventricles; the other suggests a large single "mother rotor" generating wavebreaks that propagate across the ventricles.[33] Specific triggers for initiation of IVF have been identified in the right ventricular outflow tract (RVOT) or in the Purkinje system.[34-36] Ablation of dominant triggers may reduce the recurrence of ventricular fibrillation.[34]

In patients without organic heart disease and ventricular tachycardia, the most common site of origin is the right ventricular outflow tract. The morphology of ventricular tachycardias is usually a left bundle branch block pattern with an inferior axis. The clinical course in these patients is considered to be predominantly benign. One author reported that occasionally benign PVCs originating from the RVOT may initiate ventricular fibrillation.[35] Risk factors for potentially malignant RVOT electrical activity appear to be a history of syncope, very rapid ventricular tachycardias (rates of more than 230 beats per minute), frequent PVCs (more than 20,000 per day), and ventricular ectopy with a short coupling interval.[37] However, comparison of patients with benign ventricular extrasystole and patients with PVCs that may induce IVF also shows a significant overlap of clinical parameters such as lower number of PVCs and longer coupling intervals (more than 320 ms) and QRS duration of PVCs.[35] Thus, identification of patients with potentially malignant ventricular extraystoles still remains a challenge.

The Purkinje system may be another source of triggers initiating IVF (Fig. 73-3). Haissaguerre and coworkers showed that PVCs with narrow QRS morphology and right and left bundle block pattern originating in the area of the left and right Purkinje system are involved in the development of ventricular fibrillation.[38] Elimination of focal activity by radiofrequency ablation effectively prevented further episodes of ventricular

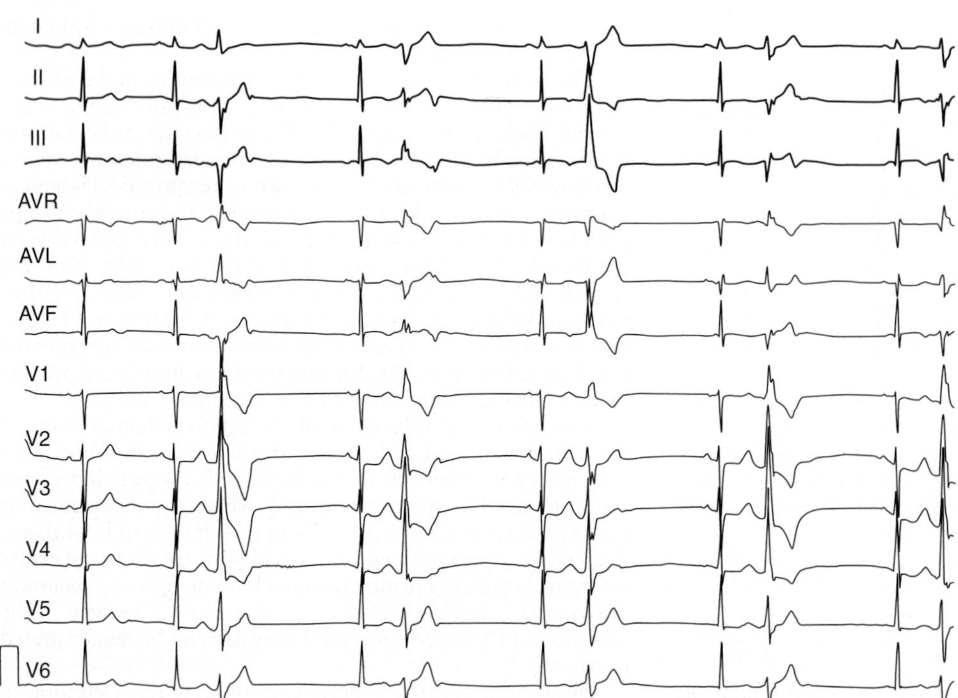

Figure 73-3 Electrocardiogram of a 34-year-old woman with a history of repetitive episodes of idiopathic ventricular fibrillation. Repetitive premature ventricular contractions suggest an origin from the left ventricular Purkinje system. Paper speed, 25 mm/second.

tachyarrhythmias. After several episodes of ventricular fibrillation (10 ± 12 episodes) in 23 patients, repetitive PVCs could be identified as triggers. After successful elimination of the foci originating in the Purkinje system, no recurrences could be documented during a follow-up period of 24 ± 28 months. This study confirmed the role of the Purkinje system in the initiation of IVF, although the exact mechanism remains unknown.[34]

In different clinical settings such as long QT syndrome, idiopathic ventricular tachycardias, and IVF, a putative role of the sympathetic system has been suggested in arrhythmogenesis.[39-41] Presynaptic catecholamine reuptake has been assessed using the norepinephrine analogue [^{123}I]meta-iodobenzylguanidine (MIBG) in either planar scintigraphy or single photon emission computed tomography (SPECT). Impairment of cardiac innervation has been found in dilated and hypertrophic cardiomyopathy, diabetes, ARVC, and ischemic heart disease. Evidence of impairment of sympathetic innervation also was found in patients with a history of IVF. The areas of the presynaptic sympathetic dysfunction were located mainly in the basal and mid-ventricular parts of the posterior wall and the inferior septum. Repetition of the [^{123}I]MIBG SPECT measurements showed a reduced event-free survival for those patients who had abnormal innervation.[42]

Follow-up and Therapy

Patients with a history of IVF have a class I indication for ICD therapy.[2,43] Data from the Unexplained Cardiac Arrest Registry

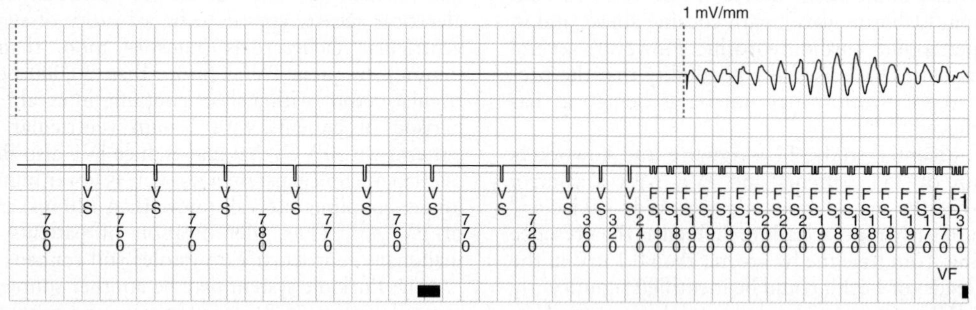

Figure 73-4 Initiation of an episode of ventricular fibrillation in a 54-year-old woman with history of idiopathic ventricular fibrillation and no clinically relevant extrasystole. The patient had been free of arrhythmic events for 6 years after resuscitation for ventricular fibrillation, when again during sleep, premature ventricular contraction triggered another episode of ventricular fibrillation, which was effectively terminated by the implantable cardioverter-debrillator (ICD) *(not shown)*. This stored endocardial electrogram was derived from the ventricular pace/sense/shock electrode. *First line*, bipolar near-field electrogram between the distal tip and ring of the electrode; *second line*, corresponding annotation of the detected events by the ICD pace/sense electrode; *third line*, cycle lengths between each sensed event in ms. FS, sensed events with cycle lengths below the programmed ventricular fibrillation zone; VS, sensed ventricular events.

of Europe (UCARE) confirmed a recurrence rate of 30% in 3 years after cardiac arrest due to IVF.[44,45]

At present, recommendations for a specific drug therapy are not available. Among the patients whose data are recorded in the UCARE registry, antiarrhythmic agents had no effect on recurrence rate. In a small group of patients with RVOT- or Purkinje system–related IVF, several antiarrhythmic drugs including beta-blockers were reported to be of no benefit in reduction of VF recurrences.[38] In a group of 34 consecutive patients with IVF, including 5 with a Brugada syndrome, 23 patients have received pharmacologic treatment after electrophysiologic testing of class IA agents. In patients on continuous treatment, predominantly with quinidine, no recurrences were reported during a mean follow-up period of 9.1 ± 5.6 years.[46]

Repetitive PVCs from the RVOT or Purkinje system may trigger episodes of ventricular fibrillation.[35,38] The elimination of the focal activity by radiofrequency ablation has been shown to be effective in preventing recurrences of further episodes of ventricular fibrillation. In a Japanese study in 16 patients with RVOT PVCs and a history of IVF, 13 patients underwent successful ablation therapy.[35] During a mean follow-up period of 54 ± 39 months, no further episodes of syncope or ventricular tachyarrhythmias were reported. Haissaguerre and coworkers described a group of 23 patients with IVF triggered by PVCs originating in the Purkinje system.[34] Radiofrequency ablation was successfully performed, with identification of a sharp potential preceding the ventricular electrogram of the premature beats as well as the sinus beats. During a follow-up period of 24 ± 28 months, no recurrent sudden deaths, syncope, or VF occurred. These same workers reported effective treatment by radiofrequency ablation in patients with long QT and Brugada syndromes with recurrent episodes of ventricular fibrillation induced by monomorphic ventricular extrasystole.[47]

A point worthy of emphasis, however, is that ablation therapy still constitutes a potential adjunct to ICD therapy, for which it is not a substitute, in patients with IVF and repetitive monomorphic PVCs, which have been identified as triggers of recurrent VF episodes (Fig. 73-4).

References

1. Huikuri HV, Castellanos A, Myerburg RJ: Sudden death due to cardiac arrhythmias. N Engl J Med 345:1473-1482, 2001.
2. Priori SG, Aliot E, Blomstrom-Lundqvist C, et al: Task Force on Sudden Cardiac Death, European Society of Cardiology. Europace 4:3-18, 2002.
3. Bonello L, Com O, Ait-Moktar O, et al: Ventricular arrhythmias during Tako-Tsubo syndrome. Int J Cardiol 128: e50-e53, 2008. Epub 2007 Aug 15.
4. Antzelevitch C, Brugada P, Borggrefe M, et al: Brugada syndrome: Report of the Second Consensus Conference: Endorsed by the Heart Rhythm Society and the European Heart Rhythm Association. Circulation 111:659-670, 2005.
5. Probst V, Denjoy I, Meregalli PG, et al: Clinical aspects and prognosis of Brugada syndrome in children. Circulation 115:2042-2048, 2007.
6. Veltmann C, Schimpf R, Echternach C, et al: A prospective study on spontaneous fluctuations between diagnostic and non-diagnostic ECGs in Brugada syndrome: Implications for correct phenotyping and risk stratification. Eur Heart J 27:2544-2552, 2006.
7. van Berlo JH, de Voogt WG, van der Kooi AJ, et al: Meta-analysis of clinical characteristics of 299 carriers of *LMNA* gene mutations: Do lamin A/C mutations portend a high risk of sudden death? J Mol Med 83:79-83, 2005.
8. Tan HL, Hofman N, van Langen IM, et al: Sudden unexplained death: Heritability and diagnostic yield of cardiological and genetic examination in surviving relatives. Circulation 112:207-213, 2005.
9. Schwartz PJ, Priori SG, Spazzolini C, et al: Genotype-phenotype correlation in the long-QT syndrome: Gene-specific triggers for life-threatening arrhythmias. Circulation 103:89-95, 2001.
10. Wilde AA, Antzelevitch C, Borggrefe M, et al: Proposed diagnostic criteria for the Brugada syndrome: Consensus report. Circulation 106:2514-2519, 2002.
11. Gussak I, Brugada P, Brugada J, et al: Idiopathic short QT interval: A new clinical syndrome? Cardiology 94:99-102, 2000.
12. Gaita F, Giustetto C, Bianchi F, et al: Short QT syndrome: A familial cause of sudden death. Circulation 108:965-970, 2003.
13. Bjerregaard P, Gussak I: Short QT syndrome: Mechanisms, diagnosis and treatment. Nat Clin Pract Cardiovasc Med 2:84-87, 2005.
14. Giustetto C, Di Monte F, Wolpert C, et al: Short QT syndrome: Clinical findings and diagnostic-therapeutic implications. Eur Heart J 27:2440-2447, 2006.
15. Anttonen O, Junttila MJ, Rissanen H, et al: Prevalence and prognostic significance of short QT interval in a middle-aged Finnish population. Circulation 116:714-720, 2007.
16. Schimpf R, Wolpert C, Gaita F, et al: Short QT syndrome. Cardiovasc Res 67:357-366, 2005.
17. Wolpert C, Schimpf R, Giustetto C, et al: Further insights into the effect of quinidine in short QT syndrome caused by a mutation in *HERG*. J Cardiovasc Electrophysiol 16:54-58, 2005.
18. Magnano AR, Holleran S, Ramakrishnan R, et al: Autonomic nervous system influences on QT interval in normal subjects. J Am Coll Cardiol 39:1820-1826, 2002.
19. Viskin S, Zeltser D, Ish-Shalom M, et al: Is idiopathic ventricular fibrillation a short QT syndrome? Comparison of QT intervals of patients with idiopathic ventricular fibrillation and healthy controls. Heart Rhythm 1:587-591, 2004.
20. Antzelevitch C, Pollevick GD, Cordeiro JM, et al: Loss-of-function mutations in the cardiac calcium channel underlie a new clinical entity characterized by ST-segment elevation, short QT intervals, and sudden cardiac death. Circulation 115:442-449, 2007.
21. Shinohara T, Takahashi N, Saikawa T, Yoshimatsu H: Characterization of J wave in a patient with idiopathic ventricular fibrillation. Heart Rhythm 3:1082-1084, 2006.
22. Gussak I, Antzelevitch C: Early repolarization syndrome: Clinical characteristics and possible cellular and ionic mechanisms. J Electrocardiol 33:299-309, 2000.
23. Parisi AF, Beckmann CH, Lancaster MC: The spectrum of ST segment elevation in the electrocardiograms of healthy adult men. J Electrocardiol 4:137-144, 1971.
24. Fujiki A, Sugao M, Nishida K, et al: Repolarization abnormality in idiopathic ventricular fibrillation: Assessment using 24-hour QT-RR and QaT-RR relationships. J Cardiovasc Electrophysiol 15:59-63, 2004.
25. Sugao M, Fujiki A, Nishida K, et al: Repolarization dynamics in patients with idiopathic ventricular fibrillation: Pharmacological therapy with bepridil and disopyramide. J Cardiovasc Pharmacol 45:545-549, 2005.
26. Tsunoda Y, Takeishi Y, Nozaki N, et al: Presence of intermittent J waves in multiple leads in relation to episode of atrial and ventricular fibrillation. J Electrocardiol 37:311-314, 2004.
27. Shu J, Zhu T, Yang L, et al: ST-segment elevation in the early repolarization syndrome, idiopathic ventricular fibrillation, and the Brugada syndrome: Cellular and clinical linkage. J Electrocardiol 38:26-32, 2005.
28. Letsas KP, Efremidis M, Pappas LK, et al: Early repolarization syndrome: Is it always benign? Int J Cardiol 114:390-392, 2007.
29. Haissaguerre M, Sacher F, Derval N, et al: Early repolarization in the inferolateral leads: A new syndrome associated with sudden cardiac death. J Interv Cardiol Electrophysiol 18:281, 2007.
30. Yan GX, Antzelevitch C: Cellular basis for the electrocardiographic J wave. Circulation 93:372-379, 1996.
31. Antzelevitch C: Cellular basis for the repolarization waves of the ECG. Ann N Y Acad Sci 1080:268-281, 2006.
32. Bloch Thomsen PE, Joergensen RM, et al: Phase 2 reentry in man. Heart Rhythm 2:797-803, 2005.

33. Nash MP, Mourad A, Clayton RH, et al: Evidence for multiple mechanisms in human ventricular fibrillation. Circulation 114:536-542, 2006.
34. Haissaguerre M, Shah DC, Jais P, et al: Role of Purkinje conducting system in triggering of idiopathic ventricular fibrillation. Lancet 359:677-678, 2002.
35. Noda T, Shimizu W, Taguchi A, et al: Malignant entity of idiopathic ventricular fibrillation and polymorphic ventricular tachycardia initiated by premature extrasystoles originating from the right ventricular outflow tract. J Am Coll Cardiol 46:1288-1294, 2005.
36. Saliba W, Abul Karim A, Tchou P, Natale A: Ventricular fibrillation: ablation of a trigger? J Cardiovasc Electrophysiol 13:1296-1299, 2002.
37. Viskin S, Antzelevitch C: The cardiologists' worst nightmare: Sudden death from "benign" ventricular arrhythmias. J Am Coll Cardiol 46:1295-1297, 2005.
38. Haissaguerre M, Shoda M, Jais P, et al: Mapping and ablation of idiopathic ventricular fibrillation. Circulation 106:962-967, 2002.
39. Kies P, Wichter T, Schafers M, et al: Abnormal myocardial presynaptic norepinephrine recycling in patients with Brugada syndrome. Circulation 110:3017-3022, 2004.
40. Wichter T, Matheja P, Eckardt L, et al: Cardiac autonomic dysfunction in Brugada syndrome. Circulation 105:702-706, 2002.
41. Oyama N, Yokoshiki H, Satoh K, et al: Iodine-123-metaiodobenzylguanidine scintigraphy of total cardiac adrenergic denervation in Brugada syndrome. Jpn Heart J 43:183-186, 2002.
42. Paul M, Schafers M, Kies P, et al: Impact of sympathetic innervation on recurrent life-threatening arrhythmias in the follow-up of patients with idiopathic ventricular fibrillation. Eur J Nucl Med Mol Imaging 33:866-870, 2006.
43. Zipes DP, Camm AJ, Borggrefe M, et al: ACC/AHA/ESC 2006 Guidelines for Management of Patients with Ventricular Arrhythmias and the Prevention of Sudden Cardiac Death—Executive Summary: A report of the American College of Cardiology/American Heart Association Task Force and the European Society of Cardiology Committee for Practice Guidelines (Writing Committee to Develop Guidelines for Management of Patients with Ventricular Arrhythmias and the Prevention of Sudden Cardiac Death). Developed in collaboration with the European Heart Rhythm Association and the Heart Rhythm Society. Eur Heart J 27:2099-2140, 2006.
44. Survivors of out-of-hospital cardiac arrest with apparently normal heart. Need for definition and standardized clinical evaluation. Consensus Statement of the Joint Steering Committees of the Unexplained Cardiac Arrest Registry of Europe and of the Idiopathic Ventricular Fibrillation Registry of the United States. Circulation 95:265-272, 1997.
45. Priori S, Crotti L: Idiopathic ventricular fibrillation. Cardiac Electrophysiol Rev 3:198-201, 1999.
46. Belhassen B, Viskin S, Fish R, et al: Effects of electrophysiologic-guided therapy with Class IA antiarrhythmic drugs on the long-term outcome of patients with idiopathic ventricular fibrillation with or without the Brugada syndrome. J Cardiovasc Electrophysiol 10:1301-1312, 1999.
47. Haissaguerre M, Extramiana F, Hocini M, et al: Mapping and ablation of ventricular fibrillation associated with long-QT and Brugada syndromes. Circulation 108:925-928, 2003.

Drug-Induced Ventricular Tachycardia 74

LARS ECKARDT AND GÜNTER BREITHARDT

CHAPTER OUTLINE

Overview

Drug-induced ventricular tachyarrhythmias may be caused by cardiovascular drugs, noncardiovascular drugs, and even nonprescription agents. They may result in arrhythmic emergencies and sudden cardiac death.[1] Development of a new arrhythmia, or aggravation of an existing arrhythmia, during therapy with a drug at a concentration usually considered not to be toxic is defined as *proarrhythmia*. This condition may occur in patients with or without structural heart disease. Major causes of proarrhythmia include direct pharmacologic effects on ion channels of the heart; cardiac glycosides, QT-prolonging agents, and sodium channel–blocking drugs all have been implicated in this proarrhythmic category. In addition, certain drugs may cause a cardiomyopathy that ultimately may lead to ventricular tachyarrhythmias—specifically, ventricular tachycardia. Others may cause coronary vasoconstriction and acute myocardial ischemia.

The proportion of patients with proarrhythmia that initially manifests as sudden death, and the extent to which proarrhythmia contributes to the overall problem of sudden death, are unknown. Nevertheless, the experience with terfenadine or cisapride and the Cardiac Arrhythmia Suppression Trial (CAST) study[2] has illustrated the potential for drugs to result in unusual severe adverse effects, which may be difficult to detect. General treatment guidelines focus on avoidance of drug treatment in high-risk patients, recognition of the syndromes of drug-induced proarrhythmia, and withdrawal of the culprit agent(s). Specific therapies often are based on anecdotal evidence or experimental studies.

Pharmacokinetic Risk Factors

Arrhythmogenic potential may become manifest in patients who are especially sensitive to the electrophysiologic effects of a particular drug ("pharmacodynamic sensitivity"). This phenomenon may be the result of overdose or drug interactions in such highly sensitive patients in whom usual drug dosages lead to extreme elevations in plasma concentration. The latter most commonly occurs when the culprit drug is eliminated by a single metabolizing pathway. If this pathway is susceptible to inhibition by the administration of a second drug, inhibited by coadministration of other drugs, or by genetic factors, marked elevation of drug concentrations and electrophysiologic toxicity may result. This was the case with terfenadine and cisapride, both of which are eliminated as noncardioactive metabolites by the intestinal and hepatic P-450 system, CYP3A4. Many commonly used drugs are potent CYP3A4 inhibitors, such as erythromycin, ketoconazole, and some calcium channel blockers, notably mibefradil, which has been withdrawn from the market. Of note, grapefruit juice markedly inhibits the activity of intestinal but not hepatic CYP3A4. Although CYP3A4 is the most important drug-metabolizing enzyme expressed in the liver and elsewhere, some drugs use other pathways. Among other members of the CYP superfamily, genetically determined polymorphisms have been described in three: CYP2D6, CYP2C9, and CYP2C19. A subset of the population absolutely lacks catalytic activity, so that plasma concentrations of substrate drugs are much higher in such "poor metabolizer" patients. The activity of the P-450 CYP2D6, for example, is absent in approximately 7% of whites and in persons of African heritage. In a situation in which CYP2D6 is the sole eliminating pathway, patients with this "poor metabolizer" trait may therefore display markedly aberrant drug concentrations.

Genetic Predisposition

Administration of a drug may unmask a subclinical (*forme fruste*) monogenic arrhythmia syndrome. Mutations in genes (*KCNQ1*, *KCNH2*, and *SCN5A*) causing congenital forms of the long QT syndrome have been identified in patients with "acquired" forms of long QT syndrome. The exact contribution and mutation frequency cannot yet be estimated. Mutations in the relevant genes play only a minor role in acquired long QT syndrome, so genetic screening should be limited to selected patients. A subclinical form of the Brugada syndrome may similarly predispose affected patients to the development of "acquired" forms of the Brugada syndrome, as a consequence of polymorphisms or mutations in *SCN5A* or other genes.[3] Exposure during provocative testing is well recognized to confer a risk for ventricular fibrillation.[4] In these monogenic syndromes, penetrance of the electrocardiographic phenotype can be highly variable, an effect often attributed to as-yet unidentified modifier genes. In addition, genetic polymorphisms may increase the risk for drug-induced sudden cardiac death. For example, approximately 10% of African Americans carry a variant in their sodium channel gene that results in a tyrosine (Y) rather than a serine

(S) at position 1103 of the protein.[5] Study of this variant protein in vitro indicates that it confers changes consistent with the sodium channel–linked variant of long QT syndrome. Similarly, the polymorphisms resulting in T8A and Q9E in the *KCNE2* gene have been associated with unusual in vitro characteristics and a higher incidence of proarrhythmia during drug therapy.

Drug-Induced Long QT Syndrome

Drug effects are the most common cause of acquired long QT syndrome. Although syncope occurring soon after the initiation of quinidine therapy was recognized as early as the 1920s, it was not until the advent of continuous electrocardiographic monitoring that "quinidine syncope" was recognized to be due to polymorphic ventricular tachycardia. In recent years, it has become apparent that in addition to antiarrhythmic drugs, a large spectrum of noncardiac drugs (Table 74-1) can cause QT prolongation and torsades de pointes. Dessertenne used the term *torsades de pointes* initially to describe this particular ventricular tachycardia in 1966.[6] This rhythm abnormality is characterized by a polymorphic, usually nonsustained, pause-dependent ventricular tachycardia that may develop in association with an excessively prolonged QT interval.[6] It may be associated with syncope or may degenerate into a sustained ventricular tachycardia or ventricular fibrillation. An electrocardiogram (ECG) recorded just before or after termination of a polymorphic ventricular tachycardia helps to distinguish torsades from other polymorphic ventricular tachycardias mainly occurring in patients with structural heart disease. Features diagnostic for torsades de pointes include a prolonged QT interval, the presence of U waves before the onset or after the termination of the arrhythmia, relatively long coupling intervals, and a typical initiating sequence: In acquired long QT syndrome, short-long-short cycle length changes constitute the typical pattern of initiation of torsades de pointes and may be regarded as a warning sign of an impending episode of torsades. Premature ventricular beats often are found to arise from exaggerated T/U waves after longer intervals, such as after extrasystolic pauses (Fig. 74-1).

Of concern is that the proarrhythmic risk for many of the drugs that may prolong repolarization, thereby causing torsades de pointes, was not detected during the developmental phase and was recognized only after such drugs had been on the market for many years.[6] Death as a direct result from acute intractable torsades de pointes occurred in up to 16% of patients in larger series. In a survey in both the United Kingdom and Italy, noncardiovascular drugs that have proarrhythmic potential (i.e., an official warning regarding risk for QT prolongation or torsades de pointes, or with published data on QT prolongation, ventricular tachycardia, or class III effect) represented 3% and 2% of total prescriptions in both countries, respectively.[7] The growing awareness of acquired long QT syndrome over the past several years has resulted in a marked increase in the number of spontaneous reports. This spontaneous reporting most likely underreports the true incidence of serious adverse reactions, so that the true incidence of drug-induced torsades de pointes is unknown. Although torsades de pointes preferentially occurs shortly after initiation of therapy, it also may develop during long-term treatment. The late occurrence has been linked to changes in dose, reinitiation of the drug after short discontinuation, and transient electrolyte disorders such as hypokalemia or hypomagnesemia. The incidence of torsades de pointes associated with sotalol has been estimated to range between 1.8% and almost 5%.

Table 74-1 Torsadogenic Potency of Drugs: A Possible Classification

Class A: High Torsadogenic Potency
Drugs that are potent blockers of currents prolonging myocardial repolarization (mainly I_{Kr}). Action potential prolongation and the induction of early afterdepolarizations have been documented. The IC_{50} for this effect is in the same range as for the IC_{50} for therapeutic action. QT prolongation has been documented at therapeutic doses and concentrations, and cases of torsades de pointes induced by the drug alone (in the absence of concomitant therapy prolonging repolarization or hypokalemia) have been documented.
Class B: Medium-High Torsadogenic Potency
Drugs that prolong myocardial repolarization (i.e., cardiac action potential duration and QT interval) at higher doses, or at normal doses with concurrent administration of drugs that inhibit drug metabolism (e.g., by inhibiting the cytochrome P-450 metabolism). Their IC_{50} for this prolongation of repolarization is above the IC_{50} for the therapeutic effect. Cases of torsades de pointes induced by the drug alone have been documented. This arrhythmia, however, usually is associated with metabolic inhibition and the presence of other risk factors.
Class C: Low Torsadogenic Potency
Drugs that prolong action potential duration and QT interval at high doses or concentrations that are clearly above the therapeutic range. Their effect on repolarization becomes manifest only with overdose or intoxication or in the presence of severe metabolic inhibition. Cases of torsades de pointes have been documented. In almost all published cases, however, several factors that are well known to increase the propensity for the development of torsades de pointes (i.e., risk factors) were present.
Class D: Torsadogenic Potential Not Clear
Drugs that block repolarizing ion currents in vitro but so far have not been shown to prolong repolarization in other in vitro models (e.g., papillary muscle fibers or isolated hearts), or the concentrations necessary for this effect were far above the clinical concentrations. Prolongation of the QT interval in humans has not been demonstrated in systematic randomized studies. Cases of torsades de pointes in association with treatment with the drug may have been reported. However, the causal relation between the event and the drug is not clear.

IC_{50}, half-maximal inhibitory concentration.

The torsadogenic potential of drugs is extremely variable, even within the same class of drugs.[8] Some drugs may provoke torsades de pointes only in the setting of overdose or with concomitant administration of other QT-prolonging drugs, or in the presence of risk factors such as hypokalemia, whereas others may induce torsades de pointes when used alone, even at therapeutic levels, and in the absence of additional risk factors. In an attempt to provide a systematic classification of QT-prolonging drugs, a classification of the torsadogenic

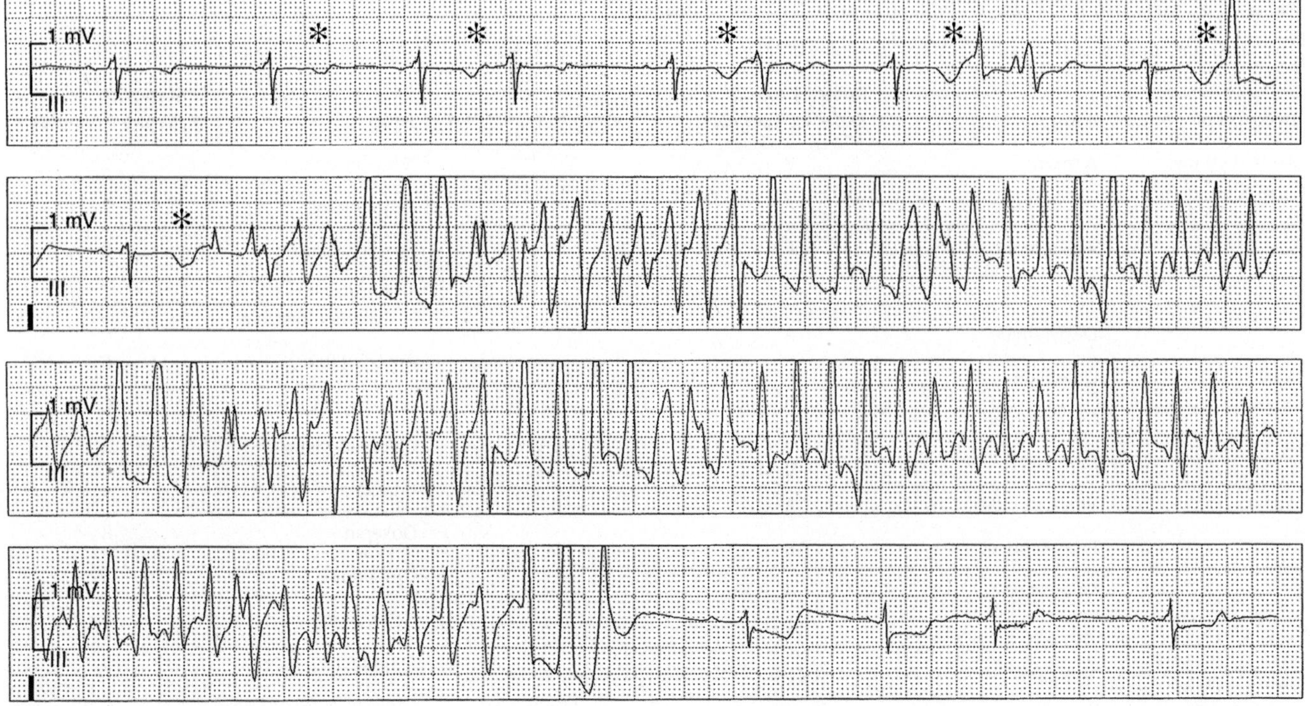

Figure 74-1 Monitor strip showing long-short ventricular cycle, pause-dependent QT prolongation with abnormal and gradually augmented T/U waves (*) leading to a self-terminating episode of torsades de pointes demonstrating the typical "twisting" morphology. Ventricular premature beats are followed by a post-extrasystolic pause. The initial beat starts from the peak of the U wave. This patient was on a combination of clarithromycin and ketoconazole.

potency of proarrhythmic drugs (Tables 74-1 and 74-2) has been proposed.[9]

Risk Factors for Torsades de Pointes

Several risk factors for the development of drug-related torsades de pointes have been proposed. Patients who developed drug-related torsades de pointes were found to have a borderline or prolonged (more than 0.44 second) QTc before drug administration. The fact that the QT interval is longer in women than in men has been suggested to account for the two- to three-fold higher incidence of abnormal QT prolongation and torsades de pointes in females. The potential mechanisms for these gender-related differences include differences in the densities of I_{Kr} and I_{K1} currents.

One hypothesis to explain the development of torsades de pointes is that normal repolarization is accomplished by multiple ion channels providing a safety reserve for repolarization. In the presence of an otherwise subclinical impairment in the repolarization mechanisms (i.e., reduced "repolarization reserve"),[10] patients may have a certain propensity for the development of torsades de pointes. Patients who have a previous history of drug-related torsades de pointes are very likely to experience further episodes on exposure to any other QT-prolonging drug. Kääb and associates[11] demonstrated that controlled exposure to sotalol successfully identified patients with normal QTc intervals but altered myocardial repolarization. Hypokalemia and hypomagnesemia prolong repolarization. A sometimes overlooked cause for hypokalemia can be ingestion of licorice.

Clinical but also experimental data reflect that potassium channel downregulation or aberrant intracellular calcium handling predispose patients to the development of arrhythmias when a QT interval–prolonging drug is superimposed. The importance of underlying structural heart disease as a potential risk factor for torsades de pointes is not clear. Acquired abnormal QT prolongation and torsades de pointes have been observed in patients with various types of heart disease as well as in patients without detectable heart disease. In larger series, arterial hypertension was present in a significant proportion of patients. In addition, clinical studies such as the Danish Investigations of Arrhythmia and Mortality on Dofetilide (DIAMOND) study provided evidence that heart failure is a risk factor for drug-induced torsades de pointes.[12] Any combination of risk factors will additionally reduce the "repolarization reserve" and thereby prolong the action potential and the QT interval. In addition, therapies used in heart failure may increase the risk. Diuretics, for example, not only decrease serum potassium but may also directly block potassium channels and thereby potentiate QT prolongation. Other risk factors that can affect repolarization and reduce the repolarization reserve, apart from the congenital long QT syndrome and drugs, are listed in Table 74-3. Knowledge of the clinical risk factors that identify patients with an increased propensity for development of drug-induced torsades de pointes and of the drugs known to provoke such arrhythmias (www.torsades.org) can help to prevent the occurrence of drug-induced proarrhythmia.

Mechanism of Acquired Torsades de Pointes

A large number of experimental and molecular studies have resulted in a better understanding of the mechanisms of torsades de pointes.[13] Prolongation of the action potential can be achieved by a reduction of the outward currents, particularly

Table 74-2 Drugs That May Cause QT Prolongation or Torsades de Pointes

This list is not comprehensive; rather, it gives examples of how drugs may be classified according to the criteria proposed in Table 74-1.

Drug Class	Drug	Potency to Provoke Torsades	Drug Class	Drug	Potency to Provoke Torsades
Antiarrhythmic drugs	Ajmaline	B		Ketoconazole	C
	Almokalant	A		Pentamidine	B
	Amiodarone	B		Sparfloxacine	B
	Azimilide	B		Trimethoprim-sulfamethoxazole	C
	Dispyramide	A	Psychiatric drugs	Amitryptiline	B
	Dofetilide	A		Chlorpromazine	C
	Dronederone	D		Chloral hydrate	B
	Ibutilide	A		Citalopram	B
	Procainamide	A		Doxepin	B
	Propafenone	B		Droperidol	B
	Quinidine	A		Haloperidol	B
	Sotalol	A		Imipramine	B
	Tedisamil	C/D		Lithium	C
Antihistaminics	Astemizole	B		Maprotiline	B
	Diphenylhydramine	B		Pimozide	B
	Loratadine	D		Sertindole	C
	Terfenadine	B		Thioridazine	B
Antimicrobial and antimalarial drugs	Amantadine	C		Zimeldine	B
	Azithromycin	C		Ziprasidone	C
	Clarithromycin	B	Vasodilators	Bepridil	A
	Chloroquine	B		Lidoflazine	A
	Erythromycin	B		Prenylamine	B
	Fluconazole	C	Miscellaneous	Cisapride	B
	Grepafloxacin	B		Domperidone	B
	Halofantrine	B		Cesium	C
	Itraconazole	C			

Data derived from a noncontrolled review of the literature. The reader is recommended to review the literature on any of these agents or drugs of the same drug group before making decisions that relate to their administration. Please see also www.torsades.org.

the outward delayed rectifier potassium currents I_{Kr} and I_{Ks} and/or enhancement of the inward currents during phases 2 and 3 of the action potential. Among the potassium currents, I_{Kr} is most susceptible to pharmacologic influence. In all known cases of drug-related acquired long QT syndrome, the blockade of I_{Kr} current is at least in part responsible for action potential prolongation and proarrhythmia. Blockade of I_{Kr} results in a reduction in the net outward current, a prolongation of the action potential, and the possible development of T/U wave abnormalities. The prolongation of repolarization may result in subsequent activation of an inward depolarization current ($I_{Ca,L}$ and I_{Na}), which may generate early afterdepolarizations and promote triggered activity at the end of repolarization.

Using high-resolution three-dimensional isochronal maps of activation and repolarization patterns, El-Sherif and coworkers[14] showed that the initial beat of torsades de pointes consistently arose as a subendocardial focal activity, whereas subsequent beats were due to successive reentrant excitation in the form of rotating scrolls. Prolongation of phase 2 repolarization, by augmenting the I_{Na} current, rather than phase 3 of repolarization, may reduce the propensity to induce early afterdepolarizations and torsades de pointes. The cardiac membrane is relatively inexcitable during phase 2 compared with phase 3, which is the phase prolonged by most drugs causing torsades de pointes. Prolongation of phase 3 allows a longer time interval for the development of early afterdepolarizations and triggered activity.

Table 74-3 Causes and Contributing Factors Leading to Acquired QT Prolongation and Torsades de Pointes (see Table 74-2)

Electrolyte abnormalities
Hypokalemia
Hypomagnesemia
Hypocalcemia
Female gender
Genetic
Asymptomatic/symptomatic carriers of long QT syndrome mutations
Genetic polymorphisms
Bradyarrhythmias
Sinus bradycardia
Atrioventricular block
"Relative" bradycardia resulting from frequent ventricular extrasystoles followed by a compensatory pause
Congestive heart failure/left ventricular dysfunction
Ventricular hypertrophy
Metabolic factors
Interaction with cytochrome P-450 system by other drugs (drug-specific)
Liver disease (drug-specific)
Kidney disease (drug-specific)
Hypothyroidism
Altered nutritional states
Anorexia nervosa
Diets, starvation
Alcoholism
Cerebrovascular diseases
Intracranial and subarachnoidal hemorrhage
Stroke
Intracranial trauma

In an in vitro model of torsades de pointes, Milberg and associates[8,15] demonstrated that QT prolongation mainly by phase 3 prolongation ("triangulation" of the action potential) corresponded to the occurrence of torsades de pointes, whereas "rectangulation" of the action potential had no proarrhythmic effects and even suppressed torsades de pointes.

Calcium channel blockade also can diminish the induction of early afterdepolarizations and torsades de pointes,[16] a property that helps explain the low torsadogenic potential of quinidine in a fixed combination with verapamil[17] and most likely of amiodarone, too. Using intravenous verapamil, Cosio and colleagues[18] successfully treated torsades de pointes in the setting of AV block in three patients. The drug effectively suppressed torsades de pointes without affecting the QT interval. In the case of amiodarone (incidence of torsades de pointes of less than 1%), the ability to diminish or eliminate dispersion or repolarization may also be important.[19]

Prevention of Acquired Torsades de Pointes

Prevention of drug-related torsades de pointes, especially by noncardiovascular drugs, is a major challenge not only for the physician but also for researchers engaged in the development of new drugs and for regulatory agencies.[6] Early identification of a potentially adverse response of the QT interval to a drug requires careful and regular observation of the ECG.[20] Apart from analysis of the QT intervals, special attention should be directed to excessive QT prolongation, QT dispersion,[21] and developing changes in T wave morphology (e.g., negative or notched or biphasic T waves and appearance of prominent U waves). Instability of repolarization also may result from interventions that affect "cardiac memory." Haverkamp and associates[22] reported on a patient in whom QT prolongation and new changes in T wave morphology developed after catheter ablation of AV reentrant tachycardia. Two days after ablation, sotalol therapy was started before torsades de pointes developed. Of note, before ablation, the patient had tolerated oral sotalol for many years. Abnormal drug-related response of repolarization also may become more apparent during episodes of bradycardia, owing to reverse use-dependent effects of I_{Kr} blockers. This explains that torsades de pointes tend to occur not during atrial fibrillation but after conversion of atrial fibrillation to sinus rhythm when sinus rhythm is slow.

Sodium Channel Blocker–Related Toxicity

Antiarrhythmic drugs are the most common precipitants, although other agents (e.g., antidepressants, cocaine) may produce some of their toxic effects through their sodium channel–blocking properties. Sodium channel–blocking drugs with slower rates of dissociation from the sodium channel (e.g., flecainide, propafenone, quinidine) tend to generate these adverse effects more commonly. These drugs tend to prolong QRS duration even at normal heart rates because of the slow dissociation rate. The drug dose does not have to be toxic but must be large enough to slow conduction velocity.

In contrast with the occurrence of torsades de pointes, which is promoted by a slow heart rate, induction of a ventricular tachycardia by a class IC drug is promoted by a fast heart rate. In the CAST study,[2] the mortality rate was higher among patients receiving flecainide for frequent ventricular ectopy after a myocardial infarction than among patients receiving placebo. Subgroup analyses of CAST data suggest that the lack of beta-blocker therapy (which avoids high rates) was accompanied by a higher mortality. Among patients in whom the index myocardial infarction was a non–Q wave event and who therefore have a very high incidence of recurrent ischemia, an 8.7-fold increase in mortality was observed, as compared with a 1.7-fold increase in patients with transmural infarctions. On the basis of CAST findings,[2] class I antiarrhythmic drugs are contraindicated in patients with a history of previous myocardial infarction. Sodium channel blockers also may "convert" atrial fibrillation to slow atrial flutter, which can show 1:1 AV conduction with wide QRS complexes. This drug-induced arrhythmia can be confused with a ventricular tachycardia. Thus, when used for atrial fibrillation, an AV node–blocking drug has to be coadministered with a sodium channel blocker to prevent rapid ventricular rates in case atrial flutter occurs.

In some patients receiving sodium channel–blocking drugs (particularly flecainide and propafenone), a slow, incessant ventricular tachycardia may develop that occasionally may be resistant to cardioversion[1] (Fig. 74-2). These tachyarrhythmias may be hemodynamically tolerated owing to the slow heart rate but also may degenerate into a hemodynamically significant ventricular tachycardia or fibrillation that can be lethal.[1] They usually are observed with high or toxic doses of the drug or in the setting of other pathophysiologic conditions that exaggerate the effects of the drug on conduction (e.g., acidosis, hyperkalemia, concomitant sodium channel blockade) but also may occur with tricyclic antidepressant overdose. In such instances, the antiarrhythmic drug should be immediately discontinued. Hypertonic saline or sodium bicarbonate may reverse the conduction slowing and terminate or accelerate the arrhythmia (see Fig. 74-2).[23] Rate slowing also may be beneficial, because the magnitude of conduction slowing is less at slower heart rates.

Acquired Brugada Syndrome

A prominent transient outward current (I_{to})-mediated action potential notch and a subsequent loss of action potential dome in the right ventricular outflow tract epicardium, but not in the endocardium, give rise to a transmural voltage gradient, resulting in ST segment elevation in surface ECG leads V_1 to V_3 and the possible induction of subsequent ventricular tachycardia through the mechanism of phase 2 reentry. Because the maintenance of the action potential dome is determined by the balance of currents active at the end of phase 1 of the action potential, any intervention that increases outward currents (e.g., I_{to}, adenosine triphosphate–sensitive potassium current [I_{KATP}], I_{Kr}, I_{Ks}) or decreases inward currents (e.g., $I_{Ca,L}$, I_{Na}) at the end of phase 1 of the action potential can accentuate or unmask ST segment elevation similar to that found in Brugada syndrome. A number of drugs and conditions that cause an outward shift in current active at the end of

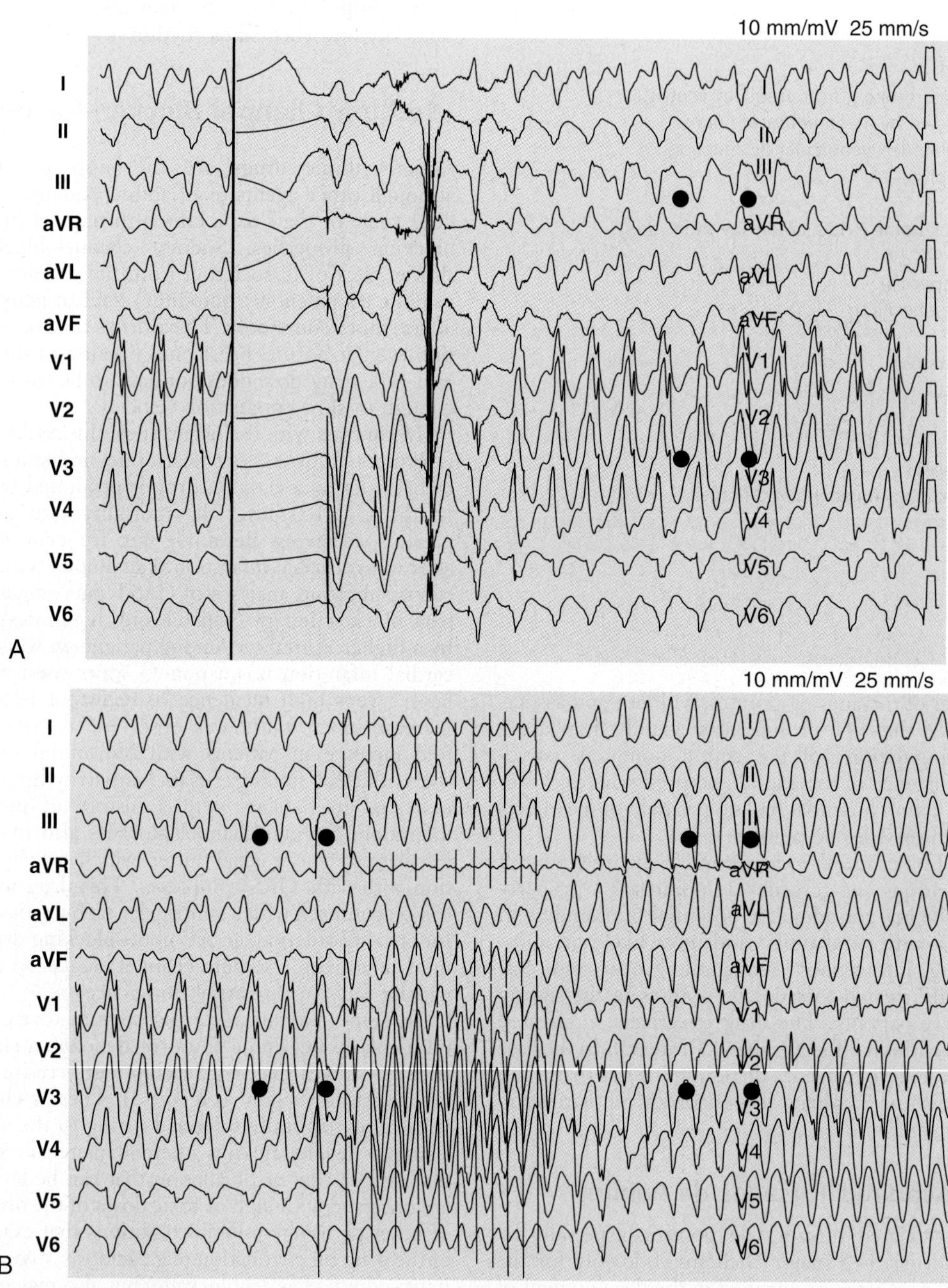

Figure 74-2 **A,** Hemodynamically stable, incessant monomorphic ventricular tachycardia (VT) in a 61-year-old man with a history of an inferior myocardial infarction 12 years earlier. Because of a recurrent monomorphic ventricular tachycardia, an implantable cardioverter-defibrillator (ICD) had been implanted 10 months previously, and amiodarone therapy was started (loading dose of 1 g/day for 10 days, then 400 mg for 8 weeks, followed by 200 mg daily). Five days before onset of the incessant VT, a cluster of ventricular tachycardias occurred; an additional 5 g of amiodarone was given, and continuous ajmaline infusion was started because of numerous recurrent VT episodes. Thereafter, the incessant VT (**A**) began. The VT immediately recurred after cardioversion or overdrive pacing (**B**).

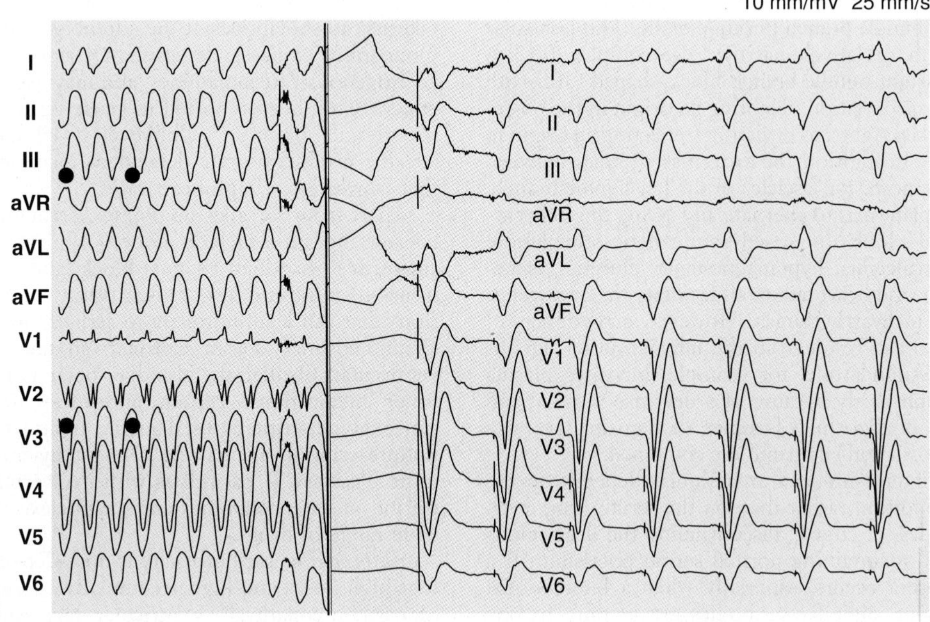

Figure 74-2 cont'd After administration of 10 mL of sodium chloride (20%), overdrive pacing converted the incessant VT into a different rapid, hemodynamically not tolerated VT, which was successfully converted into a stable sinus rhythm (**C**). Sodium chloride was given to overcome sodium channel blockade (see text for details).

phase 1 have been reported to induce transient Brugada-like ST segment elevation. Whether this "acquired" form of the Brugada syndrome unmasks clinically inapparent Brugada syndrome (*forme fruste*) or merely represents one end of a broad spectrum of responses to sodium channel–blocking drugs is not known. In a majority of reported cases of acquired Brugada syndrome, however, the characteristic type I Brugada ECG pattern disappeared after withdrawal of the drugs and could not be reproduced with subsequent flecainide testing in these patients.

Among antiarrhythmic drugs, class IC drugs most effectively amplify or unmask ST segment elevation secondary to their strong effect to block I_{Na}, and are therefore used as a diagnostic tool in Brugada patients with transient ECG abnormalities. Among the class IC drugs, pilsicainide, a pure class IC drug developed in Japan, is thought to more strongly induce ST segment elevation than flecainide. Class IA antiarrhythmic drugs (e.g., ajmaline, procainamide, disopyramide, cibenzoline), which exhibit less use-dependent blocking of I_{Na} owing to faster dissociation of the drug from the sodium channels, show weaker ST segment elevation than that caused by class IC drugs.[4] Of note, quinidine, another class IA drug, generally normalizes ST segment elevation, owing to its relatively strong I_{to}-blocking effect, and has been proposed for pharmacologic treatment of Brugada syndrome.

Several psychotropic drugs, including tricyclic antidepressants (e.g., amitryptyline, nortriptyline, despramine, clomipramine), tetracyclic antidepressants (e.g., maprotiline), phenothiazine (e.g., cyamemazine), and selective serotonin reuptake inhibitors (e.g., fluoxetine) have been reported to unmask Brugada-like ST segment elevation, secondary to block of fast I_{Na} associated with overdoses of these drugs. It has been postulated that this could be an important mechanism for drug-related sudden cardiac death in patients on chronic treatment with antidepressants and neuroleptics. One study of intoxication with tricyclic antidepressants (defined by plasma concentration greater than 1 μm/L) in a series of consecutive patients reported a Brugada electrocardiographic pattern in 15 of 98 cases (15.3%).[24] The mortality rate was slightly higher at 6.7% among patients with the Brugada ECG pattern, compared with 2.4% among patients without it, but the difference did not reach statistical significance.[24] Of note, the ECG pattern disappeared when plasma concentrations of tricyclic antidepressants were less than 1 μm/L. Cocaine intoxication (see later on) also has been reported to unmask the characteristic Brugada ECG pattern.[25] In addition, a number of case reports have demonstrated that fever (hyperthermia) can unmask Brugada-like ST segment elevation and provoke ventricular fibrillation as a result of reduced I_{Na} at high temperature.

Digitalis Toxicity

Digitalis has a very narrow therapeutic window, and the mortality associated with unrecognized digitalis intoxication is high and often unacknowledged. Digitalis inhibits the Na^+,K^+-ATPase, thereby interfering with the sodium pump; as a consequence, Na^+ accumulates within the cell, which in turn alters the Na^+-Ca^{2+} exchange. The result is an increase in Ca^{2+} concentration within the cell, which explains the positive inotropic effect of the drug. To reduce calcium transient, an electrogenic Na^+-Ca^{2+} exchange occurs. This Na^+-Ca^{2+} exchange may mediate delayed afterdepolarizations resulting in triggered activity. The latter may cause the characteristic tachycardias. Many factors determine whether a given blood level of digitalis is actually toxic and causes arrhythmias. Therefore, the serum concentrations should not be used as the only determinant for evaluating toxicity. The ECG and gastrointestinal (e.g., nausea, abdominal pain), visual (changes in color vision, reduced vision secondary to diminished accommodation), neuropsychiatric (hallucinations, nightmares, depression), and muscular (fatigue, weakness) complaints are clues to the detection of digitalis toxicity. Because of these unspecific symptoms in patients with digitalis intoxication, it is essential that ECG findings suggestive of intoxication be recognized early.

The arrhythmias of digitalis intoxication are the result of (1) a block in conduction, which may be located in the sinus or AV node, or (2) rapid impulse formation in the atrium, AV junction, and ventricular Purkinje system. In addition, severe overdose of digitalis may cause hyperkalemia and cardiac standstill. In case of abnormal impulse formation, the site of origin in the ventricle usually is located in bundle branch Purkinje tissue. This fascicular tachycardia results in a relatively narrow QRS complex (0.12 to 0.14 second) and a right bundle branch block–shaped QRS with either marked left axis deviation (denoting an origin in the posterior fascicle) or marked right axis deviation (reflecting an origin in the anterior fascicle). In addition, the focus may alternate between the anterior and the posterior fascicles of the left bundle branch, causing the frontal plane axis to alternate and giving the tachycardia a "bidirectional" look. Increased sympathetic stimulation, hypokalemia, hypercalcemia, hypomagnesemia, diuretics, ischemia and reperfusion, and heart failure all facilitate the occurrence of digitalis-related tachyarrhythmias. However, arrhythmias of digitalis toxicity also can result from the interaction of digitalis with other drugs. Amiodarone, for example, increases plasma digoxin concentration partly because of a decrease in renal and nonrenal clearance of digoxin. Clearance of digoxin dose also decreases when digoxin and verapamil are combined.

Treatment of digitalis-induced arrhythmias depends on the patient's clinical condition rather than on the serum drug level. Management includes, of course, discontinuing the drug, monitoring rhythm, and maintaining normal serum potassium. If a ventricular tachycardia occurs, especially when a bidirectional tachycardia is present, digitalis antibodies are helpful. In one series of 150 severely intoxicated patients, response was rapid (30 minutes to 4 hours). Approximately one half of the patients presenting with a cardiac arrest survived hospitalization.[26] Side effects included worsening of the underlying disease (increased ventricular rate during atrial fibrillation, exacerbation of heart failure) and hypokalemia. Digoxin concentration monitoring is unreliable after administration of antidigoxin antibody. Lidocaine and phenytoin were used in the past but have almost no role today with the available digitalis antibodies.

Other Drug-Induced Toxicity

Cocaine has both QT-prolonging (I_{Kr}-blocking) and slow-offset sodium channel–blocking properties.[27] It is a local anesthetic with potent sympathetic stimulatory effect. It blocks the reuptake of catecholamines at the adrenergic nerve endings, inhibits monoamine oxidases, desensitizes peripheral organs to the effect of exogenous catecholamines, and may exert a direct cardiotoxic effect. It has been reported to cause ventricular fibrillation and torsades de pointes.[27] Unlike class III antiarrhythmic drugs, cocaine produces a rate-dependent increase in the QT interval that is greatest at high heart rates.

Apart from torsades de pointes, arrhythmias associated with cocaine ingestion include monomorphic ventricular tachycardia suggestive of sodium channel block (and responding to sodium infusion). Cocaine also causes other cardiovascular complications that can lead indirectly to arrhythmias, notably myocarditis, and coronary spasm. Coronary spasm, which can manifest as ventricular fibrillation, also has been reported with multiple other medications: certain anticancer drugs (5-fluorouracil, capecitabine, triptans used in the treatment of migraines, and nonprescription agents (e.g., 3,4-methylenedioxymethamphetamine ["ecstasy"]), as well as with inadvertent vascular administration of catecholamines and anaphylaxis due to any one of a wide range of drugs.

Anthracycline cardiotoxicity is dose-dependent, with intermittent high doses and higher cumulative doses increasing the risk of cardiomyopathy.[28] Ventricular tachycardia and fibrillation may arise secondary to the underlying structural heart disease. This form of cardiomyopathy can occur acutely soon after treatment, within a few months of treatment (as the subacute form), or many years later. Long-term intermittent cardiac assessment of patients is therefore necessary, and cardiac decompensation should be treated conventionally. Experimental data showed that even at an early stage of anthracycline-induced cardiomyopathy, repolarization reserve is reduced.[29]

5-Fluorouracil can cause potentially fatal arrhythmias irrespective of underlying coronary disease during the acute infusion period. Onset of symptoms, with or without corresponding ECG changes demonstrating cardiac ischemia, dictates immediate discontinuation of the drug. Although this cardiotoxicity is reversible, 5-fluorouracil sensitizes the patient to such effects and should be avoided in the future if possible.

References

1. Zipes DP, Camm AJ, Borggrefe M, et al: ACC/AHA/ESC 2006 Guidelines for Management of Patients with Ventricular Arrhythmias and the Prevention of Sudden Cardiac Death: A report of the American College of Cardiology/American Heart Association Task Force and the European Society of Cardiology Committee for Practice Guidelines (Writing Committee to Develop Guidelines for Management of Patients with Ventricular Arrhythmias and the Prevention of Sudden Cardiac Death). Eur Heart J 27:2099-2144, 2006.
2. Preliminary report: Effect of encainide and flecainide on mortality in a randomized trial of arrhythmia suppression after myocardial infarction. The Cardiac Arrhythmia Suppression Trial (CAST) Investigators. N Engl J Med 321:406-412, 1989.
3. Schulze-Bahr E, Eckardt L, Breithardt G, et al: Sodium channel gene (*SCN5A*) mutations in 44 index patients with Brugada syndrome: Different incidences in familial and sporadic disease. Hum Mutat 21:651-652, 2003.
4. Rolf S, Bruns HJ, Wichter T, et al: The ajmaline challenge in Brugada syndrome: Diagnostic impact, safety, and recommended protocol. Eur Heart J 24:1104-1112, 2003.
5. Splawski I, Timothy KW, Tateyama M, et al: Variant of *SCN5A* sodium channel implicated in risk of cardiac arrhythmia. Science 297:1333-1336, 2002.
6. Haverkamp W, Breithardt G, Camm AJ, et al: The potential for QT prolongation and pro-arrhythmia by non-anti-arrhythmic drugs: Clinical and regulatory implications. Report on a Policy Conference of the European Society of Cardiology. Cardiovasc Res 47:219-233, 2000.
7. De Ponti F, Poluzzi E, Montanaro N, Ferguson J: QTc and psychotropic drugs. Lancet 356:75-76, 2000.
8. Milberg P, Eckardt L, Bruns HJ, et al: Divergent proarrhythmic potential of macrolide antibiotics despite similar QT prolongation: Fast phase 3 repolarization prevents early afterdepolarizations and torsade de pointes. J Pharmacol Exp Ther 303:218-225, 2002.
9. Haverkamp W, Eckardt L, Mönnig G, et al: Clinical aspects of ventricular arrhythmias associated with QT prolongation. Eur Heart J 3:K81-K88, 2001.
10. Roden DM: Taking the "idio" out of "idiosyncratic": Predicting torsades de pointes. Pacing Clin Electrophysiol 21:1029-1034, 1998.
11. Kääb S, Hinterseer M, Näbauer M, Steinbeck G: Sotalol testing unmasks altered repolarization in patients with suspected acquired long-QT-syndrome—a case-control pilot study using i.v. sotalol. Eur Heart J 24:649-657, 2003.
12. Torp-Pedersen C, Moller M, Bloch-Thomsen PE, et al: Dofetilide in patients with congestive heart failure and left ventricular dysfunction. Danish Investigations of Arrhythmia and Mortality on Dofetilide Study Group. N Engl J Med 341:857-865, 1999.
13. Eckardt L, Haverkamp W, Borggrefe M, Breithardt G: Experimental models of torsade de pointes. Cardiovasc Res 39:178-193, 1998.
14. El-Sherif N, Chinushi M, Caref EB, Restivo M: Electrophysiological mechanism of the characteristic electrocardiographic morphology of torsade de pointes tachyarrhythmias in the long-QT syndrome: Detailed analysis of ventricular

tridimensional activation patterns. Circulation 96:4392-4399, 1997.
15. Milberg P, Hilker E, Ramtin S, et al: Proarrhythmia as a class effect of quinolones: Increased dispersion of repolarization and triangulation of action potential predict torsades de pointes. J Cardiovasc Electrophysiol 18:647-654, 2007.
16. Milberg P, Reinsch N, Osada N, et al: Verapamil prevents torsade de pointes by reduction of transmural dispersion of repolarization and suppression of early afterdepolarizations in an intact heart model of LQT3. Basic Res Cardiol 100:365-371, 2005.
17. Fetsch T, Bauer P, Engberding R, et al: Prevention of atrial fibrillation after cardioversion: Results of the PAFAC trial. Eur Heart J 25:1385-1394, 2004.
18. Cosio FG, Goicolea A, Lopez GM, et al: Suppression of torsades de pointes with verapamil in patients with atrioventricular block. Eur Heart J 12:635-638, 1991.
19. Milberg P, Ramtin S, Mönnig G, et al: Comparison of the in vitro electrophysiologic and proarrhythmic effects of amiodarone and sotalol in a rabbit model of acute atrioventricular block. J Cardiovasc Pharmacol 44:278-286, 2004.
20. Gupta A, Lawrence AT, Krishnan K, et al: Current concepts in the mechanisms and management of drug-induced QT prolongation and torsade de pointes. Am Heart J 153:891-899, 2007.
21. Milberg P, Reinsch N, Wasmer K, et al: Transmural dispersion of repolarization as a key factor of arrhythmogenicity in a novel intact heart model of LQT3. Cardiovasc Res 65:397-404, 2005.
22. Haverkamp W, Hördt M, Breithardt G, Borggrefe M: Torsade de pointes secondary to D,L-sotalol after catheter ablation of incessant atrioventricular reentrant tachycardia—evidence for a significant contribution of the "cardiac memory". Clin Cardiol 21:55-58, 1998.
23. Winkelmann BR, Leinberger H: Life-threatening flecainide toxicity. A pharmacodynamic approach. Ann Intern Med 106:807-814, 1987.
24. Goldgran-Toledano D, Sideris G, Kevorkian JP: Overdose of cyclic antidepressants and the Brugada syndrome. N Engl J Med 346:1591-1592, 2002.
25. Bebarta VS, Summers S: Brugada electrocardiographic pattern induced by cocaine toxicity. Ann Emerg Med 49:827-829, 2007.
26. Antman EM, Wenger TL, Butler VP Jr, et al: Treatment of 150 cases of life-threatening digitalis intoxication with digoxin-specific Fab antibody fragments. Final report of a multicenter study. Circulation 81:1744-1752, 1990.
27. Karch SB: Cocaine cardiovascular toxicity. South Med J 98:794-799, 2005.
28. Appel JM, Nielsen D, Zerahn B, et al: Anthracycline-induced chronic cardiotoxicity and heart failure. Acta Oncol 46:576-580, 2007.
29. Milberg P, Fleischer D, Stypmann J, et al: Reduced repolarization reserve due to anthracycline therapy facilitates torsade de pointes induced by I_{Kr} blockers. Basic Res Cardiol 102:42-51, 2007.

Progressive Cardiac Conduction Disease 75

ARGELIA MEDEIROS-DOMINGO AND MICHAEL J. ACKERMAN

CHAPTER OUTLINE

Cardiac conduction disease is a potentially life-threatening disorder characterized by alteration of impulse propagation through the cardiac conduction system. The pathophysiologic mechanisms underlying the disease are diverse, ranging from congenital to acquired, with or without structural heart disease[1-3] (Table 75-1). Community-based studies have shown that the prevalence of cardiac conduction disease in the absence of heart disease approximates 0.75%.[3] Ventricular conduction blocks are associated with increased long-term cardiac morbidity and mortality risk, especially in the presence of left axis deviation,[1] and identifies a high-risk group of patients.

The main anatomic structures of the conduction system are the sinoatrial node, the atrioventricular (AV) node, and His-Purkinje fibers. These structures are responsible for establishing and maintaining the electrophysiologic activities in the heart. The most frequent form of cardiac conduction disease, *Lenègre-Lev disease*, exhibits a progressive deterioration of the cardiac conduction through the His-Purkinje system with right or left ventricular block, leading to complete AV block (Fig. 75-1), often culminating in syncope and sudden death. Lenègre-Lev disease, otherwise known as *progressive cardiac conduction disease* (PCCD), is considered to be a primary degenerative disease, an exaggerated aging process selectively affecting the conduction tissue, and constitutes a major indication for pacemaker implantation worldwide. Lenègre and Lev combined clinical observations, electrocardiogram (ECG) recordings, and detailed postmortem examination findings and proved the direct relationship of these two entities in the 1960s. Thus, Lenègre-Lev disease and PCCD should be viewed as referring to the same pathobiologic entity.

The first PCCD chromosomal locus was described in 1995 as 19q13.2-13.3.[4] However, the first PCCD susceptibility gene, reported in 1999,[5] was derived from a familial form of PCCD linked to chromosome 3 near the *SCN5A*-encoded cardiac sodium channel. Two different *SCN5A* mutations that cosegregated with the disease were identified; the affected members had variable expressivity of the conduction abnormalities, right bundle branch block, left bundle branch block, or AV block, and their conduction defects increased in severity with age. Supporting this discovery, the *SCN5A*-knockout model showed that the homozygous state (i.e., affecting $SCN5A^{-/-}$ mice in utero) was lethal, whereas heterozygous, $SCN5A^{+/-}$ mice exhibited normal survival and age-related lengthening of the P wave and PR and QRS interval duration, coinciding with previous observations in patients with PCCD,[6] establishing the first model for hereditary Lenègre-Lev disease due to *SCN5A* mutations. Of note, the PCCD susceptibility gene from the original chromosome 19 PCCD locus remains unknown.

Developments in molecular biology and genetics have increased the current understanding of the mechanisms of inherited cardiac conduction abnormalities. It is now known that these familial primary electrical diseases of the heart that occur in the absence of structural heart disease or systemic disease result from mutations in cardiac ion channels, whereas in the presence of structural heart disease, transcriptional factors, inborn errors of metabolism, and other structural proteins are involved. The discovery of gene mutations that are causally involved in inherited cardiac conduction disease is relatively recent. This chapter focuses on the molecular advances surrounding PCCD.

Genetic Basis of Progressive Cardiac Conduction Disease

Progressive Cardiac Conduction Disease without Structural Heart Disease

Cardiac Sodium Channel Gene *SCN5A*

SCN5A remains the principal ion channel gene associated with familial PCCD. *SCN5A* encodes the voltage-dependent sodium channel α subunit protein hNav1.5[7] and is expressed predominantly in human heart muscle, as well as in the intestinal tract. This channel is responsible for the large peak inward sodium current (I_{Na}) that underlies excitability and conduction in working myocardium (atrial and ventricular cells) and special conduction tissue (Purkinje cells and others), and also for late I_{Na}, which influences repolarization and refractoriness. Mutations that *decrease* peak I_{Na} (i.e., loss of function) (Fig. 75-2) cause several arrhythmogenic syndromes including PCCD,[5,8] type I Brugada syndrome,[9] congenital sick sinus syndrome (SSS),[10] and, more rarely, ventricular tachycardia[11-14] and dilated cardiomyopathy (DCM).[15] By contrast, mutations in *SCN5A* that *increase* late I_{Na} (i.e., gain of function) cause long QT syndrome type 3 (LQT3).[16] Of interest, these phenotypes often coexist[11,17-20] (Fig. 75-3).

Brugada syndrome type I is characterized by an ST segment elevation in the right precordial leads of the electrocardiogram and high incidence of sudden cardiac death; loss-of-function mutations in the *SCN5A* gene account for approximately 20% to 30% of cases of Brugada syndrome. An important overlap between Lenègre-Lev disease and Brugada syndrome type I has been reported[21,22]: Patients diagnosed with the latter disorder have a high incidence of bradyarrhythmias and conduction defects.[23,24] In fact, the most common phenotype among gene carriers of Brugada syndrome type I–associated *SCN5A* mutations is PCCD.[25]

Moreover, a single loss-of-function mutation in *SCN5A* may result in either a Brugada syndrome phenotype or Lenègre-Lev

Table 75-1 Summary of Progressive Cardiac Conduction Defect (PCCD) Susceptibility Genes

Gene	Protein	Rhythm and/or Conduction Disorder	Structural Heart Disease	Other Organ Involvement	Disease(s)/Syndrome(s)
CACNA1C	$Ca_V1.2$, L-type calcium channel	AVB	Patent ductus arteriosus, patent foramen ovale, ventricular septal defects, tetralogy of Fallot	Yes	Timothy syndrome
GJAS	Connexins	BBB, AF	Unknown	Yes	Atrial standstill
DAMPK	Serine-threonine protein kinase	BBB, AVB	HCM, DCM, mitral valve prolapse	Yes	Myotonic dystrophy 1
HCN4	Pacemaker I_f channel	SSS	No	No	SSS
KCNH2	I_{Kr}	AVB	No	No	LQT2, SQT1
KCNJ2	Kir2.1 channel	BBB, AVB, polymorphic VT	Bicuspid aortic valve, aorta coarctation, pulmonary valve stenosis	Yes	Andersen-Tawil syndrome, SQT3, CPVT
LAMP2	Lysosomal-associated membrane protein 2	BBB, AVB, WPW	Glycogen storage disease HCM/DCM	Yes	Danon disease
LMNA	Lamin A/C	BBB, SSS, AVB	DCM	Yes	Emery-Dreifuss and limb-girdle muscular dystrophy, Werner's syndrome, Charcot-Marie-Tooth syndrome type 2
NKX2.5	Homeobox transcription factor	AVB	Atrial septal defect, tetralogy of Fallot	No	Atrial septal defect, tetralogy of Fallot
PRKAG2	AMPK γ2 subunit	BBB, AVB, WPW	Glycogen storage disease HCM/DCM	Yes	Glycogen storage disease
*SCN5A**	$Na_V1.5$ channel	BBB, SSS, AVB, VT	Rare, DCM	No	LQT3, Brugada syndrome type I, PCCD
TBX5	T-box transcription factor	AVB	Atrial septal defect	Yes	Holt-Oram syndrome

AVB, atrioventricular block; AF, atrial fibrillation; BBB, bundle branch block; CPVT, catecholaminergic polymorphic ventricular tachycardia; DCM, dilated cardiomyopathy; HCM, hypertrophic cardiomyopathy; LQT2, long QT syndrome variant 2; SQT1, SQT3, short QT syndrome variants 1 and 3; SSS, sick sinus syndrome; VT, ventricular tachycardia; WPW, Wolff-Parkinson-White.

*Denotes the first-identified PCCD susceptibility gene, still the most common one.

disease,[26] depending on the familial branch.[22,27] Nevertheless, despite the overlap, PCCD and Brugada syndrome remain distinct clinical entities with differences in arrhythmic phenotype and in predisposition for sudden cardiac arrest. Indeed, patients with PCCD generally do not exhibit ventricular fibrillation in response to programmed electrical stimulation.[8,25]

Incomplete penetrance and variable expressivity of the disease are the norm in PCCD[11,27,28] (Fig. 75-4). *Penetrance* is an index referring to the percentage of genotype-positive subjects manifesting the characteristic electrocardiographic phenotype. In the case of PCCD and *SCN5A*, a penetrance of 40% indicates that 40% of mutation-positive subjects would have an abnormal electrocardiogram. *Expressivity* refers to the range of signs and symptoms displayed among genotype-positive subjects. Variable expressivity could stem partly from several *SCN5A* polymorphisms known to exert a modulatory effect on the phenotype. For example, the common polymorphism H558R *SCN5A* restores the trafficking defect of a Brugada syndrome type I mutation,[29,30] the polymorphism R1193Q *SCN5A* mitigates the adverse effect conferred by the nonsense mutation W1421X SCN5A,[31] and the expression of several common *SCN5A* polymorphisms, in different $Na_V1.5$ splice variants

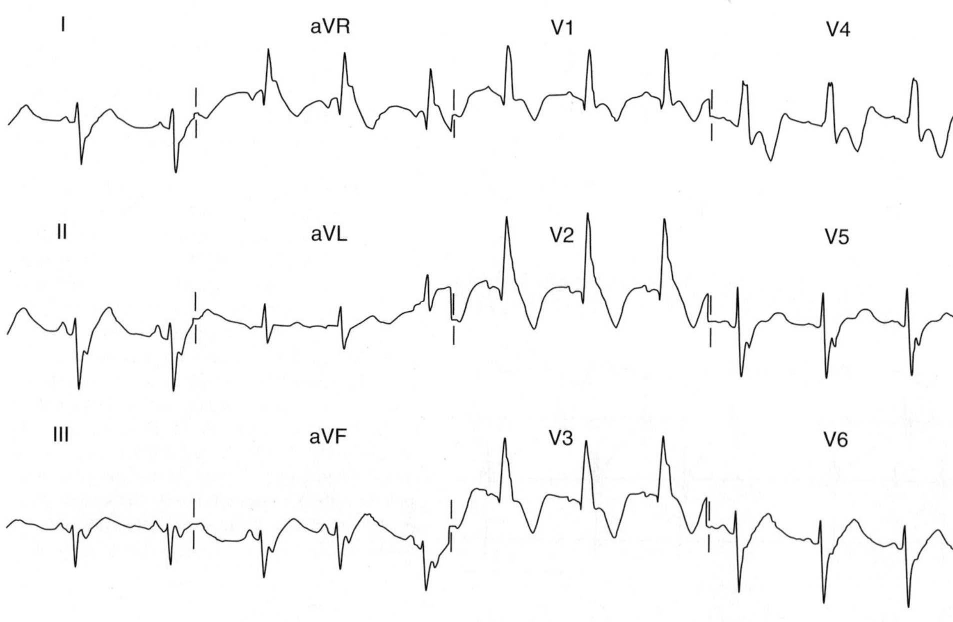

Figure 75-1 A 12-lead electrocardiogram from a patient with *SCN5A*-mediated progressive cardiac conduction disease.

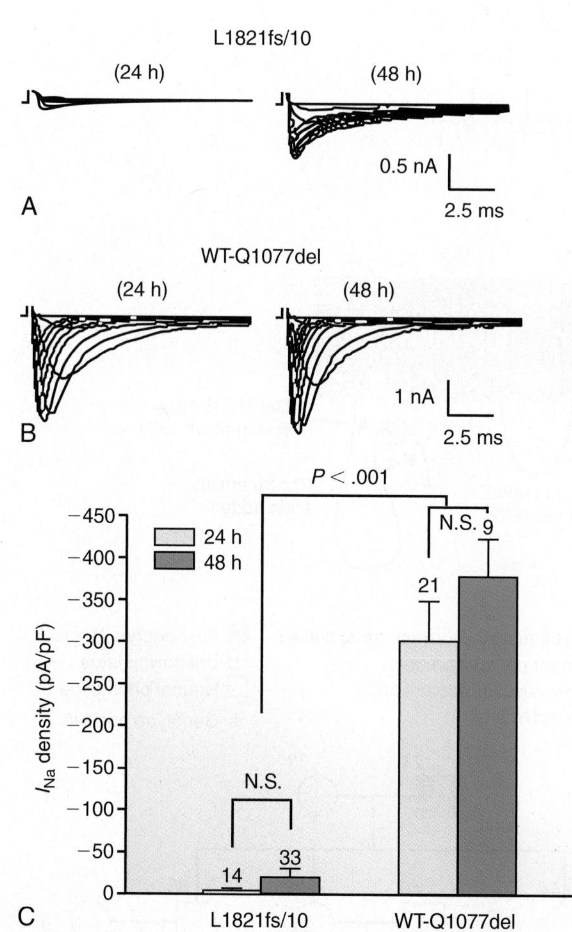

Figure 75-2 Current expression of mutant L1821fs/10 and WT in the most common splice variant *SCN5A* Q1077del background. **A** and **B**, Whole-cell current traces from representative experiments with L1821fs/10 (**A**) and WT (**B**) after 24-hour *(left)* and 48-hour *(right)* transfection. **C**, Summary of I_{Na} density in L1821fs/10 and WT after 24 hours and 48 hours of incubation, respectively. The number of experiments is indicated above the *bars*. N.S., no significant difference. (**A** to **C**, From Tan BH, Iturralde-Torres P, Medeiros-Domingo A, et al: A novel C-terminal truncation *SCN5A* mutation from a patient with sick sinus syndrome, conduction disorder and ventricular tachycardia. Cardiovasc Res 76:409-417, 2007.)

(Q1077 and Q1077del), radically modifies the sodium current density.[32-34] In vitro studies have suggested that a rightward shift in the voltage dependence of the mutant sodium channel activation curve is a common feature for *SCN5A*-mediated PCCD.[8,22]

After the initial description of *SCN5A* as a PCCD susceptibility gene, more than 30 additional mutations have been described (Fig. 75-5; Table 75-2). Seven of these 30 mutations (23%) lead to early protein truncation, whereas mis-sense mutations have shown a preferential distribution among domains I, III, and IV (DI, DII, and DIV). A majority of *SCN5A*-mediated PCCD cases exhibit a mixed phenotype. When the associated phenotype is long QT syndrome, the QRS interval usually is narrow and the conduction defect commonly is intermittent 2:1 AV block.[35-41] Intermittent functional 2:1 AV block in the setting of long QT syndrome has an incidence of 4% to 5% in pediatric series, usually is an isolated disorder, and has been associated with a high mortality rate (greater than 50%) regardless of the treatment.[42] Symptoms may appear at a very young age; neonatal paroxysmal bradycardia and hydrops fetalis are common findings. The phenomenon occurs in the setting of a very long, rate-dependent effective refractory period. Despite a very narrow QRS complex, infra-Hisian block location has been documented. Some of these LQT3 mutations in association with AV block have displayed different kinetics of fast inactivation, reduction in sodium current density, and enhancement of slower forms of inactivation.[35,42]

Mutations in Other Ion Channels

Other dysfunctional ion channels can express a cardiac conduction disease phenotype. Mutations in the *KCNH2*-encoded I_{Kr} channel cause long QT syndrome type 2 (LQT2), and occasionally, patients with LQT2 exhibit AV conduction impairment.[43] Indeed, approximately 17% of patients with complete AV block and long QT syndrome are LQT2 genotype–positive.[44] Mutations in the *CACNA1*-encoded L-type calcium channel cause Timothy syndrome, characterized by multiorgan dysfunction including QT interval prolongation and 2:1 AV block.[45] Mutations in the *KCNJ2*-encoded Kir2.1 inward rectifier potassium channel are responsible for polymorphic ventricular tachycardia and Andersen-Tawil syndrome[46]; patients often display

I
aVR
V1
V4
II
aVL
V2
V5
III
aVF
V3
V6
A
B
II
C
II
D
V1
RA
HBE
RV
1 s
E
V1
RA
RV
1 s
F

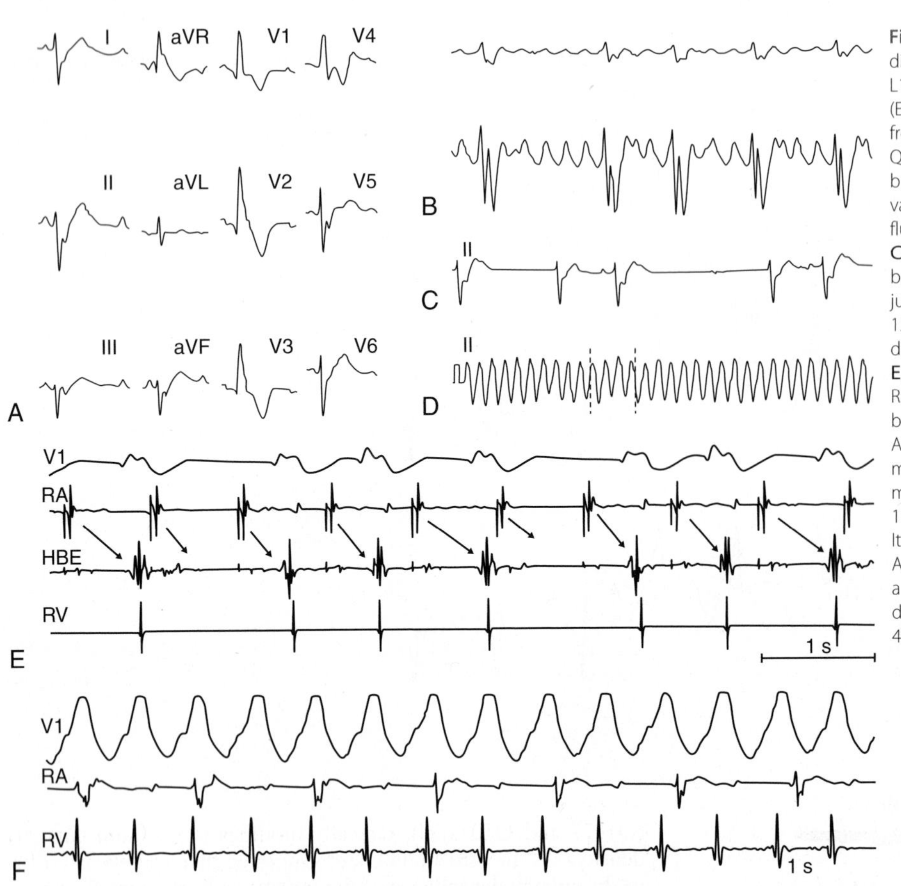

Figure 75-3 Example of mixed cardiac conduction disease phenotype conferred by a single mutation, L1821fs/10. **A,** A 12-lead surface electrocardiogram (ECG) (10 mm/mV, 25 mm/s, 71 beats per minute) from proband at 1 year of age showing a prolonged QRS duration (160 ms) with a typical right bundle branch block configuration and a prolonged QT interval. **B,** The 24-hour Holter monitor trace shows atrial flutter with 3:1 to 6:1 atrioventricular (AV) conduction. **C,** Lead II ECG (10 mm/mV, 25 mm/s) shows sinus bradycardia and sinus pause up to 3.72 seconds and junctional escapes. **D,** Lead II ECG (5 mm/mV, 12.5 mm/s) shows monomorphic ventricular tachycardia with a heart rate of 200 beats per minute. **E,** Intracardiac ECG (electrograms: V_1, V_1 surface lead; RA, RV, right atrium and right ventricular; HBE, His bundle) shows a second-degree AV block with 4:3 AV conduction during atrial pacing at 80 beats per minute. **F,** Intracardiac ECG shows an induced monomorphic ventricular tachycardia with a heart rate of 171 beats per minute. (**A** to **F,** From Tan BH, Iturralde-Torres P, Medeiros-Domingo A, et al: A novel C-terminal truncation *SCN5A* mutation from a patient with sick sinus syndrome, conduction disorder and ventricular tachycardia. Cardiovasc Res 76: 409-417, 2007.)

DI
DII
DIII
DIV
S1 S2 S3 S4 S5 S6
S1 S2 S3 S4 S5 S6
S1 S2 S3 S4 S5 S6
S1 S2 S3 S4 S5 S6
Del TCTG after
codon at no. 1821
10 new amino
acids added
Stop codon
at no. 1832
N1
A
L1821fs/10
CGATGCCCTGNNNNACNCANTNTNNN
TCTG deletion
B
SSS (bradycardia, sinus arrest, atrial flutter)
Intraventricular conduction delay
Abnormal ventricular repolarization
Ventricular tachycardia
Bradycardia
First-degree AV block
Unknown status
Normal phenotype
+ Genotype positive
74
73
I
44
40
38
35
II
17
16
13
12
10
8
4
1
III
Proband
C

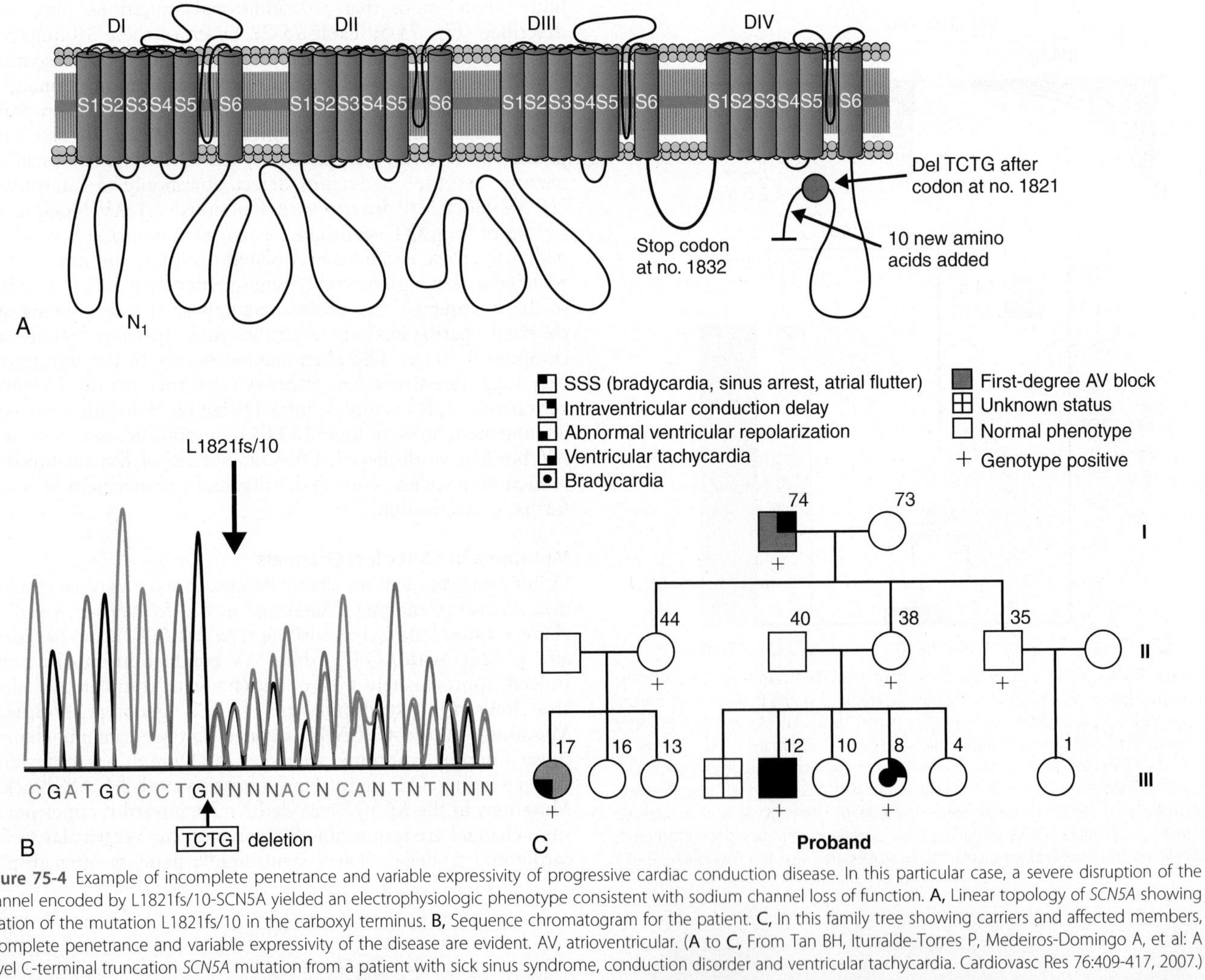

Figure 75-4 Example of incomplete penetrance and variable expressivity of progressive cardiac conduction disease. In this particular case, a severe disruption of the channel encoded by L1821fs/10-SCN5A yielded an electrophysiologic phenotype consistent with sodium channel loss of function. **A,** Linear topology of *SCN5A* showing location of the mutation L1821fs/10 in the carboxyl terminus. **B,** Sequence chromatogram for the patient. **C,** In this family tree showing carriers and affected members, incomplete penetrance and variable expressivity of the disease are evident. AV, atrioventricular. (**A** to **C,** From Tan BH, Iturralde-Torres P, Medeiros-Domingo A, et al: A novel C-terminal truncation *SCN5A* mutation from a patient with sick sinus syndrome, conduction disorder and ventricular tachycardia. Cardiovasc Res 76:409-417, 2007.)

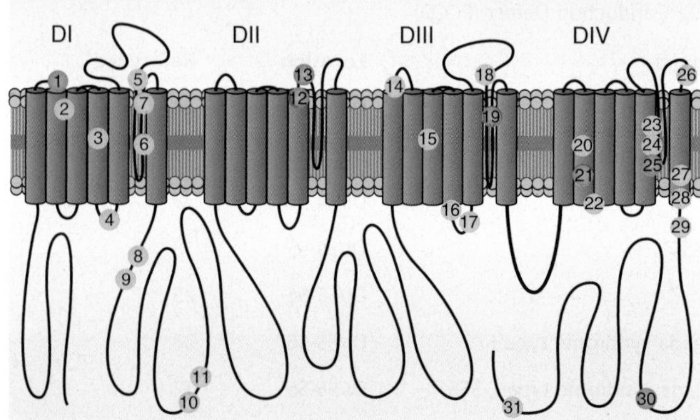

Figure 75-5 Linear channel topology of the $Na_V1.5$ encoded by *SCN5A*, with the approximate location of the pathogenic progressive cardiac conduction defect–associated *SCN5A* mutations indicated by domain (DI to DIV). *Numbers in circles* correspond to case numbers in Table 75-2. *Yellow circles* indicate mis-sense mutations; *orange circles* indicate mutations that produce a premature protein truncation.

diverse degrees of AV block and bundle branch block. The *HCN4*-encoded pacemaker current known as I_f has a key role in heart beat generation and is the major determinant of diastolic depolarization in sinus node. Mutations in *HCN4* have been associated with idiopathic sinus node dysfunction.[47]

Genetics of Cardiac Conduction Disease with Structural Heart Disease

Glycogen Storage Diseases and Cardiac Conduction Disease

The glycogen storage cardiomyopathy produced by *LAMP2* or *PRKAG2* mutations resembles hypertrophic cardiomyopathy but is distinguished by electrophysiologic abnormalities, particularly conduction disorders and ventricular preexcitation.[48]

Mutations in the *PRKAG2* gene, which encodes the regulatory γ subunit of AMP-activated protein kinase (AMPK), can give a cardiac hypertrophy phenotype[49,50] that often evolves into ventricular dilatation, associated with ventricular preexcitation or Wolff-Parkinson-White syndrome (WPW) and cardiac conduction disease. Cardiac conduction disturbances represent the major complication of *PRKAG2*-mutations and often necessitate pacemaker implantation.[51]

AMPK, a serine-threonine kinase, is a heterotrimeric complex consisting of a catalytic α subunit and two regulatory β and γ subunits. This enzyme is a key regulator of ATP levels. Activation of AMPK during acute low-energy states switches off ATP-consuming pathways and activates ATP-producing pathways, such as fatty acid oxidation and increased glucose uptake.[50] *PRKAG2* mutations lead to disequilibrium of the energetic balance. In fact, cardiomyocytes in transgenic models often exhibit vacuoles containing amylopectin, a glycogen-derived substance. The fibrous annulus of the heart can be disrupted by glycogen-filled myocytes, and these microscopic atrioventricular connections generate the ventricular preexcitation often observed in the disease. Conduction system degeneration is precipitated by affecting the phosphorylation state of several cardiac ion channels.[51]

Of interest, the phenotypes associated with *PRKAG2* mutations are diverse. Familial occurrence of right bundle branch block, sinus bradycardia, and short PR interval in absence of typical WPW or obvious structural heart disease was reported in two large families.[52] Patients with glycogen storage–associated cardiomyopathy generally have a poor prognosis owing to severe cardiac dysfunction and progressive conduction system degeneration. In terms of treatment, recent studies have shown that the glycogen storage cardiomyopathy and cardiac conduction system degeneration associated with *PRKAG2* mutation is reversible with lowering of the cardiac glycogen content by transgene regulation. Furthermore, the development of accessory electrical pathways can be prevented by inhibition of glycogen accumulation during early postnatal development.[50]

LAMP2 mutations produce Danon disease, a rare disorder inherited as an X-linked dominant trait and caused by lysosomal-associated membrane protein 2 (LAMP2) deficiency. Danon disease is characterized by either maladaptive hypertrophy or dilatation of the ventricular myocardium, cardiac conduction abnormalities, preexcitation, skeletal vacuolar myopathy, mental retardation of variable degree, and peripheral pigmentary retinopathy.[53-55] In affected females, isolated cardiomyopathy develops in adulthood, whereas males present with cardiomyopathy, myopathy, and mental retardation before the age of 20 years.[55] LAMP-2 is a highly *N*-glycosylated lysosomal membrane protein that functions in lysosomal enzyme targeting, chaperone-mediated autophagy, and lysosomal biogenesis. How a defect in this protein culminates in such a severe cardiomyopathic presentation remains unclear, but the outcome usually is fatal, and cardiac transplantation is the only effective therapeutic option.[56]

Connexins and Cardiac Conduction Disease

Connexins form intercellular conduits or gap junctions, permitting diffusion of ions and metabolites. To date, 20 different connexin genes have been identified.[57] The connexins Cx40, Cx43, and Cx45 are expressed in many different tissues but most abundantly in the heart, blood vessels, and nervous system. In heart, connexins coordinate electrical activation of the atria and ventricular conduction tissues, facilitate cell-to-cell adhesion, and provide pathways for direct intercellular communication, as connexins are the principal determinants of coupling and current conduction between adjacent myocytes. Cx45 is expressed in the AVN and proximal portion of the ventricular conduction system. Cx43 is expressed in atrial and ventricular myocardium. Replacement of Cx43 by Cx26 in transgenic mice produced slower ventricular conduction.[58] Cx40 is expressed mainly in the atrial myocardium and His-Purkinje system. Cx40-null mice have cardiac conduction abnormalities, with a very high incidence of cardiac malformations in heterozygous (18%) and homozygous (33%) animals.[59] Recently, two polymorphisms, located in the immediate upstream promoter region (−44 bp) and untranslated region (+71 bp) of the atrial Cx40 gene, causing a reduction in Cx40 gene expression in vitro have been identified in familial atrial standstill, and cardiac conduction disease[60] and somatic mutations in Cx40 predispose affected persons to idiopathic atrial fibrillation.[61]

Transcription Factors and Cardiac Conduction Disease

TBX5, *NKX2.5*, and *HF-1b* are transcription factor genes expressed broadly in the heart and support, in part, the maintenance of the conduction system.[62,63] Dominant mutations in these genes cause congenital heart defects and conduction system abnormalities, mainly AV block.[64,65] Mutations in *NKX2.5* have been found in families with secundum atrial septal defects (ASDs) and AV conduction block[66] and in some cases with tetralogy of Fallot. Nkx2.5 regulates connexin expression and the maintenance of normal cardiac conduction. Mutations in the transcription factor gene *TBX5* cause Holt-Oram syndrome, a disorder of autosomal dominant inheritance characterized by radial ray deformities of the upper limb

Table 75-2 Summary of *SCN5A* Mutations Associated with Progressive Cardiac Conduction Defect (PCCD)

Case No.*	Nucleotide Substitution	Variant	Phenotype(s)	Location	Reference
1	468 G>A	W156X	BBB, VT	DI/S1-S2	28
2	481 G>A	E161K	BBB, Brugada syndrome type I, SSS	DI/S2	19
3	672 C>T	R225W	BBB, VT	DI/S4	28
4	718 G>A	V240M	BBB, VT, SSS	DI/S4-S5	18
5	892 G>A	G298S	AVB	DI/S5-S6	35
6	1066 G>A	D356N	AVB, Brugada syndrome type I	DI/S5-S6	23
7	1127 G>A	R376H	BBB, Brugada syndrome type I, SSS	DI/S5-S6	17
8	1535 C>T	T512I	AVB	DI-DII	34
9	1541 G>T	G514C	BBB, SSS	DI-DII	8
10	1835 C>T	T612M	AVB, long QT syndrome	DI-DII	36
11	1855 C>T	L619F	AVB, long QT syndrome	DI-DII	41
12	2581-82 TTdel	F861fs/90	BBB, Brugada syndrome type I	DII/S5	21
13	2602 Cdel	L867X	BBB, Brugada syndrome type I	DII/S5-S6	21
14	3573 G>A	E1225K	BBB, Brugada syndrome type I	DIII/S1-S2	24
15	3823 G>A	D1275N	BBB, SSS, DCM	DIII/S3	20
16	T>C	IVS22+2	BBB	DIII/S4-S5	5
17	3995 C>T	P1332L	AVB, LQT3	DIII/S4-S5	37
18	4372 A>T	G1406R	BBB, Brugada syndrome type I	DIII/S5-S6	27
19	4262 G>A	W1421X	BBB, SSS, SD	DIII/S5-S6	31
20	4498-4500del	delK1500	BBB, Brugada syndrome type I, LQT3	DIII-DIV	26
21	4729 AAins	K1578Fs/52	BBB, Brugada syndrome type I, SSS	DIV/S2	23
22	4783 G>C	D1595N	AVB	DIV/S2-S3	35
23	5123 C>A	T1708N	BBB, VT, SD	DIV/S5-S6	18
24		S1710L	BBB	DIV/S5-S6	22
25	5280 Gdel	S1710Fs/65	BBB	DIV/S5-S6	5
26	5227 G>A	G1743R	BBB, Brugada syndrome type I, SSS	DIV/S5-S6	Unpublished
27	5289 G>A	V1763M	AVB, LQT3	DIV/S6	39
28	5298 A>C	M1766L	AVB, LQT3	DIV/S6	40
29	5328 G>A	V1777M	AVB, LQT3	C terminus	38
30	5464-7 TCTGdel	L1821Fs/10	BBB, AVB, SSS, VT	C terminus	12
31	6013 C>G	P2005A	AVB, LQT3	C terminus	36

*Case numbers correspond to numbers in circles in Figure 75-5.
AVB, atrioventricular block; BBB, bundle branch block; DCM, dilated cardiomyopathy; LQT3, long QT syndrome variant 3; SD, sudden death; SSS, sick sinus syndrome; VT, ventricular tachycardia.

associated with congenital heart disease, commonly secundum-type ASDs and progressive atrioventricular conduction defects.[67,68] Mutant Tbx may downregulate Cx40 and Cx45.[69] Mice deficient for HF-1b exhibit normal cardiac structure and function, with 100% penetrance of conduction system defects and increased susceptibility to sudden death.[70]

DMPK Mutations and Cardiac Conduction Disease

Myotonic dystrophy type 1 (DM1) represents the most common muscular dystrophy in adults. DM1 is a multisystem disorder of autosomal dominant inheritance that affects skeletal and cardiac muscle, eyes, and both endocrine and central nervous systems. Cardiac involvement and progressive conduction abnormalities are common and constitute the second most common cause of death among patients with DM1.[71] Atrial tachyarrhythmias are the most common rhythm disturbances, although reentrant ventricular tachycardia can also occur. Cardiac abnormalities include left ventricular hypertrophy and dilatation, systolic dysfunction, mitral valve prolapse, regional wall motion abnormalities, and left atrial dilatation.[72]

DM1 is caused by a trinucleotide (CTG) expansion in the 3′-untranslated region of the *DMPK* gene, which encodes a serine-threonine protein kinase. The magnitude of the trinucleotide expansion correlates with the severity of skeletal and cardiac myopathy in a time-dependent degenerative process.[73,74] Clear evidence in mouse models indicates that the molecular mechanisms underlying the cardiac conduction defects in DM1 stem from RNA toxicity–induced overexpression of the cardiac transcription factor Nkx2.5 and consequent downregulation of Cx40 and Cx43.[75] Almost any type of conduction anomaly can occur in DM1. Up to 40% of patients present with first-degree AV block, followed in order of frequency by left anterior fascicular block, left bundle branch block, right bundle branch block, QT interval prolongation, ST-T abnormalities, and axis deviation. In DM1 patients with a normal ECG pattern at diagnosis, repeating the ECG every 6 to 12 months is recommended, because the nature of the conduction disease usually is slow but progressive and unpredictable in any given DM1 patient.[72]

Lamin A/C and Cardiac Conduction Disease

The nuclear lamina is a filamentous structure composed of lamins that support the inner nuclear membrane. Lamins A and C function in DNA replication and nuclear envelope assembly and subserve a role in resisting mechanical stress and influencing DNA transcription and gene expression. Lamins A and C are two distinct proteins produced by alternative splicing from the same gene, *LMNA*, differing only in their carboxyl terminus. *LMNA* mutations give rise to several genetic disorders including dilated cardiomyopathy (DCM) and conduction defects,[76] commonly associated with a high risk of sudden death,[77] and a variety of neuromuscular lipodystrophy and progeria-type disorders including Emery-Dreifuss muscular dystrophy, a specific neuromuscular degenerative condition that can also manifest a severe cardiac phenotype of DCM and cardiac conduction disease.[78]

Treatment for Progressive Cardiac Conduction Disease

In general, the only effective treatment for PCCD is pacemaker implantation. However, long-term pacing therapy, especially in pediatric patients, is not without its complications, a search for novel therapeutic interventions is warranted. Extensive research is being performed on gene therapy approaches, stem cell–based therapy, and engineered tissue constructs that shows promise for future biologic alternatives to implantable electronic devices. Another possibility is the use of bone marrow–derived cardiomyocytes as biopacemakers. Genetically modified human mesenchymal stem cells can express functional cardiac pacemaker channels in vitro and in vivo[79] and are able to repair conduction block in cardiomyocyte cultures.[80] Viral gene transfer to convert heart muscle cells into pacemaker cells has been done successfully in animals.[81] Despite the encouraging results, many obstacles must be overcome before biologic pacemakers or conduction tissue regeneration techniques become viable treatment options for the patient with PCCD.

References

1. Miller WL, Hodge DO, Hammill SC: Association of uncomplicated electrocardiographic conduction blocks with subsequent cardiac morbidity in a community-based population (Olmsted County, Minnesota). Am J Cardiol 101:102-106, 2008.
2. Iturralde-Torres P, Nava-Townsend S, Gomez-Flores J, et al: Association of congenital, diffuse electrical disease in children with normal heart: Sick sinus syndrome, intraventricular conduction block, and monomorphic ventricular tachycardia. J Cardiovasc Electrophysiol 19:550-555, 2008. Epub 2007 Oct 24.
3. Chiu SN, Wang JK, Wu MH, et al: Cardiac conduction disturbance detected in a pediatric population. J Pediatr 152:85-89, 2008.
4. Brink PA, Ferreira A, Moolman JC, et al: Gene for progressive familial heart block type I maps to chromosome 19q13. Circulation 91:1633-1640, 1995.
5. Schott JJ, Alshinawi C, Kyndt F, et al: Cardiac conduction defects associate with mutations in SCN5A. Nat Genet 23:20-21, 1999.
6. Royer A, van Veen TA, Le Bouter S, et al: Mouse model of *SCN5A*-linked hereditary Lenegre's disease: Age-related conduction slowing and myocardial fibrosis. Circulation 111:1738-1746, 2005.
7. Goldin AL: Evolution of voltage-gated Na(+) channels. J Exp Biol 205:575-584, 2002.
8. Tan HL, Bink-Boelkens MT, Bezzina CR, et al: A sodium-channel mutation causes isolated cardiac conduction disease. Nature 409:1043-1047, 2001.
9. Chen Q, Kirsch GE, Zhang D, et al: Genetic basis and molecular mechanism for idiopathic ventricular fibrillation. Nature 392:293-296, 1998.
10. Benson DW, Wang DW, Dyment M, et al: Congenital sick sinus syndrome caused by recessive mutations in the cardiac sodium channel gene (*SCN5A*). J Clin Invest 112:1019-1028, 2003.
11. Tan BH, Iturralde-Torres P, Medeiros-Domingo A, et al: A novel C-terminal truncation *SCN5A* mutation from a patient with sick sinus syndrome, conduction disorder and ventricular tachycardia. Cardiovasc Res 76:409-417, 2007.
12. Papadatos GA, Wallerstein PM, Head CE, et al: Slowed conduction and ventricular tachycardia after targeted disruption of the cardiac sodium channel gene *SCN5A*. Proc Natl Acad Sci U S A 99:6210-6215, 2002.
13. Bertomeu-Gonzalez V, Ruiz-Granell R, Garcia-Civera R, et al: Syncopal monomorphic ventricular tachycardia with pleomorphism, sensitive to antitachycardia pacing in a patient with Brugada syndrome. Europace 8:1048-1050, 2006.
14. Probst V, Evain S, Gournay V, et al: Monomorphic ventricular tachycardia due to Brugada syndrome successfully treated by hydroquinidine therapy in a 3-year-old child. J Cardiovasc Electrophysiol 17:97-100, 2006.
15. Olson TM, Michels VV, Ballew JD, et al: Sodium channel mutations and susceptibility to heart failure and atrial fibrillation. JAMA 293:447-454, 2005.
16. Wang Q, Shen J, Splawski I, et al: *SCN5A* mutations associated with an inherited cardiac arrhythmia, long QT syndrome. Cell 80:805-811, 1995.
17. Rossenbacker T, Carroll SJ, Liu H, et al: Novel pore mutation in *SCN5A* manifests as a spectrum of phenotypes ranging from atrial flutter, conduction disease, and Brugada syndrome to sudden cardiac death. Heart Rhythm 1:610-615, 2004.
18. Medeiros-Domingo A, Tester JD, Iturralde-Torres P, et al: Cardiac sodium channel mutations are prevalent in a cohort of Mexican-Mestizo patients with malignant long QT syndrome. Circulation 114:505, 2006.
19. Smits JP, Koopmann TT, Wilders R, et al: A mutation in the human cardiac sodium channel (E161K) contributes to sick sinus syndrome, conduction disease and Brugada syndrome in two families. J Mol Cell Cardiol 38:969-981, 2005.
20. McNair WP, Ku L, Taylor MR, et al: *SCN5A* mutation associated with dilated cardiomyopathy, conduction disorder, and arrhythmia. Circulation 110:2163-2167, 2004.
21. Schulze-Bahr E, Eckardt L, Breithardt G, et al: Sodium channel gene (*SCN5A*) mutations in 44 index patients with Brugada

syndrome: Different incidences in familial and sporadic disease. Hum Mutat 21:651-652, 2003.

22. Shirai N, Makita N, Sasaki K, et al: A mutant cardiac sodium channel with multiple biophysical defects associated with overlapping clinical features of Brugada syndrome and cardiac conduction disease. Cardiovasc Res 53:348-354, 2002.
23. Makiyama T, Akao M, Tsuji K, et al: High risk for bradyarrhythmic complications in patients with Brugada syndrome caused by *SCN5A* gene mutations. J Am Coll Cardiol 46:2100-2106, 2005.
24. Smits JP, Eckardt L, Probst V, et al: Genotype-phenotype relationship in Brugada syndrome: Electrocardiographic features differentiate *SCN5A*-related patients from non–*SCN5A*-related patients. J Am Coll Cardiol 40:350-356, 2002.
25. Probst V, Allouis M, Sacher F, et al: Progressive cardiac conduction defect is the prevailing phenotype in carriers of a Brugada syndrome *SCN5A* mutation. J Cardiovasc Electrophysiol 17:270-275, 2006.
26. Grant AO, Carboni MP, Neplioueva V, et al: Long QT syndrome, Brugada syndrome, and conduction system disease are linked to a single sodium channel mutation. J Clin Invest 110:1201-1209, 2002.
27. Kyndt F, Probst V, Potet F, et al: Novel *SCN5A* mutation leading either to isolated cardiac conduction defect or Brugada syndrome in a large French family. Circulation 104:3081-3086, 2001.
28. Bezzina CR, Rook MB, Groenewegen WA, et al: Compound heterozygosity for mutations (W156X and R225W) in *SCN5A* associated with severe cardiac conduction disturbances and degenerative changes in the conduction system. Circ Res 92:159-168, 2003.
29. Poelzing S, Forleo C, Samodell M, et al: *SCN5A* polymorphism restores trafficking of a Brugada syndrome mutation on a separate gene. Circulation 114:368-376, 2006.
30. Ye B, Valdivia CR, Ackerman MJ, Makielski JC: A common human *SCN5A* polymorphism modifies expression of an arrhythmia causing mutation. Physiol Genomics 12:187-193, 2003.
31. Niu DM, Hwang B, Hwang HW, et al: A common *SCN5A* polymorphism attenuates a severe cardiac phenotype caused by a nonsense *SCN5A* mutation in a Chinese family with an inherited cardiac conduction defect. J Med Genet 43:817-821, 2006.
32. Makielski JC, Ye B, Valdivia CR, et al: A ubiquitous splice variant and a common polymorphism affect heterologous expression of recombinant human SCN5A heart sodium channels. Circ Res 93:821-828, 2003.
33. Tan BH, Valdivia CR, Rok BA, et al: Common human *SCN5A* polymorphisms have altered electrophysiology when expressed in Q1077 splice variants. Heart Rhythm 2:741-747, 2005.
34. Viswanathan PC, Benson DW, Balser JR: A common *SCN5A* polymorphism modulates the biophysical effects of an *SCN5A* mutation. J Clin Invest 111:341-346, 2003.
35. Wang DW, Viswanathan PC, Balser JR, et al: Clinical, genetic, and biophysical characterization of *SCN5A* mutations associated with atrioventricular conduction block. Circulation 105:341-346, 2002.
36. Shim SH, Ito M, Maher T, Milunsky A: Gene sequencing in neonates and infants with the long QT syndrome. Genet Test 9:281-284, 2005.
37. Kehl HG, Haverkamp W, Rellensmann G, et al: Images in cardiovascular medicine. Life-threatening neonatal arrhythmia: Successful treatment and confirmation of clinically suspected extreme long QT-syndrome-3. Circulation 109:e205-e206, 2004.
38. Lupoglazoff JM, Cheav T, Baroudi G, et al: Homozygous *SCN5A* mutation in long-QT syndrome with functional two-to-one atrioventricular block. Circ Res 89:E16-E21, 2001.
39. Chang CC, Acharfi S, Wu MH, et al: A novel *SCN5A* mutation manifests as a malignant form of long QT syndrome with perinatal onset of tachycardia/bradycardia. Cardiovasc Res 64:268-278, 2004.
40. Valdivia CR, Ackerman MJ, Tester DJ, et al: A novel *SCN5A* arrhythmia mutation, M1766L, with expression defect rescued by mexiletine. Cardiovasc Res 55:279-289, 2002.
41. Wehrens XH, Rossenbacker T, Jongbloed RJ, et al: A novel mutation L619F in the cardiac Na^+ channel *SCN5A* associated with long-QT syndrome (LQT3): A role for the I-II linker in inactivation gating. Hum Mutat 21:552, 2003.
42. Gorgels AP, Al Fadley F, Zaman L, et al: The long QT syndrome with impaired atrioventricular conduction: A malignant variant in infants. J Cardiovasc Electrophysiol 9:1225-1232, 1998.
43. Lupoglazoff JM, Denjoy I, Villain E, et al: Long QT syndrome in neonates: Conduction disorders associated with HERG mutations and sinus bradycardia with KCNQ1 mutations. J Am Coll Cardiol 43:826-830, 2004.
44. Chevalier P, Bellocq C, Millat G, et al: Torsades de pointes complicating atrioventricular block: Evidence for a genetic predisposition. Heart Rhythm 4:170-174, 2007.
45. Splawski I, Timothy KW, Sharpe LM, et al: Ca(V)1.2 calcium channel dysfunction causes a multisystem disorder including arrhythmia and autism. Cell 119:19-31, 2004.
46. Plaster NM, Tawil R, Tristani-Firouzi M, et al: Mutations in Kir2.1 cause the developmental and episodic electrical phenotypes of Andersen's syndrome. Cell 105:511-519, 2001.
47. Schulze-Bahr E, Neu A, Friederich P, et al: Pacemaker channel dysfunction in a patient with sinus node disease. J Clin Invest 111:1537-1545, 2003.
48. Arad M, Maron BJ, Gorham JM, et al: Glycogen storage diseases presenting as hypertrophic cardiomyopathy. N Engl J Med 352:362-372, 2005.
49. Ahmad F, Arad M, Musi N, et al: Increased alpha2 subunit-associated *AMPK* activity and *PRKAG2* cardiomyopathy. Circulation 112:3140-3148, 2005.
50. Wolf CM, Arad M, Ahmad F, et al: Reversibility of PRKAG2 glycogen-storage cardiomyopathy and electrophysiological manifestations. Circulation 117:144-154, 2008.
51. Murphy RT, Mogensen J, McGarry K, et al: Adenosine monophosphate–activated protein kinase disease mimicks hypertrophic cardiomyopathy and Wolff-Parkinson-White syndrome: Natural history. J Am Coll Cardiol 45:922-930, 2005.
52. Sternick EB, Oliva A, Magalhaes LP, et al: Familial pseudo–Wolff-Parkinson-White syndrome. J Cardiovasc Electrophysiol 17:724-732, 2006.
53. Nadeau A, Therrien C, Karpati G, Sinnreich M: Danon disease due to a novel splice mutation in the *LAMP2* gene. Muscle Nerve 37:338-342, 2008.
54. Yang Z, McMahon CJ, Smith LR, et al: Danon disease as an underrecognized cause of hypertrophic cardiomyopathy in children. Circulation 112:1612-1617, 2005.
55. Echaniz-Laguna A, Mohr M, Epailly E, et al: Novel Lamp-2 gene mutation and successful treatment with heart transplantation in a large family with Danon disease. Muscle Nerve 33:393-397, 2006.
56. Balmer C, Ballhausen D, Bosshard NU, et al: Familial X-linked cardiomyopathy (Danon disease): Diagnostic confirmation by mutation analysis of the *LAMP2* gene. Eur J Pediatr 164:509-514, 2005.
57. Willecke K, Eiberger J, Degen J, et al: Structural and functional diversity of connexin genes in the mouse and human genome. Biol Chem 383:725-737, 2002.
58. Winterhager E, Pielensticker N, Freyer J, et al: Replacement of connexin43 by connexin26 in transgenic mice leads to dysfunctional reproductive organs and slowed ventricular conduction in the heart. BMC Dev Biol 7:26, 2007.
59. Tamaddon HS, Vaidya D, Simon AM, et al: High-resolution optical mapping of the right bundle branch in connexin40 knockout mice reveals slow conduction in the specialized conduction system. Circ Res 87:929-936, 2000.
60. Groenewegen WA, Firouzi M, Bezzina CR, et al: A cardiac sodium channel mutation cosegregates with a rare connexin40 genotype in familial atrial standstill. Circ Res 92:14-22, 2003.
61. Gollob MH, Jones DL, Krahn AD, et al: Somatic mutations in the connexin 40 gene (GJA5) in atrial fibrillation. N Engl J Med 354:2677-2688, 2006.
62. Jay PY, Harris BS, Buerger A, et al: Function follows form: Cardiac conduction system defects in Nkx2.5 mutation. Anat Rec A Discov Mol Cell Evol Biol 280:966-972, 2004.
63. Jay PY, Harris BS, Maguire CT, et al: Nkx2.5 mutation causes anatomic hypoplasia of the cardiac conduction system. J Clin Invest 113:1130-1137, 2004.
64. Pashmforoush M, Lu JT, Chen H, et al: Nkx2.5 pathways and congenital heart disease: Loss of ventricular myocyte lineage specification leads to progressive cardiomyopathy and complete heart block. Cell 117:373-386, 2004.
65. Moskowitz IP, Kim JB, Moore ML, et al: A molecular pathway including Id2, Tbx5, and Nkx2.5 required for cardiac

conduction system development. Cell 129:1365-1376, 2007.

66. Schott JJ, Benson DW, Basson CT, et al: Congenital heart disease caused by mutations in the transcription factor NKX2.5. Science 281:108-111, 1998.
67. Borozdin W, Bravo Ferrer Acosta AM, Bamshad MJ, et al: Expanding the spectrum of TBX5 mutations in Holt-Oram syndrome: Detection of two intragenic deletions by quantitative real time PCR, and report of eight novel point mutations. Hum Mutat 27:975-976, 2006.
68. Moskowitz IP, Pizard A, Patel VV, et al: The T-box transcription factor Tbx5 is required for the patterning and maturation of the murine cardiac conduction system. Development 131:4107-4116, 2004.
69. Kruger O, Maxeiner S, Kim JS, et al: Cardiac morphogenetic defects and conduction abnormalities in mice homozygously deficient for connexin40 and heterozygously deficient for connexin45. J Mol Cell Cardiol 41:787-797, 2006.
70. Nguyen-Tran VT, Kubalak SW, Minamisawa S, et al: A novel genetic pathway for sudden cardiac death via defects in the transition between ventricular and conduction system cell lineages. Cell 102:671-682, 2000.
71. Bhakta D, Lowe MR, Groh WJ: Prevalence of structural cardiac abnormalities in patients with myotonic dystrophy type I. Am Heart J 147:224-227, 2004.
72. Sovari AA, Bodine CK, Farokhi F: Cardiovascular manifestations of myotonic dystrophy-1. Cardiol Rev 15:191-194, 2007.
73. Groh WJ, Lowe MR, Zipes DP: Severity of cardiac conduction involvement and arrhythmias in myotonic dystrophy type 1 correlates with age and CTG repeat length. J Cardiovasc Electrophysiol 13:444-448, 2002.
74. Salehi LB, Bonifazi E, Stasio ED, et al: Risk prediction for clinical phenotype in myotonic dystrophy type 1: Data from 2,650 patients. Genet Test 11:84-90, 2007.
75. Yadava RS, Frenzel-McCardell CD, Yu Q, et al: RNA toxicity in myotonic muscular dystrophy induces NKX2-5 expression. Nat Genet 40:61-68, 2008.
76. van Tintelen JP, Hofstra RM, Katerberg H, et al: High yield of *LMNA* mutations in patients with dilated cardiomyopathy and/or conduction disease referred to cardiogenetics outpatient clinics. Am Heart J 154:1130-1139, 2007.
77. MacLeod HM, Culley MR, Huber JM, et al: Lamin A/C truncation in dilated cardiomyopathy with conduction disease. BMC Med Genet 4:4, 2003.
78. Fatkin D, MacRae C, Sasaki T, et al: Missense mutations in the rod domain of the lamin A/C gene as causes of dilated cardiomyopathy and conduction-system disease. N Engl J Med 341:1715-1724, 1999.
79. Potapova I, Plotnikov A, Lu Z, et al: Human mesenchymal stem cells as a gene delivery system to create cardiac pacemakers. Circ Res 94:952-959, 2004.
80. Beeres SL, Atsma DE, van der Laarse A, et al: Human adult bone marrow mesenchymal stem cells repair experimental conduction block in rat cardiomyocyte cultures. J Am Coll Cardiol 46:1943-1952, 2005.
81. Miake J, Marban E, Nuss HB: Biological pacemaker created by gene transfer. Nature 419:132-133, 2002.

Sudden Infant Death Syndrome 76

JONATHAN C. MAKIELSKI

CHAPTER OUTLINE

Overview

Sudden infant death syndrome (SIDS) is the sudden unexpected death of an infant (before the age of 1 year) for which no cause is apparent. Depending on the precise definition of SIDS, the historical era, demographics, and ethnic status of the population, SIDS affects approximately 0.1 to 2 infants per 1000 live births, with a peak incidence between the ages of 2 and 5 months.[1,2] The etiologic basis for SIDS may be neurologic, endocrine, pulmonary, or cardiac. This chapter reviews the evidence that cardiac arrhythmia plays a role in SIDS, with a focus on genetic predisposition to fatal arrhythmia.[3] The literature on SIDS in general, and on the role for arrhythmia and SIDS in particular, is vast, with numerous studies, reviews, editorials, and commentaries highlighting the controversies. The focus of this chapter is on more recent studies and review papers that will lead the interested reader to this rich literature.

Linking Sudden Infant Death Syndrome and Arrhythmia

SIDS by definition occurs in infants without diagnosed or suspected disease ante mortem, and with no clear cause of death on routine postmortem examination. This lack of antemortem data has been an obstacle for the field overall and particularly for making the link to arrhythmia. Techniques to investigate the etiology of SIDS include analyses of epidemiologic data, studies of the parents and relatives of SIDS victims, and studies of infants who for one reason or another were considered to be at high risk for SIDS. Infants who came to medical attention before death, or who were resuscitated from an event (called "survivors" of SIDS, or designated as having "near miss" SIDS) also have been studied. These cases provide valuable insights into and "proof of principle" for etiologic factors in SIDS. The near-miss cases, however, do not fit the clinical and epidemiologic definition of SIDS, because the affected patients either had clinical manifestations detected ante mortem or did not die. With the discovery that mutations in ion channels and associated proteins cause long QT syndrome (Chapters 50 and 69) and other arrhythmia syndromes such as Brugada syndrome (Chapters 50 and 68) and catecholaminergic polymorphic ventricular tachycardia (CPVT) (Chapters 52 and 70), it became possible to perform a "molecular autopsy" for SIDS victims by screening candidate genes for mutations (Table 76-1).

The study of cohorts of "true" SIDS cases that meet the rigorous definition of SIDS can give an estimate of how many such cases can be explained by mutations in ion channels or related proteins (channelopathies) that cause altered electrophysiologic components. A certain semantic paradox occurs, however, in that once a cause is established, an individual case should by definition no longer be considered SIDS. This chapter focuses on recent studies showing that some cases previously considered to be SIDS can be accounted for by channelopathies and discusses the extent to which these discoveries, and as-yet undiscovered channelopathies, will lead to reclassification of SIDS cases as early deaths from channelopathies. The importance of making the diagnosis extends well beyond reclassification, because it leads to elucidation of mechanism, prevention, and possible therapy in individual patients.

It also is important to recognize that the presence of a mutation in a susceptible gene does not necessarily imply a link to causation, because mutations without functional significance may occur as common polymorphisms (affecting greater than 0.5% of the population) or as rare variants (affecting less than 0.5% of the population). The absence of the mutation in control panels provides supporting evidence for pathogenicity, but the possibility of discovering an incidental rare variant in SIDS increases as the number of genes screened increases. Traditional linkage studies in family kindreds are used to connect the genotype to the phenotype, but such studies are not possible in SIDS because the phenotype is death in infancy, and mutations may be de novo and are not present in the parents. When a mutation is found, biophysical function of the mutation can be investigated by expressing the mutated protein in heterologous expression systems, or even in myocytes, to demonstrate an abnormality consistent with known pathogenetic mechanisms for long QT syndrome, Brugada syndrome, CPVT, or other arrhythmia syndromes. If such a mutation is present, this provides strong but not conclusive evidence for pathogenicity. If it is absent, however, this does not prove nonpathogenicity because the mutation may not have been studied under the conditions necessary to elicit the dysfunction (such as reduced pH),[4,5] or that the presence of the complete macromolecular complex

Table 76-1 Summary of Studies of Channelopathies in Sudden Infant Death Syndrome (SIDS)

Study	SIDS or Other*	Gene	Mutation	Age at Diagnosis (wk)	No. of Control Alleles Affected	Biophysical Dysfunction	Known Arrhythmia Mutation†
Long QT Syndrome							
Schwartz et al, 2001 (Schwartz et al., 2000)	Near miss	*SCN5A*	S941N	6	400	↑ late I_{Na}	No
Wedekind et al, 2001[10]	Diagnosed antemortem		A1330P	9	NA	Gating shifts	No
Ackerman et al, 2001[11]	SIDS 2/93		A997S	6	800	↑ late I_{Na}	No
			R1826H	4	800	↑ late I_{Na}	No
Plant et al, 2006[4]	SIDS 3/133		S1103Y		NA	↑ late I_{Na} with ↓ pH	Yes
Arnestad et al, 2007[12]	SIDS 13/201		F1486L	1	364	↑ late I_{Na}	No
Wang et al, 2007[5]			R680H		364	↑ late I_{Na} with ↓ pH	No
			Del586		364	↑ late I_{Na} with ↓ pH	No
			T1304M		364	↑ late I_{Na}	Yes
			S216L		364	↑ late I_{Na}	No
			F2004L		364	↑ late I_{Na}	No
			F2006A		364	↑ late I_{Na}	No
			R1193Q		364	↑ late I_{Na}	Yes
			V1951L		364	↑ late I_{Na}	Yes
Cronk et al, 2007[14]	SIDS 3/134	*CAV3*	V14L	26	800	↑ late I_{Na}	No
			T78M	10	800	↑ late I_{Na}	No
			L79R	36	800	↑ late I_{Na}	No
Arnestad et al, 2007[12]	SIDS 2/201		T78M		364	↑ late I_{Na}	
			C72W		364	Unknown	
Schwartz et al, 2001[15]	SIDS	*KCNQ1*	P117L		800	Unknown	Yes
Arnestad et al, 2007[12]	SIDS 1/201		G460S		364	↓ I_{Ks}	
Christiansen et al, 2005[16]	SIDS	*KCNH2*	K101E	7	196	Unknown	No
Arnestad et al, 2007[12]	SIDS 1/201		R954C/K897T			↓ I_{Kr}	
Arnestad et al, 2007[12]	SIDS 1/201	*KCNE2*	Q9E		364	Kinetics of I_{Kr}	Yes
Brugada Syndrome							
Skinner et al, 2005[19]	Near miss	*SCN5A*	R1193Q	2		↓ I_{Na}	Yes
Van Norstrand et al, 2007[20]	SIDS 3/228	*GPD1L*	E83K	14	600	↓ I_{Na}	
			I124V	5	600	↓ I_{Na}	
			R273C	4	600	↓ I_{Na}	

*I.e., SIDS in which the cases meet the definition of "true" SIDS; for cohort studies, the number of cases positive for the given genetic defect is specified.

†I.e., whether or not the mutation was previously known to cause arrhythmia in non-SIDS cases (Yes) or was novel to SIDS (No).

Continued

Table 76-1 Summary of Studies of Channelopathies in Sudden Infant Death Syndrome (SIDS)—cont'd

Study	SIDS or Other*	Gene	Mutation	Age at Diagnosis (wk)	No. of Control Alleles Affected	Biophysical Dysfunction	Known Arrhythmia Mutation†
Catecholeminergic Polymorphic Ventricular Tachycardia							
Tester et al, 2007[21]	SIDS 2/134	*RYR2*	R2267H	28	400	"Leaky"	No
			S4565	4	400	"Leaky"	No
Short QT Syndrome							
Arnestad et al, 2007[12]	SIDS 1/228	*KCNQ1*	I274V		600	↑ I_{Ks}	No

present in myocytes but not heterologous cells is required to manifest dysfunction. To most strongly support the link between a genotype and an arrhythmic SIDS clinical phenotype, a mutation should cause biophysical dysfunction of an ion current under relevant environmental conditions that result in a cellular phenotype supporting an arrhythmogenic phenotype at the tissue and organ level (see Fig. 76-1).

Sudden Infant Death Syndrome and Long QT Syndrome

In the 1970s, Schwartz suggested that abnormalities of cardiac sympathetic innervation caused a disorder of the heart's electrical rhythm known as *long QT syndrome*, and that this also may cause SIDS.[6] Maron and associates showed a longer QT interval in parents of SIDS victims and provided evidence for a role of long QT syndrome in SIDS.[7] In a prospective trial of ECG screening in more than 34,000 infants that produced SIDS cases,[8] a long QT interval increased the risk of SIDS by factor of 41. The "proof of principle" that congenital long QT syndrome could cause SIDS came from two cases: first, a near-miss case[9] in which the infant survived, and second, a case in which the patient died in infancy but long QT syndrome was recognized ante mortem.[10] In both cases, a mutation in the gene *SCN5A* encoding the voltage-dependent cardiac sodium channel was found (see Table 76-1), and it had the characteristic biophysical phenotype of increased late sodium current associated with long QT syndrome type 3 (LQT3). These cases, however, did not meet the formal epidemiologic definition of SIDS.

In 2001 Ackerman and colleagues screened a cohort of 93 patients with defined SIDS for mutations in *SCN5A*[11] and found two novel mutations that on expression in heterologous cells showed the increased late sodium current of LQT3. Further studies in SIDS cohorts have found 10 additional

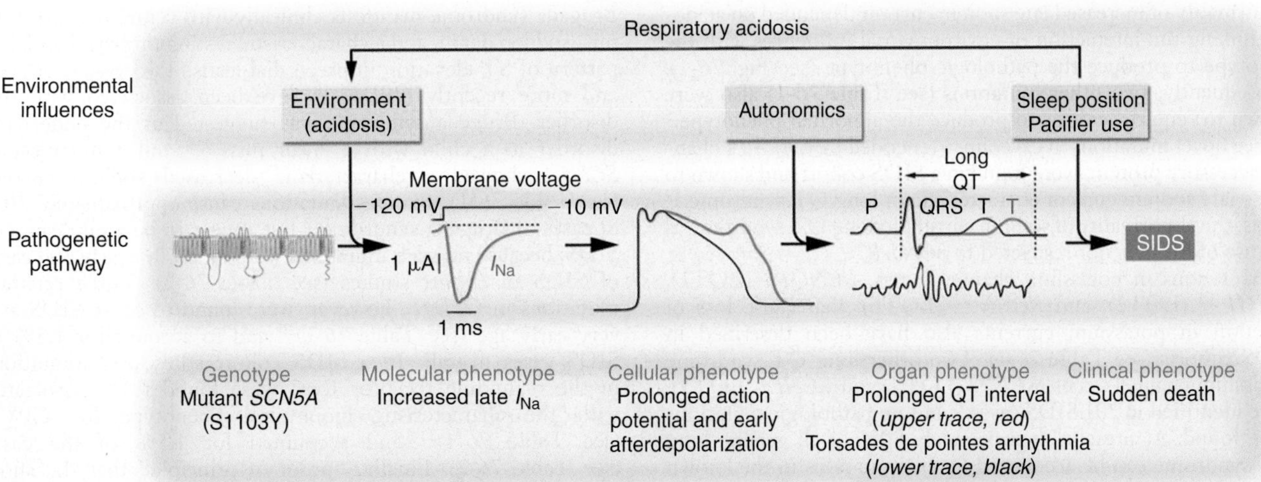

Figure 76-1 The link between genotype and phenotype in sudden infant death syndrome (SIDS) emphasizing multiple levels of phenotype and interaction with the environment. A mutation in the cardiac sodium channel gene *SCN5A* is associated with a pathologic molecular (also called biophysical) phenotypic feature of increased late sodium current, which in turn results in an abnormal cellular phenotype, in this case action potential prolongation and afterdepolarizations, which causes tissue or organ manifestations of prolonged QT interval and arrhythmia, eventuating in the clinical phenotype of SIDS. (From Makielski JC: SIDS: Genetic and environmental influences may cause arrhythmia in this silent killer. J Clin Invest 116:297, 2006.)

Table 76-2 Frequency of Channelopathies in Cohort Studies of Sudden Infant Death Syndrome (SIDS)*

Syndrome and Gene	Incidence in SIDS	Overall Frequency in SIDS	Relative Frequency In SIDS within Group	Relative Frequency In non-SIDS within Group
LQT1 *KCNQ1*	1/201	0.5%	6%	30-35%
LQT2 *KCNH2*	1/201	0.5%	6%	25-30%
LQT3 *SCN5A*	15/294	5.1%	63%	5-10%
LQT5 *KCNE1*	0/201	0.0%	0%	1%
LQT6 *KCNE2*	1/201	0.5%	6%	Rare
LQT7 *KCNJ2*	0/201	0.0%	0%	Rare
LQT9 *CAV3*	5/335	1.5%	19%	1%
Total for long QT syndrome		8.1%	100%	
Brugada syndrome type I *SCN5A*	0/294	0.0%	0%	20%
Brugada syndrome type II *GPD1L*	3/228	1.3%	100%	rare?
Total for Brugada syndrome		1.3%	100%	
CPVT1 *RYR2*	2/134	1.5%		
SQT1 *KCNQ1*	1/201	0.5%		
Total		11.4%		

*Frequency was derived from data from the cohort studies cited in Table 76-1.[11,12,14,20] Not every gene listed was tested for every cohort. The S1103Y polymorphism study was not included.[4] Relative frequency in non-SIDS citations is reported in the study by Lehnart and coworkers.[17] The percentage estimates given for non-SIDS cases include ungenotyped cases.

mutations in *SCN5A* associated with LQT3 (see Table 76-1).[4,12] Most of these were rare novel mutations, but one, S1103Y, was a common polymorphism with an allelic frequency of approximately 10% in the black population that had previously been shown to be associated with ventricular arrhythmia in adults.[13] Plant and colleagues showed that homozygosity for S1103Y increased the risk of SIDS 24-fold. Moreover, the biophysical abnormality of increased late sodium current depended on acidosis, linking the interaction of environmental influences with the genotype to produce the pathologic phenotype (see Fig. 76-1). Subsequently, two other mutations (see Table 76-1) also were shown to require acidosis to produce the abnormal phenotype.[5] Three novel mutations in caveolin-3 (encoded by *CAV3*), a channel accessory protein, were found in a SIDS cohort and shown to cause late sodium current characteristic of long QT syndrome.[14] Thus, the abnormality of sodium current in long QT syndrome as a cause of SIDS is not restricted to *SCN5A*.

Mutations in potassium channel genes, *KCNQ1*[15] (LQT1), *KCNH*[16] (LQT2), and *KCNE*[12] (LQT6), that cause loss of function in potassium currents also have been described in SIDS cohorts (see Table 76-1). Two other long QT syndrome potassium channel genes, *KCNJ2* (LQT7) and *KCNE1* (LQT5), were identified in 201 SIDS cases,[12] but no pathologic mutations were found. At present, approximately 80% of all genetic long QT syndrome can be accounted for by mutations in the known genes (for LQT1 to LQT9),[17] with the great majority of cases being caused by *KCNQ1* (LQT1) and *KCNH2* (LQT2). In SIDS, however, mutations in *SCN5A* (in LQT3) and *CAV3* (LQT9) predominate, and in the cohort studies to date they account for 83% of cases of long QT syndrome in SIDS and for 6.6% of SIDS cases overall (Table 76-2).

Sudden Infant Death Syndrome and Brugada Syndrome, Catecholaminergic Polymorphic Ventricular Tachycardia, and Short QT Syndrome

Brugada syndrome manifests clinically with ventricular arrhythmia, sudden death, and a characteristic resting or provoked ECG pattern of ST elevation in precordial leads. Two genes, *SCN5A* and more recently *GPD1L*,[18] have been associated with this disorder. Brugada syndrome was suggested as the underlying disorder in a child with a "near miss,"[19] and a mutation in *SCN5A* showed a characteristic decreased sodium current (see Table 76-1). *SCN5A* mutations cause approximately 20% of cases of Brugada syndrome[17] but appear to be a rare cause of SIDS, because no such mutations were found in nearly 300 cases of SIDS in cohort studies (see Table 76-2). Three separate mutations in *GPD1L*, however, were found to cause SIDS at a very early age (see Table 76-1)[20] and to account for 1.5% of SIDS cases overall. In a SIDS cohort study, two mutations in the ryanodine receptor Ryr2 were found to be associated with the characteristic biophysical phenotype for CPVT (see Table 76-1)[21] and accounted for 1.5% of the cases (see Table 76-2). Finally, "proof of principle" that the short QT syndrome may cause SIDS was provided by an early pediatric diagnosis in a child who did not die,[22] and subsequently a mutation in *KCNQ1* was discovered in a SIDS cohort that had the characteristic biophysical phenotype of gain of function found in short QT syndrome (see Table 76-2)[12] and accounted for 0.5% of the cases.

Congenital Arrhythmia and SIDS: How Frequent?

A comprehensive study[12] investigating seven long QT syndrome genes found mutations in 26 of 201 SIDS cases (12.9%) and concluded on the basis of molecular phenotype that 19 of these (9.5%) were pathogenic. Table 76-2 summarizes data from a total of four cohort studies,[11,12,14,20] adding Brugada syndrome, CPVT, and short QT syndrome to long QT syndrome, to bring the total incidence of channelopathies in SIDS to 11.4%. More studies are necessary to verify this number in additional, larger and diverse cohorts. This number probably represents a minimum, because new gene discoveries may increase it. In 2007 it was estimated that 75% of cases of long QT syndrome, 50% to 60% of CPVT cases, and 20% of cases of Brugada syndrome could be accounted for by the known arrhythmia genes.[17] As new arrhythmia genes are discovered for these inherited arrhythmia syndromes, they will become candidates for SIDS as well. Moreover, channelopathies unique to SIDS may be discovered. The pattern for the incidence of certain genes in SIDS already diverges sharply from that in non-SIDS congenital arrhythmia syndromes (see Table 76-2). For example, *GPD1L* mutations are very rare compared with *SCN5A* mutations as a cause of Brugada syndrome, but *GPD1L* is the only Brugada syndrome mutation discovered in SIDS. No Brugada syndrome-like *SCN5A* mutations have been found in cohort studies of SIDS despite extensive screening of SCN5A. *CAV3* mutations are a rare cause of long QT syndrome in inherited arrhythmia syndromes but are common in SIDS. *SCN5A* mutations cause only approximately 5% to 10% of cases of long QT syndrome, but in SIDS, *SCN5A* accounts for 63% of the long QT syndrome–type mutations identified (see Table 76-2). Thus, the relative frequency of genetic defects in non-SIDS inherited arrhythmia syndromes is a poor predictor of their relative frequency in SIDS. Finally, novel gene discovery in SIDS has the potential to dramatically increase the percentage of SIDS cases that may potentially be explained by channelopathies.

Congenital Arrhythmia in Sudden Infant Death Syndrome: Triple Risk Hypothesis

Are channelopathies in SIDS fundamentally different than those in non-SIDS? What accounts for their early lethality? The triple risk hypothesis[23] for SIDS states that (1) a vulnerable infant (genetically predisposed), (2) a critical development period, and (3) an environmental trigger or stressor constitute the elements that come together to cause SIDS. The explanation for increased and early lethality could potentially come in at each level of risk. A point of interest is that abnormalities in the sodium current through mutations in *SCN5A*, *GPD1L*, and *CAV3* account for approximately 70% of channelopathies in SIDS, and for nearly 8% of SIDS cases overall. What implication does this finding have for the early lethality of SIDS? At the genetic level, the severity or character of the biophysical phenotype itself may account for the early lethality. For example, common LQT3 mutations such as ΔKPQ[24] and R1623Q[25] show slow inactivation of the late sodium current which accumulates at more rapid rates, thereby mitigating QT prolongation and predisposing to arrhythmia at slower rates, when QT is longest. Two mutations unique to SIDS, A997S and R1826H,[11] however, did not show this slow inactivation, and perhaps this feature accounts for the early lethality. A unique interaction with the environment may account for a more severe biophysical phenotype, as for those mutations in *SCN5A* such as S1103Y[4] and R680H and Δ586[5] that result in an augmented late sodium current at low pH. The magnitude of the dysfunction in low pH, however, was not more severe than with defects described in non-SIDS arrhythmia mutations. Although this is an attractive hypothesis for interaction of genetic background and environment (Fig. 76-1), it alone does not account for early lethality. Overall, the studies to date suggest that the severity of the biophysical phenotypes for SIDS mutations appears to be similar to that for non-SIDS mutations. Why such early deaths in SIDS with channelopathies? Does this effect merely represent the leading edge of the non-SIDS cases? The epidemiology of SIDS (deaths concentrated in months 3 to 5) and the different distribution of channelopathies and genetic defects between SIDS and non-SIDS suggest otherwise. Nevertheless, the mechanism for early lethality at the level of biophysical dysfunction remains unknown.

The early lethality may come from other genetic interactions. The common *SCN5A* polymorphism H558R markedly affects "wild-type" *SCN5A*[26] and also modifies the function of other mutations in *SCN5A*,[27,28] and it has been associated with atrial fibrillation, Brugada syndrome, and long QTc.[29,30,31] The allelic frequency of H558R was twice that expected (44% versus 21%) in SIDS cases with *SCN5A* mutations,[12] suggesting a "double hit," but the allelic frequency of H558R was no greater in SIDS cases overall (when patients without an *SCN5A* mutation were considered). The S1103Y mutation is a common polymorphism in the black population[32] with homozygosity associated with SIDS.[4] Three common polymorphisms in potassium channel genes (K897T in *KCNH2*, R1047L in *KCNH2*, and G38S in *KCNE1*) either were no different in SIDS or, in one case (R1047L), were actually lower in SIDS cases.[12]

In addition to channelopathies, genes for serotonin transporter, the autonomic nervous system, nicotine metabolism, inflammation, metabolism, and thermoregulation[33] all have been implicated in SIDS in accordance with hypotheses generated by clinical and epidemiologic data. These data support the common view that SIDS is likely to be a heterogeneous disorder but also suggest that lethality associated with arrhythmia in infancy may involve an intersection of several genetic factors causing predisposition to SIDS and contributing to development of arrhythmia. Finally, early death by arrhythmia may be influenced by environmental factors such as respiratory acidosis (see Fig. 76-1). This association provides a rationale for the apparent success of the move to prone sleeping in the "Back to Sleep" campaign.[34] The so-called triple risk hypothesis involving complex interaction of genetic background, developmental state, and environmental triggers remains an important model for the etiology of SIDS and may link disorders of different systems in causing SIDS.

Implications for Screening, Therapy, and Further Research

Primary genetic screening of all infants for channelopathies is not yet practicable. Not only do issues of expense and low yield need to be addressed, but such screening would uncover many rare variants of unknown significance. For example, in normal populations of different racial and ethnic backgrounds, approximately 3% of screened subjects have been found to harbor a mutation in *SCN5A*.[32] The possible significance of these variants in an asymptomatic populations is not immediately apparent. On the other hand, for SIDS victims and their families, a screen for channelopathies would now appear to be useful. An important unanswered question is how often channelopathies in SIDS are sporadic or de novo in the affected infant and not present in the parents. This consideration has important implications for inheritance and recurrence in siblings.

Primary ECG screening in neonates for long QT syndrome, however, as suggested by Schwartz and colleagues[35] may be a practical and cost-effective measure.[36] Issues of sensitivity and specificity and cost-effectiveness have been raised, but with the increasing evidence for the importance of channelopathies in SIDS and the prominent role of long QT syndrome in these channelopathies, the impetus for neonatal screening is increasing.[37] With the predominance of *SCN5A* long QT syndrome mutations in SIDS, the possible effectiveness of blocking of the late sodium current[38,4] (Chapter 16) in treating the primary biophysical abnormality suggests a potential pharmacologic therapy, in addition to other therapies such as beta-blockade and use of implanted defibrillators.

This chapter has focused on ion channelopathies as a cause or contributing factor to SIDS, and such channelopathies appear to occur in 10% to 15% of defined SIDS cases, with the possibility that more channelopathies and a higher frequency of channelopathies in SIDS may be discovered as research continues. The possibility also exists that arrhythmia related not to channelopathies but to other genetic or developmental factors also may contribute to SIDS. How these channelopathies contribute to such early death compared with the non-SIDS channelopathies requires further study. Investigation of the overall contribution of channelopathies and arrhythmia in SIDS is a part of the wider search into causes for SIDS.

References

1. Task Force on SIDS: The changing concept of sudden infant death syndrome: Diagnostic coding shifts, controversies regarding the sleeping environment, and new variables to consider in reducing risk. Pediatrics 116:1245, 2005.
2. Moon RY, Horne RS, Hauck FR: Sudden infant death syndrome. Lancet 370:1578, 2007.
3. Schwartz PJ, Crotti L: Cardiac arrhythmias of genetic origin are important contributors to sudden infant death syndrome. Heart Rhythm 4:740, 2007.
4. Plant LD, Bowers PN, Liu Q, et al: A common cardiac sodium channel variant associated with sudden infant death in African Americans, *SCN5A* S1103Y. J Clin Invest 116:430, 2006.
5. Wang DW, Desai RR, Crotti L, et al: Cardiac sodium channel dysfunction in sudden infant death syndrome. Circulation 115:368, 2007.
6. Schwartz PJ: Cardiac sympathetic innervation and the sudden infant death syndrome. A possible pathogenetic link. Am J Med 60:167, 1976.
7. Maron BJ, Clark CE, Goldstein RE, et al: Potential role of QT interval prolongation in sudden infant death syndrome. Circulation 54:423, 1976.
8. Schwartz PJ, Stramba-Badiale M, Segantini A, et al: Prolongation of the QT interval and the sudden infant death syndrome. N Engl J Med 338:1709, 1998.
9. Schwartz PJ, Priori SG, Dumaine R, et al: A molecular link between the sudden infant death syndrome and the long-QT syndrome. N Engl J Med 343:262, 2000.
10. Wedekind H, Smits JP, Schulze-Bahr E, et al: De novo mutation in the *SCN5A* gene associated with early onset of sudden infant death. Circulation 104:1158, 2001.
11. Ackerman MJ, Siu BL, Sturner WQ, et al: Postmortem molecular analysis of *SCN5A* defects in sudden infant death syndrome. JAMA 286:2264, 2001.
12. Arnestad M, Crotti L, Rognum TO, et al: Prevalence of long-QT syndrome gene variants in sudden infant death syndrome. Circulation 115:361, 2007.
13. Splawski I, Timothy KW, Tateyama M, et al: Variant of *SCN5A* sodium channel implicated in risk of cardiac arrhythmia. Science 297:1333, 2002.
14. Cronk LB, Ye B, Kaku T, et al: Novel mechanism for sudden infant death syndrome: Persistent late sodium current secondary to mutations in caveolin-3. Heart Rhythm 4:161, 2007.
15. Schwartz PJ, Priori SG, Bloise R, et al: Molecular diagnosis in a child with sudden infant death syndrome. Lancet 358:1342, 2001.
16. Christiansen M, Tonder N, Larsen LA, et al: Mutations in the HERG K^+ ion channel: A novel link between long QT syndrome and sudden infant death syndrome. Am J Cardiol 95:433, 2005.
17. Lehnart SE, Ackerman MJ, Benson DW Jr, et al: Inherited arrhythmias: A National Heart, Lung, and Blood Institute and Office of Rare Diseases workshop consensus report about the diagnosis, phenotyping, molecular mechanisms, and therapeutic approaches for primary cardiomyopathies of gene mutations affecting ion channel function. Circulation 116:2325, 2007.
18. London B, Michalec M, Mehdi H, et al: Mutation in glycerol-3-phosphate dehydrogenase 1 like gene (GPD1-L) decreases cardiac Na^+ current and causes inherited arrhythmias. Circulation 116:2260, 2007.
19. Skinner JR, Chung SK, Montgomery D, et al: Near-miss SIDS due to Brugada syndrome. Arch Dis Child 90:528, 2005.
20. Van Norstrand DW, Valdivia CR, Tester DJ, et al: Molecular and functional characterization of novel glycerol-3-phosphate dehydrogenase 1 like gene (GPD1-L) mutations in sudden infant death syndrome. Circulation 116:2253, 2007.
21. Tester DJ, Dura M, Carturan E, et al: A mechanism for sudden infant death syndrome (SIDS): Stress-induced leak via ryanodine receptors. Heart Rhythm 4:733, 2007.
22. Giustetto C, Di Monte F, Wolpert C, et al: Short QT syndrome: Clinical findings and diagnostic-therapeutic implications. Eur Heart J 27:2440, 2006.
23. Filiano JJ, Kinney HC: A perspective on neuropathologic findings in victims of the sudden infant death syndrome: The triple-risk model. Biol Neonate 65:194, 1994.
24. Nagatomo T, January CT, Ye B, et al: Rate-dependent QT shortening mechanism for the LQT3 deltaKPQ mutant. Cardiovasc Res 54:624, 2002.
25. Oginosawa Y, Nagatomo T, Abe H, et al: Intrinsic mechanism of the enhanced rate-dependent QT shortening in the R1623Q mutant of the LQT3 syndrome. Cardiovasc Res 65:138, 2005.
26. Makielski JC, Ye B, Valdivia CR, et al: A ubiquitous splice variant and a common polymorphism affect heterologous expression of recombinant human *SCN5A* heart sodium channels. Circ Res 93:821, 2003.
27. Ye B, Valdivia CR, Ackerman MJ, et al: A common human *SCN5A* polymorphism modifies expression of an arrhythmia causing mutation. Physiol Genomics 12:187, 2003.
28. Viswanathan PC, Benson DW, Balser JR: A common *SCN5A* polymorphism modulates the biophysical effects of an SCN5A mutation. J Clin Invest 111:341, 2003.
29. Chen LY, Ballew JD, Herron KJ, et al: A common polymorphism in *SCN5A* is associated with lone atrial fibrillation. Clin Pharmacol Ther 81:35, 2007.
30. Gouas L, Nicaud V, Berthet M, et al: Association of KCNQ1, KCNE1, KCNH2 and *SCN5A* polymorphisms with QTc interval length in a healthy population. Eur J Hum Genet 13:1213, 2005.
31. Chen JZ, Xie XD, Wang XX, et al: Single nucleotide polymorphisms of the *SCN5A* gene in Han Chinese and their relation with Brugada syndrome. Chin Med J (Engl) 117:652, 2004.
32. Ackerman MJ, Splawski I, Makielski JC, et al: Spectrum and prevalence of cardiac sodium channel variants among black, white, Asian, and Hispanic individuals: Implications for arrhythmogenic susceptibility and Brugada/long QT syndrome genetic testing. Heart Rhythm 1:600, 2004.
33. Weese-Mayer DE, Ackerman MJ, Marazita ML, et al: Sudden infant death syndrome: Review of implicated genetic factors. Am J Med Genet A 143:771, 2007.
34. Mitchell EA, Hutchison L, Stewart AW: The continuing decline in SIDS mortality. Arch Dis Child 92:625, 2007.
35. Schwartz PJ: Pro: Newborn ECG screening to prevent sudden cardiac death. Heart Rhythm 3:1353, 2006.
36. Quaglini S, Rognoni C, Spazzolini C, et al: Cost-effectiveness of neonatal ECG screening for the long QT syndrome. Eur Heart J 27:1824, 2006.

37. Berul CI, Perry JC: Contribution of long-QT syndrome genes to sudden infant death syndrome: Is it time to consider newborn electrocardiographic screening? Circulation 115:294, 2007.

38. Nagatomo T, January CT, Makielski JC: Preferential block of late sodium current in the LQT3 (KPQ mutant by the class I(C) antiarrhythmic flecainide. Mol Pharmacol 57:101, 2000.

39. Makielski JC: SIDS: Genetic and environmental influences may cause arrhythmia in this silent killer. J Clin Invest 116:297, 2006.

Sudden Cardiac Death 77

Robert J. Myerburg and Agustin Castellanos

CHAPTER OUTLINE

Sudden cardiac death (SCD) is defined as death following cardiac arrest in a patient with or without known preexisting heart disease, in whom the mode and time of death are unexpected. Although the concept of "unexpected" is a key feature of the SCD definition, clinical markers that identify enhanced predisposition to cardiac arrest—such as heart failure or transient ischemia—have been identified. Nevertheless, a high proportion of SCD's occur as first clinical events, especially in patients with previously unrecognized ischemic heart disease or inherited arrhythmogenic disorders.

The generally accepted temporal definition is bracketed by a period of up to 1 hour between the onset of an abrupt change in clinical status and loss of consciousness.[1] This time period is more appropriate for definitions used in population studies and clinical analyses than is the absolute definition of biologic death, which may be delayed for days to a month or more by life-support interventions after central nervous system (CNS) injury that may result from the cardiac arrest. The 1-hour definition better relates to the pathophysiology leading to the ultimate death.

Sudden Cardiac Death as a Public Health Burden: Estimates of Incidence

For more than 25 years, the incidence of SCD in the United States has been estimated at 300,000 to 350,000 events per year. Unfortunately, the basis for these estimates derives not from direct epidemiologic studies but rather from observational data, such as retrospective death certificate analyses and assumptions about the proportions of cardiovascular deaths that are sudden. During the past few years, conflicting statements have been put forward regarding the current incidence of SCD. An estimate from the American Heart Association's statistical handbook,[2] based on data from the National Center For Health Statistics (NCHS) and the National Heart, Lung, and Blood Institute (NHLBI), suggested an annual incidence of less than 250,000 SCDs. An additional analysis from the Seattle, Washington, emergency medical system (EMS) database, extrapolated to total U.S. population numbers, calculated 184,000 cardiac arrests nationwide in the year 2000,[3] a significant decrease compared with 1980 statistics. Another community-based study from Oregon based on prospective medical examiner data plus other sources of data also yielded a national extrapolation of less than 200,000.[4] By contrast, a death certificate–based study, also from the NCHS, suggested that more than 50% of all cardiac deaths are sudden and estimated the total annual incidence of SCD to be in the range of 460,000.[5]

The large discrepancy between the two estimates from NCHS death certificate data stems from differences in definitions of SCD used and population sources. The American Heart Association data are derived solely from coronary heart disease cases, with narrow definitions based on selected International Classification of Diseases–Ninth Revision (ICD-9) codes (410 to 414) (Fig. 77-1A), whereas the more comprehensive NCHS study included almost all causes of SCD (see Fig. 77-1C). The much broader range of inclusion in the latter study resulted in the much larger estimate and perhaps even somewhat overestimated the true incidence. The Seattle data include only SCDs involving emergency rescue responses (see Fig. 77-1B), whereas the Oregon study population is not necessarily representative of the incidence variations within the entire U.S. population. Although the NCHS data sources also are limited by the known hazards of using death certificate data as a basis for epidemiologic estimates,[6] it is likely that the overall U.S. health burden of SCD is closer to the higher estimate than to the lower estimates. This notion is supported by the fact that the strongly emphasized reduction in age-related risk of coronary heart disease mortality during the past 40 to 50 years, when translated to total number of events and size of populations at risk for future events, cannot be interpreted to mean that absolute prevalence of disease and incidence of fatal events have decreased.[7] Rather, the population pool from which coronary events derive (patients with or without known heart disease) continues to grow with better therapies for acute coronary syndromes and longer-term therapies for chronic heart disease.[8] A prospective epidemiologic study, designed to provide accurate counts of SCDs and its specific mechanisms, would be a wise investment to help future health needs planning and clinical research designs.

A

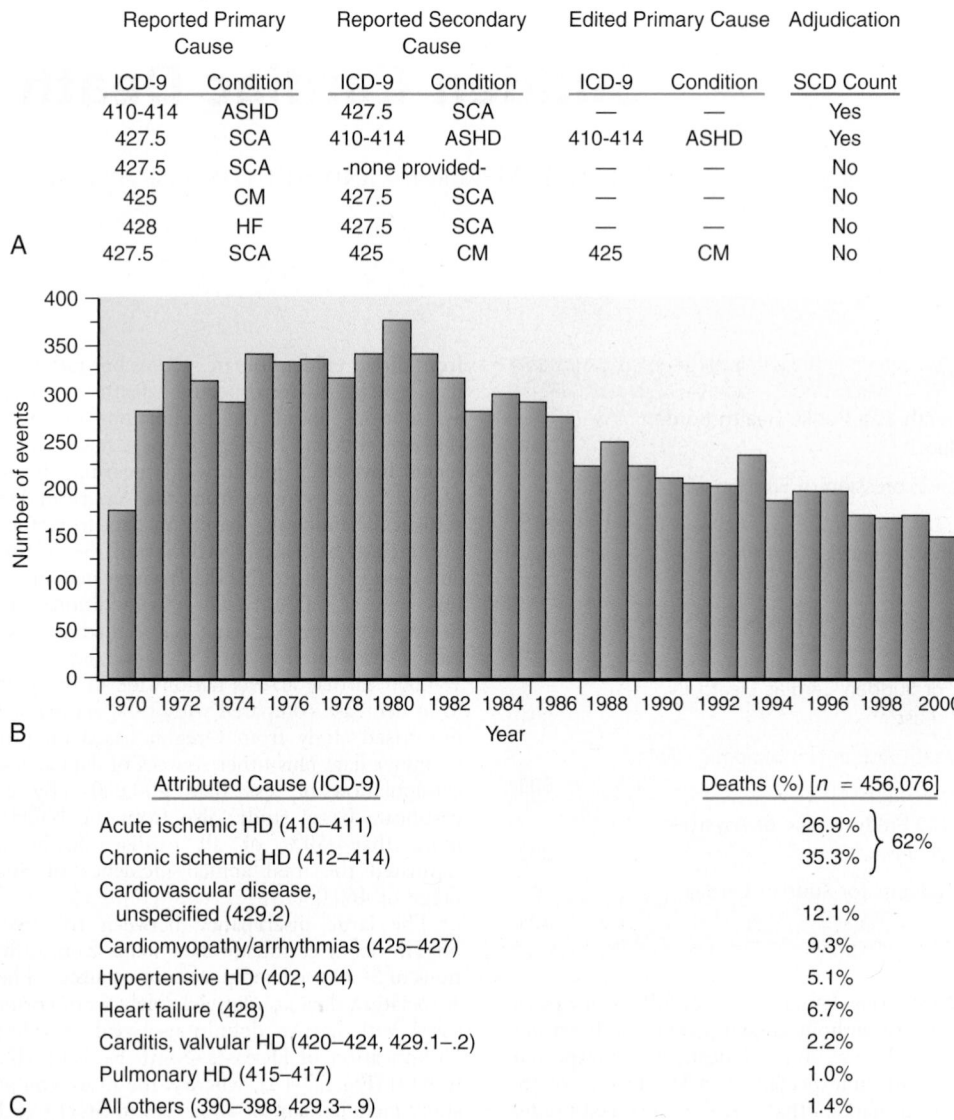

Reported Primary Cause		Reported Secondary Cause		Edited Primary Cause		Adjudication
ICD-9	Condition	ICD-9	Condition	ICD-9	Condition	SCD Count
410-414	ASHD	427.5	SCA	—	—	Yes
427.5	SCA	410-414	ASHD	410-414	ASHD	Yes
427.5	SCA	-none provided-		—	—	No
425	CM	427.5	SCA	—	—	No
428	HF	427.5	SCA	—	—	No
427.5	SCA	425	CM	425	CM	No

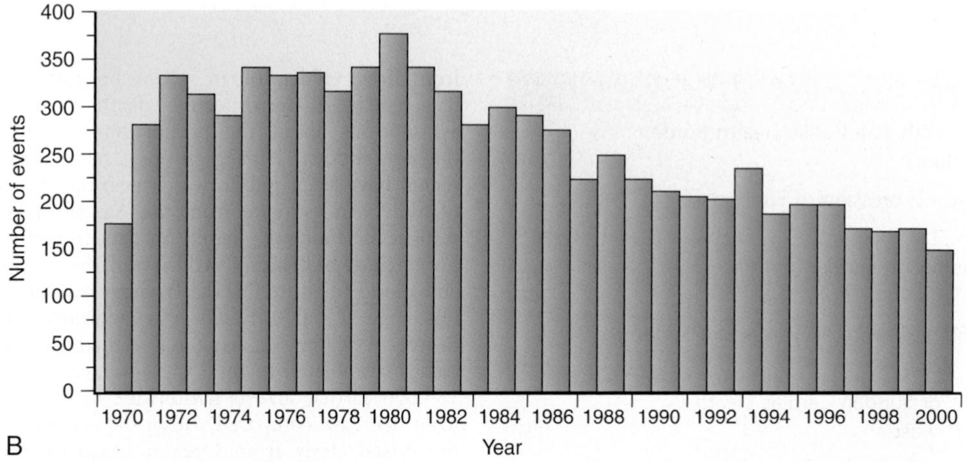

B

C

Attributed Cause (ICD-9)	Deaths (%) [n = 456,076]	
Acute ischemic HD (410–411)	26.9%	62%
Chronic ischemic HD (412–414)	35.3%	
Cardiovascular disease, unspecified (429.2)	12.1%	
Cardiomyopathy/arrhythmias (425–427)	9.3%	
Hypertensive HD (402, 404)	5.1%	
Heart failure (428)	6.7%	
Carditis, valvular HD (420–424, 429.1–.2)	2.2%	
Pulmonary HD (415–417)	1.0%	
All others (390–398, 429.3–.9)	1.4%	

Figure 77-1 Basis of conflicting estimates on the incidence of sudden cardiac death (SCD) in the United States. Recent estimates range from less than 185,000 to greater than 450,000 SCDs annually. Most of the estimates are derived from retrospective analysis of death certificate data, and none is based on a prospective analysis of a population representative of the entire country. Each study useds different inclusion criteria. In **A**, the data available in the American Heart Association (AHA) Statistical Handbook are limited to out-of-hospital cardiac arrest with a diagnosis of coronary heart disease, using specific International Classification of Diseases (ICD) codes (410 to 414). This source estimates 220,000 SCDs annually. In **B**, the annual incidence of ventricular fibrillation identified by the Seattle Emergency Rescue System is shown to have decreased between 1980 and 2000. Extrapolating these data to all cardiac arrests in the Seattle community, and then, in turn, to the nation as a whole, an incidence of 184,000 SCDs per year is estimated. In **C**, with the data reported from the National Center for Health Statistics, using a broader range of etiologic definitions for SCD (note the ICD-9 codes used), it is demonstrated that only 62% of all SCDs have a primary diagnosis using the ICD codes on which the AHA estimates are based. This source suggests an annual frequency of more than 450,000 SCDs in the United States. A prospective study using uniform criteria is desirable for clarifying the actual incidence of SCD in the United States. ASHD, arteriosclerotic heart disease; CM, cardiomyopathy; HD, heart disease; HF, heart failure; SCA, sudden cardiac arrest. (**A**, From Myerburg RJ: Scientific gaps in the prediction and prevention of sudden cardiac death. J Cardiovasc Electrophysiol 13:709-723, 2002; **B**, from Cobb LA, Fahrenbruch CE, Olsufka M, Copass MK: Changing incidence of out-of-hospital ventricular fibrillation, 1980-2000. JAMA 288:3008-3013, 2002; **C**, from Zheng ZJ, Croft JB, Giles WH, Mensah GA: Sudden cardiac death in the United States 1989 to 1998. Circulation 104:2158-2163, 2001.)

Causes and Clinical Expressions of Sudden Cardiac Death

Among the general population in the Western hemisphere, coronary heart disease is the most common etiologic basis for SCD. Although estimates vary, it is generally agreed that approximately 75% to 80% of all SCDs in the United States and western Europe are due to this one underlying etiology.[1] The second most frequent category of disorders associated with SCD is the cardiomyopathies. Most definitions of this category have included both dilated cardiomyopathy (DCM) and hypertrophic cardiomyopathy (HCM), but the hypertrophic form probably is more appropriately counted among the rare genetic syndromes associated with SCD risk, for both clinical and epidemiologic reasons. The DCMs collectively account for approximately

10% to 15% of all SCDs. Many studies of SCD risk and interventions fail to separate the DCMs into those of ischemic versus nonischemic etiology, or to distinguish between DCM as an etiology and congestive heart failure (CHF) as a clinical expression.

The various infiltrative, inflammatory, and valvular diseases constitute the underlying cause in most of the remaining SCDs. One such disorder is clinically silent myocarditis. Its frequency is uncertain because of the difficulty validating its presence, even histopathologically. It has been considered to be among the more common causes of SCD in adolescents and young adults,[9] but its incidence is debated because of inconsistent criteria for the diagnosis. More recently, the recognition of persistence of viral DNA fragments in myocytes of SCD victims, even without inflammatory markers, further confounds the issue.[10]

Only a small proportion of SCDs, occurring predominantly in adolescents and young adults (including athletes), are due to the rare genetically determined disorders, such as long QT syndrome, Brugada syndrome, HCM, right ventricular dysplasia, and other congenital disorders that are not inherited, such as aortic stenosis and anomalous coronary arteries. Cumulatively, these rare disorders account for no more than 1% to 2% of the total SCD burden, but recent information is beginning to emerge suggesting that some mutations in genes encoding ion channels, which are phenotypically normal at baseline, create a propensity to arrhythmia expression under triggering conditions.[11] Proarrhythmic responses to drugs are an example.[12,13]

The spectrum of patterns of clinical expression of the SCD syndrome ranges from anticipated events in high-risk patients with identified advanced heart disease to those persons with unrecognized or new-onset conditions in which SCD is the first clinical manifestation (Fig. 77-2). An intermediate category of patients has known heart disease but is considered to be at low risk, based on extent and stability of disease. Among the highest-risk categories are subgroups associated with low ejection fractions, based on previous myocardial infarctions or nonischemic cardiomyopathies and various other myocardial or valvular conditions, or those with high-risk arrhythmia markers after myocardial infarction or in the presence of other structural diseases. Among these groups of patients, the probability of a potentially fatal cardiac arrest is high, but the positive and negative predictive accuracies of most methods of profiling risk for individual patients is still somewhat limited.[14] At the other end of the spectrum, encompassing patients without previously identified heart disease, cardiac arrest is commonly the first clinical manifestation of the underlying disease. These subjects, and those with known heart disease but low-risk markers (ejection fractions greater than 40 percent, no heart failure, no arrhythmias) numerically constitute a large proportion of sudden cardiac deaths, but in terms of relative risk are at the low end of the spectrum of risk. Those patients with cardiac arrest as an expression of an acute coronary syndrome are of particular interest on the basis of recent data suggesting that this manifestation of acute coronary syndromes clusters in families and may have a genetic basis[15] (see later on).

Pathologic Findings in Sudden Cardiac Death Victims

Much of the information available on the pathologic anatomy in SCD victims reflects the predominance of coronary heart disease as the major underlying etiologic disorder. Both the extent of coronary artery disease and the resulting abnormalities in ventricular myocardium have been well described. It has been recognized for many years that extensive coronary atherosclerosis is the primary anatomic hallmark of coronary heart disease–related SCDs.[1] Also recognized in recent years, however, has been a close association of SCD with the presence of plaque fissuring or erosion, platelet aggregation, and acute thrombosis within the matrix of coronary atherosclerosis.[16,17] This feature of coronary artery anatomy, superimposed on chronic lesions, does not differ among the three primary expressions of acute coronary syndromes—namely, SCD, acute myocardial infarction, and unstable angina pectoris. Various studies have demonstrated the presence of one or more active coronary lesions in up to 90% of SCD victims.[18] The active plaque state and its consequences (plaque disruption with hemorrhage into the plaque or intraluminal thrombosis associated with fissuring or erosion) are more important than degree of chronic occlusion in the pathophysiology of acute coronary syndromes, including SCD.

Myocardial pathology reflects the presence and extent of chronic coronary atherosclerosis, in that myocardial scars, due to healed myocardial infarction, are common.[19] Evidence of acute myocardial infarction is far less common, probably because the pathophysiologic mechanism leading to that expression is interrupted by a fatal arrhythmia. However, even among cardiac

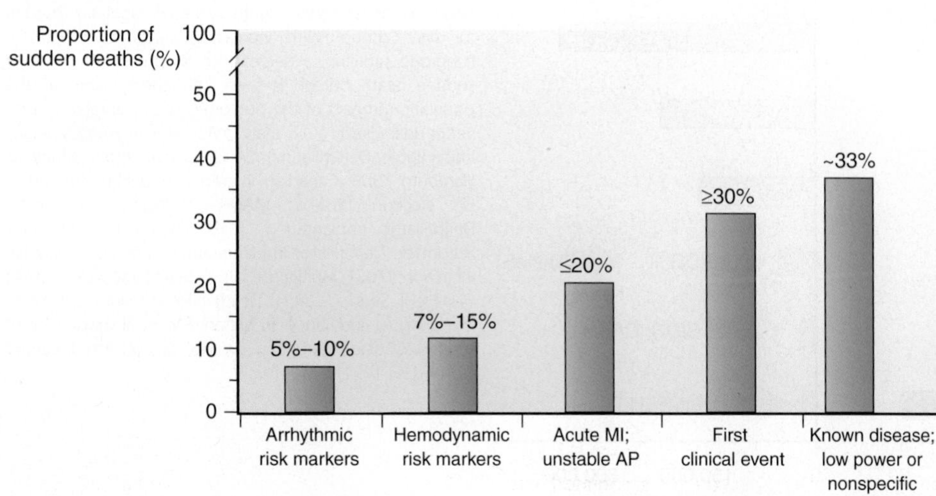

Figure 77-2 Clinical status of sudden cardiac death victims. Effectively predicting cardiac arrest among a high percentage of potential victims is difficult, because nearly two thirds of cardiac arrests occur as a first clinically manifested event or in the clinical setting of known disease in the absence of strong risk predictors. Less than 25% of the victims have high-risk markers based on arrhythmic or hemodynamic parameters. Persons at very high risk constitute a proportionately smaller segment of the population base. AP, angina pectoris; MI, myocardial infarction. (From Myerburg RJ: Sudden cardiac death: Exploring the limits of our knowledge. J Cardiovasc Electrophysiol 12:369-381, 2001.)

arrest survivors studied during the prethrombolytic or percutaneous coronary intervention (PCI) era, evolution to acute transmural myocardial infarction was less common.[20] An association between the number of involved coronary arteries and the extent of ventricular hypertrophy in SCD victims also has been recognized.[21] A correlation between extensive coronary artery disease and left ventricular hypertrophy might be a consequence of longstanding hypertension as a risk factor in coronary heart disease patients or of post–myocardial infarction remodeling. Regardless of the mechanism, both myocardial scars and left ventricular hypertrophy are considered factors in arrhythmogenesis during transient ischemia.[1,7]

Among the less common causes of SCD, pathologic anatomy reflects the underlying etiology. In the DCMs, the pathologic findings are nonspecific, characterized by interstitial fibrosis and myocyte degeneration. In HCMs, the anatomy depends on the specific form of the disease. Obstructive, nonobstructive, apical, and concentric hypertrophy patterns all are observed, some of which are dependent on the specific genetic pattern of the inherited forms.[22] One common feature observed in HCM is myocyte disarray, which is common to most but not all genetic forms of the disease. The association between HCM expression and SCD risk is complex because of patterns of inheritance involving not only multiple gene loci but mutation-specific risk.

With SCD due to myocarditis, histopathologic patterns may be variable. Acute viral myocarditis commonly is associated with high-grade inflammatory processes in the myocardium, but some forms of a viral myocarditis associated with viral DNA remnants in the cytosol may demonstrate diffuse fibrosis, without inflammatory markers.[10]

Prediction and Strategies for Prevention of Sudden Cardiac Death

The clinical usefulness and impact of SCD risk predictors are complex. Risk analysis must be divided into two general categories—population-based risk prediction and individual risk prediction. With respect to individual risk, a broad range of predictive power is characteristic, depending on the specific measures of risk used.[7,23,24] Conventional epidemiologic markers provide valuable statements about population risk, especially for the development of coronary heart disease, but individual risk prediction remains the major limitation for applying preventive strategies clinically. The inverse relationship between the incidence of SCD and absolute numbers of events in the various epidemiologic or clinical categories is important to appreciate (Fig. 77-3), especially when the intent is to use therapeutic interventions.[25] Among the general population, aged 35 years and beyond, the approximate SCD incidence of 0.1% to 0.2% per year incorporates all of the sudden deaths that occur annually in the United States. However, the low individual event rate among the general population, unselected except for age, limits the range of therapeutic approaches applicable. If patients who fall into categories of high risk for development of coronary atherosclerosis and unselected patients with established coronary heart disease are included, event rates are higher but still have limited power of individual risk prediction. By contrast, patients with heart failure or ejection fractions less than 35 percent, cardiac arrest survivors, and the specific high-risk post–myocardial infarction patients have higher event rates, but constitute decreasing absolute numbers of events and a much smaller component of the total population burden of SCD.[23] The importance of recognizing this principle relates to the magnitude of population benefit for various preventive interventions. For example, the very high-risk patient categories studied in the clinical trials of implantable defibrillators (see Fig. 77-3) constitute only a small part of the total universe of SCDs, and the reported benefits apply only to those small subgroups. This observation highlights the importance of finding specific risk markers for more general segments of the population, from which the potential for greater public health impact can emerge.

The foregoing concepts can be viewed in the context of clinical patterns preceding cardiac arrest in patients with coronary heart disease. A number of studies suggest that 30% or more of all SCDs due to coronary heart disease occur as the first clinical event, and that approximately 33% more are associated with clinical markers suggesting a low risk for an event (see Fig. 77-2). Only a small proportion of the deaths in this etiologic category are defined by high-risk markers, such as post–myocardial infarction ventricular arrhythmias, low ejection fractions, or reduced functional capacity. A major impact on SCD as a population problem will require the development of

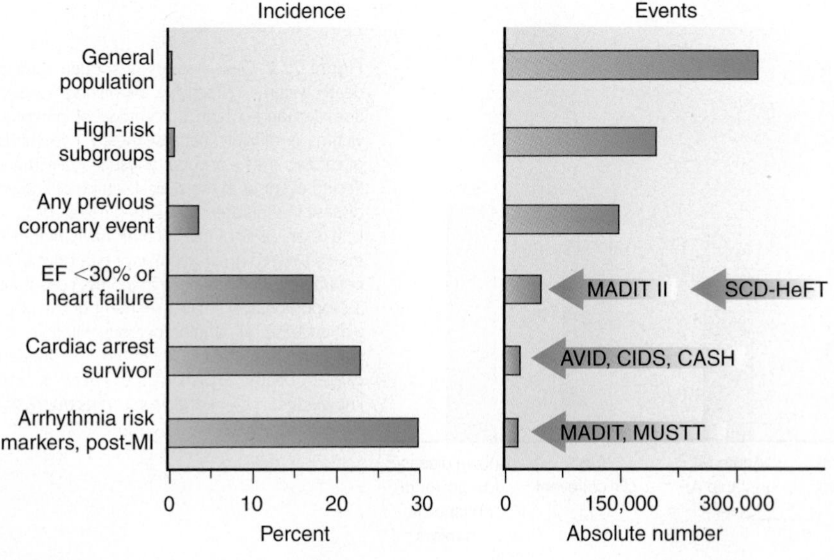

Figure 77-3 Relationship among population subsets, incidence of sudden cardiac death, and total population burden for each group. With increasing incidence, based on subgroup profiling, a decrease in proportion of the total sudden death burden is seen. This effect relates to the population impact of the outcomes of implantable cardioverter-defibrillator (ICD) trials. AVID, Antiarrhythmics versus Implantable Defibrillators; CASH, Cardiac Arrest Study of Hamburg; CIDS, Canadian Implantable Defibrillator Study; EF, ejection fraction; MADIT, Multicenter Automatic Defibrillator Implantation Trial; MADIT II, Multicenter Automatic Defibrillator Implantation Trial II; MI, myocardial infarction; MUST, Multicenter Unsustained Tachycardia Trial; SCD-HeFT, Sudden Cardiac Death in Heart Failure Trial. (From Myerburg RJ, Interian A Jr, Mitrani RM, et al: Frequency of sudden cardiac death and profiles of risk. Am J Cardiol 80:10F-19F, 1997.)

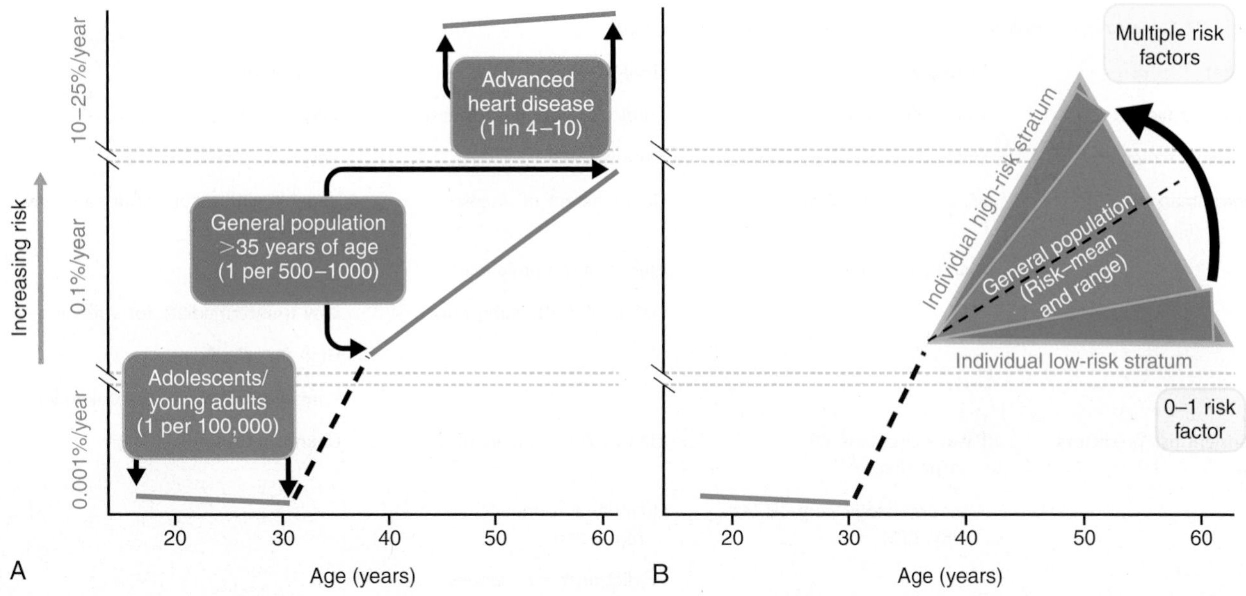

Figure 77-4 Age-related risk for sudden cardiac death (SCD). **A,** For the general population 35 years of age and older, the risk of SCD is 0.1 to 0.2 percent per year (1 per 500 to 1,000 population), and the age risk curve is steep *(middle curve)*. For the same population, subgrouped for advanced heart disease, the latter blunts the age-risk relationship *(top curve)*. Among adolescents and young adults, the risk is 1 per 100,000 population, or 0.001% per year, and the age-risk relationship is inverse *(bottom curve)*, with a higher risk at the younger end of the range because of enhanced expression of inherited disorders after puberty. **B,** The age-risk curve for the general population older than 35 years of age is an expression of the average risk among a population that reflects the cumulative effects of higher and lower risk strata. Identification of the discriminating risk factors would allow more accurate risk profiling for individual patients within the general population. (Modified from Myerburg RJ, Castellanos A: Cardiac arrest and sudden cardiac death. In Zipes D, Libby P, Bonow RO, Braunwald E [eds]: Heart Disease: A Textbook of Cardiovascular Medicine, 7th ed. Philadelphia, Saunders, 2004, 865-908.)

strategies to identify risk among more general subgroups, with a much higher level of accuracy, than is currently possible using available indices of individual risk prediction.

Magnitude of risk of SCD is a complex epidemiologic and clinic function, even within subgrouped categories of risk (Fig. 77-4A). Increasing age is a powerful risk predictor among the adult population (younger than 35 years) that becomes blunted in the presence of advanced heart disease, when it is overwhelmed by higher risk clinical factors. The general population is viewed as being composed of multiple layers of risk, the identification of which is pertinent to accurate individual risk prediction (see Fig. 77-4B). In the adolescent and younger adult population, overall risk is considerably lower than the general middle-aged adult population (1 per 100,000 per year, versus 1 to 2 per 1000 per year), with the age-risk relationship being inverse—the younger in this spectrum being at higher risk.

Prediction of Risk of Sudden Cardiac Death in Coronary Heart Disease

The evolution and expression of SCD due to coronary heart disease involves a multitiered cascade of pathophysiology, operating in different time domains (Fig. 77-5). These include initiation and progression of disease in the coronary arteries,

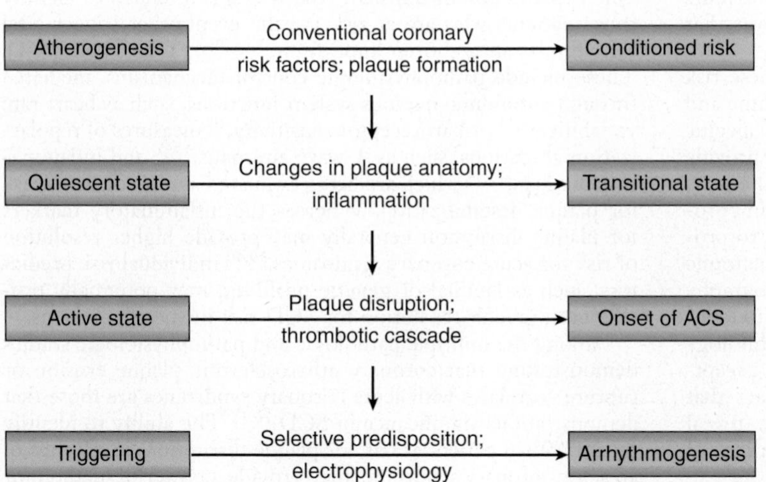

Figure 77-5 Cascade from conventional risk factors to arrhythmogenesis in sudden cardiac death due to coronary heart disease. The cascade identifies four levels of evolution of risk: (1) lesion initiation and development, (2) onset of an active state, (3) onset of acute coronary syndromes (ACSs), and (4) the specific expression of life-threatening cardiac arrhythmias. Multiple factors enter at each level, including specific risk based on genetic profiles of individual patients. (From Myerburg RJ: Scientific gaps in the prediction and prevention of sudden cardiac death. J Cardiovasc Electrophysiol 13:709-723, 2002.)

Table 77-1 Indicators of Risk for Arrhythmic Sudden Cardiac Death (SCD)*

Target	Examples	Goal	Sensitivity
ASHD risk factors	Framingham risk index	Predict evolution of disease	Very low
Anatomic screening	Electron beam tomography	Identify CAD	Very low
Clinical markers	EF; angiography; AM; EPS	Define extent of disease	Variable with extent of disease; low specificity
	AM/EPS combined with EF	Identify arrhythmia markers	
		Define high-risk subgroups	Low to intermediate for screening
			High for specific groups
			Primary predictive value unknown
Transient risk predictors	T wave alternans; QT dispersion	Identify ECG markers of risk	Unknown, potentially high
	Pathophysiologic controls (e.g., HRV, BRS)	Quantify autonomic regulation	
		Predict unstable plaques	
	Inflammatory markers		
Individual risk predictors	Familial/genetic profiles	Predict specific SCD risk before disease expression	High potential for future profiling
			Uncertain; some measures useful(?)

*The conventional risk factors and anatomic disease screening have some general use for predicting risk, but sensitivity is very low and nonspecific for arrhythmatic deaths. Transient risk predictors and individual risk predictors offer the hope for more powerful individual prediction of SCD.

From Myerburg RJ: Sudden cardiac death: Exploring the limits of our knowledge. J Cardiovasc Electrophysiol 12:369-381, 2001.

AM, ambulatory monitor; ASHD, arteriosclerotic heart disease; BRS, baroreflex sensitivity; CAD, coronary artery disease; ECG, electrocardiogram; EF, ejection fraction; EPS, electrophysiologic studies; HRV, heart rate variability; QT, QT interval.

transition of vascular lesions from quiescent to active states, initiation of acute coronary syndromes, and, finally, acute arrhythmogenesis. In the early years of attention to risk factors for SCD, the recognition of the major role played by coronary artery disease led to the use of conventional risk factors for coronary artery disease as the major focus for prediction of risk of SCD[26] (Table 77-1; see also Fig. 77-5). From a statistical and public health standpoint, this approach was (and remains) reasonable because of the large proportion and numbers of SCDs that are attributable to coronary artery disease. In fact, a recent report supports the notion that both preventive therapeutics and treatment strategies during and after coronary events contribute significantly and nearly equally to reduction of cardiovascular mortality rates,[27] including SCD.

This concept is limited, however, by the fact that these risk factors largely predict the evolution of the disease over time and identify orders of magnitude of risk that are too low for specific antiarrhythmic interventions. Furthermore, they do not provide a specific marker of risk for arrhythmic deaths. Other methods for identifying the presence of structural abnormalities in coronary arteries have been suggested as potential strategies to provide greater sensitivity and specificity. For example, anatomic disease screening using of electron beam computed tomography has been suggested as a method for large-scale screening to identify abnormal coronary arteries.[28] Although this technology identifies structural changes in coronary arteries with an acceptable degree of accuracy, its value is limited by the fact that identification of the structural abnormality does not reveal the extent and vulnerability of lesions or specific markers of arrhythmic risk.

Much of the progress that has been made to date in profiling risk of SCD has been based on clinical markers, which primarily identify the extent of disease, either at a myocardial level or at a vascular level (see Table 77-1). Ischemic cardiomyopathy identifies high risk for SCD, which is particularly notable when accompanied by a history of clinical heart failure. Although resolution of overall risk is more powerful, it is still nonspecific because of its general inability to discriminate arrhythmic death from other forms of death.

In order to achieve better profiling of arrhythmic risk, two approaches appear promising for application in future studies. One is prediction of transient risk, which is intended to identify those patients who are at risk for the events that trigger fatal arrhythmias in a shorter time frame[7,25,29-32] (see Table 77-1). These include pathophysiologic control mechanisms, mediated through autonomic nervous system functions, such as heart rate variability[24,33] or baroreceptor sensitivity,[34] measures of repolarization alterations, such as T wave alternans,[35,36] and inflammatory markers,[37,38] which are being evaluated as a predictor of risk for plaque destabilization. Whereas the inflammatory markers for plaque disruption generally may provide higher resolution of risk for acute coronary syndromes,[39,40] individual risk predictors, such as familial or genetic profiling, may potentially provide even greater resolution for SCD risk in specific persons.

Among the multiple pathologic and pathophysiologic studies demonstrating that coronary atherosclerotic plaque erosion or rupture correlates with acute coronary syndromes are those that demonstrate its significance in SCD.[16,17] The ability to identify the individual patient at risk for plaque disruption, in advance of an acute coronary syndrome, may provide a powerful method for identifying individuals at potential risk of SCD. In recent retrospective studies of men[41] and women[42] in whom both cholesterol levels and indices of inflammation could be correlated with risk of coronary events, it was observed that each appeared to provide an independent predictive value, and this combination had the strongest power of prediction of relative risk increase. However, because the outcomes were expressed as relative increases of a baseline risk among the subjects in the lowest terciles of cholesterol and inflammatory marker concentration, the absolute contribution of inflammatory markers (compared with cholesterol markers) remains to be determined. If the order of magnitude of absolute risk predicted by inflammatory markers is considerably higher than that predicted by cholesterol markers, a new marker of risk with greater potential power of resolution of risk may become available. A recent observation suggesting that complex plaques may be multiple, possibly indicating a generalized susceptibility to plaque disruption (rather than plaque-specific risk) and a higher recurrent event rate after myocardial infarction,[43] supports the notion of inflammation-based susceptibility. Other direct and indirect markers of risk of plaque destabilization from inflammatory processes also may potentially contribute to this theory of risk prediction.[44]

Familial clustering of SCD suggests a different and potentially additive benefit to risk resolution. Data from the Paris Prospective Study on risk factors for SCD[45] identified the fact that a history of parental sudden death predicted sudden death as the expression of an acute coronary event, with a nearly two-fold increase in relative risk. Family history of SCD had no impact on risk of nonsudden fatal myocardial infarction. A similar observation was reported from a retrospective analysis of cardiac arrest survivors in King County, Washington.[46] Studies from The Netherlands[14] and Finland [47] also demonstrated a familial pattern of SCD as an initial manifestation of acute coronary syndromes, in contrast with nonfatal myocardial infarctions. Family clustering may result either from cultural or environmental influences or from genetic factors. Whereas the King County study was inconclusive in regard to this distinction, the prospective study from Paris[46] and the Finnish study[47] both favored a genetic basis, because the gradient of risk increased when multiple relatives had a history of SCD.

Sudden Cardiac Death Risk in Nonischemic Dilated Cardiomyopathy

SCD among patients with nonischemic cardiomyopathies, including the familial dilated cardiomyopathies,[48] is more difficult to predict. Although left ventricular ejection fraction is a strong mortality risk predictor generally among patients who have DCM, it is not as useful for specifically predicting SCD as in coronary artery disease. A better association with functional capacity has been proposed.[49,50] For example, among patients with DCM assigned to functional class I, the risk of dying is small, but the proportional probability that a death will be sudden, if it occurs, is relatively high. The fact that this category encompasses a large number of patients at relatively low risk limits the predictive power for benefit from interventions. At the other end of the spectrum, functional class III and class IV patients are at a higher risk of death generally and at a higher risk for SCD in terms of absolute numbers of deaths,[50] although the proportional risk of sudden death is somewhat lower. Moreover, among patients who experience sudden death in this category, many have nonshockable rhythms, and some shockable rhythms are secondary to the hemodynamic state and resistant to defibrillation, possibly limiting the practical benefit of implantable cardioverter-defibrillators (ICDs) in this group as well.[51]

For this etiologic category of sudden cardiac death, discriminators of risk across the entire spectrum of disease expression, from early to advanced, are inconsistent. The importance of this limitation resides in the fact that the absolute number of SCDs counted among the relatively low-risk subgroups, which do not justify advanced interventions on a statistical basis, is disturbingly high. Future research must focus on discrimination of risk within the larger lower-risk population subsets,[52] as well as SCDs that occur in the familial forms of DCM.[48]

Tachyarrhythmic and Bradysystolic or Asystolic Cardiac Arrest Mechanisms

Ventricular tachyarrhythmias, including ventricular fibrillation and pulseless ventricular tachycardia or ventricular fibrillation–ventricular tachycardia, are the most common electrophysiologic mechanisms of cardiac arrest leading to SCD, but primary nontachyarrhythmic events also are common. The latter now appear to be even more common than indicated by the 20% to 30% rates previously estimated.[1] Nontachyarrhythmic mechanisms include pulseless electrical activity (PEA), asystole, and bradycardias severe enough to result in loss of adequate cerebral and other organ perfusion. The distinction between tachyarrhythmic mechanisms and the other (nonshockable) mechanisms is important both clinically and epidemiologically. The probability that an event will be tachyarrhythmic has an impact on the potential value of antitachycardic strategies, such as ICDs and automated external defibrillators (AEDs). Moreover, survival statistics are far more encouraging for tachyarrhythmic events in all clinical settings (i.e., both in-hospital and out-of-hospital).

Defining the initial rhythm may be difficult because of spontaneous changes between ventricular fibrillation–ventricular tachycardia and the nontachyarrhythmic mechanisms. This can confound attempts to correlate primary electrophysiologic mechanisms with outcome. For example, the time between onset of a ventricular tachycardia and deterioration to asystole or PEA may be brief, limiting the potential benefit of interventions. Conversely, an initial bradyarrhythmic event may change to ventricular fibrillation–ventricular tachycardia, with or without therapy, and in this circumstance the probability of successful defibrillation appears to be reduced.[53] Finally, data from emergency rescue responses to cardiac arrest may be misleading in regard to initial mechanisms. Observations of unexpectedly high proportions of asystole and PEA at initial contact[54] may reflect delayed 911 calls by witnesses, and shortening such delays may yield higher proportions of victims found in ventricular tachycardia at initial contact. Even among hospitalized patients, a differential survival benefit has been reported for early defibrillation, defined as occurring at 2 minutes or less after onset of the arrhythmia, compared with delayed defibrillation, defined as occurring beyond 2 minutes (39% versus 22%).[55]

Epidemiologic Paradigms for Sudden Cardiac Death Prediction

Limitations in the ability to identify *individuals* at risk of SCD from among the general population is a major reason why sudden cardiac arrest (SCA) remains an important public health problem. The variations in definition of SCD, inconsistencies in access to data, and differences in pathophysiologic mechanisms and their clinical recognition result in persisting questions about the balance between population-attributable risk and individual risk prediction. To address these limitations, conventional

Table 77-2 Epidemiologic Paradigms for Population and Individual Risk Prediction of Sudden Cardiac Death

Conventional epidemiology
- Population risk and primary prevention (e.g., atherogenesis)
- Secondary and tertiary prevention

Transient risk prediction
- Acute coronary syndrome, hemodynamic changes, electrical instability, autonomic predictors

Interventional epidemiology
- Predictors derived from clinical trials
- Long-term surveillance observations for safety

Genetic epidemiology
- Individual (personalized) risk
- Prediction of specific expression

epidemiologic concepts must be supplemented by the integration of new epidemiologic paradigms (Table 77-2). Among these are the emerging field of genetic epidemiology and interventional epidemiology, the latter being a term coined to define the population dynamics of clinical trial design and outcomes.

The Inherited Basis of Sudden Cardiac Death Risk

Interest in the genetic control of ion channel function, and in its potential role in the pathophysiology of life-threatening ventricular arrhythmias and SCD, has emerged from the identification of arrhythmogenic mutations in genes that control cardiac membrane ion channel structure and function, and of inherited cardiac structural disorders characterized by SCA risk (Table 77-3). Recognition of hereditary patterns among the uncommon familial causes of SCD, such as the congenital long QT interval syndromes, hypertrophic cardiomyopathy, right ventricular dysplasia, Brugada syndrome, and catecholaminergic ventricular tachycardia, was followed by identification of multiple specific mutations at a number of gene loci. In some, the culprit genes encode channel proteins associated with inherited arrhythmia syndromes (e.g., long QT or Brugada syndrome); in others, the genes are associated with the structural disorders linked to arrhythmic risk (e.g., hypertrophic cardiomyopathy, right ventricular dysplasia). Although most of the genetic associations provide a major advance in the understanding of the inheritance

Table 77-3 Genetic Epidemiology of Risk for Sudden Cardiac Death (SCD)

Genetically based primary arrhythmia disorders
- Congenital long QT syndrome
- Brugada syndrome
- "Idiopathic" (catecholaminergic) ventricular tachycardia/fibrillation

Inherited structural disorders with risk of arrhythmic SCD
- Hypertrophic cardiomyopathy
- Right ventricular dysplasia/cardiomyopathy

Genetic predisposition to drug- and electrolyte-induced arrhythmias and SCD
- "Acquired" long QT syndrome

Genetic modulation of complex acquired diseases
- Coronary artery disease; acute coronary syndromes
- Congestive heart failure; dilated cardiomyopathies

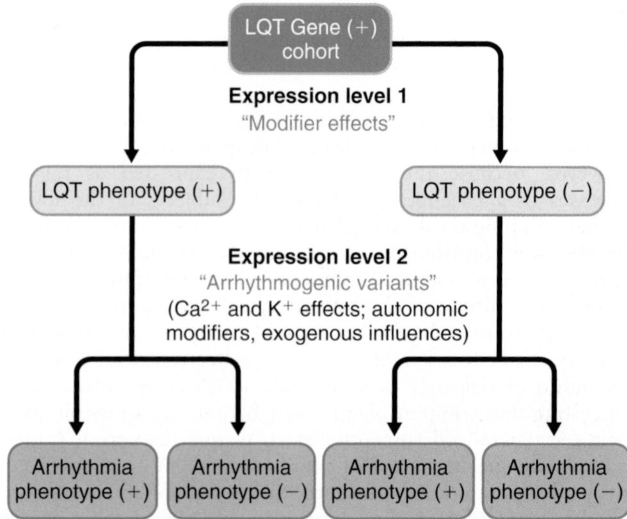

Figure 77-6 Concordant and discordant risk stratification in inherited primary arrhythmia syndromes. Among a familial cluster of patients positive for a long QT (LQT) mutation *(top)*, expression level 1 identifies the possibility for positive and negative LQT phenotypes (phenotype [+] and phenotype [−]). Phenotype-negative status among the genotype-positive cohort is thought to result from low penetrance, plus modifier effects that include modifier genes or other environmental factors. A second level of expression, expression level 2, refers to arrhythmogenic variants, and for each LQT phenotype there is the potential for both positive and negative arrhythmia phenotypes. Factors that influence arrhythmia phenotype expression may include exogenous influences, electrolyte effects, calcium handling, and autonomic modifiers. The expression level 2 concept derives from clinical observation of the relatively low rate of arrhythmia phenotype expression among LQT genotype–positive patients.

patterns for the various disorders and, to some extent, for individual risk, their contribution to elucidation of the pathophysiologic basis for these causes of sudden death remains incomplete. For example, of mutation carriers among relatives of long QT syndrome probands, only approximately 10% to 20% will experience cardiac arrest or SCD, suggesting that the inherited repolarization abnormality is a consequence of a molecular substrate that requires other variables to generate arrhythmias. These expression variables may be environmental in some cases (see Table 77-3—"acquired" long QT syndrome) or equally likely, a modifier gene that interacts with the long QT physiology (Fig. 77-6). Nonetheless, these observations provide screening tools for potentially affected persons, as well as the potential for determining specific therapeutic strategies. These gene loci also serve as candidates for investigation of the role of low-penetrance mutations or polymorphisms in SCD related to more common causes, such as coronary heart disease. An example is a genetic variant in the cardiac sodium channel gene (*SCN5A*) observed among the African-American population (carrier rate, 13.2%) that appears to predispose affected persons to the development of arrhythmias, even though it is not expressed as a long QT syndrome phenotype under control conditions.[24] Its role in predicting risk of SCD awaits clarification.

Genetic opportunities are further piqued by two recent epidemiologic studies[45,46] and by two clinical and pathologic studies[14,47] suggesting that SCD is a patient-specific response to acute coronary syndromes. Each of these studies demonstrated a pattern of familial clustering of SCD, with an excess risk of sudden death as the specific initial manifestation of an acute coronary syndrome with a family history positive for SCD in one parent and even higher when both sides of the family are

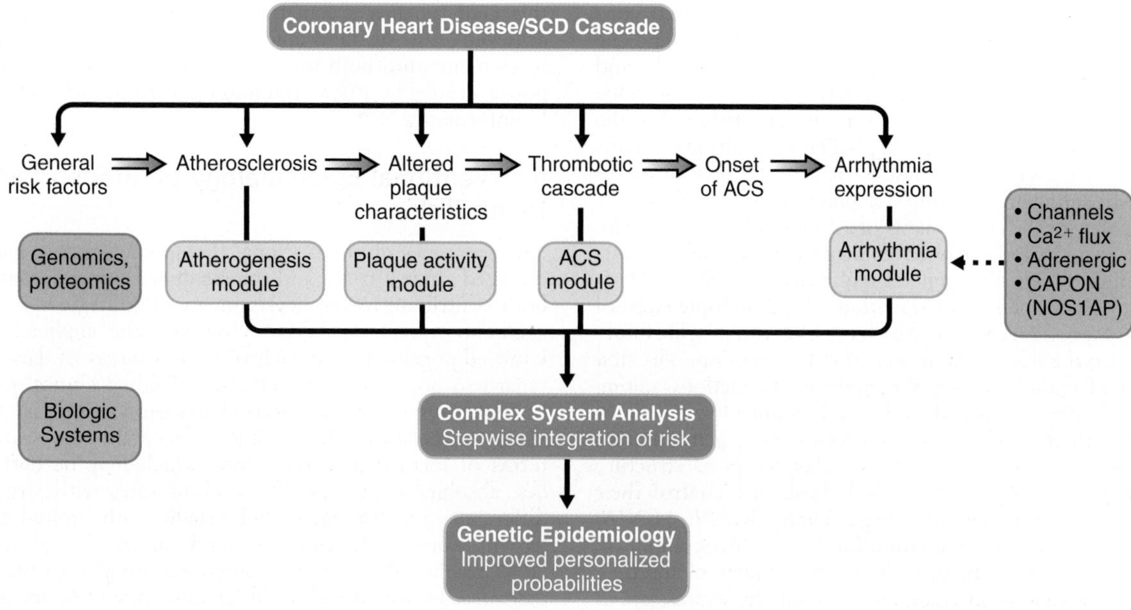

Figure 77-7 Genetic imprints on the coronary heart disease–sudden cardiac death (SCD) cascade. Genetic influences have been identified for multiple inheritance modules along the cascade from general risk factors for atherosclerosis to arrhythmic expression leading to SCD. Individual risk based on genetic profiles has been identified for atherogenesis, plaque evolution, the thrombotic cascade, and arrhythmia expression, but few of the markers identified thus far have sufficient individual predictive power to be clinically useful. Genomic and proteomic strategies may lead to stepwise integration of these modules through complex analytic methods, permitting better individual applications. Ultimately, treatment of these concepts as a biologic system may offer even greater power to the field of genetic epidemiology, leading to higher-order single-patient probabilities for predicting SCD. (Modified from Myerburg RJ: Scientific gaps in the prediction and prevention of sudden cardiac death. J Cardiovasc Electrophysiol 13:709-723, 2002.)

affected [46,47] Although familial clustering could be genetic, environmental, or a combination, studies of genetically based arrhythmia syndromes (see Table 77-3) provide a series of candidate genes, mutations, or polymorphisms that may set the stage for abnormal function in the presence of acute ischemia, even if the affected person is phenotypically normal at baseline. Support for the general concept of genetic variations that do not affect baseline phenotype but are associated with expression of effects during a transient event, has been emerging.[56]

A major paradigm shift in the epidemiology of coronary heart disease is beginning to emerge from new insights into the expression of the multiple elements in the cascade of atherosclerotic lesion formation, initiation of acute coronary syndromes, and triggering of SCD (Fig. 77-7). Genetic controls of atherogenesis,[57,58] plaque destabilization,[59] and the thrombotic cascade,[60] added to the genetics of ion channel function, have an impact on individual risks and responses to pathophysiologic states. The best genetic leads for investigation of specific SCD risk currently available reside in the realm of molecular and genetic electrophysiology. The weakest link currently centers on the basis for initiation of the atherosclerotic plaque, the epidemiology of which still depends largely on conventional risk factors, such as diabetes mellitus, hypertension, cigarette smoking, and the hyperlipidemias. Genetic markers for these basic risk factors are evolving,[61,62] but the basis for lesion initiation remains problematic. Elucidation of genetic contributions to lesion progression, transitions to active states, and activation of thrombotic cascade is progressing more rapidly.

As an expanded epidemiologic approach evolves, it will initiate a conceptual transformation of the sequential pathophysiologic cascade (see Fig. 77-7) into a complex system analysis model.[63,64] The need for this approach derives from the fundamental limitation of the ability of conventional risk factors to identify specific persons at high risk for SCD (or other manifestations of coronary artery disease) from among the general population. Because a majority of SCDs occur in people without easily identifiable high absolute risks for cardiovascular or total mortality (see Fig. 77-3), and because risk is multifactorial (see Fig. 77-7), more precise predictors of single-patient probabilities of risk of coronary heart disease generally, and SCD in particular, must be sought. This information will have to come from mathematical analyses of the interactions between multiple risks or complex system analysis.

The excess relative risk identified by single markers and the relative benefits of some interventions against specific risk factors studied in controlled interventions are impressive for selected groups of patients, but they provide limited predictive power for absolute risk reduction in individual patients. The control groups from most of the primary prevention clinical trials, such as the 3-hydroxy-3-methylglutaryl–coenzyme A (HMG-CoA) reductase trials for cholesterol lowering[65] and prophylactic use of aspirin,[66] are instructive of this problem. When the absolute mortality outcomes among the aspirin- or statin-treated and control groups in primary prevention studies are analyzed, it is evident that the absolute reduction in mortality risk for persons in the treatment groups is modest. The reported outcomes of such studies emphasize group effect (relative risk reduction), rather than their individual impact (absolute benefit).[25,65,67] Among three major primary prevention statin trials,[64] total mortality rates fell from 3.7% over 5 years to 2.8%, for a reduction of approximately 0.9%. Cardiovascular mortality benefit was 0.5% over 5 years. These figures derive from the fact that the absolute mortality risk in the placebo groups is relatively low (3.7% over 5 years, or 0.72% per year), even though the beneficial effect in a relative sense is impressively high. However, because of the absolute magnitude of the numerators and denominators in these lower-risk groups, the potential benefit of identifying persons at risk with a higher degree of precision is huge. In order to do so, however, the epidemiologic mission becomes much more complex.

When viewed from the perspective of a complex system, containing voluminous bioinformation, both the difficulty and the opportunity become evident. Genetic, environmental, and acquired pathophysiologic states all may play roles. The value of genetically based analysis of risk is the fact that it has the potential to provide predetermined predictors in advance of clinical events. Acquired characteristics may be more difficult to identify with sufficient lead time for practical interventions.

An overview of the components of a complex biologic system, leading to genetic and genomic epidemiologic models, is outlined in Figure 77-7. The general requirements include identification of polymorphisms or mutations along multiple steps of the clinical expression cascade, which together can provide information that can enhance the power of risk prediction. The first on the list of complexities is the study of interactions among genes, which may be directly related, functionally related, or integrated with remotely related functions (gene-gene interactions). The genes that control ion channel pore structure (e.g., *KVLQT1*, *HERG*, *SCN5A*) and those that control their associated modulating peptides (e.g., *MinK*, *MIRP1*, *SCN1B*) provide examples of direct relationships.[52,68-71] An example of indirect but related interactions between products of multiple genes is envisioned as interactions between the expression of ion channel gene variants and genes which modulate or modify calcium handling. Identified mutations of the latter (e.g., *RYR2* and *CASQ2*) are associated with arrhythmias.[71-73] In addition, KcLQT-1/MinK may interact with *RYR2* or *CASQ2* variations, resulting in an association between control of repolarization and calcium handling, a relationship suggested as a mechanism for arrhythmogenesis. Finally, a genetically determined influence on β-adrenergic receptor function,[74,75] interacting with the ion channel–calcium handling complex,[76] is an example of a remote but integrated gene-gene relationship.

Another component in the complex system for control of ion channel function is the interaction between genetic influences and nongene factors (gene-nongene interactions or gene-environment interactions). These include the relationships between genetic channelopathies and genetic and nongenetic β-adrenergic control, or benign polymorphisms and transient pathophysiologic modifiers.[52] The third, and most challenging, is the construct of the pathophysiologic cascade itself, leading from atherogenesis to plaque characteristics to the thrombotic cascade and then to specific arrhythmic expression. Within each compartment of the cascade reside evolving clusters of information on genetic influences, contributing to or controlling risk. These features offer the opportunity for the cascade to evolve into a complex system for simultaneous interactive analysis of multiple gene influences, rather than a sequence of independent variables. Complex systems analyses then can be used to integrate genetics into epidemiology, providing a stepwise amplification of risk prediction, based on individual probability profiles. Figure 77-7 highlights the concept of a sequence of genetic imprints on the coronary heart disease–SCD cascade. Within each element in the cascade—atherogenesis risk undergoing transition to risk for an active plaque state, followed by genetic properties of the thrombotic cascade, and finally triggering of arrhythmias—genetic influences feed into an integrated pool of characteristics that determine individual probabilities.

Higher-order or personalized single-patient probabilities (1 in 10 risk versus 1 in 1000 risk), derived from integration of properties at multiple levels of pathophysiology, will complement the power of risk expression for specific components of the SCD cascade (see Fig. 77-7, bottom). The ultimate goal is to profile individual risk at multiple steps in the SCD cascade, generating probability figures that are powerful enough to be useful for preventive strategies far in advance of clinical events. The degree to which analysis of genetic interactions can achieve this goal remains speculative. Answering the question can be achieved only by new epidemiologic models, requiring large investments into both the specialized personnel and computing power needed by a new community of science within the field of bioinformatics.[52,64]

Interventional Epidemiology of Sudden Cardiac Death Risk

The outcomes of observational therapeutic studies, and of randomized clinical trials, and the results of epidemiologic surveys both contribute to the development of strategies for the management of risk for SCD.[7] However, the application of the knowledge gained from each of these sources of data differs in regard to population impact and individual clinical effect. For example, mining of existing databases can identify risk factors or strong associations. Observations generally are expressed in terms of relative risk statements, which may be derived from low absolute event rates. Low event rates with large relative differences identify *effects*, but usually with limited individual patient impact. By contrast, randomized clinical trials with large absolute differences in outcomes are able to better define *individual* patient benefits. Observational studies are limited by their dependence on comparisons between anticipated outcomes that influence study design, rather than actual measures.

SCD in an unselected adult population includes those victims whose cardiac arrests occur as a first cardiac event, as well as those whose events can be predicted with greater accuracy because they are included in higher-risk subgroups. Based on a cumulative incidence of 1 to 2 per 1000 population (0.1% to 0.2%) per year in the United States (see Fig. 77-3), any intervention designed for the general population must be applied to the 999 in 1000 persons who will not have an event, in order to reach and possibly influence the 1 in 1000 who will. Cost and risk-benefit uncertainties limit the nature of broad-based interventions and demand a higher resolution of risk identification. With each group-specific escalation of risk, the probability of an event increases, whereas the corresponding absolute number of deaths becomes progressively smaller,[1] limiting the population impact of interventions in high-risk subgroups even though magnifying the individual benefit.

All studies of group outcomes of therapy for complex pathophysiologic states must take four factors into account: (1) relative risk reduction, (2) absolute risk reduction, (3) residual risk, and (4) cumulative benefits of multiple interventions. The primary endpoint reports for all clinical trials of ICD therapy, and for most other large clinical trials, focus largely on reduction in relative risk,[25] because this measure identifies the *effect* of the intervention. Relative risk reduction, however, does not quantify the benefit for the individual patient. To do so, a measure of absolute risk reduction is required, such as the absolute numerical difference in risk observed in the test and control groups, or calculations of a number of patients needed to be treated (NNT) in order to save a life.[67]

Other measures of group impact that do not commonly receive attention include residual risk and cumulative benefit. *Residual risk* refers to the absolute outcome among the treated group or test group in a clinical trial population, which identifies the component of total mortality risk that does not respond to the tested therapy. If residual risk is very high, the absolute and relative risk reduction benefits are correspondingly limited. *Cumulative benefit* refers to the increment in benefit from integration of multiple interventions. Despite its importance,[25,77] this is rarely stratified in clinical trial designs because it requires larger study populations, and it has not been used prospectively in any of the ICD or antiarrhythmic trials. Post hoc subgroup analysis can be used to suggest added benefit of a secondary strategy, but this does not replace stratifying the multiple interventions.

A final consideration in the epidemiology of interventions is the comparison of entry criteria against actual enrollment. In many of the ICD trials, the range of ejection fractions and functional classifications were unintentionally biased toward certain values, thereby limiting the interpretation and proper application of the outcomes. Ejection fraction entry criteria were largely in the range of 30% to 40% or less, but enrollment was dominated by lower ranges.[78] Therefore, the benefit to patients with ejection fraction values at the higher end of the range is not clear.

References

1. Myerburg RJ, Castellanos A: Cardiac arrest and sudden cardiac death. In Libby P, Bonow RO, Mann DL, Zipes DP (eds). Braunwald's Heart Disease: A Textbook of Cardiovascular Medicine, 8th ed. Oxford, UK, Elsevier, 2007, pp 933-974.
2. American Heart Association: 2001 Heart and Stroke Statistical Update. Dallas, American Heart Association, 2000.
3. Cobb LA, Fahrenbruch CE, Olsufka M, Copass MK: Changing incidence of out-of-hospital ventricular fibrillation, 1980-2000. JAMA 288:3008-3013, 2002.
4. Chugh SS, Jui J, Gunson K, et al: Current burden of sudden cardiac death: Multiple source surveillance versus retrospective death certificate–based review in a large U.S. community. J Am Coll Cardiol 44:1268-1275, 2004.
5. Zheng ZJ, Croft JB, Giles WH, Mensah GA: Sudden cardiac death in the United States, 1989 to 1998. Circulation 104:2158-2163, 2001.
6. Every NR, Parsons L, Hlatsky MA, et al: Use and accuracy of state death certificates for clarification of sudden deaths in high-risk populations. Am Heart J 134:1129-1132, 1997.
7. Myerburg RJ: Sudden cardiac death: Exploring the limits of our knowledge. J Cardiovasc Electrophysiol 12:369-381, 2001.
8. Braunwald E: Cardiovascular medicine at the turn of the millennium: Triumphs, concerns, and opportunities. N Engl J Med 337:1360-1369, 1997.
9. Myerburg RJ, Mitrani R, Interian A Jr, Castellanos A: Identification of risk of cardiac arrest and sudden cardiac death in athletes. In Estes NA, Salem DN, Estes NAM III (eds): Sudden Cardiac Death in the Athlete, Armonk, NY, Futura Publishing, 1998, pp 25-50.
10. Pauschinger M, Bowles NE, Fuentes-Garcia FJ, et al: Detection of adenoviral genome in the myocardium of adult patients with idiopathic left ventricular dysfunction. Circulation 99:1348-1354, 1999.
11. Splawski I, Timothy KW, Tateyama M, et al: Variant of *SCN5A* sodium channel implicated in risk of cardiac arrhythmia. Science 297:1333-1336, 2002.
12. Sesti F, Abbott GW, Wei J, et al: A common polymorphism associated with antibiotic-induced cardiac arrhythmia. Proc Natl Acad Sci U S A 97:10613-10618, 2000.
13. Napolitano C, Schwartz PJ, Brown AM, et al: Evidence for a cardiac ion channel mutation underlying drug-induced QT prolongation and life-threatening arrhythmias. J Cardiovasc Electrophysiol 11:691-696, 2000.
14. Myerburg RJ: Implantable cardioverter-defibrillators after myocardial infarction. New Engl J Med 359:2245-2253, 2008.
15. Dekker LR, Bezzina CR, Henriques JP, et al: Familial sudden death is an important risk factor for primary ventricular fibrillation: A case-control study in acute myocardial infarction patients. Circulation 114:1140-1145, 2006.
16. Davies MJ: Anatomic features in victims of sudden coronary death: Coronary artery pathology. Circulation 85(Suppl 1):I19-I24, 1992.
17. Taylor AJ, Burke AP, O'Malley PG, et al: A comparison of the Framingham risk index, coronary artery calcification, and culprit plaque morphology in sudden cardiac death. Circulation 101:1243-1248, 2000.
18. Mehta D, Curwin J, Gomes A, Fuster V: Sudden death in coronary artery disease: Acute ischemia versus myocardial substrate. Circulation 96:3215-3223, 1997.
19. Warnes CA, Roberts WC: Sudden coronary death: Relation of amount and distribution of coronary narrowing at necropsy to previous symptoms of myocardial ischemia, left ventricular scarring, and heart weight. Am J Cardiol 54:65-73, 1984.
20. Liberthson RR, Nagel EL, Hirschman JC, et al: Pathophysiologic observations in prehospital ventricular fibrillation and sudden cardiac death. Circulation 49:790-798, 1974.
21. Cooper RS, Simmons BE, Castaner A, et al: Left ventricular hypertrophy is associated with worse survival independent of ventricular function and number of coronary arteries severely narrowed. Am J Cardiol 65:441-445, 1990.
22. Marian AJ, Roberts R: Molecular genetic basis of hypertrophic cardiomyopathy: Genetic markers for sudden cardiac death. J Cardiovasc Electrophysiol 9:88-99, 1998.
23. Myerburg RJ, Kessler KM, Castellanos A: Sudden cardiac death: Structure, function, and time-dependence of risk. Circulation 85(Suppl I):I2-I10, 1992.
24. Huikuri HV, Castellanos A, Myerburg RJ: Sudden death due to cardiac arrhythmias. N Engl J Med 345:1473-1482, 2001.
25. Myerburg RJ, Mitrani R, Interian A Jr, Castellanos A: Interpretation of outcomes of antiarrhythmic clinical trials: Design features and population impact. Circulation 97:1514-1521, 1998.
26. Wilson PW, D'Agostino RB, Levy D, et al: Prediction of coronary heart disease using risk factor categories. Circulation 97:1837-1847, 1998.
27. Ford ES, Ajani UA, Croft JB, et al: Explaining the decrease in U.S. deaths from coronary disease, 1980-2000. N Engl J Med 356:2388-98, 2007.
28. O'Rourke RA, Brundage BH, Froelicher VF, et al: American College of Cardiology/American Heart Association Expert Consensus Document on electron-beam computed tomography for the diagnosis and prognosis of coronary artery disease. J Am Coll Cardiol 36:326-340, 2000.
29. Moss AJ, Hall WJ, Cannom DS, et al: Improved survival with an implanted defibrillator in patients with coronary disease at high risk for ventricular arrhythmia: Multicenter Automatic Defibrillator Implantation Trial Investigators. N Engl J Med 335:1933-1940, 1996.
30. A comparison of antiarrhythmic-drug therapy with implantable defibrillators in patients resuscitated from near-fatal ventricular arrhythmias: The Antiarrhythmics versus Implantable Defibrillators (AVID) Investigators. N Engl J Med 337:1576-1583, 1997.
31. Connolly SJ, Gent M, Roberts RS, et al: Canadian Implantable Defibrillator Study (CIDS): A randomized trial of the implantable cardioverter defibrillator against amiodarone. Circulation 101:1297-1302, 2000.
32. Buxton AE, Lee KL, Fisher JD, et al: A randomized study of the prevention of sudden death in patients with coronary artery disease: Multicenter Unsustained Tachycardia Trial Investigators. N Engl J Med 341:1882-1890, 1999.
33. Hartikainen JE, Malik M, Staunton A, et al: Distinction between arrhythmic and nonarrhythmic death after acute myocardial infarction based on heart rate variability, signal-averaged electrocardiogram, ventricular arrhythmias and left ventricular ejection fraction. J Am Coll Cardiol 28:296-304, 1996.
34. La Rovere MT, Bigger JT Jr, Marcus FI, et al: Baroreflex sensitivity and heart-rate variability in prediction of total cardiac mortality after myocardial infarction: ATRAMI (Autonomic Tone and Reflexes After Myocardial Infarction) Investigators. Lancet 351:478-484, 1998.
35. Rosenbaum D, Albrecht P, Cohen RJ: Predicting sudden cardiac death from T wave alternans of the surface electrocardiogram: promise and pitfalls. J Cardiovasc Electrophysiol 7:1095-1111, 1996.
36. Klingenheben T, Zabel M, D'Agostino RB, et al: Predictive value of T-wave alternans for arrhythmic events in patients with congestive heart failure. Lancet 356:651-652, 2000.
37. Ross R: Atherosclerosis: An inflammatory disease? N Engl J Med 340:115-126, 1999.
38. Ridker PM, Glynn RJ, Hennekens CH: C-reactive protein adds to the predictive value of total and HDL cholesterol in determining risk of first myocardial infarction. Circulation 97:2007-2011, 1998.
39. Koenig W, Sund M, Frohlich M, et al: C-Reactive protein, a sensitive marker of inflammation, predicts future risk of

coronary heart disease in initially healthy middle-aged men: Results from the MONICA (Monitoring Trends and Determinants in Cardiovascular Disease) Augsburg Cohort Study, 1984 to 1992. Circulation 99:237-242, 1999.

40. Ridker PM, Rifai N, Clearfield M, et al for the Air Force/Texas Coronary Atherosclerosis Prevention Study Investigators: Measurement of C-reactive protein for the targeting of statin therapy in the primary prevention of acute coronary events. N Engl J Med 344:1959-1965, 2001.
41. Ridker PM, Cushman M, Stampfer MJ, et al: Inflammation, aspirin, and the risk of cardiovascular disease in apparently healthy men. N Engl J Med 336:973-979, 1997.
42. Ridker PM, Hennekens CH, Buring JE, Rifai N: C-reactive protein and other markers of inflammation in the prediction of cardiovascular disease in women. N Engl J Med 342:836-843, 2000.
43. Goldstein JA, Demetriou D, Grines CL, et al: Multiple complex coronary plaques in patients with acute myocardial infarction. N Engl J Med 343:915-922, 2000.
44. Kuller LH, Tracy RP, Shaten J, Meilahn EN: Reaction of C-reactive protein and coronary heart disease in the MRFIT nested case-control study: Multiple Risk Factor Intervention Trial. Am J Epidemiol 144:537-547, 1996.
45. Friedlander Y, Siscovick DS, Weinmann S, et al: Family history as a risk factor for primary cardiac arrest. Circulation 97:155-160, 1998.
46. Jouven X, Desnos M, Guerot C, Ducimetiere P: Predicting sudden death in the population: The Paris Prospective Study I. Circulation 99:1978-1983, 1999.
47. Kaikkonen KS, Kortelainen ML, Linna E, Huikuri HV: Family history and the risk of sudden cardiac death as a manifestation of an acute coronary event. Circulation 114:1462-1467, 2006.
48. Burkett EL, Hershberger RE: Clinical and genetic issues in familial dilated cardiomyopathy. J Am Coll Cardiol. 45:969-981, 2005.
49. Kjekshus J: Arrhythmias and mortality in congestive heart failure. Am J Cardiol 65:42I-48I, 1990.
50. Effect of metoprolol CR/XL in chronic heart failure: Metoprolol CR/XL Randomised Intervention Trial in Congestive Heart Failure (MERIT-HF). Lancet 353:2001-2007, 1999.
51. Pires LA, Hull ML, Nino CL, et al: Sudden death in recipients of transvenous implantable cardioverter defibrillator systems: Terminal events, predictors, and potential mechanisms. J Cardiovasc Electrophysiol 10:1049-1056, 1999.
52. Myerburg RJ: Scientific gaps in the prediction and prevention of sudden cardiac death. J Cardiovasc Electrophysiol 13:709-723, 2002.
53. Kudenchuk PJ, Cobb LA, Copass MK, et al: Amiodarone for resuscitation after out-of-hospital cardiac arrest due to ventricular fibrillation. N Engl J Med 341:871-878, 1999.
54. Myerburg RJ, Fenster J, Velez M, et al: Impact of community-wide police car deployment of automated external defibrillators on survival from out-of-hospital cardiac arrest. Circulation 106:1058-1064, 2002.
55. Chan PS, Krumholz HM, Nichol G, et al: Delayed time to defibrillation after in-hospital cardiac arrest. N Engl J Med. 358:9-17, 2008.
56. Spooner PM, Albert C, Benjamin EJ, et al: Sudden cardiac death, genes, and arrhythmogenesis: Consideration of new population and mechanistic approaches from a National Heart, Lung, and Blood Institute Workshop, Part I. Circulation 103:2361-2364, 2001.
57. Marenberg MD, Risch N, Berkman LF, et al: Genetic susceptibility to death from coronary heart disease in a study of twins. N Engl J Med 330:1041-1046, 1994.
58. Smithies O, Maeda N: Gene targeting approaches to complex genetic diseases: Atherosclerosis and essential hypertension. Proc Natl Acad Sci U S A 92:5266-5272, 1995.
59. Faber BC, Cleutjens KB, Niessen RL, et al: Identification of genes potentially involved in rupture of human atherosclerotic plaques. Circ Res 89:547-554, 2001.
60. Anderson JL, King GJ, Bair BS, et al: Associations between a polymorphism in the gene encoding glycoprotein IIIa and myocardial infarction or coronary artery disease. J Am Coll Cardiol 33:727-733, 1999.
61. Arya R, Duggirala R, Almasy L, et al: Linkage of high-density lipoprotein-cholesterol concentrations to a locus on chromosome 9p in Mexican Americans. Nat Genet 30:102-105, 2002.
62. Jormsjo S, Whatling C, Walter DH, et al: Allele-specific regulation of matrix metalloproteinase-7 promoter activity is associated with coronary artery luminal dimensions among hypercholesterolemic patients. Arterioscler Thromb Vasc Biol 21:1834-1839, 2001.
63. Drew PJ, Ilstrup DM, Kerin MJ, Monson JR: Prognostic factors: Guidelines for investigation design and state of the art analytical methods. Surg Oncol 7:71-76, 1998.
64. Bonow R, Clark EB, Curfman GD, et al: Task Force on Strategic Research Direction: Clinical Science Subgroup key science topics report. Circulation 106:e162-e166, 2002.
65. Hebert PR, Gaziano JM, Chan KS, Hennekens CH: Cholesterol lowering with statin drugs, risk of stroke, and total mortality: An overview of randomized trials. JAMA 278:313-321, 1997.
66. Final report on the aspirin component of the ongoing Physicians' Health Study: Steering Committee of the Physicians' Health Study Research Group. N Engl J Med 321:129-135, 1989.
67. Laupacis A, Sackett DL, Roberts RS: An assessment of clinically useful measures of the consequences of treatment. N Engl J Med 318:1728-1733, 1988.
68. Priori SG, Barhanin J, Hauer RN, et al: Genetic and molecular basis of cardiac arrhythmias: Impact on clinical management parts I and II. Circulation 99:518-528, 1999.
69. Roden DM, Spooner PM: Inherited long QT syndromes: A paradigm for understanding arrhythmogenesis. J Cardiovasc Electrophysiol 10:1664-1683, 1999.
70. Priori SG, Napolitano C, Grillo M: Concealed arrhythmogenic syndromes: The hidden substrate of idiopathic ventricular fibrillation? Cardiovasc Res 50:218-223, 2001.
71. Marks AR, Priori S, Memmi M, et al: Involvement of the cardiac ryanodine receptor/calcium release channel in catecholaminergic polymorphic ventricular tachycardia. J Cell Physiol 190:1-6, 2002.
72. Wu Y, MacMillan LB, McNeill RB, et al: CaM kinase augments cardiac L-type Ca^{2+} current: A cellular mechanism for long Q-T arrhythmias. Am J Physiol 276: H2168-H2178, 1999.
73. Lahat H, Pras E, Olender T, et al: A missense mutation in a highly conserved region of CASQ2 is associated with autosomal recessive catecholamine-induced polymorphic ventricular tachycardia in Bedouin families from Israel. Am J Hum Genet 69:1378-1384, 2001.
74. Sosunov EA, Gainullin RZ, Moise NS, et al: beta(1) and beta(2)-adrenergic receptor subtype effects in German shepherd dogs with inherited lethal ventricular arrhythmias. Cardiovasc Res 48:211-219, 2000.
75. Podlowski S, Wenzel K, Luther HP, et al: β_1-adrenoceptor gene variations: A role in idiopathic dilated cardiomyopathy? J Mol Med 78:87-93, 2000.
76. Pogwizd SM, Schlotthauer K, Li L, et al: Arrhythmogenesis and contractile dysfunction in heart failure: Roles of sodium-calcium exchange, inward rectifier potassium current, and residual beta-adrenergic responsiveness. Circ Res 88:1159-1167, 2001.
77. Califf RM, DeMets DL: Principles from clinical trials relevant to clinical practice: Part I. Circulation 106:1015-1021, 2002.
78. Myerburg RJ, Castellanos A: Clinical research designs and implantable defibrillator indications: Spend in the beginning or pay at the end. J Am Coll Cardiol 47:108-111, 2006.

Arrhythmias in Patients with Neurologic Disorders 78

William J. Groh

CHAPTER OUTLINE

Arrhythmias occurring as a result of a neurologic disorder either are related to direct cardiac involvement or are secondary to induced neurohormonal abnormalities. In some disorders, arrhythmias can be responsible for greater morbidity and mortality than the neurologic manifestations. The chapter reviews the cardiac and arrhythmia consequences observed in muscular dystrophies, Friedreich's ataxia, periodic paralyses, mitochondrial encephalomyopathies, Guillain-Barré syndrome, myasthenia gravis, epilepsy, and acute cerebral disorders.

The Muscular Dystrophies

The muscular dystrophies are heritable disorders in which direct involvement of cardiac tissue may occur. The muscular dystrophies are classified as follows:

- X-linked: Duchenne and Becker muscular dystrophy
- Myotonic dystrophy
- Emery-Dreifuss muscular dystrophy
- Limb-girdle muscular dystrophy
- Facioscapulohumeral dystrophy

Duchenne and Becker Muscular Dystrophy

Genetics and Cardiac Pathophysiology

Both Duchenne and Becker forms of muscular dystrophy are X-linked recessive disorders caused by abnormalities in the dystrophin gene. The dystrophin protein and dystrophin-associated glycoproteins provide a structural link between the myocyte cytoskeleton and extracellular matrix. In Duchenne muscular dystrophy, dystrophin is nearly absent, whereas in Becker muscular dystrophy, dystrophin is present but reduced in molecular size or amount. This dystrophin defect leads to the characteristic rapidly progressive muscle disease in Duchenne and the more benign course in Becker muscular dystrophy.

Clinical Presentation

Duchenne muscular dystrophy is the most common inherited neuromuscular disorder. The disease becomes symptomatic before the age of 5 years, manifesting with proximal muscle weakness, with progressive weakness and death commonly occurring by the second or third decade. Use of ventilatory assist devices and spinal surgery can prolong survival. Becker muscular dystrophy is less common and has a more variable presentation of skeletal muscle weakness and a better prognosis, with a majority of the patients surviving at least to middle age.

Cardiomyopathy is a feature of virtually all cases of Duchenne muscular dystrophy, but clinical recognition may be masked by severe skeletal muscle weakness. Preclinical cardiac involvement is present in one fourth of the patients by the age of 6, with clinically apparent cardiomyopathy onset after age 10 common.[1] Predilection for involvement in the posterobasal and posterolateral left ventricle has been observed. Electrocardiographic features are abnormal in 90%, demonstrating a distinctive pattern of tall R waves and increased R/S amplitude in V1 and deep narrow Q waves in the left precordial leads related to the regional ventricular involvement.

As with the skeletal muscle weakness, cardiac involvement in Becker muscular dystrophy is more variable, ranging from none or subclinical to severe cardiomyopathy requiring transplantation.[2] Electrocardiographic abnormalities similar to those in Duchenne muscular dystrophy are present in up to 75%, with echocardiographic abnormalities in 50%. Cardiac involvement can occur at any age, with a severity that does not correlate with the degree of skeletal muscle weakness.[2]

Arrhythmia Manifestations

Cardiac involvement in Duchenne muscular dystrophy can manifest in disturbances in both rhythm and conduction. Persistent or labile sinus tachycardia is the most commonly recognized abnormality. Atrial arrhythmias including fibrillation and flutter occur commonly as a preterminal rhythm. Up to 40% of affected patients have PR intervals less than 120 ms on electrocardiogram, possibly related to atrioventricular node dystrophic changes and paradoxically enhanced conduction in remaining fibers. Prolonged infranodal conduction is evident on electrocardiograms (ECGs) in up to 10%. Complete heart block requiring pacing has been reported. Ventricular arrhythmias occur on ambulatory monitoring in 32% of patients primarily ventricular premature beats. Patients with severe skeletal muscle disease are more commonly affected. Monomorphic ventricular tachycardia has been described. The primary etiology is cardiac in approximately one fourth of persons with Duchenne muscular dystrophy who succumb, with an equal distribution of deaths from progressive heart failure and sudden deaths.[3] Sudden death occurs primarily in patients with severe skeletal muscle weakness. Whether the sudden death is arrhythmia-related is unclear. The presence of left ventricular systolic dysfunction is a risk factor for all-cause mortality.[4]

Arrhythmia manifestations in Becker muscular dystrophy correspond with the degree of associated cardiomyopathy but are poorly characterized.[5] Complete heart block has been observed. The prevalence of ventricular arrhythmias is not well documented. Bundle branch reentry tachycardia has been observed in a patient with cardiomyopathy.

Treatment and Prognosis

Duchenne muscular dystrophy is a progressive disorder, with death due to respiratory or cardiac involvement commonly occurring by the age of 20 to 30 years. Steroid derivatives have shown promise in delaying the progression of skeletal muscular weakness. Angiotensin-converting enzyme inhibitors and beta-blockers have shown promise in delaying or reversing left ventricular systolic dysfunction.[6,7] Treatment of arrhythmias, once severe skeletal and cardiac involvement is present, is unlikely to improve survival. Intravenous verapamil used for preterminal atrial arrhythmias has led to acute respiratory failure. In one report, placement of an implantable cardioverter-defibrillator (ICD) for recurrent drug-refractory ventricular tachycardia resulted in a periprocedural respiratory death.[8]

The treatment of arrhythmias in Becker muscular dystrophy is based on symptoms and the severity of cardiac involvement. Screening ECGs and echocardiograms have been recommended. A dilated cardiomyopathy develops in up to one fourth of female carriers of Duchenne or Becker muscular dystrophy.[9]

Myotonic Dystrophy

Genetics and Cardiac Pathophysiology

Myotonic dystrophy is a disease of autosomal dominant inheritance characterized by myotonia (delayed muscle relaxation after contraction), weakness and atrophy of skeletal muscles, and systemic manifestations of early balding, gonadal atrophy, cataracts, and cardiac involvement. The gene abnormality responsible for the majority of cases is an amplified and unstable trinucleotide CTG repeat (myotonic dystrophy type 1). A direct correlation has been found between the length of CTG expansion and age at onset and severity of neuromuscular disease and cardiac involvement.[10]

Myotonic dystrophy type 2 is a disorder similar to type 1 but with typically less severe muscular and systemic manifestations, including cardiac abnormalities.[11] A separate genetic locus with an unstable, amplified tetranucleotide repeat sequence, CCTG, is responsible for type 2 in a majority of affected families.[12] In type 2, the severity of disease does not correlate with the degree of repeat expansion.

The molecular mechanism by which myotonic dystrophy types 1 and 2, each with a distinct genetic basis, cause similar phenotypic presentations appears to be the toxic effect on cellular function of the repeat sequences when transcribed into RNA.

Cardiac pathology in myotonic dystrophy type 1 is common and involves degeneration of the conduction system including the sinus node, atrioventricular node, and His-Purkinje fibers. Degenerative changes are observed in other atrial and ventricular tissue, but progression to a symptomatic structural cardiomyopathy is rare.[13] Cardiac pathology in myotonic dystrophy type 2 is not as well described as in type 1. Conduction system fibrosis and a dilated cardiomyopathy have been reported in a small percentage of patients.[14]

Clinical Presentation

Myotonic dystrophy is the most common inherited muscular dystrophy manifesting in adults. Type 1 myotonic dystrophy is more common than type 2. In type 1, the age at onset of symptoms and diagnosis averages 20 to 25 years, and patients often die prematurely, typically in the fifth or sixth decade.[15,16] Patients with type 2 and less severely affected patients with type 1 live longer.

Arrhythmia Manifestations

Patients with myotonic dystrophy type 1 demonstrate a wide range of arrhythmias. On electrophysiologic study, a prolonged His-ventricular interval often is present.[17] Conduction system disease can progress to symptomatic heart block, necessitating pacing. The prevalence of permanent cardiac pacing varies widely between studies, in accordance with referral patterns and indications.[10,17] Atrial arrhythmias, primarily fibrillation and flutter, are common in myotonic dystrophy type 1.[10] An increasing prevalence of arrhythmias is reported in patients with more severe neuromuscular disease.[18] Patients with atrial arrhythmias often are asymptomatic, possibly related to a controlled ventricular response from concomitant conduction disease.

Up to one third of patients with myotonic dystrophy type 1 die suddenly.[15,18] Sudden death has been reported in young persons.[19] The mechanisms leading to sudden death are not clear but are believed to be primarily arrhythmia-related. Asystole, due to complete heart block without an appropriate escape rhythm, has been considered as a probable cause. Sudden death can occur despite pacing, implicating the potential for ventricular arrhythmias. Patients with myotonic dystrophy type 1 are at risk for bundle branch reentry tachycardia as a consequence of associated conduction disease.[20]

Arrhythmias are observed in patients with myotonic dystrophy type 2 but are both less frequent and less characterized than in type 1.[11,21] Unexplained sudden death has been reported in less than 2% of a large, genetically verified myotonic dystrophy type 2 population.[14]

Treatment and Prognosis

In patients with symptoms consistent with arrhythmias, electrophysiologic evaluation to determine an etiology is mandatory. Yearly ECGs and consideration for 24-hour ambulatory monitoring have been recommended as screening evaluations in asymptomatic patients. The American College of Cardiology/American Heart Association/Heart Rhythm Society (ACC/AHA/HRS) 2008 guideline update for implantation of cardiac pacemakers has recognized that asymptomatic conduction abnormalities, including first-degree atrioventricular block, in neuromuscular diseases such as myotonic dystrophy may warrant special consideration for pacing.[22] The severity of conduction disease at which pacing should be instituted is unclear. Electrophysiologic study for evaluation of the severity of His-Purkinje conduction disease has been recommended for guiding the consideration for pacing.[17] In patients presenting with wide complex tachycardia, electrophysiologic study with particular evaluation for bundle branch reentry tachycardia is indicated. ICD therapy in a patient with myotonic dystrophy has been reported.[23]

Anesthesia in patients with myotonic dystrophy may increase the risk of conduction block and other arrhythmias. Careful monitoring during the perioperative period with a low threshold for temporary pacing is recommended.

Emery-Dreifuss Muscular Dystrophy and Associated Disorders

Genetics and Cardiac Pathophysiology

Emery-Dreifuss muscular dystrophy is a rare disorder in which skeletal muscle weakness is mild but cardiac involvement, including arrhythmias, is common and may be life-threatening.

The disease is classically inherited as an X-linked recessive trait, with the gene abnormality responsible identified as a deficiency in the nuclear membrane protein emerin. Mutations in the *LMNA* gene encoding two other nuclear membrane proteins, lamin A and C, have been identified as responsible for a variety of other degenerative disorders with phenotypic expression related to X-linked Emery-Dreifuss muscular dystrophy.

The mechanisms by which abnormalities in emerin and lamin A and C cause cardiac involvement in Emery-Dreifuss muscular dystrophy are not clear. The nuclear membrane proteins provide structural support for the nucleus, as well as interacting with the cell's cytoskeleton. Fewer than one half of the patients with a phenotype of Emery-Dreifuss muscular dystrophy have mutations in emerin or lamin A and C; therefore, other, probably nuclear proteins are involved. Cardiac pathologic studies have shown fibrotic replacement of muscle and conduction tissue.

Clinical Presentation

A triad of early contractures of the elbow, Achilles tendon, and posterior cervical muscles, slowly progressing muscle weakness and atrophy, and cardiac involvement characterizes Emery-Dreifuss muscular dystrophy. Significant variation in the phenotypic expression of the disease is characteristic.

Cardiac involvement in Emery-Dreifuss muscular dystrophy and associated disorders most commonly is arrhythmia, but an associated dilated cardiomyopathy is increasingly being recognized, especially late after institution of pacing that prolongs survival.[24]

Arrhythmia Manifestations

Abnormalities in impulse generation and conduction are common in Emery-Dreifuss muscular dystrophy and associated disorders. ECG patterns typically are abnormal by the age of 20 to 30 years, with a typical initial manifestation of first-degree atrioventricular block. The atria are involved earlier than the ventricles, with atrial fibrillation or flutter or, more classically, permanent atrial standstill and junctional bradycardia. Need for permanent pacing is typical by age 35 to 40. Sudden death is common in Emery-Dreifuss muscular dystrophy and associated disorders, including in patients who have received pacemakers. Ventricular tachycardia and fibrillation have been reported. Female carriers of X-linked Emery-Dreifuss muscular dystrophy are at risk for cardiac conduction disease and sudden death, typically occurring late in life.

Treatment and Prognosis

Affected patients should be carefully monitored for electrocardiographic conduction abnormalities. Ambulatory electrocardiographic studies may reveal arrhythmias during sleep that are not apparent during short-term monitoring. Pacing is recommended once conduction disease is evident, although the severity that mandates pacing is not clear. Dual-chamber pacing may not be possible if atrial standstill is present. ICD therapy rather than bradycardia protection alone may be the preferred management approach.[25]

Limb-Girdle Muscular Dystrophy

Genetics and Cardiac Pathophysiology

Limb-girdle muscular dystrophy constitutes a group of disorders with a limb-shoulder and pelvic girdle distribution of weakness but otherwise with heterogeneous inheritance and clinical features.[26] Autosomal recessive (subtypes 2A to 2J), dominant (subtypes 1A to 1F), and sporadic genetic modes of inheritance have been described. Genes involved include those affecting function of the sarcomere, nuclear membrane, sarcolemma, and cytoskeleton. An autosomal dominant limb-girdle muscular dystrophy (subtype 1B) with a high prevalence of arrhythmias and late cardiomyopathy is caused by mutations encoding lamin A and C, similar to those in Emery-Dreifuss muscular dystrophy.[27] An autosomal recessive or sporadic limb-girdle muscular dystrophy, often associated with a progressive cardiomyopathy, is caused by mutations affecting the function of the dystrophin-glycoprotein complex (subtypes 2C to 2F and 2I).[26,28] Other subtypes of limb-girdle muscular dystrophy (1A, 1B, 2A, 2B, 2G, 2H, 2J) are not commonly associated with cardiac or arrhythmia abnormalities.[28]

Clinical Presentation

The onset of muscle weakness is variable but typically occurs before age 30.

Arrhythmia Manifestations

Arrhythmias occur in limb-girdle muscular dystrophy but are limited to specific genetic subtypes. Subtype 1B, similar to related Emery-Dreifuss muscular dystrophy disorders, is associated with progressive atrioventricular block, commonly requiring pacing.[27] Sudden death including in patients with a pacemaker, has been reported. A late dilated cardiomyopathy may occur.

The primary clinical manifestation of the subtypes of limb-girdle muscular dystrophy affecting the dystrophin-glycoprotein complex (subtypes 2C to 2F and 2I) is a dilated cardiomyopathy.[28] Specific arrhythmias have not been reported, but an increased risk associated with the cardiomyopathy can be anticipated.

Treatment and Prognosis

Routine screening of the ECG and echocardiogram in the subtypes of limb-girdle muscular dystrophy associated with cardiac disease is indicated. Prophylactic implantation of an ICD rather than a pacemaker has been recommended in patients with limb-girdle muscular dystrophy subtype 1B when cardiac conduction disease is present.[25] Biventricular pacing has been used in patients with limb-girdle muscular dystrophy and a dilated cardiomyopathy.[29]

Facioscapulohumeral Muscular Dystrophy

Genetics and Cardiac Pathophysiology

Facioscapulohumeral muscular dystrophy is a neuromuscular disorder of autosomal dominant inheritance in which the genetic locus has been mapped to chromosomal locus 4q35. The mechanism by which the mutation leads to the muscular dystrophy phenotype is unclear.

Clinical Presentation

Facioscapulohumeral muscular dystrophy is a common muscular dystrophy. Weakness typically follows a slowly progressive course. Serious cardiac disease including a dilated cardiomyopathy is reported but is rare.

Arrhythmia Manifestations

Arrhythmia involvement in facioscapulohumeral muscular dystrophy is reported but does not constitute as significant a problem in prevalence or severity as in other muscular dystrophies. In two series in which cardiac abnormalities were evaluated, 5% to 12% of patients were found to have arrhythmias in the absence of cardiovascular risk factors.[30,31] Arrhythmias reported included supraventricular tachycardias, atrioventricular block, and ventricular tachycardia. Many of the affected patients were asymptomatic or had mild palpitations.

Treatment and Prognosis

A screening ECG and a careful history to uncover arrhythmia-related symptoms are prudent.

Friedreich's Ataxia

Genetics and Cardiac Pathophysiology

Friedreich's ataxia is a spinocerebellar degenerative disease of autosomal recessive inheritance characterized by ataxia of the limbs and trunk, dysarthria, loss of deep tendon reflexes, sensory abnormalities, skeletal deformities, and cardiac involvement. It is linked to chromosome 9, with the gene responsible encoding a 210-amino-acid protein, frataxin. Friedreich's ataxia is associated with a concentric hypertrophic cardiomyopathy. More rarely, asymmetrical septal hypertrophy or a late dilated cardiomyopathy may develop.

Clinical Presentation

Friedreich's ataxia is the most common of the inherited ataxias. Neurologic symptoms typically manifest around puberty and almost always before the age of 25 years. Up to 95% of neurologically symptomatic patients have cardiac abnormalities, primarily findings of ventricular hypertrophy, when an ECG and an echocardiogram are done.

Arrhythmia Manifestations

Arrhythmias occur in the setting of Friedreich's ataxia but are rarer than what might be expected based on myocardial involvement. Atrial arrhythmias, including flutter and fibrillation, can be associated with progression to a dilated cardiomyopathy. Clinically relevant disorders of impulse or conduction are not frequent despite histopathologic evidence of conduction system fibrosis. Ventricular tachycardia in the setting of dilated cardiomyopathy has been observed. Sudden death can occur with a mechanism that has not been characterized.

Treatment and Prognosis

Idebenone, a free radical scavenger related to coenzyme Q10, modestly decreases cardiac hypertrophy and left ventricular mass.[32] Patients in whom a dilated cardiomyopathy develops tend to do poorly, with rapid progression to end-stage heart failure.

The Periodic Paralyses

Genetics and Cardiac Pathophysiology:

The primary periodic paralyses are rare disorders of autosomal dominant inheritance that result from abnormalities in ion channel genes. They can be classified into hypokalemic, hyperkalemic, and normokalemic periodic paralyses.[33,34] In addition, acquired hypokalemic periodic paralysis may complicate thyrotoxicosis, especially in men of Asian descent.[35]

Hypokalemic periodic paralysis is characterized by episodic attacks of flaccid paralysis in association with decreased serum potassium levels. Penetrance is complete in males and approximately 50% in females. New mutations can occur. Hypokalemic periodic paralysis is most commonly caused by mutations in the $\alpha 1$ subunit of the dihydropyridine-sensitive calcium channel. The disease is genetically heterogeneous, with a smaller number of patients having a mutation in the α subunit of the skeletal muscle sodium channel (encoded by *SCN4A*). Abnormalities in the calcium or sodium channels affect excitation-contraction coupling in skeletal muscle, leading to the characteristic paralysis.

Hyperkalemic periodic paralysis also manifests with episodic weakness but with symptoms worsening with potassium supplementation. Myotonia also may be seen. Complete penetrance is observed. Potassium levels usually are high but may be normal during an attack. Hyperkalemic periodic paralysis is due primarily to mutations in the α subunit of *SCN4A*. Multiple different mutations in this gene have been reported and appear to result in a potassium-sensitive failure of inactivation in the sodium channel.

Andersen-Tawil syndrome (also referred to as Andersen syndrome) is a distinct periodic paralysis associated with dysmorphic features of low-set ears, micrognathia, and clinodactyly, as well as a long QT interval and ventricular arrhythmias.[36] Episodic weakness can be triggered by hyper-, hypo-, or normokalemia. Response to potassium supplementation is inconsistent. Andersen-Tawil syndrome is caused by mutations in the *KCNJ2* gene encoding an inward rectifier potassium channel (Kir2.1) that is expressed in skeletal and cardiac muscle. A reduction in Kir2.1 in a ventricular myocyte model prolongs phase 3 of the action potential and induces delayed afterdepolarizations in the setting of hypokalemia.[37] Andersen-Tawil syndrome has been given an alternative nomenclature of LQT7 (long QT syndrome variant 7).

Whether and if so, what, genetic predisposition is associated with the acquired hypokalemic periodic paralyses that can complicate thyrotoxicosis is unclear.

Clinical Presentation

The primary manifestation of the periodic paralyses is episodic weakness. Attacks of weakness tend to be more severe and of longer duration with hypokalemic periodic paralysis than with hyperkalemic periodic paralysis. In both diseases, cold and rest after exercise can trigger an attack. Ingestion of carbohydrates can trigger an attack in hypokalemic periodic paralysis but may ameliorate an attack in hyperkalemic periodic paralysis.

Arrhythmia Manifestations

The periodic paralyses are associated with ventricular arrhythmias. Most arrhythmias occur with hyperkalemic periodic paralysis and Andersen-Tawil syndrome. Bidirectional ventricular tachycardia has been observed independent of digitalis intoxication. The bidirectional ventricular tachycardia occurs without relation to attacks of muscle weakness, generally does not correlate with serum potassium levels, and may convert to sinus rhythm with exercise. Ventricular ectopy often seen interspersed with bidirectional tachycardia is common.

A prolonged QT interval may be observed. In some reports, it is episodic and associated with weakness, hypokalemia, or antiarrhythmia therapy. In other cases, the prolongation may be constant. Andersen-Tawil syndrome typically is associated with a prolonged QT interval and frequent ventricular ectopy. Serious ventricular arrhythmias have been reported but are less likely in Andersen-Tawil syndrome than in the other long QT syndromes.[33]

Thyrotoxic hypokalemic periodic paralysis often manifests with the electrocardiographic findings of sinus tachycardia, prolonged QT-U intervals, and first-degree atrioventricular block.[38]

Ventricular fibrillation and sudden death have been reported in the periodic paralyses.

Treatment and Prognosis

The episodes of weakness commonly respond to measures that work to normalize potassium levels. Weakness in hyperkalemic periodic paralysis can respond to mexiletine. Weakness in hypokalemic periodic paralysis can respond to acetazolamide. Treatment of electrolytes usually does not improve arrhythmias or does so only transiently. Improvement in symptomatic nonsustained ventricular tachycardia associated with a prolonged QT interval has been reported with beta-blocker therapy.[39]

Class 1A antiarrhythmia agents can worsen muscle weakness and exacerbate arrhythmias associated with a prolonged QT interval.[40] Amiodarone has been observed to decrease episodes of sustained polymorphic ventricular tachycardia in Andersen-Tawil syndrome.[41] Normalization of thyroid indices corrects both the episodic weakness and electrocardiographic abnormalities in thyrotoxic hypokalemic periodic paralysis.

Mitochondrial Encephalomyopathies

Genetics and Cardiac Pathophysiology

The mitochondrial encephalomyopathies, so named because they cause both brain and skeletal muscle dysfunction, are a heterogeneous group of disorders resulting from abnormalities in mitochondrial function.[42] These disorders also are known as mitochondrial respiratory chain diseases. The number of distinct disorders is extensive.

Mitochondrial DNA is inherited maternally, so a majority of these disorders are transmitted from mother to offspring of both genders. Sporadic cases from new mutations can occur. Because nuclear DNA also encodes gene products used in mitochondrial function, some of the disorders are inherited in an autosomal dominant or recessive fashion. Mitochondrial encephalomyopathies manifest as several clinical phenotypes, including chronic progressive external ophthalmoplegia, which includes the Kearns-Sayre syndrome; myoclonus epilepsy with red ragged fibers (MERRF); mitochondrial myopathy, encephalopathy, lactic acidosis, and stroke-like episodes (MELAS); and Leber's hereditary optic neuropathy. Chronic progressive external ophthalmoplegia typically is a sporadic disease, whereas the others listed are maternally inherited.

Clinical Presentation

Cardiac involvement in mitochondrial encephalomyopathies is common. In the Kearns-Sayre syndrome, conduction abnormalities are typical, with a dilated cardiomyopathy reported but less common.[43] In MERRF and MELAS, left ventricular hypertrophy with systolic or diastolic dysfunction is observed.[44] Leber's hereditary optic neuropathy is characterized by painless, subacute bilateral visual loss, occurring more commonly in males than in females. A hypertrophic cardiomyopathy has been observed.[45]

Arrhythmia Manifestations

The clinical triad of progressive external ophthalmoplegia, pigmentary retinopathy, and heart block characterizes the Kearns-Sayre syndrome.[46] Symptoms usually begin in childhood. Heart block is common, typically manifesting after eye involvement becomes evident. The His-ventricular interval is prolonged. Distal conduction disease may be accompanied by a paradoxically short or normal PR interval, possibly secondary to enhanced atrioventricular node conduction. Pacing often is required before the age of 20 years. Preexcitation has been reported and can lead to the observed cases of supraventricular tachycardia.

A short PR interval and preexcitation syndromes have been observed by some but not all investigators evaluating patients with Leber's hereditary optic neuropathy.[45]

Despite the frequent presence of left ventricular hypertrophy, arrhythmias are rare in MERRF and MELAS. Preexcitation has been described with MELAS.

Treatment and Prognosis

In Kearns-Sayre syndrome, the prophylactic implantation of a pacemaker has been advocated when distal conduction disease is evident, although the severity that warrants pacing is not clear. Pacing improves survival. Ventricular arrhythmias and sudden death have been observed in patients with Kearns-Sayre syndrome. ICDs have been recommended in patients with both conduction disease and a dilated cardiomyopathy.

In Leber's hereditary optic neuropathy, a screening ECG evaluating for the presence of preexcitation is prudent.

Guillain-Barré Syndrome

Clinical Presentation

The Guillain-Barré syndrome is an acute inflammatory demyelinating neuropathy.[47] In two thirds of affected patients, a viral or bacterial infectious illness, typically respiratory or gastrointestinal, precedes the onset of symptoms by up to 6 weeks. Patients present with pain, paresthesia, and progressive weakness. One fourth of patients require assisted ventilation. Up to 15% of hospitalized patients die.

Arrhythmia Manifestations

Arrhythmias may be a feature in Guillain-Barré syndrome secondary to involvement of the autonomic nervous system.[48] Life-threatening arrhythmias occur almost exclusively in severe cases necessitating assisted ventilation. In a prospective study of 100 patients, serious arrhythmias occurred in 11 of 33 patients requiring ventilation.[49] The arrhythmias included asystole in 6, bradycardia of less than 30 beats per minute in 1, rapid atrial fibrillation in 2, and ventricular tachycardia or fibrillation in 2. Thirteen deaths occurred, 4 of which were arrhythmia-related. Asystole often was triggered by tracheal suctioning.

Treatment

In addition to supportive care, early plasmapheresis or intravenous immunoglobulin improves outcome.[47] In patients requiring ventilation, cardiac rhythm monitoring is essential. Temporary or permanent pacing may be necessary for management of patients with serious bradycardia.[49] Administration of atropine or isoproterenol before tracheal suctioning has been shown to decrease bradycardia.

Myasthenia Gravis

Clinical Presentation and Cardiac Pathophysiology

Myasthenia gravis is an autoimmune disorder of neuromuscular transmission resulting from production of antibody targeted against the nicotinic acetylcholine receptor. The primary symptom, fluctuating weakness, usually begins with the eye and facial muscles and later can involve the large limb muscles. Patients can present at any age, most commonly at a younger age in women and an older age in men. Myasthenia gravis typically is associated with hyperplasia or a tumor (thymoma) of the thymus gland. A myocarditis is associated with myasthenia gravis, especially that occurring with a thymoma. A cardiac muscle antibody may be responsible.

Arrhythmia Manifestations

In a large series of myasthenia gravis patients, 10% had arrhythmia complications not explained by another etiology.[50] Manifestations included atrial fibrillation, atrioventricular block, asystole, and unexplained sudden death. Cardiac abnormalities were more common in thymoma patients. Autopsy findings were consistent with myocarditis.

Treatment and Prognosis

Myasthenia gravis is treated with anticholinesterase and immunosuppressive agents. Anticholinesterase agents may slow heart rate and cause hypotension. Thymectomy is often recommended. Whether use of immunosuppressive agents or thymectomy improves cardiac disease is unknown.

Epilepsy

Clinical Presentation and Cardiac Pathophysiology

Epilepsy is a complex brain disorder characterized by chronic seizures. Patients with epilepsy are at an increased risk for sudden death of unknown cause that has been termed *sudden unexpected* (or *unexplained*) *death in epilepsy* (SUDEP).[51] Sudden unexpected death is responsible for 2% to 18% of all deaths in epilepsy, with a incidence ranging from 0.4 to 9.3 per 1000 patient-years, depending on the population studied.[52,53] A majority of witnessed sudden deaths occur at or in proximity to a seizure.[54] The mechanisms leading to sudden death in epilepsy are not clear but may involve apnea, excessive respiratory secretions, acute pulmonary edema, or arrhythmias.

Arrhythmia Manifestations

Severe bradycardia with sinus arrest and asystole during the peri-ictal period was documented in 4 of 19 patients with poorly controlled epilepsy undergoing long-term monitoring with an insertable loop recorder.[55] In comparison, serious bradycardia was observed in less than 0.5% of patients undergoing extensive videoelectroencephalographic monitoring at large, busy epilepsy centers.[56,57] Peri-ictal bradycardia is observed primarily in patients with temporal lobe seizures. How to correlate these disparate results and the role of bradycardia and asystole in sudden death in epilepsy is unclear.

An undiagnosed primary ventricular arrhythmia disorder such as the long QT syndrome or right ventricular dysplasia can manifest with symptoms suggestive of epilepsy and thus may potentially be responsible for a small proportion of sudden deaths.

Risk factors for sudden unexpected death in epilepsy include a higher seizure frequency, a longer duration of epilepsy, and the use of three or more antiepileptic drugs.[58]

Treatment and Prognosis

A primary arrhythmia disorder needs to be considered in the differential diagnosis of epilepsy. Patients with poorly controlled epilepsy should undergo aggressive evaluation and treatment.[52] Nighttime supervision of the epileptic patient may decrease the risk of sudden unexpected death.[59] Whether permanent pacing has any role in the management of patients with poorly controlled epilepsy is unclear.

Acute Cerebrovascular Disease

Cardiac Pathophysiology

Cardiac abnormalities, including life-threatening arrhythmias, occur in acute cerebrovascular disease encompassing subarachnoid hemorrhage, other stroke syndromes, and head injury.[60] In these entities, the mechanism responsible for cardiac involvement is an excessive autonomic central output that can accompany intracranial pathologic changes. Hypothalamic stimulation reproduces the electrocardiographic changes observed in acute cerebrovascular disease. Electrocardiographic changes associated with hypothalamic stimulation or blood in the subarachnoid space can be prevented with spinal cord transection, stellate ganglion blockade, vagolytics, and β-adrenergic receptor–blocking agents.

Arrhythmia Manifestations

Cardiac involvement with arrhythmic manifestations is most common in subarachnoid hemorrhage. Electrocardiographic abnormalities are observed in 25% to 80% of patients.[60] The risk is higher with more severe neurologic injury. Peaked and inverted T waves and a prolonged QT interval are seen in 25% to 40% of patients. Hypokalemia is observed in up to 50% of patients, increasing the likelihood of QT interval prolongation. Bradycardia related to sinoatrial block, sinus arrest, and atrioventricular block occurs in up to 10% of patients.[60] Ventricular tachycardia and fibrillation have been reported. Torsades de pointes has been observed. Prolongation of the QT interval and hypokalemia are risk factors for ventricular arrhythmias.

Stroke syndromes other than subarachnoid hemorrhage are associated with abnormal electrocardiograms, but whether these are related to the stroke syndrome or to underlying cardiac disease is unclear.[60,61] Closed head trauma may cause electrocardiographic abnormalities similar to those with subarachnoid hemorrhage, including a prolonged QT interval. Bradycardias are less common in stroke syndromes other than subarachnoid hemorrhage. Ventricular arrhythmias associated with a prolonged QT interval have been observed with closed head trauma.

Treatment and Prognosis

Life-threatening arrhythmias occur primarily in the first day after a neurologic event. Continuous electrocardiographic monitoring during this period is indicated. Monitoring of potassium levels is warranted, especially in patients with subarachnoid hemorrhage. Beta-blockers are effective in controlling both supraventricular and ventricular tachycardias and in decreasing myocardial damage associated with subarachnoid hemorrhage and head trauma. Beta-blockers can increase the likelihood of bradycardia. Stellate ganglion blockade has been reported to effectively control refractory ventricular arrhythmias.

References

1. Nigro G, Comi LI, Politano L, Bain RJ: The incidence and evolution of cardiomyopathy in Duchenne muscular dystrophy. Int J Cardiol 26:271-277, 1990.
2. Melacini P, Fanin M, Danieli GA, et al: Cardiac involvement in Becker muscular dystrophy. J Am Coll Cardiol 22:1927-1934, 1993.
3. Yanagisawa A, Miyagawa M, Yotsukura M, et al: The prevalence and prognostic significance of arrhythmias in Duchenne type muscular dystrophy. Am Heart J 124:1244-1250, 1992.
4. Corrado G, Lissoni A, Beretta S, et al: Prognostic value of electrocardiograms, ventricular late potentials, ventricular arrhythmias, and left ventricular systolic dysfunction in patients with Duchenne muscular dystrophy. Am J Cardiol 89:838-841, 2002.
5. Nigro G, Comi LI, Politano L, et al: Evaluation of the cardiomyopathy in Becker muscular dystrophy. Muscle Nerve 18:283-291, 1995.
6. Duboc D, Meune C, Lerebours G, et al: Effect of perindopril on the onset and progression of left ventricular dysfunction in Duchenne muscular dystrophy. J Am Coll Cardiol 45:855-857, 2005.
7. Jefferies JL, Eidem BW, Belmont JW, et al: Genetic predictors and remodeling of dilated cardiomyopathy in muscular dystrophy. Circulation 112:2799-2804, 2005.
8. Munoz J, Sanjuan R, Morell JS, Ibanez M: Ventricular tachycardia in Duchenne's muscular dystrophy. Int J Cardiol 54:259-262, 1996.
9. Hoogerwaard EM, Bakker E, Ippel PF, et al: Signs and symptoms of Duchenne muscular

dystrophy and Becker muscular dystrophy among carriers in the Netherlands: A cohort study. Lancet 353:2116-2119, 1999.

10. Groh WJ, Lowe MR, Zipes DP: Severity of cardiac conduction involvement and arrhythmias in myotonic dystrophy type 1 correlates with age and CTG repeat length. J Cardiovasc Electrophysiol 13:444-448, 2002.
11. Meola G, Sansone V, Marinou K, et al: Proximal myotonic myopathy: A syndrome with a favourable prognosis? J Neurol Sci 193:89-96, 2002.
12. Liquori CL, Ricker K, Moseley ML, et al: Myotonic dystrophy type 2 caused by a CCTG expansion in intron 1 of ZNF9. Science 293:864-867, 2001.
13. Bhakta D, Lowe MR, Groh WJ: The prevalence of structural heart abnormalities in myotonic dystrophy type 1. Am Heart J 147:224-227, 2004.
14. Schoser BG, Ricker K, Schneider-Gold C, et al: Sudden cardiac death in myotonic dystrophy type 2. Neurology 63:2402-2404, 2004.
15. de Die-Smulders CE, Howeler CJ, Thijs C, et al: Age and causes of death in adult-onset myotonic dystrophy. Brain 121:1557-1563, 1998.
16. Mathieu J, Allard P, Potvin L, et al: A 10-year study of mortality in a cohort of patients with myotonic dystrophy. Neurology 52:1658-1662, 1999.
17. Lazarus A, Varin J, Ounnoughene Z, et al: Relationships among electrophysiological findings and clinical status, heart function, and extent of DNA mutation in myotonic dystrophy. Circulation 99:1041-1046, 1999.
18. Phillips MF, Harper PS: Cardiac disease in myotonic dystrophy. Cardiovasc Res 33:13-22, 1997.
19. Bassez G, Lazarus A, Desguerre I, et al: Severe cardiac arrhythmias in young patients with myotonic dystrophy type 1. Neurology 63:1939-1941, 2004.
20. Merino JL, Carmona JR, Fernandez-Lozano I, et al: Mechanisms of sustained ventricular tachycardia in myotonic dystrophy: Implications for catheter ablation. Circulation 98:541-546, 1998.
21. Day JW, Ricker K, Jacobsen JF, et al: Myotonic dystrophy type 2: Molecular, diagnostic and clinical spectrum. Neurology 60:657-664, 2003.
22. Epstein AE, DiMarco JP, Ellenbogen KA, et al: ACC/AHA/HRS 2008 guidelines for device-based therapy of cardiac rhythm abnormalities. Circulation 117:2820-2840, 2008.
23. Hadian D, Lowe MR, Scott LR, Groh WJ: Use of an insertable loop recorder in a myotonic dystrophy patient. J Cardiovasc Electrophysiol 13:72-73, 2002.
24. Fatkin D, MacRae C, Sasaki T, et al: Missense mutations in the rod domain of the lamin A/C gene as causes of dilated cardiomyopathy and conduction-system disease. N Engl J Med 341:1715-1724, 1999.
25. Meune C, Van Berlo JH, Anselme F, et al: Primary prevention of sudden death in patients with lamin A/C gene mutations. N Engl J Med 354:209-210, 2006.
26. Laval SH, Bushby KMD: Limb-girdle muscular dystrophies—from genetics to molecular pathology. Neuropath Appl Neurobiol 30:91-105, 2004.
27. Muchir A, Bonne G, van der Kooi AJ, et al: Identification of mutations in the gene encoding lamins A/C in autosomal dominant limb girdle muscular dystrophy with atrioventricular conduction disturbances (*LGMD1B*). Hum Molec Genet 9:1453-1459, 2000.
28. Bushby KM, Beckmann JS: The 105th ENMC sponsored workshop: Pathogenesis in the non-sarcoglycan limb-girdle muscular dystrophies, Naarden, April 12-14, 2002. Neuromusc Disord 13:80-90, 2003.
29. Boito CA, Melacini P, Vianello A, et al: Clinical and molecular characterization of patients with limb-girdle muscular dystrophy type 2I. Arch Neurol 62:1894-1899, 2005.
30. Laforet P, de Toma C, Eymard B, et al: Cardiac involvement in genetically confirmed facioscapulohumeral muscular dystrophy. Neurology 51:1454-1456, 1998.
31. Trevisan CP, Pastorello E, Armani M, et al: Facioscapulohumeral muscular dystrophy and occurrence of heart arrhythmia. Eur Neurol 56:1-5, 2006.
32. Buyse G, Mertens L, Di Salvo G, et al: Idebenone treatment in Friedreich's ataxia: Neurological, cardiac, and biochemical monitoring. Neurology 60:1679-1681, 2003.
33. Venance SL, Cannon SC, Fialho D, et al: The primary periodic paralyses: Diagnosis, pathogenesis and treatment. Brain 129:8-17, 2006.
34. Jurkat-Rott K, Lehmann-Horn F: Paroxysmal muscle weakness: The familial periodic paralyses. J Neurol 253:1391-1398, 2006.
35. Lin S-H: Thyrotoxic periodic paralysis. Mayo Clin Proceed 80:99-105, 2005.
36. Sansone V, Griggs RC, Meola G, et al: Andersen's syndrome: A distinct periodic paralysis. Ann Neurol 42:305-312, 1997.
37. Tristani-Firouzi M, Jensen JL, Donaldson MR, et al: Functional and clinical characterization of *KCNJ2* mutations associated with LQT7 (Andersen syndrome). J Clin Invest 110:381-388, 2002.
38. Goldberger ZD: Images in Cardiovascular Medicine. An electrocardiogram triad in thyrotoxic hypokalemic periodic paralysis. Circulation 115:e179-e180, 2007.
39. Williams MJ, Hammond-Tooke GD, Restieaux NJ: Hypokalaemic periodic paralysis with cardiac arrhythmia and prolonged QT interval. Aust N Z J Med 25:549, 1995.
40. Tawil R, Ptacek LJ, Pavlakis SG, et al: Andersen's syndrome: Potassium-sensitive periodic paralysis, ventricular ectopy, and dysmorphic features. Ann Neurol 35:326-330, 1994.
41. Junker J, Haverkamp W, Schulze-Bahr E, et al: Amiodarone and acetazolamide for the treatment of genetically confirmed severe Andersen syndrome. Neurology 59:466, 2002.
42. DiMauro S, Schon EA: Mitochondrial respiratory-chain diseases. N Engl J Med 348:2656-2668, 2003.
43. Akaike M, Kawai H, Yokoi K, et al: Cardiac dysfunction in patients with chronic progressive external ophthalmoplegia. Clin Cardiol 20:239-243, 1997.
44. Vydt TG, de Coo RM, Soliman O, et al: Cardiac involvement in adults with m.3243A>G MELAS gene mutation. Am J Cardiol 99:264-269, 2007.
45. Sorajja P, Sweeney MG, Chalmers R, et al: Cardiac abnormalities in patients with Leber's hereditary optic neuropathy. Heart 89:791-792, 2003.
46. Young TJ, Shah AK, Lee MH, Hayes DL: Kearns-Sayre syndrome: A case report and review of cardiovascular complications. Pacing Clin Electrophysiol 28:454-457, 2005.
47. Hughes RA, Cornblath DR: Guillain-Barré syndrome. Lancet 366:1653-1666, 2005.
48. Zochodne DW: Autonomic involvement in Guillain-Barré syndrome: A review. Muscle Nerve 17:1145-1155, 1994.
49. Winer JB, Hughes RA: Identification of patients at risk of arrhythmia in the Guillain-Barré syndrome. Q J Med 68:735-739, 1988.
50. Hofstad H, Ohm OJ, Mork SJ, Aarli JA: Heart disease in myasthenia gravis. Acta Neurol Scand 70:176-184, 1984.
51. Ryvlin P, Montavont A, Kahane P: Sudden unexpected death in epilepsy: From mechanisms to prevention. Curr Opin Neurol 19:194-199, 2006.
52. Pedley TA, Hauser WA: Sudden death in epilepsy: A wake-up call for management. Lancet 359:1790-1791, 2002.
53. Vlooswijk MCG, Majoie HJM, De Krom MCTFM, et al: SUDEP in the Netherlands: A retrospective study in a tertiary referral center. Seizure 16:153-159, 2007.
54. Nashef L, Hindocha N, Makoff A: Risk factors in sudden death in epilepsy (SUDEP): The quest for mechanisms. Epilepsia 48:859-871, 2007.
55. Rugg-Gunn FJ, Simister RJ, Squirrell M, et al: Cardiac arrhythmias in focal epilepsy: A prospective long-term study. Lancet 364:2212-2219, 2004.
56. Britton JW, Ghearing GR, Benarroch EE, Cascino GD: The ictal bradycardia syndrome: Localization and lateralization. Epilepsia 47:737-744, 2006.
57. Schuele SU, Bermeo AC, Alexopoulos AV, et al: Video-electrographic and clinical features in patients with ictal asystole. Neurology 69:434-441, 2007.
58. Walczak TS, Leppik IE, D'Amelio M, et al: Incidence and risk factors in sudden unexpected death in epilepsy: a prospective cohort study. Neurology 56:519-525, 2001.
59. Langan Y, Nashef L, Sander JW: Case-control study of SUDEP. Neurology 64:1131-1133, 2005.
60. Sakr YL, Ghosn I, Vincent JL: Cardiac manifestations after subarachnoid hemorrhage: A systematic review of the literature. Prog Cardiovasc Dis 45:67-80, 2002.
61. Davis TP, Alexander J, Lesch M: Electrocardiographic changes associated with acute cerebrovascular disease: A clinical review. Prog Cardiovasc Dis 36:245-260, 1993.

Parasystole 79

AGUSTIN CASTELLANOS AND ROBERT J. MYERBURG

CHAPTER OUTLINE

A review of the history of cardiac arrhythmias showed that parasystole was extensively discussed from the dawn of electrocardiography to practically the end of the 20th century. At present it is of waning interest. Readers wishing to know more about it will find that the period extending from 1917 to 1973 is covered by Scherf and Schott[1]; the period between 1973 and 1995, in the encyclopedic second edition of this book[2]; and the period up to 2001, in the Surawicz and Knilans version of Chou's fifth edition.[3] Fewer than 10 papers have been published worldwide after publication of the latter. Of nine articles appearing since then,[4-12,13] four dealt with case reports,[4-8] three were experimental studies,[9,10,14] one was a review,[11] and one referred briefly to the place that parasytole occupies within the teaching of electrocardiography.[12] Only ventricular parasystole is discussed in this chapter, although it can originate in any part of the heart.

General Considerations

Any type of parasystole requires not only "focal" impulse formation but that this be surrounded by an area that protects (shield) the "focus." Although the impulses arise in the sinus node, the slower diastolic depolarization of all slower pacemakers is constantly suppressed by sinus node activity, becoming evident as an escape beat only when impulses from the originating pacemaker do not, for whatever reasons, reach the subsidiary pacemakers and suppress their activity. Under certain circumstances, this does not occur, as for example when parasystole is present. Then the latter is said to be protected from extraneous impulses.

Automaticity and protection are the hallmarks of parasystole. Experimental studies have shown that normal automaticity, abnormal automaticity, triggered acitivity produced by early and delayed afterdepolarizations and depolarized-induced automaticity can cause parasystole if the site origin is protected. Marked disagreement exists regarding the expressions and nature of this protection. In this regard, one important point is noteworthy: The original assumption of total independence (of the ventricular parasystole) from extraneous beats is no longer tenable. Most likely, any pacemaker connected to the surrounding tissues by an area of depressed excitability producing entrance conduction disturbances while allowing the impulses to exit is subject to some degree of modulation by electronic depolarizations arising in the surrounding tissues.[2,3,11]

Classic Parasystole

Pure (nonmodulated) or classic parasystole[3,6-8] is the most frequent type of ventricular parasystole discussed in books dealing with clinical cardiology and electrocardiography. The classical criteria are (Fig. 79-1) (1) varying coupling intervals, (2) mathematically related interectopic intervals, and (3) presence of fusion beats. Pure ventricular parasystole usually is classified as *continuous*, but without exit block; *continuous with exit block*; or *intermittent*.[1] Much has been said regarding the constancy of the mathematically related interectopic intervals, but irregularity of ectopic discharge is the rule rather than the exception, especially if tracings are obtained for long periods of time (as with Holter recordings). One of the most formidable obstacles to diagnosing parasystole, pure or modulated, is posed by intrinsic fluctuations or extrinsic variations in nonmodulated ectopic cycle lengths. In addition to erratic minute-to-minute (or intraminute) apparent changes in ectopic cycle lengths, 24-hour Holter recordings may show that parasystole has rate fluctuations caused by circadian variability, probably resulting from well-known changes in autonomic tone (see Fig. 79-1).[6] Also a source of debate has been how much variation in the coupling intervals is allowed for it to be considered constant. A coupling interval classically is regarded as "fixed" when it does not vary by more than 0.08 second.[3]

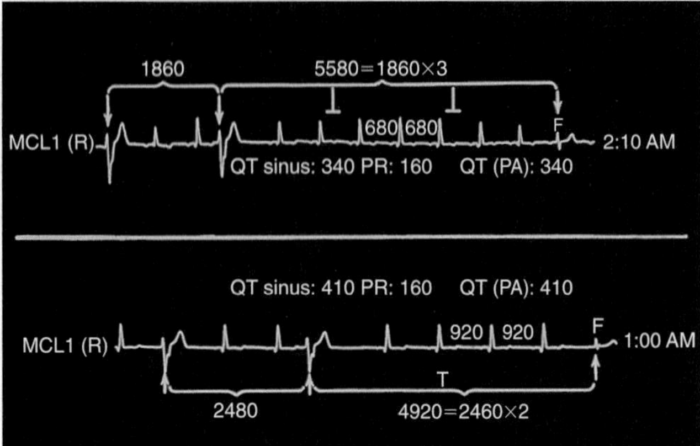

Figure 79-1 Autonomic effects on the ectopic cycle lengths of the so-called classic (nonmodulated) parasystole, as shown in standard MCL1 monitor lead. Note fulfillment of the (three) criteria for the diagnosis of this type of parasystole during an episode of nighttime sympathetic heart rate acceleration. When the sinus rates were the prevalent rates *(bottom)*, the ectopic cycle lengths were longer (2480 ms) than when the sinus rates were faster (1860 ms) *(top)*. Failure (F) of the ectopic beats to appear at the expected times was due to normal refractoriness, not to exit block. All values are expressed in milliseconds. F, fusion beats; PA, parasystole. (From Mendoza IJ, Castellanos A, Lopera G, et al: Nighttime differential autonomic modulation of sinus and idioventricular automaticity and of atrioventricular nodal conduction. Ann Noninvasive Electrocardiol 4:385-390, 1999.)

Electrocardiographic Characteristics of Modulated Ventricular Parasystole

Several investigators have observed the occurrence of modulated parasystole in clinical tracings.[2,3,11] To describe the electrocardiographic manifestations of this arrhythmia, the following nomenclature is used: X denotes a parasystolic beat; R, a nonparasystolic beat, X-X, the interval between two consecutive parasystolic beats without any interposed nonparasystolic beat (nonmodulated ectopic cycle length); X-R, the interval between a parasystolic beat and the immediately following a nonparasystolic beat; and X-R-X, the interval between consecutive parasystolic beats with a single interposed nonparasystolic beat (modulated ectopic cycle length).[2]

In the example shown in Figure 79-2 (left), all intervals were normalized as a percentage of the ectopic cycle length (which could be measured directly). It can be seen that with an ectopic cycle length of 1200 ms (100%), nonparasystolic beats occurring at X-R intervals of 42% (strip A) and 50% (strip B) lengthened the X-R-X interval to 117% and 122%, respectively. In strip C, a slight increment of the X-R interval to 53% caused an inversion of the effect, because the X-R-X interval measured 80%. In strip D, the X-R-X interval decrease was of such a magnitude that parasystolic firing occurred during the refractory period of the nonparasystolic beat. This resulted in a concealed discharge (X*) whose timing (the vertical arrow) could only be assumed by subtracting 100% from the following nonmodulated (but nevertheless manifest) parasystolic beat.

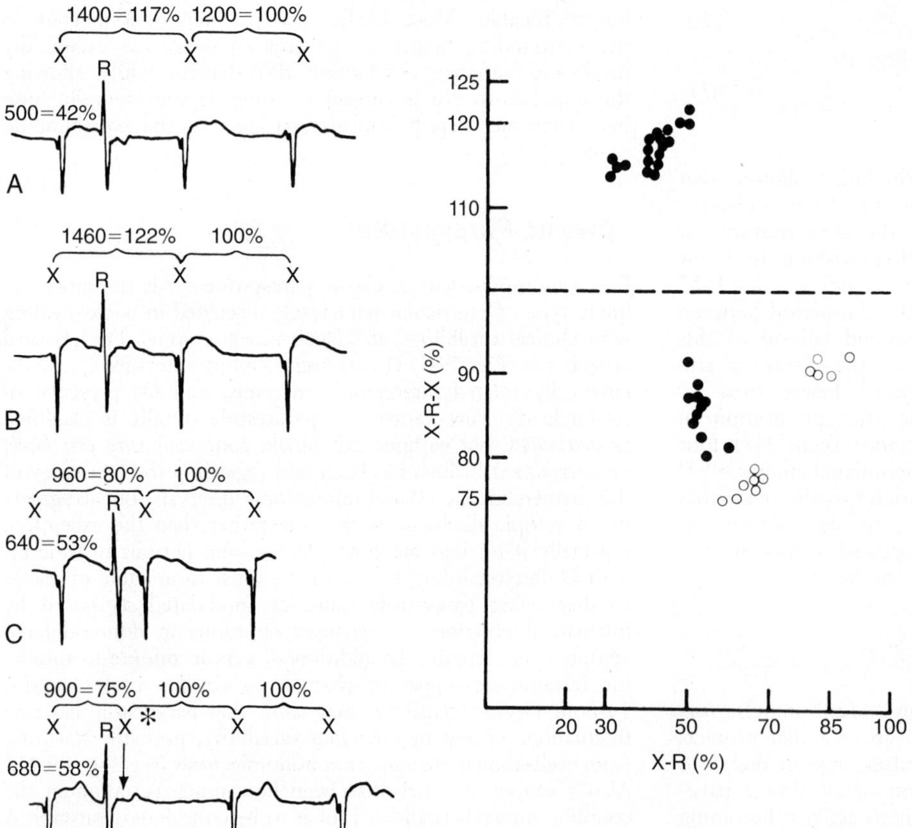

Figure 79-2 Modulated ventricular parasystole. In the corresponding biphasic phase response curve *(right)*, the X-R-X intervals (modulated parasystolic cycle lengths) are related to the X-R intervals, normalized as percentages of the ectopic cycle lengths (*broken horizontal line* at 100%). *Closed circles* represent manifest parasystolic discharges; *open circles* represent concealed parasystolic discharges; X* represents concealed modulated beat. (From Castellanos A, Luceri RM, Moleiro F, et al: Annihilation, entrainment and modulation of ventricular parasystolic rhythms. Am J Cardiol 54:317-322, 1984, copyright 1984, with permission from Excerpta Medica Inc.)

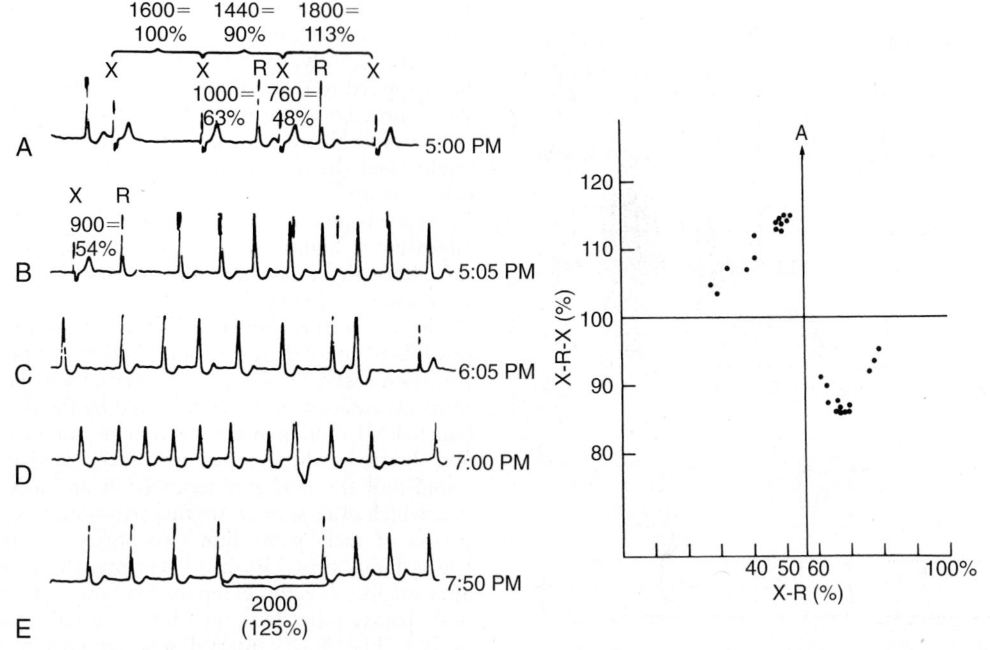

Figure 79-3 Possible pacemaker annihilation in a patient with atrial fibrillation. Note that in **A**, with an X-X interval of 1600 ms (100%), a nonparasystolic beat (NPB) occurring at an X-R interval of 760 ms (48%) increased the X-R-X interval of 1800 ms (113%), whereas one occurring at an X-R interval of 1000 ms (63%) decreased it to 90%. **B**, The NPB occurring 900 ms (56%) after a parasystolic beat apparently produced pacemaker annihilation, because no further manifest parasystolic beats (PBs) were seen during the remaining monitoring time of 8 hours (**B** to **E**), despite marked variations in supraventricular cycle lengths and the existence of NPB-NPB (R-R) intervals longer than the maximal (delayed) ectopic cycle length observed in this patient (**A**). The corresponding phase-response curve revealed that the phenomenon under consideration occurred when NPBs fell during the part of the cycle that corresponded to the reversal point (approximately 56% of the cycle). (From Castellanos A, Luceri RM, Moleiro F, et al: Annihilation, entrainment and modulation of ventricular parasystolic rhythms. Am J Cardiol 54:317-322, 1984, copyright 1984, with permission from Excerpta Medica Inc.)

As in experimental studies, the modulatory effects of nonparasystolic beats can be expressed by a phase-response curve plotting the X-R interval (abscissa) against the deviations of the X-R-X intervals from the X-X interval (ordinate). Initially described clinical phase-response curves were biphasic in relation to the horizontal line representing the X-X interval. Figure 79-3 (right) shows that as the X-R intervals were prolonged, a progressive increase occurred in the X-R-X intervals (delaying phase) until they reached their maximal value. This preceded a reversal of the curve to a point (located more or less toward the middle of the cycle) at which maximal X-R-X shortening occurred. Thereafter, the curve returned toward the horizontal line (accelerating phase). Overlapping of values usually was seen, especially close to or at the reversal point. Analysis of other published phase-response curves has shown that nonparasystolic beats falling close to the latter could produce (1) maximal delay, (2) maximal acceleration, (3) lesser effects, (4) practically no effect, and (5) pacemaker annihilation (see later). Biphasic phase-response curves may be symmetrical or asymmetrical, with the amplitude of either the delaying or shortening effect predominating.[1]

Triphasic phase-response curves are being reported with increasing frequency.[2] They are seen mainly when nonparasystolic beats falling early in the cycle capture the parasystole during its supernormal period.

Pacemaker Annihilation

Biologic oscillatory systems can display annihilation of rhythmic activity by perturbing external stimuli from their surroundings. Using the sucrose gap technique, in strips of dogs' sinoatrial node and Purkinje tissues, carefully timed subthreshold pulses applied across the gap reaching a focus at a precise time could abruptly terminate automatic activity; this phenomenon was termed "pacemaker annihilation."[2]

These findings were first interpreted in light of Winfree's theory concerning phase-resetting patterns of oscillatory systems, in which techniques of differential topology were used. Annihilation was explained in terms of repetitive firing of the Hodgkin-Huxley model at various levels of membrane depolarization. For certain ranges of depolarizing current intensity, the equations contain a "singular" point that terminates the basic rhythm. The likely clinical counterpart of these experiments is seen in Figure 79-3.

Parasystolic Entrainment

According to oscillation theory, as applied in various experimental models and in microelectrode studies of nonreentry cardiac rhythms, entrainment can be defined as the coupling of a self-sustained oscillatory system to an external forcing oscillation. With regard to modulated parasystolic rhythms, an entraining perturbation can be any recurrent nonparasystolic rhythm that is capable of modifying the parasystolic rate by an amount that depends on the instantaneous phase relation to the parasystolic period.[2] In the patient whose tracings are shown in Figure 79-4, the interaction between nonparasystolic beats and parasystolic beats led to periods of concealed and then manifest 1:1 entrainment, during which the parasystolic rate was changed so that it

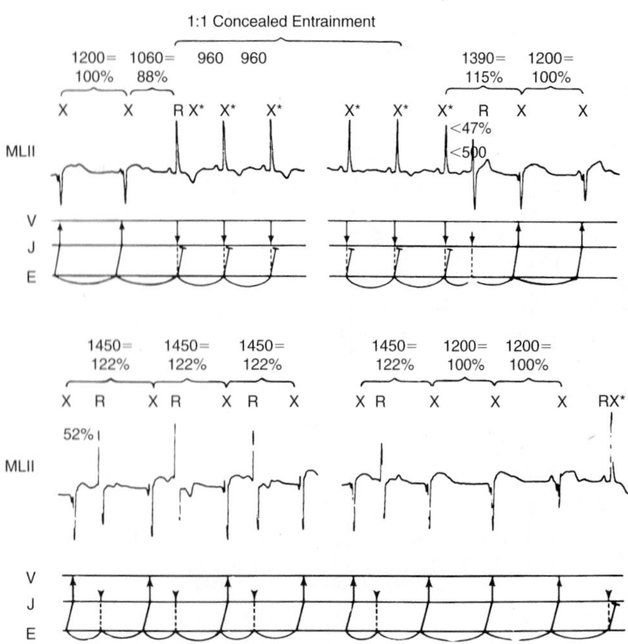

Figure 79-4 Entrainment of modulated ventricular parasystole recorded from MLII lead. *Top left*, Panel depicts the initiation of an episode of concealed 1:1 entrainment initiated by a nonparasystolic beat falling late, during the accelerating phase of the cycle. *Top right*, The termination of the episode by a nonparasystolic beat occurring in the first half of the cycle. During entrainment, the parasystolic rate is increased by the nonparasystolic beats. *Bottom*, The beginning and the end of an episode of manifest 1:1 entrainment initiated and terminated by the appearance and disappearance of a nonparasystolic beat occurring during the early, delaying part of the cycle. (From Castellanos A, Luceri RM, Moleiro F, et al: Annihilation, entrainment and modulation of ventricular parasystolic rhythms. Am J Cardiol 54:317-322, 1984, copyright 1984, with permission from Excerpta Medica Inc.)

equaled the faster and slower nonparasystolic rates. This type of entrainment is different from that occurring during overdrive of reentry tachyarrhythmias, such as atrial flutter and supraventricular and ventricular tachycardias.

Entrainment is a function of several factors: (1) the relation between parasystolic and nonparasystolic (sinus) rates, that is, of operative ectopic or nonparasystolic (sinus) cycle length ratios; (2) the amplitude of the modulating effects; (3) the location of the reversal point in the cycle; and especially (4) the moment of occurrence in the cycle (given by the X-R interval) of the first nonparasystolic beat causing the phenomenon under consideration.[2] Self-entrainment also can occur.

Intermittent Parasystole

Intermittent parasystole (not to be confused with parasystolic intermittency, as discussed later) initially was described as a type of ventricular parasystole characterized by "a periodic awakening and vanishing of an active ventricular center ... not disturbed by sinus stimuli" (apparently caused by intermittent automatic activity).[2] Thus in Figure 79-5, pure nonmodulated ventricular parasystole appears suddenly toward the end of Figure 79-5B and after "warming up" at the end of Figure 79-5C, and "cooling off" toward the middle of Figure 79-5C disappears completely (see Fig. 79-5D and E) for the rest of the monitoring time.

More recently, the term *intermittent ventricular parasystole* has been applied to cases of ventricular parasystole in which "complete" protection was limited to certain (usually the initial) parts of the cycle in such a way that critically timed sinus impulses could reset (hence effectively temporarily abolishing) parasystolic activity.[2]

At the beginning of Figure 79-6, the first three ectopic beats, appearing at slightly decreasing X-R-X intervals (1180 and 1140 ms, although expressed in hundredths of a second at the top), were associated with decreasing X-R intervals, in keeping with the inverse relation between X-R and X-R-X intervals. It is then possible to consider the ectopic rhythm as a pure nonmodulated parasystole with rates of 51 to 52 per minute. However, when the third parasystolic beat was followed by the nonparasystolic beat (labeled ^{X}R) after an interval of 810 ms, this beat was able to reset and discharge the ectopic pacemaker so that the parasystolic impulse of the next run appeared at an ^{X}R-X interval of 1180 ms, which was similar to the parasystolic cycle length. The period of early protection (see horizontal bars in Fig. 79-6) had a duration of 750 ms. Therefore, the sinus beat appearing after the fourth ectopic impulse (^{X}R) was not followed by a manifest parasystolic beat at the expected moment (indicated by X′). The ^{X}R-X′ interval was assumed to have a value of 1140 ms, similar to that of the parasystolic cycle length. Because the ventricles should have been nonrefractory at that time, type II exit block can be postulated, because the parasystolic impulse abruptly failed to traverse the periparasystolic zone to activate the ventricles.[8] However, the impulse must have created enough refractoriness in the part of the protection zone closest to the pacemaker site to block the incoming (10th) R. A similar phenomenon occurred toward the end of the strip. According to the interpretation proposed, the parasystole was not only pure but intermittent, with protection (entrance block) limited to the first part of the cycle and intermittent degrees of type II exit block.

These events also can be explained by the concept of modulation by assuming that magnitude of the early phase of delay was attenuated enough to become nondetectable in the surface eelctrocardiogram, whereas the acceleration phase was maintained at its maximum level because of the capture acceleration of the pacemaker produced by the electrotonically mediated modulations. Even with this interpretation, however, exit block has to be postulated. Phenomena such as this could perhaps be explained by the coexistence of type I and type II second-degree entrance block (without having to postulate exit block).

Intermittency of Manifest Parasystolic Activity: Recapitulation

The concept of intermittent ventricular parasystole requires recognition of other causes of parasystolic intermittency not due to "true" intermittent ventricular parasystole, including the following: (1) ventricular parasystole with the same or one-half the rate of the sinus beats with concealed discharges caused by their occurrence during the effective refractory period of the latter[2]; (2) the so-called concealed pure ventricular parasystole, so named because manifest discharges do not occur if prevented from doing so by concealed conduction of entrant sinus impulse into the zone of protection[2]; and (3) long-lasting episodes of complete exit block or of (4) total loss of entrance block (i.e., of protection). Moreover, the concept of "continuous" ventricular parasystole needs reevaluation, particularly when the diagnosis is made from Holter recordings. Although it is true

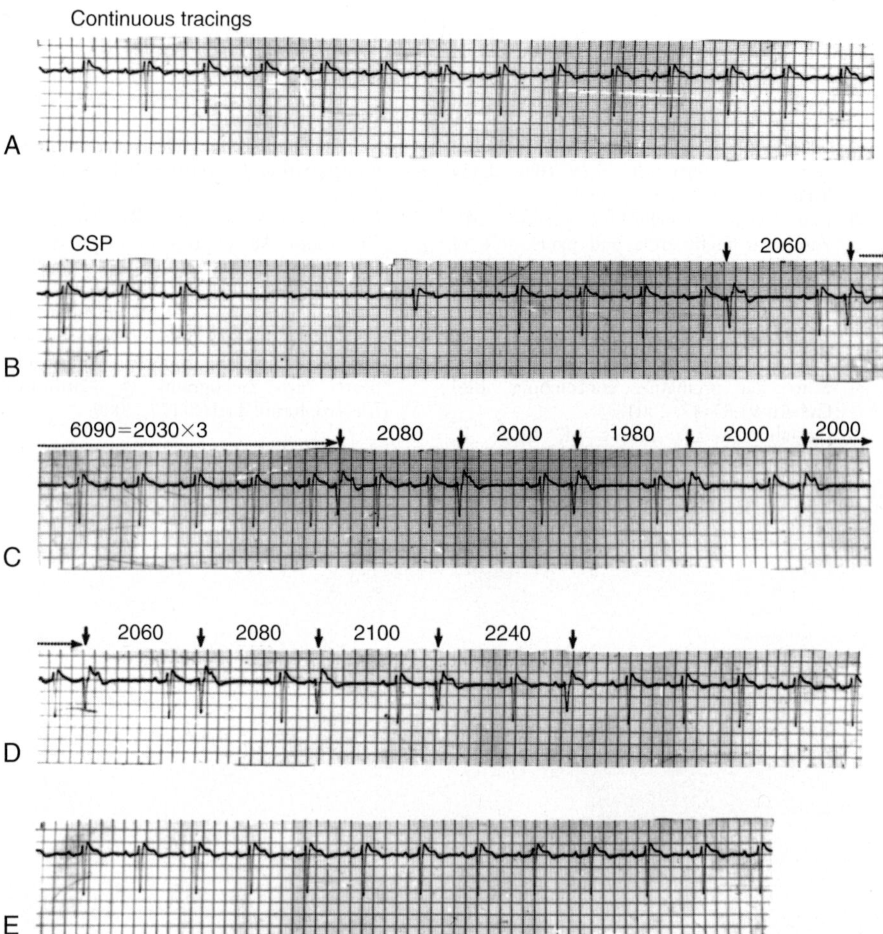

Figure 79-5 Intermittent, apparently pure, ventricular parasystole. Note that the latter appears unexpectedly (**B**) at a cycle length (2060 ms) that is shorter than the immediately preceding ventricular pause elicited by carotid sinus pressure (CSP). After "warming up" to 1980 ms (**C**), the parasystole gradually "cools off" to 2240 (**D**) before it disappears (**E**). Although several other mechanisms have been shown in other figures, variants of this type of parasystole constitute the one most frequently found when the diagnosis is made from Holter recordings. (*Arrows* indicate manifest parasystolic beats).

that some ventricular parasystoles are continuously operating for long periods of time, long-term monitoring has shown that this is the exception rather than the rule.[2] Then what is continuous? For example, if a ventricular parasystole has all of the features attributed to continuous ventricular parasystole but is apparent only from, for example, 1:00 to 3:00 PM (and absent during the remaining 22 hours of the day), should it be considered "continuous" or continuous only for 2 hours?[12] In the current world in which "consensus" medicine is predominant, no such consensus exists for ventricular parasystole.

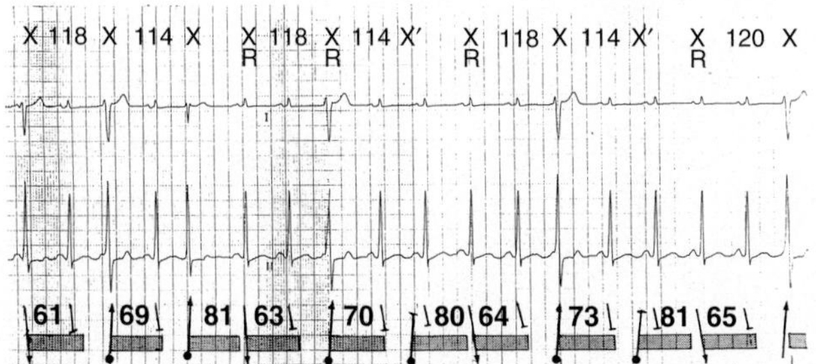

Figure 79-6 Intermittent pure ventricular parasystole having protection limited to the early parts of this cycle or continuous modulated parasystole with attenuation of the early delaying phase. In either case, exit block occurring at the moment indicated by X′ has to be postulated. *Horizontal bars* indicate the part of the cycle at which protection is absolute or electrotonic impulses cause no appreciable change (prolongation) in parasystolic cycle length. For didactic reasons, exit block is misrepresented as occurring distal to the zone of protection. (From Castellanos A, Moleiro F, Guerrero J, et al: Intermittent parasystole with exit block. J Electrocardiol 30:331-335, 1997.)

"Parasystolic Alienation" and the Withering of Parasystole

Not surprisingly, Surawicz and Knilans[3] seem to have stated what we all know intuitively: that the current incidence of ventricular parasystole is unknown. The proposed mechanisms depicted in Figures 79-1 through 79-6 have dazed interpreters to such a degree that most tend to avoid anything that has to do with ventricular parasystole, a phenomenon that we have referred to as "parasystolic alienation."[13] The use of the concept of parasystole in routine clinical cardiography has been further complicated by the recent introduction of the intellectually valuable but clinically complex technological gadgets, such as the tachometer described by Takayagani and colleagues.[14] This limitation, as well as statements that "it does not kill" and that "an accurate analysis of modulated parasystole can take more than one hour,"[12] explains why ventricular parasystole appears to be only of historical and intellectual interest.[12] The latter reference is of great importance because it deals with the place that parasystolic identification has in day-to-day electrocardiographic teaching and interpretation.

References

1. Scherf D, Schott A: Extrasystoles and Allied Arrhythmias, 2nd ed. Chicago, Year Book, 1973, pp 269-281.
2. Castellanos A, Saoudi N, Moleiro F, Myerburg RJ: Parasystole. In Zipes D, Jalife J (eds): Cardiac Electrophysiology: From Cell to Bedside, 2nd ed. Philadelphia, Saunders, 1995, pp 942-954.
3. Surawicz B, Knilans TK: Chou's Electrocardiography in Clinical Practice: Adult and Pediatric, 5th ed. Philadelphia, Saunders, 2001, pp 401-403.
4. Kinoshita S, Katoh T, Tsujimura Y, Sasaki Y: Apparent disappearance of ventricular parasystole due to a marked difference between the long form and the short form of the ectopic cycles. J Cardiovasc Med (Hagerstown) 8:192-196, 2007.
5. Skylar E, Hollander G: Is this atrial parasystole, atrial dissociation, or an artifact? J Electrocardiol 40:133-134, 2007.
6. Ono S, Ashida T, Sugiyama T, et al: Variation in parasystolic cycle length. Int Heart J 47:153-158, 2006.
7. Glancy DL: Group beating resulting from ventricular parasystole. Proc (Bayl Univ Med Cent) 16:352-353, 2003.
8. Lau EW, Marshall HG, Griffith MJ: Fascicular tachycardia and parasystole of right bundle brandh origin. Heart Rhythm 2:994-996, 2005.
9. Ikeda N, Takeuchi A, Hamada A, et al: Model of bidirectional modulated parasystole as a mechanism for cyclic bursts of ventricular premature contractions. Biol Cybern 91:37-47, 2004.
10. Grigaliuniene I, Skucas M, Lekas R, Seskevicius A: Extrapotentials and allorhythmias as an expression of experimental parasystole. Medicina (Kaunas) 40:246-252, 2004.
11. Grolleau R, Pasquie JL, Macia JC, Leclercq F: Parasystole. Arch Mal Coeur Vaiss 95:41-46, 2002.
12. Childres R: Teaching electrocardiographic interpretation. J Electrocardiol 30:426-429, 2006.
13. Castellanos A, Myerburg RJ: Parasystolic alienation: An impression or a reality? J Cardiovasc Electrophysiol 11:178-179, 2000.
14. Takayanagi K, Tanaka K, Kamishirado H, et al: Direct discrimination and full-day disclosure of ventricular parasystolic heart rate tachograms. J Cardiovasc Electrophysiol 11:168-177, 2000.

Differential Diagnosis for Wide QRS Complex Tachycardia 80

JOHN M. MILLER AND MITHILESH K. DAS

CHAPTER OUTLINE

Perspective and Definitions

"What was that criterion again?!" Clinicians looking at a sick patient's electrocardiogram (ECG) that shows a wide QRS complex tachycardia (WCT) often experience considerable frustration. Despite the existence of well-established criteria, the diagnosis of a WCT remains difficult for the practicing physician. Making the correct diagnosis is important not only for choosing appropriate initial therapy for an ongoing arrhythmia but also for subsequent management. Many physicians still assume that a WCT in a patient who is alert and hemodynamically stable must be supraventricular tachycardia (SVT), because "patients with ventricular tachycardia (VT) are always unstable." Some VTs can be terminated by administration of adenosine or verapamil, fortifying the misconception. On the other hand, verapamil administration for treatment of presumed SVT in a patient with reduced systolic function who actually has VT may cause severe and prolonged hypotension. An incorrect initial diagnosis also can set the wrong course for chronic therapy with potentially disastrous results. Thus, arriving at the correct diagnosis of the cause of WCT is more than an intellectual exercise.

Several useful sets of criteria have been developed to aid in distinguishing among causes of WCT. Although none of these systems are perfect, when properly applied they can guide the clinician to the correct diagnosis in a majority of cases. This chapter reviews the causes of WCT and the criteria that can be used to establish the correct diagnosis. It is important for diagnostic criteria to be accurate, easily applied, and readily remembered, because the clinical circumstances of patients presenting with WCT usually do not allow leisurely analysis of ECGs.

Definitions used in this chapter include the following:

wide complex tachycardia (WCT) a rhythm with a rate of 100 per minute or greater and QRS duration 120 ms or greater

ventricular tachycardia (VT) a WCT originating below the level of the His bundle

supraventricular tachycardia (SVT) a tachycardia dependent on participation of structures at or above the level of the His bundle

left bundle branch block (LBBB) morphology QRS duration 120 ms or greater, with a predominantly negative terminal deflection in ECG lead V_1

right bundle branch block (RBBB) morphology QRS duration 120 ms or greater, with a terminal positive deflection in V_1

In these definitions, *LBBB* and *RBBB* refer to the morphologic appearance of the QRS complex, without implying the actual presence of His-Purkinje disease.

Distinguishing Features of Wide QRS Complex Tachycardia

WCT has several possible causes. Broad categories include VT, SVT with abnormal (aberrant) interventricular conduction (SVT-A), and paced ventricular rhythms (Fig. 80-1):

1. *VT* is the most common cause of WCT in the general population, accounting for up to 80% of all cases of WCT. This fact has obvious implications for arriving at a diagnosis in patients with a WCT.
2. *SVT with abnormal interventricular conduction* accounts for the second largest proportion of WCT cases (15% to 30% overall) and includes several subsets:
   a. SVT with aberration is the largest subset. SVT with bundle branch block aberration (right or left bundle branch block [RBBB, LBBB]). Bundle branch block can either be permanent or *fixed* (present during the normal baseline rhythm between episodes of WCT), or *functional* (present only during WCT). Functional aberration results from a sudden increase in heart rate at a moment when a bundle branch is partially or wholly refractory.
   b. SVT with ventricular activation occurring over an anomalous atrioventricular (AV) connection (preexcited SVT in Wolff-Parkinson-White syndrome). Because these pathways almost always connect atrial and ventricular muscle at the AV valve rings, the ECG pattern in preexcited tachycardia can be indistinguishable from that in VT originating at the base of the ventricles. Thus, preexcited SVT may be considered if the ECG shows a concordant positive precordial R wave pattern (see later on), but not when a concordant negative pattern is present (with the rare exception of atriofascicular pathway-related tachycardias). Preexcited tachycardias account for a small minority of cases of WCT (1% to 5%).
   c. SVT with wide QRS complex due to abnormal muscle-to-muscle spread of impulse. In this subset, His-Purkinje conduction may be relatively normal but the baseline rhythm on ECG suggests RBBB, LBBB, or a nonspecific interventricular conduction defect (IVCD). Examples are the appearance of RBBB in patients who have undergone right ventriculotomy (e.g., repaired tetralogy of Fallot),

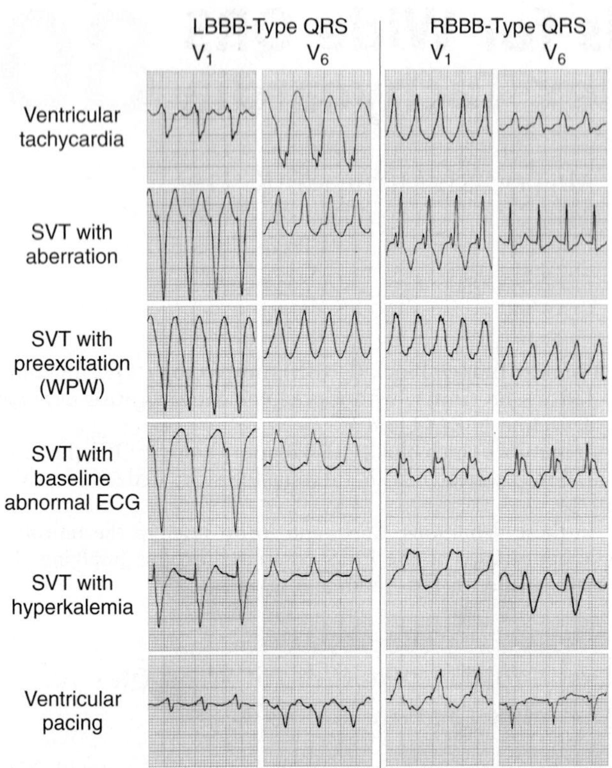

Figure 80-1 Examples of lead V_1 and V_6 traces in both left bundle branch block (LBBB) and right bundle branch block (RBBB) types of QRS complexes in different types of wide complex tachycardia. Similarities and differences can be appreciated among groups.

in which the right ventricular conduction delay is due to delayed muscle-muscle conduction in the right ventricular outflow tract (RVOT); the appearance of LBBB in patients with dilated cardiomyopathy in which the left-sided conduction delay is due to diffusely slowed muscle-muscle conduction rather than His-Purkinje disease; and other varieties of bizarre, widened QRS patterns in baseline rhythm in patients with repaired or unrepaired congenital heart disease or cardiomyopathy.

d. SVT with wide QRS complex due to drug- or electrolyte disturbance-induced changes. Sodium channel–blocking antiarrhythmic drugs can cause a nonspecific widening of the QRS complex; thus, what would otherwise have been a narrow QRS SVT can manifest with a wide QRS, or an aberrant QRS may be prolonged enough to suggest VT (see later). Drugs capable of producing this effect include class 1A agents (procainamide, quinidine, disopyramide), class IC agents (flecainide, encainide, propafenone), and amiodarone. In addition, class IC agents may provoke sustained uniform VT during exercise testing even in young healthy persons without structural heart disease or history of ventricular arrhythmias. Class IC drugs can also cause WCT by slowing the atrial rate during flutter such that 1:1 AV conduction occurs with a (drug-related) wide QRS. Recognition of these disorders is important for initiating proper therapy. Finally, hyperkalemia can widen the QRS complex enough to cause confusion about the nature of a tachycardia; this typically yields a LBBB-like appearance on the ECG, although some cases may suggest RBBB (see Fig. 80-1). Drug- and electrolyte disturbance-induced abnormalities represent rare causes of WCT, but their recognition is of critical importance for proper care of affected patients.

3. *Paced ventricular rhythms* constitute a small but growing category of WCT. Contemporary pacing systems generally require less energy for reliable ventricular capture, leading to small, almost imperceptible stimulus artifacts on the ECG. These patients may have SVT or activity-driven AV pacing without clear stimulus artifacts on ECG, resulting in a WCT that has the appearance of VT. Obviously, presence of a pacing device on physical examination is a strong clue to pacing as the cause of the WCT. Most of these WCTs have LBBB, leftward superior axis (pacing from RV apex), although an increasing number of patients have biventricular pacing devices that can produce a larger variety of ECG patterns. Because left ventricular pacing often requires higher outputs, a clear stimulus artifact provides the diagnosis. Although patients with pacemakers or implantable cardioverter-defibrillators (ICDs) can have WCT as a result of ventricular pacing, VT and SVT-A are far more likely causes.

Because most cases of WCT are either VT or SVT-A, the remainder of the discussion of distinguishing features focuses on differentiation between these two diagnoses. The distribution of WCT causes may vary in acordance with specific clinical settings; for instance, a pediatric hospital is likely to have a higher proportion of preexcited SVTs and SVT-As than of VTs.

Supraventricular Tachycardia versus Ventricular Tachycardia: History and Physical Examination

A history of heart disease—previous myocardial infarction, angina, or congestive heart failure—can serve as a rough discriminator between SVT-A and VT as the cause of WCT, each factor having a positive predictive accuracy of 95% (for VT). A majority of patients with VT have some form of structural heart disease, whereas patients with SVT-A may or may not have heart disease. Of note, however, a small subset of patients with VT has no underlying heart disease, and nothing prevents patients with significant structural heart disease from having SVT-A. Patients with VT tend to be older than those with SVT (older than 35 years). Patients with SVT-A more often have a history of previous episodes of arrhythmia; if the history includes similar episodes occurring for longer than 3 years, SVT-A is far more likely than VT. In patients who have had a previous myocardial infarction and whose first episode of WCT occurred thereafter, VT is by far the most likely diagnosis for the cause of the WCT.

The physical appearance of a patient who presents with WCT is not an accurate diagnostic point; most patients presenting with SVT-A are hemodynamically stable and do not appear very ill, as is the case for a significant proportion of patients with VT. The widespread impression that hemodynamic stability during WCT indicates a diagnosis of SVT-A is thus erroneous and can lead to potentially injurious mistreatment of these patients. As noted previously, patients with hemodynamically stable VT often become hemodynamically unstable if given verapamil to try to terminate presumed SVT.

As discussed later on, a very useful criterion in distinguishing the cause of WCT is the presence of AV dissociation. Physical findings that indicate the presence of AV dissociation include "cannon" A waves in the jugular venous waveform (due to fortuitously timed atrial contraction during ventricular systole, against a closed tricuspid valve), an S_1 of variable intensity (according to how far open or closed the tricuspid and mitral leaflets are at the time of dissociated ventricular systole), and variation in systolic blood pressure unrelated to respiration (due to variable left ventricular filling, depending on timing of the dissociated atrial contraction). AV dissociation may not be present at the time of initial examination of the patient but may be manifested by applying carotid sinus pressure or administration of adenosine. These maneuvers may cause transient retrograde block in the AV node and AV dissociation, enabling a diagnosis of VT.

Termination of WCT in response to physical maneuvers such as Valsalva or carotid sinus pressure, or medications (adenosine) strongly suggests SVT as the cause of the WCT; however, well-documented cases in which VT has been terminated by each of the aforementioned modalities generally are thought to be indicative of SVT only. Intravenous verapamil or beta-blockers can have effects similar to those noted for adenosine, but side effects from these medications (hypotension, negative inotropy) can last several minutes to an hour, so their diagnostic and therapeutic use is discouraged without a compelling reason. Several cases have been reported in which a patient with hemodynamically stable VT received intravenous verapamil, became hypotensive, and required emergency resuscitation to prevent death.

Differentiation of Supraventricular Tachycardia with Aberration from Ventricular Tachycardia: Electrocardiographic Criteria

The most reliable means of distinguishing SVT-A from VT remains the ECG. The following discussion reviews the classic ECG criteria used for this distinction, as well as their limitations. It is important for proper analysis that the clinician be provided with an adequate amount of ECG material (good-quality 12-lead ECG, long rhythm strip). Accurate recall of all of the following criteria in an emergency situation is understandably difficult. Most can, however, be distilled down to a fundamentally simple approach: If WCT is due to SVT-A, then the QRS complexes during WCT must be compatible with some form of bundle branch block or fascicular block. If no combination of bundle branch block and fascicular block could result in the QRS configuration being analyzed, then aberration probably is *not* present, and the diagnosis by default is VT. A smaller number of patterns can result from aberration than from VT arising from anywhere in the ventricles. It is thus useful for the clinician to be thoroughly familiar with what ECG patterns are possible with various forms of bundle branch block and fascicular block, permitting comparison with a WCT ECG to determine whether or not its appearance is compatible with aberration. The following ECG criteria have been suggested to distinguish between SVT-A and VT:

- QRS duration: Wellens and colleagues[1] found that 69% of VTs had QRS complex duration greater than 140 ms, whereas no cases of SVT-A had QRS duration more than 140 ms. Because the QRS duration with LBBB aberration generally is slightly longer than with RBBB, this criterion has been modified such that VT is the likely diagnosis when the QRS duration with RBBB-type morphology is more than 140 ms, but more than 160 ms with LBBB-type morphology. Antiarrhythmic drugs may nonspecifically widen the QRS complex of an SVT, potentially decreasing the utility of this criterion. Rarely, a patient exhibits QRS complexes during VT that are relatively narrow (120 to 140 ms). This is more likely to be seen in patients without structural heart disease.
- QRS axis: The more leftward the axis, the more likely the arrhythmia is VT rather than SVT-A. With true left anterior fascicular block (LAFB), the QRS axis is from −30 to −90 degrees; with left posterior fascicular block (LPFB), the axis is from +110 to +150 degrees. This leaves a quadrant of the frontal plane axis, from −90 to ±180 degrees, that cannot be achieved with any combination of bundle branch block or fascicular block. Therefore, WCTs with frontal plane axes in this rightward superior quadrant are unlikely to be SVT-A, so VT is the likely diagnosis. Some researchers have suggested that a shift in QRS axis of more than 40 degrees between the baseline rhythm and WCT ECGs suggests VT, although not strongly so.
- Specific morphologic patterns in leads V_1 and V_6 during WCT (Fig. 80-2):
  A. V_1 with "RBBB" pattern. The right ventricle does not participate in initial ventricular depolarization during a normally conducted beat, so the initial portion of the QRS complex is not affected by RBBB aberration. QRS patterns in V_1 consistent with aberration therefore include rSŕ, rŔ, rsŕ, and rSŔ. QRS patterns highly suggestive of VT include a monophasic R wave; a broad (greater than 30 ms) R with any following terminal negative QRS forces; and a qR. These latter patterns are incompatible with ventricular activation using the normal left bundle branch.
  B. V_6 with "RBBB" pattern. RBBB aberration produces a qRs, Rs, or RS (with the R/S ratio greater than 1) in V_6, reflecting ventricular activation over the LBB. Patterns differing from these, and thus suggesting VT are rS, Qrs, QS, QR, or a monophasic R wave; if an RS pattern is present, the R/S ratio is less than 1. In true RBBB aberration, delayed right ventricular activation produces

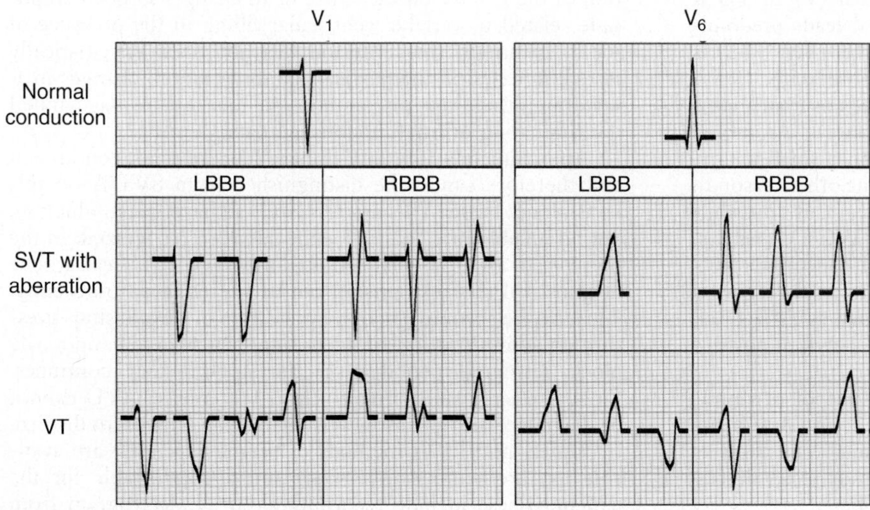

Figure 80-2 Diagrammatic representation of common QRS complex morphologic patterns encountered in ventricular tachycardia (VT) and supraventricular tachycardia with aberration (SVT-A), in lead V_1 and V_6 traces for both LBBB and RBBB QRS complexes. Note the initial portions of the QRS complex in normal and aberrant QRS complexes, contrasted with initial QRS forces in VT complexes. The "Rs" configuration can be designated as either RBBB or LBBB type (grouped with LBBB-type morphology). LBBB, left bundle branch block; RBBB, right bundle branch block.

a small S wave in V_6 because of the relatively smaller muscle mass of the right ventricle compared with the left ventricle. Because most VTs originate in the left ventricle, however, a large S wave in V_6 during VT consists of not only of the right ventricular component of ventricular activation but also depolarization of some portion of the left ventricle as activation propagates away from the location of the V_6 electrode.

C. V_1 with "LBBB" patterns. The left bundle branch mediates ventricular depolarization during a normally conducted complex, so LBBB would be expected to cause a change from the initial vector of ventricular depolarization during baseline rhythm. However, there is generally rapid penetration of the left ventricular His-Purkinje system even in the presence of LBBB, such that initial forces (mediated by the right bundle branch) are relatively preserved. This results in a QRS morphology in V_1 during LBBB aberration of either an rS or a QS, but in either case with rapid initial forces (narrow r wave and rapid, smooth descent to the nadir of the S wave). Patterns other than these during WCT, such as a broad r wave (greater than 30 ms) or deep S wave, or a QS with a slow descent to the S wave nadir (60 ms or greater), are incompatible with normal activation and thus imply VT. Additionally, the amplitude of the initial R wave in V_1 during WCT can be helpful when compared with the R wave in sinus rhythm: A taller R during WCT than in sinus rhythm suggests VT as the cause.

D. V_6 with LBBB-type pattern. During typical LBBB aberration, the QRS in V_6 lacks an initial Q wave, and instead has an RŔ or monophasic R wave. During VT, common patterns are QR, QS, QrS, and Rŕ, although patterns consistent with SVT also may be observed (RŔ, monophasic R).

E. "Ambiguous" patterns. W and Rs patterns in V_1 (see Fig. 80-2) have been variously classified as LBBB or RBBB type; because these are ambiguous in this way, they are very unlikely to represent typical aberration and are highly specific for VT.

F. Combinations of bundle branch block and axis deviation. The specific combination LBBB morphology with right axis deviation is practically always due to VT, because LBBB aberration is almost never associated with left posterior fascicular block; on the other hand, RBBB morphology with a normal axis (0 to +90 degrees) is very uncommon in VT (with less than 5% prevalence), so this combination should suggest SVT-A.

- Concordant pattern: A concordant precordial (V_1 to V_6) R wave progression pattern (i.e., all precordial leads predominantly positive or all predominantly negative) (Fig. 80-3) is uncommon in SVT-A, with the exception of preexcited tachycardia, in which ventricular activation proceeds over an anomalous AV connection (positive concordance). As noted previously, these tachycardias account for only a small minority of all WCTs (1% to 6%) and without some other reason to suspect Wolff-Parkinson-White syndrome, this possibility deserves little consideration in WCT analysis. Unfortunately, although the specificity of a concordant pattern for VT has been high (greater than 90%), its sensitivity is low; concordance is observed in only apoximately 20% of all VTs in most series, roughly equally divided between positive and negative patterns.
- Concordance of the limb leads: The presence of predominantly negative QRS complexes in leads 1, 2, and 3 also has been suggested as a criterion for diagnosing VT. This is another way of describing rightward superior axis, already noted previously to be very suggestive of VT.
- Presence of Q waves: Q waves during WCT suggest the presence of an old myocardial infarction, pointing to VT as the likely diagnosis. In general, patients with post–myocardial infarction VT maintain Q waves during WCT that had been present during baseline rhythm. These Q waves generally are in the same distribution during WCT as during baseline rhythm (i.e., a patient with an anterior myocardial infarction will have anterior Q waves during VT), although this is not always the case. Some cases of dilated cardiomyopathy also may have Q waves during VT that are not present during baseline rhythm. Finally, "pseudo Q waves" may rarely occur in some SVT-As (such AV nodal reentry with a retrograde P wave deforming the onset of the QRS, mimicking a Q wave), as well as a preexcited tachycardia in which a posterior AV connection is used for ventricular activation (resulting in pseudo inferior Q waves).
- AV dissociation (AVD): The most specific electrocardiographic feature in distinguishing VT from SVT is the AV relationship. Complete AVD occurs in 20% to 50% of all VTs and practically no SVT-As (sensitivity of 0.2 to 0.5, with specificity approaching 1.0). The wide range of prevalence of AVD may be due to (1) tachycardia rate—the more rapid a tachycardia, the less likely it is that the A:V relationship can be determined, because diastole is shortened so less opportunity is available to distinguish P waves between QRS complexes and T waves; (2) amount of ECG for analysis—AVD may be present during even relatively slow VTs but is not appreciated because of inadequate duration of ECG recordings; (3) observer experience—in some cases, P waves may be seen only by careful and experienced observers and are missed by those less experienced; or (4) observer confidence—the certainty with which the observer is willing to make the diagnosis of AVD on the basis of subtle ECG differences varies among individuals.

Although AVD is the most useful single criterion for distinguishing VT from SVT-A, an AV ratio less than 1 is equally diagnostic of VT. In addition to the 20% to 50% of VTs with AVD, 15% to 20% of VTs have second-degree ventriculoatrial block (either 2:1 retrograde conduction or Wenckebach). Although diagnostic of VT, these findings generally are more difficult to recognize on the ECG. The contour of the terminal portion of the QRS in some ECG leads may resemble P waves, leading to a diagnosis of SVT-A. Inspection of simultaneously recorded ECG leads allows comparison of the timing of the end of the QRS and can decrease suspicion of "pseudo-P waves."

Another clue to the presence of AVD is variation in QRS amplitude during WCT. This may be due to scalar summation of the P wave on the QRS, or to changes in QRS amplitude related to variable ventricular filling in the presence of AVD. Although this criterion has not been systematically tested, in cases of unequivocal AV dissociation, changes in R wave amplitude are uncommon, so this feature has limited discriminating utility (unpublished data).

Approximately 30% of VTs have 1:1 retrograde conduction and therefore cannot be distinguished from SVT-A on this basis alone. Faster VTs are less likely to have 1:1 conduction, but no reliable rate "cutoff" value has been recognized. In the presence of a 1:1 AV relationship during WCT, VT can still be diagnosed if this relationship can be altered, even transiently. This may be accomplished by application of carotid sinus pressure or administration of adenosine, which may temporarily block retrograde conduction during VT that continues. Finally, when atrial fibrillation and VT coexist, AVD cannot be diagnosed and any atrial activity may be difficult to discern.

Other, non-ECG methods of diagnosing AVD are available but are more cumbersome and uncomfortable for the patient. These include recording an atrial electrogram from

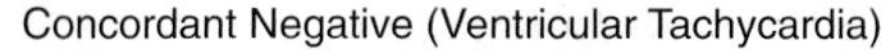

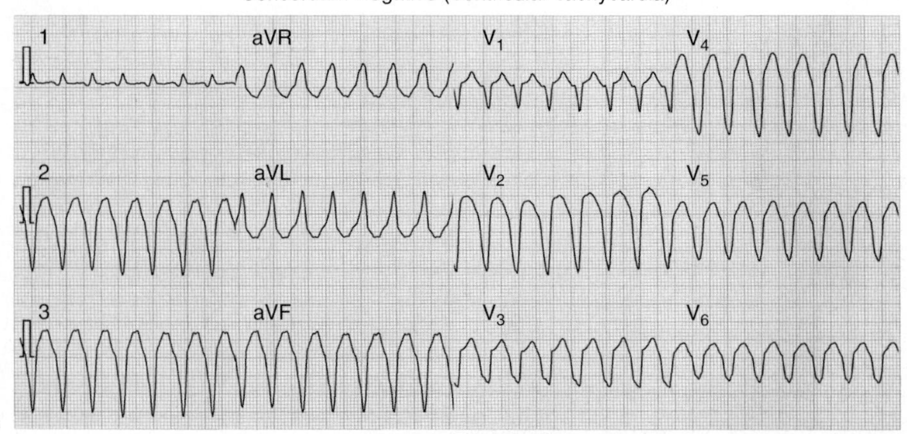

Concordant Positive (Ventricular Tachycardia)

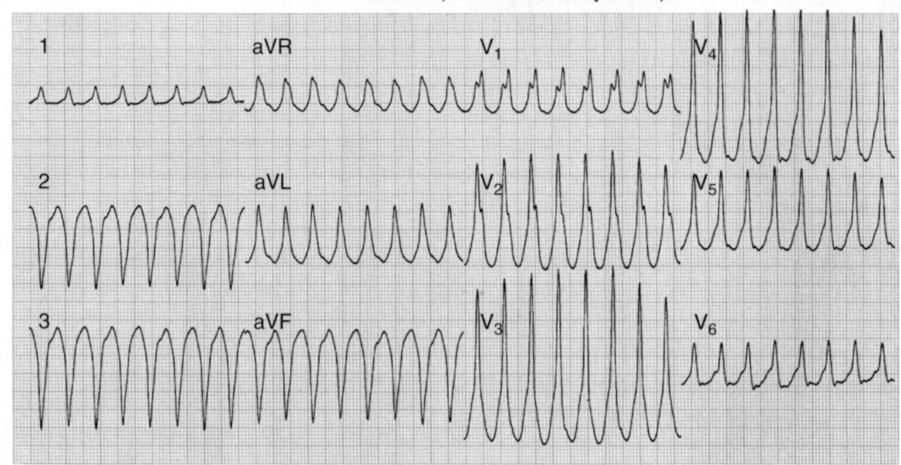

Concordant Positive (Preexcited Supraventricular Tachycardia)

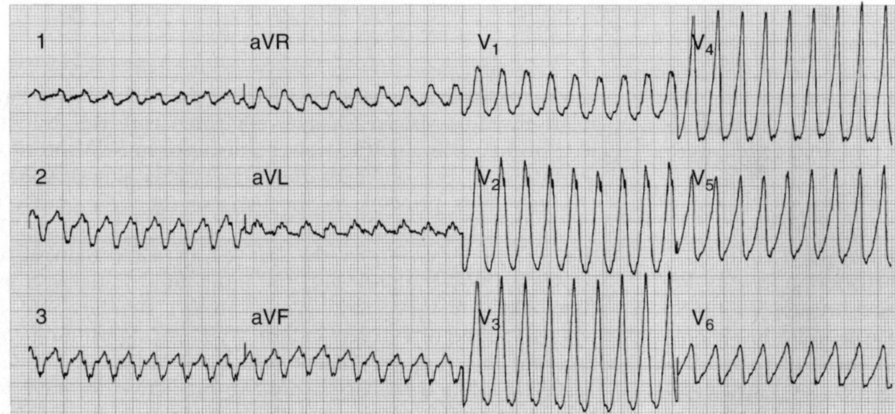

Figure 80-3 Concordant precordial patterns. **A,** Negative concordance during ventricular tachycardia (VT) in a patient with a previous anterior myocardial infarction. **B,** Positive concordance during VT in a patient with a previous inferior myocardial infarction. **C,** Positive concordance during preexcited supraventricular tachycardia in a patient with Wolff-Parkinson-White syndrome. Note similarity of electrocardiographic patterns in **B** and **C**.

an esophageal or transvenous electrode and subcostal echocardiography (evaluating right atrial contraction in relation to ventricular contraction). Although accurate, each of these methods requires time, equipment, and expertise and are therefore less attractive than ECG methods. In addition, VT with 1:1 retrograde conduction cannot be distinguished from SVT with these methods.

- Fusion beats: A fusion beat is a "hybrid" QRS complex resulting from ventricular activation from two different sources. Fusion beats during WCT imply the presence of AVD and are most frequently observed during relatively slow tachycardias, allowing time between VT QRSs for a supraventricular beat to propagate through the normal conduction system. This criterion is most reliable when the fusion beats result

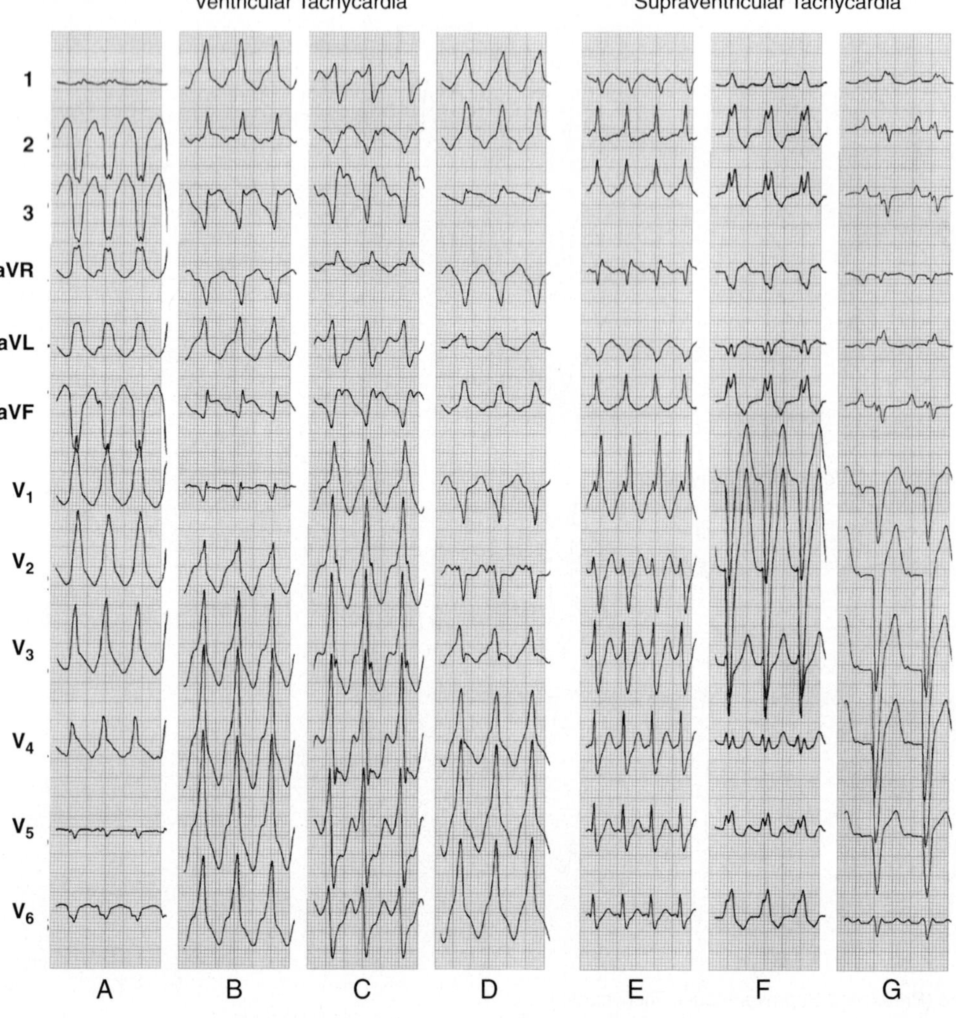

Figure 80-4 Examples of application of the "RS criteria" in several wide QRS complex tachycardias (WCTs). The 12-lead electrocardiograms are shown as labeled: **A** to **D** are from patients of ventricular tachycardia (VT); **E** and **F** are from those with supraventricular tachycardia (SVT). In **A** and **B**, none of the precordial leads show an RS complex. **C** and **D** are examples of VTs with RS complexes (V_3 to V_6 in **C**, V_2 and V_3 in **D**) with RS intervals longer than 100 ms. **E** (RBBB) and **F** (LBBB) show SVT with precordial RS complexes but RS intervals shorter than 100 ms; **G** shows an LBBB WCT without RS complexes in any precordial lead suggesting VT, but it is actually SVT. **C** also shows "pseudo P waves" (deflections in terminal QRS in leads 2, 3, and aVF); the patient had atrioventricular dissociation. LBBB, left bundle branch block; RBBB, right bundle branch block.

from the clear fusion of a supraventricular complex with a VT complex, rather than being simply a change in VT morphology for 1 beat potentially caused by a ventricular premature beat during VT. It also is possible for ventricular premature beats during SVT-A to produce fusion beats, which would erroneously be taken as evidence for a diagnosis of VT.

- The "precordial RS absent" criteria: Brugada and coworkers[2] proposed that because most SVTs with aberration have an RS complex in at least one precordial lead and because VT QRSs need not have an RS complex, the absence of an RS in *any* precordial lead would allow a diagnosis of VT. In an analysis of 554 WCTs (384 VTs, 170 SVTs), an RS complex was absent in 83 (15%), all of which were VT. In the presence of an RS complex in a precordial lead, an interval from R wave onset to S wave nadir more than 100 ms diagnosed VT. This latter finding was a feature in 175 of the remaining 471 VTs (37%). These two criteria could thus by themselves make the correct diagnosis in 258 of 554 WCTs (47%). Experience has shown that although these "RS absent" criteria can be difficult to conceptualize, they have significant practical utility; examples are shown in Figure 80-4. It should be evident that these criteria constitute an extension of the concept that, if the WCT ECG pattern does not look like aberration, it is most likely to represent VT.
- V_i/V_t ratio: Because in SVT-A, only one portion of the His-Purkinje system is blocked while another mediates initial ventricular activation, the first part of the QRS should have relatively rapid voltage changes compared with the terminal part of the QRS. In VT, slower muscle-to-muscle spread of activation at the onset of the QRS yields slower voltage changes. This principle is the basis of the V_i/V_t ratio, in which V_i is the voltage excursion in the initial 40 ms, and V_t the voltage excursion in the last 40 ms, of a biphasic or triphasic QRS complex with the most rapid initial vectors[3] (Fig. 80-5). A V_i/V_t ratio greater than 1 signifies SVT-A, whereas a ratio of 1 or less indicates VT. An algorithm incorporating this (Fig. 80-6) was recently tested in 453 WCT ECGs and found to have a positive predictive accuracy for SVT-A of 83.5%, whereas the Brugada algorithm's predictive accuracy for SVT-A was 65.2% ($P < .05$). This new criterion requires additional validation in larger numbers of WCTs.
- QRS during VT narrower than in baseline rhythm: In the presence of bundle branch block during baseline rhythm, a WCT with a QRS complex narrower than the QRS during baseline rhythm indicates VT as the cause of WCT. This is rare, occurring in less than 1% of all VTs, but would be extremely unlikely to occur during SVT-A. Of course, application of this criterion requires having a baseline ECG for comparison.
- Contralateral bundle branch block in baseline rhythm and WCT: The presence of contralateral bundle branch block

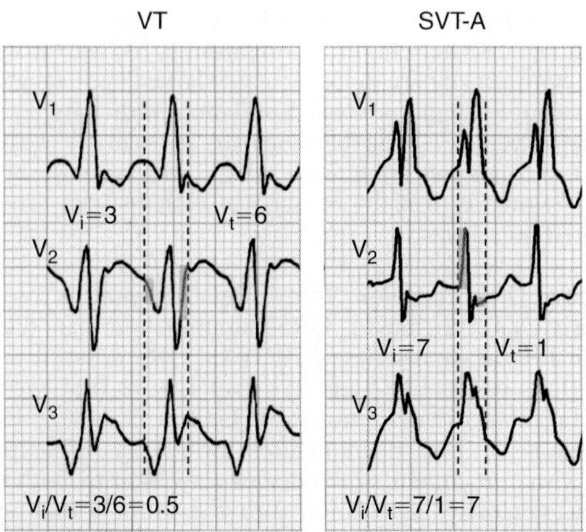

Figure 80-5 Examples of ventricular tachycardia (VT) and supraventricular tachycardia with aberration (SVT-A) diagnosed using the V_i/V_t criterion. A biphasic or triphasic QRS with a rapid initial vector is chosen for analysis. In each example, only leads V_1 to V_3 were selected; the *shaded areas* denote the initial and terminal 40 ms of the QRS complex. Voltage traversed during each 40 ms is measured and used in the equation shown. In SVT-A, initial vectors are more rapid than terminal ones; the opposite is true with VT.

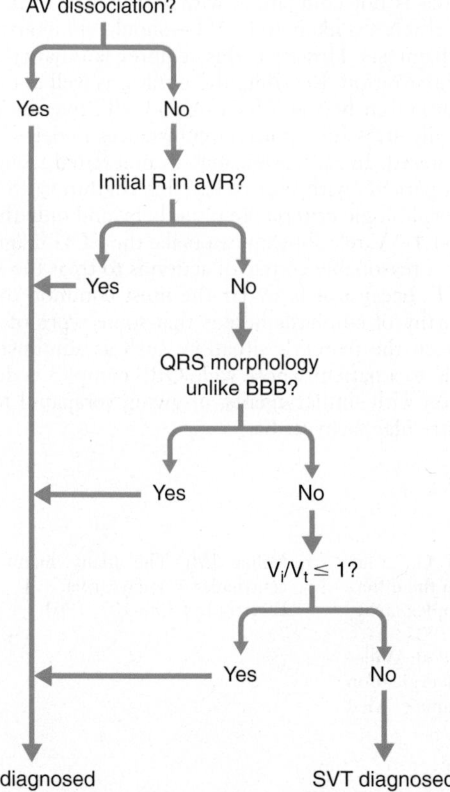

Figure 80-6 Algorithm for distinguishing ventricular tachycardia (VT) and supraventricular tachycardia with aberration (SVT-A) incorporating the V_i/V_t index. See text. (From Vereckei A, Duray G, Szenasi G, et al: Application of a new algorithm in the differential diagnosis of wide QRS complex tachycardia. Eur Heart J 28:589-600, 2007). AV, atrioventricular; BBB, bundle branch block.

during baseline rhythm and WCT strongly suggests VT. If true RBBB were present during baseline rhythm, and true LBBB developed during SVT-A, complete heart block would result. RBBB in baseline rhythm and LBBB during WCT would then strongly imply VT as the correct diagnosis for the WCT. Although intuitively obvious, this criterion is not necessarily absolute. A small proportion of both RBBBs and LBBBs are due to peripheral Purkinje blocks or to myocardial delay rather than block, so that in rare cases, contralateral bundle branch block could be present during SVT-A and baseline rhythm.

- QRS alternans: This phenomenon, defined as alternate-beat variation in the amplitude of the QRS complex greater than 0.1 mV (see Fig. 80-3), commonly is found in narrow complex SVT. Although alternans is present with nearly equal frequency in WCT due to SVT-A as well as VT (approximately 25%), a greater number of ECG leads show alternans in SVT with aberration than in VT (mean of 7 versus 4); in other series, a lower frequency of alternans has been observed. The mechanism responsible for alternans is unclear.
- Presence of multiple WCT configurations: If a patient manifests more than one QRS configuration during WCT, the diagnosis probably is VT. We analyzed a group of 861 patients with at least one WCT studied in our electrophysiology laboratory. Among 524 patients with VT, 266 (51%) had multiple QRS configurations, whereas only 31 of 392 (8%) patients with SVT-A did ($P < .001$; 55 patients had both SVT-A and VT).

Many of the foregoing morphologic criteria are much less reliable if the baseline rhythm ECG demonstrates underlying bundle branch block or axis shift. The only criterion not subject to this limitation is the non-1:1 AV relationship. Some clinicians have found that precordial concordance, rightward superior axis, and a monophasic R wave in V_1 are still reasonably reliable indicators of VT and can be applied even in the presence of preexisting bundle branch block. This is probably also true for the "precordial RS absent" criteria. The fact that these features remain useful even in the presence of an abnormal baseline rhythm ECG is in keeping with the principle that if a WCT ECG has morphologic features not compatible with bundle branch block or fascicular block, then it is probably VT. Other workers have suggested that a simple comparison of the previous ECG (showing bundle branch block) with the WCT usually can enable the correct diagnosis: If the two ECGs have identical QRS morphologic patterns, the diagnosis is SVT-A; and if different, VT. The patient in whom the baseline rhythm and VT QRS complexes are practically identical is rarely encountered. Accordingly, the only way to make a correct diagnosis of VT in such cases is to demonstrate a non-1:1 A:V relationship. All patients with identical baseline rhythm and VT ECG patterns described thus far have had RBBB with or without axis deviation in baseline rhythm.

Although comparison of the non-WCT baseline ECG with that during WCT can be helpful in making the distinction between SVT-A and VT, such a baseline ECG often is not available at the time of the WCT occurrence.

Practical Approaches to Diagnosis of Wide Complex Tachycardia

The urgent clinical circumstances usually surrounding the presentation of a patient in WCT necessitate a rapid, straightforward, and accurate means of arriving at the correct diagnosis. Complex algorithms, although having the virtue of accuracy, are difficult to recall and thus are not well suited to the quick application needed in the patient with WCT. In addition, although many criteria for distinguishing SVT from VT have been thoroughly tested, even the best criteria cannot help in determining the correct diagnosis if they cannot be accurately and reproducibly applied. For example, Isenhour and colleagues[4] asked two emergency room physicians and two cardiologists to apply the Brugada algorithm to 157 WCTs. The cardiologists' sensitivity and specificity for correct diagnoses were 85% to 91% and 55% to 60%, respectively, whereas the emergency physicians' sensitivity and specificity were 79% to 83% and 43% to 70%, respectively (the original authors achieved 98.7% and 96.5%, respectively).

With these caveats in mind, a practical approach might be to evaluate the WCT ECG for the most specific criteria in some sequence: When one such criterion is met, the diagnosis is made, as follows:

Step 1: AV relationship (if dissociated, VT is diagnosed; if not, proceed to next step)
Step 2: Rightward superior axis (if present, VT is diagnosed; if not, proceed to next step)
Step 3: V_i/V_t ratio (if greater than 1, SVT-A is diagnosed; if not, proceed to next step)
Step 4: Precordial RS pattern (if absent, VT is diagnosed; if not, proceed to next step)
Step 5: Precordial RS interval (if RS present and interval greater than 100 ms, VT is diagnosed; if not, proceed to next step)
Step 6: In LBBB type WCT, R wave less than 30 ms or R onset to S nadir less than 60 ms in V_1 (if present, SVT-A is diagnosed)

This process continues in like manner for remaining, less specific criteria.

Wide Complex Tachycardia: Special Cases

Occasionally, proper application of the rules of ECG distinction, as listed, yields an incorrect answer. As previously noted, preexcited SVTs (ventricular activation entirely or primarily over an anomalous AV connection) have an ECG configuration consistent with VT. Other situations exist in which ECG criteria suggest SVT-A, but VT is the actual diagnosis. These are discussed next.

Bundle Branch Reentry In the most common form of bundle branch reentry (BBR) VT, ventricular activation begins as the impulse exits from the right bundle branch and thereafter spreads as it does during typical LBBB. The ECG thus has an LBBB configuration and meets electrocardiographic criteria for SVT-A, although it is actually VT. The correct diagnosis can be made if AVD is present (common in these cases), despite the QRS pattern suggesting SVT-A.

Irregular Ventricular Tachycardia The regularity of a WCT generally is not helpful in distinguishing SVT-A from VT, because both usually are quite regular. Marked cycle length variability strongly suggests atrial fibrillation with bundle branch block; however, VTs can be irregular, particularly within the first 30 seconds of an episode. VTs with significant cycle length irregularity usually are seen in patients who are taking antiarrhythmic drugs.

Narrow QRS Complex Ventricular Tachycardia As noted previously, VT can have a QRS duration less than the usual cutoff of 140 ms. In a series of 702 VTs, QRS duration was less than 140 ms in 88 (12%) and less than 120 ms (not even technically fulfilling the definition of WCT) in 28 (4%).[5] Possible explanations of this phenomenon include (1) a septal VT origin, with subsequent simultaneous activation of both ventricles, and (2) early penetration into the His-Purkinje system, with subsequent relatively rapid activation of the ventricles over this network. Rarely, a patient has VT with a QRS duration narrower than that during baseline rhythm; this phenomenon was present in only 2 of 702 (less than 1%) VTs. In such cases, the relatively short QRS duration during tachycardia would ordinarily suggest SVT as the basis of the arrhythmia.

Summary

Despite the existence of adequate tools to make the correct diagnosis in a majority of cases, the distinction between VT and SVT-A remains difficult for many clinicians. Remembering a simple principle—if the QRS configuration of a wide complex tachycardia is not compatible with any known form of aberration, the rhythm is likely to be VT—should aid in arriving at the correct diagnosis. However, this requires familiarity with ECG forms of aberration. Recalling these rules, as well as other aids in ECG distinction between SVT-A and VT, may be difficult in the typically stressful clinical circumstances under which WCT is encountered. In rare cases, such as preexcited tachycardias or WCT in patients with bizarre baseline rhythm QRS configurations, morphologic criteria are of no help, and only the presence of a non-1:1 AV relationship can make the ECG diagnosis. If all else fails, a reasonable course of action is to treat the arrhythmia as for VT, because it is by far the most common diagnosis. A point worthy of emphasis here is that some types of treatments may worsen the patient's situation, such as administering procainamide to a patient whose wide QRS complex is due to overmedication with similar agents, or giving verapamil to a patient with ventricular tachycardia.

References

1. Wellens HJJ, Bär FWHM, Lie KI: The value of the electrocardiogram in the differential diagnosis of a tachycardia with a widened QRS complex. Am J Med 64:27-33, 1978.
2. Brugada P, Brugada J, Mont L, et al: A new approach to the differential diagnosis of a regular tachycardia with a wide QRS complex. Circulation 83:1649-1659, 1991.
3. Vereckei A, Duray G, Szenasi G, et al: Application of a new algorithm in the differential diagnosis of wide QRS complex tachycardia. Eur Heart J 28:589-600, 2007.
4. Isenhour JL, Craig S, Gibbs M, et al: Wide-complex tachycardia: Continued evaluation of diagnostic criteria. Acad Emerg Med 7:769-773, 2000.
5. Miller JM: The many manifestations of ventricular tachycardia. J Cardiovasc Electrophys 3:88-107, 1992.

Assessment of the Patient with a Cardiac Arrhythmia 81

MITHILESH K. DAS AND DOUGLAS P. ZIPES

CHAPTER OUTLINE

The evaluation of the patient suspected to have a cardiac rhythm disturbance is fundamental to the role of the clinical cardiac electrophysiologist. The approach followed for this evaluation varies from patient to patient and is influenced by the patient's clinical status and symptoms, but a general outline can be established, as presented in this chapter. As always, the initial evaluation begins with a careful history and physical examination.

History Taking

Significant overlap exists among the clinical features of various rhythm disturbances, imparting a degree of imprecision to the interpretation of the patient's history. Despite this drawback, the history often can provide direction and diagnostic clues as the first step in assessing the patient with, or suspected of having, a cardiac arrhythmia. It often is the most important source of information about the arrhythmia.

Symptoms and Signs

Major symptoms and signs of cardiac arrhythmias are palpitations, presyncope, syncope, and sudden cardiac death (SCD). In this setting, nonspecific symptoms such as shortness of breath, weakness, and fatigue may be due to compromise in cardiac output and prolonged duration of the arrhythmia. Elderly patients with bradycardia due to sinus node dysfunction or atrioventricular (AV) nodal block can present with altered mental status and dementia.

Palpitations

Awareness of an irregular heart beat varies greatly from patient to patient. Many patients are acutely aware of any cardiac irregularity, whereas others are oblivious even to long runs of a rapid ventricular tachycardia. Often the asymptomatic patients are those referred for evaluation of an arrhythmia noted incidentally during assessment for another reason, such as a preathletic physical examination in a youngster, a preinsurance physical examination in an adult, or a routine preoperative assessment. Those patients who do complain of symptoms most commonly note *palpitations*, defined as sensations experienced as an unpleasant awareness of forceful, irregular, or rapid beating of the heart. Patients describe these symptoms in various ways. Most frequently, they use terms such as a thumping or flip-flopping sensation in the chest; a fullness in the throat, neck, or chest; or a pause in the heart beat, "as if my heart stopped." The last is most likely to be caused by the compensatory pause after a premature ventricular complex (PVC) or the resetting of the sinus rhythm after a premature atrial complex. Presumably, the premature beat, particularly if it is a ventricular extrasystole, occurs too early to permit sufficient ventricular filling to cause a sensation when the ventricle contracts. The ventricular systole that ends the compensatory pause may be responsible for the actual palpitation and is caused by a more forceful contraction from prolonged ventricular filling or increased motion of the heart in the chest. Anxiety over such symptoms is commonly the complaint that brings the patient to the doctor's office.

Premature atrial or ventricular complexes probably constitute the most common cause of palpitations, and patients often use the term *skipped beat* or *dropped beat* to describe them. If the premature complexes are frequent or particularly if a sustained tachycardia is present, patients are more likely to complain of lightheadedness, syncope or near-syncope, chest pain, fatigue, or shortness of breath. The presence of associated cardiovascular problems influences the nature of the symptoms. For example, a supraventricular tachycardia at a rate of 180 per minute may provoke chest pain in a patient with coronary artery disease or syncope in a patient with aortic stenosis but result in only a breathless feeling in an otherwise normal youngster.

An important point is that patients with ventricular tachycardia (VT), particularly young, otherwise healthy persons, can be completely asymptomatic or experience minimal symptoms during the arrhythmic episode. The lack of significant symptoms should not exclude the diagnosis of VT. Bradyarrhythmias have their own constellation of symptoms that usually includes syncope, near-syncope, and fatigue.

Knowledge about the typical onset and termination of the tachycardia is helpful. Abrupt, paroxysmal onset is consistent with a tachycardia such as AV nodal reentrant tachycardia

Work on which this chapter is based was supported in part by the Herman C. Krannert Fund, Indianapolis.

Table 81-1 Differential Diagnosis of Palpitations

Cardiac arrhythmias
Sinus tachycardia
- Physiologic
- Inappropriate sinus tachycardia
- Postural orthostatic tachycardia syndrome
- Anxiety neurosis, thyrotoxicosis, perimenopausal syndrome, pheochromocytoma

Atrial arrhythmias
- Atrial fibrillation, atrial flutter, atrial tachycardia
- Atrial premature complexes

Supraventricular tachycardia
- Atrioventricular nodal reentry tachycardia, orthodromic atrioventricular reciprocating tachycardia, Wolff-Parkinson-White syndrome
- Permanent form of junctional reciprocating tachycardia

Junctional tachycardia
Ventricular tachycardia
- Ventricular premature complexes, ventricular couplets, nonsustained ventricular tachycardia
  Idiopathic
  Caffine intake
  Drug-induced: cocaine, QT-prolonging drugs
  Alcohol
- Sustained ventricular tachycardia

Conduction system disease
- Sinus bradycardia
- Tachycardia-bradycardia syndrome
- Heart block
- Pause-dependent torsades de pointes

Familial arrhythmia syndrome
- Long QT syndrome
- Short QT syndrome
- Catecholaminergic polymorphic ventricular tachycardia
- Brugada syndrome
- Inherited cardiomyopathy with ventricular arrhythmias, such as right ventricular cardiomyopathy

Proarrhythmia
- Antiarrhythmic agents, drugs that prolong the QT interval
- Pacemaker-mediated tachycardia

Metabolic syndromes
- Hypoglycemia
- Electrolyte imbalance

Structural heart disease
- Valvular disease
- Primary pulmonary hypertension

(AVNRT) (see Chapter 59), whereas gradual speeding and slowing are more in keeping with a sinus tachycardia (see Chapter 52). Termination by Valsalva maneuver or carotid sinus massage suggests a tachycardia incorporating nodal tissue in the reentrant pathway, such as sinus node reentry, AVNRT or AV reentrant tachycardia (AVRT) (see Chapters 58 and 59), and idiopathic right ventricular outflow tract tachycardia. It often is helpful to have the patient tap out the cadence of the perceived palpitations, from onset to termination. In this fashion, the clinician can obtain information about the nature of the beginning and end of the tachycardia, whether the ventricular rhythm is regular or irregular, and the rate of the tachycardia.

The rate of the untreated tachycardia often narrows diagnostic possibilities, and patients should be instructed in how to count their radial or carotid pulse rate. Ventricular rates of 150 beats per minute should always suggest the potential diagnosis of atrial flutter with 2:1 AV block (see Chapter 54), whereas most supraventricular tachycardias, such as those caused by AVNRT or AVRT, usually occur at rates exceeding 150 beats per minute. The rates of VTs overlap those of the supraventricular tachycardias. Palpitations, hot flashes, and sweats in a middle-aged women suggest perimenopausal syndrome. Palpitations, dizziness, and shortness of breath on mild exertion, typically in young women with structurally normal hearts, suggest the syndrome of inappropriate sinus tachycardia. Palpitations due to sinus tachycardia on standing should point toward postural hypotension. Palpitations and presyncope on standing may be symptoms of postural orthostatic tachycardia syndrome (POTS). Various possible causes of palpitations are listed in Table 81-1.

Associated Cardiac or Systemic Diseases

It also is important to establish whether the patient has structural heart disease and, if so, the diagnosis and extent of disease. Certain clinical diagnoses are linked to the presence of specific arrhythmias. For example, the occurrence of mitral stenosis should suggest the possibility of atrial fibrillation, whereas a history of a myocardial infarction or tetralogy of Fallot repair invokes VT as a distinct prospect. Thyrotoxicosis should suggest atrial arrhythmias, including sinus tachycardia. At times it may be useful to search for a family history of similar problems and to obtain electrocardiograms (ECGs) of close family members, such as parents, siblings, or children. Family history of palpitations, syncope, or SCD should be investigated carefully for inherited cardiac arrhythmias, including atrial fibrillation, long QT syndrome, short QT syndrome, catecholaminergic polymorphic VT, arrhythmogenic right ventricular dysplasia or cardiomyopathy (ARVD or ARVC) and inherited cardiomyopathy with arrhythmia.

Syncope

In the patient who complains of syncope, careful questioning about the event is often illuminating. When caused by a cardiac arrhythmia, syncope is of rapid onset and brief duration, with or without preceding aura, and usually is not followed by a postictal confusional state. It may be associated with bodily injury if the patient falls when unconscious. Seizure activity is uncommon, as is tongue biting or incontinence, but these can occur if the arrhythmia provoking the syncope, and the resulting syncope, are long in duration. A patient who has epileptiform movements within seconds of the onset of syncope is more likely to be experiencing a central nervous system problem rather than a cardiac rhythm disturbance. Palpitations preceding syncope also support an arrhythmic cause of syncope. The history of syncope should be elicited and interpreted carefully because elderly people who present with falls may deny loss of consciousness during the event, owing to a brief retrograde amnesia.

With vasodepressor and cardioinhibitory syncope, the episode usually unfolds more slowly and can be preceded by manifestations of autonomic hyperactivity such as nausea, abdominal cramping, diarrhea, sweating, or yawning. On recovery, the patient may be bradycardic, pale, sweaty, and fatigued, in contrast with the patient recovering from a Stokes-Adams attack or an episode of VT, who may be flushed and have a sinus tachycardia. Common arrhythmic causes of syncope include bradyarrhythmias caused by sinus node dysfunction or AV block and tachyarrhythmias, most often ventricular but also supraventricular on occasion. Bradycardia may follow tachycardia in patients with the bradycardia-tachycardia syndrome, and treatment of both may be necessary. Noncardiac causes of syncope such as hypoglycemia often can be excluded by careful history, whereas syncope caused by nonarrhythmic causes, such as aortic stenosis, can be excluded by a combination of history and physical examination.

Sudden Cardiac Death

SCD causes approximately 350,000 to 450,000 deaths annually in the United States. It is responsible for nearly 50% of all cardiovascular-related deaths worldwide. SCD has an incidence of 0.1% to 0.2% per year among adults older than 35 years of age. Therefore, careful evaluation of patients who are resuscitated from SCD is mandated. SCD occurs in a majority of patients without known heart disease. The life-threatening ventricular arrhythmias such as sustained VT and ventricular fibrillation are responsible for two thirds of SCDs. These arrhythmias occur unpredictably, even in high risk patients. Structural heart disease, such as coronary artery disease, cardiomyopathy, and congenital heart disease, is responsible for up to 65% to 80% cases of SCD. Approximately 5% to 10% of SCDs occur in people with primary electrical abnormalities of the heart, such as long QT syndrome, Brugada syndrome, idiopathic ventricular fibrillation, and Wolff-Parkinson-White syndrome. The remaining sudden deaths (15% to 20%) are due to noncardiac causes, such as pulmonary embolism, drugs, drowning, and sudden infant death syndrome. Therefore, careful questioning to uncover or elucidate a family history of SCD is indicated, and family screening for the suspected cardiac condition should be performed.

Precipitating Factors

While taking the history, the clinician should search for possible precipitating factors of an arrhythmia. Patients usually cannot point to a specific inciting event, but the physician should inquire about the use of potentially cardioactive drugs found in bronchodilators, histamine H_1-blocking antihistamines, some decongestants, or other over-the-counter drugs, and the ingestion of alcohol or excessive caffeine-containing foods. Knowledge about the typical onset and termination of the tachycardia is helpful. Abrupt, paroxysmal onset is consistent with a tachycardia such as AVNRT, whereas a gradual speeding and slowing is more in keeping with sinus tachycardia. In some patients, symptoms can be precipitated or exacerbated by a certain activity or occur at a certain time of day or month (e.g., associated with menses). Of interest, some patients with atrial arrhythmias may predict their recurrence by antecedent gastrointestinal symptoms. In patients with the long QT syndrome, exercise or acute emotional reactions often precipitate a ventricular arrhythmia in those with the LQT1 variant, whereas exercise, emotional upset, and sleep or rest are culprits of fairly equal frequency in LQT2, with auditory stimuli more specific precipitators and events occurring more frequently during rest in LQT3. Exercise also precipretates idiopathic right ventricular outflow tract tachycardia, exercise-induced polymorphic VT, and VT in patients with ARVD or ARVC.

Physical Examination

The physical examination offers the opportunity to gain important information about the presence of associated structural heart disease, if any, and the nature of the arrhythmia, if it is present. Although it is well known that patients with normal hearts can have supraventricular tachycardias, it is less commonly appreciated that patients without recognizable structural heart disease can also have VTs that on occasion are even life-threatening. Thus, normal results of physical examination do not preclude the diagnosis of VT, even in a young person. It is likely that at least some of these patients have structural heart disease that is not recognized.

The sex of the patient can be a clue to the nature of the tachycardia. For example, a young woman who complains of episodes of a regular tachycardia over many years is likely to have AVNRT. By contrast, a young man with a similar history is more likely to have AVRT associated with the Wolff-Parkinson-White syndrome. Symptomatic long QT syndrome is more common in females, whereas Brugada syndrome is more common in males.

Atrioventricular Dissociation

If the tachycardia is present during the physical examination, a 12-lead ECG should be obtained, if time and the patient's clinical status permit. If an ECG machine is not available, a careful physical examination can yield helpful findings. For example, the presence of regular cannon A waves in the jugular venous pulse would be consistent with a 1:1 retrograde ventriculoatrial relation, as in tachycardias such as AVRT, AVNRT, and some junctional tachycardias and VTs. By contrast, the patient may have physical features indicative of AV dissociation. These include intermittent cannon A waves in the neck, variable intensity of the first heart sound, and variable peak systolic blood pressure. Common arrhythmic causes of AV dissociation include VT and nonparoxysmal AV junctional tachycardia, naturally without retrograde capture of the atria. Ventricular or junctional tachycardias that produce retrograde 2:1 or Wenckebach block cause intermittent cannon A waves that recur at regular intervals.

Atrioventricular Block

In the patient with second-degree AV block, the study of neck veins can reveal the nature of the block, but usually the findings are too subtle to recognize. Patients with type I (Wenckebach) second-degree AV block can exhibit progressive increase in the A-C jugular venous pulse interval before the nonconducted P wave, progressive quickening of the ventricular rate, and progressive decrease in the intensity of the first heart sound. In type II second-degree heart block, the PR interval remains fixed before the block, and so do the A-C interval and intensity of S_1. The features of AV dissociation noted earlier usually are present during complete AV block.

Carotid Sinus Massage

Modulating autonomic tone by carotid sinus massage during the physical examination can be useful to expose the patient with the hypersensitive carotid sinus reflex. The clinician first needs to listen carefully over both carotids to be certain that no bruit is present, palpate lightly to determine that a normal carotid pulse is present, and then gently depress or rub the carotid sinus. Gentle massage for approximately 10 to 15 seconds or less usually is all that is necessary to produce significant periods of sinus arrest or AV block in susceptible patients.

The response to carotid sinus massage or other vagal maneuvers can be quite helpful in differentiating one tachycardia from another. In the most definitive responses, carotid sinus massage acutely terminates tachycardias such as AVRT, AVNRT, sinus node reentry, adenosine-sensitive atrial tachycardia, and idiopathic right ventricular outflow tract tachycardia. Carotid sinus massage can gradually slow a sinus tachycardia without termination and will decrease the ventricular response to atrial tachycardia, atrial flutter, and atrial fibrillation without termination, thereby exposing atrial activity. Carotid sinus massage transiently terminates the permanent form of AV junctional reciprocating tachycardia (PJRT), which then restarts when carotid massage ceases. Carotid sinus massage does not affect reentrant ventricular or junctional tachycardias. Unfortunately, not all presentations of these tachycardias behave in such "textbook" fashion, and intermediate or overlapping responses can occur.

Laboratory Tests

As indicated earlier, the initial assessment of the patient begins with a careful history and physical examination. Several noninvasive and invasive tests add to the physician's ability to obtain information about the arrhythmia. Before any test is ordered, however, it is imperative to decide whether the information provided by the test is sufficiently important to justify its risk or expense. Whenever possible, tests with maximal sensitivity, specificity, and predictive accuracy are chosen. A 12-lead ECG is obtained in all patients, and frequently a 24-hour ECG or 30-day event recording and stress test is helpful in exposing the arrhythmia. A chest roentgenogram and an echocardiogram provide information about the presence of structural heart disease. The hierarchy of steps taken to evaluate and treat a patient suspected of having an arrhythmia generally proceeds from simple, noninvasive, and inexpensive tests to more complex, expensive, and invasive studies.

The nature of the rhythm disturbance and its effects on the patient determine the order in which the tests are performed. Some rhythm disturbances, such as sustained VT or ventricular fibrillation, are hazardous in and of themselves, whereas others, such as AVRT or AVNRT, must be evaluated according to the context in which they occur. AVRT or AVNRT occurring at a rate of 180 beats per minute in a young patient who complains only of palpitations or mild anxiety is approached quite differently from such arrhythmias precipitating angina in a patient with coronary artery disease, syncope in a patient with aortic stenosis, or claudication in a patient with peripheral vascular disease. It is imperative to remember that clinical decision making must be founded on the ECG interpretation of the arrhythmia in concert with the assessment of the patient. Thus, the physician evaluates and determines treatment for a patient who has a rhythm disturbance, rather than a rhythm disturbance in isolation.

The principle in diagnosing and treating symptomatic patients with an undocumented cardiac rhythm disturbance is simple and obvious: One needs merely to record the ECG during a symptomatic episode and then document a causal relation between arrhythmia and symptoms. This often is easier said than done, however, and a variety of approaches are used to achieve that endpoint.

Long-Term Rhythm Recordings

Rhythm disturbances occurring with great frequency are naturally easier to document than those that occur sporadically. Long-term ECG recordings in the outpatient setting usually constitute one of the early diagnostic choices in the patient without a life-threatening cardiac arrhythmia The patient with a life-threatening arrhythmia may need to be hospitalized to allow these recordings to be done. A long-term ECG recording provides the most direct laboratory test to evaluate electrical abnormalities, and it, or a similar procedure, is often the first definitive, noninvasive approach taken to elucidate the nature of the electrical disturbance. Prolonged ECG recordings in patients engaged in normal daily activity provide the methodology to quantitate the frequency and complexity of the rhythm disturbance, to correlate these alterations with symptoms, and to evaluate the effect of appropriate pharmacologic therapy on the arrhythmia. In addition, such recordings can document alterations in the QRS-ST and T contour.

Unfortunately, if the arrhythmia does not occur with sufficient frequency, then a simple 24-hour, or even 48-hour, recording will not be useful. A long-term (15-day) Holter monitoring system also is commercially available. Newer Holter monitors also record a 12-channel ECG. Such studies are helpful in arrhythmia characterization as well as ST-T wave changes related to ischemia and Brugada syndrome. A 30-day event recorder often is helpful if arrhythmia occurs at least once in a month. The patient can activate these latter devices when symptoms occur, store 30 seconds or more of the ECG rhythm (a memory loop provides ECG information about the arrhythmia that transpired for some seconds before device activation), and transmit it to a central monitoring station over the telephone. Alternatively, some devices automatically record rhythms that exceed preset limits. The automatic recorder is useful in the patient who fails to perceive all symptoms associated with the arrhythmia or is unable to activate the recording system because of rapidly progressing syncope or other problems.

For the recording session to be specific, the patient must have both the arrhythmia and symptoms simultaneously. If symptoms occur without an arrhythmia, the latter can be excluded as a cause. Recording arrhythmias without symptoms precludes a definitive causal relation between symptoms and arrhythmia and reduces the specificity of the test. The sensitivity of the test is quite variable, depending on the prevalence of the arrhythmia. An implantable looop recorder placed beneath the skin can be used for monitoring of the cardiac rhythm for as long as 18 months. Use of such devices has been successful in recording bradyarrhythmias and tachyarrhythmias in patients with infrequent symptoms.

Electrophysiologic Study

Naturally, in many patients, invasive electrophysiologic testing is required to initiate the electrical abnormality (see Chapter 93). Such studies provide important information when a particular arrhythmia can be initiated that is responsible for the patient's symptoms. In some instances, however, a tachyarrhythmia present clinically cannot be induced in the electrophysiology laboratory. An important point is that failure to demonstrate a rhythm abnormality does not exclude the possibility that it may be present on another occasion and still be responsible for the patient's symptoms. Thus, the sensitivity of the electrophysiologic study may be low, depending on the nature of the rhythm disturbance. Absence of proof is not the same as proof of absence.

Ideally, the electrophysiologic study would induce only clinically and prognostically important cardiac arrhythmias in all patients who are at risk for a spontaneous arrhythmia and in no patient without such a risk. Unfortunately, this is not the case, and it is quite clear that such a study, depending on the number of extrastimuli used, can induce nonspecific tachyarrhythmias, in particular, flutter and fibrillation in both the atria and ventricles. With certain arrhythmias, the test can be very specific. For example, it would be uncommon to induce a sustained AVRT or AVNRT in a patient who does not also suffer from this arrhythmia clinically. Furthermore, it would not be likely to induce a sustained monomorphic VT in a patient who is not at risk for a clinical occurrence of such an arrhythmia.

Stress Testing and Other Noninvasive Studies

An exercise stress test can be useful, particularly in patients who experience symptoms when exercising. In response to exercise testing, approximately one third of normal subjects have ventricular ectopy, usually in the form of occasional uniform PVCs. These PVCs are more likely to occur at greater heart rates and are not reproducible from one test to the next. Multiform PVCs, pairs of PVCs, and VT infrequently develop in response to exercise in normal subjects. Because they can be recorded in normal subjects, however, their presence does not establish the existence of ischemia or heart disease. Ventricular ectopy generally appears at lower heart rates (below 130 beats per minute) in patients with coronary artery disease than in a normal population, and it often occurs in the early recovery period. Ventricular arrhythmias are more reproducible from one test to the next in patients with coronary artery disease, and more frequent PVCs (exceeding 10 per minute), polymorphic PVCs, and VT are more likely to occur in patients with coronary artery disease than in persons with normal hearts. PVCs at rest may be suppressed by exercise in patients with documented coronary disease; therefore, this observation does not necessarily imply a benign prognosis or absence of underlying structural heart disease. In normal subjects, results from consecutive exercise tests may not be reproducible, whereas in patients with coronary artery disease, the test results are more reproducible, but not dependably so. Exercise testing may be useful to expose ECG abnormalities in patients with less obvious forms of the long QT syndrome.

A variety of noninvasive tests have been developed in an attempt to identify patients at risk for sudden arrhythmic death. These include signal-averaged electrocardiography (SAECG), heart rate variability QT dispersion testing, T wave alternans assessment, and baroreflex testing. Even though these tests may help identify groups of patients at greater or lower risk for SCD, they all suffer from an inability to precisely predict the occurrence of life-threatening arrhythmias in individual patients.

Tests Indicated for Specific Symptoms

Syncope

The underlying disorder can be determined using standardized clinical evaluation in up to three fourths of patients with syncope. In unselected populations, slightly more than one third of the patients have neurocardiogenic syncope, one fourth have orthostatic hypotension, and the remaining patients have miscellaneous conditions. Evaluation of patients suspected of cardioinhibitory or vasodepressor syncope often includes tilt table testing. The yield from prolonged ECG ambulatory recordings and from electrophysiologic studies in patients experiencing syncope who do not have structural cardiac disease is in general low and unrewarding. It is important to establish the cause of the syncope, if possible, because those patients who have syncope due to a noncardiac cause usually have an excellent prognosis, whereas those who have syncope from a cardiac cause have a greater prevalence of sudden cardiac death.

Electrophysiologic testing is recommended for patients who have syncope or near-syncope that remains unexplained after a thorough evaluation, including a complete neurologic evaluation and ambulatory ECG recordings. Because both bradycardia and tachycardia can be responsible for syncope, the diagnosis or exclusion of a specific etiologic disorder should not be based on anything other than an ECG recording during the syncopal event, or replication, during an electrophysiologic study or other maneuvers, of a cardiac rhythm disturbance that produces the same or similar symptoms in the patient. For example, in the patient who has first-degree AV block and left bundle branch block, episodes of VT may be responsible for the syncope, rather than episodes of more advanced AV block.

Bradyarrhythmias

Many patients have asymptomatic bradyarrhythmias, and it is important to establish that they produce symptoms in a given patient before assuming that therapy is required. Conversely, if the patient becomes symptomatic when a spontaneous bradyarrhythmia is demonstrated, further diagnostic studies may not be necessary. It also is possible that patients may be minimally symptomatic but have arrhythmias that permit definitive therapeutic decisions. For example, in patients who have type II second-degree AV block, the demonstration of His-Purkinje block, even in the minimally symptomatic or possibly asymptomatic person, may be sufficient evidence to conclude that pacemaker therapy is indicated because of the risk for progression to complete AV block.

The patient with sinus node dysfunction can have syncope or near-syncope but also may complain of symptoms consistent with low cardiac output due to persistent bradycardia, such as fatigue or even manifestations of congestive heart failure. Some patients can have associated tachycardia—producing the aforementioned bradycardia-tachycardia syndrome. Electrophysiologic studies of sinus node function have low sensitivity but relatively high specificity. Correlation of the presence of the bradycardia with the patient's symptoms is of utmost importance. Electrophysiologic studies are indicated only when a causal relation between the appearance of the bradycardia and the patient's symptoms cannot be established despite repeated noninvasive evaluations. It is important to keep in mind that asymptomatic sinus bradycardia with heart rates of 35 to 40 beats per minute, sinus arrhythmia with pauses of 2 to 3 seconds, Wenckebach second-degree AV block (particularly during sleep), wandering atrial pacemaker, and junctional escape complexes can be completely normal, especially in young people.

In patients who have AV block, the scalar ECG is the most important laboratory test, because the site of block usually dictates the clinical course of the patient and whether a pacemaker is needed, and the site of block usually can be determined from analysis of the scalar ECG. Only infrequently is an electrophysiologic study indicated. Autonomic manipulation can be used to help establish the site of block. Atropine or isoproterenol shorten AV nodal conduction time and refractoriness, whereas vagal maneuvers prolong them. Little change occurs in the normal His-Purkinje conduction. Thus, exercise, atropine, or isoproterenol can shorten the PR interval and increase the ratio of conducted P waves during type I (Wenckebach) AV nodal block, whereas these maneuvers can increase the number of blocked P waves in type II second-degree AV block. Of note, however, important overlap between the two responses is possible.

Tachyarrhythmias

As mentioned earlier, a 12-lead ECG should be obtained during tachycardia, so long as the patient is relatively stable. If the QRS is normal and identical to that present during sinus rhythm, the tachycardia must be supraventricular, and the differential diagnosis now relates to its mechanism. The 12-lead ECG provides many diagnostic clues in this regard. Supraventricular tachycardias can be classified as short RP′ or long RP′ tachycardias, depending on the timing of the P wave in relation to the preceding R wave. When a P wave occurs closer to the preceding R wave, that is, in the first half of the R-R interval, the tachycardia is called a short RP′ tachycardia, whereas if a P wave occurs in the second half of the RR cycle, the arrhythmia is called a long RP′ tachycardia. Considerations in the differential diagnosis for a short RP′ tachycardia include AVNRT, AVRT, junctional tachycardia, and atrial tachycardia with a markedly prolonged PR interval. If no P waves or other evidence of atrial activity are apparent, and the R-R interval is regular, AVNRT is most likely. If a retrograde P wave is present in the ST segment, AVRT is most probable. Long PR tachycardias include sinus tachycardia, atypical AVNRT, PJRT, and atrial tachycardia. The presence of conduction over an accessory pathway during sinus rhythm or during tachycardia naturally suggests that the

Wolff-Parkinson-White syndrome with its associated accessory pathway is responsible for the dysrhythmia. During VT, specific QRS contours and the presence of AV dissociation are useful in making the diagnosis.

Summary

Careful evaluation of the patient who has documented or suspected cardiac arrhythmia is the prime focus of the clinical cardiac electrophysiologist. Much useful information can be gleaned noninvasively, thereby potentially sparing many patients from unnecessary electrophysiologic testing. When indicated, however, such studies, particularly when coupled with radiofrequency ablation techniques, provide the most definitive information for appropriate diagnosis and therapy.

Exercise-Induced Arrhythmias 82

MIGUEL VALDERRÁBANO

CHAPTER OUTLINE

Awareness of our own heartbeat commonly accompanies physical exercise. As part of the "fight or flight" response, our bodies are endowed with a complex machinery to enhance myocardial function at all levels in response to or in preparation for exercise. This includes a physiologic augmentation of contractility and heart rate, but the response to exercise also stresses the system to enhance pathophysiologic forms of excitability, particularly in genetically susceptible persons. Acquired forms of disease, such as myocardial ischemia, also can render affected persons prone to arrhythmogenic maladaptive responses to exercise.

This chapter reviews the mechanisms of the physiologic response to exercise, along with the molecular weak points at which the response can go awry from the electrophysiologic standpoint. A discussion on the impact of exercise in acquired forms of heart disease is presented next, followed by an overview of prognostic implications of exercise-induced arrhythmias.

Molecular, Cellular, and Physiologic Mechanisms of the Response to Exercise: Where Are the Weak Links?

Central Nervous System Control

The physiologic response to exercise starts with withdrawal of the parasympathetic tone and enhancement of sympathetic activity. The sympathetic response starts in the central nervous system, at the hypothalamus and locus coeruleus, located within the dorsal wall of the rostral pons in the lateral floor of the fourth ventricle. The norepinephrine-laden neurons of this homeostatic control center innervate the rostral ventrolateral medulla and the sympathetic neurons of the spinal cord in the intermediolateral cell column, from the first thoracic segment to the second or third lumbar segment. From there, axons leave the spinal cord and form the paravertebral ganglia or sympathetic trunks. The heart receives sympathetic influences from the stellate ganglion (Fig. 82-1).

Organ-Level Response

During exercise, sympathetic activation leads to increases in heart rate and systolic blood pressure.[1] The action potential duration (APD) shortens, which leads to shortening of the QT interval in the surface electrocardiogram. At the myocardial tissue level, consequences include increases in contractility, wall stress, and oxygen demand and consumption. These changes normally are coped with by an increased coronary artery blood flow, which relies on intact endothelial function.

Increased flow and shear stress, coupled with adrenergic platelet activation, also can trigger acute coronary syndromes due to atherosclerotic plaque rupture and platelet aggregation. Thus, coronary artery disease, the most common acquired condition, can limit the required increases in coronary blood flow, leading to ischemia-induced arrhythmogenesis, as discussed elsewhere in this book.

Molecular Mechanisms of Sympathetic Stimulation

The sympathetic modulation of cardiac function caused by exercise is mediated mostly through the effects of norepinephrine on the β-adrenergic receptor. Activation of the β-adrenergic receptor leads to G_s protein–mediated activation of adenyl cyclase,[2] which leads to the formation of cyclic adenosine monophosphate (cAMP) as a second messenger.[3] The cAMP, in turn, activates protein kinase A (PKA) or binds directly to certain ion channels. PKA is able to phosphorylate certain proteins that are key to the sympathetically mediated enhancement of myocardial function.

Direct cAMP binding enhances the hyperpolarization-activated, cyclic nucleotide–gated (HCN) channel—responsible for the I_f pacemaker current—and leads to increases in sinoatrial node activation rate and sinus tachycardia. Pathophysiologically, ectopic I_f-induced phase 4 depolarizations can lead to enhanced automaticity and extrasystoles.

The response to exercise also involves activation of α-adrenergic receptors, which have more prominent vascular than cardiac effects. The α-adrenergic receptors are coupled to G_h protein–mediated activation of phospholipase C. This in turn splits phosphatidylinositol into inositol-triphosphate (IP_3) and diacylglycerol (DAG). IP_3 has a direct effect on the sarcoplasmic reticulum to liberate calcium, generating a modest inotropic effect in the myocardium and robust vasoconstriction in the peripheral vasculature.

Augmentation of the Calcium Transient

Phosphorylation of the L-type calcium channel by PKA, at specific sites in the carboxyl-terminal (C-terminal) portion of the α subunit, leads to increased open probability of the channel and thus enhanced I_{Ca}, which in turns leads to enhanced sarcolemmal Ca^{2+} entry and calcium-induced Ca^{2+} release, generating a larger calcium transient and directly enhancing contractility.

I_{Ca} also is enhanced at rapid heart rates by a calcium-dependent mechanism (I_{Ca} staircase), which involves phosphorylation of the L-type calcium channel by calmodulin-dependent protein kinase II. This occurs when rapid heart rates lead to

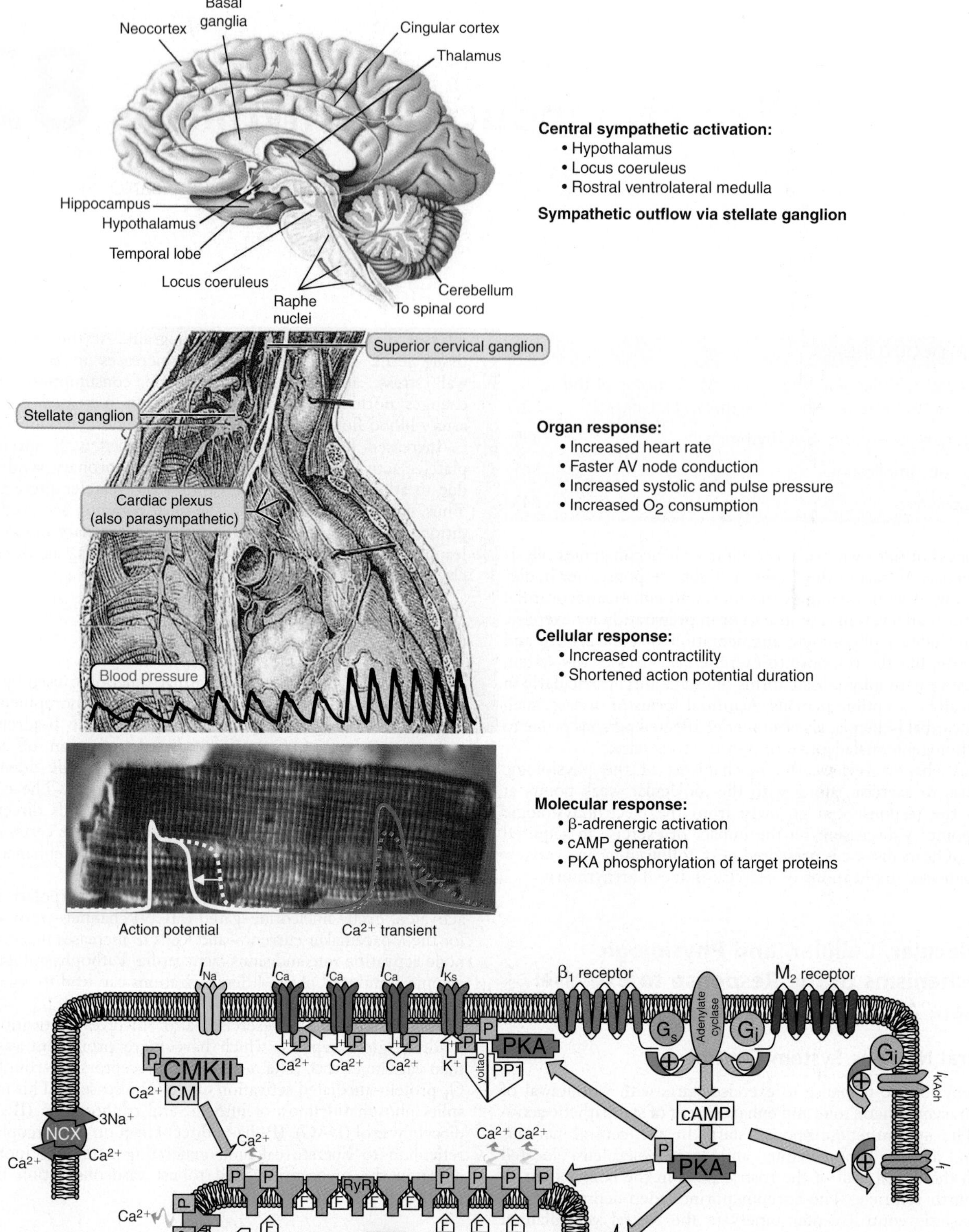

Figure 82-1 Physiologic responses to exercise. Activation of the sympathetic nervous system (and withdrawal of the parasympathetic system) follows commands from the central nervous system. The hypothalamus coordinates with the locus coeruleus to produce a widespread state of increased alertness, known as the "fight or flight response," that includes activation of the sympathetic nucleus in the rostral ventrolateral medulla and the sympathetic neurons in the spinal cord. The sympathetic outflow to the heart travels mostly through the stellate ganglion and leads to increases in heart rate, systolic blood pressure, and oxygen consumption. At the cellular level there is increased contractility (caused by higher calcium transient amplitude) and shortened action potential duration. At the molecular level, activation of the β-adrenergic receptor leads to activation of adenylate cyclase by means of G_s protein and generates cyclic adenosine monophosphate (cAMP), which activates protein kinase A (PKA). This leads to activation of I_f, which leads to faster depolarization rates in nodal tissues. PKA phosphorylates key proteins including phospholamban (which activates the sarcoplasmic reticulum [SR] Ca^{2+}-ATPase and leads to enhanced SR calcium load) and the α subunits of the calcium channel ($I_{Ca,L}$) (which leads to enhanced calcium current) and potassium channel (I_{Ks}) (which leads to enhanced current and shorter action potential duration). Increased Ca^{2+} can activate Ca^{2+}/calmodulin-dependent protein kinase II (CMKII) by way of calmodulin (CM). PKA and CMKII can phosphorylate (P) the ryanodine receptor (RyR) and make it dissociate from the FKBP12.6 protein (F). This dissociation can make the ryanodine receptor leak diastolic calcium that can lead to electrogenic (one net positive charge in) transport by the Na^+-Ca^{2+} exchanger (NCX).

increased intracellular Ca^{2+} and binding to calmodulin, which activates calmodulin-dependent protein kinase II.

However, increased Ca^{2+} release from the sarcoplasmic reticulum, and not transsarcolemmal calcium entry, accounts for the major portion of the "gain" of the system during adrenergic stimulation.[4] Such increased Ca^{2+} release is generated mostly by an increased sarcoplasmic reticulum Ca^{2+} load. β-Adrenergic stimulation leads to cAMP-PKA–induced phosphorylation of phospholamban, which in turn leads to enhanced action of the sarcoplasmic reticulum Ca^{2+}-ATPase (SERCA), with augmented Ca^{2+} uptake and increased sarcoplasmic reticulum Ca^{2+} content.

Sarcoplasmic reticulum "leakiness" can contribute to arrhythmogenesis. Normally, Ca^{2+} release from the sarcoplasmic reticulum occurs through the action of the tightly controlled ryanodine receptor complex. β-Adrenergic stimulation, through PKA activation can lead to hyperphosphorylation of the ryanodine receptor, which has been shown to lead to the dissociation of FKBP12.6 from the complex,[5] which in turn can render it prone to spontaneous Ca^{2+} release (hence the "leakiness"). This can be corrected by increasing the affinity of FKBP12.6 for the ryanodine receptor.[6] Of note, it is debated whether hyperphosphorylation and leakiness of the ryanodine receptor are truly mediated by PKA, because recent data support a predominant role of the calmodulin-dependent protein kinase II.[4,7,8] Clearly, sarcoplasmic reticulum leakiness represents another weak link in the physiologic response to exercise. Clinically, mutations in the ryanodine receptor can lead to calcium leakiness,[9] generating the phenotype of catecholaminergic polymorphic ventricular tachycardia (CPVT) (see later on). In affected persons, exercise will induce ventricular tachycardias—characteristically, bidirectional ventricular tachycardia, which recently has been shown to originate from the Purkinje system.[10] Additionally, mutations in the gene encoding calsequestrin, a calcium-binding protein in the sarcoplasmic reticulum, can replicate a similar phenotype.[11,12]

Calcium leakage from the sarcoplasmic reticulum in response to catecholamine stimulation is common in heart failure. Heart failure is a chronic hyperadrenergic state in which spontaneous Ca^{2+} release can occur by way of a hyperphosphorylated ryanodine receptor. The link between calcium leakiness and arrhythmias is provided by the Na^+-Ca^{2+} exchanger, which generates a transient inward current (for every calcium ion extruded, three sodium ions pass in, resulting in entry of one net positive charge into the cell), potentially leading to delayed afterdepolarizations[13] (Fig. 82-2). The same mechanism has been shown to operate in CPVT.[14]

Shortening of the Action Potential

PKA also phosphorylates the *KCNQ1* protein, which forms the α subunit of I_{Ks}, the slowly activating component of the delayed rectifier current. On phosphorylation, the current is enhanced, leading to shortening of the action potential (see Fig. 82-1). This is physiologically necessary to preserve diastolic filling time during rapid rates. This phosphorylation requires a macromolecular complex composed of the channel itself and the targeting protein Yotaio, which recruits PKA and a protein phosphatase 1 to the C-terminal domain of the *KCNQ1* protein.[15] Mutations in the genes encoding I_{Ks} subunits cause long QT syndrome variants 1 and 5: LQT1 (α subunit, *KCNQ1* mutations) and LQT5 (β subunit, *KCNE1* mutations). *KCNQ1* mutations not only prolong the QT interval at baseline but also impair the shortening of the APD normally associated with sympathetic activation, leading to paradoxical QT prolongation and typically sudden death during exercise. The specific arrhythmogenic mechanisms in long QT typically involve early afterdepolarizations and torsades de pointes and are described in detail elsewhere in this book.

Exercise Recovery

In some patients, arrhythmogenic activity often ensues or worsens during the recovery phase. Withdrawal of sympathetic tone, accompanied by increased parasympathetic activation, mediates slowing of the heart rate and decreases in blood pressure. Parasympathetic activation leads to a reversal of sympathetic effects by inhibition of adenyl cyclase by G_i protein on acetylcholine (ACh) binding to the M_2 muscarinic receptors (see Fig. 82-1). Additionally, ligand-operated G protein–gated potassium channels are activated, leading to an outward I_{KACh} potassium current that shortens the action potential, particularly in atrial and nodal tissues.

Although not specifically tested during exercise recovery, the combination of persistent sympathetic activation with increasing parasympathetic influences has been hypothesized to be particularly arrhythmogenic in the generation of atrial extrasystoles and atrial fibrillation.[16-18] The basic mechanism is thought to involve persistently augmented calcium transient due to sympathetic activation, with simultaneous vagally induced shortening of the action potential. Diastolic Ca^{2+} elevation in the cytosol would lead to early afterdepolarizations effected by the Na^+-Ca^{2+} exchanger (calcium transient triggering[17]).

Clinical Exercise–Induced Arrhythmias

Catecholamine-Induced Arrhythmias

Extrasystoles

As a result of the physiologic changes described previously, both enhanced automaticity (effected through phase 4 depolarization) and triggered activity (most commonly delayed afterdepolarizations due to calcium overload) can generate ectopic activations in atrial and ventricular tissue. Aside from the prognostic implications (see later on), atrial and ventricular extrasystoles can lead to the initiation of sustained tachycardias in the presence of the appropriate substrate (accessory pathway, dual–AV node physiology in the atria, or ventricular scar in the ventricles).

Outflow Tract Ventricular Tachycardias

As described elsewhere in this book in more detail, sensitivity to exercise is a prominent feature of outflow tract ventricular tachycardia (OTVT), hypothesized to be generated by focal activations arising from delayed afterdepolarizations, exacerbated by exercise-induced sympathetic stimulation. Usually associated with a left bundle branch block pattern and an inferior axis, OTVT originates most commonly in the right ventricular outflow tract, but other locations such as the left ventricular outflow tract and the aortic coronary cusps are possible. Manifestations include monomorphic ventricular tachycardia and isolated extrasystoles. The arrhythmogenic focus may be suppressed by increased sinus rates, so induction during exercise may occur only transiently or at the recovery phase. If the patient is symptomatic, treatment may include β-adrenergic receptor blockade, calcium channel blockade, or catheter ablation.

Verapamil-Sensitive Fascicular Tachycardia

Although a reentrant mechanism involving the Purkinje network neighboring the posterior fascicle[19] has become increasingly accepted, this tachycardia is known to be sensitive to exercise.[20] The mechanisms for such sensitivity are unclear. Typically manifested with a right bundle branch block pattern and left axis, this tachycardia responds to verapamil acutely, but long-term data on

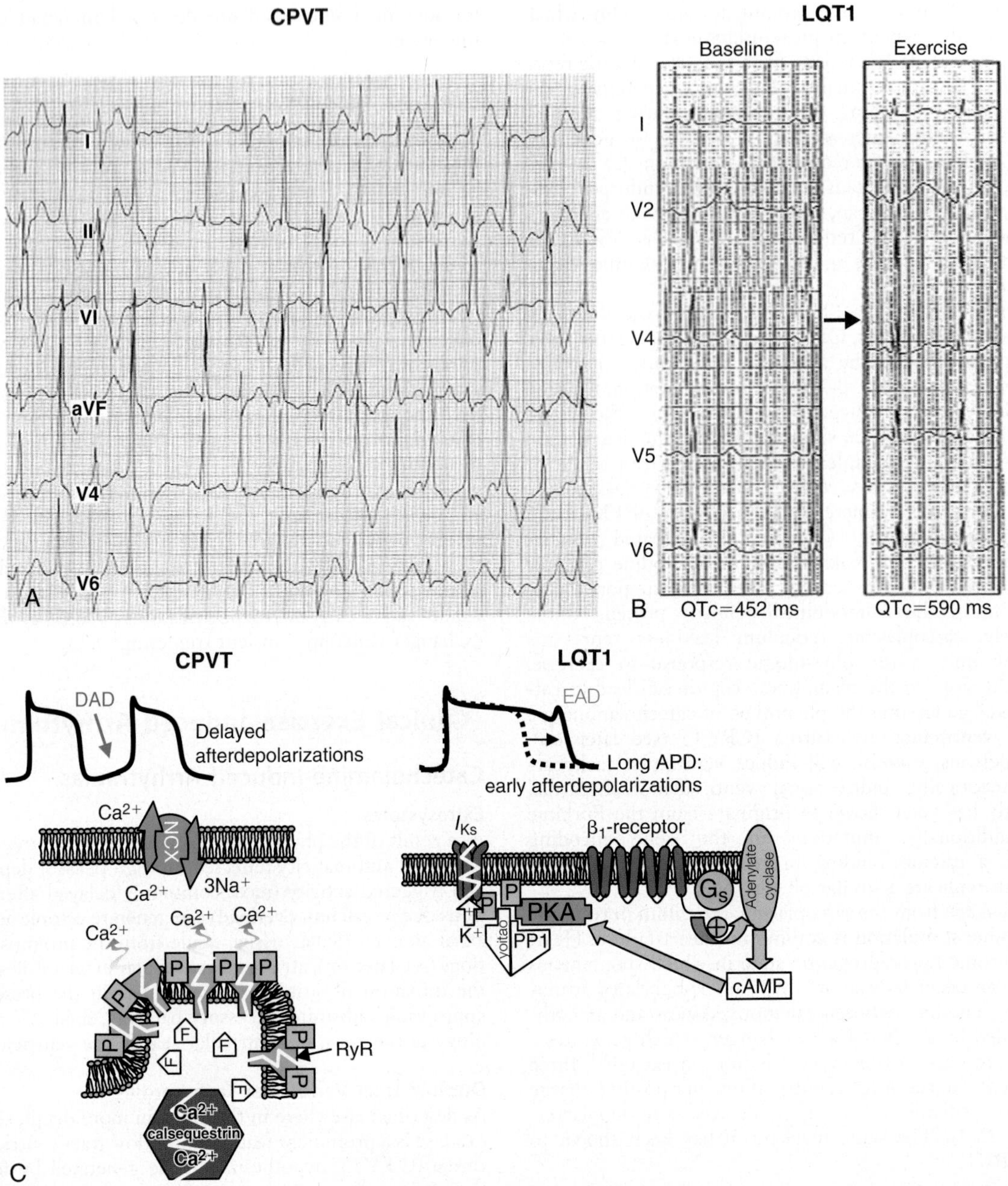

Figure 82-2 Exercise response in catecholaminergic polymorphic ventricular tachycardia (CPVT) and long QT syndrome type 1 (LQT1). **A,** Bidirectional ventricular tachycardia (alternating QRS axis) during exercise in a patient with CPVT. **B,** Paradoxical QT prolongation during exercise in a patient with LQT1. **C,** Mechanisms of arrhythmogenesis. In CPVT *(left)*, mutations *(white zigzag line)* in either the ryanodine receptor (RyR) or the calsequestrin gene make calcium leak. Excess calcium is transported by the Na^+-Ca^{2+} exchanger (NCX), which brings in 3 sodium ions for each calcium, thereby generating a slow depolarization (transient inward current) that can reach threshold and generate a delayed afterdepolarization (DAD). In long QT syndrome *(right)*, a mutated potassium channel *(zigzag line)* does not enhance I_{Ks} on phosphorylation, and the action potential prolongs, which can lead to early afterdepolarizations (EAD). APD, action potential duration; cAMP, cyclic adenosine monophosphate; PKA, protein kinase A; PP1, protein phosphatase 1. (**A,** From Francis J, Sankar V, Nair VK, Priori SG: Catecholaminergic polymorphic ventricular tachycardia. Heart Rhythm 2:550-554, 2005; **B,** from Takenaka K, Ai T, Shimizu W, et al: Exercise stress test amplifies genotype-phenotype correlation in the LQT1 and LQT2 forms of the long-QT syndrome. Circulation 107:838-844, 2003.)

its efficacy are limited. If the condition is resistant to antiarrhythmic therapy, catheter ablation is effective.

Catecholaminergic Polymorphic Ventricular Tachycardia

The molecular mechanisms (calcium leakiness) (see Figs. 82-1 and 82-2) described earlier generate a clinical phenotype characterized by highly reproducible, exercise-induced ventricular arrhythmias whose complexity and severity are proportional to the level of exercise. With increasing exercise intensity, atrial tachycardia or fibrillation, multifocal ventricular extrasystoles, bidirectional VT (see Fig. 82-2), and polymorphic VT or ventricular fibrillation may develop.[21]

The typical presentation is syncope during exercise or stress. Recently described variants of the disease, caused by certain mutations in the ryanodine receptor, combine features of CPVT with features of arrhythmogenic right ventricular dysplasia (ARVD) or dilated cardiomyopathy[22] and pose particular risk for arrhythmias during exercise owing to the concomitant presence of structural heart disease. The mainstay of therapy has been β-adrenergic blockade. However, mortality remains high, however, and implantable cardioverter-defibrillators (ICDs) are indicated for sudden death prevention. The combination of beta-blockers with calcium channel blockers appears to suppress arrhythmias effectively.[23]

Long QT Syndrome

Long QT syndrome type 1 (LQT1) typically is associated with exercise-induced syncope. As described earlier, the responsible mutations directly impair shortening of APD, which characteristically leads to paradoxical increases in QT both during epinephrine infusion[24] and with exercise.[25] In long QT syndrome, early afterdepolarizations (see Fig. 82-2) manifest as extrasystoles (R-on-T phenomenon), which can be isolated or be followed by runs of torsades de pointes. Treatment includes beta-blockade and defibrillator implantation for sudden cardiac death prevention.

Exercise-Induced Sudden Death: Structural Determinants

The issue of sudden death in the athlete is the subject of Chapter 92. A brief overview is presented here: The structural heart diseases that lead to exercise-related sudden death are diverse. In young persons, hypertrophic cardiomyopathy, coronary anomalies (anomalous origin, myocardial bridging), aortic dissection and rupture associated with connective tissue defects as in Marfan syndrome, and arrhythmogenic right ventricular cardiomyopathy (ARVC) (seemingly more common in Italy[26]) predominate. By contrast, coronary artery disease predominates in the adult population.[27,28] Exercise-induced arrhythmogenesis in hypertrophic cardiomyopathy is mechanistically complex, involving diverse hemodynamic and structural factors. In ARVC, the heterogeneous fibrofatty infiltration provides a substrate for reentrant ventricular tachyarrhythmias. In heart failure, as described earlier, sympathetic stimulation can lead to triggered ventricular tachycardias owing to calcium leakiness of the sarcoplasmic reticulum.[13]

Bradycardias

A paradoxical sinus bradycardia during exercise has been described recently in mutations of the ryanodine receptor leading to CPVT[22] and also can rarely occur in certain patients with obstructive lung disease or atherosclerotic heart disease leading to hypoxia of the sinus node.

Patients with infra-Hisian conduction disease may have rate-dependent conduction block exacerbated by exercise. This may manifest clinically as exercise-induced aberrancy of either bundle branch or as exercise-induced Mobitz II atrioventricular block.

Vagal stimulation during the recovery phase may lead to profound sinus bradycardia, which typically is transient.

Prognostic Implications

Does Exercise Increase the Risk of Sudden Death?

The evidence supporting an *acute* increase of sudden death by vigorous physical activity appears compelling.[28] Among young athletes, the incidence of sudden death was found to be 2.5 times higher than in nonathletes.[26] In adults, it is known that despite an overall reduction in coronary heart disease with regular physical activity, the rate of cardiac arrest is higher *during* vigorous exercise, and highest among previously sedentary men.[29] It also has been shown, however, that habitual vigorous exercise attenuates the relative risk of sudden death that is associated with a given episode of vigorous exertion,[30] and overall the total incidence of sudden death does decrease with increasing exercise levels.[28]

Persons with certain genetic cardiovascular diseases, including hypertrophic cardiomyopathy, ARVC, Marfan syndrome, and ion channel diseases (e.g., long QT syndrome, CPVT), are at particular risk for exercise-induced sudden death and require long-term avoidance of high-risk activity. Recommendations regarding specific exercises have been devised for specific diseases[31] (Table 82-1).

Prognostic Value of Exercise-Induced Arrhythmias

Ventricular ectopy can occur both during exercise and during the recovery phase. Data on the prognostic significance of such arrhythmias derive from cohorts of patients subjected to exercise stress testing, either those referred for clinically indicated diagnostic testing[32,33] or asymptomatic patients.[34, 35]

Among patients with clinically indicated exercise testing, earlier, smaller short-term studies failed to prove any prognostic relevance of ventricular extrasystoles. One study showed an association between frequent exercise-induced ectopy and mortality, but only after 8 years of follow-up.[33] A larger study showed an association between frequent ventricular ectopy (more than 7 beats per minute, bi- or trigeminy, ventricular tachycardia or fibrillation) *after* exercise and an increased risk of death (hazard ratio of 1.5) at a mean of 5 years of follow-up. The association was not present with ectopy *during* exercise.[32] Also, a recent study found a modest correlation between ventricular extrasystoles in the recovery phase and higher prevalence of coronary artery disease and inducible ischemia on myocardial imaging (odds ratio of 1.27 relative to patients without recovery extrasystoles).[36]

In asymptomatic patients, two large studies have suggested a prognostic significance of ventricular ectopy. Jouven and colleagues reported that frequent extrasystoles during exercise, defined as more than 10% of all ventricular beats during any 30-second recording (present in 2.2%), were associated with an increased risk of cardiovascular death over a period of 23 years (relative risk of 2.7).[34] More recently, the Framingham offspring study found that ventricular extrasystoles exceeding the median frequency (one per 4.5 minutes of exercise) were not associated with coronary artery events after a mean of 15 years but were associated with increased all-cause mortality (hazard ratio of 1.86), unrelated to severity of ectopy, occurrence at exercise or recovery, left ventricular dysfunction, or ischemia during exercise.[35]

In patients with heart failure, severe ventricular ectopy (defined as ventricular triplets, sustained or ventricular tachycardia, or polymorphic ventricular tachycardia or fibrillation) occurring *after* exercise was associated with a hazard ratio of 1.76 of death after 3 years. Of note, ventricular ectopy *during* exercise had no predictive value.[37]

Interpretation of these diverse data is difficult, but overall, a prudent approach is to recognize that exercise-induced ectopy seems to unmask a substrate that may make affected patients more vulnerable in the long term to cardiac disease.

Table 82-1 Specific Exercise Recommendations for Patients with Genetic Cardiovascular Disease

Numbers grade eligibility for exercise: 0 to 1 designate activities generally not advised or strongly discouraged, 4 to 5 indicate activities probably permitted, and 2 to 3 indicate intermediate activities, which should be assessed on an individual basis.

Intensity Level	HCM	LQTS	Marfan Syndrome	ARVC	Brugada Syndrome
High					
Basketball					
Full court	0	0	2	1	2
Half court	0	0	2	1	2
Body building	1	1	0	1	1
Ice hockey	0	0	1	0	0
Racquetball/squash	0	2	2	0	2
Rock climbing	1	1	1	1	1
Running (sprinting)	0	0	2	0	2
Skiing (downhill)	2	2	2	1	1
Skiing (cross-country)	2	3	2	1	4
Soccer	0	0	2	0	2
Tennis (singles)	0	0	3	0	2
Touch (flag) football	1	1	3	1	3
Windsurfing	1	0	1	1	1
Moderate					
Baseball/softball	2	2	2	2	4
Biking	4	4	3	2	5
Modest hiking	4	5	5	2	4
Motorcycling	3	1	2	2	2
Jogging	3	3	3	2	5
Sailing	3	3	2	2	4
Surfing	2	0	1	1	1
Swimming (lap)	5	0	3	3	4
Tennis (doubles)	4	4	4	3	4
Treadmill/stationary bicycle	5	5	4	3	5
Weightlifting (free weights)	1	1	0	1	1
Hiking	3	3	3	2	4
Low					
Bowling	5	5	5	4	5
Golf	5	5	5	4	5
Horseback riding	3	3	3	3	3
Scuba diving	0	0	0	0	0
Skating	5	5	5	4	5
Snorkeling	5	0	5	4	4
Weights (non-free weights)	4	4	0	4	4
Brisk walking	5	5	5	5	5

From Maron BJ, Chaitman BR, Ackerman MJ, et al: Recommendations for physical activity and recreational sports participation for young patients with genetic cardiovascular diseases. Circulation 109:2807-2816, 2004.

Conclusions

The physiologic adaptation to exercise is a highly orchestrated response that involves coordination of central impulses by way of the peripheral autonomic nervous system, to deliver molecular signals that mediate necessary changes to cope with the body's increased metabolic demands. The response poses a challenge to normal excitation and impulse propagation that is susceptible to deterioration toward arrhythmogenesis in the appropriate substrates. Such substrates are diverse and may be generated by molecular defects or acquired structural heart disease. In the absence of known heart disease, exercise-induced arrhythmias seem to have a nonspecific association with unfavorable prognosis, the mechanisms and relevance of which remain to be completely defined.

References

1. Fletcher GF, Balady GJ, Amsterdam EA, et al: Exercise standards for testing and training: A statement for healthcare professionals from the American Heart Association. Circulation 104:1694-1740, 2001.
2. Rockman HA, Koch WJ, Lefkowitz RJ: Seven-transmembrane-spanning receptors and heart function. Nature 415:206-212, 2002.
3. Lefkowitz RJ: G proteins in medicine. N Engl J Med 332:186-187, 1995.
4. Sipido KR: CaM or cAMP: Linking beta-adrenergic stimulation to 'leaky' RyRs. Circ Res 100:296-298, 2007.
5. Marx SO, Reiken S, Hisamatsu Y, et al: PKA phosphorylation dissociates FKBP12.6 from the calcium release channel (ryanodine receptor): Defective regulation in failing hearts. Cell 101:365-376, 2000.
6. Wehrens XH, Lehnart SE, Reiken SR, et al: Protection from cardiac arrhythmia through ryanodine receptor-stabilizing protein calstabin2. Science 304:292-296, 2004.
7. Ai X, Curran JW, Shannon TR, et al: Ca^{2+}/calmodulin-dependent protein kinase modulates cardiac ryanodine receptor phosphorylation and sarcoplasmic reticulum Ca^{2+} leak in heart failure. Circ Res 97:1314-1322, 2005.
8. Curran J, Hinton MJ, Rios E, et al: Beta-adrenergic enhancement of sarcoplasmic reticulum calcium leak in cardiac myocytes is mediated by calcium/calmodulin-dependent protein kinase. Circ Res 100: 391-398, 2007.
9. Priori SG, Napolitano C, Tiso N, et al: Mutations in the cardiac ryanodine receptor gene (hRyR2) underlie catecholaminergic polymorphic ventricular tachycardia. Circulation 103:196-200, 2001.
10. Cerrone M, Noujaim SF, Tolkacheva EG, et al: Arrhythmogenic mechanisms in a mouse model of catecholaminergic polymorphic ventricular tachycardia. Circ Res 101:1039-1048, 2007. Epub 2007 Sep 13.
11. Lahat H, Eldar M, Levy-Nissenbaum E, et al: Autosomal recessive catecholamine- or exercise-induced polymorphic ventricular tachycardia: Clinical features and assignment of the disease gene to chromosome 1p13-21. Circulation 103:2822-2827, 2001.
12. Song L, Alcalai R, Arad M, et al: Calsequestrin 2 (CASQ2) mutations increase expression of calreticulin and ryanodine receptors, causing catecholaminergic polymorphic ventricular tachycardia. J Clin Invest 117:1814-1823, 2007.
13. Pogwizd SM, Schlotthauer K, Li L, et al: Arrhythmogenesis and contractile dysfunction in heart failure: Roles of sodium-calcium exchange, inward rectifier potassium current, and residual beta-adrenergic responsiveness. Circ Res 88: 1159-1167, 2001.
14. Liu N, Colombi B, Memmi M, et al: Arrhythmogenesis in catecholaminergic polymorphic ventricular tachycardia: Insights from a RyR2 R4496C knock-in mouse model. Circ Res 99:292-298, 2006.
15. Marx SO, Kurokawa J, Reiken S, et al: Requirement of a macromolecular signaling complex for beta adrenergic receptor modulation of the *KCNQ1-KCNE1* potassium channel. Science 295:496-499, 2002.
16. Burashnikov A, Antzelevitch C: Reinduction of atrial fibrillation immediately after termination of the arrhythmia is mediated by late phase 3 early afterdepolarization-induced triggered activity. Circulation 107:2355-2360, 2003.
17. Patterson E, Lazzara R, Szabo B, et al: Sodium-calcium exchange initiated by the Ca^{2+} transient: An arrhythmia trigger within pulmonary veins. J Am Coll Cardiol 47:1196-1206, 2006.
18. Chen PS, Tan AY: Autonomic nerve activity and atrial fibrillation. Heart Rhythm 4(3 Suppl):S61-S64, 2007.
19. Ouyang F, Cappato R, Ernst S, et al: Electroanatomic substrate of idiopathic left ventricular tachycardia: Unidirectional block and macroreentry within the Purkinje network. Circulation 105:462-469, 2002.
20. Lerman BB, Stein KM, Markowitz SM: Mechanisms of idiopathic left ventricular tachycardia. J Cardiovasc Electrophysiol 8:571-583, 1997.
21. Francis J, Sankar V, Nair VK, Priori SG: Catecholaminergic polymorphic ventricular tachycardia. Heart Rhythm 2:550-554, 2005.
22. Bhuiyan ZA, van den Berg MP, van Tintelen JP, et al: Expanding spectrum of human *RYR2*-related disease: New electrocardiographic, structural, and genetic features. Circulation 116:1569-1576, 2007.
23. Rosso R, Kalman JM, Rogowski O, et al: Calcium channel blockers and beta-blockers versus beta-blockers alone for preventing exercise-induced arrhythmias in catecholaminergic polymorphic ventricular tachycardia. Heart Rhythm 4:1149-1154, 2007.
24. Vyas H, Hejlik J, Ackerman MJ: Epinephrine QT stress testing in the evaluation of congenital long-QT syndrome: Diagnostic accuracy of the paradoxical QT response. Circulation 113:1385-1392, 2006.
25. Takenaka K, Ai T, Shimizu W, et al: Exercise stress test amplifies genotype-phenotype correlation in the LQT1 and LQT2 forms of the long-QT syndrome. Circulation 107:838-844, 2003.
26. Corrado D, Basso C, Rizzoli G, et al: Does sports activity enhance the risk of sudden death in adolescents and young adults? J Am Coll Cardiol 42:1959-1963, 2003.
27. Maron BJ, Shirani J, Poliac LC, et al: Sudden death in young competitive athletes. Clinical, demographic, and pathological profiles. JAMA 276:199-204, 1996.
28. Thompson PD, Franklin BA, Balady GJ, et al: Exercise and acute cardiovascular events placing the risks into perspective: A scientific statement from the American Heart Association Council on Nutrition, Physical Activity, and Metabolism and the Council on Clinical Cardiology. Circulation 115:2358-2368, 2007.
29. Siscovick DS, Weiss NS, Fletcher RH, Lasky T: The incidence of primary cardiac arrest during vigorous exercise. N Engl J Med 311:874-877, 1984.
30. Albert CM, Mittleman MA, Chae CU, et al: Triggering of sudden death from cardiac causes by vigorous exertion. N Engl J Med 343:1355-1361, 2000.
31. Maron BJ, Chaitman BR, Ackerman MJ, et al: Recommendations for physical activity and recreational sports participation for young patients with genetic cardiovascular diseases. Circulation 109:2807-2816, 2004.
32. Frolkis JP, Pothier CE, Blackstone EH, Lauer MS: Frequent ventricular ectopy after exercise as a predictor of death. N Engl J Med 348:781-790, 2003.
33. Partington S, Myers J, Cho S, et al: Prevalence and prognostic value of exercise-induced ventricular arrhythmias. Am Heart J 145:139-146, 2003.
34. Jouven X, Zureik M, Desnos M, et al: Long-term outcome in asymptomatic men with exercise-induced premature ventricular depolarizations. N Engl J Med 343:826-833, 2000.
35. Morshedi-Meibodi A, Evans JC, Levy D, et al: Clinical correlates and prognostic significance of exercise-induced ventricular premature beats in the community: The Framingham Heart Study. Circulation 109:2417-2422, 2004.
36. Meine TJ, Patel MR, Shaw LK, Borges-Neto S: Relation of ventricular premature complexes during recovery from a myocardial perfusion exercise stress test to myocardial ischemia. Am J Cardiol 97:1570-1572, 2006.
37. O'Neill JO, Young JB, Pothier CE, Lauer MS: Severe frequent ventricular ectopy after exercise as a predictor of death in patients with heart failure. J Am Coll Cardiol 44:820-826, 2004.

The Use of Implantable Loop Recorders 83

ANDREW D. KRAHN, ALLAN C. SKANES, AND GEORGE J. KLEIN

CHAPTER OUTLINE

Overview

Ambulatory cardiac monitoring to detect arrhythmia became practical with the development of Holter monitoring and other external devices, with the feasible period of monitoring extended considerably with the development of implantable loop recorders. Clinical trials using implantable loop recorders have validated a clear role in investigation of unexplained syncope and potential usefulness in evaluation for a range of conditions including atypical epilepsy, vasovagal syncope, and post–myocardial infarction arrhythmia. Recent advances in design with the potential addition of other physiologic sensors have strengthened the capability of implantable devices and promise to translate into tools that not only detect intermittent arrhythmia in syncope, but assist in chronic disease management for common conditions such as atrial fibrillation and in post–myocardial infarction risk stratification.

Syncope represents the prototype condition that is ideally served by long-term ambulatory monitoring. The periodic and unpredictable nature of events and the high spontaneous remission rate are the major obstacles to diagnosis in most patients. Other forms of testing in unexplained syncope usually provide a context for bedside formulation of a differential diagnosis and prognosis but rarely provide a specific diagnosis. Results of provocative tilt and electrophysiologic testing may be negative, or these modalities may identify abnormalities of unknown significance, as reflected in the poor predictive value of both tests. These obvious limitations point to long-term monitoring as a step toward the ideal of comprehensive physiologic assessment performed during spontaneous symptoms. This chapter discusses the technical aspects of loop recorders, examines the established utility of loop recorders in syncope, and explores future directions for application of these devices as new designs and multiple manufacturers are emerging.

External Loop Recorders

Long-term electrocardiographic monitoring has evolved over the past decade with the availability of increasingly diverse diagnostic tools. An *external loop recorder* continuously records and stores a single external modified limb lead electrogram with a 4- to 18-minute memory buffer (Fig. 83-1). After the onset of spontaneous symptoms, the patient activates the device, which stores the previous 3 to 14 minutes, and then the following 1 to 4 minutes, of recorded information. The captured rhythm strip can subsequently be uploaded and analyzed, which often provides critical information regarding the onset and termination of the arrhythmia (Fig. 83-2). The monitoring system theoretically can be used indefinitely, but in most clinical settings its use is limited to a few weeks because of practical considerations. The recording device is attached with skin electrodes to the patient's chest wall and needs to be removed for bathing or showering and can be uncomfortable during sleep.

A randomized trial has shown diagnostic and cost-effective superiority to Holter monitors (22% yield for the Holter monitor, versus 56% for the loop recorder; $P < .01$).[1] A recent report suggests an increment in diagnostic yield when automatic activation is added to patient activation.[2] Automatic detection includes bradycardia, tachycardia and pauses, as well as atrial fibrillation based on algorithms that detect R-R irregularity. Limited data are available on the usefulness of this technology in detecting or excluding atrial fibrillation. Continuous ambulatory monitoring with data transmission to a central monitoring station staffed by health professionals (Cardionet, San Diego, California) has emerged in the United States as a useful resource to extend traditional Holter monitoring beyond 48 hours. This technique typically is used for 7 to 14 days and has shown incremental benefit over that for a standard external loop recorder in diagnosing or excluding arrhythmia.[3]

Long-term compliance with these devices can be challenging because of electrode- and skin-related problems and waning of patient motivation in the absence of recurrent symptoms. Nonetheless, some form of external monitoring generally is warranted in patients prior to proceeding with an implanted device.

Implanted Loop Recorders

The implantable loop recorder permits prolonged monitoring without external electrodes. It is ideally suited to use in patients who require more prolonged monitoring such as those with infrequent recurrent symptoms such as syncope. Similar to the external loop recorder, the device is designed to detect arrhythmia to permit specific correlation of symptoms with recorded cardiac rhythms. Its advantage over external devices is that it is implanted, thereby obviating surface electrodes and accompanying compliance issues.

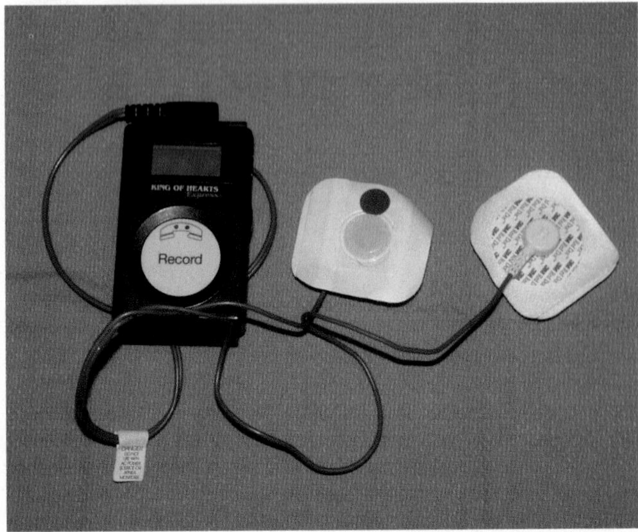

Figure 83-1 Photograph of the external loop recorder with recording electrodes *(right)*.

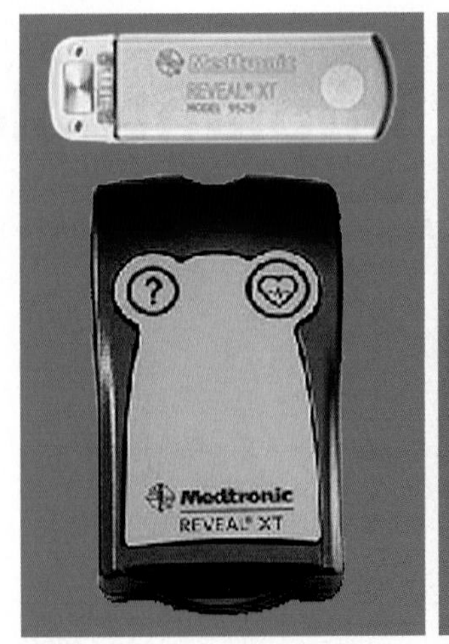

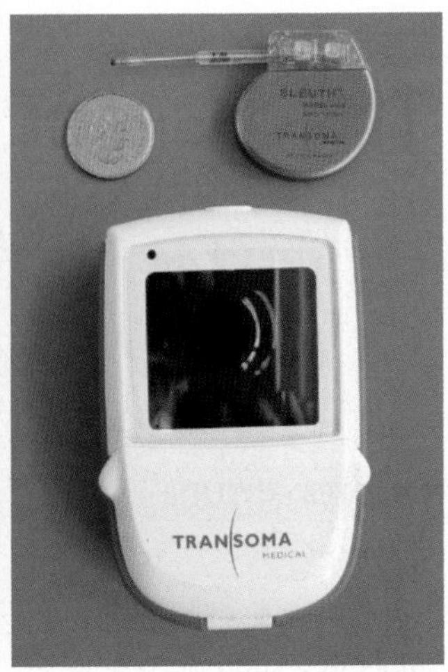

Figure 83-3 Implanted loop recorders. The Medtronic Reveal XT *(top left)* with patient activator *(bottom left)*. The Transoma Sleuth *(top right)* with patient activator *(bottom right)*. See text for discussion.

Implanted loop recorders are manufactured by Medtronic (Reveal XT Model 9529, Minneapolis, Minnesota) and Transoma Medical (Sleuth, Minneapolis) (Fig. 83-3). Both are smaller than a conventional pacemaker generator, record a single-lead electrocardiogram (ECG) without a transvenous lead, and have the potential to deliver 3 years (Medtronic) and 28 months (Transoma) of battery life. The previous-generation Medtronic implantable loop recorder (Reveal Plus Model 9525) often lasted 25% to 50% longer than the rated battery life, because it typically was left in until battery exhaustion. The new generation of devices will provide much longer monitoring capability than that for the previous 14-month device.

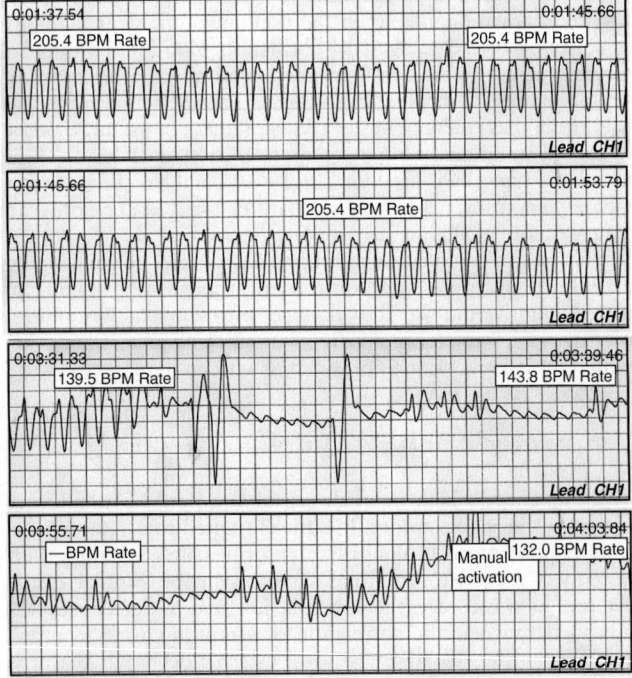

Figure 83-2 External loop recorder download from a patient with near-syncope with palpitations. Wide QRS complex tachycardia is noted at 206 beats per minute (BPM), which subsequently demonstrates underlying atrial flutter with much slower conduction, captured after patient activation.

The device typically is inserted in the left chest with use of local anesthetic, usually in a high left parasternal or medial pacemaker insertion location.[4] In principle, devices can be implanted anywhere in the chest and abdomen where an ECG can be recorded. The implantation procedure is similar to fashioning a small pacemaker pocket. An adequate signal can be obtained anywhere in the left thorax, without the need for cutaneous mapping. Mapping often is helpful to maximize signal size and the R-to-T wave ratio for optimal automatic detection. Devices have been implanted in the right parasternal location to optimize p waves, and in an inframammary or anterior axillary location for comfort or cosmetic purposes. These alternate sites typically record a lower-amplitude ECG signal. The patient, along with a spouse, family member, or friend, is instructed in the use of the activator at the time of implantation. Sterile implantation technique is essential, and use of prophylactic antibiotics generally is recommended, although the efficacy of such regimens in preventing infection has not been rigidly established. The implantation procedure has been performed by cardiologists and cardiac surgeons in various facilities including the operating room, electrophysiology laboratory, and cardiac catheterization laboratory.

Today's devices have the ability to automatically detect high and low heart rate and pause events, with recently developed features promising to recognize atrial fibrillation, ventricular ectopy, and various autonomic and risk-stratifying features such as heart rate variability. Manual activation remains possible if the patient experiences symptoms—typically, syncope, presyncope, or palpitations. The recorded bipolar ECG signal is stored in a loop buffer in any of several programmable memory bin configurations. Data storage and retrieval are influenced by the manufacturer platform. The Medtronic Reveal stores 43 minutes of ECG signal in a range of configurable memory buffers that include symptomatic and asymptomatic recordings. It retrieves data by interrogation with a standard pacemaker programmer (Medtronic Carelink Model 2090 Programmer) and promises to use remote monitoring in the future based on the Medtronic Carelink Network. The Transoma device uses a patient activator that downloads events daily through a base station that is kept in the home using an analog phone line that transmits to a staffed monitoring service. The patient activator is also the programming interface. This base station interface can potentially collect and transmit up to 10 hours of data daily but is not a continuous ECG monitoring system. At present, the ability to obtain routine ECG samples without automatic or patient activation with the device is limited. St. Jude Medical has recently released a device with similar capabilities to the Medtronic Reveal XT.

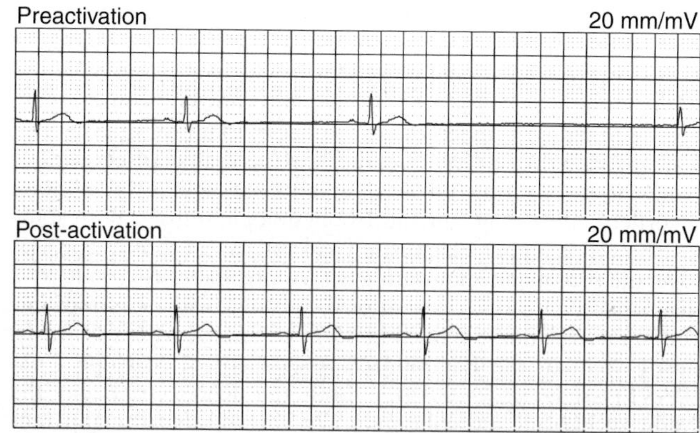

Figure 83-5 Rhythm strip from a patient with presyncope from a Transoma loop recorder, demonstrating sinus slowing followed by pause and junctional escape. These findings suggest vagal slowing but also may be compatible with sinus node disease.

Clinical Trials

Several studies have demonstrated the feasibility of establishing a symptom-rhythm correlation using an implantable loop recorder during long-term monitoring in patients with syncope.[5-10] The largest of these studies combined data from 206 patients from three clinical centers.[9] A majority of the patients had undergone previous noninvasive testing and selective invasive testing including tilt testing and electrophysiologic studies. An arrhythmia was detected in 22% of patients, was excluded in 42% of patients, and symptoms resolved without recurrence during prolonged monitoring in 31%. Bradycardia was detected more frequently than was tachycardia (17% versus 6%), usually leading to pacemaker implantation (Figs. 83-4 and 83-5). Of importance, 4% of patients failed to properly activate the device after spontaneous onset of symptoms, so symptom-rhythm correlation was not achieved in those instances. Multivariate analysis did not identify any significant preimplantation predictors of subsequent arrhythmia detection other than a weak association with advancing age and bradycardia. Unfortunately, no age group had an incidence of bradycardia greater than 30%, suggesting a limited role for empirical pacing in the unexplained syncope population.

Several studies using the implantable loop recorder have demonstrated the utility of prolonged cardiac monitoring in select populations. In the original International Study on Syncope of Uncertain Etiology (ISSUE), investigators assessed 111 patients with presumed vasovagal syncope who underwent tilt table testing and loop recorder implantation, regardless of tilt testing result.[11] Syncope recurred in 34% of patients in both the tilt-positive and the tilt-negative groups, with marked bradycardia or asystole identified as the most common recorded arrhythmia during follow-up (46% and 62%, respectively). Tilt testing failed to predict recurrence of syncope. A higher-than-expected incidence of asystole raised the possibility that detection of asystole during monitored syncope may identify a subgroup of patients responsive to permanent pacing, a tactic that has not been used in previous trials evaluating pacing in vasovagal syncope.

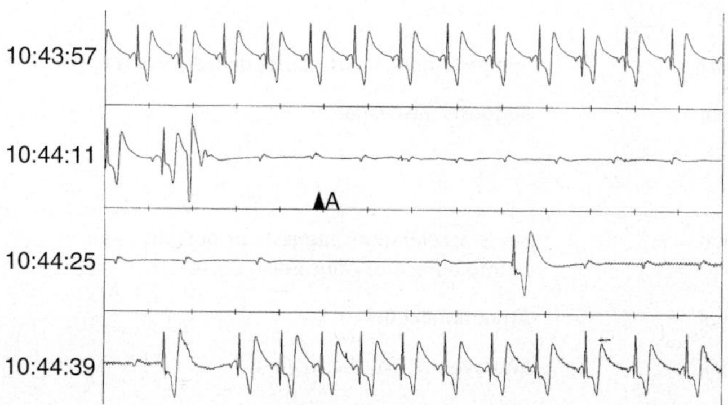

Figure 83-4 Rhythm strip from a Medtronic implanted loop recorder in a 77-year-old man with recurrent unexplained syncope and a normal baseline electrocardiogram. Note that a premature ventricular contraction induces persistent complete atrioventricular block without an escape QRS, followed by sinus slowing, suggesting a secondary cardioinhibitory vagal reaction. A, automatic activation.

In a second study, 52 patients with syncope and bundle branch block with negative results on electrophysiologic testing underwent loop recorder implantation.[12] Syncope recurred in 22 of the 52 patients. Long-term monitoring demonstrated marked bradycardia mainly attributed to complete atrioventricular (AV) block in 17, whereas it excluded AV block in 2. This study confirmed the previous view that negative electrophysiologic testing does not exclude a diagnosis of intermittent complete AV block, and that prolonged monitoring or consideration of permanent pacing is reasonable in this population. A third study examined the spontaneous rhythm in 35 patients with syncope and overt heart disease in whom electrophysiologic testing yielded a negative result.[13] The underlying heart disease was predominantly ischemic heart disease or hypertrophic cardiomyopathy with moderate left ventricular dysfunction. Although previous studies have suggested that patients with negative results on electrophysiologic testing have a better prognosis, concern remains regarding the risk of ventricular tachycardia in this group. Symptoms recurred in 19 of the 35 patients (54%), with bradycardia in 4, supraventricular tachyarrhythmia in 5, and ventricular tachycardia in only 1 patient. No sudden deaths occurred during 16 ± 11 months of follow-up.

In the ISSUE 2 study, loop recorder devices were implanted in 443 patients with recurrent syncope in the absence of structural heart disease who were presumed to have vasovagal syncope.[5] Syncope recurred in 143 patients, with a symptom-rhythm correlation in 102 patients. In those 102 patients, loop recorder–directed therapy (predominantly pacing for bradycardia) was associated with a lower risk of syncope recurrence (10% versus 41%; P = .0005). This study did not perform a randomized assessment of the benefit of pacing, but the findings raise the possibility that spontaneous cardioinhibitory syncope recorded with prolonged monitoring may identify a subgroup of patients with vasovagal syncope that benefit from pacing. This hypothesis is being tested in the ISSUE 3 trial,[14] which follows the same algorithm but randomizes patients with loop recorder–documented pauses to a regimen of pacing on or pacing off.

Two prospective randomized trials have compared early use of the loop recorder for prolonged monitoring with conventional testing in patients undergoing a cardiac workup for unexplained syncope who did not have significant structural heart disease.[6,15] Conventional testing involved monitoring with external loop recorders, tilt testing, and electrophysiologic testing. Both studies showed a higher diagnostic yield for use of loop recorders. Overall, prolonged monitoring was more likely to result in a diagnosis than was conventional testing, with a symptom-rhythm correlation obtained in 55%, compared with 19% diagnostic yield in the Randomized Assessment of Syncope Trial (RAST) study (P = .0014).[15] Both the RAST trial and the study by Farwell and colleagues also showed that the apparent upfront cost of a somewhat invasive strategy was cost-effective compared with conventional testing because of the dramatic improvement in diagnostic yield.[6,16] These data highlight the limitations of conventional diagnostic techniques. In patients who have infrequent episodes of syncope, implantable loop recorder monitoring is the diagnostic tool of choice, especially when noninvasive testing is negative and an arrhythmia is suspected.

Syncope resolves in almost one third of patients despite frequent episodes before implantation of the device.[9] This finding suggests that the cause of syncope is self-limited or may reflect a transient physiologic abnormality. All reports on use of the implantable loop recorder have suggested a low incidence of life-threatening arrhythmia or significant morbidity with a prolonged monitoring strategy.[13] Selection bias of clinicians appears to identify patients at low risk for sudden death, in whom it is appropriate to implant the device. In patients with significant structural heart disease, electrophysiologic testing or even placement of an implantable cardioverter-defibrillator (ICD) should be considered prior to a long-term monitoring strategy.

Event Classification

Interrogation of implantable loop recorders after a recurrence of syncope will often demonstrate rhythm findings that require clinical correlation and considerable judgment to interpret. Nocturnal pauses or atrial fibrillation may have different implications in patients, in accordance with their index indication for monitoring. The ISSUE investigators have proposed a useful classification system for symptomatic events in loop recorders applied to patients with syncope,[17] summarized in Table 83-1. This classification is often helpful in assigning a probable mechanism of syncope and is likely to be adopted for research purposes to create consistency in endpoints.

Table 83-1 ISSUE Classification of Detected Rhythms from the Implantable Loop Recorder

Classification	Sinus Rate	AV Node	Comment
Asystole (R-R interval >3 s)			
1A	Arrest	Normal	Progressive sinus bradycardia until sinus arrest: probably vasovagal
1B	Bradycardia	AV block	AV block with associated sinus bradycardia: probably vasovagal
1C	Normal or tachycardia	AV block	Abrupt AV block without sinus slowing: suggestive of intrinsic AV conduction disease
Bradycardia			
2A	Decrease >30%	Normal	Probably vasovagal
2B	HR <40 for >10 s	Normal	Probably vasovagal
Minimal HR change			
3A	<10% variation	Normal	Suggests noncardiac cause, unlikely vasovagal
3B	HR increase or decrease 10-30%, not <40 or >120 beats/min	Normal	Suggests vasovagal
Tachycardia			
4A	Progressive tachycardia	Normal	Sinus acceleration: suggests orthostatic intolerance or noncardiac cause
4B	N/A	Normal	Atrial fibrillation
4C	N/A	Normal	Supraventricular tachycardia
4D	N/A	Normal	Ventricular tachycardia

Adapted from Brignole M, Moya A, Menozzi C, et al: Proposed electrocardiographic classification of spontaneous syncope documented by an implantable loop recorder. Europace 7:14-18, 2005

AV, atrioventricular; HR, heart rate; ISSUE, International Study on Syncope of Uncertain Etiology; N/A, not applicable.

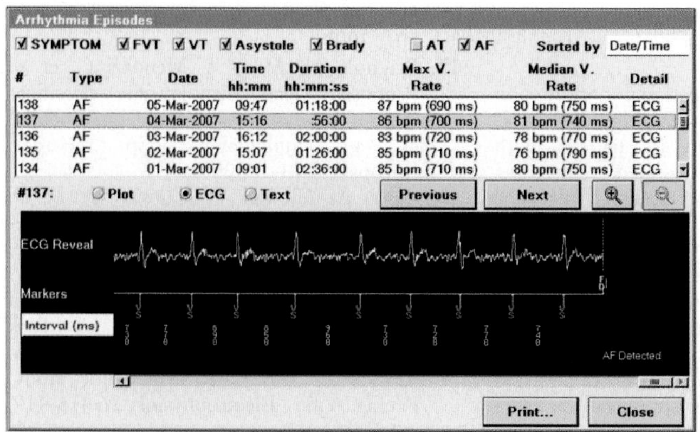

Figure 83-6 Interrogation of a Medtronic Reveal XT showing the programmer interface and rhythm strip of automatic detection of asymptomatic rate-controlled atrial fibrillation.

Additional Uses of Loop Recorders

Long-term cardiac monitoring is best suited to patients with infrequent, intermittent symptoms possibly related to arrhythmia or those in whom an infrequent "silent" arrhythmia is sought. Although investigation of syncope is a logical first application of this technology, many other clinical disease states stand to benefit from the knowledge gained from prolonged monitoring. In a study of 74 patients with ongoing seizures despite anticonvulsant therapy or unexplained recurrent seizures, Zaidi and coworkers performed cardiac assessment including tilt testing and carotid sinus massage in all patients, with implantation of the loop recorder in 10 patients.[18] Results of tilt testing were positive in 27% of the patients, and carotid sinus massage elicited seizures in 10%. Two of the 10 patients who subsequently underwent long-term monitoring demonstrated marked bradycardia preceding seizure activity—due to heart block in one patient and to sinus pauses in the second patient. This study suggested that seizures that are atypical in presentation or in response to therapy may have a cardiovascular cause in as many as 42% of patients, and that long-term cardiac monitoring has a role in select patients with atypical seizures. Several ongoing studies are assessing cardiac rhythm in a larger number of patients with atypical or unresponsive seizures.

Additional potential uses of the implantable loop recorder relate to the automatic detection feature of the device. Studies are ongoing in patients with left ventricular dysfunction to detect asymptomatic nonsustained ventricular tachycardia. A pilot study has shown promise in detection of unsuspected ventricular arrhythmia after myocardial infarction.[19] Long-term monitoring is also taking place in patients with neuromuscular diseases who are at risk for progressive conduction system disease and sudden death. Finally, strong interest in detection of atrial fibrillation has lead to several studies focusing on determining the presence of asymptomatic atrial fibrillation (Fig. 83-6).

The sensitivity and specificity of the recently devised automatic detection algorithms have not been rigorously tested in large patient populations. Previous studies have relied on elevated heart rates to detect episodes, leading to high false-positive detection rates because of overlap of atrial fibrillation and physiologic heart rates. The clinical utility of detection of atrial fibrillation will be the subject of several important clinical trials that are likely to include patients undergoing atrial fibrillation ablation and patients in whom discontinuation of warfarin is contemplated.

Future Directions

Recent advances in loop recorder design and the emergence of multiple manufacturers are indicative of rekindled interest in long-term physiologic monitoring for a variety of disease states. Enhanced data capture is likely to provide a much larger sample of data to analyze, potentially contributing novel insights into areas such as risk stratification and arrhythmia burden assessment. Improved on-board and offline diagnostic capabilities may provide an early warning or patient alert mechanism for a range of events, including recurrence of atrial fibrillation or nonsustained ventricular arrhythmia. Of greater interest is the potential to integrate a broader range of physiologic sensors into long-term monitoring devices, including those for blood pressure, oxygen saturation, chest impedance, left atrial pressure, and so on.

Conclusions

Loop recorders have significantly improved the success rate for obtaining physiologic data during spontaneous symptoms in patients with unexplained syncope. Monitoring with these devices has emerged as the assessment modality of choice in patients with problematic syncope and preserved left ventricular function. Prolonged monitoring with external and implantable loop recorders has significantly enhanced the clinician's ability to diagnose intermittent arrhythmias. Ongoing clinical trials will undoubtedly expand the use of prolonged monitoring to other disease states.

References

1. Sivakumaran S, Krahn AD, Klein GJ, et al: A prospective randomized comparison of loop recorders versus Holter monitors in patients with syncope or presyncope. Am J Med 115:1-5, 2003.
2. Reiffel JA, Schwarzberg R, Murry M: Comparison of autotriggered memory loop recorders versus standard loop recorders versus 24-hour Holter monitors for arrhythmia detection. Am J Cardiol 95:1055-1059, 2005.
3. Rothman SA, Laughlin JC, Seltzer J, et al: The diagnosis of cardiac arrhythmias: A prospective multi-center randomized study comparing mobile cardiac outpatient telemetry versus standard loop event monitoring. J Cardiovasc Electrophysiol 18:241-247, 2007.
4. Krahn AD, Klein GJ, Yee R, et al: Maturation of the sensed electrogram amplitude over time in a new subcutaneous implantable loop recorder. Pacing Clin Electrophysiol 20:1686-1690, 1997.
5. Brignole M, Sutton R, Menozzi C, et al: Early application of an implantable loop recorder allows effective specific therapy in patients with recurrent suspected neurally mediated syncope. Eur Heart J 27:1085-1092, 2006.
6. Farwell DJ, Freemantle N, Sulke N: The clinical impact of implantable loop recorders in patients with syncope. Eur Heart J 27:351-356, 2006.
7. Krahn AD, Klein GJ, Yee R, et al: Detection of asymptomatic arrhythmias in unexplained syncope. Am Heart J 148:326-332, 2004.
8. Farwell DJ, Freemantle N, Sulke AN: Use of implantable loop recorders in the diagnosis and management of syncope. Eur Heart J 25:1257-1263, 2004.
9. Krahn AD, Klein GJ, Fitzpatrick A, et al: Predicting the outcome of patients with unexplained syncope undergoing prolonged monitoring. Pacing Clin Electrophysiol 25:37-41, 2002.

10. Solano A, Menozzi C, Maggi R, et al: Incidence, diagnostic yield and safety of the implantable loop-recorder to detect the mechanism of syncope in patients with and without structural heart disease. Eur Heart J 25:1116-1119, 2004.
11. Moya A, Brignole M, Menozzi C, et al: Mechanism of syncope in patients with isolated syncope and in patients with tilt-positive syncope. Circulation 104:1261-1267, 2001.
12. Brignole M, Menozzi C, Moya A, et al: Mechanism of syncope in patients with bundle branch block and negative electrophysiological test. Circulation 104:2045-2050, 2001.
13. Menozzi C, Brignole M, Garcia-Civera R, et al: Mechanism of syncope in patients with heart disease and negative electrophysiologic test. Circulation 105:2741-2745, 2002.
14. Brignole M: International Study on Syncope of Uncertain Etiology 3 (ISSUE 3): Pacemaker therapy for patients with asystolic neurally-mediated syncope: Rationale and study design. Europace 9:25-30, 2007.
15. Krahn AD, Klein GJ, Yee R, et al: Randomized Assessment of Syncope Trial: Conventional diagnostic testing versus a prolonged monitoring strategy. Circulation 104:46-51, 2001.
16. Krahn AD, Klein GJ, Yee R, et al: Cost Implications of testing strategy in patients with syncope: Randomized Assessment of Syncope Trial. J Am Coll Cardiol 42:495-501, 2003.
17. Brignole M, Moya A, Menozzi C, et al: Proposed electrocardiographic classification of spontaneous syncope documented by an implantable loop recorder. Europace 7:14-18, 2005.
18. Zaidi A, Clough P, Cooper P, et al: Misdiagnosis of epilepsy: Many seizure-like attacks have a cardiovascular cause. J Am Coll Cardiol 36:181-184, 2000.
19. Huikuri HV, Mahaux V, Bloch-Thomsen PE: Cardiac Arrhythmias and Risk Stratification after Myocardial Infarction: Results of the CARISMA pilot study. Pacing Clin Electrophysiol 26:416-419, 2003.

High-Resolution Electrocardiography 84

Edward J. Berbari

CHAPTER OUTLINE

Background

The technique of *high-resolution electrocardiography* is defined as recording cardiac signals from the body surface that are not visible or apparent on the standard electrocardiogram (ECG). It most often implies a computer-based approach for processing the ECG and hence is not just a substitute for manual measurements made on the standard ECG. Such analysis methods may involve measurements made in either the time or the frequency domain and may include T wave alternans, cardiac late potentials, or heart rate variability. These approaches reveal electrocardiographic features that cannot be visualized or measured "by hand."

The signal-averaged ECG is the most common form of the high-resolution ECG but should not be considered as the only approach for producing a high-resolution recording. Signal averaging is a tool used primarily for improving the signal-to-noise ratio (SNR) of a noisy signal, and with a highly amplified ECG signal, the primary application has been the identification of abnormal ventricular depolarization, such as late potentials or, more recently, abnormal intra-QRS potentials. A well-established literature in this field is available, as reviewed in previous editions of this book,[1] as well as several monographs.[2-4] These late potentials quantify signals from regions of the ventricles (usually infarct border zones) that outlast the normal QRS, and the most commonly used index from these studies has been the duration of the QRS complex. Guidelines used for identifying patients in need of implantable cardioverter-defibrillator devices now include as one criterion a QRS duration greater than 120 ms. Although most work in this field has used the high-resolution ECG technique, however, the guidelines do not indicate which methodology is best for making this determination. This is still an open question.

Another method for identifying abnormalities in ventricular activation is a new technique, also based on signal-averaged electrocardiography, that measures *abnormal intra-QRS potentials* (AIQPs). Advanced signal-processing methods were used by Gomes and associates[5] to quantify changes in the "smoothness" of the QRS complex. The primary pathophysiologic rationale for this approach is that some areas of the ventricle will activate late owing to delays around or within infarct border zones, but that these signals may not prolong after the QRS complex. Activation in these small regions may not be visible at all within the QRS or at most would appear as slight slurs or notches—a concept that was studied as far back as the 1950s and is still an area of active interest today.[6] Quantifying these disruptions in the otherwise normal sequence of ventricular activation was not feasible in these earlier eras. Evidence now points to the role of passive cell facilitation of conduction, which may account for a number of abnormal QRS characteristics.[7]

Methods

The primary method used to reduce noise and identify small cardiac signals is signal averaging, which has been the subject of a number of technical and clinical reviews.[8-10] In addition, two professional society reports[11,12] have outlined the methodologies and clinical indications of the tests using the high-resolution ECG. Following is a brief overview of signal averaging and the analysis methods used to identify cardiac late potentials and the AIQP. These methods require the use of a programmed computer and are now easily implemented with the microprocessors embedded within most commercial ECG systems.

The signal-averaging method assumes several pre-conditions, including the repeating nature of the signal of interest, the randomness of the interfering noise, and the independence between the signal of interest and the interfering noise. Three sources of noise typically are encountered in performing a signal-averaged ECG: (1) the inherent noise of the electronic instrumentation; (2) power line interference (60 hertz in North America); and (3) physiologic noise primarily originating from the chest wall muscles. The electromyographic noise is the most significant noise source, whereas the others, if present, indicate a correctable technical problem such as a loose electrode.

Most implementations of high-resolution electrocardiography use uncorrected, orthogonal XYZ leads. The use of only three leads is somewhat historical in that this reduced the amount of computer processing needed in a time when such operations were costly and time-consuming. In today's technology, processing speed and the number of acquisition channels are not significant cost factors.

Figure 84-1 is a signal flow diagram of the signal-averaging method as applied to the ECG. The upper trace represents a series of stylized QRS complexes, extending out for *n* cardiac

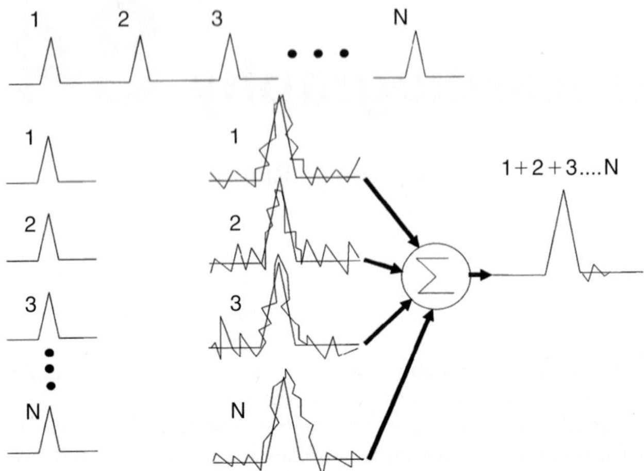

Figure 84-1 This stylized signal diagram depicts the signal averaging method graphically. Across the top are a series of triangle waves representing the QRS complexes. After digitization and application of appropriate software, these QRS complexes are time aligned, as shown on the *left*. These are then summated ($\sum$) and averaged to produce an average waveform. This process reduces the random noise that is observed after high-level amplification.

cycles. Through application of the software, each QRS complex is properly detected and accurately aligned with each other as shown in the vertically aligned complexes on the left side of the figure. The highly amplified ECG signals are represented by the nonrepetitive (random) addition of a noise signal. These aligned signals are then added together on a point-by-point basis, and the resultant average beat has a significantly reduced noise signal, allowing for the visualization of small signal previously masked by the noise. These digitized signals can analyzed and stored on a computer disk for future reference. After being averaged, the signals usually are subjected to high-pass filtration to remove low-frequency signals. This process emphasizes the higher-frequency signals that may be present; in the case of late potentials, the rationale is that conduction around and through surviving cells in an infarct region progresses in a nonuniform fashion, leading to rapid directional changes in the activation wavefront. All of the hardware and software capability of currently available ECG systems usually are sufficient to implement the signal-averaged ECG.

Ventricular Late Potentials

By far the most common application of the high-resolution ECG is to record cardiac late potentials. Late potentials are generated by tissues activated later than their usual timing in the cardiac cycle. Most often, this delay is due to depolarizing tissue within and surrounding infarct regions. Thus, the pathophysiologic basis of late potentials is the depolarizing potentials that outlast the normal end of the QRS complex. It is likely, however, that patients with an inferior infarct will have more evident late potentials than those with an anterior infarct, owing to the normal activation sequence of the ventricles. Owing to the earlier activation in the anterior regions of the ventricles, delayed depolarization potentials for this region may not outlast the QRS complex as much as delayed depolarization potentials in the posterior regions; this concept constitutes the basis for studying the AIQPs. Similarly, patients with a bundle branch block or intraventricular conduction defects have late-occurring depolarization potentials due to these conduction disorders, and infarct-related delays may not outlast the QRS complex.

Figure 84-2 illustrates the steps used to record and quantify cardiac late potentials by means of the most common approaches. Figure 84-2A shows the bipolar XYZ leads in a normal rhythm strip mode. Figure 84-2B shows a QRS complex from these three leads after proper alignment and signal averaging. The time scale was increased by a factor of 10, and the vertical scale is approximately five times greater than in Figure 84-2A. At this resolution, it is possible to visualize small inflections at the end of and after the QRS complexes. These are of relatively short duration and hence would have a higher-frequency content than the QRS complex itself. Traditional high-pass electronic filtering would be considered in separating these higher-frequency signals. The relatively large lower-frequency components of the QRS complex cannot be totally eliminated, however, and this limitation would result in considerable phase distortion of the presumed late potentials.

The method proposed by Simson and associates[13] uses software-encoded filters in the computer to filter the QRS complex in both a forward and reverse time fashion. This limits phase distortion at the beginning and end of the QRS complex at the expense of extensive phase distortion in the central part of the QRS. This is an acceptable tradeoff because most late potential parameters require accurate detection of the QRS endpoints. Figure 84-2C, further amplified by a factor of 10 compared with Figure 84-2B, shows the high-pass filtered XYZ leads. The QRS complexes are multiphasic and clipped at their extrema, but the late potentials are observed to extend as late as 148 ms after the earliest QRS onset in the Z lead. Another step and method of analysis were introduced by Simson and associates[13] and uses the vector magnitude, VM, formed by the transformation of the filtered XYZ leads using the Pythagorean theorem:

$$VM = \sqrt{X^2 + Y^2 + Z^2}$$

Figure 84-2D is the waveform that results from this vector transformation. Note that all of the waveform components are now positive. Three parameters have been used most often to characterize the late potentials: (1) The *total QRS duration* (QRSd), which includes the late potentials, is the total ventricular activation time. It is 205 ms − 67 ms = 138 ms in this example. (2) The *root-mean-square voltage* of the terminal at 40 ms (RMS40) represents the relative amplitude of the late potential component. It is depicted as the shaded region in Figure 84-2D and is 20 μV. (3) The *low-amplitude signal* (LAS) is the duration of the signal whose initial value is less than 40 μV. The bracket shows this to be 54 ms in Figure 84-2D. Many studies have used these parameters to classify patients after they have suffered a myocardial infarction. In some cases, the patients had an inducible ventricular tachycardia during an electrophysiologic study or experienced an arrhythmic event during follow-up. These cases are discussed later, but the criterion often used to classify an abnormal result on signal-averaged electrocardiography (SAECG) testing is a QRSd more than 114 ms, or RMS40 less than 20 μV, or an LAS greater than 38 ms.[11]

Figure 84-3 illustrates a weak point in the vector magnitude approach. The automatic algorithms that identify the onset and offset points of the QRS differ between the individual leads and the vector magnitude. This is true because the XYZ leads each have an independent SNR, and the resultant vector magnitude will almost always have an SNR lower than the highest SNR of the individual XYZ leads. This observation was critically examined in a study of more than 170 patients.[9] In essence, the QRSd

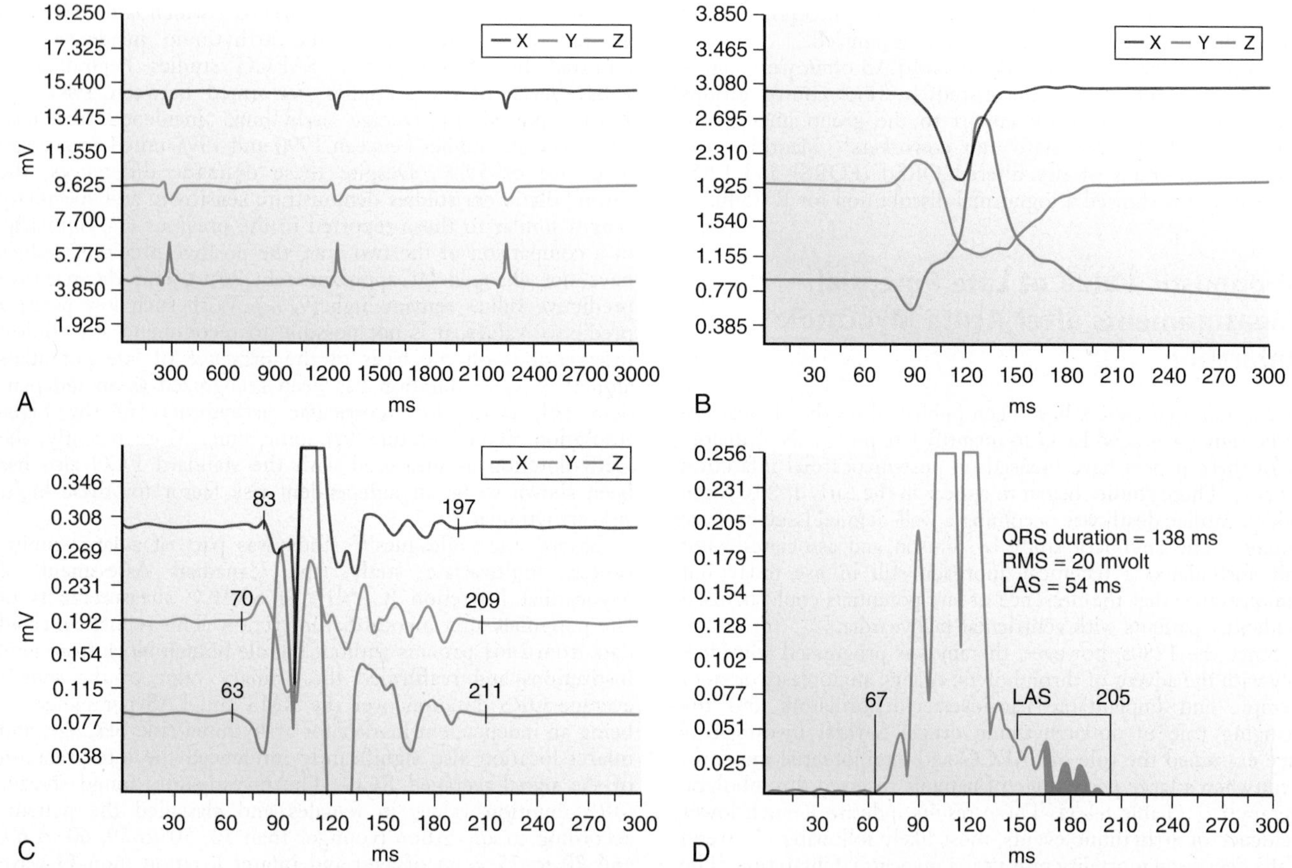

Figure 84-2 Each panel shows the progression of signal processing methods used to record the filtered vector magnitude and the late potential parameters. **A** is a rhythm strip of the XYZ lead. **B,** centered on the signal-averaged QRS complex, has a time scale one-tenth that of *A* and a vertical scale which is one-fifth that in **A. C** was obtained after high-pass filtering of the signals in **B** at 25 Hz. **D** is the filtered vector magnitude, with the three late potential parameters—QRS duration, RMS40 *(blue shaded)*, and LAS—depicted. (From Berbari EJ, Lazzara R: An introduction to high-resolution ECG recordings of cardiac late potentials. Arch Intern Med 148:1859-1863, 1988. Copyright 1988, American Medical Association. All rights reserved.)

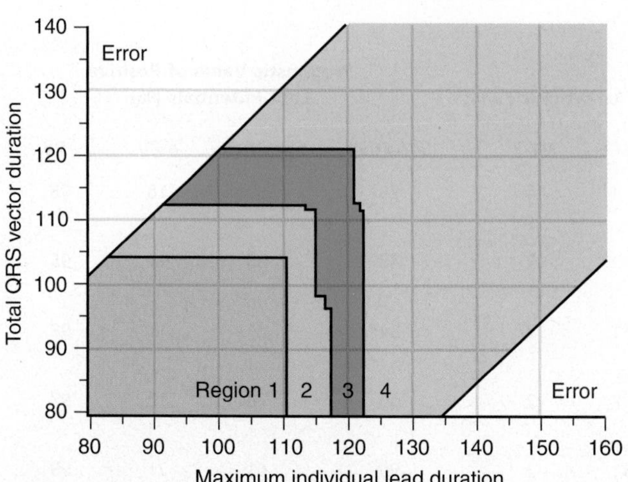

Figure 84-3 Chart of QRS vector duration versus maximum individual lead duration. Regions 1 to 4 represent normal, borderline normal, borderline abnormal, and abnormal, respectively. (From Lander P, Berbari EJ, Rajagopalan CV, et al: Critical analysis of the signal-averaged electrocardiogram: Improved identification of late potentials. Circulation 87:105-117, 1993.)

in the vector magnitude will, in general, be shorter than the longest duration in the individual XYZ leads, resulting in higher sensitivities for detecting patients with ventricular tachycardia. Using the vector magnitude alone, however, results in higher specificity when compared with the individual leads. By combining the two measurements, the chart yields five regions. The error regions are those in which at least a 20-ms discrepancy between the two measurements is found. Regions labeled 1 to 4 result in four levels of risk for future ventricular tachycardia. Regions 1 through 4 represent categories of normal, borderline normal, borderline abnormal, and abnormal, respectively. Other considerations in using this chart are described in the original study, including a complete description of the underlying statistical basis of the chart.

Other significant features of the study conducted by Lander and colleagues[9] were the lack of independence from QRSd of both the RMS and LAS measurements. This has been confirmed in many other studies, including a large multicenter study of late potentials by Savard and associates.[14] In addition, both of these studies demonstrated that compared with men, women have a lower QRS threshold for abnormal, in the range of 7 to 10 ms. This gender difference is most likely to be stem from the electrocardiographic observation that, on average, the QRS complex in females also is 7 to 10 ms shorter than that in males. Hence, the most significant and independent measure of late potentials is recognized to be the QRSd, whereas the incorporation of gender differences has not been widely recognized.

Normal values for QRDs, RMS, and LAS often were determined in the context of a clinical study in which control groups were used as a comparison cohort to the group undergoing study. A study by Nakazato and coworkers[15] identified the normal distribution of the filtered QRSd (FQRS) and LAS. The study also showed a lognormal distribution for RMS40.

Prognostic Value of Late Potential Measurements after Acute Myocardial Infarction

Several hundred papers have been published on the clinical use of the signal-averaged ECG to quantify late potentials. A majority of these papers have focused on post-myocardial infarction patients. These studies began to appear in the early 1980s, when sudden cardiac death was becoming a well-defined issue in these patients. The landmark study by Simson and associates[13] not only formulated a technical approach still in use today but demonstrated that the presence of late potentials could be used to identify patients with ventricular tachycardia.

Since the 1980s, however, therapy has progressed considerably with the advent of thrombolytic agents, angioplasty or stent therapy, and implantable cardioverter-defibrillators and the changing role of antiarrhythmic drugs. Several investigators have examined the role of SAECG and late potential measurement when a large percentage of patients received thrombolytic therapy[16-19] (Table 84-1). These results indicate a much lower incidence of arrhythmic events, most likely following the trend of the decreased mortality rate after a myocardial infarction. The reasons for this lower incidence rate are multifactorial and beyond the scope of this chapter. Also, not all patients received thrombolytic therapy in these studies, but this factor may accurately depict a general cardiology practice. The arrhythmia event rates are lower, and the size of patient populations must be substantially increased to reach statistical significance.

The study by Savard and coworkers,[14] which is described in greater detail later, charts the arrhythmic incidence rate reported by 15 prospective SAECG studies beginning in 1983. Seven of these studies performed between 1983 and 1990 reported an average arrhythmia incidence of 9.6%, whereas eight studies between 1990 and 1995 noted an average incidence of 5.8%. Despite these dramatic differences, the thrombolytic era studies demonstrate sensitivity and specificity ranges similar to those reported in the previous era. Similarly, in a comparison of the two eras, the positive predictive values have not changed (at approximately 20%), and the negative predictive values remain high (97%). With such low positive predictive values, it is not possible to recommend any clinical interventions on the basis of the presence of late potentials alone.[11,12] QRS duration has been recognized as an independent risk factor for ventricular arrhythmias in the high-resolution ECG literature for some time. More recently, the QRS duration as measured with the standard ECG also has been shown to be an independent risk factor for these high-risk arrhythmias.[20]

Savard and colleagues'[14] study was part of a large multicenter, multivariate study (the Canadian Assessment of Myocardial Infarction [CAMI]) of SAECG measurements of late potentials after myocardial infarction. This report collected data from 2461 patients without bundle branch block from nine institutions and reaffirmed the primary value of the signal-average QRS duration over the RMS and LAS parameters as being an independent marker for arrhythmia risk. Sex, age, and infarct location also significantly influenced the interpretation of the signal-averaged ECG. The investigators found shorter QRS duration values in females and classified the patients according to age group (younger than 50, 50 to 59, 60 to 69, and 70 to 75 years of age) and infarct location (non–Q wave and inferoposterior versus anterior). Figure 84-4 is a Kaplan-Meier survival plot that shows the arrhythmia-free probability for a 24-month period after sex, age, and infarct location are taken into account.[14] The differences between the SAECG-negative and SAECG-positive curves are highly significant ($P < .0001$).

Table 84-1 Prognostic Value of Late Potentials in the Thrombolytic Era

Study	Total Patients/ No. Receiving TRx	Positive for Late Potentials	Follow-up (mo)	Arrhythmic Events		Prognostic Value of Positive Late Potentials (%)			
				SCD	VT-S	Sensitivy	Specificity	+ PV	– PV
Pedretti et al, 1992[16]	174/106	41 (24%)	14	4	4	75	82	18	98
Malik et al, 1992[17]	331/130	48 (15%)	20	12	13	48	88	25	95
McClements et al, 1993[18]	301/205	61 (20%)	13	11	2	64	81	11	98
Hohnloser et al, 1994*	173/88	41 (24%)	12	7	2	56	78	12	97
Denes et al, 1994[19]	787/363	97 (12%)	10	31	2	90	61	21	98

*Data from Hohnloser SH, Franck P, Klingenheben T, et al: Open infarct artery, late potentials, and other prognostic factors in patients after acute myocardial infarction in the thrombolytic era. A prospective trial. Circulation 90:1747-1756; 1994.

PV, predictive value; SCD, sudden cardiac death; TRx, thrombolytic therapy; VT-S, sustained ventricular tachycardia.

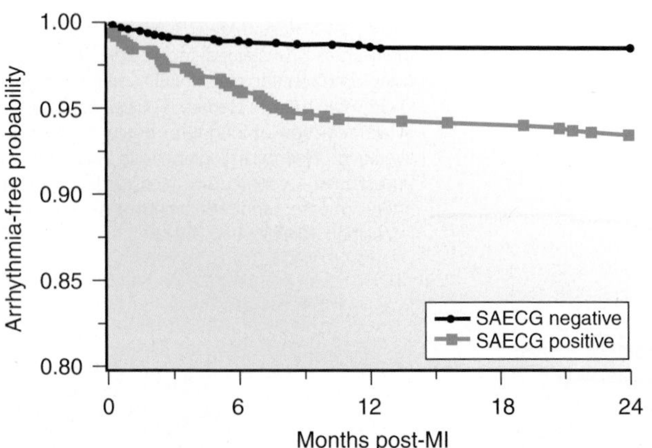

Figure 84-4 Kaplan-Meier curve of arrhythmia-free probability for 24 months of patients with positive and negative signal-averaged electrocardiography (SAECG) results after adjustment for age, sex, and infarct site. (From Savard P, Rouleau JL, Ferguson J, et al: Risk stratification after myocardial infarction using signal-averaged electrocardiographic criteria adjusted for sex, age, and myocardial infarction location. Circulation 96:202-213, 1997.)

Evaluation of Patients with Syncope of Unknown Origin

Unexplained syncope is a perplexing problem with a possible cardiac etiologic disorder of either a bradyarrhythmia or a tachyarrhythmia. As a screening tool, the SAECG measurement of late potentials can implicate a ventricular tachycardia substrate. The absence of a late potential substrate, however, does not exclude a supraventricular arrhythmia. It has been estimated that from 15% to 35% cases of syncope are due to sustained ventricular tachycardia,[10] so the use of SAECG would be helpful to identify this group of syncopal patients. Several studies have examined the role of the signal-averaged ECG in the management of syncopal patients and have shown a high level of success in identifying those with an inducible ventricular tachycardia. In syncopal patients with ischemic heart disease, the American College of Cardiology consensus document considers the signal-averaged ECG to have established value in arriving at a diagnosis for these patients.[12] The negative predictive value is the strength of the signal-averaged ECG in these cases, with values consistently above 90%.

Evaluation of Patients with Nonischemic Cardiomyopathy

The late potential substrate in patients with ischemic heart disease is localized to regions within and surrounding infarcted tissues. In nonischemic cardiomyopathy, however, the disease process usually is global, affecting the entire ventricular mass. It often is characterized as including diffuse interstitial fibrosis that leads to conduction abnormalities including bundle branch block and nonspecific intraventricular conduction defects. The degree of myocardial fibrosis determined with catheter-based biopsy has been correlated with the SAECG measures of late potentials.[21] Patients with the severest form of the disease often are candidates for heart transplantation. Studies by Mancini and colleagues[22] and Middlekauff and coworkers[23] examined the signal-averaged ECG as a means of predicting either the need for immediate transplantation or death of the patient. In the Mancini group's[22] study, survival curves over a 12-month period found the signal-averaged ECG to be a powerful predictor of either event. After 12 months, the survival of patients with normal findings on SAECG (n = 66) was 95%. Those with abnormalities on SAECG (n = 20) had a 39% survival rate after 12 months ($P < .0001$). The study by Middlekauff and colleagues,[23] however, did not find the signal-averaged ECG to be of value in predicting death in a similar setting.

Evaluation of Patients with Nonsustained Ventricular Tachycardia

Several studies have investigated the role of the signal-averaged ECG in evaluating post–myocardial infarction patients with nonsustained ventricular tachycardia. In many cases, these patients may be candidates for an electrophysiologic study to determine if they also have sustained inducible ventricular tachycardia. The usefulness of the signal-averaged ECG in these cases is the high negative predictive value (greater than 90%). Hence, it is the practice of many clinicians to use the signal-averaged ECG as a screening tool in such patients to avoid a catheterization procedure. Using a hypothetical population of 100 patients and an inducibility rate of 25%, Steinberg and Berbari[10] estimated that the signal-averaged ECG would screen out 54% of the patients and miss inducibility in two or three patients. Electrophysiologic study would correctly identify 22 patients, and an electrophysiologic study would be performed in 21 patients with noninducible arrhythmias. This conclusion, of course, assumes that the electrophysiologic study is the standard modality for predicting arrhythmic outcome.

The Multicenter Unsustained Tachycardia Trial (MUSTT)[24] focused on patients with coronary artery disease, unsustained ventricular tachycardia, and an ejection fraction less than 40%. This relatively large group of patients often have been problematic with respect to therapy. A late potential substudy was recently published that did not include those patients with bundle branch block or an intraventricular conduction defect. Thus, the study was performed in 1268 patients of the total 2202 patients enrolled in the study (66%). Patients within this group who had a prolonged QRS duration (FQRS) were much more likely to have a significantly higher event rate for cardiac arrest or arrhythmic death at both the 2- and 5-year intervals ($P < .001$). This level of significance also held for cardiac mortality and all-cause mortality. The greatest predictor was the combination of FQRS greater than 114 ms and ejection fraction (EF) less than 30%. Figure 84-5 shows the Kaplan-Meier curves for the combinations of the FQRS and EF in identifying patients with cardiac arrest or arrhythmic death.

Abnormal Intra-QRS Potentials

AIQPs are measured from the difference of the standard signal-averaged ECG, as illustrated in Figure 84-1, and a modeled version of that same recording.[5] This version is obtained from an autoregressive model of the original signal's Fourier transform representation. Figure 84-6 presents a block diagram of this approach. Basically, the modeled QRS is a smoothed version of the original QRS, and the residual represents the components of the QRS that deviate from this idealized QRS. The model can be adjusted to varying degrees by changing the number of terms in the autoregressive modeling process. An example of this process is shown in Figure 84-7. The original QRS, the modeled QRS, and the residual are shown for each case illustrated. On the

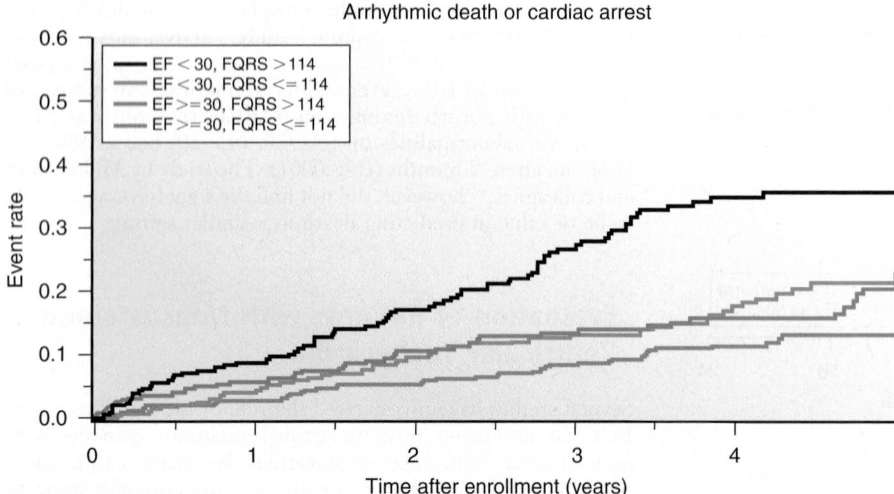

Figure 84-5 Kaplan-Meier survival curves from the Multicenter Unsustained Tachycardia Trial (MUSTT) using both ejection fraction (EF) and the prolonged QRSd (FQRS). (From Gomes JA, Cain ME, Buxton AE, et al: Prediction of long-term outcomes by signal-averaged electrocardiography in patients with unsustained ventricular tachycardia, coronary artery disease, and left ventricular dysfunction. Circulation 104:436-441, 2001.)

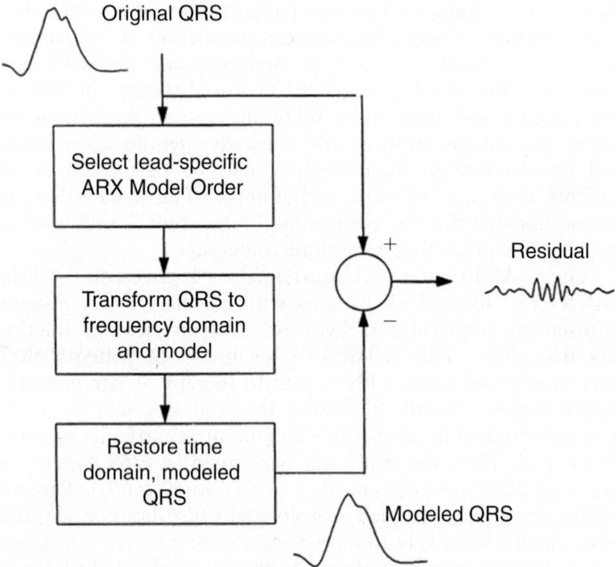

Figure 84-6 Block diagram of the abnormal intra-QRS potential (AIQP) measurement method. The modeled QRS complex is subtracted from the original signal-averaged QRS. This difference is termed the *residual* and measures the amount of change in ventricular depolarization.

left, the AIQP has a neglible voltage level; on the right, the residual voltage level is considerable. Of note, an apparently minor slur in the QRS complex is seen in the residual as a prominent signal.

Lander and colleagues[25] demonstrated the improved prediction of ventricular tachycardia this method would have in a clinical population of patients with heart disease. The AIQP method was later shown to identify transient ischemic episodes during angioplasty studies.[26] The AIQP changes were temporally linked with balloon inflation, which indicated a link between acute ischemia and ventricular activation. Another study demonstrated that AIQPs measurements in beats preceding a premature ventricular beat were anticipatory of these beats.[27] Hence, AIQP measurements are an added tool in the high-resolution methodology, which in these initial studies suggests a strong correlation with ventricular activation sequencing using standard body surface leads.

Summary

The high-resolution ECG, implemented with signal averaging, has proved to be an important development in the history of ECG analysis. Its clinical usefulness as a diagnostic tool can be considered as one of many noninvasive risk indicators.

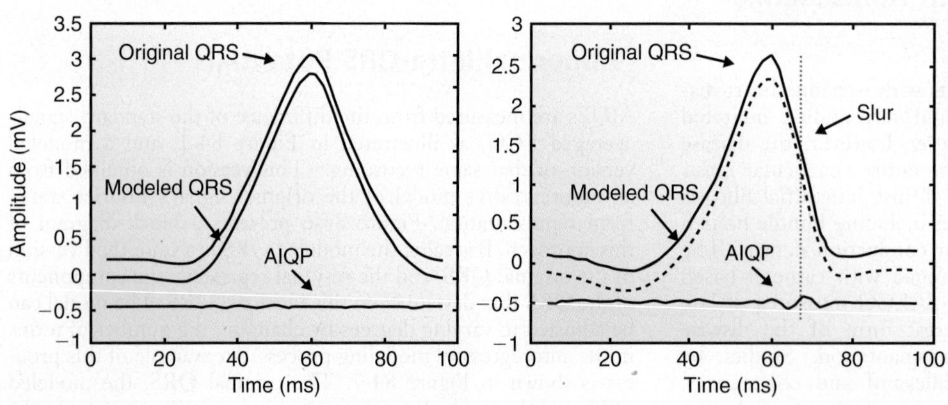

Figure 84-7 Examples of abnormal intra-QRS potential (AIQP) measurement methodology. **Left,** A case in which the AIQP voltage is negligible. **Right,** A significant AIQP voltage occurring in time coincident with a minor QRS slur, as identified by the *dotted line.*

The pathophysiologic basis of late potential signals is well established. The negative predictive value of tests for late potentials is the strength of the technique. Along with other clinical measurements, identifying high-risk groups can also be relied on. Large multicenter studies (CAMI and MUSTT) continue to demonstrate the value of this modality in identifying high-risk patients. However, the lack of a therapeutic arm that is cost-effective and safe for patients with false-positive results keeps this and other screening tools from being solely relied on to direct therapy. AIQP measurements provide a new approach to noninvasively study ventricular activation, and studies using this analysis method point to improved diagnostic criteria.

References

1. Berbari EJ: High resolution electrocardiography. In Zipes DP, Jalife J (eds): Cardiac Electrophysiology: From Cell to Bedside, 4th ed. Philadelphia, Saunders, 2004, pp 793-803.
2. El-Sherif N, Turrito G (eds): High Resolution Electrocardiography. Mt. Kisco, NY, Futura Publishing, 1992.
3. Gomes JA (ed): Signal Averaged Electrocardiography. Dordrecht, Kluwer Academic, 1993.
4. Berbari EJ, Steinberg JS: A Practical Guide to the Use of the High Resolution Electrocardiogram. Armonk, NY, Futura Publishing, 2000.
5. Gomis P, Jones DL, Caminal P, et al: Analysis of abnormal signals within the QRS complex of the high resolution ECG. IEEE Trans Biomed Eng 44:681-695, 1997.
6. Das MK, Saha C, El-Masry H, et al: Fragmented QRS on a 12-lead ECG: A predictor of mortality and cardiac events in patients with coronary artery disease. Heart Rhythm 4:1385-1392, 2007.
7. Vasquez C, Moreno AP, Berbari EJ: Modeling fibroblast mediated conduction in the ventricle. Comput Cardiol 31:349-352, 2004.
8. Lander P, Berbari EJ: Principles and signal processing techniques of the high-resolution electrocardiogram. Prog Cardiovasc Dis 35:169-188, 1992.
9. Lander P, Berbari EJ, Rajagopalan CV, et al: Critical analysis of the signal-averaged electrocardiogram: Improved identification of late potentials. Circulation 87:105-117, 1993.
10. Steinberg JS, Berbari EJ: The signal-averaged electrocardiogram: Update on clinical applications. J Cardiovasc Electrophysiol 7:972-988, 1996.
11. Breithardt G, Cain ME, El-Sherif N, et al: Standards for analysis of ventricular late potentials using high resolution or signal-averaged electrocardiography. A statement by a Task Force Committee between the European Society of Cardiology, the American Heart Association and the American College of Cardiology. Circulation 83:1481-1488, 1991.
12. Cain ME, Anderson JL, Arnsdorf MF, et al: American College of Cardiology Expert Consensus Document: Signal-averaged electrocardiography. J Am Coll Cardiol 27:238-249, 1996.
13. Simson MB, Untereker WJ, Spielman SR, et al: Relation between late potentials on the body surface and directly recorded fragmented electrograms in patients with ventricular tachycardia. Am J Cardiol 51:105-112, 1983.
14. Savard P, Rouleau JL, Ferguson J, et al: Risk stratification after myocardial infarction using signal-averaged electrocardiographic criteria adjusted for sex, age, and myocardial infarction location. Circulation 96:202-213, 1997.
15. Nakazato Y, Nakata Y, Nakazato K, et al: Normal values for time-domain, frequency-domain, and spectral turbulance analyses of signal-averaged electrocardiograms in healthy subjects. Ann Noninvasive Electrocardiol 5:139-146, 2000.
16. Pedretti R, Laporta A, Etro MD, et al: Influence of thrombolysis on signal-averaged electrocardiogram and late arrhythmic events after acute myocardial. Am J Cardiol 69:866-872, 1992.
17. Malik M, Kulakowski P, Odemuyiwa O, et al: Effect of thrombolytic therapy on the predictive value of signal-averaged electrocardiography after acute myocardial infarction. Am J Cardiol 70:21-25, 1992.
18. McClements BM, Adgey AA: Value of signal-averaged electrocardiography, radionuclide ventriculography, Holter monitoring and clinical variables for prediction of arrhythmic events in survivors of acute myocardial infarction in the thrombolytic era. J Am Coll Cardiol 21:1419-1427, 1993.
19. Denes P, El-Sherif N, Katz R, et al: Prognostic significance of signal-averaged electrocardiogram after thrombolytic therapy and/or angioplasty during acute myocardial infarction (CAST substudy). Am J Cardiol 74:216-220, 1994.
20. Kalahasti V, Nambi V, Martin DO, et al: QRS duration and prediction of mortality in patients undergoing risk stratification for ventricular arrhythmias. Am J Cardiol 92:798-803, 2003.
21. Yamada T, Fukunami M, Ohmori MD, et al: New approach to the estimation of the extent of myocardial fibrosis in patients with dilated cardiomyopathy: Use of signal-averaged electrocardiography. Am Heart J 126:626-631, 1993.
22. Mancini DM, Wong KL, Simson MB: Prognostic value of an abnormal signal-averaged electrocardiogram in patients with nonischemic congestive cardiomyopathy. Circulation 87:1083-1092, 1993.
23. Middlekauff HR, Stevenson WG, Woo MA, et al: Comparison of frequency of late potentials in idiopathic dilated cardiomyopathy and ischemic cardiomyopathy with advanced congestive heart failure and their usefulness in predicting sudden death. Am J Cardiol 66:1113-1117, 1990.
24. Gomes JA, Cain ME, Buxton AE, et al: Prediction of long-term outcomes by signal-averaged electrocardiography in patients with unsustained ventricular tachycardia, coronary artery disease, and left ventricular dysfunction. Circulation 104:436-441, 2001.
25. Lander P, Gomis P, Goyal R, et al: Analysis of intra-QRS late potentials: Improved predictive value for arrhythmic events using the signal-averaged electrocardiogram. Circulation 95:1386-1393, 1997.
26. Lander P, Gomis P, Warren S, et al: Abnormal intra-QRS potentials associated with percutaneous transluminal coronary angiography-induced transient myocardial ischemia. J. Electrocardiology 39:282-289, 2006.
27. Berbari EJ, Bock E, Chazaro AC, et al: High resolution analysis of ambulatory electrocardiograms to detect possible mechanisms of premature ventricular beats. IEEE Trans Biomed Eng 52:593-598, 2004.

Head-up Tilt Table Testing 85

DAVID G. BENDITT, SCOTT SAKAGUCHI, FEI LÜ, AND RICHARD SUTTON

CHAPTER OUTLINE

Historical Background

Head-up tilt table has been used for more than half a century by physiologists and physicians to study heart rate and blood pressure adaptations to changes in position, to model responses to hemorrhage, to assess the characteristics of orthostatic hypotension, and to evaluate hemodynamic and neuroendocrine responses in congestive heart failure, autonomic dysfunction, and hypertension. During the course of such studies, incidental observations noted that some test subjects experienced total or near-total transient loss of consciousness as a result of systemic hypotension. Furthermore, in some cases hypotension was associated with impressive degrees of bradycardia, including prolonged self-terminating asystolic periods (Fig. 85-1), and it became recognized that these reactions resembled the "common faint," or *vasovagal syncope*.

As a result of the unanticipated faints induced by head-up tilt, the concept of head-up tilt table testing as a diagnostic tool began to evolve in the early 1980s.[1,2] Initially, passive head-up tilt table testing began to be examined in earnest as a method for unmasking susceptibility to vasovagal syncope following the landmark report by Kenny and colleagues in 1986.[2] At first, prolonged periods (up to 1 hour) of passive head-up posture with the patient resting on a tilt table (usually at 60 degrees) was used as the sole means for provoking vasovagal events. Subsequently, additional interventions were introduced in an attempt to improve the sensitivity of the test (although with detrimental impact on specificity). These interventions principally included pharmacologic provocation (primarily isoproterenol or nitroglycerin, but also adenosine or edophonium). Furthermore, certain physical maneuvers including carotid sinus massage (usually in conjunction with edrophonium) were used in some laboratories. Currently, isoproterenol and nitroglycerin are the most widely used pharmacologic agents in diagnostic tilt table testing laboratries.

Ultimately, although still a controversial topic, head-up tilt table testing has become widely accepted as a valuable tool for the evaluation of susceptibility to vasovagal syncope. This chapter reviews the evolution of head-up tilt table testing as applied to evaluation of the vasovagal faint, examines its limitations, and provides a suggested methodology for use in the clinical laboratory.

Transient Loss of Consciousness and Syncope

Syncope (defined as a transient and self-terminating interruption of global cerebral activity as a result of inadequate perfusion of the brain, and resulting in loss of consciousness) is but one of many conditions that may cause transient loss of consciousness (TLOC) in humans[1] (Fig. 85-2). Consequently, before the evaluation proceeds to assessment for underlying causes in a patient with presumed syncope, careful consideration must be given to distinguishing the presenting complaint from the many other forms of TLOC or TLOC mimics. Unfortunately, physicians often are uncertain about this distinction, and the confusion has been exacerbated by imprecise writing in the medical literature.[3-7] For example, the recent scientific statement from the American College of Cardiology Foundation (ACCF) and the American Heart Association (AHA) confuses the definition of "true syncope" with the broader concept of TLOC.[3,4] Similar imprecise characterization of syncope may be found in a widely cited report from the Framingham study[5] and in a relatively recent clinical review article in the *British Medical Journal*.[6]

After it has been ascertained that the patient has experienced true TLOC, and that TLOC was indeed the result of syncope, the precise basis for the cerebral hypoperfusion leading to syncope must be determined. In this regard, a sudden cessation of cerebral blood flow for 10 seconds or longer may be sufficient to cause complete loss of consciousness. Furthermore, whatever the heart rate, either a decrease in systolic blood pressure to below 60 mm Hg (Fig. 85-3) or a fall of as little as 20% in cerebral oxygen delivery may trigger syncope. Many conditions may cause these physiologic disturbances. Neurally mediated reflex syncope, orthostatic hypotension, and tachy- or bradyarrhythmias are among the more frequent causes and are dealt with in detail elsewhere in this book.

Vasovagal syncope is the most frequent form of the neurally mediated reflex faints (others include carotid sinus syndrome and post-micturition syncope) (Table 85-1) and is the most common of all causes of syncope across all age groups. Accordingly, its recognition (and, occasionally, preventive treatment) is a problem often encountered by a wide range of medical practitioners.

Determining the basis of syncope in a given patient begins with both a careful medical history (including reports from

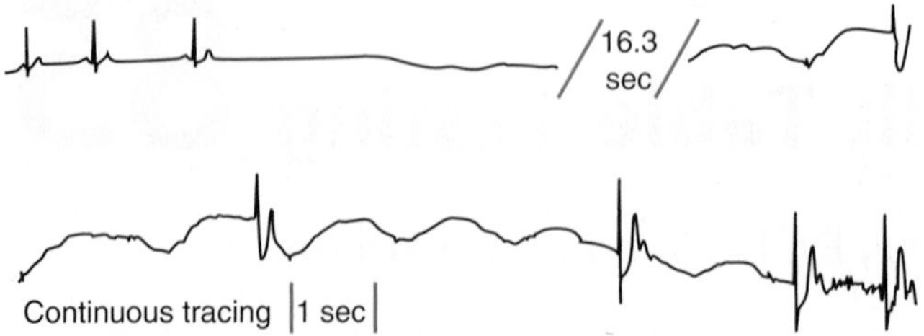

Figure 85-1 Electrocaridographic monitor recording obtained during a spontaneous vasovagal faint, illustrating a self-terminating prolonged asystolic pause. The patient was deemed to have cardioinhibitory syncope. Concomitant vasodepressor (vasodilation) also was probably present but could not be documented by current ambulatory technology.

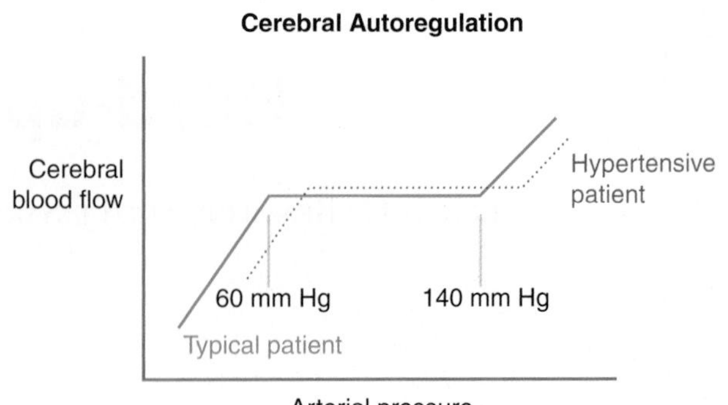

Figure 85-3 Schematic graph illustrating the relation between cerebral blood flow *(ordinate)* and systemic arterial pressure *(abscissa)* in a "typical" patient and a hypertensive patient. Cerebral flow is "autoregulated" over a wide pressure range (i.e., does not vary over this pressure range). The range is influenced by concomitant disease conditions such as hypertension, as indicated here. Below approximately 60 mm Hg, blood flow falls, which may lead to loss of consciousness.

witnesses) and a thorough physical examination, the latter incorporating orthostatic blood pressure measurements in all patients and carotid sinus massage in older persons. In the case of vasovagal syncope, the diagnosis can be established in most cases by the medical history (including bystander observations) alone,[2] and no further testing is required. When events surrounding the faint(s) are "atypical," however, even an experienced history-taker may not be certain of the diagnosis. Furthermore, it often is not possible to obtain an adequate history (especially in the elderly or the very young). In some of these latter instances, absence of reliable facts may be due to the patient's lack of insight, or (especially in the elderly) retrograde amnesia for premonitory events. Furthermore, eyewitnesses may not have been present, or their reports may not be sufficiently detailed to establish a diagnosis of the cause of the syncope. In such cases, the availability of a diagnostic test would be helpful.

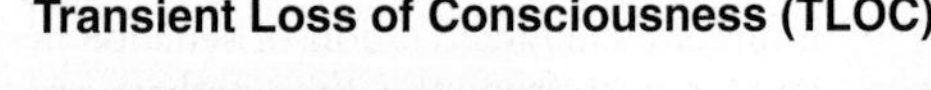

Physiologic Impact of Upright Posture

Upright posture elicits an orthostatic stress caused by the effects of gravity on the distribution of circulating blood volume in the body. Initially, as upright posture is achieved, the effects of gravity result in shifting of approximately 500 to 1000 mL of blood to the lower part of the body (Fig. 85-4). Most of this redistribution occurs in the first 10 seconds. Subsequently, in normal persons, an additional 700 mL of protein-free fluid is filtered into the interstitial space in the next 10 minutes.[8] The result of these two shifts is marked reduction of venous return and stroke volume.

In humans, the body attempts to compensate for diminution of stroke volume during movement to upright posture by both increasing heart rate and constricting resistance and capacitance vessels. Heart rate increase alone, however, is insufficient to maintain cardiac output and cerebral blood flow during these circumstances. Vasoconstriction of systemic blood vessels is crucial to maintenance of arterial blood pressure. Prevention of

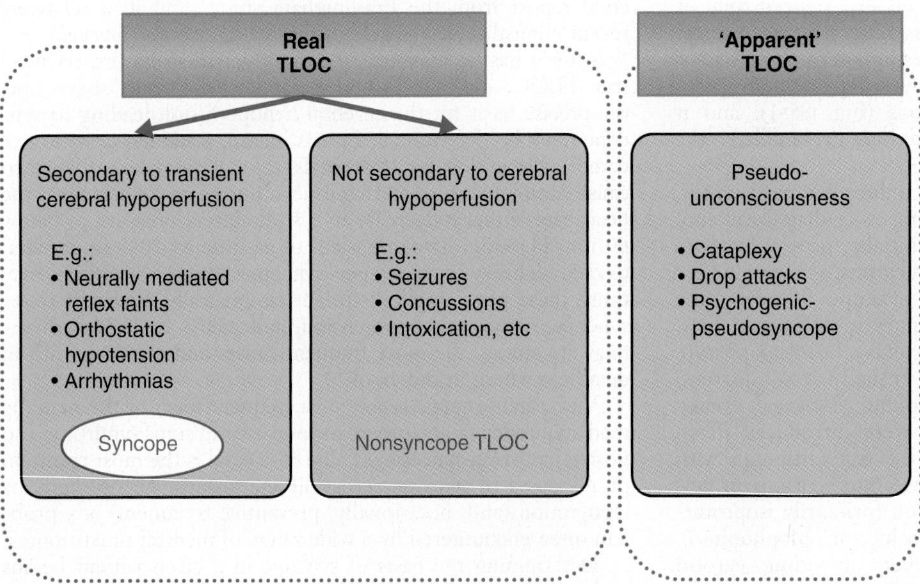

Figure 85-2 Diagram illustrating various causes of "real" versus "apparent" transient loss of consciousness (TLOC). Syncope *(left panel)* encompasses those causes of TLOC due to transient self-terminating cerebral hypoperfusion. Other nonsyncopal causes of TLOC *(middle panel)* comprise conditions such as seizures, concussions, and intoxications. Other conditions *(right panel)* may mimic TLOC but are not in fact associated with true loss of consciousness.

Table 85-1 Neurally Mediated Syncopal Syndromes

- Vasovagal syncope (common or emotional faint)
- Carotid sinus syncope
- Situational syncope
  - Micturition or post-micturition syncope
  - Airway stimulation–induced syncope
  - Cough or sneeze syncope
  - Gastrointestinal stimulation–induced syncope
  - Swallow syncope
  - Defecation syncope
  - Increased intrathoracic pressure–induced syncope
  - Trumpet playing
  - Weightlifting
  - Glossopharyngeal and trigeminal neuralgia
  - Postprandial syncope
- Miscellaneous
  - Syncope associated with aortic stenosis
  - Syncope accompanying onset of certain tachyarrhythmias (atrial fibrillation, paroxysmal supraventricular tachycardia, and possibly certain episodes of ventricular tachycardia)

syncope requires that the compensatory cardiovascular response maintain arterial pressure (in particular, systemic pressure at the level of the carotid arteries) at a value at least equal to the minimum value needed to guarantee adequate cerebral blood flow (approximately 60 mm Hg).

Short-term cardiovascular adjustments triggered by orthostatic stress are mediated primarily by the autonomic nervous system. The main sensory receptors involved in orthostatic neural reflex adjustments are the arterial mechanoreceptors (i.e., baroreceptors responding to pressure, stretch, or both) located in the aortic arch and carotid sinuses. Mechanoreceptors in the heart walls (both in the atria and in the ventricles) and the lungs (cardiopulmonary receptors) are thought to play an additional but more minor role. In the longer term, neuroendocrine compensatory mechanisms may be initiated by prolonged orthostatic stress, but these

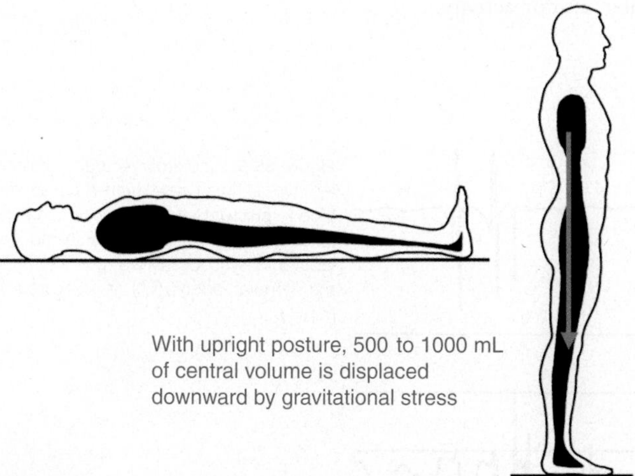

With upright posture, 500 to 1000 mL
of central volume is displaced
downward by gravitational stress

Figure 85-4 Schematic diagram illustrating qualitatively the redistribution of central blood volume that occurs with movement from the supine to upright posture.

adjustments are of lesser concern in terms of the pathophysiology of the vasovagal faint.

Reflex activation of central sympathetic outflow to the systemic blood vessels can be reinforced by local reflex mechanisms such (e.g., venoarteriolar reflex), and by more global mechanisms such as the skeletal muscle pump (even in the absence of overt movement) and the respiratory pump. Each of these may play an important adjunctive role in the maintenance of arterial pressure by promoting venous return.

Failure of compensatory adjustments to orthostatic stress may, in the absence of preexisting volume overload, result in inability to maintain central volume (the heart cannot pump what it does not receive), reduction of systemic arterial pressure, and inadequacy of cerebrovascular blood flow. If the deficits are sufficiently severe, the ultimate outcome is nearly complete or complete loss of consciousness caused by systemic hypotension. In addition, however, in susceptible persons, an inappropriate set of neural reflex responses appear to be triggered: vasodilation and severe or "relative" bradycardia—the *vasovagal response*. The precise basis for this reflex response remains speculative, but it is thought to be triggered at least in part by excessive stretch on central mechanoreceptors as intrathoracic circulating volume falls. Of note, however, although this mechanism may contribute to vasovagal faints triggered by upright posture, other common triggers (e.g., pain, emotional upset) are not readily accounted for by this explanation. In any event, it is the upright posture–triggered reflex that forms the basis for the use of tilt table testing in the evaluation of patients with suspected vasovagal syncope.[1,2,9,10]

Pathophysiology of Vasovagal Syncope

Vasovagal syncope is the most frequently occurring form of a larger group of neurally mediated reflex faints that also include carotid sinus syndrome and post-micturition syncope (see Table 85-1). In terms of pathophysiology, carotid sinus syndrome is perhaps the best-understood of the neurally mediated reflex syncope syndromes. In this case, excessive stretch on carotid baroreceptors (perhaps due to abrupt neck movements or tight collars) provides an increase of afferent signals to the central nervous system. Central processing of these signals ultimately causes an efferent neural reflex response, resulting in heart rate slowing and vascular dilatation in order to compensate for a perceived increase in central arterial pressure. In many cases, concomitant denervation of afferent proprioceptive nerves is thought to occur, thereby depriving the central nervous system of critical information indicating that neck movement was in fact the instigating trigger. Presumably, on the basis of the latter additional information, the central response to the afferent signals would be modified.

As noted earlier, the pathophysiology of the vasovagal form of neurally mediated reflex syncope remains incompletely understood. However, it can be considered in terms of four basic elements: (1) the afferent limb, (2) central nervous system processing, (3) the efferent limb, and (4) feedback loops.[11,12] A thorough discussion of these elements would be outside the scope of this chapter; a brief overview follows: Central and peripheral mechanoreceptors (see earlier) and occasionally chemoreceptors (e.g., in the presence of myocardial ischemia) are presumed to initiate afferent sensory nerve traffic to the cardiovascular modulation center (the nucleus tractus solitarius) in the medulla. The manner in which sensory processing results in an inappropriate efferent response is unknown, but the impaired response may in part relate to a lack of concordance among several afferent inputs, analogous to the situation described earlier for carotid sinus syndrome. In any event, "inappropriate" efferent sympathetic and vagal responses occur. Systemic hypotension (ultimately leading to a vasovagal faint if severe) is primarily the result of vasodilation triggered by a marked reduction in sympathetic vasoconstrictor outflow to blood vessels in skeletal muscles and substantial increase in venous capacitance, particularly in the splanchnic bed. Parasympathetically mediated bradycardia (severe, or relatively so with respect to the degree of hypotension) contributes to the process but plays a lesser role, except when prolonged asystole occurs. A poorly understood failure of baroreceptor feedback to recognize and interrupt this process also appears to be important in facilitating development of hypotension.

Impaired cerebral autoregulatory responses also may contribute to the development of vasovagal responses in some patients. It has been reported that cerebral blood flow velocity can decline before arterial pressure and cerebral vasoconstriction, and that in some cases, cerebral hypoxia may occur in the absence of systemic hypotension. The role of cerebrovascular spasm as a mechanism for transiently inadequate cerebral perfusion has been raised,[13,14] but its frequency and importance are unclear.

Several observations suggest that symptomatic hypotension-bradycardia associated with a positive result on head-up tilt table testing is comparable to spontaneous neural reflex–mediated vasovagal syncope. First, both spontaneous and induced syncopal episodes tend to be associated with similar premonitory symptoms (e.g., nausea, diaphoresis) and signs (e.g., receding tachycardia followed by relative or marked heart rate slowing, marked pallor, loss of postural tone). Second, the temporal sequence of blood pressure and heart rate changes during tilt-induced syncopal spells parallels that reported for spontaneous episodes (Fig. 85-5). Finally, measurements of plasma catecholamines before and during spontaneous and tilt-induced syncope exhibit important similarities. In particular, premonitory increases in circulating catecholamines (i.e., before evident systemic hypotension) appear to characterize both the spontaneous vasovagal faint and tilt-induced hypotension-bradycardia.

From a clinical perspective, most vasovagal fainters exhibit mixed cardioinhibitory and vasodepressor responses. In some patients, however, the observed response will be predominantly cardioinhibitory, with hypotension being caused by a prolonged asystolic pause. On rare occasions a pure vasodepressor response may be observed, although even in these cases the concomitant tachycardia is less than that expected for the severity of hyppotension.

Classification of the various types of vasovagal responses is difficult, and the clinical usefness of such classification is doubtful, because as was demonstrated in the International Study on Syncope of Uncertain Etiology (ISSUE),[15] heart rate–blood pressure features recorded during tilt-table observations only infrequently coincide with those accompanying spontaneous faints in a specific patient. In any case, the most widely accepted classification is that derived from the Vasovagal Syncope International Study (VASIS) [16,17] (Table 85-2). By definition, a pure *cardioinhibitory response* manifests as an abrupt heart rate decrease by more than 20 beats per minute (usually to rates less than 30 beats/min) with or without asystole, depressed atrioventricular (AV) conduction, or blood pressure decrease. A *vasodepressor response* is defined as significant blood pressure decrease, usually abruptly, independent of heart rate changes (less than 10%). Mixed vasovagal response may be predominantly cardioinhibitory or vasodepressor in nature. In association with these responses, patients may be asymptomatic or may experience syncope, presyncope, or other symptoms such as diaphoresis, a subjective feeling of warmth, nausea, weakness, and "seizure-like" motor activity.

Table 85-2 Characterization of Positive Responses to Tilt Testing*

- *Type 1*: Mixed. Heart rate decreases at the time of syncope, but the ventricular rate does not decrease to <40 beats per minute or decreases to <40 beats per minute for <10 seconds with or without asystole of <3 seconds. Blood pressure decreases before the heart rate does.
- *Type 2A*: Cardioinhibition without asystole. Heart rate decreases to a ventricular rate <40 beats per minute for more than 10 seconds, but asystole of >3 seconds does not occur. Blood pressure decreases before the heart rate does.
- *Type 2B*: Cardioinhibition with asystole. Asystole occurs for >3 seconds. Blood pressure decrease coincides with or occurs before the heart rate decreases.
- *Type 3*: Vasodepressor. Heart rate does not decrease >10% from its peak at the time of syncope.
- *Exception 1*: Chronotropic incompetence. No heart rate increase occurs during tilt testing (i.e., <10% from the pretilt rate).
- *Exception 2*: Excessive heart rate increase. An excessive heart rate increase occurs both at the onset of the head-up position and throughout its duration before syncope (i.e., >130 beats per minute).

*Based on Vasovagal Syncope International Study (VASIS) classification.[16,17]

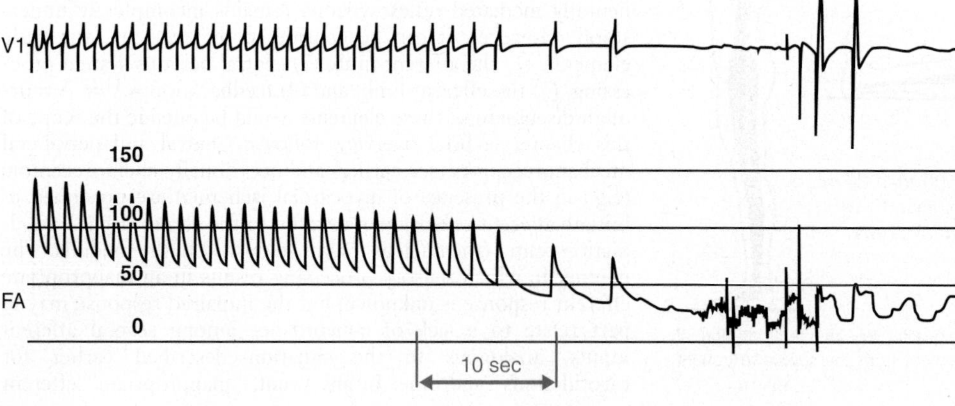

Figure 85-5 Laboratory recording illustrating typical heart rate (*upper panel*) and blood pressure (*lower panel*) changes associated with head-up tilt table–induced vasovagal syncope. Blood pressure from the femoral artery (FA) is indicated in mmHg.

The behavior of blood pressure and heart rate during the period of head-up posture that precedes the onset of the vasovagal reaction generally falls into one of two patterns. The typical pattern is characterized by an initial phase of rapid and full compensatory reflex adaptation to the head-up position, resulting in a stabilization of blood pressure and heart rate (which suggests normal baroreflex function). This scenario persists to the time of an abrupt onset of the vasovagal reaction. The patients who exhibit this pattern are largely young and healthy. A second pattern is characterized by inability to obtain a steady-state adaptation to the head-up position, so that a progressive decrease in blood pressure and heart rate occurs until the onset of symptoms. This pattern, more commonly observed in older persons, resembles a response more often seen in autonomic failure (i.e., a condition in which nervous system disease [primary or secondary to other problems such as diabetes] precludes adequate compensatory response to the gravitational stress imposed by upright posture). In this regard, an overlap between typical vasovagal syncope and more complex disturbances of the autonomic nervous system may exist in some cases but is certainly not the case in most patients.[1]

Head-Up Tilt Table Testing for Assessing Susceptibility to Vasovagal Syncope

As noted previously, the mechanisms by which upright posture triggers vasovagal faints remain incompletely understood. Nevertheless, as a result of the aforementioned early clinical observations and substantial subsequent clinical experience, head-up tilt-table testing has become the laboratory technique of choice for unmasking susceptibility to vasovagal faint in patients with unexplained syncope (Table 85-3). In this setting, tilt table testing offers the opportunity to accomplish the following:

- Assess susceptibility of patients to vasovagal reactions in a safe and well-controlled environment.
- Determine whether induced symptoms in the laboratory correspond with symptoms during spontaneous events.
- Educate patients regarding premonitory symptoms, so that they may learn to recognize warning symptoms and take appropriate evasive actions.

A subsidiary benefit of a positive result on a tilt test (i.e., one that reproduces symptoms) is that the patient may acquire greater confidence in subsequent treatment recommendations by virtue of the fact that the physician has witnessed the problem. This increased confidence in the goals and methods of treatment can be a powerful tool in the management of patients who have in many cases gone from physician to physician without receiving a satisfactory explanation for their symptoms. On the other hand, it is now generally agreed that tilt table testing should be used primarily for confirming a suspected diagnosis of vasovagal syncope, and not for assessing efficacy of pharmacologic or pacing therapy. Furthermore, tilt table testing is not considered to be useful for assessing forms of neurally mediated syncope other than the vasovagal faint (see Table 85-3).

Protocols for Head-up Tilt Table Testing

Detailed discussion of tilt-table testing protocols, test reproducibility, and estimated specificity and sensitivity is best found in the American College of Cardiology (ACC) Expert Consensus Report and the guidelines documents from the European Society of Cardiology[1,18] (Table 85-4). As a rule, the first step in a tilt test procedure is a so-called passive head-up tilt at 60 to 70 degrees, during which the patient is supported by both a footplate and gently applied body straps for a period of not less than 20 and in some laboratories for as long as 45 minutes. Use of tilt angles of less than 60 and greater than 80 degrees tends to lead to loss of test sensitivity and specificity. Subsequently, if needed, tilt table testing may be repeated immediately or at a separate time in conjunction with a drug challenge (most often isoproterenol or nitroglycerin). A less well-accepted strategy for tilt table testing entails use of provocative pharmacologic challenge from the beginning. This approach has the advantage of saving time, but concerns regarding both diminished specificity and the potential for increased frequency of adverse drug effects has limited its acceptance.

Table 85-3 Applications for Tilt Table Testing

Group I: General agreement
A. Evaluation of recurrent syncope, or single syncopal event with physical injury, motor vehicle accident, or occurring in a "high-risk" occupation or avocation setting and presumed to be vasovagal in origin
1. Patients in whom there is no history of or overt evidence for organic cardiovascular disease, and in whom the historical aspects are suggestive of vasovagal episodes
2. Patients in whom organic cardiovascular is present, but in whom historical aspects are suggestive of vasovagal episodes, and in whom other causes of syncope have not been identified by appropriate testing
B. Evaluation of unexplained syncope in settings as described earlier in subsection A
1. Patients without a history of or overt evidence for organic cardiovascular disease, and in whom vasovagal syncope may be a potential cause
2. In patients with concomitant cardiovascular disease after appropriate testing to rule out other potential causes of syncope
C. Further evaluation of patients in whom syncope has already been associated with a bradyarrhythmia, but in whom a neurally mediated origin may affect treatment
Group II: Differences of opinion
A. Differentiating "convulsive" vasovagal syncope from epilepsy
B. Recurrent "near-syncope" spells presumed to be neurally mediated in origin
C. Evaluation of exercise-induced syncope in the absence of evidence of organic heart disease
D. Evaluation to test the efficacy of prophylactic therapy to prevent syncope recurrences
Group III: Tilt table testing not usually recommended
A. Single syncopal episode, without injury and not in a high-risk setting, in which clinical features suggest vasovagal syncope
B. Syncope in which an alternative specific cause has been established, and in which the potential additional demonstration of a neurally mediated contribution to the etiology would not alter treatment plans

Passive Drug-Free Tilt Testing

In 1986, Kenny and colleagues[2] reported head-up tilt test observations in a series of patients with previous syncope. These investigators used 60 degree head-up tilt for 60 minutes and

Table 85-4 Recommended Tilt Test Protocols of European Society of Cardiology

Class I

- Supine pretilt phase of at least 5 minutes when no venous cannulation is performed, and at least 20 minutes when cannulation is undertaken.
- Tilt angle of 60 to 70 degrees.
- Passive phase of a minimum of 20 minutes and a maximum of 45 minutes.
- Use of either intravenous isoproterenol or sublingual nitroglycerin for drug provocation if passive phase has been negative. Drug challenge phase duration of 15 to 20 minutes.
- For isoproterenol, an incremental infusion rate of 1 up to 3 μg/minute to increase average heart rate by about 20% to 25% over baseline, administered without returning the patient to the supine position.
- For nitroglycerin, a fixed dose of 400 μg nitroglycerin spray sublingually administered with the patient in the head-up position.

Class II

Divergence of opinion exists in the case of induction of presyncope.

Adapted from Brignole M, Alboni P, Benditt DG, et al: Guidelines on management (diagnosis and treatment) of syncope: Update 2004. Europace 6:467-537, 2004.

The endpoint of the test is defined as induction of syncope or completion of the planned duration of tilt, including drug provocation. The test result is considered positive if syncope occurs.

observed an abnormal response to tilt testing in 10 of 15 patients with syncope of unknown origin. In essence, the test triggered a symptomatic period of hypotension and bradycardia consistent with a vasovagal reaction. By contrast, only 1 of 10 healthy control subjects without previous syncope exhibited such a response. This set of observations provided the basis for subsequent interest in tilt table testing as a diagnostic tool for evaluating patients thought to be susceptible to vasovagal faints. Since that time, tilt testing has been the subject of numerous clinical investigations and has been used widely in clinical practice.

In 1991, Fitzpatrick and colleagues[19] reported that use of a saddle or seat attached to the tilt table resulted in an excessive number of positive tests (presumably because of venous obstruction with reduced venous return from the legs). Such a tilt table configuration gave a low specificity when compared with the use of footboard support alone. These workers also showed that tilting at an angle of less than 60 degrees resulted in a low rate of positive responses. Finally, on the basis of the average time to onset of syncope in their patients (24 ± 10 minutes), they concluded that 45 minutes of passive tilting was an appropriate duration for the test. Accordingly, they proposed a protocol with 60-degree inclination for up to 45 minutes without drug provocation. With this protocol they reported a rate of positive responses for patients with syncope of unknown origin of 75% and a specificity of 93%.

The findings of Fitzpatrick and colleagues[19] were instrumental in defining a practicable tilt test protocol. Subsequently, based primarily on the reports by Almquist and associates[20] and later Natale and coworkers,[21] the angle of the table was, in most laboratories, set to the 60-70-degree range in use today. The 45-minute duration persisted, however, until acceptance of pharmacologic provocation maneuvers (particularly nitroglycerin, as used in the so-called Italian protocol) permitted introduction of shorter test durations.

Passive Tilt Testing with Pharmacologic Provocation

The first studies examining the use of pharmacologic agents to enhance the diagnostic yield of tilt-table tests were published in 1989.[20,22] In the report by Almquist and colleagues,[20] isoproterenol infusion was begun only after 10 minutes of passive tilt was nondiagnostic. Patients were returned to supine position after the first nondrug phase of the tilt test protocol, and isoproterenol infusion at initial doses of 1 mg per minute was administered. When patients achieved a stable increase in heart rate, they were tilted again. This maneuver was repeated at increasing doses of up to 5 mg per minute. With this protocol, 9 of 11 patients with syncope of unknown origin and negative electrophysiologic study exhibited hypotension and bradycardia. This same outcome was noted in only 2 of 18 control subjects.

Despite the initial popularity of isoproterenol provocation, a number of drawbacks ultimately became evident. First, some researchers argued that such provocation unduly increased the number of false-positive tests. Second, isoproterenol did cause adverse side effects in some cases, and concern arose regarding its administration to older persons who might have ischemic heart disease. Third, graded isoproterenol infusion was time-consuming. Finally, in 2000, a manufacturing problem became evident in the United States, and the drug became unavailable for a considerable time. Thus, alternative protocols, particularly those using nitroglycerin, had the opportunity to emerge.

In terms of false-positive rates with isoproterenol provocation, in 1992, Kapoor and Brant[23] reported that the addition of isoproterenol appeared to result in unacceptably low test specificity (between 45% and 65%) in certain patients. Their protocol consisted of tilt testing with the table at 80 degrees during which isoproterenol was administered in progressive doses of 1 mg up to 5 mg per minute, without returning the patient to the supine position before each dose increase. Subsequently, Morillo and colleagues[24] proposed low-dose isoproterenol tilt table testing, in which after 15 minutes of baseline tilt, incremental doses of isoproterenol (from 1 mg up to 3 mg per minute) were administered without returning patients to supine position. With this protocol, the rate of positive responses was 61%, with a specificity of 93%. This latter approach became favored in North America for some years and is still widely used.

In 1994, Raviele and coworkers[25] introduced the use of intravenous nitroglycerin infusion at progressively increasing doses as an alternative to isoproterenol for tilt test provocation. With this protocol, 21 of 40 (53%) patients with syncope of unknown origin had a positive response, with a specificity of 92%; 10 of 40 patients (25%) had progressive hypotension without bradycardia. This latter finding was considered to represent not a vasovagal response but rather an excessive hypotensive effect of the drug and was classified as "exaggerated" response. Later, Raviele and coworkers[26] used sublingual nitroglycerin instead of intravenous infusion. After 45 minutes of baseline tilting, 0.3 mg of sublingual nitroglycerin was administered. With this protocol, the overall rate of positive responses for patients with syncope of unknown origin was 51% (25% with baseline tilt test and 26% after nitroglycerin administration), with a specificity of 94%. An "exaggerated" nitroglycerin hypotensive response was observed in 14% of patients and 15% of control subjects, respectively.

Oraii and colleagues[27] compared the isoproterenol test with nitroglycerin test. The two methods resulted in approximately the same rates of positive responses and specificity, but with a lower rate of side effects with nitroglycerin. The sensitivity and specificity of the protocols were 55% and 94.7%, respectively, for nitroglycerin, compared with 58% and 89.4% for isoproterenol. Because of discordant responses in 75% of the cases, the sequential use of the tests (if one was negative) would increase the sensitivity to 84% while decreasing the specificity slightly (to 84%).

The optimal duration of the nondrug phase before administration of sublingual nitroglycerin has not been fully established. Bartoletti and colleagues[28] compared the effect of a nonpharmacologic phase of 45 minutes and that of a 5-minute phase. They found that the test with the shorter passive phase was associated with a significant reduction in the rate of positive responses. As indicated by that observation, it appears that at least 15 to 20 minutes of baseline passive unmedicated head-up tilt exposure is needed.

At present, many laboratories use a shortened head-up tilt test protocol including 0.4 mg nitroglycerin sprays administered sublingually after a 20-minute baseline phase (the "Italian protocol"). Pooled data from three studies[29-31] using this protocol and comprising 304 patients showed a positive rate of 69%. This positive response rate was similar to the positive rate of 62% for 163 patients from three other studies[26,28,32] using passive phase duration of 45 minutes and 0.4 mg nitroglycerin spray administration. Thus, a 20-minute passive phase before nitroglycerin administration appears to be an acceptable alternative to the more prolonged 45-minute drug-free passive tilt alone.

Irrespective of the protocol used, some general measures are recommended when tilt testing is performed. These recommendations were published in 1996 in an American College of Cardiology expert consensus document[18] and are summarized later (see "Head-up Tilt Table Testing Laboratory and Protocols").

Specificity of Head-up Tilt Table Testing: Studies in Healthy Subjects

Tilt table testing appears to discriminate well between symptomatic vasovagal syncope patients and asymptomatic control subjects. Initial studies in a small number of healthy subjects (fewer than 30) showed that 60- to 80-degree tilt for 10- to 60-minute duration was associated with syncope in none or less than 10% of subjects. A low false-positive test rate at baseline and during isoproterenol was later demonstrated in all age groups.

In a study comprising 202 patients with unexplained syncope,[29] tilt-induced syncope occurred in 11% of patients and in 3% of control subjects at baseline (60 degrees for 20 minutes) and in 59% of patients and in 3% of control subjects after 0.4 mg (400 μg) of sublingual nitroglycerin. False-positive response (so-called exaggerated response, as discussed earlier) was observed in 4% of patients and in 12% of control subjects. The total positive rate was 70%, with a specificity rate of 94%. A similar specificity of nitroglycerin provocation has been reported in other studies.[33]

The largest study examining the effects of head-up tilt table test exposure in healthy control subjects was reported by Natale and coworkers.[21] In 150 healthy volunteers without previous history of syncope or presyncope, tilt table testing at 60, 70, and 80 degrees for 20 minutes demonstrated specificities of 92%, 92%, and 80%, respectively.[21] Low-dose isoproterenol that increased the heart rate by an average of 20% reduced specificity to 88%, 88%, and 60%, respectively. The impact of the low isoproterenol dose (1.5 ± 0.45 mg per minute) on specificity was clinically negligible (4%). Thus, the addition of low-dose isoproterenol (1 to 2 mg per minute) to a 70-degree head-up tilt would be expected to provide a useful diagnostic yield with a high specificity (approximately 90%). However, the false-positive effect of higher dose isoproterenol is worrisome. At 3 mg and 5 mg per minute, isoproterenol infusions increased the false-positive rate to 20% and 56%, respectively.

Overall, these specificity values place tilt table testing in a comparable league with other widely accepted cardiovascular diagnostic tests (e.g., exercise stress testing for ischemic heart disease). Of note, however, tilt test specificity is substantially decreased with aggressive provocation at steeper angles, with longer tilt durations, and with greater doses of isoproterenol.[21,34]

In summary, most studies suggest that tilt table testing at angles of 60 to 70 degrees in the absence of pharmacologic provocation exhibits a specificity of approximately 90%. Sensitivity is more difficult to assess without a definitive method of diagnosis. Future studies may be designed to rely on a "classic" history as this definitive method, perhaps using the standardized diagnostic approach advocated by Sheldon and coworkers.[35] Currently, only a few observations have been made based on the classic history used for this purpose, and these suggest that sensitivity rates are relatively high. Test specificity may be reduced by pharmacologic provocation, whereas sensitivity would presumably be enhanced. If nitroglycerin or relatively low doses of isoproterenol are used, the deterioration in specificity seems to be clinically acceptable.

Pharmacologic Provocation

Pharmacologic provocation remains, in most laboratories, a secondary step to be used for eliciting susceptibility to hypotension-bradycardia during head-up tilt testing after the baseline drug-free tilt has been nondiagnostic. Currently, isoproterenol and nitroglycerin are the most frequently used agents. Adenosine and edrophonium have largely been abandoned, although further study of these and other agents may yet prove fruitful.

Isoproterenol has been the most popular provocative agent in North America, although nitroglycerin is rapidly becoming more widely used. In Europe, nitroglycerin is clearly more popular. Findings from a recently completed but as-yet unpublished survey of approximately 60 tilt test laboratories in North America and Europe are depicted in Figure 85-6 and illustrate the regional preferences for drug provocation among 34 centers that responded with their preferences.

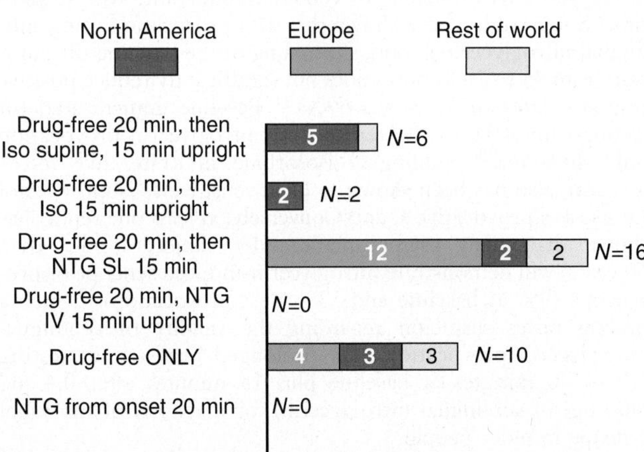

Figure 85-6 Bar graph indicating the impact of geography on preferences for tilt table testing protocols. A survey of 60 laboratories resulted in 34 responses addressing preferred tilt testing protocols. The primary protocol variants are indicated on the *left*. Color codes also are indicated. It is evident that North American centers tend to prefer isoproterenol provocation, whereas European centers lean toward the use of nitroglycerin. Iso, isoproterenol; NTG, nitroglycerin; SL, sublingual.

The mechanism underlying the utility of isoproterenol provocation is unknown. However, it is presumed to involve a combination of enhanced myocardial contractile state (i.e., a more vigorous ventricular stimulation of local mechanoreceptors), augmented mechanoreceptor sensitivity with enhanced afferent neural activity, and β-adrenergic receptor–mediated peripheral vasodilatation, reducing venous return and arterial resistance. As mentioned earlier, several approaches to isoproterenol provocation have been described:

- Isoproterenol is initiated at an infusion rate of 1 mg per minute with the patient in the supine position. The patient is again tilted for 10 minutes while drug infusion is continued. The same procedure can be repeated as needed with incremental isoproterenol at steps of 1 mg per minute, up to 3 mg per minute.
- Isoproterenol is administered during a 10- to 15-minute supine phase at doses sufficient to increase the heart rate by 20% to 30%. The tilt table testing is repeated. This approach is gaining popularity.
- Isoproterenol is given either by infusion or by bolus while the patient remains in the upright posture at the end of nondiagnostic baseline tilt, in an attempt to shorten tilt duration.
- Isoproterenol provocation is used without a period of drug-free passive tilt. This approach cannot be recommended before further validation.

The basis for the effectiveness of nitroglycerin provocation has been attributed to venous dilatation. Sublingual isosorbide dinitrate may not significantly increase venous pooling in the lower extremities, however.[36] Nitroglycerin-induced increase in epinephrine levels may contribute to nitroglycerin provocation. Both intravenous and sublingual nitroglycerin double the tilt test positivity rate from 25% to 50% while maintaining a high specificity (greater than 90%). The average time to syncope is 5 minutes (range, 2 to 9 minutes) for 0.4 mg sublingual nitroglycerin spray.[28] The positive predictive value of nitroglycerin-provoked tilt testing has been estimated at 80%, with approximate sensitivity and specificity of 80% and 85%, respectively. A positive result at a test duration longer than 18 minutes decreases specificity and should be interpreted with caution.

Compared with low-dose (1.3 ± 0.5 mg per minute) isoproterenol, nitroglycerin has similar sensitivity and specificity, but a lower rate of side effects. The main advantage of sublingual nitroglycerin is avoidance of venous cannulation; also, it saves time. Some studies have shown that with provocation using sublingual nitroglycerin sprays, shortening of the baseline tilt duration from 45 to 20 minutes does not significantly reduce positive response rates (62% versus 69%).[31] Baseline unmedicated tilt testing cannot be totally replaced by nitroglycerin provocation only, however.[28] Sublingual isosorbide dinitrate, like nitroglycerin, also has been shown to be as sensitive as isoproterenol for use as a provocative agent. Conversely, at least one report has shown that many asymptomatic older subjects (older than 60 years) will demonstrate nitroglycerin-induced syncope or presyncope (9% at baseline and 52% after provocation).[37] Such a finding raises suspicion regarding the validity of sublingual nitroglycerin provocation after prolonged head-up tilt testing (30 to 40 minutes at baseline plus 15 minutes after 0.4 mg [400 μg] of sublingual nitroglycerin) for diagnosis of vasovagal syncope in older people.

Endogenous adenosine release may be involved in the triggering mechanism of syncope.[38] Endogenous adenosine plasma levels are increased during vasovagal syncope and tend to be greater in patients with a positive tilt test result than those with a negative result. Adenosine interacts both directly (through cardiac excitatory afferent nerves) and indirectly (through vasodilatation and reflex sympathetic activation) with the autonomic nervous system. Both adenosine and adenosine triphosphate (ATP), which is a precursor of adenosine, have been reported to unmask susceptibility to neurally mediated paroxysmal AV block, and although its use is controversial, ATP has been proposed as a possible pharmacologic provocateur for evaluation of neurally mediated reflex faints.[38-45] However, ATP provocation appears to identify a separate subset of patients not usually incorporated in the neurally mediated syncope category, one that tends to be more common in older persons and is characterized by paroxysmal AV block, or marked sinus arrest, or both.[41,43-46] Therefore, ATP and isoproterenol tilt testing may have complementary roles in eliciting a positive response.

The ATP test requires the rapid injection of a 20-mg bolus of ATP during electrocardiogram (ECG) monitoring. Asystole lasting more than 6 seconds or AV block lasting more than 10 seconds is considered abnormal. Currently, ATP testing may be indicated at the end of a workup that has proved to be nondiagnostic. In view of its rapid action and high safety profile, however, ATP may have a role as an early screening tool for older patients. It has been suggested that a positive result on ATP testing is highly predictive of the need for pacemaker implantation.[45] Nevertheless, the precise role of ATP in the syncope evaluation remains unclear, and further clinical studies are needed.

Other drugs that also have been used for provocation in diagnostic tilt table testing include isosorbide dinitrate,[47,48] edrophonium,[49,50] and epinephrine.[51] Compared with isoproterenol, epinephrine is associated with a significantly lower sensitivity for reproducing the patient's symptoms.[51] This may be partly because of greater activation of peripheral α-adrenergic receptors by isoproterenol. Edrophonium is easier to administer and offers considerable saving of time compared with isoproterenol and has comparable diagnostic efficacy.[50]

Reproducibility of Head-up Tilt Table Testing Results

Tilt test reproducibility has been investigated using multiple tests on the same day, a few days apart, and a few weeks apart. In general, a relatively high (approximately 80% to 85%) concordance of test outcomes (induced syncope) has been obtained for two tilt tests repeated either on the same day or several days apart. Reproducibility with regard to the pathophysiology of the induced hypotension (i.e., cardioinhibitory versus vasodepressor characteristics) is less convincing, however. Of interest, false-positive tilt tests are associated with poorer reproducibility.[52]

Our experience suggests that the short-term reproducibility of tilt-induced vasovagal syncope is acceptable for use of this procedure as a diagnostic test.[53] Using a 10-minute, 80-degree head-up tilt protocol (using isoproterenol provocation up to 3 mg per minute as needed), the positivity or negativity of two sequential tilt tests (30 minutes apart) was concordant in 87% of cases. None of the eight patients who were tilt-negative in the first study experienced syncope on the second tilt exposure (100% concordance). A lower short-term reproducibility (67%) of tilt testing with or without isoproterenol (15-minute, 90-degree tilts) has been reported in young patients.

Reproducibility of tilt table testing with longer inter-test intervals is similar to its short-term reproducibility (70% to 80%). The tilt test reproducibility with 3- to 7-day separations was 90% in 21 patients with a protocol of 80-degree, 30-minute tilts with subsequent isoproterenol provocation if needed.[54] The level of provocation needed, however, was different between the two tests in five instances (24%). At intervals of 1 to 6 weeks between tests, findings in 46 patients using a 10-minute,

80-degree tilt protocol with graded isoproterenol provocation as needed revealed test reproducibility in 85% and 90% of patients who were initially tilt-negative and tilt-positive, respectively.[55]

The reproducibility of head-up tilt test (1 to 28 days apart) potentiated with sublingual nitroglycerin is approximately 80% for patients with unexplained syncope.[32] More than 80% of patients exhibit the same response pattern with both positive tests. Individual trough heart rates correlated well with each other between tests. Timing of onset of symptoms did not correspond well between tests, however. The reproducibility of head-up tilt testing with sublingual nitroglycerin provocation (60 degrees for 20 minutes) at a 1-week interval was reported to be 67% for a positive test and 94% for a negative test.[31]

In summary, positive tilt table testing exhibits short- and median-term reproducibility of positive response in the range of 80% whether repeat testing is conducted on the same day or somewhat later. The reproducibility of a negative study is highly reproducible, in both the shorter and the longer term. Nitroglycerin or low-dose isoproterenol does not substantially influence the reproducibility.

Risks and Complications of Head-up Tilt Table Testing

Risks associated with head-up tilt testing are minimal.[1] A rapid return to the supine position as soon as syncope occurs usually is all that is needed to prevent adverse consequences associated with loss of consciousness and to prevent potential problems associated with extended periods of hypotension. Resuscitation maneuvers are seldom needed. Because syncope and loss of consciousness can occur almost immediately on being tilted up, the patient must be gently secured before tilt to prevent falling.

Tilt-induced asystolic pauses as long as 73 seconds have been reported. Life-threatening ventricular arrhythmias associated with isoproterenol provocation also have been reported in patients with ischemic heart disease or sick sinus syndrome. Of note, however, such observations are exceedingly rare. In more than 2000 tilt studies at the University of Minnesota, we have yet to encounter such a circumstance. No complications have been published with the use of nitroglycerin. Minor side effects, such as palpitations with isoproterenol and headache with nitroglycerin, are common. Atrial fibrillation can be triggered during or after a positive result on tilt testing. The latter is a rare complication associated with a tilt-induced extreme "vagal storm." The arrhythmia usually is self-limited and self-terminating.

Head-up Tilt Table Testing Laboratory and Protocols

The tilt test protocol currently used at the University of Minnesota is summarized in this section. The most up-to-date laboratory protocol recommendations are to be found in the guidelines of the European Society of Cardiology (ESC) Task Force on Syncope[1] (see Table 85-4).

Laboratory Environment

The laboratory should be quiet, dimly lit, at a comfortable temperature, and as nonthreatening as possible. The patient should be permitted to rest in the supine position for 20 minutes or more before testing begins, particularly if venous cannulation or invasive monitoring (e.g., intravenous access, arterial line) or both are used. A briefer rest period (5 to 10 minutes) is adequate in the absence of vascular access procedures.

Patients should fast 2 to 3 hours before the test. They may continue their usual medications such as diuretics, nitrates, and antihypertensives. β-Adrenergic blockers and other medications prescribed for treatment of vasovagal syncope should be held at least 5 half-life periods before the test.

If intravenous access is available, parenteral fluid replacement to account for fasting hours is a reasonable consideration. If fasting has been brief (e.g., less than 4 hours), this step probably is unnecessary.

Recordings

Three or more simultaneous ECG leads should be recorded continuously. Optimally, the least intrusive beat-to-beat blood pressure should be recorded, such as in the finger plethysmography technique. Intra-arterial recordings are acceptable if the finger plethysmographic measurement is not available. Sphygmomanometer pressure recording is less desirable because it disturbs the patient during the procedure, is inherently less accurate at low pressures, and does not provide beat-to-beat observations.

Tilt Table Design

An appropriate electrical or manual tilt table should permit tilt angles ranging from 60 to 70 degrees over 10 to 15 seconds without wavering or loss of position during the test. Most laboratories use a 60- to 70-degree, head-up tilt angle. The table should be able to be reset quickly to the horizontal position (within 10 to 15 seconds) when the test is complete or should clinical circumstances necessitate. The patient should be gently secured to prevent falling, and footboard support should be provided.

Angle of Tilt

The physiologic effects of tilt appear to be comparable for angles of 60 to 80 degrees, whereas lesser angles (30 to 45 degrees) have a lower diagnostic yield, presumably because of inducing insufficient orthostatic stress. Tilt angles in the 60- to 70-degree range have become widely accepted. Use of a tilt angle of more than 80 degrees is discouraged.

Tilt Test Duration

A wide range of tilt test durations (ranging from 10 to 60 minutes) have been advocated at various times. Currently, absent use of pharmacologic agents, maximum test duration of 45 minutes probably is optimal. More often, however, the drug-free portion of the test is terminated at 20 minutes, and if the result is negative at that time, pharmacologic provocation is initiated.

Test Supervision

The laboratory should provide nursing staff supervision of the patient, with available technical support comparable to that in the cardiovascular exercise testing laboratory in the same institution. The presence of the physician in the tilt test room is not usually essential but may be advantageous for documenting signs and symptoms and for determining whether the test should be terminated early. In any case, the physician should be in sufficient proximity for immediate availability should a problem arise.

Factors Confounding Tilt Table Test Outcomes

Apprehension associated with exposure to a clinical laboratory environment, discomfort resulting from placement of intravenous or arterial lines (or both), or a prolonged preceding electrophysiologic procedure may affect tilt table testing outcomes. For this reason, electrophysiologic testing at the same session as for the tilt table evaluation is discouraged.

Use of Tilt Table Testing for Prediction of Treatment Effectiveness

Many investigators and clinicians have come to rely on tilt table testing to guide treatment decisions in patients with vasovagal syncope. Use of this approach for defining optimal therapy in individual patients is at best controversial, however. In this regard, the use of tilt table testing as a means of assessing therapy has been examined by clinical response to treatments during follow-up. In 535 patients receiving treatment with a wide variety of agents,[57] a negative result on tilt testing was associated with an apparently syncope-free follow-up period averaging 18 months in 91% of the patients. This finding tends to suggest that head-up tilt outcomes might predict future treatment benefit. Interpretation of this apparently favorable outcome is limited, however, by virtue of the absence of placebo or empirical treatment groups of control subjects in most studies. The few available placebo-controlled studies usually have failed to find benefit with current therapies, and tilt table outcomes generally have not been predictive.

Currently, we do not recommend assessment of treatment effectiveness based solely on repeated tilt table testing. In part, the inability of the test to predict treatment outcome is because of variability of test reproducibility. As shown in the ISSUE study,[15] however, the principal limitation is uncertainty regarding the relation of laboratory findings (i.e., the magnitude of cardioinhibitory versus vasodepressor contribution) to those during spontaneous faints.

Recommendations for Use of Head-Up Tilt Table Testing

Recommendations for tilt table testing, based on the ACC expert consensus document and the more recent ESC guidelines, are divided into three groups (see Table 85-3), as follows:

Group I: general agreement that tilt table testing is indicated
Group II: differences of opinion regarding the use of tilt table testing
Group III: tilt table testing not indicated

In addition to the applications listed in Table 85-3, a number of other conditions, seemingly unrelated to vasovagal syncope, have become of interest with respect to head-up tilt table testing. These conditions are listed here only briefly, because more study is needed to verify the use of tilt testing in these settings[57]:

- Seizures of unknown cause with negative findings on neurologic evaluation
- Chronic fatigue syndrome, in which head-up tilt table testing may help identify a subgroup of affected patients in whom therapy directed at the neurally mediated disorder may be of benefit
- Recurrent idiopathic vertigo in patients in whom clinical aspects suggest the possibility of a neurally mediated hypotension-bradycardia as a cause
- Recurrent transient ischemic attacks in some older patients in whom clinical findings are suggestive of a neurally mediated origin and appropriate studies have failed to disclose a cause
- Sudden infant death syndrome, in which a limited number of observations have led to the concept that severe bradycardic episodes may be reproduced in survivors of sudden infant death syndrome using head-up tilt table testing

In addition, head-up tilt table exposure should be considered in patients with intraventricular conduction defect or cardiac arrhythmias presenting with syncope of unknown origin when electrophysiologic study findings are inconclusive. In the patients, careful evaluation of the clinical findings may suggest the possibility that gravitational stress alone or in conjunction with a vasovagal mechanism could contribute to the faint.[58,59] In such cases, a slow or fast heart rate might not be sufficient to account for syncopal symptoms. However, concomitant susceptibility to neurally mediated reflex syncope may potentially impair vascular compensatory responses (especially if the arrhythmia is triggered with the patient in the upright posture), whereupon symptomatic hypotension could develop. This scenario has been demonstrated with both paroxysmal reentry tachycardias[60] and atrial fibrillation,[61,62] as well as certain bradycardias such as severe sinus bradycardia.[63]

Finally, tilt table–induced orthostatic stress (independent of the induction of vasovagal syncope) may be relevant to the investigation of syncope in some situations in which primary cardiac arrhythmias appear to be present but additional data are needed to connect the observed arrhythmia with syncopal symptoms.[64] In this context, tilt table orthostatic stress may make the needed diagnostic connection, thereby providing important insights that can assist in identifying more effective treatment for these patients.

Conclusions

Syncope is but one of many potential causes of TLOC in humans. It is differentiated from other causes of TLOC by its pathophysiology; in essence, syncope is TLOC caused by a self-limited inadequcy of cerebral blood flow. Determining whether TLOC is due to syncope must be the first step, before further assessment is conducted to identify or rule out the multiple possible conditions that could be responsible for syncope in a given patient.

The neurally mediated reflex syncopal syndromes, particularly the vasovagal faint, account for a large proportion of all cases of syncope (see Table 85-1). Passive drug-free, head-up tilt table testing has proved to be a useful, readily accessible, safe, and cost-effective modality for identifying susceptibility to vasovagal syncope. However, it is not considered useful for identifying or testing therapeutic interventions in most cases. Additionally, tilt table testing is not known to be useful for evaluating other forms of neurally mediated reflex syncope.

Tilt table testing has been the subject of numerous studies, resulting in the development of widely accepted protocols. These protocols offer a level of test reproducibility, sensitivity, specificity, and positive predictive value comparable with those of many other commonly accepted diagnostic cardiovascular tests (such as exercise stress testing and radionuclide myocardial imaging).

Nitroglycerin and low-dose (1 to 2 mg per minute) isoproterenol have been the most widely accepted drugs for pharmacologic interventions used in conjunction with tilt table testing. The use of these agents has enhanced the use of head-up tilt table testing by increasing the diagnostic yield while reducing test duration. A small reduction in test specificity has been an inevitable result, however.

Finally, significant progress has been made in understanding the mechanism underlying vasovagal syncope. In this regard, head-up tilt table testing has been an important contributor. For example, the application of tilt testing has permitted evaluation of treatment by physical maneuvers as an improvement over early drug therapy recommendations.[65,66] Ultimately, insights derived from such testing may further contribute to improvement in both the diagnosis and treatment of severely affected patients.

Acknowledgment

The authors thank Wendy Markuson and Barry L. S. Detloff for assistance with preparation of the manuscript.

References

1. Brignole M, Alboni P, Benditt DG, et al: Guidelines on management (diagnosis and treatment) of syncope: Update 2004. Europace 6:467-537, 2004.
2. Kenny RA, Ingram A, Bayliss J, Sutton R: Head-up tilt: A useful test for investigating unexplained syncope. Lancet 1:1352-1355, 1986.
3. Strickberger SA, Benson DW Jr, Biagggioni I, et al: AHA/ACCF scientific statement on the evaluation of syncope. J Am Coll Cardiol 47:473-484, 2006; Circulation 113:316-327, 2006.
4. Benditt DG, Olshansky B, Wieling W, on behalf of the Ad Hoc Syncope Consortium: The ACCF/AHA scientific statement on syncope needs rethinking [letter to the editor]. J Am Coll Cardiol 48:2598-2599, 2006.
5. Soteriades ES, Evans JC, Larson MG, et al: Incidence and prognosis of syncope. N Engl J Med 347:878-885, 2002.
6. Chen-Scarabelli C, Scarabelli TM: Neurocardiogenic syncope. BMJ 329:336-341, 2004.
7. Benditt DG, Brignole M: Syncope: Is a diagnosis a diagnosis? J Am Coll Cardiol 41:791-794, 2003.
8. Smit AA, Halliwill JR, Low PA, Wieling W: Pathophysiological basis of orthostatic hypotension in autonomic failure. J Physiol 519:1-10, 1999.
9. Robertson RM, Medina E, Shah N, et al: Neurally mediated syncope: Pathophysiology and implications for treatment. Am J Med Sci 317:102-109, 1999.
10. Schondorf R, Wieling W: Vasoconstrictor reserve in neurally mediated syncope. Clin Auton Res 10:53-55, 2000.
11. Benditt DG, Lurie KG, Adler SW, et al: Pathophysiology of vasovagal syncope. In Blanc JJ, Benditt DG, Sutton R (eds): Neurally Mediated Syncope: Pathophysiology, Investigation, and Treatment. Armonk, NY, Futura Publishing, 1996, pp 1-24.
12. Benditt DG: Neurally mediated syncopal syndromes: Pathophysiological concepts and clinical evaluation. PACE 20:572-584, 1997.
13. Grubb BP, Gerard G, Roush K, et al: Cerebral vasoconstriction during head-upright tilt-induced vasovagal syncope. A paradoxic and unexpected response. Circulation 84:1157-1164, 1991.
14. Grubb BP, Samoil D, Kosinski D, et al: Cerebral syncope: Loss of consciousness associated with cerebral vasoconstriction in the absence of systemic hypotension. PACE 21:652-658, 1998.
15. Moya A, Brignole M, Menozzi C, et al: Mechanism of syncope in patients with isolated syncope and in patients with tilt positive syncope. Circulation 104:1261-1267, 2001.
16. Sutton R, Petersen M, Brignole M, et al: Proposed classification for tilt induced vasovagal syncope. Eur J Cardiac Pacing Electrophysiol 3:180-188, 1992.
17. Brignole M, Menozzi C, Del Rosso A, et al: New classification of haemodynamics of vasovagal syncope: Beyond the VASIS classification. Analysis of the pre-syncopal phase of the tilt test without and with nitroglycerin challenge. Vasovagal Syncope International Study. Europace 2:66-76, 2000.
18. Benditt DG, Ferguson DW, Grubb BP, et al: Tilt table testing for assessing syncope. American College of Cardiology. J Am Coll Cardiol 28:263-275, 1996.
19. Fitzpatrick AP, Theodorakis G, Vardas P, Sutton R: Methodology of head-up tilt testing in patients with unexplained syncope. J Am Coll Cardiol 17:125-130, 1991.
20. Almquist A, Goldenberg IF, Milstein S, et al: Provocation of bradycardia and hypotension by isoproterenol and upright posture in patients with unexplained syncope. N Engl J Med 320:346-351, 1989.
21. Natale A, Akhtar M, Jazayeri M, et al: Provocation of hypotension during head-up tilt testing in subjects with no history of syncope or presyncope. Circulation 92:54-58, 1995.
22. Waxman MB, Yao L, Cameron DA, et al: Isoproterenol induction of vasodepressor-type reaction in vasodepressor-prone persons. Am J Cardiol 63:58-65, 1989.
23. Kapoor WN, Brant N: Evaluation of syncope by upright tilt testing with isoproterenol. A nonspecific test. Ann Intern Med 116:358-363, 1992.
24. Morillo CA, Klein GJ, Zandri S, Yee R: Diagnostic accuracy of a low-dose isoproterenol head-up tilt protocol. Am Heart J 129:901-906, 1995.
25. Raviele A, Gasparini G, Di Pede F, et al: Nitroglycerin infusion during upright tilt: A new test for the diagnosis of vasovagal syncope. Am Heart J 127:103-111, 1994.
26. Raviele A, Menozzi C, Brignole M, et al: Value of head-up tilt testing potentiated with sublingual nitroglycerin to assess the origin of unexplained syncope. Am J Cardiol 76:267-272, 1995.
27. Oraii S, Maleki M, Minooii M, Kafaii P: Comparing two different protocols for tilt table testing: Sublingual glyceryl trinitrate versus isoprenaline infusion. Heart 81:603-605, 1999.
28. Bartoletti A, Gaggioli G, Menozzi C, et al: Head-up tilt testing potentiated with oral nitroglycerin: A randomized trial of the contribution of a drug-free phase and a nitroglycerin phase in the diagnosis of neurally mediated syncope. Europace 1:183-186, 1999.
29. Del Rosso A, Bartoli P, Bartoletti A, et al: Shortened head-up tilt testing potentiated with sublingual nitroglycerin in patients with unexplained syncope. Am Heart J 135:564-570, 1998.
30. Natale A, Sra J, Akhtar M, et al: Use of sublingual nitroglycerin during head-up tilt-table testing in patients >60 years of age. Am J Cardiol 82:1210-1213, 1998.
31. Del Rosso A, Bartoletti A, Bartoli P, et al: Methodology of head-up tilt testing potentiated with sublingual nitroglycerin in unexplained syncope. Am J Cardiol 85:1007-1011, 2000.
32. Foglia-Manzillo G, Giada F, Beretta S, et al: Reproducibility of head-up tilt testing potentiated with sublingual nitroglycerin in patients with unexplained syncope. Am J Cardiol 84:284-288, 1999.
33. Mussi C, Tolve I, Foroni M, et al: Specificity and total positive rate of head-up tilt testing potentiated with sublingual nitroglycerin in older patients with unexplained syncope. Aging (Milano) 13:105-111, 2001.
34. Carlioz R, Graux P, Haye J, et al: Prospective evaluation of high-dose or low-dose isoproterenol upright tilt protocol for unexplained syncope in young adults. Am Heart J 133:346-352, 1997.
35. Sheldon R, Rose S, Connolly S, et al: Diagnostic criteria for vasovagal syncope based on a quantitative history. Eur Heart J 27:344-350, 2006.
36. Koole MA, Aerts A, Praet J, et al: Venous pooling during nitrate-stimulated tilt testing in patients with vasovagal syncope. Europace 2:343-345, 2000.
37. Kumar NP, Youde JH, Ruse C, et al: Responses to the prolonged head-up tilt followed by sublingual nitrate provocation in asymptomatic older adults. Age Ageing 29:419-424, 2000.
38. Sinkovec M, Grad A, Rakovec P: Role of endogenous adenosine in vasovagal syncope. Clin Auton Res 11:155-161, 2001.
39. Shen WK, Hammill SC, Munger TM, et al: Adenosine: Potential modulator for vasovagal syncope. J Am Coll Cardiol 28:146-154, 1996.
40. Mittal S, Stein KM, Markowitz SM, et al: Induction of neurally mediated syncope with adenosine. Circulation 99:1318-1324, 1999.

41. Brignole M, Menozzi C, Alboni P, et al: The effect of exogenous adenosine in patients with neurally-mediated syncope and sick sinus syndrome. PACE 17:2211-2216, 1994.
42. Brignole M, Gaggioli G, Menozzi C, et al: Adenosine-induced atrioventricular block in patients with unexplained syncope: The diagnostic value of ATP testing. Circulation 96:3921-3927, 1997.
43. Flammang D, Church T, Waynberger M, et al: Can adenosine 5′-triphosphate be used to select treatment in severe vasovagal syndrome? Circulation 96:1201-1208, 1997.
44. Flammang D, Chassing A, Donal E, et al: Reproducibility of the adenosine-5′-triphosphate test in vasovagal syndrome. J Cardiovasc Electrophysiol 9:1161-1166, 1998.
45. Flammang D, Erickson M, McCarville S, et al: Contribution of head-up tilt testing and ATP testing in assessing the mechanisms of vasovagal syndrome: Preliminary results and potential therapeutic implications. Circulation 99:2427-2433, 1999.
46. Brignole M, Gaggioli G, Menozzi C, et al: Clinical features of adenosine sensitive syncope and tilt induced vasovagal syncope. Heart 83:24-28, 2000.
47. Ammirati F, Colivicchi F, Biffi A, et al: Head-up tilt testing potentiated with low-dose sublingual isosorbide dinitrate: A simplified time-saving approach for the evaluation of unexplained syncope. Am Heart J 135:671-676, 1998.
48. Zeng C, Zhu Z, Hu W, et al: Value of sublingual isosorbide dinitrate before isoproterenol tilt test for diagnosis of neurally mediated syncope. Am J Cardiol 83:1059-1063, 1999.
49. Lurie KG, Dutton J, Mangat R, et al: Evaluation of edrophonium as a provocative agent for vasovagal syncope during head-up tilt-table testing. Am J Cardiol 72:1286-1290, 1993.
50. Voice RA, Lurie KG, Sakaguchi S, et al: Comparison of tilt angles and provocative agents (edrophonium and isoproterenol) to improve head-upright tilt-table testing. Am J Cardiol 81:346-351, 1998.
51. Calkins H, Kadish A, Sousa J, et al: Comparison of responses to isoproterenol and epinephrine during head-up tilt in suspected vasodepressor syncope. Am J Cardiol 67:207-209, 1991.
52. Sumiyoshi M, Mineda Y, Kojima S, et al: Poor reproducibility of false-positive tilt testing results in healthy volunteers. Jpn Heart J 40:71-78, 1999.
53. Chen MY, Goldenberg IF, Milstein S, et al: Cardiac electrophysiologic and hemodynamic correlates of neurally mediated syncope. Am J Cardiol 63:66-72, 1989.
54. Grubb BP, Wolfe D, Temesy-Armos P, et al: Reproducibility of head upright tilt table test results in patients with syncope. PACE 15:1477-1481, 1992.
55. Sheldon R, Splawinski J, Killam S: Reproducibility of isoproterenol tilt-table tests in patients with syncope. Am J Cardiol 69:1300-1305, 1992.
56. Benditt DG: Syncope. In Topol EJ (ed): Comprehensive Cardiovascular Medicine: Philadelphia, Lippincott-Raven, 1998, pp 2027-2051.
57. Benditt DG: Head-up tilt table testing: Rationale, methodology, and application. In Zipes DP, Jalife J (eds): Cardiac Electrophysiology: From Cell to Bedside. Philadelphia, Saunders, 2000, pp 746-753.
58. Sagrista-Sauleda J, Romero B, Permanyer-Miralda G, et al: Clinical usefulness of head-up tilt test in patients with syncope and intraventricular conduction defect. Europace 1:63-68, 1999.
59. Shinohara M, Kobayashi Y, Obara C, et al: Neurally mediated syncope and arrhythmias: A study of syncopal patients using the head-up tilt test. Jpn Circ J 63:339-342, 1999.
60. Leitch JW, Klein GJ, Yee R, et al: Syncope associated with supraventricular tachycardia. An expression of tachycardia rate or vasomotor response? Circulation 85:1064-1071, 1992.
61. Leitch J, Klein G, Yee R, et al: Neurally mediated syncope and atrial fibrillation. N Engl J Med 324:495-496, 1991.
62. Brignole M, Gianfranchi L, Menozzi C, et al: Role of autonomic reflexes in syncope associated with paroxysmal atrial fibrillation. J Am Coll Cardiol 22:1123-1129, 1993.
63. Brignole M, Menozzi C, Gianfranchi L, et al: Neurally mediated syncope detected by carotid sinus massage and head-up tilt test in sick sinus syndrome. Am J Cardiol 68:1032-1036, 1991.
64. Hammill SC, Holmes DR Jr, Wood DL, et al: Electrophysiologic testing in the upright position: Improved evaluation of patients with rhythm disturbances using a tilt table. J Am Coll Cardiol 4:65-71, 1984.
65. van Dijk N, Quartieri F, Blanc JJ, et al: Effectiveness of physical counterpressure maneuvers in preventing vasovagal syncope. The Physical Counterpressure Manoeuvres Trial (PCM-Trial). J Am Coll Cardiol 48:1652-1657, 2006.
66. Melby DP, Lu F, Sakaguchi S, et al: Increased impedance to inspiration ameliorates hemodynamic changes associated with movement to upright posture in orthostatic hypotension: A randomized pilot study. Heart Rhythm 4:128-135, 2007.

Electrocardiographic and Autonomic Testing of Cardiac Risk 86

MAREK MALIK

CHAPTER OUTLINE

Background

Reduction of mortality by means of implantable cardioverter-defibrillator (ICD) prophylaxis has been well documented in several trials in cardiac patients with compromised left ventricular function.[1-3] The results of these studies have already been incorporated into standard clinical practice.[4,5] Still, two substantial problems remain in current strategies for prophylactic ICD implantation. First, the criterion of reduced left ventricular function, assessed as a rule as a reduction of the left ventricular ejection fraction (LVEF) is not particularly specific, and many patients receive prophylactic ICDs that are never therapeutically used.[6,7] Second, the criterion of reduced LVEF also has a rather poor sensitivity. In a number of cardiac patients who die from sudden cardiac death, probably preventable by prophylactic ICD implantation, left ventricular performance is not particularly compromised.[8] Actually, more cardiac patients die suddenly among those with preserved than among those with reduced LVEF.

Hence, more accurate identification of cardiac patients who are at high arrhythmic risk for arrhythmia, and who therefore may potentially benefit from prophylactic treatment and intervention, remains an important unmet need. Accordingly, a number of studies have investigated the possibility of replacing or, in a majority of cases, complementing risk assessment based on reduced LVEF by other risk predictors and characteristics. This chapter reviews a selection of these studies that researched and used risk prediction based on the assessment of cardiac autonomic status, as well as on high-precision electrocardiographic evaluations.

Heart Rate Variability

Different expressions of heart rate variability (HRV) are used to quantify cardiac autonomic modulations. The practical utility of HRV assessment for cardiac risk stratification depends largely on the detailed methods used to measure the modulations of cardiac cycles.

Statistical and Spectral Assessment

The technology for standard statistical and spectral assessment of HRV components has not advanced much since it was reviewed by the European Society of Cardiology/National Association for Sport and Physical Education (ESC/NASPE) Task Force in the mid-1990s. Nevertheless, even in investigating populations of cardiac patients managed in accordance with contemporary standards, simple global HRV measurements are not losing their predictive power. In recent studies, global HRV—that is, the expression of overall variability of R-R intervals without any distinction between different, slower and faster modulators—maintained its predictive value in patients surviving recent myocardial infarction, in whom reduced HRV strongly predicts mortality risk even in those with reduced LVEF,[9] in those with unstable angina,[10] and in those with heart failure managed with cardiac resynchronization therapy devices,[10] as well as in other populations.[11]

Spectral analysis of HRV—that is, the distinction between modulators of cardiac periodicity operating at different frequencies— originally has been mainly seen as a tool serving physiologic studies. The spectral assessment of HRV is indeed linked to the physiology of the autonomic nervous system. Vagal afferent stimulation leads to reflex excitation of vagal efferent activity and inhibition of sympathetic efferent activity. The opposite reflex effects are mediated by the stimulation of sympathetic afferent activity. Efferent vagal activity also appears to be under "tonic" restraint by cardiac afferent sympathetic activity. Efferent sympathetic and vagal activities directed to the sinus node are characterized by discharge largely synchronous with each cardiac cycle that can be modulated by central and peripheral oscillators. These oscillators generate rhythmic fluctuations in efferent neural discharge that manifest as short- and long-term oscillation in the heart period. The efferent vagal activity is a major contributor to the so-called high-frequency component of HRV—that is, cardiac cycle modulations appearing at frequencies between 0.15 and 0.4 Hz (modulating waves lasting between approximately 2.5 to 7 seconds). Slightly more controversial is the interpretation of the low-frequency component—that is, slower modulations at frequencies between 0.05 and 0.15 Hz (modulating waves lasting between approximately 7 to 20 seconds). These modulations are considered by some investigators to constitute a marker of sympathetic modulation and by others to represent a parameter that includes both sympathetic and vagal influences.

Previously, it was believed that the distinction between the modulating frequencies of HRV components was of little importance for risk stratification. Early studies suggested that most of the predictive power was provided by much slower variations of cardiac periodicity that are not directly linked to any distinct physiologic regulatory process and that include nonperiodic responses to the environment and the circadian pattern of heart rate. Recent observations, however, suggest that

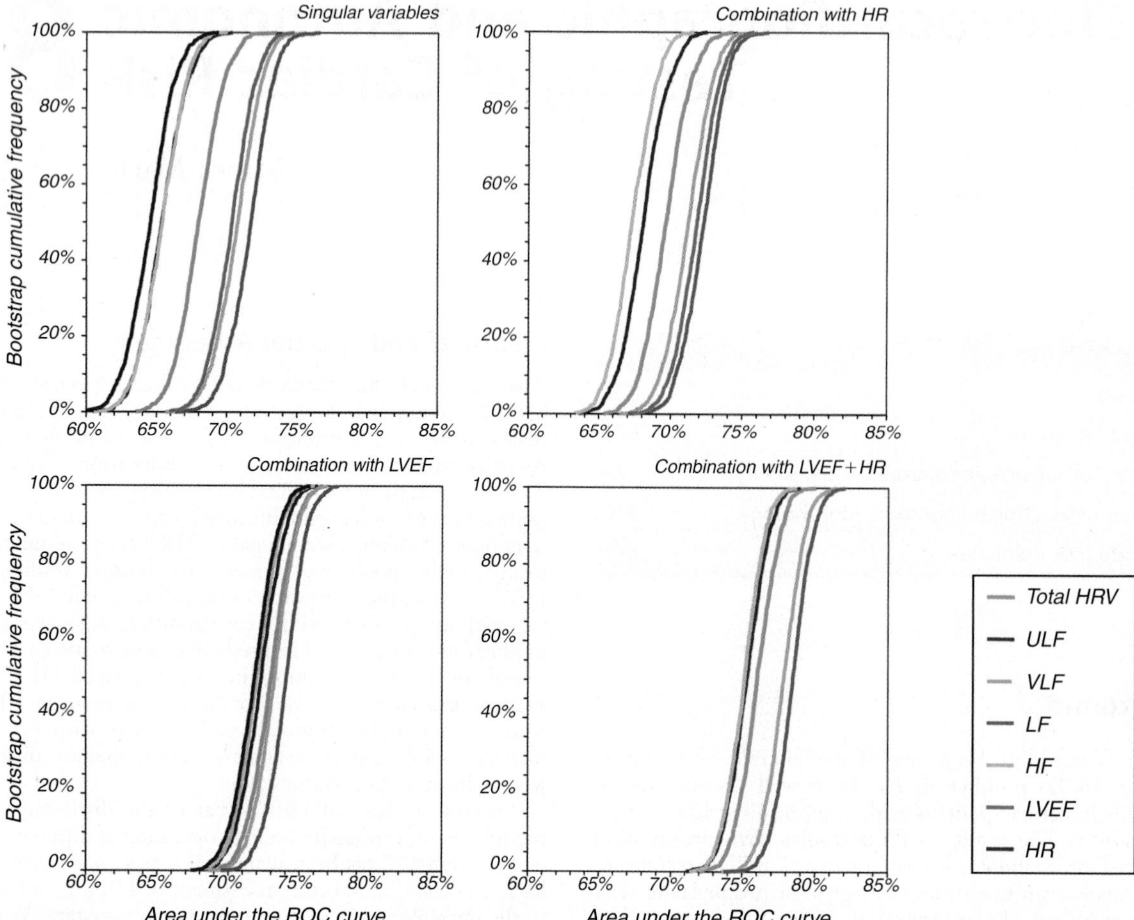

Figure 86-1 Areas under the receiver-operator characteristic (ROC) (i.e., dependency of specificity on sensitivity) curves for the prediction of 2-year all-cause mortality by different risk factors. The mortality prediction was estimated in a pool of several independent databases of survivors of acute myocardial infarction comprising a total of 4472 patients, of whom 352 died during the 2-year follow-up period. The figure shows distributions of the areas under the ROC curves that were estimated by the bootstrap method, allowing their statistical comparisons.[12] The larger the area under the ROC curve (i.e., the more rightward-shifted the distribution shown in the graphs), the stronger the risk predictor. *Top left graph*, Prediction of mortality by singular variables; *other graphs*, combination of other predictors with heart rate (HR) (*right top*), with LVEF (*left bottom*), and with LVEF and heart rate together (*right bottom*). In addition to total heart rate variability (HRV), HR, and LVEF, the graphs show the results related to four different spectral components of HRV assessed in 24-hour recordings—namely, high-frequency (HF) (spectral band 0.15 to 0.4 Hz), low-frequency (LF) (spectral band 0.05 to 0.15 Hz), very-low-frequency (VLF) (spectral band 0.00333 to 0.05 Hz), and ultra-low-frequency (ULF) (spectral band below 0.00333 Hz). Note that the low-frequency HRV components consistently provide the best risk prediction. In the evaluation of singular variables, note also that although LVEF is a more powerful predictor of total 2-year mortality than overall HRV, the low-frequency components of HRV constitute a stronger predictor than LVEF.

improvement in risk prediction can be made by concentrating on specific modulating processes—in particular, on the low-frequency modulations. This appears to be the case irrespective of whether HRV is considered separately or in combinations with other risk markers including LVEF (Fig. 86-1).

Other recent observations also suggest that risk prediction is enhanced not only by considering the amount and extent of the variations of cardiac periodicity but also by evaluating the dominant frequencies of the cardiac modulations. In particular, suggestions have been made that increased cardiac risk is characterized by faster dominant modulations within the low-frequency components[13,14]—that is, the spectral components that appear to be more important than others for the risk prediction.

Nonlinear Methods

Standard statistical and spectral characterizations of HRV use techniques that have been developed mainly for technical and engineering applications. The complex interactions between different regulatory processes that modulate heart rate lack the fixed periodicity of elementary regulatory components, thereby making the technical signal analysis somewhat unfocused. Therefore, a multitude of the so-called *nonlinear parameters* also have been investigated, aiming at more physiologically relevant description of the complex heart rate modulators. The HRV descriptors of this kind have been applied to a whole spectrum of clinical data ranging from long-term electrocardiograms (ECGs) made in patients with dilated cardiomyopathy to the recordings from hemodialyzed patients.[15-17]

Selected nonlinear measures have been shown to be capable of meaningfully stratifying risk among heart failure patients with reduced LVEF. Applying these techniques to the analysis of R-R interval series in patients with LVEF below 35% allows distinguishing among subgroups of patients who differ in their mortality risk by a factor as high as three.[18]

Nonlinear measures do not merely refine the conventional approaches to HRV assessment. Even in terms of risk prediction,

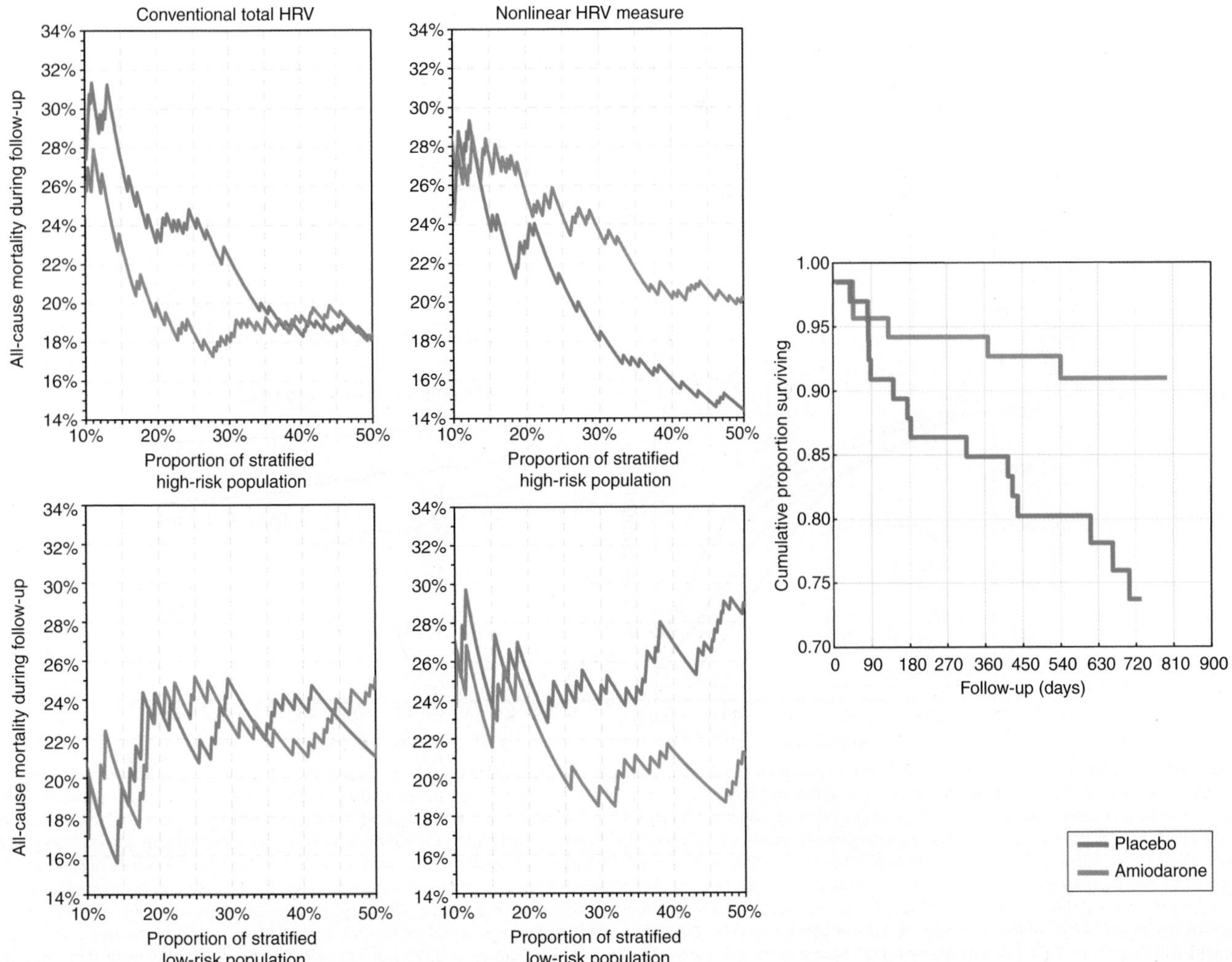

Figure 86-2 Risk prediction in the European Myocardial Infarction Amiodarone Trial (EMIAT) based on conventional and nonlinear measures of heart rate variability (HRV). The patients enrolled into the trial were classified according to the conventional total HRV[20] and according to one of the nonlinear parameters.[21] Both measures identified high-risk and low-risk subpopulations among the trial participants. The four graphs on the *left* show the mortality rates in the placebo and amiodarone arms of the trial when different proportions of high-risk and low-risk patients are selected. In the high-risk subpopulation selected by the conventional total HRV, the mortality rate for amiodarone was lower than that for placebo *(left top graph)*; the opposite was the case for the nonlinear HRV assessment *(middle top graph)*. By contrast, the patients in the low-risk population selected by the nonlinear HRV measure had lower mortality on amiodarone than on placebo *(middle bottom graph)*, but no difference between the two trial arms was observed in the low-risk population selected by the conventional total HRV *(bottom left graph)*. When "high-risk" according to conventional total HRV (selecting patients who appear to benefit from amiodarone treatment) was combined with "low-risk" according to nonlinear HRV assessment (excluding patients who might be harmed by amiodarone), a population of 135 patients was identified. Of these, 66 patients were on placebo and 69 on amiodarone. Among these patients, 16 deaths occurred during follow-up in the placebo group and 6 deaths in the amiodarone group ($P < .017$) *(far right graph)*.[21]

the nonlinear HRV measures are seen to independently complement rather than supersede the conventional HRV parameters.[19] Although the corresponding physiologic background is still to be researched, some of these measures actually seem to stratify patient groups with very different risk profiles from those identified with the conventionally assessed overall HRV. For instance, nonlinear reanalysis or de novo analysis of long-term recordings obtained in the European Myocardial Infarction Amiodarone Trial (EMIAT) appeared to identify high-risk post-infarction patients who did not benefit from amiodarone treatment—the exact opposite finding of that in the high-risk group identified by total HRV.[20,21] Combination of both measures allowed selecting patients who appeared to benefit particularly from the prophylactic pharmacologic treatment (Fig. 86-2). It remains to be investigated if similar combinations of different conventional and nonlinear HRV parameters would prove to be similarly effective in selecting patients in whom ICD prophylaxis would be greatly beneficial.

Deceleration Capacity

More recently, a new method has been reported for the analysis of the sequence of cardiac cycles with the potential to distinguish between vagal and sympathetic influences. This novel approach to HRV analysis was built with the aim of characterizing rhythm modulations associated separately with heart rate deceleration and acceleration. For this purpose, a new signal processing technique of *phase-rectified signal averaging* (PRSA) was developed.[22] The principle of the technique is identification of R-R intervals that are shorter and longer than the

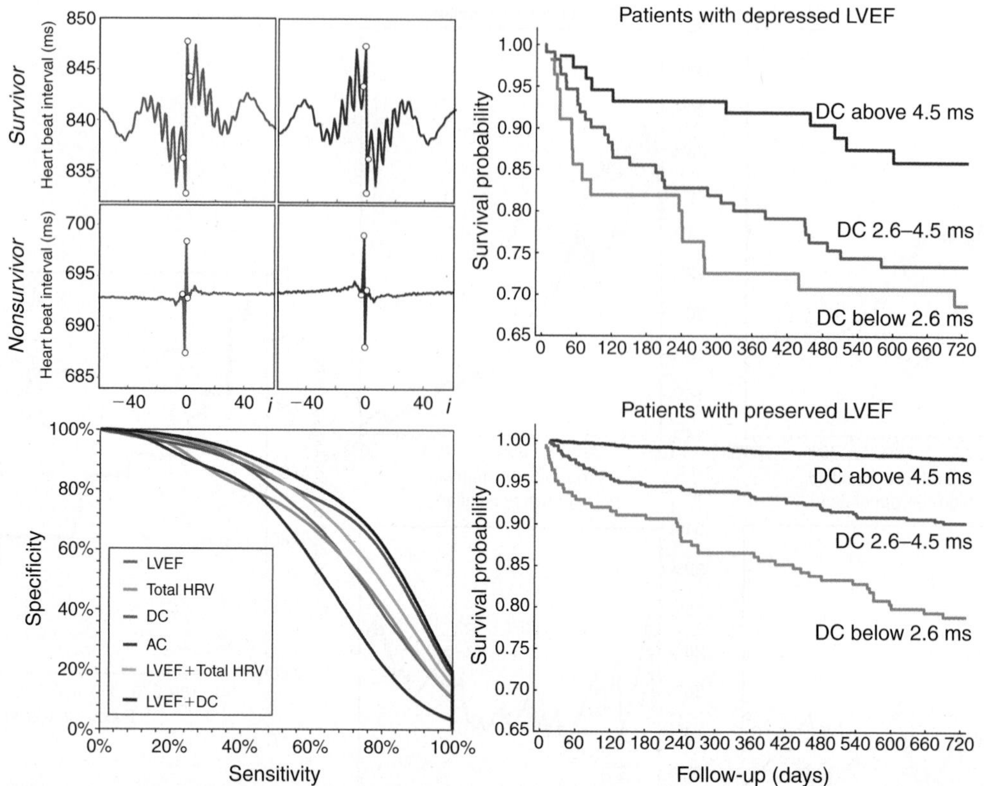

Figure 86-3 Deceleration capacity and its use in risk stratification of survivors of acute myocardial infarction.[24] The graphs at *left top* show examples of the R-R interval sequences averaged around heart rate deceleration (in *violet*) and acceleration (in *blue*) points (index *i* corresponds to the averaged R-R intervals preceding and following the beat-to-beat deceleration or acceleration points). High-risk patients also may have depressed deceleration pattern with preservation of acceleration pattern. The graph at *left bottom* shows receiver-operator characteristics (made smoother by the bootstrap technique) for a prediction of 2-year mortality rate among survivors of acute myocardial infarction. The graph shows that although acceleration capacity (AC) is a poorer predictor of mortality risk than either total conventional HRV or LVEF, the deceleration capacity (DC) is a predictor stronger than either total HRV or LVEF. DC also alone was found to be a stronger predictor than the combination of LVEF with the total conventional HRV. Combining LVEF and DC improved the risk prediction by DC alone only moderately. The graphs on the *left* show survivor curves for patients with depressed LVEF (30% or less, *top right graph*) and with preserved LVEF (above 30%) (*bottom right graph*). Comparison of the two graphs on the *right* shows that patients with depressed LVEF but well-preserved DC have a better prognosis than patients with preserved LVEF but seriously depressed DC. HRV, heart rate variability; LVEF, left ventricular ejection fraction.

immediately preceding intervals—those at which the heart rate, in terms of a beat-to-beat difference, accelerates and decelerates. Any simultaneously recorded signal can subsequently be averaged separately for the instances of heart rate acceleration and deceleration. In this way, the PRSA technique extracts periodicities from complex series that may potentially include nonstationarities, noise, and artifacts, in addition to true periodic components. Nonperiodic components are eliminated by the averaging process.[22,23]

In the first medical application, the PRSA technique was used to investigate the sequence of cardiac cycles.[24] (That is, both the identification of the acceleration and deceleration points and the averaging process used the same sequence of normal-to-normal RR intervals.) Subsequently, the averaged patterns of RR sequences surrounding the acceleration and deceleration points were quantified, which allowed the possibility of numerically characterizing the "capacity" of heart rate acceleration and deceleration. The measures of both acceleration and deceleration capacities were found to be predictors of risk in patients surviving the acute phase of myocardial infarction, but it also was found that the deceleration capacity is a substantially stronger risk predictor than the acceleration capacity. In a prospective examination of three large databases of post-infarction patients, the deceleration capacity was found be a statistically significantly stronger risk predictor not only in comparison with the overall HRV but also in comparison with LVEF[24] (Fig. 86-3). Because of the different vagal and sympathetic influences on cardiac periods, it is not implausible to speculate that deceleration capacity is an approximate measure of cardiac vagal modulations independent of sympathetic influences.

Heart Rate Turbulence and Baroreflex Sensitivity

The term *heart rate turbulence* (HRT) was introduced to describe the short-term fluctuations in sinus cycle length that follow premature ventricular complexes (PVCs).[25] In normal persons, sinus rate initially briefly accelerates and subsequently decelerates compared with the pre-PVC rate, before returning back to baseline. Although a number of other characteristics have been recently proposed, HRT still seems to be best quantified by two descriptors that were used in the seminal publication.[25] Specifically, the initial brief heart rate acceleration is measured by the so-called *turbulence onset* (TO) (expressing the percentage drop in R-R intervals immediately after the PVC compared with immediately preceding R-R intervals), whereas the subsequent and slower heart rate deceleration is quantified by the so-called *turbulence slope* (TS) (characterizing the steepest regression line between the gradually prolonging R-R intervals and their order number). The initial publication also suggested normality of these characteristics (TO less than zero and TS greater than 2.5 ms per R-R interval),[25] which has been well confirmed in subsequent clinical risk assessment studies, although much higher numbers frequently are seen in healthy subjects with occasional PVCs.[26,27]

Physiology of Heart Rate Turbulence

Already in the initial reports, HRT was suggested to be linked to baroflex.[28] Indeed, the rapid early post-PVC heart rate acceleration is consistent with vagal withdrawal in response to the missed baroreflex afferent input due to hemodynamically inefficient ventricular contraction. Different factors contribute to this hemodynamic deficiency, including incomplete electrical restitution, short and incomplete diastolic filling in the coupling interval of the PVC, and reduced efficiency and poor synchronization of ventricular contractility, as well as higher afterload during the compensatory pause. Consequently, systolic blood pressure due to the PVC contraction is considerably lower compared with normal sinus beats. Both ineffective contraction and compensatory pause cause diastolic pressure reduction. Moreover, systolic blood pressure after the first post-PVC sinus beat tends to be lower compared with the level before the PVC. Thus, both the instant hemodynamic effect of the PVC and the reduction of the systolic blood pressure during the subsequent beat activate aortic and carotid baroreceptors, thereby causing heart rate increase due to vagal inhibition. These physiologic mechanisms have been confirmed in a number of studies,[29,30] including investigations focusing on HRT changes by autonomic blockade.[31]

The HRT pattern also can be induced artificially by pacing, which has been investigated both during electrophysiologic studies[32,33] and in patients with programmable ICDs.[34] The available data suggest that the numerical characteristics obtained from induced HRT episodes are reasonably comparable to the HRT parameters assessed after spontaneous PVCs.

Rhythm disturbance also is seen after atrial premature complexes.[35,36] Although early acceleration and later deceleration are seen after PVCs, however, an abrupt heart rate deceleration occurs after atrial premature beats, with a prompt return to baseline, followed by a second and delayed transitory heart rate deceleration. The late deceleration phase of atrial HRT has the same mechanism as that of PVC-induced HRT, resulting from a baroreflex response to blood pressure dynamics after the premature contraction; the initial abrupt deceleration, however, probably is caused by sinus nodal resetting by the ectopic beat, with subsequent recovery of sinus node automaticity. Indeed, a significant intraindividual correlation has been observed between TS values of atrial and ventricular HRT.[35]

Heart Rate Turbulence–Based Risk Prediction

The strong link to baroreflex makes HRT a potent risk stratifier in patients in whom baroreflex and other autonomic abnormalities are indicative of an increased probability of poor outcome. In addition to a number of retrospective studies, two prospective trials confirmed the predictive power of HRT in survivors of acute myocardial infraction.[37,38] In risk prediction investigations, HRT most frequently is classified into three categories: In *HRT0*, both TO and TS are normal, or spontaneous VPCs are absent in long-term ECGs from which HRT assessment could be made; in *HRT1*, either TO or TS is abnormal, whereas the other is normal; and in *HRT2*, both TO and TS are abnormal. Significantly and substantially different risk profiles are associated with these categories. As with other risk stratifiers based on cardiac reflexes and autonomic regulations, HRT-based risk prediction is particularly potent in patients with preserved LVEF. In patients with LVEF above 30% over a follow-up period of 2 years, the mortality in patients with HRT 2 was increased more than eight-fold that in patients with HRT 0.[37] (Theoretically, it might be possible to classify patients without PVCs according to HRT assessed after atrial premature beats, because the atrial HRT also was found to provide risk stratification of post-infarction patients.[35] However, because the prognosis for patients without PVCs is uniformly very good, little practical value could be gained.)

Independently of etiology, patients with heart failure suffer from constant neurohumoral activation with sympathetic overdrive and progressive hemodynamic deterioration. For these reasons, patients with congestive heart failure have significantly impaired baroreflex sensitivity (as well as reduced HRV). Consequently, a high percentage of patients with cardiomyopathies or ischemic heart failure present with abnormal HRT. Strong correlations were found between the extent of heart failure and TO and TS.[39] This finding suggests that HRT assessment may potentially be a useful technique for monitoring disease progression in patients with heart failure, especially if the assessment of pacing-provoked HRT was implemented into the resynchronization devices and programmable ICDs.

The prognostic power of HRT in heart failure patients appears to be strongly dependent on the underlying mechanism of heart failure. Although HRT is a powerful predictor of mortality in patients with post-infarction heart failure, it seems to have little prognostic role in patients with nonischemic heart failure. In an investigation of patients with idiopathic dilated cardiomyopathy (Marburg Cardiomyopathy database), TO predicted transplantation-free survival, but neither TO nor TS predicted arrhythmic events.[40]

Risk Stratification Based on Other Baroreflex Tests

Data from the Autonomic Tone and Reflexes After Myocardial Infarction (ATRAMI) study provided the first large source for investigations of predictive power of the phenylephrine-induced baroreflex test in post-infarction patients. In this seminal multicenter trial, depressed baroreflex sensitivity predicted follow-up (i.e., 21-month) cardiovascular mortality in post-infarction patients but had no significant predictive power in patients with LVEF greater than 35% or patients older than 65 years of age. In a recent study that investigated modern acute treatment in a consecutive series of post-infarction patients, however, findings were not consistent with the initial ATRAMI observations. In patients with LVEF greater than 35%, phenylephrine-induced baroreflex testing was performed at approximately 1 month after the index infarction. In these patients, depressed baroreflex sensitivity showed strong association with increased follow-up (5-year) mortality. The relative risk for depressed baroreflex sensitivity was 11.4 for the overall population, 19.6 for patients of 65 years or younger, and 7.2 for patients above the age of 65 years.[41]

Whether this semi-invasive assessment of baroreflex sensitivity adds further predictive power to the fully noninvasive evaluation of HRT is not known at present. However, the observation further confirms the possibility of using autonomic tests to complement and enlarge the LVEF-based risk prediction and to improve the LVEF-based selection of candidates for prophylactic ICD implantation.

Instantaneous Electrocardiographic Morphology

Many other predictors have been proposed and investigated to improve both the sensitivity and specificity of the LVEF-based risk stratification. Of these, the electrocardiologic risk factors include heart rate recovery after exercise test, T wave alternans, and the so-called Wedensky modulation, as well as others outside the scope of this chapter. The clinical applicability of a number of these risk factors is, to some extent, limited by their practicability, which also somewhat applies to the methods based on long-term ECG described and discussed in the previous sections. Although very strong risk predictors can be derived from 24-hour Holter recording, the acquisition of such a recording may require prolonging the in-hospital stay by one extra day. Similarly, the heart rate recovery assessment and the spectral frequency–based measurement of T wave alternans require physical exercise, which clearly is not suitable for every patient.

It is therefore of substantial importance that not only meaningful but also rather strong prognostic factors may be obtained from analysis of the morphology of standard 12-lead ECGs. Although different morphologic indices were proposed and investigated, substantial experience exists with two morphologic risk factors, both of which could theoretically be obtained from the ECG recording on one single sinus beat, although in the available studies they most frequently were assessed from the representative beats of short 10-second ECGs.

Angle of the Ventricular Gradient

The concept of the so-called *ventricular gradient*—the difference in the global orientation and extent of the QRS complex and of the T wave—was introduced by Wilson as early as the 1930s. The proposed measure of the magnitude of the gradient—that is, the vector sum QRS + T—does not have any utility at present. On the contrary, the angle of the gradient—the three-dimensional angle between QRS complex and T wave loops—was found to be a surprisingly strong predictor of poor outcome in different groups of patients, including survivors of acute myocardial infarction[42] and patients with known ischemic heart disease,[43] as well as in the general population.[44,45]

Different methods were proposed to calculate the angle of the ventricular gradient. Nevertheless, it seems that because of the three-dimensional properties of the QRS complex loop, most stable results are obtained with integration of the angles between the T wave vector and different segments of the QRS loop (for statistical purposes, this frequently is expressed as cosine—the so-called total cosine R-to-T [TCRT]). In this expression, the ventricular gradient angle has been observed to predict not only all-cause mortality of survivors of acute myocardial infarction but also mortality specifically due to sudden cardiac death (Fig. 86-4).

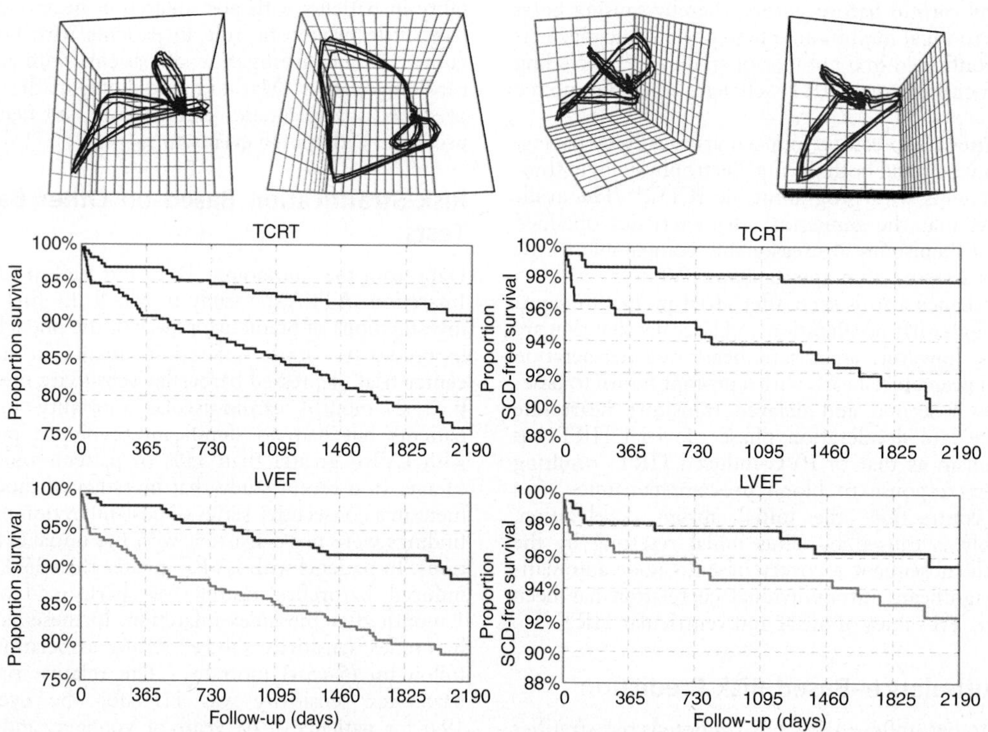

Figure 86-4 Cosine measure of the angle of the ventricular gradient and its use in risk stratification for survivors of acute myocardial infarction. The visual perception of the three-dimensional electrocardiogram (ECG) loops frequently is misleading. The *top row* shows different views on the same three-dimensional vectorcardiogram (reconstructed from 4 consecutive beats of a normal 12-lead ECG). Whereas the T wave loop is planar and has a clear three-dimensional orientation, the QRS complex loop is twisted, with a more complex three-dimensional shape, without a dominant orientation. Therefore, the calculation of the three-dimensional angle between the two loops needs to be based on integration of individual angles between T wave loop and QRS complex loop segments. The *bottom graphs* show survival curves for post-infarction patients stratified according to the total cosine of R-to-T angles (TCRT) and according to left ventricular ejection fraction (LVEF). The *left two bottom graphs* depict total survival; the *right two graphs* depict sudden cardiac death (SCD)-free survival. (For an appropriate comparison, both TCRT and LVEF were dichotomized at their median values.) The comparison of the survival curves shows that although both TCRT and LVEF are strong predictors of all-cause mortality, LVEF is a rather poor predictor of SCD (and thus probably also of implantable cardioverter-defibrillator [ICD]-preventable death). The SCD prediction by TCRT is much stronger than that by LVEF.[12]

T Wave Residuum

Numerous attempts have been made to find a noninvasive electrocardiographic measure of the heterogeneity of ventricular repolarization that could serve as an indicator of electrical instability, thereby quantifying the risk of arrhythmic complications. Some of these attempts were purely observational, without proper mechanistic links between cardiac electrophysiology and electrocardiography. A good example is the phenomenon of the so-called QT dispersion, which lost all of its appeal once it was realized that the measurements were merely reflecting artifacts due either to methodologic imprecision or to isoelectric projections of the T wave loop in different ECG leads.

Detailed ECG lead theory has been used less frequently to propose indices of repolarization heterogeneity. The T wave recording in different ECG leads is dominantly influenced by the global T wave loop that is the sum of repolarization signals from all myocardial regions and across all intramyocardial gradients. The regional repolarization differences within the myocardium—the repolarization heterogeneity—plays only a minor role in differentiating the T wave patterns recorded in different leads. Nevertheless, mathematical elaboration of the T wave signals from ECG leads is capable of separating the differences caused by the regional heterogeneity from the interlead dissimilarity due to the different projections of the three-dimensional T wave loop. Specifically, with use of a special algebraic technique, the singular value decomposition, the three-dimensional T wave loop can be reconstructed from the standard 12-lead ECG (or, more accurately, from 8 independent leads of the ECG) together with characterization of the signals that also exist in the ECG but that cannot be explained by the three-dimensional loop. Because all signals synchronized across the myocardium contribute to the three-dimensional loop, the signals that cannot be attributed to it are reflecting the true heterogeneity.

This is the principle of the so-called *T wave residuum*, which also has been investigated in different clinical populations. Although some methodologic facets still need to be perfected, increased T wave residuum was found to be another important marker of poor outcome in cardiac patients.[43,46]

Thus, together with the angle of the ventricular gradient, the predictive power of T wave residuum underlines the importance of standard short-term ECG testing in the field of risk prediction.

Multivariate Risk Prediction

Frequently, studies are reported comparing the predictive power of different risk predictors. Although such an approach is appropriate for establishing new and previously unknown risk factors, the different methodologies and clinical tests used in risk stratification should not be perceived as competing technologies. All of the different risk factors have synergy, rather than representing conflict of interest. Indeed, detailed retrospective studies of existing databases of cardiac patients suggest that very accurate identification of patients at risk may potentially be achieved if different risk factors are combined (Fig. 86-5).

In the practical setting of prospective studies, selection of dichotomies of different tests occasionally may be problematic because it is known that the conventional dichotomies of univariate prediction (e.g., LVEF below 35%) are not necessarily optimal when this approach is used in combination with other risk factors. Accordingly, in the recent multivariate studies, the strategy has been to combine different risk predictors with fairly different combinations of sensitivity and specificity. For instance, the Risk Estimation Following Infarction, Noninvasive Evaluation (REFINE) study showed that HRT might be used to select high-risk patients in combination with T wave alternans to exclude low-risk patients.[38]

Naturally, prospective evaluations of mutifactorial risk prediction strategies are requires in randomized intervention studies before clinical practice can change. Nevertheless, the need for such change seems obvious, because the prospectively verified selection of patients for ICD prophylaxis based solely on LVEF assessment both neglects substantial numbers of patients whose lives might be saved if identified properly and is economically wasteful in providing the device to far too many who never need it.

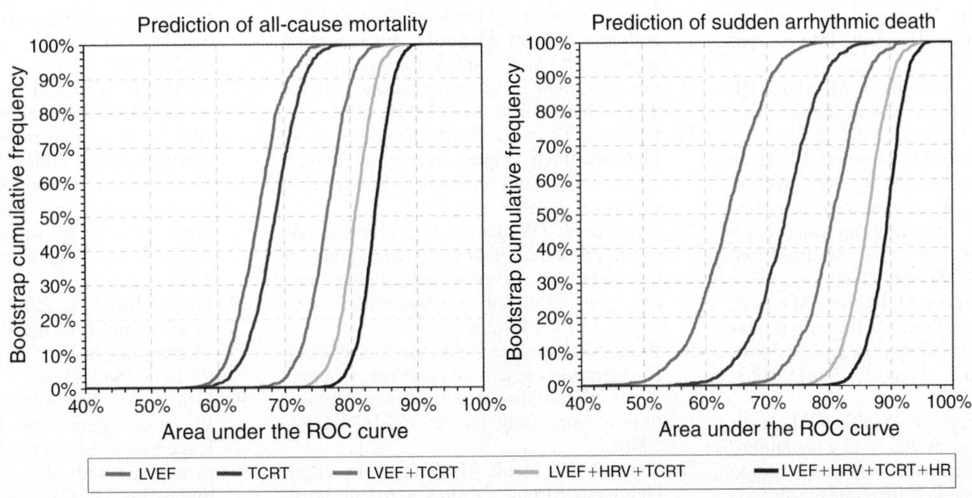

Figure 86-5 Example of multivariate risk prediction in the St. George's Hospital Medical School database of post-infarction survivors.[12] The panels show the estimates of areas under the receiver-operator characteristic (ROC) curves (see Fig. 86-1, legend) for the prediction of all-cause mortality and sudden cardiac (arrhythmic) death mortality and by different risk factors and by their combination. Univariate prediction by LVEF and TCRT is shown together with their combination, and with the combination with heart rate (HR) and global conventional HRV. Focused combination of different factors can yield even more powerful prediction of sudden cardiac death than the prediction of all-cause mortality. HRV, heart rate variability; LVEF, left ventricular ejection fraction; TCRT, total cosine of R-to-T angles.

References

1. Moss AJ, Zareba W, Hall WJ, et al: Prophylactic implantation of a defibrillator in patients with myocardial infarction and reduced ejection fraction. N Engl J Med 346:877-883, 2002.
2. Bristow MR, Saxon LA, Boehmer J, et al: Cardiac-resynchronization therapy with or without an implantable defibrillator in advanced chronic heart failure. N Engl J Med 350:2140-2150, 2004.
3. Bardy GH, Lee KL, Mark DB, et al: Amiodarone or an implantable cardioverter-defibrillator for congestive heart failure. N Engl J Med 352:225-237, 2005.
4. Gregoratos G, Abrams J, Epstein AE, et al: ACC/AHA/NASPE 2002 guideline update for implantation of cardiac pacemakers and antiarrhythmia devices: Summary article: A report of the American College of Cardiology/American Heart Association Task Force on Practice Guidelines (ACC/AHA/NASPE Committee to Update the 1998 Pacemaker Guidelines). Circulation 106:2145-2161, 2002.
5. Zipes DP, Camm AJ, Borggrefe M, et al: ACC/AHA/ESC 2006 Guidelines for Management of Patients with Ventricular Arrhythmias and the Prevention of Sudden Cardiac Death: A report of the American College of Cardiology/American Heart Association Task Force and the European Society of Cardiology Committee for Practice Guidelines (Writing Committee to Develop Guidelines for Management of Patients with Ventricular Arrhythmias and the Prevention of Sudden Cardiac Death): Developed in collaboration with the European Heart Rhythm Association and the Heart Rhythm Society. Circulation 114:e385-e484, 2006.
6. Sanders GD, Hlatky MA, Owens DK: Cost-effectiveness of implantable cardioverter-defibrillators. N Engl J Med 353:1471-1480, 2005.
7. Al-Khatib SM, Anstrom KJ, Eisenstein EL, et al: Clinical and economic implications of the Multicenter Automatic Defibrillator Implantation Trial-II. Ann Intern Med 142:593-600, 2005.
8. Huikuri HV, Castellanos A, Myerburg RJ: Sudden death due to cardiac arrhythmias. N Engl J Med 345:1473-1482, 2001.
9. Camm AJ, Pratt CM, Schwartz PJ, et al: Mortality in patients after a recent myocardial infarction: A randomized, placebo-controlled trial of azimilide using heart rate variability for risk stratification. Circulation 109:990-996, 2004.
10. Lanza GA, Cianflone D, Rebuzzi AG, et al: Prognostic value of ventricular arrhythmias and heart rate variability in patients with unstable angina. Heart 92:1055-1063, 2006.
11. Gilliam FR, Singh JP, Mullin CM, et al: Prognostic value of heart rate variability footprint and standard deviation of average 5-minute intrinsic R-R intervals for mortality in cardiac resynchronization therapy patients. J Electrocardiol 40:336-342, 2007.
12. Malik M, Hnatkova K, Batchvarov VN: Post infarction risk stratification using the 3-D angle between QRS complex and T-wave vectors. J Electrocardiol 37(Suppl): 201-208, 2004.
13. Wichterle D, Simek J, La Rovere MT, et al: Prevalent low-frequency oscillation of heart rate: Novel predictor of mortality after myocardial infarction. Circulation 110:1183-1190, 2004.
14. Kiviniemi AM, Tulppo MP, Wichterle D, et al: Novel spectral indexes of heart rate variability as predictors of sudden and non-sudden cardiac death after an acute myocardial infarction. Ann Med 39:54-62, 2007.
15. Wessel N, Voss A, Kurths J, et al: Evaluation of renormalised entropy for risk stratification using heart rate variability data. Med Biol Eng Comput 38:680-685, 2000.
16. Fukuta H, Hayano J, Ishihara S, et al: Prognostic value of nonlinear heart rate dynamics in hemodialysis patients with coronary artery disease. Kidney Int 64: 641-648, 2003.
17. Voss A, Schroeder R, Truebner S, et al: Comparison of nonlinear methods: Symbolic dynamics, detrended fluctuation, and Poincare plot analysis in risk stratification in patients with dilated cardiomyopathy. Chaos 17:015120, 2007.
18. Huikuri HV, Mäkikallio TH, Peng CK, et al: Fractal correlation properties of R-R interval dynamics and mortality in patients with depressed left ventricular function after an acute myocardial infarction. Circulation 101:47-53, 2000.
19. Stein PK, Domitrovich PP, Huikuri HV, et al: Traditional and nonlinear heart rate variability are each independently associated with mortality after myocardial infarction. J Cardiovasc Electrophysiol 16:13-20, 2005.
20. Malik M, Camm AJ, Janse MJ, et al: Depressed heart rate variability identifies postinfarction patients who might benefit from prophylactic treatment with amiodarone: A substudy of EMIAT. J Am Coll Cardiol 35:1263-1275, 2000.
21. Sassi R, Cerutti S, Hnatkova K, et al: HRV scaling exponent identifies postinfarction patients who might benefit from prophylactic treatment with amiodarone. IEEE Trans Biomed Eng 53:103-110, 2006.
22. Bauer A, Kantelhardt JW, Bunde A, et al: Phase-rectified signal averaging detects quasi-periodicities in non-stationary data. Physica A 364:423-434, 2006.
23. Kantelhardt JW, Bauer A, Schumann AY, et al: Phase-rectified signal averaging for the detection of quasi-periodicities and the prediction of cardiovascular risk. Chaos 17:015112, 2007.
24. Bauer A, Kantelhardt JW, Barthel P, et al: Deceleration capacity of heart rate as a predictor of mortality after myocardial infarction: Cohort study. Lancet 367:1674-1681, 2006.
25. Schmidt G, Malik M, Barthel P, et al: Heart-rate turbulence after ventricular premature beats as a predictor of mortality after acute myocardial infarction. Lancet 353:1390-1396, 1999.
26. Diaz J, Castellanos A, Moleiro F, et al: Relation between sinus rates preceding and following ectopic beats occurring in isolation and as episodes of bigeminy in young healthy subjects. Am J Cardiol 90:332-335, 2002.
27. Tuomainen P, Peuhkurinen K, Kettunen R, et al: Regular physical exercise, heart rate variability and turbulence in a 6-year randomized controlled trial in middle-aged men: The DNASCO study. Life Sci 77:2723-2734, 2005.
28. Malik M, Wichterle D, Schmidt G: Heart-rate turbulence. G Ital Cardiol 29:65-69, 1999.
29. Wichterle D, Melenovsky V, Simek J, et al: Hemodynamics and autonomic control of heart rate turbulence. J Cardiovasc Electrophysiol 17:286-291, 2006.
30. Watanabe MA, Schmidt G: Heart rate turbulence: A 5-year review. Heart Rhythm 1:732-738, 2004.
31. Lin LY, Lai LP, Lin JL, et al: Tight mechanism correlation between heart rate turbulence and baroreflex sensitivity: Sequential autonomic blockade analysis. J Cardiovasc Electrophysiol 13:427-431, 2002.
32. Watanabe MA, Marine JE, Sheldon R, et al: Effects of ventricular premature stimulus coupling interval on blood pressure and heart rate turbulence. Circulation 106:325-330, 2002.
33. Lee KT, Lai WT, Chu CS, et al: Effect of electrophysiologic character of ventricular premature beat on heart rate turbulence. J Electrocardiol 37:41-46, 2004.
34. Raj SR, Sheldon RS, Koshman M, et al: Role of hypotension in heart rate turbulence physiology. Heart Rhythm 2: 820-827, 2005.
35. Wichterle D, Camm AJ, Malik M: Turbulence slope after atrial premature complexes is an independent predictor of mortality in survivors of acute myocardial infarction. J Cardiovasc Electrophysiol 15:1350-1356, 2004.
36. Vikman S, Lindgren K, Makikallio TH, et al: Heart rate turbulence after atrial premature beats before spontaneous onset of atrial fibrillation. J Am Coll Cardiol 45:278-284, 2005.
37. Barthel P, Schneider R, Bauer A, et al: Risk stratification after acute myocardial infarction by heart rate turbulence. Circulation 108:1221-1226, 2003.
38. Exner DV, Kavanagh KM, Slawnych MP, et al: Noninvasive risk assessment early after a myocardial infarction the REFINE study. J Am Coll Cardiol 50:2275-2284, 2007.
39. Cygankiewicz I, Zareba W, Vazquez R, et al: Relation of heart rate turbulence to severity of heart failure. Am J Cardiol 98:1635-1640, 2006.
40. Grimm W, Schmidt G, Maisch B, et al: Prognostic significance of heart rate turbulence following ventricular premature beats in patients with idiopathic dilated cardiomyopathy. J Cardiovasc Electrophysiol 14:819-824, 2003.
41. De Ferrari GM, Sanzo A, Bertoletti A, et al. Baroreflex sensitivity predicts long-term cardiovascular mortality after myocardial infarction even in patients with preserved

left ventricular function. J Am Coll Cardiol 50:2285-2290, 2007.

42. Zabel M, Acar B, Klingenheben T, et al: Analysis of 12-lead T-wave morphology for risk stratification after myocardial infarction. Circulation 102:1252-1257, 2000.
43. Zabel M, Malik M, Hnatkova K, et al: Analysis of T-wave morphology from the 12-lead electrocardiogram for prediction of long-term prognosis in male US veterans. Circulation 105:1066-1070, 2002.
44. Kardys I, Kors JA, van der Meer IM, et al: Spatial QRS-T angle predicts cardiac death in a general population. Eur Heart J 24:1357-1364, 2003.
45. Yamazaki T, Froelicher VF, Myers J, et al: Spatial QRS-T angle predicts cardiac death in a clinical population. Heart Rhythm 2:73-78, 2005.
46. Okin PM, Malik M, Hnatkova K, et al: Repolarization abnormality for prediction of all-cause and cardiovascular mortality in American Indians: The Strong Heart Study. J Cardiovasc Electrophysiol 16:945-951, 2005.

Monophasic Action Potential Recording 87

Michael R. Franz

CHAPTER OUTLINE

Recording of monophasic action potentials (MAPs) by contact electrode catheter can be performed easily and safely in the human heart. Unlike body surface ECG recordings or standard endocardial electrograms, which produce a summative or derivative view of the heart's electrical activity, MAP recordings provide *local* information about the actual cellular depolarization and repolarization process of myocardial tissue. By giving the clinical investigator a more direct view of human myocardial electrophysiology in situ, in both normal and disease states, MAP recordings provide an important bridge between cellular and bedside electrophysiology. This chapter discusses the methodology and presents selected, clinically pertinent applications of MAP recordings. The genesis of MAPs by contact electrode technique has been described in a review[1] and also has been discussed in more recent work.[2,3]

Monophasic Action Potential Recording Devices

The MAP signal contains low-frequency components, especially during the plateau phase and during the diastolic isoelectric interval. For optimal signal fidelity, MAPs should be recorded with high-bandwidth amplifiers that can accurately reproduce a frequency range from 0 to 5000 Hz. For less rigorous signal interpretation, a bandwidth setting of 0.05 to 500 Hz is adequate and is available in most clinical electrophysiologic recording systems. Narrower bandwidths with high-pass filtering used for conventional intracardiac recordings (e.g., 30 to 300 Hz) are not suitable and will distort the MAP signal.

Monophasic Action Potential Recording Catheters for the Clinical Electrophysiology Laboratory

The design of the contact electrode catheter tip is schematically illustrated in Figure 87-1A (inset). The exploring hemispherical MAP electrode forms the catheter tip and is made of a nonpolarizable silver–silver chloride (Ag-AgCl) polymeric matrix. Another Ag-AgCl electrode is located 5 mm proximal to the tip (*close bipolar* design) and serves as the MAP reference electrode. When the catheter tip is directed axially against the endocardium, depolarization is confined to a small area subjacent to the tip electrode. The distal portion of the catheter shaft incorporates a flat spring wire that ensures stable contact between the tip electrode and the endocardium throughout the cardiac contraction-relaxation cycle. The tip electrode lead is connected to the positive input and the proximal electrode lead is connected to the negative input of the recording system.

Unlike in conventional electrode catheters, the pacing electrodes are not distal but are mounted in orthogonal position halfway between the distal (tip) and proximal (reference) MAP electrode. This electrode configuration provides for extremely low stimulus capture thresholds (0.02 to 0.25 mA; mean, 0.09 mA), resulting in minimal interference between the pacing artifact and the MAP signal.[4] This feature facilitates precise and simultaneous determinations of both the action potential duration (APD) and effective refractory period (ERP) at the same myocardial site (see Fig. 87-1B). A hands-on description of how to use the MAP catheter in the clinical electrophysiology laboratory was published recently.[5]

Monophasic Action Potential Recording in the Animal Research Laboratory

Several MAP recording techniques have been developed specifically for experimental research purposes. A spring-loaded cantilever probe that holds the MAP electrode assembly at its tip is suitable for epicardial MAP recording in open-chested dogs, pigs, or other large animals.[1] The tip electrode makes direct contact with the epicardium, and electrical continuity between the reference electrode and the heart is provided by a small plug of saline-soaked foam rubber that covers the tip assembly, including the proximal electrode. With use of a small handheld probe, MAPs can be recorded from Langendorff-perfused hearts of smaller animals such as rabbits. A multi-MAP electrode apparatus has been developed to record up to 10 epicardial and endocardial MAPs, as well as a volume-conducted 12-lead ECG, simultaneously from the isolated intact rabbit heart.[6] This capability is particularly useful for measuring dispersion of ventricular activation and repolarization—for example, to study mechanisms of ventricular defibrillation by monophasic or biphasic current shocks[7] or for visualizing early afterdepolarizations (EADs) and changes in APD and dispersion in models of the long QT syndrome.[6] This method was adopted for studying the proarrhythmic potential of antiarrhythmic[8] noncardiac drugs,[9] an extremely important issue for drug development and U.S. Food and Drug Administration (FDA) clearance. Also described and validated has been a miniaturized MAP probe with a tip electrode diameter of 0.25 mm that is suitable for MAP recordings, both endocardially and epicardially, in isolated mouse hearts.[10] This method has provided insights into electrophysiologic abnormalities in models of transgenic disease, such as mutations of *KCNQ1* (long QT syndrome type 1 [LQT1])[11] and *SCN5A* (LQT3).[12]

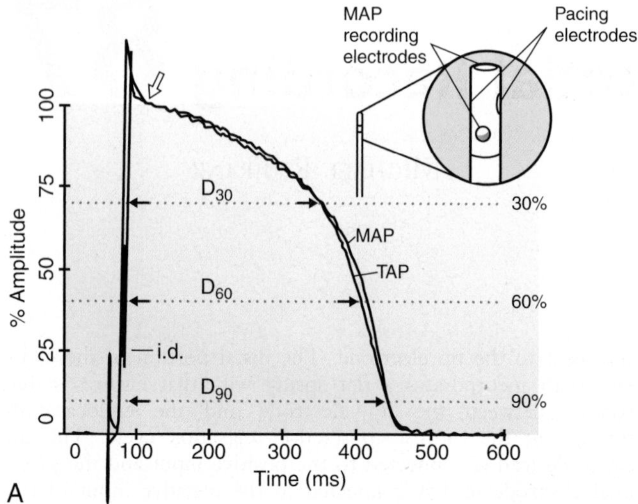

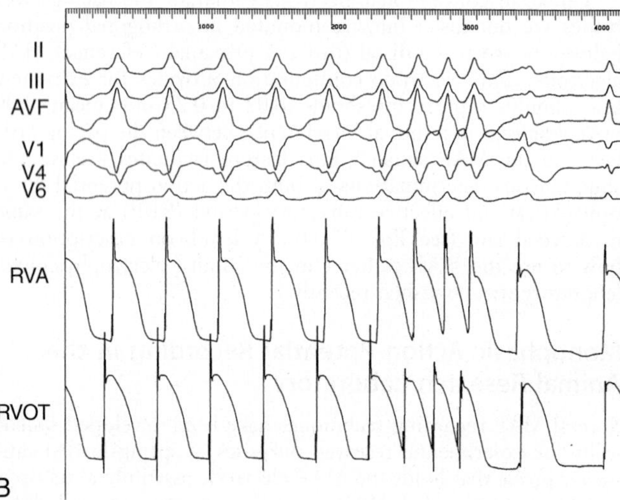

Figure 87-1 **A**, Simultaneous recordings of intracellular transmembrane action potential (TAP) and extracellular monophasic action potential (MAP) show high congruence. Repolarization is labeled at 30%, 60%, and 90% of the return from plateau to resting potential. *Inset:* Contact electrode catheter design for recording MAPs from endocardium in patients or large animals. Shown is the MAP-pacing combination catheter, which includes small pacing electrodes located 2 mm proximal to the catheter tip in an orthogonal position. This catheter incorporates a bidirectional steering feature *(not shown)*. **B**, MAP recordings from two right ventricular (RV) sites along with body surface electrocardiogram during programmed electrical stimulation. Pacing is performed at the RV outflow tract (RVOT). Note small pacing artifacts immediately preceding the MAP upstrokes. Extrastimulus responses show increasing separation between stimulus and MAP upstroke. RVA, RV apex. (**A**, From Franz MR, Burkhoff D, Yue D, Lakatta E: In vitro validation of a new cardiac catheter technique for recording monophasic action potentials. Eur Heart J 7:34-41, 1986; *inset*, adapted from Franz MR, Chin MC, Sharkey HR, et al: A new single catheter technique for simultaneous measurement of action potential duration and refractory period in vivo. J Am Coll Cardiol 16:878-886, 1990.)

Accuracy of Monophasic Action Potential Recordings

The "Franz" contact electrode MAP records the relative voltage time course of cardiac cell membranes with high fidelity (see Fig. 87-1A, inset).[13] It does not, however, reproduce the true magnitude of the transmembrane action potential (TAP), nor does the MAP render information on the absolute rise velocity (V_{max}) of the TAP upstroke. In this context, the beginning of the MAP is defined as the instance of fastest rise time of the MAP upstroke. Because the asymptotic end of repolarization makes precise measurement of total MAP duration difficult, the MAP duration usually is determined at a repolarization level of 90% (or another fraction) with respect to the MAP amplitude. The MAP amplitude is best defined as the distance from the baseline to the crest of the MAP plateau, not its upstroke peak.[1,13] As an alternative, use of the intersection between the diastolic baseline and a tangent placed on phase 3 repolarization has been suggested; this approach may produce more arbitrary results, depending on the slope of final repolarization.

Clinical Applications of Monophasic Action Potential Recording

The contact electrode MAP catheter with pacing capability (MAP-combination catheter)[4] can be used for routine electrophysiologic studies, including programmed electrical stimulation (Table 87-1). Such combination catheters have several advantages over conventional quadripolar catheters: (1) The local endocardial activation time is indicated by the MAP upstroke, which is sharp and unambiguous, in contrast with the often multiphasic deflections obtained with conventional catheters, thereby making measurements of local activation time easier and more accurate (see Fig. 87-1B). (2) Pacing thresholds with the MAP-combination catheter are extremely low and stimulus artifacts are drastically mimized,[4] providing unobscured local myocardial responses (Fig. 87-2). This feature also is useful for differentiating local stimulus response latency from "downstream" conduction delays.[14] (3) Because local repolarization is visualized by the MAP, the ERP, which usually coincides with 75% to 85% repolarization,[15] can be anticipated and confirmed quickly without prolonged extrastimulus scanning. This also helps visualize changes in the ERP that occur independently from changes in APD (see later on). (4) MAPs are recorded only when the catheter tip electrode is in close contact with the endocardium. A stable MAP verifies stable tip electrode contact, facilitates a constant stimulus threshold, and avoids confusion with intracavitary potentials as might be the case with conventional electrograms, when small signal amplitudes are the only way to suspect insufficient tissue contact. (5) With conventional electrophysiologic catheters, fractionated, double, or late potentials have been observed and interpreted as markers of abnormal conduction in scarred myocardium, which is believed to be a substrate for reentry tachycardia; however, concerns that some fractionated electrograms represent artifacts have been raised. Comparisons between MAP signals and conventional electrograms can be helpful in identifying the nature of these fractionated electrograms (see later on).

Use Dependence of Antiarrhythmic Drugs: Action Potential Duration and Refractoriness

Continuous MAP recording from the same endocardial site while pacing the heart at several steady-state cycle lengths can determine the use-dependent profile of APD-altering drugs. Use dependence is present when the APD-prolonging effect increases with the frequency of the heart beat; reverse use dependence is present when this effect diminishes during faster rates. It has been postulated that to be effective, a class III antiarrhythmic drug should increase its potential to prolong the APD during an increase in heart rate so as to self-limit the tachycardia or terminate it. So far, only amiodarone has been shown to maintain

Table 87-1 Clinical Applications of Monophasic Action Potential (MAP) Recordings

- Effects of antiarrhythmic drugs on APD and ERP/APD ratio
- Repolarization abnormalities in congenital or acquired long QT syndromes and Brugada syndrome
- Measuring dispersion of repolarization by MAP mapping techniques
- Evaluation of T wave changes and memory
- Myocardial ischemia detection and distinction between viable and nonviable myocardium
- Distinction between VT and VF during ICD testing
- Effects of rate and rhythm on APD in humans, including restitution curves
- Detection of dominant frequency in atrial fibrillation
- Targeting and monitoring radiofrequency ablation of arrhythmia substrates

APD, action potential duration; ERP, effective refractory potential; ICD, implantable cardioverter-defibrillator; VF, ventricular fibrillation; VT, ventricular tachycardia.

its APD-prolonging effect during faster rates.[16] The APD prolongation produced by amiodarone has been shown to be linear during changes in cycle length—it is neither progressive nor regressive.

A disproportionate increase in ERP relative to APD, which results in an increased ERP/APD ratio, has been linked to the antiarrhythmic efficacy of drugs, based on the rationale that ERP prolongation relative to APD provides a window of post-repolarization refractoriness. Kirchhof and associates[17] demonstrated in isolated rabbit hearts that drug-induced post-repolarization refractoriness can prevent ventricular fibrillation, allowing only ventricular tachycardia.

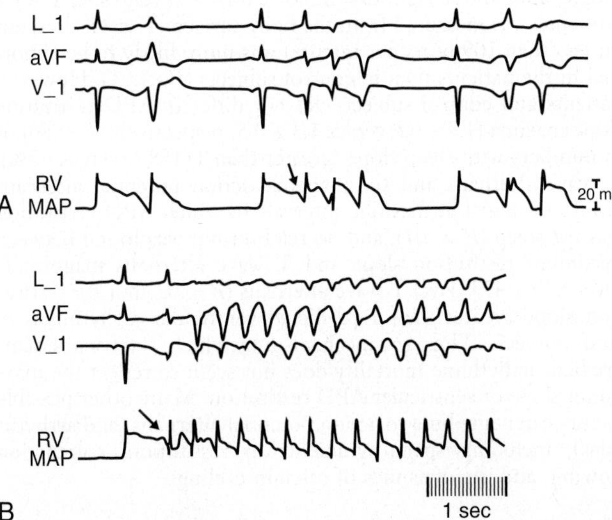

Figure 87-2 Early afterdepolarizations recorded with the monophasic action potential (MAP) catheter from right ventricular (RV) endocardium in a patient with procainamide-induced torsades de pointes. (From Habbab MA, El-Sherif N: Drug-induced torsades de pointes: Role of early afterdepolarizations and dispersion of repolarization. Am J Med 89:241-246, 1990.)

Monophasic Action Potential Recordings Detect Afterdepolarizations and Elucidate the Mechanism of Torsades de Pointes Arrhythmias: Long QT and Brugada Syndromes

Torsades de pointes arrhythmias occur in a variety of acquired and congenital long QT syndromes. Besides prolongation of the QT interval, EADs have been implicated in the genesis of ventricular tachyarrhythmias, specifically of torsades de pointes arrhythmias. Habbab and El-Sherif[18] were among the first to report clinical evidence with MAP recordings that procainamide-induced polymorphic ventricular tachycardia of the torsades de pointes type was associated with prominent EADs and U waves (see Fig. 87-2). Consistent with clinical observations on precipitating factors of torsades de pointes, EADs are enhanced by bradycardia and long pauses and are suppressed by rapid pacing. The exact electrophysiologic mechanism of torsades de pointes is still under investigation. Epinephrine challenge seems to be better suited than isoproteronol for provoking torsades de pointes. MAP durations in patients with idiopathic long QT syndrome were longer than normal at baseline and increased markedly during epinephrine infusion and exhibited EADs.[19] MAP recordings in humans also directly confirmed repolarization abnormalities underlying the Brugada syndrome.[20,21]

Monophasic Action Potential Recordings during Atrial Flutter and Fibrillation

Atrial fibrillation is characterized by rapid irregular patterns of atrial activation and repolarization. MAP recordings allow distinction between activation and repolarization and can make visible excitable gaps during atrial fibrillation. This capability has aided attempts to capture atrial myocardium during atrial fibrillation by overdrive pacing.[22] MAP recordings are useful for distinguishing among different types of atrial fibrillation and to differentiate some forms of atrial flutter from atrial fibrillation, including the transition of atrial flutter to atrial fibrillation[23,24] (Fig. 87-3). Furthermore, Narayan and associates[24] have shown that APD in the human right atrium is distributed unevenly, with abnormal prolongation and reverse rate adaptation seen in the inferior vena cava–tricuspid valve isthmus region in patients with chronic atrial flutter or fibrillation. This heterogeneous electrical remodeling may facilitate the breakup of conduction pathways if a rapid impulse generator or "driver" (atrial flutter, fast overdrive pacing, or high-frequency bursts originating from the pulmonary veins) encounters "obstacles" of prolonged refractoriness, and, through fibrillatory conduction, provokes or maintains atrial fibrillation.

Rapid drivers, representing as either high-frequency impulse discharges or rotor wave activity within the atria, are under investigation as atrial fibrillation initiators and as targets for radiofrequency ablation. Within the atria, continuous atrial fractionated electrograms (CFAEs) have been targeted as ablation sites.[25] As with other sites in which fractionation is seen in conventional bipolar electrograms, the possibility of double-counting cannot be excluded. Narayan and coworkers[23] examined atrial fibrillation cycle lengths by comparing bipolar electrograms with MAP recordings at the same sites, demonstrating greater reliability of dominant frequency (DF) measurement by MAP. The measured cycle length was represented accurately by the DF of the MAPs but, owing to double counting, not always by the DF of bipolar signals ($P = .005$).

Further interest has been directed at autonomic nerve influences on atrial APD, EAD generation, and CFAEs in initiating and maintaining atrial fibrillation, with emphasis on atrial fat

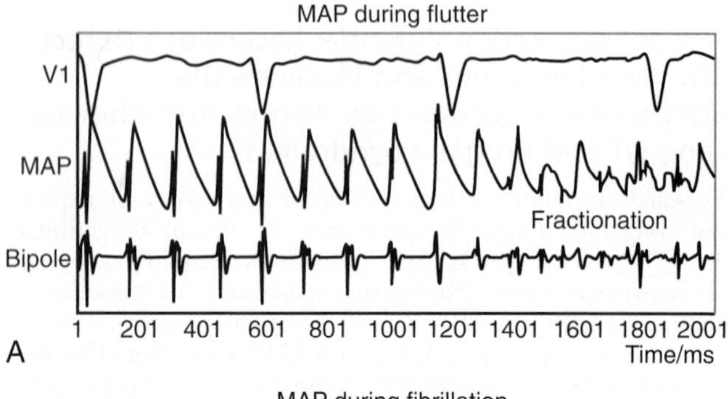

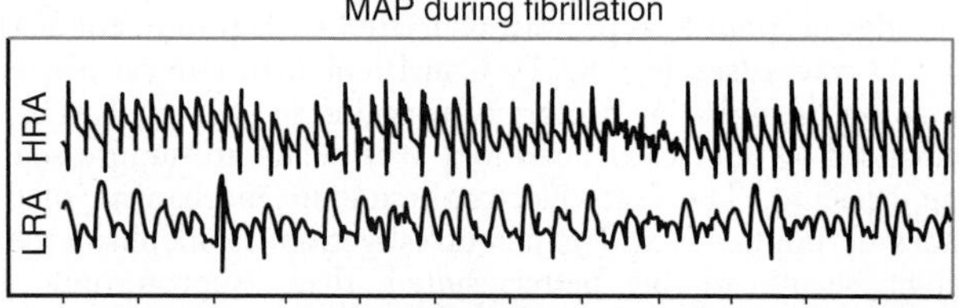

Figure 87-3 Right atrial monophasic action potential (MAP) recordings during atrial flutter (**A**) and atrial fibrillation (**B**). **A** shows simultaneous electrocardiogram (ECG), MAP, and bipolar electrogram recordings during atrial overdrive pacing demonstrating initial triangular atrial MAP waveforms and subsequent transition from atrial flutter to atrial fibrillation, evidenced by signal fractionation. **B** shows simultaneous MAP recordings from the high right atrium (HRA) and the low right atrium (LRA) during atrial fibrillation. Note continuous variations in morphology, cycle length, and regularity. (**A** and **B**, Adapted from Narayan SM, Krummen DE, Kahn AM, et al: Evaluating fluctuations in human atrial fibrillatory cycle length using monophasic action potentials. Pacing Clin Electrophysiol 29:1209-1218, 2006.)

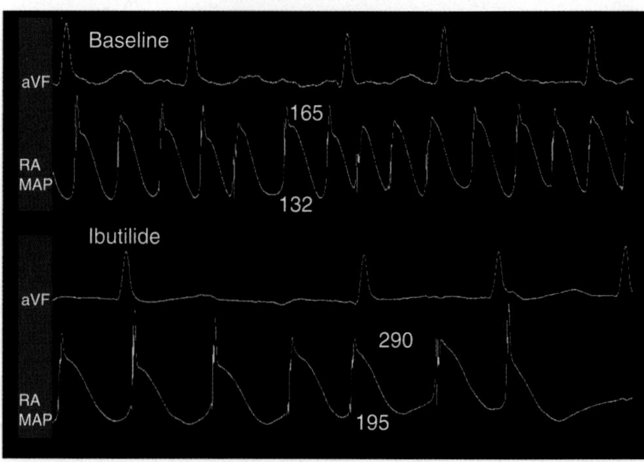

Figure 87-4 Right atrial monophasic action potential (MAP) recordings in a patient with atrial fibrillation who cardioverted during infusion of ibutilide. RA, right atrium. (From Stambler BS, Wood MA, Ellenbogen KA: Antiarrhythmic actions of intravenous ibutilide compared with procainamide during human atrial flutter and fibrillation: Electrophysiological determinants of enhanced conversion efficacy. Circulation 96: 4298-4306, 1997.)

pads that harbor ganglionic plexuses.[26] Vagal effects shorten the atrial APD at innervation sites and can be used as *local* indicators of autonomic effects, rather than using sinus bradycardia or AV block as "distant" indicators. Thus, MAP recording may portray electrophysiologic variability, fragmentation, cycle length, and APD changes for mapping and targeting atrial fibrillation substrates.

Finally, atrial MAP recording allows monitoring the effect of antiarrhythmic drugs on depolarization and repolarization, and on the excitable gap, in atrial flutter and atrial fibrillation. Two major mechanisms have been identified in halting reentry circuits in atrial fibrillation and atrial flutter: One is prolongation of APD; the other is slowing conduction velocity or enlarging pivot points (or both) at reentry curves.[27] Figure 87-4 shows MAP recordings in a patient with atrial fibrillation who received ibutilide infusion that prolonged APD and diastolic intervals, with arrest of the fibrillation.[28]

Electrical Restitution and Action Potential Alternans

MAP recordings have been instrumental in determining electrical restitution in human ventricles and atria. *Electrical restitution* refers to changes in APD or ERP during short-term interval changes. The standard restitution protocol determines the electrical restitution curve (ERC) as a function of the diastolic interval (DI) between the last regularly paced beat and a series of "extra" beats elicited at varying intervals after the last regular beat. The dynamic restitution protocol[29] uses sequential series of stepwise increased pacing rates, also plotting APD against the DI. The slope of the ERC has been implicated in susceptibility to arrhythmias.

Experimental and modeling studies showed that a slope greater than 1 is associated with action potential alternans, which may lead to wavebreak or reentry and subsequently to ventricular or atrial fibrillation, respectively. In patients undergoing electrophysiologic study, Koller and colleagues[30] showed that APD restitution was steeper for a wider range of fast rates (short DI) in patients with structural disease than in those without such disease, and that APD restitution slope greater than 1 preceded alternans at rates greater than 200 beats per minute (achieved by means of pacing or in ventricular tachycardia). Narayan and coworkers[31] studied 53 patients with left ventricular ejection fraction of 28 ± 8% and 18 control subjects with ejection fraction 58 ± 12%. APD was recorded at electrophysiologic study in the right ($n = 62$) or left ($n = 9$) ventricle; T wave alternans was measured from the body surface. T wave alternans (at less than 109 beats per minute) was more likely to be abnormal in the patients than in control subjects ($P < .01$). However, patients and control subjects did not differ in APD restitution slope maxima (1.2 ± 0.6 versus 1.3 ± 0.5, respectively, $P = .86$) or in numbers with steep slope (greater than 1) (58% versus 67%). T wave alternans and simultaneous action potential alternans always occurred at diastolic intervals in which APD restitution was *not* steep ($P < .01$), and no relationship was found between maximum restitution slope and T wave alternans magnitude. Over 829 ± 473 days, T wave alternans ($P = .02$) but *not* restitution slope greater than 1 predicted ventricular arrhythmias in study subjects. Thus, the mechanism by which T wave alternans predicts arrhythmic mortality does not seem to reflect the maximum slope of ventricular APD restitution. Many other possible factors can contribute to action potential alternans (and arrhythmias), including spatial gradients of restitution, conduction slowing, and the dynamics of calcium cycling.

Electrical Remodeling

MAP recordings have confirmed that chronic atrial fibrillation or atrial flutter causes electrical remodeling in the human heart.[32] The main effects of electrical remodeling are a

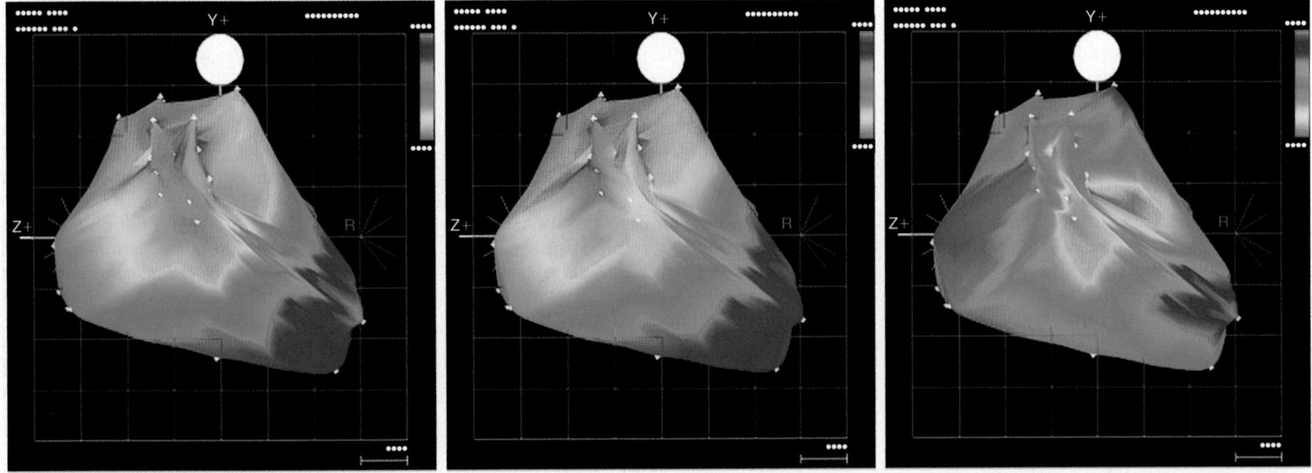

Figure 87-5 Posterior-anterior views of left ventricular maps from a patient during sustained ventricular tachycardia (VT). **Left,** The VT focus was located in the left laterobasal (*red*) area from which activation propagated toward and ended in the posteroparaseptal (*blue* and *purple*) area. **Middle,** The end-of-repolarization sequence was in principle the same as the activation sequence. **Right,** The longest monophasic action potentials (*red*) were recorded near the area activated earliest, and the shortest (*blue* and *purple*) in the area activated latest. (From Kongstad O, Yuan S, Hertervig E, et al: Global and local dispersion of ventricular repolarization: Endocardial monophasic action potential mapping in swine and humans by using an electro-anatomical mapping system. J Electrocardiol 35:159-167, 2002.)

shortening of the action potential (especially of its plateau phase) and a flattening of the relationship between APD and cycle length, with the relatively greatest shortening occurring at long cycle lengths (see Chapter 43 for a detailed discussion of the cellular and molecular basis of electrical remodeling). Although APD shortening (and its concomitant ERP shortening) is recognized to be arrhythmogenic, it is not obvious why APD shortening should be especially arrhythmogenic at *long* cycle lengths. Another important factor in promoting atrial fibrillation is electrical heterogeneity within the atria. Narayan and coworkers[24] have shown that APD in the human inferior vena cava–tricuspid valve isthmus exhibits abnormal prolongation and *reverse* rate adaptation in patients with chronic atrial flutter or fibrillation.

Repolarization Mapping, T Wave Genesis, and Cardiac Memory

The T wave polarity is concordant with the R wave in most ECG leads. This has been enigmatic and theoretically explained by assuming that ventricular sites that activate first, repolarize last. First direct evidence for this hypothesis was provided by MAP recordings in human left ventricles that showed that there is indeed a reciprocal relationship between myocardial activation and repolarization.[33] Kongstad and colleagues[34] expanded these studies by using the CARTO system to map activation and repolarization in porcine and human hearts (Fig. 87-5).

The term *cardiac memory* sometimes is applied to long-term changes in APD caused by rapid pacing ("rate memory"). However, the original definition of cardiac memory, most elegantly analyzed and described by Mauricio Rosenbaum and colleagues, referred to ectopic pacing–induced changes in the configuration of the body surface T wave (T wave memory).[35] Although rapid pacing–induced T wave changes ("memory") initially were considered an artifact caused by ischemia or cardiac nerve stimulation, it was later demonstrated (using MAP recordings in isolated rabbit hearts) that pacing from an ectopic ventricular site leads to changes in local APD and thus causes "primary" T wave changes.[36] Subsequently, Rosen and Cohen's laboratory[37] has made great strides in discerning short-term and long-term T wave memory and its molecular basis. Nam and associates[38] have verified the existence of short-term cardiac memory related to activation site in human atria in vivo using MAP recordings.[38]

Summary

Recording of MAP waveforms by contact electrode catheter has become the method of choice for evaluating repolarization of human heart tissue in vivo. It can be used easily and safely in the human heart. In contrast with surface ECG recordings and standard intracardiac electrograms, MAP recordings provide local information about the depolarization and repolarization process in myocardial tissue at the electrode-tissue contact site. This capability has been validated by showing that contact MAPs and TAPs recorded simultaneously at directly adjacent sites have virtually congruent voltage time courses. Owing to its safety and simplicity, as well as high stability and recording fidelity, the contact electrode technique has gained wide use in clinical and experimental research, including pharmacologic interventions, arrhythmia ablation, cardiac memory, electrical restitution and remodeling, and other repolarization-related phenomena in both ventricular and atrial myocardium.

References

1. Franz MR: Current status of monophasic action potential recording: Theories, measurements and interpretations. Cardiovasc Res 41:25-40, 1999.
2. Knollmann BC, Tranquillo J, Sirenko, et al: Microelectrode study of the genesis of the monophasic action potential by contact electrode technique. J Cardiovasc Electrophysiol 13:1246-1252, 2002.
3. Coronel R, de Bakker JM, Wilms-Schopman FJ, et al: Monophasic action potentials and activation recovery intervals as measures of ventricular action potential duration: Experimental evidence to resolve some controversies. Heart Rhythm 3:1043-1050, 2006.
4. Franz MR, Chin MC, Sharkey HR, et al: A new single catheter technique for

simultaneous measurement of action potential duration and refractory period in vivo. J Am Coll Cardiol 16:878-886, 1990.
5. Moore HJ, Franz MR: Monophasic action potential recordings in humans. J Cardiovasc Electrophysiol 18:787-790, 2007.
6. Zabel M, Hohnloser SH, Behrens S, et al: Electrophysiologic features of torsades de pointes: Insights from a new isolated rabbit heart model. J Cardiovasc Electrophysiol 8:1148-1158, 1997.
7. Behrens S, Li C, Kirchhof P, et al: Reduced arrhythmogenicity of biphasic versus monophasic T-wave shocks. Implications for defibrillation efficacy. Circulation 94:1974-1980, 1996.
8. Johna R, Mertens H, Haverkamp W, et al: Clofilium in the isolated perfused rabbit heart: A new model to study proarrhythmia induced by class III antiarrhythmic drugs. Basic Res Cardiol 93:127-135, 1998.
9. Milberg P, Eckardt L, Bruns HJ, et al: Divergent proarrhythmic potential of macrolide antibiotics despite similar QT prolongation: Fast phase 3 repolarization prevents early afterdepolarizations and torsade de pointes. J Pharmacol Exp Ther 303:218-225, 2002.
10. Knollmann BC, Katchman AN, Franz MR: Monophasic action potential recordings from intact mouse heart: Validation, regional heterogeneity, and relation to refractoriness. J Cardiovasc Electrophysiol 12:1286-1294, 2001.
11. Casimiro MC, Knollmann BC, Ebert SN, et al: Targeted disruption of the *KCNQ1* gene produces a mouse model of Jervell and Lange-Nielsen syndrome. Proc Natl Acad Sci U S A 98:2526-2531, 2001.
12. Fabritz L, Kirchhof P, Franz MR, et al: Effect of pacing and mexiletine on dispersion of repolarisation and arrhythmias in DeltaKPQ *SCN5A* (long QT3) mice. Cardiovasc Res 57:1085-1093, 2003.
13. Franz MR, Burkhoff D, Spurgeon H, et al: In vitro validation of a new cardiac catheter technique for recording monophasic action potentials. Eur Heart J 7:34-41, 1986.
14. Koller BS, Karasik PE, Solomon AJ, Franz MR: Prolongation of conduction time during premature stimulation in the human atrium is primarily caused by local stimulus response latency. Eur Heart J 16:1920-1924, 1995.
15. Koller BS, Karasik PE, Solomon AJ, Franz MR: The relationship between repolarization and refractoriness during programmed electrical stimulation in the human right ventricle. Implications for ventricular tachycardia induction. Circulation 91:2378-2384, 1995.
16. Zabel M, Hohnloser SH, Behrens S, et al: Differential effects of D-sotalol, quinidine, and amiodarone on dispersion of ventricular repolarization in the isolated rabbit heart. J Cardiovasc Electrophysiol 8:1239-1245, 1997.
17. Kirchhof PF, Fabritz CL, Franz MR: Postrepolarization refractoriness versus conduction slowing caused by class I antiarrhythmic drugs: Antiarrhythmic and proarrhythmic effects. Circulation 97:2567-2574, 1998.
18. Habbab MA, El-Sherif N: Drug-induced torsades de pointes: Role of early afterdepolarizations and dispersion of repolarization. Am J Med 89:241-246, 1990.
19. Urao N, Shiraishi H, Ishibashi K, et al: Idiopathic long QT syndrome with early afterdepolarization induced by epinephrine. A case report. Circ J 68:587-591, 2004.
20. Kurita T, Shimizu W, Inagaki M, et al: The electrophysiologic mechanism of ST-segment elevation in Brugada syndrome. J Am Coll Cardiol 40:330-334, 2002.
21. Narayan SM, Kim J, Tate C, Berman BJ: Steep restitution of ventricular action potential duration and conduction slowing in human Brugada syndrome. Heart Rhythm 4:1087-1089, 2007.
22. Pandozi C, Bianconi L, Villani M, et al: Local capture by atrial pacing in spontaneous chronic atrial fibrillation. Circulation 95:2416-2422, 1997.
23. Narayan SM, Krummen DE, Kahn AM, et al: Evaluating fluctuations in human atrial fibrillatory cycle length using monophasic action potentials. Pacing Clin Electrophysiol 29:1209-1218, 2006.
24. Narayan SM, Bode F, Karasik PL, Franz MR: Alternans of atrial action potentials during atrial flutter as a precursor to atrial fibrillation. Circulation 106:1968-1973, 2002.
25. Nademanee K, McKenzie J, Kosar E, et al: A new approach for catheter ablation of atrial fibrillation: Mapping of the electrophysiologic substrate. J Am Coll Cardiol 43:2044-2053, 2004.
26. Lin J, Scherlag BJ, Zhou J, et al: Autonomic mechanism to explain complex fractionated atrial electrograms (CFAE). J Cardiovasc Electrophysiol 18:1197-1205, 2007.
27. Danse PW, Garratt CJ, Allessie MA: Flecainide widens the excitable gap at pivot points of premature turning wavefronts in rabbit ventricular myocardium. J Cardiovasc Electrophysiol 12:1010-1017, 2001.
28. Stambler BS, Wood MA, Ellenbogen KA: Antiarrhythmic actions of intravenous ibutilide compared with procainamide during human atrial flutter and fibrillation: Electrophysiological determinants of enhanced conversion efficacy. Circulation 96:4298-4306, 1997.
29. Koller ML, Riccio ML, Gilmour RF Jr: Dynamic restitution of action potential duration during electrical alternans and ventricular fibrillation. Am J Physiol 275:H1635-H1642, 1998.
30. Koller ML, Maier SK, Gelzer AR, et al: Altered dynamics of action potential restitution and alternans in humans with structural heart disease. Circulation 112:1542-1548, 2005.
31. Narayan SM, Franz MR, Lalani G, et al: T-wave alternans, restitution of ventricular action potential duration, and outcome. J Am Coll Cardiol 50:2385-2392, 2007.
32. Franz MR, Karasik PL, Li C, et al: Electrical remodeling of the human atrium: Similar effects in patients with chronic atrial fibrillation and atrial flutter. J Am Coll Cardiol 30:1785-1792, 1997.
33. Franz MR, Bargheer K, Rafflenbeul W, et al: Monophasic action potential mapping in human subjects with normal electrocardiograms: Direct evidence for the genesis of the T wave. Circulation 75:379-386, 1987.
34. Kongstad O, Yuan S, Hertervig E, et al: Global and local dispersion of ventricular repolarization: Endocardial monophasic action potential mapping in swine and humans by using an electro-anatomical mapping system. J Electrocardiol 35:159-167, 2002.
35. Rosenbaum MB, Blanco HH, Elizari MV, et al: Electrotonic modulation of the T wave and cardiac memory. Am J Cardiol 50:213-222, 1982.
36. Costard-Jackle A, Goetsch B, Antz M, Franz MR: Slow and long-lasting modulation of myocardial repolarization produced by ectopic activation in isolated rabbit hearts. Evidence for cardiac "memory.". Circulation 80:1412-1420, 1989.
37. Rosen MR, Cohen IS: Cardiac memory: New insights into molecular mechanisms. J Physiol 570:209-218, 2006.
38. Nam GB, Choi KJ, Kim J, et al: Correlation of electrotonic monophasic action potential shortening with short-term memory in human atrium. Pacing Clin Electrophysiol 28:1215-1220, 2005.

T Wave Alternans 88

Stefan H. Hohnloser

CHAPTER OUTLINE

History of Cardiac Alternans

Electrical alternans is defined as beat-to-beat alterations in the shape of electrocardiographic waveforms. The occurrence of visible electrical alternans (i.e., "macrovolt" alternans) was first described by Hering in 1908.[1] Shortly thereafter, Thomas Lewis noted that alternans could occur in normal heart after marked accelerations in heart rate and also in the diseased or intoxicated myocardium.[2] In 1948, Kalter and Schwartz examined the electrocardiograms (ECGs) from 6059 patients and described an association between macroscopic T wave alternans (TWA) (observed in 5 patients) and increased mortality among the affected patients.[3] Subsequent case reports described the occurrence of visible TWA in various clinical situations such as myocardial ischemia, coronary artery spasm, and electrolyte disturbances, and particularly in the setting of congenital long QT syndrome.[4,5]

Assessment of subtle microvolt TWA (MTWA) was first reported in 1982[6] using sophisticated computerized analysis. In the 1980s, Cohen and coworkers established a close relationship between MTWA and vulnerability to ventricular fibrillation in a dog model.[6,7] Similar findings were subsequently reported by Nearing and colleagues.[8] Since the inscription of the methods for assessment of MTWA, compelling evidence for a mechanistic link between MTWA and the occurrence of ventricular tachyarrhythmias has been provided in a plethora of experimental and clinical studies. One of the nicest clinical examples of this link has recently been reported from a sophisticated clinical study.[9] By analyzing implantable cardioverter-defibrillator (ICD)-stored electrogram series, Shusterman and associates convincingly demonstrated that repolarization instability manifested by MTWA increased significantly shortly before the onset of ventricular tachyarrhythmias.

Over the past 5 to 10 years, many important new findings on the mechanisms underlying MTWA, on implementation of MTWA assessment in clinical practice, and on the prognostic value of this noninvasive ECG-derived risk marker have been reported. These findings are reviewed in this chapter.

Mechanisms Underlying T Wave Alternans

MTWA results from beat-to-beat alternation in the time course of the action potential duration (APD) at the cellular level. This was definitively established through detailed measurements of the time course of membrane voltage throughout the ventricle at a time when MTWA was elicited on the surface ECG using high-resolution optical mapping techniques in a guinea pig model of pacing-induced MTWA.[10-12] Of importance, in these studies MTWA was a consistent (in fact requisite) precursor to ventricular fibrillation. The mechanism linking action potential alternans (and therefore MTWA) to ventricular arrhythmias involves the development of spatially discordant alternans—that is, action potential alternans occurring with opposite phase between neighboring cells[10] (Fig. 88-1A). When action potential alternans is initiated, APD either prolongs or shortens simultaneously in all cells of a particular region of ventricular myocardium (i.e., concordant alternans) (Fig. 88-2A, left). After a premature impulse (* in Figure 88-2) or change in pacing rate above a critical heart rate threshold, a sequential lengthening and shortening of the action potential occurs (see Fig. 88-2A, right), with fluctuations in some regions being 180 degrees out of phase with those in other regions, such that some cells undergo a prolongation of APD while other populations of cells undergo APD shortening on the same beat (i.e., discordant alternans).[10,12] During discordant alternans (see Fig. 88-2B, right), marked spatial dispersion of APD emerges (blue bars), and discordant alternans amplifies physiologic heterogeneities of repolarization present at baseline into pathophysiologic heterogeneities of sufficient magnitude to produce conduction block and reentrant excitation (see Fig. 88-2B).[10-12] Discordant alternans also produces a substrate by which conduction block and reentrant excitation can be easily initiated by a premature stimulus (see Fig. 88-2B). When an impulse (* in Figure 88-2) propagates (from site A in the figure) into still-depolarized myocardium (i.e., in the wake of enhanced dispersion of repolarization after the long beat—blue bar in site B), conduction block, initiating reentrant excitation can occur (see Fig. 88-2B—ventricular fibrillation). Thus, discordant alternans is a mechanism linking MTWA to cardiac arrhythmogenesis, and in fact in experimental models of action potential alternans, ventricular fibrillation never occurs without discordant alternans. Under chronotropic or metabolic stress, discordant alternans leads to sufficiently large repolarization gradients to produce unidirectional block and reentry. Without a structural barrier, reentry is functional and manifests as ventricular fibrillation or polymorphic ventricular tachycardia. In the presence of structural barriers, reentry can become anatomically fixed, resulting in monomorphic ventricular tachycardia.

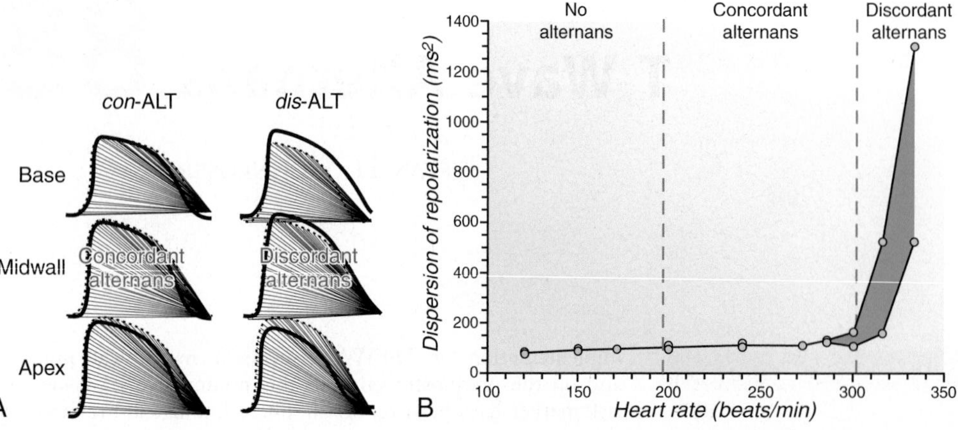

Figure 88-1 **A,** Action potential assessed by high-resolution optical mapping from epicardial cells on base, apex, and midwall of the guinea pig left ventricle during 2 consecutive beats. Above a critical heart rate, concordant alternans (*con*-ALT) is transformed to discordant alternans (*dis*-ALT) between apex and base. **B,** Amplification of spatial gradients of repolarization by discordant alternans. (Adapted from Pastore JM, Girouard SD, Laurita KR, et al: Mechanism linking T-wave alternans to the genesis of cardiac fibrillation. Circulation 99:1385-1394, 1999.)

Cellular Basis of Action Potential Alternans

Although the cellular mechanism for action potential alternans is not completely elucidated, convincing data point to a primary role of sarcoplasmic reticulum Ca^{2+} cycling in its mechanism.[13] For instance, Shimizu and Antzelevitch used a ventricular wedge preparation in which the pathophysiology mimicked that of congenital long QT syndrome.[14] In this preparation, alteration of the T wave and APD was elicited during rapid pacing; application of ryanodine or lowering the extracellular calcium concentration abolished these alterations implicating intracellular Ca^{2+} cycling in the maintenance of MTWA.[14] Other workers have shown that calcium transient alternans can occur during rapid pacing when membrane potential alternans is prevented by voltage clamping, which suggests that calcium transient alternans is the underlying trigger for voltage alternans, and not vice versa.[15,16] Furthermore, the correlation between spatial heterogeneity of calcium transients and dispersion of action potential duration during MTWA also supports this notion.[12] Thus, compelling evidence indicates that Ca^{2+}-cycling proteins in general and two general properties of sarcoplasmic reticulum Ca^{2+} handling, Ca^{2+} release and reuptake, are directly implicated in the mechanism of beat-to-beat alternans of the calcium transient. Alternans of intracellular Ca^{2+} cycling then results in cellular action potential alternans through calcium-sensitive sarcolemmal ionic currents.[17,18]

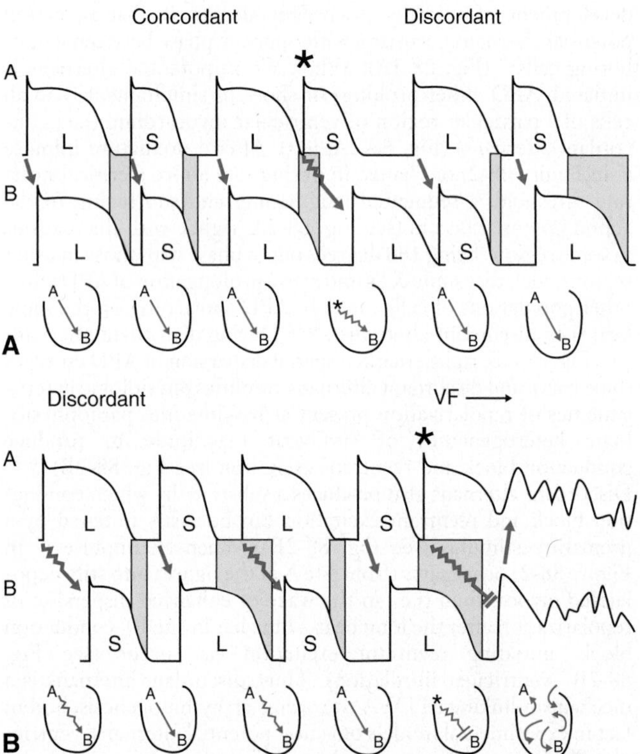

Figure 88-2 Concordant and discordant alternans and the induction of ventricular fibrillation (VF). Action potential propagation between two ventricular sites, A and B, is shown. **A,** Transition of concordant in discordant alternans following a premature impulse (*asterisk*). **B,** Occurrence of conduction block and reentrant excitation leading to ventricular fibrillation (see text for details). L, long action potential duration; S, short action potential duration. (Adapted from Wilson LD, Rosenbaum DS: Mechanisms of arrhythmogenic discordant cardiac alternans. Europace 9(Suppl 6):vi77-vi82, 2007.)

Other mechanisms involving membrane ionic and intracellular processes governing repolarization also have been proposed to explain action potential alternans.[19,20] An alternative hypothesis for the genesis of cellular alternans relates to APD restitution. *APD restitution* is the normal attenuation of APD that occurs in response to faster heart rates and is thought to be an adaptive mechanism for preserving diastole at rapid heart rates. APD restitution is presumed to cause action potential alternans because, at a constant cycle length, APD prolongation during one beat is necessarily followed by a short diastolic interval, which, according to restitution, will shorten APD on the following beat, which will then lengthen diastolic interval, causing repeated long-short-long APD cycles. The so-called restitution hypothesis states that action potential alternans will occur when the slope of the APD restitution curve exceeds unity. Although the restitution hypothesis for action potential alternans has been demonstrated primarily in modeling studies and has not been well supported experimentally,[19,20] it may nevertheless have significant impact on the spatial organization of alternans and therefore on discordant alternans in the heart, as discussed later on.

Finally, two additional, not necessarily mutually exclusive mechanisms have been proposed for discordant alternans. The first relates to spatial heterogeneities of calcium handling, which have recently been investigated as a potential mechanism underlying the spatial organization of action potential alternans and discordant alternans.[18-20] An additional mechanism contributing to susceptibility to discordant alternans has been proposed related to intracellular uncoupling.[11,21] Both of these mechanisms have been studied in computer simulation models and in experimental studies. Their precise contributions to the genesis of discordant alternans have to be yet fully elucidated. An excellent review of all of the discussed mechanisms has recently been published.[22]

Technical Aspects of Assessment of T Wave Alternans

Several computer algorithms for detection and quantification of MTWA, such as complex demodulation,[8] autocorrelation techniques,[23] and modified moving average analysis,[24] have been developed. The most widely applied technique, however, is based on the spectral method, which has been previously reported in detail.[7] This technique uses the vector magnitude ECG signal recorded from the three Frank orthogonal leads over at least 128 beats (Fig. 88-3). Each T wave is measured at the same time relative to the QRS complex. Because this spectrum is created by measurements taken once per beat, its frequencies are in units of cycles per beat. Accordingly, the point on the spectrum corresponding to 0.5 cycle per beat indicates the level of alteration of the T wave wavefront (see Fig. 88-3). The alternans power (μV^2) is defined as the difference between the power of the alternans frequency and the power at the noise frequency band (calculated over the reference frequency band between 0.44 and 0.49 cycle per beat). This is a measure of the true physiologic alternans level. The alternans voltage (V_{alt}) is simply the square root of alternans power and corresponds to the root-mean-square difference in the voltage (averaged over the T wave) between the overall mean beats and either the even-numbered or odd-numbered mean beats. A measure of the statistical significance of the alternans is defined as the alternans ratio (*K* score), calculated as the alternans power divided by the standard deviation of the noise in the reference frequency band. Alternans is considered significant if the *K* score is 3 or higher. This spectral method has been demonstrated to provide a robust measurement for MTWA.

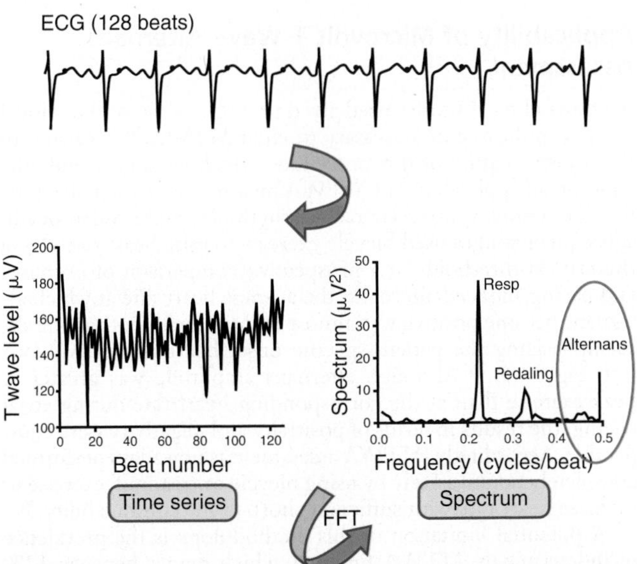

Figure 88-3 Schematic representation of microvolt T wave alternans (MTWA) assessment using the spectral method. The amplitudes of the corresponding points on the T wave are measured for 128 beats. A time series consisting of these 128 amplitudes is created. The power spectrum of this time series is computed using fast Fourier transform methods. In the power spectrum obtained from recordings during bicycle exercise, peaks corresponding to frequencies of respiration, pedaling, and alternans are illustrated. MTWA appears as a peak at exactly one-half of the beat frequency (0.5 cycle per beat). The amplitude of this peak is compared to the mean and standard deviation of the spectrum in a reference "noise band." FFT, fast Fourier transformation. (Adapted from Cohen RJ: TWA and laplacian imaging. In Zipes DP, Jalife J [eds]: Cardiac Electrophysiology: From Cell to Bedside, 3/E. Philadelphia, Saunders, 1999, pp 781-789.)

Correct assessment of MTWA depends heavily on the quality of the data collected, because MTWA is a low-amplitude and relatively low-frequency phenomenon that can be easily obscured by artifacts such as baseline wander and muscle artifacts. Accordingly, measurement of MTWA requires careful skin preparation to minimize electrode-to-skin impedance. In addition, specialized electrodes have been developed that record and process ECG signals, as well as impedance, from multiple segments of an electrode.

Determination of MTWA requires increases in heart rate. In every patient, there is a threshold heart rate above which MTWA will become apparent (see later). In the initial studies, heart rate was increased by means of atrial pacing.[25-28] Subsequently, techniques were developed to noninvasively generate an elevated heart rate by means of treadmill or bicycle exercise testing. MTWA test results obtained with both methods were highly reproducible (Fig. 88-4).[26] Currently, MTWA assessment generally is performed noninvasively.

Classification and Interpretation of Microvolt T Wave Alternans Recordings

As with every evolving new method, classification schemes for the assessment of MTWA had to be developed from the results of early clinical studies. A detailed synopsis on current guidelines for interpretation of MTWA tests has been published.[29] A brief overview follows: The presence of MTWA is defined by its magnitude, the alternans ratio (*K* score), the relationship between MTWA and heart rate, and assessment for the presence of artifacts that can cause alternans. Significant MTWA is defined as alternans having a value for V_{alt} of 1.9 μV or greater with a *K* score of 3 or higher (Table 88-1). Sustained alternans is defined as significant alternans that is at least 1 minute in duration and is consistently present above a patient-specific threshold heart rate, which is referred to as the onset heart rate.[26] Once the onset heart rate has been reached, the patient consistently has alternans until the heart rate falls below that threshold.

MTWA tracings are classified as positive, negative, or indeterminate. The classification of a MTWA tracing as positive requires only the determination of (1) whether sustained alternans is present and (2) the onset heart rate. The distinction between tracings that are negative and those that are indeterminate is made by the determination of the maximum negative heart rate as well as the maximum heart rate.

Positive tracings: If sustained alternans is present with an onset heart rate of 110 beats per minute or lower, then the tracing is classified as positive. The choice of the threshold heart rate of 110 beats per minute is based on the observation that in normal healthy subjects, alternans may develop at high heart rates, suggesting that alternans at high heart rates is not prognostically significant. If a tracing shows sustained alternans but the onset heart rate is above 110 beats per minute, then the tracing will be either negative or indeterminate, according to the patient's maximum negative heart rate (see Fig. 88-2).

Negative versus indeterminate tracings: The distinction between tracings that are negative and those that are indeterminate

Table 88-1 Classification of Microvolt T Wave Alternans Recordings

Definitions

Sustained alternans is defined as alternans that is consistently present at heart rates above a patient-specific onset heart rate (except for gaps believed to be caused by obscuring factors such as ectopics, noise or heart rate dips), in combination with:

- at least 1 minute with $V_{alt} \geq 1.9\,\mu V$
- alternans ratio ≥ 3 in any of the vector leads X, Y, Z, or VM (vector magnitude), or in a precordial lead and confirmed (with $V_{alt} \geq 1.9\,\mu V$) in an adjacent precordial lead
- some period of artifact-free data (defined below)

Alternans can be considered sustained even if the magnitude declines or disappears at heart rates above 120 beats per minute.

Interval heart rate: The lowest smoothed heart rate in a 1-minute interval.

Maximum negative heart rate: The highest interval heart rate associated with an interval without significant alternans, with noise level in the vector magnitude lead $\leq 1.8\,\mu V$ (or when the sum of the noise level plus the magnitude of alternans is $\leq 2.5\,\mu V$), with $\leq 10\%$ ectopic beats, and without lead malfunction.

Onset heart rate: The alternans onset heart rate is the smoothed heart rate above which sustained alternans is consistently present. In determining the onset heart rate, one should be prepared to read across short gaps which can be attributed to noise, ectopics, or heart rate dips.

Maximum heart rate: The highest interval heart rate.

Artifact-free data: The data are considered *artifact-free* if the following conditions are met:

- Ectopic or premature beats $\leq$ 10% of all beats
- Respiratory activity is not at 0.25 cycle per beat
- Variation in instantaneous heart rate is less than 30 beats per minute over a 128-beat segment
- Absence of R-R interval alternans level ($\geq$2 ms with alternans ratio $\geq$3)

Classification Criteria

Positive: A test is positive if it demonstrates sustained alternans with an onset heart rate $\leq$110 beats per minute, or sustained alternans at the resting heart rate, even if that is higher than 110 beats per minute.

Negative: A test is negative if it (1) does not meet the criteria for being positive and (2) maximum negative heart rate is $\geq$105 beats per minute. A test is also classified as negative if during a *maximal* exercise test the maximum heart rate $\geq$80 beats per minute and if the maximum negative heart rate $\geq$ (maximum heart rate 5 beats per minute).

Indeterminate: A test is indeterminate if it cannot be definitively classified as either positive or negative.

is based on the maximum negative heart rate, the highest heart rate on the tracing at which one is confident that alternans is not present. The original classification used prospectively in a number of studies[30,31] required that the maximum negative heart rate be 105 beats per minute or greater for a tracing to be classified as negative. For example, if a tracing has excessive levels of ectopy or noise above a heart rate of 95 beats per minute, then one cannot be confident that alternans is not present above a heart rate of 95 beats per minute, and the tracing cannot be considered to be negative. Accordingly, the maximum negative heart rate is 95 beats per minute and the tracing is classified as indeterminate. Perhaps if the ectopy or noise levels were reduced, alternans would be "unmasked" at a heart rate of 100 beats per minute. For this reason, tracings without sustained alternans and with a maximum negative heart rate less than 105 beats per minute are considered indeterminate. Similarly, tracings with sustained alternans with an onset heart rate greater than 110 beats per minute (i.e., alternans that is not prognostically significant) also are classified as indeterminate if the maximum negative heart rate is less than 105 beats per minute.

Application of this classification can result in indeterminate results in up to 25% to 30% of subjects in some populations.[30-32] Many of the tracings were classified as indeterminate because the patient's maximal heart rate was less than 105 beats per minute, so the tracing had no chance of being classified as negative (because the maximum negative heart rate cannot be greater than the maximum heart rate).

Clinical Studies on Microvolt T Wave Alternans

Applicability of Microvolt T Wave Alternans Assessment

The first clinical studies used atrial pacing to achieve the critical increase in heart rate necessary to elicit MTWA.[26-28] Owing to the invasive nature of this procedure, which would preclude the widespread applicability of MTWA measurement as a risk stratifier for serious ventricular tachyarrhythmias and sudden death, subsequent studies used bicycle exercise to raise heart rate above the critical threshold. In a prospective comparison of exercise- and pacing-induced alternans, the average heart rate at which alternans became positive was almost identical with both methods, reemphasizing the patient-specific onset heart rate of MTWA (see Fig 88-4).[26] Although alternans amplitude was greater at peak exercise than at the corresponding heart rate during atrial pacing, the results in terms of positivity and negativity were comparable. Accordingly, MTWA assessment is nowadays performed completely noninvasively by using bicycle or treadmill exercise to increase heart rate with sufficient short-term reproducibility.[33]

A potential limitation of this methodology is the prevalence of indeterminate MTWA findings, which ranges between 12% and 25%.[29-32] A high proportion of indeterminate results are due to the inability of patients to increase their heart rate above 105 beats per minute (e.g., owing to the presence of heart failure or as a result of beta-blocker therapy) or to excessive ventricular ectopy during exercise (patient factors). Other reasons for indeterminate MTWA testing include excessive noise and an exercise protocol that causes an excessively rapid rise in heart rate (technical factors). In terms of prognostic information, however, the current thinking is that an indeterminate test due to patient factors carries prognostic information similar to that obtained with a positive MTWA test result. Accordingly, newer studies

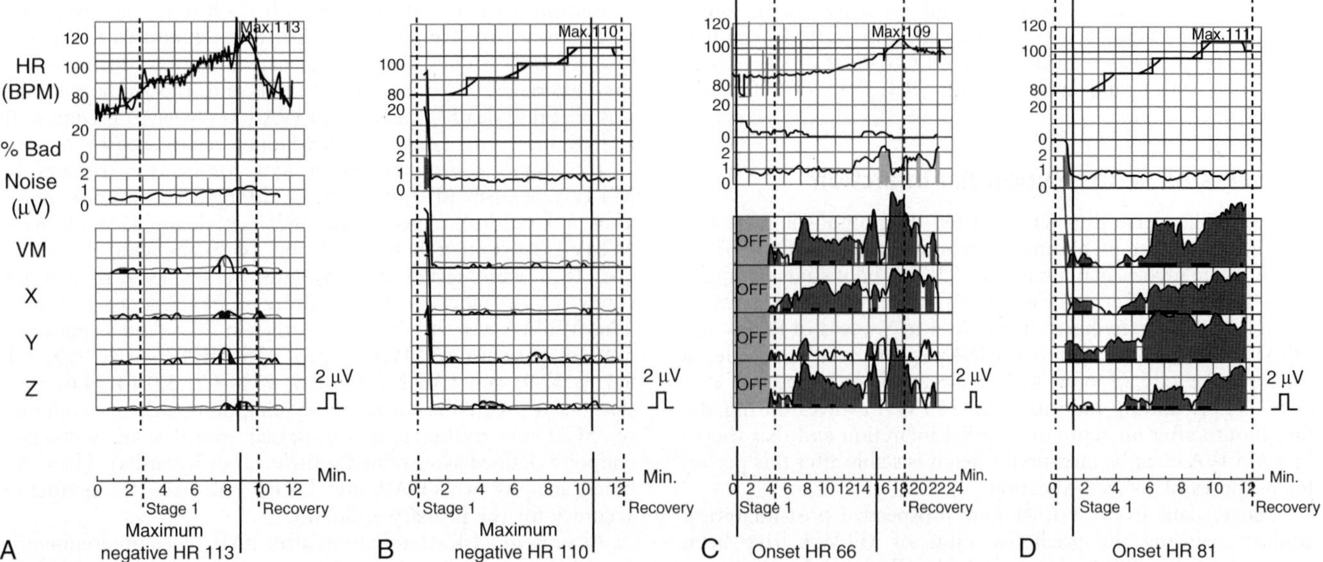

Figure 88-4 Examples of microvolt T wave alternans (MTWA) test results. *From top to bottom*: Heart rate (HR) trend; percentage of bad beats; noise level; MTWA amplitudes in vector magnitude lead VM and orthogonal leads X, Y, Z. **A**, A bicycle exercise negative MTWA test result. **B**, Atrial pacing test in the same patient as in **A** also is negative for MTWA. **C**, Bicycle exercise–induced sustained MTWA *(gray shaded area)*. **D**, Atrial pacing test in the same patient also yields MTWA-positive findings.

have differentiated "non-negative" results on testing (i.e., positive and indeterminate) from negative results. Most recently, Kaufman and associates, using data from a large prospective study, specifically looked at the prognostic yield of indeterminate MTWA test results. These workers reported that patients with dilated cardiomyopathy and an indeterminate MTWA test result had a 2-year rate for the occurrence of death or sustained ventricular tachyarrhythmias of 17.8%, compared with 12.3% in patients with a positive test result.[34]

Microvolt T Wave Alternans Assessment and Results of Invasive Electrophysiologic Testing in Patients at Risk for Ventricular Tachycardia or Fibrillation

Rosenbaum and associates carried out the first clinical landmark study of MTWA assessment in 1994.[25] In this study of 83 patients undergoing electrophysiologic testing, an excellent correlation was found between the presence of MTWA and inducibility of ventricular tachycardia or ventricular fibrillation. In fact, repolarization alternans carried a relative risk (RR) of 5.2 for susceptibility to inducible ventricular arrhythmias. Moreover, during a 20-month observation period, MTWA and inducibility of ventricular arrhythmias were significant and essentially equivalent predictors of arrhythmia-free survival ($P < .001$). A more recent multicenter study of 313 patients referred for electrophysiologic testing revealed similar results.[31] MTWA predicted the primary endpoint (composite of sudden cardiac death [SCD], sustained ventricular tachycardia, ventricular fibrillation, and appropriate ICD discharge) with an RR of 10.9, compared with 7.1 for electrophysiologic inducibility of ventricular arrhythmias. This aspect of analysis was similar to that in the Rosenbaum study[25]: The RR of MTWA for predicting electrophysiologic outcome was 5.7.

Hohnloser and associates measured MTWA in 95 consecutive patients with a history of ventricular tachyarrhythmias undergoing implantation of an ICD.[30] In addition, other conventional noninvasive risk stratifiers were assessed, and all patients underwent electrophysiologic testing. The endpoint of this study was first appropriate ICD therapy for electrogram-documented ventricular fibrillation or ventricular tachycardia during an average follow-up period of 442 days. Kaplan-Meier survival analysis revealed that MTWA ($P < .006$) and left ventricular ejection fraction (LVEF) ($P < .04$) were the only significant univariate risk stratifiers. Actually, on multivariate Cox regression analysis, only MTWA was a statistically significant independent predictor of future tachyarrhythmic events.[30] These results were subsequently confirmed in a similar study comprising 248 subjects undergoing electrophysiologic testing.[35]

Microvolt T Wave Alternans Assessment for Risk Stratification

A plethora of studies have evaluated the prognostic power of MTWA assessment in an attempt to provide risk stratification for patients prone to sudden death. The need for better assessment of risk for serious ventricular tachyarrhythmias is driven by the fact that with the implantable defibrillator, a highly efficacious tool for preventing arrhythmogenic death is available. The use of the ICD carries its own risks, however, as a result of the invasive character of this therapy, and widespread applicability is limited by the associated high costs and need for trained specialists for application. Accordingly, more accurate identification of the patient at highest risk for arrhythmogenic death is of paramount clinical importance.

Although most risk stratification studies using MTWA assessment have been conducted in survivors of acute myocardial infarction or in patients with cardiomyopathy (see later on), one recent large study evaluated the predictive power of MTWA for subsequent mortality in a general population of 1037 patients referred for a clinical exercise test.[36] These investigators from Finland used the time-domain modified moving average method to test for the presence of MTWA. The study period was 44 ± 7 months, during which time 59 deaths occurred. After adjustment for important baseline characteristics, time-domain documented

MTWA turned out to be a powerful predictor for all-cause mortality (RR, 3.3; 95% confidence interval [CI], 1.8 to 6.3; $P = .001$), cardiovascular mortality (RR, 6.0, 95% CI, 2.8 to 12.8, $P < .001$), and sudden death (RR, 7.4; 95% CI, 2.8 to 19.4; $P < .001$).

Survivors of Acute Myocardial Infarction

Several studies have thus far evaluated the prognostic power of MTWA for future arrhythmic events, including SCD in survivors of acute myocardial infarction.[37-41] In a pilot study comprising 448 patients after myocardial infarction, MTWA was tested 5 to 21 days after the heart attack. At 4 to 8 weeks of follow-up, MTWA testing was repeated in 184 patients; results revealed a concordance rate of only 67% between determinate MTWA tests.[37] This finding indicated that MTWA evolves during the first month after an acute myocardial infarction and that therefore MTWA must be measured when it is stable after this period for purposes of risk stratification.

Today, data from at least four prospective post-infarction studies analyzing the predictive value of MTWA have been reported (Table 88-2). In a study by Ikeda and colleagues, MTWA and late potentials from the signal-averaged ECG (SAECG) were assessed in 102 infarct survivors.[38] Primary percutaneous coronary intervention had been performed in 98% of the patients, but only 31% were given beta-blocking agents. During a follow-up period of 13 ± 6 months, sustained ventricular tachycardia or fibrillation developed in 15 patients. All but 1 of these 15 patients had a positive MTWA test result. The positive predictive value with respect to arrhythmic events was 28% for MTWA alone and 50% for the combination of positive MTWA and SAECG measurements.[38]

In another prospective follow-up study, MTWA and other noninvasive risk markers were assessed in 379 consecutive infarct survivors.[39] Of these, 133 (35%) had an incomplete test (inability to perform exercise in 56 patients and target heart rate below 105 beats per minute in 77 patients). A positive MTWA result was found in only 14.7% of the patients ($N = 56$), a negative test result was found in 38% ($N = 144$), and the test result was indeterminate in 12% ($N = 46$). Of note, 97% of patients received beta-blockers and 2% received amiodarone. A positive MTWA was not a predictor of all-cause mortality (primary study endpoint); however, an incomplete MTWA test was the most significant predictor of cardiac death.[39] Of note, this study suffered from two important limitations: First, MTWA was assessed only 8 days after myocardial infarction, during which time alternans is quite unstable.[37] Second, the study endpoint was all-cause death, whereas MTWA has power to predict only arrhythmic events (and not heart failure–related death).

Ikeda and colleagues tested 850 consecutive patients by MTWA assessment and SAECG during the subacute phase after infarction.[38] Specifically, 82% of patients underwent MTWA assessment between 2 and 10 weeks after the event, and 18% were tested months later. Only 13% of patients received beta-blockers at the time of MTWA assessment.[38] The MTWA test result was positive in 36% and negative in 52% of patients. MTWA (hazard ratio [HR], 11.4; 95% CI, 3.4 to 37.9) and LVEF (HR, 6.6; 95% CI, 3.0 to 14.6) were significant predictors for the study endpoints (primary endpoint of SCD or resuscitated ventricular fibrillation; secondary endpoint defined as sustained ventricular tachycardia). The combined analysis of MTWA and LVEF enhanced the predictive accuracy for the primary endpoint.

At present, risk stratification after AMI relies predominantly on the presence of reduced left ventricular function. Little is known about the value of risk markers in infarct survivors with preserved left ventricular function. Accordingly, Ikeda and colleagues measured MTWA in 1014 patients with an LVEF of 0.40 or greater at 48 ± 66 days after an acute myocardial infarction along with 10 other commonly used risk variables.[41] Over a mean period of 32 ± 14 months, a positive MTWA, nonsustained ventricular tachycardia, and ventricular late potentials were predictors of SCD or ventricular tachyarrhythmias (primary study endpoint). On multivariate analysis, a positive MTWA test result was the most significant predictor (HR, 19.7).

In conclusion, the foregoing study results indicate that MTWA assessment may yield prognostic information regarding ventricular tachyarrhythmic events in infarct survivors, even in those with preserved left ventricular function. It seems clear, however, that MTWA evolves during the subacute phase of myocardial infarction, indicating that its determination should be postponed until some weeks after the index event. Ongoing studies such as the Microvolt T Wave Alternans Testing for Risk Stratification of Post-MI Patients I (MASTER I) trial will further delineate the role of MTWA assessment in risk stratification in survivors of acute myocardial infarction.

Table 88-2 Prospective Studies Using Microvolt T Wave Alternans for Risk Stratification in Survivors of Acute Myocardial Infarction

Study (ref)	Patient Population	No. of Patients/ Follow-up (mo)	Primary Study Endpoint	% of Patients with Non-negative MTWA	Main Result
Ikeda, 2000 (38)	Survivors of AMI	102 13 ± 6 mo	Spontaneous ventricular tachyarrhythmias	n.a.	MTWA predictive of PEP (HR 16.8)
Tapanainen, 2001* (39)	Survivors of AMI	379 14 ± 8 mo	All-cause mortality	88% (31% incomplete MTWA test)	MTWA not predictive of PEP
Ikeda, 2002† (40)	Survivors of AMI	850 25 ± 13 mo	Arrhythmic death or resuscitated VF	64%	MTWA predictive of PEP (HR 5.9)
Ikeda, 2006‡ (41)	Survivors of AMI, LVEF >0.40	1041 32 ± 14 mo	Arrhythmic death or VT/VF	26%	MTWA predictive of PEP (HR 19.7)

AMI, acute myocardial infarction; HR, hazard ratio; LVEF, left ventricular ejection fraction; MTWA, microvolt T wave alternans; PEP, primary study endpoint; VT, ventricular tachycardia; VF, ventricular fibrillation.

*MTWA measured 8 ± 2 days after myocardial infarction;

†MTWA measured 2.7 ± 5.4 months after myocardial infarction;

‡MTWA measured 48 ± 66 days after myocardial infarction.

Patients with Ischemic and Nonischemic Cardiomyopathy

Dilated cardiomyopathy is a clinical condition associated with a high incidence of sudden, presumably arrhythmogenic death. Unfortunately, assessment of conventional risk stratifiers such as spontaneous ventricular arrhythmias, autonomic markers, or electrophysiologic testing has yielded insufficient predictive power for future tachyarrhythmic events. On the other hand, recent randomized controlled trials[42-44] have demonstrated that prophylactic ICD therapy in such patients improves outcome. The absolute reduction in mortality, however, was relatively small (i.e., 5.6% over 20 months in the Multicenter Automatic Defibrillator Implantation Trial *II* [MADIT II]).

In the United States, approximately 400,000 patients are diagnosed every year with coronary artery disease and advanced left ventricular dysfunction. Thus, routinely implanting defibrillators in this population would be very expensive. These considerations have prompted several studies that assessed the role of MTWA assessment in targeting ICD therapy to those patients with dilated cardiomyopathy, with or without signs of congestive heart failure, who are at highest risk for sudden death.

As summarized in Table 88-3, at least 8 published studies have addressed this issue. Hohnloser and coworkers reported the first study in which 129 MADIT II–like patients with ischemic cardiomyopathy and a negative result on MTWA testing were found to have a significantly better prognosis compared with those with a positive result on MTWA testing.[45] Bloomfield and associates confirmed these specific findings in 177 patients with ischemic cardiomyopathy and an LVEF of 0.30 or less, who constituted a subgroup of a large multicenter trial.[46] In that trial, a total of 549 patients with ischemic or nonischemic cardiomyopathy, an LVEF of 0.40 or less, and no history of sustained ventricular arrhythmias were enrolled.[47] Over a mean follow-up period of 20 ± 6 months, patients who tested MTWA-positive had an HR for the primary study endpoint (all-cause mortality or nonfatal sustained ventricular arrhythmias) of 6.5 (95% CI, 2.4 to 18.1; $P < .001$), relative to findings in MTWA-negative patients (Fig. 88-5). The largest trial published today was recently reported by Chow and coworkers.[48] These investigators identified 768 consecutive patients with ischemic cardiomyopathy and an LVEF of 0.35 or less who were classified as MTWA negative or non-negative (including MTWA-positive and -indeterminate patients[34]). After adjustment for important baseline variables, a non-negative MTWA test result was associated with a significantly higher risk for all-cause (HR, 2.24; 95% CI, 1.34 to 3.75; $P = .002$) and arrhythmic mortality (HR, 2.29; 95% CI, 1.0 to 5.25; $p = .049$). On the other hand, nonarrhythmic mortality was not significantly different in patients who tested non-negative or negative for MTWA. Accordingly, there is now convincing evidence that MTWA is a strong and independent predictor of all-cause and arrhythmic mortality, particularly in patients with ischemic cardiomyopathy. Moreover, a MTWA-based risk stratification strategy in MADIT II–like patients may actually improve the cost-effectiveness of ICD therapy, as shown by Chan and associates[49] using data from the largest MTWA study in ischemic cardiomyopathy.[49]

Table 88-3 Prospective Studies Using Microvolt T Wave Alternans for Risk Stratification in Patients with Dilated Cardiomyopathy

Study (ref)	Patient Population	No. of Patients/ Follow-up (mo)	PEP	% of Patients with Non-negative MTWA	Main Result
Klingenheben (2000) (32)	CHF, LVEF <0.45, ICMP 70%, NICMP 30%	107/14.6 mo	Arrhythmic death or VT/VF	70%	MTWA = predictor of PEP (HR ∞)
Hohnloser (2003) (45)	ICMP, LVEF <0.35	129/24 mo	Arrhythmic death	73%	MTWA = predictor of PEP (HR ∞)
Bloomfield (2004) (46)	ICMP, LVEF <0.35	177/20 ± 6 mo	2 year all-cause mortality	68%	MTWA = predictor of PEP (HR 4.8)
Hohnloser (2003) (53)	NICMP	137/14 ± 6 mo	Arrhythmic death or resuscitated VF/VT	75%	MTWA = predictor of PEP (HR 3.4)
Grimm (2003) (54)	NICMP	343/52 ± 21	Arrhythmic death or resuscitated VF/VT	n.a.	MTWA not predictive of PEP
Bloomfield (2006) (47)	ICMP (49%) NICMP (51%)	549/20 ± 6 mo	All-cause mortality or non-fatal VT/VF	66%	MTWA = predictor of PEP (HR 6.5)
Chow (2006) (48)	ICMP, LVEF <0.35	768/18 ± 10 mo	all-cause mortality	67%	MTWA = predictor of all-cause (HR 2.2) and arrhythmic mortality (HR 2.3)
Salerno-Uriarte (2007) (55)	NICMP, LVEF <0.40	446/n.a.	Cardiac death, life-threatening ventricular arrhythmias	65%	MTWA = predictor of PEP (HR 4.0)

CHF, congestive heart failure; HR, hazard ratio; ICMP, ischemic cardiomyopathy; LVEF, left ventricular ejection fraction; MTWA, microvolt T wave alternans; n.a., not available; NICMP, nonischemic cardiomyopathy; PEP, primary endpoint; VF, ventricular fibrillation; VT, ventricular tachycardia.

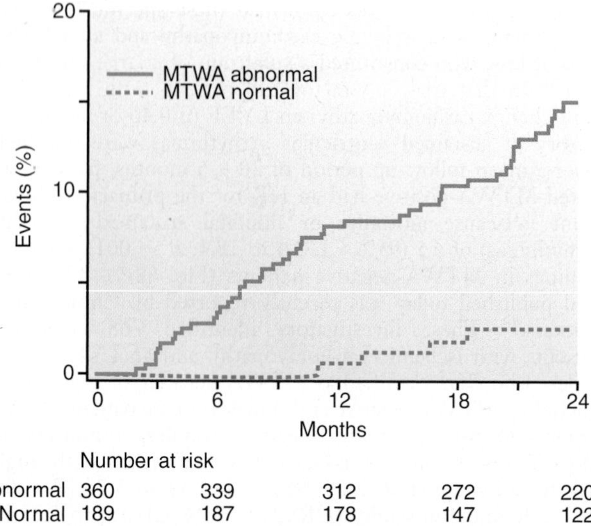

Figure 88-5 Kaplan-Meier mortality curves for patients with normal versus abnormal microvolt T wave alternans (MTWA) test results. During the 2-year follow-up period, only 4 events occurred in 189 patients with a negative MTWA result, compared with 47 in the non-negative group. Non-negative test results comprised both positive results (n = 162; 2-year event rate, 12.3%) and indeterminate results (n = 198; 2-year event rate, 17.5%). (From Bloomfield D, Bigger J, Steinman R, et al: Microvolt T-wave alternans and the risk of death or sustained ventricular arrhythmias in patients with left ventricular dysfunction. J Am Coll Cardiol 47:456-463, 2006.)

In nonischemic cardiomyopathy, the evidence is similar. Relatively small early studies[50-52] indicated that MTWA may yield predictive power for subsequent arrhythmic events in patients with nonischemic cardiomyopathy. Although two further studies by Hohnloser and associates[53] and Bloomfield[47] confirmed these findings, one additional study in 343 patients with nonischemic cardiomyopathy found no association of MTWA with future arrhythmic events.[54] The reason for this discrepant observation is not clear but may be related to methodologic differences between the studies. Most recently, preliminary results from the largest MTWA study in nonischemic cardiomyopathy were reported.[55] In an Italian multicenter trial, 446 patients with nonischemic cardiomyopathy, NYHA functional class II or III, and a, LVEF of 0.40 or less were studied and followed for the endpoint of cardiac death and life-threatening ventricular arrhythmias. Confirming results of a majority of earlier studies (see Table 88-3), an abnormal MTWA test was associated with a four-fold risk of the primary endpoint.

In summary, therefore, in patients with congestive heart failure in the setting of ischemic or nonischemic cardiomyopathy, assessment of MTWA holds promise as a clinically important risk stratifier for future tachyarrhythmic events including SCD. The results of MTWA testing (particularly its high negative predictive value) may offer the possibility of tailoring ICD therapy to those patients most likely to derive benefit from this expensive therapy.

Microvolt T Wave Alternans Assessment in the Presence of Antiarrhythmic Drug Therapy

Antiarrhythmic drug therapy may exert a modulating effect on MTWA. In particular, antiarrhythmic drugs that prolong ventricular repolarization may affect repolarization alternans. Kavesh and coworkers prospectively evaluated the effects of procainamide on MTWA in 24 patients with inducible sustained ventricular tachycardia at baseline and after acute drug loading.[56] The magnitude of MTWA amplitude decreased from 0.6 ± 0.8 to 0.3 ± 0.4 μV during sinus rhythm, from 2.0 ± 1.6 to 0.7 ± 0.7 μV during pacing at 100 beats per minute, and from 3.0 ± 2.0 to 1.7 ± 1.8 μV during pacing at 120 beats per minute ($P < .001$). This resulted in a decrease in the sensitivity of MTWA for induction of sustained ventricular tachycardia from 87% to 60% at a heart rate of 120 beats per minute.

The effects of the class III antiarrhythmic drug amiodarone on the prevalence of MTWA were evaluated in a retrospective analysis in patients fitted with an ICD.[57] In that study, a positive MTWA was found in only 1 of 9 patients (11%) receiving amiodarone, compared with 14 of 22 patients (64%) not on antiarrhythmic drug therapy. During follow-up, the presence of MTWA predicted future appropriate ICD therapy for ventricular tachyarrhythmias.

In another prospective, randomized study, 54 patients underwent repeated MTWA assessment during drug-free baseline and after acute intravenous administration of DL-sotalol or metoprolol.[58] A significant decrease in V_{alt} after drug administration was observed in the entire patient population (8.4 ± 6.4 to 4.7 ± 3.3 μV; $P < .001$), as well as in the subgroup of patients with coronary disease (8.2 ± 6.8 to 4.5 ± 3.5 μV; $P < .001$). The decrease in V_{alt} was comparable in patients receiving metoprolol (7.9 + 6.0 versus 4.9 ± 4.2 μV; $P < .001$) and in those receiving sotalol (8.6 ± 6.8 versus 4.4 ± 2.3 μV; $P = .001$). The heart rate at which MTWA became detectable was similar at baseline and at on-drug assessment in both study groups (metoprolol: 94 ± 8 versus 95 ± 7 beats per minute; $P = .86$; sotalol: 99 ± 10 versus 98 ± 12 beats per minute; $P = .83$). In 8 of 48 patients with MTWA-positive baseline ECG, MTWA turned negative after drug administration; 5 patients had received metoprolol and 3 had received sotalol. Of note, baseline V_{alt} was lower in these 8 patients than in those who remained MTWA-positive after beta-blockers (4.1 ± 1.4 versus 9.2 ± 6.7 μV; $P = .026$). Administration of beta-blockers in these patients reduced V_{alt} below 2 μV.

Somewhat different observations were recently reported by Rashba and associates in patients with ischemic cardiomyopathy and inducible ventricular tachycardia or ventricular fibrillation who underwent pacing MTWA assessment at baseline and after drug infusion.[59] After the administration of esmolol, a ultra-short-acting beta-blocker, in 20 patients, the number of MTWA-positive results was reduced, from an incidence of 70% to 35% ($P < .05$). As in the study by Klingenheben and colleagues,[58] the maximum voltage in the vector magnitude also was reduced after beta-blocker administration. The reasons why the prevalence of positive MTWA findings was significantly reduced in one[40] but not in the other[58] study are not entirely evident. It is intriguing, however, that beta-blockers, which are known to reduce risk of spontaneous ventricular arrhythmias, also tend to reduce MTWA. Because cardioactive drugs may alter MTWA and may also modulate susceptibility to spontaneous ventricular arrhythmias, it would seem to make most sense to perform MTWA testing for purposes of risk stratification while maintaining the ongoing pharmacological milieu of the patient. When the pharmacologic milieu of the patient is altered, MTWA testing should be repeated to determine if repolarization alternans status is altered.

Future Role of Microvolt T Wave Alternans Assessment

Recent years have seen a marked increase in understanding of the mechanisms underlying MTWA, its close association with malignant ventricular tachyarrhythmias, and its role as a non-invasive tool for risk stratification for arrhythmogenic complications. In multiple studies, results of MTWA recordings have been demonstrated to be predictive of the occurrence of ventricular tachyarrhythmic events, most notably in patients with ischemic or nonischemic cardiomyopathy. MTWA testing has been demonstrated to have an excellent negative predictive value in these populations, suggesting that patients with a negative result on MTWA testing generally are at low risk for sustained ventricular tachyarrhythmias and can be managed conservatively. An unanswered question relates to the problem of how often and at which time intervals MTWA-negative patients should be retested for potentially newly developed alternans. This problem needs to be prospectively studied. In summary, it appears that in the future, assessment of MTWA will help in better utilization of health care resources by directing expensive ICD therapy to those patients who are indeed at highest risk for sudden cardiac death.

References

1. Hering HE: Das Wesen des Herzalternans. Muenchner Med Wochenschr 4:1417-1421, 1908.
2. Lewis T: Notes upon alternation of the heart. Q J Med 4:141-144, 1910.
3. Kalter HH, Schwartz ML: Electrical alternans. N Y State J Med 1:1164-1166, 1948.
4. Amoundas AA, Tomaselli GF, Esperer HD: Pathophysiological basis and clinical application of T-wave alternans. J Am Coll Cardiol 40:207-217, 2002.
5. Schwartz PJ, Malliani A: Electrical alternation of the T wave: Clinical and experimental evidence of its relationship with the sympathetic nervous system and with the long-QT syndrome. Am Heart J 89:45-50, 1975.
6. Adam DR, Powell AO, Gordon H, Cohen RJ: Ventricular fibrillation and fluctuations in the magnitude of the repolarization vector. IEEE Comp Cardiol 241-244, 1982.
7. Smith JM, Clancy EA, Valeri CR, et al: Electrical alternans and cardiac electrical instability. Circulation 77:110-121, 1988.
8. Nearing B, Huang HA, Verrier RL: Dynamic tracking of cardiac vulnerability by complex demodulation of the T wave. Science 252:437-440, 1991.
9. Shusterman V, Goldberg A, London B: Upsurge in T-wave alternans and nonalternating repolarization instability precedes spontaneous initiation of ventricular tachyarrhythmias in humans. Circulation 113:2880-2887, 2006.
10. Pastore JM, Girouard SD, Laurita KR, et al: Mechanism linking T-wave alternans to the genesis of cardiac fibrillation. Circulation 99:1385-1394, 1999.
11. Pastore JM, Rosenbaum DS: Role of structural barriers in the mechanism of alternans-induced reentry. Circ Res 87:1157-1163, 2000.
12. Walker ML, Rosenbaum DS: Repolarization alternans: Implications for the mechanism and prevention of sudden cardiac death. Cardiovasc Res 57:599-614, 2003.
13. Davey P, Bryant S, Hart G: Rate-dependent electrical, contractile and restitution properties of isolated left ventricular myocytes in guinea-pig hypertrophy. Acta Physiol Scand 171:17-28, 2001.
14. Shimizu W, Antzelevitch C: Cellular and ionic basis for T-wave alternans under long-QT conditions. Circulation 99:1499-1507, 1999.
15. Chudin E, Goldhaber JI, Weiss J, Kogan B: Intracellular Ca dynamics and the stability of ventricular tachycardia. Biophys J 77:2930-2941, 1999.
16. Hüser J, Wang YG, Sheehan KA, et al: Functional coupling between glycolysis and excitation-contraction coupling underlies alternans in cat heart cells. J Physiol (Lond) 524:795-806, 2000.
17. Sato D, Shiferaw Y, Garfinkel A, et al: Spatially discordant alternans in cardiac tissue: Role of calcium cycling. Circ Res 99:520-527, 2006.
18. Weiss JN, Karma A, Shiferaw Y, et al: From pulsus to pulseless: The saga of cardiac alternans. Circ Res 98:1244-1253, 2006.
19. Pruvot EJ, Katra RP, Rosenbaum DS, Laurita KR: Role of calcium cycling versus restitution in the mechanism of repolarization alternans. Circ Res 94:1083-1090, 2004.
20. Goldhaber JI, Xie LH, Duong T, et al: Action potential duration restitution and alternans in rabbit ventricular myocytes: The key role of intracellular calcium cycling. Circ Res 96:459-466, 2005.
21. Watanabe MA, Fenton FH, Evans SJ, et al: Mechanisms for discordant alternans. J Cardiovasc Electrophysiol 12:196-206, 2001.
22. Wilson LD, Rosenbaum DS: Mechanisms of arrhythmogenic discordant cardiac alternans. Europace 9(Suppl 6):vi77-vi82, 2007.
23. Zarebra W, Moss AJ, le Cessie S, Hall WJ: T-wave alternans in idiopathic long QT syndrome. J Am Coll Cardiol 23:1541-1546, 1994.
24. Cox V, Patel M, Kim J, Liu T, et al: Predicting arrhythmia-free survival using spectral and modified-moving average analyses of T-wave alternans. PACE 30:352-358, 2007.
25. Rosenbaum DS, Jackson LE, Smith JM, et al: Electrical alternans and vulnerability to ventricular arrhythmias. N Engl J Med 330:235-241, 1994.
26. Hohnloser SH, Klingenheben T, Zabel M, et al: T wave alternans during exercise and atrial pacing in humans. J Cardiovasc Electrophysiol 8:987-993, 1997.
27. Estes MNA, Michaud G, Zipes DP, et al: Electrical alternans during rest and exercise as predictors of vulnerability to ventricular arrhythmias. Am J Cardiol 80:1314-1318, 1997.
28. Rashba EJ, Osman AF, MacMurdy K, et al: Exercise is superior to pacing for T wave alternans measurement in subjects with chronic coronary artery disease and left ventricular dysfunction. J Cardiovasc Electrophysiol 13:845-850, 2002.
29. Bloomfield DM, Hohnloser SH, Cohen RJ: Interpretation and classification of microvolt T wave alternans tests. J Cardiovasc Electrophysiol 13:502-512, 2002.
30. Hohnloser SH, Klingenheben T, Li YG, et al: T wave alternans as a predictor of recurrent ventricular tachyarrhythmias in ICD recipients: Prospective comparison with conventional risk markers. J Cardiovasc Electrophysiol 9:1258-1268, 1998.
31. Gold MR, Bloomfield DM, Anderson KP, et al: A comparison of T-wave alternans, signal averaged electrocardiography and programmed ventricular stimulation for arrhythmia risk stratification. J Am Coll Cardiol 36:2247-2253, 2000.
32. Klingenheben T, Zabel M, D'Agostino RB, et al: Predictive value of T-wave alternans for arrhythmic events in patients with congestive heart failure. Lancet 356:651-652, 2000.
33. Bloomfield DM, Ritvo BS, Parides MK, Kim MH: The immediate reproducibility of T wave alternans during bicycle exercise. PACE 25:1185-1191, 2002.
34. Kaufman E, Bloomfield D, Steinman R, et al: "Indeterminate" microvolt T-wave alternans tests predict high risk of death or sustained ventricular arrhythmias in patients with left ventricular dysfunction. J Am Coll Cardiol 48:1399-1404, 2006.
35. Tanno K, Ryu S, Watanabe N, et al: Microvolt T-wave alternans as a predictor of ventricular tachyarrhythmias. Circulation 109:1854-1858, 2004.
36. Nieminen T, Lehtimäki T, Viik J, et al: T-wave alternans predicts mortality in a apopulation undergoing a clinically indicated exercise test. Eur Heart J 28:2332-2337, 2007. Epub 2007 Jul 25.
37. Hohnloser SH, Huikuri H, Schwartz PJ, et al: T-wave alternans in post myocardial infarction patients (ACES pilot study) [abstract]. J Am Coll Cardiol 33:144A, 1999.
38. Ikeda T, Sakata T, Takami M, et al: Combined assessment of T-wave alternans and late potentials used to predict arrhythmic events after myocardial infarction. J Am Coll Cardiol 35:722-730, 2000.
39. Tapanainen JM, Still AM, Airaksinen KEJ, Huikuri HV: Prognostic significance of risk stratifiers of mortality, including T-wave alternans, after acute myocardial infarction: Results of a prospective follow-up study. J Cardiovasc Electrophysiol 12:645-652, 2001.
40. Ikeda T, Saito H, Tanno K, et al: T-wave alternans as a predictor for sudden cardiac death after myocardial infarction. Am J Cardiol 89:79-82, 2002.
41. Ikeda T, Yoshino H, Sugi K, et al: Predictive value of microvolt T-wave alternans for sudden cardiac death in patients with preserved cardiac function after acute myocardial infarction. J Am Coll Cardiol 48:2268-2274, 2006.

42. Moss AJ, Zarebra W, Jackson W, et al: Prophylactic implantation of a defibrillator in patients with myocardial infarction and reduced ejection fraction. N Engl J Med 346:877-883, 2002.
43. Kadish A, Dyer A, Daubert JP, et al: Prophylactic defibrillator implantation in patients with nonischemic dilated cardiomyopathy. N Engl J Med 350:2152-2158, 2004.
44. Bardy GH, Lee KL, Mark DB, et al: Amiodarone or an implantable cardioverter-defibrillator for congestive heart failure. N Engl J Med 352:225-237, 2005.
45. Hohnloser SH, Ikeda T, Bloomfield DM, et al: T-wave alternans negative coronary patients with low ejection fraction and benefit from defibrillator implantation. Lancet 362:125-126, 2003.
46. Bloomfield D, Steinman R, Namerow P, et al: Microvolt T-wave alternans distinguishes between patients likely and patients not likely to benefit from implanted cardiac defibrillator therapy. Circulation 110:1885-1889, 2004.
47. Bloomfield D, Bigger J, Steinman R, et al: Microvolt T-wave alternans and the risk of death or sustained ventricular arrhythmias in patients with left ventricular dysfunction. J Am Coll Cardiol 47:456-463, 2006.
48. Chow T, Kereiakes D, Bartone C, et al: Prognostic utility of microvolt T-wave alternans in risk stratification of patients with ischemic cardiomyopathy. J Am Coll Cardiol 47:1820-1827, 2006.
49. Chan P, Stein K, Chow T, et al: Cost-effectiveness of a microvolt T-wave alternans screening strategy for implantable cardioverter-defibrillator placement in the MADIT-II–eligible population. J Am Coll Cardiol 48:112-121, 2006.
50. Adachi K, Ohnishi Y, Shima T, et al: Determinant of microvolt-level T-wave alternans in patients with dilated cardiomyopathy. J Am Coll Cardiol 34:374-380, 1999.
51. Kitamura H, Ohnishi Y, Okajima K, et al: Onset heart rate of microvolt-level T-wave alternans provides clinical and prognostic value in nonischemic dilated cardiomyopathy. J Am Coll Cardiol 39:295-300, 2002.
52. Sakabe K, Ikeda T, Sakata T, et al: Comparison of T-wave alternans and QT interval dispersion to predict ventricular tachyarrhythmia in patients with dilated cardiomyopathy and without antiarrhythmic drugs: A prospective study. Jpn Heart J 42:451-457, 2001.
53. Hohnloser SH, Klingenheben T, Bloomfield D, et al: Usefulness of microvolt T-wave alternans for prediction of ventricular tachyarrhythmic events in patients with dilated cardiomyopathy: Results from a prospective study. J Am Coll Cardiol 41:2220-2224, 2003.
54. Grimm W, Christ M, Bach J, et al: Noninvasive arrhythmia risk stratification in idiopathic dilated cardiomyopathy. Circulation 108:2883-2891, 2003.
55. Salerno-Uriarte JA, Pedretti RFE, Tritto M, et al: The ALPHA study (T-wave Alternans in Patients with Heart Failure): Rationale, design and endpoints. Ital Heart J 5:587-592, 2004.
56. Kavesh NG, Shorofsky SR, Sarang SE, Gold MR: The effect of procainamide on T wave alternans. J Cardiovasc Electrophysiol 10:649-654, 1999.
57. Groh WJ, Shinn TS, Engelstein EE, Zipes DP: Amiodarone reduces the prevalence of T wave alternans in a population with ventricular tachyarrhythmias. J Cardiovasc Electrophysiol 10:1335-1339, 1999.
58. Klingenheben T, Grönefeld G, Li YG, Hohnloser SH: Effect of metoprolol and D,L-sotalol on microvolt-level T-wave alternans. J Am Coll Cardiol 38:2013-2019, 2001.
59. Rashba EJ, Cooklin M, MacMurdy K, et al: Effects of selective autonomic blockade on T-wave alternans in humans. Circulation 105:837-842, 2002.

Mapping and Imaging 89

Vias Markides, Michael Koa-Wing, and Nicholas S. Peters

CHAPTER OUTLINE

Overview

Cardiac mapping is the process of identification, characterization, and localization of an arrhythmia. With the exception of more anatomically based approaches to ablation, such as linear cavo–tricuspid isthmus ablation, the process of mapping forms the basis for guiding therapeutic intervention. The methods used for mapping can vary considerably in terms of approach, technology used, and cardiac access, all of which are largely dependent on the probable arrhythmic substrate. Thus, careful evaluation of the patient's history, the 12-lead electrocardiogram (ECG) during sinus rhythm and clinical arrhythmia, and imaging data is important to determine the mapping strategy before the procedure.

Percutaneous mapping with conventional contact electrode catheters is the most widely applied method of investigating arrhythmias. Intracardiac signal data are obtained from catheters positioned in relevant parts of the heart—for example, the high right atrium, the atrioventricular (AV) node, the tricuspid or mitral annuli (coronary sinus), the right ventricle, and sometimes the left atrium or ventricle. Normal and abnormal patterns of activation during sinus rhythm, pacing, or tachycardia can be discerned from these signals. Complementary information may then be obtained by examining the timing and morphology of electrograms and data obtained by pacing at additional sites of interest, using a roving catheter. This basic approach usually is adequate for the majority of straightforward arrhythmias. More advanced techniques using three-dimensional mapping systems may be useful in patients with structural heart disease and more complex arrhythmias.

Mapping Techniques

Conventional Mapping Techniques

Conventional mapping techniques use a combination of one or more of three main methods: activation sequence mapping, pace mapping, and entrainment mapping. These techniques are covered in greater detail in the previous edition of this book[1] and are outlined briefly here. Complementary to these methods, other potentially useful observations of the effects of causing either transient or more permanent local tissue dysfunction during tachycardia or sinus rhythm with ventricular preexcitation, such as "bumping" of an accessory or Mahaim pathway by the catheter tip, "ice-mapping" during percutaneous cryoablation, and delivery of short pulses of radiofrequency energy, also can be useful.

Activation Sequence Mapping

Activation sequence mapping compares the timing of electrograms recorded at the tip of a roving catheter with that of a reference ECG or stable intracardiac signal. As the roving catheter is moved, the timing of electrograms is continuously compared with the reference signal to identify the position of the earliest possible signal or a progression of activation around a well-defined macro-reentrant circuit. As mapping continues, with time the operator creates a mental map of the activation of the chamber or region mapped. Activation mapping is particularly useful for investigation of focal tachycardias and may be complemented by pace mapping data (as discussed next). For complex macro-reentrant circuits, mapping is greatly facilitated by displaying activation sequence data on an electroanatomic mapping system.

Pace Mapping

Pace mapping is based on the principle that pacing during sinus rhythm at the site of origin of a focal or micro-reentrant tachycardia using a cycle length similar to that of the tachycardia will result in the same activation sequence as that generated by the tachycardia. Pacing should therefore produce an identical surface ECG pattern and intracardiac activation as for the clinical tachycardia. This technique is particularly useful in patients with structurally normal hearts, such as those with focal right ventricular outflow tract tachycardias, often in combination with activation mapping.

Entrainment Mapping

Entrainment mapping involves pacing during tachycardia to characterize macro-reentrant circuits, such as in scar-related ventricular tachycardia. Entrainment provides evidence for an excitable gap, supporting reentry as the mechanism. For stable macro-reentry, entrainment mapping during tachycardia often is preferable, because regions of conduction block that define the circuit may not be present or complete during sinus rhythm. Accordingly, in such cases, pace mapping may not match the cardiac activation or ECG morphology during tachycardia, even when pacing from within the circuit. Additionally, certain aspects of entrainment mapping can help differentiate between sites that are within a critical area of the circuit, such as the diastolic pathway in a ventricular tachycardia circuit, and bystander blind alleys. Criteria for entrainment and methods of identifying whether the pacing site is within a critical part of the reentrant circuit are described in Chapter 54 of the previous edition of this book.[1]

Electrospatial Mapping

Conventional catheter mapping relies on the operator to create a mental picture of three-dimensional cardiac activation based on electrogram data and two-dimensional fluoroscopic images. This is adequate for most simple arrhythmias, but mapping of more complex arrhythmic substrates is greatly facilitated by use of three-dimensional mapping systems. These newer technologies allow nonfluoroscopic three-dimensional catheter localization and facilitate mapping within a three-dimensional model of the chamber of interest.

Technologies such as advanced three-dimensional electroanatomic mapping (CARTO), noncontact mapping (EnSite 3000), and Realtime Position Management (RPM) are capable of combining anatomic data including reconstruction of chamber geometry, three-dimensional catheter localization, and navigation with electrophysiologic data. One of the important differences among these technologies is the way in which electrophysiologic data are acquired, which is *sequential* for CARTO, NavX, and RPM and *simultaneous* for noncontact mapping. A system based on an expandable basket also allows simultaneous mapping and reconstruction of activation maps of the chamber mapped, although resolution is relatively limited.

Sequential Electrospatial Mapping

CARTO The CARTO system (Biosense Webster, Diamond Bar, California) uses a size 7F deflectable quadripolar mapping and ablation catheter (NAVI-STAR) with a magnetic field sensor and thermocouple near its tip. When placed within a magnetic field, created by an external emitter under the operating table, the catheter tip position can be located in space. The mapping catheter location is gated to a reliable point in the cardiac cycle and recorded relative to the location of an external reference patch (REF-STAR with QuikPatch) on the patient's back, allowing compensation for both cardiac and patient movement. The system can accurately record and display in real time the position of the catheter tip in three dimensions (x, y, and z), its orientation (roll, pitch, and yaw), and the local intracardiac electrograms.

Activation sequence mapping, as described previously, can be performed either in sinus rhythm or in tachycardia. At each sequential point on the endocardium, electroanatomic data such as local activation time relative to the reference signal and three-dimensional location are collected, creating a three-dimensional virtual endocardium that can then be displayed as an isochronal, propagation, peak voltage, or anatomic map of the chamber of interest (Fig. 89-1).

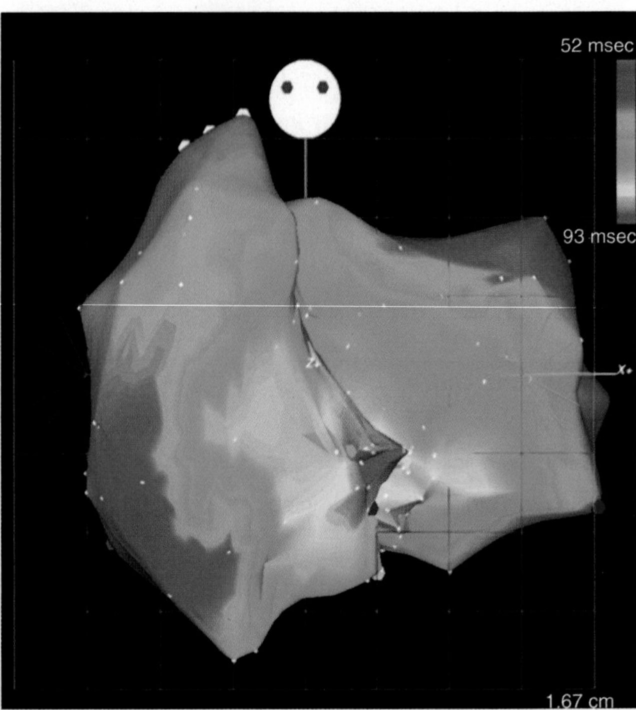

Figure 89-1 Electroanatomic activation maps of both atria, in an anteroposterior orientation, in a patient with a para-Hisian focal atrial tachycardia. The His bundle position is marked by the *amber* hexagon. *Red* denotes earliest activation, located adjacent to the His bundle potential, whereas *purple* represents latest activation.

The CARTO system has been validated and used to facilitate mapping in patients with a variety of arrhythmias in both atria and ventricles. Its use in mapping post-infarction ventricular tachycardias is complemented by its capability of displaying peak voltage maps, thus identifying areas of abnormal or scarred myocardium that can guide linear ablation at the scar border—an anatomic approach for use in cases in which mapping and ablation in tachycardia are not possible.[2] Similarly, CARTO has been used effectively to guide creation of linear lesions in the both atria and to create circumferential lesions around the ostia of the pulmonary veins in patients with atrial fibrillation.

The sequential nature of data acquisition effectively precludes use of this system in patients with short-lived, polymorphic, or hemodynamically unstable arrhythmias, except in the context of scar mapping and catheter navigation.

EnSite NavX EnSite NavX (St. Jude Medical, St. Paul, Minnesota) is an integral component of the EnSite system. The system uses three pairs of skin patches placed in orthogonal planes (x, y, and z). A 5.6-kHz signal is applied alternately across each pair of patches, creating a voltage gradient. Sensed voltages are compared to the voltage gradient in all three axes to calculate the three-dimensional position of individual electrodes on multiple catheters. The system allows simultaneous localization of up to 64 electrodes on up to 12 conventional catheters. The electrode-containing portions of any generic diagnostic or ablation catheters can be simultaneously displayed either in isolation or relative to the reconstructed three-dimensional endocardium.

Three-dimensional mapping using NavX is a two-step process. First, by moving any of the catheters to trace the endocardial contours of the chamber of interest, a virtual three-dimensional geometry is constructed. After geometry acquisition, sequential point-by-point mapping is then performed, during which the local activation time at each site is calculated with reference to a fixed intracardiac signal. The system can thereby create color-coded three-dimensional isochronal or voltage maps.

The NavX system has proved particularly useful as a nonfluoroscopic catheter navigation system in patients with atrial arrhythmias.[3,4] Reduction in radiation exposure equivalent to or even superior to that achievable with the CARTO system has been demonstrated.[5] Enhancement of geometry reconstruction based on the acquisition of multiple geometries (particularly useful around pulmonary vein–atrium junctions) and, more recently, field scaling, which uses known fixed interelectrode distances to correct for variations in transthoracic impedance in different planes, has further enhanced the usefulness of the system.

Simultaneous Electrospatial Mapping

Noncontact Mapping As discussed earlier, conventional catheter mapping and mapping using certain advanced systems such as CARTO are based on sequential acquisition of data over several cardiac cycles. This process can be time consuming and if a tachycardia is nonsustained or poorly tolerated hemodynamically the number of points that can be acquired and hence the resultant mapping resolution may be limited. Alternative systems based both on basket catheters and on noncontact mapping overcome these issues by simultaneously acquiring data from multiple sites in a cardiac chamber.

The noncontact mapping system (EnSite 3000, Endocardial Solutions Inc., St. Paul, Minnesota) comprises a multielectrode array (MEA), a proprietary recorder and amplifier system, and a workstation. The MEA consists of a 9F catheter with an 8-mL ellipsoid balloon, surrounded by a braid of 64 electrically insulated wires, all of which have a small laser-etched break in insulation that allows them to function as unipolar electrodes. A ring electrode on the proximal shaft of the array catheter in the inferior vena cava or an external reference can be used as a reference for unipolar signals. In addition to accepting signals from the MEA, the amplifier has an additional 16 inputs for data from contact catheters, as well as surface ECGs.

The far-field potentials as detected by the array are of low amplitude and frequency and are therefore mathematically enhanced and resolved. An inverse solution to the Laplace equation is used to predict how a signal detected at a remote point (a noncontact electrode) would have appeared at the source, and a boundary element method applies the inverse solution to resolve a matrix of such signals at, and originating from, the blood-endocardial boundary.

A low-current 5.68-kHz "locator" signal, passed between a conventional mapping catheter and alternately between ring electrodes on the noncontact catheter situated proximal and distal to the array, is used to locate the mapping catheter in space. The locator signal angles as determined by the system are used to identify the source of the signal. By moving the mapping catheter and tracing the contour of the endocardium, the system records the three-dimensional position of points on the endocardial surface that are used to reconstruct a three-dimensional model of the endocardium of any cardiac chamber. The same catheter localization system can also be used to navigate the mapping catheter to any point on the virtual endocardium, thereby guiding further mapping and ablation (Fig. 89-2). Software developments have allowed the system to simultaneously localize up to four electrodes on a single catheter or two pairs of electrodes on two different catheters, thus further enhancing geometry acquisition and catheter navigation.

The system reconstructs 3360 virtual endocardial electrograms responsible for creating the far-field potentials detected by the 64 electrodes of the MEA. Simultaneous acquisition of data from the entire endocardium of the chamber in which the array is placed allows analysis of endocardial activation from even a single beat of tachycardia. Data can be displayed as reconstructed virtual electrograms, as series of isopotential maps, or as isochronal maps, alongside surface ECG and contact catheter data (see Fig. 89-2).

Clinically, the system has been successfully used to map and guide ablation in all cardiac chambers. In patients with macroreentrant ventricular tachycardia complicating ischemic heart disease, noncontact mapping is effective in identifying and guiding ablation to the region of the diastolic pathway. The system also has been successfully used in procedures to ablate idiopathic left ventricular tachycardia and right ventricular outflow tract tachycardia.[6] When deployed in the left atrium, the MEA has been used to identify and guide ablation of arrhythmogenic foci responsible for initiation of atrial fibrillation, both inside pulmonary veins and in the left atrium. In the right atrium, the system has been used to map and further characterize atrial flutter and atrial fibrillation and to help localize discontinuities in linear lesions during ablation of atrial flutter.

Other Electrospatial Mapping Technologies

LocaLisa (Medtronic Inc., Minneapolis, Minnesota), a three-dimensional catheter localization-only system not in any way dependent on any dedicated consumables, has largely been superseded by the NavX system, which not only can locate multiple electrodes and catheters simultaneously but also can reconstruct three-dimensional surface contours and superimpose activation information.

The Realtime Position Management system (Cardiac Pathways, Sunnyvale, California) uses ultrasound ranging techniques to determine the position of a mapping catheter relative to two reference catheters. Two 6F multipolar fixed curve catheters are used for reference, whereas a deflectable 7F catheter used for mapping and ablation, all of which are equipped with multiple ultrasound transducers. By means of triangulation, the relative position of catheters is calculated. The system is now capable of reconstructing geometric representations of any cardiac chamber, starting with a generic three-dimensional model of the cardiac chambers that is expanded during movement of the mapping catheter, and to perform activation sequence mapping. Color-coded maps of endocardial activation are reconstructed based on the activation time of electrograms at multiple sites relative to a reference signal. Use of this version of the system has been described in atrial, junctional, and ventricular arrhythmias.[7]

Expandable basket catheters allow global and simultaneous mapping of a cardiac chamber. Mapping resolution depends on the number of splines on the basket, the number of electrodes on each spline, and the proportion of electrodes that are in contact

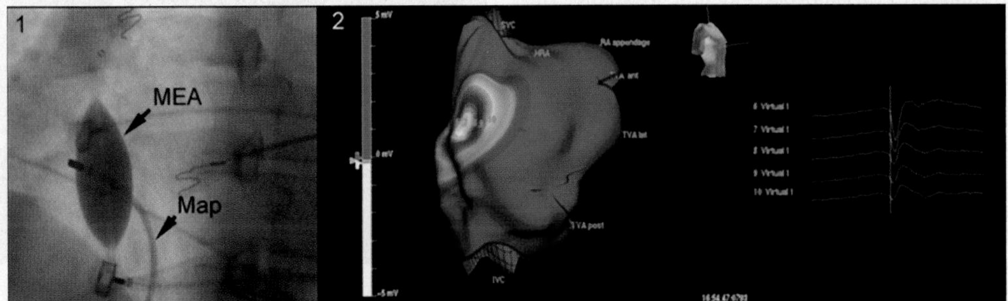

Figure 89-2 Mapping and ablation of a focal right atrial tachycardia using noncontact mapping. **1,** Left anterior oblique fluoroscopic image showing the multielectrode array (MEA) and a single mapping catheter (Map) in the right atrium. **2,** Right atrial isopotential map (right lateral projection) and corresponding unipolar virtual electrograms at sites numbered 6 to 10, as reconstructed by the noncontact mapping system. The isopotential map shows earliest endocardial activation (*white*, surrounded by other colors) at the site of origin of a focal right atrial tachycardia, surrounded by nondepolarized endocardium (*purple*). Virtual electrograms (*right*) placed over the area of the arrhythmogenic focus on the map have a QS morphology.

with the endocardium. One of the most commonly used catheters (Constellation, Cardiac Pathways-EP Technologies, Sunnyvale, California) has 64 electrodes on 8 highly flexible splines. Combined with an acquisition module and a dedicated computer, the system is capable of simultaneously processing electrogram data from a total of 56 bipoles (7 sequential bipoles from each spline), as well as electrogram data from other catheters and surface ECGs. Electrograms and color-coded activation maps can be reconstructed and displayed. The system has been successfully used to aid mapping of ventricular and atrial tachycardias and even to help mapping and ablation of atrial fibrillation–initiating foci inside pulmonary veins and the superior vena cava.[8]

Epicardial Mapping for Ventricular Tachycardia

Most ventricular tachycardias have their origin in the subendocardium. From 5% to 15% of the critical portion of these circuits is located in the subepicardial area, however, and adequate identification of these circuits is critical for therapy.

Surgical Mapping

The surgical approach has been used in the treatment of refractory ventricular arrhythmias. Epicardial mapping can be performed with relative ease in most cardiac chambers, with the chest opened, by means of hand-held probes, finger electrodes, or simultaneous multisite data acquisition systems, such as plaques or epicardial "socks." Exceptions to this indication are the posterior left atrium and the interatrial and interventricular septa, because the anatomy of these structures makes surgical mapping more difficult. Nowadays, surgery for arrhythmias is largely restricted to those that are refractory to pharmacologic and percutaneous ablative therapy or is performed in combination with other surgical procedures such as valve replacement or aneurysmectomy.

Nonsurgical Approach

Minimally invasive techniques for reaching the epicardial surface of the heart have been developed. Transvenous mapping techniques involve insertion of mapping catheters inside cardiac veins to record epicardial electrograms. Use of such techniques, which are safer and easier to perform than the surgical approach, is restricted by the anatomy of the cardiac venous system. Mapping and successful ethanol ablation of epicardial ventricular tachycardia circuits through branches of coronary arteries also have been described.[9]

The percutaneous epicardial approach involves introduction of a 7F sheath into the pericardial space after subxiphoid puncture. With the patient sedated, the epicardial surface of the heart can then be investigated using different types of mapping or ablation catheters. Advantages to this approach include avoidance of thromboembolic complications and the need for anticoagulation and the relative ease of catheter manipulation, as the pericardial space is a lubricated surface with few anatomic barriers.

Epicardial mapping uses the same electrophysiologic principles as for endocardial mapping, including identification of the earliest site of activation for focal arrhythmias or of mid-diastolic potentials and demonstration of concealed entrainment during mapping of reentrant arrhythmias. Successful radiofrequency ablation also has been performed with low risk of complications, provided that the coronary arteries are located away from the ablation site. Limitations include the inability to map epicardial septal circuits and difficulties encountered in the presence of pericardial adhesions, found particularly after previous cardiac surgery. Successful epicardial mapping and ablation of arrhythmias are well described in patients with a variety of substrates, including ischemic heart disease, Chagas' disease, right ventricular outflow tract tachycardia, and idiopathic ventricular tachycardia in pediatric populations.

Other applications of epicardial mapping include its experimental use to further current understanding of ventricular arrhythmias, including ventricular fibrillation. The possibility of covering a large part of the epicardial surface of the heart with multielectrode systems has made epicardial mapping an invaluable tool for the study of complex arrhythmia circuits. Epicardial mapping has also been used extensively to study the mechanisms of atrial fibrillation, both in animal studies and in humans undergoing cardiac surgery,[10] and to guide ablation.

Remotely Navigated Mapping

Currently, the majority of electrophysiogic procedures are performed using deflectable catheters that require operator skill to manually manoeuvre the catheter tip and maintain stability at target sites within the heart. The increasing use of anatomically based ablation strategies requires the operator to direct the catheter to sites that can be technically difficult to reach, requiring the creation of complete lines of ablation within a moving structure that is not smooth. Computer-assisted remote catheter ablation can potentially improve catheter maneuverability, precision, and stability, additionally raising the possibility of reproducible and accurate return to sites of interest during a procedure. Furthermore, when integrated with nonfluoroscopic mapping systems, remote mapping could potentially reduce radiation exposure to both patients and operators.

Magnetic Navigation

The Magnetic Navigation System (Niobe, Stereotaxis, Inc., St. Louis, Missouri) is a system that uses two permanent magnets mounted on articulating arms that are enclosed within a stationary housing with one magnet on either side of the fluoroscopy table. Between them, they create a relatively uniform magnetic field (0.08 T) inside the patient's chest. A specialized mapping and ablation catheter is equipped with multiple small permanent magnets positioned near its tip that align the catheter tip with the direction of the externally controlled magnetic field, so that it can be precisely steered. By changing the orientation of the outer magnets relative to each other by computer joystick or mouse, the orientation of the magnetic field changes, thereby leading to deflection of the catheter (Fig. 89-3). The catheter shaft can be advanced using a motorized external module (Cardiodrive, Stereotaxis, Inc). The remote magnetic navigation system also is closely integrated with CARTO-RMT (Biosense Webster), a specialized form of the CARTO electroanatomic mapping system that allows the operator to predetermine the

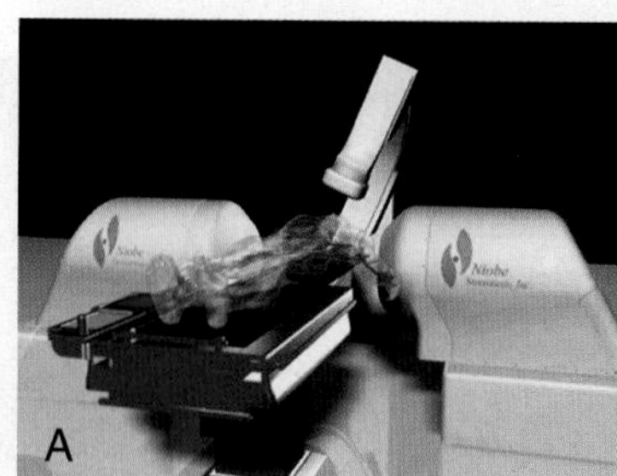

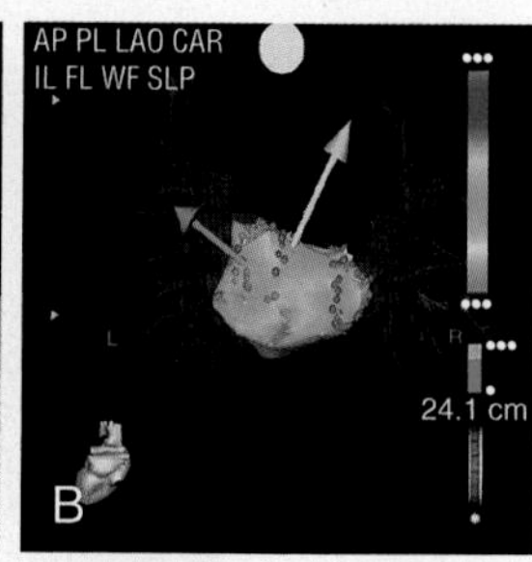

Figure 89-3 **A,** The Niobe II Stereotaxis magnetic navigation system. **B,** Image integration with CARTO-RMT nonfluoroscopic mapping system. The example shown is of an integrated left atrial computed tomography image during encirclement of the pulmonary veins. *Arrows* are moved to direct the magnets, which in turn guide the ablation catheter. *Blue dots* are ablation lesions. (**A** and **B,** Images courtesy of Stereotaxis, Inc., St. Louis, Missouri, and Biosense Webster, Diamond Bar, California.)

three-dimensional position to which the catheter should move, translating this information for the magnetic navigation system to calculate and apply the vectors required for catheter movement.

Magnetically guided remote navigation has been proved to be effective in the ablation of accessory pathways[11,12] and atrial,[13,14] nodal,[15] and ventricular arrrhythmias.[16]

Robotic Navigation

The Sensei robotic control system (Hansen Medical, Inc., Mountain View, California) is an electromechanical master-slave system that controls a steerable guide catheter (Artisan Control Catheter) that accepts any 8F or smaller mapping or ablation catheter. The system comprises three linked components: the physician's workstation, remote catheter manipulator and steerable guide catheter (Fig. 89-4). The workstation features displays for contact intracardiac electrophysiology data, three-dimensional mapping systems, and fluoroscopy, as well as an icon of the Artisan for orientation and navigation. To control the Artisan, a specialized hand-operated joystick is manipulated in combination with a control panel on the workstation. Fine movements of the joystick are translated by control computers into movement of the remote catheter manipulator (RCM); a robotic rig designed to accept and in turn control the movements of the Artisan by its internal pullwires. The Artisan is a single-use sterile guide catheter consisting of a steerable inner guide within a steerable outer guide. The outer guide catheter provides a stable base for the inner guide. Four orthogonal pull wires deflect the inner guide catheter in x and y directions, so that it can reach anywhere within a roughly toroidal workspace defined by a bend of up to 270 degrees and a 10-cm extension. Conventional mapping and ablation catheters are inserted through the inner guide and locked in place at the proximal end of the Artisan. This system has been validated and used in animals[17,18] and in limited human studies.[19]

Imaging in Cardiac Electrophysiology

With the development of anatomically guided substrate-based ablation, particularly for atrial fibrillation and ventricular tachycardias, coupled with the need to ensure safety during such procedures, imaging has acquired an increasingly important role in providing fundamental, patient-specific anatomic information and in guiding mapping and ablation.

Transesophageal Echocardiography

In the field of cardiac electrophysiology, transesophageal echocardiography (TEE) is perhaps most useful in atrial imaging.

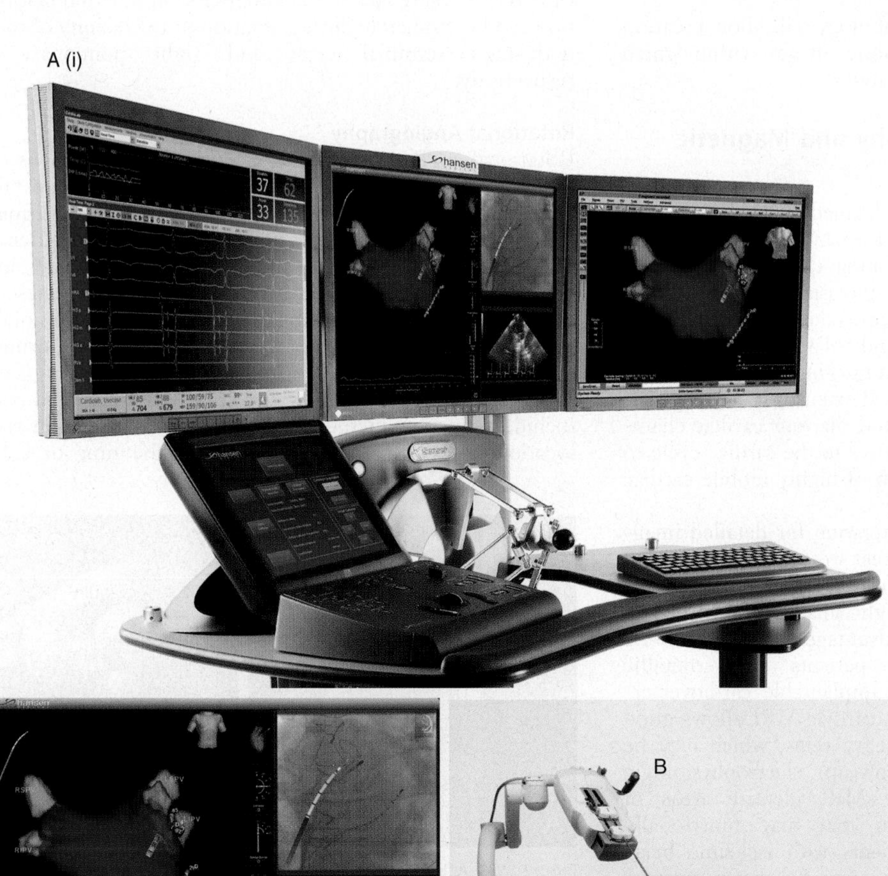

Figure 89-4 The Hansen robotic remote navigation system. **A** (i), The physician's workstation. (ii) Close-up of the workstation central display. **B**, Remote catheter manipulator with Artisan steerable guide catheter (C). (Images courtesy of Hansen Medical, Inc., Mountain View, California.)

TEE is very effective at excluding visible thrombus in the left atrium and appendage and is now routinely recommended for patients scheduled to undergo catheter ablation for atrial fibrillation.[20] TEE can easily demonstrate the presence or absence of a patent foramen ovale, accurately delineate pulmonary vein anatomy, and provide detailed information on chamber size and valvular and ventricular function. Intraoperatively, TEE can help safely guide transseptal puncture, especially in patients in whom conventional fluoroscopically guided puncture proves difficult, but this use of TEE is limited to patients under general anesthesia.

Intracardiac Echocardiography

Intracardiac echocardiography (ICE) is emerging as a powerful tool in cardiac imaging and real-time catheter guidance during electrophysiologic procedures. Several types of ICE probes are available, some of which provide basic two-dimensional imaging, whereas others can provide enhanced picture quality, color Doppler mapping, and an enhanced field of view. ICE has been used to identify important structures such as the fossa ovalis to guide transseptal puncture; to delineate true anatomy and complex structures; to guide electrophysiologic procedures such as in pulmonary vein isolation[21]; to observe catheter placement, stability, tissue contact, and lesion size, as well as to identify thrombus formation[22] and microbubble formation at the catheter tip; and to observe for other complications such as pericardial effusion.[23]

Future developments in ICE technology will allow creation of three-dimensional real-time dynamic images within which catheters can be visualized and navigated.[24]

Cardiac Computed Tomography and Magnetic Resonance Imaging

Knowledge of an individual patient's detailed cardiac anatomy is extremely important before the performance of anatomically guided ablation. Cardiac computed tomography (CT) and magnetic resonance imaging (MRI) are increasingly being used in preparation for electrophysiology procedures and in some cases can greatly facilitate mapping and ablation.

In addition to its traditional role in imaging the great vessels, more recently cardiac CT has been used extensively to image the coronary arteries, pulmonary veins, and the four cardiac chambers. Multislice CT can be gated relative to the cardiac cycle to provide detailed image reconstruction of highly mobile cardiac structures.

Cardiac MRI is a reference investigation for detailed imaging of all cardiac chambers and great vessels. Avoidance of ionizing radiation and of conventional x-ray contrast agents is a significant advantage, although image acquisition is slower than with modern CT. Disadvantages include absolute and relative contraindications in patients with metallic implants, including pacemakers and implantable cardioverter-defibrillators. In experienced centers, cardiac MRI allows good visualization of the atria and pulmonary veins, which may be relevant before and after (for follow-up) electrophysiologic procedures. Not only can cardiac MRI identify areas of hibernating ventricular myocardium that may functionally respond to revascularization in patients with ischemic heart disease, but more recent work has demonstrated that in patients with nonischemic cardiomyopathies, the presence of partial-thickness scar as identified by cardiac MRI is a powerful predictor of inducible ventricular arrhythmias.[25] The potential for cardiac imaging to identify and localize proarrhythmic myocardial substrate may become increasingly useful in coming years.

Enhanced Fluoroscopy

Angiography and fluoroscopy have long been used to directly visualize catheter placement and manipulation within the heart. Because the cardiac soft tissue structures are poorly visualized fluoroscopically, the operator has to rely on a mental image of where relevant endocardial contours may lie. Enhancement of fluoroscopic images by injection of contrast material is invaluable for visualizing the pulmonary veins and venoatrial junctions, guiding catheter placement within the left atrium.

The intimate anatomic relation between the esophagus and posterior left atrium and the potential for life-threatening complications after posterior left atrial ablation[26] have lead to the development of techniques for visualization of the esophagus during such procedures. Minimal barium swallow can help the operator to visualize the esophagus and its relation to the left atrium on fluoroscopy.[27] Alternatives include tagging the esophagus using the CARTO system (although mobility of the esophagus relative to the left atrium during a procedure limits the value of this technique) and monitoring the luminal temperature of the esophagus during posterior left atrial ablation.

Despite access to multiple imaging modalities, certain potentially vulnerable structures such as the right phrenic nerve cannot be adequately imaged during electrophysiologic procedures. In such cases, high-output electrical stimulation from the tip of a mapping catheter or circumferential pulmonary vein catheter to ensure lack of diaphragmatic stimulation before ablation can be invaluable during ablation in the vicinity of the sinus node–high terminal crest and right pulmonary veins, respectively.

Rotational Angiography

Rotational angiography uses a motorized C arm that is rotated around the patient in a continuous movement while taking a series of fluoroscopy acquisition images.[28] Acquisition data from a single rotation can be processed by computer and a high-resolution, digitally reconstructed three-dimensional model of the imaged vessel or chamber displayed. These methods have recently been applied in generating 30 images of the left atrium and esophagus[29] to be used intraoperatively during atrial fibrillation ablation (Fig. 89-5). Potential advantages of using a real-time acquisition system over CT-MRI–integrated mapping include reduction in the possible interval changes in size and location of cardiac structures between the time of CT-MRI

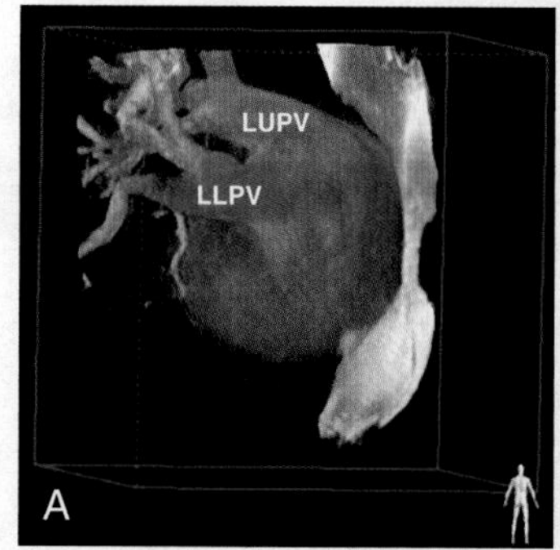

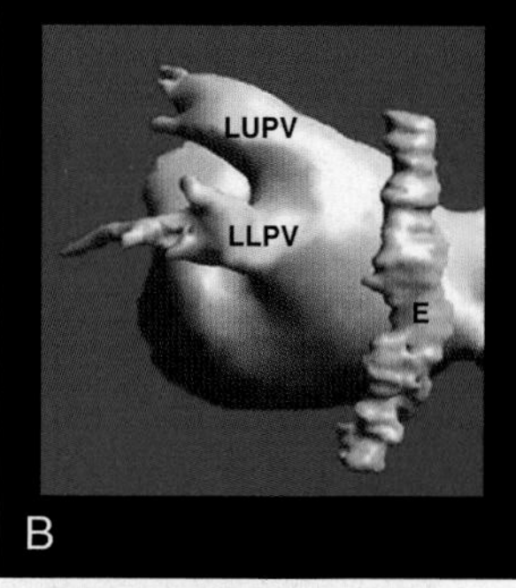

Figure 89-5 **A,** Image from a three-dimensional rotational angiogram (3DRA) of the left atrium during esophageal swallow. **B,** Reconstructed 3DRA image. Fine detail and branching of pulmonary veins (PVs) are easily seen on 3DRA, and esophageal (E) position is clearly visible. LUPV, left upper PV; LLPV, left lower PV. (**A** and **B,** Adapted from Orlov MV, Hoffmeister P, Chaudhry GM, et al: Three-dimensional rotational angiography of the left atrium and esophagus—a virtual computed tomography scan in the electrophysiology lab? Heart Rhythm 4:37- 43, 2007, with permission from Elsevier.)

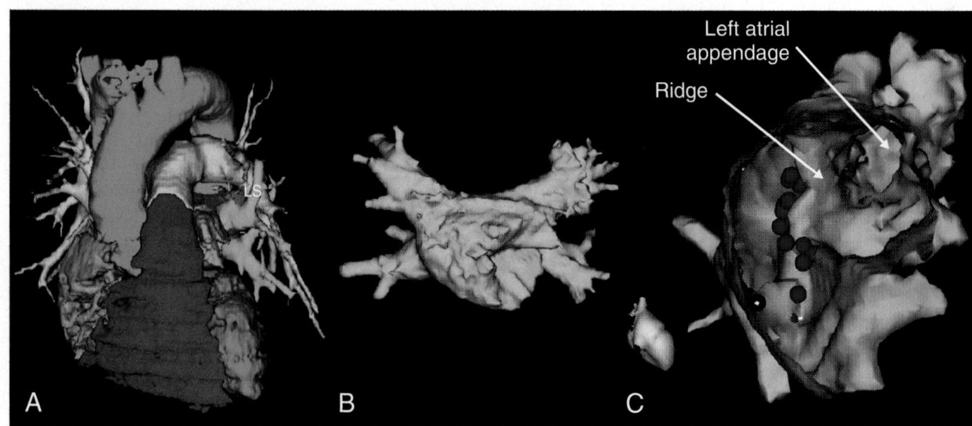

Figure 89-6 Example of CARTOMERGE computed tomography (CT) image integration. **A,** A fully segmented cardiac CT image. **B,** The chamber of interest (left atrium in anteroposterior view) can be registered with true fluoroscopic anatomy to allow catheter navigation within the three-dimensional reconstructed anatomy. **C,** Left atrial CT image in cross section, looking into the left-sided pulmonary veins. Ablation lesions in red. (**A** to **C,** Images courtesy of Biosense Webster, Diamond Bar, California.[9])

and the procedure itself and provision of three-dimensional images that are almost as good as CT images, with markedly reduced radiation exposures and accurate image registration owing to the fact that the images are acquired at the time of the procedure.[30]

Imaging-Registered Electrospatial Mapping

Developments in electroanatomic mapping systems (CARTO XP with CARTOMERGE, EnSite Verismo) now provide the capability to import cardiac CT or MRI images into a mapping study, perform segmentation of the anatomic structures, and then reconstruct an accurate three-dimensional anatomic model of the chamber of interest. Previously, this allowed rotational synchronization of the CT or MRI–derived three-dimensional model with the geometry generated from conventional electroanatomic reconstruction. Today, however, digital fusion of the two models is possible, so mapping can now be performed within an accurate three-dimensional model of a specific patient's heart (Fig. 89-6).

Both the CARTO and EnSite NavX systems require a process of image registration before the imaging-imported models can be used for nonfluoroscopic catheter navigation. Registration with CARTOMERGE involves initial "landmark registration" of a small number of easily identifiable points—for example, in the case of the left atrium, usually at the venoatrial junctions. This is followed by "surface registration," wherein a greater number of points are registered throughout the surface of the chamber to be mapped. Registration is essential, especially because changes in volume loading and cardiac rhythm that may have occurred between the time of the imaging scan and the time of the procedure may affect the actual location of the contour of the mapped chamber. CARTOMERGE has been validated[31] and shown to reduce fluoroscopy and arrhythmia recurrence in patients undergoing catheter ablation for atrial fibrillation.[32] Published experience with image-registered mapping using NavX Verismo is currently more limited.

Conclusions

Techniques and technologies for mapping of cardiac arrhythmias continue to evolve rapidly. The clinical history, previous assessment for structural heart disease, and examination of the ECG greatly facilitate the approach to and strategy for mapping. Use of three-dimensional mapping systems has become invaluable for investigation of more complex arrhythmias. In addition, developments in nonfluoroscopic catheter navigation, particularly related to advances in both CT-MRI image integration and remote navigation systems, also have an important role.

References

1. Zipes D, Jalife J (eds): Cardiac Electrophysiology: From Cell to Bedside, 4th ed. Philadelphia, Suanders, 2004.
2. Volkmer M, Outang F, Deger F, et al: Substrate mapping vs. tachycardia mapping using CARTO in patients with coronary artery disease and ventricular tachycardia: Impact on outcome of catheter ablation. Europace 8:968-976, 2006.
3. Rotter M, Takahashi Y, Sanders P, et al: Reduction of fluoroscopy exposure and procedure duration during ablation of atrial fibrillation using a novel anatomical navigation system. Eur Heart J 26:1415-1421, 2005.
4. Ventura R, Rostock T, Klemm HU, et al: Catheter ablation of common-type atrial flutter guided by three-dimensional right atrial geometry reconstruction and catheter tracking using cutaneous patches: A randomized prospective study. J Cardiovasc Electrophysiol 15:1157-1161, 2004.
5. Earley MJ, Showkathali R, Alzetani M, et al: Radiofrequency ablation of arrhythmias guided by non-fluoroscopic catheter location: A prospective randomized trial. Eur Heart J 27:1223-1229, 2006.
6. Friedman PA, Asirvatham SJ, Grice S, et al: Noncontact mapping to guide ablation of right ventricular outflow tract tachycardia. J Am Coll Cardiol 39:1808-1812, 2002.
7. Schreieck J, Ndrepepa G, Zrenner B, et al: Radiofrequency ablation of cardiac arrhythmias using a three-dimensional real-time position management and mapping system. Pacing Clin Electrophysiol 25:1699-1707, 2002.
8. Shah DC, Haissaguerre M, Jais P, et al: High-resolution mapping of tachycardia originating from the superior vena cava: Evidence of electrical heterogeneity, slow conduction, and possible circus movement reentry. J Cardiovasc Electrophysiol 13:388-392, 2002.
9. Segal OR, Wong T, Chow AW, et al: Intra-coronary guidewire mapping—a novel technique to guide ablation of human ventricular tachycardia. J Interv Card Electrophysiol 18:143-154, 2007.
10. Yamauchi S, Ogasawara H, Saji Y, et al: Efficacy of intraoperative mapping to optimize the surgical ablation of atrial fibrillation in cardiac surgery. Ann Thorac Surg 74:450-457, 2002.
11. Chun JK, Ernst S, Matthews S, Schmidt B, et al: Remote-controlled catheter ablation of accessory pathways: Results from the magnetic laboratory. Eur Heart J 28:190-195, 2007.
12. Ernst S, Hachiya H, Chun JK, et al: Remote catheter ablation of parahisian accessory pathways using a novel magnetic navigation system—a report of two cases. J Cardiovasc Electrophysiol 16:659-662, 2005.
13. Di BL, Fahmy TS, Patel D, et al: Remote magnetic navigation: Human experience in

pulmonary vein ablation. J Am Coll Cardiol 50:868-874, 2007.
14. Pappone C, Vicedomini G, Manguso F, et al: Robotic magnetic navigation for atrial fibrillation ablation. J Am Coll Cardiol 47:1390-1400, 2006.
15. Ernst S, Ouyang F, Linder C, et al: Initial experience with remote catheter ablation using a novel magnetic navigation system: Magnetic remote catheter ablation. Circulation 109:1472-1475, 2004.
16. Aryana A, d'Avila A, Heist EK, et al: Remote magnetic navigation to guide endocardial and epicardial catheter mapping of scar-related ventricular tachycardia. Circulation 115:1191-1200, 2007.
17. Al-Ahmad A, Grossman JD, Wang PJ. Early experience with a computerized robotically controlled catheter system. J Interv Card Electrophysiol 12:199-202, 2005.
18. Saliba W, Cummings JE, Oh S, et al: Novel robotic catheter remote control system: Feasibility and safety of transseptal puncture and endocardial catheter navigation. J Cardiovasc Electrophysiol 17:1102-1105, 2006.
19. Reddy VY, Neuzil P, Malchano ZJ, et al: View-synchronized robotic image-guided therapy for atrial fibrillation ablation: Experimental validation and clinical feasibility. Circulation 115:2705-2714, 2007.
20. Calkins H, Brugada J, Packer DL, et al: HRS/EHRA/ECAS expert consensus statement on catheter and surgical ablation of atrial fibrillation: Recommendations for personnel, policy, procedures and follow-up. Europace 9:335-379, 2007.
21. Mangrum JM, Mounsey JP, Kok LC, et al: Intracardiac echocardiography-guided, anatomically based radiofrequency ablation of focal atrial fibrillation originating from pulmonary veins. J Am Coll Cardiol 39:1964-1972, 2002.
22. Ren JF, Marchlinski FE, Callans DJ. Left atrial thrombus associated with ablation for atrial fibrillation: identification with intracardiac echocardiography. J Am Coll Cardiol 43:1861-1867, 2004.
23. Marrouche NF, Martin DO, Wazni O, et al: Phased-array intracardiac echocardiography monitoring during pulmonary vein isolation in patients with atrial fibrillation: Impact on outcome and complications. Circulation 107:2710-2716, 2003.
24. Knackstedt C, Franke A, Mischke K, et al: Semi-automated 3-dimensional intracardiac echocardiography: Development and initial clinical experience of a new system to guide ablation procedures. Heart Rhythm 3:1453-1459, 2006.
25. Nazarian S, Bluemke DA, Lardo AC, et al: Magnetic resonance assessment of the substrate for inducible ventricular tachycardia in nonischemic cardiomyopathy. Circulation 112:2821-2825, 2005.
26. Pappone C, Oral H, Santinelli V, et al: Atrio-esophageal fistula as a complication of percutaneous transcatheter ablation of atrial fibrillation. Circulation 109:2724-2726, 2004.
27. Good E, Oral H, Lemola K, et al: Movement of the esophagus during left atrial catheter ablation for atrial fibrillation. J Am Coll Cardiol 46:2107-2110, 2005.
28. Green NE, Chen SY, Messenger JC, et al: Three-dimensional vascular angiography. Curr Probl Cardiol 29:104-142, 2004.
29. Orlov MV, Hoffmeister P, Chaudhry GM, et al: Three-dimensional rotational angiography of the left atrium and esophagus—a virtual computed tomography scan in the electrophysiology lab? Heart Rhythm 4:37-43, 2007.
30. Oral H: Rotational angiography: A novel application of an old concept. Heart Rhythm 4:44-45, 2007.
31. Kistler PM, Earley MJ, Harris S, et al: Validation of three-dimensional cardiac image integration: Use of integrated CT image into electroanatomic mapping system to perform catheter ablation of atrial fibrillation. J Cardiovasc Electrophysiol 7:341-348, 2006.
32. Kistler PM, Rajappan K, Jahngir M, et al: The impact of CT image integration into an electroanatomic mapping system on clinical outcomes of catheter ablation of atrial fibrillation. J Cardiovasc Electrophysiol 17:1093-1101, 2006.

Noninvasive Electrocardiographic Imaging (ECGI): Clinical Applications 90

YORAM RUDY, YONG WANG, AND PHILLIP CUCULICH

CHAPTER OUTLINE

Overview

The clinical management of cardiac arrhythmias has gone through major changes over the past 20 years with the development of catheter mapping and ablation procedures, surgical approaches, and implantable pacing and defibrillation devices. Major advances also have been made in elucidation of the genetic, molecular, and cellular processes that underlie arrhythmogenesis. Yet the electrocardiogram (ECG) is still the mainstay of noninvasive diagnosis and guidance of therapy. The ECG has proved indispensable over the past 100 years. However, it is limited to measuring the reflection of cardiac electrical activation at a limited number of points on the body surface, remote from the heart.

Electrocardiographic imaging (ECGI) is a functional imaging modality that was developed in our laboratory as a noninvasive means of electroanatomic mapping of the heart.[1] After extensive validation,[2-8] it has been applied in human subjects with a variety of cardiac electrophysiologic conditions. Similar to other noninvasive imaging modalities (computed tomography [CT], magnetic resonance imaging [MRI], ultrasonography), ECGI reconstructs information on an internal organ (the heart) from external measurements. In ECGI, epicardial potentials, electrograms, activation sequences (isochrones), and repolarization patterns are reconstructed from 250 body surface ECG traces and thoracic CT images.[1] The ECGI methodology is described in Chapter 44, where images of activation and repolarization of the intact normal human heart also are provided.[9] This chapter uses previously published case reports to illustrate potential clinical applications of ECGI, with images showing relevant cardiac anatomy and conduction in patients with specific arrhythmias and abnormal electrophysiologic substrate.

Studies presented in this chapter were supported by NIH-NHLBI Merit Award R37-HL-33343 and Grant R01-HL-49054 (to Dr. Rudy). Dr. Rudy is the Fred Saigh Distinguished Professor at Washington University in St. Louis. He also chairs the scientific advisory board and holds equity in CardioInsight Technologies (CIT). CIT does not support any research conducted by Dr. Rudy, including that presented here.

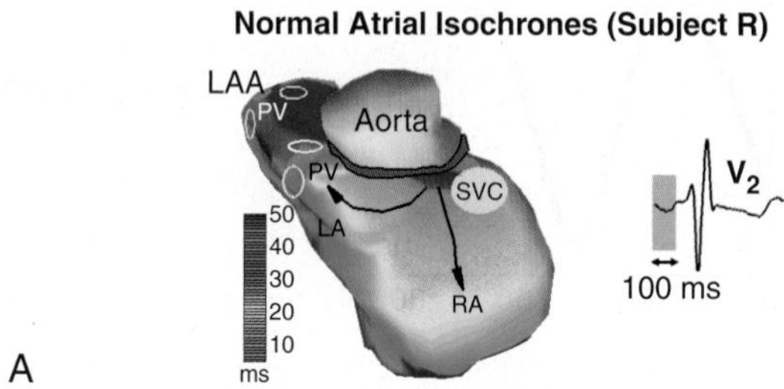

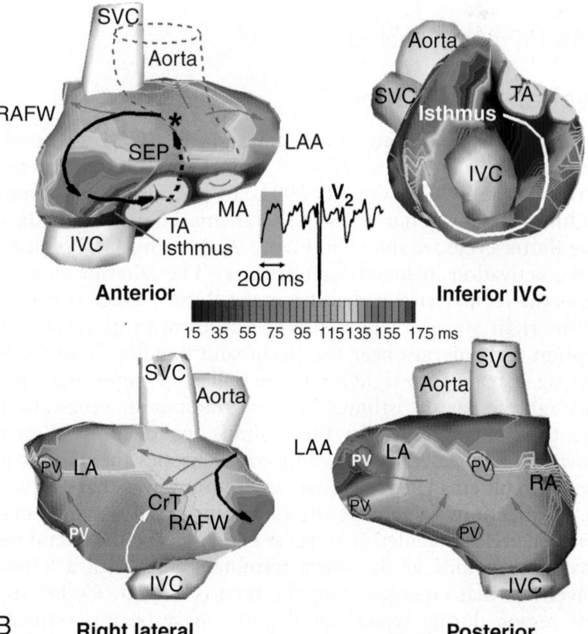

Figure 90-1 Noninvasive activation maps of typical atrial flutter. **A,** Normal atrial activation is shown for reference. Lead V_2 of the electrocardiogram (ECG) is provided for timing, with imaged P wave shaded in *blue*. **B,** Atrial flutter isochrones. Four views are shown; imaged flutter cycle is shaded *blue* on ECG lead V_2. *Black arrows* in anterior view indicate the reentrant circuit beginning from the isthmus, entering the septum *(dashed arrow)*, emerging near Bachmann bundle *(asterisk)*, and propagating down the right atrial free wall (RAFW) to reenter the isthmus. *White arrow* indicates a secondary wavefront propagating around the inferior vena cava (IVC) and up the RAFW, where it collides at the crista terminalis (CrT) with other waves *(gray arrows)* emanated from the reentry circuit. Some of the emanated waves activate the left atrium *(gray arrows)*. AF, atrial fibrillation; LA, left atrium; LAA, left atrial appendage; MA, mitral annulus; PV, pulmonary vein; RA, right atrium; SEP, septum; SVC, superior vena cava; TA, tricuspid annulus. (Adapted by permission from Macmillan Publishers Ltd: From Ramanathan C, Ghanem RN, Jia P, et al: Noninvasive electrocardiographic imaging for cardiac electrophysiology and arrhythmia. Nat Med 10:422-428, 2004.)

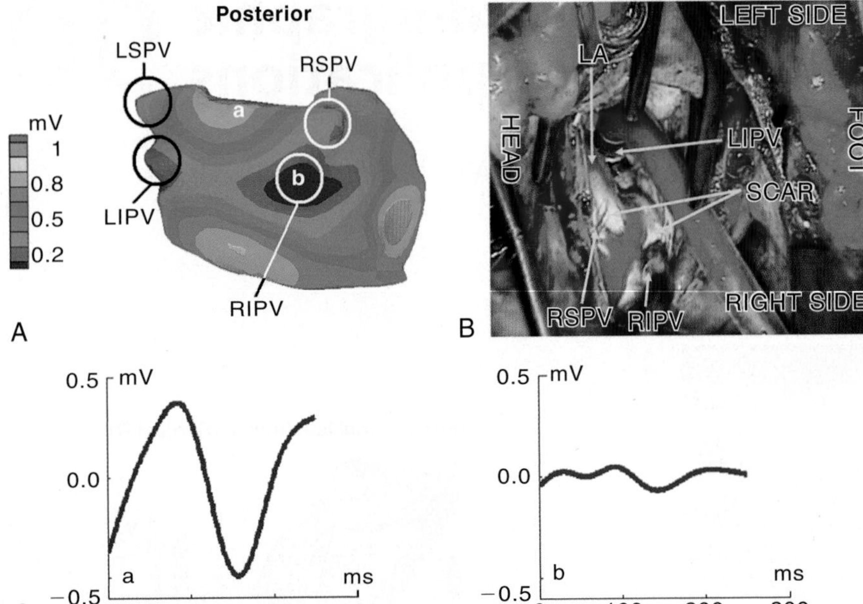

Figure 90-2 Atypical atrial flutter. **A,** Noninvasive epicardial electrogram magnitude map: posterior view. Low-potential regions (less than 0.5 mV) (*blue*) indicate scar. **B,** Photograph obtained during the Cox maze surgical procedure, showing scar (*white*). **C,** Selected reconstructed epicardial electrograms for locations remote to scar (a) and within the scar (b). LAA, left atrial appendage; LIPV, left inferior pulmonary vein; LSPV, left superior pulmonary vein; RAA, right atrial appendage; RIPV, right inferior pulmonary vein; RSPV, right superior pulmonary vein. (From Wang Y, Schuessler RB, Damiano RJ, et al: Noninvasive electrocardiographic imaging (ECGI) of scar-related atypical atrial flutter. Heart Rhythm 4:1565-1567, 2007, with permission.)

Atrial Arrhythmias

Typical Atrial Flutter

In a study by Ramanathan and colleagues,[1] ECGI was used to evaluate a patient diagnosed with typical atrial flutter (sawtooth waves on the ECG at a rate of 300 beats per minute with average width of 200 ms). Four views of ECGI-imaged isochrones during one flutter cycle are shown in Figure 90-1, with ECGI of normal atrial activation included for reference. The anterior view captures the reentry circuit that drives the flutter, which is confined to the right atrium. The reentrant wavefront propagates up the septum and emerges near the Bachmann bundle. From there it propagates down the right atrial free wall and reenters the septum through the narrow isthmus between the inferior vena cava and the tricuspid annulus. In the isthmus, conduction is greatly slowed, as indicated by crowding of isochrones there. This primary circuit emanates secondary excitation waves that propagate in all directions to activate the remaining atrial tissue. A major wave encircles the inferior vena cava and ascends the lateral right atrium to collide at the crista terminalis area with a leftward wavefront that emerges from the reentry circuit. Collisions in this region during typical atrial flutter have been described in direct mapping studies.[10,11] Other wavefronts (posterior, anterior, and right lateral views) that emanate from the reentry circuit propagate to the left atrium, with the left atrial appendage being last to activate. The ECGI-imaged counterclockwise right atrial reentry circuit and activation pattern are consistent with direct mapping of typical atrial flutter using intracardiac catheters.[11-13] The flutter was terminated by catheter ablation of the inferior vena cava–tricuspid annulus isthmus, and the patient returned to sinus rhythm.

Scar-Related Atypical Atrial Flutter

A recent study by Wang and associates[14] described the use of ECGI to investigate the basis for atypical atrial flutter in a 48-year-old man with a 2-year history of atrial fibrillation. He underwent two procedures, four months apart, of catheter-based pulmonary vein isolation, with additional ablations in the left side of the mitral isthmus, on the left atrial roof, and on the right side of the tricuspid annulus–inferior vena cava isthmus. Three months after the second procedure, persistent atypical atrial flutter developed. The patient was referred for a surgical Cox maze procedure after unsuccessful cardioversion. One day before surgery, ECGI was performed. Figure 90-2A is an electrogram magnitude map, showing low-potential regions (less than 0.5 mV peak to peak) around each of the pulmonary veins and in the left atrial appendage region. The low-potential regions corresponded well with scar areas observed during surgery (see Fig. 90-2B); they coincided with scar tissue around the pulmonary veins from the previous ablation procedures, and with extensive scarring of the left atrial appendage (caused by the underlying disease, not previous ablations).

Before the Cox maze procedure and ECGI application, the diagnosis was atrial fibrillation. However, ECGI imaged a monomorphic stable reentrant activation pattern that repeated for many beats, suggesting atrial flutter due to anatomic (rather than functional) reentry. The activation sequence for one flutter cycle is shown in Figure 90-3. The reentry circuit driving the flutter was confined mostly to the left atrium. Earliest activation occurred in the left atrium below the left inferior plumonary vein (site 1 on Fig. 90-3). It propagated posteriorly toward the right atrium (site 2) but blocked in the superior direction at a line of block between the two inferior pulmonary veins associated with a posterior scar formed by the previous catheter ablations. After a 50-ms delay due to slow conduction at the scar border around the line of block (see Fig. 90-3B), the wavefront propagated into the previously unexcited superior region (site 3) and continued toward the roof of the left atrium (site 4). From there it propagated to the anterior site 7, both directly and through the left atrial appendage (site 6). It then conducted through the mitral valve (MV) isthmus (site 8) to complete the reentry circuit. A secondary wavefront emanated from the reentry circuit; it descended from the left atrial roof (site 4′) to the inferior right atrial free wall (site 5). Thus, the flutter circuit was constrained

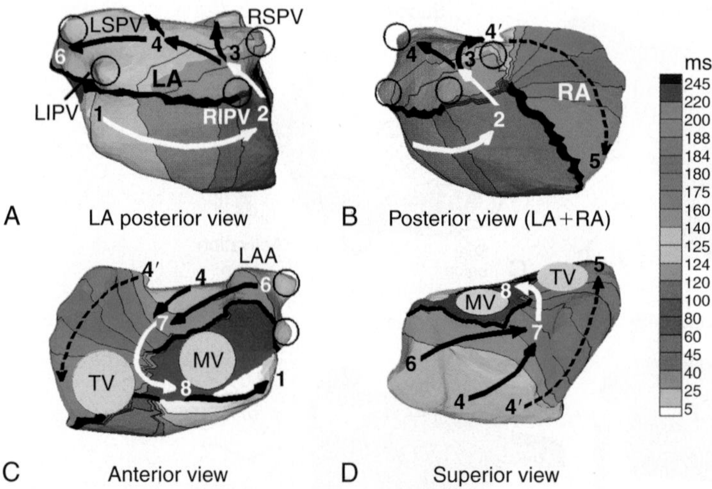

Figure 90-3 Atypical atrial flutter. Noninvasive activation (isochrone) map of the flutter cycle: four views. *Solid arrows* indicate the reentry circuit; *dashed arrows* show secondary front that emanated from the reentry circuit. The reentry sequence is 1 → 2 → 3 → 4 → (6) → 7 → 8 → 1. LA, left atrium; LAA, left atrial appendage; LIPV, left inferior pulmonary vein; LSPV, left superior pulmonary vein; MV, mitral valve; RA, right atrium; RAA, right atrial appendage; RIPV, right inferior pulmonary vein; RSPV, right superior pulmonary vein; TV, tricuspid valve. (From Wang Y, Schuessler RB, Damiano RJ, et al: Noninvasive electrocardiographic imaging (ECGI) of scar-related atypical atrial flutter. Heart Rhythm 4:1565-1567, 2007, with permission.)

by scars from the previous catheter ablation procedures. It formed around an extensive scar (identified by ECGI reconstruction of low potentials and confirmed by observation during surgery); the scar provided the anatomic substrate that stabilized the reentry. After the Cox maze procedure, the patient returned to normal sinus rhythm.

Focal Atrial Tachycardia

In another recent study reporting clinical ECGI application,[15] a 55-year-old woman presented with severe palpitations and an episode of near-syncope after two catheter-based pulmonary vein isolation procedures for longstanding atrial fibrillation. She had undergone a percutaneous valvuloplasty for rheumatic mitral valve disease 9 years before the ablation procedures. Echocardiography (transthoracic and transesophageal) showed marked left atrial enlargement, mild mitral stenosis, and moderate mitral regurgitation. During the two earlier electrophysiologic studies, low potentials were recorded throughout the left atrium. When she presented with recurring palpitations, the 12-lead ECG revealed atrial tachycardia at a rate of 136 beats per minute. The decision was made to attempt an ablation procedure.

Before the procedure, ECGI was performed to noninvasively localize the source of tachycardia. Figure 90-4 presents atrial epicardial potential maps imaged by ECGI at the onset (see Fig. 90-4A) and end (see Fig. 90-4B) of the surface P wave during the tachycardia. At P wave *onset*, a local potential minimum (see Fig. 90-4A), indicative of epicardial breakthrough and site of earliest activation, was imaged on the left atrium, near the atrial septum. At P wave *end* (see Fig. 90-4B), a repolarization pattern was imaged, with a local potential maximum replacing the potential minimum at the earlier breakthrough site. These patterns indicate an ectopic focal source of the tachycardia at the breakthrough location; they were consistent over several ECGI-imaged P waves during the tachycardia. Figure 90-4C shows an ECGI-reconstructed isochrone map for one tachycardia cycle. The earliest activation site is consistent with the ectopic focus site as determined from the potential maps (see Fig. 90-4A and B). In Figure 90-4D, the ECGI-determined ectopic focus is superimposed on a CT image; it is located on the left atrial roof between the right superior pulmonary vein and the atrial septum. Figure 90-4E shows a catheter-performed electroanatomic isochrone map (CARTO, Biosense Webster, Diamond Bar, California) constructed during the electrophysiologic study that followed ECGI. Catheter mapping identified a focal origin of the tachycardia on the superior left atrium, between the right superior pulmonary vein and atrial septum—a location consistent with the ECGI prediction. Radiofrequency energy was applied at this site and in surrounding locations. The tachycardia was terminated and did not recur with isoproterenol challenge. The patient returned to sinus rhythm at the conclusion of the procedure.

Figure 90-4F is an ECGI map of electrogram voltage magnitudes (peak to peak). Very low potentials were reconstructed on the posterior left atrium around the pulmonary veins, consistent with scarring from the previous pulmonary vein isolation procedures. In addition, diffuse low voltages also were imaged on the posterior left atrial wall, probably as a result of the patient's underlying disease (diffuse low voltages were observed during the initial electrophysiologic study, before pulmonary vein isolation).

Ventricular Arrhythmias and Abnormal Electrophysiologic Substrate

Focal Left Ventricular Tachycardia

Intini and coworkers[16] reported the case of a 29-year-old athlete with no significant medical history who had frequent asymptomatic premature ventricular complexes (PVCs) on routine (otherwise normal) ECG. During exercise testing, a spontaneous, sustained, wide QRS complex tachycardia developed. The ECG morphologic patterns of the wide complex tachycardia and the PVC were very similar (if not identical). ECGI was performed during a single PVC. The ECGI isochrone map (Fig. 90-5A) localized the origin of the PVC to the left ventricular apex, to an area of a small diverticulum (CT image in Fig. 90-5C). On the basis of the QS morphology of the reconstructed electrogram from the site of origin of the PVC (see Fig. 90-5A), it was determined that the initiation site was epicardial. Guided by the ECGI images, invasive electroanatomic mapping (CARTO) of the left ventricle was performed during PVCs (see Fig. 90-5B) and during ventricular tachycardia (induced after administration of isoproterenol). The invasive catheter maps also identified the earliest site of activation at the left ventricular apex in the region of the diverticulum,

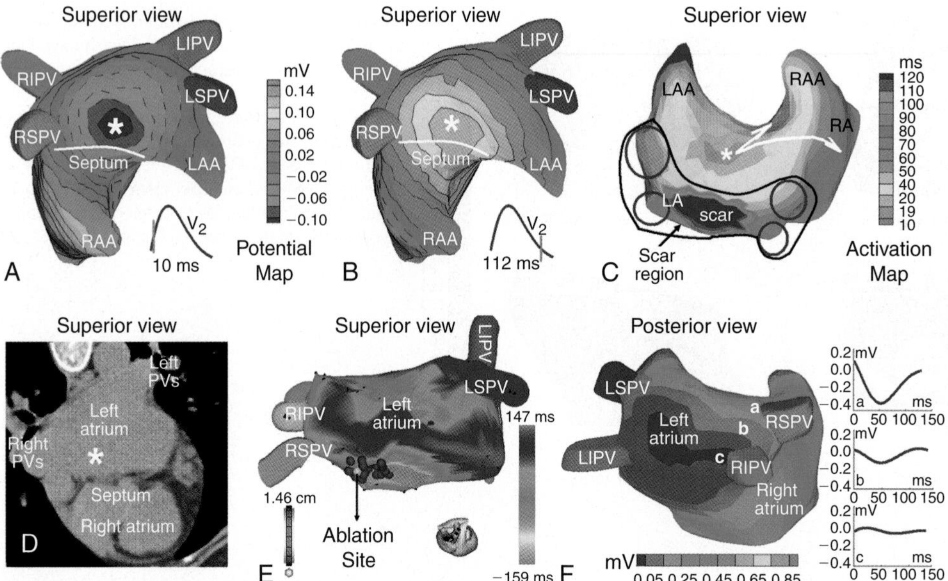

Figure 90-4 Noninvasive ECGI of focal atrial tachycardia. **A,** Atrial epicardial potential map 10 ms after onset of surface P wave (*inset* shows lead V_2 for timing). Negative minimum (*blue*) is site of epicardial breakthrough, with *asterisk* indicating site of earliest activation. **B,** Same as **A,** except during repolarization (112 ms after P wave onset). Note reversed polarity of potential pattern compared with **A,** with positive maximum (*orange*) replacing the early minimum. **C,** Noninvasive atrial activation map during one tachycardia cycle. Earliest activation region (*red*) coincides with the local potential minimum in **A** and maximum in **B.** Earliest activation site is marked by the asterisk. **D,** Earliest activation site determined by ECGI (*asterisk*) is superposed on computed tomography (CT) image of the atria. **E,** Invasive activation map obtained by catheter mapping during EP procedure. The *white marker* (*arrow*) identifies the site where ablation terminated the atrial tachycardia. *Red markers* are circumferential sites of radiofrquency energy application around the site of earliest activation. **F,** Electrogram magnitude map showing a region of low potentials (*blue*), indicative of scar. Selected electrograms outside (**a**) and inside (**b** and **c**) scar are shown. LA, left atrium; LAA, left atrial appendage; LIPV, left inferior pulmonary vein; LSPV, left superior pulmonary vein; PV, pulmonary vein; RA, right atrium; RAA, right atrial appendage; RIPV, right inferior pulmonary vein; RSPV, right superior pulmonary vein. (Adapted from Wang Y, Cuculich PS, Woodard PK, et al: Focal atrial tachycardia after pulmonary vein isolation: Noninvasive mapping with electrocardiographic imaging (ECGI). Heart Rhythm 4:1081-1084, 2007, with permission.)

consistent with the ECGI determination (compare Fig. 90-5A and Fig. 90-5B). An epicardial mapping and cryoablation procedure was performed through a subxiphoid puncture. Earliest activation of ectopic activity was localized to a region of low voltage (less than 1.45 mV) at the left ventricular apex overlying the diverticulum. Close proximity of the phrenic nerve prevented complete ablation of this region, and ventricular tachycardia recurred.

Heart Failure and Cardiac Resynchronization Therapy

In another study reported by Jia and associates,[17] ECGI was conducted in eight patients diagnosed with heart failure (six males and two females, with mean age of 72 ± 1 years and New York Heart Association [NYHA] functional class III or IV) who received cardiac resynchronization therapy (CRT) through an implanted atrial-biventricular pacing device. Ventricular activation during native rhythm and various pacing modes was imaged. Figure 90-6 shows epicardial isochrone maps during native rhythm in four of the patients—namely, patients 7, 5, 1, and 3. In all eight subjects, right ventricular epicardial activation started from a right ventricular breakthrough (RVB) site 29 ± 7 ms after body surface QRS onset (somewhat delayed relative to RVB time in normal young adults[9]). Duration of right ventricular activation was 25 ± 12 ms and activation pattern was normal.[9] Globally, all patients had delayed left ventricular activation with a left bundle branch block (LBBB) pattern. However, ECGI revealed major heterogeneity of left ventricular activation among patients. In patients 4, 7, and 8, left ventricular epicardial activation started from the septoapical region, spreading laterally and ending at the lateral or posterolateral base (see Fig. 90-6A).

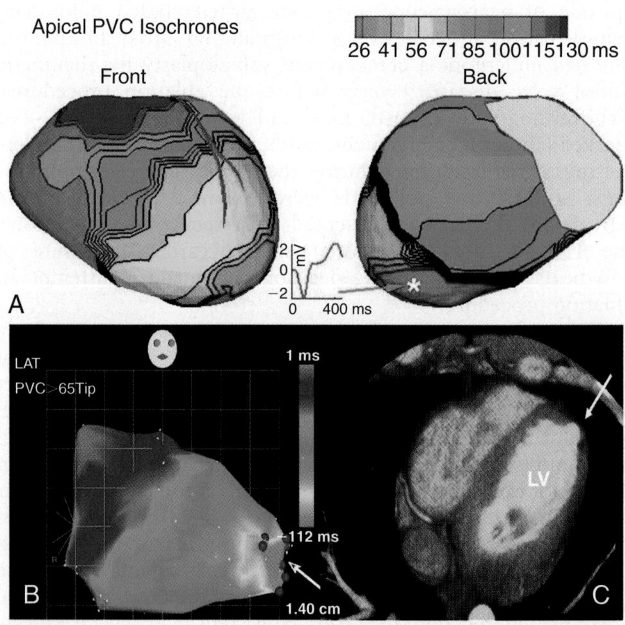

Figure 90-5 Focal left ventricular tachycardia. **A,** Noninvasive activation map during a premature ventricular contraction (PVC). Earliest activation site is marked by an *asterisk.* Electrogram from this site *(inset)* is of QS morphology, indicating epicardial origin. **B,** Invasive left ventricular endocardial activation map during a PVC using the CARTO isochrone mapping system (see text). **C,** Computed tomography scan of a cross section of the left ventricle showing the apical diverticulum *(arrow).* LV, left ventricular. (Adapted from Intini A, Goldstein RN, Jia P, et al: Electrocardiographic imaging (ECGI), a novel diagnostic modality used for mapping of focal left ventricular tachycardia in a young athlete. Heart Rhythm 2:1250-1252, 2005, with permission.)

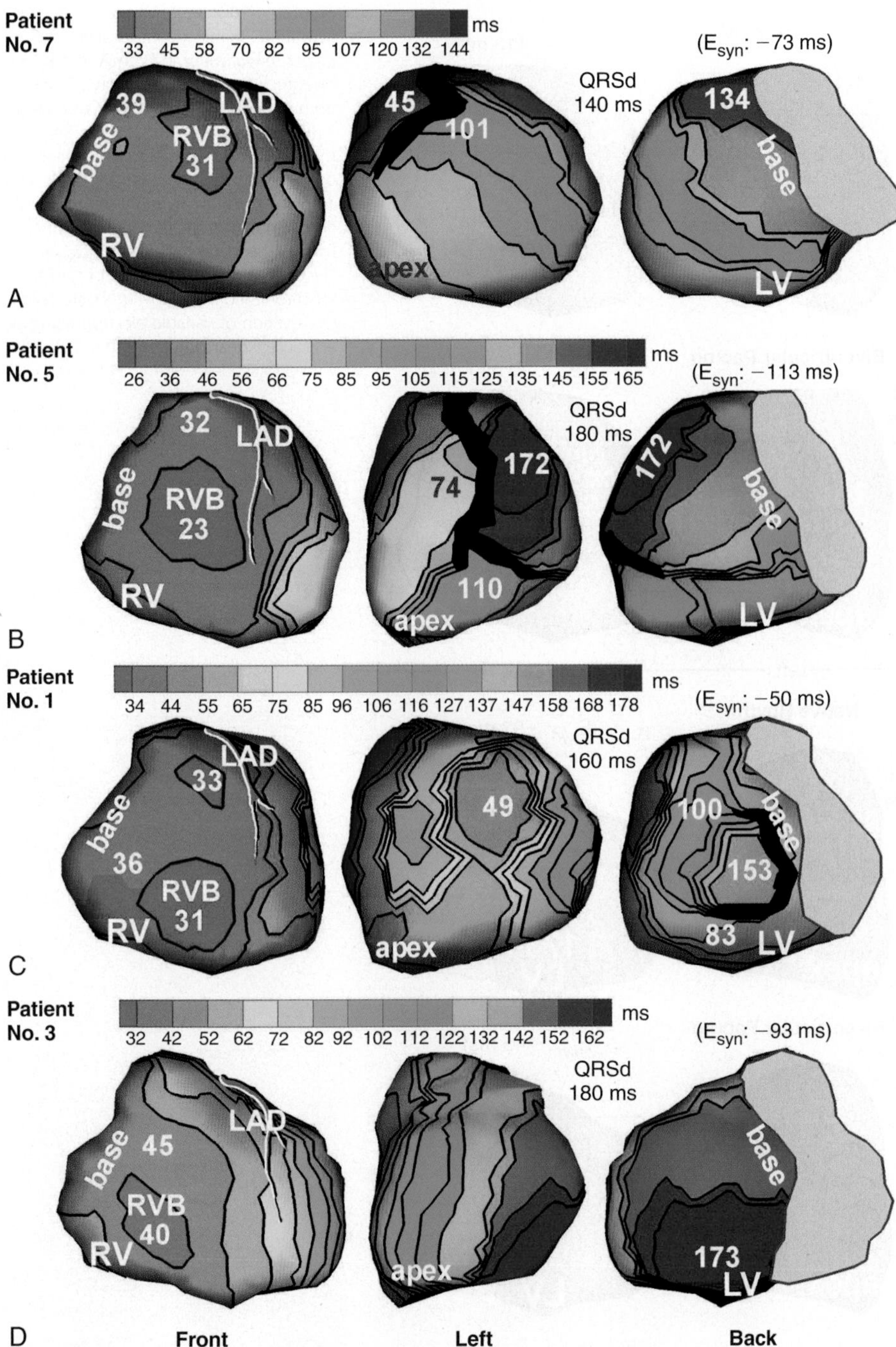

Figure 90-6 Noninvasive epicardial activation maps during native rhythm in four heart failure patients (three views each). Left anterior coronary artery (LAD) is indicated. Approximate valve region is in *gray*. *Thick black markings* indicate line or region of conduction block. Activation times (in milliseconds) of selected regions, such as right ventricular breakthrough, latest activation, and sites adjacent to block regions, are indicated on the maps. E_{syn}, electrical synchrony index (mean activation time difference between lateral right and left ventricular free walls), with smaller absolute value corresponding to greater synchrony; LV, left ventricle; QRSd, QRS complex duration; RV, right ventricle; RVB, right ventricular breakthrough. (From Jia P, Ramanathan C, Ghanem RN, et al: Electrocardiographic imaging of cardiac resynchronization therapy in heart failure: Observation of variable electrophysiologic responses. Heart Rhythm 3:296-310, 2006, with permission.)

In patient 5, activation proceeded superiorly from the inferior left ventricle, ending in the midanterolateral wall (see Fig. 90-6B). In four patients (4, 5, 7, 8), activation from the right ventricle was prevented from spreading into the left ventricle by anterior lines or regions of block; it reached the lateral wall by way of apical or inferior left ventricle in a U-shaped pattern.[18] In patient 1, wavefronts from apical, inferior, and superior left ventricle all contributed to overall left ventricular activation, which ended at the posterolateral wall (see Fig. 90-6C). In patient 3 (see Fig. 90-6D), activation slowly propagated from the right ventricle across the septum and spread inferoposteriorly from anterior left ventricle to reach the left ventriclular lateral and posterior walls. The inferoposterior base region was last to activate. Thus, the left ventricular electrophysiologic substrate varied greatly among patients, including location and geometry of block lines and regions and areas of latest activation. In contrast with the severely damaged left ventricular myocardium and left bundle branch, ECGI showed that right ventricular myocardium and right bundle preserved relatively normal function in all patients.

Figure 90-7A and B (bottom row) shows ECGI images of ventricular activation during biventricular pacing for CRT

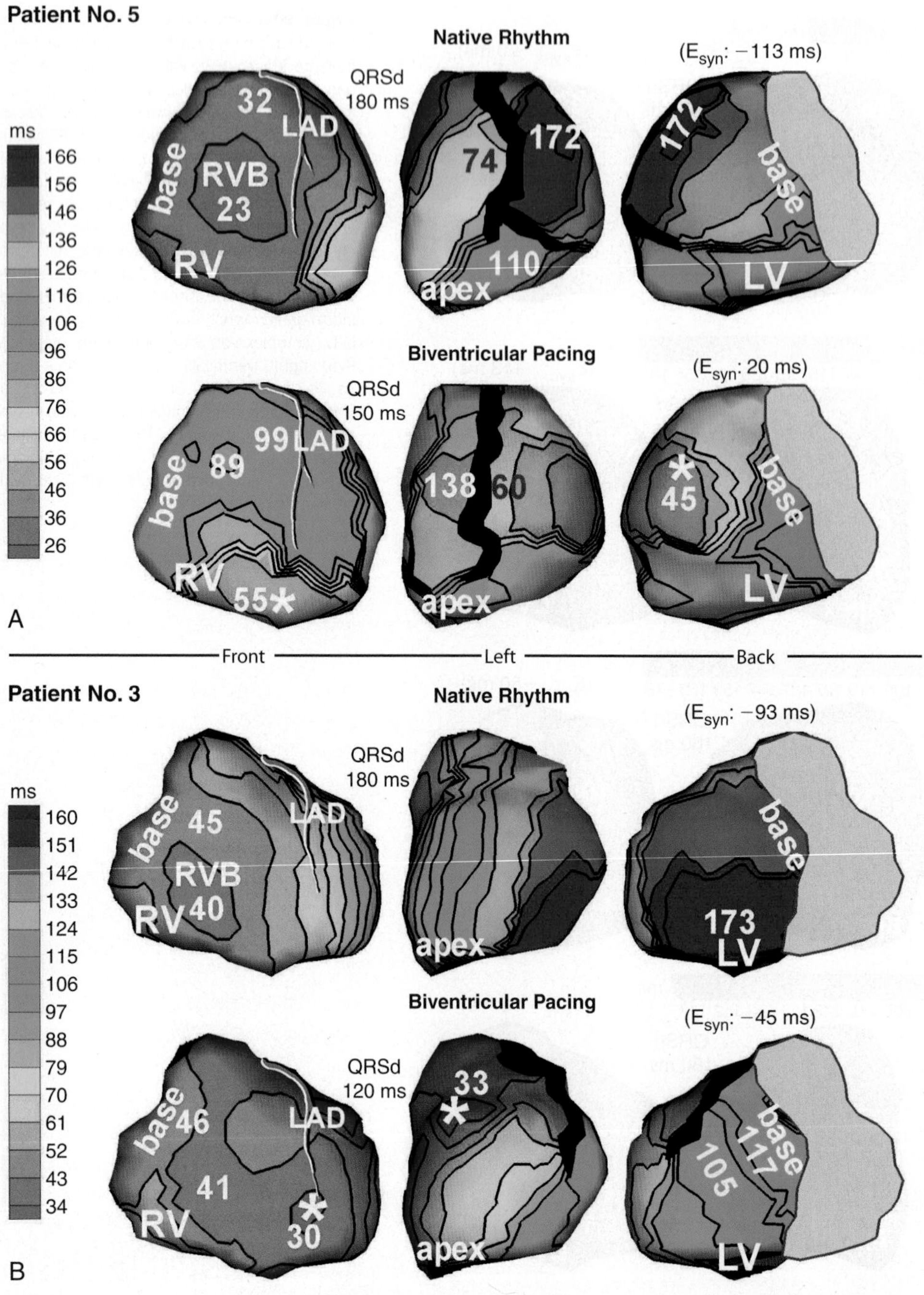

Figure 90-7 Noninvasive epicardial activation maps during native rhythm (*upper row of maps* in both **A** and **B**) and biventricular pacing (*lower row of maps* in both **A** and **B**) for patient 5 (**A**) and patient 3 (**B**) from Figure 90-6. Pacing sites are marked by *asterisks*. LAD, left anterior coronary artery; LV, left ventricle; QRSd, QRS complex duration; RV, right ventricle; RVB, right ventricular breakthrough. (From Jia P, Ramanathan C, Ghanem RN, et al: Electrocardiographic imaging of cardiac resynchronization therapy in heart failure: Observation of variable electrophysiologic responses. Heart Rhythm 3:296-310, 2006, with permission.)

from two patients (i.e., patients 5 and 3 from Fig. 90-6) who improved with therapy ("responders" as characterized by echocardiographic and other measures[17]). The native rhythm for each patient is repeated from Figure 90-6 in the top row. In patient 5, activation spread from the pacing site at the lateral wall (see Fig. 90-7A, bottom) and ended locally at basal left ventricle 110 ms after pacing. In anterior left ventricle, activation encountered a line of block, similar to that during native rhythm (see Fig. 90-7A, top). Latest activation (138 ms) was in anterior left ventricle, adjacent to the line of block. The right ventricle and most of the left ventricle were much more synchronized electrically compared with native rhythm, with E_{syn} improving from −113 to 20 ms (E_{syn} is defined in Fig. 90-6 legend). Patient 3 had an anterior left ventricular lead. Activation blocked at an anterolateral line of block (see Fig. 90-7B, bottom); it pivoted around this line and ended at lateral basal left ventricle (117 ms). E_{syn} improved from −93 to −45 ms.

Figure 90-8 shows ECGI activation maps during left ventricular pacing alone in patient 5, with increasing delay between atrial and left ventricular pacing—from top to bottom, ranging from no delay (see Fig. 90-8A) to a delay of 173 ms (see Fig. 90-8D). Increasing the delay provides more time for intrinsic excitation through the conduction system (right bundle branch) to couple to the left ventricle–paced beat progressively earlier, thereby

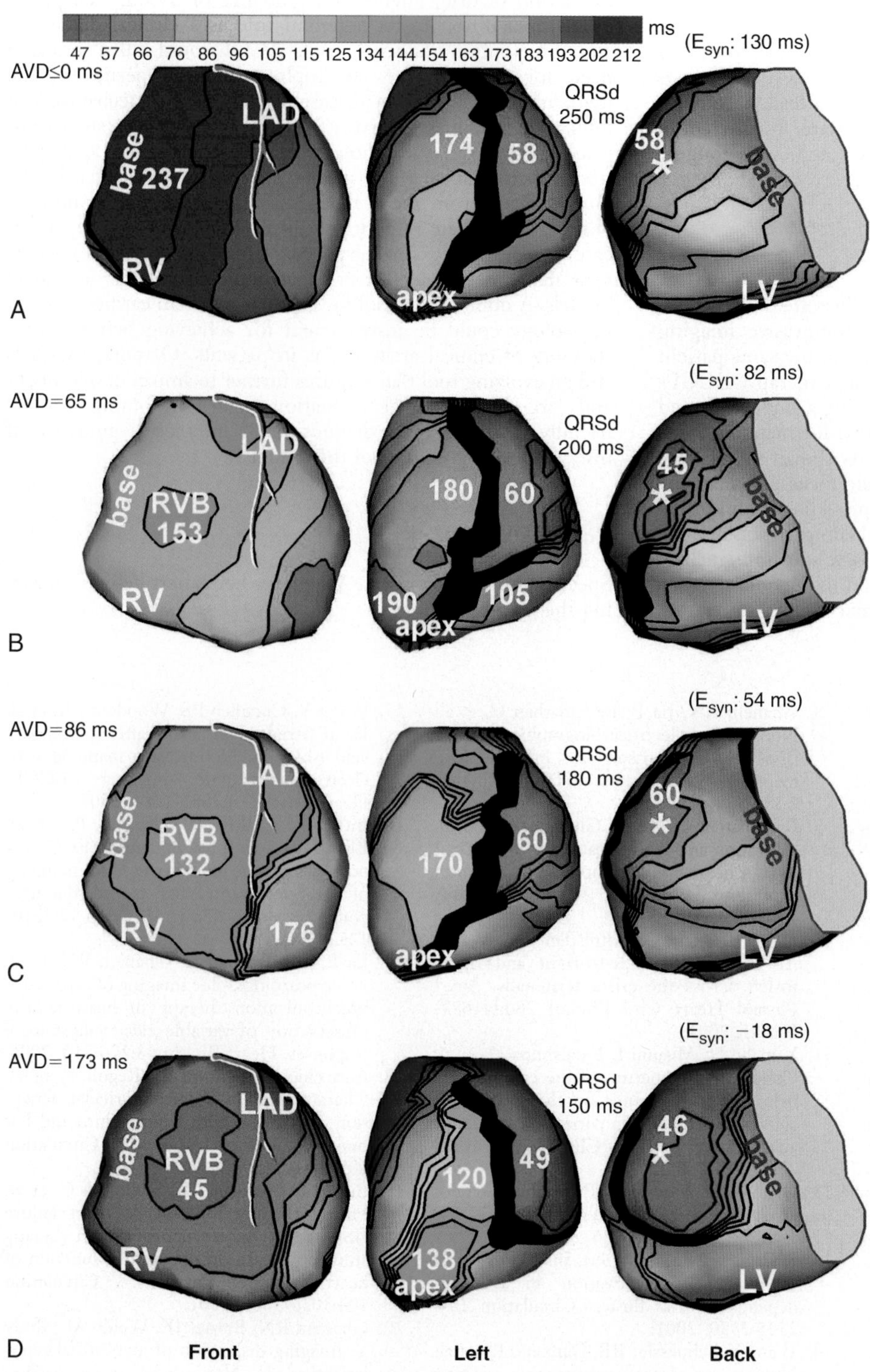

Figure 90-8 Fusion beats during left ventricular (LV) pacing alone. **A,** LV paced activation sequence without fusion from intrinsic right ventricular (RV) excitation. **B** to **D,** Fusion beats with progressively earlier intrinsic RV excitation relative to LV pacing due to increased delay between atrial and LV pacing (AVD, indicated in each panel). *Asterisks* mark LV lead location. Electrical synchrony improves with increasing degree of fusion. AVD, atrioventricular difference; LAD, left anterior coronary artery; QRSd, QRS complex duration; RVB, right ventricular breakthrough. (From Jia P, Ramanathan C, Ghanem RN, et al: Electrocardiographic imaging of cardiac resynchronization therapy in heart failure: Observation of variable electrophysiologic responses. Heart Rhythm 3:296-310, 2006, with permission.)

allowing a greater contribution to ventricular activation. The resulting fusion beat is more synchronized, with E_{syn} improving as fusion increases (see Fig. 90-8D). In this case, left ventricular pacing alone was as effective as biventricular pacing for electrical resynchronization and a right ventricular lead was not required.

These ECGI images provide useful insights. They demonstrate that patients with heart failure and an LBBB pattern on the ECG do not constitute a homogeneous group, because they display a wide range of electrical activation patterns and electrophysiologic substrates (varied regions of delayed or absent conduction and lines of conduction block). Not surprisingly, the responses to pacing and CRT among the patients described in the case examples were similarly disparate. These observations suggest that determination of optimal left ventricular lead placement should consider not only the activation sequence (i.e., pacing from the area of most delayed activation to maximize synchrony)[19] but also the electrical properties of the substrate. In particular, presence of regions of slow conduction, conduction block, and inexcitable tissue and their location relative to that of the pacing lead should be considered as well. ECGI could provide such information noninvasively for guiding lead placement. Through noninvasive imaging of the substrate, it also could facilitate proper patient selection for CRT and, with longer-term use, monitor the patient's response.

Summary

The case examples in this chapter serve to illustrate the potential clinical applications of ECGI. Being a noninvasive imaging modality, it could be applied multiple times in the same patient at different stages of disease progression and therapy. ECGI's capability of imaging cardiac activation during a single beat and on a beat-by-beat basis makes it well suited for mapping nonsustained and polymorphic arrhythmias. As shown in the case examples, ECGI can locate the arrhythmic focus and map the reentry circuit that drives an arrhythmia, providing useful information for guiding ablation and evaluating its outcome. Noninvasive imaging of the electrophysiologic substrate, including scarring, conduction abnormalities, and dispersion of repolarization,[20] could be used for arrhythmia risk stratification, evaluation of drug effects, and guidance of pacing lead placement. In addition to its potential role as a clinical diagnostic and intervention guidance tool, ECGI could fill a research need for studying the electrophysiologic properties of the human heart in different disease states and the mechanisms of human arrhythmias. At every level of the cardiac system (molecular, cellular, tissue, whole-heart), electrophysiologic properties and mechanisms are species-dependent and differ in the human heart from those in animal models (e.g., the mouse). Similarly, substrate remodeling in the human heart due to disease processes (e.g., coronary heart disease, heart failure) occurs over many years and differs substantially from that in animal models. A noninvasive tool for exploring human cardiac electrophysiology could be instrumental for achieving better understanding of clinical arrhythmias in patients. Of note, ECGI is still an evolving tool that requires further technical development and large-scale clinical evaluation before becoming a user-friendly instrument for diagnosis and interactive guidance of intervention in the hand of the clinician.

Acknowledgment

Special thanks go to Debra Adams for her expert help in preparing the manuscript.

References

1. Ramanathan C, Ghanem RN, Jia P, et al: Noninvasive electrocardiographic imaging for cardiac electrophysiology and arrhythmia. Nat Med 10:422-428, 2004.
2. Oster HS, Taccardi B, Lux RL, et al: Electrocardiographic imaging: Noninvasive localization of pacing sites simulating ectopic foci. Circulation 90:I-437, 1994.
3. Oster HS, Taccardi B, Lux RL, et al: Noninvasive electrocardiographic imaging: Reconstruction of epicardial potentials, electrograms, and isochrones and localization of single and multiple electrocardiac events. Circulation 96:1012-1024, 1997.
4. Oster HS, Taccardi B, Lux RL, et al: Electrocardiographic imaging: Noninvasive characterization of intramural myocardial activation from inverse-reconstructed epicardial potentials and electrograms. Circulation 97:1496-1507, 1998.
5. Burnes JE, Taccardi B, MacLeod RS, Rudy Y: Noninvasive ECG imaging of electrophysiologically abnormal substrates in infarcted hearts: A model study. Circulation 101:533-540, 2000.
6. Burnes JE, Taccardi B, Rudy Y: A noninvasive imaging modality for cardiac arrhythmias. Circulation 102:2152-2158, 2000.
7. Burnes JE, Taccardi B, Ershler PR, Rudy Y: Noninvasive electrocardiographic imaging of substrate and intramural ventricular tachycardia in infarcted hearts. J Am Coll Cardiol 38:2071-2078, 2001.
8. Ghanem RN, Jia P, Ramanathan C, et al: Noninvasive electrocardiographic imaging (ECGI): Comparison to intraoperative mapping in patients. Heart Rhythm 2:339-354, 2005.
9. Ramanathan C, Jia P, Ghanem RN, et al: Activation and repolarization of the normal human heart under complete physiological conditions. Proc Nat Acad Sci U S A 103:6309-6314, 2006.
10. Matsuo K, Uno K, Khrestian CM, Waldo AL: Conduction left-to-right and right-to-left across the crista terminalis. Am J Physiol Heart Circ Physiol 280:H1683-H1691, 2001.
11. Yamabe H, Misumi I, Fukushima H, et al: Conduction properties of the crista terminalis and its influence on the right atrial activation sequence in patients with typical atrial flutter. J Pacing Clin Electrophysiol 25:132-141, 2002.
12. Daoud EG, Morady F: Pathophysiology of atrial flutter. Annu Rev Med 49:77-83, 1998.
13. Rodriguez LM, Timmermans C, Nabar A, et al: Biatrial activation in isthmus-dependent atrial flutter. Circulation 104:2545-2550, 2001.
14. Wang Y, Schuessler RB, Damiano RJ, et al: Noninvasive electrocardiographic imaging (ECGI) of scar-related atypical atrial flutter. Heart Rhythm 4:1565-1567, 2007. Epub 2007 Aug 29.
15. Wang Y, Cuculich PS, Woodard PK, et al: Focal atrial tachycardia after pulmonary vein isolation: Noninvasive mapping with electrocardiographic imaging (ECGI). Heart Rhythm 4:1081-1084, 2007.
16. Intini A, Goldstein RN, Jia P, et al: Electrocardiographic imaging (ECGI), a novel diagnostic modality used for mapping of focal left ventricular tachycardia in a young athlete. Heart Rhythm 2:1250-1252, 2005.
17. Jia P, Ramanathan C, Ghanem RN, et al: Electrocardiographic imaging of cardiac resynchronization therapy in heart failure: Observation of variable electrophysiologic responses. Heart Rhythm 3:296-310, 2006.
18. Auricchio A, Fantoni C, Regoli F, et al: Characterization of left ventricular activation in patients with heart failure and left bundle branch block. Circulation 109:1133-1139, 2004.
19. Butter C, Auricchio A, Stellbrink C, et al: Pacing therapy for chronic heart failure IISG. Effect of resynchronization therapy stimulation site on the systolic function of heart failure patients. Circulation 104:3026-3029, 2001.
20. Ghanem RN, Burnes JE, Waldo AL, Rudy Y: Imaging dispersion of myocardial repolarization. II. Noninvasive reconstruction of epicardial measures. Circulation 104:1306-1312, 2001.

Syncope 91

Hugh Calkins

CHAPTER OUTLINE

Overview

Syncope (from the Greek *synkope*, "cessation, pause") is defined as a transient loss of consciousness, usually leading to falling, which results from transient inadequate cerebral perfusion.[1] The mechanism underlying the loss of consciousness is a global reversible reduction of blood flow to the reticular activating system, the neuronal network in the brainstem responsible for supporting consciousness. The metabolism of the brain, in contrast with that of many other organs, is exquisitely dependent on perfusion. Consequently, cessation of cerebral blood flow leads to loss of consciousness within approximately 10 seconds. Syncope is an important clinical problem because it is common, costly, and often disabling; may lead to injury; and may be the only warning sign before sudden cardiac death.[1-8] Patients with syncope account for up to 6% of hospital admissions and 3% of emergency room visits.

It has been estimated that more than one third of all people experience syncope at least once in their lifetime. The Framingham Study, in which biennial examinations were performed in 7814 persons, reported the incidence of a first report of syncope to be 6.2 per 1000 person-years of follow-up, with a cumulative incidence of approximately 6% over 10 years.[3] A more recent study reported a lifetime cumulative incidence of syncope of 35%, with a peak in the incidence of syncope at age 15 years.[4] The apparent disparity in the results of these studies is easily explained by the fact that the more recent study examined the lifetime cumulative incidence of syncope, whereas the earlier study reported the incidence of new-onset syncope in adults. In the United States, more than 1 million patients are evaluated each year for syncope, of whom more than 50% are admitted to the hospital. The annual cost of these admissions for syncope exceeds $2 billion, which is similar to the costs of hospitalizations in the United States for asthma, chronic obstructive lung disease, and human immunodeficiency virus.[5] The degree of functional impairment experienced by patients with syncope is similar to that in patients with chronic diseases such as chronic arthritis or recurrent moderate depressive disorder.[6]

The prognosis for patients with syncope varies greatly with the diagnosis.[1-3,8] Neurally mediated syncope generally is associated with a benign prognosis. By contrast, syncope due to a cardiac cause is associated with a more than two-fold increase in mortality.[3] Syncope also may be the only warning symptom before sudden cardiac death. This is clearly demonstrated by one recent study that reported that 42 of 162 young victims of sudden cardiac death had presented initially with syncope or presyncope.[7] For this reason, particular attention is needed to identify the subset of patients with a cardiac cause of syncope who may be at high risk for sudden death.

This chapter reviews the causes of syncope, summarizes the types and diagnostic yield of tests that may be of value in the evaluation of patients with syncope, identifies the indications for hospitalization of patients with syncope, and outlines one approach to the evaluation of patients with syncope. Because no standard method for establishing the exact cause of syncope is available, it is impossible to determine precisely the sensitivity and specificity of a diagnostic test. Only limited attention is focused on the treatment of syncope, because the approaches for treatment of cardiac arrhythmias are covered throughout this textbook.

Differential Diagnosis

The causes of apparent syncopal episodes can be broken down in several ways. One approach is to first separate patients with a real or apparent transient loss of consciousness into those with true syncope, in which the transient loss of consciousness results from cerebral hypoperfusion, and those patients with only "apparent" syncope[1] (Fig. 91-1). Because it often is difficult to distinguish true syncope from "apparent" syncope, a good beginning is to classify the causes of syncope into five primary groups—cardiac, vascular, neurologic or cerebrovascular, metabolic or miscellaneous, and syncope of unknown origin, as listed in Table 91-1. Conditions that cause only "apparent" syncope are identified as such in the table. Cardiac causes of syncope can be further subdivided into those of anatomic or arrhythmic etiology. A similar approach to subclassification of the causes of syncope can be applied to the other diagnostic groups (see Table 91-1). With current approaches to the diagnosis of syncope, a probable cause can be identified in more than 75% of patients.[1,9] By far the most common causes of syncope are reflex-mediated syncope and orthostatic hypotension. In most series, these causes of syncope are identified in more than one third of patients. Cardiac causes of syncope (particularly tachyarrhythmias and bradyarrhythmias) represent the second most common cause of syncope, accounting for 5% to 10% of the cases.

Metabolic causes of syncope are rare, accounting for less than 5% of syncopal episodes The most common metabolic causes of syncope are drug or alcohol intoxication, hypoglycemia, hypoxia,

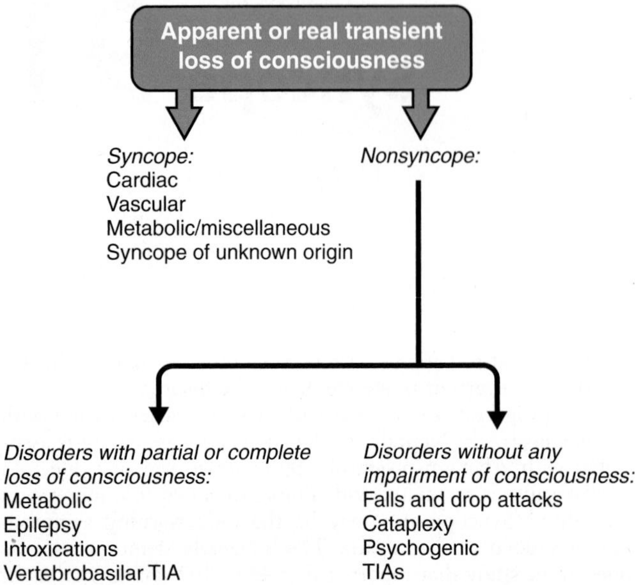

Apparent or real transient loss of consciousness

Syncope:
Cardiac
Vascular
Metabolic/miscellaneous
Syncope of unknown origin

Nonsyncope:

Disorders with partial or complete loss of consciousness:
Metabolic
Epilepsy
Intoxications
Vertebrobasilar TIA

Disorders without any impairment of consciousness:
Falls and drop attacks
Cataplexy
Psychogenic
TIAs

Figure 91-1 Approach to the differentiation of "apparent" syncope from true syncope ("real" transient loss of consciousness). TIA, transient ischemic attack.

and hyperventilation. Establishing hypoglycemia as the cause of an apparent loss of consciousness requires demonstration of hypoglycemia during the syncopal episode. Psychiatric disorders are now recognized as an important cause of apparent syncope. It is striking that several recent studies have identified a psychiatric cause of syncope in more than 80% of patients referred for evaluation of syncope of unknown origin.[10,11] The correct diagnosis of psychological causes of syncope is important because of its direct impact on further evaluation and management.

Although knowledge of the common conditions that may cause syncope is essential and will allow the clinician to arrive at a probable cause of syncope in a majority of patients, it is equally important for the clinician to be aware of several of the less common but potentially fatal causes of syncope such as the long QT syndrome,[12,13] arrhythmogenic right ventricular dysplasia (ARVD),[14] Brugada syndrome,[15-17] hypertrophic cardiomyopathy,[18] short QT syndrome,[19] and pulmonary emboli.[20] In one recent series of patients with ARVD, for example, 5 of the 31 patients who were diagnosed with ARVD on autopsy had experienced an episode of syncope an average of 1.5 years before sudden death.[14] It also is important to recognize that the distribution of the causes of syncope varies with age. Whereas neurally mediated syncope is by far the most common cause of syncope in young people, this mechanism is

Table 91-1 Differential Diagnosis of Syncope

Cardiac
- Anatomic
  - Aortic dissection
  - Aortic stenosis
  - Atrial myxoma
  - Cardiac tamponade
  - Hypertrophic cardiomyopathy (obstructuve)
  - Mitral stenosis
  - Myocardial ischemia/infarction
  - Pulmonary embolism
  - Pulmonary hypertension
- Arrhythmias
  - *Bradyarrhythmias*
    - Atrioventricular block
    - Sinus node dysfunction/bradycardia
  - *Tachyarrhythmias*
    - Supraventricular tachycardia
      - Atrial fibrillation
      - Paroxysmal supraventricular tachycardia: atrioventricular nodal reentry tachycardia,Wolff-Parkinson-White syndrome
  - Other
    - Ventricular tachycardia
- Structural heart disease
  - Inherited syndromes: arrhythmogenic reciprocating ventricular dysplasia, hypertrophic cardiomyopathy, Brugada syndrome, long QT syndrome
  - Drug-induced proarrhythmia
  - Implanted pacemaker or implantable cardioverter-defibrillator malfunction

Vascular
- Anatomic
  - Subclavian steal
- Orthostatic
  - Alcohol-induced
  - Autonomic failure
    - Primary autonomic failure syndromes: pure autonomic failure, multisystem atrophy, Parkinson's disease with autonomic failure
    - Secondary autonomic failure syndromes: diabetic neuropathy, amyloid neuropathy
  - Drug-induced
  - Idiopathic
  - Volume depletion
    - Addison's disease
    - Hemorrhage
    - Diarrhea
    - Diuretic-induced
- Reflex-mediated
  - Carotid sinus hypersensitivity
  - Glossopharyngeal and trigeminal neuralgia
  - Neurally mediated syncope: common faint, vasodepressor, neurocardiogenic, vasovagal
  - Situational: acute hemorrhage, cough, gastrointestinal stimulation (swallow, defecation, visceral pain), laugh, micturition, sneeze, postexercise, postprandial, other (e.g., brass instrument playing, weightlifting)

Neurologic/cerebrovascular*
- Arnold-Chiari malformation
- Migraine
- Seizures (partial complex, temporal lobe)
- Transient ischemic attacks/vertebrobasilar insufficiency/cerebrovascular accident)

Metabolic/miscellaneous*
- Hyperventilation with hypocapnia
- Hypoglycememia
- Hypoxemia
- Intoxication with drugs or alcohol
- Psychogenic syncope, somatization disorders

Syncope of unknown origin

*Denotes syncopal conditions that cause only "apparent" syncope but do not result from a reduction of cerebral perfusion.

unusual in elderly persons, in whom common causes include orthostatic or postprandial hypotension, medication effects, aortic stenosis, and bradyarrhythmias.[1,2]

Diagnostic Tests

Identification of the precise cause of syncope often is challenging. Because syncope usually occurs sporadically and infrequently, it is extremely difficult to either examine a patient or obtain an electrocardiogram (ECG) during an episode of syncope. For this reason, the primary goal in the evaluation of a patient with syncope is to arrive at a presumptive determination of the cause of syncope. The diagnostic tests that are available for evaluating patients with syncope and their diagnostic utility are summarized next.

History and Physical Examination

The history and physical examination are by far the most important components of the evaluation of a patient with syncope. It is well established that the probable cause of syncope can be identified on the basis of the history and physical examination alone in more than 25% of patients.[1,2,9] Maximal information can be obtained from the clinical history when it is approached in a systematic and detailed fashion. Initial evaluation should begin by determining whether the patient did in fact experience a syncopal episode. Every effort should be made to differentiate true syncope from apparent syncope with alterations in consciousness resulting from conditions such as metabolic and psychiatric disorders. Although falls can be differentiated from syncope by the absence of loss of consciousness, an overlap between symptoms of falls and syncope has been reported.[21-23] This overlap may reflect the fact that elderly persons may experience amnesia for the episode of loss of consciousness. Initial evaluation should begin by determining whether or not the patient did, in fact, experience a syncopal episode. Particular attention should then be focused on (1) determining whether or not the patient has a history of cardiac disease, or if a family history of cardiac disease, syncope, or sudden death exists; (2) identifying medications that may have played a role in syncope; (3) quantifying the number and chronicity of previous syncopal and presyncopal episodes; (4) identifying precipitating factors including body position; and (5) quantifying the type and duration of prodromal and recovery symptoms. It also is useful to obtain careful accounts from witnesses that may have been present.

Syncope due to neurally mediated hypotension generally occurs in children, adolescents, or young adults; women are affected more commonly than men. Common precipitating factors include prolonged standing, a warm environment, and emotional upset. Premonitory symptoms usually are present for longer than 5 seconds and include palpitations, nausea, a subjective feeling of warmth, constricted visual fields, diaphoresis, and lightheadedness. Patients demonstrate pallor, diaphoresis, and dilated pupils during the event. The pulse is slow and weak. Of note, that incontinence as well as brief clonic (seizure-like) movements may occur. On recovery, patients usually experience prolonged fatigue.[24,25] A recent study developed diagnostic criteria for neurally mediated syncope based on a quantitative history.[25] A point score was developed based on seven questions. This point score system had 89% sensitivity and 91% specificity for correctly diagnosing neurally mediated syncope.

Syncope resulting from cardiac arrhythmias generally occurs in persons older than 55 years of age and is more common in men than in women. Syncope may occur at rest or during exertion. A family history of sudden death should raise concern about the potential for a cardiac arrhythmias as the cause of syncope. In contrast with that due to neurally mediated hypotension, syncope due to an arrhythmia often is associated with no or only brief warning symptoms (duration less than 5 seconds). Palpitations occurring before arrhythmic syncope are rarely reported. During syncope, patients have a weak or absent pulse and appear blue. Brief clonic, seizure-like movements can occur. Recovery symptoms are uncommon unless the patient had a prolonged period of unconsciousness.

Seizures are more common in young people (i.e., before the age of 45 years) and may occur in any setting. They may be of sudden onset without warning, or patients may experience a brief aura before seizure onset. Patients who experience a seizure often exhibit frothing at the mouth with horizontal eye deviation. The blood pressure is increased and the pulse is rapid. Tongue biting is considered a fairly specific but insensitive feature of a seizure. Tonic-clonic movements are common, as is incontinence. After experiencing a seizure, patients often will be disoriented and experience a slow recovery.[26-28]

In one study, a standardized questionnaire was administered to 102 patients with seizure and 569 patients with syncope.[26] The clinical symptoms reported by patients with syncope were compared with those reported by patients with seizure. Patients with seizure were more likely to have a cut tongue, bedwetting, prodromal déjà vu, preoccupation, mood changes, hallucinations or trembling before loss of consciousness, postictal confusion, muscle pain, headaches, observed convulsive movements, head turning, unresponsiveness during loss of consciousness, and blue skin observed by a bystander. Patients with syncope were more likely to experience presyncope or have syncope associated with prolonged sitting or standing or with warm environment or exercise. Patients with syncope also were more likely to experience diaphoresis, dyspnea, chest pain, palpitations, subjective feeling of warmth, nausea, and vertigo. The study investigators then developed a simple point score of diagnostic criteria that distinguishes seizures from syncope with 85% accuracy.

It is important to recognize that syncope due to a cardiac cause and also syncope due to neurally mediated hypotension may be misdiagnosed as a seizure. One recent study reported that 13% of patients referred to an epilepsy clinic were ultimately diagnosed with neurally mediated syncope.[27] Other studies have reported similar findings.[28]

After a careful history has been obtained, evaluation should continue with a physical examination. In addition to a complete cardiac examination, particular attention should be focused on determining whether or not structural heart disease is present, defining the patient's level of hydration, and detecting the presence of significant neurologic abnormalities suggestive of a dysautonomia or cerebrovascular accident. Orthostatic vital signs are a critical component of the evaluation. The patient's blood pressure and heart rate should be obtained while he or she is supine and should then be detemined each minute for approximately 3 minutes. The two abnormalities that should be searched for are (1) early orthostatic hypotension, defined as a 20-mm Hg drop in systolic blood pressure or a 10-mm Hg drop in diastolic blood pressure within 3 minutes of standing and (2) postural orthostatic tachycardia syndrome, which is defined as an increase of 28 beats per minute or more within 5 minutes of standing with symptoms of orthostatic intolerance.[24,29-31] The significance of postural orthostatic tachycardia syndrome lies in its close overlap with neurally mediated syncope as well as the fact that it is commonly misdiagnosed as sinus tachycardia, with subsequent inappropriate treatment.[30,31]

Standard Electrocardiogram

The 12-lead ECG is another important and standard component of the initial workup of a patient with syncope.[1,2,9] The initial

ECG results in establishment of a diagnosis in approximately 5% of patients and suggests a diagnosis in another 5% of patients. In measuring the QT interval as a screen for long QT syndrome, it recently has been proposed that the maximum corrected QT interval be determined on a beat-by-beat basis and used for diagnostic and risk stratification purposes.[13] Any abnormality of the baseline ECG is an independent predictor of cardiac syncope or increased mortality and suggests the need to pursue an evaluation of cardiac causes of syncope.[1,2] Most patients with syncope have a normal ECG pattern. This finding is useful because it suggests a low likelihood of a cardiac cause of syncope and is associated with an excellent prognosis, particularly when observed in a young patient with syncope. Despite the low diagnostic yield of electrocardiography, the test is inexpensive and risk-free. For these reasons, an ECG is considered a standard part of the evaluation of virtually all patients with syncope.[1,2]

Signal-Averaged Electrocardiography

Signal-averaged electrocardiography (SAECG) is a noninvasive technique used for the detection of low-amplitude signals in the terminal portion of the QRS complex (late potentials), which are a substrate for ventricular arrhythmias. In contrast with a standard ECG, SAECG testing does not play a role in the routine evaluation of patients with syncope.[1]

Noninvasive Electrocardiographic Monitoring

Continuous ECG monitoring using telemetry or Holter monitoring, or both, is commonly performed in patients with syncope but is unlikely to identify the cause of the syncope. By contrast, the information provided by ECG monitoring at the time of syncope is extremely valuable because it allows an arrhythmic cause of syncope to be established or excluded. Because of the infrequent and sporadic nature of syncope, however, the diagnostic yield of Holter monitoring in the evaluation of patients with syncope and presyncope is extremely low. Another clinically useful finding is the detection of symptoms in the absence of an arrhythmia. This finding is observed in up to 15% of patients undergoing continuous ECG monitoring. An important point worthy of emphasis is that the absence of an arrhythmia and symptoms during continuous ECG monitoring may not exclude an arrhythmia as the cause of syncope. In patients suspected of having an arrhythmia as the cause of syncope, additional evaluation such as electrophysiologic testing or event monitoring should be considered.

Current guidelines state that in-hospital monitoring is warranted when a patient has important structural heart disease and is at high risk for a life-threatening arrhythmia. Holter monitoring is indicated in patients with syncope who have clinical or ECG features suggesting an arrhythmic cause of syncope and very frequent episodes of syncope or presyncope (e.g., more than 1 per week) (class 1).[1] ECG monitoring is considered to be diagnostic when a correlation between syncope and an electrocardiographic abnormality (brady- or tachycarrhythmia) is detected. Conversely, ECG monitoring excludes an arrhythmic cause of syncope when a correlation between syncope and sinus rhythm can be established. Other findings that can be considered to be diagnostic include (1) ventricular pauses longer than 3 seconds in an awake patient, (2) periods of Mobitz second- or third-degree atrioventricular (AV) block in an awake patient, and (3) rapid paroxysmal ventricular tachycardia.[1]

External or Implantable Event Monitors

Transtelephonic event monitors are small, portable ECG recording devices that can be activated by the patient to record a rhythm strip. The tracings can be stored and transmitted over telephone lines at a later time. Some event monitors, referred to as continuous-loop event monitors (i.e., loop recorders), (see Chapter 83) are worn continuously and allow capture of both retrospective and prospective ECG recordings. Continuous-loop event monitors are preferred when used in the evaluation of a patient with syncope. According to current guidelines, external or implantable loop recorders (see Chapter 83) are recommended in patients with clinical or ECG features suggestive of arrhythmic syncope or a history of recurrent syncope with injury when the mechanism of syncope remains undetermined after a full evaluation. External event monitors (see Chapter 83) are most likely to be diagnostic in patients with recurrent episodes of syncope or presyncope at intervals of less than 4 weeks.[1] The diagnostic findings on event monitoring are those as outlined for Holter monitoring. When event monitors are used in selected populations of patients, a diagnostic yield as high as 25% may be observed. However, a much lower diagnostic yield can be expected in less selected populations.

In some patients, episodes of syncope are extremely infrequent, occurring once or twice a year. In this population of patients, traditional event monitoring is unlikely to be diagnostic. Implantable event monitors are lightweight, small devices with a projected longevity of 18 to 24 months. These devices are implanted in the subcutaneous tissue of the chest. The ECG signal is stored in a circular buffer capable of recording up to 42 minutes of rhythm. The device can be configured to trigger automatically on the basis of programmed detection criteria as well as with a handheld activator.

The diagnostic value of the implantable event recorder is now well established. One recent study randomized patients with recurrent unexplained syncope to undergo either implantation of an implantable loop recorder or conventional evaluation. During a median follow-up period of 17 months, 43% of patients with implantable loop recorders and 6% of conventional patients received an ECG diagnosis. Patients with implantable loop recorders had fewer postrandomization investigations and fewer days in the hospital and an improved quality of life; no difference in cost or mortality was observed during follow-up, however.[32] Another recent study reported that implantable loop recorders are of higher diagnostic value in patients with syncope who are 65 years of age or older.[33] According to current guidelines, implantable loop recorders are indicated when standard 30-day event monitors are nondiagnostic because of infrequent recurrences of syncope. Implantable loop recorders also may be indicated in an initial phase of the workup of syncope in patients with preserved ventricular function who have the clinical or ECG features suggesting an arrhythmic cause of syncope.[32] Implantable loop recorders also may be useful in determining the contribution of bradycardia before cardiac pacing is instituted in patients with suspected neurally mediated syncope associated with frequent recurrences or trauma.[1,34]

Mobile cardiac outpatient telemetry is a new type of continuous event monitoring that also has been shown to be of diagnostic value in patients with syncope.[35] Telemetry devices are wireless monitoring systems that are designed to be worn by patients to allow remote monitoring 24 hours ar day.

Echocardiograms

Although echocardiograms are rarely diagnostic of the cause of syncope, they commonly are used in the evaluation of patients with syncope because they provide information about the type and severity of underlying heart disease, which may be both diagnostic of the cause of syncope and also useful for risk stratification. Not all patients with syncope, however, need to undergo echocardiography.[1] Current guidelines recommend that echocardiography be performed in patients with syncope when cardiac disease is suspected in order to stratify risk by evaluating the cardiac substrate (class 1).[1] These guidelines further state that the results of echocardiography should be considered diagnostic of the cause of syncope when either severe aortic stenosis or an atrial myxoma is identified.

Head-up Tilt Table Testing (see Chapter 85)

Tilt table testing has been used for more than 2 decades in the evaluation of patients with syncope and provides diagnostic evidence indicating susceptibility to neurally mediated syncope.[1] Upright tilt testing generally is performed for 20 to 45 minutes at an angle between 60 and 70 degrees from horizontal. The sensitivity of the test can be increased, with a corresponding fall in specificity, by the use of longer tilt durations, steeper tilt angles, and provocative agents such as isoproterenol or nitroglycerin. When isoproterenol is used as a provocative agent, it is recommended that the infusion rate be increased incrementally from 1 mg to 3 μg per minute, in order to increase the heart rate by 20% to 25% of baseline. When nitroglycerin is used, a fixed dose of 400 μg nitroglycerin spray should be administered sublingually with the patient in the upright position. The result of tilt table testing is considered positive if syncope occurs (class 1).[1] The clinical meaning of abnormal responses other than induction of syncope is not clear.

Current guidelines identify two class 1 indications for tilt table testing: (1) investigation of an unexplained single episode of syncope in high-risk settings or recurrent syncope in the absence of organic heart disease, or in the presence of organic heart disease after cardiac causes of syncope have been excluded, and (2) further evaluation of cases in which it will be of clinical value to demonstrate susceptibility to neurally mediated syncope.[1] The class 2 indications for tilt testing are (1) evaluation of cases in which an understanding of the hemodynamic pattern of syncope may alter the therapeutic approach, (2) differentiation of syncope with jerking movements from epilepsy, (3) evaluation of patients with recurrent unexplained falls, and (4) assessment for recurrent presyncope and dizziness. Tilt table testing is not indicated in patients with clear-cut neurally mediated syncope in whom demonstration of a susceptibility to neurally mediated syncope will not alter treatment, and it also is not indicated for evaluation of a single episode of syncope not associated with injury and not in a high-risk setting.

Although tilt table testing has been shown to be of great value in the evaluation of patients with syncope, it is also important to recognize its limitations in this regard. A recent article has reviewed these limitations, which include the following: (1) No definitive method of diagnosis of neurally mediated syncope is available, so tilt tests have not been evaluated against a good standard; (2) tilt testing involves the use of a complex set of methodologic variables; and (3) tilt tests have only moderate reproducibility, (4) do not have prognostic predictive power, and (5) have not been demonstrated to be useful in predicting response or in guiding treatment.[36] It also is important to recognize that identification of an asystole response at the time of a positive tilt table test does not correlate or predict the presence of an asystolic response during subsequent recurrences of neurally mediated syncope, as demonstrated in multiple studies.[34,37]

Electrophysiologic Testing

Electrophysiologic testing can provide important diagnostic and prognostic information in patients presenting with syncope. The results of such testing can be useful in establishing a diagnosis of sick sinus syndrome, carotid sinus hypersensitivity, heart block, supraventricular tachycardia, or ventricular tachycardia (VT). The indications for electrophysiologic testing in the evaluation of patients with syncope are outlined in detail in the European Society of Cardiology Task Force on Syncope guidelines and more generally in the American Heart Association/American College of Cardiology Foundation (AHA/ACCF) Scientific Statement on the Evaluation of Syncope.[1,2] An electrophysiology study is indicated in patients with syncope in whom the initial evaluation suggests an arrhythmic cause of syncope. These patients include those with ECG abnormalities or structural heart disease or syncope associated with palpitations or a family history of sudden death (class 1). Several more controversial (class 2) indications for electrophysiologic testing also are recognized. These indications include evaluation of the exact nature of an arrhythmia that has already been identified as the cause of syncope; prognostication in patients with cardiac disorders in which arrhythmia induction has a bearing on the selection of therapy; and exclusion of a cardiac cause of syncope in patients with high-risk occupations, in whom such diagnosis is critical. Electrophysiologic testing is not indicated for patients with normal findings on ECG who do not have heart disease and have not experienced palpitations (class 3).

An electrophysiology study is considered to be diagnostic of the cause of syncope when any one of the following five abnormalities is identified: (1) sinus bradycardia and a very prolonged cSNRT (less than 525 ms), (2) bifascicular block and a baseline HV interval longer than 100 ms or demonstration of second- or third-degree His-Purkinje block during incremental atrial pacing or provoked by an infusion of procainamide, (3) previous myocardial infarction and induction of sustained monomorphic VT, (4) ARVD and induction of ventricular arrhythmias, and (5) induction of a rapid supraventricular arrhythmia that reproduces hypotensive or spontaneous symptoms.[1] According to these guidelines, two findings on electrophysiologic testing have less certain diagnostic value: an HV interval greater than 70 ms but less than 100 ms and the induction of polymorphic VT or ventricular fibrillation (VF) in patients with Brugada syndrome or ARVD (or with both). In contrast with previous guidelines for evaluation of syncope, the current guidelines state that the induction of polymorphic VT or VF in patients with ischemic heart disease or dilated cardiomyopathy has a low predictive value (class 3).[1] A presumptive diagnosis can be established in approximately one third of patients referred for electrophysiologic testing to evaluate syncope of unknown origin.

Evaluation of Sinus Node Function

Sinus node function is evaluated during electrophysiologic testing primarily by determining the *sinus node recovery time* (SNRT), defined as the interval between the last paced atrial depolarization and the first spontaneous atrial depolarization resulting from activation of the sinus node. The SNRT is determined by pacing the right atrium at cycle lengths between 600 and 350 ms for 30 to 60 seconds. The SNRT is corrected for the underlying sinus cycle length (SCL) and expressed as the corrected SNRT (CSNRT = SNRT − SCL). A corrected SNRT greater than 525 ms generally is considered somewhat abnormal, and a corrected SNRT greater than 1 second is considered markedly abnormal. A *secondary pause* is defined as an inappropriately long pause among the beats that follow the first sinus recovery beat after atrial overdrive pacing. Evaluation of secondary pauses increases the sensitivity of the SNRT in the detection of sinus node dysfunction. Identification of sinus node dysfunction as the cause of syncope is uncommon during electrophysiologic testing (being seen in less than 5% of cases). A point worthy of emphasis is that the absence of evidence of sinus node dysfunction during electrophysiologic testing does not exclude a bradyarrhythmia as the cause of syncope.

Carotid Sinus Hypersensitivity

Syncope caused by carotid sinus hypersensitivity results from stimulation of carotid sinus baroreceptors, which are located in the internal carotid artery above the bifurcation of the common carotid artery. Carotid sinus hypersensitivity is diagnosed by applying gentle pressure over the maximal carotid pulsation two fingerbreadths below the angle of the jaw, where the carotid bifurcation is located. Pressure should be applied for 5 to 10 seconds during continuous electrocardiographic monitoring and blood pressure measurements. It is important to perform carotid sinus massage with the patient in both supine and upright positions. A normal response to carotid sinus massage is a transient decrease in the sinus rate or slowing of AV conduction, or both. Carotid sinus massage is considered to be positive for carotid sinus hypersensitivity if symptoms are reproduced during or immediately after the massage in the presence of asystole longer than 3 seconds or a fall in systolic blood pressure of 50 mm Hg or more. A positive response is considered to be diagnostic of the cause of syncope in the absence of any other competing diagnosis. The response to carotid sinus massage can be classified as cardioinhibitory (asystole), vasodepressive (fall in systolic blood pressure), or mixed.

The main complications associated with performing carotid sinus massage are neurologic. Because of this complication, carotid sinus massage should be avoided in patients with previous transient ischemic attacks, strokes within the past 3 months, and carotid bruits. Carotid sinus massage is recommended in patients older than 40 years of age with syncope of unknown etiology after the initial evaluation (class 1).[1] If the patient is suspected to have carotid artery disease, carotid sinus massage should be avoided.

Carotid sinus hypersensitivity is detected in approximately one third of elderly patients who present either with syncope or after nonaccidental falls.[1,21-23] It is important to recognize, however, that carotid sinus hypersensitivity also is commonly observed in asymptomatic elderly patients. Thus, the diagnosis of carotid sinus hypersensitivity should be approached cautiously after exclusion of alternative causes of syncope. Once the diagnosis is made, dual-chamber pacemaker implantation is recommended for patients with recurrent syncope or falls resulting from carotid sinus hypersensitivity. One recent study of 1624 patients who presented to the emergency department after a nonaccidental fall identified carotid sinus hypersensitivity in 34%. Patients with a cardioinhibitory response to carotid sinus massage were randomized to receive pacemaker therapy or clinical follow-up alone. Patients who underwent placement of a pacemaker were significantly less likely than control subjects to experience a recurrent fall during follow-up (odds ratio, 0.42). Syncopal events also were reduced in the follow-up period.[21]

Atrioventricular Block

During electrophysiologic testing, AV conduction is assessed by measuring the AV node–His bundle conduction time (A-H interval) and the His bundle–ventricular conduction time (H-V interval) and also by determining the response of AV conduction to incremental atrial pacing and atrial premature stimuli. Electrophysiologic features that establish AV block as the probable cause of syncope include the presence of bifascicular block and a baseline HV interval longer than 100 ms or demonstration of second- or third-degree His-Purkinje block during incremental atrial pacing or provoked by an infusion of procainamide.[1] Findings on electrophysiologic testing with less certain diagnostic value for AV block include an HV interval longer than 70 ms but shorter than 100 ms. Across studies that have reported the results of electrophysiologic testing in evaluating patients with syncope, AV block was identified as the probable cause of syncope in approximately 10% to 15% of patients. Donateo and colleagues reported the results of a systematic evaluation of patients with syncope in the setting of a bundle branch block on the baseline ECG.[38] Of 347 patients referred for evaluation of syncope, 55 had a baseline bundle branch block pattern. Systematic evaluation, including electrophysiologic testing, resulted in a diagnosis of cardiac syncope in 25 patients (45%): AV block in 20, sick sinus syndrome in 2, VT in 1, and aortic stenosis in 2. Neurally mediated syncope was diagnosed in 22 patients (40%), and syncope remained unexplained in 8 (15%).

Supraventricular Tachycardia

It is uncommon for a supraventricular tachycardia to cause syncope unless the patient has underlying heart disease, the rate is extremely rapid, or the patient has a propensity for the development of neurally mediated syncope. The typical pattern that is observed is the development of syncope or near-syncope at the onset of the supraventricular arrhythmia due to an initial drop in blood pressure. The patient often regains consciousness despite the continuation of the arrhythmia as a result of activation of a compensatory mechanism. Completion of a standard electrophysiology study allows accurate identification of most types of supraventricular arrhythmias that may cause syncope. The study should be repeated during an isoproterenol infusion to increase the sensitivity, particularly for detecting idiopathic VT or AV nodal reentrant tachycardia. Supraventriuclar tachycardia can be determined to be the cause of syncope during electrophysiologic testing if a rapid supraventricular arrhythmia is induced that reproduces hypotensive or spontaneous symptoms.[1] Supraventricular tachycardia is diagnosed as the probable cause of syncope in less than 5% of patients who undergo electrophysiologic testing for evaluation of syncope of unknown origin.

Ventricular Tachycardia

VT is the most common abnormality that is uncovered during electrophysiologic testing in patients with syncope. Among studies that have reported the results of such testing in evaluating patients with syncope, VT was identified as the probable cause of syncope in approximately 20% of patients. According to the recent update of the European Guidelines on Management of Syncope, an electrophysiology study is considered to be diagnostic for VT as the cause of syncope in patients with a previous myocardial infarction or ARVD in whom sustained monomorphic VT is induced. Also according to these guidelines, findings on electrophysiology testing with less certain diagnostic value for a ventricular arrhythmias as the cause of syncope include the induction of polymorphic VT or VF in patients with the Brugada syndrome or ARVD. The induction of polymorphic VT or VF in patients with ischemic heart disease or dilated cardiomyopathy has a low predictive value and should not be considered diagnostic of a ventricular arrhythmia as the probable cause of syncope (class 3).[1]

Significance of a Normal Response to Electrophysiologic Testing

Approximately 70% of patients referred for evaluation of syncope demonstrate a normal response to electrophysiologic testing. Although a negative result on such testing has been demonstrated in previous studies to be predictive of a low risk of sudden death, this is a controversial issue. Several studies have reported a significant incidence of sudden death among patients with markedly impaired ventricular function, despite normal findings on electrophysiologic testing. Although this issue has been debated vigorously in the past, it has lost its importance because prophylactic ICD implantation is recommended for most patients with an ischemic or nonischemic cardiomyopathy with an ejection fraction less than 0.35, regardless of symptoms.[39]

Computed Tomography Scans, Electroencephalograms, and Carotid Duplex Scans

Syncope as an isolated symptom rarely has a neurologic cause. As a result, widespread use of tests to screen for neurologic conditions is rarely diagnostic. In many institutions, computed tomography (CT) scans, electroencephalograms (EEGs), and carotid duplex scans are overused. A diagnosis is almost never uncovered that was not first suspected on the basis of findings on a careful history and neurologic examination. Transient ischemic attacks that result from carotid disease are not accompanied by loss of consciousness. No studies have suggested that carotid Doppler ultrasonography is beneficial in patients with syncope. EEGs should be obtained only in patients in whom the likelihood of epilepsy is relatively high. CT and magnetic resonance imaging should be avoided in patients with uncomplicated syncope.[1]

Stress Testing and Cardiac Catheterization

Myocardial ischemia is an unlikely cause of syncope and, when present, usually is accompanied by angina. It is for this reason that exercise testing and coronary angiography are not recommended in patients with syncope or presyncope that does not occur in association with exercise (class 3).[1]

Syncope occurring during exercise generally is considered to be suggestive of a cardiac origin. It is important to recognize, however, that not all syncopal events during exertion have a cardiac cause. Although this mechanism is uncommon, exertional syncope may in fact be neurally mediated.[40] In contrast with syncope during exercise, syncope occurring in the postexertional period almost always results from a neurally mediated mechanism or autonomic failure.

Exercise stress testing is recommended as part of the evaluation of patients who experience syncope during or shortly after exertion (class 1).[1] The test is considered to be diagnostic of the cause of syncope when ECG and hemodynamic abnormalities are present and syncope is reproduced during or immediately after exercise. The presence of Mobitz II second- or third-degree AV block is considered to be diagnostic even in the absence of syncope. Patients suspected of having severe aortic stenosis or obstructive hypertrophic cardiomyopathy should not undergo exercise stress testing because it may precipitate a cardiac arrest. Coronary angiography is recommended in patients with syncope suspected to be due, directly or indirectly, to myocardial ischemia.

Blood Tests

The routine use of blood tests, such as measurement of serum electrolytes, cardiac enzymes, and glucose and determination of hematocrit, is of low diagnostic value.[1,2] As a result, such laboratory tests are recommended only if syncope is suspected to result from a loss of circulating volume, or if a syncope-like disorder with a metabolic cause is suspected.[1]

Approach to the Evaluation of Patients with Syncope

Figure 91-2 outlines the approach to the diagnostic evaluation of a patient presenting with syncope proposed by the European Society of Cardiology Task Force on Syncope.[1] The initial evaluation begins with a careful history, physical examination, supine and upright blood pressure measurements, and a 12-lead ECG. On the basis of the findings on this initial evaluation, patients can be classified into those with true syncope and those who have not experienced true syncope. Those patients with syncope can be further divided into three main groups: (1) those in whom a certain diagnosis has been established, (2) those with a suspected diagnosis, and (3) those patients with unexplained syncope. The need for further diagnostic testing or initiation of treatment can then be determined. On the basis of this initial evaluation performed in either an emergency department or an outpatient setting, the probable cause of syncope can be identified in up to 50% of patients. When this diagnostic approach has been completed, a probable cause of syncope can be determined in more than three fourths of the patients.

Hospitalization of Patients with Syncope

Shown in Figure 91-3 is a proposed model for the evaluation of patients hospitalized with syncope. As can be appreciated from the diagram, the value of a dedicated syncope evaluation unit is increasingly recognized. In addition to attempting to establish a diagnosis, the emergency department or syncope evaluation unit physician must decide whether a patient should be admitted to the hospital for an in-patient evaluation. Table 91-2 presents the European Guidelines on Management of Syncope recommendations for hospitalization of patients with syncope.[1] Since publication of these recommendations, several studies have reported favorable outcomes when a syncope evaluation unit or standardized approach to the evaluation of syncope and decisions regarding hospitalization is used.[41-43] Brignole and associates, for example, used decision-based software to standardize the evaluation of syncope in the emergency departments of 11 general hospitals.[42] A diagnostic workup consistent with the guidelines was accomplished in 86% of patients, resulting in a presumptive diagnosis in nearly 100% of the cases evaluated. Hospitalization was deemed appropriate for evaluation of syncope in 25% of patients. Another recent study randomized patients to management in a syncope evaluation unit or to "standard" evaluation. Management in the syncope evaluation unit resulted in a diagnosis in 67% of patients, compared with 10% of patients who underwent a standard evaluation.[43] In addition to the recommendations of the European Society of Cardiology, several other guidelines or rules have been developed to aid in the identification of patients most likely to have an adverse outcome after syncope or to require hospitalization. The San Francisco Syncope Rule, for example, recommends that patients with syncope who present with ECG abnormalities, a complaint of shortness of breath, hematocrit greater than 30%, systolic blood pressure below 90 mm Hg, or a history of congestive heart failure be hospitalized for evaluation.[44] Since development of this rule, subsequent studies have shown it to be 98% sensitive and 56% specific for the prediction of serious outcomes after syncope.[45] Similar recommendations for hospital admission from the emergency department have been established by the American College of Emergency Room Physicians. The clinical policy document recommends hospital admission of patients with syncope who demonstrate (1) a history of congestive heart failure or ventricular arrhythmia, (2) associated chest pain or symptoms compatible with an acute coronary syndrome, (3) evidence of significant heart failure or valvular disease on physical examination, or (4) ECG findings of ischemia, arrhythmia, prolonged QT interval, or bundle branch block.[46]

Selected Issues Concerning the Treatment of Syncope

The approach to management of a patient with syncope depends largely on the diagnosis that is established. For example,

Transient loss of consciousness
Initial evaluation
History, physical examination, supine and upright BP, standard ECG
Syncope
Nonsyncopal attack
Confirm with specific test or specialist's consultancy
Certain diagnosis
Suspected diagnosis
Unexplained syncope
Cardiac likely
Neurally mediated or orthostatic likely
Frequent or severe episodes
Single/rare episodes
Cardiac tests
Neurally mediated tests
Neurally mediated tests
No further evaluation
Reappraisal
Reappraisal
Treatment
Treatment
Treatment
Treatment

Figure 91-2 Approach to the diagnostic evaluation of a patient presenting with syncope, as proposed by the European Society of Cardiology Task Force on Syncope.[1] BP, blood pressure; ECG, electrocardiogram.

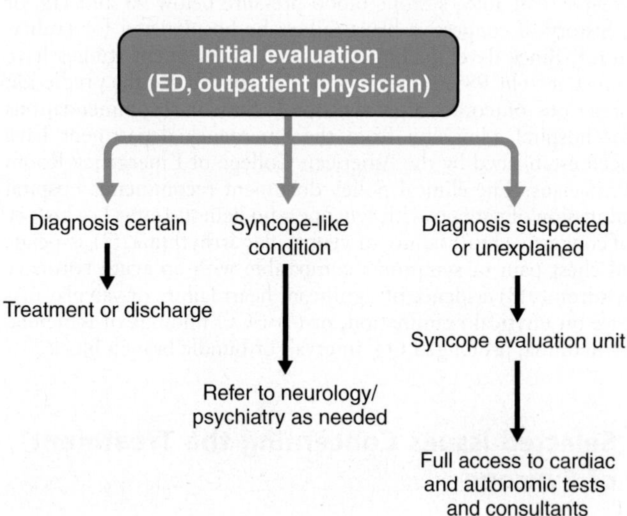

Figre 91-3 Proposed model for the evaluation of patients hospitalized with syncope. ED, emergency department.

Table 91-2 Scoring System to Determine Whether Syncope Is Due to Neurally Mediated Syncope or to Another Cause: Patient Questionnaire

Question	Scoring (points)
1. Is there a history of bifascicular block, asystole, diabetes, or supraventricular tachycardia (SVT)?	5
2. Have bystanders noted you to be blue during your passing out episode?	4
3. Did your episodes start when you were 35 years of age or older?	3
4. Do you remember anything about being unconscious?	2
5. Do you faint or have lightheaded episodes with prolonged sitting or standing?	1
6. Do you sweat or feel warm before a faint?	2
7. Do you have lightheaded spells or faint with pain in medical settings?	3

The patient has neurally mediated syncope if the point score is 2 or less (i.e., more negative).

Adapted from Sheldon R, Rose S, Connolly S, et al: Diagnostic criteria for vasovagal syncope based on a quantitative history. Eur Heart J 27:344-350, 2006.

appropriate treatment for a patient with syncope related to AV block or sick sinus syndrome probably would involve placement of a permanent pacemaker; in a patient with syncope related to the Wolff-Parkinson White syndrome, treatment probably would consist of catheter ablation; and in a patient with syncope related to VT or in the setting of an ischemic or nonischemic cardiomyopathy, treament probably would entail placement of an implantable defibrillator. For other types of syncope, optimal management may involve discontinuation of an offending pharmacologic agent, an increase in salt intake, or education of the patient.

Because neurally mediated syncope is so common, a review of treatment options seems appropriate here. Treatment of syncope due to neurally mediated hypotension begins with a careful history with particular attention focused on identifying precipitating factors, quantifying the degree of salt intake and current medication use, and determining whether the patient has a previous history of peripheral edema, hypertension, asthma, or other conditions that may alter the approach used for treatment. For most patients with neurally mediated syncope, particularly those with infrequent episodes associated with an identifiable precipitant, education and reassurance are sufficient.[1,24,29] Patients should be educated about common precipitating factors, such as dehydration, prolonged standing, alcohol, and medications such as diuretics and vasodilators. Patients also should be taught to sit or lie down at the onset of symptoms or to cross the legs (if sitting) and squeeze them together. Volume expansion by salt supplementation also is commonly recommended. Several recent studies have reported that drinking approximately 500 mL of water acutely improves orthostatic tolerance to tilt in healthy subjects and may be of value as prophylaxis for syncope in blood donors.[47,48] The effectiveness of water ingestion alone in the management of patients with recurrent neurally mediated syncope has not been well studied.

A recent important shift in the approach to treatment of neurally mediated syncope resulted from the proven effectiveness of "physical" measures and maneuvers in the treatment of patients with this condition.[24,29,49-51] It is notable that the revised European Guidelines on Management of Syncope identify the following physical measures as class 2 treatments for neurally mediated syncope: (1) tilt training, (2) head-up tilt sleeping (elevation of the head of the bed by more than 10 degrees), (3) isometric leg and arm counter-pressure maneuvers, and (4) moderate aerobic and isometric exercise.[1] One recent study, for example, reported that 2 minutes of an isometric hand grip maneuver initiated at the onset of symptoms during tilt testing rendered two thirds of patients asymptomatic.[50] Other studies have demonstrated that tilt (standing) training, which involves standing against a wall for 40 minutes twice daily, is effective in the treatment of neurally mediated syncope.[49] Although this approach has been shown to be effective in some trials, other studies have reported no impact of home tilt training on abnormal response rate for tilt table testing.[52] This lack of effect may reflect poor long-term compliance with this treatment strategy.

In contrast with physical maneuvers, which now are generally accepted to be of benefit in the management of patients with neurally mediated syncope, the value of pharmacologic agents is less certain. The medications that generally are relied on to treat neurally mediated syncope include beta-blockers, fludrocortisone, serotonin reuptake inhibitors, and midodrine. Despite the widespread use of these agents, none of these pharmacologic agents have been demonstrated to be effective in multiple large prospective randomized clinical trials. A recent small study reported that midodrine is effective.[53] Although beta-blockers are regarded by many clinicians as first-line agents, several recent studies have reported that the beta-blockers metoprolol, propranolol, and nadolol are no more effective than placebo.[54,55]

Although pacemakers also have been found to be valuable in some cases for management of neurally mediated syncope in several clinical trials, a recent large controlled trial, in which all subjects received pacemakers but pacing was activated in only 50% of the patients, showed no benefit of pacing.[56] Because of the variable results of these clinical trials and the profound implications of pacemaker implantation, considerable restraint should be exercised in considering the implantation of a pacemaker for treatment of neurally mediated syncope. The development of asystole during tilt table testing is not considered to be an absolute indication for pacemaker implantation. In fact, one recent study reported that the heart rhythm observed at the time of a positive tilt test does not correlate with the patient's heart rhythm at the time of a subsequent episode of syncope.[34] The European Guidelines on Management of Syncope state that cardiac pacing is indicated for treatment in patients with neurally mediated syncope who have a cardioinhibitory form, more than 5 episodes per year or associated severe physical injury or accident, and age older than 40 years (class 2).[1]

Summary

Syncope is a common and important clinical problem. Although the prognosis for most patients with syncope is benign, syncope may be the only warning of impending sudden cardiac death. Accordingly, a thorough evaluation is required. With use of a systematic and standardized approach to the evaluation of patients with syncope and the appropriate application of available diagnostic tools, a probable cause of syncope can be identified in more than three fourths of the patients. Once a diagnosis is established, appropriate treatment can then be initiated.

References

1. Brignole M, Alboni P, Benditt DG, et al: Guidelines on management (diagnosis and treatment) of syncope—update 2004. Eur Heart J 25:2054-2072, 2004.
2. Strickberger SA, Benson DW, Biaggioni I, et al: AHA/ACCF Scientific Statement on the Evaluation of Syncope. Circulation 113:316-327, 2006.
3. Soteriades ES, Evans JC, Larson MG, et al: Incidence and prognosis of syncope. N Engl J Med 12:878-885, 2002.
4. Ganzeboom K, Mairuhu G, Reitsma JB, et al: Lifetime cumulative incidence of syncope in the general population: A study of 549 Dutch subjects aged 35-60 years. J Cardiovasc Electrophysiol 17:1172-1176, 2006.
5. Sun BC, Emond JA, Camargo CA: Direct medical costs of syncope-related hospitalizations in the United States. Am J Cardiol 95:668-671, 2005.
6. Van Dijk N, Sprangers MA, Colman N, et al: Clinical factors associated with quality of life in patients with transient loss of consciousness. J Cardiovasc Electrophysiol 17:998-1003, 2006.
7. Wisten A, Messner T: Symptoms preceding sudden cardiac death in the young are common but often misinterpreted. Scand Cardiovasc J 39:143-149, 2005.
8. Kapoor WN, Karpf M, Wieand S, et al: A prospective evaluation and follow-up of patients with syncope. N Engl J Med 309:197-204, 1983.
9. Van Dijk N, Boer KR, Colman N, et al: High diagnostic yield and accuracy of history, physical examination, and ECG in patients with transient loss of consciousness in FAST: The Fainting Assessment Study. J Cardiovasc Electrophysiol 19:48-55, 2008.
10. Ventura R, Maas R, Ruppel R, et al: Psychiatric conditions in patients with recurrent unexplained syncope. Europace 3:311-316, 2001.

11. Benbadis SR, Chichkova R, Psychogenic pseudosyncope: An underestimated and provable diagnosis. Epilepsy Behav 9:106-110, 2006.
12. Hobbs JB, Peterson DR, Moss AJ, et al: Risk of aborted cardiac arrest or sudden cardiac death during adolescence in the long-QT syndrome. JAMA 296:1249-1254, 2006.
13. Goldenberg I, Mathew J, Moss AJ, et al: Corrected QT variability in serial electrocardiograms in long QT syndrome: The importance of the maximum corrected QT for risk stratification. J Am Coll Cardiol 48:1047-1052, 2006.
14. Dalal D, Nasir K, Bomma C, et al: Arrhythmogenic right ventricular dysplasia: A United States experience. Circulation 25:3823-3832, 2005.
15. Antzelevitch C, Brugada P, Borggrefe M, et al: Brugada syndrome: Report of the second consensus conference. Heart Rhythm 4:429-440, 2005.
16. Gehi AK, Duong TD, Metz LD, et al: Risk stratification of individuals with the Brugada electrocardiogram: A meta-analysis. J Cardiovasc Electrophysiol 17: 577-583, 2006.
17. Takagi M, Yokoyama Y, Aonuma K, et alfor the Japan Idiopathic Ventricular Fibrillation Study (J-IVFS) Investigators: Clinical characteristics and risk stratification in symptomatic and asymptomatic patients with Brugada syndrome: Multicenter study in Japan. J Cardiovasc Electrophysiol 18:1244-1251, 2007. Epub 2007 Sep 24.
18. Maron BJ, Spirito P, Shen WK, et al: Implantable cardioverter-defibrillators and prevention of sudden cardiac death in hypertrophic cardiomyopathy. JAMA 298:405-412, 2007.
19. Bjerregaard P, Gussak I: Short QT syndrome: Mechanisms, diagnosis and treatment. Nat Clin Pract Cardiovasc Med 2:84-87, 2005.
20. Calder Kirsten K, Herbert M, Henderson SO: The mortality of untreated pulmonary embolism in emergency department patients. Ann Emerg Med 45:302-310, 2005.
21. Kenny RA, Richardson DA, Bexton RS, et al: Carotid sinus syndrome: A modifiable risk factor for nonaccidental falls in older adults (SAFE PACE). J Am Coll Cardiol 38:1491-1496, 2001.
22. Parry SW, Kenny RA: Drop attacks in older adults: Systematic assessment has a high diagnostic yield. J Am Geriatr Soc 3:74-78, 2005.
23. Parry SW, Steen IN, Baptist M, Kenny RA: Amnesia for loss of consciousness in carotid sinus syndrome: Implications for presentation with falls. J Am Coll Cardiol 45:1840-1843, 2005.
24. Grubb BP: Neurocardiogenic syncope and related disorders of orthostatic intolerance. Circulation 111:2997-3006, 2005.
25. Sheldon R, Rose S, Connolly S, et al: Diagnostic criteria for vasovagal syncope based on a quantitative history. Eur Heart J 27:344-350, 2006.
26. Sheldon R, Rose S, Ritchie D, et al: Historical criteria that distinguish syncope from seizures. J Am Coll Cardiol 40:142, 2002.
27. Josephson CB, Rahey S, Sadler RM: Neurocardiogenic syncope: Frequency and consequences of its misdiagnosis as epilepsy. Can J Neurol Sci 34:221-224, 2007.
28. Zaidi A, Clough P, Cooper P, et al: Misdiagnosis of epilepsy: Many seizure-like attacks have a cardiovascular cause. J Am Coll Cardiol 36:181-184, 2000.
29. Grubb BP: Neurocardiogenic syncope. N Engl J Med 352:1004-1010, 2005.
30. Grubb BP, Kanjwal Y, Kosinski D: The postural tachycardia syndrome: A concise guide to diagnosis and management. J Cardiovasc Electrophysiol 17:108-112, 2006.
31. Thieben MJ, Sandroni P, Sletten DM, et al: Postural orthostatic tachycardia syndrome: The Mayo Clinic experience. Mayo Clin Proc 82:308-313, 2007.
32. Farwell DJ, Freemantle N, Sulke N: The clinical impact of implantable loop recorders in patients with syncope. Eur Heart J 27:351-356, 2006.
33. Brignole M, Menozzi C, Maggi R, et al: The usage and diagnostic yield of the implantable loop-recorder in detection of the mechanism of syncope and in guiding effective antiarrhythmic therapy in older people. Europace 7:273-279, 2005.
34. Deharo J, Jego C, Lanteaume A, Dijane P: An implantable loop recorder study of highly symptomatic vasovagal patients. J Am Coll Cardiol 47:587-593, 2006.
35. Olson JA, Fouts AM, Padanilam BJ, Prystowsky EN: Utility of mobile cardiac outpatient telemetry for the diagnosis of palpitations, presyncope, syncope, and the assessment of therapy efficacy. J Cardiovasc Electrophysiol 18:473-477, 2007.
36. Sheldon R: Tilt testing for syncope: A reappraisal. Curr Opin Cardiol 20:38-41, 2005.
37. Omar AR, Ng KS, Ng WL, Sutandar A: Reproducibility of tilt-table test result in patients with malignant neurocardiogenic syncope. Intern Med J 34:504-506, 2004.
38. Donateo P, Brignole M, Alboni P, et al: A standardized conventional evaluation of the mechanism of syncope in patients with bundle branch block. Europace 4:357-360, 2002.
39. Goldberger Z, Lampert R: Implantable cardioverter-defibrillators: Expanding indications and technologies. JAMA 295:809-818, 2006.
40. Krediet CT, Wilde AA, Halliwill JR, Wieling W: Syncope during exercise, documented with continuous blood pressure monitoring during ergometer testing. Clin Auton Res 15:59-62, 2005.
41. Bartoletti A, Fabiani P, Adriani P, et al: Hospital admission of patients referred to the emergency department for syncope: A single-hospital prospective study based on the application of the European Society of Cardiology Guidelines on syncope. Eur Heart J 27:83-88, 2006.
42. Brignole M, Menozzi C, Bartoletti A, et al, for the Evaluation of Guidelines in Syncope Study 2 (EGSYS-2) group: A new management of syncope: Prospective systematic guideline–based evaluation of patients referred urgently to general hospitals. Eur Heart J 27:76-82, 2006.
43. Shen WK, Decker WW, Smars PA, et al: Syncope Evaluation in the Emergency Department Study (SEEDS). A multidisciplinary approach to syncope management. Circulation 110:3636-3645, 2004.
44. Quinn JV, Stiell IG, McDermott DA, et al: Derivation of the San Francisco Syncope Rule to predict patients with short-term serious outcomes. Ann Emerg Med 43:224-232, 2004.
45. Quinn J, McDermott D, Stiell I, et al: Prospective validation of the San Francisco Syncope Rule to predict patients with serious outcomes. Ann Emerg Med 47:448-454, 2006.
46. American College of Emergency Physicians: Clinical policy: Critical issues in the evaluation and management of patients presenting with syncope. Ann Emerg Med 37:771-776, 2001.
47. Lu C, Diedrich A, Tung C, et al: Water ingestion as prophylaxis against syncope. Circulation 108:2660-2665, 2003.
48. Schroeder C, Bush VE, Norcliffe LJ, et al: Water drinking acutely improves orthostatic tolerance in healthy subjects. Circulation 106:2806-2811, 2002.
49. Abe H, Kondo S, Kohshi K, Nakashima Y: Usefulness of orthostatic self-training for the prevention of neurocardiogenic syncope. Pacing Clin Electrophysiol 25:1454-1458, 2002.
50. Brignole M, Croci F, Menozzi C, et al: Isometric arm counter-pressure maneuvers to abort impending vasovagal syncope. J Am Coll Cardiol 40:2054-2060, 2002.
51. Krediet P, van Dijk N, Linzer M, et al: Management of vasovagal syncope: Controlling or aborting faints by leg crossing and muscle tensing. Circulation 106:1684-1689, 2002.
52. On YK, Park J, Huh J, Kim JS: Is home orthostatic self-training effective in preventing neurally mediated syncope? Pacing Clin Electrophysiol 30:638-643, 2007.
53. Kaufmann H, Saadia D, Voustianiouk A: Midodrine in neurally mediated syncope: A double-blind randomized, crossover study. Ann Neurol 52:342, 2002.
54. Sheldon R, Connolly S, Rose S, et al, for the POST Investigators: Prevention of Syncope Trial (POST): A randomized, placebo-controlled study of metoprolol in the prevention of vasovagal syncope. Circulation 113:1164-1170, 2006.
55. Flevari P, Livanis EG, Theodorakis GN, et al: Vasovagal syncope. A prospective, randomized, crossover evaluation of the effect of propranolol, nadolol and placebo on syncope recurrence and patients' well-being. J Am Coll Cardiol 40:499, 2002.
56. Connolly SJ, Sheldon R, Thorpe K, et al, for the VPS II Investigators: Pacemaker therapy for prevention of syncope in patients with recurrent severe vasovagal syncope. Second Vasovagal Pacemaker Study (VPSII): A randomized trial. JAMA 289:2224, 2003.

Sudden Cardiac Deaths in Athletes, Including Commotio Cordis 92

MARK S. LINK AND N. A. MARK ESTES III

CHAPTER OUTLINE

Sudden cardiac death (SCD) in young athletes is a remarkably visible entity, despite its relative rarity. Each death of these young, healthy athletes jolts a community and spurs self-reflection and action. In the United States, the incidence of SCD averages 0.5 per 100,000 athletes a year,[1,2] similar to the current incidence in Italy.[3] This incidence has been relatively stable over time in the United States but has decreased in Italy. The incidence of SCD increases as people age, almost certainly due to the expanding prevalence of atherosclerotic coronary artery disease.

In athletes with SCD, most patients have underlying structural heart disease (Fig. 92-1). The most common of these in the United States is hypertrophic cardiomyopathy (HCM).[1] Commotio cordis, now that it has become a well-know entity, accounts for nearly 20% of SCD in athletes, the second most common etiology in the United States. Coronary artery anomalies, myocarditis, Marfan syndrome, arrhythmogenic right ventricular cardiomyopathy (ARVC), valvular disease, and dilated cardiomyopathies account for most of the remaining underlying heart disease. However, in Italian series of SCD in athletes, ARVC is the most common underlying heart disease.[3] HCM accounts for a much lower percentage, which is perhaps related to the screening process, a lower underlying genetic penetration, or less-lethal forms of the gene or disease. Anomalous coronary arteries account for a significant percentage of SCD, as does coronary artery disease. In nonathletic populations such as the military and general public, the causes of sudden death in the young are less commonly cardiomyopathies and more commonly myocarditis, anomalous coronary arteries, and coronary artery disease.[4,5] Of course, as the athletic population ages, coronary artery disease becomes more prevalent and is by far the most common underlying heart disease.

The structural heart diseases and channelopathies that underlie sudden death in athletes are extensively discussed in other chapters of this book and therefore will not be discussed individually in this chapter. Rather, the focus is on triggering of arrhythmias and remodeling of the heart by athletics, screening of athletes, recommendations for participation in competitive sports by athletes, and use of supplements in athletes. Commotio cordis, which is not covered by any other specific chapter is also discussed.

Acute Triggering of Sudden Cardiac Death with Athletic Activity

Several investigations have evaluated the relationship of acute risk of cardiovascular events such as SCD to exercise. In large-scale population studies, vigorous activity temporarily increases the risk of SCD for the time period during vigorous exertion and for 30 to 60 minutes afterwards.[6-9] This increased temporal risk of SCD is observed in both habitual exercisers and nonexercisers, although the effect is far less pronounced in people who habitually exercise vigorously. In the Physicians Health Study, Albert and colleagues found that acute exercise temporally increased the risk of SCD 11-fold in habitual exercisers and 74-fold in those who did not regularly exercise.[7] However, these studies also demonstrate the paradox of exercise: Even though acute exercise temporally increases the risk of SCD, habitual exercise reduces the risk of overall SCD and mortality.

Data are incomplete on triggering of arrhythmias in specific congenital diseases, which are the most common causes of sudden death in athletes. The temporal risk of SCD with exercise has been best documented in long-QT syndrome (LQTS).[10,11] In LQT1 and LQT2, the most common trigger of syncope and SCD was during high sympathetic states such exercise or fright. LQT1 patients, in particular, have SCD during swimming. Persons with LQT3 do not have an increased risk of cardiac events with exercise, but instead their risk is increased during sleep. This different trigger of arrhythmic events is likely related to the difference in potassium-channel versus sodium-channel defect, although the exact mechanism

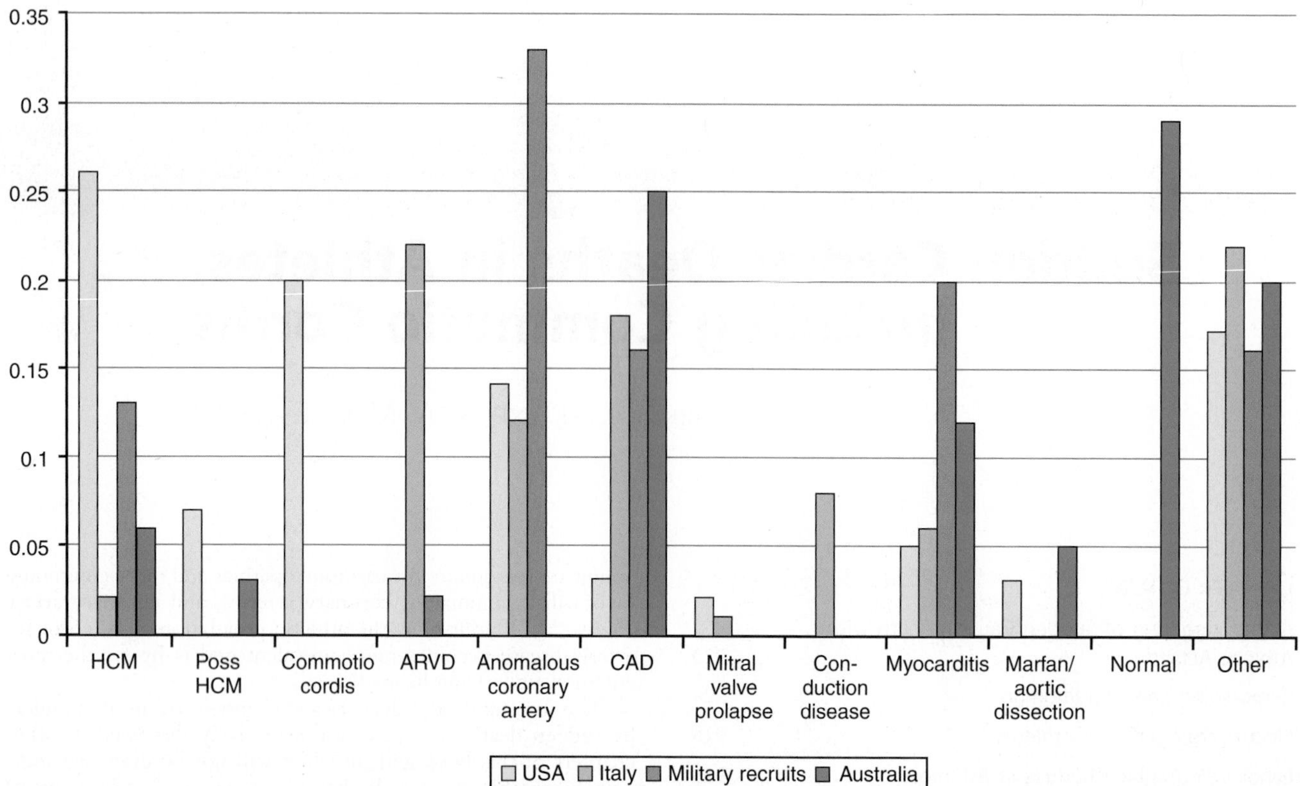

Figure 92-1 Relative incidence of underlying diseases in sudden cardiac death of athletes in United States[1] and Italy[16] and in nonathletes in the United States[4] and New Zealand.[5] Note the regional differences in the incidences of hypertrophic cardiomyopathy (HCM), commotio cordis, arrhythmogenic right ventricular cardiomyopathy (ARVC), coronary disease, and myocarditis. HCM is most commonly observed in the US athletes and ARVD is most commonly observed in Italian athletes. In nonathletic populations, anomalous coronary arteries, coronary artery disease (CAD), and myocarditis are more common causes of sudden cardiac death.

of triggering with LQTS is not yet completely elucidated. There are even data demonstrating that beta blockade, which blocks the sympathetic surge with exercise, reduces the risk of arrhythmias in LQT1 and LQT2 but does not decrease the risk in LQT3.[10,11]

The increased risk of exercise is also well documented in catecholaminergic polymorphic ventricular tachycardia (CPVT), where the disease is defined by exercise-induced arrhythmias.[12] In these patients, arrhythmias rarely occur during rest but commonly are precipitated by exercise. Beta blockade may be particularly effective in this condition. Similarly, in ARVC, most arrhythmias arise during exercise and not during rest, and beta blockade may be effective in decreasing arrhythmias.

Exercise-induced triggering of sudden death is not nearly as well documented in HCM. Although there are data showing that competitive athletes with HCM are at increased risk for SCD, it is not clear whether this increased risk is due to increased triggering of arrhythmias or remodeling of the substrate, which increases the risk of SCD. Epidemiologic data from Maron demonstrates that sudden cardiac death in athletes with HCM occurs most commonly in the afternoon, a time when training and competitive events are held. There are also multiple case reports and descriptions of athletes documenting SCD during exercise. In nonathlete HCM patients, however, the most common time for sudden cardiac death and arrhythmias for HCM patients with ICDs is during the evening and early morning.[13]

Patients with anomalous coronary arteries nearly exclusively die secondary to exercise-induced triggering of arrhythmias, quite likely mediated by acute coronary ischemia and resultant ventricular arrhythmias. Marfan syndrome is another disease for which exercise can provoke an acute trigger of dissection and sudden death. However, for many of the other conditions that underlie SCD in athletes, it is not clear that exercise can trigger arrhythmias and SCD. These include the Brugada syndrome, myocarditis, and dilated cardiomyopathies. Whether sympathetic drive affects the risk of commotio cordis is not entirely clear. In the commotio cordis registry, nearly 60% of the events are during competitive sports. It is extremely unlikely that competitive sports accounts for 60% of the incidences of being struck in the chest by balls or other objects. Thus, it is quite likely that the high adrenergic drive associated with competition in commotio cordis also increases the risk of SCD.[14]

Remodeling and Conditioning

In persons with normal hearts and those with coronary disease, there is clear evidence of a reduced risk of myocardial infarction and SCD in persons who undergo habitual, and especially high-level, vigorous exercise.[6,7] This reduced risk of cardiac events is seen with energy expenditure as minimal as walking and appears to increase with the both the time and intensity of exercise. The reduction in cardiovascular events is likely brought about by a number of beneficial effects of exercise, including decreased weight and blood pressure, improved lipids and glucose tolerance, and increased adherence to a healthy lifestyle, which includes an increased attention to diet and reduction in use of tobacco.

However, for persons with congenital heart diseases, there has never been any documentation of reduced mortality with exercise.[15] In fact, it would appear that the opposite is indeed true, that habitual exercise, and especially competitive exercise, increases the risk of sudden cardiac death.[16] This detrimental effect has not been proved, but is suggested by epidemiologic studies in which diseases such as HCM and arrhythmogenic right ventricular dysplasia (ARVD) are overrepresented in athletic populations with SCD compared to the general population. The relative contribution of triggering arrhythmias versus adverse alterations of the substrate is also not clear. In the Veneto region of Italy, Corrado and colleagues have shown that the risk of sudden cardiac death was nearly three-fold higher in competitive athletes versus nonathletes. In a 21-year period from 1979 to 1999, there were 300 cases of SCD. The incidence of SCD in athletes was 2.3/100,000 person-years compared to 0.9/100,000 person-years in nonathletes.[16] This proarrhythmic effect is possibly mediated through changes in the substrate due to ischemia, fibrosis, and nonclinical myocardial infarction.

Electrocardiograms in Athletes

Abnormalities in electrocardiograms (ECGs) of athletes are common. Whether these alterations are due to conditioning effects of sports or to underlying cardiac pathology is of critical importance (Fig. 92-2). In the Corrado screening series published in 1998, nearly 10% of their subjects who wished to

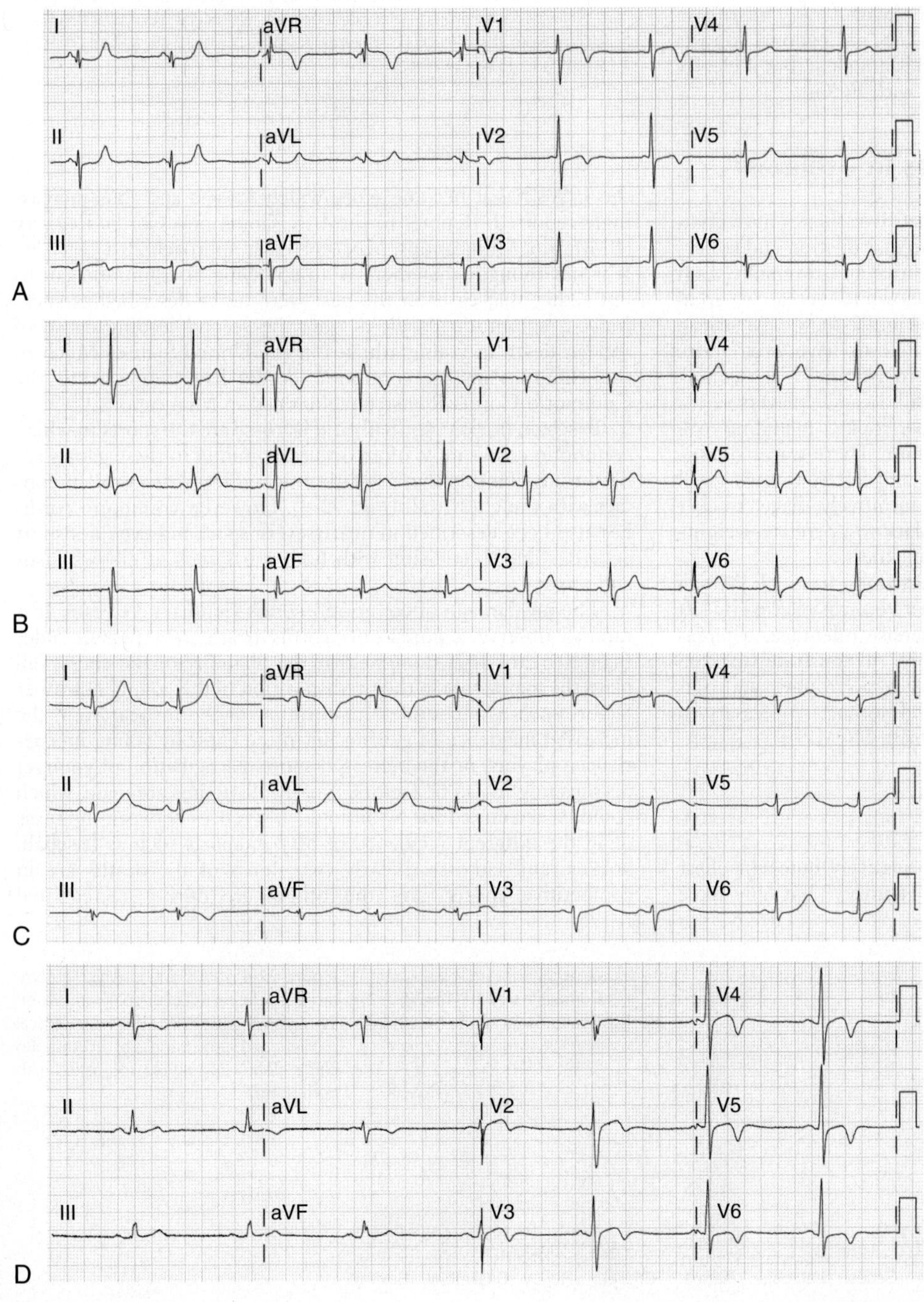

Figure 92-2 **A,** Electrocardiogram (ECG) from a 15-year-old girl with hypertrophic cardiomyopathy (HCM). Further workup on this patient demonstrated an echocardiogram with asymmetric hypertrophy and a septal thickness of 27 mm. Cardiac magnetic resonance imaging (MRI) confirmed the diagnosis and septal thickness and also revealed multiple areas of fibrosis. **B,** ECG from a 44-year-old man with arrhythmogenic right ventricular dysplasia (ARVD). He presented with palpitations and near syncope during exertion, and workup revealed an abnormal ECG with epsilon waves in lead V1. An echocardiogram revealed a dilated and hypokinetic right ventricle. At electrophysiologic study, ventricular tachycardia could be induced to which he developed hypotension. **C,** ECG from a 19-year-old woman who presented with syncope. She was taking ephedra supplements at the time. Cardiac workup demonstrated a normal echocardiogram and an ECG consistent with long QT syndrome. **D,** ECG from a 35-year-old man who presented with exertional palpitations and presyncope. A loop monitor demonstrated nonsustained ventricular flutter during symptoms. His 12-lead ECG is shown. Cardiac workup demonstrated a focal scar in the anterior wall. His coronary arteries did not demonstrate any disease, and myocarditis was diagnosed.

begin an athletic program or who were involved in an athletic program had abnormal ECGs.[17] Sinus bradycardias, first-degree heart block, and second-degree heart block are common, as are early repolarization and isolated voltage criteria for left ventricular hypertrophy.[18] These minor abnormalities are unlikely to be associated with heart disease.

However, it is clear that marked abnormalities are far less common.[19] These abnormalities include repolarization abnormalities, pathologic Q waves, conduction defects, and ventricular arrhythmias. In the analysis of the Italian screening data in high-level athletes, a markedly abnormal ECG was observed in 81 of 12,550 elite athletes. In a follow-up of nearly 10 years, five of these athletes with markedly abnormal ECGs developed heart disease,including ARVC and HCM. In U.S. series of professional football players, ECG abnormalities are seen in up to 55%, including ST abnormalities in up to 15% and IVCD in up to 20%, with an increased prevalence of abnormalities in African American compared to white players.[20,21] The reason that increased marked abnormalities in U.S. professional cohorts compared to Italian cohorts is observed is not clear, but it clearly has implications for screening athletes with ECGs.

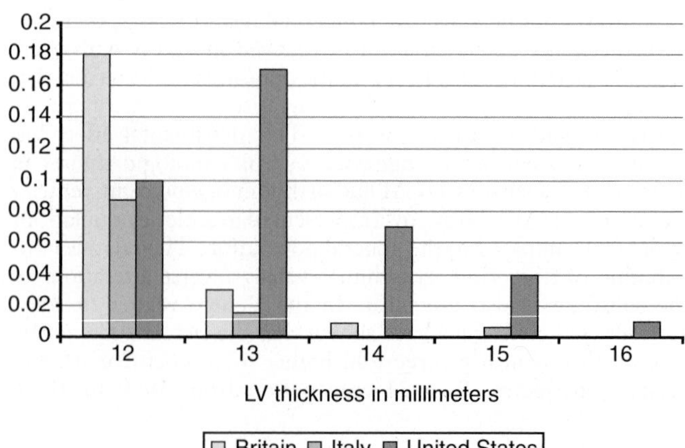

Figure 92-3 Incidence of professional athletes in Italy,[23] Britain,[22] and United States[24] with echocardiographic defined left ventricular (LV) wall thickness ≥12 mm. Note that 6% of US athletes (football players) had wall thickness of ≥15 mm, and 13% ≥14 mm.

Echocardiographic Changes in Athletes

It has been well documented that competitive athletes have myocardial remodeling, including left ventricular dilation and hypertrophy, and that these changes are adaptive and reversible. Left ventricular wall dimensions have been shown to increase to up to 14 mm in Italian and British athletes (Fig. 92-3).[22,23] American football players have been demonstrated to have even more marked myocardial hypertrophy of up to 16 mm.[24] In a cohort of 156 asymptomatic National Football League players, 23% had evidence of left ventricular hypertrophy, including 6% with wall thicknesses greater than 14 mm. There was a significant correlation between body weight and left ventricular wall thickness. Although larger athletes intuitively have thicker hearts, in fact there are insufficient data to correlate weight-based normative left ventricular wall thickness.

Differentiation of physiologic hypertrophy from HCM can be difficult. In general, physiologic hypertrophy is marked by left ventricular dilatation and excellent exercise tolerance, whereas patients with HCM more commonly demonstrate marked abnormal ECGs, bizarre patterns of hypertrophy, and left atrial enlargement. Occasionally, deconditioning is necessary to differentiate physiologic hypertrophy from HCM.[13,25]

Commotio Cordis

Commotio cordis, sudden death with relatively innocent chest wall impact, was described in the 19th century,[26] but only since the 1990s has it become more widely known and thus increasingly reported. Reports to the U.S. Commotio Cordis Registry (BJ Maron, Minneapolis, MN) currently approach 20 a year.[14,27] It is not thought that there is an epidemic of commotio cordis but rather that cases in the past were never described as such. Indeed, commotio cordis is now the second leading cause of sudden death in young athletes in the United States.[1] Much of the clinical data on commotio cordis have come from the Commotio Cordis Registry maintained in Minneapolis.[14]

Baseball, hockey, softball, and lacrosse are the sports in which commotio cordis most often occurs; common to these games are hard round objects that are airborne and thus can come in contact with the chest wall (Fig. 92-4). However, commotio cordis has also been described in nearly every sport and even nonsport activities due to collision with body parts such as elbows, fists, and knees.

The median age of commotio cordis victims is 14 years. It is rare to observe a commotio cordis death in a person older than 20 years. It is thought that the pliability of the chest wall plays the major role in the predisposition of the young, but other factors such as incomplete maturation of the myocardium, the increased incidence of getting hit in the chest by young inexperienced players, or the increased sports participation of younger persons might also be factors. Nearly all victims are male, which could be accounted for by biologic differences between the sexes or in the different incidence of play in sports such as baseball, hockey, and lacrosse. Nearly two thirds of the deaths are in competitive sports, and the others are during recreational

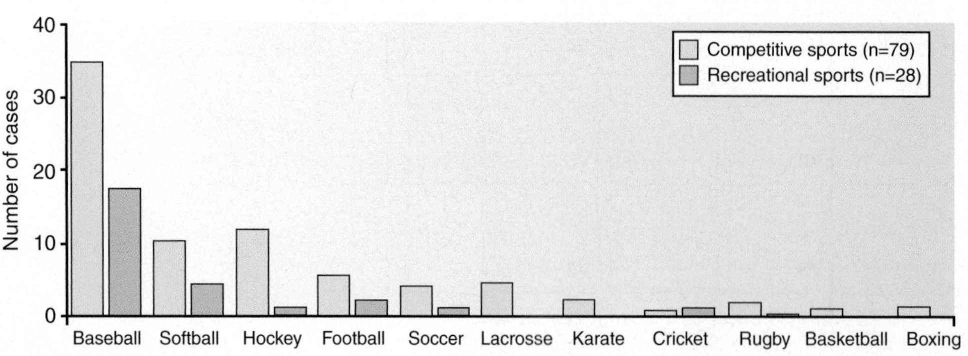

Figure 92-4 Sports during which a commotio cordis event occurred. (From Maron BJ, Gohman TE, Kyle SB, et al: Clinical profile and spectrum of commotio cordis. JAMA 287(9):1142-146, 2002, with permission.)

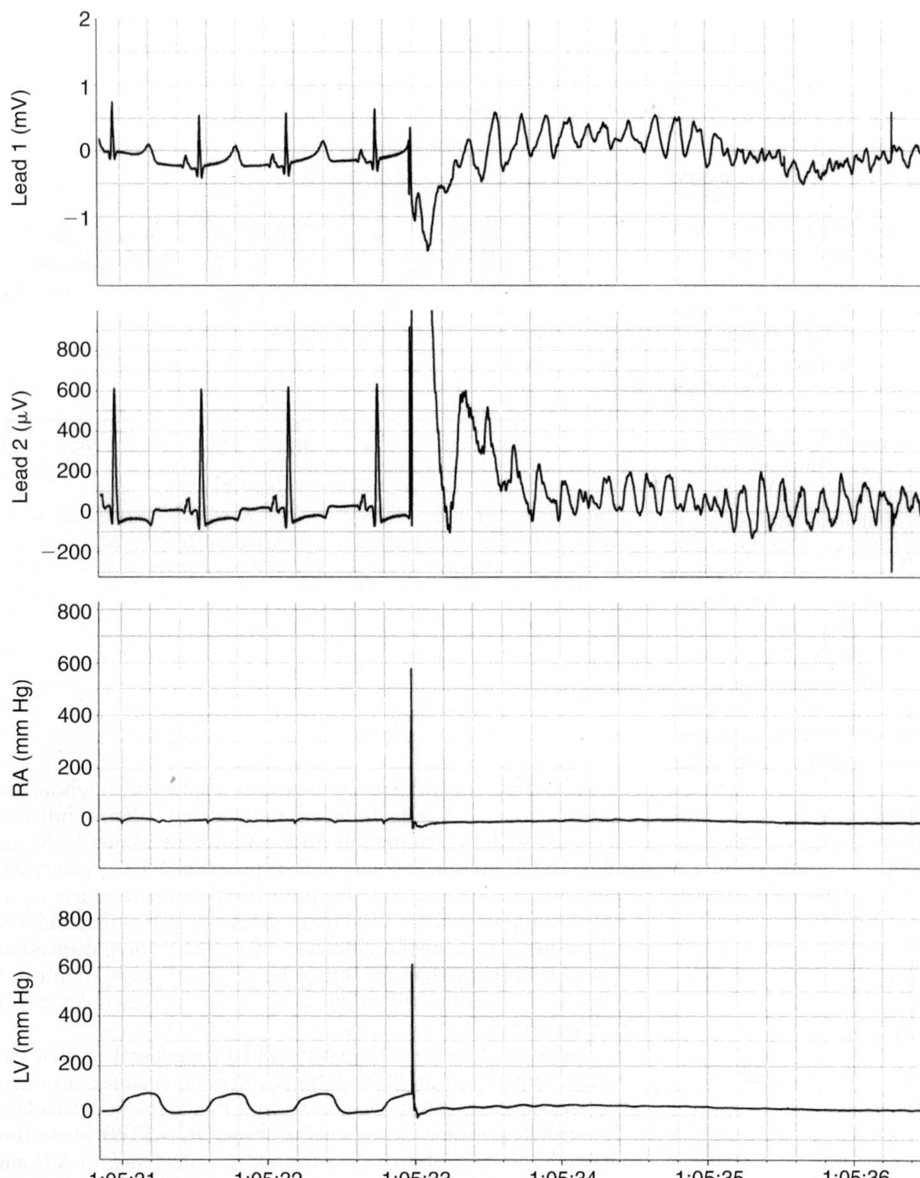

Figure 92-5 Two-lead electrocardiogram (ECG) and right atrial (RA) and left ventricular (LV) pressure tracings of a 16-kg swine undergoing chest wall impact with a 40-mph lacrosse ball. The pressure tracings recorded by Millar pressure-tip catheters demonstrate the nearly instantaneous rise in intracavitary pressures, and the ECG demonstrates immediate ventricular fibrillation.

sports and routine daily activities. Impacts occur directly over the cardiac silhouette and are thought to be of routine velocity for the age and sex of the person struck by the ball.

Approximately one half collapse instantaneously, and the others have a few seconds of lucidity before they collapse. If a defibrillator is readily available, the initial rhythms are ventricular fibrillation, and resuscitation is possible with defibrillation.[14] However, even with early defibrillation, survival is not assured.[28] As time increases from the event, the initial rhythms are increasingly found to be asystole, likely secondary to extinguished ventricular fibrillation, and resuscitation rates are markedly decreased.

In the clinical series, commotio cordis has occurred despite the use of safety baseballs and chest wall protection.[29] In two of 56 baseball-related incidents, a safety ball was reported to be the impact object.[27] In nearly one third of the players who underwent a commotio cordis event during competitive sports, a chest protector was worn.[29] In some sports, such as hockey, the arms were lifted, pulling the chest protector upward and thus exposing the chest. However, in other sports, such as lacrosse and baseball, the ball struck the chest protector, which was directly over the heart, and commotio cordis still resulted.

An animal model developed over the last 10 years has generated considerable information about the mechanisms of commotio cordis. Using juvenile anesthetized male swine, it was shown that timing the impact to the upslope of the T-wave, 10 to 30 ms before the T-peak, is one of the critical determinants of producing ventricular fibrillation (Fig. 92-5).[30] Impacts outside of this window but still on the upslope of the T-wave rarely produced VF, and impacts at all other time periods of the cardiac cycle did not produce VF, although they might cause transient heart block, ST segment elevation, or left bundle branch block. The velocity of the impact object was also crucial. When baseball impact velocity was 20 mph, VF was never produced. At 30 mph, approximately 30% of impacts caused VF, and at 40 mph nearly 70% of impacts caused VF.[31] At impact velocities of 50 mph or more, animals less commonly had VF, but now for the first time structural cardiac damage was seen, including valve rupture, cardiac rupture, and tamponade, suggesting that at these higher velocities the model was one of cardiac contusion and not commotio cordis. Impacts over the center of the cardiac silhouette are far more deadly than impacts at the base and apex.[32] Impacts outside the cardiac silhouette did not cause VF.

This experimental model has also been used to evaluate prevention of commotio cordis. With 30- and 40-mph impacts, age-appropriate safety baseballs decreased the risk of VF inversely with ball hardness.[30,33] However, commercially available chest wall protectors used in baseball and lacrosse were not found to decrease the incidence of VF with chest wall impact.[34]

The swine model and a more recently described Langendorff model offer insights into the mechanism of commotio cordis. Commotio cordis is a primary electrical event in which VF is produced directly by chest wall blow and not by ischemia or contusion. In the swine experimental model, the probability of VF induced by a chest blow is directly related to the peak LV pressure generated by the chest blow (Fig. 92-6). The threshold peak pressure necessary to produce VF is around 250 to 300 mm Hg, and the probability of VF increases with pressure increases up to 600 mm Hg. Pressure increases beyond that are associated with less VF, but increasing contusions, myocardial rupture, and pericardial tamponade. These pressure thresholds are remarkably conserved across many different experimental protocols, including sites of impact,[32] energy of impact,[31] stretch-activated channels,[35] role of the autonomic nervous system,[36] and chest wall protectors.[34]

The Langendorff model of commotio cordis has confirmed that a critical time window and energy window of pressure changes is necessary to produce VF (Fig. 92-7).[37] In this model, a fluid-filled balloon was placed in the LV of Langendorff-perfused rabbit hearts, and pressure pulses were applied throughout the cardiac cycle. VF was induced only when balloon inflation occurred within a vulnerable time window of 35 ms to 88 ms after the initiation of an action potential. This vulnerable window corresponded to the time of spontaneous increase in baseline repolarization dispersion; pressure pulses that induced VF resulted in a further increase in repolarization dispersion. Thus, it appears that the upstroke of the T wave signifies a window of potential vulnerability due to an increased dispersion of repolarization.

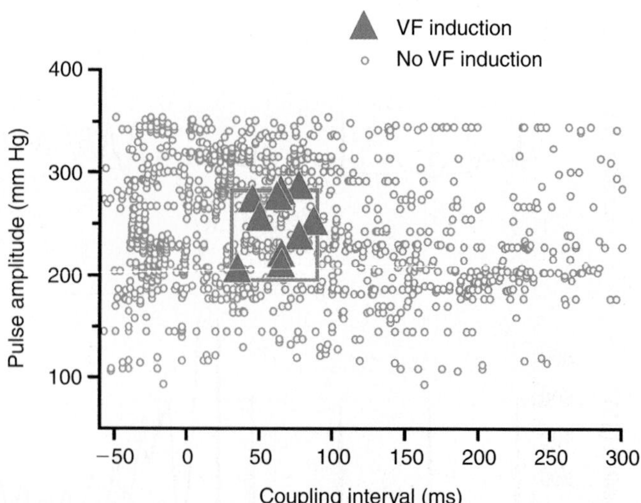

Figure 92-7 Data from Bode's Langendorff commotio cordis model. In this model, pressure impulses applied via a left ventricular balloon causes ventricular fibrillation (VF) only when a critical time and energy window of balloon inflation occurred. (From Bode F, Franz MR, Wilke I, et al: Ventricular fibrillation induced by stretch pulse: Implications for sudden death due to commotio cordis. J Cardiovasc Electrophysiol 17(9):1011-1017, 2006,with permission.)

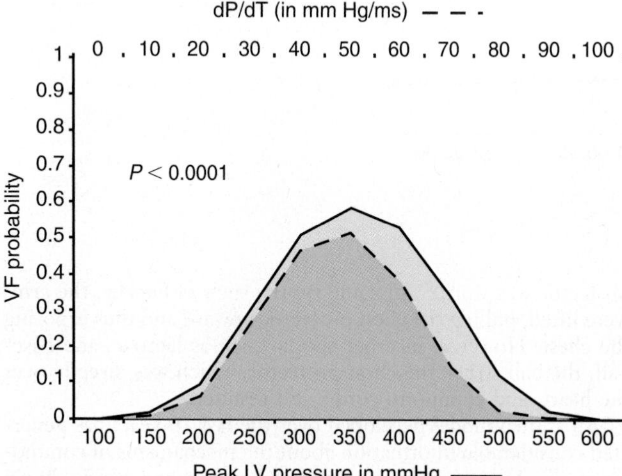

Figure 92-6 The probability of ventricular fibrillation (VF) relative to the peak left ventricular (LV) pressure and LV pressure over time (dP/dt) in 8- to 12-kg swine undergoing chest wall impacts with a baseball propelled at 20 to 70 mph. VF did not occur unless peak LV pressures generated by the chest wall blow reached 300 mm Hg. With pressures greater than 500 mm Hg, the probability of VF decreased, but myocardial damage, including contusions, myocardial ruptures, and pericardial tamponade were more evident. (From Link MS, Maron BJ, Wang PJ, et al: Upper and lower limits of vulnerability to sudden arrhythmic death with chest-wall impact (commotio cordis). J Am Coll Cardiol 41(1):99-104, 2003, with permission.)

Based on data from the swine and Langendorff models, we believe that activation of stretch-activated ion channels produces the myocardial substrate necessary for VF induction. Blockade of the stretch-sensitive adenosine triphosphate (ATP) potassium channel has been shown to decrease the incidence of VF and the magnitude of ST elevation in the experimental model.[38] Other possible channels, including the calcium stretch-activated channel, have not yet been demonstrated to be involved in commotio cordis.[35]

Screening

Screening young athletes is a particularly contentious issue, even though all agree that some elements of screening are important. The American Heart Association and the European Society of Cardiology recommend screening; they agree that a patient history—especially focused on a personal history of syncope, excess dyspnea, or chest pain—and a family history of sudden cardiac death are important elements of screening.[39,40] All agree that a physical examination for stigmata of Marfan syndrome, blood pressure measurement, femoral pulse check to rule out aortic coarctation, and evaluation for cardiac murmurs are necessary components.

Whether ECGs are warranted for screening of asymptomatic athletes is not clear. Data for including the ECG in the screening process is largely based on an observational study from the

Veneto region of Italy. This study, published in 1998, showed that by screening with an ECG and with a modified stress test, athletes with underlying cardiac pathology could be identified and prevented from participating in athletics, including not only competitive athletics but also conditioning in gymnasiums and sports clubs.[41] Of 33,735 athletes, 22 were found to have HCM and were disqualified from athletics. In addition, 238 were disqualified for rhythm and conduction abnormalities, 168 for systemic hypertension, 133 for valvular disease, and 60 for various other diseases. Thus, athletes with HCM accounted for only 3.5% of the disqualified conditions. A follow-up of this study, published in 2006, has shown that the incidence of sudden death in athletes has decreased from 3.5 per 100,000 person-years in 1979 to 1980, to 0.4 per 100,000 person-years in 2003 to 2004. The death rate in nonathletes has remained relatively stable at around 0.8 per 100,000 person-years, suggesting that the screening process reduced the incidence of SCD in athletes.[3]

No other large-scale series have replicated the Veneto series. In Japan, screening of all children in first, seventh, and 10th grades was begun in 1973, and data on this screening program were recently published.[42] In the Kagoshima region, 69,033 students were screened in seventh and 10th grade; of this group, 30,696 students subsequently moved out of the study area, leaving 37,807 students in the study. Screening included a questionnaire for the student and family and an ECG. If the questionnaire or the ECG raised concerns, the student was brought to medical attention for a workup. Of 1876 (2.7%) students brought for medical workup, nine were ultimately found to have cardiac disease, including five with HCM. In 6-year follow-up, one of the nine, a student with HCM, died while recreationally jogging. Two students, who had had normal ECGs and thus did not receive further workup also died. Autopsies were not performed, so their cardiac pathology was not known. Thus, the incidence of SCD in this screened population was 1.32 per 100,000 person-years, higher than other nonscreened populations.

Therefore, the issue of how to screen athletes remains unresolved. Whether an ECG or modified stress test, or both, should be mandated is not by any means clear at present. Ideally, a prospective randomized trial should be performed to document that potentially life-threatening diseases in athletes (or all youth for that matter) can be identified and, more importantly, that identification allows the opportunity to change the natural history of the disease. In addition, the societal and individual costs of false-positive diagnosis and restriction from sports of a potentially substantial segment of athletes must be considered.

Bethesda Guidelines for Participation in Competitive Sports

The 36th Bethesda Guidelines are the most comprehensive documents guiding physicians and athletes with regard to participation in *competitive* athletics.[43] Notably, these documents do not address participation in recreational athletics.[44] Some general themes are evident. Vigorous, aerobic competitive athletics are generally not advised for athletes with diseases that are commonly associated with sudden death in athletes. These diseases include the cardiomyopathies of HCM, ARVC, myocarditis, idiopathic dilated cardiomyopathies, and Marfan syndrome[13] and the primarily electrical diseases of LQTS (with the possible exception of LQT3), and CPVT.[11] Although there is no clear exercise-related exacerbation of SCD in Brugada syndrome, it was thought prudent to recommend these patients avoid competitive athletics. Persons with documented coronary disease likewise are advised to avoid high-level competitive athletics.[45] For persons with valvular or congenital heart disease, competitive sports are generally allowed so long as cardiovascular hemodynamics and myocardial structure and function are relatively normal.[46,47] However, as the severity of the valve or congenital heart disease and the resultant hemodynamics worsen, competitive athletics are not recommended. Persons with primary electrical diseases, including supraventricular and ventricular arrhythmias, that allow a cure with ablation are recommended to undergo such cure, after which they may return to competitive athletics.[11] Low-intensity competitive sports such as bowling or archery are allowed for nearly all persons.

The Bethesda Guidelines also specifically discuss sports participation for athletes with an implantable cardioverter-defibrillator and recommend against high-level competitive athletics for patients with an implantable cardioverter defibrillator, not only because of the underlying heart disease, for which these sports are generally prohibited, but also for the concerns of triggering of arrhythmias, failure of the implantable cardioverter-defibrillator to terminate arrhythmias in the high sympathetic state, and potential damage to the lead and generator.[11]

Supplements

Supplement use in athletes is quite common and ranges from energy drinks to more potentially hazardous substances, such as ephedra and androgenic steroids.[48-50] The true incidence of supplements used in sports is exceedingly difficult to ascertain, especially with the more illicit substances, because even if the drugs are legal athletes do not want to be tainted with the use of these agents.[51]

Energy drinks are almost certainly the most heavily used, not only by competitive but also by recreational athletes. In fact, energy drinks such as Monster and Red Bull are marketed to athletic communities all across the world. These drinks contain caffeine, taurine, and glucuronolactone. The benefits of caffeine include epinephrine release and stimulation of acetylcholine release and direct stimulation of the muscle cell. It reduces the perception of fatigue.[52] Caffeine at standard doses has little potential toxicity; however, at higher doses, agitation, tremors, and arrhythmias can result. The benefits of taurine and glucuronolactone are much less clear, as is the potential toxicity. Several deaths have been reputedly linked to these energy drinks, and thus several European countries have banned them.[48]

Creatine is a widely used supplement. Up to 41% of intercollegiate athletes admit to taking creatine.[53] Creatine is predominantly found in the muscle cell, but is also produced by the liver, pancreas, and kidneys. Exogenous supplementation reportedly increases energy levels during anaerobic activity and delays muscle fatigue. Side effects are rare at low doses, but muscle cramps, weight gain, and gastrointestinal distress can be seen, especially at higher doses.[54]

Blood doping, initially with stored blood and more recently with erythropoietin, is favored by athletes competing in sports requiring prolonged aerobic activity, such as cycling and cross-country skiing.[48-50] Oxygen-carrying capacity is increased, leading to improved skeletal-muscle performance. Adverse effects are related to the increased blood viscosity, which increases the risk of stroke and congestive heart failure.

Human growth hormone reputedly increases strength and decreases recovery time.[48-50] It is typically cycled with androgenic steroids, because human growth hormone supplementation is not currently detectable by any means. In growth hormone–deficient persons, administration clearly benefits the patient; however, whether there is truly any benefit for those without a deficiency is by no means clear. Risks associated with growth hormone include hypertension, cardiomegaly, ventricular hypertrophy, and dyslipidemia.[55]

Ephedra (ma huang) has also had a storied history and has increasingly been linked to adverse cardiovascular events.[56] Ephedra is a combination of alkaloids including ephedrine, pseudoephedrine, norephedrine, and others. Ephedra increases heart rate, blood pressure, and cardiac output.[57] It has been used to treat asthma and in weight loss and energy supplements. Several cardiovascular toxicities have been associated with ephedra use including SCD, myocardial infarction, and stroke.[56,58,59] Ephedra has been shown to increase the QTc with a single dose.[60] Although initially protected as a food supplement under the U.S. Dietary Supplement Health and Education Act of 1994, the U.S. Congress in 2004 took the extremely unusual course of banning the production and sale of ephedra in the United States.

Androgens have anabolic effects such as increase in muscle, heart, liver, and kidney mass; decrease in body fat; and stimulation of erythropoiesis, anticatabolic effects that allow faster recovery and central nervous system effects including increased aggression.[61] Androgens are therefore ideal supplements for athletes and are widely believed to possess the most beneficial results for performance enhancement. They were thus widely used by power lifters, track and field athletes, and athletes in any sport in which power and strength were a premium. However, this increased athletic prowess does not come without a cost. Androgens have been linked to cardiac toxicity including myocardial infarction, hypertrophy, and SCD; hepatocellular carcinoma; lipid abnormalities;, premature closure of growth plates; infertility; and depression.[50] The International Olympic Committee banned the use of androgens in 1975, and most sporting organizations quickly followed, based not only on the toxicity of these agents but also the unfairness they brought to the playing field.

Androstenedione was widely used in the place of androgens and is believed to be metabolized to androgens. A randomized trial and meta-analysis did not show evidence of benefit in athletic performance, but it did demonstrate that androstenedione lowered blood levels of high-density lipoprotein cholesterol.[62] Although banned by the IOC and FDA in the 1990s, it was only banned by professional baseball in 2004.

Tetrahydrogestrinone (THG) is a designer steroid solely manufactured for use by athletes. By modification from banned androgens, THG was not detectable by gas chromatography until 2003. It likely has all the beneficial effects of androgens along with the risks. THG is at the center of the controversy involving numerous professional and Olympic athletes.

Conclusion

Athletes with sudden or aborted SCD commonly have an underlying structural heart disease, with the exception of death due to commotio cordis. Athletic exercise temporally increases the risk of SCD in a person with normal heart and, by implication, also in those with abnormal hearts. Remodeling of the heart by athletics is likely beneficial in persons with normal hearts and coronary disease, but it is likely adverse in persons with HCM, ARVC, and various other genetic conditions. Screening is important; however, whether ECGs and modified stress tests are a critical part of the screen, and whether all persons should be screened or just athletes, is still unclear. Finally, performance-enhancing agents are widely used, and although randomized, controlled studies will never be performed, it is widely believed that these substances increase the risk of sudden death.

References

1. Maron BJ: Sudden death in young athletes. N Engl J Med 349(11):1064-1075, 2003.
2. Van Camp SP, Bloor CM, Mueller FO, et al: Nontraumatic sports death in high school and college athletes. Med Sci Sports Exerc 27(5):641-647, 1995.
3. Corrado D, Basso C, Pavei A, et al: Trends in sudden cardiovascular death in young competitive athletes after implementation of a preparticipation screening program. JAMA 296(13):1593-1601, 2006.
4. Eckart RE, Scoville SL, Campbell CL, et al: Sudden death in young adults: A 25-year review of autopsies in military recruits. Ann Intern Med 141(11):829-834, 2004.
5. Puranik R, Chow CK, Duflou JA, et al: Sudden death in the young. Heart Rhythm 2(12):1277-1282, 2005.
6. Siscovick DS, Weiss NS, Fletcher RH, Lasky T: The incidence of primary cardiac arrest during vigorous exercise. N Engl J Med 311:874-877, 1994.
7. Albert CM, Mittleman MA, Chae CU, et al: Triggering of sudden death from cardiac causes by vigorous exertion. N Engl J Med 343(19):1355-1361, 2000.
8. Whang W, Manson JE, Hu FB, et al: Physical exertion, exercise, and sudden cardiac death in women. JAMA 295(12):1399-1403, 2006.
9. Thompson PD, Franklin BA, Balady GJ, et al: Exercise and acute cardiovascular events placing the risks into perspective: A scientific statement from the American Heart Association Council on Nutrition, Physical Activity, and Metabolism and the Council on Clinical Cardiology. Circulation 115(17):2358-2368, 2007.
10. Kapetanopoulos A, Kluger J, Maron BJ, Thompson PD: The congenital long QT syndrome and implications for young athletes. Med Sci Sports Exerc 38(5):816-825, 2006.
11. Zipes DP, Ackerman MJ, Estes NAM III, et al: Task Force 7: Arrhythmias. 36th Bethesda Conference: Eligibility Recommendations for Competitive Athletes with Cardiovascular Abnormalities. J Am Coll Cardiol 45(8):43-52, 2005.
12. Napolitano C, Priori SG: Diagnosis and treatment of catecholaminergic polymorphic ventricular tachycardia. Heart Rhythm 4(5):675-678, 2007.
13. Maron BJ, Ackerman MJ, Nishimura RA, et al: Task Force 4: HCM and other cardiomyopathies, mitral valve prolapse, myocarditis, and Marfan syndrome. 36th Bethesda Conference: Eligibility Recommendations for Competitive Athletes with Cardiovascular Abnormalities. J Am Coll Cardiol 45(8):1340-1345, 2005.
14. Maron BJ, Gohman TE, Kyle SB, et al: Clinical profile and spectrum of commotio cordis. JAMA 287(9):1142-1146, 2002.
15. Maron BJ, Pelliccia A: The heart of trained athletes: Cardiac remodeling and the risks of sports, including sudden death. Circulation 114(15):1633-1644, 2006.
16. Corrado D, Basso C, Rizzoli G, et al: Does sports activity enhance the risk of sudden death in adolescents and young adults? J Am Coll Cardiol 42(11):1959-1963, 2003.
17. Corrado D, Basso C, Schiavon M, Thiene G: Screening for hypertrophic cardiomyopathy in young athletes. N Engl J Med 339(6):364-369, 1998.
18. Corrado D, McKenna WJ: Appropriate interpretation of the athlete's electrocardiogram saves lives as well as money. Eur Heart J 28(16):1920-1922, 2007.
19. Pelliccia A, Di Paolo FM, Quattrini FM, et al: Outcomes in athletes with marked ECG repolarization abnormalities. N Engl J Med 358(2):152-161, 2008.
20. Balady GJ, Cadigan JB, Ryan TJ: Electrocardiogram of the athlete: An analysis of 289 professional football players. Am J Cardiol 53:1339-1343, 1984.
21. Choo JK, Abernethy WB 3rd, Hutter AM Jr: Electrocardiographic observations in professional football players. Am J Cardiol 90(2):198-200, 2002.
22. Whyte GP, George K, Sharma S, et al: The upper limit of physiological cardiac hypertrophy in elite male and female athletes: The British experience. Eur J Appl Physiol 92(4-5):592-597, 2004.
23. Pelliccia A, Maron BJ, Spataro A, et al: The upper limit of physiologic cardiac hypertrophy in highly trained elite athletes. N Engl J Med 324(5):295-301, 1991.
24. Abernethy WB, Choo JK, Hutter AM Jr: Echocardiographic characteristics of professional football players. J Am Coll Cardiol 41(2):280-284, 2003.
25. Maron BJ, Douglas PS, Graham TP, et al: Task Force 1: Preparticipation screening and diagnosis of cardiovascular disease in

athletes. J Am Coll Cardiol 45(8):1322-1326, 2005.
26. Maron BJ, Doerer JJ, Haas TS, et al: Historical observation on commotio cordis. Heart Rhythm 3(5):605-606, 2006.
27. Madias C, Maron BJ, Weinstock J, et al: Commotio cordis—sudden cardiac death with chest wall impact. J Cardiovasc Electrophysiol 18(1):115-122, 2007.
28. Maron BJ, Wentzel DC, Zenovich AG, et al: Death in a young athlete due to commotio cordis despite prompt external defibrillation. Heart Rhythm 2(9):991-993, 2005.
29. Doerer JJ, Haas TS, Estes NA 3rd, et al: Evaluation of chest barriers for protection against sudden death due to commotio cordis. Am J Cardiol 99(6):857-859, 2007.
30. Link MS, Wang PJ, Pandian NG, et al: An experimental model of sudden death due to low-energy chest-wall impact (commotio cordis). N Engl J Med 338(25):1805-1811, 1998.
31. Link MS, Maron BJ, Wang PJ, et al: Upper and lower limits of vulnerability to sudden arrhythmic death with chest-wall impact (commotio cordis). J Am Coll Cardiol 41(1):99-104, 2003.
32. Link MS, Maron BJ, VanderBrink BA, et al: Impact directly over the cardiac silhouette is necessary to produce ventricular fibrillation in an experimental model of commotio cordis. J Am Coll Cardiol 37(2):649-654, 2001.
33. Link MS, Maron BJ, Wang PJ, et al: Reduced risk of sudden death from chest wall blows (commotio cordis) with safety baseballs. Pediatrics 109(5):873-877, 2002.
34. Weinstock J, Maron BJ, Song C, et al: Failure of commercially available chest wall protectors to prevent sudden cardiac death induced by chest wall blows in an experimental model of commotio cordis. Pediatrics 117(4):e656-e662, 2006.
35. Garan AR, Maron BJ, Wang PJ, et al: Role of streptomycin-sensitive stretch-activated channel in chest wall impact induced sudden death (commotio cordis). J Cardiovasc Electrophysiol 16(4):433-438, 2005.
36. Stout CW, Maron BJ, Vanderbrink BA, et al: Importance of the autonomic nervous system in an experimental model of commotio cordis. Med Sci Monit 13(1):BR11-BR15, 2007.
37. Bode F, Franz MR, Wilke I, et al: Ventricular fibrillation induced by stretch pulse: Implications for sudden death due to commotio cordis. J Cardiovasc Electrophysiol 17(9):1011-1017, 2006.
38. Link MS, Wang PJ, VanderBrink BA, et al: Selective activation of the K^{+}_{ATP} channel is a mechanism by which sudden death is produced by low-energy chest-wall impact (commotio cordis). Circulation 100(4):413-418, 1999.
39. Maron BJ, Thompson PD, Ackerman MJ, et alRecommendations and considerations related to preparticipation screening for cardiovascular abnormalities in competitive athletes: 2007 update: A scientific statement from the American Heart Association Council on Nutrition, Physical Activity, and Metabolism: Endorsed by the American College of Cardiology Foundation. Circulation 115(12):1643-1645, 2007.
40. Pelliccia A, Fagard R, Bjornstad HH, et al: Recommendations for competitive sports participation in athletes with cardiovascular disease: A consensus document from the Study Group of Sports Cardiology of the Working Group of Cardiac Rehabilitation and Exercise Physiology and the Working Group of Myocardial and Pericardial Diseases of the European Society of Cardiology. Eur Heart J 26(14):1422-1445, 2005.
41. Corrado D, Basso C, Schiavon M, Thiene G: Screening for hypertrophic cardiomyopathy in young athletes. N Engl J Med 339:364-369, 1998.
42. Tanaka Y, Yoshinaga M, Anan R, et al: Usefulness and cost effectiveness of cardiovascular screening of young adolescents. Med Sci Sports Exerc 38(1):2-6, 2006.
43. Maron BJ, Zipes DP: Introduction: Eligibility recommendations for competitive athletes with cardiovascular abnormalities—general considerations. J Am Coll Cardiol 45(8):1318-1321, 2005.
44. Maron BJ, Chaitman BR, Ackerman MJ, et al: Recommendations for physical activity and recreational sports participation for young patients with genetic cardiovascular diseases. Circulation 109(22):2807-2816, 2004.
45. Thompson PD, Balady GJ, Chaitman BR, et al: Task Force 6: Coronary artery disease. J Am Coll Cardiol 45(8):1348-1353, 2005.
46. Graham TP Jr, Driscoll DJ, Gersony WM, et al: Task Force 2: Congenital heart disease. J Am Coll Cardiol 45(8):1326-1333, 2005.
47. Bonow RO, Cheitlin MD, Crawford MH, Douglas PS: Task Force 3: Valvular heart disease. J Am Coll Cardiol 45(8):1334-1340, 2005.
48. Dhar R, Stout CW, Link MS, et al: Cardiovascular toxicities of performance-enhancing substances in sports. Mayo Clin Proc 80(10):1307-1315, 2005.
49. Bowers LD: Abuse of performance-enhancing drugs in sport. Ther Drug Monit 24(1):178-181, 2002.
50. Calfee R, Fadale P: Popular ergogenic drugs and supplements in young athletes. Pediatrics 117(3):e577-e589, 2006.
51. Alaranta A, Alaranta H, Holmila J, et al: Self-reported attitudes of elite athletes towards doping: Differences between type of sport. Int J Sports Med 27(10):842-846, 2006.
52. Bell DG, McLellan TM: Exercise endurance 1, 3, and 6 h after caffeine ingestion in caffeine users and nonusers. J Appl Physiol 93(4):1227-1234, 2002.
53. Metzl JD, Small E, Levine SR, Gershel JC: Creatine use among young athletes. Pediatrics 108(2):421-425, 2001.
54. Bohn AM, Betts S, Schwenk TL: Creatine and other nonsteroidal strength-enhancing aids. Curr Sports Med Rep 1(4):239-245, 2002.
55. Meyers DE, Cuneo RC: Controversies regarding the effects of growth hormone on the heart. Mayo Clin Proc 78(12): 1521-1526, 2003.
56. Samenuk D, Link MS, Homoud MK, et al: Adverse cardiovascular events temporally associated with ma huang, an herbal source of ephedrine. Mayo Clin Proc 77(1):12-16, 2002.
57. Jacobs I, Pasternak H, Bell DG: Effects of ephedrine, caffeine, and their combination on muscular endurance. Med Sci Sports Exerc 35(6):987-994, 2003.
58. Shekelle PG, Hardy ML, Morton SC, et al: Efficacy and safety of ephedra and ephedrine for weight loss and athletic performance: A meta-analysis. JAMA 289(12):1537-1545, 2003.
59. Haller CA, Benowitz NL: Adverse cardiovascular and central nervous system events associated with dietary supplements containing ephedra alkaloids. N Engl J Med 343(25):1833-1838, 2000.
60. McBride BF, Karapanos AK, Krudysz A, et al: Electrocardiographic and hemodynamic effects of a multicomponent dietary supplement containing ephedra and caffeine: A randomized controlled trial. JAMA 291(2):216-221, 2004.
61. Kutscher EC, Lund BC, Perry PJ: Anabolic steroids: A review for the clinician. Sports Med (Auckland) 32(5):285-296, 2002.
62. King DS, Sharp RL, Vukovich MD, et al: Effect of oral androstenedione on serum testosterone and adaptations to resistance training in young men: A randomized controlled trial. JAMA 281(21):2020-2028, 1999.

Gender Differences in Arrhythmias 93

Andrea M. Russo and Francis E. Marchlinski

CHAPTER OUTLINE

Gender differences in the incidence and risk factors for a variety of supraventricular and ventricular arrhythmias are well recognized. The mechanisms for sex differences in arrhythmias are not well established, although hormonal effects, differences in ion channel expression, and differences in autonomic tone may be contributory.

This chapter reviews gender differences in heart rate and the electrocardiogram (ECG), intracardiac electrophysiologic parameters, supraventricular tachycardia (SVT), atrial fibrillation (AF), ventricular arrhythmias and sudden cardiac death, and congenital and acquired long-QT syndromes.

Electrocardiographic Differences

In young healthy adults, resting heart rate is higher in women than men.[1-3] Gender differences in heart rate persist after autonomic blockade, suggesting intrinsic sinus node differences rather than gender differences in autonomic tone.[3] Heart rate can vary during the menstrual cycle and it appears faster during higher estrogen states.[4]

Gender differences in baseline intervals have also been demonstrated. PQ or PR interval and QRS duration are shorter in women.[1,5] In contrast, QTc is longer in women than in men.[1,2,6-8] This difference in QT interval between men and women is preserved after autonomic blockade.[8] Estrogen or progesterone effect does not appear to explain gender differences in myocardial repolarization.[8-10]

The QT interval is similar for boys and girls until puberty. The male corrected QT interval shortens at puberty and remains shorter until age 50 years.[7] This coincides with the highest androgen levels in men and suggests that male hormones (androgens) may be responsible for the shorter QTc in men.[7]

Although estrogen does not affect the QT interval in healthy women, it significantly decreases QT dispersion.[11,12] In a healthy population, QT dispersion is greater in men than in women.[2,13] It has been suggested that greater QT dispersion might increase arrhythmic events. This finding could help to explain gender differences in susceptibility to ventricular arrhythmias and changes with aging.

Heart Rate Variability

There are conflicting reports regarding gender differences in heart rate variability, and this may be related to differences in study cohorts, particularly with respect to age. In healthy subjects between the ages of 18 and 71 years, there were no differences between men and women with respect to heart rate variability indices denoting vagal activity (high-frequency power), whereas low-frequency power indices were significantly reduced in women.[14,15] This lower index for sympathetic modulation in women may be protective. For healthy young subjects (mean age 26-29 years), heart rate variability was greater in men than in women for both trained and nontrained subjects.[16] In contrast, a small study examining older men and women (mean age 50-52 years) found no differences in heart rate variability before or during recovery from exercise.[17]

Huikuri and colleagues[15] found that middle-aged women using estrogen replacement therapy had restored baroreflex sensitivity and increased heart rate variability compared to age-matched women not taking hormone therapy. This suggests that hormonal influences on autonomic tone might play a role in gender differences.

Intracardiac Electrophysiologic Measurements

Corrected sinus node recovery time is shorter in women and girls compared to their male counterparts.[18] These differences first appear in the pediatric age group and continue in adults. Atrio-His (AH) and His-ventricle (HV) intervals, effective refractory period (ERP) of the atroventricular (AV) node, and AV block cycle length are shorter in women.[19,20] Despite differences in intervals and conduction, there are no data indicating men have any greater frequency of symptomatic bradycardia or increased need for pacing compared to women.

Supraventricular Tachycardia

AV nodal reentrant tachycardia (AVNRT) has a 2:1 female-to-male predominance, and accessory pathways are twice as common in men.[21] A male predominance was seen in patients with manifest Wolff-Parkinson-White (WPW) syndrome (69%), but not in those with concealed WPW (52%).[5]

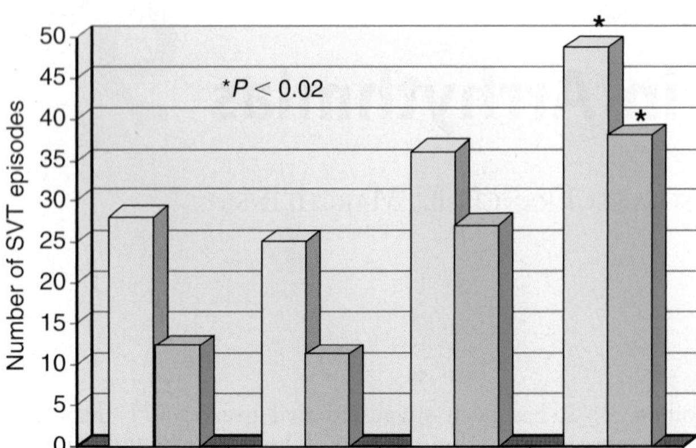

Figure 93-1 Cyclic variation of supraventricular tachycardia in women. The number of episodes of supraventricular tachycardia (SVT) are arranged as a function of the days of the menstrual cycle. It should be noted that there is a marked peak during the luteal phase. (Adapted from Rosano GMC, Leonardo F, Sorrel PM, et al: Cyclical variation in paroxysmal supraventricular tachycardia in women. Lancet 347:786-788, 1996, and Peters RW, Gold MR: The influence of gender on arrhythmias. Cardiol Rev 12:97-105, 2004.)

Women with AVNRT have shorter slow pathway refractory periods, AV block cycle lengths, and tachycardia cycle lengths than men with AVNRT.[19] There were no gender differences in fast-pathway ERP and retrograde conduction in these patients. Therefore, women have a wider tachycardia window, representing the difference between the fast and slow pathway refractory periods, which might explain the higher incidence of AVNRT in women.[19]

An increase in the number and duration of episodes of paroxysmal SVT was observed on day 28 as compared to day 7 of the menstrual cycle (Fig. 93-1).[22,23] A significant positive correlation was found between plasma progesterone and number of episodes and duration of SVT, and a significant inverse correlation was found between plasma estradiol and number of episodes and duration of SVT.[22] There might also be altered patterns of inducibility of supraventricular tachyarrhythmias during the menstrual cycle.[24] Among women with a history of perimenstrual clustering of paroxysmal SVT and among those receiving estrogen replacement therapy, scheduling elective electrophysiologic procedures at times of low estrogen levels (premenstrual or off estrogen replacement therapy) might facilitate the probability of SVT induction and a successful procedure.[24]

It has been demonstrated that there is no difference in success, complications, or recurrence rates with catheter ablation of SVT between men and women.[19,25] Success for ablation of atrial tachycardia is also similar between men and women.[26] Fluoroscopy time, radiofrequency applications, and procedure duration were also similar in women and men.[25] However, female patients are referred for ablation of reentrant SVT (AVNRT and AV reciprocating tachycardia [AVRT]) later than male patients and after receiving more antiarrhythmic drugs. This occurs even though women were more symptomatic and more women had more than one episode per month (80.3% vs. 70.3% women vs. men, $P < 0.001$).[25] Symptoms experienced by patients with paroxysmal SVT can mimic panic disorder. When SVT was initially unrecognized, women were more likely than men to have symptoms ascribed to psychiatric origins (65% vs. 32%, respectively; $P < 0.04$).[27]

Atrial Fibrillation

After adjusting for age and other risk factors, men have 1.5 times greater risk of developing AF than women (Fig. 93-2).[28] Overall, women account for 53% of patients with this arrhythmia. This is because women have a longer life expectancy, and therefore there are many more women than men older than 75 years in the general population, where the percentage of AF is the highest. A male predominance has also been seen with atrial flutter, which was shown to be 2.5 times more common in men.[29]

The reason for the increased incidence of AF in men is unclear, but it could be related to intrinsic differences in atrial electrophysiology or to gender differences in atrial size. Following induction of AF by rapid atrial pacing in patients without structural heart disease who were undergoing catheter ablation for the treatment of SVT, gender was the only significant independent predictor of spontaneous conversion back to sinus rhythm ($P = 0.005$).[30] There was no significant difference between the change in atrial ERP before and after induced AF in men and women.

Compared with men, women had a higher mean heart rate during AF.[30] Women might report more frequent and more severe clinical symptoms, with lower quality-of-life scores than men with AF, possibly due to the faster heart rates.[31-33]

Studies have also demonstrated gender differences in clinical characteristics associated with AF. At the time of initial presentation with AF, women were older, were less likely to have coronary disease, had better left ventricular function, and were more likely to have hypertension than men.[33,34]

AF was associated with an increased mortality in both men and women, after adjusting for other risk factors.[35] The odds ratio for death was 1.5 (95% confidence interval [CI], 1.2-1.8) in men and 1.9 (95% CI, 1.5-2.2) in women, and the arrhythmia decreased the female advantage in survival.

Warfarin appears to be at least as effective in women as in men in preventing stroke.[36,37] In spite of a potentially higher risk of thromboembolic complications from AF in women,[33,36] older women were half as likely to receive warfarin than older men, despite comparable risk profiles.[34]

There might also be gender differences in other outcome measures of AF management. Although there was no difference in overall cardiovascular morbidity and mortality in women

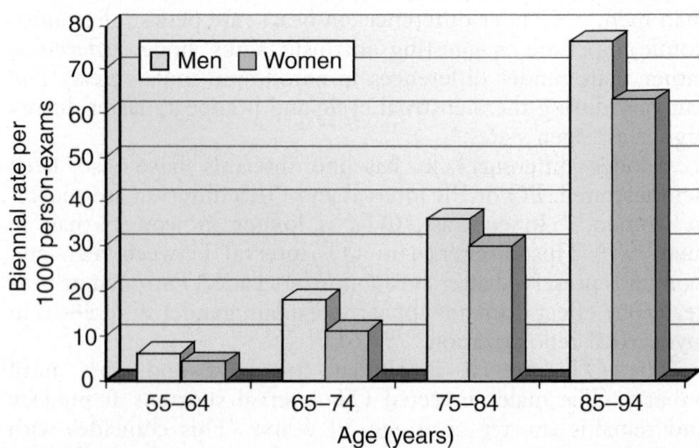

Figure 93-2 Incidence of atrial fibrillation in the Framingham Heart Study. During 38 years of follow-up, 264 men and 298 women developed atrial fibrillation. The incidence of atrial fibrillation increases with age. Men had 1.5 times greater risk of developing atrial fibrillation than women. (Adapted from Benjamin EJ, Levy D, Vaziri SM, et al: Independent risk factors for atrial fibrillation in a population-based cohort. The Framingham Heart Study. JAMA 271:840-844, 1994.)

(21%) and men (19%) in the Rate Control Versus Electrical Cardioversion (RACE) study, women who were randomized to the rhythm-control group developed more endpoints (adjusted hazard ratio [HR], 3.1; 95% CI, 1.5-6.3; $P = 0.002$), including heart failure, thromboembolic complications, and adverse effects of antiarrhythmic drugs when compared with women randomized to the rate-control group.[32] Because treatment strategy did not influence quality of life, it has been suggested, though not clearly proved, that it might be better to consider a rate-control approach in women, especially if they are asymptomatic.

One large study suggests that women are less likely than men to undergo successful electrical cardioversion (22% vs. 28%, $P < 0.001$), although there was no difference in the percentage of men and women undergoing successful pharmacologic cardioversion.[33] Following successful cardioversion of AF, arrhythmia recurrence was also more prevalent in women than in men.[38] This suggests that maintenance of sinus rhythm after cardioversion may be more difficult in women.

Women represent a minority of patients undergoing AF ablation (23%-32%).[39,40] There may be a bias in referral of women for ablation, and this under-referral does not appear to be explained by age, outcome from the procedure, or gender differences in symptoms. Acute success and complication rates appear similar in men and women, despite a higher risk profile in women, who were older and had a longer history of AF than men. A similar improvement in quality of life scores was also achieved in men and women following ablation.[40] The reduced quality of life and increased risk for antiarrhythmic drug-induced proarrhythmia could make a curative ablation strategy even more attractive for women.

Women might also be somewhat more likely than men to have nonpulmonary triggers for AF. In our experience in patients with paroxysmal AF, up to 7.5% appear to have nonpulmonary triggers as the only triggering event for their arrhythmia.

Ventricular Arrhythmias and Sudden Cardiac Death

The absolute incidence of sudden cardiac death is lower in women than men at all age groups, and the incidence in women lags behind that of men by more than 10 years (Fig. 93-3).[41,42] Studies of out-of-hospital cardiac arrest victims demonstrate that women have a lower incidence of ventricular fibrillation (VF) compared to men.[43,44] VF and ventricular tachycardia (VT) are more likely to be noted in men than in women at the time of out-of-hospital cardiac arrest, and asystole and pulseless electrical activity are more common in women.[44,45] However, resuscitation rates may be better in women (13.5% vs. 10.7%, $P = 0.005$), and women might have a slightly better survival advantage to hospital discharge.[44,45]

Gender differences in baseline characteristics have been identified in previous studies of patients presenting with sustained ventricular arrhythmias, as well as in asymptomatic patients undergoing implantation of an implantable cardioverter defibrillator (ICD) for primary prevention.[43,46-51] Women cardiac arrest survivors have a lower prevalence of coronary disease and might have a higher left ventricular ejection fraction (LVEF) than men.[46,48,51] In the Multicenter Unsustained Tachycardia Trial (MUSTT), a primary prevention trial in patients with coronary artery disease, women were older, more likely to have had an infarction within 6 months, more likely to have a history of heart failure, and more likely to have recent angina prior to enrollment compared to men.[49] In the Sudden Cardiac Death in Heart Failure Trial (SCD-HeFT), women were more likely to be nonwhite and to have class III heart failure and nonischemic heart disease.[50]

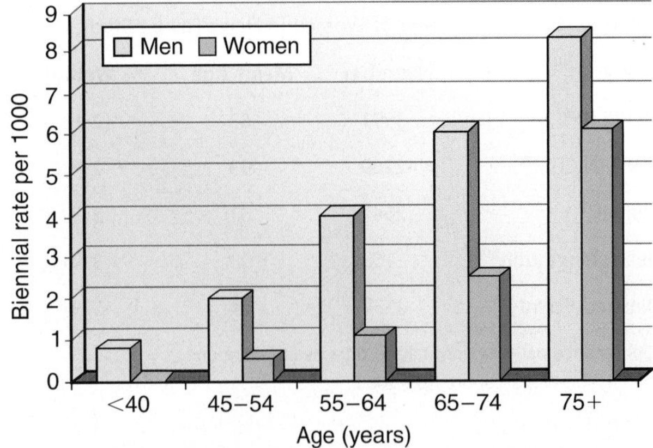

Figure 93-3 Incidence of sudden death by age and sex (in persons free of known coronary artery disease) in the Framingham study with 26 years' follow-up. The absolute incidence of sudden cardiac death increases with age in both men and women. The incidence is lower in women than men at all age groups and parallels the incidence of ischemic heart disease. (N = 5128 men and women). (Adapted from Kannel WB, Schatzkin A: Sudden death: Lessons from subsets in population studies. J Am Coll Cardiol 5:141B-149B, 1985.)

Women are also less likely to have inducible sustained ventricular arrhythmias at electrophysiologic testing.[48,49,52] This might support the hypothesis that there may be gender differences in the triggering mechanism of arrhythmias as well as the arrhythmia substrate.

Despite gender differences in the incidence of VF in out-of-hospital cardiac arrest, there was no gender difference in outcome of patients who received ICDs for secondary prevention.[46,47,53] In the Antiarrhythmics versus Implantable Defibrillators (AVID) trial, mortality was similar in women (14.4%) and men (15.5%), despite gender differences in baseline characteristics and clinical arrhythmia at the time of presentation.[46]

There are limited data regarding the influence of gender on outcome of patients receiving ICDs for primary prevention, although recent trials suggest no gender differences in outcome of patients with underlying ischemic heart disease.[49,54] Trials that include subjects with nonischemic heart disease, including SCD-HeFT and the Defibrillators in Non-Ischemic Cardiomyopathy Treatment Evaluation (DEFINITE) suggest that women might derive less relative benefit from ICD therapy than men.[50,55,56] Caution is needed with interpretation of results from post-hoc analyses, and small numbers of women were enrolled in these trials, which may be underpowered to show any benefit of ICD therapy in women.

The reasons for the smaller numbers of women enrolled in ICD trials are unclear. Compared to SCD-HeFT, which enrolled patients with both ischemic and nonischemic cardiomyopathy, a similar percentage of women (21%-24%) have been enrolled in heart failure trials (Table 93-1).[57-59] Examination of consecutive patients on a heart failure unit revealed that 31% were women.[60] In contrast, a population study based on a cohort from 1979 to 2000 in Olmsted County, Minnesota, women represented 57% of the group.[61] However, it is known that women are more likely to have diastolic dysfunction than men and would therefore not have been eligible for these primary prevention ICD trials.[62] Some contribution of bias or higher refusal rates for women cannot be excluded with certainly, but this appears less likely based on

Table 93-1 Representation of Women in Heart Failure Studies

Study	Number	Mean Age	% Women
MERIT-HF[57]	3991	63	23%
COPERNICUS[58]	2289	63	21%
CIBIS II[59]	2647	61	24%
Heart failure unit[60]*	168	68	31%
Olmsted County[61]†	4537	74	57%

*Consecutive patients hospitalized on a heart failure unit.
†Population-based cohort 1979-2000.

available data. Therefore, it is currently unclear whether or not there is truly under-representation of women in primary prevention ICD trials based on the prevalence of disease or opportunities for enrollment.

Importantly, there are no apparent gender differences in occurrence of ICD implantation complication rates in men and women undergoing implantation for secondary or primary prevention indications.[50,51] Despite population studies demonstrating gender differences in the incidence of sudden cardiac death, studies have also demonstrated no gender differences in arrhythmia occurrence or appropriate defibrillator therapy following ICD implantation in patients presenting with sustained ventricular arrhythmias or syncope with inducible sustained ventricular arrhythmias.[47,63,64] Finally, gender did not predict ventricular arrhythmia recurrence in patients with ischemic heart disease who survived an initial out-of-hospital cardiac arrest.[65]

Congenital Long-QT Syndrome

Despite an autosomal pattern of inheritance for common forms of long QT syndrome (LQTS), there is a female predominance of symptomatic patients with the congenital LQTS, with 69% of probands being female.[66] Female patients also make up 61% of symptomatic family members as identified in the International Long QT Registry.[67] Among LQTS patients, the risk of cardiac events was higher in male patients until puberty and higher in female patients during adulthood. As described earlier in this chapter, this may be due to a protective electrophysiologic effect of testosterone on the QT interval.

The postpartum period is associated with a significant increase in risk for cardiac events among patients with the long QT syndrome, but pregnancy was not associated with events.[68] After delivery, heart rate decreases and QT interval increases. Increased stress and sleep deprivation caring for a newborn might also increase the risk of cardiac events postpartum.[68]

Acquired Long-QT Syndrome: Drug-Induced Proarrhythmia

Women are more prone than men to develop drug-induced torsades de pointes. This gender difference in risk has been identified with class Ia and class III antiarrhythmic agents, as well as other cardiac and noncardiac drugs (Box 93-1).[69,70] Makkar and colleagues identified 332 cases of torsades de pointes associated with cardiovascular drug usage. Although only 44% of drug prescriptions were registered to women, 70% of cases of proarrhythmia involved women.[70]

Box 93-1 Drugs Related to Increased Risk of Torsades de Pointes in Women

ANTIANGINALS
Bepridil

ANTIARRHYTHMICS
Amiodarone
Azimilide
Disopyramide
Dofetilide
Ibutilide
Quinidine
Sotalol

ANTIBIOTICS
Erythromycin
Halofantrine
Pentamidine

ANTIHISTAMINES
Astemizole
Terfenadine

ANTIMALARIALS
Halofantrine

HYPOCHOLESTEROLEMICS
Probucol

GASTROINTESTINAL STIMULANTS
Cisapride

NARCOTICS
Methadone

Although it is well established that class III antiarrhythmic agents, such as sotalol and dofetilide, in addition to class Ia antiarrhythmic drugs, lead to an increased risk of arrhythmia in women, the proarrhythmic potential appears to be lower with amiodarone. A previous meta-analysis, however, also suggested a higher-than-expected prevalence of torsades de pointes in women than in men taking amiodarone.[70]

Experimental data support the hypothesis that gender differences in specific cardiac ion current densities are at least in part responsible for the greater susceptibility of women in developing torsades de pointes. In isolated perfused rabbit hearts (Langendorff technique), female rabbit hearts display greater drug-induced QT changes following quinidine and d-sotalol. At least two different repolarizing potassium current densities (I_{Kr} and I_{K1}) were found to be significantly lower in ventricular myocytes from female rabbits than in male rabbits.[71]

Sex hormones might also influence the activity of specific cardiac ion channels, identified in isolated rabbit preparations.[72] Following infusion of ibutilide, an increase in QTc was greater for women during menses and the ovulatory phase compared with women during the luteal phase and compared with men. Progesterone and progesterone-to-estradiol ratio were inversely correlated with ibutilide-induced QT prolongation.[73]

It has also been suggested that transmural dispersion of repolarization may be implicated in the genesis of torsades de pointes.[74-76] In one study of rabbit hearts, the monophasic action potential of the epicardium, midmyocardium, and endocardium were simultaneously recorded in male and female hearts perfused by the Langendorff method. Transmural dispersion of repolarization was significantly higher in female rabbits than in male rabbits after perfusion with D-sotalol.[75] In an isolated canine preparation, it has been demonstrated that the incidence of torsades de pointes decreases with a decrease in transmural dispersion of repolarization, despite QT prolongation.[76]

Sex differences in drug metabolism and elimination might also contribute to gender differences in drug responses. Drug metabolism in women may be affected by sex-specific factors, including menopause, pregnancy, menstruation, or oral contraceptive use. Cytochrome P-450 3A4 (CYP3A4), responsible for the metabolism of more than 50% of therapeutic drugs, exhibits higher activity in women than in men.[77] Longer QT intervals may be seen following concomitant administration of drugs that decrease CYP3A4-mediated metabolism, leading to higher concentrations and greater QT prolongation by drugs such as cisapride, suggesting that a pharmacokinetic drug interaction can contribute to an increased risk of torsades de pointes.[78,79]

Conclusions

Gender differences are apparent in the basic electrocardiographic intervals and the incidence and risk factors for a variety of supraventricular and ventricular arrhythmias. The mechanisms for these sex differences are still poorly understood, although sex hormones, autonomic tone, drug metabolism, and ion-channel differences appear contributory. Importantly, an awareness of these gender differences is essential for optimal clinical arrhythmia management in women.

References

1. Storstein L, Bjornstad H, Hals O, Meen HD: Electrocardiographic findings according to sex in athletes and controls. Cardiology 79:227-236, 1991.
2. Tran H, White CM, Chow MS, Kluger J: An evaluation of the impact of gender and age on QT dispersion in healthy subjects. Ann Noninvasive Electrocardiol 6:129-133, 2001.
3. Burke JH, Goldberger JJ, Ehlert FA, et al: Gender differences in heart rate before and after autonomic blockade: Evidence against an intrinsic gender effect. Am J Med 100:537-543, 1996.
4. Moran VH, Leathard HL, Coley J: Cardiovascular functioning during the menstrual cycle. Clin Physiol 20:496-504, 2000.
5. Liu S, Yuan S, Hertervig E, et al: Gender and atrioventricular conduction properties of patients with symptomatic atrioventricular nodal reentrant tachycardia and Wolff-Parkinson-White syndrome. J of Electrocardiol 34:295-301, 2001.
6. Luo S, Michler K, Johnston P, Macfarlane PW: A comparison of commonly used QT correction formulae: The effect of heart rate on the QTc of normal ECGs. J Electrocardiol 37:81-90, 2004.
7. Rautaharju PM, Zhou SH, Wong S, et al: Sex differences in the evolution of the electrocardiographic QT interval with age. Can J Cardiol 8:690-695, 1992.
8. Burke JH, Ehlert FA, Kruse JT, et al: Gender-specific differences in the QT interval and the effect of autonomic tone and menstrual cycle in healthy adults. Am J Cardiol 79:178-181, 1997.
9. Larsen JA, Tung RH, Sadananda R, et al: Effects of hormone replacement therapy on QT interval. Am J Cardiol 82:993-995, 1998.
10. Sbarouni E, Zarvalis E, Kyriakides ZS, Kremastinios DT: Absence of effects of short-term estrogen replacement therapy on resting and exertional QT and QTc dispersion in postmenopausal women with coronary artery disease. Pacing Clin Electrophysiol 21:2392-2395, 1998.
11. Saba S, Link MS, Homoud MK, et al: Effect of low estrogen states in healthy women on dispersion of ventricular repolarization. Am J Cardiol 87:354-356, 2001.
12. Yildirir A, Aybar F, Kabakci MG, et al: Hormone replacement therapy shortens QT dispersion in healthy postmenopausal women. Ann Noninvasive Electrocardiol 6:193-197, 2001.
13. Kassotis J, Costeas C, Bedi AK, et al: Effects of aging and gender on QT dispersion in an overtly healthy population. Pacing Clin Electrophysiol 23:1121-1126, 2000.
14. Ramaekers D, Ector H, Aubert E, et al: Heart rate variability and heart rate in healthy volunteers. Is the female autonomic nervous systym cardioprotective? Eur Heart J 19:1334-1341, 1998.
15. Huikuri HV, Pikkujämsä SM, Airaksinen KE, et al: Sex-related differences in autonomic modulation of heart rate in middle-aged subjects. Circulation 94:122-125, 1996.
16. Genovesi S, Zaccaria D, Rossi E, et al: Effects of exercise training on heart rate and QT interval in healthy young individuals: Are there gender differences? Europace 9:55-60, 2007.
17. Brown SJ, Brown JA: Resting and postexercise cardiac autonomic control in trained masters athletes. J Physiol Sci 57:23-29, 2007.
18. Sanjeev S, Karpawich PP: Developmental changes in sinus node function in growing children: An updated analysis. Pediatr Cardiol 26:585-588, 2005.
19. Liuba I, Jonsson A, Safstrom K, Walfridsson H: Gender-related differences in patients with atrioventricular nodal reentry tachycardia. Am J Cardiol 97:384-388, 2006.
20. Liu S, Yuan S, Kongstad O, Olsson SB: Gender differences in electrophysiological characteristics of atrioventricular conduction system and their clinical implications. Scand Cardiovas J 35:313-317, 2001.
21. Rodriguez LM, de Chillou C, Schlapfer J, et al: Age at onset and gender of patients with different types of supraventricular tachycardias. Am J Cardiol 70:1213-1215, 1992.
22. Rosano GMC, Leonardo F, Sorrel PM, et al: Cyclical variation in paroxysmal supraventricular tachycardia in women. Lancet 347:786-788, 1996.
23. Peters RW, Gold MR: The influence of gender on arrhythmias. Cardiol Rev 12:97-105, 2004.
24. Myerburg RJ, Cox MM, Interian A, et al: Cycling of inducibility of paroxysmal supraventricular tachycardia in women and its implications for timing of electrophysiologic procedures. Am J Cardiol 83:1049-1054, 1999.
25. Dagres N, Clague JR, Breithrd G, Borggrefe M: Significant gender-related differences in radiofrequency catheter ablation therapy. J Am Coll Cardiol 42:1103-1107, 2003.
26. Anguera I, Brugada J, Roba M, et al: Outcomes after radiofrequency catheter ablation of atrial tachycardia. Am J Cardiol 87:886-890, 2001.
27. Lessmeier TJ, Gamperling D, Johnson-Liddon V, et al: Unrecognized paroxysmal supraventricular tachycardia. Potential for misdiagnosis as panic disorder. Arch Intern Med 157:537-543, 1997.
28. Benjamin EJ, Levy D, Vaziri SM, et al: Independent risk factors for atrial fibrillation in a population-based cohort. The Framingham Heart Study. JAMA 271:840-844, 1994.
29. Granada J, Uribe W, Chyou PH, et al: Incidence and predictors of atrial flutter in the general population. J Am Coll Cardiol 36:2242-2246, 2000.
30. Tada H, Sticherling C, Chough SP, et al: Gender and age differences in induced atrial fibrillation. Am J Cardiol 88:436-438, 2001.
31. Paquette M, Roy D, Talajic M, et al: Role of gender and personality on quality-of-life impairment in intermittent atrial fibrillation. Am J Cardiol 86:764-768, 2000.
32. Rienstra M, Van Veldhuisen DJ, Hagens VE, et al: Gender-related differences in rhythm control treatment in persistent atrial fibrillation. J Am Coll Cardiol 46:1298-1306, 2005.
33. Dagres N, Nieuwlaat R, Vardas PE, et al: Gender-related differences in presentation, treatment, and outcome of patients with atrial fibrillation in Europe. J Am Coll Cardiol 49:572-577, 2007.
34. Humphries KH, Kerr CR, Connolly SJ, et al: New-onset atrial fibrillation: Sex differences in presentation, treatment, and

outcome. Circulation 103:2365-2370, 2001.
35. Benjamin EM, Wolf PA, D'Agostino RB, et al: Impact of atrial fibrillation on the risk of death: The Framingham Study. Circulation 98:946-9452, 1998.
36. Fang MC, Singer DE, Chang Y, et al: Gender differences in the risk of ischemic stroke and peripheral embolism in atrial fibrillation. The AnTicoagulation and Risk factors In Atrial fibrillation (ATRIA) Study. Circulation 112:1687-1691, 2005.
37. Risk factors for stroke and efficacy of antithrombotic therapy in atrial fibrillation. Analysis of pooled data from five randomized controlled trials. Arch Intern Med 154:1449-1457, 1994.
38. Gurevitz OT, Varadachari CJ, Ammash NM, et al: The effect of patient sex on recurrence of atrial fibrillation following successful direct current cardioversion. Am Heart J 152:155.e9-e13, 2006.
39. Gerstenfeld EP, Callans D, Dixit S, et al: Characteristics of patients undergoing atrial fibrillation ablation: Trends over a seven-year period 1999-2005. J Cardiovasc Electrophysiol 18:23-28, 2007.
40. Forleo GB, Tondo C, De Luca L, et al: Gender-related differences in catheter ablation of atrial fibrillation. Europace 9:613-620, 2007.
41. Kannel WB, Schatzkin A: Sudden death: Lessons from subsets in population studies. J Am Coll Cardiol 5:141B-149B, 1985.
42. Kannel WB, Wilson PW, D'Agostino RB, Cobb J: Sudden coronary death in women. Am Heart J 136:205-212, 1998.
43. Kim C, Fahrenbruch CE, Cobb LA, Eisenberg MS: Out-of-hospital cardiac arrest in men and women. Circulation 104:2699-2703, 2001.
44. Wigginton JG, Pepe PE, Bedolla JP, et al: Sex-related differences in the presentation and outcome of out-of-hospital cardiopulmonary arrest: A multiyear, prospective, population-based study. Crit Care Med 30(4 Suppl):S131-S136, 2002.
45. Herlitz J, Rundqvist S, Bang A, et al: Is there a difference between women and men in characteristics and outcome after in hospital cardiac arrest? Resuscitation 49:15-23, 2001.
46. Engelstein ED, Friedman PL, Yao Q, et al: Gender differences in patients with life-threatening ventricular arrhythmias: Impact on treatment and survival in the AVID Trial. Circulation 96(Suppl I):720, 1997.
47. Pires LA, Sethuraman B, Guduguntla VD, et al: Outcome of women versus men with ventricular tachyarrhythmias treated with the implantable cardioverter defibrillator. J Cardiovasc Electrophysiol 13:563-568, 2002.
48. Albert CM, McGovern BA, Newell JB, Ruskin JN: Sex differences in cardiac arrest survivors. Circulation 93:1170-1176, 1996.
49. Russo AM, Stamato NJ, Lehmann MH, et al; the MUSTT Investigators: Influence of gender on arrhythmia characteristics in the Multicenter UnSustained Tachycardia Trial. J Cardiovasc Electrophysiol 5:993-998, 2004.
50. Russo AM, Poole JE, Mark DB, et al: Primary prevention with defibrillator therapy in women: results from the Sudden Cardiac Death in Heart Failure Trial, J Cardiovasc Electrophysiol 19:720-724, 2008.
51. Kudenchuk PJ, Bardy GH, Poole JE, et al: Malignant sustained ventricular tachyarrhythmias in women: Characteristics and outcome of treatment with an implantable cardioverter defibrillator. J Cardiovasc Electrophysiol 8:2-10, 1997.
52. Buxton AE, Hafley GE, Lehmann MH, et al: Prediction of sustained ventricular tachycardia inducible by programmed stimulation in patients with coronary artery disease. Utility of clinical variables. Circulation 99:1843-1850, 1999.
53. Lampert R, McPherson CA, Clancy JF, et al: Gender differences in ventricular arrhythmia recurrence in patients with coronary artery disease and implantable cardioverter-defibrillators. J Am Coll Cardiol 43:2293-2299, 2004.
54. Moss AJ, Zareba W, Hall J, et al; the Multi-center Automatic Defibrillator Implantation II Trial Investigators: Prophylactic implantation of a defibrillator in patients with myocardial infarction and reduced ejection fraction. N Engl J Med 346:877-883, 2002.
55. Bardy GH, Lee KL, Mark DB, et al; for the Sudden Cardiac Death in Heart Failure Trial (SCD-HeFT) Investigators: Amiodarone or an implantable cardioverter-defibrillator for congestive heart failure. N Engl J Med 352:225-237, 2005.
56. Kadish A, Dyer A, Daubert JP, et al, for the Defibrillators in Non-Ischemic Cardiomyopathy Treatment Evaluation (DEFINITE) Investigators: Prophylactic defibrillator implantation in patients with nonischemic dilated cardiomyopathy. N Engl J Med 350:2151-2158, 2004.
57. Effect of metoprolol CR/XL in chronic heart failure: Metoprolol CR/XL Randomised Intervention Trial in Congestive Heart Failure (MERIT-HF). Lancet 353:2001-2007, 1999.
58. Packer M, Coats AJ, Fowler MB, et al; Carvedilol Prospective Randomized Cumulative Survival Study Group: Effect of carvedilol on survival in severe chronic heart failure. N Engl J Med 344:1651-1658, 2001.
59. Simon T, Mary-Krause M, Funck-Brentano C, Jaillon P: Sex differences in the prognosis of congestive heart failure: results from the Cardiac Insufficiency Bisoprolol Study (CIBIS II). Circulation 103:375-380, 2001.
60. Ng AC, Wong HS, Young AS, Sindone AP: Impact of gender on outcomes in chronic systolic heart failure. Int J Cardiol 117:214-221, 2007.
61. Roger VL, Weston SA, Redfield MM, et al: Trends in heart failure incidence and survival in a community-based population. JAMA 292:344-350, 2004.
62. Bursi F, Weston SA, Redfield MM, et al: Systolic and diastolic heart failure in the community. JAMA 296:2209-2216, 2006.
63. Ruppel R, Schluter CA, Boczor S, et al: Ventricular tachycardia during follow-up in patients resuscitated from ventricular fibrillation: Experience from stored electrograms of implantable cardioverter-defibrillators. J Am Coll Cardiol 32:1724-1730, 1998.
64. Pacifico A, Ferlic LL, Cedillo-Salazar FR, et al: Shocks as predictors of survival in patients with implantable cardioverter-defibrillators. J Am Coll Cardiol 34:204-210, 1999.
65. Kies P, Boersma E, Bax JJ, et al: Determinants of recurrent ventricular arrhythmia or death in 300 consecutive patients with ischemic heart disease who experienced aborted sudden death: Data from the Leiden out-of-hospital cardiac arrest study. J Cardiovasc Electrophysiol 16:1049-1056, 2005.
66. Moss AJ, Schwartz PJ, Crampton RS, et al: The long QT syndrome. Prospective longitudinal study of 328 families. Circulation 84:1136-1144, 1991.
67. Locati EH, Zareba W, Moss AJ, et al: Age- and sex-related differences in clinical manifestations in patients with congenital long-QT syndrome: Findings from the International LQTS Registry. Circulation 97:2237-2244, 1998.
68. Rashba EJ, Zareba W, Moss AJ, et al: Influence of pregnancy on the risk for cardiac events in patients with hereditary long QT syndrome. LQTS Investigators. Circulation 97:451-456, 1998.
69. Arizona Center for Education and Research on Therapeutics: Drugs with risk of torsades de pointes. Available at http://www.torsades.org/medical-pros/drug-lists/list-01.cfm?sort=Generic_name. Accessed September 20, 2008.
70. Makkar RR, Fromm BS, Steinman RT, et al: Female gender as a risk factor for torsades de pointes associated with cardiovascular drugs. JAMA 270:2590-2597, 1993.
71. Ebert SN, Liu XK, Woosley RL: Female gender as a risk factor for drug-induced cardiac arrhythmias: Evaluation of clinical and experimental evidence. J Womens Health 7:547-557, 1998.
72. Drici MD, Burklow TR, Haridasse V, et al: Sex hormones prolong the QT interval and downregulate potassium channel expression in the rabbit heart. Circulation 94:1471-1474, 1996.
73. Rodriguez I, Kilborn MJ, Liu XK, et al: Drug-induced QT prolongation in women during the menstrual cycle. JAMA 285:1322-1326, 2001.
74. Antzelevitch C: Role of transmural dispersion of repolarization in the genesis of drug-induced torsades de pointes. Heart Rhythm 2:S9-S15, 2005.
75. Ruan YF, Liu N, Zhou Q, et al: Experimental study on the mechanism of sex difference in the risk of torsades de pointes. Chin Med J 117:538-541, 2004.
76. Di Diego JM, Belardinelli L, Antzelevitch C: Cisapride-induced transmural dispersion of repolarizaton and torsades de pointes in the canine left ventricular wedge preparation

during epicardial stimulation. Circulation 108:1027-1033, 2003.

77. Tanaka E: Gender-related differences in pharmacokinetics and their clinical significance. J Clin Pharm Ther 24:339-346, 1999.

78. Wysowski DK, Corken A, Gallo-Torres H, et al: Postmarketing reports of QT prolongation and ventricular arrhythmia in association with cisapride and Food and Drug Administration regulatory actions. Am J Gastroenterol 96:1698-1703, 2001.

79. Schwartz JB: The electrocardiographic QT interval and its prolongation in response to medications: Differences between men and women. J Gend Specif Med 3:25-28, 2000.

Arrhythmias in Pediatrics 94

Mark E. Alexander

CHAPTER OUTLINE

Pediatric arrhythmias are an exceptionally broad group of disorders sharing much with adult physiology though with the important exception there are very few pediatric patients with ischemic heart disease. Developmental changes in electrophysiology, distinct natural history, technical challenges, and limited data help define current practice.

The epidemiology of virtually all the arrhythmias has a bimodal distribution, with a modest peak incidence in fetal and neonatal life. During later infancy and early childhood, these arrhythmias are less common, in part from spontaneous resolution of accessory pathways. With adolescence there is a gradual increase in symptoms, including new diagnoses and recurrence of prior symptoms.

Management of pediatric arrhythmias has a continued challenge in balancing the age-specific risk-to-benefit ratio of arrhythmia therapies. The periods of relatively infrequent symptoms and the lack of decades of personal past medical history requires considering whether fortuitous diagnoses of Wolff-Parkinson-White syndrome (WPW), hypertrophic cardiomyopathy, or long-QT syndrome (LQTS) represent asymptomatic or presymptomatic patients.

Arrhythmia management is an integrated part of the patient with congenital heart disease (Chapters 60 and 67) or cardiomyopathy. The majority of pediatric patients with arrhythmias have normal hearts, and arrhythmia is the sole source of their cardiac disability. In the Prospective Assessment of Pediatric Catheter Ablation (PAPCA) study cohorts, 8% had congenital heart disease and 2% had cardiomyopathies.[1]

After the early mortality associated with congenital malformations and sudden infant death syndrome (Chapter 76), cardiac mortality in children is rare; the risk of sudden death in adolescents is about 1 per 100,000 patients per year. This contrasts to rates of 200 to 300 per 100,000 for young adults with tetralogy of Fallot. Even in diseases like hypertrophic cardiomyopathy and LQTS, the period between ages 1 and 14 years has low, although not absent, risk. This epidemiology means there are often insufficient data regarding active management choices in children. With the feasibility of diagnostic and therapeutic approaches permitting them to be used in increasingly smaller and younger patients these realities produce a practice that is necessarily largely based on limited case series, first principles, and attempts to extrapolate from the prospective adult data.

Developmental Cardiac Electrophysiology

Current models of cardiac development identify a ring of specialized conduction system tissue that surrounds the foramen between the primitive atrial and ventricular chambers. With looping, this ring of conduction system tissue differentiates into a single atrioventricular (AV) node. Accessory pathways might represent residual conduction tissue that failed to involute. When looping is abnormal, as in levo-transposition of the great vessels and heterotaxy defects, contralateral anlage of both sinus node and AV node tissue persist or fail to form. These models help explain unusual specialized conduction system malformations such as conduction slings and twin AV nodes. NKx2.5 deficiencies have been implicated in developmental hypoplasia of AV conduction tissue. Other genetic markers (e.g., LacZ, Tbx) show progressive localization along the AV groove and concentration into the AV node, although their role in the development of accessory AV connections is not clear.[2]

Conduction velocities decrease with age and refractory periods increase with age, resulting in a shorter minimal wavelength for any reentrant tachycardia in younger patients. Rapid AV nodal conduction permits tachycardia rates of up to 300 beats per minute in the infant and fetus. With growth, AV node conduction slows from intrinsic decreases in conduction velocities and autonomic influences. The electrocardiogram (ECG) reflects the developmental physiology, with a shift from neonatal right ventricular dominance to typical adult left ventricular dominance. Heart rate decreases. With the exception of the corrected QT interval, the conduction intervals increase, reaching nearly adult levels by adolescence.

Pediatric Issues in Arrhythmias Seen in All Age Groups

Tachycardia Mediated by the Accessory Pathway

In fetal life and infancy, accessory pathway–mediated tachycardia (Chapter 58) is the most common cause of supraventricular tachycardia (SVT). More than 60% of pediatric arrhythmias managed with catheterization are mediated by the accessory pathway, and 57% of those have pre-excitation.[1]

Accessory pathway–mediated tachycardia has even higher relative incidence in the neonate.

Most cases have typical, nondecremental retrograde conduction either with antegrade pre-excitation (WPW) or without. Pre-excitation may be very subtle or latent, particularly in infants with combinations of faster sinus rates, rapid AV node conduction, and left-sided pathways. After initial symptoms in utero and in early infancy, a large percentage of patients with SVT become asymptomatic until later in childhood. Some patients lose pre-excitation or demonstrate pre-excitation that was not present in the neonatal period. Overall, SVT is not inducible with esophageal stimulation in nearly a third of infants or with prior SVT by 27 months, confirming permanent loss of the accessory pathway. The majority of children and adolescents with SVT did not have symptoms in infancy. The spontaneous resolution rate, the larger percentage who are temporarily asymptomatic, and the increased risks associated with ablation in infants combine to encourage a combination of medical therapy and expectant management for the infant and young child. A few infants with very refractory symptoms may be treated with ablation. Ablation might also be indicated in the infant and young child with congenital heart disease when the arrhythmia will complicate planned surgery or interfere with subsequent therapy.

After a period of decreased frequency, a larger secondary peak incidence begins in the school-age child, extending through adolescence. For the symptomatic patient, the consensus is to offer ablation, and ongoing debate focuses on how old is old enough. At Children's Hospital in Boston, our current practice is to try simple drug therapy or expectant management in the younger child, but as children reach 20 to 25 kg and 5 to 7 years old, we increasingly offer elective ablation.

WPW has a unique set of concerns in pediatrics, and its treatment in children is controversial. Asymptomatic pre-excitation is identified during cardiac evaluation, in screening ECGs as part of sports clearance in some countries, and increasingly before psychotropic drug management in children. Evaluating the risk of the finding involves evaluating the accuracy or risks of noninvasive (exercise), minimally invasive (esophageal stimulation), or invasive electrophysiology diagnostic studies and the effectiveness and risks of extending the study to include ablation. There are good data that children who survive cardiac arrests secondary to WPW have rapid conduction during atrial fibrillation, but there are minimal prospective historical data on asymptomatic children. An Italian study[3] reported one death and two aborted arrests in three of 27 previously asymptomatic children who had inducible orthodromic tachycardia from WPW. Other risk markers were not used. The significance of these data have been questioned[4] because the event rate was considerably higher than in larger natural history studies. At issue is our ability to determine which children are asymptomatic (estimated to be 50%-60% of WPW patients) and which are presymptomatic and will eventually have symptoms. There remains considerable practice variation, though few would recommend elective ablation in an asymptomatic child younger than 5 years.

Atypical accessory pathways, Mahaim fibers, nodoventricular fibers and decremental unidirectional retrograde pathways are observed at all ages. The often incessant tachycardia resulting from a decremental, typically posterior septal, accessory pathway is important to recognize, because it can result in curable cardiomyopathy. The term *permanent form of junctional reciprocating tachycardia* (PJRT) is a bit of a misnomer. PJRT is recognized on surface ECG by at normal PR, long RP, and inverted P waves in II, III, and F, with intermediate and somewhat variable tachycardia rates for age. Drug therapy, while challenging, is typically tried in younger patients; ablation is effective.

Atrial Arrhythmias

After the newborn period, atrial re-entry tachycardia is almost always associated with congenital heart disease (Chapter 60).

Typical atrial flutter is a relatively common arrhythmia in fetal and neonatal life, representing about 40% of sustained fetal tachycardia.[5] The baby typically presents in late pregnancy or at delivery with a fixed ventricular rate of 190 to 250 beats per minute and an atrial rate of 400 to 440 beats per minute. Adenosine or esophageal recordings confirm a 2:1 conduction pattern. Either direct current or transesophogeal pace cardioversion is typically curative, though 14% of subjects in the largest series required antiarrhythmic therapy for initial control. Although attention to identifying Ebstein's malformation and other predisposing congenital defects is required, most of these patients have normal hearts and a low risk of recurrence.[6] Because the arrhythmia is generally eliminated with a single cardioversion, there are no published data on invasive electrophysiology. Short atrial refractory periods permit atrial cycle lengths of 130 to 150 ms with P wave axis and response to pacing supporting a typical right atrial circuit. A second form of SVT contributes to the clinical course in up to 20% of these infants.

Atrial fibrillation is very rare in infancy and is nearly always associated with significantly enlarged atria. By adolescence, a small number of patients without structural disease and without WPW develop either lone atrial fibrillation or secondary atrial fibrillation. Evaluation and management mirrors that for the younger adult (see Chapter 56). There are no significant data on when these patients might benefit from ablation, though ectopic atrial tachycardia (with or without triggered atrial fibrillation) represents an ablation target.

Ectopic atrial tachycardia, chaotic atrial rhythm, and multifocal atrial tachycardia are seen both as primary arrhythmias and in the postoperative setting (Chapter 57). Each of these may be sufficiently persistent to result in tachycardia-mediated cardiomyopathy. Most of the pediatric natural history data concentrate on single-focus ectopic atrial tachycardia. Those who present in infancy and early childhood[7] and in the immediate postoperative period might not need ablation. Spontaneous resolution, typically seen over 1 to 2 years in the infant and before discharge in the postoperative patient, suggests that assertive use of drug therapy is appropriate. For the older patient, the spontaneous resolution rate is low. Low-grade ectopic atrial tachycardia may be observed or may be treated with drug therapy, but ablation is effective and the therapy of choice for those with cardiomyopathy (Fig. 94-1), significant symptoms, or triggered atrial fibrillation.

More chaotic or multifocal atrial tachycardias are significantly less common and more problematic. For the patient with refractory multifocal tachycardia, targeting a focal site might result in permanent cure.

Atrioventricular Node

AV nodal re-entry tachycardia (AVNRT; Chapter 59) is seen at all ages, but it is notably less common than accessory pathway–mediated tachycardia in the fetus and infant. By adolescence, nearly a third of ablation patients are treated for AVNRT.[1]

The physiology of the AV node has age-related transitions. Younger patients have more reliable retrograde AV node conduction and less-frequent slow pathway conduction. In the child who comes for electrophysiology study and ablation, younger patients are more likely to have continuous A1A2 curves. Like adult patients, a significant number of children do not have inducible AVNRT during electrophysiology study and need secondary markers of slow pathway

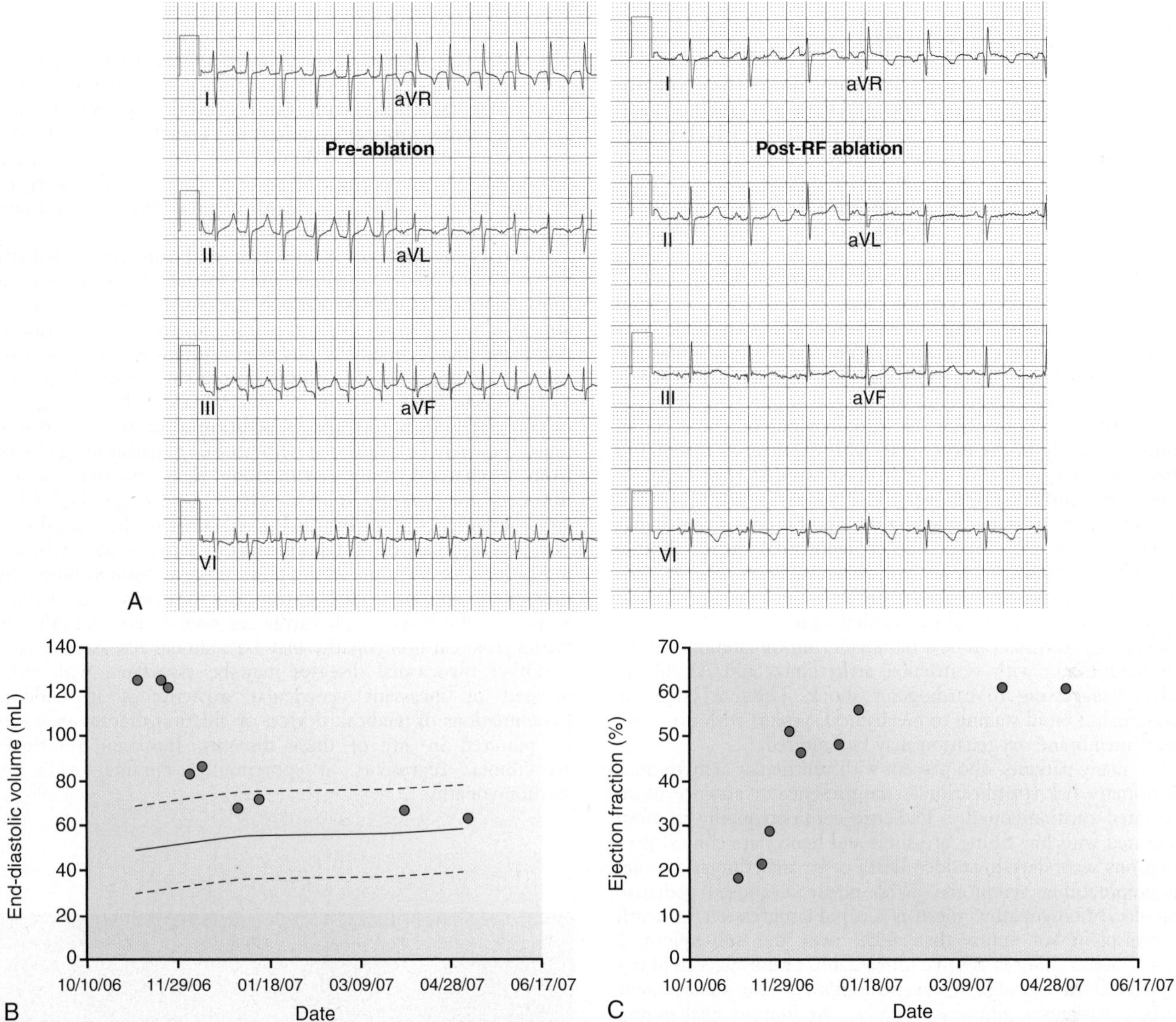

Figure 94-1 **A,** An 8-year-old presented with dilated cardiomyopathy had subsequent ablation of a 1:1 ectopic atrial tachycardia characterized by rates of about 180 beats per minute with borderline first-degree block. There was steady, but not immediate, resolution of dilated cardiomyopathy with improvement of left ventricular end diastolic volume to average age appropriate values over 7 months (B), while there was rapid normalization of left ventricular ejection fraction (C). **B** and **C,** There was steady, but not immediate, resolution of dilated cardiomyopathy and normalization of left ventricular function. RF, radiofrequency.

conduction.[8] Catheter ablation, either with radiofrequency or cryoablation, is very effective, and radiofrequency is associated with a 97% cure rate. Risks are low, but as in adult series, prospective data suggest a 1% to 2% risk of heart block with radiofrequency ablation. Cryothermal ablation has somewhat higher recurrence risks, lower acute success, and longer procedure times but lower risks of heart block.

Some patients with complex heart disease have twin node tachycardia. This variant of AV node reentry is almost always associated with complex AV connections and heterotaxy syndromes. It is recognized on surface ECG by two distinctive non-preexcited QRS patterns with pacing, SVT, or shifting atrial pacemakers. Twin node tachycardia is an SVT characterized by two functional AV nodes, with variable ventricular connections (conduction slings). These tachycardias demonstrate two distinctive and anatomically disparate His electrograms. Retrograde conduction is demonstrated through at least one of these AV nodes. In addition to drug therapy, there is the potential for successful ablation by modifying one of the AV nodes.[9]

The automatic AV node tachycardia, junctional ectopic tachycardia, seen in children has two primary patterns: acute postoperative and congenital. Acute postoperative junctional ectopic tachycardia is generally well recognized and is effectively managed with combination of overdrive atrial pacing to establish AV synchrony, cooling, intravenous procainamide, intravenous amiodarone,[10] and general supportive care.

Congenital junctional ectopic tachycardia is quite rare, and it might also be associated with progressive AV node dysfunction and AV block. It is usually managed with antiarrhythmic drug therapy, but there are several reports of successful ablation while preserving AV node function using both radiofrequency and cryoablation approaches, which may be required when there are refractory symptoms or progressive ventricular dysfunction.

Ventricular Arrhythmias

Ventricular arrhythmias are not uncommon in pediatric patients, with increased frequency in infancy and then later childhood and adolescence. They have quite variable substrates, which mirror many of those seen in adults. Broadly they can be categorized by their association with congenital heart disease (almost always postoperative), inflammatory heart disease, cardiomyopathy, myocardial tumors, ion channel defects, and idiopathic etiologies.

The incidence of ventricular arrhythmias in the immediate postoperative period is variable and is typically associated either with metabolic disturbances, residual hemodynamic concerns, or postoperative transitions. Ventricular arrhythmias are well recognized, but there are scant data regarding their long-term significance. Therapy almost always is supportive, with specific attention to optimizing the hemodynamic outcome. Serial monitoring early in the experience with the arterial switch and infant tetralogy of Fallot repairs demonstrated that many of these arrhythmias resolved over 1 to 2 years.

There are more data regarding the significance of ventricular arrhythmias during follow-up of congenital heart disease (Chapter 67). As in the adult with ischemic heart disease, ventricular arrhythmias are a primary problem and a marker of more complex hemodynamic and myocardial issues.

Acute myocarditis can be a fulminant, life-threatening condition manifesting with ventricular arrhythmias and AV block, rapidly progressing to cardiogenic shock. There is hope for recovery, but rapid staging to mechanical support with extracorporeal membrane oxygenation may be required.

For many patients who present with ventricular arrhythmias, the primary risk stratification is the presence or absence of an associated cardiomyopathy. Pediatric cardiomyopathy is often associated with low filling pressures and hence late clinical presentations secondary to sudden death or to arrhythmias appearing before other symptoms. With newly diagnosed pediatric dilated cardiomyopathy, there is a rapid progression to death or transplant for more than 40% over the subsequent 2 years.[11] Some children receive implantable cardioverter defibrillators (ICDs) as a bridge to transplantation, but the management of these patients continues to evolve. At times a challenging diagnosis, incessant atrial and ventricular arrhythmias can result in tachycardia-mediated cardiomyopathy. Once the arrhythmia is recognized, effective therapy can result in dramatic and complete recovery (see Fig. 94-1)

Hypertrophic cardiomyopathy (HCM; see Chapter 65) secondary to inborn errors has a high incidence of infant mortality.[12] For familial sarcomeric mutations, the phenotype might not manifest until adolescence or adulthood. Sudden death may be the first symptom when the disease is diagnosed in children, but most children and adolescents are asymptomatic and the absolute risk of sudden death is relatively low. There are fewer ventricular arrhythmias during exercise and Holter monitoring of children with HCM. There is little controversy regarding restriction from athletics and ICD use for secondary prevention. The combination of evolving phenotype, lower annual risks, and increased risks of inappropriate therapy or ICD failure combine to make choices regarding ICD use for primary prevention in the child and adolescent more complex.

Similar challenges exist for management of arrhythmogenic right ventricular cardiomyopathy (Chapter 64) and isolated noncompaction. There are reports of adolescents with clear arrhythmogenic right ventricular cardiomyopathy, but patients meeting task force criteria are generally adults in their fourth decade. When genetic testing becomes readily available, the diagnostic challenge in children may be resolved. Noncompaction represents another phenotype that is increasingly recognized in pediatrics. Understanding is evolving regarding when the echo observation of excessive trabeculation represents a disease or a normal variant. Initial reports were either in infants with severe disease or associated with Barth's syndrome, an X-linked systemic disease with combinations of associated ventricular dysfunction, ventricular arrhythmias, pre-excitation, and sudden death.[13] With increasing recognition, the natural history has become more variable, and many patients have no associated arrhythmias.[14]

Primary *cardiac tumors* are rare and can cause pediatric arrhythmias. Rhabdomyomas and isolated fibromas are the most common childhood cardiac tumors. Rhabdomyomas are almost always the result of tuberous sclerosis, an autosomal-dominant neurocutaneous disorder resulting typically from novel mutations of the tumor-suppressor genes *TSC1* and *TSC2*. These tumors appear in infancy and resolve substantially or completely by school age. In addition to ventricular arrhythmias, they may be associated with accessory pathways, probably from mechanical compression along their margins. Isolated fibromas are typically solitary, often quite large (Fig. 94-2), and completely intramyocardial, in contrast to the typically endocardial location of rhabdomyomas. There are no established indications for ablation attempts or surgery, though both offer therapeutic options.[15] Early enthusiasm for isolated hamartomas as a cause of incessant tachycardia has waned, though infiltrative histiocytoid cardiomyopathy may be a similar disease.

Other myocardial diseases may be associated with either isolated or incessant ventricular arrhythmias in children. Combinations of medical, device, or ablation therapy may each be required in any of these diseases. Incessant ventricular arrhythmia represents a potentially curable cause of cardiomyopathy.

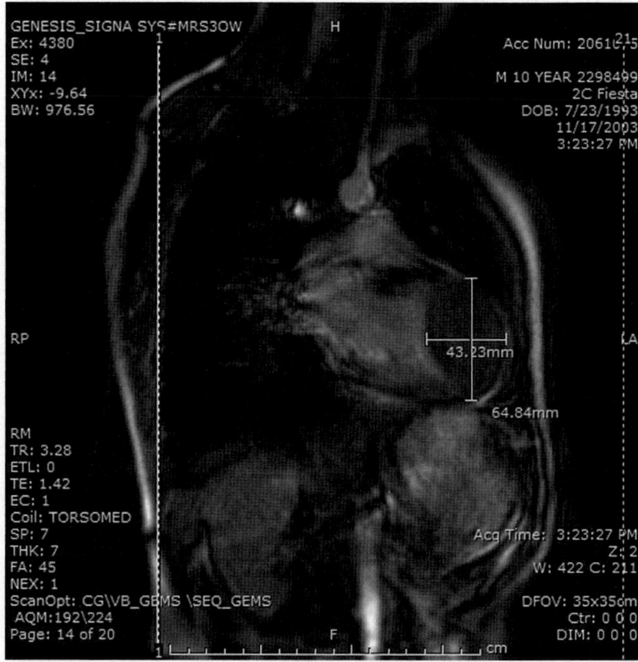

Figure 94-2 Cardiac magnetic resonance image of a 4.3 × 6.5 cm solitary cardiac fibroma identified on chest radiography. Monitoring demonstrated nonsustained ventricular tachycardia. Following resection, this patient has normal left ventricular function, a small fixed perfusion defect, and no ventricular arrhythmias on serial monitoring, exercise, or intracardiac stimulation.

All of the cardiac ion channel defects can result in recurrent polymorphic VT, sudden cardiac death, or syncope and can contribute to sudden infant death syndrome and unexplained drownings (Chapters 68 to 73). Long QT associated with LQT1, in particular, manifests at a younger age, though it appears to be highly responsive to effective beta blockade. Many adults choose ICD therapy, but that decision is often deferred in younger patients.[16] Brugada syndrome is notable for later presentation in most patients.

More than 50% of the pediatric patients with sustained or symptomatic ventricular arrhythmias have some evidence of heart disease. Although frequent, isolated premature ventricular beats are less common in children and adolescents than older adults, they are not rare. Ambulatory monitoring in normal subjects shows a bimodal pattern, with a small peak in early infancy or fetal life before a steady increase in adolescence and further increase into adulthood. Right ventricular outflow tract tachycardias (Chapter 61) and more triggered patterns of idiopathic left ventricular tachycardia are observed at all ages. Many of these patients have minimal symptoms or no more than episodic palpitations at intermediate rates.

The child with ventricular arrhythmias, without evidence of cardiomyopathy, without tumors, and without ion channel disease, generally has a favorable prognosis both in infancy and later childhood, when there is a high incidence of spontaneous resolution.[17] If ablation is considered, the success rates of initial procedures are about 60%, with a third recurring.[18] For the minimally symptomatic patient without prior heart disease, normal ventricular function, and no underlying substrate, many ventricular arrhythmias are managed expectantly.

Bradycardia

Primary sinus bradycardia is often associated with complex heart disease, particularly the polysplenia or left atrial isomerism patterns. Congenital heart surgery with extensive atrial reconstruction (Fontan operations and revisions, atrial switch operations) often result in significant and slowly progressive sinus bradycardia. Even when the sinus rates are adequate for daily activity, they may be sufficiently slow to contribute to atrial tachycardias or become symptomatic when antiarrhythmic drug therapy is needed for tachyarrhythmias. Many postoperative patients without atrial tachycardia or symptoms do appear to compensate effectively, though concerns about bradycardia-mediated remodeling keep open the decision of when to treat.[19]

Secondary bradycardia can be seen in adolescent athletes and in young people with eating disorders. The adolescent girl with anorexia-induced bradycardia typically has resting rates less than 40 to 45 beats per minute and either a body mass index less than 17 or rapid weight loss. Distinguishing the adolescent with an eating disorder from the trained athlete can be a challenge.

Atrioventricular Block

Newly recognized marked first-degree block should at least raise consideration of pathologic rhythms such as ectopic atrial tachycardia or inflammatory disease. Of the inflammatory conditions, Lyme carditis is the most common cause in much of the United States and generally responds rapidly to antibiotic therapy. In congenital heart disease, particularly in adults with atriopulmonary Fontan procedures, there may be quite prolonged PR intervals secondary to delays in atrial conduction, with normal atrioventricular conduction.

More advanced heart block can generally be classified as congenital antibody-mediated heart block, idiopathic heart block, heart block from inflammatory diseases such as Lyme or acute myocarditis, or degenerative multisystem disorders such as Kearne-Sayres, which can occur in childhood (Chapter 78).

Congenital complete heart block secondary to maternal antibodies has a variable course. Maternal antibodies (SSA and SSB or anti-Rho and anti-La) are generally identified, although most mothers do not have clinical rheumatologic disease. Recurrence risk in subsequent pregnancies is about 20%. Maternal therapy with glucocorticoids and possibly β-agonists has been advocated.[20] This approach has been criticized for the high mortality observed in the historical controls.[21] Ongoing research directed by Dr. Buyon is examining the role of steroids or intravenous immunoglobulin as preventive therapy in at-risk pregnancies. There is some in-utero demise from hydrops and postnatal mortality from cardiomyopathy, even with effective pacing. The prognosis is reasonable for those with higher heart rates and good ventricular function. There are no reliable methods for fetal pacing. After delivery, some patients have reasonable junctional rhythm (usually resting rates >55 beats per minute), good ventricular function, normal repolarization, and no symptoms, permitting expectant management until the patient receives a pacemaker in late childhood or adolescence.

Congenital heart block with structural heart disease, typically either levo-transposition or heterotaxy syndrome with atrioventricular septal defect,[22] is more problematic and results in more fetal demise. Pacemaker decisions are integrated into the surgical management. There are interesting correlations noted with familial heart disease and AV block, most notably NKx2.5, which is associated with several different forms of congenital heart disease.

A small number of children present with progressive idiopathic AV block, without clear evidence of associated disease (Chapter 75). Therapy choices generally mirror those for congenital heart block, although prognosis is better for children with idiopathic AV block.[23]

Reflex Syncope Syndromes in Childhood

Isolated syncopal events are common in toddlers and adolescents. Reflex convulsive events in children 6 months to 3 or 4 years old (variously labeled *pallid breath holding spells*, *reflex anoxic syncope*, or *white syncope*) are associated with episodic triggered sinus pauses. Ventricular pacing is not routinely needed, but it is effective in the extremely symptomatic patient.

As these children reach adolescence, the incidence of typical neurally mediated syncope increases, and more than 20% have at least a single, usually typical, episode (Chapters 85 and 91). Tilt table testing is problematic because adolescents demonstrate more orthostasis, with up to 60% of normal adolescents having syncope induced during a prolonged 80-degree tilt.

Pediatric Therapeutic Concerns

Child-specific data are being developed for ablation (Chapter 110).[1] Specific concerns include appropriate management of anesthesia or sedation, equipment that includes smaller catheters, and personnel who are skilled with appropriate imaging and interventional techniques, particularly for the child with congenital heart disease.

Infants are clearly more vulnerable to each aspect of catheter ablation. In addition to the technical challenges, there are reports of coronary damage and late lesion growth. In the initial pediatric radiofrequency registry, weight less than 15 kg was a risk factor for complications and increased mortality. When ablation is required for serious symptoms such as refractory

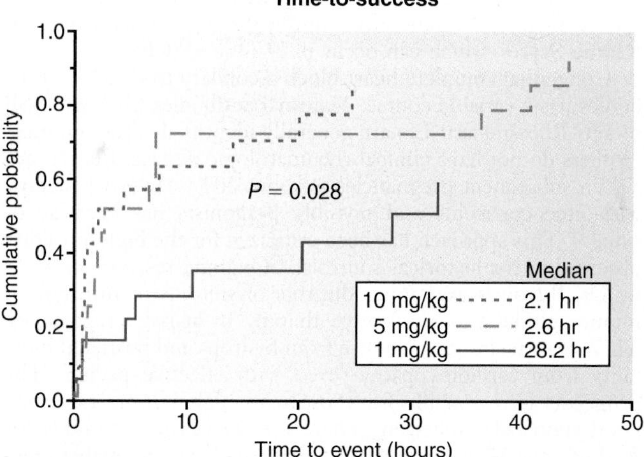

Figure 94-3 Dose-related time to effect of intravenous amiodarone administered for incessant arrhythmias. (From Saul JP, Scott WA, Brown S, et al: Intravenous amiodarone for incessant tachyarrhythmias in children: A randomized, double-blind, antiarrhythmic drug trial. Circulation 112(22):3470-3477, 2005, with permission.)

cardiomyopathy, life-threatening drug side effects, or concomitant heart disease, effective ablation is more feasible with 5-F catheters, esophageal catheters that serve as a second atrial pacing or recording site, and time- and temperature-limited lesions.

With the older child, the absolute ablation risks rapidly approach those reported in adult series. Decision making for those children depends upon local details including center-specific skills and techniques and the need for other surgical therapy.

Drug therapy in infants, small children, and particularly fetuses is based on limited reports. The possibility of extending drug patent protection for pediatric-specific data has led to some data that contribute to the care of the youngest children.

Intravenous amiodarone is a mainstay for managing life-threatening and incessant arrhythmias. With modern resuscitation guidelines, it is the first agent used in sustained ventricular arrhythmias. In a prospective double-blind, tiered-dose study of amiodarone, 5 and 10 mg/kg had faster time to success (Fig. 94-3).[10] Equally important, 87% had some adverse event, and 40% of the 5 mg/kg group had more than 1 significant event including hypotension, bradycardia, or heart block. Many small studies, without the focused methods of this study, report fewer adverse events. Subjects in those studies generally had less disease complexity, which can contribute to the more favorable risk-to-benefit balance.

A pharmacokinetic study of sotalol has refined dosing to a lower level in infants. A similar study with intravenous esmolol confirmed standard dosing. Developmental changes result in increased susceptibility to verapamil in infancy, which can result in cardiovascular collapse in the infant with depressed function.

Despite these data, most of the agents used to treat arrhythmias in pediatrics are used off label. There are commercial liquid preparations of propanolol and digoxin, but most antiarrhythmic therapy administered to infants requires extemporaneous formulations, with their intrinsic potential for error. Even benign drugs, such as propanolol, can cause toxicity from hypoglycemia in infants and psychiatric effects in older children. For acute intravenous therapy, my group commonly starts with procainamide, largely because of the favorable side-effect profile.

Pacing and Device Therapy

Areas of practice variation largely focus on technical choices in pacing, indications for ICD or multisite ventricular resynchronization therapy, and the use of antitachycardia devices. With the increased attention to adverse hemodynamic effects of right ventricular apical pacing, both experimental data and experience with multisite ventricular pacing has suggested that ventricular leads should be placed endocardially on the septum or epicardially on the left ventricle, although the impact of these changes is uncertain.[24]

More pediatric patients require epicardial pacing. Patients with lateral tunnel and older atriopulmonary connections typically have the coronary sinus in the pulmonary venous atrium, precluding all but the most creative placement for the transvenous ventricular lead.[25]

Older epicardial leads and unipolar leads in general have higher energy requirements than modern bipolar leads.[26,27] Although the failure rates of leads in pediatrics is generally higher than rates reported in large adult series, current follow-up of thin endocardial leads is comparable to the bipolar steroid-eluting epicardial leads,[26] with 5-year lead survival between 84% and 90%. Individual groups have clear lower weight limits for transvenous approaches (at Children's Hospital in Boston, that limit is ~10 kg), but committed groups report successful transvenous approaches even in infants weighing less than 3 kg. In the smallest infants, even epicardial approaches require some compromises (Fig. 94-4). There is concern that leads in the passive Fontan circulation will be prone to thrombus, and the transvenous approach is increasingly employed in that setting to avoid repeat sternotomy.[25] The presence of intracardiac shunts can result in an increased risk of embolic events.[28] Vessel occlusion is a concern, and complete occlusion was seen in 13% of a pediatric cohort.[29] These data indicate that for pacemaker leads, there will continue to be considerable practice variation.

The return of an *atrial antitachycardia pacemaker* to the market represented an attractive option for the patient who has congenital heart disease with sinus node dysfunction and atrial re-entry tachycardia. The Medtronic AT500 terminated atrial tachycardia in more than 50% of those in the initial trial. However, 1:1 AV conduction of atrial tachycardia resulted in misclassification (by the device) as ventricular tachycardia and withholding therapy for multiple episodes. These patients continue to require medications to slow AV conduction, or they use the antitachycardia device off label by plugging the ventricular port, or they might need to consider ICD devices with both atrial and ventricular therapies.

The role of chronic resynchronization therapy is established in the adult with symptomatic heart failure, left ventricular dysfunction, and left ventricular conduction delay where most patients are also candidates for ICD therapy. The role in the heterogeneous pediatric cohorts is evolving. Each of those indications is problematic: There are fewer patients with left ventricular conduction delay, symptoms develop later, and, for congenital heart disease patients, there is no clearly accepted marker for electromechanical dyssynchrony, among several barriers. Multicenter survey data suggest some improvement in ventricular function[30] and at times dramatic clinical improvement. Resynchronization of the failing right ventricle in tetralogy of Fallot may be feasible with focused lead placement,[31] though no benefit is seen with typical right ventricular apical pacing, despite preexisting right bundle branch block. For the smaller patient, an epicardial approach (Fig. 94-5) may be appropriate. Multisite pacing might also be advantageous in the acute postoperative setting.

In the younger patient and the congenital heart disease patient requiring ICD therapy, several problems contribute to

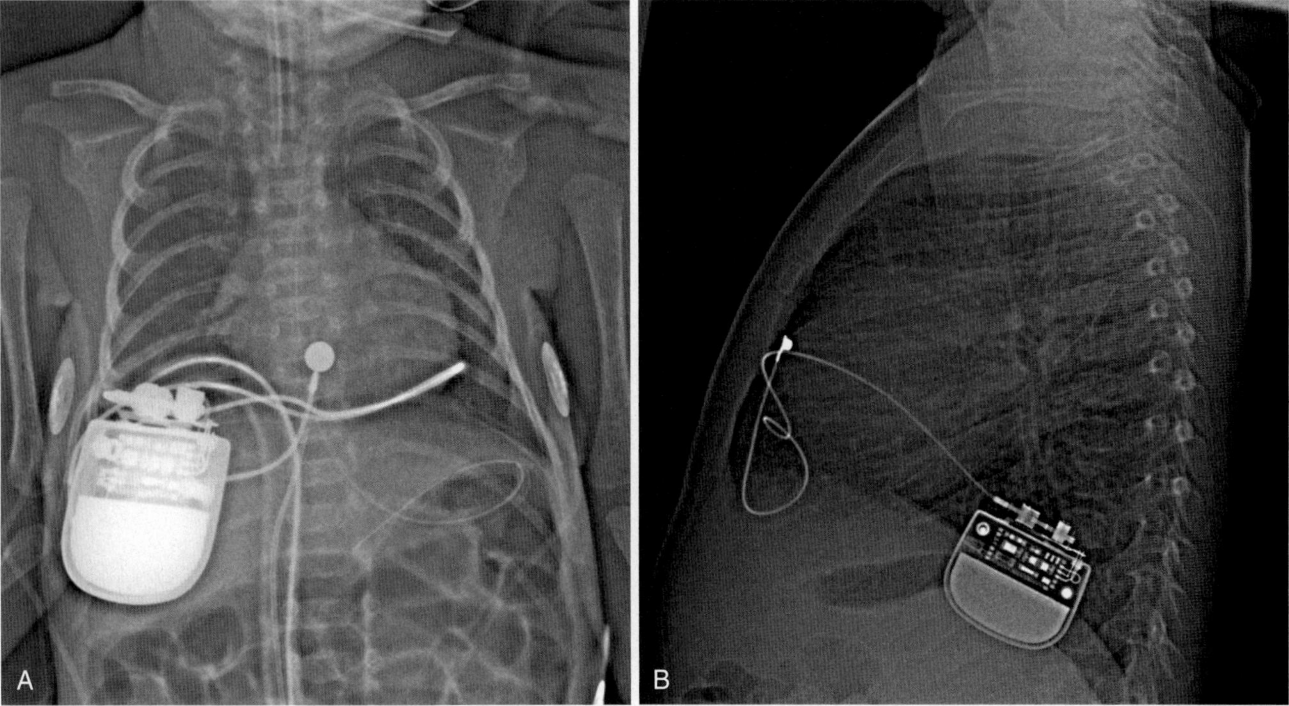

Figure 94-4 **A,** Anteroposterior radiograph of a 1.2-kg infant with congenital complete heart block. A unipolar ventricular lead is attached to a small pulse generator that placed in the right thoracic gutter. **B,** Lateral view.

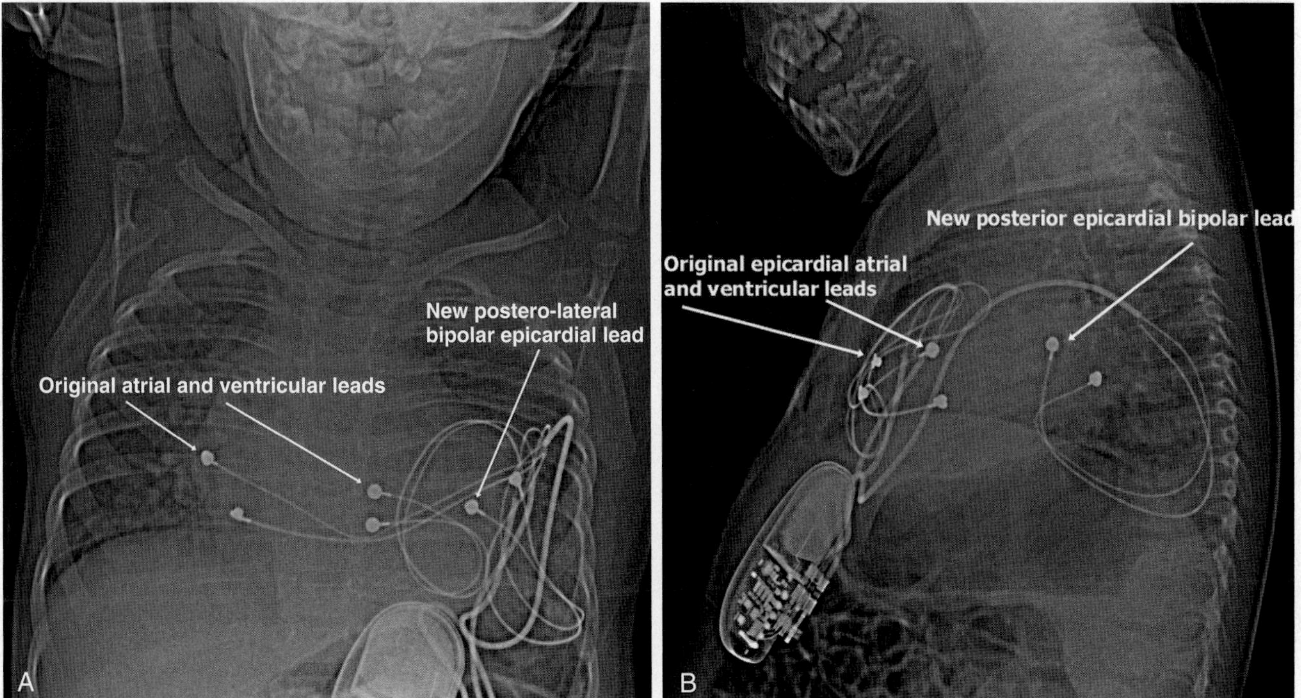

Figure 94-5 Posteroanterior **(A)** and lateral **(B)** chest radiograph of a 13-month-old patient with postoperative heart block following arterial switch for d-transposition of the great vessels. After neonatal placement of an epicardial DDD pacemaker, she was found to have significant ventricular dysfunction, apparently secondary to a septal infarct. A posterior epicardial pacing lead and upgrade to a biventricular device resulted in improved ejection fraction from 42% to 58% and decrease in ventricular end diastolic volumes.

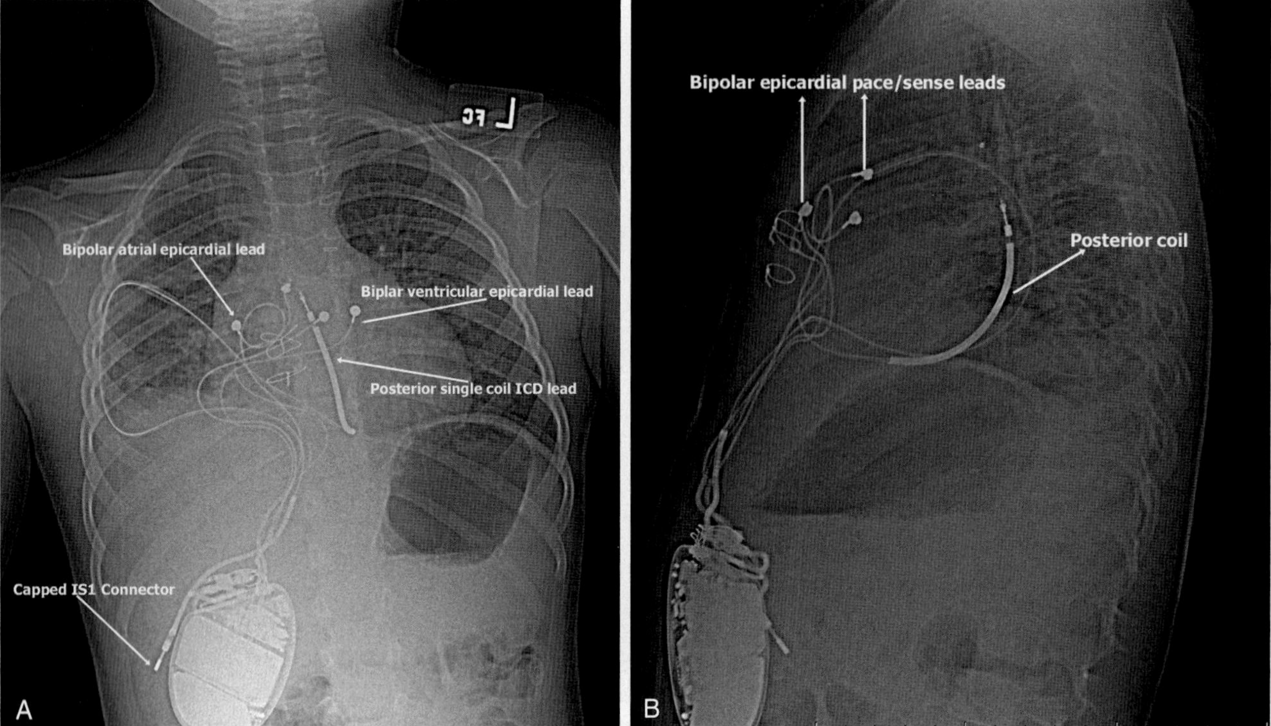

Figure 94-6 Posteroanterior **(A)** and lateral **(B)** chest radiograph of a 3-year-old patient with long QT syndrome with episodic 2:1 atrioventricular block secondary to *SCN5A* mutation, resulting in long QT. The single coil implantable cardioverter defibrillator (ICD) lead is placed in the posterior pericardial space, with the IS1 portion of the lead capped and abandoned in the pocket. Epicardial bipolar leads are used for atrial and ventricular pacing and sensing.

challenging ICD management. these include larger leads, the continued challenge of growth, higher sinus rates, concomitant supraventricular arrhythmias in congenital heart disease, and the presence of anatomic barriers, including intracardiac shunts and Fontan anatomy that has no transvenous access to the ventricle.

The incidence of inappropriate therapy secondary to sinus tachycardia, rapidly conducting atrial tachycardia, and lead fracture[32] has been comparable to the incidence of appropriate therapy, about 12%/year. Growth seems to contribute to lead failure.

In response to the anatomic and size challenges, creative nontransvenous approaches are reported with good success. Combinations of two primary techniques are used. Epicardial pace-sense leads are placed, and an ICD coil is placed posteriorly, with the ICD generator typically in a right suprahepatic subrectus pocket (Fig. 94-6). Subcutaneous arrays, a single transvenous SVC coil, or a subcutaneous SVC coil all offer additional ways of modifying the shock vector. In patients without prior congenital heart disease surgery, these may be implanted with ministernotomy or thoracoscopic techniques, limiting the acute morbidity.

Implantable event monitors are used with moderate success in pediatrics. Symptoms resolve in more than 30% of patients following placement of the device, and 50% to 60% of patients have reasonable symptom and rhythm correlation. For infrequent, frightening events without a clear diagnosis, implantable event monitors may be the most effective approach.

Special Considerations in Fetal Arrhythmias

Fetal arrhythmias are a small but important collaborative practice. With the exception of frequent atrial ectopy, which is rarely referred for therapy, the sustained fetal arrhythmias are uncommon. Physicians in multiple specialties assist with drug therapy and decision making. The technical delivery of drugs (transmaternal, transplacental, or direct fetal therapy via transuterine techniques) can be done at almost any facility, but infants and mothers have better outcome when care is transferred to a comprehensive facility.[33]

External fetal Doppler aliases at 240 beats per minute, limiting its use to monitoring typical accessory pathway mediated tachycardia. The bulk of diagnostic decision making is based on a fetal ultrasound (Fig. 94-7), which permits accurate measurement of heart rate and reasonable inference of AV and ventriculoatrial intervals. Tissue Doppler permits more detailed analysis of earliest ventricular activation. A limited number of centers have magnetocardiography,[34] which permits more prolonged monitoring and reconstruction of an ECG waveform (Fig. 94-8).

For nonsustained tachycardias with mean heart rates less than 200 beats per minute and no evidence of hydrops, expectant management may be the most appropriate approach. Similarly, for sustained tachycardia with combinations of hydrops and maternal compromise in a near-term fetus, moving toward delivery is appropriate.

The younger fetus with sustained rapid tachycardia can be expected to develop hydrops, although that takes days. Successful management has been reported with digoxin (particularly in the nonhydropic fetus), flecanide, sotalol, amiodarone,[35] and virtually all oral antiarrhythmic agents. Each approach has included fetal demise and some toxicity. Maternal renal drug clearance is increased, requiring larger doses. Although direct fetal therapy is feasible via intramuscular or uterine vessel cannulation, the fetal mortality rates seem higher than in reports that focus on administering medications to the mother.[36]

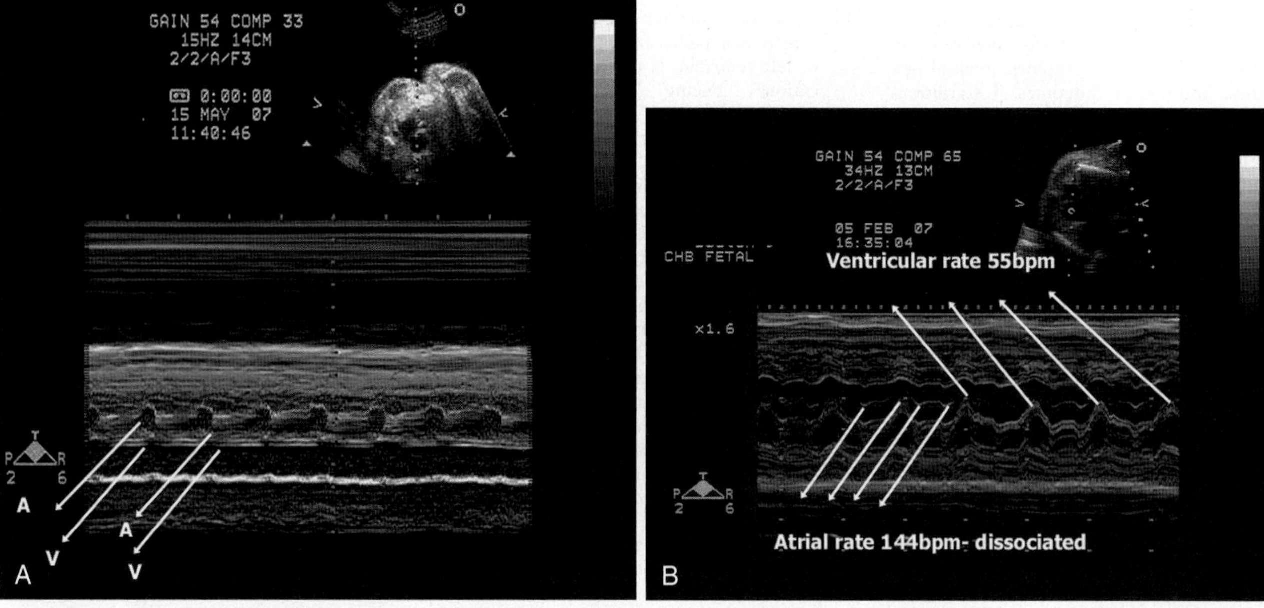

Figure 94-7 Doppler and m-mode tracing from a fetus at 32 weeks with sustained accessory pathway mediated tachycardia at 290 beats per minute (bpm) and hydrops fetalis (**A**) and congenital heart block (**B**). A, atrial beat; V, ventricular beat.

Conclusion

Arrhythmias are an important source of pediatric morbidity and mortality. Although the practice continues to evolve, management is increasingly based on data that specifically include the distinctive natural history of pediatric patients and the implications of therapy choices in those patient cohorts. With these data and continued creative practice, most of the electrophysiology diagnostic and therapeutic tools are available for even the smallest patients.

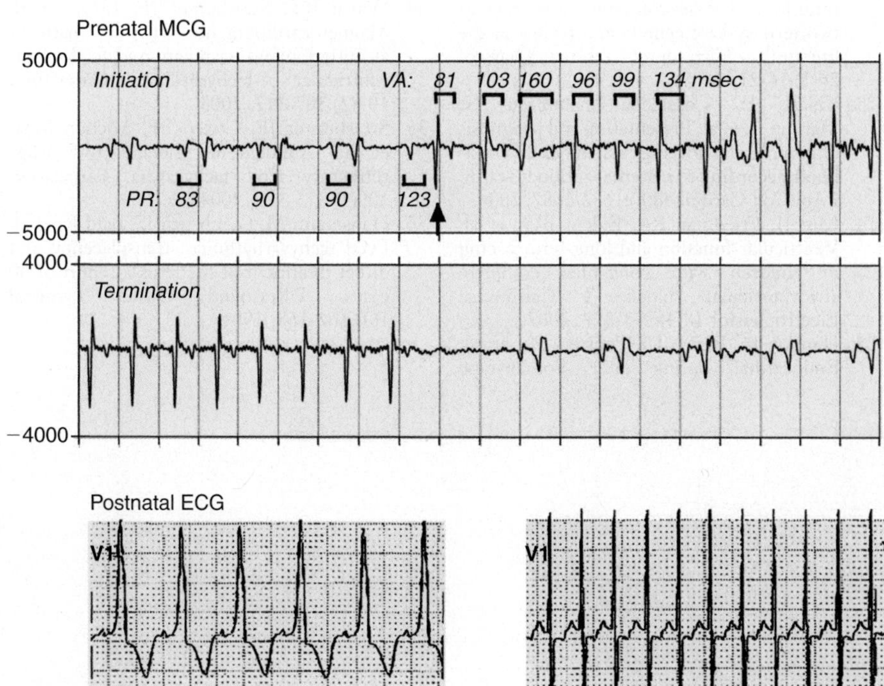

Figure 94-8 Fetal magnetocardiogram (MCG) demonstrating an atrial premature contraction, antegrade accessory pathway block, and initiation of orthodromic tachycardia with initial bundle branch aberration. Postnatal electrocargiograms (ECGs) are shown below. PR, PR interval; VA, ventricular-atrial interval. (From Wakai RT, Strasburger JF, Li Z, et al: Magnetocardiographic rhythm patterns at initiation and termination of fetal supraventricular tachycardia. Circulation 107(2):307-312, 2003, with permission.)

References

1. Van Hare GF, Javitz H, Carmelli D, et al: Prospective assessment after pediatric cardiac ablation: Demographics, medical profiles, and initial outcomes. J Cardiovasc Electrophysiol 15(7):759-770, 2004.
2. Moorman AF, Christoffels VM, Anderson RH: Anatomic substrates for cardiac conduction. Heart Rhythm 2(8):875-886, 2005.
3. Pappone C, Manguso F, Santinelli R, et al: Radiofrequency ablation in children with asymptomatic Wolff-Parkinson-White syndrome. N Engl J Med 351(12):1197-1205, 2004.
4. Triedman J, Perry J, Van HG: Risk stratification for prophylactic ablation in asymptomatic Wolff-Parkinson-White syndrome. N Engl J Med 352(1):92-93, 2005.
5. Kleinman CS, Nehgme RA: Cardiac arrhythmias in the human fetus. Pediatr Cardiol 25(3):234-251, 2004.
6. Texter KM, Kertesz NJ, Friedman RA, Fenrich AL Jr: Atrial flutter in infants. J Am Coll Cardiol 48(5):1040-1046, 2006.
7. Salerno JC, Kertesz NJ, Friedman RA, Fenrich AL Jr: Clinical course of atrial ectopic tachycardia is age-dependent: Results and treatment in children < 3 or > or =3 years of age. J Am Coll Cardiol 43(3):438-444, 2004.
8. Blurton DJ, Dubin AM, Chiesa NA, et al: Characterizing dual atrioventricular nodal physiology in pediatric patients with atrioventricular nodal reentrant tachycardia. J Cardiovasc Electrophysiol 17(6):638-644, 2006.
9. Pak HN, Hwang C, Kim YH: Twin atrioventricular node associated with interruption of the inferior vena cava and atrioventricular nodal reentrant tachycardia. J Electrocardiol 39(4):400-403, 2006.
10. Saul JP, Scott WA, Brown S, et al: Intravenous amiodarone for incessant tachyarrhythmias in children: A randomized, double-blind, antiarrhythmic drug trial. Circulation 112(22):3470-3477, 2005.
11. Towbin JA, Lowe AM, Colan SD, et al: Incidence, causes, and outcomes of dilated cardiomyopathy in children. JAMA 296(15):1867-1876, 2006.
12. Colan SD, Lipshultz SE, Lowe AM, et al: Epidemiology and cause-specific outcome of hypertrophic cardiomyopathy in children: Findings from the Pediatric Cardiomyopathy Registry. Circulation 115(6):773-781, 2007.
13. Spencer CT, Bryant RM, Day J, et al: Cardiac and clinical phenotype in Barth syndrome. Pediatrics 118(2):e337-e346, 2006.
14. Fazio G, Corrado G, Zachara E, et al: Ventricular tachycardia in non-compaction of left ventricle: Is this a frequent complication? Pacing Clin Electrophysiol 30(4):544-546, 2007.
15. Thomas-de-Montpreville V, Nottin R, Dulmet E, Serraf A: Heart tumors in children and adults: Clinicopathological study of 59 patients from a surgical center. Cardiovasc Pathol 16(1):22-28, 2007.
16. Etheridge SP, Sanatani S, Cohen MI, et al: Long QT syndrome in children in the era of implantable defibrillators. J Am Coll Cardiol 50(14):1335-1340, 2007.
17. Harris KC, Potts JE, Fournier A, et al: Right ventricular outflow tract tachycardia in children. J Pediatr 149(6):822-826, 2006.
18. Morwood JG, Triedman JK, Berul CI, et al: Radiofrequency catheter ablation of ventricular tachycardia in children and young adults with congenital heart disease. Heart Rhythm 1(3):301-308, 2004.
19. Suto F, Zhu W, Cahill SA, et al: Ventricular rate determines early bradycardic electrical remodeling. Heart Rhythm 2(3):293-300, 2005.
20. Jaeggi ET, Fouron JC, Silverman ED, et al: Transplacental fetal treatment improves the outcome of prenatally diagnosed complete atrioventricular block without structural heart disease. Circulation 110(12):1542-1548, 2004.
21. Rosenthal E, Gordon PA, Simpson JM, et al: Letter regarding article by Jaeggi et al, "Transplacental fetal treatment improves the outcome of prenatally diagnosed complete atrioventricular block without structural heart disease"; response. Circulation 111(18):e287-e288, 2005.
22. Jaeggi ET, Hornberger LK, Smallhorn JF, Fouron JC: Prenatal diagnosis of complete atrioventricular block associated with structural heart disease: combined experience of two tertiary care centers and review of the literature. Ultrasound Obstet Gynecol 26(1):16-21, 2005.
23. Villain E, Coastedoat-Chalumeau N, Marijon E, et al: Presentation and prognosis of complete atrioventricular block in childhood, according to maternal antibody status. J Am Coll Cardiol 48(8):1682-1687, 2006.
24. Kim JJ, Friedman RA, Eidem BW, et al: Ventricular function and long-term pacing in children with congenital complete atrioventricular block. J Cardiovasc Electrophysiol 18(4):373-377, 2007.
25. Hansky B, Blanz U, Peuster M, et al: Endocardial pacing after Fontan-type procedures. Pacing Clin Electrophysiol 28(2):140-148, 2005.
26. Fortescue EB, Berul CI, Cecchin F, et al: Comparison of modern steroid-eluting epicardial and thin transvenous pacemaker leads in pediatric and congenital heart disease patients. J Interv Card Electrophysiol 14(1):27-36, 2005.
27. Alexander ME: Transvenous pacing in infants: A faith based initiative? Pacing Clin Electrophysiol 27(11):1463-1465, 2004.
28. Khairy P, Landzberg MJ, Gatzoulis MA, et al: Transvenous pacing leads and systemic thromboemboli in patients with intracardiac shunts: A multicenter study. Circulation 113(20):2391-2397, 2006.
29. Bar-Cohen Y, Berul CI, Alexander ME, et al: Age, size, and lead factors alone do not predict venous obstruction in children and young adults with transvenous lead systems. J Cardiovasc Electrophysiol 17(7):754-759, 2006.
30. Dubin AM, Janousek J, Rhee E, et al: Resynchronization therapy in pediatric and congenital heart disease patients: An international multicenter study. J Am Coll Cardiol 46(12):2277-2283, 2005.
31. Janousek J, Tomek V, Chaloupecky VA, et al: Cardiac resynchronization therapy: A novel adjunct to the treatment and prevention of systemic right ventricular failure. J Am Coll Cardiol 44(9):1927-1931, 2004.
32. Alexander ME, Cecchin F, Walsh EP, et al: Implications of implantable cardioverter defibrillator therapy in congenital heart disease and pediatrics. J Cardiovasc Electrophysiol 15(1):72-76, 2004.
33. Naheed ZJ, Strasburger JF, Deal BJ, et al: Fetal tachycardia: mechanisms and predictors of hydrops fetalis. J Am Coll Cardiol 27(7):1736-1740, 1996.
34. Wakai RT, Strasburger JF, Li Z, et al: Magnetocardiographic rhythm patterns at initiation and termination of fetal supraventricular tachycardia. Circulation 107(2):307-312, 2003.
35. Strasburger JF, Cuneo BF, Michon MM, et al: Amiodarone therapy for drug-refractory fetal tachycardia. Circulation 109(3):375-379, 2004.
36. Hansmann M, Gembruch U, Bald R, et al: Fetal tachyarrhythmias: transplacental and direct treatment of the fetus-a report of 60 cases. Ultrasound Obstet Gynecol 1(3):162-168, 1991.

Sleep-Disordered Breathing and Arrhythmias 95

Apoor S. Gami, Sean M. Caples, and Virend K. Somers

CHAPTER OUTLINE

Obstructive sleep apnea (OSA) and central sleep apnea (CSA), the most common sleep-related breathing disorders, are associated with cardiac arrhythmias. This had long been recognized anecdotally, but only recently have controlled studies raised awareness of the nature and strength of this relationship. In this chapter, we discuss the pathophysiology and epidemiology of OSA and CSA; epidemiologic data supporting associations between sleep apnea and bradyarrhythmias, atrial fibrillation (AF), ventricular arrhythmias, and sudden cardiac death (SCD); the potential pathophysiologic mechanisms through which OSA and CSA can promote the initiation or maintenance of these arrhythmias; the effects of sleep apnea therapy on these relationships; and the application of our current understanding of this topic in the clinical setting, keeping in mind the limitations of the available data and the expectations for future research.

Obstructive Sleep Apnea

Pathophysiology

OSA is characterized by the failure of neuromuscular mechanisms governing upper airway patency during sleep, resulting in airway narrowing or collapse. Although apnea can occur in any position, the upper airway is more vulnerable to obstruction in the supine position due to dorsal displacement of the tongue and soft tissues. Upper airway collapse can occur during any stage of sleep, but susceptibility is greatest during rapid eye movement (REM) sleep. Heralded by atonia of skeletal muscles, including that of the pharynx and upper airway but excluding the respiratory diaphragm and extraocular muscles, REM sleep occurs cyclically (four to six times) throughout sleep and accounts for about 25% of total sleep time. Of potential pathophysiologic importance in arrhythmogenesis, REM sleep is a state of autonomic instability, marked by surges in sympathetic and vagal activity, with attendant variations in heart rate, blood pressure, and peripheral vascular resistance.[1]

Obstructive disordered breathing events are repetitive, numbering in the hundreds per night in extreme cases. Each is associated with oxyhemoglobin desaturation followed by central nervous system arousal, thereby reestablishing upper airway patency with resumption of ventilation and subsequent reoxygenation. Associated with each repetitive cycle is a cascade of acute stressors, including among others hypoxemia, surges in sympathetic neural output, production of reactive oxygen species, and fluctuations of intrathoracic and cardiac transmural pressures. The relevance of these acute pathophysiologic changes to specific arrhythmia syndromes is discussed later.

Diagnosis of OSA is by attended, in-lab multichannel polysomnography. These data generate the apnea-hypopnea index (AHI), which is the average number of apneas and hypopneas per hour of sleep. Although it is probably the best composite measurement of OSA severity, the AHI does not directly quantify other processes operative in the pathophysiology of cardiovascular disease, such as the degree and duration of oxygen desaturation or sleep disruption.

Epidemiology and Clinical Features

OSA is highly prevalent, but because overnight multichannel sleep monitoring is the standard by which the diagnosis is made, and due to regional variations in sleep lab availability, it remains under-recognized in the medical and lay community.

The best available data from population-based studies that used polysomnographic monitoring in adults provide estimates of the prevalence of OSA of between 3% and 28%.[2] Men, in part due to truncal distribution of adipose tissue and muscle, have a higher risk of OSA than women, but the sex prevalence gap narrows after menopause. Age, obesity, and increased neck circumference are additional strong risk factors for OSA.[3]

Excessive daytime sleepiness, a result of frequent nocturnal central nervous system arousals, is the most important symptom of OSA and a potential contributor to motor vehicle accidents. Yet less than 25% of persons with OSA actually report excessive sleepiness, although it is likely that subjective reporting under-represents the true symptomatic burden of OSA.[4] Daytime sleepiness, even in those with mild OSA, has been shown to correlate with the blood pressure–lowering effects of OSA therapy in patients with systemic hypertension, suggesting an important interaction between cardiovascular disease and OSA that extends beyond the absolute value of the AHI. Other typical signs and symptoms of OSA include loud snoring, interrupted and unrefreshing sleep, and pauses in breathing witnessed by a bed partner.

Central Sleep Apnea

Pathophysiology

CSA is characterized by the loss of ventilatory output from the central respiratory generator in the brainstem, resulting in interruptions of respiratory muscle output that lead to apneas and hypopneas. Generally, the maintenance of upper airway patency distinguishes CSA from OSA, although the conditions can coexist. CSA is broadly composed of a few heterogeneous disorders, such as high-altitude periodic breathing, idiopathic CSA, and some hypoventilation syndromes. The most common and studied form of CSA is Cheyne-Stokes respiration (CSA-CSR), which is most often encountered in the setting of heart failure and manifests as a characteristic waxing and waning periodicity of ventilation.

CSA-CSR reflects derangements in ventilatory control mechanisms caused by the hemodynamic consequences of left atrial hypertension and decreased cardiac output (usually due to left ventricular dysfunction). Partly because of irritant receptor stimulation by pulmonary microvascular congestion, heart failure patients chronically hyperventilate, resulting in low blood carbon dioxide tensions during wakefulness.[5] The relative hypocapnia, together with a heightened chemoreflex response to carbon dioxide and prolonged circulation time, destabilize the ventilatory control system during sleep and result in CSA-CSR. As would be expected by these mechanisms, inhalation of a carbon dioxide–enriched gas abolishes CSA.

CSA-CSR, like OSA, is diagnosed by multichannel polysomnography and is quantified by the central AHI. The characteristic waxing and waning pattern of ventilation, which also may be seen during wakefulness, is most prominent during non-REM sleep and is characteristically absent during REM sleep, where cortical influences on ventilation often override the chemoreflex. Similar to OSA, CSA-CSR is associated with repetitive cycles of acute stressors, including hypoxemia, hypercapnia, sympathetic activation, and fluctuations in heart rate and blood pressure.[6] In contrast to OSA, the influence of these processes on cardiovascular outcomes, including arrhythmias, has been relatively unexplored. Some data suggest that CSA-CSR contributes to worse cardiovascular outcomes, including mortality, in addition to what is attributable to the accompanying heart failure. What is known regarding the effect of CSA-CSR on specific arrhythmia syndromes is discussed later.

Epidemiology and Clinical Features

The prevalence of CSA-CSR in the general population or in unselected persons with left ventricular dysfunction is unknown. In two studies of more than 500 patients with predominantly New York Heart Association class II heart failure and an average left ventricular ejection fraction of about 25%, the prevalence of sleep apnea identified by polysomnography was between 33% and 40%.[7,8] The prevalence of CSA-CSR increases directly with the severity of heart failure. Like OSA, age and male sex increase the risk for CSA-CSR, with narrowing of the gender gap after menopause.

It is unclear if CSA-CSR results in symptoms independent of those related to the underlying cardiac condition. Nocturnal dyspnea attributable to cardiac dysfunction may be explained also by the hyperpneas of CSA-CSR. Even though CSA can coexist with OSA, symptoms referable to OSA are notably absent in persons with heart failure.

Mechanisms of Arrhythmias in Sleep Apnea

Obesity, diabetes, dyslipidemia, hypertension, ischemic heart disease, and systolic and diastolic heart failure all cluster with sleep apnea (Fig. 95-1).[9] Simply by association with these conditions, the risk of arrhythmias is increased in patients with OSA and CSA. The multiple pathophysiologic mechanisms by which sleep apnea can directly promote the initiation or maintenance of specific clinical arrhythmias are discussed next.

Bradyarrhythmias

It is important to recognize the mechanisms of bradycardias that occur commonly during normal sleep in healthy persons. Although sympathetic neural output and average heart rate are higher during REM sleep than during non-REM sleep, there is evidence for paroxysmal parasympathetic discharges during REM sleep that manifest as abrupt heart rate decelerations.

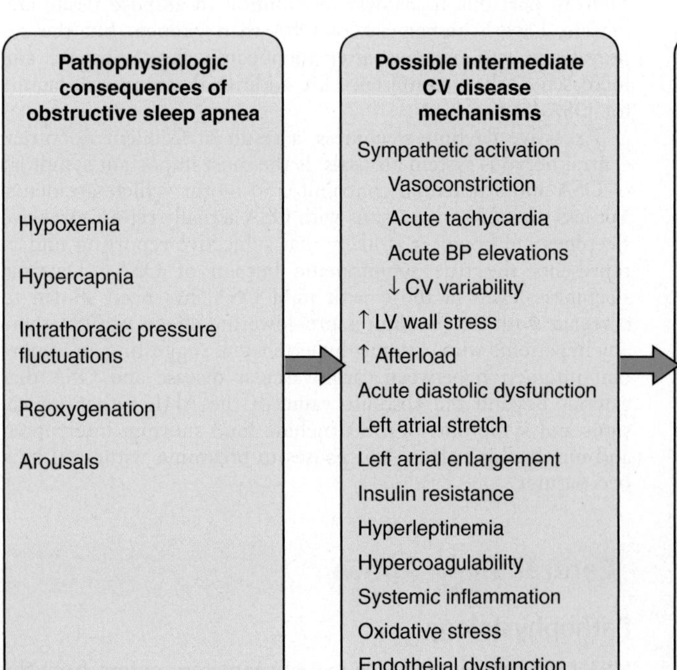

Figure 95-1 The pathophysiology of obstructive sleep apnea (OSA) may acutely and chronically elicit multiple intermediate cardiovascular disease mechanisms, which can promote the association of OSA with a number of cardiovascular (CV) conditions and diseases. BP, blood pressure; LV, left ventricle. (From Gami AS, Somers VK: Sleep apnea and cardiovascular disease. In Zipes DP (ed): Braunwald's Heart Disease: A Textbook of Cardiovascular Medicine. Philadelphia, Saunders, 2008, pp 1915-1921.)

Healthy young adults, often athletes, have periods of exaggerated vagal tone during REM sleep. This results in many benign, albeit sometimes pronounced, bradyarrhythmias, which are discussed later.

In persons with OSA, apnea and hypoxemia activate the physiologic diving reflex, so named from observations of oxygen conservation during prolonged water submersion by marine mammals. Hypoxemia, via stimulation of the carotid bodies, normally not only induces hyperventilation but also results in bradycardia. With normal breathing and hyperventilation, this heart rate slowing is attenuated by the vagolytic effects of lung inflation. This latter buffer is lost during apnea and, when coupled with the effects of oxyhemoglobin desaturation, results in marked bradycardias.[10] Electrophysiologic studies in persons with OSA and bradycardias referred for permanent pacemaker implantation showed no evidence of significant sinus, atrioventricular node, or His-Purkinje system disease, reflecting the influence of autonomic changes that occur in OSA.

Atrial Fibrillation

Several pathophysiologic mechanisms can directly link OSA and AF. Increased left atrial size is associated with OSA independently of other medical conditions.[11] Otto and colleagues compared left atrial volume indices in persons with OSA and without OSA who otherwise were completely healthy, middle-aged, men and women. They found that the left atrial volume index was normal in all subjects yet still significantly higher in the subjects with OSA. Left atrial size may be increased in persons with OSA due to its association with hypertension, for which it has been identified as a secondary cause, and diastolic dysfunction.[12] Even in otherwise healthy persons, subtle changes of diastolic dysfunction are present in those with OSA, and the severity of diastolic dysfunction correlates directly with the severity of oxygen desaturations. Concomitant obesity likely contributes to an enlarged left atrium due to larger body mass and increased total blood volume. Left atrial size might also be increased in OSA due to repetitive inspiratory efforts against an obstructed upper airway, which produce wide fluctuations in intrathoracic pressure that increase cardiac wall stress.[13] This process can also cause chronic stretching of the atrium, particularly at anchoring regions such as the pulmonary vein ostia, leading to electrical and structural remodeling. Activation of stretch-sensitive ion channels in the atrium can have implications for initiating AF.

Another potentially important mechanism of AF is the marked fluctuations in autonomic tone that occur in OSA. Cessation of breathing is associated with increases in sympathetic neural output as measured by peripheral microneurography.[14] Via the diving reflex, there can also be a concomitant rise in cardiac vagal activity.[10] Surges in sympathetic neural activity occur with each central nervous system arousal terminating an apnea. Although sleep stage–dependent mechanisms have yet to be proved in arrhythmogenesis, the influence of sleep stage on autonomic tone is well recognized. Stage II sleep is punctuated by characteristic K-complexes, which are high-amplitude EEG discharges associated with transient increases in peripheral sympathetic neural activity and a rise in blood pressure.[1] Slow-wave sleep, underrepresented in severe OSA, is a state of parasympathetic predominance. REM sleep is associated with abrupt fluctuations in both sympathetic and parasympathetic activity.

Although it is clear that the autonomic system plays a major role in the pathophysiology of AF, its specific effects are still being determined.[15] The processes that occur in OSA might lead to activation of atrial catecholamine-sensitive ion channels, which could result in focal discharges that initiate AF, and also to vagally mediated changes in atrial conduction properties that promote and maintain AF. Additionally, persons with OSA have chronically elevated sympathetic activity even during the waking period, which might have a deleterious effect on rate-control strategies for AF management.[14]

OSA is also associated with systemic inflammation, as evidenced by increased in levels of C-reactive protein, serum amyloid A, and interleukins. This association might have implications for atrial fibrosis and remodeling and AF outcomes.[16]

Ventricular Arrhythmias and Sudden Cardiac Death

Numerous pathophysiologic mechanisms might directly and indirectly link OSA to ventricular arrhythmias and SCD. The repetitive oxygen desaturations during apneic sleep are temporally associated with ventricular ectopy. This hypoxemia and the simultaneous hypercapnia activate the chemoreflex, which increases peripheral vascular sympathetic nerve activity and circulating catecholamines.[14] Tachycardia and surges in blood pressure at the end of apneas increase myocardial oxygen demand at the same time that hypoxemia decreases myocardial oxygen supply. The resultant nocturnal ischemia, whether manifest as silent ST-segment changes or nocturnal angina, has been demonstrated in persons with OSA and may be responsible for ventricular dysrhythmias during sleep.[17]

The risk of myocardial infarction and stroke, which may be the cause of SCD or lead to SCD through dysrhythmias or other complications, is increased in persons with OSA due to multiple mechanisms that promote nocturnal arterial thrombosis. In contrast to the usual diurnal variation of coagulation in healthy persons, patients with OSA have increased platelet activation and aggregation during the night. In addition, their fibrinogen levels are increased and fibrinolytic activity is decreased during sleep.

The marked autonomic dysfunction in OSA is likely an important link to SCD. Decreased heart rate variability, a risk marker for SCD, is present in patients with OSA due to abnormalities in central nervous system coupling of cardiac and ventilatory parasympathetic inputs, the arterial baroreflex, and feedback from pulmonary stretch receptors.[18] In addition, the QTc interval and QTc interval dispersion are abnormal in patients with OSA, with the latter correlating directly with the AHI and the duration of nocturnal hypoxemia.[19,20] Persons with OSA have increased sympathetic activity that persists during the awake period, which is associated with an increased risk of SCD.[14,21]

OSA is present in a large fraction of patients with heart failure, and it is implicated in chronic left ventricular dysfunction, through which it may be an important contributor to the neurohumoral response and myocardial remodeling that produce the substrate for SCD.[22]

Epidemiology of Arrhythmias in Sleep Apnea

Bradyarrhythmias

A number of factors confound an accurate description of the relationship between OSA and bradyarrhythmias, including referral biases, the presence of overt or subclinical comorbidities, variations in electrocardiographic monitoring, and the background bradycardias that exist in people without OSA. Due to the autonomic changes during normal sleep, described earlier, healthy persons commonly have nocturnal sinus bradycardia, marked sinus arrhythmia, sinus pauses or arrest, or first-degree and type I second-degree atrioventricular block. This occurs across sex and age groups and is prominent in young and older athletes.[23] This has led the American Academy of Sleep Medicine to recommend lowering the threshold heart rate for the diagnosis of bradycardia during sleep from the traditional 60 beats per minute to 40 beats per minute.[24]

The risk factors for significant bradycardias in OSA include the magnitude of oxyhemoglobin desaturation, the AHI, and REM sleep.[25] The prevalence of bradycardias in OSA patients varies widely depending upon the diagnostic strategy. Two months of recordings from an implanted loop recorder identified a prevalence of 47%, but 48 hours of ambulatory electrocardiogram monitoring found only a 13% prevalence in the same population.[26] In contrast to the majority of other data, the largest controlled study to assess nocturnal arrhythmias found no increase in bradyarrhythmias in patients with severe sleep apnea compared to persons without sleep apnea,[27] even though the group with sleep apnea was older, more obese, and had more cardiac risk factors. The reason for the discrepant finding is unclear, but it could be because OSA was not distinguished from CSA in this report.

Atrial Fibrillation

A 1983 study by Guillenminault and colleagues provided initial clues to a significant relationship between OSA and AF. Ambulatory electrocardiographic monitoring in 400 middle-aged patients with moderate or severe OSA (AHI = 25) revealed that the prevalence of nocturnal paroxysms of AF was more than 3%.[26] These findings have not received much attention, even though this prevalence was more than five times as high as the estimated prevalence of AF in middle-aged persons in the community. Also noteworthy was that all 12 of the study patients who underwent tracheostomy, which essentially cures OSA by bypassing the obstructed airway, had complete elimination of AF up to 6 months later.[26] These early observations, although not controlled or randomized data, strongly suggested that OSA might directly cause AF and that effectively treating OSA might prevent AF.

The first two controlled studies that identified a relationship between AF and sleep apnea were performed in patients with heart failure.[5,8] Together, in more than 500 patients with mostly moderate heart failure and an average ejection fraction of about 25%, the presence of sleep apnea was associated with a four-fold risk of AF, even after controlling for comorbidities. AF was present in about 20% of the patients with sleep apnea in these heart-failure populations.

Additional studies confirmed this relationship in broader groups of patients. Fifty-nine Finnish patients with lone AF (no ischemic or valvular heart disease, heart failure, sick sinus syndrome, pacemaker, hypertension, diabetes mellitus, hyperthyroidism, or acute causes of AF) underwent polysomnography, and 32% were found to have sleep apnea (AHI $\geq$15, without differentiation of OSA and CSA).[28] This was an underestimate of the true prevalence of sleep apnea in lone AF, because the standard criterion (an AHI of 5 or more) was not used. Incidentally, a control group of 56 community volunteers also had a high prevalence of sleep apnea; however, due to selective recruitment of the control group acknowledged by the investigators, a significant selection bias precluded comparisons with this group.

In another study, the prevalence of OSA was compared between 151 consecutive patients undergoing electrical cardioversion of AF and 463 consecutive patients without AF being evaluated in a general cardiology practice.[29] The groups had similar age, sex, body mass index, and prevalence of hypertension and heart failure; however, the patients with AF had a significantly higher risk of OSA (49% vs 33%), and multivariate analysis demonstrated a strong independent association between OSA and AF (odds ratio [OR], 2.2). An analysis of nocturnal arrhythmias in 566 persons undergoing polysomnography found AF in 5% of patients with severe sleep apnea and only 1% of patients without sleep apnea.[27] An additional study found that the prevalence of AF was relatively high in patients with idiopathic CSA (no heart failure) compared to patients with OSA or no sleep apnea.[30] Although it is possible that CSA in the absence of other cardiopulmonary conditions might increase the risk of AF, it also has been hypothesized and observed that the opposite cause-and-effect relationship exists, namely that AF and its hemodynamic sequelae might lead to CSA.[31]

Most convincingly, a number of longitudinal studies have identified OSA as a risk factor in the incidence or recurrence of AF. Prior to coronary artery bypass graft surgery, 121 patients underwent sleep studies; sleep apnea was diagnosed by an AHI of 5 or more or an oxygen desaturation index of 5 or more.[32] An AHI of 5 or more predicted a 32% incidence of postoperative AF requiring intervention, and an oxygen desaturation index of 5 or more predicted a 39% incidence of the same (both compared to 18% in the control groups). A prospective assessment of AF recurrence in 106 patients 1 year after electrical cardioversion found that patients with untreated OSA had a significantly higher recurrence of AF compared to those for whom OSA status was unknown (82% vs. 53%).[33] Recurrent AF was predicted independently by the severity of nocturnal oxygen desaturation and the portion of sleep time with oxygen saturation less than 90%.

The largest study to date compared the incidence of new-onset AF up to 15 years after diagnostic polysomnography in 3542 patients referred to a sleep-disorders center.[34] OSA and multiple measures of its severity, in addition to the usual clinical predictors, were significantly associated with incident AF (Fig. 95-2). In persons younger than 65 years, independent predictors of incident AF were age, male sex, coronary artery disease, body-mass index (hazard ratio [HR], 1.07) and the decrease in nocturnal oxygen saturation (HR, 3.29). This study clarified prior data that linked obesity to incident AF by revealing that obesity and OSA additively increase the risk for AF. Also, the finding that nocturnal oxygen desaturation independently predicted incident AF potentially reflects the pathophysiologic mechanism responsible for the relationship between OSA and AF. In fact, the three longitudinal studies just described that were designed to assess AF occurrence based on OSA status found that measures of nocturnal oxygen desaturation were the most powerful predictors of AF.

An additional study in 424 patients undergoing radiofrequency ablation of AF found that OSA was an independent risk factor for acute failure (i.e., within the index ablation procedure) of pulmonary vein isolation (relative risk [RR], 2.16).[35] These data suggest that it may be more difficult to achieve pulmonary vein isolation in OSA patients, possibly due to more challenging atrial anatomy or the effects of OSA on atrial fibrosis or electrical remodeling.

Ventricular Arrhythmias and Sudden Cardiac Death

Historically, clinical experience and limited observations had suggested an increased frequency of nocturnal ventricular arrhythmias and nocturnal SCD in patients with sleep apnea, particularly in those with severe OSA. A controlled multicenter study showed that nocturnal nonsustained ventricular tachycardia occurred in 5.3% and complex ventricular ectopy occurred in 25% of patients with severe sleep apnea.[27] After adjustment for comorbidities, patients with sleep apnea had a 3.4-fold risk of

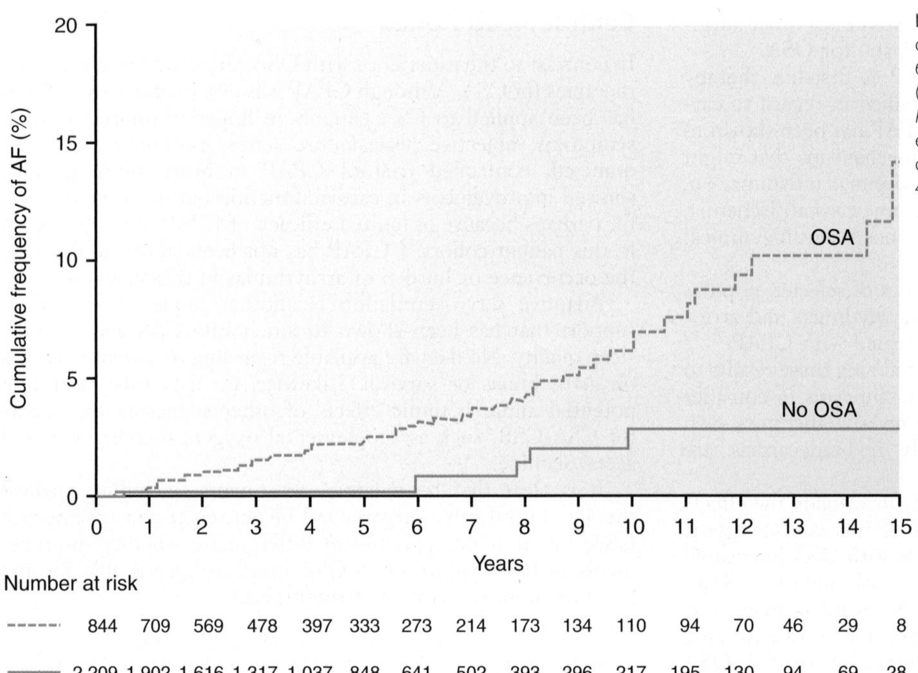

Figure 95-2 Cumulative frequency curves for incident atrial fibrillation (AF) for subjects younger than 65 years with and without obstructive sleep apnea (OSA) during an average 4.7 years of follow-up. $P = 0.002$. (From Gami AS, Hodge DO, Herges RM, et al: Obstructive sleep apnea, obesity, and the risk of incident atrial fibrillation. J Am Coll Cardiol 49(5):565-571, 2007.)

nonsustained ventricular tachycardia compared to patients without sleep apnea.

An important observation that demonstrates the acute impact of OSA on SCD is the apparent increase in nocturnal SCD in these patients.[36] The time of SCD was confirmed in 112 patients who had previously undergone polysomnography, and it was discovered that persons with OSA had a significantly increased risk of SCD from 12 midnight to 6 AM (RR, 2.57), whereas persons without OSA had a diurnal pattern of SCD similar to that expected in the general population (i.e., a peak between 6 AM and 12 noon). Nearly 50% of SCD in patients with OSA occurred during the sleeping hours, and the severity of OSA correlated directly with the risk of nocturnal SCD (Fig. 95-3).[36]

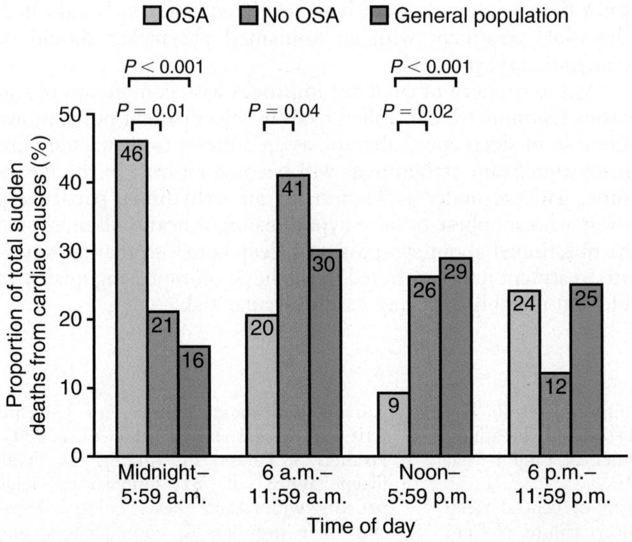

In a longitudinal study that examined the risk of SCD in patients with OSA, the rates of SCD were assessed during an average of 7.5 years in 107 OSA patients who were compliant with continuous positive airway pressure (CPAP) therapy and 61 OSA patients who had discontinued CPAP therapy. SCD occurred in four patients (7%) with untreated OSA and in no patients with treated OSA (there was one arrhythmic death in a treated patient during coronary bypass surgery).[37] These results suggest that the presence of untreated OSA might contribute to the incidence of SCD. However, these limited data do not allow inferences regarding the relative contribution of OSA vis-à-vis comorbidities to the occurrence of SCD in these patients. Additional studies are necessary to clarify the risk of SCD attributable to OSA, independently of other coexisting SCD risk factors, and the potential role of OSA therapy in modifying that risk.

Figure 95-3 Day versus night pattern of sudden cardiac death in patients with and without obstructive sleep apnea (OSA) and in the general population. (From Gami AS, Howard DE, Olson EJ, Somers VK: Day-night pattern of sudden death in obstructive sleep apnea. N Engl J Med 352(12):1206-1214, 2005. Copyright © [2005] Massachusetts Medical Society. All rights reserved.)

Sleep Apnea Therapy and Arrhythmias

Obstructive Sleep Apnea

The most immediately effective and widespread therapy for OSA is CPAP. With regular use, it relieves daytime sleepiness and improves cognitive function. Although many patients with highly symptomatic OSA adhere to CPAP therapy, those with limited symptoms may be less compliant. This poses a challenge in managing a growing population of patients with minimally symptomatic OSA and comorbid cardiovascular disease. Tracheostomy eliminates the consequences of upper airway collapse by entirely bypassing the upper airway, but it is typically regarded as a last-resort therapy in patients with debilitating or life-threatening OSA. Weight loss is also an exceedingly effective treatment for OSA, as studies of bariatric surgery have suggested, but the long-term durability of this treatment remains to be proven. There are very few controlled studies of other surgical therapies (e.g., uvulopalatopharyngoplasty) for OSA.

Given the long-standing role of CPAP as first-line therapy for OSA, it has been most extensively studied in regard to cardiovascular outcomes. Treatment with CPAP has been shown to reduce or abolish many of the putative mechanisms that might link OSA to arrhythmias, including hypoxemia, inflammation, sympathetic overactivity, hypertension, myocardial ischemia, and ventricular systolic dysfunction. Evidence regarding clinical outcomes, however, is scarce.

A number of small, observational studies of selected populations demonstrated a reduction in bradyarrhythmias and atrioventricular block in persons with OSA treated with CPAP.[25,38] Although the usual cautions apply to generalizing these results to the clinical realm, they should encourage clinicians to consider treating OSA before proceeding to more invasive therapies such as pacemaker implantation, particularly if bradycardias are asymptomatic and limited to sleep.

In the only study to date to specifically investigate the effects of OSA therapy on AF, the recurrence of AF was assessed 1 year after electrical cardioversion in 39 patients with OSA (untreated and treated by CPAP) and 79 patients with unknown OSA status.[33] AF recurred in only 42% of OSA patients effectively treated with CPAP, compared to recurrence in 82% of untreated OSA patients. Interestingly, the recurrence in treated OSA patients was even lower than that in the control group of AF patients (53%), probably because this latter group included patients with undiagnosed OSA. OSA patients without AF recurrence were three times more likely to have used effective CPAP therapy than patients with recurrence, and no differences existed between those with and without recurrence with regard to age, gender, body-mass index, or hypertension. This study showed that treatment of OSA by CPAP substantially reduces the risk of AF recurrence after electrical cardioversion and that traditional risk factors for AF do not predict recurrence in these patients as robustly as the presence or absence of CPAP therapy.

CPAP has been shown to reduce the frequency of ventricular ectopy in heart-failure patients; however this occurred in the context of concomitant improvements in global sympathetic activity, systemic blood pressure, and ventricular systolic function.[39]

No randomized, controlled trial data are available to directly address the role of OSA therapy on management of arrhythmias. Notably, studies in patients with heart failure (but not sleep apnea) demonstrated that CPAP therapy improved cardiac function in patients in sinus rhythm but worsened cardiac function in patients with AF.[40,41] Thus, assumptions cannot be made about the benefit, let alone the safety, of sleep apnea therapy on arrhythmias or other cardiovascular conditions, and this research needs to be designed cautiously. That notwithstanding, the prospect of a noninvasive, safe therapy to decrease the risk of significant clinical arrhythmias, such as AF or SCD, is enticing. Well-designed randomized, controlled trials of CPAP therapy in appropriate, high-risk OSA patients are needed.

Central Sleep Apnea

In contrast to the experience with OSA, there are few established therapies for CSA. Although CPAP was designed to treat OSA, it has been applied to CSA patients in hopes of improving their symptoms, objective heart-failure status, and survival. A randomized, controlled trial of CPAP in heart-failure patients showed improvements in cardiac function but no survival benefit, perhaps because of limited efficacy of CPAP in treating CSA in this patient cohort.[42] CPAP has not been shown to decrease the occurrence or burden of arrhythmias in these patients.

Adaptive servo-ventilation is another mode of ventilatory support that has been shown to ameliorate CSA and improve sleep quality. No data are available regarding its potential effects on arrhythmias or survival. Likewise, no data exist regarding potential antiarrhythmic effects of other suggested treatments for CSA-CSR, such as supplemental oxygen, theophylline, and acetazolamide.

It is clear that heart-failure treatments (including medical therapy, mitral valve surgery, and biventricular pacing) improve CSA, but it is not possible to differentiate whether improvements in heart failure or in CSA itself are responsible for any potential improvements in arrhythmias.[43]

Approach to the Patient

Identifying and treating sleep apnea, particularly OSA, in patients with AF or at risk or resuscitated from SCD may be an important adjunct to the overall care of these patients. Treating OSA favorably modifies the cardiovascular pathophysiologic processes that lead to these significant arrhythmias. It should be recognized, however, that currently there are limited data suggesting that effective treatment of OSA substantially reduces the burden of atrial or ventricular tachyarrhythmias. Generally, patients with benign, vagally mediated sinus node dysfunction or atrioventricular node block who remain asymptomatic during sleep do not require therapy directed at the arrhythmia. However, if the bradyarrhythmias are associated with a hypoperfusion state, ventricular dysfunction, or proarrhythmia, then treatment of OSA should be strongly considered. Also, treatment of clinically significant bradyarrhythmias by OSA therapy alone has not been validated, and if it is indicated, the usual treatment with an implanted pacemaker should be concomitantly pursued.

As the strength of evidence improves with completion of rigorous randomized, controlled trials in select patient populations, the role of sleep apnea therapy as an adjunct to managing clinically significant arrhythmias will become clearer. In the meantime, patients under evaluation for an arrhythmia, particularly those who are obese or have hypertension or heart failure, should be questioned about symptoms of sleep apnea so that appropriate treatment may be offered in the hope of improving quality of life and possibly reducing cardiovascular risk.

References

1. Somers V, Dyken M, Mark A, Abboud F: Sympathetic-nerve activity during sleep in normal subjects. N Engl J Med 328(5):303-307, 1993.
2. Young T, Peppard PE, Gottlieb DJ: Epidemiology of obstructive sleep apnea: A population health perspective. Am J Respir Crit Care Med 165(9):1217-1239, 2002.
3. Gami AS, Caples SM, Somers VK: Obesity and obstructive sleep apnea. Endocrinol Metab Clin North Am 32(4):869-894, 2003.
4. Young T, Palta M, Dempsey J, et al: The occurrence of sleep-disordered breathing among middle-aged adults. N Engl J Med 328(17):1230-1235, 1993.
5. Javaheri S: A mechanism of central sleep apnea in patients with heart failure. N Engl J Med 341(13):949-954, 1999.
6. Trinder J, Merson R, Rosenberg JI, et al: Pathophysiological interactions of ventilation, arousals, and blood pressure oscillations during Cheyne-Stokes respiration in patients with heart failure. Am J Respir Crit Care Med 162(3 Pt 1):808-813, 2000.
7. Javaheri S, Parker TJ, Liming JD, et al: Sleep apnea in 81 ambulatory male patients with stable heart failure. Types and their prevalences, consequences, and presentations. Circulation 97(21):2154-2159, 1998.
8. Sin DD, Fitzgerald F, Parker JD, et al: Risk factors for central and obstructive sleep apnea in 450 men and women with

congestive heart failure. Am J Respir Crit Care Med 160(4):1101-1106, 1999.
9. Gami AS, Somers VK: Sleep apnea and cardiovascular disease. In Zipes DP (ed): Braunwald's Heart Disease: A Textbook of Cardiovascular Medicine. Philadelphia, Saunders, 2008, pp 1915-1921.
10. Somers V, Dyken M, Mark A, Abboud F: Parasympathetic hyperresponsiveness and bradyarrhythmias during apnoea in hypertension. Clin Auton Res 2(3):171-176, 1992.
11. Otto ME, Belohlavek M, Romero-Corral A, et al: Comparison of cardiac structural and functional changes in obese otherwise healthy adults with versus without obstructive sleep apnea. Am J Cardiol 99(9):1298-1302, 2007.
12. Chobanian AV, Bakris GL, Black HR, et al: The Seventh Report of the Joint National Committee on Prevention, Detection, Evaluation, and Treatment of High Blood Pressure: the JNC 7 report. JAMA 289(19):2560-2672, 2003.
13. Virolainen J, Ventila M, Turto H, Kupari M: Effect of negative intrathoracic pressure on left ventricular pressure dynamics and relaxation. J Appl Physiol 79(2):455-460, 1995.
14. Somers VK, Dyken ME, Clary MP, Abboud FM: Sympathetic neural mechanisms in obstructive sleep apnea. J Clin Invest 96(4):1897-1904, 1995.
15. Chen PS, Douglas P. Zipes Lecture: Neural mechanisms of atrial fibrillation. Heart Rhythm 3(11):1373-1377, 2006.
16. Liu T, Li G, Li L, Korantzopoulos P: Association between C-reactive protein and recurrence of atrial fibrillation after successful electrical cardioversion: A meta-analysis. J Am Coll Cardiol 49(15):1642-1648, 2007.
17. Alonso-Fernandez A, Garcia-Rio F, Racionero MA, et al: Cardiac rhythm disturbances and ST-segment depression episodes in patients with obstructive sleep apnea–hypopnea syndrome and its mechanisms. Chest 127(1):15-22, 2005.
18. Jo JA, Blasi A, Valladares E, et al: Determinants of heart rate variability in obstructive sleep apnea syndrome during wakefulness and sleep. Am J Physiol Heart Circ Physiol 288(3):H1103-H1112, 2005.
19. Roche F, Gaspoz JM, Court-Fortune I, et al: Alteration of QT rate dependence reflects cardiac autonomic imbalance in patients with obstructive sleep apnea syndrome. Pacing Clin Electrophysiol 26(7 Pt 1):1446-1453, 2003.
20. Nakamura T, Chin K, Hosokawa R, et al: Corrected QT dispersion and cardiac sympathetic function in patients with obstructive sleep apnea–hypopnea syndrome. Chest 125(6):2107-2114, 2004.
21. Zipes DP, Rubart M: Neural modulation of cardiac arrhythmias and sudden cardiac death. Heart Rhythm 3(1):108-113, 2006.
22. Kaneko Y, Floras JS, Usui K, et al: Cardiovascular effects of continuous positive airway pressure in patients with heart failure and obstructive sleep apnea. N Engl J Med 348(13):1233-1241, 2003.
23. Brodsky M, Wu D, Denes P, et al: Arrhythmias documented by 24 hour continuous electrocardiographic monitoring in 50 male medical students without apparent heart disease. Am J Cardiol 39(3):390-395, 1977.
24. Caples SM, Rosen CL, Shen WK, et al: The scoring of cardiac events during sleep. J Clin Sleep Med 3(2):147-154, 2007.
25. Becker H, Brandenburg U, Peter JH, Von Wichert P: Reversal of sinus arrest and atrioventricular conduction block in patients with sleep apnea during nasal continuous positive airway pressure. Am J Respir Crit Care Med 151(1):215-218, 1995.
26. Guilleminault C, Conolly SJ, Winkle RA: Cardiac arrhythmia and conduction disturbances during sleep in 400 patients with sleep apnea syndrome. Am J Cardiol 52:490-494, 1983.
27. Mehra R, Benjamin EJ, Shahar E, et al: Association of nocturnal arrhythmias with sleep-disordered breathing: The Sleep Heart Health Study. Am J Respir Crit Care Med 173(8):910-916, 2006.
28. Porthan KM, Melin JH, Kupila JT, et al: Prevalence of sleep apnea syndrome in lone atrial fibrillation: A case-control study. Chest 125(3):879-885, 2004.
29. Gami AS, Pressman G, Caples SM, et al: Association of atrial fibrillation and obstructive sleep apnea. Circulation 110(4):364-367, 2004.
30. Leung RS, Huber MA, Rogge T, et al: Association between atrial fibrillation and central sleep apnea. Sleep 28(12):1543-1546, 2005.
31. Caples SM, Wolk R, Somers VK: Influence of cardiac function and failure on sleep-disordered breathing: Evidence for a causative role. J Appl Physiol 99(6):2433-2439, 2005.
32. Mooe T, Gullsby S, Rabben T, Eriksson P: Sleep-disordered breathing: A novel predictor of atrial fibrillation after coronary artery bypass surgery. Coron Artery Dis 7(6):475-478, 1996.
33. Kanagala R, Murali NS, Friedman PA, et al: Obstructive sleep apnea and the recurrence of atrial fibrillation. Circulation 107(20):2589-2594, 2003.
34. Gami AS, Hodge DO, Herges RM, et al: Obstructive sleep apnea, obesity, and the risk of incident atrial fibrillation. J Am Coll Cardiol 49(5):565-571, 2007.
35. Sauer WH, McKernan ML, Lin D, et al: Clinical predictors and outcomes associated with acute return of pulmonary vein conduction during pulmonary vein isolation for treatment of atrial fibrillation. Heart Rhythm 3(9):1024-1028, 2006.
36. Gami AS, Howard DE, Olson EJ, Somers VK: Day-night pattern of sudden death in obstructive sleep apnea. N Engl J Med 352(12):1206-1214, 2005.
37. Doherty LS, Kiely JL, Swan V, McNicholas WT: Long-term effects of nasal continuous positive airway pressure therapy on cardiovascular outcomes in sleep apnea syndrome. Chest 127(6):2076-2084, 2005.
38. Grimm W, Koehler U, Fus E, et al: Outcome of patients with sleep apnea–associated severe bradyarrhythmias after continuous positive airway pressure therapy. Am J Cardiol 86(6):688-692, A9, 2000.
39. Ryan CM, Usui K, Floras JS, Bradley TD: Effect of continuous positive airway pressure on ventricular ectopy in heart failure patients with obstructive sleep apnoea. Thorax 60(9):781-785, 2005.
40. Liston R, Deegan PC, McCreery C, et al: Haemodynamic effects of nasal continuous positive airway pressure in severe congestive heart failure. Eur Respir J 8(3):430-435, 1995.
41. Kiely JL, Deegan P, Buckley A, et al: Efficacy of nasal continuous positive airway pressure therapy in chronic heart failure: Importance of underlying cardiac rhythm. Thorax 53(11):957-962, 1998.
42. Bradley TD, Logan AG, Kimoff RJ, et al: Continuous positive airway pressure for central sleep apnea and heart failure. N Engl J Med 353(19):2025-2033, 2005.
43. Sinha AM, Skobel EC, Breithardt OA, et al: Cardiac resynchronization therapy improves central sleep apnea and Cheyne-Stokes respiration in patients with chronic heart failure. J Am Coll Cardiol 44(1):68-71, 2004.

Standard Antiarrhythmic Drugs 96

DAWOOD DARBAR

CHAPTER OUTLINE

Antiarrhythmic therapy has progressed from a handful of poorly tolerated, relatively ineffective drugs with incompletely understood mechanisms of action to more rational selection of drug and other therapies based on an improved understanding of risks and benefits derived from clinical trials and mechanistic studies. Although antiarrhythmics have improved, like many other drugs, they produce widely divergent actions in patients: The spectrum of responses ranges from suppression of highly symptomatic arrhythmias to inefficacy to provocation of life-threatening arrhythmias by the drugs themselves. The elucidation of the mechanisms underlying this striking variability in drug response has been useful not only for improving therapy with available antiarrhythmic drugs but also for delineating new mechanisms in arrhythmias and new therapies. Indeed, the development of any new drug entity with modest efficacy and yet not characterized by proarrhythmia or other side effects would represent a major advance in therapy of arrhythmias. Whether such drugs could, or should, supplant increasingly sophisticated nonpharmacologic therapies is still not clear.

The successful use of antiarrhythmic drugs necessitates knowledge of their pharmacodynamic or cellular electrophysiology, pharmacokinetic, cardiac, and extracardiac effects. Under the modified Singh and Vaughan-Williams classification, sodium channel–blocking drugs are class I, with subdivision into classes IA (prolongation of conduction and repolarization), IB (no effect on conduction and shortening of repolarization), and IC (prolongation of conduction but little effect on repolarization). The class III antiarrhythmic drugs, on the other hand, prolong the action potential duration (APD) of cardiac tissue and prevent and terminate reentrant arrhythmias. In this chapter, we first review the principles of antiarrhythmic therapy and then provide a concise overview of class I and class III antiarrhythmic drugs.

The research reported in this chapter is supported in part by grants from the U.S. Public Health Service (HL075266, HL 085690, and U01 HL65962).

Principles of Antiarrhythmic Therapy

Benefit Should Outweigh Risk

The benefits of antiarrhythmic drug therapy are evident in the acute setting, when a patient presents with a highly symptomatic, often sustained, arrhythmia that drug therapy terminates rapidly. In this setting, symptomatic benefits are obvious, and the risk is minimized because patients are monitored and exposed to the drug only for a brief period.

With chronic therapy, the balance between benefit and risk is more difficult to evaluate. Chronic therapy in a patient with heart disease may be beneficial initially, but efficacy may be lost with time due to a changing electrophysiologic substrate. Indeed, in virtually all clinical trials, chronic antiarrhythmic therapy is incompletely effective. Furthermore, the consequences of arrhythmia recurrence are clinically important (varying from recurrent hospitalization to death), and the risk of serious adverse effects appears to increase over time. Therefore, in contemporary antiarrhythmic therapy, drugs retain a primary role in the acute termination of arrhythmias and in selected chronic arrhythmia settings, notably atrial fibrillation (AF), in which arrhythmia recurrence might not be catastrophic.

By contrast, device-based and ablative therapies are more desirable from a risk-to-benefit point of view in other settings, such as ventricular tachycardia (VT), where antiarrhythmic drugs have assumed a secondary role. However, as ablative therapies for AF continue to evolve, it is possible that drugs might assume a secondary role here as well. Nevertheless, the development of new drug therapies for AF that are highly effective and, more importantly, safe during chronic therapy is also highly desirable.

Mechanism-Based Approaches

One universal principle of pharmacologic therapy is that the best treatment is that targeted specifically to disease mechanisms. In arrhythmia therapy, a good example is cure of arrhythmias in the Wolff-Parkinson-White syndrome by bypass tract ablation.

Table 96-1 Mechanism-Based Antiarrhythmic Drug Therapy

Arrhythmia	Mechanism-Based Therapy*	Mechanism Targeted†
AV nodal reentry	Adenosine	Macro-reentry using the AV node
AV reentry	Verapamil	Macro-reentry using the AV node
Outflow tract VT	β-blockers Verapamil, diltiazem	Adrenergically driven
Fascicular VT	β-blockers Verapamil, diltiazem	Reentry within the His-Purkinje system
Torsades de pointes due to drugs or bradyarrhythmias	Pacing; isoproterenol K^+ supplementation to 4.5-5 mEq/L	I_{Kr} block leading to bradycardia-dependent EADs and unstable intraventricular reentry due to heterogeneity of repolarization
Congenital long QT syndrome, type 1	β-blockers; other antisympathetic maneuvers (stellate ganglionectomy)	Failure of the adrenergically activated K^+ current I_{Ks} to maintain action potentials shortened during adrenergic activation
Congenital long QT syndrome, type 2	K^+ supplementation to 4.5-5 mEq/L; spironolactone	Abnormal AP prolongation and heterogeneity due to loss of I_{Kr} function
Congenital long QT syndrome, type 3	Sodium channel block (mexiletine, flecainide)	Abnormal AP prolongation and heterogeneity due to increased inward sodium current during the action potential plateau
Brugada syndrome	I_{to} block: quinidine	Increased heterogeneity of action repolarization due to loss of sodium channel function and maintained I_{TO}
AF, VF, or T-wave oversensing in short QT syndrome	Quinidine, sotalol	Increased outward current, leading to shortened APs, due to abnormally increased I_{Ks}, I_{Kr}, or I_{K1}.
Catecholaminergic polymorphic VT	β-blockers	Leaky SR leading to afterdepolarization-mediated arrhythmias with heart rate increases due to adrenergic stimulation

*Other therapies may be effective (e.g., magnesium for torsades de pointes) but are not listed here because their mechanisms of action are not clearly defined.

†Other mechanisms may be operative (e.g., conduction slowing in the Brugada syndrome) but these are not yet amenable to specific drug therapies.

AF, atrial fibrillation; AP, action potential; AV, atrioventricular; EADs, early afterdepolarizations; SR, sarcoplasmic reticulum; VF, ventricular fibrillation; VT, ventricular tachycardia.

As our understanding of the molecular and cellular basis of arrhythmias has evolved, so too has the list of arrhythmias for which specific mechanisms have been defined, and therefore specific antiarrhythmic drug therapies may be indicated (Table 96-1). Thus, the role of adrenergic triggering in right ventricular outflow tract VT makes β-blockers a rational mechanism-based therapy. Recognition of the critical role of slow conduction within the atrioventricular (AV) node or orthodromic reciprocating tachycardia makes adenosine a rational, mechanism-based choice of therapy for the acute termination of these arrhythmias. The recent advances in our understanding of molecular mechanisms in specific rare genetic syndromes might also prompt consideration of specific mechanism-based therapies, although the numbers of patients evaluated are small and very often the agents available are not specific.

Unfortunately, for most common arrhythmias, such as VT associated with myocardial disease or AF, arrhythmia mechanisms have been difficult to define, and so the choice of drug therapy remains empiric. In such settings, drugs shown by clinical experience or controlled trials to be effective often target multiple mechanisms, including modifying the arrhythmia-prone substrate or inhibiting known or putative trigger(s) of arrhythmias. As specific mechanisms for many arrhythmias have not been well defined, the expectation that all patients with AF or VT will respond to therapy in a similar fashion makes the assumption that underlying mechanisms are homogeneous across patients. However, as genetic, molecular, and cellular studies continue to demonstrate, this assumption is largely unfounded. Therefore, the incomplete efficacy of drugs in treating these arrhythmias, which appear to represent a spectrum of arrhythmia mechanisms, is perhaps not unexpected.

Large clinical trials provide the best evidence for choosing among drug therapies and dosages in settings like AF and VT. The use of evidence-based principles should be complemented by consideration of patient-specific characteristics that might make one drug more or less desirable than others. Thus, a remote history of myocardial infarction (MI) would argue against the use of sodium channel blockers in a patient with AF due to the risk of proarrhythmia.

Classification of Antiarrhythmic Drugs

Several approaches have been proposed to classify drugs used for treatment of cardiac arrhythmias. The earliest schemes classified

Table 96-2 Expected Effects of Blocking Antiarrhythmic Drug Targets in the Heart

Ionic Target	Blocking Drugs	Effect of Therapeutic Doses on Normal ECG	Cardiac Toxicity of Excess Block	Extracardiac Toxicity
Sodium channel	Amiodarone Quinidine Procainamide Disopyramide Propafenone Flecainide Lidocaine* Mexiletine*	QRS prolongation, exaggerated at high concentration and/or fast sinus rates PR prolongation	Slow atrial flutter, occasionally with 1:1 AV conduction Bradyarrhythmias Increased pacing threshold Increased energy requirement for defibrillation More frequent episodes of reentrant VT or SVT	Exacerbation of myasthenia gravis
L-type calcium channels†	Verapamil Diltiazem	Sinus rate slowing; PR interval prolongation	Bradyarrhythmias AV nodal block Depressed contractility	Peripheral edema
Rapid component of the delayed rectifier potassium current (I_{Kr})‡	Amiodarone‡ Quinidine Procainamide§ Disopyramide Dofetilide Sotalol Ibutilide	QT interval prolongation (sinus bradycardia can also occur)	Torsades de pointes	
β-Adrenergic receptors	β-blockers, including sotalol Propafenone¶ Amiodarone¶	Sinus rate slowing; PR interval prolongation	Bradyarrhythmias AV nodal block Depressed contractility (acutely)	Fatigue Sleep difficulties Bronchospasm Depression

*Lidocaine and mexiletine have faster rates of onset and offset of binding to the channel, and so tend to exhibit fewer of the effects (such as QRS prolongation) listed for other blockers.

†Many other drugs, notably dihydropyridines like nifedipine and amlodipine, block L-type calcium channels but not in myocardium; their effects on cardiac electrophysiology generally reflect sympathetic activation (e.g., sinus tachycardia) due to peripheral vasodilation.

‡I_{Kr} block is also the mechanism whereby many noncardiovascular drugs prolong QT interval and cause torsades de pointes. Other drugs (e.g. flecainide, verapamil) also block I_{Kr} but have such potent effects on inward currents (sodium or calcium) that the clinical effects of I_{Kr} block, prolongation of QT and risk of torsades de pointes, are not seen. Similarly, torsades de pointes is rare with amiodarone.

§QT prolongation during procainamide therapy is often due to accumulation of the active metabolite *N*-acetylprocainamide (NAPA). NAPA does not block cardiac sodium channels.

¶The β-blocking properties of propafenone are most evident clinically at high concentrations of the parent drug seen in persons deficient in cytochrome P-450 2D6 (CYP2D6) activity on a genetic basis or due to concomitant drug therapy. Unlike other drugs that competitively block β-receptors, amiodarone exhibits antiadrenergic properties by noncompetitive blockade, reducing the number of receptors available for occupancy by agonists like adrenaline.

AV, atrioventricular; ECG, electrocardiogram; SVT, supraventricular tachycardia; VT, ventricular tachycardia.

drugs into classes based on shared efficacies and toxicities. Some antiarrhythmic drugs share important electrophysiologic properties, notably block of sodium channels (class I) or of the potassium current I_{Kr} (class III), and these can provide the basis for predicting shared or class actions, including toxicities (Table 96-2). Block or enhancement of other ionic currents, such as the slow component of the delayed rectifier (I_{Ks}), the transient outward current (I_{to}), or acetylcholine-activated current ($I_{K,Ach}$) may also contribute to clinical drug actions in some cases and are not usually considered in broad classification schemes.

An alternative approach is to classify key electrophysiologic mechanisms involved in arrhythmogenesis (instead of classifying the drugs), thereby allowing specific drugs to be chosen to target the mechanisms. This is the approach adopted by the Sicilian gambit investigators and is nicely exemplified by the definition of new molecular mechanisms in congenital arrhythmia syndromes and the way these then lead naturally to mechanism-based therapies.[1,2] An evolving understanding of the molecular and cellular basis of arrhythmias should allow a more rational choice of key molecules whose targeting is likely to be safe and effective in the therapy of a particular arrhythmia.

The term *antiarrhythmic drugs* has traditionally been taken to include drugs targeting ion channels in cardiac myocytes (sodium channel blockers, calcium channel blockers, and QT-prolonging drugs, generally potassium channel blockers), β-adrenergic receptor blockers, and a series of drugs with diverse mechanisms used primarily for the therapy of arrhythmias, such as digoxin, amiodarone, magnesium, and adenosine. However, studies have demonstrated that other widely used cardiovascular therapies, such as angiotensin-converting enzyme and hydroxy-methyl-glutanyl (HMG) Co-A reductase inhibitors might also exert important antiarrhythmic effects.[3] Such effects can include not only reduction of sudden cardiac death (SCD), an arrhythmic event that represents the final common pathway for many potential disease pathways, but also prevention of AF. These studies provide new potential therapies and implicate new signaling pathways in the pathogenesis of arrhythmias and therefore as potential new targets for the development of effective antiarrhythmic

Table 96-3 Proarrhythmia Syndromes and Their Management

Syndrome	Mechanism	Clinical Presentations	Therapy*
Digitalis intoxication	Na^+-K^+ATPase inhibition → intracellular calcium overload	Ectopic activity, with suppressed sinus and AV nodal function Atrial or junctional tachycardia Bidirectional VT	Mild: observe; possible temporary pacing Serious: antidigoxin antibody
Torsades de pointes	I_{Kr} block	Pause-dependent polymorphic VT, with QT prolongation and deformity	Mild: Magnesium Serious: Pacing, isoproterenol
Sodium channel blocker toxicity	Block of cardiac sodium channels, often exacerbated by underlying tachycardia or ischemia	↑ Pacing or defibrillation threshold Atrial flutter slowing with 1:1 AV conduction Frequent or difficult to cardiovert monomorphic or polymorphic VT Incessant SVT Increase death rate during long-term therapy after myocardial infarction	Mild: no therapy or heart rate slowing (β-blocker) Serious: intravenous sodium bicarbonate
β-Blocker withdrawal	Upregulation of receptor number with chronic therapy; withdrawal → more receptors available for agonist	Sinus tachycardia, other sympathetically-mediated arrhythmia, hypertension	β-blocker
Ventricular fibrillation	Three drug-related mechanisms: Digitalis in manifest preexcitation with atrial fibrillation Coronary vasoconstriction (many drugs: cocaine, ergot) Inappropriate use of verapamil for sustained VT	VF	No specific therapy beyond drug withdrawal and resuscitation
Calcium channel blocker toxicity	Calcium channel blocker excess, often in overdose	Hypotension, bradycardia, AV block	Temporary pacing, IV calcium

ATP, adenosine triphosphate; AV, atrioventricular; IV, intravenous; SVT, supraventricular tachycardia; VF, ventricular fibrillation; VT, ventricular tachycardia.

*Therapy in all cases consists of recognition, withdrawal of the offending agent(s), and correction of any other potential exacerbating conditions (hypokalemia, hypoxia, myocardial ischemia). *Mild* refers to minimally symptomatic patients; *serious* refers to those with recurrent destabilizing arrhythmias.

interventions. The pharmacologic properties of these nontraditional antiarrhythmic agents are discussed in Chapter 98.

Proarrhythmia Syndromes

The recognition that drugs designed to suppress arrhythmias can, in some patients, actually increase arrhythmias or provoke new ones is probably the single most important factor governing the selection and use of antiarrhythmic therapy. For example, not only are drugs incompletely effective at preventing VF, but they might also increase the risk of sudden death in some patients. Therefore, many clinicians choose to use nonpharmacologic therapy, rather than drugs, as primary therapy in such patients. Proarrhythmia is not attributable to a single mechanism. Rather, numerous proarrhythmia syndromes have now been elucidated, and these are detailed in Table 96-3. Treatment of these proarrhythmia syndromes includes early recognition, withdrawal of the offending agents, and specific mechanism-based therapies.

Digitalis Toxicity

The drug that was first associated with the development of abnormal rhythms was probably digitalis. Although it is said that intoxication with digitalis glycosides can produce virtually any arrhythmia, certain arrhythmias should raise a particular suspicion. These include ectopic rhythms such as atrial tachycardia or premature ventricular contractions (PVCs), thought to be due to delayed afterdepolarization (DAD)-related triggered automaticity with sinus slowing or AV nodal block, owing to the drug's indirect vagomimetic effects. The major mechanism underlying digoxin toxicity is related to inhibition of P-glycoprotein activity, a multisubstrate drug efflux carrier, by drugs such as amiodarone, quinidine, verapamil and the azole antifungal agents. For asymptomatic arrhythmias due to digitalis toxicity, discontinuation of the drug and observation are probably sufficient. For more advanced cases, the therapy of choice is antidigoxin antibodies. Very occasionally, temporary pacing may be required.

Proarrhythmia Due to QT Prolongation

In some patients, therapy with drugs that prolong action potential, such as sotalol, quinidine, dofetilide, or ibutilide, can be associated with marked prolongation of the QT interval and induction of a morphologically distinctive polymorphic VT, torsades de pointes. Torsades de pointes can also occur during treatment with noncardiovascular drugs; common examples include terfenadine, cisapride, haloperidol, and thioridazine.[4] Many such cases are attributable to inhibition of drug elimination, and thus accumulation of drug to unusually high plasma concentrations, often due to coadministration of cytochrome

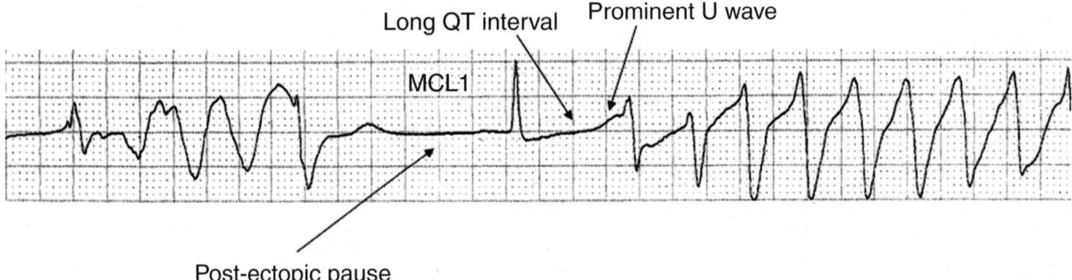

Figure 96-1 Torsades de pointes in a patient receiving sotalol. This telemetry strip shows a couple of ectopic beats followed by a pause, and a postpause sinus beat with a remarkably long and deformed QTU interval. The tachycardia starts after this U wave. This pattern of pause dependence and QTU changes is typical for drug-induced torsades de pointes.

P-450 (CYP) isoenzyme 3A4 inhibitors. Occasional cases are also unrelated to drug therapy and can be attributed to the syndrome of congenital long QT syndrome (LQTS), marked bradyarrhythmias, hypokalemia, recent conversion from AF, or acute central nervous system injury.[4] Drugs that have been associated with torsades de pointes block I_{Kr}. Mutations in genes that encode the channel responsible for I_{Kr} are now recognized as a cause of congenital LQTS, a disease associated with QT prolongation, torsades de pointes, and SCD.

Risk factors for torsades de pointes have been identified. They include female gender, hypokalemia, bradycardia, and high drug dosages or plasma concentrations of the drugs just listed.[4] An exception is quinidine, where the reaction can occur with the first dose at subtherapeutic plasma concentrations. Other data suggest that advanced heart failure, recent conversion from AF, and very rapid intravenous administration of drug can also trigger an episode of torsades de pointes.[5] Uncontrolled clinical trials suggest that potassium supplementation (to a concentration greater than 4.5 mEq/L) and intravenous magnesium should be the first approaches to therapy, because they are relatively simple and unlikely to cause harm. If these are ineffective, maneuvers to increase the heart rate to greater than 90 beats per minute are usually effective; this can be accomplished either by isoproterenol or by temporary ventricular pacing.

Most recognized cases of torsades de pointes occur shortly after starting culprit drug(s). However, a specific I_{Kr} blocker, the dextrorotatory isomer of sotalol (D-sotalol) was found in Survival with Oral D-Sotalol (SWORD), a large study with a Cardiac Arrhythmia Suppression Trial (CAST)-like design,[6] to increase long-term mortality compared to placebo in patients judged to be at risk for SCD.[7] Because the drug is not a sodium channel blocker, a mechanism different from that in CAST seems likely; torsades de pointes occurring during chronic long-term outpatient treatment is one leading possibility (Fig. 96-1).

Proarrhythmia due to Sodium Channel Block

Sodium channel block is a common mechanism underlying many well-described proarrhythmia syndromes. First, in patients with atrial flutter, sodium channel block can slow the flutter rate from (for example) 300/min to 200/min. When the atrial flutter rate is 300/min, the usual AV nodal response is 2:1 block, which is a ventricular rate of 150/min. However, when the flutter rate slows to 180 to 200/min, 1:1 AV nodal conduction can occur with a paradoxical increase in ventricular rate that was not seen before the drug was administered. Because the effects of sodium channel block increase at fast rates, patients with this syndrome often present with wide QRS complexes, making the distinction from VT difficult. Treatment includes drugs such as calcium channel blockers to increase the degree of AV nodal block.

Second, slow conduction in the edges of an old MI plays a prominent role in the pathogenesis and maintenance of sustained monomorphic VT. Use of sodium channel blockers can, in some patients, increase the frequency of episodes of this arrhythmia, likely by further slowing conduction. β-Blockers have been effective in some cases, possibly by slowing sinus rate and thereby decreasing the extent of sodium channel block. In addition, some data suggest that intravenous sodium (as bicarbonate) may be useful in treating this form of proarrhythmia.

Third, sodium channel block reduces excitability of the heart. In patients with pacemakers or implantable cardioverter defibrillators (ICDs), increased output of the devices may be required for effective function. Rarely, ventricular arrhythmias occurring in the presence of sodium channel blockers cannot be effectively terminated by internal or external direct current cardioversion and deaths have been reported.

The fourth proarrhythmia syndrome associated with treatment with sodium channel blockers is an increase in mortality during long-term treatment. This was established by the CAST, a landmark study that tested, in a placebo-controlled, randomized, double-blind fashion, the then-prevailing wisdom that suppression of PVCs in patients convalescing from an MI would reduce the incidence of SCD.[6] In CAST, patients with PVCs and a recent MI were randomly assigned to one of three sodium channel–blocker therapies, which was then titrated to the dose that appeared to suppress PVCs on a 24-hour Holter monitor. Once the effective dose and drug were established, patients were randomly assigned to continue drug or placebo. Remarkably, mortality among patients randomized to drug was two to three times that among those randomized to placebo.

The mechanism underlying this striking, and previously undefined effect of sodium channel block remains uncertain. However, conduction slowing with an increased risk of sustained ventricular arrhythmias (including VF) seems a plausible explanation. It has been argued that other sodium channel blockers might not produce the same effect as the three drugs tested in CAST (encainide [no longer available], flecainide, and moricizine). However, preclinical data suggest this may be a class action of sodium channel block, and other less well designed studies with mexiletine and with disopyramide showed a similar trend to increased mortality. Perhaps the most important implications of CAST were the recognition that surrogate endpoints (in this case, PVCs as a surrogate for arrhythmic death) should be used with extreme caution in clinical medicine unless they are well validated, and physicians should recognize that their own biases, which so often drive therapy in areas in which data are not available, may be erroneous.

More recently, it has become apparent that administration of sodium channel blockers to patients with the Brugada syndrome might not only elicit an unusual pathognomic electrocardiogram (ECG) phenotype but also rarely induce VF (Fig. 96-2).[8,9] SCD in these patients is likely related to induction of VF, usually during sleep. The latter is analogous to the situation of a patient with subclinical LQTS in whom administration of an I_{Kr}-blocker exposes the genetic defect.

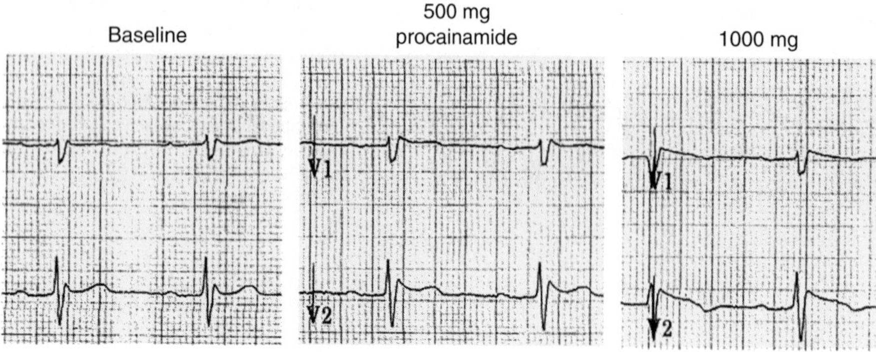

Figure 96-2 Unmasking of Brugada syndrome by intravenous infusion of a sodium channel blocker (procainamide). On the baseline tracings *(left)*, the ST-T segments in leads V1 and V2 are unremarkable. After administration of 500 mg of procainamide *(middle)*, a persistent ST elevation (saddleback) pattern develops, but the coved-type ST-segment elevation, pathognomonic for Brugada syndrome, only becomes apparent after 1000 mg of procainamide *(right)* has been administered.

Class I Antiarrhythmic Drugs

Although all class I antiarrhythmic drugs block the cardiac sodium channel, the extent of block depends on the heart rate, membrane potential, and the physicochemical characteristics of each drug that determines the rate of onset and recovery from block. This has then given rise to a subclassification of class I antiarrhythmic drugs based on the magnitude of their effects on cardiac conduction. Class IA drugs such as quinidine, procainamide, and disopyramide have intermediate effect on sodium channel block and generally only cause significant prolongation of conduction in cardiac tissue at rapid heart rates. In contrast, the class IB drugs, lidocaine and mexiletine, have minimal or no effects on the cardiac sodium channel in normal tissue but cause significant conduction slowing in depolarized tissue. Class IC drugs, flecainide and propafenone, cause significant prolongation of conduction in cardiac tissue at normal heart rates with an increase in the QRS duration on the electrocardiogram. Many class I antiarrhythmic drugs have effects on other ion channels and membrane receptors through which some of their electrophysiologic effects are mediated (Tables 96-4 and 96-5).

Class IA Antiarrhythmic Drugs

Quinidine

Pharmacodynamics

Quinidine is a component of an antimalarial extract from the bark of the cinchona plant and was developed as an antiarrhythmic by Wenckebach just after the First World War. It blocks the sodium current channel and multiple potassium currents, including I_{Kr}, I_{Ks}, and I_{to}.[10] Its kinetics of interaction with the sodium channel are intermediate. I_{Kr} block can occur at very low concentrations; in vitro, action potential prolongation by quinidine is blunted at higher concentrations, likely reflecting an additional effect of sodium channel block.[11]

Quinidine is an alpha blocker, and can thereby produce hypotension when administered intravenously. It has vagolytic actions, which make the drug occasionally useful in vasovagal syncope, and can also enhance AV nodal conduction during atrial flutter. It is a very potent inhibitor of CYP2D6, exerting this pharmacologic action at doses as low as 5 mg; low-dose quinidine has actually been used in combination with CYP2D6 substrates to increase the plasma concentrations and make them

Table 96-4 Pharmacodynamics of Class I Antiarrhythmic Drugs

Drug	Recovery from Sodium Channel Block	K⁺ Channels	Receptors
Class IA			
Disopyramide	Intermediate	$\downarrow I_{TO}$, $\downarrow I_{Kr}$, $\downarrow I_{KACh}$	Inhibits muscarinic receptors
Quinidine	Intermediate	$\downarrow I_{TO}$, $\downarrow I_{Kr}$, $\downarrow I_{Ks}$	
Procainamide, *N*-acetylprocainamide	Intermediate	$\downarrow I_{Kr}$	Inhibits β-adrenergic and muscarinic receptors
Class IB			
Lidocaine	Rapid		
Mexiletine	Rapid		
Class IC			
Flecainide	Slow	$\downarrow I_{Kr}$, $\downarrow I_{Kur}$	Inhibits β-adrenergic receptors
Propafenone	Slow	$\downarrow I_{Kr}$, $\downarrow I_{Kur}$	Inhibits β-adrenergic receptors

Table 96-5 Pharmacokinetics of Standard Antiarrhythmic Drugs

	Elimination Half-life*				Major Route of Clearance			Major Pharmacokinetic Interactions‡		
Drug	**Short**	**6-12 hours**	**Long**	**Active Metabolites†**	**Hepatic**	**Renal**	**Other**	**↑Drug concentration and effect**	**↓Drug concentration and effect**	**Effects on Other Drugs**
Adenosine	Seconds						Cellular uptake	Dipyridamole	Theophylline (receptor blocker)	
Amiodarone			Weeks	Yes	Yes (CYP3A4)					Potent inhibitor of CYP2C9 (warfarin), CYP3A4 (many drugs), P-glycoprotein (digoxin)
Disopyramide		Yes			Yes	Yes			Phenytoin Rifampin	
Dofetilide		Yes				Yes		Cimetidine Verapamil Ketoconazole		
Flecainide			12-18 hr		Yes (CYP2D6)	Yes				
Ibutilide		Yes			Yes					
Lidocaine	2 hr			Yes	Yes (CYP3A4)			Propranolol Verapamil Cimetidine		
Mexiletine		√			√				Phenytoin Rifampin	
NAPA			Yes			Yes				
Procainamide	3 hr			Yes	Yes (NAT2)	Yes				
Propafenone		Yes		Yes	Yes (CYP2D6)			Quinidine Tricyclic antidepressants Fluoxetine Paroxetine		
Quinidine		Yes		Yes	Yes (CYP3A4)				Phenytoin Rifampin	Potent inhibitor of CYP2D6 (β-blockers), P-glycoprotein (digoxin)
Sotalol		Yes				Yes				

*Elimination half-life determines the time to steady state (4-5 elimination half-lives); the actual steady state achieved is determined by clearance. Propafenone elimination half-life is highly variable due to genetic factors (see text).

†Drugs for which variability in clinical actions have been attributed to active metabolites are indicated.

‡Antiarrhythmics, β-blockers, and calcium-channel blockers interact to depress cardiac output and sinus and AV nodal function.

CYP, cytochrome P450; NAPA, *N*-acetylprocainamide; NAT2, *N*-acetyl transferase.

more uniform. Quinidine is also an inhibitor of P-glycoprotein, and as a result it decreases digoxin clearance and increases its serum concentrations and risk of toxicity.[12]

Pharmacokinetics

Quinidine is well absorbed and is 80% bound to plasma proteins including albumin and, like lidocaine, the acute phase reactant, α_1-acid glycoprotein. As with lidocaine, greater-than-usual doses (and total plasma quinidine concentrations) may be required to maintain therapeutic concentrations of free quinidine in high-stress states such as acute MI. Quinidine undergoes extensive hepatic oxidative metabolism, and about 20% is excreted unchanged by the kidneys. One metabolite, 3-hydroxyquinidine, is nearly as potent as quinidine in blocking cardiac sodium channels or prolonging the action potentials.[13] Concentrations of unbound 3-hydroxyquinidine equal to or exceeding those of quinidine are tolerated by some patients. Other metabolites are less potent than quinidine, and their plasma concentrations are lower; thus, it is unlikely that they contribute significantly to the clinical effects of quinidine.

There is substantial individual variability in the range of dosages required to achieve therapeutic plasma concentrations of 2 to 5 μg/mL. Some of this variability may be assay-dependent, because not all assays have excluded quinidine metabolites. Among patients with advanced renal disease or advanced congestive heart failure, quinidine clearance is only modestly decreased. Thus, dosage requirements in these patients are similar to those in other patients.

Quinidine is a potent inhibitor of CYP2D6.[14] As a result, the administration of quinidine to patients receiving drugs that undergo extensive CYP2D6–mediated metabolism can result in altered drug effects due to accumulation of parent drug and failure of metabolite formation. For example, inhibition of CYP 2D6–mediated metabolism of codeine to its active metabolite, morphine, results in decreased analgesia. On the other hand, inhibition of CYP2D6–mediated metabolism of propafenone results in elevated plasma propafenone concentrations and increased β-adrenergic receptor blockade. Quinidine reduces the clearance of digoxin and digitoxin; inhibition of P-glycoprotein–mediated digoxin transport has been implicated.[12] This interaction is particularly important during the initiation of quinidine therapy in patients with AF, many of whom also are receiving digoxin.

Quinidine is eliminated by CYP3A4–mediated hepatic metabolism, with a half-life of 6 to 12 hours. Its metabolism is inducible by drugs such as phenobarbital or phenytoin. In patients receiving these agents, very high doses of quinidine may be required to achieve therapeutic concentrations. If therapy with the inducing agent is then stopped, quinidine concentrations can rise to very high levels, and its dosage must be adjusted downward. Cimetidine and verapamil elevate plasma quinidine concentrations, but these usually are modest.

Adverse Effects

Quinidine is not well tolerated and so is not used as first-line therapy. Diarrhea is the most common adverse effect during quinidine therapy, occurring in 30% to 50% of patients. The mechanism is not known. Diarrhea usually occurs within the first several days of quinidine therapy, but it can occur later. In mild cases of diarrhea in which quinidine therapy is deemed vital, antidiarrheal drugs can be used. Diarrhea-induced hypokalemia can potentiate torsades de pointes due to quinidine.

A number of immunologic reactions can occur during quinidine therapy. The most common is thrombocytopenia, which can be severe but which resolves rapidly with discontinuation of the drug. Hepatitis, bone marrow depression, and a lupus syndrome occur rarely. None of these effects is related to elevated plasma quinidine concentrations.

Quinidine also can produce cinchonism, a symptom complex that includes headache and tinnitus. In contrast to other adverse effects during quinidine therapy, cinchonism usually is related to elevated plasma quinidine concentrations and can be managed by reducing the dose.

It is estimated that 2% to 5% of patients who receive quinidine therapy will develop marked QT interval prolongation and torsades de pointes. In contrast to effects of sotalol, *N*-acetyl procainamide (NAPA), and many other drugs, quinidine-associated torsades de pointes generally occurs at therapeutic, or even subtherapeutic, plasma concentrations. The reasons for individual susceptibility to this adverse effect are not known. At high plasma concentrations of quinidine, marked sodium channel block can occur, with resultant VT. This adverse effect formerly occurred when very high doses of quinidine were used to try to convert AF to normal sinus, but this aggressive approach to quinidine dosing has now been abandoned, and quinidine-induced VT due to excess sodium channel block is unusual. Quinidine can exacerbate heart failure or conduction system disease. However, in most patients with congestive heart failure, quinidine is well tolerated, perhaps because of its vasodilating actions.

Procainamide

Pharmacodynamics

Procainamide is a blocker of open sodium channels, with an intermediate time constant of recovery from block. It also prolongs cardiac action potentials in most tissues, probably by blocking I_{Kr}. Procainamide decreases automaticity, increases refractory periods, and slows conduction. The major metabolite, NAPA, lacks the sodium channel blocking activity of the parent drug but is equipotent in prolonging action potentials.[13] Because the plasma concentrations of NAPA often exceed those of procainamide, increased refractoriness and QT prolongation during chronic procainamide therapy can be attributed at least in part to the metabolite. However, it is the parent drug that slows conduction and produces QRS interval prolongation. Although hypotension can occur at high plasma concentrations, this effect usually is attributable to ganglionic blockade rather than to any negative inotropic effect, which is minimal.

Pharmacokinetics

Procainamide is rapidly eliminated (half-life, 3-4 hours) by both renal excretion of unchanged drug as well as by hepatic metabolism. The major pathway for hepatic metabolism is conjugation by *N*-acetyl transferase to form NAPA. NAPA is eliminated by renal excretion (half-life, 6-10 hours) and is not significantly converted back to procainamide. Because of the relatively rapid elimination rates of both the parent drug and its major metabolite, procainamide usually is administered as a slow-release formulation. In patients with renal failure, procainamide and NAPA can accumulate to potentially toxic plasma concentrations. Reduction of procainamide dose and dosing frequency and monitoring of plasma concentrations of both compounds are required in this situation. Because the parent drug and metabolite exert different pharmacologic effects, the practice of using the sum of their concentrations to guide therapy is inappropriate.

In patients who are slow acetylators, the procainamide-induced lupus syndrome develops more often and earlier during treatment than among rapid acetylators. In addition, the symptoms of procainamide-induced lupus resolve during treatment with NAPA. Both of these findings support results of in vivo studies suggesting that it is chronic exposure to the parent drug that results in the lupus syndrome; these findings also provided one rationale for the further development of NAPA and its analogues as antiarrhythmic agents.

Procainamide plasma concentrations should be monitored to ensure that concentrations of the parent drug remain in the range of 4 to 8 μg/mL. NAPA concentrations greater than 20 μg/mL appear to carry a higher risk of torsades de pointes. Procainamide concentrations greater than 10 μg/mL appear to carry a risk of marked QRS widening and potential arrhythmia exacerbation.

Adverse Effects

Hypotension and marked slowing of conduction are major adverse effects of high concentrations (>10 μg/mL) of procainamide, especially during intravenous use. Dose-related nausea is common during oral therapy and may be attributable in part to high plasma concentration of NAPA. Torsades de pointes can occur, particularly when plasma concentration of NAPA rise to greater than 30 μg/mL. Procainamide produces potentially fatal bone marrow aplasia in 0.2% of patients; the mechanism is not known, but high plasma drug concentrations are not suspected.

During long-term therapy, most patients develop biochemical evidence of the drug-induced lupus syndrome, such as circulating antinuclear antibodies.[15] Therapy need not be interrupted merely because of the presence of antinuclear antibodies. However, many patients, perhaps as many as 25% to 50%, eventually develop symptoms of the lupus syndrome; common early symptoms of the lupus syndrome are rash and small-joint arthralgias. Other symptoms of lupus, including pericarditis with tamponade, can occur, although renal involvement is unusual.

Disopyramide

Pharmacodynamics

Disopyramide is a sodium channel blocker with onset and offset kinetics similar to those of quinidine. It also prolongs the QT interval. Disopyramide exerts prominent anti-inotropic and anticholinergic effects at clinical dosages.

Pharmacokinetics

Disopyramide is eliminated by hepatic metabolism and renal excretion. The pathways are induced by phenytoin, suggesting participation by CYP3A4 or P-glycoprotein. The drug is administered as a racemate; the enantiomers are equally potent as sodium channel blockers, but only one, *S*-disopyramide, prolongs action potentials in vitro. The drug is variably bound to plasma proteins within the therapeutic range, and its binding is saturable; as a result, monitoring plasma concentrations of total drug is not useful.

Adverse Effects

Torsades de pointes, exacerbation of heart failure, and anticholinergic effects (constipation, urinary retention, glaucoma, dry eyes and mouth) can all occur.

Clinical Efficacy of Quinidine, Procainamide, and Disopyramide

The class IA antiarrhythmic drugs quinidine, procainamide, and disopyramide all have documented efficacy for the treatment of atrial and ventricular tachyarrhythmias.[16] However, they are less efficacious and poorly tolerated than other drugs such as amiodarone for the treatment of AF.[17,18]

The anticholinergic actions of disopyramide make it suitable for patients with vagally mediated AF; its negative inotropic effects may also be useful in managing patients with hypertrophic cardiomyopathy and outflow tract obstruction. The combination of quinidine and mexiletine has been shown to have synergistic antiarrhythmic drug efficacy for ventricular arrhythmias.[19] However, the benefits of therapy are often offset by intolerable adverse effects and the risk of ventricular proarrhythmia.[4]

These drugs are contraindicated in patients with structural heart disease, including left ventricular hypertrophy, because of the increased risk of death from proarrhythmia, and they can only be considered relatively safe in patients without structural heart disease or in patients with an ICD. Consequently, these drugs are considered second- or third-line therapy for the long-term treatment of AF and other atrial tachyarrhythmias.[18]

Intravenous procainamide can be effective in suppressing symptomatic or life-threatening ventricular arrhythmias, and the revised advanced cardiac life support (ACLS) guidelines recommend that procainamide be administered ahead of lidocaine for the initial treatment of hemodynamically stable wide complex tachycardia, especially in patients with compromised cardiac function.[20] It can also be effective in converting AF to sinus rhythm and can slow ventricular rate in patients presenting with pre-excited AF and rapid ventricular responses, although ibutilide has also recently been shown to be effective in this condition.[21] Intravenous procainamide has been used to unmask the electrocardiographic features of the Brugada syndrome.[8]

Class IB Antiarrhythmic Drugs

Lidocaine

Pharmacodynamics

Lidocaine blocks both open and inactivated cardiac sodium channels. Findings from in vivo studies suggest that lidocaine-induced block reflects an increased likelihood that the sodium channel protein assumes a nonconducting conformation in the presence of drug.[22] Recovery from block is very rapid, so lidocaine exerts greater effects in depolarized (e.g., ischemic) or rapidly driven tissues. Lidocaine is not useful in atrial arrhythmias, possibly because atrial action potentials are so short that the cardiac sodium channel is in the inactivated state only briefly compared with diastolic recovery times, which are relatively long.

Lidocaine decreases automaticity by reducing the slope of phase 4 and altering the threshold for excitability. APD usually is unaffected or is shortened; such shortening may be due to block of the few sodium channels that inactivate late during the cardiac action potential. Lidocaine usually exerts no significant effect on the PR or QRS interval duration; QT is unaltered or slightly shortened. The drug exerts little effect on hemodynamic function, although rare cases of lidocaine-associated exacerbations of heart failure have been reported, especially in patients with very poor left ventricular function.

Pharmacokinetics

Lidocaine is well absorbed, but it undergoes extensive, although variable, first-pass hepatic metabolism; thus, oral use of the drug is inappropriate. In theory, therapeutic plasma concentrations of lidocaine may be maintained by intermittent intramuscular administration, but the intravenous route is preferred. Lidocaine is cleared by CYP3A4–mediated metabolism, and two of its metabolites, glycine xylidide (GX) and monoethyl GX (MEGX), exert modest sodium channel blockade. GX and lidocaine appear to compete for access to the sodium channel, suggesting that with infusions during which GX accumulates, lidocaine efficacy may be diminished. With infusions lasting longer than 24 hours, the clearance of lidocaine falls—an effect that has been attributed to competition between parent drug and metabolites for access to hepatic drug-metabolizing enzymes.

After intravenous administration of a bolus of lidocaine, plasma concentrations decline biexponentially. The first phase is rapid, with a half-life of 8 minutes, and is attributed to rapid distribution of the drug from plasma to the periphery. Following distribution, the drug is eliminated by hepatic metabolism, with a half-life of approximately 2 hours. Thus, after initiation of a lidocaine maintenance infusion, steady-state plasma concentrations are approached in 8 to 10 hours (4-5 elimination half-lives).

Drug concentration in plasma is a reasonable guide to efficacy. To rapidly achieve therapeutic plasma concentrations, a loading regimen of 3 to 4 mg/kg is generally required. Administration as a single large bolus runs a high risk of central nervous system toxicity, notably seizures, so the loading regimen should be administered as a rapid infusion or a series of smaller intravenous boluses, such as 100 mg followed by 50 mg 5 to 10 minutes later, followed by a further 50 mg 5 to 10 minutes later. If the target arrhythmia is ongoing and suppressed by lidocaine loading, then a maintenance infusion is appropriate, whereas if the target arrhythmia persists after lidocaine loading, a maintenance infusion is unlikely to add any efficacy. A maintenance infusion of 1 to 4 mg/kg will achieve therapeutic plasma concentrations of 2 to 5 μg/mL.

In heart failure, the central volume of distribution is contracted and clearance is reduced; accordingly, the size of both the loading regimen and the maintenance infusion should be reduced. In liver disease, clearance is reduced, so a lower maintenance infusion rate is required. Lidocaine dosage does not need to be adjusted in patients with renal failure.

Efficacy

The routine use of prophylactic lidocaine in patients with acute MI is not recommended. The revised ACLS guidelines now recommend amiodarone or procainamide before lidocaine as the initial drug of choice for hemodynamically stable wide complex tachycardia.[20] Although the revised guidelines state that lidocaine remains an acceptable antiarrhythmic drug for the treatment of shock-refractory VF and pulseless VT, the evidence supporting its efficacy is limited, and lidocaine is not recommended as the first drug of choice in this setting.

Adverse Effects

Lidocaine can cause bradyarrhythmias. Prophylactic lidocaine was shown to prevent VF in acute MI in the 1970s. However, overall mortality appears to be unaffected or, in fact, increased.[23] Accordingly, the drug is no longer used for this indication. Lidocaine is cleared by CYP3A4–mediated hepatic metabolism to metabolites that exert modest antiarrhythmic effects and can mediate some of the central nervous system toxicity. Extraction of the drug is near complete during a single pass through the liver, which explains why lidocaine is not administered orally. Propranolol and cimetidine reduce lidocaine clearance, and so lower infusion rates may be required.

Mexiletine

Pharmacodynamics

Originally developed as an anticonvulsant, mexiletine is an oral congener of lidocaine used in the treatment of ventricular arrhythmias. The cardiac electrophysiologic effects of mexiletine are very similar to those of lidocaine.

Pharmacokinetics

Mexiletine is nearly completely absorbed after oral administration, and first-pass metabolism is less than 10%. It is eliminated by hepatic metabolism to inactive metabolites by the genetically variable CYP2D6 enzyme. Slow metabolizers tend to have more adverse effects. Renal excretion of mexiletine is pH sensitive; up to 35% of total clearance can be through the kidneys when the urine is acidic. Clearance is delayed markedly in cirrhosis, but little is seen in renal disease or congestive heart failure.

Efficacy

Mexiletine is effective in suppressing ventricular ectopy and VT. It is occasionally useful when added to other drugs (amiodarone, quinidine, sotalol) in patients with symptomatic VT. Mexiletine tended to increase mortality in a post-MI trial.[24] However, mexiletine has been used in the congenital LQTS, notably in the LQT3 (sodium channel–linked) subtype, where it can directly block the plateau sodium current that causes QT prolongation.[25]

Side Effects

Gastrointestinal and central nervous system side effects are the most prominent and are dose and concentration dependent. Tremor is usually the first sign of central nervous system toxicity, but blurred vision, dysarthria, ataxia, and confusion can also occur. Some of the gastrointestinal effects may be reduced by administering the drug with food, which decreases the peak plasma concentrations without affecting overall absorption.

Class IC Antiarrhythmic Drugs

Flecainide

Pharmacology

Flecainide is a potent sodium channel blocker, with slow onset and offset kinetics. It also blocks I_{Kr},[26] although reports of torsades de pointes are exceedingly rare. APD is shortened in Purkinje cells (probably due to block of late-opening Na^+ channels) but prolonged in ventricular cells, probably due to block of I_{Kr}. In atrial tissue, flecainide prolongs action potentials disproportionately at fast rates, an especially desirable antiarrhythmic drug effect and one that probably contributes to its efficacy for AF. This effect contrasts with that of quinidine, which prolongs atrial action potentials to a greater extent at slower rates. Flecainide prolongs the duration of PR, QRS, and QT intervals, even at normal heart rates.

Pharmacokinetics

Flecainide is well absorbed. The elimination half-life is shorter with urinary acidification (10 hours) than with urinary alkalinization (17 hours), but it is nevertheless sufficiently long to allow dosing twice daily. Elimination occurs by both renal excretion of unchanged drug and hepatic metabolism to inactive metabolites. The latter is mediated by the polymorphically distributed enzyme CYP2D6. However, even in patients in whom this pathway is absent because of genetic polymorphism or inhibition by other drugs (quinidine, fluoxetine), renal excretion ordinarily is sufficient to prevent drug accumulation. In the rare patient with renal dysfunction and lack of active CYP2D6, flecainide can accumulate to toxic plasma concentrations.[27] Flecainide is a racemate, but there are no differences in the electrophysiologic effects or disposition kinetics of its enantiomers. In children 1 to 12 years of age (but not younger children), elimination half-life is reduced (8 hours), often requiring dosing three times daily. Milk blocks flecainide absorption, and toxicity can result from removal of milk products from the diet.[28]

Efficacy

Flecainide is effective for managing supraventricular tachyarrhythmias including atrial tachycardia, reciprocating tachycardia involving an accessory atrioventricular bypass tract, atrial flutter, and AF.[18] Flecainide has also been used to unmask right ventricular conduction abnormalities in patients suspected of having Brugada syndrome.[29]

Adverse Effects

Flecainide produces few subjective complaints in most patients; dose-related blurred vision is the most common noncardiac adverse effect. It can exacerbate congestive heart failure in patients with depressed left ventricular performance. The most serious adverse effects are provocation or exacerbation of potentially lethal arrhythmias. CAST,[6,30] the Cardiac Arrhythmia Suppression Trial Hamburg (CASH),[31] and the Multicentre Unsustained Tachycardia Trial (MUSTT)[32] demonstrated that class IC drugs increase the risk of lethal sudden cardiovascular events in patients with ventricular arrhythmias. Therefore, class IC drugs are generally contraindicated in patients with coronary artery disease, and by extension, in patients with advanced structural heart disease.[18] Flecainide can produce atrial flutter with 1:1 AV conduction, increased pacing and defibrillating thresholds, and exacerbation of VT.

Propafenone

Pharmacodynamics

Propafenone is a potent sodium channel blocker with slow onset and offset kinetics. Some data also suggest that, like flecainide, propafenone also blocks potassium channels.[33] Its major electrophysiologic effect is to slow conduction in fast-response tissues. The drug is prescribed as a racemate; although the enantiomers do not differ in their sodium channel–blocking properties, *S*-propafenone is a β-adrenergic receptor antagonist in vitro and in some patients. Propafenone prolongs the PR and QRS interval duration.

Pharmacokinetics

Propafenone is well absorbed and is eliminated by both hepatic and renal routes. The activity of CYP2D6, an enzyme that is functionally absent in about 7% of whites and persons of African descent, is a major determinant of plasma propafenone concentrations and thus the clinical action of the drug (Chapter 53). In most subjects (extensive metabolizers), propafenone undergoes extensive first-pass hepatic metabolism to 5-hydroxy propafenone, a metabolite equipotent to propafenone as a sodium-channel blocker but much less potent as a β-adrenergic receptor antagonist. A second metabolite, *N*-desalkyl propafenone is formed by non–CYP2D6–mediated metabolism of propafenone and is a less-potent blocker of sodium channels and β-adrenergic receptors. CYP2D6–mediated metabolism of propafenone is saturable, so small increases in dose can lead to disproportionate increases in plasma propafenone concentration. In poor-metabolizer subjects, in whom functional CYP2D6 is absent, the extent of first-pass hepatic metabolism is much less than in extensive metabolizers, and plasma propafenone concentrations are much higher. The incidence of adverse effects during propafenone therapy is significantly higher in poor than in extensive metabolizers.

CYP2D6 activity can be markedly inhibited by a number of drugs, including quinidine and fluoxetine. In extensive-metabolizer subjects receiving such inhibitors or in poor-metabolizer subjects, plasma propafenone concentrations greater than 1 μg/mL are associated with clinical effects of β-adrenergic receptor blockade, such as reduction of exercise heart rate.[34] It is recommended that dosage in patients with moderate to severe liver disease should be reduced to approximately 20% to 30% of the usual dose, with careful monitoring. It is not known if propafenone doses must be decreased in patients with renal disease.

Efficacy

Propafenone is effective for managing supraventricular tachyarrhythmias including atrial tachycardia, reciprocating tachycardias involving an accessory atrioventricular bypass tract, atrial flutter, and AF.[18] Flecainide and propafenone are not recommended for treating atrial tachyarrhythmias or ventricular tachyarrhythmias in patients with structural heart disease.

Adverse Effects

Propafenone has not been formally tested in patients following MI, but it seems reasonable to assume that it might exert adverse effects in this population, as other sodium channel–blocking drugs do.[6] Therefore, it is therefore generally contraindicated in patients with coronary disease and those with advanced structural heart disease. Other adverse effects include depressed left ventricular performance, exacerbation of heart failure, atrial flutter with 1:1 AV conduction, and increased pacing and defibrillation thresholds.

Class III Antiarrhythmic Drugs

Reentry, one of the most important mechanisms underlying clinical atrial and ventricular arrhythmias, depends upon a critical balance between the conduction and refractoriness properties of a potential reentry circuit. Short refractory periods favor reentry, and longer refractory periods make reentry less likely. Because the APD is the principal determinant of refractory periods in normal working atrial and ventricular muscle and the His-Purkinje tissue, the possibility that drugs that selectively prolong the APD of cardiac tissue might prevent and terminate reentrant circuits was first suggested by Kaumann and Olson[35] in 1968. The importance of this drug action and the resultant increase in refractoriness prompted Singh and Vaughan Williams[36] in 1970 to add a new class (III) to their antiarrhythmic drug classification scheme. Since the 1990s, there has been increased attention focused on the class III antiarrhythmic drugs because the class I antiarrhythmic drugs have consistently been shown to increase mortality when used to treat atrial and ventricular arrhythmias.

Amiodarone

Pharmacodynamics

Amiodarone is certainly the "dirtiest" antiarrhythmic, interacting with multiple ion channels, cell surface receptors, and other molecules to block their function. The drug is unusually lipophilic, and this accounts for its unusual pharmacologic effects, including its very slow uptake and elimination. However, although the onset of many of the drug's effects are slow, other actions can be manifest on acute exposure; antiadrenergic actions tend to be prominent early, and changes in refractoriness can take longer to be apparent. In animal experiments, amiodarone administration appears to alter steady-state transcript levels of mRNAs encoding multiple ion channels.[37] Thus, the drug likely produces both acute and chronic effects by interacting with ion channels and other molecular targets, and it can in addition remodel the heart through an effect on transcription.

Amiodarone prolongs myocardial repolarization homogeneously (reducing dispersion of refractoriness, reentry, and proarrhythmia) via potassium channel blockade (I_{Kr} and I_{Ks}). It decreases conduction velocity by blocking cardiac sodium channels (class I effect), produces noncompetitive β-adrenergic blockade (class II effect) that can cause substantial sinus bradycardia within several days (peak, 3 months), and reduces inward L-type (slow) calcium channel activity (class IV activity) in a use-dependent manner. Inhibition of thyroxine (T_4) deiodination to triiodothyronine (T_3) can contribute to antiarrhythmic efficacy. Although amiodarone prolongs the QT interval, torsades de pointes is uncommon (incidence, <1%).[38]

Amiodarone is a potent inhibitor of many drug-metabolizing and drug-transport systems, notably CYP3A4, CYP2C9, and P-glycoprotein. The multifaceted electrophysiologic effects of amiodarone likely contribute to both safety and efficacy as an antiarrhythmic drug.

Pharmacokinetics

Amiodarone is 30% to 50% bioavailable, so intravenous doses are smaller than oral ones. The drug undergoes CYP3A4–mediated metabolism to desethylamiodarone, an active metabolite. Amiodarone has a large volume of distribution (66 L/kg), resulting in a delayed onset of action (2 days to 3 weeks for oral therapy) and long elimination half-life. For this reason, loading regimens are required when amiodarone is initiated, and dosages can often be reduced progressively during long term therapy. The therapeutic plasma range for amiodarone and desethylamiodarone is 0.5 to 2.5 μg/mL. Measured levels do not correlate well with efficacy or adverse effects.

Efficacy

Although amiodarone is approved by the USDA only for refractory ventricular arrhythmias, it is also effective in the treatment of symptomatic supraventricular arrhythmias, including AF.

A few randomized trials have found amiodarone to be more effective than other antiarrhythmic drugs at maintenance of sinus rhythm in patients with AF.[17,39] It is particularly effective at maintaining sinus rhythm in patients with congestive heart failure.[40] Due to adverse effects, however, amiodarone is recommended as second- or third-line therapy for patients with symptomatic AF.[18] Intravenous amiodarone may also be useful to slow the ventricular response rate in AF, and it has been used successfully for rate control in postoperative junctional ectopic tachycardia in children.[41]

SCD in patients with ischemic and nonischemic cardiomyopathy remains a substantial problem despite improved medical therapies. Data from several studies have demonstrated that ICD therapy is superior to medical therapy for the primary and secondary prevention of SCD in patients with ischemic and nonischemic heart disease and congestive heart failure.[42,43,44] Many patients, however, require antiarrhythmic therapy to prevent recurrent arrhythmias and ICD shocks. Amiodarone with a β-blocker proved more effective than sotalol or β-blockers alone in preventing shocks, although there was an increase in drug-related adverse effects.[45] Amiodarone might also slow rates of VT, making it more amenable to antitachycardia pacing. However, amiodarone can increase the defibrillation threshold, necessitating repeat ICD testing after initiation of therapy.

Intravenous amiodarone has been approved by the FDA for treatment and prevention of VF and hemodynamically unstable VT and for use in patients who require amiodarone therapy but are unable to take it orally. Its marginal superiority over lidocaine for out-of-hospital cardiac arrest was discussed earlier.[46]

Adverse Effects

Intravenous amiodarone can cause phlebitis and severe cellulitis if extravasated. For this reason, it is preferable to administer the drug through a large bore or central line. Hypotension is common.

During chronic therapy, PR, QRS, and QT intervals are all prolonged. Despite QT prolongation, torsades de pointes is exceedingly unusual during amiodarone therapy[38]; the likely explanation is that the drug includes among its many pharmacologic actions block of inward currents that prevent initiation of torsades de pointes. Amiodarone does not generally produce major depression of ventricular performance, an advantage compared to the class IA antiarrhythmic drugs.

The major forms of amiodarone toxicity during chronic therapy are extracardiac.[47] The most feared toxicity is pulmonary; pulmonary fibrosis (1%-17%) is the commonest manifestation, although atypical forms (which might, for example, be localized) can also occur. The cardinal laboratory manifestation of amiodarone toxicity is reduced diffusion capacity for carbon monoxide (DL_{CO}). Pulmonary toxicity does appear to be dose-related, although it can occur during chronic therapy with doses at or below 200 mg daily. Routine annual surveillance with chest x-rays and pulmonary function studies have been advocated as a method to detect early amiodarone toxicity, but the efficacy of these maneuvers is not established. Once pulmonary toxicity is suspected, further diagnostic workup may include biopsy, right heart catheterization (to eliminate a role for concomitant heart failure), and gallium scanning. None of these is specific, and biopsy often reveals foam cells but cannot make a definitive diagnosis of toxicity. If toxicity is strongly suspected, the drug should be withdrawn. Corticosteroids have been used, but their efficacy is not certain. Death from pulmonary insufficiency can occur. Risk factors for pulmonary fibrosis include underlying lung disease, amiodarone dosages greater than 400 mg/day, cumulative dosage, and recent pulmonary insults such as heart failure exacerbation, pneumonia, or general anesthesia.

Corneal microdeposits are ubiquitous during chronic amiodarone therapy, but they rarely interfere with vision; halos around lights at night may be one complaint. Much more rarely, the drug has been associated with optic neuritis.

Liver function is often abnormal, and rarely it progresses to cirrhosis. Photosensitivity is common, and patients should be warned to use sunscreen and broad-brimmed hats. Both hypothyroidism (6%) and hyperthyroidism (0.9%-2%) can occur; hypothyroidism requires thyroid supplementation, and hyperthyroidism—which can manifest as worsened arrhythmias—can require thyroid ablation or withdrawal of amiodarone. Because of the potential for toxicity, thyroid function studies and liver functions tests have been recommended every 6 months, and annual chest x-rays are recommended even in the absence of symptoms.[47]

A range of neuropsychiatric adverse effects also can occur. The most common are tremor and ataxia (3%-35%, depending on dose and duration of therapy). Peripheral neuropathy is uncommon (0.3% annually) but may be severe, requiring dose reduction or discontinuation of therapy. Insomnia, memory disturbances, and delirium also have been reported.

Dofetilide

Pharmacodynamics

Dofetilide is a potent and specific blocker of I_{Kr}, with no other significant pharmacologic actions. As a result of this specificity, it has virtually no extracardiac pharmacologic effects. Its only significant toxicity relates to QT prolongation and torsades de pointes.

Dofetilide preferentially increases the effective refractory period of the atrium compared with the ventricle. The magnitude of this difference in human beings is less than two-fold, which is substantially less than that observed in animals. Nonetheless, dofetilide's relative selectivity for the atrium likely contributes to its effectiveness in the pharmacologic conversion of atrial arrhythmias. As with many other class III antiarrhythmic agents, dofetilide's I_{Kr} block is reverse use dependent. A potential hazard of reverse use dependence in the ventricle is the development of excessive QT prolongation and risk of torsades de pointes after cardioversion. This is accentuated at slower heart rates, and the increased incidence of torsades after the restoration of sinus rhythm in part may be related to the relative bradycardia.[5]

Pharmacokinetics

Dofetilide has an absolute bioavailability that exceeds 90%. Within the therapeutic range, plasma concentrations follow a dose-related linear relation, with peak plasma concentrations achieved within 2 to 3 hours in the fasting state and 3 to 4 hours when taken with food. Dofetilide is eliminated largely by renal excretion and to a small extent by CYP3A4–mediated metabolism. Its elimination half-life (10 hours) allows twice-daily dosing. Certain drugs appear to inhibit dofetilide elimination and are contraindicated because they can thereby increase the extent of QT prolongation and risk of torsades de pointes: cimetidine, verapamil, ketoconazole, trimethoprim-sulfamethoxazole, prochlorperazine, and hydrochlorthiazide.

Efficacy

Oral administration of dofetilide is effective in pharmacologic conversion of AF in about 30% of cases at 0.5 mg twice daily, the highest dose, with less efficacy at lower doses.[48] The drug also reduces recurrence of AF following restoration of sinus rhythm.[49] Dofetilide reduces rehospitalization for heart failure, an effect that may be attributable to maintenance of sinus rhythm in patients with AF.[50] Placebo-controlled trials have failed to demonstrate efficacy of the drug in reducing the frequency of episodes of paroxysmal AF or of reducing episodes of VT or ICD discharges.

Adverse Effects

Data on incidence of torsades de pointes is available from large trials in which the drug was initiated with in-hospital monitoring. In the DIAMOND studies, dofetilide was compared to placebo in patients convalescing from MI and in patients with recent hospitalization for heart failure.[51,52] In the heart-failure arm, the incidence of torsades de pointes was 3%, and some cases were fatal. In the post-MI group the incidence was lower, 1%. Because of the risk of torsades de pointes, the drug can only be prescribed in the United States by practitioners who have been certified in its use. The drug is initiated in the hospital, and it is unique among antiarrhythmics in that the starting dose, 0.5 mg twice daily, is the highest allowable dose; downward dose adjustments are made if the QT interval is excessively long or if renal function is impaired. The drug should not be used in patients with advanced renal failure (creatinine clearance <20 mL/min).

Ibutilide

Pharmacodynamics

Ibutilide is a methanesulfonamide derivative with structural similarities to sotalol. This drug increases APD as its primary mechanism of action, largely by blocking I_{Kr}.[53] Initial studies demonstrated that the drug induced a slow sodium current during the plateau phase of the action potential. Over a limited range of stimulation rate, ibutilide can increase APD without significant reverse use dependence or loss of effect at rapid pacing rates. In humans, ibutilide causes a dose- and concentration-dependent increase in the QT interval in healthy volunteers and in patients with AF and atrial flutter. Action potential prolongation by ibutilide leads to an increase in atrial and ventricular refractoriness in vivo. Additional evidence suggests that the drug can lower the energy threshold required for VF.[54] Although administration of ibutilide can cause mild slowing of sinus rate and AV nodal conduction, there is no significant effect on heart rate, PR interval, or QRS duration.

Pharmacokinetics

Ibutilide is not available for long-term oral use because of extensive first-pass metabolism. After intravenous administration, the plasma concentration declines in a multiexponential manner, with a high systemic plasma clearance that approximates liver blood flow. The volume of distribution is large, with minimal (~40%) protein binding. Elimination half-life is variable, between 2 and 12 hours, with a mean of 6 hours. Ibutilide is extensively metabolized; the parent and at least eight metabolites are excreted largely in the urine. Although at least one of these metabolites has electrophysiologic activity, plasma concentrations during therapy are considerably less than those of ibutilide and likely do not contribute to its antiarrhythmic effect.[55] Although the metabolic pathways for ibutilide have not been completely determined, they do not appear to involve the CYP3A4 or CYP2D6 pathways, suggesting that previously described drug interaction with other agents are unlikely. Clearance is unaltered by either a reduction in creatinine clearance or left ventricular dysfunction. In patients with liver disease, there is likely reduced clearance and prolonged pharmacologic effect, necessitating longer periods of monitoring after ibutilide administration.

Efficacy

Intravenous ibutilide is effective in converting AF or atrial flutter to sinus rhythm.[56,57] It is more effective in flutter than in fibrillation, and it is more effective in recent-onset arrhythmias. Cardioversion after ibutilide administration can help maintain sinus rhythm in those in whom cardioversion alone is ineffective. Ibutilide can be safely used in patients receiving chronic amiodarone therapy. Ibutilide is also effective in patients with AF and rapid ventricular responses due to antegrade accessory pathway conduction; in this setting, it not only can convert AF but also slows conduction down the bypass tract.[21] It also improves the success of repeat direct current cardioversion after the initial failure of cardioversion.[58]

Adverse Effects

The initial dose is 1 mg over 10 minutes. If AF or atrial flutter persists 10 minutes after completion of the first dose, a second 1-mg dose may be given over 10 minutes. If the patient's weight is less than 60 kg, each dose is reduced to 0.01 mg/kg. The infusion is stopped when cardioversion occurs, marked QT prolongation develops, or torsades de pointes develops. Peak pharmacologic effects coincide roughly with the end of the infusion. Because the elimination half-life is 6 hours, patients should be observed for at least 4 hours after administration of the drug. The major adverse effect is torsades de pointes, which has been observed in 3.6% to 8.3% of patients.[57] The risk of proarrhythmia requires that ibutilide be administered in the hospital, with the necessary monitoring and resuscitation equipment. Administration of ibutilide with other drugs that prolong the APD is not recommended.

Sotalol

Pharmacodynamics

Sotalol is a class III antiarrhythmic that also has nonselective β-blocking effects (class II). This drug is a racemic mixture of its D- and L-stereoisomers. Although the D-isomer has class III effects, the L-isomer accounts for its β-blocking activity. In contrast to amiodarone, L-sotalol is a competitive β-blocker. β-Blockade is detectable at relatively low doses. The intrinsic negative inotropic effect of β-blockade is counterbalanced in vivo by a positive inotropic effect related to prolongation of the APD, which allows more time for the rise in intracellular calcium that mediates force of contraction. Clinically, sotalol produces a modest negative inotropic effect.

Both enantiomers have class III effects mediated primarily by antagonism of I_{Kr}. Sotalol does not appear to have effects on other ion channels at clinical concentrations.

The antiarrhythmic does display reverse use dependence, increasing APD at slower heart rates and diminishing effectiveness at faster heart rates. Sotalol slows the sinus rate and prolongs the PR interval, the atrio-His interval, the AV node refractory period, and the QT interval; it does not change the His-ventricle interval or QRS duration.

Pharmacokinetics

Bioavailability of sotalol is almost 100%. Peak plasma concentrations occur 2 to 4 hours after oral administration. Liver dysfunction has no appreciable effect on drug metabolism. Sotalol is eliminated by renal excretion of unchanged drug, with a half-life of 6 to 12 hours. In patients with renal dysfunction, the drug accumulates and there is a greater risk of toxicity. Administration and dosing need to be tailored to the creatinine clearance. Sotalol should be avoided in patients with creatinine clearance less than 40 mL/min. The typical oral dosing is 80 to 320 mg twice a day. Doses less than 120 mg twice a day appear to have primarily a β-blocking effect and little class III action. The benefit of higher doses must be weighed against the risk of adverse effects, particularly QT prolongation and torsades de pointes.

Efficacy

Sotalol is effective in preventing the recurrence of a wide range of supraventricular tachycardias including AV nodal reentry, AV reentry, and atrial tachycardia, but its main clinical use lies in the treatment of AF and atrial flutter.[18] In the AFFIRM trial, more than two thirds of patients in the rhythm control arm were started on either amiodarone or sotalol.[59] Both drugs had a relatively low incidence of adverse effects severe enough to cause discontinuation at 1 year (11.1% on sotalol vs 12.3% on amiodarone), whereas therapy with class I antiarrhythmics had to be stopped more often (28.1% at 1 year) due to frequent adverse effects. However, in a large randomized trial comparing sotalol, propafenone, and amiodarone for treatment of AF, amiodarone was superior to sotalol and propafenone in maintaining sinus rhythm.[17]

Although the impact of sotalol on primary prevention of SCD in patients recovering from MI has been disappointing,[7] it does appear to decrease the first defibrillation shock and death in patients with ICDs.[60] Sotalol also reduced the number of inappropriate ICD shocks, most likely due to its suppression of supraventricular arrhythmias. It, unlike amiodarone, consistently decreases the defibrillation threshold in patients with ICDs. The lowering of defibrillation threshold, along with the relative lack of noncardiac adverse effects with sotalol, makes it the first-line antiarrhythmic drug (in the absence of contraindications) for patients with ICDs.

Adverse Effects

Adverse effects are related to β-blockade and class III effects. Bradycardia, fatigue, bronchospasm, and dyspnea are related to the β-blockade. The incidence of heart failure or pulmonary edema is 3.3%.[61] The incidence of torsades de pointes is estimated be 2.4%. Most events occur within the first week after initiation of treatment or after a change in dosage. Predisposing factors for torsades de pointes include female gender, doses greater than 320 mg/day, heart failure, recent cardioversion, hypokalemia, bradycardia and elevated baseline serum creatinine level.[4]

References

1. New approaches to antiarrhythmic therapy, part I: Emerging therapeutic applications of the cell biology of cardiac arrhythmias. Circulation 104(23):2865-2873, 2001.
2. New approaches to antiarrhythmic therapy, part II: Emerging therapeutic applications of the cell biology of cardiac arrhythmias. Circulation 104(24):2990-2994, 2001.
3. Darbar D, Roden DM: Future of antiarrhythmic drugs. Curr Opin Cardiol 21(4):361-367, 2006.
4. Roden DM: Drug-induced prolongation of the QT interval. N Engl J Med 350(10):1013-1022, 2004.
5. Choy AM, Darbar D, Dell'Orto S, Roden DM: Exaggerated QT prolongation after cardioversion of atrial fibrillation. J Am Coll Cardiol 34(2):396-401, 1999.
6. The Cardiac Arrhythmia Suppression Trial (CAST) Investigators: Preliminary report: Effect of encainide and flecainide on mortality in a randomized trial of arrhythmia suppression after myocardial infarction. N Engl J Med 321(6):406-412, 1989.
7. Waldo AL, Camm AJ, deRuyter H, et al: Effect of D-sotalol on mortality in patients with left ventricular dysfunction after recent and remote myocardial infarction. The SWORD Investigators. Survival With Oral D-Sotalol. Lancet 348(9019):7-12, 1996.
8. Brugada R, Brugada J, Antzelevitch C, et al: Sodium channel blockers identify risk for sudden death in patients with ST-segment elevation and right bundle branch block but structurally normal hearts. Circulation 101(5):510-515, 2000.
9. Darbar D, Yang T, Churchwell K, et al: Unmasking of Brugada syndrome by lithium. Circulation 6:6, 2005.
10. Paul AA, Witchel HJ, Hancox JC: Inhibition of the current of heterologously expressed HERG potassium channels by flecainide and comparison with quinidine, propafenone and lignocaine. Br J Pharmacol 136(5):717-729, 2002.
11. Antzelevitch C, Shimizu W, Yan GX, et al: The M cell: Its contribution to the ECG and to normal and abnormal electrical function of the heart. J Cardiovasc Electrophysiol 10(8):1124-1152, 1999.
12. Fromm MF, Kim RB, Stein CM, et al: Inhibition of P-glycoprotein–mediated drug transport: A unifying mechanism to explain the interaction between digoxin and quinidine. Circulation 99(4):552-557, 1999.
13. Thompson KA, Murray JJ, Blair IA, et al: Plasma concentrations of quinidine, its major metabolites, and dihydroquinidine in patients with torsades de pointes. Clin Pharmacol Ther 43(6):636-642, 1988.
14. Caporaso NE, Shaw GL: Clinical implications of the competitive inhibition of the debrisoquin-metabolizing isozyme by quinidine. Arch Intern Med 151(10):1985-1992, 1991.
15. Woosley RL, Drayer DE, Reidenberg MM, et al: Effect of acetylator phenotype on the rate at which procainamide induces antinuclear antibodies and the lupus syndrome. N Engl J Med 298(21):1157-1159, 1978.
16. Grace AA, Camm AJ: Quinidine. N Engl J Med 338(1):35-45, 1998.
17. Roy D, Talajic M, Dorian P, et al: Amiodarone to prevent recurrence of atrial fibrillation. Canadian Trial of Atrial Fibrillation Investigators. N Engl J Med 342(13):913-920, 2000.
18. Fuster V, Ryden LE, Cannom DS, et al: ACC/AHA/ESC 2006 Guidelines for the Management of Patients with Atrial Fibrillation: a report of the American College of Cardiology/American Heart Association Task Force on Practice Guidelines and the European Society of Cardiology Committee for Practice Guidelines (Writing Committee to Revise the 2001 Guidelines for the Management of Patients With Atrial Fibrillation): Developed in collaboration with the European Heart Rhythm Association and the Heart Rhythm Society. Circulation 114(7):e257-e354, 2006.
19. Bonavita GJ, Pires LA, Wagshal AB, et al: Usefulness of oral quinidine-mexiletine combination therapy for sustained ventricular tachyarrhythmias as assessed by programmed electrical stimulation when quinidine monotherapy has failed. Am Heart J 127(4 Pt 1):847-851, 1994.
20. Guidelines 2000 for Cardiopulmonary Resuscitation and Emergency Cardiovascular Care. Part 6: Advanced cardiovascular life support: 7B: Understanding the algorithm approach to ACLS. The American Heart Association in collaboration with the International Liaison Committee on Resuscitation. Circulation 102(8 Suppl):I140-I141, 2000.
21. Glatter KA, Dorostkar PC, Yang Y, et al: Electrophysiological effects of ibutilide in

patients with accessory pathways. Circulation 104(16):1933-1939, 2001.

22. Balser JR, Nuss HB, Orias DW, et al: Local anesthetics as effectors of allosteric gating. Lidocaine effects on inactivation-deficient rat skeletal muscle Na channels. J Clin Invest 98(12):2874-2886, 1996.
23. MacMahon S, Collins R, Peto R, et al: Effects of prophylactic lidocaine in suspected acute myocardial infarction. An overview of results from the randomized, controlled trials. JAMA 260(13):1910-1916, 1988.
24. Impact Research Group: International mexiletine and placebo antiarrhythmic coronary trial: I. Report on arrhythmia and other findings. J Am Coll Cardiol 4(6):1148-1163, 1984.
25. Wang DW, Yazawa K, Makita N, et al: Pharmacological targeting of long QT mutant sodium channels. J Clin Invest 99(7):1714-1720, 1997.
26. Follmer CH, Colatsky TJ: Block of delayed rectifier potassium current, I_K, by flecainide and E-4031 in cat ventricular myocytes. Circulation 82(1):289-293, 1990.
27. Kroemer HK, Turgeon J, Parker RA, Roden DM: Flecainide enantiomers: Disposition in human subjects and electrophysiologic actions in vitro. Clin Pharmacol Ther 46(5):584-590, 1989.
28. Perry JC, Garson A Jr: Flecainide acetate for treatment of tachyarrhythmias in children: Review of world literature on efficacy, safety, and dosing. Am Heart J 124(6):1614-1621, 1992.
29. Rossenbacker T, Priori SG: The Brugada syndrome. Curr Opin Cardiol 22(3):163-170, 2007.
30. Echt DS, Liebson PR, Mitchell LB, et al: Mortality and morbidity in patients receiving encainide, flecainide, or placebo. The Cardiac Arrhythmia Suppression Trial. N Engl J Med 324(12):781-788, 1991.
31. Kuck KH, Cappato R, Siebels J, Ruppel R: Randomized comparison of antiarrhythmic drug therapy with implantable defibrillators in patients resuscitated from cardiac arrest: The Cardiac Arrest Study Hamburg (CASH). Circulation 102(7):748-754, 2000.
32. Wyse DG, Friedman PL, Brodsky MA, et al: Life-threatening ventricular arrhythmias due to transient or correctable causes: high risk for death in follow-up. J Am Coll Cardiol 38(6):1718-1724, 2001.
33. Cahill SA, Gross GJ: Propafenone and its metabolites preferentially inhibit I_{Kr} in rabbit ventricular myocytes. J Pharmacol Exp Ther 308(1):59-65, 2004.
34. Lee JT, Kroemer HK, Silberstein DJ, et al: The role of genetically determined polymorphic drug metabolism in the beta-blockade produced by propafenone. N Engl J Med 322(25):1764-1768, 1990.
35. Kaumann AJ, Olson CB: Temporal relation between long-lasting aftercontractions and action potentials in cat papillary muscles. Science 161(838):293-295, 1968.
36. Singh BN, Vaughan Williams EM: A third class of anti-arrhythmic action. Effects on atrial and ventricular intracellular potentials, and other pharmacological actions on cardiac muscle, of MJ 1999 and AH 3474. Br J Pharmacol 39(4):675-687, 1970.
37. Le Bouter S, El Harchi A, Marionneau C, et al: Long-term amiodarone administration remodels expression of ion channel transcripts in the mouse heart. Circulation 110(19):3028-3035, 2004.
38. Vorperian VR, Havighurst TC, Miller S, January CT: Adverse effects of low dose amiodarone: a meta-analysis. J Am Coll Cardiol 30(3):791-798, 1997.
39. Maintenance of sinus rhythm in patients with atrial fibrillation: An AFFIRM substudy of the first antiarrhythmic drug. J Am Coll Cardiol 42(1):20-29, 2003.
40. Deedwania PC, Singh BN, Ellenbogen K, et al: Spontaneous conversion and maintenance of sinus rhythm by amiodarone in patients with heart failure and atrial fibrillation: Observations from the veterans affairs congestive heart failure survival trial of antiarrhythmic therapy (CHF-STAT). The Department of Veterans Affairs CHF-STAT Investigators. Circulation 98(23):2574-2579, 1998.
41. Laird WP, Snyder CS, Kertesz NJ, et al: Use of intravenous amiodarone for postoperative junctional ectopic tachycardia in children. Pediatr Cardiol 24(2):133-137, 2003.
42. Wyse DG, Talajic M, Hafley GE, et al: Antiarrhythmic drug therapy in the Multicenter UnSustained Tachycardia Trial (MUSTT): Drug testing and as-treated analysis. J Am Coll Cardiol 38(2):344-351, 2001.
43. Bardy GH, Lee KL, Mark DB, et al: Amiodarone or an implantable cardioverter-defibrillator for congestive heart failure. N Engl J Med 352(3):225-237, 2005.
44. Zipes DP, Camm AJ, Borggrefe M, et al: ACC/AHA/ESC 2006 Guidelines for Management of Patients with Ventricular Arrhythmias and the Prevention of Sudden Cardiac Death: A report of the American College of Cardiology/American Heart Association Task Force and the European Society of Cardiology Committee for Practice Guidelines (writing committee to develop Guidelines for Management of Patients With Ventricular Arrhythmias and the Prevention of Sudden Cardiac Death): developed in collaboration with the European Heart Rhythm Association and the Heart Rhythm Society. Circulation 114(10):e385-e484, 2006.
45. Connolly SJ, Dorian P, Roberts RS, et al: Comparison of beta-blockers, amiodarone plus beta-blockers, or sotalol for prevention of shocks from implantable cardioverter defibrillators: The OPTIC Study: A randomized trial. JAMA 295(2):165-171, 2006.
46. Dorian P, Cass D, Schwartz B, et al: Amiodarone as compared with lidocaine for shock-resistant ventricular fibrillation. N Engl J Med 346(12):884-890, 2002.
47. Vassallo P, Trohman RG: Prescribing amiodarone: an evidence-based review of clinical indications. JAMA 298(11):1312-1322, 2007.
48. Norgaard BL, Wachtell K, Christensen PD, et al: Efficacy and safety of intravenously administered dofetilide in acute termination of atrial fibrillation and flutter: A multicenter, randomized, double-blind, placebo-controlled trial. Danish Dofetilide in Atrial Fibrillation and Flutter Study Group. Am Heart J 137(6):1062-1069, 1999.
49. Lenz TL, Hilleman DE. Dofetilide: A new antiarrhythmic agent approved for conversion and/or maintenance of atrial fibrillation/atrial flutter. Drugs Today (Barc) 36(11):759-771, 2000.
50. Torp-Pedersen C, Moller M, Bloch-Thomsen PE, et al: Dofetilide in patients with congestive heart failure and left ventricular dysfunction. Danish Investigations of Arrhythmia and Mortality on Dofetilide Study Group. N Engl J Med 341(12):857-865, 1999.
51. Kober L, Bloch Thomsen PE, et al: Effect of dofetilide in patients with recent myocardial infarction and left-ventricular dysfunction: A randomised trial. Lancet 356(9247):2052-2058, 2000.
52. Pedersen OD, Bagger H, Keller N, et al: Efficacy of dofetilide in the treatment of atrial fibrillation-flutter in patients with reduced left ventricular function: A Danish investigation of arrhythmia and mortality on dofetilide (DIAMOND) substudy. Circulation 104(3):292-296, 2001.
53. Yang T, Snyders DJ, Roden DM: Ibutilide, a methanesulfonanilide antiarrhythmic, is a potent blocker of the rapidly activating delayed rectifier K^+ current (I_{Kr}) in AT-1 cells. Concentration-, time-, voltage-, and use-dependent effects. Circulation 91(6):1799-1806, 1995.
54. Wesley RC Jr, Farkhani F, Morgan D, Zimmerman D: Ibutilide: enhanced defibrillation via plateau sodium current activation. Am J Physiol 264(4 Pt 2): H1269-H1274, 1993.
55. Naccarelli GV, Lee KS, Gibson JK, VanderLugt J: Electrophysiology and pharmacology of ibutilide. Am J Cardiol 78(8A):12-16, 1996.
56. Ellenbogen KA, Stambler BS, Wood MA, et al: Efficacy of intravenous ibutilide for rapid termination of atrial fibrillation and atrial flutter: A dose-response study. J Am Coll Cardiol 28(1):130-136, 1996.
57. Stambler BS, Wood MA, Ellenbogen KA, et al: Efficacy and safety of repeated intravenous doses of ibutilide for rapid conversion of atrial flutter or fibrillation. Ibutilide Repeat Dose Study Investigators. Circulation 94(7):1613-1621, 1996.
58. Oral H, Souza JJ, Michaud GF, et al: Facilitating transthoracic cardioversion of atrial fibrillation with ibutilide pretreatment. N Engl J Med 340(24):1849-1854, 1999.
59. Wyse DG, Waldo AL, DiMarco JP, et al: A comparison of rate control and rhythm control in patients with atrial fibrillation. N Engl J Med 347(23):1825-1833, 2002.
60. Pacifico A, Hohnloser SH, Williams JH, et al: Prevention of implantable-defibrillator shocks by treatment with sotalol. D,L-Sotalol Implantable Cardioverter-Defibrillator Study Group. N Engl J Med 340(24):1855-1862, 1999.
61. MacNeil DJ: The side effect profile of class III antiarrhythmic drugs: Focus on d,l-sotalol. Am J Cardiol 80(8A):90G-98G, 1997.

New Antiarrhythmic Drugs and New Concepts for Old Drugs 97

Paulus Kirchhof

CHAPTER OUTLINE

Background and Current Clinical Context

Ion channel–blocking antiarrhythmic drugs such as quinine and digitalis glycosides were among the first compounds used in modern pharmacotherapy, and their antiarrhythmic effectiveness was demonstrated in controlled clinical trials more than 35 years ago.[1] Proarrhythmic side effects of drugs that prolong the action potential have also been known for a long time, and achieving a favorable balance between anti- and proarrhythmic effects has been at the core of antiarrhythmic drug development in the past decades (see Chapters 74 and 96).[2-4]

Catheter ablation can cure many supraventricular tachycardias and some forms of ventricular tachycardia (see Chapters 105-110), and defibrillators are an effective way to prevent sudden death in high-risk patients (see Chapters 99 and 100). These fortunate therapeutic options leave two clinical areas at need for new antiarrhythmic drugs: prevention of sudden death in low-risk patients, and rhythm control treatment of atrial fibrillation (AF). Both arrhythmias are initiated and maintained by complex mechanisms. This chapter discusses new ion-channel blocking and other antiarrhythmic drugs that are under clinical development, delineates potential targets for new types of antiarrhythmic drugs, and discusses emerging concepts of patient-specific and short-term antiarrhythmic drug therapy.

Atrial Fibrillation

Targets for Antiarrhythmic Therapy in Atrial Fibrillation

AF is initiated and sustained by a variety of mechanisms that are not fully understood. AF sustains itself through AF-induced shortening of refractory period and action potential duration (electrical remodeling[5]). This may in part represent a mechanism to protect the atrial cardiomyocyte against intracellular calcium overload and programmed cell death secondary to loss of electrical diastole in AF, but it facilitates reinduction and maintenance of the arrhythmia. The AF-induced shortening of the action potential can be reversed by antiarrhythmic drugs.

Electrophysiologic triggers that initiate AF, especially paroxysmal AF, may be spontaneous or stretch-induced ectopy, often at the junction of the posterior left atrial wall with the pulmonary veins,[6] but at times early or late afterdepolarizations can trigger AF.[7]

Other changes in the atria, summarized as structural remodeling, can be a consequence of the arrhythmia itself or secondary to predisposing factors of AF such as arterial hypertension, atrial dilatation, or recurrent atrial ischemia, among others. Structural remodeling can consist of cellular hypertrophy, altered cellular calcium content and homeostasis, fibrosis, and intracellular matrix changes, as well as activation of inflammatory cells, myocardial scars, or patchy fibrosis, among others. In addition, AF causes contractile remodeling that persists several weeks after restoration of sinus rhythm. Usually, a combination of these factors initiates and maintains AF, and successful prevention of AF most likely requires modification of structural and electrical processes (Fig. 97-1).

Trigger Suppression in Atrial Fibrillation

Despite the growing impact of AF ablation, and especially of electrical isolation of the pulmonary veins (see Chapters 105 and 106), ion channel–blocking agents continue to be useful for suppressing triggers. Many sodium channel blockers, particularly slowly dissociating sodium channel blockers, or Vaughan-Williams class Ic drugs, suppress ectopy. An important, and at times under-recognized, effect of such compounds is induction of refractoriness beyond the end of the action potential. This postrepolarization refractoriness prevents ventricular fibrillation[8] and might prevent early-coupled atrial ectopy. Ranolazine, a blocker of the late inward sodium current approved for treatment of angina,[9] might induce atrial postrepolarization refractoriness[10] and reduce intracellular sodium levels by inhibiting the late sodium current. This can prevent torsades de pointes, at least in models of the long QT syndrome.[11,12] The clinical antiarrhythmic effects of ranolazine have not been systematically studied.

Inhibition of stretch-activated channels can prevent AF in experimental models.[13] Although these drugs are attractive, inhibitors of stretch-activated channels have a long way to go before they reach clinical applicability, because the only available specific inhibitor of stretch-activated channels is a peptide with all its inherent pharmacodynamic difficulties (GSMTx4).[13]

This work was supported by the Kompetenznetz Vorhofflimmern (AFNET, BMBF Gi0204), by the DFG (Ki/731/1-1), and by the Fondation LeDucq.

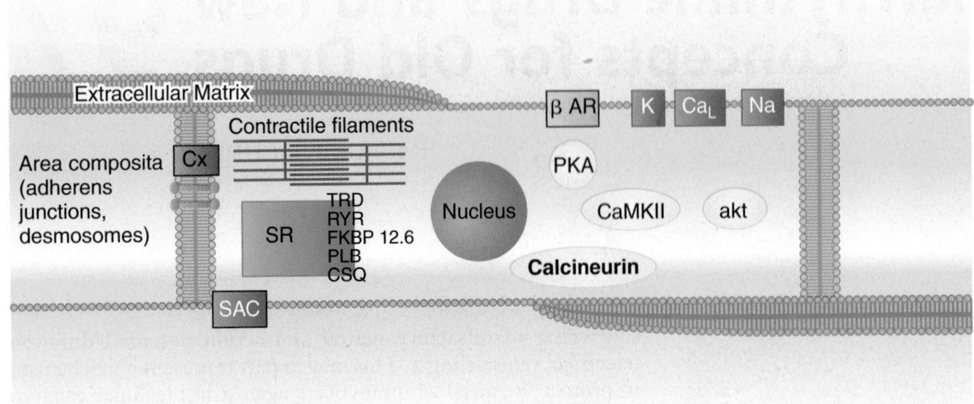

Figure 97-1 Targets for antiarrhythmic drug treatment for the prevention of atrial fibrillation and sudden death. Shown is a histologic scheme of a cardiomyocyte with some key proteins that might represent targets for antiarrhythmic drug therapy. CaMKII, akt, and calcineurin are examples for relevant protein kinases. Ca$_L$, L-type calcium channel; CaMKII, calcium-dependent calmodulin kinase II; CSQ = calsequestrin; Cx43, connexin43; FKPB 12.6 = FK506-binding protein 12.6 (an accessory protein to the ryanodine receptor); K, potassium channels; Na, sodium channel; PLB = phospholamban; RYR = ryanodine receptor; SAC = stretch-activated channel; SERCA2A = sarco-endoplasmic reticulum calcium-dependent adenosine triphosphatase (ATPase) type 2A; SR = sarcoplasmic reticulum, TRD = triadin.

Reversal of Electrical Remodeling by Prolonging Duration of Action Potential

Methods of prolonging the action potential duration are the mainstay of classic ion channel–blocking antiarrhythmic drug therapy to prevent AF.[14] Although most sodium and potassium channel–blocking drugs have been developed for ventricular arrhythmias, these drugs are in part approved, and often used, to prevent AF (see Chapter 96). Irrespective of the exact mechanism of action, both sodium and potassium channel blockers approximately double the sinus rhythm rate compared to control or placebo treatment in controlled trials of AF prevention.[14] There are many new antiarrhythmic drugs in clinical development, mainly for preventing and terminating AF, reflecting the need for such agents in the future. This field is evolving (Fig. 97-2).

When using an ion channel–blocking agent, the treatment benefit must always be weighed against the rare but potentially hazardous risk of severe ventricular proarrhythmia. Azimilide is a potassium channel blocker that mainly inhibits I_{Kr} and is, similar to other potassium channel blockers, associated with torsades de pointes proarrhythmia.[15] Its clinical antiarrhythmic efficacy appears relatively weak.[16,17] HMR1556, a novel, experimentally available substance that can convert AF in experimental models of AF, is a selective inhibitor of the slow component of the delayed rectifier current, I_{Ks}.[18] This substance does not interfere with the rapid component of the delayed rectifier current, but it appears to have a proarrhythmic potential. This might point to the relevance of the total amount of available repolarizing currents for the risk for torsades de pointes (repolarization reserve).[19]

Amiodarone appears more effective in preventing AF than are most other antiarrhythmic drugs.[20,21] Also, it is the only substance whose antiarrhythmic effects are not outweighed by proarrhythmic effects in high-risk patients, and its risk for torsades de pointes is relatively low.[22] Therefore, amiodarone has been considered a model substance for an effective and safe antiarrhythmic, ion channel–blocking drug. There are several aspects in the electrophysiologic profile of effects that could explain amiodarone's effectiveness. Some have attributed the antiarrhythmic effect of amiodarone to its nonselective inhibition of almost all types of ion channels including sodium, potassium, and calcium channels, combined with β adrenoreceptor blockade. This has resulted in the preclinical and clinical development of SSR149744C,[23] celivarone, ATI-2042, and dronedarone, multichannel blockers that have chemical properties similar to amiodarone's but that contain less iodine and hence have less iodine-dependent side effects.[24,25] In two large clinical trials (EURIDIS ADONIS), dronedarone appeared to be less effective than its mother compound[26] (but see Singh et al[20]) suggesting that other, potentially pharmacokinetic, factors favor amiodarone's effectiveness. (see later).

It is assumed that abnormal calcium release within the cardiomyocyte might provoke torsades de pointes, although the exact mechanisms initiating torsades de pointes are not well known. A fix combination of verapamil and quinidine, another form of a multichannel blocker that has been available for many years in Germany, is as effective as sotalol for preventing AF, but it appears to provoke less proarrhythmia than quinidine alone. In the PAFAC and SOPAT trials, telemetric electrocardiographic (ECG) monitoring detected one episode of ventricular tachycardia in 895 patients treated with the quinidine-verapamil combination over 1 year compared to eight episodes of torsades de pointes in 645 patients treated with sotalol over 1 year.[27,28] RSD1235 (vernakalant) is another multichannel blocker that is in clinical development for preventing AF.[29,30] AZD7009 also belongs to the class of multichannel blockers developed for rhythm-control treatment of AF.[31,32] However, AZD7009 will not become available due to unpredicted noncardiac effects. Both RSD 1235 and AZD7009 are also inhibitors of the late sodium current, similar to ranolazine (see earlier).

The outward currents that determine repolarization in the atria are slightly different than in the ventricle. In theory, inhibition of atrial-specific ion currents could be safer because such compounds would selectively prolong atrial action potentials without affecting ventricular action potentials and the QT interval (see Chapter 74 on proarrhythmia). One of the best-studied substances that attempts this approach is the relative selective inhibitor of the ultrarapid component of the outward potassium current (I_{Kur}), AVE0118. AVE0118 prevents AF effectively in preclinical studies in goats,[33,34] but there is no published record of an antiarrhythmic efficacy in patients. This compound restores atrial contractility after cardioversion.[33] RSD1235 carries properties of both multichannel blockade and atrium-specific potassium channel blockade,[29,30] similar to AZD7009.

Two inward-rectifying potassium currents, the background current I_{K1} and the acetylcholine-activated current $I_{K,ACh}$, are altered in AF, with I_{K1} being increased and $I_{K,ACh}$ becoming in part constitutively active.[35] As a consequence, the refractory period is shortened. This creates a condition that supports multiple wavelet reentry and periodic activity of sustained

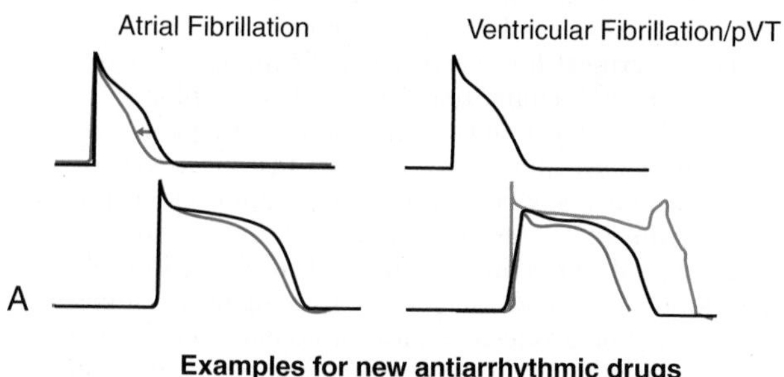

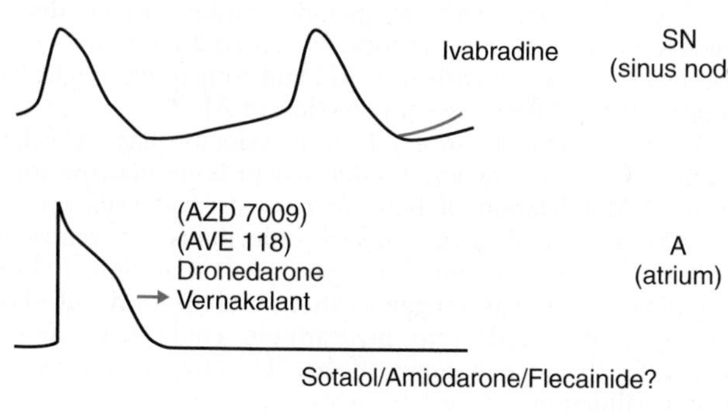

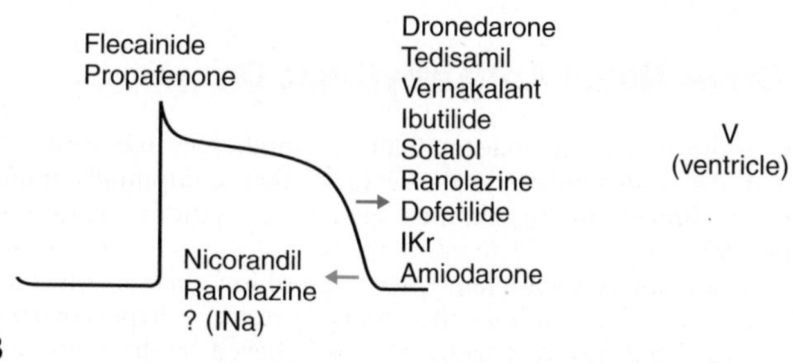

Figure 97-2 **A,** Modifications of the cardiac action potential associated with atrial fibrillation *(left)* and sudden death due to ventricular arrhythmias in inherited and acquired cardiomyopathies *(right)*. **B,** Scheme of ion channel–blocking drugs that can affect the cardiac action potential.

high-frequency functional reentry sources described as *rotors*.[36,37] In addition, a shift of the resting membrane potential toward more positive potentials might increase the chance that spontaneous depolarizations (e.g., afterdepolarizations) can activate sodium channels and thereby initiate a premature response. Restoration of normal function of these currents appears to be an attractive target for antiarrhythmic drug therapy.

Fish oil intake can prevent AF,[38] which may be related to electrophysiologic effects, namely, blockade of sarcolemmal ion channels.[39] This initial observation requires confirmation in controlled trials, similar to the initial, at present unconfirmed, suggestion that some types of unsaturated fatty acids may be helpful in preventing sudden death.

Abnormal intracellular calcium regulation is found in fibrillating human atria.[40,41] A growing body of evidence suggests that both atrial ectopy and electrical remodeling are highly calcium-dependent phenomena. Whether the calcium-stabilizing interventions that are discussed later in the context of sudden death can also be employed to prevent AF remains to be studied.

Antifibrotic Therapy and Improvement of Atrial Conduction

Slowing of atrial impulse propagation[42,43] is an important contributor to the maintenance of AF. The electrical connection between cardiomyocytes is formed by gap junctions that contain ion-channel pores, mainly formed by connexin45 (atria) or connexin43 (ventricles). Therefore, interventions that are suitable to improve the function of cardiac connexins may be used in the future as antiarrhythmic interventions for AF. Designing of such interventions may in part make use of the existing knowledge on mechanisms of sudden death (see later) but will require some additional pathophysiologic data on the genesis of AF.

It is well established that formation of fibrosis in the fibrillating atria can be prevented by angiotensin-receptor blockers in models of AF.[44] This antifibrotic effect of angiotensin receptor blockers and ACE inhibitors probably explains why these substances prevent new-onset AF in patients with heart failure[45] and in patients with preserved left ventricular function who are at risk for AF.[46] Whether this type of treatment can be used to reduce arrhythmic events in paroxysmal AF patients is currently tested in randomized trials.

Some data suggest that statins[47,48] or steroids[49] might prevent AF, especially postoperative AF. Whether anti-inflammatory interventions can really prevent postoperative or other types of AF is not yet conclusively determined, and further studies are needed to address this topic.[50]

Sudden Cardiac Death

Ventricular tachyarrhythmias after myocardial infarction often originate in zones of slow conduction that can form re-entrant circuits in the border zone of myocardial infarctions. Others are initiated by recurrent ischemic events. Therefore, rapid and complete revascularization in patients with acute myocardial infarction is an important intervention to prevent sudden cardiac death. In fact, several drugs that are used routinely in the care of survivors of a myocardial infarction and in patients with heart failure (inhibitors of platelet aggregation, statins, ACE inhibitors, and β-blockers) contribute to the prevention of sudden death.[51] Statins and antithrombotic substances (aspirin, the thienopyridines, ticlopidine) can prevent plaque rupture, acute coronary syndromes, and acute myocardial ischemia and thereby eliminate a relevant trigger for ventricular arrhythmias.

In the long run, prevention of myocardial infarctions prevents formation of myocardial scars. This in turn reduces the substrate for ventricular arrhythmias. ACE inhibitors and angiotensin receptor antagonists might contribute to limiting the substrate for ventricular arrhythmias by preventing pathologic left ventricular remodeling after myocardial infarction, by reducing myocardial stretch, and by antihypertrophic effects in the myocardium. Aldosterone antagonists such as spironolactone or eplerenone might have similar effects my modulating the activity of the renin-angiotensin-aldosterone system and by direct effects on cardiac gene expression patterns.[52,53] Any form of inhibiting the renin-angiotensin-aldosterone system will also elevate extracellular and plasma potassium levels and might thereby contribute to the prevention of ventricular arrhythmias associated with prolonged repolarization.

Modulation of Myocardial Calcium Homeostasis: A Target to Prevent Sudden Death?

Contrary to the origin of many episodes of AF at the junction of the pulmonary veins and in the posterior left atrium, initiation of ventricular fibrillation is only rarely a localized phenomenon,[54] but it is much more often a consequence of several synergistic cellular regulatory processes that combine to provoke triggered activity. Altered myocardial calcium regulation appears to be a central part of these triggers for sudden death. Targeting these processes might allow us to prevent sudden death; at present, such interventions are only available in preclinical settings. Calcium-dependent mechanisms might also be relevant for AF, although this has not been studied to the same extent as in ventricular fibrillation.

Several observations have long suggested a relevant role for calcium in sudden death: Prolongation of the ventricular action potential in hypertrophied ventricles and pause-dependence of ventricular fibrillation suggest that afterdepolarizations may be relevant for sudden death. Autonomic imbalance, and specifically excessive sympathetic stimulation, might in itself also provoke ventricular arrhythmias, most likely by catecholamine-induced increased intracellular calcium levels and facilitated calcium release from the sarcoplasmic reticulum. It is well known that diastolic calcium levels are increased in heart failure, and systolic calcium release is increased in hypertrophy. Consequently, abnormally increased systolic calcium release, at times combined with increased diastolic calcium levels, provokes ventricular fibrillation in models of cardiac hypertrophy[55,56] and might contribute to ventricular arrhythmias in other forms of pathologic cardiac hypertrophy and heart failure.[57] Abnormal diastolic calcium release from the sarcoplasmic reticulum underlies catecholaminergic ventricular tachycardias in transgenic models.[58,59] Prolonged calcium release from the contractile apparatus of cardiomyocytes might have similar effects in some forms of hypertrophic cardiomyopathy.[60]

Because intracellular calcium homeostasis is centrally involved in excitation-contraction coupling, intracellular signaling, regulation of protein function, regulation of gene expression, and potentially cell differentiation, drugs that interact with intracellular calcium homeostasis require thorough study of their acute and long-term effects. Calcium channel blockade by existing drugs (verapamil) can in selected patients suppress ventricular arrhythmias, similar to verapamil's effects in catecholaminergic ventricular tachycardia.[61] Inhibitors of the Na^+-Ca^{2+} exchanger are under preclinical evaluation for trigger suppression, but their antiarrhythmic efficacy has not yet been proved.[62,63] Inhibitors of intracellular kinases, such as CaMKII (calmodulin-dependent protein kinase II) inhibitors,[56,58,64] and possibly also phosphatase inhibitors, can acutely suppress ventricular arrhythmias in a variety of experimental models (hypertrophy, infarction). Inhibition of spontaneous diastolic calcium leaks from the sarcoplasmic reticulum (e.g., activation of FK506-binding protein ([FKBP] 12.6 by JTV519 and related substances[58]) can suppress ventricular arrhythmias associated with genetically increased calcium leak in the sarcoplasmic reticulum[40,65,66] and probably also in models with reduced calsequestrin function[67] or increased triadin function.[59,68,69] Possibly, store-operated calcium also contributes to arrhythmogenesis, either indirectly via inducing cardiac hypertrophy[70] or directly.[71,72] A thorough understanding of the subcellular calcium compartments that undergo independent calcium regulation might help researchers to devise new compounds that inhibit arrhythmogenesis while maintaining the essential effects of calcium on contractile function, regulation of protein function, and regulation of gene expression.

Improvement of Intercellular Connections to Improve Cardiac Conduction

Slowing of impulse propagation in the myocardium is one of the major proarrhythmic mechanisms after myocardial infarction. Connexins are the main pore-forming molecules that provide the electrical connections between cardiomyocytes. Reduced expression of the ventricular connexin43 is found in areas that are critical for ventricular arrhythmias after myocardial infarction.[73,74] Connexins have a high biological safety margin: Studies using inducible deletion of the gene encoding for connexin43 have convincingly shown that electrical conduction is only affected when ventricular connexin43 expression levels are reduced by more than 50%.[75] In the border zone of a myocardial infarction, such marked reduction of connexin43 levels is found, suggesting that reduced connexin43 expression may be a relevant cause of conduction slowing and ventricular arrhythmias in the border zone of an infarction.[74]

Experimentally, there are two means to improve electrical conduction of the heart via enhanced connexin function: Connexin openers, such as rotigaptide, can improve conduction velocity in experimental settings.[76,77] Altered connexin expression has also been described in AF, and rotigaptide might have antiarrhythmic effects on some models of AF.[78]

An improvement in conduction velocity has also been found in rat cardiomyocytes subjected to bone marrow stimulation.[80] Mobilization of bone marrow–derived cells into the heart is associated with reduced inducibility of ventricular arrhythmias after an anterior myocardial infarction.[74] These preliminary findings suggest that mobilization of bone marrow–derived cells into myocardium could have indirect (paracrine ?) antiarrhythmic effects. This hypothesis requires further validation.

Other Novel Antiarrhythmic Drugs

In addition to the development of antiarrhythmic drugs to treat AF and sudden death, several other compounds might be of clinical use in treating specific arrhythmia syndromes (Fig. 97-3).

Ivabradine is a completely new type of ion channel–blocking drug. Ivabradine inhibits the funny current, a hyperpolarization-activated inward current that is believed to drive impulse generation in the sinus node.[81] This current, most likely generated by ion flow through proteins coded by the HCN gene family, is an attractive drug target because the target protein isoform is predominantly expressed only in sinus node and in retina. Consequently, side effects are rare and are mainly limited to intermittent flash-like visual sensations secondary to interactions of the drug with retinal channels. These occur in 12% of treated patients, but they rarely limit therapy. Ivabradine has been approved for the treatment of patients with angina pectoris who have contraindications to β-adrenoreceptor blockade,[82,83] and the recently published BEAUTIFUL trial has confirmed the safety of the use of ivabradine in combination with β-blockers in patients with heart failure. Clinical experience with treating arrhythmias is limited, and its use as an antiarrhythmic drug is off-label at present. Nonetheless, the mode of action strongly suggests that ivabradine may be a specific and effective treatment for patients with inadequate sinus tachycardias.

Potassium channel openers like nicorandil or NS1643 may be able to reverse the action potential prolongation associated with drug-induced proarrhythmia and arrhythmias in the long-QT syndromes.[84,85] Such substances could theoretically help to acutely treat proarrhythmic situations associated with prolongation of the ventricular action potential. This might apply to patients with congenital long-QT syndromes and to those with acquired forms of torsades de pointes. An antiarrhythmic effect has been noted in case reports,[86] but it has not been tested in larger trials.

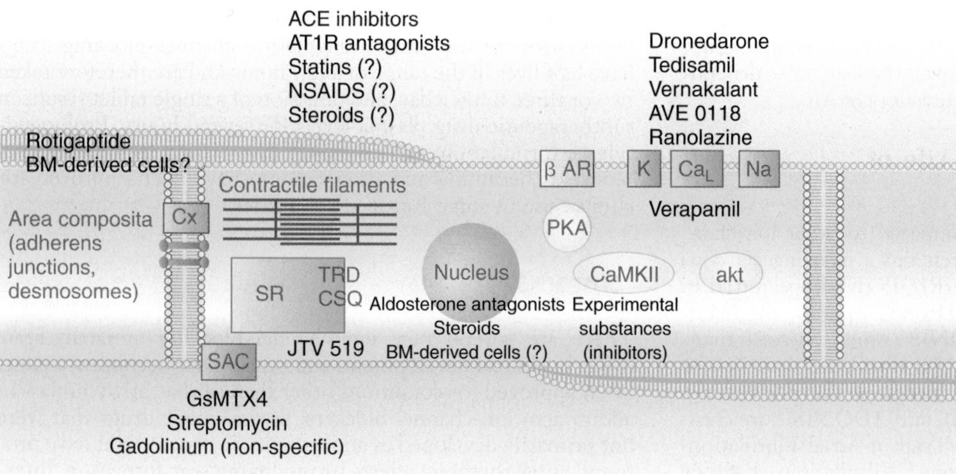

Figure 97-3 An incomplete list of new antiarrhythmic drugs. In the scheme, the substances colocalize with the putative target structures in the myocardial cell. ACE, angiotensin-converting enzyme; AT1R, angiotensin II type 1 receptor; AVE 0118, investigational potassium-channel blocker; BM, bone marrow; GsMTX4, a cationic hydrophobic peptide isolated from tarantula *(Grammostola spatulata)* venom; JTV51, investigational benzothiazepine derivative; NSAID, nonsteroidal antiinflammatory drug.

Targeted Use of Antiarrhythmic Drugs

Patient-Specific Use of Antiarrhythmic Drugs in Inherited Arrhythmogenic Cardiomyopathies

In addition to developing new compounds, clinician-researchers have identified genotype-specific or patient-specific approaches to prevent ventricular arrhythmias in patients with inherited cardiomyopathies, and others have designed and evaluated strategies to render rhythm-control treatment of AF drugs safer by limiting the duration of antiarrhythmic drug treatment. The different mechanisms that initiate ventricular fibrillation in inherited cardiomyopathies (including channelopathies[87]) open the prospect for antiarrhythmic treatments tailored to individual patients based on genotype and clinical presentation. Such patient-specific therapies have been suggested in the long-QT syndromes (LQTS).

Different genotypes might require modulation of different parts of the autonomic nervous system to prevent arrhythmias in LQTS.[88] Patients with mutations in the *KVLQT2* (LQTS2) gene might require β-adrenoreceptor blockade, and patients with mutations in the *SCN5A* gene (LQTS3) might benefit more from inhibition of the parasympathetic nervous system and from prevention of bradycardia.[89] Inhibitors of the late sodium current preferentially inhibit late opening of mutated sodium channels and shorten the QT interval in patients with mutated sodium channels.[90] A combination of β-blockers and calcium channel blockers can reduce arrhythmic events in patients with catecholaminergic ventricular tachycardias[61] and possibly also in hypertrophic cardiomyopathy patients (see earlier). Initial reports indicate that the action potential–prolonging agent quinidine might prevent arrhythmias in patients with the short-QT syndrome.[91] Whether such genotype-specific therapies really contribute to the prevention of arrhythmic events in patients with arrhythmogenic cardiomyopathies is not known.

High-level physical (endurance) training appears to provoke right ventricular tachycardias and contributes to the development of arrhythmogenic right ventricular cardiomyopathy.[92,93] Whether the proarrhythmic effects of training in patients with right ventricular arrhythmias or arrhythmogenic right ventricular cardiomyopathy—sympathetic stimulation, increased cardiac output, and pressure and volume overload—can be prevented by drug therapy has not yet been tested.

Intelligent Timing of Antiarrhythmic Drug Therapy

Clinical development of safe and effective antiarrhythmic drugs is cumbersome. An intelligent timing of antiarrhythmic drug therapy may be another, simpler way to enhance safety of antiarrhythmic drugs without reducing efficacy. Traditionally, antiarrhythmic drug therapy has been long-term therapy. During long-term antiarrhythmic drug therapy to prevent AF, 1% to 2% of patients experience (at times asymptomatic) episodes of torsades de pointes per year (see Chapter 74 and Kirchhof and Breithardt[94]). Reducing the duration of antiarrhythmic drug treatment should reduce the risk of proarrhythmia. At present, two concepts for intelligent short-term antiarrhythmic drug treatment are under clinical evaluation in patients with AF: They have been called the *pill-in-the pocket* treatment of paroxysmal AF and *targeted reversal of electrical remodeling* after cardioversion.

Pill-in-the-Pocket Treatment of Paroxysmal Atrial Fibrillation

Patients who have infrequent (fewer than 1 episode per month) symptomatic episodes of paroxysmal AF but who do not have overt structural heart disease and who have responded successfully and safely to one pharmacologic conversion of AF by sodium channel blocker administered under close in-hospital monitoring can be advised to take a single dose of a sodium channel–blocking agent (200-300 mg flecainide or 450-600 mg propafenone) *at home* as soon as AF recurs. This patient-initiated treatment converts more than 90% of AF recurrences in a controlled trial setting.[95] The duration of antiarrhythmic drug treatment was reduced by 99.2% by this type of targeted drug treatment compared to standard long-term treatment.[94]

Targeted Reversal of Electrical Remodeling after Cardioversion

AF recurrences are clustered within the first few weeks after cardioversion of persistent AF. Interestingly, the AF-induced shortening of the atrial action potential and refractory period known as *electrical remodeling*[5] is reversed after approximately 4 weeks of sinus rhythm.[96] Action potential–prolonging antiarrhythmic drugs can have reduced, if any, antiarrhythmic effects after this period. These considerations have prompted the design of the Flecainide Short-Long (Flec-SL) trial.[97] This trial systematically tests whether short-term (4-weeks) antiarrhythmic drug therapy after cardioversion is not inferior to standard long-term therapy.

The results of Flec-SL will be available in 2009. Such a short-term antiarrhythmic drug therapy after cardioversion could reduce duration of antiarrhythmic drug therapy by 66% to 92%, depending on the number and timing of recurrences of AF.

The Longer, the Better? Half-Life of Antiarrhythmic Drugs

The effectiveness of amiodarone compared to other ion channel–blocking antiarrhythmic drugs remains a puzzling yet consistent clinical finding. Results of EURIDIS (EURopean trial In atrial fibrillation patients receiving Dronedarone for the maintenance of Sinus rhythm) and ADONIS (American-Australian-African trial with Dronedarone In atrial fibrillation patients for the maintenance of Sinus rhythm) increased the puzzlement. When the main findings of EURIDIS and ADONIS[26] are compared to those of CTAF (Canadian Trial of Atrial Fibrillation) and SAFE-T (Sotalol Amiodarone Fibrillation Efficacy Trial),[20,21] it appears that amiodarone has better efficacy in preventing AF than has dronedarone, although this observation is derived from a flawed comparison of results in different populations using different rhythm outcome measures. The ion channel–blocking properties and the chemical composition of dronedarone and amiodarone are not sufficiently different to explain this supposed clinical difference.

Amiodarone has one additional unique property, however: The biologic half-life of amiodarone amounts to several months.[99] This unique pharmacokinetic profile might contribute to amiodarone's clinical efficacy. When amiodarone is not taken or not absorbed, even for several consecutive days, this interruption does not affect the therapeutic myocardial drug levels. Most of the other available ion channel–blocking drugs have half lives in the range of a few hours and are therefore taken two or three times a day, and omission of a single tablet results in subtherapeutic drug plasma levels for several hours. Prolonged-release formulations of two slowly dissociating sodium channel blockers (flecainide and propafenone) have been approved for clinical use in some European countries.

Summary

There are several new ion channel–blocking antiarrhythmic drugs in clinical development, and others have become available, often approved for conditions other than cardiac arrhythmias. In addition to ion-channel blockers, several other drugs that were not primarily developed as antiarrhythmic drugs might have profound antiarrhythmic effects by modifying scar formation, interstitial fibrosis, composition of extracellular matrix, and contact between cardiomyocytes. It is likely that these substances will be supplemented by other drugs with entirely different mechanisms of action in coming years based on subcellular and molecular pathophysiologic insights into the mechanisms of arrhythmogenesis.

Acknowledgments

I would like to thank L. Fabritz, U. Ravens, and G. Breithardt for critical review of this chapter.

References

1. Levi G, Proto C, Rovetta A: Double-blind evaluation of practolol and quinidine in the treatment of chronic atrial fibrillation. Cardiology 58:364-368, 1973.
2. Thomson GW: Quinidine as a cause of sudden death. Circulation 14:757-765, 1956.
3. Coplen SE, Antman EM, Berlin JA, et al: Efficacy and safety of quinidine therapy for maintenance of sinus rhythm after cardioversion. A meta-analysis of randomized control trials. Circulation 82:1106-1116, 1990.
4. Echt DS, Liebson PR, Mitchell LB, et al: Mortality and morbidity in patients receiving encainide, flecainide, or placebo: The Cardiac Arrhythmia Suppression Trial. N Engl J Med 324:781-788, 1991.
5. Wijffels MC, Kirchhof CJ, Dorland R, Allessie MA: Atrial fibrillation begets atrial fibrillation. A study in awake chronically instrumented goats. Circulation 92:1954-1968, 1995.
6. Haissaguerre M, Jais P, Shah DC, et al: Spontaneous initiation of atrial fibrillation by ectopic beats originating in the pulmonary veins. N Engl J Med 339:659-666, 1998.
7. Kirchhof P, Eckardt L, Monnig G, et al: A patient with "atrial torsades de pointes". J Cardiovasc Electrophysiol 11:806-811, 2000.
8. Kirchhof P, Fabritz L, Franz MR: Post-repolarization refractoriness versus conduction slowing caused by class I antiarrhythmic drugs—antiarrhythmic and proarrhythmic effects. Circulation 97:2567-2574, 1998.
9. Chaitman BR, Pepine CJ, Parker JO, et al: Effects of ranolazine with atenolol, amlodipine, or diltiazem on exercise tolerance and angina frequency in patients with severe chronic angina: A randomized controlled trial. JAMA 291:309-316, 2004.
10. Burashnikov A, Di Diego JM, Zygmunt AC, et al: Atrium-selective sodium channel block as a strategy for suppression of atrial fibrillation. Differences in sodium channel inactivation between atria and ventricles and the role of ranolazine. Circulation 116(13):1449-1457, 2007.
11. Fredj S, Sampson KJ, Liu H, Kass RS: Molecular basis of ranolazine block of LQT-3 mutant sodium channels: Evidence for site of action. Br J Pharmacol 148:16-24, 2006.
12. Antzelevitch C, Belardinelli L, Zygmunt AC, et al: Electrophysiological effects of ranolazine, a novel antianginal agent with antiarrhythmic properties. Circulation 110:904-910, 2004.
13. Bode F, Sachs F, Franz M: Tarantula peptide inhibits atrial fibrillation. Nature 409:6818-6819, 2001.
14. McNamara RL, Tamariz LJ, Segal JB, Bass EB: Management of atrial fibrillation: Review of the evidence for the role of pharmacologic therapy, electrical cardioversion, and echocardiography. Ann Intern Med 139:1018-1033, 2003.
15. Pratt CM, Al-Khalidi HR, Brum JM, et al: Cumulative experience of azimilide-associated torsades de pointes ventricular tachycardia in the 19 clinical studies comprising the azimilide database. J Am Coll Cardiol 48:471-477, 2006.
16. Page RL, Pritchett EL, Connolly S, Wilkinson WE: Azimilide for the treatment of atrial fibrillation, atrial flutter, and paroxysmal supraventricular tachycardia: Results of a randomized trial and insights on the concordance of symptoms and recurrent arrhythmias. J Cardiovasc Electrophysiol 19(2):172-177, 2008.
17. Lombardi F, Borggrefe M, Ruzyllo W, Luderitz B: Azimilide vs. placebo and sotalol for persistent atrial fibrillation: the A-COMET-II (Azimilide-CardiOversion MaintEnance Trial-II) trial. Eur Heart J 27(18):2224-2231, 2006.
18. Bauer A, Koch M, Kraft P, Becker R, et al: The new selective I_{Ks}-blocking agent HMR 1556 restores sinus rhythm and prevents heart failure in pigs with persistent atrial fibrillation. Basic Res Cardiol 100:270-278, 2005.
19. Roden DM: Taking the "idio" out of "idiosyncratic": Predicting torsades de pointes. Pacing Clin Electrophysiol 21:1029-1034, 1998.
20. Singh BN, Singh SN, Reda DJ, et al: Amiodarone versus sotalol for atrial fibrillation. N Engl J Med 352:1861-1872, 2005.
21. Roy D, Talajic M, Dorian P, et al: Amiodarone to prevent recurrence of atrial fibrillation. Canadian Trial of Atrial Fibrillation Investigators. N Engl J Med 342:913-920, 2000.
22. Singh SN, Fletcher RD, Fisher SG, et al: Amiodarone in patients with congestive heart failure and asymptomatic ventricular arrhythmia. Survival Trial of Antiarrhythmic Therapy in Congestive

Heart Failure. N Engl J Med 333:77-82, 1995.

23. Gautier P, Serre M, Cosnier-Pucheu S, et al: In vivo and in vitro antiarrhythmic effects of SSR149744C in animal models of atrial fibrillation and ventricular arrhythmias. J Cardiovasc Pharmacol 45:125-135, 2005.
24. Touboul P, Brugada J, Capucci A, et al: Dronedarone for prevention of atrial fibrillation: A dose-ranging study. Eur Heart J 24:1481-1487, 2003.
25. Thomas D, Kathofer S, Zhang W, et al: Acute effects of dronedarone on both components of the cardiac delayed rectifier K^+ current, HERG and KvLQT1/minK potassium channels. Br J Pharmacol 140:996-1002, 2003.
26. Singh BN, Connolly SJ, Crijns HJ, et al: Dronedarone for maintenance of sinus rhythm in atrial fibrillation or flutter. N Engl J Med 357:987-999, 2007.
27. Fetsch T, Bauer P, Engberding R, et al: Prevention of atrial fibrillation after cardioversion: Results of the PAFAC trial. Eur Heart J 25:1385-1394, 2004.
28. Patten M, Maas R, Bauer P, et al: Suppression of paroxysmal atrial tachyarrhythmias—results of the SOPAT trial. Eur Heart J 25:1395-1404, 2004.
29. Orth PM, Hesketh JC, Mak CK, et al: RSD1235 blocks late I_{Na} and suppresses early afterdepolarizations and torsades de pointes induced by class III agents. Cardiovasc Res 70:486-496, 2006.
30. Roy D, Rowe BH, Stiell IG, et al: A randomized, controlled trial of RSD1235, a novel anti-arrhythmic agent, in the treatment of recent onset atrial fibrillation. J Am Coll Cardiol 44:2355-2361, 2004.
31. Persson F, Andersson B, Duker G, et al: Functional effects of the late sodium current inhibition by AZD7009 and lidocaine in rabbit isolated atrial and ventricular tissue and Purkinje fibre. Eur J Pharmacol 558:133-143, 2007.
32. Crijns HJ, Van Gelder IC, Walfridsson H, et al: Safe and effective conversion of persistent atrial fibrillation to sinus rhythm by intravenous AZD7009. Heart Rhythm 3:1321-1331, 2006.
33. de Haan S, Greiser M, Harks E, et al: AVE0118, blocker of the transient outward current (I_{to}) and ultrarapid delayed rectifier current (I_{Kur}), fully restores atrial contractility after cardioversion of atrial fibrillation in the goat. Circulation 114:1234-1242, 2006.
34. Wirth KJ, Paehler T, Rosenstein B, et al: Atrial effects of the novel K^+-channel-blocker AVE0118 in anesthetized pigs. Cardiovasc Res 60:298-306, 2003.
35. Dobrev D, Friedrich A, Voigt N, et al: The G protein-gated potassium current $I_{K,ACh}$ is constitutively active in patients with chronic atrial fibrillation. Circulation 112:3697-3706, 2005.
36. Mandapati R, Skanes A, Chen J, et al: Stable microreentrant sources as a mechanism of atrial fibrillation in the isolated sheep heart. Circulation 101:194-199, 2000.
37. Atienza F, Almendral J, Moreno J, et al: Activation of inward rectifier potassium channels accelerates atrial fibrillation in humans: Evidence for a reentrant mechanism. Circulation 114:2434-2442, 2006.
38. Mozaffarian D, Psaty BM, Rimm EB, et al: Fish intake and risk of incident atrial fibrillation. Circulation 110(4):368-373, 2004.
39. Schrepf R, Limmert T, Weber CP, et al: Immediate effects of n-3 fatty acid infusion on the induction of sustained ventricular tachycardia. Lancet 363:1441-1442, 2004.
40. Vest JA, Wehrens XH, Reiken SR, et al: Defective cardiac ryanodine receptor regulation during atrial fibrillation. Circulation 111:2025-2032, 2005.
41. El-Armouche A, Boknik P, Eschenhagen T, et al: Molecular determinants of altered Ca^{2+} handling in human chronic atrial fibrillation. Circulation 114:670-680, 2006.
42. Kistler PM, Sanders P, Dodic M, et al: Atrial electrical and structural abnormalities in an ovine model of chronic blood pressure elevation after prenatal corticosteroid exposure: Implications for development of atrial fibrillation. Eur Heart J 27(24):3045-3056, 2006.
43. Gollob MH, Jones DL, Krahn AD, et al: Somatic mutations in the connexin 40 gene *(GJA5)* in atrial fibrillation. N Engl J Med 354:2677-2688, 2006.
44. Kumagai K, Nakashima H, Urata H, et al: Effects of angiotensin II type 1 receptor antagonist on electrical and structural remodeling in atrial fibrillation. J Am Coll Cardiol 41:2197-2204, 2003.
45. Pedersen OD, Bagger H, Kober L, Torp-Pedersen C: Trandolapril reduces the incidence of atrial fibrillation after acute myocardial infarction in patients with left ventricular dysfunction. Circulation 100:376-380, 1999.
46. Wachtell K, Lehto M, Gerdts E, et al: Angiotensin II receptor blockade reduces new-onset atrial fibrillation and subsequent stroke compared to atenolol: The Losartan Intervention For End Point Reduction in Hypertension (LIFE) study. J Am Coll Cardiol 45:712-719, 2005.
47. Shiroshita-Takeshita A, Schram G, Lavoie J, Nattel S: Effect of simvastatin and antioxidant vitamins on atrial fibrillation promotion by atrial-tachycardia remodeling in dogs. Circulation 110:2313-2319, 2004.
48. Patti G, Chello M, Candura D, et al: Randomized trial of atorvastatin for reduction of postoperative atrial fibrillation in patients undergoing cardiac surgery: Results of the ARMYDA-3 (Atorvastatin for Reduction of MYocardial Dysrhythmia After cardiac surgery) study. Circulation 114:1455-1461, 2006.
49. Halonen J, Halonen P, Jarvinen O, et al: Corticosteroids for the prevention of atrial fibrillation after cardiac surgery: A randomized controlled trial. JAMA 297:1562-1567, 2007.
50. Boos CJ, Anderson RA, Lip GY: Is atrial fibrillation an inflammatory disorder? Eur Heart J 27:136-149, 2006.
51. Kirchhof P, Breithardt G, Eckardt L: Primary prevention of sudden cardiac death. Heart 92:1873-1878, 2006.
52. Pitt B, Remme W, Zannad F, et al: Eplerenone, a selective aldosterone blocker, in patients with left ventricular dysfunction after myocardial infarction. N Engl J Med 348:1309-1321, 2003.
53. Pitt B, Zannad F, Remme WJ, et al: The effect of spironolactone on morbidity and mortality in patients with severe heart failure. Randomized Aldactone Evaluation Study Investigators. N Engl J Med 341:709-717, 1999.
54. Haissaguerre M, Shah DC, Jais P, et al: Role of Purkinje conducting system in triggering of idiopathic ventricular fibrillation. Lancet 359:677-678, 2002.
55. Wu Y, Temple J, Zhang R, et al: Calmodulin kinase II and arrhythmias in a mouse model of cardiac hypertrophy. Circulation 106:1288-1293, 2002.
56. Kirchhof P, Fabritz L, Begrow F, et al: Ventricular arrhythmias, increased cardiac calmodulin kinase II expression, and altered repolarization kinetics in ANP-receptor deficient mice. J Mol Cell Cardiol 36:691-700, 2004.
57. Wagner S, Dybkova N, Rasenack E, et al: Ca/calmodulin-dependent protein kinase II regulates cardiac Na channels. J Clin Invest 116:3127-3138, 2006.
58. Wehrens XH, Lehnart SE, Reiken SR, et al: Protection from cardiac arrhythmia through ryanodine receptor-stabilizing protein calstabin2. Science 304:292-296, 2004.
59. Knollmann BC, Chopra N, Hlaing T, et al: Casq2 deletion causes sarcoplasmic reticulum volume increase, premature Ca^{2+} release, and catecholaminergic polymorphic ventricular tachycardia. J Clin Invest 116:2510-2520, 2006.
60. Knollmann BC, Kirchhof P, Sirenko SG, et al: Familial hypertrophic cardiomyopathy-linked mutant troponin T causes stress-induced ventricular tachycardia and Ca^{2+}-dependent action potential remodeling. Circ Res 92:428-436, 2003.
61. Rosso R, Kalman JM, Rogowski O, et al: Calcium channel blockers and beta-blockers versus beta-blockers alone for preventing exercise-induced arrhythmias in catecholaminergic polymorphic ventricular tachycardia. Heart Rhythm 4:1149-1154, 2007.
62. Shpak B, Gofman Y, Shpak C, et al: Effects of purified endogenous inhibitor of the Na^+/Ca^{2+} exchanger on ouabain-induced arrhythmias in the atria and ventricle strips of guinea pig. Eur J Pharmacol 553:196-204, 2006.
63. Nagy ZA, Virag L, Toth A, et al: Selective inhibition of sodium-calcium exchanger by SEA-0400 decreases early and delayed after depolarization in canine heart. Br J Pharmacol 143:827-831, 2004.
64. Zhang R, Khoo MS, Wu Y, et al: Calmodulin kinase II inhibition protects against structural heart disease. Nat Med 11:409-417, 2005.
65. Wu Y, Roden DM, Anderson ME: Calmodulin kinase inhibition prevents development of the arrhythmogenic transient inward current. Circ Res 84:906-912, 1999.
66. Jiang D, Xiao B, Yang D, et al: RyR2 mutations linked to ventricular tachycardia and sudden death reduce the threshold for

store-overload-induced Ca^{2+} release (SOICR). Proc Natl Acad Sci U S A 101:13062-13067, 2004.

67. Knollmann B, Chopra N, Hlaing T, et al: Casq2 deletion causes sarcoplasmic reticulum volume increase, premature Ca^{2+} release, and catecholaminergic polymorphic ventricular tachycardia. J Clin Invest 116(9):2510-2520, 2006.
68. Terentyev D, Cala SE, Houle, et al: Triadin overexpression stimulates excitation-contraction coupling and increases predisposition to cellular arrhythmia in cardiac myocytes. Circ Res 96:651-658, 2005.
69. Kirchhof P, Klimas J, Fabritz L, et al: Stress and high heart rate provoke ventricular tachycardia in mice expressing triadin. J Mol Cell Cardiol 42:962-971, 2007.
70. Kuwahara K, Wang Y, McAnally J, et al: TRPC6 fulfills a calcineurin signaling circuit during pathologic cardiac remodeling. J Clin Invest 116:3114-3126, 2006.
71. Ju YK, Chu Y, Chaulet H, et al: Store-operated Ca^{2+} influx and expression of TRPC genes in mouse sinoatrial node. Circ Res 100:1605-1614, 2007.
72. Rosker C, Graziani A, Lukas M, et al: Ca^{2+} signaling by TRPC3 involves Na^+ entry and local coupling to the Na^+/Ca^{2+} exchanger. J Biol Chem 279:13696-13704, 2004.
73. Peters NS, Coromilas J, Severs NJ, Wit AL: Disturbed connexin43 gap junction distribution correlates with the location of reentrant circuits in the epicardial border zone of healing canine infarcts that cause ventricular tachycardia. Circulation 95:988-996, 1997.
74. Kuhlmann MT, Kirchhof P, Klocke R, et al: G-CSF/SCF reduces inducible arrhythmias in the infarcted heart potentially via increased connexin43 expression and arteriogenesis. J Exp Med 203:87-97, 2006.
75. van Rijen HV, Eckardt D, Degen J, et al: Slow conduction and enhanced anisotropy increase the propensity for ventricular tachyarrhythmias in adult mice with induced deletion of connexin43. Circulation 109:1048-1055, 2004.
76. Clarke TC, Thomas D, Petersen JS, et al: The antiarrhythmic peptide rotigaptide (ZP123) increases gap junction intercellular communication in cardiac myocytes and HeLa cells expressing connexin 43. Br J Pharmacol 147:486-495, 2006.
77. Dhein S, Larsen BD, Petersen JS, Mohr FW: Effects of the new antiarrhythmic peptide ZP123 on epicardial activation and repolarization pattern. Cell Commun Adhes 10:371-378, 2003.
78. Shiroshita-Takeshita A, Sakabe M, Haugan K, et al: Model-dependent effects of the gap junction conduction-enhancing antiarrhythmic peptide rotigaptide (ZP123) on experimental atrial fibrillation in dogs. Circulation 115:310-318, 2007.
79. Kasi VS, Xiao HD, Shang LL, et al: Cardiac-restricted angiotensin-converting enzyme overexpression causes conduction defects and connexin dysregulation. Am J Physiol Heart Circ Physiol 293:H182-H192, 2007.
80. Beeres SL, Atsma DE, van der Laarse A, et al: Human adult bone marrow mesenchymal stem cells repair experimental conduction block in rat cardiomyocyte cultures. J Am Coll Cardiol 46:1943-1952, 2005.
81. Bucchi A, Baruscotti M, DiFrancesco D: Current-dependent block of rabbit sinoatrial node I_f channels by ivabradine. J Gen Physiol 120:1-13, 2002.
82. Borer JS, Fox K, Jaillon P, Lerebours G: Antianginal and antiischemic effects of ivabradine, an I_f inhibitor, in stable angina: A randomized, double-blind, multicentered, placebo-controlled trial. Circulation 107:817-823, 2003.
83. Tardif JC, Ford I, Tendera M, et al: Efficacy of ivabradine, a new selective I_f inhibitor, compared with atenolol in patients with chronic stable angina. Eur Heart J 26:2529-2536, 2005.
84. Hansen RS, Diness TG, Christ T, et al: Activation of human ether-a-go-go–related gene potassium channels by the diphenylurea 1,3-bis-(2-hydroxy-5-trifluoromethyl-phenyl)-urea (NS1643). Mol Pharmacol 69:266-277, 2006.
85. Shimizu W, Kurita T, Matsuo K, et al: Improvement of repolarization abnormalities by a K^+ channel opener in the LQT1 form of congenital long-QT syndrome. Circulation 97:1581-1588, 1998.
86. Chang IK, Shyu MK, Lee CN, et al: Prenatal diagnosis and treatment of fetal long QT syndrome: A case report. Prenat Diagn 22:1209-1212, 2002.
87. Maron BJ, Towbin JA, Thiene G, et al: Contemporary definitions and classification of the cardiomyopathies: An American Heart Association Scientific Statement from the Council on Clinical Cardiology, Heart Failure and Transplantation Committee; Quality of Care and Outcomes Research and Functional Genomics and Translational Biology Interdisciplinary Working Groups; and Council on Epidemiology and Prevention. Circulation 113:1807-1816, 2006.
88. Schwartz PJ, Priori SG, Spazzolini C, et al: Genotype-phenotype correlation in the long-QT syndrome: Gene-specific triggers for life-threatening arrhythmias. Circulation 103:89-95, 2001.
89. Fabritz L, Kirchhof P, Franz MR, et al: Effect of pacing and mexiletine on dispersion of repolarisation and arrhythmias in hearts of SCN5A Δ-KPQ (LQT3) mice. Cardiovasc Res 57:1085-1093, 2003.
90. Windle JR, Geletka RC, Moss AJ, et al: Normalization of ventricular repolarization with flecainide in long QT syndrome patients with SCN5A:ΔKPQ mutation. Ann Noninvasive Electrocardiol 6:153-158, 2001.
91. Gaita F, Giustetto C, Bianchi F, et al: Short QT syndrome: Pharmacological treatment. J Am Coll Cardiol 43:1494-1499, 2004.
92. Kirchhof P, Fabritz L, Zwiener M, et al: Age- and training-dependent development of arrhythmogenic right ventricular cardiomyopathy in heterozygous plakoglobin-deficient mice. Circulation 114:1799-1806, 2006.
93. Heidbuchel H, Hoogsteen J, Fagard R, et al: High prevalence of right ventricular involvement in endurance athletes with ventricular arrhythmias. Role of an electrophysiologic study in risk stratification. Eur Heart J 24:1473-1480, 2003.
94. Kirchhof P, Breithardt G: New concepts for old drugs to maintain sinus rhythm in patients with atrial fibrillation. Heart Rhythm 4:790-793, 2007.
95. Alboni P, Botto GL, Baldi N, et al: Outpatient treatment of recent-onset atrial fibrillation with the "pill-in-the-pocket" approach. N Engl J Med 351:2384-2391, 2004.
96. Manios EG, Kanoupakis EM, Chlouverakis GI, et al: Changes in atrial electrical properties following cardioversion of chronic atrial fibrillation: relation with recurrence. Cardiovasc Res 47:244-253, 2000.
97. Kirchhof P, Fetsch T, Hanrath P, et al: Targeted pharmacological reversal of electrical remodeling after cardioversion—rationale and design of the Flecainide Short-Long (Flec-SL) trial. Am Heart J 150:899, 2005.
98. Shinagawa K, Shiroshita-Takeshita A, Schram G, Nattel S: Effects of antiarrhythmic drugs on fibrillation in the remodeled atrium: Insights into the mechanism of the superior efficacy of amiodarone. Circulation 107:1440-1446, 2003.
99. Connolly SJ: Evidence-based analysis of amiodarone efficacy and safety. Circulation 100:2025-2034, 1999.

Impact of Nontraditional Antiarrhythmic Drugs on Sudden Cardiac Death 98

Jeffrey J. Goldberger and Alan H. Kadish

CHAPTER OUTLINE

Although the mortality from coronary artery disease has declined in the United States, sudden cardiac death remains a major clinical problem, with an estimated 300,000 deaths occurring annually. Strategies to decrease the incidence of sudden death include the prevention of underlying structural heart disease, identification of hereditary syndromes that predispose persons to sudden death, improvements in resuscitation of patients who experience a cardiac arrest (secondary prevention), or identification of patients at high risk for sudden death and appropriate intervention.

Potential interventions to prevent sudden death include lifestyle modification, dietary changes, therapy with antiarrhythmic drugs, therapy with other cardiovascular drugs, or device therapy with implantable cardioverter defibrillators (ICDs). Results of therapy with antiarrhythmic drugs that block sodium or potassium channels for the prevention of sudden death have largely been disappointing. Other than amiodarone, these drugs have had either a neutral or deleterious effect upon mortality. ICD therapy effectively prevents sudden death in selected high-risk patients but is costly and has some associated morbidity, and thus there are challenges to applying it on a large scale to all patients who are at risk for sudden cardiac death.

Antiarrhythmic drugs have been classified using several different systems. The Vaughn-Williams classification is the oldest and most commonly used system for antiarrhythmic drugs. In this system, drugs that block sodium channels are considered class I drugs, those that block β-adrenergic receptors are considered class II drugs, those that block potassium channels are considered class III drugs, and those that block calcium channels are considered class IV drugs. β-Blockers are considered antiarrhythmic drugs based on data suggesting that they may be effective in a variety of arrhythmias. However, β-blockers have a number of effects including the prevention of myocardial ischemia, in contrast to other classic antiarrhythmic drugs whose primary mode of action is to block sodium or potassium channels. This chapter deals with the prevention of sudden death using pharmacologic agents whose primary mode of action is not to block sodium or potassium channels: nontraditional antiarrhythmic drugs.

Pathophysiology

One difficulty in interpreting the results of clinical studies on sudden cardiac death is uncertainty about the classification of the mechanism of death. In some studies, all deaths that occurred within 1 to 24 hours after the onset of symptoms were considered sudden cardiac deaths. This definition is obviously not specific for sudden arrhythmic death because many patients who die of myocardial infarction (MI) die within the first 24 hours of symptoms that may be unrelated to an arrhythmia. More recently, "events committees" have been used in clinical trials to classify the mechanism of death. Because many of these trials are large multicenter studies and the degree of information available to an even highly qualified and motivated events committee is sometimes limited, there are some limitations to the classification of the mechanism of death. Thus, in evaluating the effect of nontraditional antiarrhythmic drugs on the incidence of sudden death, we will also consider the effects on total mortality, with the understanding that it is possible that some of the mortality reduction may be due to a decreased incidence of sudden death.

Studies have suggested that the major mechanisms responsible for sudden arrhythmic death are ventricular tachycardia (VT) and ventricular fibrillation (VF). Although bradycardia or electromechanical dissociation may be more common in patients with advanced congestive heart failure or during prolonged cardiac arrest, the weight of evidence suggests that VT or VF is the major mechanism of sudden cardiac death. Thus, evaluating therapies that might alter the occurrence of VT and VF might help decrease the incidence of sudden cardiac death.

There are also data suggesting that the risk of VT and VF varies inversely with left ventricular function. In addition, left ventricular dilatation may be arrhythmogenic by altering cardiac electrophysiologic properties through contraction-excitation feedback. Thus, pharmacologic agents that alter cardiac hemodynamics may be antiarrhythmic by altering ventricular function and size even if direct antiarrhythmic activity is not present.

Despite extensive research, a coherent pathophysiologic scheme for identifying the occurrence of sudden death has not been universally accepted. Although the majority of patients who experience sudden cardiac death have coronary disease and myocardial ischemia, patients with nonischemic cardiomyopathy also have substantial risk for sudden cardiac death. In addition, even in patients with coronary disease, only a minority who experience sudden cardiac death have an acute MI. Transient autonomic and metabolic factors also contribute to sudden death.

One potential model of the pathophysiology of sudden death is shown in Figure 98-1. In this construct, transient factors interact with spontaneous arrhythmias and an underlying anatomic substrate to produce sudden cardiac death. This model recognizes that the triggering beats may be due to reentry, abnormal automaticity, or triggered activity and

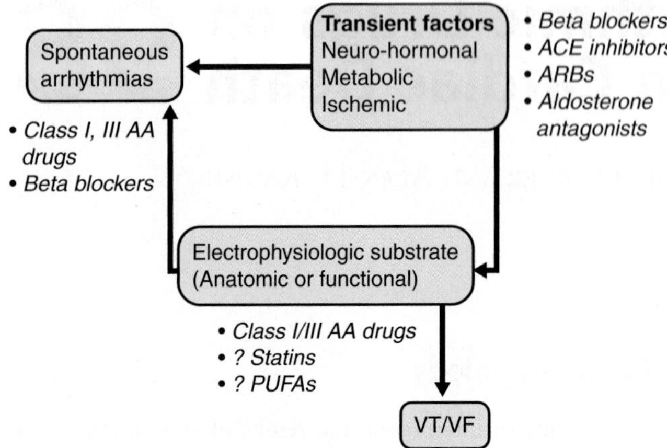

Figure 98-1 Potential mechanism of tachyarrhythmias and possible sites of action of pharmacologic interventions. AA drugs, antiarrhythmic drugs; ACE, angiotensin-converting enzyme; ARBs, adrenergic receptor blockers; PUFA, polyunsaturated fatty acid; VT/VF, ventricular tachycardia or ventricular fibrillation.

that the electrophysiologic substrate could consist of either functional or anatomic reentry. Thus, transient metabolic and autonomic factors that alter electrophysiologic properties can modulate the anatomic substrate for the occurrence of sudden death.

To target the electrophysiologic substrate that forms part of the model, it is necessary to identify a specific electrophysiologic mechanism and to identify specific ion channels that are present in the region of the myocardium that predisposes to sudden death and target those ion channels specifically. At present, antiarrhythmic drugs target sodium or potassium channels that may be present throughout the myocardium, and, therefore, are not specific for the arrhythmic mechanism (focal or reentrant) or region. Drugs such as β-blockers require fewer physiologic assumptions and do not need the specificity required of antiarrhythmic drugs. Therefore, it should not be surprising to find that nontraditional drugs that can act on more global mechanisms of arrhythmia are more effective in preventing sudden death than are drugs that indiscriminately block ion channels throughout the myocardium. Potential target sites for therapies that might reduce sudden death are shown in Figure 98-1. Table 98-1 shows interventions that might reduce mortality in patients with heart disease and the drugs that might reduce the incidence of sudden death.

β-Adrenergic Blockers

β-Adrenergic blockers (β-blockers) have emerged as important pharmacologic agents for both primary and secondary prevention of sudden cardiac death (Table 98-2). β-Blockers first were recognized as prophylactic agents for preventing sudden death in patients after MI. More recently, large-scale clinical trials have also demonstrated their efficacy in the primary prevention of sudden cardiac death in patients with congestive heart failure. There are also substantial data supporting the efficacy of β-blockers in preventing recurrences of significant ventricular tachyarrhythmias.

Efficacy of β-Blockers after Myocardial Infarction

Analysis by Freemantle and colleagues[1] of more than 50,000 patients evaluated in numerous randomized clinical trials demonstrated a substantial reduction in mortality due to β-blocker treatment (relative risk [RR], 0.77; 95% confidence interval [CI], 0.69-0.85). The largest observational report includes more than 200,000 patients in the Medicare database.[2] The benefits of β-blocker therapy have withstood the test of time despite the advent of newer therapies such as thrombolytic therapy.[3] In the Carvedilol Post-Infarct Survival Control in LV Dysfunction study (CAPRICORN), 12% mortality was seen in patients treated with carvedilol and 15% mortality in those treated with placebo (risk reduction, 23%; 95% CI, 2%-40%). Further analysis of these data[4] revealed a significant reduction in malignant ventricular arrhythmias in patients treated with carvedilol (hazard ration [HR], 0.24; 95% CI, 0.11-0.49, $P < 0.0001$).

Table 98-1 Pharmacologic Agents Shown to Decrease Mortality in Patients with Chronic Heart Disease

	Possible Mechanisms				
Agent	**Antiarrhythmic**	**Antiatherosclerotic**	**Anti-inflammatory**	**Anti-ischemic**	**Hemodynamic**
β-Blockers	x			x	
Angiotensin-converting enzyme inhibitors	?				x
Angiotensin receptor blockers	?				x
Fish oil	x	x			
Spironolactone	x				x
Aspirin			x	x	
3-Hydroxy-3-methylglutaryl		x			
Coenzyme A reductase inhibitors					
Amiodarone	x			?	
Vasodilators (hydralazine, nitrates)					x

Table 98-2 Efficacy of Drugs in Reducing Mortality and Preventing Sudden Death

Drug	Control	Study	Patients	Total N	Follow-up	Total Mortality (RR or HR) (95% CI)	SCD (RR or HR) (95% CI)
Angiotensin-Converting Enzyme Inhibitors							
Ramipril	Placebo	AIRE[16]	Post-MI + CHF	2006	15 mo	RR 0.73 (0.60-0.89)	RR 0.70 (0.53-0.92)
Ramipril	Placebo	HOPE[18]	CV disease or DM + CRF	9297	5 yr	RR 0.84 (0.75-0.95)	RR 0.62 (0.41-0.94)*
Captopril	Placebo	SAVE[48]	Post MI + EF	2231	42 mo	RR 0.81 (0.68-0.97)	NS
Enalapril	Placebo	CONSENSUS I[20]	AMI	6090	6 mo	RR 1.10 (0.93-1.29)	NS
Enalapril	Placebo	SOLVD-P[19] Prevention	EF	4228	37 mo	RR 0.92 (0.79-1.08)	RR 0.93 (0.70-1.22)
Enalapril	Hydral/isosorbide	V-Heft II[49]	CHF	804	2.5 yr	RR 0.72	RR 0.65
Zofenopril	Placebo	SMILE[50]	AMI	1556	6 wk	RR 0.78 (0.52-1.12)	RR 0.37 (0.11-1.02)
Trandolapril	Placebo	TRACE[17]	Post MI + EF	1749	24-50 mo	RR 0.78 (0.67-0.91)	RR 0.76 (0.59-0.98)
Angiotensin II Receptor Blockers							
Valsartan	Placebo	Val-Heft[51]	CHF	5010	23 mo	RR 1.02 (0.88-1.18), 98% CI	NS
Losartan	Captopril	ELITE[25]	CHF	722	48 wk	RR 0.54 (0.31-0.95)	RR 0.36 (0.14-0.97)
Losartan	Captopril	ELITE II[26]	CHF	3152	1.5 yr	HR 1.13 (0.95-1.35), 95.7% CI	HR 1.30 (1.00-1.69)
Losartan	Atenolol	LIFE[52]	HTN+LVH	9193	4.8 yr	HR 0.90 (0.78-1.03)	HR 1.91 (0.64-5.72)†
Losartan	Captopril	OPTIMAAL[27]	Post MI + CHF	5477	2.7 yr	RR 1.13 (0.99-1.28)	RR 1.19 (0.99-1.43)‡
β-Blockers							
Class	Placebo	1999 Meta-analysis[53]	Post-MI	24,974		RR 0.77 (0.69-0.85)	
Class	Placebo	Medicare Database[2]	Post-MI	201,752	2 yr	RR 0.60 (0.57-0.63)	
Carvedilol	Placebo	CAPRICORN[4]	Post-MI + EF	1959	1.3 yr	HR 0.77 (0.60-0.98)	HR 0.74 (0.51-1.06)
Metoprolol	Placebo	MERIT-HF[54]	CHF	3991	1 yr	RR 0.66 (0.53-0.81)	RR 0.59 (0.45-0.78)
Bisoprolol	Placebo	CIBIS-II[6]	CHF	2657	1.3yr	HR 0.66 (0.54-0.81)	HR 0.56 (0.39-0.80)

Note: See text for study abbreviations.

*Cardiac arrest.

†Resuscitated cardiac arrest.

‡Sudden cardiac death plus resuscitated cardiac arrest.

ACE, angiotensin-converting enzyme; AMI, acute myocardial infarction; ARB, angiotensin receptor blockers; CHF, congestive heart failure; CI, confidence interval; CRF, cardiac risk factor; CV, cardiovascular; DM, diabetes mellitus; EF, ejection fraction; HR, hazard ratio; HTN, hypertension; LVH, left ventricular hypertrophy; MI, myocardial infarction; NS, not significant; RR, relative risk; SCD, sudden cardiac death.

Efficacy of β-Blockers in Patients with Congestive Heart Failure

β-Blockers are also important agents in the prevention of sudden cardiac death in patients with congestive heart failure. In this population, carvedilol has been shown to reduce mortality.[5] Although this study was not designed as a mortality trial, carvedilol reduced total mortality by 65%. In the Cardiac Insufficiency Bisoprolol Study II (CIBIS-II),[6] the estimated annual mortality was 8.8% in patients treated with bisoprolol and 13.2% in those receiving placebo (risk reduction, 34%; 95% CI, 19%-46%). Metoprolol has also been demonstrated to improve survival in patients with congestive heart failure. In the Metoprolol CR/XL Randomized Intervention Trial in Congestive Heart Failure (MERIT-HF), 3991 patients with class II to IV (96% had class II and III) congestive heart failure (ejection fraction [EF] <40%) were randomly assigned to treatment with metoprolol ($n = 1990$) or placebo ($n = 2001$). This trial was also terminated early by the safety committee because of the benefit of β-blocker therapy. The mortality was 7.2% per patient-year of follow-up in the metoprolol group versus 11.0% in the placebo group (relative risk reduction, 34%; 95% CI, 19%-47%). In both trials, prevention of sudden death was an important component of mortality improvement.

Efficacy of β-Blockers in Secondary Prevention of Sudden Death

There are some data supporting the efficacy of β-blockers in patients known to have ventricular tachyarrhythmias. Clinical information from the Antiarrhythmics Versus Implantable Defibrillators (AVID) trial registry provides support for the role of β-blocker therapy in patients with sustained ventricular tachyarrhythmias.[7] There was an approximately 50% reduction in adjusted relative risk of mortality due to β-blocker therapy. Metoprolol has been shown to reduce the incidence of ventricular tachyarrhythmias in patients with implantable defibrillators.[8] The overwhelming majority of the study populations in all these reports were patients with coronary artery disease. Limited data suggest that β-blocker therapy in patients with nonischemic dilated cardiomyopathy and ICDs is associated with a marked reduction in appropriate therapy for ventricular tachyarrhythmias.[9] In a multivariate analysis from this study, β-blocker therapy was associated with a 0.15 relative risk (95% CI, 0.05-0.45, $P < 0.0007$) of appropriate ICD therapy. β-Blockers also have documented efficacy in treating patients with long-QT syndrome.[10]

Although β-blockers are perhaps the single most effective pharmacologic agent for preventing sudden cardiac death, it is noteworthy that there are other therapies that can provide additional benefit when added to β-blocker therapy. Steinbeck and associates[11] randomly assigned 115 patients with VT to one of two treatment approaches: β-blocker therapy or electrophysiology testing–guided therapy. Although the overall results for the two groups were similar, the 1-year recurrence rate and sudden death rate in the β-blocker group exceeded 40%. This rate was significantly greater than the recurrence rate and sudden death rate noted in patients treated with an antiarrhythmic drug proved to be efficacious by electrophysiologic testing (10% at 1 year). In both the European Myocardial Infarct Amiodarone Trial (EMIAT) and the Canadian Amiodarone Myocardial Infraction Arrhythmia Trial (CAMIAT), there appeared to be an interaction between the use of β-blockers and amiodarone; specifically, amiodarone therapy had a greater effect on mortality reduction in patients receiving β-blockers.[12] In CAMIAT, there was an 87% reduction in relative risk ($P = 0.008$) related to amiodarone therapy (versus placebo) in patients who were receiving concomitant therapy with β-blockers. Thus, although β-blocker therapy appears to be an important agent in the strategy of preventing sudden cardiac death, monotherapy with β-blockers might not be sufficient for prevention of sudden cardiac death in susceptible populations.

Mechanism of Benefit of β-Blockers

Post-MI β-blocker trials in which cause-specific mortality has been evaluated have shown that the majority of the survival benefit of β-blocker therapy is due to a reduction in sudden death.

The clinical benefits of β-blocker therapy probably stem from the important role β-adrenergic receptor signaling plays in cardiovascular control in health and in disease. Given the ubiquitous nature of these receptors throughout the heart and the pathophysiologic changes in cardiac sympathetic nerves, cardiac responsiveness to sympathetic stimulation, and circulating catecholamines that can occur in the setting of cardiac disease, adverse electrophysiologic effects may be noted that predispose to the development of life-threatening ventricular tachyarrhythmias. For example, myocardial infarction has been associated with regional denervation.[13] This can lead to denervation supersensitivity apical to the infarction. After MI, there are changes in heart rate variability and baroreflex sensitivity that can reflect abnormalities of parasympathetic and sympathetic tone.

Renin-Angiotensin-Aldosterone System

Angiotensin-Converting Enzyme Inhibitors

Angiotensin-converting enzyme (ACE) inhibitors have been extensively studied in patients at risk for sudden cardiac death, including patients with congestive heart failure and MI. Although studies involving ACE inhibitors have shown substantial reductions in total mortality (with risk reductions ranging from 8% to 40%) or cardiovascular mortality, very few have also shown similar effects with respect to arrhythmic death.

There are several possible antiarrhythmic actions of ACE inhibitors. Except in the postinfarction period, a direct antiarrhythmic effect has been reported but is inconsistent. In patients with or without heart failure, hypokalemia has been shown to be an important risk factor for ventricular arrhythmias. ACE inhibitors can raise serum potassium levels, which therefore leads to a possible beneficial effect on the myocardial substrate.[14] These results have not been consistent in other studies. However, ACE inhibitors have several direct and indirect effects on the autonomic nervous system that could modify the risk of ventricular arrhythmias. They enhance baroreflex sensitivity, thereby reducing sympathetic and increasing parasympathetic tone. Improvements in hemodynamics can also lead to a decrease in circulating catecholamines. Ventricular remodeling, a complex process involving fibrosis and dilatation of the failing heart, has been shown to have adverse effects on the electrical system of the heart, and reductions in cardiac dilatation can lead to reductions in ventricular arrhythmias.[15] Therefore, ACE-inhibitor treatment, by impeding remodeling, can lead to fewer arrhythmias and a lower incidence of sudden death.

The Acute Infarction Ramipril Efficacy study (AIRE) and the Trandolapril Cardiac Evaluation (TRACE) study have been the only two placebo-controlled trials with ACE inhibitors to show significant reductions in sudden cardiac death.[16,17] Both were conducted in patients with recent MIs. In the AIRE study, 2006 patients with a recent MI and clinical evidence of heart failure were randomly assigned to treatment with ramipril (5 mg daily) or placebo. At 15 months, the ramipril group had a 27% reduction in total mortality. There was also a 30%

reduction in sudden cardiac death (12.3%-8.9%). In the TRACE study, there was a 25% decrease in cardiovascular deaths. There was also a 26% reduction in sudden cardiac death (15.2%-12.0%). A meta-analysis of intermediate- or long-term post-MI ACE inhibitor trials (including AIRE and TRACE) involving a total of 15,104 patients showed a trend toward decreased sudden cardiac death in all of the larger trials and an overall reduction in sudden cardiac death with an odds ratio of 0.80 (95% CI, 0.70-0.92). There were also similar significant reductions in total and cardiovascular mortality.[7]

In the Heart Outcomes Prevention Evaluation (HOPE) study, more than 9000 patients with vascular disease or diabetes mellitus and a cardiac risk factor were randomly assigned to treatment with ramipril or placebo.[18] After 5 years, there was a 26% reduction in cardiovascular mortality and a 37% reduction in cardiac arrest. Sudden cardiac death was not specifically studied.

No randomized, controlled trials of an ACE inhibitor versus placebo in patients with chronic heart failure have shown a reduction in sudden cardiac death. The three major trials that have reported results for sudden death are the Cooperative New Scandinavian Enalapril Survival Study (CONSENSUS), the Studies of Left Ventricular Dysfunction (SOLVD)-Treatment, and the SOLVD-Prevention.[19,20] No clear reduction in sudden death mortality was noted. A number of other trials of ACE inhibitors have found that there is a reduction in total mortality with ACE inhibitors. However, these studies have not separated statistically sudden death mortality from other causes. Thus, it is unclear in these studies whether important mortality reductions in sudden death occurred.

Angiotensin-Receptor Blockers

Physiologically active levels of angiotensin II, a potent vasoconstrictor, persist despite long-term therapy with ACE inhibitors and might also be formed by non–ACE-dependent pathways. Possible arrhythmogenic mechanisms of angiotensin II include activation of neurohormonal agents (including norepinephrine, aldosterone, and endothelin) as well as increased conduction velocity and shorter refractory periods in cardiac myocytes.[21] Furthermore, unlike ACE inhibitors, angiotensin II receptor blockers (ARBs) do not increase bradykinin levels, which also can increase norepinephrine levels.[22] Elevated catecholamine levels theoretically could result in more ventricular arrhythmias and sudden death. Therefore, direct blockade of angiotensin II receptors might further reduce morbidity and mortality in patients requiring blockade of the renin-angiotensin-aldosterone system. These protective effects of angiotensin II may be questioned by a substudy of the Randomized Aldactone Evaluation Study (RALES) (see later). Patients with congestive heart failure treated with ACE inhibitors and randomly assigned to treatment with spironolactone had significant decreases in sudden death despite significant increases in plasma angiotensin II.[23] ARBs, as well as ACE inhibitors, increase serum potassium levels and might benefit from this potential protective mechanism as well.

ARBs have mostly been compared to ACE inhibitors in several heart failure or hypertension trials. Importantly, a meta-analysis has shown that the overall mortality rates for the two classes are similar.[24] Only one study showed a reduction in sudden death with ARBs compared with ACE inhibitors, and results of larger trials have countered these results. In the Evaluation of Losartan in the Elderly (ELITE) study, 722 patients with classes II to IV heart failure and ejection fractions 40% or less were randomly assigned to treatment with losartan or captopril.[25] At 48 weeks, the losartan group had a 45% reduction in total mortality. There was also a decrease in the number of deaths attributable to sudden cardiac death (five vs. 14 patients), with a relative risk reduction of 36%. However, in the much larger ELITE II, 3152 patients (with heart failure and ejection fraction <40%) were randomly assigned to treatment with losartan or captopril.[26] At 1.5 years, there were strong trends toward reductions in overall mortality and sudden death with captopril compared with losartan. In the Optimal Trial in Myocardial Infarction with the Angiotensin II Antagonist Losartan (OPTIMAAL), losartan and captopril were also studied in patients after MI with heart failure, and favorable results for captopril, similar to those for ELITE II, were found.[27]

Aldosterone-Receptor Antagonists

Neurohormonal suppression of the renin-angiotensin-aldosterone system by ACE inhibitors is incomplete. Therefore, aldosterone can continue to exert harmful effects on the cardiovascular system in patients with heart failure. Aldosterone promotes sodium retention, magnesium and potassium wasting, sympathetic activation, parasympathetic inhibition, myocardial and vascular fibrosis, baroreceptor dysfunction, and vascular damage, and it impairs arterial compliance.

Spironolactone, an aldosterone receptor antagonist and potassium-sparing diuretic, has gained wide acceptance for treating severe congestive heart failure. In the RALES study, 1663 patients with New York Heart Association (NYHA) class III or IV heart failure and ejection fraction 35% or less were randomly assigned to treatment with spironolactone (25 mg daily) or placebo.[28] After a mean follow-up of 24 months, cardiac death was decreased by 31%. This was due to a 36% decrease in death of progressive heart failure and a 29% reduction in sudden cardiac death.

In the Eplerenone Post Myocardial Heart Failure Efficacy and Survival Study (EPHESUS), Eplerenone was used in myocardial infarction survivors with left ventricular dysfunction. Overall mortality and sudden death mortality were reduced by eplerenone. There was a 20% reduction in sudden death mortality ($P < 0.05$). In addition, there is a 16% reduction in overall mortality that was highly significant.[29]

There are several possible mechanisms for a direct antiarrhythmic effect of aldosterone antagonists. One possible explanation is that aldosterone seems to enhance cardiac remodeling. Fibroblasts and inflammatory cells invade the perivascular space of damaged vessels, leading to fibrosis. These changes can have adverse effects on the mechanical function, vasodilatory reserve, and electrical system of the heart. A substudy of the RALES trial evaluated serum markers of collagen synthesis, which has been shown to correlate with morphologic evidence of cardiac fibrosis.[30] Spironolactone decreased the levels of these markers at 6 months, whereas the levels in the placebo group remained constant. Once again, the small increase in serum potassium levels seen with spironolactone might have a protective effect, offsetting the hypokalemia that can occur with concomitant diuretic therapy. In the spironolactone arm of the RALES study, serum potassium levels were 0.3 mEq/L higher than in the placebo arm. Several studies have shown that non–potassium-sparing diuretics are associated with an increase in sudden cardiac death and that there is a dose-response curve.

Modulators of Cholesterol and Inflammation

3-Hydroxy-3-Methylglutaryl-Coenzyme A Reductase Inhibitors

Numerous randomized, placebo-controlled clinical trials have documented the cardiovascular benefits of 3-hydroxy-3-methylglutaryl-coenzyme A reductase inhibitors, or statins.

Although these drugs are widely accepted as preventing coronary heart disease death and MI, it is much less clear whether they have antiarrhythmic properties beyond their actions in the coronary artery. Statins might exert an antiarrhythmic benefit by reducing the overall ischemic burden, as documented in many trials, with reduced ischemia and infarctions. However, statins have been shown to have beneficial effects beyond prevention of plaque progression, in that the number of clinical events is reduced as soon as 16 weeks after therapy is initiated. Actions on endothelial function, inflammation, plaque stabilization, and platelets might contribute to this early effect. It is not known whether any direct electrophysiologic effects might contribute to the beneficial effects of statins.

A potential antiarrhythmic benefit of statins was first hinted at in two secondary prevention trials. In the Scandinavian Simvastatin Survival Study (4S), 4444 patients with coronary artery disease and hypercholesterolemia were randomly assigned to receive treatment with simvastatin or placebo.[31] After 5.4 years, there was a 30% decrease in total mortality. Data on instantaneous death and death occurring within 1 hour of symptom onset were supplied but not statistically assessed. In the placebo group there were 63 sudden deaths, whereas the simvastatin group had 37. In the Long-term Intervention with Pravastatin in Ischemic Heart Disease (LIPID) study, 9014 patients with coronary artery disease and hypercholesterolemia were randomly assigned to receive treatment with pravastatin or placebo.[32] After 6.1 years, there was a 22% reduction in total mortality with pravastatin. There were 211 sudden deaths in the placebo group and 182 in the simvastatin group. Again, these results were not statistically analyzed. However, they suggest a possible antiarrhythmic benefit, but because of the length of follow-up of these trials, differences in sudden death could also be due to the ability of statins to prevent progression of atherosclerosis.

Other studies have suggested that statin therapy is associated with a reduction in ventricular tachyarrhythmias or appropriate ICD therapy in patients with coronary artery disease.[33-35] Post hoc analyses of the AVID and MADIT-II patients with coronary artery disease treated with an implantable defibrillator[33] demonstrated 40% and 28% reductions, respectively, in VT and VF episodes in patients treated with statins. Retrospective analyses[36-38] in patients with nonischemic dilated cardiomyopathy have also shown a reduction in sudden death or mortality associated with statin use. In the DEFINITE study, of 458 patients with nonischemic dilated cardiomyopathy (randomized to medical therapy versus medical therapy plus an implantable defibrillator), 110 were being treated with statins.[36] Statin use was associated with a significant reduction in total mortality (adjusted HR, 0.23; 95% CI, 0.09-0.58; $P = 0.002$). Only one arrhythmic death was noted in the 110 patients treated with statins, and 18 were noted in the 348 patients not treated with statins. Interestingly, there was no difference in the incidence of appropriate shocks in those treated versus not treated with statins.

An analysis of the SCD-HeFT study[37] showed that the mortality reduction related to statin use was identical in those with ischemic heart disease as those with nonischemic dilated cardiomyopathy (HRs, 0.69 and 0.67, respectively). If statins prevent arrhythmic events in patients with nonischemic dilated cardiomyopathy, it seems unlikely that the mechanism would be related to any anti-ischemic effects. It has therefore been assumed that this effect on arrhythmic sudden death is due to the multiple pleiotropic effects of statins. Although these data provide strong support for the possibility that statins reduce the incidence of arrhythmic sudden death, there are large-scale studies[39,40] that have not demonstrated this benefit, though this may be related to the low incidence of these events or short duration of follow-up.

Polyunsaturated Fatty Acids

Clues to the cardioprotective benefits of ω-3 polyunsaturated fatty acids (PUFAs) were originally discovered in epidemiologic studies in Inuit and Mediterranean peoples. Common to those peoples' diets were high intakes of fatty fish, which have high levels of these molecules, named for their double-bond three carbons from the N terminus. Important ω-3 PUFAs include eicosapentaenoic acid, docosahexaenoic acid, and α-linolenic acid. The cardioprotective mechanisms of ω-3 PUFAs are still being elucidated. Through their actions on I_{Na} and I_{CaL} channels, the ω-3 PUFAs cause a mild hyperpolarization of the resting membrane potential, resulting in a larger threshold voltage and stimulus and prolonging the refractory period of the cardiac cycle. These properties might explain an enhanced electrical stability in the setting of ischemia and toxins.

Several prospective cohort studies have shown an association with ω-3 PUFAs and sudden cardiac death in patients with and without known coronary disease. In the DART trial, men who recently survived an MI were randomly assigned to one of eight groups of dietary intervention.[41] In the group assigned to receive an increase in fatty fish consumption, at 2 years, there was a 33% relative decrease in deaths due to coronary heart disease, whereas there was a nonsignificant increase in the incidence of nonfatal MI. The mortality benefit was mostly seen in the first 6 months. There were eight sudden cardiac deaths in the experimental group and none in the control group. In the Nurse's Health Study,[42] food frequency questionnaires in 76,763 participating women were used to assess α-linolenic acid intake, which was inversely related to the risk of sudden cardiac death but not nonfatal MI. The GISSI-Prevenzione study, a multicenter, open-label, randomized trial, tested 11,323 patients with recent infarction.[43] At an average of 42 months of follow up, sudden death occurred in 2.7% of control subjects and 2% of patients receiving ω-3 PUFAs ($P < 0.001$) and accounted for 59% of the total mortality benefit. Also importantly, the differences in sudden death percentages approached significance by 3 months, with no change in plasma lipid levels. A further substudy[44] found that the reduction in sudden death related to ω-3 PUFAs was greater in patients with left ventricular dysfunction.

Several studies[45-47] have used a double-blind, placebo-controlled approach to prospectively evaluate the role of fish oil supplementation (1.8-2.6 g/day) in patients with ICDs. Leaf and colleagues[45] randomized 402 patients with ICDs and assessed a number of intention-to-treat and on-treatment endpoints. For the primary endpoint, time to first episode of VT and VF, there was a nonsignificant beneficial effect of fish oil supplementation (RR, 0.72; 95% CI, 0.51-1.01; $P < 0.057$). Other analyses revealed significant beneficial effects of fish oil supplementation.

Raitt and coworkers[47] studied 200 patients with ICDs. Patients receiving fish oil supplements had an increase in the red blood cell membrane ω-3 PUFAs, and patients receiving placebo did not. In this study, there were 45 episodes of VF and 901 episodes of VT over a median follow-up duration of 718 days. Fish oil supplementation did not prolong the time to first episode of VT or VF. Based on the trends observed, the authors suggested that fish oil may be proarrhythmic in this population.

The Study on Omega-3 Fatty acids and ventricular Arrhythmia (SOFA) group[46] randomized 546 patients with ICDs and found no effect of ω-3 PUFAs on time to VT or VF. While the wealth of data suggest that ω-3 PUFAs prevent sudden death, their effect on ICD therapies for VT or VF have not been demonstrated. This observed difference may be related to the specific heart disease characteristics, the type of study, clinical scenario (ischemia or infarction), and type and dose of supplementation, among others. It is also possible that ω-3 PUFAs suppress VF but not VT, accounting for a reduction in sudden death but not ICD therapies.

Conclusion

In contrast to traditional antiarrhythmic drugs that block sodium or potassium channels, drugs with antiadrenergic effects and neurohormonal effects have been shown to decrease both total and sudden death mortality in patients with underlying structural heart disease. Although amiodarone has been demonstrated to decrease sudden death in some trials, it is plausible to assume that the antiadrenergic effect of amiodarone is responsible for its efficacy because other sodium and potassium channel–blocking drugs increase or have a neutral effect on sudden death mortality.

There are two important lessons to be learned from the results of drug trials to decrease sudden death mortality. Life-threatening cardiac arrhythmias that are by nature highly sporadic or at least in part dependent on a complex series of extracardiac influences can be modulated by drugs that modify the adrenergic and the renin-angiotensin-aldosterone systems. In addition, nonspecific drugs whose primary mode of action is on cardiac ion channels are not effective at reducing sudden death. This observation suggests that despite advances in our knowledge of the basic mechanisms for cardiac arrhythmias, our current understanding of the mechanisms of sudden death are not adequate to target specific ion channels to prevent sudden death. Further studies on regional variations in ion channel properties in disease and on genetic interactions will probably be required before the development of an antiarrhythmic drug that significantly reduces sudden cardiac death. In addition, further basic research is needed to more fully understand the mechanisms of sudden death.

References

1. Freemantle N, Cleland J, Young P, et al: Beta blockade after myocardial infarction: Systematic review and meta regression analysis. BMJ 318:1730-1737, 1999.
2. Gottlieb S, McCarter R, Vogel R: Effect of beta-blockade on mortality among high-risk and low-risk patients after myocardial infarction. N Engl J Med 339:489-497, 1998.
3. Pfisterer M, Cox J, Granger C, et al: Atenolol use and clinical outcomes after thrombolysis for acute myocardial infarction: The GUSTO-I experience. J Am Coll Cardiol 32:634-640, 1998.
4. McMurray J, Køber L, Robertson M, et al: Antiarrhythmic effect of carvedilol after acute myocardial infarction: Results of the Carvedilol Post-Infarct Survival Control in Left Ventricular Dysfunction (CAPRICORN) trial. J Am Coll Cardiol 45:531-532, 2005.
5. Packer M, Bristow M, Cohn J, et al: The effect of carvedilol on morbidity and mortality in patients with chronic heart failure. N Engl J Med 334:1349-1355, 1996.
6. Lechat P, Brunhuber K, Hofmann R, et al: The cardiac insufficiency bisoprolol study II (CIBIS-II): A randomized trial. Lancet 353:9-13, 1999.
7. Domanski M, Exner D, Borkowf C, et al: Effect of angiotensin converting enzyme inhibition on sudden cardiac death in patients following acute myocardial infarction: A meta-analysis of randomized clinical trials. J Am Coll Cardiol 33:598-604, 1999.
8. Seidl K, Hauer B, Schwick N, et al: Comparison of metoprolol and sotalol in preventing ventricular tachyarrhythmias after the implantation of a cardioverter/defibrillator. Am J Cardiol 82:744-748, 1998.
9. Rankovic V, Karha J, Passman R, et al: Predictors of appropriate implantable cardioverter-defibrillator therapy in patients with idiopathic dilated cardiomyopathy. Am J Cardiol 89:1072-1076, 2002.
10. Moss A, Zareba W, Hall W, et al: Effectiveness and limitations of beta-blocker therapy in congenital long-QT syndrome. Circulation 101:616-623, 2002.
11. Steinbeck G, Andresen D, Bach P, et al: A comparison of electrophysiologically guided antiarrhythmic drug therapy with beta-blocker therapy in patients with symptomatic, sustained ventricular tachyarrhythmias. N Engl J Med 327:987-992, 1992.
12. Boutitie F, Boissel J, Connolly S, et al, and the EMIAT and CAMIAT Investigators: Amiodarone interaction with beta-blockers: Analysis of the merged EMIAT (European Myocardial Infarct Amiodarone Trial) and CAMIAT (Canadian Amiodarone Myocardial Infarction Trial) Databases. Circulation 99:2268-2275, 1999.
13. Inoue H, Zipes D: Time course of denervation of efferent sympathetic and vagal nerves after occlusion of the coronary artery in the canine heart. Circ Res 62:1111-1120, 1988.
14. Cleland J, Dargie H, Ball S, et al: Effects of enalapril in heart failure: A double-blind study of effects on exercise performance, renal function, hormones, and metabolic state. Br Heart J 54:305-312, 1985.
15. Pogwizd S: Focal mechanisms underlying ventricular tachycardia during prolonged ischemic cardiomyopathy. Circulation 90:1441-1458, 1998.
16. Cleland J, Erhardt L, Murray G, et al: Effect of ramipril on morbidity and mode of death among survivors of acute myocardial infarction with clinical evidence of heart failure. Eur Heart J 18:41-51, 1997.
17. Køber L, Torp-Pederson C, Carlsen JE, et al: A clinical trial of the angiotensin-converting-enzyme inhibitor trandolapril in patients with left ventricular dysfunction after myocardial infarction. Trandolapril Cardiac Evaluation (TRACE) Study Group. N Engl J Med 333:1670-1676, 1995.
18. Yusuf S, Sleight P, Pogue J, et al; THOPES Investigators: Effects of an angiotensin-converting-enzyme inhibitor, ramipril, on cardiovascular events in high-risk patients. N Engl J Med 342:145-153, 2002.
19. SOLVD Investigators: Effect of enalapril on mortality and the development of heart failure in asymptomatic patients with reduced left ventricular ejection fractions. N Engl J Med 327:685-691, 1992.
20. CONSENSUS Trial Study Group: Effects of enalapril on mortality in severe congestive heart failure: Results of a Cooperative North Scandinavian Enalapril Survival Study (CONSENSUS). N Engl J Med 316:1429-1435, 1987.
21. Gavras I, Gavras H: The antiarrhythmic potential of angiotensin II antagonism: Experience with losartan. Am J Hypertens 13:512-517, 2002.
22. Minisi A, Thames M: Distribution of left ventricular sympathetic afferents demonstrated by reflex responses to transmural myocardial ischemia and to intracoronary and epicardial bradykinin. Circulation 87:240-246, 1993.
23. Rousseau M, Gurne O, Duprez D, et al: Beneficial neurohormonal profile of spironolactone in severe congestive heart failure: Results from the RALES neurohormonal substudy. J Am Coll Cardiol 40:1596-1601, 2002.
24. Jong P, Demers C, McKelvie R, Liu P: Angiotensin receptor blockers in heart failure: Meta-analysis of randomized controlled trials. J Am Coll Cardiol 39:463-470, 2002.
25. Pitt B, Martinez F, Meurers G, et al: Randomized trial of losartan vs. captopril in patients $\geq$ 65 with heart failure (Evaluation of Losartan in the Elderly study, ELITE). Lancet 349:747-752, 1997.
26. Pitt B, Poole-Wilson P, Segal R, et al: Effect of losartan compared with captopril on mortality in patients with symptomatic heart failure: Randomized trial—the Losartan Heart Failure Survival Study ELITE II. Lancet 355:1582-1587, 2002.
27. Dickstein K, Kjekshus J; OPTIMAAL Steering Committee for the OPTIMAAL Study Group: Effects of losartan and captopril on mortality and morbidity in high-risk patients after acute myocardial infarction: The OPTIMAAL randomized trial. Lancet 360:752-760, 2002.
28. Pitt B, Zannad F, Remme W, et al: The effect of spironolactone on morbidity and mortality in patients with severe heart failure. N Engl J Med 341:709-717, 1999.
29. Pitt B, Remme W, Zannad F, et al: Eplerenone, a selective aldosterone blocker, in patients with left ventricular dysfunction

after myocardial infarction. N Engl J Med 348:1309-1321, 2003.
30. Zannad F, Alla F, Dousset B, et al: Limitation of excessive extracellular matrix turnover may contribute to survival benefit of spironolactone therapy in patients with congestive heart failure: insights from the randomized aldactone evaluation study (RALES). Circulation 102:2700-2706, 2000.
31. Scandinavian Simvastatin Survival Study Group: Randomized trial for cholesterol lowering in 4444 patients with coronary heart disease: The Scandinavian Simvastatin Survival Study (4S). Lancet 344:1383-1389, 1994.
32. The Long-Term Intervention with Pravastatinin Ischemic Disease (LIPID) Study Group: Prevention of cardiovascular events and death with pravastatin in patient with coronary heart disease and a broad range of initial cholesterol levels. N Engl J Med 339:1349-1357, 1998.
33. Vyas A, Guo H, Moss A, et al: Reduction in ventricular tachyarrhythmias with statins in the Multicenter Automatic Defibrillator Implantation Trial (MADIT)-II. J Am Coll Cardiol 47:769-773, 2006.
34. Chiu J, Abdelhadi R, Chung M, et al: Effect of statin therapy on risk of ventricular arrhythmia among patients with coronary artery disease and an implantable cardioverter-defibrillator. Am J Cardiol 95:490-491, 2005.
35. Mitchell L, Powell J, Gillis A, et al: Are lipid-lowering drugs also antiarrhythmic drugs? An analysis of the Antiarrhythmics versus Implantable Defibrillators (AVID) trial. J Am Coll Cardiol 42:81-87, 2003.
36. Goldberger J, Subacius H, Schaechter A, et al: Effects of statin therapy on arrhythmic events and survival in patients with nonischemic dilated cardiomyopathy. J Am Coll Cardiol 48:1228-1233, 2006.
37. Dickinson M, Ip J, Olshansky B, et al: Statin use was associated with reduced mortality in both ischemic and nonischemic cardiomyopathy and in patients with implantable defibrillators: Mortality data and mechanistic insights from the Sudden Cardiac Death in Heart Failure Trial (SCD-HeFT). Am Heart J 153:573-578, 2007.
38. Go A, Lee W, Yang J, et al: Statin therapy and risks for death and hospitalization in chronic heart failure. JAMA 296:2105-2111, 2006.
39. Schwartz G, Olsson A, Ezekowitz M, et al: Atorvastatin for acute coronary syndromes. JAMA 286:533-535, 2001.
40. Sever P, Dahlöf B, Poulter N, et al: Prevention of coronary and stroke events with atorvastatin in hypertensive patients who have average or lower-than-average cholesterol concentrations, in the Anglo-Scandinavian Cardiac Outcomes Trial—Lipid Lowering Arm (ASCOT-LLA): a multicentre randomised controlled trial. Lancet 361:1149-1158, 2003.
41. Burr M, Fehily A, Gilbert J, et al: Effects of changes in fat, fish, and fiber intakes on death and reinfarction: Diet and reinfarction trial (DART). Lancet ii:757-761, 1989.
42. Albert C, Oh K, Whang W, et al: Dietary alpha-linolenic acid intake and risk of sudden cardiac death and coronary heart disease. Circulation 112:3232-3238, 2005.
43. Marchioli R, Barzi F, Bomba E, et al: Early protection against sudden death by n-3 polyunsaturated fatty acids after myocardial infarction. Circulation 105:1903-1997, 2002.
44. Macchia A, Levantesi G, Franzosi M, et al: Left ventricular systolic dysfunction, total mortality, and sudden death in patients with myocardial infarction treated with n-3 polyunsaturated fatty acids. Eur J Heart Fail 7:904-909, 2005.
45. Leaf A, Albert C, Johnson D, et al: Prevention of fatal arrhythmias in high-risk subjects by fish oil n-3 fatty acid intakes. Circulation 112:2762-2768, 2005.
46. Brouwer I, Zock P, Camm A, et al: Effect of fish oil on ventricular tachyarrhythmia and death inpatients with implantable cardioverter defibrillators. J Am Coll Cardiol 295:2613-2619, 2006.
47. Raitt M, Connor W, Morris C, et al: Fish oil supplementation and risk of ventricular tachycardia and ventricular fibrillation in patients with implantable defibrillators: A randomized controlled trial. JAMA 293:2884-2891, 2005.
48. Pfeffer M, Braunwald E, Moyé L, et al: Effect of captopril on mortality and morbidity in patients with left ventricular dysfunction after myocardial infarction: Results of the Survival and Ventricular Enlargement Trial. N Engl J Med 327:669-677, 1992.
49. Cohn J, Johnson G, Ziesche S, et al: A comparison of enalapril with hydralazine-isosorbide dinitrate in the treatment of chronic congestive heart failure. N Engl J Med 325:303-310, 1991.
50. Ambrosioni E, Borghi C, Magnani B: The effect of the angiotensin-converting-enzyme inhibitor zofenopril on mortality and morbidity after anterior myocardial infarction. The Survival of Myocardial Infarction Long-Term Evaluation (SMILE) Study Investigators. N Engl J Med 332:80-85, 1995.
51. Cohn J, Tognoni G; Val-HeFT Investigators: A randomized trial of the angiotensin-receptor blocker valsartan in chronic heart failure. N Engl J Med 345:1667-1675, 2001.
52. Dahlof B, Devereux R, Kjeldsen S, et al: Cardiovascular morbidity and mortality in the Losartan Intervention For Endpoint reduction in hypertension study (LIFE): A randomised trial against atenolol. Lancet 359:995-1003, 2002.
53. Epstein A, Carlson M, Fogoros R, et al: Classification of death in antiarrhythmia trials. J Am Coll Cardiol 27:433-442, 1996.
54. Effect of metoprolol CR/XL in chronic heart failure: Metoprolol CR/XL randomized Intervention trial in congesitve heart failure (MERIT-HF). Lancet 353:2001-2007, 1999.

Implantable Cardioverter-Defibrillator: Technical Aspects 99

Mohamed H. Kanj and Bruce L. Wilkoff

CHAPTER OUTLINE

The accelerated rate of battery, capacitor, lead, and algorithm development of the implantable cardioverter-defibrillator (ICD) makes the job of integrating this therapy into clinical practice challenging. Although the ICD performs two basic tasks—detecting tachycardia and terminating tachycardia—most available ICDs have additional advanced pacing capabilities. This chapter outlines the technical aspects of these life-saving devices, including those of the programmer, diagnostics, and telemetry.

System Elements

The physical components of the implanted system consist of the ICD generator, the pacing and sensing electrodes, and one or more high-energy electrodes. The casing of the ICD generator usually constitutes one of the high-energy electrodes. The electrodes, or leads, attach to the generator header through sealed connectors in a manner similar to pacing leads, often using the IS-1 bradycardia connector standard for sensing and pacing leads. High-energy lead connectors consist of a 3.2-mm diameter insulator with short pin, the DF-1 connector. Usually the ICD leads divides into one IS-1 (bradycardia) and one or two DF-1 (high-energy) connectors that are inserted into the ICD generator. A new connector standard, IS-4, will be implemented in the near future that will combine the bradycardia and tachycardia electrodes into a single 3.2-mm, 4-pole connector.

Implantable Cardioverter-Defibrillator Generator

ICD generators have decreased significantly in size due to the significant advancement in battery and microprocessor technologies. The newest generations of devices have added device-initiated long-range telemetry device interrogation, automatic alert notifications, and bioimpedance measurement capability. Other improvements include additional therapies specific for ventricular tachycardia (VT), improved tachycardia discrimination algorithms, antitachycardia and bradycardia pacing, noninvasive programmed stimulation, storage of high rate counters or electrograms, and biphasic waveform shocks modification.

Current devices provide for all these options with a generator size of about 35 cm^3. The ICD generator casing is made of titanium, considered by many to be the preferred material because of its strength, biocompatability, corrosion resistance, and light weight. The casing serves mainly to protect the circuitry from the corrosive effects of body fluids, but it also serves as an active electrode in many current ICD models. The header is generally made of clear polymethyl methacrylate, so that the connections with the leads can be visually confirmed during implantation and can be inspected if ICD system troubleshooting is required for component malfunction or suspicion of failure. The lead connections gain access to the ICD circuitry through feed through wires, which penetrate the casing through sealed openings.

The interior of the ICD consists of one or more batteries, capacitors, DC-DC converter, hybrid with microprocessor, telemetry communication coil, and their connections. The sensed ventricular signals, generally 5 to 25 mV in amplitude, enter the generator through the leads, are filtered, and then are analyzed by the algorithms programmed into the hybrid. The hybrid consists of electronic circuitry embedded in a silicon wafer, specifically designed for analysis of these signals and identification of either tachycardia or fibrillation. Once the detection criteria are met, the specific programmed pacing and high-energy shock therapies are then delivered to the patient.

Battery

Unlike other batteries, ICD batteries have many performance requirements. Besides its compact size, the battery must be capable of charging the capacitors by delivering high energy (at least 50 J) within seconds and must have a low current drain on the order of milliamperes. Additionally, the battery performance over time must be predictable to allow adequate warnings before it is depleted.

The battery used by most current ICD generators is a lithium silver vanadium oxide cell (Li/SVO), which can store approximately 18,000 J of energy. At its beginning of life, this battery generates approximately 3.2 V at full charge. Some ICD generators use two of these batteries configured in series, and the initial full voltage is 6.4 V. Most defibrillators use the same battery system for all functions, including bradycardia pacing; low-voltage maintenance functions such as memory, telemetry, and powering the decision-making circuitry; and charging the capacitors for high-energy shocks.

There are two kinds of Li/SVO batteries, anode (Li) limited and cathode (SVO) limited. In anode-limited batteries, enough lithium is provided to allow the battery to discharge only to the start of the second voltage plateau of its discharge curve. This provides a cell with improved performance in an implantable defibrillator. However, anode-limited batteries have two voltage plateaus, a very early short-lived one followed by a later long-lived one. On the other hand, cathode-limited batteries are prone to voltage discharge delay resulting from accumulation of high resistant film on the lithium electrode. It usually occurs at the middle of life (MOL) period and usually results in prolonged charge times. Pulsing the battery frequently by charging the capacitors is usually sufficient in preventing this phenomenon.

The battery status is generally determined by the measured voltage. At beginning of life, an ICD battery has an open circuit voltage of approximately 3.2 V and an internal battery impedance of 300 Ω. However, as the battery is discharged, the open circuit voltage drops to a plateau of 2.7 to 2.8 V while the internal resistance increases. With further decline in open circuit voltage and a rise in internal resistance, the ability to deliver adequate current to charge the capacitors becomes impaired, causing significant prolongation in charge time, which is usually reached at 2.6 V. This is called the elective replacement indicator (ERI) or recommended replacement time (RRT). Once ERI is reached, generator replacement can be electively scheduled, usually within a few months, depending on the frequency of therapy (which determines the depletion rate). A late indicator, end of life (EOL), reflecting a lower voltage of approximately 2.2 V, indicates a more urgent need for generator replacement because of the long capacitor charge times required to achieve appropriate shock energy. In addition to voltage criteria, the time required to charge the capacitors to full energy is also used as a measurement of the battery status, and if the time required is beyond a certain value, replacement may be indicated. In certain devices, charging the capacitors stops after 20 seconds and delivers the stored energy as shock therapy. When these devices reach ERI, the stored energy may be significantly less than the programmed energy.

Fortunately, primary battery failure is rare. More often, battery depletion is caused by excessive power drain from pacing, capacitor charge, and electrogram storage. High pacing thresholds and lead insulation failure are additional causes of excessive current drain. On the other hand, repetitive capacitor charges due to nonsustained VT or temporary ventricular oversensing can cause important reductions in battery longevity.

Capacitors

The energy required for cardiac defibrillation during the few milliseconds of an ICD shock is much greater than can be delivered directly from ICD batteries. Hence, capacitors are used to store up to 30 to 40 J of energy. Capacitors are measured by their capacitance, which is a measure of the amount of electrical charge that the capacitor can store for a given voltage. Multiple capacitors are charged in the parallel configuration from the battery at 3.2 to 6.3 V through a DC-DC converter and then are connected in series to be able to deliver the stored energy but at high voltages (up to 830 V) within 10 to 20 milliseconds. As with the battery, specific criteria are required for capacitors to be useful in defibrillation. The capacitors must be able to charge up to 10 to 40 J within a clinically reasonable period of time (<10-30 seconds). Because the capacitors are not charged until the detection criteria are met and shock therapy is programmed, a prolonged charge time exposes the patient to an extended period of circulatory arrest. Animal studies, however, have demonstrated that episodes of ventricular fibrillation (VF) longer than 20 seconds are associated with an increased energy requirement. The rate with which the capacitor is being charged depends on the capacitance and the open circuitary impedance of the battery (internal resistance). As the battery ages, its internal resistance increases, resulting in prolonged charge time. Similarly, the rate with which the capacitor delivers its charge to the patient depends on its capacitance and the lead/body impedance.

To achieve high stored voltage and energy, current ICDs incorporate new designs such as capacitors with rugged surfaces to increase surface area and the use of multiple capacitors in series. Most capacitors used in the ICD industry are aluminum and tantalum electrolytic capacitors because of their ability to charge within the prescribed time limitations. However, the dielectric layer in these capacitors becomes deformed with time, causing current to flow through it (capacitor leak). This results in suboptimal charge and prolonged charge time. Capacitor reformation, where the capacitors are discharged through a high impedance circuitry to allow adequate time, usually regenerates the dielectric layer and fixes the leak.

Electrodes

There are three essential functions of defibrillator systems: detection of the tachycardia, pacing stimulation of the heart, and shock stimulation of the heart. The electrodes are the noninsulated segments of the leads that deliver these functions. The technology used for detection (sensing) and pacing is similar to that used by pacemakers. However, the bipole for sensing and pacing is sometimes from the tip of the ventricular lead to the distal shocking electrode instead of from the tip to the ring electrode. This is called an *integrated bipolar system* instead of a true bipolar system. In cardiac resynchronization therapy devices, sensing is usually restricted to the right ventricular electrodes.

High-energy shocks, however, require specialized electrodes that are capable of conducting the higher current to the heart and distributing it transvenously to the endocardium in an appropriate manner for defibrillation.

Nonthoracotomy or Transvenous Leads

The original nonthoracotomy leads (NTLs), prototypical of integrated bipolar dual-coil leads, consisted of a sensing and pacing tip electrode and two large coil electrodes (dual coil design) for delivering the high-energy shock to the heart. The proximal coil is often located in the superior vena cava or subclavian vein (usually on the left side). The ventricular electrogram is recorded between the tip electrode and the distal coil electrode. This type of sensing configuration is termed *integrated bipolar*. The next NTL to become available possessed both tip and ring electrodes for sensing (i.e., true bipolar sensing) and a single conductor coil (single coil design) just proximal to these two distal sensing electrodes. True bipolar sensing offers better sensing and pacing performances and is less susceptible to far-field oversensing and postshock undersensing. On the other hand, integrated bipolar leads can offer better defibrillation performance due to the shorter distance from tip to distal coil. The RV apical position of the right ventricular coil is important in determining the defibrillation efficacy.

ICD leads have coaxial or multilumen construction design. Coaxial design, where layered conductors are separated by layers of insulation material, is found in older ICD leads. This configuration was occasionally associated with insulation failure due to metal ion oxidation of the middle polyurethane insulation layer. This was seen in the Medtronic Transvene family of leads and was manifested by postshock oversensing. New ICD leads adopted multilumen construction design, where conductors run in parallel through a a single insulating body.

Table 99-1 Summary of Characteristics of Currently Available Nonthoracotomy Leads

Model	Conductors Pace:Sense/Coil	Electrodes Pace:Sense/Coil	Number of Coils	Sensing Configuration
Boston Scientific/Guidant				
All	MP35N/DBS	Pt-Ir/Pt coated titanium	1 or 2	Integrated bipolar
Medtronic				
Sprint Fedalis	MP35N/MP35N	TN-Pt-Ir/Pt-clad tantalum	1 or 2	True bipolar
Quattro	MP35N/MP35N-Ag	Pt-Ir/Pt-Ir clad tantalum	2	True bipolar
All others	MP35N/MP35N-Ag	Pr-Ir/Pt-Ir	1 or 2	True or integrated bipolar
St. Jude Medical				
Riata/TVL-ADX	MP35N/MP35N	TN-Pt-Ir/Pt-Ir	1 or 2	True bipolar
All others	MP35N/MP35N	Pt-Ir/Pt-Ir	1 or 2	Integrated bipolar
Biotronik				
Linox	MP35N/MP35N	Pt-Ir-Fr/Pt-Ir-Fr	1 or 2	True bipolar
Kentrox	MP35N/MP35N	Pt-Ir-Fr/Pt-Ir-Fr	1 or 2	Integrated bipolar
ELA				
Swift	MP35N/MP35N-Ag	Pr-Ir/Pt-Ir	1	Integrated bipolar

DBS, drawn brazed strand cable; MP35N, cobalt-chrome-nickel alloy; MP35N-Ag, cobalt-chrome-nickel alloy with silver core; Pt-Ir, platinum iridium alloy; Pt-Ir-Fr, platinum iridium fractal coated; TN-Pt-Ir, titanium nitride coated iridium alloy.

Compared to single-coil transvenous leads, dual-coil transvenous leads offer a small improvement in defibrillation thresholds and has been preferred by many invasive electrophysiologists. However, this small benefit needs to be weighed against the added complexity of lead construction and its potential effect on lead reliability.

Invariably, NTLs have a high-energy coil located near the distal end and lying within the right ventricular cavity. Manufacturers have released NTLs with similar construction, although some details differ (Table 99-1). The physics of DC current flow, however, requires at least one other electrode to complete the shocking circuit. The development of smaller ICD generators has allowed pectoral implantation, which has enabled the use of the outer generator casing as the second electrode (hot can). An animal study compared the defibrillation efficacy of a hot can ICD system placed in the left pectoral or subaxillary location with right pectoral, left abdominal, or right abdominal locations. The left pectoral and axillary subcutaneous positions were superior to all other locations. In addition, the right pectoral location was superior to either abdominal location. These results imply that alternative ICD implantation sites are feasible in the event of left subclavian obstruction or other reasons to avoid the left prepectoral area.

Detection of Tachyarrhythmia

The recognition of tachyarrhythmias by an ICD is a complex interaction of several dependent variables. However, the task of the ICD is more complicated because it must also recognize the lack of tachyarrhythmias. This central insight is crucial, because the patient will spend all but a small fraction of his or her life in a nontachycardiac rhythm. Obviously, it is just as important to recognize the life-threatening arrhythmias. Therefore, assuming the efficacy of the pacing and shock therapies, rhythm recognition arbitrates between quality and length of life.

Not all of the factors required for accurate rhythm recognition are potentially affected by the ICD technology. Most notably, the rate and mechanism of the arrhythmia and the programming of the ICD are major determinants of rhythm recognition and are factors that are almost completely independent of the technologic solution. However, by understanding the nature of the signals presented to the ICD, allowing the ICD to adapt to these signals, and limiting programming options, appropriate ICD function is commonly achieved.

Sensing

Tachyarrhythmia therapy is allocated on the basis of the interpretation of the signals presented to the generator. All current ICDs use ventricular heart rate as the cornerstone variable in tachycardia recognition. However, to determine heart rate, the interval between each depolarization of the ventricle must be measured. It is not interval recognition but the detection of individual electrogram events that becomes the basic building block in this process. The process begins with the placement of the sensing lead. The sensed electrogram depends on the health of the myocardium in close proximity to the lead, the far-field structures of the diaphragm and right atrium, and other electrical devices such as pacemakers, cellular phones, and other sources of electromagnetic interference.

Detection of the electrogram events completely depends on the quality of the signal, and the quality of the signal is determined only at the time of the lead placement. Because defibrillation efficacy is almost always best at the right ventricular apex, the adequacy of sensing is sometimes compromised by the apical position of the lead. Additional aspects that potentially depend on the position of the lead are measures of electrogram morphology such as electrogram event width. In dual chamber devices, the accurate recognition of arrhythmias is even more complicated with the inclusion of atrial lead data input into the generator. No longer will placement of the lead in a position to see the largest near-field electrogram minimize the chances of miscounting arrhythmias; however, the atrial lead must be positioned so that there is no discernible ventricular electrogram. Sensing is an issue not only of signal-to-noise ratio in the ventricle but also of the exclusion of all nonatrial events on the atrial lead.

Band Pass Filtering

The sense amplifier processes signals presented to the pulse generator by the leads. The amplifier allows signals of certain frequencies to be presented to the detection logic, whereas others are filtered out. This band pass filter consists of a high-frequency cutoff to filter out myopotential signals and a low-frequency cutoff to filter out T-wave signals. The mid range is intended to represent a band of frequency containing true signal events. The intent is to prevent extraneous signals from fooling the device into falsely detecting tachyarrhythmias. Unfortunately, there is some frequency overlap between repolarization and depolarization waves, atrial and ventricular events, postpacing polarization and depolarization of the ventricles, myopotentials and cardiac depolarizations, and environmental signals and cardiac events.

Frequency and Amplitude

There is a strong relation between the amplitude of the signal presented to the band pass filter and the frequencies contained within that signal. Larger signals usually improve the specificity of electrogram event detection by placing the frequency content into the center frequencies of the band pass filter. A signal that is relatively small, such as 4 to 6 mV, but that has good frequency content as represented by the slew rate measured on the pacing system analyzer of more than 1 V/sec, will probably do better than a larger signal such as 8 to 10 mV with much poorer frequency content of less than 0.1 V/sec.

Autogain and Autothreshold

One of the larger challenges presented to ICD detection algorithms is the marked variability in the amplitudes of the signal that must be accurately identified. Examples of commonly occurring situations include naturally conducted beats through the His-Purkinje system of 10 mV, paced amplitudes of 5000 mV with polarization voltage after each pacer spike, premature ventricular contractions and VT amplitudes from 2 to 25 mV, asystolic electrogram amplitudes of 0 to 0.15 mV, and VF amplitudes from 0.2 to 20 mV. The transitions between each of the rhythms must be accurately handled.

The two most difficult problems are distinguishing frequent excursions from low to high and back to low-amplitude electrogram events without oversensing large signals. The two approaches are the use of autogain and autothreshold. The autogain technique uses fixed amplitude voltage thresholds and amplifies the signal at continually varying gains according to various algorithms to single count both small and large signals. The autothreshold technique uses one amplifier gain and a continuously varying threshold to accomplish the same end. Usually the threshold varies within a single cycle, decaying after each sensed event after an adjustment proportional to the amplitude of the signal. Sometimes the floor or minimum voltage limit can be programmed to distinguish between noise on the signal and low-amplitude VF signals. After a paced beat, the autogain is usually set to maximum and the autothreshold is set to minumum.

Estimation of Adequate Amplitude

The ventricular sensing electrode is placed during a nontachycardia rhythm. Therefore, the adequacy of that placement must be determined before the VF is induced for defibrillation threshold (DFT) testing. Although there is marked variability in the average electrogram event amplitude between VF episodes and within a single VF episode, there is a relation between the amplitude of the sinus rhythm electrogram amplitude and the average, minimum, and maximum VF electrogram events of subsequently induced arrhythmias. Fortunately, it is not necessary to detect every single electrogram event in order to detect the tachyarrhythmia. As an estimate of adequacy, sinus rhythm electrograms of at least 5 mV reliably predict that less than 10% of the electrogram events will be undersensed and that failure of tachyarrhythmia detection is eliminated. Although the incidence of failed detection is rare even with sinus rhythm electrograms less than 5 mV, the amplitude of VF is much smaller and the incidence of failed detection increases significantly.

Detection Algorithms

Once an electrogram event is marked or detected, the detection algorithm interprets the pattern of the intervals between the events. The algorithms attempt to develop a hierarchy of detected rhythms that require different therapies such as bradycardia, VT requiring antitachycardia pacing, VT requiring low-energy shocks, and VF requiring higher-energy shocks. The exclusion of sinus tachycardia and atrial fibrillation with overlapping rates with ventricular arrhythmias is particularly difficult. Added to the ventricular rate criterion is the duration of the arrhythmia, the suddenness of the increase in rate, and the beat-to-beat variation of the cycle length to distinguish these rhythms. With derivatives of the electrogram morphology including templates, duration, and vector correlations, and with the addition of an atrial electrode, the pattern of the relation of the atrial and ventricular events have more recently improved the specificity of arrhythmia detection. The concern should always be how much sensitivity is sacrificed with these new algorithms. It is important that these algorithms should deliver therapy to very rapid tachycardias, irrespective of whether they originate in the atrium or the ventricle.

Sensitivity versus Specificity (Discriminating Supraventricular from Ventricular Arrhythmias)

Life-threatening arrhythmias must always be detected and terminated. However, the arrhythmia's mechanism, rate, or both do not always correlate with its hemodynamic significance. Patients can die of atrial flutter with 1:1 atrioventricular (AV) conduction and of monomorphic VT at 110 beats per minute. The lower the rate cutoff, the greater the sensitivity, but the poorer the specificity for truly life-threatening situations. The challenge is to use the algorithms to avoid the delivery of inappropriate therapy so that the ICD is better tolerated and contributes to an improved quality of life.

Rate and Duration

The primary characteristic of ventricular arrhythmias requiring treatment is the rate and duration of the arrhythmia. Slow and short-duration arrhythmias do not require therapy. However, the negative consequence of waiting to see if an arrhythmia is going to end without an intervention from the ICD increases with rapid rates. The possibility that failure to detect low-amplitude electrogram events will cause a delay or prevent detection is also a serious issue. Consequently, the faster the rhythm, the shorter the duration that should be required for detection. For VT detection, consecutive events faster than a programmed rate are appropriate; however, for VF, *X* short cycle length intervals out of a larger number of *Y* consecutive intervals facilitates the detection of these episodes. This algorithm is important because of the marked variability of electrogram amplitudes and intervals during VF.

Sudden Onset

Reentrant VT and some not clearly reentrant arrhythmias start at a rapid rate, which is usually distinct from the preceding nontachycardia rhythm. The sudden shortening of the cycle length is a factor that is somewhat useful in differentiating sinus tachycardia from slow VT. The best criterion for preventing VT detection during sinus tachycardia is programming a more rapid VT detection rate; however, when that is not possible there is some, but limited, value in using sudden onset. Unfortunately, using this approach increases the risk that the arrhythmia will not be treated if the VT arises in the setting of sinus tachycardia or exercise. In addition, this discriminator might inhibit therapies for VT that started below the programmed detection rate even when it accelerates beyond the programmed detection rate.

Cycle Length Stability

Most VTs, in distinction from the ventricular response in atrial fibrillation, have a stable cycle length with little beat-to-beat variation (<40 ms) in the interval. Unfortunately, this is not always the case, but when the ventricular response is rapid during relatively infrequent episodes of atrial fibrillation, this can be an effective tool. If there is continuous atrial fibrillation or frequent paroxysmal episodes, especially in the setting of a slow VT that also needs treatment, then AV junctional ablation with a rate-responsive pacemaker is a better choice. With the new rate-responsive, single-chambered, dual-chambered, and biventricular pacemaker-ICD combination devices, this will be a more common choice. Also, the integration of atrial cycle length in relation to ventricular cycle length greatly improves the specific detection of atrial fibrillation, but it also introduces the complex possibility of detecting dual tachycardias such as VT arising during atrial fibrillation.

Morphology and QRS Width

Electrogram width measurements, morphology criteria, and most recently morphology template matching and vector correlation techniques have been used to enhance the quickness and specificity of tachycardia detection with some success. This process is very tedious where the digital image of every tachycardia electrogram is compared to a presaved template of the baseline rhythm. Although very helpful, this discriminator is limited by numerous scenarios including physiologic rate-dependent changes in electrogram morphology and truncation and alignment errors in the digitalization process.

Atrial Lead Criteria

With placement of an atrial lead, the relation of atrial activity to the ventricular activity is available for analysis. If the data are accurate, with the caveats mentioned earlier concerning far-field signals, then AV dissociation during a rapid ventricular rhythm makes the diagnosis of VT certain. If there is a 1:1 relation, the chance that the rhythm is VT or supraventricular tachycardia (SVT) depends on the ratio of the durations of the AV to the VA interval. Unfortunately, it is still possible to have atrial tachyarrhythmia and VT at the same time. Atrial leads reduce the incidence but will not prevent inappropriate therapy because all algorithms are biased so that VF is rarely, if ever, missed.

Reconfirmation and Redetection

Detection of tachycardia, like any other test, follows Bayesian statistics. The probability of a truly positive result is directly proportional to the prevalence of the condition in the population being treated. Once a rhythm has been detected with rigorous criteria and treated, the likelihood is that a rhythm that meets the rate criteria will need to be treated again, and quickly, to prevent syncope. Thus quickness and sensitivity is enhanced during redetection by reducing the number of intervals required and by eliminating additional criteria. Conversely, it takes time to charge the ICD capacitors, during which time the arrhythmia may have terminated. For this reason, before the therapy is delivered, reconfirmation of the tachycardia is required to prevent shocks when treating patients with nonsustained tachycardia during sinus rhythm. The danger is that the autogain or autothreshold algorithm has failed to pick up very low amplitude VF during progressive hemodynamic collapse. Thus reconfirmation of rhythms in the VF zone should be used with care. Some devices permit the allocation of committed and noncommitted shocks in the VF or in the VT and VF rate zones. Redetection, on the other hand, is the process with which the ICD examines whether the programmed therapy was effective in terminating the presenting arrhyhtmia. In most ICDs except the ones manufactured by ELA Medical (Plymouth, MN), the SVT-VT discriminators are not applied during this process and redetection is based solely on the programmed rate cutoff.

Therapy for Tachyarrhythmia

Pacing Therapy

All ICDs provide bradycardia support with single-, dual-, or triple-chamber stimulation. The pacing mode, rate, and stimulation output is often separately programmable after a high-energy shock for a period to provide overdrive suppression of arrhythmias. Although most patients with ICDs receive dual-chambered rate-adaptive pacemakers, a small minority of these patients have an indication for pacing.

The Dual Chamber and VVI Implantable Defibrillator (DAVID) trial examined the effect of pacing in the DDDR mode compared with ventricular backup pacing in patients who had ICD but no pacing indications. In these patients, DDDR pacing increased the combined endpoint of hospitalization for congestive heart failure (CHF) or death.[1] In the DAVID-II trial, atrial support pacing at AAI-70 was tested and showed no significant improvement in quality-of-life outcomes compared to VVI-40.[2] Thus patients without clear indications for antibradycardia pacing should be set to ventricular backup pacing. In patients with ventricular dyssynchrony and New York Heart Association (NYHA) functional class III or IV CHF, biventricular stimulation is appropriate; however, in patients who have less-severe CHF or need for antibradycardia pacing, the appropriate choice is unclear.

Antitachycardia pacing is available in all of the current ICDs. This therapy consists of the delivery of a short burst of ventricular pacing at a (programmable) rate faster than the detected VT rate. A variety of antitachycardia pacing techniques are available, including simple bursts at a fixed rate and ramp pacing, in which each subsequent paced interval is incrementally shorter (i.e., faster) than the preceding interval. Effectiveness has been demonstrated to be 90% in terminating slower VT and and 72% in terminating fast VT using antitachycardia pacing programmed empirically. Its effectiveness was 95% when the antitachycardia pacing modality is tested before discharge from the hospital. Antitachycardia pacing was also effective in terminating supraventricular tachcyardias for which patients would have a received a shock.

A drawback to antitachycardia pacing, in some patients, is the potential for acceleration of the tachycardia to greater rates or to VF, so that high-energy shocks are required. Although 4% of patients experience acceleration of the tachycardia by antitachycardia pacing, this was not associated with any increase in mortality or incidence of syncopal events.[3,4] Generally, one or more trials of antitachycardia pacing are programmed for VT (depending on patient tolerance), followed by shock therapy. A number of safeguards are built into the treatment algorithms that enable more aggressive therapy (i.e., high-energy shocks) for prolonged, ineffective attempts at antitachycardia pacing or low-energy shocks. Once antitachycardia pacing therapy fails to terminate the tachyarrhythmia, shock therapy is delivered. In fact, in the EMPIRIC trial, standardized prespecified ICD programming with antitachcyardia pacing during slow and fast ventricular tachcyardia was at least as effective as physician-tailored programming, without an increase in mortality or shock-related morbidity.[5]

Shock Therapy

The electrical shocks delivered by ICDs arise from the discharge of the capacitors through the heart via the high-energy electrodes. Capacitor discharge follows an exponential decay (Fig. 99-1) that depends on two variables: the total capacitance within the device and the impedance of the electrode-patient body system. As either of these variables is increased, the voltage and current discharge decays more slowly, producing a flatter waveform. One to three capacitors are commonly used in each generator, each rated at about 106 to 480 μF capacitance and capable of a maximal voltage of about 350 to 830 V. These capacitors are usually charged in parallel to a programmable voltage up to the maximum. When discharged, however, these

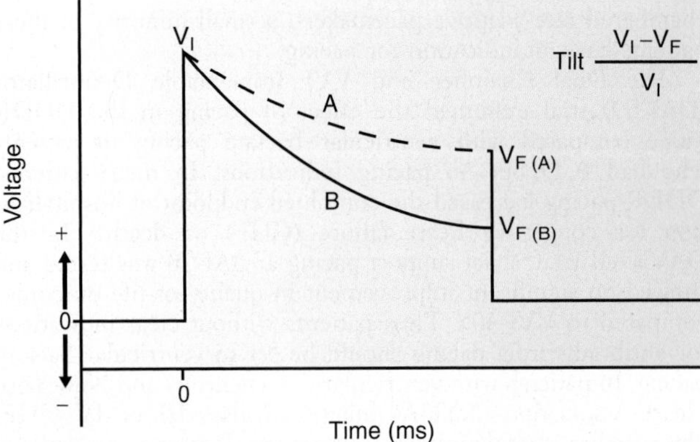

Figure 99-1 The monophasic waveform is created by truncation of a capacitor discharge and is the simplest implantable cardioverter-defibrillator (ICD) waveform. The initial voltage (V_I) is dependent on the charge placed on the capacitor. The waveform is truncated after a variable duration (depending on the manufacturer) when a certain final voltage (V_F) is reached. The rate of voltage decay (tilt) is inversely proportional to both the impedance of the lead system and the total capacitance in the ICD. Tilt is calculated according to the formula given such that waveform A demonstrates a lower tilt than waveform B.

capacitors are configured in series, so that the total voltage is doubled or tripled, depending on the number of capacitors, to a maximal voltage of 750 to 850 V. Although the voltage is multiplied in the series configuration, the capacitance is reduced by the number of capacitors used. Hence the resultant system capacitance is 120 to 150 μF for most currently available clinical devices (Table 99-2). Lowering the capacitance of the system gives a favorable clinical outcome by decreasing the discharge time. Because most lead impedance values are between 30 and 70 Ω, this results in a voltage that decreases about 60% to 90% in 20 ms. The shock waveform (see later) is generated by the discharge of the capacitors through the electrode system to the patient.

Defibrillation Threshold and Safety Margin

The main determinant of success of defibrillation is the magnitude of the electric field generated across the heart. Although the magnitude may be very hard to determine because of its dependence on numerous factors, it is usually proportional to the spatial derivative of the voltage. However, because device companies report their device outputs in energy units (Joules), it has been a trend to refer to defibrillation thresholds in the Joule unit.

The simplest measure of defibrillation effectiveness is the DFT, defined as the lowest delivered shock strength required to defibrillate. However, the clinical predictive value of defibrillation testing is limited by the probabilistic nature of defibrillation. The DFT is often determined in a step-down manner, in which shocks of progressively lower intensity are delivered, after VF is induced, and the lowest successful shock strength is defined as the DFT. Alternatively, shocks can be delivered in a step-up fashion, beginning at low energies. However, the step-up method requires several failed shocks and subsequently longer periods of circulatory arrest for the patient involved.

A third method of determining DFT has been proposed in which test shocks are delivered to the vulnerable period of the cardiac cycle, near the peak of the surface T wave.[6] Theoretically, low-energy shocks delivered during this phase of repolarization will produce VF caused by the resultant dispersion of repolarization times. If a test shock delivered during this period fails to result in VF, it is deemed to be above the DFT and, subsequently, lower shock intensities can then be tested until VF occurs. This concept is termed the *upper limit of vulnerability* (ULV) and has the advantage of inducing VF only once during the testing period. The shock of the lowest energy that does not induce VF is considered equivalent to the DFT. This method makes inductionless implants feasible in more than 80% of patients.[7,8] The disadvantage of this method is that the ability of the ICD to correctly detect VF and the subsequent decision-making algorithm to delivery VF therapy will not have been tested.

The concept of the DFT is overly simplistic, however, because electrical defibrillation is best described as a sigmoidal-shaped probability function (Fig. 99-2). Nonetheless, the step-down DFT is a convenient clinical measurement to obtain during implantation and generally correlates with a probability of success of approximately 70% to 80%. The probability-of-success approach has significant clinical relevance, because appropriate implantation of ICDs requires a high confidence that the first shock will be successful. Historically, a safety margin (a margin between the DFT and the maximum output of the ICD) of 10 J was considered minimal implantation criteria. Hence, given the 30- to 35-J outputs of most devices, 20 to 25 J has been considered the maximum acceptable DFT.

This proposed safety margin was based on the use of epicardial leads and monophasic waveforms. More recent studies have

Table 99-2 Summary of Biphasic Waveform Characteristics in Currently Available Commercial Implantable Cardioverter-Defibrillators

		Phase 1		Phase 2		Monophasic	
Model	**Capacitance**	**Characteristic**	**Programmable**	**Characteristic**	**Programmable**	**Characteristic**	**Programmable**
Boston Scientific							
Vitality HE	130-150 μF	60% Tilt	No	50% Tilt	No	80%	—
Prizm II	158 μF	60% Tilt	No	50% Tilt	No	67%	—
Medtronic							
Virtuoso/Entrust	128 μF	50% Tilt	Yes*	50% Tilt	Yes*	None	—
Gem III At	118 μF	50% Tilt	Yes*	50% Tilt	Yes*	None	—
St Jude Medical							
Photon/Atlas	106-126 μF	65% Tilt	Yes	65% Tilt	Yes	65%	Yes
		Or 5.5 ms PW	Yes	Or 5.5 ms PW	Yes		
Epic/Photon	99-102 μF	65% Tilt	Yes	65% Tilt	Yes	65%	Yes
		Or 5.5 ms PW	Yes	Or 5.5 ms PW	Yes		
ELA							
Ovatio/Alto	105-120 μF	50% Tilt	No	50% Tilt	No	None	—
Biotronik							
Lumax 340	160 μF	60% Tilt, 16 ms		50% Tilt, 10 ms	—	None	—
		Maximum PW		Maximum PW	—	—	—
Lumos	145 μF	60% Tilt, 16 ms		50% Tilt, 10 ms	—	None	—
		Maximum PW		Maximum PW	—	—	—

Note: Capacitance values can vary between models within a given manufacturer, and older models might vary from these specifications. In models in which phase parameters are programmable, the value given is the default value programmed in the factory. When a range of values is given, it refers to different models offered by the same manufacturer.

*Applies only to the atrial shock tilt; the ventricular shocks are not tilt programmable.

PW, pulse width.

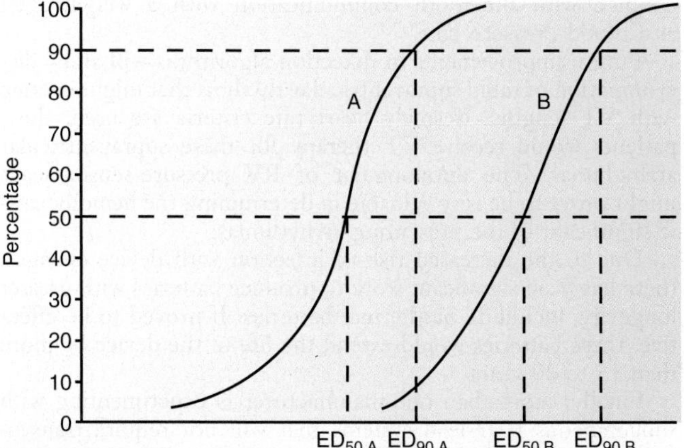

Figure 99-2 Graph shows the relation between the probability of successful defibrillation and the intensity of the shock; that is, the greater the shock intensity, the higher the probability of success. The ED_{50} and ED_{90} refer to the shock intensity that results in successful defibrillation 50% and 90% of the time, respectively. In the examples given, curves A and B represent waveforms A and B with different defibrillation efficacy. Waveform A shows a greater efficacy (lower ED_{50} and ED_{90}) than waveform B.

suggested that with biphasic shocks and NTLs, a margin of 1.9 times the DFT energy provides a 95% probability of success. Epicardial patches routinely provided good DFTs with monophasic waveforms, and a 10-J safety margin was usually obtained. However, NTLs often required additional leads or subcutaneous electrodes, or both, to ensure an adequate safety margin with monophasic waveforms.

One thing to keep in mind is that DFT testing is device and lead specific because the delivered energy is not the only parameter that ensures successful defibrillation. Other parameters, including lead impedance, waveform tilt, truncation, pulse duration, and positive- and negative-phase peak voltage, can all affect defibrillation success and are usually specific to the device or lead.[9,10] While using devices that allow the programming of the delivered energy, one has to know that these are approximate energy out that was derived from testing these devices in a nonclinical setting and often at unrealistic lead impedances.

Monophasic Waveforms

The simplest defibrillator waveform is the monophasic waveform, in which the capacitor discharge is truncated before complete discharge of the capacitor, because the terminal voltage tail might prove proarrhythmic. Monophasic waveforms were used in early ICD generators and were effective in epicardial systems. The magnitude of a monophasic (or biphasic) shock is generally described by both the amplitude (peak voltage or current) and tilt of the waveform (see Fig. 99-1). For example, a waveform whose amplitude is reduced to one half the initial value has a 50% tilt.

When the NTL was first developed and monophasic waveforms were used, the right ventricular coil electrode was configured as the cathode (negative) and the superior vena cava coil or subcutaneous patch electrode was configured as the anode (positive). This convention was carried over from pacing applications, because cathodal stimulation of the heart requires lower voltage and current than anodal stimulation. However, subsequent basic and clinical studies were performed comparing the right ventricular cathodal configuration with the right ventricular anodal configuration. Surprisingly, an anodal right ventricular electrode resulted in a significantly lower DFT in patients and a lower need for supplementary electrodes. The mechanism for this polarity difference is not yet well understood, although it has been confirmed in animal studies. Despite the additional benefit derived when monophasic waveform polarity was optimized, the defibrillation energy requirements were occasionally too high to provide an adequate degree of certainty that clinical VF could be successfully treated. This problem was largely solved when biphasic waveforms were developed.

Biphasic Waveforms

The most beneficial ICD innovation, from a viewpoint of DFT reduction, was the development of the biphasic defibrillation waveform (Fig. 99-3). This waveform consists of the capacitor discharge divided into two phases of opposite polarity. The first phase is identical to a monophasic waveform (although usually of a shorter duration) before the capacitor discharge is truncated. The electrical connection within the generator is then quickly reversed (usually within 2-3 μs) and the second phase is discharged in the opposite polarity for an additional period (usually 3-6 ms). Table 99-2 lists the biphasic waveform characteristics currently available in clinical ICDs.

Much research has been performed on optimizing the biphasic waveform to minimize the DFT energy. One study has

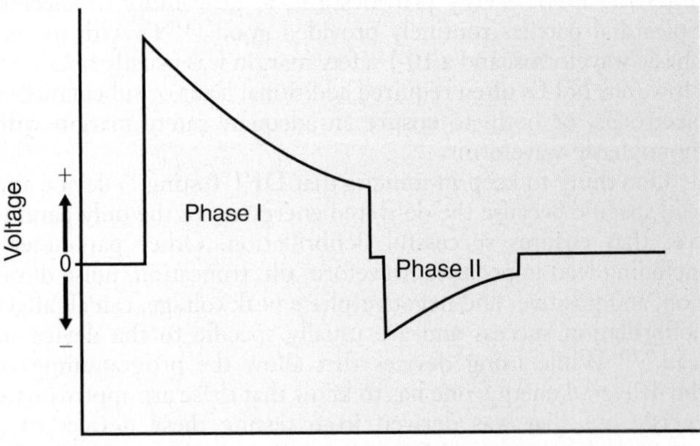

Figure 99-3 The biphasic waveform now used in all implantable defibrillators. It is composed of a capacitor discharge divided into two phases of opposite polarity. The duration of each phase depends on the manufacturer and may be programmable in some devices. The initial voltage of the second phase is equivalent to the remaining voltage on the capacitor after truncation of phase I in most cases.

extensively tested biphasic waveform characteristics in animals, identifying two factors that appear to minimize endocardial DFTs as follows: The first phase should be longer than the second phase, and the polarity of the first phase appears to be important only at phase 1 durations greater than 10 ms or when the second phase duration is greater than the first phase.

Additional studies have examined the effectiveness of other phase characteristics. One interesting modification involves doubling the second phase initial voltage by switching the capacitance from series to parallel between the first and second phases. This also reduces the capacitance of the second phase by half, resulting in an increased tilt and a more rapid decay of voltage. Animal studies have suggested that this reduces the DFT. Numerous recent studies have reported improved defibrillation thresholds with modification of the tilt percentages. The results of these studies were then used to modify the preset tilts in the current available devices. St. Jude Medical's newer devices have the capability for programing the tilt settings.

Recent and Future Directions

The combination of biphasic waveforms, hot cans, and low-polarization leads has reduced average DFTs to less than 10 J in many ICD systems. This now allows reduced maximal outputs of 20 to 25 J, which provides adequate safety margins for most patients.

The recent development of device-monitoring systems with or without wireless communication has permitted early diagnosis of arrhythmias and system malfunction. Long-distance telemetric communication in these devices is sometimes accomplished through Medical Implant Communications Service (MICS). MICS is an ultra-low power, mobile radio frequency service designed for transmitting diagnostic and therapeutic information from implanted medical devices. Its band operates at 402 to 405 MHz. This band width does not need any licensing and is shared by different manufacturers (currently Medtronic, St. Jude Medical, and Biotronik). Each manufacturer has applied mechanisms to avoid interference and cross communication with other devices. There is another frequency spectrum, the Industrial, Scientific and Medical (ISM) band (902-928 MHz) is in use for long-range telemetry by Boston Scientific. They use precisely 914 MHz for communication from the ICD to the home monitor, which is also coupled with Bluetooth communication with a weight scale and blood pressure cuff.

Future improvements in detection algorithms will allow discrimination of rapid supraventricular rhythms that might overlap with VT lengths. If solely heart rate criteria are used, these patients would receive VT therapy for these supraventricular arrhythmias. The development of RV pressure-sensor leads might prove to be very valuable in determining the hemodynamic significant of the presenting arrhythmias.

Due to the increased risk of infection with device changes, there has been significant work to produce batteries with greater longevity, including biothermal batteries. If proved to be effective, these batteries would extend the life of the device by more than 15 to 20 years.

Finally, more than one manufacturer is experimenting with subcutaneous ICD-lead systems that will not require transvenous access. This ICD is based on a single subcutaneous lead system that is tunneled from the subclavicular level to the subpectoral region and then laterally to the axillary region. This lead is then attached to a very high energy device (80 J). Tachycardia sensing is based on the far-field signal derived from the subcutaneous lead. Although this device might be appealing, this design lacks backup pacing.[11]

References

1. The DAVID Investigators: Dual-chamber pacing or ventricular backup pacing in patients with an implantable defibrillator. JAMA 288:3115-3123, 2002.
2. Wilkoff B, Kudenchuk P, Buxton A, et al: Impact of atrial pacing on quality of life in the dual chamber and VVI implantable defibrillator (DAVID) II trial. J Am Coll Cardiol (in press).
3. Wathen MS, DeGroot PJ, Sweeney MO, et al; for the PainFREE Rx II Investigators. Prospective randomized multicenter trial of empirical antitachycardia pacing versus shocks for spontaneous rapid ventricular tachycardia in patients with implantable cardioverter-defibrillators. Pacing Fast Ventricular Tachycardia Reduces Shock Therapies (PainFREE Rx II) trial results. Circulation 110:2591-2596, 2004.
4. Wathen MS, Sweeney MO, DeGroot PJ, et al: Shock reduction using antitachycardia pacing for spontaneous rapid ventricular tachycardia in patients with coronary artery disease. Circulation 104:786-801, 2001.
5. Wilkoff BL, Ousdigian KT, Sterns LD, et al; EMPIRIC Trial Investigators: A comparison of empiric to physician-tailored programming of implantable cardioverter-defibrillators: Results from the prospective randomized multicenter EMPIRIC trial. J Am Coll Cardiol 48(2):330-339, 2006.
6. Chen PS, Shibata N, Dixon EG, et al: Comparison of the defibrillation threshold and the upper limit of ventricular vulnerability. Circulation 73(5):1022-1028, 1986.
7. Swerdlow CD: Implantation of cardioverter defibrillators without induction of ventricular fibrillation. Circulation 103(17):2159-2164, 2001.
8. Day JD, Doshi RN, Belott P, et al: Inductionless or limited shock testing is possible in most patients with implantable cardioverter- defibrillators/cardiac resynchronization therapy defibrillators: Results of the multicenter ASSURE Study (Arrhythmia Single Shock Defibrillation Threshold Testing Versus Upper Limit of Vulnerability: Risk Reduction Evaluation With Implantable Cardioverter-Defibrillator Implantations). Circulation 115(18):2382-2389, 2007.
9. Sweeney MO, Natale A, Volosin KJ, et al: Prospective randomized comparison of 50/50% versus 65/65% tilt biphasic waveform on defibrillation in humans. Pacing Clin Electrophysiol 24:60-65, 2001.
10. Schauerte PN, Ziegert K, Waldmann M, et al: Effect of biphasic shock duration on defibrillation threshold with different electrode configurations and phase 2 capacitances: prediction by upper-limit-of-vulnerability determination. Circulation 99:1516-1522, 1999.
11. Grace AA, Hood MA, Smith WM, et al: Evaluation of four distinct subcutaneous implantable defibrillator (S-ICD) lead systems in humans. Heart Rhythm 27th Annual Scientific Sessions. May 2006.

Implantable Cardioverter-Defibrillator: Clinical Aspects 100

Charles Swerdlow and Paul Friedman

CHAPTER OUTLINE

Implantable cardioverter-defibrillators (ICDs) are the treatment of choice for most patients who are at high risk for ventricular fibrillation (VF) or life-threatening ventricular tachycardia (VT). This chapter on clinical aspects complements Chapter 99 on technical aspects. We address indications, implant testing, programming, follow-up, common clinical problems, psychosocial issues, electromagnetic interference, and recalls.

Indications and Use

For many years, ICDs have been the treatment of choice for secondary prevention of VT or VF if the arrhythmia is likely to recur despite other therapy. In the 21st century, most ICDs have been implanted for primary prevention in high-risk patients who have not experienced VT or VF. Primary prevention guidelines identify high risk primarily by heart failure class ($\geq$2) and left-ventricular ejection fraction ($\leq$30%-35%).[1] At present, more than 80% of ICDs are implanted for primary prevention.

Secondary prevention guidelines are supported by an overwhelming consensus of experts and practicing cardiologists. They have been widely adopted. In contrast, primary prevention guidelines are applied variably in clinical practice. Experts vary in their level of concern about comorbidities as contraindications,[2] complications, and the high number of patients who need to receive ICDs to save one life.[3,4] In 2007, *Consumer Reports* classified ICDs along with coronary stents as one of 10 most overused treatments but provided no supporting evidence.

Implant Testing

Techniques for transvenous implantation of ICD leads and pectoral placement of the generator are similar to those for pacemakers.[5] Because the pulse generator usually serves as a defibrillation electrode, placing it in the left pectoral region optimizes the shock vector for defibrillation (Fig. 100-1).

Sensing

ICD systems are tested at implantation to ensure that they will sense, detect, and defibrillate VF. ICDs use automatic adjustment of sensitivity (Fig. 100-2) to ensure reliable sensing of low- and variable-amplitude electrograms in atrial fibrillation (AF) and VF while avoiding T-wave oversensing (Fig. 100-2). To permit sensing of rapid activations, nominal blanking periods are short ($\leq$140 ms) within each chamber, and cross-chamber blanking periods are short or absent. Because short blanking periods can cause oversensing, marker channels should be inspected in both sinus and paced rhythms for evidence of oversensing P, R, and T waves. (See "Oversensing," later.) At implantation, the atrial lead should be positioned to minimize oversensing of far-field R waves.[6-8]

To test sensing during induced VF, sensitivity is programmed to an insensitive setting (~1 mV). This ensures an adequate

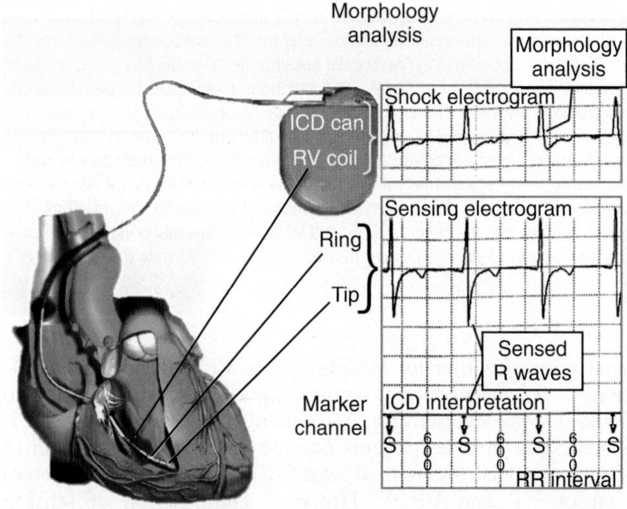

Figure 100-1 Implantable cardioverter defibrillator (ICD) leads and electrograms. An ICD system including left-pectoral active can and right ventricle (RV) lead is shown on the *left;* telemetered high-voltage (shock), far-field, and sensing near-field electrograms with annotated markers are shown on the *right.* The dual-coil lead uses true-bipolar sensing between tip and ring electrodes. *Arrows* on the marker channel denote timing of R waves sensed from the true-bipolar electrogram. ICDs measure all timing intervals from this electrogram and display them on the marker channel, which also indicates the ICD's classification of each atrial and ventricular event by letter symbols. Morphology of shock electrograms stored during detected tachycardias is useful for distinguishing ventricular tachycardia from supraventricular tachycardia. S indicates sensed ventricular events in the sinus rate zone, and numbers indicate R-R intervals.

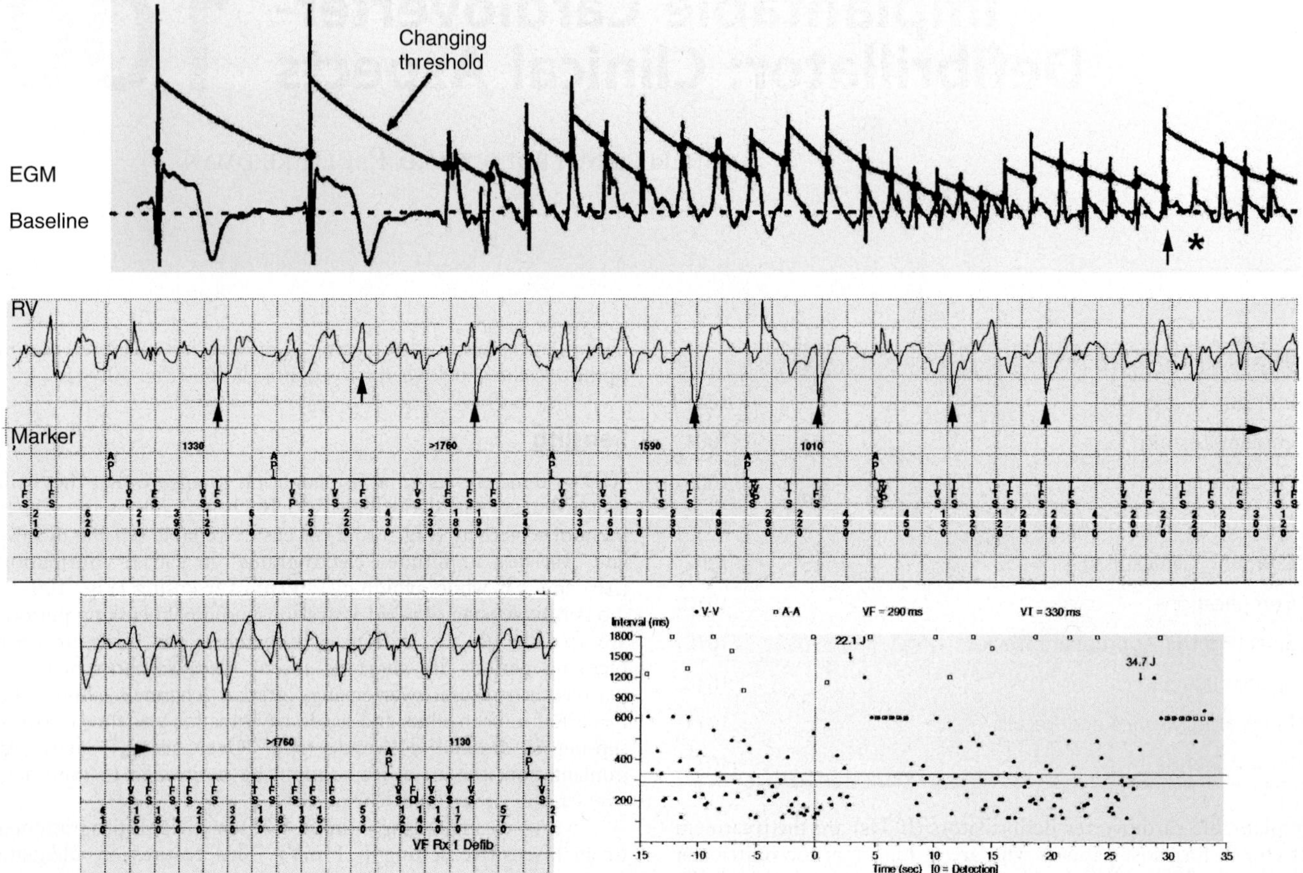

Figure 100-2 *Top,* Autoadjusting sensitivity. Real-time bipolar ventricular electrogram and sensing threshold are shown during sinus rhythm (first two beats) and spontaneous onset of ventricular fibrillation (VF). Sensing is shown by the *dots* where the signal crosses the variable threshold. The time constant for autoadjusting sensitivity is selected to prevent T-wave oversensing during sinus or paced rhythms, while permitting reliable sensing of electrograms in VF. *Asterisk* denotes low-amplitude undersensed electrogram in VF immediately following high-amplitude electrogram denoted by *arrow.* (Reprinted and modified from Olson WH: Tachyarrhythmia sensing and detection. Implantable cardioverter defibrillator. Armonk, New York, Futura, 1994, pp 71-107.) *Center and bottom left,* Appropriate detection of VF despite undersensing. Ventricular sensing electrogram (RV) is shown with dual-chamber marker channel. Electrogram is continuous from middle to lower panel. Undersensing occurs because of rapid variations in electrogram amplitude and slew rate. Low-amplitude electrograms are undersensed after each high-amplitude electrogram *(arrow)* until autoadjusting sensitivity increases. VF is detected at the end of the lower electrogram (VF Rx 1 Defib) when 18 of 24 intervals are shorter than the VF detection interval of 290 ms. The requirements to sense VF electrograms like these and to detect VF reliably despite undersensing results in oversensing and inappropriate detection of ventricular tachycardia (VT) or VF under other conditions. *Bottom right,* Interval plot shows marked variation in sensed RR intervals, with many above the VF detection interval. After the shock denoted by *22.1 J,* AV pacing resumes for six cycles, followed by recurrent VF. This shock is classified as unsuccessful because 8 consecutive sinus intervals are required to redetect sinus rhythm. The second episode of VF is therefore treated with a maximum output shock (34.7 J), which converts rhythm to AV pacing. FS, TS, and VS denote intervals in VF, VT and sinus zones, respectively. AP and VP denote atrial and ventricular pacing pulses, the latter due to ventricular undersensing or ventricular sensing immediately following atrial pacing (ventricular safety pacing).

safety margin either for sensing of fine VF with nominal sensitivity (~0.3 mV) or for programming a less-sensitive setting to avoid T-wave oversensing. Assessment of sensing during VF is unnecessary in most patients because an R wave during native rhythm or atrial pacing of at least 5-7 mV results in rapid detection of VT and VF.[9,10] However, confirmation of sensing during VF is important in specific circumstances that can impair sensing, including low-amplitude R waves, other implanted electrical stimulating devices (device-device interactions) or long ventricular blanking periods related to programmed rate-smoothing pacing in dual-chamber ICDs (intradevice interactions).[6,8,11]

Defibrillation Efficacy

At implantation, a measure of defibrillation efficacy is compared to an implantation criterion, which is the level of performance that is predicted to result in a clinically acceptable success rate for defibrillation of spontaneous VF (Fig. 100-3A). If performance that does not meet the implantation criterion, the ICD system must be revised. There is a tradeoff between the fraction of patients who are predicted to pass a given implantation criterion and subsequent success rates for defibrillation of spontaneous VF.[12]

Defibrillation efficacy can be assessed directly by defibrillation testing or indirectly by vulnerability testing. For direct testing, the defibrillation threshold (DFT) is understood to represent an estimate of a point on the patient's probability-of-success curve. Different methods of measuring the DFT approximate different points on the probability-of-success curve with varying degrees of accuracy (see Chapter 99). Vulnerability testing is based on the close relationship between the upper limit of vulnerability (ULV) and the minimum shock strength that defibrillates reliably (see Fig. 100-3B).[13] The ULV

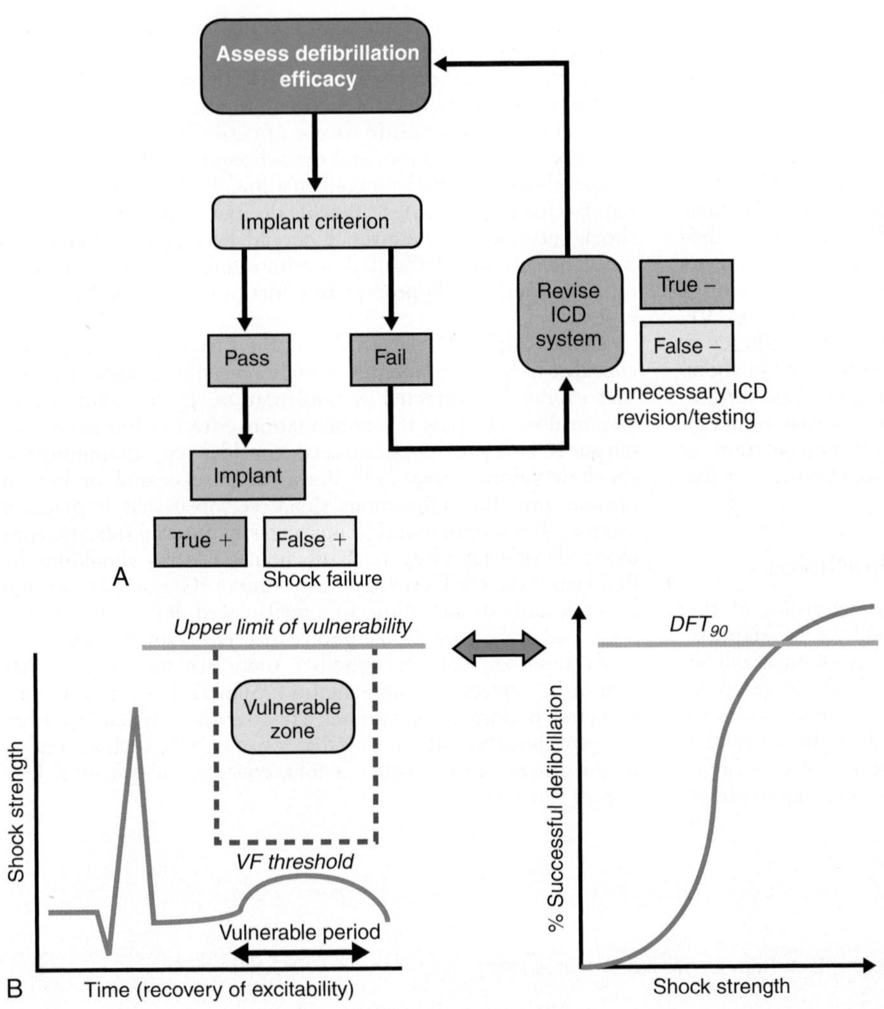

Figure 100-3 Implant testing. **A,** Role of the implant criterion for implantable cardioverter defibrillator (ICD). The implant criterion is the level of defibrillation performance predicted to result in a clinically adequate success rate for defibrillation of spontaneous ventricular fibrillation (VF). The implant criterion produces a true-positive result when patients who have reliable defibrillation of spontaneous ventricular tachycardia (VT) or VF pass the test. In a false-positive result, patients who have unreliable defibrillation pass and are placed at risk for unsuccessful defibrillation of spontaneous VT or VF. In a true-negative result, patients with unreliable defibrillation fail the implant criterion and might undergo indicated ICD system revision or retesting at a later date. In a false-negative result, patients with reliable defibrillation fail the implant criterion and undergo unnecessary system revision or retesting. **B,** Vulnerability testing. The cardiac vulnerable zone is the range of shock strengths and coupling intervals after the R wave or pacing pulse that induce VF. *Left,* The vulnerable zone is shown as a rhomboid-shaped region in a two-dimensional space defined by time (coupling interval) on the abscissa and shock strength on the ordinate. The upper border (upper limit of vulnerability, ULV) and the lower borders (VF threshold) are defined by shock strength. Note that the ULV will be identified accurately only if a shock times at the most-vulnerable interval corresponding to the peak of vulnerable zone. Because this interval cannot be determined from first principles, clinical vulnerability testing requires a scan of several shocks timed at intervals close to the peak of the T wave. The inner (left) and outer (right) borders, denoted by *dotted vertical lines,* are defined by time (coupling interval). The interval during which shocks induce VF is the vulnerable period. *Right,* An idealized defibrillation probability-of-success curve. The ULV closely approximates the shock strength that defibrillates with a probability of 90% (DFT_{90}).

is the weakest shock at which VF is not induced when it is delivered during the vulnerable period in regular rhythm. To measure the ULV, T-wave shocks must be delivered at the most vulnerable time in the vulnerable period. If a shock delivered at the peak of the vulnerable zone in regular rhythm does not induce VF, it has a 90% or greater probability of defibrillating successfully. However, because the precise timing of the peak of the vulnerable zone varies, the T wave is scanned by test shocks at several coupling intervals to ensure that shocks are delivered at the most vulnerable intervals.[13]

Both patient-specific and safety-margin strategies have been applied to defibrillation and vulnerability testing. The patient-specific strategy estimates the minimum shock strength that defibrillates reliably. The safety-margin strategy limits testing, but it only determines if there is a sufficient safety margin between the maximum output of the ICD and the shock strength required for consistent defibrillation. Vulnerability safety margin testing permits implantation without induction of VF in 80% to 95% of patients.[13,14]

Selection of Implant Testing Strategies and Methods

Defibrillation and vulnerability methods can be adapted to either patient-specific or safety-margin strategies. Both methods provide good results as assessed by conversion rates for spontaneous VT or VF.[12-14] Defibrillation testing permits assessment of sensing in VF. In comparison with the DFT, ULV testing estimates a higher point on the defibrillation probability of success and is more reproducible.[13]

A patient-specific strategy minimizes the long-term adverse effects of excessive programmed shock strength such as myocardial depression or rapid battery depletion caused by frequent delivered or aborted shocks. It is preferred to minimize the risk of syncope if long detection times are advisable in patients with frequent long episodes of nonsustained VT or VF. A safety-margin strategy reduces the number of VF episodes during testing. The vulnerability safety-margin method minimizes the risks of implant testing that are related to VF or circulatory arrest rather than to shocks (see "Complications," later).

Recommended patient-specific first-shock programming include 10 J plus DFT and 5 J plus ULV.[12] Recommended safety-margin testing includes two successful shocks at 10 J less than maximum output, one successful shock at 15 J, and no induction of VF by a four-shock T-wave scan at least 5 J less than maximum output. After safety-margin testing, the first shock is set to maximum output or 5 J above the strength of T-wave shocks that do not induce VF.[12]

Perspective

The goal of implant testing is to determine the optimal balance between implant safety and long-term benefits of ICD therapy. Since the 1980s, the value of inducing VF to ensure that ICDs will sense, detect, and defibrillate VF seemed self-evident. For current high-output, left-pectoral ICDs, the probability of passing a 10-J safety margin is sufficiently high (~95%)[12] that testing provides limited incremental information. This improved technology and use of ICDs for primary prevention have led some to question the need for either defibrillation testing or any assessment of defibrillation efficacy at ICD implantation.[15] However, most implanters, patients, and families are intolerant of sudden death caused by preventable, failed defibrillation. Experts disagree about optimal testing because data are insufficient to define the trade-off between accuracy and risk of testing. Overall, sensing and detection issues require induction of VF in about 5% of ICD recipients, testing defibrillation efficacy is required in 20% to 40%, and testing is contraindicated in about 5% because of conditions such as left atrial–appendage thrombus, inadequate anesthesia, and inadequate external rescue.[12] Currently, assessing defibrillation efficacy at implantation is the legal standard of practice and the recommendation of the Heart Rhythm Society.[16]

Patients with High Defibrillation Thresholds

Defibrillation efficacy is influenced by characteristics of the patient, ICD system, and testing method.[12] Our stepwise approach to the patient with a high DFT is summarized in Box 100-1.[12,17] Attention to preventing high DFTs (Step 0) reduces the need to troubleshoot them. This includes positioning the distal defibrillation coil accurately in the right ventricular apex (possibly against the septum) and routine use of a high-output ICD generator (≥34 J). Confirm that high-voltage connections are correct and have nominal impedances measured by low-voltage pulses.

Before troubleshooting a high DFT, the diagnosis should be confirmed to ensure that the first failure was not a chance event caused by the probabilistic nature of defibrillation. Failure of a test shock at 20 J or more and the subsequent maximum output rescue shock is sufficient confirmation, if detection of VF is rapid. However, if a test shock fails but a maximum output shock succeeds, the test shock should be repeated. Failure to meet the accepted defibrillation criterion (e.g., 10 J below maximum output) should prompt an effort to improve defibrillation efficacy.

Once a high DFT is confirmed, the first step is to apply the checklist in Step 1 to identify acutely reversible causes or causes that cannot be corrected at implantation. If the defibrillation system does not pass the implantation criterion but maximum output ICD rescue shocks succeed, consider reprogramming the shock waveform (Step 2).[18] If this is unsuccessful or not an option, alter the transvenous shock vector if that is practical (Step 3). If it is impractical or unsuccessful, insert a subcutaneous electrode or array (Step 4). A subcutaneous array should be the first step if the DFT exceeds the maximum ICD output, because programming or alterations of a well-placed, left-sided transvenous lead system are unlikely to reduce DFT sufficiently.[17]

At intervals, consider whether there are new factors that cannot be corrected at implantation (Step 1). If so, testing may be better performed on another day after the problem has been resolved, possibly with a drug that lowers DFT, such as sotalol. In the absence of reversible factors, consider an epicardial lead system (Step 5).

Box 100-1 Stepwise Approach to the Patient with a High Defibrillation Threshold

Step 0: Prevent high DFTs
- Before implant
  - Consider risks and benefits of continuing or withdrawing drugs that might increase DFT
  - Optimize medical therapy for heart failure
  - Drain left pleural effusion
- At implant
  - Position RV electrode tip at apex (before testing)
  - Ensure appropriate position of proximal coil in high SVC or innominate vein; exclude proximal coil if low in atrium
  - Set right ventricular polarity to anode for phase 1 if not nominal
  - Optimize waveform duration for shock pathway impedance if programmable
  - Use a high-output generator (≥ ~34 J)
  - Confirm high-voltage connections: Confirm correct connections of RV and SVC electrodes and integrity of current paths (nominal impedance assessed by low-voltage pulses)

Step 1: Identify and correct acutely reversible causes
- Correctable at implant
  - Metabolic: hyperkalemia, hypoxemia, hypercapnea, and acidemia due to deep sedation
  - Ischemia
  - Alternate current paths
  - Left pleural effusion or hemothorax; pericardial effusion or hemopericardium
  - Retained guidewire
  - Fragments of old intracardiac or intravascular electrodes
  - High shock pathway resistance (e.g., pneumothorax)
- Not correctable at implant
  - Myocardial depression
  - Pharmacologic (e.g., amiodarone, verapamil, lidocaine)
  - Prolonged procedure with multiple fibrillation-defibrillation episodes

Step 2: Change shock waveform if programmable (optional)
- Reprogram pulse durations for a different time constant
- For patients taking chronic amiodarone, program shorter phase 2

Step 3: Alter transvenous shock vector if defibrillation succeeds at maximum output
- Proximal coil in SVC, innominate vein, or high right atrium (exclude proximal coil if low)
- For a right-sided implant, exclude can or use cold can
- Add separate coil (e.g., innominate vein, left subclavian vein, azygous vein, coronary sinus)

Step 4: Implant subcutaneous electrode or electrode array

Step 5: Consider epicardial system

DFT, defibrillation threshold; RV, right ventricle; SVC, superior vena cava.

Programming

Appropriate programming minimizes the need for troubleshooting.[19] Optimal programming of devices that discriminate between supraventricular tachycardia (SVT) and VT reduces inappropriate therapies[20,21]; rarely, programming errors are fatal.[7,8]

Detection Zones

Detection is the algorithm by which an ICD processes (i.e. counts, measures, sorts) sensed signals to classify the rhythm and decide if therapy should be delivered. Detection of VF and hemodynamically unstable VT should be highly sensitive. Some inappropriate detection of SVT is the price of this sensitivity. Detection of hemodynamically stable VT should be more specific, and some delay in detection is acceptable.

Tiered-therapy ICDs have up to three ventricular rate-detection zones that permit programming of zone-specific therapies and SVT-VT discriminators (Fig. 100-4). The two slower zones are classified as VT zones, and the fastest one is classified as a VF zone. The sinus-VT rate boundary should be slow enough to ensure detection of all hemodynamically compromising VT. Because the upper rate limit for bradycardia pacing is about 30 ms longer than this interval in most ICDs, a long VT detection interval usually reduces the pacing upper rate limit. The boundary between the two VT zones should be based on the cycle length at which different or less antitachycardia pacing is preferred. The VT-VF rate boundary is based on the cycle length below which shocks should not be delayed for antitachycardia pacing. Typical values for these rate boundaries are 360 to 500 ms for slower VT, 340 to 300 ms for faster VT, and 280 to 240 ms for VF.

Three-zone programming is indicated in patients with clinical monomorphic VT and probably in primary prevention patients with coronary artery disease.[19] This permits different antitachycardia pacing for two distinct rates of VT and antitachycardia pacing for monomorphic VT that overlaps in rate with polymorphic VT. Two rate zones may be programmed for primary prevention with sinus-VT boundary at 340 to 320 ms. For most manufacturers, this reduces the risk of inappropriate therapy but increases that of not treating VT.

Single-zone programming may be considered for patients whose only arrhythmia is polymorphic VT or VF (e.g., long-QT syndrome).

Duration for Detection

Detection duration prior to antitachycardia pacing should not be decreased from nominal values because therapy is immediate after detection and undersensing of monomorphic VT is rare. It should be increased in patients who have long episodes of nonsustained VT.[6,8,22] Longer durations probably reduce the number of therapies and probably are safe in primary prevention patients.[23] Redetection time for VT should be increased from nominal if VT is well tolerated but antitachycardia pacing is not.

Supraventricular Tachycardia and Ventricular Tachycardia Discriminators

SVT-VT discriminators are a programmable subset of an ICD's detection algorithm for VT or VF that withhold ventricular therapy for SVT to improve specificity of therapy[6] (see Chapter 99). Some SVT discriminators should be programmed in all patients with adequate AV conduction in whom a VT zone is programmed.[19] Dual-chamber discriminators should be programmed in those with a stable, functioning atrial lead.[6-8]

SVT-VT discriminators apply in a range of cycle lengths bounded on the slower end by the VT detection interval and on the faster end by a minimum cycle length that varies among manufacturers.[6] Programming a sufficiently short minimum cycle length for SVT-VT discrimination is critical to reliable rejection of SVT. In clinical trials, about 25% of inappropriate therapy has been caused by SVT with ventricular cycle length sufficiently short that discriminators were not applied.[21]

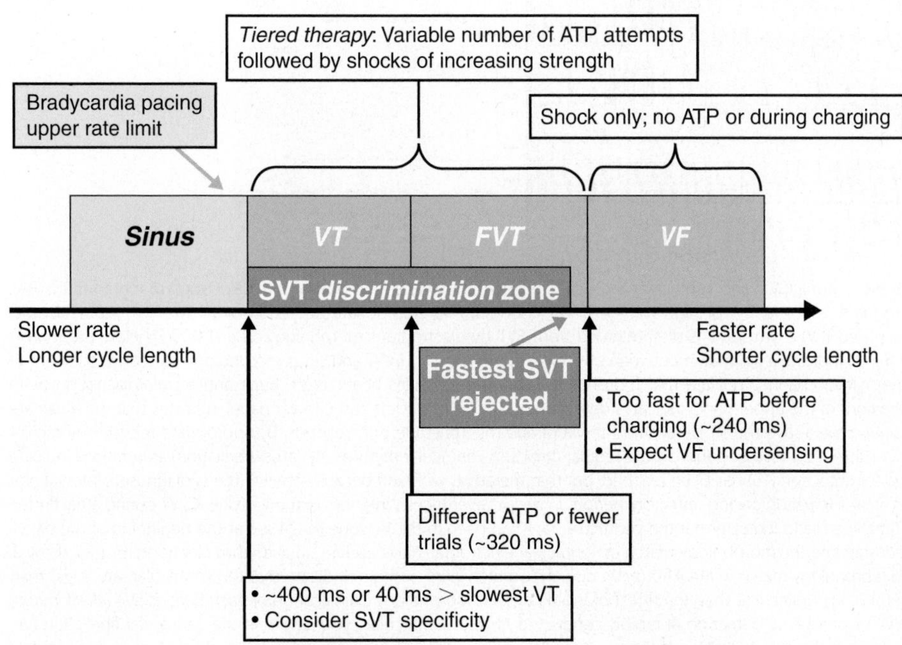

Figure 100-4 Implantable cardioverter defibrillator (ICD) rate detection zones. Some ICDs permit programming of an additional monitor-only zone. See text for details. ATP, antitachycardia pacing; FVT, fast ventricular defibrillation; SVT, supraventricular tachycardia; VF, ventricular fibrillation; VT, ventricular tachycardia.

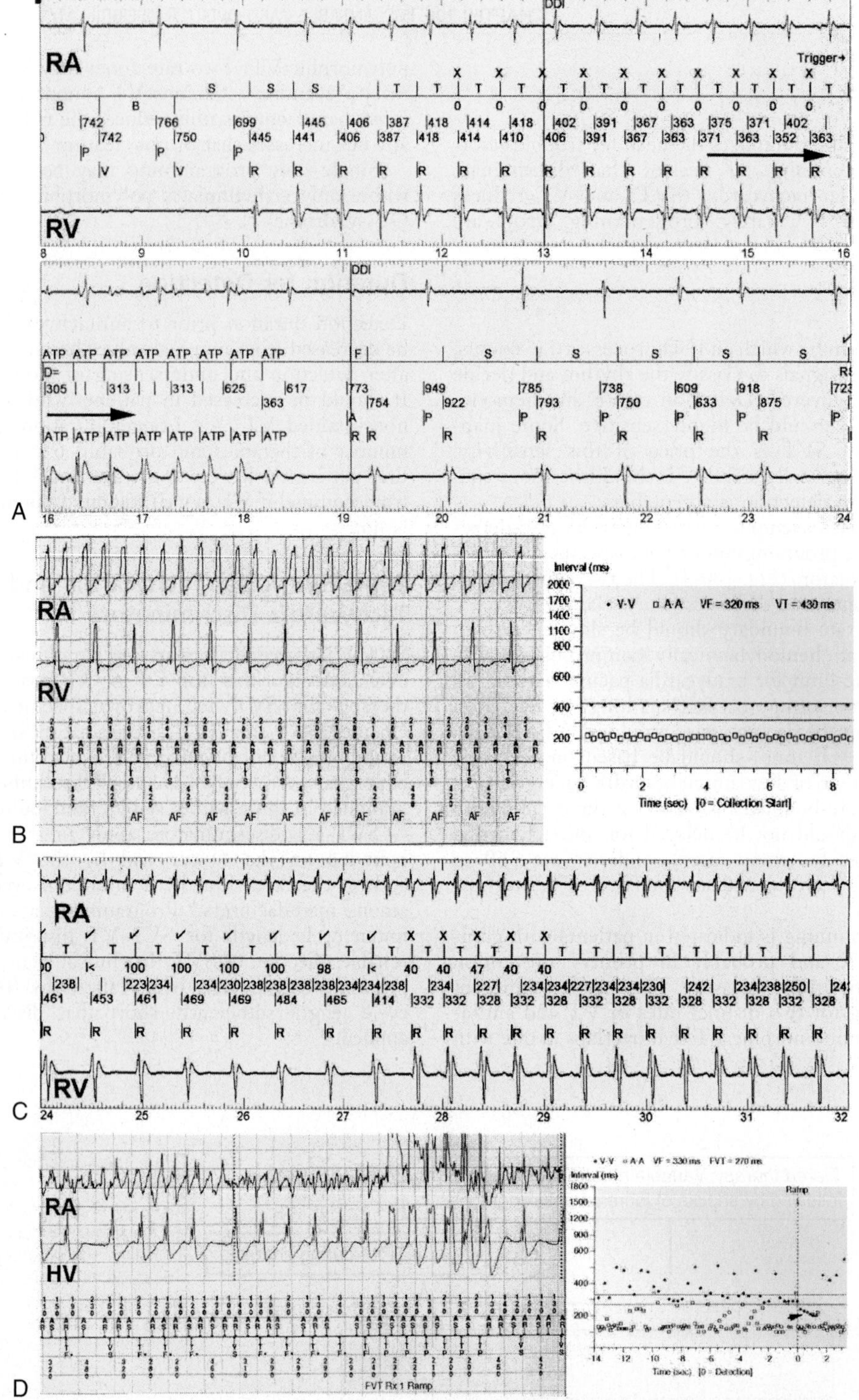

Figure 100-5 Discrimination between supraventricular tachycardia (SVT) and ventricular tachycardia (VT). Each panel shows bipolar atrial electrogram (right atrium, RA), dual-chamber marker channels, and either rate-sensing (right ventricle, RV) or high-voltage (HV) electrogram. **A,** Appropriate detection of VT with 1:1 ventriculoatrial conduction. VT begins during atrial-sensed, ventricular paced (PV) rhythm. VT is discriminated from SVT by electrogram morphology. The *0 values* below the marker channel corresponding to the electrograms in the VT zone (T) indicate a 0% match between electrogram morphology in VT and sinus morphology (R) seen at the right of the lower panel. The corresponding *X* marks above the marker channel indicate that morphology algorithm classifies beats as VT. Burst antitachycardia pacing (ATP) terminates VT at the left of the lower panel. *Trigger* at the right of the upper panel indicates detection of VT. *D* = at the left of the lower panel indicates that the atrial rate equals the ventricular rate. *S* denotes intervals in the sinus zone above the VT detection interval of 400 ms. Time line is in seconds. **B,** Appropriate rejection of rapidly conducted atrial flutter. Atrial flutter is identified by the consistent 2:1 PR association of the regular atrial and ventricular rhythms. AF (atrial fibrillation) annotations indicate that the number of intervals in the VT rate zone required for detection (16) has been reached, but that therapy is withheld because atrial flutter is diagnosed. Interval plot displays 2:1 atrioventricular (AV) association. *AR* denotes atrial intervals in pacing refractory period. *TS* denotes ventricular intervals in the VT zone. **C,** VT during atrial flutter. VT occurs during atrial flutter with 2:1 AV conduction. Time line marks indicate that the ventricular rate had been in the VT zone for 24 sec at the beginning of the panel. VT therapy is withheld because of both the 2:1 AV relationship and the morphology match of ventricular electrograms to baseline sinus rhythm electrograms (not shown). Numbers below the marker channel indicate 98%-100% morphology match in atrial flutter vs. 40%-47% match in VT. < marks indicate that the ventricular rate is less than the atrial rate. VT is detected by AV dissociation and morphology match less than the threshold value of 60%. Morphology classification of each beat as SVT *(check marks)* or VT *(X marks)* is indicated above the marker channel. **D,** Inappropriate detection of rapidly conducted AF with ventricular cycle length in the ventricular fibrillation (VF) zone. AF is detected in the fast (F) VT zone *(FVT marks)*, which is the slower portion of the VF zone. Detection in the FVT zone was programmed for 12 of 16 intervals less than the VF detection interval of 330 ms. The first inappropriate therapy (decremental ramp antitachycardia pacing) occurs toward the right of the electrogram panel *(Rx 1 Ramp)*, denoted by *TP*. A relatively long VF detection interval combined with shorter than nominal detection time increases probability of inappropriate detection of rapidly conducted AF. In the VF zone, morphology may be used to reject AF, but interval stability cannot be used because VF intervals may be irregular. Interval plot shows marked variability of RR intervals, with many longer than the VF detection interval. *Arrow* corresponds to ramp antitachycardia pacing. Long AA intervals correspond to intermittent atrial undersensing. *AS* denotes atrial sensed intervals. *VS* denotes ventricular intervals in the sinus zone.

Therapy

Painless antitachycardia pacing terminates 80% to 95% of spontaneous VT with cycle length longer than 300 to 320 ms with a low risk of acceleration (1%-5%).[24] A single trial of antitachycardia pacing can terminate 70% to 85% of fast VT (cycle length, 240-320 ms) with low rates of acceleration and syncope.[25] Usually, burst cycle lengths should be 85% to 90% of the VT cycle length for faster VTs and 70% to 80% of the VT cycle length for slower VTs.[24] Ventricular antitachycardia pacing also reduces shocks for inappropriately detected SVT, either by terminating SVT or by delaying shock therapy until SVT terminates spontaneously or slows into the sinus zone.[8] Thus antitachycardia pacing reduces both unnecessary shocks for VT and inappropriate shocks for SVT. It improves quality of life[25] and should be programmed empirically in most patients, even if its efficacy has not been assessed.[19,25]

The first shock strength for VF should be set in relation either to an established implant safety margin or to maximum output.[12] To prevent proarrhythmia caused by oversensing, it should exceed the ULV. In modern ICDs with short charge times, shocks for hemodynamically stable VT should be programmed at or above the shock strength for VF, not at a low energy. This maximizes the likelihood that a VT shock will terminate (inappropriately detected) rapidly conducted AF and minimizes the risks that it will accelerate VT, induce VF, or initiate AF if it is delivered during the atrial vulnerable period.

Monitoring and Follow-up

Remote Monitoring

The goals of ICD follow-up are to ensure appropriate device function and to provide health care professionals with access to stored diagnostic data. Historically, patients have made routine follow-up clinic visits at quarterly intervals. Remote Internet-based monitoring permits patients to transmit almost all device and clinical data obtained in a clinic visit. In some ICDs, patients actively initiate transmissions by holding an inductive telemetry wand over the pulse generator. The wand is connected to a modem, which transmits data over the Internet. ICDs with radiofrequency transmitters automatically transmit stored data to a local hub, which then resends the data over the Internet. This permits daily transmission of alerts related to ICD malfunction, spontaneous arrhythmias, and monitoring of comorbidities including heart failure. In either case, ICD data are transmitted to a secure server and then to the health care professional.[26]

Monitoring of Heart Failure and Other Comorbidities

Care of various medical conditions may be improved by home monitoring. Networks developed for remote monitoring of ICDs can be used to monitor medical conditions other than VT or VF in ICD patients if relevant data are stored in the ICD or input into the local hub from another source. Heart failure is the typical comorbidity for at least three reasons: It has a high prevalence in ICD patients, trials of home telemonitoring systems using a scale and blood pressure cuff demonstrate clinical benefit,[27] and continuous monitoring of heart failure using data stored in ICDs is technically feasible. Basic stored in ICDs include heart-rate variability and the patient's activity level estimated from the accelerometer used for rate-responsive pacing. Other data stored in cardiac resynchronization or dual chamber ICDs are useful for management of heart failure, such as percentage pacing in each chamber or frequency, duration, and ventricular rate during AF. Intrathoracic impedance can be measured using simple, low-power technology included in present ICDs. It provides an indirect measure of lung water and can detect exacerbations of heart failure with sufficient warning to permit preventive interventions.[28]

Other implanted heart-failure monitors require a special sensor. Important considerations include the relationship between the sensed parameter and heart failure, power consumption, and frequency of data acquisition. A prospective study reported the utility of a stand-alone, implantable right-ventricular pressure sensor for ambulatory monitoring of heart-failure monitoring.[29] ICD systems that include this sensor are in clinical trials.

A different approach to monitoring heart failure inputs clinical data into the ICD's remote monitoring hub from sources other than the ICD. In one system, weight and blood pressure are recorded via sensors that transmit information wirelessly to the hub.

AF is an important comorbidity that can be monitored reliably by ICDs. It can exacerbate heart failure due to loss of atrial transport or rapid ventricular rate. Identification of rapidly conducted AF during activities of daily living might permit treatment or programming interventions to prevent inappropriate shocks. Continuous ICD monitoring of patients with infrequent paroxysmal AF might permit safe with withdrawal of anticoagulation.

Common Clinical Issues

Common clinical presentations in ICD patients include shocks, ineffective therapy, and failure to deliver therapy.[7,8] Management tools include clinical data (history, chest x-ray) and ICD data (programming, lead impedance values and trends, stored electrograms, and marker channels).

Diagnosing Shocks

ICD sensing and detection is imperfect: ICD-detected VT or VF can represent either a tachycardia (SVT or VT) or oversensing of nonarrhythmic electrical signals. ICDs also discriminate tachycardias imperfectly: true SVT episodes may be classified as VT or VF, and true VT may be classified as SVT. ICDs might also deliver unnecessary shocks for VT that could be terminated by antitachycardia pacing (Fig. 100-6). The first step is to determine if therapy was delivered in response to oversensing or a tachycardia.

Oversensing

Shocks occur in the absence of tachycardias because nonarrhythmic physiologic or nonphysiologic signals are oversensed and detected as arrhythmias.[6,7] Nonphysiologic signals usually are extracardiac. Physiologic signals may be intracardiac (P, R, or T waves) or extracardiac (myopotentials) (Fig. 100-7). Oversensing accounts for approximately one third of inappropriate shocks in long-term follow-up.[30]

Oversensing of physiologic intracardiac signals results in two device-detected R waves for each cardiac cycle. P-wave oversensing and R-wave double counting occur as alternating cycle lengths. T-wave oversensing occurs as alternating morphologies.[31] P-wave oversensing can occur if the distal coil of an integrated bipolar lead is too close to the tricuspid valve. R-wave double counting occurs if the duration of the sensing electrogram exceeds the ventricular blanking period of 120 to 140 ms. It causes all VTs to be detected in the VF zone so that no VT is treated with antitachycardia pacing, regardless of its cycle length. T-wave oversensing often occurs in the setting of low-amplitude R waves. In addition to causing inappropriate therapy, T-wave oversensing can cause inappropriate inhibition of bradycardia pacing or delivery of antitachycardia pacing at the wrong rate.

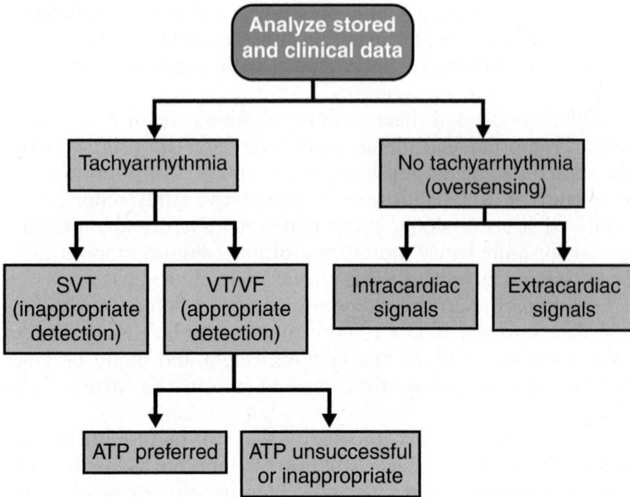

Figure 100-6 Approach to the patient who presents with implantable cardioverter defibrillator (ICD) shock(s). See text for details. ATP, antitachycardia pacing; SVT, supraventricular tachycardia; VF, ventricular fibrillation; VT, ventricular tachycardia.

The hallmark of oversensing of extracardiac signals is the replacement of the isoelectric baseline with high-frequency noise that shows no fixed relationship to the cardiac cycle. External electromagnetic interference usually is continuous. Signal amplitude is greater on the high-voltage electrogram recorded from widely spaced electrodes than on the sensing electrogram recorded from closely spaced electrodes. Oversensing due to lead or connector (header, adapter, or set-screw) problems is intermittent, occurring only during a small fraction of the cardiac cycle, and is usually associated with an abnormal pacing-lead impedance. Lead and connector signals may be limited to the sensing electrogram and might saturate the amplifier range. This type of oversensing is the most important, because the ICD system might not deliver adequate pacing or shocks.[32] Further, an inappropriate shock into a faulty lead can achieve sufficient voltage at the heart to induce VF (if applied in the vulnerable period) but insufficient voltage to defibrillate. Myopotential oversensing has variable duration. Pectoral myopotentials are more prominent on the high-voltage electrogram, and diaphragmatic myopotentials are more prominent on the sensing electrogram.

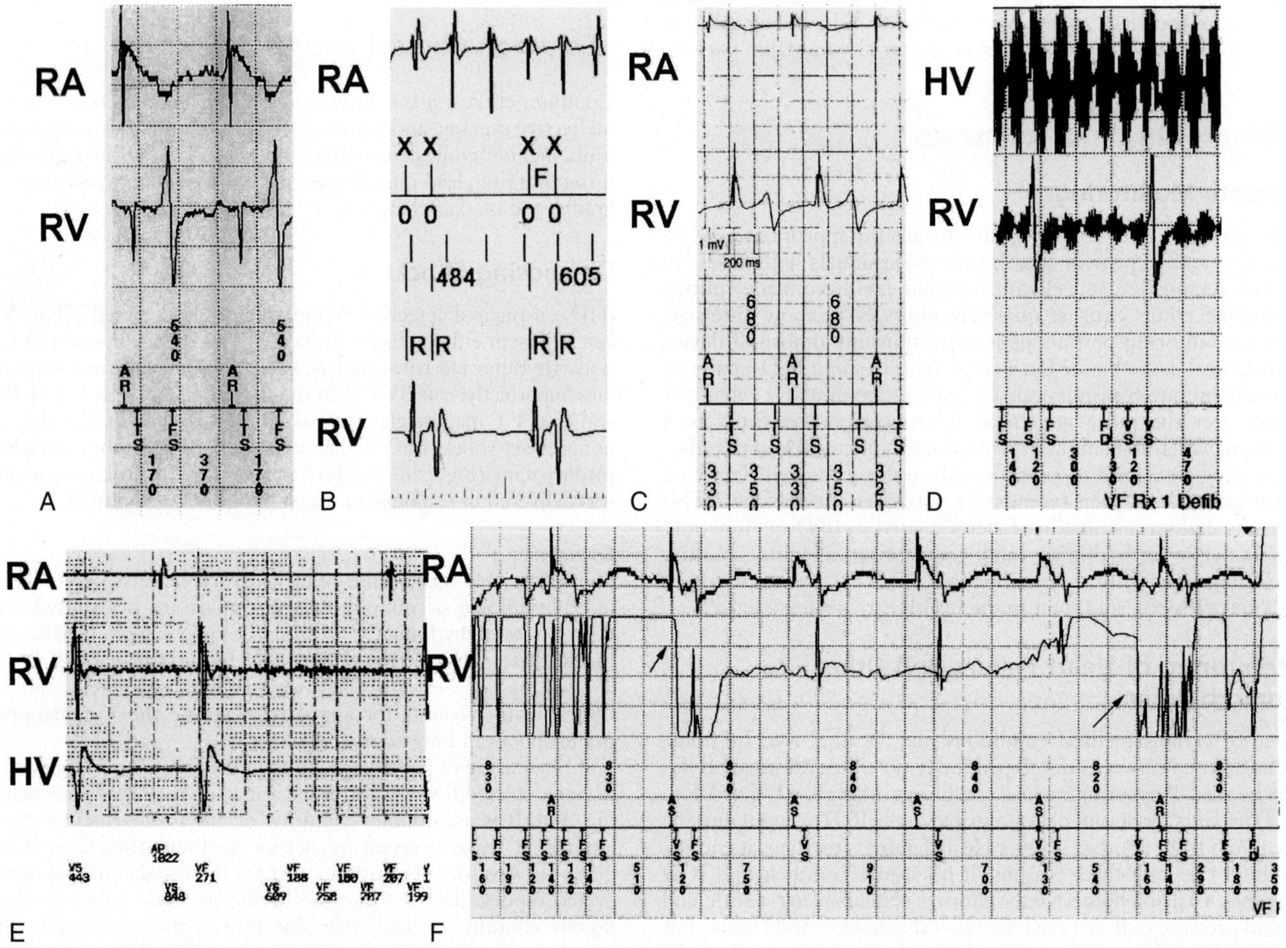

Figure 100-7 Oversensing of physiologic intracardiac signals (A to C) or extracardiac signals (D to F) resulting in inappropriate detection of ventricular fibrillation (VF). **A,** P-wave oversensing in sinus rhythm from an integrated bipolar lead with distal coil near the tricuspid valve. **B,** R-wave double-counting during conducted atrial fibrillation (AF) in a biventricular-sensing implantable cardioverter defibrillator (ICD). **C,** T-wave oversensing in a patient with low-amplitude R wave (note mV calibration marker). **D,** Electromagnetic interference from a power drill has higher amplitude on widely spaced high-voltage electrogram than on closely spaced true bipolar sensing electrogram. **E,** Diaphragmatic myopotential oversensing in a patient with an integrated bipolar lead at the right ventricle (RV) apex. Note that the noise level is constant, but oversensing does not occur until automatic gain control increases the gain sufficiently, about 600 ms after the sensed R waves. **F,** Lead fracture shows intermittent saturation of amplifier range denoted by *arrow*. HV, His-ventricle; RA, right atrium.

Ventricular Tachycardia versus Supraventricular Tachycardia

If stored electrograms indicate that a shock was delivered in response to a true tachycardia, the second step in diagnosis is to determine if the rhythm is VT or SVT. Established principles of ECG and electrogram analysis usually lead to the correct diagnosis.[6,7] For single-chamber ICDs, analysis of the tachycardia onset and the morphology and regularity of the ventricular electrogram are the cornerstones of electrogram interpretation. A real-time, reference sinus electrogram should be recorded with the patient in the same posture in which the episode occurred to facilitate analysis of electrogram morphology. For dual-chamber ICDs, analyses of the chamber of onset, atrial and ventricular rates, and AV relationships provide additional key diagnostic information.

Unnecessary Shocks for Ventricular Tachycardia

If the diagnosis of VT is confirmed, programming de novo or additional antitachycardia pacing might prevent shocks. Shocks delivered in response to self-terminating VT may be prevented by increasing the duration for detection or altering specific programming relating to shock confirmation or episode termination.[7]

Approach to the Patient with Shocks

If a patient experiences *single or infrequent* shocks, the ICD should be interrogated within 24 to 48 hours. The frequency of shocks for VT may be reduced by programming antitachycardia pacing for monomorphic VT[25,33] or by antiarrhythmic drugs. Interactions between drugs and the ICD interactions[34] are summarized in Box 100-2. Oversensing might require reprogramming, lead revision, or a new sensing lead. Inappropriate therapy of SVT may be corrected by reprogramming (rate zones or SVT-VT discriminators) or treatment with drugs or ablation. Both drugs and reprogramming can influence detection of VT. Reprogramming usually is preferred to prevent inappropriate therapy of sinus tachycardia. Other SVTs might require either approach.

Frequent or repetitive shocks constitute an emergency. If a patient receives repetitive inappropriate shocks caused by SVT or oversensing during sinus rhythm, VT or VF detection may be disabled using a programmer or magnet. The problem is corrected by the methods used for single inappropriate shocks. Repetitive shocks for VT may be caused by recurring episodes of VT after successful shock termination of VT (VT storm or cluster shocks) or by multiple unsuccessful shocks for a single episode. Therapeutic approaches differ. VT storm may be caused by acute ischemia, exacerbation of heart failure, metabolic abnormalities (e.g., hypokalemia, amiodarone-induced hyperthyroidism), and drug effects (e.g., proarrhythmia, change in prescribed drugs, or noncompliance). Diagnosis of acute coronary syndromes during VT storm is difficult, because multiple shocks can cause changes in repolarization and elevations of troponin I. Therapy may include reversing the precipitating cause, administering β-blockers or antiarrhythmic drugs (sotalolol,[35] amiodarone), and catheter ablation. Rarely, ICDs deliver unnecessary repetitive shocks for recurring self-terminating episodes of VT. Increasing the duration required for detection and redetection of VT or VF might prevent these shocks.

Unsuccessful Shocks

Because defibrillation success is probabilistic, occasional shocks fail; but failure of two maximum-output shocks is rare if the safety margin is adequate.[8,12] If an ICD classifies a shock as unsuccessful, stored electrograms must be reviewed to determine both if the shock was delivered for true VT or VF and if the shock actually failed to terminate VT or VF.

Box 100-2 Interactions between Drugs and Implantable Cardioverter Defibrillators

FREQUENCY OF VENTRICULAR TACHYCARDIA OR FIBRILLATION

Increased
- Antiarrhythmic drugs
- Drugs with proarrhythmic side effects
- Drugs that interact with proarrhythmic drugs

Decreased

DETECTION OF VENTRICULAR TACHYCARDIA OR FIBRILLATION

Programmed rate boundaries
- VT rate (decrease—class 1C, amiodarone)
- SVT ventricular rate
  - Decrease (β-blockers, amiodarone, sotalol)
  - Increase (1:1 conduction of atrial flutter on class 1C drugs)

ICD SVT-VT discrimination algorithms
- VT interval stability (more irregular on class 1C, amiodarone)
- Altered electrogram morphology

THERAPY FOR VENTRICULAR TACHYCARDIA OR FIBRILLATION

Defibrillation energy requirement
- Increase (class 1B, class 1C, chronic amiodarone, verapamil)

Decrease (III except amiodarone)

EFFECTS ON PACING

Elevated thresholds (class 1C)
- Bradycardia pacing
- Use-dependent effect during antitachycardia pacing

More pacing-induced battery drain if drug-induced sinus bradycardia or AV conduction delay

AV, atrioventricular; ICD, implantable cardioverter defibrillator; SVT, supraventricular tachycardia; VT, ventricular tachycardia.

ICDs misclassify effective therapy as ineffective if VT or VF recurs before the ICD determines that the VT or VF episode has terminated or if the postshock rhythm is SVT in the VT rate zone (catecholamine-induced sinus tachycardia or shock-induced AF). Solutions to the latter problem include applying SVT-VT discriminators to redetection of VT if programmable, increasing shock strength to prevent shock-induced AF, or administering β-blockers to slow postshock SVT.

Failure of multiple high-output shocks to terminate a regular tachycardia suggests sinus tachycardia because VT and nonsinus SVT usually are terminated by one or two shocks. Shocks from chronic ICD systems that defibrillated reliably at implant might fail to terminate true VT or VF because of patient-related or ICD system-related reasons. In chronically implanted systems, most patient-related causes of unsuccessful shocks can be reversed, but most system-related causes require operative intervention. See "Patients with High Defibrillation Thresholds" earlier for patient-related reasons.

ICD system-related causes include insufficient programmed or delivered shock strength; battery depletion; lead dislodgment; and failure of leads, device-lead connections, or generators. In evaluating stored ICD data, attention should be focused on identifying excessive detection time, excessive charge time, signs of conductor or connection failure (see Fig. 100-6), mismatch between programmed and delivered shock strength suggesting a lead short, or out-of-range high-voltage impedance.[8]

Failure to Deliver Therapy or Delayed Therapy

Delayed therapy and failure to deliver therapy may be caused by problems with either ICD programming (including human error) or the ICD system. VT or VF is not detected if the ICD is inactivated, VT is slower than the programmed detection interval, SVT-VT discriminators diagnose SVT, or sensing is impaired by device-device or intra-device interactions. VF may be undersensed due to combinations of programming (sensitivity, rate, or duration), low-amplitude electrograms, rapidly varying electrogram amplitude, drug effects, or postshock tissue changes.[8] Lead, connector or generator[36] malfunction can prevent delivery of effective therapy.

Complications

The principal surgical complications of ICDs are similar to those of pacemakers: lead dislodgment, pneumothorax, infection, and cardiac perforation. With experienced operators, these combined complications total 3% to 5%,[5] for single or dual-chamber ICDs. Additionally, the decision to implant an ICD usually adds a 1% to 3% risk of infection at each pulse generator change for the rest the patient's life.

Defibrillation testing adds risk related to shocks alone (e.g., thromboembolism), anesthesia required for shocks, and induction of VF. The latter include cerebral or myocardial ischemia, electromechanical dissociation, and refractory VF. Overall, the risk of major complications is probably about 1% and risk of death is about 0.2%.[12]

The most common late complications include inappropriate shocks and lead failures requiring reoperation. In controlled studies, the incidence of VT or VF in ICD patients exceeds that in control groups by a factor of two to three.[37,38] Recent attention has focused on ICD proarrhythmia related to pacing.[39] Proarrhythmia should be considered if the frequency of VT or VF increases after ICD implant or in association with a change in pacing mode.

Selecting the Appropriate Device

Dual Chamber versus Single Chamber

Dual-chamber ICDs provide dual-chamber pacing, diagnostics regarding atrial arrhythmias, and SVT-VT discriminators that are not available in single-chamber ICDs. Some also provide therapy of atrial arrhythmias. New dual-chamber pacing modes that minimize ventricular pacing reduce morbidity due to obligatory right ventricular pacing,[40] which might have exacerbated heart failure in patients with early dual-chamber ICDs. Disadvantages of dual-chamber ICDs include higher cost, atrial lead complications, and decreased longevity.

There are no accepted criteria to determine when a dual-chamber ICD is indicated solely for improved SVT-VT discrimination. The only randomized, controlled study showed a modest benefit of dual-chamber over single-chamber SVT-VT discrimination, but different programming between the single-chamber and dual-chamber groups might have limited the measured effect.[20] Additionally, dual-chamber stored electrograms provide higher diagnostic accuracy than single-chamber ones.

Resynchronization Pacing

In the United States, cardiac resynchronization pacing is delivered to most patients using ICDs. Cardiac resynchronization produces a major drain on ICD batteries, reducing ICD longevity. Specific technical and programming issues apply to resynchronization ICDs.[8]

Special Issues

Psychosocial and Lifestyle Issues

ICD patients might experience anxiety about shocks, but they might also feel protected from the risk of sudden death. Patients with life-threatening VT or VF have similar quality of life when treated with ICDs or antiarrhythmic drugs, but ICD shocks are associated with reduced quality of life. ICD recipients might benefit from counseling, education, and support groups.

Specific guidelines for driving and flying[41] are based on arrhythmia symptoms and frequency. Patients in whom ICDs are implanted for primary prophylaxis are not restricted from driving personal cars (as opposed to commercial vehicles). Guidelines recommend that patients refrain from all driving for 6 months after each shock and for 6 months after ICD implantation for secondary prevention. Even though most patients resume driving earlier, accidents in ICD recipients occur less often than in the general driving population.

Electromagnetic Interference

Ubiquitous electromagnetic waves can interfere with ICDs. This might result in temporary or permanent inactivation, inappropriate detection of VT or VF, or inappropriate pacing or inhibition of pacing.[42,43] Electromagnetic interference is a lesser problem for true-bipolar sensing than for integrated-bipolar sensing.[6]

Nonmedical Sources

Clinically significant electromagnetic interference is rare in daily life. Routine use of household articles should not interfere with ICD function. Activated digital cellular phones should be held to the contralateral ear and should not be carried in the ipsilateral breast pocket. ICD patients may walk through airport metal detectors and electronic article surveillance devices at a normal pace. Prolonged exposure can inhibit pacing and detection of VT or VF, cause inappropriate detection of VT or VF, or (in some ICDs) program VT or VF detection off. Some industrial sources pose sufficient risks (e.g., arc welding, power tools, large magnets) that ICD electrograms and marker channels should be recorded while the patient is operating equipment, preferably with the ICD in a monitor-only mode.

Medical Sources

Magnetic resonance imaging poses multiple risks in ICD patients and is contraindicated. If electrosurgery using a dispersive ground electrode is required, VT or VF detection should be suspended or disabled with a magnet, and the patient's rhythm should be monitored. The ICD should be interrogated and detection should be reactivated immediately following the procedure. Cardioversion of AF should be performed through the ICD. Because radiation therapy can damage ICD circuitry, ICDs should be shielded or moved to the contralateral side. Radiofrequency catheter ablation should be performed as far as possible from ICD electrodes, a temporary pacing electrode should be inserted, and VT or VF detection should be disabled. Because pacing thresholds are highest about 24 hours after ablation, outputs should be increased and thresholds should be checked several days later.

Medical Advisories and Recalls

ICDs require the highest standards of reliability. Yet all electronic devices have finite failure rates. These include random failures related to components or manufacturing and systematic failures caused by design or manufacturing flaws. Recent large recalls of ICD pulse generators and leads have focused attention on ICD reliability.[44]

An ICD malfunction occurs when it fails to meet performance specifications or otherwise perform as in tended.[44] Malfunctions can compromise therapy or involve less-critical functions such as diagnostics. Performance standards for pulse generators and leads are not uniform. Postmarket surveillance includes both passive analysis of returned products and active prospective audits.[45] The former is critical to determining the root cause of any malfunction, but it underestimates the incidence of defects because failures are underreported. Because prospective audits are performed inconsistently, usually on sample sizes that are too small to identify infrequent failure modes, postmarket surveillance is widely judged to be inadequate.[36] Internet-based remote monitoring might improve this surveillance.

Accurate communication of risk is important, both from the FDA and industry to physicians and from physicians to patients.[44] Once a malfunction is identified, the FDA may issue a safety advisory or one of three levels of recall. The Heart Rhythm Society has recommended eliminating the term *recall* because it can bias both patients and physicians toward unnecessary explants.[44]

In deciding whether to explant a recalled ICD, the physician should consider multiple patient and device factors.[44,46] These include clinical consequences of the malfunction in a specific patient (e.g., pacemaker dependent or not, probability of life-threatening VT or VF), probability and time course of the malfunction, predictability of the malfunction by clinical monitoring, effectiveness of noninvasive methods to mitigate risk (e.g. specific programming or intensified follow-up), risks of explant and replacement in a specific patient (e.g., comorbidities, anticoagulation), and patient preferences. Recalls reflect prolonged analysis of extensive data. Urgent device replacement is rarely required.

Future Trends

ICDs have evolved from a focused therapy for VT or VF to a broader platform incorporating dual- and triple-chamber pacing, therapy for atrial arrhythmias, and remote monitoring of heart failure. This trend of increasing functionality is likely to continue. ICDs under development include improved features for monitoring heart failure and other comorbidities such as ischemia. At the same time, the number of automatic, self-checking, and self-adjusting functions will increase to improve usability and reduce operator errors.

Reduction of Inappropriate Shocks

Both incremental improvements and novel technology should substantially reduce inappropriate shocks caused by oversensing and SVT. Two strategies to reduce oversensing include comparison of signals on the sensing and shock electrograms[32] and application of digital signal processing technology to discriminate true ventricular electrograms from nonphysiologic events based on frequency content. ICD pulse generators that detect lead failures and protect patients against their adverse consequences are technologically feasible.[32]

Improvements in electrogram-based methods and integration of hemodynamic sensors into the detection and therapy decision process might reduce unnecessary shocks for SVT and VT. Pressure and photoplethysmography sensors are likely to be implemented. In investigational ICD systems that include a right ventricular pressure sensor for monitoring heart failure, recorded spontaneous arrhythmias demonstrate substantial variations in pressure waveforms. Subcutaneous photoplethysmography discriminates perfusing (stable) from nonperfusing (unstable) tachycardias using an optical source and receiver on the pulse generator. Unlike endocardial pressure sensors, it does not require a special lead, but data are limited regarding long-term performance in a fibrous, chronic pocket. Assessing hemodynamic stability of tachyarrhythmias remains a challenge, but hemodynamic discrimination of oversensing in sinus rhythm from VF should be straightforward.

Information Management

Remote monitoring of ICDs might provide more raw data than can be integrated easily into effective clinical decision making. Initial efforts have been made to postprocess remotely downloaded ICD data at a central server, so that clinicians can be presented with actionable clinical knowledge rather than engineering-based data. ICD manufacturers are working to integrate these data into electronic medical records and to ensure that disparate health care providers can access meaningful information in a timely manner.

Subcutaneous Implantable Cardioverter-Defibrillators

In contrast to the dominant trend of increasing functionality, there is a counter trend favoring simplicity, motivated by awareness of the many patients who might benefit from a basic ICD for primary prevention. Morbidity associated with transvenous leads could be eliminated by an ICD that uses only subcutaneous electrodes. A subcutaneous ICD may be implanted without fluoroscopy, simplifying the implantation if testing did not require a temporary transvenous electrode to induce VF. However, subcutaneous ICDs cannot perform antitachycardia, resynchronization, or long-term bradycardia or pacing; data regarding specificity of subcutaneous sensing and detection are limited; and the fraction of patients who can be defibrillated reliably may be lower for subcutaneous than transvenous defibrillation.

References

1. Zipes DP, Camm AJ, Borggrefe M, et al: ACC/AHA/ESC 2006 Guidelines for Management of Patients with Ventricular Arrhythmias and the Prevention of Sudden Cardiac Death: A report of the American College of Cardiology/American Heart Association Task Force and the European Society of Cardiology Committee for Practice Guidelines (writing committee to develop Guidelines for Management of Patients With Ventricular Arrhythmias and the Prevention of Sudden Cardiac Death): Developed in collaboration with the European Heart Rhythm Association and the Heart Rhythm Society. Circulation 114(10):e385-e484, 2006.
2. Lee DS, Tu JV, Austin PC, et al: Effect of cardiac and noncardiac

conditions on survival after defibrillator implantation. J Am Coll Cardiol 49(25):2408-2415, 2007.
3. Stevenson LW, Desai AS: Selecting patients for discussion of the ICD as primary prevention for sudden death in heart failure. J Card Fail 12(6):407-412, 2006.
4. Stevenson LW: Implantable cardioverter-defibrillators for primary prevention of sudden death in heart failure: Are there enough bangs for the bucks? Circulation 114(2):101-103, 2006.
5. Belott P, Reynolds D: Permanent pacemaker and implantable cardioverter-defibrillator implantation. In Ellenbogen K, Kay G, Lau C, Willkoff B (eds): Clinical Cardiac Pacing, Defibrillation, and Resynchronization Therapy, 3rd ed. Philadelphia, Saunders, 2007, pp 561-652.
6. Swerdlow C, Gillberg J, Olson W: Sensing and detection. In Ellenbogen K, Kay G, Lau C, Willkoff B (eds): Clinical Cardiac Pacing, Defibrillation, and Resynchronization Therapy, 3rd ed. Philadelphia, Saunders, 2007, pp 75-160.
7. Swerdlow CD, Friedman PA: Advanced ICD troubleshooting: Part I. Pacing Clin Electrophysiol 28(12):1322-1346, 2005.
8. Swerdlow CD, Friedman PA: Advanced ICD troubleshooting: Part II. Pacing Clin Electrophysiol 29(1):70-96, 2006.
9. Ellenbogen KA, Wood MA, Stambler BS, et al: Measurement of ventricular electrogram amplitude during intraoperative induction of ventricular tachyarrhythmias. Am J Cardiol 70(11):1017-1022, 1992.
10. Swerdlow CD: Implantation of cardioverter defibrillators without induction of ventricular fibrillation. Circulation 103(17):2159-2164, 2001.
11. Glikson M, Trusty JM, Grice SK, et al: A stepwise testing protocol for modern implantable cardioverter-defibrillator systems to prevent pacemaker-implantable cardioverter-defibrillator interactions. Am J Cardiol 83(3):360-366, 1999.
12. Swerdlow CD, Russo AM, Degroot PJ: The dilemma of ICD implant testing. Pacing Clin Electrophysiol 30(5):675-700, 2007.
13. Swerdlow CD, Shehata M, Chen PS: Using the upper limit of vulnerability to assess defibrillation efficacy at implantation of ICDs. Pacing Clin Electrophysiol 30(2):258-270, 2007.
14. Day JD, Doshi RN, Belott P, et al: Inductionless or limited shock testing is possible in most patients with implantable cardioverter- defibrillators/cardiac resynchronization therapy defibrillators: Results of the multicenter ASSURE Study (Arrhythmia Single Shock Defibrillation Threshold Testing Versus Upper Limit of Vulnerability: Risk Reduction Evaluation With Implantable Cardioverter-Defibrillator Implantations). Circulation 115(18):2382-2389, 2007.
15. Strickberger SA, Klein GJ: Is defibrillation testing required for defibrillator implantation? J Am Coll Cardiol 44(1): 88-91, 2004.
16. Curtis AB, Ellenbogen KA, Hammill SC, et al: Clinical competency statement: Training pathways for implantation of cardioverter defibrillators and cardiac resynchronization devices. Heart Rhythm 1(3):371-375, 2004.
17. Mainigi SK, Callans DJ: How to manage the patient with a high defibrillation threshold. Heart Rhythm 3(4):492-495, 2006.
18. Kroll MW, Swerdlow CD: Optimizing defibrillation waveforms for ICDs. J Interv Card Electrophysiol 18(3):247-263, 2007.
19. Wilkoff BL, Ousdigian KT, Sterns LD, et al: A comparison of empiric to physician-tailored programming of implantable cardioverter-defibrillators: Results from the prospective randomized multicenter EMPIRIC trial. J Am Coll Cardiol 48(2):330-339, 2006.
20. Friedman PA, McClelland RL, Bamlet WR, et al: Dual-chamber versus single-chamber detection enhancements for implantable defibrillator rhythm diagnosis: The Detect Supraventricular Tachycardia study. Circulation 113(25):2871-2879, 2006.
21. Compton SJ, Merrill JJ, Dorian P, et al: Continuous template collection and updating for electrogram morphology discrimination in implantable cardioverter defibrillators. Pacing Clin Electrophysiol 29(3):244-254, 2006.
22. Gunderson BD, Abeyratne AI, Olson WH, Swerdlow CD: Effect of programmed number of intervals to detect ventricular fibrillation on implantable cardioverter-defibrillator aborted and unnecessary shocks. Pacing Clin Electrophysiol 30(2):157-165, 2007.
23. Wilkoff B, Williamson B, Stern R, et al: Strategic programming of detection and therapy parameters in implantable cardioverter-defibrillators reduces shocks in primary prevention patients: Results from the PREPARE (Primary Prevention Parameters Evaluation) study. J Am Coll Cardiol 52(7):541-550, 2008.
24. Sweeney MO: Antitachycardia pacing for ventricular tachycardia using implantable cardioverter defibrillators: Substrates, methods and clinical experience. Pacing Clin Electrophysiol 27:1292-1305, 2004.
25. Wathen MS, DeGroot PJ, Sweeney MO, et al: Prospective randomized multicenter trial of empirical antitachycardia pacing versus shocks for spontaneous rapid ventricular tachycardia in patients with implantable cardioverter-defibrillators: Pacing Fast Ventricular Tachycardia Reduces Shock Therapies (PainFREE Rx II) trial results. Circulation 110(17):2591-2596, 2004.
26. Reynolds D, Murrat C, Germany R: Device therapy for remote patient management. In Wilde A, Friedman F, Ackerman M, Shen W (eds): Electrical Diseases of the Heart: Genetics, Mechanisms, Treatment, Prevention. London, Springer-Verlag, 2008, pp 809-825.
27. Heart Failure Society Of America: Executive summary: HFSA 2006 Comprehensive Heart Failure Practice Guideline. J Card Fail 12(1):10-38, 2006.
28. Yu CM, Wang L, Chau E, et al: Intrathoracic impedance monitoring in patients with heart failure: Correlation with fluid status and feasibility of early warning preceding hospitalization. Circulation 112(6):841-848, 2005.
29. Bourge R, Aranda J, Aaron M, et al: Clinical outcome of a heart failure management strategy based on continuous hemodynamic monitoring [abstract]. Circulation 112:II-639, 2005.
30. Poole J, Johnson G, Callans D, et al; SCD-HeFT Investigators: Analysis of implantable defibrillator shock electrograms in the Sudden Cardiac Death—Heart Failure Trial [abstract]. Heart Rhythm 1:S178, 2004.
31. Gunderson B, Patel A, Bounds C: Automatic identification of implantable cardioverter-defibrillator lead problems using intracardiac electrograms. Comput Cardiol 29:121-124, 2002.
32. Gunderson BD, Gillberg JM, Wood MA, et al: Development and testing of an algorithm to detect implantable cardioverter-defibrillator lead failure. Heart Rhythm 3(2):155-162, 2006.
33. Sweeney MO: Antitachycardia pacing for ventricular tachycardia using implantable cardioverter defibrillators. Pacing Clin Electrophysiol 27(9):1292-1305, 2004.
34. Goldschlager N, Epstein A, Friedman P, et al: Environmental and drug effects on patients with pacemakers and implantable cardioverter/defibrillators: A practical guide to patient treatment. Arch Intern Med 161(5):649-655, 2001.
35. Pacifico A, Hohnloser SH, Williams JH, et al: Prevention of implantable-defibrillator shocks by treatment with sotalol. D,L-Sotalol Implantable Cardioverter-Defibrillator Study Group. N Engl J Med 340(24):1855-1862, 1999.
36. Hauser RG, Maron BJ: Lessons from the failure and recall of an implantable cardioverter-defibrillator. Circulation 112(13):2040-2042, 2005.
37. Germano JJ, Reynolds M, Essebag V, Josephson ME: Frequency and causes of implantable cardioverter-defibrillator therapies: Is device therapy proarrhythmic? Am J Cardiol 97(8):1255-1261, 2006.
38. Ellenbogen KA, Levine JH, Berger RD, et al: Are implantable cardioverter defibrillator shocks a surrogate for sudden cardiac death in patients with nonischemic cardiomyopathy? Circulation 113(6):776-782, 2006.
39. Sweeney MO, Ruetz LL, Belk P, et al: Bradycardia pacing-induced short-long-short sequences at the onset of ventricular tachyarrhythmias: A possible mechanism of proarrhythmia? J Am Coll Cardiol 50(7):614-622, 2007.
40. Sweeney MO, Hellkamp AS, Ellenbogen KA, et al; MOST Investigators: Adverse effect of ventricular pacing on heart failure and atrial fibrillation among patients with normal baseline QRS duration in a clinical trial of pacemaker therapy for sinus node dysfunction. Circulation 107(23):2932-2937, 2003.
41. Epstein AE, Baessler CA, Curtis AB, et al: Addendum to "Personal and public safety issues related to arrhythmias that may affect consciousness: implications for

regulation and physician recommendations: A medical/scientific statement from the American Heart Association and the North American Society of Pacing and Electrophysiology": Public safety issues in patients with implantable defibrillators: A scientific statement from the American Heart Association and the Heart Rhythm Society. Circulation 115(9):1170-1176, 2007.
42. Pinski SL, Trohman RG: Interference in implanted cardiac devices, part II. Pacing Clin Electrophysiol 25(10):1496-1509, 2002.
43. Pinski SL, Trohman RG: Interference in implanted cardiac devices, Part I. Pacing Clin Electrophysiol 25(9):1367-1381, 2002.
44. Carlson MD, Wilkoff BL, Maisel WH, et al: Recommendations from the Heart Rhythm Society Task Force on Device Performance Policies and Guidelines Endorsed by the American College of Cardiology Foundation (ACCF) and the American Heart Association (AHA) and the International Coalition of Pacing and Electrophysiology Organizations (COPE). Heart Rhythm 3(10):1250-1273, 2006.
45. Swerdlow CD, Cannom DS: ICD product reliability: Lessons from electrical overstress failures. Pacing Clin Electrophysiol 24(7):1043-1045, 2001.
46. Amin MS, Matchar DB, Wood MA, Ellenbogen KA: Management of recalled pacemakers and implantable cardioverter-defibrillators: A decision analysis model. JAMA 296(4):412-420, 2006.

Implantable Pacemakers 101

Paul J. Wang and David L. Hayes

CHAPTER OUTLINE

Use and sophistication of permanent pacemakers have increased steadily since the first pacemaker was implanted in 1958. Indications for their use have broadened as the technology has advanced, and pacemakers have become a mainstay of therapy. Those involved in arrhythmia management must have a good understanding of this discipline.

History of Pacing

Since the first epicardial pacing system was implanted in 1958, pacemaker technology has evolved rapidly. Sophistication of sensing circuitry led to the introduction of single-chamber demand pacing systems in 1963. Although atrial-synchronous systems and dual-chamber systems were described in the 1950s, clinical use of such devices did not occur for many years. In the 1970s, lithium batteries and programmability were introduced. Milestones of the 1980s include greater acceptance of dual-chamber pacing systems and the introduction of rate-adaptive pacing systems. The 1990s and the 2000s witnessed the introduction of advanced sensor technology, new pacemaker algorithms, and enhanced automaticity of many programmable features.

Pacemaker Nomenclature

Since the first introduction of a three-letter code describing basic pacemaker functions in 1974, the code has been updated periodically by a committee comprising members of the North American Society of Pacing and Electrophysiology and the British Pacing and Electrophysiology Group (NASPE/BPEG).[1] The most recent code consists of a five-letter code (Box 101-1). The first position indicates the chamber or chambers that are *stimulated:* A (atrium), V (ventricle), or D (dual chamber, both A and V). The second position indicates the chamber or chambers in which *sensing* occurs: A (atrium), V (ventricle), or D (dual chamber, both A and V). The third position indicates the *function:* I (inhibition), T (triggered), D (a dual function of atrial tracking and ventricular inhibition). The fourth position of the code indicates that *rate modulation* is present by the letter *R.* Rate modulation is the use of a sensor to meet the patient's metabolic demands, independent of intrinsic cardiac activity. The fifth position indicates whether *multisite pacing* is present: A (atrium), V (ventricle), or D (both A and V). Multisite pacing is defined as more than one stimulation site in any single chamber. In any of the positions, *O* indicates that pacing, sensing, or a function is not present.

Indications for Cardiac Pacing

Criteria established by a joint committee of the American College of Cardiology (ACC), the American Heart Association (AHA), and the Heart Rhythm Society (HRS) have categorized indications for pacing as class I, generally indicated; class II, possibly indicated; and class III, not indicated.[2] Class II has been divided into class IIa for recommendations for which there is general agreement and class IIb for which there is some disagreement. The evidence supporting the recommendations are ranked. The weight of evidence is ranked A if there are multiple randomized trials involving a large number of subjects and B if data were derived from a limited number of trials involving a relatively small number of subjects. The weight of evidence is ranked C if expert consensus is the primary source of the recommendation.[2] Although some indications for permanent pacing are relatively certain or unambiguous, others require considerable expertise and judgment. The clinician prescribing permanent pacing systems should be aware of the indications and controversies regarding indications.

Acquired Atrioventricular Block

Acquired atrioventricular (AV) block is most commonly idiopathic and related to aging, but the potential causes are many.

Class I indications for permanent pacing in patients with acquired AV block include any AV block with associated symptoms, as well as AV block after AV node ablation or persistent AV block after cardiac surgery. For some patients, heart failure may be a manifestation of AV block. In addition, some patients require medications that can cause symptomatic bradycardia and might need pacing. For postoperative AV block, the guidelines do not specify a period to wait postoperatively for recovery of conduction. Class I indications also include acquired AV block below the level of the AV node or associated with marked pauses, such as longer than 3.0 seconds or a ventricular escape rate less than 40 beats per minute. Because the cardiovascular risk is felt to be particularly high in patients with second- or third-degree

Box 101-1 The Revised NASPE/BPEG Generic Code for Antibradycardia Pacing

I: CHAMBER(S) PACED

O = None
A = Atrium
V = Ventricle
D = Dual (A+V)
S = Single (A or V) (manufacturers' designation only)

II: CHAMBER(S) SENSED

O = None
A = Atrium
V = Ventricle
D = Dual (A+V)
S = Single (A or V) (manufacturers' designation only)

III: RESPONSE TO SENSING

O = None
T = Triggered
I = Inhibited
D = Dual (T+I)

IV: RATE MODULATION

O = None
R = Rate modulation

V: MULTISITE PACING

O = None
A = Atrium
V = Ventricle
D = Dual (A+V)

BPEG, British Pacing and Electrophysiology Group; NASPE, North American Society of Pacing and Electrophysiology.

block and specific underlying conditions, permanent pacing is felt to be indicated in these patients even in the absence of symptoms. These conditions include neuromuscular diseases such as myotonic dystrophy, Kearns-Sayre syndrome, peroneal muscular atrophy, and Erb limb girdle dystrophy. Exercise-related AV block is also felt to be an indication for pacing. Advanced second-degree AV block or alternating bundle branch block in the setting of bifascicular block is considered a class I indication. Asymptomatic type II second-degree AV block with a wide QRS is a class I indication. Transient, infranodal, high-grade AV block and associated bundle branch block is a class I indication.[2]

Class IIa indications include asymptomatic type II second-degree AV block with a narrow QRS complex, and asymptomatic second-degree AV block at intra-His or infra-His levels based on electrophysiologic testing.[2] First-degree or second-degree AV block with hemodynamic compromise is also considered a class IIa indication because some patients develop pacemaker-like syndrome due to conduction delay. In patients with bifascicular block, asymptomatic severe prolongation of the His-ventricle interval (>100 ms), asymptomatic pacing-induced infra-His block that is not felt to be physiologic, or syncope when other causes such as ventricular tachycardia have been excluded are considered class IIa indications for pacing.

First-degree AV block in patients with neuromuscular disorders is considered a class IIb indication because the risk of progression to AV block is felt to be high. Another class IIb indication includes AV block that might have occurred due to drug use or toxicity, but there is a risk of recurrence of AV block. First-degree AV block in a patient with left ventricular dysfunction and congestive heart failure in whom hemodynamic improvement with AV interval optimization can be demonstrated is a class IIb indication.[2] Asymptomatic persistent second-degree or third-degree block at the AV node level is classified as a class IIb indication.[3]

Class III indications include asymptomatic first-degree AV block, asymptomatic second-degree AV block at the supra-His level or not known to be intra-His or infra-His, and AV block occurring in the setting of reversible conditions such as drug toxicity that is unlikely to recur, Lyme disease, transient increases in vagal tone, or during sleep apnea.

After a myocardial infarction, a pacemaker is generally considered to be indicated for persistent second-degree bilateral bundle branch block, third-degree AV block within or below the His bundle, or persistent symptomatic second-degree or third-degree AV block.

Congenital Complete Heart Block

Symptomatic congenital complete AV block remains a class I indication for pacing in pediatric patients.[3] In addition, in pediatric patients with congenital complete AV block, the presence of wide QRS escape rhythm, ventricular dysfunction, or complex ventricular ectopy is also a class I indication. In pediatric patients, an average heart rate less than 50 beats per minute, pauses two to three times the basic cycle length, or symptoms associated with chronotropic incompetence are considered class IIa indications. In pediatric patients with adequate rate, narrow QRS complex, and normal ventricular function, pacing is a class IIb indication.

For adult patients with congenital complete AV block, the timing and indications for permanent pacing are more controversial and continue to evolve.[4] As a result of data regarding the high incidence of unexpected syncope in adult patients with congenital complete AV block, prophylactic pacemaker implantation is often considered.[5] This has not yet been incorporated into published guidelines.

Sinus Node Dysfunction

Sinus node dysfunction may be manifested by abrupt sinus pauses or gradual sinus slowing. Symptomatic chronotropic incompetence and symptomatic sinus bradycardia occurring spontaneously or as the result of drug therapy are considered class I indications for pacing. In patients with minimal or no symptoms and chronic heart rates less than 40 beats per minute, pacing is a class IIb indication.

Class III indications for pacing include asymptomatic sinus node dysfunction. Sinus pauses occurring during sleep are generally not considered indications for pacing. Many patients, particularly trained athletes, have high levels of vagal tone and have significant pauses greater than 3 seconds and periods of sinus bradycardia. These patients do not require permanent pacing.

Neurocardiogenic Syncope

Neurocardiogenic syncope typically has both cardioinhibitory and vasodepressor components. Pacing during most episodes of neurocardiogenic syncope is still associated with a significant fall in blood pressure and symptoms because of the continued vasodepressor response. Therefore, even in the presence of signficant bradycardia, pacing is usually not considered first-line therapy. The most recent randomized trials have failed to show a substantial benefit in increasing the freedom from recurrent syncope.[6-9] As a result, neurocardiogenic syncope with documented bradycardia is considered a class IIb indication for pacing. When pacing is performed in this setting, dual-chamber pacing is necessary to preserve the atrial contribution to cardiac output.

Carotid Sinus Hypersensitivity

Carotid sinus hypersensitivity has been shown to be a cause of syncope, particularly in the elderly. However, because an abnormal response can occur even in asymptomatic persons, caution must be used when spontaneous bradycardia has not been demonstrated. In cases in which syncope has occurred during carotid sinus stimulation and carotid sinus pressure has resulted in pauses of 3 seconds or more, a class I indication is felt to be present. If such an abnormal carotid sinus pressure response is obtained but syncope did not occur in circumstances suggesting carotid sinus stimulation, a class IIa indication is present. In addition, there may be a role for pacing in patients with unexplained falls and evidence of carotid sinus hypersensitivity.[10-11]

Nonbradycardic Indications for Pacing

An increasing number of patients are receiving pacemakers for nonbradycardic indications. Cardiac resynchronization therapy for refractory congestive heart failure is the major indication in this category. Dual-chamber pacing for medically refractory symptoms of hypertrophic obstructive cardiomyopathy and pacing therapy for prevention of atrial fibrillation are no longer considered major nonbradycardic indications for pacing.

Pacing for Atrial Fibrillation

There are numerous studies that examine various pacing algorithms to prevent atrial fibrillation. Most such algorithms involve increasing the pacing rate to suppress atrial ectopy felt to trigger atrial fibrillation. Whereas most randomized studies have not demonstrated a beneficial effect, selected studies have suggested a modest decrease in the occurrence of atrial fibrillation. At present, pacing for atrial fibrillation reduction is a class III indication.[12]

Resynchronization Therapy

Numerous randomized, controlled trials have demonstrated benefit of cardiac resynchronization therapy in improving symptoms and outcomes in patients with drug-refractory heart failure. Cardiac resynchronization therapy is the pacing of the left and right ventricles to improve the hemodynamics that are impaired due to bundle branch block. These randomized studies have shown improvement in New York Heart Association (NYHA) classes, 6-minute walk time, oxygen consumption, brain natriuretic peptide levels, neurohormonal levels, ejection fraction, end-diastolic and end-systolic dimension, heart failure hospitalizations, and all-cause mortality.[13,14] The current indications for resynchonization therapy (class I) include QRS duration 120 ms or greater, left ventricular ejection fraction 35% or less, sinus rhythm, and class III or ambulatory class IV heart failure symptoms on optimal medical therapy. Because the largest randomized trial excluded patients with atrial fibrillation, the presence of atrial fibrillation results in classification as a class IIa indication.

Hypertrophic Cardiomyopathy

Early studies suggested that right ventricular apical pacing resulted in a significant reduction in outflow tract gradient and ameliorated symptoms. However, a subsequent randomized multicenter trial failed to demonstrate benefit in patients with pacing. A subset of elderly patients might have exhibited some improvement.[15] Therefore, at present, pacing in medically refractory symptomatic patients with significant resting or provoked gradient due to hypertrophic cardiomyopathy is a class IIb indication. Many such patients should be considered for a dual chamber ICD because of the risk of sudden death.

Basic Pacemaker Function and Modes

Ventricular Inhibited (VVI) Pacing

In the ventricular inhibited (VVI) pacing mode, pacemaker output is inhibited by a sensed ventricular event (Fig. 101-1). The lower rate interval determines the longest interval between any sensed or paced ventricular events. The interval from the previous sensed or paced ventricular event to the subsequent paced ventricular event is the lower rate interval. If the time interval from the last sensed ventricular event to the first paced ventricular beat is longer than the time interval between ventricular paced beats, ventricular hysteresis is present. Any ventricular event occurring after a paced or sensed ventricular event within the ventricular refractory period is not sensed and does not reset the timing cycle.

Atrial Inhibited (AAI) Pacing

Atrial inhibited (AAI) pacing incorporates the same timing cycles as VVI pacing, with the obvious difference that pacing and sensing occur in the atrium, and pacemaker output is inhibited by a sensed atrial event (Fig. 101-2). An atrial paced or sensed event initiates a refractory period during which atrial events do not reset the timing cycle. Confusion can arise when multiple ventricular events occur during atrial pacing. For example, when the atrial timing cycle ends, an atrial pacing stimulus is delivered regardless of ventricular events, because an AAI pacemaker does not sense in the ventricle. If the ventricular signal is

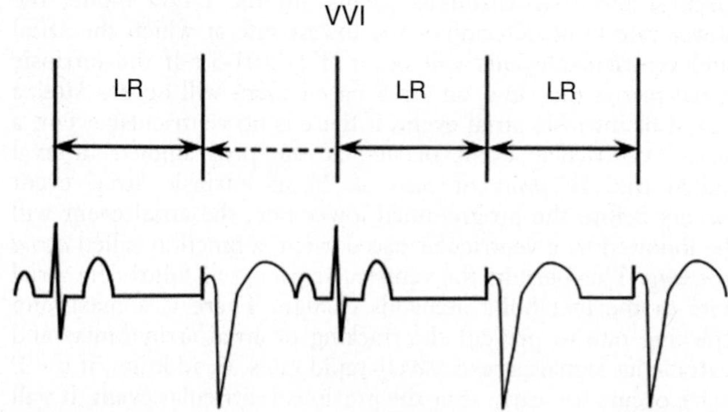

Figure 101-1 In the ventricular inhibited (VVI) pacing, the lower rate interval (LR) is the time from the last intrinsic or paced ventricular event to a ventricular paced event. When the LR interval has been completed, a ventricular paced event will occur. If an intrinsic beat occurs before the LR is completed, the ventricular output will be inhibited. The first QRS complex is intrinsic and after the LR interval is completed a second intrinsic beat has not occurred, and thus, the second QRS complex is a paced ventricular event. The third QRS complex is again intrinsic. Following the third QRS complex, intrinsic QRS complexes do not occur within the LR interval. Thus, the fourth and fifth QRS complexes are paced. The *double-headed arrows* indicate a full LR interval has transpired. The *dotted single-headed arrow* indicates that the full LR interval has not been completed and an intrinsic QRS complex inhibits ventricular pacing.

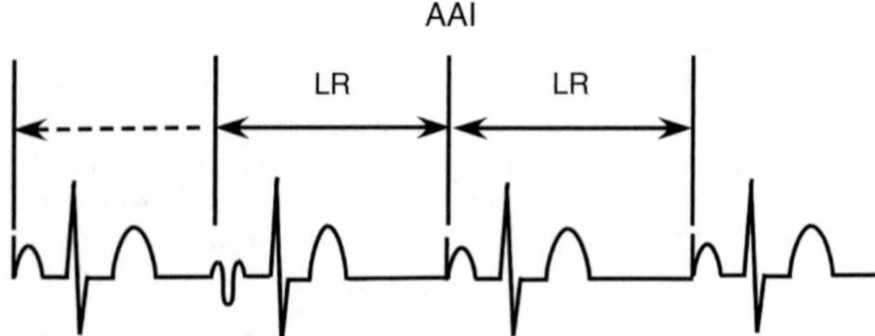

Figure 101-2 In atrial inhibited (AAI) pacing, the lower rate interval (LR) is the time from the last intrinsic or paced atrial event to an atrial paced event. When the LR interval has been completed, an atrial paced event will occur. If an intrinsic beat occurs before the LR interval is completed, the atrial output will be inhibited. The first atrial complex is paced. The second atrial complex occurs before the LR is completed. A third atrial complex does not occur spontaneously and instead, after the LR interval has been completed, an atrial paced beat occurs. The fourth atrial complex is also paced and occurs after another LR interval. The *double-headed arrows* indicate a full LR interval has transpired. The *dotted single-headed arrow* indicates that the full LR interval has not been completed and an intrinsic QRS complex inhibits ventricular pacing.

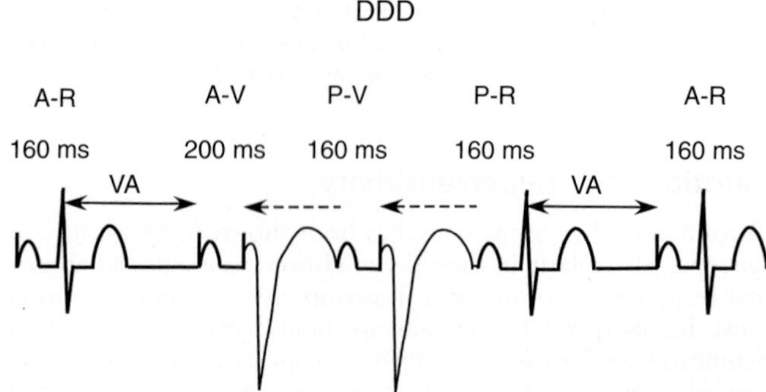

Figure 101-3 The DDD timing cycle consists of a lower rate limit interval, an atrioventricular interval (AVI), a postventricular atrial refractory period (PVARP), and an upper rate limit. In the figure, the first complex consists of an atrial paced event and an intrinsic QRS complex. Following the sensed ventricular event, a ventriculoatrial (VA) interval is created to indicate the time of the next atrial paced event if no intrinsic atrial event (after the postventricular atrial refractory period) and no intrinsic ventricular event occurs. The VA interval equals the lower rate interval minus the programmed AV interval. A completed VA interval is indicated by the *double-headed solid arrow*. In the second complex, following the atrial paced event there is no intrinsic QRS complex within the AV interval of 200 ms. Thus, a paced ventricular event occurs. If an intrinsic atrial event occurs before the VA interval is completed but after the postventricular atrial refractory period, the atrial event will be tracked or followed by a paced ventricular event (the third QRS complex). As long as the V-V interval does not occur before the upper rate limit interval is complete, the AV interval will occur after the tracked atrial event. Following the third QRS complex, an intrinsic atrial event occurs before the VA interval is complete, but an intrinsic QRS complex occurs before the AV interval is finished. Following the fourth QRS complex, the VA interval is completed and another atrial paced event occurs. The *dotted single-headed arrow* indicates that the full LR interval has not been completed and an intrinsic QRS complex inhibits ventricular pacing.

inappropriately sensed by the atrial lead (far-field sensing), the atrial timing cycle is reset. This abnormality can sometimes be corrected by making the atrial channel less sensitive or by lengthening the atrial refractory period so that a conducted ventricular complex is not sensed.

Single-chamber, rate-adaptive pacing modes (AAIR, VVIR) have timing cycles that are not markedly different from those of their non–rate-adaptive counterparts. The difference lies in the potential variability of the paced rate. Depending on the sensor incorporated and the patient's level of exertion, the basic interval shortens from the programmed lower rate limit. Shortening requires that an upper rate limit be programmed to define the absolute shortest cycle length allowable.

DDD Pacing

Four different rhythms can be seen as a result of normal DDD function: normal sinus rhythm, atrial pacing, AV sequential pacing, and P-synchronous pacing. In the DDD mode, the lower rate limit determines the lowest rate at which the atrial and ventricular events will occur (Fig. 101-3). If the intrinsic atrial rate is too slow, an atrial paced event will occur. After a paced or intrinsic atrial event, if there is no ventricular event, a paced ventricular event occurs, at the programmed interval called the *AV delay* or *interval*. If an intrinsic atrial event occurs before the programmed lower rate, the atrial event will be followed by a ventricular paced event, a function called *atrial tracking*. This permits the ventricular pacing to follow the atrial rate as the metabolic demands change. There is a maximum tracking rate to prevent the tracking of atrial arrhythmias and extraneous signals at excessively rapid rates. In addition, if the P wave occurs too early after the previous ventricular event, it will occur in the postventricular atrial refractory period (PVARP) and therefore will not be tracked. The atrial rate at which two atrial sensed events will be followed by one ventricular paced event is equal to the total atrial refractory period (TARP), which is the sum of the programmed AV delay and the PVARP.

The timing of the last ventricular beat to the next atrial paced beat is determined by the ventriculoatrial (VA) interval. This interval is determined by subtracting the AV interval (AVI) from the lower rate interval in milliseconds. Thus, the lower rate interval minus the AVI equals the VA interval. The AV interval may be adjusted based on the ventricular rate, a parameter called *rate-responsive AV interval*. In patients with AV block and rapid sinus rates that might exceed the programmed upper rate limit and 2:1 atrial tracking rate, the rate-responsive AV interval might permit much higher upper rate limit tracking rates and maximum 2:1 atrial tracking rates. The AV interval might also be extended to promote intrinsic AV conduction, a function called *positive AV hysteresis* (see the section "Intrinsic Conduction Preference," later). Negative AV hysteresis refers to a function in which the AV interval is shortened to promote ventricular pacing, which is desirable in biventricualar pacing.

Selecting the Appropriate Pacing Mode

Selection Criteria

In selecting the optimal pacing mode, the patient's overall physical condition, associated medical problems, exercise capacity, and chronotropic response to exercise must be considered, along with the underlying rhythm disturbance.[16]

VVIR pacing is indicated for patients with chronic atrial fibrillation and slow ventricular response. Although VVI pacing protects the patient from lethal bradycardia, its limitations include its inability to restore or to maintain AV synchrony and to provide rate responsiveness in the chronotropically incompetent patient. In addition, some patients with VVI pacing experience symptomatic hemodynamic deterioration with ventricular pacing. Adverse hemodynamics due to pacing are referred to as *pacemaker syndrome* if the normal coordination of atrial filling and ventricular emptying is absent due to VA

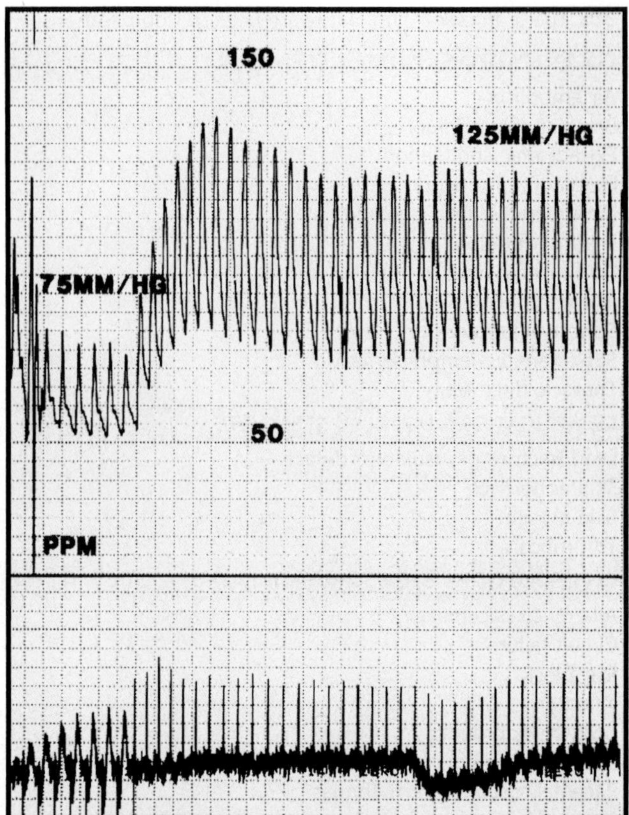

Figure 101-4 Hemodynamic tracing of a patient with pacemaker syndrome. The initial portion of the tracing shows ventricular pacing with a systolic arterial pressure of approximately 75 mm Hg. The patient's intrinsic sinus rhythm inhibits ventricular pacing, and the arterial systolic pressure increases to approximately 125 mm Hg. (From Hayes DL, Holmes DR Jr: Hemodynamics of cardiac pacing. In Furman S, Hayes DL, Holmes DR Jr [eds]: A Practice of Cardiac Pacing, 3rd ed. Mount Kisco, NY, Futura Publishing, 1993, pp 195-218. By permission of Blackwell Publishing.)

conduction or long AV conduction times. During ventricular pacing with VA conduction, the systolic blood pressure might decline (Fig. 101-4). The incidence of pacemaker syndrome depends on the definition used, and the its incidence has been estimated to be 7% to 10% of patients with VVI or VVIR pacing.[17] However, in a study of patients with DDD pacemakers who were randomly assigned to DDD or VVI pacing mode, some degree of pacemaker syndrome was present in 83%.[18] The most common symptoms reported were shortness of breath, dizziness, fatigue, pulsations in the neck or abdomen, cough, and apprehension.

AAIR pacing is appropriate for patients with sinus node dysfunction. The obvious disadvantage of atrial pacing is the lack of ventricular support if AV block occurs. If the patient with sinus node dysfunction is carefully assessed for the presence of AV node disease at the time of pacemaker implant, the occurrence of clinically significant AV node disease is very low, less than 2% per year. The concern of progression to AV block when patients are carefully selected for AAI (R) pacing has been dispelled by long-term follow-up of patients.[19] Assessment before AAI pacemaker implantation should include incremental atrial pacing with an adequate response defined as 1:1 AV nodal conduction to atrial pacing rates of 120 to 140 beats per minute. Newer pacing algorithms (discussed later) to avoid the deleterious effects of ventricular pacing allow atrial pacing to occur, and they switch to a mode that supports ventricular pacing only when necessary,

The DDD pacing mode is most appropriate for patients with normal sinus node function and AV block. DDDR pacemakers are capable of all the variations described for DDD pacemakers. In addition to use of P-synchronous pacing as a method for increasing the heart rate, the sensor incorporated in the pacemaker might also drive the increase in heart rate. The resulting rhythm may be sinus driven (alternatively called *atrial driven* or *P-synchronous*) or sensor driven.

DDDR pacing is indicated in patients with sinus node dysfunction and AV conduction disease. DDDR pacing is also appropriate for patients with pure sinus node dysfunction and when backup ventricular pacing is desired.

Effect of Pacing Mode on Morbidity and Mortality

Several large randomized, controlled trials have demonstrated benefits of physiologic (AAI(R) or DDD(R)) versus VVI(R). Andersen and associates[19] published prospective data on pacing mode and survival with the random assignment of 225 patients with sinus node dysfunction to AAI or VVI pacing. The study demonstrated a lower incidence of atrial fibrillation and thromboembolism in the AAI group than in the VVI group. The Canadian Trial of Physiologic Pacing (CTOPP)[20] randomly assigned 2568 patients to physiologic pacing (dual-chamber or AAIR) or ventricular pacing (VVI). No difference in mortality rate or quality of life was demonstrated. However, there was an 18% relative risk reduction of atrial fibrillation.

Two additional trials have examined the outcomes of physiologic pacing: PASE (Pacing Mode Selection in the Elderly)[21] and MOST (Mode Selection Trial).[22] PASE failed to demonstrate any statistically significant benefit of physiologic pacing over ventricular pacing. When the patients were separated by underlying rhythm disturbance—that is, sinus node dysfunction versus AV block—the sinus node dysfunction group had some quality-of-life improvements. In addition, there was a crossover of 26% of patients assigned to ventricular pacing because they were unable to tolerate ventricular pacing. The MOST study, like CTOPP, did not demonstrate any difference in mortality rates, but it did demonstrate a lower incidence of atrial fibrillation with physiologic pacing, reduced signs and symptoms of heart failure, and a slightly improved quality of life. The study concluded that overall dual-chamber pacing offered significant improvement compared with ventricular pacing.[22]

Taken together, these studies demonstrate the benefit of physiologic pacing with the maintenance of AV synchrony compared to ventricular only pacing in terms of atrial fibrillation and possibly quality of life.

Selecting the Appropriate Sensor for Rate-Adaptive Pacing

A variety of sensors appropriate for rate-adaptive pacing have been developed and achieve excellent responses in heart rate to exertion and changes in metabolic demand.

Activity and Accelerometer Sensors

Accelerometer sensors have replaced basic vibration-based activity sensors. Both these sensors use a piezoelectric crystal, which produces a minute electric current in response to motion. The piezoelectric vibration activity sensor senses vibration from up and down motion, and the accelerometer senses anterior and posterior motion.[23] The accelerometer is relatively free from detection of motion leading to inappropriate increases in heart rate and responds rapidly to the onset of exertion. The accelerometer is the most widely used form of rate-adaptation sensor because it is simple, easy to apply clinically, and rapid in onset of rate response.

Minute-Ventilation Sensor

Minute volume (respiratory rate × tidal volume) has an excellent correlation with metabolic demand. The transthoracic impedance, which varies with respiration, can be used to determine minute volume. Because minute ventilation maintains a predictable relation with metabolic demand, minute-ventilation values can be used to modulate the heart rate during various levels of activity for the patient.[23-26] Long-term reliability of the minute-volume sensor has been excellent.

Stimulus-T or QT-sensing Sensor

The interval from the onset of a paced QRS complex to the end of the T wave has been used for rate adaptation for many years. This stimulus-T interval is affected by autonomic activity and heart rate. The relation allows measurement of the stimulus-T interval to be used for rate adaptation. The QT-sensing, rate-adaptive pacing system has been successful clinically and responds well to mental and emotional stress.[23]

Peak Endocardial Acceleration Sensor

Using a miniature accelerometer within a pacing lead, an index called *peak endocardial acceleration* has been introduced. This sensor, placed in the right ventricular lead, provides a surrogate measure of myocardial contractility and sympathetic activation.[27,28] The sensor is also being tested as a means to optimize the AV interval and right ventricle–left ventricle timing in dual-chamber and biventricular pacing devices.

Right Ventricular Impedance-Based Sensor

Closed loop stimulation (CLS) measures impedance from the right ventricular unipolar pacing. The impedance measurements are felt to correlate with dP/dt_{max}, which is a surrogate for ventricular contractility and in turn is a reflection of autonomic activity.[29] As a reflection of autonomic activity, this sensor has the potential to respond to nonexertional stimuli.[30]

Dual-Sensor Combinations

The perfect sensor would be resistant to all nonphysiologic stimuli. A multisensor, rate-adaptive pacing system could improve specificity by having one sensor verify or cross-check the other.[23,31-33] The most widely used sensor combination is the accelerometer–minute ventilation combination or blended sensor. Using this combination, the accelerometer provides a rapid response to exertion and the minute ventilation provides an excellent physiologic response; this has been shown to mirror the normal physiologic response of the sinus node under numerous conditions.

Pacemaker Complications

Complications can occur related to the implantation procedure or because of failure of a component of the pacing system. Box 101-2 lists the most commonly encountered complications and whether they are more likely to be seen immediately or over the long term.

Box 101-2 Implant- and Hardware-Related Complications

COMPLICATIONS USUALLY SEEN EARLY

- Air embolism
- Brachial plexus injury
- Extracardiac stimulation
- Hematoma formation
- Intraoperative lead damage
- Lead perforation
- Pain or ecchymoses
- Pneumothorax
- Subclavian artery puncture
- Subcutaneous emphysema
- Thoracic duct injury

COMPLICATIONS USUALLY SEEN LATE

- Lead fracture or insulation defect
- Skin adherence
- Skin erosion
- Thrombosis

COMPLICATIONS SEEN EARLY OR LATE

- Allergy to pacemaker
- Circuit failure
- Exit block
- Infection
- Lead dislodgment
- Loose lead or connector block interface
- Pacemaker-related arrhythmias
- Pacemaker syndrome
- Twiddler syndrome

Troubleshooting Electrocardiographic Abnormalities

Electrocardiographic abnormalities in patients with pacemakers can be broadly categorized into failure to capture, failure to output, oversensing, undersensing, and inappropriate rate change.[34-36]

Failure to capture indicates that a pacing artifact is present without subsequent cardiac depolarization (Fig. 101-5; Box 101-3).

True failure to output is caused by failure to output from the pacemaker so that the electrical signal cannot reach the heart (see Box 101-3).

Oversensing is caused by the sensing of signals interpreted as the atria or ventricles deflecting in their respective channels. Sensing of signals originating in the opposite chamber is called *crosstalk*. For example, the ventricular deflection may be sensed on the atrial channel (Fig. 101-6). More seriously, the atrial stimulus may be detected on the ventricular channel, resulting in ventricular inhibition and asystole. Such an occurrence may be prevented by programming on safety pacing so that a ventricular stimulus is given if a ventricular event is sensed shortly after an atrial stimulus is delivered. The electrocardiographic hallmark of safety pacing is the presence of pacing with an shortened AV interval, ranging from 80 to 130 ms. Ventricular oversensing results in a prolonged ventricular interval, and atrial oversensing in the DDD mode results in tracking of atrial signals and rapid ventricular pacing (Fig. 101-7).

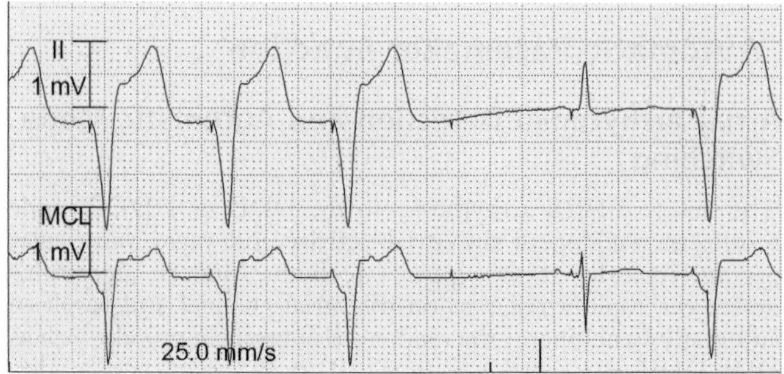

Figure 101-5 Electrocardiographic tracing demonstrating intermittent ventricular failure to capture. The first three ventricular pacing stimuli demonstrate ventricular capture. The fourth and the fifth ventricular pacing stimuli demonstrate failure to capture. The sixth ventricular stimulus results in ventricular capture. An intrinsic sinus beat occurs after the fifth ventricular pacing stimulus.

Box 101-3 Pacemaker Troubleshooting

FAILURE TO CAPTURE

Air in pocket of unipolar pacemaker
Circuit failure
Functional noncapture
High thresholds with inadequately programmed output
Impending total battery depletion
Insulation defect
Lead dislodgment or perforation
Partial conductor coil fracture
Poor or incompatible connection at connector block

FAILURE TO OUTPUT

Circuit failure
Complete or intermittent conductor coil fracture
Intermittent or permanently loose set screw
Internal insulation failure (bipolar lead)
Lack of anodal connector contact*
Oversensing any noncardiac activity
Total battery depletion

SENSING ABNORMALITIES

Battery depletion
Circuit failure
Electromagnetic interference
Lead dislodgment or poor lead positioning
Lead insulation failure
Magnet application
Malfunction of reed switch
Structure of intrinsic event different than that measured at implant

ALTERED PACING RATE

Battery depletion
Circuit failure
Crosstalk
Hysteresis
Magnet application
Malfunction of the electrocardiographic recording equipment (i.e., alteration of paper speed)
Oversensing
Runaway
Undocumented reprogramming of the pacemaker

*Examples include unipolar lead in bipolar generator, bipolar lead in pacemaker programmed unipolar, air in the pocket of a unipolar device, and unipolar pacemaker not in the pocket.

The differential diagnoses of the electrocardiographic abnormalities might overlap. For example, a ventricular lead fracture can result in failure to capture and to ventricular oversensing of noise, causing inhibition of pacing. A lead fracture can also result in undersensing.

Insulation defects similarly can manifest with oversensing or with failure to capture, although the most common presentation of insulation failure is a sensing abnormality. Lead impedance measurements are helpful in making the diagnosis, with lead fractures resulting in high impedances ($>2500\ \Omega$) and insulation breaks with low impedances ($<250\ \Omega$). As pacemaker battery power is depleted, there may be a decreased output or no output at all. This degree of battery depletion is avoidable with appropriate pacemaker follow-up. The pacemaker also might revert to VVI or VOO mode from DDD(R) mode when the replacement indicator occurs.

Sensing abnormalities can be divided into true abnormalities and functional sensing abnormalities (see Box 101-3). True abnormalities including undersensing, which is a failure to recognize normal intrinsic cardiac activity, and oversensing, which is unexpected sensing of an intrinsic or extrinsic electrical signal (Fig. 101-8). Artifact might also give the appearance of oversensing. True undersensing is most commonly caused by lead dislodgment or inadequate intrinsic amplitude. Sensing abnormalities are commonly seen secondary to insulation defects and lead fracture.

Functional undersensing is present when an intrinsic cardiac event is not sensed because it falls within a programmed refractory period. For example, if an intrinsic atrial event occurs within the postventricular atrial refractory period, the event is not sensed. However, without a thorough understanding of the timing cycle, it might appear as though true undersensing has occurred. Similarly, apparent failure to capture is noted if a pacemaker stimulus occurs during the physiologic refractory period of a spontaneous beat. This condition is referred to as *functional noncapture*.

Every pacing mode has a defined lower rate limit, and dual-chamber and rate-adaptive pacemakers also require a defined upper rate limit. One must be familiar with the timing cycle of a particular pacing mode, as well as any idiosyncrasies of the specific pacemaker, to determine whether the paced rate is appropriate. The causes of an altered pacing rate are numerous (see Box 101-3).

Drugs can affect sensing and pacing thresholds and result in electrocardiographic abnormalities.[37] Although many drugs have been reported to affect pacing thresholds, only the class IC agents commonly result in a clinical problem. If these drugs are administered to a patient with a pacemaker, especially a pacemaker-dependent patient, he or she should be monitored for an increase in pacing threshold. Class IC agents can also cause sensing abnormalities.

Electrolyte and metabolic abnormalities can also affect pacing and sensing thresholds.[24] Hyperkalemia is the most common electrolyte abnormality to cause clinically significant problems, but severe acidosis or alkalosis, hypercapnia, severe hyperglycemia, hypoxemia, and myxedema should also be considered.

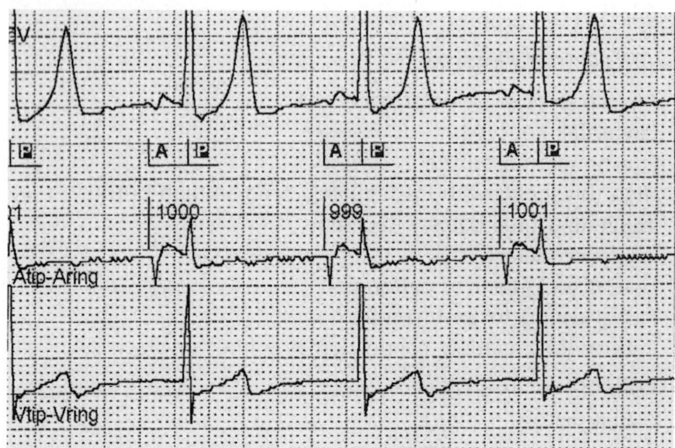

Figure 101-6 Electrocardiographic tracing demonstrating oversensing of the ventricular deflection on the atrial channel. *Top channel*, Surface electrocardiogram. *Middle channel*, Bipolar atrial electrogram (tip-ring). *Bottom channel*, Bipolar ventricular electrogram. Atrial pacing at 1000 ms cycle length occurs with intact AV conduction. There is sensing of the intrinsic ventricular deflection on the atrial channel, indicated by the *P*.

Automatic Pacemaker Function

Atrial Arrhythmia Detection and Automatic Mode Switching

The onset of atrial arrhythmias in the DDD or DDDR mode results in tracking of the atrial activity and rapid ventricular pacing, typically at the upper rate limit. Modern algorithms detect the rapid atrial rate on the atrial channel and result in automatic switching of the mode to a nontracking mode such as DDI, DDIR, VVI, or VVIR (Fig. 101-9). In any of these modes, tracking of atrial activity ceases. Once the atrial arrhythmia stops, the mode switches back to the DDD or DDDR mode.[38,39] Algorithms might also detect pacemaker-mediated tachycardia and intervene by prolonging the PVARP transiently or avoiding atrial tracking for a single cycle. Pacemaker-mediated tachycardia occurs when VA conduction is longer than the programmed PVARP and is typically induced by a premature ventricular beat or atrial failure to capture.

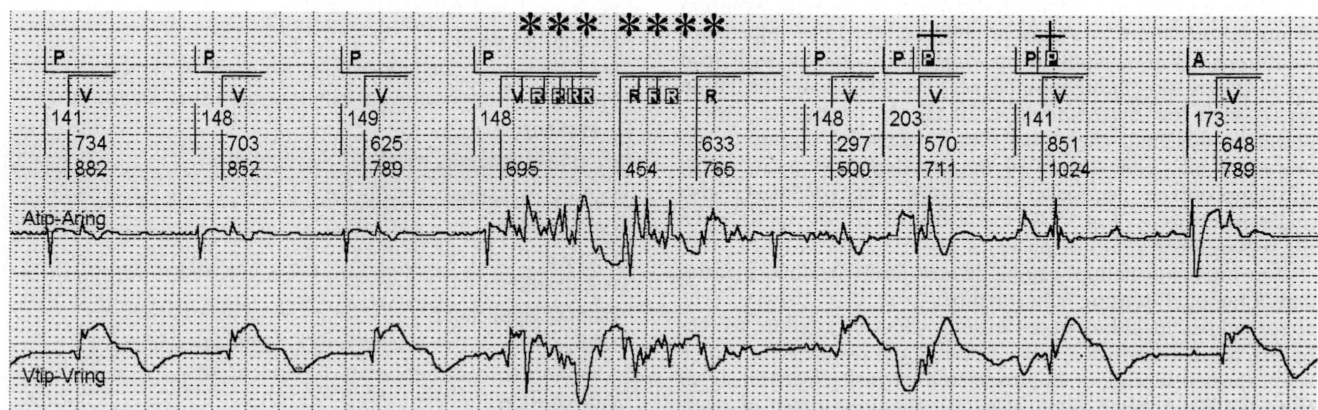

Figure 101-7 Electrograms demonstrating oversensing on the atrial and ventricular channels. *Top channel* is the marker channel. *A* indicates atrial paced event, *P* indicates intrinsic atrial activity, *V* indicates ventricular paced event, *R* indicates ventricular sensed event. *Middle channel* is the bipolar atrial electrogram. *Bottom channel* is the bipolar ventricular channel. In the first three, AV complexes represent intrinsic atrial activity (*P*) followed by ventricular paced beats (*V*). Artifact is seen on both the atrial and ventricular channels. The artifact is sensed on the ventricular channel, indicated by the *R* markers and the *asterisks*. The artifact is sensed on the atrial channel, indicated by the *P* and the *plus sign*.

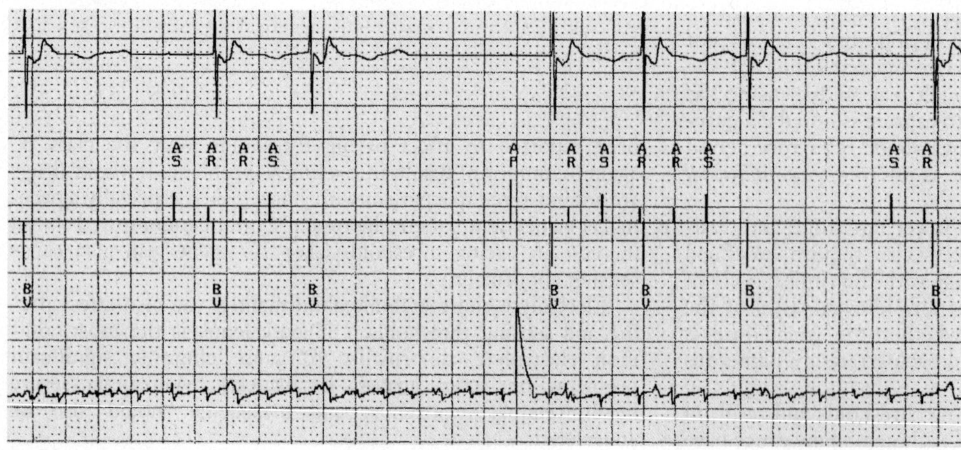

Figure 101-8 Electrogram indicating intermittent undersensing on the atrial channel of atrial fibrillation. *Top channel* is the ventricular electrogram. *Middle channel* is the marker channel. *AS* indicates an intrinsic atrial event that is sensed, *AR* indicates an intrinsic atrial event that falls within a refractory period. *BV* indicates a biventricular paced event. *Bottom channel* is the bipolar atrial electrogram. The atrial activity indicates the presence of atrial fibrillation.

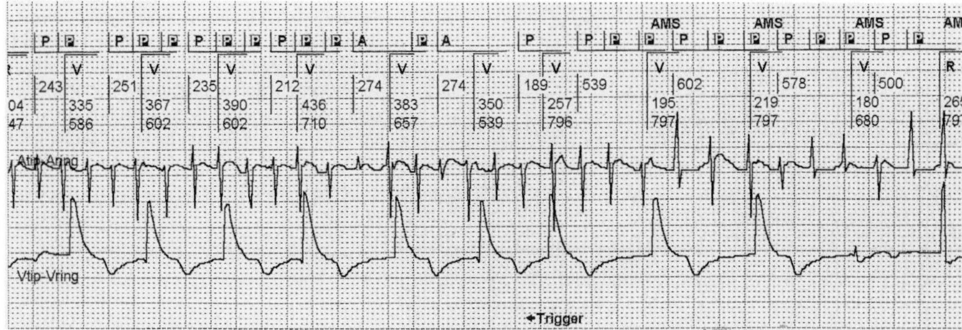

Figure 101-9 Electrogram demonstrating automatic mode switching after detection of atrial fibrillation. *Top channel* is the marker channel. *P* indicates a sensed atrial event. *A* indicates a paced atrial event. *R* indicates intrinsic ventricular event and *V* indicates a paced ventricular event. *AMS* indicates automatic mode switching from DDDR to DDIR mode. *Middle channel* is the bipolar atrial electrogram. *Bottom channel* is the bipolar ventricular electrogram. The ventricular pacing rate abruptly drops with mode switching.

Intrinsic Conduction Preference

There has been an increasing recognition that hemodynamics are improved when intrinsic ventricular conduction is permitted in the absence of bundle branch block. New algorithms have been designed to permit the automatic restoration of intrinsic conduction. These algorithms can represent a form of AV search hysteresis or mode switching from DDD or DDDR to AAI or AAIR. When ventricular pacing occurs, AV search hysteresis periodically lengthens the AV interval so that intrinsic AV conduction occurs. If AV conduction does not occur, AV pacing resumes. In mode-switching algorithms, the pacing mode is AAI or AAIR until AV block occurs and the mode switches to DDD or DDDR (Fig. 101-10). Periodically, the mode switches back to AAI or AAIR to check if AV conduction has resumed (Fig. 101-11). These algorithms are extremely successful in decreasing the incidence of ventricular pacing in patients with intact AV conduction and can decrease the incidence of atrial fibrillation.[40]

Automatic Testing and Data Storage

Many pacemakers can perform reliable automatic threshold testing of the leads. These data may be used to automatically adjust the pacing output. In addition, many pacemakers keep long-term data regarding lead thresholds, lead impedances, and R-wave and P-wave amplitudes. Such trends are extremely helpful in detecting early abnormalities in lead function and in identifying pacing abnormalities. Many pacemakers can store events that are classified as pacemaker-mediated tachycardia, atrial tachyarrhythmia, or a rapid ventricular rate.

Routine Follow-up and Remote Monitoring

Pacemakers should routinely be checked to confirm normal device and lead function and to assess the battery status. Traditionally these functions have been performed at office visits or using home transtelephonic monitoring. New technologies now permit some devices to be analyzed at home using Internet-based services. These systems can assess battery status and create alerts notifying the physician of device or lead abnormalities.

Electromagnetic Interference

Electromagnetic interference (EMI) can be defined as any signal, either biologic or nonbiologic, that falls within a frequency spectrum that may be detected by the sensing circuitry of the pacemaker. EMI can result in rate alteration, sensing abnormalities, magnet mode response, initiation of pacing algorithms, or reprogramming.

Biologic signals that may be responsible for oversensing include T waves, myopotential interference, afterpotential delay, and P waves. Isoelectric extrasystoles can give the appearance of oversensing.[37,41]

Hospital equipment that can interfere with pacemaker function includes electrocautery, cardioversion and defibrillation, magnetic resonance imaging, lithotripsy, radiofrequency ablation, electroshock therapy, and diathermy.

Potential EMI might arise from a relatively small number of sources in the nonhospital environment, including some welding equipment, degaussing equipment, conduction heaters, cellular

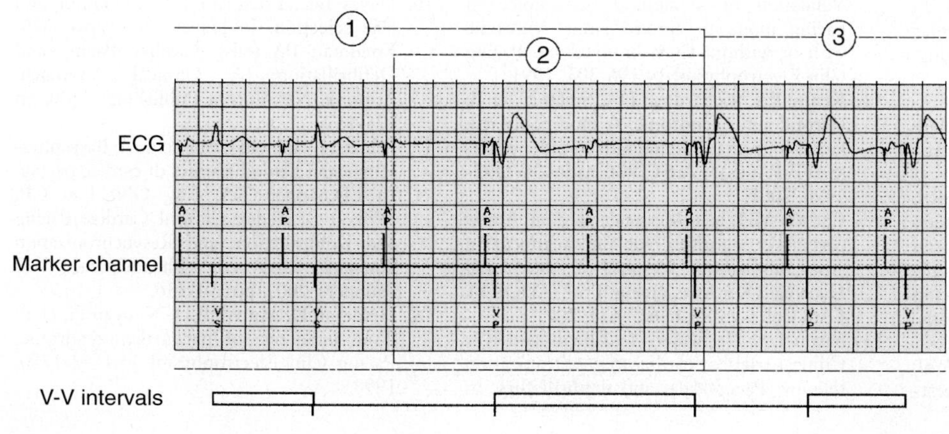

Figure 101-10 Electrocardiographic tracing reveals mode switching algorithm from AAI or AAIR to DDD or DDDR. The managed ventricular pacing algorithm significantly decreases the incidence of ventricular pacing in patients with intact AV conduction. If transient AV block occurs in the AAIR mode after an A-A interval without a ventricular sensed event, a ventricular paced event occurs 80 ms after the escape interval. If two of the four most recent A-A intervals are missing a ventricular event, the device will switch from AAIR to DDDR or from AAI to DDD. (From the Medtronic Virtuoso Device Manual.)

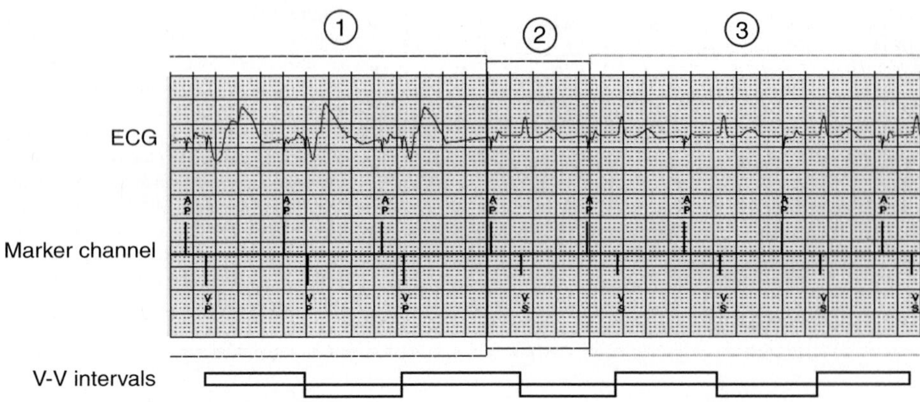

Figure 101-11 Electrocardiographic tracing reveals mode switching algorithm from DDD or DDDR to AAI or AAIR. The algorithm checks for AV conduction at progressively longer intervals, initially 1 minute in duration but increasing up to 16 hours. If AV conduction is present, the mode changes to AAIR. (From the Medtronic Virtuoso Device Manual.)

telephones, and antitheft devices. Interference due to cellular telephone use is rare, and if the patient places the phone over the pacemaker, an adverse clinical event is unlikely.[42]

Certain antitheft devices have the potential for pacemaker interference, causing pacemaker inhibition, sensing abnormalities, and induction of extrasystoles.[43] However, from a practical standpoint, if the patient walks through antitheft gates at a regular pace, clinically significant abnormalities are unlikely.[44]

Summary

Cardiac pacing has become a sophisticated and critical aspect of managing bradyarrhythmias. Recent changes in nomenclature[1] and indications[2] represent ongoing changes in the discipline of cardiac pacing and the influence of clinical trials on this practice. The future will certainly result in increasing automaticity and self-regulation of permanent pacemakers.

References

1. Bernstein AD, Daubert JC, Fletcher RD, et al: The revised NASPE/BPEG generic code for antibradycardia, adaptive-rate, and multisite pacing. Pacing Clin Electrophysiol 25:260-264, 2002.
2. Epstein AE, Dimarco JP, Ellenbogen KA, et al: ACC/AHA/HRS 2008 Guidelines for Device-Based Therapy of Cardiac Rhythm Abnormalities: Executive Summary: A Report of the American College of Cardiology/American Heart Association Task Force on Practice Guidelines (Writing Committee to Revise the ACC/AHA/NASPE 2002 Guideline Update for Implantation of Cardiac Pacemakers and Antiarrhythmia Devices). Heart Rhythm 5:1-22, 2008.
3. Serwer GA, LeRoy SS: Pediatric pacing and defibrillator use. In Ellenbogen KA, Kay GN, Lau CP, Wilkoff BL (eds): Clinical Cardiac Pacing and Defibrillation, and Resynchronization Therapy, 3rd ed. Philadelphia, WB Saunders, 2007, pp 1177-1216.
4. Michaelsson M, Jonzon A, Riesenfeld T: Isolated congenital complete atrioventricular block in adult life: A prospective study. Circulation 92:442-449, 1995.
5. Michaelsson M, Riesenfeld T, Jonzon A: Natural history of congenital complete atrioventricular block. Pacing Clin Electrophysiol 20:2098-2101, 1997.
6. Connolly SJ, Sheldon R, Roberts RS, Gent M; the Vasovagal Pacemaker Study Investigators: The North American Vasovagal Pacemaker Study (VPS): A randomized trial of permanent cardiac pacing for the prevention of vasovagal syncope. J Am Coll Cardiol 33:16-20, 1999.
7. Connolly SJ, Sheldon R, Thorpe KE, et al; the Vasovagal Pacemaker Study Investigators: Pacemaker therapy for prevention of syncope in patients with recurrent severe vasovagal syncope: Second Vasovagal Pacemaker Study (VPS II): A randomized trial. JAMA 289:2224-2229, 2003.
8. Sutton R, Brignole M, Menozzi C, et al; Vasovagal Syncope International Study (VASIS) Investigators: Dual-chamber pacing in the treatment of neurally mediated tilt-positive cardioinhibitory syncope: Pacemaker versus no therapy: A multicenter randomized study. Circulation 102:294-299, 2000.
9. Raviele A, Giada F, Menozzi C, et al; for the Vasovagal Syncope and Pacing Trial Investigators: A randomized, double-blind, placebo-controlled study of permanent cardiac pacing for the treatment of recurrent tilt-induced vasovagal syncope. The vasovagal syncope and pacing trial (SYNPACE). Eur H J 25:1741-1748, 2004.
10. Brignole M, Menozzi C, Lolli G, et al: Validation of a method for choice of pacing mode in carotid sinus syndrome with or without sinus bradycardia. Pacing Clin Electrophysiol 14:196-203, 1991.
11. Kenny RA, Richardson DA, Steen N, et al: Carotid sinus syndrome: A modifiable risk factor for nonaccidental falls in older adults (SAFE PACE). J Am Coll Cardiol 38:1491-1496, 2001.
12. Carlson MD, Ip J, Messenger J, et al: A new pacemaker algorithm for the treatment of atrial fibrillation: Results of the Atrial Dynamic Overdrive Pacing Trial (ADOPT). J Am Coll Cardiol 42:627-633, 2003.
13. Saxon LA, De Marco T, Ellenbogen KA: Clinical trials of cardiac resynchronization therapy: Pacemakers and defibrillators. In Ellenbogen KA, Kay GN, Lau CP, Wilkoff BL (eds): Clinical Cardiac Pacing and Defibrillation, and Resynchronization Therapy, 3rd ed. Philadelphia, WB Saunders, 2007, pp 385-406.
14. Bristow MR, Saxon LA, Boehmer J, et al; Comparison of Medical Therapy, Pacing, and Defibrillation in Heart Failure (COMPANION) Investigators: Cardiac-resynchronization therapy with or without an implantable defibrillator in advanced chronic heart failure. N Engl J Med 350:2140-2150, 2004.
15. Maron BJ, Nishimura RA, William J, et al; for the M-PATHY Study Investigators. Assessment of permanent dual-chamber pacing as a treatment for drug-refractory symptomatic patients with obstructive hypertrophic cardiomyopathy: A randomized, double-blind, crossover study (M-PATHY). Circulation 99:2927-2933, 1999.
16. Hayes DL, Friedman PA: Generator and lead selection. In Hayes DL, Lloyd MA, Friedman PA (eds): Cardiac Pacing and Defibrillation: A Clinical Approach. Armonk, NY, Futura Publishing, 2000, pp 125-157.
17. Prinzen F, Spinelli J, Auricchio A: Basic physiology and hemodynamics of cardiac pacing. In Ellenbogen KA, Kay GN, Lau CP, Wilkoff BL (eds): Clinical Cardiac Pacing and Defibrillation, and Resynchronization Therapy, 3rd ed. Philadelphia, WB Saunders, 2007, pp 291-336.
18. Heldman D, Mulvihill D, Nguyen H, et al: True incidence of pacemaker syndrome. Pacing Clin Electrophysiol 13:1742-1750, 1990.

19. Andersen HR, Nielsen JC, Thomsen PE, et al: Long-term follow-up of patients from a randomised trial of atrial versus ventricular pacing for sick-sinus syndrome. Lancet 350:1210-1216, 1997.
20. Connolly SJ, Kerr CR, Gent M, et al; the Canadian Trial of Physiologic Pacing Investigators: Effects of physiologic pacing versus ventricular pacing on the risk of stroke and death due to cardiovascular causes. N Engl J Med 342:1385-1391, 2000.
21. Lamas GA, Orav EJ, Stambler BS, et al; the Pacemaker Selection in the Elderly Investigators: Quality of life and clinical outcomes in elderly patients treated with ventricular pacing as compared with dual-chamber pacing. N Engl J Med 338:1097-1104, 1998.
22. Lamas GA, Lee KL, Sweeney MO, et al; the Mode Selection Trial in Sinus-Node Dysfunction: Ventricular pacing or dual-chamber pacing for sinus-node dysfunction. N Engl J Med 346:1854-1862, 2002.
23. Lau CP, Tse HF, Kay GN: Sensor driven pacing: Device specifics. In Ellenbogen KA, Kay GN, Lau CP, Wilkoff BL (eds): Clinical Cardiac Pacing and Defibrillation, and Resynchronization Therapy, 3rd ed. Philadelphia, WB Saunders, 2007, pp 499-530.
24. Alt E, Combs W, Willhaus R, et al: A comparative study of activity and dual sensors: Activity and minute ventilation pacing responses to ascending and descending stairs. Pacing Clin Electrophysiol 21:1862-1868, 1998.
25. Kay GN, Bubien RS, Epstein AE, Plumb VJ: Rate-modulated cardiac pacing based on transthoracic impedance measurements of minute ventilation: Correlation with exercise gas exchange. J Am Coll Cardiol 14:1283-1289, 1989.
26. Simon R, Ni Q, Willems R, et al: Comparison of impedance minute ventilation and direct measured minute ventilation in a rate-adaptive pacemaker. Pacing Clin Electrophysiol 26:2127-2133, 2003.
27. Deharo JC, Peyre JP, Chalvidan T, et al: Continuous monitoring of an endocardial index of myocardial contractility during head-up tilt test. Am Heart J 139:1022-1030, 2000.
28. Clementy J, Kobeissi A, Garrigue S, et al: Validation by serial standardized testing of a new rate-responsive pacemaker sensor based on variations in myocardial contractility. Europace 3:124-131, 2001.
29. Osswald S, Cron T, Grädel C, et al: Closed-loop stimulation using intracardiac impedance as a sensor principle: Correlation of right ventricular dP/dt_{max} and intracardiac impedance during dobutamine stress test. Pacing Clin Electrophysiol 23:1502-1508, 2006.
30. Chandiramani S, Cohorn LC, Chandiramani S: Heart rate changes during acute mental stress with closed loop stimulation: Report on two single-blinded, pacemaker studies. Pacing Clin Electrophysiol 30(8):976-984, 2007.
31. Padeletti L, Pieragnoli P, Di Biase L, et al: Is a dual-sensor pacemaker appropriate in patients with sino-atrial disease? Results from the DUSISLOG study. Pacing Clin Electrophyiolol 29:34-40, 2006.
32. Leung Sk, Lau CP, Tang MO, et al: An integrated dual sensor system automatically optimized by target rate histogram. Pacing Clin Electrophysiol 21:1559-1566, 1998.
33. Leung SK, Lau CP, Tang MO: Cardiac output is a sensitive indicator of difference in exercise performance between single and dual sensor pacemakers. Pacing Clin Electrophysiol 21:35-41, 1998.
34. Love CJ: Pacemaker troubleshooting and follow-up. In Ellenbogen KA, Kay GN, Lau CP, Wilkoff BL (eds): Clinical Cardiac Pacing and Defibrillation, and Resynchronization Therapy, 3rd ed. Philadelphia, WB Saunders, 2007, pp 1005-1062.
35. Hayes DL: Pacemaker timing cycles and pacemaker electrocardiography. In Hayes DL, Lloyd MA, Friedman PA (eds): Cardiac Pacing and Defibrillation: A Clinical Approach. Armonk, NY, Futura Publishing Company, 2000 pp 201-245.
36. Wang PJ, Chen H, Okamura H, et al: Timing cycles of implantable devices. In Ellenbogen KA, Kay GN, Lau CP, Wilkoff BL (eds): Clinical Cardiac Pacing and Defibrillation, and Resynchronization Therapy, 3rd ed. Philadelphia, WB Saunders, 2007, pp 969-1004.
37. Atlee JL, Bernstein AD: Cardiac rhythm management devices (part II): Perioperative management. Anesthesiology 95:1492-1506, 2001.
38. Lau CP, Leung SK, Tse HF, Barold SS: Automatic mode switching of implantable pacemakers: II. Clinical performance of current algorithms and their programming. Pacing Clin Electrophysiol 25:1094-1113, 2002.
39. Passman RS, Weinberg KM, Freher M, et al: Accuracy of mode switching algorithms for detection of atrial tachyarrhythmias. J Cardiovasc Electrophysiol 15: 773-777, 2005.
40. Sweeney MO, Bank AJ, Nash E, et al: Minimizing ventricular pacing to reduce atrial fibrillation in sinus-node disease. New Engl J Med 357:1000-1008, 2007.
41. Hayes DL: Electromagnetic interference with implantable cardiac devices. In Barold SS, Mugica J (eds): The Fifth Decade of Cardiac Pacing. Oxford, UK, Blackwell Publishing, 2003.
42. Hayes DL, Wang PJ, Reynolds DW, et al: Interference with cardiac pacemakers by cellular telephones. N Engl J Med 336:1473-1479, 1997.
43. McIvor ME, Reddinger J, Floden E, Sheppard RC: Study of Pacemaker and Implantable Cardioverter Defibrillator Triggering by Electronic Article Surveillance Devices (SPICED TEAS). Pacing Clin Electrophysiol 21:1847-1861, 1998.
44. Groh WJ, Boschee SA, Engelstein ED, et al: Interactions between electronic article surveillance systems and implantable cardioverter-defibrillators. Circulation 100:387-392, 1999.

Cardiac Resynchronization Therapy 102

Michael O. Sweeney

CHAPTER OUTLINE

A Worldwide Epidemic of Chronic Heart Failure

About 15 million people live with chronic heart failure in the United States and Europe. At least 500,000 newly diagnosed cases occur in the United States yearly, primarily in the very elderly (age >75 years), who are the most rapidly growing segment of the population in developed nations. Chronic heart failure is principally a cardiogeriatric syndrome and has become a major public health problem in the 21st century due largely to the aging population. Age-related changes throughout the cardiovascular system in combination with the high prevalence of cardiovascular diseases at older age predispose to the development of heart failure. Almost all heart failure patients have at least one acute episode with symptoms requiring hospitalization and treatment with intravenous medications. Hospital discharges with a primary diagnosis of heart failure totaled about 1 million in 2001 and have increased more than 150% from 1979. Approximately 800,000 of these patients have advanced heart failure. An additional 2 million hospitalizations with heart failure as a secondary diagnosis are recorded annually. The typical patient has approximately 10 medical contacts during the first 3 months after a heart failure hospitalization. Despite improvements in medical therapy, heart failure is associated with a poor prognosis, especially in the elderly. Heart failure hospitalization imposes the highest cost by diagnosis-related grouping and the annual costs of heart failure care in the United States are approximately $30 billion.

Electromechanical Events and Cardiac Pump Function

Optimal cardiac pump function depends on ordered mechanical events that are precisely orchestrated by electrical timing. A word applied to this electromechanical ordering is *synchrony*. This ordering of mechanical events occurs at numerous anatomic levels: between chambers, within chambers, and, of particular importance, at the level of the left ventricle (LV), within myocardial segments. The sequence of contraction at the chamber level proceeds in a descending fashion, but the relative contribution at the chamber level to overall cardiac performance is in the reverse order: ventricular pump function matters most of all.

Disrupted Electromechanical Events in Dilated Cardiomyopathy

Disruptions to electrical timing result in disordered mechanical events (desynchronization, or dyssynchrony), can occur spontaneously or be induced at any level, and can reduce pump function. Such disruptions may be induced by arrhythmia; atrial fibrillation (AF) disrupts atrial coupling (atrial desynchronization) and eliminates atrioventricular (AV) coupling (AV desynchronization). Fixed and functional disruptions to normal mechanical ordering due to conduction delay commonly accompany dilated cardiomyopathy (DCM): atrial decoupling, AV decoupling, ventricular decoupling, intraventricular conduction delay, and transmural conduction delay. These disruptions degrade pump function to different degrees and can occur in isolation or in various combinations.

Atrial Decoupling

The right atrium (RA) and left atrium (LA) are activated nearly simultaneously (within 50 to 80 milliseconds) during sinus rhythm. Preferential sites of interatrial conduction exist at the posterior-superior interatrial septum (Bachman's bundle region), fossa ovalis, and coronary sinus (CS) ostium. Significant interatrial conduction delays (up to 200 ms or greater) can occur in myopathic atria. These conduction delays can be also be induced or exacerbated by RA pacing. Delayed LA contraction can disrupt optimal left-sided AV coupling. In the most severe form of atrial decoupling, delayed LA contraction occurs simultaneously or after LV contraction, resulting in LA transport block. This causes increased LA pressures, retrograde pulmonary venous flow, and counterphysiologic neurohormonal responses.

Atrioventricular Decoupling

Optimal AV coupling contributes to ventricular pump function. The normal AV interval results in atrial contraction just before the pre-ejection (isovolumic) period of ventricular contraction that maximizes LV filling (LV end diastolic pressure, or preload) and cardiac output by the Starling mechanism. This optimal timing relationship maximizes diastolic filling, reduces diastolic mitral regurgitation (MR), and maintains mean LA pressure at low levels (Fig. 102-1).

Disruptions to AV coupling can be understood by analysis of Doppler mitral inflow patterns (Fig. 102-2). Prolonged AV

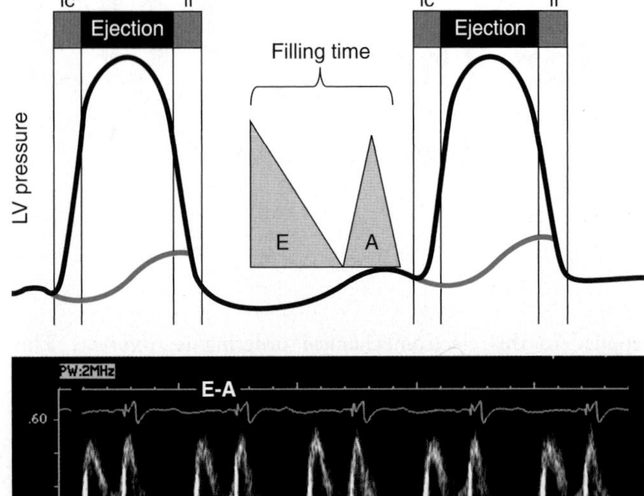

Figure 102-1 Cardiac electromechanical cycle. *Top*, Atrial contraction followed by relaxation at end diastole produces a negative transmitral pressure (TMP) gradient, initiating mitral valve closure, which is completed during isovolumetric contraction when LV $+dP/dt_{max}$ occurs. Ventricular ejection is terminated when left ventricular (LV) pressure falls below aortic pressure, closing the aortic valve. Isovolumetric relaxation follows during which LV $-dP/dt_{max}$ occurs. When LV diastolic pressure is less than left atrial (LA) pressure, a positive TMP gradient occurs, the mitral valve opens, and ventricular filling is initiated. LV pressure is shown in *black*, LA pressure is shown in *red*. *Bottom*, The mitral inflow pattern has two constituents. The initial component (E wave) is due to ventricular filling, the A wave is due to atrial contraction; the summed time is the diastolic filling period. ic, isovolumic contraction; ir, isovolumic relaxation.

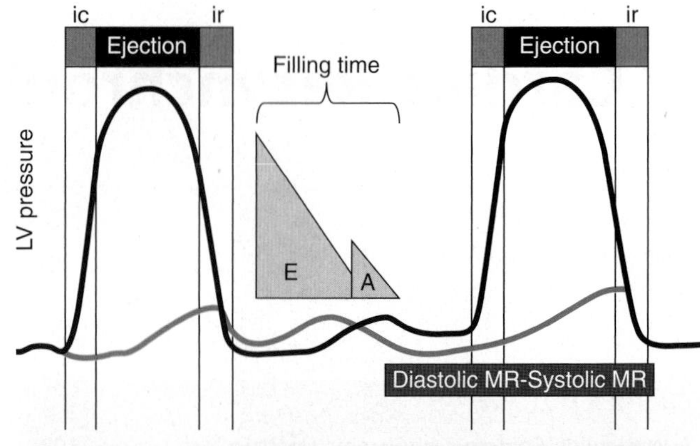

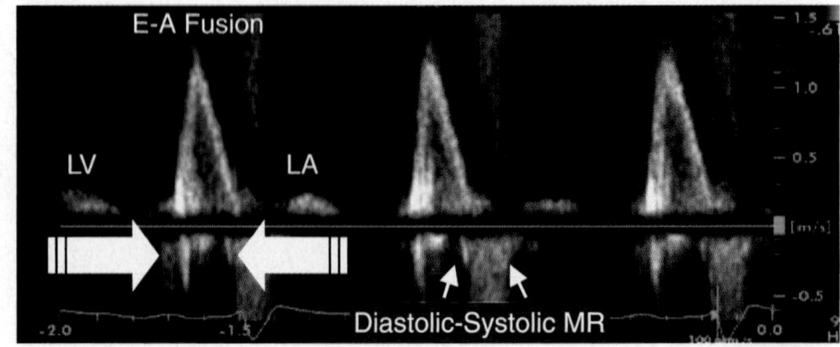

Figure 102-2 Top, Schematic representation of intracardiac pressures and mitral inflow during atrioventricular (AV) decoupling (prolonged AV interval). Left ventricular (LV) filling is displaced rightward in time due to ventricular conduction delay, and atrial contraction is displaced leftward in time due to prolonged AV conduction time. The result is fusion of filling and atrial contraction (E-A fusion). Incomplete mitral closure occurs due to delayed timing of LV contraction allowing LV diastolic pressure to exceed left atrial (LA) pressure (negative transmitral pressure [TMP] gradient) resulting in diastolic, or presystolic mitral regurgitation (MR). LV pressure is shown in *black*, LA pressure is shown in *red*. *Bottom*, Doppler mitral flow velocities displaying these relationships during ventricular and AV conduction delay.

conduction displaces atrial contraction earlier in diastole, which can occur immediately after or even within the preceding ventricular contraction. Atrial contraction before venous return is complete reduces preload stretching of the LV, which reduces ventricular volume and contractile force. Delayed AV coupling reduces diastolic filling time and can result in diastolic MR when elevated LV end-diastolic pressure exceeds LA pressure.

Ventricular Decoupling

Optimal inter- and intra-ventricular coupling is more important than AV coupling for maximum ventricular pumping function.[1,2] *Interventricular coupling* refers to coordinated contraction of the right ventricle (RV) and LV. *Interventricular decoupling* refers to a sequential RV-LV activation delay due to left bundle branch block (LBBB). Earliest ventricular depolarization is recorded over the anterior surface of the RV and latest at the posterior or posterolateral basal LV.[3,4] In canine models of LBBB, interventricular dyssynchrony disrupts ventricular interdependence primarily by reducing ventricular septal contribution to LV ejection. The hemodynamic consequences are time delay between the upslopes of LV and RV systolic pressure and reduced contractility indicated by decreases in rate of rise of LV pressure (LV $+dP/dt_{max}$) and stroke work.[1]

Intraventricular Conduction Delay

Normal LV electrical activation is rapid and homogeneous, with minimal temporal dispersion throughout the wall. This elicits a synchronous mechanical activation and ventricular contraction. The resulting coordinated myocardial segment activation maximizes ventricular pump function.

Left ventricular conduction delay, manifest as an LBBB pattern, can occur throughout the LV, may be anatomically fixed or functional, and is exhibited differently according to substrate characterization (ischemic versus nonischemic DCM). Early endocardial activation mapping studies concluded that LBBB conduction delay resided entirely within the ventricular septum and that LV endocardial activation was rapid after single point breakthrough in nonischemic DCM, whereas activation was slowed across regions of scar throughout the LV in ischemic DCM. In both situations, the posterior or posterolateral basal LV was the latest activated region. More recently, higher-resolution endocardial mapping studies have revealed that the LV septum is activated via slowly conducting LBBB or by transseptal conduction and that conduction velocities are slowed in peri-infarct regions and globally slow in nonischemic DCM.[3-5]

LBBB activation in some patients is due to a line of functional block within the LV (Fig. 102-3).[4] Anterior locations of the line of functional block were characterized by a U-shaped LV activation pattern, more prolonged QRS durations (>150 ms), and greater time to LV breakthrough. Late activation of the posterior or posterolateral basal LV occurred by wave front propagation around the line of block using the apical or inferior LV walls. Lateral locations of the line of block were characterized by less-prolonged QRS durations (<150 ms) and

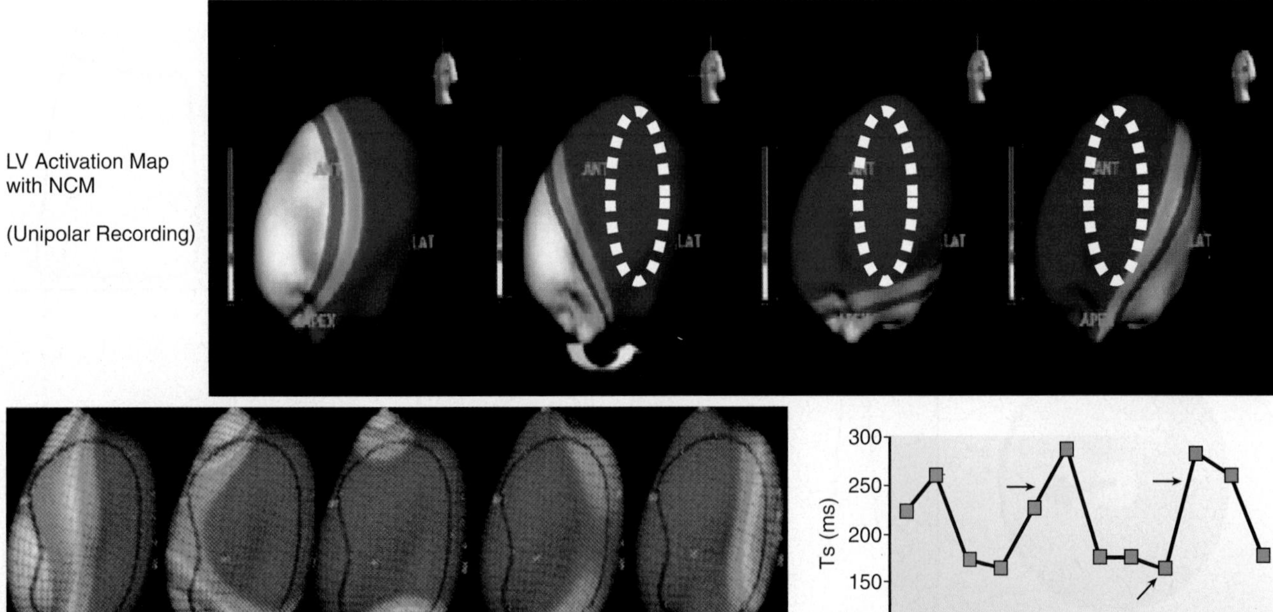

Figure 102-3 *Top*, Unipolar isopotential activation sequence shows a U-shaped LV activation wave front that rotates around the apex and activates the lateral wall late. The area of conduction block is indicated by a *dashed circle*. (Adapted from Auricchio A, Fantoni C, Regoli F, et al: Characterization of left ventricular activation in patients with heart failure and left bundle branch block. Circulation 109(9):1133-1139, 2004.) *Bottom left*, Similar area of conduction block *(black circle)*. However, the LV activation wavefront splits and rotates around the base and apex, merging on the LV lateral wall. *Bottom right*, The earliest peak systolic movement (Ts) was located at the apical septal area *(lower arrow)* and significant delay between septal and lateral LV *(upper arrows)* due to zone of block. AA, apical anterior; AL, apical lateral; AP, apical posterior segment of LV wall; AS, apical septal; BA, basal anterior; BL, basal lateral; BP, basal posterior; BS, basal septal; LV, left ventricle; MA, midanterior; ML, midlateral; MP, midposterior; MS, midseptal; NCM, noncontact mapping; Ts, time from the onset of QRS complex to peak systolic velocity in each LV segment by tissue Doppler imaging. (Adapted from Fung JW, Yu CM, Yip G, et al: Variable left ventricular activation pattern in patients with heart failure and left bundle branch block. Heart 90(1):17-19, 2004.)

shorter time to LV breakthrough. Pacing maneuvers could shift the line of block, indicating their functional nature. Noninvasive mapping of epicardial activation using body surface potentials extended these observations and demonstrated that electrical activation patterns in LBBB are highly heterogenous and unpredictable.[6]

Lines of conduction block do not correlate with regions of wall motion abnormality or scarring. Some lines of block arose only during pacing and were site-dependent (functional) whereas other lines of block could not be manipulated with pacing maneuvers, indicating these were due to slow or absent conduction (fixed). Latest activation most often occurred in the posterior or posterolateral-basal wall but was also observed in the anterior and inferior walls.

Earliest and latest sites of segmental LV activation correlate well with time to peak sustained myocardial systolic velocity, providing evidence that ventricular conduction delay is responsible for heterogenous mechanical activation (asynchrony),[5] which reduces LV pump function (see Fig. 102-3). The mechanical effect of asynchronous electrical activation is dramatic, because the various regions differ not only in the time of onset of contraction, but also in the pattern of contraction. Contraction of early activated regions cause stretching of not-yet-activated remote regions. This stretching further delays shortening of these late activation regions and increases their force of local contraction by virtue of the Frank-Starling mechanism (locally enhanced preload). Late systolic contraction at delayed sites occurs against high LV cavity pressures (locally enhanced afterload) and imposes loading on the earlier activated regions, which now undergo systolic paradoxical stretch. This reciprocated stretching of regions within the LV wall causes a less effective and energetically efficient contraction.

The hemodynamic consequences of the dyssynchronous LV contraction are reductions in contractility and relaxation. Reduced contractility occurs immediately upon induction of LBBB in animal models and is indicated by decreases in stroke volume, stroke work, LV $+dP/dt_{max}$, and a rightward shift of the LV end-systolic pressure-volume relationship, indicating that LV volumes are increased (Fig. 102-4).[1] Premature relaxation in early-activated regions and delayed contraction in others also causes abnormal relaxation expressed as decrease in LV $-dP/dt_{max}$ (maximal rate of fall of LV pressure), increase in the relaxation time constant τ, and decrease of E-wave velocity amplitude on Doppler echocardiograms. Moreover, the longer contraction and relaxation times lead to a reduction in diastolic filling time, leading to reduced preload.

Biomechanical stress due to chronic asynchronous LV activation contributes to ventricular remodeling. Regions of late activation are subject to greater wall stress and develop local myocyte hypertrophy accompanied by molecular abnormalities including reductions in sarcoplasmic reticulum calcium, adenosine triphosphatase (ATPase), and phospholamban.[7] Chronic redistribution of the mechanical load within the ventricular wall leads to reduction of blood flow and myocardial wall thickness over the site of early activation, reciprocal hypertrophy of the late activated regions, and progressive ventricular enlargement.

Ventricular conduction delay also contributes to functional MR (fMR) by inducing papillary muscle desynchronization.[8]

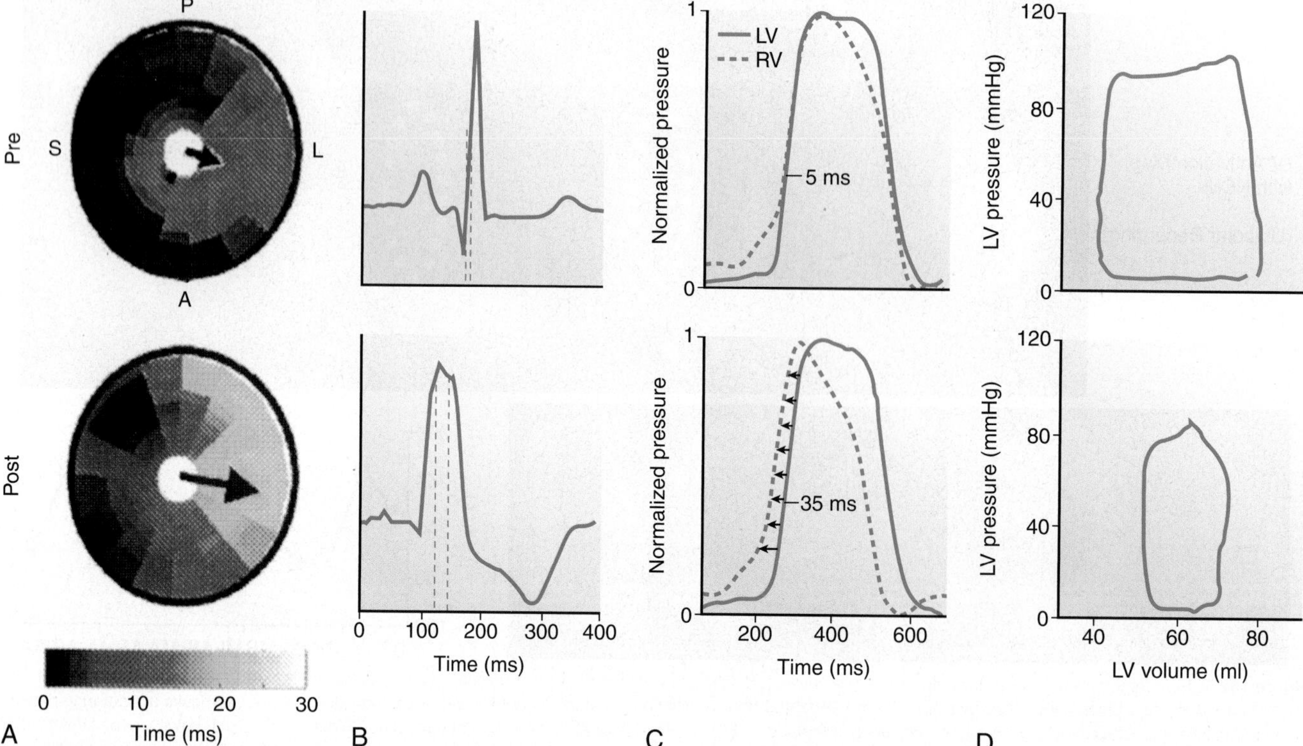

Figure 102-4 Acute reduction in pump function upon induction of left bundle branch block (LBBB). Induction of LBBB increased QRS duration and interventricular and intraventricular activation times which consistently reduced stroke volume, stroke work, dP/dt_{max}, and dP/dt_{min}. **A,** Left ventricle (LV) endocardial activation maps; the activation delay vector is indicated by *arrows*. LV endocardial activation maps are presented as bull's-eye plots, with the inner disk representing the LV apex and the outer circle disc representing the LV base. S, A, L, and P indicate the septum and anterior, lateral, and posterior walls, respectively. **B,** Electrocardiographic tracings. The earliest and latest LV endocardial activation (intraventricular activation time) are indicated by *dotted lines*. **C,** Right ventricle (RV) and LV pressure signals. RV and LV pressures are normalized to reveal timing differences (interventricular activation time). **D,** Pressure-volume loops, before and after creation of LBBB. (Adapted from Verbeek XA, Vernooy K, Peschar M: Intra-ventricular resynchronization for optimal left ventricular function during pacing in experimental left bundle branch block. J Am Coll Cardiol 42:558-567, 2003.)

Ventricular remodeling due to asynchronous contraction and fMR contribute to the progression of heart failure.

Transmural Conduction Delay

Studies of activation maps have shown different activation timing and sequence between endocardial and transmural activation. This suggests the possibility of intramural activation delay between the endocardial and myocardial layer.[4] This accounts for an LBBB pattern on the surface electrocardiogram (ECG) unaccompanied by transseptal or LV endocardial activation delay. The negative effects, if any, of intramural delay on ventricular pumping function are uncertain. However, reversal of the mural activation sequence during LV epicardial pacing is an important constituent in the mechanism of ventricular proarrhythmia.

Mechanisms

Fixed and functional disruptions to normal electromechanical ordering due to conduction delay serve as potential electrical targets for mechanical reconstitution of pump function. The basis of this therapeutic strategy is stimulation of the regionally delayed LV earlier than would have occurred because of prolonged ventricular conduction. Targeted LV pacing has two immediate effects on electromechanical ordering: ventricular activation sequence and chamber timing. The first-order effect of this intervention is positive alteration of LV activation that corrects ventricular conduction delay, which is necessary for ventricular resynchronization and reduction of contractile dyssynchrony, thereby improving ventricular pump function. The second-order effect is modulation of left-sided AV coupling, which can improve diastolic performance metrics and, indirectly, LV pumping function.

The first report of the potential hemodynamic benefit of LV pacing used epicardial leads placed on the high RA and lateral LV during surgery for aortic valve replacement in patients with LBBB.[9] de Teresa and colleagues[9] noted that LV ejection fraction was maximal when septal motion was simultaneous with free wall contraction and diminished when septal and free wall motion were dyssynchronous, such as during spontaneous activation with LBBB or during RV pacing. The term "cardiac resynchronization" was first used 10 years later when Cazeau and coworkers used epicardial leads on all four cardiac chambers to modify the ventricular activation sequence and AV coupling to improve hemodynamic performance in patients with DCM and LBBB.

First-Order Effects

Improved Ventricular Mechanics due to Reduction in Ventricular Conduction Delay

Reduction of intraventricular delay during atrial-synchronous LV or biventricular pacing has an immediate positive effect on ventricular mechanics. Instantaneous improvement in pump

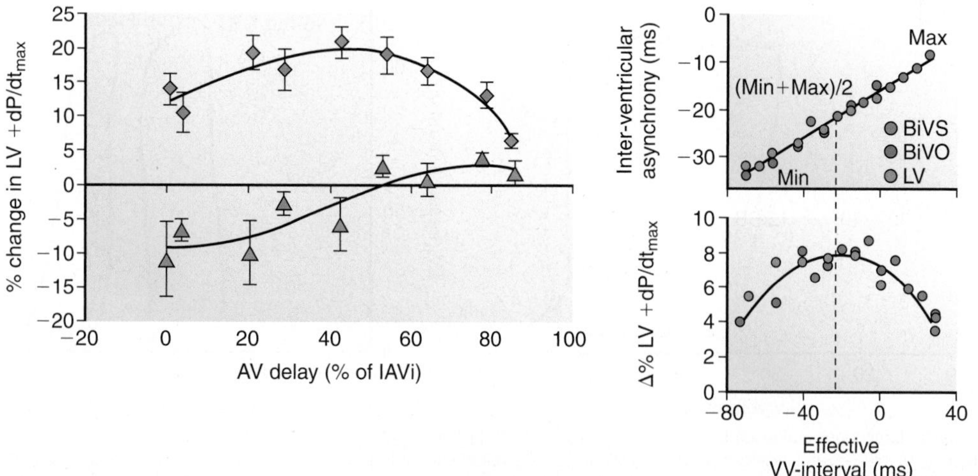

Figure 102-5 *Left*, Change in left ventricular (LV) dP/dt_{max} at various atrioventricular (AV) delays by QRS duration groups. IAVi, intrinsic AV interval. (Adapted from Auricchio A, Stellbrink C, Block M, et al: Effect of pacing chamber and atrioventricular delay on acute systolic function of paced patients with congestive heart failure. The Pacing Therapies for Congestive Heart Failure Study Group. The Guidant Congestive Heart Failure Research Group. Circulation 99(23):2993-3001, 1999; Nelson GS, Curry CW, Wyman BT, et al: Predictors of systolic augmentation from left ventricular preexcitation in patients with dilated cardiomyopathy and intraventricular conduction delay. Circulation 101(23):2703-2709, 2000; Kass DA, Chen C, Curry C, et al: Improved left ventricular mechanics from acute VDD pacing in patients with dilated cardiomyopathy and ventricular conduction delay. Circulation 99(12):1567-1573, 1999.) *Right*, Maximal improvement in LV dP/dt_{max} *(top)* coincides with midpoint of ventricle-ventricle (VV) interval (bottom). BiVO, biventricular simultaneous pacing; BiVS, biventricular sequential pacing; LV, left ventricular pacing. (Adapted from Vernooy K, Verbeek XA, Cornelussen RN, et al: Calculation of effective VV interval facilitates optimization of AV delay and VV interval in cardiac resynchronization therapy. Heart Rhythm 4(1):75-82, 2006.)

function is indicated by increases in LV $+dP/dt_{max}$, arterial pulse pressure, and peak systolic pressure. This positive contractile response is greater with single-site LV versus biventricular pacing, varies inversely with baseline contractile function, demonstrates a modestly positive correlation with increasing baseline QRS duration, and is strongly correlated with baseline mechanical dyssynchrony. Conversely, mechanical improvement does not require QRS narrowing during LV or biventricular pacing.

Early hemodynamic studies demonstrated that the relationship between AV delay and LV $+dP/dt_{max}$ among patients with an acute improvement in contractile response to LV pacing is positive and unimodal, with a peak effect at approximately 50% of the native PR interval (Fig. 102-5). LV $+dP/dt_{max}$ increases 15% to 45% across a narrow range of AV delays and declines at very short or very long AV delays. Conversely, among patients with no acute improvement in contractile response to LV pacing, LV $+dP/dt_{max}$ is greatest at AV delays closest to the native PR interval (no LV pacing) and declines progressively at shorter AV delays (increasingly early LV activation).

The relationship between AV delay and acute contractile response is explained by optimal ventricular resynchronization, not AV coupling (preload). The maximum improvement in pump function (LV $+dP/dt_{max}$ and stroke volume) occurs at minimal interventricular asynchrony (optimal resynchronization) and unchanged LV end-diastolic pressure (preload) (see Fig. 102-5).[2] Maximally effective ventricular resynchronization occurs at the midpoint of the interventricular (VV) interval, which is the conduction time from RV to LV pacing site during native activation. A single optimum AV delay will achieve maximally effective ventricular resynchronization by advancing LV activation sufficiently to minimize the VV interval (for further discussion, see "Interrelationship of AV and VV Timing," later). Therefore, the dose-response relationship between AV delay and acute contractile response shown in Figure 102-5 is interpreted as follows. The magnitude of the acute contractile response depends on the magnitude of baseline asynchrony and the AV delay, which titrates how much intrinsic activation is replaced by pacing. Patients with greater ventricular conduction delay (QRS >150 ms) benefit from near-complete replacement of intrinsic activation with biventricular or LV pacing (i.e., short AV delays). Patients with less ventricular conduction delay (QRS <150 ms) benefit from limited replacement of intrinsic activation (i.e., long AV delays). Typically, programmed short AV delays of 100 to 120 ms, although near-optimal for some patients, can result in decreased contractile function in patients with less baseline asynchrony (e.g., QRS <150 ms) because even biventricular pacing induces dyssynchrony.[10]

This acute improvement in contractility results in increased stroke work and stroke volume and reduced end-systolic volume (Fig. 102-6). However, unlike the inotropic effects of dobutamine, systolic augmentation with ventricular resynchronization does not increase detrimental myocardial oxygen consumption. These acute improvements in ventricular mechanics are maintained chronically and are accompanied by reverse volumetric remodeling of the LV (see later) (see Fig. 102-6).[11] Abrupt discontinuation of LV pacing results in immediate reduction in indices of improved contractility and regression of reverse remodeling over several weeks.[11,12]

Reduction in Functional Mitral Regurgitation

Functional MR (fMR) often accompanies DCM and results from an imbalance between the closing and tethering forces that act on the mitral leaflets that impede mitral closure (Fig. 102-7).[13] This is strongly dependent on alterations in ventricular shape because the tethering forces that act on the mitral leaflets are higher in dilated, more spherical ventricles. Ventricular dilatation and increased chamber sphericity increase the distance between the papillary muscles to the enlarged mitral annulus as well as to each other, restricting leaflet motion and increasing the force needed for effective mitral valve closure. This mitral valve closing force is determined by the difference between systolic LV pressure and LA pressure, termed the *transmitral pressure gradient*. Under these conditions, the mitral regurgitant

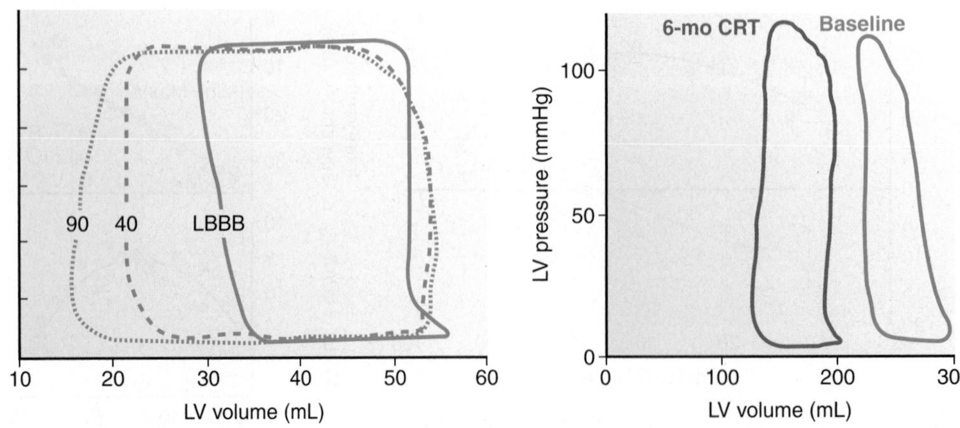

Figure 102-6 *Left*, Pressure-volume loops during left bundle branch block (LBBB) and pacing from posterolateral left ventricle (LV) at two AV delays (40 and 90 ms). Note the immediate reduction in LV volumes and increases in stroke work and stroke volume. (Adapted from Verbeek XA, Vernooy K, Peschar M: Intra-ventricular resynchronization for optimal left ventricular function during pacing in experimental left bundle branch block. J Am Coll Cardiol 42:558-567, 2003.) *Right*, LV pressure-volume loops before *(right)* and after *(left)* 6 months of cardiac resynchronization therapy. Note the sustained leftward shift of the pressure-volume relationship and the increases in stroke work, stroke volume, and dP/dt_{max}. CRT, cardiac resynchronization therapy. (Adapted from Steendijk P, Tulner SA, Bax JJ, et al: Hemodynamic effects of long-term cardiac resynchronization therapy: Analysis by pressure-volume loops. Circulation 113(10):1295-1304, 2006.)

orifice area is largely determined by the phasic changes in transmitral pressure. Increasing the transmitral pressure can reduce the effective regurgitant orifice area. When DCM is accompanied by intraventricular conduction delay, time to peak strain between papillary muscle insertion sites is increased.[8] Delayed sequential activation of the papillary muscles contributes to incomplete mitral valve closure and worsens fMR (Fig. 102-8).

There are three mechanisms by which cardiac resynchronization therapy reduces fMR. Improved contractility reduces fMR instantaneously and is quantitatively related to an increase in LV $+dP/dt_{max}$ and transmitral pressure (see Fig. 102-7).[13] Ventricular resynchronization shortens interpapillary muscle delay, which instantaneously reduces fMR due to more coordinated papillary muscle activation (see Fig. 102-8).[8] Reverse volumetric LV remodeling reduces fMR chronically by reducing LV volumes and sphericity, which reduce tethering forces on the mitral valve.

Reverse Volumetric Left Ventricular Remodeling

Mechanical resynchronization reduces mechanical load heterogeneity throughout the LV. Sustained improvement in ventricular mechanics results in regression of negative LV remodeling, termed *reverse remodeling*. This results in reductions in LV volumes and mass, reduced mitral orifice size, regression of asymmetric hypertrophy, and increased ejection fraction.[11,14,15] The magnitude of the reduction in end systolic volume ranges between 10% and 30%,[14,16] which is equivalent to or greater than the effects of β-blockers and angiotensin converting enzyme (ACE) inhibitors. Evidence of mechanical resynchronization appears to be necessary for reverse remodeling to occur, and the greater the reduction in dyssynchrony, the higher the probability of remodeling. Likewise, absence of mechanical resynchronization acutely eliminates the possibility of chronic reverse remodeling.[15] In some cases, reverse remodeling results in complete normalization of LV volumes and ejection fraction, suggesting that ventricular conduction delay may be the primary cause of DCM in some patients.

Second-Order Effects

Improved AV Coupling and Diastolic Filling

Left-sided AV decoupling can be corrected with LV pacing by reordering chamber timing. When LV contraction timing is delayed, the result is similar to a prolonged AV interval, as shown in Figure 102-2. Atrial contraction before venous return is complete reduces preload stretching of the LV, which reduces ventricular volume and contractile force. Delayed AV coupling reduces diastolic filling time and can result in diastolic MR when elevated LV end-diastolic pressure exceeds LA pressure. Conversely, when LV contraction timing is too early, LA transport block occurs.

Atrial contraction occurs simultaneously with LV contraction, resulting in increased LA pressure and loss of preload (Fig. 102-9). Ventricular and AV resynchronization results in LA contraction just before LV contraction, which increases preload and diastolic filling time (E-A separation) and reduces diastolic and systolic MR (see Fig. 102-1).

Improved Heart Rate Profile

Ventricular resynchronization favorably modifies autonomic balance as evidenced by reduced mean heart rate and increased heart rate variability, which correlate with improved functional capacity, reverse remodeling, and reduced mortality.[17]

Implantation Techniques

There are currently three approaches to achieving LV pacing. The transvenous approach uses specially designed delivery sheaths and tools for cannulating the CS in order to deliver pacing leads to the coronary veins. Epicardial LV pacing can also be achieved under direct (thoracotomy) or indirect (transcutaneous pericardial access) visualization. LV endocardial pacing via transseptal puncture has been described in the rare circumstance where neither the transvenous epicardial nor surgical options are viable. Cardiac resynchronization therapy implantation techniques have been reviewed in detail elsewhere.[18]

Approach to Transvenous Left Ventricular Lead Placement

Early attempts at LV pacing via the coronary veins used conventional endocardial pacing leads designed for RV pacing or CS leads designed for left atrial pacing and used unassisted CS cannulation, and it was technically challenging.

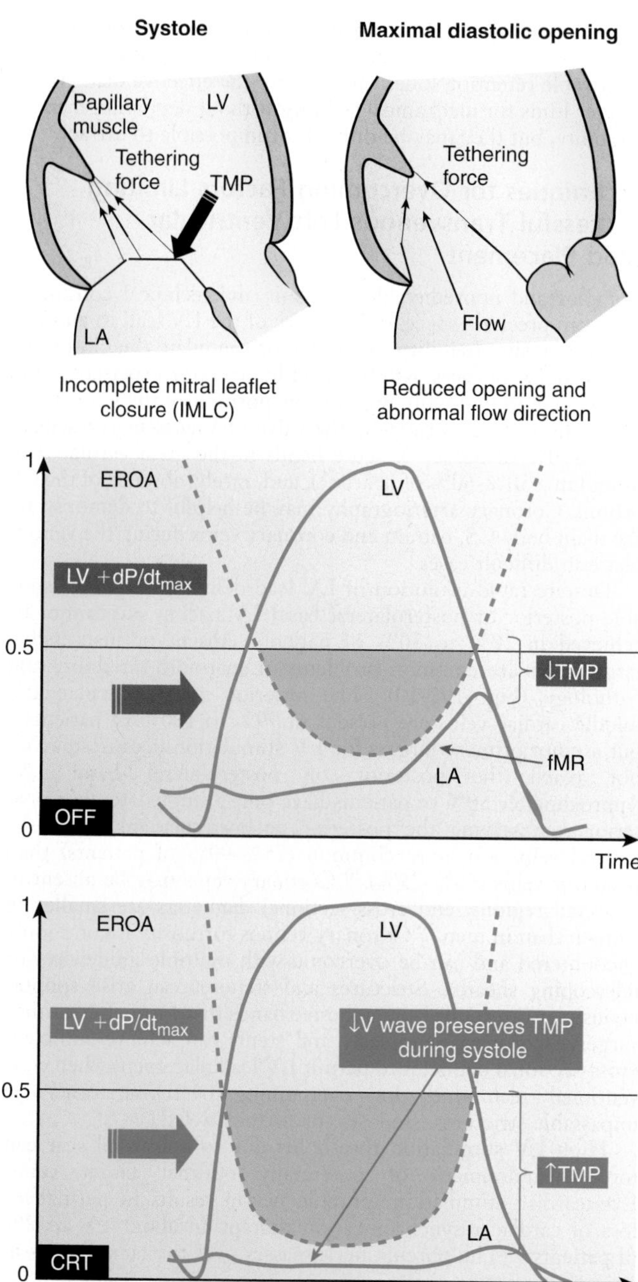

Figure 102-7 *Top*, Mechanism of functional mitral regugitation (fMR) due to augmented leaflet tethering caused by negative left ventricular (LV) volumetric remodeling. (Adapted from Otsuji Y, Gilon D, Jiang L, et al: Restricted diastolic opening of the mitral leaflets in patients with left ventricular dysfunction: Evidence for increased valve tethering. J Am Coll Cardiol 32(2):398-404, 1998.) *Middle*, CRT off. Note reduced LV dP/dt_{max}, increased left atrial (LA) pressure, and reduced transmitral pressure (TMP) gradient. *Bottom*, CRT on. Acute reduction in fMR during CRT due to increased LV dP/dt_{max} causing an accelerated rise in TMP, which counteracts increased mitral valve tethering forces and decreases effective regurgitant orifice area (EROA). *Shaded area* indicates the time EROA <50% of initial value. CRT, cardiac resynchronization therapy; TMP, transmitral pressure gradient. (Adapted from Breithardt OA, Sinha AM, Schwammenthal E, et al: Acute effects of cardiac resynchronization therapy on functional mitral regurgitation in advanced systolic heart failure. J Am Coll Cardiol 41:765-770, 2003.)

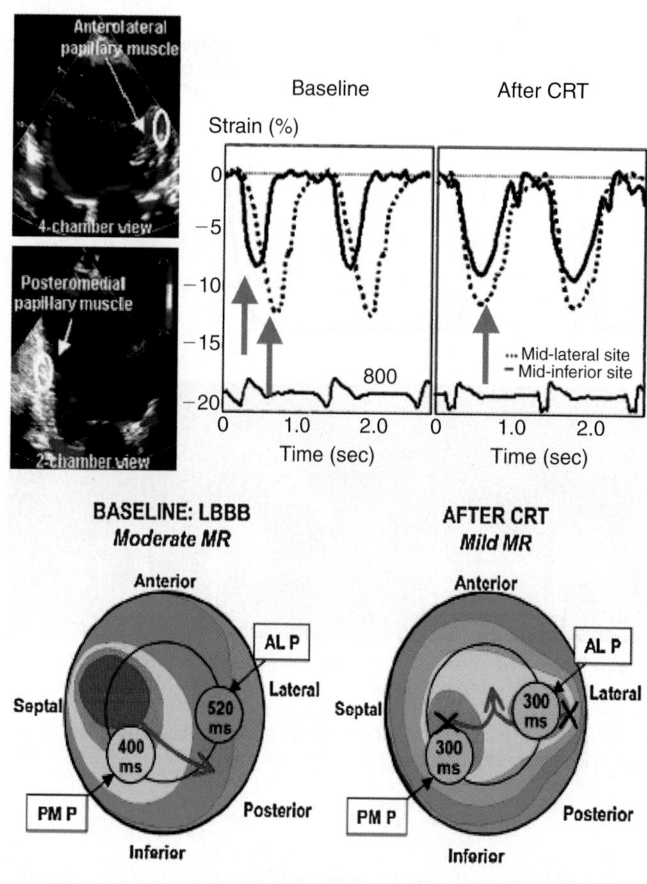

Figure 102-8 *Top*, Echocardiographic strain images demonstrate delayed sequential timing *(arrows)* of peak negative strain (contraction) at posteromedial (early) and anterosuperior (late) papillary muscles due to ventricular conduction delay. *Bottom*, Time to peak systolic strain is color coded, with lines representing isochrones of mechanical activation times at 50-ms intervals. The *X* indicates sites of lead placement, and the *arrow* indicates the direction of the propagating mechanical activation. Time to peak strain of sites adjacent to anterolateral (AL P) and posteromedial (PM P) papillary muscles are shown. Papillary muscle peak strain is time-aligned (synchronized) during biventricular stimulation. CRT, cardiac resynchronization therapy. (Adapted from Kanzaki H, Bazaz R, Schwartzman D, et al: A mechanism for immediate reduction in mitral regurgitation after cardiac resynchronization therapy: Insights from mechanical activation strain mapping. J Am Coll Cardiol 44(8):1619-1625, 2004.)

Nonetheless, successful long-term coronary venous LV pacing was achieved in 80% of patients, and 74% of leads were placed in a posterior or posterolateral basal vein.[19] Experienced implanters using currently available tools, techniques, and leads specifically designed for coronary veins can achieve reliable LV stimulation in more than 90% of cases.

Coronary Sinus Cannulation

Typically, the CS is cannulated with a specially designed sheath that serves as a workstation for retrograde coronary venography, coronary venous interventions, and LV lead placement. Such sheaths are available in a variety of diameters and shapes intended to overcome unpredictable anatomic variation in right heart chamber dimensions and orientation due to remodeling. CS cannulation is usually assisted with a deflectable electrophysiology catheter, a coronary angiography catheter, or a

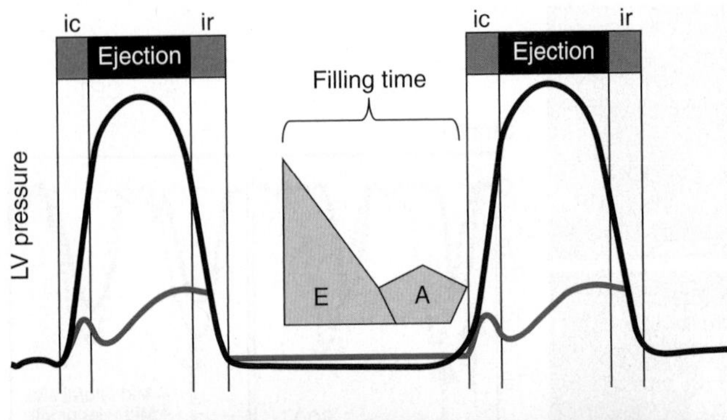

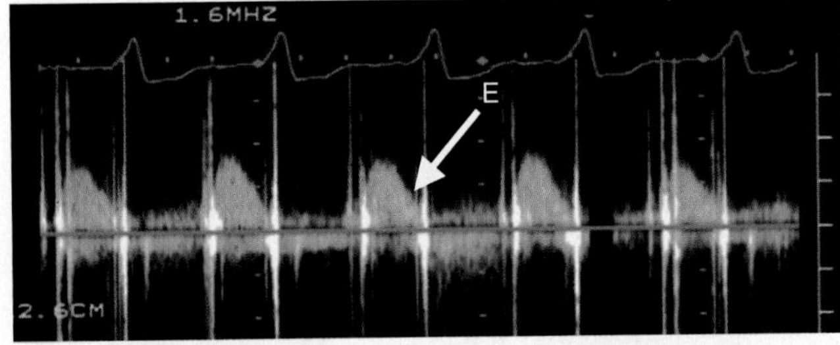

Figure 102-9 *Top,* Intracardiac pressures and mitral inflow at short atrioventricular (AV) interval. *Bottom,* Complete truncation of A wave (left atrial transport block). Diastolic filling period is shortened *(arrow)* due to premature closure of mitral valve (atrial and ventricular contraction occur simultaneously). A, a wave; E, e wave; ic, isovolumic contraction; ir, isovolumic relaxation.

hydrophilic-coated guide wire within the guiding sheath. Increasingly elaborate technologies to assist CS cannulation have been developed, including deflectable inner guides capable of contrast dye injection, ultrasound catheters, infrared imaging, and deflectable fiberoptic endoscopes.

Visualization of the Coronary Venous Circulation

Once the CS is successfully cannulated, retrograde occlusive venography is performed at multiple levels to delineate the coronary venous anatomy. A strategy of surgical planning prior to cardiac resynchronization therapy implantation using noninvasive visualization of the coronary venous circulation by fast contrast tomography (CT) or rotational coronary venous angiography has been proposed.[20] Even more elaborate image integration approaches combine left heart anatomy from CT scans and echocardiographic assessment of regional LV mechanical function. Experience with these techniques is considerably limited and the practical necessity is debatable, particularly when one considers that 80% implant success was achieved with conventional endocardial pacing leads in the coronary veins more than a decade ago.

Selecting a Left Ventricular Lead

A design advantage in one anatomic situation is almost invariably a disadvantage in another and, therefore the ideal LV lead suitable for use in all patients and anatomic situations does not exist. Several factors figure unpredictably into this lead selection, including coronary venous anatomy, extracardiac stimulation, and LV epicardial pacing thresholds. Currently available transvenous LV pacing leads may be either stylet-driven or over-the-wire (OTW). In general, the smallest diameter leads are unipolar and OTW. Larger-diameter leads may be delivered using stylets or OTW (hybrids). Some leads have multiple electrodes that can be used individually or in combinations. Most lead designs rely on passive wedging the lead tip into the target vein for fixation. Reversible self-retaining cants, S- or pigtail-shaped curves, and deployable retention lobes can increase the effective diameter of smaller leads for mechanical stability without degrading maneuverability, but they may be difficult or impossible to extract.

Techniques for Overcoming Factors Limiting Successful Transvenous Left Ventricular Lead Placement

Complex and unpredictable anatomic and technical considerations can preclude successful delivery of the LV lead to an optimal pacing site. Inability to localize or cannulate the CS occurs in 1% to 5% of cases; is influenced by operator experience; and may be due to unusually high or low position of the CS ostium, obstruction of the ostium by the valve of Vieussens (present in ~80%-90% of hearts[21]), acute bends in the great cardiac vein (found in ~50%-60% of hearts[21]), and, rarely, absence of the CS ostium. Coronary arteriography may be helpful to demonstrate the main body CS, ostium and coronary veins during the venous phase in difficult cases.

Despite rapid evolution of LV lead delivery systems, a suitable posterior or posterolateral basal LV pacing site cannot be achieved in 20% to 30% of patients. Absent or inaccessible target veins are common problems of anatomic variability and pathology (Fig. 102-10). The anterior interventricular and middle cardiac veins are present in 99% to 100% of patients[20] but are not primary targets for LV stimulation because they do not reach the posterior or posterolateral basal LV. Approximately 50% of patients have only a single lateral or posterior vein serving the posterior or posterolateral basal LV. Lateral veins are more common (75%-90% of patients) than posterior veins (50%-75%).[20] Coronary veins may be absent in infarcted regions, and cross-sectional diameters are smaller in women than in men.[20] Coronary venous tortuosity is commonly encountered and can be overcome with multiple guidewires or telescoping sheaths. Strictures and stenoses can arise spontaneously or can result from adhesive bands that form after cardiac surgery. Coronary venoplasty and stents can achieve sufficient cross-sectional diameter to permit LV lead placement when conventional techniques for overcoming overcome otherwise impassable strictures, stenoses, or tortuosity fail.

High LV stimulation thresholds due to epicardial scar can force abandonment of potentially optimal target veins. Extracardiac stimulation (phrenic nerve) results in permanent loss of cardiac resynchronization therapy in about 1% to 2% of patients.[22] The phrenic nerve passes over the lateral veins in

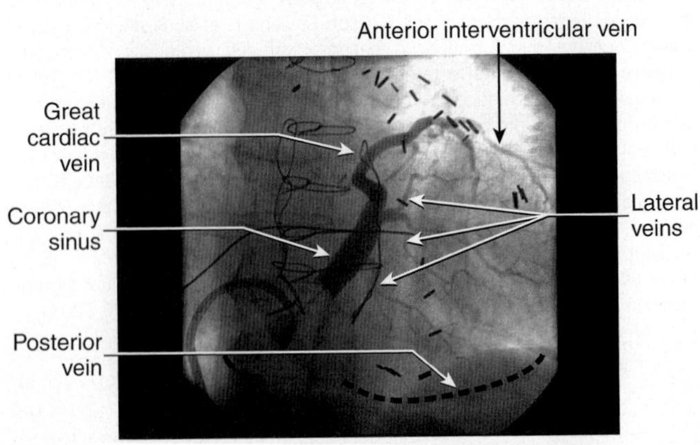

Figure 102-10 Coronary veins visualized by retrograde venography.

about 80% of specimens and over the anterior interventricular vein in the remaining 20% or so.[23] Phrenic nerve stimulation can often be overcome by repositioning the LV lead within the target vein, reducing LV voltage output in devices that permit separate RV and LV outputs, altering the LV-RV pacing vector by selecting alternate electrodes on multielectrode LV leads, or surgical placement of LV leads with careful visualization of the course of the nerve sheath.

Loss of cardiac resynchronization therapy due to LV lead dislodgment has a reported incidence of 5 to 10% in larger studies[24,25] and is influenced by implanter experience and other technical factors such as the lack of fixation mechanisms and stresses placed on the proximal portion of the lead at the junction of the right atrium and CS ostium. Lead dislodgment can be reduced by carefully matching the LV lead diameter and the luminal diameter of the target vein. Support at multiple (>2-3) positions increases mechanical stability. Nonconventional techniques for maintaining chronic LV lead stability include retained guidewires, stents, and active fixation leads. Experience with these techniques is limited, and long-term safety and performance have not been established.

Long-Term Performance of Transvenous LV Leads

Chronic capture thresholds average 1.5 to 2.0 volts, are stable for at least 6 to 30 months after implantation, and are similar across lead designs (OTW vs pre-formed shape).[26]

Acute Complications of LV Lead Placement in the Coronary Veins

Endothelial dissection of the CS is the most common complication (~6%-8%); is usually caused by guidewires, catheters, and balloons; and can force premature termination of the procedure. Endothelial dissection is easily recognized during venography as staining of the CS wall, which can track retrogradely to the ostium and pericardial space. However, pericardial tamponade virtually never occurs, unless it is accompanied by a true perforation or rupture of the vessel wall. Intimal flaps heal completely within 2 to 3 months without residual structural damage or venous remodeling. Coronary venous laceration or perforation tends to occur during lead and guidewire manipulations in small-caliber veins, is recognized by sudden free movement of the guidewire within the pericardial space, typically results in tamponade, and often requires cardiac surgery for oversewing of the culprit vessel.

Nonconventional and Alternative Approaches to Cardiac Resynchronization Therapy

Left ventricular pacing via transseptal puncture and placement of an active fixation pacing lead across the mitral valve and on the LV endocardium have been described. The major concern with this approach is thromboembolism, and permanent oral anticoagulation is mandatory.

Hardware Systems, Programming Considerations, and Troubleshooting

Optimal programming of cardiac resynchronization therapy systems requires a sophisticated understanding of the pathophysiologic electrical and mechanical substrates in DCM and is an active process that must anticipate the potential for dynamic and related changes in the patient's condition or operation of the device system. This is a critically important distinction to conventional pacemakers, which reliably provide bradycardia support with minimal need for periodic programming intervention. Similarly, though conventional implantable cardioverter defibrillators (ICDs) require a slightly higher level of surveillance, they reside primarily in a passive state for the duration of the patient's life. The hybridization of cardiac resynchronization therapy with defibrillation systems (CRT-D) invokes all of the complex considerations of cardiac resynchronization therapy and ICD programming. This introduces particularly unique challenges because the device must simultaneously exist in two fundamentally opposed states of operation, continuous delivery of ventricular pacing and continuous surveillance for ventricular arrhythmia (reviewed by Sweeney[27]).

Leads and Pulse Generators

Transvenous and epicardial LV pacing leads may be either unipolar or bipolar. Because programmed polarity settings are common to both ventricular leads and because the type (bipolar or unipolar) of these leads might not be the same, several pacing polarity configurations are possible. In a dual bipolar polarity configuration, both lead tips are the active electrodes (cathodes) and the ring(s) are the common (nonstimulating) anode. If both leads are bipolar, both rings act as the common electrode. If one lead is bipolar (RV) and the other lead is unipolar (typically LV), the ring on the bipolar lead acts as the common electrode (nonstimulating anode). This configuration results in shared-ring bipolar pacing and sensing. This hybrid bipolar-unipolar stimulation configuration (dual cathodal) is employed in most contemporary cardiac resynchronization therapy pacing systems.

A conventional dual chamber pulse generator can also be used for atrial-synchronous biventricular pacing. The single ventricular output must be divided to provide simultaneous stimulation of the RV and LV (dual cathodal system with parallel outputs). This is achieved with a Y-adaptor and results in simultaneous RV and LV sensing, which can result in ventricular double-counting and loss of cardiac resynchronization therapy or pacemaker inhibition in the case of LV lead dislodgement into the CS with sensing of atrial activity.

First-generation multisite pulse generators similarly provide a single ventricular output for simultaneous RV and LV stimulation; however, two separate ventricular channels internally connect in parallel. This connection is made for both the lead tip and ring connections and eliminates the need for a Y-adaptor. This configuration still provides simultaneous RV and LV sensing with associated limitations. Second-generation multisite pulse generators have independent ventricular ports. Each ventricular lead therefore has separate sensing and output circuits. This arrangement permits ventricular chamber-specific outputs and timing and eliminates the potential complications of biventricular sensing.

Pacing Modes

It is axiomatic that for maximal delivery of cardiac resynchronization therapy, ventricular pacing must be continuous. DDD mode (dual chamber pacing and sensing) guarantees atrial-synchronous ventricular pacing. A lower rate limit of 40 to 50 beats per minute is generally desirable to suppress atrial pacing that might otherwise induce left-sided AV desynchronization due to capture latency and interatrial conduction time. VDD mode (atrial sensing only, ventricular pacing and sensing) eliminates atrial pacing and guarantees atrial-synchronous ventricular pacing, unless the sinus rate falls below the programmed lower rate when VDD becomes operationally VVI (ventricular-only sensing and pacing).

Although conventional dual-chamber pacemakers are not designed for biventricular pacing, they are being increasingly used with short AV delays (0-30 ms) for cardiac resynchronization therapy in permanent AF. In this situation, the ventricular port is used for the RV lead and the atrial port is used for the LV lead. This permits independent ventricular outputs and VV timing by manipulation of the AV delay. The DVIR mode (dual chamber [RV + LV] pacing, single chamber [RV] sensing) is ideally suited for this arrangement because it provides absolute protection against far-field sensing of atrial activity in case of LV lead dislodgement because no sensing occurs on the atrial (LV) lead in the DVIR mode.

Interrelationship of AV and VV Timing

During LBBB, the RV is activated by intrinsic conduction before the LV and the time difference between RV and LV activation at the pacing sites is the minimally effective, or native, VV interval.[2] Short AV delays result in complete replacement of intrinsic activation with biventricular pacing, and therefore chamber timing can only be manipulated with sequential ventricular stimulation (see "Interventricular (VV) Optimization," later). Progressively longer AV delays result in RV fusion followed by intrinsic RV activation, both accompanied by LV preexcitation because intrinsic LV activation is delayed. Modification of the AV delay alone can therefore achieve biventricular fusion, LV-only fusion, and sequential VV stimulation (LV first) (Fig. 102-11).

Atrioventricular Optimization

AV coupling complements ventricular resynchronization and can be tailored by a variety of methods including invasive hemodynamic monitoring with LV pressure catheters, noninvasive hemodynamic monitoring with finger photoplethysmography, Doppler analysis of mitral inflow patterns, and regression formulas derived from intrinsic RA and RV electrogram timing. The common goal is to normalize left-sided AV coupling and maximize diastolic filling time.

Interventricular (VV) Optimization

Logically, enhancements to biventricular pacing systems might permit tailoring of ventricular stimulation by site and timing to overcome bidirectional differences in conduction times due to fixed or functional conduction blocks that degrade mechanical resynchronization. This requires separately programmable RV and LV stimulation outputs and circuitry to permit timing delay between outputs by stimulation site (VV timing) in order to achieve site-selective, sequential ventricular stimulation.

Clinical Experience with AV and VV Optimization

Acute studies have shown improvements in indices of pump function with AV and VV optimization. However, there is currently no clinical evidence that a strategy of serial AV and VV optimization improves outcome in cardiac resynchronization therapy patients.[28-30] The optimized AV delay in studies of cardiac resynchronization therapy is almost invariably in the range of 80 to 120 ms regardless of other considerations. Because of this, some have argued for empiric programming of the AV delay at ≈ 100 ms. AV coupling is dynamic, it differs as heart rate and loading conditions change, and LA mechanical transport is diminished due to myopathic processes and high LV filling pressures. Likewise, simultaneous biventricular stimulation has reproducibly been shown to be effective in the majority of patients in randomized clinical trials of cardiac resynchronization therapy. It is possible that the incremental benefits of AV and VV optimization are too small to be detected on a population scale.

Loss of Cardiac Resynchronization: Causes and Corrective Actions

Optimal cardiac resynchronization therapy operation requires 100% delivery of ventricular pacing, which is difficult to achieve. A reasonable goal is 90% to 95% cumulative LV pacing; less than 85% might negate the clinical response to cardiac resynchronization therapy.[31] Cardiac resynchronization therapy is

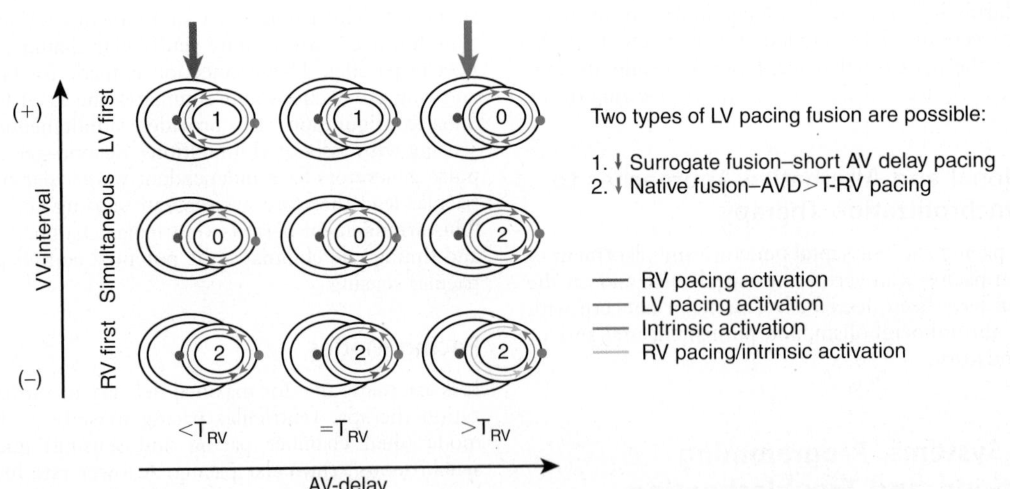

Figure 102-11 Interrelationship of atrioventricular (AV) and ventriculoventricular (VV) timing. T_{RV} is time to intrinsic right ventricle (RV) activation. During short AV delay pacing (AV delay < T_{RV}), biventricular pacing completely replaces native activation (surrogate fusion), and relative timing of ventricular activation is determined by sequential ventricular stimulation (RV first, simultaneous, left ventricle [LV] first). When AV delay = T_{RV}, RV pacing occurs simultaneously with intrinsic conduction, resulting in a combination of RV pacing and intrinsic conduction, whereas LV is still activated earlier than would have occurred due to left bundle branch block (LBBB). When AV delay > T_{RV}, LV-only pacing occurs, with true fusion of native and paced activation. The effective VV interval represents the actual time difference between the activation of the RV and LV lateral wall, either by ventricular pacing or by intrinsic activation. Positive values (+) indicate an earlier onset of LV than RV electrical activation, whereas negative values (–) indicate earlier RV activation. (Adapted from Vernooy K, Verbeek XA, Cornelussen RN, et al: Calculation of effective VV interval facilitates optimization of AV delay and VV interval in cardiac resynchronization therapy. Heart Rhythm 4(1):75-82, 2006.)

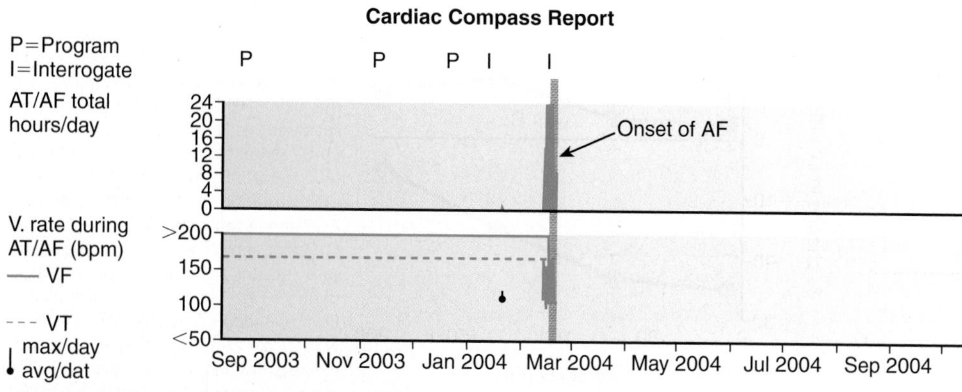

Cardiac Compass Report

P=Program
I=Interrogate

P P P I I

% Pacing/day — Atrial — Ventricular 100 75 50 25 0

Loss of CRT

Avg V. rate (bpm) — Day — Night >120 100 80 60 <40

Patient activity hours/day >8 6 4 2 0

Heart rate variability (ms) >200 160 120 80 <40

Sep 2003 Nov 2003 Jan 2004 Mar 2004 May 2004 Jul 2004 Sep 2004

Pacing	Feb 19, 2004	Aug 14, 2003	
AS-VS	99.1%	4.3%	4.3%
AS-VP	0.7% ←	95.6%	95.6%
AP-VS	<0.1%	<0.1%	<0.1%
AP-VP	0.2%	<0.1%	<0.1%
Additional counters			
Single PVCs	880	104346	104346
Runs of PVCs	104	16684	16684
V. rate stabilization paces	0	0	0
Runs of V. rate stab. paces	0	0	0

Figure 102-12 Loss of cardiac resynchronization due to atrial fibrillation (AF). Note the high percentage on the AS-VP (atrial sense–biventricular pace) counter prior to onset of AF. Onset of AF with rapid atrioventricular (AV) conduction results in a sudden loss of CRT, indicated by the high-percentage AS-VS (ventricular sense) counter. AP, atrial pace; PVC, premature ventricular contraction; VF, ventricular fibrillation; VT, ventricular tachycardia.

interrupted transiently in 36% of patients and permanently in 5% within 2 years of follow-up, and the causes are numerous.[22] Restoration of cardiac resynchronization therapy can usually be accomplished noninvasively; less commonly it requires surgical intervention.

Atrial fibrillation is the most common cause of loss of cardiac resynchronization therapy, accounting for at least 18% of all therapy interruptions.[22] Instantaneous loss of atrial, AV, and ventricular coupling results in total cardiac desynchronization accompanied by rapid ventricular cycle length irregularity, which further reduces pump function (Fig. 102-12). Pharmacologic suppression of AF and ventricular rate control is essential; the latter might require AV junction ablation to guarantee continuous ventricular pacing.[31] Specific features of pacing operation can increase the percentage of ventricular pacing during rapidly conducted AF by automatically increasing the pacing rate in alignment with the native conducted ventricular response or by triggering an immediate pacing output to both ventricles when a sensed event occurs during the AV interval. The triggered output is rendered ineffectual in the chamber where sensing occurred due to ventricular refractoriness, but it resynchronizes ventricular activation by stimulating the chamber opposite the sensed event. Loss of LV capture occurs in 1% to 10% of patients, is the second most common cause of interrupted cardiac resynchronization therapy, and is due to lead dislodgment (75%) and chronic pacing threshold elevation (25%).[22,26]

Pseudoatrial undersensing refers to loss of atrial tracking at high sinus rates with AV conduction delay that displace the P wave into the postventricular atrial refractory period (PVARP), resulting in loss of synchronous ventricular pacing. Spontaneous AV conduction emerges in the form of a preempted upper-rate Wenckebach response. Automatic shortening of the PVARP at high sinus rates is effective in preventing loss of ventricular pacing. Ventricular double-counting of the native biventricular electogram can occur in dual cathodal, parallel output configurations and can initiate and maintain pseudoatrial undersensing. The LV EGM is sensed after the RV EGM if the interventricular conduction time exceeds the blanking period initiated by RV sensing. The LV signal continuously resets the PVARP, resulting in an implied total atrial refractory period conflict and maintenance of pseudo-atrial undersensing. This is also

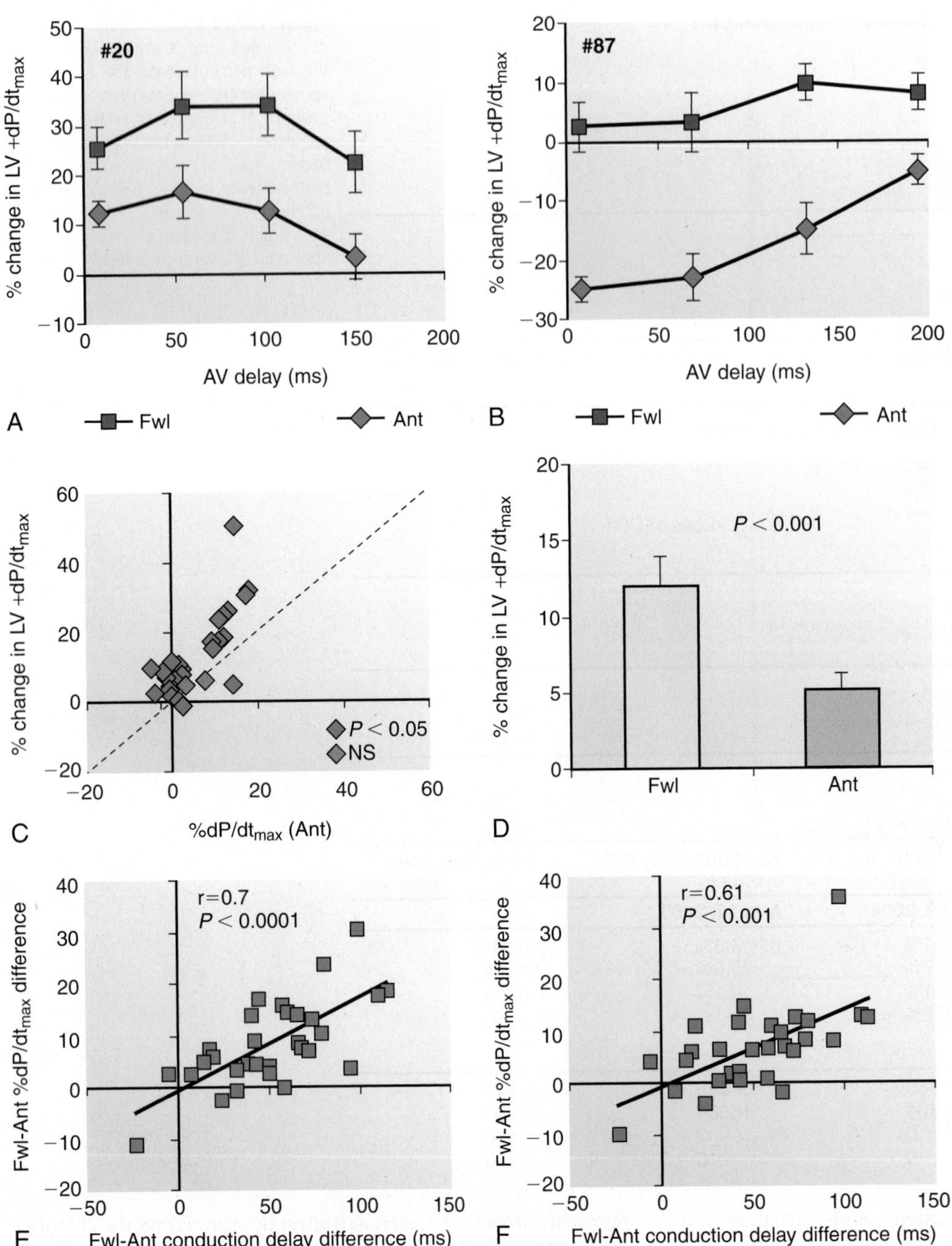

Figure 102-13 Effect of left ventricle (LV) stimulation site on acute hemodynamic response to cardiac resynchronization therapy. **A,** Free wall (Fwl) stimulation in the LV yielded significantly greater increases in LV $+dP/dt_{max}$ than anterior (Ant) stimulation at all atrioventricular (AV) delays. **B,** Fwl stimulation yielded slight increases in LV $+dP/dt_{max}$, whereas Ant stimulation worsened LV $+dP/dt_{max}$. **C,** Points above the line indicate patients with greater increase in LV $+dP/dt_{max}$ during Fwl versus Ant stimulation. **D,** In one third of patients, Ant stimulation worsened acute contractile response, whereas Fwl stimulation improved it. The opposite pattern was never observed. Correlation between Fwl and Ant intrinsic conduction delay differences and LV $+dP/dt_{max}$ response differences during Fwl and Ant stimulation for LV-only **(E)** and biventricular **(F)** pacing. Positive conduction delay differences correspond to greater LV conduction delay. Positive LV $+dP/dt_{max}$ differences correspond to a larger Fwl stimulation response (percentage change from baseline). LV, left ventricular. (Adapted from Butter C, Auricchio A, Stellbrink C, et al, for the Pacing Therapy for Chronic Heart Failure II Study Group: Effect of resynchronization therapy stimulation site on the systolic function of heart failure patients. Circulation 104(25):3026-3029, 2001.)

more likely to occur at long PVARPs, interacts with pseudo-atrial undersensing, results in loss of ventricular pacing, and can result in inappropriate therapies in CRT-D patients due to miscalculation of ventricular rate. Newer cardiac resynchronization therapy systems prevent ventricular double-counting by employing an interventricular ventricular refractory period. Ventricular sensed events (i.e. LV sensing) during the interventricular ventricular refractory period do not restart the PVARP.

Clinical Experience with Cardiac Resynchronization Therapy

CRT pacing is an effective adjunctive treatment for moderately severely symptomatic heart failure associated with DCM and ventricular conduction delay. Randomized, controlled trials involving more than 5000 patients have demonstrated modest, concordant improvements in functional class, exercise tolerance, and quality of life.[24,32,33] Heart failure hospitalizations are reduced by 29% to 52%, heart failure death by 51%, sudden cardiac death by 46%, and total mortality by 40%.[33,34]

Responders and Nonresponders

A cardiac resynchronization therapy responder is generally defined as a patient who feels better, has less heart failure morbidity, and demonstrates evidence of reverse remodeling; a nonresponder exhibits none of these. Approximately 18% to 30% of patients who meet current implant criteria are nonresponders. Techniques for selecting patients with significant ventricular dyssynchrony likely to benefit from cardiac resynchronization therapy are rapidly evolving. The optimal criteria would identify all patients with a high probability of response and reject all

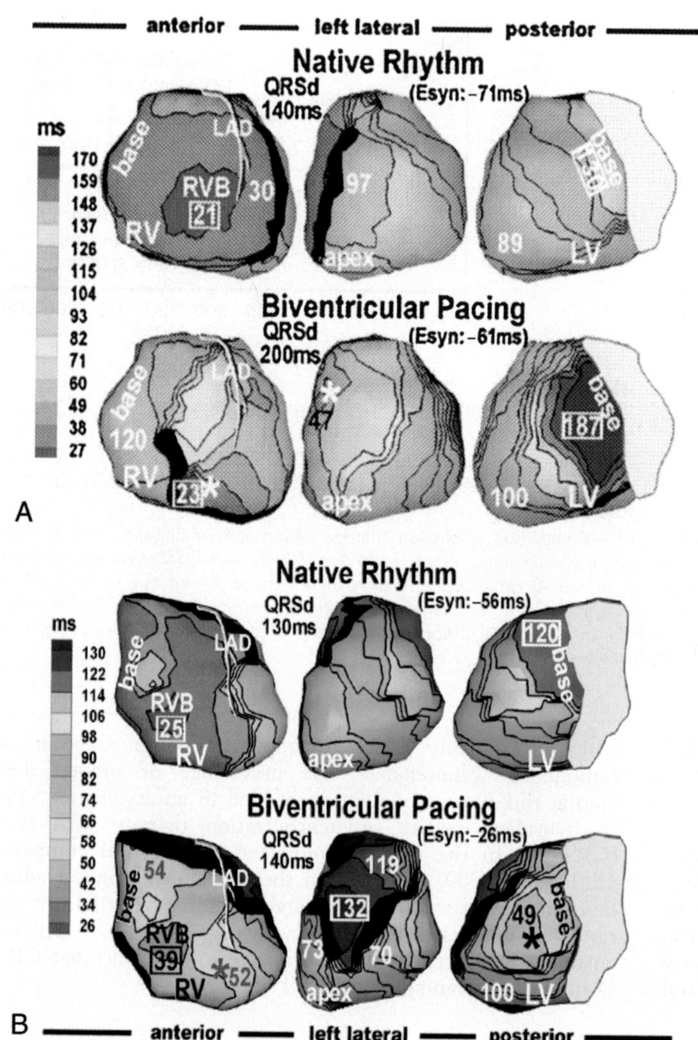

Figure 102-14 A, Worsening of left ventricle (LV) conduction delay by pacing proximal to line of functional block. Epicardial isochrone maps are shown during intrinsic activation *(top row)* and LV pacing *(bottom row)*. Activation times relative to QRS onset are color-coded with *red* earliest and *blue* latest; *framed numbers* indicate earliest and latest activated sites. During intrinsic activation (native rhythm), the right ventricle (RV) is activated earliest, and latest activation occurs at posterobasal LV. *Black line* indicates line or region of conduction block on the anterior LV wall. During biventricular pacing from an anterior wall site *(asterisk)*, LV activation was delayed relative to native activation and took twice as long to reach the posterobasal LV. This region of slow conduction only appeared during the paced beat, indicating dependence on the geometry and direction of the wave front relative to the myocardial structure (functional line of block). B, Negative effect of fixed conduction block despite regional electrical resynchronization. During intrinsic activation (native rhythm) RV is activated earliest, and latest activation occurs at posterobasal LV. During biventricular pacing, LV stimulation *(asterisk)* from a posterobasal site results in electrical synchronization of RV and LV posterobasal regions. However, due to multiple lines of block, latest activation occurred in the anterior LV, global electrical resynchronization was not achieved, and this patient was a nonresponder. Esyn, index of electrical resynchronization where negative values indicate LV activation later than RV activation; LAD, left anterior descending coronary artery; QRSd, QRS duration; RVB, right ventricular body. (Adapted from Jia P, Ramanathan C, Ghanem RN, et al: Electrocardiographic imaging of cardiac resynchronization therapy in heart failure: Observation of variable electrophysiologic responses. Heart Rhythm 3(3):296-310, 2006.)

patients with a low probability of response. The reasons for cardiac resynchronization therapy nonresponse are complex and incompletely characterized, but the likely explanation is interactions between patient-specific substrate and LV stimulation technique.

Nonresponders

Assuming heterogeneous mechanical activation is due to ventricular conduction delay, positive alteration of LV activation that corrects conduction delay should reduce contractile dyssynchrony and improve pump function. Three reasons this may fail are stimulation from the wrong site, unexpected failure to positively alter activation sequence due to ventricular conduction blocks, or new conduction blocks that arise during LV pacing, which can reduce or prevent mechanical resynchronization or induce dyssynchrony.

Stimulation at the latest electrically activated (most delayed) region of the LV is necessary for electrical resynchronization. This is usually on the posterior or posterolateral-basal wall, as demonstrated by endocardial voltage mapping[3,4] and myocardial velocity imaging.[5,35] LV stimulation at posterior or posterolateral-basal sites improves acute contractile response (Fig. 102-13), functional capacity, and possibly mortality compared to anterior sites.[36,37] LV stimulation at anterior sites worsens contractile response in some patients by exaggerating intraventricular dyssynchrony. A posterior or posterolateral basal site was obtained in only 67% to 77% of patients in randomized clnical trials of cardiac resynchronization therapy,[24] and it is likely that inadequate LV stimulation sites contribute significantly to cardiac resynchronization therapy nonresponse.

Functional block that arises only during LV pacing can worsen ventricular conduction delay (Fig. 102-14). Fixed lines of conduction block can result in large regions of delayed myocardium despite electrical resynchronization measured at the pacing sites (see Fig. 102-14). Both situations can contribute to nonresponse.[6]

Ventricular dyssynchrony, independent of QRS duration, has been shown to predict acute and chronic response (including remodeling) to cardiac resynchronization therapy.[15,38] Prolonged QRS duration might not be accompanied by mechanical dyssynchrony.[39,40] In this situation, cardiac resynchronization therapy can induce dyssynchrony and worsen pump function.[10,41]

Though QRS duration correlates poorly with ventricular asynchrony, more-severe baseline conduction delay (QRS >150 ms) is predictive of acute improvement in contractile response short-term improvements in exercise tolerance and quality of life[42] and long-term reductions in mortality and heart failure hospitalization,[25] whereas none of these benefits were consistently observed among patients with less-severe conduction delay (QRS 120-150 ms). Cardiac resynchronization therapy does not benefit patients with ventricular conduction

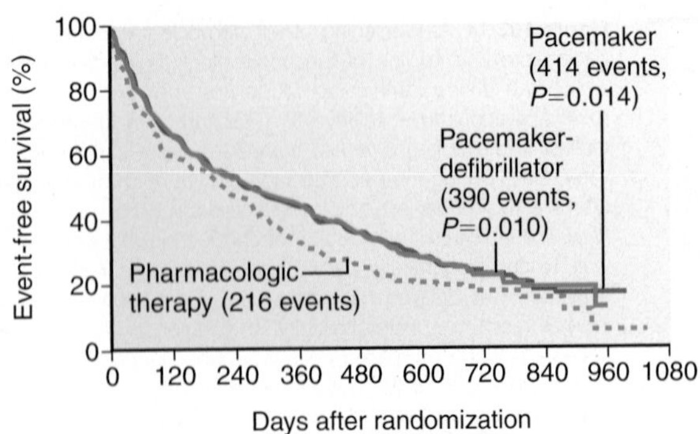

No. at risk

Pharmacologic therapy	308	176	240	72	46	24	16	6	1
Pacemaker	617	384	294	228	146	73	36	14	3
Pacemaker-defibrillator	595	385	283	217	128	61	25	8	0

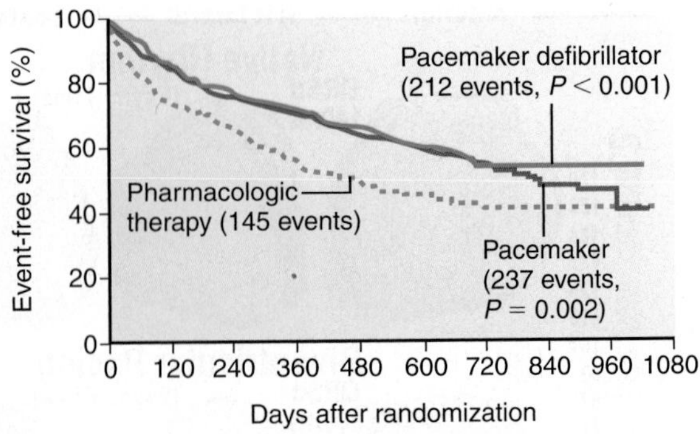

No. at risk

Pharmacologic therapy	308	216	161	118	76	39	28	11	2
Pacemaker	617	498	422	355	258	142	75	35	9
Pacemaker-defibrillator	595	497	411	343	228	131	71	27	5

Figure 102-15 *Left*, Kaplan-Meier estimates of time to death or hospitalization in the Comparison of Medical Therapy, Pacing and Defibrillation in Heart Failure (COMPANION) trial. The 12-month rates of death or hospitalization were 68% in the medical therapy group, 56% in the cardiac resynchronization therapy with pacemaker (CRT-P) group, and 56% in the cardiac resynchronization therapy with defibrillation systems (CRT-D) group. *Right*, Similarly, there were no differences between CRT-P and CRT-D for death from or hospitalization for heart failure. (From Bristow MR, Saxon LA, Boehmer J, et al; the Comparison of Medical Therapy P, and Defibrillation in Heart Failure (COMPANION) Investigators. Cardiac-resynchronization therapy with or without an implantable defibrillator in advanced chronic heart failure. N Engl J Med 350(21):2140-2150, 2004. Copyright © [2004] Massachusetts Medical Society. All rights reserved.)

delay due to right bundle branch block because significant LV asynchrony is generally absent.[25,43]

Role of Defibrillation Support

CRT-pacing (CRTP) unaccompanied by back-up defibrillation reduces sudden death and total mortality by 46% and 40%, respectively,[33,34] effects which exceed the relative mortality benefits of ICDs in overlapping patient populations and which presumably relate to improved pump function and remodeling. Nonetheless, the prevalence of sudden death among this patient population has led to an accelerated effort to hybridize cardiac resynchronization therapy with ICDs (CRT-D). In the single randomized clinical trial comparing CRT-P, CRT-D, and medical therapy, no meaningful advantages in total mortality or hospitalization for heart failure were observed for either type of device (Fig. 102-15).[25] There is currently insufficient clinical evidence to conclude that CRT-D offers an advantage over CRT-P alone.

References

1. Verbeek XA, Vernooy K, Peschar M: Intraventricular resynchronization for optimal left ventricular function during pacing in experimental left bundle branch block. J Am Coll Cardiol 42:558-567, 2003.
2. Vernooy K, Verbeek XA, Cornelussen RN, et al: Calculation of effective VV interval facilitates optimization of AV delay and VV interval in cardiac resynchronization therapy. Heart Rhythm 4(1):75-82, 2006.
3. Rodriguez LM, Timmermans C, Nabar A, et al: Variable patterns of septal activation in patients with left bundle branch block. J Cardiovasc Electrophysiol 14:135-141, 2003.
4. Auricchio A, Fantoni C, Regoli F, et al: Characterization of left ventricular activation in patients with heart failure and left bundle branch block. Circulation 109(9):1133-1139, 2004.
5. Fung JW, Yu CM, Yip G, et al: Variable left ventricular activation pattern in patients with heart failure and left bundle branch block. Heart 90(1):3-4, 2004.
6. Jia P, Ramanathan C, Ghanem RN, et al: Electrocardiographic imaging of cardiac resynchronization therapy in heart failure: Observation of variable electrophysiologic responses. Heart Rhythm 3(3):296-310, 2006.
7. Spragg DD, Leclercq C, Loghmani M, et al: Regional alterations in protein expression in the dyssynchronous failing heart. Circulation 108:929-932, 2003.
8. Kanzaki H, Bazaz R, Schwartzman D, et al: A mechanism for immediate reduction in mitral regurgitation after cardiac resynchronization therapy: Insights from mechanical activation strain mapping. J Am Coll Cardiol 44(8):1619-1625, 2004.
9. de Teresa E, Chamorro JL, Pulpon LA, et al: An even more physiologic pacing. Changing the sequence of activation. In Steinbach K, Glogar D, Laszkovics A, et al (eds): Cardiac Pacing. Proceedings of the VIIth World Symposium on Cardiac Pacing, Darmstadt, Germany, Steinkoopff, 1983, pp 395-400.
10. Wyman BT, Hunter WC, Prinzen FW, et al: Effects of single- and biventricular pacing on temporal and spatial dynamics of ventricular contraction. Am J Physiol 282:H372-H379, 2002.
11. Steendijk P, Tulner SA, Bax JJ, et al: Hemodynamic effects of long-term cardiac resynchronization therapy: Analysis by pressure-volume loops. Circulation 113(10):1295-1304, 2006.
12. Yu CM, Chau E, Sanderson EJ, et al: Tissue Doppler echocardiographic evidence of reverse remodeling and improved synchronicity by simultaneous delaying regional contraction after biventricular pacing therapy in heart failure. Circulation 105:438-445, 2002.
13. Breithardt OA, Sinha AM, Schwammenthal E, et al: Acute effects of cardiac resynchronization therapy on functional mitral regurgitation in advanced systolic heart failure. J Am Coll Cardiol 203:765-770, 2003.
14. St John Sutton MG, Plappert T, Abraham WT, et al; for the MIRACLE Study Group: Effect of cardiac resynchronization therapy on left ventricular size and function in chronic heart failure. Circulation 105(1985-1990), 2003.
15. Bleeker GB, Mollema SA, Holman ER, et al: Left ventricular resynchronization is mandatory for response to cardiac resynchronization therapy: Analysis in patients with echocardiographic evidence of left ventricular dyssynchrony at baseline. Circulation 116(13):1440-1448, 2007.
16. Bax JJ, Bleeker GB, Marwick TH, et al: Left ventricular dyssynchrony predicts response and prognosis after cardiac resynchronization therapy. J Am Coll Cardiol 44(9):1834-1840, 2004.

17. Fantoni C, Raffa S, Regoli F, et al: Cardiac resynchronization therapy improves heart rate profile and heart rate variability of patients with moderate to severe heart failure. J Am Coll Cardiol 46(10):1875-1882, 2005.
18. Sweeney MO: Implantation techniques for cardiac resynchronization therapy. In Yu CM, Hayes DL, Auricchio A (eds): Cardiac Resynchronization Therapy, Malden, MA, Blackwell, 2008, pp 175-210.
19. Daubert CJ, Ritter P, LeBreton H, et al: Permanent left ventricular pacing with transvenous leads inserted into the coronary veins. Pacing Clin Electrophysiol 21:239-345, 1998.
20. Blendea D, Shah RV, Auricchio A, et al: Variability of coronary venous anatomy in patients undergoing cardiac resynchronization therapy: A high-speed rotational venography study. Heart Rhythm 4(9): 1155-1162, 2007.
21. Ho SY, Sanchez-Quintana D, Becker AE: A review of the coronary venous system: A road less traveled. Heart Rhythm 1(1): 107-112, 2004.
22. Knight BP, Desai A, Coman J, et al: Long-term retention of cardiac resynchronization therapy. J Am Coll Cardiol 44:72-77, 2004.
23. Sanchez-Quintana D, Cabrera JA, Climent V, et al: How close are the phrenic nerves to cardiac structures? Implications for cardiac interventionalists. J Cardiovasc Electrophysiol 16:309-313, 2005.
24. Abraham WT, Fisher WG, Smith AL, et al; for the MIRACLE Study Group: Cardiac resynchronization in chronic heart failure. N Eng J Med 346(24):1845-1853, 2002.
25. Bristow MR, Saxon LA, Boehmer J, et al; the Comparison of Medical Therapy Pacing, and Defibrillation in Heart Failure (COMPANION) Investigators: Cardiac-resynchronization therapy with or without an implantable defibrillator in advanced chronic heart failure. N Engl J Med 350(21):2140-2150, 2004.
26. Leon AR, Abraham WT, Curtis AB, et al; for the MIRACLE Study Program: Safety of transvenous cardiac resynchronization system implantation in patients with chronic heart failure: Combined results of over 2,000 patients from a multicenter study program. J Am Coll Cardiol 46(12):2348-2356, 2005.
27. Sweeney MO: Programming and follow-up of CRT and CRTD devices. In Ritter P, Barold SS (eds): Cardiac Resynchronization: Technologic and Clinical Aspects. New York, Springer, 2007, pp 317-423.
28. Sawhney NS, Waggoner AD, Garhwal S, et al: Randomized prospective trial of atrioventricular delay programming for cardiac resynchronization therapy. Heart Rhythm 1:562-567, 2004.
29. Leon AR, Abraham WT, Brozena S, et al; for the InSync III Clinical Study Investigators. Cardiac resynchronization with sequential biventricular pacing for the treatment: of moderate-to-severe heart failure. J Am Coll Cardiol 46(12):2298-2304, 2005.
30. Boriani G, Muller C, Seidl K, et al: Randomized comparison of simultaneous biventricular stimulation versus optimized interventricular delay in cardiac resynchronization therapy: The Resynchronization for the HemodYnamic Treatment for Heart Failure Management II Implantable Cardioverter Defibrillator (RHYTHM II ICD) study. Am Heart J 151(5):1050-1058, 2006.
31. Gasparini M, Auricchio A, Regoli F, et al: Four-year efficacy of cardiac resynchronization therapy on exercise tolerance and disease progression: The importance of performing atrioventricular junction ablation in patients with atrial fibrillation. J Am Coll Cardiol 48(4):734-743, 2006.
32. Auricchio A, Stellbrink C, Sack S, et al; Pacing Therapies in Congestive Heart Failure (PATH-CHF) Study Group: Long-term clinical effect of hemodynamically optimized cardiac resynchronization therapy in patients with heart failure and ventricular conduction delay. J Am Coll Cardiol 39(12):2026-2033, 2002.
33. Cleland JGF, Daubert JC, Erdmann E, et al; The Cardiac Resynchronization—Heart Failure (CARE-HF) Study Investigators: The effect of cardiac resynchronization on morbidity and mortality in heart failure. N Engl J Med 352(15):1539-1549, 2005.
34. Bradley DJ, Bradley EA, Baughman KL, et al: Cardiac resynchronization and death from progressive heart failure: A meta-analysis of randomized controlled trials. JAMA 289:730-740, 2003.
35. Ansalone G, Giannantoni P, Ricci R, et al: Doppler myocardial imaging to evaluate the effectiveness of pacing sites in patients receiving biventricular pacing. J Am Coll Cardiol 39(3):489-499, 2002.
36. Butter C, Auricchio A, Stellbrink C, et al; for the Pacing Therapy for Chronic Heart Failure II Study Group: Effect of resynchronization therapy stimulation site on the systolic function of heart failure patients. Circulation 104(25):3026-3029, 2001.
37. Rossillo A, Verma A, Saad EB, et al: Impact of coronary sinus lead position on biventricular pacing: Mortality and echocardiographic evaluation during long term followup. J Cardiovasc Electrophysiol 15(10):1120-1125, 2004.
38. Yu CM, Gorscan J, Bleeker GB, et al: Usefulness of tissue Doppler velocity and strain dyssynchrony for predicting left ventricular reverse remodeling response after cardiac resynchronization therapy. Am J Cardiol 100(8):1274-1281, 2007.
39. Kerckhoffs RC, Bovendeerd PH, Kotte JC, et al: Homogeneity of cardiac contraction despite physiological asynchrony of depolarization: A model study. Ann Biomed Eng 31:536-547, 2003.
40. Bleeker GB, Schalij MJ, Molhoek SG, et al: Relationship between QRS duration and left ventricular dyssynchrony in patients with end-stage heart failure. J Cardiovasc Electrophysiol 15(5):544-549, 2004.
41. Yu Y, Kramer A, Spinelli J, et al: Biventricular mechanical asynchrony predicts hemodynamic effect of uni- and biventricular pacing. Am J Physiol Heart Circ Physiol 285:H2788-H2796, 2003.
42. Auricchio A, Stellbrink C, Butter C, et al; Pacing Therapies in Congestive Heart Failure II Study Group; Guidant Heart Failure Research Group: Clinical efficacy of cardiac resynchronization therapy using left ventricular pacing in heart failure patients stratified by severity of ventricular conduction delay. J Am Coll Cardiol 42(12):2109-2116, 2003.
43. Byrne MJ, Helm RH, Daya S, et al: Diminished left ventricular dyssynchrony and impact of resynchronization in failing hearts with right versus left bundle branch block. J Am Coll Cardiol 50(15):1484-1490, 2007.
44. Auricchio A, Stellbrink C, Block M, et al: Effect of pacing chamber and atrioventricular delay on acute systolic function of paced patients with congestive heart failure. The Pacing Therapies for Congestive Heart Failure Study Group. The Guidant Congestive Heart Failure Research Group. Circulation 99(23):2993-3001, 1999.
45. Nelson GS, Curry CW, Wyman BT, et al: Predictors of systolic augmentation from left ventricular preexcitation in patients with dilated cardiomyopathy and intraventricular conduction delay. Circulation 101(23):2703-2709, 2000.
46. Kass DA, Chen C, Curry C, et al: Improved left ventricular mechanics from acute VDD pacing in patients with dilated cardiomyopathy and ventricular conduction delay. Circulation 99(12):1567-1573, 1999.
47. Otsuji Y, Gilon D, Jiang L, et al: Restricted diastolic opening of the mitral leaflets in patients with left ventricular dysfunction: Evidence for increased valve tethering. J Am Coll Cardiol 32(2):398-404, 1998.
48. Kanzaki H, Bazaz R, Schwartzman D, et al: A mechanism for immediate reduction in mitral regurgitation after cardiac resynchronization therapy: Insights from mechanical activation strain mapping. J Am Coll Cardiol 44(8):1619-1625, 2004.

Newer Applications of Pacemakers 103

Robert W. Peters and Michael R. Gold

CHAPTER OUTLINE

Since the earliest experience with permanent pacemakers, significant changes have occurred in this technology. From primitive, asynchronous, fixed-rate single-chamber devices (VOO mode) used initially, pacemakers have undergone a major transformation in sophistication and complexity. Originally, permanent pacemakers were used primarily to provide rate support for symptomatic bradycardia. With technologic advances and improved understanding, permanent pacemakers have been suggested for a variety of additional disorders. Many of these applications are not directly related to treatment of bradycardia, but rather they use pacing to alter myocardial activation patterns, suppress tachyarrhythmias, or improve hemodynamic function. This chapter focuses on newer applications for permanent pacing.

Pacing to Improve Hemodynamics (Heart Failure)

We are in the midst of an epidemic of congestive heart failure (CHF) in the United States, with more than 550,000 new cases annually. Despite major advances in the medical therapy, mortality rates remain high. The use of cardiac transplantation has been limited by the scarcity of donor hearts. Left ventricular assist devices, although promising, are expensive, and their efficacy and applicability remains to be demonstrated. It has long been appreciated that single-chamber pacing from the right ventricular apex is suboptimal, especially in persons with impaired intraventricular conduction, and in some patients it has been associated with hemodynamic compromise (pacemaker syndrome) and heart failure exacerbation. Accordingly, there has been interest in evaluating alternative pacing techniques, especially in patients with diminished left ventricular function.

Atrioventricular Synchrony

It is estimated that a properly timed atrial contraction provides between 15% and 30% of the cardiac output in healthy persons. Although somewhat controversial, the atrial contribution may be particularly important in patients with heart failure, especially when there is any element of diastolic dysfunction. Loss of appropriate atrioventricular (AV) synchrony can have a number of adverse consequences.[1]

Accordingly, it has been suggested that manipulation of AV conduction (by reprogramming the AV delay) might provide hemodynamic benefit for patients with heart failure. Early uncontrolled studies reported benefit from dual-chamber pacing with a short AV delay, presumably by eliminating diastolic mitral regurgitation. However, these findings were not confirmed by subsequent randomized trials.[1] In fact, the results of the Dual Chamber and VVI Implantable Defibrillator (DAVID) study indicate that right ventricular apical pacing should be avoided when possible.[2] In this study, subjects undergoing implantable cardioverter defibrillator (ICD) implantation who had left ventricular systolic dysfunction and intact sinus and AV node function were randomized to DDDR pacing or backup VVI pacing. Because they had no standard pacing indication, the VVI cohort served as a control with minimal pacing. The primary endpoint of time to death or hospitalization for CHF was reached significantly earlier in the DDDR arm.

Similarly, Nahlawi and associates examined the effects of right ventricular pacing in patients with permanent pacemakers and normal left ventricular function.[3] Patients were randomized to either AAI (or, in one case, to DDD pacing with a very long AV delay, to avoid right ventricular stimulation) or standard DDD (right ventricular) pacing, using a crossover design. With standard DDD pacing, left ventricular ejection fraction decreased significantly in the first 24 hours and continued to worsen over the ensuing week. Interestingly, left ventricular function improved only gradually following cessation of right ventricular stimulation and, at 32 hours, had still not normalized. In contrast, no decrease in ejection fraction was observed with AAI pacing.

Currently, there is little enthusiasm for the general use of short AV delay pacing for hemodynamic reasons alone in patients with systolic dysfunction. In fact, based on the DAVID results, as well as other post hoc analyses, it is recommended to use programming features of pacemakers or ICDs such as AV search hysteresis, long AV delays, or AAI mode that minimize ventricular pacing. The Intrinsic RV Study Inhibition of Unnecessary RV Pacing with AVSH in ICD (Intrinsic RV) study[4] and DAVID II both showed that the deleterious effects of RV pacing can be negated with either advanced algorithms to prolong AV delay or with AAI mode, respectively. This strategy is consistent with pacemaker programming advocated in patients without left ventricular systolic dysfunction or conduction delays. In this latter group, right ventricular pacing, when compared with no or minimal pacing, is associated with worse hemodynamic function and an increased risk of developing heart failure.[1,5]

Sweeney and coworkers described an innovative pacing algorithm (managed ventricular pacing) to limit right ventricular stimulation in patients with intact AV conduction.[6,7] Using this algorithm, pacing is set in the AAIR mode while the ventricular rhythm is monitored. When ventricular asystole is sensed, a ventricularly paced backup beat is provided. With sustained loss of AV conduction (two or more P waves without accompanying QRS complexes), the pacing mode switches to DDDR for 1 minute, after which AV conduction is assessed by analyzing a single cycle. If AV conduction is still not detected, DDDR pacing is carried out for 2 minutes, then 4 minutes, then 8 minutes, and so on between assessments. Once AV conduction resumes, the mode automatically switches back to AAIR. In the event of atrial fibrillation, the device switches to DDIR. This new pacing technique is well tolerated and drastically reduces the incidence of right ventricular stimulation. However, concern has been raised that dramatic prolongation of AV delays to reduce RV pacing to less than 10% may be deleterious.

Right Ventricular Stimulation Site

Permanent pacing was initially performed from the right ventricular apex because of easy accessibility and a low incidence of lead dislodgement. There are a number of reasons that the right ventricular apex is undesirable, among them paradoxical septal motion and interference with the mitral apparatus. The development of more maneuverable catheters and passive and active fixation leads provided the option of permanent pacing from alternative right ventricular sites.[1] However, none of these methods has proved successful, and it has become increasingly clear that in general, right ventricular pacing should be avoided in the setting of left ventricular dysfunction because it increases the risk for new or worsening heart failure. In this regard, prolonging the AV delay to minimize right ventricular pacing, while still providing rate support, is preferable to shortening the AV delay to mimic AV node physiology.

Biventricular Pacing (Cardiac Resynchronization Therapy)

It is estimated that intraventricular conduction defects occur in up to 50% of patients with advanced CHF. These defects can lead to ventricular dyssynchrony, causing further hemodynamic embarrassment. Although not all patients with conduction defects demonstrate dyssynchrony, in general, the problem tends to increase with the severity of the conduction defect. In fact, mortality rates in CHF have been shown to correlate with QRS width.[1] It should also be noted that ventricular dyssynchrony can be present even without QRS widening.[1] Ventricular pacing (cardiac resynchronization therapy [CRT]) has been proposed as a means of coordinating left and right ventricular contraction, thereby improving ventricular performance. Animal studies and acute studies in patients with CHF have confirmed this hypothesis.[1]

With this background, several large clinical trials were initiated to assess the long-term effects of CRT (Table 103-1). Using a randomized single-blind crossover design, Cazeau and the Multisite Stimulation in Cardiomyopathy (MUSTIC) investigators found that CRT improved exercise tolerance and quality of life and decreased the number of hospital admissions in 67 patients with New York Heart Association (NYHA) class III heart failure and QRS duration greater than 150 ms.[8,9] Similarly, the Pacing Therapies for Congestive Heart Failure (PATH-CHF) investigators reported that CRT improved exercise capacity and functional status.[10] Subsequently, Abraham and colleagues[11] in the Multicenter INSYNCH Randomized Clinical Evaluation (MIRACLE) trial, CRT resulted in improved exercise tolerance and quality of life and a reduction in heart failure–related hospital admissions. QRS duration was shortened and there was a corresponding increase in mean ejection fraction and a decrease in end-diastolic dimension.

Many patients with CHF have standard indications for ICD therapy. Moreover, the risk of sudden death is high in the heart-failure population. Accordingly, combined ICD and CRT devices (ICD-D) were developed to address these problems, and randomized, controlled studies of these devices have confirmed the benefit of CRT, particularly in patients with NYHA class III or IV symptoms. The Comparison of Medical Therapy, Pacing and Defibrillation in Heart Failure (COMPANION) study showed that CRT (either pacing alone or in combination with an ICD) significantly reduced the composite endpoint of all-cause mortality or hospitalization in their study population.[12] A secondary analysis showed reduction in mortality rates with CRT-D devices compared with optimal medical therapy, and there was a strong but nonsignficant trend for decreased mortality with CRT-P devices.

There have been several more recent trials evaluating the use of CRT in the heart failure population. MIRACLE-ICD, using a study design similar to MIRACLE, assessed the value of adding an ICD to biventricular pacing.[13] The magnitude of improvement was similar to that seen in the original MIRACLE study. Interestingly, they found that biventricular antitachycardia pacing was more effective in terminating ventricular tachycardia than right ventricular stimulation. In MIRACLE-ICD II, it was found that quality of life and treadmill exercise duration improved with CRT.[14]

In RD-CHF (recently decompensated congestive heart failure) (upgrading from RV pacing in previously paced patients with severe heart failure and LV systolic dysfunction), patients with class III or IV heart failure and marked interventricular conduction defects were assigned to 3-month periods of CRT or right ventricular stimulation using a randomized crossover design.[14] They found that NYHA functional class, exercise capacity, and quality of life improved with CRT.

In CARE-HF (Cardiac Resynchronization in Heart Failure), CRT (without an ICD) was compared with standard medical therapy in a cohort of patients with class III or IV heart failure and systolic dysfunction.[15] CRT was associated with a significant reduction in cardiovascular morbidity and mortality as well as an improvement in various echocardiographic parameters and quality of life. CARE-HF showed that biventricular pacing without ICD backup decreased mortality in patients with advanced heart failure, QRS prolongation, and systolic dysfunction. In contrast, RETHINQ (Resynchronization Therapy in Patients with Narrow QRS) showed no benefit of CRT among patients with advanced heart failure, echocardiographic evidence of dyssynchrony without QRS prolongation.[14] Thus it appears that electrical dyssynchrony as measured electrocardiographically is necessary for a positive response to this therapy.

In summary, it is now generally accepted that CRT improves functional status and can prolong life in some patients with advanced heart failure, especially those with intraventricular conduction defects of LBBB type. The technique continues to evolve, and many of the difficulties plaguing earlier trials, such as availability of left ventricular access, have been corrected. Improvements in lead technology and delivery systems have decreased implantation

Table 103-1 Long-Term Randomized Clinical Trials of Cardiac Resynchronization Therapy for Congestive Heart Failure

Study	Population	Results
CARE-HF	NYHA III/IV, QRS >120 msec (with dyssynchrony if <150 msec)	Decreased mortality and cardiovascular hospitalizations
COMPANION	Class III-IV heart failure, EF ≤35%, QRS >120 msec	Mortality or hospitalization decreased with CRT
MIRACLE	Class III-IV heart failure, EF < 35%, QRS ≥130 msec	QOL, exercise tolerance, EF, and rehospitalization rate improved with CRT pacing
MIRACLE-ICD	LVEF <35%, LVEDD >55 mm, NYHA III/IV, QRS >130 msec, ICD indication	QOL improved
MIRACLE-ICD II	LVEF <35%, LVEDD >55 mm, NYHA II/III, QRS >130 msec, ICD indication	QOL improved
MUSTIC	Class III heart failure and IVCD	QOL and exercise tolerance improved with CRT
PATH-CHF	Class III-IV heart failure due to systolic dysfunction and IVCD	CRT associated with long-term improvement in exercise tolerance LV free wall stimulation was better than anterior wall Degree of baseline echocardiographic asynchrony predicted outcome
RETHINQ	NYHA III/IV, EF<35%, QRS <130 msec with dyssynchrony	No change in hospitalization, QOL, or LV dimensions
REVERSE	NYHA I/II, QRS >120 msec, EF <40%	Decreased heart failure hospitalizations and LV dimensions

CARE-HF, Cardiac Resynchronization in Heart Failure; COMPANION, Comparison of Medical Therapy, Pacing and Defibrillation in Heart Failure; CRT, cardiac resynchronization therapy; EF, ejection fraction; IVCD, intraventricular conduction defect; LV, left ventricular; LVEDD, left ventricular end diastolic diameter; MIRACLE, Multicenter INSYNCH Randomized Clinical Evaluation; MUSTIC, Multisite Stimulation in Cardiomyopathy; NYHA, New York Heart Association; PATH-CHF, Pacing Therapies for Congestive Heart Failure; QOL, quality of life.; RETHINQ, Resynchronization Therapy in Patients with Narrow QRS; REVERSE, Resynchronization Reverses Remodeling in Systolic Left Ventricular Dysfunction.

times and increased success. Currently, we estimate that 60% to 70% of patients benefit from CRT. Ongoing and future trials will hopefully help to identify additional subgroups that might benefit from CRT. For instance, patients with mild heart failure are being evaluated in the REVERSE (Resynchronization Reverses Remodeling in Systolic Left Ventricular Dysfunction) and MADIT-CRT (Multicenter Automatic Defibrillator Implantation Trial—Cardiac Resynchronization Therapy) trials.[16,17] It is unlikely that patients with narrow QRS will benefit from CRT because mechanical dyssynchrony in this cohort is not accompanied by conduction disturbances that can be ameliorated by pacing. Thus it was recently demonstrated that improvement in patients with CHF and chronic atrial fibrillation is comparable to that of persons with normal sinus rhythm.[18] Other approaches being evaluated include the use of echocardiographic and other imaging quantification of left ventricular dyssynchrony.[19,20] Unfortunately, preliminary results from PROSPECT suggested limited utility of echocardiographic techniques to predict clinical response.[21]

It is also anticipated that further refinements in CRT will assist in providing information about optimal AV delay,[22] use of atrial pacing versus intrinsic AV conduction, the most effective site for left ventricular stimulation, and so on,[23] as well as eliminating the problem of atrial oversensing causing inappropriate shocks. As with any relatively new technology, there is also potential for adverse effects. Biventricular pacing can alter the pattern of transmural activation, producing potentially arrhythmogenic dispersion of refractoriness.[24] Several small clinical studies have reported evidence of an arrhythmogenic response to biventricular stimulation. However, larger randomized studies have shown no increased incidence of shocks or sudden death with CRT.[1]

Among clinical trials currently under way or in planning stages are two studies comparing biventricular pacing with left ventricular stimulation, B-LEFT (Biventricular vs. Left Univentricular Pacing In Heart Failure Patients)[14] and BELIEVE (Biventricular Versus LV Pacing).[25] Studies using echocardiographic techniques to assess ventricular dyssynchrony include DESIRE (DESynchronization as Indication for Resynchronization).[14] Trials Investigating the effects of CRT in mild heart failure include BLOCK-HF (Biventricular Versus RV Pacing in Heart Failure Patients with AV Block),[14] REVERSE,[26] MADIT-CRT,[27] and BIOPACE (Biventricular pacing for AV block to prevent cardiac desynchronization).[14] These last four trials are noteworthy because they include patients with class I and class II heart failure. In fact, the only requirement for BIOPACE is a standard indication for pacing.

Atrial Fibrillation

Atrial fibrillation is the most common sustained arrhythmia encountered in clinical medicine, affecting more than 2 million people in the United States alone. Its frequency increases with age; it afflicts more than 4% of people 60 years or older. Although well tolerated by some, atrial fibrillation is associated with an increased risk for stroke, heart failure, hospitalization, and death.[1]

In patients with persistent or chronic atrial fibrillation, permanent pacemakers have traditionally been used to treat patients with slow ventricular rates. There is also evidence that permanent pacing might prevent atrial fibrillation in this population. Several large randomized clinical trials conclusively demonstrated that permanent pacing, especially dual-chamber pacing, reduces atrial fibrillation in patients with sinus node dysfunction.[1] The benefit appears largest in patients with atrial pacing alone compared with dual-chamber pacing.

Use of pacing to prevent atrial fibrillation in persons without sinus node dysfunction is less well established. It has been suggested that permanent pacing at a rate faster than the sinus rate might help to prevent atrial fibrillation by a variety of mechanisms,[1] among them suppression of atrial ectopic activity and a decrease in the dispersion in atrial refractoriness, especially after an atrial premature beat. A variety of algorithms ensure continuous atrial pacing. One approach has been the use of dynamic atrial overdrive pacing in which the atria are paced at slightly faster rates than the spontaneous sinus rate. This algorithm has been shown to reduce the number of days that patients experience symptomatic atrial fibrillation. In ADOPT (Atrial Dynamic Overdrive Pacing Trial), patients with recurrent atrial fibrillation and sinus node dysfunction were randomized to dynamic overdrive pacing or standard DDDR pacing with a base rate of 60 beats per minute.[26] They found a 25% decrease in symptomatic atrial fibrillation burden in patients in the dynamic overdrive pacing group. Additional issues to be resolved include the effect of pacing on atrial fibrillation recurrence, mortality, and incidence of CHF and thromboembolic events. Other overdrive algorithms have failed to replicate these results,[27] suggesting that the benefit of such pacing is likely limited. It is also clear that there are multiple mechanisms for triggering atrial fibrillation.[28] Pacemakers with a suite of algorithms for arrhythmia suppression have been evaluated. Preliminary results from SAFARI (Study for Atrial Fibrillation Reduction)[29] suggest a modest reduction in arrhythmia burden.

Another approach has been to pace the atrium at alternative sites. Diseased atria are often riddled with scar, interfering with impulse transmission. Pacing from the interatrial septum, the coronary sinus os, or Bachmann bundle allows simultaneous right and left atrial activation, narrowing the P wave, and might result in a lower incidence of atrial fibrillation.[30,31]

Dual-site atrial pacing provides another, perhaps more effective way of resynchronizing atrial contraction. Dual-site pacing is usually accomplished by pacing simultaneously from the right atrial appendage and coronary sinus. Preliminary results have been encouraging,[1] although problems involving insertion of two atrial leads, double-sensing of intrinsic sinus beats, and other problems remain. Subsequent large randomized clinical studies suggest that only a minority of patients benefit from this approach. One group for whom this technique may be especially applicable is patients with recent coronary artery bypass surgery, in whom the incidence of atrial fibrillation approaches 40%.[1] Leads placed directly in the left atrium may be used perioperatively, and this technique may be more effective than pacing from the ostium of the coronary sinus. Early results have been encouraging, although the longevity of epicardial leads is known to be limited.[1,32]

Because of the adverse hemodynamic effects of right ventricular pacing cited earlier, it has been hypothesized that patients with permanent pacemakers in the right ventricle may be predisposed to atrial fibrillation. Sweeney and associates, analyzing data from the MOde Selection Trial (MOST), found that the incidence of atrial fibrillation increased linearly with increasing frequency of right ventricular pacing.[33] The SAVE PACe (Search AV Extension and Managed Ventricular Pacing for Promoting Atrioventricular Conduction) trial demonstrated that managed ventricular pacing (discussed earlier) decreased the incidence of atrial fibrillation by 40% compared with DDDR pacing.[34]

It has also been predicted that the improved hemodynamics associated with biventricular pacing would lead to less atrial fibrillation. Yannopoulos and colleagues reported a decreased susceptibility to atrial tachyarrhythmias in 28 consecutive heart failure patients undergoing an upgrade from standard right ventricular stimulation to CRT.[35,36] However, the data from large randomized trials have failed to confirm this benefit of CRT (CARE-HF).[1]

Hypertrophic Cardiomyopathy

Hypertrophic cardiomyopathy is a condition characterized by disarray of myocardial fibers and myofibrils, producing excessive and inappropriate hypertrophy of the left ventricle, most often of the interventricular septum. The hypertrophy interferes with ventricular relaxation and, in up to 25% of patients, causes dynamic obstruction across the left ventricular outflow tract. Uncontrolled studies of permanent pacing have suggested regression of ventricular hypertrophy and dramatic clinical improvement.[1] However, this benefit has not been substantiated in subsequent randomized, controlled clinical trials,[1] and the technique has been largely abandoned, except when there is another indication for pacing.

Neurocardiogenic Syncope

Neurocardiogenic syncope is a common problem that accounts for approximately 6% of hospital admissions in the United States annually. Despite improved diagnostic techniques, the cause of syncope is undiagnosed in up to 50% of cases. It is likely that many of these are neurally mediated. The term *neurocardiogenic syncope* (also termed *vasovagal syncope* or *neurally mediated syncope*) is used to describe a group of related conditions that include carotid sinus hypersensitivity, post-tussive syncope, postmicturition syncope, and others. Because episodes are often accompanied by bradycardia, it has been suggested that permanent pacing may be of benefit. Unfortunately, as with hypertrophic cardiomyopathy, early uncontrolled studies suggested that permanent pacing offered major clinical benefits that have not been confirmed by subsequent randomized clinical trials.[1,37] Currently there is little clinical indication for permanent pacing in neurocardiogenic syncope.

Long-QT Syndrome

The long-QT syndrome is a heterogeneous group of disorders characterized by QT prolongation and a tendency to develop torsades de pointes and sudden cardiac death. Congenital forms of this disorder have been linked to point mutations in specific genes. Acquired forms of the long QT syndrome are usually associated with use of QT-prolonging medications (e.g., sotalol, tricyclic antidepressants), the list of which continues to grow. It is also possible that the congenital and acquired forms are actually a continuum, with some persons manifesting the abnormality in the baseline state and others requiring trigger factors to elicit QT prolongation. The pathogenesis of ventricular arrhythmias in this syndrome has not been completely elucidated but seems related to sympathetic activation and early afterdepolarizations.

Initial therapy of the long-QT disorders has traditionally been pharmacologic (β-blockers), although left stellate ganglion ablation and permanent pacing have also been advocated. The exact mechanism by which pacing exerts its beneficial effect is unclear but probably relates to preventing pauses that characteristically precede episodes of torsades de pointes, with elimination of early afterdepolarizations and decrease in dispersion of refractoriness. In addition, overdrive pacing to increase heart rate decreases the QT interval. Currently, it is standard to use an ICD in any patient with documented cardiac arrest, sustained ventricular tachycardia, or recurrent syncope refractory to β-blockers and to reserve pacing for symptomatic bradycardia.

Preventing Remodeling after Myocardial Infarction

Following myocardial infarction, there is a redistribution of cardiac workload with an increase in mechanical wall stress in the ischemic and surrounding areas. These increases in wall stress are associated with left ventricular remodeling and subsequent dysfunction, activation of cytokines, and neurohormonal factors often associated with adverse clinical outcome. It has been shown that pacing areas of high wall stress (electrical preexcitation) alters regional distribution of stroke work within the normal heart, reducing stroke work adjacent to the stimulation site and increasing stroke work in distant regions. Recently, Shuros and coworkers used a swine model to demonstrate that pacing from the peri-infarct area improves hemodynamics and attenuates cardiac remodeling.[38] Similar beneficial effects were found by Chung and colleagues among patients randomized to biventricular pacing (compared with right ventricular stimulation).[39] These observations will hopefully be confirmed by future large randomized clinical trials and lead to reduction of adverse remodeling early after myocardial infarction.

Permanent Pacing for Chronic Disorders of the Neuromuscular System

Chronic disorders of the neuromuscular system are a diverse group of chronic degenerative conditions primarily affecting skeletal muscle. It has long been appreciated that these disorders can also affect cardiac muscle, which is not surprising because of the similarities between skeletal and cardiac muscle, but there is a growing awareness that the prevalence of arrhythmias and sudden cardiac death might warrant early intervention.[40] Because these conditions are uncommon, the therapeutic guidelines are necessarily nonspecific.

In general, it can be recommended that unexplained syncope, presyncope, and other transient neurologic symptoms should be aggressively investigated using ambulatory electrocardiographic recordings, long-term event recorders and loop recorders, and, in more worrisome situations (e.g., unexplained sudden syncope precipitating a motor vehicle accident), hospitalization with inpatient monitoring. In most cases, the finding of second-degree atrioventricular block, even when asymptomatic, might warrant permanent pacemaker implantation. It should be kept in mind that ventricular tachycarrhythnias are also common in this population so, depending upon the clinical scenario, an ICD with permanent pacing capability should also be considered.

Duchenne muscular dystrophy is a progressive neuromuscular disease becoming clinically manifest in the mid-teens and usually fatal by the end of the third decade, generally from heart failure. Although cardiac involvement is the rule, the conduction system is not always involved. Permanent pacing is warranted for second- or third-degree AV block, especially in the setting of a widened QRS complex.

Becker muscular dystrophy is similar to Duchenne muscular dystrophy but more slowly progressive and with less-common cardiac involvement. The indications for permanent pacing appear similar to those for Duchenne muscular dystrophy.

In myotonic muscular dystrophy, cardiac involvement is common and usually affects the conduction system. Recent data indicate that permanent pacing is warranted with a His-ventricle interval greater than 70 ms, even in the absence of high-degree AV block.[41]

In Emery-Dreyfuss muscular dystrophy, conduction system disease is the rule. Sudden cardiac death due to high-grade AV block has been documented, and permanent pacing should be offered with the development of any unexplained transient neurologic symptoms or second- or third-degree AV block.

Limb Girdle muscular dystrophy is a heterogeneous group of disorders characterized by weakness in the pelvic musculature and upper legs. The familial form has a high incidence of conduction-system disease, and permanent pacing should be considered in anyone with a family history of heart block or sudden death.

Kearns-Sayre syndrome is a multisystem disorder of the mitochondria, with diverse clinical manifestations. Progressive conduction system disease is the rule, and permanent pacing is probably warranted for marked first-degree AV block.

Permanent Pacing for Infiltrative Diseases of the Myocardium

These are a diverse variety of disorders in which the myocardium is infiltrated and replaced by nonmyocardial tissue. Although the prognosis is usually determined more by the type and severity of the underlying disease, cardiac and conduction system involvement is not unusual and may be accompanied by potentially life-threatening brady- and tachycarrhythmias. In these situations, permanent pacemakers may be helpful symptomatically, although they might not necessarily prolong life.

Amyloidosis is characterized by deposition of an insoluble protein within the myocardium, often involving the conduction system.[42] A restrictive cardiomyopathy can develop, with death from congestive heart failure. Sinus node dysfunction and AV block are not uncommon and might require permanent pacemaker insertion if associated with symptoms.

Sarcoidosis is an infiltrative disorder characterized by noncaseating granulomas that often involve the heart and the conduction system.[43] The disease tends to be progressive, and the prognosis of a patient with extensive myocardial sarcoid is guarded. Permanent pacemakers may be implanted for symptomatic bradyarrhythmias, although the frequency of malignant ventricular tacharrhythmias often warrants an implantable cardioverter defibrillator.

In collagen vascular diseases, cardiac involvement is fairly common, especially polymyositis and systemic lupus erythematosus. Fibrosis of the conduction system can occur and the resulting AV block can require a permanent pacemaker.

Solid tumors (especially carcinoma of the breast and lung, and sarcomas) and leukemias and lymphomas can affect the heart and infiltrate the conduction system. A permanent pacemaker may be required for symptomatic bradycardia, although the prognosis is usually closely related to the extent of the underlying malignancy.

Conclusions

As techniques continue to evolve, the indications for permanent pacing will undoubtedly change. This chapter has described some newer uses of permanent pacing that are designed to improve hemodynamics or prevent arrhythmias, or both.

In particular, the technique of biventricular pacing continues to evolve, and the success of this technique has grown accordingly. Another exciting area is the concept of local stimulation adjacent to the site of acute myocardial infarction as a means of preventing ventricular remodeling. It is possible that when pacing is used in conjunction with other recently developed technologies, such as ICDs, continuous infusion pumps for pharmacologic agents, ablation techniques, and others, the role of permanent pacing will assume greater applicability and the number of potential uses might continue to expand.

References

1. Gold MR, Peters RW: Newer applications of pacemakers. In Zipes DP, Jalife J (eds): Cardiac Electrophysiology: From Cell to Bedside. Philadelphia, Saunders, 2004, pp 1011-1017.
2. The DAVID Trial Investigators: Dual-chamber pacing or ventricular backup pacing in patients with an implantable defibrillator: The Dual Chamber and VVI Implantable Defibrillator (DAVID) Trial. JAMA 288:3115-3123, 2002.
3. Nahlawi M, Waligora M, Spies SM, et al: Left ventricular function during and after right ventricular pacing. J Am Coll Cardiol 44:1883-1888, 2004.
4. Olshansky B, Day JD, Gering L, et al: Is dual-chamber programming inferior to single-chamber programming in an implantable cardioverter-defibrillator? Results of the INTRINSIC (inhibition of unnecessary RV pacing with AVSH in ICD's study. Circulation 115:9-16, 2007.
5. Sweeney M, Hellkamp A, Greenspon A, et al: Baseline QRS duration > 120 milliseconds and cumulative percent time ventricular paced predicts increased risk of heart failure, stroke, and death in DDDR-paced patients with sick sinus syndrome in MOST [abstract]. Pacing Clin Electrophysiol 25:690, 2002.
6. Sweeney MO, Ellenbogen KA, Casavant D, et al: Multicenter, prospective, randomized safety and efficacy study of a new atrial-based managed ventricular pacing mode (MVP) in dual chamber ICD's. J Cardiovasc Electrophysiol 16:1-7, 2005.
7. Sweeney MO, Shea JB, Fox V, et al: Randomized pilot study of a new atrial-based minimal ventricular pacing mode in dual-chamber implantable cardioverter-defibrillators. Heart Rhythm 1:160-167, 2004.
8. Cazeau S, Leclercq C, Lavergne T, et al: Effects of multisite biventricular pacing in patients with heart failure and intraventricular conduction delay. N Engl J Med 344:873-880, 2001.
9. Linde C, Leclercq C, Rex S, et al: Long-term benefits of biventricular pacing in congestive heart failure: Results from the Multisite Stimulation in Cardiomyopathy study. J Am Coll Cardiol 40:111-118, 2002.
10. Auricchio A, Stellbrink C, Sack S, et al: Long-term clinical effect of hemodynamically optimized cardiac resynchronization therapy in patients with heart failure and ventricular conduction delay. J Am Coll Cardiol 39:2026-2033, 2002.
11. Abraham WT, Fisher WG, Smith AL, et al: Cardiac resynchronization in chronic heart failure. N Engl J Med 346:1845-1853, 2002.
12. Bristow MR, Saxon LA, Boehmer J, et al; Comparison of Medical Therapy, Pacing, and Defibrillation in Heart Failure (COMPANION) investigators: Cardiac-resynchronization therapy with or without an implantable defibrillator in advanced chronic heart failure. N Engl J Med 350:2140-2150, 2004.
13. Young JB, Abraham WT, Smith AL, et al: Combined cardiac resynchronization and implantable cardioversion defibrillation in advanced chronic heart failure: the MIRACLE ICD Trial. JAMA 289:2685-2694, 2003.
14. Hayes DL, Abraham WT: Clinical trials—an overview. In Yu C-M, Hayes DL, Auricchio A (eds): Cardiac Resynchronization Therapy. Malden, MA, Blackwell, 2006, pp 239-256.
15. Cleleand JG, Daubert JC, Erdmann E, et al, for the CARE-HF Investigators: The effect of cardiac resynchronization on morbidity and mortality in heart failure. N Engl J Med 352:1539-1549, 2005.
16. Linde C, Gold M, Abraham WT, et al: Rationale and design of a randomized controlled clinical study to assess if cardiac resynchronization therapy can slow disease progression in mild to moderate heart failure: The Resynchronization reVerses Remodeling in aSymptomatic left vEntricular dysfunction (REVERSE) study. Am Heart J 151:288-294, 2006.
17. Moss AJ, Brown MW, Cannom DS, et al: Multicenter automatic defibrillator implantation trial—cardiac resynchronization therapy (MADIT-CRT): design and clinical protocol. Ann Noninvasive Electrocardiol 10(4 Suppl):34-43, 2005.
18. Leon AR, Greenberg JM, Kanuru N, et al: Cardiac resynchronization in patients with congestive heart failure and chronic atrial fibrillation. J Am Coll Cardiol 39:1258-1263, 2002.
19. Gorcsan J, Tanabe M, Bleeker GB, et al: Combined longitudinal and radial dyssynchrony predicts ventricular response after resynchronization therapy. J Am Coll Cardiol 50:1476-1483, 2007.
20. Yu C-M, Gorcsan J, Bleeker GB, et al: Usefulness of tissue Doppler velocity and strain dyssynchrony for predicting left ventricular reverse remodeling response after cardiac resynchronization therapy. Am J Cardiol 100:1263-1270, 2007.
21. Yu CM, Abraham WT, Bax J, et al: Predictors of response to cardiac resynchronization therapy (PROSPECT): Study design. Am Heart J 149:600-605, 2005.
22. Vidal B, Sitges M, Marigiano A, et al: Optimizing the programmation of cardiac resynchronization therapy devices in patients with heart failure and left bundle branch block. Am J Cardiol 100:1002-1006, 2007.
23. Stein KM: Left ventricular lead placement for cardiac resynchronization therapy: What you see is what you get. Heart Rhythm 4:1163-1164, 2007.
24. Roelke M: Atrial oversensing in biventricular devices: Shocked? (or inhibited?). Pacing Clin Electrophysiol 25:1411-1412, 2002.
25. Gasparini M, Bocchiardo M, Lunati M, et al: Comparison of 1-year effects of left ventricular and biventricular pacing in patients with heart failure who have ventricular arrhythmias and left bundle branch block: The Bi vs Left Ventricular Pacing: An International Pilot Evaluation on Heart Failure Patients with Ventricular arrhythmias (BELIEVE) multicenter prospective randomized pilot study. Am Heart J 152:155-157, 2006.
26. Carlson MA, Ip J, Messenger J, et al: A new treatment algorithm for the treatment of atrial fibrillation: Results of the Atrial Dynamic Overdrive Pacing Trial (ADOPT). J Am Coll Cardiol 42:627-633, 2003.
27. Padeletti L, Purerfellner H, Adler SW, et al, for the Worldwide ASPECT Investigators: Combined efficacy of atrial septal lead placement and atrial pacing algorithms for prevention of paroxysmal atrial tachycardia. J Cardiovasc Electrophysiol 14:1189-1195, 2003.
28. Hoffmann E, Sulke E, Edvardsson N, et al: New Insights into the initiation of atrial fibrillation. A detailed intraindividual and interindividual analysis of the spontaneous onset of atrial fibrillation using new diagnostic pacemaker features. Circulation 113:1933-1941, 2006.
29. Gold MR, Hoffman E: Rationale and design of a randomized clinical trial to assess the role of overdrive and triggered pacing therapies. Am Heart J 152:231-236, 2006.
30. Bailin SJ, Adler S, Giudici M, et al: Prevention of chronic atrial fibrillation by pacing in the region of Bachmann's bundle: Results of a multicenter randomized trial. J Cardiovasc Electrophysiol 12:912-917, 2001.
31. Padeletti L, Pieragnoli P, Ciapetti C, et al: Randomized crossover comparison of right atrial appendage pacing versus interatrial septum pacing for prevention of atrial fibrillation in patients with sinus bradycardia. Am Heart J 142:1047-1055, 2001.
32. Crystal E, Connolly SJ, Sleik K, et al: Interventions of prevention of postoperative atrial fibrillation in patients undergoing heart surgery: A meta-analysis. Circulation 106:75-80, 2002.
33. Sweeney MO, Hellcamp AS, Ellenbogen KA, et al: Adverse effect of ventricular pacing on heart failure and atrial fibrillation among patients with normal baseline QRS duration in a clinical trial of pacemaker therapy for sinus node dysfunction. Circulation 107:2932-2937, 2003.

34. Sweeney MO, Bank AJ, Nsah E, et al: Minimizing ventricular pacing to reduce atrial fibrillation in sinus-node disease. N Engl J Med 357:1000-1008, 2007.
35. Yannopoulos D, Lurie KG, Sakaguchi S, et al: Reduced atrial tachyarrhythmia susceptibility after upgrade of conventional implanted pulse generator to cardiac resynchronization therapy in patients with heart failure. J Am Coll Cardiol 50:1246-1251, 2007.
36. Leon AR. The class-I-cardiac resynchronization effect? 50:1252-1253, 2007.
37. Connolly SJ, Sheldon R, Thorpe KE, et al: Pacemaker therapy for prevention of syncope in patients with recurrent severe vasovagal syncope: Second vasovagal pacemaker study (VPS II): A randomized trial. JAMA 289:2224-2229, 2003.
38. Shuros AC, Salo RW, Florea VG, et al: Ventricular preexcitation modulates strain and attenuates cardiac remodeling in a swine model of myocardial infarction. Circulation 116:1-8, 2007.
39. Chung ES, Menon SG, Weiss R, et al. Feasibility of biventricular pacing in patients with recent myocardial infarction: impact on ventricular remodeling. Congestive Heart Fail 13:9-15, 2007.
40. Finsterer J, Stollberger C: The heart in human dystrophinopathies. Cardiology 99:1-19, 2003.
41. Lazarus A, Varin J, Babuty D, et al: Long-term follow-up of arrhythmias in patients with myotonic dystrophy treated by pacing: A multicenter diagnostic pacemaker study. J Am Coll Cardiol 40:1645-1652, 2002.
42. Shah KB, Inoue Y, Mahra MR: Amyloidosis and the heart. Arch Intern Med 166:1805-1813, 2006.
43. Doughan AR, Williams BR: Cardiac sarcoidosis. Heart 92:282-288, 2006.

Lesion-Forming Technologies for Catheter Ablation 104

DAVID CESARIO, NOEL G. BOYLE, AND KALYANAM SHIVKUMAR

CHAPTER OUTLINE

The ability to deliver energy into myocardial tissue in order to cause permanent lesions, thus preventing impulse generation or propagation of arrhythmias, has greatly advanced the field of clinical cardiac electrophysiology. The general goal of lesion-forming technologies is to create myocardial lesions that are effective, can be created in a reasonable time frame, and result in minimal or no collateral damage. The purpose of this chapter is to highlight the biophysical principles of lesion formation, review currently available lesion-forming technologies, and place evolving technologies for lesion formation in perspective.

Evolution of Technology

The original catheter-based energy delivered to cardiac tissue was direct current (DC) shocks. Though now mostly of historical interest, DC shocks were successfully applied from an electrode catheter percutaneously positioned adjacent to the His bundle to ablate the atrioventricular (AV) node.[1] High-energy DC shocks were delivered to the catheter from an external defibrillator to destroy cardiac tissue.[2] However, this procedure suffered from limited efficacy and collateral damage, resulting in unacceptably high in-hospital mortality rates approaching 6%.[3] It became clear that if catheter-based ablation was to advance as a therapeutic technique, safer forms of energy would need to be applied to create ablative lesions.

Biophysical Aspects of Lesion Formation

Energy sources for ablation are shown in Table 104-1. Factors in radiofrequency treatment are shown in Box 104-1.

The research reported in this chapter is supported by the American Heart Association (Grant #0430287N) and National Heart, Lung, and Blood Institute grant R01HL084261 (Dr. Shivkumar).

The Electromagnetic Spectrum

Several different wavelengths from the electromagnetic spectrum have been successfully used for ablation of cardiac arrhythmias (Fig. 104-1). Typically, electromagnetic energy is delivered via a catheter until tissue temperature increases for an adequate duration to achieve irreversible damage (see Table 104-1, Box 104-1).[4]

Radiofrequency (RF) energy was one of the first alternatives to DC shocks used for catheter ablation, has been extensively studied, has undergone only minor changes since its introduction, and is now in wide-spread clinical use.[5,6] The RF spectrum spans the range from 3 Hz to 300 GHz, with a frequency of 300 to 1000 kHz typically employed for clinical RF ablation. RF generators typically deliver unmodulated sine-wave alternating current (AC) at frequencies between 500 and 1000 kHz,[7] which are too high to depolarize the myocardium.

RF current is typically delivered in a unipolar fashion from the ablation catheter tip to a large dispersive grounding patch on the patient's skin (typically over the liver or on the thigh). The passage of AC from the ablation catheter through tissues to the grounding patch results in resistive tissue heating and lesion formation at the catheter tip. The surface area of the ablation catheter tip is relatively small compared to the dispersive patch, thus limiting resistive heating to the immediate catheter tip–tissue interface and a small rim of surrounding tissue (~1 mm). Deeper ablative lesions can be created, but they result from conductive heating of the surrounding tissues due to the virtual electrode of resistive heating. Significant tissue heating during RF delivery is associated with minor impedance drops, typically from 5 to 10 Ω.[8]

Heat Transfer to Tissue

In *resistive heating*, RF energy passes through a tissue and is dissipated as heat, usually in a unipolar mode from the tip of the catheter electrode to a grounding electrode pad usually placed over the back. The energy generated is given by the power equation:

$$W = VI = (IR)I = I^2R \quad [1]$$

where V is voltage, I is current, R is resistance, and $V = IR$ by Ohm's law.

The current disperses radially from the electrode tip, and the current density falls off with the inverse square of the distance from the catheter tip. This is specified by the current density equation for a spherical electrode:

$$Q = 1/4\pi r^2\ (Amp/cm^2) \quad [2]$$

The power or heat generated, per unit volume of tissue, will then decrease with the inverse fourth power of the distance from the catheter tip:

$$H \sim \rho/16\pi r^4 \quad [3]$$

Table 104-1 Comparison of Energy Sources for Catheter Ablation

Source	Mechanism of Injury	Catheter-based	Contact
RF	Resistive heating	Yes	Critical
Cryo	Direct cell injury	Yes	Critical
HIFU	Mechanical/heating	Yes	Not critical
Laser	Photonic heating	Yes	Not critical
Microwave	Dielectric heating	Yes	Not critical

cryo, cryotherapy; HIFU, high-intensity focused ultrasound; RF, radiofrequency.

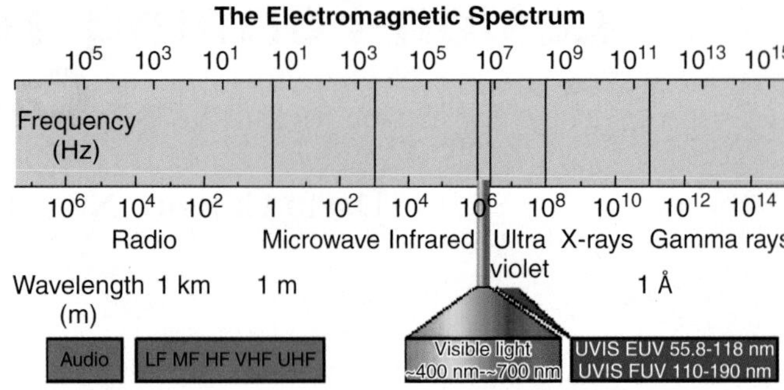

Figure 104-1 The electromagnetic spectrum as displayed in this figure is a continuum of electromagnetic waves arranged according to frequency (usually measured in Hertz) and wavelength (usually measured in meters). In catheter ablation, electromagnetic energy is delivered to the myocardium, via transvenous catheters, to create thermal lesions. Various energy sources have been used for catheter ablation of cardiac arrhythmias. Radiofrequency (RF) energy is currently the most commonly used energy source in catheter ablation of cardiac arrhythmias. Microwave energy has been investigated as another potential energy source for creating myocardial lesions. EUV, extreme ultraviolet; FUV, far ultraviolet; HF, high frequency; LF, low frequency; MF, mid frequency; UHF, ultrahigh frequency; UVIS, ultraviolet imaging spectrum; VHF, very high frequency.

where ρ = tissue resistance, r = the distance from the center of the electrode, and $I^2\rho$ = power/cm^3. Thus lesions created by RF energy are typically small and well circumscribed.[9]

As the current density decreases with the fourth power of the distance *(r)* from the electrode tip, only the 1- to 2-mm rim of tissue near the catheter tip is heated directly; the deeper tissues are heated by passive conduction. Hence, resistive heating only occurs for this small distance, with the remainder of the heating occurring via *conductive heating* from this area to the rest of the tissue. Experimental studies have shown that for tissue destruction to occur, the tissue temperature must rise above 50° C. The radius of the 50° C isotherm line in the tissue, which essentially represents the lesion boundary, increases in direct proportion to the temperature of the source. This was predicted theoretically and demonstrated experimentally by Haines.[10]

Although the tissue temperature cannot usually be monitored directly, impedance measurements have been shown to provide a usable method to estimate tissue temperature response during RF catheter ablation.[11] During the ablation procedure, the power output of the RF generator is adjusted either manually or automatically to achieve a temperature of 55° C to 70° C at the electrode tissue interface. If the temperature at the electrode tissue interface exceeds 100° C, then a coagulum or char is formed on the catheter tip, which can prevent current delivery, and it is no longer effective for ablation (see Box 104-1).

In a typical 7 F catheter (2.2 mm in diameter) with a 4-mm ablation electrode tip, the resulting lesion is 5 to 6 mm in diameter and 2 to 3 mm deep. Larger-electrode or saline-irrigated catheters result in bigger lesions. Cooling of the electrode tip allows increased power delivery, resulting in increased depth of restive heating and lesion diameter. In addition, saline irrigation results in a lower electrode-tissue interface temperature, which prevents an impedance rise and results in deeper and larger lesions. Nakagawa has found a higher temperature at up to 3.5 mm deep in the tissue when compared to the tissue interface, suggesting that direct resistive heating occurred deeper in the tissue, rather than conduction of heat from the surface.[12]

Box 104-1 Radiofrequency Treatment Factors

FACTORS AFFECTING LESION FORMATION WITH RADIOFREQUENCY

Tissue contact
Temperature
Power
Cooling: blood flow, cooled tip
Duration of energy delivery

FACTORS ASSOCIATED WITH COAGULUM ('CHAR') FORMATION WITH RADIOFREQUENCY

Poor tissue contact
High temperature
Low power

Dielectric heating occurs when the electric field produces oscillation of the water molecule dipoles in the tissue, resulting in heat generation. This occurs when microwave energies (30-3000 MHz range) are used; 915 MHz or 2450 MHz are the commercially available generators. The amount of energy absorbed in a tissue depends on the dielectric permittivity of the tissue, which varies with the water content of the tissue. The depth of penetration is also highly dependant on the water content, being up to four times greater in fat than in blood and muscle. Hence the microwave energy can propagate through tissue with low water content, such as fat, to deliver energy. As with RF energy, a conductive heating effect is also produced; however, unlike RF energy, tissue contact and a dispersive electrode are not required. Energy deposition falls of as the inverse square of the distance with microwave wavelengths compared to the inverse fourth power of the distance with RF. Hence, microwave-induced dielectric heating can penetrate to deeper distances than RF.[4]

Thermal injury, via the transfer of electrical energy to thermal energy, is the proposed major mechanism behind tissue damage during RF ablation.[10] However, additional tissue injury can result from direct effects of oscillating electromotive force on the sarcolemmal membrane of cardiac myocytes, particularly in the border zone of ablative lesions. The application of electromotive force to the cell membrane during RF delivery can cause dielectric breakdown and cellular depolarization and can result in an electrical component that contributes to myocardial tissue injury.

Myocardial tissue is irreversibly damaged at temperatures 50° C and greater.[7] Lesion depth increases proportionally to the catheter tip–tissue interface temperature, until about 100° C, at which point plasma boils, resulting in coagulum formation at the catheter tip and potentially leading to clot embolization, a sudden impedance increase, loss of thermal conductivity, and ineffective tissue heating. To avoid such excessive tissue heating, thermocouples and thermistors were added to the catheter tip to allow temperature monitoring. Subsequent RF generators have allowed titration of delivered power up or down until a chosen catheter tip temperature is reached. This is known as *temperature guided- RF ablation*.[6] Current RF generators can deliver RF in either temperature-guided or power-guided modes.

One major limitation of standard RF energy is the complex relationship between the resistive heating of tissue adjacent to the RF catheter tip during RF delivery and convective cooling caused by local blood flow. This complex interplay can result in reported RF temperature generator values underestimating local tissue temperatures.[13] In certain situations, excessive tissue heating can result in steam production, ultimately leading to an explosive steam pop, crater formation in the adjacent tissue, and even cardiac perforation.

Electrode cooling allows more effective levels of RF power to be maintained, even in areas of low blood flow (Fig. 104-2), and was initially accomplished with the development of 8- to 10-mm tip catheters. The greater surface area on 8- and 10-mm catheter tips increases convective cooling without changing blood flow. The second approach to cool the electrode tip was to infuse saline, thus allowing greater power delivery, shifting the point of maximal heating into the tissue itself, and ultimately producing deeper lesions.[13,14]

There are two basic types of irrigated catheters: closed-loop irrigation catheters, which continuously circulate saline within the electrode tip to internally cool the catheter, and open irrigation catheters, which have multiple irrigation holes through which saline is continuously flushed, providing both internal and external cooling. Yokoyama and colleagues found that open irrigated catheters resulted in greater interface cooling, lower interface temperatures, and a lower incidence of thrombus formation and steam pops than closed loop irrigated catheters.[15]

Limitations of Catheter-Based Radiofrequency Ablation

One of the problems with RF as an energy source for myocardial lesion formation continues to be interpretation of true tissue temperature. Even with relatively short applications of RF energy, tissue temperature can continue to rise after the termination of RF delivery, potentially resulting in lesion growth and collateral damage.[16] Despite the advantages of cooled-tip ablation, catheter tip and tissue temperatures can remain markedly discrepant, potentially resulting in excessive thermal injury.[17]

With the advent of percutaneous epicardial ablations, problems have arisen with the delivery of RF energy to the epicardium. Standard RF catheters often reach high temperatures quickly and thus do not deliver adequate power during RF applications. Open-loop irrigated catheters can cause excess fluid buildup in the closed pericardial space and have difficulty delivering power when pericardial access has been surgically obtained through a pericardial window and the chest is open. We have found that closed-irrigated tips often offer the best solution to epicardial RF delivery, especially in patients with open chests. Another consistent problem with standard RF catheters is the inability to form contiguous lesions and gaps in lesion lines can be proarrhythmic (Fig. 104-3).[18]

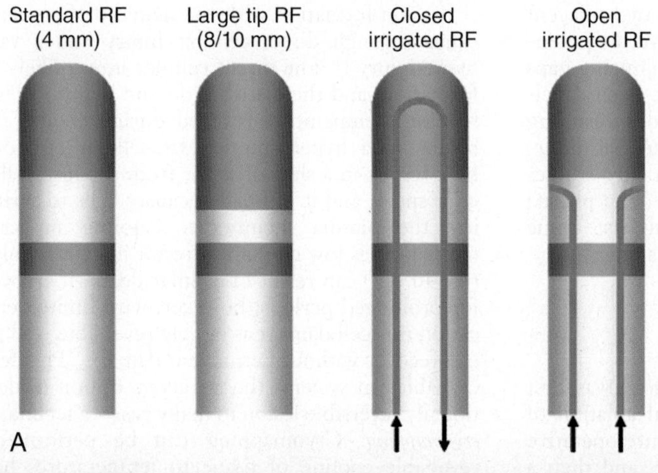

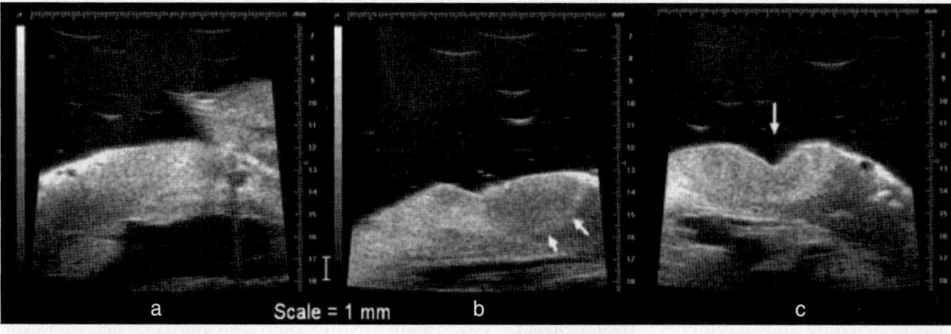

Figure 104-2 **A,** Currently available radiofrequency (RF) ablation catheter designs. Lesion depth has increased with increases in the size of the catheter tip and the development of methods for cooling the ablation electrode (irrigation). **B,** Lesion formation during RF delivery on the epicardial (*arrow*) surface of a Langendorff-perfused rabbit heart. This heart was imaged using a 30-MHz ultrasound system (VisualSonic). (Courtesy Aman Mahajan, MD, PhD, University of California at Los Angeles.)

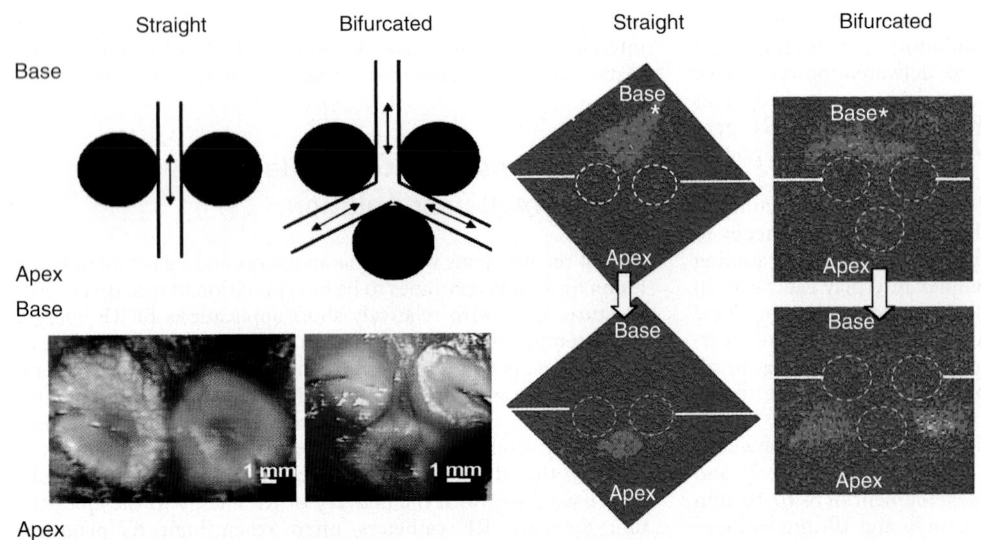

Figure 104-3 Optical mapping images of conduction through straight and bifurcated gap preparations. Radiofrequency (RF) lesions are denoted by *broken circular lines; solid straight lines* indicate the positions of incisions from the tissue edges to the RF lesions. The *top panels* demonstrate that the orange wave fronts of depolarization have propagated from the pacing sites (denoted with *asterisks*) to the openings of the gaps in RF lesions. The *lower panels* demonstrate that the orange wave fronts have emerged through both the straight and bifurcated gaps after 4 and 8 ms, respectively. Note that the bifurcated gap has resulted in the formation of two wave fronts from the two arms of the bifurcated gap. (Reproduced with permission from Scheinman MM, Morady F, Hess DS, Gonzalez R: Catheter-induced ablation of the atrioventricular junction to control refractory supraventricular arrhythmias. JAMA 248[7]:851-855, 1982.)

New Developments in Radiofrequency Ablation

Newer catheters have been designed to attempt to address some of the special obstacles encountered during RF ablation. Long linear catheters with multiple electrodes, which can ablate sequentially or simultaneously, have been developed to create more continuous linear lesions. Additionally, bipolar RF catheters have been designed to deliver current between two adjacent electrodes in a bipolar fashion.[19] Such catheters have the potential to produce longer and deeper lesions, thus minimizing gaps between lesions. Finally, phased RF catheters have been developed to deliver unipolar RF via alternating electrodes, resulting in out-of-phase sine waves of AC, producing a potential difference between electrodes similar to bipolar RF.[19] In vitro studies comparing multielectrode unipolar RF, bipolar RF, and phased RF revealed that phased RF resulted in the highest tissue temperatures and the most uniform and deepest lesions.[19]

Cryoablation

The application of cryothermal energy (cryoablation) was first described by Klein and colleagues for the surgical ablation of accessory pathways.[20] These early surgeries used intraoperative mapping to localize the arrhythmogenic substrate, and then a cryoprobe refrigerated to −60° C was applied to this site. This form of cryoablation proved to be safe and effective; however, it was time consuming and required highly invasive surgical procedures to treat arrhythmias.

Percutaneous cryoablation systems with a steerable ablation catheter and a dedicated ablation console are now available. Cryoablation catheters are capable of reaching temperatures colder than −70° C at their tip. Catheter-tip cooling is achieved by delivering a liquid refrigerant, typically nitrous oxide, under pressure, to the catheter tip. Nitrous oxide, or other refrigerant, is delivered through a hollow injection tube that runs through the entire length of the ablation catheter into a sudden luminal widening at the catheter tip. Nitrous oxide expands and decompresses within a small chamber at the catheter tip, resulting in cooling based on the Joule-Thompson effect.[21] Ultimately, a liquid-to-gas phase interface is created within the catheter tip, resulting in heat extraction from the local tissue in contact with the distal electrode. Gas is continuously removed, via vacuum, through a second coaxial lumen inside the catheter. Similar to RF catheters, cryoablation catheters have the ability to constantly monitor tip temperature on the ablation console, and in turn the nitrous oxide flow can be adjusted to obtain a preset temperature.

Lesion formation with the delivery of cryoenergy appears to occur through direct cellular injury and a vascular-mediated tissue injury.[22] The direct cellular injury likely results from ice formation, and the distribution and depth of lesions are related to tissue temperature reached during cooling.[23] Ice formation results in a hyperosmotic extracellular environment. This in turn results in a shift of water from the intracellular to extracellular space, and it ultimately causes cells to shrink, thus damaging the plasma membrane. Cooling myocardial tissue to temperatures low enough to result in extracellular ice formation (<−40° C) can result in cellular death, if cryoenergy is applied for prolonged periods; however, with limited cryoenergy application this cell damage is largely reversible, and cellular function can recover without permanent damage. This feature allows the cryoablation systems the attractive option of delivering a functionally reversible lesion in many cases, a technique referred to as *cryomapping*. Cryomapping can be performed by moderate reversible cooling of tissue to temperatures between −28° C and −32° C. For successful ablations, tissue-tip interface temperature is typically maintained at −80° C. Cooling tissue to −40° C or less results in ice formation in both the intracellular and extracellular spaces and ultimately leads to irreversible damage to the plasma membrane as well as internal organelles. Such lesions result in localized cell death and can lead to the propagation of intracellular ice between cells via intracellular channels, potentially resulting in lesion growth.

Cryoablation also results in lesion formation via vascular mediated tissue injury. Initially, the application of cryothermal energy results in vasoconstriction and decreased blood flow. As the tissue freezes, circulation eventually ceases throughout the frozen areas. This likely results in tissue damage via ischemic necrosis; however, tissue damage via ischemic necrosis cannot be easily distinguished from damage produced by intracellular ice formation. As the frozen tissue rewarms, there is a subsequent hyperemic response with increased vascular permeability and edema. Furthermore, endothelial damage can result in platelet aggregation and microthrombus formation.

In percutaneous catheter-based cryoablation systems, the coldest area is located adjacent to the catheter tip, and thus the effects of energy delivery are observed earliest at these sites. Areas located more remote from the catheter tip or at the periphery of the cryolesion are less cooled. Due to limited cooling in these outer areas, reversible tissue damage is more likely to occur, and thus effects noted late during the application of cryoenergy are likely to revert upon rewarming. In general, ablation success is correlated with early functional modification, especially if it is noted within the first 30 seconds of cryoenergy application.[23]

Cryoenergy has been used in several different forms to produce myocardial lesion formation. Surgical atrial fibrillation ablation uses the selective application of cryoenergy to isolate the pulmonary veins.[24] In this procedure, a sternotomy is performed to allow application of a T-shaped cryoprobe to the epicardial surface of the left atrium, around the pulmonary veins. This is often done in combination with endocardial cryoablation through a right-sided left atriotomy to completely isolate the left superior pulmonary vein. The use of more extensive cryoablation in combination with radiofrequency ablation, to create a lesion set similar to the Cox-Maze II procedure, has also been described with excellent results, approaching 90% maintenance of sinus rhythm at 9 months of follow-up.[25] The surgical application of cryoenergy in the treatment of cardiac arrhythmias continues to evolve. Milla and colleagues recently described the use of an argon-based cryoclamp and linear probe to epicardially isolate the pulmonary veins and left atrial appendage in the beating dog heart.[26]

The endocardial application of cryothermal energy has also been used in the treatment of several different arrhythmias via a percutaneous transvenous catheter–based approach. One of the first arrhythmias where cryoenergy was used for percutaneous catheter ablation was atrioventricular node reentrant tachycardia (AVNRT), due to concerns over inadvertent complete AV block and the potential to create cryomaps of possible ablation sites before creating permanent irreversible tissue damage. Zrenner and colleagues described a comparable acute success of 97% in patients whose arrhythmias were ablated using cryoenergy as compared to 98% in patients treated with standard RF; however, these investigators did see a higher recurrence rate in patients undergoing cryoablation (8%) as apposed to RF ablation (1%).[27] Gupta and colleagues reported both a higher primary failure rate and greater recurrence rate in patients undergoing cryoablation for AVNRT as compared with RF ablation.[28] The potential benefits of cryoablation must be weighed against the possibility that this energy source may be associated with higher recurrence and lower acute success rates. It is clear that further multicenter trials are needed to compare the short-term success rates and long-term recurrence rates for cryoablation versus RF ablation in the treatment of AVNRT.

Another potential area where cryoablation offers great promise is in the ablation of accessory pathways either located in a paraseptal location near the native conduction system or in an anatomic location, such as within the coronary sinus, where the application of RF energy could lead to unwanted collateral damage. Collins and colleagues reported an acute procedural success rate of 71% for patients with accessory pathways located within the coronary sinus, who underwent cryoablation; however, they ultimately noted a 40% recurrence rate in these patients.[29]

Cryoablation has also been used in the treatment of atrial flutter. The Cryoablation versus Radiofrequency Ablation in the Treatment of Atrial Flutter Trial (CRAAFT) randomized patients with typical atrial flutter to undergo RF ablation with an 8-mm tip RF catheter or cryoablation using an 8-mm tip cryocatheter.[30] These investigators reported a longer procedural time but improved patient tolerability in patients undergoing cryoablation as compared with RF.

Cryoablation has been investigated in the treatment of paroxysmal atrial fibrillation. In one study, complete pulmonary vein isolation was achieved in 41 of 45 veins ablated using cryothermal energy delivered via novel 7 F circular catheters, guided by circular mapping catheters, in 18 patients.[31] Further, several authors have reported using a balloon catheter to deliver cryoenergy to the pulmonary vein ostia in animal models.[32,33] Cryoablation has been successfully used inside the pulmonary veins to achieve bidirectional conduction block in patients where conduction block was not achieved after RF energy was applied around the antrum or ostia of the pulmonary veins.[34] It is clear that cryoenergy has many potential applications in the treatment of cardiac arrhythmias; however, further trials are needed to confirm whether this energy form has acute and chronic efficacy rates similar to RF ablation.

High-Intensity Focused Ultrasound

High-intensity focused ultrasound (HIFU) is a newer lesion-forming technology that has the potential to create thermal ablation lesions in subsurface regions without affecting intervening tissues and blood vessels. One of the advantages of ultrasound energy is that it can be precisely focused in a targeted tissue region to induce molecular vibration and friction, resulting in absorptive heating and ultimately necrosis of the targeted region by thermal coagulation.[35,36] Several other currently used techniques for thermal ablation, such as argon cryotherapy or interstitial laser therapy, cool or heat tissues primarily by thermal conduction and create a graded response depending on the distance from the thermal source. This mechanism for lesion formation is relatively slow, and it is thus susceptible to cooling from the nearby blood vessels. HIFU has an advantage over these techniques because it focuses ultrasonic acoustic energy into the targeted tissue by a remote transducer, allowing rapid heat ablation of the targeted tissue without damaging the intervening tissue.[35,36]

HIFU damages myocardial tissue primarily by two mechanisms.[37] Coagulative necrosis by thermal absorption is the primary mechanism for ablating tissue with focused ultrasound. Increases in tissue temperature (up to ~55-60° C) are achieved by controlling the ultrasound acoustic power and wavelength. Tissue-temperature increases are assumed to be linearly proportional to the delivered acoustic energy. The second mechanism is by cavitation-induced damage (thermal or mechanical). Cavitation-induced damage incurs much greater tissue destruction and, in the past, was generally avoided due to variable intensity values, unpredictable lesion sizes, and the potential for unwanted collateral damage. Currently, however, the idea of exploiting cavitation for the purpose of enhancing the depth of ablative lesions and reducing required exposure times is being investigated.[38,39]

The technology of focusing ultrasound into tissue to induce temperatures high enough to cause permanent tissue damage is relatively simple. The primary objective of HIFU delivery systems is to deliver frequencies that are high enough to allow significant energy absorption at the point of focus, yet not high enough to cause appreciable energy loss in the intervening tissue. HIFU is generated by a spherically curved transducer operating at frequencies approximately between 1 and 10 MHz, with most cardiac ablation procedures performed around 5 to 8 MHz.[40-42] Currently, intracardiac catheter–based technology incorporating balloons to focus the ultrasound beams is used in delivering HIFU for cardiac ablations.[40,41] Unfortunately, tissue heterogeneities can alter the intended focal point of HIFU, resulting in actual targeted tissue temperature rises that are difficult to predict. The intensity achieved at the targeted tissue varies with the procedure (range of 7-20 W/cm^2) and is usually sustained for 30 to 120 seconds.

HIFU was initially applied from outside the body to ablate tissue in internal organs. The use of HIFU on myocardial tissues was initially described in ablation of the atrioventricular (AV) junction in dogs.[43] In this study, a 7.0- MHz diagnostic ultrasound probe was affixed to a spherically focused 1.4-MHz HIFU transducer, and maximum ultrasound intensity was delivered to the AV junction during electrical diastole for a total of 30 seconds. Complete AV block was achieved in all of the dogs with an average of 6.5 30-second applications of HIFU. Histopathologic examination of these hearts revealed well-demarcated areas of necrosis and early inflammation in the areas of HIFU delivery.[43]

In another canine study, HIFU delivery to open-chest beating hearts without direct tissue contact resulted in focal myocardial lesions from 2 to 6 mm in length, depending on HIFU dose used.[44] Additionally, HIFU can be delivered via a balloon catheter designed to isolate pulmonary veins in the treatment of atrial fibrillation (Fig. 104-4). In one human study, delivery of forward-focused HIFU, from a balloon catheter located outside the pulmonary vein ostia, resulted in resolution of atrial fibrillation in 59% of patients, after a single ablation procedure, at 12 months of follow-up.[45] It was felt that new energy sources such as cryoablation and HIFU might enhance the safety and efficacy of pulmonary vein isolation. Unfortunately several major complications have been observed with HIFU delivery in the treatment of atrial fibrillation including permanent phrenic nerve palsy and formation of fatal atrioesophageal fistula.[46]

HIFU is an exciting energy source with many potential uses in the field of cardiac electrophysiology. However, further studies are needed to confirm the long-term efficacy and safety of HIFU in creating myocardial lesions.

Other Energy Sources and Approaches for Lesion Formation

Other energy sources such as lasers, microwave irradiation, and beta irradiation have been proposed for lesion formation.[47] Additionally, experimental catheters currently in the development stage will allow the electrophysiologist to image using phased-array intracardiac echocardiography and ablate through the same catheter (Fig. 104-5). Biological approaches, such as the injection of autologous fibroblasts, have also been suggested as an approach for the creation of lesions.[48] Gene-based approaches that target delivery of genes to a scar border have been successfully used for molecular ablation of ventricular tachycardia.[49]

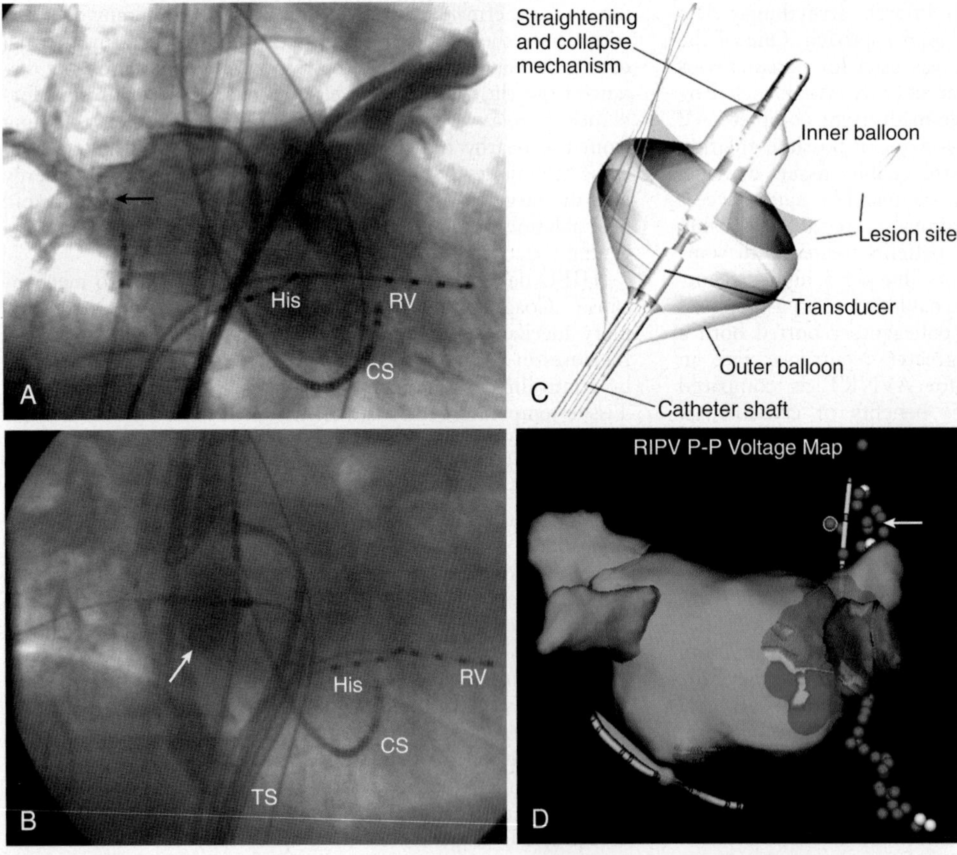

Figure 104-4 Balloon-based high-intensity focused ultrasound (HIFU) delivery panels. **A,** Left atrial and pulmonary vein angiography (*arrow* shows right inferior pulmonary vein [RIPV]). **B,** HIFU balloon engaging the RIPV. **C,** A schematic of the HIFU balloon, demonstrating its working components. **D,** A voltage map following HIFU delivery showing attenuation of voltage. *Gray* indicates voltage <0.1 mV, *purple* indicates voltage >1.5 mV). The *arrow* shows markers that represent the location of the right phrenic nerve delineated by pace mapping. CS, coronary sinus catheter; His, His bundle catheter; RV, right ventricular catheter; TS, transseptal sheath.

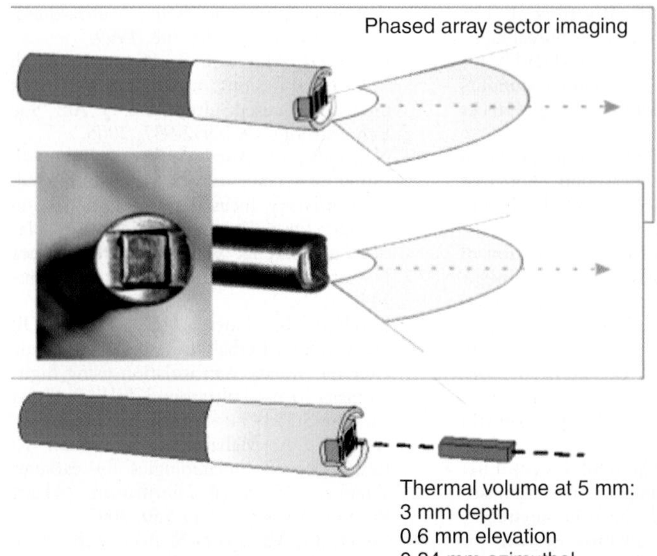

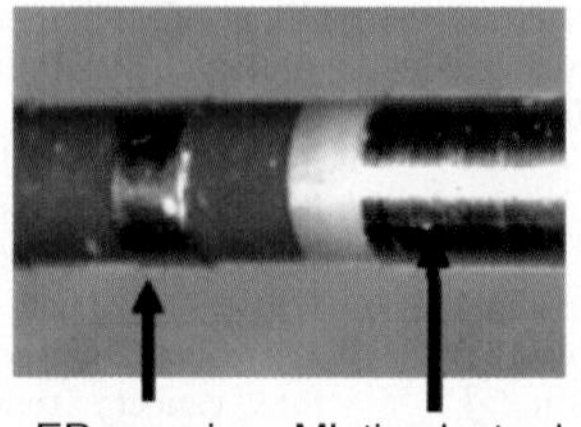

Figure 104-5 Experimental imaging/ablation microlinear catheter. This experimental catheter allows ultrasonic imaging via the catheter tip as well as the ability to ablate using the same ultrasonic array. EP, electrophysiologic; ML, microlinear. (Courtesy D. Stephens, University of California at Davis, D. Sahn, Oregon Health Sciences University, and K. Shivkumar, University of California at Los Angeles. Supported by an NIH Bioengineering Research Partnership Grant.)

References

1. Scheinman MM, Morady F, Hess DS, Gonzalez R: Catheter-induced ablation of the atrioventricular junction to control refractory supraventricular arrhythmias. JAMA 248(7):851-855, 1982.
2. Scheinman MM, Yang Y: The history of AV nodal reentry. Pacing Clin Electrophysiol 28(11):1232-1237, 2005.
3. Evans GT Jr, Scheinman MM, Bardy G, et al: Predictors of in-hospital mortality after DC catheter ablation of atrioventricular junction. Results of a prospective, international, multicenter study. Circulation 84(5):1924-1937, 1991.
4. Lin JC: Studies on microwaves in medicine and biology: From snails to humans. Bioelectromagnetics 25(3):146-159, 2004.
5. Calkins H, Yong P, Miller JM, et al: Catheter ablation of accessory pathways, atrioventricular nodal reentrant tachycardia, and the atrioventricular junction: Final results of a prospective, multicenter clinical trial. The Atakr Multicenter Investigators Group. Circulation 99(2):262-270, 1999.
6. Skanes AC, Klein GJ, Krahn AD, Yee R: Advances in energy delivery. Coron Artery Dis 14(1):15-23, 2003.
7. Haines DE: The biophysics of radiofrequency catheter ablation in the heart: The importance of temperature monitoring. Pacing Clin Electrophysiol 16(3 Pt 2):586-591, 1993.
8. Nath S, Haines DE: Biophysics and pathology of catheter energy delivery systems. Prog Cardiovasc Dis 37(4):185-204, 1995.
9. Haines DE, Watson DD, Verow AF: Electrode radius predicts lesion radius during radiofrequency energy heating. Validation of a proposed thermodynamic model. Circ Res 67(1):124-129, 1990.
10. Haines DE, Watson DD: Tissue heating during radiofrequency catheter ablation: A thermodynamic model and observations in isolated perfused and superfused canine right ventricular free wall. Pacing Clin Electrophysiol 12(6):962-976, 1989.
11. Langberg JJ, Calkins H, el-Atassi R, et al: Temperature monitoring during radiofrequency catheter ablation of accessory pathways. Circulation 86(5):1469-1474, 1992.
12. Wittkampf FH, Nakagawa H: RF catheter ablation: Lessons on lesions. Pacing Clin Electrophysiol 29(11):1285-1297, 2006.
13. Demazumder D, Mirotznik MS, Schwartzman D: Biophysics of radiofrequency ablation using an irrigated electrode. J Interv Card Electrophysiol 5(4):377-389, 2001.
14. Nakagawa H, Yamanashi WS, Pitha JV, et al: Comparison of in vivo tissue temperature profile and lesion geometry for radiofrequency ablation with a saline-irrigated electrode versus temperature control in a canine thigh muscle preparation. Circulation 91(8):2264-2273, 1995.
15. Yokoyama K, Nakagawa H, Wittkampf FH, et al: Comparison of electrode cooling between internal and open irrigation in radiofrequency ablation lesion depth and incidence of thrombus and steam pop. Circulation 113(1):11-19, 2006.
16. Wittkampf FH, Nakagawa H, Yamanashi WS, et al: Thermal latency in radiofrequency ablation. Circulation 93(6):1083-1086, 1996.
17. Bruce GK, Bunch TJ, Milton MA, et al: Discrepancies between catheter tip and tissue temperature in cooled-tip ablation: Relevance to guiding left atrial ablation. Circulation 112(7):954-960, 2005.
18. Perez FJ, Wood MA, Schubert CM: Effects of gap geometry on conduction through discontinuous radiofrequency lesions. Circulation 113(14):1723-1729, 2006.
19. Zheng X, Walcott GP, Rollins DL, et al: Comparison of the temperature profile and pathological effect at unipolar, bipolar and phased radiofrequency current configurations. J Interv Card Electrophysiol 5(4):401-410, 2001.
20. Klein GJ, Guiraudon GM, Perkins DG, et al: Surgical correction of the Wolff-Parkinson-White syndrome in the closed heart using cryosurgery: A simplified approach. J Am Coll Cardiol 3(2 Pt 1):405-409, 1984.
21. Cummings JE, Pacifico A, Drago JL, et al: Alternative energy sources for the ablation of arrhythmias. Pacing Clin Electrophysiol 28(5):434-443, 2005.
22. Gage AA, Baust J: Mechanisms of tissue injury in cryosurgery. Cryobiology 37(3):171-186, 1998.
23. De Ponti R: Cryothermal energy ablation of cardiac arrhythmias 2005: State of the art. Indian Pacing Electrophysiol J 5(1):12-24, 2005.
24. Nakamura Y, Nakano K, Nakatani H, et al: Easy pulmonary vein isolation using epicardial cryoablation. Surg Today 36(2):198-200, 2006.
25. Sternik L, Ghosh P, Luria D, et al: Mid-term results of the "hybrid maze": A combination of bipolar radiofrequency and cryoablation for surgical treatment of atrial fibrillation. J Heart Valve Dis 15(5):664-670, 2006.
26. Milla F, Skubas N, Briggs WM, et al: Epicardial beating heart cryoablation using a novel argon-based cryoclamp and linear probe. J Thorac Cardiovasc Surg 131(2):403-411, 2006.
27. Zrenner B, Dong J, Schreieck J, et al: Transvenous cryoablation versus radiofrequency ablation of the slow pathway for the treatment of atrioventricular nodal re-entrant tachycardia: A prospective randomized pilot study. Eur Heart J 25(24):2226-2231, 2004.
28. Gupta D, Al-Lamee RK, Earley MJ, et al: Cryoablation compared with radiofrequency ablation for atrioventricular nodal

re-entrant tachycardia: analysis of factors contributing to acute and follow-up outcome. Europace 8(12):1022-1026, 2006.

29. Collins KK, Rhee EK, Kirsh JA, et al: Cryoablation of accessory pathways in the coronary sinus in young patients: A multicenter study from the Pediatric and Congenital Electrophysiology Society's Working Group on Cryoablation. J Cardiovasc Electrophysiol 18(6):592-597, 2007.
30. Collins NJ, Barlow M, Varghese P, Leitch J: Cryoablation versus radiofrequency ablation in the treatment of atrial flutter trial (CRAAFT). J Interv Card Electrophysiol 16(1):1-5, 2006.
31. Cappato R, Calkins H, Chen SA, et al: Worldwide survey on the methods, efficacy, and safety of catheter ablation for human atrial fibrillation. Circulation 111(9):1100-1105, 2005.
32. Garan A, Al-Ahmad A, Mihalik T, et al: Cryoablation of the pulmonary veins using a novel balloon catheter. J Interv Card Electrophysiol 15(2):79-81, 2006.
33. Sarabanda AV, Bunch TJ, Johnson SB, et al: Efficacy and safety of circumferential pulmonary vein isolation using a novel cryothermal balloon ablation system. J Am Coll Cardiol 46(10):1902-1912, 2005.
34. Kenigsberg DN, Wood MA, Alaeddini J, Ellenbogen KA: Cryoablation inside the pulmonary vein after failure of radiofrequency antral isolation. Heart Rhythm 4(8):992-996, 2007.
35. ter Haar G: Ultrasound focal beam surgery. Ultrasound Med Biol 21(9):1089-1100, 1995.
36. Illing RO, Kennedy JE, Wu F, et al: The safety and feasibility of extracorporeal high-intensity focused ultrasound (HIFU) for the treatment of liver and kidney tumours in a Western population. Br J Cancer 93(8):890-895, 2005.
37. Hill CR, ter Haar GR: Review article: High intensity focused ultrasound—potential for cancer treatment. Br J Radiol 68(816):1296-1303, 1995.
38. Chen H, Li X, Wan M: The inception of cavitation bubble clouds induced by high-intensity focused ultrasound. Ultrasonics 44 Suppl 1:e427-e429, 2006.
39. Tran BC, Seo J, Hall TL, et al: Microbubble-enhanced cavitation for non-invasive ultrasound surgery. IEEE Trans Ultrason Ferroelectr Freq Control 50(10):1296-1304, 2003.
40. Natale A, Pisano E, Shewchik J, et al: First human experience with pulmonary vein isolation using a through-the-balloon circumferential ultrasound ablation system for recurrent atrial fibrillation. Circulation 102(16):1879-1882, 2000.
41. Meininger GR, Calkins H, Lickfett L, et al: Initial experience with a novel focused ultrasound ablation system for ring ablation outside the pulmonary vein. J Interv Card Electrophysiol 8(2):141-148, 2003.
42. Saliba W, Wilber D, Packer D, et al: Circumferential ultrasound ablation for pulmonary vein isolation: Analysis of acute and chronic failures. J Cardiovasc Electrophysiol 13:957-961, 2002.
43. Strickberger SA, Tokano T, Kluiwstra JU, et al: Extracardiac ablation of the canine atrioventricular junction by use of high-intensity focused ultrasound. Circulation 100(2):203-208, 1999.
44. Engel DJ, Muratore R, Hirata K, et al: Myocardial lesion formation using high-intensity focused ultrasound. J Am Soc Echocardiogr 19(7):932-937, 2006.
45. Nakagawa H, Antz M, Wong T, et al: Initial experience using a forward directed, high-intensity focused ultrasound balloon catheter for pulmonary vein antrum isolation in patients with atrial fibrillation. J Cardiovasc Electrophysiol 18(2):136-144, 2007.
46. Borchert B, Lawrenz T, Hansky B, Stellbrink C: Lethal atrioesophageal fistula after pulmonary vein isolation using high-intensity focused ultrasound (HIFU). Heart Rhythm 5(1):145-148, 2008.
47. Cesario DA, Mahajan A, Shivkumar K: Lesion-forming technologies for catheter ablation of atrial fibrillation. Heart Rhythm 4(3 Suppl):S44-S50, 2007.
48. Bunch TJ, Mahapatra S, Bruce GK, et al: Impact of transforming growth factor-β_1 on atrioventricular node conduction modification by injected autologous fibroblasts in the canine heart. Circulation 113(21):2485-2494, 2006.
49. Sasano T, McDonald AD, Kikuchi K, Donahue JK: Molecular ablation of ventricular tachycardia after myocardial infarction. Nat Med 12(11):1256-1258, 2006.

Atrial Substrate Ablation in Atrial Fibrillation 105

Kang Teng Lim, Sébastien Knecht, Matthew Wright, and Michel Haïssaguerre

CHAPTER OUTLINE

Pulmonary vein isolation is an effective treatment for paroxysmal atrial fibrillation (AF), but this strategy alone is inadequate for patients with persistent AF. Many experimental and clinical studies have supported the participation of the atrial myocardium in the maintenance of AF. The findings of rapid left atrial (LA) activity in comparison with the pulmonary veins have suggested that the atria might harbor critical AF drivers.[1,2] Progressive electrical remodelling of the atria, as AF progresses from paroxysmal to persistent, has been associated with shortening of atrial effective refractory period and facilitation of reentrant wavelets, leading to maintenance of AF.[3-5] Consequently, inclusion of the atrial myocardium outside the pulmonary vein region in the ablation strategy is necessary for patients with persistent AF to achieve long-term rhythm control.

The various strategies to modify atrial substrate performed in recent years can be classified broadly into electrogram-based ablation and linear ablation. Electrogram-based ablation encompasses the targeting of complex fractionated atrial electrograms,[6] high-frequency atrial activity,[7] and mapping of discrete sources that activate the atria centrifugally.[8] Linear ablation techniques modeled after the surgical maze procedure attempt to extinguish wandering atrial wavelets and macro-reentrant loops. Although the autonomic nervous system is not specifically targeted using these strategies, the ganglionic plexi also may be ablated along the trajectory of ablation lesions.

Electrogram-Guided Ablation of Atrial Substrate

The atrial ablation targets during electrogram-based ablation can differ at successive stages of AF ablation, depending on electrogram morphology, cycle length, and organization of atrial activity. During disorganized atrial activity, complex fractionated electrograms, areas of highest dominant frequency, or autonomic ganglionic plexi may be targeted. In addition, regional differences in electrogram characteristics can often be observed: Structures annexed to the LA such as the coronary sinus (CS) and left atrial appendage (LAA) often display complex fractionation and rapid atrial activity and the rest of the left atrium may be organized. Ablation at these sites has been shown to have a significant impact on the AF cycle length.[9] When the atrial activity is slower and organized, activation sequence mapping can be attempted to find localized sources of fibrillatory activity.

Atrial Ablation Targets

Complex Fractionated Electrograms

In the past few years, atrial electrograms displaying complex fractionation have been targeted for ablation. Fractionated atrial electrograms were first described as continuous activity or electrograms with fibrillatory interval of less than 100 ms and were distributed nonuniformly across the right and left atria.[7] Complex fractionated atrial electrograms (CFAEs) were subsequently described by Nademanee and colleagues as low-voltage electrograms (0.05-0.25 mV) with a cycle length shorter than 120 ms, displaying two or more deflections, or having a continuous deflection from baseline.[6,10]

CFAEs were initially thought to represent areas of slow conduction, zones of colliding wave fronts, or pivot points between different wavelets that participate actively in the AF process.[6,11] This concept encouraged many groups to target CFAEs either as a sole strategy or in combination with pulmonary vein isolation and linear ablation. However, CFAEs may be either active or passive. The passive CFAEs can result from a remote driver accelerating the local tissue beyond its refractory period or might reflect asynchronous activation of local muscle bundles during periods of short cycle length. Shortening of the AF cycle length (by at least 10 ms) has been shown to precede complex fractionation in 91% and 88% of the regions sampled in the atria and coronary sinus, respectively, implying that fractionation is a consequence of higher-frequency activity.[12] These passive CFAEs displayed nearly simultaneous activation covering only a limited part of AF cycle length, whereas active CFAEs display repetitive bursts and activities spanning the majority of AF cycle length.[12]

The relationships between CFAEs, high-frequency electrograms and the autonomic nervous system has been a subject of interest among investigators. Experiments in a sheep model of AF have shown that atrial myocardium exhibiting most fractionation occurred in areas of high-frequency activity.[11] Directly stimulating the intrinsic cardiac ganglionic plexi in dogs results in the occurrence and sustainability of CFAEs; ablation of the ganglionic plexi resulted in significant attenuation or elimination of CFAEs.[13] CFAEs have also been shown within sites with dominant high-frequency electrograms.[11] All these animal studies advocate the targeting of CFAEs during catheter ablation. However, highly fractionated electrograms can be difficult to analyze, and distinguishing active from passive CFAEs remains challenging. An alternative method to decipher these complex electrograms is to analyze them according to their frequency spectra, which allows easy and rapid identification of areas with complex fractionation and high-frequency activity.

Dominant Frequency Electrograms

Both experimental and clinical studies have shown that AF can be maintained by high-frequency sources (rotors) displaying spatially distributed frequency gradient.[1,14,14-18] Using fast Fourier transform (FFT), signals from these high-frequency electrograms can be deconstructed into sine waves. These sine waves can be quantified according to the most prevalent sine wave frequency, known as the dominant frequency (DF). Analysis of DF can be used to assess changes in activation rates and organization of AF after ablation in an attempt to understand the pathophysiology of AF even when the electrograms are fractionated or display large amplitude variability.[17,19]

Catheter ablation studies incorporating DF mapping have shown that the pulmonary veins harbor important DF sites in patients with paroxysmal AF but not in patients with persistent AF.[2,15] Ablation targeting of these DF sites was associated with slowing and termination of AF in 87% of paroxysmal AF patients.[15] The DFs in the pulmonary veins were also found to be higher among patients with paroxysmal AF compared to those with permanent AF.[2] Isolation of the pulmonary veins resulted in significant prolongation of atrial fibrillatory cycle length (AFCL) and a decrease in DF in patients with paroxysmal AF but not permanent AF: 182 ± 17 to 223 ± 41 ms ($P < 0.0001$) and 5.8 ± 1.2 Hz to 4.9 ± 0.7 Hz ($P = 0.0001$), respectively. Targeting the sites of DF in permanent AF is much less effective, possibly due to technical issues and numerous sources perpetuating AF. Inaccuracies of DF analysis may be related to complex fractionation or double potentials, resulting in multiple frequency peaks with very similar power rather than one clearly dominant frequency as seen in paroxysmal atrial fibrillation.[20]

DF mapping is currently being integrated into commercial software that computes DF from selected local atrial electrograms that can be plotted in relation to atrial geometry (Fig. 105-1). This might facilitate DF-guided ablation in the future and help to assess the efficacy of using DF analysis in patients with persistent AF. Several limitations in DF mapping

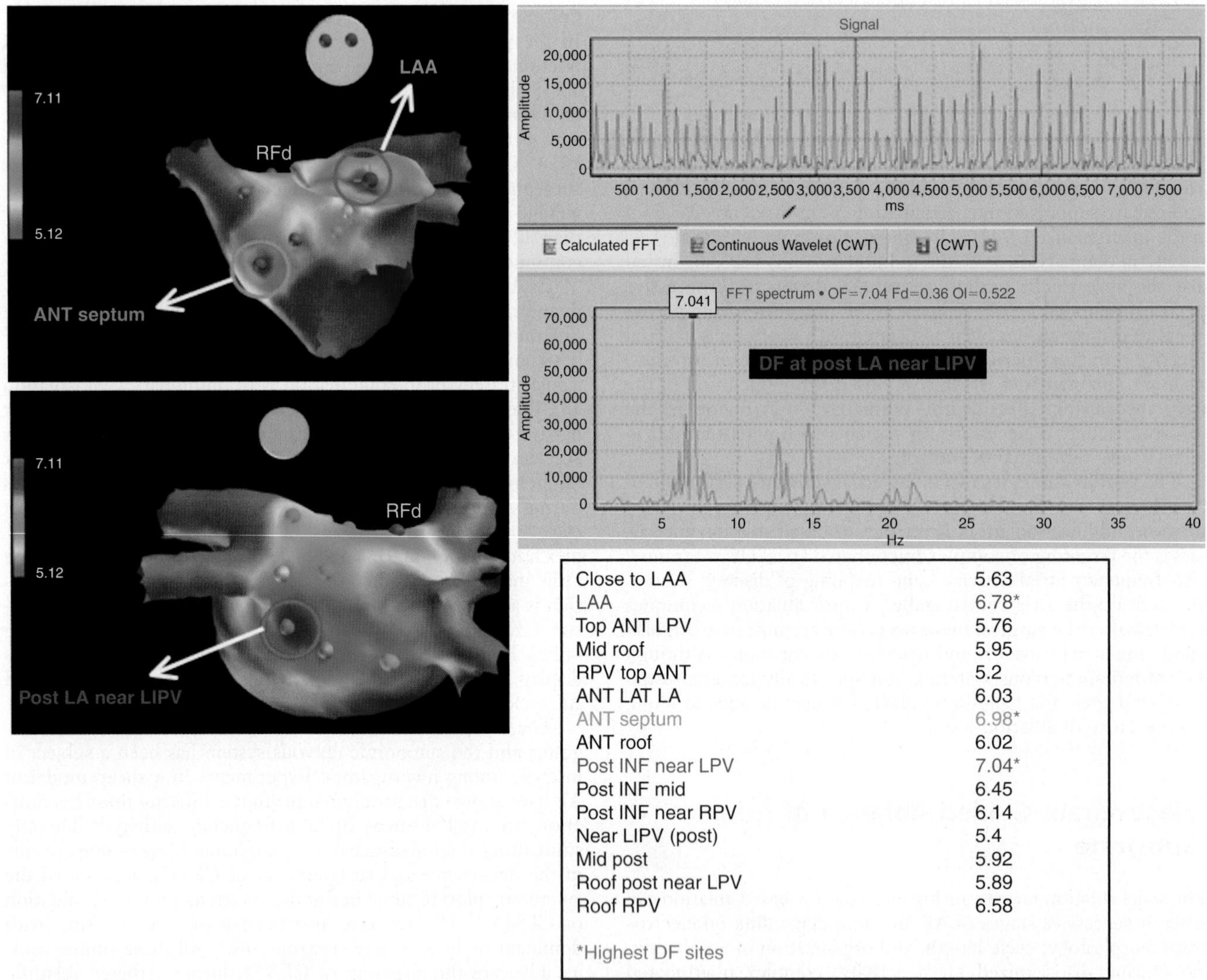

Site	DF
Close to LAA	5.63
LAA	6.78*
Top ANT LPV	5.76
Mid roof	5.95
RPV top ANT	5.2
ANT LAT LA	6.03
ANT septum	6.98*
ANT roof	6.02
Post INF near LPV	7.04*
Post INF mid	6.45
Post INF near RPV	6.14
Near LIPV (post)	5.4
Mid post	5.92
Roof post near LPV	5.89
Roof RPV	6.58

*Highest DF sites

Figure 105-1 Dominant frequency mapping using custom software. Sites with highest dominant frequency are displayed on the table and shown in the figure. Sampled signals are examined for organization and regularity, and the dominant frequency can be extrapolated based on fast Fourier transform or continuous wavelet methods. ANT, anterior; INF, inferior; LA, left atrium; LAA, left atrial appendage; LIPV, left inferior pulmonary vein; LPV, left pulmonary vein; RPV, right pulmonary vein.

ought to be recognized, such as the effects of far field electrogram, highly fractionated signals with short fibrillatory interval, confounding effects of artifacts and noise, and double potentials counting.[21]

Autonomic Ganglionic Plexi

Autonomic innervation of the heart consists of both the extrinsic and intrinsic autonomic systems. The extrinsic autonomic system innervates the heart via the vagosympathetic trunk. Innervation from the intrinsic autonomic system is via the ganglionated plexi and interganglionic axons distributed in the cardiac epicardial fat pads predominantly at the pulmonary vein antrum and superior vena cava junction.[22,23] Modulation of either extrinsic autonomic system by stimulation of vagosympathetic trunk or ganglia have both been shown to affect the heart rate and inducibility of AF.[24]

The importance of the autonomic nervous system in pulmonary vein pathophysiology have been underscored by studies demonstrating rapid firing from the pulmonary veins when the ganglia are activated by high-frequency stimulation or acetylcholine injection.[25,26,27] In addition, acceleration of the fibrillatory cycle length in the pulmonary veins due to shortening of atrial refractory period and action potential duration has also been described during vagal episodes.[28] These findings have encouraged investigators to specifically target the ganglionic plexi in patients undergoing catheter ablation of AF.

High-frequency stimulation has been used to locate clusters of ganglionic plexi in the LA outside the pulmonary vein antrum and to determine the efficacy of ganglia ablation.[29-31] Stimulation of the ganglia resulted in a vagal reflex that manifested as atrioventricular (AV) block, bradycardia (with increase in R-R interval of at least 50%), or hypotension. Although localization of clusters of ganglionic plexi is feasible using this technique, the efficacy of targeting ganglionic plexi alone, in persistent AF, is unclear. Furthermore, there is considerable overlap of the anatomic location of ganglionic plexi, CFAE, and the wide circumferential pulmonary vein ablation.[30,32]

Ablation Approach during Disorganized Atrial Activity

In persistent AF, atrial electrograms are often complex and too chaotic to allow discrete analysis of the local activation cycle length, morphology, or activation. Electrograms targeted for ablation include those displaying continuous electrical activity, complex fractionation, or rapid activity, with the aim of organizing and slowing local and subsequently global atrial activities in both right and left atria.[9]

Distinguishing passive from active sites harboring critical atrial drivers remains the most challenging part of ablation. In a prospectively randomized study, electrogram characteristics were investigated to determine their impact on AF cycle length and AF termination. The only independent predictor associated with significant prolongation of AF cycle length was atrial sites displaying continuous electrical activity (>70% of fibrillatory interval), with positive and negative predictive value of 52% and 67%, respectively.[33] Other variables such as fractionation index (number of deflections of fractionated activity in a 4-second window), electrogram voltage, or local mean cycle length were not significant predictors.

From an anatomic perspective, all atrial regions represent potential ablation targets including the LAA, inferior LA, interatrial septum around the foramen ovale, anterior LA, posterior LA, and the right atrium (RA). In particular, structures annexed to the LA, such as the base of the LAA and the inferior LA-CS interface, have been shown to have greater impact on AFCL.[9,34] The endpoint of ablation is to slow and organize local activity.

Technique of Ablating Specific Anatomic Regions

Ablation of the Left Atrial Appendage Ablation of the LAA is performed at its junction with the LA. The posterior wall separating the LAA from the left veins is a common site of complex activity. To facilitate the ablation, the catheter is advanced into the sheath and curved to ensure catheter stability before delivering RF. Ablation is performed using an irrigated-tip catheter at power settings of between 25 and 30 W, depending on the catheter contact and orientation, to avoid steam pops and subsequent perforation. Although extensive ablation around the LAA may be required to slow and organise atrial activity, complete isolation of the LAA is rare due to the presence of thick muscular connections. Care must be taken, however, to avoid electrical disconnection of the appendage, given the subsequent propensity for thrombus formation and the need for lifelong anticoagulation. Exclusion of the LAA can also affect LA transport function.[35]

Ablation of the Coronary Sinus and Inferior Left Atrium The CS might provide both the substrate and ectopic triggers for persistent AF.[9,36] Anatomically, the CS muscular sleeve extends up to 4 cm from the ostium, with connections to the adjacent inferior LA. Ablation of the inferior LA is performed by looping the ablation catheter in the LA and dragging the catheter along the posterior mitral annulus continuously, in order to interrupt the inferior LA from the CS muscular connections (see Fig. 105-2). Electrograms in the inferior LA and the CS are monitored and ablation is continued until fractionated atrial activity becomes organized. Ablation within the CS is performed with the ablation catheter positioned in the distal CS (approximately 4 o'clock in the left anterior oblique projection) and gradually dragged proximally to the CS os, with the catheter tip deflected toward the LA to minimize the risk of

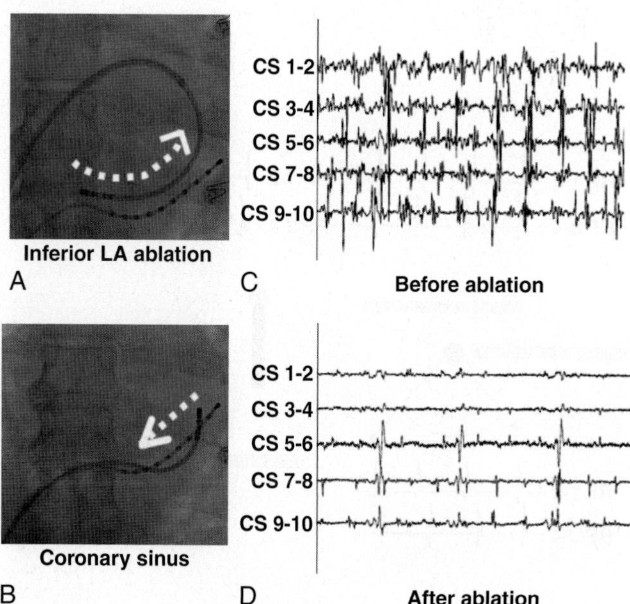

Figure 105-2 Illustration of catheter positions during ablation of inferior left atrium (LA) **(A)** and coronary sinus (CS) **(B)**. The *arrows* indicate the motion used during ablation of the respective structures. After ablation of both structures, electrograms in the coronary sinus appeared much more organized **(C** and **D)**.

circumflex coronary artery injury.[37] Power is limited to 25 W and the irrigation rate is adjusted manually to achieve temperatures between 40 and 45° C, with the highest irrigation flow rates required for ablation in the distal CS (up to 60 mL/min). Complete disconnection of this structure is not routinely attempted because minimal benefit has been demonstrated with total disconnection.[9]

Ablation of Other Left Atrial Regions Other regions within the LA are ablated point by point to eliminate sites with complex fractionation or short fibrillatory cycles. During ablation of the posterior LA, the autonomic ganglionic plexi may be inadvertently targeted along the trajectory of ablation lesions.[30,32,38,39] Based on our experience, the posterior LA (excluding the pulmonary vein antral region), is less important in maintaining persistent AF relative to other structures.

Right Atrial Ablation Targets The right atrium has an important role in perpetuating AF in a significant minority of patients. In our experience, termination of persistent AF required RA ablation in about 20% of patients, suggesting that the RA may be harboring the culprit atrial driver. The left and right atrial appendage cycle lengths (CLs) measured simultaneously at baseline and following each ablation step during the procedure offer a possible clue to the involvement of structures outside the LA, for example, the RA. Gradual prolongation of the LAA CL by ablation with persisting short AFCL in the RAA suggests a potential role for RA structures in perpetuating AF. Once the LA has been ablated, all regions within the RA, including the superior vena cava, might similarly harbor drivers perpetuating AF and are mapped using the same electrogram-guided approach as in the LA.[40,41] Care must be taken to avoid injury to the phrenic nerve and AV node during ablation in the lateral and septal RA, respectively.

Ablation Approach during Organized Atrial Activity

Organized AF is characterized by atrial electrograms displaying irregular atrial cycle length (i.e., AF) with beat-to-beat variations of at least 20 ms and discrete atrial complexes with a consistent activation sequence occurring arbitrarily for at least 75% of the time in both atria.[42] During organized AF, localized sources perpetuating AF can be identified and ablated by converging on an area displaying centrifugal activation. Animal experiments demonstrating discrete areas of high-frequency activity during pacing and acetylcholine-induced AF[43] as well as computational models of AF[44] have supported the perpetuation of AF from localized sources. Human studies have also confirmed persistent fibrillatory activity confined within isolated LA.[45,45]

Characteristics of Localized Sources Maintaining Atrial Fibrillation

Within an area of early activation, the localized source driving AF may originate from a discrete point in 58% of cases and display electrograms harboring less than 75% of the cycle length.[8] Centrifugal activation from the focal source with 1:1 conduction to the adjacent atrium allows mapping of the earliest activity. When1:1 conduction to the adjacent atrium is absent, a focal source with a short cycle length is observed.

Importantly, in 42% of cases, the source is not focal but is a small, discrete reentrant circuit with local electrical activity covering 75% to 100% of the cycle length. Depending on the reentrant circuit's size and catheter positioning, continuous activity or temporally alternating potentials between distal and proximal bipoles may be observed. High-density mapping of the source can be performed with the use of a 20-pole catheter (Pentaray, Biosense Webster, Diamond Bar, CA). A schematic diagram illustrating mapping of an AF source is shown in Figure 105-3.

Monitoring Progress of Ablation Using Atrial Fibrillatory Cycle Length

The AFCL is generally considered a surrogate for local tissue refractoriness. Earlier studies have shown that AFCL accurately tracks the shortening in local refractory periods seen with prolonged AF duration, or the lengthening in local refractory periods during antiarrhythmic drug therapy. The gradual prolongation in AFCL prior to AF termination during catheter

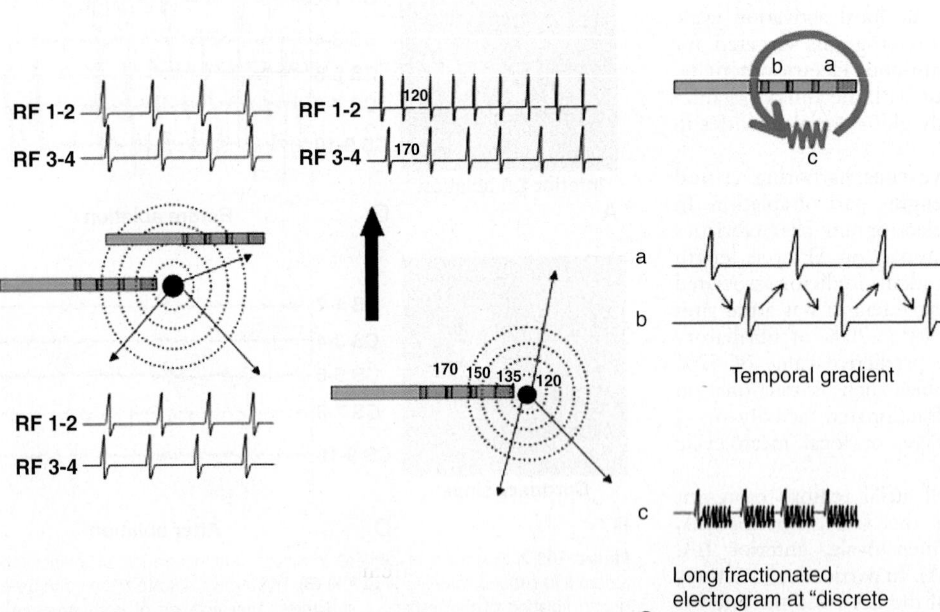

Figure 105-3 Illustration of local electrogram-based mapping of focal sources. **A**, A focal source is observed with centrifugal spread, and the recorded activation sequence corresponds to the catheter position relative to the source. **B**, Electrograms recorded with the distal catheter bipole positioned over a high-frequency source is shown. The shortest cycle length is 120 ms, with frequency gradient to surrounding tissue, as indicated by the cycle length of 170 ms recorded on the proximal bipole. **C**, A temporal gradient is observed between the distal *(a)* and proximal *(b)* bipoles when the catheter is positioned within a localized reentrant circuit, while a long fractionated activity is observed in the distal pole when the catheter tip is placed directly over a discrete isthmus *(c)*.RF, radiofrequency.

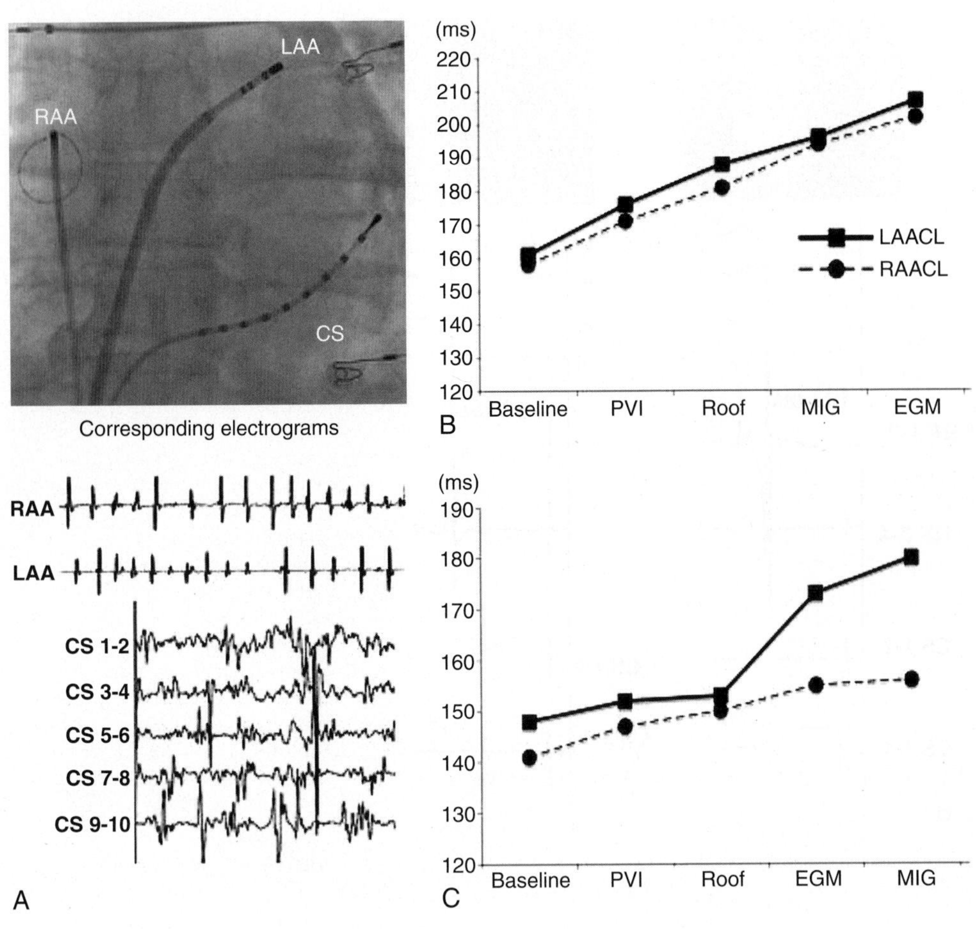

Figure 105-4 **A,** Discrete high-amplitude electrograms observed at the right atrial (RAA) and left atrial appendages (LAA) and the coronary sinus (CS). In contrast to the disorganized and fragmented electrograms in the coronary sinus, discrete electrograms in the appendages permit unambiguous measurements of AFCL (atrial fibrillatory cycle length). **B,** Increase in AFCL in both the right (RAACL) and left (LAACL) atrial appendages prior to termination of AF during left atrial ablation. **C,** A far greater increase in LAACL compared to RAACL in a patient who had termination of AF during RA ablation. Measurements of AFCL were taken after each of the ablation steps: PVI (pulmonary vein isolation), Roof, MIG (mitral isthmus), and EGM (electrogram-based ablation). (From Haissaguerre M, Hocini M, Sanders P, et al: Catheter ablation of long-lasting persistent atrial fibrillation: Clinical outcome and mechanisms of subsequent arrhythmias. J Cardiovasc Electrophysiol 16(11): 1138-1147, 2005.)

ablation supports the use of AFCL to monitor substrate modification during AF ablation.[9,46] The impact of ablation on AFCL at sites remote from ablation such as the appendages indicates changes in the substrate maintaining AF rather than changes in local refractoriness.

Measurements of the AFCL can be determined reliably by averaging 30 consecutive cycles taken from the left and right atrial appendages, where unambiguous high-voltage, discrete, and reproducible electrograms are observed. Baseline AFCL measurement has been shown to be the strongest predictor of success for persistent AF ablation of less than 5 years' duration. A longer initial AFCL is observed among patients in whom AF terminates during ablation (156 ± 23 ms vs 130 ± 14 ms).[9] AFCL of less than 140 ms is associated with AF termination in less than 69% of patients, and a longer AFCL is associated with more than 89% AF termination.

Changes in AFCL can be used to monitor the progress of substrate modification. Based on our experience, after stepwise pulmonary vein isolation, ablation of complex fractionated electrograms, and linear lesions, there is a gradual prolongation of AFCL culminating in conversion to sinus rhythm or atrial tachycardia when AFCL reaches 180 to 200 ms. In other words, more ablation is required in order to terminate AF with a lower baseline AFCL of less than 140 ms compared to an AFCL of 200 ms. Simultaneous increases in left and right atrial appendage AFCL are observed in majority of patients, but disproportionate increases in left compared to right atrial appendage AFCL occurred in 20% of patients, who eventually had AF termination during ablation in the RA. This finding highlights the role of AFCL in further defining the atrial chamber driving AF (Fig. 105-4).

Linear Ablation

Early attempts at linear ablation represented an empiric version of a catheter-based maze procedure that was limited to the right atrium to modify atrial substrate, but the results were disappointing. Although technically challenging, the primary purpose of linear ablation in the right and left atrium is to interrupt wandering reentrant wavelets or macro-reentrant loops, but secondary effects can include alteration of autonomic innervation, atrial debulking, and modification in local complex electrograms.[47,48] Verification of linear block is necessary to prevent proarrhythmia and can be easily determined using validated pacing maneuvers that will be discussed below.

Adjunctive mitral isthmus or LA roofline ablation, or both, in addition to pulmonary vein isolation have been shown to reduce AF burden in patients with paroxysmal and persistent AF.[47,47-49] In patients with paroxysmal AF, freedom from arrhythmia without antiarrhythmic therapy after 12 months of follow-up was significantly higher in patients undergoing pulmonary vein isolation and mitral isthmus ablation compared to pulmonary vein isolation alone (87% vs 69%, P = 0.002).[47] However, the incremental benefit of mitral isthmus ablation following pulmonary vein isolation is greater for patients with persistent AF compared to those with paroxysmal AF.[50] The addition of a LA roof line to pulmonary vein isolation instead of mitral isthmus line in patients with paroxysmal AF have also been associated with greater freedom from AF without antiarrhythmic therapy after 15 ± 4 months of follow-up, (87% vs 69%, respectively; P = 0.04).[48] The combination of both LA roof and mitral

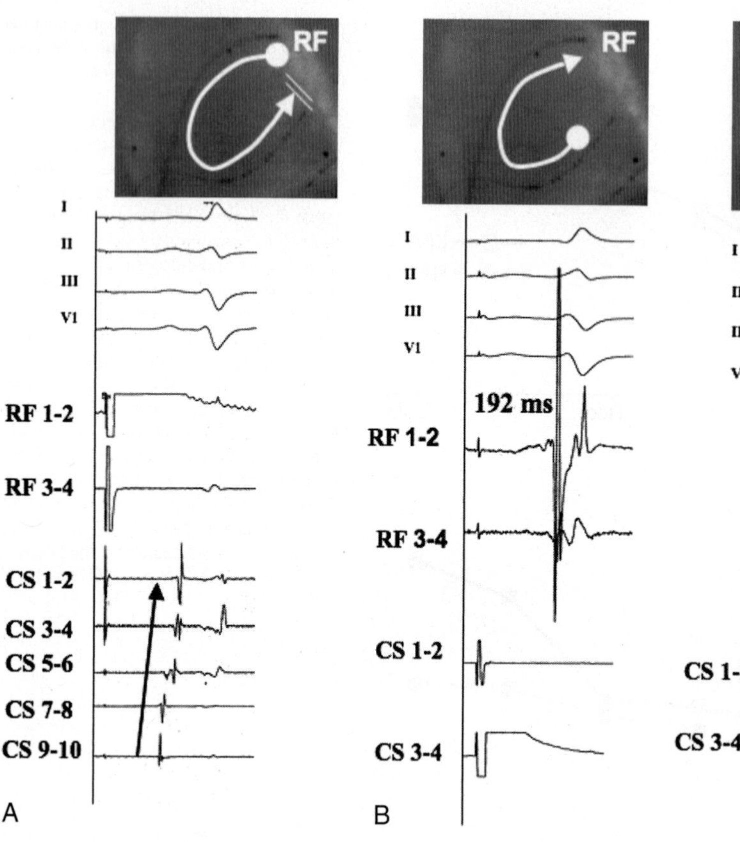

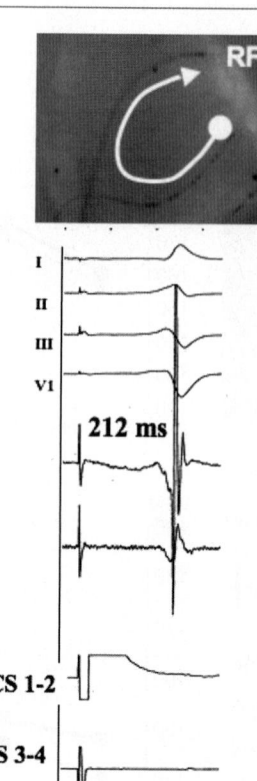

Figure 105-5 Demonstration of mitral isthmus block. **A,** During pacing lateral to the ablation line (RF 1-2 positioned in the left appendage), CS is activated proximal-to-distal while being distal-to-proximal with persistent conduction. **B,** Pacing from distal CS results in a perimitral activation delay of 212 ms, and pacing in the proximal CS results in a shorter perimitral activation delay of 192 ms. CS, coronary sinus; RF, radiofrequency.

isthmus ablation after pulmonary vein isolation has been associated with greater improvement in freedom from persistent AF after more than12 months of follow-up compared to pulmonary vein isolation alone (77% vs 44%, $P = 0.002$).[49]

Technique for Ablation of the Mitral Isthmus

The mitral line consists of linear lesions joining the posterior mitral annulus to the left inferior pulmonary vein.[47] To perform the line, an irrigated tip ablation catheter is introduced through a long sheath to facilitate catheter stability and positioned at the lateral mitral annulus, where the atrial:ventricular electrogram demonstrates a 1-2:1 ratio. The ablation line is performed, commencing at a 3- or 4-o'clock position to a 2- to 3-o'clock position at the top of the line. RF energy is typically delivered for 60 to 120 seconds at each site using a power of 30 to 37 W and temperature limited to 48° C. Care must be taken to ensure catheter stability and to avoid inadvertent displacement, which can result in high-energy delivery within the left inferior pulmonary vein or left atrial appendage. If conduction block is not achieved, potential "conduction gaps" along the line should be explored and ablated. Failing this, the lesion can be extended more superolaterally from the left inferior pulmonary vein to the base of the left atrial appendage.

In our experience, approximately two thirds of patients require ablation from within the CS in order to achieve mitral isthmus block. Ablation within the CS is performed using an irrigated tip catheter, with power delivery of 20 to 25 W, temperature limited to 48° C, and flow rates of up to 60 mL/min to reduce the risk of circumflex artery injury and cardiac tamponade. CS ablation represents an opportunistic approach in linear ablation where epicardial and endocardial ablations can be performed as a sandwich to complete a transmural lesion set.

The endpoint of ablation is confirmation of bidirectional block using criteria similar to those previously described for cavotricuspid isthmus block, namely, local corridor of widely separated double potentials, proximal to distal CS activation during pacing from the left atrial appendage, and delayed left atrial appendage activation with distal compared to proximal CS pacing. The pacing maneuvers to determine mitral isthmus block are illustrated in Figure105-5.

In 100 consecutive patients with paroxysmal AF undergoing pulmonary vein isolation and mitral isthmus ablation, mitral isthmus block was achieved in 92% of the patients, with 68% of patients requiring ablation within the CS.[47] Complete linear block was achieved with a conduction delay of 151 ± 26 ms after 20 ± 10 minutes of endocardial RF and 5 ± 4 minutes of ablation within the CS.

Technique for Ablation of the Left Atrial Roof

The LA roofline is a contiguous line of ablation lesions joining the superior pulmonary veins. An irrigated-tip ablation catheter is introduced through a long sheath to provide catheter stability, with its tip oriented toward the LA roof. Commencing at the left superior pulmonary vein, the ablation catheter is gradually dragged toward the right superior pulmonary vein by rotating the sheath and catheter assembly clockwise and posteriorly.

RF energy is typically delivered for 60 to 120 seconds at each site, with temperature limited to 48° C and power delivery guided by the catheter orientation. When the catheter tip is perpendicular to the tissue interface, power is reduced to 25 W; a power of 30 to 32 W is safe with a more parallel catheter

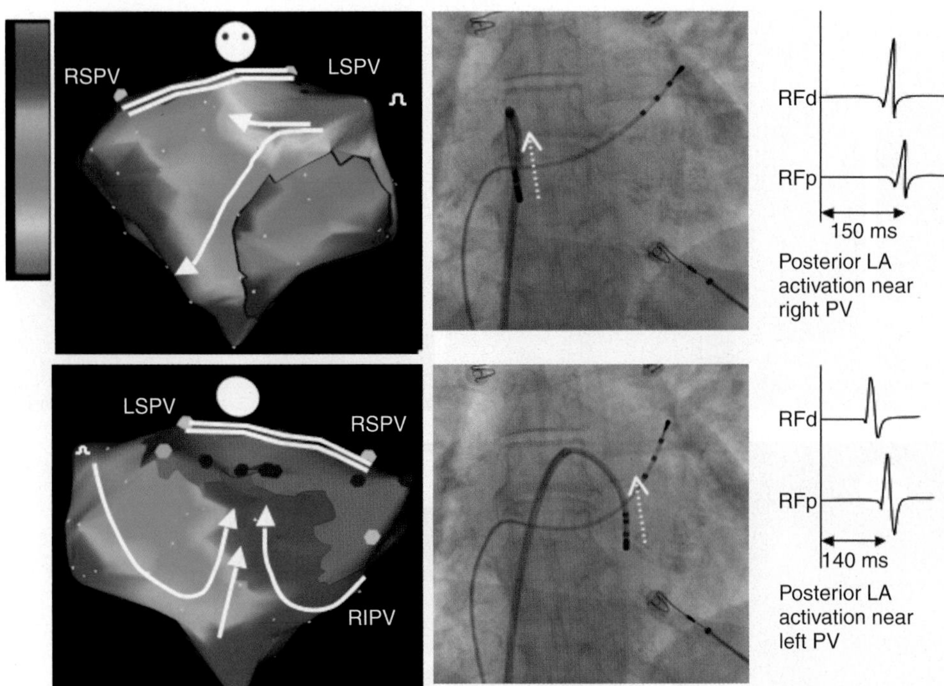

Figure 105-6 *Left,* Electroanatomic activation map during LA appendage pacing demonstrates the activation detour to the posterior LA wall. *Middle,* Series of radiographs with catheter placed in the right and left side of posterior LA and expected activation pattern in the presence of conduction block at the LA roof is also shown. *Right,* The activation in the mapping catheter is distal to proximal, indicating a low to high activation in the posterior wall. LA, left atrium; LSPV, left superior pulmonary vein; PV, pulmonary vein; RIPV, right inferior pulmonary vein; RSPV, right superior pulmonary vein.

tip position. The ablation endpoint is demonstration of a complete line of conduction block during LA appendage pacing. Conduction block is suggested by a corridor of double potential along the ablation line (not always observed) or by caudocranial activation of the posterior LA with right-to-left activation as illustrated in Figure 105-6.

In 100 consecutive paroxysmal AF patients undergoing pulmonary vein isolation and roofline ablation, conduction block was achieved in 96% of patients.[48] Complete linear block was achieved with delay of 146 ± 25 ms near the right pulmonary veins and 138 ± 15 ms near the left pulmonary veins during LAA pacing only after 12 ± 6 minutes of RF energy.

Technique for Ablation of the Anterior Line

The anterior left atrial line consists of linear lesions joining the completed LA roofline to the anterior mitral annulus as septally as possible. This line was initially performed because it was thought that left-to-right atrial connection through the Bachmann bundle perpetuated AF.[51] In order to perform the line, the ablation catheter is introduced into a long sheath and positioned at the anterior mitral annulus, where the atrioventricular electrogram demonstrates a 1-2:1 ratio. During RF delivery, a counterclockwise torque is then applied to the sheath while the catheter curvature is gradually released until the catheter reaches the completed LA roof line (Fig. 105-7).

Complete linear block is validated by demonstrating a corridor of double potentials along the line during pacing lateral to the line and by activation detour during either pacing the LA lateral to the ablation line or during high-septal RA pacing where the earliest LA activation is anteroseptal to the ablation line.

In a prospective study of 24 patients undergoing catheter ablation of AF (16 paroxysmal AF, eight chronic AF), linear block at the anterior line was achieved in only 58% of patients.[51] A delay of 158 ± 30 ms was observed during pacing lateral to the line after 14 ± 4 minutes of RF energy delivery. The anterior line is not only technically challenging to create, but it also results in significant prolongation in left atrial activation time, which can adversely affect LA transport function. As a consequence, we do not routinely perform this line as part of our catheter ablation strategy for persistent AF.

Clinical Outcomes of Atrial Substrate Ablation

Clinical outcomes of substrate modification strategies for patients with persistent atrial fibrillation are shown in Table 105-1.

Pulmonary Vein Ablation Plus Linear Ablation

Electrical isolation of the pulmonary veins (segmental or circumferential) in combination with linear ablation has been shown by many groups to increase the efficacy of catheter ablation of chronic AF. Circumferential pulmonary vein ablation alone has been proposed to modify atrial substrate by reducing local reentrant circuits and the atrial mass available to maintain AF[52] as well as interrupting autonomic ganglia along its trajectory.[32]

Pappone and colleagues performed ablation between the superior and inferior pulmonary veins and at the mitral isthmus to reduce the incidence of postablation atrial flutter.[53,54] During a follow-up of up to 12 months, they reported that up to 83% of patients with chronic AF remained in sinus rhythm without antiarrhythmic medications. Using the same approach, other authors have reported lower success rates in maintaining sinus rhythm: Oral and coworkers reported a success rate of 68% at 9 months of follow-up off drugs,[55] Bertaglia and coworkers reported 70% at 20 months[56] (64% still taking antiarrhythmics), and Beukema and coworkers reported 77% (44% on antiarrhythmics).[57]

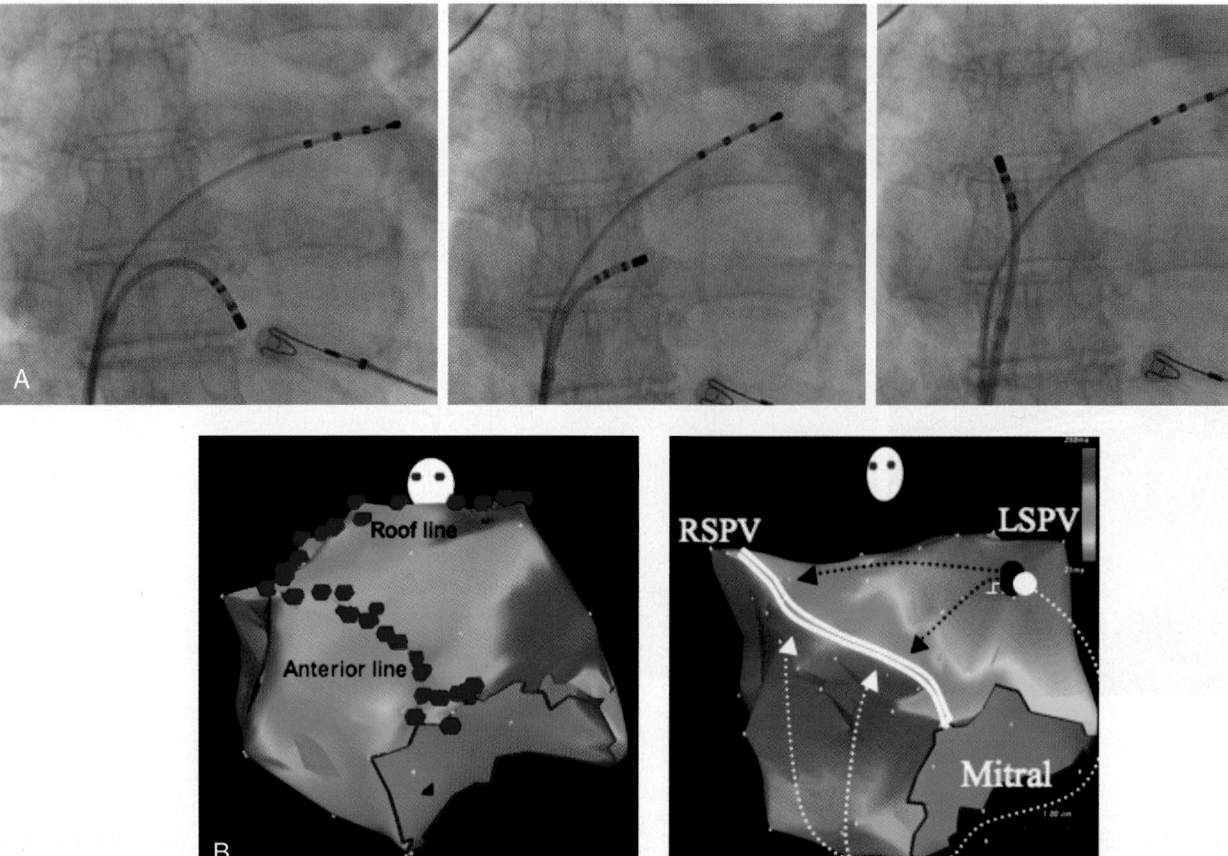

Figure 105-7 **A,** Series of radiographs showing the motion used to move the ablation catheter during ablation of the anterior line. **B,** Electroanatomic activation map during left atrial appendage pacing with complete block on the ablation line. LSPV, left superior pulmonary vein; RSPV, right superior pulmonary vein.

With the use of use of intracardiac echo to guide ablation of the pulmonary vein antrum that incorporates more of the posterior LA wall compared with wide circumferential pulmonary vein ablation, Marrouche's group has reported higher success rates of up to 90% in a combined population of paroxysmal and chronic AF patients after at least 12 months of follow-up.[58] The basis for the discrepancy in success rates between these studies is difficult to reconcile but might relate to differences in patient characteristics, duration of AF and preablation AFCL, titration of radiofrequency energy, and endpoints for ablation, use of antiarrhythmic drugs after ablation, the follow-up period, and monitoring methods.

Ablation Guided by Complex Fractionated Electrograms

The approach of targeting CFAEs as the only strategy without ablation of the LA–pulmonary vein junction (pulmonary vein isolation) was first described by Nademanee and coworkers.[6] Targeting CFAE with the use of electroanatomic mapping resulted in an AF termination rate of 95% in a mixed population of patients with paroxysmal and chronic AF. The overall success rate, defined as freedom from arrhythmia at 1 year of follow-up, was 91% after repeat ablation. Ibutilide was administered in 28% of the patients for cardioversion after ablation. Among patients with chronic AF, 88% were free of arrhythmia and 13% were taking adjunctive antiarrhythmic therapy. Using a similar approach in patients with chronic AF, Oral and colleagues reported only modest short-term efficacy, with more than 40% of patients undergoing ablation requiring a second ablation procedure and 57% of patients remaining in sinus rhythm without antiarrhythmic drugs 13 ± 7 months after the last ablation.[59] In comparison to the study by Nademanee, the acute AF termination rate was also lower, with only 12% patients converting to sinus rhythm during ablation and another 27% after ibutilide administration.

Autonomic Ganglia

Ablation of putative ganglionated plexi as evidenced by abolition of the vagal response has been associated with a reduction in AF recurrence compared to circumferential pulmonary vein ablation alone in patients with persistent AF. In patients with paroxysmal AF, Pappone's group demonstrated that vagal denervation in the 34% of patients who manifested a vagal response during wide circumferential pulmonary vein ablation was associated with significant reduction in AF recurrence during 12 months follow-up (99% vs 85%, $P = 0.0002$).[32] During a preliminary short-term follow-up of 1 to 10 months (median, 5 months), Sherlag and colleagues reported that additional ganglionic plexi ablation (localized by high-frequency stimulation) compared with conventional ablation was associated with greater freedom from AF for patients in paroxysmal AF (91% vs 71%) and persistent AF (81% vs 69%). However, in a very small recent study, the use of selective vagal denervation alone was ineffective in the seven paroxysmal AF patients studied, with only two of the seven

Table 105-1 Clinical Outcomes of Substrate Modification Strategies for Patients with Persistent Atrial Fibrillation

Study	Patients	No. of PsAF (%)	Follow-up (mo)	Technique	PVI (Confirmed)	Linear Lesions	Linear Block Confirmed	CFAE Ablation	Overall Success (PAF and PsAF)	Success in PsAF Group	% AADs in Successful PsAF Patients
Pappone et al, 2000	26	12 (46)	9 ± 3	CPVA	No	No	No	No	85%	83%	25%
Marrouche et al, 2003[58]	315	114 (36)	14 ± 5	CPVA	N/S	No	N/S	No	90% (ICE group)	N/S	N/S
Oral et al, 2005[55]	80	80 (100)	9 ± 4	CPVA	No	Yes	No	Yes		68%	0%
Hsu et al, 2004[67]	116	106 (91)	12 ± 7	PVI + linear ablation	Yes	MI, Roof	Yes	No	81%	N/S	N/S
Fassini et al, 2005[50]	187	62 (33)	12	PVI + linear ablation	Yes	MI	Yes	No	N/S	74%	50%
Willems et al, 2006[49]	32	32 (100)	14-17	PVI + linear ablation	Yes	Roof, MI	Yes, 72% MI, 44% roof	No	69%	69%	0%
Beukema et al, 2005[5]	105	53 (51)	15 ± 5	CPVA + linear ablation	No	MI	No	No	82%	77%	44%
Oral et al, 2006[68]	146	146 (100)	12	CPVA + linear ablation	No	PLA, Roof, MI	No	No	74%	74%	0%
Bertaglia et al, 2006[56]	74	74 (100)	20 ± 6	CPVA + linear ablation	No	MI	Yes	No	70%	70%	64%
Calo et al, 2006[69]	80	80 (100)	14 ± 5	CPVA + linear ablation	No	MI	No	No	73% (85% biatrial group)	73% (85% biatrial group)	60% (52% biatrial group)
Nademanee et al, 2004[6]	121	64 (53)	12	CFAE ablation	No	No	No	Yes	91%	88%	13%
Oral et al, 2007[59]	100	100 (100)	13 ± 7	CFAE ablation	No	No	No	Yes	57%	57%	0%
Haisaguerre et al, 2005[70]	60	60 (100)	11 ± 6	PVI + EGM + linear ablation	Yes	Yes	Yes	Yes	95%	95%	8%

Note: Success is defined as freedom from AF or arrhythmia.

*After the final ablation procedure.

AADs, anti-arrhythmic drugs; CFAE, complex fractionated electrograms; CPVA, circumferential pulmonary vein ablation; EGM, electrogram-based ablation; ICE, intra-cardiac echo; MI, mitral isthmus; N/S, not stated in manuscript; PAF, paroxysmal atrial fibrillation; PLA, posterior left atrium; PsAF, persistent atrial fibrillation; PVI, pulmonary vein isolation.

patients remaining asymptomatic without antiarrhythmic therapy after 8 months of follow-up.[60]

Stepwise Ablation Approach Incorporating Electrogram-Based Ablation and Linear Ablation

The stepwise ablation approach incorporates all the previously described approaches by targeting all structures potentially contributing to the initiation and maintenance of AF.[7] Using this approach, pulmonary vein isolation, electrogram-based ablation of biatrial substrate, and linear ablation were performed in patients with chronic AF. Stepwise ablation was associated with acute AF termination in 83% of patients during catheter ablation. Each region was targeted in sequence and the impact of ablation was assessed by measurements of AFCL at the right and left atrial appendages. Structures outside the left atrium (coronary sinus, superior vena cava, and right atrium) are targeted based on electrogram morphology and frequency. Measurements of AFCL during ablation demonstrated simultaneous increase in both the left and right atrial appendage in 85% of patients. In the other 15% of patients, a disparate increase in left-to-right AFCL was observed. In these patients, ablation within the RA terminated AF. Linear roof and mitral isthmus ablation was performed in cases where AF persisted, and complete linear block was assessed after restoration of sinus rhythm.

Using this approach, we evaluated long-term clinical outcomes and arrhythmia recurrence in 153 consecutive patients with persistent AF. During a mean follow-up of 21 ± 10 months, we found that recurrence of AF or new-onset atrial tachycardia depended the mode of acute AF termination during the index ablation procedure. In 58 of 66 (88%) patients with AF termination during the index procedure, atrial tachycardia was the most prevalent arrhythmia during follow-up, while recurrent AF predominated in patients in whom AF could not be terminated. After repeat ablation procedures, sinus rhythm was maintained in 123 of 129 (95%) patients with AF termination compared to 12 of 24 (50%) patients without AF termination ($P < 0.001$). Based on this experience, we propose the use of AF termination as the endpoint for catheter ablation.

Effects of Atrial Substrate Ablation on Atrial Electrical and Mechanical Properties

The main concern with using extensive ablation for substrate modification is the deleterious effect on atrial mechanical function due to replacement of healthy myocardium with scar. Takahashi and colleagues demonstrated preservation of LA contractility after a mean follow-up period of 5 months after ablation in 40 consecutive patients with chronic AF.[61] In this study, areas of scar and low-voltage atrial tissue as assessed by electroanatomic mapping accounted for 31% ± 12% and 32% ± 17% of the total LA surface area respectively. The majority of the scar burden was related to ablation around the pulmonary veins: 20% ± 4% of LA surface, that is, two thirds of all low-voltage or scar regions. In contrast, ablation in all other regions in the atrium aiming at achieving local organization and slowing of AFCL was associated with relatively preserved atrial voltages and propagation velocity as well as recovery of atrial mechanical function.

Echocardiographic evaluation of patients undergoing pulmonary vein isolation and linear ablation for chronic AF also revealed favorable reverse modeling at 12 months of follow-up, with progressive decrease in LA dimensions (from 68.4 ± 8.1 mm to 60.7 ± 6.5mm, $P < 0.05$), improvement in LA emptying volume (from 2.67 ± 1.9 mL/m^2 to 4.7 ± 2.14 mL/m^2, $P = 0.015$), LA emptying fraction (from 5.5 ± 3.6% to 21.8 ± 11%, $P < 0.05$), and LA filling fraction (from 15 ± 7% to 30 ± 5%, $P < 0.05$). Significant improvement in LV ejection fraction from 53 ± 8.5% to 63 ± 7% ($P < 0.05$), improvement in diastolic filling parameters, and decline in severity of mitral regurgitation was also observed.[62] Significant improvement of the LA ejection fraction (17 ± 6% to 22 ± 5%, $P = 0.01$) measured using cine electron-beam computed tomography have also been reported at 6 months of follow-up.[63]

Use of Three-Dimensional Nonfluoroscopic Imaging for Atrial Substrate Ablation

A variety of navigation tools, such as LocaLisa (Medtronic, Minneapolis, MN), Ensite NavX (Endocardial Solution, Inc, St Paul, MN) and CARTO (Biosense-Webster, Diamond Bar, CA), can be used to assist with the procedure. Both NavX and CARTO systems offer algorithms for the analysis of CFAEs. CFAEs detected and characterized automatically, instead of relying on the operator's analysis of CFAEs, have been studied using the CARTO system.[64] Image integration with cardiac CT or MRI might improve the understanding of atrial anatomy, especially in patients with unusual pulmonary vein anatomy and left atrial enlargement. However, the accuracy of anatomic imaging to guide ablation will depend on the patient's volume status, the effects of respiration, and the cardiac rhythm, as well as the registration process. Nevertheless, these mapping systems might help determine the position of the ablation catheter more accurately than fluoroscopy alone and could potentially aid in evaluating the completeness of linear lesions. Routine use of three-dimensional nonfluoroscopic imaging might also reduce the radiation exposure during linear ablation.[65,66]

Conclusion

AF is clearly a heterogeneous disease entity with multiple mechanistic processes. Unlike paroxysmal AF, where pulmonary vein isolation is effective, this approach has limited efficacy in persistent AF, where atrial substrate modification is also necessary. Various substrate ablation approaches have been studied, but the principal techniques consist of pulmonary vein isolation in conjunction with electrogram-based ablation and linear ablation.

Electrogram-based ablation of atrial tissue requires understanding and interpretation of complex electrograms and the ability to systematically map and ablate sources maintaining fibrillation, with the endpoint of organizing and terminating AF. The development of mapping systems and catheters that provide global and instantaneous detection of atrial arrhythmia substrate, including complex electrograms, may help guide ablation, thereby minimizing unnecessary ablation. Although linear ablation is performed on an anatomic basis without formally confirming conduction block in many centers, an incomplete line may be proarrhythmic. Hence all lines constructed must be checked for conduction block as defined by strict electrophysiologic criteria. Better mapping and ablating catheters and energy sources and better tailoring of ablation lesion sets to the individual patient will improve procedural outcomes for persistent AF in the future.

References

1. Sahadevan J, Ryu K, Peltz L, et al: Epicardial mapping of chronic atrial fibrillation in patients: Preliminary observations. Circulation 110(21):3293-3299, 2004.
2. Sanders P, Nalliah CJ, Dubois R, et al: Frequency mapping of the pulmonary veins in paroxysmal versus permanent atrial fibrillation. J Cardiovasc Electrophysiol 17(9):965-972, 2006.
3. Allessie M, Ausma J, Schotten U: Electrical, contractile and structural remodeling during atrial fibrillation. Cardiovasc Res 54(2):230-246, 2002.
4. Everett TH, Wilson EE, Verheule S, et al: Structural atrial remodeling alters the substrate and spatiotemporal organization of atrial fibrillation: A comparison in canine models of structural and electrical atrial remodeling. Am J Physiol Heart Circ Physiol 291(6):H2911-H2923, 2006.
5. Neuberger HR, Schotten U, Blaauw Y, et al: Chronic atrial dilation, electrical remodeling, and atrial fibrillation in the goat. J Am Coll Cardiol 47(3):644-653, 2006.
6. Nademanee K, McKenzie J, Kosar E, et al: A new approach for catheter ablation of atrial fibrillation: Mapping of the electrophysiologic substrate. J Am Coll Cardiol 43(11):2044-2053, 2004.
7. Jais P, O'Neill MD, Takahashi Y, et al: Regional disparities of endocardial atrial activation in paroxysmal atrial fibrillation. Pacing Clin Electrophysiol 19(11):1998-2003, 1996.
8. Haissaguerre M, Hocini M, Sanders P, et al: Localized sources maintaining atrial fibrillation organized by prior ablation. Circulation 113(5):616-625, 2006.
9. Haissaguerre M, Sanders P, Hocini M, et al: Catheter ablation of long-lasting persistent atrial fibrillation: Critical structures for termination. J Cardiovasc Electrophysiol 16(11):1125-1137, 2005.
10. Nademanee K: Trials and travails of electrogram-guided ablation of chronic atrial fibrillation. Circulation 115(20):2592-2594, 2007.
11. Kalifa J, Tanaka K, Zaitsev AV, et al: Mechanisms of wave fractionation at boundaries of high-frequency excitation in the posterior left atrium of the isolated sheep heart during atrial fibrillation. Circulation 113(5):626-633, 2006.
12. Rostock T, Rotter M, Sanders P, et al: High-density activation mapping of fractionated electrograms in the atria of patients with paroxysmal atrial fibrillation. Heart Rhythm 3(1):27-34, 2006.
13. Lin J, Scherlag BJ, Zhou J, et al: Autonomic mechanism to explain complex fractionated atrial electrograms (CFAE). J Cardiovasc Electrophysiol 18(11):1197-1205, 2007.
14. Lazar S, Dixit S, Marchlinski FE, et al: Presence of left-to-right atrial frequency gradient in paroxysmal but not persistent atrial fibrillation in humans. Circulation 110(20):3181-3186, 2004.
15. Sanders P, Berenfeld O, Hocini M, et al: Spectral analysis identifies sites of high-frequency activity maintaining atrial fibrillation in humans. Circulation 112(6): 789-797, 2005.
16. Lin YJ, Tai CT, Kao T, et al: Frequency analysis in different types of paroxysmal atrial fibrillation. J Am Coll Cardiol 47(7):1401-1407, 2006.
17. Huang JL, Tai CT, Lin YJ, et al: The mechanisms of an increased dominant frequency in the left atrial posterior wall during atrial fibrillation in acute atrial dilatation. J Cardiovasc Electrophysiol 17(2):178-188, 2006.
18. Berenfeld O, Zaitsev AV, Mironov SF, et al: Frequency-dependent breakdown of wave propagation into fibrillatory conduction across the pectinate muscle network in the isolated sheep right atrium. Circ Res 90(11):1173-1180, 2002.
19. Ryu K, Sahadevan J, Khrestian CM, et al: Use of fast Fourier transform analysis of atrial electrograms for rapid characterization of atrial activation—implications for delineating possible mechanisms of atrial tachyarrhythmias. J Cardiovasc Electrophysiol 17(2):198-206, 2006.
20. Ng J, Kadish AH, Goldberger JJ: Effect of electrogram characteristics on the relationship of dominant frequency to atrial activation rate in atrial fibrillation. Heart Rhythm 3(11):1295-1305, 2006.
21. Ng J, Kadish AH, Goldberger JJ: Technical considerations for dominant frequency analysis. J Cardiovasc Electrophysiol 18(7):757-764, 2007.
22. Chevalier P, Tabib A, Meyronnet D, et al: Quantitative study of nerves of the human left atrium. Heart Rhythm 2(5):518-522, 2005.
23. Lemery R: How to perform ablation of the parasympathetic ganglia of the left atrium. Heart Rhythm 3(10):1237-1239, 2006.
24. Hou Y, Scherlag BJ, Lin J, et al: Ganglionated plexi modulate extrinsic cardiac autonomic nerve input: Effects on sinus rate, atrioventricular conduction, refractoriness, and inducibility of atrial fibrillation. J Am Coll Cardiol 50(1):61-68, 2007.
25. Patterson E, Po SS, Scherlag BJ, Lazzara R: Triggered firing in pulmonary veins initiated by in vitro autonomic nerve stimulation. Heart Rhythm 2(6):624-631, 2005.
26. Zhou J, Scherlag BJ, Edwards J, et al: Gradients of atrial refractoriness and inducibility of atrial fibrillation due to stimulation of ganglionated plexi. J Cardiovasc Electrophysiol 18(1):83-90, 2007.
27. Po SS, Scherlag BJ, Yamanashi WS, et al: Experimental model for paroxysmal atrial fibrillation arising at the pulmonary vein-atrial junctions. Heart Rhythm 3(2):201-208, 2006.
28. Takahashi Y, Jais P, Hocini M, et al: Shortening of fibrillatory cycle length in the pulmonary vein during vagal excitation. J Am Coll Cardiol 47(4):774-780, 2006.
29. Scherlag BJ, Nakagawa H, Jackman WM, et al: Electrical stimulation to identify neural elements on the heart: Their role in atrial fibrillation. J Interv Card Electrophysiol 13(Suppl 1):37-42, 2005.
30. Lemery R, Birnie D, Tang ASL, et al: Feasibility study of endocardial mapping of ganglionated plexuses during catheter ablation of atrial fibrillation. Heart Rhythm 3(4):387-396, 2006.
31. Verma A, Saliba WI, Lakkireddy D, et al: Vagal responses induced by endocardial left atrial autonomic ganglion stimulation before and after pulmonary vein antrum isolation for atrial fibrillation. Heart Rhythm 4(9):1177-1182, 2007.
32. Pappone C, Santinelli V, Manguso F, et al: Pulmonary vein denervation enhances long-term benefit after circumferential ablation for paroxysmal atrial fibrillation. Circulation 109(3):327-334, 2004.
33. Takahashi Y, O'Neill MD, Hocini M, et al: Characterization of electrograms associated with termination of chronic atrial fibrillation by catheter ablation. J Am Coll Cardiol 51(10):1003-1010, 2008.
34. Takahashi Y, Jais P, Hocini M, et al: AB25-3: Sites of termination of chronic atrial fibrillation by catheter ablation. Heart Rhythm 3(5 Supp 1):S52, 2006.
35. Kamohara K, Popovic' ZB, Daimon M, et al: Impact of left atrial appendage exclusion on left atrial function. J Thoracic Cardiovasc Surg 133(1):174-181, 2007.
36. Haissaguerre M, Hocini M, Takahashi Y, et al: Impact of catheter ablation of the coronary sinus on paroxysmal or persistent atrial fibrillation. J Cardiovasc Electrophysiol 18(4):378-386, 2007.
37. Takahashi Y, Jais P, Hocini M, et al: Acute occlusion of the left circumflex coronary artery during mitral isthmus linear ablation. J Cardiovasc Electrophysiol 16(10):1104-1107, 2005.
38. Jalife J, Berenfeld O, Mansour M: Mother rotors and fibrillatory conduction: A mechanism of atrial fibrillation. Cardiovasc Res 54(2):204-216, 2002.
39. Arora R, Verheule S, Scott L, et al: Arrhythmogenic substrate of the pulmonary veins assessed by high-resolution optical mapping. Circulation 107(13): 1816-1821, 2003.
40. Elayi CS, Fahmy TS, Wazni OM, et al: Left superior vena cava isolation in patients undergoing pulmonary vein antrum isolation: Impact on atrial fibrillation recurrence. Heart Rhythm 3(9):1019-1023, 2006.
41. Saksena S, Skadsberg ND, Rao HB, Filipecki A: Biatrial and three-dimensional mapping of spontaneous atrial arrhythmias in patients with refractory atrial fibrillation. J Cardiovasc Electrophysiol 16(5):494-504, 2005.
42. Haissaguerre M, Hocini M, Sanders P, et al: Localized fibrillatory sources maintaining atrial fibrillation. Heart Rhythm 2(5, Supplement 1):S20, 2005.
43. Schuessler RB, Kawamoto T, Hand DE, et al: Simultaneous epicardial and endocardial activation sequence mapping in the isolated canine right atrium. Circulation 88(1):250-263, 1993.
44. Kneller J, Zou R, Vigmond EJ, et al: Cholinergic atrial fibrillation in a computer model of a two-dimensional sheet of canine atrial cells with realistic ionic properties. Circ Res 90(9):73e-87e, 2002.
45. Rostock T, Rotter M, Sanders P, et al: Fibrillating areas isolated within the left

atrium after radiofrequency linear catheter ablation. J Cardiovasc Electrophysiol 17(8):807-812, 2006.
46. Haissaguerre M, Sanders P, Hocini M, et al: Changes in atrial fibrillation cycle length and inducibility during catheter ablation and their relation to outcome. Circulation 109(24):3007-3013, 2004.
47. Jais P, Hocini M, Hsu LF, et al: Technique and results of linear ablation at the mitral isthmus. Circulation 110(19):2996-3002, 2004.
48. Hocini M, Jais P, Sanders P, et al: Techniques, evaluation, and consequences of linear block at the left atrial roof in paroxysmal atrial fibrillation: A prospective randomized study. Circulation 112(24):3688-3696, 2005.
49. Willems S, Klemm H, Rostock T, et al: Substrate modification combined with pulmonary vein isolation improves outcome of catheter ablation in patients with persistent atrial fibrillation: A prospective randomized comparison. Eur Heart J 27(23):2871-2878, 2006.
50. Fassini G, Riva S, Chiodelli R, et al: Left mitral isthmus ablation associated with PV isolation: Long-term results of a prospective randomized study. J Cardiovasc Electrophysiol 16(11):1150-1156, 2005.
51. Sanders P, Jais P, Hocini M, et al: Electrophysiologic and clinical consequences of linear catheter ablation to transect the anterior left atrium in patients with atrial fibrillation. Heart Rhythm 1(2):176-184, 2004.
52. Calkins H, Brugada J, Packer DL, et al: HRS/EHRA/ECAS expert Consensus Statement on catheter and surgical ablation of atrial fibrillation: recommendations for personnel, policy, procedures and follow-up. A report of the Heart Rhythm Society (HRS) Task Force on catheter and surgical ablation of atrial fibrillation. Heart Rhythm 4(6):816-861, 2007.
53. Pappone C, Santinelli V: Atrial fibrillation ablation: State of the art. Am J Cardiol 96(12 Suppl 1):59-64, 2005.
54. Pappone C, Manguso F, Vicedomini G, et al: Prevention of iatrogenic atrial tachycardia after ablation of atrial fibrillation: A prospective randomized study comparing circumferential pulmonary vein ablation with a modified approach. Circulation 110(19):3036-3042, 2004.
55. Oral H, Chugh A, Good E, et al: Randomized comparison of encircling and nonencircling left atrial ablation for chronic atrial fibrillation. Heart Rhythm 2(11):1165-1172, 2005.
56. Bertaglia E, Stabile G, Senatore G, et al: Long-term outcome of right and left atrial radiofrequency ablation in patients with persistent atrial fibrillation. Pacing Clin Electrophysiol 29(2):153-158, 2006.
57. Beukema WP, Elvan A, Sie HT, et al: Successful radiofrequency ablation in patients with previous atrial fibrillation results in a significant decrease in left atrial size. Circulation 112(14):2089-2095, 2005.
58. Marrouche NF, Martin DO, Wazni O, et al: Phased-array intracardiac echocardiography monitoring during pulmonary vein isolation in patients with atrial fibrillation: Impact on outcome and complications. Circulation 107(21):2710-2716, 2003.
59. Oral H, Chugh A, Good E, et al: Radiofrequency catheter ablation of chronic atrial fibrillation guided by complex electrograms. Circulation 115(20):2606-2612, 2007.
60. Scanavacca M, Pisani CF, Hachul D, et al: Selective atrial vagal denervation guided by evoked vagal reflex to treat patients with paroxysmal atrial fibrillation. Circulation 114(9):876-885, 2006.
61. Takahashi Y, O'Neill MD, Hocini M, et al: Effects of stepwise ablation of chronic atrial fibrillation on atrial electrical and mechanical properties. J Am Coll Cardiol 49(12):1306-1314, 2007.
62. Reant P, Lafitte S, Jais P, et al: Reverse remodeling of the left cardiac chambers after catheter ablation after 1 year in a series of patients with isolated atrial fibrillation. Circulation 112(19):2896-2903, 2005.
63. Verma A, Kilicaslan F, Adams JR, et al: Extensive ablation during pulmonary vein antrum isolation has no adverse impact on left atrial function: An echocardiography and cine computed tomography analysis. J Cardiovasc Electrophysiol 17(7):741-746, 2006.
64. Scherr D, Dalal D, Cheema A, et al: Automated detection and characterization of complex fractionated atrial electrograms in human left atrium during atrial fibrillation. Heart Rhythm 4(8):1013-1020, 2007.
65. Rotter M, Takahashi Y, Sanders P, et al: Reduction of fluoroscopy exposure and procedure duration during ablation of atrial fibrillation using a novel anatomical navigation system. Eur Heart J 26(14):1415-1421, 2005.
66. Takahashi Y, Rotter M, Sanders P, et al: Left atrial linear ablation to modify the substrate of atrial fibrillation using a new nonfluoroscopic imaging system. Pacing Clin Electrophysiol 28(Suppl 1):S90-S93, 2005.
67. Hsu LF, Jais P, Sanders P, et al: Catheter ablation for atrial fibrillation in congestive heart failure. N Engl J Med 351(23):2373-2383, 2004.
68. Oral H, Pappone C, Chugh A, et al: Circumferential pulmonary-vein ablation for chronic atrial fibrillation. N Engl J Med 354(9):934-941, 2006.
69. Calo L, Lamberti F, Loricchio ML, et al: Left atrial ablation versus biatrial ablation for persistent and permanent atrial fibrillation: A prospective and randomized study. J Am Coll Cardiol 47(12):2504-2512, 2006.
70. Haissaguerre M, Hocini M, Sanders P, et al: Catheter ablation of long-lasting persistent atrial fibrillation: Clinical outcome and mechanisms of subsequent arrhythmias. J Cardiovasc Electrophysiol 16(11):1138-1147, 2005.

Pulmonary Vein Isolation for Atrial Fibrillation 106

CARLO PAPPONE AND VINCENZO SANTINELLI

CHAPTER OUTLINE

The poor success of pharmacologic therapy for atrial fibrillation (AF) has encouraged many investigators to explore alternative strategies.[1-9] Recent randomized studies have demonstrated that ablation strategy is superior to antiarrhythmic drug therapy in patients with paroxysmal/persistent AF[10-12] and more recently even in patients with chronic AF.[13] Whether this superiority translates into morbidity and mortality benefits remains to be demonstrated in future multicenter trials, possibly by making ablation techniques uniform.

The number of AF ablation procedures is growing worldwide, and shorter procedure times have resulted in a move to include patients with structural heart disease and long-lasting or permanent AF. Because of the excellent success rates reported by the pioneering groups and the attractiveness of a definitive cure for AF, many patients have begun seeking this curative approach and many electrophysiologists and centers have begun to offer it according to the new guidelines for AF treatment.

From 1999 to 2007 we performed in Milan at the San Raffaele University Hospital more than 15,000 AF ablation procedures with an overall long-term success greater than 90% in paroxysmal/persistent AF and 80% in permanent AF, with an acceptably low incidence of major complications. Despite the development of newer technologies and tools, mechanisms of AF are numerous, and many of them remain unknown. In 2004, we first demonstrated the benefit of vagal denervation in patients with *paroxysmal* AF undergoing AF ablation, and these observations remain a cornerstone in the understanding of AF pathophysiology and treatment. However, at present we need to have more information on the pathophysiology of *permanent* AF to tailor or limit ablation targets because patients with long-lasting or permanent AF require an extensive ablation with repeat procedures. Data from our laboratory indicate that progression from first paroxysmal AF to persistent or permanent AF is relatively rapid and can be predicted by clinical variables.[14] As a result, identification of subjects at high risk for progression is useful for optimal timing of ablation, avoiding a late procedure when AF becomes permanent.

Currently, ablation strategies for permanent AF and associated structural heart disease are complex, time consuming, and less effective and are associated with higher risk of complications. Since 2005, pioneering groups have confirmed our previous results even in patients with permanent AF, using the stepwise tailored approach, which includes sequential additional ablation targets with repeated procedures limiting or modifying the anatomic, electrophysiologic, or autonomic substrates.[15] If elimination of the substrate is indeed crucial for the outcome, then mapping and navigation systems should be able to exactly visualize the complexity of the anatomy of the left atrium (LA) to place lesions accurately, avoiding unnecessary and dangerous radiofrequency (RF) applications to compensate for inaccuracy (Fig. 106-1).

Circumferential Pulmonary Vein Ablation

Circumferential pulmonary vein ablation (CPVA) is the standard procedure as performed in Milan at the San Raffaele University Hospital. The procedure is performed by manual catheters or remotely by magnetic soft catheters in shorter time as compared with other approaches.[16] CPVA consists of large circumferential lesion lines to perform a point-by-point tailored distal disconnection of all pulmonary veins, vagal denervation, wide encircled areas with additional standard lesion lines, and noninducibility of both AF and atrial tachycardia (AT) at the end of the procedure. Accumulating data from our laboratory indicate that among patients with paroxysmal or persistent AF without enlarged atria, the CPVA alone is associated with an excellent outcome, but in patients with long-lasting, persistent, or permanent AF and enlarged atria, further linear lesions using the least amount of ablation is necessary to achieve noninducibility.

Endpoints

The goal of catheter ablation is elimination of the trigger and modification of the substrate using the least amount of ablation necessary. Restoration of stable sinus rhythm and no inducibility of AF or AT at the end of the procedure is the gold standard of CPVA. However, in most patients with long-lasting or permanent AF, after achieving sinus rhythm at the end of the procedure, sustained AF or AT is still inducible, requiring further linear lesions in the left atrium (LA) to achieve noninducibility. Procedural endpoints of standard CPVA include pulmonary vein electrical disconnection, vagal denervation, and posterior lines with the mitral isthmus line, and further limited linear lesions, including coronary sinus (CS) disconnection, are the last targets. Endpoints are obtained with a single mapping-and-ablation catheter. At present, we do not use balloon technology because our approach is not limited to pulmonary vein disconnection alone and the achievement of multiple targets precludes its use. In addition, pulmonary veins have largely variable anatomies from patient to patient, with a wide range of diameters and the regular presence of common ostia in up to 30% of patients, which makes balloon technology challenging.

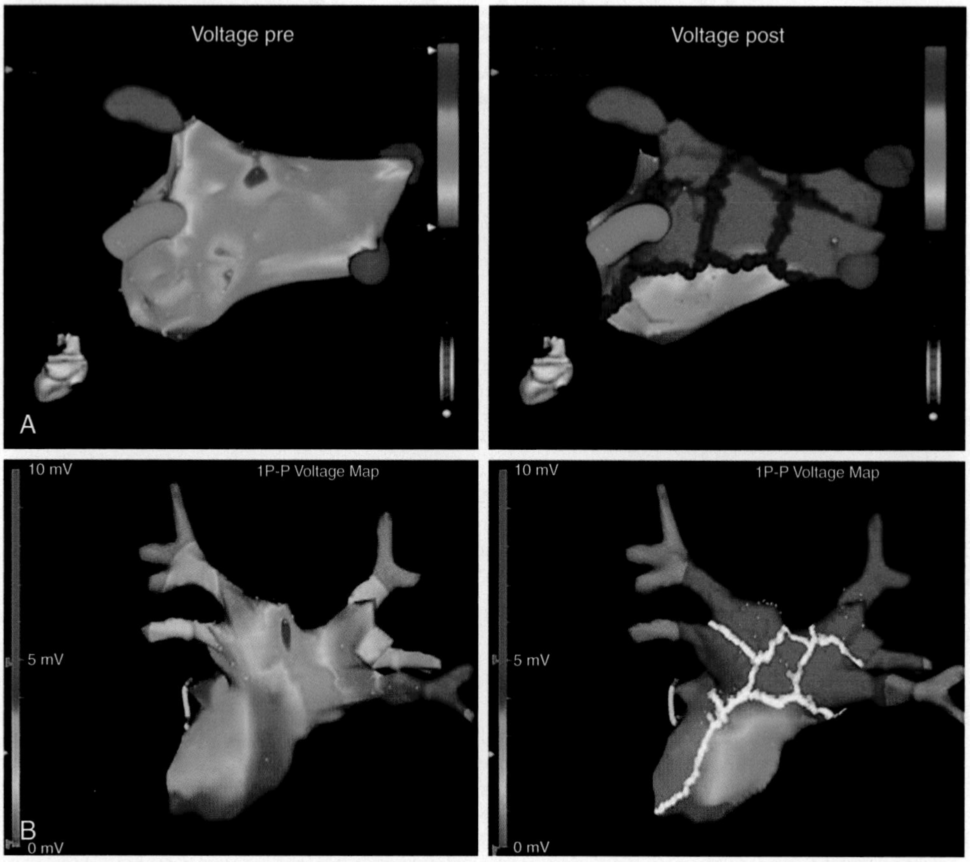

Figure 106-1 Pre- and postablation color-coded voltage maps of the left atrium by CARTO **(A)** and NavX **(B)** systems. Typical circumferential lesions as performed by circumferential pulmonary vein ablation are shown in the posteroanterior anatomic view. Note that inside *red areas* no voltage gradients are evident.

Disconnection of the Pulmonary Veins

Circumferential lines are aimed at atrial tissue *outside* the ostium of the pulmonary veins, an area often termed the *antrum* (see Fig. 106-1). The lesions are designed to encircle the left and right pulmonary veins individually or in pairs. Validation of electrical isolation with a circular mapping catheter is not performed in our laboratory because we perform a true distal electrical isolation by potential abatement (>90% reduction of electrogram amplitude) even within the encircled areas (electrogram amplitude <0.1 mV). pulmonary vein disconnection is obtained by optimal catheter stability and wall contact, which results in rapid attenuation of atrial electrograms during each RF energy application up to complete elimination for up to 50 seconds, usually within a few seconds depending on the local effect (Fig. 106-2). Partially ablated signals require further RF applications before moving on to the next ablation site.

Autonomic Targets with Vagal Denervation

When possible, elimination of vagal reflexes at innervation sites during the procedure represents one of the most important endpoints because vagal denervation is a strong predictor for long-term success (Fig. 106-3). We first demonstrated that CPVA induces a long-term but transient vagal denervation, which enhances the efficacy of the procedure in the long-term outcome.[8] These results have been confirmed by many other authors with different AF ablation approaches, and now vagal denervation constitutes a new fascinating AF ablation strategy. Our results on modification of heart-rate variability parameters after ablation add new insights for the understanding of the mechanisms of AF and its treatment.

While performing the standard CPVA lesion set, RF applications evoke vagal reflexes in up to 30% of patients. Vagal reflexes are considered to include sinus bradycardia (<40 beats per minute), asystole, atrioventricular (AV) block, and hypotension that occurs within a few seconds after the onset of RF application (see Fig. 106-3). If a reflex is elicited, RF energy is delivered until such reflexes are abolished, or for up to 30 seconds. The endpoint of ablation at these sites is termination of the reflex, followed by sinus tachycardia or AF. Failure to reproduce the reflexes with repeated RF applications is considered confirmation of denervation. Complete local vagal denervation is defined by the abolition of all vagal reflexes. Based on our experience, we always attempt to elicit and then ablate potential sites of reflexes for vagal denervation. We reported a detailed autonomic map of the LA as a target for ablation showing that, like the left superior pulmonary vein, the septal region is richly innervated.[8]

Posterior and Mitral Isthmus Lines

In the standard CPVA, additional ablation lines are placed along the back and the roof of the LA between the two sets of pulmonary veins connecting the superior and inferior pulmonary veins and the mitral valve annulus (see Fig. 106-1). The mitral isthmus line is deployed to prevent postablation macroreentrant LA tachycardias[5,16,17] and to further reduce the substrate (see Fig. 106-3). Completeness of the mitral isthmus line is an important electrophysiologic endpoint, and it is validated during CS pacing by endocardial and CS mapping, looking for widely spaced double potentials across the line of block, and confirmed by differential pacing.[5] The minimum double-potential interval at the mitral isthmus during CS pacing after block is achieved is

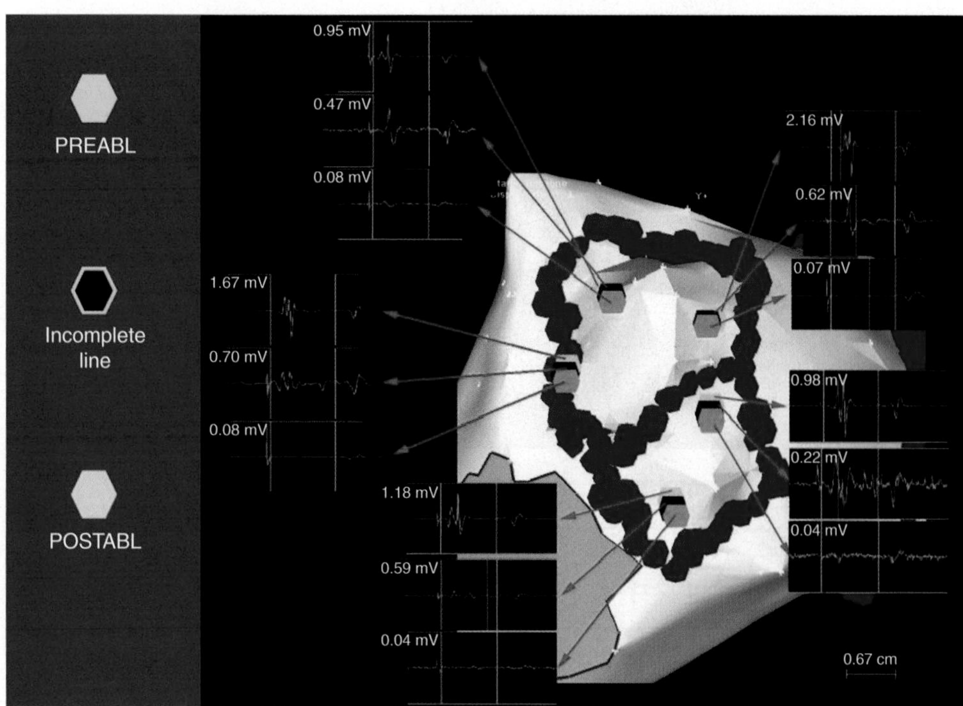

Figure 106-2 During radiofrequency applications, local atrial potentials on the lesion lines and within *encircled areas* become wider and lower *(black)*, completely disappearing *(light blue)* within 20 to 50 seconds.

150 ms, depending on the atrial dimensions and the extent of scarring and lesion creation.[5]

Cavotricuspid Isthmus Line

Patients with AF and a history of common atrial flutter or patients with permanent AF undergo ablation of the cavotricuspid isthmus line.

Noninducibility of Atrial Fibrillation and Atrial Tachycardia

If all endpoints are reached at the end of the standard CPVA and the patient is in sinus rhythm, noninducibility of AF or AT is the last endpoint.

Additional Linear Lesions and Coronary Sinus Disconnection

If AF or AT inducibility persists even after cardioversion, we revisit lesion lines and encircled areas to check for residual potentials and apply radiofrequency where needed. If necessary, adjunctive linear ablation (usually the roof, septum, or base of the LA appendage [LAA]) is performed before CS isolation, which is the last target (Fig. 106-4). Conduction block is assessed by the presence of a corridor of double potentials and demonstration of activation moving toward the line of block on both sides. A complete LA roof line may be demonstrated by activation progressing in a caudocranial direction on the posterior wall during LAA pacing. Rapid atrial activity from the musculature of the CS may be a driver for long-lasting or permanent AF. Electrical disconnection of the CS from the atrium is performed by endocardial or epicardial ablation (or both). Total elimination of CS activity is the ideal endpoint, but organization of CS activity or slowing of local rate with dissociation between CS and LA potential activity is also considered proof of CS isolation. Endocardial and epicardial CS sites are frequent ablation targets in patients with permanent AF and enlarged atria.

Postablation Remapping

Once AF and AT noninducibility has been achieved, the LA is remapped, and preablation and postablation activation maps are compared (see Fig. 106-1). In patients in sinus rhythm, postablation remapping of the LA is done using the preablation map for acquisition of new points to compare pre- and postablation bipolar voltage maps. In patients in AF, after sinus rhythm is restored, postablation remapping is performed using the anatomic map acquired during AF for accurate validation of the lesions. Incomplete block is revealed by impulse propagation across the line and requires further RF applications for completeness of the line despite noninducibility.

Ablation Procedure

Patient Selection

Patients with clear contraindications to anticoagulation (heparin or warfarin) therapy are not considered potential candidates for CPVA. CPVA may be performed in elderly patients up to 80 years of age who have permanent AF or aortic or mitral metallic prosthetic valves (or both). The procedure is indicated in symptomatic patients who have AF refractory to antiarrhythmic drug therapy or who wish an opportunity to have a long-term cure of AF, avoiding lifelong anticoagulation. Drug treatment for nonarrhythmic indications is generally continued. Although there is no consensus with regard to discontinuing antiarrhythmic drugs, to avoid confounding ablation effects, antiarrhythmic drugs except amiodarone and digoxin are discontinued for more than 5 half-lives. If symptomatic arrhythmias demand, effective antiarrhythmic drugs may be continued. A low left ventricular ejection fraction does not represent an absolute contraindication to CPVA.

Preprocedure Preparation

One month before ablation, transesophageal echocardiography (TEE) is the modality of choice to exclude LA or left atrial appendage thrombi, which are considered an absolute contraindication to the procedure. The procedure is postponed until

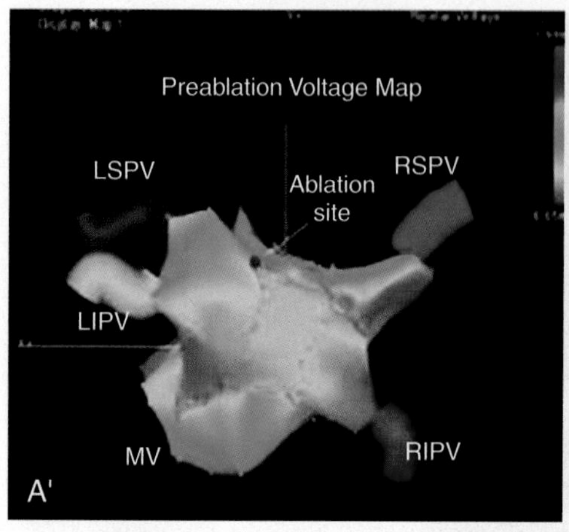

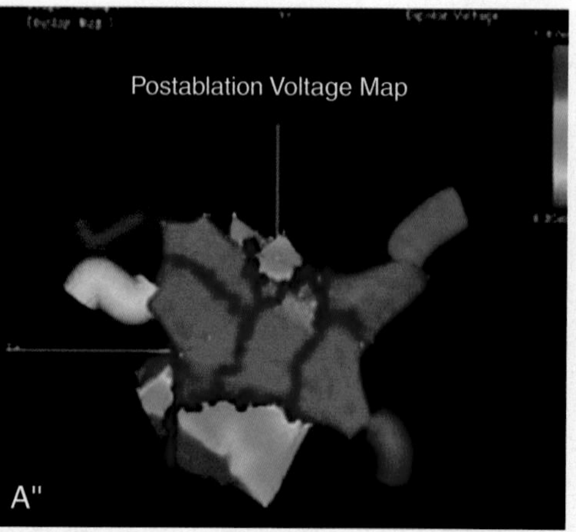

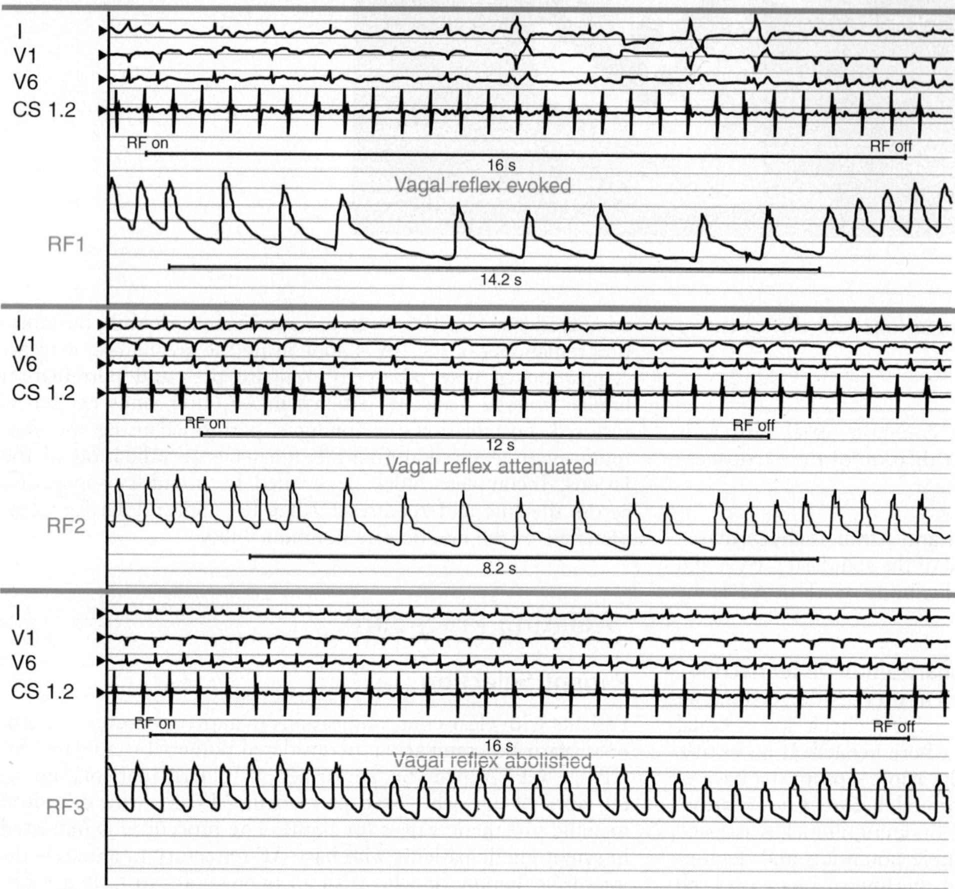

Figure 106-3 At the beginning of radiofrequency (RF) applications around the left superior pulmonary vein (ablation site on the preablation voltage map), a vagal reflex is elicited (RF1), attenuated (RF2), and then abolished (RF3). The ablation site at which the vagal reflex was evoked is included in the standard lesion set (postablation voltage map). As shown, the reflex resulted in hypotension and high-degree atrioventricular block. LIPV, left inferior pulmonary vein; LSPV, left superior pulmonary vein; MV, mitral valve; RIPV, right inferior pulmonary vein; RSPV, right superior pulmonary vein.

cardiac thrombi are excluded by a repeat TTE during anticoagulation therapy. In patients with permanent AF, an adequate and effective preablation anticoagulation therapy is necessary, and at least three consecutive international normalized ratio (INR) values ranging between 2.5 and 3.5 are required before the procedure. In addition, 24-hour Holter monitoring and daily transtelephonic random or symptom-triggered recordings are usually scheduled. A chest radiograph and laboratory tests are also required to exclude diseases that preclude anticoagulant therapy.

At admission, we perform a routine TTE. Three days before the procedure, patients taking anticoagulants stop oral anticoagulant therapy. The night before ablation, we start heparin infusion to achieve ACT (activated coagulation time) values between 200 and 250 seconds. Heparin is stopped just 2 hours before the procedure to safely perform the transseptal puncture. We also use a weight-adjusted infusion of an intravenous narcotic such as remifentanil (0.025-0.05 μg/kg per minute). Cardiac surgery should be promptly accessible to perform emergency surgical procedures as needed. Urgent bedside echocardiography in the EP laboratory should be available primarily for diagnosing pericardial tamponade. The medical personnel, nursing, and technical support staff must be appropriately trained and have adequate experience before starting AF ablation.

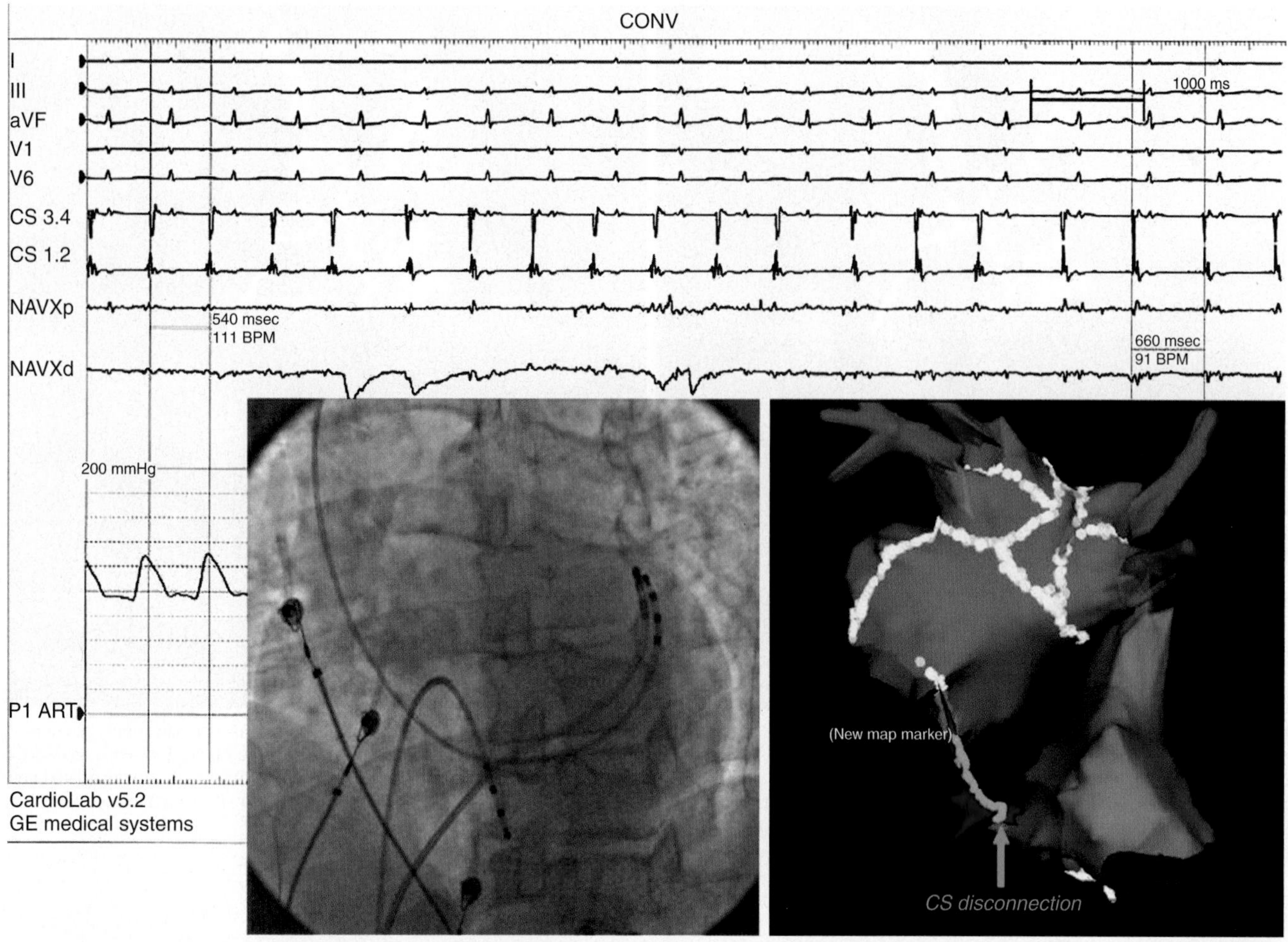

Figure 106-4 Anatomic map reconstructed by NavX guidance in a patient with permanent atrial fibrillation. After completing the standard circumferential pulmonary vein ablation lesion set, atrial fibrillation becomes more organized and slower, resembling an atrial tachycardia (cycle length, 540 ms). After coronary sinus (CS) disconnection, the arrhythmia promptly converts to sinus rhythm (cycle length, 660 ms). On the map, CS geometry is depicted in *red* and radiofrequency applications are tagged in *green*. CS disconnection is performed under electroanatomic guidance and fluoroscopy.

Procedure

Usually, before transseptal puncture, a catheter is placed into the CS to map for left atrial activity, and a multipolar catheter is placed inside the right atrium (RA) to map for right atrial activity. CPVA requires a single transseptal puncture for the mapping-ablation catheter. After transseptal access, a single bolus of intravenous heparin is administered, and two blood samples are taken every 15 minutes to monitor the activated clotting time, which needs to be 250 seconds, or more if necessary.

Identification of Ablation Targets

Accurately identifying and ablating targets in a relatively short period of time to avoid major complications is essential to successfully achieve all endpoints and an excellent long-term outcome. Currently, this is facilitated using three-dimensional (3-D) navigation and mapping systems, which provide accurate anatomic and electrophysiologic guidance. CPVA is being performed within 1 hour, but it can take longer (up to 3 hours) in patients with permanent AF and enlarged atria to achieve all endpoints, including CS disconnection and AF/AT noninducibility. We do not routinely use intracardiac echocardiography and lasso catheter.

Current Electroanatomic Mapping Systems: Advantages and Disadvantages

Generally, in evaluating the relative advantages of electroanatomic positioning systems, one must consider the need for accuracy, reproducibility, compatibility with ablation and mapping catheters, and cost issues when considering a specific system for a given patient.[16] One of the disadvantages of all catheter tracking systems is that they are operator dependent because they primarily require catheter movement to create the virtual geometry. Incomplete or inaccurate electroanatomic maps can result in deformed anatomy, difficult catheter navigation of planned ablation targets, or residual high-voltage occurrence in the lesion set. If a greater force is applied, the resulting virtual map appears to be deformed, leading to surface and volume overestimation. Better 3-D spatial resolution results in safer catheter navigation, more detailed maps, and ultimately facilitation of ablation targets at the desired endocardial sites (see Fig. 106-1). The possibility to catalog points of interest allows the operator to revisit sites of interest at any time to make contiguous and complete lesion lines.

We routinely use the CARTO (Biosense-Webster, Diamond Bar, CA) or the EnSite-NavX (St. Jude Medical, St. Paul, MN) systems for positioning of catheters in virtual 3-D space, which

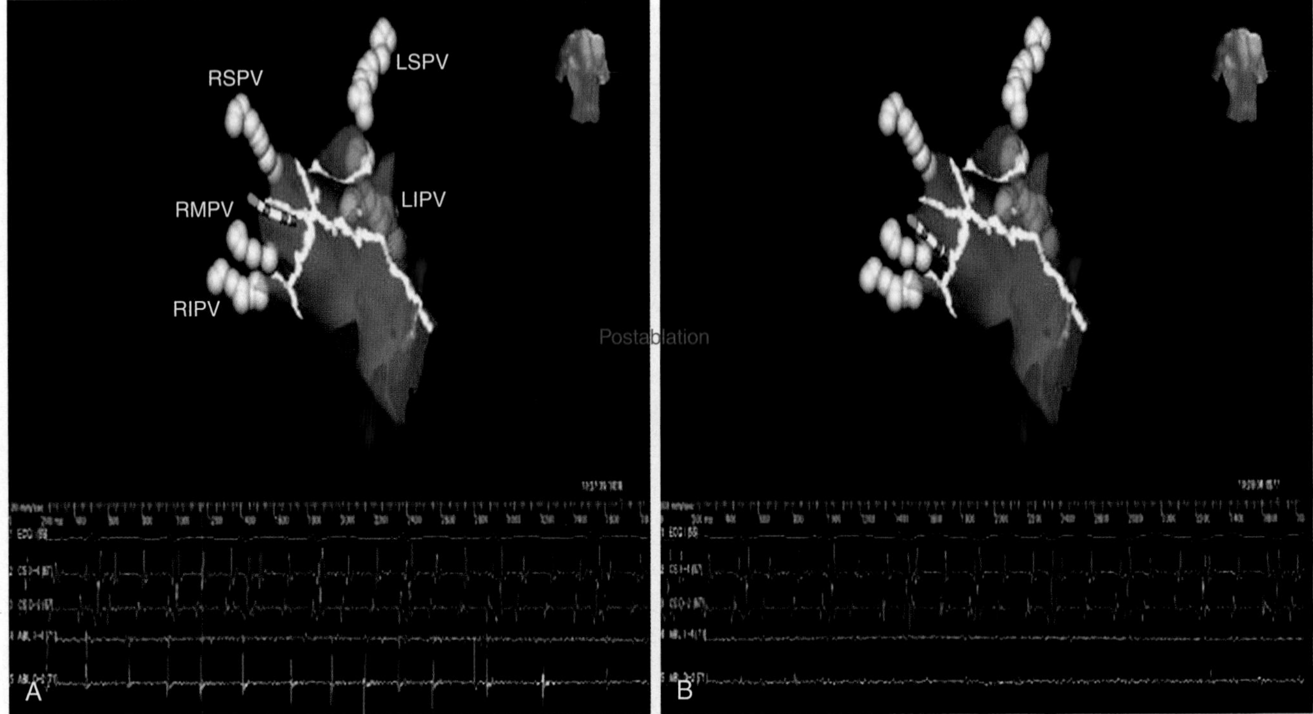

Figure 106-5 Postablation anatomic maps under NavX guidance of the left atrium with simultaneous intracardiac recordings. The coronary sinus geometry is represented in *red*. Note the shape of two catheters, one of which is inside the coronary sinus *(yellow)* as reference catheter and the other of which is around the right pulmonary vein (PV) ostium *(white with green tip)* for mapping and ablation. After ablation, local atrial potentials around the right superior PV are dissociated from the left atrium or are completely absent, indicating PV disconnection. LIPV, left inferior pulmonary vein; LSPV, left superior pulmonary vein; RIPV, right inferior pulmonary vein; RMPV, right middle pulmonary vein; RSPV, right superior pulmonary vein.

significantly shortens fluoroscopy time, enhancing safety (see Fig. 106-1). The early adoption by our group of the CARTO system many years ago allowed the first accurate reconstruction of the complex left atrial anatomy, resulting in its eventual widespread acceptance by the electrophysiologic community performing catheter ablation of AF.[2] The CARTO system localizes continuous catheter position using three ultra-low *magnetic* fields, and NavX system is based on *electrical* fields generated by three pairs orthogonal skin patches in x, y, and z axes (see Fig. 106-1).

Unlike CARTO, the recent NavX technology allows the operator to obtain a 3-D reconstruction of both the tip and the shaft of the catheter, which is particularly useful in challenging areas such as pulmonary veins ostia, the ridge, the mitral valve annulus, and the septal area. Monitoring of the ablation catheter by NavX is obtained by a proximity indicator that, based on the intensity of the color of the tip, allows the operator to monitor the optimal tissue contact of the ablation catheter, which, when associated to the atrial potential abatement, indicates the achievement of endpoints (see Fig. 106-1). During RF applications, cardiac motion, pain, and respiration all affect the stability of catheter positioning., but NavX software allows us to minimize the extent of moving targets as well as respiratory artifacts. When ablating the posterior wall, which is a vulnerable area at greater risk for cardiac perforation, pain can cause the patient to change his or her respiratory frequency, and a new respiratory compensation by NavX is useful for catheter stability. Also, NavX technology can create separately any desired anatomy for each ablation target, which results in more accurate ablation of challenging targets, particularly pulmonary veins ostia, their antrum, the posterior wall, and CS (Figs. 106-4 and 106-5). Although the Ensite NavX system allows us to collect many points rapidly and sequentially, in difficult areas we prefer to acquire points manually, as with the CARTO system.

Another important advantage of the NavX system as compared with CARTO is that patient movements during the procedure do not affect the reconstruction of the map because the reference catheter moves equally to the patches attached to the patient's body. As with the CARTO system, after ablation a voltage map is shown as color gradients to verify complete abatement on the lesion lines and within them (see Fig. 106-1). Currently, with both electroanatomic systems, in a few minutes we are able to reconstruct the LA anatomy with ablation targets. Reconstruction of pulmonary veins and their ostia represents the first step and is confirmed by simultaneous use of fluoroscopy, electrograms, and impedance gradients. Characteristically and simultaneously, once the catheter enters the pulmonary vein, the tip is seen outside cardiac shadow on fluoroscopy, the impedance values rise significantly ($\geq$4 Ω above left atrial impedance), and the atrial electrograms disappear.

Once pulmonary veins are displayed, a sequential detailed reconstruction of the LA, including the posterior and anterior walls, LAA, roof, septum, and mitral annulus with its isthmus, is performed. The septum and the channel between the LAA and the LSPV often require acquisition of many more points than other areas. The LAA, which is identified and confirmed by the presence of nonfractionated and high-amplitude atrial electrograms and large ventricular electrograms with organized electrical activity in AF, represents one of the latest areas to be mapped. The channel between LAA and LSPV shows potentials that characteristically are smaller than those of the LAA but higher and more fractionated than the rest of the LA. If this channel is not accurately reconstructed, the left-sided circumferential lesion may be deployed unsafely too close to the LAA or within the pulmonary vein ostium, which can result in poor efficacy and major complications such as LAA perforation or pulmonary vein stenosis. Although reconstruction of the roof is easier, requiring fewer points to be acquired, incorrect interpolation should be avoided when using the CARTO system.

Ablation of Desired Targets

Once the main pulmonary veins and LA have been adequately reconstructed, RF energy, which in our laboratory is the modality most commonly used for ablation, is delivered to the endocardial ablation targets to complete the lesion set while achieving the above-mentioned anatomic and electrophysiologic endpoints (see Fig. 106-1). Since 2004 we have used open-irrigation tip catheters instead of 8-mm non–irrigated-tip RF catheters; the 8-mm catheters have many limitations, including coagulum formation and insufficient power delivery in areas of low blood flow.[12] Irrigated ablation allows us to deliver adequate power to obtain larger lesion size and volume compared with traditional RF catheters, minimizing the risk of embolic events.

In our approach, efficacy of RF application is and remains important but we tailor RF applications because safety is crucial, particularly in challenging areas. Usually, at constantly lower power settings (30-50 W), we use a baseline irrigation rate of 2 mL/min (during mapping) and up to 50 mL/min depending on the location of ablation targets. RF applications are delivered at a distance at least 1 cm from the ostia (wider than 5mm, as previously used) to create circumferential lesions while reducing the risk of pulmonary vein stenosis (see Fig. 106-1). If there is an impedance rise ($\geq 10\ \Omega$) or burning pain, RF application is stopped immediately.

When ablation starts, the irrigation rate is raised from 2 to 17 mL/min, and impedance and tip temperature values are continuously monitored. Energy output is limited to 50 W and 48° C throughout the entire ablation procedure, but lower values are used in the posterior wall and into the CS to reduce the risk of injury to the surrounding structures. Usually, circumferential lesion lines are performed, starting at the lateral mitral annulus and withdrawing posteriorly, then anterior to the left-sided pulmonary vein, passing on the ridge between LSPV and LAA before completing the circumferential line on the posterior wall. The right pulmonary veins are isolated in a similar fashion, and then two posterior lines connecting the two circumferential lines are deployed. Circumferential lines are tailored according to the individual anatomy of the pulmonary vein–left atrial junction. A single large circumferential line around two ipsilateral pulmonary veins is performed in the presence of ostia less than 20 mm apart from each other, a common ostium with early branching, or separately branching pulmonary vein. If it is anatomically possible (four separate pulmonary vein ostia), we also perform a lesion line between the two pulmonary veins ostia to further reduce the electrophysiologic and anatomic substrate (see Fig. 106-1).

Characteristically, in patients with permanent AF and enlarged atria, often while delivering RF energy within the CS and before conversion of AF to sinus rhythm, we observe a gradual prolongation and stabilization of AF cycle length resembling an organized AT with uniform P-wave morphology (Fig. 106-6). With our approach there is a conversion to SR in almost all patients with permanent AF. Permanent AF converts either directly to SR or via the ablation of intermediate AT. The procedure is considered successfully completed only when all acute endpoints are fully met.

Challenging Ablation Targets

Achievement of all endpoints is crucial but it may be challenging in specific areas.[16] Usually, repeat RF applications of short duration, greater power, and higher irrigation rates are necessary around the LSPV where atrial electrogram potentials may be difficult to eliminate. Complete abatement of atrial potentials in the ridge between the LSPV and LAA also requires repeat and longer RF applications with higher-power delivery settings. If the ridge is too narrow, the ablation line is performed at the base of LAA.

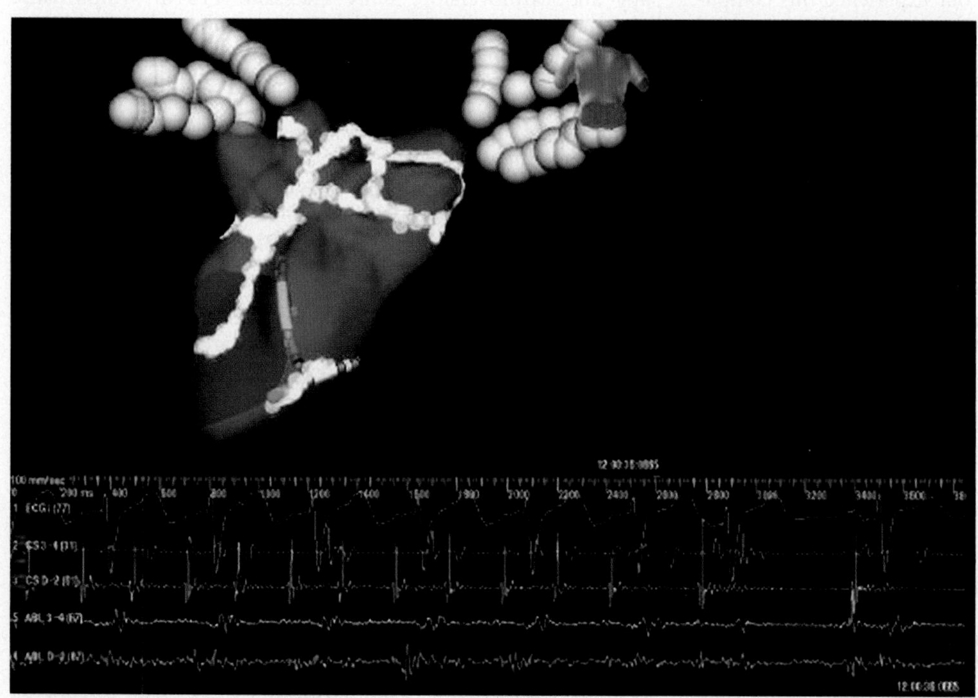

Figure 106-6 Postablation anatomic maps under NavX guidance with simultaneous intracardiac recordings in a patient with permanent atrial fibrillation. The coronary sinus shape catheter is represented in *yellow* and the tip-irrigated ablation catheter in *green*. After completing the lesion set, atrial fibrillation still persists but becomes slower and more organized. An additional ablation line to further reduce the substrate results in a further increase of the cycle length before conversion to sinus rhythm.

The right-sided pulmonary vein area and the mitral isthmus also represent two difficult sites for mapping and ablation, requiring continuous adjustment of delivery settings and irrigation rates to achieve the desired endpoint. Incomplete lesion lines, particularly the mitral isthmus line, can result in residual gaps and postablation incessant left AT.[17,18] In patients with mitral or aortic metallic prosthetic valves, mapping and ablation in the mitral area may be challenging, but no case of catheter entrapment in the mitral valve has ever occurred. The mitral isthmus line requires validation of disconnection with pacing maneuvers and, in a large minority of patients, further RF applications within CS are required.

Ablation of connection sites between CS and atrial musculature requires strict attention to lower energy settings and lower irrigation rates to avoid perforation and cardiac tamponade. Usually we deliver two short low-energy sequential RF applications (usually between 15 and 30 W) by dragging the catheter in a distal-to-proximal direction, instead of performing a single application, in order to keep the temperature down and avoid potential complications (see Fig. 106-6). The posterior wall also represents a vulnerable area for possible complications such as cardiac perforation and esophageal injury with tip-irrigated catheters. It is well known that the posterior wall is the thinnest area of the LA, and it lies in close proximity to the esophagus as well. While applying RF energy on this region, we use lower-energy delivery settings, shorter RF applications, and lower irrigation rates whenever ablation is performed.

Clinical Outcomes

Postprocedure Management and Complications

At the end of the procedure, usually we use intravenous protamine to permit removal of sheaths. Afterward, the management consists of continuing and maintaining anticoagulation by heparin and then oral anticoagulation. The possibility to tailor RF applications, energy settings, irrigation rates in vulnerable areas minimizes major complications.

Pericardial tamponade must be excluded in patients with postprocedural hypotension, but in our experience this complication is very rare if one uses a careful titration of RF power and duration delivery, particularly in challenging areas, thus reducing tissue boiling and endocardial rupture. Only a few patients have required pericardiocentesis for cardiac tamponade, and a case of nonfatal esophageal fistula has occurred. The late occurrence (6-10 days after ablation) of a febrile state with or without neurologic symptoms should prompt suspicion of an atrio-esophageal fistula, which should be excluded by contrast-enhanced spiral CT.

In our extensive experience of more than 15,000 procedures, no case of death or other major complications such as significant pulmonary vein stenosis, phrenic nerve injury, or acute coronary artery occlusion has occurred after CPVA. Minor complications occur rarely, and small, nonhemodynamically significant pericardial effusion develops in up to 4% of patients.[16] Pericarditic discomfort can occur during the first days, and aspirin is an adequate treatment.

Rhythm Outcome

The absence of symptoms might not correspond to stable restoration of sinus rhythm, and the accuracy of evaluating postablation recurrences depends mostly on the duration of ECG recording. Usually, after ablation we schedule 24- to 48-hour Holter recordings at 1, 3, 6, and 12 months and daily transtelephonic ECG monitoring, supplemented by ECG transmission, up to 1e year after the index procedure to assess the burden of asymptomatic recurrences.[12,13,16]

Efficacy

Early recurrences of AF after the index procedure usually occur within the first 2 months,[5] but in half of cases they are a transient phenomenon not requiring a revision procedure. Long-term efficacy of CPVA is more than 90% for patients with paroxysmal AF and about 85% for permanent AF once AF and AT noninducibility has been achieved at the end of the procedure. In patients with paroxysmal AF and local vagal denervation, the long-term success rate is higher. If recurrence of persistent AF or monthly episodes of symptomatic paroxysmal AF occur beyond the first month after ablation or incessant highly symptomatic left or right atrial flutter is present, then a second procedure is scheduled at 6 months after the index procedure. A maximum of three ablation procedures per patient are allowed.

Atrial Remodeling

The assessment of potential consequences of RF ablation on the LA contractility is important for a potential relationship to thromboembolic risk. After ablation, we carefully evaluate the left atrial transport function before and after the procedure and serially during the long-term follow-up. In our experience, after ablation the LA diameters decrease and LA contractile function is improved but the magnitude of this benefit mainly depends on the atrial dimensions before ablation.[12,13] In patients without recurrences and with improved atrial transport and function (reverse atrial remodeling) we discontinue chronic anticoagulation therapy.

Postablation Atrial Tachycardia

If endpoints are successfully achieved in the index procedure, postablation ATs develop in less than 5% of patients,[5] and usually they are macro- or micro-reentrant gap-related rather than focal tachycardias (Fig. 106-7). In our extensive experience, these ATs should initially be treated conservatively, with medical therapy and cardioversion. Only incessant ATs in symptomatic patients require a repeat procedure to optimize ablation therapy, which leads to a cure in most cases.[5,16,17]

Ablation should be tailored to the arrhythmia mechanism rather than performing empiric lesion lines. The 12-lead ECG with P-wave morphology and axis evaluation should be closely inspected initially because continuous activation suggests a macro-reentrant mechanism, whereas a clear isoelectric baseline between P waves suggests a focal mechanism. We routinely perform both activation and voltage maps combined with entrainment pacing maneuvers to optimize the ablation therapy. Usually, the activation map reveals earliest and latest activations in different colors relative to the reference site within a time window equal to the tachycardia cycle length. The commonest postablation AT is macroreentrant (>80% of the cycle length) mitral annular tachycardia.

Entrainment with postpacing intervals (PPI) approximately equal to the tachycardia cycle length (TCL) from three or more sites around the superior and inferior mitral annulus, with an activation time around the mitral annulus approximately equal to the AT cycle length, strongly suggests a mitral annular AT. Like the right atrial isthmus dependent flutter, the narrowest area of the circuit is between the LIPV and the mitral annulus and the most appropriate approach is to perform reablation of the mitral isthmus, looking for residual gaps. For focal micro-reentrant ATs (<80% of the cycle length) originating from reconnected pulmonary vein ostia, ablation of sites with earliest

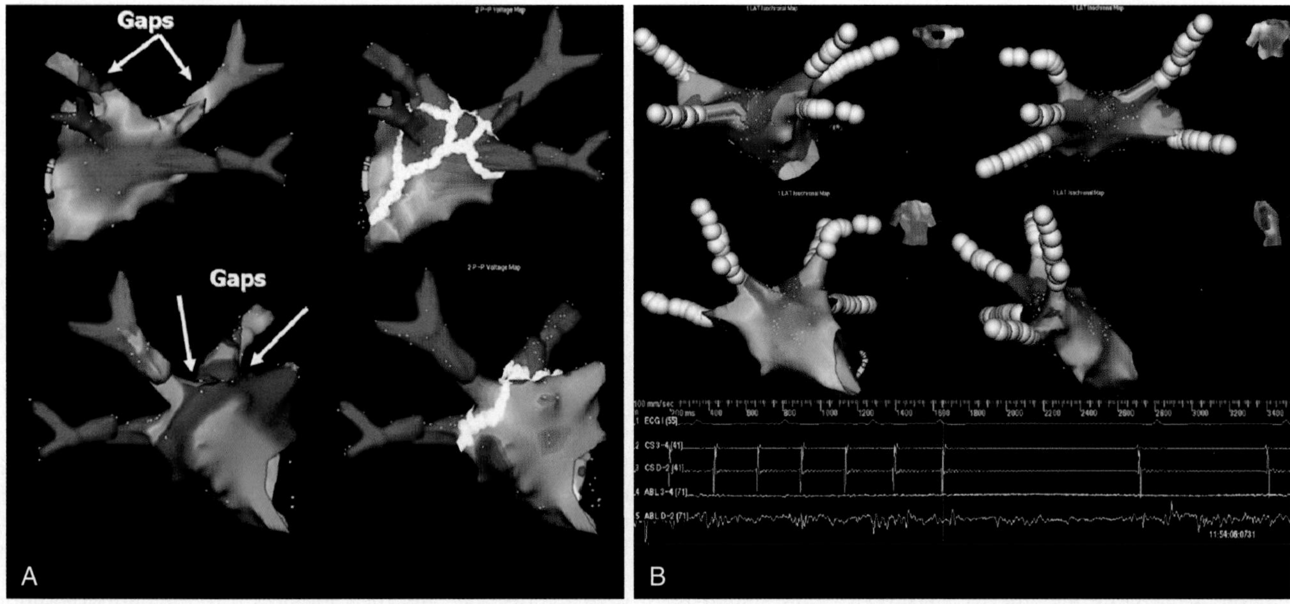

Figure 106-7 **A,** Left atrial activation maps using the NavX system in a patient with incessant postablation atrial tachycardia (AT). Activation maps demonstrated that the superior pulmonary veins (PVs) had been completely reconnected *(left)* and further radiofrequency (RF) applications on the gap *(arrows)* resulted in complete voltage abatement and AT termination with no inducibility *(right)*. **B,** Left atrial activation maps using the NavX system in another patient with postablation AT. Activation maps demonstrate that the superior right PV had been completely reconnected *(left)*. RF touch on the gap again results in AT termination and conversion to sinus rhythm *(lower panel)*.

activation that demonstrate concealed entrainment are usually successful.

Often, voltage maps show areas of preserved voltage at the site of earliest activation, suggesting areas not previously targeted or incompletely ablated during the index procedure (see Figs. 106-3 and 106-4). Reentry around left or right pulmonary veins can be demonstrated by proximal and distal CS, left atrial roof, and septal pacing. Their management requires the use of 3-D activation maps for delineating the tachycardia course and for deploying a lesion line connecting anatomic obstacles to interrupt AT circuits (see Fig. 106-7).

RF applications are delivered after critical isthmuses have been identified by detailed electroanatomic maps and concealed entrainment.[5] Usually, a few RF applications on the critical isthmus are sufficient to eliminate such tachycardias and their inducibility, but in some cases a further ablation line is required.[5,14-16] Successful ablation is defined as termination of tachycardia during ablation and noninducibility of the same tachycardia morphology with burst pacing or programmed pacing, or both.

Anticoagulation Concerns

Stroke is a potential and feared complication of AF ablation, particularly if one considers the possibility of asymptomatic ischemic events. To prevent stroke or thromboembolic events in patients not already receiving chronic anticoagulation, TEE is performed with short-term anticoagulation therapy instead of a 3-week course.

Preablation Anticoagulation Issues

Like patients with permanent AF, patients at risk (patients with persistent AF or those with paroxysmal AF or with associated risk factors) require oral anticoagulation therapy with at least 3 weeks of documented INR values and should undergo bridging with intravenous heparin or subcutaneous low molecular weight heparin before ablation. We also recommend TEE for any patient presenting in AF who has not undergone oral anticoagulation therapy with bridging before ablation.

Anticoagulation Therapy during the Ablation Procedure

Anticoagulation should be established after transseptal puncture, and in some cases ACT can be tailored up to 300 seconds if necessary to reduce sheath thrombus risk.

Postablation Anticoagulation Strategy

The best anticoagulation protocol after ablation according to the clinical characteristics and thromboembolic risk is not yet established. Due to the risk of embolic events in the early postprocedural period, all patients are maintained on oral anticoagulation during the first 4 months after CPVA. In selected patients without evidence of recurrent AF at 4 to 6 months after ablation, we discontinue warfarin and start aspirin (75-325 mg/day). However, patients at high risk for stroke according to guidelines may continue warfarin despite no AF recurrence, and those with moderate risk factors are advised to take aspirin or nothing.

Remote Mapping and Ablation with Stereotaxis

Currently, most catheter ablation procedures in patients with AF are performed with manual catheters, which requires advanced operator skills and experience with catheter manipulation and ablation. In a modern electrophysiology laboratory, the addition of remote magnetic navigation can eliminate hand motion as a variable and provide more precision, thus enhancing reproducibility of results. The feasibility of the remote system, which is not operator dependent, represents an attractive alternative approach in many laboratories to reproduce the success rates of the pioneering groups while minimizing risks.[16,19-21] The recent availability of remote-tip irrigated magnetic catheters will enhance the benefits of the remote system making deeper lesions as with manual catheters, regardless of the operator's experience. We have demonstrated that remote navigation technology can facilitate both mapping and ablation in patients with AF, independent of operator dexterity.[19]

The Magnetic Navigation System (MNS) uses soft catheters equipped with three small magnets embedded in the tip for accurate catheter orientation in the magnetic field generated by using two large magnets positioned on either side of the procedure table. This system consists of two independent but communicating components: the Niobe Stereotaxis MNS (Stereotaxis, Inc., St. Louis, MO) and an electroanatomic mapping system (CARTO-RMT, Biosense Webster, Inc., Diamond Bar, CA). The Niobe includes a computer interface system (Navigant), which is controlled by a keyboard and joystick, which in turn change the two magnets' orientation, modifying the magnetic field and thus the catheter tip orientation and location. The operator stays in a separate room, virtually at any distance from the x-ray beam and the patient's body. This system is combined with the CARTO mapping system, which has been modified to be able to function in this magnetic environment. A 4- to 8-mm tip magnetic catheter (NaviStar-RMT, Biosense Webster, Inc.) can be connected with CARTO-RMT, but tip-irrigated catheters are available now in Europe. The three magnets in the distal portion of the catheter can be deflected in any direction and steered by the magnetic field. Because magnetic fields vectors are capable of tip orientation, at present its movements can be guaranteed by a mechanical device (Cardiodrive, Stereotaxis). Magnetic field vectors for each target navigation and ablation can be stored and reapplied while the magnetic catheter is navigated automatically for autoablation (Fig. 106-8).

An accurate electroanatomic map can be performed using an automated mapping function present in the Navigant software specifically designed for mapping of the LA. Additional points can be taken manually in areas of interest, accounting for clustering of points in specific areas. Sequential acquisition of many points all around the LA by a stable wall contact of the catheter tip allows cardiac geometries to be accurately created, particularly in challenging areas, with impressive levels of detail, incredible speed, and efficiency. In our experience, remote mapping and ablation can be safely achieved in all patients undergoing AF ablation. Initially, the procedure times were a little longer than in manual cases, due to the learning curve, which at the beginning requires frequent adjustments of the tip's orientation. Ablation time to complete the lesion lines around challenging areas such as right-sided pulmonary veins is shorter remotely, which indicates that there are no difficult sites as with standard CPVA, thus avoiding unnecessary RF energy applications that may be associated with residual gaps and risk of major complications. Based on our experience, the remote mapping and ablation system has many advantages, but there are some limitations that can be overcome in the future.

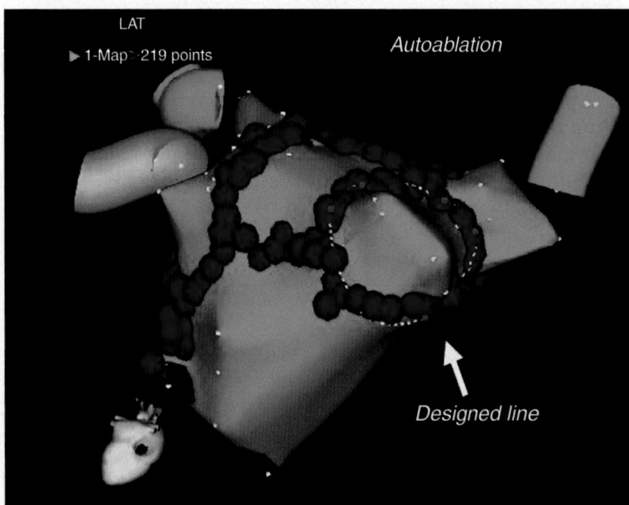

Figure 106-8 A postablation electroanatomic map using the Stereotaxis remote system in the posteroanterior projection. The automatic remote function of the system can perform an autoablation *(red tags)* according to a predesigned line around the left atrial appendage (LAA) *(white circular points).*

Advantages of the Remote System

Because its orientation is guided entirely by a magnetic field and no deflection wires are required, the RMT catheter is far softer than the traditional deflectable catheters along its distal segment. If the catheter does not reach the programmed location because of anatomic obstacles the operator simply withdraws the catheter from the obstacle, and then advances it to the desired location with additional manipulations of the magnetic field. This results in reduced endocardial trauma, and the risk of cardiac perforation is even lower. Consistent with this notion, no cardiac perforation has been reported during mapping of the thin-walled LA. The softer touch of the RMT catheter causes less deformation of cardiac chambers compared with manual mapping, which results in a more accurate reconstruction with a minimal amount of fluoroscopy. There will be further reductions in radiation exposure for both patients and operators once MNS-compatible irrigated-tip catheters become available for clinical use.

Limitations of Remote Technology

There are limitations to this system, which can be overcome rapidly by advancing technology.

The size and position of the floor magnets on either side of the patient can partially limit the fluoroscopic visual field during the procedures. However, in our experience it is possible to fluoroscopically visualize the entire atrial cavity, even in patients with dilated atrial chambers that might require a larger field of visualization. Nonetheless, this does not represent a major limitation because the need for fluoroscopy is greatly minimized by electroanatomic mapping.

The current availability of irrigated-tip catheters certainly represents an important tool, particularly in patients with permanent AF who require more extensive ablation. In the future, as irrigated catheters become compatible with the remote system, it will be possible to conduct randomized studies comparing standard and remote AF ablation.

Conclusions

It has become increasingly apparent that in patients with AF, the maintenance of a stable sinus rhythm is the ideal endpoint, and AF ablation seems to be an effective therapy and a realistic alternative to current pharmacologic therapy. However, to have the maximum long-term success and avoid complications, all acute endpoints should be safely achieved. At present, many AF ablation strategies are effective, but CPVA is one of the simplest and most effective procedures without risk of major complications. Remote navigation and ablation with irrigated catheters is an important goal to standardize lesion set, with reproducible acute and long-term results in AF catheter ablation worldwide.

References

1. Haissaguerre M, Jais P, Shah DC, et al: Spontaneous initiation of atrial fibrillation by ectopic beats originating in the pulmonary veins. N Engl J Med 339:659-666, 1998.
2. Pappone C, Oreto G, Rosanio S, et al: Atrial electroanatomic remodeling after circumferential radiofrequency pulmonary vein ablation: Efficacy of an anatomic approach in a large cohort of patients with atrial fibrillation. Circulation 104:2539-2544, 2001.
3. Oral H, Knight BP, Tada H, et al: Pulmonary vein isolation for paroxysmal and persistent atrial fibrillation. Circulation 105:1077-1081, 2002.
4. Oral H, Scharf C, Chugh A, et al: Catheter ablation for paroxysmal atrial fibrillation: Segmental pulmonary vein ostial ablation versus left atrial ablation. Circulation 108:2355-2360, 2003.
5. Pappone C, Manguso F, Vicedomini G, et al: Prevention of iatrogenic atrial tachycardia after ablation of atrial fibrillation: A prospective randomized study comparing circumferential pulmonary vein ablation with a modified approach. Circulation 110:3036-3042, 2004.
6. Nademanee K, McKenzie J, Kosar E, et al: A new approach for catheter ablation of atrial fibrillation: Mapping of the electrophysiologic substrate. J Am Coll Cardiol 43:2044-2053, 2004.
7. Ouyang F, Bansch D, Ernst S, et al: Complete isolation of left atrium surrounding the pulmonary veins: New insights from the double-lasso technique in paroxysmal atrial fibrillation. Circulation 110:2090-2096, 2004.
8. Pappone C, Santinelli V, Manguso F, et al: Pulmonary vein denervation enhances long-term benefit after circumferential ablation for paroxysmal atrial fibrillation. Circulation 109:327-334, 2004.
9. Pappone C, Rosanio S, Augello G, et al: Mortality, morbidity, and quality of life after circumferential pulmonary vein ablation for atrial fibrillation: Outcomes from a controlled nonrandomized long-term study. J Am Coll Cardiol 42:185-197, 2003.
10. Wazni OM, Marrouche NF, Martin DO, et al: Radiofrequency ablation vs antiarrhythmic drugs as first-line treatment of symptomatic atrial fibrillation: a randomized trial. JAMA 293:2634-2640, 2005.
11. Stabile G, Bertaglia E, Senatore G, et al: Catheter ablation treatment in patients with drug-refractory atrial fibrillation: A prospective, multi-centre, randomized, controlled study (Catheter Ablation For The Cure Of Atrial Fibrillation Study). Eur Heart J 27:216, 2006.
12. Pappone C, Augello G, Sala S, et al: A randomized trial of circumferential pulmonary vein ablation versus antiarrhythmic drug therapy in paroxysmal atrial fibrillation: The APAF Study. J Am Coll Cardiol 48:2340-2347, 2006.
13. Oral H, Pappone C, Chugh A, et al: Circumferential pulmonary-vein ablation for chronic atrial fibrillation. N Engl J Med 354:934-994, 2006.
14. Pappone C, Radinovic A, Manguso F, et al: Progression of atrial fibrillation in patients with a first-detected episode. A long-term prospective follow-up study. J Am Coll Cardiol 49:25A(Suppl A), 2007.
15. Haissaguerre M, Sanders P, Hocini M, et al: Catheter ablation of long-lasting persistent atrial fibrillation: Critical structures for termination. J Cardiovasc Electrophysiol 11:1125-1137, 2005.
16. Pappone C, Santinelli V: How to perform encircling ablation of the left atrium. Heart Rhythm 3:1105-1109, 2006.
17. Mesas CE, Pappone C, Lang CE, et al: Left atrial tachycardia after circumferential pulmonary vein ablation for atrial fibrillation. J Am Coll Cardiol 44:1071-1079, 2004.
18. Pappone C, Santinelli V: Towards a unified strategy for atrial fibrillation ablation? Eur Heart J 26:1687-1688, 2005.
19. Pappone C, Vicedomini G, Manguso F, et al: Robotic magnetic navigation for atrial fibrillation ablation. J Am Coll Cardiol 47:1390-1400, 2006.
20. Pappone C, Santinelli V: Remote navigation and ablation of atrial fibrillation. J Cardiovasc Electrophysiol Suppl 1:S18-S20, 2007.
21. Pappone C, and Santinelli V: Atrial fibrillation ablation: State of the art. Am J Cardiol 96:59L-64L, 2005.

Catheter Ablation of Supraventricular Arrhythmias 107

Richard L. Snowdon and Jonathan M. Kalman

CHAPTER OUTLINE

Since the 1970s, catheter ablation has developed from an experimental technique, involving the delivery of direct current shocks, into a firmly established first-line therapy for paroxysmal supraventricular tachycardia (SVT) and atrial flutter.[1] Radiofrequency catheter ablation is now routinely performed at a single sitting combined with a diagnostic EP study for patients with an undifferentiated diagnosis of regular SVT.[2] In this chapter, catheter ablation of paroxysmal and persistent regular supraventricular arrhythmias is discussed. The ablation of atrial fibrillation is covered in Chapters 105 and 106.

Ablation of Atrioventricular Node Reentrant Tachycardia

Indications

Radiofrequency (RF) ablation for cure of atrioventricular (AV) node reentrant tachycardia (AVNRT) has become an established first-line procedure for patients with recurrent or troublesome AVNRT. According to the joint American College of Cardiology (ACC) and American Heart Association (AHA) Task Force on Practice guidelines for catheter ablation, "patients with symptomatic sustained AVNRT that is drug resistant or the patient is drug intolerant or does not desire long-term drug therapy" have a class I indication for RF ablation.[2] In our experience, the vast majority of young patients with symptomatic AVNRT prefer a definitive cure to lifelong medication.

The first catheter-based approaches to cure AVNRT targeted fast pathway conduction, but pioneering these techniques were associated with now unacceptably high rates of complete AV block. Due to the risk of AV block associated with fast pathway ablation, the majority of electrophysiology departments use slow pathway ablation as the approach of choice for treatment for both typical and atypical AVNRT.

Slow Pathway Ablation

Slow pathway ablation was first described by Jackman and colleagues in a landmark paper in 1992.[3] Broadly speaking, two techniques have been adopted for successful slow pathway ablation: electrophysiologic slow pathway potential mapping and the anatomic approach.

The initial reports used electrophysiologic guidance by recording of slow pathway potentials.[3,4] Although this approach has been highly effective, the description of these potentials has been variable. Jackman and colleagues[3] recorded high amplitude, high-frequency potentials between the coronary sinus (CS) ostium (CSO) and the adjacent tricuspid annulus. During retrograde slow pathway conduction, these high-frequency potentials preceded the low-frequency atrial potential. In sinus rhythm, the reverse sequence was observed. Targeting these potentials, the authors achieved a 100% ablation success rate for a cure of AVNRT. Haissaguerre and colleagues[4] subsequently described slow pathway potentials as low-frequency, low-amplitude potentials posteroinferior to the AV node and anterior to the CSO. These potentials were located within the triangle of Koch overlying the muscular AV septum as a vertical band near the tricuspid annulus. Targeting these potentials for ablation also met with a 100% success rate for cure of the typical form of AVNRT.

The alternate method for slow pathway ablation has been to take an anatomically guided approach. This technique is based on the assumption that the slow pathway is consistently located in the inferior or posterior region of the triangle in the corridor between the tricuspid annulus and the CSO inferiorly and between the tricuspid annulus and the tendon of Todaro more superiorly. Using this technique, the catheter is located against the atrial aspect of the tricuspid annulus in between the CSO and the septal leaflet of the tricuspid valve in a region where a high-frequency atrial electrogram can be recorded but where the atrial-ventricular ratio is less than 0.5. If a series of applications in this region is unsuccessful, the catheter is gradually advanced more superiorly, and further applications of RF are delivered at each site until the endpoint is reached. Anatomic location may be inferred fluoroscopically from the position of the ablation catheter in relation to catheters in the CS (inferior) and in the His bundle position (superior). A study that compared the anatomic approach with a technique guided by recording of slow pathway potentials in a single laboratory found no differences in success rate, duration of the procedure, fluoroscopy time, or mean number of RF applications.[5]

Endpoints for Slow Pathway Ablation

A sensitive, although nonspecific, marker of successful ablation of the slow pathway is the development of junctional rhythm during the application. In one study, there was a 100% incidence of junctional rhythm in successful RF applications and a 65% incidence for unsuccessful applications.[6] Ablation was more likely to be effective if the junctional rhythm was of longer duration, with a larger number of junctional beats. However, RF ablation of the slow pathway can be successful without junctional rhythm in small percentage of cases.

After an RF application accompanied by junctional rhythm, confirmation of successful slow pathway ablation must be obtained. The most commonly accepted endpoint for cure of AVNRT using the slow-pathway approach is absence of inducibility of the arrhythmia before and during isoprenaline infusion. However, conflicting data exist as to whether elimination of all slow-pathway conduction predicts a lower incidence of late recurrence than if tachycardia is rendered noninducible but dual AV nodal physiology and single-echo beats persist. Currently, most electrophysiologic laboratories accept the presence of single-echo beats without sustained tachycardia (before and with isoproterenol) as an adequate endpoint,[3,4] and persistent dual AV nodal physiology with single echos has been reported in up to 65% of patients who have a successful long-term result.

An interesting problem occurs in patients with AVNRT and smooth AV node function curves because loss of dual AV node physiology cannot strictly be used as an endpoint. However, successful slow pathway ablation in these patients does result in loss of the tail of the curve representing the slow pathway. Similarly, significant shortening of the maximal atrial-His interval during atrial pacing after ablation suggests successful elimination of AVNRT in patients with a smooth AV nodal function curve.[7]

At the other end of the spectrum are patients who have multiple anterograde slow pathways as evidenced by the presence of multiple discontinuities in the AV node conduction curve.[8] In the majority, only one of the slow pathways is involved in sustained tachycardia, although involvement of up to three has been described. RF ablation at a single site can eliminate all slow pathway conduction in up to half of these patients but requires applications at multiple sites in the other half. Using the endpoint of noninducibility (with or without persistence of dual AV node physiology) achieved long-term clinical cure in the majority.

Risk of Atrioventricular Block during Slow Pathway Ablation

The risk of AV block during slow pathway ablation has varied according to the reported series but, in general, is less than 1%.[3,4] In cases where catheter stability is difficult to achieve and when the distance between the anterior and posterior inputs is small, a number of measures can be taken to avoid inadvertent damage to the fast pathway and compact AV node. We prefer the routine use of a long vascular sheath and, in some cases, we use general anesthesia with muscle relaxation to allow cessation of respiration during the RF application. This latter technique has proved very useful to ensure catheter stability during difficult cases.

A number of markers of impending AV block have been suggested, although universal agreement does not exist. One study found that rapid junctional rhythm during the application is predictive,[9] although other studies have not confirmed this. It is important to terminate the RF application if short cycle length junctional tachycardia occurs in order to confirm 1:1 AV conduction without prolongation of the PR interval. The anatomic location of the ablation is important and, in general, the risk of AV block appears to be higher with more anteriorly placed applications. However, the fast pathway may in some instances be located quite posteriorly and may be one cause of inadvertent AV block during posterior slow pathway ablation.[10] Perhaps the most useful sign is the presence of varying degrees of VA block in junctional rhythm during the application.[6,9] It is important to carefully monitor the VA relationship during the RF application because any increase in the VA interval or sudden development of VA block might signify imminent heart block.

Although most instances of AV block occur during the procedure, AV block can rarely present late after an apparently uncomplicated slow pathway ablation.

Cryoablation

Skanes and colleagues[11] described the use of cryoablation in 18 patients with AVNRT. Reversible loss of slow pathway conduction during ice mapping was demonstrated, and 17 of 18 patients went on to successful cryoablation of the slow pathway without recurrence over 5 months of follow-up. During cryoablation, junctional tachycardia did not occur even at successful sites and therefore could not be used to assess lesion efficacy. However, adherence of the catheter tip during cryoablation allowed a reduction in required fluoroscopy and provided the stability needed to allow atrial pacing during the application to test for slow pathway conduction. Cryoablation in the anterior region of Koch's triangle produced inadvertent loss of fast pathway conduction in two patients but was fully reversible on immediate rewarming. This technology thus allows the ability to assess the electrophysiologic outcome at specific ablation sites before producing a permanent lesion.

Noninducible Atrioventricular Node Reentrant Tachycardia

In approximately 10% of patients, the induction AVNRT is difficult and poorly reproducible despite use of standard maneuvers and the administration of isoproterenol and atropine.[12] Reasons for noninducibility of AVNRT at baseline include inability to achieve a critical atrio-His interval, fast pathway block, and slow pathway block. In some instances, isoproterenol actually renders AVNRT noninducible via a shortening of the fast pathway effective refractory period, which appears to abolish slow pathway conduction. In patients with documented SVT who have dual AV nodal pathways but whose arrythmia is noninducible at the time of study, empiric slow pathway ablation has been performed.[13] In the majority of these patients, ablation of the slow pathway resulted in clinical cure.

Ablation of Atrioventricular Reentrant Tachycardia

Indications

Radiofrequency catheter ablation is also the treatment of choice for many patients with AVRT due to a concealed or manifest accessory pathway (Wolff-Parkinson-White [WPW] syndrome), and routinely offers a cure for what was once a common, disabling, and potentially fatal medical problem.[14] Current ACC/AHA/European Society of Cardiology (ESC) practice guidelines make a class I recommend that patients with WPW syndrome (preexcitation and symptoms) undergo catheter ablation as first-line therapy. Catheter ablation is also recommended (class IIa or class I if AVRT poorly tolerated) for patients with AVRT due to a concealed accessory pathway, according to patient preference, "either as initial therapy, or for patients experiencing side effects or arrhythmia recurrence during drug therapy."[2]

Accessory Pathway Localization

The approach adopted to map and ablate an accessory pathway depends on the functional properties and the anatomic location of the accessory pathway. The locations of 2411 accessory pathways in 1969 consecutive patients are demonstrated in Figure 107-1.[15]

The electrocardiogram may be helpful for localizing manifest accessory pathways. An analysis of the delta wave vector can predict the general location of an accessory pathway to 1 of 10 sites around the tricuspid and mitral annuli or at subepicardial

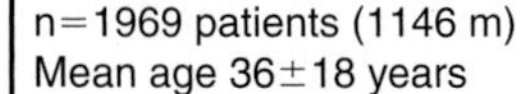

	Patients	Ebstein
	1969	40/1969
	2325 APs	86 APs
1 AP	1705	12
2 APs	193	15
3 APs	57	10
4 APs	8	1
5 APs	5	2
6 APs	1	0

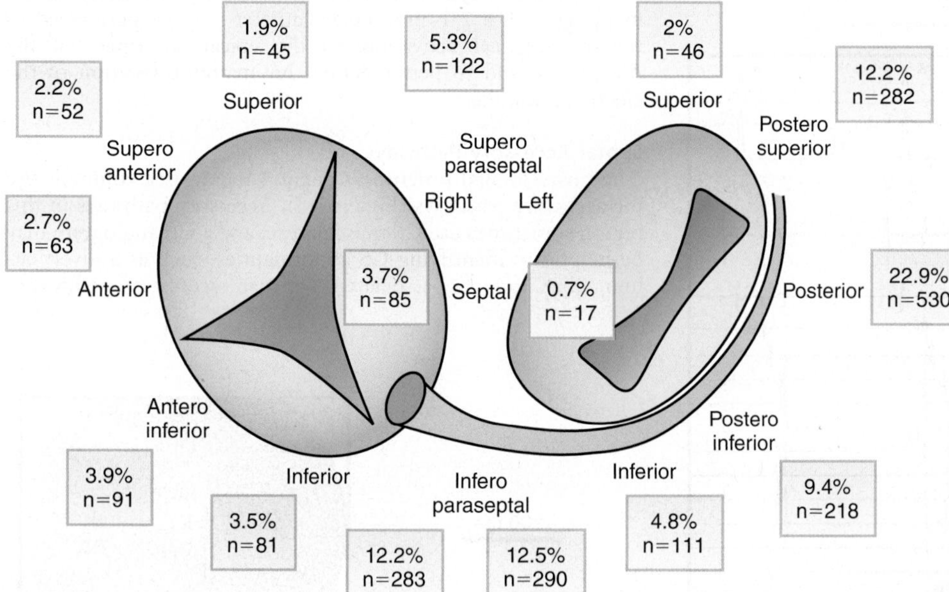

Figure 107-1 Distribution of accessory pathway location. Schematic of tricuspid and mitral atrioventricular (AV) rings, in a left anterior oblique projection, showing the locations of accessory pathways from 1969 consecutive patients. The anatomically correct terminology described by Cosio and colleagues[21] has been used. The *table* shows the number of accessory pathways per patient in those with and without the Ebstein anomaly. (From Ernst S, Ouyang F, Antz M, et al: Catheter ablation of atrioventricular reentry. In Zipes DP, Jalife J (eds): Cardiac Electrophysiology from Cell to Bedside, 4th ed. Philadelphia, WB Saunders, 2004, 1078-1086.)

locations with an overall sensitivity of 90% and specificity of 99%.[16] Precise pathway localization, however, depends on detailed mapping at EP study. Broadly, two electrophysiologic approaches may be used alone or in combination to precisely localize an accessory pathway:

The first approach is to map the earliest local ventricular or atrial electrogram. The site of earliest ventricular activation, prior to delta wave onset, usually identifies the location of the ventricular insertion of a manifest accessory pathway (Fig. 107-2). For concealed pathways (or during retrograde mapping of a manifest pathway), the site of earliest atrial activation during orthodromic tachycardia or ventricular pacing indicates the atrial insertion. This is often at a site where there is no isoelectric interval between the local ventricular and atrial electrograms (continuous electrical activity) during retrograde mapping. However, depending on the pacing site and pathway location, a late local ventricular activation and late local atrial activation can produce this appearance of continuous activity. Therefore, the absolute timing is most important.

The second approach is the direct recording of an accessory pathway potential. During anterograde conduction, an accessory pathway potential is usually assumed if a distinct bipolar potential preceding the delta wave is recorded between the local atrial and ventricular potentials. Pacing maneuvers may be used to dissociate atrial and ventricular potentials if validation of the accessory pathway potential is required. An accessory pathway potential is less often recorded during retrograde conduction, possibly due to the superimposition of a much larger ventricular potential.[15] A thorough search for an accessory pathway potential might, however, be time consuming and is not required to achieve successful ablation in many cases.[14]

Once a suitable stable ablation site has been identified, our practice is to deliver RF energy at 50 W, temperature limited to 60° C, for up to 60 seconds, via a 4 mm–tip ablation catheter. Some regions with reduced blood flow, such as under the mitral valve apparatus or in the CS, might require reduced power or the use of an irrigated-tip ablation catheter. If pathway ablation does not occur within 10 to 15 seconds of RF onset, the application is terminated and further mapping is performed.

Multiple accessory pathways occur in up to 13% of patients with WPW syndrome (see table in Fig. 107-1). Techniques for mapping multiple pathways are the same as those used for a single accessory pathway, and it might not be apparent that a second pathway is present until after successful ablation of the first. The localization of two accessory pathways that are simultaneously conducting may be more challenging, but the average number of RF applications per accessory pathway has been reported to be no different to that required to ablate a single accessory pathway.[17]

Left-Sided Accessory Pathways

Endocardial accessory pathways located on the mitral valve annulus may be approached either via the transseptal approach or the retrograde aortic approach.[14] The transseptal approach has the advantages of permitting greater catheter maneuverability and the avoidance of arterial complications,[18] such as coronary artery dissection, but it is associated with its own risks, including systemic air embolus and pericardial collection.

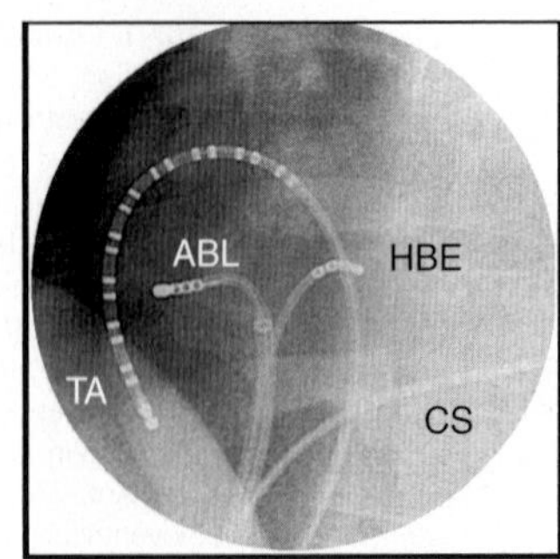

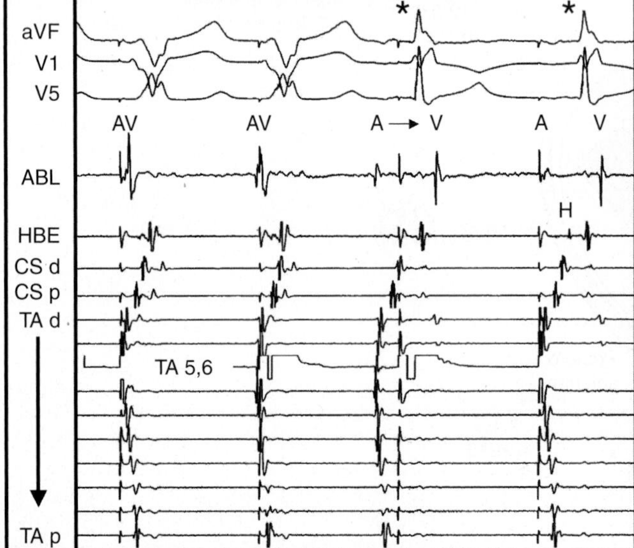

Figure 107-2 Ablation of right lateral (anterior[21]) manifest accessory pathway. *Top,* Ablation catheter (ABL) at the site of successful ablation, with a 20-pole catheter (TA) in the right atrium (RA) adjacent to the tricuspid annulus. Mapping (to earliest ventricular activation ahead of delta wave) and ablation were performed during maximal preexcitation elicited by pacing from TA 5,6. *Bottom,* Accessory pathway block with loss of preexcitation (*) after 3 seconds of radiofrequency ablation. Note the tightly fused local atrial (A) and ventricular (V) electrograms on ABL, which widely separate with pathway block. In this case, the degree of delay between A and V is accentuated by the presence of underlying right bundle branch block. Note also that the third beat is a local atrial ectopic and clearly shows the ratio of A and V electrogram amplitudes (~0.5:1). CS d, coronary sinus distal; CS p, coronary sinus proximal; HBE, His bundle electrode.

The overall success and complication rates for transseptal (85% and 6.1%) and retrograde aortic (85% and 6.7%) approaches are similar.[18] The decision as to which approach to use is therefore usually one of physician preference and familiarity.[1] Both approaches are complementary, and if one method fails, the other should be attempted.[18] It is recommended, however, that the transseptal approach be used first in children, elderly patients, and those with arterial disease.

Right Free-Wall Accessory Pathways

Achieving a stable catheter position on the right free wall of the tricuspid annulus can be technically challenging, and it contributes to a higher ablation failure rate for right free wall accessory pathways (10%-19%) compared to left free wall accessory pathways (3%-7%).[19] For this reason, we routinely use long vascular sheaths to improve ablation catheter stability when mapping the tricuspid annulus from the right femoral vein. The use of a 20-pole halo catheter positioned around the tricuspid annulus, to bracket an accessory pathway, can also aid in localizing right-sided accessory pathways and facilitate catheter stability during ablation (see Fig. 106-2).[19]

Nine percent of right sided accessory pathways are associated with Ebstein anomaly of the tricuspid valve.[20] Accessory pathway ablation in patients with Ebstein anomaly may be challenging, with 50% having multiple pathways and more than 50% of pathways lying in regions of abnormal fractionated potentials, making the identification of preexcited electrograms and accessory pathway potentials difficult.[20] If conventional mapping techniques fail, right coronary artery mapping with a 2-F multipolar catheter may be performed to record electrical activation on the epicardial aspect of the AV groove and to better define the anatomic location of the electrical annulus.[20]

Septal Accessory Pathways

The posteroseptal (inferoparaseptal[21]) region is a common site for accessory pathways (Fig. 107-3). Accessory pathways in this region sometimes use CS musculature, and a CS angiogram may be helpful in identifying CS abnormalities, such as a diverticulum, that may be associated with an accessory pathway.[22]

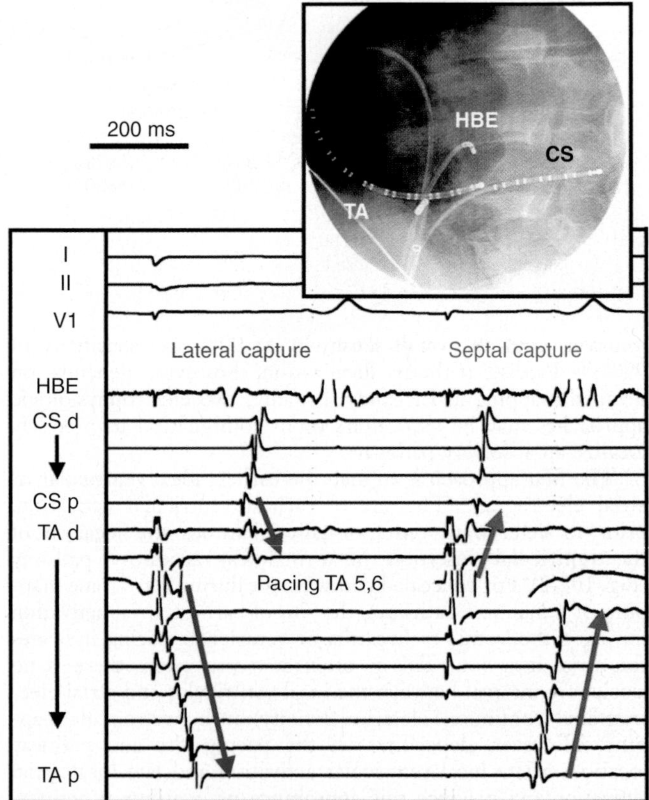

Figure 107-3 Bidirectional cavo-tricuspid isthmus (CTI) block, demonstrated by pacing and recording close to the CTI ablation line, is the endpoint of choice for ablation of typical atrial flutter. In this unusual example, pacing from tricuspid annulus (TA) 5,6, lying on the ablation line marked by the ablation catheter (*top*), alternately captures lateral then medial to the ablation line due to slight TA catheter movement with respiration. Capture lateral to the ablation line results in conduction up the right atrium free wall clockwise around the TA catheter (*blue*) and takes 190 ms to reach TA 3,4 (*medial to the line*). Note that TA 1,2 activates prior to TA 3,4, indicating conduction toward, and not across, the ablation line. With medial capture (*red*), the activation sequence is reversed and takes to 230 ms to reach TA 7,8, confirming bidirectionality of block. CS, coronary sinus; HBE, His bundle electrode.

Mapping on the right side, including from within the CS, is usually performed initially, before crossing to the left side if no suitable ablation site has been found on the right.

RF ablation for accessory pathways in septal (true septal and paraseptal[21]) locations carries a risk of causing irreversible AV block. This risk is highest for para-His and midseptal pathways, with one case series reporting a 29% risk of complete AV block.[23] The average risk is, however, probably closer to 2.5% to 5%.[24] The ability of cyroablation to suppress local cardiac electrical activity, by cooling to −30° C without producing an irreversible lesion (ice mapping), considerably reduces the risk of inadvertent permanent AV block when ablating in septal locations.[25] Pooled data from three case series of cryoablation for septal accessory pathways (45 patients) showed an initial success rate of 96% for no cases of permanent AV block, with a recurrence rate of 16%.[25]

Epicardial Accessory Pathways

Approximately 5% of accessory pathways may be mapped to an epicardial location.[15] Most of these epicardial pathways use sleeves of musculature extending into the cardiac veins (CS ~ 75%, great cardiac vein, vein of Marshal, or a CS diverticulum),[15,22] which function as a bridge between ventricular and atrial myocardium. The majority of these patients demonstrate normal coronary sinus anatomy, and only approximately 21% have a diverticulum.[22] Other rare sites for epicardial pathways include the right free wall and the right and left atrial appendages.

Ablation is usually performed by mapping within the CS, and the most common successful ablation site is within the os of a middle cardiac or posterolateral vein or within the neck of a diverticulum. Less commonly, ablation may be successful within the body of the coronary sinus. In these locations, irrigated ablation is invariably required due to low blood flow. Rarely, a transcutaneous pericardial approach is needed,[26] or the atrial insertion of an atrial appendage accessory pathway may be ablated from deep within the appendage.[26]

Accessory Pathways with Slow Decremental Conduction

Accessory pathways with decremental properties are uncommon. Most decremental atrioventricular accessory pathways are posteroseptal (inferoparaseptal[21]), and may be mapped and ablated conventionally. Decremental atriofascicular Mahaim accessory pathways, however, conduct almost exclusively anterograde and are most reliably localized by mapping an accessory pathway potential along the lateral aspect of the tricuspid annulus.[1]

Efficacy

Acute success is defined by the abolition of pathway conduction. A multicenter clinical trial of RF ablation, conducted between 1992 and 1995, reported successful ablation was achieved in 465 of 500 (93%) cases of AVRT.[24] The highest success rate was seen for left free wall accessory pathways (95%), with right free wall and posteroseptal accessory pathways being associated with lower success rates (90% and 88%, respectively). The major complication rate for AVRT in this trial included one death (0.2%), one cerebrovascular accident (0.2%), and five complete AV blocks (1%). A more-recent survey of ablation procedures (between 1997 and 2002) by Morady included pooled data from 6065 patients with AVRT and reported a long-term success rate of 98%, with a repeat procedure rate 2.2%.[1] The rate of serious complications in this survey was 0.6%, with a procedural mortality rate of 0.02%, substantially lower than the cumulative annual risk associated with WPW syndrome.[1]

Ablation of Atrial Flutter and Macro-reentrant Atrial Tachycardia

107

Indications

Cavo-tricuspid isthmus (CTI) dependent atrial flutter or typical atrial flutter accounts for 90% of macro-reentrant atrial tachycardias (ATs). The circuit of CTI atrial flutter is now well described and curative ablation, by producing bidirectional CTI conduction block, is routine. Catheter ablation for typical atrial flutter is superior to antiarrhythmic therapy, which has a low rate of maintenance of sinus rhythm (80% versus 36%, respectively, at 21 months).[27] Consequently, current ACC/AHA/ESC guidelines recommend catheter ablation for both the first episode of typical atrial flutter (class IIa) and recurrent typical atrial flutter (class I).[2] Non–CTI-dependent macro-reentrant ATs may be classified together as atypical atrial flutter. Linear ablation for atypical atrial flutter has also been shown to be highly effective, but it requires an individually tailored approach specific to the underlying substrate. Currently, catheter ablation is recommended for symptomatic atypical atrial flutter after failed antiarrhythmic therapy (Class IIa).[2]

Typical Atrial Flutter

Anatomy of Cavo-Tricuspid Isthmus

The cavo-tricuspid isthmus is composed of muscle bundles, pectinate extensions of the crista terminalis, which run longitudinally or obliquely across it.[28,29] At its narrowest point the CTI is 19 ± 4 mm wide, but it is up to 37 ± 8 mm wide in persons with a history of atrial flutter.[28] The anatomy of the CTI displays marked variability between individual patients and often contains pouch-like recesses (83%) and thick muscular ridges (37%).[29] To overcome these anatomic challenges, most centers now use large-tip, 8-mm, or externally irrigated–tip ablation catheters, which are capable of producing larger lesions than conventional 4-mm tip catheters. Irrigated-tip catheters have a theoretical advantage of maintaining power delivery in areas of poor blood flow, such as deep recesses, but studies comparing 8-mm with irrigated catheters report equally high success rates with both catheters.[30]

Approach to Isthmus Ablation

Ablation for typical atrial flutter may be performed during atrial flutter or in sinus rhythm (usually during coronary sinus pacing to facilitate identification of isthmus conduction block).

Ablation may be performed using a point-by-point approach or a continuous drag technique. In either method, diminution of the local electrogram with the appearance of a local double potential indicates successful ablation at that point. An ablation line may be created between the tricuspid annulus and the eustachian ridge at the anterior margin of the inferior vena cava. Alternatively, ablation may be performed between the tricuspid annulus and the coronary sinus ostium and then continued to the eustachian ridge if block has not yet been achieved.

An alternative approach to an uninterrupted anatomic ablation line is to perform voltage-guided ablation of the cavo-tricuspid isthmus.[31] This technique involves mapping a CTI line, then sequentially targeting high-amplitude signals in order of magnitude, regardless of position, until bidirectional block is achieved. Initial results with this technique report a reduction in the number of ablation lesions required to achieve complete CTI block and support the hypothesis that the CTI is composed of functionally discrete muscle bundles, as opposed to a continuous sheet of tissue.[31]

Endpoint for Cavo-Tricuspid Isthmus Ablation

Early studies used termination of atrial flutter and the inability to reinduce flutter by pacing as their endpoints, but reliance on these endpoints was associated with high rates of recurrence (20%-40%).[1] We now recognize that bidirectional CTI block, proved by pacing maneuvers, is the endpoint of choice, because it is associated with a recurrence rate less than 5%.[1]

Usually the presence of isthmus block can be readily appreciated by the observation of a sudden change in activation pattern in the low lateral right atrium during coronary sinus pacing. However, it is important to perform detailed mapping close to the ablation line in order to differentiate complete from incomplete CTI block with persistent slow conduction (see Fig. 107-3). The impact of pacing at sites progressively away from the ablation line on activation timing can be helpful, and pacing should also be performed from both sides of the ablation line to ensure block is bidirectional.[32] If incomplete CTI block is suspected, then the ablation line should be mapped for continuous widely spaced (>90-100 ms) double potentials.[33] Convergence of the double potentials indicates a gap in the ablation line and can be used to guide further ablation.

A survey of ablation by Morady, including pooled data from more than 7000 patients with isthmus-dependent atrial flutter, reported a long term success rate of 97% for CTI ablation.[1] Only 4% of patients require a repeat ablation procedure, and the incidence of serious complication was 0.4%.

Atypical Atrial Flutter

Nomenclature

Atypical atrial flutter is a descriptive term for an AT with an electrocardiographic pattern of continuous undulation of the atrial complex, different from typical or reverse typical flutter.[34] *Macro-reentrant AT* is an AT due to a large reentrant circuit with barriers that are fixed or functional, or both.[34] In addition to typical CTI-dependent flutter, this includes lesional or scar-mediated reentry such as circuits that occur following correction of congenital or valvular heart disease or, more recently, after surgical or catheter ablation of atrial fibrillation. These circuits are considered elsewhere. Otherwise (non-CTI dependent) macro-reentrant AT can be considered in terms of those in the left and those in the right atrium (and occasionally those that involve the septum and aspects of both the left and right atrium).

Importantly, the mechanism of reentry in many instances of (non-CTI dependent) atrial macro-reentry involves the presence of spontaneous atrial scarring. In the right atrium, the most common circuits occur in the free wall around regions of scarring.[35] Similarly, in the left atrium, atrial macro-reentry is most commonly associated with regions of spontaneous scarring and the presence of structural heart disease, such as left ventricular dysfunction or mitral valve disease.[36] The most common locations for these circuits are in relation to anatomic structures; thus perimitral flutter, reentrant loops around one or more pulmonary veins, and those in the left septum are most usually observed. Not uncommonly for both right and left atrial circuits there may be simultaneous dual-loop or figure-of-eight reentry.

Ablation of Non–Cavo-Tricuspid Isthmus Atrial Macro-reentry

The aim of ablation for atrial macro-reentry is to create a line of block that transects the path of the reentrant flutter circuit and bridges two anatomic structures. The location of such ablation depends on the path of the reentrant circuit, which is determined by the underlying anatomic substrate. RA macro-reentry is most usually ablated by creating an ablation line from an existing free wall scar to an anatomic barrier; most commonly this barrier is the inferior vena cava but at times the superior vena cava or tricuspid annulus.[35] Ablation of left atrial circuits can involve an ablation line between regions of scarring (the most common location is the posterior atrium but this is also seen in the anterior and roof regions) and a pulmonary vein or the mitral annulus. An alternative approach is a line between two anatomic structures such as the left inferior pulmonary vein and the mitral annulus (mitral isthmus), the two superior veins (roof line), the mitral annulus and a superior vein (anterior line) or the fossa ovalis and a right pulmonary vein. Left atrial (LA) flutter can involve macro-reentry around the mitral valve annulus, pulmonary veins, or scar and has been successfully treated by joining two or more of these structures together.[36] In addition, circuits can occur due to channels through a region of scarring, and in such cases, it is important to target these channels.[35]

Many patients with non-CTI dependent macro-reentry also have circuits involving the CTI, either as an obligatory component of a single flutter circuit or as part of a dual-loop reentry circuit (Fig. 107-4).[37] CTI ablation is therefore usually included as part of the ablation strategy for patients with atypical flutter.[37]

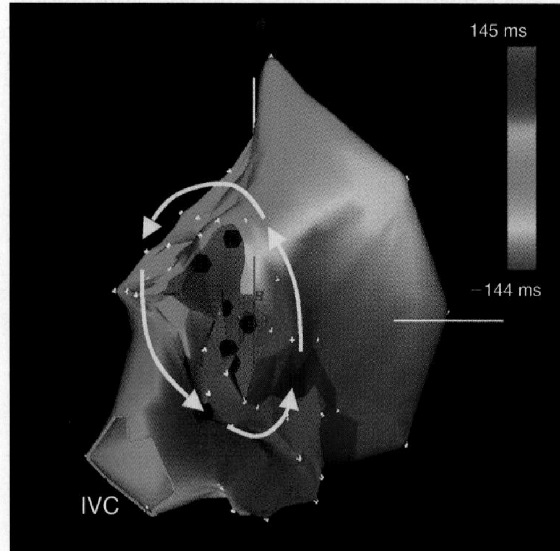

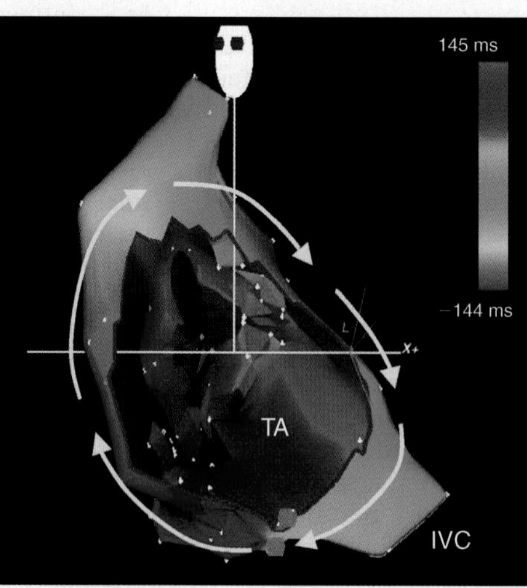

Figure 107-4 Right atrial electroanatomic isochronal map of a dual loop atypical atrial flutter. Right posterior lateral (*left*) and left anterior oblique (*right*) views are shown, with the tricuspid annulus (TA) and inferior vena cava (IVC) marked. Activation can be seen to progresses from *red* through *green* to *blue*, before arriving back at *red* where head meets tail (*dark red line*). The dual loops of the macro-reentry circuit, counter-clockwise around a right free wall scar (*gray*) and clockwise around the TA, are highlighted (*arrows*). This tachycardia was successfully treated with ablation by joining the free wall scar inferiorly to the IVC and by performing a cavotricuspid isthmus ablation.

Mapping Techniques The most commonly used techniques involve multipolar catheter activation mapping, entrainment mapping, and three-dimensional electroanatomic systems to detail the complete circuit and the anatomic location of scars and channels. In practice, these techniques are complementary, and it is usually possible to rapidly asses the circuit orientation using one or two well-positioned multipolar catheters (particularly for right atrial circuits) and entrainment from a number of widely spaced atrial sites.

Most usually, three-dimensional mapping systems, such as CARTO (Biosense Webster, Diamond Bar, CA) and EnSite (Endocardial Solutions, St. Paul, MN) are also deployed for mapping of these macro-reentrant circuits. These systems allow virtual chamber geometries to be created on to which electrophysiologic data may be displayed. These include the atrial substrate, such as anatomic structures (valve orifices and venous ostium), scar (voltage maps), and lines of conduction block (defined by double potentials); activation timing (isochronal maps), used to generate propagation maps of the flutter circuit; and ablation lesions, which can be tracked to facilitate the formation of ablation lines.

Once the flutter circuit has been defined, linear ablation is performed to transect the reentry circuit, by joining two electrically inexcitable structures on either side of a critical isthmus (see earlier). Entrainment mapping of a potential ablation line is used to confirm that the region to be ablated is indeed "in" the circuit. High-output pacing should also be performed prior to RA free wall ablation to prevent phrenic nerve damage.[38]

Efficacy

Termination of the atrial arrhythmia and noninducibility of flutter are the usual primary endpoints for ablation of these circuits. Demonstration of conduction block across the ablation line, by pacing and recording on both sides of the line, should, however be demonstrated whenever possible.[38] With currently available techniques, success rates in excess of 90% may be anticipated for ablation of these circuits.[1,36] Reported recurrence rates vary markedly from 0%[39] to 59%[37] and probably reflect differences in underlying arrhythmic substrate. Pooled data from 13 studies (192 patients) gave an average recurrence rate of 12%.[39]

Ablation of Focal Atrial Tachycardia

Indications

Focal AT is a relatively uncommon arrhythmia, yet it represents 5% to 15% of all supraventricular tachycardias in patients presenting to the electrophysiology lab for ablation.[40] This disparity reflects the low efficacy of pharmacologic antiarrhythmic therapy in the treatment of AT, and an increasing shift to a primary ablative approach for many patients with AT.[41] Current ACC/AHA/ESC guidelines make a class 1 recommendation for catheter ablation for patients with recurrent symptomatic AT or incessant AT.[2]

Anatomic Distribution of Atrial Tachycardia and P-Wave Morphology

Focal ATs are not distributed randomly throughout the atria but usually originate from preferential anatomic locations. Common sites of origin for AT include the crista terminalis, tricuspid annulus, ostium of the CS, and the perinodal region in the right atrium. In the left atrium, the majority originate from the pulmonary vein ostia, with the mitral annulus, left atrial appendage, and the left side of the septum being less-common sites.[40] The site of origin and that pattern of atrial activation determine the P-wave morphology in AT. P-wave morphology can therefore provide a useful first clue to the likely site of tachycardia origin.

Endocardial Mapping and Ablation of Atrial Tachycardia

Irrespective of the underlying arrhythmia mechanism (abnormal automaticity, triggered activity, or micro-reentry) focal ATs are ablated by targeting their site of origin. In general, stable AT or frequent atrial ectopics are a prerequisite for mapping. In the absence of adequate spontaneous atrial activity, isoprenaline infusion and atrial pacing maneuvers may be used to stimulate atrial ectopy. In our experience, the absence of adequate spontaneous atrial activity at the time of electrophysiology study, however, remains the commonest cause of procedural failure. Use of the EnSite noncontact mapping system can facilitate mapping under circumstances of infrequent atrial activity,[42] but the procedural endpoint will nevertheless remain uncertain.

Mapping Techniques

Focal tachycardias are mapped using activation mapping, which generally includes sequential point mapping with the ablation catheter, multipolar catheters to provide a broad activation picture, and the use of three-dimensional electroanatomic mapping to allow precise identification of the ablation target. Generally, an activation time of longer than 20 to 30 ms before the P wave is observed at successful sites, but this is highly variable.[41] If the onset of the P wave is obscured by the T wave, mapping can be performed to a stable intracardiac fiducial point, such as a CS catheter bipole, with a known relationship to P-wave onset.

The introduction of three-dimensional mapping systems has greatly facilitated the mapping and ablation of focal AT. The electroanatomic mapping system is based on sequential mapping technology and permits detailed reconstruction of chamber geometry and activation sequence (Fig. 107-5). A number of studies have demonstrated the ability of electroanatomic mapping to provide a high-resolution map in the region of earliest activation and to precisely locate the AT focus in relation to endocardial geometry.[41] This approach, however, still requires regular ectopics or sustained tachycardia, and as a consequence, electroanatomic maps cannot be constructed in up to 12% of patients.[43] The EnSite noncontact mapping system provides a potential solution to this problem by permitting detailed activation maps to be constructed from isolated beats and nonsustained AT. Schmitt and colleagues[42] used noncontact mapping to identify the site of earliest activation and found that the tachycardia origin could be localized from the analysis of only a few tachycardia cycles.

In general, mapping is facilitated by the targeting of likely anatomic sites. However, AT arising from closely apposed structures, such as the high RA and the right superior pulmonary vein or the perinodal and left septal areas can only be differentiated by detailed and sometimes simultaneous mapping.

Other Mapping Techniques

Paced activation sequence mapping may be used to complement activation mapping and may be helpful when the tachycardia is nonsustained or difficult to induce. This technique involves pacing from a roving ablation catheter at selected locations, with the aim of reproducing the spontaneous endocardial activation sequence on static intracardiac catheters. When this technique is combined with activation mapping for right ATs, success rates as high as 80% have been reported.[44]

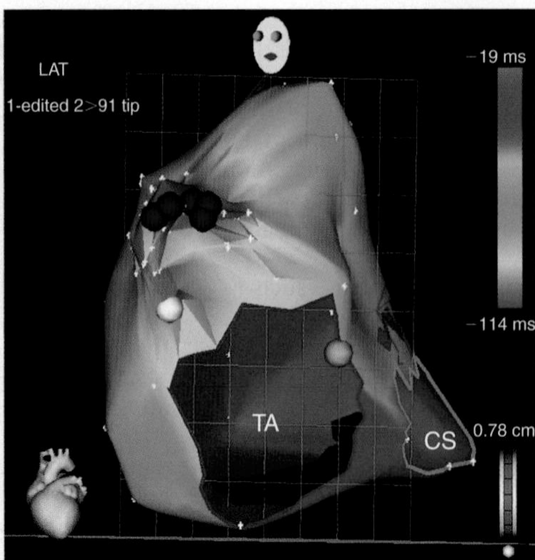

Figure 107-5 Right atrial electroanatomic activation map of an atrial tachycardia (AT) originating from the right atrial appendage. Anteroposterior (*left*) and left anterior oblique (*right*) views are shown, with the tricuspid annulus (TA), coronary sinus ostium (CS) and bundle of His (*yellow dot*) marked. The *brown dots* record the site of successful ablation of the AT in the right atrial appendage. Note the centrifugal activation from the site of origin of the AT, from *red* (early) to *blue* (late), which is precisely localized on the endocardial geometry.

Catheter pressure on an AT focus can transiently interrupt the tachycardia. Pappone and colleagues[45] evaluated the predictive value of intentionally applying pressure to identify successful ablation sites. Mechanical interruption was observed in 76% of successful ablation sites but also in 28% of unsuccessful sites, giving a sensitivity of 76%, specificity of 71%, and positive predictive value of 45%. When combined with activation or pace mapping, mechanical interruption of AT was found to improve both the specificity and positive predictive value of these mapping techniques.[45] One caveat with this technique may be an uncertain endpoint, with an operator being left in doubt as to whether a lack of AT recurrence is due to successful ablation or temporary mechanical stunning.

A study by Mohamed and colleagues[46] described the use of a novel pacing maneuver to localize focal AT. They found that when overdrive pacing from a tachycardia focus, the difference between the postpacing interval and the tachycardia cycle length was less than 20 ms (and often was 0 ms).

Signal Characteristics at Successful Ablation Site

Fractionated electrograms are often found at the successful ablation site during AT in both the right and left atria,[41] but they are not unique to the tachycardia focus. A pure negative deflection (QS pattern) on a unipolar recording, indicating activation away from the unipole, can also be used to identify the site of AT origin. When Tang and colleagues[47] analyzed the unipolar electrogram of ablation sites for focal AT, all successful sites were characterized by a QS morphology, whereas unsuccessful sites displayed an RS pattern.

Efficacy

For the majority of focal ATs, radiofrequency is the energy source of choice. Irrigated ablation may be necessary particularly in regions of low flow such as the trabeculated appendages or within the coronary sinus. Cryoablation is an important modality for ablation of foci near the AV node.[25] Successful ablation is often marked by acceleration of the AT during RF, prior to termination. Acute success is usually defined by the failure to reinitiate AT, with and without isoprenaline, during a postablation holding period of up to 45 minutes.

For patients with AT and significant symptoms, ablation is often the treatment of choice. Ablation series for AT have reported success rates of between 69% and 100%,[41] with a low incidence of complications.[41] Recurrence rates are usually low and vary between 0% and 33%.[41] In an analysis of 16 studies by Chen and colleagues,[48] the only independent predictor of successful radiofrequency ablation was a right atrial focus. Older patients and those with multiple foci or other cardiac diseases, however, were found to be at higher risk for recurrence.[48]

Conclusion

Catheter ablation for SVT has an excellent success rate and can be performed safely with low risk of complications for all forms of regular SVT. In many patients with SVT, RF ablation can be performed as a day procedure and compares very favorably on economic grounds to lifelong medical management.[2] Catheter ablation should be viewed as a first-line therapy for patients with recurrent SVT and as the treatment of choice when a cure is desired.

References

1. Morady F: Catheter ablation of supraventricular arrhythmias: State of the art. J Cardiovasc Electrophysiol 15:124-139, 2004.
2. Blomstrom-Lundqvist C, Scheinman MM, Aliot EM, et al: ACC/AHA/ESC guidelines for the management of patients with supraventricular arrhythmias—executive summary. A report of the American College of Cardiology/American Heart Association task force on practice guidelines and the European Society of Cardiology committee for practice guidelines (writing committee to develop guidelines for the management of patients with supraventricular arrhythmias) developed in collaboration with NASPE-Heart Rhythm Society. J Am Coll Cardiol 42:1493-1531, 2003.
3. Jackman WM, Beckman KJ, McClelland JH, et al: Treatment of supraventricular tachycardia due to atrioventricular nodal reentry, by radiofrequency catheter ablation of slow-pathway conduction. N Engl J Med 327:313-318, 1992.
4. Haissaguerre M, Gaita F, Fischer B, et al: Elimination of atrioventricular nodal reentrant tachycardia using discrete slow potentials to guide application of radiofrequency energy. Circulation 85:2162-2175, 1992.
5. Kalbfleisch SJ, Strickberger SA, Williamson B, et al: Randomized comparison of anatomic and electrogram mapping approaches to ablation of the slow pathway of atrioventricular node reentrant tachycardia. J Am Coll Cardiol 23:716-723, 1994.

6. Jentzer JH, Goyal R, Williamson BD, et al: Analysis of junctional ectopy during radiofrequency ablation of the slow pathway in patients with atrioventricular nodal reentrant tachycardia. Circulation 90:2820-2826, 1994.
7. Tai CT, Chen SA, Chiang CE, et al: Complex electrophysiological characteristics in atrioventricular nodal reentrant tachycardia with continuous atrioventricular node function curves. Circulation 95:2541-2547, 1997.
8. Tai CT, Chen SA, Chiang CE, et al: Multiple anterograde atrioventricular node pathways in patients with atrioventricular node reentrant tachycardia. J Am Coll Cardiol 28:725-731, 1996.
9. Thakur RK, Klein GJ, Yee R, Stites HW: Junctional tachycardia: A useful marker during radiofrequency ablation for atrioventricular node reentrant tachycardia. J Am Coll Cardiol 22:1706-1710, 1993.
10. Engelstein ED, Stein KM, Markowitz SM, Lerman BB: Posterior fast atrioventricular node pathways: Implications for radiofrequency catheter ablation of atrioventricular node reentrant tachycardia. J Am Coll Cardiol 27:1098-1105, 1996.
11. Skanes AC, Dubuc M, Klein GJ, et al: Cryothermal ablation of the slow pathway for the elimination of atrioventricular nodal reentrant tachycardia. Circulation 102:2856-2860, 2000.
12. Strickberger SA, Daoud EG, Niebauer MJ, et al: The mechanisms responsible for lack of reproducible induction of atrioventricular nodal reentrant tachycardia. J Cardiovasc Electrophysiol 7:494-502, 1996.
13. Bogun F, Knight B, Weiss R, et al: Slow pathway ablation in patients with documented but noninducible paroxysmal supraventricular tachycardia. J Am Coll Cardiol 28:1000-1004, 1996.
14. Plumb VJ: Catheter ablation of the accessory pathways of the Wolff-Parkinson-White syndrome and its variants. Prog Cardiovasc Dis 37:295-306, 1995.
15. Ernst S, Ouyang F, Antz M, et al: Catheter ablation of atrioventricular reentery. In Zipes DP, Jalife J (eds): Cardiac Electrophysiology: From Cell to Bedside. Philadelphia, Saunders, 2004, pp 1078-1086.
16. Arruda MS, McClelland JH, Wang X, et al: Development and validation of an ECG algorithm for identifying accessory pathway ablation site in Wolff-Parkinson-White syndrome. J Cardiovasc Electrophysiol 9:2-12, 1998.
17. Schluter M, Cappato R, Ouyang F, et al: Clinical recurrences after successful accessory pathway ablation: The role of "dormant" accessory pathways. J Cardiovasc Electrophysiol 8:1366-1372, 1997.
18. Lesh MD, Van Hare GF, Scheinman MM, et al: Comparison of the retrograde and transseptal methods for ablation of left free wall accessory pathways. J Am Coll Cardiol 22:542-549, 1993.
19. Wong T, Hussain W, Markides V, et al: Ablation of difficult right-sided accessory pathways aided by mapping of tricuspid annular activation using a Halo catheter: Halo-mapping of right sided accessory pathways. J Interv Card Electrophysiol 16:175-182, 2006.
20. Cappato R, Schluter M, Weiss C, et al: Radiofrequency current catheter ablation of accessory atrioventricular pathways in Ebstein's anomaly. Circulation 94:376-383, 1996.
21. Cosio FG, Anderson RH, Kuck KH, et al: Living anatomy of the atrioventricular junctions. A guide to electrophysiologic mapping. A Consensus Statement from the Cardiac Nomenclature Study Group, Working Group of Arrhythmias, European Society of Cardiology, and the Task Force on Cardiac Nomenclature from NASPE. Circulation 100:e31-e37, 1999.
22. Sun Y, Arruda M, Otomo K, et al: Coronary sinus–ventricular accessory connections producing posteroseptal and left posterior accessory pathways: Incidence and electrophysiological identification. Circulation 106:1362-1367, 2002.
23. Yeh SJ, Wang CC, Wen MS, et al: Characteristics and radiofrequency ablation therapy of intermediate septal accessory pathway. Am J Cardiol 73:50-56, 1994.
24. Calkins H, Yong P, Miller JM, et al: Catheter ablation of accessory pathways, atrioventricular nodal reentrant tachycardia, and the atrioventricular junction: Final results of a prospective, multicenter clinical trial. The Atakr Multicenter Investigators Group. Circulation 99:262-270, 1999.
25. Friedman PL: Catheter cryoablation of cardiac arrhythmias. Curr Opin Cardiol 20:48-54, 2005.
26. Lam C, Schweikert R, Kanagaratnam L, Natale A: Radiofrequency ablation of a right atrial appendage–ventricular accessory pathway by transcutaneous epicardial instrumentation. J Cardiovasc Electrophysiol 11:1170-1173, 2000.
27. Natale A, Newby KH, Pisano E, et al: Prospective randomized comparison of antiarrhythmic therapy versus first-line radiofrequency ablation in patients with atrial flutter. J Am Coll Cardiol 35:1898-1904, 2000.
28. Waki K, Saito T, Becker AE: Right atrial flutter isthmus revisited: Normal anatomy favors nonuniform anisotropic conduction. J Cardiovasc Electrophysiol 11:90-94, 2000.
29. Cabrera JA, Sanchez-Quintana D, Farre J, et al: The inferior right atrial isthmus: Further architectural insights for current and coming ablation technologies. J Cardiovasc Electrophysiol 16:402-408, 2005.
30. Sacher F, O'Neill MD, Jais P, et al: Prospective randomized comparison of 8-mm gold-tip, externally irrigated–tip and 8-mm platinum-iridium tip catheters for cavotricuspid isthmus ablation. J Cardiovasc Electrophysiol 18:709-713, 2007.
31. Redfearn DP, Skanes AC, Gula LJ, et al: Cavotricuspid isthmus conduction is dependent on underlying anatomic bundle architecture: Observations using a maximum voltage-guided ablation technique. J Cardiovasc Electrophysiol 17:832-838, 2006.
32. Shah D, Haissaguerre M, Takahashi A, et al: Differential pacing for distinguishing block from persistent conduction through an ablation line. Circulation 102:1517-1522, 2000.
33. Tada H, Oral H, Sticherling C, et al: Double potentials along the ablation line as a guide to radiofrequency ablation of typical atrial flutter. J Am Coll Cardiol 38:750-755, 2001.
34. Saoudi N, Cosio F, Waldo A, et al: Classification of atrial flutter and regular atrial tachycardia according to electrophysiologic mechanism and anatomic bases: A statement from a joint expert group from the Working Group of Arrhythmias of the European Society of Cardiology and the North American Society of Pacing and Electrophysiology. J Cardiovasc Electrophysiol 12:852-866, 2001.
35. Stevenson IH, Kistler PM, Spence SJ, et al: Scar-related right atrial macroreentrant tachycardia in patients without prior atrial surgery: Electroanatomic characterization and ablation outcome. Heart Rhythm 2:594-601, 2005.
36. Jais P, Shah DC, Haissaguerre M, et al: Mapping and ablation of left atrial flutters. Circulation 101:2928-2934, 2000.
37. Magnin-Poull I, De Chillou C, Miljoen H, et al: Mechanisms of right atrial tachycardia occurring late after surgical closure of atrial septal defects. J Cardiovasc Electrophysiol 16:681-687, 2005.
38. Cosio FG, Martin-Penato A, Pastor A, et al: Atypical flutter: A review. Pacing Clin Electrophysiol 26:2157-2169, 2003.
39. Tsai CF, Tai CT, Chen SA: Catheter ablation of atrial tachycardia. In Zipes DP, Jalife J (eds): Cardiac Electrophysiology: From Cell To Bedside. Philadelphia, Saunders, 2004, pp 1060-1068.
40. Roberts-Thomson KC, Kistler PM, Kalman JM: Focal atrial tachycardia I: Clinical features, diagnosis, mechanisms, and anatomic location. Pacing Clin Electrophysiol 29:643-652, 2006.
41. Roberts-Thomson KC, Kistler PM, Kalman JM: Focal atrial tachycardia II: Management. Pacing Clin Electrophysiol 29:769-778, 2006.
42. Schmitt H, Weber S, Schwab JO, et al: Diagnosis and ablation of focal right atrial tachycardia using a new high-resolution, non-contact mapping system. Am J Cardiol 87:1017-1021, 2001.
43. Hoffmann E, Reithmann C, Nimmermann P, et al: Clinical experience with electroanatomic mapping of ectopic atrial tachycardia. Pacing Clin Electrophysiol 25: 49-56, 2002.
44. Tracy CM, Swartz JF, Fletcher RD, et al: Radiofrequency catheter ablation of ectopic atrial tachycardia using paced activation sequence mapping. J Am Coll Cardiol 21:910-917, 1993.
45. Pappone C, Stabile G, De Simone A, et al: Role of catheter-induced mechanical trauma in localization of target sites of radiofrequency ablation in automatic atrial

tachycardia. J Am Coll Cardiol 27:1090-1097, 1996.

46. Mohamed U, Skanes AC, Gula LJ, et al: A novel pacing maneuver to localize focal atrial tachycardia. J Cardiovasc Electrophysiol 18:1-6, 2007.

47. Tang K, Ma J, Zhang S, et al: Unipolar electrogram in identification of successful targets for radiofrequency catheter ablation of focal atrial tachycardia. Chin Med J (Engl) 116:1455-1458, 2003.

48. Chen SA, Tai CT, Chiang CE, et al: Focal atrial tachycardia: Reanalysis of the clinical and electrophysiologic characteristics and prediction of successful radiofrequency ablation. J Cardiovasc Electrophysiol 9:355-365, 1998.

Catheter Ablation for Ventricular Tachycardia in Patients with Structural Heart Disease 108

William G. Stevenson and Usha Tedrow

CHAPTER OUTLINE

Ventricular tachycardia (VT) is an important cause of sudden death and morbidity in patients with structural heart disease. Implantable cardioverter defibrillators (ICDs) can terminate VT when it occurs and are the first-line therapy for most patients who are at high risk. After a spontaneous episode of VT or ventricular fibrillation (VF) and ICD implantation, 40% to 60% of patients experience recurrent VT. A first episode of VT occurs in 2.5% to 12% of patients with ICDs implanted for primary prevention of sudden death.[1-3] ICD shocks reduce quality of life and are associated with an increased risk of heart failure and death, requiring therapy to prevent episodes.[1-3] Antiarrhythmic drug therapy with amiodarone or sotalol reduces episodes of VT but with side effects and only modest efficacy.[1] Catheter ablation can reduce the frequency of VT episodes and can be life saving when VT is incessant.[4-6] Ablation is also an option for symptomatic nonsustained VT and frequent ventricular ectopy when it is symptomatic or contributing to depression of ventricular function.[6]

The type of VT and underlying heart disease direct the approach to mapping and ablation. Most VTs that are considered for ablation are monomorphic, with the same QRS complex from beat to beat indicating repetitive ventricular activation from a structural substrate or focus that can be targeted for ablation, and are due to reentry through regions of ventricular scar (Chapter 61).[7] Ablation can also be used to control recurrent polymorphic VT by targeting initiating ventricular ectopic beats.[8-11]

Preprocedure Preparation and Consideration of Risks

The procedure related mortality is approximately 2%, and most deaths are related to uncontrollable, incessant VT with hemodynamic deterioration in patients with severe disease.[12] Preprocedure planning is important to minimize risks. Underlying heart disease should be defined. The potential for myocardial ischemia should be assessed. Although acute ischemia is not usually the cause of monomorphic VT, it can contribute to hemodynamic instability and increase the risk of the procedure. It is important to consider fluid balance, electrolyte abnormalities, anemia, and metabolic abnormalities, such as hyperthyroidism, that might contribute to hemodynamic deterioration or development of uncontrollable arrhythmias during the procedure.

Cerebral or systemic embolism is reported in 0 to 2.7% of patients.[13,14] If endocardial left ventricular (LV) mapping is planned, echocardiography should be performed. A mobile LV thrombus is a contraindication to LV mapping. If laminated thrombus is suspected, a period of chronic anticoagulation with warfarin may be considered with the hope of reducing the chance that friable thrombus is present, although the efficacy of this approach is not known. During LV mapping and ablation, systemic anticoagulation is achieved with heparin. After ablation, continued anticoagulation with aspirin or warfarin is recommended depending on the extent of ablation performed.

LV access is usually achieved with a retrograde aortic approach across the aortic valve. Damage to the valve or coronary artery ostia are possible, but rare.[13] Major vascular access complications including significant bleeding, arterial dissection, and femoral AV fistulas occur in 2.1% of patients.[13] A transseptal approach to the left atrium allows access to the LV through the mitral valve for patients with peripheral vascular disease or a mechanical aortic valve or when insertion of multiple mapping catheters is desired.

Discontinuation of antiarrhythmic drug therapy is usually desirable to facilitate induction of VT and assessment of the ablation endpoint. Drug withdrawal is not always feasible or necessary in patients with frequent episodes and might precipitate electrical storm in some patients.

Electrophysiologic Evaluation

If ventricular tachycardia is incessant, mapping proceeds during VT. Otherwise, programmed stimulation is used to induce VT to confirm the diagnosis, to establish inducibility as a potential procedural endpoint, and to obtain ECG and intracardiac recordings that suggest the type of VT and its likely origin.

Most patients who have previously failed antiarrhythmic drug therapy have repeated ICD therapies, and inducible VTs are often multiple and unstable (Table 108-1). VT can be unstable for prolonged mapping (often referred to as *unmappable*) due to hemodynamic intolerance, unreliable inducibility, or induction of VT with frequent changes from one morphology to another. Substrate mapping (discussed later) or multielectrode mapping approaches have been developed for these arrhythmias.

Available mapping systems can recreate the geometry of the ventricles based on point-by-point sampling.[15,16] The recorded activation time and electrogram amplitude for each site are color

Table 108-1 Catheter Ablation of Ventricular Tachycardia in Patients with Structural Heart Disease

First Author	Year	N	Heart Disease	Age (yr)	Male	LVEF	Amio before Ablation	VTs/Pt	Unstable VTs Targeted for Ablation (% Pt)	At Least One VT Abolished	All Inducible VTs Abolished	Proc Mortality	Proc Complications	F/U (mo)	Antiarrh drug in F/U	No VT in F/U	Death in F/U
Cesario	2006	20	CAD 60%	64	75%	0.28	100%	N/A	89% of VTs	N/A	N/A	0	10% tamponade, vascular	12	100%	75%	10%
Bogun	2006	48	CAD	66	88%	0.27	79%	1.8	0	86% of VTs	N/A	0	N/A	16	≥79%	88% free of targeted VT	N/A
Segal	2005	40	CAD	65	78%	0.36	83%	3.5	N/A	N/A	73%	0	28% shock, stroke, tamponade, hemothorax AV block, vascular	36	100%	50%	32%
Deneke	2005	25	CAD	62	N/A	0.37	100%	2.4	100%	92%	70%	0	0	10	100%	84%	
Arenal	2004	26	CAD	68	N/A	0.31	N/A	N/A	N/A	96%	69%	0	0	17	N/A	73%	15%
Della Bella	2004	137	CAD	67	66%	.31-.36	99%	2-3	53%	77%	57%	0	N/A	36	99%	51%	9%
Kottkamp	2003	28	CAD	64	89%	0.29	50%	2.3	39%	86%	79%	0	3.5% TIA	15	>50%	64%	7%
Reddy	2003	11	CAD	66	N/A	0.31	64%	3.7	100%	82%	64%	0	9% tamponade	13	≥64%	81%	0
Arenal	2003	24	CAD 88%	66	92%	0.3	N/A	N/A	69%	95%	67%	0	0	9	N/A	78%	17%
Kautzner	2003	28	CAD	63	100%	0.28	71%	2.9	50%	86%	57%	0	3.5% TIA	11	N/A	79%	7%
O'Donnell	2003	112	CAD	64	85%	<0.35 in 42%	N/A	2.4	30%	72%* (more difficult to induce)	38%	0	2% tamponade	72	58%	78%	N/A
de Chillou	2002	21	CAD	66	90%	0.34	N/A	1 or 2	0	95%	57%	0	N/A	16	N/A	81%	10%
Soejima	2002	14	CAD	65	79%	0.29	N/A	N/A	N/A	86%	71%	0	0	6	93%	71%	0
van der Burg	2002	89	CAD	66	N/A	0.29	N/A	N/A	N/A	79%	N/A	2%	9% stroke, incessant VT, tamponade, AV block	34	approx 55%	73%	14%
Soejima	2001	40	CAD	66	95%	0.29	68%	3.6	83%	83%	55%	0	10% all minor vascular access	10	63%	63%	22%

Sra	2001	19	CAD	70	79%	0.27	89%	2.4	82% of targeted VTs	79%	N/A	0	5% tamponade	7	47%	66%	0%
Strickberger	2000	13	CAD	71	92%	0.33	60%	N/A	54%	77%	N/A	8%	23% tamponade, 1 stroke	1	N/A	71%	N/A
Calkins	2000	146	CAD 82%	62	92%	0.31	40%	3	0	>75%	41%	3%	8% stroke, tamponade, AV block, aortic valve injury	8	66%	54%	18%
Soejima	2004	28	DCM	54	86%	0.3	43%	2.9	64%	75%	61%	0	7% pericarditis, AV block	12	27%	64%	4%
Hsia	2003	19	DCM	61	79%	0.34	63%	3	N/A	N/A	74%	0	N/A	22	N/A	32%	21%
Marchlinski	2004	19	RVCM	47	86%	abn in 48%	N/A	3.7	84%	N/A	74%	0	0	27	N/A	84%	N/A
Satomi	2006	17	RVCM	47	76%	N/A	29%	1.5	76%	N/A	82%	0		26	53%	76%	0
Verma	2005	22	RVCM	41	68%	0.55	27%	3	100%	100%	95%	0	5% tamponade	37 median	100%	64%	0
Miljoen	2005	11	RVCM	50	73%	0.54	N/A	1	0	73%	N/A	0	0	36	N/A	73%	1 suicide
O'Donnell	2003	17	RVCM	40	65%	N/A	N/A	1.8	N/A	71%	29%	0	N/A	56	88%	52%	0
van der Burg	2002	32	RVCM	N/A	N/A	N/A	N/A	N/A	N/A	88%	N/A	0	6% tamponade	34	N/A	77%	0
Calkins*	2007	24	RVCM	36	48%	N/A	19%	3	N/A	77%	46%	2%	2% deterioration in VT	32	78%	15%	0 (2 Heart Txp for VT)

*Study had 47 procedures in 24 patients.

Modified from Stevenson WG, Soejima K: Catheter ablation for ventricular tachycardia. Circulation. 115:2750-2760, 2007.

Amio, amiodarone; Antiarrh, antiarrhythmic; CAD, coronary artery disease; DCM, dilated cardiomyopathy; F/U, follow-up; LVEF, left ventricular ejection fraction; N/A, not available; Proc, procedure; Pt, patient; RVCM, right ventricular cardiomyopathy; TIA, transient ischemic attack; Txp, transplant; VT, ventricular tachycardia.

Series from Medline search for ventricular tachycardia ablation from 2000 to 2007. Series with fewer than 10 patients with an individual diagnosis and multiple overlapping series from the same investigators are omitted.

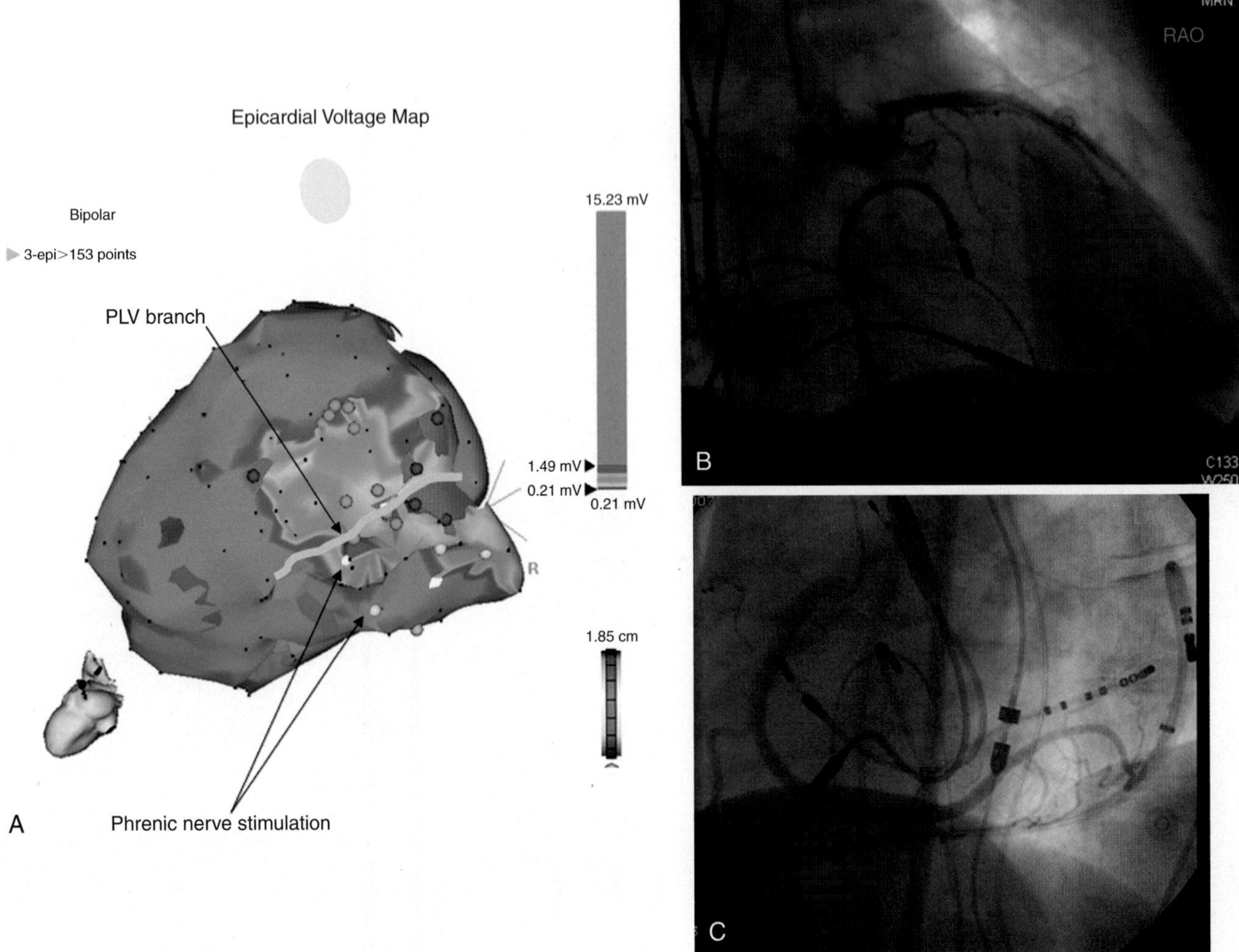

Figure 108-1 Findings from epicardial mapping during sinus rhythm for a patient with ventricular tachycardia (VT) due to idiopathic cardiomyopathy. **A,** Voltage map of the left ventricle viewed from the left posterior oblique position. *Purple* indicates a bipolar electrogram amplitude of 1.5 mV or greater; amplitude diminishes from *blue* to *red*. *Gray* indicates electrically unexcitable scar (EUS). A low amplitude region of scar is present extending along the mitral annulus. Potential obstacles to ablation are indicated. Pacing sites causing diaphragmatic stimulation are indicated in *white*, suggesting close proximity to the phrenic nerve. A *blue line* indicates the course of the posterior left ventricular (PLV) branch of the right coronary artery running through the low-voltage region. **B,** Right anterior oblique projection during left coronary angiography. The epicardial mapping catheter is at the superior border of the low-voltage scar. An implantable cardioverter defibrillator (ICD) system, coronary sinus, His and right ventricle apical catheters are also visible. **C,** Left anterior oblique view during right coronary angiography.

coded for display (Fig. 108-1). A limited map of the region of interest is often sufficient. Precise anatomic definition is limited by cardiac and respiratory motion, and fine anatomic detail, such as trabeculations and papillary muscles, are not visible. The use of intracardiac ultrasound and registration of preacquired CT or MRI images with the electrophysiologic data shows promise for improving anatomic definition.[15,17]

Epicardial Mapping and Ablation

Epicardial ablation is required for 10% to 30% of postinfarct VTs and for more than 30% of VTs due to nonischemic cardiomyopathy.[4,18-21] Percutaneous access to the pericardial space is achieved using an epidural needle under fluoroscopic imaging with contrast injection as described by Sosa and coworkers (see Fig. 108-1).[22] Due to the absence of cooling from circulating blood, low-power heating can limit creation of RF lesions. Larger lesions can likely be created with irrigated RF ablation.[23]

Several potential risks require attention. The risk of injury to an epicardial coronary artery is increased by close proximity and small vessel diameter; overlying fat is protective.[24,25] Proximity to the coronary arteries is assessed from angiography. Ablation directly on a vessel should be avoided. Experimental studies suggest that cryoablation might pose less risk of injury to adjacent coronary arteries than RF ablation, but experience is limited.[24,25] The left phrenic nerve courses down the lateral aspect of the LV and can be identified by pacing from the ablation catheter so that damage from ablation can be avoided. Phrenic nerve protection with a balloon catheter inserted into the pericardial space has been reported.[26] Pericardial bleeding can occur, but it rarely requires prolonged drainage or surgical treatment. Intra-abdominal bleeding from puncture of subdiaphragmatic vessels can also occur. After the procedure, symptoms of pericarditis are common, but they generally resolve within a few days.

Pericardial adhesions after cardiac surgery usually prevent percutaneous access, although limited access is possible in

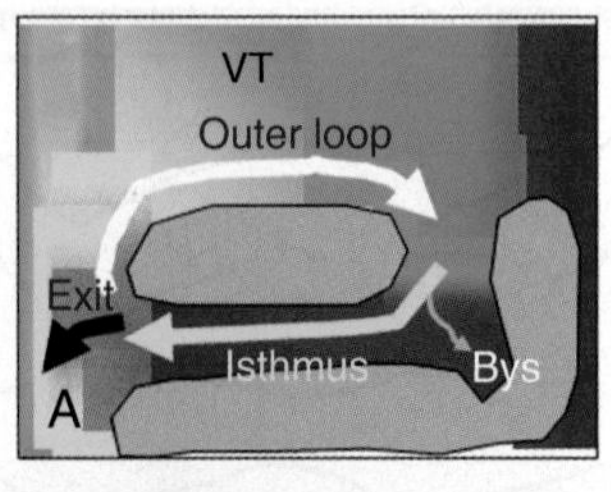

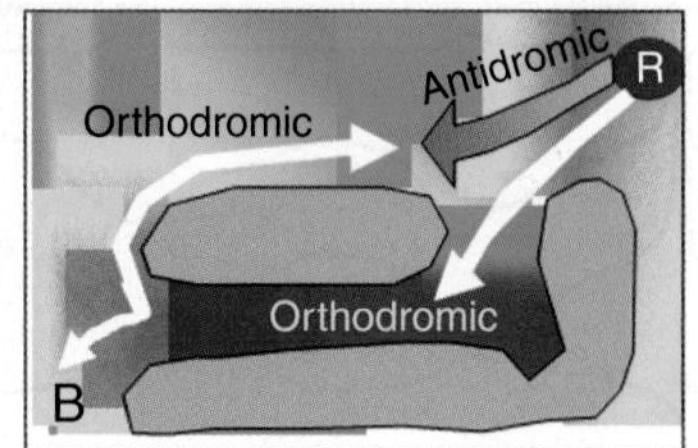

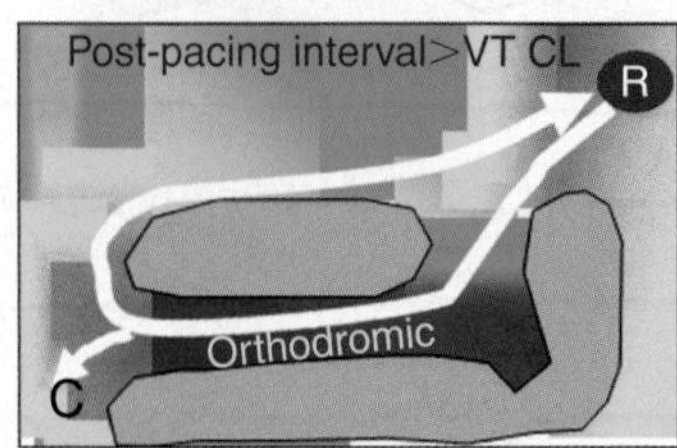

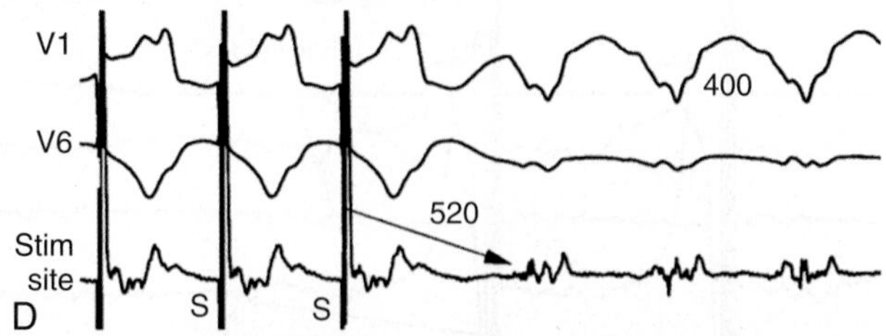

Figure 108-2 Entrainment of reentrant ventricular tachycardia (VT). **A,** Schematic of a theoretical reentry circuit with areas of dense scar *(gray)* defining the circuit. Activation sequence is indicated by arrows and the color scale. The VT circuit has an isthmus *(yellow arrow)*, outer loop along the border of the scar *(white arrow)*, and bystander region *(gray arrow)*. The QRS onset occurs when the wave front emerges from the exit region. **B,** Entrainment from a remote bystander. **C,** Activation producing the post-pacing interval (PPI). **D,** VT with a cycle length of 400 ms is present. The last three stimuli of a pacing train accelerate the QRS complexes and electrograms to the pacing cycle length with a change in QRS morphology compared to VT. The PPI is 520 ms, exceeding the VT cycle length by 120 ms, indicating that the pacing site is not in an isthmus. Bys, bystander region.

some patients.[27] A direct surgical approach to the pericardial space via a subxiphoid pericardial window or thoracotomy is often accessful in these patients.[28]

Identifying Ablation Target Sites

Scar-Related Sustained Monomorphic Ventricular Tachycardia

Reentry related to ventricular scars from prior myocardial infarction, cardiomyopathies, or surgical incisions is the most common cause of sustained monomorphic VT associated with structural heart disease. Scars include regions of dense fibrosis that create conduction block and surviving myocyte bundles that produce zones of slow conduction due to interstitial fibrosis and diminished cellular coupling.[29] The resultant reentrant circuits can be modeled as having an isthmus or channel composed of a small mass of tissue that does not contribute to the surface ECG (Figs. 108-2 and 108-3). The QRS complex begins when the excitation wave front emerges from an exit along the border of the scar and spreads across the ventricles. Scars related to VT often border a valve annulus that forms a border segment for part of the circuit.[21,30,31] Slow, stable VTs often result from relatively large macroreentry circuits spanning several centimeters.[32] Multiple VTs with different QRS morphologies can be due to multiple exits from the same region of scar or changes in activation remote from the circuit due to functional regions of block.[16,31,33] Ablation at one region often abolishes more than one VT.[33-36] Multiple reentry circuits from widely separated areas also often occur.

QRS Morphology as a Guide to the Ventricular Tachycardia Exit

The QRS morphology of VT indicates the location of the reentry circuit exit.[37] A left bundle branch block–like configuration in lead V1 indicates an exit in the right ventricle or interventricular septum; dominant R waves in V1 indicate an exit in the LV. A superiorly directed frontal plane axis indicates an inferior wall exit, and an inferiorly directed one indicates an anterior wall exit. The closer an exit is to a precordial lead, the more negative the S wave is in that lead, providing an indication of exit location between the base and apex. Apical exits generate dominant S waves in leads V3 and V4. Basal exits generate dominant R waves in these leads.

The QRS morphology is also helpful in suggesting whether epicardial ablation is likely required. Epicardial reentry circuits produce VTs that typically have a relatively long QRS duration, slow QRS upstroke, producing a pseudo-delta wave, possibly related to delayed activation of the endocardial Purkinje system as compared to endocardial VTs.[38]

It is important to recognize that the QRS morphology only suggests a starting point for localization of the VT circuit. Areas of scars, conduction block, and abnormal ventricular anatomy can render the QRS morphology misleading. Pace mapping is often helpful in suggesting whether the relation between anatomic location and anticipated QRS morphology is as expected.

Substrate Mapping—Electrograms and Pace Mapping

Substrate mapping delineates the likely arrhythmogenic substrate during a stable sinus or paced rhythm. This method often allows likely exits and channels to be identified without mapping during VT, facilitating ablation in patients with multiple and unstable VTs.[16,20,31,39]

Areas of ventricular scar are characterized by low amplitude peak-to-peak bipolar electrograms (< 1.55 mV). Electroanatomic voltage maps display this information (see Fig. 108-1).[16,39] The low voltage region is likely to contain the reentry circuit, but it is often extensive, exceeding 20 cm in circumference.[31] Ablation of the entire region might not be feasible. Additional analyses of electrograms, voltage, or pace mapping are used to refine selection of target sites.

In voltage maps, the border region extends along the scar margin defined by electrogram amplitude between 1.5 and 0.5 mV. Exit regions are usually located along the scar border (Fig. 108-4). Pacing in the exit region replicates the QRS morphology of VT,[40,41] with a short stimulus to QRS time consistent with its location in the infarct border.

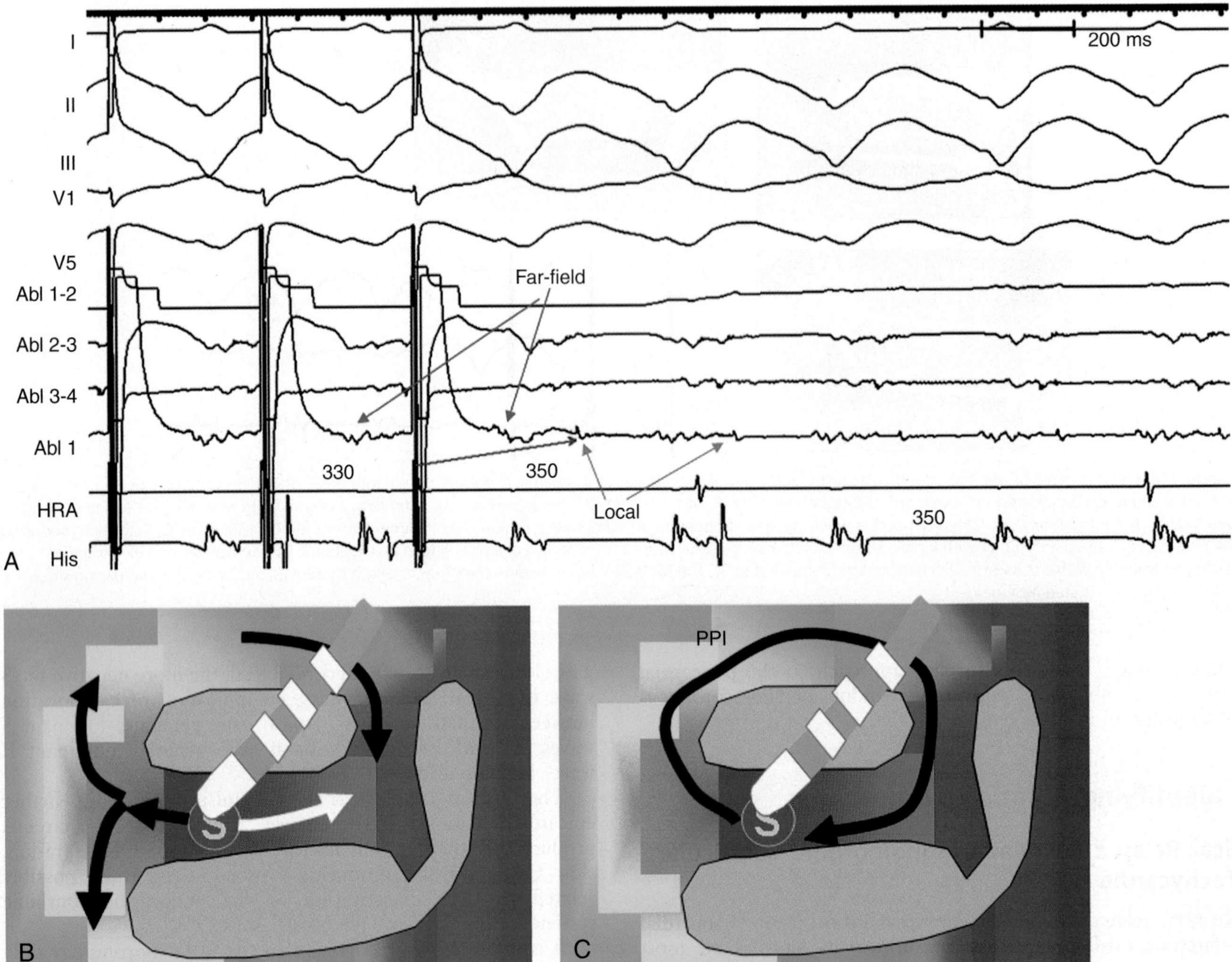

Figure 108-3 Entrainment from an epicardial isthmus site **(A)** from the patient shown in Figure 108-1 and schematics **(B** and **C)** are shown. **A,** Surface electrocardiogram (ECG) and cardiac recordings from the epicardial ablation catheter (Abl) with bipolar records from distal (1-2), mid (2-3), and proximal (3-4) electrodes and a high-pass filtered unipolar recording from electrode 1 (Abl 1), high right atrium (HRA), and His bundle region (His). Ventricular tachycardia (VT) with a cycle length (CL) of 350 ms is present. Unipolar pacing at 330 ms from the distal electrode of the ablation catheter accelerates the QRS complexes and electrograms to the pacing rate. Measurement of the postpacing interval (PPI) requires assessment of which electrogram most likely indicates the local potential. During pacing, a broad fractionated potential is visible, indicating that this is a far-field potential *(blue arrows)*. The potential that is not visible during pacing is the likely local potential *(red arrow)*. The PPI measured to the local potential is 350 ms, matching the VT cycle length. The QRS during pacing is identical to that of VT (also confirmed in the 12-lead ECG that is not shown). These findings are consistent with pacing from an isthmus in the reentry circuit as shown schematically in **B** and **C**. Stimulated orthodromic wave fronts are indicated with *black arrows*. The stimulated antidromic wave front is the *white arrow* in **B**.

An isthmus can be suggested by delayed activation during sinus or paced rhythm, creating isolated potentials inscribed after the end of the QRS.[42-46] Pacing produces a QRS that emerges after a delay (S-QRS >40 ms) due to slow conduction through the channel (see Fig. 108-4). When the stimulated wave front propagates through the channel to an exit region, the paced QRS morphology resembles VT, suggesting that the pacing site is in a reentry circuit isthmus.[40,45] If the wave front leaves the scar by another path, the paced QRS morphology might differ from VT or might resemble a different VT.

Potential channels can sometimes be exposed by assessing the relative electrogram amplitudes in a low-voltage region.[47,48] Reducing the threshold for electrogram amplitude below 1.5 mV can expose a relatively higher voltage channel bordered by lower voltage regions.

Areas of electrically unexcitable scar (EUS) that are regions of fixed conduction block can be identified from a high pacing threshold (>10 mA at 2 ms pulse width with unipolar pacing).[34] Marking EUS areas (gray area on the voltage map in Figs. 108-1 and 108-4) can create a visual map of potential VT channels. Detecting areas of EUS depends on the size of the virtual electrode produced by the pacing stimulus, relative to the dimensions of the fibrosis beneath the electrode. Narrow bands of fibrosis likely escape detection with this method. Inadequate electrode myocardial contact is also a potential source of error. EUS cannot be reliably detected based on electrogram amplitude alone. Pacing captures at the majority of sites with very low electrogram amplitude of 0.25 mV. In contrast, some EUS sites have electrogram amplitude greater than 0.5 mV due to the presence of large far-field potentials from depolarization of a substantial mass of adjacent myocardium (see Fig. 108-3). Thus, electrogram

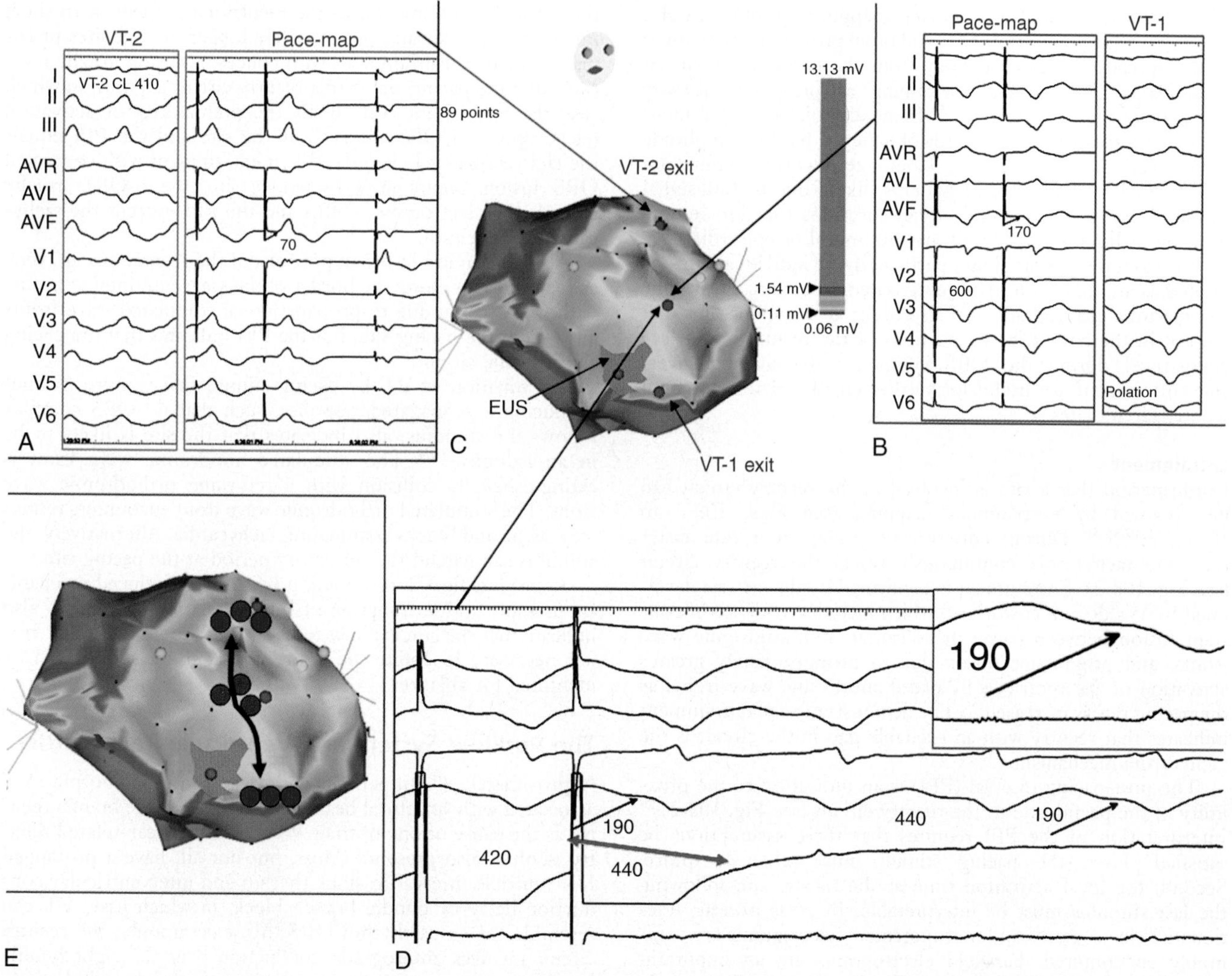

Figure 108-4 Findings from mapping in a patient with a prior anterior wall infarction. **A,** VT-2 has a right bundle branch block inferior axis configuration. Pacing at the superior aspect of the infarct *(arrow)* reproduces the VT-2 QRS morphology, indicating that the exit for VT-2 is near the pacing site. **B,** Pacing at a site in the middle of the infarct. There is a delay of 170 ms from the pacing stimulus to the QRS, indicating slow conduction through the scar to the margin of the infarct. The paced QRS has a left bundle branch block superior axis configuration that matched VT-1, suggesting that the pacing site was in a channel used by VT-1, and is confirmed by pacing during VT-1 in **D. C,** Voltage map viewed from the right anterior projection. *Purple* indicates electrogram amplitude of 1.5 mV or greater, and a *gray* region of electrically unexcitable scar is present. These are also seen in **E. D,** During VT-1 pacing at the isthmus produces entrainment with concealed fusion with a postpacing interval (PA) that matches the ventricular tachycardia (VT) cycle length. Pacing entrains tachycardia with a long stimulus to QRS interval without changing the QRS morphology and with a PPI (measured to the low-amplitude diastolic potential that is enlarged in the inset) that matches the VT cycle length. **E,** The potential channel *(black arrow)* with exits at the superior and inferior septal margin of the infarct. Potential ablation targets are the exits *(red circles)* and the channel *(dark blue circles)*. (Modified with permission from Stevenson WG, Soejima K: Catheter ablation for ventricular tachycardia. Circulation 115:2750-2760, 2007.)

characteristics and pacing techniques provide complementary information during substrate mapping.

Additional mapping and entrainment during VT can help to confirm that a candidate region is in a reentry circuit and can facilitate successful ablation with fewer ablation lesions.[31] Alternatively RF lesions can be placed through presumptive exits or channels, followed by retesting for inducible VT.[16,31,41] Even when VT is stable, substrate mapping may be used to identify regions for further evaluation during VT, minimizing the time spent in VT.

Mapping during Ventricular Tachycardia

When VT is stable for mapping, assessment of activation and electrograms and entrainment are useful for targeting the reentry circuit.[31,32,49,50] When VT is not stable for extensive mapping, these assessments might still be useful during brief episodes of tachycardia to confirm that a region identified during substrate mapping is involved in the tachycardia.[31]

Activation Mapping and Electrograms

During VT, the circuit exit and isthmus have presystolic (prior to the QRS onset) and diastolic activation (see Fig. 108-3). Isolated diastolic potentials are often recorded at isthmus sites (see Fig. 108-4D). Their timing is presystolic near the exit and progressively earlier relative to the QRS onset at sites farther from the reentry circuit isthmus. Sites that are proximal in the circuit can be activated at the end of the QRS complex, without diastolic electrical activity, but can be identified by entrainment.[51]

Multielectrode and noncontact mapping systems acquire electrograms from multiple sites and often provide an assessment of the spread of activation away from the endocardial exit or breakthrough site, usually beginning as presystolic activity along the border of a scar.[33,52-54] Some diastolic activity is identified in approximately two thirds of patients, but low-amplitude signals can escape detection. Complete reentry circuits are defined in less than 20% of patients, likely due to low signal amplitude or to endocardial circuit locations that are remote from the balloon electrodes or are intramural or epicardial.[52]

Electrogram timing alone, particularly at individual sites, is limited as an indication of a reentry circuit location. Presystolic and diastolic electrograms can also occur at bystander sites that are not in the circuit. Some portions of the reentry circuit are depolarized during the QRS complex.[55] Pacing maneuvers and entrainment are useful for further characterizing potential reentry circuit sites.

Entrainment

Confirmation that a site is involved in the reentry circuit can be obtained by entrainment mapping (see Figs. 108-2 to 108-4).[31,49,55,56] During entrainment pacing at a rate faster than the tachycardia continuously resets the reentry circuit (see Fig. 108-2). Entrainment is confirmed by the criteria developed by Waldo and coworkers, which includes evidence of constant fusion between paced orthodromic and antidromic wave fronts, and progressive fusion due to proportionately greater activation of the ventricles by paced antidromic wave fronts as the pacing rate is increased.[57] The demonstration of entrainment indicates that reentry with an excitable gap in the circuit is the tachycardia mechanism.

The post-pacing interval (PPI) is an indication of the proximity of the pacing site to the reentry circuit (see Fig. 108-2).[58] Interpretation of the PPI requires that three assumptions be satisfied. First, the pacing stimuli must reliably capture. Second, the local activation time at the pacing site following the last stimulus must be interpretable. In areas of scar, fractionated electrograms and multipotential electrograms are commonly encountered. Far-field electrograms are an important source of error interpreting the PPI, often resulting in a falsely short PPI.[59] Far-field electrograms can often be recognized by their unperturbed presence during pacing, indicating that they are the result of depolarized tissue remote from the pacing catheter (see Fig. 108-2). In contrast, the local potential is obscured by the stimulus artifact during pacing. When the local potential cannot be assessed late after the stimulus due to saturation of the recording amplifier, measuring the PPI to local electrograms recorded on the adjacent proximal electrodes agrees with the distal electrode recordings at approximately 85% of sites.[60] The $S\text{-}QRS_{n+1}$ measures can also be used.[61] The third assumption for PPI validity is that pacing does not alter conduction times in the circuit or the reentry path. Slowing of conduction, as is common in the presence of antiarrhythmic medications, falsely prolongs the PPI.

When pacing is performed at an isthmus site in the circuit, (see Fig. 108-3) the stimulated orthodromic wave fronts follow the path of the reentry circuit, emerging from the exit. The stimulated antidromic wave fronts are contained in or near the circuit by areas of block that define the isthmus and by collision with returning orthodromic wave fronts. Fusion resulting from collision of stimulated antidromic and orthodromic wave fronts occurs in or near the pacing site and is not evident as fusion in the surface ECG. The tachycardia is accelerated to the pacing rate with a QRS morphology that is identical to that of the VT. This is entrainment with concealed fusion, or a form of concealed entrainment. During entrainment with concealed fusion, the stimulus to QRS interval (S-QRS) indicates the conduction time from the pacing site to the reentry circuit exit, with short times near the exit and progressively longer ones at sites proximal to the exit. Entrainment with concealed fusion usually indicates that the pacing site is in a reentry circuit isthmus, in which case the S-QRS interval equals the prematurity of activation (electrogram to QRS interval) at the site and the PPI equals the tachycardia cycle length. When entrainment with concealed QRS fusion occurs at a bystander site, the S-QRS usually exceeds the electrogram—QRS and the PPI exceeds the tachycardia cycle length.

At sites that are in broad portions of the reentry circuit, such as reentry loops along the border of the scar, entrainment occurs with QRS fusion due to propagation of stimulated wave fronts away from the pacing site, but the PPI indicates that the pacing site is in the circuit.[62]

Termination of VT by pacing stimuli that capture without producing a propagated response, such that no QRS complex follows the stimulus, also indicates that the site is likely to be in an isthmus.[63,64] The stimulated antidromic wave front is extinguished by collision with a returning orthodromic wave front. The stimulated orthodromic wave front encounters refractory tissue and blocks terminating tachycardia. Alternatively, the stimulus can extend the refractory period at the pacing site.

Reproducible VT termination by catheter-induced mechanical pressure and termination of VT by ablation during VT also indicate that the site is likely to be in the VT circuit.[49,65,66] It is not necessary to define the entire circuit if an isthmus can be identified for ablation.

The Purkinje System and Ventricular Tachycardia

Approximately 8% of patients with sustained monomorphic VT associated with structural heart disease have bundle branch reentry as the cause of one of their VTs, although scar-related reentry is often also present.[7] Most, but not all, have a prolonged His-ventricle interval in sinus rhythm and interventricular conduction delay or bundle branch block, in which case, VT can resemble the sinus rhythm QRS. Most commonly, the reentry circuit involves anterograde conduction over the right bundle branch and retrograde conduction over the left bundle branch, giving rise to VT with a left bundle branch block configuration. The PPI at the apical septum indicates that this region is in or near the circuit.[67] A right bundle potential or His bundle electrogram preceding and linked to the QRS helps establish the diagnosis. Ablation of the right bundle branch typically eliminates this VT. Occasionally, interfascicular reentry requires ablation of left bundle fascicles. Most patients warrant implantation of an ICD due to associated depressed ventricular function, scar-related inducible VTs, and often poor infranodal conduction.

Portions of the Purkinje system can also be involved in scar-related reentry circuits, particularly after myocardial infarction.[68,69] These VTs can have a relatively narrow QRS duration of 145 ms or less, with Purkinje potentials present in the exit region.

Rarely, automaticity in the Purkinje system is the cause of VT in patients with structural heart disease. [7] VT often requires isoproterenol administration for initiation. A Purkinje potential is present at the successful ablation site.

Acute Procedural Endpoints and Outcomes

Patients with recurrent episodes of VT in reported series have generally failed drug therapy.[12,13,31,34,35,70-72] An average of three different monomorphic VTs are usually induced. Those observed to occur spontaneously are often referred to as *clinical VTs*. However, the QRS morphology of spontaneous VT is often not known when ICDs promptly terminate VT. Some *nonclinical* VTs subsequently occur spontaneously.[35,52,70]

Abolishing incessant VT and inducible clinical VT is generally considered the minimum endpoint for acute procedure success.[49,56] Some centers attempt to abolish all inducible VTs, or all inducible mappable VTs, in the hope of reducing recurrences.[16,31,35,41,71,72] Ablation lesion sets for multiple and unmappable VTs include ablation lines through exit regions, ablation through all identified isthmuses, ablation through isthmuses or exits extending to the border of the scar, and ablation of all diastolic potential sites. These strategies and endpoints have not been directly compared.

Following ablation, at least one VT is no longer inducible in 73% to 100% of patients, and no monomorphic VT of any type can be induced in 38% to 95% of patients (see Table 108-1). Remaining inducible VTs are often faster and initiated by more aggressive stimulation than the initial VTs.[31,35,72,73] Acute failure often appears to be due to anatomic obstacles, such as epicardial or intramural reentry circuits. Ablation with larger tip (8 mm) or irrigated catheters can be helpful to reach deep circuits.

When the targeted VT remains inducible after ablation, the recurrence risk exceeds 60%.[70,71] Absence of any inducible VT has been associated with a lower but still significant incidence of recurrence ranging from less than 3% to 27% in single-center reports and 44% to 51% in multicenter studies.[12,13,31,34,35,70-72] Inducible nonclinical VTs are associated with increased risk of recurrence in some studies.[72,74] Healing of initial ablation lesions and reduction of antiarrhythmic medications likely contribute to recurrences. Some patients benefit from a repeat procedure.

Major complications are reported in 5% to 10% of patients (see Table 108-1), including cardiac tamponade, shock, stroke (0 to 2.7%), AV block due to ablation of septal VTs, and major vascular access complications. The procedure mortality is in the range of 2% to 3% and is often due to failure to control VT in patients with advanced disease.[12,13]

Ablation in Specific Diseases

Prior Myocardial Infarction

Ablation is acutely successful, abolishing one or more scar-related monomorphic VTs in 77% to 95% (see Table 108-1). VT recurs in 12% to 50% of patients, but the frequency is often reduced. The annual mortality following catheter ablation ranges from 5% to more than 20%.[13,74,75] Progressive heart failure is the most common cause of death.[3] Greater age and greater LV size and dysfunction are markers for increased mortality.[74,75] The potential for ablation to adversely effect LV function is of concern. Assessment of LV ejection fraction after ablation has not shown deterioration, but is not very sensitive for detecting injury.[16,76] Confining ablation to regions of scar and attention to medical therapy for ventricular dysfunction seems prudent.

Dilated Cardiomyopathy and Valvular Heart Disease

Approximately 80% of patients with sustained monomorphic VT have scar-related reentry; in the remainder, VT is due to bundle branch reentry or has a focal origin.[20,21,77-79] Scars can be demonstrated with MR imaging and are often adjacent to a valve annulus.[21,78,80] Ablation is more difficult than for VT associated with coronary artery disease. Reentry circuits are epicardial in more than a third of patients (see Figs. 108-1 and 108-3).[20,21]

Incessant idiopathic VT or ventricular ectopy can cause tachycardia induced cardiomyopathy that improves after ablation.[77,81]

Right Ventricular Cardiomyopathies

Scar-related RV tachycardias occur in idiopathic cardiomyopathy, genetic arrhythmogenic RV dysplasia or cardiomyopathy (Chapter 64), and cardiac sarcoidosis.[30,70,82-86] Scar can be identified on delayed enhancement on MR imaging.[87,88] Reentry circuits are often adjacent to the tricuspid or pulmonic annulus.[30,85] Epicardial reentry can create endocardial breakthrough that mimics a focal origin.[85] Focal-origin VTs due to automaticity also occur. Reported series likely contain patients with heterogeneous etiologies of RV scar. Series with patients who meet criteria for genetic forms of arrhythmogenic RV dysplasia have shown a good acute success rate, but recurrence is greater than 70% during follow-up exceeding 1 year, suggesting disease progression.[84,89] Ablation for VT due to sarcoidosis has also been associated with a high recurrence rate.[83] Other series, in which the predominant disease seems less consistent with genetic arrhythmogenic RV dysplasia, have reported better outcomes.[30]

Repaired Congenital Heart Disease

Scar-related VT involving RV regions of repair also occur later after surgical correction of congenital heart disease.[90,91] In tetralogy of Fallot, VT usually involves an isthmus that can be interrupted with ablation between the tricuspid valve annulus and scar or patch material in the free wall of the RV.[91] Catheter ablation is feasible, with successful outcomes in 43% to 91% of patients reported in relatively small series with follow-up exceeding 2 years.[90,91]

Ablation for Polymorphic Ventricular Tachycardia and Ventricular Fibrillation

Recurrent polymorphic VT causing electrical storm that is not due to ongoing acute ischemia is rare, but it occurs in idiopathic ventricular fibrillation, the long QT syndrome, Brugada syndrome, and early and late after myocardial infarction.[5,8,10,11] VT is often initiated by premature beats from one or a few foci that can be targeted for ablation if they occur with sufficient frequency. Sharp potentials consistent with Purkinje activation are often recorded from foci in the left or right ventricles. Less often, a right ventricular outflow tract focus is a trigger. Arrhythmias can wax and wane. Immediate patient transport to the laboratory when the arrhythmia is active is warranted if ablation is to be attempted. Approximately 90% of selected patients are free from recurrences during follow-up.[5,8,10,11]

Summary

Catheter ablation of VT has an important role in reducing VT episodes in patients with ICDs and controlling incessant VT and electrical storms. Techniques for epicardial mapping and ablation have improved outcomes for patients with arrhythmias that are not endocardial in origin. The approach is determined by the characteristics of the arrhythmia and underlying heart disease. Present techniques enable ablation for multiple and hemodynamically unstable VTs, formerly considered unmappable. Failure is often related to anatomic obstacles that would potentially benefit from further technologic advances.

References

1. Connolly SJ, Dorian P, Roberts RS, et al: Comparison of beta-blockers, amiodarone plus beta-blockers, or sotalol for prevention of shocks from implantable cardioverter defibrillators: The OPTIC Study: A randomized trial. JAMA 295:165-171, 2006.
2. Schron EB, Exner DV, Yao Q, et al: Quality of life in the antiarrhythmics versus implantable defibrillators trial: Impact of therapy and influence of adverse symptoms and defibrillator shocks. Circulation 105:589-594, 2002.
3. Moss AJ, Greenberg H, Case RB, et al: Long-term clinical course of patients after termination of ventricular tachyarrhythmia by an implanted defibrillator. Circulation 110:3760-3765, 2004.
4. Brugada J, Berruezo A, Cuesta A, et al: Nonsurgical transthoracic epicardial radiofrequency ablation: An alternative in incessant ventricular tachycardia. J Am Coll Cardiol 41:2036-2043, 2003.
5. Bansch D, Oyang F, Antz M, et al: Successful catheter ablation of electrical storm after myocardial infarction. Circulation 108:3011-3016, 1999.
6. Zipes DP, Camm AJ, Borggrefe M, et al: ACC/AHA/ESC 2006 guidelines for management of patients with ventricular arrhythmias and the prevention of sudden cardiac death: A report of the American College of Cardiology/American Heart Association Task Force and the European Society of Cardiology Committee for Practice Guidelines (Writing Committee to Develop Guidelines for Management of Patients with Ventricular Arrhythmias and the Prevention of Sudden Cardiac Death). J Am Coll Cardiol 48:e247-e346, 2006.
7. Lopera G, Stevenson WG, Soejima K, et al: Identification and ablation of three types of ventricular tachycardia involving the His-Purkinje system in patients with heart disease. J Cardiovasc Electrophysiol 15:52-58, 2004.
8. Szumowski L, Sanders P, Walczak F, et al: Mapping and ablation of polymorphic ventricular tachycardia after myocardial infarction. J Am Coll Cardiol 44:1700-1706, 2004.
9. Noda T, Shimizu W, Taguchi A, et al: Malignant entity of idiopathic ventricular fibrillation and polymorphic ventricular tachycardia initiated by premature extrasystoles originating from the right ventricular outflow tract. J Am Coll Cardiol 46:1288-1294, 2005.
10. Haissaguerre M, Extramiana F, Hocini M, et al: Mapping and ablation of ventricular fibrillation associated with long-QT and Brugada syndromes. Circulation 108:925-928, 1999.
11. Marrouche NF, Verma A, Wazni O, et al: Mode of initiation and ablation of ventricular fibrillation storms in patients with ischemic cardiomyopathy. J Am Coll Cardiol 43:1715-1720, 2004.
12. Stevenson WG, Wilber DJ, Natale A, et al: Irrigated radiofrequency catheter ablation guided by electroanatomic mapping for recurrent ventricular tachycardia after myocardial infarction: the multicenter thermocool ventricular tachycardia ablation trial. Circulation 118:2773-2782, 2008.
13. Calkins H, Epstein A, Packer D, et al: Catheter ablation of ventricular tachycardia in patients with structural heart disease using cooled radiofrequency energy: Results of a prospective multicenter study. Cooled RF Multi Center Investigators Group. J Am Coll Cardiol 35:1905-1914, 2000.
14. Stevenson WG, Soejima K: Catheter ablation for ventricular tachycardia. Circulation 115:2750-2760, 2007.
15. Reddy VY, Malchano ZJ, Holmvang G, et al: Integration of cardiac magnetic resonance imaging with three-dimensional electroanatomic mapping to guide left ventricular catheter manipulation: Feasibility in a porcine model of healed myocardial infarction. J Am Coll Cardiol 44:2202-2213, 2004.
16. Marchlinski FE, Callans DJ, Gottlieb CD, et al: Linear ablation lesions for control of unmappable ventricular tachycardia in patients with ischemic and nonischemic cardiomyopathy. Circulation 101:1288-1296, 2007.
17. Iwai S, Cantillon DJ, Kim RJ, et al: Right and left ventricular outflow tract tachycardias: evidence for a common electrophysiologic mechanism. J Cardiovasc Electrophysiol 17:1052-1058, 2006.
18. Daniels DV, Lu YY, Morton JB, et al: Idiopathic epicardial left ventricular tachycardia originating remote from the sinus of Valsalva: Electrophysiological characteristics, catheter ablation, and identification from the 12-lead electrocardiogram. Circulation 113:1659-1666, 2006.
19. Sosa E, Scanavacca M, d'Avila A, et al: Nonsurgical transthoracic epicardial catheter ablation to treat recurrent ventricular tachycardia occurring late after myocardial infarction. J Am Coll Cardiol 35:1442-1449, 2007.
20. Cesario DA, Vaseghi M, Boyle NG, et al: Value of high-density endocardial and epicardial mapping for catheter ablation of hemodynamically unstable ventricular tachycardia. Heart Rhythm 3:1-10, 2006.
21. Soejima K, Stevenson WG, Sapp JL, et al: Endocardial and epicardial radiofrequency ablation of ventricular tachycardia associated with dilated cardiomyopathy: The importance of low-voltage scars. J Am Coll Cardiol 43:1834-1842, 2004.
22. Sosa E, Scanavacca M: Images in cardiovascular medicine. Percutaneous pericardial access for mapping and ablation of epicardial ventricular tachycardias. Circulation 115:e542-e544, 2007.
23. d'Avila A, Houghtaling C, Gutierrez P, et al: Catheter ablation of ventricular epicardial tissue: A comparison of standard and cooled-tip radiofrequency energy. Circulation 109:2363-2369, 2004.
24. D'Avila A, Gutierrez P, Scanavacca M, et al: Effects of radiofrequency pulses delivered in the vicinity of the coronary arteries: Implications for nonsurgical transthoracic epicardial catheter ablation to treat ventricular tachycardia. Pacing Clin Electrophysiol 25:1488-1495, 2002.
25. Lustgarten DL, Bell S, Hardin N, et al: Safety and efficacy of epicardial cryoablation in a canine model. Heart Rhythm 2:82-90, 2005.
26. Buch E, Vaseghi M, Cesario DA, et al: A novel method for preventing phrenic nerve injury during catheter ablation. Heart Rhythm 4:95-98, 2007.
27. Sosa E, Scanavacca M, D'Avila A, et al: Nonsurgical transthoracic epicardial approach in patients with ventricular tachycardia and previous cardiac surgery. J Interv Card Electrophysiol 10:281-288, 2004.
28. Soejima K, Couper G, Cooper JM, et al: Subxiphoid surgical approach for epicardial catheter-based mapping and ablation in patients with prior cardiac surgery or difficult pericardial access. Circulation 110:1197-1201, 2004.
29. de Bakker JM, van Capelle FJ, Janse MJ, et al: Slow conduction in the infarcted human heart. "Zigzag" course of activation. Circulation 88:915-926, 1993.
30. Marchlinski FE, Zado E, Dixit S, et al: Electroanatomic substrate and outcome of catheter ablative therapy for ventricular tachycardia in setting of right ventricular cardiomyopathy. Circulation 110:2293-2298, 2004.
31. Soejima K, Suzuki M, Maisel WH, et al: Catheter ablation in patients with multiple and unstable ventricular tachycardias after myocardial infarction: Short ablation lines guided by reentry circuit isthmuses and sinus rhythm mapping. Circulation 104:664-669, 2001.
32. de Chillou C, Lacroix D, Klug D, et al: Isthmus characteristics of reentrant ventricular tachycardia after myocardial infarction. Circulation 105:726-731, 2002.
33. Klemm HU, Ventura R, Steven D, et al: Catheter ablation of multiple ventricular tachycardias after myocardial infarction guided by combined contact and noncontact mapping. Circulation 115:2697-2704, 2007.
34. Soejima K, Stevenson WG, Maisel WH, et al: Electrically unexcitable scar mapping based on pacing threshold for identification of the reentry circuit isthmus: Feasibility for guiding ventricular tachycardia ablation. Circulation 106:1678-1683, 2002.
35. Della Bella P, Riva S, Fassini G, et al: Incidence and significance of pleomorphism in patients with postmyocardial infarction ventricular tachycardia. Acute and long-term outcome of radiofrequency catheter ablation. Eur Heart J 25:1127-1138, 2004.
36. Bogun F, Li YG, Groenefeld G, et al: Prevalence of a shared isthmus in postinfarction patients with pleiomorphic, hemodynamically tolerated ventricular tachycardias. J Cardiovasc Electrophysiol 13:237-241, 2002.
37. Josephson ME, Callans DJ: Using the twelve-lead electrocardiogram to localize the site of origin of ventricular tachycardia. Heart Rhythm 2:443-446, 2005.

38. Berruezo A, Mont L, Nava S, et al: Electrocardiographic recognition of the epicardial origin of ventricular tachycardias. Circulation 109:1842-1847, 2004.
39. Reddy VY, Neuzil P, Taborsky M, et al: Short-term results of substrate mapping and radiofrequency ablation of ischemic ventricular tachycardia using a saline-irrigated catheter. J Am Coll Cardiol 41:2228-2236, 1999.
40. Brunckhorst CB, Delacretaz E, Soejima K, et al: Identification of the ventricular tachycardia isthmus after infarction by pace mapping. Circulation 110:652-659, 2004.
41. Kottkamp H, Wetzel U, Schirdewahn P, et al: Catheter ablation of ventricular tachycardia in remote myocardial infarction: Substrate description guiding placement of individual linear lesions targeting noninducibility. J Cardiovasc Electrophysiol 14:675-681, 2003.
42. Arenal A, Glez-Torrecilla E, Ortiz M, et al: Ablation of electrograms with an isolated, delayed component as treatment of unmappable monomorphic ventricular tachycardias in patients with structural heart disease. J Am Coll Cardiol 41:81-92, 1999.
43. Harada T, Stevenson WG, Kocovic DZ, et al: Catheter ablation of ventricular tachycardia after myocardial infarction: Relation of endocardial sinus rhythm late potentials to the reentry circuit. J Am Coll Cardiol 30:1015-1023, 1997.
44. Brunckhorst CB, Stevenson WG, Jackman WM, et al: Ventricular mapping during atrial and ventricular pacing. Relationship of multipotential electrograms to ventricular tachycardia reentry circuits after myocardial infarction. Eur Heart J 23:1131-1138, 2002.
45. Bogun F, Good E, Reich S, et al: Isolated potentials during sinus rhythm and pace-mapping within scars as guides for ablation of post-infarction ventricular tachycardia. J Am Coll Cardiol 47:2013-2019, 2006.
46. Bogun F, Bender B, Li YG, et al: Analysis during sinus rhythm of critical sites in reentry circuits of postinfarction ventricular tachycardia. J Interv Card Electrophysiol 7:95-103, 2002.
47. Arenal A, del Castillo S, Gonzalez-Torrecilla E, et al: Tachycardia-related channel in the scar tissue in patients with sustained monomorphic ventricular tachycardias: influence of the voltage scar definition. Circulation 110:2568-2574, 2004.
48. Hsia HH, Lin D, Sauer WH, et al: Anatomic characterization of endocardial substrate for hemodynamically stable reentrant ventricular tachycardia: Identification of endocardial conducting channels. Heart Rhythm 3:503-512, 2006.
49. Bogun F, Kim HM, Han J, et al: Comparison of mapping criteria for hemodynamically tolerated, postinfarction ventricular tachycardia. Heart Rhythm 3:20-26, 2006.
50. Verma A, Marrouche NF, Schweikert RA, et al: Relationship between successful ablation sites and the scar border zone defined by substrate mapping for ventricular tachycardia post-myocardial infarction. J Cardiovasc Electrophysiol 16:465-471, 2005.
51. Bogun F, Knight B, Goyal R, et al: Discrete systolic potentials during ventricular tachycardia in patients with prior myocardial infarction. J Cardiovasc Electrophysiol 10:364-369, 1999.
52. Segal OR, Chow AW, Markides V, et al: Long-term results after ablation of infarct-related ventricular tachycardia. Heart Rhythm 2:474-482, 2005.
53. Della Bella P, Pappalardo A, Riva S, et al: Non-contact mapping to guide catheter ablation of untolerated ventricular tachycardia. Eur Heart J 23:742-752, 2002.
54. Strickberger SA, Knight BP, Michaud GF, et al: Mapping and ablation of ventricular tachycardia guided by virtual electrograms using a noncontact, computerized mapping system. J Am Coll Cardiol 35:414-421, 2007.
55. Delacretaz E, Stevenson WG: Catheter ablation of ventricular tachycardia in patients with coronary heart disease: Part I: Mapping. Pacing Clin Electrophysiol 24:1261-1277, 2001.
56. El-Shalakany A, Hadjis T, Papageorgiou P, et al: Entrainment/mapping criteria for the prediction of termination of ventricular tachycardia by single radiofrequency lesion in patients with coronary artery disease. Circulation 99:2283-2289, 1999.
57. Henthorn RW, Okumura K, Olshansky B, et al: A fourth criterion for transient entrainment: The electrogram equivalent of progressive fusion. Circulation 77:1003-1012, 1988.
58. Stevenson WG, Khan H, Sager P, et al: Identification of reentry circuit sites during catheter mapping and radiofrequency ablation of ventricular tachycardia late after myocardial infarction. Circulation 88:1647-1670, 1993.
59. Tung S, Soejima K, Maisel WH, et al: Recognition of far-field electrograms during entrainment mapping of ventricular tachycardia. J Am Coll Cardiol 42:110-115, 1999.
60. Hadjis TA, Harada T, Stevenson WG, et al: Effect of recording site on postpacing interval measurement during catheter mapping and entrainment of postinfarction ventricular tachycardia. J Cardiovasc Electrophysiol 8:398-404, 1997.
61. Soejima K, Stevenson WG, Maisel WH, et al: The N + 1 difference: A new measure for entrainment mapping. J Am Coll Cardiol 37:1386-1394, 2001.
62. Stevenson WG, Friedman PL, Sager PT, et al: Exploring postinfarction reentrant ventricular tachycardia with entrainment mapping. J Am Coll Cardiol 29:1180-1189, 1997.
63. Bogun F, Krishnan SC, Marine JE, et al: Catheter ablation guided by termination of postinfarction ventricular tachycardia by pacing with nonglobal capture. Heart Rhythm 1:422-426, 2004.
64. Garan H, Ruskin JN: Localized reentry. Mechanism of induced sustained ventricular tachycardia in canine model of recent myocardial infarction. J Clin Invest 74:377-392, 1984.
65. Bogun F, Good E, Han J, et al: Mechanical interruption of postinfarction ventricular tachycardia as a guide for catheter ablation. Heart Rhythm 2:687-691, 2005.
66. Soejima K, Delacretaz E, Suzuki M, et al: Saline-cooled versus standard radiofrequency catheter ablation for infarct-related ventricular tachycardias. Circulation 103:1858-1862, 2001.
67. Merino JL, Peinado R, Fernandez-Lozano I, et al: Bundle-branch reentry and the postpacing interval after entrainment by right ventricular apex stimulation: A new approach to elucidate the mechanism of wide-QRS-complex tachycardia with atrioventricular dissociation. Circulation 103:1102-1108, 2001.
68. Hayashi M, Kobayashi Y, Iwasaki YK, et al: Novel mechanism of postinfarction ventricular tachycardia originating in surviving left posterior Purkinje fibers. Heart Rhythm 3:908-918, 2006.
69. Bogun F, Good E, Reich S, et al: Role of Purkinje fibers in post-infarction ventricular tachycardia. J Am Coll Cardiol 48:2500-2507, 2006.
70. van der Burg AE, de Groot NM, van Erven L, et al: Long-term follow-up after radiofrequency catheter ablation of ventricular tachycardia: A successful approach? J Cardiovasc Electrophysiol 13:417-423, 2002.
71. O'Donnell D, Bourke JP, Furniss SS: Standardized stimulation protocol to predict the long-term success of radiofrequency ablation of postinfarction ventricular tachycardia. Pacing Clin Electrophysiol 26:348-351, 1999.
72. Deneke T, Grewe PH, Lawo T, et al: Substrate-modification using electroanatomical mapping in sinus rhythm to treat ventricular tachycardia in patients with ischemic cardiomyopathy. Z Kardiol 94:453-460, 2005.
73. Kautzner J, Cihak R, Peichl P, et al: Catheter ablation of ventricular tachycardia following myocardial infarction using three-dimensional electroanatomical mapping. Pacing Clin Electrophysiol 26:342-347, 1999.
74. Della Bella P, De Ponti R, Uriarte JA, et al: Catheter ablation and antiarrhythmic drugs for haemodynamically tolerated post-infarction ventricular tachycardia: Long-term outcome in relation to acute electrophysiological findings. Eur Heart J 23:414-424, 2002.
75. Nabar A, Rodriguez LM, Batra RK, et al: Echocardiographic predictors of survival in patients undergoing radiofrequency ablation of postinfarct clinical ventricular tachycardia. J Cardiovasc Electrophysiol 13:S118-121, 2002.
76. Khan HH, Maisel WH, Ho C, et al: Effect of radiofrequency catheter ablation of ventricular tachycardia on left ventricular function in patients with prior myocardial infarction. J Interv Card Electrophysiol 7:243-247, 2002.
77. Delacretaz E, Stevenson WG, Ellison KE, et al: Mapping and radiofrequency catheter ablation of the three types of sustained monomorphic ventricular tachycardia in nonischemic heart disease. J Cardiovasc Electrophysiol 11:11-17, 2007.
78. Hsia HH, Callans DJ, Marchlinski FE: Characterization of endocardial electrophysiological substrate in patients with nonischemic cardiomyopathy and monomorphic

ventricular tachycardia. Circulation 108:704-710, 1999.
79. Eckart RE, Hruczkowski TW, Tedrow UB, et al: Sustained ventricular tachycardia associated with corrective valve surgery. Circulation 116(18):2005-2011, 2007.
80. Nazarian S, Bluemke DA, Lardo AC, et al: Magnetic resonance assessment of the substrate for inducible ventricular tachycardia in nonischemic cardiomyopathy. Circulation 112:2821-2825, 2005.
81. Yarlagadda RK, Iwai S, Stein KM, et al: Reversal of cardiomyopathy in patients with repetitive monomorphic ventricular ectopy originating from the right ventricular outflow tract. Circulation 112:1092-1097, 2005.
82. Satomi K, Kurita T, Suyama K, et al: Catheter ablation of stable and unstable ventricular tachycardias in patients with arrhythmogenic right ventricular dysplasia. J Cardiovasc Electrophysiol 17:469-476, 2006.
83. Koplan BA, Soejima K, Baughman K, et al: Refractory ventricular tachycardia secondary to cardiac sarcoid: Electrophysiologic characteristics, mapping, and ablation. Heart Rhythm 3:924-929, 2006.
84. Verma A, Kilicaslan F, Schweikert RA, et al: Short- and long-term success of substrate-based mapping and ablation of ventricular tachycardia in arrhythmogenic right ventricular dysplasia. Circulation 111:3209-3216, 2005.
85. Miljoen H, State S, de Chillou C, et al: Electroanatomic mapping characteristics of ventricular tachycardia in patients with arrhythmogenic right ventricular cardiomyopathy/dysplasia. Europace. 7:516-524, 2005.
86. O'Donnell D, Cox D, Bourke J, et al: Clinical and electrophysiological differences between patients with arrhythmogenic right ventricular dysplasia and right ventricular outflow tract tachycardia. Eur Heart J 24:801-810, 1999.
87. Corrado D, Basso C, Leoni L, et al: Three-dimensional electroanatomic voltage mapping increases accuracy of diagnosing arrhythmogenic right ventricular cardiomyopathy/dysplasia. Circulation 111:3042-3050, 2005.
88. Tandri H, Saranathan M, Rodriguez ER, et al: Noninvasive detection of myocardial fibrosis in arrhythmogenic right ventricular cardiomyopathy using delayed-enhancement magnetic resonance imaging. J Am Coll Cardiol 45:98-103, 2005.
89. Dalal D, Jain R, Tandri H, et al: Long-term efficacy of catheter ablation of ventricular tachycardia in patients with arrhythmogenic right ventricular dysplasia/cardiomyopathy. J Am Coll Cardiol 50:432-440, 2007.
90. Morwood JG, Triedman JK, Berul CI, et al: Radiofrequency catheter ablation of ventricular tachycardia in children and young adults with congenital heart disease. Heart Rhythm 1:301-308, 2004.
91. Zeppenfeld K, Schalij M, Bartelings MM, et al: Catheter ablation of ventricular tachycardia after repair of congenital heart disease: Electroanatomical identification of the critical right ventricular isthmus. Circulation 116(20):2241-2252, 2007.

Catheter Ablation of Ventricular Arrhythmias in Patients without Structural Heart Disease 109

Hans Kottkamp and Gerhard Hindricks

CHAPTER OUTLINE

Ventricular arrhythmias in patients without structural heart disease—idiopathic ventricular arrhythmias—can arise from a variety of specific areas within both ventricles and the neighboring vessels. Two main groups can be differentiated from a clinical, mechanistic, and anatomic point of view (see also Chapter 61): arrhythmias from the ventricular outflow tract (OT) region[1] and left ventricular septal tachycardias (fascicular tachycardias).

Classifying ventricular arrhythmias as idiopathic requires a thorough and complete cardiovascular examination. For ventricular OT arrhythmias, ruling out of arrhythmogenic right ventricular cardiomyopathy (ARVC) or dysplasia may be challenging in some cases.[2] Long-term prognosis in patients with truly idiopathic ventricular arrhythmias is excellent, and only in rare cases have idiopathic ventricular arrhythmias been shown to act as triggers for malignant ventricular tachycardia (VT) or fibrillation (VF)[3,4] or to lead to tachycardiomyopathy. After exclusion of any type of structural heart disease, the indication for treatment (e.g., antiarrhythmic drugs, catheter ablation) of ventricular arrhythmias therefore is a symptomatic one.

Catheter-mapping techniques allowing the identification of critical sites for the origin or for the perpetuation of ventricular arrhythmias were originally developed for VT in patients with remote myocardial infarction (see Chapter 108). Some of these techniques can be transferred to mapping of idiopathic ventricular arrhythmias. However, successful and safe mapping and ablation of ventricular arrhythmias in patients without structural heart disease requires detailed knowledge of the peculiar anatomy of the ventricles, especially of the OT region, and of the specific electrophysiology of the distinct type of tachycardia.

In this chapter, the specific aspects of catheter ablation of OT arrhythmias and left ventricular fascicular tachycardia are described, with special emphasis on the anatomic peculiarities, the most appropriate mapping techniques, the role of three-dimensional navigation systems and imaging technologies, and clinical results.

Ventricular Outflow Tract Arrhythmias

Clinical Spectrum and Patient Selection

The clinical presentation of patients with ventricular OT arrhythmias is variable and ranges from completely asymptomatic episodes to palpitations, presyncope, or syncope. The arrhythmia episode presentation also is variable from frequent isolated premature ventricular complexes (PVCs), repetitive nonsustained VT, or recurrent episodes of sustained VT. Often, ventricular OT arrhythmias are facilitated by catecholamines, such as physical exercise or emotional stress. Patients with recurrent episodes of ventricular OT arrhythmias and corresponding symptoms that cannot be controlled by well-tolerated antiarrhythmic drugs are candidates for electrophysiologic investigation and catheter ablation. In some cases, catheter ablation can also be discussed as first-line treatment to prevent long-term antiarrhythmic drug treatment.

Outflow Tract Anatomy

The majority of OT arrhythmias arise from the right ventricular outflow tract (RVOT). The RVOT is a tube-like structure that is delimited cranially by the pulmonary valve and caudally by the level of the superior aspect of the tricuspid annulus (His bundle level). Although septal and free-wall portions of the RVOT are often described, it is important to recognize that the right ventricular infundibulum does not have a septal component.[5] The right ventricular outlet curves anterior and superior to the left ventricular outlet and is in close anatomic relation to the coronary leaflets of the aortic valve. Within the sinuses of the pulmonary valve, small areas of ventricular myocardium are enclosed.

The left ventricular outflow tract (LVOT) is bordered by the muscular ventricular septum anterosuperiorly and by the anterior leaflet of the mitral valve posteroinferiorly.[5] The two coronary sinuses of the aortic valve have ventricular muscular support, whereas the noncoronary sinus does not. Taken together, ventricular OT arrhythmias can arise from all parts of the OT region and may be approached for ablation from the endocardial RVOT or LVOT, from within the aortic or pulmonary valve sinuses, from within the coronary sinus and left ventricular veins, or from the epicardial OT area after pericardial access.

Mapping Techniques

Basics

Usually, the electrophysiologic study is performed off antiarrhythmic drugs. Sedative drugs should be applied only with caution, because sedation can exert antiarrhythmic effects, especially in patients in whom the arrhythmia is active during or after exercise or during emotional stress. In some patients, intravenous isoproterenol or epinephrine infusion is necessary to provoke the arrhythmia. Usually, OT arrhythmias can be triggered with constant-rate ventricular pacing and less often with programmed ventricular stimulation using one or multiple extrastimuli.

The morphology of OT arrhythmias is critically dependent on the proper placement of the ECG leads, especially the precordial leads V1 to V6, and the placement of the limb leads on the chest wall can influence the QRS vector in lead I. Therefore, an actual 12-lead-ECG of the OT tachycardia should be recorded at the beginning of the procedure and this should serve as the target ECG reference for mapping (see later).

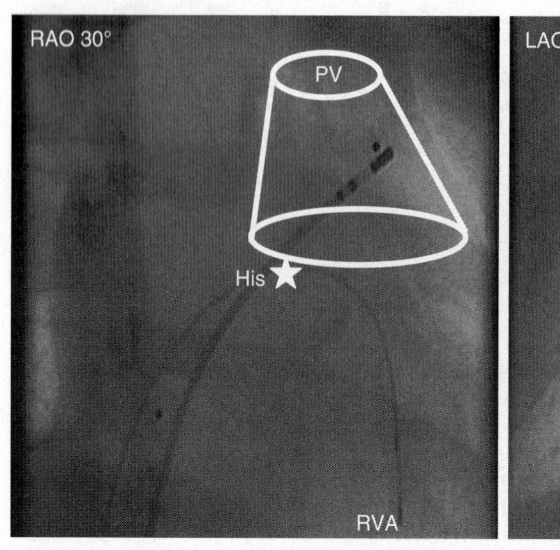

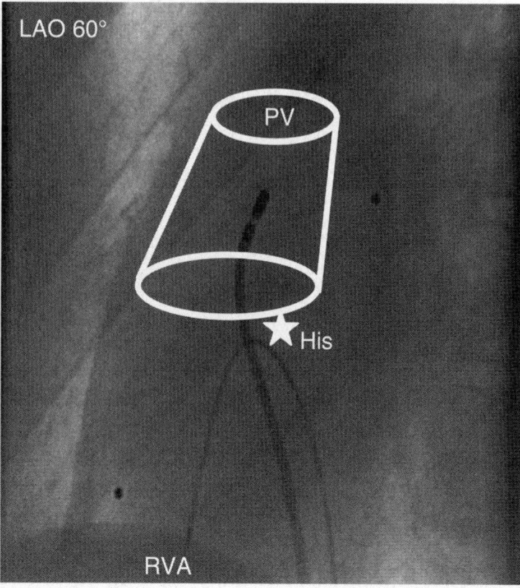

Figure 109-1 Fluoroscopic right and left anterior oblique (RAO, LAO) projections with schematic superimposition of the tube-like right ventricular outflow tract. The asterisks indicates the His bundle position. PV, pulmonary valve; RVA, right ventricular apex.

Standard Catheters and Fluoroscopy

Standard multielectrode diagnostic catheters are typically placed in the right ventricular apical region, His bundle area, and coronary sinus. For coronary sinus mapping, the very superior aspect of the mitral annulus (12 o'clock position) is most important because OT tachycardias can arise from the area of the mitral-aortic contiguity. In some laboratories, only one standard catheter in the right ventricular apex is used as an intracardiac reference catheter.

Multiplane fluoroscopy is used for navigation within the tube-like RVOT (Fig. 109-1). In our laboratories, right anterior oblique 30 degrees and left anterior oblique 60 degrees are used as standard fluoroscopic projections. Typically, mapping is started from directly underneath the pulmonary valve stepwise to more inferior sites until the area of the His bundle level is reached. In cases with positive R waves in lead I, we start at the anterior portion of the RVOT, and in cases with negative QRS in lead I, we start at the posterior (septal) portion of the RVOT. ECG algorithms have been elaborated to identify the most probable area of interest from the 12-lead-ECG.[6,7] The spatial mapping resolution is very important, and mapping steps of only a few millimetres should be used.

If the site of origin of the OT arrhythmia is not within the RVOT, mapping should be performed within the LVOT and the neighboring vessels (see later).

Techniques

RVOT arrhythmias have a *focal* origin, and *activation* mapping is the most important mapping technique. The unipolar unfiltered electrogram from the tip of the ablation catheter and the bipolar filtered electrogram from the two distal electrodes are used. The unipolar electrogram at the site of origin of an OT arrhythmia typically exerts the QS morphology, indicating that the activation spreads away directly from underneath the tip of the ablation catheter (Fig. 109-2). Importantly, no R wave is recorded at the site of origin, and the downstroke of the QS-electrogram

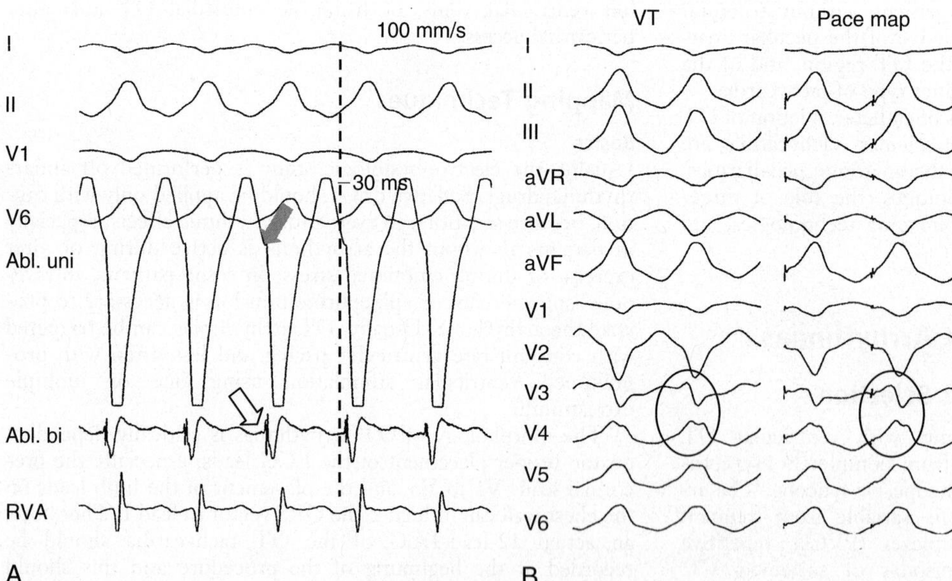

Figure 109-2 **A,** Activation mapping during right ventricular outflow tract tachycardia with unipolar and bipolar electrograms from the ablation catheter (Abl. uni, Abl. bi). The *closed arrow* indicates toward the QS morphology in the unipolar electrogram, the *open arrow* points toward the early activation time in the bipolar electrogram. RVA, right ventricular apex. **B,** Comparison of 12-lead ECG during ventricular tachycardia (VT) and pace map. Note the complete match in all leads including the R-S transition and QRS-notching *(circled)*.

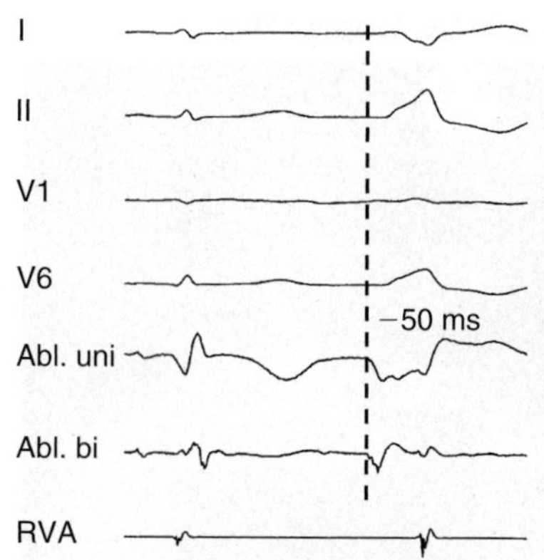

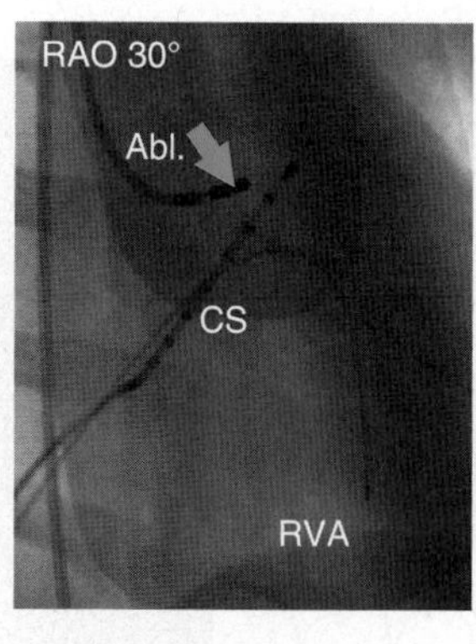

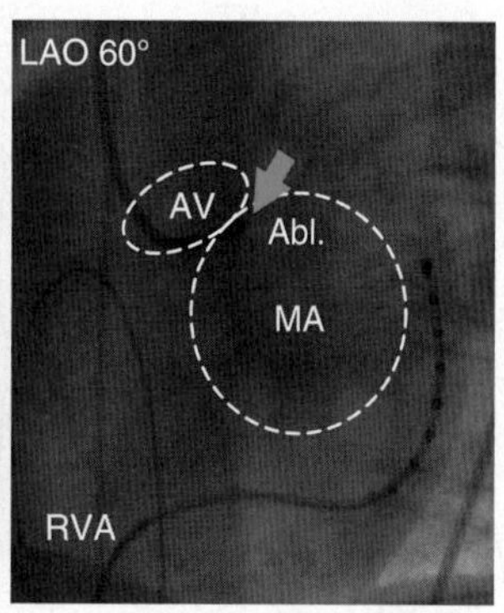

Figure 109-3 Activation mapping during outflow tract tachycardia originating from the left side with unipolar and bipolar electrograms from the ablation catheter (Abl. uni, Abl. bi), with corresponding fluoroscopic right and left anterior oblique (RAO, LAO) projections. AV, aortic valve; CS, coronary sinus; MA, mitral annulus; RVA, right ventricular apex.

should be fast and steep and not slow. The bipolar electrogram at the site of origin should have an early activation time directly at the onset of activation and—at the successful ablation site—typically precedes the onset of the QRS complex in the surface ECG by −10 to −50 ms (see Fig. 109-2).

An alternative or additive mapping technique is *pace* mapping. The 12-lead-ECG during unipolar or bipolar pacing with current strength of double threshold is compared with the 12-lead-ECG of the OT arrhythmia. Only a complete match (12 out of 12) indicates ablation success (see Fig. 109-2).[8]

Care should be taken not to mistake catheter-induced ectopic beats with the intrinsic arrhythmia. Catheter-induced ectopic beats typically exert perfect unipolar and bipolar electrogram characteristics because the site of origin is directly under the mapping electrode. In these circumstances of mechanically induced arrhythmias, comparison of the 12-lead-ECG of the mechanically induced arrhythmia with that of the intrinsic OT arrhythmia is helpful for differentiation.

Specific Outflow Tract Areas

Lead V3 is helpful to differentiate between right ventricular OT arrhythmias and those from the left side or other OT areas.[9] In cases with a R/S transition at lead V4, the site of origin usually is in the *right* ventricular OT whereas in cases with a R/S transition at lead V2, the site of origin most probably is in the *left* ventricular OT. In contrast, in cases with R/S transition in lead V3, the site of origin was found in the right ventricular OT in approximately 60% of the cases but on the left side or in the neighboring vessels in approximately 40% of the cases.[9] In rare cases of RVOT arrhythmias, the site of origin may be very inferior in close proximity to the His bundle.[10] In addition, idiopathic VT can arise from the tricuspid annulus area.[11]

As indicated earlier, OT arrhythmias can originate from the *left* ventricular OT. In these cases, the foci are often located in the area of the mitral-aortic contiguity or at the superior aspect of the mitral annulus (Fig. 109-3). In patients in whom mapping could not identify the location of the focus endocardially in the right or left ventricular OT, mapping should be continued in the neighboring vessels, specifically the aortic sinus of Valsalva[12] (Fig. 109-4) or—even less rarely—in the pulmonary trunk.[13] In addition, ablation of left ventricular *epicardial* outflow tract tachycardia has been reported from within the coronary veins (Fig. 109-5) or via transpericardial appoaches.[14,15]

Ablation

Energy Source

The most commonly applied energy source for VT ablation is radiofrequency (RF) current. Solid 4-mm tip electrodes are adequate for ablation of OT arrhythmias with power output of 20 to maximally 50 watts, maximal temperature of 60° C, and duration of 30 (to 60) seconds. Alternatively, irrigated-tip ablation may be used. However, it should be taken into account that the RVOT is thin, measuring only 2 to 4 mm in depth, and therefore energy

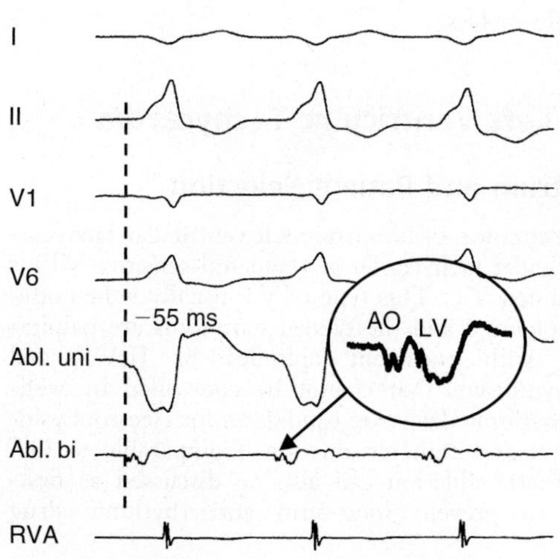

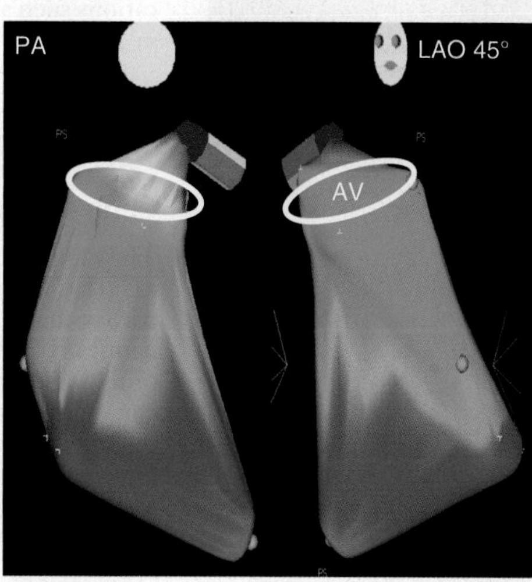

Figure 109-4 Activation mapping during outflow tract tachycardia originating from the aortic coronary cusp with unipolar and bipolar electrograms from the ablation catheter (Abl. uni, Abl. bi) with corresponding electroanatomic activation map. AO, aortic coronary cusp; AV, aortic valve; LAO, left anterior oblique; LV, left ventricle; PA posteroanterior; RVA, right ventricular apex.

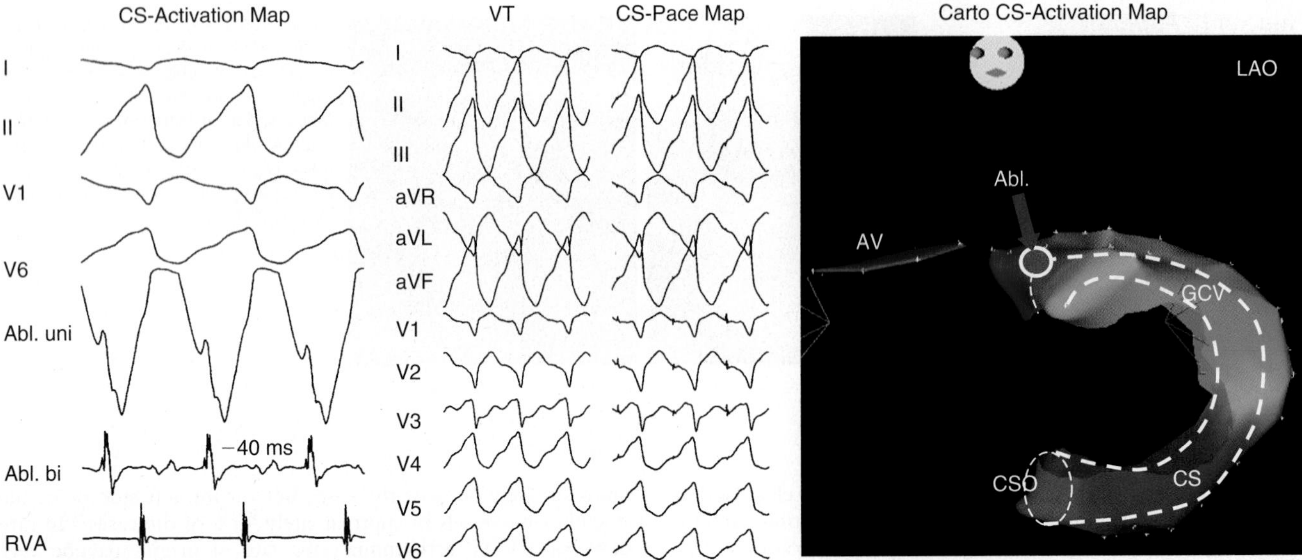

Figure 109-5 Activation and pace mapping during outflow tract tachycardia originating from the great cardiac vein with unipolar and bipolar electrograms from the ablation catheter (Abl. uni, Abl. bi) with corresponding electroanatomic activation map. AV, aortic valve; CS, coronary sinus; GCV, great cardiac vein; LAO, left anterior oblique; RVA, right ventricular apex; VT, ventricular tachycardia.

as well as application time should be limited. As an alternative energy source, the use of cryo energy has been reported with the potential advantage of absence of ablation-related pain.[16]

Localization and Imaging Technologies

In most laboratories, multiplane fluoroscopy is used as the primary localization technique within the OT. However, three-dimensional electroanatomic mapping can add further information and can help to identify the precise center of earliest activation (Fig. 109-6). For specific situations, such as ablation of epicardial foci in the vicinity of the coronary arteries or foci from the coronary aortic cusps, the integration of three-dimensional reconstruction of computed tomography imaging with three-dimensional electroanatomic mapping may be helpful with respect to procedural safety.[17,18]

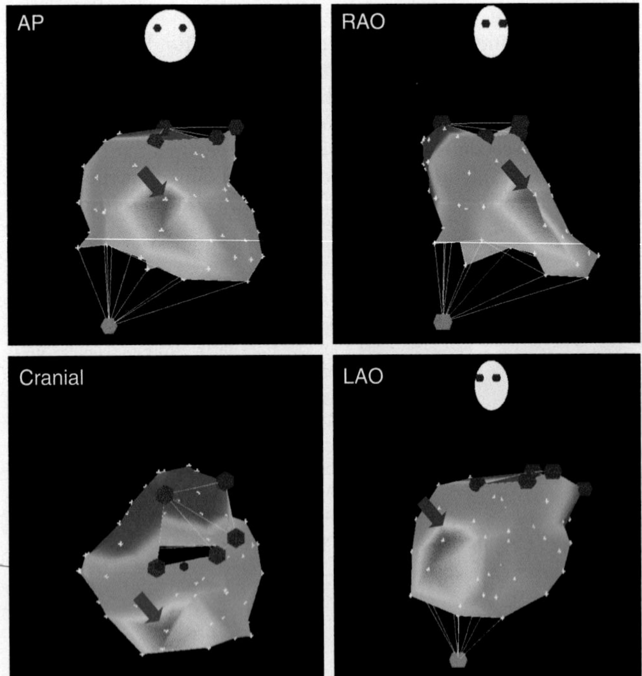

Figure 109-6 Electroanatomic map identifying the center of earliest activation during ventricular tachycardia within the tube-like three-dimensional right ventricular outflow tract. AP, anteroposterior; LAO, left anterior oblique; RAO, right anterior oblique.

Clinical Results and Complications

Successful ablation of OT arrhythmias can be achieved in about 90% of cases if focus activity during the procedure allows adequate mapping. As indicated earlier, mapping within all the specific anatomic areas of the OT region may be necessary to obtain such a high success rate. Recurrences of initially successfully ablated foci can occur in about 5% of cases, and these foci may be approached with a second procedure. Complications during ablation of OT arrhythmias are rare and are mainly related to vascular access complications. Serious cardiac complications such as tamponade or perforation are very rare and occur in 1% of the cases or less.

Idiopathic Left Ventricular Tachycardia

Clinical Spectrum and Patient Selection

The clinical presentation of idiopathic left ventricular tachycardia (ILVT) (fascicular tachycardia or verapamil-sensitive VT) is paroxysmal sustained VT. This type of VT usually is hemodynamically well tolerated and the typical symptoms are palpitations. Patients with recurrent episodes of ILVT and corresponding symptoms that cannot be controlled by well-tolerated antiarrhythmic drugs are candidates for electrophysiologic investigation and catheter ablation. Comparable to OT arrhythmias, catheter ablation can also be discussed as first-line treatment to prevent long-term antiarrhythmic drug treatment.

Anatomic Aspects

The trabeculations of the left ventricle are finer compared to those of the right ventricle.[5] Occasionally, fine muscular strands—false tendons—extend between the septum and the papillary muscles or the parietal wall and have been implicated in ILVT. The observation of false tendons, however, does not seem to be a consistent finding.

The macro-reentrant circuit of ILVT with left axis deviation is located in the area of the left posterior fascicle, and the rare variant with right axis deviation is in the area of the left anterior fascicle. Importantly, the critical structures are located subendocardially, and catheter mapping might terminate ILVT and render it transiently noninducible due to mechanical trauma. On the other hand, the subendocardial location allows curative treatment by RF ablation if critical sites of the reentrant circuit can be identified.

Mapping Techniques

Standard Catheters and Fluoroscopy

Standard multielectrode diagnostic catheters are typically placed in the right ventricular apical region and His bundle area. In some laboratories, diagnostic catheters are additionally placed in the right ventricular outflow tract or at the left ventricular septum along the left posterior fascicle.

Multiplane fluoroscopy is used for navigation within the left ventricle. In our laboratories, right anterior oblique 30 degrees and left anterior oblique 60 degrees are used as standard fluoroscopic projections (Fig. 109-7).

Techniques

Recent mapping studies indicated that macro-reentry *adjacent* to the left posterior fascicle is the underlying mechanism of ILVT, with the left posterior fascicle itself as a bystander with retrograde activation.[19-22] A slow conduction area typically exhibits a basal-to-apical septal direction during tachycardia. Typically, catheter mapping is started in the mid to apical region of the left ventricular septum in the area of the distal left posterior fascicle (see Fig. 109-7). Due to the macro-reentrant nature, *activation* mapping is the most important catheter mapping technique.

Early investigations with evidence of retrograde His bundle activation during ILVT, characteristic narrow right bundle branch block QRS morphology, and successful ablation in the area of the septal ramifications of the left posterior fascicle suggest that the arrhythmia is located within the Purkinje fiber network. Nakagawa and colleagues identified the earliest ventricular activation during right and left ventricular endocardial mapping at the posteroapical left ventricular septum.[23] In their study, earliest ventricular activation during tachycardia was preceded by specific potentials. These potentials also preceded ventricular activation during sinus rhythm, consistent with a segment of the left posterior fascicle (Purkinje potential).[23] The Purkinje potentials preceded the onset of the QRS complex during ILVT by 15 to 42 ms, and ablation was successful at the site of the earliest detectable Purkinje potential, irrespective to the timing of the ventricular electrogram component at that site.

Later, *diastolic* potentials during ILVT as well as late potentials during sinus rhythm were described. In subsequent mapping studies, diastolic and presystolic Purkinje potentials could be demonstrated as critical components in the macro-reentrant circuit of ILVT.[19,20] In the study by Tsuchiya, the mean relative activation times of late diastolic potentials, Purkinje potentials, and local ventricular potentials at the late diastolic potential recording site to the onset of the QRS complex during ILVT measured −50, −15, and 3 ms, respectively.[19] Typically, late-diastolic potentials are found in the apical third of the septum, mid-diastolic potentials in the mid septum, and early diastolic potentials in the basal third of the septum (Fig. 109-8). Importantly, basoseptal *entrance* sites with early diastolic potentials may be recorded at distances of up to 4 cm from the apicoseptal *exit* sites.

Nogami and colleagues performed entrainment pacing at sites with mid-diastolic potentials during ILVT and found that the interval from the stimulus to the mid-diastolic potential prolonged as the pacing rate increased.[20] These investigators concluded that both the diastolic potentials and the presystolic Purkinje potentials are critical components in the circuit and that normal Purkinje tissue as well as abnormal Purkinje tissue with decremental properties is involved in the macro-reentrant circuit of ILVT.[20] In our laboratories, we identify *diastolic* potentials during ILVT as primary targets for catheter ablation and

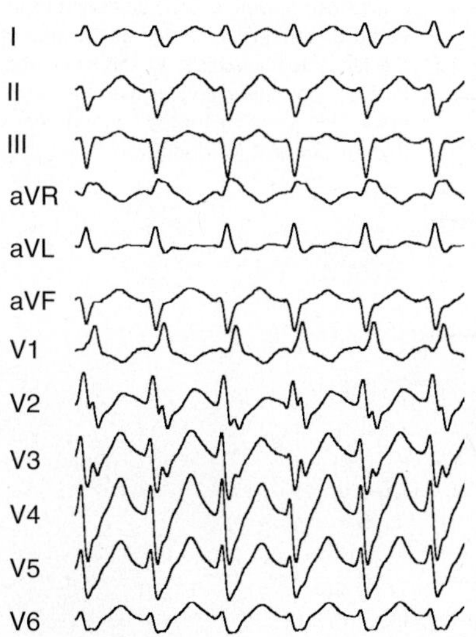

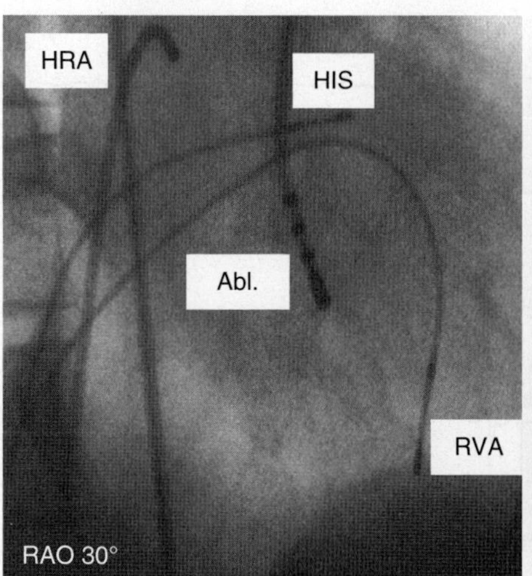

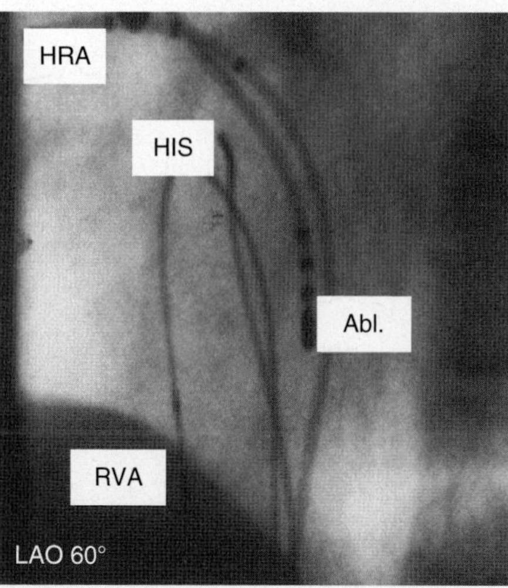

Figure 109-7 Twelve-lead ECG during idiopathic left ventricular tachycardia with left axis deviation and fluoroscopic right and left anterior oblique (RAO, LAO) projections showing diagnostic catheters in the high right atrium (HRA), His bundle area (HIS) and right ventricular apex (RVA) as well as the ablation catheter (Abl.) at the site of successful ablation.

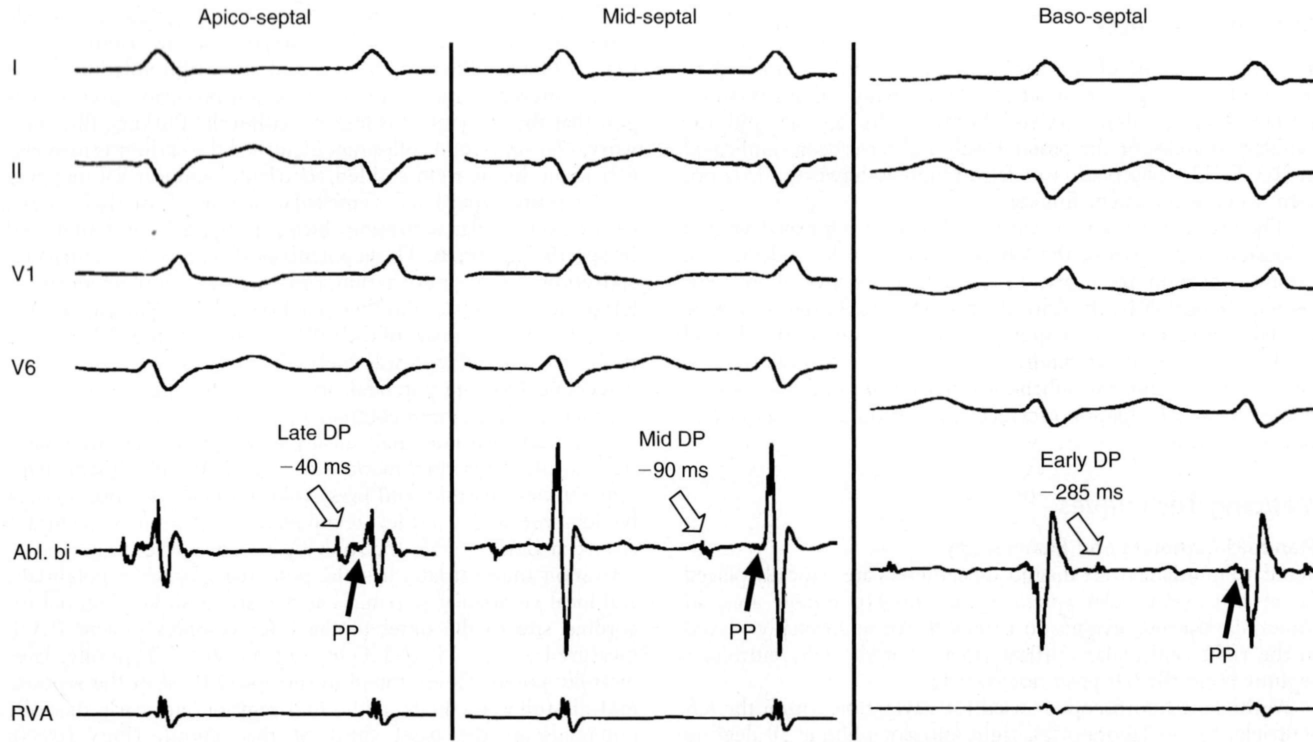

Figure 109-8 Activation mapping during idiopathic left ventricular tachycardia (ILVT) at apico-septal, mid-septal and baso-septal sites. Late, mid, and early diastolic potentials (DP) could be recorded at −40 ms, −90 ms, and −285 ms, respectively, before the onset of the QRS complex during ILVT. In addition, Purkinje potentials (PP) could be recorded at all sites. The ILVT was successfully ablated at the mid-septal site. Abl. bi, bipolar electrogram from the ablation catheter; RVA, right ventricular apex.

presystolic Purkinje potentials as secondary targets, when no stable diastolic potentials can be recorded.

Ouyang and coworkers investigated the role of abnormal late potentials (retrograde Purkinje potentials) from the left posterior Purkinje network during sinus rhythm in patients with ILVT.[21] In their study, the earliest and latest retrograde Purkinje potentials were recorded 185 ± 57 and 465 ± 37 ms after the antegrade Purkinje potential, and diastolic potentials critical for ILVT coincided with the earliest retrograde Purkinje potentials during sinus rhythm (Fig. 109-9).

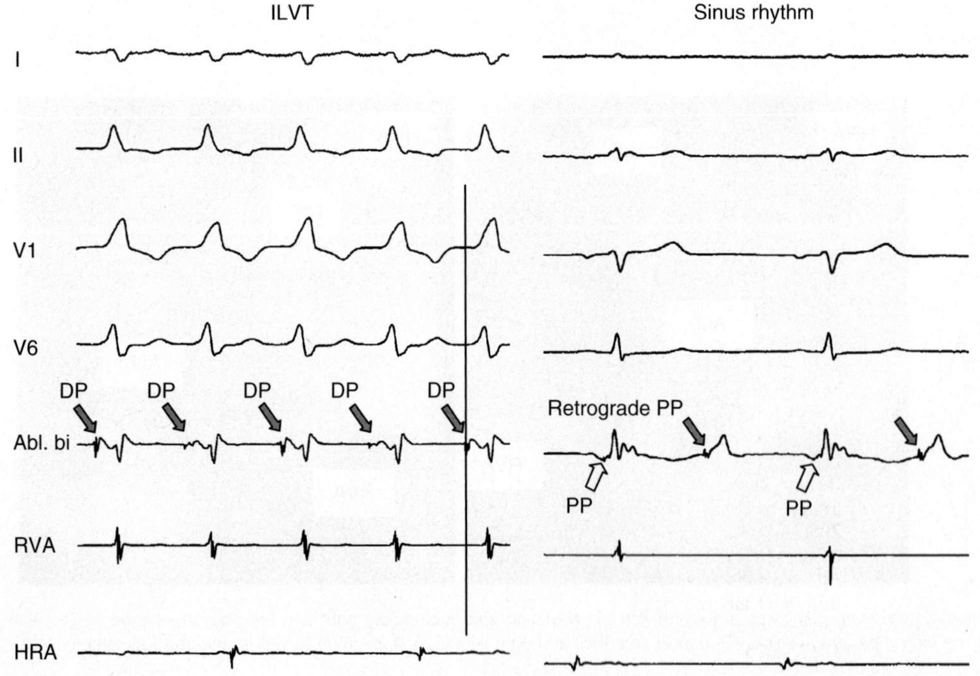

Figure 109-9 Activation mapping during idiopathic left ventricular tachycardia (ILVT) with right axis deviation and during sinus rhythm. During ILVT, diastolic potentials (DP) could be recorded at the area of the left anterior fascicle. At the same site, Purkinje potentials (PP) as well as retrograde PP were recorded during sinus rhythm. See text for discussion.

Alternatively to activation mapping, *pace mapping* may be used to identify target sites for ablation of ILVT. In the area of presystolic Purkinje potentials during ILVT, pacing during sinus rhythm can exhibit a perfect match of the 12-lead ECG compared with ILVT. However, pacing during sinus rhythm at sites with diastolic potentials during ILVT might show differing QRS morphologies because the pacing site may be several centimeters away from the exit point during ILVT.

Specific Aspects

Due to the subendocardial location of the macro-reentrant circuit, ILVT may be rendered noninducible mechanically during the mapping procedure. Ouyang and coworkers applied RF pulses to the site with the earliest retrograde Purkinje potentials during sinus rhythm in patients without inducible ILVT after sinus rhythm mapping with good clinical outcome.[21] Alternatively, Lin and colleagues investigated a linear ablation strategy for noninducible or nonsustained ILVT.[23] These authors delivered RF energy in a linear fashion approximately midway to two thirds toward the apex along the mid to inferior septum and perpendicular to the plane of the septum, and they found this strategy to be clinically effective and safe. Ma and colleagues reported on left posterior fascicular block as an endpoint of ablation of ILVT after a mean of only 1.7 ± 0.9 RF applications.[24] These findings, however, could not be confirmed by Kuo's group.[25]

Ablation

Energy Source

Comparable to OT arrhythmias, RF current is delivered via solid 4-mm tip electrodes with power output of 20 to maximally 50 watts, maximal temperature of 60° C and duration of 30 (to 60) seconds. Alternatively, irrigated-tip ablation may be used to prevent carbonization and thrombus formation at the catheter tip if several energy applications are necessary.

Localization and Imaging Technologies

In most laboratories, multiplane fluoroscopy is used as the primary localization technique at the left ventricular septum. However, three-dimensional electroanatomic mapping can add further information, facilitate renavigation to specific mapping points, and help to place a linear ablation line as proposed by Lin and colleagues.[24]

Clinical Results and Complications

Successful ablation of ILVT can be achieved in about 90% of cases, or even more if the arrhythmia is reproducibly inducible and sustained. Recurrences of initially successfully ablated ILVT occur in about 5% of the cases, and these cases may be approached with a second procedure. Complications during ablation of ILVT are rare and are mainly related to vascular access complications. Serious cardiac complications such as tamponade or perforation are very rare and occur in 1% of the cases or less.

References

1. Kim RJ, Iwai S, Markowitz SM, et al: Clinical and electrophysiological spectrum of idiopathic ventricular outflow tract arrhythmias. J Am Coll Cardiol 49:2035-2043, 2007.
2. O'Donnel D, Cox D, Bourke J, et al: Clinical and electrophysiological differences between patients with arrhythmogenic right ventricular dysplasia and right ventricular outflow tract tachycardia. Eur Heart J 24:801-810, 2003.
3. Noda T, Shimizu W, Taguchi A, et al: Malignant entity of idiopathic ventricular fibrillation and polymorphic ventricular tachycardia initiated by premature extrasystoles originating from the right ventricular outflow tract. J Am Coll Cardiol 46:1288-1294, 2005.
4. Viskin S, Rosso R, Rogowski O, Belhassen B: The "short-coupled" variant of right ventricular outflow ventricular tachycardia: A not-so-benign form of benign ventricular tachycardia? J Cardiovasc Electrophysiol 16:912-916, 2005.
5. Ho SY: Overview of cardiac anatomy relevant to catheter ablation. In Wilber DJ, Packer DL, Stevenson WG (eds): Catheter Ablation of Cardiac Arrhythmias: Basic Concepts and Clinical Applications. Malden, MA, Blackwell, 2008, pp 3-19.
6. Ito S, Tada H, Naito S, et al: Development and validation of an ECG algorithm for identifying the optimal ablation site for idiopathic ventricular outflow tract tachycardia. J Cardiovasc Electrophysiol 14:1280-1286, 2003.
7. Bala R, Marchliniski FE: Electrocardiographic recognition and ablation of outflow tract ventricular tachycardia. Heart Rhythm 4:366-370, 2007.
8. Azegami K, Wilber D, Arruda M, et al: Spatial resolution of pace mapping and activation mapping in patients with idiopathic right ventricular outflow tract tachycardia. J Cardiovasc Electrophysiol 16:823-829, 2005.
9. Tanner H, Hindricks G, Schirdewahn P, et al: Outflow tract tachycardia with R/S transition in lead V3—Six different anatomic approaches for successful ablation. J Am Coll Cardiol 45:418-423, 2005.
10. Yamauchi Y, Aonuma K, Takahashi A, et al: Electrocardiographic characteristics of repetitive monomorphic right ventricular tachycardia originating near the His-bundle. J Cardiovasc Electrophysiol 16:1041-1048, 2005.
11. Tada H, Tadokoro K, Ito S, et al: Idiopathic ventricular arrhythmias originating from the tricuspid annulus: Prevalence, electrocardiographic characteristics, and results of radiofrequency catheter ablation. Heart Rhythm 4:7-16, 2007.
12. Hachiya H, Aonuma K, Yamauchi Y, et al: How to diagnose, locate, and ablate coronary cusp ventricular tachycardia. J Cardiovasc Electrophysiol 13:551-556, 2002.
13. Sekiguchi Y, Aonuma K, Takahashi A, et al: Electrocardiographic and electrophysiologic characteristics of ventricular tachycardia originating within the pulmonary artery. J Am Coll Cardiol 45:887-895, 2005.
14. Obel OA, d'Avila A, Neuzil P, et al: Ablation of left ventricular epicardial outflow tract tachycardia from the distal great cardiac vein. J Am Coll Cardiol 48:1813-1817, 2006.
15. Daniels DV, Lu YY, Morton JB, et al: Idiopathic epicardial left ventricular tachycardia originating remote from the sinus of Valsalva. Circulation 113:1659-1666, 2006.
16. Kurzidim K, Schneider HJ, Kuniss M, et al: Cryocatheter ablation of right ventricular outflow tract tachycardia. J Cardiovasc Electrophysiol 16:366-369, 2005.
17. Zeppenfeld K, Tops LF, Bax JJ, Schalij MJ: Epicardial radiofrequency catheter ablation of ventricular tachycardia in the vicinity of coronary arteries is facilitated by fusion of 3-dimensional electroanatomical mapping with multislice computed tomography. Circulation 114:e51-e52, 2006.
18. Pasquie JL, Bortone A, Del Mazo PC, Leclercq F: Image-guided ablation of a ventricular tachycardia originating from the left aortic cusp. J Cardiovasc Electrophysiol 17:1032-1033, 2006.
19. Tsuchiya T, Okumura K, Honda T, et al: Significance of late diastolic potential preceding Purkinje potential in verapamil-sensitive idiopathic left ventricular tachycardia. Circulation 99:2408-2413, 1999.
20. Nogami A, Naito S, Tada H, et al: Demonstration of diastolic and presystolic Purkinje potentials as critical potentials in a macroreentry circuit of verapamil-sensitive idiopathic left ventricular tachycardia. J Am Coll Cardiol 36:811-823, 2000.
21. Ouyang F, Cappato R, Ernst S, et al: Electroanatomic substrate of idiopathic left ventricular tachycardia—Unidirectional block and macroreentry with the Purkinje network. Circulation 105:462-469, 2002.
22. Nakagawa H, Beckman KJ, McClelland JH, et al: Radiofrequency catheter ablation of idiopathic left ventricular tachycardia

guided by a Purkinje potential. Circulation 88:2607-2617, 1993.
23. Lin D, Hsia HH, Gerstenfeld EP, et al: Idiopathic fascicular left ventricular tachycardia: Linear ablation lesion strategy for noninducible or nonsustained tachycardia. Heart Rhythm 2:934-939, 2005.
24. Ma FS, Tang K, Han H, et al: Left posterior fascicular block: A new endpoint of ablation for verapamil-sensitive idiopathic ventricular tachycardia. Chin Med J 119:367-372, 2006.
25. Kuo JY, Tai CT, Chiang CE, et al: Is the fascicle of left bundle branch involved in the re-entrant circuit of verapamil-sensitive idiopathic left ventricular tachycardia? Pacing Clin Electrophysiol 26:1986-1992, 2003.

Catheter Ablation in Pediatric and Congenital Heart Disease Patients 110

John D. Kugler

CHAPTER OUTLINE

In previous editions of this textbook (most recently Chapter 119 of the fourth edition[1]), this chapter focused on pediatric patients undergoing radiofrequency catheter ablation (RCA). In this edition, the chapter is directed toward new information and updates for pediatric patients undergoing RCA and cryo-catheter ablation (CCA) techniques and toward adults with congenital heart disease.

Preparation for the Procedure

Discussion with the pediatric or congenital heart disease patient and family is related to several factors including age, specific underlying arrhythmia including natural history, management options including medical and surgical, type of congenital heart disease, risks of procedure, and results and follow-up considerations.[2,3] For the patient with congenital heart disease, understanding nuances and careful investigation of underlying anatomy is essential. An example of nuance includes understanding the electrocardiogram (ECG) characteristics of Ebstein's anomaly patients with preexcitation: One third of patients with preexcitation have minimal or absent typical preexcitation, so absence of the usual right bundle branch block (RBBB) pattern is a strong predictor of preexcitation.[4]

Investigation of past surgical and catheterization reports provides important anatomic detail for planning of the procedure.[2,4,6] For example, congenital heart disease patients often have a history of numerous catheterizations and operations and therefore venous access challenges that affect planning and performing the impending catheter ablation procedure.[7]

Further preprocedure preparation includes repeating and performing various imaging studies including (but not limited to) echocardiography, cardiac magnetic resonance imaging (cMRI), cardiac computed tomography (cCT), and angiography (the latter before or at the time of the catheter ablation). With the newer three-dimensional mapping electrophysiology systems, the pre-procedure cMRI and cCT images can be incorporated into the real-time mapping during the electrophysiology study at the time of the ablation procedure.[8-10]

Procedural Issues

Sedation and Anesthesia

Virtually all pediatric patients require sedation, anesthesia, or both. For congenital heart disease patients of all ages, the underlying complexity of anatomy and tachyarrhythmia is associated with long procedures, so general anesthesia is favored in most electrophysiology laboratories treating these patients.[11-13] The details of procedural anesthesia including electrophysiologic effects have been outlined in previous editions of this book.[1]

Fluoroscopy

The fluoroscopy issues were explored in the previous edition of this chapter and the confusion among studies outlined.[1] Bacher and colleagues, Campbell and colleagues, and Davies and colleagues have addressed the issues of various measurements, new technologies of radiation direct measurement, and radiation exposure reduction strategies.[14-16] In these reports, calculated effective doses in children are as high as those for adult interventional cardiology, resulting in higher radiation risks. It is important to monitor the patient dose-by-dose area product (DAP) instrumentation and to maintain records of cumulative DAP for individual patients for repeat procedures.[14-16] DAP can be reduced by using beam filtration to maintain the effective dose as low as possible.[16] Strategies to reduce radiation exposure have been proved and advocated for adults and children.[14-17]

Several factors will likely continue to decrease radiation exposure during catheter ablation in the future: ongoing replacement of older equipment with pulsed fluoroscopy (also enhanced further by using techniques such as acquisition zoom or by beam filtration), advances in alternative imaging techniques, patient selection, ongoing experience, and emphasis on patient safety. Examples of nonfluoroscopy catheter navigation techniques include intracardiac echocardiography,[18-21] three-dimensional (3-D) mapping systems,[8-10,22,23] and remote magnetic catheter techniques (Chapters 105-110).

Mapping Systems

The 3-D mapping systems are described in Chapters 104-107. The application for pediatric and congenital heart disease patients is illustrated in Figure 110-1. These systems have been extensively reviewed and described elsewhere.[10] However, they are virtually identical for adult patients, and the electroanatomic and noncontact mapping systems are especially valuable in postoperative congenital heart disease patients.[9,10,22-24]

The systems minimize fluoroscopy, thereby decreasing radiation exposure during the procedure while adding an important diagnostic component to the procedure. However, using preprocedure computed tomography (CT) images by importing and fusing them into the 3-D system considerably increases the radiation exposure, so arguably this technique is not safer in terms of radiation safety. cMRI avoids radiation exposure and can also be incorporated into the 3-D mapping systems.[10] This is especially helpful for pediatric and adult congenital heart disease patients with complex anatomy. Regardless of the specific 3-D system used, Packer has nicely outlined the goals of these systems[8]:

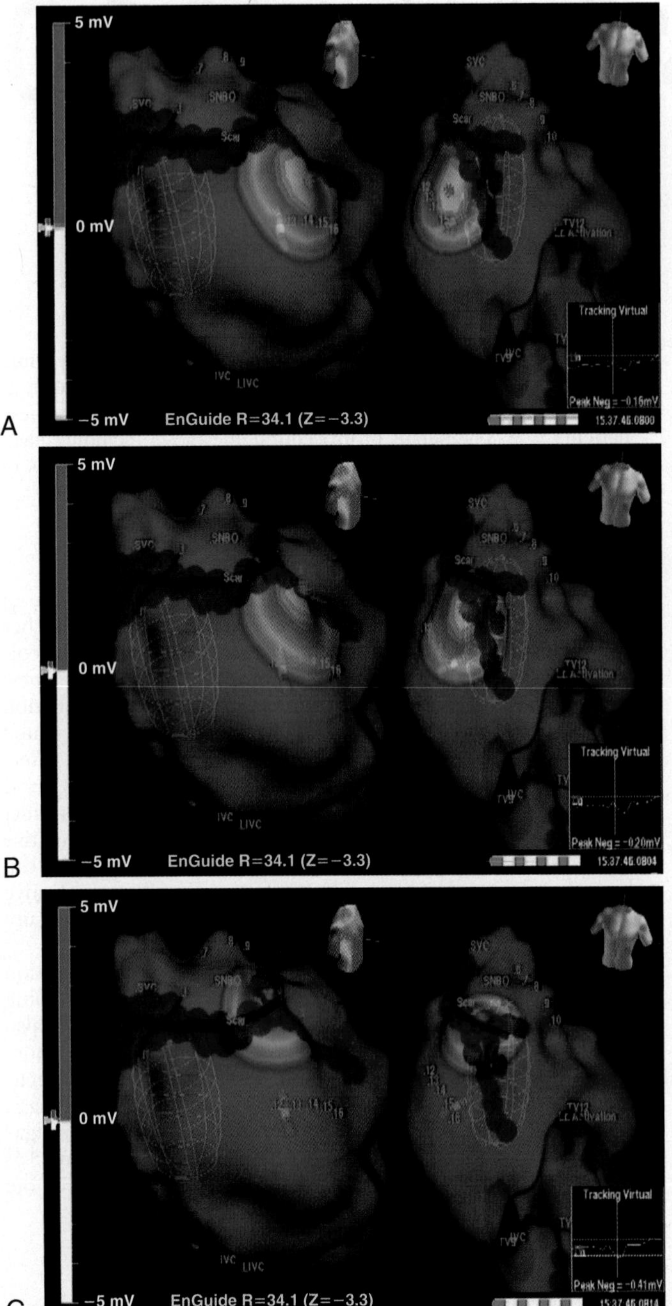

Figure 110-1 Three-dimensional (3-D), biplane noncontact map of the right atrium in an adolescent with intra-atrial reentry tachycardia (IART) due to postoperative congenital heart disease (Ebstein's anomaly). This map demonstrates the important features of a 3-D mapping system (EnSite, St. Jude Medical, St Paul MN). The rotation and view of the images are depicted by the smaller chest views at the upper right of each image. The outline of the 64-electrode mesh, mounted on the outside surface of the 18 × 40-mm inflated balloon, is shown within each image. The EnSite noncontact mapping system is summarized by Packer.[8] In this patient, a series of radiofrequency current ablation applications (each application depicted by a *small circle*) were delivered first in a line from the superior vena cava (SVC), anterior and medial to the atrial septal defect patch, because the IART circuit (not shown) was counterclockwise, which involved an area perpendicular to this line. The IART was still inducible (not shown), but the circuit changed to be more horizontal, so a second line of ablation applications was placed from the first series inferior and anterior, toward the tricuspid annulus. Although the IART was no longer inducible, atrial pacing was performed (shown here) to determine if the lines of block prevented conduction through them. **A,** The pacing catheter is shown near the outside *(blue-green)* edge of the circular activation wave of the right atrium. The atrial activation (*center*, depicted by the *red asterisk*, then earliest, indicated by *white atrial activation*) travels toward the line of scar. **B,** At 4 ms later, it reaches the ablation line. **C,** At 10 ms later, it has conducted through the ablation line to the other side. Despite placing additional ablation lesions in this area, the failure to achieve complete block persisted, but IART was not inducible and the patient is off antiarrhythmia drug therapy without IART recurrence 3 years after the procedure. (Reproduced from Kugler JD: Electrophysiologic studies. In Allen HD, Driscoll DJ, Shaddy RE, Feltes TF (eds): Moss and Adams' Heart Disease in Infants, Children, and Adolescents, 7th ed. Lippincott Williams & Wilkins, 2007, pp 275-292, with permission of Lippincott Williams & Wilkins and the author.)

accurately replicate the cardiac anatomy underlying the arrhythmia; provide a plausible representation of activation of that chamber, as linked to the specific anatomic site of data acquisition; readily capture and intelligibly display other details of physiology; and catalogue the site of interventions.

Energy Sources and Catheter Techniques

Especially for smaller and younger pediatric patients, the development of the CCA techniques has enhanced the safety of catheter ablation, particularly when the ablation target tissues are in the area of the septum, atrioventricular (AV) node and His bundle, and coronary sinus and possibly in areas where the coronary artery is vulnerable.[25-37] The CCA is appealing because safety is enhanced by the longer time to produce a smaller scar, thus allowing the surgeon more time to observe for, an limit the potential area of, undesired effects.

The technique uses a cooling system and special cryothermal catheter to achieve permanent scar in the target tissue. A cooling temperature to −75° to −80° C for 4 minutes produces a slightly smaller, more circumscribed and defined lesion compared to that from RCA. When the cryocatheter system (CryoCath Technologies Inc, Montreal) was released for commercial general use in 2004, a 4-mm tip catheter allowed two functions, mapping and ablation. The mapping function allows cooling to −25° to −30° C for 1 to 2 minutes to see if adverse effects are produced while determining if the desired effect is achieved. For example, for AV node reentry tachycardia (AVNRT), block in the slow AV node pathway can be assessed during repeated S1-S1and S1-S2 drive trains, during which slow AVN pathway conduction is demonstrated. Following mapping, ablation is performed to a maximum cooling of −75° to −80° C for 4 minutes to produce a larger, deeper permanent lesion.

Due to less-than-optimal early success and recurrence rates (see "Results of Catheter Ablation"), several aspects of CCA have undergone and continue to undergo further refinement as practitioners and investigators further explore informal and formal techniques to achieve higher success rates and lower recurrence rates. Some practitioners use 3-D mapping systems to place several more bonus lesions near the successful lesion to increase the area of scar; others use the freeze-thaw-freeze technique by immediately repeating a 4-minute application after the initial successful application, with the goal of increasing the depth and volume of the scar.[32,34,35] Drago and coworkers have also advocated using longer (7-minute) applications.[34]

Formal investigations under way involve using only 6-mm tip CCA catheters with the rationale that larger-tip catheters produce larger, deeper lesions. The mapping function is commercially available in the United States only with the 4-mm tip. Some practitioners have abandoned the 4-mm tip and only use the maximum cooling temperature. If adverse affects are noted with the 6-mm tip and maximum cooling temperature, the application is terminated. To date, no results have been reported for any of the techniques designed to theoretically increase the lesion size. It is therefore not known whether or not better success and recurrence rates can be achieved with these technique or if these techniques result in similar nearly absent complication rates of AV block for applications in the AV node and His bundle area.

Results of Catheter Ablation

The early reports of individual center series, the first report of the Pediatric and Congenital Electophysiology Society multicenter collaborative Pediatric RCA Registry data in 1994, reports from other individual centers, and the final Registry data in 2002 have been summarized in previous editions, most recently the fourth edition of this book.[1,38,39] Here, an updated review of the results of pediatric and congenital heart disease ablation is provided, focusing on three areas: the collaborative Prospective Assessment after Pediatric Cardiac Ablation (PAPCA) study, which focused on follow-up after RCA; AVNRT; and arrhythmias in patients with congenital heart disease, especially those with postoperative congenital heart disease arrhythmias.

Prospective Assessment after Pediatric Ablation

PAPCA began enrolling patients April 1, 1999, in an effort to better determine unknowns about RCA following the procedure.[40] Concerns were focused on recurrence and the development of late complications. The PAPCA study included children up to 16 years old with either accessory pathway (AP) tachycardias or AVNRT, and three reports have been published.

The first PAPCA report included 2,761patients (enrolled to May 8, 2003) and concentrated on current acute results.[40] The results mirrored the previous Registry reports. Overall acute results were high (95.7%) and were higher for left-sided (97.8%) than for right-sided (90.8%) AP. Acute complications were uncommon (approximately 4%). The complication of AV block was 1.2% of all procedures but 2.1% of AVNRT and 3.0% of septal AP procedures.

The second PAPCA study focused on recurrence up to 1 year after RCA.[41] This study involved 517 successfully ablated substrates (540 attempted, 95.7%). Loss to follow-up was disappointing—3.3% at 2 months, 10.6% at 6 months, and 21.6% at 12 months—and similar to that for the retrospective Registry follow-up recurrence data reported in 1997.[42] Recurrence rate 12 months after RCA related to substrate type (AP, AVNRT) and AP location. It was highest for right septal AP (24.6%) and lowest for left septal AP and AVNRT (both 4.8%). Recurrence rates for right and left free wall AP were in the middle range (15.8%; 9.3%, respectively).

Serial echocardiography results after RCA composed the third PAPCA study.[43] Heretofore, only anecdotal or retrospective data had been reported addressing the issue of potential cardiac structural damage (e.g. valvar regurgitation, perforation, coronary occlusion) by RCA. In the small hearts of pediatric patients, this concern especially has been prevalent among pediatric electrophysiologists and cardiologists. Of the total 481 patients (follow-up at 2, 6 and 12 months) who were recruited, moderate valve regurgitation was uncommon (0.12%). Mild valve regurgitation was common before the procedure (42.4%) and did not differ after RCA (40.5%). With exception of association of tricuspid valve regurgitation to right free wall AP and AVNRT, there was no other association of ablation targets to valve proximity. No intracardiac thrombosis or ventricular wall motion or function problems were found.

Atrioventricular Node Reentry Tachycardia

Since its recognition, electrophysiologists have been intrigued with many aspects of AVNRT. For years, pediatric electrophysiologists have reported the variability among pediatric patients with AVNRT and differences from adult patients with this tachyarrhythmia.[44] It is common to not find a typical or classically defined (as for adult patients) dual AV nodal pathway physiologic (DAVNPP) jump in the atrial-His interval of 50 ms, with a 10 ms shortening of the premature coupling interval (A1-A2 stimulation). Blurton and colleagues also found no difference in the classic jump between the pediatric group of AVNRT patients (42%) and in the controls (30%).[45] Persistent or sustained slow pathway conduction (SSPC: PR >RR during atrial pacing), however, is more common in pediatric AVNRT patients than DAVNPP.[46,47] Kannankeril and Fish showed SSPC in 75% compared with classic DAVNPP (52%) in their group of 61 young patients before RCA with also a strong age-related difference (SSPC 81% vs DAVNPP 38% in children <13 years).[47] After RCA, the ability to use SSPC as a marker for successful RCA was greater than for DAVNPP (66% vs 36%).

The effect of catheter ablation on the AV node fast pathway effective refractory period (FP-ERP) has been different with RCA and CCA. In a multicenter Pediatric Electrophysiology Society study, Van Hare and colleagues demonstrated shortening of the FP-ERP after RCA.[44] The magnitude of shortening was greater for pediatric patients than had been reported for adults. Lee and associates reported similar findings in their pediatric RCA series from Taiwan.[48] For CCA however, Miyazaki and colleagues showed prolongation of FP-ERP during the cryoapplication.[46] (After termination, the FP-ERP shortened.) These investigators suggested further studies might demonstrate the ability to use the magnitude of prolongation during CCA as a marker for successful slow pathway modification.

The development and refinement of CCA has enabled more pediatric patients who are younger and smaller and who do not have preexcitation to undergo catheter ablation for normal QRS tachycardia. Before CCA, pediatric electrophysiologists were reluctant to offer RCA in young and small patients because if AVNRT or a mid or anterior septal AP was found, then RCA was not undertaken due to the higher-than-standard risk of AV block in the small heart.

Since the inception of CCA and its subsequent widespread use, results in pediatric patients have slowly improved. Initially, success rates for AVNRT were 75% to 85%. Recurrence rates were also high (approximately 30%) although recurrence was lower when RCA was used at the procedure when CCA failed. Later, with refinement and changes in technology and technique, the results have improved. However, assessment of procedural success and recurrence rates is challenging because a mixture of various techniques, including change from CCA to RCA and vice versa within the same procedure, is common practice. This developed early on when it was evident that both success and recurrence rates were enhanced when both techniques were used. In 2005, Drago and colleagues in a pure CCA study showed a high procedural success rate of 93% for AVNRT but a high recurrence rate of 29%.[28] In the same year both Miyazaki's group and Kreibel's group reported similar cohorts of patients, but RCA was also used during the procedure when CCA failed.[26,29] Initial success rates for AVNRT also were good (96% and 85%, respectively) and recurrence rates much better at 10% and 11%, respectively.

Cryoablation of Accessory Pathways

Similar to AVNRT, the use of CCA for AP in septal locations was immediately attractive. However, the procedural success rates have been variable (early experience 50%-60%) and recurrence rates were similarly high.[30] Drago and colleagues in the CCA-only study reported an excellent 92% success rate for AP but a high recurrence rate of 36%.[28]

Advancements and experience also have led to expansion beyond the mid-septal and anterior-septal AP (as well as the rare atrial ectopic tachycardia in the AV junction) region to other anatomic areas in which higher-than-acceptable risk to nontarget tissues exists.[35-37] This includes the coronary sinus and its contiguous tissues in which potential damage to coronary arteries, higher rate of perforation, and thrombosis are found.

Bar-Cohen and colleagues in the AP CCA experience of Children's Hospital in Boston included cryoablation of AP in the coronary sinus (CS).[30] Of six within the CS system, five were successful (83% compared to historical RCA results of 41/46, 89%) Two of five (40%) had recurrence. Comparatively, the historical recurrence for RCA was 2%.

From a Pediatric and Congenital Electrophysiology Society multicenter study, Collins and coworkers reported 21 patients with AP in or near the CS who underwent catheter ablation: Six underwent CCA alone, and 15 had CCA plus RCA.[37] Despite procedural CCA success of 71% (15/21), recurrence was high (40% at a median of 17 days) and identical with that of the Children's Hospital Boston experience. The recurrences were not explained by procedural (e.g., use of 4-mm or 6-mm tip) or patient variables.

Using the same rationale as for AVNRT and septal AP substrates that are near the normal AV conduction system, CCA has been used for the substrates of junctional ectopic tachycardia and atrial ectopic tachycardia in the same region.[35,36,49] Law and coworkers reported a multicenter study of six patients who were all successfully treated with ablation using CCA. These patients had no recurrence in the short mean follow-up of only 6 weeks.[35] A case report of CCA for atrial ectopic tachycardia revealed initial success, then failure, followed by success using epicardial CCA technique.[36]

Congenital Heart Disease

Advances in mapping systems (e.g., multiple basket electrodes, three-dimensional, noncontact) and catheter technology (e.g., irrigation of the ablation catheter tip, allowing greater tissue penetration; incorporating CCA to permit further, more aggressive pursuance of previously avoided target tissues) together with experience have allowed improvement in the challenging group of patients with congenital heart disease.[5,6,7,22-24,50-67] The registry ablation data for this group of patients was not methodically studied or reported. This group can be separated into those who have underlying congenital heart disease but who have not undergone surgical intervention for it[63-67] and those who have previously undergone surgical repair.[50-62] In both groups, results have been disappointing when compared to results for patients without underlying congenital or structural heart disease. Also, reports suggest no major improvement in results despite greater experience and technologic improvements. However, it is likely that more patients who are selected now for ablation were previously not thought to be candidates, especially in the postoperative group, thus perhaps hiding major gains in the overall improvement and results.

The nonsurgical congenital heart disease group data consists primarily of those who have arrhythmia substrates similar to those without structural heart disease. The Pediatric Registry maintained data on these congenital heart disease patients, who included approximately 10% of pediatric patients with AP or AVNRT, or both, but most registry reports concentrated on those without structural heart disease. Virtually all reports that have included patients with congenital heart disease have shown that the presence of congenital heart disease is associated with lower success rates and higher recurrence rates. The most recent data from Children's Hospital in Boston revealed acute success rate for 110 AP of 77% and recurrence rate of 24%.[63] For the challenging group of Ebstein anomaly patients (27 patients, 41 procedures), success rate was 87% and recurrence rate was 29%. For the nine AVNRT patients, seven (79%) were successfully treated, with no recurrences.

Several reports of congenital heart disease ablation have focused on the unique group of patients (usually underlying single ventricle) wth twin AV nodes.[58,63] The Children's Hospital Boston series included four such patients; success was achieved in three with no recurrence.[63] The series from South Korea emphasized the challenges of these twin AV node patients in their postoperative Fontan group with supraventricular tachycardia.[58]

In the rapidly growing population of postoperative congenital heart disease patients, the intra-atrial reenty (IART), incisional reentry, and ventricular tachyarrhythmias provide a very challenging group of patients for not only pediatric electrophysiologists but also for adult electrophysiologists as these patients transition to adulthood. Individual centers are currently reporting 70% to 85% acute success rates for the more common atrial tachyarrhythmia substrates, with the greater rates in postoperative atrial baffle procedures (e.g., Mustard or Senning) or in patients with incisional IART (e.g., postoperative atrial septal defect), with the lower rates found in patients with postoperative Fontan-type anatomy.[50-62] Venous and intracardiac access to the target tissue remains a challenge, so new techniques such as transthoracic approaches have been developed. Nehgme and coworkers have used a transthoracic percutaneous approach to successfully ablate atrial ectopic tachycardia in Fontan patients.[7] As described earlier, the use of preprocedure MRI or CT images downloaded into the three-dimensional mapping systems to produce optimal anatomic delineation from the image fusion of both techniques is anticipated to further provide improvement in the results for these patients.

The arrhythmia substrate of AVNRT, although unrelated to the postoperative status, nevertheless appears in the postoperative congenital heart disease patient.[5,52,57] The congenital heart disease anatomy presents a challenge for catheter ablation of the slow AVN pathway in these patients. In patients with transposition of the great arteries who have undergone the postoperative atrial baffle (Mustard or Senning) procedure, ablation catheter access to the slow AV node pathway region can be difficult. Some patients have baffle leaks that permit access using the inferior vena caval or superior vena caval approach. In most patients, however, the arterial retrograde approach (to right ventricle then retrograde across the tricuspid valve) is required.

Complications

In 2004, the major complication rate was 3.0% and risk of death 0.1%. Two issues need emphasis: the effect of CCA on the complication of AV block and the focus on coronary artery damage.

As predicted when CCA became available, the risk of inadvertent AV block has been lowered substantially with the CCA technique. Only transient block has been reported using CCA.[25-37] This compares to the data for RFA that consistently (starting a few years after its beginning) has shown approximately 1% risk of AV block for slow AV node modification for AVNRT, 3% for ablation of anteroseptal APs, and 10% for midseptal APs.[10,41]

The concern for coronary artery damage started years ago in the animal model and has continued.[68] The close anatomic proximity of the catheter ablation to the tricuspid and mitral valve annulus, where the AP also existed, caused the most apprehension. The finding in animals of no obvious gross catheter ablation damage (e.g., stenosis or thrombosis) from the positive finding of inherently high catheter ablation blood flow that dissipated the RCA heat effects was crucial to the acceptance and eventual wide use of the technique. Subsequent clinical RCA application and results have shown, with few exceptions, no evidence of gross catheter ablation damage using standard RCA ablation techniques of AP.

However, the concern for potential catheter ablation damage issue was never completely dismissed. This was especially true in the pediatric population due to the absence of early investigative data in small animals, later findings in young pigs, and the persistent case reports of catheter ablation damage, especially in small children.[69,70] Also, further animal investigation demonstrated catheter ablation effects by more-sensitive tests such as ultrasound, suggesting that perhaps the absence of gross catheter ablation damage did not negate the potential cellular damage that could reveal clinical problems in the future, in the older pediatric population as well as in adults.

To date, no prospective studies investigating catheter ablation damage have been performed/Concerns remain that catheter ablation damage may be undetected and subclinical at the time of RCA but could become manifest in the future in some patients.

Indications

In the practical sense, when indications for any procedure are discussed, numerous factors need to be considered that may be derived from objective reports, subjective anecdotal experience, or expert opinions. Information relevant to discussion and ultimate recommendations includes natural history of the condition, symptoms and presentation, immediate and long-term risk-to-benefit ratio of the treatment modality options, potential worst-case scenarios, anecdotal experience of the physician as well as those of the patient and family, and costs. These are reviewed extensively in the elsewher.[1,2] Specific guidelines regarding indications for catheter ablation have not been published for pediatric and adult patients with congenital heart disease.

From the factors and available data detailed earlier, it appears reasonable that indications for catheter ablation in pediatric patients should vary with age and symptoms. On the basis of Van Hare's suggested approach, the 2002 NASPE Expert Consensus Conference reported guidelines for the indications of RCA in children by applying the American Heart Association (AHA) and American College of Cardiology (ACC) definitions used for other published indications: class I, class II and class III (Box 110-1).[1,2] No other guidelines for pediatric indications have been reported. However, several reports continue to stimulate opinion and discussion, especially those involving the controversial issues of the asymptomatic patient with manifest Wolff-Parkinson-White (WPW) syndrome and of catheter ablation in infants. The issue of indications for catheter ablation in children or adults with congenital heart disease also continues to be debated, especially when considering the surgical options.

Patients with asymptomatic WPW present a challenging management dilemma due to the absence of prospective randomized, controlled trials and absence of both numerator and population-based denominator data. Sarubbi and colleagues reviewed their 15-year experience in a prospective study, but mean follow-up was only 48 months and the cumulative observation period was 5.5 patient years.[71] For risk stratification, electrophysiology study (EPS) was proposed to all 57 patients and 35 accepted. Of the 57 patients (mean age 9.7 years), seven had developed intermittent preexcitation, three lost preexcitation, and five had symptomatic tachycardia (4 ORT, 1 AF); all of these 15 underwent either medical therapy or RCA. One patient (an 8-year-old who had not undergone EPS) died.

Pappone and coworkers created controversy by redefining life-threatening risk of asymptomatic WPW patients by the inducibility of orthodromic reciprocating tachycardia (ORT) or atrial fibrillation (AF).[72] In their study, after identifying ORT or AF inducibility, they randomized subjects to prophylactic ablation (n = 20) or to no treatment (n = 27). On the basis of recurrent follow-up tachyarrhythmias in one child in the ablation group and in 12 children in the nonablation group (also two children with VF in the control group), these investigators advocated prophylactic ablation if ORT or AF is inducible in asymptomatic WPW patients. This prompted criticism by Triedman and coworkers. One criticism was the use of a new definition for life-threatening risk (simply on the basis of ORT or AF inducibility). Another was the very high rate of life-threatening events in untreated asymptomatic WPW patients, which was inconsistent with previously unpublished life-threatening event rates in this population.[73] Wellens, in another editorial, mentioned the same problems with the definitions and assumptions and emphasized further the problem of identifying these patients.[74] Although screening ECGs are often performed in Italy, this is rare in other countries.

The management of asymptomatic WPW patients remains a debated topic. Consideration for changing the guidelines in adult patients was reviewed by Todd and colleagues, but their advice appears appropriate for young patients and their families also.[75] They summarized by suggesting that after a clear understanding of all the issues and risks, a "patient needs to choose between a small risk over a long period of time and a one-time risk over a short span." The most recent ACC and European Society of Cardiology (ESC) guidelines for adults list restrict catheter ablation in asymptomatic WPW patients to patients in high-risk populations and professional athletes; in these guidelines for this criterion, catheter ablation is listed as a IIA indication with a B level of evidence.[76] In the pediatric population from the 2002 NASPE Expert Consensus Conference, the indication is IIB for children older than 5 years and III for younger children.[2]

Another frequently discussed issue is ablation in infants and small children. Based on the registry data, the 2002 NASPE Expert Consensus Conference listed catheter ablation for infants

Box 110-1 Indications for Pediatric Radiofrequency

CLASS I

Wolff-Parkinson-White (WPW) syndrome following an episode of aborted sudden cardiac death

WPW syndrome associated with syncope when there is a short preexcited R-R interval during atrial fibrillation (preexcited R-R interval <250 ms) or the antegrade effective refractory period of the action potential measured during programmed electrical stimulation is <250 ms

Chronic or recurrent SVT associated with ventricular dysfunction

Recurrent VT that is associated with hemodynamic compromise and is amenable to catheter ablation

CLASS II A

Recurrent and/or symptomatic SVT refractory to conventional medical therapy and age > 4 years

Impending congenital heart surgery when vascular or chamber access may be restricted following surgery

Chronic (occurring for >6-12 mo following an initial event) or incessant SVT in the presence of normal ventricular function

Chronic or frequent recurrences of intra-atrial reentrant tachycardia

Palpitations with inducible sustained SVT during electrophysiologic testing

CLASS II B

Asymptomatic preexcitation (WPW pattern on an ECG, age >5 years, and no recognized tachycardia, when the risks and benefits of the procedure and arrhythmia have been clearly explained

SVT, age >5 years, as an alternative to chronic antiarrhythmic therapy that has been effective in controlling the arrhythmia

SVT, age <5 years (including infants), when antiarrhythmic medications, including sotalol and amiodarone, are not effective or are associated with intolerable side effects

IART, one to three episodes per year, requiring medical intervention

AV node ablation and pacemaker insertion as an alternative therapy for recurrent or intractable intra-atrial reentrant tachycardia

One episode of VT that is associated with hemodynamic compromise and that is amenable to catheter ablation

CLASS III

Asymptomatic WPW syndrome, age <5 years

SVT controlled with conventional antiarrhythmic medications, age <5 years

Nonsustained, paroxysmal VT that is not considered incessant (i.e., present on monitoring for hours at a time or on nearly all strips recorded during any 1-hour period) and where no concomitant ventricular dysfunction exists

Episodes of nonsustained SVT that do not require other therapy and/or are minimally symptomatic

Extracted from Friedman RA, Walsh EP, Silka MJ, et al: NASPE Expert Consensus Conference: Radiofrequency catheter ablation in children with and without congenital heard disease. Report of the Writing Committee. Pacing Clin Electrophysiol 25:1000-1017, 2002.

AV, atrioventricular; ECG, electrocardiogram; IART, intra-atrial reentry; SVT, supraventricular tachycardia; VT, ventricular tachycardia.

and children as acceptable in several situations (see Box 110-1): all those listed as class I, impending congenital heart disease surgery when vascular or chamber access may be restricted after congenital heart disease surgery (IIA), chronic or incessant SVT with normal ventricular function (IIA), and SVT when antiarrhythmia medications are ineffective or associated with intolerable side effects (IIB). Asymptomatic WPW and medically controlled SVT were listed as Class III for infants and young children.

More data from individual centers suggests that smaller patients appear to have a higher risk of complications, although small numbers of patients limit meaningful statistical analysis in some reports. Blaufox and colleagues showed good success rate in their 14 small patients (18 procedures) weighing less than 15 kg drawn from their total pediatric experience of 268 procedures.[77] Their success was nine out of nine for ORT, six out of seven for VT, and zero out of two in chaotic atrial tachycardia. Complications (perforation in one, mild mitral regurgitation in one, and myocardial infarction in one) were significantly associated with greater total RF application time in the smaller patients when indexed for body weight. They recommended RCA only for "dire circumstances" in this small-body-size population and, when necessary, limiting RF application duration to 20 seconds.

Aiyagari and coworkers reported their experience in two groups of patients 20 kg and under.[78] They compared patients 15 kg and smaller (group 1, n = 25) to those between 15.1 and 20 kg (group 2, n = 44). The total major complication rate (4.3%) statistically was no different (P = 0.39) for the smaller group (n = 2, 8%, two perforations) compared with the slightly larger group (n = 1, 2.3%, ventricular dysfunction). Short-term and long-term success rates were good and not different between groups 1 and 2 (96% and 91% for group 1; 86% and 89%for group 2). With these recent further data of reasonable success rates and acceptable complication rates, the prevailing approach by these authors and others to infants and young children appears to be in line with the 2002 NASPE conference indications (see Box 110-1).

The indications for catheter ablation in patients with congenital heart disease also are addressed and listed in the 2002 NASPE conference indications (see Box 110-1). Some indications apply to all patients, not just those with congenital heart disease (e.g., the third indicaiton in class I), and others are implied without specifying congenital heart disease. The latter for example includes IART, the fourth indication in Class IIB, because virtually all pediatric patients with this atrial tachyarrhythmia have underlying postoperative congenital heart disease.

It is this atrial tachyarrhythmia category that is very challenging and for which management options exist that stimulate discussion and debate. Most debated is whether or not these patients should be managed with the surgical maze procedure or catheter ablation.[3,79,80] The issue is not debated as much when the patient also has a demonstrated anatomic problem that needs surgical attention. At the same procedure, the surgical maze procedure is performed at the same setting. However, even with the dual need for arrhythmia and anatomic surgery, in some cases a catheter ablation procedure before surgery is advantageous first because the added cardiopulmonary bypass time for the maze can be a major concern or risk for very complex anatomical and arrhythmia considerations. Also, Friedman and associates reported the use of AV junction catheter ablation with pacemaker therapy in a select group (successful AV block in six of seven patients and decrease from 2.8 ± 1.5 to 0.7 ± 0.8 antiarrhythmia drugs) of postoperative Fontan patients who are not candidates for conventional catheter ablation or surgical therapy.[81]

Acknowledgment

I thank Nikki Yount for assisting me in the preparation of this chapter.

References

1. Kugler JD: Catheter ablation in pediatric patients. In Zipes DP, Jalife J (ed): Cardiac Electrophysiology: From Cell to Bedside, 4th ed. Philadelphia, WB Saunders, 2004, pp 1097-1103.
2. Friedman RA, Walsh EP, Silka MJ, et al: NASPE Expert Consensus Conference: Radiofrequency catheter ablation in children with and without congenital heard disease. Report of the Writing Committee. Pacing Clin Electrophysiol 25:1000-1017, 2002.
3. Mavroudis C, Deal BJ, Backer CL: Surgery for arrhythmias in children. Int J Cardiol 97:39-51, 2004.
4. Iturralde P, Nava S, Sálica G, et al: Electrocardiographic characteristics of patients with Ebstein's anomaly before and after ablation of an accessory atrioventricular pathway. J Cardiovasc Electrophysiol 17:1332-1336, 2006.
5. Kanter RJ, Papagiannis J, Carboni MP, et al: Radiofrequency catheter ablation of supraventricular tachycardia substrates after Mustard and Senning operations for D-transposition of the great arteries. J Am Coll Cardiol 35(2):428-441, 2000.
6. Triedman JK, Alexander ME, Love BA, et al: Influence of patient factors and ablative technologies on outcomes of radiofrequency ablation of intra-atrial re-entrant tachycardia in patients with congenital heart disease. J Am Coll Cardiol 39:1827-1835, 2002.
7. Nehgme RA, Carboni MP, Care J, Murphy JD: Transthoracic percutaneous access for electro-anatomic mapping and catheter ablation of atrial tachycardia in patients with a lateral tunnel Fontan. Heart Rhythm 3:37-43, 2006.
8. Packer DL: Three-dimensional mapping in interventional electrophysiology: Techniques and technology. J Cardiovasc Electrophysiol 16:1110-1116, 2005.
9. Tops LF, De Groot N, Bax JJ, Schalij MJ: Fusion of electroanatomical activation maps and multislice computed tomography to guide ablation of a focal atrial tachycardia in a Fontan patient. J Cardiovasc Electrophysiol 17:431-434, 2006.
10. Kugler JD: Electrophysiologic studies. In Allen HD, Driscoll DJ, Shaddy RE, Feltes TF (eds): Moss and Adams' Heart Disease in Infants, Children, and Adolescents, 7th ed. Lippincott Williams & Wilkins, 2007, pp 275-292.
11. Erb TO, Hall JM, Ing RJ, et al: Postoperative nausea and vomiting in children and adolescents undergoing radiofrequency catheter ablation: A randomized comparison of propofol and isoflurane-based anesthetics. Anesth Analg 95:1557-1581, 2002.
12. Erb TO, Kanter RJ, Hall JM, et al: Comparison of electrophysiologic effects of propofol and isoflurane-based anesthetics in children undergoing radiofrequency catheter ablation for supraventricular tachycardia. Anesthesiology 96:1386-1394, 2002.
13. Warpechowski P, Lima GG, Medeiros CM, et al: Randomized study of propofol effect on electrophysiological properties of the atrioventricular node in patients with nodal reentrant tachycardia. Pacing Clin Electrophysiology 29:1375-1382, 2006.
14. Bacher K, Bogaert E, Lapere R, et al: Patient-specific dose and radiation risk estimation in pediatric cardiac catheterization. Circulation 111(1):83-89, 2005.
15. Campbell RM, Strieper MJ, et al: Quantifying and minimizing radiation exposure during pediatric cardiac catheterization. Pediatr Cardiol 26:29-33, 2005.
16. Davies AG, Cowen AR, Kengyelics SM, et al: X-ray dose reduction in fluoroscopically guided electrophysiology procedures. Pacing Clin Electrophysiology 29:262-271, 2006.
17. Hirshfeld JW Jr, Balter S, Brinker JA, et al; American College of Cardiology Foundation; American Heart Association; American College of Physicians: ACCF/AHA/HRS/SCAI clinical competence statement on physician knowledge to optimize patient safety and image quality in fluoroscopically guided invasive cardiovascular procedures. A report of the American College of Cardiology Foundation/American Heart Association/American College of Physicians Task Force on Clinical Competence and Training. J Am Coll Cardiol 44(11):2259-2282, 2004.
18. Kedia A, Hsu PY, Holmes J, et al: Use of intracardiac echocardiography in guiding radiofrequency catheter ablation of atrial tachycardia in a patient after the Senning operation. Pacing Clin Electrophysiol 26:2178-2180, 2003.
19. Okumura Y, Watanabe I, Yamada T, et al: Comparison of coronary sinus morphology in patients with and without atrioventricular nodal reentrant tachycardia by intracardiac echocardiography. J Cardiovasc Electrophysiol 15:269-273, 2004.
20. Morton JB, Kalman JM: Intracardiac echocardiographic anatomy for the interventional electrophysiologist. J Interv Cardiavasc Electrophysiol 13:11-16, 2005.
21. Knackstedt C, Franke A, Mischke K, et al: Semi-automated 3-dimensional intracardiac echocardiography: Development and initial clinical experience of a new system to guide ablation procedures. Heart Rhythm 3:1453-1459, 2006.
22. Papagiannis J, Tsoutsinos A, Kirvassilis G, et al: Nonfluoroscopic catheter navigation for radiofrequency catheter ablation of supraventricular tachycardia in children. Pacing Clin Electrophysiol 29:971-978, 2006.
23. Abrams DJ, Earley MJ, Sporton SC, et al: Comparison of noncontact and electroanatomic mapping to identify scar and arrhythmia late after the Fontan procedure. Circulation 1738-1746, 2007.
24. Pflaumer A, Hessling G, Luis A, et al: Remote magnetic catheter mapping and ablation of permanent junctional reciprocating tachycardia in a seven-year-old child. J Cardiovasc Electrophysiol 18:882-885, 2007.
25. Kirsh JA, Gross GJ, O'Connor S, et al: Transcatheter cryoablation of tachyarrhythmias in children. J Am Coll Cardiol 45:133-136, 2007.
26. Miyazaki A, Blaufox A, Fairbrother DL, Saul JP: Cryo-ablation for septal tachycardia substrates in pediatric patients. J Am Coll Cardiol 45:581-588, 2005.
27. Gaita F, Montefusco A, Riccardi R, et al: Cryoenergy catheter ablation: A new technique for treatment of permanent junctional reciprocating tachycardia in children. J Cardiovasc Electrophysiol 15:263-268, 2004.
28. Drago F, De Santis A, Grutter G, Silvetti MS: Transvenous cryothermal catheter ablation of re-entry circuit located near the atrioventricular junction in pediatric patients: Efficacy, safety, and midterm follow-up. J Am Coll Cardiol 45:1096-1103, 2005.
29. Kriebel T, Broistedt C, Kroll M, et al: Efficacy and safety of cryoenergy in the ablation of atrioventricular reentrant tachycardia substrates in children and adolescents. J Cardiovasc Electrophysiol 16:960-968, 2005.
30. Bar-Cohen Y, Cecchin F, Alexander M, et al: Cryoabation for accessory pathways located near normal conduction tissues or within the coronary venous system in children and young adults. Heart Rhythm 3:253-258, 2006.
31. Collins KK, Dubin AM, Chiesa NA, et al: Cryoablation versus radiofrequency ablation for treatment of pediatric atrioventricular nodal reentrant tachycardia: Initial experience with 4-mm cryocatheter. Heart Rhythm 3:564-570, 2006.
32. Collins KK, Dubin AM, Chiesa NA, et al: Cryoablation in pediatric atrioventricular

nodal reentry: Electrophysiologic effects on atrioventricular nodal conduction. Heart Rhythm 3:557-563, 2006.

33. Papez AL, Al-Ahdab M, Dick M 2nd, Fischbach PS: Transcatheter Cryoablation for the treatment of supraventricular tachyarrhythmias in children: A single center experience. J Interv Cardiovasc Electrophysiol 15:191-196, 2006.
34. Drago F, Silvetti MS, De Santis A, et al: Lengthier cryoablation and a bonus cryoablation is associated with improved efficacy for cryothermal catheter ablation of supraventricular tachycardias in children. J Interv Cardiovasc Electrophysiol 16:191-198, 2006.
35. Law IH, Von Bergen NH, Gingerich JC, et al: Transcatheter cryothermal ablation of junctional ectopic tachycardia in the normal heart. Heart Rhythm 3:903-907, 2006.
36. Von Bergen NH, Abu Rasheed H, Law IH: Transcatheter cryoablation with 3-D mapping of an atrial ectopic tachycardia in a pediatric patient with tachycardia induced heart failure. J Interv Cardiovasc Electrophysiol 18:273-279, 2007.
37. Collins KK, Rhee EK, Kirsh JA, et al: Cryoablation of accessory pathways in the coronary sinus in young patients: A multicenter study from the Pediatric and Congenital Electrophysiology Society's Working Group on Cryoablation. J Cardiovasc Electrophysiol 18:592-597, 2007.
38. Kugler JD, Danford DA, Deal BJ, et al: Radiofrequency catheter ablation for tachyarrhythmias in children and adolescents. N Engl J Med 330:1481-1487, 1994.
39. Kugler JD, Danford DA, Houston K, Felix G: Pediatric radiofrequency catheter ablation registry success, fluoroscopy time, and complication rate for supraventricular tachycardia: Comparison of early and recent eras. J Cardiovasc Electrophysiol 13:336-341, 2002.
40. Van Hare GF, Javitz H, Carmelli D, et al: Prospective assessment after pediatric cardiac ablation: Demographics, medical profiles, and initial outcomes. J Cardiovasc Electrophysiol 15:759-770, 2004.
41. Van Hare GF, Javitz H, Carmelli D, et al: Prospective assessment after pediatric cardiac ablation: Recurrence at 1 year after initially successful ablation of supraventricular tachycardia. Heart Rhythm 1:188-196, 2004.
42. Kugler JD, Danford DA, Houston K, Felix G: Radiofrequency catheter ablation for paroxysmal supraventricular tachycardia in children and adolescents without structural heart disease. Am J Cardiol 80:1438-1443, 1997.
43. Van Hare GF, Colan SD, Javitz H, et al: Prospective assessment after pediatric cardiac ablation: Fate of intracardiac structure and function, as assessed by serial echocardiography. Am Heart J 153:815-820, 2007.
44. Van Hare GF, Chiesa NA, Campbell RM, et al: Atrioventricular nodal reentrant tachycardia in children: Effect of slow pathway ablation on fast pathway function. J Cardiovasc Electrophysiol 13:203-209, 2002.
45. Blurton DJ, Dubin AM, Chiesa NA, et al: Characterizing dual atrioventricular nodal physiology in pediatric patients with atrioventricular nodal reentrant tachycardia. J Cardiovasc Electrophysiol 17:638-644, 2006.
46. Miyazaki A, Blaufox AD, Fairbrother DL, Saul JP: Prolongation of the fast pathway effective refractory period during Cryoablation in children: A marker of slow pathway modification. Heart Rhythm 2:1179-1185, 2005.
47. Kannankeril PJ, Fish FA: Sustained slow pathway conduction: Superior to dual atrioventricular node physiology in young patients with atrioventricular nodal reentry tachycardia? Pacing Clin Electrophysiology 29:159-163, 2006.
48. Lee P, Hwang B, Tai C, et al: The different ablation effects on atrioventricular nodal reentrant tachycardia in children with and without dual nodal pathways. Pacing Clin Electrophysiol 29:600-606, 2006.
49. Shah MJ, Wieand T, Vetter VL: Cryoablation of congenital familial ectopic tachycardia with preservation of atrioventricular nodal function in an infant. J Cardiovasc Electrophysiol 18:773-776, 2007.
50. Mandapati R, Walsh EP, Triedman JK: Pericaval and periannular intra-atrial reentrant tachycardias in patients with congenital heart disease. J Cardiovasc Electrophysiol 14:119-125, 2003.
51. Perry JC, Boramanand NK, Ing FF: "Transseptal" technique through atrial baffles for 3-dimensional mapping and ablation of atrial tachycardia in patients with D-transposition of the great arteries. J Interv Cardiac Electrophysiol 9:365-369, 2003.
52. Khairy Paul, Seslar SP, et al: Ablation of atrioventricular nodal reentrant tachycardia in tricuspid atresia. J Cardiovasc Electrophysiol 15:719-722, 2004.
53. Verma A, Marrouche NF, Seshadri N, et al: Importance of ablating all potential right atrial flutter circuits in postcardiac surgery patients. J Am Coll Cardiol 44:409-414, 2004.
54. Morwood JG, Triedman JK, Berul CI, et al: Radiofrequency catheter ablation of ventricular tachycardia in children and young adults with congenital heart disease. Heart Rhythm 1:301-308, 2004.
55. Stevenson IH, Kistler PM, Spence SJ, et al: Scar-related right atrial macroreentrant tachycardia in patients without prior atrial surgery: Electroanatomic characterization and ablation outcome. Heart Rhythm 2:594-601, 2005.
56. Lukac P, Pedersen AK, Mortensen PT, et al: Ablation of atrial tachycardia after surgery for congenital and acquired heart disease using an electroanatomic mapping system: Which circuit to expect in which substrate? Heart Rhythm 2:64-72, 2005.
57. Greene AE, Skinner JR, Dubin AM, et al: The electrophysiology of atrioventricular nodal reentry tachycardia following the Mustard or Senning procedure and its radiofrequency ablation. Cardiol Young 15:611-616, 2005.
58. Bae E-J, Noh C-I, Choi J-Y, et al: Twin AV node and induced supraventricular tachycardia in Fontan palliation patients. Pacing Clin Electrophysiology 28:126-134, 2005.
59. Triedman JK, DeLucca JM, Alexander ME, et al: Prospective trial of electroanatomically guided, irrigated catheter ablation of atrial tachycardia in patients with congenital heart disease. Heart Rhythm 2:700-705, 2005.
60. Seslar SP, Alexander ME, Berul CI, et al: Ablation of nonautomatic focal atrial tachycardia in children and adults with congenital heart disease. J Cardiovasc Electrophysiol 17:359-365, 2006.
61. de Groot N, Zeppenfeld K, Wijffels MC, et al: Ablation of focal atrial arrhythmia in patients with congenital heart defects after surgery: Role of circumscribed areas with heterogeneous conduction. Heart Rhythm 3:526-535, 2006.
62. Khairy P, Fournier A, Mercier L-A, Dubuc M: Wolff-Parkinson-White syndrome in D-transposition of the great arteries and Mustard baffle. Heart Rhythm 3:853-856, 2006.
63. Chetaille P, Walsh EP, Triedman JK: Outcomes of radiofrequency catheter ablation of atrioventricular reciprocating tachycardia in patients with congenital heart disease. Heart Rhythm 1:168-173, 2004.
64. Shah MJ, Jones TK, Cecchin F: Improved localization of right-sided accessory pathways with microcatheter-assisted right coronary artery mapping in children. J Cardiovasc Electrophysiol 15:1238-1243, 2004.
65. Matsuoka K, Fujii E, Uchida F, et al: A combination of two simultaneous tachycardias in the right atrium close to the atrioventricular node and within the coronary sinus in a post-operative cor triatriatum patient. J Interv Card Electrophysiol 12:241-246, 2005.
66. Tuzcu V, Gonzalez Y, Gonzalez MB, Schranz D: Diagnosis of tachycardia mechanism with cryomapping in a toddler with complex congenital heart disease. J Interv Card Electrophysiol 16:59-64, 2006.
67. Rudnick AG, Deger FT, Greenberg RM: Ablation of atrioventricular conduction in corrected transposition of the great arteries. Heart Rhythm 3:598-600, 2006.
68. Aoyama H, Nakagawa H, Pitha JV, et al: Comparison of cryothermia and radiofrequency current in safety and efficacy of catheter ablation within the canine coronary sinus close to the left circumflex coronary artery. J Cardiovasc Electrophysiol 16:1218-1226, 2005.
69. Paul T, Kakavand B, Blaufox AD, Saul JP: Complete occlusion of the left circumflex coronary artery after radiofrequency catheter ablation in an infant. J Cardiovasc Electrophysiol 14:1004-1006, 2003.
70. Blaufox AD, Saul JP: Acute coronary artery stenosis during slow pathway ablation for atrioventricular nodal reentrant tachycardia in a child. J Cardiovasc Electrophysiol 15:97-100, 2004.
71. Sarubbi B, Scognamiglio G, Limongelli G, et al: Asymptomatic ventricular pre-excitation

in children and adolescents: A 15 year follow up study. Heart 89:215-217, 2003.

72. Pappone C, Manguso F, Santinelli R, et al: Radiofrequency ablation in children with asymptomatic Wolff-Parkinson-White syndrome. N Engl J Med 351:1197-1205, 2004.

73. Triedman J, Perry J, Van Hare G: Risk stratification for prophylactic ablation in asymptomatic Wolff-Parkinson-White syndrome [letter]. N Engl J Med 352:92-93, 2005.

74. Wellens HJ: Should catheter ablation be performed in asymptomatic patients with Wolff-Parkinson-White syndrome? When to perform catheter ablation in asymptomatic patients with a Wolff-Parkinson-White electrocardiogram. Circulation 112:2201-2207, 2005.

75. Todd DM, Klein GJ, Krahn AD, et al: Asymptomatic Wolff-Parkinson-White syndrome: It is time to revisit guidelines? J Am Coll Cardiol 41:245-248, 2003.

76. Blomstrom-Lundqvist C, Scheinman MM, Aliot EM, et al: for the American College of Cardiology. American Heart Association Task Force on Practice Guidelines, European Society of Cardiology Committee for Practice Guidelines. Writing Committee to Develop Guidelines for the Management of Patients with Supraventricular Arrhythmias. Circulation 108:1871-1909, 2003.

77. Blaufox AD, Paul T, Saul JP: Radiofrequency catheter ablation in small children: Relationship of complications to application dose. Pacing Clin Electrophysiology 27:224-229, 2004.

78. Aiyagari R, Etheridge SP, Bradley DJ, et al: Radiofrequency ablation for supraventricular tachycardia in children $\leq$15 kg is safe and effective. Pediatric Cardiol 26:622-626, 2005.

79. Deal BJ, Mavroudis C, Backer CL: Beyond Fontan conversion: Surgical therapy of arrhythmias including patients with associated complex congenital heart disease. Ann Thorac Surg 76:542-553, 2003.

80. Weipert J, Noebauer C, Schreiber C, et al: Occurrence and management of atrial arrhythmia after long-term Fontan circulation. J Thorac Cardiovasc Surgery 127:457-464, 2004.

81. Friedman RA, Will JC, Fenrich AL, Kertesz NJ: Atrioventricular junction ablation and pacemaker therapy in patients with drug-resistant atrial tachyarrhythmias after the Fontan operation. J Cardiovasc Electrophysiol 16:24-29, 2005.

Index

Note: Page numbers followed by **b** refer to boxes; pages numbers followed by **f** refer to figures; and page numbers followed by **t** refer to tables.

B

E

F

G

H

I

J

K

L

M

N

O

Q

S

T